AHA Guide® to the Health Care Field

2009 Edition

The body of this book is printed on 10% recycled FSC certified stock. A product group from well-managed forests, controlled sources and recycled wood or fiber.

Recycled/Recyclable

AHA Members $215
Nonmembers $330
AHA Item Number 010009
Telephone ORDERS 1–800–AHA–2626

ISSN 0094–8969
ISBN–13: 978–0–87258–841–7

Contents

Section

Section

† List supplied by The Joint Commission

Acknowledgements and Advisements

Acknowledgements

The AHA Guide® to the Health Care Field is published annually by Health Forum LLC, an affiliate of the American Hospital Association. Contributions are made by Information Systems and Technology, Member Relations, Office of the President, Office of the Secretary, Printing Services Group, AHA Resource Center and the following participants:

Stan Dziaba	Denise Loggins
DeAnn Ellis	Jennifer Pagan
Deanna Frazier	Anna Reczynski
Dyanna Gregory	Steve Reczynski
Stella Hines	Genevieve Rials
Clisby Jackson	Elsa Romero
Danny Jackson	Elaine Singh
Kimberly Jackson	Christine Wack
Peter Kralovec	Judy Williams

Health Forum LLC acknowledges the cooperation given by many professional groups and government agencies in the health care field, particularly the following: American College of Surgeons; American Medical Association; Blue Cross and Blue Shield Association; Council of Teaching Hospitals of the Association of American Medical Colleges; The Joint Commission; Commission on Accreditation of Rehabilitation Facilities; American Osteopathic Association, Centers for Medicare & Medicaid Services; and various offices within the U.S. Department of Health and Human Services.

Advisements

The data published here should be used with the following advisements: The data is based on replies to an annual survey that seeks a variety of information, not all of which is published in this book. The information gathered by the survey includes specific services, but not all of each hospital's services. Therefore, the data does not reflect an exhaustive list of all services offered by all hospitals. For information on the availability of additional data and products, please contact Health Forum LLC at 800/821–2039, or visit our web site: www.ahadata.com.

Health Forum LLC does not assume responsibility for the accuracy of information voluntarily reported by the individual institutions surveyed. **The purpose of this publication is to provide basic data reflecting the delivery of health care in the United States and associated areas, and is not to serve as an official and all inclusive list of services offered by individual hospitals. The information reflected is based on data collected as of May 31, 2008.**

Introduction

An Introduction to *AHA Guide*®

Welcome, and thank you for purchasing the 2009 edition of *AHA Guide*®. This section is designed to aid you in using the book. While the primary focus of *AHA Guide* is on hospitals, it also contains information on other areas of the health care field, divided across its three major sections:

- **A.** Hospitals
- **B.** Health care systems, networks, and alliances
- **C.** Health care organizations, agencies, and other health care providers

The information contained within this publication was compiled using AHA membership, and the AHA Annual Survey of Hospitals. *AHA Guide* is the leading hospital directory and represents hospitals with or without AHA membership.

Additional information contained in the front of AHA Guide includes:

- A section by section table of contents
- Recognition of the source of data in the *Acknowledgements and Advisements* section
- Information on AHA's history as well as a listing of our awards in *AHA Offices, Officers, Historical Data, and Awards*

2009 AHA Guide Code Chart

Sample Hospital Listing:

ANYTOWN, Universal County

ANYTOWN HOSPITAL & CLINICS (777777), (Formerly Anytown Area Community Hospital and Clinic), 100 South Main Street, Zip 12345–6789; tel. 123/456–7890 **A**9 10] ①
F10 12 23 24 29 30 31 37 39 49 51 55 57 64 65 66 68 70 71 72 77 78 83 87 88 91 96 97 106 107 110 111 113 124 **P**1 2 3 **S** Universal County Health System ⑦ ② ③
Primary Contact: Ann M. Generic, Chief Executive Officer
COO: Ann M. Generic
CFO: Michael M. Generic
CMO: Peterl Van Generic, President Medical Staff
CHR: Jerry Generic, Human Resources Director
Web address: www.website.org ④
Control: Other not–for–profit (including NFP Corporation) **Service:** General Medical and surgical ⑤

Staffed Beds: 25 **Admissions:** 892 **Census:** 9 **Outpatient Visits:** 44014 **Births:** 51 **Total Expense ($000):** 19210 **Payroll Expense ($000):** 5864 **Personnel:** 182 ⑥

ANYTOWN, Universal County

ANYTOWN HOSPITAL & CLINICS (777777), (Formerly Anytown Area Community Hospital and Clinic), 100 South Main Street, Zip 12345–6789; tel. 123/456–7890 **A**9 10

- ① = **Approval Codes**
- ② = **Physician Codes**
- ③ = **Health Care System Name**
- ④ = **Titles of Chief Administrators**
- ⑤ = **Control and Service Classifications**
- ⑥ = **Utilization Data**
- ⑦ = **Facility Codes**

Hospital, Medicare Provider Number, Address, Telephone, Approval, Facility, and Physician Codes, Health Care System

★ American Hospital Association (AHA) membership
□ The Joint Commission accreditation
○ American Osteopathic Association (AOA) accreditation
△ Commission on Accreditation of Rehabilitation Facilities (CARF) accreditation

① Approval Codes

Reported by the approving bodies specified, as of the dates noted.

- **1** Accreditation under the hospital program of The Joint Commission (May 2008).
- **2** Cancer program approved by American College of Surgeons (March 2008).
- **†3** Approval to participate in residency training, by the Accreditation Council for Graduate Medical Education (April 2008). As of June 30, 1975, internship (formerly code 4) was included under residency, code 3.
- **†5** Medical school affiliation, reported to the American Medical Association (April 2008).
- **6** Hospital–controlled professional nursing school, reported by National League for Nursing.
- **7** Accreditation by Commission on Accreditation of Rehabilitation Facilities (March 2008).
- **8** Member of Council of Teaching Hospitals of the Association of American Medical Colleges (February 2008).
- **9** Hospitals contracting or participating in a Plan, reported by the Blue Cross and Blue Shield Association (March 2008).
- **10** Certified for participation in the Health Insurance for the Aged (Medicare) Program by the Centers for Medicare and Medical Services (February 2008).
- **11** Accreditation by American Osteopathic Association (May 2008).
- **12** Internship approved by American Osteopathic Association (June 2008).
- **13** Residency approved by American Osteopathic Association (June 2008).
- **18** Critical Access Hospitals (May 2008).
- **19** Rural Referral Center (May 2008).
- **20** Sole Community Provider (May 2008).

Nonreporting indicates that the 2007 Annual Survey questionnaire for the hospital was not received prior to publication.

② Physician Codes

Actually available within, and reported by the institution; for definitions, see page A10.

(Alphabetical/Numerical Order)

- **1** Closed physician–hospital organization (PHO)
- **2** Equity model
- **3** Foundation
- **4** Group practice without walls
- **5** Independent practice association (IPA)
- **6** Integrated salary model
- **7** Management service organization (MSO)
- **8** Open physician–hospital organization (PHO)

③ Health Care System Name

The inclusion of the letter "S" (1) indicates that the hospital belongs to a health care system and (2) identifies the specific system to which the hospital belongs.

④ Titles of Chief Administrators

⑤ Control and Service Classification

For a list of control and service classifications, see page A12.

Control–The type of organization that is responsible for establishing policy for overall operation of the hospital.

Service–The type of service the hospital provides to the majority of admissions.

⑥ Utilization Data

Definitions are based on the American Hospital Association's Hospital Administration Terminology. In completing the survey, hospitals were requested to report data for a full year, in accord with their fiscal year, ending in 2007.

Beds–Number of beds regularly maintained (set up and staffed for use) for inpatients as of the close of the reporting period. Excludes newborn bassinets.

Admissions–Number of patients accepted for inpatient service during a 12–month period; does not include newborn.

Census–Average number of inpatients receiving care each day during the 12–month reporting period; does not include newborn.

Outpatient Visits–A visit by a patient who is not lodged in the hospital while receiving medical, dental, or other services. Each appearance of an outpatient in each unit constitutes one visit regardless of the number of diagnostic and/or therapeutic treatments that a patient receives.

Births–Number of infants born in the hospital and accepted for service in a newborn infant bassinet during a 12–month period; excludes stillbirths.

Expense: Expense for a 12–month period; both total expense and payroll components are shown. Payroll expenses include all salaries and wages.

Personnel: Represents personnel situations as they existed at the end of the reporting period; includes full-time equivalents of part–time personnel. Full–time equivalents were calculated on the basis that two part–time persons equal one full–time person.

†Data from the Graduate Medical Education Database, Copyright 2007, American Medical Association, Chicago, Illinois.

Getting Started: The AHA Guide Code Chart

Open the front cover and *AHA Guide* begins with the *2009 AHA Guide Code Chart*. This two page section (front and back) explains how to find and understand the most important elements of each hospital's listing. The chart is specially perforated and is meant to be extracted and used alongside Section A as a resource. The information found on these pages is repeated in the first section, so don't worry about removing the chart.

The *Code Chart* is a very useful tool to have when reading. It allows new users to become familiar with the data, and it aids returning users in understanding the new design and layout of *AHA Guide*. At the top of the chart, there is a sample listing. If you have used this publication before, you will notice the new columnar listing of all hospital entries by city. The city and county names are highlighted in gray, and all hospitals within the city follow. After the hospital name, you will find the address, telephone number, approval, facility and service codes, and health care systems to which the hospital belongs. Following this are the chief administrators and classifications for the hospital. Utilization data for the hospital is found in the box at the bottom of each hospital's entry in *AHA Guide*.

The chart further demonstrates how to understand these important elements:

1. **Approval codes** refer to certifications held by a hospital; they represent information supplied by various national approving and reporting bodies. For example, code A–3 indicates accreditation under one of the programs of the Accreditation Council for Graduate Medical Education, evidence that the hospital has been approved for participation in residency training.
2. **Physician codes** represent the different types of arrangements the hospital participates in with its physicians. In this section, code P-1 signifies a closed physician-hospital organization.
3. **Health Care System names** reference specific health care system headquarters to which the hospital belongs. The presence of a system name indicates that the hospital is a member. If no names are listed, the hospital does not belong to a system.
4. **Titles of Chief Administrators** including the Chief Executive Officer and, when available, other C-Suite officers such as the Chief Financial Officer, Chief Information Officer, Chief Medical Officer, Chief Operating Officer, and Chief Human Resources Officer.
5. **Classification** refers to two items in *AHA Guide*. **Control** classification indicates the organization that operates the hospital, and

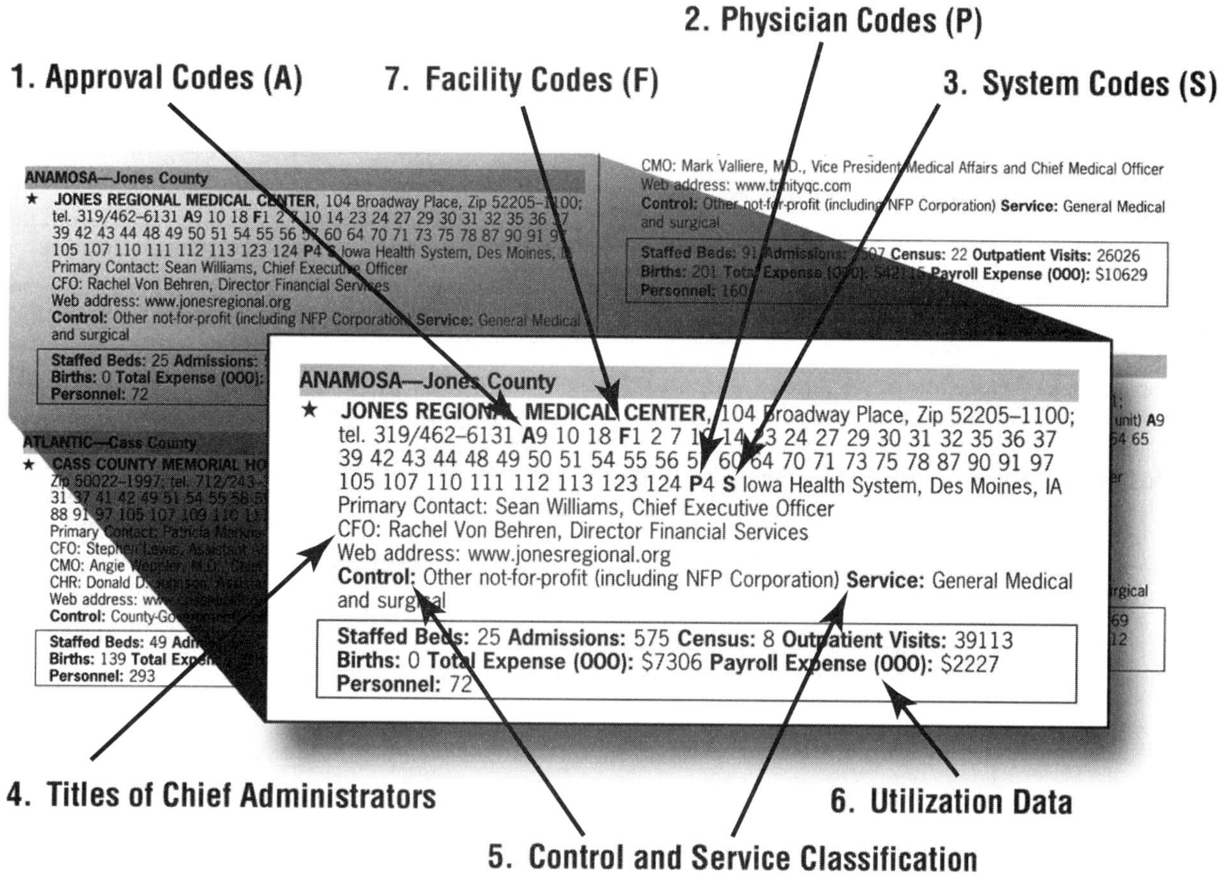

Service classification refers to the type of service the hospital offers. Previously, this section utilized numerical codes corresponding with a literal value, but the new design of *AHA Guide* bypasses the codes and instead displays the literal classifications for control and service.

- **Control:** In this section, organizations are divided among nonfederal government hospitals, nongovernment not-for-profit hospitals, investor owned for-profit hospitals, and federal government hospitals.
- **Service:** This section displays the primary type of service that a hospital offers. The most common value is general hospital. Among the other services listed in this section are specialties such as psychiatric hospitals or children's hospitals.

6. **Utilization Data** contains the statistics related to the day-to-day and cumulative operation of the hospital. The information included in this section consists of:
   - **Beds:** Number of beds regularly maintained.
   - **Admissions:** Amount of patients accepted for inpatient services over a 12-month period.
   - **Census:** Average number of patients receiving care each day.
   - **Outpatient Visits:** Amount of visits by patients not lodged in the hospital while receiving care.
   - **Births:** Number of infants born in the hospital and accepted for service in a newborn infant bassinet.
   - **Expense:** Includes all expenses (including payroll) that the hospital had over the 12-month period.
   - **Personnel:** Represents personnel situations as they existed at the end of the reporting period. In this area, full time equivalency is calculated on the basis that two part-time persons equal one full-time person.
7. **Facility codes** provide a description of the specific services offered by a hospital. Code F-14, for instance, indicates that the hospital contains a Blood Donor Center.

How To Use This Book

Section A begins with the *AHA Guide Hospital Listing Requirements*. This explains the requisite accreditations or characteristics a hospital must meet to be included in *AHA Guide*.

After this there is *An Explanation of the Hospital Listings*. These two pages review the information included in the Code Chart and are a vital resource in identifying the information, symbols, and codes for each hospital's listing.

Next up are the *Annual Survey* definitions, which go into even greater detail in explaining the facility and physician codes. Please note that these are arranged alphabetically and numerically to correspond with the code chart. Also included here are the definitions of the terms for Control and Service found in the Classification section. The listings of *Hospitals in the United States, by State* follow the definitions.

Finding Hospitals & Health Care Professionals in Section A

There are two ways to locate hospitals in the print version of *AHA Guide*. One is by the hospital's geographic classification. In Section A, hospitals are arranged alphabetically by state and then by city. The second method is through the *Hospital Index* that appears directly after the listings.

There is also an *Index of Health Care Professionals* which begins after the first index that lists key people from hospitals and health systems. Look for fold out tabs and tabs on the sides of pages that mark the indices.

AHA Membership Organizations

Section A ends with a description of the AHA Membership categories along with a listing of various AHA Membership organizations.

For more information on Systems, Networks, and Alliances, please read the introduction to Section B. Health organizations, agencies, and providers are described, prior to their listing, at the start of Section C.

AHA Offices, Officers, and Historical Data

Chicago: One North Franklin, Chicago, IL 60606–3401; tel. 312/422–3000

Washington: 325 Seventh Street, N.W., Suite 700, Washington, DC 20004; tel. 202/638–1100

Chairman of the Board of Trustees: William D. Petasnick, Froedtert and Community Health, 9200 W. Wisconsin Avenue, Milwaukee, WI 53226
Chairman–Elect of the Board of Trustees: Thomas M. Priselac, Cedars-Sinai Health System, 8700 Beverly Blvd., Room 2622, Los Angeles, CA 90048

Immediate Past Chairman of the Board of Trustees: Kevin E. Lofton, Catholic Health Initiatives, 1999 Broadway, Suite 2600, Denver, CO 80202
President & CEO: Richard J. Umbdenstock, 325 Seventh Street, N.W., Suite 700, Washington, DC 20004

Senior Vice President and Secretary: Michael P. Guerin, One North Franklin, Chicago, IL 60606–3401
Senior Vice President and Treasurer: John Evans, One North Franklin, Chicago, IL 60606–3401

Past Presidents/Chairs†

1899 ★James S. Knowles
1900 ★James S. Knowles
1901 ★Charles S. Howell
1902 ★J. T. Duryea
1903 ★John Fehrenbatch
1904 ★Daniel D. Test
1905 ★George H. M. Rowe, M.D.
1906 ★George P. Ludlam
1907 ★Renwick R. Ross, M.D.
1908 ★Sigismund S. Goldwater, M.D.
1909 ★John M. Peters, M.D.
1910 ★H. B. Howard, M.D.
1911 ★W. L. Babcock, M.D.
1912 ★Henry M. Hurd, M.D.
1913 ★F. A. Washburn, M.D.
1914 ★Thomas Howell, M.D.
1915 ★William O. Mann, M.D.
1916 ★Winford H. Smith, M.D.
1917 ★Robert J. Wilson, M.D.
1918 ★A. B. Ancker, M.D.
1919 ★A. R. Warner, M.D.
1920 ★Joseph B. Howland, M.D.
1921 ★Louis B. Baldwin, M.D.
1922 ★George O'Hanlon, M.D.
1923 ★Asa S. Bacon
1924 ★Malcolm T. MacEachern, M.D.
1925 ★E. S. Gilmore
1926 ★Arthur C. Bachmeyer, M.D.
1927 ★R. G. Brodrick, M.D.
1928 ★Joseph C. Doane, M.D.
1929 ★Louis H. Burlingham, M.D.
1930 ★Christopher G. Parnall, M.D.
1931 ★Lewis A. Sexton, M.D.
1932 ★Paul H. Fesler
1933 ★George F. Stephens, M.D.
1934 ★Nathaniel W. Faxon, M.D.
1935 ★Robert Jolly
1936 ★Robin C. Buerki, M.D.
1937 ★Claude W. Munger, M.D.
1938 ★Robert E. Neff
1939 ★G. Harvey Agnew, M.D.
1940 ★Fred G. Carter, M.D.
1941 ★B. W. Black, M.D.
1942 ★Basil C. MacLean, M.D.
1943 ★James A. Hamilton
1944 ★Frank J. Walter
1945 ★Donald C. Smelzer, M.D.
1946 ★Peter D. Ward, M.D.
1947 ★John H. Hayes
1948 ★Graham L. Davis
1949 ★Joseph G. Norby
1950 ★John N. Hatfield
1951 ★Charles F. Wilinsky, M.D.
1952 ★Anthony J. J. Rourke, M.D.
1953 ★Edwin L. Crosby, M.D.
1954 ★Ritz E. Heerman
1955 ★Frank R. Bradley
1956 ★Ray E. Brown
1957 ★Albert W. Snoke, M.D.
1958 ★Tol Terrell
1959 ★Ray Amberg
1960 ★Russell A. Nelson, M.D.
1961 ★Frank S. Groner
1962 ★Jack Masur, M.D.
1963 ★T. Stewart Hamilton, M.D.
1964 ★Stanley A. Ferguson
1965 ★Clarence E. Wonnacott
1966 ★Philip D. Bonnet, M.D.
1967 ★George E. Cartmill
1968 ★David B. Wilson, M.D.
1969 ★George William Graham, M.D.
1970 ★Mark Berke
1971 ★Jack A. L. Hahn
1972 Stephen M. Morris
1973 ★John W. Kauffman
1974 ★Horace M. Cardwell
1975 Wade Mountz
1976 H. Robert Cathcart
1977 ★John M. Stagl
1978 ★Samuel J. Tibbitts
1979 W. Daniel Barker
1980 ★Sister Irene Kraus
1981 ★Bernard J. Lachner
1982 Stanley R. Nelson
1983 Elbert E. Gilbertson
1984 Thomas R. Matherlee
1985 ★Jack A. Skarupa
1986 Scott S. Parker
1987 Donald C. Wegmiller
1988 Eugene W. Arnett
1989 Edward J. Connors
1990 David A. Reed
1991 C. Thomas Smith
1992 D. Kirk Oglesby, Jr.
1993 Larry L. Mathis
1994 Carolyn C. Roberts
1995 Gail L. Warden
1996 Gordon M. Sprenger
1997 Reginald M. Ballantyne III
1998 John G. King
1999 Fred L. Brown
2000 ★Carolyn Boone Lewis
2001 Gary A. Mecklenburg
2002 Sr. Mary Roch Rocklage
2003 Dennis R. Barry
2004 David L. Bernd
2005 George F. Lynn
January–April 2006 Richard J. Umbdenstock
April–December 2006 George F. Lynn
2007 Kevin E. Lofton

Chief Executive Officers

1917–18 ★William H. Walsh, M.D.
1919–24 ★Andrew Robert Warner, M.D.
1925–27 ★William H. Walsh, M.D.
1928–42 ★Bert W. Caldwell, M.D.
1943–54 ★George Bugbee
1954–72 ★Edwin L. Crosby, M.D.
1972 Madison B. Brown, M.D. (acting)
1972–86 J. Alexander McMahon
1986–91 Carol M. McCarthy, Ph.D., J.D.
1991 Jack W. Owen (acting)
1991–2007 Richard J. Davidson
2007 Richard J. Umbdenstock (current)

Distinguished Service Award

The award recognizes significant lifetime contributions and service to health care institutions and associations.

1934 Matthew O. Foley
1939 Malcolm T. MacEachern, M.D.
1940 Sigismund S. Goldwater, M.D.
1941 Frederic A. Washburn, M.D.
1942 Winford H. Smith, M.D.
1943 Arthur C. Bachmeyer, M.D.
1944 Rt. Rev. Msgr. Maurice F. Griffin, LL.D.
1945 Asa S. Bacon
1946 George F. Stephens, M.D.
1947 Robin C. Buerki, M.D.
1948 James A. Hamilton
1949 Claude W. Munger, M.D.
1950 Nathaniel W. Faxon, M.D.
1951 Bert W. Caldwell, M.D.
1952 Fred G. Carter, M.D.
1953 Basil C. MacLean, M.D.
1954 George Bugbee
1955 Joseph G. Norby
1956 Charles F. Wilinsky, M.D.
1957 John H. Hayes
1958 John N. Hatfield
1959 Edwin L. Crosby, M.D.
1960 Oliver G. Pratt
1961 E. M. Bluestone, M.D.
1962 Mother Loretto Bernard, S.C., R.N.
1963 Ray E. Brown
1964 Russell A. Nelson, M.D.
1965 Albert W. Snoke, M.D.
1966 Frank S. Groner
1967 Rev. John J. Flanagan, S.J.
1968 Stanley W. Martin
1969 T. Stewart Hamilton, M.D.
1970 Charles Patteson Cardwell, Jr.
1971 Mark Berke
1972 Stanley A. Ferguson
1973 Jack A. L. Hahn
1974 George William Graham, M.D.
1975 George E. Cartmill
1976 D. O. McClusky, Jr.
1977 Boone Powell
1978 Richard J. Stull
1979 Horace M. Cardwell
1980 Donald W. Cordes
1981 Sister Mary Brigh Cassidy
1982 R. Zach Thomas, Jr.
1983 H. Robert Cathcart
1984 Matthew F. McNulty, Jr., Sc.D.
1985 J. Alexander McMahon
1986 Sister Irene Kraus
1987 W. Daniel Barker
1988 Elbert E. Gilbertson
1989 Donald G. Shropshire
1990 John W. Colloton
1991 Carol M. McCarthy, Ph.D., J.D.
1992 David H. Hitt
1993 Edward J. Connors
Jack W. Owen
1994 George Adams
1995 Scott S. Parker
1996 John A. Russell
1997 D. Kirk Oglesby, Jr.
1998 Henry B. Betts, M.D.
1999 Mitchell T. Rabkin, M.D.
2000 Gail L. Warden
2001 Gordon M. Sprenger
2002 Carolyn Boone Lewis
2003 C. Thomas Smith
2004 Michael C. Waters
2005 John G. King
2006 Gary A. Mecklenburg
Sr. Mary Roch Rockage, RSM
2007 Richard J. Davidson
2008 Fred L. Brown

★Deceased
†On June 3, 1972, the House of Delegates changed the title of the chief elected officer to chairman of the Board of Trustees, and the title of president was conferred on the chief executive officer of the Association.

Award of Honor

Awarded to individuals, organizations, or groups to recognize an exemplary contribution to the health and well being of the people through leadership on a major health policy or social initiative.

1966 Senator Lister Hill
1967 Emory W. Morris, D.D.S.
1971 Special Committee on Provision of Health Services (staff also)
1982 Walter J. McNemey
1989 Ruth M. Rothstein
1990 Joyce C. Clifford, R.N.
1991 Haynes Rice
1992 Donald W. Dunn
Ira M. Lane, Jr.
1993 Elliott C. Roberts, Sr.
William A. Spencer, M.D.
1994 Robert A. Derzon
1995 Russell G. Mawby, Ph.D.
John K. Springer
1996 Stephen J. Hegarty
Mothers Against Drunk Driving (MADD)
1997 Paul B. Batalden, M.D.
Habitat for Humanity International
1998 John E. Curley, Jr.
National Civic League
1999 Joseph Cardinal Bernardin, Literacy Volunteers of America
2000 Institute for Safe Medication Practices
2001 Dennis R. Barry
2002 Donald M. Berwick, M.D.
2003 Steven A. Schroeder, M.D.
Dan S. Wilford
2004 Ron J. Anderson, M.D.
Johnson & Johnson
2005 Sr. Mary Jean Ryan
2006 Jordan J. Cohen, M.D.
James W. Varnum
2007 Edward A. Eckenhoff
Stanley F. Hupfeld
2008 Regina M. Benjamin, MD, MBA
Alfred G. Stubblefield

Justin Ford Kimball Innovators Award

Recognition to an individual who makes outstanding, innovative contributions in bringing together health care delivery and financing.

1958 E. A. van Steenwyk
1959 George A. Newbury
1960 C. Rufus Rorem, Ph.D.
1961 James E. Stuart
1962 Frank Van Dyk
1963 William S. McNary
1964 Frank S. Groner
1965 J. Douglas Colman
1967 Walter J. McNemey
1968 John W. Paynter
1970 Edwin L. Crosby, M.D.
1971 H. Charles Abbott
1972 John R. Mannix
1973 Herman M. Somers
1974 William H. Ford, Ph.D.
1975 Earl H. Kammer
1976 J. Ed McConnell
1978 Edwin R. Werner
1979 Robert M. Cunningham, Jr.
1981 Maurice J. Norby
1982 Robert E. Rinehimer
1983 John B. Morgan, Jr.
1984 Joseph F. Duplinsky
1985 David W. Stewart
1988 Ernest W. Saward, M.D.
1990 James A. Vohs
1993 John C. Lewin, M.D.
1994 Donald A. Brennan
1995 E. George Middleton, Jr.
Glenn R. Mitchell
1997 Harvey Pettry
D. David Sniff
1998 Montana Health Research and Education Foundation
1999 Kenneth W. Kizer, M.D.
2002 David M. Lawrence, M.D.
2003 Lowell C. Kruse
2006 Spencer Foreman, M.D.

Board of Trustees Award

Individuals or groups who have made substantial and noteworthy contributions to the work of the American Hospital Association.

1959 Joseph V. Friel
John H. Hayes
1960 Duncan D. Sutphen, Jr.
1963 Eleanor C. Lambertsen, R.N., Ed.D.
1964 John R. Mannix
1965 Albert G. Hahn
Maurice J. Norby
1966 Madison B. Brown, M.D.
Kenneth Williamson
1967 Alanson W. Wilcox
1968 E. Dwight Barnett, M.D.
1969 Vane M. Hoge, M.D.
Joseph H. McNinch, M.D.
1972 David F. Drake, Ph.D.
Paul W. Earle
Michael Lesparre
Andrew Pattullo
1973 Tilden Cummings
Edmond J. Lanigan
1974 James E. Hague
Sister Marybelle
1975 Helen T. Yast
1976 Boynton P. Livingston
James Ludlam
Helen McGuire
1979 Newton J. Jacobson
Edward W. Weimer
1980 Robert B. Hunter, M.D.
Samuel J. Tibbitts
1981 Vernon A. Knutson
John E. Sullivan
1982 John Bigelow
Robert W. O'Leary
Jack W. Owen
1984 Howard J. Berman
O. Ray Hurst
James R. Neely
1985 James E. Ferguson
Cleveland Rodgers
1986 Rex N. Olsen
1987 Michael Lesparre
1988 Barbara A. Donaho, R.N.
1989 Walter H. MacDonald
Donald R. Newkirk
1990 William T. Robinson
1992 Jack C. Bills
Anne Hall Davis
1993 Theodore C. Eickhoff, M.D.
Stephen W. Gamble
Yoshi Honkawa
1994 Roger M. Busfield, Jr., Ph.D.
1995 Stephen E. Dorn
William L. Yates
1996 Leigh E. Morris
John Quigley
1998 John D. Leech
1999 Sister Carol Keehan
C. Edward McCawley
Stephen Rogness
2000 Dennis May
2001 Spencer C. Johnson
Michael M. Mitchel
2002 Victor L. Campbell
Joseph A. Parker
2003 J. Richard Gaintner, M.D.
Donald A. Wilson
2004 Richard L. Clarke
Thelma Traut
2005 Merrill Gappmayer
Leo Greenawalt
2006 Robert L. Harman
Kenneth G. Stella
2007 Deborah Freund, Ph.D.
Michael D. Stephens
2008 James R. Castle

Citation for Meritorious Service

1968 F. R. Knautz
Sister Conrad Mary, R.N.
1971 Hospital Council of Southern California
1972 College of Misericordia, Dallas, PA
1973 Madison B. Brown, M.D.
Samuel J. Tibbitts
1975 Kenneth B. Babcock, M.D.
Sister Mary Maurita Sengelaube
1976 Chaiker Abbis
Susan Jenkins
Gordon McLachlan
1977 Theodore Cooper, M.D.
1979 Norman D. Burkett
John L. Quigley
William M. Whelan
1980 Sister Grace Marie Hiltz
Leo J. Gehrig, M.D.
1981 Richard Davi
Pearl S. Fryar
1982 Jorge Brull Nater
1983 David M. Kinzer
1984 Donald L. Custis, M.D.
1985 John A. D. Cooper, M.D.
Imperial Council of the Ancient Arabic Order of the Nobles of the Mystic Shrine for North America
1986 Howard F. Cook
1987 David H. Hitt
Lucile Packard

This citation is no longer awarded

AHA NOVA Awards

This award honors effective, collaborative programs focused on improving community health status.

1994

Health Partners of Philadelphi (PA): Albert Einstein Medical Center, Episcopal Hospital, Frankford Hospital, Medical College of Pennsylvania Hospital, St. Christopher's Hospital for Children, Temple University Hospital

Decker Family Development Center: Children's Hospital Medical Center of Akron (OH)

Denver (CO) School-Based Clinics: The Children's Hospital

Basic Health Plan: Dominican Network; Mount Carmel Hospital, Colville, WA; St. Joseph's Hospital, Chewelah, WA; and Holy Family Hospital, Spokane, WA

HealthLink: Lakes Region General Hospital, Laconia, NH

1995

Bladen Community Care Network: Bladen County Hospital, Elizabethtown, NC

Building a Healthier Community: Community–Kimball Health Care System, Toms River, NJ

Injury Prevention Program: Harlem Hospital Center, New York City, NY

The Community Ministries & Outreach Program: Reaching Out to Our Vickery/Meadow Neighborhood: Presbyterian Healthcare System, Dallas, TX

"CHOICES": Shriners Hospitals for Crippled Children, Tampa, FL

1996

Lincoln and Sunnyslope: John C. Lincoln Hospital and Health Center, Sunnyslope, AZ

Growing into Life Task Force: Aiken (SC) Regional Medical Centers

People Caring for People: Beatrice (NE) Community Hospital and Health Center

Injury Prevention Center of the Greater Dayton (OH) Area: The Children's Medical Center, Good Samaritan Hospital and Health Center, Grandview Hospital, Kettering Memorial Hospital, Miami Valley Hospital, and St. Elizabeth Medical Center

Family Road: Hutzel Hospital, Detroit, MI

1997

Health Promotion Schools of Excellence Program: Alliant Health System and Kosair Children's Hospital, Louisville, KY

Health, Outreach, Prevention, and Education (HOPE): Health First Holmes Regional Medical Center, Melbourne, FL

Healthy Community Initiative: Roper Care Alliance, Charleston, SC

Obstetrical Care and Prenatal Counseling Program: St. Alexius Medical Center, Bismarck, ND

HIV/AIDS Neighborhood Service Program: Yale–New Haven Hospital, New Haven, CT

1998

Partners for a Healthier Community: Evergreen Community Health Care, Group Health Cooperative of Puget Sound, Overlake Hospital Medical Center, Providence Health System/Medalia HealthCare, Seattle, WA

Glenwood–Lyndale Community Clinic: Hennepin County Medical Center, Minneapolis, MN

Greater Dallas (TX) Injury Prevention Center: Parkland Health & Hospital System, Children's Medical Center of Dallas, Baylor Health Care System, Methodist Hospitals of Dallas, and Presbyterian Healthcare System

Network of Trust: Phoebe Putney Memorial Hospital, Albany, GA

The Lauderdale Court: A Community Partnership: St. Joseph Hospital and Health Centers, Memphis, TN

1999

Making a Case for Community Health: Middletown (OH) Regional Hospital

The Family Resource Center: Mount Carmel Medical Center, Pittsburgh, KS

The Health Neighborhood Project: St. Patrick Hospital, Missoula, MT

Kids for Health: Washington Regional Medical Center, Fayetteville, AR

Children's Village: Yakima Memorial Hospital, Yakima, WA

2000

Community Healthcare Network: Columbus (GA) Regional Healthcare System

Pasadena County Asthma Project: Huntington Memorial Hospital, Pasadena, CA

Ashe County Health Council "Health Carolinias Task Force": Ashe Memorial Hospital, Jefferson, NC

Caritas–Connection Project: St. Mary's Hospital, Passaic, NJ

Correctional Health Care Program: Baystate Health System, Springfield, MA

2001

J.C. Lewis Health Center: Memorial Health and St. Joseph's Candler Health System, Savannah, GA

Project C.A.R.E.: Mercy Medical Center, Canton, OH

TeenHealthFX.com: Atlantic Health System, Florham Park, NJ

Vista ElderCARE: Vista Health, Waukegan, IL

Western Village Enterprise School: INTEGRIS Health, Oklahoma City, OK

2002

Chester Community Connections: Crozer–Keystone Health System, Springfield, PA

The Hope Street Family Center: California Hospital Medical Center, Los Angeles, CA

Mobile Health Outreach Ministry: St. Vincent's Health System, Jacksonville, FL

Operation Access: Kaiser Foundation Hospitals, Oakland; Sutter Health, Sacramento; San Francisco General Hospital, San Francisco; St. Rose Hospital, Hayward; and Santa Rosa Memorial Hospital, Santa Rosa, CA

Wilmington Health Access for Teens: New Hanover Health Network, Wilmington, NC

2003

C.O.A.C.H. for Kids: Cedars–Sinai Medical Center, Los Angeles, CA

Community Action Network: Trinity Regional Medical Center, Fort Dodge, IA

Hearts N' Health: Glendale Adventist Medical Center, Glendale, CA

Saint Joseph Health Center: Saint Joseph Regional Medical Center, South Bend, IN

St. Mary Medical Center Bensalem Ministries: St. Mary Medical Center, Langhorne, PA

2004

Better Beginnings: Brockton Hospital, Brockton, MA

Buffalo County Community Health Partners: Good Samaritan Health Systems, Kearney, NE

Quad City Health Initiative: Genesis Health System, Davenport, IA and Trinity Regional Health System, Rock Island, IL

Quality of Life in the Truckee Meadows: Washoe Health System, Reno, NV

Solano Coalition for Better Health, Inc.: NorthBay Healthcare Group, Fairfield, CA; Sutter Solano Medical Center, Vallejo, CA; and Kaiser Permanente, Martinez, CA

2005

Children's Health Connection: McKay-Dee Hospital Center, Ogden, UT

Palmetto Health's Vision Health Initiative: Palmetto Health, Columbia, SC

Project Dulce, Whittier Institute for Diabetes: Scripps Health, San Diego, CA

Toledo/Lucas County CareNet: Mercy Health Partners, ProMedica Health System, and Medical University of Ohio, all of Toledo, OH and St. Luke's Hospital, Maumee, OH

Volunteer Health Advisor (VHA) Program: Cambridge Health Alliance, Cambridge, MA

2006

Healthy Learners, Columbia, SC: Allendale County Hospital, Fairfax, SC; McLeod Medical Center–Dillon, Dillon, SC; Sisters of Charity Providence Hospitals, Columbia, SC; and Self Regional Healthcare, Greenwood, SC

Primary Care Access Network (PCAN): Health Central, Ocoee, FL; Florida Hospital, Winter Park, FL; and Orlando Regional Healthcare, Orlando, FL

ProHealth Care Community Health Outreach Initiative: ProHealth Care, Waukesha, WI

St. Joseph Mobile Health Services: Saint Joseph HealthCare Inc., Lexington, KY

Yonkers Childhood Health Initiative: St. John's Riverside, Yonkers, NY

2007

Medical-Legal Partnership for Children: Boston Medical Center, Boston, MA

NOW (Nutritional Options for Wellness) Program: Spectrum Health, Grand Rapids, MI

Richland Care: Palmetto Health, Columbia, SC

Trauma Nurses Talk Tough: Legacy Health System, Portland, OR

UMass Memorial Medical Center Healthy Youth Development Initiative: UMass Memorial Health Care, Worcester, MA

Youth Health Partnership-Patee Market Youth Dental Clinic: Heartland Health, St. Joseph, MO

2008

Partnership for Community Health: California Pacific Medical Center, San Francisco, CA

Every Child Succeeds: Cincinnati Children's Hospital Medical Center, Cincinnati, OH

Memorial Hermann Health Centers for Schools: Memorial Hermann, Houston, TX

Nutrition Center of Maine: Saint Mary's Health System, Lewiston, ME

***ENERGIZE!* Pediatric Diabetes Intervention Program:** WakeMed Health & Hospitals, Raleigh, NC

The Carolyn Boone Lewis Living the Vision Award

Organizations and individuals living AHA's vision of a society of healthy communities where all individuals reach their highest potential for health.

1998 Memorial Healthcare System, Hollywood, FL
Baptist Health System, Montgomery, AL

1999 Robert A. DeVries, Battle Creek, MI
Memorial Health System, South Bend, IN

2000 Rockingham Memorial Hospital, Harrisonburg, VA

2001 Salina Regional Health Center, Salina, KS

2002 Health Improvement Collaborative of Greater Cincinnati, Cincinnati, OH

2003 Franklin Memorial Hospital, Farmington, ME

2004 Jamaica Hospital Medical Center, Jamaica, New York

2005 Fairbanks Memorial Hospital, Fairbanks, AK
Boston Medical Center, Boston, MA

Circle of Life Award

This award celebrates innovation in palliative and end-of-life care.

2000

Improving Care through the End of Life, Franciscan Health System, Gig Harbor, WA

The Hospice of The Florida Suncoast, Largo, FL

Louisiana State Penitentiary Hospice Program, Angola, LA

2001

Department of Pain Medicine and Palliative Care, Beth Israel Medical Center, New York, NY

Palliative CareCenter & Hospice of the North Shore, Evanston , IL

St. Joseph's Manor, Trumbull, CT

2002

Children's Program of San Diego Hospice and Children's Hospital and Health Center of San Diego, San Diego, CA

Hospice of the Bluegrass, Lexington, KY

Project Safe Conduct, Hospice of the Western Reserve and Ireland Cancer Center, Cleveland, OH

Special Circle of Life Award Population–based Palliative Care Research Network (PoPCRN), Denver, CO

2003

Hospice & Palliative CareCenter, Winston–Salem, NC

Providence Health System, Portland, OR

University of California Davis Health System, Sacramento, CA

2004

Hope Hospice and Palliative Care, Fort Myers, FL

St. Mary's Healthcare System for Children, Bayside, NY

University of Texas M.D. Anderson Cancer Center Palliative Care, Houston, TX

2005

High Point Regional Health System, High Point, NC

Palliative and End-of-life Care Program, Hoag Memorial Hospital Presbyterian, Newport Beach, CA

Thomas Palliative Care Unit, VCU Massey Cancer Center, Richmond, VA

2006

Continuum Hospice Care, New York, NY

Mercy Supportive Care, St. Joseph Mercy Oakland, Pontiac, MI

Transitions and Life Choices, Fairview Health Services, Minneapolis, MN

2007

UCSF Palliative Care Program, San Francisco, CA

Covenant Hospice, Pensacola, FL

Woodwell: A Program of Presbyterian SeniorCare and Family Hospice and Palliative Care, Oakmont, PA

2008

Children's Hospitals and Clinics of Minnesota, Pain and Palliative Care Program, Minneapolis, MN

Haven Hospice, Gainesville, FL

The Pediatric Advanced Care Team, The Children's Hospital of Philadelphia, Philadelphia, PA

The American Hospital Association–McKesson Quest for Quality Prize

Honoring Leadership and Innovation in Patient Care Quality, Safety, and Commitment

2002

Missouri Baptist Medical Center, St. Louis, MO

Finalist: Fairview Hospital, Greater, Barrington, MA

Finalist: Minnesota Children's Hospital and Clinics, Minneapolis, MN

2003

Abington Memorial Hospital, Abington, PA

Finalist: Beaumont Hospitals, Royal Oak, MI

Finalist: University of Wisconsin Hospital and Clinics, Madison, WI

2004

Sentara Norfolk General Hospital, Norfolk, VA

Finalist: The Johns Hopkins Hospital, Baltimore, MD

Finalist: Mary Lanning Memorial Hospital, Hastings, NE

2005
North Mississippi Medical Center, Tupelo, MS

Finalist: El Camino Hospital, Mountain View, CA

Finalist: NewYork-Presbyterian Hospital, New York, NY

2006
Cincinnati Children's Hospital Medical Center, Cincinnati, OH

2007
Columbus Regional Hospital, Columbus, IN

Finalist: Cedars-Sinai Medical Center, Los Angeles, CA

Finalist: INTEGRIS Baptist Medical Center, Oklahoma City, OK

2008
Munson Medical Center, Traverse City, MI

Finalist: University of Michigan Hospitals & Health Centers, Ann Arbor, MI

Foster G. McGaw Prize

Honors health delivery organizations that have demonstrated exceptional commitment to community service.

1986 Lutheran Medical Center, Brooklyn, NY
1987 Copley Hospital, Morrisville, VT
Mount Sinai Hospital, Hartford, CT
1988 MetroHealth System, Cleveland, OH
1989 Greater Southeast Healthcare System, Washington, DC
1990 Mount Zion Medical Center of The University of California-San Francisco, San Francisco, CA
1991 Franklin Regional Hospital, Franklin, NH
1992 Mount Sinai Hospital Medical Center of Chicago, Chicago, IL
1993 The Cambridge Hospital, Cambridge, MA
1994 Parkland Memorial Hospital, Dallas, TX
1995 Our Lady of Lourdes Medical Center, Camden, NJ
1996 St. Mary's Hospital, Rochester, NY
1997 Bladen County Hospital Rural Health Network, Elizabethtown, NC
1998 Allina Health System, Minneapolis, MN
1999 LAC+USC Healthcare Network, Los Angeles, CA
2000 Kaweah Delta Health Care District, Visalia, CA
2001 Memorial Hospital of South Bend, South Bend, IN
2002 John C. Lincoln Health Network, Phoenix, AZ
2003 Phoebe Putney Memorial Hospital, Albany, GA
2004 Henry Ford Health System, Detroit, MI
2005 Venice Family Clinic, Venice, CA
2006 Memorial Healthcare System, Hollywood, FL
2007 Harborview Medical Center, Seattle, WA

A

Hospitals, Institutional and Associate Members

AHA Guide
Hospital Listing Requirements

An institution may be listed by the American Hospital Association as a hospital if it is accredited as a hospital by The Joint Commission or is certified as a provider of acute services under Title 18 of the Social Security Act. Membership in the American Hospital Association is not a prerequisite.

In lieu of the preceding accreditation or certification, an institution licensed as a hospital by the appropriate state agency may be registered by AHA as a hospital by meeting the following alternative requirements:

Function: The primary function of the institution is to provide patient services, diagnostic and therapeutic, for particular or general medical conditions.

1. The institution shall maintain at least six inpatient beds, which shall be continuously available for the care of patients who are nonrelated and who stay on the average in excess of 24 hours per admission.
2. The institution shall be constructed, equipped, and maintained to ensure the health and safety of patients and to provide uncrowded, sanitary facilities for the treatment of patients.
3. There shall be an identifiable governing authority legally and morally responsible for the conduct of the hospital.
4. There shall be a chief executive to whom the governing authority delegates the continuous responsibility for the operation of the hospital in accordance with established policy.
5. There shall be an organized medical staff of fully licensed physicians* that may include other licensed individuals permitted by law and by the hospital to provide patient care services independently in the hospital. The medical staff shall be accountable to the governing authority for maintaining proper standards of medical care, and it shall be governed by bylaws adopted by said staff and approved by the governing authority.
6. Each patient shall be admitted on the authority of a member of the medical staff who has been granted the privilege to admit patients to inpatient services in accordance with state law and criteria for standards of medical care established by the individual medical staff. Each patient's general medical condition is the responsibility of a qualified physician member of the medical staff. When nonphysician members of the medical staff are granted privileges to admit patients, provision is made for prompt medical evaluation of these patients by a qualified physician. Any graduate of a foreign medical school who is permitted to assume responsibilities for patient care shall possess a valid license to practice medicine, or shall be certified by the Educational Commission for Foreign Medical Graduates, or shall have qualified for and have successfully completed an academic year of supervised clinical training under the direction of a medical school approved by the Liaison Committee on GAT Medical Education.
7. Registered nurse supervision and other nursing services are continuous.
8. A current and complete medical record shall be maintained by the institution for each patient and shall be available for reference.
9. Pharmacy service shall be maintained in the institution and shall be supervised by a registered pharmacist.
10. The institution shall provide patients with food service that meets their nutritional and therapeutic requirements; special diets shall also be available.

* Physician–Term used to describe an individual with an M.D. or D.O. degree who is fully licensed to practice medicine in all its phases.

‡ The completed records in general shall contain at least the following: the patient's identifying data and consent forms, medical history, record of physical examination, physicians' progress notes, operative notes, nurses' notes, routine x–ray and laboratory reports, doctors' orders, and final diagnosis.

Types of Hospitals

In addition to meeting these 10 general requirements, hospitals are listed as one of four types of hospitals: general, special, rehabilitation and chronic disease, or psychiatric. The following definitions of function by type of hospital and special requirements are:

General

The primary function of the institution is to provide patient services, diagnostic and therapeutic, for a variety of medical conditions. A general hospital also shall provide:

- diagnostic x–ray services with facilities and staff for a variety of procedures
- clinical laboratory service with facilities and staff for a variety of procedures and with anatomical pathology services regularly and conveniently available
- operating room service with facilities and staff.

Special

The primary function of the institution is to provide diagnostic and treatment services for patients who have specified medical conditions, both surgical and nonsurgical. A special hospital also shall provide:

- such diagnostic and treatment services as may be determined by the Executive Committee of the Board of Trustees of the American Hospital Association to be appropriate for the specified medical conditions for which medical services are provided shall be maintained in the institution with suitable facilities and staff. If such conditions do not normally require diagnostic x–ray service, laboratory service, or operating room service, and if any such services are therefore not maintained in the institution, there shall be written arrangements to make them available to patients requiring them.
- clinical laboratory services capable of providing tissue diagnosis when offering pregancy termination services.

Rehabilitation and Chronic Disease

The primary function of the institution is to provide diagnostic and treatment services to handicapped or disabled individuals requiring restorative and adjustive services. A rehabilitation and chronic disease hospital also shall provide:

- arrangements for diagnostic x–ray services, as required, on a regular and conveniently available basis
- arrangements for clinical laboratory service, as required on a regular and conveniently available basis
- arrangements for operating room service, as required, on a regular and conveniently available basis
- a physical therapy service with suitable facilities and staff in the institution
- an occupational therapy service with suitable facilities and staff in the institution
- arrangements for psychological and social work services on a regular and conveniently available basis
- arrangements for educational and vocational services on a regular and conveniently available basis
- written arrangements with a general hospital for the transfer of patients who require medical, obstetrical, or surgical services not available in the institution.

Psychiatric

The primary function of the institution is to provide diagnostic and treatment services for patients who have psychiatric–related illnesses. A psychiatric hospital also shall provide:

- arrangements for clinical laboratory service, as required, on a regular and conveniently available basis
- arrangements for diagnostic x–ray services, as required on a regular and conveniently available basis
- psychiatric, psychological, and social work service with facilities and staff in the institution
- arrangements for electroencephalograph services, as required, on a regular and conveniently available basis.
- written arrangements with a general hospital for the transfer of patients who require medical, obstetrical, or surgical services not available in the institution.

The American Hospital Association may, at the sole discretion of the Executive Committee of the Board of Trustees, grant, deny, or withdraw the listing of an institution.

* Physician–Term used to describe an individual with an M.D. or D.O. degree who is fully licensed to practice medicine in all its phases.

‡ The completed records in general shall contain at least the following: the patient's identifying data and consent forms, medical history, record of physical examination, physicians' progress notes, operative notes, nurses' notes, routine x–ray and laboratory reports, doctors' orders, and final diagnosis.

Explanation of Hospital Listings

Sample Hospital Listing:

ANYTOWN, Universal County

★☐ **ANYTOWN HOSPITAL & CLINICS (777777)**, (Formerly Anytown Area Community Hospital and Clinic), 100 South Main Street, Zip 12345–6789; tel. 123/456–7890 **A**9 10] ①
F10 12 23 24 29 30 31 37 39 49 51 55 57 64 65 66 68 70 71 72 77 78 83 87 88 91 96 97 106 107 110 111 113 124 **P**1 2 3 **S** Universal County Health System ② ③ ⑦
Primary Contact: Ann M. Generic, Chief Executive Officer
COO: Ann M. Generic
CFO: Michael M. Generic
CMO: Peterl Van Generic, President Medical Staff
CHR: Jerry Generic, Human Resources Director
Web address: www.website.org ④
Control: Other not–for–profit (including NFP Corporation) **Service:** General Medical and surgical ⑤

Staffed Beds: 25 **Admissions:** 892 **Census:** 9 **Outpatient Visits:** 44014 **Births:** 51 **Total Expense ($000):** 19210 **Payroll Expense ($000):** 5864 **Personnel:** 182 ⑥

ANYTOWN, Universal County

★☐ **ANYTOWN HOSPITAL & CLINICS (777777)**, (Formerly Anytown Area Community Hospital and Clinic), 100 South Main Street, Zip 12345–6789; tel. 123/456–7890 **A**9 10

① = **Approval Codes**
② = **Physician Codes**
③ = **Health Care System Name**
④ = **Titles of Chief Administrators**
⑤ = **Control and Service Classifications**
⑥ = **Utilization Data**
⑦ = **Facility Codes**

⑥

Hospital, Medicare Provider Number, Address, Telephone, Approval, Facility, and Physician Codes, Health Care System

★ American Hospital Association (AHA) membership
☐ The Joint Commission accreditation
○ American Osteopathic Association (AOA) accreditation
△ Commission on Accreditation of Rehabilitation Facilities (CARF) accreditation

① Approval Codes

Reported by the approving bodies specified, as of the dates noted.

1 Accreditation under the hospital program of The Joint Commission (May 2008).
2 Cancer program approved by American College of Surgeons (March 2008).
†3 Approval to participate in residency training, by the Accreditation Council for Graduate Medical Education (April 2008). As of June 30, 1975, internship (formerly code 4) was included under residency, code 3.
†5 Medical school affiliation, reported to the American Medical Association (April 2008).
6 Hospital–controlled professional nursing school, reported by National League for Nursing.
7 Accreditation by Commission on Accreditation of Rehabilitation Facilities (March 2008).
8 Member of Council of Teaching Hospitals of the Association of American Medical Colleges (February 2008).
9 Hospitals contracting or participating in a Plan, reported by the Blue Cross and Blue Shield Association (March 2008).
10 Certified for participation in the Health Insurance for the Aged (Medicare) Program by the Centers for Medicare and Medical Services (February 2008).
11 Accreditation by American Osteopathic Association (May 2008).
12 Internship approved by American Osteopathic Association (June 2008).
13 Residency approved by American Osteopathic Association (June 2008).
18 Critical Access Hospitals (May 2008).
19 Rural Referral Center (May 2008).
20 Sole Community Provider (May 2008).

Nonreporting indicates that the 2007 Annual Survey questionnaire for the hospital was not received prior to publication.

② Physician Codes

Actually available within, and reported by the institution; for definitions, see page A10.

(Alphabetical/Numerical Order)

1 Closed physician–hospital organization (PHO)
2 Equity model
3 Foundation
4 Group practice without walls
5 Independent practice association (IPA)
6 Integrated salary model
7 Management service organization (MSO)
8 Open physician–hospital organization (PHO)

③ Health Care System Name

The inclusion of the letter ''S'' (1) indicates that the hospital belongs to a health care system and (2) identifies the specific system to which the hospital belongs.

④ Titles of Chief Administrators

⑤ Control and Service Classification

For a list of control and service classifications, see page A12.

Control–The type of organization that is responsible for establishing policy for overall operation of the hospital.

Service–The type of service the hospital provides to the majority of admissions.

⑥ Utilization Data

Definitions are based on the American Hospital Association's Hospital Administration Terminology. In completing the survey, hospitals were requested to report data for a full year, in accord with their fiscal year, ending in 2007.

Beds–Number of beds regularly maintained (set up and staffed for use) for inpatients as of the close of the reporting period. Excludes newborn bassinets.

Admissions–Number of patients accepted for inpatient service during a 12–month period; does not include newborn.

Census–Average number of inpatients receiving care each day during the 12–month reporting period; does not include newborn.

Outpatient Visits–A visit by a patient who is not lodged in the hospital while receiving medical, dental, or other services. Each appearance of an outpatient in each unit constitutes one visit regardless of the number of diagnostic and/or therapeutic treatments that a patient receives.

Births–Number of infants born in the hospital and accepted for service in a newborn infant bassinet during a 12–month period; excludes stillbirths.

Expense: Expense for a 12–month period; both total expense and payroll components are shown. Payroll expenses include all salaries and wages.

Personnel: Represents personnel situations as they existed at the end of the reporting period; includes full–time equivalents of part–time personnel. Full–time equivalents were calculated on the basis that two part–time persons equal one full–time person.

†Data from the Graduate Medical Education Database, Copyright 2007, American Medical Association, Chicago, Illinois.

Sample Hospital Listing:

ANYTOWN, Universal County

★□ **ANYTOWN HOSPITAL & CLINICS (777777),** (Formerly Anytown Area Community Hospital and Clinic), 100 South Main Street, Zip 12345–6789; tel. 123/456–7890 A9 10] ①
F10 12 23 24 29 30 31 37 39 49 51 55 57 64 65 66 68 70 71 72 77 78 83 87 88 91 96 97 106 107 110 111 113 124 P1 2 3 S Universal County Health System ② ③ ⑦
Primary Contact: Ann M. Generic, Chief Executive Officer
COO: Ann M. Generic
CFO: Michael M. Generic
CMO: Peterl Van Generic, President Medical Staff
CHR: Jerry Generic, Human Resources Director
Web address: www.website.org ④
Control: Other not–for–profit (including NFP Corporation) **Service:** General Medical and surgical ⑤

Staffed Beds: 25 **Admissions:** 892 **Census:** 9 **Outpatient Visits:** 44014
Births: 51 **Total Expense ($000):** 19210 **Payroll Expense ($000):** 5864
Personnel: 182 ⑥

ANYTOWN, Universal County

★□ **ANYTOWN HOSPITAL & CLINICS (777777),** (Formerly Anytown Area Community Hospital and Clinic), 100 South Main Street, Zip 12345–6789; tel. 123/456–7890 **A**9 10

① = **Approval Codes**
② = **Physician Codes**
③ = **Health Care System Name**
④ = **Titles of Chief Administrators**
⑤ = **Control and Service Classifications**
⑥ = **Utilization Data**
⑦ = **Facility Codes**

Hospital, Medicare Provider Number, Address, Telephone, Approval, Facility, and Physician Codes, Health Care System

★ American Hospital Association (AHA) membership
□ The Joint Commission accreditation
○ American Osteopathic Association (AOA) accreditation
△ Commission on Accreditation of Rehabilitation Facilities (CARF) accreditation

⑦ Facility Codes

Provided directly by the hospital; for definitions, see page A6.

(Numerical Order)

1 Acute long–term care
2 Adult Day Care program
3 Airborne infection isolation room
4 Alcoholism–drug abuse or dependency inpatient unit
5 Alcoholism–drug abuse or dependency outpatient services
6 Alzheimer Center
7 Ambulance Services
8 Ambulatory Surgery Center
9 Arthritis treatment center
10 Assisted Living
11 Auxiliary organization
12 Bariatric/weight control services
13 Birthing room–LDR room–LDRP room
14 Blood Donor Center
15 Breast cancer screening/mammograms
16 Burn care services
17 Cardiac intensive care services
18 Adult diagnostic/invasive catheterization
19 Pediatric diagnostic/invasive catheterization
20 Adult interventional cardiac catheterization
21 Pediatric interventional cardiac catheterization
22 Adult cardiac surgery
23 Pediatric cardiac surgery
24 Cardiac Rehabilitation
25 Case management
26 Chaplaincy/pastoral care services
27 Chemotherapy
28 Children wellness program
29 Chiropractic services
30 Community health reporting
31 Community health status assessment
32 Community health status based service planning
33 Community outreach
34 Complementary medicine
35 Computer assisted orthopedic surgery (CAOS)
36 Crisis Prevention
37 Dental services
38 Emergency department
39 Freestanding/Satellite Emergency Department
40 Trauma center (certified)
41 Enabling services
42 Hospice program
43 Pain management
44 Palliative care program
45 Inpatient Palliative Care Unit
46 Endoscopic ultrasound
47 Ablation of Barrett's esophagus
48 Esophageal impedance study
49 Endosopic retrograde cholangiopancreatography (ERCP)
50 Enrollment Assistance Services
51 Extracorporeal shock wave lithotripter (ESWL)
52 Fitness center
53 Freestanding outpatient care center
54 Geriatric services
55 Health fair
56 Community Health Education
57 Health screenings
58 Health Research
59 Hemodialysis
60 HIV–AIDS services
61 Home health services
62 Hospital–based outpatient care center services
63 Immunization program
64 Indigent Care Clinic
65 Intermediate nursing care
66 Linguistic/translation services
67 Meals on wheels
68 Medical surgical intensive care services
69 Mobile health services
70 Neonatal intensive care
71 Neonatal intermediate care
72 Neurological services
73 Nutrition programs
74 Obstetrics services
75 Occupational health services
76 Oncology services
77 Orthopedic services
78 Other special care
79 Outpatient surgery
80 Patient Controlled Analgesia (PCA)
81 Patient education center
82 Patient representative services
83 Pediatric intensive care services
84 Pediatric medical–surgical care
85 Physical rehabilitation inpatient services
86 Physical rehabilitation outpatient services
87 Primary care department
88 Psychiatric care
89 Psychiatric–child adolescent services
90 Psychiatric consultation–liaison services
91 Psychiatric education services
92 Psychiatric emergency services
93 Psychiatric geriatric services
94 Psychiatric outpatient services
95 Psychiatric partial hospitalization services
96 CT scanner
97 Diagnostic radioisotope facility
98 Electron beam computed tomography (EBCT)
99 Full–field digital mammography (FFDM)
100 Magnetic resonance imaging (MRI)
101 Intraoperative magnetic resonance imaging
102 Multi–slice spiral computed tomography (MSCT) (<64 slice CT)
103 Multi–slice spiral computed tomography (64 + slice CT)
104 Positron Emission Tomography (PET)
105 Positron Emission Tomography/CT (PET/CT)
106 Single Photon Emission Computerized Tomography (SPECT)
107 Ultrasound
108 Image–guided radiation therapy (IGRT)
109 Intensity–Modulated Radiation Therapy (IMRT)
110 Proton Therapy
111 Shaped beam radiation system
112 Stereotactic radiosurgery
113 Fertility Clinic
114 Genetic Testing/Counseling
115 Retirement housing
116 Robotic surgery
117 Skilled nursing
118 Sleep center
119 Social work services
120 Sports medicine
121 Support groups
122 Swing bed services
123 Teen outreach services
124 Tobacco treatment/cessation program
125 Bone marrow transplant
126 Heart transplant
127 Kidney transplant
128 Liver transplant
129 Lung transplant
130 Tissue transplant
131 Other transplant
132 Transportation to health services
133 Urgent care center
134 Virtual colonoscopy
135 Volunteer services department
136 Women's health center/services
137 Wound management services

Annual Survey

Each year, an annual survey of hospitals is conducted by the American Hospital Association through its Health Forum affiliate.

The facilities and services found below are provided by the hospital. For data products reflecting the services provided by a hospital through its health care system, or network or through a formal arrangement with another provider contact Health Forum at 800/821–2039, or visit www.ahadata.com.

The AHA Guide to the Health Care Field does not include all data collected from the 2007 Annual Survey. Requests for purchasing other Annual Survey data should be directed to Health Forum LLC, an affiliate of the American Hospital Association, One North Franklin, Chicago, IL 60606–3401, 800/821–2039.

Definitions of Facility Codes

1. **Acute long-term care.** Provides specialized acute hospital care to medically complex patients who are critically ill, have multisystem complications and/or failure, and require hospitalization averaging 25 days, in a facility offering specialized treatment programs and therapeutic intervention on a 24–hour/7 day a week basis.
2. **Adult day care program.** Program providing supervision, medical and psychological care, and social activities for older adults who live at home or in another family setting, but cannot be alone or prefer to be with others during the day. May include intake assessment, health monitoring, occupational therapy, personal care, noon meal, and transportation services.
3. **Airborne infection isolation room.** A single–occupancy room for patient care where environmental factors are controlled in an effort to minimize the transmission of those infectious agents, usually spread person to person by droplet nuclei associated with coughing and inhalation. Such rooms typically have specific ventilation requirements for controlled ventilation, air pressure and filtration.
4. **Alcoholism–drug abuse or dependency inpatient unit.** Provides, diagnosis and therapeutic services to patients with alcoholism or other drug dependencies. Includes care for inpatient/residential treatment for patients whose course of treatment involves more intensive care than provided in an outpatient setting or where patient requires supervised withdrawal.
5. **Alcoholism–drug abuse or dependency outpatient unit.** Organized hospital services that provide medical care and/or rehabilitative treatment services to outpatients for whom the primary diagnosis is alcoholism or other chemical dependency.
6. **Alzheimer Center.** Facility that offers care to persons with Alzheimer's disease and their families through an integrated program of clinical services, research, and education.
7. **Ambulance Services.** Provision of ambulance services to the ill and injured who require medical attention on a scheduled or unscheduled basis.
8. **Ambulatory Surgery Center.** Facility that provides care to patients requiring surgery who are admitted and discharged on the same day. Ambulatory surgery centers are distinct from same day surgical units within the hospital outpatient departments for purposes of Medicare payments.
9. **Arthritis treatment center.** Specifically equipped and staffed center for the diagnosis and treatment of arthritis and other joint disorders.
10. **Assisted Living.** A special combination of housing, supportive services, personalized assistance and health care designed to respond to the individual needs of those who need help in activities of daily living and instrumental activities of daily living. Supportive services are available, 24 hours a day, to meet scheduled and unscheduled needs, in a way that promotes maximum independence and dignity for each resident and encourages the involvement of a resident's family, neighbor and friends.
11. **Auxiliary organization.** A volunteer community organization formed to assist the hospital in carrying out its purpose and to serve as a link between the institution and the community.
12. **Bariatric/weight control services.** Bariatrics is the medical practice of weight reduction.
13. **Birthing room–LDR room–LDRP room.** A single room–type of maternity care with a more homelike setting for families than the traditional three–room unit (labor/delivery/recovery) with a separate postpartum area. A birthing room combines labor and delivery in one room. An LDR room accommodates three stages in the birthing process—labor, delivery, and recovery. An LDRP room accommodates all four stages of the birth process—labor, delivery, recovery and postpartum.
14. **Blood Donor Center.** A facility that performs, or is responsible for the collection, processing, testing or distribution of blood and components.
15. **Breast cancer screening/mammograms.** Mammography screening–the use of breast x–ray to detect unsuspected breast cancer in asymptomatic women. Diagnostic mammography–the x–ray imaging of breast tissue in symptomatic women who are considered to have a substantial likelihood of having breast cancer already.
16. **Burn care services.** Provides care to severely burned patients. Severely burned patients are those with any of the following: 1. Second–degree burns of more than 25% total body surface area for adults or 20% total body surface area for children; 2. Third–degree burns of more than 10% total body surface area; 3. Any severe burns of the hands, face, eyes, ears or feet or; 4. All inhalation injuries, electrical burns, complicated burn injuries involving fractures and other major traumas, and all other poor risk factors.
17. **Cardiac intensive care services.** Provides patient care of a more

specialized nature than the usual medical and surgical care, on the basis of physicians' orders and approved nursing care plans. The unit is staffed with specially trained nursing personnel and contains monitoring and specialized support or treatment equipment for patients who, because of heart seizure, open–heart surgery, or other life–threatening conditions, require intensified, comprehensive observation and care. May include myocardial infarction, pulmonary care, and heart transplant units.

18. **Adult diagnostic/invasive catheterization.** (also called coronary angiography or coronary arteriography) is used to assist in diagnosing complex heart conditions. Cardiac angiography involves the insertion of a tiny catheter into the artery in the groin then carefully threading the catheter up into the aorta where the coronary arteries originate. Once the catheter is in place, a dye is injected which allows the cardiologist to see the size, shape, and distribution of the coronary arteries. These images are used to diagnose heart disease and to determine, among other things, whether or not surgery is indicated.

19. **Pediatric diagnostic/invasive catheterization.**

20. **Adult interventional cardiac catheterization.** Non surgical procedure that utilizes the same basic principles as diagnostic catheterization and then uses advanced techniques to improve the heart's function. It can be a less–invasive alternative to heart surgery.

21. **Pediatric interventional cardiac catheterization.**

22. **Adult cardiac surgery.** Includes minimally invasive procedures that include surgery done with only a small incision or no incision at all, such as through a laparoscope or an endoscope and more invasive major surgical procedures that include open chest and open heart surgery.

23. **Pediatric cardiac surgery.**

24. **Cardiac Rehabilitation** A medically supervised program to help heart patients recover quickly and improve their overall physical and mental functioning. The goal is to reduce risk of another cardiac event or to keep an already present heart condition from getting worse. Cardiac rehabilitation programs include: counseling to patients, an exercise program, helping patients modify risk factors such as smoking and high blood pressure, providing vocational guidance to enable the patient to return to work, supplying information on physical limitations and lending emotional support.

25. **Case management.** A system of assessment, treatment planning, referral and follow–up that ensures the provision of comprehensive and continuous services and the coordination of payment and reimbursement for care.

26. **Chaplaincy/pastoral care services.** A service ministering religious activities and providing pastoral counseling to patients, their families, and staff of a health care organization.

27. **Chemotherapy.** An organized program for the treatment of cancer by the use of drugs or chemicals.

28. **Children wellness program.** A program that encourages improved health status and a healthful lifestyle of children through health education, exercise, nutrition and health promotion.

29. **Chiropractic services.** An organized clinical service including spinal manipulation or adjustment and related diagnostic and therapeutic services.

30. **Community health reporting.** Does your hospital either by itself or in conjunction with others disseminate reports to the community on the quality and costs of health care services?

31. **Community health status assessment.** Does your hospital work with other providers, public agencies, or community representatives to conduct a health status assessment of the community?

32. **Community health status based service planning.** Does your hospital use health status indicators (such as rates of health problems or surveys of self–reported health) for defined populations to design new services or modify existing services?

33. **Community outreach.** A program that systematically interacts with the community to identify those in need of services, alerting persons and their families to the availability of services, locating needed services, and enabling persons to enter the service delivery system.

34. **Complementary medicine.** Organized hospital services or formal arrangements to providers that provide care or treatment not based solely on traditional western allopathic medical teachings as instructed in most U.S. medical schools. Includes any of the following; acupuncture, chiropractic, homeopathy, osteopathy, diet and lifestyle changes, herbal medicine, massage therapy, etc.

35. **Computer assisted orthopedic surgery (CAOS).** Orthopedic surgery using computer technology, enabling three–dimensional graphic models to visualize a patient's anatomy.

36. **Crisis Prevention** Services provided in order to promote physical and mental well being and the early identification of disease and ill health prior to the onset and recognition of symptoms so as to permit early treatment.

37. **Dental services.** An organized dental service, not necessarily involving special facilities, that provides dental or oral services to inpatients or outpatients.

38. **Emergency department.** Hospital facilities for the provision of unscheduled outpatient services to patients whose conditions require immediate care. Must be staffed 24 hours a day.

39. **Freestanding/Satellite Emergency Department.** A facility owned and operated by the hospital but physically separate from the hospital for the provision of unscheduled outpatient services to patients whose conditions require.

40. **Trauma center (certified).** A facility certified to provide emergency and specialized intensive care to critically ill and injured patients.

41. **Enabling services.** A program that is designed to help the patient access health care services by offering any of the following linguistic services, transportation services, and/or referrals to local social services agencies.

42. **Hospice program.** A program providing palliative care, chiefly medical relief of pain and supportive services, addressing the emotional, social, financial, and legal needs of terminally ill patients and their families. Care can be provided in a variety of settings, both inpatient and at home.

43. **Pain management.** A hospital wide formalized program that includes staff education for the management of

chronic and acute pain based on guidelines and protocols like those developed by the agency for Health Care Policy Research, etc.

44. **Palliative care program.** An organized program providing specialized medical care, drugs or therapies for the management of acute or chronic pain and/or the control of symptoms adminstered by specially trained physicians and other clinicians; and supportive care services, such as counseling on advanced directives, spiritual care, and social services, to patients with advanced disease and their families.

45. **Inpatient palliative care unit:** An inpatient palliative care ward is a physically discreet, inpatient nursing unit where the focus is palliative care. The patient care focus is on symptom relief for complex patients who may be continuing to undergo primary treatment. Care is delivered by palliative medicine specialists.

46. **Endoscopic ultrasound:** Specially designed endoscope that incorporates an ultrasound transducer used to obtain detailed images of organs in the chest and abdomen. The endoscope can be passed through the mouth or the anus. When combined with needle biopsy the procedure can assist in diagnosis and staging of cancer.

47. **Ablation of Barrett's esophagus:** Premalignant condition that can lead to adenocarcinoma of the esophagus. The non surgical ablation of the premalignant tissue in Barrett's esophagus by the application of thermal energy or light through an endoscope passed from the mouth into the esophagus.

48. **Esophageal impedance study:** A test in which a catheter is placed through the nose into the esophagus to measure whether gas or liquids are passing from the stomach into the esophagus and causing symptoms.

49. **Endoscopic retrograde cholangiopancreatography (ERCP):** A procedure in which a catheter is introduced through an endoscope into the bile ducts and pancreatic ducts. Injection of contrast materials permits detailed x–ray of these structures. The procedure is used diagnostically as well as therapeutically to relieve obstruction or remove stones

50. **Enrollment assistance services.** A program that provides enrollment assistance for patients who are potentially eligible for public health insurance programs such as Medicaid, State Children's Health Insurance, or local/state indigent care programs. The specific services offered could include explanation of benefits, assist applicants in completing the application and locating all relevant documents, conduct eligibilty interviews, and/or forward applications and documentation to state/local social service or health agency.

51. **Extracorporeal shock wave lithotripter (ESWL).** A medical device used for treating stones in the kidney or ureter. The device disintegrates kidney stones noninvasively through the transmission of acoustic shock waves directed at the stones.

52. **Fitness Center.** Provides exercise, testing, or evaluation programs and fitness activities to the community and hospital employees.

53. **Freestanding outpatient care center.** A facility owned and operated by the hospital, but physically separate from the hospital, that provides various medical treatments on an outpatient basis only. In addition to treating minor illnesses or injuries, the center will stabilize seriously ill or injured patients before transporting them to a hospital. Laboratory and radiology services are usually available.

54. **Geriatric services.** The branch of medicine dealing with the physiology of aging and the diagnosis and treatment of disease affecting the aged. Services could include: Adult day care program; Alzheimer's diagnostic–assessment services; Comprehensive geriatric assessment; Emergency response system; Geriatric acute care unit; and/or Geriatric clinics.

55. **Health fair.** Community health education events that focus on the prevention of disease and promotion of health through such activities as audiovisual exhibits and free diagnostic services.

56. **Community Health Education:** Education that provides information to individuals and populations. Support to personal, family and community health decisions with the objective of improving health status.

57. **Health screenings.** A preliminary procedure, such as a test or examination to detect the most characteristic sign or signs of a disorder that may require further investigation.

58. **Health Research:** Organized hospital research program in any of the following areas: basic research, clinical research, community health research, and/or research on innovative health care delivery.

59. **Hemodialysis.** Provision of equipment and personnel for the treatment of renal insufficiency on an inpatient or outpatient basis.

60. **HIV–AIDS services.** Services may include one or more of the following: HIV–AIDS unit (special unit or team designated and equipped specifically for diagnosis, treatment, continuing care planning, and counseling services for HIV–AIDS patients and their families.) General inpatient care for HIV–AIDS (inpatient diagnosis and treatment for human immunodeficiency virus and acquired immunodeficiency syndrome patients, but dedicated unit is not available.) Specialized outpatient program for HIV–AIDS (special outpatient program providing diagnostic, treatment, continuing care planning, and counseling for HIV–AIDS patients and their families.)

61. **Home health services.** Service providing nursing, therapy, and health–related homemaker or social services in the patient's home.

62. **Hospital–based outpatient care center services.** Organized hospital health care services offered by appointment on an ambulatory basis. Services may include outpatient surgery, examination, diagnosis, and treatment of a variety of medical conditions on a nonemergency basis, and laboratory and other diagnostic testing as ordered by staff or outside physician referral.

63. **Immunization program:** Program that plans, coordinates and conducts immunization services in the community.

64. **Indigent Care Clinic:** Health care services for uninsured persons where care is free of charge or charged on a sliding scale. This would include "free clinics" staffed by volunteer practitioners, but could also be staffed by employees with the sponsoring health care organization and their physicians.

65. **Intermediate nursing care.** Provides health–related services (skilled nursing care and social services) to residents with a variety of physical conditions or functional disabilities.

These residents do not require the care provided by a hospital or skilled nursing facility, but do need supervision and support services.

66. **Linguistic/translation services.** Services provided by the hospital designed to make health care more accessible to non–English speaking patients and their physicians.

67. **Meals on wheels.** A hospital sponsored program which delivers meals to people, usually the elderly, who are unable to prepare their own meals. Low cost, nutritional meals are delivered to individuals' homes on a regular basis.

68. **Medical surgical intensive care services.** Provides patient care of a more intensive nature than the usual medical and surgical care, on the basis of physicians' orders and approved nursing care plans. These units are staffed with specially trained nursing personnel and contain monitoring and specialized support equipment of patients who, because of shock, trauma, or other life–threatening conditions, require intensified, comprehensive observation and care. Includes mixed intensive care units.

69. **Mobile health services.** Vans and other vehicles used to deliver primary care services.

70. **Neonatal intensive care.** A unit that must be separate from the newborn nursery providing intensive care to all sick infants including those with the very lowest birth weights (less that 1500 grams). NICU has potential for providing mechanical ventilation, neonatal surgery, and special care for the sickest infants born in the hospital or transferred from another institution. A full–time neonatologist serves as director of the NICU.

71. **Neonatal intermediate care.** A unit that must be separate from the normal newborn nursery and that provides intermediate and/or recovery care and some specialized services, including immediate resuscitation, intravenous therapy, and capacity for prolonged oxygen therapy and monitoring.

72. **Neurological services.** Services provided by the hospital dealing with the operative and nonoperative management of disorders of the central, peripheral, and autonomic nervous system.

73. **Nutrition programs.** Those services within a health care facility which are designed to provide inexpensive, nutritionally sound meals to patients.

74. **Obstetrics services.** Levels should be designated: (1) unit provides services for uncomplicated maternity and newborn cases; (2) unit provides services for uncomplicated cases, the majority of complicated problems, and special neonatal services; and (3) unit provides services for all serious illnesses and abnormalities and is supervised by a full–time maternal/fetal specialist.

75. **Occupational health services.** Includes services designed to protect the safety of employees from hazards in the work environment.

76. **Oncology services.** An organized program for the treatment of cancer by the use of drugs or chemicals.

77. **Orthopedic services.** Services provided for the prevention or correction of injuries or disorders of the skeletal system and associated muscles, joints, and ligaments.

78. **Other special care.** Provides care to patients requiring care more intensive than that provided in the acute area, yet not sufficiently intensive to require admission to an intensive care unit. Patients admitted to the area are usually transferred here from an intensive care unit once their condition has improved. These units are sometimes referred to as definitive observation, step–down, or progressive care units.

79. **Outpatient surgery.** Scheduled surgical services provided to patients who do not remain in the hospital overnight. The surgery may be performed in operating suites also used for inpatient surgery, specially designated surgical suites for outpatient surgery, or procedure rooms within an outpatient care facility.

80. **Patient Controlled Analgesia (PCA).** Patient Controlled Analgesia (PCA) is intravenously administered pain medicine under the patient's control. The patient has a button on the end of a cord than can be pushed at will, whenever more pain medicine is desired. This button will only deliver more pain medicine at pre–determined intervals, as programmed by the doctor's order.

81. **Patient education center.** Written goals and objectives for the patient and/or family related to therapeutic regimens, medical procedures, and self care.

82. **Patient representative services.** Organized hospital services providing personnel through whom patients and staff can seek solutions to institutional problems affecting the delivery of high–quality care and services.

83. **Pediatric intensive care services.** Provides care to pediatric patients that is of a more intensive nature than that usually provided to pediatric patients. The unit is staffed with specially trained personnel and contains monitoring and specialized support equipment for treatment of patients who, because of shock, trauma, or other life–threatening conditions, require intensified, comprehensive observation and care.

84. **Pediatric medical–surgical care.** Provides acute care to pediatric patients on the basis of physicians' orders and approved nursing care plans.

85. **Physical rehabilitation inpatient services.** Provides care encompassing a comprehensive array of restoration services for the disabled and all support services necessary to help patients attain their maximum functional capacity.

86. **Physical rehabilitation outpatient services.** Outpatient program providing medical, health–related, therapy, social, and/or vocational services to help disabled persons attain or retain their maximum functional capacity.

87. **Primary care department.** A unit or clinic within the hospital that provides primary care services (e.g. general pediatric care, general internal medicine, family practice and gynecology) through hospital–salaried medical and or nursing staff, focusing on evaluating and diagnosing medical problems and providing medical treatment on an outpatient basis.

88. **Psychiatric care.** Provides acute or long–term care to emotionally disturbed patients, including patients admitted for diagnosis and those admitted for treatment of psychiatric problems, on the basis of physicians' orders and approved nursing care plans. Long–term care may include intensive supervision to the chronically mentally ill, mentally disordered, or other mentally incompetent persons.

89. **Psychiatric child–adolescent services.** Provides care to emotionally disturbed children and adolescents, including those admitted for diagnosis and those admitted for treatment.

90. **Psychiatric consultation–liaison services.** Provides organized psychiatric consultation/liaison services to nonpsychiatric hospital staff and/or department on psychological aspects of medical care that may be generic or specific to individual patients.

91. **Psychiatric education services.** Provides psychiatric educational services to community agencies and workers such as schools, police, courts, public health nurses, welfare agencies, clergy and so forth. The purpose is to expand the mental health knowledge and competence of personnel not working in the mental health field and to promote good mental health through improved understanding, attitudes, and behavioral patterns.

92. **Psychiatric emergency services.** Services or facilities available on a 24–hour basis to provide immediate unscheduled outpatient care, diagnosis, evaluation, crisis intervention, and assistance to persons suffering acute emotional or mental distress.

93. **Psychiatric geriatric services.** Provides care to emotionally disturbed elderly patients, including those admitted for diagnosis and those admitted for treatment.

94. **Psychiatric outpatient services.** Provides medical care, including diagnosis and treatment of psychiatric outpatients.

95. **Psychiatric partial hospitalization services.** Organized hospital services of intensive day/evening outpatient services of three hours or more duration, distinguished from other outpatient visits of one hour.

96. **CT scanner.** Computed tomographic scanner for head and whole body scans.

97. **Diagnostic radioisotope facility.** The use of radioactive isotopes (Radiopharmaceutical) as tracers or indicators to detect an abnormal condition or disease.

98. **Electron Beam Computed Tomography (EBCT).** A high tech computed tomography scan used to detect coronary artery disease by measuring coronary calcifications. This imaging procedure uses electron beams which are magnetically steered to produce a visual of the coronary artery and the images are produced faster than conventional CT scans.

99. **Full–field digital mammography (FFDM).** Combines the x–ray generators and tubes used in analog screen–film mammography (SFM) with a detector plate that converts the x–rays into a digital signal.

100. **Magnetic resonance imaging (MRI).** The use of a uniform magnetic field and radio frequencies to study tissue and structure of the body. This procedure enables the visualization of biochemical activity of the cell in vivo without the use of ionizing radiation, radioisotopic substances, or high–frequency sound.

101. **Intraoperative magnetic resonance imaging.** An integrated surgery system which provides an MRI system in an operating room. The system allows for immediate evaluation of the degree to tumor resection while the patient is undergoing a surgical resection. Intraoperative MRI exists when a MRI (low–field or high–field) is placed in the operating theater and is used during surgical resection without moving the patient from the operating room to the diagnostic imaging suite.

102. **Multi–slice Spiral Computed Tomography (MSCT) (<64 slice CT).** A specialized computed tomography procedure that provides three–dimensional processing and allows narrower and multiple slices with increased spatial resolution and faster scanning times as compared to a regular computed tomography scan.

103. **Multi–slice spiral computed tomography (64 + slice CT).** Involves the acquisition of volumetric tomographic x–ray absorption data expressed in Hounsfield units using multiple rows of detectors. 64+ systems reconstruct the equivalent of 64 or greater slices to cover the imaged volume.

104. **Positron emission tomography scanner (PET).** is a nuclear medicine imaging technology which uses radioactive (positron emitting) isotopes created in a cyclotron or generator and computers to produce composite pictures of the brain and heart at work. PET scanning produces sectional images depicting metabolic activity or blood flow rather than anatomy.

105. **Positron Emission Tomography/CT (PET/CT).** Provides metabolic functional information for the monitoring of chemotherapy, radiotherapy and surgical planning.

106. **Single photon emission computerized tomography (SPECT).** is a nuclear medicine imaging technology that combines existing technology of gamma camera imaging with computed tomographic imaging technology to provide a more precise and clear image.

107. **Ultrasound.** The use of acoustic waves above the range of 20,000 cycles per second to visualize internal body structures.

108. **Image–guided radiation therapy (IGRT).** Automated system for image–guided radiation therapy that enables clinicians to obtain high–resolution x–ray images to pinpoint tumor sites, adjust patient positioning when necessary, and complete a treatment, all within the standard treatment time slot, allowing for more effective cancer treatments.

109. **Intensity–Modulated Radiation Therapy (IMRT).** A type of three–dimensional radiation therapy, which improves the targeting of treatment delivery in a way that is likely to decrease damage to normal tissues and allows varying intensities diagnosis of genetic diseases in newborns, children, and adults; the identification of future health risks; the prediction of drug responses; and the assessment of risks to future children.

110. **Proton Therapy:** A form of radiation therapy which administers proton beams. While producing the same biologic effects as x–ray beams, the energy distribution of protons differs from conventional x–ray beams in that they can be more precisely focused in tissue volumes in a three–dimensional pattern resulting in less surrounding tissue damage than conventional radiation therapy permitting administration of higher doses.

111. **Shaped beam radiation system.** A precise, non–invasive treatment that involves targeting beams of radiation that mirror the exact size and shape of a tumor at a specific area of a tumor to shrink or destroy cancerous cells. This procedure delivers a therapeutic dose of radiation that conforms precisely to the shape of the tumor, thus minimizing the risk to nearby tissues.

112. **Stereotactic radiosurgery.** Stereotactic radiosurgery (SRS) is a radiotherapy modality that delivers a high dosage of radiation to a discrete treatment area in as few as one treatment session. Includes gamma knife, cyberknife, etc.

113. **Fertility Clinic.** A specialized program set in an infertility center

that provides counseling and education as well as advanced reproductive techniques such as: injectable therapy, reproductive surgeries, treatment for endometriosis, male factor infertility, tubal reversals, in vitro fertilization (IVF), donor eggs, and other such services to help patients achieve successful pregnancies.

114. Genetic Testing/Counseling A service equipped with adequate laboratory facilities and directed by a qualified physician to advise parents and prospective parents on potential problems in cases of genetic defects. A genetic test is the analysis of human DNA, RNA, chromosomes, proteins, and certain metabolites in order to detect heritable disease–related genotypes, mutations, phenotypes, or karyotypes for clinical purposes. Genetic tests can have diverse purposes, including the diagnosis of genetic diseases in newborns, children, and adults; the identification of future health risks; the prediction of drug responses; and the assessment of risks to future children.

115. Retirement housing. A facility which provides social activities to senior citizens, usually retired persons, who do not require health care but some short–term skilled nursing care may be provided. A retirement center may furnish housing and may also have acute hospital and long–term care facilities, or it may arrange for acute and long term care through affiliated institutions.

116. Robotic surgery. The use of mechanical guidance devices to remotely manipulate surgical instrumentation.

117. Skilled nursing. Provides non–acute medical and skilled nursing care services, therapy, and social services under the supervision of a licensed registered nurse on a 24–hour basis.

118. Sleep Center. Specially equipped and staffed center for the diagnosis and treatment of sleep disorders.

119. Social work services. Services may include one or more of the following: Organized social work services (services that are properly directed and sufficiently staffed by qualified individuals who provide assistance and counseling to patients and their families in dealing with social, emotional, and environmental problems associated with illness or disability, often in the context of financial or discharge planning coordination.) Outpatient social work services (social work services provided in ambulatory care areas.) Emergency department social work services (social work services provided to emergency department patients by social workers dedicated to the emergency department or on call.)

120. Sports medicine. Provision of diagnostic screening and assessment and clinical and rehabilitation services for the prevention and treatment of sports–related injuries.

121. Support groups. A hospital sponsored program which allows a group of individuals with the same or similar problems who meet periodically to share experiences, problems, and solutions, in order to support each other.

122. Swing bed services. A hospital bed that can be used to provide either acute or long–term care depending on community or patients needs. To be eligible a hospital must have a Medicare provider agreement in place, have fewer than 100 beds, be located in a rural area, not have a 24 hour nursing service waiver in effect, have not been terminated from the program in the prior two years, and meet various service conditions.

123. Teen outreach services. A program focusing on the teenager which encourages an improved health status and a healthful lifestyle including physical, emotional, mental, social, spiritual and economic health through education, exercise, nutrition and health promotion.

124. Tobacco Treatment/Cessation Program. Organized hospital services with the purpose of ending tobacco–use habits of patients addicted to tobacco/nicotine.

125.–131. Transplant services. The branch of medicine that transfers an organ or tissue from one person to another or from one body part to another to replace a diseased structure or to restore function or to change appearance. Services could include: Bone marrow transplant program **(125. Bone marrow)**; heart **(126. Heart)**, kidney **(127. Kidney)**, liver **(128. Liver)** lung **(129. Lung)**, tissue **(130. Tissue Transplant)**. Please include heart/lung or other multi–transplant surgeries in other **(131. Other)**.

132. Transportation to health services. A long–term care support service designed to assist the mobility of the elderly. Some programs offer improved financial access by offering reduced rates and barrier–free buses or vans with ramps and lifts to assist the elderly or handicapped; others offer subsidies for public transport systems or operate mini–bus services exclusively for use by senior citizens.

133. Urgent care center. A facility that provides care and treatment for problems that are not life–threatening but require attention over the short term. These units function like emergency rooms but are separate from hospitals with which they may have backup affiliation arrangements.

134. Virtual colonoscopy. Noninvasive screening procedure used to visualize, analyze and detect cancerous or potentially cancerous polyps in the colon.

135. Volunteer services department. An organized hospital department responsible for coordinating the services of volunteers working within the institution.

136. Women's health center/services. An area set aside for coordinated education and treatment services specifically for and promoted by women as provided by this special unit. Services may or may not include obstetrics but include a range of services other than OB.

137. Wound management services. Services for patients with chronic wounds and non–healing wounds often resulting from diabetes, poor circulation, improper seating and immunocompromising conditions. The goals are to progress chronic wounds through stages of healing, reduce and eliminate infections, increase physical function to minimize complications from current wounds and prevent future chronic wounds. Wound management services are provided on an inpatient or outpatient basis, depending on the intensity of service needed.

Definitions of Physician Codes

1. **Closed physician–hospital organization (PHO).** A PHO that restricts physician membership to those practitioners who meet criteria for cost effectiveness and/or high quality.

2. **Equity model.** Allows established practitioners to become shareholders in a professional corporation in exchange for tangible and intangible assets of their existing practices.

3. **Foundation.** A corporation, organized either as a hospital affiliate or subsidiary, which purchases both the tangible and intangible assets of one or more medical group practices. Physicians remain in a separate corporate entity but sign a professional services agreement with the foundation.

4. **Group practice without walls.** Hospital sponsors the formation of, or provides capital to physicians to establish, a 'quasi' group to share administrative expenses while remaining independent practitioners.

5. **Independent practice association (IPA).** An IPA is a legal entity that hold managed care contracts. The IPA then contracts with physicians, usually in solo practice, to provide care either on a fee–for–services or capitated basis. The purpose of an IPA is to assist solo physicians in obtaining managed care contracts.

6. **Integrated salary model.** Physicians are salaried by the hospital or another entity of a health system to provide medical services for primary care and specialty care.

7. **Management services organization (MSO).** A corporation, owned by the hospital or a physician/hospital joint venture, that provides management services to one or more medical group practices. The MSO purchases the tangible assets of the practices and leases them back as part of a full–service management agreement, under which the MSO employs all non–physician staff and provides all supplies/administrative systems for a fee.

8. **Open physician–hospital organization (PHO).** A joint venture between the hospital and all members of the medical staff who wish to participate. The PHO can act as a unified agent in managed care contracting, own a managed care plan, own and operate ambulatory care centers or ancillary services projects, or provide administrative services to physician members.

Control and Service Classifications

Control

Government, nonfederal
State
County
City
City–county
Hospital district or authority

Nongovernment not–for–profit
Church operated
Other

Investor–owned (for–profit)
Individual
Partnership
Corporation

Government, federal
Air Force
Army
Navy
Public Health Service other than 47
Veterans Affairs
Federal other than 41–45, 47–48
Public Health Service Indian Service
Department of Justice

Osteopathic
Church operated
Other not–for–profit
Other
Individual for–profit
Partnership for–profit
Corporation for–profit

Service

General medical and surgical
Hospital unit of an institution (prison hospital, college infirmary, etc.)
Hospital unit within an institution for the mentally retarded
Surgical
Psychiatric
Tuberculosis and other respiratory diseases
Cancer
Heart
Obstetrics and gynecology
Eye, ear, nose, and throat
Rehabilitation
Orthopedic
Chronic disease
Other specialty
Children's general
Children's hospital unit of an institution
Children's psychiatric
Children's tuberculosis and other respiratory diseases
Children's eye, ear, nose, and throat
Children's rehabilitation
Children's orthopedic
Children's chronic disease
Children's other specialty
Institution for mental retardation
Long–Term Acute Care
Alcoholism and other chemical dependency
Children's Long–Term Acute Care
Children's Cancer
Children's Heart

Notes

Notes

Notes

Notes

Hospitals in the United States, by State

ALABAMA

ALABASTER—Shelby County

★□ **SHELBY BAPTIST MEDICAL CENTER (10016)**, 1000 First Street North, Zip 35007–0488; tel. 205/620–8100 **A**1 2 9 10 **F**8 11 12 13 15 17 18 20 22 24 25 26 27 30 31 32 33 35 36 38 40 41 43 49 50 52 55 56 57 59 62 65 68 70 72 73 74 75 77 79 80 82 86 90 92 96 97 99 100 102 106 107 112 116 118 119 120 121 124 135 136 137 **P**6 **S** Baptist Health System
Primary Contact: David C. Wilson, President
COO: Scott Williams, Chief Operating Officer
CFO: Lee Boles, Chief Financial Officer
CIO: Mike Nighman, Director Information Systems
CHR: Cindy Nicholson, Director Human Resources
Web address: www.bhsala.com
Control: Church–operated, Nongovernment, not–for profit **Service:** General Medical and Surgical

Staffed Beds: 176 **Admissions:** 10656 **Census:** 122 **Outpatient Visits:** 117640 **Births:** 987 **Total Expense ($000):** 112284 **Payroll Expense ($000):** 36445 **Personnel:** 878

ALEXANDER CITY—Tallapoosa County

★□ ○ **RUSSELL MEDICAL CENTER (10065)**, 3316 Highway 280, Zip 35010–3369, Mailing Address: P.O. Box 939, Zip 35011–0939; tel. 256/329–7100 **A**1 9 10 11 19 **F**3 11 13 15 18 20 24 25 26 27 28 30 31 32 33 34 38 40 49 50 51 52 55 56 57 59 62 68 71 73 74 75 76 77 78 79 80 82 84 86 96 97 99 100 102 103 104 105 106 107 109 111 118 119 120 121 132 133 135 136
Primary Contact: Luther E. Peace, III, President and Chief Executive Officer
CFO: Mike Myers, Chief Financial Officer
CIO: Joseph George, Director Information Services
CHR: Mary Shockley, Director Human Resources
Web address: www.russellmedcenter.com
Control: Other not–for–profit (including NFP Corporation) **Service:** General Medical and Surgical

Staffed Beds: 81 **Admissions:** 3805 **Census:** 33 **Outpatient Visits:** 83614 **Births:** 627 **Total Expense ($000):** 58039 **Payroll Expense ($000):** 19519 **Personnel:** 520

ANDALUSIA—Covington County

★□ **ANDALUSIA REGIONAL HOSPITAL (10036)**, 849 South Three Notch Street, Zip 36420–5325, Mailing Address: P.O. Box 760, Zip 36420–0760; tel. 334/222–8466 **A**1 9 10 **F**25 26 38 55 67 72 73 74 75 77 79 85 86 96 97 99 100 103 107 118 120 122 124 135 **S** LifePoint Hospitals, Inc.
Primary Contact: Mark J. Dooley, Chief Executive Officer
COO: Melissa Davis, Chief Operating Officer
CFO: Shirley M. Smith, Chief Financial Officer
CIO: Matthew Perry, Director Information Systems
CHR: Kaci Daughtry, Director Human Resources
Web address: www.andalusiaregionalhospital.com
Control: Corporation, Investor–owned, for–profit **Service:** General Medical and Surgical

Staffed Beds: 87 **Admissions:** 4476 **Census:** 43 **Outpatient Visits:** 34366 **Births:** 396

ANNISTON—Calhoun County

□ **LONG TERM HOSPITAL OF ANNISTON (10165)**, 400 East 10th Street, 4th Floor, Zip 36207; tel. 256/741–6141, (Nonreporting) **A**1 10 **S** Noland Health Services, Inc.
Primary Contact: Bob Notarianni, Administrator
Web address: www.nolandhealth.com
Control: Other not–for–profit (including NFP Corporation) **Service:** Long–Term Acute Care hospital

Staffed Beds: 34

★□ **NORTHEAST ALABAMA REGIONAL MEDICAL CENTER (10078)**, 400 East Tenth Street, Zip 36207–4716, Mailing Address: P.O. Box 2208, Zip 36202–2208; tel. 256/235–5121 **A**1 2 9 10 **F**3 8 11 12 13 15 17 18 20 22 24 25 26 27 30 31 32 33 38 40 41 43 46 47 48 49 50 52 53 54 55 56 57 59 60 61 62 66 68 72 74 75 76 77 79 80 81 82 84 88 92 93 94 95 96 97 100 102 104 105 107 111 118 119 121 135 136 137
Primary Contact: Allen P. Fletcher, President and Chief Executive Officer
CFO: Louis A. Bass, Vice President Finance
CMO: C. Neal Canup, M.D., Vice President Medical Affairs
CIO: Fred Wilson, Director Management Information Services
CHR: Michael S. Simms, Vice President Human Resources
Web address: www.rmccares.org
Control: Hospital district or authority, Government, nonfederal **Service:** General Medical and Surgical

Staffed Beds: 276 **Admissions:** 15746 **Census:** 202 **Outpatient Visits:** 115196 **Births:** 1552 **Total Expense ($000):** 110823 **Payroll Expense ($000):** 51978 **Personnel:** 1272

□ **STRINGFELLOW MEMORIAL HOSPITAL (10038)**, 301 East 18th Street, Zip 36207–0038, Mailing Address: P.O. Box 38, Zip 36207–0038; tel. 256/235–8900, (Nonreporting) **A**1 9 10 **S** Health Management Associates
Primary Contact: Linda P. Burdette, Chief Executive Officer
COO: Linda P. Burdette, Chief Executive Officer
CIO: Peggy Henderson, Director Health Information
CHR: Tamatha Johnson, Director Human Resources
Web address: www.stringfellowhealth.com
Control: Corporation, Investor–owned, for–profit **Service:** General Medical and Surgical

Staffed Beds: 125

ASHLAND—Clay County

★ **CLAY COUNTY HOSPITAL (10073)**, 83825 Highway 9, Zip 36251, Mailing Address: P.O. Box 1270, Zip 36251–1270; tel. 256/354–2131, (Total facility includes 83 beds in nursing home–type unit) **A**9 10 **F**10 11 15 25 26 30 31 32 38 42 50 52 54 55 56 57 61 62 65 68 75 79 81 82 85 86 96 107 117 118 119 121 122 135
Primary Contact: Linda U. Jordan, Administrator
CFO: Kerry W. Tomlin, Associate Administrator
Web address: www.claycountyhospital.com
Control: Other not–for–profit (including NFP Corporation) **Service:** General Medical and Surgical

Staffed Beds: 131 **Admissions:** 1646 **Census:** 97 **Outpatient Visits:** 28535 **Births:** 0 **Total Expense ($000):** 14567 **Payroll Expense ($000):** 6978 **Personnel:** 219

ATHENS—Limestone County

★□ **ATHENS–LIMESTONE HOSPITAL (10079)**, 700 West Market Street, Zip 35611–2457, Mailing Address: P.O. Box 999, Zip 35612–0999; tel. 256/233–9292 **A**1 9 10 **F**3 7 8 11 13 15 24 25 30 31 32 33 38 41 44 46 50 51 52 53 55 56 57 58 62 66 68 71 73 74 79 80 81 82 84 86 88 96 97 100 107 118 119 120 121 123 124 132 133 135
Primary Contact: Cary J. Payne, Chief Executive Officer
CFO: Randy Comer, Chief Financial Officer
CMO: Paul Noel, M.D., Chief of Staff
CIO: Kim Hoback, Supervisor Information Systems
CHR: Rachel Frey, Director Human Resources
Web address: www.athenslimestonehospital.com
Control: Hospital district or authority, Government, nonfederal **Service:** General Medical and Surgical

Staffed Beds: 101 **Admissions:** 4006 **Census:** 38 **Outpatient Visits:** 101016 **Births:** 460 **Payroll Expense ($000):** 19665 **Personnel:** 609

Hospital, Medicare Provider Number, Address, Telephone, Approval, Facility, and Physician Codes, Health Care System

★ American Hospital Association (AHA) membership
□ The Joint Commission accreditation
○ American Osteopathic Association (AOA) accreditation
△ Commission on Accreditation of Rehabilitation Facilities (CARF) accreditation

ATMORE—Escambia County

★ **ATMORE COMMUNITY HOSPITAL (11301)**, 401 Medical Park Drive, Zip 36502–3091; tel. 251/368–2500, (Nonreporting) **A**1 5 9 10 18 **S** Baptist Health Care Corporation
Primary Contact: Robert E. Gowing, Administrator
Web address: www.ebaptisthealthcare.org
Control: Other not–for–profit (including NFP Corporation) **Service:** General Medical and Surgical

Staffed Beds: 51

BAY MINETTE—Baldwin County

NORTH BALDWIN INFIRMARY (10129), 1815 Hand Avenue, Zip 36507–4110, Mailing Address: P.O. Box 1409, Zip 36507–1409; tel. 251/937–5521, (Nonreporting) **A**9 10 **S** Infirmary Health System
Primary Contact: William J. McLaughlin, Administrator
CFO: J. Patrick Murphy, Chief Financial Officer
Web address: www.mobileinfirmary.org
Control: Other not–for–profit (including NFP Corporation) **Service:** General Medical and Surgical

Staffed Beds: 130

BESSEMER—Jefferson County

★ **MEDICAL WEST (10114)**, 995 Ninth Avenue S.W., Zip 35022–4527; tel. 205/481–7000 **A**1 2 9 10 **F**3 8 11 13 15 18 25 26 27 30 31 32 38 40 49 50 55 56 57 63 68 72 73 74 75 76 77 78 79 80 81 85 86 88 90 91 92 93 96 97 100 107 119 121 132 135 136 137 **P**6 **S** UAB Health System
Primary Contact: Timothy J. Thornton, Chief Executive Officer
COO: Keith Pennington, Senior Vice President and Chief Operating Officer
CFO: Rita Neely, Senior Vice President and Chief Financial Officer
CMO: Frank D. Miller, M.D., President Medical Staff
CIO: Bob Duckworth, Director Information Systems
CHR: Gannon Davis, Director Human Resources
Web address: www.uabmedicalwest.org
Control: Hospital district or authority, Government, nonfederal **Service:** General Medical and Surgical

Staffed Beds: 214 **Admissions:** 9037 **Census:** 140 **Outpatient Visits:** 176388 **Births:** 683 **Total Expense ($000):** 102695 **Payroll Expense ($000):** 42936 **Personnel:** 1149

BIRMINGHAM—Jefferson County

★ **BROOKWOOD MEDICAL CENTER (10139)**, 2010 Brookwood Medical Center Drive, Zip 35209–6875; tel. 205/877–1000, (Nonreporting) **A**1 2 3 5 9 10 **S** TENET Healthcare Corporation
Primary Contact: Garry L. Gause, Chief Executive Officer
COO: Joe Stough, Chief Operating Officer
CFO: Doug Carter, Chief Financial Officer
CMO: Bradley Dennis, M.D., Chief Medical Officer
CIO: Manuel Price, Director Information Systems
CHR: Ronnelle Stewart, Vice President Human Resources
Web address: www.brookwood–medical.com
Control: Corporation, Investor–owned, for–profit **Service:** General Medical and Surgical

Staffed Beds: 586

☐ **CALLAHAN EYE FOUNDATION HOSPITAL (10018)**, 1720 University Boulevard, Zip 35233–1816; tel. 205/325–8100 **A**1 3 5 9 10 **F**31 32 33 38 55 56 57 62 64 75 79 81 119 **S** UAB Health System
Primary Contact: Raymond Butler, President
CFO: Libby Bailey, Chief Financial Officer
CMO: Robert Morris, M.D., Chief of Staff
CIO: Maxine Nichols, Director Information Systems
CHR: Karen Burleson, Assistant Vice President Human Resources
Web address: www.health.uab.edu/eyes
Control: Other not–for–profit (including NFP Corporation) **Service:** Eye, ear, nose, and throat

Staffed Beds: 20 **Admissions:** 210 **Census:** 2 **Outpatient Visits:** 18568 **Births:** 0 **Total Expense ($000):** 22623 **Payroll Expense ($000):** 7657 **Personnel:** 149

★ **COOPER GREEN HOSPITAL (10137)**, 1515 Sixth Avenue South, Zip 35233–1688; tel. 205/930–3200 **A**1 3 5 9 10 **F**3 13 15 25 26 27 31 33 38 39 40 42 43 44 45 46 49 50 53 55 56 57 58 60 62 63 64 66 68 70 71 73 74 75 76 77 79 80 81 86 87 96 97 107 119 135 136 137 **P**4 6
Primary Contact: Sandral Hullett, M.D., Chief Executive Officer and Medical Director
COO: Jamie Sullivan, Chief Operating Officer
CFO: John Garrett, Chief Financial Officer
CMO: Ryan Nash, M.D., Chief of Staff
CIO: Sri Karra, Chief Information Officer
CHR: Huberta Mayfield Howe, Director Human Resources
Control: County–Government, nonfederal **Service:** General Medical and Surgical

Staffed Beds: 141 **Admissions:** 4139 **Census:** 56 **Outpatient Visits:** 148776 **Births:** 515 **Total Expense ($000):** 81001 **Payroll Expense ($000):** 32556 **Personnel:** 581

★ **HEALTHSOUTH LAKESHORE REHABILITATION HOSPITAL (13025)**, 3800 Ridgeway Drive, Zip 35209–5599; tel. 205/868–2000 **A**1 9 10 **F**3 25 57 62 73 81 82 85 86 119 121 132 137 **P**8 **S** HEALTHSOUTH Corporation
Primary Contact: Terrence E. Brown, Chief Executive Officer
CFO: Tammy Young, Controller
CMO: Paula Stewart, M.D., Medical Director
CHR: John Estis, Director Human Resources
Web address: www.healthsouth.com
Control: Corporation, Investor–owned, for–profit **Service:** Rehabilitation

Staffed Beds: 100 **Admissions:** 1928 **Census:** 76 **Outpatient Visits:** 14351 **Births:** 0

☐ **HILL CREST BEHAVIORAL HEALTH SERVICES (14000)**, 6869 Fifth Avenue South, Zip 35212–1866; tel. 205/833–9000, (Nonreporting) **A**1 9 10 **S** Psychiatric Solutions
Primary Contact: Steve McCabe, Chief Executive Officer
CFO: Mark Teske, Chief Financial Officer
Web address: www.psysolutions.com
Control: Partnership, Investor–owned, for–profit **Service:** Psychiatric

Staffed Beds: 55

☐ **LONG TERM HOSPITAL OF BIRMINGHAM (12009)**, (Formerly Long Term Care Hospital), 50 Medical Park East Drive, 8th Floor, Zip 35235; tel. 205/808–5100, (Nonreporting) **A**1 9 10 **S** Noland Health Services, Inc.
Primary Contact: Xavier Ritchie, Administrator
Web address: www.nolandhealth.com
Control: Other not–for–profit (including NFP Corporation) **Service:** Long–Term Acute Care hospital

Staffed Beds: 23

☐ **PHYSICIANS MEDICAL CENTER – CARRAWAY (10064)**, 1600 Carraway Boulevard, Zip 35234–1990; tel. 205/502–6000 **A**1 3 5 8 9 10 **F**4 12 15 17 18 20 22 24 25 26 27 33 43 46 49 52 62 68 72 75 76 77 79 80 86 87 88 92 93 96 97 100 102 106 107 118 119 135 137
Primary Contact: Martin Nowak, FACHE, Chief Executive Officer
CFO: Peggy Allen, Chief Financial Officer
CMO: Stephen Hamburger, M.D., Senior Vice President Academic and Medical Staff Affairs
CIO: Tim Townes, Director Information Systems
CHR: Glenda Jones, Director Human Resources
Web address: www.carraway.org
Control: Corporation, Investor–owned, for–profit **Service:** General Medical and Surgical

Staffed Beds: 191 **Admissions:** 8929 **Census:** 130 **Outpatient Visits:** 119966 **Births:** 0 **Total Expense ($000):** 106885 **Payroll Expense ($000):** 44163 **Personnel:** 935

☐ **PRINCETON BAPTIST MEDICAL CENTER (10103)**, (Formerly Baptist Princeton), 701 Princeton Avenue S.W., Zip 35211–1305; tel. 205/783–3000 **A**1 2 3 5 9 10 **F**11 12 15 17 18 20 22 24 25 26 27 30 32 33 38 40 43 49 50 54 55 56 57 58 62 65 68 70 72 74 76 77 79 82 86 88 93 94 96 97 99 100 102 103 105 107 108 109 111 117 118 119 120 121 135 136 137 **S** Baptist Health System
Primary Contact: Betsy Postlethwait, Interim President
COO: Betsy Postlethwait, Chief Operating Officer
CFO: Gene Taylor, Chief Financial Officer
CMO: David Russakoff, M.D., Chief Medical Officer
Web address: www.bhsala.com
Control: Church–operated, Nongovernment, not–for profit **Service:** General Medical and Surgical

Staffed Beds: 368 **Admissions:** 13049 **Census:** 198 **Outpatient Visits:** 116558 **Births:** 421 **Total Expense ($000):** 186041 **Payroll Expense ($000):** 68778

☐ **SELECT SPECIALTY HOSPITAL–BIRMINGHAM (12008)**, 800 Montclair Road, Zip 35213; tel. 205/599–4600, (Nonreporting) **A**1 9 10 **S** Select Medical Corporation
Primary Contact: Craig L. Johnson, CHE, Chief Executive Officer
CMO: Allan Goldstein, M.D., Medical Director and Chief of Staff
Web address: www.selectmedicalcorp.com
Control: Corporation, Investor–owned, for–profit **Service:** Long–Term Acute Care hospital

Staffed Beds: 38

Many Facility Codes have changed. Please refer to the AHA Guide Code Chart.

★ **ST. VINCENT'S BIRMINGHAM (10056)**, (Formerly St Vincent's Hospital), 810 St. Vincent's Drive, Zip 35205–1695, Mailing Address: P.O. Box 12407, Zip 35202–2407; tel. 205/939–7000 **A**1 2 3 5 9 10 **F**11 13 14 15 17 18 20 22 24 25 26 27 33 34 35 38 40 43 44 50 52 55 56 57 62 64 66 68 70 72 73 74 75 76 77 79 80 81 82 84 86 87 96 97 99 100 102 107 108 109 111 116 118 119 120 135 136 137 **P**3 5 **S** Ascension Health
Primary Contact: Neeysa Biddle, President and Chief Operating Officer
COO: Neeysa Biddle, President and Chief Operating Officer
CFO: Jeffrey Rooney, Executive Vice President and Chief Financial Officer
CIO: Timothy Stettheimer, Vice President and Chief Information Officer
CHR: Katie Chamblee, Vice President Human Resources
Web address: www.stv.org
Control: Church–operated, Nongovernment, not–for profit **Service:** General Medical and Surgical

Staffed Beds: 372 **Admissions:** 24512 **Census:** 267 **Outpatient Visits:** 286077 **Births:** 4099 **Total Expense ($000):** 275933 **Payroll Expense ($000):** 90755

★ **ST. VINCENT'S EAST (10011)**, (Formerly Medical Center East), 50 Medical Park East Drive, Zip 35235–9987; tel. 205/838–3000 **A**1 2 3 5 9 10 **F**3 8 9 11 12 13 14 15 17 18 20 22 24 25 26 27 33 38 40 41 43 50 51 52 53 54 55 56 57 60 62 66 68 70 72 73 74 75 76 77 79 80 81 82 85 86 87 96 97 100 104 106 107 109 111 115 118 119 120 121 124 132 135 136 137 **S** Ascension Health
Primary Contact: Todd S. Kennedy, President and Chief Operating Officer
COO: Todd S. Kennedy, President and Chief Operating Officer
CFO: Kim Shrewsbury, Vice President Financial Services
CMO: Adeeb Thomas, M.D., Vice President Medical Affairs
CIO: Beverly Golightly, Interim Director Information Technology
CHR: Katie Chamblee, Vice President Human Resources
Web address: www.medicalcentereast.com
Control: Other not–for–profit (including NFP Corporation) **Service:** General Medical and Surgical

Staffed Beds: 282 **Admissions:** 15108 **Census:** 200 **Outpatient Visits:** 165412 **Births:** 1168 **Total Expense ($000):** 163626 **Payroll Expense ($000):** 64293

★ **THE CHILDREN'S HOSPITAL OF ALABAMA (13300)**, 1600 Seventh Avenue South, Zip 35233–1785; tel. 205/939–9100 **A**1 3 5 9 10 **F**3 7 8 11 12 16 25 26 27 28 30 31 32 33 37 38 40 43 48 49 50 53 55 56 57 58 59 60 62 63 66 70 72 73 75 76 77 78 79 80 81 82 83 84 86 87 88 89 90 91 92 94 96 97 100 102 103 106 107 114 118 119 120 121 123 125 131 132 133 135
Primary Contact: William Michael Warren, Jr., Chief Executive Officer
COO: Tom Shufflebarger, Chief Operating Officer
CFO: Mike Burgess, Chief Financial Officer
CMO: Crayton A. Fargason, M.D., Medical Director
CIO: Mike McDevitt, Chief Information Officer
CHR: Doug Dean, Chief Human Resources Officer
Web address: www.chsys.org
Control: Other not–for–profit (including NFP Corporation) **Service:** Children's general

Staffed Beds: 266 **Admissions:** 13803 **Census:** 206 **Outpatient Visits:** 629909 **Total Expense ($000):** 370461 **Payroll Expense ($000):** 155893 **Personnel:** 2923

★ **TRINITY MEDICAL CENTER (10104)**, 800 Montclair Road, Zip 35213–1984; tel. 205/592–1000, (Total facility includes 26 beds in nursing home–type unit) (Nonreporting) **A**1 2 3 5 9 10 **S** Community Health Systems, Inc.
Primary Contact: William R. Heburn, Interim Chief Executive Officer
COO: Tim McManus, Administrator and Chief Operating Officer
CFO: Paul T. Graham, CHE, CPA, Chief Financial Officer
CMO: Peter Leeson, D.O., Chief Medical Officer
CIO: Stefan Hooper, Director Information Systems
Web address: www.bhsala.com
Control: Corporation, Investor–owned, for–profit **Service:** General Medical and Surgical

Staffed Beds: 375

★ **UAB HIGHLANDS (10167)**, 1201 11th Avenue South, Zip 35205–5299; tel. 205/930–7000 **A**1 5 9 10 **F**11 25 38 43 54 59 61 63 68 77 79 80 96 100 102 107 118 119 120 **P**3 7 **S** UAB Health System
Primary Contact: Robert Cofield, Chief Operating Officer
COO: Robert Cofield, Chief Operating Officer
CFO: Mark Edwards, Controller
CMO: Annie Jackson, M.D., Chief of Staff
CIO: Joan Hicks, Chief Information Officer
CHR: Sherri Crowe, Director Human Resources
Web address: www.health.uab.edu
Control: Hospital district or authority, Government, nonfederal **Service:** General Medical and Surgical

Staffed Beds: 73 **Admissions:** 1995 **Census:** 17 **Outpatient Visits:** 48867 **Births:** 0 **Total Expense ($000):** 59766 **Payroll Expense ($000):** 19167 **Personnel:** 381

★ **UNIVERSITY OF ALABAMA HOSPITAL (10033)**, 1802 Sixth Avenue South, Zip 35249; tel. 205/934–4011 **A**1 2 3 5 8 9 10 **F**3 4 5 6 7 8 9 11 12 13 14 15 16 17 18 19 20 21 22 23 24 25 26 27 29 30 31 32 33 34 35 36 37 38 40 41 42 43 44 45 46 47 49 50 52 53 54 55 56 57 58 59 60 61 62 63 64 66 68 69 70 71 72 73 74 75 76 77 79 80 81 82 85 86 87 88 89 90 91 92 93 94 96 97 99 100 102 103 104 105 106 107 108 109 111 112 113 114 116 118 119 120 121 123 124 125 126 127 128 129 130 131 132 133 134 135 136 137 **P**3 **S** UAB Health System
Primary Contact: Michael Waldrum, M.D., Chief Executive Officer
CFO: Mary Beth Briscoe, Chief Financial Officer
CMO: Cynthia Brumfield, M.D., Chief of Staff
CIO: Joan Hicks, Chief Information Officer
CHR: Cheryl Locke, Chief Human Resources Officer
Web address: www.health.uab.edu
Control: State–Government, nonfederal **Service:** General Medical and Surgical

Staffed Beds: 908 **Admissions:** 42181 **Census:** 694 **Outpatient Visits:** 345790 **Births:** 4240 **Total Expense ($000):** 841569 **Payroll Expense ($000):** 321217 **Personnel:** 7105

★ **VETERANS AFFAIRS MEDICAL CENTER**, 700 South 19th Street, Zip 35233–1927; tel. 205/933–8101 **A**1 2 3 5 8 **F**3 5 12 17 18 20 22 24 25 26 27 31 33 36 37 38 40 41 42 43 44 45 47 50 53 54 55 56 57 58 59 60 61 62 63 64 66 68 72 73 75 76 77 79 81 82 84 86 87 90 92 93 94 96 97 100 102 106 107 118 121 124 132 135 136 137 **S** Department of Veterans Affairs
Primary Contact: Robert W. Ratliff, Ph.D., FACHE, Interim Director
CFO: Mary S. Mitchell, Chief Resource Management Services
Web address: www.va.gov/sta/guide/home.asp
Control: Veterans Affairs, Government, federal **Service:** General Medical and Surgical

Staffed Beds: 144 **Admissions:** 4617 **Census:** 89 **Outpatient Visits:** 470053 **Births:** 0 **Personnel:** 2130

BOAZ—Marshall County

★ **MARSHALL MEDICAL CENTER SOUTH (10005)**, U.S. Highway 431 North, Zip 35957–0999, Mailing Address: P.O. Box 758, Zip 35957–0758; tel. 256/593–8310, (Nonreporting) **A**1 9 10 19 **S** Marshall County Health Care Authority
Primary Contact: John D. Anderson, Administrator
CFO: Kathy Nelson, Chief Financial Officer
Web address: www.mmcs.org
Control: County–Government, nonfederal **Service:** General Medical and Surgical

Staffed Beds: 102

BREWTON—Escambia County

□ **D. W. MCMILLAN MEMORIAL HOSPITAL (10099)**, 1301 Belleville Avenue, Zip 36426–1306, Mailing Address: P.O. Box 908, Zip 36427–0908; tel. 251/867–8061 **A**1 9 10 **F**3 7 11 13 15 27 32 33 38 55 57 61 62 68 73 74 76 77 79 80 81 84 86 90 96 97 100 102 107 119 121 132 135 **P**6
Primary Contact: Christopher B. Griffin, Chief Executive Officer
CFO: Richard Owens, Chief Financial Officer
Web address: www.dwmmh.org
Control: Hospital district or authority, Government, nonfederal **Service:** General Medical and Surgical

Staffed Beds: 63 **Admissions:** 2913 **Census:** 28 **Outpatient Visits:** 32593 **Births:** 289 **Total Expense ($000):** 18747 **Payroll Expense ($000):** 9721 **Personnel:** 288

CAMDEN—Wilcox County

J. PAUL JONES HOSPITAL (10102), 317 McWilliams Avenue, Zip 36726–1610; tel. 334/682–4131 **A**9 10 20 **F**31 38 61 62 96
Primary Contact: Elizabeth M. Kennedy, Administrator
CMO: Willie White, M.D., Director Medical Staff
CIO: Jill Smith, Administrative Coordinator
CHR: Jill Smith, Administrative Coordinator
Control: City–County, Government, nonfederal **Service:** General Medical and Surgical

Staffed Beds: 32 **Admissions:** 278 **Census:** 2 **Outpatient Visits:** 12678 **Births:** 2 **Total Expense ($000):** 2688 **Payroll Expense ($000):** 1355 **Personnel:** 47

Hospital, Medicare Provider Number, Address, Telephone, Approval, Facility, and Physician Codes, Health Care System

★ American Hospital Association (AHA) membership
□ The Joint Commission accreditation
○ American Osteopathic Association (AOA) accreditation
△ Commission on Accreditation of Rehabilitation Facilities (CARF) accreditation

CARROLLTON—Pickens County

PICKENS COUNTY MEDICAL CENTER (10109), 241 Robert K. Wilson Drive, Zip 35447, Mailing Address: P.O. Box 478, Zip 35447–0478; tel. 205/367–8111, (Nonreporting) **A**9 10 20
Primary Contact: Wayne McElroy, Administrator
CFO: Janice Winters, Controller
CMO: William R. Brooke, M.D., President Medical Staff
CHR: Dottie Wilson, Director Human Resources
Web address: www.dchsystem.com
Control: County–Government, nonfederal **Service:** General Medical and Surgical

Staffed Beds: 52

CENTRE—Cherokee County

★ **CHEROKEE MEDICAL CENTER (10022)**, 400 Northwood Drive, Zip 35960–1023; tel. 256/927–5531, (Nonreporting) **A**1 9 10 **S** Community Health Systems, Inc.
Primary Contact: Jeff Noblin, FACHE, Chief Executive Officer
COO: Julie House, MSN, Chief Nursing Officer
CFO: Zac Allen, CPA, Chief Financial Officer
CIO: Joe Ford, Director Information Systems
CHR: Diane McMichen, Director Human Resources
Web address: www.cherokeemedicalcenter.com
Control: Other not–for–profit (including NFP Corporation) **Service:** General Medical and Surgical

Staffed Beds: 60

CENTREVILLE—Bibb County

BIBB MEDICAL CENTER (10058), 208 Pierson Avenue, Zip 35042–1199; tel. 205/926–4881, (Total facility includes 131 beds in nursing home–type unit) **A**9 10 **F**3 11 15 25 31 32 33 37 38 50 55 57 61 62 79 86 96 107 115 117 119 122 133 135 **P**6
Primary Contact: Terry J. Smith, Chief Executive Officer
CFO: Heather Desmond, Chief Financial Officer
CMO: John Meigs, M.D., Chief of Staff
CHR: Kim Hayes, Director Human Resources
Web address: www.bibbmedicalcenter.com
Control: County–Government, nonfederal **Service:** General Medical and Surgical

Staffed Beds: 166 **Admissions:** 559 **Census:** 124 **Outpatient Visits:** 27910 **Births:** 0 **Total Expense ($000):** 13424 **Payroll Expense ($000):** 6872 **Personnel:** 221

CHATOM—Washington County

★ **WASHINGTON COUNTY HOSPITAL AND NURSING HOME (11300)**, 14600 St. Stephens Avenue, Zip 36518–9998, Mailing Address: P.O. Box 1299, Zip 36518–1299; tel. 251/847–2223 **A**9 10 18 **F**15 25 31 38 57 62 81 84 87 96 102 107 117 122 **P**6
Primary Contact: Douglas Tanner, Administrator
CFO: Alyson Overstreet, Chief Financial Officer
CMO: Steve Donald, M.D., Chief of Staff
CHR: Ben Rich, Director Personnel Services
Web address: www.wchnh.org
Control: County–Government, nonfederal **Service:** General Medical and Surgical

Staffed Beds: 19 **Admissions:** 411 **Census:** 7 **Outpatient Visits:** 16400 **Births:** 0 **Total Expense ($000):** 4961 **Payroll Expense ($000):** 2578 **Personnel:** 95

CLANTON—Chilton County

★ **CHILTON MEDICAL CENTER (10043)**, 1010 Lay Dam Road, Zip 35045–2306; tel. 205/755–2500 **A**1 9 10 **F**3 11 15 25 32 33 38 55 56 57 61 66 79 96 97 107 119 122 124 135 **P**4 6 **S** Sunlink Health Systems
Primary Contact: Rob Followell, Chief Executive Officer
COO: David Pryor, Director Ancillary Services
CFO: Kelly Moore, Interim Controller
CHR: Joann Turpen, Director Human Resources
Web address: www.sunlinkhealth.com
Control: Corporation, Investor–owned, for–profit **Service:** General Medical and Surgical

Staffed Beds: 30 **Admissions:** 604 **Census:** 6 **Outpatient Visits:** 20701 **Births:** 0 **Total Expense ($000):** 8567 **Payroll Expense ($000):** 4106 **Personnel:** 138

CULLMAN—Cullman County

□ **CULLMAN REGIONAL MEDICAL CENTER (10035)**, 1912 Alabama Highway 157, Zip 35055, Mailing Address: P.O. Box 1108, Zip 35056–1108; tel. 256/737–2000 **A**1 2 9 10 19 **F**3 7 11 13 14 15 18 24 25 26 30 31 32 33 35 38 40 42 43 44 49 51 52 55 56 57 61 62 66 68 72 73 74 75 76 77 79 80 81 82 84 86 96 97 99 100 102 106 107 109 118 119 120 121 123 124 135 136 137
Primary Contact: James Weidner, Chief Executive Officer
COO: Jete Edmisson, Chief Operating Officer and Chief Financial Officer
CFO: Jete Edmisson, Chief Operating Officer and Chief Financial Officer
CMO: Steve Seidel, M.D., Chief of Staff
CHR: Jim Miller, Vice President Human Resources
Web address: www.crmchospital.com
Control: Other not–for–profit (including NFP Corporation) **Service:** General Medical and Surgical

Staffed Beds: 115 **Admissions:** 7213 **Census:** 75 **Outpatient Visits:** 121081 **Births:** 970 **Total Expense ($000):** 91359 **Payroll Expense ($000):** 37217 **Personnel:** 955

★ **WOODLAND MEDICAL CENTER (10143)**, 1910 Cherokee Avenue S.W., Zip 35055–5502; tel. 256/739–3500 **A**1 9 10 **F**3 11 12 14 15 24 25 26 27 38 40 41 43 46 50 54 55 56 57 61 62 68 72 73 76 77 79 80 81 82 84 86 88 89 90 91 92 93 96 97 99 102 105 107 118 119 120 121 122 124 134 135 136 137 **P**6 **S** Capella Healthcare
Primary Contact: George F. Naylor, III, FACHE, Chief Executive Officer
CFO: Margie Kipp, Chief Financial Officer
CIO: Melinda Mason, Director
CHR: Deeann Johnson, Director
Web address: www.woodlandmedicalcenter.com
Control: Corporation, Investor–owned, for–profit **Service:** General Medical and Surgical

Staffed Beds: 70 **Admissions:** 2757 **Census:** 28 **Outpatient Visits:** 34561 **Births:** 0

DADEVILLE—Tallapoosa County

LAKE MARTIN COMMUNITY HOSPITAL (10052), 201 Mariarden Road, Zip 36853–6251, Mailing Address: P.O. Box 629, Zip 36853–0629; tel. 256/825–7821, (Nonreporting) **A**9 10
Primary Contact: Michael D. Bruce, Chief Executive Officer
COO: Agnes Wages, Administrator
CHR: Karen Treadwell, Director Human Resources
Web address: www.lakemartincommunityhospital.com
Control: Partnership, Investor–owned, for–profit **Service:** General Medical and Surgical

Staffed Beds: 28

DAPHNE—Baldwin County

★ **MERCY MEDICAL (13027)**, 101 Villa Drive, Zip 36526–1090, Mailing Address: P.O. Box 1090, Zip 36526–1090; tel. 251/621–4200, (Total facility includes 131 beds in nursing home–type unit) **A**1 9 10 **F**2 6 10 24 25 26 30 31 32 33 42 43 44 54 61 62 67 73 85 86 115 117 119 121 132 135 137 **S** Catholic Health East
Primary Contact: Mary Kay Polys, President and Chief Executive Officer
CFO: Kelly Hopkins, Vice President and Chief Financial Officer
CMO: Randall Hall, M.D., Chief Medical Director
CIO: Andrew Wilhelm, Director Information Technology Services
CHR: Mary G. Lamont, Director Human Resources
Web address: www.mercymedical.com
Control: Church–operated, Nongovernment, not–for profit **Service:** Rehabilitation

Staffed Beds: 156 **Admissions:** 1884 **Census:** 100 **Outpatient Visits:** 75035 **Births:** 0 **Total Expense ($000):** 41617 **Payroll Expense ($000):** 17932 **Personnel:** 353

DECATUR—Morgan County

★ **DECATUR GENERAL HOSPITAL (10085)**, 1201 Seventh Street S.E., Zip 35601–3303, Mailing Address: P.O. Box 2239, Zip 35609–2239; tel. 256/341–2000, (Includes DECATUR GENERAL HOSPITAL–WEST, 2205 Beltline Road S.W., Zip 35601–3687, Mailing Address: P.O. Box 2240, Zip 35609–2240; tel. 256/306–4000) **A**1 2 9 10 **F**3 11 12 13 15 17 18 20 22 24 25 26 38 46 48 49 51 52 55 56 57 59 66 68 73 74 75 76 79 80 81 82 84 86 88 89 90 91 92 93 94 95 96 97 107 108 109 111 118 119 121 124 134 135 136 137
Primary Contact: James W. Hahn, President and Chief Executive Officer
COO: Dean A. Griffin, Senior Vice President and Chief Operating Officer
CFO: David Cashio, Chief Financial Officer
CMO: P. J. Reddy, M.D., President Medical Staff
CIO: Mark Megehee, Vice President and Chief Information Officer
CHR: Dean A. Griffin, Senior Vice President and Chief Operating Officer
Web address: www.decaturgeneral.org
Control: Hospital district or authority, Government, nonfederal **Service:** General Medical and Surgical

Staffed Beds: 227 **Admissions:** 11814 **Census:** 145 **Outpatient Visits:** 188800 **Births:** 1603 **Total Expense ($000):** 117338 **Payroll Expense ($000):** 47984 **Personnel:** 1105

Many Facility Codes have changed. Please refer to the AHA Guide Code Chart.

☐ **NORTH ALABAMA REGIONAL HOSPITAL (14009)**, 4218 Highway 31 South, Zip 35603–5039; tel. 256/560–2200 **A**1 10 **F**88 91 119 135
Primary Contact: J. Randall Phillips, CHE, Director
CFO: Roger Kalonick, Business Manager
CMO: Duard Bok, M.D., Clinical Director
CIO: Ronald J. Thomas, Coordinator Information Systems
CHR: Gregory Ethridge, Manager Personnel
Web address: www.narh.mh.alabama.gov
Control: State–Government, nonfederal **Service:** Psychiatric

Staffed Beds: 74 **Admissions:** 636 **Census:** 81 **Outpatient Visits:** 0 **Births:** 0 **Total Expense ($000):** 12907 **Payroll Expense ($000):** 7169 **Personnel:** 181

★☐ **PARKWAY MEDICAL CENTER (10054)**, 1874 Beltline Road S.W., Zip 35601–5509, Mailing Address: P.O. Box 2211, Zip 35609–2211; tel. 256/350–2211, (Nonreporting) **A**1 9 10 **S** Capella Healthcare
Primary Contact: Sherry J. Jones, Interim Chief Executive Officer
Web address: www.pmcrecruitment.com
Control: Corporation, Investor–owned, for–profit **Service:** General Medical and Surgical

Staffed Beds: 120

DEMOPOLIS—Marengo County

☐ **BRYAN W. WHITFIELD MEMORIAL HOSPITAL (10112)**, 105 U.S. Highway 80 East, Zip 36732–3616, Mailing Address: P.O. Box 890, Zip 36732–0890; tel. 334/289–4000, (Nonreporting) **A**1 9 10 20
Primary Contact: Michael D. Marshall, Administrator and Chief Executive Officer
CFO: Arthur D. Evans, Assistant Administrator
CHR: Danny Smith, Director Human Resources
Web address: www.bwwmh.com
Control: Hospital district or authority, Government, nonfederal **Service:** General Medical and Surgical

Staffed Beds: 99

DOTHAN—Houston County

★☐ **FLOWERS HOSPITAL (10055)**, 4370 West Main Street, Zip 36305–4000, Mailing Address: P.O. Box 6907, Zip 36302–6907; tel. 334/793–5000 **A**1 2 9 10 **F**1 3 4 12 13 15 16 17 18 20 22 24 25 27 30 32 33 38 43 46 48 49 50 51 54 55 56 57 59 60 62 65 68 72 73 74 75 76 77 78 79 80 81 82 84 85 86 87 96 97 100 103 104 105 106 107 117 118 119 123 124 135 136 137 **P**6 **S** Community Health Systems, Inc.
Primary Contact: Keith Granger, President and Chief Executive Officer
COO: Suzanne Woods, Senior Vice President
CFO: Talana Bell, Chief Financial Officer
CHR: Gayla Miskell, Director Human Resources
Web address: www.flowershospital.com
Control: Corporation, Investor–owned, for–profit **Service:** General Medical and Surgical

Staffed Beds: 235 **Admissions:** 12068 **Census:** 142 **Outpatient Visits:** 124310 **Births:** 1224 **Total Expense ($000):** 151712 **Payroll Expense ($000):** 48192 **Personnel:** 1145

★☐ **HEALTHSOUTH REHABILITATION HOSPITAL (13030)**, 1736 East Main Street, Zip 36301, Mailing Address: P.O. Box 6708, Zip 36302–6708; tel. 334/712–6333, (Nonreporting) **A**1 9 10 **S** HEALTHSOUTH Corporation
Primary Contact: Margaret A. Futch, Chief Executive Officer
CFO: Heath Watson, Controller
CMO: Stephen L. Chastain, M.D., Medical Director
CHR: Mary Beth Davis, Director Human Resources
Web address: www.healthsouth.com
Control: Corporation, Investor–owned, for–profit **Service:** Rehabilitation

Staffed Beds: 34

☐ **LAUREL OAKS BEHAVIORAL HEALTH CENTER (14013)**, 700 East Cottonwood Road, Zip 36301; tel. 334/794–7373, (Nonreporting) **A**1 9 10 **S** Psychiatric Solutions
Primary Contact: Russell C. Dean, Jr., Chief Executive Officer
CFO: Tim S. Lynch, Chief Financial Officer
CMO: Nelson Handol, M.D., Medical Director
CHR: Lorrie Evans, Director Human Resources
Web address: www.psysolutions.com
Control: Corporation, Investor–owned, for–profit **Service:** Psychiatric

Staffed Beds: 24

☐ **LONG TERM HOSPITAL OF DOTHAN (12010)**, 1108 Ross Clark Circle, 4th Floor, Zip 36302; tel. 334/699–4300, (Nonreporting) **A**1 9 10 **S** Noland Health Services, Inc.
Primary Contact: Kaye Burke, Administrator
Web address: www.nolandhealth.com
Control: Other not–for–profit (including NFP Corporation) **Service:** Long–Term Acute Care hospital

Staffed Beds: 30

★☐ **SOUTHEAST ALABAMA MEDICAL CENTER (10001)**, 1108 Ross Clark Circle, Zip 36301–3024, Mailing Address: P.O. Box 6987, Zip 36302–6987; tel. 334/793–8111 **A**1 2 9 10 19 **F**3 8 12 13 15 18 20 22 24 25 26 27 28 32 33 35 38 40 41 42 43 49 50 51 52 55 56 57 59 61 62 66 68 69 72 73 74 75 76 77 79 80 81 82 84 86 88 90 91 92 93 94 95 96 97 100 102 103 104 105 106 107 109 111 112 116 118 119 121 124 132 135 136 137 **P**6
Primary Contact: Ronald S. Owen, Chief Executive Officer
COO: Charles C. Brannen, Senior Vice President and Chief Operating Officer
CFO: Derek Miller, Senior Vice President and Chief Financial Officer
CMO: Charles Harkness, D.O., Vice President Medical Affairs
CHR: Peggy Sease, Vice President Human Resources
Web address: www.samc.org
Control: Hospital district or authority, Government, nonfederal **Service:** General Medical and Surgical

Staffed Beds: 370 **Admissions:** 20342 **Census:** 249 **Outpatient Visits:** 198591 **Births:** 1455 **Total Expense ($000):** 221882 **Payroll Expense ($000):** 90085 **Personnel:** 2219

ELBA—Coffee County

★ **ELBA GENERAL HOSPITAL (10027)**, 987 Drayton Street, Zip 36323–1494; tel. 334/897–2257, (Total facility includes 111 beds in nursing home–type unit) (Nonreporting) **A**9 10
Primary Contact: Ellen C. Briley, Administrator and Chief Executive Officer
CFO: Nicki Jinright, Chief Financial Officer
CMO: Lance K. Dyess, M.D., Chief Medical Officer
CIO: Mary Gray, R.N., Director Information Technology and Special Project
CHR: Judi Qualls, Director Human Resources
Control: Hospital district or authority, Government, nonfederal **Service:** General Medical and Surgical

Staffed Beds: 131

ENTERPRISE—Coffee County

★☐ **MEDICAL CENTER ENTERPRISE (10049)**, 400 North Edwards Street, Zip 36330; tel. 334/347–0584, (Nonreporting) **A**1 9 10 **S** Community Health Systems, Inc.
Primary Contact: Jeffrey M. Brannon, Chief Executive Officer
CFO: Greg McGilvray, Chief Financial Officer
CHR: Toni Kaminski, Director Human Resources
Web address: www.mcehospital.com
Control: Corporation, Investor–owned, for–profit **Service:** General Medical and Surgical

Staffed Beds: 117

EUFAULA—Barbour County

☐ **MEDICAL CENTER BARBOUR (10069)**, (Formerly Lakeview Community Hospital), 820 West Washington Street, Zip 36027–1899; tel. 334/688–7000 **A**1 9 10 20 **F**11 15 25 26 30 31 32 38 56 57 68 79 96 107 119 122 124 135
Primary Contact: Ralph H. Clark, Jr., FACHE, Chief Executive Officer
CFO: Terri Parsons, Chief Financial Officer
CHR: Cindy Griffin, Director Human Resources
Web address: www.medctrbarbour.org
Control: Hospital district or authority, Government, nonfederal **Service:** General Medical and Surgical

Staffed Beds: 29 **Admissions:** 1233 **Census:** 11 **Outpatient Visits:** 20969 **Births:** 0 **Total Expense ($000):** 11138 **Payroll Expense ($000):** 5072 **Personnel:** 136

EUTAW—Greene County

GREENE COUNTY HOSPITAL (10051), 509 Wilson Avenue, Zip 35462–1099; tel. 205/372–3388, (Nonreporting) **A**9 10
Primary Contact: Robert J. Coker, Jr., Administrator
Control: County–Government, nonfederal **Service:** General Medical and Surgical

Staffed Beds: 20

Hospital, Medicare Provider Number, Address, Telephone, Approval, Facility, and Physician Codes, Health Care System
★ American Hospital Association (AHA) membership
☐ The Joint Commission accreditation
○ American Osteopathic Association (AOA) accreditation
△ Commission on Accreditation of Rehabilitation Facilities (CARF) accreditation

EVERGREEN—Conecuh County

EVERGREEN MEDICAL CENTER (10148), 101 Crestview Avenue, Zip 36401–0706, Mailing Address: P.O. Box 706, Zip 36401–0706; tel. 251/578–2480 **A**9 10 **F**3 14 25 26 31 32 33 38 52 55 56 57 61 79 82 86 87 88 96 102 107 **S** Gilliard Health Services
Primary Contact: Robert J. Humphrey, Administrator
CFO: Sharon Jones, Chief Financial Officer
CMO: William Farmer, M.D., Chief of Staff
CIO: Tommy Shehan, Chief Information Officer
CHR: Alicia Donoghue, Director Human Resources
Web address: www.evergreenmedical.org
Control: Corporation, Investor–owned, for–profit **Service:** General Medical and Surgical

Staffed Beds: 44 **Admissions:** 2997 **Census:** 21 **Outpatient Visits:** 18064 **Births:** 0 **Total Expense ($000):** 12998 **Payroll Expense ($000):** 5930 **Personnel:** 167

FAIRHOPE—Baldwin County

⊛ **THOMAS HOSPITAL (10100)**, 750 Morphy Avenue, Zip 36532–1812, Mailing Address: P.O. Drawer 929, Zip 36533–0929; tel. 251/928–2375, (Nonreporting) **A**1 5 9 10 19 **S** Infirmary Health System
Primary Contact: Philip L. Cusa, Administrator
COO: Douglas Garner, Vice President
CFO: Patrick Murphy, Vice President Finance
CMO: Michael McBrearty, M.D., Vice President Medical Affairs
Web address: www.thomashospital.com
Control: Hospital district or authority, Government, nonfederal **Service:** General Medical and Surgical

Staffed Beds: 129

FAYETTE—Fayette County

☐ **FAYETTE MEDICAL CENTER (10045)**, 1653 Temple Avenue North, Zip 35555–1314, Mailing Address: P.O. Drawer 710, Zip 35555–0710; tel. 205/932–5966, (Total facility includes 122 beds in nursing home–type unit) (Nonreporting) **A**1 9 10 **S** DCH Health System
Primary Contact: Barry S. Cochran, FACHE, Administrator
CFO: Jeff Huff, Assistant Administrator Finance
CHR: Cindy Bohon, Director Human Resources
Web address: www.dchsystem.com
Control: County–Government, nonfederal **Service:** General Medical and Surgical

Staffed Beds: 169

FLORALA—Covington County

FLORALA MEMORIAL HOSPITAL (10066), 515 East Fifth Avenue, Zip 36442–0189, Mailing Address: P.O. Box 189, Zip 36442–0189; tel. 334/858–3287, (Nonreporting) **A**9 10
Primary Contact: Blair W. Henson, Administrator
Control: Corporation, Investor–owned, for–profit **Service:** General Medical and Surgical

Staffed Beds: 23

FLORENCE—Lauderdale County

⊛ **ELIZA COFFEE MEMORIAL HOSPITAL (10006)**, 205 Marengo Street, Zip 35630–6033, Mailing Address: P.O. Box 818, Zip 35631–0818; tel. 256/768–9191 **A**1 9 10 **F**3 13 15 17 18 20 22 24 25 27 31 32 38 40 44 49 51 55 57 59 62 68 72 73 74 76 77 78 79 80 82 84 86 88 96 97 102 103 104 105 106 107 118 119 134 135 137 **S** Coffee Health Group
Primary Contact: Carl W. Bailey, Administrator
CFO: Jody Pigg, Chief Financial Officer
Web address: www.chgroup.org
Control: Hospital district or authority, Government, nonfederal **Service:** General Medical and Surgical

Staffed Beds: 289 **Admissions:** 12947 **Census:** 173 **Outpatient Visits:** 101869 **Births:** 1087 **Total Expense ($000):** 134756 **Payroll Expense ($000):** 46583 **Personnel:** 1128

FOLEY—Baldwin County

⊛ **SOUTH BALDWIN REGIONAL MEDICAL CENTER (10083)**, 1613 North McKenzie Street, Zip 36535–2299; tel. 251/949–3400, (Nonreporting) **A**1 5 9 10 19 **S** Community Health Systems, Inc.
Primary Contact: Rich McAuliffe, Chief Executive Officer
CFO: Chuck Coder, Chief Financial Officer
CMO: Michael Houston, M.D., Chief Medical Officer
CIO: Justin Box, Director Information Systems
CHR: Pam Brunson, Director Human Resources
Web address: www.southbaldwinrmc.com
Control: Corporation, Investor–owned, for–profit **Service:** General Medical and Surgical

Staffed Beds: 110

FORT PAYNE—DeKalb County

⊛ **DEKALB REGIONAL MEDICAL CENTER (10012)**, 200 Medical Center Drive, Zip 35968–3415, Mailing Address: P.O. Box 680778, Zip 35968–1608; tel. 256/845–3150 **A**1 9 10 20 **F**3 8 11 12 13 15 18 20 22 24 25 30 31 32 33 38 40 46 52 55 57 61 62 68 73 74 75 77 79 82 84 86 88 93 96 97 100 107 118 135 136 **S** Community Health Systems, Inc.
Primary Contact: J. Peter Selman, Chief Executive Officer
CFO: Hugh Tobin, Chief Financial Officer
CHR: Diane McMichen, Director Human Resources
Web address: www.dekalbregional.com
Control: Corporation, Investor–owned, for–profit **Service:** General Medical and Surgical

Staffed Beds: 115 **Admissions:** 5369 **Census:** 52 **Outpatient Visits:** 62858 **Births:** 953 **Total Expense ($000):** 34129 **Payroll Expense ($000):** 14174 **Personnel:** 412

GADSDEN—Etowah County

⊛ **GADSDEN REGIONAL MEDICAL CENTER (10040)**, 1007 Goodyear Avenue, Zip 35903–1195; tel. 256/494–4000 **A**1 2 9 10 **F**11 13 15 17 18 20 22 24 25 26 27 32 38 42 47 51 55 56 57 61 62 63 68 72 74 79 86 87 88 92 93 96 97 100 102 107 109 118 135 136 **P**6 7 **S** Community Health Systems, Inc.
Primary Contact: Douglas P. DeGraaf, Chief Executive Officer
COO: Tom Moore, Chief Operating Officer
CFO: Bryan McCauley, Chief Financial Officer
CMO: James R. Phillips, M.D., Chief of Staff
CIO: Glenn Phillips, Director Information Systems
CHR: Gale H. Sanders, Director
Web address: www.gadsdenregional.com
Control: Corporation, Investor–owned, for–profit **Service:** General Medical and Surgical

Staffed Beds: 264 **Admissions:** 11429 **Census:** 172 **Outpatient Visits:** 99681 **Births:** 1008 **Total Expense ($000):** 106251 **Payroll Expense ($000):** 43237 **Personnel:** 959

⊛ **HEALTHSOUTH REHABILITATION OF GADSDEN (13032)**, 801 Goodyear Avenue, Zip 35903; tel. 256/439–5000, (Nonreporting) **A**1 9 10 **S** HEALTHSOUTH Corporation
Primary Contact: Michael W. Thompson, Chief Executive Officer
Web address: www.healthsouth.com
Control: Corporation, Investor–owned, for–profit **Service:** Rehabilitation

Staffed Beds: 40

☐ **MOUNTAIN VIEW HOSPITAL (14006)**, 3001 Scenic Highway, Zip 35901–9956, Mailing Address: P.O. Box 8406, Zip 35902–8406; tel. 256/546–9265, (Nonreporting) **A**1 9 10
Primary Contact: G. Michael Shehi, M.D., Interim Chief Executive Officer
COO: Sara Romano, Vice President
CFO: Mary Jensen, Controller
CMO: G. Michael Shehi, M.D., Medical Director
CHR: Dave Jensen, Director Human Resources, Performance Improvement and Risk Management
Web address: www.mtnviewhospital.com
Control: Corporation, Investor–owned, for–profit **Service:** Psychiatric

Staffed Beds: 108

☐ **RIVERVIEW REGIONAL MEDICAL CENTER (10046)**, 600 South Third Street, Zip 35901–5399, Mailing Address: P.O. Box 268, Zip 35999–0268; tel. 256/543–5200, (Nonreporting) **A**1 9 10 **S** Health Management Associates
Primary Contact: J. Matthew Hayes, Executive Director
COO: John Gallagher, Associate Executive Director
CFO: Rodney Ball, Associate Executive Director Finance
CMO: Ghanshyam Patel, M.D., Chief of Staff
CIO: Dennis Cantrell, Manager Management Information Systems
CHR: Dana Simpson, Manager Human Resources
Web address: www.riverviewregional.com
Control: Corporation, Investor–owned, for–profit **Service:** General Medical and Surgical

Staffed Beds: 190

GENEVA—Geneva County

★ **WIREGRASS MEDICAL CENTER (10062)**, 1200 West Maple Avenue, Zip 36340–1694; tel. 334/684–3655, (Total facility includes 96 beds in nursing home–type unit) (Nonreporting) **A**9 10 20
Primary Contact: Greg Dykes, Chief Executive Officer
CFO: Tina Segers, Accounting Officer
CMO: John Tomberlin, M.D., Medical Director
CIO: Tom Garske, Director Information Systems
CHR: Lesa Hatfield, Vice President Human Resources
Web address: www.alaweb.com/~tgarske
Control: County–Government, nonfederal **Service:** General Medical and Surgical

Staffed Beds: 163

GEORGIANA—Butler County

GEORGIANA HOSPITAL (10047), 515 Miranda Street, Zip 36033, Mailing Address: P.O. Box 548, Zip 36033–0548; tel. 334/376–2205, (Nonreporting) **A**9 10
Primary Contact: Harry Cole, Jr., Administrator
Control: Partnership, Investor–owned, for–profit **Service:** General Medical and Surgical

Staffed Beds: 22

GREENSBORO—Hale County

HALE COUNTY HOSPITAL (10095), 508 Green Street, Zip 36744–0017; tel. 334/624–3024, (Nonreporting) **A**9 10
Primary Contact: Richard M. McGill, Administrator
Control: County–Government, nonfederal **Service:** General Medical and Surgical

Staffed Beds: 39

GREENVILLE—Butler County

★□ **L. V. STABLER MEMORIAL HOSPITAL (10150)**, 29 L. V. Stabler Drive, Zip 36037–3800; tel. 334/382–2671, (Nonreporting) **A**1 9 10 **S** Community Health Systems, Inc.
Primary Contact: Bobby Ginn, Chief Executive Officer
CFO: Michael Ruff, Chief Financial Officer
CMO: Norman F. McGowin, M.D., Chief of Staff
CHR: Robert Foster, Director Human Resources
Web address: www.lvstabler.com
Control: Corporation, Investor–owned, for–profit **Service:** General Medical and Surgical

Staffed Beds: 72

GROVE HILL—Clarke County

★ **GROVE HILL MEMORIAL HOSPITAL (10091)**, 295 South Jackson Street, Zip 36451–0935, Mailing Address: P.O. Box 935, Zip 36451–0935; tel. 251/275–3191, (Nonreporting) **A**9 10
Primary Contact: Hybart D. Sewell, Administrator
CFO: Elaine Averett, Chief Financial Officer
CMO: Garrett Miller, M.D., Chief Medical Staff
CIO: Judy Payne, Health Information Officer
CHR: Emily Steadham, Administrative Assistant Human Resources and Public Relations
Control: City–Government, nonfederal **Service:** General Medical and Surgical

Staffed Beds: 50

GUNTERSVILLE—Marshall County

★□ **MARSHALL MEDICAL CENTER NORTH (10010)**, 8000 Alabama Highway 69, Zip 35976; tel. 256/753–8000, (Nonreporting) **A**1 9 10 **S** Marshall County Health Care Authority
Primary Contact: Cheryl M. Hays, FACHE, Administrator
COO: Cheryl M. Hays, FACHE, Administrator
CFO: Kathy Nelson, Chief Financial Officer
CIO: Burt Ridge, Director Information Technology
CHR: Jeff Stone, Director Human Resources
Web address: www.mmcenters.com
Control: Hospital district or authority, Government, nonfederal **Service:** General Medical and Surgical

Staffed Beds: 90

HALEYVILLE—Winston County

★□ **LAKELAND COMMUNITY HOSPITAL (10125)**, Highway 195 East, Zip 35565–9536, Mailing Address: P.O. Box 780, Zip 35565–0780; tel. 205/486–5213, (Nonreporting) **A**1 9 10 20 **S** LifePoint Hospitals, Inc.
Primary Contact: Christine R. Stewart, Chief Executive Officer
CFO: Penny Westmoreland, Chief Financial Officer
Web address: www.lifepointhospitals.com
Control: Corporation, Investor–owned, for–profit **Service:** General Medical and Surgical

Staffed Beds: 47

HAMILTON—Marion County

★□ **NORTH MISSISSIPPI MEDICAL CENTER–HAMILTON (10044)**, 1256 Military Street South, Zip 35570–5001; tel. 205/921–6200, (Nonreporting) **A**1 9 10 **S** North Mississippi Health Services, Inc.
Primary Contact: Donald J. Jones, Administrator
Web address: www.nmhs.net
Control: Other not–for–profit (including NFP Corporation) **Service:** General Medical and Surgical

Staffed Beds: 57

HARTSELLE—Morgan County

★□ **HARTSELLE MEDICAL CENTER (10009)**, 201 Pine Street N.W., Zip 35640–2309, Mailing Address: P.O. Box 969, Zip 35640–0969; tel. 256/773–6511 **A**1 9 10 **F**3 15 25 26 30 31 32 33 38 51 54 55 56 57 68 73 75 77 78 79 82 86 88 93 96 100 107 135 **S** Capella Healthcare
Primary Contact: Jeff G. Rains, Chief Executive Officer
CFO: Brent Probasco, Chief Financial Officer
CHR: Jeri Nelson, Director Human Resources
Web address: www.hartsellemedicalcenter.com
Control: Corporation, Investor–owned, for–profit **Service:** General Medical and Surgical

Staffed Beds: 120 **Admissions:** 1672 **Census:** 23 **Outpatient Visits:** 17018 **Births:** 0 **Total Expense ($000):** 17679 **Payroll Expense ($000):** 6104 **Personnel:** 155

HUNTSVILLE—Madison County

★□ **CRESTWOOD MEDICAL CENTER (10131)**, One Hospital Drive, Zip 35801–3403; tel. 256/882–3100, (Nonreporting) **A**1 9 10 **S** Community Health Systems, Inc.
Primary Contact: Pamela Hudson, M.D., Chief Executive Officer
COO: Brian N. Thomas, Chief Operating Officer
CFO: Holt Smith, Chief Financial Officer
CIO: Holt Smith, Chief Financial Officer
CHR: Lynn Dingo, Director Human Resources
Web address: www.crestwoodmedcenter.com
Control: Partnership, Investor–owned, for–profit **Service:** General Medical and Surgical

Staffed Beds: 120

★□ **HEALTHSOUTH REHABILITATION HOSPITAL OF NORTH ALABAMA (13029)**, 107 Governors Drive S.W., Zip 35801–4329; tel. 256/535–2300, (Nonreporting) **A**1 10 **S** HEALTHSOUTH Corporation
Primary Contact: Douglas H. Beverly, CHE, Chief Executive Officer
Web address: www.healthsouth.com
Control: Corporation, Investor–owned, for–profit **Service:** Rehabilitation

Staffed Beds: 50

□ **HUNTSVILLE HOSPITAL (10039)**, 101 Sivley Road, Zip 35801–4470; tel. 256/265–1000, (Includes HUNTSVILLE HOSPITAL FOR WOMEN AND CHILDREN, 911 Big Cove Road S.E., Zip 35801–3784) **A**1 2 3 5 9 10 **F**5 7 12 13 14 15 17 18 19 20 21 22 23 24 25 26 27 30 31 32 33 35 36 37 38 40 43 46 49 50 51 52 53 54 55 57 59 62 66 68 70 71 72 74 76 77 78 79 83 84 86 88 89 90 91 92 93 94 95 96 97 98 99 100 102 103 104 105 106 107 118 119 120 133 134 135 136 137
Primary Contact: David S. Spillers, Chief Executive Officer
COO: Sonya B. Greck, Chief Operating Officer
CFO: Lonnie D. Younger, Chief Financial Officer
CMO: Robert Chappell, M.D., Vice President and Chief Medical Officer
CIO: Rick Corn, Chief Information Officer
CHR: Andrea P. Rosler, Vice President Human Resources
Web address: www.huntsvillehospital.org
Control: Hospital district or authority, Government, nonfederal **Service:** General Medical and Surgical

Staffed Beds: 832 **Admissions:** 44523 **Census:** 600 **Outpatient Visits:** 609320 **Births:** 4459 **Total Expense ($000):** 568640 **Payroll Expense ($000):** 215303 **Personnel:** 4830

JACKSON—Clarke County

JACKSON MEDICAL CENTER (10128), 220 Hospital Drive, Zip 36545–2459, Mailing Address: P.O. Box 428, Zip 36545–0428; tel. 251/246–9021, (Nonreporting) **A**9 10 **S** Gilliard Health Services
Primary Contact: Teresa F. Grimes, Administrator
CFO: Amy Gibson, Chief Financial Officer
Web address: www.jacksonmedicalcenter.com
Control: Corporation, Investor–owned, for–profit **Service:** General Medical and Surgical

Staffed Beds: 26

Hospital, Medicare Provider Number, Address, Telephone, Approval, Facility, and Physician Codes, Health Care System

★ American Hospital Association (AHA) membership
□ The Joint Commission accreditation
○ American Osteopathic Association (AOA) accreditation
△ Commission on Accreditation of Rehabilitation Facilities (CARF) accreditation

JACKSONVILLE—Calhoun County

★ **JACKSONVILLE MEDICAL CENTER (10146)**, 1701 Pelham Road South, Zip 36265–3399, Mailing Address: P.O. Box 999, Zip 36265–0999; tel. 256/435–4970, (Nonreporting) **A**1 9 10 **S** Capella Healthcare
Primary Contact: Roger Collins, Chief Executive Officer
COO: Jean Ann McMurray, R.N., Chief Nursing Officer
CMO: Russell Ulrich, D.O., Chief of Staff
CIO: Richard Maust, Chief Information Officer
CHR: Amy Martin, Director Human Resources
Web address: www.jmchealth.com
Control: Corporation, Investor–owned, for–profit **Service:** General Medical and Surgical

Staffed Beds: 56

JASPER—Walker County

☐ **WALKER BAPTIST MEDICAL CENTER (10089)**, 3400 Highway 78 East, Zip 35501–8956, Mailing Address: P.O. Box 3547, Zip 35502–3547; tel. 205/387–4000 **A**1 9 10 **F**11 12 13 15 18 25 30 31 32 33 38 40 55 56 57 65 68 73 74 75 77 79 81 82 86 87 88 90 91 93 96 97 99 100 105 106 107 119 124 135 136 **S** Baptist Health System
Primary Contact: Joel W. Tate, FACHE, President
CFO: Mark Lovell, Vice President Finance
CIO: Kenny Horton, Director Information Systems
CHR: Pat Morrow, Director Human Resources
Web address: www.bhsala.com
Control: Other not–for–profit (including NFP Corporation) **Service:** General Medical and Surgical

Staffed Beds: 212 **Admissions:** 8654 **Census:** 95 **Outpatient Visits:** 219017 **Births:** 718 **Total Expense ($000):** 80331 **Payroll Expense ($000):** 25559 **Personnel:** 519

LUVERNE—Crenshaw County

CRENSHAW COMMUNITY HOSPITAL (10008), 101 Hospital Circle, Zip 36049–7317; tel. 334/335–3374, (Nonreporting) **A**9 10
Primary Contact: James McKnight, Administrator
COO: Victoria Lawrenson, Chief Operating Officer
CMO: S. Patrick Walker, M.D., Chief of Staff
CHR: Patricia Jarry, Manager Human Resources
Control: Corporation, Investor–owned, for–profit **Service:** General Medical and Surgical

Staffed Beds: 52

MADISON—Madison County

BRADFORD HEALTH SERVICES AT HUNTSVILLE, 1600 Browns Ferry Road, Zip 35758–9769, Mailing Address: P.O. Box 176, Zip 35758–0176; tel. 256/461–7272, (Nonreporting) **S** Bradford Health Services
Primary Contact: Bob Hinds, Executive Director
CFO: Bernard B. Stephens, Chief Financial Officer
CMO: Venkata S. Devabhaktuni, M.D., Medical Director
Web address: www.bradfordhealth.com
Control: Corporation, Investor–owned, for–profit **Service:** Alcoholism and other chemical dependency

Staffed Beds: 84

MOBILE—Mobile County

☐ **INFIRMARY WEST AT KNOLLWOOD (10152)**, 5600 Girby Road, Zip 36693–3398; tel. 251/660–5120, (Nonreporting) **A**1 3 5 9 10 **S** Infirmary Health System
Primary Contact: Ormond Thompson, Administrator
CFO: William B. Bush, Assistant Administrator Finance
CHR: Janice Rehm, Manager Human Resources
Web address: www.southalabama.edu/usakph/index.html
Control: State–Government, nonfederal **Service:** General Medical and Surgical

Staffed Beds: 182

☐ △ **MOBILE INFIRMARY MEDICAL CENTER (10113)**, 5 Mobile Infirmary Drive North, Zip 36607–3513, Mailing Address: P.O. Box 2144, Zip 36652–2144; tel. 251/435–2400, (Includes ROTARY REHABILITATION HOSPITAL), (Nonreporting) **A**1 2 3 5 7 9 10 **S** Infirmary Health System
Primary Contact: E. Chandler Bramlett, Jr., Chief Executive Officer
COO: D. Mark Nix, President and Chief Operating Officer
CFO: Joe Denton, Executive Vice President and Chief Financial Officer
CMO: Kenneth Brewington, M.D., Vice President Medical Administration
CIO: Eddy Stephens, Vice President Information Technology
CHR: Sheila Davidson, Vice President Human Resources
Web address: www.mobileinfirmary.org
Control: Other not–for–profit (including NFP Corporation) **Service:** General Medical and Surgical

Staffed Beds: 704

★ **PROVIDENCE HOSPITAL (10090)**, 6801 Airport Boulevard, Zip 36608–3785, Mailing Address: P.O. Box 850429, Zip 36685–0429; tel. 251/633–1000 **A**1 2 5 9 10 **F**11 13 15 17 18 20 22 24 25 26 28 31 32 33 34 36 38 41 43 44 45 49 50 51 52 53 55 56 57 58 59 60 62 63 66 68 72 73 74 75 77 78 79 80 81 82 84 86 92 96 97 99 100 102 103 105 106 107 118 119 120 121 124 135 137 **P**6 7 **S** Ascension Health
Primary Contact: Clark P. Christianson, President and Chief Executive Officer
COO: Jason P. Alexander, Executive Vice President and Chief Operating Officer
CFO: Vince N. Formica, Senior Vice President Finance and Chief Financial Officer
CMO: William M. Lightfoot, M.D., Vice President Medical Services
CIO: Cynthia Hyde, Assistant Vice President Information Systems
CHR: David G. Powell, Vice President Human Resources
Web address: www.providencehospital.org
Control: Church–operated, Nongovernment, not–for profit **Service:** General Medical and Surgical

Staffed Beds: 349 **Admissions:** 15414 **Census:** 201 **Outpatient Visits:** 112970 **Births:** 1192 **Total Expense ($000):** 167485 **Payroll Expense ($000):** 65958 **Personnel:** 1548

ROTARY REHABILITATION HOSPITAL See Mobile Infirmary Medical Center

☐ **SPRINGHILL MEMORIAL HOSPITAL (10144)**, 3719 Dauphin Street, Zip 36608–1798, Mailing Address: P.O. Box 8246, Zip 36608–8246; tel. 251/344–9630 **A**1 5 9 10 **F**11 13 15 17 18 20 22 24 25 38 43 47 49 51 55 56 68 72 73 74 75 76 77 79 80 81 82 83 84 86 96 99 100 106 107 118 119 121 135 136 137
Primary Contact: Bill A. Mason, President and Chief Executive Officer
COO: Jeffery M. St Clair, Administrator
CFO: Randy Sucher, Executive Vice President
CIO: Mark Kilborn, Director Information Systems
CHR: Daniela Batchelor, Director Human Resources
Web address: www.springhillmemorial.com
Control: Corporation, Investor–owned, for–profit **Service:** General Medical and Surgical

Staffed Beds: 232 **Admissions:** 10175 **Census:** 143 **Outpatient Visits:** 118224 **Births:** 857 **Total Expense ($000):** 121519 **Payroll Expense ($000):** 43238 **Personnel:** 1147

★ **UNIVERSITY OF SOUTH ALABAMA CHILDREN'S AND WOMEN'S HOSPITAL (13301)**, (Children and Womens Services), 1700 Center Street, Zip 36604–3301; tel. 251/415–1000 **A**1 3 5 9 10 **F**3 7 11 13 15 19 25 27 38 48 49 57 58 62 66 70 71 72 73 74 75 76 77 79 80 81 82 83 84 86 96 100 102 107 113 114 119 132 135 136 **S** University of South Alabama Hospitals
Primary Contact: Becky DeVillier, Administrator
CFO: William B. Bush, Chief Financial Officer
CMO: Richard Teplick, M.D., Chief of Staff
CIO: Thad Phillips, Director Clinical Information Systems
CHR: Janice Rehm, Manager Human Resources
Web address: www.southalabama.edu/usacwh
Control: State–Government, nonfederal **Service:** Other specialty

Staffed Beds: 198 **Admissions:** 8255 **Census:** 166 **Outpatient Visits:** 51466 **Births:** 2989 **Total Expense ($000):** 107004 **Payroll Expense ($000):** 41421 **Personnel:** 840

★ **UNIVERSITY OF SOUTH ALABAMA MEDICAL CENTER (10087)**, 2451 Fillingim Street, Zip 36617–2293; tel. 251/471–7000 **A**1 2 3 5 8 9 10 **F**3 11 16 17 18 20 22 25 27 32 38 40 46 49 55 56 57 58 59 60 62 68 72 76 77 79 80 82 96 97 100 102 103 107 119 135 137 **S** University of South Alabama Hospitals
Primary Contact: Beth Anderson, Administrator
COO: Beth Anderson, Administrator
CFO: William B. Bush, Chief Financial Officer
CMO: Richard Teplick, M.D., Chief of Staff
CIO: Thad Phillips, Director Clinical Information Systems
Web address: www.usahospitals.org
Control: State–Government, nonfederal **Service:** General Medical and Surgical

Staffed Beds: 137 **Admissions:** 6297 **Census:** 109 **Outpatient Visits:** 37147 **Births:** 0 **Total Expense ($000):** 117867 **Payroll Expense ($000):** 59423 **Personnel:** 1245

MONROEVILLE—Monroe County

★ **MONROE COUNTY HOSPITAL (10120)**, 1901 South Alabama Avenue, Zip 36460, Mailing Address: P.O. Box 886, Zip 36461–0886; tel. 251/575–3111, (Nonreporting) **A**1 9 10 20 **S** QHR
Primary Contact: Vincent B. DiFranco, Chief Executive Officer
CFO: Nellie Mason, Chief Financial Officer
CMO: David Stallworth, M.D., Chief of Staff
CHR: Tara Nowlins, Director Human Resources
Web address: www.mchcare.com
Control: County–Government, nonfederal **Service:** General Medical and Surgical

Staffed Beds: 62

MONTGOMERY—Montgomery County

★ **BAPTIST MEDICAL CENTER EAST (10149)**, 400 Taylor Road, Zip 36117–3512, Mailing Address: P.O. Box 241267, Zip 36124–1267; tel. 334/277–8330 **A**1 9 10 **F**3 13 15 25 26 31 32 38 41 43 47 49 50 54 59 62 66 68 70 71 73 74 75 77 79 80 82 86 87 96 97 99 100 102 103 107 118 119 120 121 124 135 **S** Baptist Health
Primary Contact: Mindy Burdick, Administrator
COO: Robin Barca, Senior Vice President and Chief Operating Officer
CFO: Katrina Belt, Chief Financial Officer
CHR: Kay Bennett, System Director Human Resources
Web address: www.baptistfirst.org
Control: Hospital district or authority, Government, nonfederal **Service:** General Medical and Surgical

Staffed Beds: 150 **Admissions:** 10429 **Census:** 112 **Outpatient Visits:** 57934 **Births:** 3240 **Total Expense ($000):** 74955 **Payroll Expense ($000):** 30159 **Personnel:** 756

★ **BAPTIST MEDICAL CENTER SOUTH (10023)**, 2105 East South Boulevard, Zip 36116–2498, Mailing Address: Box 11010, Zip 36111–0010; tel. 334/288–2100 **A**1 3 5 9 10 **F**3 5 8 12 13 15 17 18 20 22 24 25 26 27 30 31 32 38 41 43 49 50 54 59 60 61 62 66 68 70 72 74 76 77 79 80 82 84 86 88 90 91 92 93 94 95 96 97 99 100 102 103 107 118 119 120 121 135 137 **P**7 **S** Baptist Health
Primary Contact: Lynne Parker, Administrator
COO: Robin Barca, Senior Vice President and Chief Operating Officer
CFO: Katrina Belt, Chief Financial Officer
CHR: Kay Bennett, System Director Human Resources
Web address: www.baptistfirst.org
Control: Hospital district or authority, Government, nonfederal **Service:** General Medical and Surgical

Staffed Beds: 400 **Admissions:** 19546 **Census:** 252 **Outpatient Visits:** 128963 **Births:** 1176 **Total Expense ($000):** 223983 **Payroll Expense ($000):** 75799 **Personnel:** 1794

★ **CENTRAL ALABAMA VETERANS HEALTH CARE SYSTEM**, 215 Perry Hill Road, Zip 36109–3798; tel. 334/272–4670, (Includes MONTGOMERY DIVISION; TUSKEGEE DIVISION, 2400 Hospital Road, Tuskegee, Zip 36083–5001; tel. 334/727–0550) **A**1 3 5 **F**12 15 25 26 30 31 32 33 34 36 37 38 42 43 44 46 50 53 54 55 56 57 60 61 62 68 72 73 75 76 77 79 81 82 85 86 87 88 90 91 92 93 94 96 97 100 103 107 117 118 119 121 124 132 133 134 135 136 137 **P**6 **S** Department of Veterans Affairs
Primary Contact: N. Rao Chava, M.D., Director
CFO: Brenda Schmitz, Manager Finance
CMO: N. Rao Chava, M.D., Director
CIO: William Greer, Acting Chief Information Officer
CHR: Linda King, Chief Human Resources Management Service
Web address: www.va.gov/sta/guide/home.asp
Control: Veterans Affairs, Government, federal **Service:** General Medical and Surgical

Staffed Beds: 330 **Admissions:** 1891 **Census:** 49 **Outpatient Visits:** 330491 **Births:** 0 **Total Expense ($000):** 173116 **Payroll Expense ($000):** 77800 **Personnel:** 1448

□ **GREIL MEMORIAL PSYCHIATRIC HOSPITAL (14005)**, 2140 Upper Wetumpka Road, Zip 36107; tel. 334/262–0363, (Nonreporting) **A**1 10
Primary Contact: Allen Stewart, Director
Control: Corporation, Investor–owned, for–profit **Service:** Psychiatric

Staffed Beds: 25

★ **HEALTHSOUTH REHABILITATION HOSPITAL OF MONTGOMERY (13028)**, 4465 Narrow Lane Road, Zip 36116–2900; tel. 334/284–7700, (Nonreporting) **A**1 10 **S** HEALTHSOUTH Corporation
Primary Contact: Linda Wade, Chief Executive Officer
CFO: Heath Watson, Controller
CMO: Jeffrey Eng, M.D., Medical Director
CIO: Diane Davis, Manager Business Office
CHR: Kim McDaniel, Director Human Resources
Web address: www.healthsouth.com
Control: Corporation, Investor–owned, for–profit **Service:** Rehabilitation

Staffed Beds: 80

★ **JACKSON HOSPITAL AND CLINIC (10024)**, 1725 Pine Street, Zip 36106–1117; tel. 334/293–8000 **A**1 9 10 **F**13 17 18 22 25 26 27 30 32 38 43 44 46 50 55 56 57 62 66 68 74 75 76 77 79 80 81 82 84 86 96 97 100 102 106 107 119 120 135 136 137 **P**6
Primary Contact: Donald G. Henderson, President and Chief Executive Officer
CFO: Edward C. Scholl, Vice President Finance
CIO: Richard E. Caldwell, Vice President Informatics
Web address: www.jackson.org
Control: Other not–for–profit (including NFP Corporation) **Service:** General Medical and Surgical

Staffed Beds: 256 **Admissions:** 14068 **Census:** 171 **Outpatient Visits:** 85535 **Births:** 1631 **Personnel:** 1318

★ **LONG TERM HOSPITAL OF MONTGOMERY (12007)**, 1725 Pine Street, 5 North, Zip 36106–1109, Mailing Address: P.O. Box 11649, Zip 36111–1649; tel. 334/240–0532, (Nonreporting) **A**1 9 10 **S** Noland Health Services, Inc.
Primary Contact: Ray Owens, Administrator
Web address: www.nolandhealth.com
Control: Other not–for–profit (including NFP Corporation) **Service:** Long–Term Acute Care hospital

Staffed Beds: 36

MONTGOMERY DIVISION See Central Alabama Veterans Health Care System

MOULTON—Lawrence County

□ **LAWRENCE MEDICAL CENTER (10059)**, 202 Hospital Street, Zip 35650, Mailing Address: P.O. Box 39, Zip 35650–0039; tel. 256/974–2200, (Nonreporting) **A**1 9 10 **S** Brim Healthcare, Inc.
Primary Contact: Thomas Dunning, Chief Executive Officer
CFO: Danny Crowe, Chief Financial Officer
CIO: Jeremy Duncan, Director Information Systems
Web address: www.attentushealthcare.com/lawrencemedicalcenter.htm
Control: Corporation, Investor–owned, for–profit **Service:** General Medical and Surgical

Staffed Beds: 37

MOUNT VERNON—Mobile County

□ **SEARCY HOSPITAL (14008)**, Mailing Address: P.O. Box 1090, Zip 36560–1090; tel. 251/829–9411, (Total facility includes 142 beds in nursing home–type unit) (Nonreporting) **A**1 10
Primary Contact: Beatrice J. McLean, Director
CIO: Bobby McCarley, Director Information Management
Control: State–Government, nonfederal **Service:** Children's hospital psychiatric

Staffed Beds: 467

MUSCLE SHOALS—Colbert County

★ **SHOALS HOSPITAL (10157)**, 201 Avalon Avenue, Zip 35661–2805, Mailing Address: P.O. Box 3359, Zip 35662–3359; tel. 256/386–1600 **A**1 9 10 **F**3 15 25 26 31 32 37 38 51 55 62 66 68 73 75 76 77 79 80 82 85 96 97 100 103 107 112 135 **S** Coffee Health Group
Primary Contact: Jody Pigg, Interim Administrator
Web address: www.chgroup.org
Control: Hospital district or authority, Government, nonfederal **Service:** General Medical and Surgical

Staffed Beds: 95 **Admissions:** 2465 **Census:** 44 **Outpatient Visits:** 34233 **Births:** 0 **Total Expense ($000):** 30806 **Payroll Expense ($000):** 10673 **Personnel:** 236

NORTHPORT—Tuscaloosa County

□ **NORTHPORT MEDICAL CENTER (10145)**, (Formerly Northport Hospital–DCH), 2700 Hospital Drive, Zip 35476; tel. 205/333–4500 **A**1 9 10 **F**3 11 13 15 24 25 26 30 32 33 38 43 54 55 56 57 58 60 62 66 68 70 72 73 74 77 79 81 82 85 86 88 90 91 92 93 94 96 97 99 100 102 107 112 118 119 120 121 124 135 136 137 **P**7 8 **S** DCH Health System
Primary Contact: Luke Standeffer, Administrator
CFO: Jon Kramer, Controller and Assistant Administrator
CMO: Jerry Palmer, M.D., Assistant Administrator Medical Staff Affairs
CIO: Kim Ligon, Director Information Services
CHR: Kay Troxler, Vice President Human Resources
Web address: www.dchsystem.com
Control: Hospital district or authority, Government, nonfederal **Service:** General Medical and Surgical

Staffed Beds: 196 **Admissions:** 8450 **Census:** 141 **Outpatient Visits:** 113711 **Births:** 1515 **Total Expense ($000):** 96462 **Payroll Expense ($000):** 38052 **Personnel:** 786

Hospital, Medicare Provider Number, Address, Telephone, Approval, Facility, and Physician Codes, Health Care System

★ American Hospital Association (AHA) membership
□ The Joint Commission accreditation
○ American Osteopathic Association (AOA) accreditation
△ Commission on Accreditation of Rehabilitation Facilities (CARF) accreditation

ONEONTA—Blount County

★ **ST. VINCENT'S BLOUNT (10050)**, (Formerly Medical Center Blount), 150 Gilbreath, Zip 35121–2534, Mailing Address: P.O. Box 1000, Zip 35121–1000; tel. 205/274–3000 **A**1 9 10 **F**3 11 15 24 25 26 31 32 38 40 55 57 62 63 68 73 75 77 79 80 82 86 96 99 107 124 135 136 **S** Ascension Health
Primary Contact: Sean Tinney, President and Chief Operating Officer
Web address: www.stvhs.com
Control: Other not–for–profit (including NFP Corporation) **Service:** General Medical and Surgical

Staffed Beds: 40 **Admissions:** 1732 **Census:** 19 **Outpatient Visits:** 23568 **Births:** 2 **Total Expense ($000):** 18146 **Payroll Expense ($000):** 6924 **Personnel:** 168

OPELIKA—Lee County

★ **EAST ALABAMA MEDICAL CENTER (10029)**, 2000 Pepperell Parkway, Zip 36802–3201; tel. 334/749–3411, (Total facility includes 113 beds in nursing home–type unit) **A**1 2 9 10 19 **F**3 7 10 11 13 15 17 18 20 22 24 25 26 27 28 30 31 32 38 42 43 44 50 51 52 53 54 55 56 57 58 59 60 61 62 66 68 72 73 74 75 76 77 79 80 81 84 86 88 89 90 92 93 94 96 97 100 102 103 105 106 107 108 109 111 115 117 118 119 121 124 135 137
Primary Contact: Terry W. Andrus, President
CFO: Sam Price, Vice President Finance
CIO: Tommy Chittom, Assistant Vice President Information Services
Web address: www.eamc.org
Control: Hospital district or authority, Government, nonfederal **Service:** General Medical and Surgical

Staffed Beds: 389 **Admissions:** 15893 **Census:** 291 **Outpatient Visits:** 108542 **Births:** 1824 **Total Expense ($000):** 221401 **Payroll Expense ($000):** 92282 **Personnel:** 2367

OPP—Covington County

★ **MIZELL MEMORIAL HOSPITAL (10007)**, 702 Main Street, Zip 36467–1626, Mailing Address: P.O. Box 1010, Zip 36467–1010; tel. 334/493–3541 **A**1 9 10 **F**11 13 15 17 25 26 30 31 32 33 38 52 55 61 73 74 77 79 82 86 96 97 106 107 118 119 120 122 124 135 136 137
Primary Contact: Allen Foster, Chief Executive Officer
COO: Jana Wyatt, Chief Operating Officer and Chief Financial Officer
CFO: Jana Wyatt, Chief Financial Officer
CMO: Wheeler Gunnels, M.D., Medical Director
CIO: Elizabeth Cook, Chief Information Officer
CHR: Dianne Morrison, Director Human Resources
Web address: www.mizellmh.com
Control: Other not–for–profit (including NFP Corporation) **Service:** General Medical and Surgical

Staffed Beds: 58 **Admissions:** 2368 **Census:** 25 **Outpatient Visits:** 28930 **Births:** 117 **Total Expense ($000):** 15505 **Payroll Expense ($000):** 6528 **Personnel:** 192

OZARK—Dale County

DALE MEDICAL CENTER (10021), 100 Hospital Avenue, Zip 36360–2080; tel. 334/774–2601, (Nonreporting) **A**9 10
Primary Contact: Vernon Johnson, Administrator
CFO: Brad Hull, Chief Financial Officer
CMO: Taylor Caffey, M.D., Chief of Staff
CHR: Sheila Dunn, Assistant Administrator Human Resources
Web address: www.dalemedical.org
Control: County–Government, nonfederal **Service:** General Medical and Surgical

Staffed Beds: 69

PELL CITY—St. Clair County

★ **ST. VINCENT'S ST. CLAIR (10130)**, (Formerly St. Clair Regional Hospital), 2805 Doctor John Haynes Drive, Zip 35125–1499; tel. 205/338–3301, (Nonreporting) **A**9 10 **S** Ascension Health
Primary Contact: Terrell Vick, President and Chief Operating Officer
CIO: Susan Evans, Director Health Information Services
Web address: www.stclairregional.com
Control: Corporation, Investor–owned, for–profit **Service:** General Medical and Surgical

Staffed Beds: 72

PHENIX CITY—Russell County

★ **REGIONAL REHABILITATION HOSPITAL (13033)**, 3715 Highway 280/431 North, Zip 36867; tel. 334/732–2200 **A**1 9 10 **F**85 **S** HEALTHSOUTH Corporation
Primary Contact: Jill Jordan, Chief Executive Officer
CFO: Bobby Edmondson, Controller
CMO: Debra Schilling, M.D., Medical Director
CIO: Jacki Cuevas, Director Health Information Services
CHR: Cindy Williams, Director Human Resources
Web address: www.regionalrehabhospital.com
Control: Corporation, Investor–owned, for–profit **Service:** Rehabilitation

Staffed Beds: 38 **Admissions:** 713 **Census:** 30 **Outpatient Visits:** 2672 **Births:** 0 **Total Expense ($000):** 8860 **Payroll Expense ($000):** 4712 **Personnel:** 121

☐ **SUMMIT HOSPITAL (10168)**, 4401 Riverchase Drive, Zip 36867; tel. 334/732–3000, (Nonreporting) **A**1 9 10 **S** Ameris Health Systems
Primary Contact: Greg Griffith, Chief Executive Officer
Web address: www.summithospital.net
Control: Corporation, Investor–owned, for–profit **Service:** Surgical

Staffed Beds: 70

PRATTVILLE—Autauga County

★ **PRATTVILLE BAPTIST HOSPITAL (10108)**, 124 South Memorial Drive, Zip 36067–3619, Mailing Address: P.O. Box 681630, Zip 36067–1638; tel. 334/365–0651 **A**1 9 10 **F**3 12 15 25 26 31 32 33 38 41 43 44 49 50 54 55 56 57 62 66 68 79 80 81 82 96 100 102 118 121 135 **S** Baptist Health
Primary Contact: Ginger Henry, Administrator
CIO: B. Blaine Brown, Vice President and General Counsel
Web address: www.baptistfirst.org
Control: Hospital district or authority, Government, nonfederal **Service:** General Medical and Surgical

Staffed Beds: 50 **Admissions:** 2093 **Census:** 20 **Outpatient Visits:** 37983 **Births:** 0 **Total Expense ($000):** 21353 **Payroll Expense ($000):** 7974 **Personnel:** 209

RED BAY—Franklin County

RED BAY HOSPITAL (11302), 211 Hospital Road, Zip 35582–0490, Mailing Address: P.O. Box 490, Zip 35582–0490; tel. 256/356–9532 **A**9 10 18 **F**25 30 31 32 38 42 46 52 55 56 57 61 62 75 86 96 100 107 119 120 122 124 135 137
Primary Contact: Niles V. Floyd, Administrator
CFO: Samuel A. Strickland, Chief Financial Officer
Web address: www.redbayhospital.com
Control: Hospital district or authority, Government, nonfederal **Service:** General Medical and Surgical

Staffed Beds: 25 **Admissions:** 592 **Census:** 8 **Outpatient Visits:** 18202 **Births:** 0 **Total Expense ($000):** 7751 **Payroll Expense ($000):** 3804 **Personnel:** 118

ROANOKE—Randolph County

★ **RANDOLPH MEDICAL CENTER (11303)**, 59928 Highway 22, Zip 36274–2410, Mailing Address: P.O. Box 670, Zip 36274–0670; tel. 334/863–4111, (Nonreporting) **A**9 10 18
Primary Contact: Timothy Harlin, Chief Executive Officer
CFO: Jeff Kirkpatrick, Chief Financial Officer
CIO: Alfredia Joiner, Coordinator Information Systems
CHR: Ann Hanner, Chief Human Resources Officer
Web address: www.randolphmc.org
Control: County–Government, nonfederal **Service:** General Medical and Surgical

Staffed Beds: 25

RUSSELLVILLE—Franklin County

★ **RUSSELLVILLE HOSPITAL (10158)**, (Formerly Russellville Medical Center), 15155 Highway 43, Zip 35653–1975, Mailing Address: P.O. Box 1089, Zip 35653–1089; tel. 256/332–1611, (Nonreporting) **A**1 9 10 **S** LifePoint Hospitals, Inc.
Primary Contact: Christine R. Stewart, Chief Executive Officer
Web address: www.russellvillehospital.com
Control: Corporation, Investor–owned, for–profit **Service:** General Medical and Surgical

Staffed Beds: 100

SCOTTSBORO—Jackson County

☐ **HIGHLANDS MEDICAL CENTER (10061)**, 380 Woods Cove Road, Zip 35768–2428, Mailing Address: P.O. Box 1050, Zip 35768–1050; tel. 256/259–4444, (Nonreporting) **A**1 9 10 20
Primary Contact: Thomas O. Lackey, Chief Executive Officer
COO: Kim Bryant, Chief Operating Officer
CFO: Dan Newell, Chief Financial Officer
CIO: Doug Newby, Chief Information Officer
CHR: Susanna S. Sivley, Chief Personnel Officer
Web address: www.highlandsmedcenter.com
Control: County–Government, nonfederal **Service:** General Medical and Surgical

Staffed Beds: 85

SELMA—Dallas County

★ **VAUGHAN REGIONAL MEDICAL CENTER (10118)**, 1015 Medical Center Parkway, Zip 36701–6352; tel. 334/418–4100 **A**1 3 5 9 10 19 20 **F**8 11 15 17 18 25 26 30 38 68 74 77 79 84 96 97 100 102 103 107 118 **S** LifePoint Hospitals, Inc.
Primary Contact: Barry L. Keel, Chief Executive Officer
CFO: Don Ikner, Chief Financial Officer
Web address: www.uabsfm.org/vaughan.html
Control: Partnership, Investor–owned, for–profit **Service:** General Medical and Surgical

Staffed Beds: 149 **Admissions:** 8375 **Census:** 84 **Outpatient Visits:** 30411 **Births:** 945 **Total Expense ($000):** 22080 **Payroll Expense ($000):** 22019

Many Facility Codes have changed. Please refer to the AHA Guide Code Chart.

SHEFFIELD—Colbert County

☒ **HELEN KELLER HOSPITAL (10019)**, 1300 South Montgomery Avenue, Zip 35660–6334, Mailing Address: P.O. Box 610, Zip 35660–0610; tel. 256/386–4196 **A**1 9 10 **F**7 11 13 15 18 24 25 30 31 32 33 38 43 49 52 55 56 57 59 62 72 73 74 75 76 77 78 79 80 82 84 86 96 97 100 103 106 107 118 119 120 121 124 132 134 135
Primary Contact: William H. Anderson, President
COO: Ralph J. Wilson, Chief Operating Officer
CFO: Morris S. Strickland, Chief Financial Officer
CIO: Larry Walker, Chief Information Officer
CHR: Pam Bryant, Director Human Resources
Web address: www.helenkeller.com
Control: Hospital district or authority, Government, nonfederal **Service:** General Medical and Surgical

Staffed Beds: 159 **Admissions:** 6703 **Census:** 73 **Outpatient Visits:** 91340 **Births:** 845 **Total Expense ($000):** 59511 **Payroll Expense ($000):** 24385 **Personnel:** 722

SYLACAUGA—Talladega County

☐ **COOSA VALLEY MEDICAL CENTER (10164)**, 315 West Hickory Street, Zip 35150–2996; tel. 256/401–4000, (Nonreporting) **A**1 9 10
Primary Contact: Glenn C. Sisk, President
CFO: Pam Townsend, Vice President Finance
CIO: Sandra Murchison, Director Medical Records
CHR: Christy Knowles, Director Human Resources
Web address: www.cvhealth.net
Control: Other not–for–profit (including NFP Corporation) **Service:** General Medical and Surgical

Staffed Beds: 101

TALLADEGA—Talladega County

☐ ○ **CITIZENS BAPTIST MEDICAL CENTER (10101)**, 604 Stone Avenue, Zip 35160–2217, Mailing Address: P.O. Box 978, Zip 35161–0978; tel. 256/362–8111 **A**1 9 10 11 19 **F**3 11 13 14 15 24 25 26 30 31 32 33 38 43 52 55 56 57 59 61 62 63 65 68 72 73 74 77 79 81 83 84 85 86 96 97 99 100 101 106 107 117 120 121 124 135 **P**7 **S** Baptist Health System
Primary Contact: Steven Gautney, President
CFO: Mark Lovell, Vice President Finance
CHR: Clinton Fulton, Director Human Resources
Web address: www.bhsala.com
Control: Other not–for–profit (including NFP Corporation) **Service:** General Medical and Surgical

Staffed Beds: 106 **Admissions:** 3893 **Census:** 32 **Outpatient Visits:** 50165 **Births:** 478 **Total Expense ($000):** 27982 **Payroll Expense ($000):** 13208 **Personnel:** 353

TALLASSEE—Elmore County

★ **COMMUNITY HOSPITAL (10034)**, 805 Friendship Road, Zip 36078–1234; tel. 334/283–6541, (Nonreporting) **A**9 10
Primary Contact: Jennie R. Rhinehart, Administrator and Chief Executive Officer
Web address: www.chal.org
Control: Other not–for–profit (including NFP Corporation) **Service:** General Medical and Surgical

Staffed Beds: 69

THOMASVILLE—Clarke County

SOUTHWEST ALABAMA MEDICAL CENTER (10015), 33700 Highway 43, Zip 36784–3351; tel. 334/636–4311, (Nonreporting) **A**9 10 **S** Resurgence Health Group
Primary Contact: Anne S. Thompson, Chief Executive Officer
COO: Lisa Sims, Chief Financial Officer
CFO: David R. Pike, Chief Financial Officer
CMO: Huey Kidd, Chief Medical Officer
CHR: Holly Hutto, Director Human Resources
Web address: www.resurgencehealthgroup.com
Control: Corporation, Investor–owned, for–profit **Service:** General Medical and Surgical

Staffed Beds: 27

TROY—Pike County

☐ **TROY REGIONAL MEDICAL CENTER (10126)**, 1330 Highway 231 South, Zip 36081–1224; tel. 334/670–5000, (Nonreporting) **A**1 9 10 **S** Gilliard Health Services
Primary Contact: Russell Eldridge, Chief Executive Officer
CFO: Mike Deaton, Chief Financial Officer
CIO: Doug Calvert, Director Information Systems
CHR: Lori Austin, Director Human Resources
Control: Corporation, Investor–owned, for–profit **Service:** General Medical and Surgical

Staffed Beds: 78

TUSCALOOSA—Tuscaloosa County

☐ **BRYCE HOSPITAL (14007)**, 200 University Boulevard, Zip 35401–1294; tel. 205/759–0799, (Total facility includes 354 beds in nursing home–type unit) (Nonreporting) **A**1 5 10
Primary Contact: David Bennett, Director
COO: David Bennett, Director
CFO: Wendell Summerville, Chief Financial Officer
CMO: Cynthia Moore Sledge, M.D., Medical Director
CIO: Ronene Howell, Director Health Information Management
CHR: Jim Elliott, Director Human Resources
Control: State–Government, nonfederal **Service:** Psychiatric

Staffed Beds: 820

☐ **DCH REGIONAL MEDICAL CENTER (10092)**, 809 University Boulevard East, Zip 35401–9961; tel. 205/759–7111 **A**1 3 5 9 10 **F**3 11 12 13 15 17 18 20 22 25 26 27 30 32 33 36 38 40 43 48 49 50 51 55 57 60 61 62 64 66 68 70 72 73 74 75 76 77 79 81 82 83 84 96 97 99 100 102 103 104 105 106 107 109 118 119 121 135 136 137 **P**7 **S** DCH Health System
Primary Contact: William H. Cassels, Administrator
CFO: John W. Winfrey, Vice President Finance and Chief Financial Officer
CIO: Kim Ligon, Director Information Services
CHR: Kay Troxler, Chief Human Resources Officer
Web address: www.dchsystem.com
Control: Hospital district or authority, Government, nonfederal **Service:** General Medical and Surgical

Staffed Beds: 455 **Admissions:** 27119 **Census:** 366 **Outpatient Visits:** 395321 **Births:** 1813 **Total Expense ($000):** 277987 **Payroll Expense ($000):** 137788 **Personnel:** 2960

☐ **LONG TERM HOSPITAL OF TUSCALOOSA (10166)**, 809 Unviersity Boulevard East, 4th Floor, Zip 35401, Mailing Address: 809 University Boulevard East, 4th Floor, Zip 35401; tel. 205/759–7241, (Nonreporting) **A**1 9 10 **S** Noland Health Services, Inc.
Primary Contact: Bob Notarianni, Administrator
Web address: www.nolandhealth.com
Control: Other not–for–profit (including NFP Corporation) **Service:** Long–Term Acute Care hospital

Staffed Beds: 27

☐ **MARY S HARPER GERIATRIC PSYCHIATRIC CENTER (14012)**, 200 University Boulevard, Zip 35401; tel. 205/759–0900 **A**1 10 **F**25 26 37 43 54 73 75 88 93 119 124
Primary Contact: Beverly White, M.S., Facility Director
CFO: Sarah Mitchell, Director Finance
CMO: Robin Barton Lariscy, M.D., Medical Director
CIO: Sarah Mitchell, Director Finance
CHR: Jim Elliott, Director Human Resources
Web address: www.mh.alabama.gov
Control: State–Government, nonfederal **Service:** Psychiatric

Staffed Beds: 96 **Admissions:** 269 **Census:** 110 **Outpatient Visits:** 0 **Births:** 0 **Total Expense ($000):** 15193 **Payroll Expense ($000):** 6345 **Personnel:** 190

☐ **TAYLOR HARDIN SECURE MEDICAL FACILITY (14011)**, 1301 Jack Warner Parkway, Zip 35404; tel. 205/556–7060, (Nonreporting) **A**1 10
Primary Contact: James F. Reddoch, Jr., Director
Control: Corporation, Investor–owned, for–profit **Service:** Psychiatric

Staffed Beds: 114

Hospital, Medicare Provider Number, Address, Telephone, Approval, Facility, and Physician Codes, Health Care System
★ American Hospital Association (AHA) membership
☐ The Joint Commission accreditation
○ American Osteopathic Association (AOA) accreditation
△ Commission on Accreditation of Rehabilitation Facilities (CARF) accreditation

☒ △ **VETERANS AFFAIRS MEDICAL CENTER**, 3701 Loop Road, Zip 35404–5015; tel. 205/554–2000, (Total facility includes 198 beds in nursing home–type unit) **A**1 7 **F**4 5 25 26 31 32 37 42 43 44 45 54 57 58 61 62 66 72 73 75 81 82 86 87 88 93 94 95 96 102 117 119 121 124 135 136 137 **P**6 **S** Department of Veterans Affairs
Primary Contact: Alan J. Tyler, M.S., FACHE, Director
COO: Gary D. Trende, FACHE, Associate Director
CFO: Angelia Stevenson, Manager Finance
CMO: Mark Nissenbaum, M.D., Chief of Staff
CIO: Vicki Smallwood, Chief Information Officer
CHR: Janice Hardy, Chief Human Resources Management
Web address: www.tuscaloosa.va.gov
Control: Veterans Affairs, Government, federal **Service:** Psychiatric

Staffed Beds: 381 **Admissions:** 1161 **Census:** 323 **Outpatient Visits:** 253283 **Births:** 0 **Total Expense ($000):** 100183 **Payroll Expense ($000):** 59751 **Personnel:** 927

TUSKEGEE—Macon County

TUSKEGEE DIVISION See Central Alabama Veterans Health Care System, Montgomery

UNION SPRINGS—Bullock County

BULLOCK COUNTY HOSPITAL (10110), 102 West Conecuh Avenue, Zip 36089–1303; tel. 334/738–2140, (Nonreporting) **A**9 10 20
Primary Contact: Benton L. Busbee, Administrator
COO: Victoria Lawrenson, Chief Operating Officer
CFO: Allen J. Gamble, Comptroller
CMO: Maria Bernardo, Chief of Staff
CIO: Tony Lang, Chief Information Officer
Control: Corporation, Investor–owned, for–profit **Service:** General Medical and Surgical

Staffed Beds: 30

VALLEY—Chambers County

☐ ○ **LANIER HEALTH SERVICES (10025)**, 4800 48th Street, Zip 36854–3666; tel. 334/756–9180, (Total facility includes 103 beds in nursing home–type unit) **A**1 9 10 11 19 **F**3 11 13 15 18 24 25 26 38 46 47 48 49 51 55 56 57 61 62 66 68 72 75 76 77 79 80 81 82 86 90 92 96 97 100 106 107 112 117 119 121 122 124 135 136
Primary Contact: Kelli Powers, Chief Executive Officer and Administrator
CFO: Frank Oprandy, Chief Financial Officer
CMO: Michael A. Grossman, M.D., President Medical Staff
CIO: Kurt Leroy, Manager Information Management
CHR: Clara Pitts, Director Human Resources
Web address: www.lanierhospital.com
Control: Other not–for–profit (including NFP Corporation) **Service:** General Medical and Surgical

Staffed Beds: 173 **Admissions:** 3593 **Census:** 140 **Outpatient Visits:** 61186 **Births:** 306 **Total Expense ($000):** 37650 **Payroll Expense ($000):** 15243 **Personnel:** 524

WEDOWEE—Randolph County

★ **WEDOWEE HOSPITAL (10032)**, 209 North Main Street, Zip 36278–5138, Mailing Address: P.O. Box 307, Zip 36278–0307; tel. 256/357–2111, (Nonreporting) **A**9 10
Primary Contact: Farrell Turner, Interim Administrator
Control: County–Government, nonfederal **Service:** General Medical and Surgical

Staffed Beds: 23

WETUMPKA—Elmore County

ELMORE COMMUNITY HOSPITAL (10097), 500 Hospital Drive, Zip 36092–1625, Mailing Address: P.O. Box 130, Zip 36092–0130; tel. 334/567–4311, (Nonreporting) **A**9 10
Primary Contact: Gordon Faulk, Administrator
CFO: David Guy, Chief Financial Officer
Control: Partnership, Investor–owned, for–profit **Service:** General Medical and Surgical

Staffed Beds: 40

WINFIELD—Marion County

☒ **NORTHWEST MEDICAL CENTER (10086)**, 1530 U.S. Highway 43, Zip 35594–5056; tel. 205/487–7000, (Nonreporting) **A**1 9 10 **S** LifePoint Hospitals, Inc.
Primary Contact: Chuck Spann, Chief Executive Officer
CFO: James Gory, Chief Financial Officer
CHR: Yvonne Barker, Director Human Resources and Professional Affairs
Web address: www.northwestmedcenter.com
Control: Corporation, Investor–owned, for–profit **Service:** General Medical and Surgical

Staffed Beds: 66

YORK—Sumter County

HILL HOSPITAL OF SUMTER COUNTY (10138), 751 Derby Drive, Zip 36925; tel. 205/392–5263, (Nonreporting) **A**9 10
Primary Contact: Kathy A. Jordan, Administrator
CFO: Joyce Wedgeworth, Financial Clerk
CHR: Annette Billingsley, Director Human Resources
Control: City–County, Government, nonfederal **Service:** General Medical and Surgical

Staffed Beds: 33

Many Facility Codes have changed. Please refer to the AHA Guide Code Chart.

ALASKA

ANCHORAGE—2nd Judicial Division

★□ **ALASKA NATIVE MEDICAL CENTER (20026)**, 4315 Diplomacy Drive, Zip 99508; tel. 907/563–2662 **A**1 5 9 10 **F**3 5 7 10 11 12 13 15 18 25 26 27 28 29 30 31 32 33 34 36 37 38 40 43 48 49 50 53 54 55 56 57 58 60 61 62 63 66 68 72 73 74 75 76 77 79 80 81 82 84 86 87 90 92 94 96 97 100 102 107 114 118 119 121 122 123 124 131 132 133 135 136 137 **P**6
Primary Contact: Daniel E. Jessop, CPA, Administrator
COO: Susan M. Childers, CPA, Chief Operating Officer
CFO: Michael A. Banks, Chief Financial Officer
CMO: Edward Gilkey, M.D., Chief Physician Executive
CIO: Stephanie Morton, Chief Information Officer
CHR: Sonya Conant, Senior Director Human Resources
Web address: www.anmc.org
Control: Other not–for–profit (including NFP Corporation) **Service:** General Medical and Surgical

Staffed Beds: 150 **Admissions:** 6980 **Census:** 99 **Outpatient Visits:** 393515 **Births:** 1416 **Personnel:** 1288

□ **ALASKA PSYCHIATRIC INSTITUTE (24002)**, 2800 Providence Drive, Zip 99508–4677; tel. 907/269–7100 **A**1 9 10 **F**32 88 89 90 91 **P**1
Primary Contact: Ronald M. Adler, Chief Executive Officer
COO: Ronald M. Adler, Chief Executive Officer
CMO: Duane Hopson, M.D., Medical Director
CIO: Stephen Schneider, Manager Information Services
CHR: Elmer Goode, Administrative Manager Human Resources
Web address: www.hss.state.ak.us/dbh/API/
Control: State–Government, nonfederal **Service:** Psychiatric

Staffed Beds: 80 **Admissions:** 1231 **Census:** 65 **Outpatient Visits:** 0 **Births:** 0 **Total Expense ($000):** 23994 **Payroll Expense ($000):** 12681 **Personnel:** 225

★□ **ALASKA REGIONAL HOSPITAL (20017)**, 2801 Debarr Road, Zip 99508–2997, Mailing Address: P.O. Box 143889, Zip 99514–3889; tel. 907/264–1754 **A**1 9 10 **F**3 8 11 13 15 17 18 19 20 22 24 25 26 30 31 32 38 39 40 46 50 54 55 56 57 58 59 62 63 66 68 70 71 72 73 74 75 76 77 79 80 81 82 84 85 86 87 96 97 99 100 101 102 103 107 116 118 119 124 132 135 136 **P**5 8 **S** HCA
Primary Contact: Edward H. Lamb, FACHE, President and Chief Executive Officer
COO: Richard Davis, Chief Operating Officer
CFO: Paul G. Morris, Chief Financial Officer
CMO: Norman Wilder, M.D., Vice President Medical Affairs
CIO: Clay VanKempema, Director Information Services
CHR: Tammy McCutcheon, Director Human Resources
Web address: www.alaskaregional.com
Control: Corporation, Investor–owned, for–profit **Service:** General Medical and Surgical

Staffed Beds: 129 **Admissions:** 7689 **Census:** 64 **Outpatient Visits:** 46224 **Births:** 714 **Total Expense ($000):** 110715 **Payroll Expense ($000):** 41455 **Personnel:** 931

★□ **NORTH STAR BEHAVIORAL HEALTH SYSTEM (24001)**, 2530 DeBarr Road, Zip 99508–2948; tel. 907/258–7575, (Includes NORTH STAR BEHAVIORAL HEALTH, 1650 South Bragaw, Zip 99508–3467; tel. 907/258–7575; James Shill, Chief Executive Officer and Managing Director), (Nonreporting) **A**1 9 10 **S** Universal Health Services, Inc.
Primary Contact: James Shill, Chief Executive Officer and Managing Director
CFO: Michele Fissori, Chief Financial Officer
CMO: Arom Evans, M.D., Medical Director
CIO: Terry Thompson, Director Information Services
CHR: Patrick Higgins, Director Human Resources
Web address: www.northstarbehavioral.com
Control: Partnership, Investor–owned, for–profit **Service:** Psychiatric

Staffed Beds: 74

★□ **PROVIDENCE ALASKA MEDICAL CENTER (20001)**, 3200 Providence Drive, Zip 99508–4615, Mailing Address: P.O. Box 196604, Zip 99519–6604; tel. 907/562–2211 **A**1 2 3 5 9 10 **F**3 5 11 12 13 14 15 17 18 19 20 21 22 24 25 26 27 30 31 32 35 36 38 42 43 44 50 51 55 57 59 61 62 66 68 70 72 73 74 75 76 77 78 79 80 81 82 83 84 85 86 88 89 90 91 92 93 94 96 100 103 107 109 111 112 114 116 118 119 120 121 124 134 135 137 **P**6 8 **S** Providence Health & Services
Primary Contact: E. Al Parrish, Vice President and Chief Executive Officer
COO: Bruce Lamoureux, Administrator and Chief Operating Officer
CFO: Anthony Dorsch, Chief Financial Officer
CMO: Roy Davis, M.D., Chief Medical Officer
CIO: Stephanie Morton, Chief Information Officer
CHR: Scott Jungwirth, Chief Human Resources Officer
Web address: www.providence.org/alaska/pamc/default.htm
Control: Church–operated, Nongovernment, not–for profit **Service:** General Medical and Surgical

Staffed Beds: 364 **Admissions:** 17002 **Census:** 252 **Outpatient Visits:** 325405 **Births:** 2489 **Total Expense ($000):** 428308 **Payroll Expense ($000):** 160109

□ **ST. ELIAS SPECIALTY HOSPITAL (20028)**, 4800 Cordova Street, Zip 99503; tel. 907/561–3333, (Nonreporting) **A**1 10
Primary Contact: Chad Carpenter, Chief Executive Officer
Web address: www.st-eliashospital.com
Control: Church–operated, Nongovernment, not–for profit **Service:** Long–Term Acute Care hospital

Staffed Beds: 60

BARROW—4th Judicial Division

★□ **SAMUEL SIMMONDS MEMORIAL HOSPITAL (21312)**, 1296 Agvik Street, Zip 99723, Mailing Address: P.O. Box 29, Zip 99723; tel. 907/852–4611 **A**1 10 18 **F**3 13 15 25 32 37 38 62 99 107
Primary Contact: Michael S. Herring, Administrator
Web address: www.arcticslope.org
Control: Other not–for–profit (including NFP Corporation) **Service:** General Medical and Surgical

Staffed Beds: 14 **Admissions:** 203 **Census:** 1 **Outpatient Visits:** 18182 **Births:** 56 **Total Expense ($000):** 18517 **Payroll Expense ($000):** 8506 **Personnel:** 124

BETHEL—1st Judicial Division

★□ **YUKON–KUSKOKWIM DELTA REGIONAL HOSPITAL (20018)**, Mailing Address: P.O. Box 528, Zip 99559–3000; tel. 907/543–6300, (Nonreporting) **A**1 10
Primary Contact: Jack Crow, Vice President Health Services
CFO: Joseph DeMeo, Chief Financial Officer
CIO: David Hodges, Chief Information Officer
CHR: Edward Buckley, Director Human Resources
Web address: www.ykhc.org
Control: Other not–for–profit (including NFP Corporation) **Service:** General Medical and Surgical

Staffed Beds: 54

CORDOVA—2nd Judicial Division

★ **CORDOVA COMMUNITY MEDICAL CENTER (21307)**, 602 Chase Avenue, Zip 99574, Mailing Address: P.O. Box 160, Zip 99574; tel. 907/424–8000, (Total facility includes 10 beds in nursing home–type unit) (Nonreporting) **A**9 10 18
Primary Contact: David Bryant, Administrator and Chief Executive Officer
CFO: Mary Staab, Director Finance
CMO: Murray Buttner, M.D., Medical Director
CIO: Kim Dunn, Attorney–at–Law
CHR: Mary Staab, Director Finance
Web address: www.cityofcordova.net
Control: City–Government, nonfederal **Service:** General Medical and Surgical

Staffed Beds: 23

Hospital, Medicare Provider Number, Address, Telephone, Approval, Facility, and Physician Codes, Health Care System
★ American Hospital Association (AHA) membership
□ The Joint Commission accreditation
○ American Osteopathic Association (AOA) accreditation
△ Commission on Accreditation of Rehabilitation Facilities (CARF) accreditation

DILLINGHAM—1st Judicial Division

★ **BRISTOL BAY AREA HEALTH CORPORATION (21309)**, 6000 Kanakanak Road, Zip 99576, Mailing Address: P.O. Box 130, Zip 99576; tel. 907/842–5201, (Nonreporting) **A**1 9 10 18
Primary Contact: Darrel C. Richardson, Executive Vice President and Chief Operations Officer
COO: Darrel C. Richardson, Executive Vice President and Chief Operations Officer
CFO: Tom Berner, Vice President and Chief Financial Officer
CMO: Arnold Loera, M.D., Vice President and Medical Director
CIO: Bill Pearch, Chief Information Officer
Web address: www.bbahc.org
Control: Other not–for–profit (including NFP Corporation) **Service:** General Medical and Surgical

Staffed Beds: 15

ELMENDORF AFB—2nd Judicial Division

★ **U. S. AIR FORCE REGIONAL HOSPITAL**, 5955 Zeamer Avenue, Zip 99506–3700; tel. 907/560–6260, (Nonreporting) **A**1 5 **S** Department of the Air Force
Primary Contact: Colonel Elisha Powell, Commander
COO: Colonel Billy Cecil, Administrator
CFO: Major Mark Lamey, Flight Commander Resources Management
CMO: Lieutenant Colonel Donald Trummel, Chief Medical Staff
CIO: Captain Jeffrey Eyink, Flight Commander Medical Information Systems
Web address: www.elmendorf.af.mil/
Control: Air Force, Government, federal **Service:** General Medical and Surgical

Staffed Beds: 64

FAIRBANKS—1st Judicial Division

★ **FAIRBANKS MEMORIAL HOSPITAL (20012)**, 1650 Cowles Street, Zip 99701–5998; tel. 907/452–8181, (Total facility includes 90 beds in nursing home–type unit) **A**1 2 5 9 10 19 20 **F**3 7 11 13 15 16 18 24 25 26 27 30 31 32 33 38 43 44 46 48 49 50 52 54 55 56 57 58 59 60 61 62 65 66 68 70 72 73 74 75 76 77 79 80 81 82 84 86 88 90 91 92 93 96 99 100 103 107 108 109 117 118 119 121 124 134 135 136 137 **S** Banner Health
Primary Contact: Michael K. Powers, FACHE, Chief Executive Officer
CFO: Robert Gould, Associate Administrator and Chief Financial Officer
CIO: Carl Kegley, System Director Information Technology
CHR: Jim Lynch, Director People Resources
Web address: www.bannerhealth.com
Control: Other not–for–profit (including NFP Corporation) **Service:** General Medical and Surgical

Staffed Beds: 207 **Admissions:** 5572 **Census:** 135 **Outpatient Visits:** 307196 **Births:** 1155 **Total Expense ($000):** 156858 **Payroll Expense ($000):** 65396 **Personnel:** 1185

FORT WAINWRIGHT—1st Judicial Division

★ **BASSETT ARMY COMMUNITY HOSPITAL**, 1060 Gaffney Road, Box 7400, Zip 99703–7400, Mailing Address: 1060 Gaffney Road, Building 7440, Zip 99703–7440; tel. 907/361–5172, (Nonreporting) **A**1 **S** Department of the Army, Office of the Surgeon General
Primary Contact: Lieutenant Colonel Jeffrey Hillard, Deputy Commander for Administration
COO: Lieutenant Colonel Jeffrey Hillard, Deputy Commander for Administration
CMO: Lieutenant Colonel Vincent Barnhart, Deputy Commander Clinical Services
CIO: Michele Krause, Chief Information Management Officer
Web address: www.alaska.amedd.army.mil
Control: Army, Government, federal **Service:** General Medical and Surgical

Staffed Beds: 24

HOMER—3rd Judicial Division

★ **SOUTH PENINSULA HOSPITAL (20014)**, 4300 Bartlett Street, Zip 99603–7000; tel. 907/235–8101, (Total facility includes 25 beds in nursing home–type unit) **A**9 10 20 **F**3 11 13 15 25 26 27 30 31 32 33 38 54 56 57 61 62 65 66 68 73 74 75 77 79 80 82 84 86 87 96 100 103 107 117 119 122 137 **P**8
Primary Contact: Robert F. Letson, Chief Executive Officer
COO: Christine K. Anderson, R.N., Director Patient Care Services
CFO: MaLisa Mudgett, Assistant Administrator and Chief Financial Officer
CIO: Greg Browngoetz, Manager Information Systems
CHR: Cindy Brinkerhoff, Director Human Resources
Web address: www.sphosp.com
Control: Hospital district or authority, Government, nonfederal **Service:** General Medical and Surgical

Staffed Beds: 47 **Admissions:** 850 **Census:** 32 **Outpatient Visits:** 30758 **Births:** 136 **Total Expense ($000):** 26089 **Payroll Expense ($000):** 10060 **Personnel:** 237

JUNEAU—3rd Judicial Division

★ **BARTLETT REGIONAL HOSPITAL (20008)**, 3260 Hospital Drive, Zip 99801–7808; tel. 907/586–2611 **A**1 9 10 20 **F**3 4 5 12 13 15 24 25 26 27 30 33 38 55 66 68 69 73 74 75 79 86 88 89 90 91 92 93 94 95 96 97 100 107 112 118 119 121 124 135 137 **S** QHR
Primary Contact: Shawn Morrow, Chief Executive Officer
COO: Debbi Lehner, Chief Operating Officer
CFO: Garth Hamblin, Chief Financial Officer
CMO: Norman Thompson, M.D., Chief of Staff
CHR: Kyla Allred, Manager Human Resources
Web address: www.bartletthospital.org
Control: City–County, Government, nonfederal **Service:** General Medical and Surgical

Staffed Beds: 65 **Admissions:** 2167 **Census:** 22 **Outpatient Visits:** 33488 **Births:** 397

KETCHIKAN—3rd Judicial Division

★ **KETCHIKAN GENERAL HOSPITAL (21311)**, 3100 Tongass Avenue, Zip 99901–5746; tel. 907/225–5171, (Total facility includes 29 beds in nursing home–type unit) (Nonreporting) **A**9 10 18 **S** PeaceHealth
Primary Contact: Patrick J. Branco, Chief Executive Officer
CFO: Ken Tonjes, Vice President Finance
CMO: Peter Rice, M.D., Medical Director
CIO: Tim Walker, Manager Information Services
CHR: Lanetta Lundberg, Manager Human Resources
Web address: www.peacehealth.org
Control: Church–operated, Nongovernment, not–for profit **Service:** General Medical and Surgical

Staffed Beds: 54

KODIAK—2nd Judicial Division

★ **PROVIDENCE KODIAK ISLAND MEDICAL CENTER (21306)**, 1915 East Rezanof Drive, Zip 99615–6602; tel. 907/486–3281, (Total facility includes 19 beds in nursing home–type unit) **A**1 9 10 18 **F**3 8 11 13 15 25 26 27 30 31 32 33 36 38 45 46 55 56 57 61 62 64 65 66 68 73 74 76 77 79 80 82 84 85 86 88 89 90 91 92 93 94 96 99 100 102 107 117 119 122 135 137 **P**6 **S** Providence Health & Services
Primary Contact: Donald J. Rush, Chief Executive Officer
CFO: Timothy Hocum, Chief Financial Officer
CMO: Steve Smith, M.D., Chief Medical Staff
CIO: Fritz Ferrante, Manager Information Services
CHR: Brenda Zawacki, Manager Human Resources
Web address: www.providence.org
Control: Other not–for–profit (including NFP Corporation) **Service:** General Medical and Surgical

Staffed Beds: 25 **Admissions:** 780 **Census:** 24 **Outpatient Visits:** 8716 **Births:** 182 **Total Expense ($000):** 23750 **Payroll Expense ($000):** 11539 **Personnel:** 162

KOTZEBUE—2nd Judicial Division

★ **MANIILAQ HEALTH CENTER (21310)**, 436 5th Avenue, Zip 99752–0043, Mailing Address: P.O. Box 43, Zip 99752–0043; tel. 907/442–7344, (Nonreporting) **A**1 9 10 18
Primary Contact: Paul Hansen, Administrator
CMO: Patricia Clancy, M.D., Medical Director
CIO: Eugene Smith, Chief Information Officer
Web address: www.maniilaq.org
Control: Other not–for–profit (including NFP Corporation) **Service:** General Medical and Surgical

Staffed Beds: 17

NOME—2nd Judicial Division

★ **NORTON SOUND REGIONAL HOSPITAL (21308)**, Bering Straits, Zip 99762, Mailing Address: P.O. Box 966, Zip 99762–0966; tel. 907/443–3311, (Total facility includes 15 beds in nursing home–type unit) (Nonreporting) **A**1 9 10 18
Primary Contact: Angela Gorn, Vice President
COO: Helen Pootoogooluk, Chief Operating Officer
CFO: Nat Palaniappan, Chief Financial Officer
CMO: David Head, M.D., Chief Medical Staff
CIO: Dan Bailey, Director Information Systems
CHR: Tiffany Martinson, Director Human Resources
Web address: www.nortonsoundhealth.org
Control: Other not–for–profit (including NFP Corporation) **Service:** General Medical and Surgical

Staffed Beds: 36

Many Facility Codes have changed. Please refer to the AHA Guide Code Chart.

PALMER—3rd Judicial Division

⊠ **MAT-SU REGIONAL MEDICAL CENTER (20006)**, 2500 South Woodworth Loop, Zip 99645, Mailing Address: P.O. Box 1687, Zip 99645–1687; tel. 907/746–8600 **A**1 9 10 20 **F**3 8 13 15 18 20 24 25 26 30 31 32 33 38 42 43 44 46 51 53 55 56 57 61 62 66 68 73 74 75 76 77 79 80 81 82 86 96 97 99 100 102 103 106 107 112 118 119 122 133 135 137 **S** Community Health Systems, Inc.
Primary Contact: Norman F. Stephens, Chief Executive Officer
CFO: John Abreu, Chief Financial Officer
CMO: John Boston, D.O., Chief of Staff
CIO: Todd Lewellyn, Director Information Systems
CHR: Terry McCarty, Director Human Resources
Web address: www.matsuregional.com
Control: Partnership, Investor–owned, for–profit **Service:** General Medical and Surgical

Staffed Beds: 74 **Admissions:** 3903 **Census:** 34 **Outpatient Visits:** 64186 **Births:** 675 **Total Expense ($000):** 93814 **Payroll Expense ($000):** 35339 **Personnel:** 479

PETERSBURG—3rd Judicial Division

★ **PETERSBURG MEDICAL CENTER (21304)**, 103 Fram Street, Zip 99833, Mailing Address: Box 589, Zip 99833–0589; tel. 907/772–4291, (Total facility includes 15 beds in nursing home–type unit) **A**9 10 18 **F**1 3 13 15 17 27 28 30 31 32 38 42 53 55 56 57 61 62 65 68 74 76 79 84 87 96 99 107 117 122 136 137
Primary Contact: John F. Bringhurst, Administrator
CFO: Jan Baird, Chief Financial Officer
CMO: John Bergman, M.D., Chief of Staff
CHR: Cynthia Newman, Manager Human Resources
Control: City–Government, nonfederal **Service:** General Medical and Surgical

Staffed Beds: 27 **Admissions:** 199 **Census:** 15 **Outpatient Visits:** 15053 **Births:** 8 **Total Expense ($000):** 7393 **Payroll Expense ($000):** 4096 **Personnel:** 85

SEWARD—2nd Judicial Division

★ **PROVIDENCE SEWARD MEDICAL CENTER (21302)**, 417 First Avenue, Zip 99664, Mailing Address: P.O. Box 365, Zip 99664–0365; tel. 907/224–5205, (Nonreporting) **A**9 10 18 **S** Providence Health & Services
Primary Contact: Kathy Kloster, Administrator
CMO: Jennet Hermiston, M.D., Medical Director
Web address: www.providence.org
Control: Church–operated, Nongovernment, not–for profit **Service:** General Medical and Surgical

Staffed Beds: 6

SITKA—3rd Judicial Division

⊠ **SEARHC MT. EDGECUMBE HOSPITAL (20027)**, 222 Tongass Drive, Zip 99835–9416; tel. 907/966–2411 **A**1 9 10 **F**3 5 13 15 25 26 27 28 31 32 33 37 38 40 50 55 56 57 60 62 63 66 68 72 73 74 77 79 80 82 86 87 89 90 91 92 94 95 96 100 102 107 119 123 124 133 136 **P**6
Primary Contact: Frank Sutton, Vice President Hospital Services
COO: Martin Grasmeder, M.D., Medical Director
CFO: David Edwards, Chief Financial Officer
CMO: Susan Carlson, M.D., Medical Director
CIO: Bob Cita, Director Information Services
CHR: Melanie Millhorn, Director Human Resources
Web address: www.searhc.org
Control: Other not–for–profit (including NFP Corporation) **Service:** General Medical and Surgical

Staffed Beds: 27 **Admissions:** 1248 **Census:** 15 **Outpatient Visits:** 72836 **Births:** 71 **Personnel:** 241

★ **SITKA COMMUNITY HOSPITAL (21303)**, 209 Moller Avenue, Zip 99835–7145; tel. 907/747–3241, (Total facility includes 15 beds in nursing home–type unit) (Nonreporting) **A**9 10 18
Primary Contact: Moe Chaudry, Chief Executive Officer and Administrator
CFO: Lee W. Bennett, Chief Financial Officer
Web address: www.sitkahospital.org
Control: City–Government, nonfederal **Service:** General Medical and Surgical

Staffed Beds: 27

SOLDOTNA—3rd Judicial Division

⊠ **CENTRAL PENINSULA GENERAL HOSPITAL (20024)**, 250 Hospital Place, Zip 99669–6999; tel. 907/714–4404, (Total facility includes 58 beds in nursing home–type unit) **A**1 9 10 20 **F**3 4 5 11 13 15 24 25 26 27 30 31 32 33 34 36 38 44 49 55 56 57 66 68 73 74 75 76 77 79 80 82 86 90 95 96 97 100 102 106 107 117 118 119 120 122 124 134 135 136 137
Primary Contact: Ryan K. Smith, Chief Executive Officer
COO: Matt Dammeyer, Ph.D., Assistant Administrator
CFO: Jason Paret, Chief Financial Officer
CMO: Curt Buchholz, Chief of Staff
CIO: Mike Webb, Director Information Systems
CHR: Bonnie Nichols, Marketing and Public Relations Director
Web address: www.cpgh.org
Control: Other not–for–profit (including NFP Corporation) **Service:** General Medical and Surgical

Staffed Beds: 108 **Admissions:** 2182 **Census:** 58 **Outpatient Visits:** 62644 **Births:** 395 **Total Expense ($000):** 63628 **Payroll Expense ($000):** 29265 **Personnel:** 470

VALDEZ—3rd Judicial Division

★ **PROVIDENCE VALDEZ MEDICAL CENTER (21301)**, 911 Meals Avenue, Zip 99686–0550, Mailing Address: P.O. Box 550, Zip 99686–0550; tel. 907/835–2249, (Total facility includes 10 beds in nursing home–type unit) **A**9 10 18 **F**1 2 3 4 5 11 13 16 17 25 26 30 31 32 33 36 37 38 39 40 52 54 55 56 57 62 63 65 66 68 70 71 73 74 75 78 79 80 83 84 85 86 88 89 90 91 92 93 94 96 102 107 117 119 122 123 **P**5
Primary Contact: Sean McCallister, Administrator
CFO: Lindsie King, Manager Finance
CMO: John Cullen, M.D., Chief of Staff and Medical Director Long Term Care
CHR: Maureen Radotich, Director Human Resources
Web address: www.providence.org/alaska
Control: City–Government, nonfederal **Service:** Long–Term Acute Care hospital

Staffed Beds: 21 **Admissions:** 217 **Census:** 13 **Outpatient Visits:** 9720 **Births:** 36 **Total Expense ($000):** 9277 **Payroll Expense ($000):** 4121 **Personnel:** 76

WRANGELL—3rd Judicial Division

★ **WRANGELL MEDICAL CENTER (21305)**, First Avenue and Bennett Street, Zip 99929, Mailing Address: P.O. Box 1081, Zip 99929; tel. 907/874–7000, (Total facility includes 4 beds in nursing home–type unit) (Nonreporting) **A**9 10 18
Primary Contact: Noel Rea, Chief Executive Officer
CFO: Olinda White, Chief Financial Officer
CIO: Cathy Gross, Director Health Information Management Systems
Web address: www.wrangellmedicalcenter.com
Control: City–Government, nonfederal **Service:** General Medical and Surgical

Staffed Beds: 22

Hospital, Medicare Provider Number, Address, Telephone, Approval, Facility, and Physician Codes, Health Care System

★ American Hospital Association (AHA) membership
□ The Joint Commission accreditation
○ American Osteopathic Association (AOA) accreditation
△ Commission on Accreditation of Rehabilitation Facilities (CARF) accreditation

AZ

ARIZONA

BENSON—Cochise County

BENSON HOSPITAL (31301), 450 South Ocotillo Street, Zip 85602, Mailing Address: P.O. Box 2290, Zip 85602; tel. 520/586–2261, (Nonreporting) **A**9 10 18
Primary Contact: Ronald A. McKinnon, Chief Executive Officer
CFO: Denise Hurtado, Chief Financial Officer
Web address: www.bensonhospital.org
Control: Hospital district or authority, Government, nonfederal **Service:** General Medical and Surgical

Staffed Beds: 22

BISBEE—Cochise County

★ **COPPER QUEEN COMMUNITY HOSPITAL (31312)**, 101 Cole Avenue, Zip 85603–1399; tel. 520/432–5383, (Nonreporting) **A**9 10 18
Primary Contact: James J. Dickson, Administrator and Chief Executive Officer
COO: Ruth Kish, Director Patient Care Service
CFO: Gregory J. Was, CPA, Chief Financial Officer
CMO: Syed Azam, M.D., Chief of Staff
CIO: David Chmura, Manager Management Information Systems
CHR: Virginia Martinez, Manager Human Resources
Web address: www.cqch.org
Control: Other not–for–profit (including NFP Corporation) **Service:** General Medical and Surgical

Staffed Beds: 13

BULLHEAD CITY—Mohave County

⊞ **WESTERN ARIZONA REGIONAL MEDICAL CENTER (30101)**, 2735 Silver Creek Road, Zip 86442–8303; tel. 928/763–2273, (Nonreporting) **A**1 9 10 19 **S** Community Health Systems, Inc.
Primary Contact: Barry S. Schneider, Chief Executive Officer
Web address: www.warmc.com
Control: Corporation, Investor–owned, for–profit **Service:** General Medical and Surgical

Staffed Beds: 139

CASA GRANDE—Pinal County

⊞ △ **CASA GRANDE REGIONAL MEDICAL CENTER (30016)**, 1800 East Florence Boulevard, Zip 85222–5399; tel. 520/381–6300, (Total facility includes 64 beds in nursing home–type unit) **A**1 7 9 10 **F**3 11 13 15 18 24 25 26 27 30 32 33 35 38 43 49 50 52 55 56 57 62 66 68 72 73 74 77 79 81 82 84 85 86 88 93 94 96 97 100 102 107 118 119 124 133 134 135 137
Primary Contact: J. Marty Dernier, President and Chief Executive Officer
CFO: Karen Francis, Chief Financial Officer
CMO: Richard Stubbs, M.D., Vice President Medical Affairs
CIO: Walter Chisenski, Manager Information Technology
CHR: Cindy Wysong–Brown, Vice President Human Resources
Web address: www.casagrandehospital.com
Control: Other not–for–profit (including NFP Corporation) **Service:** General Medical and Surgical

Staffed Beds: 265 **Admissions:** 8561 **Census:** 125 **Outpatient Visits:** 66481 **Births:** 1051 **Total Expense ($000):** 101259 **Payroll Expense ($000):** 46127 **Personnel:** 756

CHANDLER—Maricopa County

ARIZONA ORTHOPEDIC SURGICAL HOSPITAL (30112), 2905 West Warner Road, Zip 85224; tel. 480/603–9000, (Nonreporting) **A**9 10 **S** United Surgical Partners International
Primary Contact: Chris Hartshorn, Chief Executive Officer
COO: Donna Simiriglia, Chief Operating Officer
Web address: www.azosh.com
Control: Corporation, Investor–owned, for–profit **Service:** Surgical

Staffed Beds: 16

⊞ **CHANDLER REGIONAL MEDICAL CENTER (30036)**, (Formerly Chandler Regional Hospital), 475 South Dobson Road, Zip 85224–4230; tel. 480/728–3000 **A**1 9 10 **F**3 11 12 13 15 17 18 20 22 24 25 26 27 28 30 31 32 33 37 38 41 42 43 44 46 47 48 49 50 51 53 55 56 57 58 59 62 63 64 66 67 68 69 71 72 73 74 76 77 79 80 81 82 86 90 96 97 100 102 107 109 110 119 121 124 132 133 135 136 137 **P**6 **S** Catholic Healthcare West
Primary Contact: David G. Covert, President
COO: Marguerite Smith, R.N., Vice President and Chief Nursing Officer
CFO: Mark Kem, Vice President Finance and Chief Financial Officer
CMO: Terry J. Happel, M.D., Medical Director Medical Staff Affairs
CHR: Renea Brunke, Vice President Human Resources
Web address: www.chandlerregional.com
Control: Church–operated, Nongovernment, not–for profit **Service:** General Medical and Surgical

Staffed Beds: 208 **Admissions:** 19119 **Census:** 178 **Outpatient Visits:** 201138 **Births:** 4922 **Total Expense ($000):** 228951 **Payroll Expense ($000):** 89175 **Personnel:** 1579

CHINLE—Apache County

⊞ **CHINLE COMPREHENSIVE HEALTH CARE FACILITY (30084)**, Highway 191, Zip 86503, Mailing Address: P.O. Drawer PH, Zip 86503; tel. 928/674–7011, (Nonreporting) **A**1 10 **S** U. S. Indian Health Service
Primary Contact: Ronald Tso, Chief Executive Officer
CMO: Kevin Rand, M.D., Clinical Director
Web address: www.ihs.gov
Control: PHS, Indian Service, Government, federal **Service:** General Medical and Surgical

Staffed Beds: 60

COTTONWOOD—Yavapai County

★ **VERDE VALLEY MEDICAL CENTER (30007)**, 269 South Candy Lane, Zip 86326–4170; tel. 928/639–6000 **A**9 10 20 **F**3 8 13 15 17 18 20 24 25 26 30 31 32 33 38 39 41 43 45 47 48 49 50 51 53 55 56 57 59 62 66 68 72 73 74 76 77 79 80 81 82 84 86 88 93 96 97 100 102 103 107 109 111 118 119 120 121 135 137 **S** Northern Arizona Healthcare
Primary Contact: James J. Sinek, President
CFO: Gregory Kuzma, Vice President and Chief Financial Officer
CMO: Michael O'Connor, M.D., Vice President Medical Affairs
CIO: John Schofield, Chief Information Officer
CHR: Michael Young, Director Human Resources
Web address: www.nahealth.com
Control: Other not–for–profit (including NFP Corporation) **Service:** General Medical and Surgical

Staffed Beds: 110 **Admissions:** 5754 **Census:** 65 **Outpatient Visits:** 144437 **Births:** 781 **Total Expense ($000):** 105233 **Payroll Expense ($000):** 41973 **Personnel:** 702

DOUGLAS—Cochise County

SOUTHEAST ARIZONA MEDICAL CENTER (31303), 2174 Oak Avenue, Zip 85607–9801; tel. 520/364–7931, (Nonreporting) **A**9 10 18
Primary Contact: Michael J. Carter, Chief Executive Officer
COO: Annie Benson, Chief Operating Officer
CMO: Alfred Wu, M.D., Chief of Staff
CIO: Lou Gallardo, Manager Computer Services
CHR: Roberta Berry, Manager Human Resources
Web address: www.samcdouglas.org
Control: Other not–for–profit (including NFP Corporation) **Service:** General Medical and Surgical

Staffed Beds: 25

FLAGSTAFF—Coconino County

★ **FLAGSTAFF MEDICAL CENTER (30023)**, 1200 North Beaver Street, Zip 86001–3198; tel. 928/779–3366 **A**9 10 19 20 **F**3 5 7 11 12 13 15 17 18 20 22 24 25 26 27 30 31 32 33 34 38 40 43 44 49 50 51 52 55 56 57 59 60 62 66 68 70 72 73 74 75 76 77 79 80 81 82 83 84 85 86 88 89 90 91 92 93 94 95 96 97 100 102 103 104 105 106 107 108 109 111 119 120 121 124 133 134 135 136 137 **S** Northern Arizona Healthcare
Primary Contact: William T. Bradel, President
COO: William T. Bradel, President
CFO: Gregory Kuzma, Vice President and Chief Financial Officer
CMO: Steven Lewis, M.D., Vice President and Chief Medical Officer
CIO: John Schofield, Chief Information Officer
CHR: Patricia Crofford, Vice President Human Resources
Web address: www.flagstaffmedicalcenter.com
Control: Other not–for–profit (including NFP Corporation) **Service:** General Medical and Surgical

Staffed Beds: 271 **Admissions:** 12849 **Census:** 163 **Outpatient Visits:** 526176 **Births:** 1591 **Total Expense ($000):** 264647 **Payroll Expense ($000):** 99499 **Personnel:** 2247

FORT DEFIANCE—Apache County

★ **FORT DEFIANCE INDIAN HEALTH SERVICE HOSPITAL (30071)**, Mailing Address: P.O. Box 649, Zip 86504–0649; tel. 928/729–8014, (Nonreporting) **A**10 **S** U. S. Indian Health Service
Primary Contact: Franklin R. Freeland, Ed.D., Chief Executive Officer
CFO: Zondra Parker, Budget Analyst and Manager Finance
CMO: David Downing, M.D., Director Clinical and Ambulatory Care
CIO: Ida McVicker, Site Manager Information Resource Management
CHR: Doris Edwards, Human Resource Specialist
Control: PHS, Indian Service, Government, federal **Service:** General Medical and Surgical

Staffed Beds: 39

FORT MOHAVE—Mohave County

★ **VALLEY VIEW MEDICAL CENTER (30117)**, 5330 South Highway 95, Zip 86426; tel. 928/788–2273 **A**9 10 **F**13 18 20 25 30 31 32 38 68 74 75 79 85 86 96 97 99 100 102 106 107 **P**4 5 **S** LifePoint Hospitals, Inc.
Primary Contact: Jim Matney, Chief Executive Officer
Web address: www.valleyviewmedicalcenter.net
Control: Corporation, Investor–owned, for–profit **Service:** General Medical and Surgical

Staffed Beds: 60 **Admissions:** 3445 **Census:** 39 **Outpatient Visits:** 25588 **Births:** 572 **Total Expense ($000):** 36749 **Payroll Expense ($000):** 13489 **Personnel:** 264

GANADO—Apache County

☐ **SAGE MEMORIAL HOSPITAL (31309)**, Highway 264, Zip 86505, Mailing Address: P.O. Box 457, Zip 86505–0457; tel. 928/755–4500, (Nonreporting) **A**1 9 10 18
Primary Contact: Ahmad Razaghi, Chief Executive Officer
COO: Perphelia Fowler, Operational Director
CFO: Charity L. Askie, Director Finance
CMO: Edmond K. Safarian, M.D., Chief of Staff
CIO: Wayne White, Director Computer Services
CHR: Clarence Chee, Manager Human Resources
Web address: www.navajosage.org
Control: Other not–for–profit (including NFP Corporation) **Service:** General Medical and Surgical

Staffed Beds: 25

GILBERT—Maricopa County

★ **BANNER GATEWAY MEDICAL CENTER (30122)**, 1900 North Higley Road, Zip 85234; tel. 480/543–2000 **A**10 **F**3 8 12 13 19 25 26 27 30 32 38 46 47 48 49 50 53 55 56 57 59 62 66 68 71 72 73 74 75 76 77 79 80 81 82 84 96 97 98 100 101 102 107 119 135 137 **P**6 8 **S** Banner Health
Primary Contact: Rebecca C. Kuhn, Chief Executive Officer
Web address: www.bannerhealth.com
Control: Other not–for–profit (including NFP Corporation) **Service:** General Medical and Surgical

Staffed Beds: 176 **Admissions:** 2436 **Census:** 65 **Outpatient Visits:** 20076 **Births:** 686 **Total Expense ($000):** 44313 **Payroll Expense ($000):** 17715 **Personnel:** 867

GILBERT HOSPITAL (30120), 5656 South Power Road, Zip 85295; tel. 480/984–2000, (Nonreporting) **A**10
Primary Contact: David S. Wanger, Chief Executive Officer
CFO: Randy Calvert, Chief Financial Officer
CMO: Timothy Johns, M.D., Medical Director
Web address: www.gilberter.com
Control: Other not–for–profit (including NFP Corporation) **Service:** General Medical and Surgical

Staffed Beds: 8

★☐ **MERCY GILBERT MEDICAL CENTER (30119)**, 3555 South Val Vista Road, Zip 85296; tel. 480/728–8000 **A**1 9 10 **F**3 11 12 13 15 18 25 26 28 30 31 32 33 37 38 41 42 43 44 49 50 55 56 57 58 59 63 66 68 71 72 73 74 77 79 80 81 82 96 100 103 107 119 121 133 135 **S** Catholic Healthcare West
Primary Contact: Laurie Eberst, RN, President and Chief Executive Officer
CFO: Mark Kem, Vice President Finance and Chief Financial Officer
CMO: Terry J. Happel, M.D., Vice President and Chief Medical Officer
CIO: Bob Campbell, Vice President Business Development and Chief Strategy Officer
CHR: Renea Brunke, Vice President Human Resources
Web address: www.mercygilbert.org
Control: Church–operated, Nongovernment, not–for profit **Service:** General Medical and Surgical

Staffed Beds: 92 **Admissions:** 7413 **Census:** 69 **Outpatient Visits:** 42358 **Births:** 1554 **Total Expense ($000):** 95811 **Payroll Expense ($000):** 34377 **Personnel:** 592

GLENDALE—Maricopa County

☐ **ARROWHEAD HOSPITAL (30094)**, 18701 North 67th Avenue, Zip 85308–5722; tel. 623/561–1000, (Nonreporting) **A**1 9 10 **S** Vanguard Health System
Primary Contact: Jonathan W. Bartlett, Chief Executive Officer
COO: Edna Nicely, Vice President
Web address: www.arrowheadhospital.com
Control: Corporation, Investor–owned, for–profit **Service:** General Medical and Surgical

Staffed Beds: 155

AURORA BEHAVIORAL HEALTH SYSTEM–GLENDALE (34024), 6015 West Peoria Avenue, Zip 85302–1201; tel. 623/344–4400, (Nonreporting) **A**9 10 **S** Aurora Behavioral Health Care
Primary Contact: Jane Blum, Interim Chief Executive Officer
COO: Jane Blum, Chief Operating Officer
CFO: Glenn Pelkey, Chief Financial Officer
CMO: Gerald Shaw, M.D., Chief Medical Officer
Web address: www.aurorabehavioral.com
Control: Corporation, Investor–owned, for–profit **Service:** Psychiatric

Staffed Beds: 90

★☐ **BANNER THUNDERBIRD MEDICAL CENTER (30089)**, 5555 West Thunderbird Road, Zip 85306–4696; tel. 602/865–5555, (Includes BANNER BEHAVIORAL HEALTH CENTER–THUNDERBIRD CAMPUS) **A**1 9 10 **F**3 5 13 15 17 18 20 22 24 25 26 27 31 32 33 34 36 38 43 46 47 49 51 55 56 57 58 59 62 65 66 68 70 72 73 74 75 76 77 79 80 81 82 84 86 88 89 92 93 94 96 97 98 99 100 102 103 105 107 108 109 111 114 116 118 119 121 123 124 132 135 136 137 **S** Banner Health
Primary Contact: Thomas C. Dickson, Chief Executive Officer
CFO: Richard Miller, Administrator Finance
CMO: Kathryn Perkins, M.D., Chief Medical Officer
CHR: Laura Witt, Administrator Human Resources
Web address: www.bannerhealth.com
Control: Other not–for–profit (including NFP Corporation) **Service:** General Medical and Surgical

Staffed Beds: 376 **Admissions:** 29189 **Census:** 324 **Outpatient Visits:** 256950 **Births:** 4821 **Total Expense ($000):** 293665 **Payroll Expense ($000):** 125854 **Personnel:** 2226

★☐ **HEALTHSOUTH VALLEY OF THE SUN REHABILITATION HOSPITAL (33032)**, 13460 North 67th Avenue, Zip 85304–1042; tel. 623/878–8800, (Nonreporting) **A**1 9 10 **S** HEALTHSOUTH Corporation
Primary Contact: Beth Bacher, Chief Executive Officer
CMO: Michael Kravetz, M.D., Medical Director
CHR: Robert Rosene, Regional Director Human Resources
Web address: www.healthsouth.com
Control: Corporation, Investor–owned, for–profit **Service:** Rehabilitation

Staffed Beds: 60

GLOBE—Gila County

★ **COBRE VALLEY COMMUNITY HOSPITAL (31314)**, 5880 South Hospital Drive, Zip 85501–9454; tel. 928/425–3261 **A**9 10 18 **F**3 11 13 15 25 26 27 30 31 32 33 38 40 54 55 56 62 68 72 73 74 76 77 79 82 86 96 97 100 106 107 119 122 124 135 **P**5 **S** Brim Healthcare, Inc.
Primary Contact: Neal Jensen, Chief Executive Officer
CIO: Sharon Bennett, Manager Information Systems
CHR: Rita Murphy, Manager Human Resources
Web address: www.cvchospital.com
Control: Other not–for–profit (including NFP Corporation) **Service:** General Medical and Surgical

Staffed Beds: 25 **Admissions:** 1367 **Census:** 12 **Outpatient Visits:** 215195 **Births:** 320 **Total Expense ($000):** 26177 **Payroll Expense ($000):** 10135 **Personnel:** 200

GOODYEAR—Maricopa County

☐ **WEST VALLEY HOSPITAL (30110)**, 13677 West McDowell Road, Zip 85338; tel. 623/882–1500, (Nonreporting) **A**1 9 10 **S** Vanguard Health System
Primary Contact: Thomas W. Keller, Chief Executive Officer
CFO: Richard Franco, Chief Financial Officer
CMO: Ron Kenneth, M.D., Chief Medical Officer
CHR: Debbie Rosenburg, Director Human Resources
Web address: www.wvhospital.com
Control: Corporation, Investor–owned, for–profit **Service:** General Medical and Surgical

Staffed Beds: 106

Hospital, Medicare Provider Number, Address, Telephone, Approval, Facility, and Physician Codes, Health Care System

★ American Hospital Association (AHA) membership
☐ The Joint Commission accreditation
○ American Osteopathic Association (AOA) accreditation
△ Commission on Accreditation of Rehabilitation Facilities (CARF) accreditation

AZ

KEAMS CANYON—Navajo County

★ **HOPI HEALTH CARE CENTER (31305)**, Mailing Address: P.O. Box 4000, Polacca, Zip 86042; tel. 928/737–6000, (Nonreporting) **A**1 10 18 **S** U. S. Indian Health Service
Primary Contact: Daryl Melvin, Chief Executive Officer
CFO: Thelma Tewahaftewa, Finance Officer
CMO: Darren Vicenti, M.D., Clinical Director
CIO: Adrian Tom, Management Information Systems Supervisor
Web address: www.ihs.gov/index.asp
Control: PHS, Indian Service, Government, federal **Service:** General Medical and Surgical

Staffed Beds: 15

KINGMAN—Mohave County

★ **KINGMAN REGIONAL MEDICAL CENTER (30055)**, 3269 Stockton Hill Road, Zip 86409–3691; tel. 928/757–2101 **A**1 9 10 12 13 20 **F**3 11 13 15 17 18 20 24 25 26 27 30 31 32 33 38 40 42 43 52 55 56 57 59 61 62 68 73 74 75 76 77 79 80 81 82 84 85 86 87 96 97 100 102 106 107 111 118 119 121 124 135 136 **P**6 7
Primary Contact: Brian Turney, Chief Executive Officer
COO: Craig A. Owens, Chief Operating Officer
CFO: Lawrence E. Lewis, Chief Financial Officer
CMO: Joseph Smith, M.D., Chief Medical Officer
CIO: Shawn Burgess, Director Information Systems
CHR: Heather Crowl, Executive Director Human Resources
Web address: www.azkrmc.com
Control: Other not–for–profit (including NFP Corporation) **Service:** General Medical and Surgical

Staffed Beds: 150 **Admissions:** 8751 **Census:** 100 **Outpatient Visits:** 193808 **Births:** 759 **Total Expense ($000):** 134953 **Payroll Expense ($000):** 51461 **Personnel:** 1116

LAKE HAVASU CITY—Mohave County

★ **HAVASU REGIONAL MEDICAL CENTER (30069)**, 101 Civic Center Lane, Zip 86403–5683; tel. 928/855–8185, (Nonreporting) **A**1 9 10 19 20 **S** LifePoint Hospitals, Inc.
Primary Contact: Ruth A. McDaniel, Interim Chief Executive Officer
COO: Jim Geist, Chief Operating Officer
CFO: Craig M. Wagner, Chief Financial Officer
CMO: Fred Scott, Chief Medical Officer
CIO: Linda Toy, Director Information Systems
CHR: Sheena Benson, Director Human Resources
Web address: www.havasuregional.com
Control: Corporation, Investor–owned, for–profit **Service:** General Medical and Surgical

Staffed Beds: 138

MESA—Maricopa County

☐ **ARIZONA SPINE AND JOINT HOSPITAL (30107)**, 4620 East Baseline Road, Zip 85206; tel. 480/832–4770, (Nonreporting) **A**1 10 **S** National Surgical Hospitals
Primary Contact: Peggy Wellman, Acting Chief Executive Officer
CFO: Brian Ebright, Chief Financial Officer
CHR: Lisa Garrett, Director Human Resources
Web address: www.azspineandjoint.com
Control: Corporation, Investor–owned, for–profit **Service:** Orthopedic

Staffed Beds: 23

★ **BANNER BAYWOOD MEDICAL CENTER (30088)**, 6644 East Baywood Avenue, Zip 85206–1797; tel. 480/321–2000 **A**1 9 10 **F**3 11 13 15 25 26 27 30 31 32 34 35 38 43 46 49 51 53 54 55 56 57 59 60 62 66 68 72 73 74 75 76 77 79 80 81 82 85 86 90 92 94 96 97 100 102 103 104 105 107 118 119 121 124 135 136 137 **P**8 **S** Banner Health
Primary Contact: Don A. Evans, FACHE, Chief Executive Officer
CFO: Sam Patterson, Chief Financial Officer
CMO: Larry Spratling, M.D., Chief Medical Officer
CIO: Michael S. Warden, Senior Vice President Information Technology
CHR: Tom Koelbl, Chief Human Resources Officer
Web address: www.bannerhealth.com
Control: Other not–for–profit (including NFP Corporation) **Service:** General Medical and Surgical

Staffed Beds: 340 **Admissions:** 20621 **Census:** 236 **Outpatient Visits:** 267715 **Births:** 2513 **Total Expense ($000):** 229486 **Payroll Expense ($000):** 98652 **Personnel:** 1837

★ **BANNER DESERT MEDICAL CENTER (30065)**, 1400 South Dobson Road, Zip 85202–9879; tel. 480/512–3000, (Includes SAMARITAN BEHAVIORAL HEALTH CENTER–DESERT SAMARITAN MEDICAL CENTER, 2225 West Southern Avenue, Zip 85202; tel. 602/464–4000) **A**1 9 10 **F**3 5 11 13 15 16 17 18 20 22 24 25 26 27 28 31 32 33 36 38 41 43 44 46 47 48 49 51 55 57 59 60 62 65 66 68 70 71 72 73 74 75 76 77 79 80 81 82 83 84 86 88 96 97 98 100 102 104 105 107 109 110 111 116 118 119 121 132 133 135 136 137 **S** Banner Health
Primary Contact: Todd S. Werner, Chief Executive Officer
CFO: Lori Linder, Chief Financial Officer
CMO: David Edwards, M.D., Chief Medical Officer
CIO: Les Licklider, Manager Information Technology Account
CHR: Joe Abdai, Interim Chief Human Resources Officer
Web address: www.bannerhealth.com
Control: Other not–for–profit (including NFP Corporation) **Service:** General Medical and Surgical

Staffed Beds: 518 **Admissions:** 41542 **Census:** 417 **Outpatient Visits:** 133208 **Births:** 7552 **Total Expense ($000):** 411041 **Payroll Expense ($000):** 179148 **Personnel:** 2932

★ **BANNER HEART HOSPITAL (30105)**, (Formerly Banner Baywood Heart Hospital), 6750 East Baywood Avenue, Zip 85206; tel. 480/854–5000 **A**1 9 10 **F**3 17 18 20 22 24 25 26 30 31 32 34 52 65 66 73 79 86 106 107 116 118 119 121 124 135 137 **P**8 **S** Banner Health
Primary Contact: John L. Harrington, Jr., FACHE, Chief Executive Officer
CFO: Dave Kaubisch, Chief Financial Officer
CMO: Mark Starling, M.D., Chief Medical Officer
CIO: Michael S. Warden, Senior Vice President and Chief Information Officer
CHR: Tom Koelbl, Chief People Resources Officer
Web address: www.bannerhealth.com
Control: Other not–for–profit (including NFP Corporation) **Service:** General Medical and Surgical

Staffed Beds: 111 **Admissions:** 6592 **Census:** 64 **Outpatient Visits:** 33069 **Births:** 0 **Total Expense ($000):** 97545 **Payroll Expense ($000):** 29558 **Personnel:** 463

SAMARITAN BEHAVIORAL HEALTH CENTER–DESERT SAMARITAN MEDICAL CENTER See Banner Desert Medical Center

NOGALES—Santa Cruz County

★ **CARONDELET HOLY CROSS HOSPITAL (31313)**, 1171 West Target Range Road, Zip 85621–2496; tel. 520/285–3000, (Total facility includes 49 beds in nursing home–type unit) **A**1 9 10 18 **F**11 13 25 26 28 30 31 32 33 38 42 44 50 51 54 55 57 59 62 66 68 73 74 75 79 81 82 84 86 92 96 100 107 117 119 121 122 123 124 135 **S** Ascension Health
Primary Contact: Richard Polheber, Chief Executive Officer
COO: Wesley E. Colvin, Chief Operating Officer
CFO: Tom Pepping, Chief Financial Officer
CMO: Guy Crawford, M.D., Chief of Staff
CIO: John Braswell, Chief Information Officer
CHR: Linda Werbylo, Vice President Human Resources
Web address: www.carondelet.org
Control: Church–operated, Nongovernment, not–for profit **Service:** General Medical and Surgical

Staffed Beds: 72 **Admissions:** 1886 **Census:** 55 **Outpatient Visits:** 38862 **Births:** 854 **Total Expense ($000):** 22017 **Payroll Expense ($000):** 11102 **Personnel:** 231

ORO VALLEY—Pima County

★ **NORTHWEST MEDICAL CENTER, ORO VALLEY (30114)**, 1551 East Tangerine Road, Zip 85737; tel. 520/901–3500 **A**1 9 10 **F**3 15 18 24 25 26 27 34 35 36 38 43 46 47 48 49 53 55 56 57 62 63 66 68 72 73 75 76 77 79 85 86 96 100 102 103 107 119 134 135 **S** Community Health Systems, Inc.
Primary Contact: Shawn G. Strash, Chief Executive Officer
CFO: Mark Hoffman, Chief Financial Officer
CMO: Paul Bejarino, M.D., Chief of Staff
Web address: www.nmcorovalley.com
Control: Corporation, Investor–owned, for–profit **Service:** General Medical and Surgical

Staffed Beds: 70 **Admissions:** 4749 **Census:** 52 **Outpatient Visits:** 81613 **Births:** 0 **Total Expense ($000):** 76424 **Payroll Expense ($000):** 24420

PAGE—Coconino County

★ **PAGE HOSPITAL (31304)**, 501 North Navajo Drive, Zip 86040, Mailing Address: P.O. Box 1447, Zip 86040–1447; tel. 928/645–2424 **A**1 9 10 18 **F**3 8 11 13 15 25 26 27 31 32 33 34 37 38 40 43 55 56 57 62 66 73 74 75 77 79 80 81 82 86 96 100 102 107 119 122 124 135 137 **S** Banner Health
Primary Contact: Sandy Haryasz, RN, Chief Executive Officer
Web address: www.bannerhealth.com
Control: Other not–for–profit (including NFP Corporation) **Service:** General Medical and Surgical

Staffed Beds: 25 **Admissions:** 614 **Census:** 4 **Outpatient Visits:** 25119 **Births:** 247 **Total Expense ($000):** 12881 **Payroll Expense ($000):** 6228 **Personnel:** 116

 Many Facility Codes have changed. Please refer to the AHA Guide Code Chart.

PARKER—La Paz County

○ **LA PAZ REGIONAL HOSPITAL (30067)**, 1200 West Mohave Road, Zip 85344–6349; tel. 928/669–9201 **A**9 10 11 20 **F**3 11 15 25 26 27 31 32 38 55 56 57 62 64 66 68 77 79 80 82 86 87 96 99 103 107 119 135
Primary Contact: M. Victoria Clark, Chief Executive Officer
CFO: Dennis Good, Chief Financial Officer
CMO: Edward Fuller, M.D., Chief of Staff
CHR: Regina Martinez, Director Human Resources
Web address: www.lapazhospital.org
Control: Other not–for–profit (including NFP Corporation) **Service:** General Medical and Surgical

Staffed Beds: 39 **Admissions:** 1071 **Census:** 10 **Outpatient Visits:** 23136 **Births:** 0 **Total Expense ($000):** 13381 **Payroll Expense ($000):** 6128 **Personnel:** 150

★□ **U. S. PUBLIC HEALTH SERVICE INDIAN HOSPITAL (31307)**, Mailing Address: Route 1, Box 12, Zip 85344; tel. 928/669–2137, (Nonreporting) **A**1 10 18 **S** U. S. Indian Health Service
Primary Contact: Timothy Taylor, Chief Executive Officer
CMO: Clare Helminiak, Clinical Director
CIO: Carol Otter, Chief Information Officer
Web address: www.ihs.gov
Control: Public Health Service, Government, federal **Service:** General Medical and Surgical

Staffed Beds: 20

PAYSON—Gila County

★□ **PAYSON REGIONAL MEDICAL CENTER (30033)**, 807 South Ponderosa Street, Zip 85541–5599; tel. 928/474–3222, (Nonreporting) **A**1 9 10 20 **S** Community Health Systems, Inc.
Primary Contact: R. Chris Wolf, Chief Executive Officer
CFO: Peter Finelli, Chief Financial Officer
CHR: David Coombes, Director Human Resources
Web address: www.paysonhospital.com
Control: Corporation, Investor–owned, for–profit **Service:** General Medical and Surgical

Staffed Beds: 44

PHOENIX—Maricopa County

□ **ARIZONA HEART HOSPITAL (30102)**, 1930 East Thomas Road, Zip 85016; tel. 602/532–1000, (Nonreporting) **A**1 9 10 **S** MedCath, Inc.
Primary Contact: James R. Resendez, Chief Executive Officer
CFO: Thomas Heywood, Vice President Finance
CMO: Edward B. Diethrich, M.D., Medical Director
Web address: www.azheart.com
Control: Partnership, Investor–owned, for–profit **Service:** Heart

Staffed Beds: 59

□ **ARIZONA STATE HOSPITAL (34021)**, 2500 East Van Buren Street, Zip 85008–6079; tel. 602/244–1331 **A**1 10 **F**26 32 37 52 57 60 66 82 88 89 91 93 119 124 132
Primary Contact: John C. Cooper, Chief Executive Officer
COO: Donna Noriega, Chief Operating Officer
CFO: Donna Noriega, Chief Operating Officer
CMO: Michael Stumpf, M.D., Chief Medical Officer
CIO: Rosleen Reynolds, Chief Quality Officer
CHR: Dennis Morgan, Director Human Resources
Web address: www.hs.state.az.us
Control: State–Government, nonfederal **Service:** Psychiatric

Staffed Beds: 338 **Admissions:** 296 **Census:** 264 **Outpatient Visits:** 0 **Births:** 0 **Total Expense ($000):** 56200 **Payroll Expense ($000):** 30565 **Personnel:** 617

★□ **BANNER ESTRELLA MEDICAL CENTER (30115)**, 9201 West Thomas Road, Zip 85037–3332; tel. 623/327–4000 **A**1 9 10 **F**3 17 18 20 22 24 25 26 27 31 32 38 46 49 66 68 71 74 76 77 79 80 96 97 100 102 103 106 107 119 135 137 **S** Banner Health
Primary Contact: Kathy Bollinger, Chief Executive Officer
CFO: Gregory Wojtal, Chief Financial Officer
CMO: Charlie M. Agee, M.D., Chief Medical Officer
CHR: Dina Steinberg, Chief People Resources Officer
Web address: www.bannerhealth.com
Control: Other not–for–profit (including NFP Corporation) **Service:** General Medical and Surgical

Staffed Beds: 172 **Admissions:** 13616 **Census:** 139 **Outpatient Visits:** 130082 **Births:** 2722 **Total Expense ($000):** 157983 **Payroll Expense ($000):** 62140 **Personnel:** 1072

★□ **BANNER GOOD SAMARITAN MEDICAL CENTER (30002)**, 1111 East McDowell Road, Zip 85006–2666, Mailing Address: P.O. Box 2989, Zip 85062–2989; tel. 602/239–2000 **A**1 2 3 5 8 9 10 **F**3 8 11 12 13 15 17 18 20 22 24 25 26 27 30 31 32 33 34 38 40 41 43 44 46 56 58 59 62 64 66 68 72 73 75 76 77 79 81 85 86 87 88 89 90 91 92 93 94 95 96 97 100 101 102 103 104 105 106 107 108 109 111 112 116 119 127 128 129 130 131 134 135 136 137 **S** Banner Health
Primary Contact: Larry E. Volkmar, Chief Executive Officer
CFO: Kathy Kotin, Chief Financial Officer
CMO: Paul Stander, M.D., Chief Medical Officer
CIO: Michael S. Warden, Senior Vice President Information Technology
CHR: Michael Fleming, Chief People Officer
Web address: www.bannerhealth.com
Control: Other not–for–profit (including NFP Corporation) **Service:** General Medical and Surgical

Staffed Beds: 601 **Admissions:** 37428 **Census:** 509 **Outpatient Visits:** 306986 **Births:** 6878 **Total Expense ($000):** 561194 **Payroll Expense ($000):** 237679 **Personnel:** 3706

CARL T. HAYDEN VETERANS AFFAIRS MEDICAL CENTER See Phoenix Veterans Affairs Health Care System

★ ○ **JOHN C. LINCOLN DEER VALLEY HOSPITAL (30092)**, 19829 North 27th Avenue, Zip 85027–4002; tel. 623/879–6100 **A**9 10 11 13 **F**3 11 15 17 18 20 22 24 25 26 27 30 31 32 33 35 38 46 49 50 55 56 59 62 66 68 72 73 75 76 77 79 80 84 85 96 97 100 102 106 107 119 121 135 137 **P**8 **S** John C. Lincoln Health Network
Primary Contact: Tim Tracy, Chief Executive Officer
CFO: David Lamparter, Chief Financial Officer
CIO: Robert Israel, Vice President and Chief Information Officer
CHR: Dale Spartz, Vice President Human Resources
Web address: www.jcl.com
Control: Other not–for–profit (including NFP Corporation) **Service:** General Medical and Surgical

Staffed Beds: 174 **Admissions:** 11167 **Census:** 119 **Outpatient Visits:** 95926 **Births:** 0 **Total Expense ($000):** 159352 **Payroll Expense ($000):** 66266 **Personnel:** 1208

★ **JOHN C. LINCOLN NORTH MOUNTAIN HOSPITAL (30014)**, 250 East Dunlap Avenue, Zip 85020–2446; tel. 602/943–2381 **A**9 10 12 **F**3 11 13 15 17 18 20 22 24 25 26 27 30 31 32 33 38 40 46 49 50 52 55 57 58 59 62 66 68 71 72 73 74 75 76 77 79 80 85 96 97 100 101 102 106 107 119 121 124 135 137 **P**8 **S** John C. Lincoln Health Network
Primary Contact: Bruce E. Pearson, Chief Executive Officer
COO: Rhonda Forsyth, Chief Executive Officer
CFO: David Lamparter, Senior Vice President and Chief Financial Officer
CMO: Lawrence Gassner, M.D., Chief of Staff
CIO: Robert Israel, Vice President and Chief Information Officer
CHR: Dale Spartz, Vice President Human Resources
Web address: www.jcl.com
Control: Other not–for–profit (including NFP Corporation) **Service:** General Medical and Surgical

Staffed Beds: 266 **Admissions:** 16822 **Census:** 188 **Outpatient Visits:** 71050 **Births:** 1701 **Total Expense ($000):** 221754 **Payroll Expense ($000):** 85826 **Personnel:** 2009

□ **KINDRED HOSPITAL ARIZONA – PHOENIX (32000)**, 40 East Indianola Avenue, Zip 85012–2059; tel. 602/280–7000, (Nonreporting) **A**1 10 **S** Kindred Healthcare
Primary Contact: Scott Floden, Chief Executive Officer
Web address: www.kindredhealthcare.com
Control: Corporation, Investor–owned, for–profit **Service:** Long–Term Acute Care hospital

Staffed Beds: 58

LOS NINOS HOSPITAL (33301), 2303 East Thomas Road, Zip 85016; tel. 602/954–7311, (Nonreporting) **A**9 10
Primary Contact: William Timmons, Chief Executive Officer
Web address: www.losninoshospital.com
Control: Other not–for–profit (including NFP Corporation) **Service:** Other specialty

Staffed Beds: 15

Hospital, Medicare Provider Number, Address, Telephone, Approval, Facility, and Physician Codes, Health Care System

★ American Hospital Association (AHA) membership
□ The Joint Commission accreditation
○ American Osteopathic Association (AOA) accreditation
△ Commission on Accreditation of Rehabilitation Facilities (CARF) accreditation

★ **MARICOPA INTEGRATED HEALTH SYSTEM (30022)**, 2601 East Roosevelt Street, Zip 85008–4956; tel. 602/344–5011 **A**1 3 5 8 9 10 **F**3 8 13 15 16 17 20 21 24 25 26 27 28 30 31 32 33 34 37 38 40 51 52 53 55 57 59 60 61 62 64 66 67 68 70 71 72 73 74 75 76 77 78 79 80 82 83 84 86 87 88 89 90 93 94 96 97 98 99 100 102 106 107 112 113 114 119 124 135 136 137 **P**1
Primary Contact: Betsey Bayless, President and Chief Executive Officer
COO: William F. Vanaskie, CHE, Chief Operating Officer
CFO: Kenneth Meinke, Chief Financial Officer
CMO: David Wisinger, M.D., Interim Vice President Medical Affairs and Chief Medical Officer
CIO: Dave Kempson, Chief Information Officer
CHR: Marshall Jones, Vice President Administrative Services
Web address: www.maricopa.gov/medcenter/mmc.html
Control: Hospital district or authority, Government, nonfederal **Service:** General Medical and Surgical

Staffed Beds: 542 **Admissions:** 17374 **Census:** 421 **Outpatient Visits:** 323370 **Births:** 4598 **Personnel:** 3213

☐ **MARYVALE HOSPITAL MEDICAL CENTER (30001)**, 5102 West Campbell Avenue, Zip 85031–1799; tel. 623/848–5000 **A**1 9 10 **F**18 20 25 26 32 33 38 43 57 66 68 71 73 74 75 77 79 80 96 100 102 107 119 135 **S** Vanguard Health System
Primary Contact: Jeff R. Egbert, Chief Executive Officer
COO: Crystal Hamilton, R.N., Chief Operating Officer and Chief Nursing Officer
CFO: Richard Franco, Chief Financial Officer
CHR: JoAnne Mengelkamp, Director Human Resources and Education
Web address: www.maryvalehospital.com
Control: Corporation, Investor–owned, for–profit **Service:** General Medical and Surgical

Staffed Beds: 226 **Admissions:** 10039 **Census:** 93 **Outpatient Visits:** 77953 **Births:** 3681 **Personnel:** 456

★ **MAYO CLINIC HOSPITAL (30103)**, 5777 East Mayo Boulevard, Zip 85054–4502; tel. 480/515–6296 **A**1 3 5 9 10 **F**3 8 12 15 18 20 22 25 26 27 32 38 43 44 46 47 48 49 51 58 59 62 66 68 72 73 75 76 77 79 80 82 85 86 96 97 100 103 106 107 108 109 111 112 116 118 119 121 124 125 126 127 128 130 131 134 135 136 137 **P**6 **S** Mayo Foundation
Primary Contact: Thomas C. Bour, Administrator
CFO: Jeffrey R. Froisland, Chief Financial Officer
CMO: Jeff T. Mueller, M.D., Medical Director
CIO: Amy Z. Vrabel, Division Information Technologist
Web address: www.mayoclinic.org
Control: Other not–for–profit (including NFP Corporation) **Service:** General Medical and Surgical

Staffed Beds: 217 **Admissions:** 13527 **Census:** 169 **Outpatient Visits:** 31630 **Births:** 0 **Total Expense ($000):** 279561 **Payroll Expense ($000):** 80704 **Personnel:** 3045

☐ **PARADISE VALLEY HOSPITAL (30083)**, 3929 East Bell Road, Zip 85032–2196; tel. 602/923–5000, (Nonreporting) **A**1 9 10 **S** Vanguard Health System
Primary Contact: Steve Sisto, Chief Executive Officer
CFO: Denise Chamberlain, Chief Financial Officer
CMO: Stephen Finberg, D.O., Chief of Staff
CHR: Michelle Wilkerson, Director Human Resources
Web address: www.paradisevalleyhospital.com
Control: Corporation, Investor–owned, for–profit **Service:** General Medical and Surgical

Staffed Beds: 142

★ **PHOENIX BAPTIST HOSPITAL (30030)**, 2000 West Bethany Home Road, Zip 85015–2110; tel. 602/249–0212 **A**1 3 5 9 10 **F**8 13 15 17 18 20 22 24 25 32 38 47 48 49 68 71 72 74 75 77 79 80 87 96 97 99 100 103 107 119 124 135 136 137 **S** Vanguard Health System
Primary Contact: Bruce F. Buchanan, FACHE, Chief Executive Officer
CFO: Julie Hastings–Smith, Interim Chief Financial Officer
CMO: James F. Wessman, M.D., Director Medical Affairs
CHR: Julia Doucette, Director Human Resources
Web address: www.phoenixbaptisthospital.com
Control: Corporation, Investor–owned, for–profit **Service:** General Medical and Surgical

Staffed Beds: 215 **Admissions:** 9663 **Census:** 94 **Outpatient Visits:** 89389 **Births:** 3891 **Total Expense ($000):** 105054 **Payroll Expense ($000):** 45851 **Personnel:** 838

★ **PHOENIX CHILDREN'S HOSPITAL (33302)**, 1919 East Thomas Road, Zip 85016; tel. 602/546–1000 **A**1 3 5 8 9 10 **F**3 8 11 19 21 23 25 26 27 28 31 32 33 36 38 41 43 50 53 55 56 57 58 59 60 62 63 64 66 69 70 71 72 73 75 76 77 79 81 82 83 84 86 87 88 89 90 91 92 94 96 97 100 102 104 105 106 107 114 119 121 123 125 127 133 135 137 **P**6
Primary Contact: Robert L. Meyer, President and Chief Executive Officer
CFO: Larry J. Smith, Chief Financial Officer
CMO: Murray Pollack, M.D., Vice President Chief Medical Officer
CIO: Bob Sarnecki, Chief Information Officer
CHR: Thomas Diederich, Vice President Human Resources
Web address: www.phoenixchildrens.com
Control: Other not–for–profit (including NFP Corporation) **Service:** Children's general

Staffed Beds: 294 **Admissions:** 11996 **Census:** 238 **Outpatient Visits:** 163019 **Births:** 0 **Total Expense ($000):** 330686 **Payroll Expense ($000):** 158678 **Personnel:** 2193

★ △ **PHOENIX VETERANS AFFAIRS HEALTH CARE SYSTEM**, (Formerly Carl T. Hayden Veterans Affairs Medical Center), 650 East Indian School Road, Zip 85012–1892; tel. 602/277–5551, (Total facility includes 104 beds in nursing home–type unit) **A**1 2 3 5 7 9 **F**1 3 4 5 8 16 17 18 24 25 26 27 29 30 32 33 35 36 37 38 41 42 43 44 46 50 51 53 54 55 56 57 59 60 61 62 63 65 66 68 70 71 72 73 74 75 76 77 78 79 80 81 82 83 84 85 86 87 88 90 92 93 94 96 102 106 107 117 118 119 121 124 132 133 134 135 136 137 **S** Department of Veterans Affairs
Primary Contact: Donald F. Moore, Medical Center Director
COO: Donald F. Moore, Medical Center Director
CFO: Christine Hollingsworth, Chief Financial Officer
CMO: Raymond Chung, M.D., Chief of Staff
CHR: Melody Mikutowski, Human Resources Officer
Web address: www.phoenix.med.va.gov
Control: Veterans Affairs, Government, federal **Service:** General Medical and Surgical

Staffed Beds: 177 **Admissions:** 7082 **Census:** 112 **Outpatient Visits:** 626237 **Births:** 0 **Total Expense ($000):** 311432 **Personnel:** 2116

PROMISE HOSPITAL OF PHOENIX (30109), (Formerly Promise Specialty Hospital of Phoenix), 1800 East Van Buren Street, 2nd Floor, Zip 85007; tel. 602/716–5000 **A**9 10 **F**1 3 25 73 **P**5 **S** Promise Healthcare
Primary Contact: Kevin Nicholson, Chief Executive Officer
Web address: www.promise–phoenix.com
Control: Corporation, Investor–owned, for–profit **Service:** Long–Term Acute Care hospital

Staffed Beds: 40 **Admissions:** 201 **Census:** 20 **Outpatient Visits:** 0 **Births:** 0 **Total Expense ($000):** 11637 **Payroll Expense ($000):** 308 **Personnel:** 79

★ **SELECT SPECIALTY HOSPITAL – PHOENIX (32001)**, 350 West Thomas Road, Zip 85013; tel. 602/406–6800, (Nonreporting) **A**1 9 10 **S** Select Medical Corporation
Primary Contact: Beth Liguori, Chief Executive Officer
Web address: www.selectmedicalcorp.com
Control: Corporation, Investor–owned, for–profit **Service:** Long–Term Acute Care hospital

Staffed Beds: 48

☐ **SELECT SPECIALTY HOSPITAL–PHOENIX DOWNTOWN**, 1012 East Willetta Street, 4th Floor, Zip 85006; tel. 602/239–6134, (Nonreporting) **A**1 9 **S** Select Medical Corporation
Primary Contact: Sharon Anthony, Chief Executive Officer
Web address: www.selectmedicalcorp.com
Control: Corporation, Investor–owned, for–profit **Service:** Long–Term Acute Care hospital

Staffed Beds: 33

★ △ **ST. JOSEPH'S HOSPITAL AND MEDICAL CENTER (30024)**, 350 West Thomas Road, Zip 85013–4496, Mailing Address: P.O. Box 2071, Zip 85001–2071; tel. 602/406–3000 **A**1 2 3 5 7 8 9 10 **F**3 6 8 10 11 13 15 17 18 19 20 21 22 23 24 25 26 27 28 30 31 32 33 36 37 38 40 41 43 44 46 47 49 50 51 53 54 55 56 57 58 59 60 62 63 64 66 68 69 70 71 72 73 74 75 76 77 80 81 82 83 84 85 86 87 89 90 92 96 97 99 100 101 102 103 106 107 108 109 111 112 114 116 119 121 123 124 129 130 132 135 136 137 **P**5 6 **S** Catholic Healthcare West
Primary Contact: Linda A. Hunt, President
COO: Patricia White, R.N., MS, Chief Operating Officer
CFO: Larry McManus, Chief Financial Officer
CMO: John Boyd, M.D., Chief Medical Officer
CHR: Maureen Sterbach, Vice President Human Resources
Web address: www.ichosestjoes.com
Control: Church–operated, Nongovernment, not–for profit **Service:** General Medical and Surgical

Staffed Beds: 690 **Admissions:** 33966 **Census:** 477 **Outpatient Visits:** 399559 **Births:** 5730 **Total Expense ($000):** 712817 **Payroll Expense ($000):** 286629 **Personnel:** 4541

☐ **ST. LUKE'S BEHAVIORAL HEALTH CENTER (34013)**, 1800 East Van Buren, Zip 85006–3742; tel. 602/251–8546, (Nonreporting) **A**1 9 10
S IASIS Healthcare
Primary Contact: Gregory L. Jahn, RN, Chief Executive Officer
COO: Gregory L. Jahn, R.N., Chief Executive Officer
CMO: Mario Tafur, M.D., Chief of Staff
CIO: Chris Ulrey, Director Management Information Systems
CHR: Trinise Thompson, Director Human Resources
Web address: www.iasishealthcare.com
Control: Corporation, Investor–owned, for–profit **Service:** Psychiatric

Staffed Beds: 85

★☐ **ST. LUKE'S MEDICAL CENTER (30037)**, 1800 East Van Buren Street, Zip 85006–3742; tel. 602/251–8100, (Nonreporting) **A**1 9 10
S IASIS Healthcare
Primary Contact: Brent A. Cope, Chief Executive Officer
CFO: Ruby Majhail, Interim Chief Financial Officer
CHR: Trinise Thompson, Director Human Resources
Web address: www.stlukesmedcenter.com
Control: Corporation, Investor–owned, for–profit **Service:** General Medical and Surgical

Staffed Beds: 225

☐ **SURGICAL SPECIALTY HOSPITAL OF ARIZONA (30108)**, 6501 North 19th Avenue, Zip 85015; tel. 602/795–6020 **A**1 9 10 **F**12 25 62 68 77 79 80
Primary Contact: Beverly Carpenter, Chief Executive Officer
COO: Carolyn Bonar, Chief Nursing Officer and Chief Operating Officer
CFO: Skip Setterlund, Chief Financial Officer
CMO: Michael Winer, M.D., Chief of Staff
CHR: Joann Lambiase, Director Human Resources
Control: Corporation, Investor–owned, for–profit **Service:** General Medical and Surgical

Staffed Beds: 33 **Admissions:** 1021 **Census:** 5 **Outpatient Visits:** 1050 **Births:** 0 **Total Expense ($000):** 16026 **Payroll Expense ($000):** 3738 **Personnel:** 75

★☐ **U. S. PUBLIC HEALTH SERVICE PHOENIX INDIAN MEDICAL CENTER (30078)**, 4212 North 16th Street, Zip 85016–5389; tel. 602/263–1200, (Nonreporting) **A**1 5 9 10 **S** U. S. Indian Health Service
Primary Contact: Vincent A. Berkley, M.D., Chief Executive Officer
COO: Charlton Wilson, M.D., Chief Operating Officer
CFO: Geraldine Harney, Chief Financial Officer
CMO: Dave Civic, M.D., Associate Director Clinical Services
CIO: Vina Montour, Director Information Technology
CHR: Betty Weston, Chief Human Resources Officer
Web address: www.ihs.gov
Control: PHS, Indian Service, Government, federal **Service:** General Medical and Surgical

Staffed Beds: 127

PRESCOTT—Yavapai County

★☐ **NORTHERN ARIZONA VA HEALTH CARE SYSTEM**, 500 Highway 89 North, Zip 86313–5000; tel. 928/445–4860, (Total facility includes 85 beds in nursing home–type unit) (Nonreporting) **A**1 9 **S** Department of Veterans Affairs
Primary Contact: Susan Angell, Ph.D., Director
COO: Wendy J. Hepker, Associate Director
CFO: Vickie Franecki, Manager Resource Management Service
CMO: A. Panneer Selvam, M.D., Chief of Staff
CIO: Roni Moore, Manager Information Technology
Web address: www.va.gov/sta/guide/home.asp
Control: Veterans Affairs, Government, federal **Service:** General Medical and Surgical

Staffed Beds: 236

★☐ **YAVAPAI REGIONAL MEDICAL CENTER (30012)**, 1003 Willow Creek Road, Zip 86301–1668; tel. 928/445–2700 **A**1 9 10 20 **F**13 14 15 18 22 24 25 26 30 31 32 33 34 42 43 44 50 52 53 55 56 57 59 61 62 66 68 72 73 74 75 76 77 79 80 81 82 86 96 97 100 102 104 105 106 107 119 120 121 124 132 135 137 **P**5
Primary Contact: Timothy Barnett, Chief Executive Officer
COO: Kevin Keighron, Chief Operating Officer
CFO: Doug Bristol, Chief Financial Officer
CMO: Joseph Goldberger, M.D., Chief Medical Officer
CIO: David Woodcock, Chief Information Officer
CHR: Andy Kresha, Director Human Resources
Web address: www.yrmc.org
Control: Hospital district or authority, Government, nonfederal **Service:** General Medical and Surgical

Staffed Beds: 169 **Admissions:** 11045 **Census:** 98 **Outpatient Visits:** 119182 **Births:** 1375 **Total Expense ($000):** 173436 **Payroll Expense ($000):** 79494 **Personnel:** 1363

PRESCOTT VALLEY—Yavapai County

MOUNTAIN VALLEY REGIONAL REHABILITATION HOSPITAL (33036), 3700 North Windsong Drive, Zip 86314; tel. 928/759–8800 **A**9 10 **F**3 25 26 33 54 55 56 57 62 66 72 77 85 86 119 121 132 137 **S** Ernest Health, Inc.
Primary Contact: Kelly Silberschlag, Chief Executive Officer
Web address: www.mvrrh.ernesthealth.com
Control: Partnership, Investor–owned, for–profit **Service:** Rehabilitation

Staffed Beds: 40 **Admissions:** 680 **Census:** 28

SACATON—Pinal County

★☐ **HUHUKAM MEMORIAL HOSPITAL (31308)**, Seed Farm and Skill Center Road, Zip 85247–0038, Mailing Address: P.O. Box 38, Zip 85247–0038; tel. 602/528–1200, (Nonreporting) **A**1 9 10 18
Primary Contact: Loren Ellery, M.P.H., Chief Executive Officer
COO: Karen Shammas, Chief Operating Officer
CFO: Corrine Wilson, Chief Financial Officer
CMO: Noel Habib, M.D., Chief Medical Officer
CHR: Michael Freeman, Director Human Resources
Web address: www.grhc.org
Control: Other not–for–profit (including NFP Corporation) **Service:** General Medical and Surgical

Staffed Beds: 12

SAFFORD—Graham County

★ **MT. GRAHAM REGIONAL MEDICAL CENTER (30068)**, 1600 20th Avenue, Zip 85546–4097; tel. 928/348–4000 **A**9 10 20 **F**3 11 13 15 25 27 30 31 32 33 38 42 44 45 46 52 53 55 56 57 58 61 62 63 66 68 73 74 76 77 79 80 82 86 96 97 99 100 103 107 118 119 121 122 123 124 130 135 **P**5
Primary Contact: Patrick Peters, Chief Executive Officer
COO: Roland Knox, Vice President and Chief Operating Officer
CIO: Roland Knox, Vice President and Chief Operating Officer
CHR: Jennifer Wilson, Vice President Human Resources and Medical Staff Services
Web address: www.mtgraham.org
Control: Other not–for–profit (including NFP Corporation) **Service:** General Medical and Surgical

Staffed Beds: 55 **Admissions:** 3563 **Census:** 26 **Outpatient Visits:** 94003 **Births:** 668 **Total Expense ($000):** 44201 **Payroll Expense ($000):** 19445 **Personnel:** 457

SAN CARLOS—Gila County

★☐ **U. S. PUBLIC HEALTH SERVICE INDIAN HOSPITAL (30077)**, Mailing Address: P.O. Box 208, Zip 85550–0208; tel. 928/475–2371, (Nonreporting) **A**1 10 **S** U. S. Indian Health Service
Primary Contact: Nella J. Ben, Chief Executive Officer
COO: Nella J. Ben, Chief Executive Officer
CFO: Shirley M. Boni, Administrative Officer
CMO: Karen Health, M.D., Clinical Director
CIO: Shirley M. Boni, Administrative Officer
CHR: Shirley M. Boni, Administrative Officer
Web address: www.ihs.gov
Control: PHS, Indian Service, Government, federal **Service:** General Medical and Surgical

Staffed Beds: 8

SCOTTSDALE—Maricopa County

★☐ **BANNER BEHAVIORAL HEALTH HOSPITAL – SCOTTSDALE (34004)**, 7575 East Earll Drive, Zip 85251–6915; tel. 480/941–7500 **A**1 9 10 **F**4 5 25 26 30 31 32 33 36 54 56 62 63 66 73 81 82 88 89 90 91 93 94 95 119 121 132 135 **P**5 **S** Banner Health
Primary Contact: Patricia A. Little–Upah, Chief Executive Officer
COO: Ross Gaetano, Chief Operating Officer
CFO: Sandy Marsh, Chief Financial Officer
CMO: James Clark, M.D., Medical Director
CIO: Erin Dwiggins, Financial Analyst
CHR: Allison Sommers, Chief Human Resources Officer
Web address: www.bannerhealth.com
Control: Other not–for–profit (including NFP Corporation) **Service:** Psychiatric

Staffed Beds: 92 **Admissions:** 2947 **Census:** 67 **Outpatient Visits:** 13146 **Births:** 0 **Total Expense ($000):** 19431 **Payroll Expense ($000):** 12346 **Personnel:** 241

Hospital, Medicare Provider Number, Address, Telephone, Approval, Facility, and Physician Codes, Health Care System

★ American Hospital Association (AHA) membership
☐ The Joint Commission accreditation
○ American Osteopathic Association (AOA) accreditation
△ Commission on Accreditation of Rehabilitation Facilities (CARF) accreditation

☒ **HEALTHSOUTH SCOTTSDALE REHABILITATION HOSPITAL (33025)**, 9630 East Shea Boulevard, Zip 85260; tel. 480/551–5400, (Nonreporting) **A**1 9 10 **S** HEALTHSOUTH Corporation
Primary Contact: Richard Schulz, Chief Executive Officer
CFO: Lisa Barrick, Controller
CMO: Carolyn L. Kinney, M.D., Medical Director
CHR: Cathy Guthrie, Director Human Resources
Web address: www.healthsouth.com
Control: Corporation, Investor–owned, for–profit **Service:** Rehabilitation

Staffed Beds: 46

☐ **KINDRED HOSPITAL ARIZONA–SCOTTSDALE**, 11250 North 92nd Street, Zip 85260; tel. 480/391–4040, (Nonreporting) **A**1 **S** Kindred Healthcare
Primary Contact: Scott Floden, Chief Executive Officer
Web address: www.kindredhealthcare.com
Control: Corporation, Investor–owned, for–profit **Service:** Long–Term Acute Care hospital

Staffed Beds: 50

☒ **SCOTTSDALE HEALTHCARE SHEA (30087)**, 9003 East Shea Boulevard, Zip 85260–6771; tel. 480/323–3000 **A**1 2 9 10 **F**3 8 11 12 13 15 17 18 20 22 24 25 26 27 28 30 31 32 33 34 37 38 40 43 44 46 50 51 52 53 54 55 56 57 59 60 61 62 66 68 70 71 72 73 74 75 76 77 79 80 81 82 84 85 86 96 97 99 100 102 103 106 107 108 109 112 113 114 116 118 119 120 121 123 124 133 135 136 137 **P**6 **S** Scottsdale Healthcare
Primary Contact: Peggy Reiley, Senior Vice President and Chief Clinical Officer
COO: Jeffrey K. Norman, Executive Vice President and Chief Operating Officer
CFO: Todd La Porte, Senior Vice President and Chief Financial Officer
CMO: James Burke, M.D., Senior Vice President and Chief Medical Officer
CIO: James R. Cramer, Vice President and Chief Information Officer
CHR: Carol Henderson, Vice President Human Resources
Web address: www.shc.org
Control: Other not–for–profit (including NFP Corporation) **Service:** General Medical and Surgical

Staffed Beds: 405 **Admissions:** 25019 **Census:** 264 **Outpatient Visits:** 74548 **Births:** 4725 **Total Expense ($000):** 353824 **Personnel:** 2249

★ **SCOTTSDALE HEALTHCARE THOMPSON PEAK (30123)**, 7400 East Thompson Peak Parkway, Zip 85255; tel. 480/324–7000, (Nonreporting) **A**10 **S** Scottsdale Healthcare
Primary Contact: Jean Knoedler, Vice President and Administrator
Web address: www.scottsdalehealthcare.org
Control: Other not–for–profit (including NFP Corporation) **Service:** General Medical and Surgical

Staffed Beds: 64

☒ **SCOTTSDALE HEALTHCARE–OSBORN (30038)**, 7400 East Osborn Road, Zip 85251–6403; tel. 480/882–4000 **A**1 2 3 5 9 10 **F**1 3 8 11 13 18 19 20 21 24 25 26 27 28 30 31 32 33 34 35 36 37 38 40 43 44 46 47 49 51 54 55 56 57 58 59 60 61 62 63 66 69 72 73 74 75 76 77 79 80 81 82 85 86 87 90 91 92 93 96 97 100 102 103 107 109 111 112 119 120 121 124 132 135 136 137 **P**6 **S** Scottsdale Healthcare
Primary Contact: Gary E. Baker, Senior Vice President and Administrator
COO: Jeffrey K. Norman, Executive Vice President and Chief Operating Officer
CFO: Todd La Porte, Senior Vice President and Chief Financial Officer
CMO: James Burke, M.D., Senior Vice President and Chief Medical Officer
CIO: James R. Cramer, Vice President and Chief Information Officer
CHR: Carol Henderson, Vice President Human Resources
Web address: www.shc.org
Control: Other not–for–profit (including NFP Corporation) **Service:** General Medical and Surgical

Staffed Beds: 337 **Admissions:** 18320 **Census:** 232 **Outpatient Visits:** 71271 **Births:** 1633 **Total Expense ($000):** 306561 **Personnel:** 2669

☐ **SELECT SPECIALTY HOSPITAL–SCOTTSDALE**, 7400 Osborn Road, 3 West, Zip 85021–6403; tel. 480/675–6040, (Nonreporting) **A**1 9 **S** Select Medical Corporation
Primary Contact: Sharon Anthony, Chief Executive Officer
Web address: www.selectmedicalcorp.com
Control: Corporation, Investor–owned, for–profit **Service:** Long–Term Acute Care hospital

Staffed Beds: 29

SELLS—Pima County

☒ **U. S. PUBLIC HEALTH SERVICE INDIAN HOSPITAL (30074)**, Mailing Address: P.O. Box 548, Zip 85634–0548; tel. 520/383–7251, (Nonreporting) **A**1 10 **S** U. S. Indian Health Service
Primary Contact: Priscilla Whitethorne, Service Unit Director
COO: Diane Shanley, Deputy Service Unit Director
CFO: Vivian Draper, Chief Financial Officer
CMO: John Kittredge, M.D., Chief Medical Officer
CIO: Karen Wade, Chief Information Officer
CHR: Richard Gerry, Director Human Resources
Web address: www.ihs.gov
Control: PHS, Indian Service, Government, federal **Service:** General Medical and Surgical

Staffed Beds: 34

SHOW LOW—Navajo County

★ **SUMMIT HEALTHCARE REGIONAL MEDICAL CENTER (30062)**, (Formerly Navapache Regional Medical Center), 2200 East Show Low Lake Road, Zip 85901–7800; tel. 928/537–4375 **A**9 10 20 **F**3 11 13 15 24 25 26 27 30 31 32 33 34 38 40 43 46 48 49 51 52 53 55 56 57 61 62 63 66 68 72 73 74 75 76 77 79 80 81 82 86 87 96 97 99 100 103 104 105 106 107 108 109 118 119 121 134 135 136 137 **P**6 **S** Brim Healthcare, Inc.
Primary Contact: Thomas D. Plantz, Chief Executive Officer
CFO: Stephen Huey, Chief Financial Officer
CMO: Jones Cavanaugh, M.D., Chief of Staff
CIO: Kent McQuillan, Chief Information Officer
CHR: Correen Bales, Director Human Resources
Web address: www.nrmc.org
Control: Other not–for–profit (including NFP Corporation) **Service:** General Medical and Surgical

Staffed Beds: 66 **Admissions:** 4589 **Census:** 34 **Outpatient Visits:** 53458 **Births:** 1140 **Total Expense ($000):** 73092 **Payroll Expense ($000):** 29471 **Personnel:** 538

SIERRA VISTA—Cochise County

☒ **SIERRA VISTA REGIONAL HEALTH CENTER (30043)**, 300 El Camino Real, Zip 85635–2899; tel. 520/458–4641 **A**1 9 10 12 13 20 **F**1 3 4 11 13 15 16 17 18 20 24 25 26 30 31 32 33 38 42 43 49 50 53 59 65 68 70 71 73 74 75 78 79 80 83 84 85 86 88 96 97 100 102 106 107 117 118 119 121 124 135 137
Primary Contact: Margaret Hepburn, President and Chief Executive Officer
COO: Rebecca McCalmont, Vice President Nursing and Chief Nursing Executive
CFO: Bruce J. Norton, Senior Vice President and Chief Financial Officer
CIO: Bruce J. Norton, Senior Vice President and Chief Financial Officer
CHR: Marie Wurth, Vice President Human Resources and Public Relations Officer
Web address: www.svrhc.org
Control: Other not–for–profit (including NFP Corporation) **Service:** General Medical and Surgical

Staffed Beds: 88 **Admissions:** 5855 **Census:** 50 **Outpatient Visits:** 85126 **Births:** 1401 **Total Expense ($000):** 71725 **Payroll Expense ($000):** 31950 **Personnel:** 701

SPRINGERVILLE—Apache County

WHITE MOUNTAIN REGIONAL MEDICAL CENTER (30099), 118 South Mountain Avenue, Zip 85938–5104; tel. 928/333–4368, (Total facility includes 64 beds in nursing home–type unit) (Nonreporting) **A**9 10 20
Primary Contact: Michael Zimmerman, Chief Executive Officer
CFO: James Hamblin, Chief Financial Officer
CMO: Scott Hamblin, M.D., President Medical Staff
Web address: www.wmrmc.com
Control: Other not–for–profit (including NFP Corporation) **Service:** General Medical and Surgical

Staffed Beds: 89

SUN CITY—Maricopa County

☒ **SUN HEALTH BOSWELL HOSPITAL (30061)**, 10401 West Thunderbird Boulevard, Zip 85351–3092, Mailing Address: P.O. Box 1690, Zip 85372–1690; tel. 623/977–7211, (Total facility includes 71 beds in nursing home–type unit) **A**1 2 9 10 **F**3 11 15 17 20 22 24 25 26 27 30 31 32 35 38 43 47 49 52 53 54 58 59 62 63 67 68 72 73 75 76 77 79 80 82 85 86 96 97 98 100 101 102 103 104 105 106 107 116 117 119 134 135 136 137 **S** Sun Health Corporation
Primary Contact: Nancy L. Burton, Chief Executive Officer
CFO: William Sellner, Vice President and Chief Financial Officer
CMO: Michel Dagher, D.O., Vice President and Chief Medical Officer
CIO: David Runt, Vice President Information Services and Chief Information Officer
Web address: www.sunhealth.org
Control: Other not–for–profit (including NFP Corporation) **Service:** General Medical and Surgical

Staffed Beds: 436 **Admissions:** 23820 **Census:** 333 **Outpatient Visits:** 105199 **Births:** 0 **Total Expense ($000):** 275791 **Payroll Expense ($000):** 109830 **Personnel:** 1730

SUN CITY WEST—Maricopa County

☒ **SUN HEALTH DEL E. WEBB HOSPITAL (30093)**, (Formerly Del E. Webb Memorial Hospital), 14502 West Meeker Boulevard, Zip 85375–5299, Mailing Address: P.O. Box 5169, Sun City, Zip 85375–5169; tel. 623/214–4000 **A**1 9 10 **F**3 5 11 13 15 18 20 24 25 26 27 31 32 33 35 38 42 43 44 45 49 59 61 62 67 68 71 72 73 74 75 76 77 79 80 82 84 85 86 88 90 91 92 93 94 95 96 97 100 102 103 106 107 119 120 121 124 133 135 136 **P**1 8 **S** Sun Health Corporation
Primary Contact: Jo Adkins, Chief Executive Officer
CFO: William Sellner, Vice President and Chief Financial Officer
CMO: Michel Dagher, D.O., Vice President and Chief Medical Officer
CIO: David Runt, Chief Information Officer
Web address: www.sunhealth.org
Control: Other not–for–profit (including NFP Corporation) **Service:** General Medical and Surgical

Staffed Beds: 332 **Admissions:** 17945 **Census:** 213 **Outpatient Visits:** 157377 **Births:** 1984 **Total Expense ($000):** 189842 **Payroll Expense ($000):** 82605 **Personnel:** 1233

Many Facility Codes have changed. Please refer to the AHA Guide Code Chart.

TEMPE—Maricopa County

□ **TEMPE ST. LUKE'S HOSPITAL (30019)**, 1500 South Mill Avenue, Zip 85281–6699; tel. 480/784–5510, (Nonreporting) **A**1 9 10 **S** IASIS Healthcare
Primary Contact: Bill R. Porter, Chief Executive Officer
CFO: Clifford Loader, Interim Chief Financial Officer
Web address: www.tempestlukehospital.com
Control: Corporation, Investor–owned, for–profit **Service:** General Medical and Surgical

Staffed Beds: 110

TUBA CITY—Coconino County

★ **TUBA CITY REGIONAL HEALTH CARE CORPORATION (30073)**, 167 Main Street, Zip 86045–0611, Mailing Address: P.O. Box 600, Zip 86045–0600; tel. 928/283–2501 **A**1 5 9 10 **F**4 5 8 13 15 24 25 27 28 30 31 32 33 37 38 39 43 53 54 55 56 57 62 63 64 66 68 71 73 74 75 77 79 80 81 82 84 85 86 87 88 90 91 92 94 96 99 102 107 112 113 114 119 121 122 123 124 132 133 135 136 137
Primary Contact: Joseph T. Engelken, Chief Executive Officer
CFO: Clifford Lee Olsson, Finance Officer
CMO: Alan Spacone, M.D., Medical Director
CHR: Laurence McGuire, Director Human Resources
Web address: www.tchealth.org
Control: Other not–for–profit (including NFP Corporation) **Service:** General Medical and Surgical

Staffed Beds: 73 **Admissions:** 3540 **Census:** 33 **Outpatient Visits:** 205979 **Births:** 540 **Total Expense ($000):** 82620 **Payroll Expense ($000):** 42139 **Personnel:** 732

TUCSON—Pima County

★ **CARONDELET ST. JOSEPH'S HOSPITAL (30011)**, 350 North Wilmot Road, Zip 85711–2678; tel. 520/296–3211 **A**1 9 10 **F**3 5 11 12 13 15 17 18 20 24 25 26 30 31 32 36 38 41 42 43 44 45 46 47 49 50 55 56 57 60 62 66 67 68 72 73 74 75 76 77 79 82 85 86 88 90 91 92 93 94 95 96 97 99 100 102 103 106 107 116 118 119 120 121 122 124 135 136 **S** Ascension Health
Primary Contact: Gregory R. Angle, Chief Executive Officer
COO: Wesley E. Colvin, Chief Operating Officer
CFO: Tom Pepping, Chief Financial Officer
CMO: Jose M. Santiago, M.D., Senior Vice President and Chief Medical Officer
CIO: Mark Amey, Chief Information Officer
CHR: Linda Werbylo, Vice President Human Resources
Web address: www.carondelet.org
Control: Church–operated, Nongovernment, not–for profit **Service:** General Medical and Surgical

Staffed Beds: 251 **Admissions:** 17673 **Census:** 211 **Outpatient Visits:** 125068 **Births:** 2634 **Total Expense ($000):** 195067 **Payroll Expense ($000):** 91658 **Personnel:** 1825

★ **CARONDELET ST. MARY'S HOSPITAL (30010)**, 1601 West St. Mary's Road, Zip 85745–2682; tel. 520/872–3000 **A**1 9 10 **F**3 5 11 15 16 17 18 20 25 26 27 30 31 32 36 38 41 42 43 44 45 47 49 50 51 54 55 56 57 59 60 62 66 68 72 75 76 77 79 82 85 86 88 90 91 92 93 94 95 96 97 99 100 102 103 104 106 107 116 118 119 121 122 124 134 135 137 **S** Ascension Health
Primary Contact: Odette Bolano, Chief Executive Officer
CFO: Tom Pepping, Chief Financial Officer
CMO: Jose M. Santiago, M.D., Senior Vice President and Chief Medical Officer
CIO: Mark Amey, Chief Information Officer
CHR: Linda Werbylo, Vice President Human Resources
Web address: www.carondelet.org
Control: Church–operated, Nongovernment, not–for profit **Service:** General Medical and Surgical

Staffed Beds: 429 **Admissions:** 18077 **Census:** 271 **Outpatient Visits:** 198123 **Births:** 0 **Total Expense ($000):** 214314 **Payroll Expense ($000):** 103137 **Personnel:** 1804

□ **CORNERSTONE HOSPITAL OF SOUTHEAST ARIZONA (32004)**, 7220 East Rosewood Drive, Zip 85710; tel. 520/546–4595, (Nonreporting) **A**1 9 10 **S** Cornerstone Healthcare Group
Primary Contact: James Mikes, Interim Chief Executive Officer
CFO: Kliff A. Rodgers, Chief Financial Officer
Web address: www.cornerstonehealthcaregroup.com
Control: Corporation, Investor–owned, for–profit **Service:** Long–Term Acute Care hospital

Staffed Beds: 54

★ **HEALTHSOUTH REHABILITATION HOSPITAL OF SOUTHERN ARIZONA (33029)**, 1921 West Hospital Drive, Zip 85704–7806; tel. 520/742–2800 **A**1 9 10 **F**3 25 33 54 55 56 57 62 67 85 86 119 132 137 **S** HEALTHSOUTH Corporation
Primary Contact: Martha Gerganoff, Chief Executive Officer
CFO: David Krogen, Controller
CMO: Susan Bulen, M.D., Medical Director
CHR: Maria Elena McElroy, Vice President Human Resources
Web address: www.healthsouth.com
Control: Corporation, Investor–owned, for–profit **Service:** Rehabilitation

Staffed Beds: 60 **Admissions:** 913 **Census:** 39 **Outpatient Visits:** 14383 **Births:** 0

★ **HEALTHSOUTH REHABILITATION INSTITUTE OF TUCSON (33028)**, 2650 North Wyatt Drive, Zip 85712–6108; tel. 520/325–1300, (Nonreporting) **A**1 9 10 **S** HEALTHSOUTH Corporation
Primary Contact: Jeffrey Christensen, Chief Executive Officer
CFO: Mary Donovan, Controller
CMO: Jon Larson, M.D., Medical Director
CHR: Dawn Mosier, Director Human Resources
Web address: www.healthsouth.com
Control: Corporation, Investor–owned, for–profit **Service:** Rehabilitation

Staffed Beds: 80

□ **KINDRED HOSPITAL – TUCSON (32002)**, 355 North Wilmot Road, Zip 85711–2635; tel. 520/584–4500 **A**1 9 10 **F**1 3 17 25 26 72 80 81 82 90 93 119 137 **S** Kindred Healthcare
Primary Contact: Heidi Miller, Chief Executive Officer
CFO: M. Troy Carpenter, Chief Financial Officer
CMO: Stuart Ouan, M.D., Medical Director
Web address: www.kindredhealthcare.com
Control: Corporation, Investor–owned, for–profit **Service:** Long–Term Acute Care hospital

Staffed Beds: 51 **Admissions:** 427 **Census:** 36 **Outpatient Visits:** 0 **Births:** 0 **Total Expense ($000):** 14246 **Payroll Expense ($000):** 7634 **Personnel:** 114

★ **NORTHWEST MEDICAL CENTER (30085)**, 6200 North La Cholla Boulevard, Zip 85741–3599; tel. 520/742–9000, (Nonreporting) **A**1 9 10 **S** Community Health Systems, Inc.
Primary Contact: Paul Kappelman, Chief Executive Officer
CFO: Ronald Patrick, Chief Financial Officer
Web address: www.northwestmedicalcenter.com
Control: Corporation, Investor–owned, for–profit **Service:** General Medical and Surgical

Staffed Beds: 244

PALO VERDE MENTAL HEALTH SERVICES See Tucson Medical Center

SIERRA TUCSON, 39580 South Lago Del Oro Parkway, Zip 85739–9637; tel. 520/624–4000, (Nonreporting)
Primary Contact: Keith Arnold, Administrator
COO: David E. Anderson, Ph.D., Chief Executive Officer
CFO: Loree Thompson, CPA, Chief Financial Officer
CMO: Michael E. Scott, M.D., Director Medical Services
CIO: Bill Rieger, Chief Information Officer
CHR: Bertha Kenny, Director Human Resources
Web address: www.sierratucson.com
Control: Corporation, Investor–owned, for–profit **Service:** Alcoholism and other chemical dependency

Staffed Beds: 95

★ △ **SOUTHERN ARIZONA VETERANS AFFAIRS HEALTH CARE SYSTEM**, 3601 South 6th Avenue, Zip 85723–0002; tel. 520/792–1450 **A**1 3 5 7 8 9 **F**3 4 5 11 12 14 18 20 22 24 25 26 27 30 32 33 36 37 38 42 43 44 45 47 48 49 50 54 55 56 57 58 59 60 61 62 63 66 68 72 73 75 76 77 78 79 80 81 82 85 86 87 88 92 93 94 96 97 100 102 104 105 107 117 118 119 121 124 132 133 135 136 137 **P**6 **S** Department of Veterans Affairs
Primary Contact: Jonathan H. Gardner, Chief Executive Officer
COO: Joan M. Ricard, R.N., FACHE, Chief Operating Officer
CFO: Larry Korn, Financial Manager
CMO: Jayendra H. Shah, M.D., Chief Medical Officer
CIO: John Walston, Chief Information Officer
CHR: Patrice Craig, Manager Human Resources
Web address: www.tucson.va.gov
Control: Veterans Affairs, Government, federal **Service:** General Medical and Surgical

Staffed Beds: 283 **Admissions:** 9041 **Census:** 220 **Outpatient Visits:** 509833 **Births:** 0 **Personnel:** 1721

Hospital, Medicare Provider Number, Address, Telephone, Approval, Facility, and Physician Codes, Health Care System

★ American Hospital Association (AHA) membership
□ The Joint Commission accreditation
○ American Osteopathic Association (AOA) accreditation
△ Commission on Accreditation of Rehabilitation Facilities (CARF) accreditation

AZ

☐ **TUCSON HEART HOSPITAL (30100)**, 4888 North Stone Avenue, Zip 85704; tel. 520/696–2328 **A**1 9 10 **F**3 17 18 20 22 25 26 30 32 33 38 50 53 57 73 79 82 96 102 121 124 137 **S** Ascension Health
Primary Contact: Edward W. Myers, Chief Executive Officer
CFO: Tom Pepping, Chief Financial Officer
CMO: Michael Hecht, M.D., Medical Director
CIO: Mark Amey, Chief Information Officer
CHR: Linda Werbylo, Vice President Human Resources
Web address: www.tucsonhearthospital.com
Control: Corporation, Investor–owned, for–profit **Service:** General Medical and Surgical

Staffed Beds: 58 **Admissions:** 4528 **Census:** 39 **Outpatient Visits:** 14355 **Births:** 0 **Total Expense ($000):** 59154 **Payroll Expense ($000):** 20352 **Personnel:** 349

★ **TUCSON MEDICAL CENTER (30006)**, 5301 East Grant Road, Zip 85712–2874; tel. 520/327–5461, (Includes PALO VERDE MENTAL HEALTH SERVICES, 2695 North Craycroft, Zip 85712–2244; tel. 520/324–4340) **A**1 3 5 9 10 **F**3 5 8 11 13 15 17 18 20 22 24 25 26 27 28 32 33 36 37 38 42 43 44 51 53 54 55 56 57 58 59 61 62 63 66 70 72 73 74 75 76 77 79 80 82 83 84 87 88 90 92 94 95 96 97 98 99 100 102 103 107 118 119 121 124 130 132 135 136 137
Primary Contact: Judy F. Rich, Executive Vice President and Administrator
CFO: Walter J. Yokobosky, Chief Financial Officer
CMO: Palmer Evans, M.D., Chief Medical Officer
CIO: Frank R. Marini, Vice President and Chief Information Officer
CHR: Peggy Bernhardt–Kadlec, Vice President Human Resources
Web address: www.tmcaz.com
Control: Other not–for–profit (including NFP Corporation) **Service:** General Medical and Surgical

Staffed Beds: 547 **Admissions:** 34427 **Census:** 405 **Outpatient Visits:** 200789 **Births:** 6689 **Total Expense ($000):** 386285 **Payroll Expense ($000):** 165676 **Personnel:** 3137

★ **UNIVERSITY MEDICAL CENTER (30064)**, 1501 North Campbell Avenue, Zip 85724–5128; tel. 520/694–0111 **A**1 3 5 8 9 10 **F**3 8 11 13 17 18 19 20 21 22 23 24 25 26 27 28 33 34 35 36 38 40 41 43 44 46 47 48 49 50 52 53 55 56 57 59 60 61 62 65 66 68 70 72 73 74 75 76 77 79 80 81 82 83 84 86 87 88 89 90 91 92 93 96 97 100 102 103 106 107 108 109 111 112 119 121 125 126 127 128 129 131 133 134 135 136 137 **P**4 6
Primary Contact: Gregory A. Pivirotto, President and Chief Executive Officer
CFO: Kevin J. Burns, Chief Financial Officer
CHR: John Marques, Vice President Human Resources
Web address: www.umcarizona.org
Control: Other not–for–profit (including NFP Corporation) **Service:** General Medical and Surgical

Staffed Beds: 351 **Admissions:** 20497 **Census:** 295 **Outpatient Visits:** 367668 **Births:** 2301 **Total Expense ($000):** 428327 **Payroll Expense ($000):** 184419 **Personnel:** 3142

☐ **UNIVERSITY PHYSICIANS HEALTHCARE HOSPITAL AT KINO CAMPUS (30111)**, 2800 East Ajo Way, Zip 85713–6289; tel. 520/874–2000, (Total facility includes 20 beds in nursing home–type unit) (Nonreporting) **A**1 9 10
Primary Contact: Norm Botsford, Chief Executive Officer
COO: Richard Mandel, M.D., Vice President and Medical Director
CMO: Richard Mandel, M.D., Vice President Operations and Medical Director
CIO: Kevin Christiansen, Director Information Technology
CHR: Tere LeBarron, Director Human Resources
Web address: www.uph.org
Control: County–Government, nonfederal **Service:** General Medical and Surgical

Staffed Beds: 114

WHITERIVER—Navajo County

★ **U. S. PUBLIC HEALTH SERVICE INDIAN HOSPITAL–WHITERIVER (31306)**, 200 West Hospital Drive, Zip 85941–0860, Mailing Address: State Route 73, Box 860, Zip 85941–0860; tel. 928/338–4911, (Nonreporting) **A**1 10 **S** U. S. Indian Health Service
Primary Contact: Michelle Martinez, Interim Chief Executive Officer
CFO: Desdemona Leslie, Finance Officer
CMO: David Yost, M.D., Clinical Director
CIO: Russell Barker, Chief Information Officer
Web address: www.ihs.gov
Control: PHS, Indian Service, Government, federal **Service:** General Medical and Surgical

Staffed Beds: 40

WICKENBURG—Maricopa County

★ **WICKENBURG COMMUNITY HOSPITAL (31300)**, 520 Rose Lane, Zip 85390–1447; tel. 928/684–5421, (Nonreporting) **A**9 10 18
Primary Contact: Dale A. Decker, Administrator
CFO: Ron Smith, Chief Financial Officer
Web address: www.wickhosp.com
Control: Other not–for–profit (including NFP Corporation) **Service:** General Medical and Surgical

Staffed Beds: 6

WILLCOX—Cochise County

★ **NORTHERN COCHISE COMMUNITY HOSPITAL (31302)**, 901 West Rex Allen Drive, Zip 85643–1009; tel. 520/384–3541, (Total facility includes 24 beds in nursing home–type unit) **A**9 10 18 **F**11 15 25 31 32 38 48 54 55 56 57 62 65 79 80 86 87 96 102 119 121 122 **P**6
Primary Contact: Chris Cronberg, Chief Executive Officer
CFO: John Hodnette, Chief Financial Officer
CIO: Peach Unrast, Chief Information Officer
CHR: Denise Linton, Director Human Resources
Web address: www.ncch.net
Control: Other not–for–profit (including NFP Corporation) **Service:** General Medical and Surgical

Staffed Beds: 48 **Admissions:** 425 **Census:** 27 **Outpatient Visits:** 18227 **Births:** 0 **Total Expense ($000):** 11033 **Payroll Expense ($000):** 5047 **Personnel:** 116

WINSLOW—Navajo County

★ **LITTLE COLORADO MEDICAL CENTER (31311)**, 1501 Williamson Avenue, Zip 86047–2797; tel. 928/289–4691 **A**9 10 18 **F**38 74 79 84 96 119 122
Primary Contact: Jeffrey J. Hamblen, Chief Executive Officer
CFO: Randy Glassman, Chief Financial Officer
CMO: Perry Mitchell, M.D., Chief of Staff
CHR: Cheryl Peterson, Director Human Resources
Web address: www.lcmcwmh.org
Control: Other not–for–profit (including NFP Corporation) **Service:** General Medical and Surgical

Staffed Beds: 25 **Admissions:** 1399 **Census:** 11 **Outpatient Visits:** 14837 **Births:** 227 **Total Expense ($000):** 16856 **Payroll Expense ($000):** 5642 **Personnel:** 166

YUMA—Yuma County

★ **YUMA REGIONAL MEDICAL CENTER (30013)**, 2400 South Avenue A, Zip 85364–7170; tel. 928/344–2000 **A**1 9 10 19 20 **F**3 8 11 13 14 15 17 18 20 22 24 25 26 27 28 31 32 33 36 37 38 43 44 46 47 48 49 50 53 55 57 58 61 62 63 66 68 69 70 72 73 74 75 77 79 80 81 82 84 96 97 100 102 103 104 106 107 118 119 121 135 136 137
Primary Contact: Robert T. Olsen, FACHE, President and Chief Executive Officer
CFO: Pat Walz, Chief Financial Officer
CMO: Stewart Hamilton, M.D., Vice President Medical Affairs and Chief Medical Officer
CIO: Gene Shaw, Chief Information Officer
CHR: Sharon Gardner, Vice President Human Resources
Web address: www.yumaregional.org
Control: Other not–for–profit (including NFP Corporation) **Service:** General Medical and Surgical

Staffed Beds: 333 **Admissions:** 18647 **Census:** 203 **Outpatient Visits:** 136687 **Births:** 3672 **Total Expense ($000):** 234970 **Payroll Expense ($000):** 91779 **Personnel:** 1880

★ **YUMA REHABILITATION HOSPITAL (33034)**, 901 West 24th Street, Zip 85364; tel. 928/726–5000 **A**1 9 10 **F**31 32 56 57 62 75 85 86 119 121 **P**5 **S** HEALTHSOUTH Corporation
Primary Contact: Steve Smith, Chief Executive Officer
CFO: Larry Barclift, Chief Executive Officer
CMO: Ronald Bontiglio, M.D., Medical Director
Web address: www.yumarehabhospital.com
Control: Corporation, Investor–owned, for–profit **Service:** Rehabilitation

Staffed Beds: 41 **Admissions:** 823 **Census:** 33 **Outpatient Visits:** 7090 **Births:** 0

ARKANSAS

ARKADELPHIA—Clark County

▣ **BAPTIST HEALTH MEDICAL CENTER–ARKADELPHIA (41321)**, 3050 Twin Rivers Drive, Zip 71923–4299; tel. 870/245–2622 **A**1 9 10 18 **F**3 7 11 13 15 24 25 31 32 38 40 42 57 60 61 67 68 74 79 86 96 100 102 107 119 122 124 **S** Baptist Health
Primary Contact: Greg Stubblefield, Interim Administrator
COO: Greg Stubblefield, Interim Administrator
CHR: Evelyn Valentine, Manager Human Resources
Web address: www.baptist-health.org
Control: Other not–for–profit (including NFP Corporation) **Service:** General Medical and Surgical

Staffed Beds: 25 **Admissions:** 1169 **Census:** 11 **Outpatient Visits:** 23373 **Births:** 218 **Total Expense ($000):** 18102 **Payroll Expense ($000):** 7629 **Personnel:** 192

ASHDOWN—Little River County

★ **LITTLE RIVER MEMORIAL HOSPITAL (41320)**, 451 West Locke Street, Zip 71822–3398; tel. 870/898–5011 **A**9 10 18 **F**3 15 25 27 30 31 32 33 38 42 55 56 57 61 62 86 96 102 107 122 137
Primary Contact: David Deaton, Administrator and Chief Executive Officer
CFO: Barbra Crow, Chief Financial Officer
Control: County–Government, nonfederal **Service:** General Medical and Surgical

Staffed Beds: 25 **Admissions:** 582 **Census:** 5 **Outpatient Visits:** 10686 **Births:** 0 **Total Expense ($000):** 8640 **Payroll Expense ($000):** 5391 **Personnel:** 123

BARLING—Sebastian County

□ **VISTA HEALTH OF FORT SMITH (44006)**, 10301 Mayo Drive, Zip 72923; tel. 479/494–5700 **A**1 9 10 **F**31 32 82 88 89 90 91 92 94 119 **P**6
Primary Contact: Kyle Naples, Chief Executive Officer
Web address: www.vistahealthservices.com
Control: Corporation, Investor–owned, for–profit **Service:** Psychiatric

Staffed Beds: 57 **Admissions:** 1056 **Census:** 49 **Outpatient Visits:** 24388 **Births:** 0 **Total Expense ($000):** 9763 **Payroll Expense ($000):** 5632 **Personnel:** 165

BATESVILLE—Independence County

★ △ **WHITE RIVER MEDICAL CENTER (40119)**, 1710 Harrison Street, Zip 72501–2197, Mailing Address: P.O. Box 2197, Zip 72503–2197; tel. 870/793–1200, (Total facility includes 12 beds in nursing home–type unit) **A**7 9 10 19 20 **F**3 8 11 12 13 15 17 18 20 24 25 26 27 30 31 32 33 38 40 41 43 47 50 51 52 54 55 56 57 61 62 66 68 72 73 74 75 76 77 79 80 81 82 85 86 88 89 90 91 93 94 96 97 100 103 105 107 109 111 117 118 119 120 121 124 133 135 136 137 **P**6
Primary Contact: Gary Bebow, FACHE, Administrator and Chief Executive Officer
COO: Tammy Gavin, Assistant Administrator and Chief Operating Officer
CFO: Gary L. Britten, Chief Financial Officer
CIO: Frank Hilbert, Chief Information Officer
CHR: Gary McDonald, Assistant Administrator Human Resources
Web address: www.wrmc.com
Control: Other not–for–profit (including NFP Corporation) **Service:** General Medical and Surgical

Staffed Beds: 189 **Admissions:** 9095 **Census:** 132 **Outpatient Visits:** 151259 **Births:** 506 **Total Expense ($000):** 120230 **Payroll Expense ($000):** 45078 **Personnel:** 1030

BENTON—Saline County

□ **RIVENDELL BEHAVIORAL HEALTH SERVICES OF ARKANSAS (44007)**, 100 Rivendell Drive, Zip 72019–9100; tel. 501/316–1255 **A**1 9 10 **F**25 30 36 53 57 62 73 88 89 90 91 92 94 95 119 121 123 **P**5 **S** Universal Health Services, Inc.
Primary Contact: Scott Williams, Administrator and Chief Executive Officer
CFO: Fred Woods, Chief Financial Officer
Web address: www.rivendellofarkansas.com
Control: Corporation, Investor–owned, for–profit **Service:** Children's hospital psychiatric

Staffed Beds: 77 **Admissions:** 1849 **Census:** 69 **Outpatient Visits:** 27440 **Births:** 0 **Total Expense ($000):** 15389 **Payroll Expense ($000):** 7031 **Personnel:** 135

▣ **SALINE MEMORIAL HOSPITAL (40084)**, 1 Medical Park Drive, Zip 72015–3354; tel. 501/776–6000, (Total facility includes 16 beds in nursing home–type unit) **A**1 9 10 **F**3 7 11 13 15 18 25 26 30 31 32 33 37 38 42 49 55 56 57 61 62 68 72 73 74 75 77 79 80 82 84 85 86 88 96 97 100 103 106 107 117 118 119 124 135 **P**8
Primary Contact: Randy Fortner, FACHE, Chief Executive Officer
COO: Steve Henson, Vice President Operations
CFO: Carla Robertson, Chief Financial Officer
CIO: Shawn Shuffield, Executive Director Information Services
CHR: Francine DelGlacco, Director Human Resources
Web address: www.salinememorial.org
Control: Other not–for–profit (including NFP Corporation) **Service:** General Medical and Surgical

Staffed Beds: 145 **Admissions:** 4944 **Census:** 61 **Outpatient Visits:** 57277 **Births:** 648 **Total Expense ($000):** 58837 **Payroll Expense ($000):** 27757 **Personnel:** 679

BENTONVILLE—Benton County

▣ **NORTHWEST MEDICAL CENTER – BENTONVILLE (40138)**, (Formerly Bates Medical Center of Benton County), 3000 Medical Center Parkway, Zip 72712; tel. 479/553–1000 **A**1 9 10 **F**1 3 11 13 15 17 18 20 22 24 25 26 30 32 38 51 52 66 68 70 71 72 73 74 75 77 79 80 82 83 84 86 87 96 100 102 103 107 119 120 124 135 136 137 **P**5 7 8 **S** Community Health Systems, Inc.
COO: Mark Bethell, Chief Operating Officer
CFO: Mary Millington, Chief Financial Officer
CMO: James McKenzie, Chief of Staff
CIO: Angela Holcomb, Chief Information Officer
CHR: Mike Meeks, Vice President Human Resources
Web address: www.northwesthealth.com
Control: Corporation, Investor–owned, for–profit **Service:** General Medical and Surgical

Staffed Beds: 91 **Admissions:** 5337 **Census:** 60 **Outpatient Visits:** 53824 **Total Expense ($000):** 53096 **Payroll Expense ($000):** 21696 **Personnel:** 385

BERRYVILLE—Carroll County

▣ **ST. JOHN'S HOSPITAL–BERRYVILLE (41329)**, 214 Carter Street, Zip 72616–4303; tel. 870/423–3355 **A**1 9 10 18 **F**3 11 13 15 24 25 26 27 30 31 32 33 38 41 48 52 55 56 57 60 62 66 68 73 74 75 76 77 79 80 81 82 86 96 97 106 107 117 118 119 120 121 122 135 136 137 **P**8 **S** Sisters of Mercy Health System
Primary Contact: Kristy K. Noble, FACHE, President
CFO: Sharon Ash, Vice President Finance
CHR: Taya James, Director
Web address: www.stjohnsberryville.com
Control: Church–operated, Nongovernment, not–for profit **Service:** General Medical and Surgical

Staffed Beds: 25 **Admissions:** 1591 **Census:** 13 **Outpatient Visits:** 22914 **Births:** 378 **Total Expense ($000):** 15209 **Payroll Expense ($000):** 7992 **Personnel:** 199

BLYTHEVILLE—Mississippi County

▣ **GREAT RIVER MEDICAL CENTER (40069)**, 1520 North Division Street, Zip 72315–1448, Mailing Address: P.O. Box 108, Zip 72316–0108; tel. 870/838–7300 **A**1 9 10 19 20 **F**1 3 4 11 13 15 16 17 24 25 27 32 38 43 52 54 55 56 57 62 65 68 70 71 74 76 77 78 79 80 83 84 85 86 87 88 93 96 97 100 102 107 108 117 118 124 136 **S** Ameris Health Systems
Primary Contact: Michael G. Layfield, Chief Executive Officer
CFO: David Lynn, Chief Financial Officer
CMO: Benjamin Boakye, M.D., Chief of Staff
CIO: Jason Pierce, Manager Information Systems
CHR: Cheri Blurton, Director Human Resources
Web address: www.greatrivermc.com
Control: Corporation, Investor–owned, for–profit **Service:** General Medical and Surgical

Staffed Beds: 111 **Admissions:** 2310 **Census:** 27 **Outpatient Visits:** 28731 **Births:** 450 **Total Expense ($000):** 21942 **Payroll Expense ($000):** 9081 **Personnel:** 246

Hospital, Medicare Provider Number, Address, Telephone, Approval, Facility, and Physician Codes, Health Care System

★ American Hospital Association (AHA) membership
□ The Joint Commission accreditation
○ American Osteopathic Association (AOA) accreditation
△ Commission on Accreditation of Rehabilitation Facilities (CARF) accreditation

BOONEVILLE—Logan County

★ **BOONEVILLE COMMUNITY HOSPITAL (41318)**, 880 West Main Street, Zip 72927–3420, Mailing Address: P.O. Box 290, Zip 72927–0290; tel. 479/675–2800 **A**9 10 18 **F**3 11 24 25 26 38 55 57 61 62 79 80 86 87 96 100 102 119 122 124 133 135 **P**6
Primary Contact: Dzaidi Daud, Chief Executive Officer
CMO: William Daniel, M.D., Chief of Staff
CIO: Aaron Albright, Chief Information Officer
CHR: Doris Whitaker, Vice President Human Resources
Web address: www.boonevillehospital.com
Control: Other not–for–profit (including NFP Corporation) **Service:** General Medical and Surgical

Staffed Beds: 25 **Admissions:** 680 **Census:** 9 **Outpatient Visits:** 9588 **Births:** 0 **Personnel:** 90

CALICO ROCK—Izard County

COMMUNITY MEDICAL CENTER OF IZARD COUNTY (41306), 103 Grasse Street, Zip 72519, Mailing Address: P.O. Box 438, Zip 72519–0438; tel. 870/297–3726 **A**9 10 18 **F**3 8 11 15 25 26 27 30 31 32 33 42 46 50 53 55 56 57 61 62 66 73 79 80 86 87 96 102 107 117 118 119 120 121 122 135 **P**4 5
Primary Contact: Angela Richmond, President and Chief Executive Officer
COO: Genna Nave, Chief Operating Officer
CMO: A. Meryl Grasse, M.D., Medical Director
CIO: Philip Hughes, Director Information Technology
Web address: www.cmcofic.org
Control: Other not–for–profit (including NFP Corporation) **Service:** General Medical and Surgical

Staffed Beds: 25 **Admissions:** 613 **Census:** 7 **Outpatient Visits:** 3408 **Births:** 0 **Total Expense ($000):** 8212 **Payroll Expense ($000):** 3802 **Personnel:** 102

CAMDEN—Ouachita County

★ **OUACHITA MEDICAL CENTER (40050)**, 638 California Street, Zip 71701–4699, Mailing Address: P.O. Box 797, Zip 71701–0797; tel. 870/836–1000 **A**1 3 5 9 10 20 **F**1 3 4 5 7 8 11 13 15 16 17 25 27 30 31 32 38 40 42 46 48 49 51 54 55 56 57 61 62 63 65 66 67 68 70 71 73 74 75 76 78 79 80 82 83 84 85 86 87 88 90 93 96 100 102 107 117 118 119 121 122 124 137 **P**8
Primary Contact: David Cicero, President
CFO: Robert Anders, Chief Financial Officer
CHR: Mary Bridges, Director Human Resources
Web address: www.ouachitamedcenter.com
Control: Other not–for–profit (including NFP Corporation) **Service:** General Medical and Surgical

Staffed Beds: 98 **Admissions:** 2769 **Census:** 31 **Outpatient Visits:** 26414 **Births:** 418 **Total Expense ($000):** 30323 **Payroll Expense ($000):** 14000 **Personnel:** 435

CLARKSVILLE—Johnson County

★ **JOHNSON REGIONAL MEDICAL CENTER (40002)**, 1100 East Poplar Street, Zip 72830–4419, Mailing Address: P.O. Box 738, Zip 72830–0738; tel. 479/754–5454 **A**9 10 **F**3 7 11 13 15 17 25 30 31 32 37 38 55 56 57 61 62 66 68 73 74 75 77 79 80 85 86 88 93 94 96 97 100 102 107 118 119 121 122 136 137
Primary Contact: Larry Morse, CHE, Chief Executive Officer and Administrator
CFO: Edward Anderson, Chief Financial Officer
CIO: Deb Bjorgum, Manager Data Processing
CHR: Maribel Baker, Director Human Resource
Web address: www.jrmc.com
Control: Other not–for–profit (including NFP Corporation) **Service:** General Medical and Surgical

Staffed Beds: 80 **Admissions:** 2585 **Census:** 36 **Outpatient Visits:** 48044 **Births:** 487 **Total Expense ($000):** 28202 **Payroll Expense ($000):** 12402 **Personnel:** 337

CLINTON—Van Buren County

★ **OZARK HEALTH MEDICAL CENTER (41313)**, Highway 65 South, Zip 72031–9045, Mailing Address: P.O. Box 206, Zip 72031–0206; tel. 501/745–7000, (Total facility includes 132 beds in nursing home–type unit) **A**9 10 18 **F**3 11 15 24 25 31 32 33 38 55 56 57 61 62 65 75 77 79 81 86 96 100 107 117 119 122 123 124 132 135
Primary Contact: Herbert K. Reamey, III, FACHE, Chief Executive Officer and Administrator
COO: Herbert K. Reamey, Chief Executive Officer
CFO: John Zeiler, Chief Financial Officer
CMO: Steve Schoettle, M.D., Chief Medical Staff
CIO: Kathy Fugitt, Chief Information Officer
CHR: Lisa Swofford, Director Administrative Services
Web address: www.ozarkhealthinc.com
Control: Other not–for–profit (including NFP Corporation) **Service:** General Medical and Surgical

Staffed Beds: 157 **Admissions:** 1071 **Census:** 115 **Outpatient Visits:** 21603 **Births:** 4 **Total Expense ($000):** 18890 **Payroll Expense ($000):** 8214 **Personnel:** 276

CONWAY—Faulkner County

★ **CONWAY REGIONAL MEDICAL CENTER (40029)**, 2302 College Avenue, Zip 72032–6297; tel. 501/329–3831 **A**1 2 9 10 **F**3 8 11 13 15 17 18 20 22 24 25 26 27 33 38 44 49 50 51 52 54 55 57 59 61 62 68 71 72 73 74 75 76 77 79 80 82 84 85 86 93 96 97 99 100 103 105 107 108 119 120 121 124 135 136 137 **P**8
Primary Contact: James M. Lambert, Chief Executive Officer
CFO: Steven P. Rose, Chief Financial Officer
CMO: Don Steely, M.D., Chief of Staff
CIO: Bob Hambuchen, Director Information Systems
CHR: Richard Tyler, Corporate Director Human Resources
Web address: www.conwayregional.org
Control: Other not–for–profit (including NFP Corporation) **Service:** General Medical and Surgical

Staffed Beds: 146 **Admissions:** 8202 **Census:** 85 **Outpatient Visits:** 93636 **Births:** 1748 **Total Expense ($000):** 98931 **Payroll Expense ($000):** 37468 **Personnel:** 924

CONWAY REGIONAL REHAB HOSPITAL (43033), 2210 Robinson Street, Zip 72032; tel. 501/932–3500 **A**9 10 **F**3 25 26 31 32 33 43 54 55 56 57 58 66 85 90 119 121 132 137
Primary Contact: Andrea LaPointe, Chief Executive Officer
Control: Partnership, Investor–owned, for–profit **Service:** Rehabilitation

Staffed Beds: 23 **Admissions:** 484 **Census:** 14 **Outpatient Visits:** 0 **Births:** 0 **Payroll Expense ($000):** 938 **Personnel:** 28

CROSSETT—Ashley County

★ **ASHLEY COUNTY MEDICAL CENTER (41323)**, 1015 Unity Road, Zip 71635–2930, Mailing Address: P.O. Box 400, Zip 71635–0400; tel. 870/364–4111 **A**9 10 18 **F**3 11 13 15 26 27 30 31 32 33 38 40 50 52 55 57 61 62 66 68 73 74 75 76 77 79 80 86 88 90 93 94 96 97 100 106 107 118 119 121 122 137
Primary Contact: Russ D. Sword, FACHE, Chief Executive Officer
CIO: Dan Austin, Manager Data Processing
CHR: Shirley White, Director Human Resources
Web address: www.acmconline.org
Control: Other not–for–profit (including NFP Corporation) **Service:** General Medical and Surgical

Staffed Beds: 33 **Admissions:** 1365 **Census:** 16 **Outpatient Visits:** 40478 **Births:** 195 **Total Expense ($000):** 18987 **Payroll Expense ($000):** 8997 **Personnel:** 193

DANVILLE—Yell County

★ **CHAMBERS MEMORIAL HOSPITAL (40011)**, Highway 10 at Detroit, Zip 72833, Mailing Address: P.O. Box 639, Zip 72833–0639; tel. 479/495–2241 **A**9 10 20 **F**3 11 25 31 32 33 38 55 61 79 96 102 107 117 119 122
Primary Contact: Scott Peek, President and Chief Executive Officer
CMO: Philip Tippin, M.D., Chief of Staff
CIO: Amber Bottoms, Director Medical Records
CHR: Stacey Lane, Executive Assistant Human Resources
Web address: www.chambershospital.com
Control: Other not–for–profit (including NFP Corporation) **Service:** General Medical and Surgical

Staffed Beds: 37 **Admissions:** 2309 **Census:** 19 **Outpatient Visits:** 26760 **Births:** 0 **Total Expense ($000):** 13697 **Payroll Expense ($000):** 5937 **Personnel:** 187

DARDANELLE—Yell County

RIVER VALLEY MEDICAL CENTER (41302), (Formerly Dardanelle Hospital), 200 North Third Street, Zip 72834–3802, Mailing Address: P.O. Box 578, Zip 72834–0578; tel. 479/229–4677 **A**9 10 18 **F**3 25 31 38 54 55 57 62 63 65 66 68 73 79 84 85 86 88 93 96 117 118 122 137 **P**5 6
Primary Contact: Joseph J. Mitchell, Chief Executive Officer
CMO: William P. Scott, M.D., Chief of Staff
CHR: Kathy Hastin, Administrative Assistant Human Resources
Control: Corporation, Investor–owned, for–profit **Service:** General Medical and Surgical

Staffed Beds: 35 **Admissions:** 271 **Census:** 3 **Outpatient Visits:** 3725 **Births:** 0 **Total Expense ($000):** 4083 **Payroll Expense ($000):** 2084 **Personnel:** 104

DE QUEEN—Sevier County

DE QUEEN MEDICAL CENTER (41319), 1306 Collin Raye Drive, Zip 71832–2198; tel. 870/584–4111 **A**9 10 18 **F**3 11 15 25 26 31 38 55 57 66 75 79 80 82 84 85 86 96 102 107 122 **S** Promise Healthcare
Primary Contact: Layne Webb, Chief Executive Officer
COO: Teresa Hodges, Assistant Administrator
CFO: Lorie Tudor, Chief Financial Officer
CHR: Teresa Hodges, Assistant Administrator
Web address: www.dequeenmedicalcenter.com
Control: Corporation, Investor–owned, for–profit **Service:** General Medical and Surgical

Staffed Beds: 35 **Admissions:** 1007 **Census:** 10 **Outpatient Visits:** 16406 **Births:** 0 **Total Expense ($000):** 6884 **Payroll Expense ($000):** 4036 **Personnel:** 123

DE WITT—Arkansas County

★ **DEWITT HOSPITAL (41314)**, Highway 1 and Madison Street, Zip 72042–9481, Mailing Address: P.O. Box 32, Zip 72042–0032; tel. 870/946–3571, (Total facility includes 60 beds in nursing home–type unit) **A**9 10 18 **F**3 7 11 25 32 38 61 62 65 86 96 107 122 **P**5 8
Primary Contact: Darren Caldwell, Chief Executive Officer
CMO: Stan Burleson, M.D., Chief Medical Staff
CIO: Christy McFerrin, Chief Information Officer
CHR: Laura Rush, Director Accounting and Human Resources
Control: Other not–for–profit (including NFP Corporation) **Service:** General Medical and Surgical

Staffed Beds: 85 **Admissions:** 480 **Census:** 59 **Outpatient Visits:** 8524 **Births:** 0 **Total Expense ($000):** 8381 **Payroll Expense ($000):** 4106 **Personnel:** 149

DUMAS—Desha County

★ **DELTA MEMORIAL HOSPITAL (41326)**, 811 South Highway 65, Zip 71639, Mailing Address: P.O. Box 887, Zip 71639–0887; tel. 870/382–4303 **A**9 10 18 **F**3 8 11 13 15 25 30 31 32 33 38 56 57 61 74 79 84 86 96 100 102 107 108 119 121 122 135 137
Primary Contact: Kent Strum, Interim Chief Executive Officer
CFO: David Jones, Interim Chief Financial Officer
CMO: Cobra Shanley–Kulik, M.D., Chief of Staff
CIO: Paula Smith, Chief Information Officer
CHR: Doris Fortenberry, Coordinator Human Resources
Web address: www.deltamem.org
Control: Other not–for–profit (including NFP Corporation) **Service:** General Medical and Surgical

Staffed Beds: 25 **Admissions:** 715 **Census:** 6 **Outpatient Visits:** 14381 **Births:** 162 **Total Expense ($000):** 11163 **Payroll Expense ($000):** 3790 **Personnel:** 112

EL DORADO—Union County

⊡ **MEDICAL CENTER OF SOUTH ARKANSAS (40088)**, 700 West Grove Street, Zip 71730–4416, Mailing Address: P.O. Box 1998, Zip 71731–1998; tel. 870/863–2000 **A**1 9 10 19 20 **F**3 11 13 15 17 18 20 22 24 25 27 30 31 32 33 38 43 54 55 57 61 62 68 70 71 72 73 74 76 77 78 79 80 84 85 86 96 97 100 102 103 107 109 117 119 135 136 **P**7 8 **S** Community Health Systems, Inc.
Primary Contact: Luther J. Lewis, FACHE, Chief Executive Officer
COO: Charles H. Long, Chief Operating Officer
CFO: Frank Canova, Chief Financial Officer
CHR: LaKeitha Davis, Director Human Resources
Web address: www.themedcenter.net
Control: Partnership, Investor–owned, for–profit **Service:** General Medical and Surgical

Staffed Beds: 140 **Admissions:** 5603 **Census:** 76 **Outpatient Visits:** 74631 **Births:** 707 **Total Expense ($000):** 73523 **Payroll Expense ($000):** 24846 **Personnel:** 596

EUREKA SPRINGS—Carroll County

★ **EUREKA SPRINGS HOSPITAL (41304)**, 24 Norris Street, Zip 72632–3541; tel. 479/253–7400 **A**9 10 18 **F**3 11 15 25 26 30 31 32 33 38 41 42 50 55 57 61 62 66 73 75 79 80 81 82 84 85 86 96 100 107 117 119 120 121 122 135 137
Primary Contact: David Wheeler, Administrator
CFO: Christina Barnes, Director Financial Services
CMO: Gregory Kresse, M.D., Chairman Medical Staff
CHR: Jodi Smith, Administrative Assistant Human Resources
Web address: www.eurekaspringshospital.com
Control: Corporation, Investor–owned, for–profit **Service:** General Medical and Surgical

Staffed Beds: 15 **Admissions:** 546 **Census:** 9 **Outpatient Visits:** 3732 **Births:** 0 **Total Expense ($000):** 4351 **Payroll Expense ($000):** 2582 **Personnel:** 79

FAYETTEVILLE—Washington County

⊡ **HEALTHSOUTH REHABILITATION HOSPITAL (43032)**, 153 East Monte Painter Drive, Zip 72703–4002; tel. 479/444–2200 **A**1 9 10 **F**30 31 32 85 **S** HEALTHSOUTH Corporation
Primary Contact: Jerry Alexander, Chief Executive Officer
CFO: Toni Hinrichs, Chief Financial Officer
CMO: Marty Hurlbut, M.D., Medical Director
CHR: Maria Altmann, Director Human Resources
Web address: www.healthsouth.com
Control: Corporation, Investor–owned, for–profit **Service:** Rehabilitation

Staffed Beds: 60 **Admissions:** 904 **Census:** 31 **Outpatient Visits:** 16490 **Births:** 0 **Total Expense ($000):** 11072 **Payroll Expense ($000):** 5410 **Personnel:** 118

⊡ **REGENCY HOSPITAL OF NORTHWEST ARKANSAS (42009)**, 1125 North College, Zip 72703; tel. 479/713–7000 **A**1 9 10 **F**1 3 25 30 31 32 66 73 80 81 82 119 137 **P**8 **S** Regency Hospital Company
Primary Contact: Michael A. McLean, Chief Executive Officer
Web address: www.regencyhospital.com
Control: Corporation, Investor–owned, for–profit **Service:** Long–Term Acute Care hospital

Staffed Beds: 25 **Admissions:** 299 **Census:** 20 **Outpatient Visits:** 0 **Births:** 0 **Personnel:** 122

⊡ **VETERANS AFFAIRS MEDICAL CENTER**, 1100 North College Avenue, Zip 72703–6995; tel. 479/443–4301 **A**1 **F**3 5 25 26 27 30 31 32 33 34 36 37 38 39 41 42 43 44 45 50 53 54 55 57 60 61 62 63 66 68 72 73 76 77 79 80 81 82 86 87 88 90 91 92 93 94 95 96 100 102 107 119 121 122 124 132 133 135 136 137 **S** Department of Veterans Affairs
Primary Contact: Kathleen R. Fogarty, M.S., Director
COO: Doris B. Cassidy, Associate Director
CFO: James Hurst, Chief Fiscal Service
CMO: Bonnie Baker, M.D., Chief Medical Services
CIO: Dale Nelson, Chief Information Officer
CHR: Kathryn L. Barker, Chief Human Resources Management
Web address: www.va.gov/sta/guide/home.asp
Control: Veterans Affairs, Government, federal **Service:** General Medical and Surgical

Staffed Beds: 70 **Admissions:** 3933 **Census:** 55 **Outpatient Visits:** 421163 **Births:** 0 **Total Expense ($000):** 84304 **Payroll Expense ($000):** 61160 **Personnel:** 1024

□ **VISTA HEALTH (44004)**, 4253 North Crossover Road, Zip 72703–4596; tel. 479/521–5731 **A**1 9 10 **F**31 32 82 88 89 90 91 92 94 119 121 **P**6
Primary Contact: Kyle Naples, Chief Executive Officer
CFO: Denise O'Dell, Controller
CMO: Norman Snyder, M.D., Medical Director
Web address: www.vistahealthservices.com
Control: Corporation, Investor–owned, for–profit **Service:** Psychiatric

Staffed Beds: 66 **Admissions:** 897 **Census:** 56 **Outpatient Visits:** 34396 **Births:** 0 **Total Expense ($000):** 17180 **Payroll Expense ($000):** 8167 **Personnel:** 239

⊡ **WASHINGTON REGIONAL MEDICAL CENTER (40004)**, 3215 North Hills Boulevard, Zip 72703–1994; tel. 479/463–1000 **A**1 2 9 10 **F**3 11 13 14 17 18 20 22 24 25 26 27 28 31 33 38 40 42 43 44 46 47 48 49 50 51 52 53 54 55 56 57 58 59 60 61 62 66 68 70 72 73 75 76 77 79 80 81 82 86 87 88 90 92 93 96 97 98 100 102 103 106 107 115 118 119 120 121 124 131 135 136 137 **P**8
Primary Contact: William L. Bradley, President and Chief Executive Officer
CFO: Dan Eckels, Chief Financial Officer
CMO: David Ratcliff, M.D., Chief Medical Affairs
CIO: Becky Magee, Chief Information Officer
CHR: Steve Percival, Director Human Resources
Web address: www.wregional.com
Control: Other not–for–profit (including NFP Corporation) **Service:** General Medical and Surgical

Staffed Beds: 256 **Admissions:** 14801 **Census:** 173 **Outpatient Visits:** 157469 **Births:** 1263 **Total Expense ($000):** 176403 **Payroll Expense ($000):** 65646 **Personnel:** 1367

FORDYCE—Dallas County

★ **DALLAS COUNTY MEDICAL CENTER (41317)**, 201 Clifton Street, Zip 71742–3099; tel. 870/352–6300 **A**9 10 18 **F**11 25 26 31 32 33 38 55 57 79 86 96 107 122
Primary Contact: Scott Kelly, Administrator
CFO: Billie Launius, Director Business Finance
CMO: Michael Payne, M.D., Chief of Staff
CHR: Audrey Allen, Coordinator Benefits
Web address: www.dcmc.org
Control: County–Government, nonfederal **Service:** General Medical and Surgical

Staffed Beds: 22 **Admissions:** 352 **Census:** 3 **Outpatient Visits:** 16027 **Births:** 0 **Total Expense ($000):** 7218 **Payroll Expense ($000):** 2324 **Personnel:** 79

Hospital, Medicare Provider Number, Address, Telephone, Approval, Facility, and Physician Codes, Health Care System

★ American Hospital Association (AHA) membership
□ The Joint Commission accreditation
○ American Osteopathic Association (AOA) accreditation
△ Commission on Accreditation of Rehabilitation Facilities (CARF) accreditation

FORREST CITY—St. Francis County

★ **FORREST CITY MEDICAL CENTER (40019)**, 1601 Newcastle Road, Zip 72335, Mailing Address: P.O. Box 667, Zip 72336–0667; tel. 870/261–0000 **A**1 9 10 20 **F**3 7 13 15 25 26 31 38 49 74 77 79 80 84 86 88 93 96 100 107 118 119 122 136 **S** Community Health Systems, Inc.
Primary Contact: Brett Kinman, Chief Executive Officer
CFO: Stephen Doherty, Chief Financial Officer
CMO: George Conner, M.D., Chief of Staff
CHR: Charles Buchert, Director Human Resources
Web address: www.chs.net
Control: Corporation, Investor–owned, for–profit **Service:** General Medical and Surgical

Staffed Beds: 70 **Admissions:** 2735 **Census:** 26 **Outpatient Visits:** 23365 **Births:** 759 **Total Expense ($000):** 20281 **Payroll Expense ($000):** 9305 **Personnel:** 220

FORT SMITH—Sebastian County

★ **ADVANCE CARE HOSPITAL OF FORT SMITH (42008)**, 7301 Rogers Avenue, 4th Floor, Zip 72917; tel. 479/314–4900 **A**9 10 **F**1 3 25 26 43 44 66 73 80 119 137 **S** Dubuis Health System
Primary Contact: Susan Legg, Administrator
Web address: www.dubuis.org
Control: Church–operated, Nongovernment, not–for profit **Service:** Long–Term Acute Care hospital

Staffed Beds: 25 **Admissions:** 234 **Census:** 20 **Outpatient Visits:** 0 **Births:** 0 **Total Expense ($000):** 7908 **Payroll Expense ($000):** 2901 **Personnel:** 74

★ **HEALTHSOUTH REHABILITATION HOSPITAL OF FORT SMITH (43028)**, 1401 South J Street, Zip 72901–5155; tel. 479/785–3300 **A**1 9 10 **F**3 9 24 25 31 32 33 34 43 54 55 56 57 62 73 75 81 82 85 86 118 119 120 121 137 **S** HEALTHSOUTH Corporation
Primary Contact: Julianne Stec, Chief Executive Officer
CFO: Kathy King, Chief Financial Officer
CHR: Penny Lensing, Director Human Resources
Web address: www.healthsouth.com
Control: Corporation, Investor–owned, for–profit **Service:** Rehabilitation

Staffed Beds: 80 **Admissions:** 1065 **Census:** 35 **Outpatient Visits:** 15420 **Births:** 0 **Total Expense ($000):** 9445 **Payroll Expense ($000):** 5416 **Personnel:** 125

☐ **SELECT SPECIALTY HOSPITAL – FORT SMITH (42006)**, 1131 South I Street, Zip 72917; tel. 479/441–3960 **A**1 9 10 **F**1 3 25 31 75 119 137 **S** Select Medical Corporation
Primary Contact: Cindy McLain, Chief Executive Officer
Web address: www.selectmedicalcorp.com
Control: Corporation, Investor–owned, for–profit **Service:** Long–Term Acute Care hospital

Staffed Beds: 34 **Admissions:** 368 **Census:** 25 **Outpatient Visits:** 0 **Births:** 0 **Total Expense ($000):** 11349 **Payroll Expense ($000):** 3632 **Personnel:** 82

★ **SPARKS REGIONAL MEDICAL CENTER (40055)**, 1311 South I Street, Zip 72901–4995, Mailing Address: P.O. Box 17006, Zip 72917–7006; tel. 479/441–4000 **A**1 2 9 10 **F**3 7 8 11 13 15 17 18 20 22 24 25 26 27 32 33 37 38 43 47 49 50 51 52 53 54 55 56 57 58 59 60 61 62 63 67 68 70 72 73 74 75 76 77 78 79 80 81 82 84 86 87 88 93 96 97 98 100 102 103 106 107 117 119 120 121 124 135 137 **P**3 8 **S** QHR
Primary Contact: Frederick D. Woodrell, FACHE, Chief Executive Officer
COO: Ronald J. Vigus, Chief Operating Officer
CFO: Dan Hamman, Chief Financial Officer
CIO: David Stone, Chief Information Officer
CHR: John Dodd, Vice President Human Resources
Web address: www.sparks.org
Control: Other not–for–profit (including NFP Corporation) **Service:** General Medical and Surgical

Staffed Beds: 303 **Admissions:** 12774 **Census:** 183 **Outpatient Visits:** 100849 **Births:** 1229 **Total Expense ($000):** 148580 **Payroll Expense ($000):** 56969 **Personnel:** 1804

★ △ **ST. EDWARD MERCY MEDICAL CENTER (40062)**, 7301 Rogers Avenue, Zip 72903–4189, Mailing Address: P.O. Box 17000, Zip 72917–7000; tel. 479/314–6000 **A**1 2 7 9 10 **F**3 11 12 13 15 17 18 20 22 24 25 26 27 30 31 32 33 37 38 41 42 43 44 45 51 52 53 55 57 59 60 61 66 68 70 71 72 73 74 75 76 77 79 80 81 82 84 85 86 96 97 99 100 102 103 106 107 109 111 116 117 118 119 124 132 135 136 137 **P**6 **S** Sisters of Mercy Health System
Primary Contact: Jerry L. Stevenson, FACHE, Chief Executive Officer
CFO: Greta Wilcher, Senior Vice President and Chief Financial Officer
CMO: Larry W. Pearce, M.D., Vice President Medical Affairs
CHR: Ron Summerhill, Vice President Human Resources
Web address: www.stedwardmercy.com
Control: Church–operated, Nongovernment, not–for profit **Service:** General Medical and Surgical

Staffed Beds: 389 **Admissions:** 15029 **Census:** 224 **Outpatient Visits:** 110013 **Births:** 2497 **Total Expense ($000):** 162129 **Payroll Expense ($000):** 61485 **Personnel:** 1289

HARRISON—Boone County

★ **NORTH ARKANSAS REGIONAL MEDICAL CENTER (40017)**, 620 North Main Street, Zip 72601–2994; tel. 870/365–2000 **A**9 10 19 20 **F**3 7 8 11 13 15 17 24 25 27 30 31 33 37 38 42 47 49 50 51 55 56 57 59 61 66 68 74 75 76 77 79 80 81 82 86 96 97 98 100 102 105 106 107 109 111 117 118 119 121 135 136 137 **P**8
Primary Contact: Timothy E. Hill, President and Chief Executive Officer
COO: Peter K. Leer, Senior Vice President and Chief Operating Officer
CFO: Debbie Henry, Vice President Financial Services
CIO: Kent Kimes, Director Information Systems
CHR: Linda Dickey Melton, Vice President Human Resources
Web address: www.narmc.com
Control: Other not–for–profit (including NFP Corporation) **Service:** General Medical and Surgical

Staffed Beds: 125 **Admissions:** 5082 **Census:** 51 **Outpatient Visits:** 76860 **Births:** 565 **Total Expense ($000):** 53229 **Payroll Expense ($000):** 25424 **Personnel:** 653

HEBER SPRINGS—Cleburne County

★ **BAPTIST HEALTH MEDICAL CENTER–HEBER SPRINGS (41312)**, 1800 Bypass Road, Zip 72543–9135; tel. 501/887–3000 **A**1 9 10 18 **F**3 8 11 15 24 25 26 27 31 32 33 38 48 55 56 57 61 62 63 66 72 73 75 76 77 79 80 86 92 96 100 102 107 118 121 122 123 124 135 **P**3 **S** Baptist Health
Primary Contact: Edward L. Lacy, FACHE, Vice President and Administrator
Web address: www.baptist–health.com
Control: Other not–for–profit (including NFP Corporation) **Service:** General Medical and Surgical

Staffed Beds: 25 **Admissions:** 830 **Census:** 8 **Outpatient Visits:** 29192 **Births:** 0 **Total Expense ($000):** 17789 **Payroll Expense ($000):** 7124 **Personnel:** 184

HELENA—Phillips County

★ **HELENA REGIONAL MEDICAL CENTER (40085)**, 1801 Martin Luther King Drive, Zip 72342, Mailing Address: P.O. Box 788, Zip 72342–0788; tel. 870/338–5800 **A**1 9 10 20 **F**3 13 15 24 25 33 38 56 57 59 61 62 68 73 74 75 79 81 82 85 86 87 96 97 100 107 119 121 122 124 133 134 135 136 137 **S** Community Health Systems, Inc.
Primary Contact: Thomas E. Fewell, Chief Executive Officer
CFO: Amy Rice, Chief Financial Officer
CIO: Jason Jaco, Director Information Technology
CHR: Juril Fonzie, Director Human Resources
Web address: www.helenarmc.com
Control: Corporation, Investor–owned, for–profit **Service:** General Medical and Surgical

Staffed Beds: 100 **Admissions:** 3458 **Census:** 32 **Outpatient Visits:** 27228 **Births:** 305 **Total Expense ($000):** 21867 **Payroll Expense ($000):** 9017 **Personnel:** 217

HOPE—Hempstead County

☐ **MEDICAL PARK HOSPITAL (40091)**, 2001 South Main Street, Zip 71801–8194; tel. 870/777–2323 **A**1 9 10 20 **F**3 8 11 13 15 25 30 31 32 38 42 43 50 54 55 56 57 62 66 68 70 71 73 74 79 80 82 86 87 93 96 97 98 100 102 106 107 118 119 122 135 136 **P**6 7 **S** Signature Hospital Corporation
Primary Contact: Faye Hughes, Interim Chief Executive Officer
COO: Faye Hughes, Chief Nursing Officer and Chief Operating Officer
CIO: Jeff Cook, Director Information Services
CHR: Vickie Barnhill–Keener, Director Human Resources
Web address: www.mphhope.com
Control: Corporation, Investor–owned, for–profit **Service:** General Medical and Surgical

Staffed Beds: 79 **Admissions:** 2406 **Census:** 25 **Outpatient Visits:** 18914 **Births:** 336 **Total Expense ($000):** 21723 **Payroll Expense ($000):** 9841 **Personnel:** 239

HOT SPRINGS—Garland County

★ △ **NATIONAL PARK MEDICAL CENTER (40078)**, 1910 Malvern Avenue, Zip 71901–7799; tel. 501/321–1000 **A**1 7 9 10 19 **F**3 11 13 15 18 20 22 24 25 26 27 31 32 33 38 46 47 48 49 54 55 56 57 61 62 68 71 72 73 74 76 77 78 79 80 82 84 85 86 96 97 100 102 107 112 117 119 120 121 124 132 135 136 137 **P**1 **S** Capella Healthcare
Primary Contact: Jerry D. Mabry, Chief Executive Officer
CFO: Robbie Pettey, Chief Financial Officer
CMO: William Cole, M.D., Chief of Staff
CIO: Thomas Elmore, Director Information System
CHR: Sandra Culliver, Director Human Resources
Web address: www.nationalparkmedical.com
Control: Corporation, Investor–owned, for–profit **Service:** General Medical and Surgical

Staffed Beds: 181 **Admissions:** 5305 **Census:** 77 **Outpatient Visits:** 21273 **Births:** 766 **Total Expense ($000):** 55424 **Payroll Expense ($000):** 22405 **Personnel:** 624

HOT SPRINGS NATIONAL PARK—Garland County

☒ **ADVANCE CARE HOSPITAL (42004)**, 300 Werner Street, 3rd Floor East, Zip 71913; tel. 501/609–4300 **A**1 9 10 **F**1 3 25 26 66 75 77 80 82 119 124 137 **P**5 **S** Dubuis Health System
Primary Contact: Keith Rogers, Administrator
CFO: Paul Veillon, CPA, Chief Financial Officer
CIO: David Hammon, Director Information Services
CHR: Deborah Farrer, Manager Human Resources
Web address: www.dubuis.org
Control: Church–operated, Nongovernment, not–for profit **Service:** Long–Term Acute Care hospital

Staffed Beds: 27 **Admissions:** 321 **Census:** 23 **Outpatient Visits:** 0 **Births:** 0 **Total Expense ($000):** 8480 **Payroll Expense ($000):** 2927 **Personnel:** 70

HEALTHPARK HOSPITAL (40142), 1636 Higdon Ferry Road, Zip 71913; tel. 501/520–2000 **A**9 10 **F**3 11 15 25 27 32 37 38 43 54 55 57 62 66 72 73 75 76 77 79 80 86 96 97 100 107 118 119 120 135 136 137
Primary Contact: Jason A. Spring, FACHE, Chief Executive Officer and Administrator
CFO: Joe Gross, Chief Financial Officer
CHR: Michael Moffit, Manager Human Resources
Web address: www.healthparkhospital.com
Control: Corporation, Investor–owned, for–profit **Service:** General Medical and Surgical

Staffed Beds: 20 **Admissions:** 1316 **Census:** 12 **Outpatient Visits:** 30443 **Births:** 0 **Total Expense ($000):** 21246 **Payroll Expense ($000):** 5032 **Personnel:** 112

HOT SPRINGS REHABILITATION CENTER (43027), 105 Reserve Avenue, Zip 71902, Mailing Address: P.O. Box 1358, Zip 71902; tel. 501/624–4411 **A**9 10 **F**3 10 11 12 25 26 36 37 41 50 62 64 66 72 73 77 82 85 86 87 89 90 91 94 119 121 132 137 **P**6
Primary Contact: Howard J. Rutenberg, Administrator
CMO: Patricia Lang, M.D., Medical Director
CIO: Dean Ulmer, Manager Information Services
Web address: www.arsinfo.org/hsrehab.html
Control: State–Government, nonfederal **Service:** Rehabilitation

Staffed Beds: 28 **Admissions:** 64 **Census:** 4 **Outpatient Visits:** 8367 **Births:** 0 **Total Expense ($000):** 4772 **Payroll Expense ($000):** 3792 **Personnel:** 125

★ **LEVI HOSPITAL (40132)**, 300 Prospect Avenue, Zip 71901–4097; tel. 501/624–1281 **A**9 10 **F**9 30 31 32 38 42 54 55 57 61 62 66 86 88 92 93 94 119 120 121 132 135
Primary Contact: Patrick G. McCabe, Jr., FACHE, President and Chief Executive Officer
CFO: Charles Oswalt, Vice President and Chief Financial Officer
CMO: P. Ross Bandy, M.D., Chief Medical Officer and Chief of Staff
Web address: www.levihospital.com
Control: Other not–for–profit (including NFP Corporation) **Service:** Psychiatric

Staffed Beds: 27 **Admissions:** 607 **Census:** 15 **Outpatient Visits:** 16696 **Births:** 0 **Total Expense ($000):** 6751 **Payroll Expense ($000):** 3448 **Personnel:** 94

☒ **ST. JOSEPH'S MERCY HEALTH CENTER (40026)**, 300 Werner Street, Zip 71913–9937, Mailing Address: P.O. Box 29001, Zip 71913–9001; tel. 501/622–1000 **A**1 2 9 10 19 **F**3 11 13 15 17 18 20 22 24 25 26 27 30 31 32 33 38 42 43 44 49 50 54 55 56 57 61 62 63 66 67 68 69 72 73 74 75 76 77 79 80 81 82 84 85 86 88 93 96 97 99 102 103 107 108 109 117 118 119 121 124 132 133 135 136 137 **P**2 7 **S** Sisters of Mercy Health System
Primary Contact: Timothy J. Johnsen, President and Chief Executive Officer
CFO: Larry D. Alford, Chief Financial Officer
CMO: Mark Larey, D.O., Vice President Medical Affairs
CIO: Judy Preuitt, Director Information Systems
CHR: Jed Liuzza, Executive Director Human Resources
Web address: www.saintjosephs.com
Control: Church–operated, Nongovernment, not–for profit **Service:** General Medical and Surgical

Staffed Beds: 264 **Admissions:** 13169 **Census:** 187 **Outpatient Visits:** 423323 **Births:** 1001 **Total Expense ($000):** 159606 **Payroll Expense ($000):** 69378 **Personnel:** 1423

JACKSONVILLE—Pulaski County

☒ **NORTH METRO MEDICAL CENTER (40074)**, (Formerly Rebsamen Medical Center), 1400 West Braden Street, Zip 72076–3788; tel. 501/985–7000 **A**1 9 10 **F**3 11 13 15 17 20 25 26 31 32 33 38 50 51 54 55 56 57 61 62 66 68 73 74 75 77 79 81 82 85 88 93 96 100 102 107 118 119 120 121 124 135 136 137 **P**1 3 **S** QHR
Primary Contact: Scott M. Landrum, Chief Executive Officer
Web address: www.rebsamenmedicalcenter.com
Control: Other not–for–profit (including NFP Corporation) **Service:** General Medical and Surgical

Staffed Beds: 111 **Admissions:** 3318 **Census:** 43 **Outpatient Visits:** 65391 **Births:** 505 **Total Expense ($000):** 38790 **Payroll Expense ($000):** 17312 **Personnel:** 368

JOHNSON—Washington County

☒ **WILLOW CREEK WOMEN'S HOSPITAL (40141)**, 4301 Greathouse Springs Road, Zip 72741–0544, Mailing Address: P.O. Box 544, Zip 72741–0544; tel. 479/684–3000 **A**1 9 10 **F**3 11 13 15 30 31 32 38 55 66 69 73 74 79 107 136 **S** Community Health Systems, Inc.
Primary Contact: Gary N. Looper, Chief Executive Officer
COO: Linda Worman, Administrator and Chief Operating Officer
CFO: Shawn Barnett, Chief Financial Officer
CIO: Shannon Williams, Chief Information Officer
CHR: Mike Meeks, Vice President Human Resources
Web address: www.northwesthealth.com
Control: Corporation, Investor–owned, for–profit **Service:** Obstetrics and gynecology

Staffed Beds: 30 **Admissions:** 3382 **Census:** 18 **Outpatient Visits:** 12122 **Births:** 2984 **Total Expense ($000):** 15989 **Payroll Expense ($000):** 7116 **Personnel:** 148

JONESBORO—Craighead County

☒ **HEALTHSOUTH REHABILITATION HOSPITAL OF JONESBORO (43029)**, 1201 Fleming Avenue, Zip 72401–4311, Mailing Address: P.O. Box 1680, Zip 72403–1680; tel. 870/932–0440 **A**1 9 10 **F**24 25 32 55 57 62 85 86 119 121 132 **S** HEALTHSOUTH Corporation
Primary Contact: Donna Harris, Chief Executive Officer
CFO: Allan Jones, Controller
CMO: Terence Braden, D.O., Medical Director
CHR: Tammy Barley, Manager Human Resources
Web address: www.healthsouth.com
Control: Corporation, Investor–owned, for–profit **Service:** Rehabilitation

Staffed Beds: 67 **Admissions:** 1186 **Census:** 39 **Outpatient Visits:** 7198 **Births:** 0 **Total Expense ($000):** 10515 **Payroll Expense ($000):** 5303 **Personnel:** 168

☒ **NEA BAPTIST MEMORIAL HOSPITAL (40118)**, (Formerly NEA Medical Center), 3024 Stadium Boulevard, Zip 72401–7493; tel. 870/972–7000 **A**1 9 10 **F**3 11 12 13 17 18 20 22 24 25 26 27 30 32 37 38 43 44 46 49 50 51 55 57 59 72 73 74 75 76 77 79 80 81 82 86 96 97 100 102 106 107 135 137 **P**8 **S** Baptist Memorial Health Care Corporation
Primary Contact: Paul Betz, Chief Executive Officer
CFO: Matthew Tulin, Chief Financial Officer
CMO: James Ameika, M.D., Chief of Staff
CHR: Kevin Thielemier, Director Human Resources
Web address: www.neamedicalcenter.com
Control: Partnership, Investor–owned, for–profit **Service:** General Medical and Surgical

Staffed Beds: 104 **Admissions:** 6073 **Census:** 63 **Outpatient Visits:** 37267 **Births:** 728 **Total Expense ($000):** 57730 **Payroll Expense ($000):** 19205 **Personnel:** 453

☐ **ST. BERNARD'S BEHAVIORAL HEALTH (44010)**, 2712 East Johnson Avenue, Zip 72401–1874; tel. 870/932–2800, (Nonreporting) **A**1 9 10
Primary Contact: George S. Fray, Administrator
CMO: Bert Price, M.D., Medical Director
CIO: Jan Lampkins, Director Medical Records
Control: Church–operated, Nongovernment, not–for profit **Service:** Psychiatric

Staffed Beds: 60

AR

Hospital, Medicare Provider Number, Address, Telephone, Approval, Facility, and Physician Codes, Health Care System
★ American Hospital Association (AHA) membership
☐ The Joint Commission accreditation
○ American Osteopathic Association (AOA) accreditation
△ Commission on Accreditation of Rehabilitation Facilities (CARF) accreditation

☒ **ST. BERNARDS MEDICAL CENTER (40020)**, 225 East Jackson Avenue, Zip 72401; tel. 870/972–4100, (Total facility includes 27 beds in nursing home–type unit) **A**1 9 10 19 **F**2 3 11 12 13 15 17 18 20 22 24 25 26 27 28 30 31 32 33 35 38 42 43 44 46 48 49 50 51 52 53 54 55 56 57 58 59 60 61 62 66 67 68 69 72 73 74 75 76 77 79 80 81 82 84 86 88 89 90 91 92 93 94 95 96 97 99 100 102 103 104 105 107 108 109 111 117 118 119 120 121 124 133 135 136 137 **P**2 6 8
Primary Contact: Chris Barber, FACHE, Administrator
CFO: Harry Hutchison, Vice President Fiscal Services
CMO: David Pyle, M.D., Vice President Medical Affairs
CIO: Charles Pigg, Chief Information Officer
CHR: Pat Overman, Vice President Human Resources
Web address: www.sbrmc.com
Control: Church–operated, Nongovernment, not–for profit **Service:** General Medical and Surgical

Staffed Beds: 375 **Admissions:** 17395 **Census:** 211 **Outpatient Visits:** 208353 **Births:** 1447 **Total Expense ($000):** 194836 **Payroll Expense ($000):** 62419 **Personnel:** 1753

SURGICAL HOSPITAL OF JONESBORO (40145), 909 Enterprise Drive, Zip 72401; tel. 870/336–1100 **A**9 10 **F**3 25 38 43 62 66 72 73 77 79 80 86 96 100 102 118
Primary Contact: Nate Miller, Chief Executive Officer
CFO: Carla Harral, Chief Financial Officer
CMO: Jason Brandt, M.D., Medical Director
CHR: Angie Stover, Administrative Assistant
Web address: www.tshj.com
Control: Partnership, Investor–owned, for–profit **Service:** General Medical and Surgical

Staffed Beds: 12 **Admissions:** 850 **Census:** 4 **Outpatient Visits:** 10813 **Births:** 0 **Total Expense ($000):** 16967 **Payroll Expense ($000):** 3080 **Personnel:** 92

LAKE VILLAGE—Chicot County

★ **CHICOT MEMORIAL HOSPITAL (41328)**, 2729 Highway 65 and 82 South, Zip 71653; tel. 870/265–5351 **A**9 10 18 **F**3 13 15 24 25 30 31 32 33 38 61 62 73 74 79 80 82 86 96 106 107 119 121 122 135 137 **S** QHR
Primary Contact: Bruce A. Bennett, Interim Chief Executive Officer
COO: Beth Holt, Chief Nursing Officer
CFO: Don Wade, Chief Financial Officer
CMO: J R Russell, Chief of Staff
CIO: David Andrews, Manager Information Systems
CHR: Rene Jones, Director Human Resources
Web address: www.chicotmemorial.com
Control: County–Government, nonfederal **Service:** General Medical and Surgical

Staffed Beds: 25 **Admissions:** 1484 **Census:** 14 **Outpatient Visits:** 15271 **Births:** 44 **Total Expense ($000):** 13478 **Payroll Expense ($000):** 5533 **Personnel:** 165

LITTLE ROCK—Pulaski County

ALLEGIANCE SPECIALTY HOSPITAL OF LITTLE ROCK (40148), 11401 Interstate 30, 2nd Floor, Zip 72209; tel. 501/455–7300, (Nonreporting) **A**9 10
Primary Contact: Richard Shelton, Chief Executive Officer
Control: Corporation, Investor–owned, for–profit **Service:** Long–Term Acute Care hospital

Staffed Beds: 40

☒ △ **ARKANSAS CHILDREN'S HOSPITAL (43300)**, 800 Marshall Street, Zip 72202–3591; tel. 501/364–1100 **A**1 3 5 7 8 9 10 **F**3 7 9 11 12 16 17 19 21 23 24 25 26 27 28 31 33 36 37 38 43 44 48 50 52 55 57 58 59 60 62 66 70 72 73 75 76 77 79 80 81 82 83 84 86 87 90 92 96 97 100 102 104 105 106 107 114 116 118 119 120 121 124 125 126 127 132 135 **P**1
Primary Contact: Jonathan R. Bates, M.D., President and Chief Executive Officer
COO: David Berry, Executive Vice President and Chief Operating Officer
CFO: Gena Wingfield, Senior Vice President and Chief Financial Officer
CMO: Bonnie Taylor, M.D., Senior Vice President and Medical Director
CIO: Darrell Leonhardt, Senior Vice President Information Systems
CHR: Andrea Trosclair, Vice President Human Resources
Web address: www.archildrens.org
Control: Other not–for–profit (including NFP Corporation) **Service:** Children's general

Staffed Beds: 295 **Admissions:** 13478 **Census:** 230 **Outpatient Visits:** 264853 **Births:** 0 **Total Expense ($000):** 370783 **Payroll Expense ($000):** 167546 **Personnel:** 3244

☐ **ARKANSAS HEART HOSPITAL (40134)**, 1701 South Shackleford Road, Zip 72211–4335; tel. 501/219–7000 **A**1 5 9 10 **F**3 11 17 18 20 22 25 26 33 38 55 56 57 58 68 73 79 81 92 96 100 102 107 119 137 **P**8 **S** MedCath, Inc.
Primary Contact: Charlie Smith, President
CFO: Bryan Nichols, Chief Financial Officer
CHR: Brent Davis, Human Resources Team Leader
Web address: www.arheart.com
Control: Corporation, Investor–owned, for–profit **Service:** General Medical and Surgical

Staffed Beds: 84 **Admissions:** 6915 **Census:** 64 **Outpatient Visits:** 7184 **Births:** 0 **Total Expense ($000):** 77590 **Payroll Expense ($000):** 25441 **Personnel:** 498

☐ **ARKANSAS STATE HOSPITAL (44011)**, 305 South Plam Street, Zip 72205–4096; tel. 501/686–9000 **A**1 3 5 9 10 **F**11 25 26 30 32 36 50 52 63 73 75 81 82 87 88 89 90 91 119 121 124 132 135 **P**6
Primary Contact: Charles Smith, Administrator
CFO: Jo Ann McDade, Assistant Administrator Finance
CMO: Albert Kittrell, M.D., Medical Director
CHR: Betty Schwartz, Director Human Resources
Web address: www.state.ar.us/dhs/dmhs
Control: State–Government, nonfederal **Service:** Psychiatric

Staffed Beds: 202 **Admissions:** 883 **Census:** 170 **Outpatient Visits:** 0 **Births:** 0 **Total Expense ($000):** 37037 **Payroll Expense ($000):** 16603 **Personnel:** 608

☒ △ **BAPTIST HEALTH MEDICAL CENTER–LITTLE ROCK (40114)**, 9601 Interstate 630, Exit 7, Zip 72205–7299; tel. 501/202–2000 **A**1 3 5 6 7 9 10 **F**3 4 5 7 8 11 12 13 15 17 18 20 22 24 25 26 27 28 30 31 32 33 34 35 36 38 41 43 49 50 53 54 55 56 57 58 59 60 61 62 63 65 66 68 70 71 72 73 74 75 76 77 79 80 81 82 84 86 88 89 90 91 92 93 94 96 97 98 100 102 103 104 106 107 116 117 118 119 120 121 123 124 126 127 132 133 135 136 137 **S** Baptist Health
Primary Contact: Steven Douglas Weeks, FACHE, Senior Vice President and Administrator
CFO: Allen F. Smith, Senior Vice President Financial Services
CMO: Philip L. Mizell, M.D., Vice President Clinical Affairs
CIO: David House, Vice President and Chief Information Officer
CHR: Anthony Kendall, Vice President Human Resources
Web address: www.baptist–health.org
Control: Other not–for–profit (including NFP Corporation) **Service:** General Medical and Surgical

Staffed Beds: 721 **Admissions:** 27627 **Census:** 424 **Outpatient Visits:** 107082 **Births:** 2932 **Total Expense ($000):** 372254 **Payroll Expense ($000):** 141655 **Personnel:** 3140

☒ △ **BAPTIST HEALTH REHABILITATION INSTITUTE (43026)**, 9601 Interstate 630, Exit 7, Zip 72205–7249; tel. 501/202–7000 **A**1 3 5 7 9 10 **F**11 25 26 30 31 32 33 50 52 62 73 77 82 85 86 119 121 132 135 **S** Baptist Health
Primary Contact: Greg Crain, Vice President
CFO: Bob Roberts, Vice President
CIO: David House, Vice President and Chief Information Officer
CHR: Anthony Kendall, Vice President Human Resources
Web address: www.baptist–health.com
Control: Other not–for–profit (including NFP Corporation) **Service:** Rehabilitation

Staffed Beds: 100 **Admissions:** 1856 **Census:** 65 **Outpatient Visits:** 162376 **Births:** 0 **Total Expense ($000):** 30738 **Payroll Expense ($000):** 15363 **Personnel:** 289

☒ △ **CENTRAL ARKANSAS VETERANS HEALTHCARE SYSTEM**, 4300 West Seventh Street, Zip 72205–5484; tel. 501/257–1000, (Includes NORTH LITTLE ROCK DIVISION, North Little Rock), (Total facility includes 152 beds in nursing home–type unit) **A**1 2 3 5 7 8 **F**2 3 5 6 15 17 18 20 24 25 26 27 31 32 33 36 37 38 43 44 46 47 48 49 50 52 54 55 56 57 58 59 60 61 62 63 66 68 72 73 75 76 77 79 80 81 82 85 86 87 88 91 92 93 94 95 96 97 100 102 106 107 110 114 117 118 119 121 124 132 133 135 136 137 **P**6 **S** Department of Veterans Affairs
Primary Contact: Michael R. Winn, Director
CFO: Debby Felton, Chief Financial Officer
CMO: Nicholas P. Lang, M.D., Chief of Staff
CIO: Jim Hall, Acting Chief Information Officer
CHR: Daniel Peterson, Chief Human Resource Management Service
Web address: www.va.gov/sta/guide/home.asp
Control: Veterans Affairs, Government, federal **Service:** General Medical and Surgical

Staffed Beds: 583 **Admissions:** 11907 **Census:** 413 **Outpatient Visits:** 620067 **Births:** 0 **Total Expense ($000):** 412582 **Payroll Expense ($000):** 171668 **Personnel:** 3156

LIVING HOPE LITTLE ROCK (44018), 600 South McKinley, Suite 400, Zip 72205; tel. 501/663–4673, (Nonreporting) **A**9 10
Primary Contact: Frank Wright, Chief Executive Officer
Control: Corporation, Investor–owned, for–profit **Service:** Psychiatric

Staffed Beds: 30

☐ **PINNACLE POINTE HOSPITAL (44013)**, 11501 Financial Center Parkway, Zip 72211–3715; tel. 501/223–3322 **A**1 9 10 **F**25 32 88 89 90 91 92 94 119 **P**5 **S** Psychiatric Solutions
Primary Contact: Lisa Evans, Chief Executive Officer
CFO: Johnny Lancaster, Chief Financial Officer
CMO: David Streett, M.D., Medical Director
CHR: James L. Howe, Chief Employee Relations
Web address: www.psysolutions.com
Control: Corporation, Investor–owned, for–profit **Service:** Children's hospital psychiatric

Staffed Beds: 102 **Admissions:** 1826 **Census:** 88 **Outpatient Visits:** 26890 **Births:** 0 **Total Expense ($000):** 15806 **Payroll Expense ($000):** 9012 **Personnel:** 212

☐ **SELECT SPECIALTY HOSPITAL–LITTLE ROCK (42000)**, 2 St. Vincent Circle, 6th Floor, Zip 72204; tel. 501/661–4198 **A**1 10 **F**1 3 25 30 32 43 72 73 75 76 77 80 81 87 90 119 137 **P**5 **S** Select Medical Corporation
Primary Contact: Maureen Henneken, Chief Executive Officer
Web address: www.selectmedicalcorp.com
Control: Corporation, Investor–owned, for–profit **Service:** Long–Term Acute Care hospital

Staffed Beds: 43 **Admissions:** 415 **Census:** 31 **Outpatient Visits:** 0 **Births:** 0 **Total Expense ($000):** 13459 **Payroll Expense ($000):** 5599 **Personnel:** 83

☐ **SOUTHWEST REGIONAL MEDICAL CENTER (40021)**, 11401 Interstate 30, Zip 72209–7056; tel. 501/455–7100 **A**1 9 10 **F**3 6 11 15 18 25 26 30 31 32 33 35 37 38 40 43 48 49 50 51 54 55 56 57 58 59 60 62 64 68 73 75 77 79 80 81 82 86 88 90 91 93 94 96 97 100 102 107 118 119 124 130 135 137 **S** Health Management Associates
Primary Contact: Nancy C. Fodi, FACHE, Chief Executive Officer
CMO: Joseph K. Buchman, M.D., Chief of Staff
CIO: Greg Hicks, Director Information Technology
CHR: Sarah Colley, Director Human Resources
Web address: www.hma–corp.com
Control: Corporation, Investor–owned, for–profit **Service:** General Medical and Surgical

Staffed Beds: 79 **Admissions:** 1368 **Census:** 21 **Outpatient Visits:** 20684 **Births:** 0 **Total Expense ($000):** 25115 **Payroll Expense ($000):** 9611 **Personnel:** 169

☒ **ST. VINCENT INFIRMARY MEDICAL CENTER (40007)**, Two St. Vincent Circle, Zip 72205–5499; tel. 501/552–3000, (Includes ST. VINCENT DOCTORS HOSPITAL, 6101 West Capitol, Zip 72205–5331; tel. 501/552–6000) **A**1 3 5 9 10 **F**3 11 12 13 15 17 18 20 22 24 25 26 27 31 32 33 35 38 40 41 43 44 50 51 52 53 54 55 56 57 59 60 61 62 66 68 70 71 72 73 74 75 76 77 79 80 81 82 85 86 87 88 93 96 97 98 99 100 102 103 104 105 106 107 112 118 119 121 124 132 134 135 136 137 **P**8 **S** Catholic Health Initiatives
Primary Contact: Peter D. Banko, FACHE, President and Chief Executive Officer
CFO: Terry L. Conrad, Interim Senior Vice President and Chief Financial Officer
CMO: David Hall, M.D., Senior Vice President and Chief Medical Affairs
CIO: Tommye Billing, Vice President and Chief Information Officer
Web address: www.stvincenthealth.com
Control: Church–operated, Nongovernment, not–for profit **Service:** General Medical and Surgical

Staffed Beds: 542 **Admissions:** 19595 **Census:** 291 **Outpatient Visits:** 176550 **Births:** 1972 **Total Expense ($000):** 237183 **Payroll Expense ($000):** 89347 **Personnel:** 2063

☒ **UAMS MEDICAL CENTER (40016)**, 4301 West Markham Street, Zip 72205–7102; tel. 501/686–7000 **A**1 3 5 8 9 10 12 13 **F**3 11 13 14 15 17 18 20 22 24 25 26 27 30 31 32 33 34 43 44 46 47 49 50 52 54 57 60 62 66 68 70 71 72 73 74 75 76 77 78 79 80 81 82 86 87 90 91 92 93 94 96 97 98 99 100 102 106 107 108 112 113 114 119 120 121 125 126 127 128 130 131 135 136 137 **P**6
Primary Contact: Richard Pierson, Executive Director
CFO: Daniel J. Riley, Chief Financial Officer
CMO: Nicholas P. Lans, M.D., Chief Medical Officer
CIO: Kari Cassel, Director Clinical Information Systems
CHR: Hosea Long, Director Human Resources
Web address: www.uams.edu/medcenter
Control: State–Government, nonfederal **Service:** General Medical and Surgical

Staffed Beds: 355 **Admissions:** 16923 **Census:** 299 **Outpatient Visits:** 458216 **Births:** 2290 **Total Expense ($000):** 363603 **Payroll Expense ($000):** 132236 **Personnel:** 2797

MAGNOLIA—Columbia County

☒ **MAGNOLIA HOSPITAL (40067)**, 101 Hospital Drive, Zip 71753–2416, Mailing Address: P.O. Box 629, Zip 71753–0629; tel. 870/235–3000 **A**1 9 10 20 **F**11 13 15 25 27 31 33 38 55 57 61 62 68 73 74 75 79 81 84 86 87 96 97 100 102 107 118 119 121 122 133 135 **S** CHRISTUS Health
Primary Contact: Terry L. Amstutz, FACHE, Chief Executive Officer
CFO: Hoye A. Bowman, Chief Financial Officer
CMO: Damon Edwards, M.D., Chief of Staff
CHR: Shawnee Hicks, Manager Human Resources
Web address: www.magnoliahospital.org
Control: City–Government, nonfederal **Service:** General Medical and Surgical

Staffed Beds: 70 **Admissions:** 1960 **Census:** 21 **Outpatient Visits:** 37998 **Births:** 211 **Total Expense ($000):** 18742 **Payroll Expense ($000):** 9338 **Personnel:** 281

MALVERN—Hot Spring County

★ **H.S.C. MEDICAL CENTER (40076)**, 1001 Schneider Drive, Zip 72104–4828; tel. 501/332–1000 **A**9 10 **F**3 8 11 15 17 25 26 31 32 33 38 50 55 56 57 61 62 68 73 75 79 82 86 88 91 92 93 96 100 102 107 118 119 121 134 135 137
Primary Contact: Sheila Williams, Interim Chief Executive Officer
CFO: Sheila Williams, Chief Financial Officer
CHR: Kelli Hopkins, Director Human Resources
Web address: www.hscmc.org
Control: Other not–for–profit (including NFP Corporation) **Service:** General Medical and Surgical

Staffed Beds: 72 **Admissions:** 2539 **Census:** 34 **Outpatient Visits:** 27833 **Births:** 0 **Total Expense ($000):** 22318 **Payroll Expense ($000):** 10709 **Personnel:** 314

AR

MAUMELLE—Pulaski County

☐ **METHODIST BEHAVIORAL HOSPITAL OF ARKANSAS (44017)**, 1601 Murphy Drive, Zip 72113, Mailing Address: P.O. Box 13340, Zip 72113; tel. 501/803–3388 **A**1 3 5 9 10 **F**26 28 30 31 32 36 50 62 73 81 82 88 89 94 **P**1
Primary Contact: Jennifer Lang, Ph.D., Administrator
Web address: www.umch.org
Control: Other not–for–profit (including NFP Corporation) **Service:** Children's hospital psychiatric

Staffed Beds: 60 **Admissions:** 724 **Census:** 52 **Outpatient Visits:** 28877 **Births:** 0 **Total Expense ($000):** 9589 **Payroll Expense ($000):** 4865 **Personnel:** 162

MCGEHEE—Desha County

★ **MCGEHEE–DESHA COUNTY HOSPITAL (41308)**, 900 South Third, Zip 71654–0351, Mailing Address: P.O. Box 351, Zip 71654–0351; tel. 870/222–5600 **A**9 10 18 **F**3 11 25 30 31 32 38 46 55 56 57 61 62 66 79 81 96 107 121 122 124 135
Primary Contact: John E. Heard, Chief Executive Officer
CFO: Sharon Morgan, Chief Financial Officer'
CMO: James Young, M.D., Chief of Staff
Web address: www.mcgeheehospital.org
Control: City–County, Government, nonfederal **Service:** General Medical and Surgical

Staffed Beds: 25 **Admissions:** 552 **Census:** 6 **Outpatient Visits:** 12798 **Births:** 3 **Total Expense ($000):** 6052 **Payroll Expense ($000):** 3396 **Personnel:** 107

MENA—Polk County

★ **MENA REGIONAL HEALTH SYSTEM (40015)**, 311 North Morrow Street, Zip 71953–2516; tel. 479/394–6100 **A**9 10 20 **F**3 11 13 15 25 27 28 33 38 50 53 54 55 56 57 62 65 66 68 73 74 75 76 77 79 81 82 85 86 87 88 89 90 91 92 93 94 96 97 100 102 107 117 118 119 122 133 135 136 **P**8 **S** QHR
Primary Contact: Leland E. Farnell, Interim Chief Executive Officer
CFO: Charles Powell, Chief Financial Officer
CHR: Mary Ellen Winters, Director Human Resources
Web address: www.menaregional.com
Control: City–Government, nonfederal **Service:** General Medical and Surgical

Staffed Beds: 65 **Admissions:** 1866 **Census:** 26 **Outpatient Visits:** 77101 **Births:** 454 **Total Expense ($000):** 21306 **Payroll Expense ($000):** 9323 **Personnel:** 262

MONTICELLO—Drew County

★ **DREW MEMORIAL HOSPITAL (40051)**, 778 Scogin Drive, Zip 71655–5728; tel. 870/367–2411 **A**9 10 20 **F**3 11 13 15 17 25 31 32 33 38 55 56 57 61 62 66 67 68 73 74 79 80 81 82 84 96 97 100 102 107 119 121 122 135
Primary Contact: Bart Millstead, Interim Chief Executive Officer
CFO: Shannon Clark, Chief Financial Officer
CMO: Jeffery Reinhart, M.D., Chief of Staff
CIO: Rusty Bryant, Director Information Technology
CHR: Rick Donham, Director Human Resources
Web address: www.drewmemorial.org
Control: County–Government, nonfederal **Service:** General Medical and Surgical

Staffed Beds: 49 **Admissions:** 2347 **Census:** 23 **Outpatient Visits:** 33578 **Births:** 233 **Total Expense ($000):** 14346 **Payroll Expense ($000):** 7567 **Personnel:** 268

Hospital, Medicare Provider Number, Address, Telephone, Approval, Facility, and Physician Codes, Health Care System
★ American Hospital Association (AHA) membership
☐ The Joint Commission accreditation
○ American Osteopathic Association (AOA) accreditation
△ Commission on Accreditation of Rehabilitation Facilities (CARF) accreditation

MORRILTON—Conway County

★ **ST. ANTHONY'S MEDICAL CENTER (41324)**, 4 Hospital Drive, Zip 72110–4510; tel. 501/977–2300 **A**9 10 18 **F**2 3 11 13 15 17 24 25 26 30 31 32 33 38 50 54 55 57 61 62 68 74 75 77 79 80 82 86 88 93 94 95 96 100 102 107 118 119 120 121 122 124 132 135 **S** Catholic Health Initiatives
Primary Contact: Christina Hockaday, FACHE, Chief Executive Officer
CFO: Tadd Richert, CPA, Chief Financial Officer
CMO: Joel Milligan, M.D., Chief of Staff
CIO: Michelle Moll, Technical Analyst
CHR: Tammy Smith, Director Human Resources
Web address: www.stanthonysmorrilton.com/
Control: Church–operated, Nongovernment, not–for profit **Service:** General Medical and Surgical

Staffed Beds: 35 **Admissions:** 1302 **Census:** 18 **Outpatient Visits:** 22027 **Births:** 81 **Total Expense ($000):** 16630 **Payroll Expense ($000):** 7426 **Personnel:** 187

MOUNTAIN HOME—Baxter County

★ **BAXTER REGIONAL MEDICAL CENTER (40027)**, 624 Hospital Drive, Zip 72653–2954; tel. 870/508–1000 **A**9 10 19 20 **F**7 11 13 15 17 18 20 22 24 25 26 27 31 32 38 42 43 44 46 47 49 52 55 57 61 62 68 69 74 75 76 77 79 80 81 82 85 86 88 93 94 96 97 100 102 103 107 112 118 119 121 124 135 136 137 **P**6 8
Primary Contact: Ron Peterson, President and Chief Executive Officer
COO: Rudy Parling, Chief Operating Officer
CFO: Ivan Holleman, Chief Financial Officer
CHR: Karen Adams, Director Human Resources
Web address: www.baxterregional.org
Control: Other not–for–profit (including NFP Corporation) **Service:** General Medical and Surgical

Staffed Beds: 263 **Admissions:** 10770 **Census:** 125 **Outpatient Visits:** 104770 **Births:** 803 **Total Expense ($000):** 131584 **Payroll Expense ($000):** 51582 **Personnel:** 1190

MOUNTAIN VIEW—Stone County

★ **STONE COUNTY MEDICAL CENTER (41310)**, 2106 East Main Street, Zip 72560, Mailing Address: P.O. Box 510, Zip 72560–0510; tel. 870/269–4361 **A**9 10 18 **F**11 15 25 27 31 32 38 50 55 56 57 62 65 66 73 75 77 79 86 96 98 100 102 107 117 119 120 122 135
Primary Contact: Karen Craft, Administrator
CFO: Gary Brittens, Chief Financial Officer
CIO: Ken Poole, Coordinator Information Systems
CHR: Gary McDonald, Assistant Administrator Human Resources
Web address: www.wrmc.com
Control: Other not–for–profit (including NFP Corporation) **Service:** General Medical and Surgical

Staffed Beds: 25 **Admissions:** 1511 **Census:** 15 **Outpatient Visits:** 18897 **Births:** 1 **Total Expense ($000):** 12250 **Payroll Expense ($000):** 4675 **Personnel:** 118

MURFREESBORO—Pike County

PIKE COUNTY MEMORIAL HOSPITAL (40081), 315 East 13th Street, Zip 71958–9541; tel. 870/285–3182 **A**9 10 **F**1 3 4 16 17 31 38 42 61 62 65 68 70 71 74 78 83 84 85 88 107 117 122 **P**5
Primary Contact: Rosemary Fritts, Administrator
Control: County–Government, nonfederal **Service:** General Medical and Surgical

Staffed Beds: 32 **Admissions:** 362 **Census:** 3 **Outpatient Visits:** 5809 **Births:** 0 **Total Expense ($000):** 1970 **Payroll Expense ($000):** 1180 **Personnel:** 54

NASHVILLE—Howard County

★ **HOWARD MEMORIAL HOSPITAL (41311)**, 800 West Leslie Street, Zip 71852–0381, Mailing Address: P.O. Box 381, Zip 71852–0381; tel. 870/845–4400 **A**9 10 18 **F**3 11 15 25 26 30 31 32 33 37 38 50 54 55 57 61 62 68 73 75 79 80 81 86 87 96 97 102 107 122 135 **S** QHR
Primary Contact: Brian E. Bickel, President and Chief Executive Officer
CFO: Chris Kuhlmann, Chief Financial Officer
CMO: Brian Oge, M.D., Chief of Staff
CIO: Steve Davis, Director Information Management
CHR: Gayla Lacefield, Director Human Resources
Control: Other not–for–profit (including NFP Corporation) **Service:** General Medical and Surgical

Staffed Beds: 25 **Admissions:** 685 **Census:** 6 **Outpatient Visits:** 40441 **Births:** 0 **Total Expense ($000):** 9709 **Payroll Expense ($000):** 4237 **Personnel:** 128

NEWPORT—Jackson County

☒ **HARRIS HOSPITAL (40080)**, 1205 McLain Street, Zip 72112–3533; tel. 870/523–8911 **A**1 9 10 20 **F**3 11 13 15 17 25 26 30 31 32 33 36 38 50 54 55 56 57 61 62 63 68 73 74 75 77 79 80 82 84 92 96 100 102 107 122 124 135 136 **P**6 **S** Community Health Systems, Inc.
Primary Contact: Claude E. Camp, III, Chief Executive Officer
CFO: Misty Gates, Chief Financial Officer
CMO: Jabez Jackson, M.D., Chief of Staff
CHR: Margaret Gates, Chief Human Resources
Web address: www.harrishospital.com
Control: Corporation, Investor–owned, for–profit **Service:** General Medical and Surgical

Staffed Beds: 83 **Admissions:** 3506 **Census:** 32 **Outpatient Visits:** 28004 **Births:** 691 **Total Expense ($000):** 21162 **Payroll Expense ($000):** 9564 **Personnel:** 255

NORTH LITTLE ROCK—Pulaski County

☐ **ARKANSAS SURGICAL HOSPITAL (40147)**, 5201 North Shore Drive, Zip 72118; tel. 501/748–8000 **A**1 9 10 **F**3 11 25 26 30 33 38 43 62 72 73 77 79 80 81 82 96 100 102 107 120 135
Primary Contact: Lyndell H. Weaks, Chief Executive Officer
CFO: Herbert Crum, Chief Financial Officer
CMO: Kenneth A. Marton, M.D., Chief of Staff
CHR: Tina Albright, Manager Human Resources
Web address: www.arksurgicalhospital.com
Control: Corporation, Investor–owned, for–profit **Service:** General Medical and Surgical

Staffed Beds: 16 **Admissions:** 2070 **Census:** 10 **Outpatient Visits:** 10028 **Births:** 0 **Total Expense ($000):** 26808 **Payroll Expense ($000):** 7220 **Personnel:** 165

☒ △ **BAPTIST HEALTH MEDICAL CENTER – NORTH LITTLE ROCK (40036)**, 3333 Springhill Drive, Zip 72117–2922; tel. 501/202–3000 **A**1 7 9 10 **F**3 8 11 13 15 17 18 20 22 24 25 26 27 28 30 31 32 33 35 36 38 46 47 49 50 52 53 54 55 56 57 59 62 63 66 68 72 73 74 75 76 77 79 80 81 82 84 85 86 87 96 97 100 105 107 112 116 118 119 121 124 132 133 135 136 137 **S** Baptist Health
Primary Contact: Harrison M. Dean, FACHE, Senior Vice President and Administrator
CFO: Allen F. Smith, Senior Vice President Financial Services
CMO: Peter Marvin, M.D., Vice President Clinical Affairs
CIO: David House, Vice President and Chief Information Officer
CHR: Anthony Kendall, Vice President Human Resources
Web address: www.baptist–health.org
Control: Other not–for–profit (including NFP Corporation) **Service:** General Medical and Surgical

Staffed Beds: 220 **Admissions:** 11989 **Census:** 141 **Outpatient Visits:** 107745 **Births:** 1675 **Total Expense ($000):** 147454 **Payroll Expense ($000):** 54877 **Personnel:** 1132

NORTH LITTLE ROCK DIVISION See Central Arkansas Veterans Healthcare System, Little Rock

☐ **THE BRIDGEWAY (44005)**, 21 Bridgeway Road, Zip 72113–9516; tel. 501/771–1500 **A**1 9 10 **F**4 32 88 89 95 **P**5 **S** Universal Health Services, Inc.
Primary Contact: Jennifer Nolan, Chief Executive Officer
CFO: Fred Woods, Chief Financial Officer
CMO: T. Stuart Harris, M.D., Medical Director
CHR: Neely Johnson, Director Human Resources
Web address: www.thebridgeway.com
Control: Corporation, Investor–owned, for–profit **Service:** Psychiatric

Staffed Beds: 98 **Admissions:** 4398 **Census:** 93 **Outpatient Visits:** 6898 **Births:** 0 **Total Expense ($000):** 14594 **Payroll Expense ($000):** 8037 **Personnel:** 134

OSCEOLA—Mississippi County

☒ **SOUTH MISSISSIPPI COUNTY REGIONAL MEDICAL CENTER (41316)**, 611 West Lee Avenue, Zip 72370–3001, Mailing Address: P.O. Box 607, Zip 72370–0607; tel. 870/563–7000 **A**1 9 10 18 **F**3 11 14 15 25 31 32 33 38 40 55 57 62 66 73 77 79 82 86 87 89 91 92 96 99 100 102 107 108 109 121 122 124 135 **P**7 **S** Ameris Health Systems
Primary Contact: Franklin G. Schupp, Chief Executive Officer
CFO: David Lynn, Chief Financial Officer
CMO: Ken Dill, Chief of Staff
CHR: Eva Middleton, Director Human Resources
Control: Corporation, Investor–owned, for–profit **Service:** General Medical and Surgical

Staffed Beds: 25 **Admissions:** 1157 **Census:** 10 **Outpatient Visits:** 17011 **Births:** 0 **Total Expense ($000):** 11089 **Payroll Expense ($000):** 4326 **Personnel:** 114

OZARK—Franklin County

★ **MERCY HOSPITAL–TURNER MEMORIAL (41303)**, 801 West River Street, Zip 72949–3000; tel. 479/667–4138 **A**9 10 18 **F**3 8 24 30 31 32 33 38 55 56 57 62 79 80 96 107 122 135 **S** Sisters of Mercy Health System
Primary Contact: Jim L. Maddox, Administrator
COO: Jim L. Maddox, Administrator
CFO: James Newman, Vice President and Chief Financial Officer
CMO: John Lachowsky, M.D., Chief Medical Officer
CIO: Tiana Bolduc, Chief Information Officer
CHR: Ron Summerhill, Vice President Human Resources
Web address: www.gravettehospital.org
Control: Church–operated, Nongovernment, not–for profit **Service:** General Medical and Surgical

Staffed Beds: 25 **Admissions:** 637 **Census:** 8 **Outpatient Visits:** 9613 **Births:** 0 **Total Expense ($000):** 6159 **Payroll Expense ($000):** 2347 **Personnel:** 52

PARAGOULD—Greene County

⊠ △ **ARKANSAS METHODIST MEDICAL CENTER (40039)**, 900 West Kingshighway, Zip 72450–5942, Mailing Address: P.O. Box 339, Zip 72451–0339; tel. 870/239–7000 **A**1 7 9 10 19 **F**3 7 11 13 15 18 20 24 25 27 30 31 32 33 37 38 40 49 50 51 52 53 55 56 57 59 61 62 66 68 73 74 76 77 79 80 81 82 84 85 86 96 97 100 102 107 118 119 120 121 122 124 135 136 137 **P**8
Primary Contact: Ronald K. Rooney, FACHE, President
COO: Barry L. Davis, Vice President Operations
CFO: Bryan Jackson, Vice President Finance
CMO: Samuel Burchfield, M.D., Chief of Staff
CIO: Mardy Holmes, Director Information Technology
CHR: Dennis Cooper, Director Human Resources
Web address: www.arkansasmethodist.org
Control: Other not–for–profit (including NFP Corporation) **Service:** General Medical and Surgical

Staffed Beds: 125 **Admissions:** 4519 **Census:** 60 **Outpatient Visits:** 99053 **Births:** 200 **Total Expense ($000):** 49839 **Payroll Expense ($000):** 20002 **Personnel:** 593

PARIS—Logan County

★ **NORTH LOGAN MERCY HOSPITAL (41300)**, 500 East Academy, Zip 72855–4099; tel. 479/963–6101 **A**9 10 18 **F**3 30 31 32 33 38 55 57 62 79 80 96 107 122 134 **S** Sisters of Mercy Health System
Primary Contact: Jim L. Maddox, Administrator
Web address: www.stedwardmercy.com
Control: Church–operated, Nongovernment, not–for profit **Service:** General Medical and Surgical

Staffed Beds: 16 **Admissions:** 307 **Census:** 4 **Outpatient Visits:** 10680 **Births:** 0 **Total Expense ($000):** 5078 **Payroll Expense ($000):** 1633 **Personnel:** 43

PIGGOTT—Clay County

★ **PIGGOTT COMMUNITY HOSPITAL (41330)**, 1206 Gordon Duckworth Drive, Zip 72454–1911; tel. 870/598–3881 **A**9 10 18 **F**3 7 11 15 25 26 38 55 57 61 62 79 86 96 100 107 118 119 121 122 132 135
Primary Contact: James L. Magee, Executive Director
CFO: Linda Ort, Chief Financial Officer
Web address: www.piggottcommunityhospital.com
Control: City–Government, nonfederal **Service:** General Medical and Surgical

Staffed Beds: 25 **Admissions:** 1018 **Census:** 14 **Outpatient Visits:** 146003 **Births:** 0 **Total Expense ($000):** 11779 **Payroll Expense ($000):** 7717 **Personnel:** 228

PINE BLUFF—Jefferson County

⊠ △ **JEFFERSON REGIONAL MEDICAL CENTER (40071)**, 1600 West 40th Avenue, Zip 71603–7089; tel. 870/541–7100 **A**1 6 7 9 10 12 13 20 **F**3 13 15 17 18 20 22 24 25 26 27 30 32 33 38 40 46 48 49 50 51 52 53 54 55 56 57 59 60 61 62 63 68 70 71 72 73 74 75 76 77 78 79 80 81 82 84 85 86 87 88 90 91 92 93 96 97 100 102 103 106 107 112 116 117 119 120 121 124 132 133 134 135 136 137 **P**7
Primary Contact: Robert P. Atkinson, FACHE, President and Chief Executive Officer
COO: Walter E. Johnson, Senior Vice President Operations and Chief Operating Officer
CFO: Nathan VanGenderen, Vice President Finance and Chief Financial Officer
CMO: George Roberson, M.D., Medical Director
CIO: Patrick Neece, Chief Information Officer
CHR: Daryl Scott, Director Human Resources
Web address: www.jrmc.org
Control: Other not–for–profit (including NFP Corporation) **Service:** General Medical and Surgical

Staffed Beds: 367 **Admissions:** 12704 **Census:** 174 **Outpatient Visits:** 163416 **Births:** 1368 **Total Expense ($000):** 157458 **Payroll Expense ($000):** 62616 **Personnel:** 1316

POCAHONTAS—Randolph County

FIVE RIVERS MEDICAL CENTER (40047), (Formerly Randolph County Medical Center), 2801 Medical Center Drive, Zip 72455–9497; tel. 870/892–6000 **A**9 10 20 **F**3 11 15 25 31 32 38 46 55 57 61 68 79 86 88 93 96 107 119 122 135
Primary Contact: John R. Tucker, Chief Executive Officer
CFO: Sharon K. Miller, Chief Financial Officer
CHR: Alvin Taylor, Chief Human Resources
Control: City–Government, nonfederal **Service:** General Medical and Surgical

Staffed Beds: 45 **Admissions:** 871 **Census:** 12 **Outpatient Visits:** 14051 **Births:** 0 **Total Expense ($000):** 12368 **Payroll Expense ($000):** 5888 **Personnel:** 154

ROGERS—Benton County

⊠ **MERCY MEDICAL CENTER (40010)**, (Formerly St Mary–Rogers Memorial Hospital), 2710 Rife Medical Lane, Zip 72758; tel. 479/338–8000 **A**1 9 10 **F**2 8 11 13 15 18 20 22 24 25 26 30 31 32 38 42 44 46 49 55 57 61 62 68 73 74 75 77 79 81 82 84 86 96 97 100 106 107 118 119 121 124 135 137 **P**6 **S** Sisters of Mercy Health System
Primary Contact: George Flynn, Chief Executive Officer
COO: Jon Vitiello, Chief Operating Officer and Chief Financial Officer
CFO: Jon Vitiello, Chief Operating Officer and Chief Financial Officer
CMO: Michael Allen, M.D., Chief of Staff
CHR: Rick Barclay, Vice President Support Services
Web address: www.mercyhealthnwa.smhs.com
Control: Church–operated, Nongovernment, not–for profit **Service:** General Medical and Surgical

Staffed Beds: 133 **Admissions:** 7345 **Census:** 65 **Outpatient Visits:** 104729 **Births:** 1267 **Total Expense ($000):** 90415 **Payroll Expense ($000):** 36938 **Personnel:** 831

RUSSELLVILLE—Pope County

⊠ △ **SAINT MARY'S REGIONAL MEDICAL CENTER (40041)**, 1808 West Main Street, Zip 72801–2724; tel. 479/968–2841, (Total facility includes 15 beds in nursing home–type unit) **A**1 7 9 10 19 **F**3 8 11 13 15 18 25 27 31 32 33 38 51 52 53 54 55 56 57 61 62 66 68 72 74 76 77 79 80 81 82 84 85 86 96 97 100 102 106 107 109 111 117 118 120 121 124 135 136 137 **S** Capella Healthcare
Primary Contact: Mike McCoy, Chief Executive Officer
CFO: Wendell VanEs, Chief Financial Officer
CMO: Chris Horan, Chief of Staff
CHR: Connie Gragg, Director Human Resources
Web address: www.saintmarysregional.com
Control: Corporation, Investor–owned, for–profit **Service:** General Medical and Surgical

Staffed Beds: 153 **Admissions:** 6158 **Census:** 75 **Outpatient Visits:** 78474 **Births:** 1178 **Total Expense ($000):** 48174 **Payroll Expense ($000):** 20659 **Personnel:** 493

SALEM—Fulton County

FULTON COUNTY HOSPITAL (41322), 679 North Main Street, Zip 72576–9122, Mailing Address: P.O. Box 517, Zip 72576–0517; tel. 870/895–2691 **A**9 10 18 **F**3 7 11 24 25 30 31 38 50 62 73 86 87 107 118 119 122 124
Primary Contact: Donna Hodges, Interim Chief Executive Officer
Control: County–Government, nonfederal **Service:** General Medical and Surgical

Staffed Beds: 25 **Admissions:** 836 **Census:** 8 **Outpatient Visits:** 27143 **Total Expense ($000):** 3269 **Payroll Expense ($000):** 2623

Hospital, Medicare Provider Number, Address, Telephone, Approval, Facility, and Physician Codes, Health Care System

★ American Hospital Association (AHA) membership
□ The Joint Commission accreditation
○ American Osteopathic Association (AOA) accreditation
△ Commission on Accreditation of Rehabilitation Facilities (CARF) accreditation

SEARCY—White County

★ **WHITE COUNTY MEDICAL CENTER (40014)**, 3214 East Race Avenue, Zip 72143–4847; tel. 501/268–6121, (Includes CENTRAL ARKANSAS HOSPITAL, 1200 South Main Street, Zip 72143–7397) **A**9 10 19 20 **F**3 11 13 17 18 20 22 25 26 27 30 31 32 33 37 38 51 53 55 56 57 60 61 62 66 68 72 73 74 75 76 77 79 81 82 84 85 86 88 90 92 96 97 100 103 107 115 118 119 120 121 123 124 135 136 137 **P**6
Primary Contact: Raymond W. Montgomery, II, President and Chief Executive Officer
CFO: Stuart Hill, Vice President and Treasurer
CMO: David Staggs, M.D., Chief of Staff
CIO: Kevin Hoofman, Director Management Information
CHR: Pam Williams, Director Human Resources
Web address: www.wcmc.org
Control: Other not–for–profit (including NFP Corporation) **Service:** General Medical and Surgical

Staffed Beds: 259 **Admissions:** 11921 **Census:** 145 **Outpatient Visits:** 74137 **Births:** 1282 **Total Expense ($000):** 132605 **Payroll Expense ($000):** 60466 **Personnel:** 1388

SHERWOOD—Pulaski County

★ **ST. VINCENT MEDICAL CENTER–NORTH (40137)**, 2215 Wildwood Avenue, Zip 72120; tel. 501/552–7100 **A**9 10 **F**3 11 15 18 25 26 27 30 31 32 33 38 43 50 51 53 55 57 62 66 68 72 76 77 79 80 92 96 97 100 102 106 107 119 132 135 **S** Catholic Health Initiatives
Primary Contact: Randall R. Cason, FACHE, Administrator and Chief Executive Officer
CMO: David Hall, M.D., Senior Vice President and Chief Medical Officer
CIO: Tommye Billing, Vice President and Chief Information Officer
CHR: Margaret Nixon, Director Human Resources
Web address: www.stvincenthealth.com
Control: Church–operated, Nongovernment, not–for profit **Service:** General Medical and Surgical

Staffed Beds: 50 **Admissions:** 2698 **Census:** 33 **Outpatient Visits:** 40000 **Births:** 0 **Total Expense ($000):** 31059 **Payroll Expense ($000):** 9572 **Personnel:** 256

⊛ **ST. VINCENT REHABILITATION HOSPITAL (43031)**, 2201 Wildwood Avenue, Zip 72120–5074, Mailing Address: P.O. Box 6930, Zip 72124–6930; tel. 501/834–1800 **A**1 9 10 **F**3 6 8 9 11 25 26 31 32 33 42 43 44 45 56 57 62 73 75 77 81 82 85 86 118 119 120 121 132 135 137
S HEALTHSOUTH Corporation
Primary Contact: Lee Frazier, Chief Executive Officer
CFO: Pat Robinson, Manager Accounting
CMO: Sean Foley, M.D., Medical Director
CHR: Sandra Pearson, Manager Human Resources
Web address: www.healthsouth.com
Control: Partnership, Investor–owned, for–profit **Service:** Rehabilitation

Staffed Beds: 60 **Admissions:** 830 **Census:** 34 **Outpatient Visits:** 8898 **Births:** 0 **Total Expense ($000):** 8741 **Payroll Expense ($000):** 4690 **Personnel:** 77

SILOAM SPRINGS—Benton County

⊛ **SILOAM SPRINGS MEMORIAL HOSPITAL (40001)**, 205 East Jefferson Street, Zip 72761–3697; tel. 479/524–4141 **A**1 9 10 **F**3 8 11 13 15 24 25 26 32 38 55 56 57 62 68 69 73 74 75 77 79 80 82 86 96 100 102 107 118 121 135 136
Primary Contact: Penny McClain, Chief Executive Officer
CFO: James E. Little, Chief Financial Officer
CMO: Dale Clemens, M.D., Chief of Staff
CHR: Julie Shearin, Director Human Resources
Web address: www.ssmh.us
Control: City–Government, nonfederal **Service:** General Medical and Surgical

Staffed Beds: 43 **Admissions:** 3046 **Census:** 25 **Outpatient Visits:** 24864 **Births:** 577 **Total Expense ($000):** 15115 **Payroll Expense ($000):** 11131 **Personnel:** 276

SPRINGDALE—Washington County

⊛ **NORTHWEST MEDICAL CENTER (40022)**, (Formerly Springdale Memorial Hospital of Washington County), 609 West Maple Avenue, Zip 72764; tel. 479/751–5711 **A**1 9 10 **F**11 12 14 15 17 18 20 22 24 25 26 27 31 33 34 38 54 55 57 61 62 66 68 69 72 73 75 76 77 79 80 81 82 84 85 86 87 96 100 102 103 107 116 118 119 120 121 133 135 137 **P**5 8 **S** Community Health Systems, Inc.
Primary Contact: Daniel E. McKay, Chief Executive Officer
COO: Lee Christenson, Administrator and Chief Operating Officer
CFO: Eddie Klein, Chief Financial Officer
CMO: Robert Petrino, M.D., Chief of Staff
CIO: Angela Cox, Chief Information Officer
CHR: Mike Meeks, Vice President Human Resources
Web address: www.northwesthealth.com
Control: Corporation, Investor–owned, for–profit **Service:** General Medical and Surgical

Staffed Beds: 179 **Admissions:** 7516 **Census:** 105 **Births:** 0 **Total Expense ($000):** 97275 **Payroll Expense ($000):** 33791 **Personnel:** 613

⊛ **REGENCY HOSPITAL OF SPRINGDALE**, 609 West Maple Avenue, 6th Floor, Zip 72764; tel. 479/757–2600 **A**1 **F**1 3 25 31 72 73 77 80 81 119 137 **P**5 **S** Regency Hospital Company
Primary Contact: Michael A. McLean, Chief Executive Officer
CMO: Gary Templeton, M.D., President Medical Staff
CHR: Missy Ross–Cole, Director Human Resources
Web address: www.regencyhospital.com
Control: Corporation, Investor–owned, for–profit **Service:** Long–Term Acute Care hospital

Staffed Beds: 25 **Admissions:** 256 **Census:** 18 **Outpatient Visits:** 0 **Births:** 0 **Total Expense ($000):** 7964 **Payroll Expense ($000):** 3874 **Personnel:** 103

STUTTGART—Arkansas County

★ **STUTTGART REGIONAL MEDICAL CENTER (40072)**, North Buerkle Road, Zip 72160–3420, Mailing Address: P.O. Box 1905, Zip 72160–1905; tel. 870/673–3511 **A**9 10 **F**3 7 11 13 15 25 26 30 31 32 33 37 38 55 56 57 62 66 68 73 74 77 79 80 82 86 87 94 96 99 100 107 117 118 119 122 124 132 135 137
Primary Contact: Bob Phillips, Interim Chief Executive Officer
CFO: Lynn Shock, Chief Financial Officer
CMO: Don Pattillo, M.D., Board Member
CIO: Warren Horton, Information and Technology Support Services Officer
CHR: Sheila Sims, Director Human Resources
Web address: www.stuttgart–medical.org
Control: Other not–for–profit (including NFP Corporation) **Service:** General Medical and Surgical

Staffed Beds: 37 **Admissions:** 2229 **Census:** 20 **Outpatient Visits:** 26839 **Births:** 212 **Total Expense ($000):** 25559 **Payroll Expense ($000):** 10327 **Personnel:** 275

TEXARKANA—Miller County

☐ **LIVING HOPE TEXARKANA (44016)**, 801 Arkansas Boulevard, Zip 71854; tel. 870/774–4673, (Nonreporting) **A**1 9 10
Primary Contact: Kimbro Stephens, President and Chief Executive Officer
CFO: Jimmy Peabody, Chief Financial Officer
CMO: Robert C. Strayhan, M.D., Medical Director
CIO: Jim Cruson, Director Information Technologies
CHR: Roberta Barkman, Chief Human Resources Officer
Web address: www.livinghope.com
Control: Corporation, Investor–owned, for–profit **Service:** Psychiatric

Staffed Beds: 62

VAN BUREN—Crawford County

⊛ **SUMMIT MEDICAL CENTER (40018)**, East Main and South 20th Streets, Zip 72956–5715, Mailing Address: P.O. Box 409, Zip 72957–0409; tel. 479/474–3401 **A**1 9 10 **F**3 11 15 22 25 26 31 37 38 40 46 50 54 55 56 57 62 63 66 68 72 73 76 77 79 80 81 82 86 90 96 97 100 102 107 119 120 121 124 133 135 137 **P**6 **S** Health Management Associates
Primary Contact: Pamela Tahan, Chief Executive Officer
CFO: Michael B. Schimming, Chief Financial Officer
CHR: James Ford, Director Human Resources
Web address: www.summitmedicalcenter.net
Control: Corporation, Investor–owned, for–profit **Service:** General Medical and Surgical

Staffed Beds: 103 **Admissions:** 1744 **Census:** 18 **Outpatient Visits:** 22513 **Births:** 0 **Total Expense ($000):** 20020 **Payroll Expense ($000):** 8817 **Personnel:** 208

WALDRON—Scott County

★ **MERCY HOSPITAL OF SCOTT COUNTY (41305)**, 1341 West 6th Street, Zip 72958–7001; tel. 479/637–4135 **A**9 10 18 **F**3 8 30 31 32 33 38 46 55 57 62 63 79 80 96 107 122 **S** Sisters of Mercy Health System
Primary Contact: Jim L. Maddox, Administrator
CFO: James Newman, Senior Vice President and Chief Financial Officer
Web address: www.stedwardmercy.com
Control: Church–operated, Nongovernment, not–for profit **Service:** General Medical and Surgical

Staffed Beds: 24 **Admissions:** 588 **Census:** 6 **Outpatient Visits:** 28907 **Births:** 0 **Total Expense ($000):** 7398 **Payroll Expense ($000):** 2351 **Personnel:** 43

 Many Facility Codes have changed. Please refer to the AHA Guide Code Chart.

WALNUT RIDGE—Lawrence County

★ **LAWRENCE MEMORIAL HOSPITAL (41309)**, 1309 West Main, Zip 72476–1430, Mailing Address: P.O. Box 839, Zip 72476–0839; tel. 870/886–1200, (Includes LAWRENCE HALL NURSING HOME), (Total facility includes 173 beds in nursing home–type unit) **A**1 9 10 18 **F**3 11 15 25 33 38 96 107 117 122 135 137
Primary Contact: George S. Fray, Interim Chief Executive Officer
CFO: Vanessa Wagner, Chief Financial Officer
CMO: Shawn Peyton, Chief of Staff
CHR: Sherri Brown, Director Human Resources
Web address: www.lawrencehealth.net
Control: County–Government, nonfederal **Service:** General Medical and Surgical

Staffed Beds: 198 **Admissions:** 1361 **Census:** 188 **Outpatient Visits:** 23585 **Births:** 0 **Total Expense ($000):** 18289 **Payroll Expense ($000):** 9642 **Personnel:** 293

WARREN—Bradley County

★ **BRADLEY COUNTY MEDICAL CENTER (41327)**, 404 South Bradley Street, Zip 71671–3493; tel. 870/226–3731 **A**9 10 18 **F**3 11 13 15 25 27 31 33 38 39 55 61 62 74 79 88 93 94 96 100 102 106 107 117 118 119 122 124 **P**8
Primary Contact: Harold E. Mitchell, Jr., Administrator and Chief Executive Officer
CMO: James W. Marsh, M.D., Chief of Staff
CHR: Debra Marshall, Director Human Resources
Web address: www.bradleycountymedicalcenter.com
Control: Other not–for–profit (including NFP Corporation) **Service:** General Medical and Surgical

Staffed Beds: 35 **Admissions:** 1823 **Census:** 17 **Outpatient Visits:** 56704 **Births:** 273 **Total Expense ($000):** 16365 **Payroll Expense ($000):** 8040 **Personnel:** 203

WEST MEMPHIS—Crittenden County

□ **CRITTENDEN MEMORIAL HOSPITAL (40042)**, 200 Tyler Avenue, Zip 72301–4223, Mailing Address: P.O. Box 2248, Zip 72303–2248; tel. 870/735–1500 **A**1 9 10 **F**3 8 11 13 15 24 25 27 30 31 32 33 38 42 46 47 55 56 57 61 62 68 73 74 75 76 77 78 79 81 82 85 86 96 97 100 101 107 119 121 124 135 **P**5
Primary Contact: James R. Carter, Jr., Chief Executive Officer
COO: Justin Vernon, Chief Operating Officer
CFO: Paul Rogers, Chief Financial Officer
Web address: www.crittendenmemorial.org
Control: Other not–for–profit (including NFP Corporation) **Service:** General Medical and Surgical

Staffed Beds: 130 **Admissions:** 4370 **Census:** 63 **Outpatient Visits:** 55883 **Births:** 818 **Total Expense ($000):** 53773 **Payroll Expense ($000):** 25115 **Personnel:** 499

WYNNE—Cross County

★ **CROSSRIDGE COMMUNITY HOSPITAL (41307)**, 310 South Falls Boulevard, Zip 72396–3013, Mailing Address: P.O. Box 590, Zip 72396–0590; tel. 870/238–3300 **A**1 9 10 18 **F**3 11 15 24 30 31 32 33 38 50 55 56 57 61 62 63 67 75 79 86 96 102 107 119 122 135
Primary Contact: Gary R. Sparks, Administrator
COO: Bryan Mattes, Associate Administrator
CFO: Janice Morris, Accountant
CIO: Gail Copeland, Director Management Information Systems
CHR: Bertha Ragle, Director Personnel
Control: Church–operated, Nongovernment, not–for profit **Service:** General Medical and Surgical

Staffed Beds: 15 **Admissions:** 755 **Census:** 8 **Outpatient Visits:** 17772 **Births:** 0 **Total Expense ($000):** 11636 **Payroll Expense ($000):** 4464 **Personnel:** 127

Hospital, Medicare Provider Number, Address, Telephone, Approval, Facility, and Physician Codes, Health Care System

★ American Hospital Association (AHA) membership
□ The Joint Commission accreditation
○ American Osteopathic Association (AOA) accreditation
△ Commission on Accreditation of Rehabilitation Facilities (CARF) accreditation

CALIFORNIA

CA

ALAMEDA—Alameda County

☐ **ALAMEDA HOSPITAL (50211)**, 2070 Clinton Avenue, Zip 94501–4397; tel. 510/522–3700, (Total facility includes 35 beds in nursing home–type unit) (Nonreporting) **A**1 9 10
Primary Contact: Stuart A. Jed, Chief Executive Officer
CFO: Gary K. Wiggins, Chief Financial Officer
CMO: Steven Lowery, M.D., President Medical Staff
CIO: Mark Moran, Director Information Systems
CHR: Bryant Welch, Director Human Resources
Web address: www.alamedahospital.org
Control: Hospital district or authority, Government, nonfederal **Service:** General Medical and Surgical

Staffed Beds: 88

ALHAMBRA—Los Angeles County

☐ **ALHAMBRA HOSPITAL MEDICAL CENTER (50281)**, 100 South Raymond Avenue, Zip 91801–3199, Mailing Address: P.O. Box 510, Zip 91802–0510; tel. 626/570–1606, (Total facility includes 26 beds in nursing home–type unit) (Nonreporting) **A**1 9 10 **S** AHMC, Inc
Primary Contact: Iris Lai, Chief Executive Officer
CFO: Linda Marsh, Vice President Financial Services and Chief Financial Officer
CIO: Kevin Chen, Director Information Systems
CHR: Elizabeth Sabandik, Director Human Resource
Web address: www.alhambrahospital.com
Control: Partnership, Investor–owned, for–profit **Service:** General Medical and Surgical

Staffed Beds: 144

ALTURAS—Modoc County

MODOC MEDICAL CENTER (50430), 228 McDowell Street, Zip 96101–3915; tel. 530/233–5131, (Total facility includes 71 beds in nursing home–type unit) (Nonreporting) **A**9 10 20
Primary Contact: Bruce R. Porter, Chief Executive Officer
CFO: Scott Mitchell, Chief Financial Officer
CMO: Ed Richert, M.D., Chief of Staff
CHR: Kimberly Crnkovic, Human Resources Generalist
Web address: www.modocmedicalcenter.com
Control: County–Government, nonfederal **Service:** General Medical and Surgical

Staffed Beds: 87

ANAHEIM—Orange County

☐ **ANAHEIM GENERAL HOSPITAL (50173)**, 3350 West Ball Road, Zip 92804–3799; tel. 714/827–6700, (Nonreporting) **A**1 9 10 **S** Pacific Health Corporation
Primary Contact: Michael Hartman, Chief Executive Officer
COO: Hassan Sharaya, Chief Nursing Officer
CFO: Mark Apodaca, Chief Financial Officer
CMO: Mir Ali, M.D., Chief Medical Staff
Control: Individual, Investor–owned, for–profit **Service:** General Medical and Surgical

Staffed Beds: 126

★ **ANAHEIM MEMORIAL MEDICAL CENTER (50226)**, 1111 West La Palma Avenue, Zip 92801–2881; tel. 714/774–1450 **A**1 2 9 10 **F**3 11 13 15 17 18 20 22 24 25 26 27 30 31 32 33 36 38 41 50 54 55 56 57 58 62 63 66 68 70 72 73 74 75 76 77 78 79 80 81 82 86 96 97 100 102 106 107 119 121 124 134 135 136 **S** Memorial Health Services
Primary Contact: Byron F. Schweigert, Interim Chief Executive Officer
CFO: Steve McNamara, Chief Financial Officer
CIO: Jeff DesRoches, Manager Information Systems
CHR: Kathy Doi, Executive Director Human Resources
Web address: www.memorialcare.org
Control: Other not–for–profit (including NFP Corporation) **Service:** General Medical and Surgical

Staffed Beds: 223 **Admissions:** 14672 **Census:** 163 **Outpatient Visits:** 91706 **Births:** 1997 **Total Expense ($000):** 161528 **Payroll Expense ($000):** 57268 **Personnel:** 829

★ **KAISER FOUNDATION HOSPITAL – ORANGE COUNTY (50609)**, 441 North Lakeview Avenue, Zip 92807–3089; tel. 714/279–4000, (Includes KAISER FOUNDATION HOSPITAL – ORANGE COUNTY, 6640 Alton Parkway, Irvine, Zip 92618; tel. 949/932–5000; Julie K. Miller–Phipps, Senior Vice President and Executive Director) **A**1 3 5 10 **F**3 8 13 14 15 17 18 20 25 26 27 28 30 31 32 33 38 41 43 44 46 47 48 49 50 53 57 60 61 62 63 66 68 70 72 73 74 76 77 78 79 80 82 84 90 96 97 100 102 107 119 124 132 135 137 **S** Kaiser Foundation Hospitals
Primary Contact: Julie K. Miller–Phipps, Senior Vice President and Executive Director
COO: Gerald A. McCall, Senior Vice President Operations
CFO: Melvin Benner, Assistant Administrator Finance
CMO: Edward Ellison, M.D., Area Associate Medical Director
CIO: Donald M. Carren, Information Technology Leader
CHR: Jean Melnikoff, Director Human Resources
Web address: www.kp.org
Control: Other not–for–profit (including NFP Corporation) **Service:** General Medical and Surgical

Staffed Beds: 176 **Admissions:** 14706 **Census:** 156 **Outpatient Visits:** 137037 **Births:** 3529 **Personnel:** 1082

☐ **WEST ANAHEIM MEDICAL CENTER (50426)**, 3033 West Orange Avenue, Zip 92804–3184; tel. 714/827–3000, (Nonreporting) **A**1 5 10 **S** Prime Healthcare Services
Primary Contact: Virgis Narbutas, Chief Executive Officer
CMO: Fariborz Shams, M.D., Chief of Staff
CIO: Debbie Horgan, Director Information Technology
CHR: Stephanie Sioson, Director Human Resource
Web address: www.westanaheimmedctr.com
Control: Partnership, Investor–owned, for–profit **Service:** General Medical and Surgical

Staffed Beds: 219

☐ **WESTERN MEDICAL CENTER ANAHEIM (50744)**, 1025 South Anaheim Boulevard, Zip 92805–5806; tel. 714/533–6220, (Nonreporting) **A**1 9 10 **S** Integrated Healthcare
Primary Contact: Josh D. Luke, Ph.D., CHE, Chief Executive Officer
CFO: Ray Rivas, Chief Financial Officer
CMO: Beena Shah, M.D., Chief Medical Officer
CIO: Nova Stewart, Chief Information Officer
CHR: Kathryn Van Dyk, Director
Web address: www.westernmedanaheim.com
Control: Corporation, Investor–owned, for–profit **Service:** General Medical and Surgical

Staffed Beds: 181

ANTIOCH—Contra Costa County

★ **SUTTER DELTA MEDICAL CENTER (50523)**, 3901 Lone Tree Way, Zip 94509–6253; tel. 925/779–7200, (Nonreporting) **A**1 9 10 **S** Sutter Health
Primary Contact: Gary D. Rapaport, Chief Executive Officer
CFO: Julie Peterson, Chief Financial Officer
CMO: Gurunath Rajapuram, M.D., Chief of Staff
CIO: Brenda Buccellato, Manager Information Technology
CHR: Christine Green, Administrative Director Human Resources
Web address: www.sutterdelta.org
Control: Other not–for–profit (including NFP Corporation) **Service:** General Medical and Surgical

Staffed Beds: 107

APPLE VALLEY—San Bernardino County

★ **ST. MARY MEDICAL CENTER (50300)**, 18300 Highway 18, Zip 92307–2206, Mailing Address: P.O. Box 7025, Zip 92307–0725; tel. 760/242–2311 **A**1 2 9 10 **F**11 13 15 18 19 20 21 22 23 24 25 26 28 30 31 32 33 38 43 44 55 56 57 59 63 66 68 69 70 74 75 76 77 79 80 82 84 86 96 97 99 100 102 106 107 112 119 121 123 124 135 136 137 **P**5 **S** St. Joseph Health System
Primary Contact: Jason Barker, President and Chief Executive Officer
CFO: James McManus, Chief Financial Officer
CIO: Dale Lepper, Director Information Services
Control: Church–operated, Nongovernment, not–for profit **Service:** General Medical and Surgical

Staffed Beds: 177 **Admissions:** 13135 **Census:** 133 **Outpatient Visits:** 89452 **Births:** 2903 **Total Expense ($000):** 160046 **Payroll Expense ($000):** 62287 **Personnel:** 1056

Many Facility Codes have changed. Please refer to the AHA Guide Code Chart.

ARCADIA—Los Angeles County

★□ **METHODIST HOSPITAL OF SOUTHERN CALIFORNIA (50238)**, 300 West Huntington Drive, Zip 91007–3473, Mailing Address: P.O. Box 60016, Zip 91066–6016; tel. 626/898–8000 **A**1 2 9 10 **F**1 3 11 12 13 15 17 18 20 22 24 25 26 27 30 31 32 33 35 36 38 46 49 54 55 56 57 58 59 62 63 66 68 70 72 73 74 75 76 77 79 80 81 82 84 85 86 96 97 100 102 103 104 105 106 107 108 109 111 114 119 121 135 136 137
Primary Contact: Dennis M. Lee, President and Chief Executive Officer
COO: Kelly Linden, Senior Vice President and Chief Operating Officer
CFO: Kay Berglund, Vice President Finance and Chief Financial Officer
CHR: Jill Underwood, Vice President Human Resources
Web address: www.methodisthospital.org
Control: Other not–for–profit (including NFP Corporation) **Service:** General Medical and Surgical

Staffed Beds: 367 **Admissions:** 17085 **Census:** 245 **Outpatient Visits:** 71375 **Births:** 2331 **Total Expense ($000):** 206021 **Payroll Expense ($000):** 97366 **Personnel:** 1836

ARCATA—Humboldt County

○ **MAD RIVER COMMUNITY HOSPITAL (50028)**, 3800 Janes Road, Zip 95521–4788, Mailing Address: P.O. Box 1115, Zip 95521–1115; tel. 707/822–3621, (Nonreporting) **A**9 10 11
Primary Contact: Douglas A. Shaw, Administrator
CFO: Michael Young, Chief Financial Officer
CMO: Charmaine Moser–Carbiener, Nurse Executive
CIO: Tom Ayotte, Chief Information Officer
CHR: Ethan Black, Manager Human Resources
Web address: www.madriverhospital.com
Control: Corporation, Investor–owned, for–profit **Service:** General Medical and Surgical

Staffed Beds: 68

ARROYO GRANDE—San Luis Obispo County

★□ **ARROYO GRANDE COMMUNITY HOSPITAL (50016)**, 345 South Halcyon Road, Zip 93420–3899; tel. 805/489–4261, (Total facility includes 12 beds in nursing home–type unit) **A**1 9 10 **F**8 11 25 26 30 31 32 33 37 38 44 50 51 55 56 57 62 66 68 73 75 76 77 79 86 90 96 97 98 99 100 102 105 106 107 117 118 119 135 **S** Catholic Healthcare West
Primary Contact: Richard Castro, President
CIO: Cyndi Lang, Director Information Services
CHR: Ami Padilla, Director Human Resources
Web address: www.arroyograndehospital.org
Control: Other not–for–profit (including NFP Corporation) **Service:** General Medical and Surgical

Staffed Beds: 65 **Admissions:** 2963 **Census:** 37 **Outpatient Visits:** 80199 **Births:** 0 **Total Expense ($000):** 40488 **Payroll Expense ($000):** 18214 **Personnel:** 268

ATASCADERO—San Luis Obispo County

□ **ATASCADERO STATE HOSPITAL**, 10333 El Camino Real, Zip 93422–7001, Mailing Address: P.O. Box 7001, Zip 93423–7001; tel. 805/468–2000, (Nonreporting) **A**1
Primary Contact: Melvin Hunter, Executive Director
Web address: www.dmh.ca.gov/statehospitals/atascadero
Control: State–Government, nonfederal **Service:** Psychiatric

Staffed Beds: 1127

AUBURN—Placer County

★ **SUTTER AUBURN FAITH HOSPITAL (50498)**, 11815 Education Street, Zip 95602–2410; tel. 530/888–4500, (Nonreporting) **A**2 9 10 **S** Sutter Health
Primary Contact: Mitchell J. Hanna, Chief Administrative Officer
CFO: Gary Hubschman, Administrative Director Finance
CMO: John Mesic, M.D., Chief Medical Officer
CHR: Lynda Dasaro, Director Human Resources
Web address: www.sutterhealth.org
Control: Other not–for–profit (including NFP Corporation) **Service:** General Medical and Surgical

Staffed Beds: 86

AVALON—Los Angeles County

CATALINA ISLAND MEDICAL CENTER (51307), 100 Falls Canyon Road, Zip 90704, Mailing Address: P.O. Box 1563, Zip 90704–1563; tel. 310/510–0700, (Total facility includes 4 beds in nursing home–type unit) **A**9 10 18 **F**3 11 31 32 33 38 50 55 56 57 61 62 63 64 66 73 86 87 96 102 107 111 117 119 122 123 124 135 **P**6
Primary Contact: Bryan M. Ballard, FACHE, Chief Executive Officer
CFO: Fred Luhman, Chief Financial Officer
CHR: Krista Steuter, Director Human Resources
Web address: www.catalinaislandmedicalcenter.org
Control: Other not–for–profit (including NFP Corporation) **Service:** General Medical and Surgical

Staffed Beds: 12 **Admissions:** 27 **Census:** 6 **Outpatient Visits:** 7631 **Births:** 0

BAKERSFIELD—Kern County

□ **BAKERSFIELD HEART HOSPITAL (50724)**, 3001 Sillect Avenue, Zip 93308–6337; tel. 661/316–6000, (Nonreporting) **A**1 10 **S** MedCath, Inc.
Primary Contact: Richard Priore, Interim Chief Executive Officer
Web address: www.bakersfieldhearthospital.com
Control: Partnership, Investor–owned, for–profit **Service:** General Medical and Surgical

Staffed Beds: 46

★□ **BAKERSFIELD MEMORIAL HOSPITAL (50036)**, 420 34th Street, Zip 93301–2237, Mailing Address: P.O. Box 1888, Zip 93303–1888; tel. 661/327–1792, (Total facility includes 24 beds in nursing home–type unit) (Nonreporting) **A**1 9 10 **S** Catholic Healthcare West
Primary Contact: Jon Van Boening, President
COO: Bruce Peters, Vice President and Chief Operating Officer
CFO: Jessica Hanson, Vice President and Chief Financial Officer
CMO: Robert Marshall, M.D., Vice President Medical Affairs
CHR: Sheri Commaianni, Vice President Human Resources
Web address: www.chw.edu
Control: Other not–for–profit (including NFP Corporation) **Service:** General Medical and Surgical

Staffed Beds: 339

□ **GOOD SAMARITAN HOSPITAL (50257)**, 901 Olive Drive, Zip 93308–4144, Mailing Address: P.O. Box 85002, Zip 93380–5002; tel. 661/399–4461, (Nonreporting) **A**1 9 10
Primary Contact: Tim Kollars, President
COO: Nick Damian, Associate Administrator and Director Mental Health and Support Services
CFO: Rick Hurst, Chief Financial Officer
CMO: Ronnie Claiborne, M.D., Chief Medical Officer
CIO: Nick Damian, Associate Administrator and Director Mental Health and Support Services
CHR: Daisy Laurino, Administrative Assistant Human Resources
Control: Corporation, Investor–owned, for–profit **Service:** General Medical and Surgical

Staffed Beds: 29

★□ **HEALTHSOUTH BAKERSFIELD REHABILITATION HOSPITAL (53031)**, 5001 Commerce Drive, Zip 93309–0689; tel. 661/323–5500, (Nonreporting) **A**1 9 10 **S** HEALTHSOUTH Corporation
Primary Contact: Sandra Hegland, Chief Executive Officer
CFO: Robert Mosesian, Controller
CMO: Chris Yoon, M.D., Medical Director
CIO: Tara DeMontgorency, Director Business Development
CHR: Tami Holden, Director Human Resources
Web address: www.healthsouth.com
Control: Corporation, Investor–owned, for–profit **Service:** Rehabilitation

Staffed Beds: 40

□ **KERN MEDICAL CENTER (50315)**, 1830 Flower Street, Zip 93305–4186; tel. 661/326–2000, (Nonreporting) **A**1 2 3 5 8 9 10
Primary Contact: Paul J. Hensler, Chief Executive Officer
COO: David Keith, Chief Operating Officer
CFO: Fred A. Plane, Chief Financial Officer
CMO: Eugene Kercher, M.D., Chief Medical Officer
CIO: Bill Fawns, Interim Manager Information Systems
CHR: Steve O'Connor, Director Human Resources
Web address: www.kernmedicalcenter.com
Control: County–Government, nonfederal **Service:** General Medical and Surgical

Staffed Beds: 180

CA

Hospital, Medicare Provider Number, Address, Telephone, Approval, Facility, and Physician Codes, Health Care System

★ American Hospital Association (AHA) membership
□ The Joint Commission accreditation
○ American Osteopathic Association (AOA) accreditation
△ Commission on Accreditation of Rehabilitation Facilities (CARF) accreditation

★ **MERCY HOSPITAL (50295)**, 2215 Truxtun Avenue, Zip 93301–3698, Mailing Address: P.O. Box 119, Zip 93302–0119; tel. 661/632–5000, (Includes MERCY SOUTHWEST HOSPITAL, 400 Old River Road, Zip 93311; tel. 661/663–6000), (Total facility includes 50 beds in nursing home–type unit) (Nonreporting) **A**1 2 9 10 **S** Catholic Healthcare West
Primary Contact: Russell V. Judd, President
COO: Kevin Klockenga, Chief Operating Officer
CFO: Rodney Winegarner, Chief Financial Officer
CMO: Mitesh Patel, M.D., Chief Medical Officer
CIO: Jeff Vague, Regional Manager Information Systems
CHR: Jay King, Vice President Human Resources
Web address: www.mercybakersfield.org
Control: Church–operated, Nongovernment, not–for profit **Service:** General Medical and Surgical

Staffed Beds: 269

★ **SAN JOAQUIN COMMUNITY HOSPITAL (50455)**, 2615 Chester Avenue, Zip 93301–2006, Mailing Address: P.O. Box 2615, Zip 93303–2615; tel. 661/395–3000, (Nonreporting) **A**1 9 10 **S** Adventist Health
Primary Contact: Robert J. Beehler, President and Chief Executive Officer
CFO: Brent Soper, Chief Financial Officer
CIO: Adrienne McReynolds, Chief Information Officer
CHR: Jack Houston, Director Human Resources
Web address: www.sanjoaquinhospital.org
Control: Church–operated, Nongovernment, not–for profit **Service:** General Medical and Surgical

Staffed Beds: 166

CA

BALDWIN PARK—Los Angeles County

★ **KAISER FOUNDATION HOSPITAL–BALDWIN PARK (50723)**, 1011 Baldwin Park Boulevard, Zip 91706–5806; tel. 626/851–1011 **A**1 10 **F**3 8 13 15 25 26 27 30 31 32 33 38 40 43 44 49 54 55 56 57 58 59 60 62 63 66 68 70 72 73 74 75 76 77 79 80 81 82 86 96 100 107 119 135 136 137 **P**6 **S** Kaiser Foundation Hospitals
Primary Contact: Margaret H. Pierce, Executive Director
CFO: Rebecca Wheeler, Director Finance
CMO: John Bigley, M.D., Medical Director
CIO: Tony Pompei, Information Technology Leader
CHR: Leesa Malcom, Director Human Resources
Web address: www.kp.org
Control: Other not–for–profit (including NFP Corporation) **Service:** General Medical and Surgical

Staffed Beds: 222 **Admissions:** 15421 **Census:** 147 **Outpatient Visits:** 221950 **Births:** 3254

VISTA SPECIALTY HOSPITAL OF SAN GABRIEL VALLEY (52045), 14148 East Francisquito Avenue, Zip 91706; tel. 626/388–2700, (Nonreporting) **A**10
Primary Contact: James Wilcox, Chief Executive Officer
Control: Corporation, Investor–owned, for–profit **Service:** Long–Term Acute Care hospital

Staffed Beds: 95

BANNING—Riverside County

★ **SAN GORGONIO MEMORIAL HOSPITAL (50054)**, 600 North Highland Springs Avenue, Zip 92220–3046; tel. 951/845–1121, (Nonreporting) **A**1 9 10 **S** Brim Healthcare, Inc.
Primary Contact: Jonathan Brenn, Chief Executive Officer
COO: Michelle Sayre, Chief Operating Officer
CFO: Johnathan Goh, Chief Financial Officer
CIO: Linda Palmer, Coordinator Medical Records
Web address: www.sgmh.org
Control: Hospital district or authority, Government, nonfederal **Service:** General Medical and Surgical

Staffed Beds: 77

BARSTOW—San Bernardino County

★ **BARSTOW COMMUNITY HOSPITAL (50298)**, 555 South Seventh Street, Zip 92311–3043; tel. 760/256–1761, (Nonreporting) **A**1 9 10 20 **S** Community Health Systems, Inc.
Primary Contact: Michael K. Stewart, Chief Executive Officer
CFO: Craig Morse, Chief Financial Officer
CIO: Ian Riggall, Manager Data Processing
CHR: Vickie Hendricks, Director Human Resources
Web address: www.barstowhospital.com
Control: Corporation, Investor–owned, for–profit **Service:** General Medical and Surgical

Staffed Beds: 56

BELLFLOWER—Los Angeles County

□ **BELLFLOWER MEDICAL CENTER (50531)**, 9542 East Artesia Boulevard, Zip 90706–6511; tel. 562/925–8355 **A**1 9 10 **F**3 12 13 15 17 25 27 33 38 68 74 79 80 84 86 88 92 96 100 107 119 135 **S** Pacific Health Corporation
Primary Contact: James Linhares, Chief Executive Officer
CFO: Clara Blom, Chief Financial Officer
CIO: Darla Kennedy, Director Information Systems
CHR: Jason Jaguez, Director Human Resources
Control: Corporation, Investor–owned, for–profit **Service:** General Medical and Surgical

Staffed Beds: 110 **Admissions:** 5227 **Census:** 72 **Outpatient Visits:** 25201 **Births:** 1707 **Total Expense ($000):** 26624 **Payroll Expense ($000):** 17715 **Personnel:** 411

★ **KAISER FOUNDATION HOSPITAL–BELLFLOWER (50139)**, 9400 East Rosecrans Avenue, Zip 90706–2246; tel. 562/461–3000 **A**1 3 5 10 **F**3 13 15 25 26 27 28 30 31 32 33 38 43 45 49 50 51 54 55 56 57 59 62 66 68 70 71 74 76 77 79 80 81 82 84 90 96 97 100 102 103 107 112 119 130 135 137 **S** Kaiser Foundation Hospitals
Primary Contact: Jane Finley, Senior Vice President and Executive Director
Web address: www.kaiserpermanente.org
Control: Other not–for–profit (including NFP Corporation) **Service:** General Medical and Surgical

Staffed Beds: 218 **Admissions:** 23231 **Census:** 187 **Outpatient Visits:** 95250 **Births:** 3419

BERKELEY—Alameda County

★ △ **ALTA BATES SUMMIT MEDICAL CENTER (50305)**, 2450 Ashby Avenue, Zip 94705–2067; tel. 510/204–4444, (Includes ALTA BATES MEDICAL CENTER–HERRICK CAMPUS, 2001 Dwight Way, Zip 94704; tel. 510/204–4444) **A**1 3 5 7 9 10 **F**3 5 8 11 12 13 15 17 18 20 24 25 26 27 30 31 32 33 34 37 38 41 43 44 46 47 49 50 54 55 56 57 58 59 60 62 63 66 68 70 71 72 73 74 75 76 77 79 80 82 85 86 88 89 90 91 92 93 94 95 96 97 99 102 104 105 106 107 108 109 110 113 114 117 119 121 124 125 132 135 136 137 **P**2 3 **S** Sutter Health
Primary Contact: Warren J. Kirk, President and Chief Executive Officer
Web address: www.altabates.com
Control: Other not–for–profit (including NFP Corporation) **Service:** General Medical and Surgical

Staffed Beds: 527 **Admissions:** 25474 **Census:** 381 **Outpatient Visits:** 346006 **Births:** 8317 **Total Expense ($000):** 493184 **Payroll Expense ($000):** 199402 **Personnel:** 1395

BIG BEAR LAKE—San Bernardino County

★ **BEAR VALLEY COMMUNITY HOSPITAL (50618)**, 41870 Garstin Road, Zip 92315, Mailing Address: P.O. Box 1649, Zip 92315–1649; tel. 909/866–6501, (Total facility includes 21 beds in nursing home–type unit) **A**9 10 20 **F**3 11 15 25 26 28 30 31 32 38 46 50 56 62 66 77 79 80 82 96 99 102 107 117 124 134 135
Primary Contact: Vi Colunga, Administrator and Chief Executive Officer
CFO: Rudy Shutta, Chief Financial Officer
CMO: Richard Baumgartner, M.D., Chief Medical Staff
CIO: Cheri Wood, Administration and Public Information Officer
CHR: Chris Birch, Director Human Resources
Web address: www.bvchd.com
Control: Hospital district or authority, Government, nonfederal **Service:** General Medical and Surgical

Staffed Beds: 30 **Admissions:** 366 **Census:** 22 **Outpatient Visits:** 19887 **Births:** 0 **Total Expense ($000):** 14168 **Payroll Expense ($000):** 6844 **Personnel:** 129

BISHOP—Inyo County

★ **NORTHERN INYO HOSPITAL (51324)**, 150 Pioneer Lane, Zip 93514–2599; tel. 760/873–5811 **A**1 9 10 **F**3 11 13 15 27 31 32 38 42 46 47 56 62 66 68 74 77 79 80 84 86 96 97 100 103 107 119
Primary Contact: John Halfen, Administrator, Chief Executive Officer and Chief Financial Officer
CFO: John Halfen, Administrator, Chief Executive Officer and Chief Financial Officer
CMO: Catherine Leja, M.D., Chief of Staff
CIO: Adam Taylor, Manager Information Technology
CHR: Gayla Blua, Director Human Resources
Web address: www.nih.org
Control: Hospital district or authority, Government, nonfederal **Service:** General Medical and Surgical

Staffed Beds: 25 **Admissions:** 1147 **Census:** 10 **Outpatient Visits:** 56468 **Births:** 218 **Total Expense ($000):** 35656 **Payroll Expense ($000):** 14148 **Personnel:** 289

Many Facility Codes have changed. Please refer to the AHA Guide Code Chart.

BLYTHE—Riverside County

★ **PALO VERDE HOSPITAL (50423)**, 250 North First Street, Zip 92225–1702; tel. 760/922–4115, (Nonreporting) **A**1 9 10 20
Primary Contact: Jeff Flood, Chief Executive Officer
CFO: Norma Hudson, Chief Financial Officer
Web address: www.paloverdehospital.org
Control: Hospital district or authority, Government, nonfederal **Service:** General Medical and Surgical

Staffed Beds: 35

BRAWLEY—Imperial County

☐ **PIONEERS MEMORIAL HEALTHCARE DISTRICT (50342)**, 207 West Legion Road, Zip 92227–7780; tel. 760/351–3333 **A**1 9 10 **F**3 11 12 13 15 25 30 32 33 38 40 50 52 53 55 56 57 62 68 70 73 75 77 79 81 86 96 97 100 102 107 119 133 135 136 137 **S** Brim Healthcare, Inc.
Primary Contact: Richard L. Mendoza, Chief Executive Officer
COO: Justina Aguirre, R.N., MSN, Associate Administrator
CFO: Daniel R. Heckathorne, Associate Administrator and Chief Financial Officer
CMO: Kestutis V. Kuraitis, M.D., Chief of Staff
CIO: Doug Darby, Director Information Systems
CHR: Robert Honaker, Associate Administrator and Chief Human Resources Officer
Web address: www.pmhd.org
Control: Hospital district or authority, Government, nonfederal **Service:** General Medical and Surgical

Staffed Beds: 107 **Admissions:** 5141 **Census:** 51 **Outpatient Visits:** 126470 **Births:** 1544 **Total Expense ($000):** 55549 **Payroll Expense ($000):** 30100 **Personnel:** 550

BREA—Orange County

☐ **KINDRED HOSPITAL–BREA (52039)**, 875 North Brea Boulevard, Zip 92821–2699; tel. 714/529–6842, (Nonreporting) **A**1 9 10 **S** Kindred Healthcare
Primary Contact: Kathleen Smith, Administrator
COO: Denise Jenkins, Chief Clinical Officer
CFO: John Browne, Assistant Administrator Finance
CMO: Jyotika Wali, M.D., Chief of Staff
Web address: www.kindredhealthcare.com
Control: Corporation, Investor–owned, for–profit **Service:** Long–Term Acute Care hospital

Staffed Beds: 48

BURBANK—Los Angeles County

★ △ **PROVIDENCE SAINT JOSEPH MEDICAL CENTER (50235)**, 501 South Buena Vista Street, Zip 91505–4866; tel. 818/843–5111, (Total facility includes 71 beds in nursing home–type unit) (Nonreporting) **A**1 2 7 9 10 **S** Providence Health & Services
Primary Contact: Barry A. Wolfman, Chief Executive
COO: Matthew S. Gerlach, Chief Administrative Officer
CFO: Dave Mast, Chief Financial Officer
CMO: Myron Berdischewsky, M.D., Chief Medical Officer
CIO: Mark Gargett, Interim Chief Information Officer
CHR: John Saavedra, Service Area Director Human Resources
Web address: www.providence.org
Control: Church–operated, Nongovernment, not–for profit **Service:** General Medical and Surgical

Staffed Beds: 448

BURLINGAME—San Mateo County

★ **MILLS–PENINSULA HEALTH SERVICES (50007)**, 1783 El Camino Real, Zip 94010–3282; tel. 650/696–5400, (Includes MILLS HOSPITAL, 100 South San Mateo Drive, San Mateo, Zip 94401; PENINSULA HOSPITAL), (Total facility includes 127 beds in nursing home–type unit) **A**1 9 10 **F**2 3 4 5 6 11 12 13 15 17 18 20 22 24 25 26 27 30 31 32 33 34 36 38 44 46 47 48 49 51 52 53 54 55 56 57 59 62 63 64 66 70 72 73 74 75 76 77 79 80 81 82 84 85 86 87 88 89 90 91 92 93 94 95 96 97 98 99 100 101 102 103 104 105 106 107 108 109 110 111 112 117 119 121 124 132 135 136 **P**5 **S** Sutter Health
Primary Contact: Robert W. Merwin, Chief Executive Officer
COO: Jeff Gerard, Chief Operating Officer
CFO: Iftikhar Hussain, Chief Financial Officer
CMO: Michael K. Wood, M.D., Chief of Staff
Web address: www.mills–peninsula.org
Control: Other not–for–profit (including NFP Corporation) **Service:** General Medical and Surgical

Staffed Beds: 389 **Admissions:** 15339 **Census:** 256 **Outpatient Visits:** 488041 **Births:** 1952 **Total Expense ($000):** 370749 **Payroll Expense ($000):** 130940 **Personnel:** 2746

CAMARILLO—Ventura County

★ **ST. JOHN'S PLEASANT VALLEY HOSPITAL (50616)**, 2309 Antonio Avenue, Zip 93010–1414; tel. 805/389–5800, (Total facility includes 92 beds in nursing home–type unit) (Nonreporting) **A**1 9 10 **S** Catholic Healthcare West
Primary Contact: Gerard Conway, President
COO: Maureen A. Malone, Chief Operating Officer
CFO: Tim Maurice, Chief Financial Officer
CMO: Eugene Fussell, M.D., Vice President Medical Affairs and Clinical Operations
CHR: John Bibi, Director Human Resources
Web address: www.catholichealthcarewest.org
Control: Other not–for–profit (including NFP Corporation) **Service:** General Medical and Surgical

Staffed Beds: 171

CAMP PENDLETON—San Diego County

★ **NAVAL HOSPITAL**, Mailing Address: Box 555191, Zip 92055–5191; tel. 760/725–1304, (Nonreporting) **A**1 3 5 **S** Bureau of Medicine and Surgery, Department of the Navy
Primary Contact: Captain Steven M. Nichols, Commanding Officer
CFO: Lieutenant Colonel S. Loberg, Director Resource Support Services
CMO: Commander C. Westropp, M.D., Director Primary Care
CIO: Colin Archibald, Chief Information Officer
CHR: Lieutenant S. Waclawski, Head Staff Administration
Web address: www.cpen.med.navy.mil
Control: Navy, Government, federal **Service:** General Medical and Surgical

Staffed Beds: 66

CANOGA PARK—Los Angeles County, See Los Angeles

CARMICHAEL—Sacramento County

★ **MERCY SAN JUAN MEDICAL CENTER (50516)**, 6501 Coyle Avenue, Zip 95608–0306, Mailing Address: P.O. Box 479, Zip 95608–0479; tel. 916/537–5000 **A**1 9 10 **F**3 8 11 12 13 15 17 18 20 22 24 25 26 27 30 31 32 33 38 40 42 43 44 52 57 61 62 66 68 70 72 73 74 75 76 77 79 80 84 86 96 97 98 99 100 102 103 104 105 106 107 112 114 118 119 121 124 133 135 136 137 **S** Catholic Healthcare West
Primary Contact: Brian K. Ivie, President
CFO: Robert Pascuzzi, Chief Financial Officer
CMO: Russ Braun, M.D., Vice President Medical Affairs
CIO: Mark Ewing, Site Manager
CHR: Donna Utley, Vice President Human Resources
Web address: www.mercysanjuan.org
Control: Church–operated, Nongovernment, not–for profit **Service:** General Medical and Surgical

Staffed Beds: 260 **Admissions:** 17400 **Census:** 207 **Outpatient Visits:** 63680 **Births:** 3258 **Total Expense ($000):** 312490 **Payroll Expense ($000):** 133702 **Personnel:** 1507

CASTRO VALLEY—Alameda County

★ **EDEN MEDICAL CENTER (50488)**, 20103 Lake Chabot Road, Zip 94546–5341; tel. 510/537–1234, (Includes SAN LEANDRO HOSPITAL, 13855 East 14th Street, San Leandro, Zip 94578–2600; tel. 510/357–6500; Ronnie Bayduza, Administrator), (Total facility includes 56 beds in nursing home–type unit) **A**1 2 9 10 **F**3 11 13 15 17 25 26 27 30 31 32 33 36 38 40 47 49 50 51 52 55 56 57 58 59 63 66 68 70 73 74 75 76 79 80 82 84 85 86 88 90 91 92 93 95 96 97 98 99 100 102 106 107 112 115 117 118 119 121 124 132 133 134 135 136 137 **P**3 5
Primary Contact: George Bischalaney, President and Chief Executive Officer
Web address: www.edenmedcenter.org
Control: Other not–for–profit (including NFP Corporation) **Service:** General Medical and Surgical

Staffed Beds: 358 **Admissions:** 13746 **Census:** 169 **Outpatient Visits:** 195650 **Births:** 1035 **Total Expense ($000):** 251839 **Payroll Expense ($000):** 101943 **Personnel:** 1281

CA

Hospital, Medicare Provider Number, Address, Telephone, Approval, Facility, and Physician Codes, Health Care System

★ American Hospital Association (AHA) membership
☐ The Joint Commission accreditation
○ American Osteopathic Association (AOA) accreditation
△ Commission on Accreditation of Rehabilitation Facilities (CARF) accreditation

CEDARVILLE—Modoc County

SURPRISE VALLEY HEALTHCARE DISTRICT (51308), 741 North Main Street, Zip 96104, Mailing Address: P.O. Box 246, Zip 96104–0246; tel. 530/279–6111, (Total facility includes 22 beds in nursing home–type unit) **A**9 10 18 **F**3 7 11 28 30 31 32 33 38 54 55 56 57 63 66 67 73 84 90 107 117 122 132 135 **P**6
Primary Contact: Wanda Grove, Chief Executive Officer
CFO: Renae Sweet, Chief Financial Officer
CMO: Chuck Colas, M.D., Medical Director
CHR: William Bostic, Administrative Assistant Human Resources
Control: Hospital district or authority, Government, nonfederal **Service:** General Medical and Surgical

Staffed Beds: 26 **Admissions:** 45 **Census:** 22 **Outpatient Visits:** 7997 **Births:** 0 **Total Expense ($000):** 3634 **Payroll Expense ($000):** 1539 **Personnel:** 94

CERRITOS—Los Angeles County

COLLEGE HOSPITAL (54055), 10802 College Place, Zip 90703–1579; tel. 562/924–9581, (Nonreporting) **A**9 10 **S** College Health Enterprises
Primary Contact: Stephen Witt, Chief Executive Officer
CFO: Roderick Bell, Chief Financial Officer
CHR: Holly Risha, Administrative Director Human Resources
Web address: www.collegehospitals.com
Control: Corporation, Investor–owned, for–profit **Service:** Psychiatric

Staffed Beds: 157

CHESTER—Plumas County

★ **SENECA HEALTHCARE DISTRICT (50333)**, 130 Brentwood Drive, Zip 96020–0737, Mailing Address: P.O. Box 737, Zip 96020–0737; tel. 530/258–2151, (Total facility includes 16 beds in nursing home–type unit) (Nonreporting) **A**9 10 20
Primary Contact: Doug Self, Chief Executive Officer
COO: Doug Self, Chief Executive Officer
CMO: David Walls, M.D., Chief of Staff
CHR: Mike Roarty, Chief Human Resources Officer
Web address: www.senecahospital.org
Control: Hospital district or authority, Government, nonfederal **Service:** General Medical and Surgical

Staffed Beds: 26

CHICO—Butte County

★ **ENLOE MEDICAL CENTER (50039)**, 1531 Esplanade, Zip 95926–3386; tel. 530/332–7300, (Includes ENLOE MEDICAL CENTER–COHASSET, 560 Cohasset Road, Zip 95926; tel. 530/332–7300) **A**9 10 **F**3 5 7 8 11 12 15 18 20 22 24 25 27 28 31 32 33 34 38 40 42 48 49 50 51 53 55 56 57 59 61 62 63 64 66 67 68 70 72 73 74 75 76 77 78 79 80 81 82 84 85 86 88 90 91 92 96 97 102 107 108 109 118 119 121 133 135 136 137 **P**7
Primary Contact: Deborah A. Yancer, RN, President and Chief Executive Officer
COO: Michael C. Wiltermood, Chief Operating Officer
CFO: Christine Sarrico, Chief Financial Officer
CMO: Daniel Thomas, M.D., Chief of Staff
CHR: Carol Linscheid, Vice President Human Resources
Web address: www.enloe.org
Control: Other not–for–profit (including NFP Corporation) **Service:** General Medical and Surgical

Staffed Beds: 263 **Admissions:** 14412 **Census:** 196 **Outpatient Visits:** 217679 **Births:** 1600 **Total Expense ($000):** 270923 **Payroll Expense ($000):** 95063 **Personnel:** 1521

CHINO—San Bernardino County

○ **CANYON RIDGE HOSPITAL (54111)**, 5353 G Street, Zip 91710–5250; tel. 909/590–3700 **A**9 10 11 **F**2 3 4 5 25 33 88 89 90 91 92 93 94 95 119 121 123 **S** Psychiatric Solutions
Primary Contact: Peggy Minnick, RN, Chief Executive Officer
COO: Jeff McDonald, Chief Operating Officer
CFO: Burt Harris, Controller
CIO: Maria Patterson, Manager Information Management
CHR: Laura Culbertson, Director Human Resources
Web address: www.psysolutions.com
Control: Corporation, Investor–owned, for–profit **Service:** Psychiatric

Staffed Beds: 59 **Admissions:** 3099 **Census:** 51 **Outpatient Visits:** 7918 **Births:** 0

○ **CHINO VALLEY MEDICAL CENTER (50586)**, 5451 Walnut Avenue, Zip 91710–2672; tel. 909/464–8600, (Nonreporting) **A**10 11 12 13 **S** Prime Healthcare Services
Primary Contact: Lex Reddy, Chief Executive Officer
CFO: Gregory Brentano, Chief Financial Officer
CMO: James M. Lally, Chief Medical Officer
CIO: Vic Mahan, Chief Information Officer
CHR: Arti Dhuper, Regional Director Human Resources
Web address: www.cvmc.com
Control: Corporation, Investor–owned, for–profit **Service:** General Medical and Surgical

Staffed Beds: 126

CHOWCHILLA—Madera County

CHOWCHILLA DISTRICT MEMORIAL HOSPITAL (50377), 1104 Ventura Avenue, Zip 93610–2298; tel. 559/665–3781, (Total facility includes 23 beds in nursing home–type unit) (Nonreporting) **A**9 10
Primary Contact: Cathy Flores, RN, Administrator and Controller
Control: Hospital district or authority, Government, nonfederal **Service:** General Medical and Surgical

Staffed Beds: 24

CHULA VISTA—San Diego County

☐ **BAYVIEW HOSPITAL AND MENTAL HEALTH SYSTEM**, 330 Moss Street, Zip 91911–2005; tel. 619/426–6310, (Nonreporting) **A**1
Primary Contact: Jack Lungu, Chief Executive Officer
CFO: Robert Bourseau, Chief Financial Officer
Web address: www.bayviewhospital.com
Control: Corporation, Investor–owned, for–profit **Service:** Psychiatric

Staffed Beds: 64

SCRIPPS MERCY HOSPITAL CHULA VISTA See Scripps Mercy Hospital, San Diego

⊠ **SHARP CHULA VISTA MEDICAL CENTER (50222)**, 751 Medical Center Court, Zip 91911–6699, Mailing Address: P.O. Box 1297, Zip 91912–1297; tel. 619/482–5800, (Total facility includes 100 beds in nursing home–type unit) **A**1 2 9 10 **F**8 11 12 13 15 18 20 22 24 25 26 27 30 31 32 33 38 42 43 47 49 51 53 55 56 57 59 62 63 68 70 73 74 75 76 77 79 81 82 86 96 97 100 102 104 106 107 109 111 117 119 132 135 136 137 **P**5 **S** Sharp Healthcare
Primary Contact: Christopher L. Boyd, Chief Executive Officer
CMO: Francisco Anguiano, M.D., Chief of Staff
CHR: Zoe Gardner, Manager Human Resources
Web address: www.sharp.com
Control: Other not–for–profit (including NFP Corporation) **Service:** General Medical and Surgical

Staffed Beds: 330 **Admissions:** 14329 **Census:** 284 **Outpatient Visits:** 80183 **Births:** 3397 **Total Expense ($000):** 192446 **Payroll Expense ($000):** 89389 **Personnel:** 1127

CLEARLAKE—Lake County

★ **REDBUD COMMUNITY HOSPITAL (51317)**, 15630 18th Avenue, Zip 95422–9339, Mailing Address: P.O. Box 6720, Zip 95422–6720; tel. 707/994–6486, (Nonreporting) **A**9 10 18 **S** Adventist Health
Primary Contact: JoAline Olson, RN, President and Chief Executive Officer
CFO: Buck McDonald, Chief Financial Officer
Web address: www.adventisthealth.org
Control: Other not–for–profit (including NFP Corporation) **Service:** General Medical and Surgical

Staffed Beds: 25

CLOVIS—Fresno County

CLOVIS COMMUNITY MEDICAL CENTER (50492), 2755 Herndon Avenue, Zip 93611–6800; tel. 559/324–4000, (Nonreporting) **A**9 10 **S** Community Medical Centers
Primary Contact: Craig Castro, Administrator
COO: Craig Waggoner, Chief Operating Officer
CFO: Tracy Kiritani, Vice President and Chief Financial Officer
CIO: George Vasquez, Chief Technology Officer
CHR: Ginny Burdick, Senior Vice President and Chief Human Resources Officer
Web address: www.communitymedical.org
Control: Other not–for–profit (including NFP Corporation) **Service:** General Medical and Surgical

Staffed Beds: 76

COALINGA—Fresno County

COALINGA REGIONAL MEDICAL CENTER (50397), 1191 Phelps Avenue, Zip 93210–9636; tel. 559/935–6400, (Total facility includes 114 beds in nursing home–type unit) **A**9 10 20 **F**15 25 33 38 55 62 80 96 99 100 102 107 117 132 **P**1
Primary Contact: Sharon A. Spurgeon, Chief Executive Officer
CFO: Sandra Earls, Chief Financial Officer
CMO: Hans Z. Wang, M.D., Medical Director
CIO: Rachael Diaz, Systems Operator
CHR: Amber Stiglianese, Manager Human Resources
Web address: www.coalingamedicalcenter.com
Control: Hospital district or authority, Government, nonfederal **Service:** General Medical and Surgical

Staffed Beds: 138 **Admissions:** 1139 **Census:** 97 **Outpatient Visits:** 19093 **Births:** 2 **Total Expense ($000):** 17316 **Payroll Expense ($000):** 6264 **Personnel:** 162

 Many Facility Codes have changed. Please refer to the AHA Guide Code Chart.

COLTON—San Bernardino County

○ **ARROWHEAD REGIONAL MEDICAL CENTER (50245)**, 400 North Pepper Avenue, Zip 92324–1819; tel. 909/580–1000 **A**2 3 5 10 11 12 13 **F**3 8 13 15 16 18 20 22 24 25 26 27 30 31 32 33 34 37 38 40 41 43 50 54 55 56 61 62 64 66 68 70 72 73 74 75 76 77 78 79 81 82 84 86 87 88 89 90 91 92 96 97 100 102 107 113 114 119 121 124 127 133 135 136 137 **P**5
Primary Contact: Patrick A. Petre, Chief Executive Officer
COO: Colene Haller, Chief Operating Officer
CFO: Frank Arambula, Chief Financial Officer
CMO: Dev GnanaDev, M.D., Medical Director
CIO: Cindie Watkins, Manager Information Systems
CHR: Christine Desko, Director Human Resources
Web address: www.arrowheadmedcenter.org
Control: County–Government, nonfederal **Service:** General Medical and Surgical

Staffed Beds: 353 **Admissions:** 22870 **Census:** 295 **Outpatient Visits:** 289573 **Births:** 3984 **Total Expense ($000):** 381715 **Payroll Expense ($000):** 139321 **Personnel:** 2675

COLUSA—Colusa County

□ **COLUSA REGIONAL MEDICAL CENTER (50434)**, 199 East Webster Street, Zip 95932–2954, Mailing Address: P.O. Box 331, Zip 95932–0331; tel. 530/458–5821, (Total facility includes 6 beds in nursing home–type unit) **A**1 9 10 20 **F**3 11 12 13 15 25 26 31 33 38 44 53 55 56 57 61 62 63 66 68 73 74 75 77 79 80 96 102 107 117 118 119 122 133 135
Primary Contact: Dale A. Kirby, Chief Executive Officer
CFO: Terry Deak, Chief Financial Officer
CMO: Samuel Medrano, M.D., Chief of Staff
CIO: Rachel Betke–Mena, Director Health Information Management
CHR: Dierdre Athenais, Director Human Resources
Web address: www.colusamedicalcenter.org
Control: Other not–for–profit (including NFP Corporation) **Service:** General Medical and Surgical

Staffed Beds: 30 **Admissions:** 1022 **Census:** 9 **Outpatient Visits:** 37181 **Births:** 220 **Total Expense ($000):** 15423 **Payroll Expense ($000):** 6189 **Personnel:** 136

CONCORD—Contra Costa County

★□ **JOHN MUIR BEHAVIORAL HEALTH (54131)**, 2740 Grant Street, Zip 94520; tel. 925/674–4100 **A**1 9 10 **F**4 5 26 30 31 32 88 89 90 91 92 93 94 95 119 121 123 132 **S** John Muir Health
Primary Contact: Elizabeth Stallings, Chief Operating Officer
COO: Elizabeth Stallings, Chief Operating Officer
CFO: Michael Moody, Senior Vice President and Chief Financial Officer
CMO: Nagui Achamallah, M.D., Chief of Staff
CIO: Eric Saff, Chief Information Officer
CHR: Alice Villanueva, Senior Vice President Human Resources
Web address: www.johnmuirhealth.com
Control: Other not–for–profit (including NFP Corporation) **Service:** Psychiatric

Staffed Beds: 70 **Admissions:** 2568 **Census:** 48 **Outpatient Visits:** 13242 **Births:** 0 **Total Expense ($000):** 23686 **Payroll Expense ($000):** 12047 **Personnel:** 95

★□ **JOHN MUIR MEDICAL CENTER, CONCORD (50496)**, 2540 East Street, Zip 94520; tel. 925/682–8200 **A**1 2 9 10 **F**3 12 15 17 18 20 22 24 25 26 27 30 31 32 33 35 38 41 43 46 47 48 49 50 53 54 55 56 57 58 62 66 68 72 73 75 76 77 78 79 80 81 82 86 90 92 96 97 99 102 106 107 108 109 111 114 116 119 121 124 132 134 135 137 **P**3 **S** John Muir Health
Primary Contact: Thomas M. Harlan, President and Chief Administrative Officer
CFO: Michael Moody, Chief Financial Officer
CMO: Randall Wenokor, M.D., Chief of Staff
CIO: Eric Saff, Vice President and Chief Information Officer
CHR: Alice Villanueva, Vice President Human Resources
Web address: www.johnmuirhealth.com
Control: Other not–for–profit (including NFP Corporation) **Service:** General Medical and Surgical

Staffed Beds: 202 **Admissions:** 9377 **Census:** 137 **Outpatient Visits:** 221421 **Births:** 3 **Total Expense ($000):** 277873 **Payroll Expense ($000):** 114417 **Personnel:** 1064

CORCORAN—Kings County

★ **CORCORAN DISTRICT HOSPITAL (50349)**, 1310 Hanna Avenue, Zip 93212–2395, Mailing Address: P.O. Box 758, Zip 93212–0758; tel. 559/992–5051, (Total facility includes 8 beds in nursing home–type unit) **A**9 10 **F**8 25 29 30 31 32 33 34 38 50 55 57 62 66 79 82 87 96 102 107 117 119 122 135
Primary Contact: David L. Hill, Chief Executive Officer
CFO: Debbie Bach, Chief Financial Officer
CMO: James Carter Thomas, M.D., Chief of Staff
CHR: Cheryl Burruss, Director Human Resources
Web address: www.cdhosp.com
Control: Hospital district or authority, Government, nonfederal **Service:** General Medical and Surgical

Staffed Beds: 32 **Admissions:** 409 **Census:** 12 **Outpatient Visits:** 33162 **Births:** 0 **Total Expense ($000):** 8942 **Payroll Expense ($000):** 3852 **Personnel:** 104

CORONA—Riverside County

□ **CORONA REGIONAL MEDICAL CENTER (50329)**, 800 South Main Street, Zip 92882–3420; tel. 951/737–4343, (Includes CORONA REGIONAL MEDICAL CENTER–REHABILITATION, 730 Magnolia Avenue, Zip 92879; tel. 951/736–7200), (Total facility includes 30 beds in nursing home–type unit) (Nonreporting) **A**1 2 9 10 **S** Universal Health Services, Inc.
Primary Contact: Kenneth I. Rivers, Chief Executive Officer
CFO: Becky Cheng, Chief Financial Officer
CIO: Rachel Sanchez, Director Information Systems
CHR: Ruth Battles, Administrative Director Human Resources
Web address: www.coronaregional.com
Control: Other not–for–profit (including NFP Corporation) **Service:** General Medical and Surgical

Staffed Beds: 228

CORONADO—San Diego County

★□ **SHARP CORONADO HOSPITAL AND HEALTH CENTER (50234)**, 250 Prospect Place, Zip 92118–1999; tel. 619/522–3600, (Total facility includes 134 beds in nursing home–type unit) **A**1 9 10 **F**3 11 15 25 26 30 32 33 34 35 37 38 42 46 51 52 55 56 57 59 62 63 66 67 68 72 73 75 77 79 80 82 86 96 100 107 117 119 121 124 135 137 **S** Sharp Healthcare
Primary Contact: Marcia K. Hall, Chief Executive Officer
COO: Susan Stone, Chief Operating Officer and Chief Nursing Officer
CFO: Tony Guerra, Chief Financial Officer
CHR: George Holtz, Manager Human Resources
Web address: www.sharp.com
Control: Other not–for–profit (including NFP Corporation) **Service:** General Medical and Surgical

Staffed Beds: 175 **Admissions:** 2691 **Census:** 143 **Outpatient Visits:** 45984 **Births:** 0 **Total Expense ($000):** 58732 **Payroll Expense ($000):** 27253 **Personnel:** 477

COSTA MESA—Orange County

□ **COLLEGE HOSPITAL COSTA MESA (50543)**, 301 Victoria Street, Zip 92627–7131; tel. 949/642–2734 **A**1 9 10 **F**30 79 80 87 88 89 90 94 95 119 132 **S** College Health Enterprises
Primary Contact: Wayne M. Lingenfelter, Ed.D., Chief Executive Officer
COO: Kara Bourne, R.N., MSN, Chief Operating Officer and Chief Nursing Officer
CFO: Dale Bracy, Chief Financial Officer
CMO: Craig A. Ross, M.D., Chief of Staff
CIO: Red Ladiana, Manager Information Systems
CHR: Sharon DuBruyne, Director Human Resources
Web address: www.collegehospitalcm.com
Control: State–Government, nonfederal **Service:** Psychiatric

Staffed Beds: 122 **Admissions:** 4197 **Census:** 102 **Births:** 0 **Total Expense ($000):** 34705 **Payroll Expense ($000):** 16199 **Personnel:** 270

COVINA—Los Angeles County

□ **AURORA CHARTER OAK HOSPITAL (54069)**, 1161 East Covina Boulevard, Zip 91724–1599; tel. 626/966–1632, (Nonreporting) **A**1 9 10 **S** Aurora Behavioral Health Care
Primary Contact: Todd A. Smith, Chief Executive Officer
COO: Sheila Cordova, Director Clinical Services and Chief Operating Officer
CFO: Cory Delello, Chief Financial Officer
CMO: Adib Bitar, M.D., Medical Director
CHR: Christine de la Paz, Director Human Resources
Web address: www.aurorabehavioral.com
Control: Corporation, Investor–owned, for–profit **Service:** Psychiatric

Staffed Beds: 82

CA

Hospital, Medicare Provider Number, Address, Telephone, Approval, Facility, and Physician Codes, Health Care System

★ American Hospital Association (AHA) membership
□ The Joint Commission accreditation
○ American Osteopathic Association (AOA) accreditation
△ Commission on Accreditation of Rehabilitation Facilities (CARF) accreditation

☐ **CITRUS VALLEY MEDICAL CENTER–INTER–COMMUNITY CAMPUS (50382)**, 210 West San Bernardino Road, Zip 91723–1901, Mailing Address: P.O. Box 6108, Zip 91722–5108; tel. 626/331–7331, (Nonreporting) **A**1 2 9 10 **S** Citrus Valley Health Partners
Primary Contact: James T. Yoshioka, President and Chief Executive Officer
COO: Elvia Foulke, Executive Vice President Healthcare Delivery and Chief Operating Officer
CFO: Lois Conyers, Senior Vice President and Chief Financial Officer
CMO: Richard Gisi, M.D., Vice President Medical Affairs
CIO: David McCobb, Chief Information Officer
CHR: Lisa Foust, Senior Vice President Human Resources
Web address: www.cvhp.org
Control: Other not–for–profit (including NFP Corporation) **Service:** General Medical and Surgical

Staffed Beds: 252

CRESCENT CITY—Del Norte County

★ **SUTTER COAST HOSPITAL (50417)**, 800 East Washington Boulevard, Zip 95531–8359; tel. 707/464–8511 **A**1 9 10 20 **F**11 13 15 25 26 30 31 32 33 38 46 47 48 53 55 58 61 68 73 74 79 80 86 96 97 100 101 106 107 121 133 135 **P**6 **S** Sutter Health
Primary Contact: John E. Menaugh, Chief Executive Officer
CFO: Judi Swartout, Chief Financial Officer
Web address: www.sutterhealth.org
Control: Other not–for–profit (including NFP Corporation) **Service:** General Medical and Surgical

Staffed Beds: 59 **Admissions:** 2431 **Census:** 24 **Outpatient Visits:** 95431 **Births:** 364 **Total Expense ($000):** 54911 **Payroll Expense ($000):** 19199 **Personnel:** 378

CULVER CITY—Los Angeles County

★ **BROTMAN MEDICAL CENTER (50752)**, 3828 Delmas Terrace, Zip 90232–6806; tel. 310/836–7000, (Total facility includes 21 beds in nursing home–type unit) **A**1 9 10 **F**3 4 5 8 12 14 17 18 20 22 25 27 31 32 33 34 35 36 38 41 43 47 49 55 56 57 58 60 62 63 66 68 72 73 75 76 77 79 82 85 86 87 88 90 91 92 93 94 95 96 97 102 106 107 117 119 120 121 122 132 135 **P**5
Primary Contact: Stanley Otake, Chief Executive Officer
COO: Diane Rafferty, Chief Operating Officer
CFO: Vincent Rubin, Chief Financial Officer
CMO: Martha Sonnenberg, M.D., Chief of Staff
CIO: Carrie Bonar, Chief Information Officer
CHR: Betty J. Harris, Director Human Resources
Web address: www.brotmanmedicalcenter.com
Control: Corporation, Investor–owned, for–profit **Service:** General Medical and Surgical

Staffed Beds: 420 **Admissions:** 8290 **Census:** 168 **Outpatient Visits:** 36971 **Births:** 0 **Total Expense ($000):** 101440 **Payroll Expense ($000):** 43023 **Personnel:** 692

DALY CITY—San Mateo County

★ **SETON MEDICAL CENTER (50289)**, 1900 Sullivan Avenue, Zip 94015–2229; tel. 650/992–4000, (Nonreporting) **A**1 2 9 10 **S** Daughters of Charity Health System
Primary Contact: Bernadette M. Smith, President and Chief Executive Officer
COO: Anne Goldfisher, Chief Operating Officer
CFO: Mark Okashima, Chief Financial Officer
CMO: Julius Zsigmond, M.D., President Medical Staff
CIO: Richard Hutsell, Vice President and Chief Information Officer
CHR: Linde Cheema, Vice President Human Resources
Web address: www.setonmedicalcenter.org
Control: Church–operated, Nongovernment, not–for profit **Service:** General Medical and Surgical

Staffed Beds: 263

DAVIS—Yolo County

★ **SUTTER DAVIS HOSPITAL (50537)**, 2000 Sutter Place, Zip 95616–6201, Mailing Address: P.O. Box 1617, Zip 95617–1617; tel. 530/756–6440, (Nonreporting) **A**1 3 5 9 10 **S** Sutter Health
Primary Contact: Janet Wagner, RN, Chief Administrative Officer
CFO: Richard SooHoo, Controller
CHR: Ann Gennuso Newton, Director Human Resources
Web address: www.sutterhealth.org
Control: Other not–for–profit (including NFP Corporation) **Service:** General Medical and Surgical

Staffed Beds: 48

DELANO—Kern County

○ **DELANO REGIONAL MEDICAL CENTER (50608)**, 1401 Garces Highway, Zip 93215–3690, Mailing Address: P.O. Box 460, Zip 93216–0460; tel. 661/725–4800, (Nonreporting) **A**9 10 11
Primary Contact: Allan G. Komarek, Ph.D., Executive Director
CFO: Bahram Ghaffari, Executive Associate Administrator and Chief Financial Officer
CIO: Sandy Bakich, Director Information Systems
CHR: Kenneth Joyner, Director Human Resources
Web address: www.drmc.com
Control: Other not–for–profit (including NFP Corporation) **Service:** General Medical and Surgical

Staffed Beds: 156

DOWNEY—Los Angeles County

☐ **DOWNEY REGIONAL MEDICAL CENTER (50393)**, 11500 Brookshire Avenue, Zip 90241–4917; tel. 562/904–5000, (Nonreporting) **A**1 9 10 12 13
Primary Contact: Kenneth Strople, President and Chief Executive Officer
COO: Robert E. Fuller, Executive Vice President and Chief Operating Officer
CMO: Bill Kim, M.D., Medical Director
Web address: www.drmci.org
Control: Other not–for–profit (including NFP Corporation) **Service:** General Medical and Surgical

Staffed Beds: 181

☐ △ **RANCHO LOS AMIGOS NATIONAL REHABILITATION CENTER (50717)**, 7601 East Imperial Highway, Zip 90242–3496; tel. 562/401–7022, (Nonreporting) **A**1 3 5 7 9 10 **S** Los Angeles County–Department of Health Services
Primary Contact: Jorge Orozco, Chief Executive Officer
CFO: Robin Bayus, Acting Chief Financial Officer
CMO: Charles A. Stewart, M.D., Acting Chief Medical Officer
CIO: Betty Romeo, Acting Chief Information Officer
CHR: Melinda Fonseca, Associate Director Human Resources
Web address: www.rancho.org
Control: County–Government, nonfederal **Service:** Rehabilitation

Staffed Beds: 207

DUARTE—Los Angeles County

★ **CITY OF HOPE NATIONAL MEDICAL CENTER (50146)**, 1500 East Duarte Road, Zip 91010–3012; tel. 626/359–8111 **A**1 2 3 5 8 9 10 **F**3 11 14 15 25 26 27 28 30 31 32 33 34 36 38 41 42 43 44 49 50 54 55 56 57 58 60 62 66 68 72 73 75 76 77 78 79 80 81 82 83 84 86 89 90 91 93 94 96 97 99 100 102 104 105 106 107 108 109 111 112 114 116 119 121 123 125 131 132 133 134 135 136 137 **P**5
Primary Contact: Michael A. Friedman, M.D., President and Chief Executive Officer
COO: Virginia A. Opipare, Chief Operating Officer
CFO: Dennis Rusch, Chief Financial Officer
CMO: Alexandra Levine, M.D., Chief Medical Officer
CIO: Jim Murry, Chief Information Officer
CHR: Patti Ossen, Interim Vice President Human Resources
Web address: www.cityofhope.org
Control: Other not–for–profit (including NFP Corporation) **Service:** Cancer

Staffed Beds: 168 **Admissions:** 5791 **Census:** 143 **Outpatient Visits:** 137832 **Births:** 0 **Total Expense ($000):** 402817 **Payroll Expense ($000):** 145029 **Personnel:** 2279

EL CENTRO—Imperial County

★ **EL CENTRO REGIONAL MEDICAL CENTER (50045)**, 1415 Ross Avenue, Zip 92243–4398; tel. 760/339–7100 **A**1 9 10 **F**3 11 13 15 25 26 31 32 38 50 51 53 55 56 57 59 60 62 66 68 70 72 73 74 75 77 79 80 81 82 84 86 96 97 100 107 119 121 132 135
Primary Contact: David R. Green, Administrator and Chief Executive Officer
CFO: Kathleen Farmer, Assistant Administrator Finance and Chief Financial Officer
CMO: Jorge F. Robles, M.D., Chief of Staff
CIO: John Gaede, Director Information Systems
CHR: Bill Moore, Chief Human Resources
Web address: www.ecrmc.org
Control: City–Government, nonfederal **Service:** General Medical and Surgical

Staffed Beds: 165 **Admissions:** 6085 **Census:** 71 **Outpatient Visits:** 127197 **Births:** 1545 **Total Expense ($000):** 75247 **Payroll Expense ($000):** 30063 **Personnel:** 690

EL MONTE—Los Angeles County

☐ **GREATER EL MONTE COMMUNITY HOSPITAL (50738)**, 1701 Santa Anita Avenue, Zip 91733–3411; tel. 626/579–7777, (Nonreporting) **A**1 9 10 **S** AHMC, Inc
Primary Contact: Philip A. Cohen, Chief Executive Officer
COO: Jose Ortega, Administrator and Chief Operating Officer
CFO: Mary Anne Monje, Chief Financial Officer
CMO: Julius Kpaduwa, M.D., Chief of Staff
CIO: Jay Geldhof, Director Information Systems
CHR: Jason Jaquez, Director Human Resources
Web address: www.greaterelmonte.com
Control: Corporation, Investor–owned, for–profit **Service:** General Medical and Surgical

Staffed Beds: 117

ELDRIDGE—Sonoma County

SONOMA DEVELOPMENTAL CENTER (50547), 15000 Arnold Drive, Zip 95431; tel. 707/938–6000, (Nonreporting) **A**10
Primary Contact: James E. Rogers, Executive Director
COO: Theresa Billeci, Director Administrative Services
CFO: Joanne S. Bender, Fiscal Officer
CMO: Judith Bjorndal, M.D., Medical Director
CIO: Karen Litzenberg, Public Information Officer
CHR: Kelly Mardell, Director Human Resources
Web address: www.dds.ca.gov/sonoma/sonoma.cfm
Control: State–Government, nonfederal **Service:** Institution for mental retardation

Staffed Beds: 1413

ENCINITAS—San Diego County

★☐ △ **SCRIPPS MEMORIAL HOSPITAL–ENCINITAS (50503)**, 354 Santa Fe Drive, Zip 92024–5182, Mailing Address: P.O. Box 230817, Zip 92023–0817; tel. 760/633–6501 **A**1 2 7 9 10 **F**3 8 11 13 15 18 25 26 27 30 31 32 33 38 43 44 49 51 55 63 66 68 70 72 73 74 75 76 77 79 80 81 82 85 86 92 96 100 102 103 107 119 121 135 136 137 **S** Scripps Health
Primary Contact: Carl J. Etter, Senior Vice President and Chief Executive
COO: Timothy Collins, Vice President Operations and Chief Operating Officer
CFO: Linda Honaker, Director Financial Services
CIO: Drexel DeFord, Vice President and Chief Information Officer
CHR: Pam Teufel, Administrative Director Human Resources
Web address: www.scrippshealth.org
Control: Other not–for–profit (including NFP Corporation) **Service:** General Medical and Surgical

Staffed Beds: 134 **Admissions:** 7927 **Census:** 108 **Outpatient Visits:** 58444 **Births:** 1573 **Total Expense ($000):** 136797 **Payroll Expense ($000):** 59135 **Personnel:** 828

ENCINO—Los Angeles County, See Los Angeles

ESCONDIDO—San Diego County

★☐ △ **PALOMAR MEDICAL CENTER (50115)**, 555 East Valley Parkway, Zip 92025–3084; tel. 760/739–3000, (Total facility includes 96 beds in nursing home–type unit) (Nonreporting) **A**1 5 7 9 10 **S** Palomar Pomerado Health
Primary Contact: Gerald E. Bracht, Chief Administrative Officer
COO: Gerald E. Bracht, Chief Administrative Officer
CFO: Robert Hemker, Chief Financial Officer
CMO: Duane Buringrud, M.D., Chief Medical and Quality Officer
CIO: Steven Tanaka, Chief Information Officer
CHR: Walter George, Chief Human Resources Officer
Web address: www.pph.org
Control: Hospital district or authority, Government, nonfederal **Service:** General Medical and Surgical

Staffed Beds: 315

EUREKA—Humboldt County

★☐ △ **ST. JOSEPH HOSPITAL (50006)**, 2700 Dolbeer Street, Zip 95501–4799; tel. 707/445–8121, (Includes GENERAL HOSPITAL, 2200 Harrison Avenue, Zip 95501–3299; tel. 707/445–5111) **A**1 2 7 9 10 19 **F**3 8 11 12 13 15 17 18 19 20 22 24 25 26 27 30 31 32 33 38 42 43 46 47 48 49 53 61 62 66 68 70 73 74 75 76 77 79 80 81 82 84 85 86 96 97 99 100 102 103 104 105 106 107 108 109 111 112 118 119 133 135 137 **P**5 **S** St. Joseph Health System
Primary Contact: Joseph M. Mark, President and Chief Executive Officer
COO: Robert C. Brannigan, Vice President, Chief Operating Officer and Chief Nursing Officer
CFO: Andrew Rybolt, Chief Financial Officer
CIO: Wendy Valdez, Area Director Information Systems
CHR: Bob Sampson, Vice President Human Resources
Web address: www.stjosepheureka.org
Control: Church–operated, Nongovernment, not–for profit **Service:** General Medical and Surgical

Staffed Beds: 125 **Admissions:** 6070 **Census:** 78 **Outpatient Visits:** 164904 **Births:** 712 **Total Expense ($000):** 133678 **Payroll Expense ($000):** 39968 **Personnel:** 840

FAIRFIELD—Solano County

★☐ **NORTHBAY MEDICAL CENTER (50367)**, 1200 B. Gale Wilson Boulevard, Zip 94533–3587; tel. 707/429–3600 **A**1 2 9 10 **F**3 11 13 18 24 25 27 28 31 32 34 38 43 46 50 53 57 62 68 70 73 74 75 76 77 78 79 80 82 84 86 87 96 97 102 103 106 107 110 119 121 135 **P**6 **S** NorthBay Healthcare System
Primary Contact: Deborah Sugiyama, President
CFO: Arthur E. DeNio, Vice President and Chief Financial Officer
CMO: Donald M. Denmark, M.D., Vice President Medical Affairs
CIO: Paul Alcala, Vice President and Chief Information Officer
CHR: Ken McCollum, Vice President Human Resources
Web address: www.northbay.org
Control: Other not–for–profit (including NFP Corporation) **Service:** General Medical and Surgical

Staffed Beds: 107 **Admissions:** 5910 **Census:** 66 **Outpatient Visits:** 116126 **Births:** 1589 **Total Expense ($000):** 166942 **Payroll Expense ($000):** 67030 **Personnel:** 609

FALL RIVER MILLS—Shasta County

★ **MAYERS MEMORIAL HOSPITAL DISTRICT (51305)**, 43563 Highway 299 East, Zip 96028–0459, Mailing Address: P.O. Box 459, Zip 96028–0459; tel. 530/336–5511, (Total facility includes 99 beds in nursing home–type unit) **A**9 10 18 **F**6 7 13 30 32 38 42 54 55 57 62 74 75 77 79 96 102 107 117 119 121 122 135 137 **P**5
Primary Contact: Katharine Ann Campbell, Administrator and Chief Executive Officer
CMO: Chris Camarata, M.D., Chief of Staff
CIO: Martha Lucero, Director Special Projects
CHR: Paul McCoy, Director Human Resources
Web address: www.mayersmemorial.com
Control: Hospital district or authority, Government, nonfederal **Service:** General Medical and Surgical

Staffed Beds: 121 **Admissions:** 696 **Census:** 91 **Outpatient Visits:** 17202 **Births:** 118 **Total Expense ($000):** 16551 **Payroll Expense ($000):** 6136 **Personnel:** 169

FALLBROOK—San Diego County

★☐ **FALLBROOK HOSPITAL (50435)**, 624 East Elder Street, Zip 92028–3099; tel. 760/728–1191, (Total facility includes 93 beds in nursing home–type unit) (Nonreporting) **A**1 9 10 20 **S** Community Health Systems, Inc.
Primary Contact: Fred Capozello, Jr., Interim Chief Executive Officer
Web address: www.fallbrookhospital.com
Control: Hospital district or authority, Government, nonfederal **Service:** General Medical and Surgical

Staffed Beds: 179

FOLSOM—Sacramento County

☐ **KINDRED HOSPITAL–SACRAMENTO (52033)**, 223 Fargo Way, Zip 95630–2961; tel. 916/351–9151, (Nonreporting) **A**1 9 10 **S** Kindred Healthcare
Primary Contact: Virginia Matthews, Chief Executive Officer
COO: Judy Lange, Chief Operating Officer
CFO: Bruce MacNeill, Chief Financial Officer
Web address: www.kindredhealthcare.com
Control: Corporation, Investor–owned, for–profit **Service:** Long–Term Acute Care hospital

Staffed Beds: 31

Hospital, Medicare Provider Number, Address, Telephone, Approval, Facility, and Physician Codes, Health Care System
★ American Hospital Association (AHA) membership
☐ The Joint Commission accreditation
○ American Osteopathic Association (AOA) accreditation
△ Commission on Accreditation of Rehabilitation Facilities (CARF) accreditation

☒ **MERCY HOSPITAL OF FOLSOM (50414)**, 1650 Creekside Drive, Zip 95630–3405; tel. 916/983–7400 **A**1 9 10 **F**3 8 11 13 15 17 25 26 30 31 32 33 34 38 43 44 46 49 51 55 56 57 62 64 66 68 72 73 74 76 77 79 80 81 86 96 97 102 103 106 107 119 121 135 136 **P**5 **S** Catholic Healthcare West
Primary Contact: Donald C. Hudson, President
CFO: Robin Rogness, Vice President and Chief Financial Officer
CMO: Russ Braun, M.D., Vice President Medical Affairs
CHR: Amy Mantell, Vice President Human Resources
Web address: www.mercyfolsom.org
Control: Church–operated, Nongovernment, not–for profit **Service:** General Medical and Surgical

Staffed Beds: 85 **Admissions:** 4652 **Census:** 43 **Outpatient Visits:** 38046 **Births:** 1089 **Total Expense ($000):** 74364 **Payroll Expense ($000):** 34513 **Personnel:** 400

FONTANA—San Bernardino County

☒ **KAISER FOUNDATION HOSPITAL – FONTANA (50140)**, 9961 Sierra Avenue, Zip 92335–6720; tel. 909/427–5000 **A**1 3 5 10 **F**3 4 5 8 13 15 17 18 24 25 26 27 30 31 32 33 38 41 42 43 44 46 48 49 50 55 58 59 61 62 63 66 68 69 70 71 72 73 74 75 76 77 79 80 81 82 84 85 92 96 97 100 102 103 105 106 107 112 119 121 124 134 135 137 **S** Kaiser Foundation Hospitals
Primary Contact: Greg Christian, Executive Director
CFO: Donald P. Bernard, Chief Financial Officer
CMO: David Quam, M.D., Area Medical Director
CIO: Jennifer Resch–Silvestri, Public Affairs Leader
CHR: Kimberly Labiaga, Human Resources Leader
Web address: www.kaiserpermanente.org
Control: Other not–for–profit (including NFP Corporation) **Service:** General Medical and Surgical

Staffed Beds: 379 **Admissions:** 31767 **Census:** 303 **Outpatient Visits:** 100440 **Births:** 4771 **Personnel:** 3961

FORT BRAGG—Mendocino County

☒ **MENDOCINO COAST DISTRICT HOSPITAL (51325)**, 700 River Drive, Zip 95437–5495; tel. 707/961–1234 **A**1 9 10 **F**3 7 11 13 15 25 26 27 30 31 32 38 42 53 55 57 61 62 63 68 73 74 75 76 77 79 86 87 96 97 100 102 106 107 119 121 122 135 137
Primary Contact: Raymond T. Hino, Chief Executive Officer
COO: Raymond T. Hino, Chief Executive Officer
CFO: Wayne Allen, Chief Financial Officer
CMO: John Kermen, D.O., Chief Medical Staff
CIO: Jeff Edwards, Manager Information Services
CHR: Scott Kidd, Director Human Resources
Web address: www.mcdh.org
Control: Hospital district or authority, Government, nonfederal **Service:** General Medical and Surgical

Staffed Beds: 25 **Admissions:** 1326 **Census:** 16 **Outpatient Visits:** 61457 **Births:** 166 **Total Expense ($000):** 32922 **Payroll Expense ($000):** 14646 **Personnel:** 225

FORT IRWIN—San Bernardino County

☒ **WEED ARMY COMMUNITY HOSPITAL**, Inner Loop Road and 4th Street, Bl 166, Zip 92310–5065, Mailing Address: P.O. Box 105109, Zip 92310–5109; tel. 760/380–3108, (Nonreporting) **A**1 **S** Department of the Army, Office of the Surgeon General
Primary Contact: Colonel Margaret Bates, Commanding Officer
CFO: Bella R. Ibanez, Budget Officer
CMO: Lieutenant Colonel John Glorioso, Deputy Commander Clinical Services
CIO: Michael Haenelt, Chief Information Management
Web address: www.irwin.amedd.army.mil
Control: Army, Government, federal **Service:** General Medical and Surgical

Staffed Beds: 27

FORTUNA—Humboldt County

☒ **REDWOOD MEMORIAL HOSPITAL (51318)**, 3300 Renner Drive, Zip 95540–3198; tel. 707/725–3361 **A**1 2 9 10 18 **F**3 11 13 15 25 26 30 31 32 33 34 38 50 55 56 57 62 66 68 73 74 75 77 79 80 81 82 86 87 96 102 107 119 121 122 135 136 **S** St. Joseph Health System
Primary Contact: Joseph M. Mark, President and Chief Executive Officer
COO: Joseph J. Rogers, Vice President and Chief Operating Officer
Web address: www.stjosepheureka.org
Control: Church–operated, Nongovernment, not–for profit **Service:** General Medical and Surgical

Staffed Beds: 25 **Admissions:** 1594 **Census:** 17 **Outpatient Visits:** 41150 **Births:** 389 **Total Expense ($000):** 28147 **Payroll Expense ($000):** 10135 **Personnel:** 203

FOUNTAIN VALLEY—Orange County

☒ **FOUNTAIN VALLEY REGIONAL HOSPITAL AND MEDICAL CENTER (50570)**, 17100 Euclid Street, Zip 92708–4043; tel. 714/966–7200, (Nonreporting) **A**1 2 3 5 9 10 **S** TENET Healthcare Corporation
Primary Contact: Deborah C. Keel, Chief Executive Officer
COO: Kathy Dowling, Chief Operating Officer
CFO: Jon Zilkow, Chief Financial Officer
CMO: Satinder Swaroop, M.D., Chief of Staff
CIO: Bill Mathiasen, Director Information Systems
CHR: Tim Howard, Chief Human Resources Officer
Web address: www.fountainvalleyhospital.com
Control: State–Government, nonfederal **Service:** General Medical and Surgical

Staffed Beds: 400

☒ **ORANGE COAST MEMORIAL MEDICAL CENTER (50678)**, 9920 Talbert Avenue, Zip 92708–5153; tel. 714/378–7000 **A**1 9 10 **F**3 11 12 13 15 18 20 25 26 27 30 31 32 33 36 38 41 43 44 46 49 50 53 54 55 56 57 58 62 63 66 68 70 72 73 74 75 76 77 79 80 81 82 86 96 97 100 102 107 119 120 121 124 132 135 136 137 **S** Memorial Health Services
Primary Contact: Marcia Manker, Chief Executive Officer
COO: Cheryl Jacob, Vice President Operations
CFO: Janice Fauchier, Chief Financial Officer
CIO: Danny Asaoka, Director Information Systems
CHR: Lorraine Booth, Executive Director Human Resources
Web address: www.memorialcare.org
Control: Other not–for–profit (including NFP Corporation) **Service:** General Medical and Surgical

Staffed Beds: 224 **Admissions:** 12409 **Census:** 122 **Outpatient Visits:** 58387 **Births:** 1511 **Total Expense ($000):** 170831 **Payroll Expense ($000):** 59592 **Personnel:** 933

FREMONT—Alameda County

☐ **FREMONT HOSPITAL (54110)**, 39001 Sundale Drive, Zip 94538–2005; tel. 510/796–1100, (Nonreporting) **A**1 9 10 **S** Psychiatric Solutions
Primary Contact: Jay R. Kellison, Chief Executive Officer
CFO: Bill Bay, Chief Financial Officer
CMO: William Barnard, M.D., Medical Director
CHR: Amy Fleming, Director Human Resources
Web address: www.fremonthospital.com
Control: Corporation, Investor–owned, for–profit **Service:** Psychiatric

Staffed Beds: 78

☒ **WASHINGTON HOSPITAL HEALTHCARE SYSTEM (50195)**, (Formerly Washington Township Health Care District), 2000 Mowry Avenue, Zip 94538–1746; tel. 510/797–1111, (Nonreporting) **A**1 2 9 10
Primary Contact: Nancy D. Farber, Chief Executive Officer
COO: Edward J. Fayen, Chief of Operations and Support
CFO: Catherine Souza, Chief Financial Officer
CMO: Ranjana Sharma, M.D., Chief of Staff
CIO: Lee Herrmann, Chief Information Officer
CHR: Kathy Hunt, Chief Human Resources
Web address: www.whhs.com
Control: Hospital district or authority, Government, nonfederal **Service:** General Medical and Surgical

Staffed Beds: 315

FRENCH CAMP—San Joaquin County

☐ **SAN JOAQUIN GENERAL HOSPITAL (50167)**, 500 West Hospital Road, Zip 95231, Mailing Address: P.O. Box 1020, Stockton, Zip 95201; tel. 209/468–6000, (Nonreporting) **A**1 3 5 9 10
Primary Contact: Kenneth B. Cohen, Director Health Care Services
CMO: Jerry Royer, M.D., Chief Medical Officer
CIO: Don Johnston, Chief Information Officer
CHR: Patricia Wright, Personal Analyst
Web address: www.sjghgeneralhospital.com
Control: County–Government, nonfederal **Service:** General Medical and Surgical

Staffed Beds: 145

FRESNO—Fresno County

☐ **COMMUNITY BEHAVIORAL HEALTH CENTER**, 7171 North Cedar Avenue, Zip 93720–3311; tel. 559/449–8000, (Nonreporting) **A**1 9 **S** Community Medical Centers
Primary Contact: Dawan Haubursin, Chief Executive Officer
COO: Patrick W. Rafferty, Executive Vice President and Chief Operating Officer
CFO: Stephen Walter, Senior Vice President and Chief Financial Officer
CMO: Thomas Utecht, M.D., Senior Vice President and Chief Quality Officer
CIO: George Vasquez, Vice President
CHR: Ginny Burdick, Vice President Human Resources
Web address: www.communitymedical.org
Control: Corporation, Investor–owned, for–profit **Service:** Psychiatric

Staffed Beds: 60

☐ **COMMUNITY REGIONAL MEDICAL CENTER (50060)**, 2823 Fresno Street, Zip 93721–1324, Mailing Address: P.O. Box 1232, Zip 93715–1232; tel. 559/459–6000, (Total facility includes 63 beds in nursing home–type unit) (Nonreporting) **A**1 2 3 5 8 9 10 **S** Community Medical Centers
Primary Contact: John M. Chubb, Chief Executive Officer
COO: Patrick W. Rafferty, Executive Vice President and Chief Operating Officer
CFO: Stephen Walter, Senior Vice President and Chief Financial Officer
CMO: Thomas Utecht, M.D., Chief Quality Officer
CIO: Craig Castro, Chief Information Officer
CHR: Ginny Burdick, Vice President Human Resources
Web address: www.communitymedical.org
Control: Other not–for–profit (including NFP Corporation) **Service:** General Medical and Surgical

Staffed Beds: 460

FRESNO HEART AND SURGICAL HOSPITAL (50732), 15 East Audubon Drive, Zip 93720; tel. 559/433–8000, (Nonreporting) **A**9 10
Primary Contact: Wanda Holderman, Chief Executive Officer
CIO: Jonathon Anderson, Director Information Technology and Telecommunications
CHR: Lynn M. Horton, Executive Director Human Resources
Web address: www.fresnoheart.com
Control: Corporation, Investor–owned, for–profit **Service:** Heart

Staffed Beds: 60

☐ **FRESNO SURGICAL HOSPITAL (50708)**, 6125 North Fresno Street, Zip 93710–5207; tel. 559/431–8000, (Nonreporting) **A**1 9 10
Primary Contact: Sheryl D. Dodds, Chief Executive Officer
CMO: Harry Joe, M.D., Medical Director
Control: Partnership, Investor–owned, for–profit **Service:** General Medical and Surgical

Staffed Beds: 16

★☐ **KAISER FOUNDATION HOSPITAL – FRESNO (50710)**, 7300 North Fresno Street, Zip 93720–2941; tel. 559/448–4500 **A**1 10 **F**3 8 12 13 15 25 26 27 30 31 32 33 38 43 44 46 47 48 49 51 52 57 62 66 68 70 71 72 74 75 76 77 79 80 81 82 86 87 92 96 97 99 100 102 105 106 107 112 119 124 133 135 137 **S** Kaiser Foundation Hospitals
Primary Contact: Susan A. Ryan, Senior Vice President and Service Area Manager
CFO: Richard Alves, Chief Financial Officer
CMO: Varouj Altebarmakian, M.D., Physician in Chief
CIO: Brad Bain, Information Systems Leader
Web address: www.kaiserpermanente.org
Control: Other not–for–profit (including NFP Corporation) **Service:** General Medical and Surgical

Staffed Beds: 169 **Admissions:** 7998 **Census:** 94 **Outpatient Visits:** 773319 **Births:** 1355 **Personnel:** 1785

★☐ **SAINT AGNES MEDICAL CENTER (50093)**, 1303 East Herndon Avenue, Zip 93720–3309; tel. 559/450–3000 **A**1 2 9 10 **F**2 3 8 11 12 13 15 17 18 20 22 24 25 26 27 30 31 32 33 34 36 38 41 42 43 44 45 46 50 51 52 54 55 56 57 60 61 62 68 72 73 74 75 76 77 79 80 81 82 86 96 99 100 102 105 106 107 108 109 111 112 114 116 118 119 120 121 135 136 137 **S** Trinity Health
Primary Contact: Thomas E. Anderson, President and Chief Executive Officer
CMO: Patrick Marabella, M.D., Chief Medical Officer
CHR: Daniel Camp, Senior Vice President Human Resources
Web address: www.samc.com
Control: Church–operated, Nongovernment, not–for profit **Service:** General Medical and Surgical

Staffed Beds: 434 **Admissions:** 25648 **Census:** 303 **Outpatient Visits:** 326691 **Births:** 3266 **Total Expense ($000):** 353186 **Payroll Expense ($000):** 151311 **Personnel:** 2363

☐ **SAN JOAQUIN VALLEY REHABILITATION HOSPITAL (53032)**, 7173 North Sharon Avenue, Zip 93720–3329; tel. 559/436–3600, (Nonreporting) **A**1 9 10 **S** Vibra Healthcare
Primary Contact: Edward C. Palacios, Chief Executive Officer
CHR: Peggy Reeve, Director Human Resources
Web address: www.sjvrehab.com
Control: Corporation, Investor–owned, for–profit **Service:** Rehabilitation

Staffed Beds: 60

★☐ **VETERANS AFFAIRS MEDICAL CENTER**, 2615 East Clinton Avenue, Zip 93703–2223; tel. 559/225–6100, (Total facility includes 60 beds in nursing home–type unit) (Nonreporting) **A**1 2 3 5 **S** Department of Veterans Affairs
Primary Contact: Alan S. Perry, Director
CFO: Holley Niethammer, Chief Business Administration
CMO: William Cahill, M.D., Chief of Staff
CIO: Byron Youngblood, Chief Information Resources Management
CHR: Pat Hilsgen, Chief Human Resources Management
Web address: www.va.gov/sta/guide/home.asp
Control: Veterans Affairs, Government, federal **Service:** General Medical and Surgical

Staffed Beds: 125

FULLERTON—Orange County

★☐ △ **ST. JUDE MEDICAL CENTER (50168)**, 101 East Valencia Mesa Drive, Zip 92835–3809; tel. 714/992–3000 **A**1 2 5 7 9 10 **F**2 3 6 8 11 13 15 17 18 20 22 24 25 26 27 28 30 31 32 33 34 37 38 41 42 43 44 46 47 48 49 50 51 52 53 54 55 56 57 58 59 62 63 64 65 66 67 68 69 70 72 73 74 75 76 77 79 80 81 82 84 85 86 90 96 97 99 100 102 104 105 106 107 108 109 111 112 114 117 118 119 120 121 124 132 135 136 137 **P**3 5 **S** St. Joseph Health System
Primary Contact: Lee Penrose, President and Chief Executive Officer
COO: Doreen Dann, R.N., Executive Vice President and Chief Operating Officer
CMO: Lytton Smith, M.D., Chief of Staff
CIO: DruAnn Copping, Director Public Affairs
CHR: Mark Jablonski, Vice President Human Resources
Web address: www.stjudemedicalcenter.org
Control: Church–operated, Nongovernment, not–for profit **Service:** General Medical and Surgical

Staffed Beds: 359 **Admissions:** 16335 **Census:** 223 **Outpatient Visits:** 265973 **Births:** 2127 **Total Expense ($000):** 301402 **Payroll Expense ($000):** 114732 **Personnel:** 2274

GARBERVILLE—Humboldt County

JEROLD PHELPS COMMUNITY HOSPITAL (51309), 733 Cedar Street, Zip 95542–3201; tel. 707/923–3921, (Total facility includes 8 beds in nursing home–type unit) (Nonreporting) **A**9 10 18
Primary Contact: Deborah Scaife, RN, M.S.N., Administrator and Director Patient Care Services
COO: Kent Scown, Director Operations and Information Services
CFO: Mike Nagle, Director Financial Services
CMO: Mark H. Phelps, M.D., Chief of Staff and Medical Director
CIO: Kent Scown, Director Operations and Information Services
CHR: Linda Feretto, Director Human Resources
Web address: www.shchd.org
Control: Hospital district or authority, Government, nonfederal **Service:** General Medical and Surgical

Staffed Beds: 17

GARDEN GROVE—Orange County

★☐ **GARDEN GROVE HOSPITAL AND MEDICAL CENTER (50230)**, 12601 Garden Grove Boulevard, Zip 92843–1908; tel. 714/537–5160 **A**1 9 10 **F**12 13 25 26 30 31 32 33 38 57 62 68 70 73 74 77 79 80 82 96 97 102 107 119 121 135 **P**8 **S** Prime Healthcare Services
Primary Contact: Maxine T. Cooper, Chief Executive Officer
COO: Karen Gulbenkian, Chief Operating Officer
CFO: Ed Salvador, Chief Financial Officer
CMO: Peter Wang, M.D., Chief of Staff
CIO: Eileen Nicodemus, Director Information Systems
CHR: Linda Lyons, Director Human Resources
Web address: www.gardengrovehospital.com
Control: Corporation, Investor–owned, for–profit **Service:** General Medical and Surgical

Staffed Beds: 74 **Admissions:** 7450 **Census:** 74 **Outpatient Visits:** 38179 **Births:** 2997 **Total Expense ($000):** 70397 **Payroll Expense ($000):** 38230 **Personnel:** 502

GARDENA—Los Angeles County

☐ **MEMORIAL HOSPITAL OF GARDENA (50468)**, 1145 West Redondo Beach Boulevard, Zip 90247–3528; tel. 310/532–4200, (Total facility includes 69 beds in nursing home–type unit) (Nonreporting) **A**1 9 10 **S** HealthPlus
Primary Contact: Steve Popkin, Chief Executive Officer
CFO: Terri Davis, Chief Financial Officer
CMO: Alfonso Baez, M.D., Chief Medical Staff
CHR: Eilene Ishizu, Director Human Resources and Administrative Services
Control: Corporation, Investor–owned, for–profit **Service:** General Medical and Surgical

Staffed Beds: 107

Hospital, Medicare Provider Number, Address, Telephone, Approval, Facility, and Physician Codes, Health Care System

★ American Hospital Association (AHA) membership
☐ The Joint Commission accreditation
○ American Osteopathic Association (AOA) accreditation
△ Commission on Accreditation of Rehabilitation Facilities (CARF) accreditation

☐ **VISTA HOSPITAL OF SOUTH BAY (52050)**, (Formerly Community Hospital of Gardena), 1246 West 155th Street, Zip 90247–4011; tel. 310/323–5330, (Total facility includes 20 beds in nursing home–type unit) (Nonreporting) **A**1 10
Primary Contact: Kevin Chavez, Chief Executive Officer
CFO: Pilar De Guzman, Chief Financial Officer
CMO: Richard Yap, M.D., Chief Clinical Officer
Web address: www.vistahealthcare.net
Control: Corporation, Investor–owned, for–profit **Service:** Long–Term Acute Care hospital

Staffed Beds: 58

GILROY—Santa Clara County

★ **ST. LOUISE REGIONAL HOSPITAL (50688)**, 9400 No Name Uno, Zip 95020–3528; tel. 408/848–2000 **A**1 9 10 **F**11 13 15 25 26 27 30 31 32 33 35 38 43 46 47 48 49 50 55 56 57 59 62 66 67 68 73 74 76 77 79 80 81 82 96 100 103 107 117 119 121 124 135 137 **S** Daughters of Charity Health System
Primary Contact: Joanne E. Allen, President and Chief Executive Officer
COO: Carol Furgurson, Chief Operating Officer
CFO: Chelva Kumar, Chief Financial Officer
CIO: Dick Hutsell, Vice President Information Technology Services
Web address: www.dochs.org
Control: Other not–for–profit (including NFP Corporation) **Service:** General Medical and Surgical

Staffed Beds: 83 **Admissions:** 3793 **Census:** 43 **Outpatient Visits:** 52730 **Births:** 615 **Total Expense ($000):** 67714 **Payroll Expense ($000):** 29830 **Personnel:** 226

GLENDALE—Los Angeles County

★ **GLENDALE ADVENTIST MEDICAL CENTER (50239)**, 1509 Wilson Terrace, Zip 91206–4098; tel. 818/409–8000, (Nonreporting) **A**1 2 3 5 9 10 **S** Adventist Health
Primary Contact: Morre Dean, President and Chief Executive Officer
CFO: Kelly Turner, Senior Vice President Finance
Web address: www.glendaleadventist.com
Control: Church–operated, Nongovernment, not–for profit **Service:** General Medical and Surgical

Staffed Beds: 396

★ **GLENDALE MEMORIAL HOSPITAL AND HEALTH CENTER (50058)**, 1420 South Central Avenue, Zip 91204–2594; tel. 818/502–1900, (Nonreporting) **A**1 9 10 **S** Catholic Healthcare West
Primary Contact: Catherine M. Pelley, President
COO: Kim Strange, Senior Vice President and Chief Operating Officer
CFO: Karen Krug, Senior Vice President Finance and Chief Financial Officer
CMO: Milton Louie, M.D., Senior Vice President Medical Affairs
CHR: Deborah Wilson, Senior Vice President Human Resources and Organizational Development
Web address: www.glendalememorial.com
Control: Other not–for–profit (including NFP Corporation) **Service:** General Medical and Surgical

Staffed Beds: 334

☐ **VERDUGO HILLS HOSPITAL (50124)**, 1812 Verdugo Boulevard, Zip 91208–1409; tel. 818/790–7100, (Nonreporting) **A**1 9 10
Primary Contact: Leonard LaBella, President and Chief Executive Officer
CFO: Cindy Trousdale, Chief Financial Officer
CHR: Paul Celuch, Vice President Human Resources and Support Services
Web address: www.verdugohillshospital.org
Control: Other not–for–profit (including NFP Corporation) **Service:** General Medical and Surgical

Staffed Beds: 124

GLENDORA—Los Angeles County

☐ **EAST VALLEY HOSPITAL MEDICAL CENTER (50205)**, 150 West Route 66, Zip 91740–6207; tel. 626/852–5000, (Nonreporting) **A**1 9 10
Primary Contact: C. Joseph Chang, President and Chief Executive Officer
CFO: Linda Reitz, Controller
CIO: Wayne Giddings, Manager Management Information Systems
CHR: Kim Bui, Director Human Resources
Control: Other not–for–profit (including NFP Corporation) **Service:** General Medical and Surgical

Staffed Beds: 118

★ **FOOTHILL PRESBYTERIAN HOSPITAL–MORRIS L. JOHNSTON MEMORIAL (50597)**, 250 South Grand Avenue, Zip 91741–4218; tel. 626/963–8411, (Nonreporting) **A**1 9 10 **S** Citrus Valley Health Partners
Primary Contact: Larry S. Fetters, Administrator
COO: Elvia Foulke, Executive Vice President and Chief Operating Officer
CFO: Lois Conyers, Senior Vice President and Chief Financial Officer
CMO: John DiMare, M.D., Medical Director
CIO: David McCobb, Chief Information Officer
CHR: Lisa Foust, Senior Vice President Human Resources
Web address: www.cvhp.org
Control: Church–operated, Nongovernment, not–for profit **Service:** General Medical and Surgical

Staffed Beds: 106

GRANADA HILLS—Los Angeles County, See Los Angeles

GRASS VALLEY—Nevada County

★ **SIERRA NEVADA MEMORIAL HOSPITAL (50150)**, 155 Glasson Way, Zip 95945–5723, Mailing Address: P.O. Box 1029, Zip 95945–1029; tel. 530/274–6000 **A**1 2 9 10 19 **F**1 3 7 11 13 15 17 18 24 25 26 27 30 31 32 38 43 44 50 51 55 56 59 61 62 63 66 68 73 74 75 76 77 79 80 81 86 96 97 99 100 104 106 107 109 111 119 121 124 133 135 137 **P**5 **S** Catholic Healthcare West
Primary Contact: Katherine Medeiros, President and Chief Executive Officer
COO: Mary L. Gish, R.N., Vice President and Chief Nursing Officer
CFO: Carolyn Canady, Chief Financial Officer
CMO: Frank Lang, M.D., Chief of Medicine
CHR: Annalise O'Connor, Director Human Resources
Web address: www.snmh.org
Control: Other not–for–profit (including NFP Corporation) **Service:** General Medical and Surgical

Staffed Beds: 121 **Admissions:** 6635 **Census:** 67 **Outpatient Visits:** 191294 **Births:** 473 **Total Expense ($000):** 89483 **Payroll Expense ($000):** 44733 **Personnel:** 555

GREENBRAE—Marin County

★ **MARIN GENERAL HOSPITAL (50360)**, 250 Bon Air Road, Zip 94904–1784, Mailing Address: P.O. Box 8010, San Rafael, Zip 94912–8010; tel. 415/925–7000, (Nonreporting) **A**1 2 9 10 **S** Sutter Health
Primary Contact: David Bradley, Chief Executive Officer
COO: Richard S. Liszewski, CHE, Chief Operating Officer
CMO: Robert MacInnes, M.D., Medical Director
CIO: Terry Mann, Director Management Information Services
Web address: www.maringeneral.sutterhealth.org
Control: Hospital district or authority, Government, nonfederal **Service:** General Medical and Surgical

Staffed Beds: 235

GRIDLEY—Butte County

BIGGS–GRIDLEY MEMORIAL HOSPITAL (51311), 240 Spruce Street, Zip 95948–2216, Mailing Address: P.O. Box 97, Zip 95948–0097; tel. 530/846–5671, (Total facility includes 7 beds in nursing home–type unit) (Nonreporting) **A**9 10 18
Primary Contact: Aaron Wood, Chief Executive Officer
COO: Ryan Quist, Administrative Assistant
CFO: Kevin Woodward, Chief Financial Officer
CMO: Henry Starkes, M.D., Medical Director
CIO: Ryan Quist, Administrative Assistant
CHR: Tresha Moreland, Vice President Human Resources
Web address: www.dmh.ca.gov/statehospitals/atascadero
Control: Other not–for–profit (including NFP Corporation) **Service:** General Medical and Surgical

Staffed Beds: 27

HANFORD—Kings County

★ **CENTRAL VALLEY GENERAL HOSPITAL (50196)**, 1025 North Douty Street, Zip 93230–3722, Mailing Address: P.O. Box 480, Zip 93232–0480; tel. 559/583–2100 **A**1 9 10 **F**26 32 33 38 53 56 57 62 74 75 79 82 86 96 97 100 102 107 118 119 121 133 135 136 **P**7 8 **S** Adventist Health
Primary Contact: Douglas L. Lafferty, Administrator
Web address: www.hanfordhealth.com
Control: Church–operated, Nongovernment, not–for profit **Service:** General Medical and Surgical

Staffed Beds: 49 **Admissions:** 888 **Census:** 28 **Outpatient Visits:** 375206 **Births:** 2254 **Total Expense ($000):** 82403 **Payroll Expense ($000):** 32214 **Personnel:** 888

★ **HANFORD COMMUNITY MEDICAL CENTER (50121)**, 450 North Greenfield Avenue, Zip 93230–3513, Mailing Address: P.O. Box 240, Zip 93232–0240; tel. 559/582–9000 **A**1 9 10 **F**3 8 11 13 15 18 20 25 26 30 31 32 33 38 42 50 55 61 62 66 68 72 73 74 75 77 79 80 81 82 86 87 96 97 100 103 107 119 121 133 135 137 **P**4 **S** Adventist Health
Primary Contact: Richard L. Rawson, President and Chief Executive Officer
COO: Richard L. Rawson, President and Chief Executive Officer
CFO: Kirby McKague, Chief Financial Officer
CMO: Nicholas Reiber, M.D., Chief of Staff
CIO: Michael Aubry, Director Information Systems
CHR: Darla Phelps, Director Human Resources
Web address: www.hanfordhealth.com
Control: Church–operated, Nongovernment, not–for profit **Service:** General Medical and Surgical

Staffed Beds: 121 **Admissions:** 4390 **Census:** 78 **Outpatient Visits:** 168308 **Births:** 1048 **Total Expense ($000):** 109195 **Payroll Expense ($000):** 48984 **Personnel:** 888

HARBOR CITY—Los Angeles County, See Los Angeles

HAWAIIAN GARDENS—Los Angeles County

☐ **TRI–CITY REGIONAL MEDICAL CENTER (50575)**, 21530 South Pioneer Boulevard, Zip 90716; tel. 562/860–0401, (Nonreporting) **A**1 10
Primary Contact: Arthur J. Gerrick, President and Chief Executive Officer
CFO: Karen Nimniyom, Director Finance
CHR: Olga Meza, Director Human Resources
Web address: www.tri-cityrmc.org
Control: Other not–for–profit (including NFP Corporation) **Service:** Other specialty

Staffed Beds: 137

HAWTHORNE—Los Angeles County

HAWTHORNE HOSPITAL See Los Angeles Metropolitan Medical Center, Los Angeles

HAYWARD—Alameda County

★ **KAISER FOUNDATION HOSPITAL – HAYWARD (50512)**, 27400 Hesperian Boulevard, Zip 94545–4235; tel. 510/784–4000, (Nonreporting) **A**1 5 10 **S** Kaiser Foundation Hospitals
Primary Contact: Colleen McKeown, Senior Vice President and Service Area Manager
COO: Kim Pardini–Keily, Chief Operating Officer
Web address: www.kaiserpermanente.org
Control: Other not–for–profit (including NFP Corporation) **Service:** General Medical and Surgical

Staffed Beds: 208

☐ **ST. ROSE HOSPITAL (50002)**, 27200 Calaroga Avenue, Zip 94545–4383; tel. 510/264–4000, (Total facility includes 22 beds in nursing home–type unit) (Nonreporting) **A**1 2 9 10
Primary Contact: Michael P. Mahoney, President and Chief Executive Officer
CFO: Michael Taylor, Vice President Financial Services and Chief Financial Officer
CMO: Charles S. Feldstein, M.D., Vice President Medical Affairs
CHR: John Davini, Vice President
Web address: www.strosehospital.org
Control: Other not–for–profit (including NFP Corporation) **Service:** General Medical and Surgical

Staffed Beds: 163

HEALDSBURG—Sonoma County

HEALDSBURG DISTRICT HOSPITAL (51321), 1375 University Street, Zip 95448–3382; tel. 707/431–6500 **A**9 10 18 **F**15 25 26 30 31 32 38 43 50 51 54 55 56 57 58 62 66 69 72 73 75 77 79 80 81 82 86 96 100 107 120 122 135 137 **P**4
Primary Contact: Evan J. Rayner, Chief Executive Officer
CFO: Dan Hull, Chief Financial Officer
CMO: Steven Vargas, M.D., Chief of Staff
CIO: Gary Crossan, Director Information Systems
CHR: George Protos, Director Human Resources
Web address: www.nschd.org
Control: Hospital district or authority, Government, nonfederal **Service:** General Medical and Surgical

Staffed Beds: 38 **Admissions:** 694 **Census:** 5 **Outpatient Visits:** 52607 **Births:** 0 **Total Expense ($000):** 19540 **Payroll Expense ($000):** 9479 **Personnel:** 207

HEMET—Riverside County

★ **HEMET VALLEY MEDICAL CENTER (50390)**, 1117 East Devonshire Avenue, Zip 92543–3083; tel. 951/652–2811, (Total facility includes 136 beds in nursing home–type unit) (Nonreporting) **A**1 9 10 **S** Valley Health System
Primary Contact: Fred M. Harder, Chief Executive Officer
CFO: Hubert U. King, Chief Financial Officer
CIO: David Pape, Chief Information Officer
CHR: Michele Bird, Chief Human Resources Officer
Web address: www.valleyhealthsystem.com
Control: Hospital district or authority, Government, nonfederal **Service:** General Medical and Surgical

Staffed Beds: 395

HOLLISTER—San Benito County

★ **HAZEL HAWKINS MEMORIAL HOSPITAL (50296)**, 911 Sunset Drive, Zip 95023–5695; tel. 831/637–5711, (Includes HAZEL HAWKINS CONVALESCENT HOSPITAL–SOUTHSIDE, 3110 Southside Road, Zip 95023; tel. 408/637–5711), (Total facility includes 93 beds in nursing home–type unit) (Nonreporting) **A**1 9 10 **S** Brim Healthcare, Inc.
Primary Contact: Ken Underwood, Chief Executive Officer
CFO: Mark Robinson, Associate Administrator and Chief Financial Officer
CIO: Julio Gil, Manager Information Services
Web address: www.hazelhawkins.com
Control: Hospital district or authority, Government, nonfederal **Service:** General Medical and Surgical

Staffed Beds: 113

HOLLYWOOD—Los Angeles County, See Los Angeles

HUNTINGTON BEACH—Orange County

☐ **HUNTINGTON BEACH HOSPITAL (50526)**, 17772 Beach Boulevard, Zip 92647–6819; tel. 714/842–1473, (Total facility includes 14 beds in nursing home–type unit) (Nonreporting) **A**1 9 10 **S** Prime Healthcare Services
Primary Contact: Sofia Abrina, Administrator and Chief Nursing Officer
CFO: Alan Smith, Chief Financial Officer
CMO: Hassan Alkhouli, M.D., Medical Director
CIO: Debbie Horgan, Director Information Technology
Web address: www.hbhospital.com
Control: Partnership, Investor–owned, for–profit **Service:** General Medical and Surgical

Staffed Beds: 145

HUNTINGTON PARK—Los Angeles County

☐ **COMMUNITY AND MISSION HOSPITALS OF HUNTINGTON PARK (50091)**, 2623 East Slauson Avenue, Zip 90255–2900; tel. 323/583–1931, (Includes MISSION HOSPITAL OF HUNTINGTON PARK, 3111 East Florence Avenue, Zip 90255; tel. 213/582–8261), (Nonreporting) **A**1 9 10
Primary Contact: Dennis E. Coleman, Chief Executive Officer
CFO: Nick Lymberopoulos, Chief Financial Officer
Web address: www.communityhosp.com
Control: Corporation, Investor–owned, for–profit **Service:** General Medical and Surgical

Staffed Beds: 157

INDIO—Riverside County

★ **JOHN F. KENNEDY MEMORIAL HOSPITAL (50534)**, 47111 Monroe Street, Zip 92201; tel. 760/347–6191, (Nonreporting) **A**1 9 10 **S** TENET Healthcare Corporation
Primary Contact: John J. Ferrelli, Chief Executive Officer
COO: Parrish Scarboro, Chief Operating Officer
CFO: Stanley Adams, Chief Financial Officer
CHR: Robert C. Taylor, Director Human Resources
Web address: www.jfkmemorialhosp.com
Control: Corporation, Investor–owned, for–profit **Service:** General Medical and Surgical

Staffed Beds: 145

CA

Hospital, Medicare Provider Number, Address, Telephone, Approval, Facility, and Physician Codes, Health Care System
★ American Hospital Association (AHA) membership
☐ The Joint Commission accreditation
○ American Osteopathic Association (AOA) accreditation
△ Commission on Accreditation of Rehabilitation Facilities (CARF) accreditation

INGLEWOOD—Los Angeles County

★ **CENTINELA HOSPITAL MEDICAL CENTER (50739)**, (Formerly Centinela Freeman Regional Medical Center, Centinela Campus), 555 East Hardy Street, Zip 90301–4011, Mailing Address: P.O. Box 720, Zip 90307–0720; tel. 310/673–4660, (Nonreporting) **A**1 9 10 **S** Prime Healthcare Services
Primary Contact: Von L. Crockett, President and Chief Executive Officer
CFO: Mark Overeem, Chief Financial Officer
CMO: Etie Moghissi, M.D., Chief Medical Staff
CIO: Vicky Morgan, Director Information Services
CHR: Margaret Morgan, Director Human Resources
Web address: www.centinelamed.com
Control: Corporation, Investor–owned, for–profit **Service:** General Medical and Surgical

Staffed Beds: 369

IRVINE—Orange County

★ **IRVINE REGIONAL HOSPITAL AND MEDICAL CENTER (50693)**, 16200 Sand Canyon Avenue, Zip 92618–3714; tel. 949/753–2000 **A**1 9 10 **F**3 13 18 20 22 25 26 27 30 32 33 37 38 41 46 49 50 54 55 56 57 62 63 68 70 72 73 74 75 76 77 79 80 81 82 84 86 90 96 97 100 102 107 119 135 136 **P**3 4 5 **S** TENET Healthcare Corporation
Primary Contact: Donald A. Lorack, Jr., Chief Executive Officer
COO: Suzanne Cannata, Chief Operating Officer
CFO: Eric Delgado, Chief Financial Officer
CIO: Dean Grippi, Director Information Systems
CHR: Sharon McKay, Director Human Resources
Web address: www.irvineregionalhospital.com
Control: Corporation, Investor–owned, for–profit **Service:** General Medical and Surgical

Staffed Beds: 176 **Admissions:** 9954 **Census:** 81 **Outpatient Visits:** 30901 **Births:** 1886 **Total Expense ($000):** 101697 **Payroll Expense ($000):** 42783 **Personnel:** 389

KAISER FOUNDATION HOSPITAL – ORANGE COUNTY See Anaheim

JACKSON—Amador County

★ **SUTTER AMADOR HOSPITAL (50014)**, 200 Mission Boulevard, Zip 95642–2132; tel. 209/223–7500 **A**1 9 10 **F**8 11 12 13 15 25 30 31 32 33 38 46 53 55 56 57 62 64 68 73 74 75 76 77 79 80 82 86 87 92 96 97 99 100 103 107 118 119 121 135 136 137 **P**4 **S** Sutter Health
Primary Contact: Anne Platt, Chief Executive Officer
CFO: Siri Nelson, Chief Financial Officer
CMO: D. Keith Kerr, M.D., Chief of Staff
CIO: Tony Jackson, Director Information Technology
CHR: Pam Santos, Director Human Resources
Web address: www.sutteramador.com
Control: Other not–for–profit (including NFP Corporation) **Service:** General Medical and Surgical

Staffed Beds: 52 **Admissions:** 2587 **Census:** 25 **Outpatient Visits:** 39782 **Births:** 374 **Total Expense ($000):** 52745 **Payroll Expense ($000):** 18397

JOSHUA TREE—San Bernardino County

★ **HI–DESERT MEDICAL CENTER (50279)**, 6601 White Feather Road, Zip 92252–6601; tel. 760/366–3711, (Total facility includes 109 beds in nursing home–type unit) **A**1 9 10 20 **F**3 11 13 15 25 26 33 38 42 50 54 55 61 62 64 65 68 72 74 77 79 80 81 82 84 86 94 96 97 100 107 117 119 121 122 132 135 **P**5 **S** Brim Healthcare, Inc.
Primary Contact: Larry L. Meyer, Interim Chief Executive Officer
CFO: Thomas J. Duda, Chief Financial Officer
CMO: Madhusudhan T. Gupta, M.D., Chief Medical Staff
CIO: Dan McClure, Chief Information Officer
CHR: Barbara Staresinc, Director Human Resources
Web address: www.hdmc.org
Control: Hospital district or authority, Government, nonfederal **Service:** General Medical and Surgical

Staffed Beds: 144 **Admissions:** 3919 **Census:** 141 **Outpatient Visits:** 84894 **Births:** 476 **Total Expense ($000):** 44825 **Payroll Expense ($000):** 18529 **Personnel:** 475

KING CITY—Monterey County

☐ **GEORGE L. MEE MEMORIAL HOSPITAL (50189)**, 300 Canal Street, Zip 93930–3431; tel. 831/385–6000, (Nonreporting) **A**1 9 10 20
Primary Contact: Walter G. Beck, Chief Executive Officer
CFO: Jonathan Marshall, Chief Financial Officer
CIO: Doug Burkhardt, Chief Information Officer
Web address: www.meememorial.com
Control: Other not–for–profit (including NFP Corporation) **Service:** General Medical and Surgical

Staffed Beds: 68

KINGSBURG—Fresno County

KINGSBURG MEDICAL CENTER (50682), 1200 Smith Street, Zip 93631–2216; tel. 559/897–5841, (Nonreporting) **A**9 10
Primary Contact: Doug Skubitz, Chief Executive Officer
COO: Stephen Ramirez, Chief Operating Officer
CFO: Luis Sierra, Chief Financial Officer
CIO: Devan Skubitz, Manager Information Services
CHR: Sylvia Munguia, Director Human Resources
Web address: www.kingsburgdh.org
Control: Hospital district or authority, Government, nonfederal **Service:** General Medical and Surgical

Staffed Beds: 35

LA JOLLA—San Diego County

★ **SCRIPPS GREEN HOSPITAL (50424)**, 10666 North Torrey Pines Road, Zip 92037–1093; tel. 858/455–9100 **A**1 2 8 9 10 **F**3 8 11 12 15 17 18 20 22 24 25 26 27 30 31 32 40 41 43 51 55 56 62 66 68 72 73 75 76 77 79 80 81 82 86 96 97 100 102 103 106 107 108 109 111 112 119 121 125 127 128 130 131 135 **P**3 **S** Scripps Health
Primary Contact: Robin Brown, Senior Vice President and Chief Executive
CMO: Brent Eastman, M.D., Chief Medical Officer
CIO: Patrick Thomas, Interim Chief Information Officer
CHR: Vic Buzachero, Vice President Human Resources
Web address: www.scrippshealth.org
Control: Other not–for–profit (including NFP Corporation) **Service:** General Medical and Surgical

Staffed Beds: 173 **Admissions:** 11073 **Census:** 104 **Outpatient Visits:** 97187 **Births:** 0 **Total Expense ($000):** 223981 **Payroll Expense ($000):** 78134 **Personnel:** 1000

★ **SCRIPPS MEMORIAL HOSPITAL–LA JOLLA (50324)**, 9888 Genesee Avenue, Zip 92037–1200, Mailing Address: P.O. Box 28, Zip 92038–0028; tel. 858/626–4123 **A**1 2 3 5 9 10 **F**3 4 5 8 12 13 15 17 18 20 22 24 25 26 27 30 31 32 33 38 40 43 46 47 48 49 50 51 52 53 55 56 57 58 62 63 66 68 72 74 75 76 77 79 80 81 82 86 89 90 91 92 93 94 96 97 99 100 101 102 103 104 105 106 107 109 111 112 119 120 121 122 123 130 131 134 135 136 **S** Scripps Health
Primary Contact: Gary G. Fybel, Senior Vice President and Chief Executive
COO: Lisa Thakur, Vice President Operations
CFO: Linda Honaker, Senior Director Finance
CMO: Brent Eastman, M.D., Chief Medical Officer
CIO: Patrick Thomas, Interim Chief Information Officer
CHR: Vic Buzachero, Senior Vice President Human Resources
Web address: www.scrippshealth.org
Control: Other not–for–profit (including NFP Corporation) **Service:** General Medical and Surgical

Staffed Beds: 301 **Admissions:** 17997 **Census:** 232 **Outpatient Visits:** 115341 **Births:** 3991 **Total Expense ($000):** 345280 **Payroll Expense ($000):** 132388 **Personnel:** 1755

LA MESA—San Diego County

★ △ **SHARP GROSSMONT HOSPITAL (50026)**, 5555 Grossmont Center Drive, Zip 91942–3019, Mailing Address: P.O. Box 158, Zip 91944–0158; tel. 619/740–6000 **A**1 2 7 9 10 **F**3 8 11 13 14 18 20 22 24 25 26 27 30 31 32 33 35 36 38 42 43 44 49 51 53 54 55 56 57 59 61 62 63 66 68 70 72 73 74 75 76 77 79 80 81 82 84 85 86 88 90 91 92 93 94 96 97 100 102 106 107 108 109 111 112 117 118 119 121 130 132 135 136 137 **P**5 **S** Sharp Healthcare
Primary Contact: Michele T. Tarbet, RN, Chief Executive Officer
CFO: Kari Cornicelli, Chief Financial Officer
CMO: Michael Long, M.D., Executive Medical Staff
CIO: William T. Spooner, Senior Vice President and Chief Information Officer
CHR: Ruth Shannon, Director Human Resources
Web address: www.sharp.com
Control: Other not–for–profit (including NFP Corporation) **Service:** General Medical and Surgical

Staffed Beds: 445 **Admissions:** 25354 **Census:** 333 **Outpatient Visits:** 314502 **Births:** 3707 **Total Expense ($000):** 387457 **Payroll Expense ($000):** 169814 **Personnel:** 2126

LA MIRADA—Los Angeles County

☐ **KINDRED HOSPITAL – LA MIRADA (52038)**, 14900 East Imperial Highway, Zip 90638; tel. 562/944–1900, (Nonreporting) **A**1 9 10
Primary Contact: Robin Rapp, Administrator
COO: Jude Sullivan, Chief Clinical Officer
CFO: Nancy V. Wilson, Chief Financial Officer
CMO: Prakash Chandra Patel, M.D., Chief of Staff
CHR: Kristen Martinez, Coordinator Human Resources
Web address: www.kindredhealthcare.com
Control: Corporation, Investor–owned, for–profit **Service:** Long–Term Acute Care hospital

Staffed Beds: 86

LA PALMA—Orange County

☒ **LA PALMA INTERCOMMUNITY HOSPITAL (50580)**, 7901 Walker Street, Zip 90623–1722, Mailing Address: P.O. Box 5850, Buena Park, Zip 90622–5850; tel. 714/670–7400 **A**1 10 **F**3 5 13 15 17 18 25 30 31 32 33 38 49 55 56 57 68 74 79 80 88 91 92 94 95 96 97 100 107 119 121 132 135 136 **S** Prime Healthcare Services
Primary Contact: Virgis Narbutas, Chief Executive Officer
CFO: Alan Smith, Chief Financial Officer
CMO: Sami Shoukair, M.D., Chief of Staff
CIO: Debbie Horgan, Director Information Technology
CHR: Stephanie Sioson, Director Human Resource
Web address: www.lapalmaintercommunityhospital.com
Control: Other not–for–profit (including NFP Corporation) **Service:** General Medical and Surgical

Staffed Beds: 141 **Admissions:** 4003 **Census:** 42 **Outpatient Visits:** 14944 **Births:** 320 **Total Expense ($000):** 53113 **Payroll Expense ($000):** 18011 **Personnel:** 241

LAGUNA BEACH—Orange County

☒ **SOUTH COAST MEDICAL CENTER (50193)**, 31872 Coast Highway, Zip 92651–6775; tel. 949/499–1311, (Nonreporting) **A**1 9 10 **S** Adventist Health
Primary Contact: Bruce C. Christian, President and Chief Executive Officer
COO: Andrea S. Kofl, R.N., Vice President Patient Care Services and Chief Nursing Officer
CFO: Larry Pugh, Chief Financial Officer
CMO: Christopher Vanley, M.D., Chief of Staff
CIO: Mindra Fielding, Director Information System Services
CHR: Donald Balli, Director Human Resources
Web address: www.southcoastmedcenter.com
Control: Church–operated, Nongovernment, not–for profit **Service:** General Medical and Surgical

Staffed Beds: 83

LAGUNA HILLS—Orange County

☒ **SADDLEBACK MEMORIAL MEDICAL CENTER (50603)**, 24451 Health Center Drive, Zip 92653–3689; tel. 949/837–4500 **A**1 2 5 9 10 **F**3 11 13 15 18 20 22 24 25 26 27 30 31 32 33 34 36 38 41 42 43 44 49 50 51 52 53 54 55 56 57 61 62 63 66 67 68 70 72 73 74 75 76 77 79 80 81 82 85 86 90 96 97 102 103 107 108 109 111 114 119 121 124 130 131 132 134 135 136 137 **P**7 **S** Memorial Health Services
Primary Contact: Steve Geidt, Chief Executive Officer
COO: LaDonna L. Butler, R.N., Chief Operating Officer
CFO: John Bishop, Vice President Finance and Chief Financial Officer
CMO: Ronald Naglie, M.D., Chief of Staff
CIO: J. Scott Joslyn, Senior Vice President and Chief Information Officer
CHR: Ron Salzberg, Executive Director Human Resources
Web address: www.memorialcare.org
Control: Other not–for–profit (including NFP Corporation) **Service:** General Medical and Surgical

Staffed Beds: 252 **Admissions:** 15961 **Census:** 172 **Outpatient Visits:** 270203 **Births:** 2898 **Total Expense ($000):** 292001 **Payroll Expense ($000):** 120015 **Personnel:** 1769

LAKE ARROWHEAD—San Bernardino County

☒ **MOUNTAINS COMMUNITY HOSPITAL (51312)**, 29101 Hospital Road, Zip 92352, Mailing Address: P.O. Box 70, Zip 92352–0070; tel. 909/336–3651, (Total facility includes 18 beds in nursing home–type unit) **A**1 9 10 18 **F**11 13 15 25 26 28 30 31 32 33 36 38 39 50 54 55 62 63 67 69 79 86 96 102 107 117 119 122 133
Primary Contact: James R. Hoss, Executive Director
CFO: Frank Adomitis, Chief Financial Officer
CMO: John Pi, M.D., Chief of Staff
CIO: Trace Kateley, Manager Information Systems
CHR: Julie Atwood, Director Human Resources
Web address: www.mchcares.com
Control: Hospital district or authority, Government, nonfederal **Service:** General Medical and Surgical

Staffed Beds: 35 **Admissions:** 554 **Census:** 25 **Outpatient Visits:** 21791 **Births:** 124 **Total Expense ($000):** 14467 **Payroll Expense ($000):** 5834 **Personnel:** 151

LAKE ISABELLA—Kern County

★ **KERN VALLEY HEALTHCARE DISTRICT (51314)**, 6412 Laurel Avenue, Zip 93240–1628, Mailing Address: P.O. Box 1628, Zip 93240–1628; tel. 760/379–2681, (Total facility includes 74 beds in nursing home–type unit) **A**9 10 18 **F**11 25 32 33 38 55 56 57 62 68 79 86 96 102 107 117 122
Primary Contact: Richard G. Carter, Chief Executive Officer
CFO: Chester Beedle, Chief Financial Officer
CMO: Gary A. Finstad, M.D., Chief of Staff
CIO: Dena Griffith, Manager Information Systems
CHR: Debra Hoffman, Manager Human Resources
Web address: www.kvhd.org
Control: Hospital district or authority, Government, nonfederal **Service:** General Medical and Surgical

Staffed Beds: 99 **Admissions:** 1171 **Census:** 81 **Outpatient Visits:** 28135 **Births:** 0 **Total Expense ($000):** 21632 **Payroll Expense ($000):** 8362 **Personnel:** 159

LAKEPORT—Lake County

☒ **SUTTER LAKESIDE HOSPITAL (50476)**, 5176 Hill Road East, Zip 95453–6300; tel. 707/262–5001 **A**1 9 10 20 **F**3 8 11 13 15 25 26 28 30 31 32 33 34 38 40 43 50 52 55 56 57 59 60 61 62 63 64 66 68 72 73 74 75 77 79 80 82 84 85 86 96 98 99 100 102 104 106 107 119 120 122 124 132 133 135 136 137 **P**8 **S** Sutter Health
Primary Contact: Kelly Mather, Chief Executive Officer
COO: Chris Chaney, Assistant Administrator
CFO: Avery Schlesenberg, Chief Financial Officer
CMO: Diane Pege, M.D., Medical Director
CIO: Jack Buell, Chief Information Officer
CHR: Laura McAndrews, Chief Human Resources Officer
Web address: www.sutterlake.org
Control: Other not–for–profit (including NFP Corporation) **Service:** General Medical and Surgical

Staffed Beds: 53 **Admissions:** 2600 **Census:** 27 **Outpatient Visits:** 98456 **Births:** 369 **Total Expense ($000):** 64807 **Payroll Expense ($000):** 24964 **Personnel:** 356

LAKEWOOD—Los Angeles County

☒ **LAKEWOOD REGIONAL MEDICAL CENTER (50581)**, 3700 East South Street, Zip 90712–1498, Mailing Address: P.O. Box 6070, Zip 90714–6070; tel. 562/531–2550 **A**1 9 10 **F**3 11 15 17 18 20 22 25 26 30 31 32 33 36 38 50 53 55 56 57 62 66 68 72 73 75 79 82 85 86 96 97 100 106 107 108 119 121 132 135 136 **S** TENET Healthcare Corporation
Primary Contact: Mark Korth, Chief Executive Officer
COO: Steve Cornejo, Chief Operating Officer
CFO: Mary Beth Formby, Chief Financial Officer
CMO: Ronald Kaufman, M.D., Chief Medical Officer
CIO: Eleanor Laneaux, Director Information Systems
CHR: Mary Okuhara, Director Human Resources
Web address: www.lakewoodregional.com
Control: Corporation, Investor–owned, for–profit **Service:** General Medical and Surgical

Staffed Beds: 157 **Admissions:** 7582 **Census:** 104 **Outpatient Visits:** 58183 **Births:** 0 **Total Expense ($000):** 100808 **Payroll Expense ($000):** 40615 **Personnel:** 577

LANCASTER—Los Angeles County

☒ **ANTELOPE VALLEY HOSPITAL (50056)**, 1600 West Avenue J, Zip 93534–2894; tel. 661/949–5000 **A**1 5 9 10 **F**1 3 4 11 13 14 16 17 18 20 22 25 26 27 30 31 32 33 36 38 43 46 47 48 49 50 51 55 56 57 61 62 63 65 66 68 69 70 71 72 73 74 75 76 77 78 79 80 81 82 83 84 85 86 87 88 89 90 91 92 93 94 95 96 97 98 99 100 101 102 104 105 106 107 108 109 117 119 121 122 124 130 132 133 135 136 137 **P**7
Primary Contact: Edward Mirzabegian, Chief Executive Officer
CFO: Dennis Empey, Chief Financial Officer
CMO: Doddanna Krishna, M.D., Chief of Staff
CIO: Humberto Quintana, Chief Information Officer
CHR: John Sullivan, Vice President Human Resources
Web address: www.avhospital.org
Control: Hospital district or authority, Government, nonfederal **Service:** General Medical and Surgical

Staffed Beds: 368 **Admissions:** 17264 **Census:** 266 **Outpatient Visits:** 164456 **Births:** 5795 **Total Expense ($000):** 252879 **Payroll Expense ($000):** 113952 **Personnel:** 1994

Hospital, Medicare Provider Number, Address, Telephone, Approval, Facility, and Physician Codes, Health Care System

★ American Hospital Association (AHA) membership
□ The Joint Commission accreditation
○ American Osteopathic Association (AOA) accreditation
△ Commission on Accreditation of Rehabilitation Facilities (CARF) accreditation

☐ **LANCASTER COMMUNITY HOSPITAL (50204)**, 43830 10th Street West, Zip 93534–4895; tel. 661/948–4781, (Nonreporting) **A**1 9 10 **S** Universal Health Services, Inc.
Primary Contact: Robert J. Trautman, Chief Executive Officer
COO: Karen Faulis, Chief Operating Officer
CFO: Kurt Broten, Chief Financial Officer
CIO: Roy Singleton, Director Computer Information Systems
CHR: Karen Hickling, Director Human Resources
Web address: www.lancastercommunityhospital.net
Control: Corporation, Investor–owned, for–profit **Service:** General Medical and Surgical

Staffed Beds: 78

LEMOORE—Kings County

★ **NAVAL HOSPITAL**, 937 Franklin Avenue, Zip 93246–5004; tel. 559/998–4201 **A**1 **F**5 7 8 13 15 25 26 28 31 37 50 52 55 57 62 63 66 73 74 75 77 79 82 86 87 89 90 91 94 96 100 124 135 136 137 **S** Bureau of Medicine and Surgery, Department of the Navy
Primary Contact: Captain Stephen Mandia, Commanding Officer
COO: Cynthia Feller, Executive Officer
CFO: Thomas M. Brui, Director Resource Management
CMO: Scott Cota, Director Medical Services
CIO: Victor Dela Torre, Command Legal Officer
CHR: Billy Newman, Department Head
Web address: www.lemoore.med.navy.mil
Control: Navy, Government, federal **Service:** General Medical and Surgical

Staffed Beds: 16 **Admissions:** 707 **Census:** 4 **Outpatient Visits:** 111329 **Births:** 443 **Total Expense ($000):** 25000 **Payroll Expense ($000):** 4643 **Personnel:** 568

LIVERMORE—Alameda County

VALLEY MEMORIAL See ValleyCare Medical Center, Pleasanton

VETERANS AFFAIRS PALO ALTO HEALTH CARE SYSTEM, LIVERMORE DIVISION See Veterans Affairs Palo Alto Health Care System, Palo Alto

LODI—San Joaquin County

★ **LODI MEMORIAL HOSPITAL (50336)**, 975 South Fairmont Avenue, Zip 95240–5179, Mailing Address: P.O. Box 3004, Zip 95241–1908; tel. 209/334–3411, (Includes LODI MEMORIAL HOSPITAL WEST, 800 South Lower Sacramento Road, Zip 95242; tel. 209/333–0211), (Total facility includes 47 beds in nursing home–type unit) (Nonreporting) **A**1 9 10
Primary Contact: Joseph P. Harrington, Chief Executive Officer
COO: Mark Sey, Vice President and Chief Administrative Officer
CFO: Ron Kreutner, Chief Financial Officer
CHR: Mark Wallace, Director Human Resources
Web address: www.lodihealth.org
Control: Other not–for–profit (including NFP Corporation) **Service:** General Medical and Surgical

Staffed Beds: 178

LOMA LINDA—San Bernardino County

★ △ **JERRY L. PETTIS MEMORIAL VETERANS MEDICAL CENTER**, 11201 Benton Street, Zip 92357; tel. 909/825–7084, (Total facility includes 108 beds in nursing home–type unit) (Nonreporting) **A**1 2 3 5 7 8 **S** Department of Veterans Affairs
Primary Contact: Dwight Evans, M.D., Acting Director
CFO: William Lysaght, Chief Financial Officer
CMO: Dwight Evans, M.D., Chief of Staff
CIO: Arlene Blas, Chief Information Technology Service
CHR: Eugene Wylie, Chief Human Resources Officer
Web address: www.lomalinda.va.gov
Control: Veterans Affairs, Government, federal **Service:** General Medical and Surgical

Staffed Beds: 205

★ △ **LOMA LINDA UNIVERSITY MEDICAL CENTER (50327)**, 11234 Anderson Street, Zip 92354–2870, Mailing Address: P.O. Box 2000, Zip 92354–0200; tel. 909/558–4000, (Includes LOMA LINDA UNIVERSITY EAST CAMPUS HOSPITAL, 25333 Barton Road, Zip 92354–3053; tel. 909/558–6000) **A**1 2 3 5 7 8 9 10 **F**2 3 8 11 13 15 17 18 19 20 21 22 23 24 25 26 27 28 30 31 32 33 38 40 43 44 46 47 48 49 50 53 55 56 57 59 61 62 63 66 70 72 73 74 75 76 77 79 80 82 83 84 85 86 96 97 99 100 101 102 103 104 105 106 107 108 109 110 111 112 116 118 119 121 123 125 126 127 128 130 131 133 135 136 137 **P**3 **S** Loma Linda University Adventist Health Sciences Center
Primary Contact: Ruthita J. Fike, Chief Executive Officer
COO: Ruthita J. Fike, Chief Executive Officer
CFO: Steve Mohr, Senior Vice President Finance and Chief Financial Officer
CMO: Daniel Giang, M.D., Vice President for Medical Administration
CIO: Richard Hergert, Chief Information Officer
CHR: Lizette Norton, Associate Vice President Human Resources Management
Web address: www.llumc.edu
Control: Other not–for–profit (including NFP Corporation) **Service:** General Medical and Surgical

Staffed Beds: 739 **Admissions:** 31255 **Census:** 567 **Outpatient Visits:** 507491 **Births:** 2806 **Total Expense ($000):** 793740 **Payroll Expense ($000):** 360613 **Personnel:** 6334

LOMPOC—Santa Barbara County

★ **LOMPOC VALLEY MEDICAL CENTER (50110)**, (Formerly Lompoc Healthcare District), 508 East Hickory Street, Zip 93436–7337, Mailing Address: P.O. Box 1058, Zip 93438–1058; tel. 805/737–3300, (Total facility includes 110 beds in nursing home–type unit) (Nonreporting) **A**1 9 10
Primary Contact: James J. Raggio, Administrator and Chief Executive Officer
CMO: Chris Lumsdoine, M.D., Chief of Staff
CIO: Jim White, Chief Information Officer
CHR: Sandi Stinson, Director Human Resources
Web address: www.lompocvmc.com
Control: Hospital district or authority, Government, nonfederal **Service:** General Medical and Surgical

Staffed Beds: 170

LONE PINE—Inyo County

★ **SOUTHERN INYO HEALTHCARE DISTRICT (51302)**, 501 East Locust Street, Zip 93545–1009, Mailing Address: P.O. Box 1009, Zip 93545–1009; tel. 760/876–5501, (Total facility includes 33 beds in nursing home–type unit) (Nonreporting) **A**9 10 18
Primary Contact: Lee Barron, Chief Executive Officer
CFO: Lee Barron, Chief Executive Officer
CIO: Patricia M. Murray, Information Officer
Web address: www.sihd.org
Control: Hospital district or authority, Government, nonfederal **Service:** General Medical and Surgical

Staffed Beds: 37

LONG BEACH—Los Angeles County

★ **COMMUNITY HOSPITAL OF LONG BEACH (50727)**, 1720 Termino Avenue, Zip 90804–2180; tel. 562/498–1000, (Nonreporting) **A**1 9 10
Primary Contact: Raymond M. Jankowski, President and Chief Executive Officer
COO: Diane DeWalsche, R.N., Chief Operating Officer
CFO: Robert Schirripa, Administrative Director Finance
CMO: Stewart Brown, M.D., Chief Medical Staff
CIO: Robert Oducado, Manager Information Systems
CHR: Elaine Garneff, Administrative Director Human Resources
Web address: www.chlb.org
Control: Other not–for–profit (including NFP Corporation) **Service:** General Medical and Surgical

Staffed Beds: 71

★ **LONG BEACH MEMORIAL MEDICAL CENTER (50485)**, 2801 Atlantic Avenue, Zip 90806–1737, Mailing Address: P.O. Box 1428, Zip 90801–1428; tel. 562/933–2000, (Total facility includes 10 beds in nursing home–type unit) **A**1 2 3 5 8 9 10 **F**3 9 11 12 14 15 17 18 20 22 24 25 26 27 30 31 32 33 34 35 36 37 38 40 41 42 43 44 45 46 47 49 50 52 54 55 56 57 58 60 61 62 63 66 68 72 73 75 76 77 79 80 81 82 85 86 87 90 91 96 97 98 100 102 107 108 109 111 112 113 114 116 117 118 119 120 121 124 130 131 132 133 135 136 137 **S** Memorial Health Services
Primary Contact: Terry A. Belmont, Chief Executive Officer
COO: M. Ross Simmonds, Chief Operating Officer
CFO: Wendy Dorchester, Ph.D., Chief Financial Officer
CMO: S. Gainer Pillsbury, M.D., Chief Medical Officer
CIO: J. Scott Joslyn, Senior Vice President and Chief Information Officer
CHR: Ron Chavira, Vice President Human Resources
Web address: www.memorialcare.org
Control: Other not–for–profit (including NFP Corporation) **Service:** General Medical and Surgical

Staffed Beds: 462 **Admissions:** 24272 **Census:** 337 **Outpatient Visits:** 191871 **Births:** 0 **Total Expense ($000):** 378858 **Payroll Expense ($000):** 158815 **Personnel:** 2915

☐ **MILLER CHILDREN'S HOSPITAL (53309)**, 2801 Atlantic Avenue, Zip 90806; tel. 562/933–5437 **A**1 9 10 **F**3 11 12 13 14 15 19 21 23 25 26 27 28 30 31 32 33 34 35 36 37 38 40 41 42 43 44 45 46 47 49 50 52 55 56 57 58 60 61 62 63 64 66 70 71 72 73 74 75 76 77 78 79 80 81 82 83 84 86 87 89 90 91 96 97 98 100 102 107 108 109 111 112 113 114 116 118 119 120 121 123 124 130 131 132 133 135 136 137 **S** Memorial Health Services
Primary Contact: Terry A. Belmont, Chief Executive Officer
Web address: www.memorialcare.org
Control: Other not–for–profit (including NFP Corporation) **Service:** Children's general

Staffed Beds: 308 **Admissions:** 15499 **Census:** 216 **Outpatient Visits:** 104354 **Births:** 5805 **Total Expense ($000):** 287633 **Payroll Expense ($000):** 126608 **Personnel:** 2424

□ **PACIFIC HOSPITAL OF LONG BEACH (50277)**, 2776 Pacific Avenue, Zip 90806–2699, Mailing Address: P.O. Box 1268, Zip 90801; tel. 562/595–1911, (Total facility includes 27 beds in nursing home–type unit) (Nonreporting) **A**1 10 12 13
Primary Contact: Michael D. Drobot, Chief Executive Officer
COO: Clark D. Todd, President and Chief Operating Officer
CFO: Jim Canedo, Chief Financial Officer
CMO: Luke Watson, M.D., Chief of Staff
CIO: David Wueste, Chief Information Officer
CHR: Tia Schiller, Vice President Human Resources
Web address: www.phlb.org
Control: Other not–for–profit (including NFP Corporation) **Service:** General Medical and Surgical

Staffed Beds: 171

REDGATE MEMORIAL HOSPITAL, 1775 Chestnut Avenue, Zip 90813–1674; tel. 562/599–8444, (Nonreporting)
Primary Contact: Lawrence Gentile, President and Chief Executive Officer
Control: Other not–for–profit (including NFP Corporation) **Service:** Alcoholism and other chemical dependency

Staffed Beds: 63

★ **ST. MARY MEDICAL CENTER (50191)**, 1050 Linden Avenue, Zip 90813, Mailing Address: P.O. Box 887, Zip 90813–0887; tel. 562/491–9000 **A**1 2 3 5 9 10 **F**1 3 4 8 12 13 15 16 17 18 20 22 24 25 26 27 28 30 31 32 33 34 37 38 40 43 44 47 49 50 54 55 56 57 58 59 60 62 63 64 65 66 67 68 70 71 72 73 74 75 76 77 78 79 80 82 83 84 85 86 88 96 97 99 100 102 106 107 111 114 115 117 119 121 123 124 130 131 132 133 135 136 **P**4 5 **S** Catholic Healthcare West
Primary Contact: Christopher DiCicco, President
COO: Gail Daly, Chief Operating Officer
CFO: Adolfo Chanez, Chief Financial Officer
CMO: Andrew Burg, M.D., Chief of Staff
CIO: Earle Johnson, Site Manager
CHR: Bob Bokern, Director President Human Resources
Web address: www.stmarymedicalcenter.org
Control: Other not–for–profit (including NFP Corporation) **Service:** General Medical and Surgical

Staffed Beds: 287 **Admissions:** 15388 **Census:** 192 **Outpatient Visits:** 77665 **Births:** 2859 **Total Expense ($000):** 185025 **Payroll Expense ($000):** 77373 **Personnel:** 1668

★ △ **VETERANS AFFAIRS LONG BEACH HEALTHCARE SYSTEM**, 5901 East Seventh Street, Zip 90822–5201; tel. 562/826–8000, (Total facility includes 99 beds in nursing home–type unit) (Nonreporting) **A**1 2 3 5 7 8 **S** Department of Veterans Affairs
Primary Contact: Isabel Duff, M.S., Acting Director
COO: Anthony DeFrancesco, Associate Director
CFO: Charles H. Feistman, Chief Financial Management Services
CMO: Sandor Szabo, M.D., Ph.D., M.P.H., Chief of Staff
CIO: Rodney Sagmit, Acting Chief Information Management
CHR: Mary Beth McCartan, Manager Human Resources
Web address: www.va.gov/sta/guide/home.asp
Control: Veterans Affairs, Government, federal **Service:** General Medical and Surgical

Staffed Beds: 333

LOS ALAMITOS—Orange County

★ **LOS ALAMITOS MEDICAL CENTER (50551)**, 3751 Katella Avenue, Zip 90720–3164; tel. 562/598–1311, (Nonreporting) **A**1 2 9 10 **S** TENET Healthcare Corporation
Primary Contact: Michele Finney, Chief Executive Officer
CFO: Dave Vickers, Chief Financial Officer
CIO: Sally Andrada, Chief Information Officer
CHR: Angie Driscoll, Director Human Resources
Web address: www.losalamitosmedctr.com
Control: Corporation, Investor–owned, for–profit **Service:** General Medical and Surgical

Staffed Beds: 167

LOS ANGELES—Los Angeles County

(Mailing Addresses - Canoga Park, Encino, Granada Hills, Harbor City, Hollywood, Mission Hills, North Hollywood, Northridge, Panorama City, San Pedro, Sepulveda, Sherman Oaks, Sun Valley, Sylmar, Tarzana, Van Nuys, West Hills, West Los Angeles, Woodland Hills)

★ **BARLOW RESPIRATORY HOSPITAL (52031)**, 2000 Stadium Way, Zip 90026–2696; tel. 213/250–4200, (Nonreporting) **A**1 9 10
Primary Contact: Margaret W. Crane, Chief Executive Officer
COO: Terry Sepulveda, Chief Operating Officer
CFO: Edward Engesser, Chief Financial Officer and Chief Information Officer
CMO: David Nelson, M.D., Medical Director
CIO: Edward Engesser, Chief Financial Officer and Chief Information Officer
CHR: Peter Kimball, Vice President Human Resources
Web address: www.barlow2000.org
Control: Other not–for–profit (including NFP Corporation) **Service:** Long–Term Acute Care hospital

Staffed Beds: 75

CA

★ **CALIFORNIA HOSPITAL MEDICAL CENTER (50149)**, 1401 South Grand Avenue, Zip 90015–3010; tel. 213/748–2411 **A**1 3 5 9 10 **F**3 8 11 25 26 27 31 32 33 38 40 43 44 46 49 50 55 56 57 63 64 66 68 70 74 77 79 80 96 99 100 102 107 109 117 119 121 132 133 137 **S** Catholic Healthcare West
Primary Contact: Mark A. Meyers, President
COO: Jerry Clute, Chief Operating Officer
CFO: David Yeager, Chief Financial Officer
CMO: Bruce A. Greenfield, M.D., Chief of Staff
CIO: Michael Minnie, Director Information Technology
Web address: www.chmcla.org
Control: Other not–for–profit (including NFP Corporation) **Service:** General Medical and Surgical

Staffed Beds: 316 **Admissions:** 17024 **Census:** 189 **Outpatient Visits:** 74339 **Births:** 4314 **Total Expense ($000):** 221528 **Payroll Expense ($000):** 99288

★ △ **CEDARS–SINAI MEDICAL CENTER (50625)**, 8700 Beverly Boulevard, Zip 90048–1865, Mailing Address: Box 48750, Zip 90048–0750; tel. 310/423–5000 **A**1 2 3 5 7 8 9 10 **F**3 5 8 11 12 13 14 15 17 18 19 20 21 22 23 24 25 26 27 28 29 30 31 32 33 34 35 36 37 38 40 41 43 44 45 46 47 48 49 50 51 52 53 54 55 56 57 58 59 60 62 63 64 66 67 68 69 70 72 73 74 75 76 77 79 80 81 82 83 84 85 86 87 88 89 90 91 92 93 94 95 96 97 98 99 100 101 102 103 104 105 106 107 108 109 110 111 112 113 114 116 119 120 121 122 125 126 127 128 129 130 131 134 135 136 137 **P**3 5 8
Primary Contact: Thomas M. Priselac, President and Chief Executive Officer
COO: Mark R. Gavens, Chief Operating Officer and Senior Vice President Clinical Care Services
CFO: Edward Prunchunas, Senior Vice President and Chief Financial Officer
CMO: Michael Langberg, M.D., Senior Vice President Medical Affairs and Chief Medical Officer
CIO: Darren Dworkin, Vice President and Chief Information Officer
CHR: Jeanne Flores, Senior Vice President Human Resources and Organizational Development
Web address: www.cedars–sinai.edu
Control: Other not–for–profit (including NFP Corporation) **Service:** General Medical and Surgical

Staffed Beds: 914 **Admissions:** 48735 **Census:** 755 **Outpatient Visits:** 416113 **Births:** 7036 **Total Expense ($000):** 1532819 **Payroll Expense ($000):** 589002 **Personnel:** 8835

□ **CHILDRENS HOSPITAL LOS ANGELES (53302)**, 4650 Sunset Boulevard, Zip 90027–6062, Mailing Address: P.O. Box 27980, Zip 90027; tel. 323/660–2450, (Nonreporting) **A**1 3 5 9 10
Primary Contact: Richard D. Cordova, President and Chief Executive Officer
COO: Rodney Hanners, Senior Vice President and Chief Operating Officer
CFO: Lannie Tonnu, Senior Vice President and Chief Financial Officer
CMO: Roberta G. Williams, M.D., Vice President Pediatrics and Academic Affairs
CIO: Steve Garske, Vice President and Chief Information Officer
CHR: Hugo Santos, Vice President Human Resources
Web address: www.childrenshospitalla.org
Control: Other not–for–profit (including NFP Corporation) **Service:** Children's other specialty

Staffed Beds: 283

Hospital, Medicare Provider Number, Address, Telephone, Approval, Facility, and Physician Codes, Health Care System
★ American Hospital Association (AHA) membership
□ The Joint Commission accreditation
○ American Osteopathic Association (AOA) accreditation
△ Commission on Accreditation of Rehabilitation Facilities (CARF) accreditation

○ **CITY OF ANGELS MEDICAL CENTER (50725)**, 1711 West Temple Street, Zip 90026; tel. 213/989–6100 **A**10 11 **F**2 12 25 30 32 33 49 77 80 86 88 94 95 107 117 119 121 132 133 137
Primary Contact: Vicki Gant, Chief Executive Officer
CFO: John Cowles, Chief Financial Officer
CMO: Louis Acosta, M.D., Chief of Staff
CIO: Scott Musack, Chief Information Officer
CHR: Sylvia Cloud, Director Human Resources
Web address: www.cofamc.org
Control: Corporation, Investor–owned, for–profit **Service:** General Medical and Surgical

Staffed Beds: 150 **Admissions:** 6281 **Census:** 101 **Outpatient Visits:** 7194 **Total Expense ($000):** 58280 **Payroll Expense ($000):** 22686 **Personnel:** 770

□ **EAST LOS ANGELES DOCTORS HOSPITAL (50641)**, 4060 East Whittier Boulevard, Zip 90023–2526; tel. 323/268–5514 **A**1 9 10 **F**3 13 15 17 25 31 32 33 38 43 62 66 72 74 75 77 79 80 84 86 96 107 117 119 132 **S** HealthPlus
Primary Contact: Araceli Lonergan, Chief Executive Officer
COO: Hector Hernandez, Chief Operating Officer
CFO: Steve K. Lopez, Chief Financial Officer
CMO: Marcos Lemor, M.D., Chief of Staff
CIO: Don Dewar, Director Information Systems
CHR: Olivia Chairez, Manager Human Resources
Web address: www.elalax.com
Control: Corporation, Investor–owned, for–profit **Service:** General Medical and Surgical

Staffed Beds: 127 **Admissions:** 3305 **Census:** 80 **Outpatient Visits:** 22201 **Births:** 794

CA

★ **ENCINO–TARZANA REGIONAL MEDICAL CENTER TARZANA CAMPUS (50601)**, 18321 Clark Street, Tarzana, Zip 91356–3521; tel. 818/881–0800 **A**1 9 10 **F**3 11 15 17 18 20 22 24 25 26 27 33 36 37 38 43 49 51 55 56 57 63 68 70 72 73 74 76 79 80 82 83 84 96 97 102 103 107 119 135 136 137
Primary Contact: Dale Surowitz, Chief Executive Officer
CFO: Nick Lymberopoulos, Chief Financial Officer
CMO: Wayne Kleinman, M.D., Medical Chief of Staff
CIO: Craig Witmer, Chief Information Officer
CHR: Jo Lewis, Director Human Resources
Web address: www.encino–tarzana.com
Control: Corporation, Investor–owned, for–profit **Service:** General Medical and Surgical

Staffed Beds: 245 **Admissions:** 11746 **Census:** 157 **Outpatient Visits:** 41832 **Births:** 2036

★ **ENCINO–TARZANA REGIONAL MEDICAL CENTER–ENCINO CAMPUS (50158)**, 16237 Ventura Boulevard, Encino, Zip 91436–2201; tel. 818/995–5000, (Total facility includes 28 beds in nursing home–type unit) **A**1 9 10 **F**3 11 17 25 26 33 35 36 38 49 55 56 57 63 68 72 73 75 77 79 80 82 85 88 93 102 103 107 117 119 121 135 137 **S** Prime Healthcare Services
Primary Contact: Dale Surowitz, Chief Executive Officer
CFO: Nick Lymberopoulos, Chief Financial Officer
CMO: Wayne Kleinman, M.D., Medical Chief of Staff
CIO: Craig Witmer, Chief Information Officer
CHR: Jo Lewis, Director Human Resources
Web address: www.encino–tarzana.com
Control: Corporation, Investor–owned, for–profit **Service:** General Medical and Surgical

Staffed Beds: 151 **Admissions:** 3450 **Census:** 72 **Outpatient Visits:** 13286 **Births:** 0

□ **GATEWAYS HOSPITAL AND MENTAL HEALTH CENTER (54028)**, 1891 Effie Street, Zip 90026–1711; tel. 323/644–2000 **A**1 10 **F**25 33 75 88 89 90 91 94 119 **P**5 6
Primary Contact: Mara Pelsman, Chief Executive Officer
CFO: Jeff Emery, Chief Financial Officer
CMO: Brian R. Holt, M.D., Medical Director
CIO: Jeff Emery, Chief Financial Officer
CHR: Jeannine Coatsworth, Vice President Human Resources and Support Services
Web address: www.gatewayshospital.org
Control: Other not–for–profit (including NFP Corporation) **Service:** Psychiatric

Staffed Beds: 55 **Admissions:** 957 **Census:** 34 **Outpatient Visits:** 79802 **Births:** 0 **Total Expense ($000):** 19017 **Payroll Expense ($000):** 10188 **Personnel:** 285

GENERAL HOSPITAL See LAC/University of Southern California Medical Center

□ △ **GOOD SAMARITAN HOSPITAL (50471)**, 1225 Wilshire Boulevard, Zip 90017–1901; tel. 213/977–2121 **A**1 2 3 5 7 9 10 **F**3 7 8 11 13 14 15 17 18 20 22 24 25 26 27 30 31 32 33 34 35 36 38 40 43 46 47 48 49 51 52 54 55 56 57 59 62 66 68 70 72 73 74 75 76 77 79 81 82 85 86 96 97 100 102 103 105 106 107 109 111 112 114 117 119 121 132 134 135 137 **P**5
Primary Contact: Andrew B. Leeka, President and Chief Executive Officer
CFO: Alan Ino, Chief Financial Officer
CIO: Cindy Moeller, Chief Information Officer
CHR: Lexie Schuster, Vice President Human Resources
Web address: www.goodsam.org
Control: Other not–for–profit (including NFP Corporation) **Service:** General Medical and Surgical

Staffed Beds: 374 **Admissions:** 17383 **Census:** 230 **Outpatient Visits:** 93563 **Births:** 5182 **Total Expense ($000):** 228033 **Payroll Expense ($000):** 83417 **Personnel:** 1384

HOLLYWOOD COMMUNITY HOSPITAL (50135), 6245 De Longpre Avenue, Zip 90028–9001; tel. 323/462–2271, (Includes HOLLYWOOD COMMUNITY HOSPITAL OF VAN NUYS, 14433 Emelita Street, Zip 91401; tel. 818/787–1511), (Nonreporting) **A**9 10 **S** Alta Healthcare System
Primary Contact: Michael Sarian, Chief Executive Officer
Web address: www.hollywoodcommunityhospital.com
Control: Corporation, Investor–owned, for–profit **Service:** General Medical and Surgical

Staffed Beds: 45

HOLLYWOOD COMMUNITY HOSPITAL OF VAN NUYS See Hollywood Community Hospital

★ **HOLLYWOOD PRESBYTERIAN MEDICAL CENTER (50063)**, 1300 North Vermont Avenue, Zip 90027–0069; tel. 323/913–4800, (Total facility includes 89 beds in nursing home–type unit) **A**1 2 9 10 **F**8 15 17 18 20 25 26 27 30 31 32 33 38 46 48 49 50 51 55 56 57 58 59 60 62 64 66 68 69 70 72 73 74 75 76 77 79 80 81 82 84 85 86 90 92 96 97 100 107 109 117 119 132 135 136 137 **P**5
Primary Contact: Jeff A. Nelson, Chief Executive Officer
CFO: Robert Allen, Chief Financial Officer
Control: Partnership, Investor–owned, for–profit **Service:** General Medical and Surgical

Staffed Beds: 443 **Admissions:** 15603 **Census:** 281 **Outpatient Visits:** 49040 **Births:** 4700 **Total Expense ($000):** 174252 **Payroll Expense ($000):** 74149 **Personnel:** 1097

★ **KAISER FOUNDATION HOSPITAL (50138)**, 4867 Sunset Boulevard, Zip 90027–5969; tel. 323/783–4011, (Includes KAISER FOUNDATION MENTAL HEALTH CENTER, 765 West College Street, Zip 90012; tel. 213/580–7200) **A**1 2 3 5 10 **F**3 8 13 14 15 17 18 19 20 21 22 23 24 25 26 27 30 31 32 33 34 36 38 41 42 43 44 46 47 49 50 51 54 59 60 61 62 63 64 66 68 70 71 72 73 74 76 77 78 79 80 81 82 83 84 87 88 89 90 91 92 93 94 95 96 97 100 102 103 106 107 108 109 110 111 112 121 133 135 136 137 **P**6 **S** Kaiser Foundation Hospitals
Primary Contact: Mark E. Costa, Executive Director
COO: Alice H. Issai, Chief Operating Officer
CFO: Daniel N. Shaw, Assistant Administrator Finance
CMO: Donald H. Marcus, M.D., Medical Director
CIO: Raymond Lowe, Information Technology Leader
CHR: Paul J. Martin, Director Human Resources
Web address: www.kaiserpermanente.org
Control: Other not–for–profit (including NFP Corporation) **Service:** General Medical and Surgical

Staffed Beds: 455 **Admissions:** 22441 **Census:** 306 **Outpatient Visits:** 76039 **Births:** 2286

★ **KAISER FOUNDATION HOSPITAL (50411)**, 25825 South Vermont Avenue, Harbor City, Zip 90710–3599; tel. 310/325–5111, (Nonreporting) **A**1 10 **S** Kaiser Foundation Hospitals
Primary Contact: Jan F. Boyd, Executive Director
Web address: www.kaiserpermanente.org
Control: Other not–for–profit (including NFP Corporation) **Service:** General Medical and Surgical

Staffed Beds: 199

★ **KAISER FOUNDATION HOSPITAL (50137)**, 13652 Cantara Street, Panorama City, Zip 91402–5497; tel. 818/375–2000, (Nonreporting) **A**1 5 10 **S** Kaiser Foundation Hospitals
Primary Contact: Dennis C. Benton, Executive Director
CFO: Mechi R. Caballero, Assistant Administrator
CMO: Virginia L. Ambrosini, M.D., Area Medical Director
CIO: Karun Kapur, Information Technology Leader
CHR: Carole L. Erken, Human Resources Leader
Web address: www.kaiserpermanente.org
Control: Other not–for–profit (including NFP Corporation) **Service:** General Medical and Surgical

Staffed Beds: 205

★ **KAISER FOUNDATION HOSPITAL (50677)**, 5601 DeSoto Avenue, Woodland Hills, Zip 91365–6701; tel. 818/719–3800 **A**1 3 5 10 **F**3 12 13 14 15 17 25 26 27 28 30 31 32 38 42 43 48 49 51 59 60 62 63 66 68 70 72 73 74 75 76 77 79 80 81 82 84 90 92 93 96 97 100 107 114 118 119 130 132 133 135 **P**6 **S** Kaiser Foundation Hospitals
Primary Contact: Cathy A. Casas, Executive Director
CFO: Marilou Cheung, Assistant Administrator Finance
CMO: Shirley Suda, M.D., Area Medical Director
CIO: Susan Ng, Director Public Affairs
CHR: Cathy Cousineau, Director Human Resources
Web address: www.kaiserpermanente.org
Control: Other not–for–profit (including NFP Corporation) **Service:** General Medical and Surgical

Staffed Beds: 218 **Admissions:** 14628 **Census:** 160 **Outpatient Visits:** 42081 **Births:** 1855 **Personnel:** 1193

★ **KAISER FOUNDATION HOSPITAL–WEST LOS ANGELES (50561)**, 6041 Cadillac Avenue, Zip 90034–1702; tel. 323/857–2201 **A**1 2 5 10 **F**3 5 8 13 15 25 26 27 28 30 31 32 33 36 38 40 43 49 53 54 56 57 59 60 61 62 63 66 68 71 72 73 74 75 76 77 79 80 81 82 84 86 87 89 90 91 92 93 94 96 97 100 102 104 105 106 107 114 119 120 121 123 124 133 135 136 137 **P**6 **S** Kaiser Foundation Hospitals
Primary Contact: Gloria Blackburn, Executive Director
CFO: Alice H. Issai, Business Strategy and Finance Leader
CMO: Fred Alexander, M.D., Medical Director
CIO: Gregory M. Sincock, Information Technology Leader
Web address: www.kaiserpermanente.org
Control: Other not–for–profit (including NFP Corporation) **Service:** General Medical and Surgical

Staffed Beds: 172 **Admissions:** 9666 **Census:** 106 **Outpatient Visits:** 1239191 **Births:** 1563 **Personnel:** 659

KAISER FOUNDATION MENTAL HEALTH CENTER See Kaiser Foundation Hospital

☐ **KINDRED HOSPITAL–LOS ANGELES (52032)**, 5525 West Slauson Avenue, Zip 90056–1067; tel. 310/642–0325 **A**1 9 10 **F**25 43 44 68 80 107 119 137 **S** Kindred Healthcare
Primary Contact: Trude Williams, RN, Administrator
CFO: Michael Gonzales, Chief Financial Officer
Web address: www.kindredhealthcare.com
Control: Corporation, Investor–owned, for–profit **Service:** General Medical and Surgical

Staffed Beds: 81 **Admissions:** 657 **Census:** 77 **Outpatient Visits:** 0 **Births:** 0 **Total Expense ($000):** 30527 **Payroll Expense ($000):** 16078

☐ **LAC–OLIVE VIEW–UCLA MEDICAL CENTER (50040)**, 14445 Olive View Drive, Sylmar, Zip 91342–1495; tel. 818/364–1555, (Nonreporting) **A**1 3 5 10 **S** Los Angeles County–Department of Health Services
Primary Contact: Gretchen McGinley, Interim Chief Executive Officer
COO: Ernest Espinoza, Interim Chief Operating Officer
CFO: Anthony Gray, Chief Financial Officer
CMO: William Loos, M.D., Chief Medical Officer
CIO: Melvin Brewster, Chief Information Officer
CHR: Thomas Beggane, Manager Human Resources
Web address: www.ladhs.org
Control: County–Government, nonfederal **Service:** General Medical and Surgical

Staffed Beds: 226

☐ **LAC/UNIVERSITY OF SOUTHERN CALIFORNIA MEDICAL CENTER (50373)**, 1200 North State Street, Zip 90033–1029; tel. 323/226–2622, (Includes GENERAL HOSPITAL, 1200 North State Street, Zip 90033; WOMEN'S AND CHILDREN'S HOSPITAL, 1240 North Mission Road, Zip 90033) **A**1 2 3 5 8 10 **F**3 8 13 14 15 16 17 18 19 20 21 22 23 25 26 27 28 30 31 32 33 37 38 40 43 46 49 50 53 54 55 56 57 58 59 60 62 63 64 66 68 69 70 72 73 74 76 77 79 81 82 83 84 86 87 88 89 90 92 93 94 95 96 97 99 107 110 111 113 114 118 119 120 133 135 136 137 **P**6 **S** Los Angeles County–Department of Health Services
Primary Contact: Pete Delgado, Chief Executive Officer
COO: Henry Ornelas, Chief Operating Officer
CFO: Andrew Shimoda, Acting Chief Financial Officer
CMO: Stephanie Hall, M.D., Chief Medical Officer
CIO: Oscar Austelli, Chief Information Officer
Web address: www.lacusc.org
Control: County–Government, nonfederal **Service:** General Medical and Surgical

Staffed Beds: 676 **Admissions:** 37623 **Census:** 619 **Outpatient Visits:** 725242 **Births:** 1437 **Total Expense ($000):** 995270 **Payroll Expense ($000):** 378511 **Personnel:** 6833

★ △ **LITTLE COMPANY OF MARY – SAN PEDRO HOSPITAL (50078)**, 1300 West Seventh Street, San Pedro, Zip 90732–3505; tel. 310/832–3311, (Total facility includes 168 beds in nursing home–type unit) **A**1 7 9 10 **F**4 5 8 11 25 26 30 31 32 33 38 43 46 55 56 57 68 73 74 75 76 77 79 80 81 82 84 85 86 87 88 89 93 94 96 97 100 106 107 117 119 121 122 132 133 135 **P**5 7 **S** Providence Health & Services
Primary Contact: Nancy Carlson, Administrator
CFO: Karl Carrier, Chief Financial Officer
CMO: Laurence Eason, M.D., Chief Medical Officer
CIO: Timothy Kirk, Chief Information Officer
CHR: Cindra Syverson, Chief Human Resources Officer
Web address: www.lcmhs.org
Control: Other not–for–profit (including NFP Corporation) **Service:** General Medical and Surgical

Staffed Beds: 335 **Admissions:** 7859 **Census:** 227 **Outpatient Visits:** 70233 **Births:** 843 **Total Expense ($000):** 108021 **Payroll Expense ($000):** 49054 **Personnel:** 795

CA

☐ **LOS ANGELES COMMUNITY HOSPITAL (50663)**, 4081 East Olympic Boulevard, Zip 90023–3330; tel. 323/267–0477, (Includes LOS ANGELES COMMUNITY HOSPITAL OF NORWALK, 13222 Bloomfield Avenue, Zip 90650; tel. 562/863–4763), (Total facility includes 30 beds in nursing home–type unit) (Nonreporting) **A**1 10 **S** Alta Healthcare System
Primary Contact: David Topper, Chief Executive Officer
CFO: Johnnette Chong, Chief Financial Officer
Control: Corporation, Investor–owned, for–profit **Service:** General Medical and Surgical

Staffed Beds: 180

LOS ANGELES COUNTY CENTRAL JAIL HOSPITAL, 441 Bauchet Street, Zip 90012–2994; tel. 213/473–6100, (Nonreporting)
Primary Contact: Tom Flaherty, Assistant Administrator
Control: County–Government, nonfederal **Service:** Hospital unit of an institution (prison hospital, college infimary, etc.)

Staffed Beds: 190

☐ **LOS ANGELES METROPOLITAN MEDICAL CENTER (50644)**, 2231 South Western Avenue, Zip 90018–1302; tel. 323/730–7300, (Includes HAWTHORNE HOSPITAL, 13300 South Hawthorne Boulevard, Zip 90250; tel. 310/679–3321), (Nonreporting) **A**1 10 **S** Pacific Health Corporation
Primary Contact: John V. Fenton, Chief Executive Officer
COO: Shannon Jones, Chief Operating Officer
CFO: Charles Natcher, Chief Financial Officer
CMO: Fred Besharat, M.D., Chief of Staff
CIO: Dean Ochoa, Chief Information Officer
CHR: Jacqueline Sanchez, Director Human Resources
Web address: www.lammc.com
Control: Corporation, Investor–owned, for–profit **Service:** General Medical and Surgical

Staffed Beds: 213

☐ **MIRACLE MILE MEDICAL CENTER (50751)**, 6000 San Vicente Boulevard, Zip 90036; tel. 323/930–1040, (Nonreporting) **A**1 10
Primary Contact: Jack Lahidjani, Chief Executive Officer
Control: Corporation, Investor–owned, for–profit **Service:** General Medical and Surgical

Staffed Beds: 17

☐ **MISSION COMMUNITY HOSPITAL–SAN FERNANDO CAMPUS (50704)**, 14850 Roscoe Boulevard, Panorama City, Zip 91402; tel. 818/787–2222, (Nonreporting) **A**1 9 10
Primary Contact: Heidi Lennartz, Chief Executive Officer
COO: Sidney Ono, Chief Operating Officer
CFO: John Holder, Chief Financial Officer
CMO: Charles Charuvastra, M.D., Medical Director
CIO: Andre Henderson, Director Information Systems
CHR: Paul Williams, Director Human Resources
Web address: www.mchonline.org
Control: Other not–for–profit (including NFP Corporation) **Service:** General Medical and Surgical

Staffed Beds: 145

Hospital, Medicare Provider Number, Address, Telephone, Approval, Facility, and Physician Codes, Health Care System

★ American Hospital Association (AHA) membership
☐ The Joint Commission accreditation
○ American Osteopathic Association (AOA) accreditation
△ Commission on Accreditation of Rehabilitation Facilities (CARF) accreditation

☐ **MOTION PICTURE AND TELEVISION FUND HOSPITAL AND RESIDENTIAL SERVICES (50552)**, 23388 Mulholland Drive, Woodland Hills, Zip 91364–2733; tel. 818/876–1888, (Total facility includes 189 beds in nursing home–type unit) (Nonreporting) **A**1 9 10
Primary Contact: David Tillman, President and Chief Executive Officer
COO: Seth Ellis, Chief Operating Officer
CFO: Frank Guarrera, Executive Vice President and Chief Financial Officer
CIO: Velma Carroll, Chief Information Officer
CHR: Jan Zlotowicz, Vice President Human Resources
Web address: www.mptvfund.org
Control: Other not–for–profit (including NFP Corporation) **Service:** General Medical and Surgical

Staffed Beds: 250

★ △ **NORTHRIDGE HOSPITAL MEDICAL CENTER–ROSCOE BOULEVARD CAMPUS (50116)**, 18300 Roscoe Boulevard, Northridge, Zip 91328–4167; tel. 818/885–8500 **A**1 2 3 5 7 9 10 **F**2 3 5 8 11 12 13 14 15 17 18 20 22 24 25 26 27 30 31 32 33 36 38 40 43 44 48 49 52 54 55 56 57 58 59 60 62 66 68 70 72 73 74 75 76 77 79 80 81 83 84 85 86 87 88 89 90 91 92 93 94 95 96 97 99 100 105 106 107 109 112 118 119 121 123 135 136 137 **P**3 5 **S** Catholic Healthcare West
Primary Contact: Michael L. Wall, President
CFO: Paul Brydon, Vice President Finance and Chief Financial Officer
CHR: George Leisher, Vice President Human Resources
Web address: www.northridgehospital.org
Control: Other not–for–profit (including NFP Corporation) **Service:** General Medical and Surgical

Staffed Beds: 371 **Admissions:** 16259 **Census:** 247 **Outpatient Visits:** 95183 **Births:** 2773 **Total Expense ($000):** 253302 **Payroll Expense ($000):** 117985 **Personnel:** 1774

★ **OLYMPIA MEDICAL CENTER (50742)**, 5900 West Olympic Boulevard, Zip 90036; tel. 310/657–5900 **A**1 9 10 **F**3 6 25 27 32 33 34 38 43 46 49 50 51 53 54 55 56 57 58 60 62 66 68 72 73 75 76 77 79 80 82 86 93 94 96 97 100 102 106 107 119 120 121 132 135 137
Primary Contact: John A. Calderone, Ph.D., Chief Executive Officer
COO: Lee Suyenaga, Chief Operating Officer
CFO: Steve Maekawa, Chief Financial Officer
CMO: James Peace, M.D., Chief of Staff
CIO: Patrick Wiseman, Director Information Systems
CHR: Lisa Valenzuela, Director Human Resources
Web address: www.olympiamc.com
Control: Corporation, Investor–owned, for–profit **Service:** General Medical and Surgical

Staffed Beds: 150 **Admissions:** 6223 **Census:** 89 **Outpatient Visits:** 35935 **Births:** 0 **Total Expense ($000):** 87427 **Payroll Expense ($000):** 41667 **Personnel:** 607

☐ △ **PACIFIC ALLIANCE MEDICAL CENTER (50018)**, 531 West College Street, Zip 90012–2315; tel. 213/624–8411, (Nonreporting) **A**1 7 9 10
Primary Contact: John R. Edwards, Administrator and Chief Executive Officer
CFO: Allan Shubin, Chief Financial Officer
CIO: John D. Brown, Director Information Systems
Web address: www.pamc.net
Control: Partnership, Investor–owned, for–profit **Service:** General Medical and Surgical

Staffed Beds: 138

☐ **PACIFICA HOSPITAL OF THE VALLEY (50378)**, 9449 San Fernando Road, Sun Valley, Zip 91352–1421; tel. 818/767–3310 **A**1 9 10 **F**1 3 8 25 27 33 38 49 50 55 57 59 63 68 74 75 77 79 84 86 88 92 96 97 100 107 119 **S** Envision Hospital Corporation
Primary Contact: Casey Fatch, Chief Executive Officer
COO: Ayman Mousa, R.N., Ph.D., Chief Operating Officer and Chief Nursing Officer
CFO: George Watkins, Chief Financial Officer
CMO: Carlos Jimenez, M.D., Chief Medical Officer
CIO: Victor Casas, Chief Information Officer
CHR: Bruno Barbaro, In–House Legal Counsel, Risk Manager and Director Human Resources
Web address: www.pacificahospital.com
Control: Corporation, Investor–owned, for–profit **Service:** General Medical and Surgical

Staffed Beds: 221 **Admissions:** 5657 **Census:** 164 **Outpatient Visits:** 18594 **Births:** 1117 **Total Expense ($000):** 65853 **Payroll Expense ($000):** 35457 **Personnel:** 526

☐ **PROMISE HOSPITAL OF EAST LOS ANGELES (52046)**, 443 South Soto Street, Zip 90033–4398; tel. 323/261–1181, (Nonreporting) **A**1 10
Primary Contact: Richard McCarthy, Chief Executive Officer
Web address: www.promiseeastla.com
Control: Corporation, Investor–owned, for–profit **Service:** Long–Term Acute Care hospital

Staffed Beds: 36

○ **SHERMAN OAKS HOSPITAL (50755)**, 4929 Van Nuys Boulevard, Sherman Oaks, Zip 91403–1702; tel. 818/981–7111 **A**10 11 **F**16 17 25 27 30 31 32 33 36 38 44 55 56 57 60 62 73 76 77 78 79 80 94 95 96 97 106 107 119 120 121 135 137 **S** Prime Healthcare Services
Primary Contact: Lex Reddy, President and Chief Executive Officer
COO: Bockhi Park, Administrator
CFO: Samuel De Nunzio, Chief Financial Officer
CMO: Michael Malamed, M.D., Chief of Staff
CHR: Rey Hernandez, Director Human Resources
Web address: www.shermanoakshospital.com
Control: Corporation, Investor–owned, for–profit **Service:** General Medical and Surgical

Staffed Beds: 112 **Admissions:** 5496 **Census:** 58 **Outpatient Visits:** 25133 **Births:** 0 **Total Expense ($000):** 69723 **Payroll Expense ($000):** 25528 **Personnel:** 505

☐ **SHRINERS HOSPITALS FOR CHILDREN, LOS ANGELES**, (pediatrics), 3160 Geneva Street, Zip 90020–1199; tel. 213/388–3151 **A**1 3 5 **F**3 30 31 33 55 56 57 58 62 66 72 73 77 80 81 82 84 86 87 107 119 120 121 132 135 **P**6 **S** Shriners Hospitals for Children
Primary Contact: Terence T. Cunningham, FACHE, Administrator
CFO: David Burkitt, Director Fiscal Services
CMO: Colin Moseley, M.D., Chief of Staff
CIO: Cecelia Thompson, Director Medical Records
CHR: Rashawn Woods, Director Human Resources
Web address: www.shrinehg.org
Control: Other not–for–profit (including NFP Corporation) **Service:** Children's other specialty

Staffed Beds: 60 **Admissions:** 1373 **Census:** 17 **Outpatient Visits:** 17852 **Births:** 0 **Personnel:** 241

★ **ST. VINCENT MEDICAL CENTER (50502)**, 2131 West Third Street, Zip 90057–7992, Mailing Address: P.O. Box 57992, Zip 90057–7992; tel. 213/484–7111, (Total facility includes 27 beds in nursing home–type unit) **A**1 2 9 10 **F**11 15 18 20 22 25 26 27 30 31 32 33 34 37 38 43 44 50 53 55 57 59 62 66 67 72 73 75 76 77 79 82 86 96 97 100 106 107 108 109 119 125 127 135 137 **P**5 **S** Daughters of Charity Health System
Primary Contact: Catherine Fickes, RN, President and Chief Executive Officer
COO: Douglas V. Kleam, Vice President and Chief Operating Officer
CFO: Michael Garko, Chief Financial Officer
CMO: Faye Montegrande, M.D., Chief of Staff
CIO: Dan Robbins, Information Technology and Account Executive
CHR: Christine Carson, Vice President Human Resources
Web address: www.stvincentmedicalcenter.com
Control: Church–operated, Nongovernment, not–for profit **Service:** General Medical and Surgical

Staffed Beds: 318 **Admissions:** 10077 **Census:** 166 **Outpatient Visits:** 68179 **Births:** 0

☐ **TEMPLE COMMUNITY HOSPITAL (50111)**, 235 North Hoover Street, Zip 90004–3672; tel. 213/382–7252, (Total facility includes 11 beds in nursing home–type unit) **A**1 10 **F**3 8 17 27 31 33 47 49 55 57 62 66 68 72 73 76 77 79 80 87 90 96 107 117 119 132
Primary Contact: Herbert G. Needman, President and Chief Executive Officer
Web address: www.templecommunityhospital.com
Control: Corporation, Investor–owned, for–profit **Service:** General Medical and Surgical

Staffed Beds: 141 **Admissions:** 2827 **Census:** 52 **Outpatient Visits:** 6200 **Births:** 0 **Personnel:** 289

★ **UNIVERSITY OF CALIFORNIA LOS ANGELES MEDICAL CENTER (50262)**, 10833 Le Conte Avenue, Zip 90095–3075; tel. 310/825–9111 **A**1 3 5 8 9 10 **F**3 7 8 11 12 13 14 15 17 18 19 20 21 22 23 24 25 26 27 28 31 32 33 34 38 40 43 44 45 46 47 48 49 51 53 54 55 56 57 58 60 61 62 63 66 68 70 72 73 74 75 76 77 79 80 81 82 83 84 85 86 87 92 96 97 99 100 101 102 103 104 105 106 107 108 109 111 112 113 114 116 119 120 121 125 126 127 128 129 131 132 134 135 136 137 **P**6 **S** University of California–Systemwide Administration
Primary Contact: David Feinberg, M.D., Chief Executive Officer
COO: Amir Dan Rubin, Chief Operating Officer
CFO: Paul Staton, Chief Financial Officer
CMO: J. Thomas Rosenthal, M.D., Chief Medical Officer
CHR: Mark Speare, Senior Associate Director Human Resources
Web address: www.uclahealth.org
Control: State–Government, nonfederal **Service:** General Medical and Surgical

Staffed Beds: 595 **Admissions:** 26434 **Census:** 484 **Outpatient Visits:** 734654 **Births:** 2004 **Total Expense ($000):** 900260 **Payroll Expense ($000):** 380090 **Personnel:** 6037

★ **UNIVERSITY OF CALIFORNIA LOS ANGELES NEUROPSYCHIATRIC HOSPITAL (54009)**, 760 Westwood Plaza, Zip 90095–8353; tel. 310/825–0511 **A**1 3 5 9 10 **F**5 11 14 25 26 30 31 32 33 36 38 39 40 54 62 66 75 81 82 86 88 89 90 91 92 93 94 95 114 119 121 123 135 **P**1 **S** University of California–Systemwide Administration
Primary Contact: Fawzy I. Fawzy, M.D., Chief Executive Officer
COO: Ruth Irwin, Associate Director Clinical Operations
CHR: Cindy Cohen, Director Human Resources
Web address: www.npi.ucla.edu
Control: State–Government, nonfederal **Service:** Psychiatric

Staffed Beds: 69 **Admissions:** 1775 **Census:** 65 **Outpatient Visits:** 17201 **Births:** 0 **Total Expense ($000):** 37210 **Payroll Expense ($000):** 20900 **Personnel:** 343

★ **UNIVERSITY OF SOUTHERN CALIFORNIA–NORRIS COMPREHENSIVE CANCER CENTER AND HOSPITAL (50660)**, 1441 Eastlake Avenue, Zip 90033–3804; tel. 323/865–3000, (Nonreporting) **A**1 2 3 5 9 10 **S** TENET Healthcare Corporation
Primary Contact: Debbie Walsh, Chief Operating Officer
CMO: Alexandra Levine, M.D., Medical Director
CIO: David Wueste, Director Information Services
Web address: www.uscnorris.com
Control: Corporation, Investor–owned, for–profit **Service:** General Medical and Surgical

Staffed Beds: 60

★ **USC UNIVERSITY HOSPITAL (50696)**, 1500 San Pablo Street, Zip 90033–4587; tel. 323/442–8500 **A**1 3 5 8 9 10 **F**3 12 17 18 20 22 25 26 30 32 33 43 46 48 49 51 56 58 59 62 66 68 72 73 75 77 79 80 81 86 88 93 96 97 100 101 102 103 106 107 112 116 119 120 121 126 127 128 129 130 131 134 135 137 **P**4 **S** TENET Healthcare Corporation
Primary Contact: Debbie Walsh, Chief Executive Officer
COO: Scott D. Evans, FACHE, Chief Operating Officer
CFO: Strawn Steele, Chief Financial Officer
CMO: Eila Skinner, M.D., Chief of Staff
CIO: Jerry Baker, Director Information Services
CHR: Susan Burrows, Director Human Resources
Web address: www.uscuh.com
Control: Corporation, Investor–owned, for–profit **Service:** General Medical and Surgical

Staffed Beds: 162 **Admissions:** 6699 **Census:** 136 **Outpatient Visits:** 42848 **Births:** 0 **Total Expense ($000):** 219958 **Payroll Expense ($000):** 83678 **Personnel:** 836

★ **VALLEY PRESBYTERIAN HOSPITAL (50126)**, 15107 Vanowen Street, Van Nuys, Zip 91405–4598; tel. 818/782–6600 **A**1 9 10 **F**3 8 14 15 18 20 22 24 25 26 27 30 32 38 41 44 49 50 53 56 57 62 63 66 68 70 72 73 74 75 76 77 79 80 82 83 84 85 96 97 107 108 111 119 121 135
Primary Contact: Albert L. Greene, President and Chief Executive Officer
CFO: Robert Allen, Chief Financial Officer
CIO: Ray Moss, Chief Information Officer
CHR: Wesley Schmidt, Director Human Resources
Web address: www.valleypres.org
Control: Other not–for–profit (including NFP Corporation) **Service:** General Medical and Surgical

Staffed Beds: 303 **Admissions:** 13654 **Census:** 173 **Outpatient Visits:** 110657 **Births:** 5719 **Total Expense ($000):** 150736 **Payroll Expense ($000):** 73130 **Personnel:** 1107

★ △ **VETERANS AFFAIRS GREATER LOS ANGELES HEALTHCARE SYSTEM**, 11301 Wilshire Boulevard, Zip 90073–1003; tel. 310/478–3711, (Total facility includes 240 beds in nursing home–type unit) (Nonreporting) **A**1 2 5 7 8 **S** Department of Veterans Affairs
Primary Contact: Donna M. Beiter, RN, M.S.N., Acting Director
COO: Lynn Carrier, Associate Director Administration and Support
CFO: Olivia Ortiz–Bitner, Acting Chief Financial Officer
CMO: Dennis Schaberg, M.D., Chief Medicine
CIO: Eugene Archey, Chief Information Technology
CHR: Harold Goings, Chief Human Resources
Web address: www.va.gov/sta/guide/home.asp
Control: Veterans Affairs, Government, federal **Service:** General Medical and Surgical

Staffed Beds: 1327

★ **WEST HILLS HOSPITAL AND MEDICAL CENTER (50481)**, 7300 Medical Center Drive, Canoga Park, Zip 91307–1910; tel. 818/676–4000, (Nonreporting) **A**1 10 **S** HCA
Primary Contact: Beverly Gilmore, President and Chief Executive Officer
COO: Janice Barnett, Chief Operating Officer
CFO: Tony Lopez, Chief Financial Officer
CMO: Alan Kuban, M.D., Chief Medical Staff
CIO: Tony Lopez, Chief Financial Officer
CHR: Mark Fisher, Vice President Human Resources
Web address: www.westhillshospital.com
Control: Corporation, Investor–owned, for–profit **Service:** General Medical and Surgical

Staffed Beds: 114

★ △ **WHITE MEMORIAL MEDICAL CENTER (50103)**, 1720 Cesar E Chavez Avenue, Zip 90033–2481; tel. 323/268–5000, (Nonreporting) **A**1 2 3 5 7 9 10 **S** Adventist Health
Primary Contact: Beth D. Zachary, President and Chief Executive Officer
CFO: John Raffoul, Senior Vice President Finance
CMO: Rosalio J. Lopez, M.D., Vice President Medical Affairs
CIO: Carl Elkins, Chief Information Officer
CHR: Natasha Milatovich, Director Human Resources
Web address: www.whitememorial.com
Control: Church–operated, Nongovernment, not–for profit **Service:** General Medical and Surgical

Staffed Beds: 277

WOMEN'S AND CHILDREN'S HOSPITAL See LAC/University of Southern California Medical Center

CA

LOS BANOS—Merced County

MEMORIAL HOSPITAL LOS BANOS See Memorial Medical Center, Modesto

LOS GATOS—Santa Clara County

★ △ **COMMUNITY HOSPITAL OF LOS GATOS (50188)**, 815 Pollard Road, Zip 95032–1438; tel. 408/378–6131 **A**1 7 9 10 **F**3 8 13 15 17 25 26 27 30 32 35 38 51 57 68 70 74 77 79 80 85 86 96 100 102 107 119 121 135 137 **S** TENET Healthcare Corporation
Primary Contact: Gary Honts, Chief Executive Officer
COO: Mary Anne McCrea, Chief Operating Officer and Chief Nursing Officer
CFO: Rollie Pirkl, Chief Financial Officer
CHR: Kathy Bailey, Director Human Resources
Web address: www.communityhospitallg.com
Control: Corporation, Investor–owned, for–profit **Service:** General Medical and Surgical

Staffed Beds: 77 **Admissions:** 4016 **Census:** 55 **Outpatient Visits:** 33942 **Births:** 696 **Total Expense ($000):** 95516 **Payroll Expense ($000):** 40629 **Personnel:** 480

LYNWOOD—Los Angeles County

★ **ST. FRANCIS MEDICAL CENTER (50104)**, 3630 East Imperial Highway, Zip 90262–2636; tel. 310/900–8900, (Nonreporting) **A**1 9 10 **S** Daughters of Charity Health System
Primary Contact: Gerald T. Kozai, President
CFO: Jesse Guevara, Senior Vice President and Chief Financial Officer
CIO: Marsha Chan, Chief Quality Officer
CHR: Laura Kato, Vice President Human Resources
Web address: www.dochs.org
Control: Church–operated, Nongovernment, not–for profit **Service:** General Medical and Surgical

Staffed Beds: 384

MADERA—Madera County

□ △ **CHILDREN'S HOSPITAL CENTRAL CALIFORNIA (53300)**, 9300 Valley Children's Place, Zip 93636–8762; tel. 559/353–3000 **A**1 3 5 7 9 10 **F**3 8 9 11 19 21 23 24 25 26 27 28 30 31 32 33 34 36 37 38 40 41 43 44 46 48 50 53 55 56 57 58 59 60 61 62 63 66 70 71 72 73 75 76 77 79 80 81 82 83 84 85 86 87 89 96 97 100 102 106 107 114 118 119 120 121 132 135 137
Primary Contact: William F. Haug, FACHE, President and Chief Executive Officer
COO: Todd Suntrapak, Executive Vice President and Chief Operating Officer
CFO: Michele Waldron, Vice President and Chief Financial Officer
CMO: James McCarty, M.D., Vice President Affairs and Chief Medical Officer
CIO: Major Mark Zielazinski, Vice President and Chief Information Officer
CHR: Marta Boyer, Vice President Human Resources
Web address: www.childrenscentralcal.org
Control: Other not–for–profit (including NFP Corporation) **Service:** Children's general

Staffed Beds: 297 **Admissions:** 11709 **Census:** 206 **Outpatient Visits:** 170511 **Births:** 0 **Total Expense ($000):** 288013 **Payroll Expense ($000):** 125239 **Personnel:** 1953

Hospital, Medicare Provider Number, Address, Telephone, Approval, Facility, and Physician Codes, Health Care System

★ American Hospital Association (AHA) membership
□ The Joint Commission accreditation
○ American Osteopathic Association (AOA) accreditation
△ Commission on Accreditation of Rehabilitation Facilities (CARF) accreditation

○ **MADERA COMMUNITY HOSPITAL (50568)**, 1250 East Almond Avenue, Zip 93637–5696, Mailing Address: P.O. Box 1328, Zip 93639–1328; tel. 559/675–5501 **A**9 10 11 19 **F**3 11 13 15 25 26 27 31 32 33 38 50 53 57 61 62 64 66 68 73 74 76 77 79 80 86 96 97 99 100 107 119 121 135 137 **P**5
Primary Contact: John W. Frye, Jr., Chief Executive Officer
CFO: Mark Foote, Chief Financial Officer
CIO: Arthur Haggerty, Director Information Systems
CHR: Christine Watts, Assistant Vice President
Web address: www.maderahospital.org
Control: Other not–for–profit (including NFP Corporation) **Service:** General Medical and Surgical

Staffed Beds: 106 **Admissions:** 5712 **Census:** 69 **Outpatient Visits:** 136799 **Births:** 2058 **Total Expense ($000):** 63180 **Payroll Expense ($000):** 30070 **Personnel:** 752

MAMMOTH LAKES—Mono County

MAMMOTH HOSPITAL (51303), 85 Sierra Park Road, Zip 93546–0660, Mailing Address: P.O. Box 660, Zip 93546–0660; tel. 760/934–3311 **A**9 10 18 **F**7 8 11 13 15 25 26 27 28 33 37 38 41 42 53 55 56 57 58 62 63 68 72 73 74 75 77 79 80 81 82 84 87 94 96 99 100 102 104 105 107 119 120 121 135 136 137 **P**5
Primary Contact: Gary Myers, Chief Executive Officer
COO: Joe Bottom, Chief Operating Officer
CFO: James L. Smith, CPA, Chief Financial Officer
CMO: Kyle Howell, M.D., Chief of Staff
CIO: Joe Bottom, Chief Operating Officer
CHR: Jeff Byberg, Manager Human Resources
Web address: www.mammothhospital.com
Control: Hospital district or authority, Government, nonfederal **Service:** General Medical and Surgical

Staffed Beds: 15 **Admissions:** 771 **Census:** 5 **Outpatient Visits:** 50532 **Births:** 125 **Total Expense ($000):** 36924 **Payroll Expense ($000):** 18024 **Personnel:** 328

MANTECA—San Joaquin County

★ **DOCTORS HOSPITAL OF MANTECA (50118)**, 1205 East North Street, Zip 95336–4900; tel. 209/823–3111 **A**1 9 10 **F**3 11 12 13 15 25 27 30 33 38 50 51 73 74 76 77 79 80 92 96 97 99 100 103 104 105 107 119 135 136 137 **S** TENET Healthcare Corporation
Primary Contact: Mark P. Lisa, FACHE, Chief Executive Officer
COO: Carmen Silva, Chief Operating Officer and Chief Nursing Officer
CFO: Tracy Roman, Chief Financial Officer
CHR: Michele Bava, Director Human Resources
Web address: www.doctorsmanteca.com
Control: Corporation, Investor–owned, for–profit **Service:** General Medical and Surgical

Staffed Beds: 73 **Admissions:** 4163 **Census:** 50 **Outpatient Visits:** 34240 **Births:** 791 **Total Expense ($000):** 56594 **Payroll Expense ($000):** 29067 **Personnel:** 331

★ **KAISER FOUNDATION HOSPITAL – MANTECA (50748)**, 1777 West Yosemite Avenue, Zip 95337–5187; tel. 209/825–3500, (Total facility includes 38 beds in nursing home–type unit) **A**1 10 **F**3 8 26 31 32 38 43 44 49 56 57 66 68 79 80 81 96 97 99 100 102 103 106 107 117 135 137 **P**3 **S** Kaiser Foundation Hospitals
Primary Contact: Corwin Harper, Senior Vice President and Service Area Manager
CMO: Andrew Jaramillo, M.D., Chief of Staff
CIO: Jeff Mazikowski, Site Manager Information Technology
CHR: Diane Formby–Renger, Manager Human Resources
Web address: www.kaiserpermanente.org
Control: Other not–for–profit (including NFP Corporation) **Service:** General Medical and Surgical

Staffed Beds: 99 **Admissions:** 3589 **Census:** 38 **Outpatient Visits:** 20000 **Births:** 0 **Personnel:** 483

MARINA DEL REY—Los Angeles County

★ **CENTINELA FREEMAN REGIONAL MEDICAL CENTER, MARINA CAMPUS (50740)**, 4650 Lincoln Boulevard, Zip 90292–6360; tel. 310/823–8911, (Nonreporting) **A**1 9 10
Primary Contact: Von L. Crockett, President and Chief Executive Officer
COO: Phyllis Buchart, Chief Operating Officer
CFO: Stephen A. Hargett, Senior Vice President and Chief Financial Officer
Web address: www.centinelafreeman.com
Control: Corporation, Investor–owned, for–profit **Service:** General Medical and Surgical

Staffed Beds: 40

MARIPOSA—Mariposa County

JOHN C. FREMONT HEALTHCARE DISTRICT (51304), 5189 Hospital Road, Zip 95338–9524, Mailing Address: P.O. Box 216, Zip 95338–0216; tel. 209/966–3631, (Total facility includes 16 beds in nursing home–type unit) (Nonreporting) **A**9 10 18
Primary Contact: Elnora George, Administrator, Chief Executive Officer and Chief Financial Officer
Web address: www.jcfhospital.com
Control: Hospital district or authority, Government, nonfederal **Service:** General Medical and Surgical

Staffed Beds: 41

MARTINEZ—Contra Costa County

□ **CONTRA COSTA REGIONAL MEDICAL CENTER (50276)**, 2500 Alhambra Avenue, Zip 94553–3156; tel. 925/370–5000 **A**1 2 3 5 10 **F**3 11 13 15 26 27 34 37 38 43 50 53 54 57 60 62 63 64 66 68 71 72 74 75 76 77 79 80 81 82 84 86 87 88 90 92 93 94 96 97 100 102 107 119 121 132 135 136 137 **P**6
Primary Contact: Jeff Smith, M.D., Executive Director
CFO: Patrick Godley, Chief Financial Officer
Web address: www.co.contra–costa.ca.us
Control: County–Government, nonfederal **Service:** General Medical and Surgical

Staffed Beds: 146 **Admissions:** 10580 **Census:** 140 **Outpatient Visits:** 436210 **Births:** 2321

KAISER FOUNDATION HOSPITAL See Kaiser Foundation Hospital, Walnut Creek

MARYSVILLE—Yuba County

□ **RIDEOUT MEMORIAL HOSPITAL (50133)**, 726 Fourth Street, Zip 95901–5600, Mailing Address: P.O. Box 2128, Zip 95901–2128; tel. 530/749–4300 **A**1 2 9 10 **F**11 13 15 17 18 20 22 24 25 26 27 30 32 38 42 57 59 60 62 66 68 70 74 75 76 79 86 96 100 107 118 119 135 136 137 **P**5 **S** Fremont–Rideout Health Group
Primary Contact: Theresa Hamilton, Chief Executive Officer
CFO: Kevin Woodward, Chief Financial Officer
CHR: Pam Norr, Director Human Resources
Web address: www.frhg.org
Control: Other not–for–profit (including NFP Corporation) **Service:** General Medical and Surgical

Staffed Beds: 222 **Admissions:** 12549 **Census:** 147 **Outpatient Visits:** 153944 **Births:** 2393 **Total Expense ($000):** 200212 **Payroll Expense ($000):** 66065 **Personnel:** 1183

MENLO PARK—San Mateo County

★ **MENLO PARK SURGICAL HOSPITAL (50754)**, 570 Willow Road, Zip 94025–2617; tel. 650/324–8500, (Nonreporting) **A**1 3 5 9 10 **S** Sutter Health
Primary Contact: Kathleen Palange, Administrator and Chief Executive Officer
CMO: Andrew Gutow, M.D., Medical Director
Web address: www.pamf.org/mpsh
Control: Other not–for–profit (including NFP Corporation) **Service:** General Medical and Surgical

Staffed Beds: 12

MERCED—Merced County

★ **MERCY MEDICAL CENTER MERCED (50444)**, 301 East 13th Street, Zip 95340–6211; tel. 209/385–7000, (Includes MERCY MEDICAL CENTER MERCED–COMMUNITY CAMPUS; MERCY MEDICAL CENTER MERCED–DOMINICAN CAMPUS, 2740 M. Street, Zip 95340–2880; tel. 209/384–6444; David S. Dunham, President), (Nonreporting) **A**1 3 5 9 10 19 **F**100 106 107 12 124 126 14 23 24 25 26 3 30 31 32 34 37 42 43 45 52 54 55 56 57 59 63 64 65 66 67 68 70 71 72 73 75 77 87 88 89 91 92 97 98 99 **S** Catholic Healthcare West
Primary Contact: David S. Dunham, President
CFO: Doreen Hartmann, Vice President and Chief Financial Officer
CMO: Robert Streeter, M.D., Vice President Medical Affairs
CIO: Noel Lee, Administrative Director and Chief Information Officer
CHR: Joe Lombardi, Vice President Human Resources
Web address: www.mercymercedcares.org
Control: Church–operated, Nongovernment, not–for profit **Service:** General Medical and Surgical

Staffed Beds: 163 **Admissions:** 10164 **Census:** 113 **Outpatient Visits:** 174727 **Births:** 2627 **Total Expense ($000):** 115778000 **Payroll Expense ($000):** 54038000 **Personnel:** 978

MISSION HILLS—Los Angeles County, See Los Angeles

MISSION VIEJO—Orange County

☐ **CHILDREN'S HOSPITAL AT MISSION (53306)**, 27700 Medical Center Road, Zip 92691–6426; tel. 949/364–1400 **A**1 9 10 **F**3 11 30 31 32 34 70 72 77 79 80 83 84 135
Primary Contact: Kimberly C. Cripe, President and Chief Executive Officer
COO: Debra Mathias, Chief Operating Officer
CFO: Kerri Ruppert, Senior Vice President and Chief Financial Officer
CMO: Maria Minon, M.D., Vice President Medical Affairs and Chief Medical Officer
CIO: Mark Headland, Chief Information Officer
CHR: Sherri Hollingsworth, Vice President Human Resources
Web address: www.choc.org
Control: Other not–for–profit (including NFP Corporation) **Service:** Children's general

Staffed Beds: 48 **Admissions:** 2348 **Census:** 27 **Outpatient Visits:** 23928 **Births:** 0 **Total Expense ($000):** 40957 **Payroll Expense ($000):** 6101 **Personnel:** 101

★ △ **MISSION HOSPITAL (50567)**, 27700 Medical Center Road, Zip 92691–6426; tel. 949/364–1400 **A**1 2 7 9 10 **F**3 8 11 13 14 15 17 18 20 22 24 25 26 27 28 30 31 32 33 38 40 41 42 43 44 46 47 48 49 50 51 52 55 56 57 58 61 62 63 64 66 68 69 72 73 74 75 76 77 78 79 80 81 82 85 86 90 92 96 97 100 102 103 106 107 112 119 120 121 123 124 132 134 135 136 137 **P**5 **S** St. Joseph Health System
Primary Contact: Peter F. Bastone, President and Chief Executive Officer
COO: Markie Cowley, Executive Vice President and Chief Operating Officer
CFO: Kenneth McFarland, Vice President Finance and Chief Financial Officer
CMO: Dennis Haghighat, M.D., Vice President Medical Affairs
CIO: Cindy Emerson, Director Information Services
CHR: Shirley Barnes, Senior Vice President Human Resources
Web address: www.mission4health.com
Control: Church–operated, Nongovernment, not–for profit **Service:** General Medical and Surgical

Staffed Beds: 284 **Admissions:** 16673 **Census:** 187 **Outpatient Visits:** 121874 **Births:** 3002 **Total Expense ($000):** 275634 **Payroll Expense ($000):** 95310 **Personnel:** 1565

MODESTO—Stanislaus County

★ **DOCTORS MEDICAL CENTER (50464)**, 1441 Florida Avenue, Zip 95350–4418, Mailing Address: P.O. Box 4138, Zip 95352–4138; tel. 209/578–1211 **A**1 2 3 5 9 10 **F**3 7 13 17 18 20 22 25 26 27 31 32 33 38 40 43 51 59 64 66 68 70 72 74 76 77 78 79 80 84 86 88 96 97 100 102 103 107 118 119 121 135 136 137 **P**4 **S** TENET Healthcare Corporation
Primary Contact: Dennis M. Litos, Chief Executive Officer
COO: Mike King, Chief Operating Officer
CFO: Greg Berry, Chief Financial Officer
CMO: Eric Ramos, M.D., Chief Medical Officer
CIO: Debbie Fuller, Director Health Information Systems and Chief Information Officer
CHR: Michele West, Director Human Resources
Web address: www.dmc–modesto.com
Control: Corporation, Investor–owned, for–profit **Service:** General Medical and Surgical

Staffed Beds: 456 **Admissions:** 18784 **Census:** 281 **Outpatient Visits:** 87103 **Births:** 4797 **Total Expense ($000):** 277079 **Payroll Expense ($000):** 136825 **Personnel:** 1730

★ **MEMORIAL MEDICAL CENTER (50557)**, Mailing Address: P.O. Box 942, Zip 95353–0942; tel. 209/526–4500, (Includes MEMORIAL HOSPITAL LOS BANOS, 520 West I. Street, Los Banos, Zip 93635; tel. 209/826–0591; MEMORIAL MEDICAL CENTER, 1700 Coffee Road, Zip 95355) **A**1 2 9 10 **F**8 11 12 13 15 18 20 22 24 25 26 27 30 31 32 33 38 40 55 56 57 59 61 68 71 72 73 74 75 76 77 79 80 81 84 96 97 100 102 103 106 107 119 135 137 **S** Sutter Health
Primary Contact: David P. Benn, Chief Executive Officer
COO: Steve Mitchell, Chief Operating Officer
CFO: Joe Hirt, Chief Financial Officer
CIO: Jennifer Sierras, Chief Information Officer
CHR: Susan Donker, Vice President Human Resources
Web address: www.memorialmedicalcenter.org
Control: Other not–for–profit (including NFP Corporation) **Service:** General Medical and Surgical

Staffed Beds: 417 **Admissions:** 19034 **Census:** 262 **Outpatient Visits:** 178116 **Births:** 2090 **Total Expense ($000):** 378610 **Payroll Expense ($000):** 138893 **Personnel:** 2401

STANISLAUS SURGICAL HOSPITAL (50726), 1421 Oakdale Road, Zip 95355–3359; tel. 209/572–2700, (Nonreporting) **A**3 5 9 10
Primary Contact: Timothy J. Noakes, Chief Executive Officer
CFO: Timothy J. Noakes, Chief Executive Officer and Chief Financial Officer
CMO: Michael B. Purnell, M.D., Chief of Staff
CIO: Terry Renner, Manager Information Technology
CHR: Laura Boyles, Director Human Resources
Web address: www.stanislaussurgical.com
Control: Individual, Investor–owned, for–profit **Service:** General Medical and Surgical

Staffed Beds: 23

MONTCLAIR—San Bernardino County

☐ **MONTCLAIR HOSPITAL MEDICAL CENTER (50584)**, 5000 San Bernardino Street, Zip 91763–2326; tel. 909/625–5411, (Nonreporting) **A**1 10 **S** Prime Healthcare Services
Primary Contact: Gregory Brentano, Chief Executive Officer
Web address: www.dhmcm.com
Control: Corporation, Investor–owned, for–profit **Service:** General Medical and Surgical

Staffed Beds: 102

CA

MONTEBELLO—Los Angeles County

☐ **BEVERLY HOSPITAL (50350)**, 309 West Beverly Boulevard, Zip 90640–4308; tel. 323/726–1222, (Nonreporting) **A**1 9 10
Primary Contact: Gary V. Kiff, President and Chief Executive Officer
CFO: Narci Egan, Vice President and Chief Financial Officer
CIO: Ronnie O. Cobarrubias, Director Information Systems
Web address: www.beverly.org
Control: Other not–for–profit (including NFP Corporation) **Service:** General Medical and Surgical

Staffed Beds: 223

MONTEREY—Monterey County

★ **COMMUNITY HOSPITAL OF THE MONTEREY PENINSULA (50145)**, 23625 Holman Highway, Zip 93940–5902, Mailing Address: Box 'HH', Zip 93942–1085; tel. 831/624–5311, (Total facility includes 28 beds in nursing home–type unit) **A**1 2 9 10 **F**5 11 12 13 14 15 17 18 20 22 24 25 26 27 30 31 32 33 38 41 42 43 44 47 49 51 53 55 56 57 59 60 62 66 68 71 72 73 74 75 76 77 79 80 81 82 84 86 88 89 90 91 92 93 94 95 96 97 98 100 102 103 104 105 107 108 109 111 112 117 118 119 121 123 124 134 135 137 **P**7
Primary Contact: Steven J. Packer, M.D., Chief Executive Officer
CFO: Laura Zehm, Vice President and Chief Financial Officer
CMO: Anthony D. Chavis, M.D., Vice President Medical Affairs
CIO: Tom McNamara, Director Information Technology
CHR: Joanne Webster, Director Human Resources
Web address: www.chomp.org
Control: Other not–for–profit (including NFP Corporation) **Service:** General Medical and Surgical

Staffed Beds: 233 **Admissions:** 12027 **Census:** 169 **Outpatient Visits:** 285012 **Births:** 1358 **Total Expense ($000):** 370156 **Payroll Expense ($000):** 135427 **Personnel:** 1811

MONTEREY PARK—Los Angeles County

☐ **GARFIELD MEDICAL CENTER (50737)**, 525 North Garfield Avenue, Zip 91754–1205; tel. 626/573–2222 **A**1 9 10 **F**3 11 13 15 17 18 20 22 24 25 30 32 38 41 55 57 59 66 68 70 74 77 79 81 85 86 96 97 107 119 132 134 135 137 **S** AHMC, Inc
Primary Contact: Philip A. Cohen, Chief Executive Officer
COO: Erik Jiang, Chief Operating Officer
CFO: Harold Way, Chief Financial Officer
CMO: Joseph Kuei, M.D., Chief of Staff
CIO: James Ricketts, Director Information Systems
CHR: Jocelyn Herrera, Director Human Resources
Web address: www.garfieldmedicalcenter.com
Control: Partnership, Investor–owned, for–profit **Service:** General Medical and Surgical

Staffed Beds: 210 **Admissions:** 12275 **Census:** 176 **Outpatient Visits:** 42664 **Births:** 3691 **Personnel:** 1048

Hospital, Medicare Provider Number, Address, Telephone, Approval, Facility, and Physician Codes, Health Care System

★ American Hospital Association (AHA) membership
☐ The Joint Commission accreditation
○ American Osteopathic Association (AOA) accreditation
△ Commission on Accreditation of Rehabilitation Facilities (CARF) accreditation

★ **MONTEREY PARK HOSPITAL (50736)**, 900 South Atlantic Boulevard, Zip 91754–4780; tel. 626/570–9000 **A**1 9 10 **F**15 25 30 31 32 33 38 50 55 56 57 59 68 74 79 81 82 84 96 102 107 119 131 132 135 **S** AHMC, Inc
Primary Contact: Philip A. Cohen, Chief Executive Officer
COO: Ericka Smith, Chief Operating Officer
CFO: Harold Way, Chief Financial Officer
CMO: Azucena Porral, M.D., Chief of Staff
CIO: James Ricketts, Director Information Systems
CHR: Jocelyn Herrera, Director Human Resources
Web address: www.montereyparkhosp.com
Control: Partnership, Investor–owned, for–profit **Service:** General Medical and Surgical

Staffed Beds: 101 **Admissions:** 5303 **Census:** 56 **Outpatient Visits:** 18995 **Total Expense ($000):** 45963 **Payroll Expense ($000):** 18708 **Personnel:** 284

MORENO VALLEY—Riverside County

★ **MORENO VALLEY COMMUNITY HOSPITAL (50694)**, 27300 Iris Avenue, Zip 92555–4800; tel. 951/243–0811, (Nonreporting) **A**1 9 10 **S** Valley Health System
Primary Contact: Corey A. Seale, Administrator
CFO: Michael Garko, Chief Financial Officer
Web address: www.valleyhealthsystem.com
Control: Hospital district or authority, Government, nonfederal **Service:** General Medical and Surgical

Staffed Beds: 101

★ **RIVERSIDE COUNTY REGIONAL MEDICAL CENTER (50292)**, 26520 Cactus Avenue, Zip 92555–3911; tel. 951/486–4000 **A**1 3 5 10 12 13 **F**3 8 11 13 25 26 27 28 30 31 32 33 37 38 40 41 43 47 49 50 54 55 57 58 59 62 63 64 66 68 69 70 71 72 73 74 75 76 77 79 80 82 83 84 86 87 88 90 96 97 100 102 106 107 119 124 132 135 136 137 **P**6
Primary Contact: Douglas D. Bagley, Chief Executive Officer
COO: Ellie Bennett, Chief Operating Officer
CFO: David Runke, Chief Financial Officer
CMO: Arnold Tabuenca, M.D., Medical Director
CIO: Ed Papp, Chief Information Officer
Web address: www.rcrmc.org
Control: County–Government, nonfederal **Service:** General Medical and Surgical

Staffed Beds: 367 **Admissions:** 22329 **Census:** 288 **Outpatient Visits:** 228803 **Births:** 3406 **Personnel:** 2748

MOSS BEACH—San Mateo County

★ **SETON MEDICAL CENTER COASTSIDE**, 600 Marine Boulevard, Zip 94038–9641; tel. 650/563–7100, (Total facility includes 116 beds in nursing home–type unit) (Nonreporting) **A**1 9 **S** Daughters of Charity Health System
Primary Contact: Bernadette M. Smith, President and Chief Executive Officer
COO: Anne Goldfisher, Chief Operating Officer
CFO: Mark Okashima, Vice President and Chief Financial Officer
CHR: Linde Cheema, Vice President Human Resources
Web address: www.setonmedicalcenter.com/coastside
Control: Church–operated, Nongovernment, not–for profit **Service:** Chronic disease

Staffed Beds: 121

MOUNT SHASTA—Siskiyou County

★ **MERCY MEDICAL CENTER MOUNT SHASTA (51319)**, 914 Pine Street, Zip 96067–2143; tel. 530/926–6111, (Total facility includes 47 beds in nursing home–type unit) **A**1 9 10 18 **F**1 3 11 12 13 15 25 26 27 31 32 33 38 40 42 43 44 50 52 54 55 57 61 62 65 66 68 73 74 75 76 77 79 86 96 97 100 102 106 107 109 117 118 119 120 121 122 124 132 135 137 **S** Catholic Healthcare West
Primary Contact: Chuck Gersdorf, President
CMO: Peter Halt, M.D., Chief of Staff
CHR: Gary Blevins, Director Human Resources
Web address: www.mercy.org
Control: Other not–for–profit (including NFP Corporation) **Service:** General Medical and Surgical

Staffed Beds: 80 **Admissions:** 1747 **Census:** 46 **Outpatient Visits:** 35073 **Births:** 185 **Total Expense ($000):** 40754 **Payroll Expense ($000):** 17610 **Personnel:** 262

MOUNTAIN VIEW—Santa Clara County

★ △ **EL CAMINO HOSPITAL (50308)**, 2500 Grant Road, Zip 94040, Mailing Address: P.O. Box 7025, Zip 94039–7025; tel. 650/940–7000, (Total facility includes 30 beds in nursing home–type unit) **A**1 7 9 10 **F**1 3 8 11 12 13 15 17 18 20 22 24 25 26 27 31 32 33 34 36 38 43 44 45 46 50 52 53 54 55 56 57 58 59 62 63 66 68 70 72 73 74 75 76 77 79 81 82 84 86 88 91 92 93 94 95 96 97 99 100 101 102 103 106 107 108 109 111 112 114 116 119 121 122 124 132 134 135 136
Primary Contact: Kenneth D. Graham, FACHE, Chief Executive Officer
CFO: Marla Gularte, Chief Financial Officer
CMO: Eric Pifer, M.D., Chief Medical Information Officer
CIO: Greg Walton, Chief Information Officer
CHR: Charlene Gliniecki, Vice President Human Resources
Web address: www.elcaminohospital.org
Control: Hospital district or authority, Government, nonfederal **Service:** General Medical and Surgical

Staffed Beds: 215 **Admissions:** 16531 **Census:** 206 **Outpatient Visits:** 617315 **Births:** 4805 **Total Expense ($000):** 326143 **Payroll Expense ($000):** 135660 **Personnel:** 1379

MURRIETA—Riverside County

□ **RANCHO SPRINGS MEDICAL CENTER (50701)**, 25500 Medical Center Drive, Zip 92562–5965; tel. 951/696–6000, (Nonreporting) **A**1 9 10 **S** Universal Health Services, Inc.
Primary Contact: Linda Bradley, Chief Executive Officer and Managing Director
COO: Richard Ellis, Chief Operating Officer
CFO: Barry Thorfinnson, Chief Financial Officer
CMO: Atalanta Olito, M.D., Chief of Staff
CHR: Shannon Weidauer, Director Human Resources
Web address: www.swhcs.com
Control: Corporation, Investor–owned, for–profit **Service:** General Medical and Surgical

Staffed Beds: 51

NAPA—Napa County

□ **NAPA STATE HOSPITAL (54122)**, 2100 Napa–Vallejo Highway, Zip 94558–6293; tel. 707/253–5000 **A**1 3 5 10 **F**26 32 37 52 54 57 60 65 66 75 81 88 93 117 119 121 124 135 **P**6
Primary Contact: Edward Foulk, Executive Director
COO: Edward Foulk, Executive Director
Control: State–Government, nonfederal **Service:** Psychiatric

Staffed Beds: 1196 **Admissions:** 494 **Census:** 1168 **Outpatient Visits:** 0 **Births:** 0 **Total Expense ($000):** 179577 **Payroll Expense ($000):** 133470 **Personnel:** 2122

★ **QUEEN OF THE VALLEY MEDICAL CENTER (50009)**, 1000 Trancas Street, Zip 94558–2906, Mailing Address: P.O. Box 2340, Zip 94558–2340; tel. 707/252–4411, (Total facility includes 12 beds in nursing home–type unit) **A**1 2 9 10 **F**3 11 13 15 17 18 20 22 24 25 26 27 30 31 32 33 38 40 41 50 51 52 54 55 56 57 59 60 62 66 68 70 71 73 74 75 76 77 79 80 81 82 85 86 87 96 97 99 100 102 103 104 105 106 107 108 109 111 112 116 117 119 121 124 132 133 135 136 137 **S** St. Joseph Health System
Primary Contact: Dennis Sisto, President and Chief Executive Officer
CFO: Donald Miller, Vice President and Chief Financial Officer
CMO: Vincent Morgese, M.D., Vice President Medical Affairs
CIO: Vincent Morgese, M.D., Vice President Medical Affairs
CHR: Ron Scott, Vice President Human Resources
Web address: www.thequeen.org
Control: Church–operated, Nongovernment, not–for profit **Service:** General Medical and Surgical

Staffed Beds: 179 **Admissions:** 8752 **Census:** 129 **Outpatient Visits:** 230053 **Births:** 985 **Total Expense ($000):** 207112 **Payroll Expense ($000):** 82574 **Personnel:** 1415

NATIONAL CITY—San Diego County

□ △ **PARADISE VALLEY HOSPITAL (50024)**, 2400 East Fourth Street, Zip 91950–2099; tel. 619/470–4321, (Nonreporting) **A**1 7 10 **S** Prime Healthcare Services
Primary Contact: Luis Leon, Chief Executive Officer
CFO: Janet L. Baker, Vice President Finance
CMO: John Videen, Chief of Staff
CHR: Denton Gruzensky, Director Human Resources
Web address: www.paradisevalleyhospital.org
Control: Corporation, Investor–owned, for–profit **Service:** General Medical and Surgical

Staffed Beds: 301

NEEDLES—San Bernardino County

★ **COLORADO RIVER MEDICAL CENTER (51323)**, 1401 Bailey Avenue, Zip 92363–3103; tel. 760/326–4531, (Nonreporting) **A**1 9 10
Primary Contact: Jim Matney, Chief Executive Officer
CFO: Greg Schultz, Chief Financial Officer
CMO: Brad Barth, M.D., Chief of Staff
Control: Corporation, Investor–owned, for–profit **Service:** General Medical and Surgical

Staffed Beds: 53

NEWPORT BEACH—Orange County

★ **HOAG MEMORIAL HOSPITAL PRESBYTERIAN (50224)**, One Hoag Drive, Zip 92663–4120, Mailing Address: P.O. Box 6100, Zip 92658–6100; tel. 949/764–4624 **A**1 2 9 10 **F**3 4 5 8 11 13 14 15 17 18 19 20 22 24 25 26 27 31 32 33 34 35 38 43 44 46 49 50 53 55 56 57 59 62 66 68 70 72 73 74 75 76 77 79 80 81 82 84 86 96 97 99 100 102 103 106 107 108 109 111 112 116 118 119 121 124 132 134 135 136 137 **P**5 7
Primary Contact: Richard Afable, M.D., President and Chief Executive Officer
CFO: Jennifer C. Mitzner, Vice President Finance and Chief Financial Officer
CMO: Jack Cox, M.D., Chief Quality Officer
CIO: Mary Kay Payne, Vice President and Chief Information Officer
Web address: www.hoaghospital.org
Control: Other not–for–profit (including NFP Corporation) **Service:** General Medical and Surgical

Staffed Beds: 419 **Admissions:** 27909 **Census:** 314 **Outpatient Visits:** 337210 **Births:** 5240 **Total Expense ($000):** 573874 **Payroll Expense ($000):** 205611 **Personnel:** 3433

NEWPORT BAY HOSPITAL (54135), 1501 East 16th Street, Zip 92663–5924; tel. 949/650–9750, (Nonreporting) **A**10
Primary Contact: James E. Parkhurst, President and Chief Executive Officer
Web address: www.newportbayhospital.com
Control: Corporation, Investor–owned, for–profit **Service:** Psychiatric

Staffed Beds: 34

NORTH HOLLYWOOD—Los Angeles County, See Los Angeles

NORTHRIDGE—Los Angeles County, See Los Angeles

NORWALK—Los Angeles County

★ ○ **COAST PLAZA DOCTORS HOSPITAL (50219)**, 13100 Studebaker Road, Zip 90650–2531; tel. 562/868–3751, (Nonreporting) **A**1 10 11
Primary Contact: Craig B. Garner, Chief Executive Officer
COO: Craig B. Garner, Chief Executive Officer
CFO: Mihi Lee, Chief Financial Officer
CMO: Galal S. Gough, M.D., Chief of Staff
CIO: Linda K. Roman, Administrator
CHR: Matthew Kempiak, Director Human Resources
Web address: www.coastplaza.com
Control: Partnership, Investor–owned, for–profit **Service:** General Medical and Surgical

Staffed Beds: 126

LOS ANGELES COMMUNITY HOSPITAL OF NORWALK See Los Angeles Community Hospital, Los Angeles

□ **METROPOLITAN STATE HOSPITAL (54133)**, 11401 Bloomfield Avenue, Zip 90650; tel. 562/863–7011, (Nonreporting) **A**1 10
Primary Contact: Sharon Smith–Nevins, Executive Director
COO: William G. Silva, Executive Director
CFO: Benilda Ramos, Senior Accounting Officer
CMO: Sarath Gunatilake, M.D., DPH, Medical Director
CIO: Paul Mello, Manager Data Processing
CHR: Denise Bates, Director Human Resources
Web address: www.dmh.cahwnet.gov/statehospitals/metro
Control: State–Government, nonfederal **Service:** Psychiatric

Staffed Beds: 740

NOVATO—Marin County

★ **NOVATO COMMUNITY HOSPITAL (50131)**, 180 Rowland Way, Zip 94945–5009, Mailing Address: P.O. Box 1108, Zip 94948–1108; tel. 415/209–1300, (Nonreporting) **A**1 9 10 **S** Sutter Health
Primary Contact: Anne L. Hosfeld, Chief Administrative Officer
CMO: Barbara Nylund, M.D., Chief of Staff
CIO: Kathryn Graham, Director Communications and Community Relations
CHR: Diana G. Johnson, Acting Chief Human Resources Officer
Web address: www.novatocommunity.sutterhealth.org
Control: Other not–for–profit (including NFP Corporation) **Service:** General Medical and Surgical

Staffed Beds: 47

OAKDALE—Stanislaus County

★ **OAK VALLEY HOSPITAL DISTRICT (50067)**, 350 South Oak Street, Zip 95361–3519; tel. 209/847–3011, (Total facility includes 115 beds in nursing home–type unit) (Nonreporting) **A**1 9 10 **S** Catholic Healthcare West
Primary Contact: John P. Friel, President and Chief Executive Officer
CFO: Wayne Mills, Chief Financial Officer
CMO: Bob Peterson, M.D., Chief of Staff
CIO: David Rodrigues, Manager Information Systems
CHR: Kim Bukhari, Manager Human Resources
Web address: www.oakvalleycares.org
Control: Church–operated, Nongovernment, not–for profit **Service:** General Medical and Surgical

Staffed Beds: 150

OAKLAND—Alameda County

□ **ALAMEDA COUNTY MEDICAL CENTER-HIGHLAND CAMPUS (50320)**, 1411 East 31st Street, Zip 94602–1018; tel. 510/437–4800, (Total facility includes 109 beds in nursing home–type unit) (Nonreporting) **A**1 3 5 10 **S** Alameda Medical Center
Primary Contact: Wright L. Lassiter, III, Chief Executive Officer
CFO: Peter Praetz, Chief Financial Officer
CIO: Bob Woods, Chief Information Officer
CHR: Jeanette Louden Corbett, Chief Human Resources Officer
Web address: www.acmedctr.org
Control: Hospital district or authority, Government, nonfederal **Service:** General Medical and Surgical

Staffed Beds: 399

★ **ALTA BATES SUMMIT MEDICAL CENTER – SUMMIT CAMPUS (50043)**, 350 Hawthorne Avenue, Zip 94609–3100; tel. 510/655–4000 **A**1 2 9 10 **F**3 4 11 12 15 17 18 20 22 24 25 26 27 30 31 32 33 34 37 38 41 43 44 46 47 49 50 53 54 55 56 57 58 59 60 62 63 66 68 73 75 76 77 79 80 81 82 86 87 90 96 97 99 100 102 107 108 109 110 116 117 119 121 124 134 135 137 **P**2 3 5 **S** Sutter Health
Primary Contact: Warren J. Kirk, President and Chief Executive Officer
CFO: Robert Petrina, Chief Financial Officer
CMO: John Gentile, M.D., Vice President Medical Affairs
CHR: Mark Beiting, Vice President Human Resources
Web address: www.altabatessummit.com
Control: Other not–for–profit (including NFP Corporation) **Service:** General Medical and Surgical

Staffed Beds: 408 **Admissions:** 15550 **Census:** 258 **Outpatient Visits:** 254676 **Births:** 0 **Total Expense ($000):** 356336 **Payroll Expense ($000):** 144966 **Personnel:** 1172

□ **CHILDREN'S HOSPITAL AND RESEARCH CENTER AT OAKLAND (53301)**, (Pediatric), 747 52nd Street, Zip 94609–1809; tel. 510/428–3000 **A**1 3 5 9 10 **F**3 11 19 21 23 25 26 27 28 29 30 31 32 33 34 36 38 40 43 44 45 48 50 53 55 56 57 58 60 62 63 64 66 70 72 73 75 76 77 79 81 82 83 84 85 86 87 89 90 91 92 94 96 97 100 102 106 107 114 118 119 120 121 123 125 132 135 137 **P**5 8
Primary Contact: Frank Tiedemann, President and Chief Executive Officer
CFO: Doug Myers, Senior Vice President and Chief Financial Officer
CMO: Vipul Mankad, M.D., Senior Vice President and Chief Medical Officer
CIO: Don Livsey, Vice President and Chief Information Officer
Web address: www.childrenshospitaloakland.org
Control: Other not–for–profit (including NFP Corporation) **Service:** Children's other specialty

Staffed Beds: 190 **Admissions:** 10413 **Census:** 150 **Outpatient Visits:** 227930 **Births:** 0 **Total Expense ($000):** 310907 **Payroll Expense ($000):** 149558 **Personnel:** 1555

CA

Hospital, Medicare Provider Number, Address, Telephone, Approval, Facility, and Physician Codes, Health Care System

★ American Hospital Association (AHA) membership
□ The Joint Commission accreditation
○ American Osteopathic Association (AOA) accreditation
△ Commission on Accreditation of Rehabilitation Facilities (CARF) accreditation

★ **KAISER FOUNDATION HOSPITAL (50075)**, 280 West MacArthur Boulevard, Zip 94611–5693; tel. 510/752–1000, (Nonreporting) **A**1 3 5 8 10 **S** Kaiser Foundation Hospitals
Primary Contact: Bettie L. Coles, RN, Senior Vice President and Area Manager
CFO: David S. McGrew, Area Finance Officer
CMO: John Loftus, M.D., Chief of Staff
CIO: Johnny Law, Director Area Technology
CHR: Robert Scott, Business Partner Human Resources
Web address: www.kaiserpermanente.org
Control: Other not–for–profit (including NFP Corporation) **Service:** General Medical and Surgical

Staffed Beds: 341

OCEANSIDE—San Diego County

★ **TRI–CITY MEDICAL CENTER (50128)**, 4002 Vista Way, Zip 92056–4506; tel. 760/724–8411 **A**1 2 3 5 9 10 **F**3 7 11 13 14 15 17 18 20 22 24 25 26 27 28 30 31 32 33 38 42 43 46 47 49 50 51 53 55 56 57 58 61 62 63 65 66 68 70 72 73 75 76 77 79 80 81 82 84 85 86 88 90 91 92 94 95 96 97 99 100 105 106 107 119 121 122 123 124 132 133 134 135 136 137
Primary Contact: Arthur A. Gonzalez, Dr.P.h., FACHE, President and Chief Executive Officer
COO: Suellyn Ellerbe, Chief Operating Officer and Chief Nursing Executive
CFO: Robert D. Wardwell, Vice President and Chief Financial Officer
CIO: Mark Facuri, Director Information Systems
Web address: www.tricitymed.org
Control: Hospital district or authority, Government, nonfederal **Service:** General Medical and Surgical

Staffed Beds: 330 **Admissions:** 17995 **Census:** 215 **Outpatient Visits:** 209637 **Births:** 3764 **Total Expense ($000):** 257511 **Payroll Expense ($000):** 116529 **Personnel:** 1832

ONTARIO—San Bernardino County

★ **KINDRED HOSPITAL–ONTARIO (52037)**, 550 North Monterey Avenue, Zip 91764–3399; tel. 909/391–0333, (Nonreporting) **A**1 9 10 **S** Kindred Healthcare
Primary Contact: Peter J. Adamo, Chief Executive Officer
COO: Curtis Powell, Assistant Administrator
CFO: John Browne, Assistant Administrator Finance
Web address: www.kindredhealthcare.com
Control: Corporation, Investor–owned, for–profit **Service:** General Medical and Surgical

Staffed Beds: 91

ORANGE—Orange County

□ **CHAPMAN MEDICAL CENTER (50745)**, 2601 East Chapman Avenue, Zip 92869–3206; tel. 714/633–0011, (Total facility includes 27 beds in nursing home–type unit) (Nonreporting) **A**1 9 10 **S** Integrated Healthcare
Primary Contact: Doug Norris, Chief Executive Officer
COO: Ada Yeh, Chief Operating Officer and Chief Nursing Officer
CFO: Jason McLaughlin, Chief Financial Officer
CMO: Norman Harris, M.D., Chief of Staff
CIO: Nova Stewart, Chief Information Officer
CHR: Gretchen Lindeman, Director Human Resources
Web address: www.chapmanmedicalcenter.com
Control: Corporation, Investor–owned, for–profit **Service:** General Medical and Surgical

Staffed Beds: 114

□ **CHILDREN'S HOSPITAL OF ORANGE COUNTY (53304)**, 455 South Main Street, Zip 92868–3874, Mailing Address: P.O. Box 5700, Zip 92863–5700; tel. 714/997–3000 **A**1 2 3 5 9 10 **F**3 14 17 19 21 23 25 26 27 30 31 32 33 50 55 56 57 58 60 62 63 64 66 69 70 72 73 75 76 77 79 80 81 82 83 84 86 87 94 114 116 118 119 121 123 125 135 **P**5
Primary Contact: Kimberly C. Cripe, President and Chief Executive Officer
COO: Debra Mathias, Chief Operating Officer
CFO: Kerri Ruppert, Senior Vice President and Chief Financial Officer
CMO: Maria Minon, M.D., Vice President Medical Affairs and Chief Medical Officer
CIO: Mark Headland, Chief Information Officer
CHR: Sherri Hollingsworth, Vice President Human Resources
Web address: www.choc.org
Control: Other not–for–profit (including NFP Corporation) **Service:** Children's general

Staffed Beds: 202 **Admissions:** 10305 **Census:** 149 **Outpatient Visits:** 188309 **Births:** 0 **Total Expense ($000):** 295778 **Payroll Expense ($000):** 95600 **Personnel:** 1937

□ **HEALTHBRIDGE CHILDRENS REHABILITATION HOSPITAL (53308)**, 393 South Tustin Street, Zip 92868; tel. 714/289–2400, (Nonreporting) **A**1 9 10 **S** Nexus Health Systems
Primary Contact: Ronelo Mysburgh, Administrator
Web address: www.nhsltd.com/HealthBridge–Orange/Default.htm
Control: Corporation, Investor–owned, for–profit **Service:** Rehabilitation

Staffed Beds: 6

★ **ST. JOSEPH HOSPITAL (50069)**, 1100 West Stewart Drive, Zip 92668–3891, Mailing Address: P.O. Box 5600, Zip 92613–5600; tel. 714/633–9111 **A**1 2 5 9 10 **F**3 8 11 12 13 14 15 17 18 19 20 21 22 23 24 25 26 27 30 31 32 33 34 35 37 38 41 43 44 47 49 50 51 53 55 56 57 58 59 62 63 64 66 67 68 69 72 73 74 75 76 77 78 79 80 81 82 86 88 90 92 94 95 96 97 99 100 102 104 106 107 109 111 112 116 118 119 120 121 124 125 127 130 135 136 137 **P**2 3 5 **S** St. Joseph Health System
Primary Contact: Larry K. Ainsworth, President and Chief Executive Officer
COO: Alan Garrett, Executive Vice President and Chief Operating Officer
CFO: Tina Mycroft, Vice President and Chief Financial Officer
CMO: Raymond Cosciari, M.D., Chief Medical Officer
CIO: Tina Mycroft, Vice President and Chief Financial Officer
CHR: Mary Leahy, Vice President Human Resources
Web address: www.sjo.org
Control: Other not–for–profit (including NFP Corporation) **Service:** General Medical and Surgical

Staffed Beds: 366 **Admissions:** 21361 **Census:** 236 **Outpatient Visits:** 257577 **Births:** 5009 **Total Expense ($000):** 447783 **Payroll Expense ($000):** 155972 **Personnel:** 3520

★ **UNIVERSITY OF CALIFORNIA, IRVINE MEDICAL CENTER (50348)**, 101 The City Drive, Zip 92868–3298; tel. 714/456–6011 **A**1 2 3 5 8 9 10 **F**3 6 11 12 13 14 15 16 17 18 19 20 21 22 25 26 27 28 30 31 32 33 34 35 37 38 40 41 43 44 46 47 49 50 51 53 54 55 56 57 58 59 60 62 63 64 66 68 69 70 71 72 73 74 75 76 77 78 79 80 81 82 83 84 85 86 87 88 89 90 91 92 93 94 95 96 97 99 100 101 102 104 105 106 107 109 111 112 114 116 118 119 121 124 127 130 131 134 135 136 137 **S** University of California–Systemwide Administration
Primary Contact: Maureen Zehntner, RN, Interim Chief Executive Officer
COO: Maureen Zehntner, R.N., Chief Operating Officer
CFO: Ron King, Chief Financial Officer
CMO: Eugene Spiritus, M.D., Chief Medical Officer
CIO: Joy Grosser, Chief Information Officer
CHR: Patricia Thatcher, Executive Director Human Resources and Customer Services
Web address: www.ucihealth.com
Control: State–Government, nonfederal **Service:** General Medical and Surgical

Staffed Beds: 348 **Admissions:** 16682 **Census:** 282 **Outpatient Visits:** 527358 **Births:** 1174 **Total Expense ($000):** 442313 **Payroll Expense ($000):** 201778 **Personnel:** 3399

OROVILLE—Butte County

OROVILLE HOSPITAL (50030), 2767 Olive Highway, Zip 95966–6118; tel. 530/533–8500, (Total facility includes 20 beds in nursing home–type unit) **A**9 10 **F**3 11 13 15 24 25 26 27 28 29 30 31 33 36 37 38 40 43 46 47 49 50 51 54 56 57 59 60 61 62 63 64 66 68 72 73 74 75 76 77 79 80 81 82 86 87 96 97 100 102 106 107 113 114 117 118 119 133 135 136 137
Primary Contact: Robert J. Wentz, President and Chief Executive Officer
COO: Scott Chapple, Chief Operating Officer
CFO: Ashok Khanchandani, Chief Financial Officer
CMO: Mark T. Heinrich, D.O., President Medical Staff
CIO: Denise LeFevre, Chief Information Officer
CHR: Scott Chapple, Chief Operating Officer
Web address: www.orovillehospital.com
Control: Other not–for–profit (including NFP Corporation) **Service:** General Medical and Surgical

Staffed Beds: 128 **Admissions:** 7974 **Census:** 101 **Outpatient Visits:** 306877 **Births:** 612 **Total Expense ($000):** 88153 **Payroll Expense ($000):** 39463 **Personnel:** 903

OXNARD—Ventura County

★ **ST. JOHN'S REGIONAL MEDICAL CENTER (50082)**, 1600 North Rose Avenue, Zip 93030–3723; tel. 805/988–2500, (Nonreporting) **A**1 9 10 **S** Catholic Healthcare West
Primary Contact: T. Michael Murray, President
CFO: Tim Maurice, Chief Financial Officer
CMO: Eugene Fussell, M.D., Vice President Medical Affairs and Clinical Operations
CIO: Jeff Perry, Site Manager Information Technology
CHR: John Bibi, Vice President Human Resources
Web address: www.chw.edu
Control: Other not–for–profit (including NFP Corporation) **Service:** General Medical and Surgical

Staffed Beds: 230

PALM SPRINGS—Riverside County

★ **DESERT REGIONAL MEDICAL CENTER (50243)**, 1150 North Indian Canyon Drive, Zip 92262–4872, Mailing Address: P.O. Box 2739, Zip 92263–2739; tel. 760/323–6511, (Total facility includes 30 beds in nursing home–type unit) **A**1 2 9 10 **F**3 8 9 11 12 13 15 17 18 20 22 24 25 26 27 30 31 32 33 35 38 40 42 44 45 49 52 55 56 57 58 60 62 68 70 72 73 74 75 76 77 79 80 81 82 84 85 86 96 97 99 100 102 103 106 107 108 109 112 116 117 119 120 121 124 135 137 **S** TENET Healthcare Corporation
Primary Contact: Karolee M. Sowle, RN, Chief Executive Officer
Web address: www.desertmedctr.com
Control: Corporation, Investor–owned, for–profit **Service:** General Medical and Surgical

Staffed Beds: 331 **Admissions:** 18048 **Census:** 229 **Outpatient Visits:** 174187 **Births:** 3647 **Total Expense ($000):** 251076 **Payroll Expense ($000):** 90994 **Personnel:** 1306

PALO ALTO—Santa Clara County

★ **LUCILE SALTER PACKARD CHILDREN'S HOSPITAL AT STANFORD (53305)**, 725 Welch Road, Zip 94304–1601; tel. 650/497–8000 **A**1 3 5 9 10 **F**3 11 12 13 17 23 24 25 26 27 28 30 31 32 33 34 36 41 43 44 49 50 53 55 56 57 58 59 60 62 63 64 66 69 70 71 72 73 74 75 76 77 78 79 80 81 82 83 84 86 87 89 90 94 96 100 103 107 114 116 118 119 120 121 123 125 126 127 128 129 130 131 133 134 135 137 **S** Stanford Health Care
Primary Contact: Christopher G. Dawes, President and Chief Executive Officer
COO: Susan Flanagan, Chief Operating Officer
CFO: Timothy W. Carmack, Chief Financial Officer
CMO: Kenneth Cox, M.D., Chief Medical Officer
CIO: James McCaughey, Chief Strategy Officer
CHR: Greg Souza, Vice President Human Resources
Web address: www.lpch.org
Control: Other not–for–profit (including NFP Corporation) **Service:** Children's general

Staffed Beds: 264 **Admissions:** 13877 **Census:** 221 **Outpatient Visits:** 125095 **Births:** 5418 **Total Expense ($000):** 512482 **Payroll Expense ($000):** 201002 **Personnel:** 2103

★ **STANFORD HOSPITAL AND CLINICS (50441)**, 300 Pasteur Drive, Zip 94304–2299; tel. 650/723–4000 **A**1 3 5 8 9 10 **F**3 4 11 12 14 15 17 18 19 20 21 22 23 24 25 26 27 30 31 32 33 34 35 36 37 38 40 41 43 44 46 49 50 53 55 56 57 58 59 60 62 65 66 68 72 73 75 76 77 79 80 81 82 85 86 87 88 89 90 91 92 93 94 96 97 99 100 102 103 104 105 106 107 108 109 111 112 113 116 118 119 120 121 124 125 126 127 128 129 130 131 132 133 135 136 137 **P**6 **S** Stanford Health Care
Primary Contact: Martha H. Marsh, President and Chief Executive Officer
COO: Mike Peterson, Chief Operating Officer
CIO: Carolyn Byerly, Chief Information Officer
Web address: www.stanfordhospital.com/
Control: Other not–for–profit (including NFP Corporation) **Service:** General Medical and Surgical

Staffed Beds: 467 **Admissions:** 23234 **Census:** 364 **Outpatient Visits:** 719549 **Births:** 0 **Total Expense ($000):** 1372847 **Payroll Expense ($000):** 450379 **Personnel:** 6034

★ △ **VETERANS AFFAIRS PALO ALTO HEALTH CARE SYSTEM**, 3801 Miranda Avenue, Zip 94304–1207; tel. 650/493–5000, (Includes PALO ALTO DIVISION; VETERANS AFFAIRS PALO ALTO HEALTH CARE SYSTEM, LIVERMORE DIVISION, 4951 Arroyo Road, Livermore, Zip 94550; tel. 510/447–2560), (Total facility includes 393 beds in nursing home–type unit) (Nonreporting) **A**1 2 3 5 7 8 **S** Department of Veterans Affairs
Primary Contact: Elizabeth Joyce Freeman, Director
COO: John Sisty, Associate Director
CFO: Mel Niese, Chief Fiscal Service
CMO: Lawrence Leung, M.D., Chief of Staff
CIO: Terence Gant, Acting Chief Information Officer
CHR: Lori Peery, Chief Human Resource Management Services
Web address: www.va.gov/sta/guide/home.asp
Control: Veterans Affairs, Government, federal **Service:** General Medical and Surgical

Staffed Beds: 967

PANORAMA CITY—Los Angeles County, See Los Angeles

PARADISE—Butte County

★ **FEATHER RIVER HOSPITAL (50225)**, 5974 Pentz Road, Zip 95969–5509; tel. 530/877–9361, (Total facility includes 21 beds in nursing home–type unit) **A**1 9 10 **F**3 11 13 15 18 24 25 26 27 28 29 30 33 37 42 43 44 45 46 49 50 53 55 56 57 61 62 63 64 66 67 73 74 75 76 77 79 80 82 94 96 97 98 100 102 103 104 105 106 107 108 109 115 117 118 119 121 124 135 137 **S** Adventist Health
Primary Contact: A. Wayne Ferch, President and Chief Executive Officer
CFO: Dan Gordon, Chief Financial Officer
CMO: Helmuth Jones, M.D., Chief Medical Staff
CIO: Dan Gordon, Chief Financial Officer
CHR: Don Williams, Director Human Resources
Web address: www.frhosp.org
Control: Church–operated, Nongovernment, not–for profit **Service:** General Medical and Surgical

Staffed Beds: 101 **Admissions:** 4628 **Census:** 56 **Outpatient Visits:** 128114 **Births:** 832 **Total Expense ($000):** 107777 **Payroll Expense ($000):** 46183 **Personnel:** 877

CA

PARAMOUNT—Los Angeles County

☐ **PROMISE HOSPITAL OF EAST LOS ANGELES, SUBURBAN MEDICAL CENTER CAMPUS**, 16453 South Colorado Avenue, Zip 90723–5000; tel. 562/531–3110, (Total facility includes 34 beds in nursing home–type unit) (Nonreporting) **A**1 9 **S** Promise Healthcare
Primary Contact: Richard McCarthy, Chief Executive Officer
COO: Cynthia Duque, R.N., Chief Operating Officer
CMO: Mojtaba Sabahi, M.D., Chief of Staff
CIO: Jim Wilson, Vice President Information Technology
CHR: Sylvia Munoz, Director Human Resources
Web address: www.promiseeastla.com
Control: Corporation, Investor–owned, for–profit **Service:** General Medical and Surgical

Staffed Beds: 182

PASADENA—Los Angeles County

☐ **AURORA LAS ENCINAS HOSPITAL (54078)**, 2900 East Del Mar Boulevard, Zip 91107–4399; tel. 626/795–9901, (Nonreporting) **A**1 10 **S** Aurora Behavioral Health Care
Primary Contact: Linda Parks, Chief Executive Officer
COO: Brenda Nocon, Chief Operating Officer
CFO: Paul Smith, Chief Financial Officer
CMO: Daniel Suzuki, M.D., Medical Director
CIO: Eric Kim, Chief Information Officer
CHR: Sarah Keever, Director Human Resources
Web address: www.lasencinashospital.com
Control: Corporation, Investor–owned, for–profit **Service:** Psychiatric

Staffed Beds: 138

★ **HUNTINGTON MEMORIAL HOSPITAL (50438)**, 100 West California Boulevard, Zip 91105–3097, Mailing Address: P.O. Box 7013, Zip 91109–7013; tel. 626/397–5000 **A**1 2 3 5 8 9 10 **F**3 8 11 12 13 14 15 17 18 20 22 24 25 26 27 30 31 32 33 35 38 40 41 43 44 46 47 48 49 51 52 54 56 57 58 59 60 62 63 64 66 68 70 72 73 74 75 76 77 79 81 83 84 85 86 88 90 91 92 93 94 95 96 97 100 102 106 107 109 111 112 116 118 119 121 135 137 **P**3
Primary Contact: Stephen A. Ralph, President and Chief Executive Officer
CFO: James S. Noble, Vice President Finance and Chief Financial Officer
CMO: Paula Verrette, M.D., Vice President Quality and Performance Improvement
CIO: Scott Cebula, Vice President and Chief Information Officer
CHR: Debra Ortega, Vice President Human Resources
Web address: www.huntingtonhospital.com
Control: Other not–for–profit (including NFP Corporation) **Service:** General Medical and Surgical

Staffed Beds: 522 **Admissions:** 26471 **Census:** 377 **Outpatient Visits:** 251207 **Births:** 3456 **Total Expense ($000):** 400771 **Payroll Expense ($000):** 171658 **Personnel:** 3118

IMPACT DRUG AND ALCOHOL TREATMENT CENTER, 1680 North Fair Oaks Avenue, Zip 91103–1642; tel. 323/681–2575, (Nonreporting)
Primary Contact: James M. Stillwell, Director
Web address: www.impacthouse.com
Control: Other not–for–profit (including NFP Corporation) **Service:** Alcoholism and other chemical dependency

Staffed Beds: 130

Hospital, Medicare Provider Number, Address, Telephone, Approval, Facility, and Physician Codes, Health Care System

★ American Hospital Association (AHA) membership
☐ The Joint Commission accreditation
○ American Osteopathic Association (AOA) accreditation
△ Commission on Accreditation of Rehabilitation Facilities (CARF) accreditation

PATTON—San Bernardino County

□ **PATTON STATE HOSPITAL**, 3102 East Highland Avenue, Zip 92369; tel. 909/425–7000, (Nonreporting) **A**1
Primary Contact: William L. Summers, Executive Director
CFO: Diane Keel, Fiscal Officer
CIO: Cindy Barrett, Administrative Assistant
Web address: www.dmh.cahwnet.gov/statehospitals/patton
Control: State–Government, nonfederal **Service:** Psychiatric

Staffed Beds: 1510

PETALUMA—Sonoma County

★ **PETALUMA VALLEY HOSPITAL (50136)**, 400 North McDowell Boulevard, Zip 94954–2369; tel. 707/778–1111 **A**1 9 10 **F**3 11 13 15 25 26 30 31 32 33 36 38 41 42 43 50 51 55 56 59 60 62 66 67 68 73 74 75 76 77 79 81 82 86 87 96 100 106 107 109 119 135 137 **S** St. Joseph Health System
Primary Contact: George Perez, President and Chief Executive Officer
CFO: Mich Riccioni, Chief Financial Officer
CMO: Gary Greensweig, D.O., Chief Medical Officer
CIO: Patrick Wylie, Director Information Systems
CHR: Debra Miller, Senior Vice President Human Resources
Web address: www.stjosephhealth.org/petalumavalley
Control: Other not–for–profit (including NFP Corporation) **Service:** General Medical and Surgical

Staffed Beds: 59 **Admissions:** 3385 **Census:** 37 **Outpatient Visits:** 56430 **Births:** 542 **Total Expense ($000):** 69943 **Payroll Expense ($000):** 29453 **Personnel:** 406

PLACENTIA—Orange County

★ **PLACENTIA–LINDA HOSPITAL (50589)**, 1301 North Rose Drive, Zip 92870–3899; tel. 714/993–2000 **A**1 9 10 **F**3 11 15 17 25 26 27 30 32 38 43 46 47 48 49 55 56 57 63 68 73 77 79 80 82 86 96 97 100 106 107 108 119 120 121 124 134 135 **P**5 **S** TENET Healthcare Corporation
Primary Contact: Kent G. Clayton, President and Chief Executive Officer
COO: Pat Swaller, R.N., Chief Operating Officer
CFO: Kristi Liberatore, Chief Financial Officer
CMO: Christopher Lundquist, M.D., Chief of Staff
CIO: Gary Morrisette, Director Information Systems
CHR: Diane McCluskey, Director Human Resources
Web address: www.placentialinda.com
Control: Corporation, Investor–owned, for–profit **Service:** General Medical and Surgical

Staffed Beds: 114 **Admissions:** 4048 **Census:** 39 **Outpatient Visits:** 34490 **Births:** 2 **Total Expense ($000):** 49125 **Payroll Expense ($000):** 23412 **Personnel:** 333

PLACERVILLE—El Dorado County

★ **MARSHALL HOSPITAL CENTER (50254)**, 1100 Marshall Way, Zip 95667–6599; tel. 530/622–1441, (Total facility includes 14 beds in nursing home–type unit) **A**1 2 9 10 **F**3 8 11 24 25 26 27 30 31 32 33 35 38 43 44 45 49 51 53 56 57 58 59 61 62 66 68 73 74 75 76 77 79 81 82 86 87 96 97 100 104 105 107 117 119 135 137
Primary Contact: James Whipple, Administrator
CFO: Laurie Eldridge, Chief Financial Officer
CMO: Rene Orona, M.D., Chief of Staff
CIO: Mike Jones, Director Information Services
CHR: Scott Comer, Director Administrative Services
Web address: www.marshallmedical.org
Control: Other not–for–profit (including NFP Corporation) **Service:** General Medical and Surgical

Staffed Beds: 105 **Admissions:** 6424 **Census:** 79 **Outpatient Visits:** 160478 **Births:** 630 **Total Expense ($000):** 136848 **Payroll Expense ($000):** 55224 **Personnel:** 869

PLEASANTON—Alameda County

VALLEY MEMORIAL See ValleyCare Medical Center

★ **VALLEYCARE MEDICAL CENTER (50283)**, 5555 West Las Positas Boulevard, Zip 94588–4000; tel. 925/847–3000, (Includes VALLEY MEMORIAL, 1111 East Stanley Boulevard, Livermore, Zip 94550–4115; tel. 925/447–7000), (Total facility includes 20 beds in nursing home–type unit) **A**1 2 9 10 **F**3 8 9 11 12 13 15 17 18 20 22 24 25 26 27 30 31 32 33 35 38 43 44 50 52 53 54 55 56 57 62 63 67 68 69 71 73 74 75 76 77 79 80 81 82 84 85 86 88 93 96 100 102 107 117 119 120 121 122 133 134 135 136 137 **P**5
Primary Contact: Marcy L. Feit, President and Chief Executive Officer
COO: Cindy Noonan, Chief Operating Officer
CFO: Ken Jensen, Chief Financial Officer
CMO: Michael Alper, M.D., Chief of Staff
CIO: Bob Woods, Chief Information Officer
CHR: Ron Bickert, Director Human Resources
Web address: www.valleycare.com
Control: Other not–for–profit (including NFP Corporation) **Service:** General Medical and Surgical

Staffed Beds: 177 **Admissions:** 8074 **Census:** 114 **Outpatient Visits:** 184103 **Births:** 1563 **Total Expense ($000):** 195015 **Payroll Expense ($000):** 85444 **Personnel:** 1080

POMONA—Los Angeles County

★ △ **CASA COLINA HOSPITAL FOR REHABILITATIVE MEDICINE (53027)**, 255 East Bonita Avenue, Zip 91767–1933, Mailing Address: P.O. Box 6001, Zip 91769–6001; tel. 909/596–7733, (Total facility includes 26 beds in nursing home–type unit) (Nonreporting) **A**1 7 9 10
Primary Contact: Felice L. Loverso, Ph.D., President and Chief Executive Officer
CMO: David Patterson, M.D., Medical Director
CIO: Ross Lesins, Chief Information Officer
CHR: Karen Du Pont, Director Human Resources
Web address: www.casacolina.org
Control: Other not–for–profit (including NFP Corporation) **Service:** Rehabilitation

Staffed Beds: 64

LANTERMAN DEVELOPMENTAL CENTER (50545), 3530 Pomona Boulevard, Zip 91768–3238, Mailing Address: P.O. Box 100, Zip 91769–0100; tel. 909/444–7200, (Total facility includes 97 beds in nursing home–type unit) (Nonreporting) **A**10
Primary Contact: Pamela Meeker, Executive Director
COO: Ignacio Pina, Director Administrative Services
CFO: Rosie Flores–Ramirez, Director Fiscal Services
CMO: Hao Nguyen, M.D., Medical Director
CIO: George Oliva, Associate Information Systems Analyst
CHR: Mark Kaufman, Director Human Resources
Web address: www.dds.ca.gov
Control: State–Government, nonfederal **Service:** Hospital unit within an institution for the mentally retarded

Staffed Beds: 561

★ **POMONA VALLEY HOSPITAL MEDICAL CENTER (50231)**, 1798 North Garey Avenue, Zip 91767–2918; tel. 909/865–9500 **A**1 2 3 5 9 10 **F**3 11 13 15 17 18 20 22 24 25 26 27 28 31 32 33 38 42 43 44 49 50 51 52 53 55 56 57 58 59 60 62 63 64 66 67 68 69 70 72 73 74 75 76 77 79 80 81 82 84 86 87 96 97 98 99 100 103 104 105 106 107 108 109 111 112 114 116 117 118 119 120 121 123 124 133 134 135 136 137 **P**5
Primary Contact: Richard E. Yochum, President and Chief Executive Officer
COO: Kurt Weinmeister, Executive Vice President and Chief Operating Officer
CFO: Michael Nelson, Executive Vice President and Chief Financial Officer
CMO: Kenneth Nakamoto, M.D., Vice President Medical Affairs
CIO: Kent Hoyos, Chief Information Officer
CHR: Ray Inge, Vice President Human Resources
Web address: www.pvhmc.org
Control: Other not–for–profit (including NFP Corporation) **Service:** General Medical and Surgical

Staffed Beds: 453 **Admissions:** 23295 **Census:** 307 **Outpatient Visits:** 415957 **Births:** 8117 **Total Expense ($000):** 350733 **Payroll Expense ($000):** 177408 **Personnel:** 2714

PORTERVILLE—Tulare County

PORTERVILLE DEVELOPMENTAL CENTER (50546), 26501 Avenue 140, Zip 93257–9430, Mailing Address: Box 2000, Zip 93258–2000; tel. 559/782–2222, (Nonreporting) **A**10
Primary Contact: John Sawyer, Executive Director
COO: Larry Harris, Director Administrative Services
CFO: Karen Warren, Fiscal Officer
CMO: Rajachandran Srinivasan, M.D., Medical Director
CIO: Vincent Chandler, Director Information Services
CHR: Roger Wright, Director Human Resources
Web address: www.pdc.dds.ca.gov
Control: State–Government, nonfederal **Service:** Institution for mental retardation

Staffed Beds: 805

□ **SIERRA VIEW DISTRICT HOSPITAL (50261)**, 465 West Putnam Avenue, Zip 93257–3320; tel. 559/784–1110, (Total facility includes 35 beds in nursing home–type unit) **A**1 9 10 **F**3 13 15 25 26 27 30 31 32 33 37 38 55 56 57 59 63 66 68 73 74 76 77 79 80 82 84 86 90 96 97 100 102 107 109 111 119 121 124 135 136
Primary Contact: Dennis F. Coleman, President and Chief Executive Officer
CFO: Douglas Dickson, Vice President Finance
CMO: Bindusagar H. Reddy, M.D., Chief of Staff
CIO: Lisa Flores, Director Information Technology
CHR: Sharon White, Director Human Resources
Web address: www.sierra–view.com
Control: Hospital district or authority, Government, nonfederal **Service:** General Medical and Surgical

Staffed Beds: 145 **Admissions:** 8423 **Census:** 128 **Outpatient Visits:** 166824 **Births:** 2210 **Total Expense ($000):** 105645 **Payroll Expense ($000):** 37964 **Personnel:** 820

PORTOLA—Plumas County

★ **EASTERN PLUMAS DISTRICT HOSPITAL (51300)**, 500 First Avenue, Zip 96122–9406; tel. 530/832–6500, (Total facility includes 27 beds in nursing home–type unit) (Nonreporting) **A**9 10 18
Primary Contact: Charles R. Guenther, Chief Executive Officer
COO: Kathy Valladon, Chief Operating Officer
CFO: Jeri Nelson, Chief Financial Officer
CMO: Eric Bugna, M.D., Chief of Staff
CHR: Cathy Conant, Chief Human Resources and Personnel
Web address: www.ephc.org
Control: Hospital district or authority, Government, nonfederal **Service:** General Medical and Surgical

Staffed Beds: 36

POWAY—San Diego County

★□ **POMERADO HOSPITAL (50636)**, 15615 Pomerado Road, Zip 92064–2460; tel. 858/613–4000, (Total facility includes 129 beds in nursing home–type unit) (Nonreporting) **A**1 9 10 **S** Palomar Pomerado Health
Primary Contact: David A. Tam, M.D., FACHE, Chief Administrative Officer
CFO: Robert Hemker, Chief Financial Officer
CMO: Benjamin Kanter, M.D., Chief of Staff
CIO: Steven Tanaka, Chief Information Officer
CHR: Wallie George, Chief Human Resources Officer
Web address: www.pph.org
Control: Hospital district or authority, Government, nonfederal **Service:** General Medical and Surgical

Staffed Beds: 204

QUINCY—Plumas County

□ **PLUMAS DISTRICT HOSPITAL (50148)**, 1065 Bucks Lake Road, Zip 95971–9599; tel. 530/283–2121 **A**1 9 10 **F**3 7 13 15 26 28 31 37 38 42 43 55 60 62 66 73 79 80 96 100 102 107
Primary Contact: Richard D. Hathaway, Chief Executive Officer
CFO: John Nadone, Chief Financial Officer
CMO: Lawrence Price, M.D., Chief of Staff
CIO: Chase Harding, Coordinator Information Systems
CHR: Denise Harding, Manager Human Resources
Web address: www.pdh.org
Control: Hospital district or authority, Government, nonfederal **Service:** General Medical and Surgical

Staffed Beds: 25 **Admissions:** 604 **Census:** 4 **Outpatient Visits:** 79186 **Births:** 93 **Total Expense ($000):** 18357 **Payroll Expense ($000):** 7897 **Personnel:** 223

RANCHO MIRAGE—Riverside County

★□ **EISENHOWER MEDICAL CENTER (50573)**, 39000 Bob Hope Drive, Zip 92270–3221; tel. 760/340–3911 **A**1 2 5 9 10 **F**2 3 9 11 15 17 18 20 22 24 25 26 27 31 32 33 35 38 50 52 53 54 55 56 57 59 62 63 66 68 72 73 75 76 77 79 81 82 84 86 96 97 99 100 107 108 109 111 112 118 119 121 135 137 **P**7
Primary Contact: G. Aubrey Serfling, President and Chief Executive Officer
COO: Thomas J. Tokheim, Senior Vice President and Chief Operating Officer
CFO: Caryn Conklin–Hawthorne, Vice President and Chief Financial Officer
CMO: Robert Waterbor, M.D., Chief Medical Officer
CIO: David Perez, Chief Information Officer
CHR: Liz Guignier, Vice President Human Resources
Web address: www.emc.org
Control: Other not–for–profit (including NFP Corporation) **Service:** General Medical and Surgical

Staffed Beds: 289 **Admissions:** 18993 **Census:** 223 **Outpatient Visits:** 238238 **Births:** 0 **Total Expense ($000):** 319168 **Payroll Expense ($000):** 116900 **Personnel:** 1826

RED BLUFF—Tehama County

★□ **ST. ELIZABETH COMMUNITY HOSPITAL (50042)**, 2550 Sister Mary Columba Drive, Zip 96080–4397; tel. 530/529–8000 **A**1 9 10 20 **F**3 7 11 13 15 25 26 28 30 31 32 33 38 40 42 43 44 51 53 55 61 62 66 68 73 74 79 80 84 86 96 97 99 100 102 107 119 121 122 132 134 135 137 **S** Catholic Healthcare West
Primary Contact: Jon W. Halfhide, President
CFO: Tim Panks, Chief Financial Officer
CIO: Henry Niessink, Senior Manager Information Technology Systems
CHR: Ellie Delucchi, Director Human Resources
Web address: www.mercy.org
Control: Church–operated, Nongovernment, not–for profit **Service:** General Medical and Surgical

Staffed Beds: 65 **Admissions:** 3996 **Census:** 31 **Outpatient Visits:** 57070 **Births:** 706 **Total Expense ($000):** 65074 **Payroll Expense ($000):** 25689 **Personnel:** 386

REDDING—Shasta County

★□ **MERCY MEDICAL CENTER REDDING (50280)**, 2175 Rosaline Avenue, Zip 96001–2509, Mailing Address: P.O. Box 496009, Zip 96049–6009; tel. 530/225–6000, (Nonreporting) **A**1 2 3 5 9 10 **S** Catholic Healthcare West
Primary Contact: Richard J. Barnett, President
CFO: Tim Panks, Regional Vice President Finance and Chief Financial Officer
CMO: James DeSoto, M.D., Vice President Medical Affairs
CIO: Henry Niessink, Regional Director Information Technology Services
CHR: Stephan Hosler, Vice President Human Resources
Web address: www.mercy.org
Control: Church–operated, Nongovernment, not–for profit **Service:** General Medical and Surgical

Staffed Beds: 250

NORTHERN CALIFORNIA REHABILITATION HOSPITAL (52047), 2801 Eureka Way, Zip 96001; tel. 530/246–9000, (Total facility includes 20 beds in nursing home–type unit) **A**9 10 **F**1 25 73 75 86 117 119 135 137 **S** Vibra Healthcare
Primary Contact: Chris Jones, Chief Executive Officer
COO: Lisa Stevens, Chief Clinical Officer and Chief Operating Officer
CFO: Kraig Couture, Chief Financial Officer
CMO: Nanda Kumar, M.D., Chief of Staff
CIO: Mark Cardenas, Director Plant Operations
CHR: Wendy Tempest, Director Human Resources
Web address: www.norcalrehab.com
Control: Corporation, Investor–owned, for–profit **Service:** General Medical and Surgical

Staffed Beds: 76 **Admissions:** 588 **Census:** 35 **Outpatient Visits:** 3398 **Births:** 0 **Total Expense ($000):** 20545 **Payroll Expense ($000):** 8270 **Personnel:** 201

PATIENT'S HOSPITAL OF REDDING (50697), 2900 Eureka Way, Zip 96001; tel. 530/225–8700 **A**9 10 **F**72 77 79
Primary Contact: Lori Wenham, Administrator
COO: Lori Wenham, Administrator
CFO: Jacky Gregore, Director Business Relations and Human Resources
CMO: Bruce Kittrick, M.D., Chief of Staff
CIO: Kim Cameron, Manager Health Information Services
CHR: Jacky Gregore, Director Human Resources
Web address: www.patientshospital.com
Control: Individual, Investor–owned, for–profit **Service:** General Medical and Surgical

Staffed Beds: 10 **Admissions:** 351 **Census:** 2 **Outpatient Visits:** 3175 **Births:** 0

★□ **SHASTA REGIONAL MEDICAL CENTER (50733)**, 1100 Butte Street, Zip 96001–0853, Mailing Address: P.O. Box 496072, Zip 96049–6072; tel. 530/244–5400, (Nonreporting) **A**1 2 9 10 **S** Hospital Partners of America
Primary Contact: Philip G. Dionne, Chief Executive Officer
Control: Corporation, Investor–owned, for–profit **Service:** General Medical and Surgical

Staffed Beds: 125

REDLANDS—San Bernardino County

□ **LOMA LINDA UNIVERSITY BEHAVIORAL MEDICINE CENTER (54093)**, 1710 Barton Road, Zip 92373–5304; tel. 909/558–9200 **A**1 5 9 10 **F**4 5 25 26 30 32 33 55 56 82 88 89 90 91 92 93 94 95 119 121 **P**7 **S** Loma Linda University Adventist Health Sciences Center
Primary Contact: Ruthita J. Fike, Chief Executive Officer
COO: Ruthita J. Fike, Chief Executive Officer
CFO: Steve Mohr, Senior Vice President Finance and Chief Financial Officer
CIO: Richard Hergert, Vice President and Chief Information Officer
Web address: www.llu.edu
Control: Other not–for–profit (including NFP Corporation) **Service:** Psychiatric

Staffed Beds: 89 **Admissions:** 4366 **Census:** 79 **Outpatient Visits:** 23332 **Births:** 0 **Total Expense ($000):** 24095 **Payroll Expense ($000):** 11760 **Personnel:** 276

★□ **REDLANDS COMMUNITY HOSPITAL (50272)**, 350 Terracina Boulevard, Zip 92373–4897, Mailing Address: P.O. Box 3391, Zip 92373–3391; tel. 909/335–5500, (Total facility includes 31 beds in nursing home–type unit) (Nonreporting) **A**1 9 10
Primary Contact: James R. Holmes, President and Chief Executive Officer
Web address: www.redlandshospital.org
Control: Other not–for–profit (including NFP Corporation) **Service:** General Medical and Surgical

Staffed Beds: 172

Hospital, Medicare Provider Number, Address, Telephone, Approval, Facility, and Physician Codes, Health Care System

★ American Hospital Association (AHA) membership
□ The Joint Commission accreditation
○ American Osteopathic Association (AOA) accreditation
△ Commission on Accreditation of Rehabilitation Facilities (CARF) accreditation

CA

REDWOOD CITY—San Mateo County

★ **KAISER FOUNDATION HOSPITAL (50541)**, 1150 Veterans Boulevard, Zip 94063–2037; tel. 650/299–2000, (Nonreporting) **A**1 3 5 10 **S** Kaiser Foundation Hospitals
Primary Contact: Linda Jensen, Senior Vice President and Area Manager
COO: Maureen O'Brien, Chief Operating Officer
CFO: Doug Reynolds, Chief Financial Officer
CIO: Angel Shew, Director Area Technology
CHR: Sharon Barncord, Business Partner Human Resources
Web address: www.kaiserpermanente.org
Control: Other not–for–profit (including NFP Corporation) **Service:** General Medical and Surgical

Staffed Beds: 168

★ **SEQUOIA HOSPITAL (50197)**, 170 Alameda De Las Pulgas, Zip 94062–2799; tel. 650/369–5811, (Total facility includes 44 beds in nursing home–type unit) **A**1 9 10 **F**11 12 13 15 18 20 22 24 25 26 27 31 32 33 38 44 45 46 49 50 52 55 56 57 59 62 66 68 72 73 74 75 76 77 79 81 82 86 88 96 97 99 100 102 103 106 107 109 111 117 118 119 121 124 135 136 137 **P**3 **S** Catholic Healthcare West
Primary Contact: Glenna L. Vaskelis, President and Administrator
COO: Kathy Romano, Chief Operating Officer
CFO: Gratia Barton, Chief Financial Officer
CMO: Leonard Valentino, M.D., President Professional Staff
CIO: Jason Chang, Chief Information Officer
CHR: Sharon Henderson, Director Human Resources
Web address: www.sequoiahospital.org
Control: Other not–for–profit (including NFP Corporation) **Service:** General Medical and Surgical

Staffed Beds: 205 **Admissions:** 8614 **Census:** 117 **Outpatient Visits:** 126714 **Births:** 1310 **Total Expense ($000):** 186082 **Payroll Expense ($000):** 74498 **Personnel:** 896

REEDLEY—Fresno County

☐ **SIERRA–KINGS DISTRICT HOSPITAL (50192)**, 372 West Cypress Avenue, Zip 93654–2199; tel. 559/638–8155, (Nonreporting) **A**1 9 10
Primary Contact: Pamela Ott, RN, Chief Executive Officer
CFO: Barbara Jennings, Chief Financial Officer
CMO: Robert Fernandez, M.D., Chief Medical Staff
CIO: Angela Kim, Executive Assistant
CHR: Barbara Maselli, Director Human Resources
Web address: www.skdh.org
Control: Hospital district or authority, Government, nonfederal **Service:** General Medical and Surgical

Staffed Beds: 44

RIDGECREST—Kern County

★ **RIDGECREST REGIONAL HOSPITAL (50448)**, 1081 North China Lake Boulevard, Zip 93555–3198; tel. 760/446–3551 **A**1 9 10 20 **F**3 8 11 13 15 17 24 25 26 33 55 61 67 68 74 77 79 82 84 86 96 100 107 119 135 137 **P**3
Primary Contact: David A. Mechtenberg, Chief Executive Officer
CFO: David Recupero, Chief Financial Officer
CMO: Iresha Goonesinghe, M.D., Chief of Staff
CHR: Davie Shary, Director Human Resources
Web address: www.rrh.org
Control: Other not–for–profit (including NFP Corporation) **Service:** General Medical and Surgical

Staffed Beds: 55 **Admissions:** 2626 **Census:** 25 **Outpatient Visits:** 56437 **Births:** 555 **Total Expense ($000):** 43804 **Payroll Expense ($000):** 16737

RIVERSIDE—Riverside County

★ **KAISER FOUNDATION HOSPITAL–RIVERSIDE (50686)**, 10800 Magnolia Avenue, Zip 92505–3000; tel. 951/353–2000, (Nonreporting) **A**1 3 5 10 **S** Kaiser Foundation Hospitals
Primary Contact: Vita M. Willett, Executive Director
CFO: Elizabeth Farnum, Assistant Administrator Finance
CMO: Richard Rajatatnam, M.D., Area Medical Director
CHR: Wendy Sander, Human Res Leader
Web address: www.kaiserpermanente.org
Control: Other not–for–profit (including NFP Corporation) **Service:** General Medical and Surgical

Staffed Beds: 215

☐ **PARKVIEW COMMUNITY HOSPITAL MEDICAL CENTER (50102)**, 3865 Jackson Street, Zip 92503–3998; tel. 951/688–2211 **A**1 9 10 **F**3 8 12 13 15 25 26 27 32 33 38 41 44 55 56 57 59 62 66 68 70 74 75 77 79 80 81 82 84 96 97 100 102 107 119 135
Primary Contact: Douglas Drumwright, Chief Executive Officer
COO: Ann Marie Miller, R.N., Chief Operating Officer, Chief Nursing Officer and Director Quality Services
CFO: Patti Lepe, Chief Financial Officer
CMO: Kaustubh Patankar, M.D., Chief of Staff
CIO: John Ciccarelli, Chief Information Officer
Web address: www.pchmc.org
Control: Other not–for–profit (including NFP Corporation) **Service:** General Medical and Surgical

Staffed Beds: 193 **Admissions:** 8489 **Census:** 98 **Outpatient Visits:** 50233 **Births:** 1963 **Total Expense ($000):** 92294 **Payroll Expense ($000):** 38884 **Personnel:** 760

★ **RIVERSIDE COMMUNITY HOSPITAL (50022)**, 4445 Magnolia Avenue, Zip 92501–4199, Mailing Address: P.O. Box 1669, Zip 92502–1669; tel. 951/788–3000 **A**1 9 10 **F**3 11 13 15 17 18 20 22 25 30 31 32 38 40 57 67 68 70 74 76 79 80 81 84 86 96 97 106 107 111 119 121 127 131 135 136 **P**5 **S** HCA
Primary Contact: Michael A. Rembis, FACHE, President and Chief Executive Officer
COO: Gregory A. Seiler, Chief Operating Officer
CFO: Dan Houghton, Chief Financial Officer
CIO: Tracy Dallarda, Vice President Marketing
CHR: Paul Woerz, Vice President Human Resources
Web address: www.riversidecommunityhospital.com
Control: Corporation, Investor–owned, for–profit **Service:** General Medical and Surgical

Staffed Beds: 373 **Admissions:** 19518 **Census:** 249 **Outpatient Visits:** 102921 **Births:** 3661 **Total Expense ($000):** 183249 **Payroll Expense ($000):** 99679 **Personnel:** 1566

ROSEMEAD—Los Angeles County

☐ **ALHAMBRA HOSPITAL (54032)**, 4619 North Rosemead Boulevard, Zip 91770–1478, Mailing Address: P.O. Box 369, Zip 91770–0369; tel. 626/286–1191, (Nonreporting) **A**1 5 9 10 **S** Psychiatric Solutions
Primary Contact: Peggy Minnick, RN, Chief Executive Officer
CFO: Michelle Jackson, Chief Financial Officer
CMO: Carlos Figueroa, M.D., Medical Director
CIO: Debbie Irvin, Director Health Information Management
CHR: Venus Taylor, Administrative Assistant and Human Resources Representative
Web address: www.ardenthealth.com
Control: Corporation, Investor–owned, for–profit **Service:** Psychiatric

Staffed Beds: 85

ROSEVILLE—Placer County

★ **SUTTER ROSEVILLE MEDICAL CENTER (50309)**, One Medical Plaza, Zip 95661–3037; tel. 916/781–1000, (Nonreporting) **A**1 2 5 9 10 **S** Sutter Health
Primary Contact: Patrick R. Brady, Chief Executive Officer
CFO: Gary Hubschman, Administrative Director Finance
CIO: Nancy Turner, Director Communications
CHR: Lynda Dasaro, Director Human Resources
Web address: www.sutterroseville.org
Control: Other not–for–profit (including NFP Corporation) **Service:** General Medical and Surgical

Staffed Beds: 172

SACRAMENTO—Sacramento County

☐ **HERITAGE OAKS HOSPITAL (54104)**, 4250 Auburn Boulevard, Zip 95841–4164; tel. 916/489–3336, (Nonreporting) **A**1 9 10 **S** Psychiatric Solutions
Primary Contact: Kenneth A. Meibert, Chief Executive Officer
CFO: Dino Quarante, Chief Financial Officer
CMO: Joseph Sison, M.D., Medical Director
CHR: Lisa Myers, Director Human Resources
Web address: www.psysolutions.com/facilities/heritageoaks/index.html
Control: Corporation, Investor–owned, for–profit **Service:** Psychiatric

Staffed Beds: 76

★ **KAISER FOUNDATION HOSPITAL (50425)**, 2025 Morse Avenue, Zip 95825–2115; tel. 916/973–5000, (Nonreporting) **A**1 3 5 10 **S** Kaiser Foundation Hospitals
Primary Contact: Deborah Aspling, Senior Vice President and Service Area Manager
COO: Sandy Sharon, Chief Operating Officer
CFO: David J. Connor, Area Finance Officer
CMO: Chris Palkowski, M.D., Physician in Chief
CIO: Phillip Fasano, Chief Information Officer
CHR: Gay Westfall, Senior Vice President Human Resources
Web address: www.kp.org
Control: Other not–for–profit (including NFP Corporation) **Service:** General Medical and Surgical

Staffed Beds: 410

★ **KAISER FOUNDATION HOSPITAL (50674)**, 6600 Bruceville Road, Zip 95823–4671; tel. 916/688–2430 **A**1 3 5 10 **F**3 8 13 15 17 25 26 27 30 31 32 33 38 42 43 49 56 60 61 62 63 66 68 71 73 74 75 76 79 80 81 82 86 87 90 94 96 97 100 102 103 107 119 133 135 136 **P**4 **S** Kaiser Foundation Hospitals
Primary Contact: Max Villalobos, Area Manager and Chief Operating Officer
CFO: Jim Eldridge, Business, Strategy and Financial Leader
CIO: Kathleen McKenna, Public Affairs Leader
Web address: www.kp.org
Control: Other not–for–profit (including NFP Corporation) **Service:** General Medical and Surgical

Staffed Beds: 161 **Admissions:** 13102 **Census:** 135 **Outpatient Visits:** 69398 **Births:** 3649

★ **MERCY GENERAL HOSPITAL (50017)**, 4001 J Street, Zip 95819–3600; tel. 916/453–4545, (Total facility includes 38 beds in nursing home–type unit) **A**1 2 3 5 9 10 **F**3 11 13 15 17 18 20 22 24 25 26 27 30 31 32 33 35 38 40 43 44 45 46 50 51 54 55 57 62 64 66 68 72 73 74 75 76 77 79 80 81 82 85 86 96 97 100 102 103 106 107 117 119 121 124 132 135 137 **P**3 5 **S** Catholic Healthcare West
Primary Contact: Denny W. Powell, President
COO: Anna Cheung, Chief Operating Officer
CFO: Ronald Kroll, Chief Financial Officer
CMO: Dan Ferguson, M.D., Chief Medical Officer
CHR: Cyndi kirch, Vice President Human Resources
Web address: www.mercygeneral.org
Control: Church–operated, Nongovernment, not–for profit **Service:** General Medical and Surgical

Staffed Beds: 342 **Admissions:** 18123 **Census:** 230 **Outpatient Visits:** 94737 **Births:** 2615 **Total Expense ($000):** 337806 **Payroll Expense ($000):** 128341 **Personnel:** 1584

★ **METHODIST HOSPITAL OF SACRAMENTO (50590)**, 7500 Hospital Drive, Zip 95823–5477; tel. 916/423–3000, (Total facility includes 171 beds in nursing home–type unit) (Nonreporting) **A**1 9 10 **S** Catholic Healthcare West
Primary Contact: Timothy M. Moran, President
COO: Veronica Knudson, Chief Operating Officer and Chief Nursing Executive
CHR: Christopher Joyce, Vice President Human Resources
Web address: www.methodistsacramento.org
Control: Other not–for–profit (including NFP Corporation) **Service:** General Medical and Surgical

Staffed Beds: 326

□ **SHRINERS HOSPITALS FOR CHILDREN, NORTHERN CALIFORNIA (53310)**, 2425 Stockton Boulevard, Zip 95817–2215; tel. 916/453–2000, (Nonreporting) **A**1 3 5 10 **S** Shriners Hospitals for Children
Primary Contact: Margaret Bryan, Administrator
COO: Margaret Bryan, Administrator
CFO: William Dalby, Director Fiscal Services
CIO: John Bevel, Manager Information Systems
CHR: Debbie Rubens, Director Human Resources
Web address: www.shrinershq.org
Control: Other not–for–profit (including NFP Corporation) **Service:** Children's general

Staffed Beds: 40

□ **SIERRA VISTA HOSPITAL (54087)**, 8001 Bruceville Road, Zip 95823–2329; tel. 916/288–0300, (Nonreporting) **A**1 9 10 **S** Psychiatric Solutions
Primary Contact: Nancy Purtell, Chief Executive Officer
CFO: Irene McMillan, Chief Financial Officer
CMO: Andrea Bates, M.D., Medical Director
CIO: Mark Grip, Executive Director Business Development
CHR: David Lish, Director Human Resources
Control: Corporation, Investor–owned, for–profit **Service:** Psychiatric

Staffed Beds: 72

★ **SUTTER CENTER FOR PSYCHIATRY (54096)**, 7700 Folsom Boulevard, Zip 95826–2608; tel. 916/386–3000 **A**1 9 10 **F**30 31 32 88 89 90 91 93 94 95 **P**5 **S** Sutter Health
Primary Contact: Diane Gail Stewart, Chief Administrative Officer
COO: Diane Gail Stewart, Chief Administrative Officer
CFO: Marcus Armstrong, Director Finance
CMO: Richard Bowdle, M.D., Medical Director Service Line
CIO: Jonathan L. Manis, Vice President and Chief Information Officer
CHR: Lisa Love, Coordinator Human Resources
Web address: www.sutterpsychiatry.org
Control: Other not–for–profit (including NFP Corporation) **Service:** Psychiatric

Staffed Beds: 69 **Admissions:** 2102 **Census:** 45 **Outpatient Visits:** 14784 **Births:** 0 **Total Expense ($000):** 19455 **Payroll Expense ($000):** 9820 **Personnel:** 154

★ **SUTTER MEDICAL CENTER, SACRAMENTO (50108)**, 5151 F Street, Zip 95819–3295; tel. 916/454–3333, (Includes SUTTER GENERAL HOSPITAL, 2801 L. Street, Zip 95816; tel. 916/454–2222), (Total facility includes 89 beds in nursing home–type unit) **A**1 2 9 10 **F**3 5 8 11 12 15 17 18 19 20 21 22 23 24 25 26 27 30 31 32 33 35 38 43 44 46 47 48 49 54 56 58 59 60 62 66 68 70 72 73 74 75 76 77 79 80 81 83 84 86 88 89 90 91 92 93 94 95 96 97 98 99 100 101 102 103 107 112 113 114 116 117 118 119 121 123 124 125 126 127 133 135 136 137 **P**5 **S** Sutter Health
Primary Contact: Thomas C. Gagen, Chief Executive Officer
CFO: Richard SooHoo, Chief Financial Officer
CMO: Mark Leibenhaut, M.D., Chief of Staff
CIO: Julie Montera, Director Information Technology
CHR: Laurie Rose, Director Human Resources
Web address: www.sutterhealth.org
Control: Other not–for–profit (including NFP Corporation) **Service:** General Medical and Surgical

Staffed Beds: 659 **Admissions:** 30314 **Census:** 413 **Outpatient Visits:** 164111 **Births:** 5819 **Total Expense ($000):** 628769 **Payroll Expense ($000):** 221357 **Personnel:** 3202

CA

★ **UNIVERSITY OF CALIFORNIA, DAVIS MEDICAL CENTER (50599)**, 2315 Stockton Boulevard, Zip 95817–2282; tel. 916/734–2011 **A**1 2 3 5 8 9 10 **F**3 6 8 9 11 12 13 15 16 17 18 19 20 21 22 23 24 25 26 27 28 31 32 33 36 37 38 40 41 42 43 44 46 47 48 49 50 51 53 54 55 56 57 58 59 60 61 62 63 66 68 69 70 72 73 74 75 76 77 79 80 81 82 83 84 85 86 87 90 91 94 96 97 99 100 102 104 105 106 107 108 109 111 112 113 114 116 118 119 120 121 124 125 127 128 130 131 132 133 134 135 136 137 **P**6 **S** University of California–Systemwide Administration
Primary Contact: Ann Madden Rice, Chief Executive Officer
CFO: William H. McGowan, Chief Financial Officer
CMO: Allan Siefkin, M.D., Chief Medical Officer
CIO: Guy Koppel, Chief Information Officer
CHR: Gloria Alvarado, Associate Director Human Resources
Web address: www.ucdmc.ucdavis.edu
Control: State–Government, nonfederal **Service:** General Medical and Surgical

Staffed Beds: 565 **Admissions:** 28677 **Census:** 457 **Outpatient Visits:** 984912 **Births:** 2633 **Total Expense ($000):** 856956 **Payroll Expense ($000):** 421822 **Personnel:** 6477

SAINT HELENA—Napa County

★ **ST. HELENA HOSPITAL (50013)**, 10 Woodland Road, Zip 94574; tel. 707/963–3611 **A**1 9 10 **F**5 15 18 20 22 24 25 26 27 30 32 33 34 38 52 55 57 61 62 68 72 74 75 76 77 79 81 82 86 88 89 92 94 95 96 99 103 107 118 119 120 121 124 131 132 135 136 137 **S** Adventist Health
Primary Contact: JoAline Olson, RN, President and Chief Executive Officer
CFO: Edward A. McDonald, Senior Vice President and Chief Financial Officer
CIO: Mons Jensen, Information Systems Team Leader
CHR: Mark Fowler, Executive Director Human Resources
Web address: www.sthelenahospital.org
Control: Other not–for–profit (including NFP Corporation) **Service:** General Medical and Surgical

Staffed Beds: 140 **Admissions:** 5965 **Census:** 103 **Outpatient Visits:** 96511 **Births:** 282 **Total Expense ($000):** 113173 **Payroll Expense ($000):** 50106 **Personnel:** 605

SALINAS—Monterey County

★ **NATIVIDAD MEDICAL CENTER (50248)**, 1441 Constitution Boulevard, Zip 93906–3100, Mailing Address: P.O. Box 81611, Zip 93912–1611; tel. 831/755–4111 **A**1 3 5 9 10 **F**3 13 15 25 26 32 33 38 49 50 55 60 62 66 68 70 74 77 79 80 82 84 85 86 87 88 90 92 96 97 100 102 107 119 122 135 **P**6
Primary Contact: William T. Foley, Chief Executive Officer
COO: William T. Foley, Chief Executive Officer
CFO: Harry Weis, Chief Financial Officer
CMO: Jan R. Radke, M.D., Chief Medical Officer
CIO: Michael Jobin, Chief Information Officer
CHR: Janine Bouyea, Director Human Resources
Web address: www.natividad.com
Control: County–Government, nonfederal **Service:** General Medical and Surgical

Staffed Beds: 136 **Admissions:** 7404 **Census:** 83 **Outpatient Visits:** 53410 **Births:** 2541 **Total Expense ($000):** 120873 **Payroll Expense ($000):** 43635 **Personnel:** 664

Hospital, Medicare Provider Number, Address, Telephone, Approval, Facility, and Physician Codes, Health Care System
★ American Hospital Association (AHA) membership
□ The Joint Commission accreditation
○ American Osteopathic Association (AOA) accreditation
△ Commission on Accreditation of Rehabilitation Facilities (CARF) accreditation

★ **SALINAS VALLEY MEMORIAL HEALTHCARE SYSTEM (50334)**, 450 East Romie Lane, Zip 93901–4098; tel. 831/757–4333 **A**1 2 9 10 **F**3 8 11 13 17 18 20 22 24 25 26 27 30 31 32 33 35 37 38 39 42 43 44 45 46 49 52 53 54 55 56 57 58 59 62 63 66 68 70 72 73 74 75 76 77 79 80 81 82 84 87 96 97 98 100 102 103 104 105 106 107 112 118 119 121 122 123 124 134 135 136 137 **P**8
Primary Contact: Samuel W. Downing, President and Chief Executive Officer
COO: Bev Ranzenberger, Senior Vice President Operations
CFO: John Fletcher, Senior Vice President Finance and Information Technology
CMO: David Perrott, M.D., Senior Vice President and Medical Director
CIO: Audrey Parks, Director Information Technology
CHR: Wendy Crawford, Interim Director Human Resources
Web address: www.svmh.com
Control: Hospital district or authority, Government, nonfederal **Service:** General Medical and Surgical

Staffed Beds: 269 **Admissions:** 13173 **Census:** 162 **Outpatient Visits:** 76507 **Births:** 2550 **Total Expense ($000):** 298214 **Payroll Expense ($000):** 142256 **Personnel:** 1383

CA

SAN ANDREAS—Calaveras County

★ **MARK TWAIN ST. JOSEPH'S HOSPITAL (50366)**, 768 Mountain Ranch Road, Zip 95249–9707; tel. 209/754–3521 **A**1 9 10 20 **F**3 15 24 25 26 30 31 32 38 43 44 46 55 56 57 63 68 75 79 80 86 96 107 117 122 135 **S** Catholic Healthcare West
Primary Contact: Feliciano Jiron, President
CFO: Jacob Lewis, Chief Financial Officer
CMO: Peter Gierke, M.D., Chief of Staff
CHR: Lori Tribble, Director Human Resources
Web address: www.marktwainhospital.com
Control: Other not–for–profit (including NFP Corporation) **Service:** General Medical and Surgical

Staffed Beds: 26 **Admissions:** 1711 **Census:** 18 **Outpatient Visits:** 85393 **Births:** 51 **Total Expense ($000):** 37983 **Payroll Expense ($000):** 17263 **Personnel:** 240

SAN BERNARDINO—San Bernardino County

★ **COMMUNITY HOSPITAL OF SAN BERNARDINO (50089)**, 1805 Medical Center Drive, Zip 92411–1214; tel. 909/887–6333, (Total facility includes 99 beds in nursing home–type unit) (Nonreporting) **A**1 9 10 **S** Catholic Healthcare West
Primary Contact: Diane Nitta, Administrator
CFO: Ed Sorenson, Chief Financial Officer and Vice President Finance
Web address: www.chsb.org
Control: Other not–for–profit (including NFP Corporation) **Service:** General Medical and Surgical

Staffed Beds: 292

□ △ **ROBERT H. BALLARD REHABILITATION HOSPITAL (53037)**, 1760 West 16th Street, Zip 92411; tel. 909/473–1200, (Nonreporting) **A**1 7 9 10 **S** Sun Healthcare Group
Primary Contact: Robert Herrick, Chief Executive Officer
Web address: www.ballardhospital.com
Control: Corporation, Investor–owned, for–profit **Service:** Rehabilitation

Staffed Beds: 60

★ **ST. BERNARDINE MEDICAL CENTER (50129)**, 2101 North Waterman Avenue, Zip 92404–4836; tel. 909/883–8711 **A**1 2 9 10 **F**5 8 11 12 13 14 15 17 18 20 22 24 25 26 27 28 30 31 32 33 36 38 41 43 44 50 51 52 53 55 56 57 59 60 62 66 68 70 72 73 74 75 76 77 79 80 81 82 84 86 96 97 98 99 100 102 104 107 112 119 120 121 123 124 135 136 **P**5 **S** Catholic Healthcare West
Primary Contact: Steven R. Barron, President
COO: Jack Ivie, Chief Operating Officer
CFO: Darryl VandenBosch, Senior Vice President and Chief Financial Officer
CMO: Jean–Claude Hage, M.D., Chief of Staff
CIO: James Croker, Director Information Systems
CHR: Dee Webb, Vice President Human Resources
Web address: www.stbernardinemedicalcenter.com
Control: Other not–for–profit (including NFP Corporation) **Service:** General Medical and Surgical

Staffed Beds: 250 **Admissions:** 15467 **Census:** 202 **Outpatient Visits:** 66217 **Births:** 2222 **Total Expense ($000):** 207028 **Payroll Expense ($000):** 91691

SAN CLEMENTE—Orange County

★ **SADDLEBACK MEMORIAL MEDICAL CENTER – SAN CLEMENTE CAMPUS**, 654 Camino De Los Mares, Zip 92673–2827; tel. 949/496–1122 **A**1 9 **F**3 11 15 24 25 26 27 30 31 32 33 34 36 38 41 42 43 44 49 50 55 57 61 63 66 68 72 73 75 76 77 79 80 81 82 86 90 96 100 102 107 119 121 124 130 131 135 136 137 **S** Memorial Health Services
Primary Contact: Liz Bear, Administrator
CFO: John Bishop, Chief Financial Officer
CMO: Ronald Saltzman, M.D., Chief of Staff
Web address: www.sanclementehospital.com
Control: Other not–for–profit (including NFP Corporation) **Service:** General Medical and Surgical

Staffed Beds: 73 **Admissions:** 2652 **Census:** 25 **Outpatient Visits:** 45959 **Births:** 0 **Personnel:** 238

SAN DIEGO—San Diego County

★ **ALVARADO HOSPITAL MEDICAL CENTER (50583)**, 6655 Alvarado Road, Zip 92120–5208; tel. 619/287–3270, (Includes SAN DIEGO REHABILITATION INSTITUTE, 6645 Alvarado Road, Zip 92120; tel. 619/287–3270) **A**1 2 9 10 **F**3 7 8 11 12 15 17 18 20 22 24 25 26 27 30 31 32 33 34 38 42 43 44 46 53 54 56 59 62 66 68 72 73 75 76 77 79 80 81 82 85 86 87 96 97 100 102 106 107 108 109 111 112 117 118 119 121 135 137
Primary Contact: Harris Koenig, Chief Executive Officer
COO: Darlene Wetton, Chief Operating Officer
CHR: Floss Manning, Director Human Resources
Control: Corporation, Investor–owned, for–profit **Service:** General Medical and Surgical

Staffed Beds: 134 **Admissions:** 8281 **Census:** 133 **Outpatient Visits:** 46290 **Births:** 0 **Total Expense ($000):** 138744 **Payroll Expense ($000):** 57741 **Personnel:** 876

□ **AURORA SAN DIEGO HOSPITAL (54095)**, 11878 Avenue of Industry, Zip 92128–3423; tel. 858/487–3200, (Nonreporting) **A**1 9 10 **S** Aurora Behavioral Health Care
Primary Contact: James S. Plummer, Chief Executive Officer
COO: Peggy McGowan, Director Nursing
CFO: Cory Delello, Chief Financial Officer
CMO: Thomas Flanagan, M.D., Medical Director
CIO: Alain Azcona, Director Business Development
CHR: Susan Haas, Director Human Resources
Web address: www.aurorasandiego.com
Control: Corporation, Investor–owned, for–profit **Service:** Psychiatric

Staffed Beds: 80

★ **CONTINENTAL REHABILITATION HOSPITAL (52044)**, 555 Washington Street, Zip 92103; tel. 619/260–8300, (Nonreporting) **A**1 9 10 **S** Sun Healthcare Group
Primary Contact: Nancy Wiewiora, Interim Chief Executive Officer
COO: Nancy Wiewiora, Chief Operating Officer
CMO: John Fox, M.D., Chief Medical Officer
CHR: Wes Burns, Director Human Resources
Web address: www.continentalrehab.com
Control: Corporation, Investor–owned, for–profit **Service:** Long–Term Acute Care hospital

Staffed Beds: 110

★ **KAISER FOUNDATION HOSPITAL – SAN DIEGO (50515)**, 4647 Zion Avenue, Zip 92120–2507; tel. 619/528–5000, (Nonreporting) **A**1 3 5 10 **S** Kaiser Foundation Hospitals
Primary Contact: Nathaniel L. Oubre, Jr., Senior Vice President and Executive Director
COO: Anthony G. Minks, Chief Operating Officer
CFO: Lorna Curtis, Assistant Administrator Finance
CMO: Arthur M. Flippin, M.D., Medical Director
CIO: Alexis Sgouros, Information Technology Leader
CHR: Cherie L. Sampson, Human Resources Leader
Web address: www.kaiserpermanente.org
Control: Other not–for–profit (including NFP Corporation) **Service:** General Medical and Surgical

Staffed Beds: 392

□ **KINDRED HOSPITAL–SAN DIEGO (52036)**, 1940 El Cajon Boulevard, Zip 92104–1096; tel. 619/543–4500, (Nonreporting) **A**1 9 10 **S** Kindred Healthcare
Primary Contact: Natalie Germuska, Chief Executive Officer
COO: Patricia Cavaness, Chief Clinical Officer
CFO: Geoffrey Blomely, Chief Financial Officer
CMO: Davies Wong, M.D., Medical Director
Web address: www.kindredsandiego.com
Control: Corporation, Investor–owned, for–profit **Service:** General Medical and Surgical

Staffed Beds: 70

★ **NAVAL MEDICAL CENTER**, 34800 Bob Wilson Drive, Zip 92134–5000; tel. 619/532–6400 **A**1 2 3 5 **F**4 5 8 12 13 14 15 17 18 19 20 21 22 23 24 25 26 27 28 29 32 33 36 37 38 43 45 46 47 48 49 50 52 53 55 56 57 58 59 60 62 63 66 68 70 71 72 73 74 75 76 77 78 79 80 81 82 83 84 86 87 88 89 90 91 92 94 95 96 97 98 99 100 106 107 108 109 111 112 118 119 120 121 124 133 135 136 137 **S** Bureau of Medicine and Surgery, Department of the Navy
Primary Contact: Captain Christine S. Hunter, Commander
CFO: Captain O. G. Haugen, Director Resources
CMO: Captain John Thiringer, M.D., Chief Medical Officer
CIO: Lieutenant D. V. Gonzales, Head Information Technology Management
Web address: www.nmcsd.med.navy.mil
Control: Navy, Government, federal **Service:** General Medical and Surgical

Staffed Beds: 285 **Admissions:** 15753 **Census:** 162 **Outpatient Visits:** 565032 **Births:** 3658 **Personnel:** 6144

□ **PROMISE HOSPITAL OF SAN DIEGO (50447)**, 5550 University Avenue, Zip 92105–2307, Mailing Address: P.O. Box 5587, Zip 92105–5507; tel. 619/582–3516, (Nonreporting) **A**1 10
Primary Contact: Timothy R. Patten, Chief Executive Officer
CFO: Jim McCabe, Chief Financial Officer
CMO: Joseph Baran, M.D., Chief of Staff
CIO: Jim Wilson, Vice President Information Technology
CHR: Stacia Rasina, Director Human Resources
Web address: www.promisesandiego.com
Control: Partnership, Investor–owned, for–profit **Service:** Psychiatric

Staffed Beds: 100

★ **RADY CHILDREN'S HOSPITAL AND HEALTH CENTER (53303)**, 3020 Children's Way, Zip 92123–4282; tel. 858/576–1700, (Total facility includes 65 beds in nursing home–type unit) **A**1 3 5 9 10 **F**1 3 7 8 10 11 12 19 21 23 25 26 27 28 30 31 32 33 34 36 37 38 40 43 45 46 47 48 50 53 55 56 57 58 59 61 62 63 66 70 72 73 75 76 77 78 79 80 81 82 83 84 85 86 89 90 91 92 94 96 97 100 102 103 106 107 114 117 118 119 120 121 122 123 124 125 127 128 130 132 133 135 **P**5 7
Primary Contact: Kathleen Ann Sellick, President and Chief Executive Officer
COO: Meg Norton, Senior Vice President and Chief Operating Officer
CFO: Roger Roux, Senior Vice President Financial Affairs and Chief Financial Officer
CMO: Irvin A. Kaufman, M.D., Senior Vice President Health Affairs and Chief Medical Officer
CIO: Albert Oriol, Vice President Information Management
CHR: Robert Braithwaite, Vice President Personnel Development and Services
Web address: www.rchsd.org
Control: Other not–for–profit (including NFP Corporation) **Service:** Children's general

Staffed Beds: 309 **Admissions:** 13748 **Census:** 245 **Outpatient Visits:** 286625 **Births:** 0 **Personnel:** 2440

□ **SAN DIEGO COUNTY PSYCHIATRIC HOSPITAL (54114)**, 3853 Rosecrans Street, Zip 92110–3115, Mailing Address: P.O. Box 85524, Zip 92138–5524; tel. 619/692–8211, (Nonreporting) **A**1 10
Primary Contact: Janet Seawell, Administrator
Control: County–Government, nonfederal **Service:** Psychiatric

Staffed Beds: 357

★ **SAN DIEGO HOSPICE & PALLIATIVE CARE (50698)**, 4311 Third Avenue, Zip 92103–7499; tel. 619/688–1600, (Nonreporting) **A**10
Primary Contact: Janet E. Cetti, President and Chief Executive Officer
CFO: Kathleen Jones, Vice President Finance and Chief Financial Officer
CMO: Laurel Herbst, M.D., Vice President Medical Affairs
CIO: Barbara Radice, Vice President and Chief Information Officer
Web address: www.sdhospice.org
Control: Other not–for–profit (including NFP Corporation) **Service:** Other specialty

Staffed Beds: 23

★ **SCRIPPS MERCY HOSPITAL (50077)**, 4077 Fifth Avenue, Zip 92103–2105; tel. 619/294–8111, (Includes SCRIPPS MERCY HOSPITAL CHULA VISTA, 435 H. Street, Chula Vista, Zip 91912–6617, Mailing Address: P.O. Box 1537, Zip 91910–1537; tel. 619/691–7000) **A**1 2 3 5 9 10 **F**2 3 8 9 11 12 13 14 15 17 18 20 22 24 25 26 27 28 30 31 32 33 34 37 38 40 41 43 44 45 46 49 51 53 54 55 56 57 58 60 62 63 64 66 68 70 72 73 74 75 76 77 79 81 82 86 87 88 89 90 91 92 93 94 95 96 97 100 106 107 116 118 119 120 121 123 124 130 133 135 137 **P**5 7 **S** Scripps Health
Primary Contact: Thomas A. Gammiere, Senior Vice President and Chief Executive
COO: Leanne M. Hunstock, R.N., Vice President and Chief Operations Executive
CFO: Edward Turk, Vice President Finance
CMO: Davis Cracroft, M.D., Senior Director Medical Affairs
CIO: Drexel DeFord, Chief Information Officer
Web address: www.scrippshealth.org
Control: Other not–for–profit (including NFP Corporation) **Service:** General Medical and Surgical

Staffed Beds: 420 **Admissions:** 30215 **Census:** 393 **Outpatient Visits:** 171743 **Births:** 4368 **Total Expense ($000):** 428260 **Payroll Expense ($000):** 190495 **Personnel:** 2938

★ **SHARP MARY BIRCH HOSPITAL FOR WOMEN (50722)**, 3003 Health Center Drive, Zip 92123; tel. 858/939–3400, (Nonreporting) **A**1 9 10 **S** Sharp Healthcare
Primary Contact: Mary Henrikson, Senior Vice President and Chief Executive Officer
CFO: Kevin Thompson, Chief Financial Officer
CMO: Allan Bombard, M.D., Chief Medical Officer
CIO: William T. Spooner, Senior Vice President and Chief Information Officer
CHR: Connie Duquette, Director Human Resources
Web address: www.sharp.com
Control: Other not–for–profit (including NFP Corporation) **Service:** Other specialty

Staffed Beds: 169

★ △ **SHARP MEMORIAL HOSPITAL (50100)**, 7901 Frost Street, Zip 92123–2701; tel. 858/939–3400, (Includes SHARP MESA VISTA HOSPITAL, 7850 Vista Hill Avenue, Zip 92123–2717; tel. 858/694–8300; Karenlee Robinson, Chief Operating Officer), (Total facility includes 76 beds in nursing home–type unit) (Nonreporting) **A**1 2 7 9 10 **S** Sharp Healthcare
Primary Contact: Tim Smith, Chief Executive Officer
CFO: Kevin Thompson, Chief Financial Officer
CMO: Richard Santore, M.D., Chief Medical Officer
CIO: William T. Spooner, Senior Vice President and Chief Information Officer
CHR: Diane Delaney, Vice President
Web address: www.sharp.com
Control: Other not–for–profit (including NFP Corporation) **Service:** General Medical and Surgical

Staffed Beds: 488

★ **UNIVERSITY OF CALIFORNIA SAN DIEGO MEDICAL CENTER (50025)**, 200 West Arbor Drive, Zip 92103–8970; tel. 619/543–6222 **A**1 2 3 5 8 9 10 **F**3 6 9 11 12 13 15 16 17 18 20 22 25 26 27 31 32 34 35 38 40 41 43 44 46 47 48 49 50 54 55 56 57 58 59 60 62 63 64 66 68 70 72 73 74 75 76 77 78 79 80 81 82 86 87 88 89 92 93 96 99 100 102 106 107 108 109 111 112 114 116 118 119 120 121 125 127 128 129 130 131 133 134 135 136 137 **P**1 **S** University of California–Systemwide Administration
Primary Contact: Richard Liekweg, Chief Executive Officer
COO: Mona Sonnenshein, Chief Operating Officer
CFO: Robert Hogan, Chief Financial Officer
CMO: Angela Scioscia, M.D., Chief Medical Officer
CIO: Ed Babakanian, Chief Information Officer
CHR: Ann Skinner, Director Human Resources
Web address: www.health.ucsd.edu
Control: State–Government, nonfederal **Service:** General Medical and Surgical

Staffed Beds: 519 **Admissions:** 21694 **Census:** 363 **Outpatient Visits:** 536656 **Births:** 2933 **Total Expense ($000):** 580188 **Payroll Expense ($000):** 225768 **Personnel:** 4306

★ △ **VETERANS AFFAIRS SAN DIEGO HEALTHCARE SYSTEM**, 3350 LaJolla Village Drive, Zip 92161–0002; tel. 858/552–8585, (Nonreporting) **A**1 2 3 5 7 8 **S** Department of Veterans Affairs
Primary Contact: Gary J. Rossio, Director
COO: Cynthia Abair, Associate Director
CFO: Deborah Stiles, Acting Chief Financial Officer
CMO: Jacqueline G. Parthemore, M.D., Chief of Staff
CIO: Debra Dyer, Chief Information Officer
CHR: Stephanie Wright, Director Human Resources Management
Web address: www.sandiego.va.gov
Control: Veterans Affairs, Government, federal **Service:** General Medical and Surgical

Staffed Beds: 238

Hospital, Medicare Provider Number, Address, Telephone, Approval, Facility, and Physician Codes, Health Care System

★ American Hospital Association (AHA) membership
□ The Joint Commission accreditation
○ American Osteopathic Association (AOA) accreditation
△ Commission on Accreditation of Rehabilitation Facilities (CARF) accreditation

SAN DIMAS—Los Angeles County

★ **SAN DIMAS COMMUNITY HOSPITAL (50588)**, 1350 West Covina Boulevard, Zip 91773–3219; tel. 909/599–6811 **A**1 9 10 **F**3 13 15 17 25 26 30 31 32 38 49 55 56 57 58 63 66 68 74 77 79 86 96 97 100 103 107 119 134 135 **S** Prime Healthcare Services
Primary Contact: Dan Bowers, Chief Executive Officer
COO: David Batista, Chief Operating Officer
CFO: Frederick J. Drewette, Chief Financial Officer
CMO: Dinesh Samant, M.D., Chief Medical Staff
CIO: Gerald Martin, Director Information Services
CHR: Tamera Jones, Director Human Resources
Web address: www.sandimashospital.com
Control: Corporation, Investor–owned, for–profit **Service:** General Medical and Surgical

Staffed Beds: 64 **Admissions:** 3893 **Census:** 38 **Outpatient Visits:** 27756 **Births:** 769 **Personnel:** 267

SAN FERNANDO—Los Angeles County

CA

★ △ **PROVIDENCE HOLY CROSS MEDICAL CENTER (50278)**, 15031 Rinaldi Street, Zip 91346–9600; tel. 818/365–8051, (Total facility includes 48 beds in nursing home–type unit) (Nonreporting) **A**1 2 7 9 10 **S** Providence Health & Services
Primary Contact: Kerry Carmody, Chief Executive
CFO: Dave Mast, Chief Financial Officer
CMO: Bernard Klein, M.D., Chief Medical Officer
CIO: Mark Garett, Regional Chief Information Officer
CHR: Cindra Syverson, Regional Chief Human Resources Officer
Web address: www.providence.org/losangeles/facilities/providence_holy_cross/
Control: Church–operated, Nongovernment, not–for profit **Service:** General Medical and Surgical

Staffed Beds: 254

SAN FRANCISCO—San Francisco County

★ △ **CALIFORNIA PACIFIC MEDICAL CENTER (50047)**, 2333 Buchanan Street, Zip 94115–1925, Mailing Address: P.O. Box 7999, Zip 94120–7999; tel. 415/563–4321, (Includes CALIFORNIA PACIFIC MEDICAL CENTER–DAVIES CAMPUS, Castro and Duboce Streets, Zip 94114; tel. 415/565–6000) **A**1 2 3 5 7 8 9 10 **F**2 6 8 12 13 15 17 18 19 20 21 22 23 24 25 26 27 28 30 31 32 33 34 36 37 38 42 43 44 46 51 54 56 57 59 60 63 66 68 70 71 72 74 75 76 79 80 81 82 83 84 85 86 87 88 91 92 93 94 96 97 99 100 102 103 106 107 109 113 114 116 117 119 121 122 124 126 127 128 130 132 133 134 135 136 137 **S** Sutter Health
Primary Contact: Martin Brotman, M.D., President and Chief Executive Officer
CFO: Michael P. Holdsworth, Vice President Finance and Chief Financial Officer
CMO: Morris Flaum, M.D., Vice President Medical Affairs
CIO: Jerry Padavano, Chief Information Officer
Web address: www.cpmc.org
Control: Other not–for–profit (including NFP Corporation) **Service:** General Medical and Surgical

Staffed Beds: 798 **Admissions:** 28700 **Census:** 483 **Outpatient Visits:** 729035 **Total Expense ($000):** 845127 **Payroll Expense ($000):** 326504 **Personnel:** 6597

★ **CHINESE HOSPITAL (50407)**, 845 Jackson Street, Zip 94133–4899; tel. 415/982–2400 **A**1 9 10 **F**3 8 11 15 25 26 27 30 31 33 38 47 49 50 55 56 57 59 62 63 68 73 75 76 77 79 81 82 87 96 97 99 106 107 119 121 124 134 135 136 **P**5
Primary Contact: Brenda Yee, RN, M.S.N., Chief Executive Officer
CFO: Thomas Bolger, Chief Financial Officer
CMO: Joseph Woo, M.D., Chief of Staff
CIO: Helen Lee, Manager Information Systems
CHR: Karen Chow, Director Human Resources
Web address: www.chinesehospital–sf.org
Control: Other not–for–profit (including NFP Corporation) **Service:** General Medical and Surgical

Staffed Beds: 54 **Admissions:** 2400 **Census:** 35 **Outpatient Visits:** 68531 **Births:** 0 **Total Expense ($000):** 72258 **Payroll Expense ($000):** 19500 **Personnel:** 291

★ **KAISER FOUNDATION HOSPITAL (50076)**, 2200 O'Farrell Street, Zip 94115–3358; tel. 415/833–2000, (Nonreporting) **A**1 3 5 10 **S** Kaiser Foundation Hospitals
Primary Contact: Christine Robisch, Senior Vice President and Service Area Manager
CFO: Jim Phillips, Business Strategy and Finance Leader
CMO: Bruce Blumberg, M.D., Physician in Chief
CIO: Beverly Seyfert, Information Technology Leader
CHR: Michael H. Sweet, Human Resources Business Partner
Web address: www.kaiserpermanente.org
Control: Other not–for–profit (including NFP Corporation) **Service:** General Medical and Surgical

Staffed Beds: 264

★ **LAGUNA HONDA HOSPITAL AND REHABILITATION CENTER (50668)**, 375 Laguna Honda Boulevard, Zip 94116–1499; tel. 415/759–2300, (Total facility includes 1030 beds in nursing home–type unit) (Nonreporting) **A**10
Primary Contact: John Kanaley, Chief Executive Officer
COO: Robert Christmas, Chief Operating Officer
CFO: Nancy Arata, Chief Financial Officer
CIO: Pat Skala, Chief Information Officer
Web address: www.dph.sf.ca.us/chn/lagunahondahosp/rehabilitation.shtml
Control: City–County, Government, nonfederal **Service:** Other specialty

Staffed Beds: 1065

★ △ **SAINT FRANCIS MEMORIAL HOSPITAL (50152)**, 900 Hyde Street, Zip 94109–4899, Mailing Address: P.O. Box 7726, Zip 94120–7726; tel. 415/353–6000, (Nonreporting) **A**1 2 7 9 10 **S** Catholic Healthcare West
Primary Contact: Thomas G. Hennessy, President
COO: James Jackson, Chief Operating Officer
CFO: Alan Fox, Chief Financial Officer
CHR: Richard Mead, Senior Director Human Resources
Web address: www.saintfrancismemorial.org
Control: Other not–for–profit (including NFP Corporation) **Service:** General Medical and Surgical

Staffed Beds: 210

★ **SAN FRANCISCO GENERAL HOSPITAL MEDICAL CENTER (50228)**, 1001 Potrero Avenue, Zip 94110–3594; tel. 415/206–8000 **A**1 2 3 5 8 10 **F**2 3 13 15 17 18 20 25 26 31 33 34 36 37 38 40 41 43 46 47 48 49 50 55 56 57 58 59 60 62 63 66 68 69 70 72 73 74 75 76 77 79 81 82 84 86 87 88 89 90 92 95 96 97 99 100 107 117 118 119 120 121 124 133 135 136 137
Primary Contact: Gene Marie O'Connell, Executive Administrator
COO: Sue Currin, Chief Nursing Officer
CFO: Valerie Inouye, Chief Financial Officer
CMO: John Luce, M.D., Chief Medical Officer
CIO: Robert Brody, M.D., Chief Information Officer
Web address: www.dph.sf.ca.us/chn/SFGH/sfghmenu.htm
Control: City–County, Government, nonfederal **Service:** General Medical and Surgical

Staffed Beds: 521 **Admissions:** 15734 **Census:** 401 **Outpatient Visits:** 506150 **Births:** 1249 **Total Expense ($000):** 519522 **Payroll Expense ($000):** 234128 **Personnel:** 4297

★ **ST. LUKE'S HOSPITAL (50055)**, 3555 Cesar Chavez Street, Zip 94110–4490; tel. 415/647–8600 **A**1 5 9 10 **F**3 11 12 13 15 17 18 22 25 26 27 30 31 32 33 34 38 43 44 55 56 57 63 68 71 74 75 76 77 79 80 83 86 94 95 96 100 107 117 119 121 135 136 **S** Sutter Health
Primary Contact: Martin Brotman, M.D., President and Chief Executive Officer
CMO: Jerome Franz, M.D., Chief Medical Staff
CIO: Rob Seide, Manager Marketing and Communications
CHR: Linda Isaacs, Vice President Human Resources
Web address: www.stlukes–sf.org
Control: Other not–for–profit (including NFP Corporation) **Service:** General Medical and Surgical

Staffed Beds: 229 **Admissions:** 4968 **Census:** 130 **Outpatient Visits:** 24167 **Total Expense ($000):** 123119 **Payroll Expense ($000):** 47833 **Personnel:** 261

★ **ST. MARY'S MEDICAL CENTER (50457)**, 450 Stanyan Street, Zip 94117–1079; tel. 415/668–1000, (Total facility includes 32 beds in nursing home–type unit) **A**1 3 5 9 10 **F**2 3 11 12 15 17 18 20 22 24 25 26 27 30 31 32 33 38 42 43 44 48 49 52 53 54 55 56 57 58 59 60 62 63 64 66 68 69 72 73 75 76 77 79 82 85 86 87 88 89 90 91 92 93 94 95 96 97 100 103 107 117 119 120 121 123 124 132 135 136 137 **S** Catholic Healthcare West
Primary Contact: Anna Cheung, Interim President
CFO: Eric Brettner, Interim Vice President and Chief Financial Officer
CMO: Richard Podolin, M.D., Chief Medical Staff
CHR: Phill Moss, Vice President Human Resources
Web address: www.stmarysmedicalcenter.com
Control: Other not–for–profit (including NFP Corporation) **Service:** General Medical and Surgical

Staffed Beds: 232 **Admissions:** 6955 **Census:** 115 **Outpatient Visits:** 93116 **Births:** 0 **Total Expense ($000):** 168924 **Payroll Expense ($000):** 80536 **Personnel:** 883

★ **UCSF MEDICAL CENTER (50454)**, 500 Parnassus Avenue, Zip 94143–0296, Mailing Address: 500 Parnassus Avenue, Box 0296, Zip 94143–0296; tel. 415/476–1000 **A**1 2 3 5 8 9 10 **F**3 6 7 8 9 11 12 13 14 15 17 18 19 20 21 22 23 25 26 27 28 31 33 34 35 37 38 43 44 45 46 47 48 49 50 51 52 53 54 55 56 57 58 59 60 61 62 63 64 66 68 70 72 73 74 75 76 77 79 80 81 82 83 84 86 87 90 92 96 97 98 99 100 101 102 103 104 105 106 107 108 109 111 112 113 114 116 118 119 120 121 123 124 125 126 127 128 129 130 131 132 133 134 135 136 137 **P**6 **S** University of California–Systemwide Administration
Primary Contact: Mark R. Laret, Chief Executive Officer
COO: Tomi S. Ryba, Chief Operating Officer
CFO: Ken M. Jones, Chief Financial Officer
CMO: Ernest Ring, M.D., Chief Medical Officer
CIO: Larry Lotenero, Chief Information Officer
CHR: David Odato, Executive Director Patient and Staff Services
Web address: www.ucsfhealth.org
Control: Other not–for–profit (including NFP Corporation) **Service:** General Medical and Surgical

Staffed Beds: 642 **Admissions:** 27847 **Census:** 489 **Outpatient Visits:** 746808 **Births:** 1901 **Total Expense ($000):** 1283918 **Payroll Expense ($000):** 516897 **Personnel:** 6063

★ **VETERANS AFFAIRS MEDICAL CENTER**, 4150 Clement Street, Zip 94121–1598; tel. 415/221–4810, (Total facility includes 112 beds in nursing home–type unit) (Nonreporting) **A**1 2 3 5 **S** Department of Veterans Affairs
Primary Contact: Sheila M. Cullen, Director
CFO: Del Lewis, Chief Fiscal Services
CIO: Roy Chaney, Chief Information Management Service
CHR: Marie Boland, Chief Human Resource Management Service
Web address: www.va.gov/sta/guide/home.asp
Control: Veterans Affairs, Government, federal **Service:** General Medical and Surgical

Staffed Beds: 244

SAN GABRIEL—Los Angeles County

★ **SAN GABRIEL VALLEY MEDICAL CENTER (50132)**, 438 West Las Tunas Drive, Zip 91776–1216, Mailing Address: P.O. Box 1507, Zip 91778–1507; tel. 626/289–5454, (Total facility includes 41 beds in nursing home–type unit) (Nonreporting) **A**1 9 10 **S** AHMC, Inc
Primary Contact: Makoto Nakayama, Chief Executive Officer
CFO: Daniel Song, Chief Financial Officer
CIO: Bernie Sauer, Director Information Technology
CHR: Edwin Dewees, Director Human Resources
Web address: www.sgvmc.org
Control: Other not–for–profit (including NFP Corporation) **Service:** General Medical and Surgical

Staffed Beds: 231

SAN JOSE—Santa Clara County

★ **GOOD SAMARITAN HOSPITAL (50380)**, 2425 Samaritan Drive, Zip 95124–3997, Mailing Address: P.O. Box 240002, Zip 95154–2402; tel. 408/559–2011 **A**1 2 9 10 **F**3 5 8 11 12 13 15 17 18 20 22 24 25 26 27 30 32 33 35 36 37 38 42 43 44 46 47 48 49 53 55 56 57 58 59 62 66 68 70 72 73 74 75 76 77 79 80 81 82 84 85 86 88 91 92 94 95 96 97 100 102 103 104 105 106 107 108 109 111 112 116 119 121 124 135 **S** HCA
Primary Contact: William K. Piche, Chief Executive Officer
COO: Paul Beaupre, M.D., Chief Operating Officer and Chief Medical Officer
CFO: Darrel Neuenschwander, Chief Financial Officer
CMO: Stephen Jackson, M.D., Chief of Staff
CIO: Ravi Ramaswamy, Director Information Services
CHR: Carolyn DeLeon, Vice President Human Resources
Web address: www.goodsamsanjose.com
Control: Corporation, Investor–owned, for–profit **Service:** General Medical and Surgical

Staffed Beds: 328 **Admissions:** 18235 **Census:** 233 **Outpatient Visits:** 134407 **Births:** 3629 **Total Expense ($000):** 304110 **Payroll Expense ($000):** 137327 **Personnel:** 1092

★ **KAISER FOUNDATION HOSPITAL – SAN JOSE MEDICAL CENTER (50604)**, (Formerly Kaiser Foundation Hospital – Santa Teresa), 250 Hospital Parkway, Zip 95119–1199; tel. 408/972–7000, (Nonreporting) **A**1 10 **S** Kaiser Foundation Hospitals
Primary Contact: Terry L. Austen, Senior Vice President and Area Manager
COO: Terry L. Austen, Senior Vice President and Area Manager
CFO: Colin Tran, Interim Area Finance Officer
CMO: Raj Bhandari, M.D., Physician–in–Chief
CIO: Ernie Japec, Area Director Technology
CHR: Susan Franzella, Human Resource Business Partner
Web address: www.kaiserpermanente.org
Control: Other not–for–profit (including NFP Corporation) **Service:** General Medical and Surgical

Staffed Beds: 228

★ **O'CONNOR HOSPITAL (50153)**, 2105 Forest Avenue, Zip 95128–1471; tel. 408/947–2500, (Total facility includes 24 beds in nursing home–type unit) **A**1 2 9 10 **F**68 70 74 84 117 **S** Daughters of Charity Health System
Primary Contact: Robert H. Curry, President and Chief Executive Officer
COO: Ronald J. Galonsky, Chief Operating Officer
CFO: Bonnie Liang, Chief Financial Officer
CMO: George Block, M.D., Chief Medical Officer
CIO: Richard Hutsell, Vice President and Chief Information Officer
CHR: Julie Hatcher, Vice President Human Resources
Web address: www.oconnorhospital.org
Control: Church–operated, Nongovernment, not–for profit **Service:** General Medical and Surgical

Staffed Beds: 248 **Admissions:** 16299 **Census:** 179 **Outpatient Visits:** 132185 **Births:** 3763

★ **REGIONAL MEDICAL CENTER OF SAN JOSE (50125)**, 225 North Jackson Avenue, Zip 95116–1691; tel. 408/259–5000, (Nonreporting) **A**9 10 **S** HCA
Primary Contact: William L. Gilbert, Chief Executive Officer
COO: Brian J. Knecht, Chief Operating Officer
CFO: Raju Iyer, Chief Financial Officer
CMO: William Scott, M.D., Vice President Medical Affairs
CIO: Shirley Joyal, Director Information Systems
CHR: Nancy Clark, Vice President Human Resources
Web address: www.regionalmedicalsanjose.com
Control: Partnership, Investor–owned, for–profit **Service:** General Medical and Surgical

Staffed Beds: 184

□ △ **SANTA CLARA VALLEY MEDICAL CENTER (50038)**, 751 South Bascom Avenue, Zip 95128–2604; tel. 408/885–5000, (Nonreporting) **A**1 3 5 7 9 10
Primary Contact: Michael J. Skehan, Director
CFO: Nancy Kaatz, Chief Financial Officer
CMO: Alfonso Banuelos, M.D., Chief Medical Officer
CIO: Dennis Kotecki, Chief Information Officer
CHR: David Manson, Manager Human Resources
Web address: www.scvmed.org
Control: County–Government, nonfederal **Service:** General Medical and Surgical

Staffed Beds: 574

SAN LEANDRO—Alameda County

□ **ALAMEDA COUNTY MEDICAL CENTER–FAIRMONT CAMPUS**, 15400 Foothill Boulevard, Zip 94578–1009; tel. 510/895–4200, (Total facility includes 113 beds in nursing home–type unit) (Nonreporting) **A**1 **S** Alameda Medical Center
Primary Contact: Wright L. Lassiter, III, Chief Executive Officer
COO: Bill Manns, Chief Operating Officer
CFO: Geoff Daugherty, Chief Financial Officer
CMO: David Altman, M.D., Chief Medical Officer
CIO: Ed Dullard, Chief Information Officer
CHR: Jeanette Louden Corbett, Chief Human Resources Officer
Web address: www.acmedctr.org
Control: County–Government, nonfederal **Service:** General Medical and Surgical

Staffed Beds: 399

★ **KINDRED HOSPITAL–SAN FRANCISCO BAY AREA (52034)**, 2800 Benedict Drive, Zip 94577–6840; tel. 510/357–8300, (Nonreporting) **A**1 9 10 **S** Kindred Healthcare
Primary Contact: Michael P. Lawson, FACHE, Chief Executive Officer
COO: Mary Schwind, R.N., MS, Chief Clinical Officer
CFO: Ziba Aflak, Chief Financial Officer
CMO: Aamir Faruqui, M.D., Medical Director
CHR: Linda Scharber, Coordinator Human Resources
Web address: www.kindredhospitalsfba.com
Control: Corporation, Investor–owned, for–profit **Service:** Long–Term Acute Care hospital

Staffed Beds: 80

SAN LUIS OBISPO—San Luis Obispo County

CALIFORNIA MENS COLONY HOSPITAL, Highway 1, Zip 93409–8101, Mailing Address: P.O. Box 8101, Zip 93409–8101; tel. 805/547–7913, (Nonreporting)
Primary Contact: Galen Kirn, Administrator
CFO: William Cook, Associate Warden Business Service
CIO: Terry Knight, Public Information Officer and Administrative Assistant
Web address: www.yaca.ca.gov/visitors/fac_prison_cmc.html
Control: State–Government, nonfederal **Service:** Hospital unit of an institution (prison hospital, college infimary, etc.)

Staffed Beds: 39

Hospital, Medicare Provider Number, Address, Telephone, Approval, Facility, and Physician Codes, Health Care System
★ American Hospital Association (AHA) membership
□ The Joint Commission accreditation
○ American Osteopathic Association (AOA) accreditation
△ Commission on Accreditation of Rehabilitation Facilities (CARF) accreditation

▣ **FRENCH HOSPITAL MEDICAL CENTER (50232)**, 1911 Johnson Avenue, Zip 93401–4131; tel. 805/543–5353 **A**1 9 10 **F**11 15 18 20 22 24 25 26 30 31 32 33 38 44 45 50 55 56 57 62 66 68 73 74 75 76 79 82 84 86 88 96 97 100 102 107 112 119 121 135 136 **S** Catholic Healthcare West
Primary Contact: Alan Iftiniuk, President
CFO: Sue Andersen, Chief Financial Officer
CMO: Paul Christensen, M.D., Chief of Staff
CIO: Cyndi Lang, Director Information Services
CHR: Adrienne Tuttle, Manager Human Resources
Web address: www.frenchmedicalcenter.org
Control: Other not–for–profit (including NFP Corporation) **Service:** General Medical and Surgical

Staffed Beds: 112 **Admissions:** 4335 **Census:** 42 **Outpatient Visits:** 110010 **Births:** 814 **Total Expense ($000):** 61648 **Payroll Expense ($000):** 26100 **Personnel:** 377

▣ **SIERRA VISTA REGIONAL MEDICAL CENTER (50506)**, 1010 Murray Street, Zip 93405–8800, Mailing Address: P.O. Box 1367, Zip 93406–1367; tel. 805/546–7600 **A**1 9 10 19 **F**1 3 4 11 13 15 16 17 18 20 22 25 27 31 32 33 37 38 44 45 46 50 55 56 62 65 68 70 71 72 73 74 75 76 77 78 79 80 81 83 84 85 88 96 102 103 107 117 119 120 121 134 135 136 137 **S** TENET Healthcare Corporation
Primary Contact: Candace L. Markwith, Chief Executive Officer
COO: Joseph DeSchryver, Chief Operating Officer
CFO: Richard Phillips, Chief Financial Officer
CIO: Robert Leonard, Director Information Services
CHR: Betty Baker, Director Human Resources
Web address: www.sierravistaregional.com
Control: Corporation, Investor–owned, for–profit **Service:** General Medical and Surgical

Staffed Beds: 165 **Admissions:** 6487 **Census:** 86 **Outpatient Visits:** 78182 **Births:** 1319 **Personnel:** 564

SAN MATEO—San Mateo County

MILLS HOSPITAL See Mills–Peninsula Health Services, Burlingame

☐ **SAN MATEO MEDICAL CENTER (50113)**, 222 West 39th Avenue, Zip 94403–4398; tel. 650/573–2222, (Total facility includes 260 beds in nursing home–type unit) (Nonreporting) **A**1 3 5 9 10
Primary Contact: Sang–ick Chang, M.D., M.P.H., Chief Executive Officer
CFO: David Spitler, Chief Financial Officer
CMO: Susan Ehrlich, M.D., Vice President and Medical Director Ambulatory and Medical Services
CIO: Michael Araton, M.D., Chief Information Officer
CHR: Heather Ruiz, Manager Human Resources
Web address: www.sanmateomedicalcenter.org
Control: City–County, Government, nonfederal **Service:** General Medical and Surgical

Staffed Beds: 367

SAN PABLO—Contra Costa County

▣ **DOCTORS MEDICAL CENTER–SAN PABLO CAMPUS (50079)**, 2000 Vale Road, Zip 94806–3808; tel. 510/970–5000, (Nonreporting) **A**1 2 9 10
Primary Contact: Joseph A. Stewart, Chief Executive Officer
CFO: Dev Mahadevan, Chief Financial Officer
CMO: John Rampulla, M.D., President Medical Staff
CIO: Viki Lampert, Director Information Systems and Data Center
CHR: Melissa Ridlon, Vice President Human Resources
Web address: www.doctorsmedicalcenter.org
Control: Hospital district or authority, Government, nonfederal **Service:** General Medical and Surgical

Staffed Beds: 131

SAN PEDRO—Los Angeles County, See Los Angeles

SAN RAFAEL—Marin County

▣ **KAISER FOUNDATION HOSPITAL (50510)**, 99 Montecillo Road, Zip 94903–3308; tel. 415/444–2000, (Nonreporting) **A**1 10 **S** Kaiser Foundation Hospitals
Primary Contact: Judy Coffey, Senior Vice President and Service Area Manager
COO: Jill Magri, Chief Operating Officer
CFO: Connie Giuliano, Area Financial Officer
CIO: Stanley Dobrawa, Director Information Technology
CHR: Rudy Collins, Human Resources Business Partner
Web address: www.kaiserpermanente.org
Control: Other not–for–profit (including NFP Corporation) **Service:** General Medical and Surgical

Staffed Beds: 107

★ **KENTFIELD REHABILITATION AND SPECIALTY HOSPITAL (52043)**, 1125 Sir Francis Drake Boulevard, Zip 94904–1455; tel. 415/456–9680, (Nonreporting) **A**9 10 **S** Vibra Healthcare
Primary Contact: Ann Gors, Chief Executive Officer
CFO: Kraig Couture, Chief Financial Officer
CMO: Curtis Roebken, M.D., Chief Medical Staff
CHR: Helen Herman, Director Human Resources
Web address: www.kentfieldrehab.com
Control: Corporation, Investor–owned, for–profit **Service:** Rehabilitation

Staffed Beds: 60

SAN RAMON—Contra Costa County

▣ **SAN RAMON REGIONAL MEDICAL CENTER (50689)**, 6001 Norris Canyon Road, Zip 94583–5400; tel. 925/275–9200, (Nonreporting) **A**1 9 10 **S** TENET Healthcare Corporation
Primary Contact: Gary Sloan, Chief Executive Officer
COO: Susan C. Micheletti, Chief Operating Officer
CFO: Beenu Chadha, Chief Financial Officer
CMO: Paul Wotowic, M.D., Chief of Staff
CIO: Jonathan Eakin, Director Information Systems
CHR: Dennis Mills, Director Human Resources
Web address: www.sanramonmedctr.com
Control: Corporation, Investor–owned, for–profit **Service:** General Medical and Surgical

Staffed Beds: 123

SANTA ANA—Orange County

☐ **COASTAL COMMUNITIES HOSPITAL (50747)**, 2701 South Bristol Street, Zip 92704–6201; tel. 714/754–5454, (Nonreporting) **A**1 9 10 **S** Integrated Healthcare
Primary Contact: Craig G. Myers, Chief Executive Officer
CFO: Patricia Henry, Chief Financial Officer
CHR: Margaret Ettenheim, Director Human Resources
Web address: www.coastalcommhospital.com
Control: Corporation, Investor–owned, for–profit **Service:** General Medical and Surgical

Staffed Beds: 178

☐ **KINDRED HOSPITAL SANTA ANA**, 1901 North College Avenue, Zip 92706–2334; tel. 714/564–7800, (Nonreporting) **A**1 9 **S** Kindred Healthcare
Primary Contact: Diana C. Hanyak, Administrator
COO: Gem Lindsay, Chief Clinical Officer
CFO: Nancy V. Wilson, Chief Financial Officer
CHR: Becca Steinhoff, Director Human Resources
Web address: www.kindredhealthcare.com
Control: Corporation, Investor–owned, for–profit **Service:** Long–Term Acute Care hospital

Staffed Beds: 54

☐ **WESTERN MEDICAL CENTER–SANTA ANA (50746)**, 1001 North Tustin Avenue, Zip 92705–3577; tel. 714/835–3555, (Nonreporting) **A**1 3 5 9 10 **S** Integrated Healthcare
Primary Contact: Daniel Brothman, Chief Executive Officer
COO: S. Sean Fowler, Chief Operating Officer
CFO: Kathy Hammack, Chief Financial Officer
CMO: Brian Cross, M.D., Chief of Staff
CIO: Nova Stewart, Chief Information Officer
CHR: Gwen Chambers, Director Human Resources
Web address: www.westernmedicalcenter.com
Control: Corporation, Investor–owned, for–profit **Service:** General Medical and Surgical

Staffed Beds: 287

SANTA BARBARA—Santa Barbara County

COTTAGE REHABILITATION HOSPITAL See Santa Barbara Cottage Hospital

▣ **GOLETA VALLEY COTTAGE HOSPITAL (50357)**, 351 South Patterson Avenue, Zip 93111–2496, Mailing Address: Box 6306, Zip 93160–6306; tel. 805/967–3411, (Total facility includes 55 beds in nursing home–type unit) (Nonreporting) **A**1 9 10 **S** Cottage Health System
Primary Contact: Ronald C. Werft, President and Chief Executive Officer
Web address: www.sbch.org
Control: Other not–for–profit (including NFP Corporation) **Service:** General Medical and Surgical

Staffed Beds: 177

REHABILITATION INSTITUTE AT SANTA BARBARA See Santa Barbara Cottage Hospital

★ △ **SANTA BARBARA COTTAGE HOSPITAL (50396)**, Pueblo at Bath Streets, Zip 93105–4390, Mailing Address: P.O. Box 689, Zip 93102–0689; tel. 805/682–7111, (Includes COTTAGE REHABILITATION HOSPITAL, 2415 De la Vina Street, Zip 93105–3819; tel. 805/687–7444; Melinda Staveley, President and Chief Executive Officer) **A**1 2 3 5 7 9 10 **F**3 4 5 11 12 13 15 17 18 20 22 24 25 26 27 31 32 33 38 40 43 44 52 53 55 56 57 59 62 66 68 70 72 73 74 76 77 79 81 82 83 84 85 86 88 90 92 93 94 96 100 102 103 107 116 119 121 124 135 137 **S** Cottage Health System
Primary Contact: Ronald C. Werft, President and Chief Executive Officer
COO: Steven A. Fellows, Executive Vice President and Chief Operating Officer
CFO: Joan Bricher, Senior Vice President Finance and Chief Financial Officer
CMO: Robert E. Reid, M.D., Director Medical Affairs
CIO: Alberto Kywi, Chief Information Officer
CHR: Patrice Ryan, Vice President Human Resources
Web address: www.cottagehealthsystem.org
Control: Other not–for–profit (including NFP Corporation) **Service:** General Medical and Surgical

Staffed Beds: 353 **Admissions:** 18966 **Census:** 216 **Outpatient Visits:** 119722 **Births:** 2501 **Total Expense ($000):** 292349 **Payroll Expense ($000):** 119187 **Personnel:** 2223

SANTA CLARA—Santa Clara County

★ **KAISER FOUNDATION HOSPITAL (50071)**, 700 Lawrence Expressway, Zip 75051–5173; tel. 408/236–6400, (Nonreporting) **A**1 3 5 10 **S** Kaiser Foundation Hospitals
Primary Contact: Mary Ann Barnes, Vice President and Service Area Manager
COO: Susan G. Murphy, Chief Operating Officer
CFO: Jerry L. Yu, Area Finance Officer
CMO: Bernadette Loftus, M.D., Physician–in–Chief
CIO: Theodore Persinger, Director Area Technology
CHR: Steve Bartz, Business Partner Human Resources
Web address: www.kaiserpermanente.org
Control: Other not–for–profit (including NFP Corporation) **Service:** General Medical and Surgical

Staffed Beds: 286

SANTA CRUZ—Santa Cruz County

★ **DOMINICAN HOSPITAL (50242)**, 1555 Soquel Drive, Zip 95065–1794; tel. 831/462–7700, (Nonreporting) **A**1 9 10 **S** Catholic Healthcare West
Primary Contact: Nanette Mickiewicz, M.D., President and Chief Medical Officer
COO: Chris Wernke, Chief Operating Officer
CFO: Rick Harron, Chief Financial Officer
CMO: Nanette Mickiewicz, M.D., President and Chief Medical Officer
CIO: Lee Vanderpool, Vice President
CHR: Vicki Miranda, Vice President Human Resources
Web address: www.dominicanhospital.org
Control: Church–operated, Nongovernment, not–for profit **Service:** General Medical and Surgical

Staffed Beds: 281

★ **SUTTER MATERNITY AND SURGERY CENTER OF SANTA CRUZ (50714)**, 2900 Chanticleer Avenue, Zip 95065–1816; tel. 831/477–2200, (Nonreporting) **A**1 9 10 **S** Sutter Health
Primary Contact: Richard Nichols, Administrator
CFO: Sharon Kutis, Chief Financial Officer
CMO: Steven Roberts, M.D., Chief of Staff
CHR: Al Nocella, Vice President Human Resources
Web address: www.suttermatsurg.org
Control: Other not–for–profit (including NFP Corporation) **Service:** Obstetrics and gynecology

Staffed Beds: 28

SANTA MARIA—Santa Barbara County

★ **MARIAN MEDICAL CENTER (50107)**, 1400 East Church Street, Zip 93454–5906; tel. 805/739–3000, (Total facility includes 95 beds in nursing home–type unit) **A**1 9 10 **F**3 8 11 13 15 17 18 20 22 24 25 26 27 30 31 32 33 34 37 38 42 43 44 45 46 49 50 52 53 54 55 56 57 59 61 62 64 66 72 73 74 75 76 77 79 80 81 82 84 86 87 90 96 97 99 100 102 106 107 116 117 119 121 123 132 133 135 136 137 **S** Catholic Healthcare West
Primary Contact: Charles J. Cova, President
CFO: Sue Andersen, Chief Financial Officer
CMO: Chuck Merrill, M.D., Vice President Medical Affairs
CIO: Patricia Haase, Director Information Technology and Communications
CHR: Mary Michael, Vice President Human Resources
Web address: www.marianmedicalcenter.org
Control: Church–operated, Nongovernment, not–for profit **Service:** General Medical and Surgical

Staffed Beds: 262 **Admissions:** 11244 **Census:** 187 **Outpatient Visits:** 166107 **Births:** 3067 **Total Expense ($000):** 151628 **Payroll Expense ($000):** 71186 **Personnel:** 1101

SANTA MONICA—Los Angeles County

★ **SAINT JOHN'S HEALTH CENTER (50290)**, 1328 Twenty Second Street, Zip 90404–2091; tel. 310/829–5511, (Nonreporting) **A**1 2 9 10 **S** Sisters of Charity of Leavenworth Health System
Primary Contact: Lourdes Lazatin, President and Chief Executive Officer
COO: Eleanor Ramirez, R.N., Chief Operating Officer
CFO: Michelle Mok, Interim Chief Financial Officer
CMO: Charles Pietrafesa, M.D., Executive Medical Director
CIO: Karen Oi, Chief Information Officer
CHR: Stephen Sharrer, Vice President
Web address: www.stjohns.org
Control: Church–operated, Nongovernment, not–for profit **Service:** General Medical and Surgical

Staffed Beds: 228

★ **SANTA MONICA–UCLA MEDICAL CENTER AND ORTHOPAEDIC HOSPITAL (50112)**, 1250 16th Street, Zip 90404; tel. 310/319–4000 **A**1 3 5 9 10 **F**3 11 12 13 15 18 20 22 25 26 27 31 32 33 38 43 44 54 55 57 58 62 63 66 68 70 72 73 74 76 77 79 80 82 84 86 92 96 97 99 100 102 103 106 107 113 114 118 119 120 134 135 136 **P**6 **S** University of California–Systemwide Administration
Primary Contact: Posie Carpenter, RN, M.S.N., Chief Administrative Officer
COO: Posie Carpenter, R.N., MSN, Chief Administrative Officer
CFO: Paul Staton, Chief Financial Officer
CMO: Michael Herbst, M.D., Medical Director
CIO: Mitchell Creem, Associate Vice Chancellor and Chief Financial Officer
CHR: Mark Speare, Senior Associate Director Patient Relations and Human Resources
Web address: www.healthcare.ucla.edu
Control: State–Government, nonfederal **Service:** General Medical and Surgical

Staffed Beds: 236 **Admissions:** 11052 **Census:** 156 **Outpatient Visits:** 114455 **Births:** 1370 **Total Expense ($000):** 175810 **Payroll Expense ($000):** 81680 **Personnel:** 1115

SANTA ROSA—Sonoma County

★ **KAISER FOUNDATION HOSPITAL (50690)**, 401 Bicentennial Way, Zip 95403–2192; tel. 707/571–4000 **A**1 10 **F**3 25 26 27 28 30 31 32 33 38 43 44 50 52 53 54 55 56 57 60 61 62 63 66 68 69 70 72 73 74 75 76 77 79 80 81 82 84 86 87 89 90 91 92 94 96 97 99 100 107 113 114 118 119 120 121 123 124 132 133 135 136 137 **S** Kaiser Foundation Hospitals
Primary Contact: Judy Coffey, Senior Vice President and Service Area Manager
COO: Susan Janvrin, R.N., Chief Operating Officer
CFO: Connie Giuliano, Area Financial Officer
CMO: Robert Schultz, M.D., Physician–in–Chief
CIO: Stanley Dobrawa, Director Information Technology
CHR: Rudy Collins, Human Resources Business Partner
Web address: www.kaiserpermanente.org
Control: Other not–for–profit (including NFP Corporation) **Service:** General Medical and Surgical

Staffed Beds: 117 **Admissions:** 8406 **Census:** 850 **Outpatient Visits:** 34397 **Births:** 1816

★ **SANTA ROSA MEMORIAL HOSPITAL (50174)**, 1165 Montgomery Drive, Zip 95405–4897, Mailing Address: P.O. Box 522, Zip 95402–0522; tel. 707/546–3210 **A**1 2 9 10 **F**1 3 8 11 13 15 18 19 20 22 25 26 27 28 30 31 32 33 37 38 40 42 43 44 45 46 53 54 55 57 59 62 68 69 70 72 73 74 75 76 77 79 81 84 86 87 88 92 93 94 95 96 97 100 102 106 107 117 120 121 132 133 135 137 **S** St. Joseph Health System
Primary Contact: George Perez, President and Chief Executive Officer
COO: Michael Glasberg, Chief Operating Officer
CFO: Mich Riccioni, Chief Financial Officer
CMO: Gary Greensweig, D.O., Chief Medical Officer
CIO: Patrick Wylie, Director Information Systems
CHR: Carol Aaron, Senior Vice President Human Resources
Web address: www.stjosephhealth.org
Control: Other not–for–profit (including NFP Corporation) **Service:** General Medical and Surgical

Staffed Beds: 337 **Admissions:** 15493 **Census:** 218 **Outpatient Visits:** 186845 **Births:** 1271 **Total Expense ($000):** 304412 **Payroll Expense ($000):** 131390 **Personnel:** 1846

CA

Hospital, Medicare Provider Number, Address, Telephone, Approval, Facility, and Physician Codes, Health Care System
★ American Hospital Association (AHA) membership
□ The Joint Commission accreditation
○ American Osteopathic Association (AOA) accreditation
△ Commission on Accreditation of Rehabilitation Facilities (CARF) accreditation

☒ **SUTTER MEDICAL CENTER OF SANTA ROSA, CHANATE CAMPUS (50291)**, 3325 Chanate Road, Zip 95404–1707; tel. 707/576–4000, (Includes WARRACK CAMPUS, 2449 Summerfield Road, Zip 95405–7815; tel. 707/576–4200), (Total facility includes 10 beds in nursing home–type unit) (Nonreporting) **A**1 3 5 9 10 **S** Sutter Health
Primary Contact: Michael J. Cohill, Chief Executive Officer
COO: F. Dana Ellerbe, Assistant Administrator
CFO: Avery Schlesenberg, Chief Financial Officer
CMO: Robert Heckey, M.D., Chief of Staff
CHR: Steve Morales, Director Human Resources
Web address: www.sutterhealth.org
Control: Other not–for–profit (including NFP Corporation) **Service:** General Medical and Surgical

Staffed Beds: 143

SEBASTOPOL—Sonoma County

○ **PALM DRIVE HOSPITAL (50385)**, 501 Petaluma Avenue, Zip 95472–4281; tel. 707/823–8511, (Total facility includes 10 beds in nursing home–type unit) (Nonreporting) **A**9 10 11
Primary Contact: James T. Sato, Chief Executive Officer
CFO: David M. Semple, Chief Financial Officer
CMO: Terri L. Turner, D.O., Chief of Staff
CHR: Julane Gonnella, Chief Human Resources Officer
Web address: www.palmdrivehospital.com
Control: Other not–for–profit (including NFP Corporation) **Service:** General Medical and Surgical

Staffed Beds: 49

SELMA—Fresno County

☒ **SELMA COMMUNITY HOSPITAL (50470)**, 1141 Rose Avenue, Zip 93662–3241; tel. 559/891–1000, (Total facility includes 14 beds in nursing home–type unit) (Nonreporting) **A**1 10 **S** Adventist Health
Primary Contact: Richard L. Rawson, President and Chief Executive Officer
COO: Richard L. Rawson, President and Chief Executive Officer
Web address: www.selmahospital.org
Control: Other not–for–profit (including NFP Corporation) **Service:** General Medical and Surgical

Staffed Beds: 57

SEPULVEDA—Los Angeles County, See Los Angeles

SHERMAN OAKS—Los Angeles County, See Los Angeles

SIMI VALLEY—Ventura County

☒ **SIMI VALLEY HOSPITAL AND HEALTH CARE SERVICES (50236)**, 2975 North Sycamore Drive, Zip 93065–1201; tel. 805/955–6000, (Includes SIMI VALLEY HOSPITAL AND HEALTH CARE SERVICES–SOUTH CAMPUS, 1850 Heywood Street, Zip 93065; tel. 805/955–7000), (Total facility includes 34 beds in nursing home–type unit) (Nonreporting) **A**1 2 9 10 **S** Adventist Health
Primary Contact: Gary G. Irish, President and Chief Executive Officer
CFO: John Beaman, Chief Financial Officer
CMO: Jonathan Kurohara, M.D., Chief of Staff
CIO: Orville Beach, Director Information Systems
CHR: Wesley Schmidt, Director Human Resources
Web address: www.simivalleyhospital.com
Control: Church–operated, Nongovernment, not–for profit **Service:** General Medical and Surgical

Staffed Beds: 181

SOLVANG—Santa Barbara County

☒ **SANTA YNEZ VALLEY COTTAGE HOSPITAL (50478)**, 2050 Viborg Road, Zip 93463–2295; tel. 805/688–6431 **A**1 9 10 20 **F**8 15 24 38 55 79 80 96 107 122 132 135 **S** Cottage Health System
Primary Contact: Wende Cappetta, Administrator
Web address: www.cottagehealthsystem.org
Control: Other not–for–profit (including NFP Corporation) **Service:** General Medical and Surgical

Staffed Beds: 20 **Admissions:** 311 **Census:** 3 **Outpatient Visits:** 31755 **Births:** 0 **Total Expense ($000):** 9398 **Payroll Expense ($000):** 4686 **Personnel:** 80

SONOMA—Sonoma County

☐ **SONOMA VALLEY HOSPITAL (50090)**, 347 Andrieux Street, Zip 95476–6811, Mailing Address: P.O. Box 600, Zip 95476–0600; tel. 707/935–5000, (Nonreporting) **A**1 9 10
Primary Contact: Carl H. Gerlach, President and Chief Executive Officer
COO: Mary Kelly, Chief Nursing Officer
CFO: James M. McSweeney, Chief Financial Officer
CMO: Robert Cohen, M.D., President Medical Staff
CIO: Fe Sandaydiego, Manager Information Systems
CHR: Paula M. Davis, Director Human Resources
Web address: www.svh.com
Control: Hospital district or authority, Government, nonfederal **Service:** General Medical and Surgical

Staffed Beds: 67

SONORA—Tuolumne County

☒ **SONORA REGIONAL MEDICAL CENTER (50335)**, 1000 Greenley Road, Zip 95370–4819; tel. 209/536–5000, (Total facility includes 64 beds in nursing home–type unit) (Nonreporting) **A**1 9 10 19 **S** Adventist Health
Primary Contact: Lary Davis, President and Chief Executive Officer
CFO: David Larsen, Vice President Finance
CMO: Eugene Margolis, M.D., Chief of Staff
CIO: Doug Duffield, Vice President Business Planning and Marketing
CHR: Donn Swartz, Director Human Resources
Web address: www.sonorahospital.org
Control: Church–operated, Nongovernment, not–for profit **Service:** General Medical and Surgical

Staffed Beds: 147

☐ **TUOLUMNE GENERAL HOSPITAL (50325)**, 101 Hospital Road, Zip 95370–5297; tel. 209/533–7100, (Total facility includes 42 beds in nursing home–type unit) (Nonreporting) **A**1 9 10
Primary Contact: John M. Wilson, Interim Chief Executive Officer
COO: Jack D. McCue, M.D., Chief Operating Officer and Chief Medical Officer
CFO: Rebecca Bales, Interim Chief Financial Officer
CMO: Tracey Roe, M.D., Coordinator Medical Staff
CIO: Dan Baldree, System Analyst
CHR: Tracie Riggs, Human Resources Officer
Web address: www.tghospital.com
Control: County–Government, nonfederal **Service:** General Medical and Surgical

Staffed Beds: 79

SOUTH LAKE TAHOE—El Dorado County

☒ **BARTON HEALTHCARE SYSTEM (50352)**, 2170 South Avenue, Zip 96150–7008, Mailing Address: P.O. Box 9578, Zip 96158; tel. 530/541–3420, (Total facility includes 48 beds in nursing home–type unit) **A**1 9 10 20 **F**1 3 4 10 11 13 15 16 17 25 26 27 28 30 31 32 33 34 36 37 38 41 42 43 44 45 46 48 49 50 53 54 55 56 57 60 61 62 63 64 65 66 68 70 71 72 73 74 75 77 78 79 80 81 82 83 84 85 86 87 88 90 92 93 96 97 98 99 100 102 103 107 112 117 118 119 120 121 122 124 132 133 135 136 137
Primary Contact: John G. Williams, Chief Executive Officer
CFO: Richard P. Derby, Chief Financial Officer
CIO: Rob Quadri, Director Management Information Systems
CHR: LeAnne Kankel, Director Human Resources
Web address: www.bartonhealth.org
Control: Other not–for–profit (including NFP Corporation) **Service:** General Medical and Surgical

Staffed Beds: 119 **Admissions:** 3356 **Census:** 73 **Outpatient Visits:** 154461 **Births:** 524 **Total Expense ($000):** 108378 **Payroll Expense ($000):** 45450 **Personnel:** 681

SOUTH SAN FRANCISCO—San Mateo County

☒ **KAISER FOUNDATION HOSPITAL (50070)**, 1200 El Camino Real, Zip 94080–3299; tel. 650/742–2000, (Nonreporting) **A**1 10 **S** Kaiser Foundation Hospitals
Primary Contact: Linda Jensen, Senior Vice President and Service Area Manager
Web address: www.kaiserpermanente.org
Control: Other not–for–profit (including NFP Corporation) **Service:** General Medical and Surgical

Staffed Beds: 105

STOCKTON—San Joaquin County

☐ **DAMERON HOSPITAL (50122)**, 525 West Acacia Street, Zip 95203–2484; tel. 209/944–5550, (Nonreporting) **A**1 9 10
Primary Contact: Christopher Arismendi, M.D., Chief Executive Officer
COO: Nicholas Arismendi, Chief Operating Officer
CFO: Cyrus E. Dah, Chief Financial Officer
CMO: Alfredo Leon, M.D., Chief of Staff
CIO: Glenn Whipple, Director
CHR: Annette Lorenzi, Director Human Resources
Web address: www.dameronhospital.org
Control: Other not–for–profit (including NFP Corporation) **Service:** General Medical and Surgical

Staffed Beds: 188

☒ **ST. JOSEPH'S BEHAVIORAL HEALTH CENTER (54123)**, 2510 North California Street, Zip 95204–5502; tel. 209/461–2000 **A**1 9 10 **F**4 5 25 26 30 31 32 36 54 57 66 73 82 88 90 91 92 93 94 95 119 121 132 135 **S** Catholic Healthcare West
Primary Contact: Paul Rains, President
CFO: Wayne Silveria, Chief Financial Officer
CMO: Michael Smith, M.D., Medical Director
CHR: Debbie Murillo, Vice President Human Resources
Web address: www.stjosephscanhelp.org
Control: Church–operated, Nongovernment, not–for profit **Service:** Psychiatric

Staffed Beds: 35 **Admissions:** 1756 **Census:** 36 **Outpatient Visits:** 7246 **Total Expense ($000):** 8833 **Payroll Expense ($000):** 4941 **Personnel:** 90

Many Facility Codes have changed. Please refer to the AHA Guide Code Chart.

★ **ST. JOSEPH'S MEDICAL CENTER (50084)**, 1800 North California Street, Zip 95204–6019, Mailing Address: P.O. Box 213008, Zip 95213–3008; tel. 209/943–2000, (Total facility includes 21 beds in nursing home–type unit) **A**1 2 9 10 **F**3 13 17 18 20 22 24 25 26 27 30 31 32 33 38 43 44 53 56 59 61 62 68 69 70 72 73 74 75 76 79 80 82 84 86 96 97 99 106 107 109 117 119 121 133 137 **P**5 **S** Catholic Healthcare West
Primary Contact: Donald J. Wiley, President
COO: Michael Ricks, Chief Operating Officer
CFO: Wayne Silveria, Chief Financial Officer
CMO: Sandon Saffier, M.D., Vice President
CHR: Debbie Murillo, Vice President Human Resources
Web address: www.stjosephsCARES.org
Control: Church–operated, Nongovernment, not–for profit **Service:** General Medical and Surgical

Staffed Beds: 294 **Admissions:** 18222 **Census:** 234 **Outpatient Visits:** 486131 **Births:** 2509 **Total Expense ($000):** 260627 **Payroll Expense ($000):** 122009 **Personnel:** 2054

SUN CITY—Riverside County

★ **MENIFEE VALLEY MEDICAL CENTER (50684)**, 28400 McCall Boulevard, Zip 92585–9537; tel. 951/679–8888, (Nonreporting) **A**1 9 10 **S** Valley Health System
Primary Contact: Thomas E. Dougherty, Administrator
CFO: Michael Garko, Chief Financial Officer
CHR: Michele Bird, Chief Human Resources Officer
Web address: www.valleyhealthsystem.com
Control: Hospital district or authority, Government, nonfederal **Service:** General Medical and Surgical

Staffed Beds: 82

SUN VALLEY—Los Angeles County, See Los Angeles

SUSANVILLE—Lassen County

★ **BANNER LASSEN MEDICAL CENTER (51320)**, 1800 Spring Ridge Drive, Zip 96130–4809; tel. 530/252–2000 **A**1 9 10 18 **F**3 11 13 15 25 27 30 31 32 33 38 50 54 55 56 57 62 66 73 75 76 77 79 80 82 96 97 100 102 106 107 118 119 135 137 **S** Banner Health
Primary Contact: Richard L. Smith, Chief Executive Officer
CFO: Shelby Diede, Chief Financial Officer
CHR: Charlotte Luhring, Director People Resources
Web address: www.bannerhealth.com
Control: Other not–for–profit (including NFP Corporation) **Service:** General Medical and Surgical

Staffed Beds: 25 **Admissions:** 1268 **Census:** 12 **Outpatient Visits:** 53504 **Births:** 238 **Total Expense ($000):** 27932 **Payroll Expense ($000):** 11615 **Personnel:** 198

SYLMAR—Los Angeles County, See Los Angeles

TARZANA—Los Angeles County, See Los Angeles

TEHACHAPI—Kern County

★ **TEHACHAPI VALLEY HEALTHCARE DISTRICT (51301)**, 115 West E Street, Zip 93561, Mailing Address: P.O. Box 1900, Zip 93581–1900; tel. 661/823–3000 **A**9 10 18 **F**15 25 32 38 55 56 63 75 86 96 102 107 117 119 122 124 132 135 **P**3 5
Primary Contact: Alan J. Burgess, FACHE, Chief Executive Officer
CFO: Joe Demont, Chief Financial Officer
CMO: Terry Warsaw, M.D., Chief of Staff
CIO: Alan J. Burgess, FACHE, Chief Executive Officer
CHR: Debbie Thebeau, Director Human Resources
Web address: www.tvhd.org
Control: Hospital district or authority, Government, nonfederal **Service:** General Medical and Surgical

Staffed Beds: 24 **Admissions:** 104 **Census:** 19 **Outpatient Visits:** 33622 **Births:** 0 **Total Expense ($000):** 11869 **Payroll Expense ($000):** 5367 **Personnel:** 149

TEMPLETON—San Luis Obispo County

★ **TWIN CITIES COMMUNITY HOSPITAL (50633)**, 1100 Las Tablas Road, Zip 93465–9704; tel. 805/434–3500 **A**1 9 10 **F**13 18 25 31 32 33 35 38 55 56 57 62 68 73 74 75 76 77 79 96 97 107 119 121 135 **P**5 **S** TENET Healthcare Corporation
Primary Contact: Richard D. Lyons, Chief Executive Officer
COO: Joe Badalian, Chief Operating Officer
CFO: Paul Posmoga, Chief Financial Officer
CMO: Terry Ann Murphy, Chief Nursing Officer
CIO: Scott Harrison, Director Information Systems
CHR: Eloise Rendon, Director Human Resources
Web address: www.twincitieshospital.com
Control: Corporation, Investor–owned, for–profit **Service:** General Medical and Surgical

Staffed Beds: 114 **Admissions:** 5089 **Census:** 60 **Outpatient Visits:** 43824 **Births:** 690 **Total Expense ($000):** 53562 **Payroll Expense ($000):** 26035 **Personnel:** 414

THOUSAND OAKS—Los Angeles County

★ **LOS ROBLES HOSPITAL AND MEDICAL CENTER (50549)**, 215 West Janss Road, Zip 91360–1847; tel. 805/497–2727, (Total facility includes 42 beds in nursing home–type unit) **A**1 2 9 10 **F**3 13 14 17 18 20 22 24 25 26 27 30 31 32 37 38 40 43 46 47 48 49 53 54 55 57 68 70 72 73 74 75 76 77 79 80 82 84 86 88 92 93 96 97 100 102 107 117 119 121 124 135 136 137 **S** HCA
Primary Contact: Jim Sherman, President and Chief Executive Officer
COO: Don Kreitz, Chief Operating Officer
CFO: Debra J. Herwaldt, Chief Financial Officer
CMO: Barry Thall, M.D., Medical Director
CIO: Dan Isozaki, Director Information Management
CHR: Dayle Dalton, Vice President Human Resources
Web address: www.losrobleshospital.com
Control: Corporation, Investor–owned, for–profit **Service:** General Medical and Surgical

Staffed Beds: 273 **Admissions:** 13157 **Census:** 201 **Outpatient Visits:** 87774 **Births:** 2083 **Total Expense ($000):** 188220 **Payroll Expense ($000):** 82187 **Personnel:** 1276

THOUSAND OAKS SURGICAL HOSPITAL (50749), 401 East Rolling Oaks Drive, Zip 91361; tel. 805/777–7750 **A**9 10 **F**12 25 30 32 37 51 52 56 62 73 77 79 80 135
Primary Contact: Michael D. Bass, M.D., Chief Executive Officer and Administrator
CFO: Craig Corley, Chief Financial Officer
CMO: Steven Bansbach, M.D., Medical Director
CIO: Michael Lashley, Network Administrator
CHR: Jean Callahan, Manager Human Resources
Web address: www.toshospital.com
Control: Partnership, Investor–owned, for–profit **Service:** General Medical and Surgical

Staffed Beds: 21 **Admissions:** 865 **Census:** 5 **Outpatient Visits:** 6278 **Births:** 0 **Total Expense ($000):** 22510 **Payroll Expense ($000):** 5502 **Personnel:** 86

TORRANCE—Los Angeles County

□ **DEL AMO HOSPITAL (54053)**, 23700 Camino Del Sol, Zip 90505–5000; tel. 310/530–1151, (Nonreporting) **A**1 9 10 **S** Universal Health Services, Inc.
Primary Contact: Lisa K. Montes, Chief Executive Officer and Managing Director
Web address: www.delamohospital.com
Control: Corporation, Investor–owned, for–profit **Service:** Psychiatric

Staffed Beds: 70

□ **LAC–HARBOR–UNIVERSITY OF CALIFORNIA AT LOS ANGELES MEDICAL CENTER (50376)**, 1000 West Carson Street, Zip 90502–2004; tel. 310/222–2345 **A**1 2 3 5 8 10 **F**3 11 12 13 14 15 17 18 20 22 23 25 26 27 30 31 32 33 37 38 40 41 43 46 47 49 50 53 54 55 56 57 59 60 62 63 64 66 68 70 72 74 75 76 77 79 80 81 82 83 84 86 87 88 89 90 92 94 95 96 97 103 106 107 113 114 118 119 120 121 123 124 127 133 134 135 136 137 **P**3 6 **S** Los Angeles County–Department of Health Services
Primary Contact: Miguel Ortiz–Marroquin, Interim Chief Executive Officer
COO: Miguel Ortiz–Marroquin, Chief Operating Officer
CFO: Jody Nakasuji, Chief Financial Officer
CMO: Gail Anderson, M.D., Chief Medical Officer
CIO: Sandy Mungovan, Chief Information Officer
CHR: Karyl Smith, Director Human Resources
Web address: www.humc.edu
Control: County–Government, nonfederal **Service:** General Medical and Surgical

Staffed Beds: 343 **Admissions:** 21617 **Census:** 340 **Outpatient Visits:** 357081 **Births:** 1128 **Total Expense ($000):** 486695 **Payroll Expense ($000):** 209768 **Personnel:** 3175

Hospital, Medicare Provider Number, Address, Telephone, Approval, Facility, and Physician Codes, Health Care System

★ American Hospital Association (AHA) membership
□ The Joint Commission accreditation
○ American Osteopathic Association (AOA) accreditation
△ Commission on Accreditation of Rehabilitation Facilities (CARF) accreditation

★ **LITTLE COMPANY OF MARY HOSPITAL (50353)**, 4101 Torrance Boulevard, Zip 90503–4698; tel. 310/540–7676, (Total facility includes 78 beds in nursing home–type unit) **A**1 2 9 10 **F**11 13 14 17 18 20 22 24 25 26 30 31 32 33 38 43 46 55 56 57 61 62 67 68 70 72 73 74 75 76 77 79 80 81 82 84 86 87 96 97 100 104 105 106 107 116 117 119 121 122 132 133 134 135 136 137 **P**5 7 **S** Providence Health & Services
Primary Contact: Michael Hunn, Administrator
COO: Michael Hunn, Administrator
CFO: Karl Carrier, Regional Chief Financial Officer
CMO: James Mollenkamp, M.D., Chief of Staff
CIO: Timothy Kirk, Regional Chief Information Officer
CHR: Pam Stahl, Service Area Director Human Resources
Web address: www.lcmweb.org
Control: Other not–for–profit (including NFP Corporation) **Service:** General Medical and Surgical

Staffed Beds: 272 **Admissions:** 18047 **Census:** 241 **Outpatient Visits:** 199675 **Births:** 2609 **Total Expense ($000):** 224328 **Payroll Expense ($000):** 84628 **Personnel:** 1448

CA

★ **TORRANCE MEMORIAL MEDICAL CENTER (50351)**, 3330 Lomita Boulevard, Zip 90505–5002; tel. 310/325–9110 **A**1 2 9 10 **F**3 5 8 11 12 13 14 15 16 17 18 20 22 24 25 26 27 30 31 32 33 35 38 42 43 44 45 46 49 50 51 53 55 56 57 58 59 60 61 62 68 70 72 73 74 75 76 77 79 80 81 82 84 86 87 96 97 98 99 100 102 104 105 106 107 109 111 116 117 118 119 121 123 132 133 134 135 136 137 **P**2
Primary Contact: Craig Leach, President and Chief Executive Officer
CFO: Douglas Klebe, Chief Financial Officer
CMO: David Rand, M.D., Chief of Staff
CIO: Robert Proto, Director Information Systems
CHR: Lois Michael, Vice President Human Resources
Web address: www.torrancememorial.org
Control: Other not–for–profit (including NFP Corporation) **Service:** General Medical and Surgical

Staffed Beds: 272 **Admissions:** 22918 **Census:** 271 **Outpatient Visits:** 256565 **Births:** 3900 **Total Expense ($000):** 351919 **Payroll Expense ($000):** 149379 **Personnel:** 2392

TRACY—San Joaquin County

★ **SUTTER TRACY COMMUNITY HOSPITAL (50313)**, 1420 North Tracy Boulevard, Zip 95376–3497; tel. 209/835–1500 **A**1 9 10 **F**3 11 13 15 17 25 26 27 30 31 32 33 38 43 46 49 50 53 55 56 57 59 62 66 68 72 73 74 75 76 77 79 80 84 86 96 97 99 100 107 119 121 124 135 137 **S** Sutter Health
Primary Contact: David M. Thompson, Chief Executive Officer
COO: Fred Ford, Assistant Administrator
CFO: Eric Dalton, Chief Financial Officer
CIO: Karen Mudd, Director Marketing and Public Affairs
CHR: Vanessa Dega, Manager Human Resources
Web address: www.suttertracy.org
Control: Other not–for–profit (including NFP Corporation) **Service:** General Medical and Surgical

Staffed Beds: 82 **Admissions:** 4435 **Census:** 50 **Outpatient Visits:** 86507 **Births:** 744 **Total Expense ($000):** 78680 **Payroll Expense ($000):** 29211 **Personnel:** 483

TRAVIS AFB—Solano County

★ **DAVID GRANT MEDICAL CENTER**, 101 Bodin Circle, Zip 94535–1800; tel. 707/423–7300, (Nonreporting) **A**1 3 5 **S** Department of the Air Force
Primary Contact: Colonel Michael R. Skidmore, Administrator
Control: Air Force, Government, federal **Service:** General Medical and Surgical

Staffed Beds: 84

TRUCKEE—Nevada County

○ **TAHOE FOREST HOSPITAL DISTRICT (50494)**, 10121 Pine Avenue, Zip 96161–4856, Mailing Address: P.O. Box 759, Zip 96160–0759; tel. 530/587–6011, (Total facility includes 35 beds in nursing home–type unit) (Nonreporting) **A**9 10 11 20 **S** Tahoe Forest Health System
Primary Contact: Robert A. Schapper, Chief Executive Officer
COO: Janet Van Gelder, Chief Operating Officer and Chief Nursing Officer
CMO: Larry Danto, M.D., Chief Of Staff
Web address: www.tfhd.com
Control: Hospital district or authority, Government, nonfederal **Service:** General Medical and Surgical

Staffed Beds: 61

TULARE—Tulare County

★ **TULARE LOCAL HEALTH CARE DISTRICT (50359)**, 869 Cherry Street, Zip 93274–2207; tel. 559/688–0821 **A**1 9 10 **F**3 11 13 15 18 25 26 27 30 32 38 49 50 52 56 57 61 63 66 68 69 70 72 73 74 76 77 79 80 81 84 86 96 97 99 100 102 107 118 119 120 121 135
Primary Contact: Shawn Bolouki, Chief Executive Officer
CFO: John C. Church, Chief Financial Officer
CMO: Gary Walter, M.D., Chief Medical Staff
CHR: Brooke Brown, Director Human Services
Web address: www.tdhs.org
Control: Hospital district or authority, Government, nonfederal **Service:** General Medical and Surgical

Staffed Beds: 116 **Admissions:** 6047 **Census:** 55 **Outpatient Visits:** 98899 **Births:** 1218 **Total Expense ($000):** 61132 **Payroll Expense ($000):** 26032 **Personnel:** 632

TURLOCK—Stanislaus County

★ **EMANUEL MEDICAL CENTER (50179)**, 825 Delbon Avenue, Zip 95382–2016, Mailing Address: P.O. Box 819005, Zip 95381–9005; tel. 209/667–4200, (Total facility includes 145 beds in nursing home–type unit) **A**1 9 10 **F**3 8 10 11 13 15 24 25 26 27 32 33 37 38 42 43 47 48 49 53 57 59 61 62 66 67 68 71 73 74 75 76 77 79 84 86 96 97 100 102 103 106 107 108 109 111 117 119 121 132 133 135 136 137 **P**7
Primary Contact: John R. Sigsbury, President and Chief Executive Officer
COO: Michael T. Iltis, Vice President Professional Services
CFO: Margaret Lera, Chief Financial Officer
CIO: Wendy Burns, Assistant Vice President and Interim Chief Information Officer
CHR: Terry Gray, Vice President Human Resources
Web address: www.emanuelmed.org
Control: Church–operated, Nongovernment, not–for profit **Service:** General Medical and Surgical

Staffed Beds: 366 **Admissions:** 13481 **Census:** 259 **Outpatient Visits:** 81431 **Births:** 2872 **Total Expense ($000):** 143602 **Payroll Expense ($000):** 68467 **Personnel:** 1254

TUSTIN—Orange County

★ **HEALTHSOUTH TUSTIN REHABILITATION HOSPITAL (53034)**, 14851 Yorba Street, Zip 92780–2925; tel. 714/832–9200 **A**1 9 10 **F**85 **S** HEALTHSOUTH Corporation
Primary Contact: David Mulhern, Chief Executive Officer
CFO: Susan Wilson, Controller
CMO: Wilfredo Escober, M.D., President of Staff
CHR: Tobi Williams, Director Human Resources
Web address: www.healthsouth.com
Control: Corporation, Investor–owned, for–profit **Service:** Rehabilitation

Staffed Beds: 48 **Admissions:** 963 **Census:** 30 **Outpatient Visits:** 5824 **Births:** 0 **Total Expense ($000):** 14918 **Payroll Expense ($000):** 7871

□ **TUSTIN HOSPITAL AND MEDICAL CENTER (50720)**, 14662 Newport Avenue, Zip 92680–6064; tel. 714/838–9600, (Total facility includes 42 beds in nursing home–type unit) (Nonreporting) **A**1 9 10 **S** Pacific Health Corporation
Primary Contact: R. Michael Hartman, Chief Executive Officer
COO: Daniel J. Davis, Chief Operating Officer
CMO: N. Charle Morcos, M.D., Chief of Staff
CIO: Ruben DeGuzman, Director Information Services
CHR: Toni Wright, Director Human Resources
Web address: www.tustinhospital.com
Control: Corporation, Investor–owned, for–profit **Service:** General Medical and Surgical

Staffed Beds: 64

TWENTYNINE PALMS—San Bernardino County

★ **NAVAL HOSPITAL**, Mailing Address: Box 788250, MCAGCC, Zip 92278–8250; tel. 760/830–2190, (Nonreporting) **A**1 **S** Bureau of Medicine and Surgery, Department of the Navy
Primary Contact: Captain Don Albia, Commanding Officer
COO: Captain Bruce Laverly, Executive Officer
CFO: Lieutenant Holly Lee, Comptroller
CMO: Captain Charles Nixon, M.D., Chief Medical Officer
CIO: Lieutenant Colonel Michael Klemann, Head Information
CHR: Virginia Ward, Human Resources Officer
Web address: www.nhtp.med.navy.mil/nhtp
Control: Navy, Government, federal **Service:** General Medical and Surgical

Staffed Beds: 29

Many Facility Codes have changed. Please refer to the AHA Guide Code Chart.

UKIAH—Mendocino County

★ **UKIAH VALLEY MEDICAL CENTER (50301)**, 275 Hospital Drive, Zip 95482–4531; tel. 707/462–3111 **A**1 9 10 **F**3 8 11 12 13 15 25 26 27 28 30 31 32 33 34 38 41 46 48 49 50 51 53 54 55 56 57 62 63 66 68 70 73 75 76 77 79 80 81 82 86 87 90 91 92 96 97 99 100 102 103 104 105 106 107 108 119 121 124 133 134 135 136 137 **P**1 **S** Adventist Health
Primary Contact: Terry M. Burns, President and Chief Executive Officer
CFO: Rodney Grainger, Chief Financial Officer
CHR: Rick Dodds, Administrative Director Human Resources and Employee Health Job Care
Web address: www.adventisthealth.org
Control: Church–operated, Nongovernment, not–for profit **Service:** General Medical and Surgical

Staffed Beds: 65 **Admissions:** 3887 **Census:** 33 **Outpatient Visits:** 109331 **Births:** 860 **Total Expense ($000):** 66903 **Payroll Expense ($000):** 26517 **Personnel:** 537

UPLAND—San Bernardino County

★ **SAN ANTONIO COMMUNITY HOSPITAL (50099)**, 999 San Bernardino Road, Zip 91786–4920, Mailing Address: Box 5001, Zip 91785–5001; tel. 909/985–2811 **A**1 2 9 10 **F**3 8 11 13 15 17 18 20 22 24 25 27 31 32 33 36 38 43 44 45 49 50 53 55 57 59 60 62 63 67 68 70 72 73 74 75 76 77 78 79 80 81 82 84 86 96 97 100 102 103 106 107 109 111 112 119 121 135 136 137
Primary Contact: Steven C. Moreau, President and Chief Executive Officer
CFO: Roger Parsons, Senior Vice President Finance
CMO: Naveen Gupta, M.D., President Medical Staff
CIO: Perry Strength, Director Information Services
CHR: Lynn Kelly, Vice President Human Resources
Web address: www.sach.org
Control: Other not–for–profit (including NFP Corporation) **Service:** General Medical and Surgical

Staffed Beds: 279 **Admissions:** 15094 **Census:** 153 **Outpatient Visits:** 212089 **Births:** 2304 **Total Expense ($000):** 222960 **Payroll Expense ($000):** 97523 **Personnel:** 1557

VACAVILLE—Solano County

CALIFORNIA MEDICAL FACILITY, 1600 California Drive, Zip 95696–2000; tel. 707/448–6841, (Nonreporting)
Primary Contact: Brenda Green, RN, Correctional Health Services Administrator II
COO: Nadim K. Khoury, M.D., Chief Deputy Clinical Services
CFO: Vickie Flandi, Associate Warden
CMO: Raymond Andreasen, M.D., Chief Medical Officer–Inpatient
CIO: Tammi Godard, Public Information Officer
Web address: www.cya.ca.gov/visitors/fac_prison_cmf.html
Control: State–Government, nonfederal **Service:** Hospital unit of an institution (prison hospital, college infimary, etc.)

Staffed Beds: 215

★ **NORTHBAY VACAVALLEY HOSPITAL (50680)**, 1000 Nut Tree Road, Zip 95687–4100; tel. 707/446–4000 **A**1 9 10 **F**3 11 25 31 32 38 46 49 50 62 68 73 75 77 78 79 80 82 86 87 96 97 106 107 110 119 121 135 137 **P**6 **S** NorthBay Healthcare System
Primary Contact: Deborah Sugiyama, President
CFO: Arthur E. DeNio, Chief Financial Officer
CMO: Donald M. Denmark, M.D., Vice President Medical Affairs
CIO: Paul Alcala, Vice President and Chief Information Officer
CHR: Ken McCollum, Vice President Human Resources
Web address: www.northbay.org
Control: Other not–for–profit (including NFP Corporation) **Service:** General Medical and Surgical

Staffed Beds: 48 **Admissions:** 2642 **Census:** 37 **Outpatient Visits:** 63764 **Births:** 0 **Total Expense ($000):** 73916 **Payroll Expense ($000):** 28956 **Personnel:** 254

VALENCIA—Los Angeles County

□ **HENRY MAYO NEWHALL MEMORIAL HOSPITAL (50624)**, 23845 McBean Parkway, Zip 91355–2083; tel. 661/253–8000, (Total facility includes 27 beds in nursing home–type unit) **A**1 2 9 10 **F**1 3 4 7 8 11 15 16 17 25 26 27 30 31 32 33 38 40 46 48 49 53 55 56 57 59 62 65 68 70 71 72 74 75 76 77 78 79 80 81 82 83 84 85 86 88 92 94 96 97 99 100 102 103 106 107 117 119 121 124 135 136 137 **P**5
Primary Contact: Roger E. Seaver, President and Chief Executive Officer
COO: John V. Schleif, Senior Vice President and Chief Operating Officer
CFO: C. R. Hudson, Senior Vice President and Chief Financial Officer
CMO: Chand Khanna, M.D., Chief of Staff
CIO: Cindy Peterson, Chief Information Officer
CHR: Mark Puleo, Chief Human Resources Officer
Web address: www.henrymayo.com
Control: Other not–for–profit (including NFP Corporation) **Service:** General Medical and Surgical

Staffed Beds: 217 **Admissions:** 11779 **Census:** 162 **Outpatient Visits:** 66955 **Births:** 1301 **Total Expense ($000):** 130458 **Payroll Expense ($000):** 46764 **Personnel:** 926

VALLEJO—Solano County

★ △ **KAISER FOUNDATION HOSPITAL AND REHABILITATION CENTER (50073)**, 975 Sereno Drive, Zip 94589–2441; tel. 707/651–1000 **A**1 3 5 7 10 **F**5 8 13 15 17 25 26 27 30 31 32 33 38 42 43 44 45 46 47 48 49 55 56 57 58 59 60 61 62 63 66 68 70 72 73 74 75 76 77 79 80 81 85 86 87 94 96 97 100 102 103 106 107 118 119 124 133 135 136 137 **S** Kaiser Foundation Hospitals
Primary Contact: Steven Stricker, M.D., Administrator and Chief Executive Officer
COO: Mariann White, Chief Operating Officer
CFO: Pamela Booher, Area Finance Officer
CIO: Brad Pfeifer, Director Area Technology
CHR: Mike McClure, Director Human Resources
Web address: www.kaiserpermanente.org
Control: Other not–for–profit (including NFP Corporation) **Service:** General Medical and Surgical

Staffed Beds: 270 **Admissions:** 15188 **Census:** 226 **Outpatient Visits:** 726751 **Births:** 2499 **Personnel:** 1555

★ **ST. HELENA HOSPITAL–CENTER FOR BEHAVIORAL HEALTH (54074)**, 525 Oregon Street, Zip 94590–3201; tel. 707/648–2200, (Nonreporting) **A**1 9 10 **S** Adventist Health
Primary Contact: JoAline Olson, RN, President and Chief Executive Officer
CFO: Edward A. McDonald, Chief Financial Officer
Web address: www.sthelenahospital.org/Behavioral/
Control: Church–operated, Nongovernment, not–for profit **Service:** Psychiatric

Staffed Beds: 61

★ **SUTTER SOLANO MEDICAL CENTER (50101)**, 300 Hospital Drive, Zip 94589–2517, Mailing Address: P.O. Box 3189, Zip 94589–3189; tel. 707/554–4444, (Total facility includes 9 beds in nursing home–type unit) (Nonreporting) **A**1 2 9 10 **S** Sutter Health
Primary Contact: Theresa Glubka, Chief Executive Officer
CFO: Cynthia Landerfelt, Chief Financial Officer
CHR: Jean Willhite, Director Human Resources
Web address: www.suttersolano.org
Control: Other not–for–profit (including NFP Corporation) **Service:** General Medical and Surgical

Staffed Beds: 111

VAN NUYS—Los Angeles County, See Los Angeles

VENTURA—Ventura County

□ **AURORA VISTA DEL MAR HOSPITAL (54077)**, 801 Seneca Street, Zip 93001–1411; tel. 805/653–6434 **A**1 9 10 **F**25 88 89 91 92 94 95 119 121 **S** Aurora Behavioral Health Care
Primary Contact: Mayla Krebsbach, Chief Executive Officer
COO: Theresa Berkin, Chief Operating Officer
CFO: Cory Delello, Chief Financial Officer
CMO: Robert M. Carvalho, M.D., Medical Director
Web address: www.vistadelmarhospital.com
Control: Corporation, Investor–owned, for–profit **Service:** Psychiatric

Staffed Beds: 87 **Admissions:** 3145 **Census:** 63 **Outpatient Visits:** 2522 **Births:** 0 **Total Expense ($000):** 14284 **Payroll Expense ($000):** 7556 **Personnel:** 153

Hospital, Medicare Provider Number, Address, Telephone, Approval, Facility, and Physician Codes, Health Care System

★ American Hospital Association (AHA) membership
□ The Joint Commission accreditation
○ American Osteopathic Association (AOA) accreditation
△ Commission on Accreditation of Rehabilitation Facilities (CARF) accreditation

★ **COMMUNITY MEMORIAL HEALTH SYSTEM**, 147 North Brent Street, Zip 93003–2854; tel. 803/652–5011, (Includes COMMUNITY MEMORIAL HOSPITAL, 147 North Brent Street, tel. 805/652–5011; OJAI VALLEY COMMUNITY HOSPITAL, 1306 Maricopa Highway, Ojai, Zip 93023–3163; tel. 805/646–1401; Mary Jo Garrett, Vice President Operations and Administrative Officer) **A**1 9 10 **F**3 11 12 13 15 17 18 20 22 24 26 27 31 32 37 38 52 53 55 57 59 68 70 72 74 75 76 77 79 80 84 86 87 96 97 99 100 106 107 116 119 121 124 133 **P**7
Primary Contact: Gary Wilde, Chief Executive Officer
COO: Adam Thunell, Chief Operating Officer and Vice President Operations
CFO: David Glyer, Vice President Finance
CMO: Peter Gaal, M.D., Medical Director
CIO: Nick Pappas, Manager Information Systems
CHR: Diany Klein, Vice President Human Resources
Control: Other not–for–profit (including NFP Corporation) **Service:** General Medical and Surgical

Staffed Beds: 244 **Admissions:** 13047 **Census:** 148 **Outpatient Visits:** 321169 **Births:** 3026 **Total Expense ($000):** 189194 **Payroll Expense ($000):** 76162 **Personnel:** 1390

CA

☐ **VENTURA COUNTY MEDICAL CENTER (50159)**, 3291 Loma Vista Road, Zip 93003–3099; tel. 805/652–6000, (Nonreporting) **A**1 5 9 10
Primary Contact: Michael Powers, Director
COO: Christina Thielst, Chief Operating Officer
CFO: Catherine Rodriguez, Chief Financial Officer
CMO: Robert Gonzalez, M.D., Medical Director
CIO: David Herzog, Chief Information Officer
CHR: Maria Teran, Personnel Officer
Web address: www.vchca.org
Control: County–Government, nonfederal **Service:** General Medical and Surgical

Staffed Beds: 208

VICTORVILLE—San Bernardino County

○ **DESERT VALLEY HOSPITAL (50709)**, 16850 Bear Valley Road, Zip 92395; tel. 760/241–8000 **A**10 11 **F**3 13 15 20 25 26 38 43 55 56 57 62 68 72 73 74 75 77 79 82 96 99 100 107 119 135 137 **P**4 **S** Prime Healthcare Services
Primary Contact: Lex Reddy, President and Chief Executive Officer
CFO: Roger Krissman, Chief Financial Officer
CIO: Sreekant Gotti, Director Information Systems
CHR: Arti Dhuper, Regional Director Human Resources
Web address: www.dvmc.com
Control: Corporation, Investor–owned, for–profit **Service:** General Medical and Surgical

Staffed Beds: 83 **Admissions:** 7352 **Census:** 67 **Outpatient Visits:** 65371 **Births:** 484 **Total Expense ($000):** 63495 **Payroll Expense ($000):** 25663

VICTOR VALLEY COMMUNITY HOSPITAL (50517), 15248 Eleventh Street, Zip 92395; tel. 760/245–8691, (Nonreporting) **A**9 10
Primary Contact: Margaret R. Peterson, Ph.D., Chief Executive Officer
CFO: Emma Macaraeg, Chief Financial Officer
CHR: Brent Nielsen, Chief Human Resources Officer
Web address: www.vvch.org
Control: Other not–for–profit (including NFP Corporation) **Service:** General Medical and Surgical

Staffed Beds: 115

VISALIA—Tulare County

★ △ **KAWEAH DELTA HEALTH CARE DISTRICT (50057)**, 400 West Mineral King Boulevard, Zip 93291–6263; tel. 559/624–2000, (Includes SOUTH CAMPUS, 1633 South Court Street, Zip 93277; tel. 559/624–6090), (Total facility includes 53 beds in nursing home–type unit) **A**1 2 7 9 10 **F**3 5 13 15 18 20 22 24 25 26 27 30 31 32 33 38 42 43 44 46 49 50 51 52 53 54 55 56 57 59 61 62 63 66 68 71 72 73 74 75 76 77 79 80 81 82 84 85 86 87 88 89 90 91 92 93 94 96 97 99 100 102 104 105 106 107 111 112 117 118 119 120 121 123 124 133 135 136 137 **P**7
Primary Contact: Lindsay K. Mann, Chief Executive Officer
CFO: Gary Herbst, Senior Vice President and Chief Financial Officer
CMO: Mark Garfield, M.D., Vice President and Chief Medical Officer
CIO: Dave Gravender, Vice President and Chief Information Officer
CHR: Jean Haskell, Vice President Human Resources
Web address: www.kaweahdelta.org
Control: Hospital district or authority, Government, nonfederal **Service:** General Medical and Surgical

Staffed Beds: 353 **Admissions:** 20175 **Census:** 327 **Outpatient Visits:** 464862 **Births:** 4184 **Total Expense ($000):** 301632 **Payroll Expense ($000):** 141299 **Personnel:** 2994

WALNUT CREEK—Contra Costa County

★ **JOHN MUIR MEDICAL CENTER, WALNUT CREEK (50180)**, 1601 Ygnacio Valley Road, Zip 94598–3194; tel. 925/939–3000 **A**1 2 9 10 **F**3 11 13 15 17 18 20 22 24 25 26 27 30 31 32 33 35 37 38 40 41 43 46 47 49 50 53 54 55 56 57 59 61 62 63 66 68 70 72 73 74 75 76 77 79 80 81 82 84 85 86 90 92 96 99 106 107 108 109 111 112 114 119 121 124 134 135 136 137 **P**3 4 5 **S** John Muir Health
Primary Contact: Jane Willemsen, Chief Administrative Officer
Web address: www.jmmdhs.com/index.php/jmmdhs_jmmc.html
Control: Other not–for–profit (including NFP Corporation) **Service:** General Medical and Surgical

Staffed Beds: 324 **Admissions:** 17453 **Census:** 248 **Outpatient Visits:** 234329 **Births:** 2897 **Total Expense ($000):** 575098 **Payroll Expense ($000):** 213689 **Personnel:** 1765

★ **KAISER FOUNDATION HOSPITAL (50072)**, 1425 South Main Street, Zip 94596–5300; tel. 925/295–4000, (Includes KAISER FOUNDATION HOSPITAL, 200 Muir Road, Martinez, Zip 94553–4696; tel. 510/372–1000), (Nonreporting) **A**1 5 10 **S** Kaiser Foundation Hospitals
Primary Contact: Sandra H. Small, RN, Senior Vice President and Service Area Manager
CFO: Yakesun Wing, Business Strategy and Finance Leader
CMO: Don Palmer, M.D., Chief of Staff
CIO: Kevin Wheeler, Information Technology Leader
Web address: www.kaiserpermanente.org
Control: Other not–for–profit (including NFP Corporation) **Service:** General Medical and Surgical

Staffed Beds: 257

WATSONVILLE—Santa Cruz County

★ **WATSONVILLE COMMUNITY HOSPITAL (50194)**, 75 Nielson Street, Zip 95076–2468; tel. 831/724–4741, (Nonreporting) **A**1 9 10 **S** Community Health Systems, Inc.
Primary Contact: Jae Dale, Interim Chief Executive Officer
CFO: Jae Dale, Chief Financial Officer
CMO: Ali Khademi, M.D., Chief Medical Staff
CIO: Sergio Nell, Director Information Systems
CHR: Jeri Gilbert, Director Human Resources
Web address: www.watsonvillehospital.com
Control: Other not–for–profit (including NFP Corporation) **Service:** General Medical and Surgical

Staffed Beds: 74

WEAVERVILLE—Trinity County

TRINITY HOSPITAL (51315), (Formerly Mountain Community Medical Services), 60 Easter Avenue, Zip 96093, Mailing Address: P.O. Box 1229, Zip 96093–1229; tel. 530/623–5541, (Total facility includes 26 beds in nursing home–type unit) **A**9 10 18 **F**3 11 25 26 30 31 32 37 38 47 55 56 61 62 80 81 96 107 117
Primary Contact: Claire M. Kuczkowski, Chief Executive Officer
CFO: Thomas Pyper, Chief Financial Officer
CMO: Dale Stemple, M.D., Chief of Staff
CHR: Tamara Harris, Director Human Resources
Web address: www.mcmedical.org
Control: Hospital district or authority, Government, nonfederal **Service:** General Medical and Surgical

Staffed Beds: 51 **Admissions:** 402 **Census:** 26 **Outpatient Visits:** 11031 **Births:** 2

WEST COVINA—Los Angeles County

☐ **CITRUS VALLEY MEDICAL CENTER–QUEEN OF THE VALLEY CAMPUS (50369)**, 1115 South Sunset Avenue, Zip 91790–3940, Mailing Address: P.O. Box 1980, Zip 91793–1980; tel. 626/962–4011, (Nonreporting) **A**1 9 10 **S** Citrus Valley Health Partners
Primary Contact: James T. Yoshioka, President and Chief Executive Officer
COO: Elvia Foulke, Executive Vice President Healthcare Delivery
CFO: Lois Conyers, Senior Vice President and Chief Financial Officer
CMO: Richard Gisi, M.D., Vice President Medical Affairs
CIO: David McCobb, Senior Vice President and Chief Information Officer
CHR: Lisa Foust, Senior Vice President Human Resources
Web address: www.cvhp.org
Control: Other not–for–profit (including NFP Corporation) **Service:** General Medical and Surgical

Staffed Beds: 263

☐ **DOCTORS HOSPITAL OF WEST COVINA (50096)**, 725 South Orange Avenue, Zip 91790–2614; tel. 626/338–8481, (Total facility includes 27 beds in nursing home–type unit) (Nonreporting) **A**1 9 10
Primary Contact: Gerald H. Wallman, Administrator
CFO: Frank Bumgardner, Chief Financial Officer
CMO: Nashat Ateia, M.D., Chief of Staff
CHR: Lourdes Meza, Coordinator Human Resources
Control: Corporation, Investor–owned, for–profit **Service:** General Medical and Surgical

Staffed Beds: 51

 Many Facility Codes have changed. Please refer to the AHA Guide Code Chart.

☐ **KINDRED HOSPITAL SAN GABRIEL VALLEY**, 845 North Lark Ellen Avenue, Zip 91791–1069; tel. 626/339–5451, (Nonreporting) **A**1 9 **S** Kindred Healthcare
Primary Contact: Norman J. Andrews, Administrator
Web address: www.kindredhealthcare.com
Control: Partnership, Investor–owned, for–profit **Service:** Long–Term Acute Care hospital

Staffed Beds: 76

WEST HILLS—Los Angeles County, See Los Angeles

WEST LOS ANGELES—Los Angeles County, See Los Angeles

WESTMINSTER—Orange County

☐ **KINDRED HOSPITAL–WESTMINSTER (52035)**, 200 Hospital Circle, Zip 92683–3910; tel. 714/893–4541, (Nonreporting) **A**1 9 10 **S** Kindred Healthcare
Primary Contact: Adam Darvish, M.P.H., Executive Director
COO: Jack Boggess, Chief Operating Officer
CFO: Dale Wagner, Chief Financial Officer
Web address: www.kindredhealthcare.com
Control: Corporation, Investor–owned, for–profit **Service:** Long–Term Acute Care hospital

Staffed Beds: 99

WHITTIER—Los Angeles County

★☐ **PRESBYTERIAN INTERCOMMUNITY HOSPITAL (50169)**, 12401 Washington Boulevard, Zip 90602–1099; tel. 562/698–0811, (Total facility includes 35 beds in nursing home–type unit) **A**1 2 3 5 9 10 **F**3 11 13 14 15 17 18 20 22 24 25 26 27 30 31 32 33 34 35 38 40 42 43 44 45 46 52 53 54 55 56 57 58 59 60 61 62 63 64 66 67 68 69 70 71 72 73 74 75 76 77 79 80 81 82 84 85 86 87 96 97 99 100 102 106 107 109 117 119 121 123 124 135 136 137 **P**3 5
Primary Contact: James R. West, CHE, President and Chief Executive Officer
COO: Todd Salnas, Vice President Operations
CFO: Mitchell T. Thomas, Chief Financial Officer
CMO: Rosalio J. Lopez, M.D., Senior Vice President and Chief Medical Officer
CIO: Peggy Chulack, Chief Administrative Officer and Chief Information Officer
CHR: Lon Orey, Vice President Human Resources
Web address: www.whittierpres.com
Control: Other not–for–profit (including NFP Corporation) **Service:** General Medical and Surgical

Staffed Beds: 444 **Admissions:** 20189 **Census:** 238 **Outpatient Visits:** 119813 **Births:** 3725 **Total Expense ($000):** 305534 **Payroll Expense ($000):** 127310 **Personnel:** 2635

☐ **WHITTIER HOSPITAL MEDICAL CENTER (50735)**, 9080 Colima Road, Zip 90605–1600; tel. 562/945–3561, (Total facility includes 22 beds in nursing home–type unit) **A**1 9 10 **F**25 31 33 34 38 55 56 57 62 64 66 67 68 74 79 86 96 97 107 117 119 132 135 **P**5 **S** AHMC, Inc
Primary Contact: Howard Ternes, Chief Executive Officer
CFO: Mary Anne Monje, Chief Financial Officer
CIO: Jay Geldhof, Director Information Systems
CHR: Jason Jaquez, Director Human Resources
Web address: www.whittierhospital.com
Control: Corporation, Investor–owned, for–profit **Service:** General Medical and Surgical

Staffed Beds: 104 **Admissions:** 9348 **Census:** 104 **Outpatient Visits:** 40951 **Births:** 2126 **Total Expense ($000):** 78822 **Payroll Expense ($000):** 33402 **Personnel:** 531

WILDOMAR—Riverside County

☐ **INLAND VALLEY MEDICAL CENTER**, 36485 Inland Valley Drive, Zip 92595–9700; tel. 951/677–1111, (Nonreporting) **A**1 9 **S** Universal Health Services, Inc.
Primary Contact: Dennis M. Knox, Chief Executive Officer
COO: Linda Bradley, Chief Executive Officer and Managing Director
CFO: Barry Thorfinnson, Chief Financial Officer
CMO: Kevin Flaig, M.D., Chief Medical Officer
CHR: Shannon Weidauer, Director Human Resources
Web address: www.ivrmc–rsmc.com
Control: Corporation, Investor–owned, for–profit **Service:** General Medical and Surgical

Staffed Beds: 80

VICTOR VALLEY COMMUNITY HOSPITAL See Victorville

WILLITS—Mendocino County

★ **FRANK R. HOWARD MEMORIAL HOSPITAL (51310)**, One Madrone Street, Zip 95490–4225; tel. 707/459–6801 **A**9 10 18 **F**11 15 25 26 31 32 33 38 42 43 44 55 61 62 68 73 77 79 86 96 99 100 102 107 122 135 137 **S** Adventist Health
Primary Contact: Kevin R. Erich, President and Chief Executive Officer
CFO: Carlton Jacobson, Vice President Finance
CHR: Anthony Stahl, Director Human Resources
Web address: www.howardhospital.com
Control: Church–operated, Nongovernment, not–for profit **Service:** General Medical and Surgical

Staffed Beds: 25 **Admissions:** 1248 **Census:** 13 **Outpatient Visits:** 26932 **Births:** 0 **Total Expense ($000):** 32167 **Payroll Expense ($000):** 14160 **Personnel:** 226

WILLOWS—Glenn County

GLENN MEDICAL CENTER (51306), 1133 West Sycamore Street, Zip 95988–2745; tel. 530/934–1800 **A**9 10 18 **F**8 29 32 38 57 72 77 79 96 100 107 118 122 133 136
Primary Contact: Woody J. Laughnan, Jr., Administrator
CFO: Gary Pea, Chief Financial Officer
CMO: Jared Garrison, D.O., Chief of Staff
CHR: Deborah McMillan, Director Human Resources
Web address: www.glennmed.org
Control: Other not–for–profit (including NFP Corporation) **Service:** General Medical and Surgical

Staffed Beds: 15 **Admissions:** 371 **Census:** 3 **Outpatient Visits:** 23329 **Births:** 0 **Total Expense ($000):** 10487 **Payroll Expense ($000):** 4492 **Personnel:** 101

WOODLAND—Yolo County

★☐ **WOODLAND HEALTHCARE (50127)**, (Formerly Woodland Memorial Hospital), 1325 Cottonwood Street, Zip 95695–5199; tel. 530/662–3961, (Nonreporting) **A**1 9 10 **S** Catholic Healthcare West
Primary Contact: H. Kevin Vaziri, President
Web address: www.woodlandhealthcare.org
Control: Other not–for–profit (including NFP Corporation) **Service:** General Medical and Surgical

Staffed Beds: 111

WOODLAND HILLS—Los Angeles County, See Los Angeles

YOUNTVILLE—Napa County

VETERANS HOME OF CALIFORNIA (50667), 100 California Drive, Zip 94599–1411; tel. 707/944–4500, (Nonreporting) **A**10
Primary Contact: Marcella M. McCormack, Administrator
Control: State–Government, nonfederal **Service:** Hospital unit of an institution (prison hospital, college infimary, etc.)

Staffed Beds: 431

YREKA—Siskiyou County

FAIRCHILD MEDICAL CENTER (51316), 444 Bruce Street, Zip 96097–3450; tel. 530/842–4121 **A**9 10 18 **F**3 11 13 15 26 31 32 33 38 50 51 55 57 62 68 73 74 77 79 81 82 84 86 96 97 102 106 107 118 119 121 122 135 137
Primary Contact: Dwayne Jones, Chief Executive Officer
CFO: Kelly Martin, Controller
CMO: Dan Purtzer, M.D., Chief of Staff
CIO: Joan Munson, Manager Information Systems
CHR: Joann Sarmento, Manager Human Resources
Web address: www.fairchildmed.org
Control: Other not–for–profit (including NFP Corporation) **Service:** General Medical and Surgical

Staffed Beds: 25 **Admissions:** 1853 **Census:** 15 **Outpatient Visits:** 59851 **Births:** 235 **Total Expense ($000):** 34665 **Payroll Expense ($000):** 14530 **Personnel:** 340

YUBA CITY—Sutter County

☐ **FREMONT MEDICAL CENTER**, 989 Plumas Street, Zip 95991–4087; tel. 530/751–4000, (Nonreporting) **A**1 3 5 9 **S** Fremont–Rideout Health Group
Primary Contact: Theresa Hamilton, Chief Executive Officer
CFO: Kevin Woodward, Chief Financial Officer
CMO: Robert Plass, M.D., Chief Medical Officer
CHR: Tresha Moreland, Vice President Human Resources
Web address: www.frhg.org
Control: Other not–for–profit (including NFP Corporation) **Service:** General Medical and Surgical

Staffed Beds: 90

CA

Hospital, Medicare Provider Number, Address, Telephone, Approval, Facility, and Physician Codes, Health Care System
★ American Hospital Association (AHA) membership
☐ The Joint Commission accreditation
○ American Osteopathic Association (AOA) accreditation
△ Commission on Accreditation of Rehabilitation Facilities (CARF) accreditation

COLORADO

ALAMOSA—Alamosa County

★ **SAN LUIS VALLEY REGIONAL MEDICAL CENTER (60008)**, 106 Blanca Avenue, Zip 81101–2393; tel. 719/589–2511 **A**1 9 10 20 **F**3 7 11 12 15 26 27 38 51 68 73 74 76 77 79 80 82 85 96 100 102 118 119 120 135 136 137 **P**6
Primary Contact: Russell Johnson, Chief Executive Officer
COO: Henry Garvin, Vice President Operations
CFO: David Freshour, Vice President Finance
CIO: Kathy Rogers, Vice President Development
CHR: Leonard Snow, Vice President Human Resources, Quality and Compliance
Web address: www.slvrmc.org
Control: Other not–for–profit (including NFP Corporation) **Service:** General Medical and Surgical

Staffed Beds: 59 **Admissions:** 3323 **Census:** 22 **Outpatient Visits:** 55918 **Births:** 616 **Total Expense ($000):** 41841 **Payroll Expense ($000):** 20744 **Personnel:** 461

CO

ASPEN—Pitkin County

★ **ASPEN VALLEY HOSPITAL DISTRICT (61324)**, 401 Castle Creek Road, Zip 81611–1159; tel. 970/925–1120, (Nonreporting) **A**1 9 10 18
Primary Contact: David R. Ressler, Chief Executive Officer
COO: Natalie Booker, Chief Nursing Officer
CFO: Terry Collins, Chief Financial Officer
CMO: Steve Ayers, D.O., President Medical Staff
CIO: Ginny Dyche, Director Community Relations
CHR: Alicia Miller, Director Human Resources
Web address: www.avhaspen.org
Control: Hospital district or authority, Government, nonfederal **Service:** General Medical and Surgical

Staffed Beds: 25

AURORA—Adams and Arapahoe County

★ **MEDICAL CENTER OF AURORA (60100)**, 1501 South Potomac Street, Zip 80012–5499; tel. 303/695–2600, (Includes MEDICAL CENTER OF AURORA NORTH, 700 Potomac Street, Zip 80011–6792; tel. 303/363–7200; SOUTH CAMPUS, Zip 80012) **A**1 2 9 10 **F**3 4 8 11 13 15 22 24 25 26 27 30 32 33 35 37 38 39 40 43 44 46 47 48 49 52 53 54 55 56 62 66 68 70 72 73 74 75 76 77 79 80 81 82 84 88 93 96 97 99 100 102 103 105 106 107 118 119 121 124 135 136 137 **P**6 **S** HCA
Primary Contact: John Hill, President and Chief Executive Officer
COO: Mary Berrigan, Chief Operating Officer
CFO: Bill Voloch, Chief Financial Officer
Web address: www.auroramed.com
Control: Partnership, Investor–owned, for–profit **Service:** General Medical and Surgical

Staffed Beds: 314 **Admissions:** 15096 **Census:** 194 **Outpatient Visits:** 134963 **Births:** 2400 **Total Expense ($000):** 212745 **Payroll Expense ($000):** 82855 **Personnel:** 1244

★ △ **SPALDING REHABILITATION HOSPITAL (63027)**, 900 Potomac Street, Zip 80011–6716; tel. 303/367–1166, (Nonreporting) **A**1 7 10 **S** HCA
Primary Contact: Cynthia Kreutz, President and Chief Executive Officer
COO: Debbie Petersen, Chief Operating Officer
CFO: Joyce Webber, Chief Financial Officer
CHR: Donna Greeley, Director Human Resources
Web address: www.spaldingrehab.com
Control: Partnership, Investor–owned, for–profit **Service:** Rehabilitation

Staffed Beds: 50

★ **THE CHILDREN'S HOSPITAL (63301)**, 13123 East 16th Avenue, Zip 80045; tel. 720/777–1234 **A**1 3 5 8 9 10 **F**3 8 11 14 17 19 21 23 25 26 27 28 30 31 32 33 34 36 37 38 39 40 42 43 44 46 49 50 52 53 56 57 58 59 60 62 63 64 66 69 70 72 73 75 76 77 79 80 81 82 83 84 86 87 88 89 90 91 92 94 95 96 97 100 102 104 105 107 114 116 118 119 120 121 123 125 126 127 128 130 133 134 135
Primary Contact: James E. Shmerling, President and Chief Executive Officer
COO: Jena Hausmann, Executive Vice President and Chief Operating Officer
CFO: Len Dryer, Chief Financial Officer
CMO: Joan Bothner, M.D., Chief Medical Officer
CIO: Mary Ann Leach, Vice President and Chief Information Officer
CHR: Michael Wukitsch, Vice President Human Resources
Web address: www.thechildrenshospital.org
Control: Other not–for–profit (including NFP Corporation) **Service:** Children's general

Staffed Beds: 270 **Admissions:** 10253 **Census:** 187 **Outpatient Visits:** 349433 **Births:** 0 **Total Expense ($000):** 422959 **Payroll Expense ($000):** 180191 **Personnel:** 2866

□ **TRIUMPH HOSPITAL AURORA (62013)**, 700 Potomac Street, Zip 80012; tel. 720/857–8333, (Nonreporting) **A**1 9 10 **S** Triumph HealthCare
Primary Contact: Jay Quebedeaux, Chief Executive Officer
Web address: www.triumph–healthcare.com
Control: Corporation, Investor–owned, for–profit **Service:** Long–Term Acute Care hospital

Staffed Beds: 29

★ **UNIVERSITY OF COLORADO HOSPITAL (60024)**, 12401 East 17th Avenue, Zip 80045; tel. 720/848–0000 **A**1 2 3 5 8 9 10 **F**3 4 5 8 9 12 13 14 15 16 17 18 20 22 24 25 26 27 29 30 31 32 33 34 35 36 37 38 40 43 44 46 47 48 49 50 53 54 55 56 57 58 59 60 62 63 66 68 70 72 73 74 75 76 77 79 80 81 82 85 86 87 88 89 90 92 93 94 96 97 99 100 102 103 105 106 107 108 109 111 112 113 114 119 120 121 124 125 126 127 128 129 130 131 135 136 137 **P**3
Primary Contact: Bruce Schroffel, Chief Executive Officer
COO: John Harney, Chief Operating Officer
CFO: Anthony C. Defurio, Vice President and Chief Financial Officer
CMO: Greg Stiegmann, M.D., Vice President Clinical Affairs
CIO: Steve Clark, Vice President Information Services
CHR: Darryl Varnado, Vice President Human Resources
Web address: www.uch.edu
Control: Hospital district or authority, Government, nonfederal **Service:** General Medical and Surgical

Staffed Beds: 415 **Admissions:** 19057 **Census:** 316 **Outpatient Visits:** 604994 **Births:** 3097 **Total Expense ($000):** 601609 **Payroll Expense ($000):** 218387 **Personnel:** 3093

BOULDER—Boulder County

★ △ **BOULDER COMMUNITY HOSPITAL (60027)**, 1100 Balsam Avenue, Zip 80304–3496, Mailing Address: P.O. Box 9019, Zip 80301–9019; tel. 303/440–2273 **A**1 2 7 9 10 **F**3 5 8 9 11 13 15 18 20 22 24 25 26 27 30 31 32 34 35 36 38 39 40 41 42 43 44 50 51 52 53 54 56 57 59 60 61 62 66 68 70 72 73 74 75 76 77 79 80 81 82 84 85 86 87 88 89 90 91 92 93 94 95 97 99 100 102 103 104 106 107 108 109 111 112 118 119 120 121 123 133 135 136 137
Primary Contact: David P. Gehant, President and Chief Executive Officer
CFO: Bill Munson, Vice President and Chief Financial Officer
Web address: www.bch.org
Control: Other not–for–profit (including NFP Corporation) **Service:** General Medical and Surgical

Staffed Beds: 186 **Admissions:** 9197 **Census:** 112 **Outpatient Visits:** 405862 **Births:** 1554 **Total Expense ($000):** 237504 **Payroll Expense ($000):** 99608 **Personnel:** 2362

BRIGHTON—Adams County

★ **PLATTE VALLEY MEDICAL CENTER (60004)**, 1600 Prairie Center Parkway, Zip 80601–4006; tel. 303/498–1600 **A**1 9 10 **F**3 13 15 17 20 24 25 26 27 31 32 33 36 38 40 43 46 49 50 56 66 68 70 73 74 75 76 77 79 80 81 82 84 86 87 96 97 99 100 102 103 106 107 119 120 121 135 136 137 **P**5
Primary Contact: John R. Hicks, President and Chief Executive Officer
COO: Cheryl Bentley, Vice President Operations
CFO: Harold Dupper, Chief Financial Officer
CMO: Tillman Farley, M.D., Chief of Staff
CIO: Randy Ferguson, Director Information Systems
CHR: Jackie Dunkin, Director Human Resources
Web address: www.pvmc.org
Control: Other not–for–profit (including NFP Corporation) **Service:** General Medical and Surgical

Staffed Beds: 79 **Admissions:** 3456 **Census:** 27 **Outpatient Visits:** 58049 **Births:** 1065 **Total Expense ($000):** 60123 **Payroll Expense ($000):** 23376 **Personnel:** 441

BRUSH—Morgan County

★ **EAST MORGAN COUNTY HOSPITAL (61303)**, 2400 West Edison Street, Zip 80723–1640; tel. 970/842–6200 **A**9 10 18 **F**8 11 15 25 26 27 30 31 32 33 34 38 40 49 50 52 55 57 62 66 73 75 76 77 78 79 80 82 86 87 96 97 99 100 102 107 118 119 120 121 122 133 135 137 **P**6 **S** Banner Health
Primary Contact: Christopher J. Rogers, Chief Executive Officer
CFO: Linda Thorpe, Chief Financial Officer
CIO: Michael S. Warden, Senior Vice President and Chief Information Officer
CHR: Randy Brigham, Human Resource Generalist
Web address: www.emchbrush.com
Control: Other not–for–profit (including NFP Corporation) **Service:** General Medical and Surgical

Staffed Beds: 15 **Admissions:** 380 **Census:** 5 **Outpatient Visits:** 52021 **Births:** 0 **Total Expense ($000):** 12460 **Payroll Expense ($000):** 6080 **Personnel:** 116

 Many Facility Codes have changed. Please refer to the AHA Guide Code Chart.

BURLINGTON—Kit Carson County

★ **KIT CARSON COUNTY MEMORIAL HOSPITAL (61313)**, 286 16th Street, Zip 80807–1697; tel. 719/346–5311, (Nonreporting) **A**9 10 18
Primary Contact: James Jordan, Chief Executive Officer
COO: Regina Korsvold, R.N., Chief Operating Officer
CFO: Mona Ebsen, Chief Financial Officer
CMO: Sacremento Pimentel, M.D., Chief Medical Officer
CIO: Arlan Tanner, Chief Information Officer
CHR: Robin Konecne, Manager Human Resources
Web address: www.kccmh.org
Control: Hospital district or authority, Government, nonfederal **Service:** General Medical and Surgical

Staffed Beds: 25

CANON CITY—Fremont County

☒ **ST. THOMAS MORE HOSPITAL (60016)**, 1338 Phay Avenue, Zip 81212–2221; tel. 719/285–2000, (Nonreporting) **A**1 9 10 20 **S** Catholic Health Initiatives
Primary Contact: Diane Swagger, RN, President and Chief Executive Officer
COO: Mark Hartman, Vice President Operations
CFO: Sheri Trahern, Chief Financial Officer
CMO: Victoria King, M.D., Chief Medical Officer
CIO: Jennifer Kemp, Director Marketing and Public Relations
CHR: Stan Miller, Executive Director Human Resources
Web address: www.stmhospital.org
Control: Other not–for–profit (including NFP Corporation) **Service:** General Medical and Surgical

Staffed Beds: 49

CHEYENNE WELLS—Cheyenne County

★ **KEEFE MEMORIAL HOSPITAL (60043)**, 602 North 6th Street West, Zip 80810, Mailing Address: P.O. Box 578, Zip 80810–0578; tel. 719/767–5661, (Nonreporting) **A**9 10 20
Primary Contact: Steve Carty, Chief Executive Officer
CFO: Kara Hoover, Controller and Director Human Resources
CMO: Christopher Williams, M.D., Chief of Staff
CHR: Kara Hoover, Controller and Director Human Resources
Web address: www.keefememorialhospital.org
Control: County–Government, nonfederal **Service:** General Medical and Surgical

Staffed Beds: 12

COLORADO SPRINGS—El Paso County

☐ **CEDAR SPRINGS BEHAVIORAL HEALTH SYSTEM (64009)**, 2135 Southgate Road, Zip 80906–2693; tel. 719/633–4114 **A**1 9 10 **F**4 5 25 62 73 88 89 90 91 92 93 94 119 **S** Psychiatric Solutions
Primary Contact: Elaine Crnkovic, Chief Executive Officer
CFO: Melissa Bodin, Chief Financial Officer
CMO: Larry Shores, M.D., Executive Medical Director
CIO: Lynn Threlfall, Director Medical Records
CHR: Amy Tomlin, Director Human Resources
Web address: www.psysolutions.com
Control: Corporation, Investor–owned, for–profit **Service:** Psychiatric

Staffed Beds: 110 **Admissions:** 2339 **Census:** 85 **Outpatient Visits:** 5952 **Births:** 0 **Personnel:** 187

☒ **HEALTHSOUTH REHABILITATION HOSPITAL OF COLORADO SPRINGS (63030)**, 325 Parkside Drive, Zip 80910; tel. 719/630–8000, (Nonreporting) **A**1 10 **S** HEALTHSOUTH Corporation
Primary Contact: William B. Mohon, Chief Executive Officer
CFO: Michele Osika, Controller
CHR: Jennifer Venendaal, Manager Human Resources
Web address: www.healthsouth.com
Control: Corporation, Investor–owned, for–profit **Service:** Rehabilitation

Staffed Beds: 64

☒ △ **MEMORIAL HEALTH SYSTEM (60022)**, 1400 East Boulder Street, Zip 80909–5599, Mailing Address: P.O. Box 1326, Zip 80901–1326; tel. 719/365–5000, (Nonreporting) **A**1 2 7 9 10
Primary Contact: Lawrence McEvoy, M.D., Chief Executive Officer
CMO: Lawrence McEvoy, M.D., Chief Executive Officer
CIO: Thomas Kerwin, Vice President and Chief Information Officer
CHR: Carlene Crall, Senior Vice President and Chief Human Resources Officer
Web address: www.memorialhealthsystem.com
Control: City–Government, nonfederal **Service:** General Medical and Surgical

Staffed Beds: 384

☒ **PENROSE–ST. FRANCIS HEALTH SERVICES (60031)**, 2215 North Cascade Avenue, Zip 80907–6799, Mailing Address: P.O. Box 7021, Zip 80933–7021; tel. 719/776–5000, (Includes PENROSE COMMUNITY HOSPITAL, 3205 North Academy Boulevard, Zip 80917; tel. 719/776–5000; PENROSE HOSPITAL; ST FRANCIS HEALTH CENTER, 825 East Pikes Peak Avenue, Zip 80903; tel. 719/776–5000) **A**1 2 9 10 19 **F**3 5 11 12 13 14 15 17 18 20 22 24 25 26 27 30 31 32 33 34 36 37 38 39 40 41 43 44 46 47 48 49 50 52 53 54 55 56 57 60 61 62 63 66 68 69 70 72 73 74 75 76 77 79 80 81 82 84 85 86 87 88 89 90 91 92 93 94 96 97 101 102 103 106 107 108 109 111 112 113 114 116 118 119 120 121 124 133 135 136 137 **S** Catholic Health Initiatives
Primary Contact: Philip Shaw, Interim Chief Executive Officer
COO: Andrea C. Coleman, Chief Operating Officer
CFO: Michael A. Scialdone, Chief Financial Officer
CMO: Jeffrey C. Oram–Smith, M.D., Chief Medical Officer
CIO: Tanya Bell, Public Information Officer
CHR: James Humphrey, Director Human Resource and Educational Resources
Web address: www.penrosestfrancis.org
Control: Church–operated, Nongovernment, not–for profit **Service:** General Medical and Surgical

Staffed Beds: 443 **Admissions:** 23258 **Census:** 261 **Outpatient Visits:** 218629 **Births:** 3031 **Total Expense ($000):** 278000 **Payroll Expense ($000):** 99512 **Personnel:** 1976

☐ **SELECT LONG TERM CARE HOSPITAL OF COLORADO SPRINGS (62016)**, 825 Pikes Peak Avenue, Zip 80903; tel. 719/667–1009, (Nonreporting) **A**1 10
Primary Contact: Valerie Brickell, Chief Executive Officer
Web address: www.selectmedicalcorp.com
Control: Corporation, Investor–owned, for–profit **Service:** Long–Term Acute Care hospital

Staffed Beds: 30

CORTEZ—Montezuma County

☒ **SOUTHWEST MEMORIAL HOSPITAL (60018)**, 1311 North Mildred Road, Zip 81321–2299; tel. 970/565–6666, (Nonreporting) **A**1 9 10 20 **S** QHR
Primary Contact: Nelson Toebbe, Interim Chief Executive Officer
COO: Liz Sellers, R.N., Chief Clinical Officer
CFO: Daniel L. Jessup, Chief Financial Officer
CIO: David Cabana, Director Management Information Systems
CHR: Gary Wallace, Director Human Resources
Web address: www.swhealth.org
Control: Other not–for–profit (including NFP Corporation) **Service:** General Medical and Surgical

Staffed Beds: 49

CRAIG—Moffat County

☒ **MEMORIAL HOSPITAL (61314)**, 785 Russell Street, Zip 81625–9906; tel. 970/824–9411 **A**1 9 10 18 **F**7 11 12 13 15 25 30 31 32 33 38 40 57 68 73 74 79 80 82 86 87 92 96 100 103 107 118 122 135 137 **S** QHR
Primary Contact: George A. Rohrich, Chief Executive Officer
COO: Robert A. Lindberg, Chief Clinical Officer
CFO: Barry Bergman, Chief Financial Officer
CMO: Allan Reishus, M.D., Chief of Staff
CIO: Samantha Johnston, Service Excellence Officer
Web address: www.thememorialhospital.com
Control: County–Government, nonfederal **Service:** General Medical and Surgical

Staffed Beds: 25 **Admissions:** 816 **Census:** 9 **Outpatient Visits:** 18078 **Births:** 83 **Total Expense ($000):** 16751 **Payroll Expense ($000):** 6814 **Personnel:** 136

DEL NORTE—Rio Grande County

★ **RIO GRANDE HOSPITAL (61301)**, 310 County Road 14, Zip 81132; tel. 719/657–2510 **A**9 10 18 **F**30 31 32 38 40 51 54 55 56 62 63 64 79 86 87 96 102 122 **P**6
Primary Contact: Arlene Harms, Chief Executive Officer
CFO: Greg Porter, Chief Financial Officer
Control: Other not–for–profit (including NFP Corporation) **Service:** General Medical and Surgical

Staffed Beds: 17 **Admissions:** 345 **Census:** 3 **Outpatient Visits:** 38472 **Births:** 0 **Total Expense ($000):** 9164 **Payroll Expense ($000):** 3533 **Personnel:** 92

CO

Hospital, Medicare Provider Number, Address, Telephone, Approval, Facility, and Physician Codes, Health Care System
★ American Hospital Association (AHA) membership
☐ The Joint Commission accreditation
○ American Osteopathic Association (AOA) accreditation
△ Commission on Accreditation of Rehabilitation Facilities (CARF) accreditation

DELTA—Delta County

★ **DELTA COUNTY MEMORIAL HOSPITAL (60071)**, 1501 East 3rd Street, Zip 81416–2297, Mailing Address: P.O. Box 10100, Zip 81416–5003; tel. 970/874–7681 **A**1 9 10 **F**3 13 24 26 27 30 31 38 40 55 61 68 73 74 76 77 79 80 82 86 96 100 102 103 107 118 124 135 137 **P**5 8
Primary Contact: Tom Mingen, Chief Executive Officer
COO: Veronica Franco, Chief Clinical Officer
CFO: Bev Carlson, Chief Financial Officer
CMO: Lee Bules, Chief Medical Staff
CIO: Mitch Van Scoyk, Manager
CHR: Cindy Winzenburg, Director Human Resources
Web address: www.deltahospital.org
Control: Hospital district or authority, Government, nonfederal **Service:** General Medical and Surgical

Staffed Beds: 49 **Admissions:** 3066 **Census:** 27 **Outpatient Visits:** 88652 **Births:** 273 **Total Expense ($000):** 44749 **Payroll Expense ($000):** 19778 **Personnel:** 450

DENVER—Denver, Adams and Arapahoe Counties

☐ **COLORADO ACUTE LONG TERM HOSPITAL (62012)**, 1601 North Lowell Boulevard, Zip 80204–1545; tel. 303/899–5166, (Nonreporting) **A**1 9 10 **S** LifeCare Management Services
Primary Contact: Kent Ashley, Chief Executive Officer
Web address: www.lifecare–hospitals.com
Control: Other not–for–profit (including NFP Corporation) **Service:** Long–Term Acute Care hospital

Staffed Beds: 24

CO

☐ **COLORADO MENTAL HEALTH INSTITUTE AT FORT LOGAN (64003)**, 3520 West Oxford Avenue, Zip 80236–3197; tel. 303/761–0220, (Nonreporting) **A**1 10
Primary Contact: Elizabeth M. Stillman, Acting Director
CFO: Bob Fries, Director Fiscal Services
CIO: Billie Busby, Assistant Director
Web address: www.cdhs.state.co.us/cmhifl
Control: State–Government, nonfederal **Service:** Psychiatric

Staffed Beds: 297

☐ **DENVER HEALTH MEDICAL CENTER (60011)**, 777 Bannock Street, Zip 80204–4507; tel. 303/436–6000 **A**1 3 5 9 10 **F**3 4 5 7 8 11 12 13 15 18 20 24 25 26 27 28 30 31 32 33 35 36 37 38 40 41 43 46 49 50 52 53 54 55 56 57 58 59 60 62 63 64 66 68 69 70 72 73 74 75 76 77 78 79 80 81 82 83 84 85 86 87 88 89 90 92 93 94 96 97 100 102 107 113 114 118 119 120 121 123 124 132 133 135 136 137 **P**6
Primary Contact: Patricia A. Gabow, M.D., Chief Executive Officer
COO: Stephanie Thomas, Chief Operating Officer
CFO: Peg Burnette, Chief Financial Officer
CMO: Philip Mehler, M.D., Chief Medical Officer
CIO: Bobbi Barrow, Chief Communications Officer
CHR: Greg Rossman, Chief Human Resource Officer
Web address: www.denverhealth.org
Control: Hospital district or authority, Government, nonfederal **Service:** General Medical and Surgical

Staffed Beds: 379 **Admissions:** 18902 **Census:** 260 **Outpatient Visits:** 444569 **Births:** 3439 **Total Expense ($000):** 532415 **Payroll Expense ($000):** 273337 **Personnel:** 4590

★ **EXEMPLA SAINT JOSEPH HOSPITAL (60028)**, 1835 Franklin Street, Zip 80218–1191; tel. 303/837–7111 **A**1 2 3 5 9 10 **F**3 12 13 14 15 18 20 22 24 25 26 27 33 35 38 40 42 44 51 57 59 60 62 66 68 69 70 72 73 74 75 76 77 78 79 81 82 86 87 92 96 97 100 102 103 106 107 109 119 135 136 **P**6 **S** Exempla Healthcare, Inc.
Primary Contact: Robert A. Minkin, CHE, President and Chief Executive Officer
COO: Margo A. Karsten, Chief Operating Officer
CFO: Brad Ludford, Vice President Finance
CMO: Sheldon Stadnyk, M.D., Vice President Medical Affairs and Chief Medical Officer
CHR: Vanita Bellen, Vice President Human Resources
Web address: www.exempla.org
Control: Other not–for–profit (including NFP Corporation) **Service:** General Medical and Surgical

Staffed Beds: 436 **Admissions:** 21166 **Census:** 243 **Outpatient Visits:** 124589 **Births:** 5133

☐ **KINDRED HOSPITAL–DENVER (62009)**, 1920 High Street, Zip 80218–1213; tel. 303/320–5871, (Nonreporting) **A**1 9 10 **S** Kindred Healthcare
Primary Contact: April Myers, Chief Executive Officer
CFO: Tim Stecker, Chief Financial Officer
CMO: Eric Yeager, M.D., Medical Director
Web address: www.kh–denver.com
Control: Corporation, Investor–owned, for–profit **Service:** Long–Term Acute Care hospital

Staffed Beds: 55

★ **NATIONAL JEWISH MEDICAL AND RESEARCH CENTER (60107)**, (Resp/Immunologic), 1400 Jackson Street, Zip 80206–2762; tel. 303/388–4461 **A**1 3 5 9 10 **F**3 9 11 12 24 25 26 28 30 33 48 50 52 56 57 58 60 62 64 66 73 75 81 82 84 86 89 90 94 96 97 102 106 107 118 119 121 123 124 132 133 135 **P**6
Primary Contact: Michael Salem, M.D., President and Chief Executive Officer
COO: J. Verne Singleton, Chief Administrative Officer
CFO: Christine Forkner, Chief Financial Officer
CIO: Jim Harbin, Director Information Systems
CHR: Susan Roll, Chief Human Resources
Web address: www.nationaljewish.org
Control: Other not–for–profit (including NFP Corporation) **Service:** Other specialty

Staffed Beds: 46 **Admissions:** 125 **Census:** 1 **Outpatient Visits:** 39980 **Births:** 0 **Total Expense ($000):** 130310 **Payroll Expense ($000):** 68224 **Personnel:** 1079

★ **PORTER ADVENTIST HOSPITAL (60064)**, 2525 South Downing Street, Zip 80210–5876; tel. 303/778–1955 **A**1 2 9 10 **F**3 15 18 20 22 24 25 26 27 30 31 32 34 35 38 44 45 52 53 56 58 59 62 68 72 73 75 76 77 79 81 82 85 86 88 90 91 92 93 94 95 96 97 99 100 102 103 104 106 107 109 114 116 118 119 120 124 127 128 135 137 **P**6 **S** Adventist Health System Sunbelt Health Care Corporation
Primary Contact: James W. Boyle, Chief Executive Officer
COO: Mark LaRose, Chief Operating Officer
CFO: Michael Blair, Chief Financial Officer
CMO: Diane McCallister, M.D., Chief Medical Officer
Web address: www.centura.org
Control: Church–operated, Nongovernment, not–for profit **Service:** General Medical and Surgical

Staffed Beds: 220 **Admissions:** 10633 **Census:** 145 **Outpatient Visits:** 73254 **Births:** 0 **Total Expense ($000):** 182090 **Payroll Expense ($000):** 69125 **Personnel:** 1430

★ △ **PRESBYTERIAN–ST. LUKE'S MEDICAL CENTER (60014)**, 1719 East 19th Avenue, Zip 80218–1281; tel. 303/839–6000, (Nonreporting) **A**1 2 7 9 10 **S** HCA
Primary Contact: Madeleine Roberson, President and Chief Executive Officer
CFO: Douglas A. Zehner, Chief Financial Officer
CIO: Mark Chankij, Director Information Services
CHR: Eric Artis, Director Human Resources
Web address: www.pslmc.com
Control: Partnership, Investor–owned, for–profit **Service:** General Medical and Surgical

Staffed Beds: 400

★ **ROSE MEDICAL CENTER (60032)**, 4567 East Ninth Avenue, Zip 80220–3941; tel. 303/320–2121 **A**1 2 3 5 9 10 **F**3 8 9 11 12 13 15 18 20 22 24 25 26 27 28 30 31 32 33 35 38 40 41 43 44 46 50 52 53 55 56 57 59 60 62 64 66 68 69 70 72 73 74 75 76 77 79 80 81 82 84 86 87 92 96 97 98 99 100 101 102 103 104 105 107 108 109 110 113 114 116 118 119 120 122 124 125 132 134 135 136 137 **P**5 6 8 **S** HCA
Primary Contact: Kenneth H. Feiler, President and Chief Executive Officer
CFO: Jack Connelly, Chief Financial Officer
CIO: Maureen Murphy, Director Information Systems
Web address: www.rosebabies.com
Control: Corporation, Investor–owned, for–profit **Service:** General Medical and Surgical

Staffed Beds: 294 **Admissions:** 13745 **Census:** 150 **Outpatient Visits:** 138220 **Births:** 3886 **Total Expense ($000):** 164174 **Payroll Expense ($000):** 63835 **Personnel:** 1498

☐ **SELECT SPECIALTY HOSPITAL – DENVER (62015)**, 1719 East 19th Avenue, 5th Floor, Zip 80218; tel. 303/563–3700, (Nonreporting) **A**1 9 10 **S** Select Medical Corporation
Primary Contact: Lynn Dawson, Chief Executive Officer
Web address: www.selectmedicalcorp.com
Control: Corporation, Investor–owned, for–profit **Service:** Long–Term Acute Care hospital

Staffed Beds: 65

★ **ST. ANTHONY CENTRAL HOSPITAL (60015)**, 4231 West 16th Avenue, Zip 80204–4098; tel. 303/629–3511 **A**1 2 3 5 9 10 **F**3 7 11 12 13 17 18 20 22 24 25 26 27 30 31 32 33 34 38 40 46 47 48 49 50 52 54 55 57 62 66 68 70 72 73 74 75 76 77 79 80 82 85 86 87 92 96 97 102 106 107 109 111 112 118 119 121 122 123 124 135 136 **S** Catholic Health Initiatives
Primary Contact: Peter E. Makowski, Chief Executive Officer
CFO: David Thompson, Chief Financial Officer
CMO: Jodi Chambers, M.D., Chief Medical Officer
CIO: Dana Moore, Senior Vice President Information Services
CHR: Gary Jones, Vice President Human Resources
Web address: www.stanthonyhosp.org
Control: Church–operated, Nongovernment, not–for profit **Service:** General Medical and Surgical

Staffed Beds: 265 **Admissions:** 13337 **Census:** 170 **Outpatient Visits:** 55761 **Births:** 1001 **Total Expense ($000):** 219023 **Payroll Expense ($000):** 67012 **Personnel:** 996

UNIVERSITY OF COLORADO HOSPITAL See Aurora

 Many Facility Codes have changed. Please refer to the AHA Guide Code Chart.

☒ △ **VETERANS AFFAIRS EASTERN COLORADO HEALTH CARE SYSTEM**, 1055 Clermont Street, Zip 80220–3877; tel. 303/399–8020, (Nonreporting) **A**1 3 5 7 8 **S** Department of Veterans Affairs
Primary Contact: Lynette A. Roff, Director
COO: Terry S. Atienza, Associate Director
CFO: Eliott R. Vanderstek, Chief Fiscal Service
CMO: Ellen Mangione, M.D., Chief of Staff
CIO: Don Huckaby, Chief Information Management Service
CHR: Lorene Connel, Chief Human Resources Management Service
Web address: www.va.gov/sta/guide/home.asp
Control: Veterans Affairs, Government, federal **Service:** General Medical and Surgical

Staffed Beds: 222

DURANGO—La Plata County

ANIMAS SURGICAL HOSPITAL (60117), 575 Rivergate Lane, Zip 81301; tel. 970/247–3537, (Nonreporting) **A**9 10
Primary Contact: Brett Gosney, Chief Executive Officer
Web address: www.animassurgical.com/index.htm
Control: Corporation, Investor–owned, for–profit **Service:** Surgical

Staffed Beds: 12

☒ **MERCY REGIONAL MEDICAL CENTER (60013)**, 1010 Three Springs Boulevard, Zip 81301–5089; tel. 970/247–4311 **A**1 2 9 10 20 **F**11 13 15 18 20 24 25 26 27 30 31 32 33 34 38 40 44 50 57 59 60 64 68 70 71 74 75 77 79 80 84 96 100 103 107 118 119 120 121 124 135 136 137 **P**6 **S** Catholic Health Initiatives
Primary Contact: Kirk Dignum, Ph.D., President and Chief Executive Officer
CFO: George Sprinkel, Financial Officer
CMO: John A K Boyd, M.D., Executive Director Mission and Chief Medical Officer
CIO: Neil Stock, Director Information Services
CHR: Cathy Roberts, Director Human Resources
Web address: www.mercydurango.org
Control: Church–operated, Nongovernment, not–for profit **Service:** General Medical and Surgical

Staffed Beds: 82 **Admissions:** 4583 **Census:** 41 **Outpatient Visits:** 113743 **Births:** 1047 **Total Expense ($000):** 84136 **Payroll Expense ($000):** 31792 **Personnel:** 582

EADS—Kiowa County

★ **WEISBROD MEMORIAL COUNTY HOSPITAL (61300)**, (Critical Access Hospital), 1208 Luther Street, Zip 81036, Mailing Address: P.O. Box 817, Zip 81036–0817; tel. 719/438–5401, (Total facility includes 34 beds in nursing home–type unit) **A**9 10 18 **F**38 43 56 57 61 62 63 64 65 66 85 86 87 119 122 **P**6
Primary Contact: Warren Yule, Administrator and Chief Executive Officer
CFO: Shannon Dixon, Manager Business Office
CMO: Jeff Waggoner, M.D., Chief of Staff
CHR: Shannon Dixon, Manager Business Office
Web address: www.weisbrod.org
Control: County–Government, nonfederal **Service:** Other specialty

Staffed Beds: 42 **Admissions:** 68 **Census:** 19 **Outpatient Visits:** 8823 **Births:** 0 **Personnel:** 80

ENGLEWOOD—Arapahoe County

☒ **CRAIG HOSPITAL (62011)**, 3425 South Clarkson Street, Zip 80113–2899; tel. 303/789–8000 **A**1 3 5 9 10 **F**25 26 30 33 34 41 50 52 53 56 58 62 66 72 73 75 79 81 82 85 86 119 121 135 137
Primary Contact: Dennis O'Malley, President
COO: Kelly Johnson, Chief Operating Officer
CFO: Ron Branish, Vice President Finance
CMO: Daniel P. Lammertse, M.D., Medical Director
Web address: www.craighospital.org
Control: Other not–for–profit (including NFP Corporation) **Service:** Rehabilitation

Staffed Beds: 78 **Admissions:** 426 **Census:** 74 **Outpatient Visits:** 5213 **Births:** 0 **Total Expense ($000):** 60840 **Payroll Expense ($000):** 27941 **Personnel:** 587

☒ **SWEDISH MEDICAL CENTER (60034)**, 501 East Hampden Avenue, Zip 80113; tel. 303/788–5000 **A**1 2 3 5 9 10 **F**3 7 8 11 12 13 15 17 18 20 22 25 26 27 30 31 32 33 36 37 38 39 40 41 43 44 47 48 49 50 52 53 55 56 57 58 59 62 64 66 68 70 71 72 73 74 75 76 77 79 80 81 82 83 84 85 87 96 97 98 100 102 103 104 105 106 107 108 109 110 111 112 113 114 116 118 119 120 121 135 136 137 **S** HCA
Primary Contact: Mary M. White, President and Chief Executive Officer
CFO: Kathy Ashenfelter, Chief Financial Officer
CMO: Matthew Fleishman, M.D., President Medical Staff
CIO: Robert Hollowell, Director Information Systems
Web address: www.swedishhospital.com
Control: Partnership, Investor–owned, for–profit **Service:** General Medical and Surgical

Staffed Beds: 350 **Admissions:** 16372 **Census:** 222 **Outpatient Visits:** 106710 **Births:** 2169 **Personnel:** 1288

ESTES PARK—Larimer County

★ **ESTES PARK MEDICAL CENTER (61312)**, 555 Prospect Avenue, Zip 80517–2740, Mailing Address: P.O. Box 2740, Zip 80517–2740; tel. 970/586–2317, (Total facility includes 45 beds in nursing home–type unit) **A**9 10 18 **F**3 7 8 13 15 25 26 27 32 38 40 42 46 54 55 56 61 62 73 74 75 77 79 80 81 82 86 87 96 115 117 119 121 122 132 133 135 137 **P**7
Primary Contact: Robert S. Austin, FACHE, Chief Executive Officer
COO: Marcia L. DePriest, R.N., Chief Clinical Officer
CFO: Shirley Holt, Chief Financial Officer
CMO: Bruce Woolman, M.D., Chief of Staff
CHR: Tim Coakley, Director Human Resources
Web address: www.epmedcenter.com
Control: Hospital district or authority, Government, nonfederal **Service:** General Medical and Surgical

Staffed Beds: 61 **Admissions:** 539 **Census:** 43 **Outpatient Visits:** 57564 **Births:** 71 **Total Expense ($000):** 23362 **Payroll Expense ($000):** 10247 **Personnel:** 226

FORT CARSON—El Paso County

☒ **EVANS U. S. ARMY COMMUNITY HOSPITAL**, 1650 Cochrane Circle, Building 7500, Zip 80913–5101; tel. 719/526–7200, (Nonreporting) **A**1 2 **S** Department of the Army, Office of the Surgeon General
Primary Contact: Colonel John Cho, Commander
COO: Lieutenant Colonel Noel J. Cardenas, Chief Operating Officer
CFO: Major Bradley Robinson, Chief Financial Officer
CMO: Colonel James Terrio, M.D., Chief Medical Officer
CIO: Major Barry Ryle, Chief Information Officer
CHR: Lieutenant Colonel Lory Gurr, Chief Human Resources Division
Web address: www.evans.amedd.army.mil
Control: Army, Government, federal **Service:** General Medical and Surgical

Staffed Beds: 78

FORT COLLINS—Larimer County

☒ **POUDRE VALLEY HOSPITAL (60010)**, 1024 South Lemay Avenue, Zip 80524–3998; tel. 970/495–7000, (Includes MOUNTAIN CREST HOSPITAL, 4601 Corbett Drive, Zip 80525; tel. 970/270–4800) **A**1 2 9 10 **F**3 5 7 11 12 13 14 15 18 20 22 24 25 26 27 28 30 32 33 36 37 38 40 43 44 45 47 49 50 52 53 56 57 58 59 60 62 63 66 67 68 72 73 74 75 76 77 78 79 80 81 82 84 85 86 87 88 89 90 91 92 93 94 95 96 97 100 102 106 107 108 109 112 116 118 119 120 121 123 124 133 135 136 137 **S** Poudre Valley Health System
Primary Contact: Kevin L. Unger, FACHE, President and Chief Executive Officer
COO: Dan Robinson, Vice President Operations
CFO: Stephanie Doughty, Chief Financial Officer
CMO: William Neff, M.D., Chief Medical Officer
CIO: Russ Branzell, Chief Information Officer
CHR: Patti Oakes, Director Human Resources
Web address: www.pvhs.org
Control: Other not–for–profit (including NFP Corporation) **Service:** General Medical and Surgical

Staffed Beds: 233 **Admissions:** 15821 **Census:** 171 **Outpatient Visits:** 442986 **Births:** 2566 **Total Expense ($000):** 291656 **Payroll Expense ($000):** 134016 **Personnel:** 2760

CO

Hospital, Medicare Provider Number, Address, Telephone, Approval, Facility, and Physician Codes, Health Care System

★ American Hospital Association (AHA) membership
☐ The Joint Commission accreditation
○ American Osteopathic Association (AOA) accreditation
△ Commission on Accreditation of Rehabilitation Facilities (CARF) accreditation

FORT MORGAN—Morgan County

⊠ **COLORADO PLAINS MEDICAL CENTER (60044)**, 1000 Lincoln Street, Zip 80701–3298; tel. 970/867–3391 **A**1 9 10 20 **F**11 13 15 24 25 26 27 30 31 32 33 34 38 40 43 51 52 54 55 56 57 61 62 66 68 69 73 74 75 77 79 80 82 86 87 88 90 91 93 96 100 102 104 105 107 108 109 119 120 122 124 132 135 136 137 **P**6 **S** LifePoint Hospitals, Inc.
Primary Contact: Michael A. Anaya, Sr., FACHE, Chief Executive Officer
CFO: Michael Patterson, Chief Financial Officer
CHR: Lorna Fulton, Director Human Resources
Web address: www.coloradoplainsmedicalcenter.com
Control: Corporation, Investor–owned, for–profit **Service:** General Medical and Surgical

Staffed Beds: 50 **Admissions:** 1908 **Census:** 14 **Outpatient Visits:** 23387 **Births:** 373 **Total Expense ($000):** 22187 **Payroll Expense ($000):** 9579

FRISCO—Summit County

⊠ **ST. ANTHONY SUMMIT MEDICAL CENTER (60118)**, 340 Peak One Drive, Zip 80443, Mailing Address: P.O. Box 738, Zip 80443–0738; tel. 970/668–3300, (Includes ST. ANTHONY GRANBY MEDICAL CENTER, 480 East Agate, Granby, Zip 80446, Mailing Address: P.O. Box 397, Zip 80446; tel. 970/887–7400; Paul J. Chodkowski, Chief Executive Officer) **A**1 9 10 **F**13 25 26 30 31 32 33 34 38 39 40 43 44 55 56 57 66 68 73 74 75 77 79 80 85 90 96 100 102 107 119 121 133 135 136 **S** Catholic Health Initiatives
Primary Contact: Paul J. Chodkowski, Chief Executive Officer
CFO: David Thompson, Chief Financial Officer
CHR: Dana Laverdiere, Generalist
Web address: www.summitmedicalcenter.org
Control: Church–operated, Nongovernment, not–for profit **Service:** General Medical and Surgical

Staffed Beds: 22 **Admissions:** 1322 **Census:** 10 **Outpatient Visits:** 19296 **Births:** 331 **Total Expense ($000):** 31078 **Payroll Expense ($000):** 10071 **Personnel:** 130

FRUITA—Mesa County

★ **FAMILY HEALTH WEST (61302)**, 228 North Cherry Street, Zip 81521–2101, Mailing Address: P.O. Box 130, Zip 81521–0130; tel. 970/858–9871, (Total facility includes 352 beds in nursing home–type unit) (Nonreporting) **A**9 10 18
Primary Contact: Dennis E. Ficklin, Chief Executive Officer
COO: Errol Snider, Chief Operating Officer
CFO: Dennis E. Ficklin, Chief Executive Officer
Web address: www.familyhealthwest.org
Control: Other not–for–profit (including NFP Corporation) **Service:** General Medical and Surgical

Staffed Beds: 358

GLENWOOD SPRINGS—Garfield County

⊠ **VALLEY VIEW HOSPITAL (60075)**, 1906 Blake Avenue, Zip 81601–4259, Mailing Address: P.O. Box 1970, Zip 81602–1970; tel. 970/945–6535 **A**1 9 10 20 **F**3 4 11 12 13 14 15 18 20 24 25 26 27 30 31 32 33 34 35 38 40 41 42 43 44 46 47 48 49 51 53 54 55 56 57 62 66 67 68 71 72 73 74 75 76 77 79 80 81 82 85 86 87 96 97 99 100 103 106 107 118 119 120 121 124 134 135 136 **P**6
Primary Contact: Gary L. Brewer, Chief Executive Officer
COO: Deb Wiepking, Chief Clinical Officer
CFO: Larry L. Dupper, Chief Financial Officer
CMO: Drew Werner, M.D., Chief of Staff
CIO: Ron Hines, Director Information Technology
CHR: Daniel Biggs, Director Human Resources
Web address: www.vvh.org
Control: Other not–for–profit (including NFP Corporation) **Service:** General Medical and Surgical

Staffed Beds: 76 **Admissions:** 3147 **Census:** 32 **Outpatient Visits:** 123977 **Births:** 843 **Total Expense ($000):** 86966 **Payroll Expense ($000):** 33666 **Personnel:** 366

GRANBY—Grand County

ST. ANTHONY GRANBY MEDICAL CENTER See St. Anthony Summit Medical Center, Frisco

GRAND JUNCTION—Mesa County

⊠ ○ **COMMUNITY HOSPITAL (60054)**, 2021 North 12th Street, Zip 81501–2999; tel. 970/242–0920, (Nonreporting) **A**1 9 10 11 **S** QHR
Primary Contact: Wesley White, President
COO: Gary Wallace, Chief Operating Officer
CFO: Robert Elberfeld, Interim Chief Financial Officer
CIO: Mike Kansgen, Director Information Services
CHR: Paula Kocherar, Human Resources Leader
Web address: www.gjhosp.org
Control: Other not–for–profit (including NFP Corporation) **Service:** General Medical and Surgical

Staffed Beds: 40

⊠ **ST. MARY'S HOSPITAL AND MEDICAL CENTER (60023)**, 2635 North 7th Street, Zip 81501–8204, Mailing Address: P.O. Box 1628, Zip 81502–1628; tel. 970/244–2273 **A**1 2 3 5 9 10 19 20 **F**3 13 14 15 17 18 19 20 21 22 24 25 26 27 28 30 31 32 33 34 35 36 38 40 41 43 49 50 51 52 53 55 56 57 58 59 60 62 66 67 68 70 71 72 73 74 75 76 77 79 80 81 82 84 85 86 87 90 94 96 97 98 99 100 102 103 104 105 106 107 109 111 112 116 118 119 120 121 124 135 136 137 **P**6 **S** Sisters of Charity of Leavenworth Health System
Primary Contact: Robert W. Ladenburger, President and Chief Executive Officer
COO: Cherie Gorby, R.N., MSN, Executive Vice President and Chief Operating Officer
CFO: Forest Binder, Vice President Finance
CMO: John C. Beeson, M.D., Vice President Medical Affairs
CIO: Jane Wild, Director Information Technology
CHR: Terry Stefaniak, Director Human Resources
Web address: www.stmarygj.com
Control: Church–operated, Nongovernment, not–for profit **Service:** General Medical and Surgical

Staffed Beds: 280 **Admissions:** 13419 **Census:** 163 **Outpatient Visits:** 353033 **Births:** 2322 **Total Expense ($000):** 228352 **Payroll Expense ($000):** 98916 **Personnel:** 1652

⊠ **VETERANS AFFAIRS MEDICAL CENTER**, 2121 North Avenue, Zip 81501–6499; tel. 970/242–0731, (Total facility includes 30 beds in nursing home–type unit) **A**1 9 **F**3 5 11 12 24 25 26 30 31 32 33 34 36 37 41 42 43 44 49 50 53 54 55 56 57 60 61 62 64 68 72 73 75 76 77 79 80 81 82 86 87 88 90 91 92 93 94 95 96 100 102 103 107 117 119 121 124 134 135 136 137 **P**6 **S** Department of Veterans Affairs
Primary Contact: William R. Berryman, M.D., Acting Director
COO: Patricia A. Hitt, Associate Director
CFO: Laquita Gruver, Fiscal Officer
CMO: William R. Berryman, M.D., Chief of Staff
CIO: Craig Frerichs, Chief Information Technology Service
CHR: William Chester, Manager Human Resources
Web address: www.va.gov/sta/guide/home.asp
Control: Veterans Affairs, Government, federal **Service:** General Medical and Surgical

Staffed Beds: 53 **Admissions:** 1659 **Census:** 42 **Outpatient Visits:** 94668 **Births:** 0 **Total Expense ($000):** 63601 **Payroll Expense ($000):** 25641 **Personnel:** 410

GREELEY—Weld County

⊠ **NORTH COLORADO MEDICAL CENTER (60001)**, 1801 16th Street, Zip 80631–5199; tel. 970/352–4121 **A**1 2 9 10 **F**3 4 5 11 12 13 14 15 16 18 20 22 24 25 26 27 28 30 31 32 33 35 37 38 40 43 46 48 49 50 51 52 53 54 55 56 57 60 61 62 66 68 69 70 72 73 74 75 76 77 78 79 80 81 82 84 85 86 87 88 89 90 91 92 93 94 95 96 97 99 100 102 103 104 105 106 107 108 109 111 112 116 117 118 119 120 121 124 131 132 134 135 136 137 **P**6 7 8 **S** Banner Health
Primary Contact: Richard O. Sutton, Chief Executive Officer
CFO: Mary McCabe, Chief Financial Officer
CMO: George Liesmann, M.D., Chief Medical Officer
CIO: Paul Panico, Associate Administrator
CHR: Lucy Dupree, Chief Human Resources Officer
Web address: www.ncmcgreeley.com
Control: Other not–for–profit (including NFP Corporation) **Service:** General Medical and Surgical

Staffed Beds: 282 **Admissions:** 16489 **Census:** 181 **Outpatient Visits:** 517004 **Births:** 2356 **Total Expense ($000):** 285879 **Payroll Expense ($000):** 109360 **Personnel:** 1777

GUNNISON—Gunnison County

★ **GUNNISON VALLEY HOSPITAL (61320)**, 711 North Taylor Street, Zip 81230–2296; tel. 970/641–1456 **A**9 10 18 **F**3 7 11 13 15 24 25 26 27 30 31 32 33 38 40 54 55 56 57 61 62 66 68 74 75 76 77 79 80 82 86 96 100 102 107 118 121 122 124 135 136 137
Primary Contact: M. Randell Phelps, Chief Executive Officer
COO: Betsy Bair, Chief Operating Officer
CFO: Tim Cashman, Chief Financial Officer
CMO: John S. Tarr, M.D., Chief of Staff
CIO: Trevor Smith, Chief Management Information Services
CHR: Elaine Crumpton, Director Human Resources
Web address: www.gvh-colorado.org
Control: County–Government, nonfederal **Service:** General Medical and Surgical

Staffed Beds: 24 **Admissions:** 596 **Census:** 4 **Outpatient Visits:** 41221 **Births:** 161 **Total Expense ($000):** 17156 **Payroll Expense ($000):** 7135 **Personnel:** 138

 Many Facility Codes have changed. Please refer to the AHA Guide Code Chart.

HAXTUN—Phillips County

★ **HAXTUN HOSPITAL DISTRICT (61304)**, 235 West Fletcher Street, Zip 80731–0308; tel. 970/774–6123, (Total facility includes 32 beds in nursing home–type unit) (Nonreporting) **A**9 10 18
Primary Contact: Natalie Lamberton, Chief Executive Officer
COO: Lona Salyards, Director Health Information Management and Business Office
CFO: Sandra Lambrecht, Chief Financial Officer
CMO: Paul Simmons, M.D., Chief of Staff
CHR: Brenda Lechman, Director Human Resources
Web address: www.haxtunhealth.org
Control: Hospital district or authority, Government, nonfederal **Service:** General Medical and Surgical

Staffed Beds: 57

HIGHLANDS RANCH—Adams County

HIGHLANDS BEHAVIORAL HEALTH SYSTEM (64024), 8565 South Poplar Way, Zip 80130; tel. 720/348–2800, (Nonreporting) **A**10 **S** Universal Health Services, Inc.
Web address: www.highlandsbhs.com
Control: Corporation, Investor–owned, for–profit **Service:** Psychiatric

Staffed Beds: 86

HOLYOKE—Phillips County

★ **MELISSA MEMORIAL HOSPITAL (61305)**, 1001 East Johnson Street, Zip 80734; tel. 970/854–2241, (Nonreporting) **A**9 10 18
Primary Contact: John J. Ayoub, FACHE, Administrator
CFO: Shelly Larson, Chief Financial Officer
CMO: Dennis Jelden, M.D., Chief of Staff
CHR: Sharon Greenman, Director Human Resources
Web address: www.melissamemorial.org
Control: Hospital district or authority, Government, nonfederal **Service:** General Medical and Surgical

Staffed Beds: 19

HUGO—Lincoln County

★ **LINCOLN COMMUNITY HOSPITAL AND NURSING HOME (61306)**, 111 6th Street, Zip 80821–0248, Mailing Address: P.O. Box 248, Zip 80821–0248; tel. 719/743–2421, (Total facility includes 35 beds in nursing home–type unit) (Nonreporting) **A**9 10 18
Primary Contact: Herman Schreivogel, Chief Executive Officer
CFO: Herman Schreivogel, Chief Executive Officer
CMO: John E. Fox, M.D., Chief of Staff
Control: County–Government, nonfederal **Service:** General Medical and Surgical

Staffed Beds: 50

JOHNSTOWN—Weld County

★☐ **NORTHERN COLORADO REHABILITATION HOSPITAL (63033)**, 4401 Union Street, Zip 80534; tel. 970/619–3400 **A**1 10 **F**25 26 33 41 56 62 85 **S** Ernest Health, Inc.
Primary Contact: Dennis R. Shelby, Chief Executive Officer
Web address: www.ncrh.ernesthealth.com
Control: State–Government, nonfederal **Service:** Rehabilitation

Staffed Beds: 40 **Admissions:** 719 **Census:** 29 **Outpatient Visits:** 4672 **Births:** 0

JULESBURG—Sedgwick County

SEDGWICK COUNTY HEALTH CENTER (61310), 900 Cedar Street, Zip 80737–1199; tel. 970/474–3323, (Total facility includes 52 beds in nursing home–type unit) **A**9 10 18 **F**10 13 15 27 30 31 32 38 40 52 55 57 62 63 65 74 79 84 96 102 107 117 121 122 **P**6
Primary Contact: David Garnas, Chief Executive Officer
COO: David Garnas, Chief Executive Officer
CFO: Karla Dunker, Director Finance
CMO: Donald Regier, M.D., Chief of Staff
CHR: Sonja Bell, Coordinator Human Resources
Control: County–Government, nonfederal **Service:** General Medical and Surgical

Staffed Beds: 64 **Admissions:** 217 **Census:** 47 **Outpatient Visits:** 13115 **Births:** 24 **Total Expense ($000):** 6882 **Payroll Expense ($000):** 3154 **Personnel:** 89

KREMMLING—Grand County

★ **KREMMLING MEMORIAL HOSPITAL (61318)**, 214 South Fourth Street, Zip 80459, Mailing Address: P.O. Box 399, Zip 80459–0399; tel. 970/724–3442 **A**9 10 18 **F**1 3 11 15 24 25 30 31 34 38 40 41 52 53 55 57 62 63 65 66 68 73 74 75 76 77 79 80 81 82 84 85 86 87 96 97 98 99 107 117 119 120 122 124 **P**6
Primary Contact: Bill Widener, Administrator and Chief Executive Officer
CFO: Amy Butler, Director Finance
CMO: Lynn Telck, M.D., Medical Director
CIO: Eric Murray, Director Community Relations
CHR: Marianne Hayes, Director Human Resources
Web address: www.kremmlinghospital.org
Control: Hospital district or authority, Government, nonfederal **Service:** General Medical and Surgical

Staffed Beds: 19 **Admissions:** 167 **Census:** 7 **Outpatient Visits:** 24303 **Births:** 1 **Total Expense ($000):** 8579 **Payroll Expense ($000):** 4246 **Personnel:** 108

LA JARA—Conejos County

★ **CONEJOS COUNTY HOSPITAL (61308)**, 19021 U.S. Highway 285, Zip 81140–0639, Mailing Address: P.O. Box 639, Zip 81140–0639; tel. 719/274–5121, (Total facility includes 4 beds in nursing home–type unit) (Nonreporting) **A**9 10 18
Primary Contact: Thomas Henton, Chief Executive Officer
CFO: Pat Cooper, Comptroller
CMO: Vaughn Jackson, M.D., Chief of Staff
CIO: Kathy Rogers, Vice President Marketing
CHR: Delilah Chavez, Human Resources Assistant
Web address: www.cchoo.org
Control: Hospital district or authority, Government, nonfederal **Service:** General Medical and Surgical

Staffed Beds: 21

LA JUNTA—Otero County

★☐ **ARKANSAS VALLEY REGIONAL MEDICAL CENTER (60036)**, 1100 Carson Avenue, Zip 81050–2799; tel. 719/383–6000, (Total facility includes 102 beds in nursing home–type unit) **A**1 9 10 20 **F**3 8 11 13 15 25 27 30 31 33 38 40 44 45 46 50 55 56 57 61 62 65 66 68 73 74 75 76 79 80 81 82 84 86 87 96 100 102 106 107 117 118 119 121 124 134 136 137 **P**6 **S** QHR
Primary Contact: Lynn Crowell, Chief Executive Officer
CFO: Janette Bender, Chief Financial Officer
CMO: Jason Sims, D.O., Chief of Staff
CIO: Rocky Ackelson, Director Information Services
CHR: Kerri Kimsey, Director Human Resources
Web address: www.avrmc.org
Control: Other not–for–profit (including NFP Corporation) **Service:** General Medical and Surgical

Staffed Beds: 155 **Admissions:** 2232 **Census:** 112 **Outpatient Visits:** 43954 **Births:** 285 **Total Expense ($000):** 29784 **Payroll Expense ($000):** 15162 **Personnel:** 388

LAFAYETTE—Boulder County

★☐ **EXEMPLA GOOD SAMARITAN MEDICAL CENTER (60116)**, 200 Exempla Circle, Zip 80026; tel. 303/689–4000 **A**1 10 **F**12 13 14 15 17 18 20 24 25 26 27 33 34 38 40 42 44 55 57 59 62 66 70 72 73 74 75 76 77 78 79 80 81 82 84 86 92 96 97 100 102 103 107 119 121 132 134 135 136 137 **P**6 **S** Exempla Healthcare, Inc.
Primary Contact: David Hamm, President and Chief Executive Officer
CFO: John Higgins, Director Finance
CMO: Robert Billerbeck, M.D., Chief Medical Officer
CIO: David C. Pecoraro, Vice President and Chief Information Officer
CHR: Amy Pacey, Director Human Resources
Web address: www.exempla.org
Control: Other not–for–profit (including NFP Corporation) **Service:** General Medical and Surgical

Staffed Beds: 150 **Admissions:** 10631 **Census:** 113 **Outpatient Visits:** 84429 **Births:** 2073

CO

Hospital, Medicare Provider Number, Address, Telephone, Approval, Facility, and Physician Codes, Health Care System
★ American Hospital Association (AHA) membership
☐ The Joint Commission accreditation
○ American Osteopathic Association (AOA) accreditation
△ Commission on Accreditation of Rehabilitation Facilities (CARF) accreditation

LAMAR—Prowers County

★ **PROWERS MEDICAL CENTER (61323)**, 401 Kendall Drive, Zip 81052–3993; tel. 719/336–4343 **A**9 10 18 **F**3 11 13 15 25 27 31 32 33 38 54 55 56 57 61 62 63 66 73 74 75 76 79 80 86 87 96 100 107 119 122 135 136 137 **P**4 5 **S** QHR
Primary Contact: Theodore Kubicki, Chief Executive Officer
COO: Karen Bryant, Chief Support Services Officer
CFO: Randy Nightengale, Chief Financial Officer
CMO: Andrew Saueracker, M.D., Chief of Staff
CIO: Vince Yoder, Manager Information Technology
CHR: Karen Bryant, Chief Support Services Officer
Web address: www.prowersmedical.com
Control: Hospital district or authority, Government, nonfederal **Service:** General Medical and Surgical

Staffed Beds: 25 **Admissions:** 1104 **Census:** 12 **Outpatient Visits:** 8542 **Births:** 191 **Total Expense ($000):** 22525 **Payroll Expense ($000):** 9374 **Personnel:** 188

LEADVILLE—Lake County

ST. VINCENT GENERAL HOSPITAL DISTRICT (61319), 822 West 4th Street, Zip 80461–3897; tel. 719/486–0230 **A**9 10 18 **F**1 3 4 7 8 13 15 16 17 25 33 38 61 65 68 70 71 74 78 79 83 84 85 87 88 96 107 117
Primary Contact: David Zaitz, Chief Executive Officer
CFO: Rhonda Koehn, Chief Financial Officer
CMO: William Bradshaw, M.D., Chief of Staff
CHR: Dawn Nelson, Director Human Resources
Web address: www.svghd.org
Control: Hospital district or authority, Government, nonfederal **Service:** General Medical and Surgical

Staffed Beds: 25 **Admissions:** 452 **Census:** 19 **Outpatient Visits:** 2014 **Births:** 0 **Total Expense ($000):** 8938 **Payroll Expense ($000):** 5772 **Personnel:** 147

CO

LITTLETON—Arapahoe County

⊡ **LITTLETON ADVENTIST HOSPITAL (60113)**, 7700 South Broadway Street, Zip 80122–2628; tel. 303/730–8900, (Nonreporting) **A**1 9 10 **S** Adventist Health System Sunbelt Health Care Corporation
Primary Contact: Kenneth J. Bacon, Chief Executive Officer
CMO: Tom Fawell, M.D., Chief Medical Officer
CHR: Deb Canales, Senior Vice President Human Resources
Web address: www.centura.org
Control: Church–operated, Nongovernment, not–for profit **Service:** General Medical and Surgical

Staffed Beds: 134

LONE TREE—Douglas County

⊡ **SKY RIDGE MEDICAL CENTER (60112)**, 10101 Ridge Gate Parkway, Zip 80124; tel. 720/225–1000 **A**1 9 10 **F**3 11 12 13 15 18 20 22 25 26 27 30 31 32 33 34 37 38 40 46 47 48 49 54 55 56 57 60 62 68 70 72 73 74 75 76 77 79 80 81 82 84 86 87 96 97 100 102 103 106 107 109 111 118 119 120 124 135 136 137 **S** HCA
Primary Contact: Maureen Tarrant, Chief Executive Officer
COO: Susan Hicks, Chief Operating Officer
CFO: Craig Sammons, Chief Financial Officer
CMO: Brian Gill, M.D., President Medical Staff
CIO: William Baker, Director Information Technology and Systems
CHR: Carol Haun, Vice President Human Resources
Web address: www.skyridgemedcenter.com
Control: Corporation, Investor–owned, for–profit **Service:** General Medical and Surgical

Staffed Beds: 150 **Admissions:** 10480 **Census:** 107 **Outpatient Visits:** 43949 **Births:** 2973 **Total Expense ($000):** 137167 **Payroll Expense ($000):** 46189 **Personnel:** 643

LONGMONT—Boulder County

⊡ **LONGMONT UNITED HOSPITAL (60003)**, 1950 West Mountain View Avenue, Zip 80501–3162, Mailing Address: P.O. Box 1659, Zip 80502–1659; tel. 303/651–5111, (Total facility includes 15 beds in nursing home–type unit) **A**1 2 9 10 **F**2 3 11 13 15 18 20 22 24 25 26 27 30 31 32 33 34 37 38 40 41 43 44 46 50 52 53 54 55 56 57 60 62 66 68 71 72 73 74 75 76 77 79 80 81 82 84 86 88 90 91 92 93 95 96 97 100 102 106 107 109 111 117 118 119 120 121 124 135 137 **P**6
Primary Contact: Mitchell C. Carson, President and Chief Executive Officer
CFO: Neil W. Bertrand, Chief Financial Officer
CMO: Mary Faini, M.D., Chief of Staff
CIO: John Peterson, Vice President Information Systems
CHR: Warren Laughlin, Vice President Human Resources
Web address: www.luhcares.org
Control: Other not–for–profit (including NFP Corporation) **Service:** General Medical and Surgical

Staffed Beds: 168 **Admissions:** 10221 **Census:** 115 **Outpatient Visits:** 107363 **Births:** 1491 **Total Expense ($000):** 133400 **Payroll Expense ($000):** 57971 **Personnel:** 1040

LOUISVILLE—Boulder County

⊡ **AVISTA ADVENTIST HOSPITAL (60103)**, 100 Health Park Drive, Zip 80027–9583; tel. 303/673–1000 **A**1 9 10 **F**8 13 15 18 20 25 26 30 31 32 34 35 36 38 40 41 50 51 53 56 57 59 62 68 70 71 73 74 75 77 79 81 82 84 86 96 100 103 107 118 119 120 135 137 **P**1 **S** Adventist Health System Sunbelt Health Care Corporation
Primary Contact: John Sackett, Chief Executive Officer
COO: David A. Smith, Vice President and Chief Operating Officer
CFO: Cheryl Curry, Vice President Finance
CMO: David Ehrenberger, M.D., Chief Medical Officer
CHR: Derek Morgan, Director Human Resources
Web address: www.avistahosp.org
Control: Church–operated, Nongovernment, not–for profit **Service:** General Medical and Surgical

Staffed Beds: 85 **Admissions:** 5382 **Census:** 44 **Outpatient Visits:** 47956 **Births:** 2676 **Total Expense ($000):** 67800 **Payroll Expense ($000):** 26300 **Personnel:** 607

□ **CENTENNIAL PEAKS HOSPITAL (64007)**, 2255 South 88th Street, Zip 80027–9716; tel. 303/673–9990, (Nonreporting) **A**1 9 10
Primary Contact: Andrew Braun, Executive Director
CFO: Tim Ryan, Director Finance
CMO: Daniel Fisher, M.D., Chief of Staff
CHR: Laura Hobbs, Director Human Resources
Web address: www.centennialpeaks.com
Control: Other not–for–profit (including NFP Corporation) **Service:** Psychiatric

Staffed Beds: 72

LOVELAND—Larimer County

⊡ **MCKEE MEDICAL CENTER (60030)**, 2000 Boise Avenue, Zip 80538–4281, Mailing Address: P.O. Box 830, Zip 80539–0830; tel. 970/669–4640 **A**1 2 9 10 **F**2 3 8 11 12 13 15 18 20 25 26 27 30 31 32 33 36 38 40 43 46 49 50 53 54 55 56 57 59 60 61 62 66 68 72 73 74 75 76 77 79 80 81 82 86 87 94 96 97 99 100 102 107 109 111 117 118 119 121 122 123 124 133 135 136 137 **P**1 6 **S** Banner Health
Primary Contact: Richard O. Sutton, Chief Executive Officer
COO: Marilyn Schock, Associate Administrator
CFO: Lori Sehrt, Chief Financial Officer
CMO: Bert Honea, M.D., Medical Director
CIO: Steve Rains, Director Information Services
CHR: Darlene Alvis, Manager People Resources
Web address: www.mckeeloveland.com
Control: Other not–for–profit (including NFP Corporation) **Service:** General Medical and Surgical

Staffed Beds: 132 **Admissions:** 6428 **Census:** 62 **Outpatient Visits:** 246281 **Births:** 1002 **Total Expense ($000):** 107627 **Payroll Expense ($000):** 42137 **Personnel:** 838

★ **MEDICAL CENTER OF THE ROCKIES (60119)**, 2500 Rocky Mountain Avenue, Zip 80538; tel. 970/624–2500 **A**9 10 **F**3 17 18 20 22 24 25 26 30 31 32 38 40 49 50 55 59 66 68 72 73 74 77 78 79 80 81 82 84 96 97 100 102 106 107 116 119 135 136 137 **S** Poudre Valley Health System
Primary Contact: George E. Hayes, Chief Executive Officer
Web address: www.medctrrockies.org
Control: Other not–for–profit (including NFP Corporation) **Service:** General Medical and Surgical

Staffed Beds: 136 **Admissions:** 4084 **Census:** 47 **Outpatient Visits:** 34112 **Births:** 208 **Total Expense ($000):** 133113 **Payroll Expense ($000):** 40171 **Personnel:** 811

MEEKER—Rio Blanco County

★ **PIONEERS MEDICAL CENTER (60041)**, (Formerly Pioneers Hospital of Rio Blanco County), 345 Cleveland Street, Zip 81641–3238; tel. 970/878–5047, (Includes WALBRIDGE MEMORIAL CONVALESCENT WING), (Total facility includes 32 beds in nursing home–type unit) **A**9 10 20 **F**1 15 30 31 38 55 61 67 86 96 107 119 122 132 **P**6 **S** QHR
Primary Contact: Robert W. Omer, FACHE, Chief Executive Officer
CFO: Roger White, Chief Financial Officer
CMO: Victor Mihal, M.D., Chief of Staff
CIO: Curtis Cooper, Manager Information Systems
CHR: Twyla Jensen, Director Human Resources
Web address: www.pioneershospital.com
Control: Hospital district or authority, Government, nonfederal **Service:** General Medical and Surgical

Staffed Beds: 47 **Admissions:** 188 **Census:** 30 **Outpatient Visits:** 28463 **Births:** 0 **Total Expense ($000):** 9227 **Payroll Expense ($000):** 5336 **Personnel:** 114

Many Facility Codes have changed. Please refer to the AHA Guide Code Chart.

MONTROSE—Montrose County

★ **MONTROSE MEMORIAL HOSPITAL (60006)**, 800 South Third Street, Zip 81401–4291; tel. 970/249–2211 **A**1 9 10 20 **F**3 13 15 17 18 20 24 25 26 27 30 31 32 33 38 40 46 51 55 56 64 68 71 72 73 74 76 77 79 80 83 84 85 86 96 97 100 102 107 118 119 120 **P**5 8 **S** QHR
Primary Contact: Kenneth E. S. Platou, Chief Executive Officer
COO: Mary E. Snyder, Associate Administrator Operations
CFO: Connie Prewitt, Chief Financial Officer
CMO: Michael Brezinsky, M.D., Chief of Staff
CIO: Mother Superior Carlos Lovera, Director Information Systems
CHR: Tom Sams, Assistant Administrator Human Resources
Web address: www.montrosehospital.com
Control: County–Government, nonfederal **Service:** General Medical and Surgical

Staffed Beds: 63 **Admissions:** 3433 **Census:** 30 **Outpatient Visits:** 93647 **Births:** 604 **Total Expense ($000):** 59686 **Payroll Expense ($000):** 21183 **Personnel:** 448

PARKER—Douglas County

★ **PARKER ADVENTIST HOSPITAL (60114)**, 9395 Crown Crest Boulevard, Zip 80138; tel. 303/269–4000, (Nonreporting) **A**1 9 10 **S** Adventist Health System Sunbelt Health Care Corporation
Primary Contact: Terry Forde, Chief Executive Officer
Web address: www.parkerhospital.org
Control: Other not–for–profit (including NFP Corporation) **Service:** General Medical and Surgical

Staffed Beds: 10

PUEBLO—Pueblo County

□ **COLORADO MENTAL HEALTH INSTITUTE AT PUEBLO (60115)**, 1600 West 24th Street, Zip 81003–1499; tel. 719/546–4000, (Nonreporting) **A**1 3 5 10
Primary Contact: John R. DeQuardo, M.D., Superintendent
CFO: Jim Duff, Chief Financial Officer
CMO: Al Singleton, M.D., Chief Psychiatry and Chief Medical Staff
CIO: Eunice Wolther, Public Information Officer
CHR: Mary Young, Director Human Resources
Web address: www.cdhs.state.co.us/cmhip
Control: State–Government, nonfederal **Service:** Psychiatric

Staffed Beds: 514

★ △ **PARKVIEW MEDICAL CENTER (60020)**, 400 West 16th Street, Zip 81003–2781; tel. 719/584–4000 **A**1 7 9 10 **F**2 3 4 5 11 13 15 18 20 22 24 25 26 27 30 31 32 33 35 36 38 40 43 44 46 50 52 54 55 57 58 61 62 68 72 73 74 76 77 79 80 81 82 84 85 86 88 89 90 91 92 93 94 96 97 100 102 103 104 106 107 112 117 118 119 121 124 135 136 137 **P**6 8 **S** QHR
Primary Contact: C. W. Smith, President and Chief Executive Officer
COO: Mike Baxter, Chief Operating Officer
CFO: William Patterson, Chief Financial Officer
CMO: Steve Nafziger, M.D., Vice President Medical Affairs
CHR: Darrin Smith, Vice President Human Resources
Web address: www.parkviewmc.org
Control: Other not–for–profit (including NFP Corporation) **Service:** General Medical and Surgical

Staffed Beds: 293 **Admissions:** 13702 **Census:** 182 **Outpatient Visits:** 151482 **Births:** 1680 **Total Expense ($000):** 161401 **Payroll Expense ($000):** 75399 **Personnel:** 1558

★ **ST. MARY–CORWIN MEDICAL CENTER (60012)**, 1008 Minnequa Avenue, Zip 81004–3798; tel. 719/560–4000, (Nonreporting) **A**1 2 9 10 12 19 **S** Catholic Health Initiatives
Primary Contact: Michael J. Stenger, Chief Executive Officer
CFO: Kimberly Monjesky, CPA, Chief Financial Officer and Chief Operating Officer
CMO: Stephen Brown, M.D., Chief Medical Officer
CHR: Rudy Krasovec, Director Human Resources
Web address: www.centura.org
Control: Church–operated, Nongovernment, not–for profit **Service:** General Medical and Surgical

Staffed Beds: 254

RANGELY—Rio Blanco County

★ **RANGELY DISTRICT HOSPITAL (61307)**, 511 South White Avenue, Zip 81648–2104; tel. 970/675–5011, (Nonreporting) **A**9 10 18
Primary Contact: Jason McCormick, Chief Executive Officer
CFO: Sue Broughton, CPA, Vice President and Chief Financial Officer
Web address: www.rangelyhospital.com
Control: Hospital district or authority, Government, nonfederal **Service:** General Medical and Surgical

Staffed Beds: 25

RIFLE—Garfield County

★ **GRAND RIVER HOSPITAL DISTRICT (61317)**, 501 Airport Road, Zip 81650–2970, Mailing Address: P.O. Box 912, Zip 81650–0912; tel. 970/625–1510, (Total facility includes 57 beds in nursing home–type unit) **A**9 10 18 **F**3 117
Primary Contact: Martie Wisdom, Chief Executive Officer
COO: Mary Desormeau, Director Patient Care Services
CFO: James Coombs, Chief Financial Officer
CMO: Gary Meyer, M.D., Chief of Staff
CIO: Diana Murray, Director Information Systems
CHR: Michael Weerts, Director Human Resources
Web address: www.grhd.org
Control: Hospital district or authority, Government, nonfederal **Service:** General Medical and Surgical

Staffed Beds: 71 **Admissions:** 717 **Census:** 58 **Outpatient Visits:** 79394 **Births:** 0 **Total Expense ($000):** 30169 **Payroll Expense ($000):** 14253

SALIDA—Chaffee County

★ **HEART OF THE ROCKIES REGIONAL MEDICAL CENTER (61322)**, 1000 Rush Drive, Zip 81201–0429, Mailing Address: P.O. Box 429, Zip 81201–0429; tel. 719/530–2200 **A**9 10 18 **F**3 11 13 15 17 24 25 26 27 30 31 38 40 48 53 54 55 62 66 68 73 74 75 76 77 79 80 82 84 85 86 87 92 96 100 102 107 117 118 119 122 124 136 137
Primary Contact: Kenneth W. Leisher, Chief Executive Officer
CFO: Lesley Fagerberg, Vice President Fiscal Services
CHR: Barbara Abel, Vice President Human Resources
Web address: www.hrrmc.com
Control: Hospital district or authority, Government, nonfederal **Service:** General Medical and Surgical

Staffed Beds: 25 **Admissions:** 973 **Census:** 10 **Outpatient Visits:** 36773 **Births:** 135 **Total Expense ($000):** 20212 **Payroll Expense ($000):** 7688 **Personnel:** 227

SPRINGFIELD—Baca County

★ **SOUTHEAST COLORADO HOSPITAL DISTRICT (61311)**, 373 East Tenth Avenue, Zip 81073–1699; tel. 719/523–4501, (Total facility includes 56 beds in nursing home–type unit) **A**9 10 18 **F**3 6 7 11 25 27 30 31 32 33 38 42 50 54 55 61 64 65 79 86 87 96 117 122 136 137
Primary Contact: Donna R. Walker, Administrator
COO: Donna R. Walker, Administrator
CFO: James L. Forrest, Controller
CMO: Antonio Manalo, M.D., Chief of Staff
CHR: Sherrilyn Turner, Director Human Resources
Web address: www.sechosp.org
Control: Hospital district or authority, Government, nonfederal **Service:** General Medical and Surgical

Staffed Beds: 79 **Admissions:** 356 **Census:** 56 **Outpatient Visits:** 42481 **Births:** 0 **Total Expense ($000):** 9547 **Payroll Expense ($000):** 4726 **Personnel:** 140

STEAMBOAT SPRINGS—Routt County

★ **YAMPA VALLEY MEDICAL CENTER (60049)**, 1024 Central Park Drive, Zip 80487–5010; tel. 970/879–1322, (Total facility includes 59 beds in nursing home–type unit) **A**1 9 10 20 **F**3 11 13 15 24 25 26 27 32 33 34 38 40 43 49 51 52 55 56 57 62 66 68 71 73 74 75 77 79 80 81 82 84 86 96 100 102 107 117 118 119 120 121 122 124 132 135 136
Primary Contact: Karl B. Gills, Chief Executive Officer
CFO: Frank May, Chief Financial Officer
CMO: Larry Bookman, Chief Medical Officer
CIO: Laura Kaster, Chief Information Officer
CHR: Michael Turner, Director Human Resources
Web address: www.yvmc.org
Control: Other not–for–profit (including NFP Corporation) **Service:** General Medical and Surgical

Staffed Beds: 88 **Admissions:** 1983 **Census:** 71 **Outpatient Visits:** 52871 **Births:** 404 **Total Expense ($000):** 54517 **Payroll Expense ($000):** 19502 **Personnel:** 387

CO

Hospital, Medicare Provider Number, Address, Telephone, Approval, Facility, and Physician Codes, Health Care System

★ American Hospital Association (AHA) membership
□ The Joint Commission accreditation
○ American Osteopathic Association (AOA) accreditation
△ Commission on Accreditation of Rehabilitation Facilities (CARF) accreditation

STERLING—Logan County

☒ **STERLING REGIONAL MEDCENTER (60076)**, 615 Fairhurst Street, Zip 80751–0500; tel. 970/522–0122 **A**1 9 10 20 **F**3 13 15 24 25 26 27 28 30 32 38 40 41 43 51 55 56 57 59 62 66 67 68 73 74 75 76 77 79 80 81 82 86 87 96 97 99 100 102 106 107 118 119 120 135 137 **P**6
S Banner Health
Primary Contact: Michelle L. Joy, Chief Executive Officer
CFO: Pamela Stieb, Manager Finance
Web address: www.bannerhealth.com
Control: Other not–for–profit (including NFP Corporation) **Service:** General Medical and Surgical

Staffed Beds: 36 **Admissions:** 1715 **Census:** 17 **Outpatient Visits:** 138438 **Births:** 231 **Total Expense ($000):** 40066 **Payroll Expense ($000):** 16429 **Personnel:** 309

THORNTON—Adams County

☒ **NORTH SUBURBAN MEDICAL CENTER (60065)**, 9191 Grant Street, Zip 80229–4341; tel. 303/451–7800 **A**1 9 10 **F**1 3 4 11 12 13 15 16 17 18 20 24 25 26 30 31 32 33 38 40 43 44 55 57 62 65 66 68 70 71 72 74 77 78 79 80 82 83 84 85 88 96 97 100 103 107 117 118 119 121 124 135 **P**2 **S** HCA
Primary Contact: Todd Steward, President and Chief Executive Officer
COO: Jennifer Alderfer, Chief Operating Officer
CFO: Kevin Corcoran, Chief Financial Officer
CHR: Stacie Robertson, Director Human Resources
Web address: www.northsuburban.com
Control: Corporation, Investor–owned, for–profit **Service:** General Medical and Surgical

Staffed Beds: 118 **Admissions:** 6546 **Census:** 66 **Outpatient Visits:** 81286 **Births:** 1832 **Total Expense ($000):** 86756 **Payroll Expense ($000):** 36392 **Personnel:** 501

☐ **NORTH VALLEY HOSPITALS (62014)**, 8451 Pearl Street, Zip 80229–4804; tel. 303/288–3000, (Nonreporting) **A**1 9 10 **S** Vibra Healthcare
Primary Contact: Kathleen Cahill, Chief Executive Officer
CFO: Mark Ninke, Chief Financial Officer
CHR: Jerri Cain, Director Human Resources
Web address: www.northvalleyrehab.com
Control: Corporation, Investor–owned, for–profit **Service:** Long–Term Acute Care hospital

Staffed Beds: 117

TRINIDAD—Las Animas County

☒ **MT. SAN RAFAEL HOSPITAL (61321)**, 410 Benedicta Avenue, Zip 81082–2093; tel. 719/846–9213 **A**1 9 10 18 **F**3 11 15 30 31 32 38 40 55 75 77 79 80 86 96 107 118 122 137 **S** QHR
Primary Contact: James Robertson, Chief Executive Officer
CFO: Rich Armentrout, Chief Financial Officer
CMO: Douglas McFarland, M.D., Chief Medical Officer
CHR: Lori Silva, Director Human Resources
Web address: www.msrhc.org
Control: Other not–for–profit (including NFP Corporation) **Service:** General Medical and Surgical

Staffed Beds: 25 **Admissions:** 1038 **Census:** 14 **Outpatient Visits:** 33571 **Births:** 0 **Total Expense ($000):** 16837 **Payroll Expense ($000):** 6674 **Personnel:** 148

USAF ACADEMY—El Paso County

☒ **U. S. AIR FORCE ACADEMY HOSPITAL**, 4102 Pinion Drive, Zip 80840–4000; tel. 719/333–5102, (Nonreporting) **A**1 **S** Department of the Air Force
Primary Contact: Colonel Alan B. Berg, Commander
CIO: Captain James Hughes, Information Systems Flight Commander
Web address: www.usafa.af.mil
Control: Air Force, Government, federal **Service:** General Medical and Surgical

Staffed Beds: 27

VAIL—Eagle County

☒ **VAIL VALLEY MEDICAL CENTER (60096)**, 181 West Meadow Drive, Zip 81657–5059, Mailing Address: P.O. Box 40000, Zip 81658; tel. 970/476–2451 **A**1 3 5 9 10 20 **F**3 11 13 15 24 25 27 31 32 33 35 38 39 40 42 43 50 51 53 55 56 57 61 62 64 66 68 71 73 74 75 76 77 79 80 81 82 86 96 97 99 100 103 107 109 111 118 119 120 132 135 136 137
Primary Contact: John Cassin, Chief Executive Officer
COO: Thomas L. Kyllo, Executive Vice President
CFO: Shaun J. Scanlon, Senior Vice President Finance and Chief Financial Officer
CMO: John Woodland, M.D., Medical Director
CIO: Dave Pluta, Chief Information Officer
CHR: David Blackwell, Vice President Human Resources
Web address: www.vvmc.com
Control: Other not–for–profit (including NFP Corporation) **Service:** General Medical and Surgical

Staffed Beds: 58 **Admissions:** 2918 **Census:** 20 **Outpatient Visits:** 122690 **Births:** 702 **Total Expense ($000):** 133086 **Payroll Expense ($000):** 44247 **Personnel:** 648

WALSENBURG—Huerfano County

★ **SPANISH PEAKS REGIONAL HEALTH CENTER (61316)**, 23500 U.S. Highway 160, Zip 81089–9524; tel. 719/738–5100, (Nonreporting) **A**9 10 18
Primary Contact: Steven J. Perkins, President and Chief Executive Officer
CFO: Richard L. Corradino, Chief Finance Officer
CHR: L. Anthony Marostica, Director Human Resources
Web address: www.sprhc.org
Control: Hospital district or authority, Government, nonfederal **Service:** General Medical and Surgical

Staffed Beds: 25

WESTMINSTER—Jefferson County

CLEO WALLACE CENTERS HOSPITAL, 8405 Church Ranch Boulevard, Zip 80021–3918; tel. 303/466–7391, (Nonreporting) **A**9
Primary Contact: Michael J. Montgomery, President and Chief Executive Officer
CFO: Jonelle A. Roberts, Chief Finance Officer
Web address: www.devereux.org
Control: Other not–for–profit (including NFP Corporation) **Service:** Children's hospital psychiatric

Staffed Beds: 61

☒ **ST. ANTHONY NORTH HOSPITAL (60104)**, 2551 West 84th Avenue, Zip 80031; tel. 303/426–2151 **A**1 9 10 **F**11 13 15 18 20 24 25 26 27 30 31 32 33 38 40 44 46 49 55 56 59 62 66 68 70 72 73 74 75 76 77 79 80 82 86 87 92 96 97 102 106 107 118 119 135 136 **S** Catholic Health Initiatives
Primary Contact: James F. Dover, FACHE, Chief Executive Officer
CFO: Barbara Carveth, Chief Financial Officer
CMO: Patrick Sankovitz, M.D., Chief Medical Officer
CHR: Ginny Arndt, Director Human Resources
Web address: www.stanthonynorth.org
Control: Church–operated, Nongovernment, not–for profit **Service:** General Medical and Surgical

Staffed Beds: 123 **Admissions:** 6706 **Census:** 77 **Outpatient Visits:** 61345 **Births:** 487 **Total Expense ($000):** 87666 **Payroll Expense ($000):** 31257 **Personnel:** 628

WHEAT RIDGE—Jefferson County

☒ **EXEMPLA LUTHERAN MEDICAL CENTER (60009)**, 8300 West 38th Avenue, Zip 80033–6005; tel. 303/425–4500, (Includes EXEMPLA WEST PINES, 3400 Lutheran Parkway, Zip 80033; tel. 303/467–4000), (Total facility includes 120 beds in nursing home–type unit) **A**1 2 9 10 **F**4 5 6 10 11 13 14 15 17 18 20 22 24 25 26 27 33 34 38 40 42 43 44 50 53 54 57 59 62 66 68 70 72 73 74 75 76 77 79 80 81 82 84 86 87 88 89 90 91 92 93 94 95 96 97 100 102 105 106 107 109 111 115 117 118 119 121 122 124 135 136 137 **P**6 7 **S** Exempla Healthcare, Inc.
Primary Contact: Robert H. Malte, President and Chief Executive Officer
COO: Peggy Cain Price, Vice President and Chief Operating Officer
CFO: Karen Scremin, Vice President Finance
CMO: David Munch, M.D., Vice President and Chief Clinical and Quality Officer
CIO: David C. Pecoraro, Vice President Information Services
CHR: Scott Day, Vice President Human Resources
Web address: www.exempla.org
Control: Other not–for–profit (including NFP Corporation) **Service:** General Medical and Surgical

Staffed Beds: 543 **Admissions:** 21349 **Census:** 372 **Outpatient Visits:** 159352 **Births:** 2820

WRAY—Yuma County

★ **WRAY COMMUNITY DISTRICT HOSPITAL (61309)**, 1017 West 7th Street, Zip 80758–1420; tel. 970/332–4811, (Nonreporting) **A**9 10 18
Primary Contact: Edward Finley, Administrator
CFO: Jennie Sullivan, Director Finance
CMO: Monte Uyemura, M.D., Chief of Staff
Web address: www.wcdh.org
Control: Hospital district or authority, Government, nonfederal **Service:** General Medical and Surgical

Staffed Beds: 16

YUMA—Yuma County

★ **YUMA DISTRICT HOSPITAL (61315)**, 1000 West 8th Avenue, Zip 80759–2641; tel. 970/848–5405 **A**9 10 18 **F**3 11 13 15 24 26 27 30 31 32 33 34 38 40 41 43 50 52 55 56 57 61 62 63 66 72 73 74 75 76 77 79 82 86 87 92 96 100 103 107 122 132 137 **P**6
Primary Contact: John Gardner, Chief Executive Officer
COO: Lyndia Loppe, Chief Operating Officer
CFO: Cathy Wolff, Vice President Financial Services and Chief Financial Officer
CMO: Doug Everson, M.D., Chief Medical Staff
CHR: Gini Adams, Director Employee and Public Relations
Web address: www.yumahospital.org
Control: Hospital district or authority, Government, nonfederal **Service:** General Medical and Surgical

Staffed Beds: 12 **Admissions:** 272 **Census:** 2 **Outpatient Visits:** 48016 **Births:** 21 **Total Expense ($000):** 14597 **Payroll Expense ($000):** 6194 **Personnel:** 142

Many Facility Codes have changed. Please refer to the AHA Guide Code Chart.

CONNECTICUT

BETHLEHEM—Litchfield County

WELLSPRING FOUNDATION, 21 Arch Bridge Road, Zip 06751–0370, Mailing Address: P.O. Box 370, Zip 06751–0370; tel. 203/266–7235, (Nonreporting)
Primary Contact: Richard E. Beauvais, Ph.D., Chief Executive Officer
CFO: Richard E. Beauvais, Ph.D., Chief Executive Officer
Web address: www.wellspring.org
Control: Other not–for–profit (including NFP Corporation) **Service:** Psychiatric

Staffed Beds: 36

BRANFORD—New Haven County

□ **THE CONNECTICUT HOSPICE (70038)**, 100 Double Beach Road, Zip 06405–4096; tel. 203/315–7500, (Nonreporting) **A**1 10
Primary Contact: Rosemary Johnson Hurzeler, President and Chief Executive Officer
Web address: www.hospice.com
Control: Other not–for–profit (including NFP Corporation) **Service:** Other specialty

Staffed Beds: 52

BRIDGEPORT—Fairfield County

★ **BRIDGEPORT HOSPITAL (70010)**, 267 Grant Street, Zip 06610–0120, Mailing Address: P.O. Box 5000, Zip 06610–5000; tel. 203/384–3000 **A**1 2 3 5 6 8 9 10 **F**3 8 11 13 15 16 18 20 22 24 25 26 27 28 30 31 32 33 34 36 38 40 41 42 43 44 46 49 50 51 54 55 56 57 58 60 62 63 64 66 68 70 72 73 74 75 76 77 78 79 80 81 82 83 84 85 86 87 88 89 90 91 92 93 94 95 96 97 102 104 105 106 107 109 111 114 116 118 119 120 121 123 124 133 134 135 136 137 **P**6 8 **S** Yale New Haven Health System
Primary Contact: Robert J. Trefry, President and Chief Executive Officer
COO: Hope Juckel–Regan, R.N., Executive Vice President and Chief Operating Officer
CFO: Patrick McCabe, Senior Vice President Finance and Chief Financial Officer
CMO: Bruce M. McDonald, M.D., Senior Vice President Medical Affairs
CIO: Mark Tepping, Chief Information Officer
CHR: Joseph Janell, Senior Vice President Human Resources
Web address: www.bridgeporthospital.org
Control: Other not–for–profit (including NFP Corporation) **Service:** General Medical and Surgical

Staffed Beds: 354 **Admissions:** 17268 **Census:** 270 **Outpatient Visits:** 218680 **Births:** 2623 **Total Expense ($000):** 299185 **Payroll Expense ($000):** 119613 **Personnel:** 1971

SOUTHWEST CONNECTICUT MENTAL HEALTH SYSTEM (74012), 97 Middle Street, Zip 6604; tel. 203/551–7400 **A**9 10 **F**4 25 26 33 36 50 57 88 90 91 92 94 119 121 124 132 **S** Connecticut Department of Mental Health and Addiction Services
Primary Contact: James M. Pisciotta, Chief Executive Officer
COO: James M. Pisciotta, Chief Executive Officer
CFO: Magnus Ezeji, Chief Financial Officer
CMO: Stephen R. Atkins, M.D., Medical Director
CIO: Daniel Wartenberg, Director Quality Improvement Services
CHR: Michael McGarthy, Director Human Resources
Control: State–Government, nonfederal **Service:** Psychiatric

Staffed Beds: 62 **Admissions:** 873 **Census:** 57 **Outpatient Visits:** 57265 **Births:** 0

★ **ST. VINCENT'S MEDICAL CENTER (70028)**, 2800 Main Street, Zip 06606–4292; tel. 203/576–5454, (Includes HALL–BROOKE HOSPITAL, A DIVISION OF HALL–BROOKE BEHAVIORAL HEALTH SERVICES, 47 Long Lots Road, Westport, Zip 06880–3800; tel. 203/221–8802; James McCreath, Ph.D., President and Chief Executive Officer) **A**1 2 3 5 9 10 **F**2 3 5 8 11 12 13 15 16 17 18 20 22 24 25 26 27 28 30 31 32 33 34 36 38 39 40 41 42 43 44 45 46 49 50 52 53 54 55 56 57 58 60 62 63 64 66 68 69 72 73 74 75 76 77 78 79 80 81 82 85 86 87 88 89 90 91 92 93 94 95 96 97 99 100 103 107 108 109 111 114 118 119 121 123 124 132 133 134 135 136 **S** Ascension Health
Primary Contact: Susan L. Davis, RN, Ed.D., President and Chief Executive Officer
CFO: John Gleckler, Chief Financial Officer
CMO: Jose Missri, M.D., Chief Medical Officer
CIO: Betsy Thornquist, Chief Information Officer
CHR: Pamela Tarulli, Corporate Vice President Human Resources
Web address: www.stvincents.org
Control: Other not–for–profit (including NFP Corporation) **Service:** General Medical and Surgical

Staffed Beds: 312 **Admissions:** 18207 **Census:** 266 **Outpatient Visits:** 193981 **Births:** 1302 **Total Expense ($000):** 267789 **Payroll Expense ($000):** 119336 **Personnel:** 1522

BRISTOL—Hartford County

★ △ **BRISTOL HOSPITAL (70029)**, Brewster Road, Zip 6011; tel. 860/585–3000, (Nonreporting) **A**1 2 5 7 9 10
Primary Contact: Kurt A. Barwis, FACHE, CPA, President and Chief Executive Officer
COO: Marc D. Edelman, Vice President Operations
CFO: Michael Orr, Vice President Finance and Chief Financial Officer
CMO: Valerie Vitale, M.D., Chief of Staff
CIO: David Rackliffe, Assistant Vice President Information Services
Web address: www.bristolhospital.org
Control: Other not–for–profit (including NFP Corporation) **Service:** General Medical and Surgical

Staffed Beds: 128

DANBURY—Fairfield County

★ **DANBURY HOSPITAL (70033)**, 24 Hospital Avenue, Zip 06810–6099; tel. 203/739–7000 **A**1 2 3 5 8 9 10 **F**3 5 8 9 12 13 14 15 17 18 20 22 24 25 26 27 28 29 30 31 32 33 34 35 36 37 38 40 41 43 44 45 46 47 48 49 50 51 52 53 54 55 56 57 58 59 60 62 63 64 66 68 69 70 72 73 74 75 76 77 79 80 81 82 84 85 86 87 88 89 90 91 92 93 94 95 96 97 98 99 100 101 102 103 104 105 106 107 108 109 111 112 114 118 119 120 121 123 124 133 134 135 136 137
Primary Contact: Frank J. Kelly, President and Chief Executive Officer
CMO: Matthew Miller, M.D., Vice President Medical Affairs
CIO: Peter Courtway, Chief Information Officer
CHR: Phyllis Zappala, Vice President Human Resources
Web address: www.danburyhospital.org
Control: Other not–for–profit (including NFP Corporation) **Service:** General Medical and Surgical

Staffed Beds: 339 **Admissions:** 18480 **Census:** 227 **Outpatient Visits:** 157800 **Births:** 2444 **Total Expense ($000):** 370680 **Payroll Expense ($000):** 156644 **Personnel:** 2346

DERBY—New Haven County

★ **GRIFFIN HOSPITAL (70031)**, 130 Division Street, Zip 06418–1326; tel. 203/735–7421 **A**1 2 9 10 **F**3 5 8 13 15 24 25 27 30 31 32 33 34 36 38 43 44 49 50 51 52 54 55 56 57 58 59 62 63 66 68 69 72 73 74 75 76 77 79 80 81 82 86 87 88 89 90 91 92 93 94 95 96 97 100 102 106 107 118 119 121 123 124 133 135 136 137
Primary Contact: Patrick Charmel, President and Chief Executive Officer
CFO: James J. Moylan, Vice President Finance
CMO: Kenneth V. Schwartz, M.D., Medical Director
CIO: George Tomas, Director Information Services
CHR: Steve Mordecai, Director Human Resources
Web address: www.griffinhealth.org
Control: Other not–for–profit (including NFP Corporation) **Service:** General Medical and Surgical

Staffed Beds: 111 **Admissions:** 7062 **Census:** 88 **Outpatient Visits:** 167304 **Births:** 797 **Total Expense ($000):** 105611 **Payroll Expense ($000):** 49888 **Personnel:** 816

CT

Hospital, Medicare Provider Number, Address, Telephone, Approval, Facility, and Physician Codes, Health Care System

★ American Hospital Association (AHA) membership
□ The Joint Commission accreditation
○ American Osteopathic Association (AOA) accreditation
△ Commission on Accreditation of Rehabilitation Facilities (CARF) accreditation

FARMINGTON—Hartford County

★ **UNIVERSITY OF CONNECTICUT HEALTH CENTER, JOHN DEMPSEY HOSPITAL (70036)**, 263 Farmington Avenue, Zip 06032–1941; tel. 860/679–2000 **A**1 2 3 5 8 9 10 12 **F**5 7 8 9 11 12 13 15 18 20 22 25 26 27 30 31 32 33 34 36 37 38 43 50 51 54 56 57 58 59 60 62 66 68 70 72 73 74 75 76 77 79 81 82 86 88 89 90 91 92 93 94 95 96 97 100 102 103 104 105 106 107 108 109 113 114 118 119 120 121 132 135 136 **P**6
Primary Contact: James H. Thornton, Director
CFO: Daniel Upton, Chief Financial Officer
CMO: Richard Simon, M.D., Chief of Staff
CIO: Sandra Armstrong, Vice Chancellor Information Technology
CHR: Brian Eaton, Associate Vice President
Web address: www.uchc.edu
Control: State–Government, nonfederal **Service:** General Medical and Surgical

Staffed Beds: 153 **Admissions:** 9147 **Census:** 153 **Outpatient Visits:** 291378 **Births:** 854 **Total Expense ($000):** 221637 **Payroll Expense ($000):** 86379 **Personnel:** 2467

GREENWICH—Fairfield County

★ **GREENWICH HOSPITAL (70018)**, 5 Perryridge Road, Zip 06830–4697; tel. 203/863–3000 **A**1 2 3 5 9 10 **F**4 17 65 68 70 74 78 84 **S** Yale New Haven Health System
Primary Contact: Frank A. Corvino, President and Chief Executive Officer
COO: Quinton J. Friesen, Executive Vice President and Chief Operating Officer
CFO: Eugene Colucci, Vice President Finance
CMO: A. Michael Marino, M.D., Senior Vice President Medical Administration
CIO: James Weeks, Chief Information Officer
Web address: www.greenhosp.org
Control: Other not–for–profit (including NFP Corporation) **Service:** General Medical and Surgical

Staffed Beds: 174 **Admissions:** 10567 **Census:** 113 **Outpatient Visits:** 419387 **Births:** 2212

CT

HARTFORD—Hartford County

★ **CONNECTICUT CHILDREN'S MEDICAL CENTER (73300)**, 282 Washington Street, Zip 06106–3322; tel. 860/545–9000, (Nonreporting) **A**1 3 5 9 10
Primary Contact: Martin J. Gavin, President and Chief Executive Officer
COO: Wendy Warring, Vice President and Chief Operating Officer
CFO: Gerald J. Boisvert, Senior Vice President and Chief Financial Officer
CMO: Paul Dworkin, M.D., Physician–in–Chief
CHR: Elizabeth Rudden, Vice President Human Resources
Web address: www.ccmckids.org
Control: Other not–for–profit (including NFP Corporation) **Service:** Children's general

Staffed Beds: 114

★ △ **HARTFORD HOSPITAL (70025)**, 80 Seymour Street, Zip 06102–5037, Mailing Address: P.O. Box 5037, Zip 06102–5037; tel. 860/545–5000, (Includes INSTITUTE OF LIVING, 400 Washington Street, Zip 06106–3392; tel. 860/545–7000) **A**1 2 3 5 7 8 9 10 **F**2 3 4 5 8 10 11 12 13 15 17 18 20 22 24 25 26 27 30 31 32 33 34 36 37 38 40 42 43 44 45 46 48 49 51 52 53 54 55 56 57 58 59 60 62 63 64 66 67 68 69 72 73 74 75 76 77 79 80 81 82 85 86 87 88 89 90 91 92 93 94 95 96 97 99 100 101 102 103 104 105 106 107 109 111 112 113 114 115 116 118 119 120 121 124 125 126 127 128 129 130 131 134 135 136 137 **P**5 6 8
Primary Contact: Elliot T. Joseph, President and Chief Executive Officer
COO: Jeffrey A. Flaks, Executive Vice President and Chief Operating Officer
CMO: Joseph Klimek, M.D., Vice President Medical Affairs
CIO: Stephan O'Neill, Vice President Information Services
CHR: Richard McAloon, Vice President Human Resources
Web address: www.harthosp.org
Control: Other not–for–profit (including NFP Corporation) **Service:** General Medical and Surgical

Staffed Beds: 552 **Admissions:** 35449 **Census:** 552 **Outpatient Visits:** 190917 **Births:** 3977 **Total Expense ($000):** 604771 **Payroll Expense ($000):** 309602 **Personnel:** 5109

★ **MOUNT SINAI REHABILITATION HOSPITAL (73025)**, 490 Blue Hills Avenue, Zip 6112; tel. 860/714–3500 **A**1 10 **F**30 31 32 85 86 120 **P**8 **S** Saint Francis Care, Inc.
Primary Contact: Christopher M. Dadlez, President and Chief Executive Officer
Web address: www.stfranciscare.org
Control: Other not–for–profit (including NFP Corporation) **Service:** Rehabilitation

Staffed Beds: 46 **Admissions:** 677 **Census:** 25 **Outpatient Visits:** 17277 **Births:** 0 **Total Expense ($000):** 11759 **Payroll Expense ($000):** 7169 **Personnel:** 163

★ **SAINT FRANCIS HOSPITAL AND MEDICAL CENTER (70002)**, 114 Woodland Street, Zip 06105–1208; tel. 860/714–4000 **A**1 2 3 5 8 9 10 **F**3 11 12 13 15 17 18 20 22 24 25 26 27 28 30 31 32 33 34 36 37 38 40 42 43 44 45 46 47 49 50 52 53 54 55 56 57 58 60 61 62 63 64 66 68 69 70 72 73 74 75 76 77 79 80 81 82 86 87 88 89 90 91 92 93 96 97 100 102 103 106 107 108 109 110 111 112 116 118 119 120 121 123 124 133 134 135 136 137 **P**8 **S** Saint Francis Care, Inc.
Primary Contact: Christopher M. Dadlez, President and Chief Executive Officer
COO: Amit K. Mody, M.D., Executive Vice President and Chief Operating Officer
CFO: Steven Rosenberg, Senior Vice President and Chief Financial Officer
CMO: Rolf W. Knoll, M.D., Senior Vice President Medical Affairs
CIO: Kathleen DeMatteo, Chief Information Officer and Vice President Information Systems
CHR: Jeffrey Chitester, Vice President Human Resources
Web address: www.saintfranciscare.com
Control: Church–operated, Nongovernment, not–for profit **Service:** General Medical and Surgical

Staffed Beds: 542 **Admissions:** 28831 **Census:** 425 **Outpatient Visits:** 373493 **Births:** 3019 **Total Expense ($000):** 511874 **Payroll Expense ($000):** 212173 **Personnel:** 4047

MANCHESTER—Hartford County

★ **MANCHESTER MEMORIAL HOSPITAL (70027)**, 71 Haynes Street, Zip 06040–4188; tel. 860/646–1222 **A**1 2 5 9 10 **F**3 5 11 13 15 24 25 26 27 28 30 31 33 36 37 38 41 42 48 49 50 55 56 57 58 62 68 70 72 73 74 75 76 77 78 79 80 81 82 84 86 88 89 90 91 92 93 94 95 96 97 99 100 102 106 107 118 119 120 121 123 124 133 134 135 137 **P**1 5 6 **S** Eastern Connecticut Health Network
Primary Contact: Peter J. Karl, President and Chief Executive Officer
COO: Kathleen Sims, Vice President Operations
CFO: Kevin G. Murphy, Senior Vice President Finance and Chief Financial Officer
CMO: Joel R. Reich, M.D., Senior Vice President Medical Affairs
CIO: Charles Covin, Chief Information Officer
CHR: Deborah Gogliettino, Senior Vice President Human Resources
Web address: www.echn.org
Control: Other not–for–profit (including NFP Corporation) **Service:** General Medical and Surgical

Staffed Beds: 148 **Admissions:** 7981 **Census:** 114 **Outpatient Visits:** 327779 **Births:** 1110 **Total Expense ($000):** 153544 **Payroll Expense ($000):** 70319 **Personnel:** 1199

MANSFIELD CENTER—Tolland County

☐ **NATCHAUG HOSPITAL (74008)**, 189 Storrs Road, Zip 06250–0260; tel. 860/456–1311 **A**1 9 10 **F**3 4 5 30 31 32 88 89 90 91 93 94 95 119 121
Primary Contact: Stephen W. Larcen, Ph.D., President and Chief Executive Officer
COO: Ellen Buffington, MSN, Vice President Operations
CFO: Paul V. Maloney, Chief Financial Officer
CMO: Craig Martin, M.D., Medical Director
CIO: Brian Jaworowski, Director Management Information Systems
CHR: Janet Keown, Director Human Resources
Web address: www.natchaug.org
Control: Other not–for–profit (including NFP Corporation) **Service:** Psychiatric

Staffed Beds: 57 **Admissions:** 1674 **Census:** 47 **Outpatient Visits:** 50708 **Births:** 0 **Total Expense ($000):** 34162 **Payroll Expense ($000):** 20825 **Personnel:** 387

MERIDEN—New Haven County

★ **MIDSTATE MEDICAL CENTER (70017)**, 435 Lewis Avenue, Zip 06451–2101; tel. 203/694–8200 **A**1 2 9 10 **F**3 11 12 13 15 18 24 25 26 27 30 31 32 33 36 37 38 41 42 43 46 48 49 50 51 52 53 54 55 56 57 60 61 62 66 68 72 73 74 76 77 79 80 81 82 87 88 92 96 97 99 100 102 103 105 106 107 109 111 112 118 119 120 121 133 134 135 136 137 **P**5 7
Primary Contact: Lucille A. Janatka, President and Chief Executive Officer
CFO: Ralph W. Becker, Chief Financial Officer
CMO: Paul Zimmering, M.D., Chief of Staff
CIO: Jennifer Comerford, Manager Information Services
CHR: Ken Cesca, Vice President Human Resources
Web address: www.midstatemedical.org
Control: Other not–for–profit (including NFP Corporation) **Service:** General Medical and Surgical

Staffed Beds: 123 **Admissions:** 8586 **Census:** 114 **Outpatient Visits:** 143613 **Births:** 1051 **Total Expense ($000):** 144250 **Payroll Expense ($000):** 54604 **Personnel:** 927

MIDDLETOWN—Middlesex County

☐ **CONNECTICUT VALLEY HOSPITAL (74003)**, Eastern Drive, Zip 06457–3947, Mailing Address: P.O. Box 351, Zip 06457–0351; tel. 860/262–5000, (Includes WHITING FORENSIC DIVISION OF CONNECTICUT VALLEY HOSPITAL, O'Brien Drive, Zip 06457, Mailing Address: Box 70, Zip 06457–3942; tel. 203/344–2541) **A**1 3 5 9 10 **F**3 4 26 30 33 37 52 54 55 59 66 73 81 82 88 90 91 93 119 124 132 135 **S** Connecticut Department of Mental Health and Addiction Services
Primary Contact: Luis B. Perez, Chief Executive Officer
COO: C Michael Niman, Ph.D., Chief Operating Officer
CIO: Dan Eley, Chief Information Technology
Control: State–Government, nonfederal **Service:** Psychiatric

Staffed Beds: 537 **Admissions:** 1968 **Census:** 528 **Outpatient Visits:** 0 **Births:** 0 **Total Expense ($000):** 168267 **Payroll Expense ($000):** 102732 **Personnel:** 1429

★ **MIDDLESEX HOSPITAL (70020)**, 28 Crescent Street, Zip 06457–3650; tel. 860/358–6000 **A**1 2 3 5 9 10 **F**3 5 12 13 15 17 18 20 22 24 25 26 27 30 31 32 33 34 36 38 39 42 43 44 45 49 50 51 53 55 56 57 58 59 60 61 62 63 66 68 72 73 74 75 76 77 78 79 80 81 82 84 86 87 88 89 90 91 92 93 94 95 96 97 100 102 103 104 105 106 107 109 111 114 118 119 120 121 122 123 124 134 135 136 137 **P**5 6
Primary Contact: Robert Gerard Kiely, President and Chief Executive Officer
COO: Vincent Capece, Chief Operating Officer
CFO: Susan Martin, Vice President Finance
CMO: Arthur V. McDowell, M.D., Chairman, Board of Directors
CIO: Ludwig Johnson, Vice President Information Technology
CHR: Gregory B. Nokes, Vice President Human Resources
Web address: www.middlesexhospital.org
Control: Other not–for–profit (including NFP Corporation) **Service:** General Medical and Surgical

Staffed Beds: 199 **Admissions:** 12606 **Census:** 146 **Outpatient Visits:** 1232650 **Births:** 1166 **Total Expense ($000):** 256715 **Payroll Expense ($000):** 126725 **Personnel:** 1724

☐ **RIVERVIEW HOSPITAL FOR CHILDREN AND YOUTH**, (Formerly Riverview Hospital for Children), 915 River Road, Zip 06457–2792, Mailing Address: P.O. Box 2792, Zip 06457–2792; tel. 860/704–4000, (Nonreporting) **A**1 3 5
Primary Contact: Melodie J. Peet, Superintendent
CFO: Connie Tessarzik, Business Manager
CMO: Lesley Siegel, M.D., Medical Director
CIO: Andrew J A Kass, M.D., Assistant Superintendent
Control: State–Government, nonfederal **Service:** Children's hospital psychiatric

Staffed Beds: 102

WHITING FORENSIC DIVISION OF CONNECTICUT VALLEY HOSPITAL See Connecticut Valley Hospital

MILFORD—New Haven County

★ **MILFORD HOSPITAL (70019)**, 300 Seaside Avenue, Zip 06460–4603; tel. 203/876–4000 **A**1 9 10 **F**3 8 11 13 15 18 25 26 27 28 30 31 32 33 35 38 39 40 42 43 45 46 49 50 55 56 57 58 62 66 68 72 73 76 77 79 80 82 92 96 97 100 102 104 105 106 107 119 121 124 133 134 135 136
Primary Contact: Paul E. Moss, President
CFO: Joseph Pelaccia, Vice President Finance
Web address: www.milfordhospital.org
Control: Other not–for–profit (including NFP Corporation) **Service:** General Medical and Surgical

Staffed Beds: 87 **Admissions:** 4477 **Census:** 57 **Outpatient Visits:** 76362 **Births:** 547 **Total Expense ($000):** 77739 **Payroll Expense ($000):** 34377 **Personnel:** 644

NEW BRITAIN—Hartford County

★ △ **HOSPITAL FOR SPECIAL CARE (72004)**, 2150 Corbin Avenue, Zip 06053–2298; tel. 860/223–2761 **A**1 5 7 10 **F**3 11 25 26 30 31 32 33 37 43 52 54 62 66 72 73 75 85 86 90 119 120 121 124 135 137 **P**6
Primary Contact: David Crandall, FACHE, President and Chief Executive Officer
CFO: Laurie A. Whelan, Vice President Finance and Chief Financial Officer
CMO: Mervet Elkair, M.D., Chief Medicine
CIO: Stan Jankowski, Corporate Manager Information Technology
Web address: www.hfsc.org
Control: Other not–for–profit (including NFP Corporation) **Service:** Rehabilitation

Staffed Beds: 219 **Admissions:** 538 **Census:** 202 **Outpatient Visits:** 21757 **Births:** 0 **Total Expense ($000):** 77643 **Payroll Expense ($000):** 41466 **Personnel:** 695

★ **THE HOSPITAL OF CENTRAL CONNECTICUT (70035)**, 100 Grand Street, Zip 06052–2017, Mailing Address: P.O. Box 100, Zip 06050–0100; tel. 860/224–5011, (Includes BRADLEY MEMORIAL HOSPITAL AND HEALTH CENTER, 81 Meriden Avenue, Southington, Zip 06489–3297; tel. 860/276–5000; Clarence J. Silvia, President and Chief Executive Officer; NEW BRITAIN GENERAL HOSPITAL) **A**1 2 3 5 9 10 **F**2 3 4 11 12 13 15 17 18 20 24 25 26 27 31 32 33 36 38 41 42 43 44 49 50 51 52 53 55 56 57 58 59 60 61 62 63 64 66 68 70 72 73 74 75 76 77 79 80 81 82 84 86 87 88 89 90 91 92 93 94 95 96 97 100 102 104 105 106 107 109 111 113 118 119 120 121 124 131 132 133 135 136 137 **P**6
Primary Contact: Laurence A. Tanner, President and Chief Executive Officer
COO: Clarence J. Silvia, Senior Vice President Operations and Chief Operating Officer
CFO: David R. Newton, Senior Vice President Finance and Chief Financial Officer
CMO: Steven D. Hanks, M.D., Senior Vice President Medical Affairs and Chief Medical Officer
CIO: Frank Pinto, Chief Information Officer
CHR: Elizabeth A. Lynch, Vice President Human Resources
Web address: www.thocc.org
Control: Other not–for–profit (including NFP Corporation) **Service:** General Medical and Surgical

Staffed Beds: 330 **Admissions:** 20837 **Census:** 232 **Outpatient Visits:** 372257 **Births:** 1960 **Total Expense ($000):** 323173 **Payroll Expense ($000):** 132106 **Personnel:** 2223

NEW CANAAN—Fairfield County

☐ **SILVER HILL HOSPITAL (74014)**, 208 Valley Road, Zip 06840–3899; tel. 203/966–3561 **A**1 9 10 **F**4 5 25 26 31 32 33 34 52 56 57 66 73 88 89 90 91 93 94 95 119 121 135 **P**1
Primary Contact: Sigurd H. Ackerman, M.D., President and Chief Executive Officer
COO: Elizabeth Moore, Chief Operating Officer
CFO: Ruurd Leegstra, Chief Financial Officer
CMO: Sigurd H. Ackerman, M.D., President and Chief Executive Officer
CIO: Maria Klinga, Director Management Information Systems
CHR: Rich Juliana, Director Human Resources
Web address: www.silverhillhospital.org
Control: Other not–for–profit (including NFP Corporation) **Service:** Psychiatric

Staffed Beds: 60 **Admissions:** 2024 **Census:** 42 **Outpatient Visits:** 11070 **Births:** 0 **Total Expense ($000):** 26410 **Payroll Expense ($000):** 13675 **Personnel:** 216

NEW HAVEN—New Haven County

☐ **CONNECTICUT MENTAL HEALTH CENTER (74011)**, 34 Park Street, Zip 06508–1842, Mailing Address: P.O. Box 1842, Zip 06508–1842; tel. 203/974–7144 **A**1 3 5 9 10 **F**4 5 26 36 88 90 91 92 94 95 117 **S** Connecticut Department of Mental Health and Addiction Services
Primary Contact: Selby Jacobs, M.D., Director
COO: Robert Cole, Chief Operating Officer
CFO: Robert Cole, Chief Operating Officer
CMO: Jeanne Steines, D.O., Medical Director
CIO: Paul Moore, Chief Information Officer
CHR: Carolyn Wallace, Director Human Resources
Web address: www.dmhas.state.ct.us/lmha.htm
Control: State–Government, nonfederal **Service:** Psychiatric

Staffed Beds: 33 **Admissions:** 176 **Census:** 29 **Births:** 0 **Total Expense ($000):** 41641 **Payroll Expense ($000):** 15523 **Personnel:** 275

★ **HOSPITAL OF SAINT RAPHAEL (70001)**, 1450 Chapel Street, Zip 06511–1450; tel. 203/789–3000 **A**1 2 3 5 8 9 10 **F**3 5 11 12 13 15 17 18 20 22 24 25 26 27 28 31 32 33 34 36 37 38 40 41 43 44 46 47 49 50 51 54 55 56 57 58 59 60 62 63 64 66 68 69 71 72 73 74 75 76 77 79 80 81 82 84 85 86 87 88 89 90 91 92 93 94 95 96 97 99 100 102 104 105 106 107 108 109 111 112 116 119 121 123 124 133 135 136 137 **P**6
Primary Contact: David W. Benfer, FACHE, President and Chief Executive Officer
COO: Charles Hollander, M.D., Vice President and Chief Operating Officer
CIO: Gary Davidson, Vice President and Chief Information Officer
CHR: Elizabeth Conrad, Vice President Human Resources
Web address: www.srhs.org
Control: Church–operated, Nongovernment, not–for profit **Service:** General Medical and Surgical

Staffed Beds: 442 **Admissions:** 25245 **Census:** 362 **Births:** 1359 **Total Expense ($000):** 414539 **Payroll Expense ($000):** 184744 **Personnel:** 2682

CT

Hospital, Medicare Provider Number, Address, Telephone, Approval, Facility, and Physician Codes, Health Care System
★ American Hospital Association (AHA) membership
☐ The Joint Commission accreditation
○ American Osteopathic Association (AOA) accreditation
△ Commission on Accreditation of Rehabilitation Facilities (CARF) accreditation

★ **YALE–NEW HAVEN HOSPITAL (70022)**, 20 York Street, Zip 06510–3202; tel. 203/688–4242, (Includes YALE–NEW HAVEN CHILDREN'S HOSPITAL, 1 Park Street, Zip 06504–8901; tel. 203/688–4242; Michael Apkon, M.D., Vice President and Executive Director; YALE–NEW HAVEN PSYCHIATRIC HOSPITAL, 184 Liberty Street, Zip 06519–1625; tel. 203/688–9704; Paul Haeberle, Executive Director) **A**1 2 3 5 8 9 10 **F**3 5 8 11 12 13 15 17 18 19 20 21 22 23 25 26 27 28 30 31 32 33 34 36 37 38 39 40 41 43 44 46 47 48 49 50 51 53 54 55 56 57 58 60 62 64 66 68 69 70 72 73 74 75 76 77 78 79 80 81 82 83 84 86 87 88 89 90 91 92 93 94 95 96 97 99 100 102 103 104 105 106 107 108 109 111 112 113 114 116 118 119 120 121 122 123 124 125 126 127 128 131 132 133 134 135 136 137 **P**4 5 **S** Yale New Haven Health System
Primary Contact: Marna P. Borgstrom, President and Chief Executive Officer
COO: Richard D'Aquila, Executive Vice President and Chief Operating Officer
CFO: James Staten, Senior Vice President Finance
CMO: Peter N. Herbert, M.D., Senior Vice President Medical Affairs and Chief of Staff
CIO: Mark Andersen, Senior Vice President Information Systems and Chief Information Officer
CHR: Kevin A. Myatt, Senior Vice President Human Resources
Web address: www.ynhh.org
Control: Other not–for–profit (including NFP Corporation) **Service:** General Medical and Surgical

Staffed Beds: 881 **Admissions:** 46913 **Census:** 658 **Outpatient Visits:** 320545 **Births:** 4592 **Total Expense ($000):** 941064 **Payroll Expense ($000):** 380796 **Personnel:** 6939

CT

NEW LONDON—New London County

★ △ **LAWRENCE & MEMORIAL HOSPITAL (70007)**, 365 Montauk Avenue, Zip 06320–4769; tel. 860/442–0711 **A**1 2 3 5 7 9 10 **F**3 8 11 13 15 17 18 20 24 25 26 27 28 30 31 32 33 34 36 37 38 39 42 43 44 45 46 47 48 49 50 51 52 53 54 55 56 57 58 59 60 62 63 64 66 68 70 72 73 74 75 76 77 79 80 81 82 84 85 86 88 89 90 91 92 93 94 96 97 100 102 104 106 107 109 112 118 119 120 121 123 124 133 135 136 137 **P**6
Primary Contact: Bruce D. Cummings, President and Chief Executive Officer
COO: Cynthia B. Kane, Executive Vice President and Chief Operating Officer
CFO: Elwin Bresette, Vice President and Chief Financial Officer
CIO: Randy Scarpati, Chief Information Officer
Web address: www.lmhospital.org
Control: Other not–for–profit (including NFP Corporation) **Service:** General Medical and Surgical

Staffed Beds: 252 **Admissions:** 13032 **Census:** 180 **Outpatient Visits:** 167680 **Births:** 1665 **Total Expense ($000):** 244442 **Payroll Expense ($000):** 121960 **Personnel:** 1790

NEW MILFORD—Litchfield County

★ ○ **NEW MILFORD HOSPITAL (70015)**, 21 Elm Street, Zip 06776–2993; tel. 860/355–2611 **A**1 9 10 11 19 **F**3 8 13 14 15 17 18 24 25 26 27 30 31 32 33 34 36 37 38 42 43 44 49 51 55 56 57 58 60 66 68 72 73 74 76 77 79 80 84 92 94 96 97 99 100 102 105 106 107 108 109 111 114 118 119 120 121 124 134 135 136
Primary Contact: Joseph Frolkis, M.D., President and Chief Executive Officer
COO: Susan Iovino, Chief Operating Officer and Chief Nursing Officer
CFO: Joseph Hart, Controller and Chief Financial Officer
CMO: Joan Puglia, M.D., President Medical Staff
CIO: Stephen Veillette, Director Management Information Systems
CHR: Robert Sommer, Vice President Human Resources
Web address: www.newmilfordhospital.org
Control: Other not–for–profit (including NFP Corporation) **Service:** General Medical and Surgical

Staffed Beds: 62 **Admissions:** 2551 **Census:** 29 **Outpatient Visits:** 105919 **Births:** 294 **Total Expense ($000):** 84330 **Payroll Expense ($000):** 35112 **Personnel:** 519

NEWINGTON—Hartford County

☐ **CEDARCREST HOSPITAL (74009)**, 525 Russell Road, Zip 06111–1595; tel. 860/666–4613 **A**1 10 **F**3 4 5 31 32 66 88 119 135 136 **P**6 **S** Connecticut Department of Mental Health and Addiction Services
Primary Contact: Brenda Thorington, Chief Executive Officer
CFO: Rosemarie Peshka, Fiscal Officer
CMO: Thomas Pisano, Chief Professional Services
CIO: Stephen Janik, Ph.D., Director Information Systems
CHR: Cheryl Thompson, Director Human Resources
Control: State–Government, nonfederal **Service:** Psychiatric

Staffed Beds: 145 **Admissions:** 1730 **Census:** 138 **Outpatient Visits:** 0 **Births:** 0 **Total Expense ($000):** 52093 **Payroll Expense ($000):** 30154 **Personnel:** 417

NORWALK—Fairfield County

★ △ **NORWALK HOSPITAL (70034)**, 34 Maple Street, Zip 06850–3894; tel. 203/852–2000, (Nonreporting) **A**1 2 7 9 10
Primary Contact: Geoffrey F. Cole, President and Chief Executive Officer
CFO: Thomas Breen, Vice President Finance
CMO: Michael Marks, M.D., Chief of Staff
CIO: Christian Randon, Chief Information Officer and Vice President Information Technology
CHR: Anthony Aceto, Vice President Human Resources
Web address: www.norwalkhosp.org
Control: Other not–for–profit (including NFP Corporation) **Service:** General Medical and Surgical

Staffed Beds: 269

NORWICH—New London County

★ **THE WILLIAM W. BACKUS HOSPITAL (70024)**, 326 Washington Street, Zip 06360–2733; tel. 860/889–8331 **A**1 2 9 10 **F**3 9 11 13 15 18 24 25 26 27 30 31 32 33 34 38 40 42 43 44 46 49 51 53 55 56 57 58 59 60 61 62 63 68 69 72 73 74 75 76 77 79 80 81 82 84 86 87 88 90 91 92 93 94 95 96 97 99 100 102 104 105 106 107 108 109 119 121 122 123 124 133 134 135 136 137
Primary Contact: Thomas P. Pipicelli, President and Chief Executive Officer
COO: Mark A. Santamaria, Senior Vice President and Chief Operating Officer
CFO: Daniel E. Lohr, Senior Vice President and Chief Financial Officer
CMO: Peter H. Shea, M.D., Medical Director
CIO: Pamela M. Muccilli, Vice President and Chief Information Officer
CHR: Theresa L. Buss, Director Human Resources
Web address: www.backushospital.org
Control: Other not–for–profit (including NFP Corporation) **Service:** General Medical and Surgical

Staffed Beds: 184 **Admissions:** 10987 **Census:** 132 **Outpatient Visits:** 371132 **Births:** 1057 **Total Expense ($000):** 200872 **Payroll Expense ($000):** 87441 **Personnel:** 1413

PUTNAM—Windham County

★ **DAY KIMBALL HOSPITAL (70003)**, 320 Pomfret Street, Zip 06260–0901, Mailing Address: P.O. Box 6001, Zip 06260–6001; tel. 860/928–6541 **A**1 9 10 **F**3 5 8 13 15 25 26 27 28 30 31 33 38 42 43 44 54 56 57 61 62 63 68 72 74 75 76 79 84 86 88 92 94 96 100 103 105 106 107 118 119 121 135 136
Primary Contact: Robert E. Smanik, FACHE, President and Chief Executive Officer
CFO: Crista Durand, Senior Vice President Finance and Chief Financial Officer
CMO: Douglas Waite, M.D., Vice President Medical Affairs
CIO: Carl Gentry, Vice President Management Information Systems and Chief Information Officer
CHR: Rita Conrad, Interim Manager Human Resources
Web address: www.daykimball.org
Control: Other not–for–profit (including NFP Corporation) **Service:** General Medical and Surgical

Staffed Beds: 63 **Admissions:** 4998 **Census:** 52 **Outpatient Visits:** 421200 **Births:** 338 **Total Expense ($000):** 91555 **Payroll Expense ($000):** 40291

ROCKY HILL—Hartford County

VETERANS HOME AND HOSPITAL (72006), 287 West Street, Zip 06067–3501; tel. 860/529–2571, (Nonreporting) **A**10
Primary Contact: Margaret Concannon, Acting Administrator
CFO: Gregory J. Gioia, Chief Fiscal and Administrative Services
CMO: Michael M. Cebrik, M.D., Director Medical Staff
Web address: www.state.ct.us/ctva/
Control: State–Government, nonfederal **Service:** Long–Term Acute Care hospital

Staffed Beds: 215

SHARON—Litchfield County

☐ **SHARON HOSPITAL (70004)**, 50 Hospital Hill Road, Zip 06069–0789, Mailing Address: P.O. Box 789, Zip 06069–0789; tel. 860/364–4141, (Nonreporting) **A**1 2 9 10 20 **S** Essent Healthcare
Primary Contact: Charles Therrien, Chief Executive Officer
CMO: Evan Provisor, M.D., Chief of Staff
CIO: Daniel Rego, Director Information Management
CHR: Kathleen Berlinghoff, Director Human Resources
Web address: www.sharonhospital.com
Control: Corporation, Investor–owned, for–profit **Service:** General Medical and Surgical

Staffed Beds: 78

SOMERS—Tolland County

CONNECTICUT DEPARTMENT OF CORRECTION'S HOSPITAL, 100 Bilton Road, Zip 6071, Mailing Address: P.O. Box 100, Zip 06071–0100; tel. 860/749–8391, (Nonreporting)
Primary Contact: Edward A. Blanchette, M.D., Director
Control: State–Government, nonfederal **Service:** Hospital unit of an institution (prison hospital, college infimary, etc.)

Staffed Beds: 29

SOUTHINGTON—Hartford County

BRADLEY MEMORIAL HOSPITAL AND HEALTH CENTER See The Hospital of Central Connecticut, New Britain

STAFFORD SPRINGS—Tolland County

★ **JOHNSON MEMORIAL HOSPITAL (70008)**, 201 Chestnut Hill Road, Zip 06076–4005; tel. 860/684–4251 **A**1 9 10 **F**3 5 8 11 13 15 24 25 27 30 31 32 33 36 38 42 43 44 51 53 54 55 56 57 59 60 62 66 68 72 73 74 76 77 79 80 81 82 84 86 87 88 90 91 92 94 95 96 97 98 99 100 102 103 104 105 106 107 118 119 120 121 133 135 136 **P**5
Primary Contact: Peter Betts, Interim President and Chief Executive Officer
COO: Peter Kuzmickas, Vice President Operations
CMO: Herbert J. DiMeola, M.D., Vice President Medical Affairs
CIO: Mark Rivard, Director Information Services
CHR: Robert van Heiningen, Vice President Human Resources
Web address: www.johnsonhealthnetwork.com
Control: Other not–for–profit (including NFP Corporation) **Service:** General Medical and Surgical

Staffed Beds: 92 **Admissions:** 4149 **Census:** 66 **Outpatient Visits:** 107752 **Births:** 289 **Total Expense ($000):** 61159 **Payroll Expense ($000):** 28594 **Personnel:** 491

STAMFORD—Fairfield County

★ **STAMFORD HOSPITAL (70006)**, 30 Shelburne Road, Zip 6902, Mailing Address: P.O. Box 9317, Zip 06904–9317; tel. 203/276–1000 **A**1 2 3 5 8 9 10 **F**2 3 7 8 11 13 15 18 20 22 24 25 26 27 28 31 32 33 34 36 38 39 40 41 43 44 46 49 50 52 53 54 55 56 57 58 59 60 62 63 64 66 68 69 70 72 73 74 75 76 77 79 80 81 82 84 85 86 87 88 90 91 92 93 94 95 96 97 98 99 100 102 103 106 107 108 109 113 114 118 119 120 121 124 133 134 135 136 137 **P**6
Primary Contact: Brian G. Grissler, President and Chief Executive Officer
COO: Kathleen A. Silard, Executive Vice President Operations and Chief Operating officer
CMO: John Rodis, M.D., Senior Vice President Medical Affairs
CIO: David Taylor, Vice President Information Systems and Chief Information Officer
CHR: Elaine Guglielmo, Vice President Human Resources and Organizational Development
Web address: www.stamhealth.org
Control: Other not–for–profit (including NFP Corporation) **Service:** General Medical and Surgical

Staffed Beds: 277 **Admissions:** 14018 **Census:** 184 **Outpatient Visits:** 303556 **Births:** 2662 **Total Expense ($000):** 306587 **Payroll Expense ($000):** 123207 **Personnel:** 1734

TORRINGTON—Litchfield County

★ **THE CHARLOTTE HUNGERFORD HOSPITAL (70011)**, 540 Litchfield Street, Zip 06790–0988, Mailing Address: P.O. Box 988, Zip 06790–0988; tel. 860/496–6666 **A**1 2 9 10 **F**3 5 11 13 15 17 24 25 26 27 28 31 32 33 34 36 38 39 40 42 43 50 51 52 53 55 56 57 60 62 66 68 72 73 74 76 77 79 80 81 82 84 88 89 90 91 92 93 94 95 96 97 100 104 106 107 109 118 119 121 124 133 135 136 137 **P**6
Primary Contact: Daniel J. McIntyre, President and Chief Executive Officer
CFO: Gary J. DePaul, Vice President Finance and Treasurer
CMO: Mark Prete, M.D., Vice President Medical Affairs
CIO: Jonathan Trask, Director Management Information Services
CHR: R. James Elliott, Vice President Human Resources
Web address: www.charlottesweb.hungerford.org
Control: Other not–for–profit (including NFP Corporation) **Service:** General Medical and Surgical

Staffed Beds: 105 **Admissions:** 6145 **Census:** 75

VERNON ROCKVILLE—Hartford County

★ **ROCKVILLE GENERAL HOSPITAL (70012)**, 31 Union Street, Zip 06066–3160; tel. 860/872–0501 **A**1 9 10 **F**3 11 13 15 18 24 25 26 30 31 33 37 38 41 42 46 49 50 51 54 55 56 57 60 62 64 68 72 73 74 77 79 80 81 82 84 86 96 97 100 106 107 112 119 120 121 124 133 135 137 **P**1 5 6 **S** Eastern Connecticut Health Network
Primary Contact: Peter J. Karl, President and Chief Executive Officer
CFO: Kevin G. Murphy, Senior Vice President Finance and Chief Financial Officer
CMO: Joel R. Reich, M.D., Senior Vice President Medical Affairs
CIO: Charles Covin, Chief Information Officer
CHR: Mary Kohanski, Senior Vice President Human Resources
Web address: www.echn.org
Control: Other not–for–profit (including NFP Corporation) **Service:** General Medical and Surgical

Staffed Beds: 59 **Admissions:** 3156 **Census:** 38 **Outpatient Visits:** 136591 **Births:** 466 **Total Expense ($000):** 61563 **Payroll Expense ($000):** 28332 **Personnel:** 432

WALLINGFORD—New Haven County

□ △ **GAYLORD HOSPITAL (72003)**, Gaylord Farm Road, Zip 06492–7048, Mailing Address: P.O. Box 400, Zip 06492–0400; tel. 203/284–2800 **A**1 5 7 10 **F**1 25 26 33 62 75 86 96 118 119 135 137
Primary Contact: James J. Cullen, President and Chief Executive Officer
CFO: Janine L. Epright, Vice President and Chief Financial Officer
CMO: Jerrold L. Kaplan, M.D., Vice President and Medical Director
CIO: Brian Richards, Director Information Technology
CHR: Bruce Dalstrom, Vice President Human Resources
Web address: www.gaylord.org
Control: Other not–for–profit (including NFP Corporation) **Service:** Long–Term Acute Care hospital

Staffed Beds: 107 **Admissions:** 1352 **Census:** 99 **Outpatient Visits:** 67371 **Births:** 0 **Total Expense ($000):** 68989 **Payroll Expense ($000):** 38087 **Personnel:** 501

★ **MASONIC HEALTHCARE CENTER (70039)**, 22 Masonic Avenue, Zip 06492–3048, Mailing Address: P.O. Box 70, Zip 06492–7002; tel. 203/679–5900 **A**5 10 **F**29 33 37 42 54 56 57 62 63 65 75 77 86 88 93 94 96 107 117 119 135 137
Primary Contact: William C. Piper, President
COO: James F. Standish, Chief Financial Officer
CFO: James F. Standish, Chief Financial Officer
CMO: Ronald Schwartz, M.D., Medical Director
CIO: James Albert, Director Information Services
CHR: Douglas T. Barrett, Senior Vice President Human Resources
Web address: www.masonicare.org
Control: Other not–for–profit (including NFP Corporation) **Service:** General Medical and Surgical

Staffed Beds: 447 **Admissions:** 1640 **Census:** 403 **Total Expense ($000):** 57937 **Payroll Expense ($000):** 27909 **Personnel:** 577

WATERBURY—New Haven County

★ **SAINT MARY'S HOSPITAL (70016)**, 56 Franklin Street, Zip 06706–1281; tel. 203/709–6000 **A**1 2 3 5 9 10 **F**3 5 8 11 12 13 15 17 18 20 22 24 25 26 27 30 31 32 33 34 35 37 38 40 42 43 49 50 53 55 56 57 62 68 70 72 73 74 75 76 77 78 79 80 82 84 85 86 87 88 90 92 94 95 96 97 99 100 101 102 106 107 118 119 121 124 135 **P**3 6 7 8
CFO: Robert Halko, Vice President and Chief Financial Officer
CMO: Steve Holland, M.D., Chief Medical Officer
CIO: Carolyn Orrell, Chief Information Officer
CHR: M. Clark Kearney, Vice President Human Resources
Web address: www.stmh.org
Control: Church–operated, Nongovernment, not–for profit **Service:** General Medical and Surgical

Staffed Beds: 202 **Admissions:** 12052 **Census:** 158 **Outpatient Visits:** 208437 **Births:** 1265 **Total Expense ($000):** 169018 **Payroll Expense ($000):** 69635 **Personnel:** 1348

★ **WATERBURY HOSPITAL (70005)**, 64 Robbins Street, Zip 06708–2600; tel. 203/573–6000 **A**1 2 3 5 9 10 **F**3 5 9 13 15 17 18 20 22 24 25 26 30 31 32 33 36 38 40 41 43 47 49 50 51 52 55 56 57 60 62 66 68 71 72 73 74 75 77 79 80 81 82 84 87 88 89 90 91 92 93 94 95 96 97 99 100 103 106 107 114 118 119 120 121 134 135 137
Primary Contact: John H. Tobin, President and Chief Executive Officer
COO: Mary Prybylo, Vice President Patient Care Services and Chief Operating Officer
CFO: Colleen M. Scott, Vice President Finance
CIO: James Olson, Chief Information Officer
CHR: Kathy Mulston, Vice President Human Resources
Web address: www.waterburyhospital.org
Control: Other not–for–profit (including NFP Corporation) **Service:** General Medical and Surgical

Staffed Beds: 235 **Admissions:** 13726 **Census:** 188 **Outpatient Visits:** 179153 **Births:** 1293 **Total Expense ($000):** 174896 **Payroll Expense ($000):** 105736 **Personnel:** 1557

CT

Hospital, Medicare Provider Number, Address, Telephone, Approval, Facility, and Physician Codes, Health Care System

★ American Hospital Association (AHA) membership
□ The Joint Commission accreditation
○ American Osteopathic Association (AOA) accreditation
△ Commission on Accreditation of Rehabilitation Facilities (CARF) accreditation

WEST HARTFORD—Hartford County

★ **HEBREW HOME AND HOSPITAL (70040)**, (Formerly Hebrew Health Care), (Comprehensive Geriatric Health), 1 Abrahms Boulevard, Zip 06117–1525; tel. 860/523–3800, (Total facility includes 287 beds in nursing home–type unit) **A**3 5 10 **F**1 2 6 10 11 24 25 26 29 32 36 37 43 44 45 54 61 62 67 73 75 76 85 86 87 88 93 115 117 119 121 132 135 137 **P**5
Primary Contact: Bonnie B. Gauthier, President and Chief Executive Officer
COO: Kathy Mon, Vice President Operations
CFO: David Houle, Executive Vice President and Chief Financial Officer
CMO: Henry Schneiderman, M.D., Vice President Medical Services and Physician in Chief
CHR: Nancy J. Williams, Manager Human Resources
Web address: www.hebrewhealthcare.org
Control: Other not–for–profit (including NFP Corporation) **Service:** Other specialty

Staffed Beds: 332 **Admissions:** 1095 **Census:** 298 **Outpatient Visits:** 319
Births: 0 **Total Expense ($000):** 41071 **Payroll Expense ($000):** 23102
Personnel: 462

WEST HAVEN—New Haven County

★ **VETERANS AFFAIRS CONNECTICUT HEALTHCARE SYSTEM–NEW HAVEN DIVISION**, 950 Campbell Avenue, Zip 06516–2770; tel. 203/932–5711, (Includes WEST HAVEN DIVISION), (Total facility includes 40 beds in nursing home–type unit) (Nonreporting) **A**1 2 3 5 8 **S** Department of Veterans Affairs
Primary Contact: Roger L. Johnson, Director
CFO: Joseph LaMadeleine, Chief Financial Officer
CMO: Michael Ebert, M.D., Chief of Staff
CIO: Joseph Erdos, M.D., Chief Information Officer
CHR: Mark Bain, Chief Human Resources
Web address: www.va.gov/sta/guide/home.asp
Control: Veterans Affairs, Government, federal **Service:** General Medical and Surgical

Staffed Beds: 200

CT

WESTPORT—Fairfield County

HALL–BROOKE HOSPITAL, A DIVISION OF HALL–BROOKE BEHAVIORAL HEALTH SERVICES See St. Vincent's Medical Center, Bridgeport

WILLIMANTIC—Windham County

★ **WINDHAM COMMUNITY MEMORIAL HOSPITAL (70021)**, 112 Mansfield Avenue, Zip 06226–2040; tel. 860/456–9116 **A**1 9 10 19 **F**3 8 11 13 14 15 17 24 25 26 27 30 32 33 34 38 43 45 50 51 55 56 57 60 64 66 67 68 72 73 74 75 76 77 79 81 84 85 86 96 97 100 103 104 106 107 118 119 120 121 124 133 135 136
Primary Contact: Richard A. Brvenik, FACHE, President and Chief Executive Officer
CFO: James Papadakos, Vice President Finance and Chief Financial Officer
CMO: Anthea Woodley, M.D., Chief of Staff
CIO: Kevin Tupper, Director Information Technology
CHR: Marty Levine, Vice President Human Resources
Web address: www.windhamhospital.org
Control: Other not–for–profit (including NFP Corporation) **Service:** General Medical and Surgical

Staffed Beds: 79 **Admissions:** 5281 **Census:** 57 **Outpatient Visits:** 144377
Births: 456 **Total Expense ($000):** 76141 **Payroll Expense ($000):** 36047
Personnel: 633

DELAWARE

DOVER—Kent County

★ △ **BAYHEALTH MEDICAL CENTER (80004)**, 640 South State Street, Zip 19901–3597; tel. 302/674–4700, (Includes BAYHEALTH MEDICAL CENTER AT KENT GENERAL; BAYHEALTH MEDICAL CENTER, MILFORD MEMORIAL HOSPITAL, 21 West Clarke Avenue, Milford, Zip 19963–1840; tel. 302/430–5738) **A**1 2 7 9 10 **F**3 11 13 15 17 18 20 22 24 25 26 27 28 30 31 32 33 36 38 40 41 43 44 47 48 49 50 51 52 53 55 56 57 59 60 61 62 65 66 68 70 71 72 73 74 75 76 77 79 80 81 82 83 84 85 86 88 89 90 91 92 93 94 95 96 97 98 100 102 103 104 105 106 107 109 111 118 119 120 121 123 124 133 135 136 **P**6 8
Primary Contact: Dennis E. Klima, President and Chief Executive Officer
COO: Terry Murphy, Executive Vice President and Chief Operating Officer
CFO: Earl P. Tanis, Senior Vice President Financial Operations
CMO: Gary M. Siegelman, M.D., Ph.D., Senior Vice President and Chief Medical Officer
CIO: Terry Feinour, Senior Vice President Corporate Services
CHR: Jon McDowell, Vice President
Web address: www.bayhealth.org
Control: Other not–for–profit (including NFP Corporation) **Service:** General Medical and Surgical

Staffed Beds: 345 **Admissions:** 18954 **Census:** 281 **Outpatient Visits:** 403657 **Births:** 2312 **Total Expense ($000):** 301083 **Payroll Expense ($000):** 127527 **Personnel:** 2501

DOVER BEHAVIORAL HEALTH SYSTEM (84004), 725 Horsepond Road, Zip 19901; tel. 302/741–0140, (Nonreporting) **A**10 **S** Universal Health Services, Inc.
Web address: www.doverbehavioral.com
Control: Corporation, Investor–owned, for–profit **Service:** Psychiatric

Staffed Beds: 56

LEWES—Sussex County

★ **BEEBE MEDICAL CENTER (80007)**, 424 Savannah Road, Zip 19958–0226; tel. 302/645–3300, (Total facility includes 89 beds in nursing home–type unit) **A**1 2 6 9 10 19 **F**2 11 13 15 17 18 20 22 24 25 26 27 28 30 31 32 33 34 36 38 39 40 50 51 53 54 55 56 57 58 59 60 61 62 65 66 68 73 74 75 76 77 79 80 82 86 87 90 92 96 97 98 100 102 104 105 106 107 109 111 117 118 119 121 123 132 135 136 137 **P**6 7
Primary Contact: Jeffrey M. Fried, FACHE, President and Chief Executive Officer
COO: Thomas Steiner, Chief Operating Officer
CFO: James W. Bartle, Vice President Finance
CMO: Andrejs Strauss, M.D., Interim Vice President Medical Affairs
CIO: Barbara P. Vugrinec, Vice President Information Systems
CHR: Catherine Halen, Vice President Human Resources
Web address: www.beebemed.org
Control: Other not–for–profit (including NFP Corporation) **Service:** General Medical and Surgical

Staffed Beds: 205 **Admissions:** 9718 **Census:** 175 **Outpatient Visits:** 370220 **Births:** 976 **Total Expense ($000):** 173670 **Payroll Expense ($000):** 66996 **Personnel:** 1350

MILFORD—Sussex County

BAYHEALTH MEDICAL CENTER, MILFORD MEMORIAL HOSPITAL See Bayhealth Medical Center, Dover

NEW CASTLE—New Castle County

☐ **DELAWARE PSYCHIATRIC CENTER (84001)**, 1901 North Dupont Highway, Zip 19720–1199; tel. 302/255–2700, (Total facility includes 35 beds in nursing home–type unit) (Nonreporting) **A**1 10
Primary Contact: Susan Watson Robinson, Director
CFO: Bruce Ashbaugh, Senior Fiscal Administrative Officer
CIO: James Nau, Manager Computer and Applications Support
Web address: www.dhss.delaware.gov
Control: State–Government, nonfederal **Service:** Psychiatric

Staffed Beds: 270

☐ **MEADOW WOOD BEHAVIORAL HEALTH SYSTEM (84003)**, 575 South Dupont Highway, Zip 19720–4600; tel. 302/328–3330, (Nonreporting) **A**1 9 10 **S** Horizon Health Corporation
Primary Contact: Kim Whitelock, Chief Executive Officer
CFO: John Greenly, Chief Financial Officer
Web address: www.horizonhealth.com
Control: State–Government, nonfederal **Service:** Psychiatric

Staffed Beds: 53

NEWARK—New Castle County

CHRISTIANA HOSPITAL See Christiana Care Health System, Wilmington

☐ **ROCKFORD CENTER (84002)**, 100 Rockford Drive, Zip 19713–2121; tel. 302/996–5480 **A**1 9 10 **F**31 32 54 88 89 93 95 119 **P**6 8 **S** Universal Health Services, Inc.
Primary Contact: John F. McKenna, Chief Executive Officer and Managing Director
COO: Shawn Walsh, Chief Operating Officer
CFO: Kumar Purohit, Chief Financial Officer
CHR: Jessi Jeppi, Director Human Resources
Web address: www.rockfordcenter.com
Control: Corporation, Investor–owned, for–profit **Service:** Psychiatric

Staffed Beds: 92 **Admissions:** 3677 **Census:** 82 **Outpatient Visits:** 12178 **Births:** 0 **Total Expense ($000):** 15003 **Payroll Expense ($000):** 8834 **Personnel:** 144

SEAFORD—Sussex County

★ **NANTICOKE MEMORIAL HOSPITAL (80006)**, 801 Middleford Road, Zip 19973–3698; tel. 302/629–6611, (Total facility includes 110 beds in nursing home–type unit) **A**1 2 9 10 19 **F**3 11 13 15 18 24 25 26 27 28 32 33 38 40 43 44 49 51 55 56 57 66 68 72 73 74 75 76 77 79 80 82 84 86 96 97 100 102 107 109 111 117 118 119 121 124 135 137
Primary Contact: Mark J. Rappaport, President and Chief Executive Officer
COO: Catherine Kenny, Vice President Operations
CFO: Darr Hall, Chief Financial Officer
CIO: Susan Godesky, Chief Information Officer
CHR: Theresa Drye, Vice President Human Resources
Web address: www.nanticoke.org
Control: Other not–for–profit (including NFP Corporation) **Service:** General Medical and Surgical

Staffed Beds: 234 **Admissions:** 6398 **Census:** 182 **Outpatient Visits:** 108396 **Births:** 950 **Total Expense ($000):** 103808 **Payroll Expense ($000):** 39691 **Personnel:** 732

WILMINGTON—New Castle County

★ △ **ALFRED I. DUPONT HOSPITAL FOR CHILDREN (83300)**, (Formerly duPont Hospital for Children), 1600 Rockland Road, Zip 19803–3616, Mailing Address: Box 269, Zip 19899–0269; tel. 302/651–4000, (Nonreporting) **A**1 3 5 7 10
Primary Contact: Thomas P. Ferry, Chief Executive Officer
COO: Paul D. Kempinski, Chief Operating Officer
CFO: William N. Britton, Associate Administrator Finance
CMO: Bernard J. Clark, M.D., Medical Director
CIO: Ann Altoe, Senior Director Information Systems and Security Officer
CHR: Terri Young, Vice President Human Resources
Web address: www.nemours.org
Control: Other not–for–profit (including NFP Corporation) **Service:** Children's general

Staffed Beds: 166

DE

Hospital, Medicare Provider Number, Address, Telephone, Approval, Facility, and Physician Codes, Health Care System

★ American Hospital Association (AHA) membership
☐ The Joint Commission accreditation
○ American Osteopathic Association (AOA) accreditation
△ Commission on Accreditation of Rehabilitation Facilities (CARF) accreditation

★ **CHRISTIANA CARE HEALTH SYSTEM (80001)**, 501 West 14th Street, Zip 19801; tel. 302/428–2570, (Includes CHRISTIANA HOSPITAL, 4755 Ogletown–Stanton Road, Newark, Zip 19718; tel. 302/428–2570; WILMINGTON HOSPITAL, 501 West 14th Street, Mailing Address: Box 1668, Zip 19899; tel. 302/733–1000), (Total facility includes 93 beds in nursing home–type unit) **A**1 2 3 5 8 9 10 12 13 **F**2 3 6 8 11 12 13 15 17 18 20 22 24 25 26 27 28 30 31 32 33 34 35 36 37 38 40 41 43 44 46 47 49 50 52 53 54 55 56 57 58 59 60 61 62 63 64 65 66 68 70 72 73 74 75 76 77 78 79 80 81 82 83 84 85 86 87 88 89 90 91 92 93 94 95 96 97 99 100 102 103 104 105 106 107 108 109 111 112 114 116 117 118 119 120 121 123 124 125 127 134 135 136 **P**6 **S** Christiana Care Health System
Primary Contact: Robert J. Laskowski, M.D., President and Chief Executive Officer
COO: Gary W. Ferguson, Executive Vice President and Chief Operating Officer
CFO: Thomas L. Corrigan, Senior Vice President Finance, Managed Care and Chief Financial Officer
CMO: James H. Newman, M.D., Chief Medical Officer
CIO: Steve Hess, Chief Information Officer
CHR: Benjamin T. Shaw, Senior Vice President Human Resources
Web address: www.christianacare.org
Control: Other not–for–profit (including NFP Corporation) **Service:** General Medical and Surgical

Staffed Beds: 1011 **Admissions:** 56145 **Census:** 885 **Outpatient Visits:** 382091 **Births:** 7100 **Total Expense ($000):** 1009640 **Payroll Expense ($000):** 480788 **Personnel:** 8488

DUPONT HOSPITAL FOR CHILDREN See Alfred I. duPont Hospital for Children

☐ **SELECT SPECIALTY HOSPITAL WILMINGTON (82000)**, 7 Clayton Street, 5th Floor, Zip 19801; tel. 302/421–4545, (Nonreporting) **A**1 10 **S** Select Medical Corporation
Primary Contact: Carol Chrisman, Chief Executive Officer
Web address: www.selectmedicalcorp.com
Control: Corporation, Investor–owned, for–profit **Service:** Long–Term Acute Care hospital

Staffed Beds: 35

DE

★ **ST. FRANCIS HOSPITAL (80003)**, Seventh and Clayton Streets, Zip 19805–0500, Mailing Address: P.O. Box 2500, Zip 19805–0500; tel. 302/421–4100, (Total facility includes 104 beds in nursing home–type unit) **A**1 2 3 5 9 10 **F**7 12 13 15 18 20 22 24 25 26 27 30 31 32 33 38 43 46 47 49 50 53 55 56 57 61 62 66 68 69 70 72 73 75 76 77 79 82 85 96 100 107 116 117 118 119 124 135 136 137 **S** Catholic Health East
Primary Contact: Clarence R. LaLiberty, Jr., President and Chief Executive Officer
COO: Ernest Baptiste, Chief Operating Officer
CFO: David Capone, Chief Financial Officer
CMO: Valentine Burroughs, M.D., Medical Director
CIO: Paul W. Rowe, Director Information Technology
CHR: Charlene J. Wilson, Vice President Human Resources
Web address: www.stfrancishealthcare.org
Control: Other not–for–profit (including NFP Corporation) **Service:** General Medical and Surgical

Staffed Beds: 298 **Admissions:** 7587 **Census:** 202 **Outpatient Visits:** 167874 **Births:** 974 **Total Expense ($000):** 131077 **Payroll Expense ($000):** 60388 **Personnel:** 886

★ **VETERANS AFFAIRS MEDICAL CENTER**, 1601 Kirkwood Highway, Zip 19805–4989; tel. 302/994–2511, (Total facility includes 60 beds in nursing home–type unit) **A**1 2 3 5 8 **F**3 5 9 12 25 26 27 33 34 36 37 38 41 43 44 50 51 52 53 54 55 56 57 58 59 60 61 62 63 64 66 68 72 73 75 76 77 79 80 81 82 86 87 90 91 92 93 94 96 97 102 106 107 117 119 124 132 133 135 136 137 **P**6 **S** Department of Veterans Affairs
Primary Contact: Charles M. Dorman, FACHE, Director
CFO: Lori Barbanel, Resource Management Center Leader
CMO: Morris D. Kerstein, M.D., Chief of Staff
CIO: Scott Vlars, Chief Information Technology Services
CHR: William Hucker, Manager Administrative Support
Web address: www.va.gov/wilmington
Control: Veterans Affairs, Government, federal **Service:** General Medical and Surgical

Staffed Beds: 120 **Admissions:** 2639 **Census:** 41 **Outpatient Visits:** 187459 **Births:** 0

WILMINGTON HOSPITAL See Christiana Care Health System

Many Facility Codes have changed. Please refer to the AHA Guide Code Chart.

DISTRICT OF COLUMBIA

WASHINGTON—District of Columbia County

★ **CHILDREN'S NATIONAL MEDICAL CENTER (93300)**, 111 Michigan Avenue N.W., Zip 20010–2970; tel. 202/476–5000 **A**1 3 5 8 9 10 **F**3 7 8 9 14 17 18 19 20 21 22 23 24 25 26 27 28 30 31 32 33 35 37 38 40 41 43 44 50 53 55 56 57 58 59 60 62 63 64 66 69 70 72 73 75 76 77 79 80 81 82 83 84 86 87 88 89 90 91 92 94 95 96 97 100 102 106 107 112 114 118 119 120 121 122 123 124 125 126 127 131 132 133 135 137 **P**6
Primary Contact: Edwin K. Zechman, Jr., President and Chief Executive Officer
COO: Jody Burdell, Vice President and Chief Operating Officer
CMO: Peter Holbrook, M.D., Chief Medical Officer
CIO: Joseph O' Connor, Chief Information Officer
CHR: Carole Schor, Vice President Human Resources
Web address: www.childrensnational.org
Control: Other not–for–profit (including NFP Corporation) **Service:** Children's general

Staffed Beds: 230 **Admissions:** 13047 **Census:** 205 **Outpatient Visits:** 366051 **Births:** 0 **Total Expense ($000):** 440912 **Payroll Expense ($000):** 210650 **Personnel:** 4104

★ △ **GEORGE WASHINGTON UNIVERSITY HOSPITAL (90001)**, 900 23rd Street N.W., Zip 20037–2377; tel. 202/715–4000, (Nonreporting) **A**1 2 3 5 7 8 9 10 **S** Universal Health Services, Inc.
Primary Contact: Trent Crable, Interim Chief Executive Officer
COO: Trent Crable, Chief Operating Officer
CFO: Richard Davis, Chief Financial Officer
CMO: Carlos Silva, M.D., Medical Director
CIO: Gretchen Tegethoff, Vice President Information Resources
CHR: Karen Frazier, Director Human Resources
Web address: www.gwhospital.com
Control: Partnership, Investor–owned, for–profit **Service:** General Medical and Surgical

Staffed Beds: 326

GREATER SOUTHEAST COMMUNITY HOSPITAL See United Medical Center

HADLEY MEMORIAL HOSPITAL See Specialty Hospitals of Washington–Hadley

★ **HOWARD UNIVERSITY HOSPITAL (90003)**, 2041 Georgia Avenue N.W., Zip 20060–0002; tel. 202/865–6100 **A**1 2 3 5 8 9 10 **F**1 3 4 6 7 8 11 12 13 15 16 17 18 20 22 24 25 26 27 28 30 31 32 33 34 36 37 38 40 41 43 44 46 50 52 53 54 55 56 57 58 59 60 62 63 64 65 66 68 69 70 71 72 73 74 75 76 77 78 79 80 81 82 83 84 85 86 87 88 89 90 91 92 93 94 96 97 99 100 102 103 106 107 111 112 114 117 118 119 120 121 123 124 125 127 132 133 135 136 137 **P**4
Primary Contact: Larry Warren, Chief Executive Officer
COO: Paul Musgrove, Chief Operating Officer
CFO: Joel Celestin, Assistant Executive Director and Chief Financial Officer
CMO: Thomas E. Gaiter, M.D., Chief Medical Officer
CIO: Alem Moges, Interim Director Management Information Systems
CHR: Renee Inman, JD, Chief Human Resources Officer
Web address: www.huhosp.org
Control: Other not–for–profit (including NFP Corporation) **Service:** General Medical and Surgical

Staffed Beds: 305 **Admissions:** 11419 **Census:** 174 **Outpatient Visits:** 108716 **Births:** 758 **Total Expense ($000):** 296146 **Payroll Expense ($000):** 113630 **Personnel:** 2448

★ **MEDSTAR–GEORGETOWN MEDICAL CENTER (90004)**, 3800 Reservoir Road N.W., Zip 20007–2197; tel. 202/444–3000 **A**1 2 3 5 8 9 10 **F**3 5 6 9 13 15 18 24 25 26 27 28 30 31 32 33 34 35 36 38 41 43 44 46 47 49 50 51 53 54 55 56 57 58 59 60 62 63 64 66 68 69 70 72 73 74 75 76 77 78 79 80 81 82 83 84 86 87 88 89 90 91 92 93 94 95 96 97 99 100 102 104 105 106 107 108 109 111 112 114 118 119 120 121 123 124 125 127 128 130 131 132 134 135 136 137 **P**6 **S** MedStar Health
Primary Contact: M. Joy Drass, M.D., President
COO: Joyce E. Johnson, R.N., Senior Vice President Operations
CFO: Paul Warda, Chief Financial Officer
CMO: Richard L. Goldberg, M.D., Vice President Medical Affairs and Medical Director
CIO: Catherine Szenczy, Senior Vice President and Chief Information Officer
CHR: Michael McFadden, Chief Human Resources Officer
Web address: www.georgetownuniversityhospital.org
Control: Other not–for–profit (including NFP Corporation) **Service:** General Medical and Surgical

Staffed Beds: 390 **Admissions:** 15943 **Census:** 314 **Outpatient Visits:** 705508 **Births:** 1373 **Total Expense ($000):** 586303 **Payroll Expense ($000):** 257726 **Personnel:** 3697

★ △ **NATIONAL REHABILITATION HOSPITAL (93025)**, 102 Irving Street N.W., Zip 20010–2949; tel. 202/877–1000 **A**1 3 5 7 9 10 **F**3 9 24 25 26 31 33 34 36 43 46 53 58 62 66 72 73 77 81 82 85 86 107 113 118 119 120 121 132 135 136 **P**6 **S** MedStar Health
Primary Contact: Edward A. Eckenhoff, President and Chief Executive Officer
COO: John D. Rockwood, Senior Vice President Operations
CFO: Dennis Werner, Chief Financial Officer
CMO: Edward B. Healton, M.D., Senior Vice President and Medical Director
CHR: Deborah Lewis, Vice President Human Resources
Web address: www.nrhrehab.org
Control: Other not–for–profit (including NFP Corporation) **Service:** Rehabilitation

Staffed Beds: 137 **Admissions:** 2194 **Census:** 100 **Outpatient Visits:** 187408 **Births:** 0 **Total Expense ($000):** 72893 **Payroll Expense ($000):** 39991 **Personnel:** 925

★ **PROVIDENCE HOSPITAL (90006)**, 1150 Varnum Street N.E., Zip 20017–2180; tel. 202/269–7000, (Total facility includes 250 beds in nursing home–type unit) **A**1 2 3 5 9 10 **F**3 4 5 12 13 15 17 18 20 25 26 27 30 31 32 33 38 39 40 42 43 44 46 49 50 52 53 54 55 57 58 60 62 63 64 66 67 68 70 72 73 74 75 76 77 79 80 81 82 86 87 88 92 93 94 95 96 97 100 102 106 107 116 117 118 119 120 121 123 124 132 133 135 136 137 **P**6 **S** Ascension Health
Primary Contact: Julius D. Spears, Jr., President and Chief Executive Officer
COO: Paul Grenaldo, Executive Vice President and Chief Operating Officer
CFO: David G. Sparks, Senior Vice President Finance
CMO: Robert Simmons, M.D., Senior Vice President Medical Affairs
CIO: Tom Anderson, Vice President General Services
CHR: LaVerne Street, Vice President Human Resources
Web address: www.provhosp.org
Control: Other not–for–profit (including NFP Corporation) **Service:** General Medical and Surgical

Staffed Beds: 533 **Admissions:** 14415 **Census:** 412 **Outpatient Visits:** 130805 **Births:** 2372 **Total Expense ($000):** 205171 **Payroll Expense ($000):** 103512 **Personnel:** 2007

DC

□ **PSYCHIATRIC INSTITUTE OF WASHINGTON (94004)**, 4228 Wisconsin Avenue N.W., Zip 20016–2138; tel. 202/885–5600 **A**1 5 9 10 **F**5 82 88 89 90 91 92 93 94 95 119 **P**6
Primary Contact: Kenneth F. Courage, Chief Executive Officer and Chairman of the Board
COO: Carol Desjeunes, Chief Operating Officer
CFO: Charles J. Baumgardner, Vice President Corporate Operations
CMO: Howard Hoffman, M.D., Medical Director
CIO: Hector Benedi, Coordinator Information Systems
CHR: Randy Kellar, Director Human Resources
Web address: www.psychinstitute.com
Control: Corporation, Investor–owned, for–profit **Service:** Psychiatric

Staffed Beds: 104 **Admissions:** 2384 **Census:** 76 **Outpatient Visits:** 3108 **Births:** 0 **Total Expense ($000):** 17976 **Payroll Expense ($000):** 10526 **Personnel:** 222

★ **SIBLEY MEMORIAL HOSPITAL (90005)**, 5255 Loughboro Road N.W., Zip 20016–2695; tel. 202/537–4000, (Total facility includes 45 beds in nursing home–type unit) **A**1 2 3 5 9 10 **F**3 6 10 12 13 14 15 17 18 20 25 26 27 30 31 32 33 38 43 44 52 54 55 56 57 59 61 62 66 68 71 72 73 74 75 76 77 79 80 81 82 86 88 90 92 93 95 96 97 99 100 102 103 105 106 107 109 111 117 118 119 120 121 124 130 134 135 136 137
Primary Contact: Robert L. Sloan, President and Chief Executive Officer
COO: Jerry L. Price, Executive Vice President and Chief Operating Officer
CFO: Stephen C. McDonnell, Senior Vice President and Chief Financial Officer
CIO: Lorraine Fordham, Chief Information Officer
CHR: Queenie Plater, Vice President and Human Resources Officer
Web address: www.sibley.org
Control: Other not–for–profit (including NFP Corporation) **Service:** General Medical and Surgical

Staffed Beds: 271 **Admissions:** 12447 **Census:** 156 **Outpatient Visits:** 88029 **Births:** 3505 **Total Expense ($000):** 192644 **Payroll Expense ($000):** 89972 **Personnel:** 1404

Hospital, Medicare Provider Number, Address, Telephone, Approval, Facility, and Physician Codes, Health Care System
★ American Hospital Association (AHA) membership
□ The Joint Commission accreditation
○ American Osteopathic Association (AOA) accreditation
△ Commission on Accreditation of Rehabilitation Facilities (CARF) accreditation

SPECIALTY HOSPITAL OF WASHINGTON (92002), 700 Constitution Avenue N.E., Zip 20002–6058; tel. 202/546–5700, (Total facility includes 117 beds in nursing home–type unit) **A**10 **F**1 25 43 44 46 54 73 80 117 119 135 137 **P**5 **S** Specialty Hospitals of America, LLC
Primary Contact: Susan P. Bailey, RN, Chief Executive Officer
Web address: www.specialtyhospitalofwashington.com
Control: Corporation, Investor–owned, for–profit **Service:** Long–Term Acute Care hospital

Staffed Beds: 177 **Admissions:** 768 **Census:** 170 **Outpatient Visits:** 0 **Births:** 0 **Total Expense ($000):** 39540 **Payroll Expense ($000):** 16901 **Personnel:** 380

☐ **SPECIALTY HOSPITALS OF WASHINGTON–HADLEY (92003)**, (Formerly Hadley Memorial Hospital), 4601 Martin Luther King Jr. Avenue, S.W., Zip 20032–1199; tel. 202/574–5700, (Nonreporting) **A**1 10 **S** Specialty Hospitals of America, LLC
Primary Contact: Irving B. Sawyers, Jr., Chief Executive Officer
CFO: Ronald Davis, Chief Financial Officer
CMO: Samir Al–Khouri, M.D., Medical Director
CHR: Bing Lechoco, Director Human Resources
Control: Corporation, Investor–owned, for–profit **Service:** General Medical and Surgical

Staffed Beds: 82

★ **ST. ELIZABETHS HOSPITAL (94001)**, 2700 Martin Luther King Jr. Avenue S.E., Zip 20032–2698; tel. 202/562–4000, (Nonreporting) **A**3 5 10
Primary Contact: Patrick Canavan, Chief Executive Officer
CFO: Gerald Tolliver, Associate Director Finance and Administration
CMO: Rizwan Malik, M.D., Acting Associate Director Medical Affairs
Control: City–Government, nonfederal **Service:** Psychiatric

Staffed Beds: 817

⊠ △ **THE HSC PEDIATRIC CENTER**, 1731 Bunker Hill Road N.E., Zip 20017–3096; tel. 202/832–4400 **A**1 7 9 **F**25 26 31 32 37 44 45 62 66 73 75 78 81 82 85 86 119 132 135 137 **P**6
Primary Contact: Bruce Goldman, Chief Operating Officer
COO: Bruce Goldman, Chief Operating Officer
CFO: Nancy J. Southers, Vice President and Chief Financial Officer
CMO: Karen Smith, M.D., Chief Medical Officer
CIO: Eugene Greer, Chief Information Officer
CHR: Lynne Hostetter, Director Human Resources
Web address: www.hfscsite.org
Control: Other not–for–profit (including NFP Corporation) **Service:** Children's rehabilitation

Staffed Beds: 101 **Admissions:** 508 **Census:** 45 **Outpatient Visits:** 3595 **Births:** 0 **Total Expense ($000):** 34926 **Payroll Expense ($000):** 15222 **Personnel:** 213

☐ **UNITED MEDICAL CENTER (90008)**, (Formerly Greater Southeast Community Hospital), 1310 Southern Avenue S.E., Zip 20032–4699; tel. 202/574–6000, (Nonreporting) **A**1 9 10 **S** Specialty Hospitals of America, LLC
Primary Contact: Gary L. Rowe, Chief Executive Officer
COO: James Jacobs, Chief Operating Officer
CFO: Barry Harding, Chief Financial Officer
CIO: Richard Holsclaw, Chief Information Officer
CHR: Jackie Johnson, Vice President Human Resources
Web address: www.greatersoutheast.org
Control: Corporation, Investor–owned, for–profit **Service:** General Medical and Surgical

Staffed Beds: 303

⊠ △ **VETERANS AFFAIRS MEDICAL CENTER**, 50 Irving Street N.W., Zip 20422–0002; tel. 202/745–8100, (Nonreporting) **A**1 3 5 7 8 9 **S** Department of Veterans Affairs
Primary Contact: Fernando O. Rivera, Director
CFO: Frank Filosa, Fiscal Manager
CIO: Amanda Graves, Chief Information Systems
Web address: www.va.gov/sta/guide/home.asp
Control: Veterans Affairs, Government, federal **Service:** General Medical and Surgical

Staffed Beds: 291

⊠ **WALTER REED ARMY MEDICAL CENTER**, 6900 Georgia Avenue N.W., Zip 20307–5001; tel. 202/782–6395, (Nonreporting) **A**1 2 3 5 12 13 **S** Department of the Army, Office of the Surgeon General
Primary Contact: Colonel Patricia Horoho, Commander
CFO: Lieutenant Colonel James Hawkins, Comptroller
CMO: Colonel Felicia Pehrson, M.D., Chief Medical Staff
CIO: Lieutenant Colonel Paul Lavan, Chief Information Management Division
CHR: Adrian Morales, Chief Human Resources
Web address: www.wramc.amedd.army.mil
Control: Army, Government, federal **Service:** General Medical and Surgical

Staffed Beds: 256

⊠ **WASHINGTON HOSPITAL CENTER (90011)**, 110 Irving Street N.W., Zip 20010–2975; tel. 202/877–7000 **A**1 2 3 5 8 9 10 **F**3 5 7 8 11 12 13 14 15 16 17 18 20 22 24 25 26 27 30 31 32 33 35 36 37 38 40 41 43 44 45 46 47 48 49 50 51 54 55 56 57 58 59 60 62 63 66 68 69 70 71 72 73 74 75 76 77 79 80 81 82 86 87 88 90 91 92 93 94 95 96 97 99 100 102 103 104 105 106 107 108 109 111 112 113 114 116 119 120 121 123 124 126 127 130 131 132 133 135 136 137 **P**1 6 **S** MedStar Health
Primary Contact: James F. Caldas, President
COO: Dennis Pullin, Senior Vice President and Chief Operating Officer
CFO: Thomas Marchozzi, Senior Vice President Finance and Chief Financial Officer
CMO: Janis M. Orlowski, M.D., Senior Vice President Medical Affairs and Chief Medical Officer
CIO: Kenda Tavakoli, Vice President Information Systems
CHR: Christina Younger, Senior Vice President Human Resources
Web address: www.whcenter.org
Control: Other not–for–profit (including NFP Corporation) **Service:** General Medical and Surgical

Staffed Beds: 841 **Admissions:** 41849 **Census:** 669 **Outpatient Visits:** 389795 **Births:** 4556 **Total Expense ($000):** 914474 **Payroll Expense ($000):** 432097 **Personnel:** 5480

FLORIDA

ALTAMONTE SPRINGS—Seminole County

FLORIDA HOSPITAL–ALTAMONTE See Florida Hospital, Orlando

APALACHICOLA—Franklin County

GEORGE E. WEEMS MEMORIAL HOSPITAL (101305), 135 Avenue G., Zip 32320–1613, Mailing Address: P.O. Box 580, Zip 32329–0580; tel. 850/653–8853, (Nonreporting) **A**9 10 18
Primary Contact: Charles C. Colvert, Chief Executive Officer
CFO: James Robinson, Chief Financial Officer
CIO: Dennis Peterson, Chief Information Officer
CHR: Ginny Grimer, Director Human Resources
Control: Partnership, Investor–owned, for–profit **Service:** General Medical and Surgical

Staffed Beds: 25

APOPKA—Orange County

FLORIDA HOSPITAL–APOPKA See Florida Hospital, Orlando

ARCADIA—De Soto County

□ **DESOTO MEMORIAL HOSPITAL (100175)**, 900 North Robert Avenue, Zip 34266–8765, Mailing Address: P.O. Box 2180, Zip 34265–2180; tel. 863/494–3535 **A**1 9 10 20 **F**3 11 13 15 25 30 31 32 33 38 42 46 48 50 51 53 55 56 57 61 62 63 66 68 73 75 79 80 86 87 96 97 100 102 107 119 124 135 **P**6
Primary Contact: Vincent A. Sica, President and Chief Executive Officer
CFO: Nancy L. Frisby, CPA, Senior Vice President and Chief Financial Officer
CMO: Wael Alokeh, M.D., Chief of Staff
CIO: Annie Curnow, Coordinator Medical Staff and Public Relations
CHR: Lois Hilton, Director Human Resources
Web address: www.dmh.org
Control: Other not–for–profit (including NFP Corporation) **Service:** General Medical and Surgical

Staffed Beds: 49 **Admissions:** 2240 **Census:** 20 **Outpatient Visits:** 43775 **Births:** 650 **Total Expense ($000):** 27317 **Payroll Expense ($000):** 12695 **Personnel:** 250

ATLANTIS—Palm Beach County

★□ **J. F. K. MEDICAL CENTER (100080)**, 5301 South Congress Avenue, Zip 33462–1197; tel. 561/965–7300 **A**1 2 3 5 9 10 **F**3 12 15 17 18 20 22 24 25 26 27 30 31 32 33 35 38 43 46 49 51 54 55 56 57 58 59 62 63 66 68 72 73 75 76 77 79 80 81 82 86 96 97 99 100 102 103 106 107 109 111 118 119 120 121 124 134 135 136 137 **S** HCA
Primary Contact: Gina Melby, Chief Executive Officer
COO: Robbin M. Lee, Chief Operating Officer
CFO: Lynn Dick, Chief Financial Officer
CMO: Charles Posternack, M.D., Chief Medical Officer
CIO: Jane Stewart, Director Information Services
CHR: Trudy Bromley, Vice President Human Resources
Web address: www.jfkmc.com
Control: Corporation, Investor–owned, for–profit **Service:** General Medical and Surgical

Staffed Beds: 424 **Admissions:** 25101 **Census:** 338 **Outpatient Visits:** 116954 **Births:** 0 **Total Expense ($000):** 324457 **Payroll Expense ($000):** 109203 **Personnel:** 1649

AVENTURA—Dade County

★□ **AVENTURA HOSPITAL AND MEDICAL CENTER (100131)**, 20900 Biscayne Boulevard, Zip 33180–1407; tel. 305/682–7000, (Nonreporting) **A**1 2 9 10 **S** HCA
Primary Contact: Heather J. Rohan, Chief Executive Officer
CFO: Lester Eljaiek, Chief Financial Officer
CMO: Natarajan Rajagopalan, M.D., Chief of Staff
CHR: Maria Naranjo, Director Human Resources
Web address: www.aventurahospital.com
Control: Corporation, Investor–owned, for–profit **Service:** General Medical and Surgical

Staffed Beds: 359

BARTOW—Polk County

□ **BARTOW REGIONAL MEDICAL CENTER (100121)**, 2200 Osprey Boulevard, Zip 33830–3308, Mailing Address: P.O. Box 1050, Zip 33830–1050; tel. 863/533–8111 **A**1 9 10 **F**3 11 15 18 25 26 31 32 38 46 55 56 57 65 68 72 73 77 79 80 96 97 100 102 107 135 **P**5 **S** Health Management Associates
Primary Contact: Justin Davis, Chief Executive Officer
COO: Tonja Mosley, Chief Financial Officer
Web address: www.bartowregional.com
Control: Corporation, Investor–owned, for–profit **Service:** General Medical and Surgical

Staffed Beds: 72 **Admissions:** 4261 **Census:** 48 **Outpatient Visits:** 57394 **Births:** 0 **Total Expense ($000):** 34709 **Payroll Expense ($000):** 15694 **Personnel:** 376

BAY PINES—Pinellas County

★□ △ **VETERANS AFFAIRS MEDICAL CENTER**, 10000 Bay Pines Boulevard, Zip 33744, Mailing Address: P.O. Box 5005, Zip 33744–5005; tel. 727/398–6661, (Total facility includes 142 beds in nursing home–type unit) **A**1 2 3 5 7 **F**1 2 3 4 5 8 12 15 16 17 18 20 24 25 26 27 32 33 34 35 36 37 38 41 42 43 44 45 46 48 50 52 53 54 55 56 57 58 59 60 61 62 63 65 66 68 69 70 71 72 73 74 75 76 77 78 79 80 81 82 83 84 85 86 87 88 90 91 92 93 94 95 96 97 99 100 101 102 103 104 105 106 107 117 118 119 121 124 132 133 135 136 137 **S** Department of Veterans Affairs
Primary Contact: Wallace M. Hopkins, FACHE, Director
COO: Kaye Green, FACHE, Associate Director
CFO: Jeanine Ergle, Chief Financial Officer
CMO: George F. Van Buskirk, M.D., Chief of Staff
CIO: John Williams, Facility Chief Information Officer
CHR: Barry M. Kevin, Human Resources Officer
Web address: www.baypines.va.gov/
Control: Veterans Affairs, Government, federal **Service:** General Medical and Surgical

Staffed Beds: 461 **Admissions:** 10655 **Census:** 461 **Outpatient Visits:** 1086394 **Births:** 0 **Total Expense ($000):** 447892 **Payroll Expense ($000):** 189676 **Personnel:** 3174

BELLE GLADE—Palm Beach County

★□ **GLADES GENERAL HOSPITAL (100130)**, 1201 South Main Street, Zip 33430–4911; tel. 561/996–6571 **A**1 9 10 **F**3 11 13 15 25 33 38 55 68 74 79 84 86 96 97 100 102 107 119
Primary Contact: Ron Wiewora, M.D., Interim Chief Executive Officer
CFO: David C. Chapman, Interim Chief Financial Officer
CMO: Ron Wiewora, M.D., Chief Medical Officer
CIO: Adam Levenson, Manager Information Systems
CHR: Donna Grieve, Director Human Resources
Web address: www.gladesgeneral.org
Control: Hospital district or authority, Government, nonfederal **Service:** General Medical and Surgical

Staffed Beds: 73 **Admissions:** 3340 **Census:** 32 **Births:** 395 **Total Expense ($000):** 21298 **Payroll Expense ($000):** 14162

BLOUNTSTOWN—Calhoun County

★□ **CALHOUN–LIBERTY HOSPITAL (101304)**, 20370 N.E. Burns Avenue, Zip 32424–1097, Mailing Address: P.O. Box 419, Zip 32424–0419; tel. 850/674–5411 **A**1 9 10 18 **F**32 38 57 96 107 122
Primary Contact: Ronald M. Gilliard, FACHE, Chief Executive Officer
CFO: Haley Green, Controller
CHR: Lynn Pitts, Director Human Resources
Control: Other not–for–profit (including NFP Corporation) **Service:** General Medical and Surgical

Staffed Beds: 25 **Admissions:** 499 **Census:** 4 **Outpatient Visits:** 15918 **Births:** 0 **Total Expense ($000):** 3604 **Payroll Expense ($000):** 2330 **Personnel:** 76

FL

Hospital, Medicare Provider Number, Address, Telephone, Approval, Facility, and Physician Codes, Health Care System

★ American Hospital Association (AHA) membership
□ The Joint Commission accreditation
○ American Osteopathic Association (AOA) accreditation
△ Commission on Accreditation of Rehabilitation Facilities (CARF) accreditation

BOCA RATON—Palm Beach County

★ **BOCA RATON COMMUNITY HOSPITAL (100168)**, 800 Meadows Road, Zip 33486–2368; tel. 561/955–7100, (Nonreporting) **A**1 2 9 10
Primary Contact: Richard Van Lith, President and Chief Executive Officer
CFO: Kenneth Meinke, Vice President and Chief Financial Officer
CMO: Richard A. Greenwald, M.D., Vice President Medical Affairs
CIO: Robin Hildwein, Chief Information Officer
CHR: Mindy Raymond, Vice President Human Resources
Web address: www.brch.com
Control: Other not–for–profit (including NFP Corporation) **Service:** General Medical and Surgical

Staffed Beds: 394

★ **WEST BOCA MEDICAL CENTER (100268)**, 21644 State Road 7, Zip 33428–1899; tel. 561/488–8000, (Nonreporting) **A**1 9 10 **S** TENET Healthcare Corporation
Primary Contact: Walt Mickens, Chief Executive Officer
COO: Larry Coomes, Chief Operating Officer
CFO: Brook Thomas, Chief Financial Officer
CHR: Stephanie Sherman, Director Human Resources
Web address: www.westbocamedctr.com
Control: Corporation, Investor–owned, for–profit **Service:** Other specialty

Staffed Beds: 185

BONIFAY—Holmes County

DOCTORS MEMORIAL HOSPITAL (101307), 2600 Hospital Drive, Zip 32425–3007, Mailing Address: P.O. Box 188, Zip 32425–0188; tel. 850/547–8000, (Nonreporting) **A**9 10 18
Primary Contact: Robert E. Winkler, Chief Executive Officer
COO: Ruby Gardner, Controller
CFO: Ruby Gardner, Controller
CMO: Herbert Brooks, Chief of Staff
CIO: Ruby Gardner, Controller
CHR: Christy Booth, Chief Human Resources Officer
Web address: www.doctorsmemorialhospital.com
Control: Other not–for–profit (including NFP Corporation) **Service:** General Medical and Surgical

Staffed Beds: 25

BOYNTON BEACH—Palm Beach County

★ **BETHESDA MEMORIAL HOSPITAL (100002)**, 2815 South Seacrest Boulevard, Zip 33435–7995; tel. 561/737–7733 **A**1 2 9 10 **F**3 8 11 12 13 18 24 25 26 27 32 33 38 46 49 50 51 54 56 58 59 60 62 66 68 70 72 73 74 75 76 77 79 80 81 82 83 84 85 86 97 98 99 100 107 108 109 111 112 118 119 120 121 132 135 137 **P**6
Primary Contact: Robert B. Hill, President and Chief Executive Officer
COO: Robert B. Hill, President and Chief Executive Officer
CFO: Joanne Aquilina, Vice President Finance and Chief Financial Officer
CMO: Albert Biehl, M.D., Vice President Medical Affairs
CIO: Leslie Durham, Vice President Information Systems
CHR: Regina Crafa, Vice President Human Resources
Web address: www.bethesdahealthcare.com
Control: Other not–for–profit (including NFP Corporation) **Service:** General Medical and Surgical

Staffed Beds: 390 **Admissions:** 18676 **Census:** 273 **Outpatient Visits:** 201997 **Births:** 3431 **Total Expense ($000):** 196965 **Payroll Expense ($000):** 76100 **Personnel:** 1685

BRADENTON—Manatee County

★ △ **BLAKE MEDICAL CENTER (100213)**, 2020 59th Street West, Zip 34209–4669; tel. 941/792–6611 **A**1 2 7 9 10 **F**3 11 12 15 17 18 20 22 24 25 26 27 30 31 32 33 38 46 48 49 55 57 62 68 72 73 75 76 77 79 80 81 82 85 86 96 97 99 100 102 103 106 107 112 118 119 120 121 134 135 **S** HCA
Primary Contact: Daniel J. Friedrich, III, Chief Executive Officer
COO: Maureen Greenway, Chief Operating Officer
CFO: Priscilla Parrish, Chief Financial Officer
CMO: Lawrence Lieberman, M.D., Medical Director
CIO: Shannon Piatkowski, Director Information Technology
CHR: Veronica Lequeux, Vice President Human Resources
Web address: www.blakemedicalcenter.com
Control: Corporation, Investor–owned, for–profit **Service:** General Medical and Surgical

Staffed Beds: 263 **Admissions:** 12552 **Census:** 173 **Outpatient Visits:** 40172 **Births:** 0 **Total Expense ($000):** 127845 **Payroll Expense ($000):** 45120 **Personnel:** 754

□ **LAKEWOOD RANCH MEDICAL CENTER (100299)**, 8330 Lakewood Ranch Boulevard, Zip 34202; tel. 941/782–2100, (Nonreporting) **A**1 9 10 **S** Universal Health Services, Inc.
Primary Contact: Linda S. Widra, FACHE, Ph.D., RN, Interim Chief Executive Officer
COO: Linda S. Widra, FACHE, Ph.D., R.N., Chief Operating Officer
CFO: Gerald Christine, Chief Financial Officer
CHR: Trish Morales, Director Human Resources
Web address: www.lakewoodranchmedicalcenter.com
Control: Corporation, Investor–owned, for–profit **Service:** Long–Term Acute Care hospital

Staffed Beds: 120

MANATEE GLENS HOSPITAL (104040), 2020 26th Avenue East, Zip 34208, Mailing Address: P.O. Box 9478, Zip 34208; tel. 941/741–3117, (Nonreporting) **A**9 10
Primary Contact: Mary Ruiz, Chief Executive Officer
COO: Deborah Kostroun, Chief Operating Officer
CFO: John Denaro, Chief Financial Officer
CMO: Jose Zaglul, M.D., Chief Medical Officer
CIO: Chris Mitchell, Director Information Systems
CHR: Chris McKenna, Director Human Resources
Web address: www.manateeglens.org
Control: Other not–for–profit (including NFP Corporation) **Service:** Psychiatric

Staffed Beds: 27

□ **MANATEE MEMORIAL HOSPITAL (100035)**, 206 Second Street East, Zip 34208–1000; tel. 941/746–5111, (Total facility includes 10 beds in nursing home–type unit) (Nonreporting) **A**1 2 5 9 10 **S** Universal Health Services, Inc.
Primary Contact: Moody L. Chisholm, Chief Executive Officer
COO: Roy Orr, Chief Operating Officer
CFO: Jerry Christine, Chief Financial Officer
CMO: George Van Buren, M.D., Chief of Staff
CIO: Ken Lubben, Director Information Services
CHR: Sheree Threewits, Director Human Resources
Web address: www.manateememorial.com
Control: Corporation, Investor–owned, for–profit **Service:** General Medical and Surgical

Staffed Beds: 512

BRANDON—Hillsborough County

★ **BRANDON REGIONAL HOSPITAL (100243)**, 119 Oakfield Drive, Zip 33511–5799; tel. 813/681–5551 **A**1 5 9 10 **F**3 11 12 13 15 17 18 20 22 24 25 27 30 31 32 38 43 46 47 48 49 51 55 57 59 62 66 68 70 71 72 73 74 75 76 77 79 80 83 84 86 87 96 97 100 102 106 107 121 135 136 137 **S** HCA
Primary Contact: Michael M. Fencel, Chief Executive Officer
CFO: Michael T. Terrell, Chief Financial Officer
CMO: John Butterick, M.D., Medical Advisor
CIO: Scott Morrison, Director Information Systems
CHR: Jay Kuhns, Vice President Human Resources
Web address: www.brandonhospital.com
Control: Corporation, Investor–owned, for–profit **Service:** General Medical and Surgical

Staffed Beds: 367 **Admissions:** 21407 **Census:** 257 **Outpatient Visits:** 98148 **Births:** 3619 **Total Expense ($000):** 173879 **Payroll Expense ($000):** 77289 **Personnel:** 1067

BROOKSVILLE—Hernando County

□ **BROOKSVILLE REGIONAL HOSPITAL (100071)**, 17240 Cortez Boulevard, Zip 34601, Mailing Address: P.O. Box 37, Zip 34605–0037; tel. 352/796–5111, (Nonreporting) **A**1 9 10 **S** Health Management Associates
Primary Contact: Kathy A. Burke, Chief Executive Officer
COO: Corey Lively, Chief Operating Officer
CFO: Alan Archbold, Chief Financial Officer
CMO: Raja L. Rao, M.D., Chief of Staff
CIO: Deb Otis, Director
Web address: www.brooksvilleregionalhospital.org
Control: Corporation, Investor–owned, for–profit **Service:** General Medical and Surgical

Staffed Beds: 91

★ **HEALTHSOUTH REHABILITATION HOSPITAL OF SPRING HILL (103042)**, 12440 Cortez Boulevard, Zip 34613–2628; tel. 352/592–4250, (Nonreporting) **A**1 9 10 **S** HEALTHSOUTH Corporation
Primary Contact: Lori Bedard, Chief Executive Officer
CFO: Debbie Punzirudu, Controller
CMO: Charles Dempsey, M.D., Medical Director
CIO: Myra Merillo, Supervisor Health Information Management
CHR: Ava McLellan, Coordinator Human Resources
Web address: www.healthsouth.com
Control: Corporation, Investor–owned, for–profit **Service:** Rehabilitation

Staffed Beds: 60

★ **OAK HILL HOSPITAL (100264)**, 11375 Cortez Boulevard, Zip 34613, Mailing Address: P.O. Box 5300, Spring Hill, Zip 34611–5300; tel. 352/596–6632 **A**1 2 10 **F**3 15 17 18 20 22 25 26 27 31 32 33 38 43 49 50 51 54 55 56 57 59 62 66 68 72 73 75 76 77 79 80 84 86 96 97 100 102 107 135 137 **S** HCA
Primary Contact: Mickey Smith, Chief Executive Officer
COO: Sonia I. Gonzalez, R.N., Chief Operating Officer
CFO: Robert Grace, Chief Financial Officer
CMO: Mallik Pidurm, M.D., Chief of Staff
CIO: Kristen Foxx, Chief Information Officer
CHR: Charles Snider, Vice President Human Resources
Web address: www.oakhillhospital.com
Control: Corporation, Investor–owned, for–profit **Service:** General Medical and Surgical

Staffed Beds: 204 **Admissions:** 11978 **Census:** 151 **Outpatient Visits:** 39528 **Births:** 0 **Total Expense ($000):** 107365 **Payroll Expense ($000):** 40415 **Personnel:** 755

□ **SPRING HILL REGIONAL HOSPITAL (100280)**, 10461 Quality Drive, Zip 34609–9634; tel. 352/688–8200, (Nonreporting) **A**1 9 10 **S** Health Management Associates
Primary Contact: Jason N. Roeback, Chief Executive Officer
COO: Ricardo Diaz, Chief Operating Officer
CFO: Marc Nakagawa, Chief Financial Officer
CMO: Naresh Menezes, M.D., Chief of Staff
CIO: Deb Otis, Director
CHR: Linda Campo, Director of Human Resources
Web address: www.springhillregionalhospital.org
Control: Corporation, Investor–owned, for–profit **Service:** General Medical and Surgical

Staffed Beds: 75

□ **SPRINGBROOK HOSPITAL (104057)**, 7007 Grove Road, Zip 34609–8610; tel. 352/596–4306, (Nonreporting) **A**1 9 10
Primary Contact: James E. O'Shea, Administrator
Control: Other not–for–profit (including NFP Corporation) **Service:** Psychiatric

Staffed Beds: 50

CAPE CORAL—Lee County

□ **CAPE CORAL HOSPITAL (100244)**, 636 Del Prado Boulevard, Zip 33990–2695; tel. 239/574–2323, (Nonreporting) **A**1 9 10 **S** Lee Memorial Health System
Primary Contact: James R. Nathan, President
COO: Donna Giannuzzi, R.N., Chief Nurse Executive
CFO: John Weist, Chief Financial Officer
CMO: Chuck Krivenko, M.D., Chief Medical Officer
CIO: Mike Smith, Chief Information Officer
CHR: Jon C. Cecil, Chief Human Resource Officer
Web address: www.leememorial.org
Control: Other not–for–profit (including NFP Corporation) **Service:** General Medical and Surgical

Staffed Beds: 209

CELEBRATION—Osceola County

FLORIDA HOSPITAL CELEBRATION HEALTH See Florida Hospital, Orlando

CHATTAHOOCHEE—Gadsden County

FLORIDA STATE HOSPITAL (104000), U.S. Highway 90 East, Zip 32324–1000, Mailing Address: P.O. Box 1000, Zip 32324–1000; tel. 850/663–7536, (Nonreporting) **A**10
Primary Contact: Diane R. James, Administrator
CFO: Denise Smith, Director Financial Services
Web address: www.dcf.state.fl.us/institutions/fsh
Control: State–Government, nonfederal **Service:** Psychiatric

Staffed Beds: 987

CHIPLEY—Washington County

★ **NORTHWEST FLORIDA COMMUNITY HOSPITAL (101308)**, 1360 Brickyard Road, Zip 32428–6303, Mailing Address: P.O. Box 889, Zip 32428–0889; tel. 850/638–1610, (Total facility includes 34 beds in nursing home–type unit) **A**1 9 10 18 **F**2 3 11 15 25 26 30 31 32 33 38 50 54 55 56 57 60 61 66 73 79 80 81 82 87 93 94 96 102 107 117 118 119 122 124 135
Primary Contact: Patrick A. Schlenker, President
COO: Gregg Moreau, Chief Operating Officer and Chief Financial Officer
CFO: Gregg Moreau, Chief Operating Officer and Chief Financial Officer
CMO: Samuel E. Ward, M.D., Chief of Staff
CHR: Carrie Jantti, Coordinator Hum Resources
Web address: www.nfch.org
Control: Corporation, Investor–owned, for–profit **Service:** General Medical and Surgical

Staffed Beds: 59 **Admissions:** 648 **Census:** 40 **Outpatient Visits:** 26617 **Births:** 0 **Total Expense ($000):** 10603 **Payroll Expense ($000):** 5302 **Personnel:** 180

CLEARWATER—Pinellas County

★ **MORTON PLANT HOSPITAL (100127)**, 300 Pinellas Street, Zip 33756–3825, Mailing Address: P.O. Box 210, Zip 34657–0210; tel. 727/462–7000, (Nonreporting) **A**1 2 3 5 9 10 **S** Morton Plant Mease Health Care
Primary Contact: Philip K. Beauchamp, FACHE, President and Chief Executive Officer
COO: Hal Ziecheck, Chief Operating Officer
CMO: Donald Pocock, M.D., Chief Medical Officer
CHR: Sharon Collotta, Director Human Resources
Web address: www.mortonplant.com
Control: Other not–for–profit (including NFP Corporation) **Service:** General Medical and Surgical

Staffed Beds: 742

□ **WINDMOOR HEALTHCARE OF CLEARWATER (104017)**, 11300 U.S. 19 North, Zip 33764; tel. 727/541–2646 **A**1 9 10 **F**4 5 25 31 32 33 36 56 73 88 91 92 93 94 95 119 121 132 **S** Psychiatric Solutions
Primary Contact: Wendy Merson, Chief Executive Officer
Web address: www.windmoor–healthcare.com
Control: Corporation, Investor–owned, for–profit **Service:** Psychiatric

Staffed Beds: 100 **Admissions:** 1859 **Census:** 70 **Outpatient Visits:** 5833 **Births:** 0 **Total Expense ($000):** 13362 **Payroll Expense ($000):** 7268 **Personnel:** 154

CLERMONT—Lake County

□ **SOUTH LAKE HOSPITAL (100051)**, 1099 Citrus Tower Boulevard, Zip 34711–2787; tel. 352/394–4071 **A**1 9 10 **F**3 11 12 13 15 18 20 25 26 27 30 31 32 33 38 42 43 49 51 52 55 56 57 61 62 64 66 68 72 73 74 76 77 78 79 80 81 82 84 86 96 99 100 102 103 105 107 120 121 124 135 136 **P**6 **S** Orlando Health
Primary Contact: Leslie Longacre, Chief Executive Officer
COO: John Moore, Chief Operating Officer
CFO: Lance Sewell, Chief Financial Officer
CHR: Sue Brown, Administrator, Human Resources
Web address: www.southlakehospital.com
Control: Hospital district or authority, Government, nonfederal **Service:** General Medical and Surgical

Staffed Beds: 104 **Admissions:** 6600 **Census:** 73 **Outpatient Visits:** 88296 **Births:** 705 **Total Expense ($000):** 93713 **Payroll Expense ($000):** 38084 **Personnel:** 838

CLEWISTON—Hendry County

★ **HENDRY REGIONAL MEDICAL CENTER (101309)**, 524 West Sagamore Avenue, Zip 33440–3094; tel. 863/983–9121 **A**9 10 18 **F**3 11 15 25 26 27 33 38 50 57 62 66 68 73 75 79 86 96 97 100 107 121 122 **S** QHR
Primary Contact: Craig R. Cudworth, Chief Executive Officer
CFO: Joe Denno, Chief Financial Officer
CMO: James Forbes, M.D., Chief Medical Director
CIO: Arland J. Pappas, Director Information Systems
CHR: Lisa Miller, Director Human Resources
Web address: www.hendryregional.org
Control: Hospital district or authority, Government, nonfederal **Service:** General Medical and Surgical

Staffed Beds: 25 **Admissions:** 1091 **Census:** 12 **Births:** 0 **Total Expense ($000):** 14458 **Payroll Expense ($000):** 6902

FL

Hospital, Medicare Provider Number, Address, Telephone, Approval, Facility, and Physician Codes, Health Care System
★ American Hospital Association (AHA) membership
□ The Joint Commission accreditation
○ American Osteopathic Association (AOA) accreditation
△ Commission on Accreditation of Rehabilitation Facilities (CARF) accreditation

COCOA BEACH—Brevard County

★ **CAPE CANAVERAL HOSPITAL (100177)**, 701 West Cocoa Beach Causeway, Zip 32931–5595, Mailing Address: P.O. Box 320069, Zip 32932–0069; tel. 321/799–7111 **A**1 2 9 10 **F**3 11 13 15 18 25 26 27 30 31 32 33 38 41 43 44 49 51 53 54 55 56 57 59 61 62 66 68 72 73 74 76 77 79 80 81 82 86 96 97 98 99 100 102 106 107 118 119 121 124 135 136 137 **P**6 7 **S** Health First, Inc.
Primary Contact: Roy Wright, FACHE, President and Chief Executive Officer
CFO: Robert Galloway, Senior Vice President Finance and Chief Financial Officer
CMO: Rodney Moore, M.D., Vice President Medical Affairs
CIO: Rich Rogers, Senior Vice President Support Services and Chief Information Officer
CHR: Robert Suttles, Vice President Human Resources
Web address: www.health–first.org
Control: Other not–for–profit (including NFP Corporation) **Service:** General Medical and Surgical

Staffed Beds: 145 **Admissions:** 6844 **Census:** 84 **Outpatient Visits:** 193440 **Births:** 778 **Total Expense ($000):** 111211 **Payroll Expense ($000):** 52544 **Personnel:** 958

CORAL GABLES—Dade County

★ **CORAL GABLES HOSPITAL (100183)**, 3100 Douglas Road, Zip 33134–6990; tel. 305/445–8461, (Nonreporting) **A**1 9 10 **S** TENET Healthcare Corporation
Primary Contact: Jay S. Miranda, Chief Executive Officer
COO: Caridad Nieves, Chief Nursing Officer and Chief Operating Officer
Web address: www.coralgableshospital.com
Control: Corporation, Investor–owned, for–profit **Service:** General Medical and Surgical

Staffed Beds: 256

★ **DOCTORS HOSPITAL (100296)**, 5000 University Drive, Zip 33146–2094; tel. 305/308–3000 **A**1 3 5 9 10 **F**3 25 26 27 30 32 35 38 42 43 44 47 49 52 56 68 72 73 75 76 77 78 79 80 82 86 96 97 100 102 107 112 116 119 120 121 132 135 **P**6 **S** Baptist Health South Florida
Primary Contact: Lincoln S. Mendez, Chief Executive Officer
CFO: Seth Van Essendelft, Chief Financial Officer
Web address: www.baptisthealth.net
Control: Other not–for–profit (including NFP Corporation) **Service:** General Medical and Surgical

Staffed Beds: 148 **Admissions:** 7843 **Census:** 118 **Outpatient Visits:** 52224 **Births:** 0 **Total Expense ($000):** 150574 **Payroll Expense ($000):** 45270 **Personnel:** 860

FL

□ **KINDRED HOSPITAL SOUTH FLORIDA–CORAL GABLES**, 5190 S.W. Eighth Street, Zip 33134–2495; tel. 305/445–1364, (Nonreporting) **A**1 9 **S** Kindred Healthcare
Primary Contact: Charles Doten, Chief Executive Officer
Web address: www.kindredhealthcare.com
Control: Corporation, Investor–owned, for–profit **Service:** Other specialty

Staffed Beds: 53

CORAL SPRINGS—Broward County

★ **CORAL SPRINGS MEDICAL CENTER (100276)**, 3000 Coral Hills Drive, Zip 33065; tel. 954/344–3000 **A**1 9 10 **F**3 11 12 13 15 17 25 27 31 32 33 38 42 43 44 48 51 55 56 57 58 60 62 64 66 68 70 72 73 74 75 76 77 78 79 80 81 82 83 84 86 96 97 99 100 102 103 106 107 114 118 119 120 121 132 135 136 137 **P**6 **S** Broward Health
Primary Contact: Patrick Maloney, Chief Executive Officer
COO: Drew Grossman, Chief Operating Officer
CFO: Arthur Wallace, Chief Financial Officer
CMO: Kutty Chandran, M.D., Chief of Staff
CHR: Robert Diano, Vice President Human Resources
Web address: www.browardhealth.org
Control: Hospital district or authority, Government, nonfederal **Service:** General Medical and Surgical

Staffed Beds: 182 **Admissions:** 11876 **Census:** 128 **Outpatient Visits:** 110680 **Births:** 2152 **Total Expense ($000):** 119116 **Payroll Expense ($000):** 50056 **Personnel:** 814

CRESTVIEW—Okaloosa County

★ **NORTH OKALOOSA MEDICAL CENTER (100122)**, 151 Redstone Avenue S.E., Zip 32539–6026; tel. 850/689–8100, (Nonreporting) **A**1 9 10 **S** Community Health Systems, Inc.
Primary Contact: David S. Sanders, Chief Executive Officer
CFO: Jim Andrews, Chief Financial Officer
CIO: Jenny Zeitler, Network Administrator
Web address: www.northokaloosa.com
Control: Corporation, Investor–owned, for–profit **Service:** General Medical and Surgical

Staffed Beds: 110

CRYSTAL RIVER—Citrus County

□ **SEVEN RIVERS REGIONAL MEDICAL CENTER (100249)**, 6201 North Suncoast Boulevard, Zip 34428–6712; tel. 352/795–6560, (Nonreporting) **A**1 9 10 19 **S** Health Management Associates
Primary Contact: Joyce Brancato, Chief Executive Officer
COO: Christian Stroucken, Chief Operating Officer
CFO: Dima Didenko, Chief Financial Officer
CHR: Joann Mramor, Director Human Resources
Web address: www.srrmc.com
Control: Corporation, Investor–owned, for–profit **Service:** General Medical and Surgical

Staffed Beds: 128

DADE CITY—Pasco County

□ **PASCO REGIONAL MEDICAL CENTER (100211)**, 13100 Fort King Road, Zip 33525–5294; tel. 352/521–1100 **A**1 9 10 **F**3 12 13 15 18 25 30 34 38 41 43 46 48 50 51 52 55 57 59 62 66 68 73 74 75 76 77 79 80 84 90 91 93 96 97 100 103 107 118 119 135 136 137 **P**6 **S** Health Management Associates
Primary Contact: Stan Holm, Chief Executive Officer
CFO: Linda Stockton, Chief Financial Officer
CMO: Joseph Hubaykah, M.D., Chief of Staff
CHR: Angela Giese, Director Human Resources
Web address: www.pascoregionalmc.com
Control: Corporation, Investor–owned, for–profit **Service:** General Medical and Surgical

Staffed Beds: 90 **Admissions:** 5127 **Census:** 45 **Outpatient Visits:** 50198 **Births:** 321 **Total Expense ($000):** 40908 **Payroll Expense ($000):** 16441 **Personnel:** 356

DAVENPORT—Polk County

□ **HEART OF FLORIDA REGIONAL MEDICAL CENTER (100137)**, 40100 Highway 27, Zip 33837–5902, Mailing Address: P.O. Box 67, Haines City, Zip 33845–0067; tel. 863/422–4971 **A**1 9 10 **F**3 8 11 12 13 15 18 25 26 30 31 32 33 36 38 43 45 50 51 55 56 57 59 62 66 68 72 73 74 75 76 77 79 80 81 82 86 90 96 97 100 102 106 107 112 119 120 121 134 135 136 137 **S** Health Management Associates
Primary Contact: James R. Beatty, Chief Executive Officer
COO: Rebecca Brewer, Chief Operating Officer
CFO: Tonja Mosley, Chief Financial Officer
CMO: Kulmeet Kundlas, M.D., Chief of Staff
CIO: Louis Jones, Director Management Information Systems
CHR: Joan Allard, Director Human Resources
Web address: www.heartofflorida.com
Control: Corporation, Investor–owned, for–profit **Service:** General Medical and Surgical

Staffed Beds: 142 **Admissions:** 11197 **Census:** 117 **Outpatient Visits:** 47046 **Births:** 1118 **Personnel:** 641

DAYTONA BEACH—Volusia County

★ **HALIFAX HEALTH MEDICAL CENTER (100017)**, (Formerly Halifax Community Health System), 303 North Clyde Morris Boulevard, Zip 32114–2700; tel. 386/254–4000, (Includes HALIFAX BEHAVIORAL SERVICES, 841 Jimmy Ann Drive, Zip 32117–4599; tel. 904/274–5333; HALIFAX HOSPITAL PORT ORANGE, 1041 Dunlawton Avenue, Port Orange, Zip 32127; tel. 386/322–4700; Ann Martorano, Administrator) **A**1 2 3 5 9 10 **F**17 18 20 22 24 25 26 27 31 32 38 39 40 46 47 48 49 50 52 58 59 63 68 74 75 76 77 79 80 81 82 83 84 88 89 90 91 92 93 96 97 100 102 103 106 107 108 109 111 112 114 116 119 120 121 124 127 135 136 137
Primary Contact: Jeff Feasel, Chief Executive Officer
CFO: Eric Peburn, Interim Chief Financial Officer
CIO: Lori Delone, Chief Technology Officer
CHR: Albert Alexander, Chief Human Resources Officer
Web address: www.halifax.org
Control: Hospital district or authority, Government, nonfederal **Service:** General Medical and Surgical

Staffed Beds: 562 **Admissions:** 29560 **Census:** 404 **Outpatient Visits:** 338388 **Births:** 2580 **Total Expense ($000):** 339792 **Payroll Expense ($000):** 178008 **Personnel:** 3948

Many Facility Codes have changed. Please refer to the AHA Guide Code Chart.

DE LAND—Union County

★ **FLORIDA HOSPITAL – DE LAND (100045)**, 701 West Plymouth Avenue, Zip 32720; tel. 386/943–4522 **A**1 9 10 **F**3 4 11 13 15 18 24 25 26 27 30 31 32 33 35 38 43 44 51 52 55 56 57 59 66 68 72 73 74 76 77 79 80 81 82 84 86 88 92 96 100 102 104 105 107 118 119 121 124 135 136 137
S Adventist Health System Sunbelt Health Care Corporation
Primary Contact: Daryl Tol, President and Chief Executive Officer
COO: Steve Otto, Chief Operating Officer
CFO: Nigel Hinds, Chief Financial Officer
CMO: Hendrik Dinkla, M.D., Chief of Staff
CIO: Mike Freeland, Regional Director
CHR: Opal Howard, Director Human Resources
Web address: www.fhdeland.org
Control: Other not–for–profit (including NFP Corporation) **Service:** General Medical and Surgical

Staffed Beds: 156 **Admissions:** 8099 **Census:** 92 **Outpatient Visits:** 96983 **Births:** 1117 **Total Expense ($000):** 86976 **Payroll Expense ($000):** 34038 **Personnel:** 713

DEERFIELD BEACH—Broward County

★ △ **NORTH BROWARD MEDICAL CENTER (100086)**, 201 Sample Road, Zip 33064–3502; tel. 954/941–8300 **A**1 2 7 9 10 **F**3 6 11 15 17 18 25 26 27 31 32 33 35 38 40 42 43 44 45 49 51 54 55 56 57 58 59 60 62 64 66 68 72 73 75 76 77 78 79 80 81 82 85 86 96 97 100 102 105 106 107 111 112 114 118 119 120 121 132 134 135 136 137 **P**6 **S** Broward Health
Primary Contact: Pauline Grant, Chief Executive Officer
COO: Kevin Fusco, Chief Operating Officer
CFO: Robert Bugg, Chief Financial Officer
CMO: Joel Silverman, D.O., Chief of Staff
CIO: Doris Crain, Vice President and Chief Information Officer
CHR: Grace King, Regional Director
Web address: www.nbhd.org
Control: Hospital district or authority, Government, nonfederal **Service:** General Medical and Surgical

Staffed Beds: 360 **Admissions:** 15274 **Census:** 239 **Outpatient Visits:** 117455 **Births:** 0 **Total Expense ($000):** 185611 **Payroll Expense ($000):** 76975 **Personnel:** 1226

DEFUNIAK SPRINGS—Walton County

HEALTHMARK REGIONAL MEDICAL CENTER (100081), 4413 U.S. Highway 331 South, Zip 32435; tel. 850/951–4500 **A**9 10 **F**3 31 32 38 50 61 62 68 75 79 82 96 102 107 137
Primary Contact: James H. Thompson, Ph.D., Owner and Chief Executive Officer
COO: Gerald C. Beard, Chief Operating Officer
CFO: Jim Brewer, Chief Financial Officer
CMO: Robert L. Titelbaum, M.D., Chief of Staff
CHR: Phyllis Watts, Director Personnel
Web address: www.healthmarkregional.com
Control: Corporation, Investor–owned, for–profit **Service:** General Medical and Surgical

Staffed Beds: 50 **Admissions:** 1292 **Census:** 13 **Outpatient Visits:** 23972 **Births:** 0 **Total Expense ($000):** 10990 **Payroll Expense ($000):** 4723 **Personnel:** 129

DELRAY BEACH—Palm Beach County

★ **DELRAY MEDICAL CENTER (100258)**, 5352 Linton Boulevard, Zip 33484–6580; tel. 561/498–4440, (Includes FAIR OAKS PAVILION, 5440 Linton Boulevard, Zip 33484–6578; tel. 561/495–1000), (Nonreporting) **A**1 9 10
S TENET Healthcare Corporation
Primary Contact: Robert M. Krieger, Chief Executive Officer
COO: Matt Heywod, Chief Operating Officer
CFO: Ralph Decerbo, Chief Financial Officer
CIO: Cathy Christiansen, Director Information Systems
CHR: Veronica Leque, Director Human Resources
Web address: www.delraymedicalctr.com
Control: Corporation, Investor–owned, for–profit **Service:** General Medical and Surgical

Staffed Beds: 403

□ △ **PINECREST REHABILITATION HOSPITAL (103030)**, 5360 Linton Boulevard, Zip 33484–6538; tel. 561/495–0400, (Nonreporting) **A**1 7 10
S TENET Healthcare Corporation
Primary Contact: Robert M. Krieger, Chief Executive Officer
COO: Ruth Stewart, Chief Operating Officer
CFO: Ralph Decerbo, Chief Financial Officer
CMO: Jeffrey Farber, M.D., Medical Director
Web address: www.pinecrestrehab.com
Control: Corporation, Investor–owned, for–profit **Service:** Rehabilitation

Staffed Beds: 90

DESTIN—Walton County

★ **SACRED HEART HOSPITAL ON THE EMERALD COAST (100292)**, 7800 Highway 98 West, Zip 32550; tel. 850/278–3000 **A**1 9 10 **F**3 15 18 24 25 26 30 31 32 33 34 38 41 49 51 52 53 55 56 57 62 66 68 73 76 77 78 79 80 81 82 86 87 96 97 98 99 100 102 106 107 119 124 135 136 137
S Ascension Health
Primary Contact: Roger L. Hall, Chief Executive Officer
Web address: www.sacredheartemerald.org
Control: Other not–for–profit (including NFP Corporation) **Service:** General Medical and Surgical

Staffed Beds: 50 **Admissions:** 2420 **Census:** 25 **Outpatient Visits:** 66503 **Births:** 0 **Total Expense ($000):** 45268 **Payroll Expense ($000):** 16017 **Personnel:** 350

SACRED HEART HOSPITAL ON THE EMERALD COAST See

DUNEDIN—Pinellas County

□ **MEASE HOSPITAL DUNEDIN (100043)**, 601 Main Street, Zip 34698–5891, Mailing Address: P.O. Box 760, Zip 34697–0760; tel. 727/733–1111, (Total facility includes 20 beds in nursing home–type unit) (Nonreporting) **A**1 9 10
S Morton Plant Mease Health Care
Primary Contact: Philip K. Beauchamp, FACHE, President and Chief Executive Officer
COO: Lou Galdieri, Chief Operating Officer and Administrator
CMO: Donald Pocock, M.D., Chief Medical Officer
CHR: Sharon Collotta, Director Human Resources
Web address: www.mpmhealth.com
Control: Other not–for–profit (including NFP Corporation) **Service:** General Medical and Surgical

Staffed Beds: 258

EGLIN AFB—Okaloosa County

★ **U. S. AIR FORCE REGIONAL HOSPITAL**, 307 Boatner Road, Suite 114, Zip 32542–1282; tel. 850/883–8221, (Nonreporting) **A**1 3 5 **S** Department of the Air Force
Primary Contact: Tama Van Decar, M.D., Commander
Web address: www.eglin.af.mil
Control: Air Force, Government, federal **Service:** General Medical and Surgical

Staffed Beds: 61

ENGLEWOOD—Sarasota County

★ **ENGLEWOOD COMMUNITY HOSPITAL (100267)**, 700 Medical Boulevard, Zip 34223–3978; tel. 941/475–6571 **A**1 9 10 **F**15 18 25 30 31 32 33 38 43 48 49 50 51 54 55 56 57 62 63 68 72 73 76 77 79 80 82 86 96 100 102 107 121 122 124 132 135 136 137 **S** HCA
Primary Contact: Wendy H. Brandon, Chief Executive Officer
CFO: James Ayersman, Chief Financial Officer
CHR: Linda V. Smith, Director Human Resources
Web address: www.englewoodcommunityhospital.com
Control: Corporation, Investor–owned, for–profit **Service:** General Medical and Surgical

Staffed Beds: 100 **Admissions:** 3412 **Census:** 40 **Outpatient Visits:** 38349 **Births:** 0 **Total Expense ($000):** 35615 **Payroll Expense ($000):** 14657 **Personnel:** 251

FERNANDINA BEACH—Nassau County

★ **BAPTIST MEDICAL CENTER NASSAU (100140)**, 1250 South 18th Street, Zip 32034–3098; tel. 904/321–3500 **A**1 9 10 **F**3 11 13 15 25 26 32 33 38 43 46 48 68 74 79 86 96 97 100 102 103 107 112 118 135 137
S Baptist Health
Primary Contact: Jim L. Mayo, FACHE, Administrator
CFO: Patricia K. Hausauer, Director Finance
CHR: Katie Howard, Director Human Resources
Web address: www.e–baptisthealth.com
Control: Other not–for–profit (including NFP Corporation) **Service:** General Medical and Surgical

Staffed Beds: 32 **Admissions:** 2267 **Census:** 27 **Outpatient Visits:** 61270 **Births:** 406 **Total Expense ($000):** 33727 **Payroll Expense ($000):** 14788 **Personnel:** 298

FL

Hospital, Medicare Provider Number, Address, Telephone, Approval, Facility, and Physician Codes, Health Care System

★ American Hospital Association (AHA) membership
□ The Joint Commission accreditation
○ American Osteopathic Association (AOA) accreditation
△ Commission on Accreditation of Rehabilitation Facilities (CARF) accreditation

FORT LAUDERDALE—Broward County

☐ **ATLANTIC SHORES HOSPITAL (104065)**, 4545 North Federal Highway, Zip 33308–5274; tel. 954/771–2711, (Nonreporting) **A**1 9 10 **S** Psychiatric Solutions
Primary Contact: Steve Shell, Administrator
Web address: www.atlanticshoreshospital.com
Control: Individual, Investor–owned, for–profit **Service:** Psychiatric

Staffed Beds: 86

★ **BROWARD GENERAL MEDICAL CENTER (100039)**, 1600 South Andrews Avenue, Zip 33316–2510; tel. 954/355–4400 **A**1 2 3 5 9 10 12 13 **F**3 11 12 13 15 17 18 19 20 21 22 23 24 25 26 27 31 32 33 36 38 40 42 43 44 46 49 51 52 54 55 56 57 60 62 63 64 66 68 70 71 72 73 74 75 76 77 78 79 80 81 82 83 84 86 88 89 90 92 94 95 96 97 99 100 102 103 105 106 107 109 111 112 114 118 119 120 121 128 132 135 136 **P**6 **S** Broward Health
CFO: Louis FungSang, Chief Financial Officer
CMO: Wilfred McKenzie, M.D., Chief of Staff
CIO: Doris Crain, Vice President Information Services
CHR: Dionne Wong, Vice President and Chief Human Resources Officer
Web address: www.nbhd.org
Control: Hospital district or authority, Government, nonfederal **Service:** General Medical and Surgical

Staffed Beds: 640 **Admissions:** 27640 **Census:** 453 **Outpatient Visits:** 233228 **Births:** 3787 **Total Expense ($000):** 388386 **Payroll Expense ($000):** 158999 **Personnel:** 2703

★ **FLORIDA MEDICAL CENTER (100210)**, 5000 West Oakland Park Boulevard, Zip 33313–1585; tel. 954/735–6000, (Nonreporting) **A**1 9 10 **S** TENET Healthcare Corporation
Primary Contact: Robert Haley, Chief Executive Officer
Web address: www.floridamedicalctr.com
Control: Partnership, Investor–owned, for–profit **Service:** General Medical and Surgical

Staffed Beds: 459

☐ **FORT LAUDERDALE HOSPITAL (104026)**, 1601 East Las Olas Boulevard, Zip 33301–2393; tel. 954/463–4321, (Nonreporting) **A**1 9 10 **S** Psychiatric Solutions
Primary Contact: Ali A. Elhaj, Ph.D., Chief Executive Officer
Web address: www.psysolutions.com
Control: Corporation, Investor–owned, for–profit **Service:** Psychiatric

Staffed Beds: 100

★ △ **HEALTHSOUTH SUNRISE REHABILITATION HOSPITAL (103028)**, 4399 Nob Hill Road, Zip 33351–5899; tel. 954/749–0300, (Nonreporting) **A**1 7 9 10 **S** HEALTHSOUTH Corporation
Primary Contact: Kevin R. Conn, Chief Executive Officer
CFO: Ruth Goodstein, Controller
CMO: Scott Tannenbaum, M.D., Medical Director
CIO: Angela Crippen, Director Health Information Services
CHR: Barbara Dunkiel, Director Human Resources
Web address: www.healthsouth.com
Control: Corporation, Investor–owned, for–profit **Service:** Rehabilitation

Staffed Beds: 116

★ **HOLY CROSS HOSPITAL (100073)**, 4725 North Federal Highway, Zip 33308–4668, Mailing Address: P.O. Box 23460, Zip 33307–3460; tel. 954/771–8000 **A**1 2 9 10 **F**3 8 11 12 13 14 15 17 18 20 22 24 25 26 27 31 32 33 34 35 38 43 44 46 49 50 52 53 54 55 56 57 58 60 61 62 63 64 65 66 68 70 72 73 74 75 76 77 79 80 81 82 85 86 87 96 97 99 100 102 103 105 107 109 111 116 118 119 120 121 123 124 132 133 134 135 136 137 **P**6 **S** Catholic Health East
Primary Contact: John C. Johnson, Chief Executive Officer
COO: Patrick Taylor, M.D., Executive Vice President, Chief Operating Officer and Medical Director
CFO: Linda Wilford, Chief Financial Officer
CMO: Patrick Taylor, M.D., Executive Vice President, Chief Operating Officer and Medical Director
Web address: www.holy–cross.com
Control: Church–operated, Nongovernment, not–for profit **Service:** General Medical and Surgical

Staffed Beds: 436 **Admissions:** 16522 **Census:** 253 **Outpatient Visits:** 158197 **Births:** 1410 **Total Expense ($000):** 330918 **Payroll Expense ($000):** 137052 **Personnel:** 2027

★ **IMPERIAL POINT MEDICAL CENTER (100200)**, 6401 North Federal Highway, Zip 33308–1495; tel. 954/776–8500 **A**1 9 10 **F**3 11 12 15 18 25 27 31 32 33 38 42 43 44 51 52 55 56 57 58 60 62 64 66 68 72 73 75 76 77 78 79 80 81 82 86 88 90 92 94 95 96 97 99 100 102 103 106 107 114 118 119 120 121 132 135 136 137 **P**6 **S** Broward Health
Primary Contact: Calvin E. Glidewell, Jr., Chief Executive Officer
CFO: Susan Newton, Chief Financial Officer
CHR: Sybil Henry, Region Director Human Resources
Web address: www.browardhealth.org
Control: Hospital district or authority, Government, nonfederal **Service:** General Medical and Surgical

Staffed Beds: 180 **Admissions:** 7419 **Census:** 106 **Outpatient Visits:** 81442 **Births:** 0 **Total Expense ($000):** 82634 **Payroll Expense ($000):** 35953 **Personnel:** 612

☐ **KINDRED HOSPITAL SOUTH FLORIDA–FORT LAUDERDALE (102010)**, (Formerly Kindred Hospital–Fort Lauderdale), 1516 East Las Olas Boulevard, Zip 33301–2399; tel. 954/764–8900, (Nonreporting) **A**1 9 10 **S** Kindred Healthcare
Primary Contact: Theodore L. Welding, Chief Executive Officer
CFO: Dean Card, Chief Financial Officer
Web address: www.kindredhealthcare.com
Control: Corporation, Investor–owned, for–profit **Service:** Long–Term Acute Care hospital

Staffed Beds: 64

FORT MYERS—Lee County

★ ○ **GULF COAST HOSPITAL (100279)**, 13681 Doctors Way, Zip 33912–4309; tel. 239/768–5000, (Nonreporting) **A**1 9 10 11 **S** Lee Memorial Health System
Primary Contact: James R. Nathan, President and Chief Executive Officer
COO: Douglas R. Luckett, Chief Executive Officer
CFO: John K. Wiest, Chief Financial Officer
CMO: Marilyn Kole, M.D., Medical Director
CIO: Mike Smith, Chief Information Officer
CHR: Jon C. Cecil, Chief Human Resource Officer
Web address: www.gulfcoasthospital.com
Control: Corporation, Investor–owned, for–profit **Service:** General Medical and Surgical

Staffed Beds: 107

★ △ **LEE MEMORIAL HOSPITAL (100012)**, 2776 Cleveland Avenue, Zip 33901–5855, Mailing Address: P.O. Box 2218, Zip 33902–2218; tel. 239/332–1111, (Includes HEALTHPARK MEDICAL CENTER, 9981 South HealthPark Drive, Zip 33908; tel. 239/433–7799; THE CHILDREN'S HOSPITAL, 9981 South HealthPark Drive, Zip 33908; tel. 239/433–7799; THE REHABILITATION HOSPITAL), (Total facility includes 112 beds in nursing home–type unit) **A**1 2 7 9 10 **F**17 30 31 32 68 70 71 74 78 79 83 84 85 117 **S** Lee Memorial Health System
Primary Contact: James R. Nathan, President and Chief Executive Officer
CFO: John K. Wiest, Chief Financial and Institutional Service Officer
CMO: Chuck Krivenko, M.D., Chief Medical Officer, Clinical and Quality Services
CIO: Mike Smith, Chief Information Officer
CHR: Jon C. Cecil, Chief Human Resource Officer
Web address: www.leememorial.org
Control: Hospital district or authority, Government, nonfederal **Service:** General Medical and Surgical

Staffed Beds: 1574 **Admissions:** 67855 **Census:** 963 **Outpatient Visits:** 1108206 **Births:** 8225 **Total Expense ($000):** 779451 **Payroll Expense ($000):** 411060 **Personnel:** 6904

★ **SOUTHWEST FLORIDA REGIONAL MEDICAL CENTER (100220)**, 2727 Winkler Avenue, Zip 33901–9396; tel. 239/939–1147, (Nonreporting) **A**1 2 9 10 **S** Lee Memorial Health System
Primary Contact: Douglas R. Luckett, Chief Executive Officer
CFO: Robert F. Carrel, Chief Financial Officer
CMO: Douglas Savage, M.D., President Medical Staff
CIO: Keith Brooks, Director Information and Technology Services
CHR: Peggy Hanover, Vice President Human Resources
Web address: www.swfrmc.com
Control: Corporation, Investor–owned, for–profit **Service:** General Medical and Surgical

Staffed Beds: 279

FORT PIERCE—St. Lucie County

★ **LAWNWOOD REGIONAL MEDICAL CENTER (100246)**, 1700 South 23rd Street, Zip 34950–0188; tel. 772/461–4000, (Includes LAWNWOOD PAVILION, 1860 North Lawnwood Circle, Zip 34950; tel. 361/466–1500) **A**1 9 10 **F**3 11 13 15 17 18 20 22 24 25 27 31 32 33 36 38 43 46 47 48 49 55 57 58 59 60 62 63 66 68 72 73 74 75 76 77 79 80 84 85 86 88 90 91 92 93 96 97 98 100 101 102 106 107 112 116 119 135 **S** HCA
Primary Contact: Thomas R. Pentz, President and Chief Executive Officer
COO: Brian P. Baumgardner, Chief Operating Officer
CFO: Robert Dunwoody, Chief Financial Officer
CIO: Eric Castle, Director Information Services
CHR: Pam Burchell, Director Human Resources
Web address: www.lawnwoodmed.com
Control: Corporation, Investor–owned, for–profit **Service:** General Medical and Surgical

Staffed Beds: 331 **Admissions:** 14802 **Census:** 225 **Outpatient Visits:** 67399 **Births:** 1318 **Total Expense ($000):** 159011 **Payroll Expense ($000):** 61275 **Personnel:** 1023

FORT WALTON BEACH—Okaloosa County

★ △ **FORT WALTON BEACH MEDICAL CENTER (100223)**, 1000 Mar–Walt Drive, Zip 32547–6795; tel. 850/862–1111 **A**1 2 7 9 10 **F**3 11 13 15 17 18 20 22 24 25 26 27 30 31 32 33 35 36 37 38 39 47 51 55 56 57 59 62 66 68 70 71 72 73 74 75 76 77 79 80 82 84 85 88 90 91 92 93 94 96 97 99 100 102 103 104 105 106 107 108 109 111 119 121 135 136 137 **P**6 **S** HCA
Primary Contact: Wayne F. Campbell, Chief Executive Officer
CFO: Vincent N. Wyatt, Chief Financial Officer
Web address: www.fwbmedicalcenter.com
Control: Corporation, Investor–owned, for–profit **Service:** General Medical and Surgical

Staffed Beds: 257 **Admissions:** 12079 **Census:** 178 **Outpatient Visits:** 113602 **Births:** 1466 **Total Expense ($000):** 110729 **Payroll Expense ($000):** 40832 **Personnel:** 723

GAINESVILLE—Alachua County

★ **MALCOM RANDALL VETERANS AFFAIRS MEDICAL CENTER**, 1601 S.W. Archer Road, Zip 32608–1197; tel. 352/376–1611, (Total facility includes 240 beds in nursing home–type unit) (Nonreporting) **A**1 3 5 8 **S** Department of Veterans Affairs
Primary Contact: Frederick L. Malphurs, Director
COO: Thomas Sutton, Associate Director
CFO: Jim Taylor, Chief Business Office
CMO: Brad Bender, M.D., Chief of Staff
CIO: Deborah Michel–Ogborn, Chief Information Resource Management
CHR: Michelle Manderino, Chief Human Resources
Web address: www.va.gov/visn8/nfsg
Control: Veterans Affairs, Government, federal **Service:** General Medical and Surgical

Staffed Beds: 535

★ **NORTH FLORIDA REGIONAL MEDICAL CENTER (100204)**, 6500 Newberry Road, Zip 32605–4392, Mailing Address: P.O. Box 147006, Zip 32614–7006; tel. 352/333–4000, (Nonreporting) **A**1 2 9 10 **S** HCA
Primary Contact: James R. Thomas, Chief Executive Officer
COO: Matt Davis, Chief Operating Officer
CFO: Eric Lawson, Chief Financial Officer
CIO: Deborah Bush, Director Information Services
CHR: William Coorpender, Assistant Vice President Human Resources
Web address: www.nfrmc.com
Control: Corporation, Investor–owned, for–profit **Service:** General Medical and Surgical

Staffed Beds: 278

★ **SHANDS AGH**, 801 S.W. Second Avenue, Zip 32601–6289; tel. 352/733–0111, (Total facility includes 30 beds in nursing home–type unit) (Nonreporting) **A**1 3 5 9 **S** Shands HealthCare
Primary Contact: Francis A. Pommett, Jr., Administrator
COO: Jodi J. Mansfield, Executive Vice President and Chief Operating Officer
CFO: Elizabeth Matthews, Director Finance
CIO: William L. Montgomery, Senior Vice President and Chief Information Officer
CHR: Edie Parker, Director Human Resources
Web address: www.shands.org/hospitals/agh
Control: Other not–for–profit (including NFP Corporation) **Service:** General Medical and Surgical

Staffed Beds: 269

★ **SHANDS AT THE UNIVERSITY OF FLORIDA (100113)**, 1600 S.W. Archer Road, Zip 32610–0326, Mailing Address: P.O. Box 100326, Zip 32610–0326; tel. 352/265–0111 **A**1 2 3 5 8 9 10 **F**2 3 4 5 6 7 8 11 12 13 15 16 17 18 19 20 21 22 23 24 25 26 27 28 30 31 32 33 34 35 36 37 38 40 41 43 44 46 47 49 50 51 52 53 54 55 56 57 58 59 60 61 62 63 66 67 68 70 71 72 73 74 75 76 77 78 79 80 81 82 83 84 85 86 87 88 89 90 91 92 93 94 95 96 97 99 100 102 103 104 105 106 107 108 109 111 112 113 116 118 119 120 121 123 124 125 126 127 128 129 130 131 132 134 135 136 137 **P**1 6 **S** Shands HealthCare
Primary Contact: Timothy J. Goldfarb, Chief Executive Officer
COO: Jodi J. Mansfield, Executive Vice President and Chief Operating Officer
CFO: William J. Robinson, Senior Vice President and Treasurer
CMO: Michael L. Good, M.D., Chief of Staff
CIO: Joan Hovhanesian, Vice President and Chief Information Officer
Web address: www.shands.org
Control: Other not–for–profit (including NFP Corporation) **Service:** General Medical and Surgical

Staffed Beds: 734 **Admissions:** 29764 **Census:** 600 **Outpatient Visits:** 685676 **Births:** 2731 **Total Expense ($000):** 720131 **Payroll Expense ($000):** 273543 **Personnel:** 5437

★ △ **SHANDS REHAB HOSPITAL**, 4101 N.W. 89th Boulevard, Zip 32606–3813; tel. 352/265–5491, (Nonreporting) **A**1 7 **S** Shands HealthCare
Primary Contact: Marina T. Cecchini, Administrator
CFO: William J. Robinson, Senior Vice President and Chief Financial Officer
Web address: www.shands.org
Control: Other not–for–profit (including NFP Corporation) **Service:** Psychiatric

Staffed Beds: 121

GRACEVILLE—Jackson County

CAMPBELLTON GRACEVILLE HOSPITAL (101302), (Critical Access Hospital), 5429 College Drive, Zip 32440–1897; tel. 850/263–4431 **A**9 10 18 **F**38 54 55 56 57 62 64 65 75 85 96 107 118 119 120 122 135 **P**4
Primary Contact: Jimmy Rigsby, Chief Executive Officer
CMO: Jack Sanders, M.D., Chief Medical Officer
CHR: Judy Austin, Director Human Resources
Web address: www.pahn.org/cgh.cfm
Control: Hospital district or authority, Government, nonfederal **Service:** Other specialty

Staffed Beds: 25 **Admissions:** 475 **Census:** 5 **Outpatient Visits:** 10385 **Births:** 0

GREEN COVE SPRINGS—Clay County

☐ **KINDRED HOSPITAL NORTH FLORIDA (102015)**, 801 Oak Street, Zip 32043–4317; tel. 904/284–9230 **A**1 9 10 **F**1 3 25 26 43 59 68 72 73 75 80 82 96 107 119 137 **S** Kindred Healthcare
Primary Contact: Tim Simpson, Executive Director
CFO: Joyce Caltrider, Chief Financial Officer
CMO: Eugene McCoskey, M.D., Chief of Staff
CIO: Rick Chapman, Chief Information Officer
Web address: www.khnorthflorida.com
Control: Corporation, Investor–owned, for–profit **Service:** Long–Term Acute Care hospital

Staffed Beds: 60 **Admissions:** 511 **Census:** 54 **Outpatient Visits:** 86 **Births:** 0 **Personnel:** 253

GULF BREEZE—Santa Rosa County

★ **GULF BREEZE HOSPITAL (100266)**, 1110 Gulf Breeze Parkway, Zip 32561; tel. 850/934–2000 **A**1 9 10 **F**3 8 11 15 25 26 27 30 31 32 34 38 41 43 46 50 53 55 57 62 66 68 72 73 76 77 79 80 81 86 96 97 100 102 107 109 111 119 120 121 132 135 136 **P**6 **S** Baptist Health Care Corporation
Primary Contact: Robert Harriman, Administrator
CFO: Joseph G. Felkner, Chief Financial Officer
Web address: www.e–baptisthealthcare.org
Control: Other not–for–profit (including NFP Corporation) **Service:** General Medical and Surgical

Staffed Beds: 60 **Admissions:** 3659 **Census:** 41 **Outpatient Visits:** 105723 **Births:** 0 **Total Expense ($000):** 57787 **Payroll Expense ($000):** 17797 **Personnel:** 381

FL

Hospital, Medicare Provider Number, Address, Telephone, Approval, Facility, and Physician Codes, Health Care System

★ American Hospital Association (AHA) membership
☐ The Joint Commission accreditation
○ American Osteopathic Association (AOA) accreditation
△ Commission on Accreditation of Rehabilitation Facilities (CARF) accreditation

HIALEAH—Dade County

★ **HIALEAH HOSPITAL (100053)**, 651 East 25th Street, Zip 33013–3878; tel. 305/693–6100, (Nonreporting) **A**1 9 10 **S** TENET Healthcare Corporation
Primary Contact: Ralph A. Aleman, Chief Executive Officer
COO: Steven Burghart, Chief Operating Officer
CFO: Arthur West, Chief Financial Officer
CHR: Yamila Castro, Director Human Resources
Web address: www.hialeahhosp.com
Control: Corporation, Investor–owned, for–profit **Service:** General Medical and Surgical

Staffed Beds: 378

☐ **PALM SPRINGS GENERAL HOSPITAL (100050)**, 1475 West 49th Street, Zip 33012–3275, Mailing Address: P.O. Box 2804, Zip 33012–2804; tel. 305/558–2500, (Nonreporting) **A**1 10
Primary Contact: Tony Mazzorano, Chief Executive Officer
CFO: Tony Milian, Chief Financial Officer
CHR: Lourdes Anton, Director Human Resources
Control: Corporation, Investor–owned, for–profit **Service:** General Medical and Surgical

Staffed Beds: 190

★ **PALMETTO GENERAL HOSPITAL (100187)**, 2001 West 68th Street, Zip 33016–1898; tel. 305/823–5000, (Nonreporting) **A**1 9 10 12 13 **S** TENET Healthcare Corporation
Primary Contact: Ana J. Mederos, Chief Executive Officer
COO: Alex Contreras–Soto, Chief Operating Officer
CFO: Oscar Vicente, Chief Financial Officer
CMO: Jose Gamez, M.D., Chief of Staff
Web address: www.palmettogeneral.com
Control: Corporation, Investor–owned, for–profit **Service:** General Medical and Surgical

Staffed Beds: 360

SOUTHERN WINDS HOSPITAL See Westchester General Hospital, Miami

HOLLYWOOD—Broward County

☐ **HOLLYWOOD PAVILION (104015)**, 1201 North 37th Avenue, Zip 33021–5498; tel. 954/962–1355, (Nonreporting) **A**1 9 10
Primary Contact: Karen Kallen–Zury, Chief Executive Officer
COO: Christopher Gabel, Chief Operating Officer
CFO: Harold Mandelbaum, Controller
Web address: www.hollywoodpavilion.net
Control: Corporation, Investor–owned, for–profit **Service:** Psychiatric

Staffed Beds: 46

☐ **KINDRED HOSPITAL SOUTH FLORIDA–HOLLYWOOD (102010)**, 1859 Van Buren Street, Zip 33020–5127; tel. 954/920–9000, (Nonreporting) **A**1 9 10 **S** Kindred Healthcare
Primary Contact: Chris Clements, Chief Executive Officer
COO: Carlene Nugent, Chief Clinical Officer
CFO: Donald Gemmel, Controller
CMO: James Stern, M.D., Senior Vice President Medical Staff
CIO: Linda McQuade, Director Information Management
Web address: www.kindredhealthcare.com
Control: Corporation, Investor–owned, for–profit **Service:** General Medical and Surgical

Staffed Beds: 124

★ △ **MEMORIAL REGIONAL HOSPITAL (100038)**, 3501 Johnson Street, Zip 33021–5421; tel. 954/987–2000, (Includes JOE DIMAGGIO CHILDREN'S HOSPITAL) **A**1 2 3 5 7 9 10 **F**2 3 4 7 11 12 13 15 17 18 19 20 21 22 23 24 25 26 27 28 30 31 32 36 38 40 41 43 46 47 48 49 50 51 52 53 54 55 56 57 58 59 60 61 62 63 64 66 68 69 70 71 72 73 74 75 76 77 79 80 81 82 83 84 85 86 87 88 89 90 91 92 93 94 95 96 97 98 99 100 101 102 106 107 108 109 111 112 114 116 117 118 119 120 121 124 132 134 135 136 137 **S** Memorial Healthcare System
Primary Contact: Rodney E. Miller, Sr., Administrator
COO: Deborah Tedder, Chief Operating Officer and Chief Nursing Officer
CFO: David Smith, Chief Financial Officer
CMO: Stanley Marks, M.D., Chief Medical Officer
CIO: Forest Blanton, Administrator Process Engineering
CHR: Ray Kendrick, Chief Human Resources Officer
Web address: www.mhs.net
Control: Hospital district or authority, Government, nonfederal **Service:** General Medical and Surgical

Staffed Beds: 690 **Admissions:** 38642 **Census:** 569 **Outpatient Visits:** 369721 **Births:** 4920 **Total Expense ($000):** 448685 **Payroll Expense ($000):** 230902 **Personnel:** 3725

★ △ **MEMORIAL REGIONAL HOSPITAL SOUTH (100225)**, 3600 Washington Street, Zip 33021–8216; tel. 954/966–4500 **A**1 7 9 10 **F**2 3 11 15 25 26 30 31 32 33 38 42 44 45 46 49 50 51 53 54 55 56 57 59 62 66 68 72 73 75 77 79 80 81 82 85 96 97 99 100 102 107 118 119 120 121 122 134 135 136 137 **S** Memorial Healthcare System
Primary Contact: Douglas Zaren, FACHE, Administrator
CFO: David Smith, Chief Financial Officer
Web address: www.memorialregionalsouth.com
Control: Hospital district or authority, Government, nonfederal **Service:** General Medical and Surgical

Staffed Beds: 120 **Admissions:** 1294 **Census:** 45 **Outpatient Visits:** 9020 **Births:** 0 **Total Expense ($000):** 18451 **Payroll Expense ($000):** 8826 **Personnel:** 370

☐ **SOUTH FLORIDA STATE HOSPITAL (104001)**, 800 East Cypress Drive, Zip 33025–4543; tel. 954/392–3000, (Nonreporting) **A**1 5 10
Primary Contact: Sal A. Barbera, FACHE, Administrator
Web address: www.sfsh.org
Control: State–Government, nonfederal **Service:** Psychiatric

Staffed Beds: 355

HOMESTEAD—Dade County

★ **HOMESTEAD HOSPITAL (100125)**, 975 Baptist Way, Zip 33033–7600; tel. 786/243–8000 **A**1 9 10 **F**3 8 11 13 15 25 26 27 30 31 32 33 38 42 43 44 47 49 50 51 52 53 55 56 57 59 62 66 68 73 74 76 77 79 80 82 84 86 96 97 100 107 118 119 121 123 124 133 134 135 136 137 **S** Baptist Health South Florida
Primary Contact: Bill Duquette, Chief Executive Officer
CFO: Erik Long, Controller
CMO: Jorge Mejia, M.D., Chief of Staff
CIO: Mimi Taylor, Corporate Vice President Information Technology
Web address: www.baptisthealth.net
Control: Other not–for–profit (including NFP Corporation) **Service:** General Medical and Surgical

Staffed Beds: 120 **Admissions:** 8502 **Census:** 107 **Outpatient Visits:** 70148 **Births:** 1418 **Total Expense ($000):** 124302 **Payroll Expense ($000):** 44695 **Personnel:** 810

HUDSON—Pasco County

★ **REGIONAL MEDICAL CENTER–BAYONET POINT (100256)**, 14000 Fivay Road, Zip 34667–7199; tel. 727/863–2411 **A**2 9 10 **F**3 15 17 18 20 22 24 25 26 27 30 31 32 38 46 47 48 49 50 55 56 57 59 62 68 72 73 75 76 77 79 80 82 86 96 97 100 102 103 107 118 121 124 135 137 **S** HCA
Primary Contact: Stephen A. Rector, Chief Executive Officer
CFO: Patrick Long, Chief Financial Officer
CMO: Marshall DeSantis, M.D., Chief of Staff
CIO: Stephen Goldstein, Director Information Systems
CHR: Andrea Pinion, Vice President
Web address: www.rmchealth.com
Control: Corporation, Investor–owned, for–profit **Service:** General Medical and Surgical

Staffed Beds: 280 **Admissions:** 12038 **Census:** 173 **Outpatient Visits:** 58010 **Total Expense ($000):** 130838 **Payroll Expense ($000):** 51122 **Personnel:** 819

INVERNESS—Citrus County

★ **CITRUS MEMORIAL HEALTH SYSTEM (100023)**, (Formerly Citrus Memorial Hospital), 502 West Highland Boulevard, Zip 34452–4754; tel. 352/726–1551 **A**1 9 10 19 **F**3 8 11 13 15 17 18 20 22 24 25 26 27 30 31 32 33 38 41 47 48 49 50 53 55 56 57 61 62 66 67 68 73 74 75 76 77 79 80 81 84 85 86 87 96 97 99 100 102 103 106 107 119 121 133 135 136 **P**6
Primary Contact: Ryan D. Beaty, President and Chief Executive Officer
COO: Jerrald Deloach, Chief Operating Officer
CFO: Emery Hensley, Chief Financial Officer
CHR: Lee Glotzback, Director Human Resources
Web address: www.citrusmh.com
Control: Other not–for–profit (including NFP Corporation) **Service:** General Medical and Surgical

Staffed Beds: 198 **Admissions:** 13345 **Census:** 156 **Outpatient Visits:** 183833 **Births:** 644 **Total Expense ($000):** 147720 **Payroll Expense ($000):** 46221 **Personnel:** 1145

FL

Many Facility Codes have changed. Please refer to the AHA Guide Code Chart.

JACKSONVILLE—Duval County

★ **BAPTIST MEDICAL CENTER (100088)**, 800 Prudential Drive, Zip 32207–8203; tel. 904/202–2000, (Includes BAPTIST MEDICAL CENTER SOUTH, 14550 St. Augustine Road, Zip 32258–2160; tel. 904/821–6000; Ronald G. Robinson, Administrator) **A**1 2 3 5 9 10 **F**3 5 11 13 15 17 18 19 20 21 22 23 24 25 26 27 28 30 31 32 33 34 36 37 38 41 43 46 47 49 50 51 52 53 55 56 57 58 59 60 61 62 66 68 70 71 72 73 74 75 76 77 78 79 80 81 82 83 84 86 88 89 90 91 92 93 94 95 96 97 98 99 100 102 103 104 105 107 108 109 112 114 116 118 119 120 121 124 125 130 134 135 136 137 **P**6 **S** Baptist Health
Primary Contact: Joseph M. Mitrick, FACHE, Administrator
COO: John F. Wilbanks, FACHE, Chief Operating Officer
CFO: Mike Lukaszewski, Chief Financial Officer
CMO: Keith L. Stein, M.D., Senior Vice President Medical Affairs and Chief Medical Officer
CIO: Roland Garcia, Senior Vice President and Chief Information Officer
CHR: Beth Mehaffey, Vice President Human Resources
Web address: www.e–baptisthealth.com
Control: Other not–for–profit (including NFP Corporation) **Service:** General Medical and Surgical

Staffed Beds: 579 **Admissions:** 30323 **Census:** 454 **Outpatient Visits:** 381689 **Births:** 2419 **Total Expense ($000):** 482507 **Payroll Expense ($000):** 172549 **Personnel:** 4389

★ △ **BROOKS REHABILITATION HOSPITAL (103039)**, 3599 University Boulevard South, Zip 32216–4252; tel. 904/858–7600 **A**1 7 10 **F**3 11 25 26 43 62 85 86 119 121 135
Primary Contact: Douglas Baer, Chief Executive Officer
COO: Michael Spigel, Chief Operating Officer
CFO: Becky Chaudoin, Assistant Administrator
CMO: Deborah G. Stewart, M.D., Chief Medical Officer and Medical Director
CIO: Karen Green, Chief Information Officer
CHR: Elizabeth Figura, Vice President Human Resources
Web address: www.brookshealth.org
Control: Other not–for–profit (including NFP Corporation) **Service:** Rehabilitation

Staffed Beds: 127 **Admissions:** 2605 **Census:** 116

★ **MAYO CLINIC JACKSONVILLE (100151)**, 4500 San Pablo Road, Zip 32224; tel. 904/953–2000 **A**1 3 5 8 9 10 **F**3 8 11 12 13 18 20 22 24 25 26 27 30 31 32 38 42 43 44 46 49 51 59 66 68 70 72 74 76 77 79 80 82 96 100 106 107 112 116 119 124 125 126 127 128 129 135 137 **S** Mayo Foundation
Primary Contact: Hilary G. Mathews, Administrator
COO: Hilary G. Mathews, Administrator
CFO: Mary Hoffman, Chief Financial Officer
CMO: Charles Burger, M.D., President Medical Staff
CIO: Cheryl Croft, Chairman Information Services
CHR: Michael Estes, Chair Human Resources
Web address: www.mayoclinic.org
Control: Other not–for–profit (including NFP Corporation) **Service:** General Medical and Surgical

Staffed Beds: 313 **Admissions:** 17106 **Census:** 240 **Outpatient Visits:** 36668 **Births:** 1402 **Total Expense ($000):** 331810 **Payroll Expense ($000):** 87889 **Personnel:** 1786

★ **MEMORIAL HOSPITAL JACKSONVILLE (100179)**, (Formerly Memorial Hospital of Jacksonville), 3625 University Boulevard South, Zip 32216–4240, Mailing Address: P.O. Box 16325, Zip 32216–6325; tel. 904/399–6111 **A**1 2 9 10 **F**3 11 12 13 15 17 18 20 22 24 25 26 27 30 32 33 35 36 38 40 46 47 52 53 54 55 56 57 58 59 62 68 70 72 74 76 77 78 79 80 81 82 87 96 97 99 100 101 102 104 106 107 108 109 112 113 114 119 120 121 134 135 136 137 **P**6 8 **S** HCA
Primary Contact: James B. Wood, President and Chief Executive Officer
COO: Eric Goldman, Chief Operating Officer
CFO: Rodney Van Pelt, Chief Financial Officer
Web address: www.memorialhospitaljax.com
Control: Corporation, Investor–owned, for–profit **Service:** General Medical and Surgical

Staffed Beds: 353 **Admissions:** 20113 **Census:** 290 **Outpatient Visits:** 124528 **Births:** 2509 **Total Expense ($000):** 211509 **Payroll Expense ($000):** 78931 **Personnel:** 1433

★ **NAVAL HOSPITAL**, 2080 Child Street, Zip 32214–5000; tel. 904/542–7300, (Nonreporting) **A**1 3 5 **S** Bureau of Medicine and Surgery, Department of the Navy
Primary Contact: Captain Raquel Bono, Commanding Officer
COO: Captain Kathy Pierce, Executive Officer
CFO: Lieutenant Commander David Breier, Comptroller
CMO: Commander David Weiss, Director Medical Services
CIO: Lieutenant Commander Mike Haytaian, Head Director Information Resources Management
CHR: Commander Darin Rogers, Director Administration
Web address: www.navalhospitaljax.com
Control: Navy, Government, federal **Service:** General Medical and Surgical

Staffed Beds: 76

★ **SHANDS JACKSONVILLE MEDICAL CENTER (100001)**, 655 West Eighth Street, Zip 32209–6595; tel. 904/244–0411, (Total facility includes 40 beds in nursing home–type unit) **A**1 2 3 5 8 9 10 **F**3 7 8 11 12 13 15 17 18 20 22 23 24 25 26 27 28 30 31 32 33 34 35 36 37 38 40 41 43 44 46 49 50 51 53 54 55 56 57 58 59 60 61 62 63 64 66 68 69 70 71 72 73 74 75 76 77 78 79 80 81 82 83 84 86 87 88 89 90 91 92 93 94 95 96 97 98 99 100 102 103 104 105 106 107 108 109 111 113 114 117 118 119 120 121 122 123 124 127 133 134 135 136 137 **P**1 **S** Shands HealthCare
Primary Contact: James R. Burkhart, FACHE, President and Chief Executive Officer
COO: James R. Burkhart, FACHE, President and Chief Executive Officer
CMO: David Vukich, M.D., Senior Vice President and Chief Medical Officer
CHR: Lesli Ward, Vice President Human Resources
Web address: www.shandsjacksonville.org
Control: Other not–for–profit (including NFP Corporation) **Service:** General Medical and Surgical

Staffed Beds: 599 **Admissions:** 27273 **Census:** 458 **Outpatient Visits:** 410053 **Births:** 3648 **Total Expense ($000):** 494911 **Payroll Expense ($000):** 173372 **Personnel:** 3508

★ **SPECIALTY HOSPITAL JACKSONVILLE (102012)**, 4901 Richard Street, Zip 32207–7328; tel. 904/737–3120, (Nonreporting) **A**1 9 10 **S** HCA
Primary Contact: Barbara Walsh, Chief Executive Officer
CMO: Wendell H. Williams, M.D., Medical Director
CIO: Liz Rhodes, Director Information Services
CHR: Lisa Ayala, R.N., Director Human Resources
Web address: www.specialtyhospitaljax.com
Control: Corporation, Investor–owned, for–profit **Service:** General Medical and Surgical

Staffed Beds: 62

□ **ST. LUKE'S HOSPITAL**, 4201 Belfort Road, Zip 32216; tel. 904/296–3700, (Nonreporting) **A**1 9 10 **S** Ascension Health
Primary Contact: Michael D. Holmes, Chief Operating Officer
Web address: www.stlukesjax.com
Control: Other not–for–profit (including NFP Corporation) **Service:** General Medical and Surgical

Staffed Beds: 214

★ **ST. VINCENT'S MEDICAL CENTER (100040)**, 1 Shircliff Way, Zip 32204–2982, Mailing Address: P.O. Box 2982, Zip 32203–2982; tel. 904/308–7300 **A**1 2 3 5 9 10 12 13 **F**3 8 11 13 15 17 18 20 22 24 25 26 27 30 31 32 33 35 37 38 41 43 46 48 49 50 52 53 54 55 56 57 58 59 60 62 63 64 66 68 69 71 72 73 74 75 76 77 79 80 81 82 86 92 96 97 100 102 104 105 106 107 109 111 118 119 120 121 124 131 132 133 135 136 137 **P**6 **S** Ascension Health
Primary Contact: Scott Whalen, Ph.D., Chief Executive Officer
COO: Gene K. Miyamoto, Chief Operating Officer
CFO: Daniel Curran, Chief Financial Officer
CMO: Phil Perry, M.D., Chief Medical Officer
CIO: Ann Carey, Vice President and Chief Information Officer
CHR: Jan Lipsky, Vice President Organizational Effectiveness
Web address: www.jaxhealth.com
Control: Church–operated, Nongovernment, not–for profit **Service:** General Medical and Surgical

Staffed Beds: 455 **Admissions:** 26432 **Census:** 364 **Outpatient Visits:** 142464 **Births:** 2230 **Total Expense ($000):** 346503 **Payroll Expense ($000):** 126648 **Personnel:** 3458

□ **TEN BROECK HOSPITAL JACKSONVILLE (104016)**, 6300 Beach Boulevard, Zip 32216–2782; tel. 904/724–9202, (Nonreporting) **A**1 9 10 **S** United Medical Corporation
Primary Contact: Paul Andrews, Chief Executive Officer
CFO: Jenni Stackhouse, Chief Financial Officer
CIO: Bill Willis, Director Information Technology
CHR: Cathy Calhoun, Director Human Resources
Web address: www.tenbroeck.com
Control: Corporation, Investor–owned, for–profit **Service:** Psychiatric

Staffed Beds: 99

FL

Hospital, Medicare Provider Number, Address, Telephone, Approval, Facility, and Physician Codes, Health Care System

★ American Hospital Association (AHA) membership
□ The Joint Commission accreditation
○ American Osteopathic Association (AOA) accreditation
△ Commission on Accreditation of Rehabilitation Facilities (CARF) accreditation

JACKSONVILLE BEACH—Duval County

★ **BAPTIST MEDICAL CENTER BEACHES (100117)**, 1350 13th Avenue South, Zip 32250–3205; tel. 904/627–2900 **A**1 9 10 **F**3 11 13 15 24 25 26 27 30 31 32 34 38 40 43 49 50 52 53 55 57 60 62 72 73 74 75 76 77 78 79 80 81 86 96 97 99 100 102 106 107 118 119 135 137 **S** Baptist Health
Primary Contact: Mark F. Slyter, FACHE, Administrator
COO: John F. Wilbanks, FACHE, Chief Operating Officer
CFO: Mike Lukaszewski, Chief Financial Officer
CMO: Keith L. Stein, M.D., Chief Medical Officer
CIO: Roland Garcia, Senior Vice President and Chief Information Officer
CHR: Dana Voiselle, Director Human Resources
Web address: www.e–baptisthealth.com
Control: Other not–for–profit (including NFP Corporation) **Service:** General Medical and Surgical

Staffed Beds: 146 **Admissions:** 7186 **Census:** 92 **Outpatient Visits:** 92107 **Births:** 1057 **Total Expense ($000):** 82123 **Payroll Expense ($000):** 33026 **Personnel:** 887

JASPER—Hamilton County

TRINITY COMMUNITY HOSPITAL (100108), 506 N.W. Fourth Street, Zip 32052–6603; tel. 386/792–7200, (Nonreporting) **A**9 10
Primary Contact: Christina Ortega, Administrator
COO: Christina Ortega, Administrator
CIO: Natalie Krasnow, Chief Information Officer
CHR: Angela Cohen, Director Human Resources
Control: Corporation, Investor–owned, for–profit **Service:** General Medical and Surgical

Staffed Beds: 42

JAY—Santa Rosa County

★ **JAY HOSPITAL (100048)**, 14114 South Alabama Street, Zip 32565–1070; tel. 850/675–8000, (Total facility includes 27 beds in nursing home–type unit) **A**9 10 **F**15 25 26 30 31 32 33 38 41 46 48 50 55 56 57 62 75 77 79 80 86 96 100 102 107 119 121 122 135 **S** Baptist Health Care Corporation
Primary Contact: Michael T. Hutchins, Administrator
CFO: Keith Strickling, Chief Accountant
CMO: Bascom Raney, M.D., Chief of Staff
CHR: Chanda Gay, Manager Human Resources
Web address: www.bhcpns.org/jayhospital/
Control: Other not–for–profit (including NFP Corporation) **Service:** General Medical and Surgical

Staffed Beds: 56 **Admissions:** 1262 **Census:** 26 **Outpatient Visits:** 28767 **Births:** 0 **Total Expense ($000):** 12113 **Payroll Expense ($000):** 4571 **Personnel:** 132

FL

JUPITER—Palm Beach County

★ **JUPITER MEDICAL CENTER (100253)**, 1210 South Old Dixie Highway, Zip 33458–7299; tel. 561/747–2234, (Total facility includes 120 beds in nursing home–type unit) **A**1 2 9 10 **F**3 11 12 13 15 24 25 26 27 30 31 32 33 38 41 43 44 47 49 50 52 53 55 56 57 62 68 72 73 74 75 76 77 79 80 81 82 86 96 97 98 99 100 102 103 105 106 107 108 109 110 111 112 114 117 118 119 121 124 132 135 136 137 **P**6
Primary Contact: Paul Dell Uomo, President and Chief Executive Officer
CFO: Stephen J. Grigsby, Chief Financial Officer
CMO: James P. Ketterhagen, M.D., Vice President Medical Affairs and Chief Quality Officer
CIO: Mike Fehr, Director Information Systems
CHR: John Wolf, Chief Human Resources Officer
Web address: www.jupitermed.com
Control: Other not–for–profit (including NFP Corporation) **Service:** General Medical and Surgical

Staffed Beds: 283 **Admissions:** 11085 **Census:** 235 **Outpatient Visits:** 142831 **Births:** 1174 **Total Expense ($000):** 152730 **Payroll Expense ($000):** 60257 **Personnel:** 1316

KEY WEST—Monroe County

☐ **LOWER KEYS MEDICAL CENTER (100150)**, 5900 College Road, Zip 33040–4396, Mailing Address: P.O. Box 9107, Zip 33041–9107; tel. 305/294–5531, (Includes DE POO HOSPITAL, 1200 Kennedy Drive, Zip 33041; tel. 305/294–4692; FLORIDA KEYS MEMORIAL HOSPITAL), (Nonreporting) **A**1 9 10 19 20 **S** Health Management Associates
Primary Contact: Nicki Will, Ph.D., President and Chief Executive Officer
COO: Meylan Love–Watler, Chief Operating Officer
CFO: Ronald L. Brown, Chief Financial Officer
CMO: Jerome Covington, M.D., Chief Medical Officer
CIO: Les Jackson, Manager Information Systems
CHR: Donald Canalejo, Director Human Resources
Web address: www.lkmc.com
Control: Corporation, Investor–owned, for–profit **Service:** General Medical and Surgical

Staffed Beds: 100

KISSIMMEE—Osceola County

FLORIDA HOSPITAL KISSIMMEE See Florida Hospital, Orlando

★ **OSCEOLA REGIONAL MEDICAL CENTER (100110)**, 700 West Oak Street, Zip 34741–4996; tel. 407/846–2266, (Nonreporting) **A**1 9 10 **S** HCA
Primary Contact: E. Tim Cook, Chief Executive Officer
COO: Randy Gross, Chief Operating Officer
CFO: Peter Mercer, Chief Financial Officer
CHR: Sylvia Lollis, Director Human Resources
Web address: www.osceolaregional.com
Control: Corporation, Investor–owned, for–profit **Service:** General Medical and Surgical

Staffed Beds: 156

LAKE BUTLER—Union County

LAKE BUTLER HOSPITAL HAND SURGERY CENTER (101303), 850 East Main Street, Zip 32054–1335, Mailing Address: P.O. Box 748, Zip 32054–0748; tel. 386/496–2323 **A**9 10 18 **F**25 31 32 38 50 55 56 57 75 79 119 122
Primary Contact: Pamela B. Howard, Administrator
CFO: Paula Webb, Chief Financial Officer
CMO: Cynthia Larimer, M.D., Medical Director Emergency Room
CIO: Jennifer Thomas, Director Public Relations
CHR: Diane Cason, Supervisor Personnel and Payroll
Web address: www.lakebutlerhospital.com
Control: Corporation, Investor–owned, for–profit **Service:** General Medical and Surgical

Staffed Beds: 25 **Admissions:** 153 **Census:** 2 **Outpatient Visits:** 6947 **Births:** 0 **Total Expense ($000):** 6272 **Payroll Expense ($000):** 3729 **Personnel:** 85

RECEPTION AND MEDICAL CENTER, (Formerly North Florida Reception Center Hospital), State Road 231 South, Zip 32054, Mailing Address: P.O. Box 628, Zip 32054–0628; tel. 386/496–6000, (Nonreporting)
Primary Contact: Marinell Brown, Administrator
Control: State–Government, nonfederal **Service:** Hospital unit of an institution (prison hospital, college infirmary, etc.)

Staffed Beds: 133

LAKE CITY—Columbia County

★ **LAKE CITY MEDICAL CENTER (100156)**, 340 N.W. Commerce Drive, Zip 32055–3718; tel. 386/719–9000 **A**1 9 10 **F**3 11 15 18 25 26 27 30 31 32 33 38 47 49 51 52 54 55 57 62 66 68 73 75 76 77 79 80 81 82 86 96 97 99 100 102 104 105 107 118 119 135 **S** HCA
Primary Contact: John Deardorff, Chief Executive Officer
COO: Jennifer B. Adams, Chief Operating Officer and Chief Financial Officer
CFO: Jennifer B. Adams, Chief Operating Officer and Chief Financial Officer
CMO: Vernon Montoya, M.D., Chief of Medicine
CIO: Taylor Dickerson, Chief Information Officer
CHR: Steve Gordon, Director Human Resources
Web address: www.lakecitymedical.com
Control: Corporation, Investor–owned, for–profit **Service:** General Medical and Surgical

Staffed Beds: 67 **Admissions:** 3806 **Census:** 47 **Outpatient Visits:** 50501 **Births:** 0 **Personnel:** 299

★ **SHANDS LAKE SHORE (100102)**, 368 N.E. Franklin Street, Zip 32055–3047; tel. 386/754–8000 **A**1 9 10 **F**3 11 13 15 25 27 30 31 32 33 38 41 53 54 55 56 57 62 66 68 73 74 75 76 77 78 79 80 81 82 84 86 96 97 100 102 107 119 120 124 137 **P**6 **S** Shands HealthCare
Primary Contact: Rhonda Kay Sherrod, RN, M.S.N., Administrator
CMO: Ricardo Rosato, M.D., President Medical Staff
CHR: Janice Jackson, Director Human Resources
Web address: www.shands.org
Control: Other not–for–profit (including NFP Corporation) **Service:** General Medical and Surgical

Staffed Beds: 94 **Admissions:** 5082 **Census:** 52 **Outpatient Visits:** 101717 **Births:** 706 **Total Expense ($000):** 43571 **Payroll Expense ($000):** 20085 **Personnel:** 400

★ **VETERANS AFFAIRS MEDICAL CENTER**, 619 South Marion Avenue, Zip 32025–5898; tel. 386/755–3016, (Total facility includes 180 beds in nursing home–type unit) (Nonreporting) **A**1 **S** Department of Veterans Affairs
Primary Contact: Thomas A. Cappello, M.P.H., FACHE, Director
CIO: James Hudson, Assistant Chief Information Resource Management
Web address: www.va.gov/sta/guide/home.asp
Control: Veterans Affairs, Government, federal **Service:** General Medical and Surgical

Staffed Beds: 360

Many Facility Codes have changed. Please refer to the AHA Guide Code Chart.

LAKE WALES—Polk County

★ □ **LAKE WALES MEDICAL CENTERS (100099)**, 410 South 11th Street, Zip 33853–4256; tel. 863/676–1433 **A**1 9 10 **F**3 11 15 18 25 38 43 49 50 55 56 57 68 72 73 77 79 80 84 86 96 97 99 102 107 118 120 121 135 137 **S** Community Health Systems, Inc.
Primary Contact: Michael Yungmann, Chief Executive Officer
CFO: Thomas Chaundy, Chief Financial Officer
CMO: Caroline Honculada, M.D., Chief Medical Staff
CIO: Erwin Jaropillo, Director Information Systems
CHR: Renee Latterner, Director Human Resources
Web address: www.lakewalesmedicalcenter.com
Control: Corporation, Investor–owned, for–profit **Service:** General Medical and Surgical

Staffed Beds: 126 **Admissions:** 5600 **Census:** 50 **Outpatient Visits:** 39979 **Births:** 0 **Total Expense ($000):** 42856 **Payroll Expense ($000):** 16552 **Personnel:** 361

LAKELAND—Polk County

★ □ **LAKELAND REGIONAL MEDICAL CENTER (100157)**, 1324 Lakeland Hills Boulevard, Zip 33805–4543, Mailing Address: P.O. Box 95448, Zip 33804–5448; tel. 863/687–1100 **A**1 2 3 5 9 10 **F**3 4 5 6 11 13 15 17 18 20 22 24 25 26 27 30 31 32 33 36 38 40 41 43 44 45 46 49 54 55 56 57 58 59 60 62 63 68 70 72 73 74 75 76 77 79 80 81 82 83 84 88 89 90 91 92 93 94 95 96 97 98 100 102 106 107 112 114 116 119 121 123 124 132 133 135 136 137 **P**6
Primary Contact: Jack T. Stephens, Jr., President and Chief Executive Officer
CFO: Paul A. Powers, Vice President
CMO: Edwin Sammer, M.D., Vice President and Chief Medical Officer
CIO: Mary Ford, Vice President and Chief Information Officer
CHR: Jeffery Payne, Vice President Human Resources
Web address: www.lrmc.com
Control: Other not–for–profit (including NFP Corporation) **Service:** General Medical and Surgical

Staffed Beds: 762 **Admissions:** 37082 **Census:** 514 **Outpatient Visits:** 180091 **Births:** 3674 **Total Expense ($000):** 451670 **Payroll Expense ($000):** 188480 **Personnel:** 3902

LANTANA—Palm Beach County

A. G. HOLLEY STATE HOSPITAL (102000), 1199 West Lantana Road, Zip 33462–1514, Mailing Address: P.O. Box 3084, Zip 33465–3084; tel. 561/582–5666, (Nonreporting) **A**10
Primary Contact: David Ashkin, M.D., Medical Executive Director
CFO: Doreen Thomas, Director Administrative Services
Web address: www.doh.state.fl.us/agholley/index.html
Control: State–Government, nonfederal **Service:** Long–Term Acute Care hospital

Staffed Beds: 50

LARGO—Pinellas County

★ □ **HEALTHSOUTH REHABILITATION HOSPITAL (103037)**, 901 North Clearwater–Largo Road, Zip 33770–4126; tel. 727/586–2999, (Nonreporting) **A**1 9 10 **S** HEALTHSOUTH Corporation
Primary Contact: Elaine D. Ebaugh, Chief Executive Officer
CFO: Judith Johnson, Controller
CMO: Richard A. Liles, M.D., Medical Director
CHR: Jackie Chalk, Director Human Resources
Web address: www.healthsouth.com
Control: Corporation, Investor–owned, for–profit **Service:** Rehabilitation

Staffed Beds: 60

★ □ **LARGO MEDICAL CENTER (100248)**, 201 14th Street S.W., Zip 33770–3133, Mailing Address: P.O. Box 2905, Zip 33779–2905; tel. 727/588–5200, (Total facility includes 13 beds in nursing home–type unit) (Nonreporting) **A**1 2 5 9 10 **S** HCA
Primary Contact: Richard H. Satcher, President and Chief Executive Officer
COO: Lawrence W. Kaufman, Administrator and Chief Operating Officer
CFO: Robert E. Billings, Chief Financial Officer
CIO: Silvia Padro, Director Information Services
CHR: Debra Dennis, Director Human Resources
Web address: www.largomedical.com
Control: Corporation, Investor–owned, for–profit **Service:** General Medical and Surgical

Staffed Beds: 243

□ ○ **SUN COAST HOSPITAL (100015)**, 2025 Indian Rocks Road, Zip 33774–1096, Mailing Address: P.O. Box 2025, Zip 33779–2025; tel. 727/581–9474, (Total facility includes 14 beds in nursing home–type unit) (Nonreporting) **A**1 9 10 11 12 13
Primary Contact: Darrell Lentz, Chief Executive Officer
COO: Nita Kasan, Chief Operating and Nursing Officer
CIO: George Evans, Vice President and Chief Information Officer
Web address: www.suncoasthealthcare.com
Control: Other not–for–profit (including NFP Corporation) **Service:** General Medical and Surgical

Staffed Beds: 300

LAUDERDALE LAKES—Broward County

△ **ST. ANTHONY'S REHABILITATION HOSPITAL (103027)**, 3485 N.W. 30th Street, Zip 33311; tel. 954/739–6233 **A**7 9 10 **F**5 9 43 52 55 56 62 73 81 85 119
Primary Contact: Joe Catania, Chief Executive Officer
Control: Corporation, Investor–owned, for–profit **Service:** Rehabilitation

Staffed Beds: 26 **Admissions:** 600 **Census:** 21 **Outpatient Visits:** 2237 **Births:** 0 **Total Expense ($000):** 8064 **Payroll Expense ($000):** 2893

LEESBURG—Lake County

★ □ △ **LEESBURG REGIONAL MEDICAL CENTER (100084)**, 600 East Dixie Avenue, Zip 34748–5999; tel. 352/323–5762, (Total facility includes 120 beds in nursing home–type unit) **A**1 2 7 9 10 19 **F**3 8 11 13 15 17 18 20 22 24 25 26 27 30 31 32 33 38 46 49 50 52 53 55 56 57 61 64 68 72 73 74 75 76 77 79 80 81 82 84 85 86 96 97 100 103 107 117 119 121 124 133 135 137
Primary Contact: Lee S. Huntley, President and Chief Executive Officer
CFO: Dale E. Hocking, Chief Financial Officer
CMO: Daniel Carlson, M.D., President Medical Staff
CIO: Nancy Vester, Vice President Information Technology
CHR: Darlene Stone, Vice President Human Resources
Web address: www.Leesburgregional.org
Control: Other not–for–profit (including NFP Corporation) **Service:** General Medical and Surgical

Staffed Beds: 429 **Admissions:** 18499 **Census:** 317 **Outpatient Visits:** 93507 **Births:** 1550 **Total Expense ($000):** 224322 **Payroll Expense ($000):** 82486 **Personnel:** 2024

LEHIGH ACRES—Lee County

□ **LEHIGH REGIONAL MEDICAL CENTER (100107)**, 1500 Lee Boulevard, Zip 33936–4897; tel. 239/369–2101 **A**1 10 **F**3 8 15 25 26 38 39 46 55 65 67 68 75 77 79 82 86 96 97 100 102 107 118 120 135 137 **P**6 **S** Health Management Associates
Primary Contact: Jose Morillo, Chief Executive Officer
COO: Rodney Majors, Chief Operating Officer
CFO: Jeff McMullen, Chief Financial Officer
CMO: Robert Strathman, M.D., President Medical Staff
CIO: Jeff Hampton, Director Information Systems
CHR: Carmen Bech de Garcia, Director Human Resources
Web address: www.lehighregional.com
Control: Corporation, Investor–owned, for–profit **Service:** General Medical and Surgical

Staffed Beds: 71 **Admissions:** 3759 **Census:** 38 **Outpatient Visits:** 46662 **Births:** 0 **Total Expense ($000):** 35451 **Payroll Expense ($000):** 15123

FL

LIVE OAK—Suwannee County

★ □ **SHANDS LIVE OAK (101301)**, 1100 S.W. 11th Street, Zip 32060–3608; tel. 386/362–0800 **A**1 9 10 18 **F**3 11 15 25 26 30 31 32 33 38 41 43 44 50 53 54 55 56 57 60 62 63 66 72 73 79 81 82 86 87 92 96 102 107 119 124 135 137 **P**6 **S** Shands HealthCare
Primary Contact: Russell A. Test, Administrator
Web address: www.shands.org
Control: Other not–for–profit (including NFP Corporation) **Service:** General Medical and Surgical

Staffed Beds: 15 **Admissions:** 741 **Census:** 6 **Outpatient Visits:** 81536 **Births:** 0 **Total Expense ($000):** 14748 **Payroll Expense ($000):** 7911 **Personnel:** 148

LONGWOOD—Seminole County

ORLANDO REGIONAL SOUTH SEMINOLE HOSPITAL, 555 West State Road 434, Zip 32750–4999; tel. 407/767–1200, (Nonreporting) **A**9 **S** Orlando Health
Primary Contact: Stephen M. Glazier, President
CIO: Rick Schooler, Vice President Information Services
Web address: www.orhs.org
Control: Partnership, Investor–owned, for–profit **Service:** General Medical and Surgical

Staffed Beds: 206

Hospital, Medicare Provider Number, Address, Telephone, Approval, Facility, and Physician Codes, Health Care System

★ American Hospital Association (AHA) membership
□ The Joint Commission accreditation
○ American Osteopathic Association (AOA) accreditation
△ Commission on Accreditation of Rehabilitation Facilities (CARF) accreditation

LOXAHATCHEE—Palm Beach County

★ **PALMS WEST HOSPITAL (100269)**, 13001 Southern Boulevard, Zip 33470–1150; tel. 561/798–3300, (Nonreporting) **A**1 9 10 12 13 **S** HCA
Primary Contact: Bland Eng, Chief Executive Officer
COO: Michael Patterson, Chief Operating Officer
CFO: Robert Preato, Chief Financial Officer
CIO: Fariba Borjian, Chief Information Officer
CHR: Robbie Tatum, Director Human Resources
Web address: www.palmswesthospital.com
Control: Corporation, Investor–owned, for–profit **Service:** General Medical and Surgical

Staffed Beds: 175

MACCLENNY—Baker County

ED FRASER MEMORIAL HOSPITAL AND BAKER COMMUNITY HEALTH CENTER (100134), 159 North Third Street, Zip 32063–0484, Mailing Address: P.O. Box 484, Zip 32063–0484; tel. 904/259–3151, (Total facility includes 62 beds in nursing home–type unit) (Nonreporting) **A**9 10 20
Primary Contact: Dennis R. Markos, Chief Executive Officer
CFO: Maria Allen, Chief Financial Officer
CMO: Mark Hardin, M.D., Medical Director
Control: Other not–for–profit (including NFP Corporation) **Service:** General Medical and Surgical

Staffed Beds: 68

MADISON—Madison County

MADISON COUNTY MEMORIAL HOSPITAL (101311), 309 N.E. Marion Street, Zip 32340–2561; tel. 850/973–2271, (Nonreporting) **A**9 10 18
Primary Contact: David Abercrombie, Chief Executive Officer
COO: Tammy Stevens, Chief Compliance Officer
CFO: Patrick McGee, Chief Financial Officer
CMO: Michael Stick, M.D., Chief Medical Staff
CIO: Melissa Meyer, Business Office Manager and Chief Information Officer
CHR: Cindi King, Director Human Resources
Control: Other not–for–profit (including NFP Corporation) **Service:** General Medical and Surgical

Staffed Beds: 25

MARATHON—Monroe County

□ **FISHERMEN'S HOSPITAL (100024)**, 3301 Overseas Highway, Zip 33050–0068; tel. 305/743–5533, (Nonreporting) **A**1 9 10 20 **S** Health Management Associates
Primary Contact: Kim Bassett, Chief Executive Officer
CFO: Ted Quinn, Chief Financial Officer
CMO: Scott Burns, M.D., Chief of Staff
CIO: Joe Brake, Director Information Services
CHR: Michele Teller, Director Human Resources
Web address: www.fishermenshospital.com
Control: Corporation, Investor–owned, for–profit **Service:** General Medical and Surgical

Staffed Beds: 46

MARGATE—Broward County

★ **NORTHWEST MEDICAL CENTER (100189)**, 2801 North State Road 7, Zip 33063; tel. 954/978–4000 **A**1 9 10 **F**3 8 11 12 13 15 18 20 25 27 30 31 32 38 42 43 45 46 49 50 51 52 54 55 56 57 59 60 62 63 66 68 71 72 73 74 75 76 77 78 79 80 81 82 84 86 96 97 100 102 103 105 106 107 113 118 119 120 121 124 135 136 137 **S** HCA
Primary Contact: Dianne Aleman, Chief Executive Officer
COO: Stacy Modlin, Chief Operating Officer
CFO: Gary Mervak, Chief Financial Officer
CMO: Peter Gach, M.D., Chief of Staff
CIO: Mother Superior Andres Blanco, Director Information Systems
CHR: Scott Mazo, Vice President Human Resources
Web address: www.northwestmed.com
Control: Corporation, Investor–owned, for–profit **Service:** General Medical and Surgical

Staffed Beds: 215 **Admissions:** 12238 **Census:** 130 **Outpatient Visits:** 70834 **Births:** 1934 **Total Expense ($000):** 99349 **Payroll Expense ($000):** 45299 **Personnel:** 806

MARIANNA—Jackson County

★ **JACKSON HOSPITAL (100142)**, 4250 Hospital Drive, Zip 32446–1939, Mailing Address: P.O. Box 1608, Zip 32447–1608; tel. 850/526–2200 **A**1 9 10 20 **F**3 11 13 15 25 26 31 32 33 38 42 50 51 68 73 74 77 79 81 82 86 96 97 100 102 107 118 119 120 121 122 135 **S** QHR
Primary Contact: David L. Hample, Chief Executive Officer
CFO: Kevin Rovito, Interim Chief Financial Officer
CMO: Joe Gay, M.D., Chief Medical Officer
CIO: Beth Medlock, Manager Information Technology
CHR: Brooke Donaldson, Assistant Administrator Human Resources
Web address: www.jacksonhosp.com
Control: Hospital district or authority, Government, nonfederal **Service:** General Medical and Surgical

Staffed Beds: 62 **Admissions:** 3084 **Census:** 35 **Outpatient Visits:** 66285 **Births:** 588 **Total Expense ($000):** 37508 **Payroll Expense ($000):** 17781 **Personnel:** 422

MELBOURNE—Brevard County

□ **CIRCLES OF CARE (104024)**, 400 East Sheridan Road, Zip 32901–3184; tel. 321/722–5200, (Nonreporting) **A**1 9 10
Primary Contact: James B. Whitaker, President
CFO: David L. Feldman, Executive Vice President and Treasurer
CMO: Jose Alvarez, M.D., Chief Medical Staff
CHR: Linda Brannon, Vice President Human Resources
Web address: www.circlesofcare.org
Control: Other not–for–profit (including NFP Corporation) **Service:** Psychiatric

Staffed Beds: 134

DEVEREUX HOSPITAL AND CHILDREN'S CENTER OF FLORIDA, 8000 Devereux Drive, Zip 32940–7907; tel. 321/242–9100, (Nonreporting) **A**9 **S** Devereux
Primary Contact: Mark Halal, Administrator
COO: Amy Blakely, Assistant Executive Director Operations
CFO: Pamela Griffith, Director Administrative Services
CMO: Emilio Roig, M.D., Network Medical Director
CIO: Rob Fensterer, Director Information Services
Web address: www.devereux.org
Control: Other not–for–profit (including NFP Corporation) **Service:** Children's hospital psychiatric

Staffed Beds: 100

★ **HEALTHSOUTH SEA PINES REHABILITATION HOSPITAL (103034)**, 101 East Florida Avenue, Zip 32901–9966; tel. 321/984–4600, (Nonreporting) **A**1 9 10 **S** HEALTHSOUTH Corporation
Primary Contact: Denise B. McGrath, Chief Executive Officer
CMO: Stuart P. Miller, M.D., Medical Director
CHR: Donna Anderson, Director Human Resources
Web address: www.healthsouthseapines.com
Control: Corporation, Investor–owned, for–profit **Service:** Rehabilitation

Staffed Beds: 90

★ **HOLMES REGIONAL MEDICAL CENTER (100019)**, 1350 South Hickory Street, Zip 32901–3276; tel. 321/434–7000 **A**1 2 9 10 **F**3 11 13 15 17 18 20 22 24 25 26 27 30 31 32 35 38 40 49 51 52 55 56 57 59 66 68 70 72 73 74 75 76 77 79 80 81 82 84 86 96 97 98 99 100 101 102 103 104 105 106 107 119 120 121 122 123 124 132 135 137 **P**6 7 **S** Health First, Inc.
Primary Contact: Jerry Senne, FACHE, President
COO: Judy Killebrew, Chief Operating Officer
CFO: Robert Galloway, Senior Vice President Finance and Chief Financial Officer
CMO: Scott Gettings, Chief Medical Officer
CIO: Rich Rogers, Vice President Information Technology
CHR: Robert Suttles, Vice President Human Resources
Web address: www.health–first.org
Control: Other not–for–profit (including NFP Corporation) **Service:** General Medical and Surgical

Staffed Beds: 514 **Admissions:** 28995 **Census:** 415 **Outpatient Visits:** 178210 **Births:** 2735 **Total Expense ($000):** 389853 **Payroll Expense ($000):** 155565 **Personnel:** 2742

□ **WUESTHOFF MEDICAL CENTER – MELBOURNE (100291)**, 250 North Wickham Road, Zip 32935; tel. 321/752–1200 **A**1 9 10 **F**3 11 13 15 18 25 26 30 31 32 36 38 49 51 55 57 59 62 66 68 72 73 74 75 77 78 79 80 82 84 86 92 96 97 100 102 107 119 120 121 124 133 135 136 137 **S** Wuesthoff Health System
Primary Contact: Donald McKenna, Administrator
Web address: www.wuesthoff.org
Control: Other not–for–profit (including NFP Corporation) **Service:** General Medical and Surgical

Staffed Beds: 115 **Admissions:** 5979 **Census:** 67 **Outpatient Visits:** 59729 **Births:** 554 **Total Expense ($000):** 61754 **Payroll Expense ($000):** 20829 **Personnel:** 385

FL

Many Facility Codes have changed. Please refer to the AHA Guide Code Chart.

MIAMI—Dade County

★ △ **BAPTIST HOSPITAL OF MIAMI (100008)**, 8900 North Kendall Drive, Zip 33176–2197; tel. 786/596–1960 **A**1 2 7 9 10 **F**3 8 11 13 14 15 17 18 20 22 24 25 26 27 28 30 31 32 33 38 39 42 43 44 49 52 53 54 55 56 57 59 60 61 62 65 66 68 70 71 72 73 74 75 76 77 79 80 81 82 83 84 85 86 87 90 92 96 97 98 99 100 103 104 105 106 107 108 109 111 112 116 118 119 121 124 133 134 135 136 137 **P**6 **S** Baptist Health South Florida
Primary Contact: Bo Boulenger, Chief Executive Officer
COO: Randall Lee, Vice President and Chief Operating Officer
CFO: Ralph E. Lawson, Executive Vice President and Chief Financial Officer
CMO: Mark J. Hauser, M.D., Chief Medical Officer
CIO: Mimi Taylor, Corporate Vice President
CHR: Kathryn Fisk, Corporate Vice President Employee Services and Human Resources
Web address: www.baptisthealth.net
Control: Other not–for–profit (including NFP Corporation) **Service:** General Medical and Surgical

Staffed Beds: 584 **Admissions:** 32522 **Census:** 479 **Outpatient Visits:** 264521 **Births:** 4385 **Total Expense ($000):** 614134 **Payroll Expense ($000):** 205436 **Personnel:** 3684

★ **BASCOM PALMER EYE INSTITUTE–ANNE BATES LEACH EYE HOSPITAL (100240)**, 900 N.W. 17th Street, Zip 33136–1199, Mailing Address: Box 016880, Zip 33101–6880; tel. 305/326–6000, (Nonreporting) **A**1 3 5 9 10
Primary Contact: Michael B. Gittelman, Administrator
COO: Michael B. Gittelman, Administrator
CFO: Dean Cocchi, Chief Financial Officer
CMO: Eduardo Alfonso, Chairman Ophthalmology
CHR: Paul Hudgins, Associate Vice President Human Resources
Web address: www.bascompalmer.org
Control: Other not–for–profit (including NFP Corporation) **Service:** Eye, ear, nose, and throat

Staffed Beds: 56

CEDARS MEDICAL CENTER See University of Miami Hospital

★ **HEALTHSOUTH REHABILITATION HOSPITAL (103038)**, 20601 Old Cutler Road, Zip 33189–2400; tel. 305/251–3800, (Nonreporting) **A**1 9 10 **S** HEALTHSOUTH Corporation
Primary Contact: Elizabeth L. Izquierdo, CPA, Chief Executive Officer
CFO: Myriam Torres, Chief Financial Officer
CHR: Susan Riley, Director Human Resources
Web address: www.healthsouthmiami.com
Control: Corporation, Investor–owned, for–profit **Service:** Rehabilitation

Staffed Beds: 60

HIGHLAND PARK HOSPITAL See Jackson Health System

★ △ **JACKSON HEALTH SYSTEM (100022)**, 1611 N.W. 12th Avenue, Zip 33136–1094; tel. 305/585–1111, (Includes HIGHLAND PARK HOSPITAL, 1695 N.W. Ninth Avenue, Zip 33136; tel. 305/355–8234; JACKSON MEMORIAL HOSPITAL, 1611 N.W. 12th Avenue, Zip 33136; tel. 305/585–6661; JACKSON NORTH MEDICAL CENTER, 160 N.W. 170th Street, North Miami Beach, Zip 33169–5576; tel. 305/651–1100; Sandy Sears, Senior Vice President and Chief Administrative Officer; JACKSON SOUTH COMMUNITY HOSPITAL, 9333 S.W. 152nd Street, Zip 33157–1780; tel. 305/251–2500; Stuart Podolnick, Chief Administrative Officer), (Total facility includes 324 beds in nursing home–type unit) **A**1 2 3 5 7 8 9 10 13 **F**1 3 4 5 11 12 13 14 15 16 17 18 19 20 21 22 23 25 26 27 28 30 31 32 33 34 36 37 38 40 41 43 49 50 51 54 55 56 57 58 59 60 62 63 64 66 68 69 70 71 72 73 74 75 76 77 78 79 80 81 82 83 84 85 86 87 88 89 90 91 92 93 94 95 96 97 100 102 103 104 105 106 107 109 111 112 114 116 117 118 119 120 121 124 125 126 127 128 129 130 131 135 136 137
Primary Contact: Marvin O'Quinn, President and Chief Executive Officer
COO: Steven M. Klein, Executive Vice President and Chief Operating Officer
CFO: Frank Barrett, Executive Vice President Corporate Affairs and Chief Financial Officer
CMO: Gerard A. Kaiser, M.D., Senior Vice President
CIO: James Sandy Phillips, Vice President and Chief Information Officer
CHR: Trummell Valdera, Senior Vice President and Chief Human Resources Officer
Web address: www.um–jmh.org
Control: County–Government, nonfederal **Service:** General Medical and Surgical

Staffed Beds: 2157 **Admissions:** 70764 **Census:** 1653 **Outpatient Visits:** 637711 **Births:** 9085 **Total Expense ($000):** 1721920 **Payroll Expense ($000):** 757789 **Personnel:** 11604

JACKSON SOUTH COMMUNITY HOSPITAL See Jackson Health System

★ **KENDALL REGIONAL MEDICAL CENTER (100209)**, 11750 Bird Road, Zip 33175–3530; tel. 305/223–3000, (Nonreporting) **A**1 9 10 **S** HCA
Primary Contact: Mauricio E. Sirvent, Chief Executive Officer
COO: Georgina Diaz, Chief Operating Officer
CMO: Braulio Sabates, M.D., Chief of Staff
CIO: Carlos Bitar, Assistant Administrator
CHR: Lazara Marchante, Director Human Resources
Web address: www.kendallmed.com
Control: Partnership, Investor–owned, for–profit **Service:** General Medical and Surgical

Staffed Beds: 300

★ △ **MERCY HOSPITAL (100061)**, 3663 South Miami Avenue, Zip 33133–4237; tel. 305/854–4400 **A**1 2 6 7 9 10 **F**3 8 11 12 13 15 17 18 20 22 24 25 26 27 30 31 32 33 34 35 38 42 49 53 55 57 58 59 60 61 62 63 64 66 68 70 72 73 74 75 76 77 79 80 82 85 86 88 90 91 92 93 96 97 102 103 104 105 106 107 108 109 111 112 118 119 120 132 133 135 136 137 **S** Catholic Health East
Primary Contact: John E. Matuska, President and Chief Executive Officer
CFO: Jerry Mashburn, Senior Vice President and Chief Financial Officer
CMO: Manuel P. Anton, M.D., Senior Vice President and Medical Director
CIO: Camille Rivera, Interim Chief Information Officer
CHR: Eduard Rundle, Vice President Human Resources
Web address: www.mercymiami.com
Control: Church–operated, Nongovernment, not–for profit **Service:** General Medical and Surgical

Staffed Beds: 357 **Admissions:** 19698 **Census:** 277 **Outpatient Visits:** 92710 **Births:** 1422 **Total Expense ($000):** 260298 **Payroll Expense ($000):** 102278 **Personnel:** 1949

□ **METROPOLITAN HOSPITAL OF MIAMI (100076)**, 5959 N.W. Seventh Street, Zip 33126–3198; tel. 305/264–1000 **A**1 9 10 **F**3 8 15 17 25 27 38 54 62 72 75 76 79 82 86 96 97 102 107 111 119 122 124 132 135 137
Primary Contact: Sandra Sosa–Guerrero, Chief Executive Officer
COO: Sandra Sosa–Guerrero, Chief Operating Officer
CFO: Vivian Acevedo, Chief Financial Officer
CIO: Frank Canovaca, Director Management Information Systems
CHR: Ana Carrocera, Director Human Resources
Control: Corporation, Investor–owned, for–profit **Service:** General Medical and Surgical

Staffed Beds: 146 **Admissions:** 5295 **Census:** 80 **Outpatient Visits:** 33012 **Births:** 0 **Total Expense ($000):** 46819 **Payroll Expense ($000):** 20846 **Personnel:** 516

★ **MIAMI CHILDREN'S HOSPITAL (103301)**, 3100 S.W. 62nd Avenue, Zip 33155–3009; tel. 305/666–6511 **A**1 2 3 5 9 10 12 13 **F**3 7 9 17 18 19 20 21 23 25 26 27 28 31 33 34 36 37 38 39 40 41 43 46 50 52 53 55 56 57 58 59 60 62 63 64 66 68 69 70 71 72 73 75 76 77 78 79 80 81 82 83 84 86 87 88 89 90 91 92 94 95 96 97 100 102 104 105 106 107 114 118 119 120 121 123 125 133 135 **P**6
Primary Contact: M. Narendra Kini, M.D., President and Chief Executive Officer
COO: Kevin R. Hammeran, Executive Vice President and Chief Operating Officer
CFO: Pedro Alfaro, Vice President and Chief Financial Officer
CMO: Christain C. Patrick, M.D., Ph.D., Chief Medical Officer and Senior Vice President Medical Affairs
CHR: Ana Poveda, Chief Talent Management Officer
Web address: www.mch.com
Control: Other not–for–profit (including NFP Corporation) **Service:** Children's general

Staffed Beds: 250 **Admissions:** 12346 **Census:** 189 **Outpatient Visits:** 267052 **Births:** 0 **Total Expense ($000):** 341329 **Payroll Expense ($000):** 159631 **Personnel:** 2291

★ **MIAMI JEWISH HOME AND HOSPITAL FOR AGED (100277)**, 5200 N.E. Second Avenue, Zip 33137–2706; tel. 305/751–8626, (Nonreporting) **A**3 5 10
CFO: Lourdes Boue, Chief Financial Officer
CMO: Michael Silverman, M.D., Medical Director
CIO: David Wolff, Director Information Technology
CHR: Larry McDonald, Director Human Resources
Web address: www.mjhha.org
Control: Other not–for–profit (including NFP Corporation) **Service:** General Medical and Surgical

Staffed Beds: 32

FL

Hospital, Medicare Provider Number, Address, Telephone, Approval, Facility, and Physician Codes, Health Care System

★ American Hospital Association (AHA) membership
□ The Joint Commission accreditation
○ American Osteopathic Association (AOA) accreditation
△ Commission on Accreditation of Rehabilitation Facilities (CARF) accreditation

★ **NORTH SHORE MEDICAL CENTER (100029)**, 1100 N.W. 95th Street, Zip 33150–2098; tel. 305/835–6000, (Nonreporting) **A**1 2 9 10 **S** TENET Healthcare Corporation
Primary Contact: Manuel Linares, Chief Executive Officer
CFO: Jennifer Pittman, Chief Financial Officer
CMO: Andrew Nullman, M.D., Chief of Staff
CIO: Luis Estrada, Director Multifacility Information Systems
Web address: www.northshoremedical.com
Control: Corporation, Investor–owned, for–profit **Service:** General Medical and Surgical

Staffed Beds: 357

□ **SELECT SPECIALTY HOSPITAL OF MIAMI (102001)**, 955 N.W. 3rd Street, Zip 33128; tel. 305/416–5700, (Nonreporting) **A**1 9 10 **S** Select Medical Corporation
Primary Contact: Dionisio Bencomo, Chief Executive Officer
Web address: www.selectmedicalcorp.com
Control: Corporation, Investor–owned, for–profit **Service:** Long–Term Acute Care hospital

Staffed Beds: 40

□ **SISTER EMMANUEL HOSPITAL FOR CONTINUING CARE (102016)**, 3663 South Miami Avenue, 4th Floor, Zip 33133, Mailing Address: 3663 South Miami Avenue, 4th Floor, Zip 33133; tel. 305/285–2939 **A**1 9 10 **F**1 3 25 27 33 43 58 72 73 80 81 82 119 121 124 137
Primary Contact: Shed Boren, Administrator and Chief Executive Officer
COO: Beverlin Allen, Chief Nursing Officer
CFO: Miguel Vasquez, Chief Financial Officer
CMO: Hugo Gonzalez, M.D., Chief Medical Officer
CIO: Macarena Restrepo, Manager Business Office
CHR: Kathy Mainieri, Human Resource Generalist
Control: Church–operated, Nongovernment, not–for profit **Service:** Long–Term Acute Care hospital

Staffed Beds: 29 **Admissions:** 315 **Census:** 25 **Outpatient Visits:** 0 **Births:** 0 **Total Expense ($000):** 10458 **Payroll Expense ($000):** 4929 **Personnel:** 86

★ △ **SOUTH MIAMI HOSPITAL (100154)**, 6200 S.W. 73rd Street, Zip 33143–9990; tel. 786/662–4000 **A**1 2 7 9 10 **F**3 4 5 8 11 12 13 15 17 18 20 22 24 25 26 27 30 31 33 34 38 39 43 44 46 48 50 51 52 55 56 57 59 60 62 66 68 70 72 73 74 75 76 77 79 80 81 82 85 86 96 97 98 99 100 102 103 105 106 107 108 109 111 112 113 116 118 119 121 124 132 133 135 136 137 **P**6 **S** Baptist Health South Florida
Primary Contact: Javier Hernandez–Lichtl, Chief Executive Officer
CFO: Berta Rufat, Controller
CMO: Rodney Benjamin, M.D., President Medical Staff
CHR: Mercedes del Rey, Director Human Resources
Web address: www.baptisthealth.net
Control: Other not–for–profit (including NFP Corporation) **Service:** General Medical and Surgical

Staffed Beds: 324 **Admissions:** 19218 **Census:** 260 **Outpatient Visits:** 102577 **Births:** 4251 **Total Expense ($000):** 337351 **Payroll Expense ($000):** 113638 **Personnel:** 2136

FL

★ **UNIVERSITY OF MIAMI HOSPITAL (100009)**, (Formerly Cedars Medical Center), 1400 N.W. 12th Avenue, Zip 33136–1003; tel. 305/325–5511 **A**1 2 3 5 9 10 **F**3 11 12 15 17 18 20 22 25 26 27 30 31 32 33 38 41 43 46 48 49 51 57 58 59 62 66 68 72 76 77 78 79 80 81 82 86 88 92 93 96 97 100 107 109 111 116 118 119 130 135 137 **P**6
Primary Contact: Anthony M. Degina, Jr., Chief Executive Officer
COO: Susie Lambert, Chief Operating Officer and Chief Nursing Officer
CFO: Darryl Caulton, Chief Financial Officer
CMO: Francisco Kerdel, M.D., President Medical Staff
CIO: Craig Scott, Interim Director, Management Information Systems
CHR: Errol Douglas, Director Human Resources
Web address: www.umiamihospital.com
Control: Partnership, Investor–owned, for–profit **Service:** General Medical and Surgical

Staffed Beds: 525 **Admissions:** 15764 **Census:** 265 **Outpatient Visits:** 53799 **Births:** 0 **Total Expense ($000):** 181265 **Payroll Expense ($000):** 72422 **Personnel:** 1101

★ **UNIVERSITY OF MIAMI HOSPITAL AND CLINICS (100079)**, 1475 N.W. 12th Avenue, Zip 33136–1002; tel. 305/243–1000 **A**1 2 3 5 9 10 **F**3 9 11 12 15 25 26 27 30 31 32 33 34 36 41 43 46 47 49 53 55 56 57 58 60 62 66 72 73 75 76 77 79 80 81 82 87 90 93 94 96 97 99 100 102 103 105 106 107 108 109 111 119 121 130 135 137 **P**6
Primary Contact: Michael B. Gittelman, Administrator
COO: Lazara Pagan, Chief Operating Officer
CFO: Harry Rohrer, Chief Financial Officer
CMO: W. Jarrad Goodwin, M.D., Director
CHR: Paul Hudgins, Associate Vice President Human Resources
Web address: www.sylvester.org
Control: Other not–for–profit (including NFP Corporation) **Service:** General Medical and Surgical

Staffed Beds: 40 **Admissions:** 1581 **Census:** 23 **Outpatient Visits:** 196895 **Births:** 0 **Total Expense ($000):** 197255 **Payroll Expense ($000):** 52817 **Personnel:** 986

★ △ **VETERANS AFFAIRS MEDICAL CENTER**, 1201 N.W. 16th Street, Zip 33125–1624; tel. 305/575–7000, (Total facility includes 58 beds in nursing home–type unit) (Nonreporting) **A**1 3 5 7 8 **S** Department of Veterans Affairs
Primary Contact: Mary D. Berrocal, Director
COO: Paul D. Magalian, Associate Director
CFO: Rick Hunter, Chief Financial Officer
CMO: John Vara, M.D., Chief of Staff
CIO: Bill Tyson, Chief Information Officer
CHR: Larry Brinkman, Chief Human Resources
Web address: www.va.gov/miami
Control: Veterans Affairs, Government, federal **Service:** General Medical and Surgical

Staffed Beds: 339

★ △ **WEST GABLES REHABILITATION HOSPITAL (103036)**, 2525 S.W. 75th Avenue, Zip 33155; tel. 305/262–6800 **A**1 7 9 10 **F**31 32 73 75 85 86 **S** RehabCare Group, Inc.
Primary Contact: Ismael Roque–Velasco, M.D., Chief Executive Officer
Web address: www.rehabcare.com/portfolio/long_term_acute_care/westgables.htm
Control: Corporation, Investor–owned, for–profit **Service:** Rehabilitation

Staffed Beds: 60 **Admissions:** 1135 **Census:** 40 **Outpatient Visits:** 8818 **Payroll Expense ($000):** 8469 **Personnel:** 198

○ **WESTCHESTER GENERAL HOSPITAL (100284)**, 2500 S.W. 75th Avenue, Zip 33155–9947; tel. 305/264–5252, (Includes SOUTHERN WINDS HOSPITAL, 4225 West 20th Street, Hialeah, Zip 33012–5835; tel. 305/558–9700) **A**9 10 11 12 13 **F**15 25 30 31 38 49 54 63 68 72 73 75 76 77 79 82 88 90 92 93 96 97 99 102 107 119
Primary Contact: Gilda Baldwin, Chief Executive Officer
CFO: Kevin Loudy, Chief Financial Officer
CMO: Rogelio Zaldivar, M.D., Medical Director
CHR: Alicia Lund, Director Human Resources
Web address: www.westchesterhospital.com
Control: Corporation, Investor–owned, for–profit **Service:** General Medical and Surgical

Staffed Beds: 197 **Admissions:** 6637 **Census:** 124 **Outpatient Visits:** 21426 **Births:** 0 **Total Expense ($000):** 60258 **Payroll Expense ($000):** 24901 **Personnel:** 486

MIAMI BEACH—Dade County

MIAMI HEART CAMPUS AT MOUNT SINAI MEDICAL CENTER See Mount Sinai Medical Center

□ △ **MOUNT SINAI MEDICAL CENTER (100034)**, 4300 Alton Road, Zip 33140–2800; tel. 305/674–2121, (Includes MIAMI HEART CAMPUS AT MOUNT SINAI MEDICAL CENTER, 4701 North Meridian Avenue, Zip 33140–2910; tel. 305/672–1111) **A**1 2 3 5 7 8 9 10 12 13 **F**6 8 12 13 15 18 20 22 24 25 26 27 30 31 32 33 38 39 41 43 51 53 54 55 56 57 58 59 60 62 63 64 66 68 70 71 72 73 74 75 76 77 79 81 82 84 85 86 87 88 90 91 92 93 96 97 98 99 100 102 103 104 105 106 107 108 109 111 112 118 119 120 121 132 134 135 136 137
Primary Contact: Steven D. Sonenreich, President and Chief Executive Officer
COO: Amy Perry, Senior Vice President and Chief Operating Officer
CFO: Alex A. Mendez, Senior Vice President and Chief Financial Officer
CMO: Robert Goldszer, M.D., Senior Vice President and Chief Medical Officer
CIO: Tom Gillette, Vice President and Chief Information Officer
CHR: Georgia McLean, Director Human Resources
Web address: www.msmc.com
Control: Other not–for–profit (including NFP Corporation) **Service:** General Medical and Surgical

Staffed Beds: 712 **Admissions:** 22240 **Census:** 407 **Outpatient Visits:** 172699 **Births:** 1793 **Total Expense ($000):** 432816 **Payroll Expense ($000):** 161230 **Personnel:** 3250

MILTON—Santa Rosa County

□ **SANTA ROSA MEDICAL CENTER (100124)**, 1450 Berryhill Road, Zip 32570–4028, Mailing Address: P.O. Box 648, Zip 32572–0648; tel. 850/626–7762 **A**1 9 10 **F**3 13 15 25 26 32 33 38 43 46 51 53 55 56 57 59 62 66 68 72 73 74 75 77 79 82 86 87 96 97 98 99 100 102 103 107 118 119 120 121 124 134 135 136 137 **S** Health Management Associates
Primary Contact: M. P. Gandy, Jr., Chief Executive Officer
CFO: Kay Burns, Chief Financial Officer
CIO: Rick Payne, Director Information Systems
Web address: www.santarosamedicalcenter.org
Control: Corporation, Investor–owned, for–profit **Service:** General Medical and Surgical

Staffed Beds: 129 **Admissions:** 4860 **Census:** 51 **Outpatient Visits:** 67200 **Births:** 444

Many Facility Codes have changed. Please refer to the AHA Guide Code Chart.

MIRAMAR—Broward County

★ **MEMORIAL HOSPITAL MIRAMAR (100285)**, 1901 S.W. 172nd Avenue, Zip 33029; tel. 954/538–5000 **A**1 9 10 **F**3 13 15 25 26 30 31 32 38 47 49 55 56 57 60 62 68 72 73 74 76 77 79 80 81 82 86 96 97 99 100 101 102 107 119 124 134 135 137 **S** Memorial Healthcare System
Primary Contact: Aurelio Fernandez, Administrator
CFO: Judy Sada, Chief Financial Officer
CMO: Stanley Marks, M.D., Chief Medical Officer
CHR: Ray Kendrick, Chief Human Resources Officer
Web address: www.mhs.net
Control: Hospital district or authority, Government, nonfederal **Service:** General Medical and Surgical

Staffed Beds: 128 **Admissions:** 6860 **Census:** 64 **Outpatient Visits:** 79983 **Births:** 2333 **Total Expense ($000):** 77561 **Payroll Expense ($000):** 36491 **Personnel:** 617

NAPLES—Collier County

★ △ **NAPLES COMMUNITY HOSPITAL (100018)**, 350 Seventh Street North, Zip 34102–4746, Mailing Address: P.O. Box 413029, Zip 34101–3029; tel. 239/436–5000 **A**1 2 7 9 10 **F**3 7 11 13 14 17 18 20 22 24 25 26 27 28 30 31 32 35 38 43 49 50 52 53 54 55 56 57 62 66 68 70 72 73 74 75 76 77 79 80 81 82 84 85 86 88 90 92 93 94 96 97 100 102 107 108 109 112 116 118 119 120 121 124 132 133 135 136 **P**8
Primary Contact: Allen S. Weiss, M.D., President and Chief Executive Officer
COO: Phillip C. Dutcher, Chief Operating Officer
CFO: Vicki Hale, Chief Financial Officer
CMO: Aurora Estevez, M.D., Chief Medical Officer
CIO: Susan Wolff, Chief Information Officer
CHR: Brian Settle, Chief Human Resources Officer
Web address: www.nchmd.org
Control: Other not–for–profit (including NFP Corporation) **Service:** General Medical and Surgical

Staffed Beds: 681 **Admissions:** 32757 **Census:** 412 **Outpatient Visits:** 303840 **Births:** 4291 **Total Expense ($000):** 356978 **Payroll Expense ($000):** 153280 **Personnel:** 3243

★ **PHYSICIANS REGIONAL MEDICAL CENTER – PINE RIDGE (100286)**, 6101 Pine Ridge Road, Zip 34119; tel. 239/348–4000, (Includes PHYSICIANS REGIONAL MEDICAL CENTER, 8300 Collier Boulevard, Zip 34114; tel. 239/354–6000; J. Michael Mastej, Chief Executive Officer), (Nonreporting) **A**1 9 10 **S** Health Management Associates
Primary Contact: Geoffrey D. Moebius, Chief Executive Officer
CIO: Lisa Gardiner, Director Marketing and Public Relations
CHR: Maureen Mino, Director Human Resources
Web address: www.physiciansregional.com
Control: Corporation, Investor–owned, for–profit **Service:** General Medical and Surgical

Staffed Beds: 70

WILLOUGH HEALTHCARE SYSTEM (104063), 9001 Tamiami Trail East, Zip 34113–3316; tel. 239/775–4500, (Nonreporting) **A**9 10
Primary Contact: James E. O'Shea, Administrator
CFO: Steve Baldwin, Vice President Finance
Control: Corporation, Investor–owned, for–profit **Service:** Psychiatric

Staffed Beds: 80

NEW PORT RICHEY—Pasco County

★ **COMMUNITY HOSPITAL (100191)**, 5637 Marine Parkway, Zip 34652–4331, Mailing Address: P.O. Box 996, Zip 34656–0996; tel. 727/848–1733, (Nonreporting) **A**1 2 5 9 10 **S** HCA
Primary Contact: Kathryn Gillette, Chief Executive Officer
COO: Mary Ann Knight, Chief Operating Officer
CFO: Glenn Romig, Chief Financial Officer
CIO: Kurt Hornung, Director
CHR: Jay Kuhns, Director Human Resources
Web address: www.communityhospitalnpr.com
Control: Corporation, Investor–owned, for–profit **Service:** General Medical and Surgical

Staffed Beds: 267

★ △ **MORTON PLANT NORTH BAY HOSPITAL (100063)**, 6600 Madison Street, Zip 34652–1900; tel. 727/842–8468, (Nonreporting) **A**1 7 9 10 **S** Morton Plant Mease Health Care
Primary Contact: Philip K. Beauchamp, FACHE, President and Chief Executive Officer
CFO: Linda Wolfe, Manager Finance
Web address: www.mpmhealth.com
Control: Other not–for–profit (including NFP Corporation) **Service:** General Medical and Surgical

Staffed Beds: 122

NEW SMYRNA BEACH—Volusia County

★ **BERT FISH MEDICAL CENTER (100014)**, 401 Palmetto Street, Zip 32168–7399; tel. 386/424–5000 **A**1 9 10 **F**3 11 12 15 18 24 25 26 27 33 34 38 41 43 50 54 55 57 59 60 61 62 68 73 75 76 77 79 80 81 82 86 90 96 97 99 100 102 106 107 119 121 124 128 135 136 137
Primary Contact: Robert B. Williams, Chief Executive Officer
COO: Steven W. Harrell, CHE, Chief Operating Officer
CFO: Al W. Allred, Chief Financial Officer
CMO: Raj Ailani, M.D., Chief of Staff
CIO: Debbie Burgess, Director Information Services
CHR: Nancy Evoiga, Vice President
Web address: www.bertfish.com
Control: Hospital district or authority, Government, nonfederal **Service:** General Medical and Surgical

Staffed Beds: 112 **Admissions:** 4951 **Census:** 62 **Births:** 0 **Total Expense ($000):** 76206 **Payroll Expense ($000):** 30013

NICEVILLE—Okaloosa County

★ **TWIN CITIES HOSPITAL (100054)**, 2190 Highway 85 North, Zip 32578–1045; tel. 850/678–4131, (Nonreporting) **A**1 9 10 **S** HCA
Primary Contact: David Whalen, Chief Executive Officer
CFO: Mark Day, Chief Financial Officer
CHR: Cyndi Ronca, Director Human Resources
Web address: www.tchealthcare.com
Control: Corporation, Investor–owned, for–profit **Service:** General Medical and Surgical

Staffed Beds: 65

NORTH MIAMI—Dade County

□ △ **ST. CATHERINE'S REHABILITATION HOSPITAL (103026)**, 1050 N.E. 125th Street, Zip 33161–5881; tel. 305/357–1735, (Nonreporting) **A**1 7 9 10
Primary Contact: Jaime Gonzalez, Administrator
COO: Jim Ball, Chief Operating Officer
CFO: Mary Jo Frick, Director Finance
CMO: Miriam Feliz, M.D., Medical Director
Web address: www.catholichealthservices.org
Control: Church–operated, Nongovernment, not–for profit **Service:** Rehabilitation

Staffed Beds: 272

NORTH MIAMI BEACH—Dade County

JACKSON NORTH MEDICAL CENTER See Jackson Health System, Miami

OCALA—Marion County

KINDRED HOSPITAL OCALA (102019), 1500 S.W. 1st Avenue, Zip 34474; tel. 352/369–0513 **A**10 **F**1 25 26 30 31 43 59 72 73 75 82 119 137 **S** Kindred Healthcare
Primary Contact: Angelica Cotshott, Administrator
COO: Karen Elmore, Director Nursing Services
CFO: Joyce Caltrider, Chief Financial Officer
Web address: www.kindredhealthcare.com
Control: Corporation, Investor–owned, for–profit **Service:** Long–Term Acute Care hospital

Staffed Beds: 31 **Admissions:** 287 **Census:** 21 **Outpatient Visits:** 0 **Births:** 0

★ **MUNROE REGIONAL MEDICAL CENTER (100062)**, 1500 S.W. 1st Avenue, Zip 34471–4059, Mailing Address: P.O. Box 6000, Zip 34478–6000; tel. 352/351–7200 **A**1 5 9 10 **F**11 12 13 15 17 18 20 22 24 25 26 27 28 30 31 32 33 34 35 38 39 43 52 54 55 56 57 58 59 60 62 63 68 72 73 74 75 77 79 80 81 82 84 86 87 96 97 100 102 107 108 112 116 118 119 120 121 124 133 135 136 137
Primary Contact: Stephen A. Purves, FACHE, President and Chief Executive Officer
COO: Paul Clark, Chief Operating Officer
CFO: Richard Mutarelli, Chief Financial Officer
CIO: Carl Candullo, Chief Information Officer
CHR: Pamela W. Michell, Vice President Munroe Heart
Web address: www.munroeregional.com
Control: Hospital district or authority, Government, nonfederal **Service:** General Medical and Surgical

Staffed Beds: 364 **Admissions:** 25259 **Census:** 298 **Outpatient Visits:** 146575 **Births:** 3017 **Total Expense ($000):** 229810 **Payroll Expense ($000):** 100224 **Personnel:** 2187

FL

Hospital, Medicare Provider Number, Address, Telephone, Approval, Facility, and Physician Codes, Health Care System

★ American Hospital Association (AHA) membership
□ The Joint Commission accreditation
○ American Osteopathic Association (AOA) accreditation
△ Commission on Accreditation of Rehabilitation Facilities (CARF) accreditation

★ **OCALA REGIONAL MEDICAL CENTER (100212)**, 1431 S.W. First Avenue, Zip 34474–4058, Mailing Address: P.O. Box 2200, Zip 34478–2200; tel. 352/401–1000, (Includes WEST MARION COMMUNITY HOSPITAL, 4600 S.W. 46th Court, Zip 34471; tel. 352/291–3000; Rex Etheredge, Chief Executive Officer), (Nonreporting) **A**1 2 9 10 **S** HCA
Primary Contact: H. Rex Etheredge, President and Chief Executive Officer
CFO: Jeffrey D. Baiocco, Chief Financial Officer
CIO: Taylor Dickerson, Director Information Services
CHR: Wayne Nielsen, Director Human Resources
Web address: www.ocalaregional.com
Control: State–Government, nonfederal **Service:** General Medical and Surgical

Staffed Beds: 270

OCOEE—Orange County

★ **HEALTH CENTRAL (100030)**, 10000 West Colonial Drive, Zip 34761–3499; tel. 407/296–1000, (Total facility includes 228 beds in nursing home–type unit) **A**1 9 10 **F**3 7 8 11 12 13 15 17 18 24 25 26 27 30 31 32 33 38 43 46 50 51 53 55 56 57 58 59 60 62 63 68 72 73 74 75 76 77 79 80 81 82 84 86 96 97 100 102 103 106 107 116 117 118 119 121 124 132 133 135 136 137
Primary Contact: Richard M. Irwin, Jr., President and Chief Executive Officer
CFO: Michael E. Mueller, Chief Financial Officer
CMO: W. Kevin Cox, M.D., Chief of Staff
CIO: Robert B. Williams, Chief Information Officer
CHR: John Sullivan, Vice President Human Resources
Web address: www.healthcentral.org
Control: Hospital district or authority, Government, nonfederal **Service:** General Medical and Surgical

Staffed Beds: 399 **Admissions:** 11000 **Census:** 336 **Outpatient Visits:** 108466 **Births:** 1251 **Total Expense ($000):** 49479 **Payroll Expense ($000):** 58017 **Personnel:** 1247

OKEECHOBEE—Okeechobee County

★ **RAULERSON HOSPITAL (100252)**, 1796 Highway 441 North, Zip 34972–1918, Mailing Address: P.O. Box 1307, Zip 34973–1307; tel. 863/763–2151 **A**1 9 10 20 **F**3 11 12 15 25 38 41 42 50 52 62 66 68 73 75 77 79 81 82 84 86 96 97 100 102 107 118 135 137 **S** HCA
Primary Contact: Robert H. Lee, President
CFO: Heather Garvey, Chief Financial Officer
CMO: Mohammad Riaz, M.D., Chief of Staff
CIO: Doug Schneider, Director Information Systems
CHR: Janis Stevens, Director Human Resources
Web address: www.raulersonhospital.com
Control: Corporation, Investor–owned, for–profit **Service:** General Medical and Surgical

Staffed Beds: 100 **Admissions:** 4450 **Census:** 60 **Births:** 0 **Total Expense ($000):** 33618 **Payroll Expense ($000):** 15975

FL

ORANGE CITY—Volusia County

★ **FLORIDA HOSPITAL FISH MEMORIAL (100072)**, 1055 Saxon Boulevard, Zip 32763–8468; tel. 386/917–5000 **A**1 9 10 **F**3 11 15 18 24 25 26 27 31 32 33 35 38 43 55 57 61 62 68 72 73 75 76 77 79 80 82 86 90 96 97 99 100 102 103 104 105 106 107 108 109 118 119 121 124 133 135 136 137 **P**8 **S** Adventist Health System Sunbelt Health Care Corporation
Primary Contact: Joe Johnson, President and Chief Executive Officer
COO: Evie Lowe, R.N., Chief Operating Officer
CFO: Michael Lukens, Chief Financial Officer
CMO: Rajendra Hippal, M.D., Chief of Staff
CIO: Trish Stebbins, Director Management Information Systems
CHR: Bonne Barrows–MacPherson, Director Human Resources
Web address: www.fhfishmemorial.org
Control: Church–operated, Nongovernment, not–for profit **Service:** General Medical and Surgical

Staffed Beds: 139 **Admissions:** 9001 **Census:** 103 **Outpatient Visits:** 106721 **Births:** 0 **Total Expense ($000):** 107620 **Payroll Expense ($000):** 43090 **Personnel:** 1007

ORANGE PARK—Clay County

★ **ORANGE PARK MEDICAL CENTER (100226)**, 2001 Kingsley Avenue, Zip 32073–5156; tel. 904/276–8500 **A**1 2 9 10 **F**8 11 13 15 18 20 24 25 26 27 31 33 38 43 46 49 53 54 56 57 59 66 72 73 75 76 77 79 80 81 82 86 90 91 92 93 94 96 97 100 102 103 104 107 119 133 135 136 137 **S** HCA
Primary Contact: Thomas R. Pentz, President and Chief Executive Officer
COO: Marsha A. Easley, Chief Operating Officer
CFO: Bryce DeHaven, Chief Financial Officer
CIO: Karen Parish, Director Information Systems
CHR: Paula Shields, Director Human Resources
Web address: www.opmedical.com
Control: Corporation, Investor–owned, for–profit **Service:** General Medical and Surgical

Staffed Beds: 230 **Admissions:** 13465 **Census:** 176 **Outpatient Visits:** 132752 **Births:** 2021 **Total Expense ($000):** 119068 **Payroll Expense ($000):** 52125 **Personnel:** 792

ORLANDO—Orange County

ARNOLD PALMER CHILDREN'S HOSPITAL See Orlando Regional Medical Center

★ ○ △ **FLORIDA HOSPITAL (100007)**, 601 East Rollins Street, Zip 32803–1489; tel. 407/303–6611, (Includes FLORIDA HOSPITAL CELEBRATION HEALTH, 400 Clebration Place, Celebration, Zip 34747; tel. 407/303–4000; Monica Reed, M.D., Administrator; FLORIDA HOSPITAL EAST ORLANDO, 7727 Lake Underhill Drive, Zip 32822; tel. 407/277–8110; Ed Noseworthy, Administrator; FLORIDA HOSPITAL KISSIMMEE, 2450 North Orange Blossom Trai, Kissimmee, Zip 34741; tel. 407/846–4343; William Haupt, Administrator; FLORIDA HOSPITAL–ALTAMONTE, 601 East Altamonte Drive, Altamonte Springs, Zip 32701; tel. 407/830–4321; Rob Fulbright, Administrator; FLORIDA HOSPITAL–APOPKA, 201 North Park Avenue, Apopka, Zip 32703; tel. 407/889–2566; Verbelee Neilsen Swanson, Administrator; WINTER PARK MEMORIAL HOSPITAL, 200 North Lakemont Avenue, Winter Park, Zip 32792–3273; tel. 407/646–7000; Kenneth Bradley, Administrator) **A**1 2 3 5 7 9 10 11 **F**3 7 9 11 12 13 14 15 17 18 19 20 22 24 25 26 27 28 30 31 32 33 34 35 36 37 38 41 43 44 45 46 47 48 49 50 51 52 53 54 55 56 57 58 59 60 61 62 63 64 66 68 69 70 71 72 73 74 75 76 77 78 79 80 81 82 83 84 85 86 87 88 90 91 92 93 94 96 97 98 99 100 102 103 104 105 106 107 108 109 111 112 116 118 119 120 121 123 124 125 127 128 130 131 134 135 136 137 **P**1 6 8 **S** Adventist Health System Sunbelt Health Care Corporation
Primary Contact: Lars D. Houmann, President
CFO: Eddie Soler, Chief Financial Officer
CMO: David Moorhead, M.D., Senior Medical Officer
CIO: Andy Crowder, Chief Information Officer
CHR: Richard M. Tibbits, Chief People Officer
Web address: www.flhosp.org
Control: Other not–for–profit (including NFP Corporation) **Service:** General Medical and Surgical

Staffed Beds: 1906 **Admissions:** 108560 **Census:** 1401 **Outpatient Visits:** 816025 **Births:** 8491 **Total Expense ($000):** 1925979 **Payroll Expense ($000):** 643591 **Personnel:** 13860

★ △ **ORLANDO REGIONAL MEDICAL CENTER (100006)**, 1414 Kuhl Avenue, Zip 32806–2093; tel. 407/841–5111, (Includes ARNOLD PALMER CHILDREN'S HOSPITAL, 92 West Miller Street, Zip 32806; tel. 407/649–6960; John Bozard, President; ORLANDO REGIONAL–LUCERNE, 818 Main Lane, Zip 32801–3727; tel. 321/841–4200; Karen Frenier, Executive Director; WINNIE PALMER HOSPITAL FOR WOMEN AND BABIES, 83 West Miller Street, Zip 32806; tel. 321/843–2201; Kathy Swanson, President) **A**1 2 5 7 8 9 10 **F**2 3 4 5 6 8 12 13 15 16 17 18 19 20 21 22 23 24 25 26 27 28 30 31 32 33 34 38 40 43 44 45 46 49 50 51 52 54 55 56 57 58 59 60 61 62 63 66 68 69 70 71 72 73 74 75 76 77 78 79 80 81 82 83 84 85 86 88 89 90 91 92 93 94 95 96 97 100 102 103 104 105 106 107 108 109 111 112 114 116 119 120 121 123 124 132 135 136 137 **P**6 **S** Orlando Health
Primary Contact: Sherrie Sitarik, President
CFO: Paul Goldstein, Vice President Finance and Chief Financial Officer
CMO: Timothy Bullard, M.D., Chief of Staff
CIO: Rick Schooler, Vice President and Chief Information Officer
CHR: Nancy Dinon, Vice President Human Resources
Web address: www.orhs.org
Control: Other not–for–profit (including NFP Corporation) **Service:** General Medical and Surgical

Staffed Beds: 1387 **Admissions:** 81413 **Census:** 1081 **Outpatient Visits:** 464820 **Births:** 15554 **Total Expense ($000):** 1204614 **Payroll Expense ($000):** 510312 **Personnel:** 11767

□ **SELECT SPECIALTY HOSPITAL OF ORLANDO (102003)**, 2250 Bedford Road, Zip 32803; tel. 407/303–7869, (Nonreporting) **A**1 9 10 **S** Select Medical Corporation
Primary Contact: Rose O'Neil, Chief Executive Officer
Web address: www.selectmedicalcorp.com
Control: Corporation, Investor–owned, for–profit **Service:** Long–Term Acute Care hospital

Staffed Beds: 35

WINNIE PALMER HOSPITAL FOR WOMEN AND BABIES See Orlando Regional Medical Center

ORMOND BEACH—Volusia County

★ **FLORIDA HOSPITAL–ORMOND MEMORIAL (100068)**, 875 Sterthaus Avenue, Zip 32174–5197; tel. 386/676–6000, (Includes FLORIDA HOSPITAL–OCEANSIDE, 264 South Atlantic Avenue, Zip 32176–8192; tel. 386/672–4161; Dan Wolcott, Administrator), (Nonreporting) **A**1 2 9 10 **S** Adventist Health System Sunbelt Health Care Corporation
Primary Contact: Darlinda Copeland, Chief Operating Officer
COO: Darlinda Copeland, Chief Operating Officer
CFO: Deborah Thomas, Chief Financial Officer
CHR: Connie Schott, Administrative Assistant
Web address: www.memorial–health.com
Control: Church–operated, Nongovernment, not–for profit **Service:** General Medical and Surgical

Staffed Beds: 324

 Many Facility Codes have changed. Please refer to the AHA Guide Code Chart.

PALATKA—Putnam County

★ **PUTNAM COMMUNITY MEDICAL CENTER (100232)**, Highway 20 West, Zip 32177–8118, Mailing Address: P.O. Box 778, Zip 32178–0778; tel. 386/328–5711, (Total facility includes 10 beds in nursing home–type unit) (Nonreporting) **A**1 9 10 19 **S** LifePoint Hospitals, Inc.
Primary Contact: Bruce A. Baldwin, Chief Executive Officer
CFO: James McGonnell, Chief Financial Officer
CMO: Hussein Zabad, M.D., Chief of Staff
CHR: Kay Svendsen, Director Human Resources
Web address: www.pcmcfl.com
Control: Corporation, Investor–owned, for–profit **Service:** General Medical and Surgical

Staffed Beds: 141

PALM BEACH GARDENS—Palm Beach County

★ **PALM BEACH GARDENS MEDICAL CENTER (100176)**, 3360 Burns Road, Zip 33410–4304; tel. 561/622–1411, (Nonreporting) **A**1 9 10 **S** TENET Healthcare Corporation
Primary Contact: David A. Pettit, Chief Executive Officer
COO: Ruth Stewart, Chief Operating Officer
CFO: Judi Stimson–Rusin, Chief Financial Officer
CIO: John Crump, Director Information Systems
CHR: Lisa Oremus, Director Human Resources
Web address: www.pbgmc.com
Control: Corporation, Investor–owned, for–profit **Service:** General Medical and Surgical

Staffed Beds: 199

PALM COAST—Flagler County

★ **FLORIDA HOSPITAL–FLAGLER (100118)**, 60 Memorial Medical Parkway, Zip 32164; tel. 386/586–2000 **A**1 9 10 **F**11 15 18 24 25 26 27 33 38 42 43 52 53 54 55 56 57 60 61 62 68 73 75 76 77 79 81 82 86 87 96 97 100 104 105 107 109 111 119 120 121 124 133 135 136 137 **S** Adventist Health System Sunbelt Health Care Corporation
Primary Contact: David Ottati, President and Chief Executive Officer
CFO: Valerie Ziesmer, Chief Financial Officer
Web address: www.fhms.com
Control: Church–operated, Nongovernment, not–for profit **Service:** General Medical and Surgical

Staffed Beds: 99 **Admissions:** 5396 **Census:** 61 **Births:** 0 **Payroll Expense ($000):** 23580

PANAMA CITY—Bay County

★ **BAY MEDICAL CENTER (100026)**, 615 North Bonita Avenue, Zip 32401–3600, Mailing Address: P.O. Box 59515, Zip 32402–2515; tel. 850/769–1511 **A**1 2 9 10 **F**3 7 8 11 13 14 15 17 18 20 22 24 25 26 27 30 31 32 33 38 43 49 52 53 55 56 57 58 59 60 62 63 66 68 72 73 74 75 76 77 78 79 82 84 86 88 89 90 91 92 94 95 96 97 98 100 102 107 109 111 116 118 119 120 121 123 124 132 133 135 136 137
Primary Contact: Steven M. Johnson, President and Chief Executive Officer
COO: Kathy Wilder, Vice President Clinical Operations
CFO: Daniel R. Morgan, Chief Financial Officer
CMO: Gregory M. England, M.D., President Medical Staff
CIO: Tom Bialorvcki, Chief Information Officer
CHR: Donna Vincent, Vice President Corporate Services
Web address: www.baymedical.org
Control: Hospital district or authority, Government, nonfederal **Service:** General Medical and Surgical

Staffed Beds: 346 **Admissions:** 18305 **Census:** 233 **Outpatient Visits:** 183146 **Births:** 544 **Total Expense ($000):** 215819 **Payroll Expense ($000):** 84042 **Personnel:** 1550

★ **GULF COAST MEDICAL CENTER (100242)**, 449 West 23rd Street, Zip 32405–4593, Mailing Address: P.O. Box 15309, Zip 32406–5309; tel. 850/769–8341 **A**1 2 9 10 **F**1 3 4 8 12 13 15 16 17 18 25 26 27 30 31 32 35 37 38 46 48 49 51 53 54 55 56 57 59 62 65 66 68 70 71 72 73 74 75 76 77 78 79 80 81 82 83 84 85 86 88 96 97 98 100 102 104 105 106 107 117 119 120 121 124 133 135 136 137 **P**5 **S** HCA
Primary Contact: Todd Gallati, Chief Executive Officer
COO: Nancy Dodson, Chief Operating Officer
CFO: Donald Murphy, Chief Financial Officer
CHR: Wanda Salley, Administrative Director Human Resources
Web address: www.egulfcoastmedical.com
Control: Corporation, Investor–owned, for–profit **Service:** General Medical and Surgical

Staffed Beds: 176 **Admissions:** 10487 **Census:** 109 **Outpatient Visits:** 109728 **Births:** 2273 **Total Expense ($000):** 100875 **Payroll Expense ($000):** 33938 **Personnel:** 624

★ △ **HEALTHSOUTH EMERALD COAST REHABILITATION HOSPITAL (103040)**, 1847 Florida Avenue, Zip 32405–4640; tel. 850/914–8600 **A**1 7 9 10 **F**3 25 32 36 41 43 52 53 55 56 57 61 62 75 81 82 85 86 118 120 121 124 135 137 **P**5 **S** HEALTHSOUTH Corporation
Primary Contact: Tony N. Bennett, Chief Executive Officer
CFO: Angela Eddins, Manager Finance
CMO: Michael Hennigan, M.D., Medical Director
CHR: Michelle Liesemeyer, Manager Human Resources
Web address: www.healthsouthpanamacity.com
Control: State–Government, nonfederal **Service:** Rehabilitation

Staffed Beds: 75 **Admissions:** 1033 **Census:** 42 **Outpatient Visits:** 16006 **Births:** 0 **Total Expense ($000):** 12038 **Payroll Expense ($000):** 6484 **Personnel:** 244

□ **SELECT SPECIALTY HOSPITAL OF PANAMA CITY (102017)**, 615 North Bonita Avenue, 3rd Floor, Zip 32401; tel. 850/767–3180 **A**1 9 10 **F**1 3 85 **S** Select Medical Corporation
Primary Contact: Debra R. Gibson, Chief Executive Officer
CMO: Amir Manzoor, M.D., Medical Director
Web address: www.selectmedicalcorp.com
Control: Corporation, Investor–owned, for–profit **Service:** General Medical and Surgical

Staffed Beds: 30 **Admissions:** 332 **Census:** 23 **Births:** 0 **Total Expense ($000):** 10090 **Payroll Expense ($000):** 4564

PEMBROKE PINES—Broward County

★ **MEMORIAL HOSPITAL PEMBROKE (100230)**, 7800 Sheridan Street, Zip 33024–2536; tel. 954/962–9650 **A**1 9 10 **F**3 6 11 15 17 25 26 30 31 32 38 43 49 50 51 54 55 57 58 59 62 63 66 68 72 73 75 77 79 80 81 82 86 96 100 101 102 107 112 114 116 118 119 121 133 134 135 137 **S** Memorial Healthcare System
Primary Contact: Zeff Ross, Interim Administrator
CFO: Joseph Stuczynski, Assistant Administrator Finance and Support
CMO: Stanley Marks, M.D., Chief Medical Officer
CIO: Robert Reiss, Chief Information Officer
CHR: Margie Vargas, Director Human Resources
Web address: www.mhs–net.com
Control: Hospital district or authority, Government, nonfederal **Service:** General Medical and Surgical

Staffed Beds: 149 **Admissions:** 7387 **Census:** 86 **Outpatient Visits:** 126227 **Births:** 0 **Total Expense ($000):** 65495 **Payroll Expense ($000):** 44523 **Personnel:** 683

★ **MEMORIAL HOSPITAL WEST (100281)**, 703 North Flamingo Road, Zip 33028–1014; tel. 954/436–5000 **A**1 2 9 10 **F**3 13 15 17 18 20 24 25 26 27 30 31 32 38 43 46 47 49 52 54 55 56 57 59 60 62 66 68 70 72 73 74 76 77 79 80 82 84 86 96 97 99 100 102 103 106 107 108 109 111 114 119 120 121 134 135 136 137 **S** Memorial Healthcare System
Primary Contact: Kennon Hetlage, Chief Executive Officer Administrator
COO: Sue E. Bradford, R.N., Chief Operating Officer
CFO: Walter Bussell, Chief Financial Officer
CMO: Miguel Venereo, M.D., Director Medical Staff
CIO: Forest Blanton, Chief Information Officer
CHR: Christopher Perry, Director Human Resources
Web address: www.mhs.net
Control: Hospital district or authority, Government, nonfederal **Service:** General Medical and Surgical

Staffed Beds: 299 **Admissions:** 22602 **Census:** 246 **Outpatient Visits:** 261749 **Births:** 4923 **Total Expense ($000):** 256068 **Payroll Expense ($000):** 109296 **Personnel:** 1700

PENSACOLA—Escambia County

★ **BAPTIST HOSPITAL (100093)**, 1000 West Moreno, Zip 32501–2393, Mailing Address: P.O. Box 17500, Zip 32522–7500; tel. 850/434–4011 **A**1 2 9 10 **F**3 7 11 12 13 15 17 18 20 22 24 25 26 27 30 31 32 33 34 36 38 40 41 42 43 44 46 47 48 49 50 51 53 54 55 56 57 58 59 60 61 62 66 68 72 73 74 75 76 77 79 80 81 82 86 88 89 90 91 92 93 94 95 96 97 100 102 103 104 105 106 107 108 109 111 112 113 114 116 118 119 120 121 132 133 135 136 137 **P**6 **S** Baptist Health Care Corporation
Primary Contact: Mark Faulkner, Administrator
COO: David Wildebrandt, Vice President Operations
CFO: Joseph G. Felkner, Chief Financial Officer and Senior Vice President Finance
CMO: David Di Loreto, M.D., Senior Vice President Medical Affairs
CIO: Robert Johnson, Vice President and Chief Information Officer
CHR: Celeste Norris, Vice President Human Resources
Web address: www.ebaptisthealthcare.org
Control: Other not–for–profit (including NFP Corporation) **Service:** General Medical and Surgical

Staffed Beds: 435 **Admissions:** 15725 **Census:** 221 **Outpatient Visits:** 283319 **Births:** 1261 **Total Expense ($000):** 213929 **Payroll Expense ($000):** 73392 **Personnel:** 1492

FL

Hospital, Medicare Provider Number, Address, Telephone, Approval, Facility, and Physician Codes, Health Care System

★ American Hospital Association (AHA) membership
□ The Joint Commission accreditation
○ American Osteopathic Association (AOA) accreditation
△ Commission on Accreditation of Rehabilitation Facilities (CARF) accreditation

★ **NAVAL HOSPITAL**, 6000 West Highway 98, Zip 32512–0003; tel. 850/505–6413 **A**1 3 5 **F**3 5 13 15 18 25 26 28 29 33 36 37 38 43 49 50 55 56 57 62 66 68 72 73 74 75 77 79 80 81 82 86 87 90 91 92 94 96 97 98 99 100 101 102 107 118 119 120 124 135 136 137 **S** Bureau of Medicine and Surgery, Department of the Navy
Primary Contact: Captain Maryalice Morro, Commanding Officer
Web address: www.psaweb.pcola.med.navy.mil
Control: Navy, Government, federal **Service:** General Medical and Surgical

Staffed Beds: 30 **Admissions:** 2326 **Census:** 18 **Outpatient Visits:** 434194 **Births:** 589 **Total Expense ($000):** 32453 **Payroll Expense ($000):** 25634 **Personnel:** 1014

REHABILITATION INSTITUTE OF WEST FLORIDA See West Florida Hospital

★ **SACRED HEART HOSPITAL OF PENSACOLA (100025)**, 5151 North Ninth Avenue, Zip 32504–8795, Mailing Address: P.O. Box 2700, Zip 32513–2700; tel. 850/416–7000 **A**1 2 3 5 9 10 **F**3 7 8 11 12 13 15 17 18 20 22 24 25 26 27 28 30 31 32 33 37 38 40 43 44 46 49 50 52 53 54 55 56 57 58 61 62 66 68 69 70 71 72 73 74 75 76 77 78 79 80 81 82 83 84 86 87 96 97 98 99 100 102 103 104 105 106 107 108 109 111 112 119 120 121 124 133 135 136 137 **S** Ascension Health
Primary Contact: Debbie Bostic, President
CFO: Buddy Elmore, Chief Financial Officer
CMO: Paul T. Baroco, Senior Vice President Medical Affairs
CIO: Bill Winter, Director Information Technology
Web address: www.sacred–heart.org
Control: Other not–for–profit (including NFP Corporation) **Service:** General Medical and Surgical

Staffed Beds: 458 **Admissions:** 24262 **Census:** 312 **Outpatient Visits:** 325602 **Births:** 3715 **Total Expense ($000):** 277670 **Payroll Expense ($000):** 99149 **Personnel:** 2182

★ **WEST FLORIDA HOSPITAL (100231)**, 8383 North Davis Highway, Zip 32514–6088; tel. 850/494–4000, (Includes REHABILITATION INSTITUTE OF WEST FLORIDA, tel. 850/494–6000; THE PAVILION, tel. 904/494–5000), (Nonreporting) **A**1 9 10 **S** HCA
Primary Contact: Dennis A. Taylor, Chief Executive Officer
COO: Robert Peterson, Chief Operating Officer
CFO: Randy Butler, Chief Financial Officer
CMO: Louis Perillo, M.D., Senior Vice President Medical Affairs
CIO: Jeff Amerson, Director Information System
CHR: Karen Oliver, Vice President Human Resources
Web address: www.westfloridahospital.com
Control: Corporation, Investor–owned, for–profit **Service:** General Medical and Surgical

Staffed Beds: 339

PERRY—Taylor County

DOCTOR'S MEMORIAL HOSPITAL (100106), 333 North Byron Butler Parkway, Zip 32347–2104; tel. 850/584–0800 **A**9 10 20 **F**3 7 11 15 25 26 31 32 38 55 56 57 61 68 79 80 84 86 96 100 107 118 119 121 122
Primary Contact: Charles Darcy, Chief Executive Officer
CMO: Bilah Khodr, M.D., Chief of Staff
CIO: Kyle Wright, Chief Information Officer
CHR: Diana McRory, Director Human Resources
Web address: www.doctorsmemorial.com
Control: Other not–for–profit (including NFP Corporation) **Service:** General Medical and Surgical

Staffed Beds: 48 **Admissions:** 2101 **Census:** 18 **Outpatient Visits:** 41237 **Births:** 0 **Total Expense ($000):** 21369 **Payroll Expense ($000):** 13020 **Personnel:** 268

PLANT CITY—Hillsborough County

★ **SOUTH FLORIDA BAPTIST HOSPITAL (100132)**, 301 North Alexander Street, Zip 33563–9058, Mailing Address: Drawer H, Zip 33564–9058; tel. 813/757–1200, (Nonreporting) **A**1 9 10 **S** Catholic Health East
Primary Contact: Isaac Mallah, President and Chief Executive Officer
CFO: Cathy Yoder, Chief Financial Officer
CMO: Mark Vaaler, M.D., Chief Medical Officer
CHR: Juanita Radford, Coordinator Team Resource
Web address: www.sjbhealth.org
Control: Other not–for–profit (including NFP Corporation) **Service:** General Medical and Surgical

Staffed Beds: 147

PLANTATION—Broward County

★ **PLANTATION GENERAL HOSPITAL (100167)**, 401 N.W. 42nd Avenue, Zip 33317–2882; tel. 954/587–5010, (Nonreporting) **A**1 9 10 **S** HCA
Primary Contact: Barbara Simmons, RN, Chief Executive Officer
COO: Shana Sappington, Chief Operating Officer
CFO: David L. Hughes, Chief Financial Officer
CIO: Patrick Adesso, Director Management Information Systems
CHR: Ben Bittner, Vice President Human Resources
Web address: www.plantationgeneral.com
Control: Corporation, Investor–owned, for–profit **Service:** General Medical and Surgical

Staffed Beds: 264

★ **WESTSIDE REGIONAL MEDICAL CENTER (100228)**, 8201 West Broward Boulevard, Zip 33324–9937; tel. 954/473–6600, (Nonreporting) **A**1 2 9 10 **S** HCA
Primary Contact: MaryLynn Swartz, Chief Executive Officer
COO: Scott A. Cihak, Chief Operating Officer
CFO: Michael Houston, Chief Financial Officer
CMO: Joel Shulman, M.D., Chief of Staff
CIO: Trish Campbell, Director Management Information Systems
CHR: Amy Paces, Director Human Resources
Web address: www.westsideregional.com
Control: Corporation, Investor–owned, for–profit **Service:** General Medical and Surgical

Staffed Beds: 204

POMPANO BEACH—Broward County

CORAL SPRINGS MEDICAL CENTER See Coral Springs

NORTH BROWARD MEDICAL CENTER See Deerfield Beach

PORT CHARLOTTE—Charlotte County

★ △ **FAWCETT MEMORIAL HOSPITAL (100236)**, 21298 Olean Boulevard, Zip 33952–6765, Mailing Address: P.O. Box 494960, Punta Gorda, Zip 33949–4960; tel. 941/629–1181, (Nonreporting) **A**1 7 9 10 **S** HCA
Primary Contact: Thomas J. Rice, President and Chief Executive Officer
COO: Thomas J. Rice, President and Chief Executive Officer
CFO: James P. Burns, Vice President and Chief Financial Officer
CHR: Linda V. Smith, Director Human Resources
Web address: www.fawcetthospital.com
Control: Corporation, Investor–owned, for–profit **Service:** General Medical and Surgical

Staffed Beds: 238

☐ **PEACE RIVER REGIONAL MEDICAL CENTER (100077)**, 2500 Harbor Boulevard, Zip 33952–5396; tel. 941/766–4122, (Total facility includes 104 beds in nursing home–type unit) **A**1 5 9 10 **F**3 12 13 15 18 25 26 27 30 31 32 38 45 46 47 48 49 51 54 59 61 63 68 72 73 74 75 76 77 78 79 80 82 84 85 86 96 97 98 100 102 103 107 117 133 135 136 **S** Health Management Associates
Primary Contact: David McCormack, Chief Executive Officer
COO: Eric Barber, Chief Operating Officer
CFO: Robert Stiekes, Chief Financial Officer
CIO: Ted Bailey, Vice President Information Systems
Web address: www.peaceriverregional.com
Control: Corporation, Investor–owned, for–profit **Service:** General Medical and Surgical

Staffed Beds: 296 **Admissions:** 9043 **Census:** 105 **Outpatient Visits:** 98772 **Births:** 1336

PORT ST. LUCIE—St. Lucie County

★ **ST. LUCIE MEDICAL CENTER (100260)**, 1800 S.E. Tiffany Avenue, Zip 34952–7580; tel. 772/335–4000, (Nonreporting) **A**1 2 9 10 **S** HCA
Primary Contact: Gary Cantrell, President and Chief Executive Officer
CFO: Steve Barnhill, Chief Financial Officer
Web address: www.stluciemed.com
Control: Corporation, Investor–owned, for–profit **Service:** General Medical and Surgical

Staffed Beds: 194

PUNTA GORDA—Charlotte County

☐ **CHARLOTTE REGIONAL MEDICAL CENTER (100047)**, 809 East Marion Avenue, Zip 33950–3898, Mailing Address: P.O. Box 51–1328, Zip 33951–1328; tel. 941/639–3131, (Nonreporting) **A**1 9 10 **S** Health Management Associates
Primary Contact: Brad K. Nurkin, Chief Executive Officer
CFO: Cheryl Tibbett, Chief Financial Officer
CHR: Shelley Baker, Director Human Resources
Web address: www.charlotteregional.com
Control: Corporation, Investor–owned, for–profit **Service:** General Medical and Surgical

Staffed Beds: 208

FL

ROCKLEDGE—Brevard County

☐ **WUESTHOFF MEDICAL CENTER – ROCKLEDGE (100092)**, 110 Longwood Avenue, Zip 32955–2887, Mailing Address: P.O. Box 565002, Mail Stop 1, Zip 32956–5002; tel. 321/636–2211 **A**1 2 9 10 **F**3 11 13 15 17 18 20 22 24 25 26 27 30 31 32 35 38 43 44 45 49 51 53 54 55 56 57 59 60 61 62 66 68 70 72 73 74 75 76 77 79 80 81 82 84 86 88 90 91 92 96 97 100 102 103 107 118 119 120 121 124 133 134 135 136 **S** Wuesthoff Health System
Primary Contact: Chantal Leconte, Administrator
CFO: George Fayer, Chief Financial Officer
CIO: David Barnhart, Director Information Systems
CHR: Marchita Marino, Vice President Human Resources
Web address: www.wuesthoff.org
Control: Other not–for–profit (including NFP Corporation) **Service:** General Medical and Surgical

Staffed Beds: 291 **Admissions:** 13424 **Census:** 182 **Outpatient Visits:** 274579 **Births:** 695 **Total Expense ($000):** 140619 **Payroll Expense ($000):** 55074 **Personnel:** 1079

SAFETY HARBOR—Pinellas County

☐ **MEASE COUNTRYSIDE HOSPITAL (100265)**, 3231 McMullen–Booth Road, Zip 34695–1098, Mailing Address: P.O. 1098, Zip 34695–1098; tel. 727/725–6111, (Nonreporting) **A**1 2 9 10 **S** Morton Plant Mease Health Care
Primary Contact: Philip K. Beauchamp, FACHE, President and Chief Executive Officer
COO: Lou Galdieri, Chief Operating Officer and Administrator
CMO: Donald Pocock, M.D., Chief Medical Officer
CHR: Sharon Collotta, Director Human Resources
Web address: www.mpmhealth.com
Control: Other not–for–profit (including NFP Corporation) **Service:** General Medical and Surgical

Staffed Beds: 100

SAINT AUGUSTINE—St. Johns County

☐ **FLAGLER HOSPITAL (100090)**, 400 Health Park Boulevard, Zip 32086–5779; tel. 904/819–5155 **A**1 2 9 10 **F**3 11 13 15 18 20 22 24 25 26 30 31 32 38 46 49 51 52 53 55 56 57 63 64 68 72 74 75 77 79 80 84 86 87 88 96 97 100 102 107 118 119 121 124 135 137
Primary Contact: Joseph S. Gordy, President
CFO: Lynda I. Kirker, Chief Financial Officer
CMO: Douglas Dew, M.D., President Medical Staff
CIO: Rollie McNeil, Director
CHR: Jeff Hurley, Director Human Resources
Web address: www.flaglerhospital.com
Control: Other not–for–profit (including NFP Corporation) **Service:** General Medical and Surgical

Staffed Beds: 316 **Admissions:** 14156 **Census:** 184 **Outpatient Visits:** 170330 **Births:** 1228 **Total Expense ($000):** 155454 **Payroll Expense ($000):** 59553 **Personnel:** 1388

SAINT CLOUD—Lowndes County

☐ **ST. CLOUD REGIONAL MEDICAL CENTER (100302)**, 2906 17th Street, Zip 34769–6099; tel. 407/892–2135 **A**1 9 10 **F**3 11 15 25 26 33 38 46 49 50 51 54 55 56 57 59 62 66 68 72 73 75 77 79 80 81 82 86 96 97 98 100 102 103 106 107 119 121 124 135 136 137 **P**6 **S** Health Management Associates
Primary Contact: Thomas D. Barb, Chief Executive Officer
COO: Ronald R. Beer, CHE, Chief Operating Officer
CFO: Eric Smith, Chief Financial Officer
CMO: Charles Powers, M.D., Chief Medical Director
CIO: Edju Ewasko, Director Information Systems
CHR: Cheryl Paolillo, Director Human Resources
Web address: www.stcloudregional.com
Control: State–Government, nonfederal **Service:** General Medical and Surgical

Staffed Beds: 84 **Admissions:** 4045 **Census:** 49 **Outpatient Visits:** 48152 **Births:** 0 **Total Expense ($000):** 33906 **Payroll Expense ($000):** 17450

SAINT PETERSBURG—Pinellas County

⊠ **ALL CHILDREN'S HOSPITAL (103300)**, 801 Sixth Street South, Zip 33701–4899; tel. 727/898–7451 **A**1 3 5 8 9 10 **F**3 7 11 18 19 20 21 22 23 25 26 27 28 30 31 32 33 34 35 37 38 40 41 43 44 48 49 50 51 53 57 58 59 60 62 63 66 70 72 73 75 76 77 78 79 80 81 82 83 84 86 87 89 90 94 96 97 100 102 106 107 114 116 118 119 120 121 123 125 126 131 133 135 137 **P**1
Primary Contact: Gary Carnes, President and Chief Executive Officer
CFO: Arnold Stenberg, Senior Vice President and Chief Financial Officer
CMO: Michael Epstein, M.D., Senior Vice President Medical Affairs
CIO: Cal Popovich, Vice President Information Technology
Web address: www.allkids.org
Control: Other not–for–profit (including NFP Corporation) **Service:** Children's general

Staffed Beds: 216 **Admissions:** 8646 **Census:** 170 **Outpatient Visits:** 245607 **Births:** 0 **Total Expense ($000):** 248232 **Payroll Expense ($000):** 102596 **Personnel:** 2029

⊠ △ **BAYFRONT MEDICAL CENTER (100032)**, 701 Sixth Street South, Zip 33701–4891; tel. 727/823–1234 **A**1 2 3 5 7 9 10 **F**3 8 11 13 15 17 18 20 22 24 25 26 27 31 32 33 34 36 38 40 43 44 46 49 50 52 53 54 55 56 57 58 60 61 62 63 66 68 71 72 73 74 75 76 77 79 80 81 82 85 86 87 96 97 98 100 102 106 107 109 111 112 118 119 120 121 124 133 135 136 137 **P**6
Primary Contact: Sue G. Brody, President and Chief Executive Officer
COO: Eric Feder, Chief Operating Officer
CFO: Bob Thornton, Chief Financial Officer
CMO: Paul McRae, M.D., Chief of Staff
CIO: John McLendon, Chief Information Officer
CHR: Deborah Menendez, Director Human Resources
Web address: www.bayfront.org
Control: Other not–for–profit (including NFP Corporation) **Service:** General Medical and Surgical

Staffed Beds: 382 **Admissions:** 17908 **Census:** 253 **Outpatient Visits:** 200976 **Births:** 3383 **Total Expense ($000):** 231628 **Payroll Expense ($000):** 89004 **Personnel:** 1852

⊠ **EDWARD WHITE HOSPITAL (100239)**, 2323 Ninth Avenue North, Zip 33713–6898, Mailing Address: P.O. Box 12018, Zip 33733–2018; tel. 727/323–1111, (Nonreporting) **A**1 5 9 10 **S** HCA
Primary Contact: Roland Metivier, Chief Executive Officer
COO: Richard S. Frank, Vice President Operations
CFO: Peggy Gatliff, Chief Financial Officer
CMO: Fadi Saba, M.D., Chief of Staff
CIO: Donna Leitenberger, Director Information Services
CHR: Bonnie O'Laskey, Vice President Human Resources
Web address: www.edwardwhitehospital.com
Control: Corporation, Investor–owned, for–profit **Service:** General Medical and Surgical

Staffed Beds: 113

☐ **KINDRED HOSPITAL–BAY AREA ST. PETERSBURG**, (Formerly Kindred Hospital–St. Petersburg), 3030 Sixth Street South, Zip 33705–3720; tel. 727/894–8719, (Nonreporting) **A**1 9 **S** Kindred Healthcare
Primary Contact: Pamela M. Riter, RN, Chief Executive Officer
CFO: John Miner, Chief Financial Officer
Web address: www.kindredstpete.com
Control: Corporation, Investor–owned, for–profit **Service:** General Medical and Surgical

Staffed Beds: 112

★ ○ **NORTHSIDE HOSPITAL AND HEART INSTITUTE (100238)**, 6000 49th Street North, Zip 33709–2145; tel. 727/521–4411 **A**9 10 11 12 13 **F**3 17 18 20 22 24 25 26 33 38 50 62 68 72 75 76 77 79 80 86 87 96 97 100 102 103 107 135 **S** HCA
Primary Contact: Ward Boston, III, Chief Executive Officer
COO: Betsy Bomar, Chief Operating Officer
CFO: Shalin Shah, Chief Financial Officer
CIO: Steve McDonald, Director Information Systems
CHR: Maggie Miklos, Director Human Resources
Web address: www.northsidehospital.com
Control: Corporation, Investor–owned, for–profit **Service:** General Medical and Surgical

Staffed Beds: 288 **Admissions:** 10045 **Census:** 167 **Births:** 0 **Total Expense ($000):** 97624 **Payroll Expense ($000):** 36994

FL

Hospital, Medicare Provider Number, Address, Telephone, Approval, Facility, and Physician Codes, Health Care System

★ American Hospital Association (AHA) membership
☐ The Joint Commission accreditation
○ American Osteopathic Association (AOA) accreditation
△ Commission on Accreditation of Rehabilitation Facilities (CARF) accreditation

☐ **PALMS OF PASADENA HOSPITAL (100126)**, 1501 Pasadena Avenue South, Zip 33707–3798; tel. 727/381–1000, (Total facility includes 13 beds in nursing home–type unit) (Nonreporting) **A**1 2 5 9 10 **S** IASIS Healthcare
Primary Contact: James E. Purcell, III, Chief Executive Officer
CFO: Linda Stockton, Chief Financial Officer
CMO: David Long, M.D., Chief of Staff
CIO: Ron Truitt, Director Information Services
CHR: Karen Casteel, Director Human Resources
Web address: www.palmspasadena.com
Control: Corporation, Investor–owned, for–profit **Service:** General Medical and Surgical

Staffed Beds: 307

★ **ST. ANTHONY'S HOSPITAL (100067)**, 1200 Seventh Avenue North, Zip 33705–1388, Mailing Address: P.O. Box 12588, Zip 33733–2588; tel. 727/825–1100, (Total facility includes 30 beds in nursing home–type unit) (Nonreporting) **A**1 2 9 10 **S** Catholic Health East
Primary Contact: William G. Ulbricht, President
COO: Ronald J. Colaguori, Vice President Operations
CFO: Carl Tremonti, Chief Financial Officer
CMO: Teresa Bradley, M.D., Vice President Medical Affairs
CIO: Lindsey Jarrell, Vice President Information Services
CHR: Jim Bacon, Director Team Resources
Web address: www.stanthonys.org
Control: Other not–for–profit (including NFP Corporation) **Service:** General Medical and Surgical

Staffed Beds: 370

★ **ST. PETERSBURG GENERAL HOSPITAL (100180)**, 6500 38th Avenue North, Zip 33710–1629; tel. 727/384–1414 **A**1 5 9 10 12 13 **F**3 11 13 15 18 22 25 26 27 33 38 43 54 55 57 62 68 72 73 74 75 76 77 79 80 96 97 102 104 105 106 107 118 119 120 121 124 135 136 137 **S** HCA
Primary Contact: Robert B. Conroy, Jr., Chief Executive Officer
COO: Stephanie Sanderson, Chief Operating Officer
CFO: Andrew Smith, Chief Financial Officer
CHR: Guy Samuel, Director Human Resources
Web address: www.stpetegeneral.com
Control: Corporation, Investor–owned, for–profit **Service:** General Medical and Surgical

Staffed Beds: 219 **Admissions:** 7691 **Census:** 104 **Births:** 1609 **Total Expense ($000):** 59913 **Payroll Expense ($000):** 27762

FL

SANFORD—Seminole County

★ **CENTRAL FLORIDA REGIONAL HOSPITAL (100161)**, 1401 West Seminole Boulevard, Zip 32771–6764; tel. 407/321–4500, (Total facility includes 18 beds in nursing home–type unit) (Nonreporting) **A**1 9 10 **S** HCA
Primary Contact: Rodney R. Smith, Chief Executive Officer
CFO: Ashley F. Johnson, Chief Financial Officer
CIO: Nancy Ryerson, Director Information Systems
CHR: Karla Langlotz, Director Human Resources
Web address: www.centralfloridaregional.com
Control: Corporation, Investor–owned, for–profit **Service:** General Medical and Surgical

Staffed Beds: 226

SARASOTA—Sarasota County

★ **DOCTORS HOSPITAL OF SARASOTA (100166)**, 5731 Bee Ridge Road, Zip 34233–5056; tel. 941/342–1100 **A**1 9 10 **F**3 11 18 24 25 26 27 38 51 52 57 59 62 68 72 73 75 76 77 78 79 96 97 100 102 107 135 137 **S** HCA
Primary Contact: Robert C. Meade, Chief Executive Officer
COO: Linda Lemon–Steiner, Chief Operating Officer
CFO: Charles Schwaner, Chief Financial Officer
CHR: Theresa Levering, Director Human Resources
Web address: www.doctorsofsarasota.com
Control: Corporation, Investor–owned, for–profit **Service:** General Medical and Surgical

Staffed Beds: 168 **Admissions:** 6425 **Census:** 72 **Births:** 0 **Total Expense ($000):** 76635 **Payroll Expense ($000):** 26056

★ **HEALTHSOUTH REHABILITATION HOSPITAL OF SARASOTA (103031)**, 6400 Edgelake Drive, Zip 34240–8813; tel. 941/921–8600, (Nonreporting) **A**1 9 10 **S** HEALTHSOUTH Corporation
Primary Contact: Daniel A. Eppley, FACHE, Chief Executive Officer
CFO: Barbara Bierut, Chief Financial Officer
CMO: Alexander De Jesus, M.D., Medical Director
Web address: www.healthsouthsarasota.com
Control: Corporation, Investor–owned, for–profit **Service:** Rehabilitation

Staffed Beds: 76

★ △ **SARASOTA MEMORIAL HOSPITAL (100087)**, 1700 South Tamiami Trail, Zip 34239–3555; tel. 941/917–9000 **A**1 2 5 7 9 10 **F**3 5 6 7 11 12 13 15 17 18 20 22 24 25 26 27 28 30 31 32 33 34 35 36 37 38 41 43 44 46 47 48 49 50 51 52 53 54 55 56 57 58 59 62 64 66 68 70 71 72 73 74 75 76 77 78 79 80 81 82 84 85 86 88 89 90 91 92 93 94 95 96 97 99 100 102 103 106 107 112 114 116 118 119 120 121 124 132 133 134 135 136 137
Primary Contact: Gwen MacKenzie, RN, Chief Executive Officer
COO: Michael L. Harrington, Chief Operating Officer
CFO: David Verinder, Chief Financial Officer
CMO: Parlane Reid, M.D., Chief Medical Officer
CIO: Denis Baker, Chief Information Officer
CHR: Laurie Bennett, Director Human Resources
Web address: www.smh.com
Control: Hospital district or authority, Government, nonfederal **Service:** General Medical and Surgical

Staffed Beds: 613 **Admissions:** 27337 **Census:** 372 **Outpatient Visits:** 353368 **Births:** 3641 **Total Expense ($000):** 355591 **Payroll Expense ($000):** 150034 **Personnel:** 3232

SEBASTIAN—Indian River County

☐ **SEBASTIAN RIVER MEDICAL CENTER (100217)**, 13695 North U.S. Highway 1, Zip 32958–3230, Mailing Address: Box 780838, Zip 32978–0838; tel. 772/589–3186, (Nonreporting) **A**1 9 10 **S** Health Management Associates
Primary Contact: Emily Holliman, Chief Executive Officer
COO: Brian Gibbons, Chief Operating Officer
CFO: John McEachern, Controller
CMO: Ralph Geiger, M.D., Chief of Staff
CHR: Kam Storey, Director Human Resources
Web address: www.sebastianrivermedical.com
Control: Corporation, Investor–owned, for–profit **Service:** General Medical and Surgical

Staffed Beds: 119

SEBRING—Highlands County

★ **FLORIDA HOSPITAL HEARTLAND MEDICAL CENTER (100109)**, 4200 Sun'n Lake Boulevard, Zip 33872–1986, Mailing Address: P.O. Box 9400, Zip 33871–9400; tel. 863/314–4466 **A**1 9 10 19 **F**11 13 15 18 20 24 25 26 30 31 32 33 35 38 41 43 49 50 51 52 53 55 56 57 61 62 68 73 74 77 79 81 82 84 88 89 90 91 93 94 96 97 99 100 102 104 106 107 118 119 121 122 123 134 135 136 137 **P**6 **S** Adventist Health System Sunbelt Health Care Corporation
Primary Contact: Timothy W. Cook, President and Chief Executive Officer
COO: Isaac Palmer, Chief Executive Officer
CFO: Todd Goodman, Vice President and Chief Financial Officer
CHR: Douglas Harcombe, Director Human Resources
Web address: www.flhosp–heartland.org
Control: Church–operated, Nongovernment, not–for profit **Service:** General Medical and Surgical

Staffed Beds: 234 **Admissions:** 12093 **Census:** 143 **Outpatient Visits:** 128789 **Births:** 1211 **Total Expense ($000):** 121207 **Payroll Expense ($000):** 47342 **Personnel:** 1052

☐ **HIGHLANDS REGIONAL MEDICAL CENTER (100049)**, 3600 South Highlands Avenue, Zip 33870–5495, Mailing Address: Drawer 2066, Zip 33871–2066; tel. 863/471–5800, (Nonreporting) **A**1 9 10 19 **S** Health Management Associates
Primary Contact: Robert Mahaffey, Chief Executive Officer
COO: Allison Mulholland, Chief Operating Officer
CFO: San Juana Garza, Chief Financial Officer
CMO: Vinod Thakker, M.D., Chief of Staff
CIO: Felix Garcia, Director Health Information Services
CHR: Shawn Korzep, Director Human Resources
Web address: www.highlandsregional.com
Control: Corporation, Investor–owned, for–profit **Service:** General Medical and Surgical

Staffed Beds: 126

SOUTH MIAMI—Dade County

☐ **LARKIN COMMUNITY HOSPITAL (100181)**, 7031 S.W. 62nd Avenue, Zip 33143–4781; tel. 305/284–7500, (Nonreporting) **A**1 10
Primary Contact: Jack J. Michel, M.D., President and Chief Executive Officer
COO: Jack J. Michel, M.D., President and Chief Executive Officer
CFO: Edgar Castillo, Chief Financial Officer
CMO: Pauline Radix, M.D., Director Physician Relations
CIO: Carlos Siu, Director Information Technology
CHR: Carmen Martinez, Director Human Resources
Web address: www.larkinhospital.com
Control: Corporation, Investor–owned, for–profit **Service:** General Medical and Surgical

Staffed Beds: 122

STARKE—Bradford County

★ **SHANDS STARKE (101310)**, 922 East Call Street, Zip 32091–3699; tel. 904/368–2300 **A**1 9 10 18 **F**3 11 15 25 30 31 32 38 41 50 55 56 57 62 66 73 79 81 86 87 96 100 102 107 118 124 137 **P**6 **S** Shands HealthCare
Primary Contact: Jeannie Baker, Administrator
Web address: www.shands.org
Control: Other not–for–profit (including NFP Corporation) **Service:** General Medical and Surgical

Staffed Beds: 25 **Admissions:** 1158 **Census:** 10 **Outpatient Visits:** 99646 **Births:** 0 **Total Expense ($000):** 20988 **Payroll Expense ($000):** 11077 **Personnel:** 205

STUART—Martin County

★ **MARTIN MEMORIAL HEALTH SYSTEMS (100044)**, 200 S.E. Hospital Avenue, Zip 34994, Mailing Address: P.O. Box 9010, Zip 34995–9010; tel. 772/287–5200, (Includes MARTIN MEMORIAL HOSPITAL SOUTH, 2100 S.E. Salerno Road, Zip 34997; tel. 772/223–2300) **A**1 2 9 10 **F**3 8 11 12 13 15 17 18 20 22 24 25 26 27 28 33 34 35 38 43 44 50 52 54 59 62 66 68 70 72 73 74 75 76 77 79 80 81 82 84 86 92 96 97 100 102 103 105 106 107 108 109 111 112 114 118 119 121 135 136 **P**6
Primary Contact: Richmond M. Harman, President and Chief Executive Officer
COO: Mark E. Robitaille, Senior Vice President and Chief Operating Officer
CFO: Mark Cocorullo, Senior Vice President and Chief Financial Officer
CMO: Howard M. Robbins, M.D., Senior Vice President and Chief Medical Officer
CIO: Chuck Cleaver, Acting Chief Information Officer
CHR: Amy Barry, Vice President and Chief Human Resources Officer
Web address: www.mmhs.com
Control: Other not–for–profit (including NFP Corporation) **Service:** General Medical and Surgical

Staffed Beds: 309 **Admissions:** 17588 **Census:** 214 **Outpatient Visits:** 80375 **Births:** 2118 **Total Expense ($000):** 262577 **Payroll Expense ($000):** 108083 **Personnel:** 1792

SUN CITY CENTER—Hillsborough County

★ **SOUTH BAY HOSPITAL (100259)**, 4016 State Road 674, Zip 33573–5298; tel. 813/634–3301, (Nonreporting) **A**1 9 10 **S** HCA
Primary Contact: Stephen J. Daugherty, Chief Executive Officer
COO: Louis Caputo, Chief Operating Officer
CFO: Russ Young, Chief Financial Officer
CIO: Melissa Morgan, Director Public Relations and Marketing
CHR: Christena Miano, Director Human Resources
Web address: www.southbayhospital.com
Control: Corporation, Investor–owned, for–profit **Service:** General Medical and Surgical

Staffed Beds: 112

TALLAHASSEE—Leon County

★ **CAPITAL REGIONAL MEDICAL CENTER (100254)**, 2626 Capital Medical Boulevard, Zip 32308–4499; tel. 850/325–5000 **A**1 9 10 **F**3 8 11 13 15 17 18 20 22 24 25 26 27 30 31 32 33 35 38 43 46 49 50 54 55 57 59 62 68 72 73 74 76 77 79 80 86 96 97 98 100 102 103 107 108 109 111 112 119 135 136 137 **S** HCA
Primary Contact: Sharon L. Roush, Chief Executive Officer
COO: Dale Neely, Chief Operating Officer
CFO: Michael Gordian, Chief Financial Officer
CMO: William Yahr, M.D., Director Medical Affairs
CIO: Robert A. Steed, Director Information Systems
CHR: Kevin Caracciolo, Director Human Resources
Web address: www.capitalregionalmedicalcenter.com
Control: Corporation, Investor–owned, for–profit **Service:** General Medical and Surgical

Staffed Beds: 177 **Admissions:** 8777 **Census:** 114 **Outpatient Visits:** 81450 **Births:** 1019 **Total Expense ($000):** 96545 **Payroll Expense ($000):** 31783 **Personnel:** 587

★ **HEALTHSOUTH REHABILITATION HOSPITAL OF TALLAHASSEE (103033)**, 1675 Riggins Road, Zip 32308–5315; tel. 850/656–4800, (Nonreporting) **A**1 9 10 **S** HEALTHSOUTH Corporation
Primary Contact: Robert F. Jernigan, Jr., Chief Executive Officer
CFO: Jennifer Spooner, Controller
CMO: Robert Rowland, M.D., Medical Director
CIO: Charles O'Keefe, Director Health Information Services
CHR: Shelia Schiefelbein, Director Human Resources
Web address: www.healthsouth.com
Control: Corporation, Investor–owned, for–profit **Service:** Rehabilitation

Staffed Beds: 70

★ **TALLAHASSEE MEMORIAL HEALTHCARE (100135)**, 1300 Miccosukee Road, Zip 32308–5093; tel. 850/431–1155, (Total facility includes 42 beds in nursing home–type unit) **A**1 2 3 5 9 10 **F**2 3 5 6 8 11 12 15 17 18 20 22 24 25 26 27 30 31 32 33 38 43 44 45 46 47 48 49 50 51 52 53 54 55 56 57 58 59 60 61 62 63 66 68 70 71 72 73 74 75 76 77 78 79 80 81 82 83 84 86 87 88 89 90 91 92 94 96 97 98 99 102 106 107 109 111 112 116 117 119 120 121 124 133 135 136 137 **P**6
Primary Contact: Mark O'Bryant, President and Chief Executive Officer
CFO: William A. Giudice, Vice President and Chief Financial Officer
CMO: John P. Mahoney, M.D., Chief Medical Officer
CIO: Don Lindsey, Vice President and Chief Information Officer
CHR: Steve W. Adriaanse, Vice President and Chief Human Resources Officer
Web address: www.tmh.org
Control: Other not–for–profit (including NFP Corporation) **Service:** General Medical and Surgical

Staffed Beds: 495 **Admissions:** 23655 **Census:** 344 **Outpatient Visits:** 364287 **Births:** 4245 **Total Expense ($000):** 323019 **Payroll Expense ($000):** 141404 **Personnel:** 2818

TAMARAC—Broward County

★ **UNIVERSITY HOSPITAL AND MEDICAL CENTER (100224)**, 7201 North University Drive, Zip 33321–2996; tel. 954/721–2200, (Includes UNIVERSITY PAVILION, 7425 North University Drive, Zip 33328; tel. 305/722–9933), (Nonreporting) **A**1 9 10 **S** HCA
Primary Contact: Lee B. Chaykin, Chief Executive Officer
CFO: Nicole Slaughter, Chief Financial Officer
CMO: Nicholas Katz, M.D., Chief of Staff
CIO: Tom Scharff, Director Information Services
Web address: www.uhmchealth.com
Control: Corporation, Investor–owned, for–profit **Service:** General Medical and Surgical

Staffed Beds: 271

TAMPA—Hillsborough County

★ **H. LEE MOFFITT CANCER CENTER AND RESEARCH INSTITUTE (100271)**, 12902 Magnolia Drive, Zip 33612–9497; tel. 813/972–4673 **A**1 2 3 5 8 9 10 **F**3 15 25 26 27 30 31 32 33 34 41 42 43 44 45 46 47 48 49 50 53 54 55 56 57 58 59 62 66 68 69 72 73 75 76 79 80 81 82 86 90 91 93 94 96 97 98 99 100 101 102 103 104 105 106 107 108 109 111 112 114 119 121 123 124 125 130 132 135 136 137 **P**1
Primary Contact: William S. Dalton, M.D., Ph.D., Chief Executive Officer and Director
COO: John A. Kolosky, Executive Vice President Planning, Finance and Chief Financial Officer
CFO: John A. Kolosky, Executive Vice President Planning, Finance and Chief Financial Officer
CMO: W. Michael Alberts, M.D., Chief Medical Officer
CHR: Yvette Tremonti, Vice President Human Resources
Web address: www.moffitt.usf.edu
Control: Other not–for–profit (including NFP Corporation) **Service:** Cancer

Staffed Beds: 158 **Admissions:** 7261 **Census:** 124 **Outpatient Visits:** 264533 **Births:** 0 **Total Expense ($000):** 350587 **Payroll Expense ($000):** 116828 **Personnel:** 3023

★ △ **JAMES A. HALEY VETERANS HOSPITAL**, 13000 Bruce B. Downs Boulevard, Zip 33612–4798; tel. 813/972–2000, (Total facility includes 228 beds in nursing home–type unit) (Nonreporting) **A**1 3 5 7 8 **S** Department of Veterans Affairs
Primary Contact: Stephen M. Lucas, FACHE, Director
COO: Steven W. Young, Associate Director
CFO: James Skidmore, Manager Finance
CMO: Thomas Bowen, M.D., Chief of Staff
CIO: Jose Seymour, Chief Information Resource Management
CHR: Victoria Rosas, Chief Human Resources
Web address: www.va.gov/visn8/tampa
Control: Veterans Affairs, Government, federal **Service:** General Medical and Surgical

Staffed Beds: 321

☐ **KINDRED HOSPITAL – CENTRAL TAMPA (102013)**, 4801 North Howard Avenue, Zip 33603–1484; tel. 813/874–7575, (Nonreporting) **A**1 9 10 **S** Kindred Healthcare
Primary Contact: Brian L. Pugh, Interim Chief Executive Officer
CFO: Cindee Herlocker, Chief Financial Officer
CMO: Dennis Alfonso, M.D., President Medical Staff
Web address: www.kindredhealthcare.com
Control: Corporation, Investor–owned, for–profit **Service:** Long–Term Acute Care hospital

Staffed Beds: 73

FL

Hospital, Medicare Provider Number, Address, Telephone, Approval, Facility, and Physician Codes, Health Care System
★ American Hospital Association (AHA) membership
☐ The Joint Commission accreditation
○ American Osteopathic Association (AOA) accreditation
△ Commission on Accreditation of Rehabilitation Facilities (CARF) accreditation

☐ **KINDRED HOSPITAL BAY AREA –TAMPA (102009)**, 4555 South Manhattan Avenue, Zip 33611–2397; tel. 813/839–6341, (Nonreporting) **A**1 10
S Kindred Healthcare
Primary Contact: Sally Hoffmann, Chief Executive Officer
CFO: Robert Morrissey, Controller
CHR: Michael Grimes, Manager Human Resources
Web address: www.kindredhealthcare.com
Control: Corporation, Investor–owned, for–profit **Service:** Long–Term Acute Care hospital

Staffed Beds: 73

☐ **MEMORIAL HOSPITAL OF TAMPA (100206)**, 2901 Swann Avenue, Zip 33609–4057; tel. 813/873–6400 **A**1 5 9 10 **F**3 12 15 18 24 25 38 57 60 62 66 68 72 75 76 77 79 80 86 88 92 93 96 100 102 105 106 107 119 121 135 137 **S** IASIS Healthcare
Primary Contact: John J. Mainieri, Chief Executive Officer
CFO: Shelley V. Kolseth, Chief Financial Officer
CIO: John Riton, Director Information Services
Web address: www.memorialhospitaltampa.com
Control: Partnership, Investor–owned, for–profit **Service:** General Medical and Surgical

Staffed Beds: 180 **Admissions:** 6211 **Census:** 85 **Births:** 0 **Payroll Expense ($000):** 21551

☐ **SHRINERS HOSPITALS FOR CHILDREN, TAMPA**, 12502 USF Pine Drive, Zip 33612–9499; tel. 813/972–2250 **A**1 3 5 **F**84 **P**6 **S** Shriners Hospitals for Children
Primary Contact: Alice Reed Lanford, RN, M.S.N., FACHE, Administrator
COO: Cary Burcham, Director Patient Services
CFO: Ruth Gregos, Director Finance
CMO: Dennis Grogan, M.D., Chief of Staff
Web address: www.shrinershq.org
Control: Other not–for–profit (including NFP Corporation) **Service:** Children's orthopedic

Staffed Beds: 60 **Admissions:** 1169 **Census:** 12 **Births:** 0 **Personnel:** 306

★ **ST. JOSEPH'S HOSPITAL (100075)**, 3001 West Dr. Martin Luther King Jr. Boulevard, Zip 33607–6387, Mailing Address: P.O. Box 4227, Zip 33677–4227; tel. 813/870–4000, (Includes ST. JOSEPH'S CHILDREN'S HOSPITAL OF TAMPA, 3001 Dr. Martin Luther King Jr. Boulevard, Zip 33607; tel. 813/554–8500; Michael D. Aubin, Chief Operating Officer; ST. JOSEPH'S WOMEN'S HOSPITAL – TAMPA, 3030 West Dr. Martin L. King Boulevard, Zip 33607–6394; tel. 813/872–2950; Kimberly Guy, Chief Operating Officer), (Nonreporting) **A**1 2 5 9 10 **S** Catholic Health East
Primary Contact: Isaac Mallah, President and Chief Executive Officer
COO: Lorraine Lutton, Chief Operating Officer
CFO: Cathy Yoder, Chief Financial Officer
CMO: Mark Vaaler, M.D., Vice President Medical Staff Affairs
CIO: Lindsey Jarrell, Vice President Information Services
CHR: Pat Teeuwen, Director Team Resources
Web address: www.sjbhealth.org
Control: Church–operated, Nongovernment, not–for profit **Service:** General Medical and Surgical

Staffed Beds: 883

FL

★ △ **TAMPA GENERAL HOSPITAL (100128)**, 2 Columbia Drive, Zip 33606–3508, Mailing Address: P.O. Box 1289, Zip 33601–1289; tel. 813/844–7000 **A**1 7 8 9 10 **F**3 7 8 11 12 13 15 16 17 18 20 22 24 25 26 27 28 30 31 32 33 34 35 36 37 38 40 41 43 44 46 47 48 49 50 51 52 53 54 55 56 57 58 59 60 62 63 64 66 68 70 71 72 73 74 75 76 77 78 79 80 81 82 83 84 85 86 87 88 90 91 92 93 96 97 100 102 103 106 107 113 114 118 119 120 121 123 124 126 127 128 129 130 131 132 133 134 135 136 137
Primary Contact: Ronald A. Hytoff, President and Chief Executive Officer
COO: Deana Nelson, R.N., Executive Vice President Patient Care Services
CFO: Steve Short, Executive Vice President Finance and Administration
CMO: Sally Houston, Senior Vice President and Chief Medical Officer
CIO: Ginger Oliver, Vice President Information Systems
CHR: Chris Roederer, Vice President Human Resources
Web address: www.tgh.org
Control: Other not–for–profit (including NFP Corporation) **Service:** General Medical and Surgical

Staffed Beds: 877 **Admissions:** 36173 **Census:** 651 **Outpatient Visits:** 244368 **Births:** 5454 **Total Expense ($000):** 722781 **Payroll Expense ($000):** 266613 **Personnel:** 5304

☐ **TOWN AND COUNTRY HOSPITAL (100255)**, 6001 Webb Road, Zip 33615–3291; tel. 813/888–7060, (Total facility includes 15 beds in nursing home–type unit) (Nonreporting) **A**1 5 9 10 **S** IASIS Healthcare
Primary Contact: Michael J. Landry, Chief Executive Officer
CFO: Linda Stockton, Chief Financial Officer
CMO: Hernan Giraldo, M.D., Chief of Staff
CIO: Larry Mohammed, Director Information Systems
CHR: Jill Spencer, Director Human Resources
Web address: www.townandcountryhospital.com
Control: Partnership, Investor–owned, for–profit **Service:** General Medical and Surgical

Staffed Beds: 200

☐ **UNIVERSITY COMMUNITY HOSPITAL (100173)**, 3100 East Fletcher Avenue, Zip 33613–4688; tel. 813/971–6000 **A**1 2 3 5 9 10 **F**3 8 11 12 13 15 17 18 20 22 24 25 26 27 30 31 32 33 34 37 38 41 43 50 52 53 54 55 56 57 58 60 61 62 66 68 69 70 71 72 73 74 75 76 77 78 79 81 82 83 84 85 86 87 96 97 100 102 106 107 109 118 119 120 121 132 133 135 136 137 **P**6 **S** University Community Health
Primary Contact: Larry J. Archbell, Chief Executive Officer
COO: Jeffrey Oskin, Vice President Ancillary and Support Services
CFO: Marvin A. Kurtz, Senior Vice President Finance and Chief Financial Officer
CMO: Brad Bjornstad, M.D., Vice President and Chief Medical Officer
CIO: George Evans, Vice President and Chief Information Officer
CHR: James Hackman, Corporate Vice President Human Resources
Web address: www.uch.org
Control: Other not–for–profit (including NFP Corporation) **Service:** General Medical and Surgical

Staffed Beds: 306 **Admissions:** 24294 **Census:** 306 **Outpatient Visits:** 128393 **Births:** 3124

☐ **UNIVERSITY COMMUNITY HOSPITAL–CARROLLWOOD (100069)**, 7171 North Dale Mabry Highway, Zip 33614–2699; tel. 813/932–2222 **A**1 9 10 **F**3 8 11 15 25 26 27 30 31 32 33 38 41 43 48 49 50 52 53 54 55 56 57 58 59 60 61 62 63 66 68 72 73 75 76 77 78 79 80 81 82 86 87 96 100 102 107 119 120 121 132 133 135 137 **S** University Community Health
Primary Contact: Norman V. Stein, Interim Chief Executive Officer
CFO: Bill Woeltjen, Vice President Fiscal Services
CIO: George Evans, Vice President and Chief Information Officer
Web address: www.uch.org
Control: Other not–for–profit (including NFP Corporation) **Service:** General Medical and Surgical

Staffed Beds: 57 **Admissions:** 5276 **Census:** 57 **Outpatient Visits:** 55235 **Births:** 0

TARPON SPRINGS—Pinellas County

☐ **HELEN ELLIS MEMORIAL HOSPITAL (100055)**, 1395 South Pinellas Avenue, Zip 34689–3721; tel. 727/942–5000, (Total facility includes 18 beds in nursing home–type unit) **A**1 5 9 10 **F**3 8 11 13 15 17 18 20 24 25 26 27 33 38 49 51 55 56 57 61 68 73 74 75 76 77 79 80 81 86 96 100 107 117 118 135 136 137 **S** University Community Health
Primary Contact: Donald D. Evans, Chief Executive Officer
COO: Margaret Perreira, Chief Operating Officer and Chief Nursing Officer
CMO: Thomas E. Carson, M.D., President Medical Staff
CIO: Paul Shafer, Director Information Services
CHR: Vernon Elarbee, Director Human Resources
Web address: www.hemh.com
Control: Other not–for–profit (including NFP Corporation) **Service:** General Medical and Surgical

Staffed Beds: 168 **Admissions:** 6197 **Census:** 79 **Outpatient Visits:** 38949 **Births:** 733 **Total Expense ($000):** 72256 **Payroll Expense ($000):** 27227 **Personnel:** 409

TAVARES—Lake County

★ **FLORIDA HOSPITAL WATERMAN (100057)**, 1000 Waterman Way, Zip 32778–5266; tel. 352/253–3333, (Nonreporting) **A**1 2 9 10 19 **S** Adventist Health System Sunbelt Health Care Corporation
Primary Contact: Kenneth R. Mattison, President and Chief Executive Officer
COO: Carrie Fish, Senior Vice President and Chief Operating Officer
CFO: Frances H. Crunk, Vice President and Chief Financial Officer
CMO: Rosemary A. Cirelli, M.D., Chief of Staff
CIO: Mike Freeland, Regional Manager
CHR: Madge Springer, Director Human Resources
Web address: www.fhwat.org
Control: Church–operated, Nongovernment, not–for profit **Service:** General Medical and Surgical

Staffed Beds: 182

TAVERNIER—Monroe County

★ **MARINERS HOSPITAL (100160)**, 91500 Overseas Highway, Zip 33070–2547; tel. 305/434–1582 **A**1 9 10 20 **F**3 8 11 15 24 25 30 31 32 38 44 52 55 57 62 68 73 77 79 80 81 82 86 96 97 99 100 102 106 107 118 119 121 124 135 136 137 **P**1 6 **S** Baptist Health South Florida
Primary Contact: Nelson Lazo, Chief Executive Officer
CFO: Erik Long, Controller
CIO: Mimi Taylor, Vice President Information Technology
CHR: Staci Fulper, Human Resources Site Specialist
Web address: www.baptisthealth.net
Control: Other not–for–profit (including NFP Corporation) **Service:** General Medical and Surgical

Staffed Beds: 42 **Admissions:** 1022 **Census:** 13 **Outpatient Visits:** 29641 **Births:** 0 **Total Expense ($000):** 35793 **Payroll Expense ($000):** 12119 **Personnel:** 191

Many Facility Codes have changed. Please refer to the AHA Guide Code Chart.

TEQUESTA—Martin County

SANDYPINES, 11301 S.E. Tequesta Terrace, Zip 33469–8146; tel. 561/744–0211 **F**30 31 32 88 89 **P**6 **S** Psychiatric Solutions
Primary Contact: John W. Thompson, Ph.D., Chief Executive Officer
Web address: www.psysolutions.com
Control: Corporation, Investor–owned, for–profit **Service:** Children's hospital psychiatric

Staffed Beds: 80 **Admissions:** 166 **Census:** 70 **Outpatient Visits:** 0 **Births:** 0 **Total Expense ($000):** 9269 **Payroll Expense ($000):** 4058 **Personnel:** 106

THE VILLAGES—Sumter County

★ **THE VILLAGES REGIONAL HOSPITAL (100290)**, 1451 El Camino Real, Zip 32159; tel. 352/751–8000 **A**1 9 10 **F**3 8 11 25 26 27 30 31 32 33 38 47 49 50 53 55 56 57 68 72 73 75 76 77 79 80 81 96 97 100 103 107 118 121 124 135
Primary Contact: Timothy P. Menton, Administrator
CFO: Dale E. Hocking, Chief Financial Officer
CMO: Daniel Carlson, M.D., President Medical Staff
CIO: Nancy Vester, Vice President and Chief Information Officer
CHR: Darlene Stone, Vice President Human Resources
Web address: www.tvrh.org
Control: Other not–for–profit (including NFP Corporation) **Service:** General Medical and Surgical

Staffed Beds: 72 **Admissions:** 5744 **Census:** 67 **Outpatient Visits:** 37563 **Births:** 0 **Total Expense ($000):** 54220 **Payroll Expense ($000):** 22137 **Personnel:** 602

TITUSVILLE—Brevard County

★ **PARRISH MEDICAL CENTER (100028)**, 951 North Washington Avenue, Zip 32796–2194; tel. 321/268–6111 **A**1 2 10 **F**3 11 13 15 18 20 24 25 26 33 38 43 44 51 52 55 56 57 59 61 68 72 73 74 76 77 79 81 82 84 86 96 100 103 104 105 106 107 116 118 119 120 121 124 135 136 137
Primary Contact: George Mikitarian, Jr., Chief Executive Officer
CFO: Timothy K. Skeldon, Senior Vice President and Chief Financial Officer
CHR: Roberta Chaildin, Manager Human Resources
Web address: www.parrishmed.com
Control: Hospital district or authority, Government, nonfederal **Service:** General Medical and Surgical

Staffed Beds: 210 **Admissions:** 8606 **Census:** 104 **Births:** 885 **Total Expense ($000):** 140894 **Payroll Expense ($000):** 45213

VENICE—Sarasota County

☐ **VENICE REGIONAL MEDICAL CENTER (100070)**, 540 The Rialto, Zip 34285–2900; tel. 941/485–7711, (Total facility includes 120 beds in nursing home–type unit) (Nonreporting) **A**1 2 9 10 **S** Health Management Associates
Primary Contact: Melody Trimble, Chief Executive Officer
COO: Darcey O'Brien, Chief Operating Officer
CFO: Fred Ashworth, Chief Financial Officer
CHR: Dana Wheeler, Director Human Resources
Web address: www.veniceregional.com
Control: Other not–for–profit (including NFP Corporation) **Service:** General Medical and Surgical

Staffed Beds: 394

VERO BEACH—Indian River County

★ **HEALTHSOUTH TREASURE COAST REHABILITATION HOSPITAL (103032)**, 1600 37th Street, Zip 32960–6549; tel. 772/778–2100, (Nonreporting) **A**1 9 10 **S** HEALTHSOUTH Corporation
Primary Contact: Patricia Parden, Chief Executive Officer
CFO: Kevin Hardy, Chief Financial Officer
CMO: Jimmy Wayne Lockhart, M.D., Medical Director
CHR: Barbara Papagni, Director Human Resources
Web address: www.healthsouthtreasurecoast.com
Control: Corporation, Investor–owned, for–profit **Service:** Rehabilitation

Staffed Beds: 90

★ **INDIAN RIVER MEDICAL CENTER (100105)**, (Formerly Indian River Memorial Hospital), 1000 36th Street, Zip 32960–6592; tel. 772/567–4311, (Total facility includes 35 beds in nursing home–type unit) **A**1 2 9 10 **F**3 11 12 13 15 17 18 20 22 24 25 26 27 30 31 32 33 35 38 41 43 44 49 50 51 55 56 57 58 59 60 62 68 72 73 74 75 76 77 78 79 80 81 82 84 86 87 88 89 90 91 92 93 94 96 97 98 100 102 103 106 107 108 109 111 112 117 118 119 120 121 124 135 136 137 **P**6 8
Primary Contact: Jeffrey L. Susi, President and Chief Executive Officer
COO: W. Carl Martin, Senior Vice President and Chief Operating Officer
CFO: Greg Gardner, Senior Vice President and Chief Financial Officer
CHR: Barbara Horne, R.N., Vice President and Chief Human Resource Development Officer
Web address: www.irmc.cc
Control: Other not–for–profit (including NFP Corporation) **Service:** General Medical and Surgical

Staffed Beds: 265 **Admissions:** 15143 **Census:** 216 **Outpatient Visits:** 133038 **Births:** 1298 **Total Expense ($000):** 170094 **Payroll Expense ($000):** 73808 **Personnel:** 1372

WAUCHULA—Hardee County

★ **FLORIDA HOSPITAL WAUCHULA (101300)**, 533 West Carlton Street, Zip 33873; tel. 863/773–3101, (Nonreporting) **A**1 9 10 18 **S** Adventist Health System Sunbelt Health Care Corporation
Primary Contact: Linda Adler, Administrator
COO: Isaac Palmer, Chief Executive Officer
CFO: Todd Goodman, Vice President and Chief Financial Officer
CHR: Douglas Harcombe, Director Human Resources
Web address: www.flhosp–heartland.org/Facilities/Wauchula.htm
Control: Church–operated, Nongovernment, not–for profit **Service:** General Medical and Surgical

Staffed Beds: 25

WEST PALM BEACH—Palm Beach County

CHILDREN'S HOSPITAL AT ST. MARY'S MEDICAL CENTER See St. Mary's Medical Center

★ ○ **COLUMBIA HOSPITAL (100234)**, 2201 45th Street, Zip 33407–2069; tel. 561/842–6141 **A**1 9 10 11 12 13 **F**3 8 15 25 30 31 32 33 36 38 43 44 49 50 51 54 57 59 60 62 68 72 73 75 76 77 79 80 86 87 88 89 90 91 92 93 94 95 96 97 100 102 107 112 118 119 135 136 137 **S** HCA
Primary Contact: Valerie A. Jackson, Chief Executive Officer
COO: Suzanne Beauvoir, Chief Operating Officer
CFO: Oon Soo Ung, Chief Financial Officer
CMO: Martin Frisosky, M.D., Chief of Staff
CIO: Martha Stinson, Director
CHR: Donna Boyle, Director
Web address: www.columbiahospital.com
Control: Corporation, Investor–owned, for–profit **Service:** General Medical and Surgical

Staffed Beds: 250 **Admissions:** 9186 **Census:** 119 **Outpatient Visits:** 40520 **Births:** 0 **Total Expense ($000):** 68478 **Payroll Expense ($000):** 27106 **Personnel:** 476

★ **GOOD SAMARITAN MEDICAL CENTER (100287)**, Flagler Drive at Palm Beach Lakes Boulevard, Zip 33401–3499; tel. 561/655–5511, (Nonreporting) **A**1 2 9 10 **S** TENET Healthcare Corporation
Primary Contact: Mark Nosacka, Chief Executive Officer
COO: Mary T. Bazzicalupo, Chief Operating Officer
CFO: Oscar J. Fernandez, Chief Financial Officer
CIO: Candace Helms, Director Information Services
CHR: Nancy Bentley, Director Human Resources
Web address: www.goodsamaritanmc.com
Control: Corporation, Investor–owned, for–profit **Service:** General Medical and Surgical

Staffed Beds: 174

HOSPICE OF PALM BEACH COUNTY, 5300 East Avenue, Zip 33407–2352; tel. 561/848–5200, (Nonreporting)
Primary Contact: David Fielding, Chief Executive Officer
Web address: www.hpbc.com
Control: Other not–for–profit (including NFP Corporation) **Service:** Other specialty

Staffed Beds: 24

Hospital, Medicare Provider Number, Address, Telephone, Approval, Facility, and Physician Codes, Health Care System

★ American Hospital Association (AHA) membership
☐ The Joint Commission accreditation
○ American Osteopathic Association (AOA) accreditation
△ Commission on Accreditation of Rehabilitation Facilities (CARF) accreditation

FL

OAKWOOD CENTER OF THE PALM BEACHES, INC. (104008), 1041 45th Street, Zip 33407–2494; tel. 561/383–8000, (Nonreporting) **A**9 10
Primary Contact: Linda De Piano, Ph.D., Chief Executive Officer
CFO: Pat Priola, Chief Financial Officer
CMO: Suresh Rajpara, M.D., Chief Medical Officer
CIO: Michael DiBartolo, Director Information Services
CHR: Russ Bowers, Director Human Resources
Web address: www.oakwoodcenter.org
Control: Other not–for–profit (including NFP Corporation) **Service:** Psychiatric

Staffed Beds: 44

★ △ **ST. MARY'S MEDICAL CENTER (100288)**, 901 45th Street, Zip 33407–2495, Mailing Address: P.O. Box 24620, Zip 33416–4620; tel. 561/844–6300, (Includes CHILDREN'S HOSPITAL AT ST. MARY'S MEDICAL CENTER, 901 45th Street, Zip 33407; tel. 561/844–6300) **A**1 7 9 10 **F**3 6 7 8 11 13 15 18 25 26 27 30 31 32 33 37 38 40 45 46 49 50 51 53 55 56 57 58 59 62 63 68 70 72 73 74 75 76 77 79 80 81 82 83 84 85 86 88 90 91 92 95 96 97 98 99 100 102 107 108 109 114 119 120 121 124 135 137 **P**6 7 **S** TENET Healthcare Corporation
Primary Contact: Davide M. Carbone, Chief Executive Officer
COO: G. Scott Manis, Chief Operating Officer
CFO: Tom Schlemmer, Chief Financial Officer
CIO: Rich Avato, Director
CHR: Sandy Wyant, Director Human Resources
Web address: www.stmarysmc.com
Control: Corporation, Investor–owned, for–profit **Service:** General Medical and Surgical

Staffed Beds: 463 **Admissions:** 17024 **Census:** 283 **Outpatient Visits:** 103595 **Births:** 4020 **Total Expense ($000):** 203836 **Payroll Expense ($000):** 88592 **Personnel:** 1397

★ △ **VETERANS AFFAIRS MEDICAL CENTER**, 7305 North Military Trail, Zip 33410–6400; tel. 561/422–8262, (Total facility includes 98 beds in nursing home–type unit) (Nonreporting) **A**1 7 **S** Department of Veterans Affairs
Primary Contact: Charleen R. Szabo, FACHE, Director
CFO: Randall Sommer, Chief Business Office
CIO: Karen Gabaldon, Chief Management Information Systems
Web address: www.va.gov/sta/guide/home.asp
Control: Veterans Affairs, Government, federal **Service:** General Medical and Surgical

Staffed Beds: 231

FL

□ ○ **WELLINGTON REGIONAL MEDICAL CENTER (100275)**, 10101 Forest Hill Boulevard, Zip 33414–6199; tel. 561/798–8500, (Nonreporting) **A**1 2 9 10 11 12 13 **S** Universal Health Services, Inc.
Primary Contact: Kevin DiLallo, Chief Executive Officer and Managing Director
CFO: Woody White, Chief Financial Officer
CMO: Gordon Johnson, M.D., Chief of Staff
CIO: Pierre Bergeron, Director Information Services
CHR: Mary Jo Garski, Director Human Resources
Web address: www.wellingtonregional.com
Control: Corporation, Investor–owned, for–profit **Service:** General Medical and Surgical

Staffed Beds: 108

WESTON—Broward County

★ **CLEVELAND CLINIC FLORIDA (100289)**, 3100 Weston Road, Zip 33331–3602; tel. 954/689–5000 **A**1 3 5 9 10 **F**3 8 12 15 18 20 22 24 25 26 27 30 31 32 33 34 35 38 43 46 47 49 50 54 55 56 57 58 59 60 62 63 66 68 72 73 75 76 77 79 80 81 82 86 87 90 91 96 97 99 100 102 103 104 105 107 113 114 116 118 119 120 121 124 135 136 137 **S** Cleveland Clinic Health System
Primary Contact: Bernardo Fernandez, M.D., Chief Executive Officer
COO: Marilyn Sargeant, Chief Operating Officer
CFO: Scott Campbell, Chief Financial Officer
CMO: Juan Nogueras, Chief of Staff
CIO: John Santangelo, Director Information Technology
CHR: Paula Adamson, Manager Human Resources
Web address: www.clevelandclinic.org/florida
Control: Other not–for–profit (including NFP Corporation) **Service:** General Medical and Surgical

Staffed Beds: 150 **Admissions:** 9551 **Census:** 107 **Outpatient Visits:** 29953 **Births:** 0 **Total Expense ($000):** 121013 **Payroll Expense ($000):** 44988 **Personnel:** 1483

WILLISTON—Levy County

NATURE COAST REGIONAL HOSPITAL (100139), 125 S.W. Seventh Street, Zip 32696–2403; tel. 352/528–2801 **A**9 10 **F**3 25 30 31 33 38 50 53 55 56 57 62 66 75 82 84 86 87 96 97 107 117 119 120 122 135 **P**4 **S** Cypress Health Systems
Primary Contact: Kim B. Bird, Administrator
COO: Alan Bird, Administrator
CFO: Barbara Miller, Manager Business Office
CMO: Jeremie Young, M.D., Chief of Staff
CHR: Karla Dass, Director Human Resources
Web address: www.cypress–of–fl.com
Control: Corporation, Investor–owned, for–profit **Service:** General Medical and Surgical

Staffed Beds: 40 **Admissions:** 1212 **Census:** 11 **Outpatient Visits:** 11736 **Births:** 0 **Total Expense ($000):** 5669 **Payroll Expense ($000):** 1935 **Personnel:** 52

WINTER HAVEN—Polk County

★ △ **WINTER HAVEN HOSPITAL (100052)**, 200 Avenue F. N.E., Zip 33881–4193; tel. 863/293–1121 **A**1 7 9 10 **F**3 8 11 13 14 15 17 18 20 22 24 25 26 27 30 31 32 34 38 43 44 55 56 57 58 62 66 68 70 71 72 73 75 76 77 79 80 81 82 85 86 88 90 91 92 93 94 96 97 100 102 106 107 109 111 113 119 121 124 133 135 136 137 **P**6
Primary Contact: Lance W. Anastasio, President
CFO: David MacDougall, Vice President Finance
CMO: Charles C. Inman, M.D., President Medical Staff
CIO: Pat Mongoven, Director Information Systems
Web address: www.winterhavenhospital.org
Control: Other not–for–profit (including NFP Corporation) **Service:** General Medical and Surgical

Staffed Beds: 519 **Admissions:** 16647 **Census:** 215 **Outpatient Visits:** 308414 **Births:** 1942 **Total Expense ($000):** 219576 **Payroll Expense ($000):** 105432 **Personnel:** 2444

WINTER PARK—Orange County

WINTER PARK MEMORIAL HOSPITAL See Florida Hospital, Orlando

ZEPHYRHILLS—Pasco County

★ **FLORIDA HOSPITAL ZEPHYRHILLS (100046)**, 7050 Gall Boulevard, Zip 33541–1399; tel. 813/788–0411, (Nonreporting) **A**1 5 9 10 **S** Adventist Health System Sunbelt Health Care Corporation
Primary Contact: John R. Harding, President and Chief Executive Officer
COO: Kevan Metcalfe, Chief Administrative Officer
CFO: Donald E. Welch, Chief Financial Officer
CMO: William Sangster, M.D., Chief of Staff
CIO: Kelley Sasser, Director Information Systems
CHR: Sylvia Seals–Brown, Vice President Human Resources
Web address: www.fhzep.org
Control: Church–operated, Nongovernment, not–for profit **Service:** General Medical and Surgical

Staffed Beds: 154

 Many Facility Codes have changed. Please refer to the AHA Guide Code Chart.

GEORGIA

ADEL—Cook County

☐ **MEMORIAL HOSPITAL OF ADEL (110101)**, 706 North Parrish Avenue, Zip 31620–0677; tel. 229/896–8000, (Total facility includes 95 beds in nursing home–type unit) (Nonreporting) **A**1 9 10 **S** Sunlink Health Systems
Primary Contact: William Hawley, Chief Executive Officer
COO: Kim Wills, Chief Operating Officer
CFO: John Jeter, Chief Financial Officer
CMO: Thomas Fausett, M.D., Chief of Staff
CIO: Barry Medley, Director Information Systems
CHR: Shirley Padgett, Director Human Resources
Web address: www.sunlinkhealth.com
Control: Corporation, Investor–owned, for–profit **Service:** General Medical and Surgical

Staffed Beds: 155

ALBANY—Dougherty County

★☐ **PALMYRA MEDICAL CENTERS (110163)**, 2000 Palmyra Road, Zip 31702–1908, Mailing Address: P.O. Box 1908, Zip 31702–1908; tel. 229/434–2000 **A**1 9 10 **F**3 12 17 25 30 31 32 38 40 43 46 51 54 55 56 59 62 68 72 73 75 77 79 85 86 96 100 102 107 119 120 121 135 137 **P**5 **S** HCA
Primary Contact: Bud Wethington, Chief Executive Officer
COO: David Nicely, Chief Operating Officer
CFO: Karen Hayes, Chief Financial Officer
Web address: www.palmyramedicalcenters.com
Control: Corporation, Investor–owned, for–profit **Service:** General Medical and Surgical

Staffed Beds: 170 **Admissions:** 3867 **Census:** 65 **Outpatient Visits:** 48997 **Births:** 0 **Total Expense ($000):** 59240 **Payroll Expense ($000):** 21466 **Personnel:** 291

★☐ **PHOEBE PUTNEY MEMORIAL HOSPITAL (110007)**, 417 Third Avenue, Zip 31701–1828, Mailing Address: P.O. Box 1828, Zip 31703–1828; tel. 229/883–1800 **A**1 2 3 5 9 10 **F**3 5 7 11 13 15 17 18 20 22 24 25 26 27 30 31 32 33 36 38 41 42 43 44 46 49 50 51 52 53 54 55 56 57 58 59 61 62 66 68 69 70 71 72 73 74 75 76 77 79 80 81 82 84 85 86 87 88 90 91 92 93 94 95 96 97 99 100 102 106 107 108 109 111 115 118 119 120 121 122 123 124 125 132 133 135 136 137 **P**1 6 7 **S** Phoebe Putney Health System
Primary Contact: Joel Wernick, President and Chief Executive Officer
COO: Jim Hobson, Executive Vice President and Chief Operating Officer
CFO: Kerry Loudermilk, Senior Vice President and Chief Financial Officer
CMO: Douglas Patten, M.D., Director Medical Affairs
CIO: Jesse Diaz, Chief Information Officer
CHR: Dave Baranski, Vice President Human Resources
Web address: www.phoebeputney.com
Control: Other not–for–profit (including NFP Corporation) **Service:** General Medical and Surgical

Staffed Beds: 439 **Admissions:** 20245 **Census:** 308 **Outpatient Visits:** 788335 **Births:** 3264 **Total Expense ($000):** 405775 **Payroll Expense ($000):** 137066 **Personnel:** 3087

ALMA—Bacon County

★☐ **BACON COUNTY HOSPITAL AND HEALTH SYSTEM (111327)**, 302 South Wayne Street, Zip 31510–2997, Mailing Address: P.O. Drawer 1987, Zip 31510–1987; tel. 912/632–8961, (Total facility includes 88 beds in nursing home–type unit) (Nonreporting) **A**1 9 10 18
Primary Contact: Cindy R. Turner, Chief Executive Officer
COO: Cindy R. Turner, Chief Executive Officer
CFO: Harry Bennett, Chief Financial Officer
CMO: Lou Ellen Hutcheson, M.D., Chief of Staff
CHR: Jackie Lewis, Director Human Resources
Web address: www.baconcountyhospital.com
Control: Other not–for–profit (including NFP Corporation) **Service:** General Medical and Surgical

Staffed Beds: 113

AMERICUS—Sumter County

★☐ △ **SUMTER REGIONAL HOSPITAL (110044)**, 1048 East Forsyth Street, Zip 31709; tel. 229/924–6011, (Nonreporting) **A**1 2 7 9 10
Primary Contact: David H. Seagraves, President and Chief Executive Officer
COO: Stephen J. Machen, Senior Vice President and Chief Operations Officer
CFO: Troy Hammett, Vice President Finance and Chief Financial Officer
CMO: Gatewood Dudley, M.D., Vice President Medical Staff Services
Web address: www.sumterregional.org/
Control: City–County, Government, nonfederal **Service:** General Medical and Surgical

Staffed Beds: 76

ARLINGTON—Calhoun County

CALHOUN MEMORIAL HOSPITAL (111309), 209 Academy and Carswell Streets, Zip 31713, Mailing Address: Drawer R, Zip 31713; tel. 229/725–4272, (Nonreporting) **A**9 10 18
Primary Contact: Peggy Pierce, Administrator
Control: Hospital district or authority, Government, nonfederal **Service:** General Medical and Surgical

Staffed Beds: 25

ATHENS—Clarke County

★☐ **ATHENS REGIONAL MEDICAL CENTER (110074)**, 1199 Prince Avenue, Zip 30606–2793; tel. 706/475–7000 **A**1 2 9 10 **F**7 8 11 13 15 17 18 20 22 24 25 26 27 33 34 38 44 45 46 51 53 54 55 56 57 59 61 62 66 68 70 71 72 74 75 76 77 78 79 80 81 82 84 86 88 93 95 96 97 99 100 104 105 107 112 118 119 120 121 124 133 134 135 136 137
Primary Contact: John A. Drew, President and Chief Executive Officer
COO: Gary L. Phelps, Senior Vice President and Chief Operating Officer
CFO: W. Larry Webb, Senior Vice President and Chief Financial Officer
CMO: Stephen K. Lucas, M.D., Senior Vice President and Chief Medical Officer
CIO: Tim Penning, Vice President and Chief Information Officer
CHR: Kevin Thigpen, Vice President Human Resources
Web address: www.armc.org
Control: Other not–for–profit (including NFP Corporation) **Service:** General Medical and Surgical

Staffed Beds: 315 **Admissions:** 18326 **Census:** 218 **Births:** 2684 **Personnel:** 2400

★☐ △ **ST. MARY'S HEALTH CARE SYSTEM (110006)**, 1230 Baxter Street, Zip 30606–3791; tel. 706/389–3000, (Nonreporting) **A**1 7 9 10 **S** Catholic Health East
Primary Contact: Thomas E. Fitz, Jr., FACHE, President and Chief Executive Officer
COO: Brenda Duggar, Senior Vice President Patient Care Services
CFO: Marty Hutson, Chief Financial Officer
CIO: Kerry Vaughn, Director Information Services
CHR: Jeff English, Vice President Human Resources
Web address: www.stmarysathens.com
Control: Other not–for–profit (including NFP Corporation) **Service:** General Medical and Surgical

Staffed Beds: 188

ATLANTA—Fulton and De Kalb Counties

☐ **ANCHOR HOSPITAL (114032)**, 5454 Yorktowne Drive, Zip 30349–5305; tel. 770/991–6044, (Nonreporting) **A**1 9 10 **S** Universal Health Services, Inc.
Primary Contact: Jennifer Morgan, Chief Executive Officer and Managing Director
COO: Jennifer Morgan, Chief Executive Officer and Managing Director
CMO: Joel Kirson, M.D., Medical Director
Web address: www.anchorhospital.com
Control: Corporation, Investor–owned, for–profit **Service:** Alcoholism and other chemical dependency

Staffed Beds: 74

GA

Hospital, Medicare Provider Number, Address, Telephone, Approval, Facility, and Physician Codes, Health Care System

★ American Hospital Association (AHA) membership
☐ The Joint Commission accreditation
○ American Osteopathic Association (AOA) accreditation
△ Commission on Accreditation of Rehabilitation Facilities (CARF) accreditation

★ **ATLANTA MEDICAL CENTER (110115)**, 303 Parkway Drive N.E., Zip 30312–1212; tel. 404/265–4000 **A**1 2 3 5 8 9 10 **F**11 12 13 15 17 18 20 22 24 25 26 27 30 32 33 35 36 38 40 41 46 50 51 52 53 54 55 56 57 59 60 62 63 64 66 68 70 71 72 73 74 75 76 77 79 80 81 82 85 86 87 88 90 91 92 93 94 96 97 100 102 107 109 118 119 121 133 135 136 137 **P**8
S TENET Healthcare Corporation
Primary Contact: William T. Moore, Chief Executive Officer
COO: William J. Masterton, Chief Operating Officer
CFO: Lisa Napier, Chief Financial Officer
CMO: Steven Saltzman, M.D., Senior Vice President and Medical Director
CIO: Maryland McCarty, Director Information Systems
CHR: Troy Bond, Chief Human Resources Officer
Web address: www.atlantamedcenter.com
Control: Corporation, Investor–owned, for–profit **Service:** General Medical and Surgical

Staffed Beds: 403 **Admissions:** 15130 **Census:** 248 **Outpatient Visits:** 76438 **Births:** 4090 **Total Expense ($000):** 237828 **Payroll Expense ($000):** 85805 **Personnel:** 1509

□ △ **CHILDREN'S HEALTHCARE OF ATLANTA (113300)**, 1600 Tullie Circle, N.E., Zip 30329–2303; tel. 404/325–6000, (Includes CHILDREN'S HEALTHCARE OF ATLANTA AT EGLESTON; CHILDREN'S HEALTHCARE OF ATLANTA AT SCOTTISH RITE, 1001 Johnson Ferry Road N.E., Zip 30342–1600; tel. 404/256–5252) **A**1 3 5 7 8 9 10 **F**3 7 8 11 12 17 19 21 23 25 26 27 28 32 33 35 37 38 40 41 43 46 50 53 55 56 57 58 59 60 62 63 66 70 72 73 75 76 77 78 79 80 81 82 83 84 85 86 87 90 96 97 100 101 102 103 106 107 114 118 119 120 121 125 126 127 128 130 133 135 137 **P**8
Primary Contact: James E. Tally, Ph.D., President and Chief Executive Officer
COO: Donna Hyland, Chief Operating Officer
CFO: Ruth Fowler, Senior Vice President Finance and Chief Financial Officer
CMO: Jay Berkelhamer, M.D., Senior Vice President Medical Affairs
CIO: Praveen Chopra, Chief Information and Supply Chain Officer
CHR: Linda Matzigkeit, Senior Vice President Human Resources
Web address: www.choa.org
Control: Other not–for–profit (including NFP Corporation) **Service:** Children's general

Staffed Beds: 455 **Admissions:** 22569 **Census:** 373 **Outpatient Visits:** 476018 **Births:** 0 **Total Expense ($000):** 706165 **Payroll Expense ($000):** 336478 **Personnel:** 6696

★ **EMORY CRAWFORD LONG HOSPITAL (110078)**, 550 Peachtree Street N.E., Zip 30308; tel. 404/686–4411 **A**1 2 3 5 8 9 10 **F**3 11 12 13 15 17 18 20 22 24 25 26 27 30 32 33 36 38 41 43 44 45 46 50 51 53 55 56 57 58 59 60 62 63 66 68 70 72 73 74 76 77 78 79 80 81 82 86 90 92 94 96 97 99 100 102 104 106 107 108 109 111 112 113 114 119 120 121 124 135 136 137 **S** Emory Healthcare
Primary Contact: John T. Fox, Chief Executive Officer
CFO: Mark Aycock, Chief Financial Officer
CMO: Jay Steinberg, M.D., Chief Medical Officer
CIO: Debra Cantrell, Chief Information Officer
CHR: Margaret A. Bloomquist, Chief Human Resources
Web address: www.emoryhealthcare.org
Control: Other not–for–profit (including NFP Corporation) **Service:** General Medical and Surgical

Staffed Beds: 439 **Admissions:** 22775 **Census:** 323 **Outpatient Visits:** 157138 **Births:** 4218 **Total Expense ($000):** 398740 **Payroll Expense ($000):** 131289 **Personnel:** 2431

GA

★ △ **EMORY UNIVERSITY HOSPITAL (110010)**, 1364 Clifton Road N.E., Zip 30322–1102; tel. 404/712–2000 **A**1 2 3 5 7 8 9 10 **F**3 11 12 15 17 18 20 22 24 25 26 27 32 33 36 38 41 43 44 45 46 47 49 50 55 56 57 58 59 60 62 63 66 68 72 73 75 76 77 79 80 81 82 85 86 88 89 90 91 92 93 94 96 97 99 100 102 103 104 105 106 107 108 109 111 112 114 119 120 121 124 125 126 127 128 129 130 131 135 136 137 **S** Emory Healthcare
Primary Contact: John T. Fox, Chief Executive Officer
COO: Robert J. Bachman, Chief Operating Officer
CFO: Mark Aycock, Chief Financial Officer
CMO: Ira Horowitz, M.D., Chief Medical Officer
CIO: Dedra Cantrell, Chief Information Officer
CHR: Margaret A. Bloomquist, Assistant Administrator Human Resources
Web address: www.emoryhealthcare.org
Control: Other not–for–profit (including NFP Corporation) **Service:** General Medical and Surgical

Staffed Beds: 548 **Admissions:** 23494 **Census:** 433 **Outpatient Visits:** 81919 **Births:** 0 **Total Expense ($000):** 523163 **Payroll Expense ($000):** 177876 **Personnel:** 3113

★ **GRADY MEMORIAL HOSPITAL (110079)**, 80 Jesse Hill Jr. Drive S.E., Zip 30303, Mailing Address: P.O. Box 26189, Zip 30303–3801; tel. 404/616–4307, (Total facility includes 260 beds in nursing home–type unit) (Nonreporting) **A**1 3 5 8 9 10
Primary Contact: Pamela S. Stephenson, President and Chief Executive Officer
COO: Craig Tindall, Interim Executive Vice President and Chief Operating Officer
CFO: Michael D. Ayres, Chief Financial Officer
CMO: Curtis Lewis, M.D., Chief of Staff
CHR: Michael Black, Vice President Human Resources
Web address: www.gradyhealthsystem.org
Control: Hospital district or authority, Government, nonfederal **Service:** General Medical and Surgical

Staffed Beds: 927

HILLSIDE HOSPITAL, 690 Courtney Drive N.E., Zip 30306–0206, Mailing Address: P.O. Box 8247, Zip 31106–0247; tel. 404/875–4551, (Nonreporting)
Primary Contact: Teresa Stoker, Chief Executive Officer
CFO: Harry Frazer, Chief Financial Officer
CMO: Edward Gotlieb, M.D., Medical Director
CHR: Stacey Gilber, Manager Human Resources
Web address: www.hside.org
Control: Other not–for–profit (including NFP Corporation) **Service:** Children's hospital psychiatric

Staffed Beds: 74

□ **KINDRED HOSPITAL–ATLANTA (112004)**, 705 Juniper Street N.E., Zip 30365–2500; tel. 404/873–2871, (Nonreporting) **A**1 9 10
S Kindred Healthcare
Primary Contact: Tim E. Merritt, Chief Executive Officer
CFO: Shayne Olmstead, Controller
CMO: David DeRuyter, M.D., President Medical Staff
Web address: www.kindredhealthcare.com
Control: Partnership, Investor–owned, for–profit **Service:** Long–Term Acute Care hospital

Staffed Beds: 70

★ **NORTHSIDE HOSPITAL (110161)**, 1000 Johnson Ferry Road N.E., Zip 30342–1611; tel. 404/851–8000 **A**1 2 9 10 **F**3 5 11 12 13 15 17 18 24 25 26 27 30 31 32 33 38 41 43 48 49 50 51 53 55 56 57 58 59 62 66 68 70 71 72 73 74 75 76 77 78 79 80 81 82 86 90 94 95 96 97 100 102 106 107 108 109 111 116 118 119 121 124 125 134 135 136 **P**6
Primary Contact: Robert Quattrocchi, President and Chief Executive Officer
CFO: Debbie Mitcham, Chief Financial Officer
CIO: Tina Wakim, Vice President Operations
CHR: Dwight Hill, Vice President Human Resources
Web address: www.northside.com
Control: Other not–for–profit (including NFP Corporation) **Service:** General Medical and Surgical

Staffed Beds: 567 **Admissions:** 40080 **Census:** 463 **Outpatient Visits:** 381553 **Births:** 17994 **Total Expense ($000):** 627168 **Payroll Expense ($000):** 246596 **Personnel:** 4566

□ **PEACHFORD BEHAVIORAL HEALTH SYSTEM (114010)**, 2151 Peachford Road, Zip 30338–6599; tel. 770/455–3200, (Nonreporting) **A**1 9 10 **S** Universal Health Services, Inc.
Primary Contact: Matthew Crouch, Chief Executive Officer and Managing Director
COO: Sharon Stackhouse, Assistant Administrator and Director Risk Management
CFO: April Hughes, Chief Financial Officer
CMO: Asaf Aleem, M.D., Medical Director
CHR: Clay Boyles, Director Human Resources
Web address: www.peachfordhospital.com
Control: Corporation, Investor–owned, for–profit **Service:** Psychiatric

Staffed Beds: 224

★ △ **PIEDMONT HOSPITAL (110083)**, 1968 Peachtree Road N.W., Zip 30309–1231; tel. 404/605–5000 **A**1 2 3 5 7 9 10 **F**3 11 13 15 17 18 20 22 24 25 26 27 30 31 32 33 38 42 43 44 46 47 48 49 50 51 52 53 54 55 56 57 58 59 62 63 66 68 70 71 72 73 74 75 76 77 79 80 81 82 85 86 96 97 99 100 102 103 104 105 106 107 108 109 111 112 114 118 119 120 121 124 127 128 131 132 135 136 137 **S** Piedmont Healthcare
Primary Contact: Robert W. Maynard, President and Chief Executive Officer
COO: Gregory A. Hurst, Executive Vice President and Chief Operating Officer
CFO: Thomas Arnold, Chief Financial Officer
CMO: Steve Taylor, M.D., Executive Vice President and Chief Medical Officer
CIO: John Hilliard, Vice President Information Systems
CHR: Joseph W. Herzberg, Vice President Human Resources
Web address: www.piedmonthospital.org
Control: Other not–for–profit (including NFP Corporation) **Service:** General Medical and Surgical

Staffed Beds: 441 **Admissions:** 25909 **Census:** 367 **Outpatient Visits:** 261420 **Births:** 3557 **Personnel:** 3576

★ **SAINT JOSEPH'S HOSPITAL OF ATLANTA (110082)**, 5665 Peachtree Dunwoody Road N.E., Zip 30342–1764; tel. 404/851–7001 **A**1 2 9 10 **F**3 11 15 17 18 20 22 24 25 26 27 30 31 32 33 38 41 43 44 46 47 49 50 55 56 57 58 59 60 62 66 68 72 73 75 76 77 79 80 81 82 86 96 97 99 100 102 103 105 107 109 111 112 116 119 121 124 126 134 135 136 137 **P**2 8
S Catholic Health East
Primary Contact: Kirk G. Wilson, President and Chief Executive Officer
COO: Kim Sharkey, Vice President Medicine and Chief Nursing Officer
CFO: Kevin Brenan, Chief Financial Officer
CMO: Paul Scheinberg, Chief of Staff
CIO: Scott Rattray, Vice President and Chief Information Officer
CHR: Audra Farish, Vice President Human Resources
Web address: www.stjosephsatlanta.org
Control: Other not–for–profit (including NFP Corporation) **Service:** General Medical and Surgical

Staffed Beds: 410 **Admissions:** 21647 **Census:** 291 **Outpatient Visits:** 174692 **Births:** 0 **Total Expense ($000):** 340988 **Payroll Expense ($000):** 121061 **Personnel:** 2502

SELECT SPECIALTY HOSPITAL–ATLANTA (112009), 550 Peachtree Street N.E., Zip 30327; tel. 404/350–4623, (Nonreporting) **A**9 10 **S** Select Medical Corporation
Primary Contact: Phil Greenhill, Chief Executive Officer
Web address: www.selectmedicalcorp.com
Control: Corporation, Investor–owned, for–profit **Service:** Long–Term Acute Care hospital

Staffed Beds: 30

□ △ **SHEPHERD CENTER (112003)**, 2020 Peachtree Road N.W., Zip 30309–1465; tel. 404/352–2020, (Nonreporting) **A**1 7 9 10
Primary Contact: Gary R. Ulicny, Ph.D., President and Chief Executive Officer
CFO: Stephen B. Holleman, Chief Financial Officer
CMO: Donald P. Leslie, M.D., Medical Director
CIO: Michael L. Jones, Ph.D., Chief Information Officer
CHR: Betsy Fox, Director Human Resources
Web address: www.shepherd.org
Control: Other not–for–profit (including NFP Corporation) **Service:** Rehabilitation

Staffed Beds: 100

★ **SOUTH FULTON MEDICAL CENTER (110219)**, 1170 Cleveland Avenue, Zip 30344–3665; tel. 404/466–1170, (Total facility includes 28 beds in nursing home–type unit) (Nonreporting) **A**1 2 3 5 9 10 **S** TENET Healthcare Corporation
Primary Contact: James Clements, Chief Executive Officer
COO: Jennifer Eslinger, Chief Operating Officer
CMO: Albert Barrocas, Chief Medical Officer
CHR: Detra Bickerstaff, Chief Human Resources Officer
Web address: www.southfultonmedicalcenter.com
Control: Corporation, Investor–owned, for–profit **Service:** General Medical and Surgical

Staffed Beds: 260

★ **WESLEY WOODS CENTER OF EMORY UNIVERSITY (110203)**, (Multi–Discip Geri Hospital), 1821 Clifton Road N.E., Zip 30329–5102; tel. 404/728–6200, (Total facility includes 210 beds in nursing home–type unit) **A**1 3 5 9 10 **F**1 2 3 6 10 11 25 26 33 36 37 41 43 44 50 53 54 56 57 58 59 62 63 65 66 72 73 75 80 81 82 85 86 87 88 90 91 92 93 94 95 96 107 115 117 118 119 121 132 135 137 **S** Emory Healthcare
Primary Contact: Albert K. Blackwelder, FACHE, Chief Operating Officer
COO: Albert K. Blackwelder, FACHE, Chief Operating Officer
CFO: Mark Aycock, Chief Financial Officer
CIO: Dedra Cantrell, Chief Information Officer
CHR: Dallis Howard, Senior Vice President Human Resources
Web address: www.emory.org
Control: Other not–for–profit (including NFP Corporation) **Service:** Other specialty

Staffed Beds: 344 **Admissions:** 2908 **Census:** 239 **Outpatient Visits:** 37584 **Births:** 0 **Total Expense ($000):** 56458 **Payroll Expense ($000):** 29539 **Personnel:** 570

WESLEY WOODS LONG TERM CARE HOSPITAL (112005), (Multi–Discip Geri Hospital), 1821 Clifton Road N.E., 2nd Floor, Zip 30329, Mailing Address: 1821 Clifton Road N.E., 2nd Floor, Zip 30329; tel. 404/728–6200 **A**10 **F**1 3 6 11 25 26 30 31 32 33 36 37 41 43 50 53 54 56 57 62 65 66 69 72 73 75 80 81 82 85 86 87 88 90 91 92 93 94 95 96 107 117 118 119 121 132 135 137
Primary Contact: William Such, Administrator
CFO: Theodore Saunders, Director Finance
CMO: Gerald W. Staton, M.D., Medical Director
Web address: www.emoryhealthcare.org
Control: Other not–for–profit (including NFP Corporation) **Service:** Other specialty

Staffed Beds: 18 **Admissions:** 207 **Census:** 16 **Outpatient Visits:** 0 **Births:** 0 **Total Expense ($000):** 8782 **Payroll Expense ($000):** 2324 **Personnel:** 570

AUGUSTA—Richmond County

★ **DOCTORS HOSPITAL (110177)**, 3651 Wheeler Road, Zip 30909–6426; tel. 706/651–3232, (Nonreporting) **A**1 5 9 10 **S** HCA
Primary Contact: C. Shayne George, President and Chief Executive Officer
COO: Kenneth Wicker, Chief Operating Officer
CFO: Terence Van Arkel, Chief Financial Officer
CMO: Lee Gray, M.D., Vice President Medical Affairs
CIO: Dona Hornung, Director Information and Technology Services
CHR: Leigh Mangum, Vice President Human Resources
Web address: www.doctors–hospital.net
Control: Corporation, Investor–owned, for–profit **Service:** General Medical and Surgical

Staffed Beds: 242

□ **EAST CENTRAL REGIONAL HOSPITAL (114029)**, 3405 Mike Padgett Highway, Zip 30906–3897; tel. 706/792–7000, (Includes EAST CENTRAL REGIONAL HOSPITAL, 100 Myrtle Boulevard, Gracewood, Zip 30812–1299; tel. 706/790–2011), (Total facility includes 450 beds in nursing home–type unit) **A**1 3 5 9 10 **F**25 30 32 36 37 56 57 62 63 65 73 75 81 82 88 90 91 94 117 119 132 **P**6
Primary Contact: Gail C. Jackson, M.D., Chief Executive Officer
CFO: Terry Tribble, Chief Financial Officer
Web address: www.augustareg.dhr.state.ga.us
Control: State–Government, nonfederal **Service:** Psychiatric

Staffed Beds: 585 **Admissions:** 1738 **Census:** 542 **Outpatient Visits:** 150 **Births:** 0 **Total Expense ($000):** 65141 **Payroll Expense ($000):** 37342 **Personnel:** 1357

★ **MEDICAL COLLEGE OF GEORGIA HEALTH (110034)**, 1120 15th Street, Zip 30912–5000; tel. 706/721–0211 **A**1 2 3 5 8 9 10 12 13 **F**1 2 3 6 11 12 13 14 15 17 18 19 20 21 22 23 24 25 26 27 28 30 31 32 33 34 36 37 38 40 41 43 44 46 48 49 50 51 53 54 55 56 57 58 59 60 62 63 64 65 66 68 70 71 72 73 74 75 76 77 79 80 81 82 83 84 86 87 88 89 90 91 92 93 94 96 97 100 102 104 105 106 107 108 109 111 112 114 118 119 120 121 123 124 125 127 130 131 132 134 135 136 137 **P**3 7
Primary Contact: Donald F. Snell, President and Chief Executive Officer
COO: Patricia Sodomka, FACHE, Senior Vice President Patient and Family Center Care
CFO: Dennis Roemer, Senior Vice President and Chief Financial Officer
CMO: Ralph Caruana, M.D., Senior Vice President and Chief Medical Officer
CIO: Harold Scott, Vice President Information Systems and Chief Information Officer
CHR: William G. Hayes, Vice President Human Resources
Web address: www.mcghealth.org
Control: Other not–for–profit (including NFP Corporation) **Service:** General Medical and Surgical

Staffed Beds: 474 **Admissions:** 19349 **Census:** 310 **Outpatient Visits:** 413677 **Births:** 1673 **Total Expense ($000):** 361359 **Payroll Expense ($000):** 154528 **Personnel:** 2950

□ **SELECT SPECIALTY HOSPITAL (112013)**, 1537 Walton Way, Zip 30901; tel. 706/774–7101, (Nonreporting) **A**1 9 10 **S** Select Medical Corporation
Primary Contact: Brian Davis, Chief Executive Officer
COO: Jeffrey Fenn, Chief Operating Officer
CHR: Terrie Richardson, Coordinator Human Resources
Web address: www.selectmedicalcorp.com
Control: Corporation, Investor–owned, for–profit **Service:** Long–Term Acute Care hospital

Staffed Beds: 30

★ **TRINITY HOSPITAL OF AUGUSTA (110039)**, 2260 Wrightsboro Road, Zip 30904–4726; tel. 706/481–7000, (Nonreporting) **A**1 5 9 10 **S** Community Health Systems, Inc.
Primary Contact: James A. Cruickshank, Chief Executive Officer
COO: Janie Sinacore–Jaberg, R.N., MS, FACHE, Chief Operating Officer
CFO: Eric Lachance, Interim Chief Financial Officer
CMO: Danny Newman, M.D., Chief of Staff
CIO: Charlotte Choate, Director Information Systems
CHR: Connie Martin, Director Human Resources
Web address: www.trinityofaugusta.com
Control: Corporation, Investor–owned, for–profit **Service:** General Medical and Surgical

Staffed Beds: 105

★ **UNIVERSITY HEALTH CARE SYSTEM (110028)**, 1350 Walton Way, Zip 30901–2629; tel. 706/722–9011 **A**1 2 3 5 9 10 **F**3 12 13 15 17 18 20 22 24 25 26 27 28 30 31 32 33 35 36 38 41 43 44 45 48 49 50 52 53 54 55 56 57 59 60 61 62 64 66 68 70 71 72 73 74 75 76 77 78 79 80 81 82 84 86 87 90 96 97 100 102 103 104 106 107 118 119 120 121 123 124 133 135 136 137 **P**8
Primary Contact: J. Larry Read, President and Chief Executive Officer
COO: Jason H. Moore, Chief Operating Officer
CFO: David Belkoski, Chief Financial Officer
CMO: William L. Farr, M.D., Chief Medical Officer
CIO: William Colbert, Chief Information Officer
CHR: Richard J. Roche, Vice President Human Resources
Web address: www.universityhealth.org
Control: Other not–for–profit (including NFP Corporation) **Service:** General Medical and Surgical

Staffed Beds: 510 **Admissions:** 21685 **Census:** 327 **Outpatient Visits:** 296983 **Births:** 3179 **Total Expense ($000):** 352330 **Payroll Expense ($000):** 140109 **Personnel:** 2551

GA

Hospital, Medicare Provider Number, Address, Telephone, Approval, Facility, and Physician Codes, Health Care System

★ American Hospital Association (AHA) membership
□ The Joint Commission accreditation
○ American Osteopathic Association (AOA) accreditation
△ Commission on Accreditation of Rehabilitation Facilities (CARF) accreditation

★ △ **VETERANS AFFAIRS MEDICAL CENTER**, (primary care), 1 Freedom Way, Zip 30904–6285; tel. 706/733–0188, (Total facility includes 132 beds in nursing home–type unit) **A**1 2 3 5 7 8 **F**1 3 4 5 8 12 17 18 20 24 25 26 27 29 33 36 37 38 41 42 43 44 45 46 47 48 49 50 51 52 53 54 55 57 58 59 60 61 62 63 64 66 68 69 72 73 75 76 77 79 80 81 82 85 86 87 88 90 91 92 93 94 95 96 97 100 101 102 107 118 119 121 124 133 135 136 137 **P**6
S Department of Veterans Affairs
Primary Contact: John S. Goldman, Associate Director
CFO: Earline Corder, Chief Fiscal
CMO: Thomas Kiernan, M.D., Chief of Staff
CIO: Susan Lloyd, Chief Health Information Management and Revenue Administration
CHR: Linda Dailey, Acting Chief
Web address: www.va.gov/sta/guide/home.asp
Control: Veterans Affairs, Government, federal **Service:** Other specialty

Staffed Beds: 470 **Admissions:** 7205 **Census:** 270 **Outpatient Visits:** 340916 **Births:** 0 **Personnel:** 1917

☐ △ **WALTON REHABILITATION HOSPITAL (113026)**, 1355 Independence Drive, Zip 30901–1037; tel. 706/724–7746, (Nonreporting) **A**1 3 5 7 9 10
Primary Contact: Dennis B. Skelley, President and Chief Executive Officer
COO: Bob Orsini, Chief Operating Officer
CFO: Mike Harrell, Chief Financial Officer
CMO: Pamela Salazar, M.D., Chief of Staff
CHR: Larry Stroud, Director Human Resources
Web address: www.wrh.org
Control: Other not–for–profit (including NFP Corporation) **Service:** Rehabilitation

Staffed Beds: 58

AUSTELL—Cobb County

★ △ **WELLSTAR COBB HOSPITAL (110143)**, 3950 Austell Road, Zip 30106–1121; tel. 770/732–4000 **A**1 2 7 9 10 **F**3 4 11 12 13 15 17 18 20 22 24 25 26 27 30 31 32 33 35 36 38 41 42 44 46 47 48 49 50 53 55 56 57 60 61 62 64 66 68 70 71 72 73 74 75 76 77 78 79 80 81 82 84 85 86 88 90 91 92 93 96 97 99 100 102 103 106 107 119 121 123 124 135 136 137 **P**1 6 **S** WellStar Health System
Primary Contact: Randy Cook, Senior Vice President and Administrator
CFO: Marsha Burke, Senior Vice President and Chief Financial Officer
CMO: Don Campbell, M.D., Senior Vice President and Chief Medical Officer
CIO: Leigh Cox, Chief Information Officer
CHR: Alma Stanfield, Director Human Resources
Web address: www.wellstar.org
Control: Other not–for–profit (including NFP Corporation) **Service:** General Medical and Surgical

Staffed Beds: 378 **Admissions:** 22491 **Census:** 298 **Outpatient Visits:** 207365 **Births:** 5610 **Personnel:** 2269

GA

BAINBRIDGE—Decatur County

★ **MEMORIAL HOSPITAL AND MANOR (110132)**, 1500 East Shotwell Street, Zip 39819–4256; tel. 229/246–3500, (Total facility includes 107 beds in nursing home–type unit) (Nonreporting) **A**1 9 10
Primary Contact: James G. Peak, Chief Executive Officer
COO: Lee Harris, Assistant Administrator Support Services
CFO: Billy Walker, Chief Financial Officer
CIO: Nelda Moore, Director Data Processing
CHR: Cathy Willis, Director Human Resources
Web address: www.mh–m.org
Control: Hospital district or authority, Government, nonfederal **Service:** General Medical and Surgical

Staffed Beds: 211

BAXLEY—Appling County

★ **APPLING HEALTHCARE SYSTEM (110071)**, 163 East Tollison Street, Zip 31513–2898; tel. 912/367–9841, (Total facility includes 101 beds in nursing home–type unit) (Nonreporting) **A**1 9 10
Primary Contact: Dale Spell, Chief Executive Officer
COO: Dale Spell, Chief Executive Officer
CFO: Greg Jones, Chief Financial Officer
CIO: Brian Snow, Manager Information Systems
Web address: www.appling–hospital.org
Control: Other not–for–profit (including NFP Corporation) **Service:** General Medical and Surgical

Staffed Beds: 140

BLAIRSVILLE—Union County

★ **UNION GENERAL HOSPITAL (110051)**, 214 Hospital Drive, Zip 30512–6538; tel. 706/745–2111, (Total facility includes 150 beds in nursing home–type unit) **A**1 9 10 20 **F**3 7 8 11 13 15 25 26 27 37 38 55 57 65 68 74 75 76 77 79 80 81 84 86 96 97 99 100 102 107 117 119 122 132
Primary Contact: Rebecca T. Dyer, Administrator
COO: Mike Gowder, Assistant Administrator
CFO: Tim Henry, Chief Financial Officer
CMO: Andre Schaeffer, M.D., Chief of Staff
CHR: Kathy Hood, Administrative Assistant
Web address: www.uniongeneralhospital.com
Control: Hospital district or authority, Government, nonfederal **Service:** General Medical and Surgical

Staffed Beds: 195 **Admissions:** 1583 **Census:** 161 **Outpatient Visits:** 48968 **Births:** 311 **Personnel:** 481

BLAKELY—Early County

★ **EARLY MEMORIAL HOSPITAL (111314)**, 11740 Columbia Street, Zip 39823–9604; tel. 229/723–4241, (Total facility includes 127 beds in nursing home–type unit) **A**1 9 10 18 **F**3 7 13 15 25 26 30 31 32 33 38 50 54 55 56 57 62 66 73 74 75 80 81 82 86 92 96 100 107 117 119 121 122 124 132 135 137 **P**6 **S** Archbold Medical Center
Primary Contact: Robin Rau, Administrator
CFO: William H. Sellers, Senior Vice President
Web address: www.archbold.org
Control: Hospital district or authority, Government, nonfederal **Service:** General Medical and Surgical

Staffed Beds: 152 **Admissions:** 504 **Census:** 119 **Outpatient Visits:** 15680 **Births:** 0 **Total Expense ($000):** 14460 **Payroll Expense ($000):** 6672 **Personnel:** 190

BLUE RIDGE—Fannin County

★ **FANNIN REGIONAL HOSPITAL (110189)**, 2855 Old Highway 5, Zip 30513–6248; tel. 706/632–3711 **A**1 9 10 **F**3 11 13 15 24 25 26 30 31 32 33 37 38 43 50 52 54 55 57 62 66 68 73 74 75 77 79 80 81 82 84 86 96 97 100 107 112 118 119 121 122 123 124 135 136 137 **P**6 **S** Community Health Systems, Inc.
Primary Contact: Scott M. Smith, Chief Executive Officer
CFO: Keith Newton, Chief Financial Officer
CHR: Terrasina Ensley, Director Human Resources
Web address: www.fanninregionalhospital.com
Control: Corporation, Investor–owned, for–profit **Service:** General Medical and Surgical

Staffed Beds: 50 **Admissions:** 2608 **Census:** 20 **Outpatient Visits:** 25278 **Births:** 433 **Total Expense ($000):** 27790 **Payroll Expense ($000):** 10359 **Personnel:** 224

BREMEN—Haralson County

★ **HIGGINS GENERAL HOSPITAL (111320)**, 200 Allen Memorial Drive, Zip 30110–2012, Mailing Address: P.O. Box 655, Zip 30110–0655; tel. 770/537–5851, (Nonreporting) **A**1 9 10 18 **S** Tanner Health System
Primary Contact: Michael Alexander, Administrator
CFO: Lee Sherseth, Chief Financial Officer
CIO: Dianne Reed, Director Information Systems
CHR: Vivian Barr, Director Human Resources
Web address: www.tanner.org
Control: Other not–for–profit (including NFP Corporation) **Service:** General Medical and Surgical

Staffed Beds: 25

BRUNSWICK—Glynn County

☐ **SOUTHEAST GEORGIA HEALTH SYSTEM BRUNSWICK CAMPUS (110025)**, 2415 Parkwood Drive, Zip 31520–4252, Mailing Address: P.O. Box 1518, Zip 31521–1518; tel. 912/466–7000, (Nonreporting) **A**1 2 9 10 19 20
S Southeast Georgia Health System
Primary Contact: Gary R. Colberg, FACHE, President and Chief Executive Officer
CFO: Michael D. Scherneck, Executive Vice President and Chief Financial Officer
CMO: T. Wayne Rentz, M.D., Chief of Staff
CIO: Chuck Bumgardner, Director Information Systems
CHR: Patrick Ebri, Ph.D., Vice President Human Resources
Web address: www.sghs.org
Control: City–County, Government, nonfederal **Service:** General Medical and Surgical

Staffed Beds: 273

Many Facility Codes have changed. Please refer to the AHA Guide Code Chart.

CAIRO—Grady County

★ **GRADY GENERAL HOSPITAL (110121)**, 1155 Fifth Street S.E., Zip 39828–0360, Mailing Address: P.O. Box 360, Zip 39828–0360; tel. 229/377–1150 **A**1 9 10 **F**3 11 13 15 24 25 30 31 32 33 38 46 50 55 56 57 62 66 68 73 74 75 77 79 80 81 82 86 92 96 100 107 119 122 124 135 **S** Archbold Medical Center
Primary Contact: LaDon Toole, Administrator
CFO: Bill Sellers, Chief Financial Officer
CIO: William Zimmermann, Chief Information Officer
Web address: www.archbold.org
Control: Hospital district or authority, Government, nonfederal **Service:** General Medical and Surgical

Staffed Beds: 48 **Admissions:** 1602 **Census:** 21 **Outpatient Visits:** 32645 **Births:** 300 **Total Expense ($000):** 15811 **Payroll Expense ($000):** 6996 **Personnel:** 173

CALHOUN—Gordon County

★ ○ **GORDON HOSPITAL (110023)**, 1035 Red Bud Road, Zip 30701–2082, Mailing Address: P.O. Box 12938, Zip 30703–7013; tel. 706/629–2895 **A**1 9 10 11 19 **F**3 7 11 13 15 25 26 27 30 31 33 35 38 43 46 55 57 61 62 68 69 73 74 75 76 77 79 80 81 86 96 97 100 102 107 118 119 124 133 135 136 **P**1 6 **S** Adventist Health System Sunbelt Health Care Corporation
Primary Contact: Carlene Jamerson, President and Chief Executive Officer
CFO: Cory Reeves, Chief Financial Officer
CMO: Will Theus, M.D., Chief of Staff
CHR: Jeni Hasselbrack, Director Human Resources
Web address: www.gordonhospital.com
Control: Church–operated, Nongovernment, not–for profit **Service:** General Medical and Surgical

Staffed Beds: 69 **Admissions:** 3768 **Census:** 41 **Outpatient Visits:** 81698 **Births:** 668 **Total Expense ($000):** 48485 **Payroll Expense ($000):** 22088 **Personnel:** 484

CAMILLA—Mitchell County

★ **MITCHELL COUNTY HOSPITAL (111331)**, 90 Stephens Street, Zip 31730, Mailing Address: P.O. Box 639, Zip 31730–0639; tel. 229/336–5284, (Total facility includes 156 beds in nursing home–type unit) **A**9 10 18 **F**15 25 26 30 31 32 33 38 50 54 55 56 57 62 66 73 75 77 79 80 81 82 86 92 96 100 107 117 119 122 124 135 **P**6 **S** Archbold Medical Center
Primary Contact: Mark E. Kimball, Administrator
CFO: J. William Sellers, Senior Vice President and Chief Financial Officer
CMO: Melvin Hartsfield, M.D., Vice President Medical Affairs
CIO: William Zimmermann, Chief Information Officer
CHR: Vickie County, Coordinator Human Resources
Web address: www.archbold.org
Control: Hospital district or authority, Government, nonfederal **Service:** General Medical and Surgical

Staffed Beds: 181 **Admissions:** 650 **Census:** 171 **Outpatient Visits:** 25831 **Births:** 59 **Total Expense ($000):** 22039 **Payroll Expense ($000):** 9901 **Personnel:** 235

CANTON—Cherokee County

★ **NORTHSIDE HOSPITAL – CHEROKEE (110008)**, 201 Hospital Road, Zip 30114–2408, Mailing Address: P.O. Box 906, Zip 30114–0906; tel. 770/720–5100 **A**1 9 10 **F**3 11 13 15 24 25 26 27 30 31 32 33 38 41 50 53 55 56 57 62 66 68 71 73 74 76 77 79 80 81 82 86 96 97 100 107 118 119 121 135 136 **P**6
Primary Contact: William M. Hayes, Chief Executive Officer
CFO: Steve Hudson, Chief Financial Officer
CMO: Michael Hulse, M.D., Chief of Staff
Web address: www.northside.com
Control: Other not–for–profit (including NFP Corporation) **Service:** General Medical and Surgical

Staffed Beds: 81 **Admissions:** 5030 **Census:** 47 **Outpatient Visits:** 71832 **Births:** 1070 **Total Expense ($000):** 67628 **Payroll Expense ($000):** 27206 **Personnel:** 549

CARROLLTON—Carroll County

★ **TANNER MEDICAL CENTER (110011)**, 705 Dixie Street, Zip 30117–3818; tel. 770/836–9666, (Total facility includes 20 beds in nursing home–type unit) (Nonreporting) **A**1 9 10 **S** Tanner Health System
Primary Contact: Loy M. Howard, President and Chief Executive Officer
COO: Richard L. McConahy, Chief Operating Officer
CFO: Lee Sherseth, Chief Financial Officer
CHR: Vivian Barr, Director Human Resources
Web address: www.tanner.org
Control: Other not–for–profit (including NFP Corporation) **Service:** General Medical and Surgical

Staffed Beds: 176

CARTERSVILLE—Bartow County

★ **CARTERSVILLE MEDICAL CENTER (110030)**, 960 Joe Frank Harris Parkway, Zip 30120–2129, Mailing Address: P.O. Box 200008, Zip 30120–9001; tel. 770/382–1530, (Nonreporting) **A**1 9 10 **S** HCA
Primary Contact: Keith Sandlin, Chief Executive Officer
Web address: www.cartersvillemedical.com
Control: Corporation, Investor–owned, for–profit **Service:** General Medical and Surgical

Staffed Beds: 80

CEDARTOWN—Polk County

★ **POLK MEDICAL CENTER (111330)**, 424 North Main Street, Zip 30125–2698; tel. 770/748–2500 **A**1 9 10 18 **F**3 15 25 30 31 32 38 50 55 56 57 62 66 75 86 93 96 103 107 118 119 120 121 122 135 137 **S** HCA
Primary Contact: Steven C. Hoelscher, Chief Executive Officer
CFO: Jon Riggs, Controller
CHR: Jeanna Smith, Administrative Assistant and Human Resources Officer
Web address: www.polkmedicalcenter.com
Control: Corporation, Investor–owned, for–profit **Service:** General Medical and Surgical

Staffed Beds: 18 **Admissions:** 486 **Census:** 5 **Outpatient Visits:** 35925 **Total Expense ($000):** 13914 **Payroll Expense ($000):** 5216 **Personnel:** 89

CHATSWORTH—Murray County

□ **MURRAY MEDICAL CENTER (110050)**, 707 Old Dalton Ellijay Road, Zip 30705–2060, Mailing Address: P.O. Box 1406, Zip 30705–1406; tel. 706/695–4564 **A**1 9 10 **F**3 8 11 15 25 31 38 46 55 56 57 68 73 75 79 96 100 102 107 119 124 135
Primary Contact: James Hazel, M.D., Chief Executive Officer
CFO: Jana Briley, Financial Services Director
CMO: Robert T. Cook, Chief of Staff
CIO: Cynthia Austin, Manager Health Information and Utilization Management
CHR: Jason Hopkins, Director Human Resources
Web address: www.hamiltonhealth.com/hhcs/
Control: Hospital district or authority, Government, nonfederal **Service:** General Medical and Surgical

Staffed Beds: 36 **Admissions:** 1111 **Census:** 11 **Outpatient Visits:** 39793 **Births:** 0 **Total Expense ($000):** 17289 **Payroll Expense ($000):** 8689 **Personnel:** 155

CLAXTON—Evans County

★ **EVANS MEMORIAL HOSPITAL (110142)**, 200 North River Street, Zip 30417–1659, Mailing Address: P.O. Box 518, Zip 30417–0518; tel. 912/739–5000, (Total facility includes 160 beds in nursing home–type unit) **A**1 9 10 **F**3 15 38 52 55 57 66 73 74 75 77 79 86 96 97 100 103 106 107 117 124 134 135 136
Primary Contact: Martha F. Tatum, Chief Executive Officer
CFO: John Wiggins, Vice President Finance and Chief Financial Officer
CMO: Randy Hawkins, M.D., Chief of Staff
CIO: Steve Schmidt, Director Information Systems
CHR: Gina Waters, Director Human Resources
Web address: www.evansmemorialhospital.org
Control: Other not–for–profit (including NFP Corporation) **Service:** General Medical and Surgical

Staffed Beds: 187 **Admissions:** 2115 **Census:** 165 **Outpatient Visits:** 31610 **Births:** 250 **Total Expense ($000):** 25236 **Payroll Expense ($000):** 13593 **Personnel:** 343

CLAYTON—Rabun County

RABUN COUNTY HOSPITAL (111336), 196 Ridgecrest Circle, Zip 30525–4111; tel. 706/782–4233, (Nonreporting) **A**9 10 18
Primary Contact: Christopher Bonham, Chief Executive Officer
Web address: www.rabunhospital.com
Control: Hospital district or authority, Government, nonfederal **Service:** General Medical and Surgical

Staffed Beds: 25

COCHRAN—Bleckley County

□ **BLECKLEY MEMORIAL HOSPITAL (111302)**, 408 Peacock Street, Zip 31014–1559, Mailing Address: P.O. Box 536, Zip 31014–0536; tel. 478/934–6211, (Nonreporting) **A**1 9 10 18
Primary Contact: Cary Martin, Administrator
Control: Hospital district or authority, Government, nonfederal **Service:** General Medical and Surgical

Staffed Beds: 25

GA

Hospital, Medicare Provider Number, Address, Telephone, Approval, Facility, and Physician Codes, Health Care System
★ American Hospital Association (AHA) membership
□ The Joint Commission accreditation
○ American Osteopathic Association (AOA) accreditation
△ Commission on Accreditation of Rehabilitation Facilities (CARF) accreditation

COLQUITT—Miller County

★ **MILLER COUNTY HOSPITAL (111305)**, 209 North Cuthbert Street, Zip 39837, Mailing Address: P.O. Box 7, Zip 39837; tel. 229/758–3385, (Total facility includes 97 beds in nursing home–type unit) (Nonreporting) **A**9 10 18
Primary Contact: Thomas Meadows, Chief Executive Officer
COO: Shawn Whittaker, Chief Nursing Officer
CFO: Thomas Meadows, Chief Executive Officer
CMO: Lamar Brand, M.D., Chief of Staff
CIO: Keith Lovering, Information Technician
CHR: Debbie Wittmer, Director Human Resources
Web address: www.millercountyhospital.com
Control: Hospital district or authority, Government, nonfederal **Service:** General Medical and Surgical

Staffed Beds: 124

COLUMBUS—Muscogee County

BRADLEY CENTER OF ST. FRANCIS See St. Francis Hospital

★ **COLUMBUS SPECIALTY HOSPITAL (112012)**, 710 Center Street, 9th Floor, Zip 31901; tel. 706/321–6712 **A**9 10 **F**1 3 25 26
Primary Contact: Greg Thomsen, Ed.D., FACHE, Chief Executive Officer
COO: Vivian F. Lee, R.N., Chief Operating Officer and Chief Nursing Executive
CHR: Melissa Lassiter, Coordinator Human Resources
Web address: www.columbusspecialtyhospital.com
Control: Other not–for–profit (including NFP Corporation) **Service:** Long–Term Acute Care hospital

Staffed Beds: 30 **Admissions:** 296 **Census:** 23 **Outpatient Visits:** 0 **Births:** 0 **Total Expense ($000):** 8662 **Payroll Expense ($000):** 3430 **Personnel:** 82

⊡ **DOCTORS HOSPITAL OF COLUMBUS (110186)**, 616 19th Street, Zip 31901–1528, Mailing Address: P.O. Box 2188, Zip 31902–2188; tel. 706/494–4262 **A**1 9 10 **F**3 11 13 15 18 25 27 30 31 32 33 38 43 50 55 56 57 60 68 72 73 74 76 77 79 82 87 96 97 100 102 107 118 119 121 132 135 136 137 **S** Columbus Regional Healthcare System
Primary Contact: Lance B. Duke, FACHE, Interim Chief Executive Officer
COO: K. Dale Neely, Chief Operating Officer
CFO: Bill Saller, Chief Financial Officer
CMO: Thomas L. Theus, M.D., Chief of Medicine
CIO: David Cornelius, Director Information Services
CHR: Louise Truitt, Director Human Resources
Web address: www.doctorshospital.net
Control: Corporation, Investor–owned, for–profit **Service:** General Medical and Surgical

Staffed Beds: 171 **Admissions:** 5361 **Census:** 63 **Outpatient Visits:** 52120 **Births:** 1439 **Total Expense ($000):** 54067 **Payroll Expense ($000):** 23594 **Personnel:** 465

GA

⊡ **HUGHSTON ORTHOPEDIC HOSPITAL (110200)**, 100 Frist Court, Zip 31908–7188, Mailing Address: P.O. Box 7188, Zip 31908–7188; tel. 706/576–2101 **A**1 9 10 **F**3 25 26 31 33 57 62 66 68 75 77 79 81 82 85 86 96 97 100 107 119 120 **S** HCA
Primary Contact: Donald R. Avery, FACHE, President and Chief Executive Officer
COO: Melanie Salsgiver, R.N., Chief Operating Officer and Chief Nursing Officer
CFO: Michael Hoskins, Vice President and Chief Financial Officer
CMO: Carlton G. Savory, M.D., President Medical Staff
Web address: www.hughstonsports.com
Control: Corporation, Investor–owned, for–profit **Service:** Orthopedic

Staffed Beds: 100 **Admissions:** 3260 **Census:** 44 **Outpatient Visits:** 3217 **Births:** 0 **Total Expense ($000):** 55666 **Payroll Expense ($000):** 16813 **Personnel:** 277

⊡ **ST. FRANCIS HOSPITAL (110129)**, 2122 Manchester Expressway, Zip 31904–6878, Mailing Address: P.O. Box 7000, Zip 31908–7000; tel. 706/596–4000, (Includes BRADLEY CENTER OF ST. FRANCIS, 2000 16th Avenue, Zip 31906–0308; tel. 706/320–3700) **A**1 9 10 **F**2 4 10 11 15 17 18 20 22 24 25 26 27 30 33 37 38 47 48 49 51 55 56 57 59 62 63 68 72 73 75 76 77 79 85 86 88 89 90 92 93 94 95 96 99 100 102 104 107 118 136 137 **P**6
Primary Contact: Robert P. Granger, Chief Executive Officer
CFO: Matthew Moore, Senior Vice President and Chief Financial Officer
CMO: Bobbi Farber, M.D., Chief Medical Officer
CIO: David Steele, Vice President and Chief Information Officer
CHR: Monika Sanders, Vice President Human Resources
Web address: www.sfhga.com
Control: Other not–for–profit (including NFP Corporation) **Service:** General Medical and Surgical

Staffed Beds: 272 **Admissions:** 12539 **Census:** 183 **Outpatient Visits:** 121402 **Births:** 0 **Total Expense ($000):** 174523 **Payroll Expense ($000):** 76636 **Personnel:** 1703

⊡ **THE MEDICAL CENTER (110064)**, 710 Center Street, Zip 31901–1527, Mailing Address: P.O. Box 951, Zip 31902–0951; tel. 706/571–1000, (Total facility includes 128 beds in nursing home–type unit) **A**1 2 3 5 9 10 12 13 **F**5 11 13 15 18 25 26 27 31 32 33 38 40 41 43 49 50 54 55 56 57 59 60 62 64 66 68 69 70 71 72 73 74 75 76 77 79 81 82 83 84 86 87 88 90 91 92 96 97 100 102 104 106 107 109 111 117 118 119 121 123 124 133 135 136 137 **P**6 8 **S** Columbus Regional Healthcare System
Primary Contact: Lance B. Duke, FACHE, President and Chief Executive Officer
CFO: Roland Thacker, Senior Vice President and Chief Financial Officer
CMO: Andrew P. Morley, M.D., Senior Vice President and Chief Medical Officer
CIO: Joseph T. Wood, Vice President and Chief Information Officer
CHR: Wayne Joiner, Vice President Human Resources
Web address: www.columbusregional.com
Control: Other not–for–profit (including NFP Corporation) **Service:** General Medical and Surgical

Staffed Beds: 497 **Admissions:** 14601 **Census:** 293 **Outpatient Visits:** 167178 **Births:** 3292 **Total Expense ($000):** 242191 **Payroll Expense ($000):** 100344 **Personnel:** 1863

☐ **WEST CENTRAL GEORGIA REGIONAL HOSPITAL (114013)**, 3000 Schatulga Road, Zip 31995–3117, Mailing Address: P.O. Box 12435, Zip 31995–2435; tel. 706/568–5000, (Nonreporting) **A**1 9 10
Primary Contact: John L. Robertson, Administrator
COO: Larmar Cunningham, Chief Operating Officer
CMO: Mark Stracks, M.D., Clinical Director
CIO: Ron Buchanan, Director Information Services
CHR: Carolyn Mitchell, Human Resources Lead
Web address: www.wcgrh.org
Control: State–Government, nonfederal **Service:** Psychiatric

Staffed Beds: 145

COMMERCE—Jackson County

⊡ **BJC MEDICAL CENTER (110040)**, 70 Medical Center Drive, Zip 30529–9989; tel. 706/335–1000, (Total facility includes 167 beds in nursing home–type unit) (Nonreporting) **A**1 9 10
Primary Contact: James Yarborough, FACHE, Chief Executive Officer
CFO: Bill Williams, Chief Financial Officer
CMO: Narasimhulu Neelagaru, M.D., Chief of Staff
CIO: Greg Fields, Manager Systems Support
CHR: Marilyn Anglin, Director Human Resources
Web address: www.bjcmc.org
Control: Hospital district or authority, Government, nonfederal **Service:** General Medical and Surgical

Staffed Beds: 257

CONYERS—Rockdale County

⊡ **ROCKDALE MEDICAL CENTER (110091)**, 1412 Milstead Avenue N.E., Zip 30012; tel. 770/918–3000 **A**1 2 9 10 **F**3 11 13 15 18 24 25 26 27 30 31 32 38 43 46 47 55 56 57 61 62 66 68 70 71 72 73 74 76 77 79 80 81 86 96 97 100 102 106 107 119 120 121 123 124 134 135 136 137 **P**1 5 **S** Brim Healthcare, Inc.
Primary Contact: Michael S. Potter, FACHE, Chief Executive Officer
CFO: Sandra Albrecht, Chief Financial Officer
CMO: George Isshak, Chief of Staff
CHR: Marianne Freeman, Vice Human Resources
Web address: www.rockdalemedicalcenter.org
Control: Other not–for–profit (including NFP Corporation) **Service:** General Medical and Surgical

Staffed Beds: 154 **Admissions:** 8357 **Census:** 89 **Outpatient Visits:** 110872 **Births:** 2288 **Total Expense ($000):** 100785 **Payroll Expense ($000):** 37842 **Personnel:** 783

CORDELE—Crisp County

⊡ **CRISP REGIONAL HOSPITAL (110104)**, 902 North Seventh Street, Zip 31015–5007; tel. 229/276–3100, (Total facility includes 143 beds in nursing home–type unit) **A**1 9 10 20 **F**3 10 11 13 15 24 25 26 27 30 31 33 38 41 42 43 44 48 50 51 53 54 55 56 57 58 59 60 61 62 63 66 68 73 74 75 76 79 80 81 82 84 85 86 87 96 97 103 106 115 117 118 119 121 124 133 135 136 137 **P**2 8
Primary Contact: D. Wayne Martin, President and Chief Executive Officer
CFO: Charlotte Vestal, Chief Financial Officer
CIO: Mark Dose, Manager Marketing and Outpatient Services
Web address: www.crispregional.org
Control: County–Government, nonfederal **Service:** General Medical and Surgical

Staffed Beds: 208 **Admissions:** 3248 **Census:** 156 **Outpatient Visits:** 124850 **Births:** 483 **Personnel:** 570

 Many Facility Codes have changed. Please refer to the AHA Guide Code Chart.

COVINGTON—Newton County

★☐ **NEWTON MEDICAL CENTER (110018)**, 5126 Hospital Drive, Zip 30014–2567; tel. 770/786–7053 **A**1 9 10 **F**7 11 13 15 18 20 24 25 26 30 31 33 38 43 49 52 55 57 61 62 63 68 72 73 74 77 79 80 82 84 86 87 96 97 100 102 107 112 119 121 131 132 135 136 **P**8
Primary Contact: James F. Weadick, Administrator and Chief Executive Officer
CFO: Troy Brooks, Assistant Administrator Fiscal Services
CMO: A. Steven McIntosh, M.D., Chief of Staff
CIO: Robert Guyton, Director
CHR: Greg Richardson, Director Human Resources
Web address: www.newtonmedical.com
Control: Other not–for–profit (including NFP Corporation) **Service:** General Medical and Surgical

Staffed Beds: 97 **Admissions:** 6187 **Census:** 55 **Outpatient Visits:** 101450 **Births:** 740 **Total Expense ($000):** 64449 **Payroll Expense ($000):** 30710 **Personnel:** 665

CUMMING—Forsyth County

★☐ **NORTHSIDE HOSPITAL FORSYTH (110005)**, 1200 Northside Forsyth Drive, Zip 30041–7659; tel. 770/844–3200 **A**1 9 10 **F**3 11 15 24 25 26 27 30 31 32 33 38 41 43 49 50 52 55 56 57 59 62 66 68 73 77 79 80 81 82 86 96 97 100 102 107 118 119 121 124 135 137 **P**6
Primary Contact: Lynn Jackson, Administrator
CFO: Mitch Logan, Director Finance
Web address: www.northside.com
Control: Other not–for–profit (including NFP Corporation) **Service:** General Medical and Surgical

Staffed Beds: 100 **Admissions:** 6987 **Census:** 77 **Outpatient Visits:** 104261 **Births:** 0 **Total Expense ($000):** 103214 **Payroll Expense ($000):** 37863 **Personnel:** 811

CUTHBERT—Randolph County

★ **SOUTHWEST GEORGIA REGIONAL MEDICAL CENTER (111300)**, 109 Randolph Street, Zip 39840–1338; tel. 229/732–2181, (Total facility includes 80 beds in nursing home–type unit) (Nonreporting) **A**9 10 18
Primary Contact: Keith J. Petersen, Chief Executive Officer
CFO: Susan Rakel, Chief Financial Officer
Control: Hospital district or authority, Government, nonfederal **Service:** General Medical and Surgical

Staffed Beds: 105

DAHLONEGA—Lumpkin County

☐ **CHESTATEE REGIONAL HOSPITAL (110187)**, 227 Mountain Drive, Zip 30533–1606; tel. 706/864–6136 **A**1 9 10 **F**3 13 15 25 26 31 32 33 38 43 51 53 55 57 62 63 72 74 75 77 79 80 82 96 97 100 102 106 107 112 118 119 122 133 134 136 **P**1 **S** Sunlink Health Systems
Primary Contact: Alan E. George, Chief Executive Officer
CFO: Julia Berndt, Chief Financial Officer
CMO: David Hochschild, M.D., Chief of Staff
Web address: www.chestateeregionalhospital.com
Control: Corporation, Investor–owned, for–profit **Service:** General Medical and Surgical

Staffed Beds: 49 **Admissions:** 1856 **Census:** 17 **Outpatient Visits:** 12274 **Births:** 186 **Total Expense ($000):** 21090 **Payroll Expense ($000):** 8972 **Personnel:** 156

DALLAS—Paulding County

★☐ **WELLSTAR PAULDING HOSPITAL (110042)**, 600 West Memorial Drive, Zip 30132–1335; tel. 770/445–4411, (Total facility includes 182 beds in nursing home–type unit) **A**1 2 9 10 **F**3 11 15 25 26 30 31 32 33 35 36 38 41 43 46 47 48 49 50 55 56 57 60 62 65 66 68 73 75 77 79 80 81 82 86 92 96 97 99 102 106 107 117 119 121 123 135 **P**1 6 **S** WellStar Health System
Primary Contact: John Law, Administrator
CFO: Marsha Burke, Senior Vice President Financial Services
Web address: www.wellstar.org
Control: Other not–for–profit (including NFP Corporation) **Service:** General Medical and Surgical

Staffed Beds: 216 **Admissions:** 1572 **Census:** 189 **Outpatient Visits:** 55947 **Births:** 0 **Personnel:** 449

DALTON—Whitfield County

★☐ **HAMILTON MEDICAL CENTER (110001)**, 1200 Memorial Drive, Zip 30720–2529, Mailing Address: P.O. Box 1168, Zip 30722–1168; tel. 706/272–6000 **A**1 2 9 10 19 **F**2 4 5 8 12 13 15 18 20 24 25 26 27 28 31 32 33 36 38 40 41 42 43 49 50 51 52 53 55 56 57 60 61 62 66 68 69 71 72 73 74 75 76 77 79 80 81 82 84 86 88 89 90 91 92 93 94 95 96 97 99 100 102 103 105 106 107 108 109 111 118 119 120 121 124 135 136 137 **P**8
Primary Contact: John S. Bowling, President and Chief Executive Officer
COO: Karen J. Wisdom, Chief Operating Officer and Senior Vice President
CFO: Gary L. Howard, Chief Financial Officer
CMO: Carlton Lancaster, M.D., Medical Consultant
CIO: John M. Forrester, Director Information Services
CHR: Steven Pound, Vice President Human Resources
Web address: www.hamiltonhealth.com
Control: Other not–for–profit (including NFP Corporation) **Service:** General Medical and Surgical

Staffed Beds: 256 **Admissions:** 11240 **Census:** 126 **Outpatient Visits:** 186880 **Births:** 2528 **Personnel:** 1160

DECATUR—De Kalb County

★☐ **DEKALB MEDICAL CENTER (110076)**, 2701 North Decatur Road, Zip 30033–5995; tel. 404/501–1000 **A**1 2 9 10 **F**3 4 8 11 12 13 15 18 25 26 27 30 31 32 33 34 35 38 40 46 50 51 52 55 56 57 58 59 61 62 65 66 70 71 72 73 74 75 76 77 79 80 81 82 84 85 86 88 90 96 97 100 105 109 118 119 120 121 132 135 136 **P**1 6 **S** DeKalb Regional Health System
Primary Contact: Eric P. Norwood, President and Chief Executive Officer
COO: John Shelton, Executive Vice President and Chief Operating Officer
CFO: Diane P. Harden, Chief Financial Officer
CMO: Duane Barclay, M.D., Vice President Physician Support Services
CIO: Mark Trocino, Chief Information Officer
CHR: Tom Crawford, Vice President Human Resources
Web address: www.dekalbmedicalcenter.org
Control: Other not–for–profit (including NFP Corporation) **Service:** General Medical and Surgical

Staffed Beds: 417 **Admissions:** 19135 **Census:** 260 **Outpatient Visits:** 187510 **Births:** 4767 **Total Expense ($000):** 259812 **Payroll Expense ($000):** 98801 **Personnel:** 2153

☐ **DEKALB MEDICAL CENTER AT DECATUR (112006)**, 450 North Candler Street, Zip 30030–2671; tel. 404/501–6700, (Nonreporting) **A**1 9 10 **S** DeKalb Regional Health System
Primary Contact: Brent Robinson, Vice President
COO: John Shelton, Executive Vice President and Chief Operating Officer
CFO: Diane P. Harden, Chief Financial Officer
CMO: David Snyder, M.D., Chief of Staff
CHR: Tom Crawford, Vice President Human Resources
Web address: www.dekalbmedicalcenter.org
Control: Other not–for–profit (including NFP Corporation) **Service:** General Medical and Surgical

Staffed Beds: 76

☐ **GEORGIA REGIONAL HOSPITAL AT ATLANTA (114019)**, 3073 Panthersville Road, Zip 30034–3828; tel. 404/243–2100, (Total facility includes 77 beds in nursing home–type unit) **A**1 3 5 9 10 **F**11 25 26 37 41 56 57 64 65 75 82 88 89 91 92 93 117 119 124 **P**6
Primary Contact: Susan Trueblood, Chief Executive Officer
COO: Sonny Slate, Chief Operating Officer
CFO: Reginald Jones, Business Manager
CMO: Emile Risby, Clinical Director
CIO: Elfie Early, Manager Data Services
CHR: Lorraine Farr, Manager Human Resources
Web address: www.atlantareg.dhr.state.ga.us
Control: State–Government, nonfederal **Service:** Psychiatric

Staffed Beds: 319 **Admissions:** 3486 **Census:** 318 **Outpatient Visits:** 3533 **Births:** 0 **Total Expense ($000):** 34898 **Payroll Expense ($000):** 26130 **Personnel:** 737

★☐ △ **VETERANS AFFAIRS MEDICAL CENTER**, 1670 Clairmont Road, Zip 30033–4004; tel. 404/321–6111, (Nonreporting) **A**1 2 3 5 7 8 **S** Department of Veterans Affairs
Primary Contact: Thomas A. Cappello, M.P.H., FACHE, Director
COO: Orlando Dunson, Assistant Director
CFO: Gregg Becker, Chief Financial Officer
CMO: David Bower, M.D., Chief of Staff
CIO: Linda Feaselman, Chief Information Officer
CHR: Neal Falkner, Chief Human Resources
Web address: www.va.gov/sta/guide/home.asp
Control: Other, Government, federal **Service:** General Medical and Surgical

Staffed Beds: 239

GA

Hospital, Medicare Provider Number, Address, Telephone, Approval, Facility, and Physician Codes, Health Care System

★ American Hospital Association (AHA) membership
☐ The Joint Commission accreditation
○ American Osteopathic Association (AOA) accreditation
△ Commission on Accreditation of Rehabilitation Facilities (CARF) accreditation

DEMOREST—Habersham County

★ **HABERSHAM COUNTY MEDICAL CENTER (110041)**, 541 Historic Highway 441, Zip 30535–3118, Mailing Address: P.O. Box 37, Zip 30535–0037; tel. 706/754–2161, (Total facility includes 106 beds in nursing home–type unit) **A**1 9 10 **F**3 7 10 11 13 15 24 25 26 30 31 32 33 36 38 41 43 52 53 55 57 61 62 66 68 73 74 75 77 79 80 81 82 84 86 96 97 100 102 104 105 107 112 117 118 119 120 121 122 124 135 136 **P**7 **S** QHR
Primary Contact: C. Richard Dwozan, Chief Executive Officer
CFO: James Peterson, Senior Vice President Finance
CMO: Nancy Watson, M.D., Chief of Staff
CIO: Roger Ivester, Manager Information Systems
CHR: Wanda Hardman, Director Human Resources
Web address: www.hcmcmed.org
Control: Hospital district or authority, Government, nonfederal **Service:** General Medical and Surgical

Staffed Beds: 159 **Admissions:** 2539 **Census:** 117 **Outpatient Visits:** 89027 **Births:** 419 **Total Expense ($000):** 40379 **Payroll Expense ($000):** 19879 **Personnel:** 486

DONALSONVILLE—Seminole County

☐ **DONALSONVILLE HOSPITAL (110194)**, 102 Hospital Circle, Zip 39845–1199; tel. 229/524–5217, (Total facility includes 75 beds in nursing home–type unit) **A**1 9 10 **F**13 30 31 32 38 46 55 56 57 62 66 74 75 79 82 86 96 97 99 102 107 117 122 136 137
Primary Contact: Charles H. Orrick, Administrator
CFO: James Moody, Chief Financial Officer
CMO: C. O. Walker, M.D., Chief of Staff
CHR: Jo Adams, Director Human Resources
Control: Other not–for–profit (including NFP Corporation) **Service:** General Medical and Surgical

Staffed Beds: 140 **Admissions:** 2370 **Census:** 77 **Outpatient Visits:** 107663 **Births:** 329 **Total Expense ($000):** 23547 **Payroll Expense ($000):** 10139 **Personnel:** 248

DOUGLAS—Coffee County

★ **COFFEE REGIONAL MEDICAL CENTER (110089)**, 1101 Ocilla Road, Zip 31533–3617, Mailing Address: P.O. Box 1287, Zip 31534–1287; tel. 912/384–1900 **A**9 10 20 **F**3 7 11 13 15 24 25 26 27 28 30 31 32 33 36 38 43 46 49 50 52 53 54 55 56 57 60 61 63 66 68 73 74 76 77 79 80 81 82 84 86 87 96 97 99 100 102 107 119 120 121 124 132 133 135 136 **P**8
Primary Contact: George L. Heck, III, President and Chief Executive Officer
CFO: Donald C. Lewis, Vice President and Chief Financial Officer
CIO: George L. Heck, President and Chief Executive Officer
CHR: Laura Bloom, Director Human Resources
Web address: www.coffeeregional.org
Control: Other not–for–profit (including NFP Corporation) **Service:** General Medical and Surgical

Staffed Beds: 88 **Admissions:** 5598 **Census:** 54 **Outpatient Visits:** 83576 **Births:** 691 **Total Expense ($000):** 60667 **Payroll Expense ($000):** 26793 **Personnel:** 634

DOUGLASVILLE—Douglas County

INNER HARBOUR, 4685 Dorsett Shoals Road, Zip 30135–4999; tel. 770/942–2391 **F**5 72 82 88 89 90 91 94 95 119 121 135 **P**5 6
Primary Contact: Ron Scroggy, Chief Executive Officer
CFO: J. Steve Lewis, Director Finance
CMO: Yolanda Graham, M.D., Medical Director
CIO: Laura Sellers, Director Information Systems
CHR: Sherry Kollmeyer, Vice President Human Resources
Web address: www.innerharbour.org
Control: Other not–for–profit (including NFP Corporation) **Service:** Children's hospital psychiatric

Staffed Beds: 177 **Admissions:** 462 **Census:** 177 **Outpatient Visits:** 1397 **Births:** 0 **Total Expense ($000):** 23491 **Payroll Expense ($000):** 14556 **Personnel:** 338

★ **WELLSTAR DOUGLAS HOSPITAL (110184)**, 8954 Hospital Drive, Zip 30134–2282; tel. 770/949–1500 **A**1 2 9 10 **F**3 11 13 15 24 25 26 27 30 31 32 33 35 36 38 41 43 46 47 48 49 50 53 55 56 57 60 62 66 68 72 73 74 75 77 79 80 81 82 84 86 92 96 97 99 100 102 106 107 118 119 121 123 135 136 **P**1 6 **S** WellStar Health System
Primary Contact: J. Michael Poore, Vice President and Administrator
COO: Paul Johnson, Executive Vice President Operations
CFO: Marsha Burke, Senior Vice President and Chief Financial Officer
CMO: Richard Hart, M.D., Executive Vice President and Chief Medical Officer
CIO: Leigh Cox, Chief Information Officer
CHR: Bobby DeCoux, Director Human Resources
Web address: www.wellstar.org
Control: Other not–for–profit (including NFP Corporation) **Service:** General Medical and Surgical

Staffed Beds: 98 **Admissions:** 5728 **Census:** 67 **Outpatient Visits:** 106402 **Births:** 452 **Personnel:** 633

DUBLIN—Laurens County

★ **CARL VINSON VETERANS AFFAIRS MEDICAL CENTER**, 1826 Veterans Boulevard, Zip 31021–3620; tel. 478/272–1210, (Total facility includes 161 beds in nursing home–type unit) (Nonreporting) **A**1 **S** Department of Veterans Affairs
Primary Contact: Kelly O. Duke, Acting Director
CFO: Marcy Chambless, Manager Business Office
CMO: Eva Martin, M.D., Chief of Staff
CIO: Sandra Clem, Manager Information Management
CHR: Teresa L. Lindsey, Supervisor Human Resources
Web address: www.va.gov/sta/guide/home.asp
Control: Veterans Affairs, Government, federal **Service:** General Medical and Surgical

Staffed Beds: 339

★ **FAIRVIEW PARK HOSPITAL (110125)**, 200 Industrial Boulevard, Zip 31021–2997, Mailing Address: P.O. Box 1408, Zip 31040–1408; tel. 478/275–2000 **A**1 9 10 19 **F**3 8 11 13 15 17 18 24 25 27 30 31 32 33 38 40 49 52 54 55 57 62 68 72 73 74 75 76 77 79 80 81 84 85 86 96 97 100 102 106 107 118 119 120 121 124 135 136 137 **S** HCA
Primary Contact: Donald R. Avery, FACHE, President and Chief Executive Officer
COO: Brad Griffin, Chief Operating Officer
CFO: Ted Short, Chief Financial Officer
CMO: Sandeep D'Souza, M.D., President Medical Staff
CIO: Marsha Morris, Manager Information Services
CHR: Jeff Bruton, Director Human Resources
Web address: www.fairviewparkhospital.com
Control: Partnership, Investor–owned, for–profit **Service:** General Medical and Surgical

Staffed Beds: 168 **Admissions:** 6988 **Census:** 71 **Outpatient Visits:** 73450 **Births:** 1300 **Total Expense ($000):** 65786 **Payroll Expense ($000):** 23806 **Personnel:** 460

DULUTH—Gwinnett County

GWINNETT MEDICAL CENTER–DULUTH See Gwinnett Hospital System, Lawrenceville

JOAN GLANCY MEMORIAL HOSPITAL See Gwinnett Hospital System, Lawrenceville

EAST POINT—Fulton County

★ **REGENCY HOSPITAL OF SOUTH ATLANTA (112014)**, 1170 Cleveland Avenue, 4th Floor, Zip 30344; tel. 404/466–6250 **A**1 10 **F**1 3 25 33 56 75 82 107 119 137 **P**5 **S** Regency Hospital Company
Primary Contact: Paul C. Miller, Chief Executive Officer
Web address: www.regencyhospital.com
Control: Partnership, Investor–owned, for–profit **Service:** Long–Term Acute Care hospital

Staffed Beds: 37 **Admissions:** 371 **Census:** 34 **Outpatient Visits:** 0 **Births:** 0 **Total Expense ($000):** 20279 **Payroll Expense ($000):** 7757 **Personnel:** 115

EASTMAN—Dodge County

☐ **DODGE COUNTY HOSPITAL (110092)**, 901 Griffin Avenue, Zip 31023–2223, Mailing Address: P.O. Box 4309, Zip 31023–4309; tel. 478/374–4000 **A**1 9 10 **F**3 7 11 15 25 26 27 31 38 52 55 57 62 67 68 73 74 75 77 79 80 81 82 86 96 97 98 100 102 106 107 119 122 124 135 137
Primary Contact: Kevin Bierschenk, Chief Executive Officer
CFO: Michael Hester, Chief Financial Officer
CIO: Debra Lewis, Manager Business Office
Web address: www.dodgecountyhospital.com
Control: Hospital district or authority, Government, nonfederal **Service:** General Medical and Surgical

Staffed Beds: 72 **Admissions:** 2272 **Census:** 25 **Outpatient Visits:** 51591 **Births:** 196 **Total Expense ($000):** 23218 **Payroll Expense ($000):** 9508 **Personnel:** 225

EATONTON—Putnam County

☐ **PUTNAM GENERAL HOSPITAL (111313)**, 101 Lake Oconee Parkway, Zip 31024; tel. 706/485–2711 **A**1 9 10 18 **F**3 11 15 24 25 30 31 32 38 51 55 62 73 77 79 81 86 96 100 102 107 118 122 135 **P**2
Primary Contact: Darrell M. Oglesby, Administrator
CFO: Brenda Jarrett, Chief Financial Officer
CMO: Ajay Kumar, Chief of Staff
CIO: Steven Cason, Chief Information Officer
CHR: Marsha Bergmann, Director Human Resources
Web address: www.putnamgeneral.com
Control: Hospital district or authority, Government, nonfederal **Service:** General Medical and Surgical

Staffed Beds: 25 **Admissions:** 893 **Census:** 6 **Outpatient Visits:** 20137 **Births:** 0 **Total Expense ($000):** 13051 **Payroll Expense ($000):** 5282 **Personnel:** 121

GA

Many Facility Codes have changed. Please refer to the AHA Guide Code Chart.

ELBERTON—Elbert County

★ **ELBERT MEMORIAL HOSPITAL (110026)**, 4 Medical Drive, Zip 30635–1897; tel. 706/283–3151, (Nonreporting) **A**1 9 10 **S** QHR
Primary Contact: Mark LeNeave, Chief Executive Officer
CFO: Walter Mitchell, Interim Chief Financial Officer
CIO: Cynthia Johanson, Director Information Technology
CHR: Georgian Walton, Director Human Resources
Web address: www.emhcare.net
Control: Hospital district or authority, Government, nonfederal **Service:** General Medical and Surgical

Staffed Beds: 52

ELLIJAY—Gilmer County

□ **NORTH GEORGIA MEDICAL CENTER (110205)**, 1362 South Main Street, Zip 30540–0346, Mailing Address: P.O. Box 2239, Zip 30540–0346; tel. 706/276–4741, (Total facility includes 100 beds in nursing home–type unit) (Nonreporting) **A**1 9 10 **S** Sunlink Health Systems
Primary Contact: Jeffrey Dunn, Chief Executive Officer
COO: Jeffrey Dunn, Chief Executive Officer
CFO: Debbie Self, Chief Financial Officer
CMO: Anne B. Todd, M.D., Chief of Staff
CHR: Faron Barton, Manager Human Resources
Web address: www.northgeorgiamedicalcenter.com
Control: Corporation, Investor–owned, for–profit **Service:** General Medical and Surgical

Staffed Beds: 150

FAYETTEVILLE—Fayette County

★ **PIEDMONT FAYETTE HOSPITAL (110215)**, 1255 Highway 54 West, Zip 30214; tel. 770/719–7000 **A**1 9 10 **F**3 11 13 15 17 18 24 25 26 27 30 31 32 33 38 39 44 46 47 48 51 52 55 56 57 71 72 73 74 75 76 77 79 82 86 96 97 100 102 103 104 105 107 118 119 121 124 135 136 137 **S** Piedmont Healthcare
Primary Contact: W. Darrell Cutts, President and Chief Executive Officer
COO: Michael Burnett, Chief Operating Officer
CFO: John Miles, Chief Financial Officer
CMO: Richard Mitchell, M.D., Vice President Medical Affairs
CIO: John Hilliard, Vice President Information Services
CHR: Catherine Crisler, Executive Director Human Resources
Web address: www.fayettehospital.org
Control: Other not–for–profit (including NFP Corporation) **Service:** General Medical and Surgical

Staffed Beds: 106 **Admissions:** 8232 **Census:** 88 **Outpatient Visits:** 157425 **Births:** 852

FITZGERALD—Ben Hill County

□ **DORMINY MEDICAL CENTER (110073)**, Perry House Road, Zip 31750, Mailing Address: P.O. Box 1447, Zip 31750–1447; tel. 229/424–7100 **A**1 9 **F**3 11 13 15 25 26 30 32 33 38 42 43 44 50 55 57 59 62 66 68 73 74 79 82 84 85 86 96 100 107 118 119 122
Primary Contact: Bruce Shepard, Administrator
COO: Debbie Thomas, Chief Operating Officer
CFO: Paige Wynn, Chief Financial Officer
CMO: Don Smith, M.D., Chief of Staff
CIO: Mike James, Director Management Information Systems
CHR: Denise Steverson, Director Human Resources
Web address: www.dorminymedical.org
Control: Hospital district or authority, Government, nonfederal **Service:** General Medical and Surgical

Staffed Beds: 61 **Admissions:** 2106 **Census:** 19 **Outpatient Visits:** 28652 **Births:** 216 **Total Expense ($000):** 19770 **Payroll Expense ($000):** 9283 **Personnel:** 291

FOLKSTON—Charlton County

CHARLTON MEMORIAL HOSPITAL (111315), 1203 North Third Street, Zip 31537–1303, Mailing Address: P.O. Box 188, Zip 31537–0188; tel. 912/496–2531, (Nonreporting) **A**9 10 18
Primary Contact: Dee McKrow, Administrator
COO: Dee McKrow, Administrator
CFO: Ray Leadbetter, Controller
CMO: Richard Eaton, M.D., Chief of Staff
Control: Hospital district or authority, Government, nonfederal **Service:** General Medical and Surgical

Staffed Beds: 25

FORSYTH—Monroe County

□ **MONROE COUNTY HOSPITAL (111318)**, 88 Martin Luther King Jr. Drive, Zip 31029–1682, Mailing Address: P.O. Box 1068, Zip 31029–1068; tel. 478/994–2521 **A**1 9 10 18 **F**3 11 15 25 30 31 33 38 55 57 66 73 79 96 100 102 107 121 122 135 137 **P**1 2
Primary Contact: Oliver J. Booker, Chief Executive Officer
CFO: Becky Firster, Controller
CIO: Donna Hogg, Supervisor Medical Records
CHR: Deborah Flowers, Director Human Resources
Web address: www.monroehospital.org
Control: Hospital district or authority, Government, nonfederal **Service:** General Medical and Surgical

Staffed Beds: 25 **Admissions:** 724 **Census:** 8 **Outpatient Visits:** 20885 **Births:** 0 **Total Expense ($000):** 7858 **Payroll Expense ($000):** 4323 **Personnel:** 119

FORT BENNING—Muscogee County

★ **MARTIN ARMY COMMUNITY HOSPITAL**, 7950 Martin Loop, Zip 31905–6100; tel. 706/544–2516 **A**1 3 5 **F**5 7 12 13 14 15 25 26 28 29 32 33 37 38 50 52 53 55 57 58 60 62 63 68 72 73 75 77 79 80 81 82 86 87 88 90 92 94 96 102 107 113 114 118 119 120 124 135 **P**6 **S** Department of the Army, Office of the Surgeon General
Primary Contact: Colonel Margaret Rivera, Commander
COO: Colonel Margaret Rivera, Commander
CFO: Major Sean Casperson, Chief Resource Management
CMO: Colonel Sonja Thompson, Deputy Commander Clinical Services
CIO: Major Tony Cromer, Chief Information Management
CHR: Major Bernita Hightower, Chief Human Resources
Web address: www.martin.amedd.army.mil
Control: Army, Government, federal **Service:** General Medical and Surgical

Staffed Beds: 57 **Admissions:** 4086 **Census:** 36 **Outpatient Visits:** 705872 **Births:** 837 **Total Expense ($000):** 111447 **Payroll Expense ($000):** 36951

FORT GORDON—Richmond County

★ **DWIGHT DAVID EISENHOWER ARMY MEDICAL CENTER**, Hospital Drive, Zip 30905–5650; tel. 706/787–5811 **A**1 2 3 5 **F**3 4 5 7 8 9 11 12 14 15 18 20 22 24 25 26 27 29 32 33 35 36 37 38 40 41 50 53 54 55 56 57 58 59 62 63 66 68 72 73 75 76 77 79 80 81 82 84 85 86 87 88 89 90 91 92 94 95 96 97 100 102 104 105 107 118 119 120 121 123 124 132 133 134 135 136 137 **P**6 **S** Department of the Army, Office of the Surgeon General
Primary Contact: Brigadier General Donald M. Bradshaw, Commander
COO: Lieutenant Colonel David P. Budinger, Deputy Chief Administration
CMO: Colonel James M. Baunchalk, Deputy Chief Clinical Services
CIO: Major Joseph A. Ponce, Chief Information Management
CHR: Elizabeth Shelt, Civilian Personnel Officer
Web address: www.ddeamc.amedd.army.mil
Control: Army, Government, federal **Service:** General Medical and Surgical

Staffed Beds: 95 **Admissions:** 4794 **Census:** 49 **Outpatient Visits:** 712724 **Births:** 0 **Personnel:** 2153

FORT OGLETHORPE—Catoosa County

□ **HUTCHESON MEDICAL CENTER (110004)**, 100 Gross Crescent Circle, Zip 30742–3669; tel. 706/858–2000, (Total facility includes 109 beds in nursing home–type unit) **A**1 9 10 **F**3 7 8 11 13 15 17 18 24 25 26 27 30 33 38 41 42 43 50 55 56 57 59 61 62 66 68 69 70 75 76 77 79 80 81 82 86 96 97 100 106 107 109 111 117 119 120 121 124 133 135 136 **P**5 6
Primary Contact: Charles L. Stewart, President and Chief Executive Officer
COO: Gerald Faircloth, Chief Operating Officer
CFO: Douglas R. Volinski, Chief Financial Officer
CMO: Radian Florea, M.D., Chief of Staff
CIO: Don Williams, Director Information Systems
CHR: Jim Treglown, Chief President Human Resources
Web address: www.hutcheson.org
Control: Hospital district or authority, Government, nonfederal **Service:** General Medical and Surgical

Staffed Beds: 294 **Admissions:** 6367 **Census:** 184 **Outpatient Visits:** 112738 **Births:** 992 **Total Expense ($000):** 92180 **Payroll Expense ($000):** 42853 **Personnel:** 1114

GA

Hospital, Medicare Provider Number, Address, Telephone, Approval, Facility, and Physician Codes, Health Care System

★ American Hospital Association (AHA) membership
□ The Joint Commission accreditation
○ American Osteopathic Association (AOA) accreditation
△ Commission on Accreditation of Rehabilitation Facilities (CARF) accreditation

FORT VALLEY—Peach County

★ **PEACH REGIONAL MEDICAL CENTER (111310)**, 601 Blue Bird Boulevard, Zip 31030–4599, Mailing Address: P.O. Box 1799, Zip 31030–1799; tel. 478/825–8691, (Nonreporting) **A**1 9 10 18
Primary Contact: Nancy Peed, Administrator and Chief Executive Officer
COO: Kathy Louth, Chief Operating Officer
CFO: Lisa Urbistondo, Chief Financial Officer
CMO: Crystal Brown, M.D., Medical Director
CHR: Priscilla B. Yaughn, Manager Human Resources
Web address: www.peachregional.org
Control: Hospital district or authority, Government, nonfederal **Service:** General Medical and Surgical

Staffed Beds: 25

GAINESVILLE—Hall County

★ △ **NORTHEAST GEORGIA MEDICAL CENTER (110029)**, 743 Spring Street N.E., Zip 30501–3899; tel. 770/535–3553, (Total facility includes 285 beds in nursing home–type unit) (Nonreporting) **A**1 2 7 9 10 19
Primary Contact: Jim Gardner, President and Chief Executive Officer
COO: Carol H. Burrell, Executive Vice President and Chief Operating Officer
CFO: Tony Herdener, Vice President Systems and Finance
CIO: Mark Jennings, Director Information Systems
CHR: Jack Fulbright, Vice President Human Resources
Web address: www.nghs.com
Control: Other not–for–profit (including NFP Corporation) **Service:** General Medical and Surgical

Staffed Beds: 418

GLENWOOD—Wheeler County

☐ **WHEELER COUNTY HOSPITAL (111321)**, 111 Third Street, Zip 30428–2301, Mailing Address: P.O. Box 398, Zip 30428–0398; tel. 912/523–5113, (Nonreporting) **A**1 9 10 18 **S** Accord Health Care Corporation
Primary Contact: William Posey, Administrator
CFO: Lynan Fowler, Director Patient Financial Services
CHR: June Adcock, Chief Human Resources Officer
Control: Corporation, Investor–owned, for–profit **Service:** General Medical and Surgical

Staffed Beds: 25

GRACEWOOD—Richmond County

EAST CENTRAL REGIONAL HOSPITAL See East Central Regional Hospital, Augusta

GREENSBORO—Greene County

☐ **MINNIE G. BOSWELL MEMORIAL HOSPITAL (111329)**, 1201 Siloam Highway, Zip 30642–2811; tel. 706/453–7331 **A**1 9 10 18 **F**3 15 25 30 31 32 38 66 75 79 86 96 99 107 119 122 124 132 137
Primary Contact: Michael H. Huff, Chief Executive Officer
CMO: Dave Ringer, M.D., Chief of Staff
CHR: Terrie Franklin, Chief Human Resources Officer
Web address: www.mgbmh.com
Control: Corporation, Investor–owned, for–profit **Service:** General Medical and Surgical

Staffed Beds: 25 **Admissions:** 530 **Census:** 8 **Outpatient Visits:** 14496 **Births:** 0 **Total Expense ($000):** 9653 **Payroll Expense ($000):** 4514 **Personnel:** 81

GRIFFIN—Spalding County

★ **SPALDING REGIONAL MEDICAL CENTER (110031)**, 601 South Eighth Street, Zip 30224–4294, Mailing Address: P.O. Drawer V, Zip 30224–1168; tel. 770/228–2721 **A**1 2 9 10 **F**3 7 11 13 15 18 20 25 26 27 30 31 32 33 38 50 51 52 53 55 57 62 65 68 71 72 73 74 75 76 77 79 80 84 86 96 97 100 102 107 112 118 119 120 124 132 133 135 136 137 **P**8 **S** TENET Healthcare Corporation
Primary Contact: John A. Quinn, Chief Executive Officer
COO: Christopher Locke, Chief Operating Officer
CFO: Tamara Ison, Chief Financial Officer
CIO: Steven E. Brown, Director Information Systems
CHR: Amanda Moore–Remington, Director Human Resources
Web address: www.spaldingregional.com
Control: Corporation, Investor–owned, for–profit **Service:** General Medical and Surgical

Staffed Beds: 160 **Admissions:** 9086 **Census:** 107 **Outpatient Visits:** 90603 **Births:** 1041 **Total Expense ($000):** 80356 **Payroll Expense ($000):** 36660 **Personnel:** 666

HARTWELL—Hart County

★ **HART COUNTY HOSPITAL (110059)**, Gibson and Cade Streets, Zip 30643–0280, Mailing Address: P.O. Box 280, Zip 30643–0280; tel. 706/856–6100, (Total facility includes 92 beds in nursing home–type unit) **A**1 9 10 **F**3 11 25 26 30 31 32 33 38 50 54 55 56 57 62 68 73 75 77 79 82 84 86 96 97 103 107 117 119 120 122 135 **S** Ty Cobb Healthcare System, Inc.
Primary Contact: Jerry R. Wise, Administrator and Vice President
Web address: www.tycobbhealthcare.org
Control: Other not–for–profit (including NFP Corporation) **Service:** General Medical and Surgical

Staffed Beds: 174 **Admissions:** 1228 **Census:** 111 **Outpatient Visits:** 22662 **Births:** 0 **Total Expense ($000):** 19766 **Payroll Expense ($000):** 8231 **Personnel:** 288

HAWKINSVILLE—Pulaski County

☐ **TAYLOR REGIONAL HOSPITAL (110135)**, Macon Highway, Zip 31036, Mailing Address: P.O. Box 1297, Zip 31036–1297; tel. 478/783–0200, (Nonreporting) **A**1 9 10
Primary Contact: Dan S. Maddock, President
CFO: Lisa Halliday, Director Accounting Services
CMO: Al Baggett, M.D., Interim Chief of Staff
CIO: Dawn Warnock, Director Medical Records
Web address: www.taylorregional.org
Control: Other not–for–profit (including NFP Corporation) **Service:** General Medical and Surgical

Staffed Beds: 55

HAZLEHURST—Jeff Davis County

☐ **JEFF DAVIS HOSPITAL (111333)**, 1215 South Tallahassee Street, Zip 31539–2921, Mailing Address: P.O. Box 1690, Zip 31539–1690; tel. 912/375–7781, (Nonreporting) **A**1 9 10 18
Primary Contact: Rich McClements, Administrator
Control: Hospital district or authority, Government, nonfederal **Service:** General Medical and Surgical

Staffed Beds: 25

HIAWASSEE—Towns County

CHATUGE REGIONAL HOSPITAL AND NURSING HOME (111324), 110 Main Street, Zip 30546–2212, Mailing Address: P.O. Box 509, Zip 30546–0509; tel. 706/896–2222, (Total facility includes 112 beds in nursing home–type unit) (Nonreporting) **A**9 10 18
Primary Contact: R. Lewis Kelley, Administrator
CFO: Tim Henry, Accountant
CMO: Robert F. Stahlkuppe, M.D., Chief of Staff
CIO: Walt Stafford, Director Information Technology
CHR: Rita Bradshaw, Director Human Resources
Web address: www.chatugeregionalhospital.org
Control: County–Government, nonfederal **Service:** General Medical and Surgical

Staffed Beds: 137

HINESVILLE—Liberty County

☐ **LIBERTY REGIONAL MEDICAL CENTER (111335)**, 462 East G. Miles Parkway, Zip 31313, Mailing Address: P.O. Box 919, Zip 31313; tel. 912/369–9438, (Total facility includes 108 beds in nursing home–type unit) **A**1 9 10 18 **F**3 6 7 13 15 24 25 26 27 28 30 31 32 33 34 36 38 43 46 50 55 56 57 63 64 66 73 74 75 76 77 79 80 81 82 86 87 96 97 99 100 102 103 104 105 107 112 117 118 119 120 121 122 124 132 135 136 137 **P**1
Primary Contact: H. Scott Kroell, Jr., Chief Executive Officer
CFO: Martha F. Traylor, Chief Financial Officer
Web address: www.libertyregional.org
Control: Hospital district or authority, Government, nonfederal **Service:** General Medical and Surgical

Staffed Beds: 133 **Admissions:** 1975 **Census:** 115 **Outpatient Visits:** 29160 **Births:** 503 **Total Expense ($000):** 14175 **Payroll Expense ($000):** 15260 **Personnel:** 404

★ **WINN ARMY COMMUNITY HOSPITAL**, 1061 Harmon Avenue, Zip 31314–5611; tel. 912/435–6965, (Nonreporting) **A**1 3 5 **S** Department of the Army, Office of the Surgeon General
Primary Contact: Colonel John P. Collins, Commander
Web address: www.winn.amedd.army.mil/
Control: Army, Government, federal **Service:** General Medical and Surgical

Staffed Beds: 79

GA

HOMERVILLE—Clinch County

★ **CLINCH MEMORIAL HOSPITAL (111308)**, 282 Carswell Street, Zip 31634–1507, Mailing Address: P.O. Box 516, Zip 31634–0516; tel. 912/487–5211, (Nonreporting) **A**9 10 18
Primary Contact: Phillip Cook, Administrator
CFO: Sandra Hughes, Chief Financial Officer
CMO: Roger Huelsnitz, M.D., Chief of Staff
CIO: Shelly Studebaker, Director Management Information Systems
Web address: www.sgmc.org/healthsystem/clinchmemorial.htm
Control: County–Government, nonfederal **Service:** General Medical and Surgical

Staffed Beds: 25

JACKSON—Butts County

★ **SYLVAN GROVE HOSPITAL (111319)**, 1050 McDonough Road, Zip 30233–1599; tel. 770/775–7861 **A**9 10 18 **F**15 25 30 31 32 33 38 50 55 57 66 75 86 96 107 118 119 122 124 137 **S** TENET Healthcare Corporation
Primary Contact: John A. Quinn, Chief Executive Officer
COO: Edward J. Whitehouse, Chief Operating Officer
CFO: Tamara Ison, Chief Financial Officer
CIO: Steve Brown, Information Officer
CHR: Amanda Moore–Remington, Director Human Resources
Web address: www.sylvangrovehospital.com
Control: Corporation, Investor–owned, for–profit **Service:** General Medical and Surgical

Staffed Beds: 21 **Admissions:** 478 **Census:** 11 **Outpatient Visits:** 21491 **Births:** 0 **Total Expense ($000):** 8073 **Payroll Expense ($000):** 4472 **Personnel:** 68

JASPER—Pickens County

★ **PIEDMONT MOUNTAINSIDE HOSPITAL (110225)**, 1266 Highway 515 South, Zip 30143; tel. 706/692–2441 **A**1 9 10 **F**3 11 13 15 25 26 31 32 33 38 46 47 49 57 62 68 73 74 77 79 80 81 82 84 96 97 102 107 119 122 124 137 **S** Piedmont Healthcare
Primary Contact: Ed Lovern, President and Chief Executive Officer
COO: Mike Robertson, Vice President Operations
CFO: Sheryl Klink, Chief Financial Officer
CMO: Folsom Proctor, President Medical Staff
CHR: Christy Sims, Manager Human Resources
Web address: www.piedmontmountainsidehospital.org
Control: Other not–for–profit (including NFP Corporation) **Service:** General Medical and Surgical

Staffed Beds: 48 **Admissions:** 2663 **Census:** 27 **Outpatient Visits:** 45155 **Births:** 332 **Total Expense ($000):** 35483 **Payroll Expense ($000):** 13559 **Personnel:** 258

JESUP—Wayne County

★ **WAYNE MEMORIAL HOSPITAL (110124)**, 865 South First Street, Zip 31598–0210, Mailing Address: P.O. Box 410, Zip 31598–0410; tel. 912/427–6811 **A**1 9 10 20 **F**3 11 13 15 24 25 26 30 31 33 35 40 51 55 56 68 73 74 75 77 79 80 82 86 96 100 102 103 107 135
Primary Contact: Joseph P. Ierardi, Chief Executive Officer
CFO: Greg Jones, Chief Financial Officer
CMO: William Headley, M.D., Chief of Staff
CIO: Deborah Six, Coordinator Data Processing
CHR: John McIwain, Director Human Resources
Web address: www.wmhweb.com
Control: Hospital district or authority, Government, nonfederal **Service:** General Medical and Surgical

Staffed Beds: 83 **Admissions:** 3162 **Census:** 35 **Outpatient Visits:** 49966 **Births:** 514 **Total Expense ($000):** 38429 **Payroll Expense ($000):** 16622 **Personnel:** 440

JOHNS CREEK—De Kalb County

★ **EMORY JOHNS CREEK HOSPITAL (110172)**, 6325 Hospital Parkway, Zip 30097; tel. 678/474–7000 **A**1 10 **F**3 11 12 13 15 25 26 27 30 31 32 33 38 43 46 47 49 51 55 56 57 59 66 70 72 73 75 76 77 79 86 96 100 103 107 119 121 **S** HCA
Primary Contact: John Quinlivan, Chief Executive Officer
COO: Kavita Narayan, Chief Operating Officer
CFO: JoAnn Manning, Chief Financial Officer
CMO: Alan Wang, M.D., Chief Medical Officer
CIO: Hope Jackson, Director Information Systems
CHR: Pat Hack, Director Human Resources
Web address: www.emoryjohnscreek.com
Control: Corporation, Investor–owned, for–profit **Service:** General Medical and Surgical

Staffed Beds: 76 **Admissions:** 2816 **Census:** 29 **Outpatient Visits:** 23157 **Births:** 371 **Personnel:** 402

KENNESAW—Cobb County

DEVEREUX GEORGIA TREATMENT NETWORK, 1291 Stanley Road N.W., Zip 30152–4359, Mailing Address: P.O. Box 1688, Zip 30156–8688; tel. 770/427–0147 **F**25 30 31 32 73 88 89 135 **S** Devereux
Primary Contact: Mario Bolivar, Executive Director
COO: John Zdencanovic, Assistant Executive Director
CFO: Teresa Carter, Director Administrative Services
CMO: Yassar Kanawati, M.D., Medical Director
CIO: Kerry Shepherd, Coordinator Information Systems
CHR: Rudie Delien, Director Human Resources
Web address: www.devereuxga.org
Control: Other not–for–profit (including NFP Corporation) **Service:** Children's hospital psychiatric

Staffed Beds: 187 **Admissions:** 133 **Census:** 68 **Outpatient Visits:** 0 **Births:** 0 **Total Expense ($000):** 17382 **Payroll Expense ($000):** 3944 **Personnel:** 404

LA GRANGE—Troup County

★ **WEST GEORGIA HEALTH SYSTEM (110016)**, 1514 Vernon Road, Zip 30240–4199; tel. 706/882–1411, (Total facility includes 264 beds in nursing home–type unit) **A**1 2 9 10 19 **F**2 3 8 11 13 15 18 20 24 25 26 27 30 31 32 33 37 38 42 43 44 47 49 50 51 52 53 54 55 56 57 58 59 61 62 64 66 68 71 72 73 74 76 77 78 79 80 81 82 84 86 92 96 97 102 107 117 118 119 121 124 135
Primary Contact: Gerald N. Fulks, President and Chief Executive Officer
COO: Charis Acree, Senior Vice President
CFO: Paul R. Perrotti, CPA, Chief Financial Officer
CHR: Tommy Britt, Director Human Resources
Web address: www.wghs.org
Control: Hospital district or authority, Government, nonfederal **Service:** General Medical and Surgical

Staffed Beds: 413 **Admissions:** 7774 **Census:** 331 **Outpatient Visits:** 95150 **Births:** 1123 **Total Expense ($000):** 116335 **Payroll Expense ($000):** 49673 **Personnel:** 1189

LAKELAND—Lanier County

★ **LOUIS SMITH MEMORIAL HOSPITAL (111326)**, (Sub–Acute), 852 West Thigpen Avenue, Zip 31635–1099; tel. 229/482–3110, (Total facility includes 62 beds in nursing home–type unit) **A**9 10 18 **F**3 7 30 31 38 54 75 86 96 100 102 107 117 119 122 132
Primary Contact: Neil W. Ginty, Administrator
CFO: David Zammit, Chief Financial Officer
CMO: Bruce Herrington, Chief Medical Officer
CIO: Lucile Mann, Chief Information Officer
CHR: Vicki Dinkins, Director Human Resources
Web address: www.sgmc.org
Control: Hospital district or authority, Government, nonfederal **Service:** Other specialty

Staffed Beds: 87 **Admissions:** 589 **Census:** 71 **Outpatient Visits:** 12737 **Births:** 0 **Total Expense ($000):** 9536 **Payroll Expense ($000):** 3634 **Personnel:** 120

LAWRENCEVILLE—Gwinnett County

★ **GWINNETT HOSPITAL SYSTEM (110087)**, Mailing Address: P.O. Box 348, Zip 30246–0348; tel. 678/312–4321, (Includes GWINNETT MEDICAL CENTER, 1000 Medical Center Boulevard, Zip 30245; GWINNETT MEDICAL CENTER–DULUTH, 3620 Howell Ferry Road, Duluth, Zip 30096; tel. 678/312–6800), (Total facility includes 89 beds in nursing home–type unit) **A**1 2 9 10 **F**3 4 5 8 11 13 15 18 24 25 26 27 31 32 33 34 36 38 40 41 43 44 48 49 50 53 54 55 56 57 58 62 63 64 65 66 68 69 70 71 72 73 74 75 76 77 79 80 81 82 84 85 86 88 89 90 91 92 93 94 95 96 97 99 100 102 103 106 107 117 118 119 120 121 123 124 135 136 137 **P**8
Primary Contact: Philip R. Wolfe, President and Chief Executive Officer
COO: Jeffrey D. Nowlin, Executive Vice President and Chief Operating Officer
CFO: Thomas Y. McBride, Vice President and Chief Financial Officer
CMO: Alan Bier, M.D., Executive Vice President and Chief Medical Officer
CIO: Ed Brown, Chief Information Officer
CHR: Steve Nadeau, Vice President Human Resources
Web address: www.gwinnettmedicalcenter.org
Control: Other not–for–profit (including NFP Corporation) **Service:** General Medical and Surgical

Staffed Beds: 524 **Admissions:** 28627 **Census:** 451 **Outpatient Visits:** 234374 **Births:** 6206 **Total Expense ($000):** 449073 **Payroll Expense ($000):** 202142 **Personnel:** 3344

GA

Hospital, Medicare Provider Number, Address, Telephone, Approval, Facility, and Physician Codes, Health Care System

★ American Hospital Association (AHA) membership
□ The Joint Commission accreditation
○ American Osteopathic Association (AOA) accreditation
△ Commission on Accreditation of Rehabilitation Facilities (CARF) accreditation

LITHONIA—De Kalb County

☐ **DEKALB MEDICAL CENTER AT HILLANDALE (110226)**, 2801 DeKalb Medical Parkway, Zip 30058; tel. 404/501–8700 **A**1 9 10 **F**3 8 11 13 15 25 26 30 31 32 33 38 40 46 50 59 66 68 71 72 73 74 75 77 79 80 82 96 100 107 119 135 **S** DeKalb Regional Health System
Primary Contact: Clay Fowler, Vice President and Administrator
Web address: www.dekalbmedicalcenter.org
Control: Other not–for–profit (including NFP Corporation) **Service:** General Medical and Surgical

Staffed Beds: 100 **Admissions:** 4354 **Census:** 48 **Outpatient Visits:** 84934 **Births:** 1421 **Personnel:** 0

LOUISVILLE—Jefferson County

☐ **JEFFERSON HOSPITAL (110100)**, 1067 Peachtree Street, Zip 30434–1599; tel. 478/625–7000 **A**1 9 10 20 **F**27 38 52 53 55 56 57 62 63 64 76 79 86 87 96 98 102 107 122 **P**6
Primary Contact: Heyward Wells, III, Administrator
Control: City–County, Government, nonfederal **Service:** General Medical and Surgical

Staffed Beds: 37 **Admissions:** 1141 **Census:** 11 **Outpatient Visits:** 71168 **Births:** 0 **Total Expense ($000):** 11049 **Payroll Expense ($000):** 6352 **Personnel:** 137

MACON—Bibb County

★ **CENTRAL GEORGIA REHABILITATION HOSPITAL (113029)**, 3351 Northside Drive, Zip 31210–2591; tel. 478/201–6500 **A**1 9 10 **F**25 31 32 33 59 66 85 86 118 120 121 131 132 137
Primary Contact: Elbert T. McQueen, President and Chief Executive Officer
CFO: Beverly Owens, Controller
CHR: Carla Coates, Director Human Resources
Web address: www.centralgarehab.com
Control: Hospital district or authority, Government, nonfederal **Service:** Rehabilitation

Staffed Beds: 58 **Admissions:** 1038 **Census:** 38 **Outpatient Visits:** 13031 **Births:** 0 **Total Expense ($000):** 11962 **Payroll Expense ($000):** 6430 **Personnel:** 188

★ **COLISEUM MEDICAL CENTERS (110164)**, 350 Hospital Drive, Zip 31217–3871; tel. 478/765–7000 **A**1 2 9 10 **F**3 13 15 17 18 20 22 24 25 26 27 31 32 33 38 46 49 51 53 55 56 57 59 62 68 70 71 72 73 74 75 76 77 79 80 81 82 85 86 96 97 100 103 107 114 119 121 132 135 136 137 **S** HCA
Primary Contact: Allen Golson, Chief Executive Officer
COO: David A. Portwood, Chief Operating Officer
CFO: Roger Simmons, Chief Financial Officer
CIO: Joan Morstad, Director Information Systems
CHR: Pat Lattrell, Director Human Resources
Web address: www.coliseumhealthsystem.com
Control: Corporation, Investor–owned, for–profit **Service:** General Medical and Surgical

Staffed Beds: 227 **Admissions:** 9632 **Census:** 143 **Outpatient Visits:** 79996 **Births:** 1284 **Personnel:** 736

★ **COLISEUM NORTHSIDE HOSPITAL (110201)**, (Formerly Macon Northside Hospital), 400 Charter Boulevard, Zip 31210–4853, Mailing Address: P.O. Box 4627, Zip 31208–4627; tel. 478/757–8200, (Nonreporting) **A**1 9 10 **S** HCA
Primary Contact: Mark Nichols, FACHE, Chief Executive Officer
CFO: Roger Simmons, Chief Financial Officer
CHR: Pat Luttrell, Director Human Resources
Web address: www.coliseumhealthsystem.com
Control: Corporation, Investor–owned, for–profit **Service:** General Medical and Surgical

Staffed Beds: 103

★ **COLISEUM PSYCHIATRIC CENTER (114015)**, 340 Hospital Drive, Zip 31217–8002; tel. 478/741–1355 **A**1 9 10 **F**4 5 25 26 30 31 32 33 36 73 88 90 91 92 93 94 95 119 121 **S** HCA
Primary Contact: James W. Eyler, FACHE, Chief Executive Officer
CFO: Roger Simmons, Chief Financial Officer
Web address: www.coliseumhealthsystem.com
Control: Corporation, Investor–owned, for–profit **Service:** Psychiatric

Staffed Beds: 34 **Admissions:** 1336 **Census:** 26 **Outpatient Visits:** 3174 **Births:** 0 **Personnel:** 83

★ **MEDICAL CENTER OF CENTRAL GEORGIA (110107)**, 777 Hemlock Street, Zip 31201–2155, Mailing Address: P.O. Box 6000, Zip 31208–6000; tel. 478/633–1000 **A**1 2 3 5 8 9 10 **F**1 3 5 7 8 11 12 13 14 15 17 18 20 22 24 25 26 27 28 30 31 32 33 34 37 38 40 42 43 44 45 46 47 48 49 50 52 53 54 55 56 57 58 59 60 61 62 63 64 66 68 70 71 72 73 74 75 76 77 79 81 82 83 84 86 87 88 89 90 91 92 93 94 96 97 99 100 102 103 104 105 106 107 114 116 119 121 124 132 133 134 135 136 137 **P**1
Primary Contact: A. Donald Faulk, Jr., FACHE, President
COO: Joseph D. Lavelle, Executive Vice President and Chief Operating Officer
CFO: Rhonda Perry, Chief Financial Officer
CMO: James M. Cunningham, M.D., Senior Vice President Medical Affairs
CIO: Madison Mock, Vice President Information Services
Web address: www.mccg.org
Control: Hospital district or authority, Government, nonfederal **Service:** General Medical and Surgical

Staffed Beds: 597 **Admissions:** 29900 **Census:** 446 **Outpatient Visits:** 398879 **Births:** 3115 **Total Expense ($000):** 549272 **Payroll Expense ($000):** 225985 **Personnel:** 4607

★ **REGENCY HOSPITAL OF CENTRAL GEORGIA (112016)**, 700 Spring Street, Zip 31201; tel. 478/633–8260 **A**1 10 **F**1 3 25 30 31 32 55 59 75 82 119 121 137 **P**5 **S** Regency Hospital Company
Primary Contact: Susan Smith, RN
Web address: www.regencyhospital.com
Control: Corporation, Investor–owned, for–profit **Service:** Long–Term Acute Care hospital

Staffed Beds: 34 **Admissions:** 321 **Census:** 34 **Outpatient Visits:** 0 **Births:** 0 **Total Expense ($000):** 18205 **Payroll Expense ($000):** 7388 **Personnel:** 187

MADISON—Morgan County

☐ **MORGAN MEMORIAL HOSPITAL (111304)**, 1077 South Main Street, Zip 30650, Mailing Address: P.O. Box 860, Zip 30650–0860; tel. 706/342–1667, (Total facility includes 21 beds in nursing home–type unit) (Nonreporting) **A**1 9 10 18
Primary Contact: H. D. Cannington, Chief Executive Officer
CFO: Darlene Kinnett, Chief Financial Officer
CMO: Eduardo M. Cossio, M.D., Chief of Staff
CIO: Patrick Cook, Vice President Support Services
CHR: Melissa Malcolm, Director Human Resources
Web address: www.mmh.org
Control: Hospital district or authority, Government, nonfederal **Service:** General Medical and Surgical

Staffed Beds: 46

MARIETTA—Cobb County

★ △ **WELLSTAR KENNESTONE HOSPITAL (110035)**, 677 Church Street, Zip 30060–1148; tel. 770/793–5000 **A**1 2 3 5 7 9 10 **F**3 10 11 12 13 15 17 18 20 22 24 25 26 27 30 31 32 33 35 36 38 41 43 44 46 47 48 49 50 52 53 55 56 57 58 60 62 63 64 66 68 70 71 72 73 74 75 76 77 78 79 80 81 82 84 85 86 90 92 96 97 99 100 102 103 105 106 107 109 111 112 115 119 121 123 124 135 136 137 **P**1 6 **S** WellStar Health System
Primary Contact: Candice Saunders, Senior Vice President and Administrator
COO: Linda A. Clark, Executive Vice President and Administrator
CFO: Jim Budzinski, Vice President and Chief Financial Officer
CMO: Barry Nedoba, M.D., Medical Director
CIO: Ronald Strachan, Chief Information Officer
CHR: David W. Anderson, Executive Vice President Human Resources and Chief Compliance Officer
Web address: www.wellstar.org
Control: Other not–for–profit (including NFP Corporation) **Service:** General Medical and Surgical

Staffed Beds: 604 **Admissions:** 33446 **Census:** 464 **Outpatient Visits:** 356507 **Births:** 6426 **Personnel:** 3677

★ **WELLSTAR WINDY HILL HOSPITAL (112007)**, 2540 Windy Hill Road, Zip 30067–8632; tel. 770/644–1000 **A**1 2 9 10 **F**1 3 5 11 15 25 26 30 31 32 33 36 41 46 47 48 49 50 51 55 56 57 60 62 66 73 75 77 79 80 81 82 86 91 94 95 96 97 99 100 102 106 107 118 119 121 124 135 137 **P**1 6 **S** WellStar Health System
Primary Contact: Lou Little, Vice President and Administrator
COO: Paul Johnson, Executive Vice President Operations
CFO: Marsha Burke, Senior Vice President and Chief Financial Officer
CMO: Larry Haldeman, M.D., Executive Vice President and Chief Medical Officer
CIO: Leigh Cox, Chief Information Officer
Web address: www.wellstar.org
Control: Other not–for–profit (including NFP Corporation) **Service:** Long–Term Acute Care hospital

Staffed Beds: 42 **Admissions:** 281 **Census:** 30 **Outpatient Visits:** 29676 **Births:** 0 **Personnel:** 283

GA

MCRAE—Telfair County

☐ **TAYLOR–TELFAIR REGIONAL HOSPITAL (111301)**, U.S. 341 South, Zip 31055, Mailing Address: P.O. Box 150, Zip 31055–0150; tel. 229/868–5621, (Nonreporting) **A**1 9 10 18
Primary Contact: Joan Hartley, Chief Executive Officer and Administrator
CIO: Shirley Ashley, Director Health Information Management Systems
Control: Other not–for–profit (including NFP Corporation) **Service:** General Medical and Surgical

Staffed Beds: 25

METTER—Candler County

☐ **CANDLER COUNTY HOSPITAL (111334)**, 400 Cedar Street, Zip 30439–3338, Mailing Address: P.O. Box 597, Zip 30439–0597; tel. 912/685–5741, (Nonreporting) **A**1 9 10 18
Primary Contact: Danny B. Moxley, Chief Executive Officer
Web address: www.candlercountyhospital.com
Control: Hospital district or authority, Government, nonfederal **Service:** General Medical and Surgical

Staffed Beds: 25

MILLEDGEVILLE—Baldwin County

CENTRAL STATE HOSPITAL (114018), 620 Broad Street, Zip 31062–0001; tel. 478/445–4128, (Total facility includes 536 beds in nursing home–type unit) **A**9 10 **F**15 26 30 37 41 52 57 65 73 75 81 82 87 88 89 90 93 96 97 99 100 107 117 119 **P**6
Primary Contact: Marvin Bailey, Chief Executive Officer
COO: Terry McGee, Chief Operations Officer
CMO: Scott VanSant, M.D., Chief Medical Officer
CIO: Betsy Bradley, Coordinator Performance Improvement
CHR: Myra Holloway, Director Human Resources Management
Web address: www.centralstatehospital.org
Control: State–Government, nonfederal **Service:** Psychiatric

Staffed Beds: 852 **Admissions:** 2927 **Census:** 791 **Outpatient Visits:** 0 **Births:** 0 **Total Expense ($000):** 105721 **Payroll Expense ($000):** 58823 **Personnel:** 2031

☐ **OCONEE REGIONAL MEDICAL CENTER (110150)**, 821 North Cobb Street, Zip 31061–2351, Mailing Address: P.O. Box 690, Zip 31061–0690; tel. 478/454–3500, (Total facility includes 7 beds in nursing home–type unit) **A**1 9 10 19 **F**11 13 15 25 26 30 32 33 38 40 46 47 48 49 50 51 52 55 56 57 62 66 68 74 77 78 79 82 84 86 96 97 98 100 102 104 107 108 109 112 117 118 135 136 **S** Oconee Regional Health System
Primary Contact: Jean Aycock, President and Chief Executive Officer
Web address: www.oconeeregional.com
Control: Other not–for–profit (including NFP Corporation) **Service:** General Medical and Surgical

Staffed Beds: 106 **Admissions:** 4943 **Census:** 54 **Outpatient Visits:** 98633 **Births:** 742 **Total Expense ($000):** 70082 **Payroll Expense ($000):** 27864 **Personnel:** 557

MILLEN—Jenkins County

JENKINS COUNTY HOSPITAL (111311), 931 East Winthrope Avenue, Zip 30442–1839; tel. 478/982–4221, (Nonreporting) **A**9 10 18
Primary Contact: Pete Mills, Chief Executive Officer
Control: Hospital district or authority, Government, nonfederal **Service:** General Medical and Surgical

Staffed Beds: 25

MONROE—Walton County

☐ **WALTON REGIONAL MEDICAL CENTER (110046)**, 330 Alcovy Street, Zip 30655–2140, Mailing Address: P.O. Box 1346, Zip 30655–1346; tel. 770/267–8461, (Total facility includes 58 beds in nursing home–type unit) (Nonreporting) **A**1 9 10 **S** Health Management Associates
Primary Contact: Gary Lang, Chief Executive Officer
COO: Blake Watts, Chief Operating Officer
CFO: Jeff Grimsley, Chief Financial Officer
CMO: Mark Shaffer, DPM, Chief of Staff
CHR: Michele Monsrud, Director Human Resources
Web address: www.walton.org
Control: Corporation, Investor–owned, for–profit **Service:** General Medical and Surgical

Staffed Beds: 115

MONTEZUMA—Macon County

☐ **FLINT RIVER COMMUNITY HOSPITAL (110190)**, 509 Sumter Street, Zip 31063–0770, Mailing Address: P.O. Box 770, Zip 31063–0770; tel. 478/472–3100, (Nonreporting) **A**1 9 10 **S** Resurgence Health Group
Primary Contact: Laurie Hair, Chief Executive Officer and Chief Financial Officer
CFO: Laurie Hair, Chief Executive Officer and Chief Financial Officer
CMO: Douglas Joyner, M.D., Chief of Staff
CIO: La Tonya Henderson, Director Information Management
CHR: Judd Conner, Coordinator Human Resources
Web address: www.resurgencehealthgroup.com
Control: Corporation, Investor–owned, for–profit **Service:** General Medical and Surgical

Staffed Beds: 49

MONTICELLO—Jasper County

JASPER MEMORIAL HOSPITAL (111303), 898 College Street, Zip 31064–1298; tel. 706/468–6411, (Total facility includes 55 beds in nursing home–type unit) **A**9 10 18 **F**11 25 38 55 56 57 62 63 75 86 87 96 100 102 107 117 119 122 135 137 **P**6 **S** Oconee Regional Health System
Primary Contact: David J. Owens, Chief Executive Officer
CFO: Laura Hammonds, Controller
Web address: www.jaspermemorialhospital.org
Control: Other not–for–profit (including NFP Corporation) **Service:** General Medical and Surgical

Staffed Beds: 67 **Admissions:** 184 **Census:** 45 **Outpatient Visits:** 13860 **Births:** 0 **Total Expense ($000):** 8875 **Payroll Expense ($000):** 4631 **Personnel:** 120

MOULTRIE—Colquitt County

★ ○ **COLQUITT REGIONAL MEDICAL CENTER (110105)**, 3131 South Main Street, Zip 31768–6701, Mailing Address: P.O. Box 40, Zip 31776–0040; tel. 229/985–3420 **A**9 10 11 20 **F**3 7 11 13 15 17 18 25 26 27 28 30 31 32 33 37 38 42 43 48 49 54 55 56 57 59 60 61 63 66 68 72 73 74 75 76 77 79 80 81 82 84 86 87 96 97 100 102 106 107 118 119 120 121 124 132 133 135 136 137
Primary Contact: James R. Lowry, FACHE, Chief Executive Officer
COO: Madis Spires, Vice President Patient Services
CFO: W. Larry Sims, Chief Financial Officer and Vice President Financial Services
CMO: D. W. Adcock, M.D., Medical Director
CIO: Mitch Hiers, Director Information Services
CHR: Dawn Johns, Director Human Resources
Web address: www.colquittregional.com
Control: Hospital district or authority, Government, nonfederal **Service:** General Medical and Surgical

Staffed Beds: 73 **Admissions:** 3975 **Census:** 43 **Outpatient Visits:** 108704 **Births:** 779 **Total Expense ($000):** 65076 **Payroll Expense ($000):** 26349 **Personnel:** 657

TURNING POINT HOSPITAL (110209), 3015 Veterans Parkway S.E., Zip 31768–6705, Mailing Address: P.O. Box 1177, Zip 31776–1177; tel. 229/985–4815 **A**9 10 **F**4 5 73 82 94 95 119 124 132 **P**6 **S** Universal Health Services, Inc.
Primary Contact: Ben Marion, Chief Executive Officer and Managing Director
CFO: Edwin Bennett, Controller
Web address: www.turningpointcare.com
Control: Corporation, Investor–owned, for–profit **Service:** Alcoholism and other chemical dependency

Staffed Beds: 59 **Admissions:** 1222 **Census:** 13 **Outpatient Visits:** 11574 **Births:** 0 **Total Expense ($000):** 6532 **Payroll Expense ($000):** 3372 **Personnel:** 82

NASHVILLE—Berrien County

☐ **BERRIEN COUNTY HOSPITAL (110112)**, 1221 East McPherson Avenue, Zip 31639–2326, Mailing Address: P.O. Box 665, Zip 31639–0665; tel. 229/543–7100, (Total facility includes 108 beds in nursing home–type unit) (Nonreporting) **A**1 9 10 **S** Associated Healthcare Systems, Inc.
Primary Contact: James D. Janek, Chief Executive Officer
CFO: Stephanie Fletcher, Chief Financial Officer
Web address: www.berrienhospital.com
Control: Corporation, Investor–owned, for–profit **Service:** General Medical and Surgical

Staffed Beds: 171

Hospital, Medicare Provider Number, Address, Telephone, Approval, Facility, and Physician Codes, Health Care System

★ American Hospital Association (AHA) membership
☐ The Joint Commission accreditation
○ American Osteopathic Association (AOA) accreditation
△ Commission on Accreditation of Rehabilitation Facilities (CARF) accreditation

NEWNAN—Coweta County

★ **PIEDMONT NEWNAN HOSPITAL (110020)**, 60 Hospital Road, Zip 30263–1210, Mailing Address: P.O. Box 997, Zip 30264–0997; tel. 770/253–1912, (Total facility includes 143 beds in nursing home–type unit) (Nonreporting) **A**1 9 10 **S** Piedmont Healthcare
Primary Contact: G. Michael Bass, President and Chief Executive Officer
COO: Nathan Nipper, Chief Operating Officer
CFO: G. Michael Bass, President and Chief Executive Officer
CIO: Henry Scott, Director Management Information Systems
CHR: Virginia Lyles, Vice President Human Resources
Web address: www.newnanhospital.org
Control: Other not–for–profit (including NFP Corporation) **Service:** General Medical and Surgical

Staffed Beds: 271

OCILLA—Irwin County

★ **IRWIN COUNTY HOSPITAL (110130)**, 710 North Irwin Avenue, Zip 31774–1098; tel. 229/468–3800, (Total facility includes 30 beds in nursing home–type unit) **A**1 9 10 **F**3 13 15 31 38 50 62 66 73 79 80 96 102 107 117 119 124
Primary Contact: Sue Spivey, Administrator
CFO: Tami Gray, Chief Financial Officer
CMO: Ashfaq Saiyed, M.D., Medical Director
CHR: Becky Edwards, Manager Human Resources
Web address: www.irwincntyhospital.com
Control: Hospital district or authority, Government, nonfederal **Service:** General Medical and Surgical

Staffed Beds: 64 **Admissions:** 1416 **Census:** 40 **Outpatient Visits:** 11578 **Births:** 655 **Total Expense ($000):** 11298 **Payroll Expense ($000):** 5596 **Personnel:** 205

PERRY—Houston County

★ **PERRY HOSPITAL (110153)**, 1120 Morningside Drive, Zip 31069–2906; tel. 478/987–3600 **A**1 9 10 **F**3 11 15 25 26 30 31 32 33 37 38 43 48 49 50 54 55 56 57 58 60 66 68 73 77 79 80 81 82 84 90 96 102 107 119 120 121 122 123 124 135 136 137
Primary Contact: Lora Davis, Administrator
CFO: Frank R. Powell, Chief Financial Officer
CIO: Beth Benefield, Director Information Systems
Web address: www.hhc.org
Control: Hospital district or authority, Government, nonfederal **Service:** General Medical and Surgical

Staffed Beds: 39 **Admissions:** 2220 **Census:** 26 **Outpatient Visits:** 37175 **Births:** 0 **Total Expense ($000):** 22318 **Payroll Expense ($000):** 9624 **Personnel:** 181

QUITMAN—Brooks County

★ **BROOKS COUNTY HOSPITAL (111332)**, 903 North Court Street, Zip 31643–1315, Mailing Address: P.O. Box 5000, Zip 31643–5000; tel. 229/263–4171 **A**1 9 10 18 **F**11 15 25 26 30 31 32 33 38 50 55 56 57 73 75 81 82 86 92 96 100 107 119 122 124 135 **P**6 **S** Archbold Medical Center
Primary Contact: LaDon Toole, Administrator
COO: LaDon Toole, Administrator
CFO: LaDon Toole, Administrator
CMO: Michael Sopt, M.D., Chief of Staff
CHR: Janet Eldridge, Director Human Resources and Personnel
Web address: www.archbold.org
Control: Hospital district or authority, Government, nonfederal **Service:** General Medical and Surgical

Staffed Beds: 25 **Admissions:** 795 **Census:** 18 **Outpatient Visits:** 16973 **Births:** 0 **Total Expense ($000):** 9859 **Payroll Expense ($000):** 4502 **Personnel:** 100

REIDSVILLE—Tattnall County

TATTNALL COMMUNITY HOSPITAL (111323), 247 South Main Street, Zip 30453; tel. 912/557–1000, (Nonreporting) **A**9 10 18
Primary Contact: Karen O'Neal, Chief Executive Officer
Web address: www.resurgencehealthgroup.com
Control: Hospital district or authority, Government, nonfederal **Service:** General Medical and Surgical

Staffed Beds: 25

RICHLAND—Stewart County

STEWART–WEBSTER HOSPITAL (111322), 300 Alston Street, Zip 31825–1406, Mailing Address: P.O. Box 190, Zip 31825–0190; tel. 229/887–3366, (Nonreporting) **A**9 10 18 **S** Accord Health Care Corporation
Primary Contact: Stephen H. Noble, President
CFO: Randy Stigleman, Chief Financial Officer
Control: Corporation, Investor–owned, for–profit **Service:** General Medical and Surgical

Staffed Beds: 25

RIVERDALE—Clayton County

★ **SOUTHERN CRESCENT HOSPITAL FOR SPECIALTY CARE (112015)**, 11 Upper Riverdale Road S.W., 6th Floor, Zip 30274; tel. 770/897–7603 **A**1 10 **F**1 25 26 30 31 32 33 41 43 44 73 75 82 137 **P**8 **S** Dubuis Health System
Primary Contact: Janice Hamilton–Crawford, Administrator
Control: Other not–for–profit (including NFP Corporation) **Service:** Long–Term Acute Care hospital

Staffed Beds: 30 **Admissions:** 265 **Census:** 20 **Outpatient Visits:** 0 **Births:** 0 **Total Expense ($000):** 8867 **Payroll Expense ($000):** 3137 **Personnel:** 72

★ **SOUTHERN REGIONAL MEDICAL CENTER (110165)**, 11 Upper Riverdale Road S.W., Zip 30274–2615; tel. 770/991–8000, (Nonreporting) **A**1 2 9 10
Primary Contact: Edward J. Bonn, President and Chief Executive Officer
COO: Mary Kay Gardenier, Senior Vice President Operations and Chief Operating Officer
CFO: Richard G. Stovall, Senior Vice President Fiscal Services and Chief Financial Officer
CMO: Willie Cochran, M.D., Chief of Staff
CIO: Karen Moore, Vice President Information Technology and Chief Information Officer
CHR: Norma Adams, Director Human Resources
Web address: www.southernregional.org
Control: Other not–for–profit (including NFP Corporation) **Service:** General Medical and Surgical

Staffed Beds: 329

ROME—Floyd County

★ △ **FLOYD MEDICAL CENTER (110054)**, 304 Turner McCall Boulevard, Zip 30165–2734, Mailing Address: P.O. Box 233, Zip 30162–0233; tel. 706/509–5000 **A**1 2 3 5 7 9 10 12 13 19 **F**1 3 4 5 6 7 8 9 11 12 13 15 17 18 24 25 26 27 28 30 31 32 33 34 35 36 37 38 40 41 42 43 44 46 48 49 50 51 52 53 54 55 56 57 58 60 61 62 63 64 66 68 70 71 72 73 74 75 76 77 79 80 81 82 83 84 85 86 87 88 90 91 92 93 94 95 96 97 99 100 102 106 107 108 109 111 118 119 120 121 123 124 132 133 135 136 137
Primary Contact: Kurt Stuenkel, FACHE, President and Chief Executive Officer
COO: Sonny Rigas, Senior Vice President and Chief Operating Officer
CFO: Rick Sheerin, Vice President Fiscal Services
CMO: Dee B. Russell, M.D., Chief Executive Officer
CIO: Brian Barnette, Chief Information Officer
CHR: Rick Tew, Director Human Resources
Web address: www.floyd.org
Control: Other not–for–profit (including NFP Corporation) **Service:** General Medical and Surgical

Staffed Beds: 304 **Admissions:** 12450 **Census:** 172 **Outpatient Visits:** 273697 **Births:** 2635 **Total Expense ($000):** 203157 **Payroll Expense ($000):** 89756 **Personnel:** 1894

☐ **NORTHWEST GEORGIA REGIONAL HOSPITAL (114014)**, 1305 Redmond Circle, Zip 30165–1393; tel. 706/295–6011, (Nonreporting) **A**1 9 10
Primary Contact: Karl H. Schwarzkopf, Regional Administrator
COO: Frank L. Davis, Assistant Superintendent
CFO: Jerry Jacobs, Business Manager
CMO: Thomas W. Muller, M.D., Clinical Director
Web address: www.nwgrh.dhr.state.ga.us
Control: State–Government, nonfederal **Service:** Psychiatric

Staffed Beds: 297

★ **REDMOND REGIONAL MEDICAL CENTER (110168)**, 501 Redmond Road, Zip 30165–7001, Mailing Address: Box 107001, Zip 30164–7001; tel. 706/291–0291 **A**1 2 9 10 19 **F**3 7 12 15 17 18 20 22 24 25 26 27 32 38 43 46 47 48 49 50 55 56 57 60 62 66 68 72 73 75 76 77 79 80 81 82 85 86 96 97 99 100 102 103 106 107 118 119 120 121 132 135 136 137 **S** HCA
Primary Contact: Brenda M. Waltz, FACHE, Chief Executive Officer
COO: Carlton Ulmer, Chief Operating Officer
CFO: Danny Smith, Chief Financial Officer
CMO: Ted Pennel, M.D., Chief Medical Officer
CIO: Brad Treglown, Director Information Systems
CHR: Patsy Adams, Director Human Resources
Web address: www.redmondregional.com
Control: Corporation, Investor–owned, for–profit **Service:** General Medical and Surgical

Staffed Beds: 230 **Admissions:** 12571 **Census:** 156 **Outpatient Visits:** 75843 **Total Expense ($000):** 147829 **Payroll Expense ($000):** 52451 **Personnel:** 973

SPECIALTY HOSPITAL (112010), 304 Turner McCall Boulevard, Zip 30162; tel. 706/802–4100 **A**9 10 **F**1 3 25 75
Primary Contact: Mark Fall, Chief Executive Officer
Control: Other not–for–profit (including NFP Corporation) **Service:** Long–Term Acute Care hospital

Staffed Beds: 24 **Admissions:** 236 **Census:** 20 **Outpatient Visits:** 0 **Births:** 0 **Total Expense ($000):** 8001 **Payroll Expense ($000):** 2707 **Personnel:** 57

Many Facility Codes have changed. Please refer to the AHA Guide Code Chart.

ROSWELL—Fulton County

★□ **NORTH FULTON REGIONAL HOSPITAL (110198)**, 3000 Hospital Boulevard, Zip 30076–3899; tel. 770/751–2500 **A**1 9 10 **F**3 11 12 13 15 17 18 24 25 26 27 30 31 32 33 38 40 47 48 49 50 53 55 56 57 62 68 70 72 73 74 76 77 79 80 82 85 86 96 97 100 102 106 107 124 135 136 137 **S** TENET Healthcare Corporation
Primary Contact: Joe Austin, Chief Executive Officer
COO: Ilona Wozniak, Chief Operating Officer
CFO: Wesley James, Chief Financial Officer
CHR: Susan Brown, Chief Human Resources Officer
Web address: www.northfultonregional.com
Control: Corporation, Investor–owned, for–profit **Service:** General Medical and Surgical

Staffed Beds: 195 **Admissions:** 9537 **Census:** 123 **Outpatient Visits:** 70075 **Births:** 2263 **Total Expense ($000):** 114314 **Payroll Expense ($000):** 43993 **Personnel:** 813

ROYSTON—Franklin County

□ **COBB MEMORIAL HOSPITAL (110027)**, 521 Franklin Springs Street, Zip 30662–3909, Mailing Address: P.O. Box 589, Zip 30662–0589; tel. 706/245–5071, (Includes BROWN MEMORIAL CONVALESCENT CENTER, COBB HEALTH CARE CENTER AND THE GABLES), (Total facility includes 260 beds in nursing home–type unit) **A**1 9 10 **F**3 11 13 15 25 26 30 31 32 33 38 46 50 55 56 57 62 65 67 68 73 74 77 79 82 84 86 96 97 99 100 102 107 117 119 120 122 124 **S** Ty Cobb Healthcare System, Inc.
Primary Contact: John M. Herron, Administrator
CFO: Kimberly Massey, Controller
Web address: www.tycobbhealthcare.org
Control: Other not–for–profit (including NFP Corporation) **Service:** General Medical and Surgical

Staffed Beds: 331 **Admissions:** 2311 **Census:** 286 **Outpatient Visits:** 28803 **Births:** 351 **Total Expense ($000):** 31952 **Payroll Expense ($000):** 13200 **Personnel:** 482

SAINT MARYS—Camden County

□ **SOUTHEAST GEORGIA HEALTH SYSTEM CAMDEN CAMPUS (110146)**, 2000 Dan Proctor Drive, Zip 31558–3810; tel. 912/576–6200, (Nonreporting) **A**1 9 10 20 **S** Southeast Georgia Health System
Primary Contact: Howard W. Sepp, Jr., FACHE, Vice President and Administrator
CFO: Michael D. Scherneck, Executive Vice President
CHR: Patrick Ebri, Ph.D., Vice President Human Resources
Web address: www.sghs.org
Control: Other not–for–profit (including NFP Corporation) **Service:** General Medical and Surgical

Staffed Beds: 40

SAINT SIMONS ISLAND—Glynn County

□ **FOCUS BY–THE–SEA (114016)**, 2927 Demere Road, Zip 31522–1620; tel. 912/638–1999, (Nonreporting) **A**1 9 10 **S** Horizon Health Corporation
Primary Contact: Ronald Mays, Chief Executive Officer
CMO: Kim Masters, M.D., Medical Director
CIO: Chisty Mosely, Director Information Management
Web address: www.focushealthcare.com
Control: Corporation, Investor–owned, for–profit **Service:** Psychiatric

Staffed Beds: 101

SANDERSVILLE—Washington County

□ **WASHINGTON COUNTY REGIONAL MEDICAL CENTER (110086)**, 610 Sparta Road, Zip 31082–1362, Mailing Address: P.O. Box 636, Zip 31082–0636; tel. 478/240–2000, (Total facility includes 60 beds in nursing home–type unit) (Nonreporting) **A**1 9 10 20
Primary Contact: H. Thomas Brown, Chief Executive Officer
CFO: Cythia Parker, Fiscal Director
CMO: Robert Wright, M.D., Chief of Staff
CHR: Gayle Prince, Director Human Resources
Web address: www.wcrmc.com
Control: Hospital district or authority, Government, nonfederal **Service:** General Medical and Surgical

Staffed Beds: 116

SAVANNAH—Chatham County

COASTAL HARBOR TREATMENT CENTER (114008), 1150 Cornell Avenue, Zip 31406–2797; tel. 912/354–3911 **A**9 10 **F**25 88 89 92 95 119 **S** Universal Health Services, Inc.
Primary Contact: Ray Heckerman, Chief Executive Officer and Managing Director
CFO: Garry Ege, Chief Financial Officer
CMO: Ed Merves, M.D., Medical Director
CHR: Beth Thompson, Director Human Resources
Web address: www.coastalharbor.com
Control: Corporation, Investor–owned, for–profit **Service:** Children's hospital psychiatric

Staffed Beds: 132 **Admissions:** 486 **Census:** 123 **Outpatient Visits:** 4817 **Births:** 0 **Total Expense ($000):** 16167 **Payroll Expense ($000):** 7906 **Personnel:** 225

□ **GEORGIA REGIONAL HOSPITAL AT SAVANNAH (114028)**, 1915 Eisenhower Drive, Zip 31406–5098; tel. 912/356–2011 **A**1 9 10 **F**30 31 32 37 88 92 119 135
Primary Contact: Charles Li, M.D., Regional Administrator
COO: Thomas F. Kurtz, Chief Operating Officer
CFO: Janet Edenfield, Director Financial Services
CMO: Francine Friedman, Clinical Dir
CHR: Jamekia Powers, Assistant Director Human Resources
Web address: www.garegionalsavannah.com
Control: State–Government, nonfederal **Service:** Psychiatric

Staffed Beds: 105 **Admissions:** 2201 **Census:** 105 **Outpatient Visits:** 0 **Births:** 0 **Total Expense ($000):** 20400 **Payroll Expense ($000):** 16584 **Personnel:** 420

★□ △ **MEMORIAL HEALTH (110036)**, 4700 Waters Avenue, Zip 31404–6283, Mailing Address: P.O. Box 23089, Zip 31403–3089; tel. 912/350–8000 **A**1 2 3 5 7 8 9 10 **F**3 11 12 13 15 17 18 20 22 24 25 26 27 30 31 32 33 34 35 37 38 40 41 43 44 45 46 49 50 52 53 54 55 56 57 58 59 60 62 63 66 68 69 70 71 72 73 74 76 77 79 80 81 82 83 84 85 86 87 88 90 91 92 93 94 96 99 100 102 103 106 107 108 109 111 112 113 114 118 119 120 121 124 133 135 136 137
Primary Contact: Robert A. Colvin, President and Chief Executive Officer
COO: Margaret Gill, Senior Vice President Operations
CFO: Margaret Gill, Senior Vice President Operations and Interim Chief Financial Officer
CMO: Ramon V. Meguiar, M.D., Senior Vice President and Chief Medical Officer
CIO: Patty Massey, Chief Information Officer
CHR: David Thaeler, Vice President Human Resources
Web address: www.memorialhealth.com
Control: Hospital district or authority, Government, nonfederal **Service:** General Medical and Surgical

Staffed Beds: 504 **Admissions:** 24499 **Census:** 370 **Outpatient Visits:** 267926 **Births:** 2789 **Total Expense ($000):** 449222 **Payroll Expense ($000):** 178575 **Personnel:** 3376

GA

□ **SELECT SPECIALTY HOSPITAL OF SAVANNAH (112011)**, 5353 Reynolds Street, 4 South, Zip 31405; tel. 912/819–7972, (Nonreporting) **A**1 9 10 **S** Select Medical Corporation
Primary Contact: John Heffner, Chief Executive Officer
Web address: www.selectmedicalcorp.com
Control: Corporation, Investor–owned, for–profit **Service:** Long–Term Acute Care hospital

Staffed Beds: 40

★□ △ **ST. JOSEPH'S/CANDLER, CANDLER HOSPITAL (110024)**, 5353 Reynolds Street, Zip 31405–6013; tel. 912/819–6000, (Total facility includes 11 beds in nursing home–type unit) **A**1 7 9 10 **F**3 8 11 13 15 18 20 24 25 26 27 28 30 31 32 33 34 35 36 37 38 41 43 44 46 48 49 50 55 56 57 58 59 60 61 63 66 68 69 71 72 73 74 75 76 77 79 80 81 82 84 85 86 90 96 97 99 100 102 105 106 107 117 118 119 120 121 124 132 135 136 137
Primary Contact: Paul P. Hinchey, President and Chief Executive Officer
COO: Paul P. Hinchey, President and Chief Executive Officer
CFO: Gregory J. Schaack, Vice President and Chief Financial Officer
CMO: James Jackson, M.D., Vice President Medical Affairs
CIO: John Adkins, Vice President and Chief Information Officer
Web address: www.sjchs.org
Control: Church–operated, Nongovernment, not–for profit **Service:** General Medical and Surgical

Staffed Beds: 289 **Admissions:** 10147 **Census:** 172 **Outpatient Visits:** 198833 **Births:** 3009 **Total Expense ($000):** 173664 **Payroll Expense ($000):** 74363 **Personnel:** 1547

Hospital, Medicare Provider Number, Address, Telephone, Approval, Facility, and Physician Codes, Health Care System

★ American Hospital Association (AHA) membership
□ The Joint Commission accreditation
○ American Osteopathic Association (AOA) accreditation
△ Commission on Accreditation of Rehabilitation Facilities (CARF) accreditation

□ △ **ST. JOSEPH'S/CANDLER, ST. JOSEPH'S HOSPITAL (110043)**, 11705 Mercy Boulevard, Zip 31419–1791; tel. 912/925–4100, (Total facility includes 11 beds in nursing home–type unit) **A**1 2 7 9 10 **F**3 8 11 15 17 18 20 22 24 25 26 27 30 31 32 33 34 35 36 37 38 41 43 44 46 48 49 50 51 54 55 56 57 58 59 60 62 63 66 68 72 73 75 76 77 78 79 80 81 82 85 86 90 96 97 100 102 103 106 107 116 117 119 120 121 124 135 137
Primary Contact: Paul P. Hinchey, President and Chief Executive Officer
CFO: Gregory J. Schaack, Vice President and Chief Financial Officer
CMO: James Jackson, M.D., Vice President Medical Affairs
CIO: John Adkins, Vice President and Chief Information Officer
CHR: Don Stubbs, Vice President Human Resources
Web address: www.sjchs.org
Control: Church–operated, Nongovernment, not–for profit **Service:** General Medical and Surgical

Staffed Beds: 225 **Admissions:** 10185 **Census:** 167 **Outpatient Visits:** 83736 **Births:** 0 **Total Expense ($000):** 161437 **Payroll Expense ($000):** 62079 **Personnel:** 1206

SMYRNA—Cobb County

★ **EMORY–ADVENTIST HOSPITAL (110183)**, 3949 South Cobb Drive S.E., Zip 30080–6300; tel. 770/434–0710, (Nonreporting) **A**1 9 10 **S** Adventist Health System Sunbelt Health Care Corporation
Primary Contact: Dennis Kiley, President
COO: Peggy Seckler, Chief Operating Officer
CFO: Carol Hazen, Vice President Finance
Web address: www.emoryadventist.org
Control: Church–operated, Nongovernment, not–for profit **Service:** General Medical and Surgical

Staffed Beds: 57

★ **RIDGEVIEW INSTITUTE (114012)**, 3995 South Cobb Drive S.E., Zip 30080–6397; tel. 770/434–4567 **A**1 9 10 **F**4 5 31 33 36 73 82 88 89 90 91 92 93 94 95 119 121 136 **P**8
Primary Contact: Paul Hackman, Chief Executive Officer
CFO: Jerry Magnison, Vice President Finance
CMO: James Vargo, M.D., Medical Director
CIO: Lynn Leger, Director Information Systems
CHR: Betty Sonderman, Manager Human Resources
Web address: www.ridgeviewinstitute.com
Control: Other not–for–profit (including NFP Corporation) **Service:** Psychiatric

Staffed Beds: 92 **Admissions:** 4050 **Census:** 67 **Outpatient Visits:** 38876 **Births:** 0 **Total Expense ($000):** 28066 **Payroll Expense ($000):** 14585 **Personnel:** 343

SNELLVILLE—Gwinnett County

★ **EMORY EASTSIDE MEDICAL CENTER (110192)**, 1700 Medical Way, Zip 30078–2195, Mailing Address: P.O. Box 587, Zip 30078–0587; tel. 770/979–0200 **A**1 2 9 10 **F**3 11 13 15 18 24 25 26 27 30 31 32 35 37 38 43 49 50 54 55 56 57 62 68 70 71 72 73 74 75 76 77 79 80 81 82 85 86 88 91 93 94 96 97 99 100 102 106 107 112 118 119 121 133 135 136 137 **S** HCA
Primary Contact: Kimberly Ryan, Chief Executive Officer
COO: Dustin Greene, Chief Operating Officer
CFO: Greg Caples, Chief Financial Officer
CMO: Michael Heisler, M.D., Chief Medical Officer
CIO: Sheila C. Adcock, Director Marketing and Public Relations
CHR: Scott Lowe, Director Human Resources
Web address: www.emoryeastside.com
Control: Corporation, Investor–owned, for–profit **Service:** General Medical and Surgical

Staffed Beds: 218 **Admissions:** 11372 **Census:** 175 **Outpatient Visits:** 128333 **Births:** 2525 **Total Expense ($000):** 113272 **Payroll Expense ($000):** 53566 **Personnel:** 1039

SPRINGFIELD—Effingham County

★ **EFFINGHAM HOSPITAL (111306)**, 459 Highway 119 South, Zip 31329–3021, Mailing Address: P.O. Box 386, Zip 31329–0386; tel. 912/754–6451, (Total facility includes 105 beds in nursing home–type unit) **A**1 9 10 18 **F**11 15 24 25 38 46 50 53 54 57 62 63 65 79 81 82 87 117 119 122 132 133 135
Primary Contact: Norma J. Morgan, Chief Executive Officer
CFO: Ed Brown, Chief Financial Officer
CMO: George W. Brelsford, M.D., Chief Medical Staff
CIO: Bart Hunter, Manager Information Technology
CHR: Vicky B. Edwards, Director Human Resources
Web address: www.effinghamhospital.com
Control: Hospital district or authority, Government, nonfederal **Service:** General Medical and Surgical

Staffed Beds: 130 **Admissions:** 222 **Census:** 106 **Outpatient Visits:** 29276 **Births:** 0

STATESBORO—Bulloch County

□ **EAST GEORGIA REGIONAL MEDICAL CENTER (110075)**, 1499 Fair Road, Zip 30458, Mailing Address: P.O. Box 1048, Zip 30459–1048; tel. 912/486–1000 **A**1 9 10 19 **F**3 13 15 18 25 26 27 30 31 32 33 38 43 46 48 49 55 57 65 68 72 73 74 76 77 79 80 82 84 86 93 96 97 100 101 102 103 104 105 106 107 118 121 135 137 **P**5 **S** Health Management Associates
Primary Contact: Robert F. Bigley, Chief Executive Officer
COO: Spencer Thomas, Chief Operating Officer
CFO: Scott Whittemore, Chief Financial Officer
CMO: Thomas D. Carico, M.D., Chief of Staff
CIO: Marisa Smith, Director Information Services
CHR: Jim Reames, Director Human Resources
Web address: www.egrmc.com
Control: Corporation, Investor–owned, for–profit **Service:** General Medical and Surgical

Staffed Beds: 150 **Admissions:** 7464 **Census:** 80 **Outpatient Visits:** 91337 **Births:** 1593 **Total Expense ($000):** 67196 **Payroll Expense ($000):** 26406 **Personnel:** 631

WILLINGWAY HOSPITAL, 311 Jones Mill Road, Zip 30458–4765; tel. 912/764–6236, (Nonreporting) **A**9
Primary Contact: Jimmy Mooney, Chief Executive Officer
CFO: Barbara S. Reid, Chief Financial Officer
CMO: Robert W. Mooney, M.D., Medical Director
Web address: www.willingway.com
Control: Corporation, Investor–owned, for–profit **Service:** Alcoholism and other chemical dependency

Staffed Beds: 40

STOCKBRIDGE—Henry County

★ **HENRY MEDICAL CENTER (110191)**, 1133 Eagle's Landing Parkway, Zip 30281–5099; tel. 678/604–1000, (Total facility includes 89 beds in nursing home–type unit) **A**1 2 9 10 **F**3 8 11 12 13 15 18 24 25 26 27 30 32 33 38 43 46 49 53 55 56 57 60 62 68 71 72 73 74 75 76 77 79 80 81 84 86 90 96 97 99 100 102 103 106 107 112 117 119 121 124 133 135 136 137
Primary Contact: Charles F. Scott, President and Chief Executive Officer
CFO: Claude Carruth, Vice President and Chief Financial Officer
CMO: Jorge Spinolo, M.D., Chief of Staff
CIO: Terry Wilk, Chief Information Officer
CHR: Maribeth Ledford, Director Human Resources
Web address: www.henrymedical.com
Control: Hospital district or authority, Government, nonfederal **Service:** General Medical and Surgical

Staffed Beds: 289 **Admissions:** 11636 **Census:** 217 **Outpatient Visits:** 123349 **Births:** 2246 **Total Expense ($000):** 130050 **Payroll Expense ($000):** 54550 **Personnel:** 1089

SWAINSBORO—Emanuel County

□ **EMANUEL MEDICAL HOSPITAL (110109)**, 117 Kite Road, Zip 30401–3231, Mailing Address: P.O. Box 879, Zip 30401–0879; tel. 478/237–9911, (Total facility includes 49 beds in nursing home–type unit) **A**1 9 10 20 **F**4 7 13 15 25 26 31 38 55 57 62 68 74 77 79 80 82 96 100 107 112 117 118 119 121 122 124 135 **S** Brim Healthcare, Inc.
Primary Contact: Leonard W. Daugherty, Chief Executive Officer
Web address: www.emanuelmedical.org
Control: Hospital district or authority, Government, nonfederal **Service:** General Medical and Surgical

Staffed Beds: 108 **Admissions:** 2772 **Census:** 76 **Outpatient Visits:** 30156 **Births:** 214 **Total Expense ($000):** 19827 **Payroll Expense ($000):** 12082 **Personnel:** 339

SYLVANIA—Screven County

★ **SCREVEN COUNTY HOSPITAL (111312)**, 215 Mims Road, Zip 30467–2097; tel. 912/564–7426 **A**9 10 18 **F**3 11 15 25 30 31 32 33 38 50 57 62 64 73 77 79 86 87 96 107 119 122 135
Primary Contact: George H. St. George, FACHE, Chief Executive Officer
CFO: Marsha Carroll, Director Financial Services
Control: Hospital district or authority, Government, nonfederal **Service:** General Medical and Surgical

Staffed Beds: 25 **Admissions:** 573 **Census:** 6 **Outpatient Visits:** 17070 **Births:** 0 **Total Expense ($000):** 6575 **Payroll Expense ($000):** 3285 **Personnel:** 90

GA

SYLVESTER—Worth County

★ **PHOEBE WORTH MEDICAL CENTER (111328)**, 807 South Isabella Street, Zip 31791–0545, Mailing Address: P.O. Box 545, Zip 31791–0545; tel. 229/776–6961 **A**1 9 10 18 **F**3 7 11 25 26 27 31 32 33 38 55 57 62 73 75 76 79 82 86 96 107 118 119 122 132 135 137 **P**6 **S** Phoebe Putney Health System
Primary Contact: Keith J. Petersen, Chief Executive Officer
COO: Keith J. Petersen, Chief Executive Officer
CFO: John Graham, Interim Chief Financial Officer
CMO: Natu M. Patel, M.D., Chief of Staff
CHR: Chris Foreman, Director
Web address: www.phobeputney.com
Control: Other not–for–profit (including NFP Corporation) **Service:** General Medical and Surgical

Staffed Beds: 25 **Admissions:** 501 **Census:** 12 **Outpatient Visits:** 14831 **Births:** 0 **Total Expense ($000):** 11872 **Payroll Expense ($000):** 6084 **Personnel:** 190

THOMASTON—Upson County

★ **UPSON REGIONAL MEDICAL CENTER (110002)**, 801 West Gordon Street, Zip 30286–2831, Mailing Address: P.O. Box 1059, Zip 30286–1059; tel. 706/647–8111 **A**1 2 9 10 19 20 **F**3 7 11 13 15 24 25 26 27 30 31 32 33 37 38 43 49 50 51 52 55 56 57 62 68 73 75 76 77 78 79 80 81 82 86 92 96 97 100 103 106 107 112 118 119 120 121 122 124 133 135 137 **P**5 6 **S** Brim Healthcare, Inc.
Primary Contact: Gene B. Wright, Chief Executive Officer
CFO: John Williams, Chief Financial Officer
CIO: George Curtis, Director Information Technology Services
CHR: Celeste Johnson, Director Human Resources
Web address: www.urmc.org
Control: Other not–for–profit (including NFP Corporation) **Service:** General Medical and Surgical

Staffed Beds: 115 **Admissions:** 4484 **Census:** 45 **Outpatient Visits:** 83506 **Births:** 643 **Total Expense ($000):** 46047 **Payroll Expense ($000):** 23626 **Personnel:** 619

THOMASVILLE—Thomas County

★ **JOHN D. ARCHBOLD MEMORIAL HOSPITAL (110038)**, Gordon Avenue at Mimosa Drive, Zip 31792–6113, Mailing Address: P.O. Box 1018, Zip 31799–1018; tel. 229/228–2000, (Total facility includes 64 beds in nursing home–type unit) **A**1 2 9 10 19 **F**3 4 5 8 11 13 15 17 18 20 24 25 26 27 30 31 32 33 34 36 38 40 43 46 48 49 50 53 54 55 56 57 59 60 62 63 66 68 72 73 74 75 76 77 79 80 81 82 84 85 86 88 89 90 91 92 93 94 95 96 97 100 102 103 105 106 107 109 111 112 117 118 119 120 121 123 124 132 133 135 136 137 **P**8 **S** Archbold Medical Center
Primary Contact: J. Perry Mustian, President and Chief Executive Officer
COO: Kevin Taylor, Chief Operating Officer
CFO: Skip Hightower, Interim Chief Financial Officer
CMO: Charles M. Tomlinson, M.D., Vice President Medical Affairs
CIO: William Zimmermann, Vice President Information Services
CHR: Zach Wheeler, Vice President Human Resources
Web address: www.archbold.org
Control: Other not–for–profit (including NFP Corporation) **Service:** General Medical and Surgical

Staffed Beds: 328 **Admissions:** 11136 **Census:** 218 **Outpatient Visits:** 245361 **Births:** 1024 **Total Expense ($000):** 179905 **Payroll Expense ($000):** 66447 **Personnel:** 1622

☐ **SOUTHWESTERN STATE HOSPITAL (114021)**, Pine Tree Boulevard, Zip 31792, Mailing Address: P.O. Box 1378, Zip 31799–1378; tel. 229/227–2833, (Total facility includes 20 beds in nursing home–type unit) (Nonreporting) **A**1 9 10
Primary Contact: Beverly Bajerski, Regional Administrator
CFO: Susie Oates, Assistant Superintendent for Administration
CMO: Joseph B. LeRoy, M.D., Clinical Director
CIO: Loma Owens, Data Manager
CHR: Robert Moore, Director Personnel
Control: State–Government, nonfederal **Service:** Psychiatric

Staffed Beds: 236

THOMSON—McDuffie County

★ **MCDUFFIE REGIONAL MEDICAL CENTER (110111)**, 521 Hill Street S.W., Zip 30824–2199; tel. 706/595–1411, (Nonreporting) **A**1 9 10 **S** QHR
Primary Contact: Douglas C. Keir, Chief Executive Officer
CFO: Pat Parris, Chief Financial Officer
CIO: Lisa Tucker, Chief Information Officer
Web address: www.mrmc.org
Control: Hospital district or authority, Government, nonfederal **Service:** General Medical and Surgical

Staffed Beds: 35

TIFTON—Tift County

★ **TIFT REGIONAL MEDICAL CENTER (110095)**, 901 East 18th Street, Zip 31794–3648, Mailing Address: Drawer 747, Zip 31793–0747; tel. 229/382–7120, (Total facility includes 15 beds in nursing home–type unit) **A**1 2 9 10 19 **F**3 8 9 11 13 15 18 20 24 25 27 30 31 32 33 38 40 42 43 46 47 49 50 53 55 56 57 59 62 66 68 72 73 74 75 76 77 79 80 81 82 84 85 86 87 96 97 99 100 102 107 109 111 117 118 119 121 132 135 136 137 **P**6
Primary Contact: William T. Richardson, President and Chief Executive Officer
COO: Sarah Thompson, Vice President Operations
CFO: Dennis L. Crum, Vice President and Chief Financial Officer
CMO: Raymond Moreno, M.D., Vice President Medical Affairs
CIO: Guy McAllister, Chief Information Officer
CHR: Ellen Eaton, Director Human Resources
Web address: www.tiftregional.com
Control: Hospital district or authority, Government, nonfederal **Service:** General Medical and Surgical

Staffed Beds: 191 **Admissions:** 10045 **Census:** 113 **Outpatient Visits:** 136905 **Births:** 1267 **Total Expense ($000):** 137831 **Payroll Expense ($000):** 57083 **Personnel:** 1318

TOCCOA—Stephens County

★ **STEPHENS COUNTY HOSPITAL (110032)**, 163 Hospital Drive, Zip 30577–9700; tel. 706/282–4200, (Total facility includes 82 beds in nursing home–type unit) **A**1 9 10 20 **F**3 7 10 11 13 15 26 30 31 32 33 38 43 51 55 56 57 59 62 66 68 71 73 74 75 77 79 80 81 84 86 96 99 100 102 107 115 118 119 124 131 134 135 137
Primary Contact: Edward C. Gambrell, Jr., Administrator
CFO: Jeff Laird, Controller
CHR: Diane Hardeman, Director Personnel
Web address: www.stephenscountyhospital.com
Control: Hospital district or authority, Government, nonfederal **Service:** General Medical and Surgical

Staffed Beds: 178 **Admissions:** 3664 **Census:** 103 **Outpatient Visits:** 43764 **Births:** 667 **Total Expense ($000):** 44180 **Payroll Expense ($000):** 20605 **Personnel:** 506

VALDOSTA—Lowndes County

★ **SMITH NORTHVIEW HOSPITAL (110212)**, 4280 North Valdosta Road, Zip 31602, Mailing Address: P.O. Box 10010, Zip 31604; tel. 229/671–2000, (Nonreporting) **A**1 9 10 **S** Ameris Health Systems
Primary Contact: Larry R. Jeter, Chief Executive Officer
CFO: Shamb Purohit, Chief Financial Officer
CMO: Dennis Thomas, M.D., Chief of Staff
CHR: Paula Goff, Assistant Administrator Human Resources
Web address: www.smithhospital.com
Control: Partnership, Investor–owned, for–profit **Service:** General Medical and Surgical

Staffed Beds: 31

★ △ **SOUTH GEORGIA MEDICAL CENTER (110122)**, 2501 North Patterson Street, Zip 31602–1735, Mailing Address: P.O. Box 1727, Zip 31603–1727; tel. 229/333–1000, (Includes GREENLEAF CENTER, 2209 Pineview Drive, Zip 31602–7316; tel. 229/247–4357) **A**1 2 7 9 10 19 **F**3 4 5 7 11 13 15 17 18 20 22 24 25 26 27 28 30 31 32 33 34 36 37 38 40 46 49 50 51 53 54 55 56 57 59 60 62 68 69 72 73 74 75 76 77 79 80 81 82 84 85 86 87 88 89 90 91 92 93 94 95 96 97 98 100 102 104 105 106 107 108 109 111 112 118 119 120 121 124 132 133 135 136 137 **P**5
Primary Contact: James McGahee, Administrator and Chief Executive Officer
COO: Randy Sauls, Chief Operating Officer
CFO: Greg Hembree, Chief Financial Officer
CMO: Bill Gee, M.D., Chief Medical Officer
CIO: Bob Foster, Chief Information Officer
CHR: Charles Eidson, Assistant Administrator Human Resources
Web address: www.sgmc.org
Control: Hospital district or authority, Government, nonfederal **Service:** General Medical and Surgical

Staffed Beds: 335 **Admissions:** 14641 **Census:** 192 **Outpatient Visits:** 188130 **Births:** 1803 **Total Expense ($000):** 194340 **Payroll Expense ($000):** 84970 **Personnel:** 2069

GA

Hospital, Medicare Provider Number, Address, Telephone, Approval, Facility, and Physician Codes, Health Care System

★ American Hospital Association (AHA) membership
☐ The Joint Commission accreditation
○ American Osteopathic Association (AOA) accreditation
△ Commission on Accreditation of Rehabilitation Facilities (CARF) accreditation

VIDALIA—Toombs County

★ **MEADOWS REGIONAL MEDICAL CENTER (110128)**, 1703 Meadows Lane, Zip 30474–8915, Mailing Address: P.O. Box 1048, Zip 30475–1048; tel. 912/537–8921, (Total facility includes 35 beds in nursing home–type unit) **A**1 9 10 20 **F**11 13 15 18 25 26 27 30 31 32 33 38 50 51 52 53 55 57 60 62 66 68 73 74 75 76 77 79 86 87 96 97 100 102 103 104 106 107 117 118 119 120 135
Primary Contact: Alan Kent, Chief Executive Officer
CFO: Ron Peterson, Vice President Finance
CIO: Craig Floyd, Director Management Information System
Web address: www.meadowsregional.org
Control: Other not–for–profit (including NFP Corporation) **Service:** General Medical and Surgical

Staffed Beds: 104 **Admissions:** 4417 **Census:** 63 **Outpatient Visits:** 55829 **Births:** 559 **Total Expense ($000):** 57959 **Payroll Expense ($000):** 23865 **Personnel:** 523

VILLA RICA—Carroll County

★ **TANNER MEDICAL CENTER–VILLA RICA (110015)**, 601 Dallas Road, Zip 30180–1202, Mailing Address: P.O. Box 638, Zip 30180–0638; tel. 770/456–3100, (Nonreporting) **A**1 9 10 **S** Tanner Health System
Primary Contact: Larry N. Steed, FACHE, Administrator
CFO: Lee Sherseth, Chief Financial Officer
Web address: www.tanner.org
Control: Other not–for–profit (including NFP Corporation) **Service:** General Medical and Surgical

Staffed Beds: 39

WARM SPRINGS—Meriwether County

☐ **ROOSEVELT WARM SPRINGS INSTITUTE FOR REHABILITATION (113028)**, 6135 Roosevelt Highway, Zip 31830, Mailing Address: P.O. Box 1000, Zip 31830–1000; tel. 706/655–5000, (Nonreporting) **A**1 9 10
Primary Contact: Greg Schmieg, Executive Director
CFO: David Cawthon, Director Financial Services
CMO: Duan Huang, M.D., Chief of Staff
CIO: Martin Harmon, Director Public Relations
CHR: Bill Bulloch, Director Human Resources
Web address: www.rooseveltrehab.org
Control: State–Government, nonfederal **Service:** Long–Term Acute Care hospital

Staffed Beds: 64

★ **WARM SPRINGS MEDICAL CENTER (111316)**, 5995 Spring Street, Zip 31830–2149, Mailing Address: P.O. Box 8, Zip 31830–0008; tel. 706/655–3331, (Total facility includes 79 beds in nursing home–type unit) **A**1 9 10 18 **F**11 15 25 26 31 38 53 55 62 66 77 86 96 100 107 117 119 122 135
Primary Contact: Harry J. Carr, Chief Executive Officer
CFO: Robert Steckley, Chief Financial Officer
CMO: Alan Thompson, M.D., President Medical Staff
CIO: Milo Varnadoe, Systems Director
CHR: Barbara Nolan, Coordinator Human Resources
Web address: www.warmspringsmc.org
Control: Hospital district or authority, Government, nonfederal **Service:** General Medical and Surgical

Staffed Beds: 104 **Admissions:** 650 **Census:** 83 **Outpatient Visits:** 16375 **Births:** 0 **Total Expense ($000):** 13082 **Payroll Expense ($000):** 5663 **Personnel:** 79

WARNER ROBINS—Houston County

★ **HOUSTON MEDICAL CENTER (110069)**, 1601 Watson Boulevard, Zip 31093–3431, Mailing Address: P.O. Box 2886, Zip 31099–2886; tel. 478/922–4281 **A**1 9 10 **F**3 11 13 15 25 26 27 30 31 32 33 36 37 38 43 48 49 50 52 53 54 55 56 57 58 60 62 66 68 71 72 73 74 75 76 77 79 80 81 82 84 86 88 90 91 92 93 96 97 100 101 102 103 106 107 118 119 120 121 123 124 133 135 136 137
Primary Contact: Anthony Alford, D.O., FACHE, Chief Executive Officer
CFO: Frank R. Powell, Chief Financial Officer
CIO: Beth Benefield, Executive Director Information Systems
CHR: Linda Watson, Executive Director Human Resources
Web address: www.hhc.org
Control: Hospital district or authority, Government, nonfederal **Service:** General Medical and Surgical

Staffed Beds: 186 **Admissions:** 11532 **Census:** 138 **Outpatient Visits:** 208240 **Births:** 1993 **Total Expense ($000):** 136472 **Payroll Expense ($000):** 56895 **Personnel:** 1118

WASHINGTON—Wilkes County

★ **WILLS MEMORIAL HOSPITAL (111325)**, 120 Gordon Street, Zip 30673–1602, Mailing Address: P.O. Box 370, Zip 30673–0370; tel. 706/678–2151 **A**1 9 10 18 **F**30 32 33 37 38 54 55 56 57 68 73 75 77 79 80 81 86 96 107 122 135 137
Primary Contact: T. Marvin Goldman, Chief Executive Officer
CFO: Cliff Cooper, Chief Financial Officer
CHR: Tom Urban, Director Human Resources
Web address: www.willsmemorialhospital.com
Control: Hospital district or authority, Government, nonfederal **Service:** General Medical and Surgical

Staffed Beds: 25 **Admissions:** 1188 **Census:** 16 **Outpatient Visits:** 16958 **Births:** 0 **Total Expense ($000):** 10007 **Payroll Expense ($000):** 5409 **Personnel:** 170

WAYCROSS—Ware County

★ **SATILLA REGIONAL MEDICAL CENTER (110003)**, 410 Darling Avenue, Zip 31501–5246, Mailing Address: P.O. Box 139, Zip 31502–0139; tel. 912/283–3030 **A**1 3 5 10 19 20 **F**3 13 15 17 18 24 25 26 30 31 32 33 38 49 51 55 56 57 59 68 71 72 73 74 75 76 77 78 79 80 82 84 85 86 88 96 97 100 102 104 105 107 118 119 121 124 135 **P**6
Primary Contact: Robert M. Trimm, President and Chief Executive Officer
COO: Windell Smith, Chief Operating Officer
CFO: Katrina Wheeler, Chief Financial Officer
CMO: John Butler, M.D., Director Medical Staff
CIO: Barry Rudd, Chief Information Officer
CHR: David Pritchett, Director Human Resources
Web address: www.satilla.org
Control: Other not–for–profit (including NFP Corporation) **Service:** General Medical and Surgical

Staffed Beds: 206 **Admissions:** 6924 **Census:** 82 **Outpatient Visits:** 126799 **Births:** 733 **Total Expense ($000):** 95005 **Payroll Expense ($000):** 36841 **Personnel:** 941

WAYNESBORO—Burke County

☐ **BURKE MEDICAL CENTER (110113)**, 351 Liberty Street, Zip 30830–9686; tel. 706/554–4435, (Nonreporting) **A**1 9 10
Primary Contact: Jennifer A. Royal, Administrator
CFO: Dianne Stewart, Controller
CHR: Danette Highsmith, Director Human Resources
Web address: www.burkemedical.net
Control: Hospital district or authority, Government, nonfederal **Service:** General Medical and Surgical

Staffed Beds: 40

WILDWOOD—Dade County

WILDWOOD LIFESTYLE CENTER AND HOSPITAL, 435 Lifestyle Lane, Zip 30757–4128, Mailing Address: P.O. Box 129, Zip 30757–0129; tel. 706/820–1493, (Nonreporting)
Primary Contact: Larry E. Clements, Administrator
Web address: www.wildwoodlsc.org
Control: Other not–for–profit (including NFP Corporation) **Service:** General Medical and Surgical

Staffed Beds: 13

WINDER—Barrow County

☐ **BARROW REGIONAL MEDICAL CENTER (110045)**, 316 North Broad Street, Zip 30680–2150, Mailing Address: P.O. Box 688, Zip 30680–0688; tel. 770/867–3400, (Nonreporting) **A**1 9 10 **S** Health Management Associates
Primary Contact: Joe Clancy, Chief Executive Officer
COO: Brent Burish, Chief Operating Officer
CFO: Cassie Ball, Chief Financial Officer
CMO: Drew Xenos, DPM, Chief of Staff
CIO: Ed Stanley, Director Information Systems
CHR: Michele Monsrud, Director Human Resources
Web address: www.barrowregional.com
Control: Corporation, Investor–owned, for–profit **Service:** General Medical and Surgical

Staffed Beds: 56

GA

Many Facility Codes have changed. Please refer to the AHA Guide Code Chart.

HAWAII

AIEA—Honolulu County

★ **KAPIOLANI MEDICAL CENTER AT PALI MOMI (120026)**, 98–1079 Moanalua Road, Zip 96701–4713; tel. 808/486–6000 **A**1 2 3 5 9 10 **F**3 15 18 25 27 33 38 43 46 49 50 55 57 62 68 72 73 75 76 77 79 81 86 96 97 99 100 103 107 119 135 136 137 **S** Hawaii Pacific Health
Primary Contact: Raymond Vara, Chief Executive Officer
COO: Jen Chahanovich, Chief Operating Officer
CFO: David Okabe, Executive Vice President, Chief Financial Officer and Treasurer
CMO: Hugh Hazenfield, M.D., Chief of Staff
CIO: Steve Robertson, Senior Vice President
CHR: Gail Lerch, R.N., Vice President Human Resources
Web address: www.kapiolani.org
Control: Other not–for–profit (including NFP Corporation) **Service:** General Medical and Surgical

Staffed Beds: 116 **Admissions:** 5690 **Census:** 94 **Outpatient Visits:** 100418 **Births:** 0 **Total Expense ($000):** 98711 **Payroll Expense ($000):** 36852 **Personnel:** 607

EWA BEACH—Honolulu County

★ **HAWAII MEDICAL CENTER–WEST (120027)**, (Formerly St. Francis Medical Center–West), 91–2141 Fort Weaver Road, Zip 96706–1993; tel. 808/678–7000, (Nonreporting) **A**1 5 9 10 **S** Sisters of Saint Francis
Primary Contact: Danelo R. Canete, M.D., Chief Executive Officer
COO: Malcolm J. Tom, Chief Operations Officer
CFO: Suanne Morikuni, Executive Director Finance
CIO: Jerry Correa, Vice President Information Services
CHR: Jessica Sphar, Director Human Resources
Web address: www.sfhs–hi.org
Control: Church–operated, Nongovernment, not–for profit **Service:** General Medical and Surgical

Staffed Beds: 102

★ **KAHI MOHALA BEHAVIORAL HEALTH (124001)**, 91–2301 Old Fort Weaver Road, Zip 96706–3602; tel. 808/671–8511 **A**1 9 10 **F**5 25 30 32 33 88 89 90 91 94 95 **S** Sutter Health
Primary Contact: Leonard Licina, Chief Executive Officer
CFO: Rose Choy, Controller
CMO: Steven Chaplin, M.D., Interim Medical Director
CHR: Christina Enoka, Director Human Resources
Web address: www.kahi.org
Control: Other not–for–profit (including NFP Corporation) **Service:** Psychiatric

Staffed Beds: 88 **Admissions:** 697 **Census:** 59 **Outpatient Visits:** 4112 **Births:** 0 **Total Expense ($000):** 18598 **Payroll Expense ($000):** 9764 **Personnel:** 172

HILO—Hawaii County

★ **HILO MEDICAL CENTER (120005)**, 1190 Waianuenue Avenue, Zip 96720–2095; tel. 808/974–4700, (Total facility includes 112 beds in nursing home–type unit) **A**1 5 9 10 20 **F**1 3 13 17 25 26 27 30 31 32 49 51 55 56 57 61 62 65 68 73 74 75 76 77 79 80 84 85 88 90 91 92 93 96 100 102 107 117 119 124 135 137 **S** Hawaii Health Systems Corporation
Primary Contact: Ronald J. Schurra, Regional Chief Executive Officer
CFO: Money Atwal, Chief Financial Officer
CIO: Money Atwal, Chief Information Officer
CHR: Holly Ka'Akimaka, Director Human Resources
Web address: www.hmc.hhsc.org
Control: State–Government, nonfederal **Service:** General Medical and Surgical

Staffed Beds: 271 **Admissions:** 7613 **Census:** 240 **Outpatient Visits:** 68101 **Births:** 1185 **Total Expense ($000):** 109893 **Payroll Expense ($000):** 44084 **Personnel:** 893

HONOKAA—Hawaii County

★ **HALE HO'OLA HAMAKUA (121307)**, 45–547 Plumeria Street, Zip 96727–6902; tel. 808/775–7211, (Total facility includes 48 beds in nursing home–type unit) (Nonreporting) **A**3 5 9 10 18 **S** Hawaii Health Systems Corporation
Primary Contact: Jeanne Abe, Administrator
CFO: Felisa Rosario, Accountant
Web address: www.hhsc.org
Control: State–Government, nonfederal **Service:** General Medical and Surgical

Staffed Beds: 52

HONOLULU—Honolulu County

□ **HAWAII MEDICAL CENTER EAST (120010)**, 2230 Liliha Street, Zip 96817–9979, Mailing Address: P.O. Box 30100, Zip 96820–0100; tel. 808/547–6011, (Total facility includes 52 beds in nursing home–type unit) (Nonreporting) **A**1 2 3 5 9 10 **S** Sisters of Saint Francis
Primary Contact: Danelo R. Canete, M.D., Chief Executive Officer
COO: Catherine Tanaka, Chief Operating Officer
CFO: Suanne Morikuni, Executive Director Finance
CMO: Patricia Blanchette, M.D., Chief Medical Officer
CIO: Jerry Correa, Chief Information Officer
CHR: Jessica Sphar, Director Human Resources
Web address: www.stfrancishawaii.org
Control: Church–operated, Nongovernment, not–for profit **Service:** General Medical and Surgical

Staffed Beds: 240

★ **KAISER PERMANENTE MEDICAL CENTER (120011)**, 3288 Moanalua Road, Zip 96819–1469; tel. 808/432–0000 **A**1 3 5 10 **F**3 12 13 15 17 18 19 20 22 24 25 26 27 28 30 31 32 34 35 36 38 41 43 44 46 47 49 50 54 57 59 60 61 62 66 68 70 71 72 73 74 75 76 77 78 79 80 82 83 84 96 97 100 102 106 107 112 116 119 121 123 135 136 137 **P**3 **S** Kaiser Foundation Hospitals
Primary Contact: Susan R. Murray, Regional Administrator
COO: Patricia Rodriguez, Chief Operating Officer and Chief Nursing Officer
CFO: David P. Delaney, Chief Financial Officer
CMO: James Griffith, M.D., Chief of Staff
CIO: Brian Yoshii, Chief Information Officer
CHR: Winona White, Vice President Human Resources
Web address: www.kaiserpermanente.org
Control: Other not–for–profit (including NFP Corporation) **Service:** General Medical and Surgical

Staffed Beds: 217 **Admissions:** 10326 **Census:** 177 **Outpatient Visits:** 54697 **Births:** 1699 **Personnel:** 1881

□ **KAPIOLANI MEDICAL CENTER FOR WOMEN & CHILDREN (123300)**, 1319 Punahou Street, Zip 96826–1032; tel. 808/983–6000, (Nonreporting) **A**1 3 5 9 10 **S** Hawaii Pacific Health
Primary Contact: Raymond Vara, Chief Executive Officer
COO: Martha Smith, Chief Operating Officer
CFO: David Okabe, Senior Vice President, Chief Financial Officer and Treasurer
CIO: Steve Robertson, Vice President
CHR: Gail Lerch, R.N., Vice President
Web address: www.kapiolani.org
Control: Other not–for–profit (including NFP Corporation) **Service:** Obstetrics and gynecology

Staffed Beds: 225

★ **KUAKINI MEDICAL CENTER (120007)**, 347 North Kuakini Street, Zip 96817–2381; tel. 808/536–2236 **A**1 2 3 5 9 10 **F**3 11 15 17 18 20 22 24 25 27 30 31 32 33 34 38 43 44 46 49 55 56 57 59 66 68 72 73 75 76 77 79 80 81 82 96 97 99 100 102 106 107 109 112 118 119 120 121 134 135 136 137 **P**1
Primary Contact: Gary K. Kajiwara, President and Chief Executive Officer
COO: Gregg Oishi, Senior Vice President and Chief Operating Officer
CFO: Gregg Oishi, Interim Chief Financial Officer
CMO: Nobuyuki Miki, M.D., Vice President Medical Affairs
CIO: Gary K. Kajiwara, President and Chief Executive Officer
Web address: www.kuakini.org
Control: Other not–for–profit (including NFP Corporation) **Service:** General Medical and Surgical

Staffed Beds: 115 **Admissions:** 5605 **Census:** 113 **Outpatient Visits:** 64369 **Births:** 0 **Total Expense ($000):** 114447 **Payroll Expense ($000):** 53113 **Personnel:** 1004

Hospital, Medicare Provider Number, Address, Telephone, Approval, Facility, and Physician Codes, Health Care System

★ American Hospital Association (AHA) membership
□ The Joint Commission accreditation
○ American Osteopathic Association (AOA) accreditation
△ Commission on Accreditation of Rehabilitation Facilities (CARF) accreditation

HI

★ **LEAHI HOSPITAL (122001)**, (SNF/ICF; Acute TB Inpatient), 3675 Kilauea Avenue, Zip 96816–2398; tel. 808/733–8000, (Total facility includes 179 beds in nursing home–type unit) **A**9 10 **F**2 3 26 30 32 33 41 42 43 50 54 56 62 65 66 73 75 82 86 117 119 122 135 137 **S** Hawaii Health Systems Corporation
Primary Contact: Vincent H. S. Lee, FACHE, Regional Chief Executive Officer
CFO: Nathan Yim, Regional Chief Financial Officer
CMO: Albert Yazawa, M.D., Regional Medical Director
CHR: Glenn Sakumoto, Regional Director Human Resources
Web address: www.hhsc.org
Control: State–Government, nonfederal **Service:** Other specialty

Staffed Beds: 190 **Admissions:** 155 **Census:** 177 **Outpatient Visits:** 0 **Births:** 0 **Total Expense ($000):** 21310 **Payroll Expense ($000):** 12043 **Personnel:** 292

▣ **QUEEN'S MEDICAL CENTER (120001)**, 1301 Punchbowl Street, Zip 96813–2499; tel. 808/538–9011, (Total facility includes 26 beds in nursing home–type unit) **A**1 2 3 5 9 10 **F**3 5 11 12 13 15 17 18 20 22 25 26 27 30 31 32 33 36 37 38 40 41 42 43 44 50 51 54 55 57 59 60 62 64 66 68 71 72 73 74 75 76 77 79 80 81 82 86 87 88 89 90 91 92 93 94 95 96 97 100 102 103 104 105 106 107 108 109 114 117 118 119 121 124 125 132 133 135 136 137 **S** Queen's Health Systems
Primary Contact: Arthur A. Ushijima, President
COO: Paula Yoshioka, Chief Administrative Officer
CFO: Rix Maurer, Vice President Finance and Chief Financial Officer
CMO: Gerard Akaka, M.D., Vice President Medical Affairs
CIO: David Starr, Vice President Information Technology and Chief Information Officer
CHR: Bert Kido, Vice President Human Resources
Web address: www.queens.org
Control: Other not–for–profit (including NFP Corporation) **Service:** General Medical and Surgical

Staffed Beds: 470 **Admissions:** 21131 **Census:** 397 **Outpatient Visits:** 275077 **Births:** 2270 **Total Expense ($000):** 509174 **Payroll Expense ($000):** 208747 **Personnel:** 3129

▣ **REHABILITATION HOSPITAL OF THE PACIFIC (123025)**, 226 North Kuakini Street, Zip 96817–9881; tel. 808/531–3511, (Total facility includes 20 beds in nursing home–type unit) **A**1 9 10 **F**3 11 25 30 31 32 43 53 62 66 72 73 75 77 85 86 117 119 120 121 132 135 137
Primary Contact: Clair Jones, President and Chief Executive Officer
CFO: Sue Ann Moriwaki, Vice President Finance and Chief Financial Officer
CMO: Gary Okamoto, M.D., Chief Medical Executive
CIO: Dave Orme, Chief Information Officer
CHR: Faye Miyamoto, Vice President Human Resources
Web address: www.rehabhospital.org
Control: Other not–for–profit (including NFP Corporation) **Service:** Rehabilitation

Staffed Beds: 100 **Admissions:** 1961 **Census:** 67 **Outpatient Visits:** 68332 **Births:** 0 **Total Expense ($000):** 36398 **Payroll Expense ($000):** 19001 **Personnel:** 322

□ **SHRINERS HOSPITALS FOR CHILDREN, HONOLULU**, 1310 Punahou Street, Zip 96826–1099; tel. 808/941–4466, (Nonreporting) **A**1 3 5 **S** Shriners Hospitals for Children
Primary Contact: Stanley B. Berry, FACHE, Administrator
CFO: Quin Ogawa, Director Fiscal Service
CMO: Ellen Raney, M.D., Chief of Staff
CIO: Ross Imoda, Director Information Systems
CHR: Derek Ito, Director Human Resources
Web address: www.shrinershq.org
Control: Other not–for–profit (including NFP Corporation) **Service:** Children's other specialty

Staffed Beds: 40

STRAUB CLINIC & HOSPITAL (120022), 888 South King Street, Zip 96813–3083; tel. 808/522–4000 **A**2 3 5 9 10 **F**3 9 12 15 16 17 18 19 20 21 22 25 26 27 30 31 32 38 43 44 49 53 54 55 56 57 62 63 66 68 72 73 75 76 77 79 80 81 82 86 87 94 96 97 99 100 102 107 108 112 118 119 120 121 124 132 135 137 **P**6 **S** Hawaii Pacific Health
Primary Contact: Raymond Vara, Chief Executive Officer
COO: Art Gladstone, Chief Operating Officer
CFO: David Okabe, Executive Vice President, Chief Financial Officer and Treasurer
CMO: Kenneth Robbins, M.D., Chief Medical Officer
CIO: Steve Robertson, Vice President
CHR: Gail Lerch, R.N., Executive Vice President Human Resources
Web address: www.straubhealth.org
Control: Other not–for–profit (including NFP Corporation) **Service:** General Medical and Surgical

Staffed Beds: 143 **Admissions:** 6252 **Census:** 104 **Outpatient Visits:** 558184 **Births:** 0 **Total Expense ($000):** 245619 **Payroll Expense ($000):** 105980 **Personnel:** 1352

▣ **TRIPLER ARMY MEDICAL CENTER**, 1 Jarret White Road, Zip 96859–5000; tel. 808/433–6661 **A**1 2 3 5 9 **F**3 5 7 8 12 13 14 15 17 18 19 20 21 22 24 25 26 27 28 29 30 31 32 33 34 36 37 38 42 43 44 50 51 52 53 54 55 56 57 58 59 60 62 63 68 70 72 73 74 75 76 77 78 79 80 81 82 83 84 86 87 88 89 90 91 92 94 96 97 100 102 104 105 106 107 108 109 111 113 119 120 121 124 133 135 136 137 **S** Department of the Army, Office of the Surgeon General
CFO: Lieutenant Colonel David Petray, Chief Resource Management
CMO: Captain Christopher Culp, Deputy Commander Clinical Services
CIO: Lieutenant Colonel Ralph A. Franco, Chief Information Management Division
CHR: Colonel Paul W. Wingo, Troop Commander
Web address: www.tamc.amedd.army.mil
Control: Army, Government, federal **Service:** General Medical and Surgical

Staffed Beds: 180 **Admissions:** 12989 **Census:** 130 **Outpatient Visits:** 863040 **Births:** 2143 **Personnel:** 2994

KAHUKU—Honolulu County

△ **KAHUKU HOSPITAL (121304)**, 56–117 Pualalea Street, Zip 96731–2052; tel. 808/293–9221, (Nonreporting) **A**7 9 10 18
Primary Contact: Stephany Vaioleti, Interim Administrator
CFO: Francis Daquioag, Controller
CMO: P. Douglas Nielson, M.D., Chief of Staff
Control: Other not–for–profit (including NFP Corporation) **Service:** General Medical and Surgical

Staffed Beds: 13

KAILUA—Honolulu County

▣ **CASTLE MEDICAL CENTER (120006)**, 640 Ulukahiki Street, Zip 96734–4498; tel. 808/263–5500 **A**1 9 10 **F**12 13 15 20 24 25 26 27 30 31 32 33 38 51 56 57 61 62 66 68 69 73 74 75 76 77 79 88 89 92 100 102 107 121 124 135 136 **P**8 **S** Adventist Health
Primary Contact: Kevin Roberts, President and Chief Executive Officer
COO: A. John Monge, Vice President Operations
CFO: Dale Northrop, Vice President Finance
CMO: Ramsey Hasan, M.D., Chief of Staff
CIO: Brian Rothe, Site Director Information Systems
CHR: Adele Hoe, Director Human Resources
Web address: www.castlemed.com
Control: Church–operated, Nongovernment, not–for profit **Service:** General Medical and Surgical

Staffed Beds: 160 **Admissions:** 6300 **Census:** 91 **Outpatient Visits:** 119332 **Births:** 834 **Total Expense ($000):** 96736 **Payroll Expense ($000):** 44875 **Personnel:** 627

KAMUELA—Hawaii County

▣ △ **NORTH HAWAII COMMUNITY HOSPITAL (120028)**, 67–1125 Mamalahoa Highway, Zip 96743; tel. 808/885–4444 **A**1 5 7 9 10 20 **F**3 13 15 25 27 31 32 33 34 38 52 55 57 61 62 66 68 74 75 76 77 79 82 86 96 97 100 102 103 107 118 119 120 135 136 137 **P**6
Primary Contact: W. Jefferson Comer, Jr., Chief Executive Officer
CFO: Nick Braccino, Interim Vice President Finance
CMO: Sheila Cooper, M.D., Co–Chief of Staff
CIO: Victor Gouge, Information Systems Leader
CHR: Delsa Bentelmann, Human Resources Leader
Web address: www.northhawaiicommunityhospital.org
Control: Other not–for–profit (including NFP Corporation) **Service:** General Medical and Surgical

Staffed Beds: 40 **Admissions:** 2166 **Census:** 21 **Outpatient Visits:** 31597 **Births:** 627 **Total Expense ($000):** 45632 **Payroll Expense ($000):** 21545 **Personnel:** 298

KANEOHE—Honolulu County

□ **HAWAII STATE HOSPITAL**, 45–710 Keaahala Road, Zip 96744–3597; tel. 808/236–8237 **A**1 3 5 **F**31 32 54 56 60 82 88 90 91 93 119 121 132
Primary Contact: Mark Fridovich, Ph.D., Administrator
COO: William T. Elliott, Associate Administrator Administrative and Support Services
CFO: Elnora Guieb, Business Manager
CMO: William Sheehan, M.D., Medical Director
CIO: John Jansen, Management Information Specialist
CHR: Karen Hara, Personnel Management Specialist
Web address: www.hshweb.health.state.hi.us
Control: State–Government, nonfederal **Service:** Psychiatric

Staffed Beds: 202 **Admissions:** 217 **Census:** 187 **Outpatient Visits:** 0 **Births:** 0 **Total Expense ($000):** 56564 **Payroll Expense ($000):** 31006 **Personnel:** 565

KAPAA—Kauai County

★ **SAMUEL MAHELONA MEMORIAL HOSPITAL (121306)**, 4800 Kawaihau Road, Zip 96746–1998; tel. 808/822–4961, (Nonreporting) **A**9 10 18 **S** Hawaii Health Systems Corporation
Primary Contact: Orianna A. Skomoroch, Regional Chief Executive Officer
CFO: Michael Perel, Regional Chief Financial Officer
CMO: Gerald Tomory, M.D., Regional Medical Director
CIO: Sandra McMaster, Regional Chief Information Officer
CHR: Lani Aranio, Regional Director Human Resources
Web address: www.smmh.hhsc.org
Control: State–Government, nonfederal **Service:** Long–Term Acute Care hospital

Staffed Beds: 14

KAUNAKAKAI—Maui County

☒ **MOLOKAI GENERAL HOSPITAL (121303)**, Mailing Address: P.O. Box 408, Zip 96748–0408; tel. 808/553–5331, (Total facility includes 2 beds in nursing home–type unit) **A**1 5 9 10 18 **F**13 15 25 27 31 32 33 38 42 43 44 57 62 65 66 67 73 74 75 82 86 96 107 119 122 136 137 **S** Queen's Health Systems
Primary Contact: Janice Kalanihuia, President
CMO: William Thomas, M.D., Medical Director Clinical and Internal Affairs
CIO: Randy Lite, Vice President
CHR: Lei Mokiao, Coordinator Human Resources
Web address: www.queens.org
Control: Other not–for–profit (including NFP Corporation) **Service:** General Medical and Surgical

Staffed Beds: 15 **Admissions:** 146 **Census:** 4 **Outpatient Visits:** 16748 **Births:** 30 **Total Expense ($000):** 8689 **Payroll Expense ($000):** 3242 **Personnel:** 67

KEALAKEKUA—Hawaii County

☒ **KONA COMMUNITY HOSPITAL (120019)**, 79–1019 Haukapila Street, Zip 96750–7920; tel. 808/322–9311, (Total facility includes 34 beds in nursing home–type unit) **A**1 5 9 10 20 **F**3 8 11 13 26 27 30 31 32 33 38 46 47 49 51 53 54 55 57 65 66 68 73 74 75 76 77 79 82 84 86 88 92 93 96 97 99 100 102 104 107 109 111 117 119 131 134 135 136 137 **S** Hawaii Health Systems Corporation
Primary Contact: Earl Greenia, Regional Chief Executive Officer
CFO: Raymond Liu, Chief Financial Officer
CMO: Barry Blum, M.D., Medical Director
CIO: Ed Heaukulani, Manager Information Technology
CHR: Karen Sandrock, Director Human Resources
Web address: www.kch.hhsc.org
Control: State–Government, nonfederal **Service:** General Medical and Surgical

Staffed Beds: 88 **Admissions:** 3248 **Census:** 36 **Outpatient Visits:** 26740 **Births:** 554 **Total Expense ($000):** 47537 **Payroll Expense ($000):** 22268 **Personnel:** 414

KOHALA—Hawaii County

★ **KOHALA HOSPITAL (121302)**, 54–383 Hospital Road, Zip 96755, Mailing Address: P.O. Box 10, Kapaau, Zip 96755–0010; tel. 808/889–6211, (Total facility includes 22 beds in nursing home–type unit) (Nonreporting) **A**9 10 18 **S** Hawaii Health Systems Corporation
Primary Contact: Donald Lewis, Administrator
CFO: Eugene Amar, Chief Financial Officer
CMO: Silvia Sonnenschein, M.D., Chief of Staff
Web address: www.koh.hhsc.org
Control: State–Government, nonfederal **Service:** General Medical and Surgical

Staffed Beds: 26

KULA—Maui County

★ **KULA HOSPITAL (121308)**, 100 Keokea Place, Zip 96790–7450; tel. 808/878–1221, (Nonreporting) **A**5 9 10 18 **S** Hawaii Health Systems Corporation
Primary Contact: Lee Johnson, Administrator
CFO: Lloyd Kawabata, Chief Financial Officer
Web address: www.hhsc.org
Control: State–Government, nonfederal **Service:** General Medical and Surgical

Staffed Beds: 5

LANAI CITY—Maui County

★ **LANAI COMMUNITY HOSPITAL (121305)**, 628 Seventh Street, Zip 96763–0650, Mailing Address: P.O. Box 630650, Zip 96763–0650; tel. 808/565–6411 **A**9 10 18 **F**38 **S** Hawaii Health Systems Corporation
Primary Contact: John Schaumburg, Administrator
Web address: www.lch.hhsc.org
Control: State–Government, nonfederal **Service:** General Medical and Surgical

Staffed Beds: 14 **Admissions:** 1142 **Census:** 7 **Births:** 0 **Total Expense ($000):** 3655 **Payroll Expense ($000):** 1398 **Personnel:** 39

LIHUE—Kauai County

☐ **WILCOX MEMORIAL HOSPITAL (120014)**, 3–3420 Kuhio Highway, Zip 96766–1099; tel. 808/245–1100 **A**1 5 9 10 20 **F**2 3 11 13 15 25 26 30 31 32 38 40 43 57 59 60 62 66 68 73 74 75 79 80 86 96 97 100 107 119 122 124 135 137 **S** Hawaii Pacific Health
Primary Contact: Kathleen Clark, President and Chief Executive Officer
CFO: David Okabe, Executive Vice President, Chief Financial Officer and Treasurer
CMO: Christopher Jordan, M.D., President Medical Staff
CIO: Steve Robertson, Senior Vice President Revenue Cycle Management and Chief Information Officer
CHR: Teri Gomez, Supervisor Human Resources Operations
Web address: www.wilcoxhealth.org
Control: Other not–for–profit (including NFP Corporation) **Service:** General Medical and Surgical

Staffed Beds: 71 **Admissions:** 4101 **Census:** 48 **Outpatient Visits:** 27520 **Births:** 566 **Total Expense ($000):** 66783 **Payroll Expense ($000):** 20664 **Personnel:** 435

PAHALA—Hawaii County

★ **KAU HOSPITAL (121301)**, 1 Kamani Street, Zip 96777, Mailing Address: P.O. Box 40, Zip 96777–0040; tel. 808/928–8331, (Total facility includes 16 beds in nursing home–type unit) (Nonreporting) **A**9 10 18 **S** Hawaii Health Systems Corporation
Primary Contact: Merilyn Harris, Administrator
CFO: Russell Morinaga, Accountant
CMO: Carol Wilder, M.D., Medical Director
Web address: www.hhsc.org
Control: State–Government, nonfederal **Service:** General Medical and Surgical

Staffed Beds: 21

WAHIAWA—Honolulu County

☒ **WAHIAWA GENERAL HOSPITAL (120004)**, 128 Lehua Street, Zip 96786–2036; tel. 808/621–8411 **A**1 3 5 9 10 **F**3 8 11 13 15 25 27 31 38 54 61 65 68 73 74 75 76 77 79 80 81 82 86 93 96 97 98 99 103 107 117 119 121 135 137 **P**8
Primary Contact: R. Don Olden, Chief Executive Officer
COO: R. Don Olden, Chief Executive Officer
CMO: Timothy Whiteside, M.D., Chief of Staff
CIO: Jason Fujinaka, Manager Information System
CHR: Richard Aea, Director Human Resources
Web address: www.wahiawageneral.org
Control: Other not–for–profit (including NFP Corporation) **Service:** General Medical and Surgical

Staffed Beds: 162 **Admissions:** 1895 **Census:** 135 **Births:** 0 **Total Expense ($000):** 32789 **Payroll Expense ($000):** 15597 **Personnel:** 358

WAILUKU—Maui County

☒ **MAUI MEMORIAL MEDICAL CENTER (120002)**, 221 Mahalani Street, Zip 96793–2581; tel. 808/244–9056, (Nonreporting) **A**1 5 9 10 20 **S** Hawaii Health Systems Corporation
Primary Contact: Wesley Lo, Regional Chief Executive Officer
CIO: Dana Mendoza, Chief Information Officer
Web address: www.mmmc.hhsc.org
Control: State–Government, nonfederal **Service:** General Medical and Surgical

Staffed Beds: 203

HI

Hospital, Medicare Provider Number, Address, Telephone, Approval, Facility, and Physician Codes, Health Care System
★ American Hospital Association (AHA) membership
☐ The Joint Commission accreditation
○ American Osteopathic Association (AOA) accreditation
△ Commission on Accreditation of Rehabilitation Facilities (CARF) accreditation

WAIMEA—Kauai County

★ **KAUAI VETERANS MEMORIAL HOSPITAL (121300)**, Waimea Canyon Road, Zip 96796, Mailing Address: P.O. Box 337, Zip 96796–0337; tel. 808/338–9431, (Total facility includes 20 beds in nursing home–type unit) **A**1 9 10 18 **F**11 13 15 17 65 68 74 75 77 79 84 96 99 102 107 117 119 135 136 **S** Hawaii Health Systems Corporation
Primary Contact: Orianna A. Skomoroch, Regional Chief Executive Officer
CFO: Michael Perel, Regional Chief Financial Officer
CMO: Gerald Tomory, M.D., Regional Medical Director
CIO: Sandra McMaster, Regional Chief Information Officer
CHR: Solette Perry, Regional Director Human Resources
Web address: www.kvmh.hhsc.org
Control: State–Government, nonfederal **Service:** General Medical and Surgical

Staffed Beds: 45 **Admissions:** 1027 **Census:** 28 **Births:** 221 **Total Expense ($000):** 27866 **Payroll Expense ($000):** 10960 **Personnel:** 220

HI

IDAHO

AMERICAN FALLS—Power County

★ **HARMS MEMORIAL HOSPITAL DISTRICT (131304)**, 510 Roosevelt Road, Zip 83211–0420, Mailing Address: P.O. Box 420, Zip 83211–0420; tel. 208/226–3200, (Total facility includes 31 beds in nursing home–type unit) **A**9 10 18 **F**2 31 38 57 63 75 86 96 99 107 117 122 **P**5
Primary Contact: Dallas Clinger, Administrator
CFO: Cheryl Reas, Manager Accounting
CMO: Bret Timmons, M.D., Chief Medical Staff
CIO: Mindy Earl, Administrator Health Information Systems
CHR: Norma Hartley, Director Human Resources
Web address: www.harmsmemorial.org
Control: Hospital district or authority, Government, nonfederal **Service:** General Medical and Surgical

Staffed Beds: 41 **Admissions:** 81 **Census:** 26 **Outpatient Visits:** 9998 **Births:** 0

ARCO—Butte County

LOST RIVERS DISTRICT HOSPITAL (131324), 551 Highland Drive, Zip 83213–9771, Mailing Address: P.O. Box 145, Zip 83213–0145; tel. 208/527–8206, (Total facility includes 29 beds in nursing home–type unit) (Nonreporting) **A**9 10 18
Primary Contact: Kim Dahlman, Administrator
COO: Kim Dahlman, Administrator
CFO: Kim Dahlman, Administrator
CMO: Jeffrey Haskell, M.D., Chief Medical Staff
CIO: Doug Hymas, Information Technologist
CHR: Leann Wartchow, Director Human Resources and Assistant Chief Executive Officer
Web address: www.lostriverhospital.com
Control: Hospital district or authority, Government, nonfederal **Service:** General Medical and Surgical

Staffed Beds: 43

BLACKFOOT—Bingham County

▣ **BINGHAM MEMORIAL HOSPITAL (131325)**, 98 Poplar Street, Zip 83221–1799; tel. 208/785–4100, (Total facility includes 75 beds in nursing home–type unit) **A**1 9 10 18 **F**2 3 13 15 25 30 31 32 33 38 40 50 54 55 56 57 62 64 68 69 73 74 75 77 79 80 81 82 86 96 100 103 107 117 119 120 121 122 123 124 135 136 137 **P**1
Primary Contact: Louis D. Kraml, CHE, Chief Executive Officer
COO: Dan Cochran, Chief Operating Officer
CFO: Charlie Button, Chief Financial Officer
CIO: Justin Hansen, Director Information Systems
Web address: www.binghammemorial.org
Control: Other not–for–profit (including NFP Corporation) **Service:** General Medical and Surgical

Staffed Beds: 100 **Admissions:** 1752 **Census:** 65 **Outpatient Visits:** 37929 **Births:** 379 **Total Expense ($000):** 41137 **Payroll Expense ($000):** 18104 **Personnel:** 344

MOUNTAIN RIVER BIRTHING AND SURGERY CENTER (130067), 350 North Meridian Street, Zip 83221; tel. 208/782–0300, (Nonreporting) **A**9 10
Control: Corporation, Investor–owned, for–profit **Service:** Obstetrics and gynecology

Staffed Beds: 8

☐ **STATE HOSPITAL SOUTH (134010)**, 700 East Alice Street, Zip 83221–0400, Mailing Address: Box 400, Zip 83221–0400; tel. 208/785–1200, (Total facility includes 29 beds in nursing home–type unit) (Nonreporting) **A**1 9 10
Primary Contact: Tracy J. Farnsworth, Administrator
COO: Dennis Larsen, Director Physical Plant
CFO: Duane Klomp, Chief Financial Officer
CIO: Marv Perry, Director Performance Improvement
CHR: Heidi Anderson, Human Resources Specialist
Control: State–Government, nonfederal **Service:** Psychiatric

Staffed Beds: 165

BOISE—Ada County

★ △ **IDAHO ELKS REHABILITATION HOSPITAL (133025)**, 600 North Robbins Road, Zip 83702–4597, Mailing Address: P.O. Box 1100, Zip 83701–1100; tel. 208/489–4444 **A**7 9 10 **F**53 73 85 86 117 119 132 135 137
Primary Contact: Joseph P. Caroselli, Administrator
CFO: Doug Lewis, Chief Financial Officer
CMO: Robert Friedman, M.D., Medical Director
CHR: Jim Atkins, Director Employee Services
Web address: www.idahoelksrehab.org
Control: Other not–for–profit (including NFP Corporation) **Service:** Rehabilitation

Staffed Beds: 71 **Admissions:** 1236 **Census:** 40 **Outpatient Visits:** 9515 **Births:** 0 **Total Expense ($000):** 22510 **Payroll Expense ($000):** 12366 **Personnel:** 568

☐ **INTERMOUNTAIN HOSPITAL (134002)**, 303 North Allumbaugh Street, Zip 83704–9266; tel. 208/377–8400, (Nonreporting) **A**1 10
S Psychiatric Solutions
Primary Contact: Richard A. Bangert, Chief Executive Officer
CMO: Harry Silsby, M.D., Medical Director
CHR: Angela Billingsley, Director Human Resources
Web address: www.psysolutions.com
Control: Corporation, Investor–owned, for–profit **Service:** Psychiatric

Staffed Beds: 140

▣ △ **SAINT ALPHONSUS REGIONAL MEDICAL CENTER (130007)**, 1055 North Curtis Road, Zip 83706–1370; tel. 208/367–2121 **A**1 2 3 5 7 9 10 **F**3 5 7 8 9 11 12 13 14 15 17 18 20 22 24 25 26 27 28 29 30 31 32 33 34 35 36 37 38 41 42 43 44 45 48 49 50 53 54 55 56 57 58 59 60 62 63 66 68 69 70 72 73 74 75 76 77 79 80 81 82 84 85 86 87 88 89 90 91 92 94 96 97 100 102 103 106 107 108 109 111 112 114 116 117 118 119 120 121 123 124 133 134 135 136 137 **P**5 6 7 **S** Trinity Health
Primary Contact: Sandra B. Bruce, President and Chief Executive Officer
COO: Janelle Reilly, Chief Operating Officer
CFO: Kenneth Fry, Chief Financial Officer
CMO: J. Robert Polk, M.D., Vice President Quality and Patient Safety Officer
CHR: Susan Gibson, Vice President Human Resources and Mission Services
Web address: www.saintalphonsus.org
Control: Church–operated, Nongovernment, not–for profit **Service:** General Medical and Surgical

Staffed Beds: 351 **Admissions:** 17560 **Census:** 236 **Outpatient Visits:** 510230 **Births:** 1630 **Total Expense ($000):** 350712 **Payroll Expense ($000):** 141955 **Personnel:** 2953

▣ **ST. LUKE'S REGIONAL MEDICAL CENTER (130006)**, 190 East Bannock Street, Zip 83712–6298; tel. 208/381–2222, (Nonreporting) **A**1 2 3 5 9 10
S St. Luke's Health System
Primary Contact: Gary Fletcher, Chief Executive Officer
COO: Chris Roth, Chief Operating Officer
CFO: Jeff Taylor, Vice President Finance
CMO: Bart Hill, M.D., Vice President Medical Affairs
CHR: Maureen O'Keeffe, Regional Vice President Human Resources and Strategic Planning
Web address: www.slrmc.org
Control: Other not–for–profit (including NFP Corporation) **Service:** General Medical and Surgical

Staffed Beds: 475

SUNHEALTH BEHAVIORAL HEALTH SYSTEM FOR BOISE (134009), 8050 Northview Street, Zip 83704; tel. 208/327–0504 **A**10 **F**6 54 62 88 93 94 119 **P**5 **S** Sun Healthcare Group
Primary Contact: Phil Herink, Chief Executive Officer
CFO: Phil Herink, Chief Executive Officer
CMO: David Kent, M.D., Chief Medical Officer
CIO: Debra Alexander, Chief Information Officer
Control: Corporation, Investor–owned, for–profit **Service:** Psychiatric

Staffed Beds: 22 **Admissions:** 387 **Census:** 17 **Outpatient Visits:** 7761 **Births:** 0 **Total Expense ($000):** 3235 **Payroll Expense ($000):** 2610 **Personnel:** 74

ID

Hospital, Medicare Provider Number, Address, Telephone, Approval, Facility, and Physician Codes, Health Care System
★ American Hospital Association (AHA) membership
☐ The Joint Commission accreditation
○ American Osteopathic Association (AOA) accreditation
△ Commission on Accreditation of Rehabilitation Facilities (CARF) accreditation

★ **TREASURE VALLEY HOSPITAL (130063)**, 8800 West Emerald Street, Zip 83704; tel. 208/373–5000, (Nonreporting) **A**1 9 10
Primary Contact: Nick Genna, Administrator
CMO: Jeffrey Hessing, M.D., Medical Director
CHR: Kathleen Phelps, Director Human Resources
Control: Corporation, Investor–owned, for–profit **Service:** General Medical and Surgical

Staffed Beds: 9

★ **VETERANS AFFAIRS MEDICAL CENTER**, 500 West Fort Street, Zip 83702–4598; tel. 208/422–1000, (Total facility includes 40 beds in nursing home–type unit) (Nonreporting) **A**1 3 5 9 **S** Department of Veterans Affairs
Primary Contact: Dewayne Hamlin, Director
CFO: Ron Blanton, Chief Fiscal Services
Web address: www.va.gov/directory/guide/home.asp
Control: Veterans Affairs, Government, federal **Service:** General Medical and Surgical

Staffed Beds: 176

BONNERS FERRY—Boundary County

★ **BOUNDARY COMMUNITY HOSPITAL (131301)**, 6640 Kaniksu Street, Zip 83805–7532; tel. 208/267–3141, (Includes BOUNDARY COUNTY NURSING HOME), (Total facility includes 36 beds in nursing home–type unit) **A**9 10 18 **F**3 11 15 31 32 33 38 50 54 55 73 75 77 79 80 82 86 96 100 102 107 117 119 122 124 132 137
Primary Contact: Craig A. Johnson, Chief Executive Officer and Chief Financial Officer
CFO: Craig A. Johnson, Chief Executive Officer and Chief Financial Officer
CHR: Ann Coughlin, Director Human Resources
Web address: www.boundaryhospital.org
Control: County–Government, nonfederal **Service:** General Medical and Surgical

Staffed Beds: 56 **Admissions:** 261 **Census:** 38 **Outpatient Visits:** 19659 **Births:** 0 **Total Expense ($000):** 9384 **Payroll Expense ($000):** 4823 **Personnel:** 151

BURLEY—Cassia County

★ **CASSIA REGIONAL MEDICAL CENTER (131326)**, 1501 Hiland Avenue, Zip 83318–2648; tel. 208/678–4444, (Nonreporting) **A**1 9 10 18 **S** Intermountain Healthcare, Inc.
Primary Contact: Kenneth Harman, Administrator
CFO: Brian Hickenlooper, Assistant Administrator Finance and Chief Financial Officer
CMO: Fred Wood, M.D., Medical Director
CIO: Carie Call, Chief Computer Support
CHR: Keri Perrigot, Assistant Administrator Human Resources
Web address: www.ihc.com
Control: Other not–for–profit (including NFP Corporation) **Service:** General Medical and Surgical

Staffed Beds: 25

CALDWELL—Canyon County

★ **WEST VALLEY MEDICAL CENTER (130014)**, 1717 Arlington, Zip 83605–4864; tel. 208/459–4641, (Nonreporting) **A**1 9 10 **S** HCA
Primary Contact: Kathy D. Moore, Chief Executive Officer
COO: Deanna Martin, MSN, Chief Nursing Officer and Chief Operating Officer
CFO: Scott Davis, Chief Financial Officer
CIO: Lance Christiansen, Chief Information Officer
CHR: Terry Peoples, Director Human Resources
Web address: www.westvalleymedctr.com
Control: Corporation, Investor–owned, for–profit **Service:** General Medical and Surgical

Staffed Beds: 122

CASCADE—Valley County

★ **CASCADE MEDICAL CENTER (131308)**, 402 Old State Highway, Zip 83611, Mailing Address: P.O. Box 1330, Zip 83611–1330; tel. 208/382–4242 **A**9 10 18 **F**11 25 28 38 52 55 56 57 62 63 65 84 86 87 92 117 120 122 136 **P**6 **S** Trinity Health
Primary Contact: William C. Behnke, Jr., Administrator
CMO: Douglas Hill, M.D., Medical Director
Control: Hospital district or authority, Government, nonfederal **Service:** General Medical and Surgical

Staffed Beds: 10 **Admissions:** 22 **Census:** 3 **Outpatient Visits:** 2425 **Births:** 1 **Total Expense ($000):** 2428 **Payroll Expense ($000):** 1213 **Personnel:** 23

COEUR D'ALENE—Kootenai County

★ **KOOTENAI MEDICAL CENTER (130049)**, 2003 Lincoln Way, Zip 83814–2677; tel. 208/666–2000, (Includes NORTH IDAHO BEHAVIORAL HEALTH, DIVISION OF KOOTENAI MEDICAL CENTER, 2301 North Ironwood Place, Zip 83814–2650; tel. 208/765–4800) **A**1 2 9 10 19 **F**1 2 3 4 5 8 11 12 13 15 16 17 18 20 22 24 25 26 27 30 31 32 33 37 38 40 42 43 44 45 46 47 49 50 51 52 55 56 57 58 59 62 63 65 66 68 70 71 72 73 74 75 76 77 78 79 81 82 83 84 85 86 88 89 90 91 92 93 94 95 101 102 103 104 107 108 109 114 117 118 119 121 123 124 132 135
Primary Contact: Joseph E. Morris, Chief Executive Officer
CFO: Tom Legel, Vice President and Chief Financial Officer
CMO: Joseph Bujak, M.D., Vice President Medical Affairs
CIO: Tom Legel, Vice President and Chief Financial Officer
CHR: Daniel Klocko, Vice President Human Resources
Web address: www.kmc.org
Control: Hospital district or authority, Government, nonfederal **Service:** General Medical and Surgical

Staffed Beds: 246 **Admissions:** 13161 **Census:** 153 **Outpatient Visits:** 154239 **Births:** 1625 **Total Expense ($000):** 180421 **Payroll Expense ($000):** 73286 **Personnel:** 1369

COTTONWOOD—Idaho County

★ **ST. MARY'S HOSPITAL (131321)**, Lewiston and North Streets, Zip 83522–9750, Mailing Address: P.O. Box 137, Zip 83522–0137; tel. 208/962–3251, (Total facility includes 10 beds in nursing home–type unit) (Nonreporting) **A**9 10 18 **S** Essentia Health
Primary Contact: Casey Meza, Chief Executive Officer
Web address: www.stmaryshospital.net
Control: Other not–for–profit (including NFP Corporation) **Service:** General Medical and Surgical

Staffed Beds: 28

DRIGGS—Teton County

★ **TETON VALLEY HOSPITAL AND SURGICENTER (131313)**, 120 East Howard Street, Zip 83422–5112; tel. 208/354–2383, (Nonreporting) **A**9 10 18
Primary Contact: Floyd D. Bounds, Chief Executive Officer
CHR: Carla Romero–Erlanson, Director Human Resources
Web address: www.tvhcare.org
Control: County–Government, nonfederal **Service:** General Medical and Surgical

Staffed Beds: 13

EMMETT—Gem County

★ **WALTER KNOX MEMORIAL HOSPITAL (131318)**, 1202 East Locust Street, Zip 83617–2715; tel. 208/365–3561 **A**9 10 18 **F**3 8 11 13 25 27 33 38 43 55 56 57 62 79 80 82 96 102 107 122 133
Primary Contact: Max Long, FACHE, Chief Executive Officer
CFO: Larry Droppers, Chief Financial Officer
CHR: Susan Vahlberg, Director Employee and Community Relations
Web address: www.wkmh.org
Control: County–Government, nonfederal **Service:** General Medical and Surgical

Staffed Beds: 16 **Admissions:** 536 **Census:** 3 **Outpatient Visits:** 19846 **Births:** 81 **Total Expense ($000):** 7611 **Payroll Expense ($000):** 2963 **Personnel:** 67

GOODING—Gooding County

★ **GOODING COUNTY MEMORIAL HOSPITAL (131302)**, 1120 Montana Street, Zip 83330–1858; tel. 208/934–4433 **A**9 10 18 **F**3 11 15 25 26 28 31 32 33 38 41 42 43 47 48 49 50 52 53 55 56 57 62 66 73 75 79 80 82 86 96 100 107 118 119 120 122 124 135 **S** St. Luke's Health System
Primary Contact: Earl Fitzpatrick, Chief Executive Officer
CFO: Rod Larsen, Chief Financial Officer
CMO: Samantha Marshal, M.D., Chief of Staff
CIO: Paul Castronova, Chief Information Officer
CHR: Sara Otto, Director Human Resources
Web address: www.goodinghospital.org
Control: Hospital district or authority, Government, nonfederal **Service:** General Medical and Surgical

Staffed Beds: 14 **Admissions:** 704 **Census:** 6 **Outpatient Visits:** 19425 **Births:** 0 **Total Expense ($000):** 8153 **Payroll Expense ($000):** 2597 **Personnel:** 113

GRANGEVILLE—Idaho County

★ **SYRINGA GENERAL HOSPITAL (131315)**, 607 West Main Street, Zip 83530–1396; tel. 208/983–1700 **A**9 10 18 **F**25 26 30 31 32 33 38 42 53 55 56 57 61 62 66 75 79 96 107 122
Primary Contact: Joseph Cladouhos, Chief Executive Officer
CFO: Betty A. Watson, Chief Financial Officer
CHR: Katy Eimers, Human Resources Officer
Web address: www.syringahospital.org
Control: Hospital district or authority, Government, nonfederal **Service:** General Medical and Surgical

Staffed Beds: 15 **Admissions:** 387 **Census:** 3 **Outpatient Visits:** 17798 **Births:** 52 **Total Expense ($000):** 8412 **Payroll Expense ($000):** 3764 **Personnel:** 98

ID

Many Facility Codes have changed. Please refer to the AHA Guide Code Chart.

IDAHO FALLS—Bonneville County

☒ **EASTERN IDAHO REGIONAL MEDICAL CENTER (130018)**, 3100 Channing Way, Zip 83404–7533, Mailing Address: P.O. Box 2077, Zip 83403–2077; tel. 208/529–6111, (Total facility includes 16 beds in nursing home–type unit) **A**1 2 9 10 19 **F**3 7 11 12 13 15 18 19 20 21 22 24 25 26 27 30 31 32 33 34 37 38 40 41 43 46 50 51 52 55 56 57 62 63 65 66 68 70 72 73 74 75 76 77 79 80 81 82 84 85 86 88 89 90 92 96 97 100 102 106 107 108 109 111 117 118 119 120 121 124 135 136 137 **P**5 **S** HCA
Primary Contact: Douglas Crabtree, Chief Executive Officer
COO: Jordan Herget, Chief Operating Officer
CFO: Derek Lythgoe, Chief Financial Officer
CMO: Dave Chamberlain, M.D., President Medical Staff
CHR: Nate Bigler, Director Human Resources
Web address: www.eirmc.com
Control: Corporation, Investor–owned, for–profit **Service:** General Medical and Surgical

Staffed Beds: 294 **Admissions:** 11188 **Census:** 181 **Outpatient Visits:** 178157 **Births:** 1434 **Total Expense ($000):** 145783 **Payroll Expense ($000):** 55996 **Personnel:** 1114

IDAHO FALLS RECOVERY CENTER (130062), 1957 East 17th Street, Zip 83404–6429; tel. 208/529–5285, (Nonreporting) **A**9 10
Primary Contact: Lindee Hokanson, Administrator
COO: Lindee Hokanson, Administrator
Web address: www.ifrecoverycenter.com
Control: Other not–for–profit (including NFP Corporation) **Service:** General Medical and Surgical

Staffed Beds: 10

MOUNTAIN VIEW HOSPITAL (130065), 2325 Coronado Street, Zip 83404; tel. 208/557–2700, (Nonreporting) **A**9 10
Primary Contact: James Adamson, Chief Executive Officer
COO: Peter Fabrick, Vice President Clinical Operations
CFO: Jeff Sayer, President and Chief Financial Officer
CHR: Eilene Horne, Manager Human Resources
Web address: www.mountainviewhospital.org
Control: Corporation, Investor–owned, for–profit **Service:** General Medical and Surgical

Staffed Beds: 22

JEROME—Jerome County

★ **ST. BENEDICTS FAMILY MEDICAL CENTER (131310)**, 709 North Lincoln Street, Zip 83338–1851, Mailing Address: P.O. Box 586, Zip 83338–0586; tel. 208/324–4301, (Total facility includes 40 beds in nursing home–type unit) (Nonreporting) **A**9 10 18 **S** Essentia Health
Primary Contact: Alan Stevenson, Administrator
COO: Curtis Maier, Assistant Administrator
CFO: Mark Christensen, Chief Financial Officer
CMO: James Irwin, M.D., Director Medical Staff Affairs
CIO: Curtis Maier, Assistant Administrator
CHR: Dee Hartzell, Manager Human Resources
Web address: www.stbenshospital.org
Control: Other not–for–profit (including NFP Corporation) **Service:** General Medical and Surgical

Staffed Beds: 65

KELLOGG—Shoshone County

★ **SHOSHONE MEDICAL CENTER (131314)**, 25 Jacobs Gulch, Zip 83837–2096; tel. 208/784–1221 **A**9 10 18 **F**25 26 33 38 50 52 56 57 63 66 73 75 77 79 82 86 96 100 102 107 118 122 124 135 **S** QHR
Primary Contact: David B. Selman, FACHE, Chief Executive Officer
CFO: Jerry Brantz, Chief Financial Officer
CMO: Tony Branz, M.D., Chief Of Staff
CIO: Russ Allred, Manager Information Systems
CHR: Joanna Radford, Chief Human Resources Officer
Web address: www.shomed.org
Control: Hospital district or authority, Government, nonfederal **Service:** General Medical and Surgical

Staffed Beds: 25 **Admissions:** 529 **Census:** 6 **Outpatient Visits:** 15131 **Births:** 0 **Total Expense ($000):** 10345 **Payroll Expense ($000):** 3447 **Personnel:** 92

KETCHUM—Blaine County

☒ **ST. LUKE'S WOOD RIVER MEDICAL CENTER (131323)**, 100 Hospital Drive, Zip 83340, Mailing Address: P.O. Box 100, Zip 83340; tel. 208/727–8800 **A**1 9 10 18 **F**3 8 11 13 15 25 26 27 30 32 33 38 40 43 52 55 56 57 62 66 68 73 74 77 79 80 81 96 100 107 119 122 123 134 135 136 **S** St. Luke's Health System
Primary Contact: Bruce C. Jensen, Chief Executive Officer
CFO: Carl Hollingsworth, Chief Financial Officer
CHR: Stacey Doby, Director Human Resources
Web address: www.slrmc.org
Control: Other not–for–profit (including NFP Corporation) **Service:** General Medical and Surgical

Staffed Beds: 25 **Admissions:** 1112 **Census:** 8 **Outpatient Visits:** 32407 **Births:** 294 **Total Expense ($000):** 33277 **Payroll Expense ($000):** 14894 **Personnel:** 255

LEWISTON—Nez Perce County

☒ **ST. JOSEPH REGIONAL MEDICAL CENTER (130003)**, 415 Sixth Street, Zip 83501–0816; tel. 208/743–2511, (Total facility includes 16 beds in nursing home–type unit) **A**1 2 9 10 19 **F**3 11 13 15 18 25 26 27 28 30 31 32 33 35 36 37 38 40 42 43 44 45 46 48 49 50 51 52 54 55 56 57 60 61 62 63 66 68 69 72 73 74 75 76 77 79 80 81 82 84 86 88 90 91 92 93 94 96 97 99 100 103 104 106 107 109 111 117 118 119 120 121 124 130 133 135 136 137 **P**6 **S** Ascension Health
Primary Contact: Howard A. Hayes, President and Chief Executive Officer
CFO: Douglas C. Johnson, Vice President and Chief Financial Officer
CMO: Lyndal Stoutin, M.D., Chief of Staff
CIO: Collin Lamb, Director Management Information Systems
CHR: Brenda Forge, Vice President Human Resources
Web address: www.sjrmc.org
Control: Church–operated, Nongovernment, not–for profit **Service:** General Medical and Surgical

Staffed Beds: 149 **Admissions:** 5436 **Census:** 63 **Outpatient Visits:** 97227 **Births:** 709 **Total Expense ($000):** 92597 **Payroll Expense ($000):** 35549 **Personnel:** 625

MALAD CITY—Oneida County

ONEIDA COUNTY HOSPITAL (131303), 150 North 200 West, Zip 83252–0126, Mailing Address: Box 126, Zip 83252–0126; tel. 208/766–2231, (Total facility includes 41 beds in nursing home–type unit) **A**9 10 18 **F**2 11 30 32 33 38 40 50 54 55 56 57 61 63 64 66 67 73 77 79 80 82 87 96 97 117 122 132 135 137 **P**6
Primary Contact: Todd Winder, Administrator and Chief Executive Officer
CFO: Cindy Howard, Director Financial Services
Web address: www.oneidahospital.com
Control: County–Government, nonfederal **Service:** General Medical and Surgical

Staffed Beds: 52 **Admissions:** 171 **Census:** 30 **Outpatient Visits:** 5161 **Births:** 0 **Total Expense ($000):** 6053 **Payroll Expense ($000):** 2913 **Personnel:** 102

MCCALL—Valley County

★ **MCCALL MEMORIAL HOSPITAL (131312)**, 1000 State Street, Zip 83638–3704; tel. 208/634–2221 **A**9 10 18 **F**3 11 13 15 26 27 28 30 31 32 33 34 36 37 38 41 43 47 48 50 55 56 57 62 68 74 79 80 81 82 84 87 96 102 107 119 121 122 123 124 130 135 136 137 **P**6 7 **S** St. Luke's Health System
Primary Contact: Karen J. Kellie, RN, President and Administrator
CFO: Guy Rivers, Vice President Finance and Information Services
CIO: Guy Rivers, Vice President Finance and Information Services
Web address: www.mccallhosp.org
Control: Hospital district or authority, Government, nonfederal **Service:** General Medical and Surgical

Staffed Beds: 15 **Admissions:** 537 **Census:** 3 **Outpatient Visits:** 27999 **Births:** 127 **Total Expense ($000):** 14184 **Payroll Expense ($000):** 5162 **Personnel:** 102

MONTPELIER—Bear Lake County

★ **BEAR LAKE MEMORIAL HOSPITAL (131316)**, 164 South Fifth Street, Zip 83254–1597; tel. 208/847–1630, (Total facility includes 37 beds in nursing home–type unit) (Nonreporting) **A**9 10 18
Primary Contact: Rodney D. Jacobson, Administrator
Web address: www.blmhospital.com
Control: State–Government, nonfederal **Service:** General Medical and Surgical

Staffed Beds: 58

ID

Hospital, Medicare Provider Number, Address, Telephone, Approval, Facility, and Physician Codes, Health Care System

★ American Hospital Association (AHA) membership
□ The Joint Commission accreditation
○ American Osteopathic Association (AOA) accreditation
△ Commission on Accreditation of Rehabilitation Facilities (CARF) accreditation

MOSCOW—Latah County

☒ **GRITMAN MEDICAL CENTER (131327)**, 700 South Main Street, Zip 83843–3047; tel. 208/882–4511 **A**1 9 10 18 **F**2 3 8 11 13 15 24 25 26 31 32 33 34 35 38 42 43 44 46 49 51 53 54 55 56 57 61 62 63 68 73 74 75 77 79 80 81 82 84 86 89 96 97 100 102 107 118 119 120 121 124 132 135 136 137 **P**3 5 **S** QHR
Primary Contact: Jeffrey W. Martin, Chief Executive Officer
CFO: Kara Besst, Chief Financial Officer
CMO: Sara Lawrence, M.D., Chief Medical Staff
CIO: Kane Francetich, Chief Information Officer
CHR: Dennis Cockrell, Director Human Resources
Web address: www.gritman.org
Control: Other not–for–profit (including NFP Corporation) **Service:** General Medical and Surgical

Staffed Beds: 25 **Admissions:** 1779 **Census:** 16 **Outpatient Visits:** 64246 **Births:** 414 **Total Expense ($000):** 36488 **Payroll Expense ($000):** 15623 **Personnel:** 361

MOUNTAIN HOME—Elmore County

★ **ELMORE MEDICAL CENTER (131311)**, 895 North Sixth East Street, Zip 83647–2207, Mailing Address: P.O. Box 1270, Zip 83647–1270; tel. 208/587–8401, (Total facility includes 45 beds in nursing home–type unit) **A**9 10 18 **F**3 11 13 25 26 31 33 38 55 62 73 74 79 84 96 100 102 107 117 119 122 135 **S** St. Luke's Health System
Primary Contact: Gregory L. Maurer, Administrator
COO: Betty Van Gheluwe, Chief Operating Officer
CFO: Tricia Senger, Chief Financial Officer
Web address: www.elmoremedicalcenter.org
Control: Hospital district or authority, Government, nonfederal **Service:** General Medical and Surgical

Staffed Beds: 63 **Admissions:** 751 **Census:** 33 **Outpatient Visits:** 43995 **Births:** 94 **Total Expense ($000):** 16436 **Payroll Expense ($000):** 6260 **Personnel:** 193

NAMPA—Canyon County

☒ △ **MERCY MEDICAL CENTER (130013)**, 1512 12th Avenue Road, Zip 83686–6008; tel. 208/463–5000 **A**1 7 9 10 **F**12 13 15 18 20 25 26 27 30 31 32 35 38 40 42 49 59 61 67 68 74 77 79 84 96 97 102 103 107 118 119 124 132 **S** Catholic Health Initiatives
Primary Contact: Joseph Messmer, President and Chief Executive Officer
CFO: B. Lannie Checketts, Vice President Finance and Chief Financial Officer
CIO: Major Daniel Wright, Director Information Technology
CHR: Audra Pratt, Vice President Human Resources and Chief Administrative Officer
Web address: www.mercynampa.org
Control: Church–operated, Nongovernment, not–for profit **Service:** General Medical and Surgical

Staffed Beds: 118 **Admissions:** 6248 **Census:** 49 **Outpatient Visits:** 113548 **Births:** 1563 **Total Expense ($000):** 70074 **Payroll Expense ($000):** 29284 **Personnel:** 645

OROFINO—Clearwater County

★ **CLEARWATER VALLEY HOSPITAL AND CLINICS (131320)**, 301 Cedar, Zip 83544–9029; tel. 208/476–4555, (Nonreporting) **A**9 10 18 **S** Essentia Health
Primary Contact: Casey Meza, Chief Executive Officer
Web address: www.smh–cvhc.org
Control: Other not–for–profit (including NFP Corporation) **Service:** General Medical and Surgical

Staffed Beds: 23

STATE HOSPITAL NORTH, 300 Hospital Drive, Zip 83544–9034; tel. 208/476–4511 **A**9 **F**30 88 119 **P**6
Primary Contact: Debra Manfull, Acting Administrative Director
CFO: Debra Manfull, Assistant Administrator
CMO: Fraun Flerchinger, M.D., Clinical Director
CIO: James Sarbacher, Chief Information Officer
CHR: Sharon Larson, Human Resource Specialist
Control: State–Government, nonfederal **Service:** Psychiatric

Staffed Beds: 50 **Admissions:** 231 **Census:** 48 **Outpatient Visits:** 62 **Births:** 0 **Total Expense ($000):** 7181 **Payroll Expense ($000):** 4094 **Personnel:** 103

POCATELLO—Bannock County

BEACON HOSPITAL AND REHABILITATION OF POCATELLO (134011), 1200 Hospital Way, Zip 83201; tel. 208/232–2570, (Nonreporting) **A**10
Primary Contact: Josiah Dahlstrom, Administrator
Control: Individual, Investor–owned, for–profit **Service:** Rehabilitation

Staffed Beds: 12

☒ **PORTNEUF MEDICAL CENTER (130028)**, 651 Memorial Drive, Zip 83201–4004; tel. 208/239–1000 **A**1 2 9 10 **F**3 7 11 13 14 15 17 18 20 22 24 25 26 27 31 32 33 37 38 41 43 48 49 50 51 53 55 56 57 58 59 60 62 66 68 69 70 72 73 74 75 76 77 79 80 81 82 83 84 85 86 87 88 90 91 92 93 94 95 96 97 98 99 100 102 103 104 105 106 107 109 111 118 119 121 124 132 133 135 136 137 **P**6 8
Primary Contact: Patrick M. Hermanson, FACHE, President and Chief Executive Officer
COO: Callen Northam, Executive Vice President and Chief Operating Officer
CFO: John Wilker, Vice President and Chief Financial Officer
CMO: Gary Hart, M.D., Vice President Medical Affairs
CHR: Dale Mapes, Vice President Human Resources and Support Services
Web address: www.portmed.org
Control: County–Government, nonfederal **Service:** General Medical and Surgical

Staffed Beds: 161 **Admissions:** 7859 **Census:** 82 **Outpatient Visits:** 282091 **Births:** 1641 **Total Expense ($000):** 123710 **Payroll Expense ($000):** 50455 **Personnel:** 978

POST FALLS—Kootenai County

☐ **NORTHWEST SPECIALTY HOSPITAL (130066)**, 1593 East Polston Avenue, Zip 83854; tel. 208/262–2300, (Nonreporting) **A**1 9 10 **S** National Surgical Hospitals
Web address: www.northwestspecialtyhospital.com
Control: Corporation, Investor–owned, for–profit **Service:** Other specialty

Staffed Beds: 12

PRESTON—Franklin County

★ **FRANKLIN COUNTY MEDICAL CENTER (131322)**, 44 North First East Street, Zip 83263–1399; tel. 208/852–0137, (Total facility includes 45 beds in nursing home–type unit) **A**9 10 18 **F**2 3 11 13 27 33 38 42 43 55 61 66 73 77 79 86 96 102 107 117 119 122 135 **P**1
Primary Contact: Michael G. Andrus, Administrator and Chief Executive Officer
CFO: Paul Smart, CPA, Chief Financial Officer
CHR: Courtney Dursteler, Chief Human Resources Officer
Web address: www.fcmc.org
Control: County–Government, nonfederal **Service:** General Medical and Surgical

Staffed Beds: 65 **Admissions:** 599 **Census:** 41 **Outpatient Visits:** 3721 **Births:** 98 **Total Expense ($000):** 9923 **Payroll Expense ($000):** 5140 **Personnel:** 173

REXBURG—Madison County

★ **MADISON MEMORIAL HOSPITAL (130025)**, 450 East Main Street, Zip 83440–2048, Mailing Address: P.O. Box 310, Zip 83440–0310; tel. 208/356–3691 **A**9 10 **F**3 11 13 17 24 25 26 27 28 29 30 31 33 37 38 43 55 56 57 63 64 68 71 73 74 75 76 77 79 80 81 82 84 86 96 97 100 106 107 118 119 120 121 124 135 **P**1 5 6
Primary Contact: David B. Rowe, Chief Executive Officer
CFO: Calvin Carey, Assistant Administrator and Chief Financial Officer
CMO: Michael Packer, M.D., Chief Medical Staff
Web address: www.madisonhospital.org
Control: County–Government, nonfederal **Service:** General Medical and Surgical

Staffed Beds: 49 **Admissions:** 4070 **Census:** 27 **Outpatient Visits:** 48129 **Births:** 1557 **Total Expense ($000):** 38803 **Payroll Expense ($000):** 16168 **Personnel:** 385

RUPERT—Minidoka County

★ **MINIDOKA MEMORIAL HOSPITAL AND EXTENDED CARE FACILITY (131319)**, 1224 Eighth Street, Zip 83350–1599; tel. 208/436–0481, (Total facility includes 59 beds in nursing home–type unit) **A**9 10 18 **F**3 7 11 15 25 26 30 31 32 33 38 42 43 44 45 50 54 55 56 57 61 62 63 66 68 73 75 76 77 79 80 81 82 84 87 96 97 100 102 107 117 119 120 121 122 132 135 136 137 **P**1 3 5
Primary Contact: Carl Hanson, Administrator
COO: Joel Rogers, Chief Operating Officer
CFO: Jason Gibbons, Chief Financial Officer
CMO: Margo Saunders, M.D., Chief of Staff
CHR: Tammy Hanks, Director Human Resources
Web address: www.minidokamemorial.com
Control: County–Government, nonfederal **Service:** General Medical and Surgical

Staffed Beds: 88 **Admissions:** 870 **Census:** 60 **Outpatient Visits:** 12096 **Births:** 0 **Total Expense ($000):** 15280 **Payroll Expense ($000):** 7492 **Personnel:** 226

ID

SAINT MARIES—Benewah County

★ **BENEWAH COMMUNITY HOSPITAL (131317)**, 229 South Seventh Street, Zip 83861–1803; tel. 208/245–5551 **A**9 10 18 **F**8 13 15 25 26 27 30 31 32 33 38 42 43 44 55 56 57 62 73 74 76 77 79 80 86 87 96 100 102 107 119 120 122 **P**4 6 **S** QHR
Primary Contact: Brian Nall, Chief Executive Officer
CFO: Lori Stoltz, Interim Chief Financial Officer
CMO: Richard Thurston, M.D., Chief of Staff
CHR: Debbie Kerns, Director Human Resources
Web address: www.bchmed.org
Control: County–Government, nonfederal **Service:** General Medical and Surgical

Staffed Beds: 19 **Admissions:** 643 **Census:** 5 **Outpatient Visits:** 20022 **Births:** 64 **Total Expense ($000):** 12474 **Payroll Expense ($000):** 4850 **Personnel:** 112

SALMON—Lemhi County

★ **STEELE MEMORIAL MEDICAL CENTER (131305)**, 203 South Daisy, Zip 83467–4109, Mailing Address: P.O. Box 700, Zip 83467–0700; tel. 208/756–5600 **A**9 10 18 **F**3 11 13 15 24 25 26 27 30 33 38 46 55 56 57 62 63 66 74 75 77 79 80 85 86 87 96 100 103 107 118 120 122 124 134 135 136 137 **P**6 **S** QHR
Primary Contact: Victoria A. Alexander, Chief Executive Officer
COO: Linda Astalos, R.N., MSN, Chief Operating Officer and Chief Nursing Officer
CFO: Preston Becker, Chief Financial Officer
CMO: David Yanoff, M.D., Chief of Staff
CIO: Abner King, Director Information Systems
CHR: Kathryn Leavitt, Manager Human Resources
Web address: www.steelemh.org
Control: County–Government, nonfederal **Service:** General Medical and Surgical

Staffed Beds: 18 **Admissions:** 503 **Census:** 3 **Outpatient Visits:** 45774 **Births:** 72 **Total Expense ($000):** 12495 **Payroll Expense ($000):** 6138 **Personnel:** 148

SANDPOINT—Bonner County

🞸 **BONNER GENERAL HOSPITAL (130024)**, 520 North Third Avenue, Zip 83864–0877, Mailing Address: Box 1448, Zip 83864–0877; tel. 208/263–1441 **A**1 9 10 20 **F**3 11 13 15 17 24 25 32 33 38 42 46 47 48 53 55 56 57 61 62 66 73 74 75 77 78 79 80 81 82 86 92 96 97 100 102 106 107 119 120 122 131 133 135 **P**8
Primary Contact: Sheryl Rickard, Chief Executive Officer
CFO: Norilina Harvel, Chief Financial Officer
CIO: Bob Hess, Chief Information Officer
CHR: Diane Ross, Director Human Resources
Web address: www.bonnergen.org
Control: Other not–for–profit (including NFP Corporation) **Service:** General Medical and Surgical

Staffed Beds: 41 **Admissions:** 2482 **Census:** 18 **Outpatient Visits:** 57209 **Births:** 400 **Total Expense ($000):** 37390 **Payroll Expense ($000):** 15160 **Personnel:** 312

SODA SPRINGS—Caribou County

★ **CARIBOU MEMORIAL HOSPITAL AND LIVING CENTER (131309)**, 300 South Third West, Zip 83276–1598; tel. 208/547–3341, (Total facility includes 37 beds in nursing home–type unit) **A**9 10 18 **F**1 11 13 17 25 30 31 32 33 38 50 52 54 55 56 57 63 65 68 74 75 77 79 80 81 82 86 90 94 96 100 102 107 119
Primary Contact: John L. Hoopes, Chief Executive Officer
CFO: Leota Carver, Manager Finance
CMO: John K. Fransen, M.D., Chief Medical Staff
CHR: Michael D. Peck, Assistant Administrator
Web address: www.cariboumemorial.org
Control: City–County, Government, nonfederal **Service:** General Medical and Surgical

Staffed Beds: 62 **Admissions:** 364 **Census:** 31 **Outpatient Visits:** 10777 **Births:** 45 **Total Expense ($000):** 8321 **Personnel:** 118

TWIN FALLS—Twin Falls County

🞸 **ST. LUKE'S MAGIC VALLEY REGIONAL MEDICAL CENTER (130002)**, 650 Addison Avenue West, Zip 83301–5444, Mailing Address: P.O. Box 409, Zip 83303–0409; tel. 208/737–2000 **A**1 2 9 10 19 20 **F**3 4 5 7 11 13 15 18 20 24 25 26 27 31 32 33 34 35 37 38 42 44 48 49 51 55 56 57 59 61 62 66 68 71 72 73 74 75 76 77 79 80 84 85 87 88 89 90 91 92 93 94 96 97 100 102 103 105 107 118 119 124 136 137 **P**4 5 7 **S** St. Luke's Health System
Primary Contact: Mark Schwartz, Chief Executive Officer
COO: Kent Loosle, Chief Operating Officer
CFO: John Groesbeck, Chief Financial Officer
CIO: R'Nee Mullen, Chief Information Officer
Web address: www.mvrmc.org
Control: Other not–for–profit (including NFP Corporation) **Service:** General Medical and Surgical

Staffed Beds: 191 **Admissions:** 10061 **Census:** 111 **Outpatient Visits:** 148446 **Births:** 1707 **Total Expense ($000):** 152681 **Payroll Expense ($000):** 58753 **Personnel:** 1037

WEISER—Washington County

★ **WEISER MEMORIAL HOSPITAL (131307)**, 645 East Fifth Street, Zip 83672–2202; tel. 208/549–0370 **A**9 10 18 **F**3 11 13 26 38 55 56 57 62 74 77 79 96 107 120 121 122 124 135 137
Primary Contact: Wade Johnson, Chief Executive Officer
CFO: Tom Murphy, Chief Financial Officer
CMO: Lore Wooton, M.D., Chief of Staff
CHR: Terri Kautz, Manager Human Resources
Web address: www.weisermemorialhospital.org
Control: Hospital district or authority, Government, nonfederal **Service:** General Medical and Surgical

Staffed Beds: 25 **Admissions:** 408 **Census:** 3 **Outpatient Visits:** 12061 **Births:** 82 **Total Expense ($000):** 7616 **Payroll Expense ($000):** 2965 **Personnel:** 71

ID

Hospital, Medicare Provider Number, Address, Telephone, Approval, Facility, and Physician Codes, Health Care System
★ American Hospital Association (AHA) membership
□ The Joint Commission accreditation
○ American Osteopathic Association (AOA) accreditation
△ Commission on Accreditation of Rehabilitation Facilities (CARF) accreditation

ILLINOIS

ALEDO—Mercer County

★ **MERCER COUNTY HOSPITAL (141304)**, 409 N.W. Ninth Avenue, Zip 61231–1296; tel. 309/582–5301, (Total facility includes 14 beds in nursing home–type unit) **A**9 10 18 **F**11 15 25 26 31 32 33 38 54 56 57 61 62 67 77 79 82 86 87 96 106 107 117 122 136
Primary Contact: Timothy Putnam, Administrator and Chief Executive Officer
COO: Myron Higgins, Director Operations
CFO: Jodie Criswell, Chief Financial Officer
CMO: Julio Santiago, M.D., Chief of Staff
CHR: Myron Higgins, Director Operations
Web address: www.mercercountyhosp.org
Control: County–Government, nonfederal **Service:** General Medical and Surgical

Staffed Beds: 39 **Admissions:** 300 **Census:** 14 **Outpatient Visits:** 17487 **Births:** 0 **Total Expense ($000):** 10575 **Payroll Expense ($000):** 5168 **Personnel:** 107

ALTON—Madison County

⊛ **ALTON MEMORIAL HOSPITAL (140002)**, One Memorial Drive, Zip 62002–6722; tel. 618/463–7311, (Total facility includes 62 beds in nursing home–type unit) **A**1 2 9 10 **F**3 5 7 11 13 15 18 20 24 25 26 27 30 31 32 33 36 37 38 50 55 56 57 59 62 66 68 72 73 74 75 76 77 79 80 84 86 88 96 100 102 103 104 106 107 109 117 118 119 120 121 124 135 137 **P**6 7 **S** BJC HealthCare
Primary Contact: David A. Braasch, President
COO: David A. Braasch, President
CFO: Brad Goacher, Director Finance
CMO: David Burnside, M.D., Chief Medical Officer
CIO: David Weiss, Vice President Information System
CHR: Tina Kristoff, Manager Human Resources
Web address: www.altonmemorialhospital.org
Control: Other not–for–profit (including NFP Corporation) **Service:** General Medical and Surgical

Staffed Beds: 240 **Admissions:** 6504 **Census:** 145 **Outpatient Visits:** 72686 **Births:** 562 **Total Expense ($000):** 100029 **Payroll Expense ($000):** 36184 **Personnel:** 755

☐ **ALTON MENTAL HEALTH CENTER (144016)**, 4500 College Avenue, Zip 62002–5099; tel. 618/474–3800, (Nonreporting) **A**1 10
Primary Contact: Kay Greenwood, RN, M.S., Administrator
CFO: Susan Shobe, Director Administration and Support Services
CMO: Claudia Kachigion, M.D., Medical Director
Control: State–Government, nonfederal **Service:** Psychiatric

Staffed Beds: 165

⊛ △ **SAINT ANTHONY'S HEALTH CENTER (140052)**, 1 Saint Anthony's Way, Zip 62002–4579, Mailing Address: P.O. Box 340, Zip 62002–0340; tel. 618/465–2571, (Includes SAINT CLARE'S HOSPITAL, 915 East Fifth Street, Zip 62002–6434; tel. 618/463–5151), (Total facility includes 38 beds in nursing home–type unit) **A**1 2 7 9 10 **F**2 3 6 8 10 11 13 14 15 18 20 24 25 26 27 28 30 31 32 33 34 36 37 38 42 43 44 50 51 53 54 55 56 57 59 60 61 62 64 65 66 68 72 73 74 75 76 77 79 80 81 84 85 86 87 90 91 92 93 94 95 96 97 100 102 104 105 106 107 109 112 117 118 119 120 121 124 134 135 136 137 **P**8 **S** Hospital Sisters Health System
Primary Contact: Mark F. Weber, FACHE, President
COO: E. J. Kuiper, Executive Vice President and Chief Operating Officer
CFO: Mike Nelson, Executive Vice President and Chief Financial Officer
CMO: Larry Reed, M.D., Medical Director
CIO: Noncy J. Dooling, Vice President Finance
CHR: William D. Baiocchi, Senior Vice President
Web address: www.sahc.org
Control: Other not–for–profit (including NFP Corporation) **Service:** General Medical and Surgical

Staffed Beds: 229 **Admissions:** 5369 **Census:** 87 **Outpatient Visits:** 137084 **Births:** 572 **Total Expense ($000):** 89533 **Payroll Expense ($000):** 32943 **Personnel:** 762

ANNA—Union County

☐ **CHOATE MENTAL HEALTH CENTER (144038)**, 1000 North Main Street, Zip 62906–1699; tel. 618/833–5161 **A**1 5 10 **F**25 26 30 31 32 37 82 88 89 90 91 92 93 119 **P**6
Primary Contact: Sarah H. Andrew, Ph.D., Administrator
COO: Sarah H. Andrew, Ph.D., Administrator
CMO: J. S R Van, M.D., Medical Director
CIO: Cindy Flamm, Manager Quality
CHR: Aaron Phelps, Director Human Resources
Control: State–Government, nonfederal **Service:** Psychiatric

Staffed Beds: 79 **Admissions:** 561 **Census:** 66 **Outpatient Visits:** 0 **Births:** 0 **Personnel:** 160

⊛ **UNION COUNTY HOSPITAL (141342)**, 517 North Main Street, Zip 62906–1696; tel. 618/833–4511, (Total facility includes 22 beds in nursing home–type unit) **A**1 9 10 18 **F**3 11 15 24 25 26 30 31 32 33 38 50 55 56 57 61 62 65 66 73 75 79 80 82 84 86 87 96 102 107 119 122 135 **P**6 **S** Community Health Systems, Inc.
Primary Contact: James R. Farris, CHE, Chief Executive Officer
COO: Jeanette Hook, Chief Nursing Officer
CFO: Terry Paligo, Chief Financial Officer
CMO: Brian J. Reach, M.D., Chief of Staff
CIO: Bill Hinchcliff, Director Information Systems
CHR: Tammy Samuels, Director Human Resources
Web address: www.unioncountyhospital.com
Control: Corporation, Investor–owned, for–profit **Service:** General Medical and Surgical

Staffed Beds: 47 **Admissions:** 1147 **Census:** 29 **Outpatient Visits:** 24044 **Births:** 0 **Total Expense ($000):** 12779 **Payroll Expense ($000):** 6354 **Personnel:** 167

ARLINGTON HEIGHTS—Cook County

⊛ **NORTHWEST COMMUNITY HOSPITAL (140252)**, (Formerly Northwest Community Healthcare), 800 West Central Road, Zip 60005–2392; tel. 847/618–1000 **A**1 2 9 10 **F**2 3 4 5 13 15 17 18 20 22 24 25 26 27 28 30 31 32 36 38 40 41 46 47 49 50 53 54 55 56 57 58 59 61 62 63 66 68 71 72 73 74 75 76 77 79 80 81 82 84 86 88 89 90 91 92 93 94 95 96 97 99 100 102 103 104 105 106 107 108 109 111 116 118 119 120 121 124 132 134 135 136 137 **P**5 8
Primary Contact: Bruce K. Crowther, President and Chief Executive Officer
COO: Michael B. Zenn, Executive Vice President and Chief Operating Officer
CFO: Gail Finn, Vice President Finance and Chief Financial Officer
CMO: Leighton B. Smith, M.D., Vice President Medical Affairs
CIO: George Morris, Vice President Information Technology and Chief Information Officer
CHR: Mark Lusson, Vice President Human Resources
Web address: www.nch.org
Control: Other not–for–profit (including NFP Corporation) **Service:** General Medical and Surgical

Staffed Beds: 441 **Admissions:** 25158 **Census:** 276 **Outpatient Visits:** 551588 **Births:** 3246 **Total Expense ($000):** 401673 **Payroll Expense ($000):** 171695 **Personnel:** 2782

AURORA—Du Page and Kane Counties County

⊛ **PROVENA MERCY MEDICAL CENTER (140174)**, 1325 North Highland Avenue, Zip 60506–1449; tel. 630/859–2222 **A**1 2 9 10 **F**3 5 11 12 13 15 18 20 22 24 25 26 27 30 31 32 33 36 38 40 43 46 49 54 55 56 57 60 63 66 68 71 73 74 75 76 77 79 80 81 82 84 86 87 88 89 90 91 92 93 94 95 96 100 102 103 107 119 121 124 133 135 136 **P**5 **S** Provena Health
Primary Contact: William A. Brown, FACHE, President and Chief Executive Officer
COO: Mary Mong, R.N., Chief Operating Officer
CFO: Paul E. Belter, Vice President Finance and Chief Financial Officer
CMO: Daniel Hatcher, M.D., Vice President Medical Affairs
CHR: Diane Hargreaves, Vice President Human Resources
Web address: www.provenamercy.com
Control: Other not–for–profit (including NFP Corporation) **Service:** General Medical and Surgical

Staffed Beds: 261 **Admissions:** 10532 **Census:** 124 **Outpatient Visits:** 197360 **Births:** 1178 **Total Expense ($000):** 147762 **Payroll Expense ($000):** 50378 **Personnel:** 925

⊛ △ **RUSH–COPLEY MEDICAL CENTER (140029)**, 2000 Ogden Avenue, Zip 60504–4206; tel. 630/978–6200 **A**1 2 3 5 7 9 10 **F**3 9 13 15 17 18 20 22 24 25 26 27 28 29 30 31 32 33 34 36 37 38 40 41 43 44 46 47 49 50 52 53 54 55 56 57 58 59 61 62 63 64 66 68 70 71 72 73 74 75 76 77 79 80 81 82 84 85 86 87 96 97 100 102 103 105 106 107 109 111 112 113 114 119 120 121 123 124 132 133 134 135 136 137 **P**6 **S** Rush University Medical Center
Primary Contact: Barry C. Finn, President and Chief Executive Officer
COO: John A. Diederich, Senior Vice President Operations and Chief Operating Officer
CFO: Macario Salazar, Senior Vice President Finance and Chief Financial Officer
CMO: Steve B. Lowenthal, M.D., M.P.H., FACS, Senior Vice President Medical Affairs and Chief Medical Officer
CIO: Dennis DeMasie, Vice President Information Systems and Chief Information Officer
CHR: Darla Mullner, Director Human Resources
Web address: www.rushcopley.com
Control: Other not–for–profit (including NFP Corporation) **Service:** General Medical and Surgical

Staffed Beds: 157 **Admissions:** 13972 **Census:** 118 **Outpatient Visits:** 170101 **Births:** 3795 **Total Expense ($000):** 189287 **Payroll Expense ($000):** 70258 **Personnel:** 1254

Many Facility Codes have changed. Please refer to the AHA Guide Code Chart.

BARRINGTON—Lake County

▣ **ADVOCATE GOOD SHEPHERD HOSPITAL (140291)**, 450 West Highway 22, Zip 60010–1901; tel. 847/381–0123, (Nonreporting) **A**1 2 9 10 **S** Advocate Health Care
Primary Contact: Karen A. Lambert, President
COO: Doug Ryder, Vice President Operations
CFO: George Teufel, Vice President Finance
CMO: Barry Rosen, M.D., Vice President Medical Management
CIO: Wolfgang Anderle, Chief Information Officer
CHR: Christine Kass, Vice President Human Resources
Web address: www.advocatehealth.com
Control: Church–operated, Nongovernment, not–for profit **Service:** General Medical and Surgical

Staffed Beds: 142

BELLEVILLE—St. Clair County

★ ○ **MEMORIAL HOSPITAL (140185)**, 4500 Memorial Drive, Zip 62226–5399; tel. 618/233–7750, (Total facility includes 96 beds in nursing home–type unit) **A**9 10 11 **F**2 3 11 13 15 18 20 22 24 25 26 27 31 32 37 38 41 43 44 46 49 51 52 53 55 56 57 59 60 61 62 68 72 73 74 75 77 79 80 81 82 84 86 90 94 96 97 99 100 103 106 107 117 118 119 120 121 124 134 135 136 137 **P**8
Primary Contact: Mark J. Turner, President and Chief Executive Officer
CFO: Joe Lanius, Vice President Finance
CMO: William Casperson, M.D., Vice President Medical Affairs
CIO: Jennifer Meinkoth, Director Information Systems
CHR: Ed French, Vice President
Web address: www.memhosp.com
Control: Other not–for–profit (including NFP Corporation) **Service:** General Medical and Surgical

Staffed Beds: 378 **Admissions:** 16161 **Census:** 232 **Outpatient Visits:** 308286 **Births:** 1600 **Total Expense ($000):** 190335 **Payroll Expense ($000):** 83761 **Personnel:** 1802

▣ ○ △ **ST. ELIZABETH'S HOSPITAL (140187)**, 211 South Third Street, Zip 62220–1998; tel. 618/234–2120 **A**1 3 5 7 9 10 11 **F**3 4 5 11 13 15 17 18 20 22 24 25 26 27 28 30 31 32 33 37 38 43 44 46 49 50 52 53 54 55 57 59 60 61 62 63 66 68 72 73 74 75 76 77 79 80 81 82 85 86 87 88 90 91 92 93 94 95 96 97 100 103 104 105 106 107 109 112 118 119 120 121 123 124 133 135 136 137 **P**8 **S** Hospital Sisters Health System
Primary Contact: Kevin Shrake, Interim President and Chief Executive Officer
COO: Jean M. Jensen, Interim Chief Operating Officer
CFO: Daniel D. Powell, Interim Assistant Administrator Finance
CMO: Salil Gupta, M.D., Medical Director
CIO: Illa David, Director Information Technology
CHR: Margaret Luna, Director Human Resources
Web address: www.steliz.org
Control: Church–operated, Nongovernment, not–for profit **Service:** General Medical and Surgical

Staffed Beds: 260 **Admissions:** 14026 **Census:** 173 **Outpatient Visits:** 281459 **Births:** 1230 **Total Expense ($000):** 173488 **Payroll Expense ($000):** 59753 **Personnel:** 1391

BELVIDERE—Boone County

□ **NORTHWEST SUBURBAN COMMUNITY HOSPITAL (140205)**, 1625 South State Street, Zip 61008–5900; tel. 815/547–5441, (Nonreporting) **A**1 9 10
Primary Contact: David Schuetz, President and Chief Executive Officer
Control: Other not–for–profit (including NFP Corporation) **Service:** General Medical and Surgical

Staffed Beds: 69

BENTON—Franklin County

★ **FRANKLIN HOSPITAL (141321)**, 201 Bailey Lane, Zip 62812–1999; tel. 618/439–3161 **A**10 18 **F**11 15 25 26 31 32 33 38 54 55 56 57 64 73 75 79 86 87 96 107 121 122 133 **P**6 **S** Alliant Management Services
Primary Contact: Hervey E. Davis, Chief Executive Officer
COO: Frank T. Caruso, Chief Operating Officer
CFO: Frank T. Caruso, Chief Operating Officer
CMO: Julia Bancroft, D.O., Chief Medical Staff
CIO: David Williams, Director Information Technology
CHR: Nancy Seibert, Director Human Resources
Web address: www.franklinhospital.net
Control: Hospital district or authority, Government, nonfederal **Service:** General Medical and Surgical

Staffed Beds: 25 **Admissions:** 587 **Census:** 5 **Outpatient Visits:** 23042 **Births:** 0 **Total Expense ($000):** 12792 **Payroll Expense ($000):** 5816 **Personnel:** 160

BERWYN—Cook County

▣ **MACNEAL HOSPITAL (140054)**, 3249 South Oak Park Avenue, Zip 60402–0715; tel. 708/783–9100, (Nonreporting) **A**1 2 3 5 8 9 10 12 13 **S** Vanguard Health System
Primary Contact: Brian J. Lemon, Chief Executive Officer
COO: J. Scott Steiner, Chief Operating Officer
CFO: Mary E. Cleary, Interim Chief Financial Officer
CMO: Charles Bareis, M.D., Medical Director
CIO: Thomas Crawford, Market Chief Information Officer
CHR: John Zubiena, Director Human Resources
Web address: www.macneal.com
Control: Corporation, Investor–owned, for–profit **Service:** General Medical and Surgical

Staffed Beds: 240

BLOOMINGTON—McLean County

▣ **OSF ST. JOSEPH MEDICAL CENTER (140162)**, 2200 East Washington Street, Zip 61701–4323; tel. 309/662–3311, (Total facility includes 12 beds in nursing home–type unit) **A**1 2 9 10 **F**3 11 13 15 18 20 22 24 25 26 27 30 31 32 33 35 38 39 40 44 53 55 56 57 59 60 62 63 64 66 68 72 73 74 75 76 77 79 80 81 82 84 86 87 96 97 100 102 103 106 107 117 119 120 121 124 133 135 136 137 **P**6 **S** OSF Healthcare System
Primary Contact: Kenneth J. Natzke, President and Chief Executive Officer
COO: Lawrence E. Wills, Vice President Operations
CFO: John R. Zell, Chief Financial Officer
CMO: Paul E. Pedersen, M.D., Vice President and Chief Medical Officer
CHR: Sue Herriott, Director
Web address: www.osfstjoseph.org
Control: Church–operated, Nongovernment, not–for profit **Service:** General Medical and Surgical

Staffed Beds: 157 **Admissions:** 6430 **Census:** 68 **Outpatient Visits:** 278803 **Births:** 780 **Total Expense ($000):** 116338 **Payroll Expense ($000):** 43195 **Personnel:** 795

BLUE ISLAND—Cook County

▣ **ST. FRANCIS HOSPITAL & HEALTH CENTER (140118)**, 12935 South Gregory Street, Zip 60406–2470; tel. 708/597–2000 **A**1 9 10 **F**3 11 13 15 18 20 22 24 25 26 27 30 32 33 38 43 46 47 48 49 50 52 55 56 57 58 60 62 66 68 71 72 73 74 75 76 77 79 80 81 84 86 90 96 97 100 102 106 107 118 119 121 124 135 136 137 **P**5 **S** SSM Health Care
Primary Contact: Colleen Kannaday, FACHE, President
COO: David Cemate, Executive Vice President and Chief Operating Officer
CFO: David Nelson, Vice President Finance and Chief Financial Officer
CHR: Cheryl Burenski–Champoux, Vice President Human Resource Management and Development
Web address: www.stfrancisblueisland.com
Control: Church–operated, Nongovernment, not–for profit **Service:** General Medical and Surgical

Staffed Beds: 282 **Admissions:** 13572 **Census:** 164 **Outpatient Visits:** 98367 **Births:** 1272 **Total Expense ($000):** 157125 **Payroll Expense ($000):** 63975 **Personnel:** 1104

BREESE—Clinton County

▣ **ST. JOSEPH'S HOSPITAL (140145)**, 9515 Holy Cross Lane, Zip 62230–0099; tel. 618/526–4511 **A**1 9 10 **F**3 11 13 15 24 25 26 28 30 31 32 33 38 40 41 50 52 54 55 56 57 62 66 68 71 73 74 77 79 80 84 86 93 94 95 96 97 103 106 107 118 119 120 121 123 124 135 **S** Hospital Sisters Health System
Primary Contact: Lowell Jones, Interim Administrator
CFO: Dennis G. Herzig, Chief Financial Officer
CIO: Dennis G. Herzig, Chief Financial Officer
CHR: Kathryn Mines, Director Human Resources
Web address: www.stjoebreese.com
Control: Church–operated, Nongovernment, not–for profit **Service:** General Medical and Surgical

Staffed Beds: 60 **Admissions:** 2087 **Census:** 20 **Outpatient Visits:** 85077 **Births:** 511 **Total Expense ($000):** 32425 **Payroll Expense ($000):** 13194

Hospital, Medicare Provider Number, Address, Telephone, Approval, Facility, and Physician Codes, Health Care System

★ American Hospital Association (AHA) membership
□ The Joint Commission accreditation
○ American Osteopathic Association (AOA) accreditation
△ Commission on Accreditation of Rehabilitation Facilities (CARF) accreditation

CANTON—Fulton County

☒ **GRAHAM HOSPITAL (140001)**, 210 West Walnut Street, Zip 61520–2497; tel. 309/647–5240, (Total facility includes 54 beds in nursing home–type unit) **A**1 6 9 10 20 **F**3 11 13 15 24 25 26 28 30 31 32 33 34 38 42 51 52 53 54 55 56 57 61 62 63 65 66 68 69 73 74 75 77 79 80 82 84 86 87 96 97 99 100 103 107 112 117 118 119 120 121 124 132 135 **P**3
Primary Contact: Robert G. Senneff, FACHE, President and Chief Executive Officer
CFO: Jim Stratton, Vice President Finance
CHR: Chris Duvendack, Vice President Clinic Operations and Medical Staff Affairs
Web address: www.grahamhospital.org
Control: Other not–for–profit (including NFP Corporation) **Service:** General Medical and Surgical

Staffed Beds: 105 **Admissions:** 3399 **Census:** 74 **Outpatient Visits:** 200202 **Births:** 297 **Total Expense ($000):** 59204 **Payroll Expense ($000):** 21151 **Personnel:** 662

CARBONDALE—Jackson County

☐ **MEMORIAL HOSPITAL OF CARBONDALE (140164)**, 405 West Jackson Street, Zip 62901–1467, Mailing Address: P.O. Box 10000, Zip 62902–9000; tel. 618/549–0721 **A**1 2 3 5 9 10 12 13 19 **F**3 11 13 15 18 20 22 24 25 26 27 30 31 32 33 38 48 49 50 55 56 57 62 66 68 70 72 73 74 76 77 79 80 81 82 84 96 97 100 102 103 106 107 108 109 119 120 121 124 134 135 136 **S** Southern Illinois Hospital Services
Primary Contact: George Maroney, Senior Vice President and Administrator
CFO: Rex P. Budde, Senior Vice President and Chief Financial Officer
CIO: Frank Sears, Vice President Information Services
Web address: www.sih.net
Control: Other not–for–profit (including NFP Corporation) **Service:** General Medical and Surgical

Staffed Beds: 142 **Admissions:** 8710 **Census:** 89 **Outpatient Visits:** 104759 **Births:** 1960 **Total Expense ($000):** 149667 **Payroll Expense ($000):** 42614 **Personnel:** 1016

CARLINVILLE—Macoupin County

★ **CARLINVILLE AREA HOSPITAL (141347)**, 1001 East Morgan Street, Zip 62626–1499; tel. 217/854–3141 **A**9 10 18 **F**11 15 24 25 33 38 62 75 79 86 96 118 122 133 **S** Brim Healthcare, Inc.
Primary Contact: Kenneth G. Reid, President and Chief Executive Officer
CFO: Greg Ward, Vice President and Chief Financial Officer
CMO: Julie Fleischer, M.D., President Medical Staff
CIO: Jerod Cottingham, Director Information Systems
CHR: Tracy Koster, Director Human Resources
Web address: www.cahcare.com
Control: Other not–for–profit (including NFP Corporation) **Service:** General Medical and Surgical

Staffed Beds: 25 **Admissions:** 609 **Census:** 10 **Outpatient Visits:** 21128 **Births:** 0 **Total Expense ($000):** 10584 **Payroll Expense ($000):** 4329 **Personnel:** 102

CARROLLTON—Greene County

THOMAS H. BOYD MEMORIAL HOSPITAL (141300), 800 School Street, Zip 62016–1498; tel. 217/942–6946, (Includes REISCH MEMORIAL NURSING HOME), (Total facility includes 40 beds in nursing home–type unit) (Nonreporting) **A**9 10 18
Primary Contact: Deborah Campbell, Administrator
CFO: Howard Schou, Chief Financial Officer
CHR: Lisa Eldridge, Human Resources Officer
Control: Other not–for–profit (including NFP Corporation) **Service:** General Medical and Surgical

Staffed Beds: 65

CARTHAGE—Hancock County

☐ **MEMORIAL HOSPITAL (141305)**, 402 South Adams Street, Zip 62321–1600, Mailing Address: P.O. Box 160, Zip 62321–0160; tel. 217/357–3131 **A**1 9 10 18 **F**11 13 15 24 25 26 27 30 31 32 43 55 56 62 73 74 78 79 96 97 107 118 119 121 122 135
Primary Contact: Ada Bair, Chief Executive Officer
CFO: Teresa Smith, Chief Financial Officer
CIO: Syndi Horn, Director Information Systems
CHR: Ann Dunham, Director Human Resources
Web address: www.mhtlc.org
Control: Other not–for–profit (including NFP Corporation) **Service:** General Medical and Surgical

Staffed Beds: 15 **Admissions:** 670 **Census:** 9 **Outpatient Visits:** 15011 **Births:** 98 **Total Expense ($000):** 14339 **Payroll Expense ($000):** 6989 **Personnel:** 146

CENTRALIA—Marion County

☒ **ST. MARY'S HOSPITAL (140034)**, 400 North Pleasant Avenue, Zip 62801–3091; tel. 618/436–8000 **A**1 2 9 10 19 **F**3 5 11 13 15 18 20 24 25 26 27 30 31 32 33 36 38 41 43 44 46 50 55 56 57 62 66 68 71 72 73 74 75 76 77 79 80 81 82 84 86 88 90 91 92 93 94 95 96 97 100 102 106 107 109 111 118 119 120 121 124 134 135 136 137 **P**8 **S** SSM Health Care
Primary Contact: Bruce Merrell, FACHE, President
CFO: Kay Tinsley, Vice President Finance
CIO: Ralph Caudill, Director Information Systems
Web address: www.smgsi.com
Control: Church–operated, Nongovernment, not–for profit **Service:** General Medical and Surgical

Staffed Beds: 114 **Admissions:** 7266 **Census:** 77 **Outpatient Visits:** 126790 **Births:** 397 **Total Expense ($000):** 81536 **Payroll Expense ($000):** 30456 **Personnel:** 765

CHAMPAIGN—Champaign County

☐ **THE PAVILION (144029)**, 809 West Church Street, Zip 61820–3399; tel. 217/373–1700, (Nonreporting) **A**1 9 10 **S** Universal Health Services, Inc.
Primary Contact: Joseph Sheehy, Chief Executive Officer and Managing Director
CFO: Edith Frasca, Controller and Chief Financial Officer
Web address: www.info@pavilionhospital.com
Control: Corporation, Investor–owned, for–profit **Service:** Psychiatric

Staffed Beds: 46

CHESTER—Randolph County

☐ **CHESTER MENTAL HEALTH CENTER**, Chester Road, Zip 62233–0031, Mailing Address: Box 31, Zip 62233–0031; tel. 618/826–4571 **A**1 3 5 **F**25 26 37 81 88 119
Primary Contact: Brian E. Thomas, Administrator
Control: State–Government, nonfederal **Service:** Psychiatric

Staffed Beds: 302 **Admissions:** 197 **Census:** 286 **Outpatient Visits:** 0 **Births:** 0 **Total Expense ($000):** 36021 **Payroll Expense ($000):** 27404 **Personnel:** 496

☐ **MEMORIAL HOSPITAL (141338)**, 1900 State Street, Zip 62233–0609, Mailing Address: P.O. Box 609, Zip 62233–0609; tel. 618/826–4581 **A**1 9 10 18 **F**3 5 8 11 15 27 31 32 38 55 56 57 62 67 68 72 73 76 77 79 80 86 94 96 97 102 107 118 119 121 122 124 134 135
Primary Contact: Eric Freeburg, Administrator
CFO: Gail Miesner, Chief Financial Officer
CMO: Alan Liefer, M.D., President Medical Staff
CIO: Becky Bunselmeyer, Director Information Services
CHR: May Rose, Director Human Resources
Web address: www.mhchester.com
Control: Hospital district or authority, Government, nonfederal **Service:** General Medical and Surgical

Staffed Beds: 25 **Admissions:** 1252 **Census:** 12 **Outpatient Visits:** 33714 **Births:** 0 **Total Expense ($000):** 16997 **Payroll Expense ($000):** 7266 **Personnel:** 202

CHICAGO—Cook County

☒ **ADVOCATE BETHANY HOSPITAL (142012)**, 3435 West Van Buren Street, Zip 60624–3399; tel. 773/265–7700 **A**1 9 10 **F**1 11 15 25 26 27 30 31 32 33 38 53 55 56 57 66 68 75 76 79 82 86 96 99 102 107 119 137 **S** Advocate Health Care
Primary Contact: Lena Dobbs–Johnson, President
CFO: James Riggio, Vice President Finance
CMO: Joseph Rosman, M.D., Chief Medical Director
CIO: Linda Peterson, Director Information Systems
CHR: Menai Edwards, Manager Human Resources
Web address: www.advocatehealth.com
Control: Other not–for–profit (including NFP Corporation) **Service:** Long–Term Acute Care hospital

Staffed Beds: 54 **Admissions:** 459 **Census:** 40 **Outpatient Visits:** 5178 **Births:** 0 **Total Expense ($000):** 44595 **Payroll Expense ($000):** 15911 **Personnel:** 251

☒ △ **ADVOCATE ILLINOIS MASONIC MEDICAL CENTER (140182)**, 836 West Wellington Avenue, Zip 60657–5193; tel. 773/975–1600 **A**1 2 3 5 7 8 9 10 12 13 **F**3 5 13 14 15 17 18 20 22 24 25 26 27 28 29 30 31 32 33 34 36 37 38 40 41 42 43 44 49 50 52 53 54 55 56 57 58 59 60 61 62 64 66 68 69 70 71 72 73 74 75 76 77 79 80 81 82 83 84 85 86 87 88 89 90 91 92 93 94 95 96 99 100 102 106 107 109 111 113 114 116 119 121 123 124 132 135 136 **P**6 8 **S** Advocate Health Care
Primary Contact: Susan Nordstrom Lopez, President
CFO: Jack Gilbert, Vice President Finance
CMO: Robert Zadylak, M.D., Vice President Medical Management
CIO: Ann Malinowski, Director Information Systems
CHR: Marc Senesac, Vice President Human Resources
Web address: www.advocatehealth.com
Control: Other not–for–profit (including NFP Corporation) **Service:** General Medical and Surgical

Staffed Beds: 348 **Admissions:** 18229 **Census:** 248 **Outpatient Visits:** 145427 **Births:** 2926 **Total Expense ($000):** 296960 **Payroll Expense ($000):** 121380 **Personnel:** 2345

IL

☒ **ADVOCATE TRINITY HOSPITAL (140048)**, 2320 East 93rd Street, Zip 60617–9984; tel. 773/967–2000, (Nonreporting) **A**1 9 10 **S** Advocate Health Care
Primary Contact: Jonathan R. Bruss, Interim Administrator
CFO: Maureen Morrison, Vice President Financial Services
CMO: Michael Davenport, Vice President Medical Management
CIO: Tracy C. Owens, Director Communications and Government Relations
CHR: Narin Trent, Vice President Human Resources
Web address: www.advocatehealth.com/trinity
Control: Church–operated, Nongovernment, not–for profit **Service:** General Medical and Surgical

Staffed Beds: 195

☐ **AURORA CHICAGO LAKESHORE HOSPITAL (144005)**, (Formerly Chicago Lakeshore Hospital), 4840 North Marine Drive, Zip 60640–4296; tel. 773/878–9700 **A**1 3 5 9 10 **F**5 31 32 88 89 94 95 119 121 **S** Aurora Behavioral Health Care
Primary Contact: C. Alan Eaks, Chief Executive Officer
COO: Pam Mazzini, Director Clinical Services
CFO: Carol Peart, Chief Financial Officer
CMO: Peter Nierman, M.D., Chief Medical Officer
CHR: Johanne Jeanty, Director Human Resources
Web address: www.chicagolakeshorehospital.com
Control: Corporation, Investor–owned, for–profit **Service:** Psychiatric

Staffed Beds: 108 **Admissions:** 3001 **Census:** 78 **Outpatient Visits:** 7102 **Births:** 0 **Personnel:** 157

BERNARD MITCHELL HOSPITAL See University of Chicago Medical Center

CHICAGO LYING–IN HOSPITAL See University of Chicago Medical Center

☐ **CHICAGO–READ MENTAL HEALTH CENTER (144010)**, 4200 North Oak Park Avenue, Zip 60634–1457; tel. 773/794–4000, (Nonreporting) **A**1 10
Primary Contact: Thomas Simpatico, M.D., Facility Director and Network System Manager
Control: State–Government, nonfederal **Service:** Psychiatric

Staffed Beds: 200

☒ **CHILDREN'S MEMORIAL HOSPITAL (143300)**, 2300 Children's Plaza, Zip 60614–3394; tel. 773/880–4000 **A**1 2 3 5 8 9 10 **F**3 7 8 9 11 12 14 19 21 23 25 26 27 28 30 31 32 33 34 35 36 37 38 40 41 42 43 44 45 49 50 51 53 55 56 57 58 59 60 62 63 64 66 70 72 73 75 76 77 78 79 80 81 82 83 84 86 87 88 89 90 91 92 94 95 96 97 100 102 103 104 105 106 107 114 118 119 120 121 123 125 126 127 128 131 132 133 135 137 **P**6
Primary Contact: Patrick M. Magoon, President and Chief Executive Officer
COO: Gordon B. Bass, Chief Operating Officer
CFO: Paula Noble, Chief Financial Officer and Treasurer
CMO: Edward S. Ogata, M.D., Chief Medical Officer
CIO: Stan Krok, Chief Information Officer
CHR: Barbara Bowman, Chief Human Resource Officer
Web address: www.childrensmemorial.org
Control: Other not–for–profit (including NFP Corporation) **Service:** Children's general

Staffed Beds: 247 **Admissions:** 9549 **Census:** 181 **Outpatient Visits:** 394042 **Births:** 0 **Total Expense ($000):** 482863 **Payroll Expense ($000):** 193765 **Personnel:** 3520

☐ **HARTGROVE HOSPITAL (144026)**, 520 North Ridgeway Avenue, Zip 60624–1299; tel. 773/722–3113, (Nonreporting) **A**1 9 10 **S** Universal Health Services, Inc.
Primary Contact: Steven Airhart, Chief Executive Officer and Managing Director
CIO: Len Servidio, Director Information Management
Web address: www.uhsinc.com
Control: Corporation, Investor–owned, for–profit **Service:** Psychiatric

Staffed Beds: 128

★ ○ **HOLY CROSS HOSPITAL (140133)**, 2701 West 68th Street, Zip 60629–1882; tel. 773/884–9000, (Nonreporting) **A**9 10 11
Primary Contact: Wayne M. Lerner, XDPH, President and Chief Executive Officer
CFO: Gary Zmrhal, Vice President and Chief Financial Officer
CMO: Catherine Kallal, M.D., Chief Medical Officer
CIO: Ken Slawkowski, Interim Director Information Systems
CHR: Doris Gutierrez, Director Human Resources
Web address: www.holycrosshospital.org
Control: Other not–for–profit (including NFP Corporation) **Service:** General Medical and Surgical

Staffed Beds: 282

☐ **JACKSON PARK HOSPITAL AND MEDICAL CENTER (140177)**, 7531 Stony Island Avenue, Zip 60649–3993; tel. 773/947–7500, (Nonreporting) **A**1 9 10
Primary Contact: Merritt J. Hasbrouck, President
COO: Jay Silha, Chief Operating Officer
CFO: Nelson Vasquez, Vice President Finance
CMO: Bangalore Murthy, M.D., Director Medical Staff
CIO: Thomas Pankow, Chief Information Officer
CHR: Tracey Jones, Director Human Resources
Web address: www.jacksonparkhospital.org
Control: Other not–for–profit (including NFP Corporation) **Service:** General Medical and Surgical

Staffed Beds: 225

☒ △ **JESSE BROWN VETERANS AFFAIRS CHICAGO HEALTH CARE SYSTEM**, 820 South Damen, Zip 60612–3776; tel. 312/569–8387, (Includes VETERANS AFFAIRS CHICAGO HEALTH CARE SYSTEM, 333 East Huron Street, Zip 60611–3004; tel. 312/640–2100) **A**1 3 5 7 8 9 **F**4 17 18 20 22 24 25 26 27 33 36 37 38 40 42 43 44 45 46 47 48 49 50 51 52 53 54 55 56 57 58 59 60 61 62 63 64 66 68 72 73 75 76 77 78 79 80 81 82 85 86 87 88 90 91 92 93 94 95 96 97 100 106 107 118 119 121 124 132 133 135 136 137 **S** Department of Veterans Affairs
Primary Contact: James S. Jones, Medical Center Director
COO: Michelle Blakely, Associate Director
CFO: Raleigh Beard, Chief Fiscal Services
CMO: Wendy W. Brown, M.D., M.P.H., Chief of Staff
CIO: Howard Loewenstein, Chief Information Resource Management Services
CHR: Wayne Davis, Manager Human Resources
Web address: www.va.gov/sta/guide/home.asp
Control: Veterans Affairs, Government, federal **Service:** General Medical and Surgical

Staffed Beds: 241 **Admissions:** 6618 **Census:** 129 **Outpatient Visits:** 494750 **Births:** 0 **Personnel:** 1693

☒ **JOHN H. STROGER JR. HOSPITAL OF COOK COUNTY (140124)**, 1901 West Harrison Street, Zip 60612–3785; tel. 312/864–6000 **A**1 2 3 5 8 9 10 12 13 **F**3 5 11 13 15 16 17 18 20 22 24 25 26 27 30 31 32 33 34 36 37 38 40 43 44 45 46 47 48 49 53 58 59 60 62 63 66 68 70 72 73 74 75 76 77 79 80 81 82 83 84 86 87 89 90 91 92 93 94 96 100 102 107 113 114 118 119 121 123 124 135 136 **P**6 **S** Cook County Bureau of Health Services
Primary Contact: Johnny C. Brown, Chief Operating Officer
COO: Johnny C. Brown, Chief Operating Officer
CFO: John R. Morales, Chief Financial Officer
CMO: Bradley Langer, M.D., Interim Medical Director
CIO: Dan Howard, Chief Information Officer
CHR: Cecil Marchand, Associate Administrator and Director Administrative Staff Services
Web address: www.ccbhs.org
Control: County–Government, nonfederal **Service:** General Medical and Surgical

Staffed Beds: 460 **Admissions:** 22808 **Census:** 318 **Outpatient Visits:** 699415 **Births:** 946 **Total Expense ($000):** 364193 **Payroll Expense ($000):** 322404 **Personnel:** 4603

JOHNSTON R. BOWMAN HEALTH CENTER See Rush University Medical Center

☐ **KINDRED CHICAGO CENTRAL HOSPITAL (142009)**, 4058 West Melrose Street, Zip 60641–4797; tel. 773/736–7000, (Nonreporting) **A**1 9 10 **S** Kindred Healthcare
Primary Contact: Sandra Yule, Administrator
COO: Joanne Garcia, Chief Operating Officer
CFO: Mary Treacy Shiff, Chief Financial Officer
Web address: www.kindredhealthcare.com
Control: Corporation, Investor–owned, for–profit **Service:** Long–Term Acute Care hospital

Staffed Beds: 76

☐ **KINDRED CHICAGO LAKESHORE**, 6130 North Sheridan Road, Zip 60660; tel. 773/381–1222, (Nonreporting) **A**1
Primary Contact: Diane Otteman, Chief Executive Officer
Web address: www.kindredhealthcare.com
Control: Corporation, Investor–owned, for–profit **Service:** Other specialty

Staffed Beds: 103

☐ **KINDRED HOSPITAL CHICAGO NORTH**, 2544 West Montrose Avenue, Zip 60618–1589; tel. 773/267–2622, (Nonreporting) **A**1 **S** Kindred Healthcare
Primary Contact: Larry Foster, Chief Executive Officer
CFO: Jay Schweikart, Chief Financial Officer
Web address: www.kindredhealthcare.com
Control: Corporation, Investor–owned, for–profit **Service:** Other specialty

Staffed Beds: 164

Hospital, Medicare Provider Number, Address, Telephone, Approval, Facility, and Physician Codes, Health Care System

★ American Hospital Association (AHA) membership
☐ The Joint Commission accreditation
○ American Osteopathic Association (AOA) accreditation
△ Commission on Accreditation of Rehabilitation Facilities (CARF) accreditation

★ **LA RABIDA CHILDREN'S HOSPITAL (143301)**, East 65th Street at Lake Michigan, Zip 60649–1395; tel. 773/363–6700 **A**1 3 5 9 10 **F**3 12 24 25 26 28 33 38 43 50 55 56 57 58 62 63 73 75 77 80 81 82 84 86 87 119 121 132 133 135 137 **P**6
Primary Contact: Paula Kienberger Jaudes, M.D., President and Chief Executive Officer
COO: Brenda J. Wolf, Executive Vice President and Chief Operating Officer
CFO: Mark Renfree, Chief Financial Officer
CMO: Dilek Bishku, M.D., Vice President Medical Affairs
CIO: Timothy Diamond, Chief Information Officer
CHR: Frances Lefkow, Director Human Resources
Web address: www.larabida.org
Control: Other not–for–profit (including NFP Corporation) **Service:** Children's chronic disease

Staffed Beds: 49 **Admissions:** 1078 **Census:** 30 **Outpatient Visits:** 34705 **Births:** 0 **Total Expense ($000):** 44703 **Payroll Expense ($000):** 21211 **Personnel:** 433

□ **LINCOLN PARK HOSPITAL (140207)**, 550 Webster Avenue, Zip 60614–9980; tel. 773/883–2000, (Nonreporting) **A**1 9 10 **S** Merit Health Systems
Primary Contact: Frank G. DeLisi, III, CHE, Chief Executive Officer
COO: Jess Taylor, Chief Operating Officer
CFO: John Ansorge, Chief Financial Officer
CMO: Sukhjit Gill, M.D., President Medical Staff
CIO: Karen Gill, Director Information Systems
CHR: Gladys Abarca–Lopez, Director Human Resources
Web address: www.lincolnparkhospital.com
Control: Corporation, Investor–owned, for–profit **Service:** General Medical and Surgical

Staffed Beds: 158

□ **LORETTO HOSPITAL (140083)**, 645 South Central Avenue, Zip 60644–9987; tel. 773/626–4300, (Nonreporting) **A**1 9 10
Primary Contact: Steve C. Drucker, President and Chief Executive Officer
COO: Lee Marie Kotnour, Chief Operating Officer and Chief Nursing Officer
CFO: John Valles, Senior Vice President and Chief Financial Officer
CMO: Natu R. Patel, M.D., President Medical Staff
CIO: Eva McMiller, Director Information Systems
CHR: Ruby Isom, Associate Vice President Human Resources
Web address: www.lorettohospital.org
Control: Other not–for–profit (including NFP Corporation) **Service:** General Medical and Surgical

Staffed Beds: 172

★ **LOUIS A. WEISS MEMORIAL HOSPITAL (140082)**, 4646 North Marine Drive, Zip 60640–1501; tel. 773/878–8700, (Nonreporting) **A**1 2 3 5 9 10 **S** Vanguard Health System
Primary Contact: Frank L. Molinaro, Chief Executive Officer
COO: Marianne Araujo, R.N., FACHE, Chief Operating Officer and Chief Nursing Officer
CFO: Jeffrey L. Meigs, Chief Financial Officer
CMO: Martin Siglin, M.D., Vice President Medical Affairs
CHR: Keoni Nader, Director Human Resources
Web address: www.weisshospital.com
Control: Corporation, Investor–owned, for–profit **Service:** General Medical and Surgical

Staffed Beds: 172

★ **MERCY HOSPITAL AND MEDICAL CENTER (140158)**, 2525 South Michigan Avenue, Zip 60616–2477; tel. 312/567–2000 **A**2 3 5 9 10 **F**3 4 5 12 13 15 17 18 20 22 24 25 26 27 28 30 31 32 33 34 38 41 43 49 50 51 52 53 54 55 56 57 60 62 63 64 68 71 72 74 75 76 77 79 80 81 82 84 85 86 87 88 89 90 91 92 93 94 95 96 97 100 102 103 107 109 111 112 113 119 121 122 123 124 132 133 134 135 136 137 **P**5
Primary Contact: Sister Sheila Lyne, President and Chief Executive Officer
COO: Richard Cerceo, Executive Vice President and Chief Operating Officer
CFO: Thomas J. Garvey, Chief Financial Officer
CMO: Warren Furey, M.D., Chairman, Department of Medicine
CIO: Kevin Lane, Chief Information Officer
CHR: Nancy L. Hill–Davis, Vice President Human Resources and Risk Management
Web address: www.mercy–chicago.org
Control: Church–operated, Nongovernment, not–for profit **Service:** General Medical and Surgical

Staffed Beds: 270 **Admissions:** 14775 **Census:** 171 **Outpatient Visits:** 344967 **Births:** 3072 **Total Expense ($000):** 194352 **Payroll Expense ($000):** 77409 **Personnel:** 1446

○ **METHODIST HOSPITAL OF CHICAGO (140197)**, 5025 North Paulina Street, Zip 60640–2797; tel. 773/271–9040, (Total facility includes 17 beds in nursing home–type unit) (Nonreporting) **A**9 10 11
Primary Contact: Steven H. Friedman, Ph.D., Executive Vice President
CFO: Harold Reisler, Controller
CIO: Bernie Ziegler, Manager Information Systems
Web address: www.bethanymethodist.org
Control: Other not–for–profit (including NFP Corporation) **Service:** General Medical and Surgical

Staffed Beds: 189

□ △ **MICHAEL REESE HOSPITAL AND MEDICAL CENTER (140075)**, 2929 South Ellis Avenue, Zip 60616–3376; tel. 312/791–2000, (Nonreporting) **A**1 2 3 5 7 9 10 **S** Envision Hospital Corporation
Primary Contact: Enrique Beckmann, M.D., Ph.D., Chief Executive Officer
CMO: Glenn Beard, M.D., President Medical Staff
CIO: John Ulett, Chief Information Officer
CHR: Barbara Fideli, Director Human Resources
Web address: www.michaelreesehospital.com
Control: Corporation, Investor–owned, for–profit **Service:** General Medical and Surgical

Staffed Beds: 364

★ △ **MOUNT SINAI HOSPITAL (140018)**, California Avenue and 15th Street, Zip 60608–1610; tel. 773/542–2000 **A**1 2 3 5 7 8 9 10 12 **F**3 11 13 15 17 18 20 22 25 26 27 30 31 32 33 35 36 37 38 40 41 42 43 44 49 50 54 55 57 58 59 60 61 62 66 68 70 71 72 73 74 75 76 77 79 80 81 82 83 84 87 88 89 90 92 93 94 96 97 100 102 103 107 109 111 113 114 118 119 120 124 133 135 136 137 **P**3 **S** Sinai Health System
Primary Contact: Alan H. Channing, President and Chief Executive Officer
COO: Karen Teitelbaum, Executive Vice President and Chief Operating Officer
CFO: Charles Weis, Chief Financial Officer
CMO: Robert Parker, M.D., Chief Medical Officer
CIO: Peter Ingram, Vice President and Chief Information Officer
CHR: Andrew Wissel, Director Human Resources
Web address: www.sinai.org
Control: Other not–for–profit (including NFP Corporation) **Service:** General Medical and Surgical

Staffed Beds: 291 **Admissions:** 18468 **Census:** 221 **Outpatient Visits:** 345687 **Births:** 3794 **Total Expense ($000):** 296235 **Payroll Expense ($000):** 95413 **Personnel:** 1512

★ **NORTHWESTERN MEMORIAL HOSPITAL (140281)**, 251 East Huron Street, Zip 60611–2908; tel. 312/926–2000, (Includes NORMAN AND IDA STONE INSTITUTE OF PSYCHIATRY, 320 East Huron Street, Zip 60611; PRENTICE WOMEN'S HOSPITAL, 333 East Superior Street, Zip 60611) **A**1 2 3 5 8 9 10 **F**3 4 5 6 9 11 12 13 14 15 17 18 19 20 21 22 24 25 26 27 28 29 31 32 33 34 35 36 37 38 40 41 42 43 44 45 46 47 48 49 50 51 52 53 54 55 56 57 58 59 60 61 62 63 64 66 68 70 71 72 73 74 75 76 77 78 79 80 81 82 86 87 88 89 90 91 92 93 94 95 96 97 99 100 102 103 104 106 107 108 109 111 112 113 114 116 118 119 120 121 123 124 125 126 127 128 130 131 132 133 135 136 137 **P**5 6
Primary Contact: Dean M. Harrison, President and Chief Executive Officer
COO: Dennis Murphy, Executive Vice President and Chief Operating Officer
CFO: Pete McCanna, Senior Vice President Administration and Chief Financial Officer
CMO: Charles M. Watts, M.D., Senior Vice President Medical Affairs
CIO: Tim Zoph, Vice President Information Services
CHR: Dean Manheimer, Senior Vice President Human Resources
Web address: www.nmh.org
Control: Other not–for–profit (including NFP Corporation) **Service:** General Medical and Surgical

Staffed Beds: 787 **Admissions:** 47055 **Census:** 642 **Outpatient Visits:** 495823 **Births:** 10766 **Total Expense ($000):** 1168949 **Payroll Expense ($000):** 390414 **Personnel:** 6928

□ **NORWEGIAN AMERICAN HOSPITAL (140206)**, Mailing Address: 1044 North Francisco Avenue, Zip 60622–2794; tel. 773/292–8200, (Nonreporting) **A**1 9 10
Primary Contact: Michael J. O'Grady, Jr., President and Chief Executive Officer
CFO: William E. Groeper, Chief Financial Officer
CMO: Joseph Villalona, M.D., Medical Director
CHR: Russ Dickow, Vice President Human Resources
Web address: www.nahospital.org
Control: Other not–for–profit (including NFP Corporation) **Service:** General Medical and Surgical

Staffed Beds: 230

OUR LADY OF THE RESURRECTION MEDICAL CENTER (140251), 5645 West Addison Street, Zip 60634–4455; tel. 773/282–7000, (Total facility includes 46 beds in nursing home–type unit) (Nonreporting) **A**9 10 **S** Resurrection Health Care
Primary Contact: Ivette Estrada, Executive Vice President and Chief Executive Officer
COO: Mary Hillard, Vice President Patient Care Services
CFO: Thomas Capobianco, Senior Vice President Finance
CIO: George Chessum, Vice President Information Systems and Chief Information Officer
CHR: Aletha Ottlinger, Director Human Resources
Web address: www.reshealthcare.org
Control: Other not–for–profit (including NFP Corporation) **Service:** General Medical and Surgical

Staffed Beds: 237

PRENTICE WOMEN'S HOSPITAL See Northwestern Memorial Hospital

☒ **PROVIDENT HOSPITAL OF COOK COUNTY (140300)**, 500 East 51st Street, Zip 60615–2494; tel. 312/572–2000, (Nonreporting) **A**1 3 5 9 10 **S** Cook County Bureau of Health Services
Primary Contact: Sidney Thomas, Chief Operating Officer
COO: Michele T. Thompson, Deputy Chief Operating Officer
CFO: Barbara Patterson, Chief Financial Officer
CMO: Aaron Hamb, M.D., Chief Medical Officer
CIO: Donna Hart, Chief Information Officer
Web address: www.ccbhs.org/pages/ProvidentHospitalofCookCounty.htm
Control: County–Government, nonfederal **Service:** General Medical and Surgical

Staffed Beds: 119

☒ △ **REHABILITATION INSTITUTE OF CHICAGO (143026)**, 345 East Superior Street, Zip 60611–4496; tel. 312/238–1000 **A**1 3 5 7 9 10 **F**9 24 25 26 29 30 31 32 33 34 43 52 53 54 56 57 58 62 66 75 77 81 85 86 107 119 120 121 123 132 135 136 137 **P**6
Primary Contact: Joanne C. Smith, M.D., President and Chief Executive Officer
CFO: Ed Case, Executive Vice President and Chief Financial Officer
CMO: Elliot J. Roth, M.D., Senior Vice President and Medical Director
CIO: Tim McKula, Vice President Information Systems and Chief Information Officer
Web address: www.ric.org
Control: Other not–for–profit (including NFP Corporation) **Service:** Rehabilitation

Staffed Beds: 165 **Admissions:** 2373 **Census:** 134 **Outpatient Visits:** 93616 **Births:** 0 **Personnel:** 1150

★ ○ △ **RESURRECTION MEDICAL CENTER (140117)**, 7435 West Talcott Avenue, Zip 60631–3746; tel. 773/774–8000 **A**2 3 5 7 9 10 11 12 13 **F**3 9 11 13 15 17 18 20 22 24 25 26 27 30 31 32 33 34 37 38 42 43 44 47 49 50 52 54 55 56 57 58 59 62 63 64 68 71 72 73 74 75 76 77 79 80 81 82 84 85 86 87 96 97 100 102 104 105 106 107 108 109 111 114 116 119 120 121 124 132 135 136 **P**1 5 **S** Resurrection Health Care
Primary Contact: Sister Donna Marie Wolowicki, Executive Vice President and Chief Executive Officer
COO: James Hill, Executive Vice President
CFO: Thomas Capobianco, Executive Vice President Finance
CMO: Linda Henriksen, M.D., President Medical Staff
CIO: George Chessum, Senior Vice President Information Systems and Chief Information Officer
CHR: James P. Hill, Executive Vice President Administrative Services
Web address: www.reshealthcare.org
Control: Church–operated, Nongovernment, not–for profit **Service:** General Medical and Surgical

Staffed Beds: 406 **Admissions:** 18910 **Census:** 263 **Outpatient Visits:** 201822 **Births:** 1386 **Total Expense ($000):** 251820 **Payroll Expense ($000):** 100123 **Personnel:** 1891

★ ○ **ROSELAND COMMUNITY HOSPITAL (140068)**, 45 West 111th Street, Zip 60628–4294; tel. 773/995–3000, (Nonreporting) **A**9 10 11
Primary Contact: Ian McFadden, President and Chief Executive Officer
COO: Anthony Tedeschi, M.D., Chief Operating Officer
CFO: Maurice Washington, Director Controls and Accountability
CMO: Rogelio Cave, M.D., Medical Director
CHR: Brenda Mitchell, Director Human Resources
Web address: www.roselandcommunityhospital.org
Control: Other not–for–profit (including NFP Corporation) **Service:** General Medical and Surgical

Staffed Beds: 100

☒ △ **RUSH UNIVERSITY MEDICAL CENTER (140119)**, 1653 West Congress Parkway, Zip 60612–3833; tel. 312/942–5000, (Includes JOHNSTON R. BOWMAN HEALTH CENTER, 700 South Paulina, Zip 60612; tel. 312/942–7000) **A**1 2 3 5 7 8 9 10 **F**3 6 8 9 11 12 13 14 15 17 18 19 20 21 22 23 25 26 27 28 33 34 36 37 38 40 41 42 43 44 46 47 48 49 50 51 54 55 56 57 58 59 60 62 63 64 66 68 70 71 72 73 74 75 76 77 78 79 80 81 82 83 84 85 86 87 88 89 90 91 92 93 94 95 96 97 100 102 103 104 106 107 109 111 112 113 114 115 116 118 119 120 121 123 124 125 126 127 128 130 131 134 135 136 137 **P**8 **S** Rush University Medical Center
Primary Contact: Larry J. Goodman, M.D., President and Chief Executive Officer
COO: Peter W. Butler, Executive Vice President and Chief Operating Officer
CFO: Catherine A. Jacobson, Senior Vice President Finance
CMO: David A. Ansell, M.D., Vice President and Chief Medical Officer
CIO: Lac Tran, Senior Vice President Information Services
CHR: Sheri Marker, Vice President Human Resources
Web address: www.rush.edu
Control: Other not–for–profit (including NFP Corporation) **Service:** General Medical and Surgical

Staffed Beds: 676 **Admissions:** 30012 **Census:** 465 **Outpatient Visits:** 364203 **Births:** 2149 **Total Expense ($000):** 708742 **Payroll Expense ($000):** 246404 **Personnel:** 6752

○ **SACRED HEART HOSPITAL (140151)**, 3240 West Franklin Boulevard, Zip 60624–1599; tel. 773/722–3020, (Nonreporting) **A**9 10 11
Primary Contact: Edward Novak, President and Chief Executive Officer
CFO: Roy Payawal, Executive Vice President Finance
Control: Corporation, Investor–owned, for–profit **Service:** General Medical and Surgical

Staffed Beds: 96

☒ **SAINT ANTHONY HOSPITAL (140095)**, 2875 West 19th Street, Zip 60623–3596; tel. 773/484–1000 **A**1 3 5 9 10 **F**3 13 15 25 26 27 28 32 33 38 50 54 55 56 57 62 66 68 72 74 76 77 79 82 84 86 87 88 94 95 96 97 100 103 107 119 120 121 122 124 132 135 **P**4 **S** Ascension Health
Primary Contact: Guy Medaglia, President and Chief Executive Officer
COO: Gwenn A. Rausch, Chief Operating Officer
CFO: Charles R. Brobst, Chief Financial Officer
CMO: Rolando Lara, M.D., Medical Director
CIO: Ray Gonzalez, Director Information Systems
CHR: Margaret Loisel, Vice President
Web address: www.saintanthonyhospital.org
Control: Church–operated, Nongovernment, not–for profit **Service:** General Medical and Surgical

Staffed Beds: 151 **Admissions:** 7149 **Census:** 91 **Outpatient Visits:** 120110 **Births:** 2088

★ ○ **SAINT JOSEPH HOSPITAL (140224)**, 2900 North Lake Shore Drive, Zip 60657–6274; tel. 773/665–3000, (Total facility includes 26 beds in nursing home–type unit) **A**2 3 5 9 10 11 **F**3 4 5 11 13 15 17 18 20 22 24 25 26 27 28 29 30 31 32 33 34 37 38 43 44 46 49 50 52 53 54 55 56 57 58 59 60 61 62 63 64 66 68 70 72 73 74 75 76 77 79 80 81 82 84 85 86 87 88 90 91 92 93 94 96 97 100 102 105 107 109 112 117 119 120 121 124 134 135 136 137 **P**6 8 **S** Resurrection Health Care
Primary Contact: Ronald E. Struxness, Chief Executive Officer
CFO: Donna Pareti, Controller
CMO: Jack Lyons, M.D., President Medical Staff
CIO: George Chessum, Senior Vice President Information Systems and Chief Information Officer
CHR: Denise Brown, Vice President Human Resources
Web address: www.reshealth.org
Control: Church–operated, Nongovernment, not–for profit **Service:** General Medical and Surgical

Staffed Beds: 347 **Admissions:** 15317 **Census:** 224 **Outpatient Visits:** 200784 **Births:** 1703 **Total Expense ($000):** 180095 **Payroll Expense ($000):** 77668 **Personnel:** 1293

○ **SAINTS MARY & ELIZABETH MEDICAL CENTER, CLAREMONT AVENUE (140094)**, 1431 North Claremont Avenue, Zip 60622–1791; tel. 773/278–2000, (Total facility includes 25 beds in nursing home–type unit) (Nonreporting) **A**9 10 11 **S** Resurrection Health Care
Primary Contact: Margaret McDermott, Chief Executive Officer
COO: Martin Judd, Vice President Professional Service
CFO: Thomas Capobianco, Chief Financial Officer
CIO: George Chessum, Senior Vice President Information Systems and Chief Information Officer
Web address: www.reshealthcare.org
Control: Other not–for–profit (including NFP Corporation) **Service:** General Medical and Surgical

Staffed Beds: 246

★ **SAINTS MARY & ELIZABETH MEDICAL CENTER, DIVISION STREET (140180)**, 2233 West Division Street, Zip 60622–3086; tel. 312/770–2000, (Nonreporting) **A**2 9 10 **S** Resurrection Health Care
Primary Contact: Margaret McDermott, Chief Executive Officer
CFO: Kenneth A. Kautzer, Senior Vice President Finance and Treasurer
CIO: Steven Smith, Chief Information Officer
Web address: www.stmaryofnazareth.org
Control: Other not–for–profit (including NFP Corporation) **Service:** General Medical and Surgical

Staffed Beds: 313

IL

Hospital, Medicare Provider Number, Address, Telephone, Approval, Facility, and Physician Codes, Health Care System
★ American Hospital Association (AHA) membership
□ The Joint Commission accreditation
○ American Osteopathic Association (AOA) accreditation
△ Commission on Accreditation of Rehabilitation Facilities (CARF) accreditation

★ △ **SCHWAB REHABILITATION HOSPITAL (143025)**, (Formerly Schwab Rehabilitation Hospital and Care Network), 1401 South California Boulevard, Zip 60608–1612; tel. 773/522–2010 **A**1 7 9 10 **F**9 25 26 32 33 50 55 58 66 72 73 75 77 81 82 85 86 107 117 120 121 135 137 **P**6 **S** Sinai Health System
Primary Contact: Alan H. Channing, President and Chief Executive Officer
COO: Karen Teitelbaum, Executive Vice President and Chief Operating Officer
CFO: Charles Weis, Chief Financial Officer
CMO: Susan Rayner, M.D., M.P.H., Executive Vice President
CIO: Peter Ingram, Vice President and Chief Information Officer
CHR: Andrew Wissel, Director Human Resources
Web address: www.schwabrehab.org
Control: Other not–for–profit (including NFP Corporation) **Service:** Rehabilitation

Staffed Beds: 75 **Admissions:** 1756 **Census:** 70 **Outpatient Visits:** 38018 **Births:** 0 **Total Expense ($000):** 34921 **Payroll Expense ($000):** 18173 **Personnel:** 297

★ **SHRINERS HOSPITALS FOR CHILDREN–CHICAGO**, 2211 North Oak Park Avenue, Zip 60707–3392; tel. 773/622–5400 **A**1 3 5 **F**3 8 9 25 28 31 32 33 50 62 64 66 72 73 75 77 79 80 81 83 84 85 86 107 119 120 121 123 132 135 137 **P**6 **S** Shriners Hospitals for Children
Primary Contact: James Cohick, Administrator
CFO: Philip Magid, Director Fiscal Services
CMO: Peter F. Sturm, M.D., Chief of Staff
CIO: Robert Gilb, Director Information Services
CHR: James E. Pawlowicz, Director Human Resources
Web address: www.shrinershospitals.org
Control: Other not–for–profit (including NFP Corporation) **Service:** Children's orthopedic

Staffed Beds: 36 **Admissions:** 1794 **Census:** 20 **Outpatient Visits:** 14121 **Births:** 0 **Total Expense ($000):** 38586 **Payroll Expense ($000):** 17522 **Personnel:** 343

★ **SOUTH SHORE HOSPITAL (140181)**, 8012 South Crandon Avenue, Zip 60617–1199; tel. 773/768–0810 **A**1 9 10 **F**3 4 5 11 15 25 27 30 31 32 33 38 46 50 53 54 55 56 57 60 62 63 68 76 77 79 80 81 82 86 96 97 103 107 118 119 132 134 135 137
Primary Contact: Jesus M. Ong, President
CFO: Timothy Caveney, Chief Financial Officer
CMO: C. Tyson, M.D., President Medical Staff
CIO: Jim Ritchie, Director Management Information Systems
CHR: Roger Rak, Director Human Resources
Web address: www.southshorehospital.com
Control: Other not–for–profit (including NFP Corporation) **Service:** General Medical and Surgical

Staffed Beds: 125 **Admissions:** 5306 **Census:** 85 **Outpatient Visits:** 20412 **Births:** 0 **Total Expense ($000):** 41326 **Payroll Expense ($000):** 20621 **Personnel:** 438

□ **ST. BERNARD HOSPITAL AND HEALTH CARE CENTER (140103)**, 326 West 64th Street, Zip 60621–3146; tel. 773/962–3900, (Nonreporting) **A**1 10
Primary Contact: Sister Elizabeth Van Straten, President and Chief Executive Officer
COO: Janet G. Nohos, Executive Vice President
CFO: Guy Alton, Chief Financial Officer
CIO: Guy Alton, Chief Financial Officer
CHR: Donna Nemeth, Director Human Resources
Web address: www.stbernardhospital.com
Control: Church–operated, Nongovernment, not–for profit **Service:** General Medical and Surgical

Staffed Beds: 194

★ ○ **SWEDISH COVENANT HOSPITAL (140114)**, 5145 North California Avenue, Zip 60625–3688; tel. 773/878–8200 **A**2 9 10 11 12 13 **F**3 12 13 15 18 20 22 24 25 26 27 28 31 32 33 34 36 37 38 40 43 44 46 50 54 55 56 57 58 59 61 62 66 68 72 73 74 75 76 77 79 80 81 82 84 85 86 87 88 90 91 92 93 94 95 96 97 100 102 105 106 107 109 111 117 118 119 120 121 123 124 132 135 136 137 **P**1 5 7
Primary Contact: Mark Newton, President and Chief Executive Officer
CFO: Gary M. Krugel, Senior Vice President Operations and Chief Financial Officer
CIO: Karen Sheehan, Director Information Systems
CHR: Anthony Guaccio, Senior Vice President Operations and Chief Human Resource Officer
Web address: www.schosp.org
Control: Church–operated, Nongovernment, not–for profit **Service:** General Medical and Surgical

Staffed Beds: 324 **Admissions:** 16212 **Census:** 231 **Outpatient Visits:** 257569 **Births:** 2424 **Total Expense ($000):** 221169 **Payroll Expense ($000):** 91535 **Personnel:** 2006

□ **THE NEUROLOGIC AND ORTHOPEDIC INSTITUTE OF CHICAGO (140303)**, 4501 North Winchester Avenue, Zip 60640; tel. 773/250–0000, (Nonreporting) **A**1 10
Primary Contact: Tom Hodson, Acting Chief Executive Officer
Web address: www.neuro–ortho.org
Control: Corporation, Investor–owned, for–profit **Service:** Orthopedic

Staffed Beds: 90

○ **THOREK MEMORIAL HOSPITAL (140115)**, 850 West Irving Park Road, Zip 60613–3099; tel. 773/525–6780 **A**9 10 11 **F**3 15 18 27 30 31 38 47 49 54 55 57 60 62 63 68 72 76 77 79 80 82 87 96 97 99 100 102 107 109 119 132 137
Primary Contact: Frank A. Solare, President and Chief Executive Officer
CFO: Edward Budd, Chief Financial Officer
CIO: Ron Krol, Chief Information Officer
Web address: www.thorek.org
Control: Other not–for–profit (including NFP Corporation) **Service:** General Medical and Surgical

Staffed Beds: 134 **Admissions:** 7127 **Census:** 75 **Outpatient Visits:** 161637 **Births:** 0 **Total Expense ($000):** 50106 **Payroll Expense ($000):** 19295 **Personnel:** 333

UNIVERSITY OF CHICAGO COMER CHILDREN'S HOSPITAL See University of Chicago Medical Center

★ **UNIVERSITY OF CHICAGO MEDICAL CENTER (140088)**, (Formerly University of Chicago Hospitals), 5841 South Maryland Avenue, Zip 60637–1470; tel. 773/702–1000, (Includes BERNARD MITCHELL HOSPITAL; CHICAGO LYING–IN HOSPITAL; UNIVERSITY OF CHICAGO COMER CHILDREN'S HOSPITAL) **A**1 2 3 5 8 9 10 **F**3 4 5 6 7 9 11 12 13 14 15 16 17 18 19 20 21 22 23 24 25 26 27 28 30 31 32 33 34 35 36 37 38 40 41 42 43 44 45 46 47 48 49 50 51 52 53 54 55 56 57 58 59 60 61 62 63 66 68 69 70 71 72 73 74 75 76 77 78 79 80 81 82 83 84 86 87 88 89 90 91 92 93 94 96 97 99 100 102 103 104 105 106 107 108 109 111 112 113 114 116 118 119 120 121 123 124 125 126 127 128 129 130 131 132 133 134 135 136 137 **P**1
Primary Contact: James L. Madara, M.D., Chief Executive Officer
CFO: Lawrence Furnstahl, Chief Financial Officer, Vice President Strategic Planning and Treasurer
CMO: Harvey Golomb, M.D., Dean Clinical Affairs
CIO: Eric Yablonka, Vice President and Chief Information Officer
CHR: Maya Bordeaux, Interim Vice President and Chief Human Resource Officer
Web address: www.uchospitals.edu
Control: Other not–for–profit (including NFP Corporation) **Service:** General Medical and Surgical

Staffed Beds: 553 **Admissions:** 26377 **Census:** 455 **Outpatient Visits:** 702841 **Births:** 2680 **Total Expense ($000):** 970702 **Payroll Expense ($000):** 356583 **Personnel:** 7174

★ △ **UNIVERSITY OF ILLINOIS MEDICAL CENTER AT CHICAGO (140150)**, 1740 West Taylor Street, Zip 60612–7236; tel. 312/996–7000 **A**1 2 3 5 7 8 9 10 **F**3 9 12 13 14 15 17 18 19 20 21 22 23 24 25 26 27 28 30 31 32 33 36 37 38 39 40 41 43 46 49 50 53 54 55 56 57 58 59 60 62 63 64 66 68 70 71 72 73 74 75 76 77 79 80 81 82 83 84 85 86 87 88 89 90 91 92 93 94 95 96 97 98 100 102 103 104 106 107 109 111 112 113 114 116 118 119 120 121 123 124 125 127 128 130 131 133 134 135 136 137 **P**4
Primary Contact: John J. DeNardo, Executive Director
COO: Bernadette Biskup, Chief Operating Officer
CFO: William Devoney, Chief Financial Officer
CMO: William Chamberlin, M.D., Chief Medical Officer
CIO: Rose Ann Laureto, Chief Information Officer
CHR: Sherry Hearn, Interim Chief Human Resource Officer
Web address: www.uillinoismedcenter.org
Control: State–Government, nonfederal **Service:** General Medical and Surgical

Staffed Beds: 456 **Admissions:** 19384 **Census:** 336 **Outpatient Visits:** 480919 **Births:** 2732 **Total Expense ($000):** 527175 **Payroll Expense ($000):** 241831 **Personnel:** 3981

VETERANS AFFAIRS CHICAGO HEALTH CARE SYSTEM See Jesse Brown Veterans Affairs Chicago Health Care System

CHICAGO HEIGHTS—Cook County

ST. JAMES HOSPITAL AND HEALTH CENTERS – CHICAGO HEIGHTS CAMPUS See St. James Hospital and Health Centers, Olympia Fields

CLINTON—Dewitt County

★ **DR. JOHN WARNER HOSPITAL (141303)**, 422 West White Street, Zip 61727–2199; tel. 217/935–9571 **A**9 10 18 **F**3 7 11 12 15 24 31 38 57 62 68 73 79 80 87 96 119 121 122 124 135 **P**6
Primary Contact: Patricia A. Luker, Chief Executive Officer and Administrator
CFO: Donna Wisner, Chief Financial Officer
CMO: Britt Williams, M.D., President Medical Staff
CIO: Larry Schleicher, Manager Information Services
CHR: Belinda Rittenhouse, Director Human Resources
Web address: www.djwhospital.org
Control: City–Government, nonfederal **Service:** General Medical and Surgical

Staffed Beds: 25 **Admissions:** 488 **Census:** 5 **Outpatient Visits:** 15372 **Births:** 0 **Total Expense ($000):** 11725 **Payroll Expense ($000):** 5050 **Personnel:** 168

IL

 Many Facility Codes have changed. Please refer to the AHA Guide Code Chart.

DANVILLE—Vermilion County

★ **PROVENA UNITED SAMARITANS MEDICAL CENTER (140093)**, 812 North Logan, Zip 61832–3788; tel. 217/443–5000 **A**1 2 9 10 19 **F**3 11 13 15 18 24 25 26 27 30 31 32 33 38 43 46 47 49 50 55 56 57 62 66 68 72 73 74 75 76 77 79 80 81 82 84 86 92 94 95 96 97 99 100 102 106 107 108 109 118 119 121 124 135 136 137 **P**7 **S** Provena Health
Primary Contact: David Bertauski, President and Chief Executive Officer
COO: Michael L. Brown, Chief Operating Officer and Chief Nursing Executive
CFO: Judy Brown, Chief Financial Officer
CIO: Michael Boyd, Manager Information Systems
CHR: Janet S. Payne, Vice President Human Resources
Web address: www.provenausmc.org
Control: Church–operated, Nongovernment, not–for profit **Service:** General Medical and Surgical

Staffed Beds: 158 **Admissions:** 7664 **Census:** 81 **Outpatient Visits:** 226019 **Births:** 848 **Total Expense ($000):** 98652 **Payroll Expense ($000):** 32803 **Personnel:** 692

★ △ **VETERANS AFFAIRS ILLIANA HEALTH CARE SYSTEM**, 1900 East Main Street, Zip 61832–5198; tel. 217/554–3000, (Total facility includes 217 beds in nursing home–type unit) **A**1 3 5 7 9 **F**2 3 5 6 7 8 25 26 29 30 31 32 33 34 36 37 38 43 44 45 49 50 52 53 54 56 57 58 60 61 62 64 68 72 73 75 77 79 80 81 82 86 87 88 90 91 92 93 94 95 96 97 100 102 106 107 117 118 119 121 124 132 133 134 135 136 137 **P**6 **S** Department of Veterans Affairs
Primary Contact: Michael E. Hamilton, Director
COO: Diana Carranza, Associate Director
CFO: Becky Tissier, Chief Fiscal Service
CMO: Sarita Prabhudesai, M.D., Chief of Staff
CIO: Sherry Boone, Chief Information Resource Management
CHR: Karla McIntosh, Chief Human Resources
Web address: www.va.gov/sta/guide/home.asp
Control: Veterans Affairs, Government, federal **Service:** General Medical and Surgical

Staffed Beds: 346 **Admissions:** 2651 **Census:** 215 **Outpatient Visits:** 250347 **Births:** 0 **Total Expense ($000):** 234825 **Payroll Expense ($000):** 72600 **Personnel:** 1291

DE KALB—De Kalb County

★ **KISHWAUKEE COMMUNITY HOSPITAL (140286)**, One Kish Hospital Drive, Zip 60115–4939, Mailing Address: P.O. Box 707, Zip 60115–0707; tel. 815/756–1521 **A**1 2 9 10 **F**3 8 11 12 13 15 24 25 26 27 30 31 32 33 34 35 38 43 45 46 48 49 51 55 57 58 59 66 68 71 72 73 74 75 76 77 79 80 81 82 84 86 88 92 96 99 100 102 105 107 118 119 120 121 122 124 132 134 135 136 137 **P**8 **S** Kish Health System
Primary Contact: Brad Copple, Administrator
CFO: Loren Foelske, Vice President Finance
CIO: Heath Bell, Chief Information Officer
CHR: Mark Thate, Director Human Resources
Web address: www.kishhospital.org
Control: Other not–for–profit (including NFP Corporation) **Service:** General Medical and Surgical

Staffed Beds: 100 **Admissions:** 5699 **Census:** 56 **Outpatient Visits:** 133736 **Births:** 847 **Total Expense ($000):** 94699 **Payroll Expense ($000):** 27655 **Personnel:** 584

DECATUR—Macon County

★ **DECATUR MEMORIAL HOSPITAL (140135)**, 2300 North Edward Street, Zip 62526–4192; tel. 217/876–8121, (Total facility includes 54 beds in nursing home–type unit) (Nonreporting) **A**1 2 3 5 9 10 12 13 19
Primary Contact: Kenneth L. Smithmier, President and Chief Executive Officer
COO: Timothy D. Stone, Executive Vice President and Chief Operating Officer
CFO: Gary Peacock, Senior Vice President and Chief Financial Officer
CIO: Jim Edwards, Director Information Systems
CHR: Mark Gates, Director Human Resources
Web address: www.dmhcares.org
Control: Other not–for–profit (including NFP Corporation) **Service:** General Medical and Surgical

Staffed Beds: 258

★ **ST. MARY'S HOSPITAL (140166)**, 1800 East Lake Shore Drive, Zip 62521–3883; tel. 217/464–2966, (Total facility includes 40 beds in nursing home–type unit) **A**1 3 5 9 10 **F**2 3 5 11 13 15 18 20 24 25 26 27 30 31 32 33 38 43 44 46 47 48 49 50 53 54 55 56 57 62 64 68 72 73 74 75 76 77 79 80 81 82 84 86 88 89 90 91 92 93 94 95 96 97 100 102 103 106 107 117 118 119 121 130 131 135 137 **P**7 **S** Hospital Sisters Health System
Primary Contact: Kevin F. Kast, President and Chief Executive Officer
COO: Theresa Rutherford, R.N., MS, Chief Operating Officer
CFO: Adam Cumbo, Chief Financial Officer
CHR: Terri Kuhle, Director Human Resources
Web address: www.stmarys-hospital.com
Control: Church–operated, Nongovernment, not–for profit **Service:** General Medical and Surgical

Staffed Beds: 226 **Admissions:** 7579 **Census:** 109 **Outpatient Visits:** 108449 **Births:** 646 **Total Expense ($000):** 85467 **Payroll Expense ($000):** 31479 **Personnel:** 855

DES PLAINES—Cook County

○ **HOLY FAMILY MEDICAL CENTER (142011)**, 100 North River Road, Zip 60016–1255; tel. 847/297–1800, (Nonreporting) **A**9 10 11 **S** Resurrection Health Care
Primary Contact: John D. Baird, Chief Executive Officer
CFO: Thomas Capobianco, Executive Vice President Finance and Chief Financial Officer
CMO: Timothy Cahill, D.O., President Medical Staff
CIO: George Chessum, Senior Vice President Information Systems and Chief Information Officer
CHR: Paul Skiem, Senior Vice President Human Resources
Web address: www.reshealth.org
Control: Church–operated, Nongovernment, not–for profit **Service:** Long–Term Acute Care hospital

Staffed Beds: 165

□ **MARYVILLE SCOTT NOLAN CENTER**, (Formerly Maryville Academy Scott A Nolan Center), 555 Wilson Lane, Zip 60016; tel. 847/768–5430 **A**1 9 **F**88 89 94 95 119
Primary Contact: Teresa Maganzini, Administrator
CFO: Timothy J. Morgan, Chief Financial Officer
CMO: Lerwut Wongsarnpigoon, M.D., Medical Director
CIO: Richard Arceo, Director Information Technology
CHR: Betty Barnes, Director Human Resources
Control: Church–operated, Nongovernment, not–for profit **Service:** Psychiatric

Staffed Beds: 40 **Admissions:** 451 **Census:** 19 **Outpatient Visits:** 1286 **Births:** 0 **Total Expense ($000):** 4322 **Payroll Expense ($000):** 1867 **Personnel:** 70

DIXON—Lee County

★ **KATHERINE SHAW BETHEA HOSPITAL (140012)**, 403 East First Street, Zip 61021–3187; tel. 815/288–5531 **A**9 10 **F**2 5 11 13 15 18 20 24 25 26 27 28 29 30 31 32 33 34 36 38 40 41 42 43 44 46 49 50 53 54 55 56 57 61 62 63 64 66 67 68 69 72 73 74 75 76 77 79 80 81 82 84 86 87 88 89 90 91 92 93 94 95 96 97 100 103 106 107 113 117 118 119 120 121 122 123 124 133 135 136 137 **P**6
Primary Contact: Darryl L. Vandervort, President and Chief Executive Officer
COO: David Schreiner, Chief Operating Officer
CFO: Vernon Farrell, Vice President and Chief Financial Officer
CIO: Timothy W. Broos, Vice President and Chief Information Officer
CHR: Julie Mann, Director Human Resources
Web address: www.ksbhospital.com
Control: Other not–for–profit (including NFP Corporation) **Service:** General Medical and Surgical

Staffed Beds: 84 **Admissions:** 4138 **Census:** 42 **Outpatient Visits:** 163637 **Births:** 404 **Total Expense ($000):** 92584 **Payroll Expense ($000):** 45637 **Personnel:** 765

Hospital, Medicare Provider Number, Address, Telephone, Approval, Facility, and Physician Codes, Health Care System
★ American Hospital Association (AHA) membership
□ The Joint Commission accreditation
○ American Osteopathic Association (AOA) accreditation
△ Commission on Accreditation of Rehabilitation Facilities (CARF) accreditation

DOWNERS GROVE—Du Page County

★ **ADVOCATE GOOD SAMARITAN HOSPITAL (140288)**, 3815 Highland Avenue, Zip 60515–1590; tel. 630/275–5900 **A**1 2 5 9 10 **F**3 5 11 13 15 17 18 20 22 24 25 26 27 28 31 32 33 34 36 38 40 41 42 43 44 46 47 49 50 52 53 54 55 56 57 62 66 68 70 72 73 74 75 76 77 79 80 81 82 84 86 88 90 91 92 93 94 95 96 97 98 99 100 102 103 107 108 109 111 112 114 118 119 120 121 124 133 134 135 136 137 **P**8 **S** Advocate Health Care
Primary Contact: David S. Fox, President
CFO: Peter Bury, Vice President Finance
CMO: Michael McKenna, M.D., Vice President Medical Management
CIO: Pete Caboor, Manager Information Systems
CHR: Sandra Norton, Vice President Human Resources
Web address: www.advocatehealth.com
Control: Church–operated, Nongovernment, not–for profit **Service:** General Medical and Surgical

Staffed Beds: 325 **Admissions:** 17654 **Census:** 215 **Outpatient Visits:** 190320 **Births:** 1640 **Total Expense ($000):** 292036 **Payroll Expense ($000):** 108937 **Personnel:** 1961

DU QUOIN—Perry County

★ **MARSHALL BROWNING HOSPITAL (141331)**, 900 North Washington Street, Zip 62832–1230, Mailing Address: P.O. Box 192, Zip 62832–0192; tel. 618/542–2146 **A**1 9 10 18 **F**11 15 24 25 33 38 55 57 67 79 86 96 102 107 115 118 122
Primary Contact: William J. Huff, Chief Executive Officer
CFO: Brice Harsy, Chief Financial Officer
CHR: Sarah Dickey, Manager Personnel
Web address: www.marshallbrowninghospital.com
Control: Other not–for–profit (including NFP Corporation) **Service:** General Medical and Surgical

Staffed Beds: 25 **Admissions:** 861 **Census:** 9 **Outpatient Visits:** 23495 **Births:** 0 **Total Expense ($000):** 13807 **Payroll Expense ($000):** 5905 **Personnel:** 137

EAST SAINT LOUIS—St. Clair County

☐ **KENNETH HALL REGIONAL HOSPITAL (140066)**, 129 North Eighth Street, Zip 62201–2917; tel. 618/274–1900, (Nonreporting) **A**1 9 10
Primary Contact: Michael T. McManus, Chief Operating Officer
COO: Michael T. McManus, Chief Operating Officer
CFO: Steve Lawrence, Chief Financial Officer and Chief Information Officer
CMO: Leyland Thomas, M.D., President Medical Staff
CIO: Michael Nichols, Corporate Vice President Information Technology
CHR: Wardell Sullivan, Director Human Resources
Web address: www.khrh.org
Control: Other not–for–profit (including NFP Corporation) **Service:** General Medical and Surgical

Staffed Beds: 119

TOUCHETTE REGIONAL HOSPITAL (140077), 5900 Bond Avenue, Zip 62207–2397; tel. 618/332–3060, (Nonreporting) **A**9 10
Primary Contact: Robert Klutts, Chief Executive Officer
COO: Michael T. McManus, Chief Operating Officer
CFO: Steve Lawrence, Chief Financial Officer and Chief Information Officer
CMO: Tom Mikkelson, M.D., Vice President Medical Affairs
CIO: Michael Nichols, Corporate Vice President Information Technology
CHR: Wardell Sullivan, Director Human Resources
Web address: www.touchette.org
Control: Other not–for–profit (including NFP Corporation) **Service:** General Medical and Surgical

Staffed Beds: 105

EFFINGHAM—Effingham County

★ **ST. ANTHONY'S MEMORIAL HOSPITAL (140032)**, 503 North Maple Street, Zip 62401–2099; tel. 217/342–2121, (Total facility includes 13 beds in nursing home–type unit) **A**1 2 9 10 19 **F**3 8 11 13 15 24 26 30 31 32 35 38 43 55 57 61 62 66 68 74 77 79 80 84 86 96 97 102 106 107 109 117 118 119 121 134 135 137 **S** Hospital Sisters Health System
Primary Contact: Daniel J. Woods, President and Chief Executive Officer
COO: Robert W. Esker, Assistant Administrator
CFO: Dave Storm, Director Business Support
CHR: Kal Keitel, Manager Personnel Services
Web address: www.stanthonyshospital.org
Control: Church–operated, Nongovernment, not–for profit **Service:** General Medical and Surgical

Staffed Beds: 146 **Admissions:** 7387 **Census:** 79 **Outpatient Visits:** 197584 **Births:** 840 **Total Expense ($000):** 77079 **Payroll Expense ($000):** 27194 **Personnel:** 641

ELDORADO—Saline County

★ **FERRELL HOSPITAL COMMUNITY FOUNDATION (141324)**, 1201 Pine Street, Zip 62930–1634; tel. 618/273–3361 **A**9 10 18 **F**1 4 11 15 16 17 24 25 31 32 33 38 55 56 57 65 68 70 71 78 79 80 81 83 84 85 88 96 107 117 118 119 122 **S** Alliant Management Services
Primary Contact: William Hartley, FACHE, President and Chief Executive Officer
CFO: James Fraser, Chief Financial Officer
CIO: Doug Rash, Director Information Technology
CHR: Beth Anderton, Vice President Human Resources
Web address: www.ferrellhosp.org
Control: Other not–for–profit (including NFP Corporation) **Service:** General Medical and Surgical

Staffed Beds: 25 **Admissions:** 943 **Census:** 9 **Outpatient Visits:** 7236 **Births:** 0 **Total Expense ($000):** 12459 **Payroll Expense ($000):** 5067 **Personnel:** 149

ELGIN—Kane County

☐ **ELGIN MENTAL HEALTH CENTER (144037)**, 750 South State Street, Zip 60123–7692; tel. 847/742–1040, (Nonreporting) **A**1 3 5 10
Primary Contact: Charles F. Hoffman, Interim Executive Director
CMO: Malini Patel, M.D., Medical Director
CIO: Kelly Callahan, Public Information Officer
CHR: Darek Williams, Director Human Resources
Web address: www.dhs.state.il.us
Control: State–Government, nonfederal **Service:** Psychiatric

Staffed Beds: 500

★ △ **PROVENA SAINT JOSEPH HOSPITAL (140217)**, 77 North Airlite Street, Zip 60123–4912; tel. 847/695–3200 **A**1 2 5 7 9 10 **F**1 5 11 12 13 15 17 18 20 22 24 25 26 27 30 31 32 33 34 35 36 38 39 40 41 42 43 44 49 50 52 53 54 55 56 57 58 59 60 61 62 63 66 67 68 72 73 74 75 76 77 79 80 81 82 86 87 88 89 90 91 92 93 94 95 96 97 100 102 103 104 105 107 108 109 111 112 119 121 123 124 132 133 134 135 136 137 **P**5 **S** Provena Health
Primary Contact: William A. Brown, FACHE, President and Chief Executive Officer
COO: Michael Wright, Chief Operating Officer
CFO: Paul E. Belter, Chief Financial Officer
CIO: Trevor O'Malley, Site Manager
CHR: Diane Hargreaves, Vice President Human Resources
Web address: www.provenahealth.com
Control: Other not–for–profit (including NFP Corporation) **Service:** General Medical and Surgical

Staffed Beds: 179 **Admissions:** 9220 **Census:** 135 **Outpatient Visits:** 198359 **Births:** 483 **Total Expense ($000):** 142924 **Payroll Expense ($000):** 51734 **Personnel:** 995

★ **SHERMAN HOSPITAL (140030)**, 934 Center Street, Zip 60120–2198; tel. 847/742–9800 **A**1 2 9 10 **F**3 4 8 11 13 15 17 18 20 22 24 25 26 27 28 30 32 33 38 40 41 43 49 53 54 55 56 57 59 60 62 63 66 68 69 70 71 72 73 74 75 76 77 79 80 81 82 83 85 86 87 90 96 97 100 102 103 106 107 116 118 119 121 123 132 133 135 136 137 **P**6 8
Primary Contact: Richard B. Floyd, President and Chief Executive Officer
COO: Linda Deering, R.N., Executive Vice President, Chief Operating Officer and Chief Nursing Officer
CFO: Eric Krueger, Vice President and Chief Financial Officer
CHR: Katie Bata, Vice President Human Resources
Web address: www.shermanhealthsystems.com
Control: Other not–for–profit (including NFP Corporation) **Service:** General Medical and Surgical

Staffed Beds: 254 **Admissions:** 13091 **Census:** 145 **Outpatient Visits:** 207625 **Births:** 2613 **Total Expense ($000):** 203847 **Payroll Expense ($000):** 76673 **Personnel:** 1218

ELK GROVE VILLAGE—Cook County

★ △ **ALEXIAN BROTHERS MEDICAL CENTER (140258)**, 800 Biesterfield Road, Zip 60007–3397; tel. 847/437–5500, (Includes ALEXIAN REHABILITATION HOSPITAL, 935 Beisner Road, Zip 60007; tel. 847/640–5600; Mark A. Frey, Senior Vice President), (Nonreporting) **A**1 2 5 7 9 10 **S** Alexian Brothers Health System
Primary Contact: John P. Werrbach, Acting President and Chief Executive Officer
Web address: www.alexian.org
Control: Church–operated, Nongovernment, not–for profit **Service:** General Medical and Surgical

Staffed Beds: 348

IL

ELMHURST—Du Page County

★□ **ELMHURST MEMORIAL HOSPITAL (140200)**, 200 Berteau Avenue, Zip 60126–2989; tel. 630/833–1400, (Total facility includes 38 beds in nursing home–type unit) **A**1 2 9 10 **F**5 8 11 12 13 15 16 18 20 22 24 25 26 27 30 32 33 38 39 40 42 43 44 45 49 52 53 54 55 56 57 58 59 60 61 62 63 66 68 70 72 73 74 75 76 77 79 80 81 82 84 86 87 88 89 90 91 92 93 94 95 96 97 98 99 100 102 103 104 105 107 108 109 110 111 117 118 119 120 121 124 133 134 135 136 137 **P**2 4 5 7 8
Primary Contact: Leo F. Fronza, Jr., President and Chief Executive Officer
CFO: James F. Doyle, Senior Vice President Finance and Chief Financial Officer
CMO: Lawrence Barr, M.D., President Medical Staff
CHR: Lois Grubb, Vice President Human Resources
Web address: www.emhc.org
Control: Other not–for–profit (including NFP Corporation) **Service:** General Medical and Surgical

Staffed Beds: 335 **Admissions:** 17353 **Census:** 230 **Outpatient Visits:** 372546 **Births:** 1609 **Total Expense ($000):** 264829 **Payroll Expense ($000):** 118762 **Personnel:** 2090

EUREKA—Woodford County

□ **EUREKA COMMUNITY HOSPITAL (141309)**, 101 South Major Street, Zip 61530; tel. 309/467–2371 **A**1 9 10 18 **F**3 11 15 24 25 26 27 30 31 32 33 36 38 41 43 47 48 50 55 56 57 62 65 66 73 76 77 79 80 81 82 86 96 102 107 117 119 120 122 133 135 **P**8
COO: Gary Hagens, Chief Operating Officer and Vice President Medical Affairs
CFO: Penny Cermak, Vice President and Chief Financial Officer
CMO: Steven K. Jones, M.D., Medical Director
CIO: Vincent Vitali, Interim Chief Information Officer
CHR: Diane Crutcher, Director Human Resources
Web address: www.bromenn.org
Control: Church–operated, Nongovernment, not–for profit **Service:** General Medical and Surgical

Staffed Beds: 25 **Admissions:** 513 **Census:** 7 **Outpatient Visits:** 38431 **Births:** 0 **Total Expense ($000):** 7796 **Payroll Expense ($000):** 4597 **Personnel:** 102

EVANSTON—Cook County

★□ **EVANSTON NORTHWESTERN HEALTHCARE (140010)**, 1301 Central Street, Zip 60201–1613; tel. 847/570–2000, (Includes EVANSTON HOSPITAL, 2650 Ridge Avenue, Zip 60201–1797; tel. 847/570–2000; GLENBROOK HOSPITAL, 2100 Pfingsten Road, Glenview, Zip 60025; tel. 847/657–5800; HIGHLAND PARK HOSPITAL, 718 Glenview Avenue, Highland Park, Zip 60035–2497; tel. 847/432–8000), (Total facility includes 27 beds in nursing home–type unit) **A**1 2 3 5 8 9 10 **F**2 3 4 5 6 8 9 11 12 13 14 15 17 18 20 22 24 25 26 27 28 30 31 32 33 34 35 36 37 38 40 41 42 43 44 45 46 47 48 49 50 53 54 55 56 57 58 59 60 61 62 64 66 68 70 72 73 74 75 76 77 79 80 81 82 84 85 86 87 88 89 90 91 92 93 94 95 96 97 98 99 100 102 103 104 105 106 107 108 109 110 111 112 113 114 116 117 118 119 120 121 123 124 125 134 135 136 137
Primary Contact: Mark R. Neaman, President and Chief Executive Officer
COO: Jeffrey H. Hillebrand, Chief Operating Officer
CFO: Gary Weiss, Chief Financial Officer
CIO: Thomas Smith, Chief Information Officer
CHR: Bill Luehrs, Chief Human Resources Officer
Web address: www.enh.org
Control: Other not–for–profit (including NFP Corporation) **Service:** General Medical and Surgical

Staffed Beds: 608 **Admissions:** 33981 **Census:** 452 **Outpatient Visits:** 1694379 **Births:** 4840 **Total Expense ($000):** 835972 **Payroll Expense ($000):** 293998 **Personnel:** 6035

○ **SAINT FRANCIS HOSPITAL (140080)**, 355 Ridge Avenue, Zip 60202–3399; tel. 847/316–4000, (Total facility includes 20 beds in nursing home–type unit) (Nonreporting) **A**2 3 5 9 10 11 **S** Resurrection Health Care
Primary Contact: Jeffrey J. Murphy, Executive Vice President and Chief Executive Officer
CFO: Thomas Capobianco, Chief Financial Officer
CIO: George Chessum, Vice President Information Systems
CHR: Paul Skiem, Senior Vice President Human Resources
Web address: www.reshealth.org
Control: Church–operated, Nongovernment, not–for profit **Service:** General Medical and Surgical

Staffed Beds: 232

EVERGREEN PARK—Cook County

□ **LITTLE COMPANY OF MARY HOSPITAL AND HEALTH CARE CENTERS (140179)**, 2800 West 95th Street, Zip 60805–2795; tel. 708/422–6200 **A**1 2 9 10 **F**2 5 11 12 13 15 20 21 25 26 27 30 31 32 33 38 42 43 44 45 49 53 55 56 57 59 61 62 68 69 70 73 74 76 77 79 82 83 84 88 91 94 95 96 97 100 102 107 109 116 118 119 121 124 133 135 136 137 **P**6 7 8
S American Province of Little Company of Mary Sisters
Primary Contact: Dennis A. Reilly, President and Chief Executive Officer
COO: Mary Freyer, Chief Operating Officer
CFO: Randy Ruther, Vice President Finance and Chief Financial Officer
CMO: Irving Fuld, M.D., President Medical Staff
CIO: Darryl Mazzuca, Director Management Information Systems
CHR: Colleen Rohan, Director Human Resources
Web address: www.lcmh.org
Control: Other not–for–profit (including NFP Corporation) **Service:** General Medical and Surgical

Staffed Beds: 294 **Admissions:** 15789 **Census:** 191 **Outpatient Visits:** 139776 **Births:** 1294 **Total Expense ($000):** 170154 **Payroll Expense ($000):** 77770 **Personnel:** 1535

FAIRFIELD—Wayne County

★□ **FAIRFIELD MEMORIAL HOSPITAL (141311)**, 303 N.W. 11th Street, Zip 62837–1203; tel. 618/842–2611, (Total facility includes 104 beds in nursing home–type unit) **A**1 9 10 18 **F**3 11 13 15 24 26 27 30 31 32 36 38 54 55 56 57 61 62 67 68 73 74 76 79 82 86 93 94 96 97 100 104 107 117 118 119 121 124 134 135 **S** Alliant Management Services
Primary Contact: Katherine Bunting, Chief Executive Officer
CFO: Michael J. Brown, Chief Financial Officer
CMO: Patrick Molt, M.D., President Medical Staff
CHR: Mary Harvey, Director Human Resources
Web address: www.fairfieldmemorial.org
Control: Other not–for–profit (including NFP Corporation) **Service:** General Medical and Surgical

Staffed Beds: 163 **Admissions:** 1672 **Census:** 113 **Outpatient Visits:** 35711 **Births:** 155 **Total Expense ($000):** 20938 **Payroll Expense ($000):** 9344 **Personnel:** 299

FLORA—Clay County

★ **CLAY COUNTY HOSPITAL (141351)**, 911 Stacy Burk Drive, Zip 62839–1823, Mailing Address: P.O. Box 280, Zip 62839–0280; tel. 618/662–2131, (Nonreporting) **A**9 10 18 **S** BJC HealthCare
Primary Contact: Susan G. Batchelor, President
CFO: Mike Stoverink, Chief Financial Officer
CMO: Ashok Kumar, M.D., Chief of Staff
CHR: C. L. Halsey, Director Human Resources and Marketing
Web address: www.claycountyhospital.org
Control: County–Government, nonfederal **Service:** General Medical and Surgical

Staffed Beds: 22

FOREST PARK—Cook County

★□ **RIVEREDGE HOSPITAL (144009)**, 8311 West Roosevelt Road, Zip 60130–2500; tel. 708/771–7000, (Nonreporting) **A**1 5 9 10
S Psychiatric Solutions
Primary Contact: Carey Carlock, Chief Executive Officer
COO: Michael D. Gara, PsyD, Chief Operating Officer
CFO: Robert Maziarka, Chief Financial Officer
CMO: Shiraz Butt, M.D., Executive Medical Director
CIO: Kyle Heinze, Coordinator Information Technology
CHR: Nancy Bourque, Director Human Resources
Web address: www.psysolutions.com
Control: Corporation, Investor–owned, for–profit **Service:** Psychiatric

Staffed Beds: 210

Hospital, Medicare Provider Number, Address, Telephone, Approval, Facility, and Physician Codes, Health Care System

★ American Hospital Association (AHA) membership
□ The Joint Commission accreditation
○ American Osteopathic Association (AOA) accreditation
△ Commission on Accreditation of Rehabilitation Facilities (CARF) accreditation

FREEPORT—Stephenson County

★ **FHN MEMORIAL HOSPITAL (140160)**, 1045 West Stephenson Street, Zip 61032–4899; tel. 815/599–6000, (Total facility includes 18 beds in nursing home–type unit) **A**2 9 10 19 **F**3 11 12 13 14 15 17 18 24 25 26 27 28 30 31 32 36 38 42 43 44 46 47 48 49 50 51 52 55 56 57 60 61 62 63 66 67 72 73 74 75 76 77 79 80 81 82 84 86 87 89 90 91 92 93 94 96 97 98 100 102 107 117 118 119 120 121 124 130 135 **P**6 8
Primary Contact: Michael R. Perry, M.D., President and Chief Executive Officer
COO: Sharon K. Summers, R.N., Executive Vice President and Chief Operating Officer
CFO: Michael Clark, Vice President Finance
CMO: Robert D. Geller, M.D., Vice President Medical Affairs
CIO: Phil Wasson, Vice President and Chief Information Officer
CHR: Len Carter, Vice President Human Resources
Web address: www.fhn.org
Control: Other not–for–profit (including NFP Corporation) **Service:** General Medical and Surgical

Staffed Beds: 157 **Admissions:** 6257 **Census:** 76 **Outpatient Visits:** 169773 **Births:** 565 **Total Expense ($000):** 90309 **Payroll Expense ($000):** 27631 **Personnel:** 613

GALENA—Jo Daviess County

★ **MIDWEST MEDICAL CENTER (141302)**, (Formerly Galena–Stauss Hospital and Healthcare Center), One Medical Center Drive, Zip 61036–1697; tel. 815/777–1340, (Total facility includes 57 beds in nursing home–type unit) **A**9 10 18 **F**2 10 11 15 31 32 38 52 55 56 63 65 66 79 96 101 107 117 118 119 121 122 **P**5
Primary Contact: Jeff Hill, Chief Executive Officer
COO: Steve Busch, Chief Operating Officer
CFO: Tracy Bauer, Chief Financial Officer
CMO: Grant Westenfelder, M.D., Chief Medical Officer
CIO: Patricia Allvin, Information Specialist
CHR: Melissa Conley, Director Human Resources
Web address: www.midwestmedicalcenter.org
Control: Other not–for–profit (including NFP Corporation) **Service:** General Medical and Surgical

Staffed Beds: 82 **Admissions:** 409 **Census:** 59 **Outpatient Visits:** 21991 **Births:** 0 **Total Expense ($000):** 10184 **Payroll Expense ($000):** 4478 **Personnel:** 81

GALESBURG—Knox County

⊡ **GALESBURG COTTAGE HOSPITAL (140040)**, 695 North Kellogg Street, Zip 61401–2885; tel. 309/343–8131, (Total facility includes 31 beds in nursing home–type unit) (Nonreporting) **A**1 9 10 19 **S** Community Health Systems, Inc.
Primary Contact: Kenneth Hutchenrider, Chief Executive Officer
CMO: Angelo Soyangco, M.D., President Medical Staff
CIO: Teresa Mach, Manager Information Technology
CHR: Steven Hogberg, Director Human Resources
Web address: www.cottagehospital.com
Control: Other not–for–profit (including NFP Corporation) **Service:** General Medical and Surgical

Staffed Beds: 150

⊡ **OSF ST. MARY MEDICAL CENTER (140064)**, 3333 North Seminary Street, Zip 61401–1299; tel. 309/344–3161 **A**1 9 10 19 **F**3 11 15 18 24 25 26 27 30 31 32 37 38 40 42 44 46 49 51 52 54 55 56 57 58 60 61 66 68 72 73 74 75 76 77 79 80 81 82 84 86 87 96 99 100 104 105 107 118 119 121 124 134 135 136 **P**1 6 **S** OSF Healthcare System
Primary Contact: Richard S. Kowalski, Administrator and Chief Executive Officer
CFO: Curt Lipe, Chief Financial Officer
CMO: James M. Nesselroad, M.D., President Medical Staff
CIO: Becky Lynch, Manager Business Entity Management and Information Systems
CHR: Roxanna Crosser, Senior Assistant Administrator Staff Services
Web address: www.osfstmary.org
Control: Church–operated, Nongovernment, not–for profit **Service:** General Medical and Surgical

Staffed Beds: 99 **Admissions:** 5491 **Census:** 62 **Outpatient Visits:** 101676 **Births:** 398 **Total Expense ($000):** 70027 **Payroll Expense ($000):** 28493 **Personnel:** 564

GENESEO—Henry County

⊡ **HAMMOND–HENRY HOSPITAL (141319)**, 600 North College Avenue, Zip 61254–1099; tel. 309/944–4625, (Total facility includes 57 beds in nursing home–type unit) **A**1 9 10 18 **F**11 13 15 17 25 31 32 33 38 40 55 56 57 61 62 65 68 74 75 76 77 79 82 83 84 86 96 100 107 117 118 119 120 121 122 135 **S** Brim Healthcare, Inc.
Primary Contact: Bradley Solberg, FACHE, Chief Executive Officer
CFO: Bill Murdock, Vice President Fiscal Services
CIO: Heather Henry, Manager Information Systems
CHR: Margaret Chavez, Manager Human Resources
Web address: www.hammondhenry.com
Control: Hospital district or authority, Government, nonfederal **Service:** General Medical and Surgical

Staffed Beds: 80 **Admissions:** 1031 **Census:** 47 **Outpatient Visits:** 48408 **Births:** 124 **Total Expense ($000):** 22211 **Payroll Expense ($000):** 9140 **Personnel:** 245

GENEVA—Kane County

⊡ **DELNOR–COMMUNITY HOSPITAL (140211)**, 300 Randall Road, Zip 60134–4200; tel. 630/208–3000 **A**1 2 9 10 **F**3 11 13 15 18 20 24 25 26 27 28 30 31 32 33 34 37 38 40 41 49 55 56 57 61 62 63 66 68 72 73 75 76 77 79 80 81 82 86 92 94 96 97 99 100 103 106 107 108 109 114 118 119 120 121 124 132 134 135 136 137
Primary Contact: Craig A. Livermore, President and Chief Executive Officer
Web address: www.delnor.com
Control: Other not–for–profit (including NFP Corporation) **Service:** General Medical and Surgical

Staffed Beds: 159 **Admissions:** 9590 **Census:** 98 **Outpatient Visits:** 211066 **Births:** 1659 **Total Expense ($000):** 174292 **Payroll Expense ($000):** 71968 **Personnel:** 1320

GIBSON CITY—Ford County

⊡ **GIBSON AREA HOSPITAL AND HEALTH SERVICES (141317)**, 1120 North Melvin Street, Zip 60936, Mailing Address: P.O. Box 429, Zip 60936–0429; tel. 217/784–4251, (Includes GIBSON COMMUNITY HOSPITAL NURSING HOME), (Total facility includes 42 beds in nursing home–type unit) **A**1 9 10 18 **F**3 7 11 13 15 24 27 30 31 32 33 38 40 41 42 49 50 52 54 55 57 62 63 66 67 68 73 74 77 79 80 82 86 96 97 99 100 102 107 117 118 120 121 122 132 135 136 137 **P**1 7 **S** QHR
Primary Contact: Robert C. Schmitt, II, Chief Executive Officer
CFO: Gary Abrams, Chief Financial Officer
CMO: David J. Hagan, M.D., President Medical Staff
CIO: Sean Patrick, Director Information Technology
CHR: Ty Royal, Director Human Resources
Web address: www.gibsonhospital.org
Control: Other not–for–profit (including NFP Corporation) **Service:** General Medical and Surgical

Staffed Beds: 67 **Admissions:** 936 **Census:** 48 **Outpatient Visits:** 56537 **Births:** 168 **Total Expense ($000):** 31105 **Payroll Expense ($000):** 13338 **Personnel:** 323

GLENDALE HEIGHTS—Du Page County

⊡ **ADVENTIST GLENOAKS HOSPITAL (140292)**, 701 Winthrop Avenue, Zip 60139–1403; tel. 630/545–8000 **A**1 9 10 **F**3 11 13 15 17 18 20 25 26 27 28 31 32 33 36 38 40 43 49 55 56 57 58 60 62 66 68 70 72 73 74 76 77 79 80 81 82 86 87 88 89 90 91 92 93 94 95 96 97 100 102 106 107 118 119 120 121 123 124 135 136 137 **P**7 8 **S** Adventist Health System Sunbelt Health Care Corporation
Primary Contact: Brinsley B. Lewis, Chief Executive Officer
CFO: Shane Cox, Chief Financial Officer
CMO: Joseph Lagattuta, Assistant Director Medical Affairs
CIO: Russell Soliman, Regional Director Information Services
CHR: Donald Russell, Vice President
Web address: www.keepingyouwell.com
Control: Church–operated, Nongovernment, not–for profit **Service:** General Medical and Surgical

Staffed Beds: 141 **Admissions:** 5092 **Census:** 73 **Outpatient Visits:** 31226 **Births:** 713 **Total Expense ($000):** 56725 **Payroll Expense ($000):** 24470 **Personnel:** 464

GLENVIEW—Cook County

GLENBROOK HOSPITAL See Evanston Northwestern Healthcare, Evanston

GRANITE CITY—Madison County

☐ **GATEWAY REGIONAL MEDICAL CENTER (140125)**, 2100 Madison Avenue, Zip 62040–4799; tel. 618/798–3000 **A**1 9 **F**3 11 13 15 18 20 24 25 38 42 43 46 47 48 49 50 51 52 55 56 57 59 61 62 66 68 72 73 74 75 77 79 82 85 86 87 88 89 93 94 96 99 100 107 117 118 120 124 135 136 **S** Community Health Systems, Inc.
Primary Contact: John W. Sanders, Chief Executive Officer
Web address: www.gatewayregional.net
Control: Corporation, Investor–owned, for–profit **Service:** General Medical and Surgical

Staffed Beds: 327 **Admissions:** 8837 **Census:** 148 **Outpatient Visits:** 80342 **Births:** 351

GREENVILLE—Bond County

⊡ **GREENVILLE REGIONAL HOSPITAL (140137)**, 200 Healthcare Drive, Zip 62246–1156; tel. 618/664–1230, (Includes FAIR OAKS), (Total facility includes 108 beds in nursing home–type unit) **A**1 9 10 **F**1 2 4 7 11 13 15 16 17 24 25 27 30 31 32 38 43 49 50 54 55 56 57 62 65 66 68 70 71 73 74 75 76 77 78 79 80 81 82 83 84 85 86 88 89 90 93 94 96 100 102 107 115 117 118 119 120 121 122 124 135 **P**5
Primary Contact: James M. Hayes, President and Chief Executive Officer
CFO: Jerald Graber, Senior Manager Finance
Web address: www.greenvilleregionalhospital.com
Control: Other not–for–profit (including NFP Corporation) **Service:** General Medical and Surgical

Staffed Beds: 150 **Admissions:** 1960 **Census:** 107 **Outpatient Visits:** 41489 **Births:** 101 **Total Expense ($000):** 28460 **Payroll Expense ($000):** 11155 **Personnel:** 334

IL

 Many Facility Codes have changed. Please refer to the AHA Guide Code Chart.

HARRISBURG—Saline County

★ **HARRISBURG MEDICAL CENTER (140210)**, 100 Drive Warren Tuttle Drive, Zip 62946, Mailing Address: P.O. Box 428, Zip 62946–0428; tel. 618/253–7671 **A**1 9 10 20 **F**3 8 11 15 24 25 26 27 28 31 32 38 50 54 55 56 57 60 61 62 73 75 76 77 79 80 82 84 86 88 89 90 91 92 93 94 95 96 97 99 100 107 118 119 120 122 135 137
Primary Contact: Vincent Ashley, Chief Executive Officer
CFO: Barbara Vickery, Chief Financial Officer
CIO: Rick Pyle, Supervisor Data Processing
CHR: Rodney Smith, Director Human Resources and Development
Web address: www.harrisburgmedicalcenter.com
Control: Other not–for–profit (including NFP Corporation) **Service:** General Medical and Surgical

Staffed Beds: 74 **Admissions:** 3447 **Census:** 40 **Outpatient Visits:** 39969 **Births:** 0 **Total Expense ($000):** 33978 **Payroll Expense ($000):** 16707 **Personnel:** 405

HARVARD—McHenry County

★ **MERCY HARVARD HOSPITAL (141335)**, 901 Grant Street, Zip 60033–1898, Mailing Address: P.O. Box 850, Zip 60033–0850; tel. 815/943–5431, (Total facility includes 34 beds in nursing home–type unit) **A**1 9 10 18 **F**3 11 12 15 24 25 26 30 31 32 33 38 43 46 52 55 57 62 67 68 73 75 77 79 80 82 86 87 96 97 98 107 117 118 119 121 132 135 **P**6
Primary Contact: Sue Ripsch, Chief Operating Officer
COO: Sue Ripsch, Chief Operating Officer
CFO: John Cook, Chief Financial Officer
Web address: www.mercyhealthsystem.org
Control: Other not–for–profit (including NFP Corporation) **Service:** General Medical and Surgical

Staffed Beds: 54 **Admissions:** 664 **Census:** 32 **Outpatient Visits:** 47476 **Births:** 0 **Total Expense ($000):** 19276 **Payroll Expense ($000):** 7750 **Personnel:** 127

HARVEY—Cook County

★ △ **INGALLS MEMORIAL HOSPITAL (140191)**, One Ingalls Drive, Zip 60426–3591; tel. 708/333–2300 **A**1 2 7 9 10 **F**3 4 5 8 11 12 13 15 17 18 20 22 24 25 26 27 28 30 31 32 33 35 36 37 38 39 42 43 44 46 47 49 50 51 53 54 55 56 57 58 59 61 62 63 64 66 68 71 72 73 74 75 76 77 78 79 80 81 82 84 85 86 87 88 91 92 93 94 96 97 100 102 103 104 105 106 107 108 109 111 112 114 118 119 120 121 122 124 133 135 136 137 **P**8
Primary Contact: Kurt E. Johnson, President and Chief Executive Officer
CFO: Vincent Pryor, Chief Financial Officer
CIO: Doug Buffone, Director Information Services
CHR: Aletha Ross, Director Human Resources
Web address: www.ingallshealthsystem.org
Control: Other not–for–profit (including NFP Corporation) **Service:** General Medical and Surgical

Staffed Beds: 419 **Admissions:** 19169 **Census:** 255 **Outpatient Visits:** 301355 **Births:** 1447 **Total Expense ($000):** 248611 **Payroll Expense ($000):** 105722 **Personnel:** 1904

HAVANA—Mason County

★ **MASON DISTRICT HOSPITAL (141313)**, 615 North Promenade Street, Zip 62644–0530, Mailing Address: P.O. Box 530, Zip 62644–0530; tel. 309/543–4431, (Nonreporting) **A**1 9 10 18
Primary Contact: Harry Wolin, Administrator and Chief Executive Officer
CFO: Robert J. Stolba, Chief Financial Officer
CHR: Anne Davis, Director Human Resources
Web address: www.masondistricthospital.org
Control: Hospital district or authority, Government, nonfederal **Service:** General Medical and Surgical

Staffed Beds: 25

HAZEL CREST—Cook County

★ **ADVOCATE SOUTH SUBURBAN HOSPITAL (140250)**, 17800 South Kedzie Avenue, Zip 60429–0989; tel. 708/799–8000, (Total facility includes 40 beds in nursing home–type unit) (Nonreporting) **A**1 2 9 10 **S** Advocate Health Care
Primary Contact: Ann Errichetti, M.D., President
CFO: Brian Kelly, Vice President Finance
CMO: Stewart Reingold, M.D., Vice President Medical Management
CIO: Beth Tyrek, Site Manager Information Systems
CHR: Jason Spigner, Vice President Human Resources
Web address: www.advocatehealth.com/ssub/
Control: Other not–for–profit (including NFP Corporation) **Service:** General Medical and Surgical

Staffed Beds: 240

HERRIN—Williamson County

□ **HERRIN HOSPITAL (140011)**, 201 South 14th Street, Zip 62948–3631; tel. 618/942–2171 **A**1 9 10 **F**3 11 15 24 25 26 30 31 32 33 38 47 49 53 54 55 56 57 58 62 68 72 73 75 76 77 79 80 81 85 86 90 96 97 102 107 119 120 121 124 132 135 136 137 **S** Southern Illinois Hospital Services
Primary Contact: Becky Ashton, Administrator
CFO: Rex P. Budde, Senior Vice President and Chief Financial Officer
CMO: Terrence Glennon, M.D., President Medical Staff
CIO: Frank Sears, Vice President and Chief Information Officer
Web address: www.sih.net
Control: Other not–for–profit (including NFP Corporation) **Service:** General Medical and Surgical

Staffed Beds: 94 **Admissions:** 4728 **Census:** 68 **Outpatient Visits:** 77749 **Births:** 0 **Total Expense ($000):** 67800 **Payroll Expense ($000):** 23722 **Personnel:** 554

HIGHLAND—Madison County

★ **ST. JOSEPH'S HOSPITAL (141336)**, 1515 Main Street, Zip 62249–1656; tel. 618/654–7421, (Total facility includes 30 beds in nursing home–type unit) **A**1 9 10 18 **F**15 24 25 26 33 38 40 42 55 57 62 66 67 68 73 75 77 79 86 87 96 97 102 107 117 118 119 121 122 132 135 **P**6 **S** Hospital Sisters Health System
Primary Contact: Claudio Fort, Executive Vice President and Administrator
CFO: James Johnson, Chief Financial Officer
CMO: A. Greg Miranda, D.O., President Medical Staff
Web address: www.stjosephshighland.com
Control: Church–operated, Nongovernment, not–for profit **Service:** General Medical and Surgical

Staffed Beds: 55 **Admissions:** 1396 **Census:** 29 **Outpatient Visits:** 31928 **Births:** 0 **Total Expense ($000):** 20086 **Payroll Expense ($000):** 8199 **Personnel:** 212

HIGHLAND PARK—Lake County

HIGHLAND PARK HOSPITAL See Evanston Northwestern Healthcare, Evanston

HILLSBORO—Montgomery County

★ **HILLSBORO AREA HOSPITAL (141332)**, 1200 East Tremont Street, Zip 62049–1900; tel. 217/532–6111, (Total facility includes 40 beds in nursing home–type unit) **A**1 9 10 18 **F**3 10 15 25 26 30 31 32 33 38 40 54 55 56 57 61 62 63 73 75 77 79 80 81 82 84 86 87 96 99 102 115 117 118 119 120 122 124 135 137 **S** Brim Healthcare, Inc.
Primary Contact: Rex H. Brown, Chief Executive Officer
CFO: Terri L. Carroll, Vice President Financial Services
CHR: Sharon Clark, Director Human Resources
Web address: www.hillsboroareahospital.org
Control: Other not–for–profit (including NFP Corporation) **Service:** General Medical and Surgical

Staffed Beds: 65 **Admissions:** 875 **Census:** 28 **Outpatient Visits:** 28915 **Births:** 0 **Total Expense ($000):** 15749 **Payroll Expense ($000):** 6510 **Personnel:** 176

HINES—Cook County

□ **JOHN J. MADDEN MENTAL HEALTH CENTER (144028)**, 1200 South First Avenue, Zip 60141; tel. 708/338–7202 **A**1 5 10 **F**30 32 88 119 135 **P**1
Primary Contact: Fred Nirde, Administrator
CFO: Patricia Madden, Administrator
Control: State–Government, nonfederal **Service:** Psychiatric

Staffed Beds: 150 **Admissions:** 4268 **Census:** 136 **Outpatient Visits:** 0 **Births:** 0 **Total Expense ($000):** 29324 **Payroll Expense ($000):** 22332

IL

Hospital, Medicare Provider Number, Address, Telephone, Approval, Facility, and Physician Codes, Health Care System
★ American Hospital Association (AHA) membership
□ The Joint Commission accreditation
○ American Osteopathic Association (AOA) accreditation
△ Commission on Accreditation of Rehabilitation Facilities (CARF) accreditation

★ △ **VETERANS AFFAIRS EDWARD HINES, JR. HOSPITAL**, Fifth Avenue and Roosevelt Road, Zip 60141–5000, Mailing Address: P.O. Box 5000, Zip 60141–5000; tel. 708/202–8387, (Total facility includes 199 beds in nursing home–type unit) **A**1 2 3 5 7 8 9 **F**1 2 3 4 5 6 7 8 9 10 11 12 14 15 17 18 20 22 24 25 26 27 31 32 33 34 35 36 37 38 40 41 42 43 44 45 46 47 48 49 50 52 53 54 55 56 57 58 59 60 61 62 63 64 66 68 72 73 75 76 77 79 80 81 82 85 86 87 88 90 91 92 93 94 95 96 97 98 99 100 101 102 103 106 107 108 109 110 111 112 113 114 115 118 119 121 124 132 133 135 136 137 **P**6 **S** Department of Veterans Affairs
Primary Contact: Nathan L. Geraths, Director
COO: Nathan L. Geraths, Director
CFO: Raleigh Beard, Chief Fiscal Services
CMO: Barbara Temeck, M.D., Chief of Staff
CIO: Gordon Brown, Chief Information Resources Management
CHR: Clare Hadjuk, Director Human Resources
Web address: www.va.gov/sta/guide/home.asp
Control: Veterans Affairs, Government, federal **Service:** General Medical and Surgical

Staffed Beds: 484 **Admissions:** 7380 **Census:** 346 **Outpatient Visits:** 546455 **Births:** 0 **Total Expense ($000):** 392755 **Payroll Expense ($000):** 183652 **Personnel:** 2941

HINSDALE—Du Page and Cook Counties

★ △ **ADVENTIST HINSDALE HOSPITAL (140122)**, 120 North Oak Street, Zip 60521–3890; tel. 630/856–9000 **A**1 2 3 5 7 9 10 **F**3 5 8 11 12 13 14 15 17 18 20 22 24 25 26 27 31 32 33 36 37 38 39 40 41 42 43 49 53 54 55 56 57 58 60 61 62 66 68 70 71 72 73 74 76 77 79 80 81 82 83 84 85 86 87 88 89 91 92 93 94 95 96 97 100 102 106 107 109 111 112 113 114 118 119 120 121 124 125 130 135 136 137 **P**7 8 **S** Adventist Health System Sunbelt Health Care Corporation
Primary Contact: David Crane, President and Chief Executive Officer
COO: Alan Schneider, Chief Operating Officer
CFO: Steve Chen, Chief Financial Officer
CMO: Gary Lipinski, M.D., Regional Vice President and Chief Medical Officer
CIO: Russell Soliman, Regional Director Information Services
CHR: Donald Russell, Regional Vice President Human Resources
Web address: www.keepingyouwell.com
Control: Church–operated, Nongovernment, not–for profit **Service:** General Medical and Surgical

Staffed Beds: 353 **Admissions:** 14469 **Census:** 177 **Outpatient Visits:** 282899 **Births:** 2422 **Total Expense ($000):** 276790 **Payroll Expense ($000):** 102430 **Personnel:** 1935

★ **R M L SPECIALTY HOSPITAL (142010)**, 5601 South County Line Road, Zip 60521–8900; tel. 630/286–4000 **A**1 5 9 10 **F**1 3 12 25 26 38 49 50 55 56 57 59 62 66 73 75 82 96 107 119 121 137
Primary Contact: James R. Prister, President and Chief Executive Officer
CFO: Tom Pater, Chief Financial Officer
CMO: John Brofman, M.D., Medical Director
CIO: Julie Ames, Chief Information Officer
CHR: John Landstrom, Director Human Resources
Web address: www.rmlspecialtyhospital.org
Control: Other not–for–profit (including NFP Corporation) **Service:** General Medical and Surgical

Staffed Beds: 83 **Admissions:** 777 **Census:** 69 **Outpatient Visits:** 1544 **Births:** 0 **Total Expense ($000):** 39508 **Payroll Expense ($000):** 19567 **Personnel:** 356

HOFFMAN ESTATES—Cook County

★ **ALEXIAN BROTHERS BEHAVIORAL HEALTH HOSPITAL (144031)**, 1650 Moon Lake Boulevard, Zip 60194–5000; tel. 847/882–1600, (Nonreporting) **A**1 5 9 10 **S** Alexian Brothers Health System
Primary Contact: Bruce Anderson, President and Chief Executive Officer
COO: Francine McGouey, Chief Operating Officer
CFO: David Jones, Chief Financial Officer
CMO: Anthony D'Agostino, M.D., Medical Director
Web address: www.abbhh.org
Control: Church–operated, Nongovernment, not–for profit **Service:** Psychiatric

Staffed Beds: 94

★ **ST. ALEXIUS MEDICAL CENTER (140290)**, 1555 Barrington Road, Zip 60194–1018; tel. 847/843–2000 **A**1 2 5 9 10 **F**3 8 11 12 13 15 17 18 20 25 26 27 28 30 31 32 33 35 37 38 39 40 42 43 46 47 48 49 55 56 57 62 68 71 72 73 74 75 76 77 78 79 80 81 82 83 84 86 87 92 96 97 100 102 103 107 108 109 112 114 119 121 124 133 134 135 136 137 **S** Alexian Brothers Health System
Primary Contact: Edward M. Goldberg, President and Chief Executive Officer
CFO: Robin Chopp, Vice President and Chief Financial Officer
CIO: Kathleen Davis, Chief Information Officer
CHR: Linda Baker, Director Human Resources
Web address: www.stalexius.org
Control: Church–operated, Nongovernment, not–for profit **Service:** General Medical and Surgical

Staffed Beds: 211 **Admissions:** 17242 **Census:** 184 **Outpatient Visits:** 219061 **Births:** 2879 **Total Expense ($000):** 243914 **Payroll Expense ($000):** 91436 **Personnel:** 1490

HOOPESTON—Vermilion County

☐ **HOOPESTON REGIONAL HEALTH CENTER (141316)**, 701 East Orange Street, Zip 60942–1871; tel. 217/283–5531, (Total facility includes 75 beds in nursing home–type unit) (Nonreporting) **A**1 10 18
Primary Contact: John Crawford, Chief Executive Officer
COO: Jacqueline Johnson, Chief Clinical Officer
CFO: Bob Robertson, Chief Financial Officer
CIO: Bernie McCarty, Manager Information Technology
CHR: Betsy Morgenroth, Chief Support Officer
Web address: www.hoopestonhospital.org
Control: Other not–for–profit (including NFP Corporation) **Service:** General Medical and Surgical

Staffed Beds: 100

HOPEDALE—Tazewell County

HOPEDALE MEDICAL COMPLEX (141330), 107 Tremont Street, Zip 61747; tel. 309/449–3321, (Total facility includes 52 beds in nursing home–type unit) (Nonreporting) **A**9 10 18
Primary Contact: Alfred N. Rossi, M.D., Chief Executive Officer
COO: Mark F. Rossi, Chief Operating Officer and General Counsel
Web address: www.hopedalemedicalcomplex.com
Control: Other not–for–profit (including NFP Corporation) **Service:** General Medical and Surgical

Staffed Beds: 77

JACKSONVILLE—Morgan County

★ **PASSAVANT AREA HOSPITAL (140058)**, 1600 West Walnut Street, Zip 62650–1136; tel. 217/245–9541, (Total facility includes 15 beds in nursing home–type unit) **A**1 2 9 10 19 20 **F**3 8 11 12 13 15 17 24 25 26 31 32 33 38 43 49 51 55 56 57 62 63 64 66 67 68 73 74 75 77 79 80 81 82 84 85 86 87 89 90 92 94 96 97 98 100 103 106 107 117 118 119 120 121 133 135 137 **P**6
Primary Contact: Chester A. Wynn, President and Chief Executive Officer
COO: Joanne K. Condi, Vice President and Chief Operating Officer
CFO: Larry Ragel, Vice President and Chief Financial Officer
CMO: James Hinchen, M.D., President Medical Staff
CIO: Marc Steinberg, Vice President Community Relations and Physician Recruitment
CHR: Rick Mogler, Director Human Resources
Web address: www.passavanthospital.com
Control: Other not–for–profit (including NFP Corporation) **Service:** General Medical and Surgical

Staffed Beds: 112 **Admissions:** 4044 **Census:** 50 **Outpatient Visits:** 82457 **Births:** 397 **Total Expense ($000):** 74380 **Payroll Expense ($000):** 31481 **Personnel:** 716

JERSEYVILLE—Jersey County

★ **JERSEY COMMUNITY HOSPITAL (140059)**, 400 Maple Summit Road, Zip 62052–2028, Mailing Address: P.O. Box 426, Zip 62052–0426; tel. 618/498–6402 **A**1 9 10 **F**3 7 8 11 13 15 24 25 27 28 30 31 32 33 34 36 38 51 52 54 55 56 57 59 60 62 63 66 67 68 72 73 74 75 76 77 79 80 82 84 86 96 97 100 107 114 117 118 119 120 121 122 124 132 135 136 137
Primary Contact: Lawrence P. Bear, Administrator
COO: Lawrence P. Bear, Administrator
CFO: David Kennett, Chief Financial Officer
CIO: Bob Bray, Chief Information Officer
Web address: www.jch.org
Control: Hospital district or authority, Government, nonfederal **Service:** General Medical and Surgical

Staffed Beds: 67 **Admissions:** 1883 **Census:** 17 **Outpatient Visits:** 66783 **Births:** 208 **Total Expense ($000):** 0 **Payroll Expense ($000):** 11027 **Personnel:** 281

JOLIET—Will County

★ △ **PROVENA SAINT JOSEPH MEDICAL CENTER (140007)**, 333 North Madison Street, Zip 60435–6595; tel. 815/725–7133 **A**1 2 3 5 7 9 10 **F**3 5 11 12 13 15 17 18 20 22 24 25 26 27 28 30 31 32 33 34 35 36 37 38 40 41 43 46 47 48 49 50 52 53 54 55 56 57 58 59 60 62 63 66 68 70 71 72 73 74 75 76 77 79 80 81 82 83 84 85 86 87 88 89 90 91 92 93 94 95 96 99 100 101 102 103 106 107 108 109 111 112 116 118 119 120 121 123 124 132 133 134 135 136 137 **P**8 **S** Provena Health
Primary Contact: Jeffrey Brickman, President and Chief Executive Officer
COO: Beth Hughes, Executive Vice President and Chief Operating Officer
CFO: Patricia Keel, Regional Chief Financial Officer
CMO: Lon McPherson, M.D., Vice President Medical Affairs
CIO: Dana Nylen, Director Medical Records
CHR: Edward Malindzak, Regional Vice President Human Resources
Web address: www.provenasaintjoe.org
Control: Church–operated, Nongovernment, not–for profit **Service:** General Medical and Surgical

Staffed Beds: 462 **Admissions:** 23894 **Census:** 297 **Outpatient Visits:** 479701 **Births:** 1923 **Total Expense ($000):** 302963 **Payroll Expense ($000):** 113211 **Personnel:** 2029

Many Facility Codes have changed. Please refer to the AHA Guide Code Chart.

☒ △ **SILVER CROSS HOSPITAL (140213)**, 1200 Maple Road, Zip 60432–1497; tel. 815/740–1100 **A**1 2 7 9 10 **F**5 7 11 12 13 15 18 20 24 25 26 27 28 30 31 32 33 35 36 38 40 41 43 49 50 52 55 56 57 59 61 62 66 68 72 73 74 75 76 77 79 80 84 85 86 88 90 91 92 93 94 95 96 97 100 102 103 106 107 119 120 121 123 124 135 136 137 **P**1 5
Primary Contact: Paul Pawlak, President and Chief Executive Officer
COO: Mary Bakken, Chief Operating Officer
CFO: William R. Brownlow, Senior Vice President Finance
CMO: Umesh Sharma, Chief of Staff
CIO: Matthew Ebaugh, Vice President Information Systems
CHR: Mark Jepson, Vice President
Web address: www.silvercross.org
Control: Other not–for–profit (including NFP Corporation) **Service:** General Medical and Surgical

Staffed Beds: 245 **Admissions:** 17010 **Census:** 174 **Outpatient Visits:** 186162 **Total Expense ($000):** 183407 **Payroll Expense ($000):** 68909 **Personnel:** 1116

KANKAKEE—Kankakee County

☒ **PROVENA ST. MARY'S HOSPITAL (140155)**, 500 West Court Street, Zip 60901–3661; tel. 815/937–2400 **A**1 2 9 10 **F**3 5 11 12 13 15 18 20 24 25 26 27 28 30 31 32 33 34 36 37 38 40 43 44 48 49 50 51 52 53 54 55 56 57 58 59 60 62 63 66 68 72 73 74 75 76 77 79 80 81 82 84 86 87 88 89 90 91 92 93 94 95 96 97 100 102 104 107 118 119 120 121 124 132 135 136 137 **P**7 **S** Provena Health
Primary Contact: Jeffrey Brickman, President and Chief Executive Officer
COO: Michael J. Arno, Executive Vice President and Chief Operating Officer
CFO: Patricia Keel, Regional Chief Financial Officer
CMO: Gary Plundo, D.O., Chief Medical Officer
CIO: Patricia Freeland, Director Information Systems
CHR: Edward Malindzak, Regional Vice President Human Resources
Web address: www.provena–stmarys.com
Control: Church–operated, Nongovernment, not–for profit **Service:** General Medical and Surgical

Staffed Beds: 143 **Admissions:** 7061 **Census:** 77 **Outpatient Visits:** 212781 **Births:** 398 **Total Expense ($000):** 115933 **Payroll Expense ($000):** 34001 **Personnel:** 724

☒ **RIVERSIDE MEDICAL CENTER (140186)**, 350 North Wall Street, Zip 60901–0749; tel. 815/933–1671 **A**1 2 5 9 10 **F**3 4 5 6 7 8 9 10 11 12 13 15 17 18 20 22 24 25 26 27 28 30 31 32 33 34 36 37 38 40 41 43 44 46 47 48 49 50 51 52 54 55 56 57 60 61 62 63 64 66 67 68 69 72 73 74 75 76 77 79 80 81 82 84 85 86 87 88 89 90 91 92 93 94 95 96 97 99 100 102 103 105 106 107 108 109 111 113 114 115 116 118 119 120 121 123 124 130 131 132 133 134 135 136 137 **P**6 7 8
Primary Contact: Phillip M. Kambic, Chief Executive Officer
COO: David Duda, Senior Vice President and Chief Nursing Officer
CFO: Bill Douglas, Chief Financial Officer
CMO: John Jurica, M.D., Vice President Medical Affairs
CIO: Wayne Kelsheimer, Corporate Director Information Systems
CHR: Becky Hinrichs, Vice President Human Resources
Web address: www.riversidehealthcare.org
Control: Other not–for–profit (including NFP Corporation) **Service:** General Medical and Surgical

Staffed Beds: 285 **Admissions:** 13786 **Census:** 178 **Outpatient Visits:** 329424 **Births:** 1300 **Total Expense ($000):** 185572 **Payroll Expense ($000):** 76780 **Personnel:** 1550

KEWANEE—Henry County

★ **KEWANEE HOSPITAL (141325)**, 1051 West South Street, Zip 61443–2711, Mailing Address: P.O. Box 747, Zip 61443–0747; tel. 309/852–7500 **A**9 10 18 **F**3 11 13 15 25 26 27 28 30 31 32 33 34 36 38 42 43 44 45 50 52 55 56 57 61 62 66 68 73 74 75 76 77 79 80 81 82 84 86 87 96 102 107 118 119 120 121 122 124 135 136 137 **P**6
Primary Contact: Margaret Gustafson, Chief Executive Officer
COO: Lynn Fulton, Chief Operating Officer
CFO: Jennifer Coombes, Chief Financial Officer
CMO: Julio Ramos, M.D., Chief of Staff
CIO: Rob Coombes, Network Administrator
CHR: Renee Salisbury, Executive Director Human Resources
Web address: www.kewaneehospital.com
Control: Other not–for–profit (including NFP Corporation) **Service:** General Medical and Surgical

Staffed Beds: 25 **Admissions:** 1231 **Census:** 11 **Outpatient Visits:** 39082 **Births:** 151 **Total Expense ($000):** 30807 **Payroll Expense ($000):** 12693 **Personnel:** 261

LA GRANGE—Cook County

☒ **ADVENTIST LA GRANGE MEMORIAL HOSPITAL (140065)**, 5101 South Willow Spring Road, Zip 60525–2680; tel. 708/245–9000 **A**1 2 3 5 9 10 **F**3 12 13 15 17 18 20 22 24 25 26 27 31 32 33 35 37 38 40 41 43 49 54 55 56 57 58 60 62 66 68 71 72 73 74 76 77 79 80 81 82 84 86 87 90 96 97 99 100 102 103 106 107 109 111 118 119 120 121 135 136 137 **P**7 8 **S** Adventist Health System Sunbelt Health Care Corporation
Primary Contact: Rick Wright, FACHE, CPA, Chief Executive Officer
COO: Edward Gervain, Chief Operating Officer
CFO: Paul Ziegele, Chief Financial Officer
CMO: Gary Lipinski, M.D., Regional Vice President and Chief Medical Officer
CIO: Russ Solimon, Chief Information Officer
CHR: Patty Sanchez, Site Manager Human Resources
Web address: www.keepingyouwell.com
Control: Church–operated, Nongovernment, not–for profit **Service:** General Medical and Surgical

Staffed Beds: 180 **Admissions:** 8654 **Census:** 109 **Outpatient Visits:** 117228 **Births:** 834 **Total Expense ($000):** 144236 **Payroll Expense ($000):** 51592 **Personnel:** 879

LAKE FOREST—Lake County

☒ **LAKE FOREST HOSPITAL (140130)**, 660 North Westmoreland Road, Zip 60045–1696; tel. 847/234–5600, (Total facility includes 68 beds in nursing home–type unit) **A**1 2 9 10 **F**2 3 9 11 12 13 15 18 20 24 25 26 27 28 30 31 32 33 34 35 37 38 40 41 43 44 49 50 51 52 53 54 55 56 57 61 62 68 69 71 72 73 74 75 76 77 79 80 81 82 84 86 87 96 97 99 100 102 103 104 105 106 107 109 111 113 117 118 119 120 121 124 133 135 136 137 **P**8
Primary Contact: Thomas J. McAfee, President
CFO: Matthew J. Flynn, Vice President and Chief Financial Officer
CMO: Michael Ankin, M.D., Vice President Medical Affairs
CHR: Marsha Oberrieder, Vice President
Web address: www.lfh.org
Control: Other not–for–profit (including NFP Corporation) **Service:** General Medical and Surgical

Staffed Beds: 205 **Admissions:** 9738 **Census:** 140 **Outpatient Visits:** 335254 **Births:** 2254 **Total Expense ($000):** 195001 **Payroll Expense ($000):** 80312 **Personnel:** 1289

LAWRENCEVILLE—Lawrence County

★ **LAWRENCE COUNTY MEMORIAL HOSPITAL (141344)**, 2200 West State Street, Zip 62439–1853; tel. 618/943–1000 **A**9 10 18 **F**3 7 11 15 17 24 26 31 38 57 68 73 79 86 88 93 96 119 121 122 132 135 **P**6 **S** QHR
Primary Contact: Doug Florkowski, Chief Executive Officer
CFO: Jerry Klein, Chief Financial Officer
CHR: Kim Kendall, Director Human Resources
Control: County–Government, nonfederal **Service:** General Medical and Surgical

Staffed Beds: 35 **Admissions:** 1061 **Census:** 12 **Outpatient Visits:** 18242 **Births:** 0 **Total Expense ($000):** 11389 **Payroll Expense ($000):** 4040 **Personnel:** 112

LIBERTYVILLE—Lake County

☒ **CONDELL MEDICAL CENTER (140202)**, 801 South Milwaukee Avenue on Condell Drive, Zip 60048–3199; tel. 847/362–2900 **A**1 2 10 **F**2 3 8 11 12 13 15 17 18 20 22 24 25 26 27 28 30 32 33 35 38 40 42 43 46 48 49 51 52 53 54 55 56 57 59 60 61 62 63 66 68 70 71 72 73 74 75 76 77 79 80 81 82 83 84 86 95 96 97 99 100 102 103 105 106 107 109 111 116 118 119 120 121 124 132 133 135 136 137 **P**1 5
Primary Contact: Dennis C. Millirons, FACHE, President and Chief Executive Officer
COO: Mark Pelletier, Senior Vice President and Chief Operating Officer
CFO: Andrew Stefo, Chief Financial Officer
CMO: Joan Boomsma, M.D., Vice President Medical Affairs and Chief Medical Officer
CIO: Michael Devore, Chief Information Officer
CHR: Gwenn Leschke, Vice President Human Resources
Web address: www.condell.org
Control: Other not–for–profit (including NFP Corporation) **Service:** General Medical and Surgical

Staffed Beds: 283 **Admissions:** 18226 **Census:** 199 **Outpatient Visits:** 639360 **Births:** 2353 **Total Expense ($000):** 294732 **Payroll Expense ($000):** 113605 **Personnel:** 2167

IL

Hospital, Medicare Provider Number, Address, Telephone, Approval, Facility, and Physician Codes, Health Care System
★ American Hospital Association (AHA) membership
□ The Joint Commission accreditation
○ American Osteopathic Association (AOA) accreditation
△ Commission on Accreditation of Rehabilitation Facilities (CARF) accreditation

LINCOLN—Logan County

★ **ABRAHAM LINCOLN MEMORIAL HOSPITAL (141322)**, 315 8th Street, Zip 62656–2698; tel. 217/732–2161 **A**1 5 9 10 18 **F**13 15 24 30 31 32 33 38 43 55 57 62 68 69 73 74 75 76 79 82 84 86 96 97 100 107 118 119 121 122 132 133 135 **P**5 **S** Memorial Health System
Primary Contact: Dolan Dalpoas, President and Chief Executive Officer
COO: Kathleen Vipond, Assistant Administrator and Director
CFO: Andrew Costic, Regional Chief Financial Officer
CMO: Thomas Zwilling, M.D., President Medical Staff
CHR: Holley Tygrett, Director Human Resources
Web address: www.almh.org
Control: Other not–for–profit (including NFP Corporation) **Service:** General Medical and Surgical

Staffed Beds: 25 **Admissions:** 1295 **Census:** 12 **Outpatient Visits:** 54012 **Births:** 253 **Total Expense ($000):** 32828 **Payroll Expense ($000):** 10583 **Personnel:** 248

LITCHFIELD—Montgomery County

★ **ST. FRANCIS HOSPITAL (141350)**, 1215 Franciscan Drive, Zip 62056–1799, Mailing Address: P.O. Box 1215, Zip 62056–1215; tel. 217/324–2191, (Total facility includes 11 beds in nursing home–type unit) **A**1 9 10 18 **F**11 12 13 15 24 25 26 30 33 34 38 41 43 46 50 54 55 56 57 62 66 68 72 73 74 75 76 77 79 80 81 82 86 96 100 106 107 117 118 119 120 121 122 124 135 136 137 **S** Hospital Sisters Health System
Primary Contact: Daniel L. Perryman, President and Chief Executive Officer
CFO: Diane Lindsay, Chief Financial Officer
Web address: www.stfrancis–litchfield.org
Control: Church–operated, Nongovernment, not–for profit **Service:** General Medical and Surgical

Staffed Beds: 36 **Admissions:** 2002 **Census:** 27 **Outpatient Visits:** 51805 **Births:** 339 **Total Expense ($000):** 28416 **Payroll Expense ($000):** 11014 **Personnel:** 234

MACOMB—McDonough County

★ **MCDONOUGH DISTRICT HOSPITAL (140089)**, 525 East Grant Street, Zip 61455–3318; tel. 309/833–4101, (Total facility includes 16 beds in nursing home–type unit) **A**1 2 9 10 20 **F**2 3 5 7 11 13 15 24 25 26 27 31 33 38 41 42 43 44 52 54 55 56 57 61 62 68 73 74 75 76 77 79 80 81 82 84 86 90 91 92 93 94 96 97 106 107 117 118 119 120 121 124 135 137 **P**6 7 8
Primary Contact: Stephen R. Hopper, President and Chief Executive Officer
COO: Lori Moon, Vice President Clinical Operations
CFO: Linda Dace, Vice President Finance
CMO: Michelle Reeves, M.D., President Medical Staff
CIO: Harlan T. Baker, Director Information Systems
CHR: Sue Dexter, Administrative Director Human Resources
Web address: www.mdh.org
Control: Hospital district or authority, Government, nonfederal **Service:** General Medical and Surgical

Staffed Beds: 91 **Admissions:** 3169 **Census:** 39 **Outpatient Visits:** 59643 **Births:** 378 **Total Expense ($000):** 46569 **Payroll Expense ($000):** 21045 **Personnel:** 460

MARION—Williamson County

★ **HEARTLAND REGIONAL MEDICAL CENTER (140184)**, 3333 West DeYoung, Zip 62959; tel. 618/998–7000 **A**1 10 **F**3 11 13 15 18 20 22 24 25 26 27 33 38 43 55 56 57 59 68 73 74 75 76 77 79 80 82 84 86 96 97 100 102 103 106 107 118 121 122 135 **P**4 6 **S** Community Health Systems, Inc.
Primary Contact: Timothy E. Schmidt, Chief Executive Officer
Web address: www.heartlandregional.com
Control: Corporation, Investor–owned, for–profit **Service:** General Medical and Surgical

Staffed Beds: 92 **Admissions:** 7101 **Census:** 66 **Outpatient Visits:** 74081 **Births:** 1100 **Total Expense ($000):** 78693 **Payroll Expense ($000):** 27681 **Personnel:** 456

★ **VETERANS AFFAIRS MEDICAL CENTER**, 2401 West Main Street, Zip 62959–1194; tel. 618/997–5311, (Total facility includes 60 beds in nursing home–type unit) (Nonreporting) **A**1 5 **S** Department of Veterans Affairs
Primary Contact: Robert D. Morrel, Director
CFO: Wayne Morris, Chief Financial Officer
CMO: Joseph Herman, M.D., Chief of Staff
CIO: Clint Bishop, Program Manager
CHR: Tonya Floyd, Manager Human Resources
Web address: www.va.gov/sta/guide/home.asp
Control: Veterans Affairs, Government, federal **Service:** General Medical and Surgical

Staffed Beds: 115

MARYVILLE—Madison County

★ △ **ANDERSON HOSPITAL (140289)**, 6800 State Route 162, Zip 62062–8500; tel. 618/288–5711 **A**1 7 9 10 **F**3 11 13 15 18 24 25 26 27 30 31 32 33 36 37 38 40 43 49 51 53 54 55 56 57 61 62 67 68 72 73 74 76 77 79 80 81 82 85 86 96 97 100 102 103 107 108 112 118 119 120 121 124 133 134 135 136 137
Primary Contact: Keith Allen Page, President and Chief Executive Officer
CFO: Michael Marshall, Vice President Finance and Chief Financial Officer
CMO: Rodney L. Greeling, D.O., President Medical Staff
CIO: Michael Ward, Director Information Services
CHR: Robin Steinmann, Administrative Director Human Resources
Web address: www.andersonhospital.org
Control: Other not–for–profit (including NFP Corporation) **Service:** General Medical and Surgical

Staffed Beds: 135 **Admissions:** 9695 **Census:** 91 **Outpatient Visits:** 134206 **Births:** 1782 **Total Expense ($000):** 90352 **Payroll Expense ($000):** 36635 **Personnel:** 797

MATTOON—Coles County

★ **SARAH BUSH LINCOLN HEALTH CENTER (140189)**, 1000 Health Center Drive, Zip 61938–0372, Mailing Address: P.O. Box 372, Zip 61938–0372; tel. 217/258–2525, (Total facility includes 13 beds in nursing home–type unit) **A**1 2 9 10 20 **F**2 3 11 13 15 18 24 25 26 27 28 30 32 33 34 36 37 38 41 42 43 47 48 49 50 53 54 55 56 57 60 61 62 63 64 66 68 69 72 73 74 75 76 77 79 80 81 82 84 86 87 88 90 91 92 93 94 95 96 97 99 100 102 103 107 108 109 111 117 118 119 120 121 123 134 135 136 137 **P**6
Primary Contact: Gary L. Barnett, President and Chief Executive Officer
COO: Dennis Pluard, Vice President Operations
CFO: Craig Sheagren, Vice President Finance
CMO: James Hildebrandt, D.O., President Medical Staff
CIO: Mike DeLuca, Vice President Information Systems
CHR: Eric Benson, Vice President Human Resources
Web address: www.sarahbush.org
Control: Other not–for–profit (including NFP Corporation) **Service:** General Medical and Surgical

Staffed Beds: 132 **Admissions:** 7424 **Census:** 72 **Outpatient Visits:** 377200 **Births:** 855 **Total Expense ($000):** 146208 **Payroll Expense ($000):** 71709 **Personnel:** 1234

MAYWOOD—Cook County

☐ △ **LOYOLA UNIVERSITY MEDICAL CENTER (140276)**, 2160 South First Avenue, Zip 60153–5585; tel. 708/216–9000 **A**1 2 3 5 7 8 9 10 **F**1 3 5 6 7 8 9 11 12 13 14 15 16 17 18 19 20 21 22 23 24 25 26 27 28 30 31 32 33 34 36 37 38 40 41 42 43 44 46 47 49 50 51 52 53 54 55 56 57 58 59 60 61 62 63 64 66 68 69 70 71 72 73 74 75 76 77 78 79 80 81 82 83 84 85 86 87 88 89 90 91 92 93 94 96 97 99 100 102 103 104 106 107 109 111 112 114 116 118 119 120 121 123 124 125 126 127 128 129 130 131 133 134 135 136 137 **P**3
Primary Contact: Paul K. Whelton, M.D., President and Chief Executive Officer
COO: Martin Massiello, Executive Vice President
CFO: Michael Scheer, Senior Vice President, Chief Financial Officer and Treasurer
CMO: William Dannon, M.D., Chief of Staff
CIO: Arthur J. Krumrey, Chief Information Officer
CHR: Vicky Piper, Vice President Human Resources
Web address: www.lumc.edu
Control: Other not–for–profit (including NFP Corporation) **Service:** General Medical and Surgical

Staffed Beds: 507 **Admissions:** 25650 **Census:** 366 **Outpatient Visits:** 1100961 **Births:** 1563 **Total Expense ($000):** 669743 **Payroll Expense ($000):** 273152 **Personnel:** 5463

MCHENRY—McHenry County

★ **CENTEGRA NORTHERN ILLINOIS MEDICAL CENTER (140116)**, 4201 Medical Center Drive, Zip 60050–9506; tel. 815/344–5000 **A**1 2 3 5 9 10 **F**3 11 13 15 18 20 22 24 25 26 27 30 31 32 33 36 38 40 41 42 43 44 47 49 50 55 56 57 62 66 67 68 72 73 74 75 76 77 79 80 81 82 84 85 86 96 97 99 100 102 106 107 109 111 112 119 121 132 135 136 137 **P**5 **S** Centegra Health System
Primary Contact: Michael S. Eesley, President and Chief Executive Officer
COO: Jason Sciarro, Chief Operating Officer
CFO: Robert Rosenberger, Chief Financial Officer
CMO: Ted Lorenc, M.D., Vice President Medical Affairs
CIO: Paul Solverson, Director Information Systems
CHR: Barbara Jo Johnson, Senior Vice President Human Resources
Web address: www.centegra.org
Control: Other not–for–profit (including NFP Corporation) **Service:** General Medical and Surgical

Staffed Beds: 156 **Admissions:** 10854 **Census:** 116 **Outpatient Visits:** 124980 **Births:** 854 **Total Expense ($000):** 178989 **Payroll Expense ($000):** 76487 **Personnel:** 1108

IL

Many Facility Codes have changed. Please refer to the AHA Guide Code Chart.

MCLEANSBORO—Hamilton County

HAMILTON MEMORIAL HOSPITAL DISTRICT (141326), 611 South Marshall Avenue, Zip 62859–0429; tel. 618/643–2361, (Total facility includes 60 beds in nursing home–type unit) **A**9 10 18 **F**11 15 25 31 38 40 55 61 62 65 79 84 86 96 97 102 107 119 122
Primary Contact: Randall W. Dauby, Chief Executive Officer
COO: Bradley Futrell, Chief Operating Officer
CFO: Kent Mitchell, Chief Financial Officer
Web address: www.hmhospital.org
Control: Hospital district or authority, Government, nonfederal **Service:** General Medical and Surgical

Staffed Beds: 85 **Admissions:** 1107 **Census:** 68 **Outpatient Visits:** 27693 **Births:** 0 **Total Expense ($000):** 11020 **Payroll Expense ($000):** 5878 **Personnel:** 186

MELROSE PARK—Cook County

★□ **GOTTLIEB MEMORIAL HOSPITAL (140008)**, 701 West North Avenue, Zip 60160–1692; tel. 708/681–3200, (Total facility includes 32 beds in nursing home–type unit) **A**1 9 10 **F**2 3 4 8 9 11 12 13 15 18 20 22 24 25 26 27 30 31 32 33 36 38 40 41 42 43 44 50 54 55 56 57 58 60 61 62 63 66 68 70 71 72 73 74 75 76 77 79 80 81 82 84 86 93 96 97 100 102 106 107 117 118 119 120 121 132 135 136 137 **P**8
Primary Contact: John Morgan, President
CFO: Andrew Knauf, Vice President Finance
CMO: Brian Proctor, D.O., President Medical Staff
CIO: Maurita Adler, Director Information Services
CHR: Brett Wakefield, Vice President Human Resources
Web address: www.gottliebhospital.org
Control: Other not–for–profit (including NFP Corporation) **Service:** General Medical and Surgical

Staffed Beds: 266 **Admissions:** 8883 **Census:** 140 **Outpatient Visits:** 155485 **Births:** 573 **Total Expense ($000):** 123267 **Payroll Expense ($000):** 53716 **Personnel:** 830

○ △ **WESTLAKE HOSPITAL (140240)**, 1225 Lake Street, Zip 60160–4000; tel. 708/681–3000 **A**3 5 7 9 10 11 **F**3 8 13 15 17 18 20 22 25 26 27 30 31 32 33 38 43 46 49 50 52 53 54 55 56 57 62 64 66 68 71 72 73 74 76 77 79 80 81 82 84 85 86 87 88 90 92 96 97 99 100 103 106 107 118 119 120 121 123 135 136 137 **P**5 6 **S** Resurrection Health Care
Primary Contact: Patricia Shehorn, Chief Executive Officer
CFO: Thomas Capobianco, Chief Financial Officer
CIO: George Chessum, Chief Information Officer
Web address: www.reshealth.org
Control: Church–operated, Nongovernment, not–for profit **Service:** General Medical and Surgical

Staffed Beds: 181 **Admissions:** 7824 **Census:** 110 **Outpatient Visits:** 21037 **Births:** 1383 **Total Expense ($000):** 108536 **Payroll Expense ($000):** 35465 **Personnel:** 639

MENDOTA—La Salle County

★□ **MENDOTA COMMUNITY HOSPITAL (141310)**, 1315 Memorial Drive, Zip 61342–1496; tel. 815/539–7461 **A**1 9 10 18 **F**3 11 15 24 25 27 30 31 32 33 38 49 55 56 57 61 62 67 68 73 75 79 80 81 82 86 96 102 118 119 121 122 134 135 **P**6
Primary Contact: Lynn E. Klein, Administrator
CFO: Larry Peach, Assistant Administrator and Chief Financial Officer
CMO: David Scholl, M.D., President Medical Staff
CIO: Gilbert Hermosillo, Manager Information Services
CHR: Kimberly Kennedy, Manager Human Resources
Web address: www.mendotahospital.org
Control: Other not–for–profit (including NFP Corporation) **Service:** General Medical and Surgical

Staffed Beds: 25 **Admissions:** 1517 **Census:** 18 **Outpatient Visits:** 46429 **Births:** 0 **Total Expense ($000):** 24417 **Payroll Expense ($000):** 10432 **Personnel:** 226

METROPOLIS—Massac County

★ **MASSAC MEMORIAL HOSPITAL (141323)**, 28 Chick Street, Zip 62960, Mailing Address: P.O. Box 850, Zip 62960–0850; tel. 618/524–2176 **A**9 10 18 **F**3 7 15 24 25 26 31 32 33 38 55 56 57 62 73 79 84 86 87 96 97 100 102 107 118 122 **P**5
Primary Contact: Sharon Mumford, RN, M.S.N., Chief Executive Officer
COO: Melanie Koch, Chief Clinical Officer
CFO: Chelle Keplinger, Chief Financial Officer
CHR: Joel Foster, Director Human Resources
Web address: www.massachealth.com
Control: Hospital district or authority, Government, nonfederal **Service:** General Medical and Surgical

Staffed Beds: 25 **Admissions:** 1022 **Census:** 10 **Outpatient Visits:** 23056 **Births:** 0 **Total Expense ($000):** 16836 **Payroll Expense ($000):** 7213 **Personnel:** 153

MOLINE—Rock Island County

TRINITY MEDICAL CENTER–SEVENTH STREET See Trinity Medical Center–West, Rock Island

MONMOUTH—Warren County

OSF HOLY FAMILY MEDICAL CENTER (141318), (Formerly Community Medical Center at Western Illinois), 1000 West Harlem Avenue, Zip 61462–1099; tel. 309/734–3141, (Total facility includes 45 beds in nursing home–type unit) **A**9 10 18 **F**11 15 24 25 26 30 31 32 33 34 38 42 43 46 54 55 56 57 62 63 65 73 75 77 79 80 82 86 87 96 97 100 103 106 107 117 119 121 122 124 134 135 137 **P**6
Primary Contact: Donald G. Brown, Chief Executive Officer
CFO: Theresa Springer, Vice President Finance
CMO: James R. Battenburg, M.D., President Medical Staff
CIO: Lew McCann, Director Management Information Systems
CHR: Irene Kress, Director Human Resources
Web address: www.osfholyfamily.org
Control: Church–operated, Nongovernment, not–for profit **Service:** General Medical and Surgical

Staffed Beds: 68 **Admissions:** 443 **Census:** 41 **Outpatient Visits:** 23079 **Births:** 0 **Total Expense ($000):** 10009 **Payroll Expense ($000):** 4896 **Personnel:** 224

MONTICELLO—Piatt County

★□ **JOHN AND MARY KIRBY HOSPITAL (141301)**, 1111 North State Street, Zip 61856–1116; tel. 217/762–2115, (Nonreporting) **A**1 9 10 18
Primary Contact: Steve Tenhouse, Chief Executive Officer
CFO: C. David Harms, Chief Financial Officer
CMO: Narain Mandhan, M.D., President Medical Staff
CIO: Rocky Winterbottom, Chief Information Officer
Web address: www.kirbyhospital.org
Control: Other not–for–profit (including NFP Corporation) **Service:** General Medical and Surgical

Staffed Beds: 21

MORRIS—Grundy County

★□ **MORRIS HOSPITAL & HEALTHCARE CENTERS (140101)**, 150 West High Street, Zip 60450–1497; tel. 815/942–2932 **A**1 2 9 10 **F**3 11 13 15 18 20 24 31 32 38 40 47 49 50 53 55 56 57 62 64 67 68 72 73 74 75 76 77 79 80 81 82 84 86 92 96 97 100 102 103 106 107 109 111 119 121 122 124 132 135 **P**6
Primary Contact: Clifford L. Corbett, President and Chief Executive Officer
CFO: Tom Meyer, Vice President Finance
Web address: www.morrishospital.org
Control: Other not–for–profit (including NFP Corporation) **Service:** General Medical and Surgical

Staffed Beds: 86 **Admissions:** 4839 **Census:** 45 **Outpatient Visits:** 205314 **Births:** 694 **Total Expense ($000):** 85686 **Payroll Expense ($000):** 36467 **Personnel:** 602

MORRISON—Whiteside County

★ **MORRISON COMMUNITY HOSPITAL (141329)**, 303 North Jackson Street, Zip 61270–3042; tel. 815/772–4003, (Total facility includes 35 beds in nursing home–type unit) (Nonreporting) **A**9 10 18 **S** Trinity Health
Primary Contact: John R. Perushek, Chief Executive Officer
COO: Pam Pfister, Chief Operating Officer
CMO: Duncan Dinkha, M.D., Chief of Staff
CIO: Pam Pfister, Chief Operating Officer
CHR: Pam Pfister, Chief Operating Officer
Control: Hospital district or authority, Government, nonfederal **Service:** General Medical and Surgical

Staffed Beds: 60

IL

Hospital, Medicare Provider Number, Address, Telephone, Approval, Facility, and Physician Codes, Health Care System
★ American Hospital Association (AHA) membership
□ The Joint Commission accreditation
○ American Osteopathic Association (AOA) accreditation
△ Commission on Accreditation of Rehabilitation Facilities (CARF) accreditation

MOUNT CARMEL—Wabash County

★ **WABASH GENERAL HOSPITAL DISTRICT (141327)**, 1418 College Drive, Zip 62863–2638; tel. 618/262–8621, (Nonreporting) **A**1 9 10 18 **S** Alliant Management Services
Primary Contact: Jay Purvis, Administrator
CFO: Steve McGill, Chief Financial Officer
Web address: www.wabashgeneral.com
Control: Hospital district or authority, Government, nonfederal **Service:** General Medical and Surgical

Staffed Beds: 25

MOUNT VERNON—Jefferson County

★ **CROSSROADS COMMUNITY HOSPITAL (140294)**, 8 Doctors Park Road, Zip 62864–6224; tel. 618/244–5500 **A**1 9 10 **F**3 8 11 15 25 26 30 31 33 38 42 51 52 53 54 55 56 57 61 62 66 68 72 73 75 77 79 80 86 96 97 102 107 118 122 135 136 **S** Community Health Systems, Inc.
Primary Contact: M. Edward Cunningham, Chief Executive Officer
CFO: Brian Schneider, Chief Financial Officer
CMO: Norman Cohen, M.D., Chief Medical Officer
CIO: Regina Garrett, Director Health Information Management
CHR: Reva Weems, Director Human Resources
Web address: www.crossroadscommunityhospital.com
Control: Corporation, Investor–owned, for–profit **Service:** General Medical and Surgical

Staffed Beds: 41 **Admissions:** 1828 **Census:** 19 **Outpatient Visits:** 102108 **Births:** 0 **Total Expense ($000):** 30281 **Payroll Expense ($000):** 13301 **Personnel:** 211

★ **GOOD SAMARITAN REGIONAL HEALTH CENTER (140046)**, 605 North 12th Street, Zip 62864–2899; tel. 618/242–4600 **A**1 2 9 10 19 **F**3 11 13 15 18 20 22 24 25 26 27 30 31 32 33 36 37 38 41 42 43 44 50 53 55 56 57 60 61 62 66 68 72 73 74 75 76 77 79 80 81 82 84 85 86 96 97 100 102 106 107 118 119 121 124 134 135 136 137 **P**6 8 **S** SSM Health Care
Primary Contact: Leo F. Childers, Jr., FACHE, President
COO: Wayne Grote, Vice President Operations
CFO: Kay Tinsley, Vice President Fiscal Services
CMO: Daniel Hoffman, M.D., Administrative Medical Director
CIO: Steve Murphy, Director Networks
CHR: Thomas Blythe, Vice President Human Resources
Web address: www.smgsi.com
Control: Church–operated, Nongovernment, not–for profit **Service:** General Medical and Surgical

Staffed Beds: 139 **Admissions:** 7965 **Census:** 89 **Outpatient Visits:** 91254 **Births:** 781 **Total Expense ($000):** 102492 **Payroll Expense ($000):** 36421 **Personnel:** 883

MURPHYSBORO—Jackson County

★ **ST. JOSEPH MEMORIAL HOSPITAL (141334)**, 2 South Hospital Drive, Zip 62966–3333; tel. 618/684–3156 **A**9 10 18 **F**3 11 15 24 25 26 30 31 32 33 38 50 54 55 56 57 62 73 75 76 77 79 80 81 86 96 102 107 118 119 121 122 124 135 136 **S** Southern Illinois Hospital Services
Primary Contact: Scott Seaborn, Administrator
CFO: Rex P. Budde, Senior Vice President and Chief Financial Officer
CMO: Terry N. Brown, M.D., President Medical Staff
CIO: Frank Sears, Vice President Information Services
CHR: Kelly Stevens, Manager Human Resources
Web address: www.sih.net
Control: Other not–for–profit (including NFP Corporation) **Service:** General Medical and Surgical

Staffed Beds: 25 **Admissions:** 1190 **Census:** 12 **Outpatient Visits:** 28422 **Births:** 0 **Total Expense ($000):** 23304 **Payroll Expense ($000):** 9222 **Personnel:** 199

IL

NAPERVILLE—Du Page County

★ **EDWARD HOSPITAL (140231)**, 801 South Washington Street, Zip 60540–7499; tel. 630/527–3000 **A**1 2 9 10 **F**3 13 15 17 18 20 22 24 25 26 27 28 30 31 32 33 35 36 38 40 43 44 49 50 53 55 56 57 60 61 62 66 68 70 71 72 73 74 75 76 77 79 80 81 82 83 84 86 87 92 96 97 98 99 100 102 103 104 105 106 107 108 109 111 112 118 119 120 121 124 133 135 136 137 **P**6 7 8
Primary Contact: Pamela Meyer Davis, President and Chief Executive Officer
COO: Trish Anen, Vice President Operations and Nursing
CFO: John P. Mordach, Senior Vice President and Chief Financial Officer
CMO: Alan Kaplan, M.D., Vice President and Chief Medical Officer
CHR: Maggie Shontz, Vice President Human Resources
Web address: www.edward.org
Control: Other not–for–profit (including NFP Corporation) **Service:** General Medical and Surgical

Staffed Beds: 301 **Admissions:** 22803 **Census:** 237 **Outpatient Visits:** 492526 **Births:** 4121 **Total Expense ($000):** 418338 **Payroll Expense ($000):** 140900 **Personnel:** 2445

★ **LINDEN OAKS HOSPITAL AT EDWARD (144035)**, 852 West Street, Zip 60540–6400; tel. 630/305–5500 **A**1 5 9 10 **F**4 5 25 26 30 31 32 33 36 54 55 56 57 62 66 73 82 88 89 90 91 93 94 95 119 121 123 **P**6
Primary Contact: Mary Lou Mastro, Chief Executive Officer
COO: Paul M. Teodo, Chief Operating Officer
CFO: Gina Sharp, Controller
CMO: Barry Rabin, M.D., Medical Director
CIO: Hugh Siddiqui, System Specialist
CHR: Maggie Shontz, Vice President Human Resources
Web address: www.edward.org
Control: Other not–for–profit (including NFP Corporation) **Service:** Psychiatric

Staffed Beds: 96 **Admissions:** 3376 **Census:** 65 **Outpatient Visits:** 26902 **Births:** 0 **Total Expense ($000):** 27537 **Payroll Expense ($000):** 14377 **Personnel:** 309

NASHVILLE—Washington County

★ **WASHINGTON COUNTY HOSPITAL (141308)**, 705 South Grand Avenue, Zip 62263–1534; tel. 618/327–8236, (Total facility includes 33 beds in nursing home–type unit) **A**1 9 10 18 **F**8 11 13 15 24 25 27 30 31 32 33 38 49 54 55 56 57 63 73 74 75 76 77 79 80 81 86 92 96 97 100 104 107 110 117 122 124 136 137 **P**5
Primary Contact: Nancy M. Newby, Ph.D., President and Chief Executive Officer
CFO: Elaine Matzenbacher, Chief Financial Officer
CMO: Marc Zerbe, M.D., President Medical Staff
CIO: Kim Larkin, Chief Information Officer
CHR: Melodie Wilkey, Director Human Resources
Web address: www.washingtoncountyhospital.org
Control: Hospital district or authority, Government, nonfederal **Service:** General Medical and Surgical

Staffed Beds: 58 **Admissions:** 359 **Census:** 33 **Outpatient Visits:** 38501 **Births:** 28 **Total Expense ($000):** 11938 **Payroll Expense ($000):** 5939 **Personnel:** 140

NORMAL—McLean County

★ **BROMENN HEALTHCARE SYSTEM (140127)**, 1304 Franklin Avenue, Zip 61761, Mailing Address: P.O. Box 2850, Bloomington, Zip 61702–2850; tel. 309/454–1400, (Includes BROMENN REGIONAL MEDICAL CENTER, tel. 309/454–1400) **A**1 2 9 10 12 13 **F**2 3 4 5 11 13 15 17 18 20 22 24 25 26 27 28 30 31 32 33 36 38 40 41 42 43 44 49 50 54 55 56 57 60 61 62 63 64 66 68 69 72 73 74 75 76 77 79 80 81 82 84 85 86 87 88 90 91 92 93 96 97 100 102 103 106 107 119 120 121 123 124 135 136 137 **P**8
Primary Contact: Roger S. Hunt, Chief Executive Officer
COO: Gary Hagens, Chief Operating Officer and Vice President Medical Affairs
CFO: Penny Cermak, Vice President and Chief Financial Officer
CMO: Gary Hagens, Vice President Medical Affairs and Chief Operating Officer
CHR: Alex Horvath, Vice President Human Resources
Web address: www.bromenn.org
Control: Church–operated, Nongovernment, not–for profit **Service:** General Medical and Surgical

Staffed Beds: 213 **Admissions:** 10119 **Census:** 115 **Outpatient Visits:** 177900 **Births:** 1754 **Total Expense ($000):** 158736 **Payroll Expense ($000):** 59861 **Personnel:** 1201

NORTH CHICAGO—Lake County

★ △ **VETERANS AFFAIRS MEDICAL CENTER**, 3001 Green Bay Road, Zip 60064–3049; tel. 847/688–1900, (Total facility includes 180 beds in nursing home–type unit) **A**1 3 5 7 **F**1 3 5 8 11 15 24 26 27 32 33 36 37 38 42 43 44 49 50 53 54 55 56 57 58 59 60 61 62 63 66 68 72 73 75 76 77 79 80 81 82 86 87 88 90 91 92 93 94 95 96 97 100 102 103 117 118 119 121 124 132 135 136 137 **P**6 **S** Department of Veterans Affairs
Primary Contact: Patrick L. Sullivan, Director
COO: Marianne Semrad, Associate Director Administrative Services
CMO: Tariq Hassan, M.D., Chief of Staff
CIO: Bradford P. Nystrom, Chief Informatics Program
CHR: Wayne Davis, Chief Human Resources
Web address: www.va.gov/sta/guide/home.asp
Control: Veterans Affairs, Government, federal **Service:** General Medical and Surgical

Staffed Beds: 103 **Admissions:** 4584 **Census:** 331 **Outpatient Visits:** 242520 **Births:** 0 **Total Expense ($000):** 164258 **Payroll Expense ($000):** 79152

NORTHLAKE—Cook County

☐ **KINDRED HOSPITAL CHICAGO NORTHLAKE (142008)**, 365 East North Avenue, Zip 60164–2628; tel. 708/345–8100, (Nonreporting) **A**1 9 10 **S** Kindred Healthcare
Primary Contact: Timothy Page, Chief Executive Officer
COO: Sandra Buckhoy, Chief Clinical Officer
CFO: Jay Schweikart, Chief Financial Officer
CMO: Maher Najjar, M.D., Medical Director
Web address: www.kindredhealthcare.com
Control: Corporation, Investor–owned, for–profit **Service:** Long–Term Acute Care hospital

Staffed Beds: 86

Many Facility Codes have changed. Please refer to the AHA Guide Code Chart.

OAK FOREST—Cook County

★□ △ **OAK FOREST HOSPITAL OF COOK COUNTY (140301)**, 15900 South Cicero Avenue, Zip 60452–4006; tel. 708/687–7200, (Total facility includes 340 beds in nursing home–type unit) **A**1 3 5 7 9 10 **F**3 25 26 27 33 34 37 38 43 44 54 60 62 63 65 66 68 72 75 76 77 79 82 85 86 87 90 96 107 117 119 121 124 132 133 135 137 **P**6 **S** Cook County Bureau of Health Services
Primary Contact: Sylvia Edwards, Chief Operating Officer
CMO: Judith Frigo, M.D., Medical Director
CIO: Jet Boulware, Director Information and Technology Services
CHR: Lori Jordan, Director Human Resources Services
Web address: www.cookcountygov.com
Control: County–Government, nonfederal **Service:** General Medical and Surgical

Staffed Beds: 456 **Admissions:** 2972 **Census:** 192 **Outpatient Visits:** 89963 **Births:** 0 **Total Expense ($000):** 115999 **Payroll Expense ($000):** 72305 **Personnel:** 995

OAK LAWN—Cook County

★□ △ **ADVOCATE CHRIST MEDICAL CENTER (140208)**, 4440 West 95th Street, Zip 60453–2699; tel. 708/684–8000, (Includes ADVOCATE HOPE CHILDREN'S HOSPITAL) **A**1 2 3 5 7 8 9 10 12 13 **F**8 11 13 14 15 17 18 19 20 21 22 23 24 25 26 27 28 29 30 31 32 33 34 35 36 38 40 43 44 45 46 48 49 54 55 56 57 59 66 67 68 69 70 72 73 74 75 76 77 79 83 84 85 86 88 89 90 91 92 93 94 95 96 97 98 99 100 102 103 106 107 108 109 111 112 114 116 118 119 121 124 126 135 136 137 **S** Advocate Health Care
Primary Contact: Kenneth W. Lukhard, President
CFO: Robert Pekofske, Vice President Finance
CMO: Robert Stein, M.D., Vice President Medical Management
CIO: Brian Banbury, Site Manager Information Technology
Web address: www.advocatehealth.com/christ
Control: Church–operated, Nongovernment, not–for profit **Service:** General Medical and Surgical

Staffed Beds: 678 **Admissions:** 40416 **Census:** 565 **Outpatient Visits:** 325985 **Births:** 4236 **Total Expense ($000):** 670025 **Payroll Expense ($000):** 246719 **Personnel:** 5368

OAK PARK—Cook County

★□ △ **RUSH OAK PARK HOSPITAL (140063)**, 520 South Maple Avenue, Zip 60304–1097; tel. 708/383–9300, (Total facility includes 36 beds in nursing home–type unit) **A**1 5 7 9 10 **F**3 15 18 25 26 30 31 32 33 38 42 43 47 49 50 54 55 56 57 59 62 66 68 72 73 75 77 79 80 81 82 85 86 87 96 97 100 102 106 107 117 119 135 137 **P**5 8 **S** Wheaton Franciscan Healthcare
Primary Contact: Bruce M. Elegant, President and Chief Executive Officer
COO: James Kaese, Vice President Administration
CFO: Deborah Wilberding, Controller
CMO: Michael R. Silver, M.D., Vice President Medical Affairs
CIO: Dewey Gosnell, Manager
CHR: Cristina Diaz, Director
Web address: www.roph.org
Control: Church–operated, Nongovernment, not–for profit **Service:** General Medical and Surgical

Staffed Beds: 177 **Admissions:** 4318 **Census:** 78 **Outpatient Visits:** 93499 **Births:** 0 **Total Expense ($000):** 82883 **Payroll Expense ($000):** 38784 **Personnel:** 752

○ **WEST SUBURBAN MEDICAL CENTER (140049)**, 3 Erie Court, Zip 60302–2599; tel. 708/383–6200, (Nonreporting) **A**2 3 5 9 10 11 12 13 **S** Resurrection Health Care
Primary Contact: Jay E. Kreuzer, FACHE, President and Chief Executive Officer
COO: Joan Ormsby, Senior Vice President and Chief Operating Officer
CFO: Thomas Capobianco, Chief Financial Officer
CMO: Kevin Cullinane, M.D., President Medical Staff
CIO: George Chessum, Chief Information Officer
CHR: Cliff Van Dyke, Director Human Resources
Web address: www.wsmc.reshealth.org
Control: Other not–for–profit (including NFP Corporation) **Service:** General Medical and Surgical

Staffed Beds: 152

OLNEY—Richland County

★□ **RICHLAND MEMORIAL HOSPITAL (140147)**, 800 East Locust Street, Zip 62450–2553; tel. 618/395–2131, (Total facility includes 34 beds in nursing home–type unit) (Nonreporting) **A**1 9 10
Primary Contact: David B. Allen, Interim Chief Executive Officer
CFO: David B. Allen, Executive Director Fiscal and Support Services
CMO: Robert Nash, M.D., Chief of Staff
CIO: Tim Gillespie, Manager Information Systems
CHR: Jill Van Hyning, Director Human Resources
Web address: www.richlandmemorial.com
Control: Other not–for–profit (including NFP Corporation) **Service:** General Medical and Surgical

Staffed Beds: 112

OLYMPIA FIELDS—Cook County

○ **ST. JAMES HOSPITAL AND HEALTH CENTERS (140172)**, (Includes ST. JAMES HOSPITAL AND HEALTH CENTERS – CHICAGO HEIGHTS CAMPUS, 1423 Chicago Road, Chicago Heights, Zip 60411–3483; tel. 708/756–1000; ST. JAMES HOSPITALS AND HEALTH CENTERS – OLYMPIA FIELDS CAMPUS, 20201 South Crawford Avenue, Zip 60461–1080; tel. 708/747–4000), (Nonreporting) **A**9 10 11 12 13 **S** Sisters of St. Francis Health Services, Inc.
Primary Contact: Seth C. R. Warren, President
CIO: Stephen Maes, Director Information Systems
Web address: www.stjameshhc.org
Control: Other not–for–profit (including NFP Corporation) **Service:** General Medical and Surgical

Staffed Beds: 494

OTTAWA—La Salle County

★□ **OTTAWA REGIONAL HOSPITAL AND HEALTHCARE CENTER (140110)**, (Formerly Community Hospital of Ottawa), 1100 East Norris Drive, Zip 61350–1687; tel. 815/433–3100 **A**1 9 10 19 **F**2 3 11 13 15 24 26 27 31 33 34 36 38 40 42 43 44 46 49 52 54 55 56 57 61 66 68 72 73 74 75 76 77 79 80 81 82 84 86 88 89 90 91 92 93 94 95 96 97 99 102 106 107 119 120 121 124 132 135 136 137
Primary Contact: Robert A. Chaffin, President and Chief Executive Officer
COO: Judy A. Christiansen, R.N., Chief Operating Officer
CMO: Robert B. Maguire, M.D., President Medical Staff
CIO: John Maynard, Director Information Systems
CHR: Robert Gibson, Senior Director Operating Services
Web address: www.ottawaregional.org
Control: Other not–for–profit (including NFP Corporation) **Service:** General Medical and Surgical

Staffed Beds: 113 **Admissions:** 4217 **Census:** 41 **Outpatient Visits:** 185978 **Births:** 298 **Total Expense ($000):** 61298 **Payroll Expense ($000):** 25413 **Personnel:** 524

PALOS HEIGHTS—Cook County

★□ **PALOS COMMUNITY HOSPITAL (140062)**, 12251 South 80th Avenue, Zip 60463–0930; tel. 708/923–4000 **A**1 2 9 10 **F**3 4 5 13 15 17 18 20 22 24 25 26 27 28 30 31 32 33 34 36 38 42 49 53 54 55 56 57 60 61 62 67 68 72 73 74 76 77 79 80 82 84 86 88 89 90 92 93 94 95 96 97 99 102 106 107 119 121 124 133 135 137
Primary Contact: Sister Margaret Wright, President
CFO: Hugh Rose, Vice President Fiscal Management
CIO: Peggy Carroll, Chief Information Officer
CHR: Mary Denisienko, Vice President Human Resources
Web address: www.paloscommunityhospital.org
Control: Other not–for–profit (including NFP Corporation) **Service:** General Medical and Surgical

Staffed Beds: 369 **Admissions:** 20950 **Census:** 253 **Outpatient Visits:** 422907 **Births:** 1673 **Total Expense ($000):** 286999 **Payroll Expense ($000):** 148404 **Personnel:** 2137

PANA—Christian County

★ **PANA COMMUNITY HOSPITAL (141341)**, 101 East Ninth Street, Zip 62557–1785; tel. 217/562–2131, (Nonreporting) **A**9 10 18
Primary Contact: Roland R. Carlson, President and Chief Executive Officer
CFO: Trina Casner, Chief Financial Officer
Web address: www.panahospital.com
Control: Other not–for–profit (including NFP Corporation) **Service:** General Medical and Surgical

Staffed Beds: 25

IL

Hospital, Medicare Provider Number, Address, Telephone, Approval, Facility, and Physician Codes, Health Care System

★ American Hospital Association (AHA) membership
□ The Joint Commission accreditation
○ American Osteopathic Association (AOA) accreditation
△ Commission on Accreditation of Rehabilitation Facilities (CARF) accreditation

PARIS—Edgar County

★ **PARIS COMMUNITY HOSPITAL (141320)**, 721 East Court Street, Zip 61944–2420; tel. 217/465–4141 **A**1 9 10 18 **F**3 15 24 25 26 27 31 32 33 38 43 55 57 62 63 65 67 72 73 75 76 79 80 82 84 85 86 96 97 102 107 117 119 120 121 122 124 135 137 **P**6 **S** Alliant Management Services
Primary Contact: Randy Simmons, President and Chief Executive Officer
CFO: Terry Brinkley, Vice President Finance
CIO: Gary Taylor, Manager Information Services
CHR: Ollie Smith, Vice President Human Resources
Web address: www.pariscommunityhospital.com
Control: Other not–for–profit (including NFP Corporation) **Service:** General Medical and Surgical

Staffed Beds: 25 **Admissions:** 688 **Census:** 19 **Outpatient Visits:** 97636 **Births:** 0 **Total Expense ($000):** 26781 **Payroll Expense ($000):** 12552 **Personnel:** 215

PARK RIDGE—Cook County

★ △ **ADVOCATE LUTHERAN GENERAL HOSPITAL (140223)**, 1775 Dempster Street, Zip 60068–1174; tel. 847/723–2210 **A**1 2 3 5 7 8 9 10 12 13 **F**2 3 5 6 8 9 11 12 13 14 15 17 18 19 20 21 22 23 24 25 26 27 28 29 30 31 32 33 34 35 36 37 38 40 41 42 43 44 46 47 49 50 51 52 53 54 55 56 57 58 59 60 62 63 64 66 67 68 70 72 73 74 76 77 78 79 80 81 82 83 84 85 86 87 88 89 90 91 92 93 94 95 96 97 99 100 101 102 103 104 105 106 107 108 109 111 112 114 116 118 119 120 121 123 124 125 130 132 133 134 135 136 137 **P**6 8 **S** Advocate Health Care
Primary Contact: Bruce C. Campbell, President
COO: Julie W. Schaffner, R.N., Chief Operating Officer and Chief Nurse Executive
CFO: Susan Nibbe, Vice President Finance
CMO: Kris Narasimhan, M.D., Vice President Medical Management
CHR: Penny Pilarczyk, Vice President Human Resources
Web address: www.advocatehealth.com
Control: Other not–for–profit (including NFP Corporation) **Service:** General Medical and Surgical

Staffed Beds: 584 **Admissions:** 28075 **Census:** 403 **Outpatient Visits:** 294789 **Births:** 3713 **Total Expense ($000):** 519643 **Payroll Expense ($000):** 196092 **Personnel:** 3297

PEKIN—Tazewell County

★ **PEKIN HOSPITAL (140120)**, 600 South 13th Street, Zip 61554–5098; tel. 309/347–1151 **A**1 9 10 **F**3 8 11 13 15 18 20 24 25 26 27 30 31 32 33 38 46 47 48 49 50 51 52 55 56 57 59 61 66 68 72 73 74 76 77 79 80 81 82 84 90 96 97 102 103 107 117 119 121 124 133 135 136 137 **P**1 **S** QHR
Primary Contact: Kevin R. Andrews, Chief Executive Officer
CFO: Alan Nerone, Chief Financial Officer
CMO: John E. Lovell, M.D., President Medical Staff
CHR: Anne Dierker, Vice President Human Resources
Web address: www.pekinhospital.org
Control: Other not–for–profit (including NFP Corporation) **Service:** General Medical and Surgical

Staffed Beds: 110 **Admissions:** 4486 **Census:** 56 **Outpatient Visits:** 109533 **Births:** 464 **Total Expense ($000):** 66727 **Payroll Expense ($000):** 25756 **Personnel:** 672

PEORIA—Peoria County

★ △ **METHODIST MEDICAL CENTER OF ILLINOIS (140209)**, 221 N.E. Glen Oak Avenue, Zip 61636–4310; tel. 309/672–5522 **A**1 2 3 5 6 7 9 10 **F**3 8 11 12 13 15 17 18 20 22 24 25 26 27 28 30 31 32 33 36 38 40 41 42 43 44 46 49 50 52 53 54 55 56 57 58 59 61 62 66 68 72 73 74 75 76 77 79 80 81 82 84 85 86 88 89 90 91 92 93 94 95 96 97 99 100 102 103 104 105 106 107 109 116 118 119 121 123 124 125 132 133 134 135 136 137 **P**8
Primary Contact: W. Michael Bryant, President and Chief Executive Officer
COO: Debbie Simon, Senior Vice President Operations and Chief Nursing Officer
CFO: Calvin R. MacKay, Chief Financial Officer
CMO: Richard A. Anderson, M.D., Senior Vice President Medical Affairs and Chief Medical Officer
CIO: Ellen T. Swoger, Vice President Information Technology
Web address: www.mmci.org
Control: Other not–for–profit (including NFP Corporation) **Service:** General Medical and Surgical

Staffed Beds: 296 **Admissions:** 15659 **Census:** 220 **Outpatient Visits:** 447458 **Births:** 1875 **Total Expense ($000):** 283732 **Payroll Expense ($000):** 111864 **Personnel:** 2061

★ △ **OSF SAINT FRANCIS MEDICAL CENTER (140067)**, 530 N.E. Glen Oak Avenue, Zip 61637–0001; tel. 309/655–2000 **A**1 2 3 5 6 7 8 9 10 **F**3 8 9 11 12 13 14 15 17 18 19 20 21 22 23 24 25 26 27 28 30 31 32 33 34 35 36 38 40 43 44 45 46 48 49 50 51 53 54 55 56 57 58 59 62 63 64 66 68 70 71 72 73 74 75 76 77 79 80 82 83 84 85 86 87 92 94 95 96 97 98 99 100 101 102 103 104 105 106 107 108 109 111 112 116 118 119 121 124 127 129 131 133 135 136 137 **P**6 **S** OSF Healthcare System
Primary Contact: Keith E. Steffen, President and Chief Executive Officer
COO: Susan C. Wozniak, R.N., Senior Vice President and Chief Operating Officer
CFO: Ken Harbaugh, Vice President and Chief Financial Officer
CMO: Tim C. Miller, M.D., Vice President, Chief Medical Officer and Director Academy Affairs
CHR: Lynn Gillespie, Assistant Administrator
Web address: www.osfsaintfrancis.org
Control: Church–operated, Nongovernment, not–for profit **Service:** General Medical and Surgical

Staffed Beds: 566 **Admissions:** 27485 **Census:** 424 **Outpatient Visits:** 761717 **Births:** 2544 **Total Expense ($000):** 622646 **Payroll Expense ($000):** 246903 **Personnel:** 4720

□ **PROCTOR HOSPITAL (140013)**, 5409 North Knoxville Avenue, Zip 61614–5094; tel. 309/691–1000, (Total facility includes 20 beds in nursing home–type unit) **A**1 9 10 **F**3 4 5 11 13 15 18 20 22 24 25 26 30 31 32 38 49 52 55 56 57 61 62 63 68 72 73 74 77 79 80 81 82 84 86 96 97 100 103 106 107 117 118 119 124 134 135 137
Primary Contact: Norman H. LaConte, President and Chief Executive Officer
CFO: David M. Underwood, Vice President Finance
CMO: R. Parker McRae, M.D., President Medical Staff
CIO: Darrell Johnston, Vice President Information Services and Chief Information Officer
CHR: Linda Buck, Vice President Human Resources
Web address: www.proctor.org
Control: Other not–for–profit (including NFP Corporation) **Service:** General Medical and Surgical

Staffed Beds: 163 **Admissions:** 7011 **Census:** 97 **Outpatient Visits:** 159934 **Births:** 589 **Total Expense ($000):** 89370 **Payroll Expense ($000):** 34281 **Personnel:** 856

PERU—La Salle County

★ **ILLINOIS VALLEY COMMUNITY HOSPITAL (140234)**, 925 West Street, Zip 61354–2757; tel. 815/223–3300 **A**9 10 **F**3 11 13 15 24 25 26 27 30 31 32 33 36 38 43 44 49 51 53 54 55 56 57 62 63 66 67 68 72 73 74 75 76 77 79 80 81 82 84 86 96 97 100 103 106 107 118 119 120 121 122 124 132 135 136 137 **P**8
Primary Contact: Tommy Hobbs, Chief Executive Officer
COO: Monica Gustafson, Chief Operating Officer
CFO: Stephen Davis, Chief Financial Officer
CMO: Joel Leifheit, M.D., Chief of Staff and President Medical Staff
CIO: Nancy McDonnell, Manager Information Systems
CHR: Mark Batty, Assistant Administrator Human Resources
Web address: www.ivch.org
Control: Other not–for–profit (including NFP Corporation) **Service:** General Medical and Surgical

Staffed Beds: 72 **Admissions:** 3686 **Census:** 35 **Outpatient Visits:** 119964 **Births:** 459 **Total Expense ($000):** 48912 **Payroll Expense ($000):** 18315 **Personnel:** 508

PINCKNEYVILLE—Perry County

★ **PINCKNEYVILLE COMMUNITY HOSPITAL (141307)**, 101 North Walnut Street, Zip 62274–1099; tel. 618/357–2187, (Total facility includes 50 beds in nursing home–type unit) **A**9 10 18 **F**15 25 27 30 31 32 38 40 42 50 52 55 61 65 76 78 79 86 87 96 97 107 117 119 122 137 **P**6
Primary Contact: Thomas J. Hudgins, FACHE, Administrator and Chief Executive Officer
CFO: Kara Jo Carson, Chief Financial Officer
CIO: Bill Doerflein, Director Information Technology
Control: Hospital district or authority, Government, nonfederal **Service:** General Medical and Surgical

Staffed Beds: 75 **Admissions:** 1071 **Census:** 55 **Outpatient Visits:** 60050 **Births:** 0 **Total Expense ($000):** 19603 **Payroll Expense ($000):** 9019 **Personnel:** 255

PITTSFIELD—Pike County

★ ○ **ILLINI COMMUNITY HOSPITAL (141315)**, 640 West Washington Street, Zip 62363–1397; tel. 217/285–2113 **A**9 10 11 18 **F**3 15 17 24 26 27 30 31 32 38 46 50 56 57 62 63 66 67 68 73 76 77 79 80 82 84 87 96 103 107 118 119 122 130 135 137
Primary Contact: Connie L. Schroeder, Chief Executive Officer
CFO: Sandra Purcell, Administrative Director Finance
CMO: Cris Del Rosario, M.D., President Medical Staff
CHR: Danny Holland, Administrative Director Human Resources
Web address: www.illinihospital.org
Control: Other not–for–profit (including NFP Corporation) **Service:** General Medical and Surgical

Staffed Beds: 25 **Admissions:** 665 **Census:** 7 **Outpatient Visits:** 7458 **Births:** 0 **Total Expense ($000):** 14244 **Payroll Expense ($000):** 5474 **Personnel:** 149

PONTIAC—Livingston County

★ **OSF SAINT JAMES – JOHN W. ALBRECHT MEDICAL CENTER (140161)**, 2500 West Reynolds, Zip 61764–2194; tel. 815/842–2828 **A**1 9 10 20 **F**3 8 11 13 15 24 25 26 28 30 31 32 33 38 50 54 55 56 57 62 66 68 73 74 75 77 79 80 81 82 84 86 87 96 99 100 102 103 105 106 107 119 120 121 122 124 135 136 **P**7 **S** OSF Healthcare System
Primary Contact: David T. Ochs, President and Chief Executive Officer
CFO: Paula Corrigan, Vice President and Chief Financial Officer
CHR: Kenneth Beutke, Vice President, Organization Development and Planning
Web address: www.osfsaintjames.org
Control: Church–operated, Nongovernment, not–for profit **Service:** General Medical and Surgical

Staffed Beds: 42 **Admissions:** 1772 **Census:** 16 **Outpatient Visits:** 158926 **Births:** 225 **Total Expense ($000):** 51461 **Payroll Expense ($000):** 19695 **Personnel:** 335

PRINCETON—Bureau County

PERRY MEMORIAL HOSPITAL (141337), 530 Park Avenue East, Zip 61356–2598; tel. 815/875–2811 **A**9 10 18 **F**3 11 13 15 24 25 26 27 30 31 32 33 34 36 38 40 43 44 49 50 54 55 56 57 62 66 67 68 73 74 75 76 77 79 81 82 86 96 97 100 102 104 107 118 119 120 121 122 124 134 135 136 137 **P**8
Primary Contact: Rex D. Conger, FACHE, President and Chief Executive Officer
CMO: Edward Doran, M.D., Chief of Staff
CIO: Karen Behrens, Director Technology Services
CHR: Karen Russell, Director Human Resources
Web address: www.perry–memorial.org
Control: City–Government, nonfederal **Service:** General Medical and Surgical

Staffed Beds: 25 **Admissions:** 1546 **Census:** 13 **Outpatient Visits:** 63846 **Births:** 149 **Total Expense ($000):** 27769 **Payroll Expense ($000):** 11469 **Personnel:** 228

QUINCY—Adams County

★ △ **BLESSING HOSPITAL (140015)**, Broadway at 11th Street, Zip 62305–7005, Mailing Address: P.O. Box 7005, Zip 62305–7005; tel. 217/223–1200, (Includes BLESSING HOSPITAL, Broadway & 14th Street), (Total facility includes 20 beds in nursing home–type unit) **A**1 2 3 5 7 9 10 19 20 **F**3 5 8 11 13 15 17 18 20 22 25 26 27 28 30 31 32 33 38 40 41 42 43 44 48 49 50 52 54 55 56 57 58 59 60 61 62 64 66 68 71 72 73 74 75 76 77 79 80 81 82 84 85 86 88 89 90 91 92 93 94 96 97 99 100 102 103 106 107 108 109 111 117 118 119 120 121 124 133 135 136 137 **P**8
Primary Contact: Maureen A. Kahn, President and Chief Executive Officer
COO: Tim Moore, Chief Accounting Officer
CFO: Patrick M. Gerveler, Vice President Finance and Chief Financial Officer
CMO: Tom Diller, M.D., Chief Medical Officer
CIO: Patrick Dillon, Chief Information Officer
CHR: Zigrida Brown, Vice President Human Resources
Web address: www.blessinghospital.org
Control: Other not–for–profit (including NFP Corporation) **Service:** General Medical and Surgical

Staffed Beds: 337 **Admissions:** 14085 **Census:** 181 **Outpatient Visits:** 336720 **Births:** 1300 **Total Expense ($000):** 194858 **Payroll Expense ($000):** 80380 **Personnel:** 1792

RED BUD—Randolph County

★ **RED BUD REGIONAL HOSPITAL (141348)**, 325 Spring Street, Zip 62278–1194; tel. 618/282–3831, (Total facility includes 115 beds in nursing home–type unit) **A**1 9 10 18 **F**3 15 25 32 38 46 54 55 56 57 61 62 77 79 80 86 96 102 106 107 119 122 135 137 **P**5 7 **S** Community Health Systems, Inc.
Primary Contact: Robert Honeycutt, Chief Executive Officer
COO: Shane Watson, Assistant Administrator
CFO: Roseann M. Devault, Chief Financial Officer
CMO: Steven Elster, M.D., President Medical Staff
CIO: Casey Baldridge, Supervisor Information Technology
CHR: Kathleen Wilson, Director Human Resources
Web address: www.redbudhospital.com
Control: Corporation, Investor–owned, for–profit **Service:** General Medical and Surgical

Staffed Beds: 140 **Admissions:** 1310 **Census:** 118 **Outpatient Visits:** 22395 **Births:** 0 **Total Expense ($000):** 16127 **Payroll Expense ($000):** 6992 **Personnel:** 268

ROBINSON—Crawford County

★ **CRAWFORD MEMORIAL HOSPITAL (141343)**, 1000 North Allen Street, Zip 62454–1167; tel. 618/544–3131, (Total facility includes 40 beds in nursing home–type unit) **A**1 9 10 18 **F**3 8 11 13 15 24 26 27 31 32 38 52 54 57 61 62 74 75 76 77 78 79 80 86 96 97 100 107 117 118 119 121 122 135 136 **P**6 **S** QHR
Primary Contact: Donald E. Annis, Chief Executive Officer
CFO: Richard Carlson, Chief Financial Officer
CMO: David Rotman, M.D., Chief of Staff
CHR: Kristi Zane, Chief Human Resources Officer
Web address: www.crawfordmh.com
Control: Hospital district or authority, Government, nonfederal **Service:** General Medical and Surgical

Staffed Beds: 65 **Admissions:** 1283 **Census:** 37 **Outpatient Visits:** 44911 **Births:** 144 **Total Expense ($000):** 28239 **Payroll Expense ($000):** 13288 **Personnel:** 291

ROCHELLE—Ogle County

★ **ROCHELLE COMMUNITY HOSPITAL (141312)**, 900 North Second Street, Zip 61068–0330; tel. 815/562–2181 **A**1 9 10 18 **F**3 15 25 26 27 33 38 43 52 55 56 57 62 68 72 73 75 76 77 79 80 81 82 86 87 96 97 100 103 107 118 119 121 122 124 133 135 **P**6
Primary Contact: Bruce D. Peterson, Chief Executive Officer
CFO: John M. Ross, Vice President Finance and Chief Financial Officer
CMO: Michael Monfils, M.D., Chief Medical Staff
CIO: Scott Stewart, Manager Information Services
CHR: Robert Johns, Senior Vice President Administration
Web address: www.rcha.net
Control: Other not–for–profit (including NFP Corporation) **Service:** General Medical and Surgical

Staffed Beds: 25 **Admissions:** 812 **Census:** 7 **Outpatient Visits:** 34277 **Births:** 0 **Total Expense ($000):** 20567 **Payroll Expense ($000):** 7369 **Personnel:** 179

ROCK ISLAND—Rock Island County

★ △ **TRINITY MEDICAL CENTER–WEST (140280)**, 2701 17th Street, Zip 61201–5393; tel. 309/779–5000, (Includes TRINITY MEDICAL CENTER–SEVENTH STREET, 500 John Deere Road, Moline, Zip 61265; tel. 309/779–5000), (Total facility includes 29 beds in nursing home–type unit) **A**1 2 7 9 10 **F**3 4 5 7 8 11 12 13 15 18 20 22 24 25 26 27 28 30 31 32 33 35 36 38 40 43 49 54 55 56 57 58 62 63 68 72 73 74 75 76 77 79 80 81 82 84 85 86 87 88 89 90 91 92 93 94 95 96 97 102 107 108 109 111 117 118 119 121 123 124 132 133 135 136 137 **P**6 **S** Iowa Health System
Primary Contact: Andrea Y. Coleman, President and Chief Executive Officer
COO: Florence Spyrow, Vice President Operations
CFO: Kevin Vermeer, Chief Financial Officer
CMO: Morris H. Seligman, M.D., Vice President Medical Affairs and Chief Medical Officer
CHR: Jeffery Stolze, Vice President Human Resources
Web address: www.trinityqc.com
Control: Other not–for–profit (including NFP Corporation) **Service:** General Medical and Surgical

Staffed Beds: 314 **Admissions:** 17540 **Census:** 217 **Outpatient Visits:** 293761 **Births:** 1498 **Total Expense ($000):** 230290 **Payroll Expense ($000):** 82472 **Personnel:** 1957

ROCKFORD—Winnebago County

□ **H. DOUGLAS SINGER MENTAL HEALTH AND DEVELOPMENTAL CENTER (144023)**, 4402 North Main Street, Zip 61103–1278; tel. 815/987–7096, (Nonreporting) **A**1 10
Primary Contact: Gail Tennant, Director
Control: State–Government, nonfederal **Service:** Psychiatric

Staffed Beds: 162

IL

Hospital, Medicare Provider Number, Address, Telephone, Approval, Facility, and Physician Codes, Health Care System

★ American Hospital Association (AHA) membership
□ The Joint Commission accreditation
○ American Osteopathic Association (AOA) accreditation
△ Commission on Accreditation of Rehabilitation Facilities (CARF) accreditation

★ **OSF SAINT ANTHONY MEDICAL CENTER (140233)**, 5666 East State Street, Zip 61108–2472; tel. 815/226–2000 **A**1 2 5 9 10 **F**3 11 13 15 16 17 18 20 22 24 25 26 27 30 31 32 33 34 35 36 37 38 40 41 43 44 46 49 50 51 52 54 55 56 57 58 62 64 68 71 72 73 74 75 76 77 79 80 81 82 84 86 96 97 99 100 102 103 104 105 106 107 108 109 111 114 118 119 120 121 124 133 135 136 137 **P**6 **S** OSF Healthcare System
Primary Contact: David A. Schertz, Administrator
CFO: David Stenerson, Assistant Administrator Fiscal Services and Chief Financial Officer
CMO: Eric Benink, M.D., Assistant Administrator Medical Affairs
CIO: Mary Madden, Director Information Services
CHR: Karen C. Brown, Assistant Director Strategic Human Resources
Web address: www.osfhealth.com
Control: Church–operated, Nongovernment, not–for profit **Service:** General Medical and Surgical

Staffed Beds: 238 **Admissions:** 11259 **Census:** 150 **Outpatient Visits:** 193915 **Births:** 748 **Total Expense ($000):** 253626 **Payroll Expense ($000):** 94275 **Personnel:** 1764

★ **ROCKFORD MEMORIAL HOSPITAL (140239)**, 2400 North Rockton Avenue, Zip 61103–3692; tel. 815/971–5000 **A**1 2 5 10 13 **F**3 11 13 17 18 20 22 24 25 26 27 28 31 32 33 35 36 37 38 40 41 42 43 49 50 52 53 55 56 57 62 66 68 69 70 72 73 74 75 76 77 78 79 80 81 82 83 84 86 87 88 89 90 91 92 93 96 97 100 102 103 106 107 109 111 112 114 116 118 119 121 124 135 136 137
Primary Contact: Gary E. Kaatz, President and Chief Executive Officer
COO: Earl J. Tamar, Chief Operating Officer
CFO: Henry Seybold, Senior Vice President and Chief Financial Officer
CMO: Milton G. Schmitt, M.D., Chief Medical Officer
CIO: Dennis P. L'Heureux, Chief Information Officer
CHR: Dan Parod, Vice President Human Resources
Web address: www.rhsnet.org
Control: Other not–for–profit (including NFP Corporation) **Service:** General Medical and Surgical

Staffed Beds: 286 **Admissions:** 14633 **Census:** 206 **Outpatient Visits:** 406476 **Births:** 1906 **Total Expense ($000):** 251291 **Payroll Expense ($000):** 99791 **Personnel:** 1891

★ **SWEDISHAMERICAN HOSPITAL (140228)**, 1401 East State Street, Zip 61104–2315; tel. 815/968–4400 **A**1 2 3 5 9 10 **F**3 13 15 17 18 20 22 24 25 26 27 28 30 31 32 33 34 35 36 37 38 40 41 44 46 49 50 54 55 56 57 58 60 62 63 66 67 68 70 72 73 74 76 77 79 80 81 82 84 86 88 89 90 91 92 93 95 96 97 100 102 103 105 106 107 109 111 118 119 121 124 135 136 137 **P**6 7
Primary Contact: William R. Gorski, M.D., President and Chief Executive Officer
COO: Richard Walsh, Executive Vice President and Chief Operating Officer
CFO: Don Haring, Vice President Finance and Treasurer
CMO: Kathleen Kelly, M.D., Chief Medical Officer and Chief Quality Officer
CIO: Phil Wasson, Chief Information Officer
CHR: Harvey Lightbody, Vice President Human Resources
Web address: www.swedishamerican.org
Control: Other not–for–profit (including NFP Corporation) **Service:** General Medical and Surgical

Staffed Beds: 284 **Admissions:** 15455 **Census:** 183 **Outpatient Visits:** 201731 **Births:** 2443 **Total Expense ($000):** 241364 **Payroll Expense ($000):** 90243 **Personnel:** 1815

★ △ **VAN MATRE HEALTHSOUTH REHABILITATION HOSPITAL (143028)**, 950 South Mulford Road, Zip 61108; tel. 815/381–8500 **A**1 7 9 10 **F**25 30 31 32 43 62 66 72 73 81 85 86 119 120 121 137 **S** HEALTHSOUTH Corporation
Primary Contact: Daniel B. Woloszyn, Chief Executive Officer
CFO: Mark Lundvall, Controller
CMO: Scott Craig, M.D., Medical Director
CIO: Dianne Miller, Director Health Information Management
CHR: Lisa Vitale, Director Human Resources
Web address: www.healthsouth.com
Control: Partnership, Investor–owned, for–profit **Service:** Rehabilitation

Staffed Beds: 40 **Admissions:** 1190 **Census:** 38 **Outpatient Visits:** 7192 **Births:** 0 **Total Expense ($000):** 12636 **Payroll Expense ($000):** 7206 **Personnel:** 131

IL

ROSICLARE—Hardin County

★ **HARDIN COUNTY GENERAL HOSPITAL (141328)**, Ferrell Road, Zip 62982; tel. 618/285–6634 **A**9 10 18 **F**3 11 15 25 38 87 96 107 118 119 122
Primary Contact: Roby D. Williams, Administrator
CFO: Janie Parker, Director Fiscal Services
CMO: Marcos N. Sunga, M.D., Chief of Staff
CHR: Joyce Shelby, Manager Human Resources
Control: Other not–for–profit (including NFP Corporation) **Service:** General Medical and Surgical

Staffed Beds: 25 **Admissions:** 843 **Census:** 10 **Outpatient Visits:** 22409 **Births:** 0 **Total Expense ($000):** 8437 **Payroll Expense ($000):** 4555 **Personnel:** 126

RUSHVILLE—Schuyler County

★ **SARAH D. CULBERTSON MEMORIAL HOSPITAL (141333)**, 238 South Congress Street, Zip 62681–1472; tel. 217/322–4321, (Total facility includes 30 beds in nursing home–type unit) **A**9 10 18 **F**11 15 30 38 57 67 76 79 96 102 107 115 122
Primary Contact: D. David Sniff, Administrator
COO: Lynn E. Stambaugh, R.N., Chief Operating Officer
CFO: Jerry Bartlett, Chief Financial Officer
CMO: S. K. Kanthila, M.D., President Medical Staff
Web address: www.cmhospital.com
Control: Hospital district or authority, Government, nonfederal **Service:** General Medical and Surgical

Staffed Beds: 53 **Admissions:** 513 **Census:** 27 **Births:** 0 **Total Expense ($000):** 11699 **Payroll Expense ($000):** 4775 **Personnel:** 163

SALEM—Marion County

★ ○ **SALEM TOWNSHIP HOSPITAL (141345)**, 1201 Ricker Drive, Zip 62881–6250; tel. 618/548–3194 **A**9 10 11 18 **F**3 11 15 24 25 31 32 38 46 50 55 56 57 61 62 68 79 80 87 96 97 99 102 103 107 118 121 122 134
Primary Contact: Richelle Rennegarbe, Ph.D., RN, President
COO: Stephanie Hilton–Siebert, Chief Operating Officer
CFO: Teresa Fuhrhop, Chief Financial Officer
CIO: Steve Turner, Director Information Technology
CHR: Diane Boswell, Director Human Resources and Marketing
Web address: www.sthcares.org
Control: City–County, Government, nonfederal **Service:** General Medical and Surgical

Staffed Beds: 25 **Admissions:** 1105 **Census:** 12 **Outpatient Visits:** 38239 **Births:** 0 **Total Expense ($000):** 16492 **Payroll Expense ($000):** 6319 **Personnel:** 183

SANDWICH—De Kalb County

★ **VALLEY WEST COMMUNITY HOSPITAL (141340)**, 11 East Pleasant Avenue, Zip 60548–0901; tel. 815/786–8484 **A**1 9 10 18 **F**3 11 13 15 24 25 26 27 30 31 32 33 38 46 49 51 55 56 57 58 66 68 73 74 75 76 77 79 80 82 86 96 100 102 106 107 119 120 121 124 135 136 **S** Kish Health System
Primary Contact: Brad Copple, Administrator
COO: Michael Muzzillo, Assistant Administrator
CFO: Loren Foelske, Vice President Finance
CMO: David L. Faulk, M.D., Chief of Staff
CIO: Heath Bell, Chief Information Officer
CHR: Mark Thate, Director Human Resources
Web address: www.vwch.org
Control: Other not–for–profit (including NFP Corporation) **Service:** General Medical and Surgical

Staffed Beds: 25 **Admissions:** 1460 **Census:** 11 **Outpatient Visits:** 37083 **Births:** 252 **Total Expense ($000):** 30611 **Payroll Expense ($000):** 7668 **Personnel:** 139

SCOTT AFB—St. Clair County

★ **SCOTT MEDICAL CENTER**, 310 West Losey Street, Zip 62225–5252; tel. 618/256–7000, (Nonreporting) **S** Department of the Air Force
Primary Contact: Colonel Diane C. Ritter, Commanding Officer
COO: Lieutenant Colonel Leslie Dixon, Administrator
CFO: Major Gregory Cullison, Flight Commander Resource Management
CMO: Colonel James H. Heriot, M.D., Chief Medical Staff
Web address: www.public.scott.amc.af.mil
Control: Air Force, Government, federal **Service:** General Medical and Surgical

Staffed Beds: 18

SHELBYVILLE—Shelby County

★ **SHELBY MEMORIAL HOSPITAL (140019)**, 200 South Cedar Street, Zip 62565–1899; tel. 217/774–3961, (Total facility includes 15 beds in nursing home–type unit) **A**1 9 10 20 **F**3 15 24 25 38 56 57 61 62 79 86 96 97 106 107 117 121 122 **P**5
Primary Contact: John Bennett, President and Chief Executive Officer
CFO: Marilyn Sears, Chief Financial Officer
CMO: Arnold Agapito, M.D., President Medical Staff
CHR: Amy Koehler, Director Human Resources
Control: Other not–for–profit (including NFP Corporation) **Service:** General Medical and Surgical

Staffed Beds: 45 **Admissions:** 1526 **Census:** 26 **Outpatient Visits:** 26963 **Births:** 0 **Total Expense ($000):** 15547 **Payroll Expense ($000):** 5478 **Personnel:** 155

Many Facility Codes have changed. Please refer to the AHA Guide Code Chart.

SILVIS—Rock Island County

★ **GENESIS MEDICAL CENTER, ILLINI CAMPUS (140275)**, 801 Illini Drive, Zip 61282–1893; tel. 309/792–9363 **A**1 10 **F**3 7 11 13 15 18 20 24 25 26 27 30 31 32 33 36 38 40 41 42 43 46 47 48 50 52 53 55 56 57 62 66 68 72 73 74 75 76 77 79 80 82 84 86 87 96 99 100 102 104 107 115 118 119 120 121 124 133 135 136 **S** Genesis Health System
Primary Contact: Charles E. Bruhn, Administrator
CFO: Mark G. Rogers, Interim Vice President Finance and Chief Financial Officer
CMO: Peter Metcalf, M.D., President Medical Staff
CIO: Robert Frieden, Vice President Information Systems
CHR: Jerry McCormick, Vice President Human Resources
Web address: www.genesishealth.com
Control: Other not–for–profit (including NFP Corporation) **Service:** General Medical and Surgical

Staffed Beds: 110 **Admissions:** 4432 **Census:** 40 **Outpatient Visits:** 93594 **Births:** 707 **Total Expense ($000):** 61419 **Payroll Expense ($000):** 18824 **Personnel:** 532

SKOKIE—Cook County

★ **RUSH NORTH SHORE MEDICAL CENTER (140051)**, 9600 Gross Point Road, Zip 60076–1257; tel. 847/677–9600 **A**1 2 3 5 9 10 **F**3 8 13 15 18 20 22 24 25 26 27 30 31 32 33 35 36 37 38 40 41 43 46 48 49 50 54 55 56 57 58 62 63 66 67 68 72 73 74 75 76 77 79 80 81 82 84 86 88 90 91 92 93 97 99 106 107 113 114 119 120 121 135 136 137 **P**1 **S** Rush University Medical Center
Primary Contact: James T. Frankenbach, President and Chief Executive Officer
COO: Anthony Di Lorenzo, Vice President Operations
CFO: Greg Pagliuzza, Interim Vice President Finance
CMO: Michael Raymond, M.D., Chief Medical Officer
CIO: Kerry Kerlin, Vice President Information Technology
CHR: Richard J. Casey, Assistant Vice President Operations
Web address: www.rnsmc.org
Control: Other not–for–profit (including NFP Corporation) **Service:** General Medical and Surgical

Staffed Beds: 234 **Admissions:** 10937 **Census:** 145 **Outpatient Visits:** 179228 **Births:** 529 **Total Expense ($000):** 173558 **Payroll Expense ($000):** 71480 **Personnel:** 1128

SPARTA—Randolph County

★ **SPARTA COMMUNITY HOSPITAL (141349)**, 818 East Broadway Street, Zip 62286–0297, Mailing Address: P.O. Box 297, Zip 62286–0297; tel. 618/443–2177 **A**1 9 10 18 **F**3 11 13 15 24 30 31 33 38 52 57 61 66 74 75 79 84 86 96 107 119 122 132 135 **P**5
Primary Contact: Joann Emge, Chief Executive Officer
COO: Joann Emge, Chief Executive Officer
CFO: Steve Bricker, Chief Financial Officer
CMO: Russell Coulter, M.D., Chief Medical Staff
CIO: Susan Gutjahr, Reimbursement Specialist
CHR: Darla Shawgo, Director Human Resources
Web address: www.spartahospital.com
Control: Hospital district or authority, Government, nonfederal **Service:** General Medical and Surgical

Staffed Beds: 25 **Admissions:** 1090 **Census:** 10 **Outpatient Visits:** 37419 **Births:** 178 **Total Expense ($000):** 21765 **Payroll Expense ($000):** 10040 **Personnel:** 259

SPRING VALLEY—Bureau County

ST. MARGARET'S HOSPITAL (140143), 600 East First Street, Zip 61362–2034; tel. 815/664–5311 **A**9 10 **F**3 11 13 15 24 25 26 27 28 30 31 32 33 36 38 41 42 43 46 49 52 55 56 57 58 68 73 74 75 77 79 80 82 84 85 86 96 107 117 118 119 120 121 122 124 132 135 136 137 **P**6 8 **S** Sisters of Mary of the Presentation Health System
Primary Contact: Tim Muntz, President and Chief Executive Officer
CFO: Kim D. Santman, Chief Financial Officer
Web address: www.st–margarets.com
Control: Church–operated, Nongovernment, not–for profit **Service:** General Medical and Surgical

Staffed Beds: 86 **Admissions:** 3395 **Census:** 39 **Outpatient Visits:** 229904 **Births:** 371

SPRINGFIELD—Sangamon County

□ **ANDREW MCFARLAND MENTAL HEALTH CENTER (144021)**, 901 Southwind Road, Zip 62703–5195; tel. 217/786–6994, (Nonreporting) **A**1 5 10
Primary Contact: G. Scott Viniard, Administrator
CFO: Beverly McCurley, Business Administrator
CMO: Brad S. Hughes, M.D., Medical Director
CHR: Robert Braasch, Human Resources Administrator
Control: State–Government, nonfederal **Service:** Psychiatric

Staffed Beds: 122

★ △ **MEMORIAL MEDICAL CENTER (140148)**, 701 North First Street, Zip 62781–0001; tel. 217/788–3000 **A**1 2 3 5 7 8 9 10 **F**3 8 11 12 13 14 15 16 17 18 20 22 24 25 26 27 28 30 31 32 33 34 35 38 40 41 42 43 44 46 49 50 51 53 55 56 57 58 59 60 62 66 67 68 72 73 74 75 76 77 79 80 81 82 84 85 86 87 88 89 90 91 92 93 94 95 96 99 100 102 103 104 105 106 107 108 109 111 112 118 119 120 121 124 127 130 131 133 134 135 136 137 **P**3 5 **S** Memorial Health System
Primary Contact: Edgar J. Curtis, RN, Executive Vice President and Chief Operating Officer
COO: Douglas L. Rahn, Senior Vice President and Chief Operating Officer
CFO: Robert W. Kay, Senior Vice President and Chief Financial Officer
CMO: Mark Weaver, M.D., Chief Medical Officer
CIO: Steven Riney, Senior Vice President and Chief Information Officer
CHR: Forrest G. Hester, Senior Vice President and Chief People Officer
Web address: www.memorialmedical.com
Control: Other not–for–profit (including NFP Corporation) **Service:** General Medical and Surgical

Staffed Beds: 446 **Admissions:** 24170 **Census:** 310 **Outpatient Visits:** 465250 **Births:** 1732 **Total Expense ($000):** 411361 **Payroll Expense ($000):** 138370 **Personnel:** 2617

★ **ST. JOHN'S HOSPITAL (140053)**, 800 East Carpenter Street, Zip 62769–0002; tel. 217/544–6464 **A**1 2 3 5 8 9 10 **F**2 3 11 13 15 17 18 19 20 21 22 23 24 25 26 27 28 30 31 32 33 34 37 38 40 41 42 43 44 45 47 48 49 50 51 52 54 55 56 57 58 59 60 61 62 64 65 66 68 70 72 73 74 75 76 77 79 80 81 82 83 84 86 88 90 91 92 93 94 96 97 99 100 102 103 105 106 107 108 109 110 111 112 116 117 118 119 120 121 124 135 136 137 **S** Hospital Sisters Health System
Primary Contact: Robert P. Ritz, Chief Executive Officer
COO: John Short, Chief Operating Officer
CFO: J. Steven Eavenson, Chief Financial Officer
CMO: Craig Backs, M.D., Medical Director
CIO: Robert Milner, Chief Information Officer
CHR: Joe Bretz, Director Human Resources
Web address: www.st–johns.org
Control: Church–operated, Nongovernment, not–for profit **Service:** General Medical and Surgical

Staffed Beds: 465 **Admissions:** 20911 **Census:** 293 **Outpatient Visits:** 246792 **Total Expense ($000):** 378734 **Payroll Expense ($000):** 125519 **Personnel:** 2651

STAUNTON—Macoupin County

★ **COMMUNITY MEMORIAL HOSPITAL (141306)**, 400 Caldwell Street, Zip 62088–1499; tel. 618/635–2200 **A**9 10 18 **F**3 11 15 24 25 27 31 38 43 56 61 62 67 72 73 76 77 79 80 81 82 86 87 96 107 119 121 122 135 137 **S** QHR
Primary Contact: Susie Campbell, Chief Executive Officer
CFO: Donald Brunnworth, Chief Financial Officer
CMO: Bryan Siegfried, M.D., President Medical Staff
CIO: Cheryl Horner, Data Processing Supervisor
CHR: Marilyn Herbeck, Coordinator Human Resources
Web address: www.stauntonhospital.org
Control: Other not–for–profit (including NFP Corporation) **Service:** General Medical and Surgical

Staffed Beds: 25 **Admissions:** 567 **Census:** 6 **Outpatient Visits:** 26207 **Births:** 0 **Total Expense ($000):** 12226 **Payroll Expense ($000):** 4830 **Personnel:** 127

STERLING—Whiteside County

★ **CGH MEDICAL CENTER (140043)**, 100 East LeFevre Road, Zip 61081–1279; tel. 815/625–0400 **A**1 2 9 10 **F**3 7 8 11 13 15 18 20 24 25 26 27 30 31 32 33 38 47 49 50 51 55 56 57 61 62 66 68 72 74 76 77 79 80 81 82 84 86 87 96 97 100 102 103 106 107 112 118 119 121 122 124 134 135 **P**6
Primary Contact: Edward Andersen, President and Chief Executive Officer
COO: Norm Deets, Chief Operating Officer
CFO: Krystal Claymore, Chief Financial Officer
CMO: Mark Schmelzel, Medical Director
CIO: Raymond Sharp, Vice President and Chief Information Officer
CHR: Tom McCawley, Manager Human Resources
Web address: www.cghmc.com
Control: City–Government, nonfederal **Service:** General Medical and Surgical

Staffed Beds: 99 **Admissions:** 5270 **Census:** 47 **Outpatient Visits:** 113007 **Births:** 621 **Total Expense ($000):** 88821 **Payroll Expense ($000):** 33935 **Personnel:** 875

IL

Hospital, Medicare Provider Number, Address, Telephone, Approval, Facility, and Physician Codes, Health Care System

★ American Hospital Association (AHA) membership
□ The Joint Commission accreditation
○ American Osteopathic Association (AOA) accreditation
△ Commission on Accreditation of Rehabilitation Facilities (CARF) accreditation

STREAMWOOD—Cook County

★ **STREAMWOOD HOSPITAL (144034)**, 1400 East Irving Park Road, Zip 60107–3203; tel. 630/837–9000 **A**1 9 10 **F**5 25 26 30 31 32 33 36 55 56 62 73 75 81 82 88 89 90 91 92 94 95 119 121 123 **P**6
S Psychiatric Solutions
Primary Contact: Cynthia A. Meyer, Chief Executive Officer
CFO: Nancy Costello, Chief Financial Officer
CMO: Joseph McNally, M.D., Medical Director
CHR: Carolyn Paganoni, Director Human Resources
Web address: www.streamwoodhospital.com
Control: Corporation, Investor–owned, for–profit **Service:** Children's hospital psychiatric

Staffed Beds: 134 **Admissions:** 1859 **Census:** 104 **Outpatient Visits:** 16679 **Births:** 0 **Total Expense ($000):** 22951 **Payroll Expense ($000):** 14546 **Personnel:** 291

STREATOR—La Salle County

★ **ST. MARY'S HOSPITAL (140026)**, 111 Spring Street, Zip 61364–3399; tel. 815/673–2311, (Total facility includes 30 beds in nursing home–type unit) **A**1 9 10 **F**2 3 11 13 15 24 25 26 27 30 31 32 33 38 44 50 54 55 56 57 61 62 68 73 74 75 76 77 79 81 82 84 86 97 103 106 107 117 119 120 121 124 132 135 137 **P**8 **S** Hospital Sisters Health System
Primary Contact: Richard J. Carlson, Interim President and Chief Executive Officer
COO: Robert V. Gubbels, Chief Operating Officer
CFO: Karen S. Clark, Chief Financial Officer
CIO: Georgene Lansford, Manager Information Systems
CHR: David Smith, Director Human Resources
Web address: www.stmaryshospital.org
Control: Church–operated, Nongovernment, not–for profit **Service:** General Medical and Surgical

Staffed Beds: 116 **Admissions:** 3686 **Census:** 53 **Outpatient Visits:** 47370 **Births:** 246 **Total Expense ($000):** 45085 **Payroll Expense ($000):** 17618 **Personnel:** 386

SYCAMORE—De Kalb County

☐ **KINDRED HOSPITAL–SYCAMORE (142006)**, 225 Edward Street, Zip 60178–2197; tel. 815/895–2144 **A**1 10 **F**1 3 25 31 38 59 78 119 137
S Kindred Healthcare
Primary Contact: Cindy Smith, Chief Executive Officer
CFO: Jay Schweikart, Chief Financial Officer
CMO: Thomas Liske, M.D., Chief Medical Officer
CHR: Eileen Strachan, Coordinator Human Resources
Web address: www.kindredhealthcare.com
Control: Corporation, Investor–owned, for–profit **Service:** Long–Term Acute Care hospital

Staffed Beds: 69 **Admissions:** 483 **Census:** 45 **Outpatient Visits:** 0 **Births:** 0 **Total Expense ($000):** 14813 **Payroll Expense ($000):** 6997 **Personnel:** 142

TAYLORVILLE—Christian County

★ **TAYLORVILLE MEMORIAL HOSPITAL (141339)**, (Formerly St. Vincent Memorial Hospital), 201 East Pleasant Street, Zip 62568–1597; tel. 217/824–3331, (Total facility includes 20 beds in nursing home–type unit) **A**1 9 10 18 **F**3 11 13 15 22 24 25 26 28 30 31 32 33 34 36 38 42 43 50 54 55 56 57 61 62 63 66 67 68 73 74 75 76 77 79 81 82 84 86 87 96 97 102 106 107 117 118 119 121 122 124 134 135 136 137 **S** Memorial Health System
Primary Contact: Daniel J. Raab, President and Chief Executive Officer
CFO: Sue Hill, Director Finance
CHR: Todd Ray, Director Operations and Human Resources
Web address: www.taylorvillememorial.org
Control: Other not–for–profit (including NFP Corporation) **Service:** General Medical and Surgical

Staffed Beds: 45 **Admissions:** 2100 **Census:** 33 **Outpatient Visits:** 70202 **Births:** 108 **Total Expense ($000):** 29245 **Payroll Expense ($000):** 13537 **Personnel:** 279

TINLEY PARK—Cook County

☐ **TINLEY PARK MENTAL HEALTH CENTER (144019)**, 7400 West 183rd Street, Zip 60477–3695; tel. 708/614–4000, (Nonreporting) **A**1 10
Primary Contact: Brenda Hampton, Network Manager
CFO: Ruth Doyle, Business Administrator
CMO: Lambros Chrones, M.D., Medical Director
Control: State–Government, nonfederal **Service:** Psychiatric

Staffed Beds: 150

URBANA—Champaign County

★ △ **CARLE FOUNDATION HOSPITAL (140091)**, 611 West Park Street, Zip 61801–2595; tel. 217/383–3311 **A**1 2 3 5 7 9 10 12 13 **F**3 7 8 11 12 13 17 18 20 22 24 25 26 27 32 33 35 38 40 42 43 44 48 49 50 51 52 54 55 56 57 58 59 60 61 62 63 66 68 69 70 72 73 74 76 77 78 79 80 81 82 84 85 86 118 119 120 121 124 135 137 **P**5
Primary Contact: James C. Leonard, M.D., President and Chief Executive Officer
COO: John T. Snyder, Executive Vice President
CFO: Robert Tonkinson, Vice President Finance
CMO: Napoleon Knight, M.D., Vice President Medical Affairs
CIO: Rick Rinehart, Chief Information Officer
CHR: Phillip Kubow, Vice President Human Resources
Web address: www.carle.com/hospital
Control: Other not–for–profit (including NFP Corporation) **Service:** General Medical and Surgical

Staffed Beds: 276 **Admissions:** 17093 **Census:** 203 **Outpatient Visits:** 245142 **Births:** 2104 **Total Expense ($000):** 322497 **Payroll Expense ($000):** 94935 **Personnel:** 1806

★ △ **PROVENA COVENANT MEDICAL CENTER (140113)**, 1400 West Park Street, Zip 61801–2396; tel. 217/337–2000 **A**1 3 5 7 9 10 **F**3 7 11 13 15 18 19 20 22 23 24 25 26 27 30 31 32 33 36 38 42 43 44 45 49 50 54 55 56 57 60 62 63 66 68 72 73 74 75 76 77 79 80 81 82 84 85 86 88 90 91 92 93 96 97 99 100 102 107 109 111 118 119 121 124 132 135 136 137
S Provena Health
Primary Contact: David Bertauski, President and Chief Executive Officer
COO: Patricia A. Schulte, Chief Operations Officer and Chief Nursing Executive
CFO: Judy Brown, Chief Financial Officer
CIO: Paula Keele, Manager Information Systems
CHR: Janet S. Payne, Vice President Human Resources
Web address: www.provenacovenant.org
Control: Church–operated, Nongovernment, not–for profit **Service:** General Medical and Surgical

Staffed Beds: 202 **Admissions:** 9780 **Census:** 107 **Outpatient Visits:** 241389 **Births:** 1231 **Total Expense ($000):** 133158 **Payroll Expense ($000):** 42143 **Personnel:** 885

VANDALIA—Fayette County

★ **FAYETTE COUNTY HOSPITAL (141346)**, 650 West Taylor Street, Zip 62471–1296; tel. 618/283–1231, (Total facility includes 85 beds in nursing home–type unit) (Nonreporting) **A**1 9 10 18 **S** Alliant Management Services
Primary Contact: Gregory D. Starnes, Chief Executive Officer
CFO: Jolyn Feller, Chief Financial Officer
Web address: www.fayettecountyhospital.org
Control: Hospital district or authority, Government, nonfederal **Service:** General Medical and Surgical

Staffed Beds: 110

WATSEKA—Iroquois County

☐ **IROQUOIS MEMORIAL HOSPITAL AND RESIDENT HOME (140167)**, 200 Fairman Avenue, Zip 60970–1644; tel. 815/432–5841, (Total facility includes 35 beds in nursing home–type unit) (Nonreporting) **A**1 9 10 20
Primary Contact: Stephen O. Leurck, President and Chief Executive Officer
COO: Chuck Bohlmann, Vice President
CIO: Angela Rathburn, Director Information Systems
Web address: www.iroquoismemorial.com
Control: Other not–for–profit (including NFP Corporation) **Service:** General Medical and Surgical

Staffed Beds: 84

WAUKEGAN—Lake County

★ **VISTA MEDICAL CENTER EAST (140084)**, 1324 North Sheridan Road, Zip 60085–2181; tel. 847/360–4000 **A**1 2 10 **F**12 13 15 18 20 22 24 25 26 27 30 31 32 33 36 38 40 43 46 49 57 59 66 68 72 74 76 77 79 80 86 92 96 100 102 103 104 107 118 119 121 135 136 137 **P**6 **S** Community Health Systems, Inc.
Primary Contact: Barbara J. Martin, RN, President and Chief Executive Officer
CFO: John Kerndl, Vice President Finance and Chief Financial Officer
CMO: Robert Thain, M.D., President Medical Staff
CIO: Cathy Adler–Marks, Director Information Technology
CHR: Robin Matsil, Director Human Resources
Web address: www.vistahealth.com
Control: Corporation, Investor–owned, for–profit **Service:** General Medical and Surgical

Staffed Beds: 209 **Admissions:** 11457 **Census:** 118 **Outpatient Visits:** 105439 **Births:** 2035 **Total Expense ($000):** 122405 **Payroll Expense ($000):** 45640 **Personnel:** 840

★ △ **VISTA MEDICAL CENTER WEST (140033)**, 2615 Washington Street, Zip 60085–4988; tel. 847/249–3900 **A**1 7 10 **F**25 26 30 31 32 33 36 38 57 62 66 85 88 89 91 92 94 95 119 121 **P**6 **S** Community Health Systems, Inc.
Primary Contact: Barbara J. Martin, RN, President and Chief Executive Officer
CFO: John Kerndl, Vice President Finance and Chief Financial Officer
CMO: Robert Thain, M.D., President Medical Staff
CIO: Cathy Adler–Marks, Director Information Technology
CHR: Robin Matsil, Director Human Resources
Web address: www.vistahealth.com
Control: Corporation, Investor–owned, for–profit **Service:** Psychiatric

Staffed Beds: 67 **Admissions:** 2174 **Census:** 43 **Outpatient Visits:** 14969 **Births:** 0 **Total Expense ($000):** 15763 **Payroll Expense ($000):** 6690 **Personnel:** 113

WHEATON—Du Page County

★ △ **MARIANJOY REHABILITATION HOSPITAL (143027)**, 26 West 171 Roosevelt Road, Zip 60187–0795, Mailing Address: P.O. Box 795, Zip 60189–0795; tel. 630/909–8000 **A**1 3 5 7 9 10 **F**11 25 26 30 31 33 34 54 55 56 57 62 73 81 82 85 86 121 132 135 **P**6 **S** Wheaton Franciscan Healthcare
Primary Contact: Kathleen C. Yosko, President and Chief Executive Officer
CFO: Michael Hedderman, Senior Vice President Finance and Chief Financial Officer
CMO: Noel Rao, M.D., Medical Director
CIO: Pat Orrison, Director Information Services
CHR: Teresa Chapman, Vice President Human Resources
Web address: www.marianjoy.org
Control: Church–operated, Nongovernment, not–for profit **Service:** Rehabilitation

Staffed Beds: 120 **Admissions:** 2428 **Census:** 101 **Outpatient Visits:** 49378 **Births:** 0 **Total Expense ($000):** 56300 **Payroll Expense ($000):** 28387 **Personnel:** 709

WINFIELD—Du Page County

★ **CENTRAL DUPAGE HOSPITAL (140242)**, 25 North Winfield Road, Zip 60190; tel. 630/933–1600, (Includes BEHAVIORAL HEALTH CENTER, 27 West 350 High Lake Road, tel. 630/653–4000) **A**1 2 5 9 10 **F**3 4 5 8 11 12 13 15 17 18 20 22 24 25 26 27 30 31 32 33 34 35 36 37 38 39 40 41 43 44 46 47 48 49 50 53 55 56 57 58 59 62 66 68 70 71 72 73 74 76 77 78 79 80 81 82 83 84 86 88 89 90 91 92 93 94 95 96 97 100 102 103 104 105 106 107 114 116 118 119 120 121 124 130 132 133 135 136 137
Primary Contact: Luke McGuinness, President
CFO: James Spear, Executive Vice President and Chief Financial Officer
CMO: Kevin Most, D.O., Vice President Medical Affairs
CIO: David Printz, Vice President and Chief Information Officer
Web address: www.cdh.org
Control: Other not–for–profit (including NFP Corporation) **Service:** General Medical and Surgical

Staffed Beds: 337 **Admissions:** 21767 **Census:** 242 **Outpatient Visits:** 454320 **Births:** 3029 **Total Expense ($000):** 397104 **Payroll Expense ($000):** 138990 **Personnel:** 1953

WOODSTOCK—McHenry County

★ **CENTEGRA MEMORIAL MEDICAL CENTER (140176)**, 3701 Doty Road, Zip 60098–3797, Mailing Address: P.O. Box 1990, Zip 60098–1990; tel. 815/338–2500 **A**1 2 9 10 **F**3 4 5 11 12 13 15 24 25 26 27 30 31 32 33 36 38 40 41 42 43 44 47 49 50 55 56 57 62 66 67 68 72 73 74 76 77 79 80 81 82 84 86 88 89 90 91 92 93 94 95 96 97 100 102 103 106 107 111 112 117 118 119 121 123 132 135 136 137 **P**5 **S** Centegra Health System
Primary Contact: Michael S. Eesley, President and Chief Executive Officer
COO: Jason Sciarro, Chief Operating Officer
CFO: Robert Rosenberger, Interim Chief Financial Officer
CMO: Z. Ted Lorenc, M.D., Chief Medical Officer
CIO: Paul Solverson, Interim Chief Information Officer
CHR: Barbara Jo Johnson, Senior Vice President Human Resources
Web address: www.centegra.org
Control: Other not–for–profit (including NFP Corporation) **Service:** General Medical and Surgical

Staffed Beds: 145 **Admissions:** 8959 **Census:** 109 **Outpatient Visits:** 90797 **Births:** 1248 **Total Expense ($000):** 120115 **Payroll Expense ($000):** 55387 **Personnel:** 853

ZION—Lake County

□ **MIDWESTERN REGIONAL MEDICAL CENTER (140100)**, 2520 Elisha Avenue, Zip 60099–2587; tel. 847/872–4561, (Nonreporting) **A**1 2 5 9 10 **S** Cancer Treatment Centers of America
Primary Contact: Roger C. Cary, President and Chief Executive Officer
CFO: Cecilia Taylor, Director Finance
CMO: Edgar Staren, M.D., Senior Vice President Medical Affairs
CIO: Chad Eckes, Chief Information Officer
CHR: Scott Gallo, Director Human Resources
Web address: www.cancercenter.com
Control: Corporation, Investor–owned, for–profit **Service:** General Medical and Surgical

Staffed Beds: 73

IL

Hospital, Medicare Provider Number, Address, Telephone, Approval, Facility, and Physician Codes, Health Care System

★ American Hospital Association (AHA) membership
□ The Joint Commission accreditation
○ American Osteopathic Association (AOA) accreditation
△ Commission on Accreditation of Rehabilitation Facilities (CARF) accreditation

INDIANA

ANDERSON—Madison County

☐ **COMMUNITY HOSPITAL OF ANDERSON AND MADISON COUNTY (150113)**, 1515 North Madison Avenue, Zip 46011–3453; tel. 765/298–4242, (Total facility includes 30 beds in nursing home–type unit) **A**1 2 9 **F**3 6 11 13 15 18 20 22 24 25 26 27 28 30 31 32 33 38 41 49 50 51 53 54 55 56 57 58 60 62 65 66 68 70 72 73 74 75 76 77 79 80 81 82 84 86 96 97 100 102 107 118 119 121 124 132 135 136 137 **S** Community Health Network
Primary Contact: William C. Vanness, II, M.D., President
Web address: www.ecommunity.org
Control: Other not–for–profit (including NFP Corporation) **Service:** General Medical and Surgical

Staffed Beds: 173 **Admissions:** 7077 **Census:** 80 **Outpatient Visits:** 146018 **Births:** 1043 **Total Expense ($000):** 104293 **Payroll Expense ($000):** 47968 **Personnel:** 990

★ **SAINT JOHN'S HEALTH SYSTEM (150088)**, 2015 Jackson Street, Zip 46016–4339; tel. 765/649–2511, (Total facility includes 20 beds in nursing home–type unit) **A**1 2 9 10 **F**3 4 5 8 11 13 14 15 18 24 25 26 27 28 30 31 32 33 36 37 38 40 41 42 43 44 50 51 53 55 56 57 58 59 60 61 62 63 64 66 68 72 73 74 75 76 77 79 80 81 82 84 85 86 88 89 90 91 92 93 94 95 96 97 99 100 102 104 105 106 107 108 109 111 117 118 119 121 123 124 133 134 135 136 137 **P**7 **S** Ascension Health
Primary Contact: Thomas J. VanOsdol, Interim President
COO: Thomas J. VanOsdol, Vice President
CFO: Donald L. Apple, Chief Financial Officer
CMO: Gary Brazel, M.D., Chief Medical Officer
CIO: Roger Strange, Chief Information Officer
CHR: Glenn Fields, Vice President Human Resources
Web address: www.stjohnshealthsystem.org
Control: Church–operated, Nongovernment, not–for profit **Service:** General Medical and Surgical

Staffed Beds: 209 **Admissions:** 7784 **Census:** 138 **Outpatient Visits:** 330931 **Births:** 464 **Total Expense ($000):** 150866 **Payroll Expense ($000):** 68980 **Personnel:** 1378

ANGOLA—Steuben County

★ △ **CAMERON MEMORIAL COMMUNITY HOSPITAL (151315)**, 416 East Maumee Street, Zip 46703–2015; tel. 260/665–2141 **A**7 9 10 18 **F**3 5 10 11 13 15 24 26 30 31 32 42 43 44 61 64 66 68 74 79 80 82 86 96 99 102 103 107 108 111 119 122 124 133 135
Primary Contact: Ellen Bisson, Interim Chief Executive Officer
CFO: Darryl Faye, Vice President Finance
Web address: www.cameronmch.com
Control: Other not–for–profit (including NFP Corporation) **Service:** General Medical and Surgical

Staffed Beds: 25 **Admissions:** 1007 **Census:** 8 **Outpatient Visits:** 115202 **Births:** 232 **Total Expense ($000):** 32988 **Payroll Expense ($000):** 12512 **Personnel:** 327

AUBURN—De Kalb County

★ **DEKALB MEMORIAL HOSPITAL (150045)**, 1316 East Seventh Street, Zip 46706–2515, Mailing Address: P.O. Box 542, Zip 46706–0542; tel. 260/925–4600 **A**9 10 **F**3 7 11 13 15 24 25 28 30 31 32 33 34 38 42 43 44 52 54 55 56 57 61 62 68 73 74 75 77 79 80 81 82 86 87 96 97 100 102 106 107 118 119 121 124 135 137 **P**6 8
Primary Contact: Jack M. Corey, President
CFO: Craig Polkow, Chief Financial Officer
CMO: James Buchanan, M.D., Chief Medical Officer
CIO: Ed Hobbs, Director Information Services
CHR: Deb Arend Sinclair, Director Human Resources
Web address: www.dekalbmemorial.com
Control: Other not–for–profit (including NFP Corporation) **Service:** General Medical and Surgical

Staffed Beds: 48 **Admissions:** 2131 **Census:** 16 **Outpatient Visits:** 89572 **Births:** 527 **Total Expense ($000):** 37944 **Payroll Expense ($000):** 16853 **Personnel:** 377

AVON—Marion County

★ **CLARIAN WEST MEDICAL CENTER (150158)**, 1111 North Ronald Reagan Parkway, Zip 46123; tel. 317/217–3000 **A**1 5 9 10 **F**13 15 18 20 25 26 31 38 40 68 72 74 79 80 82 84 86 96 100 107 109 118 119 124 135 136 **S** Clarian Health
Primary Contact: Alfonso W. Gatmaitan, Chief Executive Officer
COO: Doug Puckett, Chief Operating Officer and Chief Financial Officer
CFO: Doug Puckett, Chief Operating Officer and Chief Financial Officer
CMO: James Fesenmeier, M.D., Chief of Staff
CHR: Lana Funkhouser, Vice President Human Resources
Web address: www.clarian.org
Control: Corporation, Investor–owned, for–profit **Service:** General Medical and Surgical

Staffed Beds: 86 **Admissions:** 4354 **Census:** 45 **Outpatient Visits:** 80407 **Births:** 1212 **Total Expense ($000):** 88548 **Payroll Expense ($000):** 28244 **Personnel:** 520

BATESVILLE—Ripley County

★ **MARGARET MARY COMMUNITY HOSPITAL (151329)**, 321 Mitchell Avenue, Zip 47006–0226, Mailing Address: P.O. Box 226, Zip 47006–0226; tel. 812/934–6624 **A**1 9 10 18 **F**3 13 15 24 27 30 31 32 33 34 37 38 42 50 53 54 56 57 61 62 63 67 68 73 74 76 77 79 80 81 82 86 96 97 100 102 106 107 109 111 118 119 120 121 124 135 137
Primary Contact: James L. Amos, President
CFO: Brian Daeger, Vice President Financial Services
CMO: Charles McGovern, M.D., Chief of Staff
CIO: Donna Nobbe, Director Information Systems
CHR: Tate Shepard, Vice President Human Resources
Web address: www.mmch.org
Control: Other not–for–profit (including NFP Corporation) **Service:** General Medical and Surgical

Staffed Beds: 25 **Admissions:** 1713 **Census:** 15 **Outpatient Visits:** 272268 **Births:** 379 **Total Expense ($000):** 45784 **Payroll Expense ($000):** 18379 **Personnel:** 384

BEDFORD—Lawrence County

★ **BEDFORD REGIONAL MEDICAL CENTER (151328)**, 2900 West 16th Street, Zip 47421–3583; tel. 812/275–1200 **A**1 2 9 10 18 **F**3 7 11 13 15 24 25 26 27 30 31 32 33 34 35 37 38 41 43 44 46 49 50 51 55 56 57 61 62 63 66 68 69 72 73 74 75 76 77 79 80 81 82 84 85 86 87 90 92 94 96 97 100 102 103 105 106 107 118 119 120 121 122 123 124 133 134 135 136 137 **P**6 **S** Clarian Health
Primary Contact: Bradford W. Dykes, President and Chief Executive Officer
COO: James Pittman, Vice President Operations
CFO: Charles L. Shetler, CPA, Chief Financial Officer
CIO: Becky Johnson, Director Management Information Systems
CHR: Cindy Smale, Director Human Resources
Web address: www.brmchealthcare.com
Control: Other not–for–profit (including NFP Corporation) **Service:** General Medical and Surgical

Staffed Beds: 25 **Admissions:** 1648 **Census:** 18 **Outpatient Visits:** 73272 **Births:** 90 **Total Expense ($000):** 46281 **Payroll Expense ($000):** 23934 **Personnel:** 471

DUNN MEMORIAL HOSPITAL (151335), 1600 23rd Street, Zip 47421–4704; tel. 812/275–3331 **A**9 10 18 **F**7 11 13 17 18 20 24 25 30 31 32 33 38 43 46 53 54 55 56 57 61 62 68 74 75 77 79 85 86 88 93 96 100 107 120 124 135 137 **P**3 5
Primary Contact: Michael W. Cooper, Chief Executive Officer
COO: Debra Bruner, Chief Operating Officer
CMO: Deborah Craton, M.D., Chief Medical Staff
CIO: Chad Damon, Chief Information Officer
CHR: Darci Medlock, Manager Human Resources
Web address: www.dunnmemorial.org
Control: County–Government, nonfederal **Service:** General Medical and Surgical

Staffed Beds: 25 **Admissions:** 1956 **Census:** 23 **Outpatient Visits:** 50066 **Births:** 360 **Personnel:** 515

BEECH GROVE—Marion County

☐ **SELECT SPECIALTY HOSPITAL OF BEECH GROVE (152013)**, 1600 Albany Street, Suite 200, Zip 46107; tel. 317/783–8913 **A**1 10 **F**1 3 25 26 27 30 31 32 37 59 73 80 82 119 132 137 **S** Select Medical Corporation
Primary Contact: Cheryl G. Gentry, Chief Executive Officer
Web address: www.selectmedicalcorp.com
Control: Corporation, Investor–owned, for–profit **Service:** Long–Term Acute Care hospital

Staffed Beds: 40 **Admissions:** 463 **Census:** 35 **Outpatient Visits:** 0 **Births:** 0 **Total Expense ($000):** 19086 **Payroll Expense ($000):** 7412 **Personnel:** 127

IN

○ **ST. FRANCIS HOSPITAL AND HEALTH CENTERS – NORTH CAMPUS (150033)**, 1600 Albany Street, Zip 46107–1593; tel. 317/787–3311, (Total facility includes 35 beds in nursing home–type unit) (Nonreporting) **A**2 3 5 9 10 11 **S** Sisters of St. Francis Health Services, Inc.
Primary Contact: Robert J. Brody, President and Chief Executive Officer
COO: Keith Jewell, Chief Operating Officer
CFO: Jay R. Brehm, Regional Chief Financial Officer
CMO: Alan Gillespie, Vice President Medical Affairs
CIO: Barbara Coulter, Director Information Systems
CHR: John Ross, Vice President Human Resources
Web address: www.stfrancishospitals.org
Control: Church–operated, Nongovernment, not–for profit **Service:** General Medical and Surgical

Staffed Beds: 434

BLOOMINGTON—Monroe County

★□ **BLOOMINGTON HOSPITAL (150051)**, 601 West Second Street, Zip 47403–2317, Mailing Address: P.O. Box 1149, Zip 47402–1149; tel. 812/336–6821 **A**1 2 5 9 10 19 **F**3 6 7 8 11 12 13 15 17 18 20 22 24 25 26 27 30 31 32 33 36 38 39 40 42 43 44 46 48 49 50 52 53 55 56 57 59 60 61 62 63 68 69 71 72 73 74 75 76 77 79 80 81 82 84 85 86 88 90 91 92 93 94 95 96 97 100 102 103 107 108 109 118 119 120 121 124 132 133 135 136 137 **P**6
Primary Contact: Mark E. Moore, President and Chief Executive Officer
COO: Larry Bailey, Vice President and Chief Operating Officer
CFO: Jim Myers, Chief Financial Officer
CIO: Mark W. McMath, Chief Information Officer
CHR: Steven Deckard, Vice President Human Resources
Web address: www.bloomingtonhospital.org
Control: Other not–for–profit (including NFP Corporation) **Service:** General Medical and Surgical

Staffed Beds: 280 **Admissions:** 13583 **Census:** 166 **Outpatient Visits:** 283955 **Births:** 2174 **Total Expense ($000):** 247308 **Payroll Expense ($000):** 108644 **Personnel:** 2177

□ **MEADOWS HOSPITAL (154041)**, 3600 North Prow Road, Zip 47404; tel. 812/331–8000 **A**1 10 **F**4 50 88 89 91 92 119 **P**6 **S** Psychiatric Solutions
Primary Contact: Kurt A. Isaacson, Chief Executive Officer
Web address: www.psysolutions.com
Control: Partnership, Investor–owned, for–profit **Service:** Psychiatric

Staffed Beds: 66 **Admissions:** 1080 **Census:** 45 **Outpatient Visits:** 207 **Births:** 0 **Total Expense ($000):** 7506 **Payroll Expense ($000):** 4923 **Personnel:** 129

MONROE HOSPITAL (150164), 4011 South Tiwari Boulevard, Zip 47403; tel. 812/825–1111 **A**9 10 **F**3 18 20 25 30 31 32 38 51 55 56 57 62 63 68 77 79 80 96 100 102 107 119 124 **P**2 5 6
Primary Contact: Fred Price, Interim Chief Executive Officer
Web address: www.monroehospital.com
Control: Corporation, Investor–owned, for–profit **Service:** General Medical and Surgical

Staffed Beds: 20 **Admissions:** 884 **Census:** 8 **Outpatient Visits:** 21972 **Births:** 1 **Total Expense ($000):** 24076 **Payroll Expense ($000):** 8383 **Personnel:** 213

BLUFFTON—Wells County

★□ **BLUFFTON REGIONAL MEDICAL CENTER (150075)**, 303 South Main Street, Zip 46714–2529; tel. 260/824–3210, (Total facility includes 13 beds in nursing home–type unit) **A**1 2 9 10 **F**3 5 9 12 13 15 17 24 25 26 27 30 31 32 33 37 38 43 48 49 53 54 55 57 61 62 63 66 68 73 74 75 76 77 79 81 82 84 86 87 96 99 100 107 117 118 119 121 124 135 **P**8 **S** Community Health Systems, Inc.
Primary Contact: Thomas A. Clark, Chief Executive Officer
COO: Vicki Hanselman, Chief Operating Officer
CFO: Larry DeBolt, Chief Financial Officer
CMO: Carol Butler, M.D., President Medical Staff
CIO: Vicki Hanselman, Chief Operating Officer
Web address: www.blufftonregional.com
Control: Corporation, Investor–owned, for–profit **Service:** General Medical and Surgical

Staffed Beds: 79 **Admissions:** 2767 **Census:** 38 **Outpatient Visits:** 49156 **Births:** 274 **Total Expense ($000):** 41988 **Payroll Expense ($000):** 14405 **Personnel:** 307

BOONVILLE—Warrick County

★□ **ST. MARY'S WARRICK HOSPITAL (151325)**, 1116 Millis Avenue, Zip 47601–0629, Mailing Address: P.O. Box 629, Zip 47601–0629; tel. 812/897–4800 **A**1 9 10 18 **F**3 11 15 24 25 26 30 33 38 50 52 54 55 57 60 62 68 75 77 79 84 86 87 88 93 96 100 102 107 117 119 122 124 135 **S** Ascension Health
Primary Contact: Carol Godsey, Administrator
CHR: Lisa Hodges, Executive Director Ancillary Services
Web address: www.stmarys.org
Control: Other not–for–profit (including NFP Corporation) **Service:** General Medical and Surgical

Staffed Beds: 35 **Admissions:** 1135 **Census:** 18 **Outpatient Visits:** 29162 **Births:** 1 **Total Expense ($000):** 13257 **Payroll Expense ($000):** 6367 **Personnel:** 154

BRAZIL—Clay County

★□ **ST. VINCENT CLAY HOSPITAL (151309)**, 1206 East National Avenue, Zip 47834–2797, Mailing Address: P.O. Box 489, Zip 47834–0489; tel. 812/442–2500, (Nonreporting) **A**1 9 10 18 **S** Ascension Health
Primary Contact: Jerry Laue, Administrator
CFO: Wayne Knight, Director Finance
CMO: Craig Johnson, D.O., Medical Director
CHR: Jennifer French, Director Organizational Quality
Web address: www.stvincent.org
Control: Hospital district or authority, Government, nonfederal **Service:** General Medical and Surgical

Staffed Beds: 25

BREMEN—Marshall County

★ **COMMUNITY HOSPITAL OF BREMEN (151300)**, 1020 High Road, Zip 46506, Mailing Address: P.O. Box 8, Zip 46506–0008; tel. 574/546–2211 **A**9 10 18 **F**3 11 13 15 24 25 30 31 32 33 38 42 43 50 55 56 57 62 63 64 66 67 73 74 75 77 79 84 86 87 96 100 102 107 117 118 119 121 122 124 135 **P**1
Primary Contact: Scott R. Graybill, President and Chief Executive Officer
CFO: Debra Kipfer, Chief Financial Officer
CMO: Paul Gettinger, M.D., President Medical Staff
CIO: Linda Barrett, Director Information Systems
CHR: Patricia Board, Vice President Human Resources
Web address: www.bremenhospital.com
Control: Other not–for–profit (including NFP Corporation) **Service:** General Medical and Surgical

Staffed Beds: 24 **Admissions:** 436 **Census:** 5 **Outpatient Visits:** 27086 **Births:** 81 **Total Expense ($000):** 12986 **Payroll Expense ($000):** 6147 **Personnel:** 128

CARMEL—Hamilton County

★□ **CLARIAN NORTH MEDICAL CENTER (150161)**, 11700 North Meridian Avenue, Zip 46032; tel. 317/688–2000 **A**1 9 10 **F**3 12 13 15 18 20 25 26 27 30 32 33 34 35 37 38 40 49 55 56 57 59 62 66 68 70 72 73 74 76 77 79 80 82 83 84 86 96 97 99 100 103 107 113 114 116 118 119 121 124 135 136 137 **S** Clarian Health
Primary Contact: Jonathan R. Goble, President and Chief Executive Officer
COO: Randall C. Yust, Chief Operating Officer and Chief Financial Officer
CFO: Randall C. Yust, Chief Operating Officer and Chief Financial Officer
CMO: Lynda Ann Smirz, M.D., Chief Medical Officer
CIO: Terry Baker, Manager Information Services
CHR: Angela S. Thompson, Vice President Human Resources and Support Services
Web address: www.clariannorth.com
Control: Partnership, Investor–owned, for–profit **Service:** General Medical and Surgical

Staffed Beds: 154 **Admissions:** 6766 **Census:** 71 **Outpatient Visits:** 68965 **Births:** 2128 **Total Expense ($000):** 154517 **Payroll Expense ($000):** 50685 **Personnel:** 938

★□ **ST. VINCENT CARMEL HOSPITAL (150157)**, 13500 North Meridian Street, Zip 46032; tel. 317/582–7000 **A**1 9 **F**3 11 12 13 15 25 26 27 30 31 32 33 37 38 41 46 48 49 50 52 55 56 57 59 66 67 68 72 73 74 75 77 79 80 81 82 90 92 96 99 100 102 107 118 119 120 121 124 132 134 135 136 137 **P**6 8 **S** Ascension Health
Primary Contact: Michael D. Chittenden, President
Web address: www.stvincent.org
Control: Church–operated, Nongovernment, not–for profit **Service:** General Medical and Surgical

Staffed Beds: 104 **Admissions:** 6095 **Census:** 63 **Outpatient Visits:** 52811 **Births:** 1272 **Total Expense ($000):** 95166 **Payroll Expense ($000):** 39658 **Personnel:** 762

IN

Hospital, Medicare Provider Number, Address, Telephone, Approval, Facility, and Physician Codes, Health Care System

★ American Hospital Association (AHA) membership
□ The Joint Commission accreditation
○ American Osteopathic Association (AOA) accreditation
△ Commission on Accreditation of Rehabilitation Facilities (CARF) accreditation

CHARLESTOWN—Clark County

☐ **SAINT CATHERINE REGIONAL HOSPITAL (150163)**, 2200 Market Street, Zip 47111–0009, Mailing Address: P.O. Box 9, Zip 47111–0009; tel. 812/256–3301, (Nonreporting) **A**1 9 10 **S** Saint Catherine Healthcare, LLC
Primary Contact: Michael J. Funk, President and Chief Executive Officer
CMO: William Garner, M.D., Chief Medical Officer
CIO: Kevin McLaughlin, Director Information Systems
Web address: www.stchc.com/scrh/
Control: Corporation, Investor–owned, for–profit **Service:** General Medical and Surgical

Staffed Beds: 77

CLINTON—Vermillion County

○ **WEST CENTRAL COMMUNITY HOSPITAL (151326)**, 801 South Main Street, Zip 47842–0349; tel. 765/832–2451 **A**9 10 11 18 **F**13 15 25 30 31 32 33 37 38 46 52 55 62 66 68 72 73 74 75 76 77 79 81 82 84 86 87 96 102 103 107 119 122 135 **P**6
Primary Contact: Terri L. Hill, Administrator
COO: Scott Teffeteller, Vice President and Chief Operating Officer
CFO: Wayne Hutson, Chief Financial Officer
CMO: Greg Brock, D.O., Chief of Staff
CIO: Kym Pfrank, Vice President Information Systems
CHR: Sally Zuel, Vice President Human Resources
Web address: www.uhhg.org/wcch/index.html
Control: Other not–for–profit (including NFP Corporation) **Service:** General Medical and Surgical

Staffed Beds: 25 **Admissions:** 1344 **Census:** 10 **Outpatient Visits:** 47365 **Births:** 122 **Total Expense ($000):** 18979 **Payroll Expense ($000):** 8377 **Personnel:** 174

COLUMBIA CITY—Whitley County

⊠ **PARKVIEW WHITLEY HOSPITAL (150101)**, 353 North Oak Street, Zip 46725–1623; tel. 260/248–9000, (Total facility includes 81 beds in nursing home–type unit) **A**1 9 10 **F**3 7 8 13 15 24 25 30 31 32 33 34 36 38 43 50 53 55 56 57 62 67 68 73 74 77 79 80 84 86 96 97 100 102 107 115 117 118 121 124 133 135 137 **S** Parkview Health
Primary Contact: John K. Meister, Chief Operating Officer
COO: John K. Meister, Chief Operating Officer
CFO: Lisa Peppler, Financial and Operations Analyst
CMO: Jeff Brookes, M.D., Medical Director
Web address: www.parkview.com
Control: Other not–for–profit (including NFP Corporation) **Service:** General Medical and Surgical

Staffed Beds: 118 **Admissions:** 1837 **Census:** 85 **Outpatient Visits:** 48010 **Births:** 277 **Total Expense ($000):** 30280 **Payroll Expense ($000):** 14537 **Personnel:** 249

COLUMBUS—Bartholomew County

★ ○ **COLUMBUS REGIONAL HOSPITAL (150112)**, 2400 East 17th Street, Zip 47201–5360; tel. 812/379–4441 **A**2 9 10 11 19 **F**3 7 8 11 12 13 15 17 18 20 22 24 25 26 27 28 30 31 32 33 34 36 37 38 43 44 46 49 50 51 52 55 56 57 58 62 64 66 68 71 72 73 74 75 76 77 79 80 81 82 84 85 86 88 90 91 92 93 96 97 99 100 102 106 107 108 109 111 118 119 120 121 124 132 133 135 136 137 **P**3 8
Primary Contact: James Bickel, Chief Executive Officer
CFO: Marlene Weatherwax, Vice President and Chief Financial Officer
CMO: Thomas Sonderman, M.D., Vice President and Chief Medical Officer
CIO: Diana Boyer, Chief Information Officer
CHR: Joseph Turco, Director Human Resources
Web address: www.crh.org
Control: County–Government, nonfederal **Service:** General Medical and Surgical

Staffed Beds: 251 **Admissions:** 9318 **Census:** 109 **Outpatient Visits:** 218595 **Births:** 1377 **Total Expense ($000):** 177715 **Payroll Expense ($000):** 70208 **Personnel:** 1497

CONNERSVILLE—Fayette County

★ ○ **FAYETTE REGIONAL HEALTH SYSTEM (150064)**, 1941 Virginia Avenue, Zip 47331–9990; tel. 765/825–5131 **A**9 10 11 **F**3 7 8 11 13 15 18 20 24 25 26 27 31 32 38 42 46 49 52 55 56 57 61 68 72 73 74 75 76 77 79 80 82 85 88 89 90 91 92 94 96 100 102 107 109 111 112 118 119 120 121 124 133 135 136
Primary Contact: David R. Brandon, Chief Executive Officer
CFO: John Jeffries, Chief Financial Officer
CMO: William McDonald, M.D., Chief of Staff
CIO: Roy Cupp, Director Management Information Systems
CHR: Rhonda McPherson, Vice President Human Resources
Web address: www.fayetteregional.org
Control: State–Government, nonfederal **Service:** General Medical and Surgical

Staffed Beds: 118 **Admissions:** 2118 **Census:** 43 **Outpatient Visits:** 94953 **Births:** 257 **Total Expense ($000):** 51709 **Payroll Expense ($000):** 25710 **Personnel:** 584

CORYDON—Harrison County

★ ○ **HARRISON COUNTY HOSPITAL (151331)**, 1141 Hospital Drive North W., Zip 47112–1774; tel. 812/738–4251 **A**9 10 11 18 **F**7 13 15 24 25 27 30 31 32 33 38 57 61 62 66 68 73 74 75 76 79 81 82 86 96 97 99 100 103 105 106 107 118 121 124 132 133 135 **P**7
Primary Contact: Steven L. Taylor, Chief Executive Officer
CFO: Jeff Davis, Chief Financial Officer
CIO: Chuck Wiley, Manager Information Systems
CHR: Angie Phelps Sells, Manager Human Resources
Web address: www.hchin.org
Control: County–Government, nonfederal **Service:** General Medical and Surgical

Staffed Beds: 25 **Admissions:** 1435 **Census:** 15 **Outpatient Visits:** 45112 **Births:** 215 **Total Expense ($000):** 33045 **Payroll Expense ($000):** 14986 **Personnel:** 327

CRAWFORDSVILLE—Montgomery County

○ **ST. CLARE MEDICAL CENTER (150022)**, 1710 Lafayette Road, Zip 47933–1099; tel. 765/362–2800, (Total facility includes 17 beds in nursing home–type unit) (Nonreporting) **A**9 10 11 **S** Sisters of St. Francis Health Services, Inc.
Primary Contact: Jim Siemers, Chief Executive Officer
COO: Nancy Sennett, Vice President Nursing Services
CFO: Keith Lauter, Vice President Finance
Web address: www.stclaremedical.org
Control: Other not–for–profit (including NFP Corporation) **Service:** General Medical and Surgical

Staffed Beds: 83

CROWN POINT—Lake County

○ **ST. ANTHONY MEDICAL CENTER (150126)**, 1201 South Main Street, Zip 46307–8483; tel. 219/738–2100, (Nonreporting) **A**2 9 10 11 **S** Sisters of St. Francis Health Services, Inc.
Primary Contact: David Ruskowski, President
COO: Lawrence O. Leaman, Executive Vice President and Chief Operating Officer
CFO: Larry Stazinski, Vice President Finance
CMO: John T. King, M.D., Vice President Medical Staff Affairs
CIO: Michael Worden, Director
CHR: Janet Slaven–Allen, Vice President Human Resources
Web address: www.stanthonymedicalcenter.com
Control: Church–operated, Nongovernment, not–for profit **Service:** General Medical and Surgical

Staffed Beds: 234

DANVILLE—Hendricks County

★ ○ **HENDRICKS REGIONAL HEALTH (150005)**, 1000 East Main Street, Zip 46122–0409, Mailing Address: P.O. Box 409, Zip 46122–0409; tel. 317/745–4451 **A**2 9 10 11 **F**3 8 11 13 15 18 24 25 26 27 28 30 31 32 33 38 53 54 55 56 57 60 62 64 67 68 72 73 74 75 76 77 79 80 81 82 84 86 87 88 90 91 92 93 96 97 99 100 102 105 106 107 108 109 111 114 118 119 120 121 124 133 135 136 137 **P**6
Primary Contact: Dennis W. Dawes, FACHE, President
CFO: John Komenda, Chief Financial Officer
CMO: John Sparzo, M.D., Vice President Medical Affairs
CIO: Lowell Nicodemus, Director Information Systems
CHR: Gary Lenard, Director Human Resources
Web address: www.hendrickshospital.org
Control: County–Government, nonfederal **Service:** General Medical and Surgical

Staffed Beds: 137 **Admissions:** 5811 **Census:** 62 **Outpatient Visits:** 302935 **Births:** 957 **Total Expense ($000):** 143240 **Payroll Expense ($000):** 65167 **Personnel:** 1240

DECATUR—Adams County

★ **ADAMS MEMORIAL HOSPITAL (151330)**, 1100 Mercer Avenue, Zip 46733–2311, Mailing Address: P.O. Box 151, Zip 46733–0151; tel. 260/724–2145 **A**9 10 18 **F**2 3 5 7 8 13 14 15 24 25 26 27 28 30 31 32 33 36 38 42 43 44 45 50 52 54 55 56 57 61 62 63 64 66 68 73 75 76 77 79 80 81 82 86 87 88 90 91 92 93 94 95 96 97 100 102 107 117 118 119 122 124 132 133 135 136 137
Primary Contact: Marvin L. Baird, Executive Director
CFO: William G. Seck, Chief Financial Officer
Web address: www.adamshospital.com
Control: County–Government, nonfederal **Service:** General Medical and Surgical

Staffed Beds: 50 **Admissions:** 2436 **Census:** 33 **Outpatient Visits:** 67781 **Births:** 202 **Total Expense ($000):** 39929 **Payroll Expense ($000):** 14814 **Personnel:** 386

DYER—Lake County

SAINT MARGARET MERCY HEALTHCARE CENTERS–SOUTH CAMPUS See Saint Margaret Mercy Healthcare Centers, Hammond

 Many Facility Codes have changed. Please refer to the AHA Guide Code Chart.

EAST CHICAGO—Lake County

☒ **REGENCY HOSPITAL OF NORTHWEST INDIANA (152024)**, 4321 Fir Street, 4th Floor, Zip 46312; tel. 219/392–7790, (Nonreporting) **A**1 10 **S** Regency Hospital Company
Primary Contact: Beverly Foster, Chief Executive Officer
Web address: www.regencyhospital.com
Control: Corporation, Investor–owned, for–profit **Service:** Long–Term Acute Care hospital

Staffed Beds: 25

□ △ **ST. CATHERINE HOSPITAL (150008)**, 4321 Fir Street, Zip 46312–3097; tel. 219/392–7000 **A**1 5 7 9 10 **F**1 3 5 11 13 15 18 20 22 24 25 26 27 31 32 33 38 43 49 50 53 55 56 57 58 59 60 61 62 66 68 73 74 75 76 77 78 79 80 81 82 84 86 88 89 90 91 92 93 94 96 97 100 102 107 108 117 118 119 121 124 135 136 137 **P**1 **S** Community Healthcare System
Primary Contact: JoAnn Birdzell, President and Chief Executive Officer
CFO: Joseph Winterhaler, Chief Financial Officer
CMO: John Griep, M.D., Chief Medical Director
CIO: Vernon Groeber, Chief Information Officer
Web address: www.stcatherinehospital.org
Control: Other not–for–profit (including NFP Corporation) **Service:** General Medical and Surgical

Staffed Beds: 200 **Admissions:** 7811 **Census:** 108 **Outpatient Visits:** 115746 **Births:** 777 **Total Expense ($000):** 127216 **Payroll Expense ($000):** 43704 **Personnel:** 885

ELKHART—Elkhart County

★ ○ △ **ELKHART GENERAL HOSPITAL (150018)**, 600 East Boulevard, Zip 46514–2499, Mailing Address: P.O. Box 1329, Zip 46515–1329; tel. 574/294–2621 **A**2 5 7 9 10 11 **F**3 11 12 13 14 15 17 18 20 22 24 25 26 27 30 31 32 33 34 38 43 46 49 50 51 55 56 57 59 60 61 62 66 67 70 72 73 74 75 76 77 79 80 81 82 84 85 86 88 89 90 92 94 95 96 97 99 100 102 103 106 107 108 109 118 119 121 123 124 135 136 137 **P**8
Primary Contact: Gregory W. Lintjer, President
COO: Greg Losasso, Vice President Operations
CFO: Kevin Higdon, Vice President Finance
CMO: Kenneth L. Gammon, M.D., Chief of Staff
CIO: Wade Patrick, Director Information Systems
CHR: Kurt A. Meyer, Vice President Human Resources
Web address: www.egh.org
Control: Other not–for–profit (including NFP Corporation) **Service:** General Medical and Surgical

Staffed Beds: 297 **Admissions:** 12340 **Census:** 158 **Outpatient Visits:** 438768 **Births:** 1342 **Total Expense ($000):** 246605 **Payroll Expense ($000):** 86256 **Personnel:** 1778

ELWOOD—Madison County

☒ **ST. VINCENT MERCY HOSPITAL (151308)**, 1331 South A Street, Zip 46036–1942; tel. 765/552–4600 **A**1 2 9 10 18 **F**3 5 8 11 15 24 25 26 27 30 31 32 33 38 40 41 43 46 50 53 54 55 56 57 58 62 63 66 68 72 73 75 76 77 79 80 81 82 86 87 89 91 94 96 97 100 102 107 117 118 119 120 121 122 123 124 130 132 135 137 **P**6 **S** Ascension Health
Primary Contact: Deborah Y. Rasper, FACHE, Administrator
COO: Ann C. Yates, R.N., Director Patient Care and Clinical Services
CFO: Lora A. Webber, Director Financial Services
CMO: Stephen Berghofer, M.D., Chief Medical Officer
CHR: Barbara Whitenack, Manager Human Resources
Web address: www.stvincent.org
Control: Church–operated, Nongovernment, not–for profit **Service:** General Medical and Surgical

Staffed Beds: 25 **Admissions:** 859 **Census:** 13 **Outpatient Visits:** 45747 **Births:** 0 **Total Expense ($000):** 23838 **Payroll Expense ($000):** 11465 **Personnel:** 241

EVANSVILLE—Vanderburgh County

☒ **DEACONESS HOSPITAL (150082)**, 600 Mary Street, Zip 47747–0001; tel. 812/450–5000, (Includes DEACONESS CROSS POINTE CENTER, 7200 East Indiana Street, Zip 47715; tel. 812/476–7200; Cheryl Rietman, Chief Administrative Officer), (Total facility includes 48 beds in nursing home–type unit) **A**1 2 3 5 9 10 **F**3 5 11 12 17 18 20 22 24 25 26 27 30 31 32 33 34 36 37 38 40 41 42 43 46 49 50 52 53 54 55 56 57 58 59 60 61 62 63 64 66 67 68 69 72 73 75 76 77 79 80 81 82 83 84 87 88 89 90 91 92 94 95 96 97 100 102 103 106 107 108 109 111 117 118 119 121 124 132 133 134 135 137 **P**1 **S** Deaconess Health System
Primary Contact: Harry L. Smith, Jr., President and Chief Executive Officer
COO: Shawn W. McCoy, Chief Administrative Officer
CFO: Richard M. Stivers, Senior Vice President and Chief Financial Officer
CMO: James Porter, M.D., Vice President Medical Affairs
CIO: James Kloosterman, Chief Information Officer
CHR: Larry Pile, Director Human Resources
Web address: www.deaconess.com
Control: Other not–for–profit (including NFP Corporation) **Service:** General Medical and Surgical

Staffed Beds: 541 **Admissions:** 25066 **Census:** 376 **Outpatient Visits:** 262440 **Births:** 0 **Total Expense ($000):** 393376 **Payroll Expense ($000):** 153711 **Personnel:** 2914

□ **EVANSVILLE STATE HOSPITAL**, 3400 Lincoln Avenue, Zip 47714–0146; tel. 812/469–6800, (Nonreporting) **A**1
Primary Contact: Robert M. Spear, Superintendent
CFO: Janet Kelsey, Director Business
CMO: Melba Briones, M.D., Medical Director
CHR: Cheryl Lutey, Director Human Resources
Control: State–Government, nonfederal **Service:** Psychiatric

Staffed Beds: 168

☒ **HEALTHSOUTH DEACONESS REHABILITATION HOSPITAL (153025)**, 4100 Covert Avenue, Zip 47714–5567, Mailing Address: P.O. Box 5349, Zip 47716–5349; tel. 812/476–9983, (Total facility includes 12 beds in nursing home–type unit) **A**1 9 10 **F**24 25 30 31 32 62 66 73 82 85 86 117 119 121 132 137 **S** HEALTHSOUTH Corporation
Primary Contact: Barbara Butler, Chief Executive Officer
CFO: Diane Riley, Controller
CMO: Ashok Dhingra, M.D., Executive Medical Director
CHR: Sue Nolte, Director Human Resources
Web address: www.healthsouth.com
Control: Corporation, Investor–owned, for–profit **Service:** Rehabilitation

Staffed Beds: 80 **Admissions:** 1195 **Census:** 46 **Outpatient Visits:** 6486 **Births:** 0 **Total Expense ($000):** 11364 **Payroll Expense ($000):** 6100 **Personnel:** 146

□ **SELECT SPECIALTY HOSPITAL OF EVANSVILLE (152014)**, 600 Mary Street, Suite 3325, Zip 47747; tel. 812/450–5270 **A**1 10 **F**1 3 25 27 59 137 **S** Select Medical Corporation
Primary Contact: Tracy Conroy, Chief Executive Officer
Web address: www.selectmedicalcorp.com
Control: Corporation, Investor–owned, for–profit **Service:** Long–Term Acute Care hospital

Staffed Beds: 60 **Admissions:** 556 **Census:** 40 **Outpatient Visits:** 0 **Births:** 0 **Total Expense ($000):** 20066 **Payroll Expense ($000):** 7675 **Personnel:** 202

☒ △ **ST. MARY'S MEDICAL CENTER OF EVANSVILLE (150100)**, 3700 Washington Avenue, Zip 47750–0002; tel. 812/485–4000 **A**1 2 3 5 7 9 10 **F**3 8 11 12 13 15 17 18 20 22 23 24 25 26 27 28 30 32 33 34 35 37 38 40 43 44 46 49 50 51 52 53 54 55 56 57 59 60 62 63 64 66 68 69 70 71 72 73 74 75 76 77 78 79 80 81 82 83 84 85 86 87 88 90 93 96 97 99 100 102 103 104 105 106 107 111 112 114 118 119 120 121 124 132 133 135 136 137 **P**6 **S** Ascension Health
Primary Contact: Timothy A. Flesch, President and Chief Executive Officer
CFO: Michael P. Browning, Senior Vice President and Chief Financial Officer
CMO: John Gallagher, M.D., Chief Medical Officer
CHR: Claudia Richardt, Director Human Resources and Organization Development
Web address: www.stmarys.org
Control: Church–operated, Nongovernment, not–for profit **Service:** General Medical and Surgical

Staffed Beds: 455 **Admissions:** 14996 **Census:** 223 **Outpatient Visits:** 282505 **Births:** 1476 **Total Expense ($000):** 287875 **Payroll Expense ($000):** 102064 **Personnel:** 2229

IN

Hospital, Medicare Provider Number, Address, Telephone, Approval, Facility, and Physician Codes, Health Care System

★ American Hospital Association (AHA) membership
□ The Joint Commission accreditation
○ American Osteopathic Association (AOA) accreditation
△ Commission on Accreditation of Rehabilitation Facilities (CARF) accreditation

FORT WAYNE—Allen County

★ **DUPONT HOSPITAL (150150)**, 2520 East Dupont Road, Zip 46825; tel. 260/416–3000 **A**1 9 10 **F**3 13 15 25 26 30 31 32 33 38 43 54 55 56 57 62 63 66 68 70 71 72 73 74 77 79 80 81 82 84 96 97 100 101 102 103 107 112 118 120 121 124 130 134 135 136 **P**1 5 **S** Community Health Systems, Inc.
Primary Contact: Michael H. Schatzlein, M.D., Chief Executive Officer
COO: Dawn Rudolph, Chief Operating Officer
CFO: Craig Polkow, Chief Financial Officer
CMO: Theodore Wagner, M.D., President Medical Staff
CIO: Michael H. Schatzlein, M.D., Chief Executive Officer
CHR: Stacy Junk, Director Human Resources
Web address: www.theduponthospital.com
Control: Partnership, Investor–owned, for–profit **Service:** General Medical and Surgical

Staffed Beds: 122 **Admissions:** 5764 **Census:** 53 **Outpatient Visits:** 97864 **Births:** 2374 **Total Expense ($000):** 69066 **Payroll Expense ($000):** 26349 **Personnel:** 492

★ **LUTHERAN HOSPITAL OF INDIANA (150017)**, 7950 West Jefferson Boulevard, Zip 46804–1677; tel. 260/435–7001, (Nonreporting) **A**1 2 3 5 9 10 **S** Community Health Systems, Inc.
Primary Contact: Joseph M. Dorko, Chief Executive Officer
COO: Joseph M. Dorko, Vice President Operations
CMO: Michael Musgrave, M.D., Chief Medical Officer
CIO: Randy Cox, Chief Information Officer
CHR: Bruce Hamilton, Vice President Human Resources
Web address: www.lutheran–hosp.com
Control: Corporation, Investor–owned, for–profit **Service:** General Medical and Surgical

Staffed Beds: 435

★ △ **PARKVIEW HOSPITAL (150021)**, 2200 Randallia Drive, Zip 46805–4699; tel. 260/373–4000, (Includes PARKVIEW NORTH HOSPITAL, 11115 Parkview Plaza Drive, Zip 46845; tel. 260/672–4000), (Total facility includes 28 beds in nursing home–type unit) **A**1 2 3 5 7 9 10 **F**3 4 5 7 11 13 14 15 17 18 20 22 24 25 26 27 28 30 31 32 33 38 40 41 42 43 44 46 49 50 52 53 55 56 57 58 59 60 61 62 63 66 67 68 70 71 72 73 74 76 77 78 79 80 81 82 83 84 85 86 88 89 90 91 92 93 94 95 96 97 98 100 102 103 106 107 108 109 112 114 116 117 118 119 120 121 124 130 135 136 137 **S** Parkview Health
Primary Contact: Sue Ehinger, Chief Operating Officer
COO: Sue Ehinger, Chief Operating Officer
CFO: Mark A. Nafziger, Chief Financial Officer
CMO: Thomas Bono, President Medical Staff
CIO: Ron Double, Chief Information Officer
CHR: Catherine Wilcox, Senior Vice President and General Counsel
Web address: www.parkview.com
Control: Other not–for–profit (including NFP Corporation) **Service:** General Medical and Surgical

Staffed Beds: 673 **Admissions:** 23100 **Census:** 362 **Outpatient Visits:** 272937 **Births:** 2190 **Total Expense ($000):** 455016 **Payroll Expense ($000):** 173015 **Personnel:** 2897

★ △ **REHABILITATION HOSPITAL OF FORT WAYNE (153030)**, 7970 West Jefferson Boulevard, Zip 46804–4140; tel. 260/435–6100 **A**7 9 10 **F**25 26 85 86 119 121 135 **P**5 **S** Community Health Systems, Inc.
Primary Contact: Ted Scholten, Interim Chief Operating Officer
COO: Ted Scholten, Interim Chief Operating Officer
CFO: Stephen R. Miller, Senior Vice President and Chief Financial Officer
CMO: William Hedrick, M.D., Chief Medical Officer
CIO: Randy Cox, Chief Information Officer
CHR: Deborah Giardina, Director Human Resources and Medical Staff Services
Web address: www.rehabhospital.com
Control: Corporation, Investor–owned, for–profit **Service:** Rehabilitation

Staffed Beds: 36 **Admissions:** 539 **Census:** 20 **Outpatient Visits:** 7 **Births:** 0 **Total Expense ($000):** 8230 **Payroll Expense ($000):** 4345 **Personnel:** 92

□ **SELECT SPECIALTY HOSPITAL (152016)**, 700 Broadway, 7th Floor, Zip 46802; tel. 260/425–3810 **A**1 10 **F**1 3 12 25 50 73 80 119 137 **S** Select Medical Corporation
Primary Contact: Darlene Degener, Chief Executive Officer
CHR: Donna Leaman, Coordinator Human Resources
Web address: www.selectmedicalcorp.com
Control: Corporation, Investor–owned, for–profit **Service:** Long–Term Acute Care hospital

Staffed Beds: 32 **Admissions:** 320 **Census:** 26 **Outpatient Visits:** 0 **Births:** 0 **Total Expense ($000):** 14724 **Payroll Expense ($000):** 5494 **Personnel:** 101

★ **ST. JOSEPH HOSPITAL (150047)**, 700 Broadway, Zip 46802–1493; tel. 260/425–3000, (Total facility includes 21 beds in nursing home–type unit) **A**1 3 5 9 10 **F**3 4 5 8 13 15 16 17 18 20 22 24 25 26 27 30 31 32 33 37 38 41 43 44 46 49 50 54 55 56 57 59 61 62 66 67 68 69 70 73 74 75 77 79 80 81 82 86 87 88 90 91 92 93 94 95 96 97 102 107 117 118 119 130 135 137 **P**8 **S** Community Health Systems, Inc.
Primary Contact: Kirk M. Ray, Chief Executive Officer
COO: Chad Towner, Chief Operating Officer
CFO: Tom Fox, Chief Financial Officer
CIO: Randy Cox, Chief Information Officer
CHR: Charlee Hakes, Director Human Resources
Web address: www.stjoehospital.com
Control: Corporation, Investor–owned, for–profit **Service:** General Medical and Surgical

Staffed Beds: 201 **Admissions:** 5932 **Census:** 93 **Outpatient Visits:** 87003 **Births:** 584 **Total Expense ($000):** 92420 **Payroll Expense ($000):** 33394 **Personnel:** 788

★ **VETERANS AFFAIRS NORTHERN INDIANA HEALTH CARE SYSTEM**, 2121 Lake Avenue, Zip 46805–5347; tel. 260/460–1310, (Includes VETERANS AFFAIRS NORTHERN INDIANA HEALTH CARE SYSTEM–MARION CAMPUS, 1700 East 38th Street, Marion, Zip 46953–4589; tel. 765/674–3321), (Total facility includes 150 beds in nursing home–type unit) **A**1 **F**4 5 8 25 26 27 29 33 34 36 37 38 42 43 44 45 50 52 53 54 55 56 57 58 59 60 61 62 63 64 68 72 73 75 76 77 79 80 81 82 86 87 91 92 93 94 95 96 97 102 107 117 119 121 124 132 133 135 136 **P**6 **S** Department of Veterans Affairs
Primary Contact: Cathi Spivey–Paul, Director
CIO: David Troyer, Manager Information Resources Management
Web address: www.va.gov/sta/guide/home.asp
Control: Veterans Affairs, Government, federal **Service:** General Medical and Surgical

Staffed Beds: 255 **Admissions:** 2323 **Census:** 183 **Outpatient Visits:** 264411 **Births:** 0 **Total Expense ($000):** 165656 **Payroll Expense ($000):** 66406 **Personnel:** 1272

FRANKFORT—Clinton County

★ **ST. VINCENT FRANKFORT HOSPITAL (151316)**, 1300 South Jackson Street, Zip 46041–3394, Mailing Address: P.O. Box 669, Zip 46041–0669; tel. 765/656–3000 **A**1 2 9 10 18 **F**3 8 11 13 15 24 25 26 27 30 31 32 33 38 50 55 57 62 66 68 72 73 75 76 77 79 80 81 82 86 87 94 96 100 102 107 121 122 124 137 **S** Ascension Health
Primary Contact: Thomas Crawford, Chief Executive Officer
CFO: Jerry Marks, Chief Financial Officer
CMO: Stephen Tharp, M.D., Medical Director
CHR: Krista Wright, Director Human Resources
Web address: www.stvincent.org
Control: Church–operated, Nongovernment, not–for profit **Service:** General Medical and Surgical

Staffed Beds: 25 **Admissions:** 1134 **Census:** 11 **Outpatient Visits:** 38424 **Births:** 299 **Total Expense ($000):** 19937 **Payroll Expense ($000):** 7642 **Personnel:** 153

FRANKLIN—Johnson County

★ ○ **JOHNSON MEMORIAL HOSPITAL (150001)**, 1125 West Jefferson Street, Zip 46131–2140, Mailing Address: P.O. Box 549, Zip 46131–0549; tel. 317/736–3300, (Total facility includes 25 beds in nursing home–type unit) **A**2 9 10 11 **F**12 13 15 24 25 26 27 30 31 32 33 34 38 41 49 50 53 55 56 57 61 62 66 68 72 73 74 75 76 77 79 80 82 85 86 87 96 97 100 101 103 104 105 106 107 109 111 117 118 119 120 121 123 124 133 135 136 **P**1
Primary Contact: Larry Heydon, President and Chief Executive Officer
COO: Steve Wohlford, Chief Operating Officer
CFO: Elizabeth A. Hedden, Chief Financial Officer
CMO: Gaston Dana, D.O., Chief of Staff
CIO: Al Godsoe, Director Information Systems
CHR: Judy Ware, Director Human Resources
Web address: www.johnsonmemorial.org
Control: County–Government, nonfederal **Service:** General Medical and Surgical

Staffed Beds: 125 **Admissions:** 4061 **Census:** 60 **Outpatient Visits:** 149432 **Births:** 635 **Total Expense ($000):** 72534 **Payroll Expense ($000):** 32387 **Personnel:** 675

IN

GARY—Lake County

★ ○ △ **METHODIST HOSPITALS (150002)**, 600 Grant Street, Zip 46402–6099; tel. 219/886–4000, (Includes SOUTHLAKE CAMPUS, 8701 Broadway, Merrillville, Zip 46410; tel. 219/738–5500), (Total facility includes 30 beds in nursing home–type unit) **A**1 2 3 5 7 9 10 11 **F**3 11 12 13 15 18 20 22 24 25 26 27 28 31 32 33 36 38 40 42 43 48 49 50 51 53 55 56 57 61 62 66 68 70 71 72 73 74 75 76 77 79 80 81 82 84 85 86 87 88 89 90 91 92 93 94 95 96 97 100 104 105 106 107 109 112 114 117 118 119 121 122 135 136 137 **P**6
Primary Contact: Claude D. Watts, Jr., Interim President and Chief Executive Officer
COO: Clint Matthews, Chief Operating Officer
CFO: Al Mansfield, Chief Financial Officer
CMO: Charles O. Davidson, M.D., Vice President Medical Affairs
CIO: Shaw Collins, Director Information Technology
CHR: Joyce McGlory, Vice President Human Resources
Web address: www.methodisthospitals.org
Control: Other not–for–profit (including NFP Corporation) **Service:** General Medical and Surgical

Staffed Beds: 534 **Admissions:** 19897 **Census:** 322 **Outpatient Visits:** 164965 **Births:** 1460 **Total Expense ($000):** 310066 **Payroll Expense ($000):** 116023 **Personnel:** 1867

GOSHEN—Elkhart County

★ **GOSHEN GENERAL HOSPITAL (150026)**, 200 High Park Avenue, Zip 46526–4899, Mailing Address: P.O. Box 139, Zip 46527–0139; tel. 574/533–2141 **A**1 2 9 10 **F**3 11 12 13 15 18 20 24 25 26 27 28 30 31 32 33 34 38 40 41 42 43 44 46 47 49 50 51 53 54 55 56 57 58 61 62 65 66 68 69 72 73 74 76 77 78 79 80 81 82 84 86 96 97 99 100 102 105 106 107 108 109 111 112 116 118 119 121 124 135 136 137 **P**8
S Clarian Health
Primary Contact: James O. Dague, President and Chief Executive Officer
COO: Paulette Brown, Chief Operating Officer
CFO: Randal Christophel, Executive Vice President and Chief Financial Officer
CMO: Randall Cammenga, M.D., Vice President Medical Affairs
CIO: Dolph Voelker, Director Information Services
CHR: Alan Weldy, Vice President Human Resources, Compliance and Legal Services
Web address: www.goshenhealth.org
Control: Other not–for–profit (including NFP Corporation) **Service:** General Medical and Surgical

Staffed Beds: 123 **Admissions:** 5758 **Census:** 57 **Outpatient Visits:** 152163 **Births:** 1606 **Total Expense ($000):** 135838 **Payroll Expense ($000):** 49712 **Personnel:** 985

OAKLAWN PSYCHIATRIC CENTER (154031), 330 Lakeview Drive, Zip 46528–9365, Mailing Address: P.O. Box 809, Zip 46527–0809; tel. 574/533–1234, (Nonreporting) **A**9 10
Primary Contact: Laurie N. Nafziger, President and Chief Executive Officer
CFO: Lynn J. Miller, Vice President Financial Services
CMO: Daniel Kinsey, M.D., Medical Director
CIO: Gloria Holub, Manager Communications
CHR: Mary Coursey, Director Human Resources
Web address: www.oaklawn.org
Control: Other not–for–profit (including NFP Corporation) **Service:** Psychiatric

Staffed Beds: 16

GREENCASTLE—Putnam County

★ ○ **PUTNAM COUNTY HOSPITAL (151333)**, 1542 Bloomington Street, Zip 46135–2297; tel. 765/653–5121, (Nonreporting) **A**2 9 10 11 18
Primary Contact: Dennis Weatherford, Chief Executive Officer
CFO: Kevin Fowler, Director Finance
Control: County–Government, nonfederal **Service:** General Medical and Surgical

Staffed Beds: 25

GREENFIELD—Hancock County

★ ○ **HANCOCK REGIONAL HOSPITAL (150037)**, 801 North State Street, Zip 46140–1270, Mailing Address: P.O. Box 827, Zip 46140–0827; tel. 317/462–5544 **A**5 9 10 11 **F**3 11 13 15 17 18 20 24 25 26 27 28 30 31 32 33 34 36 38 41 42 43 44 47 48 49 50 52 53 54 55 56 57 60 61 62 64 66 67 68 72 73 74 75 76 77 79 80 81 82 84 85 86 88 93 96 100 107 118 119 120 121 123 124 133 135 136 137 **P**8
Primary Contact: Robert C. Keen, Ph.D., FACHE, President and Chief Executive Officer
CFO: Rick Edwards, Vice President Finance and Business Services
CMO: Tom O'Connor, M.D., President Medical Staff
CIO: Jon Miller, Team Leader Accounting and Information Services
CHR: Dave Holmes, Vice President Support Services
Web address: www.hancockregional.org
Control: County–Government, nonfederal **Service:** General Medical and Surgical

Staffed Beds: 95 **Admissions:** 3960 **Census:** 57 **Outpatient Visits:** 182402 **Births:** 578 **Total Expense ($000):** 71892 **Payroll Expense ($000):** 33381 **Personnel:** 694

GREENSBURG—Decatur County

★ **DECATUR COUNTY MEMORIAL HOSPITAL (151332)**, 720 North Lincoln Street, Zip 47240–1398; tel. 812/663–4331, (Total facility includes 15 beds in nursing home–type unit) **A**2 9 10 18 **F**2 3 7 8 13 15 24 25 27 28 30 31 33 38 50 53 54 55 56 57 61 62 63 66 67 68 73 74 75 76 77 79 80 81 82 84 86 87 96 97 99 100 102 105 106 107 118 119 120 121 122 124 134 135 136 137 **P**6
Primary Contact: William R. Alloy, President and Chief Executive Officer
CFO: Michael R. Ruckel, Vice President Finance
CIO: Kathy Dickman, Director Information Systems
CHR: Robin Meyer, Vice President Support Services
Web address: www.dcmh.net
Control: County–Government, nonfederal **Service:** General Medical and Surgical

Staffed Beds: 25 **Admissions:** 1361 **Census:** 23 **Outpatient Visits:** 68951 **Births:** 265 **Total Expense ($000):** 30788 **Payroll Expense ($000):** 15885 **Personnel:** 341

GREENWOOD—Johnson County

□ **KINDRED HOSPITAL INDIANAPOLIS SOUTH (152008)**, 607 Greenwood Spring Drive, Zip 46143–1400; tel. 317/888–8155, (Nonreporting) **A**1 9 10
S Kindred Healthcare
Primary Contact: Mona Euler, Chief Executive Officer
COO: Kristy Walden, Chief Clinical Officer
CFO: William Brenner, Chief Financial Officer
Web address: www.kindredhealthcare.com
Control: Corporation, Investor–owned, for–profit **Service:** Long–Term Acute Care hospital

Staffed Beds: 36

□ **SELECT SPECIALTY HOSPITAL OF INDIANAPOLIS (152010)**, 1701 North Senate Boulevard, Building C, 7th Floor, Zip 46143; tel. 317/884–2599 **A**1 10 **F**1 3 25 27 30 31 32 33 43 59 72 73 75 76 77 80 81 82 93 119 137
S Select Medical Corporation
Primary Contact: Mary L. Jackson–Boustani, Chief Executive Officer
Web address: www.selectmedicalcorp.com
Control: Corporation, Investor–owned, for–profit **Service:** Long–Term Acute Care hospital

Staffed Beds: 54 **Admissions:** 448 **Census:** 33 **Outpatient Visits:** 0 **Births:** 0 **Total Expense ($000):** 18515 **Payroll Expense ($000):** 4904 **Personnel:** 106

□ **VALLE VISTA HOSPITAL (154024)**, 898 East Main Street, Zip 46143–1400; tel. 317/887–1348, (Total facility includes 42 beds in nursing home–type unit) (Nonreporting) **A**1 9 10 **S** Psychiatric Solutions
Primary Contact: David Bell, Chief Executive Officer
COO: Cheryl Stultz, Chief Operating Officer
CFO: Anne Knapp, Chief Financial Officer
CMO: Vicki Burdine, M.D., Medical Director
CIO: Karen Hayden, Director Health Information Services
CHR: Ismael Santos, Director Human Resources
Web address: www.vallevistahospital.com
Control: Corporation, Investor–owned, for–profit **Service:** Psychiatric

Staffed Beds: 98

Hospital, Medicare Provider Number, Address, Telephone, Approval, Facility, and Physician Codes, Health Care System

★ American Hospital Association (AHA) membership
□ The Joint Commission accreditation
○ American Osteopathic Association (AOA) accreditation
△ Commission on Accreditation of Rehabilitation Facilities (CARF) accreditation

HAMMOND—Lake County

○ △ **SAINT MARGARET MERCY HEALTHCARE CENTERS (150004)**, 5454 Hohman Avenue, Zip 46320–1999; tel. 219/933–2074, (Includes SAINT MARGARET MERCY HEALTHCARE CENTERS–NORTH CAMPUS, tel. 219/932–2300; SAINT MARGARET MERCY HEALTHCARE CENTERS–SOUTH CAMPUS, 24 Joliet Street, Dyer, Zip 46311–1799; tel. 219/865–2141), (Total facility includes 67 beds in nursing home–type unit) (Nonreporting) **A**2 7 9 10 11 **S** Sisters of St. Francis Health Services, Inc.
Primary Contact: Thomas J. Gryzbek, President
CFO: Jim Lipinski, Chief Financial Officer
Web address: www.smmhc.com
Control: Church–operated, Nongovernment, not–for profit **Service:** General Medical and Surgical

Staffed Beds: 624

□ **SELECT SPECIALTY HOSPITAL OF NORTHWEST INDIANA (152012)**, 5454 Hohman Avenue, 5th Floor, Zip 46320; tel. 219/937–9900 **A**1 10 **F**1 3 4 16 17 25 30 65 66 68 70 71 72 74 78 80 82 83 84 85 88 117 119 137 **S** Select Medical Corporation
Primary Contact: Scott Deig, Interim Chief Executive Officer
Web address: www.selectmedicalcorp.com
Control: Corporation, Investor–owned, for–profit **Service:** Long–Term Acute Care hospital

Staffed Beds: 70 **Admissions:** 533 **Census:** 39 **Outpatient Visits:** 0 **Births:** 0 **Total Expense ($000):** 20393 **Payroll Expense ($000):** 5909 **Personnel:** 132

HARTFORD CITY—Blackford County

★ **BLACKFORD COMMUNITY HOSPITAL (151302)**, 410 Pilgrim Boulevard, Zip 47348–1897; tel. 765/348–0300 **A**9 10 18 **F**3 7 11 15 24 25 30 33 38 41 43 50 55 56 57 62 79 80 81 86 96 107 118 119 121 122 124 132 **S** Cardinal Health System
Primary Contact: Steven J. West, Chief Executive Officer
CFO: Walter Soptelean, Chief Financial Officer
CHR: John Crosbie, Director Support Services
Web address: www.blackfordcommunityhospital.org
Control: Other not–for–profit (including NFP Corporation) **Service:** General Medical and Surgical

Staffed Beds: 15 **Admissions:** 685 **Census:** 9 **Outpatient Visits:** 25579 **Births:** 0 **Total Expense ($000):** 14541 **Payroll Expense ($000):** 4217 **Personnel:** 122

HOBART—Lake County

□ △ **ST. MARY MEDICAL CENTER (150034)**, 1500 South Lake Park Avenue, Zip 46342–6699; tel. 219/942–0551 **A**1 7 9 10 **F**3 8 11 13 15 18 20 22 24 25 26 27 30 31 32 33 36 37 38 43 47 49 50 51 53 55 56 57 58 61 62 63 68 72 73 74 76 77 78 79 80 81 82 84 86 96 97 99 100 102 106 107 109 111 118 119 121 123 124 135 136 137 **P**6 8 **S** Community Healthcare System
Primary Contact: Janice Ryba, Administrator
CFO: Mary Sudicky, Chief Financial Officer
CIO: Vernon Groeber, Vice President Information Technology and Chief Information Officer
CHR: Tony Ferracane, Vice President Human Resources
Web address: www.comhs.org
Control: Other not–for–profit (including NFP Corporation) **Service:** General Medical and Surgical

Staffed Beds: 186 **Admissions:** 10387 **Census:** 140 **Outpatient Visits:** 82564 **Births:** 629 **Total Expense ($000):** 135024 **Payroll Expense ($000):** 48663 **Personnel:** 808

HUNTINGTON—Huntington County

★ **PARKVIEW HUNTINGTON HOSPITAL (150091)**, 2001 Stults Road, Zip 46750–3696; tel. 260/355–3000 **A**1 9 10 **F**3 7 8 13 15 24 25 26 27 28 30 31 32 33 34 36 37 38 41 46 50 52 54 55 56 57 62 66 67 68 73 74 75 76 77 79 80 81 82 86 87 96 97 100 107 119 120 121 123 124 135 137 **S** Parkview Health
Primary Contact: Darlene Garrett, Chief Operating Officer
COO: Darlene Garrett, Chief Operating Officer
Web address: www.parkview.com
Control: Other not–for–profit (including NFP Corporation) **Service:** General Medical and Surgical

Staffed Beds: 36 **Admissions:** 1667 **Census:** 14 **Outpatient Visits:** 44232 **Births:** 336 **Total Expense ($000):** 27195 **Payroll Expense ($000):** 12797 **Personnel:** 218

INDIANAPOLIS—Marion County

★ **CLARIAN HEALTH PARTNERS (150056)**, I–65 at 21st Street, Zip 46202–5250, Mailing Address: P.O. Box 1367, Zip 46206–1367; tel. 317/962–2000, (Includes INDIANA UNIVERSITY HOSPITAL, 550 North University Boulevard, Zip 46202–5262; tel. 317/274–5000; Samuel L. Odle, President and Chief Executive Officer; METHODIST HOSPITAL, 1701 North Senate Boulevard, Zip 46202, Mailing Address: 1701 North Senate Boulevard, Zip 46202; tel. 317/962–2000; Samuel L. Odle, President and Chief Executive Officer; RILEY HOSPITAL FOR CHILDREN, 702 Barnhill Drive, Zip 46202–5225; tel. 317/274–5000; Ora Pescovitz, M.D., President and Chief Executive Officer) **A**1 2 3 5 8 9 10 **F**3 5 7 8 9 11 12 13 15 16 17 18 19 20 21 22 23 24 25 26 27 28 30 31 32 33 34 35 36 37 38 40 41 42 43 44 45 46 47 48 49 50 51 52 53 54 55 56 57 58 59 60 61 62 63 66 67 68 69 70 72 73 74 75 76 77 78 79 80 81 82 83 84 86 87 88 89 90 91 92 93 94 95 96 97 98 99 100 101 102 103 104 105 106 107 108 109 110 111 112 113 114 116 118 119 120 121 123 124 125 126 127 128 129 130 133 134 135 136 137 **P**6 **S** Clarian Health
Primary Contact: Daniel F. Evans, Jr., President and Chief Executive Officer
CFO: Marvin G. Pember, Executive Vice President and Chief Financial Officer
CMO: Richard Graffis, M.D., Executive Vice President and Chief Medical Officer
CIO: Richard F. Johnson, Senior Vice President and Chief Information Officer
CHR: Steve Wantz, Senior Vice President Human Resources and Administration
Web address: www.clarian.org
Control: Other not–for–profit (including NFP Corporation) **Service:** General Medical and Surgical

Staffed Beds: 1380 **Admissions:** 47894 **Census:** 895 **Outpatient Visits:** 860847 **Births:** 3896 **Total Expense ($000):** 1754572 **Payroll Expense ($000):** 616643 **Personnel:** 9903

□ △ **COMMUNITY HOSPITAL EAST (150074)**, 1500 North Ritter Avenue, Zip 46219–3095; tel. 317/355–1411 **A**1 2 3 5 7 9 10 **F**3 11 13 17 18 20 24 25 26 27 28 30 31 32 33 34 38 41 42 44 49 50 51 52 55 56 57 58 59 62 63 66 67 68 72 73 74 75 76 77 78 79 80 81 82 85 86 96 97 99 100 102 103 107 108 109 111 118 119 120 124 133 135 137 **P**6 **S** Community Health Network
Primary Contact: Anita J. Harden, Administrator
Web address: www.ecommunity.org
Control: Other not–for–profit (including NFP Corporation) **Service:** General Medical and Surgical

Staffed Beds: 233 **Admissions:** 10269 **Census:** 153 **Outpatient Visits:** 293582 **Births:** 936 **Total Expense ($000):** 260015 **Payroll Expense ($000):** 90556 **Personnel:** 2213

□ **COMMUNITY HOSPITAL NORTH**, 7150 Clearvista Drive, Zip 46256; tel. 317/621–6262 **A**1 9 **F**3 11 12 13 25 26 27 28 30 31 32 33 34 36 38 41 42 44 46 47 48 49 50 51 52 55 56 57 58 59 62 63 66 67 68 70 72 73 74 76 77 78 79 80 81 82 84 86 88 89 90 91 92 93 94 95 96 97 100 102 103 107 108 109 111 113 114 116 118 119 120 124 135 137 **P**6 **S** Community Health Network
Primary Contact: Barbara Summers, Chief Executive Officer
Web address: www.ecommunity.org
Control: Other not–for–profit (including NFP Corporation) **Service:** General Medical and Surgical

Staffed Beds: 389 **Admissions:** 15971 **Census:** 226 **Outpatient Visits:** 746532 **Births:** 2580 **Total Expense ($000):** 314817 **Payroll Expense ($000):** 83273 **Personnel:** 1186

□ **COMMUNITY HOSPITAL SOUTH (150128)**, 1402 East County Line Road South, Zip 46227; tel. 317/887–7000 **A**1 9 10 **F**3 11 12 13 15 18 20 24 25 26 28 30 31 32 33 34 38 41 42 44 49 50 51 55 56 57 58 59 62 63 66 67 68 72 73 74 76 77 79 80 81 82 86 96 97 99 100 102 107 118 119 120 124 135 137 **P**6 **S** Community Health Network
Primary Contact: Michael Blanchet, President
Web address: www.ecommunity.com
Control: Other not–for–profit (including NFP Corporation) **Service:** General Medical and Surgical

Staffed Beds: 108 **Admissions:** 6743 **Census:** 68 **Outpatient Visits:** 87041 **Births:** 819 **Total Expense ($000):** 118857 **Payroll Expense ($000):** 28642 **Personnel:** 504

FAIRBANKS (154034), 8102 Clearvista Parkway, Zip 46256–4698; tel. 317/849–8222 **A**9 10 **F**4 5 90 119 121 124 135 **P**8
Primary Contact: Helene M. Cross, President and Chief Executive Officer
COO: Cindy Leigh, Chief Operating Officer
CFO: Barb Elliott, Chief Financial Officer
CMO: Timothy J. Kelly, M.D., Medical Director
CIO: Cindy Leigh, Chief Operating Officer
CHR: Sharon Baker, Assistant Administrator Support Services
Web address: www.fairbankscd.org
Control: Other not–for–profit (including NFP Corporation) **Service:** Alcoholism and other chemical dependency

Staffed Beds: 86 **Admissions:** 3413 **Census:** 51 **Outpatient Visits:** 17702 **Births:** 0 **Total Expense ($000):** 13140 **Payroll Expense ($000):** 6837 **Personnel:** 194

Many Facility Codes have changed. Please refer to the AHA Guide Code Chart.

□ **INDIANA HEART HOSPITAL (150154)**, 8075 North Shadeland Avenue, Zip 46256; tel. 317/621–8000, (Nonreporting) **A**1 9 10 **S** Community Health Network
Primary Contact: Thomas A. Malasto, Chief Executive Officer
Web address: www.hearthospital.com
Control: Other not–for–profit (including NFP Corporation) **Service:** General Medical and Surgical

Staffed Beds: 56

INDIANA ORTHOPAEDIC HOSPITAL (150160), 8400 Northwest Boulevard, Zip 46278; tel. 317/956–1180, (Nonreporting) **A**9 10
Primary Contact: Jane Keller, Chief Executive Officer
Web address: www.orthoindy.com
Control: Corporation, Investor–owned, for–profit **Service:** Orthopedic

Staffed Beds: 37

INDIANA UNIVERSITY HOSPITAL See Clarian Health Partners

□ **KINDRED HOSPITAL–INDIANAPOLIS (152007)**, 1700 West 10th Street, Zip 46222–3802; tel. 317/636–4400 **A**1 9 10 **F**1 3 32 59 73 80 96 107 119 137 **S** Kindred Healthcare
Primary Contact: Dennis Nicely, Administrator
COO: Napntali B. Edge, Chief Clinical Officer
CFO: William Brenner, Chief Financial Officer
CMO: Kalpana Jindal, M.D., Medical Director
CHR: Linda Russell, Director Human Resources
Web address: www.kindredhealthcare.com
Control: Corporation, Investor–owned, for–profit **Service:** Long–Term Acute Care hospital

Staffed Beds: 59 **Admissions:** 405 **Census:** 30 **Outpatient Visits:** 0 **Births:** 0 **Total Expense ($000):** 15803 **Payroll Expense ($000):** 5631 **Personnel:** 154

□ **LARUE D. CARTER MEMORIAL HOSPITAL (154008)**, 2601 Cold Spring Road, Zip 46222–2273; tel. 317/941–4000, (Nonreporting) **A**1 3 5 10
Primary Contact: Alan D. Schmetzer, M.D., Superintendent
COO: Lisa Kellum, Chief Operating Officer
CFO: Norene Briggs, Chief Financial Officer
CMO: Jeffrey J. Kellams, M.D., Chief Medical Officer
CIO: Paul Wagner, M.D., Director Performance Improvement
CHR: Patricia Clift, Director Human Resources
Control: State–Government, nonfederal **Service:** Psychiatric

Staffed Beds: 146

METHODIST HOSPITAL See Clarian Health Partners

□ △ **REHABILITATION HOSPITAL OF INDIANA (153028)**, 4141 Shore Drive, Zip 46254–2607; tel. 317/329–2000, (Nonreporting) **A**1 3 5 7 9 10
Primary Contact: Dennis Armington, Chief Executive Officer
Web address: www.rhin.com
Control: Other not–for–profit (including NFP Corporation) **Service:** Rehabilitation

Staffed Beds: 80

★ △ **RICHARD L. ROUDEBUSH VETERANS AFFAIRS MEDICAL CENTER**, 1481 West Tenth Street, Zip 46202–2884; tel. 317/554–0000, (Nonreporting) **A**1 2 3 5 7 8 **S** Department of Veterans Affairs
Primary Contact: Thomas Mattice, Director
CFO: Paul Pessagno, Chief Financial Officer
CMO: Ken Klotz, M.D., Chief of Staff
CIO: General Kearney, Chief Information Officer
CHR: Annie Herbert, Chief Human Resources Management Services
Web address: www.va.gov/sta/guide/home.asp
Control: Veterans Affairs, Government, federal **Service:** General Medical and Surgical

Staffed Beds: 144

RILEY HOSPITAL FOR CHILDREN See Clarian Health Partners

SELECT SPECIALTY HOSPITAL OF INDIANAPOLIS See Greenwood

★ **ST VINCENT SETON SPECIALTY HOSPITAL (152020)**, 8050 Township Line Road, Zip 46260; tel. 317/415–8353, (Nonreporting) **A**1 9 10 **S** Ascension Health
Primary Contact: Peter H. Alexander, Administrator
COO: Troy T. Reiff, Corporate Director Operations
CFO: David M. Girten, Corporate Director Financial Services
CHR: Terry A. Wignall, Director Human Resources
Control: Church–operated, Nongovernment, not–for profit **Service:** Long–Term Acute Care hospital

Staffed Beds: 74

○ **ST. FRANCIS HOSPITAL AND HEALTH CENTERS – SOUTH CAMPUS (150162)**, 8111 South Emerson Avenue, Zip 46217, (Nonreporting) **A**9 10 11
Control: Church–operated, Nongovernment, not–for profit **Service:** General Medical and Surgical

Staffed Beds: 50

○ **ST. VINCENT HEART CENTER OF INDIANA (150153)**, 10580 North Meridian Street, Zip 46290; tel. 317/583–5000 **A**9 10 11 **F**3 17 18 20 22 25 26 30 31 32 33 38 46 55 57 68 73 79 80 82 96 100 103 107 119 124 **P**2 **S** Ascension Health
Primary Contact: John Stewart, Chief Executive Officer
COO: Mike Schroyer, M.D., Chief Operating Officer
CFO: Becky Jacobson, Vice President Finance
CMO: William Storer, M.D., Medical Director
CIO: Alec Williams, Chief Information Officer
CHR: Jane Richardson, Vice President Human Resources
Web address: www.theheartcenter.com
Control: Partnership, Investor–owned, for–profit **Service:** Heart

Staffed Beds: 80 **Admissions:** 6069 **Census:** 59 **Outpatient Visits:** 8837 **Births:** 0 **Total Expense ($000):** 100908 **Payroll Expense ($000):** 25651 **Personnel:** 403

★ △ **ST. VINCENT INDIANAPOLIS HOSPITAL (150084)**, 2001 West 86th Street, Zip 46260–1991, Mailing Address: P.O. Box 40970, Zip 46240–0970; tel. 317/338–2345, (Includes PEYTON MANNING CHILDREN'S HOSPITAL AT ST. VINCENT, 2001 West 86th Street, Zip 46260; tel. 317/415–8111; Anne Coleman, Administrator; ST. VINCENT STRESS CENTER, 8401 Harcourt Road, Zip 46260, Mailing Address: P.O. Box 80160, Zip 46280; tel. 317/338–4600; Sheila Mishler, Chief Executive Officer) **A**1 2 3 5 7 8 9 10 **F**2 3 4 5 9 11 13 15 17 18 19 20 21 22 23 24 25 26 27 28 30 31 32 33 35 36 37 38 40 41 42 43 44 46 47 48 49 50 51 52 53 54 55 56 57 58 60 61 62 64 66 68 69 70 72 73 74 76 77 79 80 81 82 83 84 86 87 88 89 90 91 92 93 94 95 96 97 99 100 102 103 104 105 106 107 108 109 111 112 116 118 119 120 121 123 124 125 126 132 133 135 136 137 **P**6 8 **S** Ascension Health
Primary Contact: Kyle De Fur, FACHE, President
COO: Michael Wiemann, M.D., Senior Vice President and Chief Medical Officer
CFO: Terry Hamilton, Executive Director Finance
CMO: Michael Wiemann, M.D., Senior Vice President and Chief Medical Officer
CIO: Greg Jones, Interim Chief Information Officer
CHR: Marty Du Rall, Executive Director Human Resources
Web address: www.stvincent.org
Control: Church–operated, Nongovernment, not–for profit **Service:** General Medical and Surgical

Staffed Beds: 744 **Admissions:** 33307 **Census:** 505 **Outpatient Visits:** 679435 **Births:** 4211 **Total Expense ($000):** 697948 **Payroll Expense ($000):** 293599 **Personnel:** 5478

★ △ **ST. VINCENT PEDIATRIC REHABILITATION CENTER (153300)**, 1707 West 86th Street, Zip 46240, Mailing Address: P.O. Box 40407, Zip 46240; tel. 317/415–5500, (Nonreporting) **A**1 7 9 10 **S** Ascension Health
Primary Contact: Anne Coleman, Administrator
Control: Church–operated, Nongovernment, not–for profit **Service:** Children's rehabilitation

Staffed Beds: 20

★ **ST. VINCENT WOMEN'S HOSPITAL**, 8111 Township Line Road, Zip 46260–8043; tel. 317/415–8111, (Nonreporting) **A**1 9 10 **S** Ascension Health
Primary Contact: Anne Coleman, Administrator
CIO: Ken Meyer, Head Information Systems
Web address: www.stvincent.org
Control: Corporation, Investor–owned, for–profit **Service:** Obstetrics and gynecology

Staffed Beds: 60

○ **WESTVIEW HOSPITAL (150129)**, 3630 Guion Road, Zip 46222–1699; tel. 317/924–6661, (Nonreporting) **A**9 10 11 12 13
Primary Contact: Jerry L. Porter, Chief Executive Officer
CFO: Jon P. Anderson, CPA, Executive Vice President
CHR: Emily Rogers, Manager Human Resources
Web address: www.westviewhospital.org
Control: Hospital district or authority, Government, nonfederal **Service:** General Medical and Surgical

Staffed Beds: 95

IN

Hospital, Medicare Provider Number, Address, Telephone, Approval, Facility, and Physician Codes, Health Care System

★ American Hospital Association (AHA) membership
□ The Joint Commission accreditation
○ American Osteopathic Association (AOA) accreditation
△ Commission on Accreditation of Rehabilitation Facilities (CARF) accreditation

WISHARD HEALTH SERVICES (150024), 1001 West 10th Street, Zip 46202–2879; tel. 317/630–7033, (Total facility includes 202 beds in nursing home–type unit) **A**3 5 8 9 10 **F**3 5 7 10 12 13 14 15 16 18 19 20 24 25 26 27 28 30 31 32 33 34 36 37 38 40 41 42 43 44 47 48 50 53 54 55 56 57 60 62 63 64 65 66 68 69 70 72 73 74 75 76 77 79 80 81 82 84 85 86 87 88 89 90 91 92 93 94 95 96 99 100 104 105 106 107 112 117 119 121 123 124 132 133 134 135 136 137 **P**5
Primary Contact: Lisa E. Harris, M.D., Chief Executive Officer and Medical Director
CFO: Lee Livin, Chief Financial Officer
CMO: Lisa E. Harris, M.D., Chief Executive Officer and Medical Director
CIO: David Shaw, Vice President Information Systems
CHR: Kimberly Harper, Vice President Human Resources and Public Affairs
Web address: www.wishard.edu
Control: County–Government, nonfederal **Service:** General Medical and Surgical

Staffed Beds: 528 **Admissions:** 16914 **Census:** 427 **Outpatient Visits:** 1187210 **Births:** 3211 **Total Expense ($000):** 322657 **Payroll Expense ($000):** 169768 **Personnel:** 3208

JASPER—Dubois County

★ **MEMORIAL HOSPITAL AND HEALTH CARE CENTER (150115)**, 800 West Ninth Street, Zip 47546–2516; tel. 812/482–2345, (Total facility includes 20 beds in nursing home–type unit) **A**1 2 9 10 19 **F**3 7 11 12 13 15 18 20 24 25 26 27 33 36 38 43 44 48 51 53 54 55 56 57 61 62 64 66 68 72 73 74 75 76 77 79 80 81 82 84 85 86 87 88 90 91 92 93 94 96 97 100 103 106 107 109 117 119 120 121 124 132 133 135 136 137 **P**6 **S** American Province of Little Company of Mary Sisters
Primary Contact: Raymond W. Snowden, President and Chief Executive Officer
CFO: E. Kyle Bennett, Executive Vice President
CMO: Scott Beckman, President Medical Staff
CIO: Todd Mehringer, Director Information Systems
CHR: Diane Denk, Director Human Resources
Web address: www.mhhcc.org
Control: Church–operated, Nongovernment, not–for profit **Service:** General Medical and Surgical

Staffed Beds: 129 **Admissions:** 6757 **Census:** 76 **Outpatient Visits:** 172861 **Births:** 998 **Total Expense ($000):** 95773 **Payroll Expense ($000):** 44141 **Personnel:** 953

JEFFERSONVILLE—Clark County

★ **CLARK MEMORIAL HOSPITAL (150009)**, 1220 Missouri Avenue, Zip 47130–3743, Mailing Address: P.O. Box 69, Zip 47131–0069; tel. 812/282–6631, (Total facility includes 18 beds in nursing home–type unit) **A**1 2 3 5 9 10 **F**3 5 8 11 12 13 15 17 18 20 24 25 26 27 28 30 31 32 33 38 39 43 50 52 53 54 55 56 57 61 62 68 72 73 74 75 76 77 79 80 81 82 87 88 90 91 92 93 94 95 96 97 100 102 103 107 117 118 119 121 124 134 135 136 137 **P**6 **S** Jewish Hospital & St. Mary's HealthCare
Primary Contact: Martin Padgett, President and Chief Executive Officer
CFO: Kirk Strack, Vice President and Chief Financial Officer
CMO: William Templeton, M.D., Medical Director
CIO: Larry Reverman, Director Information Systems
CHR: Fred Horlander, Vice President
Web address: www.clarkmemorial.org
Control: County–Government, nonfederal **Service:** General Medical and Surgical

Staffed Beds: 241 **Admissions:** 11775 **Census:** 129 **Outpatient Visits:** 160795 **Births:** 1406 **Total Expense ($000):** 117801 **Payroll Expense ($000):** 51053 **Personnel:** 1207

☐ **WELLSTONE REGIONAL HOSPITAL (154051)**, 2700 Vissing Park Road, Zip 47130; tel. 812/284–8000, (Nonreporting) **A**1 9 10 **S** Psychiatric Solutions
Primary Contact: Dean T. Saling, President and Chief Executive Officer
Web address: www.psysolutions.com/facilities/wellstone/
Control: Corporation, Investor–owned, for–profit **Service:** Psychiatric

Staffed Beds: 100

KENDALLVILLE—Noble County

★ **PARKVIEW NOBLE HOSPITAL (150146)**, 401 Sawyer Road, Zip 46755–2293, Mailing Address: P.O. Box 728, Zip 46755–0728; tel. 260/347–8700 **A**1 9 10 **F**3 7 11 13 15 25 26 30 31 32 33 38 46 47 50 55 56 57 62 68 72 73 74 77 79 80 82 86 87 96 97 100 102 106 107 118 119 121 124 134 135 136 137 **S** Parkview Health
Primary Contact: David C. Hunter, Chief Operating Officer
COO: David C. Hunter, Chief Operating Officer
CFO: Mark A. Nafziger, Chief Financial Officer
CMO: Ron Sloan, M.D., Chief of Staff
CIO: Cynthia Davis, Chief Information Officer
CHR: Peter Ford, Director Human Resources
Web address: www.parkview.com
Control: Other not–for–profit (including NFP Corporation) **Service:** General Medical and Surgical

Staffed Beds: 31 **Admissions:** 1677 **Census:** 15 **Outpatient Visits:** 62568 **Births:** 323 **Total Expense ($000):** 31429 **Payroll Expense ($000):** 12765 **Personnel:** 207

KNOX—Starke County

★ **STARKE MEMORIAL HOSPITAL (150102)**, 102 East Culver Road, Zip 46534–2299, Mailing Address: P.O. Box 339, Zip 46534–0339; tel. 574/772–6231 **A**1 10 **F**24 38 42 61 68 74 79 80 86 96 97 100 104 106 119 122 **S** LifePoint Hospitals, Inc.
Primary Contact: Michael J. Meadows, Chief Executive Officer
CFO: Vickie Magurean, Chief Financial Officer
CMO: A. N. Damodaran, M.D., President Medical Staff
CIO: Ashley Norem, Chief Information Systems
CHR: Doug Jesch, Director Human Resources
Web address: www.starkememorial.com
Control: Corporation, Investor–owned, for–profit **Service:** General Medical and Surgical

Staffed Beds: 49 **Admissions:** 1191 **Census:** 11 **Outpatient Visits:** 27794 **Births:** 54 **Total Expense ($000):** 16632 **Payroll Expense ($000):** 8557 **Personnel:** 218

KOKOMO—Howard County

★ **HOWARD REGIONAL HEALTH SYSTEM (150007)**, 3500 South Lafountain Street, Zip 46904–9011, Mailing Address: P.O. Box 9011, Zip 46904–9011; tel. 765/453–0702, (Nonreporting) **A**1 2 9 10 **S** Howard Regional Health System
Primary Contact: James P. Alender, President and Chief Executive Officer
COO: Theodore Brown, Chief Operating Officer
CFO: Thom Cook, Chief Financial Officer
CIO: Sharon Miller, Chief Information Officer
CHR: Michael L. Williams, Vice President Human Resources
Web address: www.howardregional.org
Control: County–Government, nonfederal **Service:** General Medical and Surgical

Staffed Beds: 150

★ **HOWARD REGIONAL HEALTH SYSTEM WEST CAMPUS SPECIALTY HOSPITAL (153039)**, 829 North Dixon Road, Zip 46901–7709; tel. 765/452–6700 **A**1 9 10 **F**25 30 31 32 82 85 86 118 132 **S** Howard Regional Health System
Primary Contact: Michelle L. Russell, Vice President and Administrator
CFO: Julie Pena, Director Finance
CMO: Brad Vossberg, M.D., Chief Rehabilitation
CHR: Kathy Leonard, Manager Human Resources
Web address: www.howardregional.org
Control: Corporation, Investor–owned, for–profit **Service:** Rehabilitation

Staffed Beds: 30 **Admissions:** 657 **Census:** 20 **Outpatient Visits:** 42296 **Births:** 0 **Total Expense ($000):** 13347 **Payroll Expense ($000):** 6861 **Personnel:** 177

★ **ST. JOSEPH HOSPITAL (150010)**, 1907 West Sycamore Street, Zip 46901–4197, Mailing Address: P.O. Box 9010, Zip 46904–9010; tel. 765/452–5611 **A**9 10 **F**3 4 5 7 8 13 15 18 24 25 26 27 30 31 32 33 34 38 41 43 49 50 55 56 57 62 64 66 67 68 71 72 73 74 75 76 77 79 80 82 84 85 86 87 88 89 90 91 92 93 94 95 96 97 98 100 102 106 107 108 109 111 118 119 120 121 124 132 133 134 135 136 137 **S** Ascension Health
Primary Contact: Kathlene A. Young, M.S., FACHE, Interim President
COO: Kathleen Peoples, Vice President Nursing
CFO: Dennis Ressler, Chief Financial Officer
CMO: David L. Williams, M.D., Chief Medical Officer
CIO: Roger Strange, Chief Information Officer
CHR: Cindy Babb, Director Human Resources
Web address: www.stjosephhospital.net
Control: Church–operated, Nongovernment, not–for profit **Service:** General Medical and Surgical

Staffed Beds: 136 **Admissions:** 4739 **Census:** 66 **Outpatient Visits:** 121147 **Births:** 589 **Total Expense ($000):** 80456 **Payroll Expense ($000):** 32749 **Personnel:** 710

LA PORTE—La Porte County

★ **LA PORTE REGIONAL HEALTH SYSTEM (150006)**, 1007 Lincolnway, Zip 46350–3201, Mailing Address: P.O. Box 250, Zip 46352–0250; tel. 219/326–1234, (Total facility includes 55 beds in nursing home–type unit) **A**1 2 5 9 10 19 **F**3 5 11 13 15 17 18 20 22 24 25 26 27 28 31 32 33 34 36 37 38 41 42 43 44 46 49 50 51 52 53 54 55 56 57 59 60 61 62 64 65 66 67 68 72 73 74 75 76 77 78 79 80 81 82 84 85 86 87 88 90 91 92 93 94 96 97 98 99 100 102 103 104 105 107 109 111 117 118 119 120 121 124 134 135 136 137 **S** Clarian Health
Primary Contact: Michael E. Haley, President and Chief Executive Officer
CFO: Mark Rafalski, Vice President Finance and Chief Financial Officer
CMO: William J. Houston, M.D., Medical Director
CIO: Earl Adams, Chief Information Officer
CHR: Connie Ford, Vice President Human Resources
Web address: www.laportehealth.org
Control: Other not–for–profit (including NFP Corporation) **Service:** General Medical and Surgical

Staffed Beds: 227 **Admissions:** 6241 **Census:** 107 **Outpatient Visits:** 100764 **Births:** 781 **Total Expense ($000):** 136769 **Payroll Expense ($000):** 55902 **Personnel:** 1216

LAFAYETTE—Tippecanoe County

ST VINCENT SETON SPECIALTY HOSPITAL (152021), (Formerly Seton Specialty Hospital), 1907 West Sycamore Street, 4th Floor, Zip 47904; tel. 765/236–8900 **A**9 10 **F**1 25 26 27 30 31 32 33 41 43 50 59 60 66 72 73 76 80 81
Primary Contact: Peter H. Alexander, Administrator
Web address: www.stvincent.org
Control: Other not–for–profit (including NFP Corporation) **Service:** Long–Term Acute Care hospital

Staffed Beds: 30 **Admissions:** 189 **Census:** 15 **Outpatient Visits:** 0 **Births:** 0 **Total Expense ($000):** 9548 **Payroll Expense ($000):** 5205 **Personnel:** 71

○ **ST. ELIZABETH REGIONAL HEALTH (150109)**, 2400 South Street, Zip 47904–3027; tel. 765/447–6811, (Includes LAFAYETTE HOME HOSPITAL; ST. ELIZABETH MEDICAL CENTER, 1501 Hartford Street, Zip 47904–2126; tel. 765/423–6011), (Total facility includes 23 beds in nursing home–type unit) (Nonreporting) **A**2 6 9 10 11 **S** Sisters of St. Francis Health Services, Inc.
Primary Contact: Terrance E. Wilson, President and Chief Executive Officer
CFO: Keith Lauter, Chief Financial Officer
CMO: Donald B. Edelen, M.D., Vice President Medical Services and Quality Initiatives
CIO: Lisa K. Decker, Division Director Public Relations and Marketing
CHR: Jan Garvin, Vice President Human Resources
Web address: www.ste.org
Control: Other not–for–profit (including NFP Corporation) **Service:** General Medical and Surgical

Staffed Beds: 451

LAGRANGE—LaGrange County

★ **PARKVIEW LAGRANGE HOSPITAL (151323)**, 207 North Townline Road, Zip 46761–1325; tel. 260/463–2143 **A**1 9 10 18 **F**3 7 13 15 25 26 30 31 32 33 38 42 43 44 45 55 56 57 62 68 73 74 77 79 80 81 82 84 86 96 102 107 117 118 119 122 135 137 **S** Parkview Health
Primary Contact: Robert T. Myers, Chief Operating Officer
COO: Robert T. Myers, Chief Operating Officer
CFO: Vickie Stanski, Financial Analyst
CMO: Jeffrey Brookes, M.D., President Medical Staff
CHR: Bob Pruitt, Director Human Resources
Web address: www.parkview.com
Control: Other not–for–profit (including NFP Corporation) **Service:** General Medical and Surgical

Staffed Beds: 25 **Admissions:** 1114 **Census:** 12 **Outpatient Visits:** 21109 **Births:** 327 **Total Expense ($000):** 16681 **Payroll Expense ($000):** 8290 **Personnel:** 145

LAWRENCEBURG—Dearborn County

★ ○ **DEARBORN COUNTY HOSPITAL (150086)**, 600 Wilson Creek Road, Zip 47025–1199; tel. 812/537–1010, (Total facility includes 12 beds in nursing home–type unit) **A**9 10 11 **F**3 11 13 15 18 24 26 27 30 32 33 35 38 40 41 42 44 46 49 50 55 56 57 61 62 68 73 74 75 76 77 79 80 81 82 84 86 96 97 100 102 104 105 106 107 117 119 120 121 135 137 **P**6
Primary Contact: Peter V. Resnick, Executive Director
CFO: Philip A. Meyer, Director Finance
CHR: Pat Sutton, Director Human Resources
Web address: www.dch.org
Control: County–Government, nonfederal **Service:** General Medical and Surgical

Staffed Beds: 95 **Admissions:** 4641 **Census:** 55 **Outpatient Visits:** 144168 **Births:** 557 **Total Expense ($000):** 66015 **Payroll Expense ($000):** 29406 **Personnel:** 611

LEBANON—Boone County

★ **WITHAM MEMORIAL HOSPITAL (150104)**, 2605 North Lebanon Street, Zip 46052, Mailing Address: P.O. Box 1200, Zip 46052–3005; tel. 765/485–8000 **A**1 9 10 **F**3 7 8 13 15 18 20 24 25 26 31 32 38 50 53 54 55 56 57 59 62 63 66 67 68 73 74 75 77 79 80 81 82 86 87 88 93 96 97 100 102 106 107 118 119 121 124 133 135 136 137 **P**1
Primary Contact: Raymond V. Ingham, Ph.D., President and Chief Executive Officer
COO: Diane Feder, Senior Vice President and Chief Operating Officer
CFO: George Pogas, Senior Vice President and Chief Financial Officer
CMO: Robert Watt, M.D., Chief of Staff
CIO: Glenn Davis, Director Information Systems
CHR: Gary A. Deater, Vice President Administrative and Support Services
Web address: www.witham.org
Control: County–Government, nonfederal **Service:** General Medical and Surgical

Staffed Beds: 48 **Admissions:** 2322 **Census:** 25 **Outpatient Visits:** 102974 **Births:** 352 **Total Expense ($000):** 59761 **Payroll Expense ($000):** 24170 **Personnel:** 433

LINTON—Greene County

★ **GREENE COUNTY GENERAL HOSPITAL (151317)**, Rural Route 1, Box 1000, Zip 47441–9457; tel. 812/847–2281 **A**1 9 10 18 **F**3 11 13 15 17 26 27 31 32 38 55 56 57 61 62 68 73 74 75 76 77 79 80 84 86 96 97 99 102 107 119 122 124 134 135 137
Primary Contact: Jonas S. Uland, Executive Director
COO: Jonas S. Uland, Executive Director
CFO: Timothy Norris, Chief Financial Officer
CMO: Owen A. Batterton, M.D., Chief of Staff
CIO: Steve Phillips, Information Officer
Web address: www.greenecountyhospital.com
Control: County–Government, nonfederal **Service:** General Medical and Surgical

Staffed Beds: 25 **Admissions:** 1230 **Census:** 11 **Outpatient Visits:** 380318 **Births:** 111 **Total Expense ($000):** 20625 **Payroll Expense ($000):** 8928 **Personnel:** 224

LOGANSPORT—Cass County

□ **LOGANSPORT STATE HOSPITAL**, 1098 South State Road 25, Zip 46947–9699; tel. 574/737–3633, (Nonreporting) **A**1
Primary Contact: Todd B. Graybill, Chief Executive Officer
COO: Robert Clover, Assistant Superintendent
CFO: Misty Moss, Assistant Superintendent Business Administration
CMO: Rohit Borkhetaria, M.D., Acting Medical Director
CIO: Joe McIntosh, Director Management Information Systems
CHR: Dianne Renner, Director Human Resources
Web address: www.lshonline.org
Control: State–Government, nonfederal **Service:** Psychiatric

Staffed Beds: 396

★ ○ **MEMORIAL HOSPITAL (150072)**, 1101 Michigan Avenue, Zip 46947–7013, Mailing Address: P.O. Box 7013, Zip 46947–7013; tel. 574/753–7541, (Total facility includes 21 beds in nursing home–type unit) **A**1 9 10 11 20 **F**3 7 11 13 15 24 25 26 28 31 32 33 34 38 41 48 49 50 51 55 56 57 62 63 66 67 68 73 74 75 76 77 79 80 81 82 86 87 96 97 99 100 102 106 107 112 117 118 119 121 124 135 **P**6
Primary Contact: Brian T. Shockney, FACHE, President and Chief Executive Officer
COO: Alan W. Biggs, Chief Operating Officer
CFO: Chad Higgins, Chief Financial Officer
CMO: Charles Montgomery, M.D., Medical Director
CIO: Beth Jump, Chief Information Officer
CHR: Lynda Murphy, Vice President Human Resources
Web address: www.logansportmemorial.org
Control: County–Government, nonfederal **Service:** General Medical and Surgical

Staffed Beds: 104 **Admissions:** 2400 **Census:** 26 **Outpatient Visits:** 91278 **Births:** 491 **Total Expense ($000):** 46088 **Payroll Expense ($000):** 20814 **Personnel:** 480

MADISON—Jefferson County

★ ○ **KING'S DAUGHTERS' HOSPITAL AND HEALTH SERVICES (150069)**, One King's Daughters' Drive, Zip 47250–3357, Mailing Address: P.O. Box 447, Zip 47250–0447; tel. 812/265–5211 **A**2 9 10 11 19 **F**3 7 13 15 24 25 26 27 28 30 31 32 33 38 41 42 43 48 49 50 51 54 55 56 57 61 62 63 66 68 72 73 74 75 76 77 79 80 81 82 84 86 87 96 97 100 103 107 109 111 118 119 120 121 123 133 135 137 **P**6
Primary Contact: Roger J. Allman, Chief Executive Officer
CFO: Steve Meacham, Vice President Finance
CMO: Steve Vorhies, President Medical Staff
CIO: Linda Darnell, Director Management Information Systems
CHR: Susie Poling, Director Human Resources
Web address: www.kdhhs.org
Control: Other not–for–profit (including NFP Corporation) **Service:** General Medical and Surgical

Staffed Beds: 82 **Admissions:** 4324 **Census:** 51 **Outpatient Visits:** 177438 **Births:** 430 **Total Expense ($000):** 94697 **Payroll Expense ($000):** 50798 **Personnel:** 910

□ **MADISON STATE HOSPITAL (154019)**, 711 Green Road, Zip 47250–2199; tel. 812/265–2611 **A**1 10 **F**26 31 32 37 54 88 91 93 119 135 **P**6
Primary Contact: Peggy Stephens, M.D., Superintendent and Medical Director
COO: Peggy Stephens, M.D., Superintendent and Medical Director
CFO: Carolyn Copeland, Business Administrator
CMO: Peggy Stephens, M.D., Superintendent and Medical Director
CIO: Ric Martin, Information Specialist
Web address: www.in.gov/fssa/msh
Control: State–Government, nonfederal **Service:** Psychiatric

Staffed Beds: 150 **Admissions:** 27 **Census:** 136 **Outpatient Visits:** 0 **Births:** 0 **Total Expense ($000):** 24616 **Payroll Expense ($000):** 16244 **Personnel:** 471

Hospital, Medicare Provider Number, Address, Telephone, Approval, Facility, and Physician Codes, Health Care System

★ American Hospital Association (AHA) membership
□ The Joint Commission accreditation
○ American Osteopathic Association (AOA) accreditation
△ Commission on Accreditation of Rehabilitation Facilities (CARF) accreditation

MARION—Grant County

★ ○ **MARION GENERAL HOSPITAL (150011)**, 441 North Wabash Avenue, Zip 46952–2690; tel. 765/662–1441 **A**2 9 10 11 19 20 **F**3 7 8 11 13 14 15 18 20 24 25 26 27 30 31 32 33 38 43 50 53 55 56 57 58 62 63 66 67 68 72 73 74 75 76 77 78 79 80 81 82 84 85 86 87 96 97 99 100 101 102 106 107 112 118 119 121 124 133 134 135 136 137 **P**6
Primary Contact: Paul Usher, Interim Chief Executive Officer, Vice President Finance and Chief Financial Officer
COO: Larry P. Burns, Vice President Operations
CFO: Paul Usher, Vice President Finance and Chief Financial Officer
CMO: Paul D. Wolfe, M.D., Chief of Staff
CIO: Emmanuel Ndow, Administrative Director Information Technology
CHR: Bruce J. Tisdale, Administrative Director Human Resources
Web address: www.mgh.net
Control: Other not–for–profit (including NFP Corporation) **Service:** General Medical and Surgical

Staffed Beds: 168 **Admissions:** 5572 **Census:** 55 **Outpatient Visits:** 193789 **Births:** 783 **Total Expense ($000):** 111353 **Payroll Expense ($000):** 37916 **Personnel:** 1035

VETERANS AFFAIRS NORTHERN INDIANA HEALTH CARE SYSTEM–MARION CAMPUS See Veterans Affairs Northern Indiana Health Care System, Fort Wayne

MARTINSVILLE—Morgan County

⊛ **MORGAN HOSPITAL AND MEDICAL CENTER (150038)**, 2209 John R. Wooden Drive, Zip 46151–1840, Mailing Address: P.O. Box 1717, Zip 46151–1717; tel. 765/342–8441 **A**1 2 9 10 **F**3 8 11 13 15 24 25 27 30 31 32 33 38 54 55 56 57 62 63 67 68 72 73 74 75 76 77 79 80 81 84 85 86 87 88 93 96 97 100 102 104 107 108 109 114 118 119 120 121 124 133 135 136 **P**6 8
Primary Contact: Thomas W. Laux, President and Chief Executive Officer
COO: Vicky Reed, Chief Operating Officer and Chief Nursing Executive
CFO: Susan Havers, Vice President and Chief Financial Officer
CMO: Warren L. Gray, M.D., Chief of Staff
CIO: Karon E. Perkins, Vice President Physician Practice Operations and Corporate Compliance Officer
CHR: Charlene Hall, Vice President Human Resources and Guest Support Services
Web address: www.morganhospital.org
Control: County–Government, nonfederal **Service:** General Medical and Surgical

Staffed Beds: 93 **Admissions:** 2361 **Census:** 26 **Outpatient Visits:** 77570 **Births:** 194 **Total Expense ($000):** 42554 **Payroll Expense ($000):** 16326 **Personnel:** 396

MERRILLVILLE—Lake County

SOUTHLAKE CAMPUS See Methodist Hospitals, Gary

MICHIGAN CITY—La Porte County

○ **SAINT ANTHONY MEMORIAL (150015)**, 301 West Homer Street, Zip 46360–4358; tel. 219/879–8511, (Nonreporting) **A**2 9 10 11 19 **S** Sisters of St. Francis Health Services, Inc.
Primary Contact: James Callaghan, III, M.D., President
CFO: Jim Lipinski, Regional Chief Financial Officer
CIO: Terry Veith, Director Management Information Systems
CHR: Susan King–Schreiber, Vice President Human Resources
Web address: www.saintanthonymemorial.org
Control: Church–operated, Nongovernment, not–for profit **Service:** General Medical and Surgical

Staffed Beds: 168

MISHAWAKA—St. Joseph County

⊛ **SAINT JOSEPH REGIONAL MEDICAL CENTER–MISHAWAKA CAMPUS (150029)**, 215 West Fourth Street, Zip 46544–1999; tel. 574/259–2431 **A**1 9 10 13 **F**13 15 17 18 19 20 21 22 23 24 25 26 30 31 32 33 38 46 50 53 55 56 57 62 66 68 69 72 73 74 77 79 82 84 86 96 97 103 107 108 109 110 111 112 117 119 121 135 137 **S** Trinity Health
Primary Contact: Steven A. Rose, RN, Executive Vice President
COO: Lori Price, Chief Operating Officer
CFO: Terry Heck, Chief Financial Officer
CMO: Thomas F. Lavelle, M.D., Chief Medical Officer
CIO: Gary L. Miller, Regional Director Information Systems
CHR: Aaron Austin, Vice President Human Resources
Web address: www.sjmed.com
Control: Church–operated, Nongovernment, not–for profit **Service:** General Medical and Surgical

Staffed Beds: 78 **Admissions:** 3335 **Census:** 48 **Outpatient Visits:** 87041 **Births:** 608 **Total Expense ($000):** 58643 **Payroll Expense ($000):** 19182 **Personnel:** 363

MONTICELLO—White County

★ ○ **WHITE COUNTY MEMORIAL HOSPITAL (151312)**, 1101 O'Connor Boulevard, Zip 47960–1698; tel. 574/583–7111 **A**9 10 11 18 **F**3 11 13 15 25 26 27 31 32 33 34 38 43 53 55 56 57 61 62 68 72 73 74 75 76 77 79 80 81 82 86 87 96 97 100 102 107 117 118 119 120 121 122 124 134 136
Primary Contact: Paul Cardwell, Chief Executive Officer
COO: David Bailey, Vice President Operations
CFO: Annette Eichholz, Chief Financial Officer
CIO: Chanel Kyle, Director Information Systems
Web address: www.whitecmh.org
Control: County–Government, nonfederal **Service:** General Medical and Surgical

Staffed Beds: 25 **Admissions:** 1071 **Census:** 14 **Outpatient Visits:** 30733 **Births:** 204 **Total Expense ($000):** 23190 **Payroll Expense ($000):** 9687 **Personnel:** 251

MOORESVILLE—Morgan County

○ **ST. FRANCIS HOSPITAL–MOORESVILLE (150057)**, 1201 Hadley Road N.W., Zip 46158–1789; tel. 317/831–1160, (Nonreporting) **A**9 10 11 **S** Sisters of St. Francis Health Services, Inc.
Primary Contact: D. Keith Jewell, Interim Executive Director
COO: D. Keith Jewell, Senior Vice President and Chief Operating Officer
CFO: Greg Anderson, Vice President Finance
CMO: Donald Kerner, M.D., Vice President Medical Affairs
CIO: Barbara Coulter, Director Information Systems
CHR: John Ross, Vice President
Control: Church–operated, Nongovernment, not–for profit **Service:** General Medical and Surgical

Staffed Beds: 54

MUNCIE—Delaware County

⊛ △ **BALL MEMORIAL HOSPITAL (150089)**, 2401 University Avenue, Zip 47303–3499; tel. 765/747–3111, (Total facility includes 30 beds in nursing home–type unit) **A**1 2 3 5 7 8 9 10 19 **F**3 8 11 12 13 15 17 18 20 22 24 25 26 27 28 30 31 32 33 37 38 42 43 49 50 51 53 55 56 57 58 62 63 67 68 70 71 72 73 74 75 76 77 78 79 80 81 82 84 85 86 87 90 91 92 93 96 99 100 102 103 105 106 107 108 109 111 112 113 114 116 117 118 119 120 121 135 136 137 **P**6 8 **S** Cardinal Health System
Primary Contact: Brent L. Batman, President
CFO: Robert E. Gildersleeve, Executive Vice President and Chief Financial Officer
CMO: Thomas K. Gardiner, M.D., Executive Vice President Clinical Development
CIO: Tom Powers, Vice President Information Systems and Chief Information Systems
CHR: Terry Allen, Senior Vice President Human Resources
Web address: www.accesschs.org
Control: Other not–for–profit (including NFP Corporation) **Service:** General Medical and Surgical

Staffed Beds: 356 **Admissions:** 17489 **Census:** 235 **Outpatient Visits:** 322604 **Births:** 1666 **Total Expense ($000):** 264622 **Payroll Expense ($000):** 92617 **Personnel:** 1887

☐ **RENAISSANCE SPECIALTY HOSPITAL OF CENTRAL INDIANA (152025)**, 3400 West Community Drive, Zip 47304; tel. 765/282–5822, (Nonreporting) **A**1 10
Primary Contact: Brian Couch, Chief Executive Officer
Control: Corporation, Investor–owned, for–profit **Service:** Long–Term Acute Care hospital

Staffed Beds: 32

MUNSTER—Lake County

☐ △ **COMMUNITY HOSPITAL (150125)**, 901 MacArthur Boulevard, Zip 46321–2959; tel. 219/836–1600 **A**1 2 5 7 9 10 **F**3 11 13 15 17 18 20 22 24 25 27 31 32 33 37 38 43 49 50 51 52 53 55 56 57 58 61 62 66 68 70 72 73 74 75 76 77 78 79 80 81 82 84 85 86 96 97 99 100 102 103 105 107 108 109 111 112 118 119 121 124 133 135 136 137 **P**6 **S** Community Healthcare System
Primary Contact: Donald P. Fesko, Administrator
CFO: Lou Molina, Chief Financial Officer
CIO: Vernon Groeber, Chief Information Officer
CHR: Mike Graham, Chief Human Resources Officer
Web address: www.comhs.org
Control: Other not–for–profit (including NFP Corporation) **Service:** General Medical and Surgical

Staffed Beds: 367 **Admissions:** 21070 **Census:** 285 **Outpatient Visits:** 312097 **Births:** 2250 **Total Expense ($000):** 288158 **Payroll Expense ($000):** 122584 **Personnel:** 2233

○ **FRANCISCAN PHYSICIANS HOSPITAL (150147)**, (Formerly Heartland Memorial Hospital), 701 Superior Avenue, Zip 46321–4029; tel. 219/924–1300 **A**9 10 11 **F**3 8 15 17 18 20 22 25 26 30 37 43 46 62 68 77 80 96 100 102 107 118 119 124 133 **S** Sisters of St. Francis Health Services, Inc.
Primary Contact: Barbara M. Greene, President
CFO: Harold E. Collins, JD, Chief Financial Officer
CMO: Vijay D. Gupta, M.D., President and Chief Executive Officer
CIO: Steven Krause, Manager Information Technology
Web address: www.heartlandmemorial.org
Control: Partnership, Investor–owned, for–profit **Service:** General Medical and Surgical

Staffed Beds: 32 **Admissions:** 520 **Census:** 7 **Outpatient Visits:** 4278 **Births:** 0 **Total Expense ($000):** 13932 **Payroll Expense ($000):** 4998 **Personnel:** 126

NEW ALBANY—Floyd County

★ ○ **FLOYD MEMORIAL HOSPITAL AND HEALTH SERVICES (150044)**, 1850 State Street, Zip 47150–4997; tel. 812/949–5500 **A**2 3 5 9 10 11 **F**8 11 13 15 17 18 20 22 24 25 26 27 30 31 32 33 38 40 43 49 50 54 55 56 57 61 62 68 69 72 73 74 75 76 77 78 79 80 81 82 84 86 90 96 97 99 100 102 103 106 107 108 109 111 118 119 120 121 124 133 135 136 137
Primary Contact: Mark D. Shugarman, President and Chief Executive Officer
COO: Jerri Quillman, Executive Vice President
CFO: Ted Miller, Chief Financial Officer
CMO: Joseph A. Bruckman, M.D., Medical Director
CIO: Mother Superior Barry Grover, Director Information Systems
CHR: Mike Ford, Vice President Human Resources
Web address: www.floydmemorial.com
Control: County–Government, nonfederal **Service:** General Medical and Surgical

Staffed Beds: 206 **Admissions:** 12569 **Census:** 133 **Outpatient Visits:** 277791 **Births:** 1079 **Total Expense ($000):** 154456 **Payroll Expense ($000):** 60309 **Personnel:** 1347

☒ △ **SOUTHERN INDIANA REHABILITATION HOSPITAL (153037)**, 3104 Blackiston Boulevard, Zip 47150–9579; tel. 812/941–8300, (Total facility includes 22 beds in nursing home–type unit) **A**1 7 9 10 **F**25 30 31 32 33 54 55 57 72 73 77 81 82 85 86 117 119 121 124 132 135 137 **S** Jewish Hospital & St. Mary's HealthCare
Primary Contact: Randy L. Napier, President and Chief Executive Officer
CFO: Cathy Kidd, Controller
CMO: John C. Shaw, M.D., Medical Director
Web address: www.sirh.org
Control: Other not–for–profit (including NFP Corporation) **Service:** Rehabilitation

Staffed Beds: 60 **Admissions:** 932 **Census:** 31 **Outpatient Visits:** 26848 **Births:** 0 **Total Expense ($000):** 15628 **Payroll Expense ($000):** 7952 **Personnel:** 170

NEW CASTLE—Henry County

★ ○ **HENRY COUNTY HOSPITAL (150030)**, 1000 North 16th Street, Zip 47362–4319, Mailing Address: P.O. Box 490, Zip 47362–0490; tel. 765/521–0890 **A**9 10 11 **F**3 8 10 11 13 15 24 26 33 38 42 43 46 50 51 52 55 57 61 62 66 68 72 73 74 75 77 79 84 86 87 96 100 103 106 107 118 119 120 121 124 133 135 136 137 **P**1
Primary Contact: Blake A. Dye, President and Chief Executive Officer
CFO: Paul Janssen, Senior Vice President and Chief Financial Officer
CMO: Daniel House, M.D., Chief of Staff
CIO: Mike Spencer, Chief Information Officer
CHR: Deanna Malott, Director Human Resources
Web address: www.hcmhcares.org
Control: County–Government, nonfederal **Service:** General Medical and Surgical

Staffed Beds: 87 **Admissions:** 3515 **Census:** 38 **Outpatient Visits:** 135557 **Births:** 439 **Total Expense ($000):** 57321 **Payroll Expense ($000):** 24565 **Personnel:** 638

NEWBURGH—Warrick County

☒ **THE WOMEN'S HOSPITAL (150149)**, 4199 Gateway Boulevard, Zip 47630; tel. 812/842–4200, (Includes DEACONESS GATEWAY HOSPITAL, 4011 Gateway Boulevard, Zip 47630–8947; tel. 812/842–2000) **A**1 9 10 **F**3 13 25 26 30 31 32 41 50 52 55 56 57 63 70 73 74 75 79 80 81 82 107 113 114 119 121 123 124 135 136 **P**6 **S** Deaconess Health System
Primary Contact: Christina M. Ryan, Chief Executive Officer
CFO: Martha McClain, Controller
CIO: Liz Adams, Manager Informatics
CHR: Susie Traylor, Manager Human Resources
Web address: www.deaconess.com
Control: Partnership, Investor–owned, for–profit **Service:** Obstetrics and gynecology

Staffed Beds: 74 **Admissions:** 4621 **Census:** 48 **Outpatient Visits:** 7097 **Births:** 3417 **Total Expense ($000):** 42456 **Payroll Expense ($000):** 16192 **Personnel:** 383

NOBLESVILLE—Hamilton County

☒ △ **RIVERVIEW HOSPITAL (150059)**, 395 Westfield Road, Zip 46060–1425, Mailing Address: P.O. Box 220, Zip 46061–0220; tel. 317/773–0760 **A**1 7 9 10 **F**3 11 13 15 17 18 20 22 24 25 26 27 30 31 32 33 36 37 38 42 43 44 46 47 48 49 50 52 53 54 55 56 57 59 61 62 63 64 66 68 72 73 74 75 76 77 79 80 81 82 84 85 86 87 90 92 96 97 99 100 102 104 105 106 107 108 109 111 117 118 119 120 121 122 124 132 133 135 136 137 **P**2 6 8
Primary Contact: Patricia K. Fox, President and Chief Executive Officer
CFO: James P. Porter, CPA, Vice President and Chief Financial Officer
CMO: John Paris, M.D., Chief Medical Officer
CIO: Randy Cox, Chief Information Officer
CHR: Karol Bonine, Executive Director Human Resources
Web address: www.riverview.org
Control: County–Government, nonfederal **Service:** General Medical and Surgical

Staffed Beds: 156 **Admissions:** 5691 **Census:** 81 **Outpatient Visits:** 296434 **Births:** 1016 **Total Expense ($000):** 131104 **Payroll Expense ($000):** 52940 **Personnel:** 953

NORTH VERNON—Jennings County

☒ **ST. VINCENT JENNINGS HOSPITAL (151303)**, 301 Henry Street, Zip 47265–1097; tel. 812/352–4200 **A**1 9 10 18 **F**3 15 25 26 28 30 31 32 33 34 38 41 45 46 47 50 54 55 56 57 62 63 64 72 75 77 79 80 86 87 96 100 102 107 112 121 122 124 133 135 137 **P**4 **S** Ascension Health
Primary Contact: Joseph E. Roche, Administrator
CFO: John Lines, Chief Financial Officer
CMO: Jennifer Stanley, M.D., President Medical Staff
CHR: Kathryn Johnson, Manager Human Resources, Marketing and Public Relations
Web address: www.stvincent.org
Control: Other not–for–profit (including NFP Corporation) **Service:** General Medical and Surgical

Staffed Beds: 25 **Admissions:** 569 **Census:** 6 **Outpatient Visits:** 89679 **Births:** 1 **Total Expense ($000):** 21877 **Payroll Expense ($000):** 10428 **Personnel:** 209

PAOLI—Orange County

□ **BLOOMINGTON HOSPITAL OF ORANGE COUNTY (151306)**, 642 West Hospital Road, Zip 47454–0499, Mailing Address: P.O. Box 499, Zip 47454–0499; tel. 812/723–2811 **A**1 9 10 18 **F**3 7 13 15 25 26 31 32 33 38 44 50 55 57 62 66 74 75 76 77 79 80 84 86 96 100 107 118 121 122 124 135 137
Primary Contact: Gene Perry, Chief Executive Officer
COO: Candy Isom, Chief Operating Officer
CFO: Sue Brock, Chief Financial Officer
CMO: Dan O'Brien, D.O., Medical Director
CHR: Jessica Fortner, Director Human Resources
Web address: www.bhhs.org
Control: Other not–for–profit (including NFP Corporation) **Service:** General Medical and Surgical

Staffed Beds: 24 **Admissions:** 599 **Census:** 5 **Outpatient Visits:** 26702 **Births:** 174 **Total Expense ($000):** 17568 **Payroll Expense ($000):** 8853 **Personnel:** 279

PERU—Miami County

☒ **DUKES MEMORIAL HOSPITAL (151318)**, 275 West 12th Street, Zip 46970–1698; tel. 765/472–8000 **A**1 9 10 18 **F**3 7 13 15 24 25 26 30 31 32 38 43 50 51 54 55 57 62 66 67 68 73 74 75 77 79 80 82 85 86 96 97 100 102 106 107 118 119 120 122 124 133 135 136 137 **P**6 **S** Community Health Systems, Inc.
Primary Contact: Debra Close, Chief Executive Officer
COO: Elena McNutt, Chief Nursing Officer
CMO: Neil Stalker, M.D., Chief of Staff
CHR: Kim Black, Manager Human Resources
Web address: www.dukesmemorialhosp.com
Control: Corporation, Investor–owned, for–profit **Service:** General Medical and Surgical

Staffed Beds: 25 **Admissions:** 1503 **Census:** 13 **Outpatient Visits:** 52515 **Births:** 418 **Total Expense ($000):** 37197 **Payroll Expense ($000):** 16372 **Personnel:** 355

Hospital, Medicare Provider Number, Address, Telephone, Approval, Facility, and Physician Codes, Health Care System

★ American Hospital Association (AHA) membership
□ The Joint Commission accreditation
○ American Osteopathic Association (AOA) accreditation
△ Commission on Accreditation of Rehabilitation Facilities (CARF) accreditation

PLYMOUTH—Marshall County

MICHIANA BEHAVIORAL HEALTH CENTER (154047), 1800 North Oak Road, Zip 46563–3492; tel. 574/936–3784, (Nonreporting) **A**9 10 **S** Horizon Health Corporation
Primary Contact: Bryan W. Lett, Chief Executive Officer
COO: Terrance Cook, Chief Financial Officer
CFO: Terrance Cook, Chief Financial Officer
CMO: John Haskin, M.D., Medical Director
CIO: Bob Kedalis, Director Business Development
CHR: Becky Nowicki, Director Human Resources
Web address: www.michianabhc.com
Control: Corporation, Investor–owned, for–profit **Service:** Psychiatric

Staffed Beds: 76

★ **SAINT JOSEPH REGIONAL MEDICAL CENTER–PLYMOUTH CAMPUS (150076)**, 1915 Lake Avenue, Zip 46563–9905, Mailing Address: P.O. Box 670, Zip 46563–9905; tel. 574/936–3181 **A**1 9 10 **F**13 15 25 26 27 30 31 32 33 38 46 50 53 55 56 57 66 68 72 73 74 76 77 79 82 86 96 97 103 107 108 109 110 111 112 114 118 119 121 135 **S** Trinity Health
Primary Contact: Nancy R. Hellyer, Chief Executive Officer
COO: Lori Price, Chief Operating Officer
CFO: Terry Heck, Vice President Finance and Chief Financial Officer
CMO: Thomas F. Lavelle, M.D., Chief Medical Officer
CIO: Gary L. Miller, Regional Director Information Systems
CHR: Aaron Austin, Vice President Human Resources
Web address: www.sjmed.com
Control: Church–operated, Nongovernment, not–for profit **Service:** General Medical and Surgical

Staffed Beds: 45 **Admissions:** 2569 **Census:** 25 **Outpatient Visits:** 79722 **Births:** 354 **Total Expense ($000):** 40393 **Payroll Expense ($000):** 15968 **Personnel:** 250

PORTAGE—Porter County

★ **REGENCY HOSPITAL OF PORTER COUNTY**, 3630 Willow Road, Zip 46368; tel. 219/364–3800, (Nonreporting) **A**1 9 **S** Regency Hospital Company
Primary Contact: Beverly Foster, Chief Executive Officer
Web address: www.regencyhospital.com
Control: Corporation, Investor–owned, for–profit **Service:** Long–Term Acute Care hospital

Staffed Beds: 23

PORTLAND—Jay County

★ **JAY COUNTY HOSPITAL (151320)**, 500 West Votaw Street, Zip 47371–1322; tel. 260/726–7131 **A**1 9 10 18 **F**3 8 11 13 15 24 26 32 33 38 55 56 57 66 68 73 74 75 77 79 80 81 82 93 96 97 100 102 107 118 119 121 122 123 124 135 **S** Cardinal Health System
Primary Contact: Joe Johnston, Chief Executive Officer
CFO: Don Michael, Chief Financial Officer
CIO: Jeff Horn, Coordinator Information Systems
CHR: Jerry Bozell, Administrative Director Human Resources
Web address: www.jaycountyhospital.com
Control: County–Government, nonfederal **Service:** General Medical and Surgical

Staffed Beds: 35 **Admissions:** 1213 **Census:** 18 **Outpatient Visits:** 34374 **Births:** 92 **Total Expense ($000):** 18339 **Payroll Expense ($000):** 8076 **Personnel:** 197

PRINCETON—Gibson County

★ **GIBSON GENERAL HOSPITAL (151319)**, 1808 Sherman Drive, Zip 47670–1043; tel. 812/385–3401, (Total facility includes 45 beds in nursing home–type unit) **A**1 9 10 18 **F**3 5 11 15 24 25 26 30 31 32 33 36 38 40 53 54 55 56 57 61 62 66 68 73 75 77 79 84 86 87 89 90 91 92 93 94 96 100 103 107 117 118 119 120 121 122 135 136 137 **P**6 **S** Alliant Management Services
Primary Contact: Emmett C. Schuster, President and Chief Executive Officer
CFO: Gregory Schulten, Vice President and Chief Financial Officer
CIO: Steve Rausch, Director Information Services
CHR: Mike Logan, Director Human Resources
Web address: www.gibsongeneral.com
Control: Other not–for–profit (including NFP Corporation) **Service:** General Medical and Surgical

Staffed Beds: 70 **Admissions:** 903 **Census:** 50 **Outpatient Visits:** 39111 **Births:** 13 **Total Expense ($000):** 19476 **Payroll Expense ($000):** 9143 **Personnel:** 311

RENSSELAER—Jasper County

★ **JASPER COUNTY HOSPITAL (151324)**, 1104 East Grace Street, Zip 47978–3296; tel. 219/866–5141, (Total facility includes 17 beds in nursing home–type unit) **A**9 10 18 **F**3 11 13 15 24 25 26 27 30 31 33 37 38 42 43 48 49 50 51 52 53 54 55 56 57 61 62 63 66 67 68 73 74 75 76 77 79 80 82 86 92 96 97 100 102 106 107 117 118 119 120 121 122 124 137
Primary Contact: Timothy M. Schreeg, President and Chief Executive Officer
CFO: Jeffrey D. Webb, CPA, Controller
CIO: Kirby Reed, Director Information Systems
CHR: Deana Brown, Director Administrative Services
Web address: www.jchh.com
Control: County–Government, nonfederal **Service:** General Medical and Surgical

Staffed Beds: 42 **Admissions:** 1373 **Census:** 31 **Outpatient Visits:** 88895 **Births:** 166 **Total Expense ($000):** 28112 **Payroll Expense ($000):** 14513 **Personnel:** 380

RICHMOND—Wayne County

★ ○ **REID HOSPITAL AND HEALTH CARE SERVICES (150048)**, 1401 Chester Boulevard, Zip 47374–1986; tel. 765/983–3000 **A**2 5 9 10 11 19 20 **F**3 5 11 13 15 17 18 20 22 24 25 26 27 28 30 31 32 33 37 38 40 41 42 43 44 49 50 51 54 55 56 57 59 60 62 66 68 72 73 74 75 76 77 79 80 81 82 84 85 86 88 90 91 92 93 94 96 97 99 100 102 103 106 107 108 109 111 118 119 120 121 124 135 136 137 **P**7 8
Primary Contact: Barry S. MacDowell, President
CFO: Craig Kinyon, Vice President Finance and Chief Financial Officer
CMO: Thomas Huth, M.D., Vice President Medical Affairs
CIO: Eric Synnestvedt, Director Information Services
Web address: www.reidhosp.com
Control: Other not–for–profit (including NFP Corporation) **Service:** General Medical and Surgical

Staffed Beds: 214 **Admissions:** 11263 **Census:** 133 **Outpatient Visits:** 140516 **Births:** 775 **Total Expense ($000):** 200771 **Payroll Expense ($000):** 75833 **Personnel:** 1343

□ **RICHMOND STATE HOSPITAL (154018)**, 498 N.W. 18th Street, Zip 47374–2898; tel. 765/966–0511 **A**1 10 **F**4 25 26 37 73 75 82 88 89 90 91 92 93 119 121 124 132 **P**6
Primary Contact: Jeffrey Butler, Superintendent
COO: Max Callis, Director Physical Plant
CFO: Dave Shelford, Assistant Superintendent
CMO: Anthony Siegel, M.D., Medical Director
CIO: Robert Boatman, Director Information Technology
CHR: Sarah Witt, Director Human Resources
Web address: www.richmondstatehospital.org
Control: State–Government, nonfederal **Service:** Psychiatric

Staffed Beds: 312 **Admissions:** 460 **Census:** 279 **Outpatient Visits:** 0 **Births:** 0 **Personnel:** 618

ROCHESTER—Fulton County

★ **WOODLAWN HOSPITAL (151313)**, 1400 East Ninth Street, Zip 46975–8937; tel. 574/223–3141 **A**1 9 10 18 **F**3 7 11 13 15 25 26 27 38 43 46 54 55 57 61 63 67 68 73 74 75 76 77 79 82 86 87 96 97 100 103 105 107 118 119 121 122 124 135 137 **P**6
Primary Contact: John L. Alley, Chief Executive Officer
CFO: Dave Cholger, Chief Financial Officer
CHR: Deb Lemasters, Director Human Resources
Web address: www.woodlawnhospital.com
Control: County–Government, nonfederal **Service:** General Medical and Surgical

Staffed Beds: 25 **Admissions:** 976 **Census:** 8 **Outpatient Visits:** 73667 **Births:** 220 **Total Expense ($000):** 31095 **Payroll Expense ($000):** 14623 **Personnel:** 255

RUSHVILLE—Rush County

★ **RUSH MEMORIAL HOSPITAL (151304)**, 1300 North Main Street, Zip 46173–1198, Mailing Address: P.O. Box 608, Zip 46173–0608; tel. 765/932–4111, (Nonreporting) **A**9 10 18
Primary Contact: Brad Smith, Chief Executive Officer
CFO: Karen Meyer, Chief Financial Officer
CMO: Raz Kedd, M.D., Chief Medical Officer and Chief of Staff
CIO: Jim Boyer, Director Information Systems
CHR: Pam RenneKamp, Director Human Resources
Web address: www.rushmemorial.com
Control: County–Government, nonfederal **Service:** General Medical and Surgical

Staffed Beds: 25

IN

Many Facility Codes have changed. Please refer to the AHA Guide Code Chart.

SALEM—Washington County

▣ **WASHINGTON COUNTY MEMORIAL HOSPITAL (151314)**, 911 North Shelby Street, Zip 47167–1694; tel. 812/883–5881 **A**1 9 10 18 **F**3 5 7 8 11 13 15 24 25 26 27 31 32 33 36 38 43 47 48 49 50 55 56 57 62 63 68 72 73 74 76 77 79 86 88 89 90 91 92 93 94 95 96 100 102 106 107 118 119 120 121 122 124 132 134 135 136 **P**6
Primary Contact: Randy Lindauer, President and Chief Executive Officer
COO: James J. Steggeman, Chief Operating Officer
CFO: Tricia Ellison, Director Financial and Support Services
CMO: S. E. Kemker, M.D., President Medical Staff
CIO: Cale Kearschner, Manager Information Systems
CHR: Betsey Johnson, Director Human Resources
Web address: www.wcmhospital.org
Control: County–Government, nonfederal **Service:** General Medical and Surgical

Staffed Beds: 35 **Admissions:** 947 **Census:** 17 **Outpatient Visits:** 36679 **Births:** 88 **Total Expense ($000):** 22798 **Payroll Expense ($000):** 14179 **Personnel:** 251

SCOTTSBURG—Scott County

▣ **SCOTT MEMORIAL HOSPITAL (151334)**, 1415 North Gardner Street, Zip 47170–0430, Mailing Address: Box 430, Zip 47170–0430; tel. 812/752–3456 **A**1 9 10 18 **F**3 11 13 15 24 25 26 30 31 32 33 38 55 56 57 62 66 68 72 74 75 77 79 80 81 87 96 97 100 102 107 118 121 124 133 135 136 **P**6 **S** Jewish Hospital & St. Mary's HealthCare
Primary Contact: Clifford D. Nay, Executive Director
CFO: Angela Doan, Chief Financial Officer
Web address: www.scottmemorial.com
Control: County–Government, nonfederal **Service:** General Medical and Surgical

Staffed Beds: 25 **Admissions:** 1528 **Census:** 15 **Outpatient Visits:** 43958 **Births:** 186 **Total Expense ($000):** 20979 **Payroll Expense ($000):** 10680 **Personnel:** 208

SEYMOUR—Jackson County

▣ **SCHNECK MEDICAL CENTER (150065)**, 411 West Tipton Street, Zip 47274–5000, Mailing Address: P.O. Box 2349, Zip 47274–2349; tel. 812/522–2349 **A**1 2 9 10 **F**3 11 12 13 15 24 25 26 27 30 32 33 34 38 42 43 44 46 49 50 51 55 56 57 58 61 62 67 68 73 74 75 76 77 79 80 81 82 84 86 93 94 96 99 100 102 106 107 108 109 111 112 118 119 120 121 122 124 135 136 137 **P**6 8
Primary Contact: Gary A. Meyer, President and Chief Executive Officer
CFO: Warren Forgey, Vice President Fiscal Services
CIO: Vickie Burrell, Director Management Information Systems
CHR: William Lewis, Vice President Human Resources
Web address: www.schneckmed.org
Control: County–Government, nonfederal **Service:** General Medical and Surgical

Staffed Beds: 108 **Admissions:** 3628 **Census:** 40 **Outpatient Visits:** 93000 **Births:** 680 **Total Expense ($000):** 70024 **Payroll Expense ($000):** 31610 **Personnel:** 679

SHELBYVILLE—Shelby County

★ ○ **MAJOR HOSPITAL (150097)**, 150 West Washington Street, Zip 46176–1236; tel. 317/392–3211 **A**9 10 11 **F**3 11 12 13 15 24 25 27 30 31 32 34 38 57 61 62 66 68 71 73 74 75 76 79 80 82 84 86 87 96 97 99 100 102 105 107 108 109 111 112 118 119 120 121 124 135 136 137 **P**4 7
Primary Contact: Anthony B. Lennen, President and Chief Executive Officer
CFO: Robin Nichols, Vice President and Chief Financial Officer
CIO: John M. Horner, Vice President and Chief Information Officer
CHR: Nicki Sparling, Manager Human Resources
Web address: www.majorhospital.com
Control: City–County, Government, nonfederal **Service:** General Medical and Surgical

Staffed Beds: 62 **Admissions:** 2882 **Census:** 27 **Outpatient Visits:** 124236 **Births:** 389 **Total Expense ($000):** 60853 **Payroll Expense ($000):** 24744 **Personnel:** 522

SOUTH BEND—St. Joseph County

MADISON CENTER AND HOSPITAL (154040), 403 East Madison, Zip 46617; tel. 574/234–0061 **A**9 10 **F**4 5 6 25 31 32 33 36 38 50 53 54 56 57 58 73 81 88 89 90 91 92 93 94 95 119 121 123 **P**6
Primary Contact: Jack Roberts, Chief Executive Officer
COO: Wendy Chapman, Senior Vice President Administration
CFO: Andrew J. Poole, Chief Financial Officer
CMO: John Zwerneman, M.D., Chief Medical Officer
CHR: Jill Seifer, Director Human Resources
Web address: www.madison.org
Control: Other not–for–profit (including NFP Corporation) **Service:** Psychiatric

Staffed Beds: 91 **Admissions:** 952 **Census:** 53 **Outpatient Visits:** 771294 **Births:** 0 **Total Expense ($000):** 59326 **Payroll Expense ($000):** 32754 **Personnel:** 1021

▣ △ **MEMORIAL HOSPITAL OF SOUTH BEND (150058)**, 615 North Michigan Street, Zip 46601–9986; tel. 574/647–1000 **A**1 2 3 5 7 9 10 **F**7 8 9 12 13 15 17 18 20 22 24 25 26 27 30 31 32 33 36 38 40 43 44 46 49 50 52 54 59 60 62 65 66 68 70 72 73 74 75 76 77 79 80 81 82 83 84 85 86 96 97 102 103 104 105 107 109 112 116 118 119 120 121 123 124 132 134 135 136 137 **P**8
Primary Contact: Philip A. Newbold, President and Chief Executive Officer
COO: Kreg Gruber, Chief Operating Officer
CFO: Jeff Costello, Chief Financial Officer
CIO: Steve Huffman, Interim Vice President Information Systems
Web address: www.qualityoflife.org
Control: Other not–for–profit (including NFP Corporation) **Service:** General Medical and Surgical

Staffed Beds: 325 **Admissions:** 20924 **Census:** 224 **Outpatient Visits:** 161302 **Births:** 3309 **Total Expense ($000):** 319258 **Payroll Expense ($000):** 115849 **Personnel:** 2147

□ **OUR LADY OF PEACE HOSPITAL (152018)**, 801 East LaSalle Avenue, Zip 46617; tel. 574/237–7457 **A**1 9 10 **F**1 3 25 30 80
Primary Contact: Christine T. Voorde, Chief Executive Officer
CFO: Jeff Calvin, Financial Officer
CIO: Gary L. Miller, Regional Director Information Systems
CHR: Aaron Austin, Vice President Human Resources
Web address: www.ourladyofpeacehospital.org
Control: Other not–for–profit (including NFP Corporation) **Service:** Long–Term Acute Care hospital

Staffed Beds: 32 **Admissions:** 309 **Census:** 24 **Outpatient Visits:** 0 **Births:** 0 **Total Expense ($000):** 9636 **Payroll Expense ($000):** 3085 **Personnel:** 57

RIVERSIDE HOSPITAL (154049), 533 North Niles Avenue, Zip 46617; tel. 574/283–1104 **A**9 10 **F**31 73 88 90 119 **P**6
Primary Contact: Jack Roberts, Chief Executive Officer
COO: Wendy Chapman, Senior Vice President Administration
CFO: Andrew J. Poole, Chief Financial Officer
CMO: John Zwerneman, M.D., Chief Medical Officer
CHR: Jill Seifer, Director Human Resources
Web address: www.madison.org
Control: Other not–for–profit (including NFP Corporation) **Service:** Psychiatric

Staffed Beds: 16 **Admissions:** 462 **Census:** 13 **Outpatient Visits:** 0 **Births:** 0 **Total Expense ($000):** 1779

▣ △ **SAINT JOSEPH REGIONAL MEDICAL CENTER (150012)**, 801 East LaSalle, Zip 46617–2800; tel. 574/237–7111 **A**1 2 3 5 7 9 10 **F**13 15 17 18 19 20 21 22 23 24 25 26 27 30 31 32 33 38 46 47 48 49 50 53 55 56 57 59 64 66 68 70 71 72 73 74 76 77 79 82 84 85 86 96 97 103 105 107 108 109 111 112 114 118 119 120 121 124 135 136 137 **S** Trinity Health
Primary Contact: Lori Price, Chief Operating Officer
COO: Lori Price, Chief Operating Officer
CFO: Terry Heck, Vice President Finance and Chief Financial Officer
CMO: Thomas F. Lavelle, M.D., Chief Medical Officer
CIO: Gary L. Miller, Regional Director Information Systems
CHR: Aaron Austin, Vice President Human Resources
Web address: www.sjmed.com
Control: Other not–for–profit (including NFP Corporation) **Service:** General Medical and Surgical

Staffed Beds: 267 **Admissions:** 11996 **Census:** 149 **Outpatient Visits:** 116089 **Births:** 1147 **Total Expense ($000):** 184713 **Payroll Expense ($000):** 57645 **Personnel:** 1171

IN

Hospital, Medicare Provider Number, Address, Telephone, Approval, Facility, and Physician Codes, Health Care System
★ American Hospital Association (AHA) membership
□ The Joint Commission accreditation
○ American Osteopathic Association (AOA) accreditation
△ Commission on Accreditation of Rehabilitation Facilities (CARF) accreditation

SULLIVAN—Sullivan County

★ ○ **SULLIVAN COUNTY COMMUNITY HOSPITAL (151327)**, 2200 North Section Street, Zip 47882, Mailing Address: P.O. Box 10, Zip 47882–0010; tel. 812/268–4311 **A**9 10 11 18 **F**3 8 13 15 24 25 28 31 33 38 41 47 52 54 55 56 57 60 61 67 68 73 74 75 76 77 79 81 82 86 87 96 100 119 120 122 135 136 137 **P**8 **S** QHR
Primary Contact: Michelle Sly–Smith, Chief Executive Officer
CFO: Alan J. Montella, Assistant Administrator Finance
CMO: Gene Bourgasser, M.D., Chief of Staff
CIO: Hap Beckes, Director Information Systems
CHR: Denise Brashear, Director Human Resources
Web address: www.schosp.com
Control: County–Government, nonfederal **Service:** General Medical and Surgical

Staffed Beds: 25 **Admissions:** 1132 **Census:** 10 **Outpatient Visits:** 56828 **Births:** 113 **Total Expense ($000):** 18043 **Payroll Expense ($000):** 7642 **Personnel:** 190

TELL CITY—Perry County

★ ○ **PERRY COUNTY MEMORIAL HOSPITAL (151322)**, 1 Hospital Road, Zip 47586–0362; tel. 812/547–7011 **A**9 10 11 18 **F**3 7 11 13 15 24 25 26 27 32 33 36 38 42 50 54 55 56 57 61 62 66 68 73 74 75 76 77 79 81 82 86 92 96 97 99 100 102 106 107 118 119 121 122 124 135 136 **S** Alliant Management Services
Primary Contact: Joseph A. Stuber, President and Chief Executive Officer
COO: Becky Elder, Vice President Clinical Services
CFO: Kathy Clayton, Chief Financial Officer
CMO: Anastacia Lagunzad, Chief of Staff
CIO: Debbie Kleeman, Manager Information Systems
CHR: Sheila Gaynor, Director Human Resources
Web address: www.pchospital.org
Control: County–Government, nonfederal **Service:** General Medical and Surgical

Staffed Beds: 25 **Admissions:** 1391 **Census:** 11 **Outpatient Visits:** 58981 **Births:** 78 **Total Expense ($000):** 27016 **Payroll Expense ($000):** 8085 **Personnel:** 252

TERRE HAUTE—Vigo County

HAMILTON CENTER (154009), 620 Eighth Avenue, Zip 47804–0323; tel. 812/231–8323, (Nonreporting) **A**9 10
Primary Contact: Galen Goode, Chief Executive Officer
COO: Robb Johnson, Director Operations
CFO: Susie Thompson, Executive Director Fiscal Services
CMO: David Hilton, Medical Director
CIO: Mel Burks, Executive Director Administrative Services
CHR: Mel Burks, Executive Director Administrative Services
Web address: www.hamiltoncenter.org
Control: Other not–for–profit (including NFP Corporation) **Service:** Psychiatric

Staffed Beds: 16

☒ **TERRE HAUTE REGIONAL HOSPITAL (150046)**, 3901 South Seventh Street, Zip 47802–4299; tel. 812/232–0021 **A**1 2 5 9 10 **F**3 13 15 18 20 22 24 25 26 27 31 32 33 38 42 45 46 47 49 50 51 52 54 55 56 57 59 66 67 68 72 73 74 75 76 77 79 80 81 82 84 85 86 88 90 92 96 97 98 99 100 103 107 108 109 111 121 133 134 135 136 137 **P**8 **S** HCA
Primary Contact: Christopher J. Hill, Chief Executive Officer
COO: Lea Ann Klarner, Chief Operating Officer
CFO: Brian Bauer, Chief Financial Officer
CMO: Divyesh Purohit, President Medical Staff
CIO: Mike Kuckewich, Director Information Systems
CHR: Aaron Garofola, Director Human Resources
Web address: www.regionalhospital.com
Control: Corporation, Investor–owned, for–profit **Service:** General Medical and Surgical

Staffed Beds: 231 **Admissions:** 6951 **Census:** 93 **Outpatient Visits:** 61341 **Births:** 789 **Total Expense ($000):** 77935 **Payroll Expense ($000):** 32796 **Personnel:** 641

★ ○ △ **UNION HOSPITAL (150023)**, 1606 North Seventh Street, Zip 47804–2780; tel. 812/238–7000 **A**2 3 5 7 9 10 11 19 **F**3 8 9 13 15 17 18 20 22 24 25 26 27 30 31 32 33 34 37 38 43 44 45 46 49 50 52 53 55 56 57 60 62 64 66 68 70 71 72 73 74 75 76 77 79 80 81 82 84 85 86 87 96 99 100 101 102 103 106 107 108 109 111 119 120 121 124 135 136 137 **P**5 6
Primary Contact: David R. Doerr, Chief Executive Officer
COO: Scott Teffeteller, Vice President and Chief Operating Officer
CFO: Wayne Hutson, Chief Financial Officer
CMO: Ronald Leach, M.D., Medical Director
CIO: Kym Pfrank, Vice President Information Systems
CHR: Sally Zuel, Assistant Vice President Human Resources
Web address: www.uhhg.org
Control: Other not–for–profit (including NFP Corporation) **Service:** General Medical and Surgical

Staffed Beds: 278 **Admissions:** 15131 **Census:** 191 **Outpatient Visits:** 361770 **Births:** 1503 **Total Expense ($000):** 286200 **Payroll Expense ($000):** 92165 **Personnel:** 1770

TIPTON—Tipton County

☒ **TIPTON HOSPITAL (151311)**, 1000 South Main Street, Zip 46072–9799; tel. 765/675–8500 **A**1 2 9 10 18 **F**3 10 11 15 24 25 26 27 30 33 38 49 52 55 56 57 62 67 68 72 73 75 76 77 79 81 82 86 87 92 94 96 100 102 106 107 118 119 120 121 122 124 135 **P**7 **S** Clarian Health
Primary Contact: Michael Harlowe, President and Chief Executive Officer
COO: Carl Pafford, M.D., Vice President Operations and Business Development
CFO: Vern J. Schmaltz, Vice President Finance
Web address: www.tiptonhospital.org
Control: County–Government, nonfederal **Service:** General Medical and Surgical

Staffed Beds: 25 **Admissions:** 1482 **Census:** 18 **Outpatient Visits:** 46212 **Births:** 0 **Total Expense ($000):** 33304 **Payroll Expense ($000):** 13724 **Personnel:** 311

VALPARAISO—Porter County

☒ **PORTER–VALPARAISO HOSPITAL CAMPUS (150035)**, 814 La Porte Avenue, Zip 46383–5898; tel. 219/263–4600 **A**1 9 10 **F**3 7 8 11 13 15 17 18 20 22 24 25 26 27 28 30 31 32 33 34 36 38 39 43 44 53 55 56 57 59 62 64 66 67 68 69 70 71 72 73 74 76 77 78 79 80 81 82 87 96 97 98 99 100 102 103 107 108 112 119 120 121 123 124 130 133 135 136 137 **S** Community Health Systems, Inc.
Primary Contact: Jonathan Nalli, Chief Executive Officer
COO: William H. Cummins, Chief Operations Officer
CFO: Cheryl A. Harmon, Chief Financial Officer
CMO: Ramireddy K. Tummuru, M.D., Chief Medical Officer
CHR: Angie Hampton, Director Human Resources
Web address: www.porterhealth.org
Control: Corporation, Investor–owned, for–profit **Service:** General Medical and Surgical

Staffed Beds: 276 **Admissions:** 7801 **Census:** 95 **Outpatient Visits:** 171530 **Births:** 925 **Total Expense ($000):** 138927 **Payroll Expense ($000):** 53306 **Personnel:** 1538

VINCENNES—Knox County

☒ △ **GOOD SAMARITAN HOSPITAL (150042)**, 520 South Seventh Street, Zip 47591–1098; tel. 812/882–5220 **A**1 2 7 9 10 19 **F**3 5 8 11 13 15 17 18 20 22 24 25 26 27 28 30 31 32 33 34 36 37 38 40 42 46 48 49 51 52 55 56 57 59 64 65 66 68 71 72 73 74 75 76 77 79 80 81 82 84 85 86 88 89 90 91 92 93 94 95 96 97 99 100 103 106 107 109 111 112 118 119 121 123 124 133 134 135 136 137 **P**6
Primary Contact: Matthew D. Bailey, FACHE, President and Chief Executive Officer
COO: Gerald E. Waldroup, Senior Vice President
CFO: Robert McLin, Vice President Finance
CMO: Charles C. Hedde, M.D., Vice President Medical Affairs
CIO: Charles Christian, Director Information Systems
CHR: Dean Wagoner, Director Human Resources
Web address: www.gshvin.org/goodsamaritan
Control: County–Government, nonfederal **Service:** General Medical and Surgical

Staffed Beds: 232 **Admissions:** 8337 **Census:** 101 **Outpatient Visits:** 335190 **Births:** 587 **Total Expense ($000):** 135227 **Payroll Expense ($000):** 56331 **Personnel:** 1238

WABASH—Wabash County

☒ **WABASH COUNTY HOSPITAL (151310)**, 710 North East Street, Zip 46992–1924, Mailing Address: P.O. Box 548, Zip 46992–0548; tel. 260/563–3131, (Total facility includes 25 beds in nursing home–type unit) **A**1 2 9 10 18 **F**3 11 15 24 25 26 27 28 30 32 33 38 42 43 44 52 54 55 56 57 58 61 62 63 66 67 68 73 75 76 77 79 80 81 82 86 87 96 97 99 100 102 103 107 112 117 120 121 122 124 135 136 **S** Alliant Management Services
Primary Contact: Marilyn J. Custer–Mitchell, President and Chief Executive Officer
CFO: Kent H. Giles, Director Finance
CMO: Jeff Miller, M.D., Chief Medical Officer
CIO: Kent H. Giles, Director Finance
CHR: Kim Shininger, Director Human Resources
Web address: www.wchospital.com
Control: County–Government, nonfederal **Service:** General Medical and Surgical

Staffed Beds: 50 **Admissions:** 933 **Census:** 24 **Outpatient Visits:** 49781 **Births:** 0 **Total Expense ($000):** 32044 **Payroll Expense ($000):** 13172 **Personnel:** 302

IN

WARSAW—Kosciusko County

☒ **KOSCIUSKO COMMUNITY HOSPITAL (150133)**, 2101 East Dubois Drive, Zip 46580–3288; tel. 574/267–3200 **A**1 2 9 10 19 **F**3 12 13 15 24 25 26 27 30 31 32 38 41 43 51 52 55 56 57 62 66 68 73 74 75 76 77 79 80 81 86 96 97 100 103 104 105 106 107 108 109 118 119 120 121 124 133 135 136 137 **P**6 **S** Community Health Systems, Inc.
Primary Contact: Stephen R. Miller, Chief Executive Officer
COO: Joan Darr, Chief Operating Officer
CFO: Doug BeMent, Chief Financial Officer
CMO: Michael Williams, M.D., Medical Director
CIO: Tammy Lukens, Director
CHR: Joe Jarboe, Director Human Resources
Web address: www.kch.com
Control: Corporation, Investor–owned, for–profit **Service:** General Medical and Surgical

Staffed Beds: 72 **Admissions:** 3709 **Census:** 30 **Outpatient Visits:** 95050 **Total Expense ($000):** 48755 **Payroll Expense ($000):** 20361 **Personnel:** 811

OTIS R BOWEN CENTER FOR HUMAN SERVICES (154014), 850 North Harrison Street, Zip 46580–3163; tel. 574/267–7169 **A**10 **F**4 25 36 88 89 90 91 92 93 94 95
Primary Contact: Kurt Carlson, Chief Executive Officer
Web address: www.bowencenter.org
Control: Other not–for–profit (including NFP Corporation) **Service:** Psychiatric

Staffed Beds: 16 **Admissions:** 689 **Census:** 8 **Outpatient Visits:** 193000 **Births:** 0 **Total Expense ($000):** 23955 **Personnel:** 466

WASHINGTON—Daviess County

☒ △ **DAVIESS COMMUNITY HOSPITAL (150061)**, 1314 East Walnut Street, Zip 47501–2198, Mailing Address: P.O. Box 760, Zip 47501–0760; tel. 812/254–2760 **A**1 7 9 10 **F**3 11 13 15 24 25 26 27 28 30 31 32 33 38 42 46 54 55 56 57 61 62 64 66 68 73 74 75 76 77 79 80 81 82 84 85 86 87 88 93 94 95 96 99 100 107 118 119 121 122 124 134 135 136 137 **P**8 **S** QHR
Primary Contact: Louis H. Bremer, Jr., Interim Chief Executive Officer
COO: Don Kelso, Director Human Resources
CFO: Brad Hardcastle, Chief Financial Officer
CMO: Stephen Cullen, Chief of Staff
CHR: Richard Pea, Director Human Resources
Web address: www.dchosp.org
Control: County–Government, nonfederal **Service:** General Medical and Surgical

Staffed Beds: 80 **Admissions:** 2845 **Census:** 34 **Outpatient Visits:** 176001 **Births:** 492 **Total Expense ($000):** 42361 **Payroll Expense ($000):** 19563 **Personnel:** 495

WEST LAFAYETTE—Tippecanoe County

WABASH VALLEY HOSPITAL (154005), 2900 North River Road, Zip 47906–3766; tel. 765/463–2555, (Nonreporting) **A**10
Primary Contact: Rick Crawley, Administrator and Chief Executive Officer
CFO: Douglas A. Lane, Chief Financial Officer
CMO: Richard Rahdert, M.D., Medical Director
CHR: Jan Shaw, Director Personnel
Web address: www.wvhmhc.org
Control: Other not–for–profit (including NFP Corporation) **Service:** Psychiatric

Staffed Beds: 70

WILLIAMSPORT—Warren County

☒ **ST. VINCENT WILLIAMSPORT HOSPITAL (151307)**, 412 North Monroe Street, Zip 47993–0215; tel. 765/762–4000, (Nonreporting) **A**1 9 10 18 **S** Ascension Health
Primary Contact: Jane Craigin, Chief Executive Officer
CFO: Janet Merritt, Chief Financial Officer
Web address: www.stvincent.org
Control: Other not–for–profit (including NFP Corporation) **Service:** General Medical and Surgical

Staffed Beds: 16

WINAMAC—Pulaski County

★ ○ **PULASKI MEMORIAL HOSPITAL (151305)**, 616 East 13th Street, Zip 46996–1117, Mailing Address: P.O. Box 279, Zip 46996–0279; tel. 574/946–2100, (Nonreporting) **A**9 10 11 18
Primary Contact: Richard H. Mynark, Chief Executive Officer
CFO: Gregg Malott, Chief Financial Officer
CMO: Brian Johnson, M.D., Medical Staff President
CIO: Kevin Trusty, Director Information Technology and Manager Materials
CHR: Amy A. Bean, Director Human Resources
Web address: www.pulaskimemorial.com
Control: County–Government, nonfederal **Service:** General Medical and Surgical

Staffed Beds: 25

WINCHESTER—Randolph County

☒ **ST. VINCENT RANDOLPH HOSPITAL (151301)**, 473 Greenville Avenue, Zip 47394–2235, Mailing Address: P.O. Box 407, Zip 47394–0407; tel. 765/584–0004 **A**1 9 10 18 **F**3 11 13 15 24 25 26 28 30 31 32 33 38 50 54 55 56 57 62 63 66 73 74 75 76 77 79 80 81 82 84 86 96 100 102 107 112 118 119 120 121 122 123 124 135 136 137 **S** Ascension Health
Primary Contact: Francis G. Albarano, Administrator
CFO: John Arthur, Chief Financial Officer
CMO: Daniel Wegg, M.D., Medical Director
CIO: Brandy Ralls, Chief Information Officer
CHR: Darlene Hart, Human Resource Assistant
Web address: www.stvincent.org
Control: Church–operated, Nongovernment, not–for profit **Service:** General Medical and Surgical

Staffed Beds: 20 **Admissions:** 1105 **Census:** 10 **Outpatient Visits:** 45536 **Births:** 214 **Total Expense ($000):** 19182 **Payroll Expense ($000):** 8410 **Personnel:** 178

IN

Hospital, Medicare Provider Number, Address, Telephone, Approval, Facility, and Physician Codes, Health Care System

★ American Hospital Association (AHA) membership
□ The Joint Commission accreditation
○ American Osteopathic Association (AOA) accreditation
△ Commission on Accreditation of Rehabilitation Facilities (CARF) accreditation

IOWA

ALBIA—Monroe County

★ **MONROE COUNTY HOSPITAL (161342)**, 6580 165th Street, Zip 52531–8793; tel. 641/932–2134 **A**9 10 18 **F**7 11 15 24 25 27 30 31 32 33 38 42 55 57 62 79 80 96 107 122 124
Primary Contact: Gregory A. Paris, CHE, Chief Executive Officer
Web address: www.mchalbia.com
Control: County–Government, nonfederal **Service:** General Medical and Surgical

Staffed Beds: 25 **Admissions:** 449 **Census:** 12 **Outpatient Visits:** 25959 **Births:** 0 **Total Expense ($000):** 11793 **Payroll Expense ($000):** 4632 **Personnel:** 129

ALGONA—Kossuth County

★ **KOSSUTH REGIONAL HEALTH CENTER (161353)**, 1515 South Phillips Street, Zip 50511–3649; tel. 515/295–2451 **A**9 10 18 **F**11 13 15 17 24 25 26 27 28 31 32 33 38 40 42 43 44 50 54 55 56 57 61 62 63 65 66 68 73 74 75 76 79 81 82 84 85 86 87 96 102 107 117 118 119 120 121 122 124 135 136 **P**8 **S** Trinity Health
Primary Contact: Scott A. Curtis, Administrator and Chief Executive Officer
CFO: Dan Myers, Controller
CMO: Manasi Nadkarni, M.D., Chief of Staff
CIO: Nancy Erickson, Administrator Information Systems
Web address: www.krhc.com
Control: County–Government, nonfederal **Service:** General Medical and Surgical

Staffed Beds: 22 **Admissions:** 841 **Census:** 9 **Outpatient Visits:** 26625 **Births:** 103 **Total Expense ($000):** 19428 **Payroll Expense ($000):** 6432 **Personnel:** 168

AMES—Story County

☒ **MARY GREELEY MEDICAL CENTER (160030)**, 1111 Duff Avenue, Zip 50010–5745; tel. 515/239–2011, (Total facility includes 11 beds in nursing home–type unit) **A**1 2 9 10 19 **F**3 7 8 11 12 13 15 17 18 24 25 26 27 30 31 32 33 34 36 37 38 40 42 43 46 49 50 52 54 55 56 57 58 59 60 61 62 63 66 67 68 70 72 73 74 75 76 77 79 80 81 84 85 86 88 89 90 91 92 93 94 95 96 97 100 102 103 106 107 109 111 114 117 118 119 120 121 124 135 137
Primary Contact: Lynn V. Whisler, Interim Chief Executive Officer
CFO: Brian Dieter, Vice President and Chief Financial Officer
CIO: JaNelle Anderson, Director
CHR: Toni Shropshire, Vice President
Web address: www.mgmc.org
Control: City–Government, nonfederal **Service:** General Medical and Surgical

Staffed Beds: 198 **Admissions:** 10113 **Census:** 113 **Outpatient Visits:** 138028 **Births:** 1334 **Total Expense ($000):** 131171 **Payroll Expense ($000):** 50591 **Personnel:** 1038

ANAMOSA—Jones County

★ **JONES REGIONAL MEDICAL CENTER (161306)**, 104 Broadway Place, Zip 52205–1100; tel. 319/462–6131 **A**9 10 18 **F**1 7 11 15 24 25 30 31 32 33 36 37 38 40 43 44 50 54 55 56 57 62 65 66 69 73 79 80 82 84 87 89 90 91 92 93 94 96 99 100 107 117 119 121 122 124 134 135 **P**4 **S** Iowa Health System
Primary Contact: Sean J. Williams, Chief Executive Officer
CFO: Rachel Von Behren, Director Financial Services
CMO: Victor Salas, M.D., President Medical Staff
CHR: Donna Condry, Director Human Resources
Web address: www.jonesregional.org
Control: Other not–for–profit (including NFP Corporation) **Service:** General Medical and Surgical

Staffed Beds: 25 **Admissions:** 541 **Census:** 6 **Outpatient Visits:** 44734 **Births:** 0 **Total Expense ($000):** 9023 **Payroll Expense ($000):** 2886 **Personnel:** 86

ATLANTIC—Cass County

★ **CASS COUNTY MEMORIAL HOSPITAL (161376)**, 1501 East Tenth Street, Zip 50022–1997; tel. 712/243–3250 **A**9 10 18 **F**11 13 15 24 25 30 32 38 42 43 55 57 61 62 67 68 73 74 76 79 86 88 89 91 92 93 94 95 96 97 100 107 112 117 118 119 121 122 124 137 **P**8
Primary Contact: Patricia A. Markham, Administrator
CFO: Stephen Lewis, Assistant Administrator and Chief Financial Officer
CMO: Robert Beck, M.D., Chief of Staff
CIO: Arthur Kirsher, Chief Information Officer
CHR: Donald D. Johnson, Assistant Administrator Human Resources
Web address: www.casshealth.org
Control: County–Government, nonfederal **Service:** General Medical and Surgical

Staffed Beds: 43 **Admissions:** 1431 **Census:** 17 **Outpatient Visits:** 50358 **Births:** 150 **Total Expense ($000):** 24198 **Payroll Expense ($000):** 11266 **Personnel:** 298

AUDUBON—Audubon County

AUDUBON COUNTY MEMORIAL HOSPITAL (161330), 515 Pacific Street, Zip 50025–1052; tel. 712/563–2611 **A**9 10 18 **F**3 11 15 24 27 31 32 38 40 52 57 62 76 77 79 86 107 122 124
Primary Contact: Thomas G. Smith, Administrator and Chief Executive Officer
CFO: Karen McGuire, Chief Financial Officer
CIO: Kelli Burgin, Director Information Technology
Web address: www.acmhhosp.org
Control: County–Government, nonfederal **Service:** General Medical and Surgical

Staffed Beds: 25 **Admissions:** 277 **Census:** 3 **Outpatient Visits:** 15970 **Births:** 0 **Total Expense ($000):** 7751 **Payroll Expense ($000):** 2673 **Personnel:** 69

BELMOND—Wright County

★ **BELMOND MEDICAL CENTER (161301)**, 403 First Street S.E., Zip 50421–1201; tel. 641/444–3223 **A**9 10 18 **F**7 11 15 24 30 31 32 38 40 42 52 56 57 62 66 73 75 79 80 84 86 87 96 118 119 122 135 137 **P**8 **S** Trinity Health
Primary Contact: Nancy Gabrielson, Administrator
CFO: Greg Polzin, Chief Financial Officer
CMO: Donald Woodhouse, M.D., Chief Medical Staff
CHR: Reagan Swisher, Director Human Resources
Web address: www.belmondmedicalcenter.com
Control: City–Government, nonfederal **Service:** General Medical and Surgical

Staffed Beds: 22 **Admissions:** 251 **Census:** 4 **Outpatient Visits:** 9138 **Births:** 0 **Total Expense ($000):** 5730 **Payroll Expense ($000):** 1965 **Personnel:** 64

BETTENDORF—Scott County

☒ ○ **TRINITY AT TERRACE PARK (160104)**, 4500 Utica Ridge Road, Zip 52722–1626; tel. 563/742–5000 **A**1 9 10 11 12 13 **F**8 11 12 13 15 18 20 25 26 30 31 32 33 34 35 38 42 54 55 56 57 62 63 68 73 74 75 77 79 80 81 82 86 87 96 97 102 107 118 119 121 124 135 136 137 **S** Iowa Health System
Primary Contact: Andrea Y. Coleman, President and Chief Executive Officer
COO: Florence Spyrow, Vice President Operations
CFO: Kevin Vermeer, Chief Financial Officer
CMO: Morris H. Seligman, M.D., Vice President Medical Affairs and Chief Medical Officer
CHR: Jeffery Stolze, Vice President Human Resources
Web address: www.trinityqc.com
Control: Other not–for–profit (including NFP Corporation) **Service:** General Medical and Surgical

Staffed Beds: 69 **Admissions:** 3290 **Census:** 25 **Outpatient Visits:** 32079 **Births:** 357 **Total Expense ($000):** 52105 **Payroll Expense ($000):** 14177 **Personnel:** 192

BLOOMFIELD—Davis County

★ **DAVIS COUNTY HOSPITAL (161327)**, 507 North Madison Street, Zip 52537–1271; tel. 641/664–2145, (Total facility includes 32 beds in nursing home–type unit) **A**9 10 18 **F**7 11 13 15 24 25 28 30 31 32 33 38 41 42 50 55 56 57 60 61 62 63 65 66 67 73 74 76 77 79 81 82 86 87 96 107 122 135 **P**6
Primary Contact: Deborah Herzberg, RN, M.S., CHE, Chief Executive Officer
COO: Debbie Scott, Chief Operating Officer
CFO: Gary R. Foll, Chief Financial Officer
CIO: Deb Barker, Communications and Information Specialist
CHR: Lois Westercamp, Manager Human Resources
Web address: www.daviscountyhospital.org
Control: County–Government, nonfederal **Service:** General Medical and Surgical

Staffed Beds: 57 **Admissions:** 758 **Census:** 40 **Outpatient Visits:** 16676 **Births:** 70 **Total Expense ($000):** 13484 **Payroll Expense ($000):** 5542 **Personnel:** 177

BOONE—Boone County

★ **BOONE COUNTY HOSPITAL (161372)**, 1015 Union Street, Zip 50036–4821; tel. 515/432–3140, (Total facility includes 14 beds in nursing home–type unit) **A**9 10 18 **F**2 7 11 13 15 24 26 27 30 31 32 33 38 40 50 55 57 61 62 63 67 68 73 74 75 76 77 79 81 86 96 100 102 107 117 121 122 134 135 136 137 **P**6 **S** QHR
Primary Contact: Joseph S. Smith, Chief Executive Officer
CFO: David Mellett, Chief Financial Officer
CMO: Sascha Parsons, M.D., Chief of Staff
CHR: Veronica Burke, Director Human Resources
Web address: www.boonehospital.com
Control: County–Government, nonfederal **Service:** General Medical and Surgical

Staffed Beds: 39 **Admissions:** 1594 **Census:** 18 **Outpatient Visits:** 63500 **Births:** 106 **Total Expense ($000):** 29730 **Payroll Expense ($000):** 12780 **Personnel:** 308

BRITT—Hancock County

★ **HANCOCK COUNTY MEMORIAL HOSPITAL (161307)**, 532 First Street N.W., Zip 50423; tel. 641/843–5000 **A**9 10 18 **F**8 11 15 24 25 27 30 31 32 33 34 38 40 42 46 52 54 55 56 57 62 63 67 73 76 79 80 86 87 96 102 107 118 119 121 122 135 **P**1 **S** Trinity Health
Primary Contact: Vance Jackson, FACHE, Administrator and Chief Executive Officer
CFO: Julie Damm, Chief Financial Officer
CMO: Anne Boileau, M.D., Chief Medical Staff
CIO: Julie Damm, Chief Financial Officer
CHR: Denise Jakoubeck, Director Human Resources
Web address: www.hancockmemhospital.com
Control: County–Government, nonfederal **Service:** General Medical and Surgical

Staffed Beds: 25 **Admissions:** 350 **Census:** 6 **Outpatient Visits:** 16565 **Births:** 0 **Total Expense ($000):** 9944 **Payroll Expense ($000):** 3419 **Personnel:** 99

CARROLL—Carroll County

★ **ST. ANTHONY REGIONAL HOSPITAL (160005)**, 311 South Clark Street, Zip 51401–3038, Mailing Address: P.O. Box 628, Zip 51401–0628; tel. 712/792–3581, (Total facility includes 79 beds in nursing home–type unit) **A**9 10 19 20 **F**2 6 11 13 15 24 25 26 27 30 31 32 33 35 36 37 38 40 41 42 43 44 46 50 51 54 55 56 57 59 60 61 62 63 65 66 67 68 72 73 74 75 76 77 79 80 81 82 84 86 87 88 89 90 91 92 93 94 96 97 100 102 106 115 118 119 120 121 122 123 124 134 135 136 137 **P**6
Primary Contact: Gary P. Riedmann, FACHE, President and Chief Executive Officer
CFO: Edward H. Smith, Vice President and Chief Financial Officer
CMO: Michael Slattery, M.D., Chief of Staff
CIO: Randy Eischeid, Director Information Systems
CHR: Gina Ramaekers, Director Human Resources
Web address: www.stanthonyhospital.org
Control: Church–operated, Nongovernment, not–for profit **Service:** General Medical and Surgical

Staffed Beds: 155 **Admissions:** 2771 **Census:** 113 **Outpatient Visits:** 95867 **Births:** 418 **Total Expense ($000):** 44445 **Payroll Expense ($000):** 19147 **Personnel:** 469

CEDAR FALLS—Black Hawk County

★□ **SARTORI MEMORIAL HOSPITAL (160040)**, 515 College Street, Zip 50613–2500; tel. 319/268–3000, (Total facility includes 16 beds in nursing home–type unit) **A**1 9 10 **F**3 7 11 12 15 25 26 32 33 38 41 46 52 55 57 62 66 68 73 75 79 86 87 88 93 96 107 109 117 119 120 121 132 135 **P**1 6 **S** Wheaton Franciscan Healthcare
Primary Contact: Sherri Greenwood, Administrator
COO: David Olejniczak, Chief Operating Officer
CFO: Shelli Panicucci, Chief Financial Officer
CIO: Todd Richardson, Regional Vice President Information Services
CHR: Vicki L. Parsons, Regional Vice President Human Resources
Web address: www.covhealth.com
Control: Church–operated, Nongovernment, not–for profit **Service:** General Medical and Surgical

Staffed Beds: 66 **Admissions:** 1977 **Census:** 26 **Outpatient Visits:** 50981 **Births:** 0 **Total Expense ($000):** 27401 **Payroll Expense ($000):** 10386 **Personnel:** 218

CEDAR RAPIDS—Linn County

★□ **MERCY MEDICAL CENTER (160079)**, 701 Tenth Street S.E., Zip 52403–1292; tel. 319/398–6011, (Total facility includes 76 beds in nursing home–type unit) **A**1 3 5 9 10 **F**3 5 11 13 15 17 18 20 24 25 26 27 28 30 31 32 33 36 38 40 41 42 43 44 49 50 52 54 55 56 57 59 60 61 62 63 65 66 68 69 70 72 73 74 75 76 77 79 80 81 82 83 84 85 86 88 89 90 91 92 93 94 96 97 98 99 100 102 103 104 105 106 107 108 109 111 112 114 117 118 119 120 121 124 132 134 135 136 137 **P**7 8
Primary Contact: Timothy L. Charles, President and Chief Executive Officer
COO: Karl Keeler, Senior Vice President and Operations Officer Service Development
CFO: Philip Peterson, Executive Vice President and Chief Financial Officer
CMO: Mark Valliere, M.D., Senior Vice President and Chief Medical Officer
CIO: Jeff Cash, Vice President and Chief Information Officer
CHR: Kathy Krusie, Senior Vice President and Operations Officer Administrative and Support Services
Web address: www.mercycare.org
Control: Church–operated, Nongovernment, not–for profit **Service:** General Medical and Surgical

Staffed Beds: 314 **Admissions:** 10977 **Census:** 187 **Outpatient Visits:** 299973 **Births:** 805 **Total Expense ($000):** 177326 **Payroll Expense ($000):** 72820 **Personnel:** 1745

★□ △ **ST. LUKE'S HOSPITAL (160045)**, 1026 A Avenue N.E., Zip 52402–3026, Mailing Address: P.O. Box 3026, Zip 52406–3026; tel. 319/369–7211, (Total facility includes 21 beds in nursing home–type unit) **A**1 3 5 7 9 10 **F**3 5 11 12 13 14 15 17 18 20 22 24 25 26 27 28 30 31 32 33 34 35 37 38 40 41 42 43 44 49 50 52 53 54 55 56 57 59 60 61 64 66 68 70 72 73 74 75 76 77 79 80 81 82 83 84 85 86 87 88 89 90 91 92 93 94 95 96 97 99 100 102 103 104 106 107 116 117 118 119 120 121 123 124 135 136 137 **P**6 8 **S** Iowa Health System
Primary Contact: Theodore E. Townsend, President and Chief Executive Officer
COO: John C. Sheehan, Executive Vice President and Chief Operating Officer
CHR: Sue Slattery, Director Human Resources
Web address: www.crstlukes.org
Control: Other not–for–profit (including NFP Corporation) **Service:** General Medical and Surgical

Staffed Beds: 390 **Admissions:** 17255 **Census:** 245 **Outpatient Visits:** 433765 **Births:** 2663 **Total Expense ($000):** 240382 **Payroll Expense ($000):** 98847 **Personnel:** 2241

CENTERVILLE—Appanoose County

★ **MERCY MEDICAL CENTER–CENTERVILLE (161377)**, 1 St. Joseph's Drive, Zip 52544–8055; tel. 641/437–4111, (Total facility includes 29 beds in nursing home–type unit) **A**9 10 18 **F**3 7 8 11 13 15 24 25 26 27 32 38 42 46 50 51 52 53 55 56 57 59 61 62 65 68 73 74 75 76 77 79 80 81 82 86 87 96 100 102 105 106 107 117 119 121 122 124 **P**6 **S** Catholic Health Initiatives
Primary Contact: Clinton J. Christianson, President and Chief Executive Officer
CFO: Lori Rathbun, Vice President Operations
CIO: Ann Young, Vice President Community and Staff Relations
CHR: Tonya Clawson, Manager Human Resources
Web address: www.mercycenterville.org
Control: Church–operated, Nongovernment, not–for profit **Service:** General Medical and Surgical

Staffed Beds: 54 **Admissions:** 1217 **Census:** 32 **Outpatient Visits:** 73563 **Births:** 141 **Total Expense ($000):** 18423 **Payroll Expense ($000):** 8001 **Personnel:** 181

CHARITON—Lucas County

★ **LUCAS COUNTY HEALTH CENTER (161341)**, 1200 North Seventh Street, Zip 50049–1258; tel. 641/774–3000 **A**9 10 18 **F**2 3 5 7 13 15 24 25 27 30 31 32 36 38 40 41 45 47 49 50 56 57 62 66 68 73 74 79 81 82 84 85 86 96 102 107 117 119 120 121 122 124 132 134 135 137
Primary Contact: Veronica Fuhs, Chief Executive Officer
CFO: Denise Hook, Controller
CMO: Greg McKernan, M.D., Chief Medical Staff
CIO: Richard Eikelboom, Network Manager
CHR: Lana Kuball, Director Administrative Services
Web address: www.lchcia.com
Control: County–Government, nonfederal **Service:** General Medical and Surgical

Staffed Beds: 25 **Admissions:** 535 **Census:** 4 **Outpatient Visits:** 39090 **Births:** 83 **Total Expense ($000):** 12578 **Payroll Expense ($000):** 5335 **Personnel:** 148

Hospital, Medicare Provider Number, Address, Telephone, Approval, Facility, and Physician Codes, Health Care System

★ American Hospital Association (AHA) membership
□ The Joint Commission accreditation
○ American Osteopathic Association (AOA) accreditation
△ Commission on Accreditation of Rehabilitation Facilities (CARF) accreditation

CHARLES CITY—Floyd County

FLOYD COUNTY MEDICAL CENTER (161347), (Formerly Floyd County Memorial Hospital), 800 Eleventh Street, Zip 50616–3499; tel. 641/228–6830 **A**9 10 18 **F**3 11 13 15 24 25 27 30 31 33 38 48 50 55 56 57 62 67 73 74 75 77 79 80 84 86 87 96 103 107 119 121 122 135 137 **S** Mayo Foundation
Primary Contact: Bill D. Faust, Administrator
CFO: Ron James, Chief Financial Officer
CHR: Don Nosbisch, Director Human Resources
Control: County–Government, nonfederal **Service:** General Medical and Surgical

Staffed Beds: 25 **Admissions:** 1074 **Census:** 12 **Outpatient Visits:** 51185 **Births:** 102 **Total Expense ($000):** 17124 **Payroll Expense ($000):** 6777 **Personnel:** 170

CHEROKEE—Cherokee County

★ **CHEROKEE REGIONAL MEDICAL CENTER (161362)**, 300 Sioux Valley Drive, Zip 51012–1205; tel. 712/225–5101 **A**9 10 18 **F**7 11 13 15 17 24 25 30 31 32 33 38 40 42 44 52 54 55 56 57 61 62 63 65 66 67 73 74 75 76 79 81 82 84 86 87 96 105 107 115 117 118 119 120 121 122 124 135 136 137 **P**6
Primary Contact: John M. Comstock, Chief Executive Officer
CFO: Joan Bierman, Vice President Finance
Web address: www.cherokeermc.org
Control: Other not–for–profit (including NFP Corporation) **Service:** General Medical and Surgical

Staffed Beds: 25 **Admissions:** 1198 **Census:** 11 **Outpatient Visits:** 40304 **Births:** 130 **Total Expense ($000):** 14467 **Payroll Expense ($000):** 6414 **Personnel:** 177

□ **MENTAL HEALTH INSTITUTE (164002)**, 1251 West Cedar Loop, Zip 51012–1599; tel. 712/225–2594 **A**1 9 10 **F**3 25 27 30 31 32 62 66 73 81 88 89 90 91 94 95 119 124 132 **P**6
Primary Contact: Daniel Gillette, M.D., CHE, Clinical Director
CFO: Tony Morris, Business Manager
CMO: Daniel Gillette, M.D., CHE, Clinical Director
CHR: Mary Ann Hanson, Dir Personnel
Web address: www.dhs.state.ia.us
Control: State–Government, nonfederal **Service:** Psychiatric

Staffed Beds: 58 **Admissions:** 584 **Census:** 40 **Outpatient Visits:** 92 **Births:** 0 **Total Expense ($000):** 15697 **Payroll Expense ($000):** 9839 **Personnel:** 228

CLARINDA—Page County

★ **CLARINDA REGIONAL HEALTH CENTER (161352)**, 823 South 17th Street, Zip 51632, Mailing Address: P.O. Box 217, Zip 51632–0217; tel. 712/542–2176 **A**9 10 18 **F**3 7 11 15 24 25 27 30 31 34 38 40 50 55 56 57 61 62 63 64 67 72 73 75 76 77 79 80 81 82 86 87 96 100 102 106 107 112 117 118 119 120 121 122 132 135 137 **P**6
Primary Contact: Keith E. Heuser, Chief Executive Officer
COO: Elaine Otte, Chief Operating Officer
CFO: Alan Palo, Chief Financial Officer
CHR: Tammi Driftmier, Director Human Resources
Web address: www.clarindahealth.com
Control: City–Government, nonfederal **Service:** General Medical and Surgical

Staffed Beds: 25 **Admissions:** 734 **Census:** 7 **Outpatient Visits:** 58027 **Births:** 0 **Total Expense ($000):** 16029 **Payroll Expense ($000):** 7488 **Personnel:** 190

MENTAL HEALTH INSTITUTE (164005), Mailing Address: P.O. Box 338, Zip 51632–0338; tel. 712/542–2161, (Total facility includes 35 beds in nursing home–type unit) **A**9 10 **F**1 4 26 30 37 65 88 91 117 119 135 **P**6
Primary Contact: Mark Lund, Superintendent
CFO: Randy Bengard, Business Manager
CMO: Teresa Rosales, M.D., Clinical Director
CIO: Phil Jorgensen, Compliance Officer
Web address: www.dhs.state.ia.us
Control: State–Government, nonfederal **Service:** Psychiatric

Staffed Beds: 55 **Admissions:** 200 **Census:** 46 **Outpatient Visits:** 0 **Births:** 0 **Total Expense ($000):** 8495 **Payroll Expense ($000):** 5207 **Personnel:** 99

CLARION—Wright County

★ **WRIGHT MEDICAL CENTER (161302)**, 1316 South Main Street, Zip 50525–2019; tel. 515/532–2811 **A**9 10 18 **F**11 13 15 24 25 27 30 31 33 38 40 42 43 54 55 56 57 62 63 66 67 73 74 75 77 79 80 82 86 87 96 100 102 105 107 112 115 118 120 121 122 124 135 137 **P**6
Primary Contact: Steven J. Simonin, Chief Executive Officer
COO: Annette Odland, Clinical Services Leader
CFO: Amy McDaniel, Chief Financial Officer
CMO: Charles B. Brindle, M.D., Chief of Staff
CHR: Pat Kirstein, Human Resources Leader
Web address: www.wrightmed.com
Control: City–Government, nonfederal **Service:** General Medical and Surgical

Staffed Beds: 25 **Admissions:** 1317 **Census:** 12 **Outpatient Visits:** 87189 **Births:** 178 **Total Expense ($000):** 31664 **Payroll Expense ($000):** 11638 **Personnel:** 335

CLINTON—Clinton County

⊛ **MERCY MEDICAL CENTER–CLINTON (160080)**, 1410 North Fourth Street, Zip 52732–2940; tel. 563/244–5555, (Includes MERCY SERVICES FOR AGING, 600 14th Avenue North, Zip 52732; tel. 563/244–3888), (Total facility includes 183 beds in nursing home–type unit) **A**1 9 10 19 20 **F**3 11 13 15 17 18 20 24 25 26 27 31 32 33 34 36 38 41 42 43 44 49 50 52 54 55 56 57 59 60 61 62 65 66 68 72 73 74 75 76 77 78 79 80 82 84 85 86 88 89 90 91 92 93 96 97 99 102 106 107 109 111 117 118 119 121 135 **S** Trinity Health
Primary Contact: Donna M. Oliver, President and Chief Executive Officer
CFO: Paul Mangin, Vice President Finance
Web address: www.mercyclinton.com
Control: Church–operated, Nongovernment, not–for profit **Service:** General Medical and Surgical

Staffed Beds: 341 **Admissions:** 6877 **Census:** 219 **Outpatient Visits:** 58952 **Births:** 569 **Total Expense ($000):** 76263 **Payroll Expense ($000):** 33802 **Personnel:** 799

CORNING—Adams County

★ **ALEGENT HEALTH MERCY HOSPITAL (161304)**, 603 Rosary Drive, Zip 50841–1685, Mailing Address: P.O. Box 368, Zip 50841–0368; tel. 641/322–3121 **A**9 10 18 **F**3 11 15 24 27 30 31 32 38 40 50 52 54 55 56 57 61 62 65 67 73 79 96 107 117 118 122 135 137 **S** Alegent Health
Primary Contact: James C. Ruppert, Regional Administrator
CMO: Maeo Haddadin, M.D., President Medical Staff
CHR: Sandra Lammers, Coordinator Human Resources and Finance
Web address: www.alegent.com
Control: Church–operated, Nongovernment, not–for profit **Service:** General Medical and Surgical

Staffed Beds: 22 **Admissions:** 394 **Census:** 6 **Outpatient Visits:** 29385 **Births:** 19 **Total Expense ($000):** 11125 **Payroll Expense ($000):** 3943 **Personnel:** 132

CORYDON—Wayne County

★ **WAYNE COUNTY HOSPITAL (161358)**, 417 South East Street, Zip 50060–1860, Mailing Address: P.O. Box 305, Zip 50060–0305; tel. 641/872–2260 **A**9 10 18 **F**7 10 11 13 15 26 30 31 33 34 37 38 40 54 55 56 57 59 62 67 68 73 74 75 79 82 84 86 87 96 102 107 115 117 119 120 121 122 132 135 **P**6
Primary Contact: Brian D. Burnside, Chief Executive Officer
CFO: Mark Raven, Chief Financial Officer
CHR: Dave Carlyle, Director Human Resources
Web address: www.waynecountyhospital.org
Control: County–Government, nonfederal **Service:** General Medical and Surgical

Staffed Beds: 25 **Admissions:** 600 **Census:** 6 **Outpatient Visits:** 25775 **Births:** 92 **Total Expense ($000):** 10816 **Payroll Expense ($000):** 4802 **Personnel:** 148

COUNCIL BLUFFS—Pottawattamie County

⊛ **ALEGENT HEALTH MERCY HOSPITAL (160028)**, 800 Mercy Drive, Zip 51503–3128, Mailing Address: P.O. Box 1C, Zip 51502–3001; tel. 712/328–5000 **A**1 9 10 **F**3 5 11 12 13 15 20 24 25 26 27 28 30 31 32 33 36 37 38 40 41 43 44 50 53 54 55 56 57 59 60 61 62 63 66 68 73 74 75 76 77 79 80 81 82 84 86 87 88 89 90 91 92 93 94 95 96 97 100 102 103 106 107 118 119 121 123 124 132 133 135 136 **P**6 8 **S** Alegent Health
Primary Contact: Marie E. Knedler, RN, Vice President and Chief Operating Officer
COO: Marie E. Knedler, R.N., Vice President and Chief Operating Officer
CFO: Amy Knott, Chief Financial Officer
CMO: Fred Hosler, M.D., Senior Vice President and Chief Medical Officer
CIO: Kenneth Lawonn, Senior Vice President and Chief Information Officer
CHR: Margaret Breen, Senior Vice President Human Resources
Web address: www.alegent.com/mercy
Control: Church–operated, Nongovernment, not–for profit **Service:** General Medical and Surgical

Staffed Beds: 147 **Admissions:** 7932 **Census:** 83 **Outpatient Visits:** 55751 **Births:** 602 **Total Expense ($000):** 87060 **Payroll Expense ($000):** 32555 **Personnel:** 681

⊛ **JENNIE EDMUNDSON HOSPITAL (160047)**, 933 East Pierce Street, Zip 51503–4652, Mailing Address: P.O. Box 2C, Zip 51502–3002; tel. 712/396–6000 **A**1 2 5 9 10 **F**3 5 11 13 15 18 20 24 25 26 27 31 32 33 37 38 40 43 49 55 56 57 58 60 66 68 72 73 74 76 77 79 80 81 82 84 86 88 89 90 91 92 93 94 95 96 97 99 100 102 106 107 111 118 119 120 121 124 132 133 134 135 136 137 **P**8 **S** Nebraska Methodist Health System, Inc.
Primary Contact: Steven P. Baumert, President and Chief Executive Officer
COO: Evan Ray, Vice President
CFO: Linda K. Burt, Corporate Vice President Finance
CMO: Michael A. Romano, M.D., Vice President Medical Affairs
CIO: Dennis Weeks, Director Information Services
CHR: Carmen Lester, Vice President Human Resources
Web address: www.bestcare.org
Control: Other not–for–profit (including NFP Corporation) **Service:** General Medical and Surgical

Staffed Beds: 118 **Admissions:** 6168 **Census:** 73 **Outpatient Visits:** 124030 **Births:** 506 **Total Expense ($000):** 80041 **Payroll Expense ($000):** 33205 **Personnel:** 613

Many Facility Codes have changed. Please refer to the AHA Guide Code Chart.

CRESCO—Howard County

★ **REGIONAL HEALTH SERVICES OF HOWARD COUNTY (161328)**, 235 Eighth Avenue West, Zip 52136–1098; tel. 563/547–2101 **A**9 10 18 **F**7 11 13 15 24 25 27 31 38 40 41 42 55 56 57 58 61 62 63 66 73 74 75 77 78 79 80 81 82 86 96 102 117 119 121 122 135 137 **P**8 **S** Trinity Health
Primary Contact: David Hartberg, Chief Executive Officer
CFO: Brenda Moser, Chief Financial Officer
CMO: Tanya Vreeke, D.O., Chief of Staff
CHR: Connie Kuennen, Director Human Resources and Community Relations
Web address: www.rhshc.com
Control: County–Government, nonfederal **Service:** General Medical and Surgical

Staffed Beds: 25 **Admissions:** 350 **Census:** 5 **Outpatient Visits:** 20940 **Births:** 93 **Total Expense ($000):** 11836 **Payroll Expense ($000):** 5100 **Personnel:** 90

CRESTON—Union County

★ **GREATER REGIONAL MEDICAL CENTER (161365)**, 1700 West Townline, Zip 50801–1099; tel. 641/782–7091 **A**9 10 18 **F**7 11 13 15 24 25 26 27 30 31 32 33 36 38 42 43 44 52 54 55 56 57 59 61 62 63 66 67 68 73 74 75 76 77 79 81 86 88 96 97 102 103 107 108 109 112 115 118 119 121 122 124 135 137 **P**6 **S** Iowa Health System
Primary Contact: Monte Neitzel, Administrator and Chief Executive Officer
CFO: Dave Brokaw, Chief Financial Officer
CMO: Louise Connery, M.D., Chief Medical Officer
CIO: Karla Winn, Chief Information Officer
CHR: Lisa Morgan, Human Resources Officer
Web address: www.greaterregional.org
Control: County–Government, nonfederal **Service:** General Medical and Surgical

Staffed Beds: 34 **Admissions:** 1532 **Census:** 16 **Outpatient Visits:** 29320 **Births:** 248 **Total Expense ($000):** 24292 **Payroll Expense ($000):** 9882 **Personnel:** 234

DAVENPORT—Scott County

☒ △ **GENESIS MEDICAL CENTER–DAVENPORT (160033)**, 1227 East Rusholme Street, Zip 52803–2498; tel. 563/421–1000, (Includes GENESIS MEDICAL CENTER–EAST CAMPUS; GENESIS MEDICAL CENTER–WEST CAMPUS, 1401 West Central Park, Zip 52804–1769; tel. 563/421–1000) **A**1 2 3 5 7 9 10 **F**3 4 5 11 12 13 15 18 20 22 24 25 26 27 30 31 32 33 35 36 38 40 41 42 43 46 47 48 49 50 52 55 56 57 58 59 62 68 70 72 73 74 75 76 77 79 80 81 82 84 85 86 87 88 89 90 91 92 93 94 95 96 99 100 102 104 106 107 109 111 112 118 119 120 121 124 133 135 136 137 **P**6 **S** Genesis Health System
Primary Contact: Douglas P. Cropper, Chief Executive Officer
CFO: Mark G. Rogers, Interim Vice President Finance and Chief Financial Officer
CMO: Frank Claudy, M.D., Vice President Medical Staff Affairs
CIO: Robert Frieden, Vice President Information Systems
CHR: Jerry McCormick, Vice President Human Resources
Web address: www.genesishealth.com
Control: Other not–for–profit (including NFP Corporation) **Service:** General Medical and Surgical

Staffed Beds: 414 **Admissions:** 22787 **Census:** 283 **Outpatient Visits:** 188617 **Births:** 2395 **Total Expense ($000):** 280344 **Payroll Expense ($000):** 89078 **Personnel:** 1879

☐ **SELECT SPECIALTY HOSPITAL–QUAD CITIES (160155)**, 1111 West Kimberly Road, Zip 52806–5711; tel. 563/468–2000 **A**1 10 **F**1 3 25 30 41 72 73 75 77 78 80 82 90 107 119 137 **S** Select Medical Corporation
Primary Contact: Kerry McLane, Interim Chief Executive Officer
Web address: www.selectmedicalcorp.com
Control: Corporation, Investor–owned, for–profit **Service:** Long–Term Acute Care hospital

Staffed Beds: 50 **Admissions:** 211 **Census:** 18 **Outpatient Visits:** 0 **Births:** 0 **Total Expense ($000):** 11909 **Payroll Expense ($000):** 4251 **Personnel:** 87

DE WITT—Clinton County

☒ **GENESIS MEDICAL CENTER, DEWITT (161313)**, 1118 11th Street, Zip 52742–1296; tel. 563/659–4200, (Total facility includes 75 beds in nursing home–type unit) **A**1 9 10 18 **F**7 11 15 25 26 27 30 31 32 33 36 38 40 41 50 52 55 56 57 62 72 73 75 76 77 79 80 82 86 87 96 99 100 107 117 118 119 120 121 122 124 133 **S** Genesis Health System
Primary Contact: Jeffrey M. Cooper, Vice President, DeWitt Operations
CMO: Tom Snyder, M.D., President Medical Staff
CHR: Brandi Tiesman, Coordinator Human Resources
Web address: www.genesishealth.com
Control: Other not–for–profit (including NFP Corporation) **Service:** General Medical and Surgical

Staffed Beds: 86 **Admissions:** 333 **Census:** 71 **Outpatient Visits:** 33862 **Births:** 0 **Total Expense ($000):** 12519 **Payroll Expense ($000):** 4623 **Personnel:** 169

DECORAH—Winneshiek County

★ **WINNESHIEK MEDICAL CENTER (161371)**, 901 Montgomery Street, Zip 52101–2325; tel. 563/382–2911 **A**9 10 18 **F**7 11 13 15 17 24 25 27 30 31 32 33 38 42 43 55 57 60 61 62 67 73 74 75 77 79 86 96 102 107 119 120 122 135
Primary Contact: Daniel J. Werner, Chief Administrative Officer
CFO: Lynn Luloff, Chief Financial Officer
CMO: Kurt Carlson, M.D., Chief Medical Officer
CHR: Laurie Bulman, Director Human Resources
Web address: www.winmedical.org
Control: County–Government, nonfederal **Service:** General Medical and Surgical

Staffed Beds: 25 **Admissions:** 1167 **Census:** 12 **Outpatient Visits:** 55716 **Births:** 302 **Total Expense ($000):** 34179 **Payroll Expense ($000):** 13314 **Personnel:** 330

DENISON—Crawford County

★ **CRAWFORD COUNTY MEMORIAL HOSPITAL (161369)**, 2020 First Avenue South, Zip 51442–2299; tel. 712/263–5021 **A**9 10 18 **F**7 8 11 13 15 17 24 30 32 33 38 54 55 57 62 65 68 73 74 79 84 86 87 96 107 117 122 132 **P**6
Primary Contact: Mark Rinehardt, Administrator
CFO: Larry Brown, Chief Financial Officer
CHR: Tara Jepsen, Director Human Resources and Community Relations
Web address: www.ccmhia.com
Control: County–Government, nonfederal **Service:** General Medical and Surgical

Staffed Beds: 25 **Admissions:** 919 **Census:** 8 **Outpatient Visits:** 34232 **Births:** 126 **Total Expense ($000):** 15613 **Payroll Expense ($000):** 7514 **Personnel:** 146

DES MOINES—Polk County

☒ **BROADLAWNS MEDICAL CENTER (160101)**, 1801 Hickman Road, Zip 50314–1597; tel. 515/282–2200 **A**1 3 5 9 10 **F**2 3 5 8 11 13 15 25 26 27 28 30 31 32 33 36 37 38 40 41 43 50 51 52 54 55 56 57 58 59 62 63 64 66 68 72 73 74 75 77 79 80 82 86 87 88 89 90 91 92 93 94 95 96 97 103 107 119 120 121 124 132 133 135 136 137 **P**6
Primary Contact: Jody Jenner, President and Chief Executive Officer
CFO: Al White, Senior Vice President Business Services
CMO: Vincent Mandracchia, DPM, Chief Medical Officer
Web address: www.broadlawns.org
Control: County–Government, nonfederal **Service:** General Medical and Surgical

Staffed Beds: 89 **Admissions:** 4436 **Census:** 47 **Outpatient Visits:** 163718 **Births:** 469 **Total Expense ($000):** 68225 **Payroll Expense ($000):** 42081 **Personnel:** 774

DES MOINES DIVISION See Veterans Affairs Central Iowa Health Care System

☒ **IOWA LUTHERAN HOSPITAL (160024)**, 700 East University Avenue, Zip 50316–2392; tel. 515/263–5612, (Total facility includes 16 beds in nursing home–type unit) **A**1 3 5 9 10 **F**3 4 5 11 12 13 15 18 20 22 24 25 26 27 30 31 32 33 36 37 38 40 41 43 44 49 50 52 54 55 56 57 58 59 60 62 63 64 66 68 69 71 72 73 74 76 77 79 80 81 82 86 87 88 89 90 91 92 93 94 95 96 97 99 100 102 106 107 117 118 119 121 123 124 130 135 136 137 **P**6 **S** Iowa Health System
Primary Contact: Eric T. Crowell, President and Chief Executive Officer
COO: David A. Stark, Chief Operating Officer
CFO: Joe Corfits, Chief Financial Officer
CMO: Mark Purtle, M.D., Vice President Medical Affairs
CHR: Sue Allyn, Vice President Human Resources
Web address: www.iowahealth.org
Control: Other not–for–profit (including NFP Corporation) **Service:** General Medical and Surgical

Staffed Beds: 219 **Admissions:** 10149 **Census:** 140 **Outpatient Visits:** 58931 **Births:** 955 **Total Expense ($000):** 110950 **Payroll Expense ($000):** 50904 **Personnel:** 964

Hospital, Medicare Provider Number, Address, Telephone, Approval, Facility, and Physician Codes, Health Care System

★ American Hospital Association (AHA) membership
☐ The Joint Commission accreditation
○ American Osteopathic Association (AOA) accreditation
△ Commission on Accreditation of Rehabilitation Facilities (CARF) accreditation

☒ △ **IOWA METHODIST MEDICAL CENTER (160082)**, 1200 Pleasant Street, Zip 50309–9976; tel. 515/241–6212, (Includes POWELL CONVALESCENT CENTER; RAYMOND BLANK MEMORIAL HOSPITAL FOR CHILDREN; YOUNKER MEMORIAL REHABILITATION CENTER) **A**1 2 7 8 9 10 **F**3 7 8 11 12 13 17 18 20 22 25 26 27 28 30 31 32 33 37 38 40 41 43 44 49 50 52 53 54 55 56 57 58 59 60 62 63 66 68 70 72 73 74 75 76 77 79 80 81 82 83 84 85 86 87 90 96 97 100 102 103 104 105 106 107 109 111 112 116 118 119 121 123 124 127 130 131 135 136 137 **P**6 **S** Iowa Health System
Primary Contact: Eric T. Crowell, President and Chief Executive Officer
COO: David A. Stark, Executive Vice President and Chief Operating Officer
CFO: Joseph Corfits, Senior Vice President Finance
CMO: Mark Purtle, M.D., Vice President Medical Affairs
CHR: Sue Allyn, Vice President Human Resources
Web address: www.iowahealth.org
Control: Other not–for–profit (including NFP Corporation) **Service:** General Medical and Surgical

Staffed Beds: 444 **Admissions:** 23060 **Census:** 331 **Outpatient Visits:** 206672 **Births:** 3543 **Total Expense ($000):** 378795 **Payroll Expense ($000):** 158913 **Personnel:** 3160

☐ **MERCY CAPITOL**, 603 East 12th Street, Zip 50309–5515; tel. 515/643–1000 **A**1 **F**3 7 11 12 13 15 18 20 25 26 30 31 32 38 40 41 50 52 54 60 61 62 63 66 68 73 74 75 77 79 80 81 82 85 86 96 97 102 106 107 119 121 124 132 135 **S** Catholic Health Initiatives
Primary Contact: David H. Vellinga, FACHE, President and Chief Executive Officer
COO: Jackie Frost–Kunnen, Senior Vice President Operations
CFO: Steven F. Kukla, Senior Vice President and Chief Financial Officer
CIO: Cristina Thomas, Vice President and Chief Information Officer
CHR: Robyn Wilkinson, Vice President Human Resources
Control: Church–operated, Nongovernment, not–for profit **Service:** General Medical and Surgical

Staffed Beds: 62 **Admissions:** 1495 **Census:** 27 **Outpatient Visits:** 61981 **Births:** 2 **Total Expense ($000):** 15354 **Payroll Expense ($000):** 8185 **Personnel:** 279

☒ △ **MERCY MEDICAL CENTER–DES MOINES (160083)**, 1111 6th Avenue, Zip 50314–2611; tel. 515/247–3121, (Includes MERCY FRANKLIN CENTER, 1818 48th Street, Zip 50310; tel. 515/271–6000), (Total facility includes 35 beds in nursing home–type unit) **A**1 2 3 5 7 9 10 12 13 **F**2 3 4 5 6 7 8 9 10 11 13 15 16 17 18 19 20 21 22 23 24 25 26 27 28 30 31 32 33 34 36 37 38 40 41 42 43 44 46 48 49 50 52 53 54 55 56 57 58 59 60 61 62 63 64 66 68 70 71 72 73 74 75 76 77 79 80 81 82 83 84 85 86 87 88 89 90 91 92 93 94 95 96 97 98 100 102 103 104 105 106 107 108 109 111 112 115 116 117 118 119 120 121 123 124 127 130 131 132 133 134 135 136 137 **P**6 **S** Catholic Health Initiatives
Primary Contact: David H. Vellinga, FACHE, President and Chief Executive Officer
COO: Jackie Frost–Kunnen, Senior Vice President Operations
CFO: Steven F. Kukla, Senior Vice President and Chief Financial Officer
CMO: Dale Andres, D.O., Interim Vice President Medical Affairs
CIO: Cristina Thomas, Vice President and Chief Information Officer
CHR: Robyn Wilkinson, Senior Vice President Human Resources
Web address: www.mercydesmoines.org
Control: Church–operated, Nongovernment, not–for profit **Service:** General Medical and Surgical

Staffed Beds: 584 **Admissions:** 30454 **Census:** 405 **Outpatient Visits:** 954157 **Births:** 4448 **Total Expense ($000):** 443174 **Payroll Expense ($000):** 178606 **Personnel:** 5311

☒ **VETERANS AFFAIRS CENTRAL IOWA HEALTH CARE SYSTEM**, 3600 30th Street, Zip 50310–5774; tel. 515/699–5999, (Includes DES MOINES DIVISION, 3600 30th Street; KNOXVILLE DIVISION, 1515 West Pleasant, Knoxville, Zip 50138–3399; tel. 515/842–3101), (Total facility includes 156 beds in nursing home–type unit) **A**1 2 3 5 9 **F**2 3 4 5 11 15 18 20 24 25 26 27 29 31 32 33 34 36 37 38 41 42 43 44 45 46 50 54 55 56 57 60 61 62 63 64 65 68 72 73 75 76 77 79 80 81 82 85 86 87 88 90 91 92 93 94 95 96 97 106 107 117 118 119 121 124 133 135 136 137 **S** Department of Veterans Affairs
Primary Contact: Donald C. Cooper, Director
COO: Marjorie Hedstrom, Associate Director Operations
CFO: Ronald Larson, Chief Fiscal Services
CMO: Fredrick Bahls, M.D., Chief of Staff
CIO: James Danuser, Chief Information Officer
CHR: Sabrina Owen, Human Resources Officer
Web address: www.va.centra/iowa.va.gov
Control: Veterans Affairs, Government, federal **Service:** General Medical and Surgical

Staffed Beds: 227 **Admissions:** 3044 **Census:** 172 **Outpatient Visits:** 296741 **Births:** 0 **Total Expense ($000):** 169649 **Payroll Expense ($000):** 73397 **Personnel:** 1160

DUBUQUE—Dubuque County

☒ △ **FINLEY HOSPITAL (160117)**, 350 North Grandview Avenue, Zip 52001–6392; tel. 563/582–1881, (Total facility includes 16 beds in nursing home–type unit) **A**1 2 7 9 10 **F**11 12 13 15 24 25 26 27 28 30 31 32 33 37 38 40 41 43 48 49 50 52 54 55 56 57 59 60 61 62 67 68 70 72 73 74 75 76 77 79 80 81 82 85 86 87 88 93 96 97 100 102 104 105 106 107 108 109 111 113 117 118 119 120 121 124 132 133 135 136 137 **P**1 5 **S** Iowa Health System
Primary Contact: John E. Knox, FACHE, President and Chief Executive Officer
Web address: www.finleyhospital.org
Control: Other not–for–profit (including NFP Corporation) **Service:** General Medical and Surgical

Staffed Beds: 137 **Admissions:** 5036 **Census:** 65 **Outpatient Visits:** 97795 **Births:** 709 **Total Expense ($000):** 75070 **Payroll Expense ($000):** 29625 **Personnel:** 674

☒ △ **MERCY MEDICAL CENTER–DUBUQUE (160069)**, 250 Mercy Drive, Zip 52001–7360; tel. 563/589–8000, (Total facility includes 40 beds in nursing home–type unit) **A**1 7 9 10 **F**3 4 5 8 11 13 15 18 20 22 24 25 26 27 28 31 32 33 34 36 37 38 40 41 49 50 51 52 54 55 56 57 58 60 61 62 63 65 66 68 70 72 73 74 75 76 77 78 79 80 81 82 84 85 86 87 88 89 90 91 92 93 94 96 97 100 102 104 107 117 118 119 120 121 123 124 132 133 135 136 137 **P**8 **S** Trinity Health
Primary Contact: Russell M. Knight, President and Chief Executive Officer
CFO: Gary Guetzko, Vice President Finance
CIO: Matt Trimmer, Director Information Services
Web address: www.mercydubuque.com
Control: Church–operated, Nongovernment, not–for profit **Service:** General Medical and Surgical

Staffed Beds: 303 **Admissions:** 9204 **Census:** 142 **Outpatient Visits:** 37141 **Births:** 963 **Total Expense ($000):** 119054 **Payroll Expense ($000):** 40042 **Personnel:** 962

DYERSVILLE—Dubuque County

★ **MERCY MEDICAL CENTER–DYERSVILLE (161378)**, 1111 Third Street S.W., Zip 52040; tel. 319/875–7101 **A**9 10 18 **F**11 15 31 32 33 34 37 38 41 50 54 55 56 57 62 63 66 73 77 79 80 81 86 107 119 120 121 122 123 124 135 136 **P**8 **S** Trinity Health
Primary Contact: Russell M. Knight, President and Chief Executive Officer
CFO: Gary Guetzko, Vice President Finance
Web address: www.mercydubuque.com/dyersville
Control: Church–operated, Nongovernment, not–for profit **Service:** General Medical and Surgical

Staffed Beds: 25 **Admissions:** 119 **Census:** 4 **Outpatient Visits:** 4526 **Births:** 0 **Total Expense ($000):** 4228 **Payroll Expense ($000):** 2179 **Personnel:** 58

ELKADER—Clayton County

★ **CENTRAL COMMUNITY HOSPITAL (161319)**, 901 Davidson Street N.W., Zip 52043–9015; tel. 563/245–7000 **A**9 10 18 **F**7 11 15 17 24 30 31 32 33 38 40 54 55 56 57 62 63 65 66 68 73 79 80 81 82 84 92 96 102 117 119 121 122 123 132 **S** Trinity Health
Primary Contact: Frances J. Zichal, Chief Executive Officer
CFO: Lisa Manson, Chief Financial Officer
Web address: www.centralcommunityhospital.com
Control: Other not–for–profit (including NFP Corporation) **Service:** General Medical and Surgical

Staffed Beds: 16 **Admissions:** 237 **Census:** 3 **Outpatient Visits:** 9288 **Births:** 0 **Total Expense ($000):** 4846 **Payroll Expense ($000):** 1572 **Personnel:** 57

EMMETSBURG—Palo Alto County

★ **PALO ALTO COUNTY HEALTH SYSTEM (161357)**, 3201 First Street, Zip 50536; tel. 712/852–5500, (Total facility includes 22 beds in nursing home–type unit) **A**9 10 18 **F**3 7 11 14 15 24 25 27 30 31 32 33 38 42 43 44 50 55 56 57 61 62 63 65 66 67 68 73 74 75 77 79 80 81 82 86 96 97 107 115 119 121 122 124 132 135 **P**6 **S** Trinity Health
Primary Contact: Thomas J. Lee, Chief Executive Officer
CFO: Renay Hauswirth, Chief Financial Officer
CMO: Daunyale Sporaa, D.O., President Medical Staff
CIO: Randy Beaver, Chief Information Officer
CHR: Lisa Mart, Director Human Resources
Web address: www.pachs.com
Control: County–Government, nonfederal **Service:** General Medical and Surgical

Staffed Beds: 47 **Admissions:** 651 **Census:** 25 **Outpatient Visits:** 22069 **Births:** 109 **Total Expense ($000):** 16618 **Payroll Expense ($000):** 6357 **Personnel:** 156

IA

ESTHERVILLE—Emmet County

★ **AVERA HOLY FAMILY HEALTH (161351)**, 826 North Eighth Street, Zip 51334–1598; tel. 712/362–2631 **A**9 10 18 **F**3 11 13 15 24 25 26 27 31 33 38 42 57 61 62 66 67 68 73 74 75 76 77 79 80 81 82 86 87 96 102 107 115 119 121 122 135 **P**4 **S** Avera Health
Primary Contact: William Bumgarner, Chief Executive Officer
CFO: Deb Rosburg, Finance Manager
CMO: Randy Asman, M.D., Chief of Staff
CHR: Janette Jensen, Manager Human Resources
Web address: www.avera–holyfamily.org
Control: Church–operated, Nongovernment, not–for profit **Service:** General Medical and Surgical

Staffed Beds: 25 **Admissions:** 984 **Census:** 9 **Outpatient Visits:** 37634
Births: 75 **Total Expense ($000):** 13531 **Payroll Expense ($000):** 5293
Personnel: 171

FAIRFIELD—Jefferson County

★ **JEFFERSON COUNTY HOSPITAL (161364)**, 400 Highland Avenue, Zip 52556–3713, Mailing Address: P.O. Box 588, Zip 52556–0588; tel. 641/472–4111, (Total facility includes 36 beds in nursing home–type unit) **A**9 10 18 **F**11 15 24 26 27 30 31 32 33 34 38 40 55 57 66 68 73 75 76 77 79 80 84 86 92 96 107 118 121 122 124 132
Primary Contact: Ralph Paulding, Chief Executive Officer
CFO: Gene Irwin, Chief Financial Officer
CHR: Nanette Conger, Manager Human Resources and Administrative Assistant
Web address: www.jchospital.org
Control: County–Government, nonfederal **Service:** General Medical and Surgical

Staffed Beds: 61 **Admissions:** 916 **Census:** 48 **Outpatient Visits:** 25551
Births: 0 **Total Expense ($000):** 17399 **Payroll Expense ($000):** 7220
Personnel: 195

FORT DODGE—Webster County

☒ **TRINITY REGIONAL MEDICAL CENTER (160016)**, 802 Kenyon Road, Zip 50501–5795; tel. 515/573–3101 **A**1 2 9 10 19 20 **F**3 5 7 8 11 12 13 15 18 20 22 24 25 26 27 28 30 31 32 33 34 38 40 42 43 50 51 55 56 57 59 61 62 66 68 71 73 74 75 76 77 79 81 82 84 86 94 95 96 97 100 102 105 106 107 118 119 120 121 124 135 137 **S** Iowa Health System
Primary Contact: Tom Tibbitts, President
CFO: Brian Wegener, Chief Financial Officer
Web address: www.trmc.org
Control: Other not–for–profit (including NFP Corporation) **Service:** General Medical and Surgical

Staffed Beds: 133 **Admissions:** 6358 **Census:** 67 **Outpatient Visits:** 134329
Births: 631 **Total Expense ($000):** 96162 **Payroll Expense ($000):** 39649
Personnel: 818

FORT MADISON—Lee County

☒ **FORT MADISON COMMUNITY HOSPITAL (160122)**, 5445 Avenue O, Zip 52627–0174, Mailing Address: P.O. Box 174, Zip 52627–0174; tel. 319/372–6530 **A**1 9 10 **F**3 11 13 15 24 25 27 30 31 32 38 40 50 51 52 55 56 57 61 62 65 66 68 72 73 74 75 76 77 79 80 81 82 85 86 87 89 90 91 92 93 94 96 97 99 100 102 104 105 106 107 113 114 117 118 119 120 121 122 132 133 134 135 136 137 **P**6 **S** QHR
Primary Contact: C. James Platt, Chief Executive Officer
CFO: Bradley J. Kokjohn, Chief Financial Officer
CMO: David Wenger–Keller, M.D., Chief of Staff
CIO: Shane Tapper, Director Management Information Systems
CHR: Vicki Kokjohn, Director Employee Relations
Web address: www.fmchosp.com
Control: Other not–for–profit (including NFP Corporation) **Service:** General Medical and Surgical

Staffed Beds: 50 **Admissions:** 2323 **Census:** 23 **Outpatient Visits:** 59963
Births: 294 **Total Expense ($000):** 39880 **Payroll Expense ($000):** 17466
Personnel: 380

GREENFIELD—Adair County

ADAIR COUNTY MEMORIAL HOSPITAL (161310), 609 S.E. Kent Street, Zip 50849–9454; tel. 641/743–2123 **A**9 10 18 **F**7 11 15 25 27 30 31 32 33 34 38 40 48 55 56 57 61 62 63 67 68 73 75 77 79 84 86 87 96 97 100 102 107 117 118 119 122 135 137 **P**6
Primary Contact: Myrna Erb–Gundel, Administrator
CFO: Lisa Blazek, Chief Financial Officer
CMO: Melissa Thompson, M.D., Chief Medical Officer
CIO: Andy Christie, Chief Information Technology
CHR: Angie Lilly, Director Human Resources
Web address: www.adaircountyhealthsystem.org
Control: County–Government, nonfederal **Service:** General Medical and Surgical

Staffed Beds: 22 **Admissions:** 365 **Census:** 4 **Outpatient Visits:** 10282
Births: 0 **Total Expense ($000):** 7466 **Payroll Expense ($000):** 3051
Personnel: 92

GRINNELL—Poweshiek County

★ **GRINNELL REGIONAL MEDICAL CENTER (160147)**, 210 Fourth Avenue, Zip 50112–1833; tel. 641/236–7511 **A**9 10 **F**3 11 12 13 15 24 25 26 27 28 30 31 32 33 34 35 36 37 38 40 41 42 43 44 50 52 53 54 55 56 57 60 61 62 63 64 68 72 73 74 75 76 77 79 80 81 82 84 86 87 96 97 100 102 106 107 118 119 120 121 122 123 124 132 135 136 137 **P**7
Primary Contact: Todd C. Linden, President and Chief Executive Officer
COO: Suzanne Cooner, Vice President Operations
CFO: Todd Nelson, Vice President Finance
CMO: David C. Cranston, M.D., Vice President Medical Staff Affairs
Web address: www.grmc.us
Control: Other not–for–profit (including NFP Corporation) **Service:** General Medical and Surgical

Staffed Beds: 49 **Admissions:** 2455 **Census:** 22 **Outpatient Visits:** 53176
Births: 195 **Total Expense ($000):** 46049 **Payroll Expense ($000):** 21831
Personnel: 448

GRUNDY CENTER—Grundy County

★ **GRUNDY COUNTY MEMORIAL HOSPITAL (161303)**, 201 East J Avenue, Zip 50638–2096; tel. 319/824–5421, (Total facility includes 55 beds in nursing home–type unit) **A**9 10 18 **F**15 24 25 30 31 32 33 38 40 42 55 56 57 65 73 76 77 79 81 82 86 96 100 102 107 117 118 119 120 121 122 124 135 137 **S** Iowa Health System
Primary Contact: Pamela K. Delagardelle, Chief Executive Officer
COO: Ryan Bingman, Director Operations
CFO: Lisa Zinkula, Chief Financial Officer
CMO: William Durbin, M.D., Chief Medical Officer
CIO: Ryan Bingman, Director Operations
CHR: Nathan Stucky, Manager Human Resources
Web address: www.grundyhospital.com
Control: County–Government, nonfederal **Service:** General Medical and Surgical

Staffed Beds: 80 **Admissions:** 383 **Census:** 56 **Outpatient Visits:** 21960
Births: 0 **Total Expense ($000):** 8439 **Payroll Expense ($000):** 3659
Personnel: 116

GUTHRIE CENTER—Guthrie County

★ **GUTHRIE COUNTY HOSPITAL (161314)**, 710 North 12th Street, Zip 50115–1544; tel. 641/332–2201 **A**9 10 18 **F**11 15 24 25 27 31 33 34 38 40 52 54 55 57 62 67 72 73 75 76 77 79 80 86 96 99 107 117 119 122 132 **P**5 **S** Iowa Health System
Primary Contact: Gerald D. Neal, Chief Executive Officer and Administrator
COO: Danielle Navarro, R.N., Chief Nursing Officer
CFO: Melinda Alt, Chief Financial Officer
CIO: Jeff Cobb, Information Technologist
CHR: Mark Cautin, Director Human Resources
Web address: www.gcho.org
Control: County–Government, nonfederal **Service:** General Medical and Surgical

Staffed Beds: 25 **Admissions:** 443 **Census:** 5 **Outpatient Visits:** 26402
Births: 0 **Total Expense ($000):** 8231 **Payroll Expense ($000):** 4410
Personnel: 95

IA

Hospital, Medicare Provider Number, Address, Telephone, Approval, Facility, and Physician Codes, Health Care System
★ American Hospital Association (AHA) membership
☐ The Joint Commission accreditation
○ American Osteopathic Association (AOA) accreditation
△ Commission on Accreditation of Rehabilitation Facilities (CARF) accreditation

GUTTENBERG—Clayton County

★ **GUTTENBERG MUNICIPAL HOSPITAL (161312)**, 200 Main Street, Zip 52052–0550, Mailing Address: P.O. Box 550, Zip 52052–0550; tel. 563/252–1121 **A**9 10 18 **F**7 8 11 13 15 24 30 31 32 33 38 40 50 52 57 62 66 68 74 79 80 84 86 92 96 107 117 119 121 122 137 **P**5 6 **S** Iowa Health System
Primary Contact: Kimberley A. Gau, Chief Executive Officer
CMO: Andrew Smith, M.D., Chief Medical Staff
CHR: Leigh Ann Judge, Manager Human Resources
Web address: www.guttenberghospital.org
Control: City–Government, nonfederal **Service:** General Medical and Surgical

Staffed Beds: 23 **Admissions:** 608 **Census:** 6 **Outpatient Visits:** 18780 **Births:** 30 **Total Expense ($000):** 6709 **Payroll Expense ($000):** 2510 **Personnel:** 81

HAMBURG—Fremont County

GRAPE COMMUNITY HOSPITAL (161324), 2959 U.S. Highway 275, Zip 51640–5067; tel. 712/382–1515, (Total facility includes 5 beds in nursing home–type unit) **A**9 10 18 **F**11 15 24 27 31 38 40 43 52 56 57 61 62 63 73 75 76 77 79 86 96 103 107 117 119 122 135 **P**8
Primary Contact: James L. Clough, Administrator
COO: Randy Upton, Assistant Administrator
CFO: Dan Schonlan, CPA, Chief Financial Officer
CMO: Kelli Woltemath, D.O., Chief Medical Staff
CIO: Nancy Tiemeyer, Director Health Information Management
CHR: Jackie Wertz, Director Human Resources
Web address: www.grapehospital.com
Control: Other not–for–profit (including NFP Corporation) **Service:** General Medical and Surgical

Staffed Beds: 25 **Admissions:** 407 **Census:** 11 **Outpatient Visits:** 35792 **Births:** 0 **Total Expense ($000):** 10477 **Payroll Expense ($000):** 4712 **Personnel:** 153

HAMPTON—Franklin County

★ **FRANKLIN GENERAL HOSPITAL (161308)**, 1720 Central Avenue East, Zip 50441–1859; tel. 641/456–5000, (Total facility includes 52 beds in nursing home–type unit) **A**9 10 18 **F**7 11 15 24 26 27 28 30 31 32 37 38 42 43 55 56 57 62 63 65 66 73 75 79 80 81 84 85 86 87 96 97 100 102 107 117 118 119 121 122 124 135 137 **P**8 **S** Trinity Health
Primary Contact: Mark Klosterman, Chief Executive Officer
CFO: Michelle Craighton, Manager Finance
CHR: Victoria Kruse, Manager Human Resources
Web address: www.franklingeneral.com
Control: County–Government, nonfederal **Service:** General Medical and Surgical

Staffed Beds: 77 **Admissions:** 394 **Census:** 54 **Outpatient Visits:** 16073 **Births:** 0 **Total Expense ($000):** 11446 **Payroll Expense ($000):** 5196 **Personnel:** 137

HARLAN—Shelby County

★ **MYRTUE MEDICAL CENTER (161374)**, 1213 Garfield Avenue, Zip 51537–2057; tel. 712/755–5161 **A**9 10 18 **F**11 12 13 15 24 25 27 28 30 31 32 33 34 36 38 42 52 55 56 57 61 62 63 66 67 73 74 75 76 77 79 80 86 87 89 91 92 94 96 102 107 118 120 121 122 124 135 137 **P**6 8
Primary Contact: Mark Woodring, Administrator
CFO: Barry Jacobsen, Chief Financial Officer
CMO: Don Klitgaard, M.D., Chief of Staff
CIO: Khristine Jacobsen, Chief Information Officer
CHR: Donna Christensen–Mores, Director Human Resources
Web address: www.myrtuemedical.org
Control: County–Government, nonfederal **Service:** General Medical and Surgical

Staffed Beds: 25 **Admissions:** 1536 **Census:** 16 **Outpatient Visits:** 75256 **Births:** 84 **Total Expense ($000):** 22195 **Payroll Expense ($000):** 9269 **Personnel:** 278

HAWARDEN—Sioux County

★ **HAWARDEN COMMUNITY HOSPITAL (161311)**, 1111 11th Street, Zip 51023–1999; tel. 712/551–3100 **A**9 10 18 **F**1 4 11 15 16 17 24 25 27 30 31 38 40 52 54 55 56 57 62 65 68 70 71 73 74 75 78 79 83 84 85 86 88 96 97 107 117 118 121 122 135 137 **P**7 **S** Trinity Health
Primary Contact: Chad Markham, Chief Executive Officer
CHR: Amy Miller, Human Resources Assistant
Web address: www.hawardencommunityhospital.org
Control: City–Government, nonfederal **Service:** General Medical and Surgical

Staffed Beds: 18 **Admissions:** 190 **Census:** 2 **Outpatient Visits:** 17717 **Births:** 0 **Total Expense ($000):** 4621 **Payroll Expense ($000):** 1809 **Personnel:** 54

HUMBOLDT—Humboldt County

★ **HUMBOLDT COUNTY MEMORIAL HOSPITAL (161334)**, 1000 North 15th Street, Zip 50548–1008; tel. 515/332–4200, (Total facility includes 28 beds in nursing home–type unit) **A**9 10 18 **F**1 4 7 10 11 14 15 16 17 24 25 27 28 30 31 32 38 40 42 43 44 50 51 57 61 63 65 67 68 70 71 73 75 76 77 78 79 82 83 84 85 86 88 96 100 104 105 107 115 117 119 122 123 **S** Iowa Health System
Primary Contact: Steven Colerick, Chief Executive Officer
CFO: Betty Etherington, Chief Financial Officer
CHR: Mary Moritz, Administrator Human Resources
Web address: www.humboldthospital.org
Control: County–Government, nonfederal **Service:** General Medical and Surgical

Staffed Beds: 49 **Admissions:** 401 **Census:** 32 **Outpatient Visits:** 51475 **Births:** 0 **Total Expense ($000):** 10838 **Payroll Expense ($000):** 4870 **Personnel:** 142

IDA GROVE—Ida County

★ **HORN MEMORIAL HOSPITAL (161354)**, 701 East Second Street, Zip 51445–1699; tel. 712/364–3311 **A**9 10 18 **F**8 11 13 15 24 27 30 31 32 33 38 40 42 43 44 55 56 57 61 62 67 74 75 76 77 79 80 84 86 87 94 96 99 100 102 107 117 118 119 121 122 123 124 134 135 136 **P**2
Primary Contact: Dan Ellis, Administrator
CFO: Gary Teut, Assistant Administrator
Web address: www.hornmemorialhospital.org
Control: Other not–for–profit (including NFP Corporation) **Service:** General Medical and Surgical

Staffed Beds: 25 **Admissions:** 909 **Census:** 12 **Outpatient Visits:** 27230 **Births:** 75 **Total Expense ($000):** 11533 **Payroll Expense ($000):** 4709 **Personnel:** 111

INDEPENDENCE—Buchanan County

★ **BUCHANAN COUNTY HEALTH CENTER (161335)**, 1600 First Street East, Zip 50644–3155; tel. 319/332–0999, (Total facility includes 59 beds in nursing home–type unit) **A**9 10 18 **F**11 15 24 25 28 30 31 32 33 34 38 40 43 52 54 55 56 57 60 62 63 65 68 73 75 77 79 81 82 86 87 96 97 99 102 107 115 119 120 121 122 124 135 136 137
Primary Contact: Robert J. Richard, FACHE, Administrator
CFO: Ronald Timpe, Associate Administrator
CHR: Amber Youngblut, Manager Human Resources
Web address: www.bchealth.info
Control: County–Government, nonfederal **Service:** General Medical and Surgical

Staffed Beds: 84 **Admissions:** 599 **Census:** 53 **Outpatient Visits:** 44398 **Births:** 0 **Total Expense ($000):** 12695 **Payroll Expense ($000):** 5847 **Personnel:** 196

□ **MENTAL HEALTH INSTITUTE (164003)**, 2277 Iowa Avenue, Zip 50644–9106; tel. 319/334–2583 **A**1 9 10 **F**26 30 32 37 63 88 89 91 92 119 132 135 **P**6
Primary Contact: Bhasker J. Dave, M.D., Superintendent
Web address: www.dhs.state.ia.us
Control: State–Government, nonfederal **Service:** Psychiatric

Staffed Beds: 95 **Admissions:** 351 **Census:** 86 **Outpatient Visits:** 13 **Births:** 0 **Total Expense ($000):** 20892 **Payroll Expense ($000):** 13271 **Personnel:** 286

IOWA CITY—Johnson County

⊠ **MERCY IOWA CITY (160029)**, 500 East Market Street, Zip 52245–2689; tel. 319/339–0300, (Total facility includes 16 beds in nursing home–type unit) **A**1 2 9 10 **F**3 11 13 15 18 20 22 24 25 26 27 30 31 32 33 36 38 40 41 50 51 54 55 56 57 58 61 62 68 70 71 72 73 74 75 76 77 79 80 81 82 84 87 88 95 96 97 99 100 102 106 107 117 119 121 124 134 135 137 **P**1
Primary Contact: Ronald R. Reed, President and Chief Executive Officer
COO: Catherine H. Abrams, R.N., MS, Vice President Nursing
CFO: Michael G. Heinrich, Senior Vice President Finance and Chief Financial Officer
CMO: Peter D. Wallace, M.D., Vice President Medical Staff Affairs
CIO: Paul Foelsch, Vice President Information Services and Chief Information Officer
CHR: Marie Peeters, Director Human Resources
Web address: www.mercyiowacity.org
Control: Church–operated, Nongovernment, not–for profit **Service:** General Medical and Surgical

Staffed Beds: 240 **Admissions:** 8413 **Census:** 108 **Outpatient Visits:** 371735 **Births:** 1240 **Total Expense ($000):** 128308 **Payroll Expense ($000):** 54222 **Personnel:** 987

IA

☒ **UNIVERSITY OF IOWA HOSPITALS AND CLINICS (160058)**, 200 Hawkins Drive, Zip 52242–1009; tel. 319/356–1616, (Includes CHEMICAL DEPENDENCY CENTER, tel. 319/384–8765; STATE PSYCHIATRIC HOSPITAL, tel. 319/356–4658; UNIVERSITY HOSPITAL SCHOOL, tel. 319/353–6456) **A**1 2 3 5 8 9 10 **F**3 5 6 7 8 9 11 12 13 14 15 16 17 18 19 20 21 22 23 24 25 26 27 28 30 31 32 33 34 35 36 37 38 40 41 42 43 44 46 47 48 49 50 51 53 54 55 56 57 58 59 60 61 62 63 64 66 68 70 71 72 73 74 75 76 77 78 79 80 81 82 83 84 85 86 87 88 89 90 91 92 93 94 95 96 97 99 100 102 103 104 105 106 107 108 109 111 112 113 114 116 118 119 120 121 124 125 126 127 128 129 130 131 132 133 134 135 136 137 **P**1 7
Primary Contact: Gordon D. Williams, Interim Chief Executive Officer
COO: Eric Dickson, M.D., Interim Chief Operating Officer
CFO: Kenneth Fisher, Associate Vice President Finance and Chief Financial Officer
CIO: Lee Carmen, Director Health Care Information Systems
CHR: Diana Leventry, Director Human Resources
Web address: www.uihealthcare.com
Control: State–Government, nonfederal **Service:** General Medical and Surgical

Staffed Beds: 653 **Admissions:** 27829 **Census:** 500 **Outpatient Visits:** 917770 **Births:** 1808 **Total Expense ($000):** 767668 **Payroll Expense ($000):** 298252 **Personnel:** 6375

☒ **VETERANS AFFAIRS MEDICAL CENTER**, 601 Highway 6 West, Zip 52246–2208; tel. 319/338–0581 **A**1 3 5 8 9 **F**3 5 8 17 18 20 25 26 27 30 31 33 37 38 40 41 42 43 44 45 47 53 54 55 57 58 59 60 61 62 63 68 72 73 75 76 77 79 81 82 86 87 88 90 92 93 94 96 97 100 102 103 106 107 118 119 121 124 127 132 133 135 136 137 **S** Department of Veterans Affairs
Primary Contact: Barry Sharp, Director
CIO: Antonio Razavi, Chief Information Officer
Web address: www.va.gov/sta/guide/home.asp
Control: Veterans Affairs, Government, federal **Service:** General Medical and Surgical

Staffed Beds: 93 **Admissions:** 3224 **Census:** 48 **Outpatient Visits:** 245784 **Births:** 0 **Total Expense ($000):** 177958 **Payroll Expense ($000):** 66351 **Personnel:** 1427

IOWA FALLS—Hardin County

★ **ELLSWORTH MUNICIPAL HOSPITAL (161380)**, 110 Rocksylvania Avenue, Zip 50126–2400; tel. 641/648–4631 **A**9 10 18 **F**5 8 11 13 15 24 25 26 33 34 38 40 52 55 56 57 62 73 74 75 79 80 81 82 86 88 89 90 91 92 94 95 96 107 118 119 120 121 122 124 132 **P**6 **S** Trinity Health
Primary Contact: John O'Brien, Administrator
CFO: Betty Riley, Chief Financial Officer
CMO: Kathleen Haverkamp, M.D., Chief Medical Officer
CHR: Cheri Geitz, Director Human Resources
Web address: www.emhia.com
Control: City–Government, nonfederal **Service:** General Medical and Surgical

Staffed Beds: 35 **Admissions:** 1795 **Census:** 19 **Outpatient Visits:** 56344 **Births:** 105 **Total Expense ($000):** 17273 **Payroll Expense ($000):** 7969 **Personnel:** 220

JEFFERSON—Greene County

★ **GREENE COUNTY MEDICAL CENTER (161325)**, 1000 West Lincolnway, Zip 50129–1697; tel. 515/386–2114, (Total facility includes 72 beds in nursing home–type unit) **A**9 10 18 **F**11 13 15 24 25 31 32 33 34 38 42 43 46 54 57 61 62 63 65 66 73 74 76 79 80 86 96 102 107 115 117 119 120 121 122 124 **P**5 6 **S** Iowa Health System
Primary Contact: Karen L. Bossard, FACHE, Administrator and Chief Executive Officer
CFO: William Steussy, Chief Financial Officer
CMO: Steven Karber, M.D., Medical Director
CIO: Kevin Kibby, Manager Information Systems
Web address: www.gcmchealth.com
Control: County–Government, nonfederal **Service:** General Medical and Surgical

Staffed Beds: 97 **Admissions:** 629 **Census:** 73 **Outpatient Visits:** 24576 **Births:** 66 **Total Expense ($000):** 16712 **Payroll Expense ($000):** 8373 **Personnel:** 202

KEOKUK—Lee County

☒ **KEOKUK AREA HOSPITAL (160008)**, 1600 Morgan Street, Zip 52632–3456; tel. 319/524–7150 **A**1 9 10 **F**3 13 15 17 24 30 31 32 33 38 40 46 55 56 57 61 62 66 74 77 79 80 81 82 84 85 86 88 90 91 92 96 97 102 103 106 107 118 120 121 122 135 **P**6
Primary Contact: Allan Zastrow, FACHE, Chief Executive Officer
COO: Richard Thomason, Chief Operating Officer
CFO: Walter Winkler, Chief Financial Officer
CMO: James W. Holsinger, M.D., Chief of Staff
CIO: Linda Shaffner, Chief Information Officer
CHR: Rhonda Schreck, Director Human Resources
Web address: www.keokukhealthsystems.org
Control: Other not–for–profit (including NFP Corporation) **Service:** General Medical and Surgical

Staffed Beds: 83 **Admissions:** 3059 **Census:** 32 **Outpatient Visits:** 43389 **Births:** 231 **Total Expense ($000):** 29696 **Payroll Expense ($000):** 13390 **Personnel:** 408

KEOSAUQUA—Van Buren County

★ **VAN BUREN COUNTY HOSPITAL (161337)**, 304 Franklin, Zip 52565; tel. 319/293–3171 **A**9 10 18 **F**3 7 10 11 13 15 24 25 27 30 31 32 33 38 40 46 50 55 56 57 61 62 63 68 69 73 74 75 76 77 79 80 81 82 84 86 87 92 96 102 107 117 118 119 121 122 124 135 136 137 **P**6
Primary Contact: Lisa Schnedler, Chief Executive Officer and Administrator
CFO: Kara McEntee, Chief Financial Officer
CIO: Chris McEntee, Network Specialist
Web address: www.vbch.org
Control: County–Government, nonfederal **Service:** General Medical and Surgical

Staffed Beds: 25 **Admissions:** 742 **Census:** 12 **Outpatient Visits:** 16255 **Births:** 49 **Total Expense ($000):** 10836 **Payroll Expense ($000):** 4506 **Personnel:** 151

KNOXVILLE—Marion County

KNOXVILLE DIVISION See Veterans Affairs Central Iowa Health Care System, Des Moines

★ **KNOXVILLE HOSPITAL & CLINICS (161355)**, 1002 South Lincoln Street, Zip 50138–3155; tel. 641/842–2151 **A**9 10 18 **F**3 11 13 15 24 25 30 31 32 38 40 55 57 62 63 66 73 74 75 77 79 80 81 86 87 92 96 97 100 102 106 107 118 119 121 122 124 135 **P**6 **S** QHR
Primary Contact: Ann M. Helwig, Chief Executive Officer
COO: Ann M. Helwig, Chief Executive Officer
CFO: Michael Creary, Chief Financial Officer
CMO: David Kobliska, M.D., President Medical Staff
CHR: Brenda Maddison, Director Human Resources
Web address: www.kach.org
Control: Other not–for–profit (including NFP Corporation) **Service:** General Medical and Surgical

Staffed Beds: 25 **Admissions:** 756 **Census:** 8 **Outpatient Visits:** 48353 **Births:** 80 **Total Expense ($000):** 17137 **Payroll Expense ($000):** 7326 **Personnel:** 170

LAKE CITY—Calhoun County

★ **STEWART MEMORIAL COMMUNITY HOSPITAL (161350)**, 1301 West Main, Zip 51449–1585; tel. 712/464–3171 **A**9 10 18 **F**7 11 12 13 15 24 25 26 27 31 38 40 42 56 57 61 62 63 67 68 73 74 75 76 79 81 86 96 107 119 122 124 136 **P**5 6
Primary Contact: Leah Marxen, Chief Executive Officer
CFO: Jim Henkenius, Chief Financial Officer
Web address: www.stewartmemorial.org
Control: Other not–for–profit (including NFP Corporation) **Service:** General Medical and Surgical

Staffed Beds: 25 **Admissions:** 785 **Census:** 9 **Outpatient Visits:** 38388 **Births:** 80 **Total Expense ($000):** 21845 **Payroll Expense ($000):** 9089 **Personnel:** 191

IA

Hospital, Medicare Provider Number, Address, Telephone, Approval, Facility, and Physician Codes, Health Care System

★ American Hospital Association (AHA) membership
□ The Joint Commission accreditation
○ American Osteopathic Association (AOA) accreditation
△ Commission on Accreditation of Rehabilitation Facilities (CARF) accreditation

LE MARS—Plymouth County

★ **FLOYD VALLEY HOSPITAL/AVERA HEALTH (161368)**, 714 Lincoln Street N.E., Zip 51031–0010, Mailing Address: P.O. Box 10, Zip 51031–0010; tel. 712/546–7871 **A**9 10 18 **F**3 10 11 13 15 17 24 25 26 27 28 31 32 33 38 40 52 55 56 57 61 62 63 65 68 74 76 77 78 79 80 81 82 84 96 102 107 117 121 122 124 135 137 **P**5 **S** Avera Health
Primary Contact: Michael T. Donlin, Administrator
CFO: Daryl Friedenbach, Director Fiscal Services
CMO: Steven Meis, M.D., President Medical Staff
CHR: Mary Helen McManus, Director Human Resources
Web address: www.floydvalleyhospital.org
Control: City–Government, nonfederal **Service:** General Medical and Surgical

Staffed Beds: 25 **Admissions:** 1273 **Census:** 11 **Outpatient Visits:** 45546 **Births:** 120 **Total Expense ($000):** 20565 **Payroll Expense ($000):** 7278 **Personnel:** 179

LEON—Decatur County

★ **DECATUR COUNTY HOSPITAL (161340)**, 1405 N.W. Church Street, Zip 50144–1299; tel. 641/446–4871 **A**9 10 18 **F**7 11 15 24 27 38 42 52 55 57 61 62 65 66 73 76 77 79 80 84 86 96 100 102 107 117 119 122
Primary Contact: Lynn Milnes, Chief Executive Officer
CFO: Missy Walter, Chief Financial Officer
CMO: Larry Richard, M.D., Chief Medical Staff
CHR: Jo Beth Smith, Director Support Services
Web address: www.decaturcountyhospital.org
Control: County–Government, nonfederal **Service:** General Medical and Surgical

Staffed Beds: 25 **Admissions:** 392 **Census:** 7 **Outpatient Visits:** 13014 **Births:** 0 **Total Expense ($000):** 7798 **Payroll Expense ($000):** 3092 **Personnel:** 87

MANCHESTER—Delaware County

★ **REGIONAL MEDICAL CENTER (161343)**, (Formerly Regional Medical Center of Northeast Iowa and Delaware County), 709 West Main Street, Zip 52057–0359, Mailing Address: P.O. Box 359, Zip 52057–0359; tel. 563/927–3232 **A**9 10 18 **F**3 7 11 13 15 17 24 25 30 31 32 33 34 36 38 40 41 42 44 50 52 55 56 57 61 62 63 64 66 68 73 74 75 79 80 81 82 84 86 89 90 91 92 93 94 96 97 100 102 107 117 118 119 120 121 122 135 137
Primary Contact: Lon D. Butikofer, RN, Ph.D., Chief Executive Officer
CFO: Danette Kramer, Vice President Finance and Chief Financial Officer
CIO: Julie Bente, Vice President Human and Facility Resources
CHR: Julie Bente, Vice President Human and Facility Resources
Web address: www.regmedctr.org
Control: County–Government, nonfederal **Service:** General Medical and Surgical

Staffed Beds: 25 **Admissions:** 776 **Census:** 8 **Outpatient Visits:** 91986 **Births:** 149 **Total Expense ($000):** 20287 **Payroll Expense ($000):** 9098 **Personnel:** 216

MANNING—Carroll County

★ **MANNING REGIONAL HEALTHCARE CENTER (161332)**, 410 Main Street, Zip 51455–1093; tel. 712/655–2072, (Total facility includes 56 beds in nursing home–type unit) **A**9 10 18 **F**3 4 5 11 13 15 27 30 31 32 33 34 36 38 40 43 50 51 54 55 56 57 60 61 66 69 73 74 75 76 77 79 80 82 84 86 96 97 100 102 106 107 117 119 121 122 124 135 **P**5
Primary Contact: Darrell E. Vondrak, Interim Chief Executive Officer
CFO: Abbey Stangl, Chief Financial Officer
CMO: Tracy Kahl, M.D., Chief Medical Officer
CIO: Kim Jahn, Director Support Services
CHR: Shelli Lorenzen, Director Human Resources
Web address: www.mrhcia.com
Control: Other not–for–profit (including NFP Corporation) **Service:** General Medical and Surgical

Staffed Beds: 73 **Admissions:** 317 **Census:** 52 **Outpatient Visits:** 9136 **Births:** 19 **Total Expense ($000):** 9635 **Payroll Expense ($000):** 4052 **Personnel:** 130

MAQUOKETA—Jackson County

🟆 **JACKSON COUNTY REGIONAL HEALTH CENTER (161329)**, 700 West Grove Street, Zip 52060–0910; tel. 563/652–2474, (Total facility includes 18 beds in nursing home–type unit) **A**1 9 10 18 **F**3 7 11 13 15 24 26 27 30 31 32 33 38 40 52 56 57 59 61 62 63 65 67 68 73 74 79 80 82 84 86 96 102 107 117 119 121 122 135 **S** Iowa Health System
Primary Contact: Curt Coleman, CHE, FACHE, Chief Executive Officer
CFO: Donna Roeder, Chief Financial Officer
CHR: Shannon Langenberg, Director Human Resources
Web address: www.jcrhc.org
Control: County–Government, nonfederal **Service:** General Medical and Surgical

Staffed Beds: 43 **Admissions:** 587 **Census:** 23 **Outpatient Visits:** 21436 **Births:** 79 **Total Expense ($000):** 13090 **Payroll Expense ($000):** 5837 **Personnel:** 159

MARENGO—Iowa County

★ **MARENGO MEMORIAL HOSPITAL (161317)**, 300 West May Street, Zip 52301–1261, Mailing Address: P.O. Box 228, Zip 52301–0228; tel. 319/642–5543 **A**9 10 18 **F**3 7 8 24 25 30 31 32 33 38 40 41 50 55 57 59 62 67 73 79 80 82 86 96 102 119 121 122 135 137 **P**6
Primary Contact: Genice Maroc, FACHE, Chief Executive Officer
COO: Terry Brecht, Chief Operating Officer and Director Ambulance Services
CFO: Nancy Kohrt, Chief Financial Officer
CMO: Malcolm Findlater, M.D., Chief Medical Staff
CHR: Lesa Waddell, Director Human Resources
Web address: www.marengohospital.org
Control: City–Government, nonfederal **Service:** General Medical and Surgical

Staffed Beds: 25 **Admissions:** 304 **Census:** 12 **Outpatient Visits:** 17739 **Births:** 0 **Total Expense ($000):** 12001 **Payroll Expense ($000):** 5562 **Personnel:** 172

MARSHALLTOWN—Marshall County

★ **MARSHALLTOWN MEDICAL & SURGICAL CENTER (160001)**, 3 South Fourth Avenue, Zip 50158–2998; tel. 641/754–5151, (Total facility includes 26 beds in nursing home–type unit) **A**9 10 19 20 **F**3 7 11 13 15 18 20 24 26 27 30 32 33 34 38 40 41 43 50 52 53 55 57 61 62 63 65 66 68 69 72 73 74 75 76 77 79 80 81 82 84 86 87 96 97 103 105 106 107 117 118 119 120 121 135 136 137
Primary Contact: Robert Cooper, Chief Executive Officer
COO: LaRae Schelling, Vice President Operations and Chief Nursing Officer
CFO: Robert Downey, Vice President Finance
CMO: Gary Peasley, M.D., President Medical Staff
CIO: Robert Downey, Vice President Finance
CHR: Colleen Springer, Director Human Resources
Web address: www.everydaychampions.org
Control: Other not–for–profit (including NFP Corporation) **Service:** General Medical and Surgical

Staffed Beds: 105 **Admissions:** 3629 **Census:** 37 **Outpatient Visits:** 212525 **Births:** 622 **Total Expense ($000):** 49566 **Payroll Expense ($000):** 22169 **Personnel:** 485

MASON CITY—Cerro Gordo County

🟆 **MERCY MEDICAL CENTER–NORTH IOWA (160064)**, 1000 Fourth Street S.W., Zip 50401–2800; tel. 641/422–7000 **A**1 2 3 5 9 10 19 20 **F**3 11 12 13 15 17 18 20 22 24 25 26 27 28 30 31 32 33 34 36 37 38 40 41 42 43 44 47 48 49 50 52 54 55 56 57 59 60 61 62 64 66 68 69 70 72 73 74 75 76 77 79 80 81 82 84 85 86 87 88 89 90 91 92 93 94 95 96 97 100 102 105 106 107 108 109 111 115 117 118 119 120 121 122 123 124 133 135 136 137 **P**1 6 **S** Trinity Health
Primary Contact: James G. FitzPatrick, President and Chief Executive Officer
COO: Scott Leighty, Chief Operating Officer
CFO: Rod G. Schlader, Chief Financial Officer
CIO: Randy Haskins, Director Information Systems
CHR: Diane Fischels, Vice President Operations and Chief Human Resource Officer
Web address: www.mercynorthiowa.com
Control: Church–operated, Nongovernment, not–for profit **Service:** General Medical and Surgical

Staffed Beds: 241 **Admissions:** 12923 **Census:** 140 **Outpatient Visits:** 453673 **Births:** 1099 **Total Expense ($000):** 264026 **Payroll Expense ($000):** 117911 **Personnel:** 2303

MISSOURI VALLEY—Harrison County

★ **ALEGENT HEALTH COMMUNITY MEMORIAL HOSPITAL (161309)**, 631 North Eighth Street, Zip 51555–1199; tel. 712/642–2784 **A**9 10 18 **F**3 8 11 15 24 25 26 27 30 31 32 33 38 40 50 53 57 62 73 75 76 77 79 80 84 86 89 90 92 94 96 102 107 117 118 119 121 122 135 **P**8 **S** Alegent Health
Primary Contact: Robert R. Sellers, Regional Administrator
CFO: Sue Blake, Operations Director Finance and Support Services
CMO: Jean C. Griesel, D.O., Chief of Staff
CIO: Alicia Leapley, Information System Liaison and Coordinator Registration
CHR: Julie Brown, Human Resources Assistant
Web address: www.alegent.org
Control: Other not–for–profit (including NFP Corporation) **Service:** General Medical and Surgical

Staffed Beds: 25 **Admissions:** 719 **Census:** 9 **Outpatient Visits:** 29967 **Births:** 0 **Total Expense ($000):** 16657 **Payroll Expense ($000):** 6283 **Personnel:** 149

MOUNT AYR—Ringgold County

RINGGOLD COUNTY HOSPITAL (161373), 211 Shellway Drive, Zip 50854–1299; tel. 641/464–3226 **A**9 10 18 **F**7 8 11 15 24 25 27 30 32 33 36 38 54 55 57 59 62 63 65 79 86 96 107 117 122 137 **P**6
Primary Contact: Gordon W. Winkler, Administrator
CFO: Teresa Roberts, Chief Financial Officer
CIO: Jan Lyons, Regional Director Health Improvement Management
CHR: Mitzi Hymbaugh, Chief Personnel
Web address: www.rchmtayr.org
Control: County–Government, nonfederal **Service:** General Medical and Surgical

Staffed Beds: 25 **Admissions:** 499 **Census:** 6 **Outpatient Visits:** 25046 **Births:** 0 **Total Expense ($000):** 9585 **Payroll Expense ($000):** 4572 **Personnel:** 110

MOUNT PLEASANT—Henry County

★ **HENRY COUNTY HEALTH CENTER (161356)**, 407 South White Street, Zip 52641–2299; tel. 319/385–3141, (Total facility includes 49 beds in nursing home–type unit) **A**9 10 18 **F**7 11 13 15 24 25 27 28 31 32 33 38 40 50 54 55 56 57 62 65 66 68 73 74 75 76 77 79 80 81 84 86 92 96 97 99 102 103 107 117 118 119 120 121 122 124 132 134 135 137 **P**8
Primary Contact: Daniel F. Sheehan, Chief Executive Officer
CFO: David Muhs, Chief Financial Officer
CMO: James Widmer, M.D., Chief of Staff
CHR: Jim Carson, Manager Human Resources
Web address: www.hchc.org
Control: County–Government, nonfederal **Service:** General Medical and Surgical

Staffed Beds: 74 **Admissions:** 1313 **Census:** 59 **Outpatient Visits:** 149963 **Births:** 140 **Total Expense ($000):** 24628 **Payroll Expense ($000):** 10543 **Personnel:** 230

MENTAL HEALTH INSTITUTE (164004), 1200 East Washington Street, Zip 52641–1898; tel. 319/385–7231 **A**9 10 **F**4 5 88 119 121
Primary Contact: James A. Carter, Superintendent
CFO: Sandy Scheib, Business Manager
CMO: Josephine Hizon, M.D., Clinical Director
CHR: Janice Creighton, Human Resources Associate
Web address: www.dhs.state.ia.us
Control: State–Government, nonfederal **Service:** Alcoholism and other chemical dependency

Staffed Beds: 79 **Admissions:** 726 **Census:** 57 **Outpatient Visits:** 4 **Births:** 0 **Total Expense ($000):** 7949 **Payroll Expense ($000):** 4966 **Personnel:** 95

MUSCATINE—Muscatine County

★☐ **UNITY HEALTHCARE (160013)**, 1518 Mulberry Avenue, Zip 52761–3499; tel. 563/264–9100, (Total facility includes 8 beds in nursing home–type unit) **A**1 9 10 20 **F**3 11 13 15 24 31 32 38 40 46 50 54 57 60 62 66 67 68 73 74 77 79 80 82 84 86 92 96 97 99 106 107 117 118 119 137
Primary Contact: Jill Kordick, Interim Chief Executive Officer
CMO: Steven Paulsrud, D.O., Chief of Staff
CIO: Blake Jones, Director Information Technology
CHR: Dena Brockhouse, Director Human Resources
Web address: www.unityiowa.org
Control: Other not–for–profit (including NFP Corporation) **Service:** General Medical and Surgical

Staffed Beds: 64 **Admissions:** 1754 **Census:** 17 **Outpatient Visits:** 93915 **Births:** 352 **Total Expense ($000):** 32906 **Payroll Expense ($000):** 12508 **Personnel:** 278

NEVADA—Story County

★ **STORY COUNTY MEDICAL CENTER (161333)**, 630 Sixth Street, Zip 50201–2266; tel. 515/382–2111, (Total facility includes 60 beds in nursing home–type unit) **A**9 10 18 **F**7 11 24 25 27 28 31 33 34 38 40 50 52 55 57 62 66 67 73 75 76 77 79 80 86 87 96 102 119 120 121 122 124 132 135 **P**6
Primary Contact: Todd Willert, Administrator
CFO: Pamela Kluender, Chief Financial Officer
Web address: www.scmcnevada.org
Control: County–Government, nonfederal **Service:** General Medical and Surgical

Staffed Beds: 78 **Admissions:** 368 **Census:** 67 **Outpatient Visits:** 25033 **Births:** 0 **Total Expense ($000):** 12847 **Payroll Expense ($000):** 6224 **Personnel:** 111

NEW HAMPTON—Chickasaw County

★☐ **MERCY MEDICAL CENTER–NEW HAMPTON (161331)**, 308 North Maple Avenue, Zip 50659–1142; tel. 641/394–4121 **A**1 9 10 18 **F**3 11 13 15 24 25 26 27 30 31 32 33 34 38 40 48 54 55 56 57 62 66 72 73 74 75 77 79 80 86 96 102 107 120 121 122 135 137 **P**8 **S** Trinity Health
Primary Contact: Bruce Roesler, Chief Executive Officer
COO: Jodi Geerts, Chief Nursing Officer
CFO: Jennifer Rapenske, Manager Financial Services
CMO: Mary Sharon Peraud, M.D., President Medical Staff
CIO: Randy Haskins, Director Information Systems
CHR: Lisa Heller, Manager Human Resources and Payroll
Web address: www.mercynewhampton.com
Control: Church–operated, Nongovernment, not–for profit **Service:** General Medical and Surgical

Staffed Beds: 18 **Admissions:** 489 **Census:** 5 **Outpatient Visits:** 19272 **Births:** 29 **Total Expense ($000):** 11007 **Payroll Expense ($000):** 4336 **Personnel:** 98

NEWTON—Jasper County

★ ○ **SKIFF MEDICAL CENTER (160032)**, 204 North Fourth Avenue East, Zip 50208–3100, Mailing Address: P.O. Box 1006, Zip 50208–1006; tel. 641/792–1273 **A**9 10 11 **F**3 11 13 15 24 25 26 27 28 31 33 34 38 40 41 42 44 55 56 57 61 62 63 67 68 73 74 75 76 77 79 80 86 92 96 97 99 100 102 106 107 119 120 121 122 124 135 136 137 **P**6
Primary Contact: Kris Baumgart, Chief Executive Officer
CFO: Cheryl Ritter, Vice President and Chief Financial Officer
CMO: Tammara Chance, D.O., Medical Director
CHR: Gena Garber, Director Human Resources
Web address: www.skiffmed.com
Control: City–Government, nonfederal **Service:** General Medical and Surgical

Staffed Beds: 52 **Admissions:** 2549 **Census:** 26 **Outpatient Visits:** 76089 **Births:** 220 **Total Expense ($000):** 34003 **Payroll Expense ($000):** 16929 **Personnel:** 358

OAKDALE—Johnson County

IOWA MEDICAL AND CLASSIFICATION CENTER, Highway 965, Zip 52319, Mailing Address: IMCC, Box A, Zip 52319; tel. 319/626–2391 **F**88
Primary Contact: Lowell Brandt, Warden
Control: State–Government, nonfederal **Service:** Psychiatric

Staffed Beds: 15 **Admissions:** 63 **Census:** 16 **Outpatient Visits:** 0 **Births:** 0 **Total Expense ($000):** 1603 **Personnel:** 25

OELWEIN—Fayette County

★ **MERCY HOSPITAL OF FRANCISCAN SISTERS (161338)**, 201 Eighth Avenue S.E., Zip 50662–2447; tel. 319/283–6000, (Total facility includes 39 beds in nursing home–type unit) **A**9 10 18 **F**7 8 11 15 25 26 31 33 38 54 55 57 67 68 73 79 81 82 87 96 100 107 117 119 121 122 124 135 **S** Wheaton Franciscan Healthcare
Primary Contact: Katherine Hintz, Administrator
COO: David Olejniczak, Chief Operating Officer
CFO: Timothy Huber, Manager Financial Support
CIO: Todd Richardson, Regional Vice President Information Services
CHR: Vicki L. Parsons, Regional Vice President Human Resources
Web address: www.covhealth.com
Control: Church–operated, Nongovernment, not–for profit **Service:** General Medical and Surgical

Staffed Beds: 62 **Admissions:** 814 **Census:** 42 **Outpatient Visits:** 34627 **Births:** 0 **Total Expense ($000):** 13154 **Payroll Expense ($000):** 5558 **Personnel:** 122

ONAWA—Monona County

★ **BURGESS HEALTH CENTER (161359)**, 1600 Diamond Street, Zip 51040–1548; tel. 712/423–2311 **A**9 10 18 **F**3 7 11 13 15 24 25 27 30 31 32 33 38 42 54 55 56 57 61 62 63 68 73 74 75 76 77 79 80 86 87 90 93 94 96 102 107 119 121 122 124 135 137 **P**6
Primary Contact: Francis Tramp, President
CFO: Shawn Gosch, Chief Financial Officer
CMO: John Garred, M.D., Chief Medical Officer
CIO: Kim Norby, Chief Information Officer
CHR: Denise Trukenmiller, Director Human Resources
Web address: www.burgesshc.org
Control: Other not–for–profit (including NFP Corporation) **Service:** General Medical and Surgical

Staffed Beds: 25 **Admissions:** 1301 **Census:** 15 **Outpatient Visits:** 50286 **Births:** 77 **Total Expense ($000):** 19394 **Payroll Expense ($000):** 7593 **Personnel:** 193

ORANGE CITY—Sioux County

★ **ORANGE CITY AREA HEALTH SYSTEM (161360)**, 1000 Lincoln Circle S.E., Zip 51041–1398; tel. 712/737–4984, (Total facility includes 79 beds in nursing home–type unit) **A**9 10 18 **F**7 10 11 13 14 15 24 25 27 30 31 33 38 42 43 52 54 56 57 59 61 62 65 66 67 68 73 74 75 76 77 79 80 81 82 84 86 87 96 99 100 102 105 107 108 115 119 120 121 122 135 136 137 **P**6 **S** Sanford Health
Primary Contact: Martin W. Guthmiller, Chief Executive Officer
COO: Daniel P. McCarty, Chief Operating Officer
CFO: Dina Baas, Director Financial Services
CHR: Shari Baker, Director Human Resources
Web address: www.ochealthsystem.org
Control: City–Government, nonfederal **Service:** General Medical and Surgical

Staffed Beds: 104 **Admissions:** 1088 **Census:** 89 **Outpatient Visits:** 73534 **Births:** 209 **Total Expense ($000):** 31112 **Payroll Expense ($000):** 13478 **Personnel:** 383

IA

Hospital, Medicare Provider Number, Address, Telephone, Approval, Facility, and Physician Codes, Health Care System

★ American Hospital Association (AHA) membership
☐ The Joint Commission accreditation
○ American Osteopathic Association (AOA) accreditation
△ Commission on Accreditation of Rehabilitation Facilities (CARF) accreditation

OSAGE—Mitchell County

★ **MITCHELL COUNTY REGIONAL HEALTH CENTER (161323)**, 616 North Eighth Street, Zip 50461–1498; tel. 641/732–6000 **A**9 10 18 **F**7 11 13 15 24 30 31 32 38 40 55 57 62 73 74 79 80 86 96 102 107 119 121 122 135 **P**8 **S** Trinity Health
Primary Contact: Sandy Leggett, Chief Executive Officer
COO: Kay Gabriel, R.N., Assistant Administrator and Chief Nursing Officer
CMO: Kelly Ross, M.D., Chief of Staff
CHR: Kerry Knudsen, Director Human Resources
Web address: www.mitchellcohospital–clinics.com
Control: County–Government, nonfederal **Service:** General Medical and Surgical

Staffed Beds: 25 **Admissions:** 688 **Census:** 7 **Outpatient Visits:** 60622 **Births:** 34 **Total Expense ($000):** 15470 **Payroll Expense ($000):** 4802 **Personnel:** 159

OSCEOLA—Clarke County

★ **CLARKE COUNTY HOSPITAL (161348)**, 800 South Fillmore Street, Zip 50213–1619; tel. 641/342–2184 **A**9 10 18 **F**7 11 15 24 25 27 32 33 38 52 55 57 62 65 69 73 79 84 85 86 96 100 103 106 107 117 118 122 **S** Iowa Health System
Primary Contact: Brian Evans, Chief Executive Officer
CFO: Michael Thilges, Chief Operating Officer and Chief Financial Officer
CMO: George Fotiadis, M.D., Chief of Staff
CIO: Nathan Pieken, Chief Information Officer
CHR: Kate Emanuel, Director Human Resources
Web address: www.clarkehosp.org
Control: County–Government, nonfederal **Service:** General Medical and Surgical

Staffed Beds: 25 **Admissions:** 361 **Census:** 16 **Outpatient Visits:** 18549 **Births:** 0 **Total Expense ($000):** 12666 **Payroll Expense ($000):** 4669 **Personnel:** 123

OSKALOOSA—Mahaska County

★ **MAHASKA HEALTH PARTNERSHIP (161379)**, 1229 C Avenue East, Zip 52577–4298; tel. 641/672–3100 **A**1 9 10 18 **F**5 7 8 11 13 15 24 25 26 27 30 31 32 33 34 35 38 40 42 43 50 53 54 55 57 61 62 66 67 68 73 74 75 76 77 79 80 81 82 86 87 88 89 90 91 92 93 94 96 100 103 106 107 118 119 120 121 122 123 124 134 135 136 137 **P**6 7
Primary Contact: Jay Christensen, Administrator
COO: David Leighton, Chief Operating Officer
CFO: Susan Horras, Chief Financial Officer
CMO: Tim Breon, M.D., Chief Medical Officer
CHR: Jacky Bresnahan, Director Human Resources
Web address: www.mahaskahospital.com
Control: County–Government, nonfederal **Service:** General Medical and Surgical

Staffed Beds: 33 **Admissions:** 1594 **Census:** 22 **Outpatient Visits:** 82109 **Births:** 231 **Total Expense ($000):** 26632 **Payroll Expense ($000):** 13775 **Personnel:** 252

OTTUMWA—Wapello County

★ **OTTUMWA REGIONAL HEALTH CENTER (160089)**, 1001 Pennsylvania Avenue, Zip 52501–2186; tel. 641/684–2300 **A**1 2 9 10 19 20 **F**3 4 5 7 11 13 15 24 25 26 27 30 31 32 33 38 40 43 46 47 48 51 53 54 55 56 57 61 62 66 67 68 70 71 73 74 75 76 77 78 79 80 81 82 84 85 86 88 89 90 91 92 93 94 95 97 99 100 101 106 107 118 119 121 123 124 134 135 136 137 **P**6
Primary Contact: Thomas R. Siemers, Chief Executive Officer
CFO: Dan Porter, Vice President and Chief Financial Officer
CHR: JoEllen Randall, Vice President Human Resources
Web address: www.orhc.com
Control: Other not–for–profit (including NFP Corporation) **Service:** General Medical and Surgical

Staffed Beds: 135 **Admissions:** 4746 **Census:** 54 **Outpatient Visits:** 142938 **Births:** 731 **Total Expense ($000):** 73908 **Payroll Expense ($000):** 34792 **Personnel:** 829

PELLA—Marion County

★ **PELLA REGIONAL HEALTH CENTER (161367)**, 404 Jefferson Street, Zip 50219–1257; tel. 641/628–3150, (Total facility includes 128 beds in nursing home–type unit) **A**9 10 18 **F**3 6 11 13 15 25 26 27 30 31 32 33 38 40 42 48 50 56 59 61 62 63 65 68 73 74 75 76 77 79 80 81 82 86 87 96 97 99 100 102 107 112 118 119 120 121 122 130 133 135 137 **P**6
Primary Contact: Robert D. Kroese, Chief Executive Officer
COO: Robert D. Kroese, Chief Executive Officer
CFO: Ron Wauters, Chief Financial Officer
CIO: Kurt Teare, Manager Information Systems
CHR: Jennifer Savage, Chief Human Resources
Web address: www.pellahealth.org
Control: Other not–for–profit (including NFP Corporation) **Service:** General Medical and Surgical

Staffed Beds: 153 **Admissions:** 2166 **Census:** 138 **Outpatient Visits:** 126772 **Births:** 370 **Total Expense ($000):** 40114 **Payroll Expense ($000):** 17834 **Personnel:** 610

PERRY—Dallas County

★ **DALLAS COUNTY HOSPITAL (161322)**, 610 10th Street, Zip 50220–2221; tel. 515/465–3547 **A**9 10 18 **F**3 10 11 15 24 25 27 31 32 33 34 38 40 42 54 55 57 59 62 66 73 75 76 77 79 84 86 92 96 102 107 115 117 118 119 121 122 124 135 **P**6 **S** Iowa Health System
Primary Contact: Laurie A. Conner, Chief Executive Officer
COO: Donna J. Vandehaar, R.N., Chief Clinical Officer
CFO: Sandra Christensen, Chief Financial Officer
CMO: Eric Ash, M.D., Chief of Staff
CHR: Michelle Corwin, Human Resources Officer
Web address: www.dallascohospital.org
Control: County–Government, nonfederal **Service:** General Medical and Surgical

Staffed Beds: 25 **Admissions:** 330 **Census:** 4 **Outpatient Visits:** 25477 **Births:** 0 **Total Expense ($000):** 12676 **Payroll Expense ($000):** 3674 **Personnel:** 96

POCAHONTAS—Pocahontas County

★ **POCAHONTAS COMMUNITY HOSPITAL (161305)**, 606 N.W. Seventh, Zip 50574–1099; tel. 712/335–3501 **A**9 10 18 **F**7 11 15 17 24 25 27 32 33 38 40 42 57 61 62 65 68 73 75 76 77 78 79 84 85 86 96 107 117 119 121 122 124 135 **P**6 **S** Iowa Health System
Primary Contact: James D. Roetman, President and Chief Executive Officer
CFO: Lynn Raveling, Chief Financial Officer
Web address: www.pocahontashospital.org
Control: City–Government, nonfederal **Service:** General Medical and Surgical

Staffed Beds: 20 **Admissions:** 280 **Census:** 3 **Outpatient Visits:** 32302 **Births:** 0 **Total Expense ($000):** 6280 **Payroll Expense ($000):** 2294 **Personnel:** 71

PRIMGHAR—Obrien County

★ **BAUM HARMON MERCY HOSPITAL (161300)**, 255 North Welch Avenue, Zip 51245–1034, Mailing Address: P.O. Box 528, Zip 51245–0528; tel. 712/957–2300 **A**9 10 18 **F**11 15 24 25 26 27 28 31 33 38 52 55 56 57 62 65 68 73 75 76 79 84 92 107 117 121 122 124 **P**8 **S** Trinity Health
Primary Contact: Robert Monical, Chief Executive Officer and Administrator
CFO: Sue E. McCauley, Director Finance
CMO: Shailesh Desai, M.D., Chief of Staff
Web address: www.baumharmon.org
Control: Church–operated, Nongovernment, not–for profit **Service:** General Medical and Surgical

Staffed Beds: 13 **Admissions:** 219 **Census:** 2 **Outpatient Visits:** 25635 **Births:** 0 **Total Expense ($000):** 6203 **Payroll Expense ($000):** 3126 **Personnel:** 64

RED OAK—Montgomery County

★ **MONTGOMERY COUNTY MEMORIAL HOSPITAL (161363)**, 2301 Eastern Avenue, Zip 51566–1300, Mailing Address: P.O. Box 498, Zip 51566–0498; tel. 712/623–7000 **A**9 10 18 **F**11 13 15 24 25 27 31 33 38 41 42 43 50 52 55 56 57 61 62 66 67 68 73 74 75 76 79 80 81 82 86 96 99 100 102 106 107 118 119 122 124 135 136 137
Primary Contact: Allen E. Pohren, Administrator
CFO: Rick Leinen, Chief Financial Officer
CMO: Michael Mahoney, M.D., Chief of Staff
CIO: Ron Kloewer, Chief Information Officer
Web address: www.mcmh.org
Control: County–Government, nonfederal **Service:** General Medical and Surgical

Staffed Beds: 25 **Admissions:** 1424 **Census:** 18 **Outpatient Visits:** 45439 **Births:** 118 **Total Expense ($000):** 20324 **Payroll Expense ($000):** 9925 **Personnel:** 238

ROCK RAPIDS—Lyon County

★ **SANFORD MERRILL MEDICAL CENTER (161321)**, (Formerly Merrill Pioneer Community Hospital), 801 South Greene Street, Zip 51246–1998; tel. 712/472–2591 **A**9 10 18 **F**11 13 24 27 31 38 52 55 57 74 75 79 84 87 107 119 122 124 **P**6 **S** Sanford Health
Primary Contact: Gordon U. Smith, Chief Executive Officer
CFO: Stanley Knobloch, Chief Financial Officer
CMO: David Springer, M.D., President Medical Staff
Web address: www.merrillpioneer.org
Control: Other not–for–profit (including NFP Corporation) **Service:** General Medical and Surgical

Staffed Beds: 16 **Admissions:** 322 **Census:** 4 **Outpatient Visits:** 9617 **Births:** 31 **Total Expense ($000):** 6270 **Payroll Expense ($000):** 2999 **Personnel:** 68

Many Facility Codes have changed. Please refer to the AHA Guide Code Chart.

ROCK VALLEY—Sioux County

★ **HEGG MEMORIAL HEALTH CENTER/AVERA HEALTH (161336)**, 1202 21st Avenue, Zip 51247–1497; tel. 712/476–8000, (Total facility includes 60 beds in nursing home–type unit) **A**9 10 18 **F**10 11 13 15 24 25 27 30 31 33 38 40 52 55 57 61 62 65 66 68 73 74 75 79 84 86 87 96 100 102 107 115 119 120 122 124 135 137 **P**5 **S** Avera Health
Primary Contact: Glenn Zevenbergen, Chief Executive Officer
CFO: Kari Hoogendoorn, Chief Financial Officer
CMO: Roy Slice, M.D., Chief Medical Officer
CHR: Tammy Faber, Director Human Resources
Web address: www.heggmemorialhealthcenter.org
Control: Other not–for–profit (including NFP Corporation) **Service:** General Medical and Surgical

Staffed Beds: 85 **Admissions:** 433 **Census:** 64 **Outpatient Visits:** 32788 **Births:** 94 **Total Expense ($000):** 9636 **Payroll Expense ($000):** 4413 **Personnel:** 98

SAC CITY—Sac County

★ **LORING HOSPITAL (161370)**, 211 Highland Avenue, Zip 50583–0217; tel. 712/662–7105 **A**9 10 18 **F**3 11 15 24 25 26 27 28 30 31 32 33 38 40 42 54 55 56 57 61 62 66 72 73 75 76 77 79 81 82 86 92 93 94 96 107 115 117 118 119 120 121 122 135 137 **S** Iowa Health System
Primary Contact: Michael S. Ketcham, President and Chief Executive Officer
CFO: Angie Fischer, Chief Financial Officer
CIO: Kathy Veit, Director Health Information Services
Web address: www.loringhospital.org
Control: Other not–for–profit (including NFP Corporation) **Service:** General Medical and Surgical

Staffed Beds: 50 **Admissions:** 1178 **Census:** 18 **Outpatient Visits:** 20650 **Births:** 0 **Total Expense ($000):** 8944 **Payroll Expense ($000):** 4104 **Personnel:** 123

SHELDON—Obrien County

★ **SANFORD SHELDON MEDICAL CENTER (161381)**, 118 North Seventh Avenue, Zip 51201–1235, Mailing Address: P.O. Box 250, Zip 51201–0250; tel. 712/324–5041, (Total facility includes 70 beds in nursing home–type unit) **A**9 10 18 **F**6 11 13 15 24 25 27 30 31 32 33 38 42 43 44 50 52 54 55 57 61 62 63 65 66 67 72 73 75 76 77 79 81 82 86 96 102 103 107 118 119 120 121 122 124 135 137 **P**6 **S** Sanford Health
Primary Contact: Charles R. Miller, Chief Executive Officer
CFO: Stanley Knobloch, Chief Financial Officer
CIO: Scott Moffitt, Director Information Systems
CHR: Dianne Wolthuizen, Director Human Resources
Web address: www.nwiowahealthcenter.org
Control: Other not–for–profit (including NFP Corporation) **Service:** General Medical and Surgical

Staffed Beds: 95 **Admissions:** 1030 **Census:** 73 **Outpatient Visits:** 32952 **Births:** 125 **Total Expense ($000):** 18975 **Payroll Expense ($000):** 9460 **Personnel:** 232

SHENANDOAH—Page County

★ **SHENANDOAH MEDICAL CENTER (161366)**, 300 Pershing Avenue, Zip 51601–2397; tel. 712/246–1230, (Total facility includes 53 beds in nursing home–type unit) **A**9 10 18 **F**3 10 11 13 15 24 27 30 31 32 34 38 40 42 52 54 55 56 57 61 62 65 66 67 68 73 74 75 76 77 79 80 86 89 93 94 96 97 100 102 103 105 106 107 118 119 121 122 124 135 136 137 **P**6
Primary Contact: Susan A. McGough, Chief Executive Officer
CFO: Sandra Chesshire, Chief Financial Officer
CMO: Jerry Schaaf, M.D., Chief Medical Officer
Web address: www.shenandoahmedcenter.com
Control: Other not–for–profit (including NFP Corporation) **Service:** General Medical and Surgical

Staffed Beds: 78 **Admissions:** 892 **Census:** 49 **Outpatient Visits:** 118360 **Births:** 107 **Total Expense ($000):** 19217 **Payroll Expense ($000):** 9685 **Personnel:** 234

SIBLEY—Osceola County

★ **OSCEOLA COMMUNITY HOSPITAL (161345)**, Ninth Avenue North, Zip 51249–0258, Mailing Address: P.O. Box 258, Zip 51249–0258; tel. 712/754–2574 **A**9 10 18 **F**3 6 8 9 10 11 13 15 17 24 25 27 28 30 31 32 33 34 38 40 43 44 45 46 49 52 54 55 56 57 60 61 62 63 65 66 68 73 74 75 76 77 79 80 81 82 84 86 96 97 107 115 117 118 119 120 121 122 124 132 133 134 135 136 137 **P**5 **S** Avera Health
Primary Contact: Janet Dykstra, Administrator
CFO: Jerri Palsrok, Business Office Manager
CMO: Douglas J. Miedema, D.O., Chief Medical Officer
CIO: Sherry McElroy, Director Health Information Management
Web address: www.osceolacommunityhospital.org
Control: Other not–for–profit (including NFP Corporation) **Service:** General Medical and Surgical

Staffed Beds: 25 **Admissions:** 438 **Census:** 6 **Outpatient Visits:** 19330 **Births:** 37 **Total Expense ($000):** 7739 **Payroll Expense ($000):** 3025 **Personnel:** 85

SIGOURNEY—Keokuk County

KEOKUK COUNTY HEALTH CENTER (161315), 23019 Highway 149, Zip 52591; tel. 641/622–2720 **A**9 10 18 **F**3 7 11 12 24 25 26 30 31 32 33 36 38 40 42 43 44 46 50 54 55 57 62 63 73 75 82 85 86 87 102 119 121 122 123 124 133 135 137 **P**5 6
Primary Contact: Ray Brownsworth, Chief Executive Officer
CFO: Matthew Ives, Chief Financial Officer
CMO: John Buckingham, M.D., Chief Medical Staff
CIO: Matthew Ives, Chief Financial Officer
CHR: Larry Driscoll, Director Human Resources
Web address: www.kchc.net
Control: Hospital district or authority, Government, nonfederal **Service:** General Medical and Surgical

Staffed Beds: 14 **Admissions:** 183 **Census:** 8 **Outpatient Visits:** 5932 **Births:** 0 **Personnel:** 70

SIOUX CENTER—Sioux County

★ **SIOUX CENTER COMMUNITY HOSPITAL/HEALTH CENTER (161346)**, 605 South Main Avenue, Zip 51250–1398; tel. 712/722–1271, (Total facility includes 69 beds in nursing home–type unit) **A**9 10 18 **F**3 8 10 13 15 17 24 25 26 27 30 31 33 34 38 42 43 44 45 55 57 61 62 65 66 72 73 74 75 76 77 79 81 84 86 87 96 97 102 105 107 115 117 119 120 121 122 124 132 133 135 136 137 **P**6 **S** Avera Health
Primary Contact: Wayne Muth, Interim Chief Executive Officer
COO: Marla Toering, Chief Operating Officer
CFO: Nancy Carlson, Director Finance
CHR: Gail Vonk, Director Human Resources and Marketing
Web address: www.schospital.org
Control: Other not–for–profit (including NFP Corporation) **Service:** General Medical and Surgical

Staffed Beds: 90 **Admissions:** 723 **Census:** 76 **Outpatient Visits:** 51052 **Births:** 196 **Total Expense ($000):** 24126 **Payroll Expense ($000):** 11489 **Personnel:** 307

SIOUX CITY—Woodbury County

★□ **MERCY MEDICAL CENTER–SIOUX CITY (160153)**, 801 Fifth Street, Zip 51101–1326, Mailing Address: P.O. Box 3168, Zip 51102–3168; tel. 712/279–2010 **A**1 2 3 5 9 10 **F**3 5 11 13 15 17 18 20 22 24 25 26 28 30 31 32 33 34 35 36 38 40 41 43 44 49 50 54 55 56 57 60 62 63 66 67 68 69 72 73 74 75 76 77 79 80 81 82 84 85 86 87 88 89 90 91 92 93 94 95 96 97 100 102 107 112 113 114 117 118 119 121 123 124 133 135 137 **P**6 7 8 **S** Trinity Health
Primary Contact: Paul Dougherty, President and Chief Executive Officer
COO: Mari Kaptain–Dahlen, Chief Operating Officer
CFO: Mel Goin, Chief Financial Officer
CMO: Larry W. Sellers, M.D., Chief Medical Officer
CIO: Steve Larson, Director Information Systems
CHR: Julie Anfinson, Director Human Resources
Web address: www.mercysiouxcity.com
Control: Church–operated, Nongovernment, not–for profit **Service:** General Medical and Surgical

Staffed Beds: 258 **Admissions:** 11563 **Census:** 158 **Outpatient Visits:** 327655 **Births:** 543 **Total Expense ($000):** 183938 **Payroll Expense ($000):** 80525 **Personnel:** 1525

IA

Hospital, Medicare Provider Number, Address, Telephone, Approval, Facility, and Physician Codes, Health Care System

★ American Hospital Association (AHA) membership
□ The Joint Commission accreditation
○ American Osteopathic Association (AOA) accreditation
△ Commission on Accreditation of Rehabilitation Facilities (CARF) accreditation

★ **ST. LUKE'S REGIONAL MEDICAL CENTER (160146)**, 2720 Stone Park Boulevard, Zip 51104–2000; tel. 712/279–3500 **A**1 3 5 9 10 **F**3 11 13 15 18 20 24 25 26 28 30 31 32 33 37 38 42 43 44 49 50 51 53 55 56 57 59 61 62 66 68 70 71 72 73 74 75 76 77 79 81 83 84 85 86 87 88 92 95 96 97 100 102 106 107 118 119 120 121 124 131 134 135 136 **P**6 **S** Iowa Health System
Primary Contact: Peter W. Thoreen, President and Chief Executive Officer
COO: Patricia Denzer, Senior Vice President and Chief Operating Officer
CFO: Mark Johnson, Vice President and Chief Financial Officer
CMO: Richard D. Hildebrand, M.D., Vice President Medical Affairs and Chief Medical Officer
CIO: Mark Johnson, Vice President and Chief Financial Officer
CHR: Gary Johnson, Director Human Resources
Web address: www.stlukes.org
Control: Other not–for–profit (including NFP Corporation) **Service:** General Medical and Surgical

Staffed Beds: 146 **Admissions:** 8755 **Census:** 98 **Outpatient Visits:** 78665 **Births:** 2072 **Total Expense ($000):** 104182 **Payroll Expense ($000):** 41104 **Personnel:** 889

SPENCER—Clay County

★ **SPENCER HOSPITAL (160112)**, 1200 First Avenue East, Zip 51301; tel. 712/264–6111 **A**9 10 **F**7 8 11 13 15 24 25 26 27 30 31 32 33 38 40 42 43 44 50 52 54 55 56 57 59 61 62 67 68 73 74 75 76 79 81 82 86 88 89 90 91 92 93 94 95 96 97 98 100 101 106 107 109 118 119 120 121 122 124 135 137 **P**5
Primary Contact: Douglas Doorn, President and Chief Executive Officer
COO: Jason Harrington, Vice President
CFO: Lois Morris, Chief Financial Officer
CIO: Matt Wrather, Director Information Systems
Web address: www.spencerhospital.org
Control: City–Government, nonfederal **Service:** General Medical and Surgical

Staffed Beds: 80 **Admissions:** 3330 **Census:** 39 **Outpatient Visits:** 35874 **Births:** 272 **Total Expense ($000):** 51534 **Payroll Expense ($000):** 19434 **Personnel:** 480

SPIRIT LAKE—Dickinson County

LAKES REGIONAL HEALTHCARE (160124), Highway 71 South, Zip 51360–6810, Mailing Address: P.O. Box AB, Zip 51360–6810; tel. 712/336–1230 **A**9 10 **F**7 11 13 15 24 27 30 31 32 33 38 40 42 55 57 61 62 63 67 68 73 74 75 76 77 79 80 86 96 100 102 107 118 119 121 122 132 135 137
Primary Contact: Richard C. Kielman, President and Chief Executive Officer
CFO: Gordon Larson, Senior Vice President
Web address: www.lakeshealth.org
Control: County–Government, nonfederal **Service:** General Medical and Surgical

Staffed Beds: 28 **Admissions:** 1588 **Census:** 16 **Outpatient Visits:** 31021 **Births:** 178 **Total Expense ($000):** 21840 **Payroll Expense ($000):** 8806 **Personnel:** 195

STORM LAKE—Buena Vista County

★ **BUENA VISTA REGIONAL MEDICAL CENTER (161375)**, 1525 West Fifth Street, Zip 50588–0309, Mailing Address: P.O. Box 309, Zip 50588–0309; tel. 712/732–4030 **A**1 9 10 18 **F**3 7 8 11 13 15 24 25 26 27 30 31 32 38 42 43 44 52 56 57 61 62 66 68 72 73 74 75 76 77 79 81 82 86 88 93 96 97 99 100 102 105 106 107 118 119 120 121 122 124 135 136 137 **S** Iowa Health System
Primary Contact: Todd Hudspeth, Chief Executive Officer
CFO: Mike Dewerff, Chief Financial Officer
CMO: Mark Schultz, M.D., Chief Medical Staff
CIO: Stan Spack, Director Information Technology
CHR: Carrie Turnquist, Director Human Resources
Web address: www.bvrmc.org
Control: County–Government, nonfederal **Service:** General Medical and Surgical

Staffed Beds: 35 **Admissions:** 1867 **Census:** 24 **Outpatient Visits:** 71979 **Births:** 270 **Total Expense ($000):** 27601 **Payroll Expense ($000):** 12373 **Personnel:** 322

SUMNER—Bremer County

★ **COMMUNITY MEMORIAL HOSPITAL (161320)**, 909 West First Street, Zip 50674–1203, Mailing Address: P.O. Box 148, Zip 50674–0148; tel. 563/578–3275 **A**9 10 18 **F**3 11 15 24 25 31 32 38 55 56 57 62 79 80 81 87 96 117 118 120 122 124 137 **P**5 6 **S** Iowa Health System
Primary Contact: Mary Wells, Administrator
CFO: Sara Trainor, Chief Financial Officer
CMO: Mary Pat Rosman, Chief Medical Staff
CHR: Robin Elliott, Personnel Officer
Control: Other not–for–profit (including NFP Corporation) **Service:** General Medical and Surgical

Staffed Beds: 25 **Admissions:** 257 **Census:** 3 **Outpatient Visits:** 11137 **Births:** 0 **Total Expense ($000):** 6915 **Payroll Expense ($000):** 2844 **Personnel:** 71

VINTON—Benton County

★ **VIRGINIA GAY HOSPITAL (161349)**, 502 North Ninth Avenue, Zip 52349–2299; tel. 319/472–6200, (Total facility includes 50 beds in nursing home–type unit) **A**9 10 18 **F**24 25 26 30 31 32 33 38 40 54 55 57 61 62 63 64 73 75 79 80 81 86 87 96 102 115 119 120 121 122 124 132 **P**6
Primary Contact: Michael J. Riege, Chief Executive Officer
CFO: Julia Meadows, Chief Financial Officer
CMO: Brian Meeker, D.O., President Medical Staff
CHR: Kim Frank, Chief Human Resources Officer
Web address: www.vghinc.com
Control: Other not–for–profit (including NFP Corporation) **Service:** General Medical and Surgical

Staffed Beds: 83 **Admissions:** 453 **Census:** 107 **Outpatient Visits:** 82872 **Births:** 0 **Total Expense ($000):** 13975 **Payroll Expense ($000):** 5134 **Personnel:** 165

WASHINGTON—Washington County

★ **WASHINGTON COUNTY HOSPITAL (161344)**, 400 East Polk Street, Zip 52353, Mailing Address: P.O. Box 909, Zip 52353–0909; tel. 319/653–5481, (Total facility includes 43 beds in nursing home–type unit) **A**9 10 18 **F**3 13 15 24 25 26 30 38 40 43 44 55 56 57 62 65 66 67 73 74 79 80 81 86 96 102 113 114 119 122 135 136 **P**6
Primary Contact: Donald E. Patterson, Chief Executive Officer
CFO: Greg Seubert, Chief Financial Officer
CIO: Jennifer Durst, Director Information Services
CHR: Tracy Ousey, Director Human Resources
Web address: www.wchc.org
Control: County–Government, nonfederal **Service:** General Medical and Surgical

Staffed Beds: 68 **Admissions:** 2029 **Census:** 56 **Outpatient Visits:** 43887 **Births:** 83 **Total Expense ($000):** 17716 **Payroll Expense ($000):** 8609 **Personnel:** 205

WATERLOO—Black Hawk County

★ **ALLEN MEMORIAL HOSPITAL (160110)**, 1825 Logan Avenue, Zip 50703–1916; tel. 319/235–3941, (Total facility includes 24 beds in nursing home–type unit) **A**1 3 5 9 10 **F**3 5 8 11 13 15 17 18 20 22 24 25 26 27 30 32 33 34 37 38 40 43 48 49 51 52 53 54 55 56 57 61 62 64 66 68 70 72 73 74 75 76 77 79 80 81 82 83 84 86 87 88 89 90 91 92 93 94 95 96 97 100 102 106 107 113 117 118 119 121 123 124 132 135 136 137 **P**6 8 **S** Iowa Health System
Primary Contact: Richard A. Seidler, FACHE, Chief Executive Officer
COO: Sara Poling, Senior Vice President and Chief Operating Officer
CFO: Renee Rasmussen, Senior Vice President and Chief Financial Officer
CMO: Jeff Crandall, M.D., Chief Medical Officer
Web address: www.allenhospital.org
Control: Other not–for–profit (including NFP Corporation) **Service:** General Medical and Surgical

Staffed Beds: 225 **Admissions:** 11287 **Census:** 120 **Outpatient Visits:** 270805 **Births:** 1075 **Total Expense ($000):** 162328 **Payroll Expense ($000):** 66957 **Personnel:** 1316

★ △ **COVENANT MEDICAL CENTER (160067)**, 3421 West Ninth Street, Zip 50702–5499; tel. 319/272–8000, (Includes KIMBALL–RIDGE CENTER, 2101 Kimball Avenue, Zip 50702), (Total facility includes 44 beds in nursing home–type unit) **A**1 2 3 5 7 9 10 **F**3 4 5 7 8 11 13 15 18 20 24 25 26 27 29 30 31 32 33 34 36 37 38 40 41 43 44 46 49 52 55 56 57 59 60 61 62 66 68 69 70 72 73 74 75 76 77 79 81 84 85 86 87 88 89 90 91 92 94 95 96 97 100 102 106 107 117 118 119 120 121 123 124 132 133 135 136 137 **P**1 6 **S** Wheaton Franciscan Healthcare
Primary Contact: Jack Dusenbery, President and Chief Executive Officer
COO: David Olejniczak, Chief Operating Officer
CFO: Michele Panicucci, Senior Vice President and Chief Financial Officer
CMO: Paul Franke, M.D., Vice President Medical Affairs
CIO: Todd Richardson, Regional Director Information Services
CHR: Vicki L. Parsons, Regional Vice President Human Resources
Web address: www.covhealth.com
Control: Church–operated, Nongovernment, not–for profit **Service:** General Medical and Surgical

Staffed Beds: 275 **Admissions:** 10179 **Census:** 134 **Outpatient Visits:** 728799 **Births:** 1583 **Total Expense ($000):** 232324 **Payroll Expense ($000):** 108760 **Personnel:** 2060

WAUKON—Allamakee County

VETERANS MEMORIAL HOSPITAL (161318), 40 First Street S.E., Zip 52172–2099; tel. 563/568–3411 **A**9 10 18 **F**7 11 13 15 24 27 30 31 32 33 38 46 55 56 57 61 62 73 74 76 77 79 96 120 121 122 123 133 135
Primary Contact: Michael D. Myers, Chief Executive Officer
COO: Fred Mathews, Purchasing Director
CFO: Scott Knode, Chief Financial Officer
CHR: Erin Berns, Director Human Resources
Web address: www.vmhospital.com
Control: City–Government, nonfederal **Service:** General Medical and Surgical

Staffed Beds: 25 **Admissions:** 701 **Census:** 7 **Outpatient Visits:** 48514 **Births:** 92 **Total Expense ($000):** 10302 **Payroll Expense ($000):** 4662 **Personnel:** 131

Many Facility Codes have changed. Please refer to the AHA Guide Code Chart.

WAVERLY—Bremer County

☒ **WAVERLY HEALTH CENTER (161339)**, 312 Ninth Street S.W., Zip 50677–2999; tel. 319/352–4120 **A**1 9 10 18 **F**3 7 8 11 13 15 24 30 33 38 40 42 52 55 56 57 61 62 66 73 74 75 79 80 81 96 100 102 107 119 121 122 123 124 135 136 **P**6
Primary Contact: Michael D. Trachta, Chief Executive Officer
COO: Elly Steffen, Chief Operating Officer
CFO: Lisa Bennett, CPA, Chief Financial Officer
CIO: Jerry Tiedt, Director Information Systems
CHR: Karen Buls, Director Human Resources
Web address: www.waverlyhealthcenter.org
Control: City–Government, nonfederal **Service:** General Medical and Surgical

Staffed Beds: 25 **Admissions:** 1213 **Census:** 11 **Outpatient Visits:** 58436 **Births:** 215 **Total Expense ($000):** 32645 **Payroll Expense ($000):** 13166 **Personnel:** 249

WEBSTER CITY—Hamilton County

★ **HAMILTON HOSPITAL (161361)**, 800 Ohio Street, Zip 50595–2824, Mailing Address: P.O. Box 430, Zip 50595–0430; tel. 515/832–9400 **A**9 10 18 **F**3 7 11 13 15 24 25 31 32 33 36 38 40 41 42 43 57 62 68 73 74 75 77 79 80 81 82 84 86 96 107 118 119 121 122 124 135 136
Primary Contact: Palmer Schneider, Administrator
CFO: Alice Heinrichs, CPA, Chief Financial Officer
CMO: J. X. Latella, M.D., Chief of Staff
CIO: Dave Dawson, Director Information Services
CHR: Douglas Crimmins, Director Human Resources
Web address: www.hamiltonhospital.com
Control: County–Government, nonfederal **Service:** General Medical and Surgical

Staffed Beds: 25 **Admissions:** 1256 **Census:** 13 **Outpatient Visits:** 15521 **Births:** 108 **Total Expense ($000):** 15543 **Payroll Expense ($000):** 7018 **Personnel:** 163

WEST BURLINGTON—Des Moines County

☒ △ **GREAT RIVER MEDICAL CENTER (160057)**, 1221 South Gear Avenue, Zip 52655–1681; tel. 319/768–1000, (Total facility includes 165 beds in nursing home–type unit) **A**1 7 9 10 19 **F**3 5 11 13 15 18 20 24 25 26 28 30 31 32 33 34 36 38 40 42 43 44 50 52 55 56 57 59 61 62 65 66 67 68 71 73 74 75 76 77 79 80 81 82 84 85 86 88 89 90 91 92 93 94 96 97 99 100 102 106 107 109 111 116 117 118 119 120 121 132 135 136 137 **P**6
Primary Contact: Mark D. Richardson, President and Chief Executive Officer
CFO: Todd J. Sladky, Chief Financial Officer
CMO: Carl Hays, M.D., Chief of Staff
CIO: Gary Davis, Director Information Systems
CHR: Ron Halligan, Vice President Human Resources
Web address: www.greatrivermedical.org
Control: Other not–for–profit (including NFP Corporation) **Service:** General Medical and Surgical

Staffed Beds: 378 **Admissions:** 8307 **Census:** 225 **Outpatient Visits:** 225000 **Births:** 652 **Total Expense ($000):** 125877 **Payroll Expense ($000):** 54121 **Personnel:** 942

WEST UNION—Fayette County

★ **PALMER LUTHERAN HEALTH CENTER (161316)**, 112 Jefferson Street, Zip 52175–1022; tel. 563/422–3811 **A**9 10 18 **F**3 8 11 13 15 24 25 26 27 31 32 38 40 42 43 54 55 56 57 61 62 63 66 68 74 75 76 77 79 80 81 86 96 100 102 107 117 118 119 120 121 122 124 133 135 137
Primary Contact: Debrah Chensvold, President and Chief Executive Officer
CFO: Joni Gisleson, Director Finance
CMO: Chaudri Rasool, M.D., Chief of Staff
CIO: Kurt Chicken, Director Support Services
CHR: Cheryl Meyer, Director Human Resources
Web address: www.palmerlutheran.org
Control: Other not–for–profit (including NFP Corporation) **Service:** General Medical and Surgical

Staffed Beds: 25 **Admissions:** 554 **Census:** 6 **Outpatient Visits:** 46365 **Births:** 108 **Total Expense ($000):** 14053 **Payroll Expense ($000):** 6172 **Personnel:** 166

WINTERSET—Madison County

★ **MADISON COUNTY HEALTHCARE SYSTEM (161326)**, (Formerly Madison County Memorial Hospital), 300 Hutchings Street, Zip 50273–2199; tel. 515/462–2373 **A**9 10 18 **F**4 5 15 24 27 30 32 33 38 40 42 55 57 61 68 76 79 84 86 87 89 91 92 93 94 96 102 107 117 118 119 120 121 122 123 124 135 **P**6
Primary Contact: Marcia Harris, Chief Executive Officer
CFO: Rebekah Mitchell, Chief Financial Officer
CMO: Amy Kimball, D.O., Chief of Staff
CHR: Jennifer Hannon, Manager Human Resources
Web address: www.madisonhealth.com
Control: County–Government, nonfederal **Service:** General Medical and Surgical

Staffed Beds: 22 **Admissions:** 702 **Census:** 9 **Outpatient Visits:** 68600 **Births:** 1 **Total Expense ($000):** 13721 **Payroll Expense ($000):** 6228 **Personnel:** 145

IA

Hospital, Medicare Provider Number, Address, Telephone, Approval, Facility, and Physician Codes, Health Care System
★ American Hospital Association (AHA) membership
☐ The Joint Commission accreditation
○ American Osteopathic Association (AOA) accreditation
△ Commission on Accreditation of Rehabilitation Facilities (CARF) accreditation

KANSAS

ABILENE—Dickinson County

★ **MEMORIAL HEALTH SYSTEM (171381)**, 511 N.E. Tenth Street, Zip 67410; tel. 785/263–2100, (Total facility includes 72 beds in nursing home–type unit) **A**9 10 18 **F**3 7 13 15 24 25 27 31 38 42 52 55 56 57 61 62 66 67 69 73 74 75 76 77 79 80 82 84 86 88 93 96 97 100 102 107 117 119 120 121 122 124 132 135 137
Primary Contact: Mark A. Miller, Chief Executive Officer
COO: Robert Brazil, Chief Operating Officer
CFO: Elgin Glanzer, Chief Financial Officer
CMO: W L Short, M.D., Chairman
CIO: Blaine Cappel, Director Information Systems
CHR: Robert Brazil, Chief Operating Officer
Web address: www.mhsks.org
Control: Hospital district or authority, Government, nonfederal **Service:** General Medical and Surgical

Staffed Beds: 107 **Admissions:** 1215 **Census:** 82 **Outpatient Visits:** 22223 **Births:** 98 **Total Expense ($000):** 16580 **Payroll Expense ($000):** 8571 **Personnel:** 272

ANDOVER—Butler County

KANSAS MEDICAL CENTER (170197), 1124 West 21st Street, Zip 67002; tel. 316/300–4000 **A**10 **F**3 18 20 22 25 26 31 32 38 43 49 62 68 73 77 79 80 82 103 107 119 134 135
Primary Contact: Badr Idbeis, M.D., Chief Executive Officer
COO: Daryl W. Thornton, Chief Operating Officer
Control: Corporation, Investor–owned, for–profit **Service:** General Medical and Surgical

Staffed Beds: 35 **Admissions:** 1944 **Census:** 23 **Outpatient Visits:** 6685 **Births:** 0 **Personnel:** 186

ANTHONY—Harper County

★ **HOSPITAL DISTRICT NUMBER SIX OF HARPER COUNTY (171346)**, 1101 East Spring Street, Zip 67003–2122; tel. 620/842–5111 **A**9 10 18 **F**27 31 32 38 48 52 55 62 65 75 76 79 86 87 96 107 117 122 **P**6
Primary Contact: J. Bryant Anderson, Administrator and Chief Executive Officer
CFO: Lori Allen, Chief Financial Officer
CHR: Kim Barwick, Administrative Assistant
Control: Hospital district or authority, Government, nonfederal **Service:** General Medical and Surgical

Staffed Beds: 25 **Admissions:** 270 **Census:** 13 **Outpatient Visits:** 23603 **Births:** 0 **Total Expense ($000):** 7079 **Payroll Expense ($000):** 3565 **Personnel:** 99

ARKANSAS CITY—Cowley County

★ **SOUTH CENTRAL KANSAS REGIONAL MEDICAL CENTER (170150)**, 216 West Birch Avenue, Zip 67005–1598, Mailing Address: P.O. Box 1107, Zip 67005–1107; tel. 620/442–2500 **A**9 10 **F**11 13 15 25 26 33 37 38 43 55 57 61 62 66 67 68 73 74 75 77 79 82 86 87 92 96 97 99 100 101 102 107 118 119 122 134 137
Primary Contact: Phyllis Macy–Mills, Administrator and Chief Executive Officer
CFO: Pam Jackson, CPA, Chief Financial Officer
CMO: Rhonda Green, M.D., Chief Medical Staff
Web address: www.sckrmc.com
Control: City–Government, nonfederal **Service:** General Medical and Surgical

Staffed Beds: 33 **Admissions:** 1006 **Census:** 12 **Outpatient Visits:** 66458 **Births:** 136 **Total Expense ($000):** 11951 **Payroll Expense ($000):** 5617 **Personnel:** 155

ASHLAND—Clark County

★ **ASHLAND HEALTH CENTER (171304)**, 709 Oak Street, Zip 67831–0188, Mailing Address: P.O. Box 188, Zip 67831–0188; tel. 620/635–2241, (Total facility includes 35 beds in nursing home–type unit) **A**9 10 18 **F**2 26 38 52 56 57 61 62 65 66 80 82 86 96 117 122 132 **P**6 **S** Great Plains Health Alliance, Inc.
Primary Contact: Daryl Marshall, Administrator
CFO: Debbie Filson, Chief Financial Officer and Manager Business Office
Web address: www.ashlandks.com/healthserv.htm
Control: Hospital district or authority, Government, nonfederal **Service:** General Medical and Surgical

Staffed Beds: 47 **Admissions:** 169 **Census:** 25 **Outpatient Visits:** 19411 **Births:** 0 **Total Expense ($000):** 4157 **Payroll Expense ($000):** 1898 **Personnel:** 61

ATCHISON—Atchison County

★ ○ **ATCHISON HOSPITAL (171382)**, 1301 North Second Street, Zip 66002–1297; tel. 913/367–2131 **A**9 10 11 18 **F**3 7 8 11 12 13 15 24 25 26 27 30 31 32 33 38 42 43 50 55 56 57 61 62 66 68 74 75 77 79 80 82 84 86 87 96 97 100 106 107 118 119 120 121 122 124 135 136 **P**6
Primary Contact: John L. Jacobson, President and Chief Executive Officer
CFO: Lorne J. Archer, Vice President Finance and Chief Financial Officer
CMO: Dina Seibert, D.O., Chief of Staff
CIO: Mike Boos, Manager Information Systems
CHR: Shari Boos, Director Human Resources
Web address: www.atchisonhospital.org
Control: Other not–for–profit (including NFP Corporation) **Service:** General Medical and Surgical

Staffed Beds: 25 **Admissions:** 1279 **Census:** 10 **Outpatient Visits:** 37412 **Births:** 157 **Total Expense ($000):** 22927 **Payroll Expense ($000):** 11470 **Personnel:** 234

ATWOOD—Rawlins County

★ **RAWLINS COUNTY HEALTH CENTER (171307)**, 707 Grant Street, Zip 67730–4700, Mailing Address: P.O. Box 47, Zip 67730–4700; tel. 785/626–3211 **A**9 10 18 **F**3 24 26 30 31 32 38 55 62 73 79 80 86 96 115 117 122 124 135 137 **P**6 **S** Great Plains Health Alliance, Inc.
Primary Contact: Deanna Freeman, Administrator and Chief Executive Officer
CFO: Heather Prideaux, Director Finance
Web address: www.rchc.us
Control: County–Government, nonfederal **Service:** General Medical and Surgical

Staffed Beds: 24 **Admissions:** 375 **Census:** 4 **Outpatient Visits:** 17370 **Births:** 0 **Total Expense ($000):** 4752 **Payroll Expense ($000):** 2350 **Personnel:** 57

BELLEVILLE—Republic County

⊠ **REPUBLIC COUNTY HOSPITAL (171361)**, 2420 G Street, Zip 66935–2400; tel. 785/527–2254, (Total facility includes 38 beds in nursing home–type unit) **A**1 9 10 18 **F**3 13 15 24 25 26 27 30 31 33 37 38 54 55 62 65 66 73 74 75 76 77 79 80 81 82 84 86 96 97 107 117 119 120 122 **S** Great Plains Health Alliance, Inc.
Primary Contact: Blaine K. Miller, Administrator
CFO: Barry Bottger, Chief Financial Officer
Web address: www.rphospital.org
Control: Other not–for–profit (including NFP Corporation) **Service:** General Medical and Surgical

Staffed Beds: 63 **Admissions:** 1297 **Census:** 51 **Outpatient Visits:** 12162 **Births:** 58 **Total Expense ($000):** 10841 **Payroll Expense ($000):** 5154 **Personnel:** 168

BELOIT—Mitchell County

★ **MITCHELL COUNTY HOSPITAL HEALTH SYSTEMS (171375)**, 400 West Eighth, Zip 67420–1605, Mailing Address: P.O. Box 399, Zip 67420–0399; tel. 785/738–2266, (Total facility includes 40 beds in nursing home–type unit) **A**9 10 18 **F**11 13 15 24 25 30 31 33 38 42 43 50 54 61 62 65 66 67 75 79 81 86 88 93 96 100 102 107 119 121 122 124 137
Primary Contact: David Dick, Chief Executive Officer
CFO: Eldon Koepke, Chief Financial Officer
CIO: Mark Marihugh, Director Information Technology
CHR: Phyllis Oetting, Director Human Resources
Web address: www.mchks.com
Control: Other not–for–profit (including NFP Corporation) **Service:** General Medical and Surgical

Staffed Beds: 75 **Admissions:** 1463 **Census:** 51 **Outpatient Visits:** 16801 **Births:** 98 **Total Expense ($000):** 18754 **Payroll Expense ($000):** 7867 **Personnel:** 229

BURLINGTON—Coffey County

★ **COFFEY COUNTY HOSPITAL (170094)**, 801 North Fourth Street, Zip 66839–0189, Mailing Address: P.O. Box 189, Zip 66839–0189; tel. 620/364–2121, (Total facility includes 42 beds in nursing home–type unit) **A**9 10 20 **F**3 7 10 11 13 15 17 26 27 30 31 32 38 55 57 61 62 65 68 73 74 75 76 77 79 80 82 96 100 102 107 117 119 122 135 **P**6
Primary Contact: Dennis L. George, Chief Executive Officer
CFO: James H. Garner, Chief Financial Officer
CHR: Larry V. Gales, Director Human Resources
Web address: www.coffeyhealth.org
Control: County–Government, nonfederal **Service:** General Medical and Surgical

Staffed Beds: 78 **Admissions:** 1467 **Census:** 47 **Outpatient Visits:** 18891 **Births:** 101 **Total Expense ($000):** 20107 **Payroll Expense ($000):** 8942 **Personnel:** 205

Many Facility Codes have changed. Please refer to the AHA Guide Code Chart.

CALDWELL—Sumner County

★ **SUMNER COUNTY HOSPITAL DISTRICT ONE (171329)**, 601 South Osage Street, Zip 67022–1654; tel. 620/845–6492 **A**9 10 18 **F**7 11 38 55 61 65 73 79 86 96 100 107 118 122 **P**5
Primary Contact: Virgil Watson, Administrator
CFO: Paul Bowerman, CPA, Certified Public Accountant
CMO: Jim Blunk, D.O., Chief Medical Officer
CIO: Jennifer Marcrun, Chief Financial Officer
CHR: Tammy Albright, Director Human Resources and Quality Assurance
Web address: www.schd1.com
Control: Hospital district or authority, Government, nonfederal **Service:** General Medical and Surgical

Staffed Beds: 25 **Admissions:** 156 **Census:** 4 **Outpatient Visits:** 5256 **Births:** 0 **Total Expense ($000):** 4152 **Payroll Expense ($000):** 1930 **Personnel:** 62

CHANUTE—Neosho County

★ **NEOSHO MEMORIAL REGIONAL MEDICAL CENTER (171380)**, 629 South Plummer, Zip 66720–0426, Mailing Address: P.O. Box 426, Zip 66720–0426; tel. 620/431–4000 **A**9 10 18 **F**3 7 11 13 15 24 25 30 31 38 42 52 55 61 62 68 74 75 77 79 80 84 86 96 97 100 102 107 117 118 119 122 124 132 135 **P**8 **S** QHR
Primary Contact: Dennis Franks, FACHE, Chief Executive Officer
CFO: Nancy Woodyard, Chief Financial Officer
CMO: Robert Thomen, M.D., Chief Medical Officer
CIO: Gretchen Keller, Director Health Information
CHR: R. C. Rowan, Director Human Resources
Web address: www.nmrmc.com
Control: County–Government, nonfederal **Service:** General Medical and Surgical

Staffed Beds: 25 **Admissions:** 2223 **Census:** 19 **Outpatient Visits:** 23817 **Births:** 376 **Total Expense ($000):** 26063 **Payroll Expense ($000):** 11216 **Personnel:** 276

CLAY CENTER—Clay County

★ **CLAY COUNTY MEDICAL CENTER (171371)**, 617 Liberty Street, Zip 67432–0512, Mailing Address: P.O. Box 512, Zip 67432–0512; tel. 785/632–2144 **A**9 10 18 **F**13 15 24 26 27 30 31 32 38 42 43 44 50 51 52 57 62 65 66 68 72 73 74 75 76 77 79 80 81 82 83 84 86 97 100 102 107 117 119 121 122 137
Primary Contact: Ron Bender, Chief Executive Officer
CFO: Jim Brinkman, Chief Financial Officer
CIO: Jim Seley, Chief Information Officer
CHR: Cindy Rush, Director Human Resources
Web address: www.ccmcks.org
Control: County–Government, nonfederal **Service:** General Medical and Surgical

Staffed Beds: 25 **Admissions:** 1054 **Census:** 13 **Outpatient Visits:** 43651 **Births:** 65 **Total Expense ($000):** 13363 **Payroll Expense ($000):** 6316 **Personnel:** 182

COFFEYVILLE—Montgomery County

★□ **COFFEYVILLE REGIONAL MEDICAL CENTER (170145)**, 1400 West Fourth, Zip 67337–0856; tel. 620/251–1200, (Total facility includes 20 beds in nursing home–type unit) **A**1 2 9 10 **F**3 11 13 15 24 25 26 27 30 31 32 38 54 55 56 57 61 66 68 73 74 75 76 77 79 85 86 88 89 93 96 97 102 103 107 117 119 121 124 136 **P**1 8 **S** QHR
Primary Contact: Gerald J. Marquette, Jr., Chief Executive Officer
COO: Gerald J. Marquette, Chief Executive Officer
CFO: John C. Hester, Chief Financial Officer
CIO: Doug Stacy, Chief Information Officer
CHR: Becky McCune, Director Human Resources, Community Relations and Education
Web address: www.crmcinc.com
Control: Other not–for–profit (including NFP Corporation) **Service:** General Medical and Surgical

Staffed Beds: 105 **Admissions:** 4520 **Census:** 56 **Outpatient Visits:** 44849 **Births:** 235 **Total Expense ($000):** 37653 **Payroll Expense ($000):** 16171 **Personnel:** 439

COLBY—Thomas County

CITIZENS MEDICAL CENTER (171362), 100 East College Drive, Zip 67701–3799; tel. 785/462–7511, (Total facility includes 68 beds in nursing home–type unit) **A**9 10 18 **F**3 10 11 13 15 24 26 27 30 32 38 56 62 65 72 74 75 77 79 80 81 82 86 87 96 97 100 102 107 119 122 135 137 **P**6
Primary Contact: Janice McCart, Chief Executive Officer
CFO: Kevan Trenkle, Chief Financial Officer
CMO: Bruce Kellogg, D.O., Chief Medical Staff
CIO: Rod Williams, Director Information Systems
CHR: Margaret Kummer, Director Human Resources
Web address: www.nwkshealthcare.com
Control: Other not–for–profit (including NFP Corporation) **Service:** General Medical and Surgical

Staffed Beds: 93 **Admissions:** 1304 **Census:** 78 **Outpatient Visits:** 11790 **Births:** 158 **Total Expense ($000):** 18406 **Payroll Expense ($000):** 8036 **Personnel:** 215

COLDWATER—Comanche County

★ **COMANCHE COUNTY HOSPITAL (171312)**, 202 South Frisco Street, Zip 67029, Mailing Address: HC 65, Box 8A, Zip 67029; tel. 620/582–2144 **A**9 10 18 **F**11 27 31 38 52 57 60 61 66 73 75 76 86 92 117 122 **P**6 **S** Great Plains Health Alliance, Inc.
Primary Contact: Nancy Zimmerman, RN, Administrator
CMO: Daniel Schowengerdt, M.D., Chief of Staff
CIO: LaNell Wagnon, Director Medical Records
Web address: www.gpha.com
Control: County–Government, nonfederal **Service:** General Medical and Surgical

Staffed Beds: 14 **Admissions:** 167 **Census:** 4 **Outpatient Visits:** 10410 **Births:** 0 **Total Expense ($000):** 2879 **Payroll Expense ($000):** 1758 **Personnel:** 43

COLUMBUS—Cherokee County

★ **ST. JOHN'S MAUDE NORTON MEMORIAL HOSPITAL (171308)**, 220 North Pennsylvania Street, Zip 66725–1110; tel. 620/429–2545 **A**9 10 18 **F**11 15 31 32 37 38 55 57 75 79 86 107 122 134 **S** Catholic Health Initiatives
Primary Contact: Cindy Neely, Administrator
CMO: Darcy Selenke, M.D., Chief of Staff
Control: Church–operated, Nongovernment, not–for profit **Service:** General Medical and Surgical

Staffed Beds: 18 **Admissions:** 147 **Census:** 2 **Outpatient Visits:** 9958 **Births:** 0 **Total Expense ($000):** 2714 **Payroll Expense ($000):** 1275 **Personnel:** 43

CONCORDIA—Cloud County

CLOUD COUNTY HEALTH CENTER (171349), 1100 Highland Drive, Zip 66901–3923; tel. 785/243–1234 **A**9 10 18 **F**11 13 15 24 27 31 33 38 43 54 55 57 62 63 72 73 74 75 77 79 80 81 82 84 86 87 92 96 97 102 106 107 119 120 121 122 135 137 **P**6
Primary Contact: James E. Wahlmeier, President and Chief Executive Officer
CFO: Patricia M. Moyer, Chief Financial Officer
CMO: Maria Jindra, Chief Medical Staff
CIO: Jerad Monzon, Network Administrator
CHR: Nicole Nelson, Director Human Resources
Web address: www.cchc.com
Control: Other not–for–profit (including NFP Corporation) **Service:** General Medical and Surgical

Staffed Beds: 25 **Admissions:** 910 **Census:** 10 **Outpatient Visits:** 21240 **Births:** 35 **Total Expense ($000):** 11264 **Payroll Expense ($000):** 6042 **Personnel:** 148

COUNCIL GROVE—Morris County

★ **MORRIS COUNTY HOSPITAL (171379)**, 600 North Washington Street, Zip 66846–0275, Mailing Address: P.O. Box 275, Zip 66846–0275; tel. 620/767–6811 **A**9 10 18 **F**7 11 13 15 24 27 30 31 32 33 38 57 62 63 68 74 75 79 82 86 96 119 121 122 135 137 **P**5
Primary Contact: James H. Reagan, Jr., Ph.D., Chief Executive Officer
COO: Beth Voorhees, Chief Nursing Officer
CFO: Ron Christenson, Chief Financial Officer
CMO: Joel Hornuug, M.D., Chief Medical Officer
CIO: Bill Lauer, Chief Information Officer
CHR: Don Zimmerman, Director Human Resources
Web address: www.mrcohosp.com
Control: County–Government, nonfederal **Service:** General Medical and Surgical

Staffed Beds: 25 **Admissions:** 548 **Census:** 6 **Outpatient Visits:** 14450 **Births:** 54 **Total Expense ($000):** 6153 **Payroll Expense ($000):** 2391 **Personnel:** 76

Hospital, Medicare Provider Number, Address, Telephone, Approval, Facility, and Physician Codes, Health Care System

★ American Hospital Association (AHA) membership
□ The Joint Commission accreditation
○ American Osteopathic Association (AOA) accreditation
△ Commission on Accreditation of Rehabilitation Facilities (CARF) accreditation

KS

DIGHTON—Lane County

★ **LANE COUNTY HOSPITAL (171303)**, 235 West Vine, Zip 67839–0969, Mailing Address: P.O. Box 969, Zip 67839–0969; tel. 620/397–5321, (Total facility includes 21 beds in nursing home–type unit) **A**9 10 18 **F**26 38 54 65 75 80 86 87 117 120 122 **P**6 **S** Great Plains Health Alliance, Inc.
Primary Contact: Donna McGowan, Administrator
CFO: Marilyn James, Chief Financial Officer
CMO: Paul Chinburg, M.D., Medical Director
Web address: www.gpha.com
Control: County–Government, nonfederal **Service:** General Medical and Surgical

Staffed Beds: 31 **Admissions:** 200 **Census:** 21 **Outpatient Visits:** 10725
Births: 0 **Total Expense ($000):** 3695 **Payroll Expense ($000):** 1655
Personnel: 38

DODGE CITY—Ford County

★ **WESTERN PLAINS MEDICAL COMPLEX (170175)**, 3001 Avenue A, Zip 67801–6508, Mailing Address: P.O. Box 1478, Zip 67801–1478; tel. 620/225–8400 **A**1 9 10 20 **F**3 11 13 15 18 20 24 25 26 30 31 32 33 38 40 51 57 68 71 72 73 74 75 77 79 80 81 82 83 84 86 96 97 100 103 106 107 118 119 120 122 135 136 137 **S** LifePoint Hospitals, Inc.
Primary Contact: John E. Walker, President and Chief Executive Officer
CFO: Scott Hankinson, Chief Financial Officer
CMO: R. C. Trotter, M.D., Chief Medical Staff
CIO: Shawna Culver, Director Information Systems
CHR: Donna Metcalf, Director Human Resources
Web address: www.westernplainsmc.com
Control: Corporation, Investor–owned, for–profit **Service:** General Medical and Surgical

Staffed Beds: 99 **Admissions:** 3633 **Census:** 32 **Outpatient Visits:** 23509
Births: 742 **Personnel:** 282

EL DORADO—Butler County

★ **SUSAN B. ALLEN MEMORIAL HOSPITAL (170017)**, 720 West Central Avenue, Zip 67042–2112; tel. 316/321–3300 **A**1 9 10 **F**3 11 13 15 24 26 38 57 59 61 67 68 74 79 80 88 93 96 97 100 103 107 109 111 119 122 135 137
Primary Contact: Gayle Arnett, President and Chief Executive Officer
COO: David Shaw, Vice President and Chief Operating Officer
CFO: Gayle Arnett, Vice President and Chief Financial Officer
CIO: Mark Rooker, Director Information Systems
CHR: Gay Kimble, Director Human Resources
Web address: www.sbamh.com
Control: Other not–for–profit (including NFP Corporation) **Service:** General Medical and Surgical

Staffed Beds: 87 **Admissions:** 2759 **Census:** 32 **Outpatient Visits:** 82340
Births: 335 **Total Expense ($000):** 40393 **Payroll Expense ($000):** 17165
Personnel: 377

ELKHART—Morton County

★ **MORTON COUNTY HEALTH SYSTEM (170166)**, 445 Hilltop Street, Zip 67950–0937, Mailing Address: P.O. Box 937, Zip 67950–0937; tel. 620/697–2141, (Total facility includes 80 beds in nursing home–type unit) **A**9 10 20 **F**11 15 25 27 31 38 53 54 55 56 57 62 65 66 68 73 75 79 81 82 86 87 88 89 90 91 92 93 94 96 100 102 107 118 119 120 121 122 132 135 136 137 **P**5 6
Primary Contact: Leonard Hernandez, Chief Executive Officer
CFO: Jeff Weaver, Chief Financial Officer
CHR: Sonja May, Director Human Resources
Web address: www.mchswecare.com
Control: County–Government, nonfederal **Service:** General Medical and Surgical

Staffed Beds: 130 **Admissions:** 1351 **Census:** 93 **Outpatient Visits:** 21203
Births: 0 **Total Expense ($000):** 14178 **Payroll Expense ($000):** 8415
Personnel: 207

ELLINWOOD—Barton County

★ **ELLINWOOD DISTRICT HOSPITAL (171301)**, 605 North Main Street, Zip 67526–1440; tel. 620/564–2548 **A**9 10 18 **F**11 38 62 63 67 96 117 122 134 **P**6 **S** Great Plains Health Alliance, Inc.
Primary Contact: Joyce Schulte, Chief Executive Officer
CFO: Penny Stephenson, Chief Financial Officer
CHR: Deanna Hulse, Human Resources Officer
Web address: www.ellinwood.org
Control: Other not–for–profit (including NFP Corporation) **Service:** General Medical and Surgical

Staffed Beds: 25 **Admissions:** 108 **Census:** 9 **Outpatient Visits:** 9805
Births: 0 **Total Expense ($000):** 3702 **Payroll Expense ($000):** 1566
Personnel: 49

ELLSWORTH—Ellsworth County

★ **ELLSWORTH COUNTY MEDICAL CENTER (171327)**, 1604 Aylward Street, Zip 67439–0087, Mailing Address: P.O. Box 87, Zip 67439–0087; tel. 785/472–3111 **A**9 10 18 **F**3 11 30 31 33 38 47 52 55 65 75 80 81 82 86 96 102 107 117 119 122 124 135
Primary Contact: Roger W. Pearson, Administrator
CFO: Danny D. Urban, Chief Financial
Web address: www.ewmed.com
Control: County–Government, nonfederal **Service:** General Medical and Surgical

Staffed Beds: 20 **Admissions:** 1061 **Census:** 11 **Outpatient Visits:** 13066
Births: 0 **Total Expense ($000):** 12199 **Payroll Expense ($000):** 5743
Personnel: 151

EMPORIA—Lyon County

EMPORIA SURGICAL HOSPITAL (170193), 1602 West 15th Street, Zip 66801; tel. 620/342–8822, (Nonreporting) **A**9 10
Primary Contact: Joseph Conroy, Administrator
Control: Corporation, Investor–owned, for–profit **Service:** Surgical

Staffed Beds: 6

★ ○ **NEWMAN REGIONAL HEALTH (170001)**, 1201 West 12th Avenue, Zip 66801–2597; tel. 620/343–6800 **A**9 10 11 20 **F**3 5 11 13 24 25 26 27 31 32 37 38 42 43 44 51 52 55 57 60 61 62 63 66 68 74 75 76 77 79 80 81 82 84 85 86 90 92 96 97 100 102 106 107 118 119 120 121 122 124 135 136 137 **S** QHR
Primary Contact: Joyce Grove–Hein, Interim Chief Executive Officer
CFO: Holly French, Chief Financial Officer
CMO: James Geitz, M.D., Chief of Staff
CIO: Sheri Rawlings, Information Systems and Security Officer
CHR: Kathy Orear, Director Human Resources
Web address: www.newmanrh.org
Control: County–Government, nonfederal **Service:** General Medical and Surgical

Staffed Beds: 122 **Admissions:** 3897 **Census:** 49 **Outpatient Visits:** 45224
Births: 569 **Total Expense ($000):** 49181 **Payroll Expense ($000):** 20213
Personnel: 472

EUREKA—Greenwood County

★ **GREENWOOD COUNTY HOSPITAL (171339)**, 100 West 16th Street, Zip 67045–1064; tel. 620/583–7451 **A**9 10 18 **F**3 11 15 30 38 55 56 61 75 79 86 96 97 107 **P**5
Primary Contact: Bruce K. Birchell, Administrator and Chief Executive Officer
CFO: Janel Palmer, Chief Financial Officer
CIO: Filiberto J. Ojeda, Director Quality Improvement, Risk Management and Information System
Web address: www.gwch.org
Control: City–County, Government, nonfederal **Service:** General Medical and Surgical

Staffed Beds: 25 **Admissions:** 652 **Census:** 5 **Outpatient Visits:** 14030
Births: 0 **Total Expense ($000):** 11029 **Payroll Expense ($000):** 5067
Personnel: 140

FORT SCOTT—Bourbon County

★ △ **MERCY HEALTH CENTER–FORT SCOTT (170058)**, 401 Woodland Hills Boulevard, Zip 66701–8797; tel. 620/223–2200 **A**7 9 10 **F**3 7 11 13 15 24 26 31 32 33 38 45 52 55 56 57 61 68 70 73 74 75 77 79 85 86 87 96 97 99 100 102 107 119 120 121 122 132 135 137 **P**6 **S** Sisters of Mercy Health System
Primary Contact: John T. Woodrich, Chief Executive Officer
COO: Reta Baker, Chief Operating Officer
CFO: Terri Del Chiaro, Chief Financial Officer
CMO: Robert R. Nichols, M.D., Vice President Medical Affairs
CHR: Eric Ammons, Director Rehabilitation Services and Physical Therapy
Web address: www.mercykansas.com
Control: Church–operated, Nongovernment, not–for profit **Service:** General Medical and Surgical

Staffed Beds: 72 **Admissions:** 2706 **Census:** 30 **Outpatient Visits:** 52715
Births: 287 **Total Expense ($000):** 33530 **Payroll Expense ($000):** 15632
Personnel: 379

FREDONIA—Wilson County

★ **FREDONIA REGIONAL HOSPITAL (171374)**, 1527 Madison Street, Zip 66736–1751, Mailing Address: P.O. Box 579, Zip 66736–0579; tel. 620/378–2121 **A**9 10 18 **F**7 11 15 26 30 31 38 61 79 80 86 88 93 96 107 117 122 **S** Great Plains Health Alliance, Inc.
Primary Contact: Terry Deschaine, Chief Executive Officer
CFO: Bryan Coffey, Chief Financial Officer
CHR: Debbie Marr, Director Human Resources
Web address: www.gpha.com
Control: City–Government, nonfederal **Service:** General Medical and Surgical

Staffed Beds: 34 **Admissions:** 1372 **Census:** 21 **Outpatient Visits:** 13211
Births: 0 **Total Expense ($000):** 9634 **Payroll Expense ($000):** 3737
Personnel: 106

GARDEN CITY—Finney County

☐ **ST. CATHERINE HOSPITAL (170023)**, 401 East Spuce Street, Zip 67846–5679; tel. 620/272–2561 **A**1 5 9 10 20 **F**3 13 15 25 26 30 31 32 33 38 42 43 44 55 56 57 61 62 66 68 71 72 73 74 75 77 79 80 81 82 84 86 87 88 90 92 96 97 98 100 103 106 107 108 109 110 111 112 114 118 119 121 124 130 135 **P**5 6 7 **S** Catholic Health Initiatives
Primary Contact: Scott J. Taylor, President and Chief Executive Officer
CFO: Amanda Vaughan, Chief Financial Officer
CMO: James W. Bruno, Chief Medical Officer
CIO: Victor Hawkins, Executive Director Marketing and Development
CHR: Bennie Salkil, Executive Director Human Resources
Web address: www.stcath–hosp.org
Control: Church–operated, Nongovernment, not–for profit **Service:** General Medical and Surgical

Staffed Beds: 101 **Admissions:** 4215 **Census:** 51 **Outpatient Visits:** 140936 **Births:** 900 **Total Expense ($000):** 73680 **Payroll Expense ($000):** 27489 **Personnel:** 630

GARDNER—Johnson County

MEADOWBROOK REHABILITATION HOSPITAL (170180), 427 West Main Street, Zip 66030–1183; tel. 913/856–8747, (Total facility includes 40 beds in nursing home–type unit) **A**10 **F**85 86 117 119 132 137
Primary Contact: Sharon L. Bingham, Administrator
COO: Pam Hall, Chief Operating Officer
CFO: Carla Nagy, Business Manager
CMO: Alan Berman, M.D., Medical Director
Web address: www.meadowbrookrehab.com
Control: Partnership, Investor–owned, for–profit **Service:** Rehabilitation

Staffed Beds: 74 **Admissions:** 395 **Census:** 61 **Outpatient Visits:** 0 **Births:** 0 **Total Expense ($000):** 9118 **Payroll Expense ($000):** 4103 **Personnel:** 135

GARNETT—Anderson County

ANDERSON COUNTY HOSPITAL (171316), 421 South Maple, Zip 66032–1334, Mailing Address: P.O. Box 309, Zip 66032–0309; tel. 785/448–3131, (Total facility includes 32 beds in nursing home–type unit) **A**9 10 18 **F**7 11 15 30 31 38 55 57 61 62 79 86 87 96 97 119 122 **P**6 **S** Saint Luke's Health System
Primary Contact: Dennis A. Hachenberg, FACHE, Chief Executive Officer
CFO: Vicki L. Mills, Chief Financial Officer
CMO: George A. Pagels, M.D., Senior Vice President and Chief Medical Officer
CHR: Karen Gillespie, Director Human Resources
Web address: www.saint–lukes.org
Control: Other not–for–profit (including NFP Corporation) **Service:** General Medical and Surgical

Staffed Beds: 47 **Admissions:** 278 **Census:** 35 **Outpatient Visits:** 34021 **Births:** 0 **Total Expense ($000):** 11596 **Payroll Expense ($000):** 5602 **Personnel:** 156

GIRARD—Crawford County

★ **HOSPITAL DISTRICT NUMBER 1 OF CRAWFORD COUNTY (171376)**, 302 North Hospital Drive, Zip 66743–2000; tel. 620/724–8291 **A**9 10 18 **F**3 11 15 24 31 32 33 38 47 49 55 57 61 62 73 75 79 86 96 97 117 121 122 132 135 137
Primary Contact: Kenneth Boyd, Jr., Administrator
CFO: Holly Koch, Chief Financial Officer
CIO: Pat Holt, Chief Information Officer
CHR: Mary Ann Holloway, Manager Human Resources
Web address: www.girardmedicalcenter.com
Control: Hospital district or authority, Government, nonfederal **Service:** General Medical and Surgical

Staffed Beds: 25 **Admissions:** 947 **Census:** 11 **Outpatient Visits:** 27604 **Births:** 0 **Total Expense ($000):** 11618 **Payroll Expense ($000):** 5466 **Personnel:** 134

GOODLAND—Sherman County

GOODLAND REGIONAL MEDICAL CENTER (171370), 220 West Second Street, Zip 67735–1602; tel. 785/890–3625 **A**9 10 18 **F**3 7 11 13 15 24 26 27 31 33 38 46 55 56 57 62 63 65 67 73 74 75 76 77 79 80 82 84 86 87 90 96 107 117 119 121 122 132 135 **P**6
Primary Contact: Jay P. Jolly, Chief Executive Officer
CFO: James Precht, Chief Financial Officer
CIO: Kevin Sanderson, Director Information Systems
CHR: Dale Schields, Director Human Resources
Web address: www.goodlandregional.com
Control: County–Government, nonfederal **Service:** General Medical and Surgical

Staffed Beds: 25 **Admissions:** 620 **Census:** 8 **Outpatient Visits:** 39482 **Births:** 50 **Total Expense ($000):** 11785 **Payroll Expense ($000):** 5244 **Personnel:** 123

GREAT BEND—Barton County

☐ **CENTRAL KANSAS MEDICAL CENTER (170033)**, 3515 Broadway Street, Zip 67530–3633; tel. 620/792–2511 **A**1 9 10 20 **F**3 13 15 24 25 26 27 30 31 32 34 38 40 41 42 43 44 45 50 61 62 67 68 69 71 73 74 75 76 77 79 80 81 82 84 85 86 87 96 97 100 102 106 107 109 111 112 118 119 120 121 122 132 135 137 **P**6 **S** Catholic Health Initiatives
Primary Contact: Sharon Lind, President and Chief Executive Officer
COO: Larry E. Brown, Chief Operating Officer and Director Nursing
CMO: Steven Tyree, M.D., Chief Medical Staff
CIO: Pete Billinger, Director Information Systems
CHR: Shelly Gompf, Vice President Human Resources
Web address: www.ckmc.org
Control: Church–operated, Nongovernment, not–for profit **Service:** General Medical and Surgical

Staffed Beds: 61 **Admissions:** 2446 **Census:** 30 **Outpatient Visits:** 85240 **Births:** 445 **Total Expense ($000):** 37615 **Payroll Expense ($000):** 15581 **Personnel:** 386

SURGICAL AND DIAGNOSTIC CENTER OF GREAT BEND (170191), 514 Cleveland Street, Zip 67530; tel. 620/792–8833 **A**9 10 **F**79
Primary Contact: Pamela Chambers, Chief Executive Officer
CFO: Paula Mauler, Manager Business Officer
Control: Partnership, Investor–owned, for–profit **Service:** Surgical

Staffed Beds: 9 **Admissions:** 325 **Census:** 3 **Outpatient Visits:** 4283 **Births:** 0 **Personnel:** 48

HANOVER—Washington County

★ **HANOVER HOSPITAL (171365)**, 205 South Hanover, Zip 66945–0038, Mailing Address: P.O. Box 38, Zip 66945–0038; tel. 785/337–2214 **A**9 10 18 **F**7 38 52 61 67 79 100 122 **P**5
Primary Contact: Roger D. Warren, M.D., Administrator
CFO: Sheryl Adan, Office Manager
CMO: Roger D. Warren, M.D., Administrator
Control: Hospital district or authority, Government, nonfederal **Service:** General Medical and Surgical

Staffed Beds: 25 **Admissions:** 133 **Census:** 4 **Outpatient Visits:** 1083 **Births:** 8 **Total Expense ($000):** 2788 **Payroll Expense ($000):** 1390 **Personnel:** 44

HARPER—Harper County

★ **HOSPITAL DISTRICT NUMBER FIVE OF HARPER COUNTY (171366)**, 1204 Maple Street, Zip 67058–1438; tel. 620/896–7324 **A**9 10 18 **F**3 10 12 25 26 28 30 31 32 33 38 40 44 46 50 52 55 56 57 61 62 63 66 67 73 75 77 79 82 86 87 96 100 102 107 115 118 119 122 124 135 136 137
Primary Contact: Kim Cinelli, Administrator and Chief Executive Officer
CFO: Sandra Owen, Director Fiscal and Accounting
CMO: Ralph Bellar, M.D., Chief of Staff
CIO: Cindi Beadman, Director Medical Records
CHR: Vicki Longbine, Director Human Resources
Web address: www.harperhosp.com
Control: Hospital district or authority, Government, nonfederal **Service:** General Medical and Surgical

Staffed Beds: 25 **Admissions:** 517 **Census:** 15 **Outpatient Visits:** 9099 **Births:** 0 **Total Expense ($000):** 6558 **Payroll Expense ($000):** 3622 **Personnel:** 123

HAYS—Ellis County

☐ **HAYS MEDICAL CENTER (170013)**, 2220 Canterbury Drive, Zip 67601–2342, Mailing Address: P.O. Box 8100, Zip 67601–8100; tel. 785/623–5000 **A**1 2 9 10 19 20 **F**3 11 12 13 15 18 20 22 24 25 26 27 28 30 31 32 33 34 35 36 37 38 42 43 44 46 49 51 52 54 55 56 57 59 62 63 64 66 67 68 69 70 72 73 74 75 76 78 79 80 81 82 84 85 86 87 91 92 96 97 99 100 103 106 107 108 109 118 119 120 121 124 132 135 136 137 **P**6
Primary Contact: John H. Jeter, M.D., President and Chief Executive Officer
COO: Bryce Young, Chief Operating Officer
CFO: Bill Overbey, Chief Financial Officer and Chief Information Officer
CIO: Bill Overbey, Chief Financial Officer and Chief Information Officer
CHR: Bruce Whittington, Vice President Human Resources
Web address: www.haysmed.com
Control: Other not–for–profit (including NFP Corporation) **Service:** General Medical and Surgical

Staffed Beds: 147 **Admissions:** 5886 **Census:** 73 **Outpatient Visits:** 279779 **Births:** 708 **Total Expense ($000):** 129905 **Payroll Expense ($000):** 53442 **Personnel:** 894

Hospital, Medicare Provider Number, Address, Telephone, Approval, Facility, and Physician Codes, Health Care System

★ American Hospital Association (AHA) membership
☐ The Joint Commission accreditation
○ American Osteopathic Association (AOA) accreditation
△ Commission on Accreditation of Rehabilitation Facilities (CARF) accreditation

HERINGTON—Dickinson County

HERINGTON MUNICIPAL HOSPITAL (171340), 100 East Helen Street, Zip 67449–1606; tel. 785/258–2207 **A**9 10 18 **F**11 15 24 25 38 55 62 65 75 79 80 86 87 96 115 117 122 137
Primary Contact: Richard Q. Bergling, Chief Executive Officer
CFO: Mark Schlesener, Chief Financial Officer
CMO: John Mosier, M.D., Chief of Staff
CHR: Traci Alt, Human Resources Officer
Web address: www.heringtonhospital.org
Control: City–Government, nonfederal **Service:** General Medical and Surgical

Staffed Beds: 25 **Admissions:** 381 **Census:** 6

HIAWATHA—Brown County

★ **HIAWATHA COMMUNITY HOSPITAL (171341)**, 300 Utah Street, Zip 66434–2314; tel. 785/742–2131 **A**9 10 18 **F**8 13 15 24 38 61 67 68 74 77 79 96 100 102 107 119 122 135 **P**6
Primary Contact: John Moore, Administrator
CIO: Cheryl Wenger, Manager Health Information
CHR: Stephanie Gaudreau, Director Human Resources
Web address: www.hiawathacommunityhospital.org
Control: Other not–for–profit (including NFP Corporation) **Service:** General Medical and Surgical

Staffed Beds: 25 **Admissions:** 1170 **Census:** 13 **Outpatient Visits:** 28726 **Births:** 127 **Total Expense ($000):** 15196 **Payroll Expense ($000):** 6409 **Personnel:** 175

HILL CITY—Graham County

★ **GRAHAM COUNTY HOSPITAL (171325)**, 304 West Prout Street, Zip 67642–1435, Mailing Address: P.O. Box 339, Zip 67642–0339; tel. 785/421–2121 **A**9 10 18 **F**2 3 11 15 24 30 31 32 38 42 46 52 55 56 61 62 67 73 79 80 81 86 96 102 107 122 134 **P**6
Primary Contact: Shaun Keef, Administrator and Chief Executive Officer
CFO: Julie Williams, Chief Financial Officer
CHR: Donella Belleau, Director Human Resources
Web address: www.grahamcountyhospital.org
Control: County–Government, nonfederal **Service:** General Medical and Surgical

Staffed Beds: 25 **Admissions:** 707 **Census:** 9 **Outpatient Visits:** 50281 **Births:** 0 **Total Expense ($000):** 7523 **Payroll Expense ($000):** 4112 **Personnel:** 95

HILLSBORO—Marion County

★ **HILLSBORO COMMUNITY MEDICAL CENTER (171357)**, 701 South Main Street, Zip 67063–1595; tel. 620/947–3114, (Total facility includes 59 beds in nursing home–type unit) **A**9 10 18 **F**2 6 11 25 26 30 31 32 33 38 50 54 55 56 57 62 63 73 75 79 81 86 96 102 115 117 119 121 122 135 **P**5
Primary Contact: Michael J. Ryan, Chief Executive Officer
COO: Brenda Brown, Director Nursing
CFO: Marion Regier, Chief Financial Officer
CIO: Marsha Setzkorn–Meyer, Director Public Relations and Marketing
CHR: Wendy McCarty, Director Human Resources
Web address: www.hcmcks.org
Control: Other not–for–profit (including NFP Corporation) **Service:** General Medical and Surgical

Staffed Beds: 76 **Admissions:** 356 **Census:** 54 **Outpatient Visits:** 9622 **Births:** 0 **Total Expense ($000):** 5381 **Payroll Expense ($000):** 2685 **Personnel:** 95

HOISINGTON—Barton County

CLARA BARTON HOSPITAL (171333), 250 West Ninth Street, Zip 67544–1706; tel. 620/653–2114 **A**9 10 18 **F**3 11 13 24 25 31 33 34 38 50 51 57 62 64 66 67 73 74 75 79 81 82 84 86 87 96 102 107 117 119 120 122 137 **P**3
Primary Contact: W. Charles Waters, President and Chief Executive Officer
CFO: James Blackwell, Vice President and Chief Financial Officer
CMO: Cameron Knackstedt, M.D., Chief of Staff
CHR: Gloria J. Walsh, Director Human Resources
Web address: www.clarabartonhospital.org
Control: Other not–for–profit (including NFP Corporation) **Service:** General Medical and Surgical

Staffed Beds: 25 **Admissions:** 559 **Census:** 6 **Outpatient Visits:** 49931 **Births:** 0 **Total Expense ($000):** 13615 **Payroll Expense ($000):** 6253 **Personnel:** 189

HOLTON—Jackson County

★ **HOLTON COMMUNITY HOSPITAL (171319)**, 1110 Columbine Drive, Zip 66436–1545; tel. 785/364–2116 **A**9 10 18 **F**3 11 13 15 24 31 38 42 61 62 73 74 75 79 86 96 107 119 120 121 122 135 137
Primary Contact: Ron Marshall, Interim Chief Executive Officer
CFO: Marlene Kranz, Controller
CIO: Cindy Watkins, Director Health Information Management
CHR: Gretchen Snavely, Director Human Resources
Web address: www.holtonhospital.com
Control: Other not–for–profit (including NFP Corporation) **Service:** General Medical and Surgical

Staffed Beds: 12 **Admissions:** 336 **Census:** 2 **Outpatient Visits:** 35324 **Births:** 21 **Total Expense ($000):** 10191 **Payroll Expense ($000):** 4652 **Personnel:** 118

HORTON—Brown County

HORTON COMMUNITY HOSPITAL (171320), (Formerly Northeast Kansas Center for Health and Wellness), 240 West 18th Street, Zip 66439–1245; tel. 785/486–2642 **A**9 10 18 **F**7 11 15 25 38 62 76 77 79 86 96 117 122 132 **P**6
Primary Contact: Dale A. White, Chief Executive Officer
CFO: Sue Kidd, Chief Financial Officer
CMO: Galen Seymour, M.D., Chief of Staff
Control: Other not–for–profit (including NFP Corporation) **Service:** General Medical and Surgical

Staffed Beds: 25 **Admissions:** 420 **Census:** 5 **Outpatient Visits:** 1606 **Births:** 0 **Total Expense ($000):** 6740 **Payroll Expense ($000):** 2800 **Personnel:** 80

HOXIE—Sheridan County

SHERIDAN COUNTY HEALTH COMPLEX (171347), 826 18th Street, Zip 67740–0167, Mailing Address: P.O. Box 167, Zip 67740–0167; tel. 785/675–3281, (Total facility includes 38 beds in nursing home–type unit) **A**9 10 18 **F**2 3 10 25 26 31 32 38 55 62 67 79 86 117 122 **P**6
Primary Contact: Joe Stratton, Chief Executive Officer
CFO: Kristine Niblock, Chief Financial Officer
CMO: John France, M.D., Chief of Staff
Control: County–Government, nonfederal **Service:** General Medical and Surgical

Staffed Beds: 64 **Admissions:** 225 **Census:** 33 **Outpatient Visits:** 8722 **Births:** 0 **Total Expense ($000):** 5370 **Payroll Expense ($000):** 2988 **Personnel:** 104

HUGOTON—Stevens County

STEVENS COUNTY HOSPITAL (171335), 1006 South Jackson Street, Zip 67951–2842, Mailing Address: P.O. Box 10, Zip 67951–0010; tel. 620/544–8511, (Total facility includes 58 beds in nursing home–type unit) **A**9 10 18 **F**1 3 6 11 15 24 25 26 34 38 43 54 55 56 57 61 62 63 65 79 85 86 96 97 107 117 119 122 135
Primary Contact: Linda Stalcup, Chief Executive Officer
CMO: Samer Al–hashmi, Chief Medical Staff
Web address: www.healthcarefor the heartland.org
Control: County–Government, nonfederal **Service:** General Medical and Surgical

Staffed Beds: 83 **Admissions:** 252 **Census:** 2 **Outpatient Visits:** 12651 **Births:** 0 **Total Expense ($000):** 9554 **Payroll Expense ($000):** 5076 **Personnel:** 160

HUTCHINSON—Reno County

★ **HUTCHINSON HOSPITAL CORPORATION (170020)**, 1701 East 23rd Avenue, Zip 67502–1191; tel. 620/665–2000, (Total facility includes 70 beds in nursing home–type unit) **A**3 5 9 10 19 20 **F**3 7 10 11 13 18 20 22 24 25 26 27 31 32 38 42 43 44 45 48 49 50 51 59 61 62 65 66 68 72 73 74 75 76 77 79 80 84 85 86 88 92 93 96 97 100 107 108 109 111 115 117 118 119 135 137
Primary Contact: Linda Harrison, President
CFO: Gary Witham, Vice President Finance
CMO: Verlin Janzen, M.D., Chief of Staff
CIO: Bob Lies, Chief Information Officer
CHR: Loretta Fletchall, Vice President Human Resources
Web address: www.hutchinsonhospital.com
Control: Other not–for–profit (including NFP Corporation) **Service:** General Medical and Surgical

Staffed Beds: 211 **Admissions:** 10022 **Census:** 197 **Outpatient Visits:** 115671 **Births:** 875 **Total Expense ($000):** 112634 **Payroll Expense ($000):** 42797 **Personnel:** 1105

SUMMIT SURGICAL, LLC (170198), 1818 East 23rd Avenue, Zip 67502; tel. 620/663–4800, (Nonreporting) **A**9 10
Primary Contact: Gordon Funk, Chief Executive Officer
Control: Corporation, Investor–owned, for–profit **Service:** Surgical

Staffed Beds: 6

 Many Facility Codes have changed. Please refer to the AHA Guide Code Chart.

INDEPENDENCE—Montgomery County

🞖 **MERCY HOSPITAL – INDEPENDENCE (170010)**, 800 West Myrtle Street, Zip 67301–9980, Mailing Address: P.O. Box 388, Zip 67301–0388; tel. 620/331–2200 **A**1 9 10 **F**3 11 13 15 24 25 26 31 32 38 44 52 57 61 63 68 74 75 77 79 86 87 96 97 99 100 102 106 107 119 122 132 135 **P**6
Primary Contact: John T. Woodrich, Chief Executive Officer
COO: Reta Baker, Chief Operating Officer
CFO: Terri Del Chiaro, Vice President and Chief Financial Officer
CMO: Robert R. Nichols, M.D., Vice President Medical Affairs
CHR: Eric Ammons, Corporate Director Human Resources
Web address: www.mercykansas.com
Control: Church–operated, Nongovernment, not–for profit **Service:** General Medical and Surgical

Staffed Beds: 40 **Admissions:** 1679 **Census:** 17 **Outpatient Visits:** 60163 **Births:** 320 **Total Expense ($000):** 23517 **Payroll Expense ($000):** 10387 **Personnel:** 235

IOLA—Allen County

🞖 **ALLEN COUNTY HOSPITAL (171373)**, 101 South First Street, Zip 66749–3505, Mailing Address: P.O. Box 540, Zip 66749–0540; tel. 620/365–1000 **A**1 9 10 18 **F**3 11 13 15 25 26 27 30 31 32 33 38 42 43 44 50 54 55 57 61 62 66 68 74 75 76 77 79 80 81 82 84 86 87 96 97 107 117 118 119 121 122 124 135 136 137 **S** HCA
Primary Contact: Joyce Heismeyer, Chief Executive Officer
CFO: Larry Peterson, Chief Financial Officer
CMO: David King, D.O., Chief of Staff
CHR: Paula Sell, Director Human Resources
Web address: www.allencountyhospital.com
Control: Corporation, Investor–owned, for–profit **Service:** General Medical and Surgical

Staffed Beds: 25 **Admissions:** 1199 **Census:** 12 **Outpatient Visits:** 20533 **Births:** 115 **Total Expense ($000):** 14175 **Payroll Expense ($000):** 6190 **Personnel:** 111

JETMORE—Hodgeman County

★ **HODGEMAN COUNTY HEALTH CENTER (171369)**, 809 Bramley Street, Zip 67854–9320, Mailing Address: P.O. Box 310, Zip 67854–0310; tel. 620/357–8361, (Total facility includes 15 beds in nursing home–type unit) **A**9 10 18 **F**38 52 79 96 115 117 119 122 132
Primary Contact: Phillip W. Lowe, Chief Executive Officer
Web address: www.hchconline.org
Control: County–Government, nonfederal **Service:** General Medical and Surgical

Staffed Beds: 30 **Admissions:** 379 **Census:** 21 **Outpatient Visits:** 29841 **Births:** 0 **Total Expense ($000):** 5559 **Payroll Expense ($000):** 2470 **Personnel:** 92

JOHNSON—Stanton County

STANTON COUNTY HEALTH CARE FACILITY (171343), 404 North Chestnut Street, Zip 67855–0779, Mailing Address: P.O. Box 779, Zip 67855–0779; tel. 620/492–6250, (Total facility includes 26 beds in nursing home–type unit) **A**9 10 18 **F**1 3 4 16 17 30 31 32 38 50 55 56 57 65 66 68 70 71 73 74 78 79 81 82 83 84 85 86 87 88 96 117 119 121 122 132 135 **P**6
Primary Contact: Shae Veach, Administrator
CFO: Barbara Anderson, Chief Financial Officer
CMO: Bill Troup, M.D., Chief of Staff
CHR: Peggy Carrithers, Director Human Resources
Web address: www.stantoncountyhospital.com
Control: County–Government, nonfederal **Service:** General Medical and Surgical

Staffed Beds: 44 **Admissions:** 152 **Census:** 26 **Outpatient Visits:** 9286 **Births:** 52 **Total Expense ($000):** 3971 **Payroll Expense ($000):** 1953 **Personnel:** 71

JUNCTION CITY—Geary County

🞖 **GEARY COMMUNITY HOSPITAL (170074)**, 1102 St. Mary's Road, Zip 66441–4196, Mailing Address: P.O. Box 490, Zip 66441–0490; tel. 785/238–1204 **A**1 3 5 9 10 **F**3 11 12 13 15 24 25 26 31 32 33 38 54 60 61 62 66 68 73 74 75 77 79 81 82 84 85 87 88 93 100 102 106 107 118 119 121 122 124 136 137
Primary Contact: David K. Bradley, FACHE, Chief Executive Officer
CFO: Darren K. Rumford, Chief Financial Officer
Web address: www.gchks.org
Control: County–Government, nonfederal **Service:** General Medical and Surgical

Staffed Beds: 69 **Admissions:** 1920 **Census:** 21 **Outpatient Visits:** 177525 **Births:** 345 **Total Expense ($000):** 29377 **Payroll Expense ($000):** 16721 **Personnel:** 385

🞖 **IRWIN ARMY COMMUNITY HOSPITAL**, 600 Caisson Hill Road, Zip 66442–5037; tel. 785/239–7000 **A**1 2 5 **F**3 5 7 8 13 14 15 25 26 28 30 31 32 33 35 36 37 38 40 50 52 54 55 56 57 62 63 66 73 74 75 77 78 79 80 81 82 84 86 87 89 90 91 92 93 94 96 100 102 107 119 121 124 135 136 **P**1 **S** Department of the Army, Office of the Surgeon General
Primary Contact: Colonel Dawn Smith, Chief Executive Officer
CFO: Janice Mailen, Chief Resource Management Division
CIO: May Garlick, Chief Information Management Officer
CHR: Dianna Kallenberger, Chief Manpower Branch
Web address: www.iach.amedd.army.mil/
Control: Army, Government, federal **Service:** General Medical and Surgical

Staffed Beds: 44 **Admissions:** 2688 **Census:** 15 **Outpatient Visits:** 282613 **Births:** 816 **Personnel:** 834

KANSAS CITY—Wyandotte County

🞖 **PROVIDENCE MEDICAL CENTER (170146)**, 8929 Parallel Parkway, Zip 66112–1636; tel. 913/596–4000 **A**1 2 9 10 **F**3 13 15 17 18 20 22 24 25 26 27 30 31 32 33 38 41 43 44 46 54 55 56 57 60 61 62 66 68 71 72 73 74 75 76 77 78 79 80 81 84 86 87 96 97 100 102 103 106 107 108 109 111 112 118 119 120 121 124 135 136 137 **P**6 **S** Sisters of Charity of Leavenworth Health System
Primary Contact: Michael A. Dorsey, President and Chief Executive Officer
CFO: Juanita Roy, Vice President Finance
CIO: Robert Boysen, Vice President Information Systems
CHR: Carolyn Bowmer, Vice President Human Resources
Web address: www.providence–health.org
Control: Church–operated, Nongovernment, not–for profit **Service:** General Medical and Surgical

Staffed Beds: 257 **Admissions:** 11031 **Census:** 134 **Outpatient Visits:** 116547 **Births:** 1419 **Total Expense ($000):** 144314 **Payroll Expense ($000):** 61238 **Personnel:** 965

□ **RAINBOW MENTAL HEALTH FACILITY (174010)**, 2205 West 36th Avenue, Zip 66103–2107; tel. 913/384–4706 **A**1 10 **F**11 30 50 73 82 88 89 92 119 **P**6
Primary Contact: Gregory Valentine, Superintendent
COO: Susan Flora, Director Operations
CFO: Donna Dean, Chief Financial Officer
CMO: Maria Gustilo, M.D., Medical Director
CHR: Marilyn Williamson, Director Human Resources
Control: State–Government, nonfederal **Service:** Psychiatric

Staffed Beds: 50 **Admissions:** 671 **Census:** 41 **Outpatient Visits:** 0 **Births:** 0 **Total Expense ($000):** 8011 **Payroll Expense ($000):** 4451 **Personnel:** 78

🞖 △ **UNIVERSITY OF KANSAS HOSPITAL (170040)**, 3901 Rainbow Boulevard, Zip 66160–7200; tel. 913/588–5000 **A**1 2 3 5 7 8 9 10 **F**3 6 8 9 11 12 13 14 15 16 17 18 20 22 24 25 26 27 28 30 31 32 33 34 35 36 37 38 40 41 43 44 45 46 47 48 49 50 51 52 53 54 55 56 57 58 59 60 62 63 64 66 68 70 72 73 74 75 76 77 79 80 81 82 83 84 85 86 87 88 89 90 91 92 93 94 96 97 99 100 102 103 104 105 106 107 109 111 112 113 114 116 118 119 120 121 124 125 127 128 130 131 133 134 135 136 137 **P**6
Primary Contact: Bob Page, Chief Executive Officer
COO: Tammy Peterman, Chief Operating Officer and Chief Nursing Officer
CFO: Scott Glasrud, Senior Vice President and Chief Financial Officer
CMO: H. William Barkman, M.D., Chief of Staff
CHR: Dwight Kasperbauer, Vice President Human Resources
Web address: www.kumc.edu
Control: Hospital district or authority, Government, nonfederal **Service:** General Medical and Surgical

Staffed Beds: 508 **Admissions:** 19922 **Census:** 324 **Outpatient Visits:** 270537 **Births:** 1467 **Total Expense ($000):** 558447 **Payroll Expense ($000):** 215141 **Personnel:** 4061

KINGMAN—Kingman County

★ **NINNESCAH VALLEY HEALTH SYSTEM (171378)**, 750 Avenue D West, Zip 67068–0376, Mailing Address: P.O. Box 376, Zip 67068–0376; tel. 620/532–3147 **A**9 10 18 **F**3 11 15 17 24 25 27 30 31 32 33 38 54 55 56 57 61 62 65 67 68 73 75 76 79 81 82 84 85 86 87 96 102 107 117 119 121 122 134 135 137
Primary Contact: Gary L. Tiller, Chief Executive Officer
CIO: Jay Gehring, Director Information Systems
CHR: Nancy Stucky, Director Human Resources and Public Relations
Web address: www.nvhsinc.com
Control: Other not–for–profit (including NFP Corporation) **Service:** General Medical and Surgical

Staffed Beds: 25 **Admissions:** 830 **Census:** 12 **Outpatient Visits:** 30120 **Births:** 0 **Total Expense ($000):** 9132 **Payroll Expense ($000):** 4070 **Personnel:** 126

Hospital, Medicare Provider Number, Address, Telephone, Approval, Facility, and Physician Codes, Health Care System

★ American Hospital Association (AHA) membership
□ The Joint Commission accreditation
○ American Osteopathic Association (AOA) accreditation
△ Commission on Accreditation of Rehabilitation Facilities (CARF) accreditation

KINSLEY—Edwards County

EDWARDS COUNTY HOSPITAL AND HEALTHCARE CENTER (171317), 620 West Eighth Street, Zip 67547–2329, Mailing Address: P.O. Box 99, Zip 67547–0099; tel. 620/659–3621 **A**9 10 18 **F**38 52 55 56 79 86 96 122 135
Primary Contact: Ann Zielinski, Chief Executive Officer
CFO: McKay Perry, Chief Financial Officer
CHR: Kitrinia Craft, Director Human Resources
Web address: www.edcohospital.com
Control: County–Government, nonfederal **Service:** General Medical and Surgical

Staffed Beds: 12 **Admissions:** 118 **Census:** 5 **Outpatient Visits:** 8818 **Births:** 0 **Total Expense ($000):** 3834 **Payroll Expense ($000):** 1932 **Personnel:** 64

KIOWA—Barber County

★ **KIOWA DISTRICT HOSPITAL AND MANOR (171331)**, 810 Drumm Street, Zip 67070–1626; tel. 620/825–4131, (Total facility includes 40 beds in nursing home–type unit) **A**9 10 18 **F**1 4 16 17 25 30 31 32 38 62 65 66 68 70 71 78 79 80 83 84 85 86 87 88 107 117 119 122 **P**6
Primary Contact: Bryan Stacey, Chief Executive Officer
CFO: Robin Lewis, Chief Financial Officer
CMO: Paul Wilhelm, M.D., Chief of Staff
CHR: Tara Girty, Director Human Resources
Control: Hospital district or authority, Government, nonfederal **Service:** General Medical and Surgical

Staffed Beds: 64 **Admissions:** 209 **Census:** 35 **Outpatient Visits:** 6847 **Births:** 0 **Total Expense ($000):** 4199 **Payroll Expense ($000):** 2111 **Personnel:** 39

LA CROSSE—Rush County

★ **RUSH COUNTY MEMORIAL HOSPITAL (171342)**, 801 Locust Street, Zip 67548–9673, Mailing Address: P.O. Box 520, Zip 67548–0520; tel. 785/222–2545, (Total facility includes 25 beds in nursing home–type unit) **A**9 10 18 **F**30 31 38 42 52 62 79 86 87 96 100 107 122
Primary Contact: George Stover, Administrator and Chief Executive Officer
CFO: Carol Larkin, Chief Financial Officer
CMO: Kristine Arano, M.D., Chief of Staff
Control: County–Government, nonfederal **Service:** General Medical and Surgical

Staffed Beds: 49 **Admissions:** 214 **Census:** 21 **Outpatient Visits:** 5839 **Births:** 0 **Total Expense ($000):** 4004 **Payroll Expense ($000):** 1919 **Personnel:** 59

LAKIN—Kearny County

KEARNY COUNTY HOSPITAL (171313), 500 Thorpe Street, Zip 67860; tel. 620/355–7111, (Total facility includes 75 beds in nursing home–type unit) **A**9 10 18 **F**2 3 6 10 13 24 28 33 38 41 50 54 55 56 57 61 62 65 66 73 74 79 80 81 82 84 86 87 96 115 117 120 121 122 132 **P**6
Primary Contact: John Loebl, Chief Executive Officer
CFO: Joe Meyer, Chief Financial Officer
CHR: Donna Winright, Director Human Resources and Senior Services
Web address: www.kearnycountyhospital.com
Control: County–Government, nonfederal **Service:** General Medical and Surgical

Staffed Beds: 100 **Admissions:** 266 **Census:** 41 **Outpatient Visits:** 18832 **Births:** 126 **Total Expense ($000):** 10659 **Payroll Expense ($000):** 5636 **Personnel:** 153

LARNED—Pawnee County

☐ **LARNED STATE HOSPITAL (174006)**, Mailing Address: Rural Route 3, P.O. Box 89, Zip 67550–9365; tel. 620/285–2131 **A**1 10 **F**26 30 50 52 55 60 66 73 75 81 82 88 89 91 92 93 119 121 132 135
Primary Contact: Mark E. Schutter, Ph.D., Superintendent
CFO: Mary Odom, Accountant
CIO: Sid Smith, Director Information Resources
CHR: Adele Dunn, Director Human Resources
Web address: www.larnedstatehospital.org
Control: State–Government, nonfederal **Service:** Psychiatric

Staffed Beds: 466 **Admissions:** 1411 **Census:** 414 **Outpatient Visits:** 0 **Births:** 0 **Total Expense ($000):** 51045 **Payroll Expense ($000):** 31760 **Personnel:** 989

★ **ST. JOSEPH MEMORIAL HOSPITAL (171345)**, 923 Carroll Avenue, Zip 67550; tel. 620/285–3161, (Total facility includes 30 beds in nursing home–type unit) **A**9 10 18 **F**2 15 24 25 26 30 31 32 38 54 55 73 75 79 85 86 107 119 122 124 135 136 **P**6 **S** Catholic Health Initiatives
Primary Contact: Teri Thomas, Administrator
CMO: David Sanger, M.D., Chief Medical Officer
CHR: Scharolette Sampson, Vice President Human Resources
Web address: www.ckmc.org
Control: Church–operated, Nongovernment, not–for profit **Service:** General Medical and Surgical

Staffed Beds: 55 **Admissions:** 253 **Census:** 28 **Outpatient Visits:** 21967 **Births:** 0 **Total Expense ($000):** 8438 **Payroll Expense ($000):** 3685 **Personnel:** 72

LAWRENCE—Douglas County

☒ △ **LAWRENCE MEMORIAL HOSPITAL (170137)**, 325 Maine Street, Zip 66044–1389; tel. 785/749–6100, (Total facility includes 12 beds in nursing home–type unit) **A**1 7 9 10 20 **F**3 11 13 15 18 20 24 25 26 27 30 31 32 34 36 38 41 43 44 50 51 53 55 56 57 60 62 66 67 68 72 73 74 75 76 77 79 80 81 82 84 85 86 90 92 96 97 100 102 103 104 105 106 107 117 118 119 121 124 134 135 136 137 **P**6
Primary Contact: Eugene W. Meyer, President and Chief Executive Officer
CFO: Simon Scholtz, Vice President and Chief Financial Officer
CMO: Michael Thompson, M.D., Chief of Staff
CIO: Jane Maskus, Chief Information Officer
CHR: Deborah Thompson, Vice President Human Resources
Web address: www.lmh.org
Control: City–Government, nonfederal **Service:** General Medical and Surgical

Staffed Beds: 137 **Admissions:** 6612 **Census:** 65 **Outpatient Visits:** 211832 **Births:** 1149 **Total Expense ($000):** 115571 **Payroll Expense ($000):** 48850 **Personnel:** 976

LEAVENWORTH—Leavenworth County

☐ **CUSHING MEMORIAL HOSPITAL (170133)**, 711 Marshall Street, Zip 66048–3235; tel. 913/684–1100 **A**1 9 10 **F**11 13 15 24 25 30 32 38 43 46 50 51 55 57 62 68 73 74 79 80 82 86 88 90 91 92 93 96 97 100 102 107 118 119 124 135 137 **S** Saint Luke's Health System
Primary Contact: Ronald L. Baker, Chief Executive Officer
CFO: Judy Scott, Chief Financial Officer
CMO: John Reifschneider, M.D., President
CHR: Bertt Matthews, Director Human Resources
Web address: www.cushinghospital.org
Control: Other not–for–profit (including NFP Corporation) **Service:** General Medical and Surgical

Staffed Beds: 49 **Admissions:** 2251 **Census:** 28 **Outpatient Visits:** 38114 **Births:** 82 **Total Expense ($000):** 27947 **Payroll Expense ($000):** 12325 **Personnel:** 263

DWIGHT D. EISENHOWER VETERANS AFFAIRS MEDICAL CENTER See Veterans Affairs Eastern Kansas Health Care System, Topeka

☒ **SAINT JOHN HOSPITAL (170009)**, 3500 South Fourth Street, Zip 66048–5043; tel. 913/680–6000 **A**1 9 10 **F**3 8 13 15 25 26 30 31 32 33 38 41 43 44 46 53 54 55 56 57 60 61 62 63 68 72 73 74 75 76 77 79 80 86 88 93 96 102 106 107 119 121 122 124 135 136 137 **P**6 **S** Sisters of Charity of Leavenworth Health System
Primary Contact: Greg Madsen, Administrator
Web address: www.providence–health.org/sjh
Control: Church–operated, Nongovernment, not–for profit **Service:** General Medical and Surgical

Staffed Beds: 43 **Admissions:** 2513 **Census:** 34 **Outpatient Visits:** 42389 **Births:** 254 **Total Expense ($000):** 30429 **Payroll Expense ($000):** 14615 **Personnel:** 176

LEAWOOD—Johnson County

☐ **DOCTOR'S HOSPITAL (170194)**, 4901 College Boulevard, Zip 66211; tel. 913/529–1801 **A**1 5 10 **F**30 79 96 100 102
Primary Contact: Phil Harness, Chief Executive Officer
Web address: www.dshospital.net
Control: Partnership, Investor–owned, for–profit **Service:** General Medical and Surgical

Staffed Beds: 10 **Admissions:** 166 **Census:** 1 **Outpatient Visits:** 5681 **Births:** 0 **Total Expense ($000):** 8357 **Payroll Expense ($000):** 1642 **Personnel:** 36

LENEXA—Johnson County

☐ **MINIMALLY INVASIVE SURGERY CENTER**, (Bariatric), 11217 Lakeview Avenue, Zip 66219; tel. 913/322–7401 **A**1 **F**12 32 96
Primary Contact: Parajeet Sabharrwal, Administrator
Control: Corporation, Investor–owned, for–profit **Service:** Other specialty

Staffed Beds: 9 **Admissions:** 91 **Census:** 1 **Births:** 0 **Personnel:** 13

LEOTI—Wichita County

★ **WICHITA COUNTY HEALTH CENTER (171306)**, 211 East Earl Street, Zip 67861–9620; tel. 620/375–2233, (Includes WICHITA COUNTY HOSPITAL LONG TERM CARE), (Total facility includes 24 beds in nursing home–type unit) **A**9 10 18 **F**2 3 11 13 25 33 34 38 43 54 55 62 65 74 81 82 84 86 87 96 117 119 122 134 **P**3 6
Primary Contact: Victoria J. Hahn, Administrator and Chief Executive Officer
CFO: Janice Campas, Chief Financial Officer
CHR: Patti Whalen, Manager Human Resources
Web address: www.phn.org
Control: County–Government, nonfederal **Service:** General Medical and Surgical

Staffed Beds: 37 **Admissions:** 173 **Census:** 23 **Outpatient Visits:** 17459 **Births:** 4 **Total Expense ($000):** 5126 **Payroll Expense ($000):** 2759 **Personnel:** 86

LIBERAL—Seward County

☒ **SOUTHWEST MEDICAL CENTER (170068)**, 315 West 15th Street, Zip 67901–1340, Mailing Address: Box 1340, Zip 67905–1340; tel. 620/624–1651, (Total facility includes 18 beds in nursing home–type unit) **A**1 9 10 19 20 **F**3 11 13 15 25 27 32 38 48 55 66 68 71 74 75 77 79 80 82 84 86 88 93 94 96 97 100 102 106 107 117 118 119 134
Primary Contact: Norman Lambert, Chief Executive Officer
CFO: DeLany Fawkes, Vice President and Chief Financial Officer
Web address: www.swmedcenter.com
Control: County–Government, nonfederal **Service:** General Medical and Surgical

Staffed Beds: 101 **Admissions:** 3290 **Census:** 39 **Outpatient Visits:** 43639 **Births:** 847 **Total Expense ($000):** 36510 **Payroll Expense ($000):** 14806 **Personnel:** 357

LINCOLN—Lincoln County

LINCOLN COUNTY HOSPITAL (171360), 624 North Second Street, Zip 67455–1738, Mailing Address: P.O. Box 406, Zip 67455–0406; tel. 785/524–4403 **A**9 10 18 **F**11 38 67 107 122 **P**6
Primary Contact: Greg R. McNeil, Chief Executive Officer
Control: County–Government, nonfederal **Service:** General Medical and Surgical

Staffed Beds: 14 **Admissions:** 325 **Census:** 3 **Outpatient Visits:** 5580 **Births:** 0 **Total Expense ($000):** 4245 **Payroll Expense ($000):** 2252 **Personnel:** 59

LINDSBORG—McPherson County

★ **LINDSBORG COMMUNITY HOSPITAL (171358)**, 605 West Lincoln Street, Zip 67456–2328; tel. 785/227–3308 **A**9 10 18 **F**3 15 24 25 31 38 52 57 65 67 73 79 86 96 107 117 119 122 **P**6
Primary Contact: Larry VanDer Wege, Administrator and Chief Executive Officer
CFO: Laraine Gengler, Chief Financial Officer
CMO: Bryce Loder, M.D., Chief of Staff
CHR: Brad Malm, Director Human Resources and Marketing
Web address: www.lindsborghospital.org
Control: Other not–for–profit (including NFP Corporation) **Service:** General Medical and Surgical

Staffed Beds: 25 **Admissions:** 459 **Census:** 5 **Outpatient Visits:** 20375 **Births:** 0 **Total Expense ($000):** 5080 **Payroll Expense ($000):** 2619 **Personnel:** 73

LYONS—Rice County

★ **HOSPITAL DISTRICT NUMBER ONE OF RICE COUNTY (171330)**, (Formerly Rice County Hospital District Number One), 619 South Clark Street, Zip 67554–0828, Mailing Address: P.O. Box 828, Zip 67554–0828; tel. 620/257–5173 **A**9 10 18 **F**10 11 13 25 26 31 32 33 38 55 56 73 74 79 96 115 122
Primary Contact: Robert L. Mullen, Chief Executive Officer
Web address: www.rch–lyons.com
Control: Hospital district or authority, Government, nonfederal **Service:** General Medical and Surgical

Staffed Beds: 25 **Admissions:** 495 **Census:** 17 **Outpatient Visits:** 10016 **Births:** 68 **Total Expense ($000):** 7139 **Payroll Expense ($000):** 3659 **Personnel:** 102

MANHATTAN—Riley County

MANHATTAN SURGICAL CENTER (170190), 1829 College Avenue, Zip 66502; tel. 785/776–5100 **A**9 10 **F**30 51 77 79 118 119
Primary Contact: Scott Chapman, Administrator
Web address: www.manhattansurgical.com
Control: Corporation, Investor–owned, for–profit **Service:** Surgical

Staffed Beds: 7 **Admissions:** 446 **Census:** 2 **Outpatient Visits:** 5761 **Births:** 0 **Personnel:** 49

★ ○ **MERCY REGIONAL HEALTH CENTER (170142)**, 1823 College Avenue, Zip 66502, Mailing Address: P.O. Box 1289, Zip 66505–1289; tel. 785/776–3322, (Includes MEMORIAL HOSPITAL, 1105 Sunset Avenue, tel. 785/776–3300; SAINT MARY HOSPITAL) **A**9 10 11 19 **F**3 11 12 13 15 18 20 24 25 26 27 30 31 32 33 35 38 41 43 46 48 49 52 55 56 57 66 68 71 73 74 75 76 77 78 79 80 81 82 84 85 86 88 89 90 91 92 93 94 96 97 99 100 103 106 107 118 119 120 121 122 132 134 135 136 137 **S** Via Christi Health System
Primary Contact: Richard L. Allen, President and Chief Executive Officer
COO: James Murguia, Chief Operating Officer and Chief Financial Officer
CFO: James Murguia, Chief Operating Officer and Chief Financial Officer
CMO: Joseph Philipp, M.D., Chief Medical Officer
CIO: Andy Gagnon, Director Information Systems
CHR: Floyd Chasse, Vice President Human Resources
Web address: www.mercyregional.org
Control: Other not–for–profit (including NFP Corporation) **Service:** General Medical and Surgical

Staffed Beds: 121 **Admissions:** 5710 **Census:** 61 **Outpatient Visits:** 110927 **Births:** 1014 **Total Expense ($000):** 76556 **Payroll Expense ($000):** 31038 **Personnel:** 770

MANKATO—Jewell County

JEWELL COUNTY HOSPITAL (171309), 100 Crestvue Avenue, Zip 66956–2407, Mailing Address: P.O. Box 327, Zip 66956–0327; tel. 785/378–3137, (Total facility includes 34 beds in nursing home–type unit) **A**9 10 18 **F**24 25 28 31 32 38 50 53 73 86 96 122 **P**6
Primary Contact: Doyle McKimmy, Administrator
Control: County–Government, nonfederal **Service:** General Medical and Surgical

Staffed Beds: 46 **Admissions:** 117 **Census:** 32 **Outpatient Visits:** 3009 **Births:** 0 **Personnel:** 70

MARION—Marion County

★ **ST. LUKE HOSPITAL AND LIVING CENTER (171356)**, 535 South Freeborn, Zip 66861–1299; tel. 620/382–2177, (Total facility includes 32 beds in nursing home–type unit) **A**9 10 18 **F**3 11 15 25 27 38 43 54 61 62 68 76 79 96 97 102 106 122 135 137 **S** QHR
Primary Contact: Jeremy Armstrong, CHE, Chief Executive Officer
CMO: Don Hodson, M.D., Chief Medical Officer
CIO: Jeff Methuen, Manager Information Technology
CHR: Sharon Zogelman, Director Human Resources
Web address: www.slhmarion.org
Control: Hospital district or authority, Government, nonfederal **Service:** General Medical and Surgical

Staffed Beds: 42 **Admissions:** 386 **Census:** 47 **Outpatient Visits:** 42400 **Births:** 0 **Total Expense ($000):** 6611 **Payroll Expense ($000):** 2864 **Personnel:** 90

MARYSVILLE—Marshall County

★ **COMMUNITY MEMORIAL HEALTHCARE (171363)**, 708 North 18th Street, Zip 66508–1338; tel. 785/562–2311 **A**9 10 18 **F**3 11 13 24 25 26 27 30 31 32 33 38 50 55 56 57 61 62 66 67 73 74 75 76 77 79 82 86 87 96 97 102 117 118 119 120 121 122 124 135 136 137 **P**6
Primary Contact: Curtis R. Hawkinson, Chief Executive Officer
CFO: Therese Landoll, Interim Chief Financial Officer
CMO: John Haefele, M.D., Chief Medical Staff
CHR: Jessie Schneider, Director Human Resources
Web address: www.cmhcare.org
Control: Other not–for–profit (including NFP Corporation) **Service:** General Medical and Surgical

Staffed Beds: 27 **Admissions:** 801 **Census:** 6 **Outpatient Visits:** 27610 **Births:** 92 **Total Expense ($000):** 16911 **Payroll Expense ($000):** 7884 **Personnel:** 211

MCPHERSON—McPherson County

★ **MEMORIAL HOSPITAL (170105)**, 1000 Hospital Drive, Zip 67460–2321; tel. 620/241–2250 **A**9 10 **F**3 7 11 13 15 24 31 38 43 52 55 57 62 63 68 73 74 75 77 79 80 87 96 97 102 107 121 122 135 **P**6
Primary Contact: James R. Chromik, Interim Administrator
COO: Terri Gehring, Vice President Operations
CFO: Cindy Brown, Vice President Finance
CHR: Jill Wenger, Vice President Human Resources
Web address: www.mcphersonmemorial.org
Control: Other not–for–profit (including NFP Corporation) **Service:** General Medical and Surgical

Staffed Beds: 41 **Admissions:** 1456 **Census:** 15 **Outpatient Visits:** 52814 **Births:** 196 **Total Expense ($000):** 22710 **Payroll Expense ($000):** 10675 **Personnel:** 256

Hospital, Medicare Provider Number, Address, Telephone, Approval, Facility, and Physician Codes, Health Care System
★ American Hospital Association (AHA) membership
□ The Joint Commission accreditation
○ American Osteopathic Association (AOA) accreditation
△ Commission on Accreditation of Rehabilitation Facilities (CARF) accreditation

MEADE—Meade County

★ **MEADE DISTRICT HOSPITAL (171321)**, 510 East Carthage Street, Zip 67864–0820, Mailing Address: P.O. Box 820, Zip 67864–0820; tel. 620/873–2141, (Total facility includes 57 beds in nursing home–type unit) **A**9 10 18 **F**3 15 24 25 31 32 33 38 52 54 55 56 57 61 79 80 86 93 96 97 99 102 105 106 107 117 119 120 122 137 **P**8
Primary Contact: Michael P. Thomas, Administrator
CFO: Lori Smith, Chief Financial Officer
CIO: Leighton Miller, Chief Information Officer
Web address: www.meadehospital.com
Control: Hospital district or authority, Government, nonfederal **Service:** General Medical and Surgical

Staffed Beds: 77 **Admissions:** 487 **Census:** 52 **Outpatient Visits:** 13062 **Births:** 0 **Total Expense ($000):** 12795 **Payroll Expense ($000):** 6600 **Personnel:** 153

MEDICINE LODGE—Barber County

★ **MEDICINE LODGE MEMORIAL HOSPITAL (171334)**, 710 North Walnut Street, Zip 67104–1019; tel. 620/886–3771 **A**9 10 18 **F**7 11 31 32 38 41 52 54 62 79 86 96 107 117 122 137 **P**6 **S** Great Plains Health Alliance, Inc.
Primary Contact: Kevin A. White, Administrator
CFO: Thomas G. Lee, Chief Financial Officer
CHR: Erin Jones, Director Human Resources
Control: Hospital district or authority, Government, nonfederal **Service:** General Medical and Surgical

Staffed Beds: 25 **Admissions:** 457 **Census:** 15 **Outpatient Visits:** 24083 **Births:** 0 **Total Expense ($000):** 7446 **Payroll Expense ($000):** 3971 **Personnel:** 99

MINNEAPOLIS—Ottawa County

★ **OTTAWA COUNTY HEALTH CENTER (171328)**, 215 East Eighth, Zip 67467–1999, Mailing Address: P.O. Box 290, Zip 67467–0290; tel. 785/392–2122, (Total facility includes 27 beds in nursing home–type unit) **A**9 10 18 **F**10 24 26 30 31 32 33 37 38 52 54 61 62 65 67 80 81 86 96 117 119 122 132 **S** Great Plains Health Alliance, Inc.
Primary Contact: Joy Johnson, RN, Administrator
CFO: Cheryl Lanoue, Chief Financial Officer
CIO: Linda Wright, Director Information
Web address: www.ottawacountyhealthcenter.com
Control: Other not–for–profit (including NFP Corporation) **Service:** General Medical and Surgical

Staffed Beds: 52 **Admissions:** 390 **Census:** 38 **Outpatient Visits:** 5220 **Births:** 0 **Total Expense ($000):** 5066 **Payroll Expense ($000):** 2641 **Personnel:** 88

MINNEOLA—Clark County

★ **MINNEOLA DISTRICT HOSPITAL (171368)**, 212 Main Street, Zip 67865–0127, Mailing Address: P.O. Box 127, Zip 67865–0127; tel. 620/885–4264, (Total facility includes 36 beds in nursing home–type unit) **A**9 10 18 **F**2 13 25 30 38 45 46 54 55 62 63 65 74 79 86 92 96 117 119 122 137 **P**6 **S** Great Plains Health Alliance, Inc.
Primary Contact: Cynthia K. Schneider, Interim Administrator and Chief Executive Officer
CFO: Tanga Mayfield, Chief Financial Officer
CMO: Tony Luna, M.D., Chief of Staff
CHR: Vena Harris, Director Human Resources
Web address: www.minneolakansas.com
Control: Hospital district or authority, Government, nonfederal **Service:** General Medical and Surgical

Staffed Beds: 54 **Admissions:** 636 **Census:** 42 **Outpatient Visits:** 25235 **Births:** 38 **Total Expense ($000):** 9001 **Payroll Expense ($000):** 4924 **Personnel:** 134

MOUNDRIDGE—McPherson County

★ **MERCY HOSPITAL (170075)**, 218 East Pack Street, Zip 67107–0180, Mailing Address: P.O. Box 180, Zip 67107–0180; tel. 620/345–6391 **A**9 10 **F**31 32 38 54 74 79 84 122
Primary Contact: Doyle K. Johnson, Administrator
CFO: Royce Holdeman, Chief Financial Officer
Control: Church–operated, Nongovernment, not–for profit **Service:** General Medical and Surgical

Staffed Beds: 21 **Admissions:** 466 **Census:** 5 **Outpatient Visits:** 9088 **Births:** 27 **Total Expense ($000):** 2597 **Payroll Expense ($000):** 1155 **Personnel:** 38

NEODESHA—Wilson County

★ **WILSON MEDICAL CENTER (171344)**, (Formerly Wilson County Hospital), 2600 Ottawa Road, Zip 66757–1817, Mailing Address: P.O. Box 360, Zip 66757–0360; tel. 620/325–2611 **A**9 10 18 **F**11 31 32 33 38 52 55 56 62 79 80 86 88 117 122 137
Primary Contact: Deanna Pittman, Chief Executive Officer
CFO: John Gutschenritter, Chief Financial Officer
CIO: Julie Quanstrom, Director Information Systems and Reimbursement Specialist
CHR: Susie Olson, Director Human Resources
Web address: www.wilsonmedical.org
Control: County–Government, nonfederal **Service:** General Medical and Surgical

Staffed Beds: 28 **Admissions:** 394 **Census:** 6 **Outpatient Visits:** 11441 **Births:** 0 **Total Expense ($000):** 6789 **Payroll Expense ($000):** 3857 **Personnel:** 97

NESS CITY—Ness County

★ **NESS COUNTY HOSPITAL (171336)**, 312 Custer Street, Zip 67560–1654; tel. 785/798–2291, (Total facility includes 43 beds in nursing home–type unit) **A**9 10 18 **F**3 7 15 24 31 38 61 65 79 96 100 107 115 117 122 134 **P**6
Primary Contact: Kyle Hahn, Administrator
CMO: Mikhail Imseis, M.D., Chief of Staff
CIO: Vicki Howe, Chief Information Officer
CHR: Susie C. Schlegel, Director Human Resources
Control: Hospital district or authority, Government, nonfederal **Service:** General Medical and Surgical

Staffed Beds: 63 **Admissions:** 309 **Census:** 45 **Outpatient Visits:** 6599 **Births:** 0 **Total Expense ($000):** 5804 **Payroll Expense ($000):** 3001 **Personnel:** 100

NEWTON—Harvey County

★ ○ **NEWTON MEDICAL CENTER (170103)**, Mailing Address: P.O. Box 308, Zip 67114–0308; tel. 316/283–2700 **A**9 10 11 **F**3 8 13 15 24 25 26 31 32 38 49 51 55 57 62 66 68 71 73 74 75 79 80 81 85 86 96 97 99 100 102 106 107 119 122 135 136 **P**6
Primary Contact: Steven G. Kelly, President and Chief Executive Officer
COO: J. Michael Keller, Vice President Operations
CFO: Paul Lavender, Vice President Finance
Web address: www.newtonmedicalcenter.com
Control: Other not–for–profit (including NFP Corporation) **Service:** General Medical and Surgical

Staffed Beds: 106 **Admissions:** 4149 **Census:** 50 **Outpatient Visits:** 66038 **Births:** 508 **Total Expense ($000):** 46164 **Payroll Expense ($000):** 20103 **Personnel:** 521

□ **PRAIRIE VIEW (174016)**, 1901 East First Street, Zip 67114–0467, Mailing Address: P.O. Box 467, Zip 67114–0467; tel. 316/284–6400, (Nonreporting) **A**1 9 10
Primary Contact: Jessie Kaye, Chief Executive Officer
CFO: Dan Evans, Vice President Business and Finance
CMO: John Marker, Vice President Hospital Services
CIO: Joel Loflin, Director Information Services
CHR: Joy Robb, Vice President Human Resources
Web address: www.prairieview.org
Control: Other not–for–profit (including NFP Corporation) **Service:** Psychiatric

Staffed Beds: 38

NORTON—Norton County

★ **NORTON COUNTY HOSPITAL (171348)**, 102 East Holme, Zip 67654–0250, Mailing Address: P.O. Box 250, Zip 67654–0250; tel. 785/877–3351 **A**9 10 18 **F**3 13 15 24 27 30 31 32 38 43 55 56 57 62 65 67 74 76 79 84 86 96 107 117 119 122
Primary Contact: Richard Miller, Administrator and Chief Executive Officer
CFO: Ryan Stover, Chief Financial Officer
CHR: Shannan Hempler, Director Human Resources
Web address: www.ntcohosp.com
Control: County–Government, nonfederal **Service:** General Medical and Surgical

Staffed Beds: 25 **Admissions:** 776 **Census:** 11 **Outpatient Visits:** 49645 **Births:** 49 **Total Expense ($000):** 7856 **Payroll Expense ($000):** 4165 **Personnel:** 105

OAKLEY—Logan County

LOGAN COUNTY HOSPITAL (171326), 211 Cherry Street, Zip 67748–1201; tel. 785/672–3211, (Total facility includes 46 beds in nursing home–type unit) **A**9 10 18 **F**24 32 38 50 62 65 67 79 86 96 119 122 132 137 **P**5
Primary Contact: Scott Buck, Administrator
CFO: Darcy Howard, Chief Financial Officer
CMO: Charles Zerr, M.D., Chief of Staff
CHR: Vicky Joseph, Director Human Resources
Web address: www.logancountyhospital.org
Control: County–Government, nonfederal **Service:** General Medical and Surgical

Staffed Beds: 71 **Admissions:** 536 **Census:** 39 **Outpatient Visits:** 13428 **Births:** 0 **Total Expense ($000):** 7074 **Payroll Expense ($000):** 3674 **Personnel:** 139

OBERLIN—Decatur County

★ **DECATUR COUNTY HOSPITAL AND CEDAR LIVING CENTER (171352)**, 810 West Columbia Street, Zip 67749–2450, Mailing Address: P.O. Box 268, Zip 67749–0268; tel. 785/475–2208, (Total facility includes 36 beds in nursing home–type unit) **A**9 10 18 **F**3 13 15 24 30 31 32 38 42 44 52 54 55 60 61 62 67 73 74 76 78 79 80 81 86 96 102 106 107 109 119 122 **P**5
Primary Contact: Lynn Doeden, Chief Executive Officer
CFO: Dave Nichols, Manager Finance
CMO: Elizabeth Sliter, Chairman Medical Staff
CHR: Amanda Farr, Manager Business Office and Human Resources
Web address: www.decaturhealthsystems.org
Control: Other not–for–profit (including NFP Corporation) **Service:** General Medical and Surgical

Staffed Beds: 60 **Admissions:** 396 **Census:** 35 **Outpatient Visits:** 3818 **Births:** 17 **Total Expense ($000):** 6092 **Payroll Expense ($000):** 3072 **Personnel:** 96

OLATHE—Johnson County

☐ **OLATHE MEDICAL CENTER (170049)**, 20333 West 151st Street, Zip 66061–5350; tel. 913/791–4200 **A**1 2 5 9 10 **F**3 8 11 12 13 15 18 20 22 24 25 26 27 30 31 32 33 38 42 43 46 49 53 54 55 56 57 58 61 62 63 66 68 72 73 74 75 76 77 79 80 81 82 84 86 96 97 99 100 102 103 107 118 119 120 121 124 133 134 135 136 137 **P**8
Primary Contact: Frank H. Devocelle, President and Chief Executive Officer
CFO: Tierney Grasser, Senior Vice President Finance
CIO: Peggy Donovan, Chief Information Officer
CHR: David Klimek, Director Human Resources
Web address: www.ohsi.com
Control: Other not–for–profit (including NFP Corporation) **Service:** General Medical and Surgical

Staffed Beds: 228 **Admissions:** 11164 **Census:** 121 **Outpatient Visits:** 266515 **Births:** 1552 **Personnel:** 1330

ONAGA—Pottawatomie County

★ **COMMUNITY HEALTH CARE SYSTEM (171354)**, 120 West Eighth Street, Zip 66521–0120; tel. 785/889–4272, (Total facility includes 82 beds in nursing home–type unit) **A**9 10 18 **F**2 3 5 10 11 12 13 15 24 25 27 28 30 31 32 33 34 38 40 43 44 50 52 54 56 57 61 62 63 65 68 72 73 74 75 76 77 78 79 81 82 84 86 87 96 102 107 115 117 119 120 121 122 123 132 133 135 136 137 **P**6
Primary Contact: Greg Unruh, Chief Executive Officer
COO: Marcia S. Walsh, M.P.H., Chief Operating Officer
CFO: Becky Meyer, CPA, Chief Financial Officer
CMO: Nancy Zidek, Chief of Staff
CIO: Mary Matzke, Chief Information Officer
CHR: Terry Bernatis, Manager Human Resources
Web address: www.chcs–ks.org
Control: Other not–for–profit (including NFP Corporation) **Service:** General Medical and Surgical

Staffed Beds: 176 **Admissions:** 1098 **Census:** 84 **Outpatient Visits:** 83716 **Births:** 132 **Total Expense ($000):** 19760 **Payroll Expense ($000):** 11425 **Personnel:** 264

OSAWATOMIE—Miami County

☐ **OSAWATOMIE STATE HOSPITAL (174004)**, 500 State Hospital Drive, Zip 66064–0500, Mailing Address: P.O. Box 500, Zip 66064–0500; tel. 913/755–7000 **A**1 10 **F**11 26 41 50 73 82 88 92 93 119 121 124 135 **P**6
Primary Contact: Gregory Valentine, Superintendent
COO: Susan Flora, Director Operations
CFO: Donna Dean, Business Manager
CMO: Maria Gustilo, M.D., Clinical Director
CIO: Lester Vohs, Chief Information Management
CHR: Marilyn Williamson, Director Human Resources
Web address: www.srskansas.org
Control: State–Government, nonfederal **Service:** Psychiatric

Staffed Beds: 176 **Admissions:** 1969 **Census:** 170 **Outpatient Visits:** 41 **Births:** 0 **Total Expense ($000):** 19594 **Payroll Expense ($000):** 13447 **Personnel:** 461

OSBORNE—Osborne County

★ **OSBORNE COUNTY MEMORIAL HOSPITAL (171364)**, 424 West New Hampshire Street, Zip 67473–0070, Mailing Address: P.O. Box 70, Zip 67473–0070; tel. 785/346–2121 **A**9 10 18 **F**3 11 13 38 62 67 74 79 96 107 117 122 **S** Great Plains Health Alliance, Inc.
Primary Contact: Kiley Floyd, Administrator
CFO: Linda Murphy, Chief Financial Officer
CMO: Barbara Brown, D.O., Chief of Staff
CIO: Kiley Floyd, Administrator
Web address: www.ocmh.org
Control: County–Government, nonfederal **Service:** General Medical and Surgical

Staffed Beds: 25 **Admissions:** 381 **Census:** 5 **Outpatient Visits:** 7736 **Births:** 18 **Total Expense ($000):** 3603 **Payroll Expense ($000):** 1729 **Personnel:** 50

OSWEGO—Labette County

★ **OSWEGO MEDICAL CENTER (171302)**, 800 Barker Drive, Zip 67356–9033; tel. 620/795–2921 **A**9 10 18 **F**31 38 55 62 75 85 86 93 94 96 117 119 122 **P**8 **S** Hospital Management Consulting, LLC
Primary Contact: Daniel Hiben, Chief Executive Officer
CFO: Bill Owens, Chief Financial Officer
CMO: Stanley W. Haag, M.D., Medical Director
CHR: Paula Adler, Director Human Resources
Web address: www.oswegomedical.com
Control: Corporation, Investor–owned, for–profit **Service:** General Medical and Surgical

Staffed Beds: 12 **Admissions:** 181 **Census:** 5 **Outpatient Visits:** 1910 **Births:** 0 **Total Expense ($000):** 2379 **Payroll Expense ($000):** 1163 **Personnel:** 33

OTTAWA—Franklin County

★☐ **RANSOM MEMORIAL HOSPITAL (170014)**, 1301 South Main Street, Zip 66067–3598; tel. 785/229–8200 **A**1 9 10 **F**3 11 13 15 24 26 30 31 32 33 34 38 43 52 54 55 57 61 62 68 73 74 75 77 79 80 81 84 86 96 97 100 103 106 107 118 119 120 121 122 123 124 135 136 137 **P**8
Primary Contact: Larry A. Felix, FACHE, Administrator
CFO: Dean Ohmart, Assistant Administrator and Chief Financial Officer
Web address: www.ransom.org
Control: County–Government, nonfederal **Service:** General Medical and Surgical

Staffed Beds: 47 **Admissions:** 1619 **Census:** 15 **Outpatient Visits:** 94169 **Births:** 181 **Total Expense ($000):** 20296 **Payroll Expense ($000):** 12236 **Personnel:** 271

OVERLAND PARK—Johnson County

☐ **CHILDREN'S MERCY SOUTH (173300)**, (Pediatric Hospital), 5808 West 110th Street, Zip 66211; tel. 913/696–8000 **A**1 9 10 **F**3 9 25 26 28 31 32 33 34 41 43 48 50 57 61 62 66 73 75 77 79 80 82 84 86 89 90 94 96 100 102 107 118 119 120 121 123 133 135 137 **P**6 8
Primary Contact: Randall L. O'Donnell, Ph.D., President and Chief Executive Officer
CFO: Sandra A J Lawrence, Executive Vice President and Chief Financial Officer
CMO: Charles Roberts, M.D., Medical Director
CIO: Jean Ann Breedlove, Chief Information Officer
CHR: Dan Wright, Vice President Human Resources
Web address: www.childrens–mercy.org
Control: Other not–for–profit (including NFP Corporation) **Service:** Children's other specialty

Staffed Beds: 35 **Admissions:** 2232 **Census:** 13 **Outpatient Visits:** 90672 **Births:** 0 **Total Expense ($000):** 36666 **Payroll Expense ($000):** 24125 **Personnel:** 435

☐ **HEARTLAND SPINE & SPECIALTY HOSPITAL (170195)**, 10720 Nall Avenue, Zip 66211; tel. 913/754–5000 **A**1 9 10 **F**3 12 25 30 38 40 43 62 72 77 79 80 84 96 100 102 107 120 121 **P**8
Primary Contact: Mary Nan Holley, Chief Executive Officer
CFO: Jeff Van Horn, Chief Financial Officer
CMO: Alexander Bailey, M.D., Medical Director
CIO: Matt Czugala, Manager Information Systems
CHR: Don Ehbauer, Director Human Resources
Web address: www.hssh.org
Control: Corporation, Investor–owned, for–profit **Service:** General Medical and Surgical

Staffed Beds: 29 **Admissions:** 1998 **Census:** 6 **Outpatient Visits:** 10386 **Births:** 0 **Total Expense ($000):** 34588 **Payroll Expense ($000):** 7811 **Personnel:** 159

Hospital, Medicare Provider Number, Address, Telephone, Approval, Facility, and Physician Codes, Health Care System

★ American Hospital Association (AHA) membership
☐ The Joint Commission accreditation
○ American Osteopathic Association (AOA) accreditation
△ Commission on Accreditation of Rehabilitation Facilities (CARF) accreditation

KS

☒ **MENORAH MEDICAL CENTER (170182)**, 5721 West 119th Street, Zip 66209–3722; tel. 913/498–6000 **A**1 2 9 10 **F**3 12 13 15 17 18 20 22 24 25 26 27 30 31 32 33 36 38 43 46 47 49 55 56 57 58 59 62 63 66 68 70 71 72 73 74 75 76 77 79 80 81 82 85 86 87 92 96 97 99 100 102 104 105 107 109 112 114 118 119 120 121 124 134 135 136 **P**5 **S** HCA
Primary Contact: Steven D. Wilkinson, President and Chief Executive Officer
COO: Sheilahn Davis–Wyatt, Chief Operating Officer
CFO: Deborah Gafford, Chief Financial Officer
CHR: Nikki Johnson, Director Nursing
Web address: www.menorahmedicalcenter.com
Control: Corporation, Investor–owned, for–profit **Service:** General Medical and Surgical

Staffed Beds: 158 **Admissions:** 7078 **Census:** 82 **Outpatient Visits:** 54215 **Births:** 1554 **Total Expense ($000):** 119441 **Payroll Expense ($000):** 33997 **Personnel:** 631

☒ **OVERLAND PARK REGIONAL MEDICAL CENTER (170176)**, 10500 Quivira Road, Zip 66215–2306, Mailing Address: P.O. Box 15959, Zip 66215–5959; tel. 913/541–5000 **A**1 5 9 10 **F**3 13 15 18 20 22 24 25 26 27 31 32 33 35 38 40 43 44 45 50 54 55 56 57 59 60 62 63 65 68 70 72 73 74 75 76 77 79 80 81 82 86 96 97 100 102 107 118 119 120 124 132 133 134 135 136 **S** HCA
Primary Contact: Steven M. Anderson, CHE, Chief Executive Officer
COO: Jacqueline DeSouza, Chief Operating Officer
CFO: Shari Collier, Chief Financial Officer
CHR: Connie Miller, Director Human Resources
Web address: www.oprmc.com
Control: Corporation, Investor–owned, for–profit **Service:** General Medical and Surgical

Staffed Beds: 244 **Admissions:** 9821 **Census:** 131 **Outpatient Visits:** 35311 **Births:** 3201 **Total Expense ($000):** 112209 **Payroll Expense ($000):** 44152 **Personnel:** 712

☒ **SAINT LUKE'S SOUTH HOSPITAL (170185)**, 12300 Metcalf Avenue, Zip 66213; tel. 913/317–7000 **A**1 9 10 **F**3 8 13 15 17 18 20 24 25 26 30 31 32 38 43 55 57 62 68 70 71 72 73 74 75 77 79 80 82 85 86 96 97 100 102 107 114 118 119 120 121 135 137 **S** Saint Luke's Health System
Primary Contact: Julie Quirin, Chief Executive Officer
CFO: Amy Nachtigal, Chief Financial Officer
CMO: Susan Lee, President Medical Staff
CIO: Deborah Gash, Chief Information Officer
CHR: Donna Kunz, Manager Human Resources
Web address: www.saint–lukes.org
Control: Church–operated, Nongovernment, not–for profit **Service:** General Medical and Surgical

Staffed Beds: 95 **Admissions:** 5874 **Census:** 57 **Outpatient Visits:** 72809 **Births:** 1395 **Total Expense ($000):** 78729 **Payroll Expense ($000):** 30959 **Personnel:** 517

☐ **SELECT SPECIALTY HOSPITAL – KANSAS CITY (172005)**, 10550 Quivira Road, Zip 66215; tel. 913/541–5886 **A**1 9 10 **F**1 3 25 43 80 119 137 **P**5 **S** Select Medical Corporation
Primary Contact: Sheryl Laing, Interim Administrator
Web address: www.selectmedicalcorp.com
Control: Corporation, Investor–owned, for–profit **Service:** Long–Term Acute Care hospital

Staffed Beds: 40 **Admissions:** 434 **Census:** 31 **Outpatient Visits:** 0 **Births:** 0 **Total Expense ($000):** 16593 **Payroll Expense ($000):** 6257 **Personnel:** 103

☐ **SPECIALTY HOSPITAL OF MID–AMERICA (172004)**, 6509 West 103rd Street, Zip 66212–1728; tel. 913/649–3701, (Total facility includes 52 beds in nursing home–type unit) **A**1 9 10 **F**1 78 85 132 **S** Fundamental Long Term Care Holdings, LLC
Primary Contact: Karen Leverich, Chief Executive Officer
CFO: William Scott, Chief Financial Officer
CHR: Darren Enochs, Director Human Resources
Web address: www.thicare.com/SpecHospOfMidAmerica/
Control: Corporation, Investor–owned, for–profit **Service:** Long–Term Acute Care hospital

Staffed Beds: 108 **Admissions:** 410 **Census:** 72 **Outpatient Visits:** 0 **Births:** 0 **Total Expense ($000):** 9036 **Payroll Expense ($000):** 6504 **Personnel:** 126

PAOLA—Miami County

☐ **MIAMI COUNTY MEDICAL CENTER (170109)**, 2100 Baptiste Drive, Zip 66071–0365, Mailing Address: P.O. Box 365, Zip 66071–0365; tel. 913/294–2327 **A**1 9 10 **F**3 11 15 26 32 38 43 57 60 62 66 73 75 76 77 79 80 82 84 85 86 87 92 96 97 100 102 107 118 119 120 135 137 **P**8
Primary Contact: Gerald Wiesner, Administrator
Web address: www.ohsi.com
Control: Other not–for–profit (including NFP Corporation) **Service:** General Medical and Surgical

Staffed Beds: 20 **Admissions:** 854 **Census:** 7 **Outpatient Visits:** 38273 **Births:** 0 **Personnel:** 149

PARSONS—Labette County

★ **LABETTE HEALTH (170120)**, 1902 South U.S. Highway 59, Zip 67357–7404, Mailing Address: P.O. Box 956, Zip 67357–0956; tel. 620/421–4880 **A**9 10 19 20 **F**3 7 11 13 15 24 26 32 33 38 54 55 57 61 62 68 73 74 75 77 79 81 85 86 96 100 107 118 119 120 121 122 124 132 133 135 137 **P**4 6 7
Primary Contact: William K. Mahoney, Chief Executive Officer
COO: Derek Vance, Vice President Business Development and Operations
CFO: Thomas Macaronas, Chief Financial Officer
CHR: Christina Sykes, Director Human Resources
Web address: www.lcmc.com
Control: County–Government, nonfederal **Service:** General Medical and Surgical

Staffed Beds: 67 **Admissions:** 3066 **Census:** 32 **Outpatient Visits:** 67144 **Births:** 290 **Total Expense ($000):** 44449 **Payroll Expense ($000):** 19741 **Personnel:** 460

PARSONS STATE HOSPITAL AND TRAINING CENTER, 2601 Gabriel Avenue, Zip 67357–0738, Mailing Address: P.O. Box 738, Zip 67357–0738; tel. 620/421–6550 **F**1 33 37 89 90 91 93 94 119 135
Primary Contact: Jerry A. Rea, Ph.D., Superintendent
CFO: John Spare, Accountant
CMO: Rema Menon, M.D., Clinical Director
CIO: Ron Malmstrom, Information Research Specialist
CHR: Tim Posch, Business Manager and Director Personnel
Web address: www.pshtc.org
Control: State–Government, nonfederal **Service:** Institution for mental retardation

Staffed Beds: 200 **Admissions:** 29 **Census:** 198 **Outpatient Visits:** 0 **Births:** 0 **Total Expense ($000):** 23234 **Payroll Expense ($000):** 15028 **Personnel:** 467

PHILLIPSBURG—Phillips County

★ **PHILLIPS COUNTY HOSPITAL (171353)**, 1150 State Street, Zip 67661–1799, Mailing Address: P.O. Box 607, Zip 67661–0607; tel. 785/543–5226, (Total facility includes 33 beds in nursing home–type unit) **A**9 10 18 **F**2 3 11 13 15 24 26 27 31 37 38 57 62 65 66 74 76 79 82 86 96 107 117 119 122 134 135 137 **P**6 **S** Great Plains Health Alliance, Inc.
Primary Contact: Heather L. Harper, Administrator
CFO: Dennis Fredrickson, Chief Financial Officer
Web address: www.phillipshospital.org
Control: Other not–for–profit (including NFP Corporation) **Service:** General Medical and Surgical

Staffed Beds: 58 **Admissions:** 512 **Census:** 38 **Outpatient Visits:** 24596 **Births:** 7 **Total Expense ($000):** 8922 **Payroll Expense ($000):** 4356 **Personnel:** 124

PITTSBURG—Crawford County

☒ △ **MT. CARMEL REGIONAL MEDICAL CENTER (170006)**, 1102 East Centennial Drive, Zip 66762–6643; tel. 620/232–0109 **A**1 2 7 9 10 **F**3 18 20 25 26 27 30 31 32 33 38 44 47 50 51 52 55 56 57 61 67 68 69 72 74 75 76 77 78 79 80 82 84 85 86 88 96 97 99 100 103 104 105 107 109 111 117 118 119 120 121 124 132 134 135 136 137 **P**8 **S** Via Christi Health System
Primary Contact: Jonathan S. Davis, FACHE, President and Chief Executive Officer
COO: Drew Talbott, Vice President Operations and Corporate Compliance
CFO: Deb Bainbridge, Chief Financial Officer
CIO: Troy Mascher, Director Information Systems
CHR: Connie McCune, Vice President Human Resources
Web address: www.mtcarmel.org
Control: Church–operated, Nongovernment, not–for profit **Service:** General Medical and Surgical

Staffed Beds: 129 **Admissions:** 4917 **Census:** 63 **Outpatient Visits:** 94957 **Births:** 539 **Total Expense ($000):** 69285 **Payroll Expense ($000):** 31559 **Personnel:** 665

PLAINVILLE—Rooks County

★ **ROOKS COUNTY HEALTH CENTER (171311)**, 304 South Colorado Avenue, Zip 67663–0389; tel. 785/434–4553 **A**9 10 18 **F**3 11 13 24 38 55 57 63 67 74 79 86 96 102 107 115 122 132 135
Primary Contact: Julie Price, Chief Executive Officer and Chief Financial Officer
COO: William D. Stahl, Chief Operating Officer
CFO: Julie Price, Chief Executive Officer and Chief Financial Officer
CMO: Lynn Fisher, M.D., Chief of Staff
CIO: Kathy Ramsay, R.N., Director Communications and Development
CHR: Cindi Knipp, Director Human Resources
Web address: www.rookscountyhealthcenter.com
Control: Hospital district or authority, Government, nonfederal **Service:** General Medical and Surgical

Staffed Beds: 20 **Admissions:** 371 **Census:** 5 **Outpatient Visits:** 14431 **Births:** 19 **Total Expense ($000):** 6337 **Payroll Expense ($000):** 2999 **Personnel:** 111

Many Facility Codes have changed. Please refer to the AHA Guide Code Chart.

PRATT—Pratt County

★ **PRATT REGIONAL MEDICAL CENTER (170027)**, 200 Commodore Street, Zip 67124–2903; tel. 620/672–7451, (Total facility includes 47 beds in nursing home–type unit) **A**9 10 20 **F**3 11 13 15 26 27 30 31 32 38 49 52 53 54 55 56 57 60 61 62 67 68 73 74 75 77 79 80 81 82 84 86 96 97 102 106 107 119 120 121 122 134 135 136 137 **P**6
Primary Contact: Susan M. Page, President and Chief Executive Officer
CFO: Hilary Dolbee, Vice President Fiscal Services
CIO: Amy Cox, Director Health Information Services
CHR: Ken Brown, Vice President Human Services
Web address: www.prmc.org
Control: Other not–for–profit (including NFP Corporation) **Service:** General Medical and Surgical

Staffed Beds: 85 **Admissions:** 1725 **Census:** 57 **Outpatient Visits:** 100387 **Births:** 235 **Total Expense ($000):** 31855 **Payroll Expense ($000):** 15463 **Personnel:** 333

QUINTER—Gove County

GOVE COUNTY MEDICAL CENTER (171367), 520 West Fifth Street, Zip 67752–0129, Mailing Address: P.O. Box 129, Zip 67752–0129; tel. 785/754–3341, (Total facility includes 49 beds in nursing home–type unit) **A**9 10 18 **F**11 13 24 27 38 55 56 61 65 79 86 96 107 122 132
Primary Contact: Paul Davis, Administrator
CFO: Joy Bretz, Chief Financial Officer
CHR: Stacy Abel, Director Human Resources
Control: County–Government, nonfederal **Service:** General Medical and Surgical

Staffed Beds: 70 **Admissions:** 849 **Census:** 55 **Outpatient Visits:** 10835 **Births:** 65 **Total Expense ($000):** 9128 **Payroll Expense ($000):** 4316 **Personnel:** 139

RANSOM—Ness County

★ **GRISELL MEMORIAL HOSPITAL DISTRICT ONE (171300)**, 210 South Vermont Avenue, Zip 67572; tel. 785/731–2231, (Total facility includes 34 beds in nursing home–type unit) **A**9 10 18 **F**3 38 54 65 67 80 86 87 117 122 **P**6 **S** Great Plains Health Alliance, Inc.
Primary Contact: Kristine Ochs, RN, Administrator
CMO: Allen McLain, M.D., Chief of Staff
Web address: www.gpha.com
Control: Hospital district or authority, Government, nonfederal **Service:** General Medical and Surgical

Staffed Beds: 46 **Admissions:** 100 **Census:** 23 **Outpatient Visits:** 9533 **Births:** 0 **Total Expense ($000):** 3766 **Payroll Expense ($000):** 2061 **Personnel:** 69

RUSSELL—Russell County

★ **RUSSELL REGIONAL HOSPITAL (171350)**, 200 South Main Street, Zip 67665–2997; tel. 785/483–3131, (Total facility includes 26 beds in nursing home–type unit) **A**9 10 18 **F**3 7 11 15 25 26 28 30 31 38 50 54 55 56 57 62 64 66 67 73 75 79 81 82 86 90 96 99 102 119 122 135 136 137 **P**6
Primary Contact: Shelley Boden, Administrator and Chief Executive Officer
CFO: Duane Fields, Controller
CMO: Charlie Joslin, M.D., Chief of Staff
CIO: Scott Glassman, Director Information Systems
CHR: Sharon Collins, Director Human Resources
Web address: www.russellhospital.org
Control: Other not–for–profit (including NFP Corporation) **Service:** General Medical and Surgical

Staffed Beds: 51 **Admissions:** 543 **Census:** 31 **Outpatient Visits:** 20474 **Births:** 0 **Total Expense ($000):** 11725 **Payroll Expense ($000):** 6683 **Personnel:** 163

SABETHA—Nemaha County

★ **SABETHA COMMUNITY HOSPITAL (171338)**, 14th and Oregon Streets, Zip 66534–0229, Mailing Address: P.O. Box 229, Zip 66534–0229; tel. 785/284–2121 **A**9 10 18 **F**3 11 13 15 24 31 32 33 38 42 54 55 57 61 62 73 74 75 76 77 79 81 86 96 102 107 117 119 122 137 **P**6 **S** Great Plains Health Alliance, Inc.
Primary Contact: Lora Key, Chief Executive Officer
CFO: Lori Lackey, Chief Financial Officer
CIO: Sheli White, Director Health Information
Web address: www.sabethahospital.com
Control: Other not–for–profit (including NFP Corporation) **Service:** General Medical and Surgical

Staffed Beds: 25 **Admissions:** 523 **Census:** 7 **Outpatient Visits:** 41242 **Births:** 53 **Total Expense ($000):** 9147 **Payroll Expense ($000):** 4245 **Personnel:** 92

SAINT FRANCIS—Cheyenne County

★ **CHEYENNE COUNTY HOSPITAL (171310)**, 210 West First Street, Zip 67756–0547, Mailing Address: P.O. Box 547, Zip 67756–0547; tel. 785/332–2104 **A**9 10 18 **F**3 8 11 13 24 27 31 32 38 55 57 63 64 74 76 79 80 84 86 87 96 117 122 **P**6 **S** Great Plains Health Alliance, Inc.
Primary Contact: Leslie Lacy, Administrator
CFO: Heidi Tice, Chief Financial Officer
CHR: Sandi Murray, Director Human Resources
Web address: www.cheyennecountyhospital.com
Control: Other not–for–profit (including NFP Corporation) **Service:** General Medical and Surgical

Staffed Beds: 16 **Admissions:** 350 **Census:** 4 **Outpatient Visits:** 18826 **Births:** 2 **Total Expense ($000):** 5937 **Payroll Expense ($000):** 2816 **Personnel:** 70

SALINA—Saline County

★ ○ **SALINA REGIONAL HEALTH CENTER (170012)**, 400 South Santa Fe Avenue, Zip 67401–4198, Mailing Address: P.O. Box 5080, Zip 67401–5080; tel. 785/452–7000, (Includes SALINA REGIONAL HEALTH CENTER– PENN CAMPUS, 139 North Penn Street, Zip 67401; SALINA REGIONAL HEALTH CENTER–SANTA FE CAMPUS) **A**2 9 10 11 19 **F**3 11 13 15 18 20 22 24 25 26 27 30 31 32 33 36 37 38 41 42 43 44 46 49 50 51 52 54 55 56 57 58 59 60 62 66 68 70 71 72 73 74 75 76 77 79 80 81 82 84 85 86 88 89 90 91 92 93 94 95 96 97 99 100 102 107 108 109 111 118 119 120 121 124 132 135 136 137
Primary Contact: Micheal Terry, President and Chief Executive Officer
CFO: Cheryl Mason, Vice President Finance
CIO: Larry Barnes, Vice President Information Technology
CHR: David Moody, Vice President Human Resources
Web address: www.srhc.com
Control: Other not–for–profit (including NFP Corporation) **Service:** General Medical and Surgical

Staffed Beds: 219 **Admissions:** 9371 **Census:** 108 **Outpatient Visits:** 161656 **Births:** 1134 **Total Expense ($000):** 120213 **Payroll Expense ($000):** 51717 **Personnel:** 959

SALINA SURGICAL HOSPITAL (170187), 401 South Sante Fe, Zip 67401–2697; tel. 785/827–0610 **A**9 10 **F**25 31 49 51 72 77 79 80
Primary Contact: Jim Sergeant, Administrator
Control: Partnership, Investor–owned, for–profit **Service:** Surgical

Staffed Beds: 16 **Admissions:** 649 **Census:** 4 **Outpatient Visits:** 7247 **Births:** 0 **Personnel:** 85

SATANTA—Haskell County

★ **SATANTA DISTRICT HOSPITAL (171324)**, 401 South Cheyenne Street, Zip 67870–0159, Mailing Address: P.O. Box 159, Zip 67870–0159; tel. 620/649–2761, (Total facility includes 44 beds in nursing home–type unit) **A**9 10 18 **F**3 11 31 38 43 62 65 66 73 79 82 86 94 96 107 117 119 122 **P**4 **S** Great Plains Health Alliance, Inc.
Primary Contact: Curt Colson, Administrator
CFO: Carlene Linnebur, Chief Financial Officer
CMO: Juvenal Jabel, M.D., Chief Medical Officer
CHR: Tammy Oxford, Manager Human Resources
Web address: www.satantahospital.org
Control: Hospital district or authority, Government, nonfederal **Service:** General Medical and Surgical

Staffed Beds: 57 **Admissions:** 151 **Census:** 38 **Outpatient Visits:** 19563 **Births:** 0 **Total Expense ($000):** 10554 **Payroll Expense ($000):** 4296 **Personnel:** 123

SCOTT CITY—Scott County

★ **SCOTT COUNTY HOSPITAL (171372)**, 310 East Third Street, Zip 67871–1203; tel. 620/872–5811 **A**9 10 18 **F**7 11 13 15 25 26 27 30 33 38 50 55 57 61 62 65 66 67 72 73 74 75 76 77 79 80 86 96 107 117 119 122 **P**6
Primary Contact: Mark Burnett, President and Chief Executive Officer
COO: Karma Huck, Chief Operating Officer
CFO: Joe Meyer, Chief Financial Officer
CMO: Elizabeth Hineman, M.D., Chief Medical Staff
CHR: Pam Wheeler, Manager Human Resources
Web address: www.scotthospital.net
Control: Other not–for–profit (including NFP Corporation) **Service:** General Medical and Surgical

Staffed Beds: 23 **Admissions:** 563 **Census:** 6 **Outpatient Visits:** 12280 **Births:** 57 **Total Expense ($000):** 9483 **Payroll Expense ($000):** 5241 **Personnel:** 166

Hospital, Medicare Provider Number, Address, Telephone, Approval, Facility, and Physician Codes, Health Care System

★ American Hospital Association (AHA) membership
□ The Joint Commission accreditation
○ American Osteopathic Association (AOA) accreditation
△ Commission on Accreditation of Rehabilitation Facilities (CARF) accreditation

SEDAN—Chautauqua County

SEDAN CITY HOSPITAL (171318), 300 North Street, Zip 67361–0427, Mailing Address: P.O. Box C, Zip 67361–0427; tel. 620/725–3115 **A**9 10 18 **F**25 30 31 32 38 52 86 117 119 122
Primary Contact: Ron Dunkle, Administrator
CFO: Ron Dunkle, Administrator
CMO: James McDermott, M.D., Chief of Staff
Control: City–Government, nonfederal **Service:** General Medical and Surgical

Staffed Beds: 25 **Admissions:** 270 **Census:** 3 **Outpatient Visits:** 4273 **Births:** 0 **Personnel:** 34

SENECA—Nemaha County

★ **NEMAHA VALLEY COMMUNITY HOSPITAL (171315)**, 1600 Community Drive, Zip 66538–9739; tel. 785/336–6181 **A**9 10 18 **F**11 12 13 15 24 27 31 32 38 44 54 55 57 62 73 74 75 76 77 79 80 84 86 96 100 102 107 118 119 120 121 122 **P**6
Primary Contact: Stan Regehr, President and Chief Executive Officer
CFO: Connie Ingwerson, Chief Financial Officer
CHR: Jan Lueb, Coordinator Human Resources
Web address: www.nemvch.org
Control: Other not–for–profit (including NFP Corporation) **Service:** General Medical and Surgical

Staffed Beds: 24 **Admissions:** 412 **Census:** 5 **Outpatient Visits:** 16792 **Births:** 37 **Total Expense ($000):** 8306 **Payroll Expense ($000):** 4035 **Personnel:** 99

SHAWNEE MISSION—Johnson County

DOCTORS SPECIALTY HOSPITAL (170194), 4901 College Boulevard, Zip 66211; tel. 913/529–1801, (Nonreporting) **A**10
Primary Contact: Douglas C. Palzer, Administrator
Web address: www.dshospital.net
Control: Corporation, Investor–owned, for–profit **Service:** General Medical and Surgical

Staffed Beds: 10

KANSAS CITY ORTHOPAEDIC INSTITUTE (170188), 3651 College Boulevard, Zip 66211; tel. 913/319–7586 **A**10 **F**8 25 30 66 77 79 80 82 85 100 111
Primary Contact: Paul Kerens, Administrator
CIO: Jim Leveling, Director Information Technology
CHR: Laura Sinclair, Director Human Resources
Web address: www.kcoi.com
Control: Partnership, Investor–owned, for–profit **Service:** Orthopedic

Staffed Beds: 9 **Admissions:** 588 **Census:** 5 **Outpatient Visits:** 8646 **Births:** 0 **Personnel:** 93

⊛ **MID–AMERICA REHABILITATION HOSPITAL (173026)**, 5701 West 110th Street, Zip 66211–2503; tel. 913/491–2400 **A**1 10 **F**25 30 31 32 55 57 62 76 81 82 85 86 90 107 119 121 132 **S** HEALTHSOUTH Corporation
Primary Contact: Kristen De Hart, Chief Executive Officer
CFO: Richard Lane, Chief Financial Officer
CMO: Cielo Dehning, M.D., Medical Director
CHR: Holly Ray, Director Human Resources
Web address: www.healthsouth.com
Control: Corporation, Investor–owned, for–profit **Service:** Rehabilitation

Staffed Beds: 80 **Admissions:** 1456 **Census:** 55 **Outpatient Visits:** 8365 **Births:** 0 **Total Expense ($000):** 13542 **Payroll Expense ($000):** 7731 **Personnel:** 202

⊛ **SHAWNEE MISSION MEDICAL CENTER (170104)**, 9100 West 74th Street, Zip 66204–4004, Mailing Address: Box 2923, Zip 66201–1323; tel. 913/676–2000 **A**1 2 5 9 10 **F**3 4 5 8 12 13 15 18 20 22 24 25 26 27 28 30 31 32 33 34 38 43 44 48 49 53 54 55 56 57 59 60 61 62 68 70 71 72 73 74 75 76 77 79 80 81 82 84 86 88 90 91 92 93 94 95 96 97 100 102 106 107 113 114 116 118 119 120 121 124 133 135 136 **P**6 **S** Adventist Health System Sunbelt Health Care Corporation
Primary Contact: Samuel H. Turner, Sr., Chief Executive Officer
COO: Joyce Portela, Executive Vice President and Chief Operating Officer
CFO: Jack W. Wagner, Executive Vice President and Chief Financial Officer
CMO: Kevin Koch, M.D., President Medical Staff
CIO: Steve Burns, Director Information Services
CHR: Brad Hoffman, Administrative Director
Web address: www.shawneemission.org
Control: Church–operated, Nongovernment, not–for profit **Service:** General Medical and Surgical

Staffed Beds: 317 **Admissions:** 19140 **Census:** 211 **Outpatient Visits:** 405208 **Births:** 3188 **Total Expense ($000):** 261741 **Payroll Expense ($000):** 99484 **Personnel:** 1940

SMITH CENTER—Smith County

★ **SMITH COUNTY MEMORIAL HOSPITAL (171377)**, 614 South Main Street, Zip 66967–0349, Mailing Address: P.O. Box 349, Zip 66967–0349; tel. 785/282–6845, (Total facility includes 28 beds in nursing home–type unit) **A**9 10 18 **F**2 13 15 24 26 27 31 38 52 62 65 66 67 73 74 79 86 96 107 117 122 **P**6 **S** Great Plains Health Alliance, Inc.
Primary Contact: Carolyn K. Hess, RN, Administrator
CFO: Laura Zabel, Chief Financial Officer
CHR: Jody Maxwell, Manager Business Office
Web address: www.gpha.com
Control: Other not–for–profit (including NFP Corporation) **Service:** General Medical and Surgical

Staffed Beds: 53 **Admissions:** 463 **Census:** 32 **Outpatient Visits:** 28396 **Births:** 21 **Total Expense ($000):** 7356 **Payroll Expense ($000):** 3554 **Personnel:** 117

STAFFORD—Stafford County

★ **STAFFORD DISTRICT HOSPITAL (171323)**, 502 South Buckeye Street, Zip 67578–2035, Mailing Address: P.O. Box 190, Zip 67578–0190; tel. 620/234–5221 **A**9 10 18 **F**31 32 38 61 65 117 122
Primary Contact: Vernon Minnis, Administrator and Chief Executive Officer
CFO: Janell Goodno, Chief Financial Officer
Control: Hospital district or authority, Government, nonfederal **Service:** General Medical and Surgical

Staffed Beds: 25 **Admissions:** 74 **Census:** 1 **Outpatient Visits:** 25793 **Births:** 0 **Total Expense ($000):** 3074 **Payroll Expense ($000):** 1387 **Personnel:** 41

SYRACUSE—Hamilton County

HAMILTON COUNTY HOSPITAL (171322), East Avenue G and Huser Street, Zip 67878–0948, Mailing Address: P.O. Box 948, Zip 67878–0948; tel. 620/384–7461, (Total facility includes 44 beds in nursing home–type unit) **A**9 10 18 **F**30 31 38 41 50 54 55 62 64 66 73 79 86 87 119 122 137 **P**6
Primary Contact: Todd Burch, Administrator and Chief Executive Officer
COO: Jeff Colburn, Chief Operating Officer
CFO: Phyllis Horning, Chief Financial Officer
CHR: Angela Talbot, Manager Human Resources
Web address: www.phn.org
Control: County–Government, nonfederal **Service:** General Medical and Surgical

Staffed Beds: 54 **Admissions:** 154 **Census:** 41 **Outpatient Visits:** 5399 **Total Expense ($000):** 5742 **Payroll Expense ($000):** 2878 **Personnel:** 91

TOPEKA—Shawnee County

COLMERY–O'NEIL VETERANS AFFAIRS MEDICAL CENTER See Veterans Affairs Eastern Kansas Health Care System

KANSAS NEUROLOGICAL INSTITUTE, 3107 West 21st Street, Zip 66604–3298; tel. 785/296–5301 **F**37 65 119 135 **P**6
Primary Contact: Ray Dalton, Superintendent
COO: Ray Dalton, Superintendent
CFO: Sara Watson, Accountant
CIO: Cheryl Fuller, Director Information Resources
CHR: Virginia Galvin, Director Personnel
Web address: www.srskansas.org/kni/
Control: State–Government, nonfederal **Service:** Institution for mental retardation

Staffed Beds: 166 **Admissions:** 3 **Census:** 163 **Outpatient Visits:** 0 **Births:** 0 **Total Expense ($000):** 27084 **Payroll Expense ($000):** 17154 **Personnel:** 537

⊛ **KANSAS REHABILITATION HOSPITAL (173025)**, 1504 S.W. Eighth Avenue, Zip 66606–1632; tel. 785/235–6600, (Total facility includes 19 beds in nursing home–type unit) **A**1 9 10 **F**3 25 26 31 52 53 61 62 75 85 86 117 119 120 121 132 **S** HEALTHSOUTH Corporation
Primary Contact: Paul Livingston, Chief Executive Officer
CFO: Lori Finney, Chief Financial Officer
CMO: Edward Wood, M.D., Chief Medical Staff
CHR: Cheryl Menges, Coordinator Human Resources
Web address: www.kansasrehab.com
Control: Corporation, Investor–owned, for–profit **Service:** Rehabilitation

Staffed Beds: 79 **Admissions:** 1024 **Census:** 42 **Outpatient Visits:** 16441 **Births:** 0 **Total Expense ($000):** 12355 **Payroll Expense ($000):** 6306 **Personnel:** 161

□ **SELECT SPECIALTY HOSPITAL – TOPEKA (172006)**, 1700 S.W. Seventh Street, Suite 840, Zip 66606–1660; tel. 785/295–5551 **A**1 9 10 **F**1 3 25 32 75 80 82 119 137 **P**8 **S** Select Medical Corporation
Primary Contact: Mark Davis, Chief Executive Officer
Web address: www.selectmedicalcorp.com
Control: Corporation, Investor–owned, for–profit **Service:** Long–Term Acute Care hospital

Staffed Beds: 34 **Admissions:** 293 **Census:** 20 **Outpatient Visits:** 0 **Births:** 0 **Total Expense ($000):** 9640 **Payroll Expense ($000):** 3824 **Personnel:** 70

Many Facility Codes have changed. Please refer to the AHA Guide Code Chart.

☒ △ **ST. FRANCIS HEALTH CENTER (170016)**, 1700 West Seventh Street, Zip 66606–1690; tel. 785/295–8000 **A**1 2 3 5 7 9 10 **F**3 5 11 13 15 18 20 22 24 25 26 27 30 31 32 33 35 37 38 43 44 47 49 50 51 52 55 57 58 60 61 62 66 68 72 73 74 75 76 77 79 80 81 82 84 85 86 87 92 96 97 99 100 102 103 104 105 106 107 109 111 116 118 119 120 121 123 124 135 137 **P**8 **S** Sisters of Charity of Leavenworth Health System
Primary Contact: Michael E. Schrader, President and Chief Executive Officer
CFO: Mike Kongs, Vice President Finance and Information Services
CIO: Jeff Hall, Director Information Services
CHR: Jeanne Hippe, Director
Web address: www.stfrancistopeka.org
Control: Church–operated, Nongovernment, not–for profit **Service:** General Medical and Surgical

Staffed Beds: 283 **Admissions:** 10276 **Census:** 127 **Outpatient Visits:** 380761 **Births:** 979 **Total Expense ($000):** 182615 **Payroll Expense ($000):** 76338 **Personnel:** 1398

☒ **STORMONT–VAIL HEALTHCARE (170086)**, 1500 S.W. Tenth Avenue, Zip 66604–1353; tel. 785/354–6000 **A**1 3 5 9 10 **F**3 11 12 13 15 17 18 19 20 22 24 25 26 27 30 31 32 33 35 38 39 40 44 45 47 49 50 51 52 54 55 56 57 58 59 60 62 63 66 67 68 69 70 72 73 74 75 76 77 79 80 81 82 84 86 87 88 89 91 92 93 94 95 96 97 100 101 102 103 105 107 108 109 111 118 119 120 121 124 132 133 134 135 136 137 **P**6
Primary Contact: Maynard F. Oliverius, President and Chief Executive Officer
COO: Janet Stanek, Senior Vice President Hospital Operations
CFO: Vernon Long, Vice President and Chief Financial Officer
CMO: Kent Palmberg, M.D., Senior Vice President and Chief Medical Officer
CIO: Judy Corzine, Administrative Director and Chief Information Officer
CHR: Bernard Becker, Vice President and Chief Human Resources Officer
Web address: www.stormontvail.org
Control: Other not–for–profit (including NFP Corporation) **Service:** General Medical and Surgical

Staffed Beds: 348 **Admissions:** 15814 **Census:** 183 **Outpatient Visits:** 91344 **Births:** 2277 **Total Expense ($000):** 336708 **Payroll Expense ($000):** 166913 **Personnel:** 3020

☒ **VETERANS AFFAIRS EASTERN KANSAS HEALTH CARE SYSTEM**, (Med/Surg/Psych), 2200 Gage Boulevard, Zip 66622–0002; tel. 785/350–3111, (Includes COLMERY–O'NEIL VETERANS AFFAIRS MEDICAL CENTER; DWIGHT D. EISENHOWER VETERANS AFFAIRS MEDICAL CENTER, 4101 South Fourth Street Trafficway, Leavenworth, Zip 66048–5055; tel. 913/682–2000), (Total facility includes 138 beds in nursing home–type unit) **A**1 3 5 **F**3 5 9 11 25 26 27 30 32 33 34 36 37 38 40 41 42 43 44 50 52 53 54 55 57 58 60 62 63 65 68 69 72 73 75 76 77 79 80 81 82 85 86 87 88 90 91 92 93 94 95 96 97 98 102 106 107 118 119 121 124 125 126 127 128 129 130 131 132 133 135 136 137 **S** Department of Veterans Affairs
Primary Contact: Marie L. Weldon, FACHE, Director
COO: Karen Glotzbach, Acting Associate Director
CMO: Rajeev Trehan, M.D., M.P.H., Chief of Staff
CIO: Joni Davin, Director Information and Business Management Service Line
Web address: www.va.gov/sta/guide/home.asp
Control: Veterans Affairs, Government, federal **Service:** Other specialty

Staffed Beds: 351 **Admissions:** 4334 **Census:** 205 **Outpatient Visits:** 354443 **Births:** 0 **Personnel:** 1627

TRIBUNE—Greeley County

★ **GREELEY COUNTY HEALTH SERVICES (171359)**, 506 Third Street, Zip 67879–0338, Mailing Address: P.O. Box 338, Zip 67879–0338; tel. 620/376–4221, (Total facility includes 32 beds in nursing home–type unit) **A**9 10 18 **F**2 3 13 15 24 27 31 34 38 49 56 57 61 65 67 74 79 80 84 85 86 96 107 115 117 120 121 122 136
Primary Contact: Todd Burch, Administrator and Chief Executive Officer
COO: Chris Ekrem, Chief Operating Officer
CFO: Jeremy Clingenpeel, Chief Financial Officer
CMO: Robert Moser, M.D., Chief Medical Staff
Web address: www.phn.org
Control: County–Government, nonfederal **Service:** General Medical and Surgical

Staffed Beds: 52 **Admissions:** 663 **Census:** 36 **Outpatient Visits:** 10252 **Births:** 27 **Total Expense ($000):** 7514 **Payroll Expense ($000):** 3767 **Personnel:** 97

ULYSSES—Grant County

★ **BOB WILSON MEMORIAL GRANT COUNTY HOSPITAL (170110)**, 415 North Main Street, Zip 67880–2133; tel. 620/356–1266 **A**9 10 20 **F**11 13 15 25 26 31 33 36 38 55 61 62 63 68 73 78 79 81 82 86 96 107 119 120 122 123 135 136 **P**6
Primary Contact: Robert B. Ohlen, Chief Executive Officer
CFO: Belinda Moody, Manager Business Officer
CIO: Jerry Horton, Chief Information Officer
CHR: Jay Tusten, Vice President Human Resources
Web address: www.bobwilsonmemorial.org
Control: County–Government, nonfederal **Service:** General Medical and Surgical

Staffed Beds: 44 **Admissions:** 727 **Census:** 8 **Outpatient Visits:** 9789 **Births:** 107 **Total Expense ($000):** 10433 **Payroll Expense ($000):** 5565 **Personnel:** 122

WAKEENEY—Trego County

★ **TREGO COUNTY–LEMKE MEMORIAL HOSPITAL (171355)**, 320 North 13th Street, Zip 67672–2099; tel. 785/743–2182, (Total facility includes 37 beds in nursing home–type unit) **A**9 10 18 **F**3 8 10 11 15 24 31 32 38 55 61 65 79 81 86 96 107 117 119 122 132 137 **P**6 **S** Great Plains Health Alliance, Inc.
Primary Contact: Jean Dean, Administrator
CFO: Gail Jensen, Chief Financial Officer
CMO: David Bolling, M.D., Chief of Staff
CIO: Jolene Schuster, Director Information Technology
CHR: Sherrie String, Vice President Human Resources
Web address: www.tclmh.com
Control: County–Government, nonfederal **Service:** General Medical and Surgical

Staffed Beds: 62 **Admissions:** 931 **Census:** 45 **Outpatient Visits:** 25789 **Births:** 0 **Total Expense ($000):** 10393 **Payroll Expense ($000):** 4283 **Personnel:** 143

WAMEGO—Pottawatomie County

★ **WAMEGO CITY HOSPITAL (171337)**, 711 Genn Drive, Zip 66547–1179; tel. 785/456–2295 **A**9 10 18 **F**3 11 15 25 28 31 32 33 38 56 57 75 79 84 86 87 93 96 107 118 119 121 122 132 135 136 137
Primary Contact: John R. Broberg, Interim Chief Executive Officer
CFO: Pam Allen, Chief Financial Officer and Administrative Director Decision Support
Web address: www.wamegocityhospital.com
Control: Other not–for–profit (including NFP Corporation) **Service:** General Medical and Surgical

Staffed Beds: 18 **Admissions:** 424 **Census:** 6 **Outpatient Visits:** 22705 **Births:** 0 **Total Expense ($000):** 6334 **Payroll Expense ($000):** 2878 **Personnel:** 58

WASHINGTON—Washington County

WASHINGTON COUNTY HOSPITAL (171351), 304 East Third Street, Zip 66968–2033; tel. 785/325–2211 **A**9 10 18 **F**2 3 11 13 15 24 25 27 30 31 33 38 52 55 62 65 68 74 79 80 84 86 96 117 119 122 137 **P**5
Primary Contact: Everett Lutjemeier, Administrator
CFO: Linda Rettig, Director Financial Services
Web address: www.washingtoncountyhospital.com
Control: County–Government, nonfederal **Service:** General Medical and Surgical

Staffed Beds: 25 **Admissions:** 259 **Census:** 7 **Outpatient Visits:** 3280 **Births:** 16 **Total Expense ($000):** 2621 **Payroll Expense ($000):** 1200 **Personnel:** 43

WELLINGTON—Sumner County

★ **SUMNER REGIONAL MEDICAL CENTER (170039)**, 1323 North A Street, Zip 67152–4350; tel. 620/326–7451, (Total facility includes 13 beds in nursing home–type unit) **A**9 10 **F**10 11 13 15 27 30 32 33 38 54 55 56 57 62 63 67 74 75 76 77 79 80 86 87 88 93 96 102 106 107 108 117 119 124 137 **P**8
Primary Contact: Robert H. Bean, Ph.D., President and Chief Executive Officer
CFO: Stephan Wilson, CPA, Chief Financial Officer
CIO: Kathie Henton, Manager Information Management
CHR: Allen Keller, Director Human Resources
Web address: www.srmcks.org
Control: City–Government, nonfederal **Service:** General Medical and Surgical

Staffed Beds: 61 **Admissions:** 1149 **Census:** 17 **Outpatient Visits:** 27162 **Births:** 144 **Total Expense ($000):** 12239 **Payroll Expense ($000):** 5108 **Personnel:** 143

Hospital, Medicare Provider Number, Address, Telephone, Approval, Facility, and Physician Codes, Health Care System

★ American Hospital Association (AHA) membership
□ The Joint Commission accreditation
○ American Osteopathic Association (AOA) accreditation
△ Commission on Accreditation of Rehabilitation Facilities (CARF) accreditation

WICHITA—Sedgwick County

GALICHIA HEART HOSPITAL (170192), 2610 North Woodlawn, Zip 67220; tel. 316/858–2610 **A**10 **F**3 16 17 18 20 22 25 26 30 31 32 33 37 38 40 47 55 56 57 62 68 73 77 78 79 80 82 96 103 107 116 119 121
Primary Contact: Stephen J. Harris, Chief Executive Officer
Web address: www.ghhospital.com
Control: Partnership, Investor–owned, for–profit **Service:** General Medical and Surgical

Staffed Beds: 85 **Admissions:** 4186 **Census:** 45 **Outpatient Visits:** 18909 **Births:** 0 **Total Expense ($000):** 44668 **Payroll Expense ($000):** 16089 **Personnel:** 318

KANSAS HEART HOSPITAL (170186), 3601 North Webb Road, Zip 67226; tel. 316/630–5000 **A**10 **F**3 17 18 20 22 24 26 31 62 79 81 97 107 119 **P**7
Primary Contact: Thomas L. Ashcom, M.D., Ph.D., Chief Executive Officer
COO: I. Lynn Jeane, Chief Operating Officer
CFO: Steve Smith, Chief Financial Officer
Web address: www.kansasheart.com
Control: Corporation, Investor–owned, for–profit **Service:** Heart

Staffed Beds: 54 **Admissions:** 2386 **Census:** 29 **Outpatient Visits:** 8107 **Births:** 0 **Personnel:** 208

KANSAS SPINE HOSPITAL (170196), 3333 North Webb Road, Zip 67226; tel. 316/462–5000 **A**10 **F**3 25 30 32 79 80 82 96 100 102
Primary Contact: Thomas Schmitt, Chief Executive Officer
CIO: Michael Knocke, Chief Information Officer
CHR: Jean Marie Jurczewsky, Coordinator Human Resources
Web address: www.ksspine.com
Control: Corporation, Investor–owned, for–profit **Service:** Surgical

Staffed Beds: 30 **Admissions:** 1344 **Census:** 9 **Outpatient Visits:** 4782 **Births:** 0 **Personnel:** 88

KANSAS SURGERY AND RECOVERY CENTER (170183), 2770 North Webb Road, Zip 67226–8112; tel. 316/634–0090 **A**9 10 **F**35 51 62 66 79 80 82 96 100 102 107 **S** Via Christi Health System
Primary Contact: Ely Bartal, M.D., Chief Executive Officer
CFO: Ashley Simon, Chief Financial Officer
Web address: www.ksrc.org
Control: Partnership, Investor–owned, for–profit **Service:** General Medical and Surgical

Staffed Beds: 32 **Admissions:** 1613 **Census:** 12 **Outpatient Visits:** 8369 **Births:** 0 **Total Expense ($000):** 22549 **Payroll Expense ($000):** 5631 **Personnel:** 120

★ **ROBERT J. DOLE VETERANS AFFAIRS MEDICAL CENTER**, 5500 East Kellogg, Zip 67218; tel. 316/685–2221, (Total facility includes 40 beds in nursing home–type unit) (Nonreporting) **A**1 3 5 **S** Department of Veterans Affairs
Primary Contact: Thomas J. Sanders, CHE, Director
COO: Thomas J. Sanders, CHE, Director
CFO: Ronald Dreher, Finance Officer
CMO: Kent Murray, M.D., Chief of Staff
CIO: Sharon Williamson, Chief Information Technology
CHR: Nancy Gerstner, Manager Human Resources
Web address: www.va.gov/sta/guide/home.asp
Control: Veterans Affairs, Government, federal **Service:** General Medical and Surgical

Staffed Beds: 81

☐ **SELECT SPECIALTY HOSPITAL – WICHITA CENTRAL (172007)**, 929 North St. Francis Street, 5 S.W., Zip 67208, Mailing Address: 929 North St. Francis Street, 5 S.W., Zip 67208; tel. 316/268–5593 **A**1 9 10 **F**1 3 25 31 119 137 **S** Select Medical Corporation
Primary Contact: David Cross, Chief Executive Officer
Web address: www.selectmedicalcorp.com
Control: Corporation, Investor–owned, for–profit **Service:** Long–Term Acute Care hospital

Staffed Beds: 60 **Admissions:** 426 **Census:** 34 **Outpatient Visits:** 0 **Births:** 0 **Total Expense ($000):** 16876 **Payroll Expense ($000):** 5965 **Personnel:** 90

☐ **SELECT SPECIALTY HOSPITAL OF WICHITA (172007)**, 3243 East Murdock, Suite 103, Zip 67208; tel. 316/688–3900, (Nonreporting) **A**1 9 10 **S** Select Medical Corporation
Primary Contact: David Cross, Chief Executive Officer
Web address: www.selectmedicalcorp.com
Control: Corporation, Investor–owned, for–profit **Service:** Long–Term Acute Care hospital

Staffed Beds: 35

★ ○ **VIA CHRISTI REGIONAL MEDICAL CENTER (170122)**, 929 North St. Francis Street, Zip 67214–3882; tel. 316/268–5000, (Includes GOOD SHEPHERD CAMPUS, 8901 East Orme, Zip 67207; tel. 316/858–0333; ST. FRANCIS CAMPUS; ST. JOSEPH CAMPUS, 3600 East Harry Street, Zip 67218–3713; tel. 316/685–1111) **A**1 2 3 5 9 10 11 12 13 **F**3 5 11 12 13 15 16 17 18 20 22 24 25 26 27 28 30 31 32 33 36 38 40 41 43 44 46 47 48 49 50 51 53 54 55 56 57 58 59 60 62 66 68 70 72 73 74 75 76 77 79 80 81 82 83 84 86 87 88 89 90 91 92 93 94 95 96 97 99 100 102 103 104 106 107 109 111 112 116 119 120 121 124 125 126 127 131 134 135 136 137 **P**6 **S** Via Christi Health System
Primary Contact: Laurie Labarca, Interim President and Chief Executive Officer
COO: Laurie Labarca, Executive Vice President and Chief Operating Officer
CFO: Mike Wegner, Chief Financial Officer
CMO: Hewitt Goodpasture, M.D., Chief Medical Officer
CIO: Diana Hilburn, Vice President Information Technology and Chief Information Officer
Web address: www.via–christi.org
Control: Church–operated, Nongovernment, not–for profit **Service:** General Medical and Surgical

Staffed Beds: 749 **Admissions:** 38276 **Census:** 506 **Outpatient Visits:** 306161 **Births:** 2942 **Total Expense ($000):** 460928 **Payroll Expense ($000):** 188230 **Personnel:** 3818

☐ △ **VIA CHRISTI REHABILITATION CENTER (173028)**, 1151 North Rock Road, Zip 67206–1262; tel. 316/634–3400 **A**1 7 9 10 **F**25 26 30 31 32 33 50 54 55 57 62 66 72 73 75 77 81 85 86 90 118 119 120 121 132 135 137 **P**2 **S** Via Christi Health System
Primary Contact: Laurie Labarca, Chief Operating Officer
CMO: Kevin Rieg, M.D., President Medical Staff
Web address: www.via–christi.org
Control: Other not–for–profit (including NFP Corporation) **Service:** Rehabilitation

Staffed Beds: 60 **Admissions:** 859 **Census:** 31 **Outpatient Visits:** 103602 **Births:** 0 **Total Expense ($000):** 22608 **Payroll Expense ($000):** 12084 **Personnel:** 240

★ **WESLEY MEDICAL CENTER (170123)**, 550 North Hillside, Zip 67214–4976; tel. 316/962–2000 **A**1 3 5 9 10 **F**3 7 11 13 15 17 18 20 22 24 25 26 27 30 32 33 37 38 39 40 41 48 49 50 51 54 55 56 57 58 59 62 63 66 68 70 71 72 74 76 77 79 80 81 82 83 84 86 87 90 92 96 97 100 102 103 107 109 111 112 118 119 120 121 124 132 135 136 137 **P**6 **S** HCA
Primary Contact: Hugh C. Tappan, President and Chief Executive Officer
COO: G. B. Serrill, Chief Operating Officer
CFO: David A. Busatti, Chief Financial Officer
CMO: Francie H. Ekengren, M.D., Chief Medical Officer
CIO: Larry Forsyth, Director Information System
CHR: Don Morris, Vice President Human Resources
Web address: www.wesleymc.com
Control: Corporation, Investor–owned, for–profit **Service:** General Medical and Surgical

Staffed Beds: 529 **Admissions:** 26229 **Census:** 334 **Outpatient Visits:** 250577 **Births:** 6475 **Total Expense ($000):** 29170 **Payroll Expense ($000):** 116114 **Personnel:** 2217

★ **WESLEY REHABILITATION HOSPITAL (173027)**, 8338 West 13th Street North, Zip 67212–2984; tel. 316/729–9999 **A**1 9 10 **F**25 30 32 33 61 62 85 86 136 137 **S** HEALTHSOUTH Corporation
Primary Contact: Pamela Stanberry, Chief Executive Officer
CFO: Bob Peck, Supervisor Accounting
CMO: Pastor Causin, M.D., Medical Director
CIO: Debbie Patterson, Director Health Information Management
CHR: Betty Shuman, Director Human Resources
Web address: www.wesleyrehabhospital.com
Control: Corporation, Investor–owned, for–profit **Service:** Rehabilitation

Staffed Beds: 65 **Admissions:** 860 **Census:** 35 **Outpatient Visits:** 20678 **Births:** 0 **Total Expense ($000):** 14256 **Payroll Expense ($000):** 5737 **Personnel:** 152

★ **WICHITA SPECIALTY HOSPITAL (172003)**, 8080 East Pawnee Street, Zip 67207–5475; tel. 316/682–0004 **A**1 9 10 **F**1 25 32 75 85 86 132 137 **S** Fundamental Long Term Care Holdings, LLC
Primary Contact: Phyllis Williams, Chief Executive Officer
CFO: Myra Dick, Business Office Manager
CIO: Michelle Bradley, Director Health Information Management
CHR: Adrienne Burkholder, Director Human Resources
Web address: www.fundltc.com
Control: Corporation, Investor–owned, for–profit **Service:** Long–Term Acute Care hospital

Staffed Beds: 26 **Admissions:** 235 **Census:** 16 **Outpatient Visits:** 0 **Births:** 0 **Total Expense ($000):** 5283 **Payroll Expense ($000):** 2135 **Personnel:** 65

Many Facility Codes have changed. Please refer to the AHA Guide Code Chart.

WINCHESTER—Jefferson County

JEFFERSON COUNTY MEMORIAL HOSPITAL (171314), 408 Delaware Street, Zip 66097–4003; tel. 913/774–4340, (Total facility includes 55 beds in nursing home–type unit) **A**9 10 18 **F**3 10 26 31 32 38 54 57 65 73 86 119 122 **P**1 8
Primary Contact: LaMont Cook, Administrator
CFO: Mary Hoffman, Manager Business Office
CMO: Larry Campbell, D.O., Chief of Staff
Web address: www.jcmhospital.org
Control: Other not–for–profit (including NFP Corporation) **Service:** General Medical and Surgical

Staffed Beds: 80 **Admissions:** 78 **Census:** 37 **Outpatient Visits:** 3769
Births: 0 **Total Expense ($000):** 3388 **Payroll Expense ($000):** 2114
Personnel: 74

WINFIELD—Cowley County

★ **WILLIAM NEWTON HOSPITAL (171383)**, 1300 East Fifth Street, Zip 67156–2407; tel. 620/221–2300 **A**9 10 18 **F**3 11 13 15 24 28 30 33 36 37 38 41 43 51 55 56 57 61 62 63 66 68 72 73 74 75 76 77 79 80 81 82 86 92 96 97 99 100 102 106 107 109 111 118 119 120 121 122 124 135 136 137
Primary Contact: Richard H. Vaught, Administrator
CFO: Danny Huckvale, Assistant Administrator and Chief Financial Officer
CMO: Ben Short, M.D., Chief of Staff
CIO: Randy Mayo, Director Information Technology
CHR: Cathy McClurg, Director Human Resources
Web address: www.wnmh.org
Control: City–Government, nonfederal **Service:** General Medical and Surgical

Staffed Beds: 25 **Admissions:** 1544 **Census:** 12 **Outpatient Visits:** 67064
Births: 279 **Total Expense ($000):** 20233 **Payroll Expense ($000):** 10332
Personnel: 261

Hospital, Medicare Provider Number, Address, Telephone, Approval, Facility, and Physician Codes, Health Care System

★ American Hospital Association (AHA) membership
□ The Joint Commission accreditation
○ American Osteopathic Association (AOA) accreditation
△ Commission on Accreditation of Rehabilitation Facilities (CARF) accreditation

KS

KENTUCKY

ALBANY—Clinton County

CLINTON COUNTY HOSPITAL (180106), 723 Burkesville Road, Zip 42602–1654; tel. 606/387–6421 **A**9 10 20 **F**7 15 25 26 31 38 68 79 96 99 107 119 122 135 **P**1
Primary Contact: Randel Flowers, Ph.D., Administrator
CHR: Pat Beard, Director Human Resources
Web address: www.clintoncountyhospital.com
Control: Other not–for–profit (including NFP Corporation) **Service:** General Medical and Surgical

Staffed Beds: 42 **Admissions:** 1874 **Census:** 22 **Outpatient Visits:** 20041 **Births:** 0 **Total Expense ($000):** 11706 **Payroll Expense ($000):** 5315 **Personnel:** 170

ASHLAND—Boyd County

★ △ **KING'S DAUGHTERS MEDICAL CENTER (180009)**, 2201 Lexington Avenue, Zip 41101–2874, Mailing Address: P.O. Box 151, Zip 41105–0151; tel. 606/408–4000, (Total facility includes 151 beds in nursing home–type unit) **A**1 2 7 9 10 **F**3 8 11 12 13 15 17 18 20 22 24 25 26 27 30 31 32 33 36 38 43 46 47 48 49 51 53 55 56 57 58 59 60 61 62 63 66 68 69 70 72 73 74 75 76 77 79 80 81 82 84 85 86 87 88 90 91 92 93 96 97 99 100 102 103 104 105 106 107 113 116 117 118 119 120 121 123 124 133 135 136 137 **P**8
Primary Contact: Fred L. Jackson, FACHE, Chief Executive Officer
COO: Bob Lucas, Vice President Operations
CFO: Paul L. McDowell, Vice President Finance and Chief Financial Officer
CMO: Phil Fioret, M.D., Vice President Medical Affairs
CIO: David Oliver, Director Information Systems
CHR: Larry Higgins, Vice President Human Resources
Web address: www.kdmc.com
Control: Other not–for–profit (including NFP Corporation) **Service:** General Medical and Surgical

Staffed Beds: 536 **Admissions:** 24499 **Census:** 445 **Outpatient Visits:** 394269 **Births:** 1706 **Total Expense ($000):** 382720 **Payroll Expense ($000):** 139376 **Personnel:** 2933

★ **OUR LADY OF BELLEFONTE HOSPITAL (180036)**, St. Christopher Drive, Zip 41101–7071, Mailing Address: P.O. Box 789, Zip 41105–0789; tel. 606/833–3333 **A**1 2 9 10 12 13 **F**3 4 5 8 11 12 15 18 20 22 24 25 26 27 30 32 33 34 36 38 39 41 43 44 49 50 51 52 53 55 56 57 59 61 62 63 66 67 68 69 72 73 75 76 77 79 80 81 82 84 86 87 88 90 91 94 95 96 97 100 102 103 106 107 118 119 120 121 124 132 133 135 136 137 **P**1 6 **S** Bon Secours Health System, Inc.
Primary Contact: Mark M. Gordon, Chief Executive Officer
COO: Kevin Halter, Vice President Planning and Operations
CFO: Angela Foltz, Chief Financial Officer
CMO: Craigan Gray, M.D., Vice President Medical Affairs
CIO: Shelli Ferguson, Site Manager Medical Information Systems
CHR: Judy Daniels, Vice President Human Resources
Web address: www.olbh.com
Control: Church–operated, Nongovernment, not–for profit **Service:** General Medical and Surgical

Staffed Beds: 214 **Admissions:** 7299 **Census:** 83 **Outpatient Visits:** 171163 **Births:** 0 **Total Expense ($000):** 115238 **Payroll Expense ($000):** 42356 **Personnel:** 879

BARBOURVILLE—Knox County

★ **KNOX COUNTY HOSPITAL (181328)**, 80 Hospital Drive, Zip 40906–1317, Mailing Address: P.O. Box 10, Zip 40906–0160; tel. 606/546–4175, (Total facility includes 16 beds in nursing home–type unit) (Nonreporting) **A**9 10 18 **S** Pacer Health Corporation
Primary Contact: Rebecca Lewis, Chief Executive Officer
COO: Brenda Graham, Director Nursing
CFO: Kris Partin, Chief Financial Officer
CMO: Richard Carter, M.D., Chief Medical Staff
CIO: Evan Davis, Director Technology and Environmental Services
CHR: Janet Wilder, Coordinator Human Resources
Web address: www.knoxcohospital.com
Control: Corporation, Investor–owned, for–profit **Service:** General Medical and Surgical

Staffed Beds: 41

BARDSTOWN—Nelson County

★ **FLAGET MEMORIAL HOSPITAL (180025)**, 4305 New Shepherdsville Road, Zip 40004; tel. 502/350–5000, (Total facility includes 12 beds in nursing home–type unit) **A**1 9 10 **F**3 13 15 24 25 26 27 30 33 38 42 43 53 55 56 57 65 66 68 73 74 75 76 77 79 80 82 86 90 96 100 107 117 118 119 121 124 133 135 136 137 **S** Catholic Health Initiatives
Primary Contact: Bruce A. Klockars, CHE, President
CFO: John Bradford, Vice President Finance
CMO: Mark Abramovich, M.D., Chief of Staff
CHR: Deborah Cowles, Vice President Human Resources
Web address: www.flaget.com
Control: Other not–for–profit (including NFP Corporation) **Service:** General Medical and Surgical

Staffed Beds: 52 **Admissions:** 2884 **Census:** 32 **Outpatient Visits:** 97447 **Births:** 325 **Total Expense ($000):** 44507 **Payroll Expense ($000):** 16055 **Personnel:** 391

BENTON—Marshall County

★ **MARSHALL COUNTY HOSPITAL (181327)**, 503 George McClain Drive, Zip 42025–1399, Mailing Address: P.O. Box 630, Zip 42025–0630; tel. 270/527–4800, (Total facility includes 34 beds in nursing home–type unit) **A**1 9 10 18 **F**3 7 11 15 24 25 30 31 32 33 38 51 55 57 61 75 77 79 80 84 85 86 96 97 107 117 121 122 124 **P**6 **S** QHR
Primary Contact: Kathy Long, Chief Executive Officer
CFO: Janice Kelley, Chief Financial Officer
CMO: Glen Van Loon, M.D., Chief of Staff
CHR: Brian York, Director Human Resources
Web address: www.marshallcountyhospital.org
Control: County–Government, nonfederal **Service:** General Medical and Surgical

Staffed Beds: 59 **Admissions:** 1039 **Census:** 48 **Outpatient Visits:** 8447 **Births:** 0 **Total Expense ($000):** 13738 **Payroll Expense ($000):** 6773 **Personnel:** 96

BEREA—Madison County

★ **SAINT JOSEPH BEREA (181329)**, 305 Estill Street, Zip 40403–1909; tel. 859/986–3151 **A**5 9 10 18 **F**11 15 25 26 27 30 31 32 38 55 62 68 73 75 77 79 82 86 96 97 100 102 107 118 122 135 136 **P**6 **S** Catholic Health Initiatives
Primary Contact: Eugene A. Woods, President and Chief Executive Officer
CMO: Patrick Kelleher, M.D., Chief Medical Staff
CIO: Katie Heckman, Director Community Relations
CHR: Renee Bullock, Vice President Human Resources
Web address: www.bereahospital.com
Control: Church–operated, Nongovernment, not–for profit **Service:** General Medical and Surgical

Staffed Beds: 25 **Admissions:** 1808 **Census:** 15 **Outpatient Visits:** 53981 **Births:** 0 **Total Expense ($000):** 17232 **Payroll Expense ($000):** 10665 **Personnel:** 245

BOWLING GREEN—Warren County

COMMONWEALTH REGIONAL SPECIALTY HOSPITAL (182005), 250 Park Drive, 5th Floor, Zip 42101, Mailing Address: P.O. Box 90010, Zip 42101; tel. 270/796–6200 **A**9 10 **F**1 3 25 26 30 31 32 119
Primary Contact: Joe Murrell, Administrator
Web address: www.commonwealthregionalspecialtyhospital.org
Control: Other not–for–profit (including NFP Corporation) **Service:** Long–Term Acute Care hospital

Staffed Beds: 28 **Admissions:** 278 **Census:** 20 **Outpatient Visits:** 0 **Births:** 0 **Personnel:** 68

★ **GREENVIEW REGIONAL HOSPITAL (180124)**, 1801 Ashley Circle, Zip 42104–3384; tel. 270/793–1000 **A**1 2 9 10 19 **F**3 8 11 15 17 18 20 25 26 27 30 31 32 33 35 37 38 40 43 46 48 49 50 51 55 56 57 59 62 63 66 68 72 73 75 76 77 79 80 81 82 96 97 100 102 104 105 107 112 118 119 120 121 122 124 134 135 **S** HCA
Primary Contact: Mark A. Marsh, Chief Executive Officer
COO: Jarrett Millsaps, Chief Operating Officer
CFO: Joe Jeans, Chief Financial Officer
CMO: Michael Boggess, M.D., Chief of Staff
CHR: Judy Fulkerson, Director Human Resources
Web address: www.greenviewhospital.com
Control: Corporation, Investor–owned, for–profit **Service:** General Medical and Surgical

Staffed Beds: 211 **Admissions:** 3553 **Census:** 38 **Outpatient Visits:** 39586 **Births:** 0 **Personnel:** 379

☐ **RIVENDELL BEHAVIORAL HEALTH (184017)**, 1035 Porter Pike, Zip 42103; tel. 270/843–1199 **A**1 9 10 **F**5 25 26 30 31 32 73 88 89 91 92 95 119 **P**5 **S** Universal Health Services, Inc.
Primary Contact: Janice Richardson, Chief Executive Officer and Managing Director
Web address: www.rivendellbehavioral.com
Control: Corporation, Investor–owned, for–profit **Service:** Children's hospital psychiatric

Staffed Beds: 84 **Admissions:** 501 **Census:** 79 **Outpatient Visits:** 457 **Births:** 0 **Total Expense ($000):** 10534 **Payroll Expense ($000):** 4901 **Personnel:** 132

☐ △ **SOUTHERN KENTUCKY REHABILITATION HOSPITAL (183029)**, 1300 Campbell Lane, Zip 42104–4162; tel. 270/782–6900 **A**1 7 9 10 **F**24 25 30 31 32 33 62 73 77 85 119 121 124 137 **S** Vibra Healthcare
Primary Contact: Joanna Thomas, Chief Executive Officer
COO: Dana Lewis, Director Clinical Services
CFO: Stuart Locke, Chief Financial Officer
CMO: Jim Farrage, M.D., Medical Director
CHR: Suzanne Cornett, Director Human Resources
Web address: www.skyrehab.com
Control: Corporation, Investor–owned, for–profit **Service:** Rehabilitation

Staffed Beds: 60 **Admissions:** 1336 **Census:** 38 **Outpatient Visits:** 309 **Births:** 0 **Personnel:** 175

★☐ **THE MEDICAL CENTER AT BOWLING GREEN (180013)**, 250 Park Street, Zip 42101–1795, Mailing Address: P.O. Box 90010, Zip 42102–9010; tel. 270/745–1000 **A**1 2 9 10 19 **F**1 3 7 13 15 17 18 20 22 24 25 26 27 28 31 32 33 35 37 38 43 44 46 50 51 54 55 56 57 59 61 62 66 68 70 72 73 74 76 77 78 79 80 81 82 84 86 88 90 92 93 94 95 96 97 99 100 102 104 105 107 109 111 118 119 121 124 134 135 136 137
Primary Contact: Connie Smith, Chief Executive Officer
CFO: Ron Sowell, Executive Vice President
CIO: Jean Cherry, Executive Vice President and Chief Information Officer
CHR: Lynn Williams, Vice President Human Resources
Web address: www.themedicalcenter.org
Control: Other not–for–profit (including NFP Corporation) **Service:** General Medical and Surgical

Staffed Beds: 330 **Admissions:** 15450 **Census:** 195 **Outpatient Visits:** 103962 **Births:** 2043 **Personnel:** 1495

BURKESVILLE—Cumberland County

★ **CUMBERLAND COUNTY HOSPITAL (181317)**, Highway 90 West, Zip 42717–0280, Mailing Address: P.O. Box 280, Zip 42717–0280; tel. 270/864–2511, (Nonreporting) **A**9 10 18
Primary Contact: Richard Neikirk, Chief Executive Officer
CFO: Rick Capps, Interim Chief Financial Officer
CMO: Christian Konsavage, M.D., Chief of Staff
CHR: Martha Young, Director Human Resources
Web address: www.cchospital.org
Control: Other not–for–profit (including NFP Corporation) **Service:** General Medical and Surgical

Staffed Beds: 25

CADIZ—Trigg County

★ **TRIGG COUNTY HOSPITAL (181304)**, 254 Main Street, Zip 42211–9153, Mailing Address: P.O. Box 312, Zip 42211–0312; tel. 270/522–3215 **A**9 10 18 **F**3 7 8 11 15 25 30 31 32 38 50 53 55 56 57 61 73 75 79 82 86 87 96 100 102 107 122 124 132 **P**6
Primary Contact: Alisa Coleman, Chief Executive Officer
CFO: Bethany Goss, Chief Financial Officer
CHR: Audra Hodges, Director Human Resources
Web address: www.trigghospital.org
Control: County–Government, nonfederal **Service:** General Medical and Surgical

Staffed Beds: 25 **Admissions:** 481 **Census:** 6 **Outpatient Visits:** 31016 **Births:** 0 **Total Expense ($000):** 8081 **Payroll Expense ($000):** 3885 **Personnel:** 112

CAMPBELLSVILLE—Taylor County

★☐ **TAYLOR REGIONAL HOSPITAL (180087)**, 1700 Old Lebanon Road, Zip 42718–9600; tel. 270/465–3561 **A**1 2 9 10 **F**3 11 13 15 18 24 25 26 27 30 33 34 37 38 40 42 44 45 46 48 49 50 51 55 56 57 59 61 62 66 68 73 74 75 76 77 79 80 81 86 90 96 97 98 100 102 103 106 107 109 110 118 119 121 124 132 133 135 136 137 **S** Jewish Hospital & St. Mary's HealthCare
Primary Contact: Jane Wheatley, Chief Executive Officer
CFO: David Massengale, Chief Financial Officer
CIO: Gary Neat, Director Information Management Systems
CHR: Andrea Settle, Director Human Resources
Web address: www.trhosp.org
Control: Hospital district or authority, Government, nonfederal **Service:** General Medical and Surgical

Staffed Beds: 90 **Admissions:** 3037 **Census:** 34 **Outpatient Visits:** 76184 **Births:** 318 **Total Expense ($000):** 48895 **Payroll Expense ($000):** 19012 **Personnel:** 487

CARLISLE—Nicholas County

NICHOLAS COUNTY HOSPITAL (181303), 2323 Concrete Road, Zip 40311–9721, Mailing Address: P.O. Box 232, Zip 40311–0232; tel. 859/289–7181, (Includes JOHNSON–MATHERS NURSING HOME), (Total facility includes 104 beds in nursing home–type unit) **A**9 10 18 **F**3 11 15 31 32 38 55 57 75 79 86 96 103 107 119 122 124 **P**1
Primary Contact: Doris Ecton, Administrator and Chief Executive Officer
CFO: Wesley Berry, Chief Financial Officer
CMO: Stephen Besson, M.D., Chief Medical Staff
CIO: Trish Stone, Chief Information Officer
CHR: Wendy Price, Manager Human Resources
Web address: www.johnsonmathers.org
Control: Other not–for–profit (including NFP Corporation) **Service:** General Medical and Surgical

Staffed Beds: 122 **Admissions:** 848 **Census:** 101 **Outpatient Visits:** 16896 **Births:** 0 **Total Expense ($000):** 9577 **Payroll Expense ($000):** 5025 **Personnel:** 151

CARROLLTON—Carroll County

★ **CARROLL COUNTY MEMORIAL HOSPITAL (181310)**, 309 11th Street, Zip 41008–1400; tel. 502/732–4321, (Nonreporting) **A**9 10 18
Primary Contact: Kanute Rarey, Chief Executive Officer
CFO: Joe McCullum, Manager Finance
Web address: www.nortonhealthcare.com
Control: County–Government, nonfederal **Service:** General Medical and Surgical

Staffed Beds: 25

COLUMBIA—Adair County

WESTLAKE REGIONAL HOSPITAL (180149), 901 Westlake Drive, Zip 42728–1149, Mailing Address: P.O. Box 1269, Zip 42728–1269; tel. 270/384–4753, (Nonreporting) **A**9 10
Primary Contact: Rex A. Tungate, Administrator
Web address: www.westlake–healthcare.org
Control: Hospital district or authority, Government, nonfederal **Service:** General Medical and Surgical

Staffed Beds: 25

CORBIN—Whitley County

★☐ **BAPTIST REGIONAL MEDICAL CENTER (180080)**, 1 Trillium Way, Zip 40701–8420; tel. 606/528–1212 **A**1 9 10 19 **F**1 3 4 5 11 13 15 18 25 26 30 31 32 33 36 38 47 48 49 52 53 55 57 62 66 68 71 74 77 79 80 81 84 85 86 88 89 90 91 92 93 94 95 96 97 99 100 102 106 107 119 121 122 124 134 135 136 137 **S** Baptist Healthcare System
Primary Contact: John S. Henson, President
CFO: John Burgett, Team Leader
CMO: Stephen Toadvine, M.D., Vice President Medical Staff Services
CIO: Jackie Lucas, Vice President Information Systems
CHR: Tim Perry, Coordinator Human Resources
Web address: www.baptistregional.com
Control: Other not–for–profit (including NFP Corporation) **Service:** General Medical and Surgical

Staffed Beds: 263 **Admissions:** 9932 **Census:** 131 **Outpatient Visits:** 82279 **Births:** 883 **Total Expense ($000):** 99456 **Payroll Expense ($000):** 40390 **Personnel:** 1003

Hospital, Medicare Provider Number, Address, Telephone, Approval, Facility, and Physician Codes, Health Care System

★ American Hospital Association (AHA) membership
☐ The Joint Commission accreditation
○ American Osteopathic Association (AOA) accreditation
△ Commission on Accreditation of Rehabilitation Facilities (CARF) accreditation

OAK TREE HOSPITAL (182006), One Trillium Way, Lower Level, Zip 40701; tel. 606/523–5150 **A**9 10 **F**1 3 25 26 27 37 43 46 47 48 49 59 76 77 79 100 102 103 107 119 137
Primary Contact: Alan Coppock, Administrator
Control: Corporation, Investor–owned, for–profit **Service:** Long–Term Acute Care hospital

Staffed Beds: 32 **Admissions:** 376 **Census:** 25 **Outpatient Visits:** 0 **Births:** 0

COVINGTON—Kenton County

HEALTHSOUTH NORTHERN KENTUCKY REHABILITATION HOSPITAL See Edgewood

NORTHKEY COMMUNITY CARE (184006), (Formerly Children's Psychiatric Hospital), 502 Farrell Drive, Zip 41011–3799, Mailing Address: P.O. Box 2680, Zip 41012–2680; tel. 859/578–3200 **A**9 10 **F**88 90 91 92 94 95 119
Primary Contact: Edward G. Muntel, Ph.D., President and Chief Executive Officer
CFO: John Metzger, Controller
Web address: www.northkey.org
Control: Other not–for–profit (including NFP Corporation) **Service:** Children's hospital psychiatric

Staffed Beds: 25 **Admissions:** 384 **Census:** 17 **Outpatient Visits:** 0 **Births:** 0 **Total Expense ($000):** 3714 **Payroll Expense ($000):** 2306 **Personnel:** 54

★ **ST. ELIZABETH MEDICAL CENTER–SOUTH (180035)**, 1 Medical Village Drive, Zip 41017–3403; tel. 859/301–2000, (Includes ST. ELIZABETH MEDICAL CENTER–NORTH, 401 East 20th Street, Zip 41014–1585; tel. 859/292–4000), (Total facility includes 19 beds in nursing home–type unit) **A**1 2 3 5 9 10 **F**3 5 8 11 12 13 14 15 17 18 20 22 24 25 26 27 30 31 32 33 34 36 38 40 41 42 43 44 45 46 49 50 53 55 56 57 58 59 61 62 66 68 69 70 72 73 74 75 76 77 79 80 84 86 87 88 91 92 93 94 95 96 97 98 99 100 101 102 103 104 105 106 107 108 109 111 112 114 117 118 119 120 121 123 124 130 131 132 134 135 136 137 **P**6
Primary Contact: Joseph W. Gross, FACHE, President and Chief Executive Officer
CFO: Garren Colvin, Senior Vice President and Chief Financial Officer
CMO: Allen Zobay, M.D., Vice President Medical Affairs
CIO: Alex Rodriguez, Vice President and Chief Information Officer
CHR: Martin Oscadal, Vice President Human Resources
Web address: www.stelizabeth.com
Control: Church–operated, Nongovernment, not–for profit **Service:** General Medical and Surgical

Staffed Beds: 501 **Admissions:** 29923 **Census:** 350 **Outpatient Visits:** 538901 **Births:** 3256 **Total Expense ($000):** 441789 **Payroll Expense ($000):** 192004 **Personnel:** 3117

CYNTHIANA—Harrison County

★ **HARRISON MEMORIAL HOSPITAL (180079)**, 1210 KY Highway 36E, Zip 41031–7498; tel. 859/234–2300 **A**1 9 10 **F**3 11 13 15 24 25 26 27 30 31 32 33 34 37 38 41 49 50 52 55 56 57 60 62 66 67 68 72 73 74 75 76 77 79 80 81 82 84 86 87 96 97 102 106 107 119 120 121 122 124 135 136 137 **P**1
Primary Contact: Darwin E. Root, Chief Executive Officer
COO: Sheila Currans, Chief Operating Officer
CFO: Charles Duffy, Chief Financial Officer
CIO: Martha Sullivan, Director Information Services
CHR: Janice Ogden, Director Human Resource Management
Web address: www.harrisonmemhosp.com
Control: Other not–for–profit (including NFP Corporation) **Service:** General Medical and Surgical

Staffed Beds: 49 **Admissions:** 1725 **Census:** 16 **Outpatient Visits:** 50334 **Births:** 245 **Total Expense ($000):** 25507 **Payroll Expense ($000):** 10075 **Personnel:** 227

DANVILLE—Boyle County

★ **EPHRAIM MCDOWELL REGIONAL MEDICAL CENTER (180048)**, 217 South Third Street, Zip 40422–9983; tel. 859/239–1000, (Total facility includes 18 beds in nursing home–type unit) **A**1 5 9 10 19 **F**3 11 15 17 20 24 25 26 27 38 43 55 56 57 59 64 68 69 71 72 73 74 75 76 77 79 80 81 82 84 86 88 90 91 92 93 96 100 102 105 107 112 117 118 121 122 124 135 137 **P**5 7 8
Primary Contact: L. Clark Taylor, Jr., Chief Executive Officer
COO: Vick Darnell, Executive Vice President and Chief Operating Officer
CFO: William R. Snapp, Vice President and Chief Financial Officer
CMO: Jonathan Ricker, M.D., President Medical Staff
CIO: Allen Levi, Director Information Services
CHR: Carl Metz, Vice President Human Resources
Web address: www.emrmc.org
Control: Other not–for–profit (including NFP Corporation) **Service:** General Medical and Surgical

Staffed Beds: 160 **Admissions:** 8420 **Census:** 121 **Outpatient Visits:** 119086 **Births:** 784 **Total Expense ($000):** 93529 **Payroll Expense ($000):** 39918 **Personnel:** 1015

EDGEWOOD—Kenton County

★ **HEALTHSOUTH NORTHERN KENTUCKY REHABILITATION HOSPITAL (183027)**, 201 Medical Village Drive, Zip 41017–3407; tel. 859/341–2044, (Nonreporting) **A**1 9 10 **S** HEALTHSOUTH Corporation
Primary Contact: Brenda Gosney, Chief Executive Officer
CFO: Lisa McGue, Manager Accounting
CMO: Neal Moser, M.D., Medical Director
CHR: Diane Goldschmidt, Manager Human Resources
Web address: www.healthsouth.com
Control: Corporation, Investor–owned, for–profit **Service:** Rehabilitation

Staffed Beds: 40

ELIZABETHTOWN—Hardin County

★ **HARDIN MEMORIAL HOSPITAL (180012)**, 913 North Dixie Avenue, Zip 42701; tel. 270/737–1212, (Total facility includes 15 beds in nursing home–type unit) **A**1 2 9 10 19 **F**3 8 11 12 13 15 17 18 20 22 24 25 26 27 28 30 31 32 33 35 37 38 41 43 48 49 50 51 55 56 57 61 62 66 68 69 71 72 73 74 75 76 77 78 79 80 81 82 84 86 88 92 96 97 100 102 103 105 106 107 108 109 113 117 118 119 120 121 123 124 133 135 136 137 **S** Baptist Healthcare System
Primary Contact: David L. Gray, President
COO: Diane Logsdon, Vice President
CFO: Elmer Cummings, Vice President and Chief Financial Officer
CIO: Mark Brookman, Director Information Technology
CHR: Ann Kelley, Director Human Resources
Web address: www.hmh.net
Control: County–Government, nonfederal **Service:** General Medical and Surgical

Staffed Beds: 268 **Admissions:** 12492 **Census:** 169 **Outpatient Visits:** 251917 **Births:** 1695 **Total Expense ($000):** 154610 **Payroll Expense ($000):** 64391 **Personnel:** 1373

★ **HEALTHSOUTH REHABILITATION HOSPITAL OF CENTRAL KENTUCKY (183028)**, (Formerly Lakeview Rehabilitation Hospital), 134 Heartland Drive, Zip 42701–2778; tel. 270/769–3100, (Nonreporting) **A**1 9 10 **S** HEALTHSOUTH Corporation
Primary Contact: Eileen Nelson, Chief Executive Officer
CFO: James Hutcherson, Supervisor Accounting
CMO: Vickie Lowe, M.D., Medical Director
CHR: Janet Morris, Coordinator Human Resources
Web address: www.healthsouth.com
Control: Corporation, Investor–owned, for–profit **Service:** Rehabilitation

Staffed Beds: 40

FLEMINGSBURG—Fleming County

★ **FLEMING COUNTY HOSPITAL (180053)**, 920 Elizaville Avenue, Zip 41041, Mailing Address: P.O. Box 388, Zip 41041–0388; tel. 606/849–5000 **A**1 9 10 **F**3 11 15 25 26 27 30 31 32 33 38 46 55 56 57 68 72 73 75 76 77 79 80 81 82 86 96 97 99 100 102 107 117 118 119 122 124 135 **S** QHR
Primary Contact: David R. Sirk, Chief Executive Officer
CFO: Ron Harrington, Chief Financial Officer
CMO: Michael Dunaway, M.D., Chief of Staff
CIO: Don Daugherty, Director Information Systems
CHR: Marsha Mitchell, Director Human Resources
Web address: www.flemingcountyhospital.org
Control: County–Government, nonfederal **Service:** General Medical and Surgical

Staffed Beds: 52 **Admissions:** 2145 **Census:** 30 **Outpatient Visits:** 41045 **Births:** 0 **Total Expense ($000):** 17547 **Payroll Expense ($000):** 8176 **Personnel:** 261

FLORENCE—Boone County

☐ **GATEWAY REHABILITATION HOSPITAL (183030)**, 5940 Merchant Street, Zip 41042; tel. 859/426–2400, (Nonreporting) **A**1 9 10 **S** United Rehab Corporation
Primary Contact: Jim Burcham, Chief Executive Officer
Web address: www.gatewaylouisville.com
Control: Corporation, Investor–owned, for–profit **Service:** Rehabilitation

Staffed Beds: 40

★ **ST. LUKE HOSPITAL WEST (180045)**, 7380 Turfway Road, Zip 41042–1337; tel. 859/212–5200, (Total facility includes 16 beds in nursing home–type unit) **A**1 9 10 **F**3 5 11 12 13 15 18 24 25 26 27 28 30 31 32 33 34 38 40 41 43 46 48 49 50 52 54 55 56 57 59 60 62 66 69 71 72 73 74 75 76 77 78 79 80 81 82 84 86 87 88 90 91 92 93 94 95 96 100 102 103 106 107 113 114 117 118 119 120 121 123 124 133 135 136
Primary Contact: Nancy Kremer, Senior Vice President
COO: Nancy Kremer, Senior Vice President
CMO: Nannette Bernales, M.D., Medical Staff President
CIO: Alex Rodriguez, Vice President Information Systems Technology
CHR: Janet Patterson, Director Human Resources
Web address: www.stlukeshospitals.com
Control: Other not–for–profit (including NFP Corporation) **Service:** General Medical and Surgical

Staffed Beds: 177 **Admissions:** 9106 **Census:** 118 **Outpatient Visits:** 133429 **Births:** 1094 **Total Expense ($000):** 83549 **Payroll Expense ($000):** 38441 **Personnel:** 732

Many Facility Codes have changed. Please refer to the AHA Guide Code Chart.

FORT CAMPBELL—Christian County

★ **COLONEL FLORENCE A. BLANCHFIELD ARMY COMMUNITY HOSPITAL,** 650 Joel Drive, Zip 42223; tel. 270/798–8040, (Nonreporting) **A**1 5 **S** Department of the Army, Office of the Surgeon General
Primary Contact: Colonel Richard Thomas, Commander
CMO: Lieutenant Colonel Michael Place, M.D., Deputy Commander Clinical Services
CIO: Gloria K. Davis, Chief Information Management
CHR: Major Travis Burchett, Troop Commander Human Resources
Web address: www.campbell.amedd.army.mil/
Control: Army, Government, federal **Service:** General Medical and Surgical

Staffed Beds: 66

FORT KNOX—Hardin County

★ **IRELAND ARMY COMMUNITY HOSPITAL,** 289 Ireland Avenue, Zip 40121–5111; tel. 502/624–0467, (Nonreporting) **A**1 5 9 **S** Department of the Army, Office of the Surgeon General
Primary Contact: Colonel Rhonda Earls, Commander
Web address: www.iach.knox.amedd.army.mil/
Control: Army, Government, federal **Service:** General Medical and Surgical

Staffed Beds: 76

FORT THOMAS—Campbell County

□ **CARDINAL HILL SPECIALTY HOSPITAL (182004),** 85 North Grand Avenue, Zip 41075; tel. 859/572–3880 **A**1 9 10 **F**1 3 25 26 27 30 31 32 37 43 44 50 60 72 73 76 77 80 81 82 90 119 137 **P**5 **S** Cardinal Hill Healthcare System
Primary Contact: Janice Bauer, Administrator
Web address: www.iglou.com/cardinalhill/ltach.html
Control: Other not–for–profit (including NFP Corporation) **Service:** Long–Term Acute Care hospital

Staffed Beds: 32 **Admissions:** 210 **Census:** 17 **Outpatient Visits:** 0 **Births:** 0 **Total Expense ($000):** 7787 **Payroll Expense ($000):** 2950 **Personnel:** 65

★ **ST. LUKE HOSPITAL EAST (180001),** 85 North Grand Avenue, Zip 41075–1796; tel. 859/572–3100, (Total facility includes 26 beds in nursing home–type unit) **A**1 2 9 10 **F**3 4 11 12 13 15 17 18 24 25 26 27 28 30 31 32 33 34 37 38 40 41 46 49 50 52 54 55 56 57 59 60 62 66 68 69 71 72 73 74 75 76 77 78 79 80 81 82 86 87 90 96 97 100 102 103 106 107 112 113 117 118 119 120 121 123 124 133 135 136
Primary Contact: Nancy Kremer, President and Chief Executive Officer
COO: Nancy Kremer, President and Chief Executive Officer
CFO: James Sommerkamp, Director Financial Services
CMO: James Devitt, M.D., President Medical Staff
CHR: Ernie Prater, Interim Director Human Resources
Web address: www.health–alliance.com
Control: Other not–for–profit (including NFP Corporation) **Service:** General Medical and Surgical

Staffed Beds: 249 **Admissions:** 8363 **Census:** 124 **Outpatient Visits:** 114366 **Births:** 960 **Total Expense ($000):** 77258 **Payroll Expense ($000):** 37704 **Personnel:** 709

FRANKFORT—Franklin County

★ **FRANKFORT REGIONAL MEDICAL CENTER (180127),** 299 King's Daughters Drive, Zip 40601–4186; tel. 502/875–5240, (Nonreporting) **A**1 9 10 19 **S** HCA
Primary Contact: Chip Peal, Chief Executive Officer
CFO: Richard Patterson, Chief Financial Officer
CMO: Willis P. McKee, M.D., Chief Medical Officer
CIO: Bill Knapke, Director Information Technology and Systems
CHR: Bev Young, Director Human Resources
Web address: www.frankfortregional.com
Control: Corporation, Investor–owned, for–profit **Service:** General Medical and Surgical

Staffed Beds: 148

FRANKLIN—Simpson County

□ **THE MEDICAL CENTER AT FRANKLIN (181318),** 1100 Brookhaven Road, Zip 42134–2746; tel. 270/598–4800 **A**1 9 10 18 **F**3 15 24 25 26 28 30 31 32 33 38 46 55 56 57 62 66 73 75 79 81 82 86 96 100 102 107 119 122 124 135 137
Primary Contact: Clara M. Sumner, Chief Executive Officer
CFO: Ron Sowell, Executive Vice President
CIO: Jean Cherry, Executive Vice President
Web address: www.themedicalcenterfranklin.org
Control: Other not–for–profit (including NFP Corporation) **Service:** General Medical and Surgical

Staffed Beds: 25 **Admissions:** 947 **Census:** 14 **Outpatient Visits:** 17547 **Births:** 0 **Personnel:** 91

FULTON—Fulton County

★ **PARKWAY REGIONAL HOSPITAL (180117),** 2000 Holiday Lane, Zip 42041–8468; tel. 270/472–2522, (Nonreporting) **A**1 9 10 **S** Community Health Systems, Inc.
Primary Contact: Stephen Lunn, Chief Executive Officer
CFO: Dana Lawrence, Chief Financial Officer
CMO: F. Gregory Cox, M.D., Chief of Staff
CHR: Janice Bone, Director Human Resources
Web address: www.parkwayregionalhospital.com
Control: Corporation, Investor–owned, for–profit **Service:** General Medical and Surgical

Staffed Beds: 70

GEORGETOWN—Scott County

★ **GEORGETOWN COMMUNITY HOSPITAL (180101),** 1140 Lexington Road, Zip 40324–9362; tel. 502/868–1100 **A**1 5 9 10 **F**3 8 11 12 13 15 24 25 26 38 51 55 56 57 67 68 72 73 74 75 77 79 80 82 86 96 97 98 99 100 102 103 118 119 120 121 122 135 136 **P**5 **S** LifePoint Hospitals, Inc.
Primary Contact: Barry A. Papania, Chief Executive Officer
COO: Carrie H. Johnson, Chief Nursing Officer
CFO: Patrick C. Bolander, Chief Financial Officer
CMO: Ray Depa, M.D., President Medical Staff
CHR: Sandy Hickey, Director Human Resources
Web address: www.georgetowncommunityhospital.com
Control: Corporation, Investor–owned, for–profit **Service:** General Medical and Surgical

Staffed Beds: 75 **Admissions:** 2634 **Census:** 22 **Outpatient Visits:** 27111 **Births:** 541 **Total Expense ($000):** 33051 **Payroll Expense ($000):** 13230 **Personnel:** 243

GLASGOW—Barren County

★ **T. J. SAMSON COMMUNITY HOSPITAL (180017),** 1301 North Race Street, Zip 42141–3483; tel. 270/651–4444, (Total facility includes 16 beds in nursing home–type unit) **A**1 3 5 9 10 19 **F**2 3 11 13 15 18 20 22 24 25 26 27 30 31 32 38 42 43 55 56 57 59 61 62 68 69 70 72 73 74 75 76 77 79 80 81 82 84 86 87 96 99 100 101 102 103 107 112 117 118 119 121 124 135 137
Primary Contact: Bill Kindred, Interim Chief Executive Officer
COO: Larry Morgan, Controller
CFO: Anthony G. Sudduth, CPA, Chief Financial Officer
CMO: Matt Rose, M.D., Chief of Staff
CIO: Debbie Caudel–Logsdon, Director Information System
CHR: LaDonna Rogers, Director Human Resources
Web address: www.tjsamson.org
Control: Other not–for–profit (including NFP Corporation) **Service:** General Medical and Surgical

Staffed Beds: 196 **Admissions:** 7841 **Census:** 76 **Outpatient Visits:** 89371 **Births:** 1146 **Total Expense ($000):** 95054 **Payroll Expense ($000):** 45044 **Personnel:** 1046

GREENSBURG—Green County

JANE TODD CRAWFORD HOSPITAL (181325), 202–206 Milby Street, Zip 42743–1100, Mailing Address: P.O. Box 220, Zip 42743–0220; tel. 270/932–4211, (Total facility includes 20 beds in nursing home–type unit) (Nonreporting) **A**9 10 18
Primary Contact: Rex A. Tungate, Administrator
CMO: James G. Bland, M.D., Chief of Staff
Control: County–Government, nonfederal **Service:** General Medical and Surgical

Staffed Beds: 45

GREENVILLE—Muhlenberg County

★ **MUHLENBERG COMMUNITY HOSPITAL (180004),** 440 Hopkinsville Street, Zip 42345–1172, Mailing Address: P.O. Box 387, Zip 42345–0387; tel. 270/338–8000 **A**1 9 10 **F**3 7 8 11 13 15 25 26 33 37 38 46 47 48 51 55 56 57 61 62 68 73 74 75 77 79 82 84 87 96 97 98 99 100 101 102 107 112 117 118 119 120 121 124 134 135 136 **S** Alliant Management Services
Primary Contact: George E. Walz, CHE, Interim Chief Executive Officer
CFO: John R. Clements, Chief Financial Officer
CMO: Marty Casebier, M.D., President Medical Staff
CIO: Clarice Guy, Director Health Information Management
CHR: Lisa R. Hope, Director Human Resources
Web address: www.mchky.org
Control: Other not–for–profit (including NFP Corporation) **Service:** General Medical and Surgical

Staffed Beds: 135 **Admissions:** 3600 **Census:** 70 **Births:** 300

Hospital, Medicare Provider Number, Address, Telephone, Approval, Facility, and Physician Codes, Health Care System

★ American Hospital Association (AHA) membership
□ The Joint Commission accreditation
○ American Osteopathic Association (AOA) accreditation
△ Commission on Accreditation of Rehabilitation Facilities (CARF) accreditation

HARDINSBURG—Breckinridge County

★ **BRECKINRIDGE MEMORIAL HOSPITAL (181319)**, 1011 Old Highway 60, Zip 40143–2597; tel. 270/756–7000, (Total facility includes 18 beds in nursing home–type unit) **A**1 9 10 18 **F**3 11 15 24 25 26 32 33 38 42 43 52 54 55 56 57 61 62 63 66 73 75 77 79 82 86 90 96 107 119 121 122 123 124 135 **P**6 **S** Alliant Management Services
Primary Contact: John E. Monnahan, President and Chief Executive Officer
CFO: David R. Hayes, Vice President and Chief Financial Officer
CMO: Shannon Elliot, M.D., President Medical Staff
CIO: Virginia D. Bradley, Chief Information Officer
CHR: Clara Cordelia Hall, Chief Human Resources Officer
Web address: www.breckhealth.org
Control: Other not–for–profit (including NFP Corporation) **Service:** General Medical and Surgical

Staffed Beds: 43 **Admissions:** 986 **Census:** 31 **Outpatient Visits:** 26120 **Births:** 0 **Total Expense ($000):** 12410 **Payroll Expense ($000):** 5044 **Personnel:** 163

HARLAN—Harlan County

☐ **HARLAN ARH HOSPITAL (180050)**, 81 Ball Park Road, Zip 40831–1792; tel. 606/573–8100 **A**1 9 10 19 **F**3 11 13 15 24 25 26 30 31 32 33 38 43 50 53 55 56 57 61 62 65 68 73 74 75 77 79 80 81 82 84 85 86 87 88 92 96 97 102 106 107 118 119 121 135 136 **P**6 **S** Appalachian Regional Healthcare
Primary Contact: Dan Stone, Chief Executive Officer
CFO: Pam Sutherland, Chief Financial Officer
CMO: Abdullah Dahhan, M.D., Chief of Staff
CHR: Sabra Howard, Manager Human Resources
Web address: www.arh.org
Control: Other not–for–profit (including NFP Corporation) **Service:** General Medical and Surgical

Staffed Beds: 130 **Admissions:** 4520 **Census:** 45 **Outpatient Visits:** 71028 **Births:** 301 **Total Expense ($000):** 43262 **Payroll Expense ($000):** 16017 **Personnel:** 452

HARRODSBURG—Mercer County

★ **THE JAMES B. HAGGIN MEMORIAL HOSPITAL (181302)**, 464 Linden Avenue, Zip 40330–1862; tel. 859/734–5441, (Total facility includes 34 beds in nursing home–type unit) (Nonreporting) **A**1 5 9 10 18 **S** Alliant Management Services
Primary Contact: Earl J. Motzer, Ph.D., FACHE, Chief Executive Officer
CFO: Tony Patterson, Chief Financial Officer
Web address: www.hagginhosp.org
Control: Other not–for–profit (including NFP Corporation) **Service:** General Medical and Surgical

Staffed Beds: 59

HARTFORD—Ohio County

★ **OHIO COUNTY HOSPITAL (181323)**, 1211 Main Street, Zip 42347–1619; tel. 270/298–7411 **A**1 9 10 18 **F**3 11 15 17 24 25 26 27 30 31 32 33 34 36 38 40 42 43 44 48 49 52 53 55 56 57 62 68 72 73 75 76 77 79 81 86 87 96 100 107 119 120 121 122 124 135 **P**8 **S** QHR
Primary Contact: Blaine Pieper, Chief Executive Officer
Web address: www.ohiocountyhospital.com
Control: Other not–for–profit (including NFP Corporation) **Service:** General Medical and Surgical

Staffed Beds: 25 **Admissions:** 1329 **Census:** 14 **Outpatient Visits:** 30809 **Births:** 0 **Total Expense ($000):** 18507 **Payroll Expense ($000):** 8637 **Personnel:** 226

HAZARD—Perry County

☐ **HAZARD ARH REGIONAL MEDICAL CENTER (180029)**, 100 Medical Center Drive, Zip 41701–1000; tel. 606/439–6600 **A**1 2 3 5 9 10 19 **F**3 11 13 15 17 18 20 22 24 25 26 27 30 31 32 33 38 40 43 50 53 55 56 57 61 62 68 71 72 73 74 75 76 77 79 80 81 82 84 85 86 87 88 92 96 97 100 103 106 107 118 119 121 135 136 137 **P**6 **S** Appalachian Regional Healthcare
Primary Contact: Donald R. Fields, Senior Community Chief Executive Officer
COO: Donald R. Fields, Senior Community Chief Executive Officer
CMO: J. D. Miller, M.D., Chief Medical Officer
CIO: Jeff Brady, Director Information Systems
CHR: Sheila Cornett, Human Resources Manager
Web address: www.arh.org
Control: Other not–for–profit (including NFP Corporation) **Service:** General Medical and Surgical

Staffed Beds: 308 **Admissions:** 13066 **Census:** 221 **Outpatient Visits:** 98443 **Births:** 381 **Total Expense ($000):** 95147 **Payroll Expense ($000):** 32605 **Personnel:** 1006

HENDERSON—Henderson County

☐ △ **METHODIST HOSPITAL (180056)**, 1305 North Elm Street, Zip 42420–2775, Mailing Address: P.O. Box 48, Zip 42420–0048; tel. 270/827–7700 **A**1 7 9 10 12 13 **F**3 5 7 11 13 15 18 25 26 27 28 30 31 32 33 36 37 38 47 51 52 53 55 56 57 61 62 64 66 68 71 72 73 74 75 76 77 79 80 81 82 84 85 86 87 88 92 96 97 99 100 104 105 107 118 119 120 121 124 135 136 137 **P**8
Primary Contact: Bruce D. Begley, Executive Director
CFO: Gregory P. Hebbeler, Chief Financial Officer
CMO: James M. Stearns, M.D., Chief of Staff
CIO: Gregory P. Hebbeler, Chief Financial Officer
CHR: Karen Freeman, Director Human Resources
Web address: www.methodisthospital.net
Control: Church–operated, Nongovernment, not–for profit **Service:** General Medical and Surgical

Staffed Beds: 216 **Admissions:** 6692 **Census:** 80 **Outpatient Visits:** 313889 **Births:** 748 **Total Expense ($000):** 94891 **Payroll Expense ($000):** 41710 **Personnel:** 1041

HOPKINSVILLE—Christian County

☐ **CUMBERLAND HALL HOSPITAL (184014)**, 210 West 17th Street, Zip 42240–1999; tel. 270/886–1919, (Nonreporting) **A**1 9 10 **S** Psychiatric Solutions
Primary Contact: Catherine Willner, Chief Executive Officer
CFO: Greg Francois, Chief Financial Officer
CMO: Deepak Patel, M.D., Medical Director
CIO: Patricia Gray, Director Health Information Management
CHR: Kelly Hagy, Director Human Resources
Web address: www.psysolutions.com
Control: Corporation, Investor–owned, for–profit **Service:** Psychiatric

Staffed Beds: 48

★ **JENNIE STUART MEDICAL CENTER (180051)**, 320 West 18th Street, Zip 42241–2400, Mailing Address: P.O. Box 2400, Zip 42241–2400; tel. 270/887–0100 **A**1 2 9 10 **F**11 13 15 17 18 24 25 31 32 33 38 40 43 48 49 55 57 61 62 68 70 72 73 74 75 76 77 78 79 81 84 86 96 97 100 104 106 107 118 119 120 124 133 135 137 **P**8 **S** QHR
Primary Contact: Terry Peeples, Chief Executive Officer
COO: Eric A. Lee, Vice President Development and Operations
CFO: Samuel L. Brown, Vice President Financial Services
CMO: Dan Perkins, M.D., President Medical Staff
CIO: Jerry Houston, Director Information Systems
CHR: Austin Moss, Vice President Human Resources
Web address: www.jsmc.org
Control: Other not–for–profit (including NFP Corporation) **Service:** General Medical and Surgical

Staffed Beds: 139 **Admissions:** 7169 **Census:** 83 **Outpatient Visits:** 140884 **Births:** 882 **Total Expense ($000):** 82640 **Payroll Expense ($000):** 30716 **Personnel:** 832

☐ **WESTERN STATE HOSPITAL (184002)**, Russellville Road, Zip 42240–3017, Mailing Address: P.O. Box 2200, Zip 42241–2200; tel. 270/889–6025, (Nonreporting) **A**1 10
Primary Contact: Stephen P. Wiggins, Director
CFO: Jessica Cates, Fiscal Manager
CMO: Nayyar Iqbal, Medical Staff Director
CIO: Valerie Majors, Director Information Services
CHR: James L. Hayes, Director Human Resources
Control: State–Government, nonfederal **Service:** Psychiatric

Staffed Beds: 222

HORSE CAVE—Hart County

★ **CAVERNA MEMORIAL HOSPITAL (181314)**, 1501 South Dixie Street, Zip 42749–1477; tel. 270/786–2191 **A**9 10 18 **F**3 15 31 32 38 55 57 62 68 79 80 84 96 100 102 107 117 122 **S** Alliant Management Services
Primary Contact: Alan B. Alexander, Chief Executive Officer
CFO: Debra Riggs, Chief Financial Officer
CHR: Cathy Szabo, Director Human Resources
Web address: www.cavernahospital.com
Control: Other not–for–profit (including NFP Corporation) **Service:** General Medical and Surgical

Staffed Beds: 25 **Admissions:** 643 **Census:** 8 **Outpatient Visits:** 19609 **Births:** 0 **Total Expense ($000):** 8158 **Payroll Expense ($000):** 3316 **Personnel:** 112

HYDEN—Leslie County

MARY BRECKINRIDGE HOSPITAL (181316), 130 Kate Ireland Drive, Zip 41749–0000, Mailing Address: P.O. Box 447–A, Zip 41749–0000; tel. 606/672–2901 **A**9 10 18 **F**3 11 13 15 25 30 31 32 38 55 62 74 79 82 84 96 107 119 122 **P**6
Primary Contact: Mallie S. Noble, Administrator
COO: Nathan W. Lee, Chief Executive Officer
CFO: Robert Besten, Chief Financial Officer
CMO: Roy Varghese, M.D., Chief of Staff
CIO: Frank Baker, Chief Information Officer
CHR: Beulah Couch, Director Human Resources
Web address: www.frontiernursing.org
Control: Other not–for–profit (including NFP Corporation) **Service:** General Medical and Surgical

Staffed Beds: 25 **Admissions:** 1246 **Census:** 10 **Outpatient Visits:** 9760 **Births:** 94 **Total Expense ($000):** 16873 **Payroll Expense ($000):** 5712 **Personnel:** 189

IRVINE—Estill County

★ **MARCUM AND WALLACE MEMORIAL HOSPITAL (181301)**, 60 Mercy Court, Zip 40336–1331; tel. 606/723–2115 **A**9 10 18 **F**3 11 15 25 26 30 32 33 34 38 44 55 56 57 79 84 86 87 96 102 106 107 122 136 **P**6 **S** Catholic Healthcare Partners
Primary Contact: Susan Starling, President and Chief Executive Officer
CFO: Della Deerfield, Vice President Finance
CMO: James Foster, M.D., Medical Director
CIO: Elizabeth Walling, Coordinator Mission and Quality
CHR: Dana Stepp, Human Resources Officer
Web address: www.marcumandwallace.org
Control: Church–operated, Nongovernment, not–for profit **Service:** General Medical and Surgical

Staffed Beds: 25 **Admissions:** 849 **Census:** 8 **Outpatient Visits:** 51907 **Births:** 0 **Total Expense ($000):** 10587 **Payroll Expense ($000):** 4592 **Personnel:** 131

JACKSON—Breathitt County

★☐ **KENTUCKY RIVER MEDICAL CENTER (180139)**, 540 Jett Drive, Zip 41339–9620; tel. 606/666–6000, (Nonreporting) **A**1 9 10 20 **S** Community Health Systems, Inc.
Primary Contact: Donald Rentfro, Chief Executive Officer
CFO: Michael Ackley, Chief Financial Officer
CMO: Eunice Johnson, M.D., Chief Medical Staff
CIO: Diana Tyra, Director Health Information
CHR: Naomi Mitchell, Director Human Resources
Web address: www.kentuckyrivermc.com
Control: Corporation, Investor–owned, for–profit **Service:** General Medical and Surgical

Staffed Beds: 54

JENKINS—Letcher County

☐ **JENKINS COMMUNITY HOSPITAL (181326)**, Main Street, Zip 41537–9614, Mailing Address: P.O. Box 472, Zip 41537–0472; tel. 606/832–2171, (Nonreporting) **A**1 9 10 18 **S** Wellmont Health System
Primary Contact: Sherrie L. Newcomb, Administrator
CFO: Barbara Collins, Controller
CMO: Adil Warsy, M.D., Chief Medical Officer
CIO: Ursla Scott, Chief Information Officer
Control: Corporation, Investor–owned, for–profit **Service:** General Medical and Surgical

Staffed Beds: 25

LA GRANGE—Oldham County

★☐ **BAPTIST HOSPITAL NORTHEAST (182006)**, 1025 New Moody Lane, Zip 40031–0559; tel. 502/222–5388, (Total facility includes 18 beds in nursing home–type unit) **A**1 9 10 **F**3 11 13 15 24 25 26 31 32 33 34 38 40 43 46 49 50 54 55 56 57 62 66 68 72 73 74 75 77 79 80 81 82 86 96 97 100 102 107 117 118 119 120 121 122 124 135 136 137 **P**6 **S** Baptist Healthcare System
Primary Contact: Dennis B. Johnson, Administrator
CFO: Susanne Haynes, Executive Director Finance
CMO: Joshua Honaker, M.D., Chief Medical Officer
CIO: Jackie Lucas, Vice President Information Systems
CHR: Jean Harden, Executive Director Human Resources
Web address: www.baptistnortheast.com
Control: Other not–for–profit (including NFP Corporation) **Service:** General Medical and Surgical

Staffed Beds: 82 **Admissions:** 3303 **Census:** 48 **Outpatient Visits:** 44604 **Births:** 423 **Total Expense ($000):** 37983 **Payroll Expense ($000):** 17907 **Personnel:** 306

LEBANON—Marion County

★☐ **SPRING VIEW HOSPITAL (180024)**, 320 Loretto Road, Zip 40033–0320; tel. 270/692–3161 **A**1 9 10 **F**3 11 13 15 25 26 31 32 33 38 48 49 50 51 55 56 57 62 66 68 73 74 75 77 79 81 82 85 86 96 97 100 102 107 119 120 122 124 135 136 137 **P**6 **S** LifePoint Hospitals, Inc.
Primary Contact: Michael T. Sherrod, Chief Executive Officer
CFO: Denise Thomas, Chief Financial Officer
CIO: Douglas Bland, Manager Information Services
CHR: Ann Dabney, Manager Human Resources
Web address: www.springviewhospital.com
Control: Corporation, Investor–owned, for–profit **Service:** General Medical and Surgical

Staffed Beds: 60 **Admissions:** 2055 **Census:** 19 **Outpatient Visits:** 43300 **Births:** 432 **Total Expense ($000):** 20567 **Payroll Expense ($000):** 9688 **Personnel:** 231

LEITCHFIELD—Grayson County

★☐ **TWIN LAKES REGIONAL MEDICAL CENTER (180070)**, 910 Wallace Avenue, Zip 42754–1499; tel. 270/259–9400 **A**1 9 10 **F**3 11 13 15 24 25 26 27 32 38 52 55 56 57 61 66 68 74 76 77 79 80 81 82 84 86 96 97 102 106 107 118 119 121 122 124 135 **P**6 **S** Alliant Management Services
Primary Contact: Stephen L. Meredith, Chief Executive Officer
COO: Deneace Clemons, Chief Operating Officer
CFO: Scott Arndell, Chief Financial Officer
CMO: Darren Lyle, M.D., President Medical Staff
CIO: Pam McCrady, Director Information Systems
CHR: Mandy Bryant, Director Human Resources
Web address: www.tlrmc.com
Control: Other not–for–profit (including NFP Corporation) **Service:** General Medical and Surgical

Staffed Beds: 75 **Admissions:** 2592 **Census:** 30 **Outpatient Visits:** 71053 **Births:** 353 **Total Expense ($000):** 26206 **Payroll Expense ($000):** 11220 **Personnel:** 317

LEXINGTON—Fayette County

★ △ **CARDINAL HILL REHABILITATION HOSPITAL (183026)**, 2050 Versailles Road, Zip 40504–1499; tel. 859/254–5701 **A**3 5 7 9 10 **F**2 3 9 11 25 26 28 30 31 32 33 34 36 41 43 44 50 52 54 55 56 57 58 61 63 64 66 72 73 75 77 81 82 85 86 107 119 120 121 123 135 137 **S** Cardinal Hill Healthcare System
Primary Contact: Kerry G. Gillihan, FACHE, President and Chief Executive Officer
COO: Beth Monarch, Executive Vice President and Chief Operating Officer
CFO: Timothy Wilson, Vice President Finance and Chief Financial Officer
CMO: William Lester, M.D., Vice President Medical Affairs
CIO: Steve Kincaid, Manager Information Systems
CHR: Laban Miller, Ph.D., Vice President Human Resources
Web address: www.cardinalhill.org
Control: Other not–for–profit (including NFP Corporation) **Service:** Rehabilitation

Staffed Beds: 108 **Admissions:** 2215 **Census:** 92 **Outpatient Visits:** 58257 **Births:** 0 **Total Expense ($000):** 44138 **Payroll Expense ($000):** 25789 **Personnel:** 534

★☐ **CENTRAL BAPTIST HOSPITAL (180103)**, 1740 Nicholasville Road, Zip 40503–1499; tel. 859/260–6100 **A**1 2 9 10 **F**3 11 13 15 17 18 20 22 24 25 26 27 30 31 32 33 34 35 38 41 42 43 44 45 49 52 53 55 56 57 58 59 61 62 66 68 70 72 73 74 75 76 77 79 80 81 82 84 86 96 97 99 100 101 102 103 105 106 107 108 109 112 114 118 119 120 121 124 135 136 137 **P**5 **S** Baptist Healthcare System
Primary Contact: William G. Sisson, President
CFO: Bobbie L. Prather, Chief Financial Officer
CMO: Preston Nunelley, M.D., Chief Medical Officer
CIO: Ty Knox, Director Information Services
CHR: Lynette Walker, Director Human Resources
Web address: www.centralbap.com
Control: Other not–for–profit (including NFP Corporation) **Service:** General Medical and Surgical

Staffed Beds: 347 **Admissions:** 18885 **Census:** 225 **Outpatient Visits:** 175569 **Births:** 3700 **Total Expense ($000):** 295217 **Payroll Expense ($000):** 100339 **Personnel:** 1966

★ **CONTINUING CARE HOSPITAL (182002)**, 150 North Eagle Creek Drive, 5th Floor, Zip 40509; tel. 859/967–5744 **A**9 10 **F**1 3 25 26 31 32 34 66 **S** Catholic Health Initiatives
Primary Contact: Tonja Williams, President and Chief Executive Officer
Control: Other not–for–profit (including NFP Corporation) **Service:** Long–Term Acute Care hospital

Staffed Beds: 30 **Admissions:** 424 **Census:** 27 **Outpatient Visits:** 0 **Births:** 0 **Total Expense ($000):** 10140 **Payroll Expense ($000):** 3391 **Personnel:** 74

Hospital, Medicare Provider Number, Address, Telephone, Approval, Facility, and Physician Codes, Health Care System

★ American Hospital Association (AHA) membership
☐ The Joint Commission accreditation
○ American Osteopathic Association (AOA) accreditation
△ Commission on Accreditation of Rehabilitation Facilities (CARF) accreditation

☐ **EASTERN STATE HOSPITAL (184004)**, 627 West Fourth Street, Zip 40508–1294; tel. 859/246–7000, (Nonreporting) **A**1 3 5 9 10
Primary Contact: Joseph A. Toy, President and Chief Executive Officer
COO: Susan M. Griffith, Chief Operations
CFO: Tambara Nalle, Chief Financial Officer
CMO: Enedino R. Corales, M.D., Chief Medical Staff
CIO: Bud Stone, Director Information Systems
CHR: Kimberly White, Director Employee Relations
Web address: www.bluegrass.org
Control: State–Government, nonfederal **Service:** Psychiatric

Staffed Beds: 197

FEDERAL MEDICAL CENTER, 3301 Leestown Road, Zip 40511–8799; tel. 859/255–6812, (Nonreporting)
Primary Contact: Stephen DeWalt, Warden
CFO: Mike Kinsel, Controller
CMO: Michael Growse, M.D., Clinical Director
Control: Department of Justice, Government, federal **Service:** Hospital unit of an institution (prison hospital, college infimary, etc.)

Staffed Beds: 22

☐ **RIDGE BEHAVIORAL HEALTH SYSTEM (184009)**, 3050 Rio Dosa Drive, Zip 40509–9990; tel. 859/269–2325, (Nonreporting) **A**1 3 5 9 10 **S** Universal Health Services, Inc.
Primary Contact: Nina W. Eisner, Chief Executive Officer and Managing Director
CFO: Richard McDowell, Chief Financial Officer
CMO: Saeed Hamid, M.D., Medical Director
CHR: Lori Redding, Director Human Resources
Web address: www.ridgebhs.com
Control: Corporation, Investor–owned, for–profit **Service:** Psychiatric

Staffed Beds: 110

★ **SAINT JOSEPH HOSPITAL (180010)**, One St. Joseph Drive, Zip 40504–3754; tel. 859/278–3436 **A**1 2 3 5 9 10 **F**1 3 11 15 17 18 20 22 24 25 26 27 28 30 31 32 33 34 38 43 44 50 53 54 55 57 60 61 62 66 67 68 72 73 75 76 77 78 79 80 81 82 86 92 96 97 100 102 103 104 105 106 107 118 119 120 121 124 135 137 **P**3 **S** Catholic Health Initiatives
Primary Contact: Eugene A. Woods, President and Chief Executive Officer
CFO: Gary J. Ermers, Vice President Finance and Chief Financial Officer
CIO: Janie Fergus, Director and Chief Information Officer
Web address: www.sjhlex.org
Control: Church–operated, Nongovernment, not–for profit **Service:** General Medical and Surgical

Staffed Beds: 366 **Admissions:** 16504 **Census:** 227 **Outpatient Visits:** 104880 **Births:** 0 **Total Expense ($000):** 250465 **Payroll Expense ($000):** 84710 **Personnel:** 1891

★ **SAINT JOSEPH HOSPITAL EAST (180143)**, 150 North Eagle Creek Drive, Zip 40509–1807; tel. 859/268–4800 **A**1 5 9 10 **F**1 3 11 12 13 15 18 20 25 26 28 30 31 32 38 43 50 53 54 55 57 60 62 66 70 72 73 74 75 76 77 79 80 81 82 84 86 92 96 97 100 102 103 107 118 119 120 121 124 135 136 **S** Catholic Health Initiatives
Primary Contact: Eric Gilliam, Administrator
CFO: Gary J. Ermers, Vice President Finance and Chief Financial Officer
CIO: Janie Fergus, Director and Chief Information Officer
CHR: Rick Tolson, Vice President Human Resources
Web address: www.sjhlex.org
Control: Church–operated, Nongovernment, not–for profit **Service:** General Medical and Surgical

Staffed Beds: 144 **Admissions:** 8302 **Census:** 87 **Outpatient Visits:** 79466 **Births:** 2039 **Total Expense ($000):** 92087 **Payroll Expense ($000):** 33961 **Personnel:** 722

SAMARITAN HOSPITAL See UK HealthCare Good Samaritan Hospital

☐ **SELECT SPECIALTY HOSPITAL OF LEXINGTON (182003)**, 310 South Limeston Street, 3rd Floor, Zip 40509; tel. 859/226–7178, (Nonreporting) **A**1 9 10 **S** Select Medical Corporation
Primary Contact: Seth A. Sauve, Chief Executive Officer
Web address: www.selectmedicalcorp.com
Control: Corporation, Investor–owned, for–profit **Service:** Long–Term Acute Care hospital

Staffed Beds: 41

☐ **SHRINERS HOSPITALS FOR CHILDREN–LEXINGTON**, 1900 Richmond Road, Zip 40502–1298; tel. 859/266–2101, (Nonreporting) **A**1 3 5 **S** Shriners Hospitals for Children
Primary Contact: Tony Lewgood, Administrator
CFO: Robert Montgomery, Chief Financial Officer
CMO: Chester Tylkowski, M.D., Chief of Staff
CIO: David Brian, Director Information Services
Web address: www.shrinershq.com
Control: Other not–for–profit (including NFP Corporation) **Service:** Children's orthopedic

Staffed Beds: 50

★ **UK HEALTHCARE GOOD SAMARITAN HOSPITAL (180007)**, (Formerly Samaritan Hospital), 310 South Limestone Street, Zip 40508–3008; tel. 859/226–7000, (Nonreporting) **A**1 3 5 9 10 **S** UK HealthCare
Primary Contact: Frank Beirne, Chief Executive Officer
COO: Mark Armstrong, Chief Operating Officer
CMO: Tadarro J. Richardson, M.D., Chief of Staff
CHR: Pat Imerman, Director Human Resources
Web address: www.samaritanhospital.com
Control: Other not–for–profit (including NFP Corporation) **Service:** General Medical and Surgical

Staffed Beds: 271

★ **UNIVERSITY OF KENTUCKY HOSPITAL (180067)**, 800 Rose Street, N100, Zip 40536–0293; tel. 859/323–5000 **A**1 2 3 5 8 9 10 **F**3 5 6 7 8 11 12 13 15 16 17 18 19 20 21 22 23 25 26 27 28 30 31 32 33 34 35 36 37 38 40 41 43 46 47 48 49 50 54 55 56 57 58 59 60 62 63 64 66 68 70 72 73 74 75 76 77 79 80 81 82 83 84 86 87 88 89 90 91 92 93 94 96 97 99 100 102 106 107 109 111 112 113 114 116 119 120 121 123 124 125 126 127 128 129 130 131 135 136 137 **P**6 **S** UK HealthCare
Primary Contact: Murray B. Clark, Jr., Associate Vice President Operations and Hospital Administration
CFO: Sergio L. Melgar, Chief Financial Officer
CMO: Richard Lofgren, M.D., Chief Medical Officer
CIO: Zed Day, Chief Information Officer
CHR: Kimberly P. Wilson, Director Human Resources
Web address: www.ukhealthcare.uky.edu
Control: State–Government, nonfederal **Service:** General Medical and Surgical

Staffed Beds: 473 **Admissions:** 27331 **Census:** 406 **Outpatient Visits:** 476103 **Births:** 2040 **Total Expense ($000):** 529274 **Payroll Expense ($000):** 167078 **Personnel:** 4084

★ **VETERANS AFFAIRS MEDICAL CENTER–LEXINGTON**, 1101 Veterans Drive, Zip 40502; tel. 859/233–4511, (Total facility includes 61 beds in nursing home–type unit) **A**1 3 5 8 **F**3 4 5 17 18 20 24 25 26 27 37 38 42 43 44 49 52 53 54 55 56 57 58 59 60 62 66 68 69 72 73 75 76 77 79 80 82 86 87 88 90 92 93 94 96 97 100 102 106 107 117 118 119 121 124 135 136 137 **P**6 **S** Department of Veterans Affairs
Primary Contact: Sandy Nielsen, Director
COO: Donna K. Jacobs, Associate Director
CFO: Walter Zawisza, Chief Fiscal Service
CMO: Walter A. Divers, M.D., Chief of Staff
CIO: Karen Merrill, Chief Information Officer
CHR: Laura Faulkner, Chief Human Resource Management Service
Web address: www.va.gov/sta/guide/home.asp
Control: Veterans Affairs, Government, federal **Service:** General Medical and Surgical

Staffed Beds: 199 **Admissions:** 6017 **Census:** 152 **Outpatient Visits:** 337159 **Births:** 0 **Total Expense ($000):** 215096 **Payroll Expense ($000):** 85689 **Personnel:** 1558

LIBERTY—Casey County

☐ **CASEY COUNTY HOSPITAL (181309)**, 187 Wolford Avenue, Zip 42539; tel. 606/787–6275, (Nonreporting) **A**1 9 10 18
Primary Contact: Rex A. Tungate, Administrator
Control: County–Government, nonfederal **Service:** General Medical and Surgical

Staffed Beds: 24

LONDON—Laurel County

★ **SAINT JOSEPH – LONDON (180011)**, (Formerly Marymount Medical Center), 310 East Ninth Street, Zip 40741–1299; tel. 606/878–6520 **A**1 9 10 19 **F**11 13 15 18 20 22 25 26 27 31 32 33 37 38 42 43 44 45 49 50 51 55 56 57 58 59 61 62 63 68 69 72 73 74 75 76 77 79 81 82 96 97 100 107 119 121 124 135 **S** Catholic Health Initiatives
Primary Contact: Virginia B. Dempsey, Chief Executive Officer
CFO: Robert Brock, Chief Financial Officer
CMO: Marc Briere, M.D., President Medical Staff
CIO: Debbie Mullins, Director
CHR: Richard Huck, Vice President Human Resources
Web address: www.marymount.com
Control: Church–operated, Nongovernment, not–for profit **Service:** General Medical and Surgical

Staffed Beds: 89 **Admissions:** 6971 **Census:** 70 **Outpatient Visits:** 131945 **Births:** 702 **Total Expense ($000):** 83826 **Payroll Expense ($000):** 41050 **Personnel:** 704

LOUISA—Lawrence County

★ **THREE RIVERS MEDICAL CENTER (180128)**, Highway 644, Zip 41230–9632, Mailing Address: P.O. Box 769, Zip 41230–0769; tel. 606/638–9451 **A**1 9 10 **F**3 12 13 15 17 25 30 31 32 38 51 55 56 57 61 68 74 75 77 79 80 81 82 86 87 88 92 93 94 96 100 107 119 121 122 135 **S** Community Health Systems, Inc.
Primary Contact: Greg Kiser, Chief Executive Officer
CFO: Marcus Conley, Chief Financial Officer
CHR: Pat Hart, Director Human Resources and Marketing
Web address: www.threeriversmedicalcenter.com
Control: Corporation, Investor–owned, for–profit **Service:** General Medical and Surgical

Staffed Beds: 80 **Admissions:** 5037 **Census:** 48 **Outpatient Visits:** 32073 **Births:** 195 **Total Expense ($000):** 38950 **Personnel:** 321

LOUISVILLE—Jefferson County

★ △ **BAPTIST HOSPITAL EAST (180130)**, 4000 Kresge Way, Zip 40207–4676; tel. 502/897–8100 **A**1 2 5 7 9 10 **F**3 5 11 13 15 17 18 20 22 24 25 26 27 30 31 32 33 34 36 38 41 43 44 45 49 50 51 52 53 54 55 56 57 61 62 66 68 70 72 73 74 76 77 79 80 81 82 84 85 86 88 89 90 91 92 93 94 95 96 97 99 100 102 103 105 106 107 108 109 111 112 118 119 121 123 124 135 136 137 **S** Baptist Healthcare System
Primary Contact: Susan Stout Tamme, FACHE, President
CFO: Steve Warren, Vice President Finance
CMO: Thomas Dedman, M.D., Medical Director
CHR: Anthony Bohn, Vice President Human Resources
Web address: www.baptisteast.com
Control: Other not–for–profit (including NFP Corporation) **Service:** General Medical and Surgical

Staffed Beds: 407 **Admissions:** 26761 **Census:** 348 **Outpatient Visits:** 190097 **Births:** 3529 **Total Expense ($000):** 329381 **Payroll Expense ($000):** 139371 **Personnel:** 2705

□ **CENTRAL STATE HOSPITAL (184015)**, 10510 LaGrange Road, Zip 40223–1228; tel. 502/253–7000 **A**1 3 5 10 **F**26 81 82 88 119 **P**6
Primary Contact: Patricia Brodie, Chief Executive Officer
CFO: Bernie Babione, Chief Financial Officer
Control: State–Government, nonfederal **Service:** Psychiatric

Staffed Beds: 116 **Admissions:** 1143 **Census:** 110 **Outpatient Visits:** 0 **Births:** 0 **Total Expense ($000):** 32589 **Payroll Expense ($000):** 3558 **Personnel:** 493

★ △ **FRAZIER REHAB INSTITUTE**, 220 Abraham Flexner Way, Zip 40202–1887; tel. 502/582–7400 **A**1 3 5 7 9 **F**24 25 26 30 32 33 43 44 50 53 54 55 56 57 58 62 66 72 73 75 76 77 80 81 82 85 86 90 119 120 121 135 137 **P**6 **S** Jewish Hospital & St. Mary's HealthCare
Primary Contact: Joanne Berryman, Senior Vice President
COO: Deborah Molnar, Senior Vice President and Chief Operating Officer
CFO: Stephen Scannell, Vice President Finance and Associate Chief Financial Officer
CMO: David R. Watkins, M.D., Chief of Staff
CIO: Maria Russo, Vice President and Chief Information Officer
CHR: Lisa Burris, Manager Human Resources
Web address: www.frazierrehab.org
Control: Other not–for–profit (including NFP Corporation) **Service:** Rehabilitation

Staffed Beds: 135 **Admissions:** 1870 **Census:** 78 **Outpatient Visits:** 114341 **Births:** 0 **Total Expense ($000):** 47938 **Payroll Expense ($000):** 20747 **Personnel:** 467

★ **JEWISH HOSPITAL (180040)**, 200 Abraham Flexner Way, Zip 40202–1886; tel. 502/587–4011 **A**1 2 3 5 9 10 **F**1 3 8 11 14 15 17 18 20 22 24 25 26 27 30 32 33 35 37 38 39 40 42 43 44 46 48 49 50 53 54 55 56 57 58 59 60 62 66 68 69 72 73 75 76 77 78 79 80 81 82 87 90 96 97 99 100 102 103 104 106 107 116 118 119 120 121 124 126 127 128 129 130 131 134 135 136 137 **P**6 **S** Jewish Hospital & St. Mary's HealthCare
Primary Contact: Martin J. Bonick, President and Chief Executive Officer
COO: Deborah Molnar, Senior Vice President and Chief Operating Officer
CFO: Douglas Davenport, Interim Chief Financial Officer
CMO: Lynn Simon, M.D., Senior Vice President and Chief Medical Officer
CIO: Jim Basham, Interim Chief Information Officer
CHR: Ed Farmer, Vice President and Chief People Officer
Web address: www.jewishhospital.org
Control: Other not–for–profit (including NFP Corporation) **Service:** General Medical and Surgical

Staffed Beds: 442 **Admissions:** 21092 **Census:** 341 **Outpatient Visits:** 548819 **Births:** 1 **Total Expense ($000):** 460883 **Payroll Expense ($000):** 148641 **Personnel:** 2976

KINDRED HOSPITAL LOUISVILLE AT JEWISH HOSPITAL (182001), 200 Abraham Flexner Way, 2nd Floor, Zip 40202; tel. 502/587–3999, (Nonreporting) **A**9 10 **S** Kindred Healthcare
Primary Contact: Jack Nicholson, Chief Executive Officer
Web address: www.kindredhealthcare.com
Control: Corporation, Investor–owned, for–profit **Service:** Long–Term Acute Care hospital

Staffed Beds: 30

□ **KINDRED HOSPITAL–LOUISVILLE (182001)**, 1313 St. Anthony Place, Zip 40204–1765; tel. 502/587–7001, (Total facility includes 37 beds in nursing home–type unit) (Nonreporting) **A**1 5 9 10 **S** Kindred Healthcare
Primary Contact: Lourene Money, Interim Chief Executive Officer
CFO: Debra Michalek, Chief Financial Officer
Web address: www.kindredhealthcare.com
Control: Partnership, Investor–owned, for–profit **Service:** Long–Term Acute Care hospital

Staffed Beds: 156

KOSAIR CHILDREN'S HOSPITAL See Norton Hospital

★ **NORTON AUDUBON HOSPITAL**, One Audubon Plaza Drive, Zip 40217–1397, Mailing Address: P.O. Box 17550, Zip 40217–0550; tel. 502/636–7111 **A**1 2 3 5 9 **F**3 9 11 15 17 18 20 22 25 26 27 30 31 32 33 36 38 43 46 49 50 54 55 56 57 62 68 72 73 76 77 79 80 81 82 86 87 96 97 99 100 102 107 118 119 121 124 135 136 **S** Norton Healthcare
Primary Contact: Thomas D. Kmetz, President
COO: Jon Cooper, Associate Vice President Operations
CFO: Jeff Lilly, Associate Vice President Finance
CMO: Steven Hester, M.D., Vice President Medical Affairs
CIO: Joseph DeVenuto, Vice President and Chief Information Officer
CHR: Larry Callahan, Vice President Human Resources
Web address: www.nortonhealthcare.org
Control: Other not–for–profit (including NFP Corporation) **Service:** General Medical and Surgical

Staffed Beds: 268 **Admissions:** 13266 **Census:** 196 **Outpatient Visits:** 126727 **Births:** 0 **Total Expense ($000):** 203488 **Payroll Expense ($000):** 75034 **Personnel:** 1234

★ **NORTON HOSPITAL (180088)**, 200 East Chestnut Street, Zip 40202–1800, Mailing Address: P.O. Box 35070, Zip 40232–5070; tel. 502/629–8000, (Includes KOSAIR CHILDREN'S HOSPITAL, tel. 502/629–6000; Douglas J. Eighmey, Administrator; NORTON HEALTHCARE PAVILION, 315 East Broadway, Zip 40202–1703; tel. 502/629–2000) **A**1 2 3 5 9 10 **F**3 11 12 13 15 16 17 18 19 20 21 22 23 24 25 26 27 28 30 31 32 33 34 36 37 38 40 43 44 50 51 52 54 55 56 57 62 66 68 70 71 72 73 74 76 77 79 81 82 83 84 86 88 89 90 91 92 94 96 97 99 100 101 102 105 106 107 113 114 116 118 119 121 125 126 127 132 135 136 137 **S** Norton Healthcare
Primary Contact: Kevin S. Wardell, President
COO: Gregg Davis, Associate Vice President Operations
CFO: Carl Amorose, Associate Vice President Finance
CMO: Steven Hester, M.D., Vice President Medical Affairs
CIO: Joseph DeVenuto, Vice President Information Services and Chief Information Officer
CHR: Elizabeth Hanckel, Vice President Human Resources
Web address: www.nortonhealthcare.org
Control: Other not–for–profit (including NFP Corporation) **Service:** General Medical and Surgical

Staffed Beds: 649 **Admissions:** 27606 **Census:** 435 **Outpatient Visits:** 225068 **Births:** 2433 **Total Expense ($000):** 507465 **Payroll Expense ($000):** 167233 **Personnel:** 3048

★ **NORTON SUBURBAN HOSPITAL**, 4001 Dutchmans Lane, Zip 40207–4799; tel. 502/893–1000 **A**1 2 5 9 **F**3 8 11 12 13 15 18 20 22 25 26 27 30 31 32 33 34 36 38 41 43 50 51 54 55 56 57 62 68 70 71 72 73 74 76 77 79 80 81 82 86 87 96 97 100 102 107 108 109 111 113 119 120 121 132 135 136 137 **S** Norton Healthcare
Primary Contact: John D. Harryman, President
COO: Allyn Simmons, Associate Vice President Operations
CFO: Mark Kircher, Associate Vice President Finance
CMO: Steven Hester, M.D., Vice President Medical Affairs
CIO: Joseph DeVenuto, Vice President and Chief Information Officer
Web address: www.nortonhealthcare.com
Control: Other not–for–profit (including NFP Corporation) **Service:** General Medical and Surgical

Staffed Beds: 348 **Admissions:** 17526 **Census:** 219 **Outpatient Visits:** 112402 **Births:** 5995 **Total Expense ($000):** 191356 **Payroll Expense ($000):** 68661 **Personnel:** 1172

Hospital, Medicare Provider Number, Address, Telephone, Approval, Facility, and Physician Codes, Health Care System

★ American Hospital Association (AHA) membership
□ The Joint Commission accreditation
○ American Osteopathic Association (AOA) accreditation
△ Commission on Accreditation of Rehabilitation Facilities (CARF) accreditation

★ **OUR LADY OF PEACE**, 2020 Newburg Road, Zip 40205–1879; tel. 502/451–3330, (Nonreporting) **A**1 9 **S** Jewish Hospital & St. Mary's HealthCare
Primary Contact: JoAnne D. Maamry, Chief Executive Officer
CMO: Gerald Moore, M.D., Medical Director
Web address: www.jhsmh.org
Control: Other not–for–profit (including NFP Corporation) **Service:** Psychiatric

Staffed Beds: 206

★ **STS. MARY & ELIZABETH HOSPITAL**, 1850 Bluegrass Avenue, Zip 40215–1199; tel. 502/361–6000, (Total facility includes 33 beds in nursing home–type unit) **A**1 9 **F**3 8 11 12 15 18 24 25 26 27 30 31 32 33 38 39 40 43 47 49 50 51 52 53 55 56 57 59 62 67 68 72 73 76 77 79 81 82 86 96 97 99 100 102 103 106 107 117 118 119 121 124 135 137 **S** Jewish Hospital & St. Mary's HealthCare
Primary Contact: Thomas Gessel, Chief Executive Officer
COO: Kenneth Johnson, Vice President
CFO: Elaine Hayes, Controller
CMO: Lawrence Goldberg, M.D., Medical Director
CIO: Maria Russo, Vice President and Chief Information Officer
CHR: Julie McGregor, Director Human Resources
Web address: www.jhsmh.org
Control: Other not–for–profit (including NFP Corporation) **Service:** General Medical and Surgical

Staffed Beds: 236 **Admissions:** 12609 **Census:** 183 **Outpatient Visits:** 165089 **Total Expense ($000):** 125812 **Payroll Expense ($000):** 51210 **Personnel:** 1029

☐ **TEN BROECK DUPONT (184007)**, 1405 Browns Lane, Zip 40207; tel. 502/896–0495, (Nonreporting) **A**1 9 10 **S** United Medical Corporation
Primary Contact: John Hollinsworth, Executive Director
Control: Corporation, Investor–owned, for–profit **Service:** Psychiatric

Staffed Beds: 66

☐ **TEN BROECK HOSPITAL (184008)**, 8521 Old LaGrange Road, Zip 40242–3800; tel. 502/426–6380 **A**1 5 9 10 **F**4 5 30 31 54 62 88 89 90 91 92 93 94 95 119 **P**5 **S** United Medical Corporation
Primary Contact: John Hollinsworth, Executive Director
COO: Kim Peabody, Chief Operating Officer
CFO: Glenn Brewer, Chief Financial Officer
CMO: Timothy Burke, M.D., Medical Director
CIO: Joel Roy, Manager Information Systems
CHR: Sean Davenport, Director Human Resources
Web address: www.tenbroeck.com
Control: Corporation, Investor–owned, for–profit **Service:** Psychiatric

Staffed Beds: 94 **Admissions:** 1618 **Census:** 91 **Outpatient Visits:** 14346 **Births:** 0 **Total Expense ($000):** 13841 **Payroll Expense ($000):** 7150

★ **UNIVERSITY OF LOUISVILLE HOSPITAL (180141)**, 530 South Jackson Street, Zip 40202–3611; tel. 502/562–3000 **A**1 2 3 5 8 9 10 **F**3 13 15 16 17 18 20 22 25 26 27 30 31 32 33 35 37 38 40 44 46 47 48 49 50 54 55 56 57 58 60 62 63 66 68 69 70 71 72 73 74 76 77 78 79 80 81 82 86 88 90 92 93 96 97 99 100 102 103 105 106 107 108 109 111 112 118 119 121 124 125 133 135 **P**4
Primary Contact: James H. Taylor, FACHE, President and Chief Executive Officer
CFO: Robert P. Barbier, Chief Financial Officer
CMO: Kristine Krueger, M.D., Chief of Staff
CIO: Troy May, Chief Information Officer
CHR: Gary Bensing, Vice President Human Resources
Web address: www.ulh.org
Control: Other not–for–profit (including NFP Corporation) **Service:** General Medical and Surgical

Staffed Beds: 325 **Admissions:** 16019 **Census:** 286 **Outpatient Visits:** 196767 **Births:** 2282 **Total Expense ($000):** 348791 **Payroll Expense ($000):** 113700 **Personnel:** 2460

★ **VETERANS AFFAIRS MEDICAL CENTER–LOUISVILLE**, 800 Zorn Avenue, Zip 40206–1499; tel. 502/287–4000, (Nonreporting) **A**1 2 3 5 8 **S** Department of Veterans Affairs
Primary Contact: Wayne L. Pfeffer, FACHE, Director
COO: Beth Brown, Associate Director
CFO: Barbara Roberts, Chief Financial Officer
CMO: Marylee Rothschild, M.D., Chief of Staff
CIO: Augustine Bittner, Chief Information Officer
CHR: Angela Dutton, Chief Human Resources Management Service
Web address: www.louisville.va.gov
Control: Veterans Affairs, Government, federal **Service:** General Medical and Surgical

Staffed Beds: 110

MADISONVILLE—Hopkins County

★ **REGIONAL MEDICAL CENTER OF HOPKINS COUNTY (180093)**, 900 Hospital Drive, Zip 42431–1694; tel. 270/825–5100 **A**1 2 3 5 9 10 19 20 **F**3 8 11 13 14 18 20 22 24 25 26 27 30 31 32 33 38 41 42 49 51 52 55 56 57 58 59 61 62 66 68 71 74 76 77 79 80 82 83 84 85 86 96 97 98 100 102 105 106 107 109 117 118 119 120 121 135 137
Primary Contact: E. Berton Whitaker, Chief Executive Officer
CFO: David Cauble, Chief Financial Officer
CMO: Mark Browne, M.D., Vice President Medical Affairs
CIO: Terry Jackson, Director Information System
CHR: David Lang, Vice President Human Resources
Web address: www.troverfoundation.org
Control: Other not–for–profit (including NFP Corporation) **Service:** General Medical and Surgical

Staffed Beds: 223 **Admissions:** 10677 **Census:** 132 **Outpatient Visits:** 232854 **Births:** 1011 **Total Expense ($000):** 115351 **Payroll Expense ($000):** 51531 **Personnel:** 1488

MANCHESTER—Clay County

★ ○ **MANCHESTER MEMORIAL HOSPITAL (180043)**, 210 Marie Langdon Drive, Zip 40962–9156; tel. 606/598–5104 **A**1 9 10 11 19 20 **F**3 13 15 25 26 28 30 31 32 33 38 52 55 56 57 61 66 68 73 74 75 77 79 86 96 97 100 107 124 135 **P**5 6 **S** Adventist Health System Sunbelt Health Care Corporation
Primary Contact: Dennis Meyers, President and Chief Executive Officer
COO: Helen Wilson, Chief Operating Officer
CFO: Gary Carlson, Chief Financial Officer
CHR: Joe Skula, Director Human Resources
Web address: www.manchestermemorial.com
Control: Church–operated, Nongovernment, not–for profit **Service:** General Medical and Surgical

Staffed Beds: 63 **Admissions:** 3020 **Census:** 32 **Outpatient Visits:** 54085 **Births:** 155 **Total Expense ($000):** 44123 **Payroll Expense ($000):** 17946 **Personnel:** 472

MARION—Crittenden County

★ **CRITTENDEN COUNTY HOSPITAL (180095)**, 520 West Gum Street, Zip 42064–6201, Mailing Address: P.O. Box 386, Zip 42064–0386; tel. 270/965–5281 **A**1 9 10 20 **F**7 11 15 17 25 26 38 50 55 57 61 75 79 86 96 100 102 107 118 122 **P**6 **S** QHR
Primary Contact: Jim Christensen, Chief Executive Officer
CFO: Joseph A. Swab, Chief Financial Officer
CIO: Reese Baker, Director Information Systems
CHR: Jan Gregory, Vice President Human Resources
Web address: www.crittenden–health.org
Control: Other not–for–profit (including NFP Corporation) **Service:** General Medical and Surgical

Staffed Beds: 48 **Admissions:** 2021 **Census:** 20 **Outpatient Visits:** 14344 **Births:** 0 **Total Expense ($000):** 14877 **Payroll Expense ($000):** 7296 **Personnel:** 189

MARTIN—Floyd County

★ **OUR LADY OF THE WAY HOSPITAL (181305)**, 11203 Main Street, Zip 41649–0910; tel. 606/285–6400 **A**1 9 10 18 **F**3 15 25 26 30 31 32 33 38 50 55 56 57 73 75 79 80 87 96 107 119 122 123 124 135 **P**6 **S** Catholic Health Initiatives
Primary Contact: Kathy Stumbo, Chief Executive Officer
CFO: Robert Brock, Chief Financial Officer
CMO: Bill Webb, D.O., President Medical Staff
CIO: Chris Dye, Director Information Systems
Web address: www.olwh.org
Control: Church–operated, Nongovernment, not–for profit **Service:** General Medical and Surgical

Staffed Beds: 25 **Admissions:** 995 **Census:** 11 **Outpatient Visits:** 66118 **Births:** 0 **Total Expense ($000):** 18423 **Payroll Expense ($000):** 9546

MAYFIELD—Graves County

★ **JACKSON PURCHASE MEDICAL CENTER (180116)**, 1099 Medical Center Circle, Zip 42066–1179; tel. 270/251–4100 **A**1 9 10 19 **F**1 3 4 8 11 12 13 15 16 17 18 20 24 25 26 27 31 32 33 35 38 40 47 49 50 51 54 55 56 57 62 65 66 68 70 71 72 73 74 75 77 78 79 80 81 82 83 84 85 86 87 88 96 100 103 105 107 112 117 118 119 120 121 122 124 135 136 137 **P**7 **S** LifePoint Hospitals, Inc.
Primary Contact: Mary Jo Lewis, Chief Executive Officer
CFO: Dirk Morgan, Chief Financial Officer
Web address: www.jacksonpurchase.com
Control: Corporation, Investor–owned, for–profit **Service:** General Medical and Surgical

Staffed Beds: 107 **Admissions:** 4939 **Census:** 54 **Outpatient Visits:** 76256 **Births:** 462 **Total Expense ($000):** 37228 **Payroll Expense ($000):** 14333 **Personnel:** 428

MAYSVILLE—Mason County

★ **MEADOWVIEW REGIONAL MEDICAL CENTER (180019)**, 989 Medical Park Drive, Zip 41056–8750; tel. 606/759–5311 **A**1 9 10 **F**1 3 4 8 13 15 16 17 18 20 25 26 27 30 31 32 33 34 36 38 43 49 54 55 56 57 62 63 65 68 70 71 73 74 76 77 78 79 80 81 82 83 84 85 86 87 88 96 102 103 107 112 117 118 119 120 121 122 124 135 136 **S** LifePoint Hospitals, Inc.
Primary Contact: Chad Patrick, Chief Executive Officer
CFO: Teresa Daniel, Chief Financial Officer
CIO: Lori Moore, Director Information Services
CHR: Diana Kennedy, Director Human Resources
Web address: www.meadowviewregional.com
Control: Corporation, Investor–owned, for–profit **Service:** General Medical and Surgical

Staffed Beds: 101 **Admissions:** 3848 **Census:** 31 **Outpatient Visits:** 32012 **Births:** 535 **Total Expense ($000):** 27545 **Payroll Expense ($000):** 11843 **Personnel:** 256

MCDOWELL—Floyd County

MCDOWELL ARH HOSPITAL (181331), Route 122, Zip 41647, Mailing Address: P.O. Box 247, Zip 41647–0247; tel. 606/377–3400, (Total facility includes 10 beds in nursing home–type unit) **A**9 10 18 **F**3 11 15 17 25 26 30 31 32 33 38 43 50 55 56 57 61 62 63 65 68 71 73 75 79 81 82 84 85 86 87 88 96 102 107 117 119 122 135 **P**6 **S** Appalachian Regional Healthcare
Primary Contact: Russel Barker, Community Chief Executive Officer
COO: Russel Barker, Community Chief Executive Officer
CFO: Chris Ellington, Chief Financial Officer
CMO: Mary A. Hall, Chief Medical Staff
CIO: Jeff Brady, Director Information Systems
CHR: Stephanie Owens, Manager Human Resources
Web address: www.arh.org
Control: Other not–for–profit (including NFP Corporation) **Service:** General Medical and Surgical

Staffed Beds: 35 **Admissions:** 1074 **Census:** 15 **Outpatient Visits:** 34810 **Births:** 0 **Total Expense ($000):** 13578 **Payroll Expense ($000):** 5683 **Personnel:** 127

MIDDLESBORO—Bell County

☐ **MIDDLESBORO APPALACHIAN REGIONAL HOSPITAL (180020)**, 3600 West Cumberland Avenue, Zip 40965–2614, Mailing Address: P.O. Box 340, Zip 40965–0340; tel. 606/242–1100 **A**1 9 10 **F**3 11 13 15 17 25 26 30 31 32 33 37 38 50 55 56 57 61 62 68 73 74 75 77 79 80 81 82 84 85 86 87 96 97 100 102 106 107 119 122 135 136 137 **P**6 **S** Appalachian Regional Healthcare
Primary Contact: Susan Roman, Community Chief Executive Officer
CFO: Greg Giles, Assistant Administrator and Community Chief Financial Officer
CMO: Rogelio Uy, M.D., Chief of Staff
CIO: Lisa Dooley, Health Information Officer
CHR: Edie Kelley, Human Resources Representative
Web address: www.arh.org/middlesboro
Control: Other not–for–profit (including NFP Corporation) **Service:** General Medical and Surgical

Staffed Beds: 96 **Admissions:** 3593 **Census:** 37 **Outpatient Visits:** 64380 **Births:** 351 **Total Expense ($000):** 28751 **Payroll Expense ($000):** 11430 **Personnel:** 295

MONTICELLO—Wayne County

WAYNE COUNTY HOSPITAL (181321), 166 Hospital Street, Zip 42633–2416; tel. 606/348–9343, (Nonreporting) **A**9 10 18
Primary Contact: John L. Osborne, Administrator
CFO: Anne Sawyer, Chief Financial Officer
CMO: Cory Ryan, M.D., Chief of Staff
CIO: Angela Griffin, Privacy Officer
CHR: Mollie Dick, Coordinator Human Resources
Web address: www.waynehospital.org
Control: Other not–for–profit (including NFP Corporation) **Service:** General Medical and Surgical

Staffed Beds: 25

MOREHEAD—Rowan County

★ **ST. CLAIRE REGIONAL MEDICAL CENTER (180018)**, 222 Medical Circle, Zip 40351–1180; tel. 606/783–6500, (Total facility includes 10 beds in nursing home–type unit) **A**1 2 3 5 9 10 19 **F**3 5 11 13 15 18 24 25 26 27 30 31 32 33 36 37 38 40 42 43 44 48 49 50 53 54 55 56 57 58 59 60 61 62 63 66 68 72 73 74 75 76 77 79 80 81 82 84 85 86 87 88 89 90 91 92 93 94 96 97 100 103 106 107 117 118 119 121 124 135 136 137 **P**6
Primary Contact: Mark J. Neff, FACHE, President and Chief Executive Officer
CFO: Sonny Jones, Vice President Finance and Chief Financial Officer
CMO: Kim Williams, M.D., Vice President Medical Affairs
CIO: Randy McCleese, Chief Information Officer
CHR: Travis Bailey, Vice President Administration
Web address: www.st–claire.org
Control: Church–operated, Nongovernment, not–for profit **Service:** General Medical and Surgical

Staffed Beds: 133 **Admissions:** 5377 **Census:** 55 **Outpatient Visits:** 232634 **Births:** 501 **Total Expense ($000):** 99729 **Payroll Expense ($000):** 48319 **Personnel:** 1092

MORGANFIELD—Union County

★ **METHODIST HOSPITAL UNION COUNTY (181306)**, 4604 Highway 60 West, Zip 42437–9570; tel. 270/389–5000, (Total facility includes 16 beds in nursing home–type unit) **A**1 9 10 18 **F**3 7 11 15 25 26 31 32 38 55 62 73 75 79 80 86 96 107 117 119 122 124 135
Primary Contact: Patrick Donahue, Administrator
CFO: Gregory P. Hebbeler, Chief Financial Officer
Web address: www.methodisthospitaluc.net
Control: Church–operated, Nongovernment, not–for profit **Service:** General Medical and Surgical

Staffed Beds: 41 **Admissions:** 785 **Census:** 25 **Outpatient Visits:** 18818 **Births:** 0 **Total Expense ($000):** 11210 **Payroll Expense ($000):** 4724 **Personnel:** 124

MOUNT STERLING—Montgomery County

★ **SAINT JOSEPH MOUNT STERLING (180064)**, (Formerly Gateway Regional Health System), 50 Sterling Avenue, Zip 40353–1158, Mailing Address: P.O. Box 7, Zip 40353–0007; tel. 859/497–6000 **A**1 5 9 10 **F**3 13 15 17 24 25 31 32 33 38 46 55 56 57 62 68 72 73 74 75 76 77 79 81 82 86 96 97 102 107 118 119 121 122 124 136 137 **P**6 **S** Catholic Health Initiatives
Primary Contact: James F. Heitzenrater, President
CFO: Janelle Pugh, Vice President Finance and Operations
CMO: Danielle King, M.D., President Medical Staff
CIO: Jeff Ryder, Director Information Systems
CHR: Cindy Clark, Human Resource Consultant
Web address: www.sjhlex.org
Control: Other not–for–profit (including NFP Corporation) **Service:** General Medical and Surgical

Staffed Beds: 56 **Admissions:** 1713 **Census:** 19 **Outpatient Visits:** 55551 **Births:** 368 **Total Expense ($000):** 23693 **Payroll Expense ($000):** 9656 **Personnel:** 317

MOUNT VERNON—Rockcastle County

★ **ROCKCASTLE HOSPITAL AND RESPIRATORY CARE CENTER (180115)**, 145 Newcomb Avenue, Zip 40456–2733, Mailing Address: P.O. Box 1310, Zip 40456–1310; tel. 606/256–2195, (Total facility includes 79 beds in nursing home–type unit) **A**1 9 10 **F**3 12 15 24 27 30 31 32 33 38 52 55 56 57 61 62 66 73 79 82 84 86 96 100 103 106 107 117 119 122 124 135 136 **P**8
Primary Contact: Stephen A. Estes, Chief Executive Officer
CFO: Charles Black, Chief Financial Officer
CMO: Jon A. Arvin, M.D., Chief Medical Officer
CIO: Maleigha Amyx, Chief Information Officer
CHR: Carmen Poynter, Director Human Resources
Web address: www.rockcastlehospital.org
Control: Other not–for–profit (including NFP Corporation) **Service:** General Medical and Surgical

Staffed Beds: 105 **Admissions:** 1583 **Census:** 87 **Outpatient Visits:** 26915 **Births:** 0 **Total Expense ($000):** 30669 **Payroll Expense ($000):** 14722 **Personnel:** 434

Hospital, Medicare Provider Number, Address, Telephone, Approval, Facility, and Physician Codes, Health Care System

★ American Hospital Association (AHA) membership
☐ The Joint Commission accreditation
○ American Osteopathic Association (AOA) accreditation
△ Commission on Accreditation of Rehabilitation Facilities (CARF) accreditation

MURRAY—Calloway County

★ **MURRAY–CALLOWAY COUNTY HOSPITAL (180027)**, 803 Poplar Street, Zip 42071–2432; tel. 270/762–1100, (Total facility includes 218 beds in nursing home–type unit) **A**1 2 9 10 19 **F**2 3 7 11 13 14 15 18 24 25 26 27 30 31 32 33 38 42 50 51 52 55 56 57 61 62 64 65 66 68 69 72 73 74 75 76 77 79 80 82 85 86 96 97 100 102 107 109 117 118 119 120 121 124 135 136
Primary Contact: Keith E. Bailey, Chief Executive Officer
COO: Mark B. Steadham, Vice President Operations
CFO: Brad Bloemer, Vice President Finance
CMO: Richard Crouch, M.D., Chief Medical Officer
CIO: Ed Mohrman, Director Information Systems
CHR: John R. Wilson, Director Human Resources
Web address: www.murrayhospital.org
Control: City–County, Government, nonfederal **Service:** General Medical and Surgical

Staffed Beds: 323 **Admissions:** 5384 **Census:** 252 **Outpatient Visits:** 92603 **Births:** 586 **Total Expense ($000):** 77812 **Payroll Expense ($000):** 31968 **Personnel:** 879

OWENSBORO—Daviess County

★ △ **OWENSBORO MEDICAL HEALTH SYSTEM (180038)**, 811 East Parrish Avenue, Zip 42303, Mailing Address: P.O. Box 20007, Zip 42304–0007; tel. 270/688–2000, (Includes HEALTHPARK, 1006 Ford Avenue, Zip 42301; tel. 270/688–5433), (Total facility includes 30 beds in nursing home–type unit) **A**2 5 7 9 10 19 20 **F**3 5 11 12 13 15 17 18 20 22 25 26 27 28 30 31 32 33 38 39 42 43 44 45 46 47 49 52 53 54 55 56 57 58 60 61 62 64 68 71 72 74 75 76 77 79 80 81 82 84 85 86 88 90 91 92 93 94 95 96 97 99 100 102 103 106 107 108 109 110 111 112 117 119 120 121 124 133 135 136 **P**4 6 8
Primary Contact: Jeffrey B. Barber, Dr.P.h., FACHE, President and Chief Executive Officer
COO: Greg Strahan, Chief Operating Officer
CFO: John Hackbarth, CPA, CHE, Senior Vice President Finance and Chief Financial Officer
CIO: Gordon Rohweder, Chief Information Officer
CHR: Mia Suter, Senior Vice President Organizational Development
Web address: www.omhs.org
Control: Other not–for–profit (including NFP Corporation) **Service:** General Medical and Surgical

Staffed Beds: 358 **Admissions:** 18662 **Census:** 234 **Outpatient Visits:** 301575 **Births:** 1856 **Total Expense ($000):** 245093 **Payroll Expense ($000):** 92573 **Personnel:** 2437

RIVERVALLEY BEHAVIORAL HEALTH HOSPITAL (184013), 1000 Industrial Drive, Zip 42301–8715; tel. 270/689–6500 **A**9 10 **F**25 88 89 90 92 95 119 **P**6
Primary Contact: Gayle DiCesare, President and Chief Executive Officer
CFO: J. Michael Mountain, Chief Financial Officer
Web address: www.rvbh.com
Control: Other not–for–profit (including NFP Corporation) **Service:** Children's hospital psychiatric

Staffed Beds: 80 **Admissions:** 647 **Census:** 45 **Outpatient Visits:** 0 **Births:** 0 **Total Expense ($000):** 8158 **Payroll Expense ($000):** 3836 **Personnel:** 146

OWENTON—Owen County

★ ○ **NEW HORIZONS HEALTH SYSTEMS, INC. (181312)**, 330 Roland Avenue, Zip 40359–1502; tel. 502/484–3663 **A**9 10 11 18 **F**3 26 30 31 32 33 38 50 55 57 62 79 80 86 87 96 102 107 122 124 **P**6
Primary Contact: Bernard T. Poe, Administrator
COO: Bernard T. Poe, Administrator
CFO: Roger Williams, Chief Financial Officer
CMO: Douglas Smalara, M.D., Medical Director
CIO: Edward Seale, Chief Information Officer
CHR: Ruth Middleton, Director Human Resources
Web address: www.newhorizonsmedicalcenter.com
Control: Other not–for–profit (including NFP Corporation) **Service:** General Medical and Surgical

Staffed Beds: 25 **Admissions:** 522 **Census:** 5 **Outpatient Visits:** 17593 **Births:** 0 **Total Expense ($000):** 9678 **Payroll Expense ($000):** 4573 **Personnel:** 90

PADUCAH—McCracken County

★ △ **LOURDES HOSPITAL (180102)**, 1530 Lone Oak Road, Zip 42003–7900, Mailing Address: P.O. Box 7100, Zip 42002–7100; tel. 270/444–2444, (Total facility includes 20 beds in nursing home–type unit) **A**1 7 9 10 19 **F**3 10 11 12 13 15 17 18 20 22 24 25 26 27 30 31 32 33 34 38 40 41 42 43 44 50 51 52 54 55 56 57 60 61 63 66 68 71 72 73 74 75 76 77 78 79 80 81 82 84 85 86 88 90 91 92 93 94 95 96 99 100 104 105 107 117 118 119 121 124 132 133 134 135 136 **S** Catholic Healthcare Partners
Primary Contact: Steven Grinnell, President and Chief Executive Officer
COO: Nicholas P. Lewis, Chief Operating Officer
CFO: John F. Dempsey, Vice President Finance and Chief Financial Officer
CHR: Kevin McVeigh, Chief Human Resources Officer
Web address: www.lourdes–pad.org
Control: Church–operated, Nongovernment, not–for profit **Service:** General Medical and Surgical

Staffed Beds: 256 **Admissions:** 12123 **Census:** 178 **Births:** 430 **Personnel:** 984

★ **WESTERN BAPTIST HOSPITAL (180104)**, 2501 Kentucky Avenue, Zip 42003–3200; tel. 270/575–2100, (Total facility includes 24 beds in nursing home–type unit) (Nonreporting) **A**1 2 9 10 19 **S** Baptist Healthcare System
Primary Contact: Larry O. Barton, FACHE, President
CFO: Jim Carmain, Vice President Financial and Information Services
CHR: Dick Thomas, Executive Director Human Resources
Web address: www.westernbaptist.com
Control: Church–operated, Nongovernment, not–for profit **Service:** General Medical and Surgical

Staffed Beds: 288

PAINTSVILLE—Johnson County

□ **PAUL B. HALL REGIONAL MEDICAL CENTER (180078)**, 625 James S Trimble Boulevard, Zip 41240–0000; tel. 606/789–3511, (Nonreporting) **A**1 9 10 **S** Health Management Associates
Primary Contact: Deborah L. Trimble, Chief Executive Officer
CFO: Pattie Major, Controller
CMO: F. K. Belhasen, M.D., Medical Director
CHR: Samantha Castle, Human Resource Officer
Web address: www.pbhrmc.com
Control: Corporation, Investor–owned, for–profit **Service:** General Medical and Surgical

Staffed Beds: 72

PARIS—Bourbon County

★ **BOURBON COMMUNITY HOSPITAL (180046)**, 9 Linville Drive, Zip 40361–2196; tel. 859/987–3600 **A**1 9 10 **F**15 25 30 31 32 33 36 37 38 41 42 49 50 51 54 55 56 57 62 66 68 72 73 75 77 79 81 82 86 88 89 90 91 92 96 97 100 102 107 118 119 122 135 137 **S** LifePoint Hospitals, Inc.
Primary Contact: Ronald Tyrer, Interim Chief Executive Officer
COO: Donna Davis, Chief Nursing Officer
CMO: Robert Casey Wilson, M.D., Chief of Staff
CIO: David Alward, Director Information Technology
CHR: Marrianne Slonina, Director Human Resources
Web address: www.bourbonhospital.com
Control: Corporation, Investor–owned, for–profit **Service:** General Medical and Surgical

Staffed Beds: 58 **Admissions:** 1676 **Census:** 20 **Outpatient Visits:** 19753 **Births:** 0 **Total Expense ($000):** 17336 **Payroll Expense ($000):** 8339 **Personnel:** 189

PIKEVILLE—Pike County

□ **PIKEVILLE MEDICAL CENTER (180044)**, 911 Bypass Road, Zip 41501–1595; tel. 606/218–3500 **A**1 2 9 10 12 13 20 **F**5 11 13 15 18 20 22 24 25 26 27 28 33 37 38 43 49 50 51 52 55 56 57 59 60 61 62 64 66 67 68 70 72 73 74 75 76 77 79 80 81 82 84 85 86 87 96 97 99 100 103 104 105 106 107 109 111 112 118 119 121 124 132 133 135 136 137
Primary Contact: Walter E. May, President and Chief Executive Officer
COO: Deborah Puckett, Chief Operating Officer
CFO: Danny Harris, Chief Financial Officer
CMO: William Johnson, M.D., Chief Medical Director
CIO: Bernie Galla, Director Information Services
CHR: Juanita Deskins, Vice President Human Resources
Web address: www.pikevillehospital.org
Control: Other not–for–profit (including NFP Corporation) **Service:** General Medical and Surgical

Staffed Beds: 232 **Admissions:** 8692 **Census:** 119 **Outpatient Visits:** 233132 **Births:** 923 **Total Expense ($000):** 189809 **Payroll Expense ($000):** 69542 **Personnel:** 1609

PINEVILLE—Bell County

☒ **PINEVILLE COMMUNITY HOSPITAL ASSOCIATION (180021)**, 850 Riverview Avenue, Zip 40977–0850; tel. 606/337–3051, (Total facility includes 30 beds in nursing home–type unit) **A**1 9 10 **F**3 13 15 25 26 30 32 38 40 46 55 57 61 62 68 73 74 75 79 80 82 84 87 96 97 102 107 117 119
Primary Contact: J. Milton Brooks, III, Administrator
CFO: Colan Kelly, Chief Financial Officer
CMO: Steven Morgan, M.D., Chief Medical Officer
CIO: David Hall, Chief Information Officer
CHR: Greg Nunnelley, Director Human Resources
Web address: www.pinevillehospital.com
Control: Other not–for–profit (including NFP Corporation) **Service:** General Medical and Surgical

Staffed Beds: 150 **Admissions:** 4191 **Census:** 72 **Outpatient Visits:** 34822 **Births:** 243 **Total Expense ($000):** 27122 **Payroll Expense ($000):** 12079 **Personnel:** 319

PRESTONSBURG—Floyd County

☒ **HIGHLANDS REGIONAL MEDICAL CENTER (180005)**, 5000 Kentucky Route 321, Zip 41653–1273, Mailing Address: P.O. Box 668, Zip 41653–0668; tel. 606/886–8511 **A**1 2 5 9 10 12 13 19 **F**3 9 11 13 15 18 26 31 32 38 40 51 52 53 55 56 57 61 62 63 66 68 73 74 75 76 77 79 80 81 82 84 86 88 90 91 92 93 96 97 100 102 103 107 112 117 119 121 124 135
Primary Contact: Harold C. Warman, Jr., FACHE, President and Chief Executive Officer
COO: Chris Hoffman, Chief Operating Officer
CFO: Jack Blackwell, Chief Financial Officer
CIO: J. D. Jackson, Chief Information Officer
CHR: Susan Ellis, R.N., MSN, Vice President Human Resources
Web address: www.hrmc.org
Control: Other not–for–profit (including NFP Corporation) **Service:** General Medical and Surgical

Staffed Beds: 139 **Admissions:** 6994 **Census:** 80 **Outpatient Visits:** 87205 **Births:** 868 **Total Expense ($000):** 57717 **Payroll Expense ($000):** 16881 **Personnel:** 470

PRINCETON—Caldwell County

☒ **CALDWELL COUNTY HOSPITAL (181322)**, 101 Hospital Drive, Zip 42445–0410; tel. 270/365–0300 **A**1 9 10 18 **F**11 15 25 30 31 32 33 38 55 56 57 61 75 79 80 96 97 100 106 107 118 122 124 135 **S** QHR
Primary Contact: Charles D. Lovell, Jr., President and Chief Executive Officer
CFO: Shane Whittington, Chief Financial Officer
CHR: Terri Brasher, Director Human Resources
Web address: www.caldwellhosp.org
Control: Other not–for–profit (including NFP Corporation) **Service:** General Medical and Surgical

Staffed Beds: 25 **Admissions:** 762 **Census:** 7 **Outpatient Visits:** 25361 **Births:** 0 **Total Expense ($000):** 13841 **Payroll Expense ($000):** 5477 **Personnel:** 151

RADCLIFF—Hardin County

☐ **LINCOLN TRAIL BEHAVIORAL HEALTH SYSTEM (184012)**, 3909 South Wilson Road, Zip 40160–9714, Mailing Address: P.O. Box 369, Zip 40159–0369; tel. 270/351–9444, (Nonreporting) **A**1 9 10 **S** Universal Health Services, Inc.
Primary Contact: Charles L. Webb, Jr., Administrator
CFO: Debbie Ditto, CPA, Controller
Web address: www.lincolnbehavioral.com
Control: Corporation, Investor–owned, for–profit **Service:** Psychiatric

Staffed Beds: 67

RICHMOND—Madison County

☒ **PATTIE A. CLAY REGIONAL MEDICAL CENTER (180049)**, 801 Eastern Bypass, Zip 40475–2405, Mailing Address: P.O. Box 1600, Zip 40476–2603; tel. 859/623–3131 **A**1 9 10 19 **F**3 11 13 15 18 24 25 26 30 31 32 33 38 46 48 49 50 51 55 56 57 59 63 66 72 73 74 75 77 78 79 82 86 90 96 97 98 100 102 106 107 112 118 119 121 124 133 135 136 137
Primary Contact: Robert J. Hudson, President and Chief Executive Officer
CMO: Doug Owen, M.D., Chief of Staff
CHR: Joy Benedict, Director Human Resources
Web address: www.pattieaclay.org
Control: Other not–for–profit (including NFP Corporation) **Service:** General Medical and Surgical

Staffed Beds: 69 **Admissions:** 3797 **Census:** 39 **Outpatient Visits:** 97776 **Births:** 946 **Total Expense ($000):** 53082 **Payroll Expense ($000):** 21319 **Personnel:** 497

RUSSELL SPRINGS—Russell County

★ **RUSSELL COUNTY HOSPITAL (181330)**, 153 Dowell Road, Zip 42642–4236, Mailing Address: P.O. Box 1610, Zip 42642–1610; tel. 270/866–4141 **A**9 10 18 **F**3 11 15 24 25 26 28 30 31 32 33 34 36 37 38 41 42 48 50 52 53 55 56 57 62 66 68 79 80 81 86 90 96 97 107 119 121 122 124 135 137 **P**6
Primary Contact: Gary L. DelForge, President and Chief Executive Officer
CFO: Ken Kimsal, Chief Financial Officer
CMO: Jerry Westerfield, M.D., Chief of Staff
CIO: Monte Monsanto, Chief Information Systems
CHR: Tammy Lee, Director Human Resources
Web address: www.russellcohospital.org
Control: County–Government, nonfederal **Service:** General Medical and Surgical

Staffed Beds: 25 **Admissions:** 1079 **Census:** 11 **Outpatient Visits:** 36256 **Births:** 2 **Personnel:** 189

RUSSELLVILLE—Logan County

☒ **LOGAN MEMORIAL HOSPITAL (180066)**, 1625 South Nashville Road, Zip 42276–8834, Mailing Address: P.O. Box 10, Zip 42276–0010; tel. 270/726–4011, (Nonreporting) **A**1 9 10 **S** LifePoint Hospitals, Inc.
Primary Contact: Greg Moore, Chief Executive Officer
CFO: Katrina Kie, Chief Financial Officer
CMO: Kamal Singh, M.D., Chief Medical Staff
CIO: Kim Richardson, Information Systems Director
CHR: Courtney Jackson, Director Human Resources
Web address: www.loganmemorial.com
Control: Corporation, Investor–owned, for–profit **Service:** General Medical and Surgical

Staffed Beds: 92

SALEM—Livingston County

★ **LIVINGSTON HOSPITAL AND HEALTHCARE SERVICES (181320)**, 131 Hospital Drive, Zip 42078–8043; tel. 270/988–2299 **A**9 10 18 **F**1 3 4 15 16 17 25 26 31 32 33 38 46 50 54 55 56 57 61 62 65 68 70 71 73 75 78 79 82 83 84 85 88 93 96 100 102 103 107 117 118 119 121 122 124 134 135 136 137
Primary Contact: Michael J. Budnick, FACHE, Chief Executive Officer
CFO: Dale Kromminga, Controller and Chief Financial Officer
CMO: Michael P. Gavin, M.D., President Medical Staff
CIO: Shannan Landreth, Chief Information Technology
CHR: Carla Wiggins, Director Human Resources
Web address: www.lhhs.org
Control: Other not–for–profit (including NFP Corporation) **Service:** General Medical and Surgical

Staffed Beds: 25 **Admissions:** 1201 **Census:** 10 **Outpatient Visits:** 13862 **Births:** 0 **Total Expense ($000):** 11975 **Payroll Expense ($000):** 5241 **Personnel:** 129

SCOTTSVILLE—Allen County

☐ **MEDICAL CENTER AT SCOTTSVILLE (181324)**, 456 Burnley Road, Zip 42164–6355; tel. 270/622–2800, (Total facility includes 110 beds in nursing home–type unit) **A**1 9 10 18 **F**3 15 24 25 26 31 38 54 55 57 62 66 69 72 73 77 79 80 81 82 85 86 87 92 94 96 100 102 107 117 119 121 122 132 135 137
Primary Contact: Eric Hagan, RN, Vice President and Administrator
Web address: www.mcbg.org/scottsville
Control: Other not–for–profit (including NFP Corporation) **Service:** General Medical and Surgical

Staffed Beds: 135 **Admissions:** 817 **Census:** 121 **Outpatient Visits:** 19019 **Births:** 0 **Personnel:** 165

SHELBYVILLE—Shelby County

☒ **JEWISH HOSPITAL–SHELBYVILLE (180016)**, 727 Hospital Drive, Zip 40065–1699; tel. 502/647–4000, (Total facility includes 6 beds in nursing home–type unit) **A**1 9 10 **F**15 24 25 26 30 32 33 38 46 48 49 55 56 57 66 68 72 73 75 77 79 80 82 86 87 96 97 99 100 102 106 107 117 118 124 135 136 137 **P**6 **S** Jewish Hospital & St. Mary's HealthCare
Primary Contact: Michael L. Collins, President and Chief Executive Officer
CFO: Erika McGimsey, Controller
CMO: Dale Senior, M.D., Chief Medical Officer
CIO: Toby Clark, Manager Physician Advocates
CHR: Cindy Stewart Rattray, Human Resources Director
Web address: www.jhsmh.org
Control: Other not–for–profit (including NFP Corporation) **Service:** General Medical and Surgical

Staffed Beds: 76 **Admissions:** 2597 **Census:** 33 **Outpatient Visits:** 61336 **Births:** 0 **Total Expense ($000):** 32963 **Payroll Expense ($000):** 14827 **Personnel:** 295

Hospital, Medicare Provider Number, Address, Telephone, Approval, Facility, and Physician Codes, Health Care System

★ American Hospital Association (AHA) membership
☐ The Joint Commission accreditation
○ American Osteopathic Association (AOA) accreditation
△ Commission on Accreditation of Rehabilitation Facilities (CARF) accreditation

SOMERSET—Pulaski County

★ **LAKE CUMBERLAND REGIONAL HOSPITAL (180132)**, 305 Langdon Street, Zip 42501–2750, Mailing Address: P.O. Box 620, Zip 42502–2750; tel. 606/679–7441, (Total facility includes 12 beds in nursing home–type unit) **A**1 2 9 10 19 20 **F**3 8 11 13 15 17 18 20 22 24 25 26 27 30 31 32 33 38 42 43 47 49 53 54 55 56 57 60 62 63 66 68 71 72 73 74 75 76 77 78 79 80 81 82 84 85 86 88 92 93 96 97 98 99 100 102 103 107 109 112 117 118 119 120 121 124 135 136 137 **P**4 **S** LifePoint Hospitals, Inc.
Primary Contact: Jeffrey G. Seraphine, CHE, Chief Executive Officer
COO: Robert Parker, Assistant Administrator
CFO: Steve Sloan, Chief Financial Officer
CMO: Michael Citak, M.D., Chief Medical Officer
CIO: Thomas Gilbert, Director Information Technology Services
CHR: James Hughes, Director Human Resources
Web address: www.lakecrmc.com
Control: Corporation, Investor–owned, for–profit **Service:** General Medical and Surgical

Staffed Beds: 259 **Admissions:** 12383 **Census:** 176 **Outpatient Visits:** 106956 **Births:** 1643 **Total Expense ($000):** 105521 **Payroll Expense ($000):** 42922 **Personnel:** 1074

SOUTH WILLIAMSON—Pike County

□ **WILLIAMSON ARH HOSPITAL (180069)**, 260 Hospital Drive, Zip 41503–4072; tel. 606/237–1710, (Total facility includes 50 beds in nursing home–type unit) **A**1 9 10 19 **F**3 11 13 15 25 26 30 31 32 33 38 40 43 50 55 56 57 61 62 65 68 72 73 74 75 77 79 80 81 82 84 85 86 87 96 97 106 107 117 119 121 123 135 136 **P**6 **S** Appalachian Regional Healthcare
Primary Contact: Timothy A. Hatfield, Community Chief Executive Officer
CFO: Chris Ellington, Chief Financial Officer
CMO: J. D. Miller, M.D., Vice President Medical Affairs
CIO: Jeff Brady, Chief Information Officer
Web address: www.arh.org
Control: Other not–for–profit (including NFP Corporation) **Service:** General Medical and Surgical

Staffed Beds: 138 **Admissions:** 3389 **Census:** 70 **Outpatient Visits:** 42079 **Births:** 156 **Total Expense ($000):** 33686 **Payroll Expense ($000):** 12784 **Personnel:** 314

STANFORD—Lincoln County

★ **FORT LOGAN HOSPITAL (181315)**, 124 Portman Avenue, Zip 40484–1200; tel. 606/365–2187 **A**9 10 18 **F**3 11 13 15 25 26 30 31 32 33 38 44 55 56 57 74 79 82 96 99 107 119 122 124 135 **P**5
Primary Contact: Mike Jackson, President and Chief Executive Officer
CFO: William R. Snapp, Vice President and Chief Financial Officer
CMO: Rod Bates, M.D., Chief of Staff
CIO: Sharon McWhorter, Information Systems Director
Web address: www.fortloganhospital.org
Control: Other not–for–profit (including NFP Corporation) **Service:** General Medical and Surgical

Staffed Beds: 25 **Admissions:** 919 **Census:** 8 **Outpatient Visits:** 20331 **Births:** 230 **Total Expense ($000):** 9446 **Payroll Expense ($000):** 4861 **Personnel:** 146

TOMPKINSVILLE—Monroe County

★ **MONROE COUNTY MEDICAL CENTER (180105)**, 529 Capp Harlan Road, Zip 42167–1840; tel. 270/487–9231 **A**1 9 10 **F**2 3 7 15 25 26 30 31 32 38 55 57 61 62 80 86 96 100 107 121 **P**8 **S** QHR
Primary Contact: Vicky McFall, Chief Executive Officer
CFO: Rickie F. Brown, Chief Financial Officer
CHR: Sue Page, Director Human Resources
Web address: www.mcmccares.com
Control: Other not–for–profit (including NFP Corporation) **Service:** General Medical and Surgical

Staffed Beds: 49 **Admissions:** 2564 **Census:** 28 **Outpatient Visits:** 47595 **Births:** 0 **Total Expense ($000):** 14846 **Payroll Expense ($000):** 7045 **Personnel:** 212

VERSAILLES—Woodford County

★ **BLUEGRASS COMMUNITY HOSPITAL (181308)**, 360 Amsden Avenue, Zip 40383–1286; tel. 859/873–3111 **A**9 10 18 **F**8 11 15 25 26 32 38 51 55 57 62 63 66 68 73 75 77 79 80 81 82 84 86 96 97 100 107 118 119 120 121 122 124 135 137 **S** LifePoint Hospitals, Inc.
Primary Contact: Kathy Love, Chief Executive Officer
Web address: www.lifepointhospitals.com
Control: Corporation, Investor–owned, for–profit **Service:** General Medical and Surgical

Staffed Beds: 25 **Admissions:** 473 **Census:** 5 **Outpatient Visits:** 26686 **Births:** 0 **Total Expense ($000):** 12625 **Payroll Expense ($000):** 4893 **Personnel:** 95

WEST LIBERTY—Morgan County

□ **MORGAN COUNTY APPALACHIAN REGIONAL HOSPITAL (181307)**, 476 Liberty Road, Zip 41472–2049, Mailing Address: P.O. Box 579, Zip 41472–0579; tel. 606/743–3186 **A**1 9 10 18 **F**11 15 25 26 30 31 32 33 38 42 43 53 55 56 57 61 62 73 81 82 86 87 96 102 107 118 119 121 122 135 **P**6 **S** Appalachian Regional Healthcare
Primary Contact: Stephen M. Gavalchik, Community Chief Executive Officer
CFO: Chris Ellington, Vice President Fiscal Affairs and Chief Financial Officer
CMO: J. D. Miller, M.D., Vice President Medical Affairs
CIO: Jeff Brady, Director Information Systems
CHR: Lisa Redding, Manager Human Resources
Web address: www.arh.org
Control: Other not–for–profit (including NFP Corporation) **Service:** General Medical and Surgical

Staffed Beds: 25 **Admissions:** 1090 **Census:** 11 **Outpatient Visits:** 30842 **Births:** 0 **Total Expense ($000):** 11459 **Payroll Expense ($000):** 4559 **Personnel:** 104

WHITESBURG—Letcher County

WHITESBURG APPALACHIAN REGIONAL HOSPITAL (180002), 240 Hospital Road, Zip 41858–1254; tel. 606/633–3600 **A**9 10 **F**3 11 13 15 25 26 30 31 32 33 38 40 43 50 55 56 57 61 62 68 73 74 75 79 80 81 82 84 85 86 87 96 97 100 102 106 107 118 119 122 135 136 **P**6 **S** Appalachian Regional Healthcare
Primary Contact: Ellen Wright, Community Chief Executive Officer
COO: Joseph Grossman, Vice President Administration
CFO: Chris Ellington, Vice President Fiscal Affairs
CMO: Robert Buck, M.D., Chief of Staff
CIO: Jeff Brady, Chief Information Officer
CHR: Daniel Fitzpatrick, Director Human Resources
Web address: www.arh.org/whitesburg
Control: Other not–for–profit (including NFP Corporation) **Service:** General Medical and Surgical

Staffed Beds: 82 **Admissions:** 3678 **Census:** 38 **Outpatient Visits:** 49602 **Births:** 481 **Total Expense ($000):** 28981 **Payroll Expense ($000):** 11101 **Personnel:** 277

WILLIAMSTOWN—Grant County

★ **ST. ELIZABETH MEDICAL CENTER–GRANT COUNTY (181311)**, 238 Barnes Road, Zip 41097–9460; tel. 859/824–8240, (Nonreporting) **A**1 9 10 18
Primary Contact: Chris Carle, Administrator
Web address: www.stelizabeth.com
Control: Church–operated, Nongovernment, not–for profit **Service:** General Medical and Surgical

Staffed Beds: 15

WINCHESTER—Clark County

★ ○ **CLARK REGIONAL MEDICAL CENTER (180092)**, 1107 West Lexington Avenue, Zip 40391–1138; tel. 859/745–3500, (Total facility includes 25 beds in nursing home–type unit) **A**5 9 10 11 **F**11 13 15 24 25 26 27 30 31 32 38 43 52 53 54 55 56 57 62 74 77 79 81 82 85 86 96 97 100 107 117 118 119 120 121 122 124 133 135 136 **P**5
Primary Contact: Robert D. Fraraccio, CHE, Chief Executive Officer
CFO: Carolyn Allen, Chief Financial Officer
CMO: Michael Kuduk, M.D., President Medical Staff
CHR: Barry Lindeman, Director Human Resources
Web address: www.clarkhospital.org
Control: County–Government, nonfederal **Service:** General Medical and Surgical

Staffed Beds: 100 **Admissions:** 3055 **Census:** 46 **Outpatient Visits:** 66853 **Births:** 679 **Total Expense ($000):** 41756 **Payroll Expense ($000):** 17664 **Personnel:** 477

LOUISIANA

ABBEVILLE—Vermilion Parish

★ **ABBEVILLE GENERAL HOSPITAL (190034)**, 118 North Hospital Drive, Zip 70510–4077, Mailing Address: P.O. Box 580, Zip 70511–0580; tel. 337/893–5466 **A**1 9 10 **F**11 13 15 25 26 30 31 32 38 43 50 53 57 59 62 64 68 73 74 77 79 82 84 87 88 93 95 96 97 102 107 117 119 122 135 **P**6
Primary Contact: Ray A. Landry, Chief Executive Officer
CFO: Troy Hair, Chief Financial Officer
CIO: John Trahan, Director Information Systems
Web address: www.abbgen.net
Control: Hospital district or authority, Government, nonfederal **Service:** General Medical and Surgical

Staffed Beds: 60 **Admissions:** 2652 **Census:** 42 **Outpatient Visits:** 49425 **Births:** 161 **Personnel:** 294

ALEXANDRIA—Rapides Parish

★ **CHRISTUS ST. FRANCES CABRINI HOSPITAL (190019)**, 3330 Masonic Drive, Zip 71301–3899; tel. 318/487–1122 **A**1 2 9 10 **F**11 13 15 18 20 22 24 25 26 27 28 30 31 32 33 38 40 42 43 44 47 49 50 51 52 55 56 57 58 59 62 66 68 69 70 72 73 74 76 77 79 80 82 84 85 86 96 97 100 102 103 104 105 106 107 108 109 111 118 119 120 121 124 132 133 135 136 137 **P**6 **S** CHRISTUS Health
Primary Contact: Stephen F. Wright, President and Chief Executive Officer
COO: Bruce J. Tassin, Senior Vice President and Administrator
CFO: Scott Merryman, Chief Financial Officer
CMO: Jonathan Weisul, M.D., Vice President Medical Affairs and Chief Medical Officer
CIO: Ron Dekeyzer, Chief Information Officer and Vice President Planning
Web address: www.christushealth.org/sfcabrini
Control: Church–operated, Nongovernment, not–for profit **Service:** General Medical and Surgical

Staffed Beds: 246 **Admissions:** 14265 **Census:** 193 **Outpatient Visits:** 230078 **Births:** 1074 **Total Expense ($000):** 185111 **Payroll Expense ($000):** 65333 **Personnel:** 1592

□ **CROSSROADS REGIONAL HOSPITAL (194022)**, 110 John Eskew Drive, Zip 71303; tel. 318/445–5111, (Nonreporting) **A**1 9 10
Primary Contact: Tracy Griffin, Chief Executive Officer
Web address: www.crossroadshospital.com
Control: Corporation, Investor–owned, for–profit **Service:** Psychiatric

Staffed Beds: 70

★ **DUBUIS HOSPITAL OF ALEXANDRIA (192012)**, 3330 Masonic Drive, 4th Floor, Zip 71301; tel. 318/448–6505 **A**1 10 **F**1 3 25 33 73 119 137 **S** Dubuis Health System
Primary Contact: Michelle Hamilton, Administrator
Web address: www.dubuis.org
Control: Church–operated, Nongovernment, not–for profit **Service:** Long–Term Acute Care hospital

Staffed Beds: 33 **Admissions:** 271 **Census:** 19 **Outpatient Visits:** 0 **Births:** 0 **Total Expense ($000):** 7964 **Payroll Expense ($000):** 2903 **Personnel:** 82

★ **HEALTHSOUTH REHABILITATION HOSPITAL OF ALEXANDRIA (193031)**, 104 North Third Street, Zip 71301–8581; tel. 318/449–1370, (Nonreporting) **A**1 10 **S** HEALTHSOUTH Corporation
Primary Contact: William Bush, Interim Chief Executive Officer
CFO: Bobby Bouillion, Chief Financial Officer
CMO: Vasudeva Dhulipala, M.D., Medical Director
CHR: Suzie Wagner, Human Resource Director
Web address: www.healthsouth.com
Control: Partnership, Investor–owned, for–profit **Service:** Rehabilitation

Staffed Beds: 47

★ **RAPIDES REGIONAL MEDICAL CENTER (190026)**, 211 Fourth Street, Zip 71301; tel. 318/473–3000 **A**1 2 3 5 9 10 **F**3 11 13 15 17 18 20 22 24 25 26 27 28 30 31 32 33 34 36 38 40 41 42 43 44 46 47 48 49 50 51 53 55 56 57 59 60 62 63 66 68 70 72 73 74 75 76 77 79 80 81 82 83 84 86 87 96 97 99 100 102 103 107 108 109 111 112 113 114 118 119 120 121 124 133 135 136 137 **P**8 **S** HCA
Primary Contact: A. C. Buchanan, President and Chief Executive Officer
COO: Cheryl A. Wilson, Chief Operating Officer
CFO: Daniel E. Davis, Chief Financial Officer
CMO: Francis Brian, M.D., Senior Vice President Medical Affairs
CHR: Allen Crain, Director Human Resources
Web address: www.rapidesregional.com
Control: Partnership, Investor–owned, for–profit **Service:** General Medical and Surgical

Staffed Beds: 343 **Admissions:** 16975 **Census:** 217 **Outpatient Visits:** 128163 **Births:** 2234 **Total Expense ($000):** 167190 **Payroll Expense ($000):** 63097 **Personnel:** 1506

★ **RIVERSIDE HOSPITAL OF LOUISIANA (192043)**, (Formerly HEALTHSOUTH Riverside Hospital of Alexandria), 211 Fourth Street, 5th Floor, Zip 71301; tel. 318/767–2900, (Nonreporting) **A**1 10
Primary Contact: Douglas Boulware, Chief Executive Officer
Control: Corporation, Investor–owned, for–profit **Service:** Long–Term Acute Care hospital

Staffed Beds: 27

AMITE—Tangipahoa Parish

★ **HOOD MEMORIAL HOSPITAL (191309)**, 301 West Walnut Street, Zip 70422–2098; tel. 985/748–9485, (Nonreporting) **A**9 10 18
Primary Contact: Claude J. Jones, Jr., Administrator
Control: Hospital district or authority, Government, nonfederal **Service:** General Medical and Surgical

Staffed Beds: 25

ARCADIA—Bienville Parish

★ **BIENVILLE MEDICAL CENTER (191320)**, 1175 Pine Street, Suite 200, Zip 71001; tel. 318/263–4700, (Nonreporting) **A**9 18
Primary Contact: Marc B. Pearce, Administrator
Control: Other not–for–profit (including NFP Corporation) **Service:** General Medical and Surgical

Staffed Beds: 21

BASTROP—Morehouse Parish

BASTROP REHABILITATION HOSPITAL (193058), 323 West Walnut Street, Zip 71220, Mailing Address: P.O. Box 1531, Zip 71221–1531; tel. 318/556–1191, (Nonreporting) **A**10
Primary Contact: William H. Means, Jr., Administrator
COO: Tena Hughes, Program Director and Director Nursing
Control: Corporation, Investor–owned, for–profit **Service:** Rehabilitation

Staffed Beds: 15

LIVERTY HEALTHCARE SYSTEMS (194074), (Formerly Lillian Louise Behavioral Health Hospital), 4673 Eugene Ware Boulevard, Zip 71220–1425; tel. 318/281–2448, (Nonreporting) **A**9 10
Primary Contact: Toby Tubbs, RN, Administrator
Control: Corporation, Investor–owned, for–profit **Service:** Psychiatric

Staffed Beds: 60

★ **MOREHOUSE GENERAL HOSPITAL (190116)**, 323 West Walnut Avenue, Zip 71220–4521, Mailing Address: P.O. Box 1060, Zip 71221–1060; tel. 318/283–3600, (Nonreporting) **A**9 10
Primary Contact: Cheryl Faulkenberry, RN, Administrator and Chief Executive Officer
CFO: James Allbritton, Chief Financial Officer
CMO: John Coats, M.D., Chief Medical Staff
CIO: David Berry, Director Information Systems
CHR: Debbie Spann, Interim Director Human Resources
Web address: www.mghospital.com
Control: Hospital district or authority, Government, nonfederal **Service:** General Medical and Surgical

Staffed Beds: 60

Hospital, Medicare Provider Number, Address, Telephone, Approval, Facility, and Physician Codes, Health Care System

★ American Hospital Association (AHA) membership
□ The Joint Commission accreditation
○ American Osteopathic Association (AOA) accreditation
△ Commission on Accreditation of Rehabilitation Facilities (CARF) accreditation

BATON ROUGE—East Baton Rouge Parish

★ **BATON ROUGE GENERAL MEDICAL CENTER (190065)**, 3600 Florida Street, Zip 70806–3889, Mailing Address: P.O. Box 2511, Zip 70821–2511; tel. 225/387–7000, (Includes BATON ROUGE GENERAL MEDICAL CENTER–BLUEBONNET, 8585 Picardy Avenue, Zip 70809–3679, Mailing Address: P.O. Box 84330, Zip 70884–4330; tel. 225/763–4000) **A**1 2 3 5 6 8 9 10 **F**1 8 11 12 13 14 15 16 17 18 20 22 24 25 26 27 30 31 33 36 38 43 46 50 54 55 56 57 58 59 60 62 63 66 68 70 72 73 74 75 76 77 79 81 82 83 84 85 86 87 88 91 92 93 96 97 100 102 105 106 107 108 109 114 117 118 119 120 121 124 132 133 135 136 137 **P**6
Primary Contact: William R. Holman, FACHE, President and Chief Executive Officer
COO: Edgardo Tenreiro, Chief Operating Officer
CFO: Dionne Viator, CPA, FACHE, Senior Vice President and Chief Financial Officer
CMO: Floyd Roberts, M.D., Chief Medical Officer
CIO: David Hastings, Director Information Technology
CHR: Paul Douglas, Vice President Human Resources
Web address: www.brgeneral.org
Control: Other not–for–profit (including NFP Corporation) **Service:** General Medical and Surgical

Staffed Beds: 460 **Admissions:** 20170 **Census:** 310 **Outpatient Visits:** 141365 **Births:** 1945 **Total Expense ($000):** 252028 **Payroll Expense ($000):** 92981 **Personnel:** 2003

BENTON REHABILITATION HOSPITAL (193070), 4660 Convention Street, Zip 70806; tel. 225/336–1000 **A**10 **F**32 85 119 **P**6
Primary Contact: Scott McClelland, Administrator
Control: Corporation, Investor–owned, for–profit **Service:** Rehabilitation

Staffed Beds: 8 **Admissions:** 45 **Census:** 1 **Outpatient Visits:** 0 **Births:** 0

CYPRESS PSYCHIATRIC HOSPITAL (194071), 4363 Convention Street, Suite A., Zip 70806; tel. 225/336–8940, (Nonreporting) **A**10
Primary Contact: Kenneth O'Rourke, Administrator
Control: Corporation, Investor–owned, for–profit **Service:** Psychiatric

Staffed Beds: 30

★ **EARL K. LONG MEDICAL CENTER (190122)**, 5825 Airline Highway, Zip 70805–2498; tel. 225/358–1000 **A**1 3 5 9 10 **F**3 15 25 27 33 38 49 50 53 56 57 60 62 64 68 70 71 73 74 76 77 79 86 87 96 97 100 103 107 114 119 135 136 137 **S** LSU Health Sciences Center
Primary Contact: Kathy A. Viator, Interim Administrator
CFO: Sue Tolbert, Chief Financial Officer
CIO: Kevin Bolds, Director Information Technology
Web address: www.lsuhsc.edu
Control: State–Government, nonfederal **Service:** General Medical and Surgical

Staffed Beds: 146 **Admissions:** 6342 **Census:** 119 **Outpatient Visits:** 199459 **Births:** 662

GREATER BATON ROUGE SURGICAL HOSPITAL (190273), 7855 Howell Place Boulevard, Zip 70807; tel. 225/358–4900, (Nonreporting) **A**9 10
Primary Contact: Robert D. Blair, Administrator
Web address: www.gbrsh.com
Control: Corporation, Investor–owned, for–profit **Service:** Surgical

Staffed Beds: 10

★ **HEALTHSOUTH REHABILITATION HOSPITAL OF BATON ROUGE (193028)**, 8595 United Plaza Boulevard, Zip 70809–2251; tel. 225/927–0567, (Nonreporting) **A**1 10 **S** HEALTHSOUTH Corporation
Primary Contact: David M. Snyder, Chief Executive Officer
CFO: Andrea Smart, Area Controller
CMO: Lisa Diehl, M.D., Medical Director
CHR: Gayle Courtney, Director Human Resources
Web address: www.healthsouth.com
Control: Corporation, Investor–owned, for–profit **Service:** Rehabilitation

Staffed Beds: 80

★ **OCHSNER MEDICAL CENTER–BATON ROUGE (190202)**, 17000 Medical Center Drive, Zip 70816–3224; tel. 225/752–2470 **A**1 9 10 **F**3 11 15 18 20 22 25 26 27 31 32 33 35 38 43 46 48 49 50 54 55 56 57 68 72 73 76 77 79 80 82 87 88 92 96 99 100 102 104 105 107 116 118 119 120 124 135 137 **S** Ochsner Health System
Primary Contact: Mitch Wasden, Chief Executive Officer
CFO: Barry M. Chambers, CPA, Chief Financial Officer
CMO: F. Ralph Dauterive, M.D., Vice President Medical Affairs
Web address: www.ochsner.org/page.cfm?id=103
Control: Corporation, Investor–owned, for–profit **Service:** General Medical and Surgical

Staffed Beds: 164 **Admissions:** 6151 **Census:** 76 **Outpatient Visits:** 61215 **Births:** 0 **Total Expense ($000):** 69911 **Payroll Expense ($000):** 23650 **Personnel:** 611

★ **OUR LADY OF THE LAKE REGIONAL MEDICAL CENTER (190064)**, 5000 Hennessy Boulevard, Zip 70808–4350; tel. 225/765–6565, (Total facility includes 380 beds in nursing home–type unit) **A**1 2 5 8 9 10 **F**1 2 3 4 5 11 14 15 16 17 18 19 20 21 22 24 25 26 27 33 36 37 38 43 44 46 50 52 53 54 55 56 57 60 62 64 65 66 68 69 70 71 72 73 74 75 76 77 78 79 80 81 82 83 84 85 86 87 88 89 90 91 92 93 94 95 96 97 100 102 103 106 107 115 117 118 119 120 121 124 125 132 135 137 **P**2 6 **S** Franciscan Missionaries of Our Lady Health System, Inc.
Primary Contact: K. Scott Wester, FACHE, President and Chief Executive Officer
COO: Terrie P. Sterling, Chief Operating Officer
CFO: Robert Ramsey, Chief Financial Officer
CMO: Ronald A. Radzikowski, M.D., Chief Medical Officer
CIO: Gary Jump, Vice President Information and Materials Systems
CHR: Terry Bowman, Vice President Human Resources
Web address: www.ololrmc.com
Control: Church–operated, Nongovernment, not–for profit **Service:** General Medical and Surgical

Staffed Beds: 1006 **Admissions:** 33763 **Census:** 787 **Outpatient Visits:** 288939 **Births:** 0 **Total Expense ($000):** 451808 **Payroll Expense ($000):** 181988

PROMISE HOSPITAL OF BATON ROUGE (192049), (Formerly Promise Specialty Hospital of Baton Rouge), 17000 Medical Center Drive, 3rd Floor, Zip 70816; tel. 225/236–5440, (Nonreporting) **A**10 **S** Promise Healthcare
Primary Contact: Craig Boudreaux, Jr., Chief Executive Officer
COO: Michael J. Nolan, Chief Operating Officer
CFO: Christopher A. Stegall, Chief Financial Officer
Web address: www.promise–batonrouge.com
Control: Corporation, Investor–owned, for–profit **Service:** Long–Term Acute Care hospital

Staffed Beds: 29

☐ **SAGE REHABILITATION INSTITUTE (193078)**, 8225 Summa Avenue, Zip 70809, Mailing Address: P.O. Box 82681, Zip 70884; tel. 225/819–0703, (Nonreporting) **A**1 10
Primary Contact: Kenneth Ivy, Chief Executive Officer
Web address: www.aboutseniorhealthcare.com/sage/
Control: Individual, Investor–owned, for–profit **Service:** Rehabilitation

Staffed Beds: 22

SOUTH BATON ROUGE REHABILITATION HOSPITAL (193089), 170 West Washington Street, Zip 70802; tel. 225/303–0572, (Nonreporting) **A**10
Primary Contact: Ralph McEldowney, Administrator
Control: Corporation, Investor–owned, for–profit **Service:** Rehabilitation

Staffed Beds: 12

☐ **SURGICAL SPECIALTY CENTRE (190251)**, 8080 Bluebonnet Boulevard, Zip 70810; tel. 225/408–8080 **A**1 9 10 **F**30 31 32 43 55 56 79 96 100 102 118
Primary Contact: Shannon McConnell, Chief Executive Officer
Control: Corporation, Investor–owned, for–profit **Service:** General Medical and Surgical

Staffed Beds: 14 **Admissions:** 456 **Census:** 2 **Outpatient Visits:** 28859 **Births:** 0 **Total Expense ($000):** 26100 **Payroll Expense ($000):** 7303 **Personnel:** 158

THE NEURO MEDICAL CENTER SURGICAL HOSPITAL (190266), (Formerly Neuro Medical Center Rehabilitation Hospital), 10101 Park Row Avenue, Suite 6000, Zip 70810; tel. 225/763–9900, (Nonreporting) **A**9 10
Primary Contact: Patti Clement, Chief Executive Officer
CFO: Amanda Hymel, Chief Financial Officer
CMO: Thomas Flynn, M.D., Medical Director
CHR: Carol Caddy, Human Resources Representative
Web address: www.theneuromedicalcenter.com
Control: Corporation, Investor–owned, for–profit **Service:** Other specialty

Staffed Beds: 23

VISTA SURGICAL HOSPITAL OF BATON ROUGE (190249), 9032 Perkins Road, Zip 70810; tel. 225/819–4100, (Nonreporting) **A**10 **S** Dynacq Healthcare, Inc.
Primary Contact: Alan A. Beauchamp, Chief Executive Officer
Web address: www.dynacq.com
Control: Corporation, Investor–owned, for–profit **Service:** Other specialty

Staffed Beds: 39

VITAL SOURCE SPECIALTY HOSPITAL (192045), 8225 Summa Avenue, Suite A., Zip 70809; tel. 225/766–5001, (Nonreporting) **A**10
Primary Contact: Sherry Mix, Chief Executive Officer
Control: Corporation, Investor–owned, for–profit **Service:** Long–Term Acute Care hospital

Staffed Beds: 22

Many Facility Codes have changed. Please refer to the AHA Guide Code Chart.

★ □ **WOMAN'S HOSPITAL (190128)**, 9050 Airline Highway, Zip 70815–4192, Mailing Address: P.O. Box 95009, Zip 70895–5009; tel. 225/927–1300 **A**1 2 9 10 **F**3 11 13 15 27 28 30 31 32 33 34 36 50 52 53 55 56 57 58 60 61 62 63 66 68 69 70 71 72 73 74 75 76 79 80 81 82 86 96 99 100 102 107 119 121 123 124 135 136 **P**6
Primary Contact: Teri G. Fontenot, FACHE, President and Chief Executive Officer
CFO: Julia Lively, Vice President Finance
CMO: Kenneth Brown, M.D., Medical Director
CIO: Paul Kirk, Vice President
CHR: Jamie Haeuser, Senior Vice President
Web address: www.womans.org
Control: Other not–for–profit (including NFP Corporation) **Service:** Obstetrics and gynecology

Staffed Beds: 229 **Admissions:** 13464 **Census:** 155 **Outpatient Visits:** 133271 **Births:** 8333 **Total Expense ($000):** 180449 **Payroll Expense ($000):** 95522 **Personnel:** 1545

BERNICE—Union Parish

TRI–WARD GENERAL HOSPITAL (191326), 409 First Street, Zip 71222–0697, Mailing Address: P.O. Box 697, Zip 71222–0697; tel. 318/285–9066, (Nonreporting) **A**9 10 18
Primary Contact: Charolette Thompson, Chief Executive Officer and Chief Financial Officer
COO: Beth Jones, Chief Operating Officer
CFO: Charolette Thompson, Chief Executive Officer and Chief Financial Officer
CMO: R. Brian Harris, M.D., Chief of Staff
Control: Hospital district or authority, Government, nonfederal **Service:** General Medical and Surgical

Staffed Beds: 11

BOGALUSA—Washington Parish

GULF STATES LONG TERM ACUTE CARE OF WASHINGTON/ST. TAMMANY–BOGALUSA CAMPUS (192046), 433 Plaza Street, Zip 70427; tel. 985/730–7040, (Nonreporting) **A**10
Primary Contact: Tara Roberts, RN, Administrator
Web address: www.gulfstateshs.com
Control: Partnership, Investor–owned, for–profit **Service:** General Medical and Surgical

Staffed Beds: 40

★ □ **LSU BOGALUSA MEDICAL CENTER (190095)**, (Formerly Bogalusa Medical Center), 433 Plaza Street, Zip 70427–3793; tel. 985/730–6700, (Includes BOGALUSA COMMUNITY MEDICAL CENTER, 433 Plaza Street, tel. 985/730–6700; WASHINGTON–ST. TAMMANY REGIONAL MEDICAL CENTER, 400 Memphis Street, Zip 70427–0040, Mailing Address: P.O. Box 40, Zip 70429–0040) **A**1 9 10 **F**3 8 11 15 24 25 26 28 30 31 32 33 38 50 53 54 55 56 57 58 60 62 64 68 73 79 80 81 82 86 87 88 96 97 100 102 107 119 124 130 135 137 **P**6 **S** LSU Health Sciences Center
Primary Contact: Kurt M. Scott, FACHE, Administrator
CFO: Bryan Lahaye, Chief Financial Officer
CMO: Lee Roy Joyner, M.D., Medical Director
CIO: Betina Owens, Chief Information Officer
CHR: Elizabeth Pounds, Human Resources Director
Control: State–Government, nonfederal **Service:** General Medical and Surgical

Staffed Beds: 66 **Admissions:** 2647 **Census:** 45 **Outpatient Visits:** 89085 **Births:** 0 **Total Expense ($000):** 41301 **Payroll Expense ($000):** 21140 **Personnel:** 527

BOSSIER CITY—Bossier Parish

BOSSIER SPECIALTY HOSPITAL (190258), 2105 Airline Drive, Zip 71111; tel. 318/549–2011, (Nonreporting) **A**9 10
Primary Contact: Lee McLendon, Chief Executive Officer
Control: Corporation, Investor–owned, for–profit **Service:** Other specialty

Staffed Beds: 12

CHRISTUS SCHUMPERT BOSSIER See CHRISTUS Schumpert Health System, Shreveport

□ **CORNERSTONE HOSPITAL OF BOSSIER CITY (192006)**, 4900 Medical Drive, Zip 71112–4596; tel. 318/747–9500, (Nonreporting) **A**1 10 **S** Cornerstone Healthcare Group
Primary Contact: Sheri Burnette, RN, Chief Executive Officer and Administrator
CFO: Amy Hardy, Chief Financial Officer
CMO: James Jackson, M.D., Chief of Staff
Web address: www.cornerstonehealthcaregroup.com
Control: Corporation, Investor–owned, for–profit **Service:** Long–Term Acute Care hospital

Staffed Beds: 54

RED RIVER BEHAVIORAL CENTER (194079), 2800 Melrose Avenue, Zip 71111; tel. 318/549–2033, (Nonreporting) **A**9 10
Primary Contact: Linda K. Ellis, Administrator
Control: State–Government, nonfederal **Service:** Psychiatric

Staffed Beds: 20

□ △ **WILLIS–KNIGHTON BOSSIER HEALTH CENTER (190236)**, 2400 Hospital Drive, Zip 71111; tel. 318/212–7000, (Nonreporting) **A**1 7 9 10
S Willis–Knighton Health System
Primary Contact: Cliff LeBlanc, Administrator
Web address: www.wkhs.com/wkb/
Control: Other not–for–profit (including NFP Corporation) **Service:** Rehabilitation

Staffed Beds: 115

BREAUX BRIDGE—St. Martin Parish

ST. MARTIN HOSPITAL (191302), 210 Champagne Boulevard, Zip 70517–3852, Mailing Address: P.O. Box 357, Zip 70517–0357; tel. 337/332–2178, (Nonreporting) **A**9 10 18
Primary Contact: Burton Dupuis, Chief Executive Officer
CIO: Rena B. Mouisset, Administrative Assistant
Control: Hospital district or authority, Government, nonfederal **Service:** General Medical and Surgical

Staffed Beds: 25

BROUSSARD—Lafayette Parish

□ **OCEANS BEHAVIORAL HOSPITAL – BROUSSARD (194073)**, 811 Martin Luther King Jr. Drive, Zip 70518; tel. 337/237–6444, (Nonreporting) **A**1 9 10
Primary Contact: Rebecca Theriot, Administrator
Control: Corporation, Investor–owned, for–profit **Service:** Psychiatric

Staffed Beds: 20

BUNKIE—Avoyelles Parish

★ **BUNKIE GENERAL HOSPITAL (191311)**, 427 Evergreen Highway, Zip 71322–3901, Mailing Address: P.O. Box 380, Zip 71322–0380; tel. 318/346–6681, (Nonreporting) **A**9 10 18
Primary Contact: Linda F. Deville, Chief Executive Officer
COO: Lonnie L. Dufour, Chief Operating Officer, Chief Information Officer and Director Human Resources
CFO: Layla Chase, Chief Financial Officer
CMO: Mohit Srivastava, M.D., Chief of Staff
CIO: Lonnie L. Dufour, Chief Operating Officer, Chief Information Officer and Director Human Resources
CHR: Lonnie L. Dufour, Chief Operating Officer, Chief Information Officer and Director Human Resource
Web address: www.bunkiegeneral.com
Control: Hospital district or authority, Government, nonfederal **Service:** General Medical and Surgical

Staffed Beds: 25

CHURCH POINT—Acadia Parish

ACADIA–ST. LANDRY HOSPITAL (191319), 810 South Broadway Street, Zip 70525–4497; tel. 337/684–5435, (Total facility includes 15 beds in nursing home–type unit) (Nonreporting) **A**9 10 18
Primary Contact: F. Peter Savoy, III, Chief Executive Officer
CFO: Judy Young, Chief Financial Officer
CMO: Ward Bellard, M.D., Chief of Staff
CHR: Judy Young, Chief Financial Officer
Web address: www.aslh.org
Control: Other not–for–profit (including NFP Corporation) **Service:** General Medical and Surgical

Staffed Beds: 40

CLINTON—East Feliciana Parish

□ **GULF STATES LONG TERM ACUTE CARE OF FELICIANA (192041)**, 9725 Grace Lane, Zip 70722; tel. 225/683–1600, (Nonreporting) **A**1 10
Primary Contact: Dun Stockwell, Administrator
Web address: www.gulfstateshs.com
Control: Corporation, Investor–owned, for–profit **Service:** Long–Term Acute Care hospital

Staffed Beds: 16

Hospital, Medicare Provider Number, Address, Telephone, Approval, Facility, and Physician Codes, Health Care System
★ American Hospital Association (AHA) membership
□ The Joint Commission accreditation
○ American Osteopathic Association (AOA) accreditation
△ Commission on Accreditation of Rehabilitation Facilities (CARF) accreditation

COLUMBIA—Caldwell Parish

CALDWELL MEMORIAL HOSPITAL (190190), 411 Main Street, Zip 71418, Mailing Address: P.O. Box 899, Zip 71418–0899; tel. 318/649–6111, (Nonreporting) **A**9 10
Primary Contact: Heather Clark, Chief Executive Officer
CFO: Cathie Clifford, Chief Financial Officer
Control: Corporation, Investor–owned, for–profit **Service:** Long–Term Acute Care hospital

Staffed Beds: 25

CITIZENS MEDICAL CENTER (190184), 7939 U.S. Highway 165, Zip 71418–1079, Mailing Address: P.O. Box 1079, Zip 71418–1079; tel. 318/649–6106, (Nonreporting) **A**9 10
Primary Contact: Steve Barbo, RN, Administrator
Control: Hospital district or authority, Government, nonfederal **Service:** General Medical and Surgical

Staffed Beds: 40

COUSHATTA—Red River Parish

★ **CHRISTUS COUSHATTA HEALTH CARE CENTER (191312)**, 1635 Marvel Street, Zip 71019–9022, Mailing Address: P.O. Box 589, Zip 71019–0589; tel. 318/932–2000 **A**1 9 10 18 **F**2 3 7 8 14 15 25 26 33 37 38 50 53 54 55 57 62 64 73 75 79 82 86 87 96 99 100 102 107 118 119 122 137 **P**6 **S** CHRISTUS Health
Primary Contact: Karen Mixon, RN, Administrator
CFO: Scott Merryman, Chief Financial Officer
CMO: Jonathan Weisul, M.D., Vice President Medical Affairs and Chief Medical Officer
CIO: Bruce Honea, Director Information Services
CHR: Donnette Craig, Director Human Resources
Web address: www.christuscoushatta.org
Control: Church–operated, Nongovernment, not–for profit **Service:** General Medical and Surgical

Staffed Beds: 25 **Admissions:** 1433 **Census:** 12 **Outpatient Visits:** 6202 **Births:** 0 **Personnel:** 104

SPECIALTY REHABILITATION HOSPITAL (193080), (Formerly Community Rehabilitation Hospital of Coushatta), 1110 Ringgold Avenue, Suite B., Zip 71019; tel. 318/932–1770, (Nonreporting) **A**10
Primary Contact: Craig Ball, Chief Executive Officer
COO: Charlie Ball, Chief Operating Officer
CFO: Connie Ball, Chief Financial Officer
CMO: Jalal Houdeh, M.D., Chief Medical Officer
CHR: Denise Logan, Director Human Resources
Control: Individual, Investor–owned, for–profit **Service:** Rehabilitation

Staffed Beds: 12

COVINGTON—St. Tammany Parish

☐ **FAIRWAY MEDICAL CENTER (190267)**, 67252 Industry Lane, Zip 70433; tel. 985/809–9888, (Nonreporting) **A**1 9 10
Primary Contact: David J. Guzan, Chief Executive Officer
COO: Colleen Gollnick, Chief Operating Officer
CFO: Sandy Badinger, Chief Financial Officer
CMO: William Preau, M.D., Medical Director
CHR: Pam Collins, Director Human Resources
Web address: www.fairwaymedical.com
Control: Corporation, Investor–owned, for–profit **Service:** General Medical and Surgical

Staffed Beds: 21

GREENBRIER HOSPITAL (194069), 201 Greenbrier Boulevard, Zip 70433; tel. 985/893–2970, (Nonreporting) **A**10
Primary Contact: Robert J. Guasco, Administrator
CMO: Jason Coe, M.D., Medical Director
Control: Corporation, Investor–owned, for–profit **Service:** Other specialty

Staffed Beds: 58

☐ **GULF STATES LONG TERM ACUTE CARE OF COVINGTON (192048)**, 20050 Crestwood Boulevard, Zip 70433; tel. 985/875–7525, (Nonreporting) **A**1 10
Primary Contact: Herman Frank, CHE, Administrator
Web address: www.gulfstateshs.com
Control: Corporation, Investor–owned, for–profit **Service:** Long–Term Acute Care hospital

Staffed Beds: 58

★ **LAKEVIEW REGIONAL MEDICAL CENTER (190177)**, 95 East Fairway Drive, Zip 70433–7507; tel. 985/867–3800 **A**1 9 10 **F**11 12 13 15 18 20 22 24 25 30 31 32 33 38 49 55 56 57 62 66 68 73 74 75 76 79 80 84 86 88 92 93 96 97 99 100 102 103 107 119 121 132 133 135 136 **S** HCA
Primary Contact: Jason E. Cobb, FACHE, Chief Executive Officer
CFO: Tim Breslin, Chief Financial Officer
CMO: George Barnes, M.D., Medical Director
CIO: Debra Willie, Director Medical Records
CHR: Lyle Theriot, Director Human Resources
Web address: www.lakeviewregional.com
Control: Corporation, Investor–owned, for–profit **Service:** General Medical and Surgical

Staffed Beds: 159 **Admissions:** 6876 **Census:** 90 **Outpatient Visits:** 54022 **Births:** 990 **Total Expense ($000):** 75028 **Payroll Expense ($000):** 28382 **Personnel:** 498

★ **REGENCY HOSPITAL OF COVINGTON (192051)**, 195 Highland Park Entrance, Zip 70433; tel. 985/867–3977, (Nonreporting) **A**1 10 **S** Regency Hospital Company
Primary Contact: Timothy Burke, Chief Executive Officer
CMO: Merrill Laurent, M.D., Medical Director
CHR: Beth Sayler, Director Human Resources
Web address: www.regencyhospital.com
Control: Corporation, Investor–owned, for–profit **Service:** Long–Term Acute Care hospital

Staffed Beds: 38

★ **ST. TAMMANY PARISH HOSPITAL (190045)**, 1202 South Tyler Street, Zip 70433–2394; tel. 985/898–4000 **A**1 2 9 10 **F**3 8 11 12 13 15 17 18 20 22 24 25 26 27 28 30 31 32 33 35 38 40 42 43 44 48 49 50 52 53 55 56 57 61 62 63 67 68 70 73 74 75 76 77 79 80 81 82 84 85 86 87 96 97 100 102 103 107 112 116 118 119 121 124 133 135 136 137 **P**8
Primary Contact: Patti M. Ellish, President and Chief Executive Officer
COO: Sharon A. Toups, Senior Vice President and Chief Operating Officer
CFO: David L. Mabe, Senior Vice President and Chief Financial Officer
CMO: Robert Capitelli, M.D., Senior Vice President and Chief Medical Officer
CHR: Judy Gracia, Vice President Human Resources
Web address: www.stph.org
Control: Hospital district or authority, Government, nonfederal **Service:** General Medical and Surgical

Staffed Beds: 223 **Admissions:** 12539 **Census:** 151 **Outpatient Visits:** 237058 **Births:** 1654 **Total Expense ($000):** 148467 **Payroll Expense ($000):** 71916 **Personnel:** 1512

CROWLEY—Acadia Parish

★ **AMERICAN LEGION HOSPITAL (190044)**, 1305 Crowley Rayne Highway, Zip 70526; tel. 337/783–3222 **A**9 10 **F**13 15 25 31 32 38 57 68 73 74 77 79 84 88 93 96 107 119 **P**5
Primary Contact: Terry W. Osborne, CPA, Chief Executive Officer
CFO: Charmaine Vidrine, CPA, Chief Financial Officer
CMO: Paul B. Stringfellow, M.D., Chief of Staff
Control: Other not–for–profit (including NFP Corporation) **Service:** General Medical and Surgical

Staffed Beds: 178 **Admissions:** 4823 **Census:** 58 **Outpatient Visits:** 39580 **Births:** 553 **Total Expense ($000):** 30133 **Payroll Expense ($000):** 13549 **Personnel:** 337

CROWLEY REHABILITATION HOSPITAL (192050), 713 North Avenue L., Zip 70526; tel. 337/783–2859, (Nonreporting) **A**10
Primary Contact: Gil Pinac, Chief Executive Officer
Control: Partnership, Investor–owned, for–profit **Service:** General Medical and Surgical

Staffed Beds: 15

CUT OFF—Lafourche Parish

★ **LADY OF THE SEA GENERAL HOSPITAL (191325)**, 200 West 134th Place, Zip 70345–4145; tel. 985/632–6401, (Nonreporting) **A**9 10 18 **S** Brim Healthcare, Inc.
Primary Contact: Don Werner, Chief Executive Officer
CFO: Randy Tabor, Chief Financial Officer
CHR: Bennie Smith, Director Human Resources and Risk Management
Web address: www.losgh.org
Control: Hospital district or authority, Government, nonfederal **Service:** General Medical and Surgical

Staffed Beds: 25

 Many Facility Codes have changed. Please refer to the AHA Guide Code Chart.

DE RIDDER—Beauregard Parish

★ **BEAUREGARD MEMORIAL HOSPITAL (190050)**, 600 South Pine Street, Zip 70634–4998, Mailing Address: P.O. Box 730, Zip 70634–0730; tel. 337/462–7100 **A**1 9 10 **F**3 11 13 15 17 18 24 25 26 27 33 38 46 50 52 55 61 62 68 73 74 76 77 79 80 84 86 96 97 102 107 119 122 135 137 **P**5
Primary Contact: Theodore J. Badger, Jr., CHE, Chief Executive Officer
CFO: Darrell L. Kingham, CPA, Vice President Finance
CMO: Charlotte Fowler, D.O., President Medical Staff
CIO: Meg Jackson, Director Biomedical and Management Information Systems
CHR: Hope Leedom, Director Human Resources
Web address: www.beauregard.org
Control: Hospital district or authority, Government, nonfederal **Service:** General Medical and Surgical

Staffed Beds: 60 **Admissions:** 2857 **Census:** 32 **Outpatient Visits:** 38569 **Births:** 339 **Total Expense ($000):** 26988 **Payroll Expense ($000):** 12999 **Personnel:** 336

DELHI—Richland Parish

RICHLAND PARISH HOSPITAL (191323), 407 Cincinnati Street, Zip 71232–3009; tel. 318/878–5171, (Nonreporting) **A**9 10 18
Primary Contact: Michael W. Carroll, Administrator
CIO: Barbra Hutchison, Director Medical Records
CHR: Patsy Stout, Personnel Director
Web address: www.delhihospital.com
Control: Hospital district or authority, Government, nonfederal **Service:** General Medical and Surgical

Staffed Beds: 25

DENHAM SPRINGS—Livingston Parish

□ **GULF STATES LONG TERM ACUTE CARE OF DENHAM SPRINGS (192008)**, 8375 Florida Boulevard, Zip 70726; tel. 225/665–2664, (Nonreporting) **A**1 10
Primary Contact: Richard Daughdrill, RN, Administrator
Web address: www.gulfstateshs.com
Control: Corporation, Investor–owned, for–profit **Service:** Long–Term Acute Care hospital

Staffed Beds: 117

DEQUINCY—Calcasieu Parish

DEQUINCY MEMORIAL HOSPITAL (191307), 110 West Fourth Street, Zip 70633–3508, Mailing Address: P.O. Box 1166, Zip 70633–1166; tel. 337/786–1200, (Nonreporting) **A**9 10 18 **S** Promise Healthcare
Primary Contact: Michael Ashford, Administrator
CFO: Brandy Maddox, Chief Financial Officer
CMO: Jalal Joudeh, M.D., Chief of Staff
Web address: www.dequincyhospital.com
Control: City–Government, nonfederal **Service:** General Medical and Surgical

Staffed Beds: 19

□ **REHABILITATION HOSPITAL OF DEQUINCY**, 110 West Fourth Street, Zip 70633; tel. 337/786–6100, (Nonreporting) **A**1
Web address: www.triparishrehab.com
Control: Corporation, Investor–owned, for–profit **Service:** Rehabilitation

Staffed Beds: 13

DONALDSONVILLE—Ascension Parish

★ **PREVOST MEMORIAL HOSPITAL (191308)**, 301 Memorial Drive, Zip 70346–4376; tel. 225/473–7931 **A**1 9 10 18 **F**3 11 15 25 38 55 57 117 118 119 122 135 **P**4
Primary Contact: Vincent A. Cataldo, Administrator
CFO: Jane Arboneaux, Chief Financial Officer
CMO: Michel Y. Hirsch, M.D., Chief Medical Staff
CHR: Linda Cataldo, Human Resources Secretary
Web address: www.prevosthospital.com
Control: Hospital district or authority, Government, nonfederal **Service:** General Medical and Surgical

Staffed Beds: 25 **Admissions:** 155 **Census:** 1 **Outpatient Visits:** 22595 **Births:** 0 **Total Expense ($000):** 4783 **Personnel:** 55

EUNICE—St. Landry Parish

★ **ACADIAN MEDICAL CENTER (190078)**, 3501 Highway 190 East, Zip 70535–3628; tel. 337/580–7500, (Nonreporting) **A**1 9 10 **S** LifePoint Hospitals, Inc.
Primary Contact: James P. Frazier, III, M.D., Chief Executive Officer
CFO: Melissa Bordelon, Chief Financial Officer
CMO: Randy Miller, M.D., Chief Medical Staff
CIO: Ariana Pommier, Health Information Management Director
CHR: Dawn Buckley, Director Human Resources
Web address: www.acadianmedicalcenter.com
Control: Corporation, Investor–owned, for–profit **Service:** General Medical and Surgical

Staffed Beds: 42

FARMERVILLE—Union Parish

LIBERTY HEALTHCARE SYSTEMS (194074), (Formerly Lillian Louise Behavioral Health Hospital), 309 North Main, Zip 71241; tel. 318/368–0110, (Nonreporting) **A**9 10
Primary Contact: William P. Gunther, Administrator
Control: Corporation, Investor–owned, for–profit **Service:** Psychiatric

Staffed Beds: 18

UNION GENERAL HOSPITAL (191301), 901 James Avenue, Zip 71241–0398, Mailing Address: P.O. Box 398, Zip 71241–0398; tel. 318/368–9751, (Nonreporting) **A**9 10 18
Primary Contact: Evalyn Ormond, Administrator
CFO: William Adcock, Chief Financial Officer
CHR: Juanita Sanford, Comptroller and Director Human Resources
Web address: www.uniongen.com
Control: Other not–for–profit (including NFP Corporation) **Service:** General Medical and Surgical

Staffed Beds: 25

FERRIDAY—Concordia Parish

□ **PROMISE HOSPITAL OF MISS LOU (192028)**, (Formerly Promise Specialty Hospital of Miss Lou), 6818–A Highway 84, Zip 71334–5101; tel. 318/757–7575, (Nonreporting) **A**1 10 **S** Promise Healthcare
Primary Contact: Lee Huckaby, Chief Executive Officer
COO: Howard B. Koslow, President and Chief Executive Officer
CFO: Larry Leder, Chief Financial Officer
CMO: Barry Tillman, M.D., Chief Medical Staff
CIO: Elizabeth Carpenter, Director Quality Assurance and Quality Improvement and Assistant Administrator
CHR: Roxan Houghton, Director Human Resources
Web address: www.camelothealthcare.net
Control: Corporation, Investor–owned, for–profit **Service:** Long–Term Acute Care hospital

Staffed Beds: 40

RIVERLAND MEDICAL CENTER (191318), 1700 North E 'E' Wallace Boulevard, Zip 71334–0111, Mailing Address: P.O. Box 111, Zip 71334–0111; tel. 318/757–6551 **A**9 10 18 **F**3 8 11 15 25 26 30 31 32 38 46 50 55 56 57 62 63 79 80 82 86 87 96 107 122
Primary Contact: Vernon R. Stevens, Jr., Administrator
CFO: Jerry Daye, Financial Officer
CIO: Rebecca Gaspard, Medical Records Director
CHR: Norma Jean Price, Personnel Manager
Control: Hospital district or authority, Government, nonfederal **Service:** General Medical and Surgical

Staffed Beds: 25 **Admissions:** 1043 **Census:** 10 **Outpatient Visits:** 20813 **Births:** 0 **Total Expense ($000):** 9133 **Payroll Expense ($000):** 5705 **Personnel:** 169

FORT POLK—Vernon Parish

★ **BAYNE–JONES ARMY COMMUNITY HOSPITAL**, 1585 Third Street, Zip 71459–5110; tel. 337/531–3928, (Nonreporting) **A**1 9 **S** Department of the Army, Office of the Surgeon General
Primary Contact: Colonel William K. Statz, Commander
COO: Lieutenant Colonel Steven Hale, Deputy Commander for Administration
CFO: Major Karl Devlin, Chief, Resource Management Division
CMO: Lieutenant Colonel Alfonso Alarcon, Deputy Commander Clinical Services
CIO: Thomas Baker, Chief Information Management Division
CHR: Major Karl Devlin, Chief Resource Management Division
Web address: www.polk.amedd.army.mil
Control: Army, Government, federal **Service:** General Medical and Surgical

Staffed Beds: 44

Hospital, Medicare Provider Number, Address, Telephone, Approval, Facility, and Physician Codes, Health Care System
★ American Hospital Association (AHA) membership
□ The Joint Commission accreditation
○ American Osteopathic Association (AOA) accreditation
△ Commission on Accreditation of Rehabilitation Facilities (CARF) accreditation

FRANKLIN—St. Mary Parish

★ **FRANKLIN FOUNDATION HOSPITAL (191310)**, 1097 Northwest Boulevard, Zip 70538–3724, Mailing Address: P.O. Box 577, Zip 70538–0577; tel. 337/828–0760, (Nonreporting) **A**1 9 10 18 **S** QHR
Primary Contact: Cindy Bradley, Interim Chief Executive Officer
CFO: Gary Marti, Chief Financial Officer
CMO: Donna Tesi, M.D., Chief of Staff
CIO: Hal Goree, Chief Information Officer
CHR: David Williamson, Director Human Resources
Web address: www.franklinfoundation.org
Control: Hospital district or authority, Government, nonfederal **Service:** General Medical and Surgical

Staffed Beds: 25

FRANKLINTON—Washington Parish

★ **RIVERSIDE MEDICAL CENTER (191313)**, 1900 Main Street, Zip 70438–3688; tel. 985/839–4431 **A**1 9 10 18 **F**3 11 15 25 27 30 31 32 38 47 54 55 56 57 62 66 68 73 75 76 79 80 86 87 96 97 100 102 107 119 121 122 124 135 **P**6
Primary Contact: Conrad G. Flowers, Chief Executive Officer
CFO: Patricia A. Mizell, Chief Financial Officer
CMO: Mark James, M.D., Chief of Staff
CIO: Herman Ingram, Director
CHR: John Seal, Director Human Resources
Web address: www.rmchospital.com
Control: Hospital district or authority, Government, nonfederal **Service:** General Medical and Surgical

Staffed Beds: 25 **Admissions:** 943 **Census:** 9 **Outpatient Visits:** 28725 **Total Expense ($000):** 21556 **Payroll Expense ($000):** 8524 **Personnel:** 214

GONZALES—Ascension Parish

☐ **PROMISE HOSPITAL OF ASCENSION (192004)**, 615 East Worthey Road, Zip 70737–4240; tel. 225/621–1248, (Nonreporting) **A**1 9 10
Primary Contact: Craig Boudreaux, Jr., Area Vice President and Chief Executive Officer
COO: Christopher A. Stegall, Regional Chief Financial Officer and Chief Operating Officer
CFO: Christopher A. Stegall, Regional Chief Financial Officer and Chief Operating Officer
CMO: Peter J. Monteyne, M.D., Chief Medical Staff
CHR: Wendy Cobbs, Manager Human Resources
Web address: www.promisehealthcare.com
Control: Hospital district or authority, Government, nonfederal **Service:** Long–Term Acute Care hospital

Staffed Beds: 54

★ **ST. ELIZABETH HOSPITAL (190242)**, 1125 West Highway 30, Zip 70737; tel. 225/647–5000, (Nonreporting) **A**1 9 10 **S** Franciscan Missionaries of Our Lady Health System, Inc.
Primary Contact: Dolores LeJeune, Chief Executive Officer
CFO: Sue Knight, Vice President Finance and Operations
CMO: Craig Vitrano, M.D., Medical Director
CIO: Kevin Bolds, Director Information Technology
CHR: Victor Vidaurre, Assistant Vice President Compliance and Human Resources
Web address: www.steh.com
Control: Church–operated, Nongovernment, not–for profit **Service:** General Medical and Surgical

Staffed Beds: 66

GREENSBURG—St. Helena Parish

ST. HELENA PARISH HOSPITAL (191300), 16874 Highway 43, Zip 70441, Mailing Address: P.O. Box 337, Zip 70441–0337; tel. 225/222–6111, (Nonreporting) **A**9 10 18
Primary Contact: Alcus Trahan, Administrator and Chief Executive Officer
CFO: Dennis Maciasz, Certified Public Accountant
CMO: Jrveshwar Kumar, Chief of Staff
Web address: www.sthelenaparishhospital.com
Control: Other not–for–profit (including NFP Corporation) **Service:** General Medical and Surgical

Staffed Beds: 25

GRETNA—Jefferson Parish

★ **OCHSNER MEDICAL CENTER – WEST BANK (190275)**, 2500 Belle Chase Highway, Zip 70056–7196; tel. 504/392–3131 **A**1 9 10 **S** Ochsner Health System
Primary Contact: Michael O'Bryan, M.D., Chief Executive Officer
COO: DeAnna Davis, Vice President Operations
CMO: Yvens LaBorde, M.D., Vice President Medical Affairs
CIO: Bryan Clarke, Director Information Systems
CHR: Wendy Willis, Assistant Vice President Human Resources
Web address: www.ochsner.org/westbank
Control: Other not–for–profit (including NFP Corporation) **Service:** General Medical and Surgical

Staffed Beds: 132 **Admissions:** 7553 **Census:** 116 **Outpatient Visits:** 52439 **Births:** 1522 **Total Expense ($000):** 92808 **Payroll Expense ($000):** 41598

UNITED MEDICAL HEALTHWEST–NEW ORLEANS (193074), (Formerly Healthwest Rehabilitation Hospital), 3201 Wall Boulevard, Suite B., Zip 70056; tel. 504/433–5551, (Nonreporting) **A**10
Primary Contact: Michele Desport, RN, Administrator
Control: Individual, Investor–owned, for–profit **Service:** Rehabilitation

Staffed Beds: 15

HAMMOND—Tangipahoa Parish

☐ **GULF STATES LONG TERM ACUTE CARE OF HAMMOND (192036)**, 42074 Veterans Avenue, Zip 70403; tel. 985/902–8148, (Nonreporting) **A**1 10
Primary Contact: Michael Rabalais, Interim Chief Executive Officer
Web address: www.gulfstateshs.com
Control: Corporation, Investor–owned, for–profit **Service:** Long–Term Acute Care hospital

Staffed Beds: 20

★ △ **NORTH OAKS MEDICAL CENTER (190015)**, 15790 Paul Vega, M. D. Drive, Zip 70403–1436, Mailing Address: P.O. Box 2668, Zip 70404–2668; tel. 985/345–2700 **A**1 7 9 10 19 **F**3 13 15 17 18 20 22 24 25 26 27 28 30 32 38 42 43 44 49 50 53 54 55 56 57 58 62 65 66 68 70 71 72 73 74 75 76 77 79 80 81 82 84 86 88 92 93 96 97 99 100 102 103 105 106 107 114 118 119 120 121 124 132 133 135 136 137 **P**6
Primary Contact: James E. Cathey, Jr., Chief Executive Officer
COO: Michele K. Sutton, Operations Officer
CFO: Shirley Hsing, Chief Financial Officer
CMO: James Nelson, M.D., Chief Medical Officer
CIO: Bach Nguyen, Information Systems Director
CHR: Carolyn Adema, Human Resources Officer
Web address: www.northoaks.org
Control: Hospital district or authority, Government, nonfederal **Service:** General Medical and Surgical

Staffed Beds: 196 **Admissions:** 14551 **Census:** 203 **Outpatient Visits:** 224555 **Births:** 1803 **Total Expense ($000):** 190307 **Payroll Expense ($000):** 99484 **Personnel:** 1993

☐ **NORTH OAKS REHABILITATION HOSPITAL (193044)**, 1900 South Morrison Boulevard, Zip 70403; tel. 504/230–5700 **A**1 9 10 **F**25 30 32 54 73 75 81 82 85 93 119 121 132 135
Primary Contact: Sybil Paulson, RN, Administrator
Web address: www.northoaks.org
Control: Hospital district or authority, Government, nonfederal **Service:** Rehabilitation

Staffed Beds: 27 **Admissions:** 447 **Census:** 15 **Outpatient Visits:** 0 **Births:** 0 **Total Expense ($000):** 10668 **Payroll Expense ($000):** 2610 **Personnel:** 57

UNITED MEDICAL REHABILITATION HOSPITAL (193079), 15717 Belle Drive, Zip 70403; tel. 985/340–5998, (Nonreporting) **A**10
Web address: www.umrhospital.com
Control: Corporation, Investor–owned, for–profit **Service:** Rehabilitation

Staffed Beds: 20

HOMER—Claiborne Parish

HOMER MEMORIAL HOSPITAL (190114), 620 East College Street, Zip 71040–3202; tel. 318/927–2024 **A**9 10 **F**3 13 15 25 26 30 31 32 33 38 43 48 54 55 57 61 62 63 68 73 74 79 81 82 84 88 91 93 96 97 107 117 119 121 122 132 137
Primary Contact: Douglas P. Efferson, Administrator
CFO: Amy H. Legendre, Chief Financial Officer
CMO: Clint Butler, M.D., Chief of Staff
CIO: Vance Robinson, Chief Information Officer
CHR: Theola A. Corley, Human Resources Officer
Web address: www.homerhospital.com
Control: City–Government, nonfederal **Service:** General Medical and Surgical

Staffed Beds: 60 **Admissions:** 2102 **Census:** 35 **Outpatient Visits:** 20627 **Births:** 40 **Total Expense ($000):** 13354 **Payroll Expense ($000):** 6595 **Personnel:** 227

HOUMA—Terrebonne Parish

★☐ **LEONARD J. CHABERT MEDICAL CENTER (190183)**, 1978 Industrial Boulevard, Zip 70363–7094; tel. 985/873–2200 **A**1 3 5 9 10 **F**11 15 18 26 27 30 31 32 36 37 38 43 49 50 51 57 58 59 60 62 64 66 68 70 72 73 74 76 77 79 80 82 84 87 88 92 96 97 99 100 103 107 114 119 124 135 136 137 **P**5 **S** LSU Health Sciences Center
Primary Contact: Rhonda G. Green, Administrator
CFO: Elizabeth Callais, Chief Fiscal Officer
CMO: Michael Garcia, M.D., Medical Director
CIO: Susan Arceneaux, R.N., Coordinator Information Technology
CHR: Donna Duplantis, Director Human Resources
Web address: www.lsuhsc.edu/hcsd/ljc
Control: State–Government, nonfederal **Service:** General Medical and Surgical

Staffed Beds: 85 **Admissions:** 5354 **Census:** 72 **Outpatient Visits:** 160915 **Births:** 577 **Total Expense ($000):** 91446 **Payroll Expense ($000):** 33979 **Personnel:** 867

PHYSICIANS SURGICAL SPECIALTY HOSPITAL (190241), 218 Corporate Drive, Zip 70360–2764; tel. 985/853–1390, (Nonreporting) **A**9 10
Primary Contact: Connie Martin, Administrator
Web address: www.obesitysurgeryhouma.com
Control: Corporation, Investor–owned, for–profit **Service:** Other specialty

Staffed Beds: 10

★☐ △ **TERREBONNE GENERAL MEDICAL CENTER (190008)**, 8166 Main Street, Zip 70360–3498, Mailing Address: P.O. Box 6037, Zip 70361–6037; tel. 985/873–4141, (Total facility includes 16 beds in nursing home–type unit) **A**1 7 9 10 **F**8 11 13 14 15 17 18 20 22 25 26 27 30 31 32 33 38 41 42 43 49 50 55 56 57 58 62 63 66 68 70 72 73 74 75 76 77 79 80 81 82 84 85 86 96 97 98 99 100 102 103 105 106 107 112 117 118 119 121 123 124 135 136 137 **P**6
Primary Contact: Phyllis Peoples, M.S.N., RN, President and Chief Executive Officer
COO: Diane Yeates, Chief Operating Officer
CFO: Dean Verret, Vice President Financial Services
CMO: Mary Eschete, M.D., Chief of Staff
CHR: Mickie Rousseau, Director Human Resources
Web address: www.tgmc.com
Control: Hospital district or authority, Government, nonfederal **Service:** General Medical and Surgical

Staffed Beds: 333 **Admissions:** 11172 **Census:** 134 **Outpatient Visits:** 112608 **Births:** 2111 **Total Expense ($000):** 157061 **Payroll Expense ($000):** 58505 **Personnel:** 1184

INDEPENDENCE—Tagipahoa Parish

★☐ **LALLIE KEMP MEDICAL CENTER (191321)**, 52579 Highway 51 South, Zip 70443–2231; tel. 985/878–9421 **A**1 9 10 18 **F**3 15 25 27 30 32 33 38 40 50 54 55 56 57 60 62 63 64 68 73 75 76 77 79 80 81 82 87 96 97 102 107 119 121 122 124 135 136 137 **P**6 **S** LSU Health Sciences Center
Primary Contact: Sherre Pack–Hookfin, Administrator
COO: Sherre Pack–Hookfin, Administrator
CFO: Chad Thompson, Chief Financial Officer
CMO: Kathy Willis, M.D., Medical Director
CIO: Charles Tate, Director Information Technology
CHR: Wanda Hoffman, Director Human Resources
Web address: www.lsuhospitals.org
Control: State–Government, nonfederal **Service:** General Medical and Surgical

Staffed Beds: 25 **Admissions:** 996 **Census:** 11 **Outpatient Visits:** 109855 **Births:** 0 **Total Expense ($000):** 38700 **Payroll Expense ($000):** 16500 **Personnel:** 426

JACKSON—East Feliciana Parish

☐ **EASTERN LOUISIANA MENTAL HEALTH SYSTEM (194008)**, 4502 Highway 951, Zip 70748–5842, Mailing Address: P.O. Box 498, Zip 70748–0498; tel. 225/634–0100 **A**1 10 **F**11 26 32 33 37 50 57 66 72 73 81 82 88 89 90 94 95 119 124 135 **P**6 **S** Louisiana State Hospitals
Primary Contact: Mark Anders, Chief Executive Officer
COO: Hampton P S Lea, Chief Operating Officer
CFO: Janet O'Dell, Administrative Director
CMO: John W. Thompson, M.D., Chief of Staff
CIO: Deborah Brandon, Director
CHR: Anita Knighton, Director Human Resources
Web address: www.dhh.louisiana.gov/offices/locations.asp?ID=62&Detail=126
Control: State–Government, nonfederal **Service:** Psychiatric

Staffed Beds: 515 **Admissions:** 1319 **Census:** 562 **Outpatient Visits:** 0 **Births:** 0 **Total Expense ($000):** 70391 **Personnel:** 1357

VILLA FELICIANA MEDICAL COMPLEX (190199), 5002 Highway 10, Zip 70748–3627, Mailing Address: P.O. Box 438, Zip 70748–0438; tel. 225/634–4000, (Total facility includes 185 beds in nursing home–type unit) **A**10 **F**3 12 37 73 80 90 119 132 137
Primary Contact: James R. O'Rear, Administrator
CMO: John F. Piker, M.D., Medical Director
CIO: Robert McCollough, Information Systems Network Technician
CHR: Sandra Delatte, Director Human Resources
Web address: www.dhh.state.la.us/
Control: State–Government, nonfederal **Service:** General Medical and Surgical

Staffed Beds: 195 **Admissions:** 52 **Census:** 149 **Outpatient Visits:** 835 **Births:** 0 **Total Expense ($000):** 18015 **Payroll Expense ($000):** 9527 **Personnel:** 303

JENA—La Salle Parish

★ **LASALLE GENERAL HOSPITAL (190145)**, 187 Ninth Street, Zip 71342–2780, Mailing Address: P.O. Box 2780, Zip 71342–2780; tel. 318/992–9200 **A**9 10 **F**7 11 25 30 38 52 55 57 61 62 69 79 84 86 96 97 107 119 122 **P**5 6
Primary Contact: Mary B. Moffett, CPA, Administrator
CFO: Allyson Fannin, CPA, Chief Financial Officer
CMO: I. C. Turnley, M.D., Chief of Staff
Web address: www.lasallegeneralhospital.com
Control: Hospital district or authority, Government, nonfederal **Service:** General Medical and Surgical

Staffed Beds: 60 **Admissions:** 1848 **Census:** 32 **Outpatient Visits:** 21756 **Births:** 0 **Total Expense ($000):** 15949 **Payroll Expense ($000):** 8035 **Personnel:** 239

JENNINGS—Jefferson Davis Parish

☐ **JENNINGS AMERICAN LEGION HOSPITAL (190053)**, 1634 Elton Road, Zip 70546–3614; tel. 337/616–7000, (Nonreporting) **A**1 9 10
Primary Contact: Terry J. Terrebonne, Chief Executive Officer
COO: Dana Williams, Chief Operating Officer
CFO: Pam Primeaux, Chief Financial Officer
CIO: Gary Courrege, Chief Information Officer
Web address: www.jalh.com
Control: Other not–for–profit (including NFP Corporation) **Service:** General Medical and Surgical

Staffed Beds: 60

WESTEND HOSPITAL (194075), 1530 Highway 90 West, Zip 70546; tel. 337/616–8122, (Nonreporting) **A**10
Primary Contact: Stacey G. Wilson, Administrator
Web address: www.westendhospital.com
Control: Corporation, Investor–owned, for–profit **Service:** Psychiatric

Staffed Beds: 20

JONESBORO—Jackson Parish

JACKSON PARISH HOSPITAL (191317), 165 Beech Springs Road, Zip 71251–2059; tel. 318/259–4435, (Nonreporting) **A**9 10 18
Primary Contact: L. J. Pecot, Administrator
CFO: David Sanders, Chief Financial Officer
CMO: Abraham Jacob, M.D., President Medical Staff
CHR: Elizabeth Cheatwood, Administrative Assistant and Human Resource Director
Web address: www.jacksonparishhospital.com
Control: Hospital district or authority, Government, nonfederal **Service:** General Medical and Surgical

Staffed Beds: 25

KAPLAN—Vermilion Parish

ABROM KAPLAN MEMORIAL HOSPITAL (191322), 1310 West Seventh Street, Zip 70548–2998; tel. 337/643–8300, (Nonreporting) **A**9 10 18
Primary Contact: Lyman Trahan, Chief Executive Officer
CFO: Mary Melancon, Chief Financial Officer
CMO: Alton Romero, M.D., Chief Medical Staff
Web address: www.lafayettegeneral.com
Control: Hospital district or authority, Government, nonfederal **Service:** General Medical and Surgical

Staffed Beds: 20

Hospital, Medicare Provider Number, Address, Telephone, Approval, Facility, and Physician Codes, Health Care System

★ American Hospital Association (AHA) membership
☐ The Joint Commission accreditation
○ American Osteopathic Association (AOA) accreditation
△ Commission on Accreditation of Rehabilitation Facilities (CARF) accreditation

LA

KENNER—Jefferson Parish

☒ **OCHSNER MEDICAL CENTER – KENNER (190274)**, (Formerly Kenner Regional Medical Center), 180 West Esplanade Avenue, Zip 70065–6001; tel. 504/468–8600 **A**1 3 5 8 9 10 **F**3 13 14 15 18 20 22 24 25 26 30 31 32 33 35 38 50 52 55 56 57 59 62 66 68 74 75 77 79 80 82 86 96 97 100 102 107 112 118 119 120 124 135 137 **S** Ochsner Health System
Primary Contact: Paolo Zambito, Chief Executive Officer
COO: Paolo Zambito, Chief Executive Officer
CFO: Mark Eckert, Chief Financial Officer
Web address: www.ochsner.org/body.cfm?id=1397
Control: Other not–for–profit (including NFP Corporation) **Service:** General Medical and Surgical

Staffed Beds: 106 **Admissions:** 4136 **Census:** 57 **Outpatient Visits:** 58063 **Births:** 65 **Total Expense ($000):** 69170 **Payroll Expense ($000):** 26079 **Personnel:** 531

KENTWOOD—Tangipahoa Parish

SOUTHEAST REGIONAL MEDICAL CENTER (192040), 719 Avenue G., Zip 70444–2601; tel. 985/229–9193, (Nonreporting) **A**10
Primary Contact: Lionel Murphy, Chief Executive Officer
Control: Corporation, Investor–owned, for–profit **Service:** Long–Term Acute Care hospital

Staffed Beds: 14

KINDER—Allen Parish

★ **ALLEN PARISH HOSPITAL (190133)**, 108 North Sixth Avenue, Zip 70648–3519, Mailing Address: P.O. Box 1670, Zip 70648–1670; tel. 337/738–2527 **A**9 10 **F**4 25 30 31 32 33 38 46 49 50 55 56 57 61 62 63 75 86 87 88 91 92 96 100 107 117 119 121 122 **P**6
Primary Contact: Scott G. Barrilleaux, FACHE, Chief Executive Officer and Administrator
COO: Brandy Fontenot, Chief Operating Officer
CFO: Chad Guidry, Chief Financial Officer
CMO: Ejiro Ughouwa, M.D., Chief of Staff
CIO: Bill Marcantel, Chief Information Officer
CHR: Amand Lambert, Director Human Resources
Web address: www.allenparishhospital.com
Control: Hospital district or authority, Government, nonfederal **Service:** General Medical and Surgical

Staffed Beds: 49 **Admissions:** 1265 **Census:** 27 **Outpatient Visits:** 26889 **Births:** 0 **Total Expense ($000):** 8541 **Payroll Expense ($000):** 4868 **Personnel:** 175

LA PLACE—St. John the Baptist Parish

☐ **LA PLACE REHABILITATION HOSPITAL (193064)**, 508 West 5th Street, Zip 70068; tel. 985/653–8447, (Nonreporting) **A**1 10
Primary Contact: Peter J. Jolet, Administrator
Web address: www.gulfstateshs.com
Control: Corporation, Investor–owned, for–profit **Service:** Rehabilitation

Staffed Beds: 21

☒ **RIVER PARISHES HOSPITAL (190175)**, 500 Rue de Sante, Zip 70068–5420; tel. 985/652–7000, (Nonreporting) **A**1 9 10 **S** LifePoint Hospitals, Inc.
Primary Contact: Charlotte W. Dupre', Chief Executive Officer
CFO: Tim Matney, Chief Financial Officer
CHR: Katherine Trepagnier, Director Human Resources
Web address: www.riverparisheshospital.com
Control: Corporation, Investor–owned, for–profit **Service:** General Medical and Surgical

Staffed Beds: 72

LACOMBE—St. Tammany Parish

☐ **LOUISIANA MEDICAL CENTER AND HEART HOSPITAL (190250)**, (Formerly Louisiana Heart Hospital), 64030 Highway 434, Zip 70445; tel. 985/690–7500, (Nonreporting) **A**1 9 10 **S** MedCath, Inc.
Primary Contact: William W. Fox, III, President
Web address: www.louisianahearthospital.com
Control: Corporation, Investor–owned, for–profit **Service:** Heart

Staffed Beds: 58

LAFAYETTE—Lafayette Parish

★ **ACADIA VERMILION HOSPITAL (194044)**, 2520 North University Avenue, Zip 70507–5306; tel. 337/234–5614 **A**9 10 **F**2 5 88 92 94 95 **P**8
Primary Contact: Craig S. Juengling, Chief Executive Officer
COO: Luis Betances, Chief Operating Officer
CFO: James Todd, Chief Financial Officer
CMO: Bob Winston, M.D., Medical Director
CHR: Cassie O'Neal, Director Human Resources
Web address: www.vermilionhospital.com
Control: Corporation, Investor–owned, for–profit **Service:** Psychiatric

Staffed Beds: 44 **Admissions:** 1531 **Census:** 33 **Outpatient Visits:** 1950 **Births:** 0 **Total Expense ($000):** 8721 **Payroll Expense ($000):** 4697 **Personnel:** 113

COMMUNITY SPECIALTY HOSPITAL (192020), 811 Martin Luther King Jr. Drive, Zip 70501–7129; tel. 337/234–4031, (Nonreporting) **A**10
Primary Contact: John E. Jumonville, III, Administrator
Control: Corporation, Investor–owned, for–profit **Service:** Rehabilitation

Staffed Beds: 36

☐ **HEART HOSPITAL OF LAFAYETTE (190263)**, 1105 Kaliste Saloom, Zip 70508; tel. 337/521–1000 **A**1 9 10 **F**3 17 18 20 22 25 26 31 32 33 38 46 55 56 57 62 66 73 79 80 96 97 103 107 137 **S** MedCath, Inc.
Primary Contact: Karen O. Wyble, Interim President
Web address: www.hearthospitaloflafayette.com
Control: Partnership, Investor–owned, for–profit **Service:** General Medical and Surgical

Staffed Beds: 32 **Admissions:** 2262 **Census:** 20 **Outpatient Visits:** 8326 **Births:** 0 **Total Expense ($000):** 36788 **Payroll Expense ($000):** 8928 **Personnel:** 196

☒ **LAFAYETTE GENERAL MEDICAL CENTER (190002)**, 1214 Coolidge Avenue, Zip 70503–2696, Mailing Address: P.O. Box 52009 OCS, Zip 70505–2009; tel. 337/289–7991, (Nonreporting) **A**1 2 9 10
Primary Contact: Patrick W. Gandy, President and Chief Executive Officer
COO: Patrick W. Gandy, Chief Operating Officer
CFO: Roger Mattke, Chief Financial Officer
CIO: Edwina Mallery, Vice President Information Systems
CHR: Gary Lacaze, Assistant Vice President Human Resources
Web address: www.lafayettegeneral.org
Control: Other not–for–profit (including NFP Corporation) **Service:** General Medical and Surgical

Staffed Beds: 294

LAFAYETTE GENERAL SURGICAL HOSPITAL (190268), 1000 West Pinhook Road, Zip 70503; tel. 337/289–8088, (Nonreporting) **A**9 10
Primary Contact: Katherine Hebert, Administrator and Chief Executive Officer
Web address: www.lgsh.us
Control: Partnership, Investor–owned, for–profit **Service:** General Medical and Surgical

Staffed Beds: 10

☐ **LAFAYETTE SURGICAL SPECIALTY HOSPITAL (190259)**, 1101 Kaliste Saloom Road, Zip 70508; tel. 337/769–4100, (Nonreporting) **A**1 9 10
Primary Contact: Gary I. Keller, Chief Executive Officer
Web address: www.lafayettesurgical.com
Control: Corporation, Investor–owned, for–profit **Service:** Other specialty

Staffed Beds: 20

LONG TERM ACUTE CARE OF ACADIANA (192029), 310 Youngsville Highway, Zip 70508; tel. 337/839–9880, (Nonreporting) **A**10
Primary Contact: James H. Morgan, Chief Executive Officer
CFO: Jessica McGee, Chief Financial Officer
CMO: Roderick V. Clark, M.D., Chief Medical Officer
CHR: Heather Lamarche, Manager Human Resources
Control: Individual, Investor–owned, for–profit **Service:** General Medical and Surgical

Staffed Beds: 23

LOUISIANA EXTENDED CARE HOSPITAL OF LAFAYETTE (192032), 1214 Coolidge Boulevard, 8th Floor, Zip 70503–2621, Mailing Address: 1214 Coolidge Boulelvard, 8th Floor, Zip 70503–2621; tel. 337/984–4224, (Nonreporting) **A**10
Primary Contact: Stuart Archer, Administrator
Web address: www.lhcgroup.com
Control: County–Government, nonfederal **Service:** Long–Term Acute Care hospital

Staffed Beds: 10

☒ **MEADOWBROOK SPECIALTY HOSPITAL OF LAFAYETTE (192033)**, 204 Energy Parkway, Zip 70508; tel. 337/232–1905 **A**1 10 **F**3 25 33 62 73 75 86 119 132 137 **S** RehabCare Group, Inc.
Primary Contact: R. Christopher Fox, Chief Executive Officer and Administrator
Web address: www.rehabcare.com
Control: Corporation, Investor–owned, for–profit **Service:** Long–Term Acute Care hospital

Staffed Beds: 70 **Admissions:** 554 **Census:** 38 **Outpatient Visits:** 0 **Births:** 0 **Total Expense ($000):** 17060 **Payroll Expense ($000):** 7481

★ **OUR LADY OF LOURDES REGIONAL MEDICAL CENTER (190102)**, 611 St. Landry Street, Zip 70506–4627, Mailing Address: P.O. Box 4027, Zip 70502–4027; tel. 337/289–2000 **A**1 2 9 10 **F**3 9 11 12 15 17 18 20 22 24 25 26 27 28 32 33 38 39 40 43 44 47 49 50 51 52 53 55 57 58 59 62 64 65 66 68 72 73 75 76 77 79 80 82 85 86 96 97 99 100 102 103 106 107 112 118 119 121 124 132 133 135 136 137 **S** Franciscan Missionaries of Our Lady Health System, Inc.
Primary Contact: William F. Barrow, II, President and Chief Executive Officer
COO: Robert Davis, Chief Operating Officer
CFO: Kim Hebert, Chief Financial Officer
CMO: Gary Arnold, M.D., Physician Executive
CIO: Nona Mire, Director Information Systems
CHR: Kevin Domingue, Director Human Resources and Medical Affairs
Web address: www.lourdes.net
Control: Church–operated, Nongovernment, not–for profit **Service:** General Medical and Surgical

Staffed Beds: 217 **Admissions:** 9918 **Census:** 156 **Outpatient Visits:** 113420 **Births:** 0 **Total Expense ($000):** 147493 **Payroll Expense ($000):** 52761 **Personnel:** 1118

PARK PLACE SURGICAL HOSPITAL (190255), 901 Wilson Street, Zip 70503; tel. 337/237–8119, (Nonreporting) **A**9 10
Primary Contact: Brandon Moore, CHE, Administrator and Chief Executive Officer
Control: Corporation, Investor–owned, for–profit **Service:** Other specialty

Staffed Beds: 10

★ **SOUTHWEST MEDICAL CENTER (190205)**, 2810 Ambassador Caffery Parkway, Zip 70506; tel. 337/981–2949 **A**1 9 10 **F**3 12 15 18 20 22 24 25 26 27 30 31 32 35 38 42 43 44 46 49 55 57 62 63 68 72 73 75 77 79 80 81 82 85 86 87 96 97 102 106 107 135 137 **S** HCA
Primary Contact: Kyle J. Viator, Chief Executive Officer
CFO: Penny Hutson, Chief Financial Officer
CHR: Wendy Alexander, Director Human Resources
Web address: www.southwestmc.com
Control: Corporation, Investor–owned, for–profit **Service:** General Medical and Surgical

Staffed Beds: 142 **Admissions:** 5207 **Census:** 72 **Outpatient Visits:** 54127 **Births:** 0 **Total Expense ($000):** 60261 **Payroll Expense ($000):** 17691 **Personnel:** 326

ST. LUKE'S SPECIALTY HOSPITAL OF SUNSET (192053), 2500 East Simcoe Street, Zip 70501; tel. 337/233–2864 **A**10 **F**1
Primary Contact: Gary Chaney, Administrator
Control: Partnership, Investor–owned, for–profit **Service:** Long–Term Acute Care hospital

Staffed Beds: 16 **Admissions:** 128 **Census:** 9 **Personnel:** 28

★ **UNIVERSITY MEDICAL CENTER (190006)**, 2390 West Congress Street, Zip 70506–4298, Mailing Address: P.O. Box 69300, Zip 70596–9300; tel. 337/261–6001, (Nonreporting) **A**1 2 3 5 9 10 **S** LSU Health Sciences Center
Primary Contact: Lawrence T. Dorsey, Administrator
COO: Glenn L. Craig, Chief Operating Officer
CFO: Karen Gardiner, Director Fiscal Services
CMO: James B. Falterman, M.D., Medical Director
CIO: J. Barry Daigle, Manager Information Systems
CHR: Jennifer Simms, Director Human Resources
Web address: www.lsuhospitals.org
Control: State–Government, nonfederal **Service:** General Medical and Surgical

Staffed Beds: 124

□ **UNIVERSITY MEDICAL CENTER–PSYCHIATRIC UNIT**, 302 Dulles Drive, Zip 70506–3008; tel. 337/262–4190, (Nonreporting) **A**1
Primary Contact: George Diggs, M.D., Medical Director
Control: State–Government, nonfederal **Service:** Psychiatric

Staffed Beds: 20

★ **WOMEN'S AND CHILDREN'S HOSPITAL (190196)**, 4600 Ambassador Caffery Parkway, Zip 70508–6923, Mailing Address: P.O. Box 88030, Zip 70598–8030; tel. 337/521–9100 **A**1 9 10 **F**3 8 13 15 25 26 27 30 31 32 33 37 38 50 55 57 66 68 70 72 73 74 75 77 79 80 81 82 83 84 86 96 99 100 102 107 113 114 118 119 121 135 136 **S** HCA
Primary Contact: Kathy J. Bobbs, Chief Executive Officer
COO: Patricia Monczewski, Chief Operating Officer
CFO: James Miller, Chief Financial Officer
CIO: James Gahn, Director Information Systems
CHR: Jane Fuller, Director Human Resources
Web address: www.womens–childrens.com
Control: Corporation, Investor–owned, for–profit **Service:** Obstetrics and gynecology

Staffed Beds: 161 **Admissions:** 7219 **Census:** 87 **Outpatient Visits:** 68390 **Births:** 3509 **Total Expense ($000):** 50505 **Payroll Expense ($000):** 22432 **Personnel:** 510

LAKE CHARLES—Calcasieu Parish

★ △ **CHRISTUS ST. PATRICK HOSPITAL OF LAKE CHARLES (190027)**, 524 South Ryan Street, Zip 70601–5799, Mailing Address: P.O. Box 3401, Zip 70602–3401; tel. 337/436–2511 **A**1 2 7 9 10 **F**3 5 11 12 15 17 18 20 22 24 25 26 27 28 30 31 32 33 36 37 38 41 44 46 47 48 49 50 54 55 56 57 60 62 63 66 68 72 73 76 77 79 80 81 82 84 85 86 88 90 91 92 93 94 95 96 97 99 106 107 108 109 110 111 112 116 119 121 123 124 132 135 136 137 **P**8 **S** CHRISTUS Health
Primary Contact: Ellen M. Jones, President and Chief Executive Officer
COO: Dianne P. Teal, Chief Operating Officer
CFO: Bill Hecht, Chief Financial Officer
CMO: Darrell Dixon, M.D., Vice President Medical Affairs
CIO: Allen Abshire, Director Information Services
CHR: Shelly Welch, Assistant Administrator Human Resources
Web address: www.stpatrickhospital.org
Control: Church–operated, Nongovernment, not–for profit **Service:** General Medical and Surgical

Staffed Beds: 288 **Admissions:** 9987 **Census:** 141 **Outpatient Visits:** 136498 **Births:** 0 **Total Expense ($000):** 130565 **Payroll Expense ($000):** 45554 **Personnel:** 865

★ **DUBUIS HOSPITAL OF LAKE CHARLES (192024)**, 524 South Ryan, 5th Floor, Zip 70601–5725; tel. 337/491–7752 **A**1 10 **F**1 3 25 33 73 119 137 **S** Dubuis Health System
Primary Contact: Ronald E. Hand, Administrator
CMO: Ron Lewis, M.D., Medical Director
Control: Church–operated, Nongovernment, not–for profit **Service:** Long–Term Acute Care hospital

Staffed Beds: 24 **Admissions:** 178 **Census:** 16 **Outpatient Visits:** 0 **Births:** 0 **Total Expense ($000):** 7092 **Payroll Expense ($000):** 2286 **Personnel:** 62

EXTENDED CARE OF SOUTHWEST LOUISIANA (192019), 2837 Ernest Street, Building B., Zip 70601; tel. 337/436–6111, (Nonreporting) **A**10
Primary Contact: Mark D. Severns, Chief Executive Officer
Web address: www.lcmh.com/extcare.htm
Control: Other not–for–profit (including NFP Corporation) **Service:** Long–Term Acute Care hospital

Staffed Beds: 28

★ **LAKE CHARLES MEMORIAL HOSPITAL (190060)**, 1701 Oak Park Boulevard, Zip 70601; tel. 337/494–3000, (Nonreporting) **A**1 2 3 5 9 10 12
Primary Contact: Larry M. Graham, CHE, President and Chief Executive Officer
COO: David Usher, Vice President Operations
CFO: Charles P. Whitson, CPA, Vice President Finance
CMO: Paul Comeaux, M.D., Director Medical Staff
CIO: Belinda Sommers, Chief Information Officer
CHR: Ginger Consigney, Director Human Resources
Web address: www.lcmh.com
Control: Other not–for–profit (including NFP Corporation) **Service:** General Medical and Surgical

Staffed Beds: 298

★ **WALTER OLIN MOSS REGIONAL MEDICAL CENTER (190161)**, 1000 Walters Street, Zip 70605–4647; tel. 337/475–8100 **A**9 10 **F**3 8 11 15 25 27 30 32 37 38 50 55 57 58 60 62 64 66 68 73 76 79 80 81 82 87 88 90 92 93 96 99 102 107 119 135 136 137 **P**3 4 **S** LSU Health Sciences Center
Primary Contact: Patrick C. Robinson, M.D., Administrator
CFO: Ranelda Benoit, Administrative Manager and Fiscal Officer
CMO: Ben Darby, M.D., Medical Director
CIO: Steve Demourelle, Chief Information Officer
CHR: Sharon Powell, Director Human Resources
Control: State–Government, nonfederal **Service:** General Medical and Surgical

Staffed Beds: 36 **Admissions:** 1435 **Census:** 25 **Outpatient Visits:** 106199 **Births:** 0 **Total Expense ($000):** 41059 **Payroll Expense ($000):** 15109 **Personnel:** 405

★ **WOMEN AND CHILDREN'S HOSPITAL (190201)**, 4200 Nelson Road, Zip 70605–4118; tel. 337/474–6370, (Nonreporting) **A**1 9 10 **S** Community Health Systems, Inc.
Primary Contact: William L. Willis, Chief Executive Officer
CFO: Dawn Johnson–Hatcher, Chief Financial Officer
CMO: Lloyd Guidry, M.D., Medical Director
CIO: Tracy Leger, Director Information Systems
CHR: Kasey Cormier, Director Human Resources
Web address: www.women–childrens.com
Control: Corporation, Investor–owned, for–profit **Service:** Other specialty

Staffed Beds: 118

Hospital, Medicare Provider Number, Address, Telephone, Approval, Facility, and Physician Codes, Health Care System
★ American Hospital Association (AHA) membership
□ The Joint Commission accreditation
○ American Osteopathic Association (AOA) accreditation
△ Commission on Accreditation of Rehabilitation Facilities (CARF) accreditation

LAKE PROVIDENCE—East Carroll Parish

EAST CARROLL PARISH HOSPITAL (190208), 336 North Hood Street, Zip 71254–2194; tel. 318/559–2441, (Nonreporting) **A**9 10
Primary Contact: Ladonna Englerth, Administrator
Control: Hospital district or authority, Government, nonfederal **Service:** Other specialty

Staffed Beds: 11

LEESVILLE—Vernon Parish

☒ **BYRD REGIONAL HOSPITAL (190164)**, 1020 Fertitta Boulevard, Zip 71446–4697; tel. 337/239–9041 **A**1 9 10 **F**1 3 4 13 16 17 18 25 27 31 32 38 48 49 50 55 56 57 59 65 68 70 71 73 74 76 77 78 79 80 81 82 83 84 85 88 96 97 100 102 103 107 117 118 120 122 134 135 136 **P**7 **S** Community Health Systems, Inc.
Primary Contact: Roger C. LeDoux, Chief Executive Officer
CFO: Wendell Wilkes, Chief Financial Officer
CMO: Hanna Lubbos, M.D., Chief of Staff
CHR: Karolyne Christian, Director Human Resources
Web address: www.byrdregional.com
Control: Corporation, Investor–owned, for–profit **Service:** General Medical and Surgical

Staffed Beds: 60 **Admissions:** 4296 **Census:** 42 **Outpatient Visits:** 46070 **Births:** 396 **Personnel:** 317

☐ **LEESVILLE REHABILITATION HOSPITAL (193086)**, 900 South Sixth Street, Zip 71446; tel. 337/392–8118 **A**1 10 **F**30 31 85
Primary Contact: Jack M. Causey, Administrator
Web address: www.leesvillerehab.com
Control: Partnership, Investor–owned, for–profit **Service:** Rehabilitation

Staffed Beds: 16 **Admissions:** 304 **Census:** 12 **Outpatient Visits:** 0 **Births:** 0 **Total Expense ($000):** 3876 **Payroll Expense ($000):** 1277 **Personnel:** 41

LULING—St. Charles Parish

LULING REHABILITATION HOSPITAL (193060), 1125 Paul Maillard Road, Zip 70070, Mailing Address: P.O. Box 243, Zip 70070–0243; tel. 985/331–2281, (Nonreporting) **A**10
Primary Contact: Juanita Bates, Administrator
Web address: www.lulingrehab.com
Control: County–Government, nonfederal **Service:** Rehabilitation

Staffed Beds: 16

☐ **ST. CHARLES PARISH HOSPITAL (190079)**, 1057 Paul Maillard Road, Zip 70070, Mailing Address: P.O. Box 87, Zip 70070; tel. 985/785–6242 **A**1 9 10 **F**3 7 11 15 24 25 27 30 31 33 38 54 55 56 57 59 62 63 68 72 73 75 76 77 79 81 86 88 90 91 92 93 96 99 100 102 107 119 120 121 135 137 **P**5
Primary Contact: Fred Martinez, Jr., Chief Executive Officer
COO: Karen Guillot, R.N., Chief Operating Officer
CMO: Martin Belanger, M.D., Chief Medical Staff
CIO: Angela Duet, Director Information Technology
CHR: Carolyn Faucheaux, Director Human Resources
Web address: www.stch.net
Control: Hospital district or authority, Government, nonfederal **Service:** General Medical and Surgical

Staffed Beds: 56 **Admissions:** 1931 **Census:** 36 **Outpatient Visits:** 31912 **Births:** 0 **Total Expense ($000):** 29602 **Payroll Expense ($000):** 14315 **Personnel:** 385

LUTCHER—St. James Parish

ST. JAMES BEHAVIORAL HEALTH HOSPITAL (194063), 2471 Louisiana Avenue, Zip 70071; tel. 225/869–3788, (Nonreporting) **A**10
Primary Contact: Candy Lewis, Administrator
COO: Wendell Smith, Chief Operating Officer
CFO: Gopinath Gopalam, Chief Financial Officer
CMO: Lance Bullock, M.D., Medical Director
CIO: Candy Lewis, Administrator
CHR: Charla Burchfield, Manager Human Resources
Control: Corporation, Investor–owned, for–profit **Service:** Psychiatric

Staffed Beds: 10

☒ **ST. JAMES PARISH HOSPITAL (191305)**, 1645 Lutcher Avenue, Zip 70071; tel. 225/869–5512 **A**1 9 10 18 **F**15 25 26 30 31 32 33 38 55 56 57 62 73 79 82 86 96 97 107 117 118 121 122 124 137
Primary Contact: Mary Ellen Pratt, Chief Executive Officer
CFO: Tracy L. George, Chief Financial Officer
CIO: Kim Scharwath, Director Medical Records
CHR: Lisa Faucheux, Director Human Resources
Web address: www.stjamesparishhospital.com
Control: Hospital district or authority, Government, nonfederal **Service:** General Medical and Surgical

Staffed Beds: 16 **Admissions:** 417 **Census:** 7 **Outpatient Visits:** 21821 **Births:** 0 **Total Expense ($000):** 8445 **Payroll Expense ($000):** 4318 **Personnel:** 121

MAMOU—Evangeline Parish

☒ **SAVOY MEDICAL CENTER (190025)**, 801 Poinciana Avenue, Zip 70554–2298; tel. 337/468–5261, (Nonreporting) **A**1 9 10 **S** HCA
Primary Contact: Cristina Rivera, Chief Executive Officer
COO: Gerald Fuselier, Chief Operating Officer
CFO: Melissa Schatzle, Chief Financial Officer
CMO: Brent Ardoin, M.D., Chief Medical Officer
CIO: Daniel Lahaye, Manager
CHR: Annette Thibodeaux, Director Human Resources
Web address: www.savoymedicalcenter.com
Control: Corporation, Investor–owned, for–profit **Service:** General Medical and Surgical

Staffed Beds: 180

MANDEVILLE—St. Tammany Parish

☐ **SOUTHEAST LOUISIANA HOSPITAL (194007)**, 23515 Highway 190, Zip 70448–5612, Mailing Address: P.O. Box 3850, Zip 70470–3850; tel. 985/626–6300 **A**1 3 5 10 **F**26 30 31 32 36 73 81 82 88 89 **S** Louisiana State Hospitals
Primary Contact: Patricia Gonzales, Chief Executive Officer
CFO: Denise Businelle, Account Administrator
CMO: Hossam Abou–Taleb, M.D., Medical Director
CIO: Mike Ziemba, Information Technology Project Lead
CHR: Daphne Stewart, Director Human Resources
Web address: www.dhh.state.la.us/offices/?ID=335
Control: State–Government, nonfederal **Service:** Psychiatric

Staffed Beds: 151 **Admissions:** 563 **Census:** 134 **Outpatient Visits:** 0 **Births:** 0 **Total Expense ($000):** 38079 **Payroll Expense ($000):** 19264 **Personnel:** 536

MANSFIELD—De Soto Parish

★ **DE SOTO REGIONAL HEALTH SYSTEM (190118)**, 207 Jefferson Street, Zip 71052–2603, Mailing Address: P.O. Box 1636, Zip 71052–2603; tel. 318/871–3100, (Nonreporting) **A**9 10 20 **S** Brim Healthcare, Inc.
Primary Contact: John Domansky, Interim Chief Executive Officer
CFO: Norbert Crafts, Chief Financial Officer
CMO: Leigh Dillard, Chief of Staff
CHR: Rhonda Potter, Director Human Resources
Web address: www.desotoregional.com
Control: Other not–for–profit (including NFP Corporation) **Service:** General Medical and Surgical

Staffed Beds: 49

MANY—Sabine Parish

SABINE MEDICAL CENTER (190218), 240 Highland Drive, Zip 71449–3718; tel. 318/256–7383 **A**9 10 20 **F**3 15 25 27 30 31 32 38 40 50 55 57 62 79 84 96 99 103 107 117 119 122 134 **S** Associated Healthcare Systems, Inc.
Primary Contact: Patrick W. Gandy, Chief Executive Officer
CFO: Frances F. Hopkins, Chief Financial Officer
Web address: www.sabinemedicalcenter.net
Control: Corporation, Investor–owned, for–profit **Service:** General Medical and Surgical

Staffed Beds: 44 **Admissions:** 1343 **Census:** 12 **Outpatient Visits:** 21000 **Births:** 0 **Total Expense ($000):** 9101 **Payroll Expense ($000):** 4387 **Personnel:** 124

MARKSVILLE—Avoyelles Parish

☒ **AVOYELLES HOSPITAL (190099)**, 4231 Highway 1192, Zip 71351, Mailing Address: P.O. Box 249, Zip 71351–0249; tel. 318/253–8611 **A**1 9 10 **F**3 11 15 25 26 30 38 46 55 62 66 68 73 79 80 84 96 102 107 119 122 124 135 **S** HCA
Primary Contact: David M. Mitchel, Chief Executive Officer
CFO: Craig A. Roy, Chief Financial Officer
CMO: Allen McClure, M.D., Chief of Staff
CIO: Billy Tingle, Director Information Systems and Respiratory Therapy
CHR: Sheila Kight, Director Human Resources
Web address: www.avoyelleshospital.com
Control: Partnership, Investor–owned, for–profit **Service:** General Medical and Surgical

Staffed Beds: 47 **Admissions:** 1639 **Census:** 18 **Outpatient Visits:** 41308 **Births:** 0 **Total Expense ($000):** 15530 **Payroll Expense ($000):** 6882 **Personnel:** 176

MARRERO—Jefferson Parish

★ **LOUISIANA SPECIALTY HOSPITAL (192007)**, 1111 Medical Center Boulevard, 7th Floor, Zip 70072, Mailing Address: 1111 Medical Center Boulecvard, 7th Floor, Zip 70072; tel. 504/349–2584, (Nonreporting) **A**10 **S** RehabCare Group, Inc.
Primary Contact: Stephanie T. Wells, CPA, Chief Executive Officer
Web address: www.rehabcare.com
Control: Corporation, Investor–owned, for–profit **Service:** Long–Term Acute Care hospital

Staffed Beds: 56

Many Facility Codes have changed. Please refer to the AHA Guide Code Chart.

★ △ **WEST JEFFERSON MEDICAL CENTER (190039)**, 1101 Medical Center Boulevard, Zip 70072–3191; tel. 504/347–5511, (Nonreporting) **A**1 2 3 5 7 9 10
Primary Contact: Nancy R. Cassagne, Chief Executive Officer
COO: Erie J. Hebert, FACHE, Senior Vice President
CFO: Christopher W. Daniel, Chief Financial Officer
CMO: Alfred E. Abaunza, M.D., Chief Medical Officer
CHR: Maureen Morris, Director Human Resources
Web address: www.wjmc.org
Control: Hospital district or authority, Government, nonfederal **Service:** General Medical and Surgical

Staffed Beds: 307

METAIRIE—Jefferson Parish

★ △ **EAST JEFFERSON GENERAL HOSPITAL (190146)**, 4200 Houma Boulevard, Zip 70011–2996; tel. 504/454–4000, (Includes DOCTORS HOSPITAL OF JEFFERSON, 4320 Houma Boulevard, Zip 70006–2973; tel. 504/849–4000) **A**1 2 3 5 7 9 10 **F**2 3 7 8 11 13 14 15 17 18 20 22 24 25 26 27 30 31 32 33 38 40 43 44 46 49 52 54 55 56 57 59 62 66 68 70 71 72 73 74 75 76 77 79 80 82 85 86 88 90 92 93 96 97 99 100 102 103 105 106 107 108 109 111 112 116 117 118 119 120 121 132 135 136 137 **P**4 6 8
Primary Contact: Mark J. Peters, M.D., President and Chief Executive Officer
COO: Janice Kishner, Chief Operating Officer and Nurse Executive
CFO: Bruce Naremore, Chief Financial Officer
CMO: Frannie R. Kronenberg, M.D., MSC, Chief Medical Officer
CIO: Bernie Clement, Chief Information Officer
CHR: Donna Ammons, Director Human Resources
Web address: www.ejgh.org
Control: Hospital district or authority, Government, nonfederal **Service:** General Medical and Surgical

Staffed Beds: 435 **Admissions:** 19282 **Census:** 337 **Outpatient Visits:** 246506 **Births:** 2565 **Total Expense ($000):** 341886 **Payroll Expense ($000):** 145515 **Personnel:** 2436

☐ **ST. THERESA SPECIALTY HOSPITAL (192030)**, (Formerly Select Specialty Hospital–Jefferson Parish), 4200 Houma Boulevard, Zip 70006; tel. 504/780–3020, (Nonreporting) **A**1 10
Primary Contact: Sam Kurz, Chief Executive Officer
Control: Corporation, Investor–owned, for–profit **Service:** Long–Term Acute Care hospital

Staffed Beds: 31

★ **TULANE–LAKESIDE HOSPITAL**, 4700 I–10 Service Road, Zip 70001–1269; tel. 504/780–8282, (Nonreporting) **A**1 9 **S** HCA
Primary Contact: Stephen Robinson, Administrator
COO: Andre duPlessis, Chief Operating Officer
Web address: www.hcahealthcare.com
Control: Corporation, Investor–owned, for–profit **Service:** General Medical and Surgical

Staffed Beds: 116

MINDEN—Webster Parish

★ **MINDEN MEDICAL CENTER (190144)**, 1 Medical Plaza, Zip 71055–3330, Mailing Address: P.O. Box 5003, Zip 71058–5003; tel. 318/377–2321 **A**1 9 10 19 **F**11 13 15 18 20 25 26 30 31 32 38 43 46 54 55 56 57 61 62 68 69 73 74 75 76 77 79 82 84 85 86 88 93 96 100 103 107 118 119 121 135 136 **S** LifePoint Hospitals, Inc.
Primary Contact: George E. French, III, CHE, Chief Executive Officer
CFO: Jim Williams, Chief Financial Officer
CMO: G. Max Steel, M.D., Medical Director
CIO: Renae Simmons, Director Information Systems
CHR: Mary Winget, Director Human Resources
Web address: www.mindenmedicalcenter.com
Control: Corporation, Investor–owned, for–profit **Service:** General Medical and Surgical

Staffed Beds: 159 **Admissions:** 5185 **Census:** 57 **Outpatient Visits:** 35467 **Births:** 790 **Total Expense ($000):** 34506 **Payroll Expense ($000):** 16698 **Personnel:** 437

MONROE—Ouachita Parish

☐ **E. A. CONWAY MEDICAL CENTER (190011)**, 4864 Jackson Street, Zip 71202–6497, Mailing Address: P.O. Box 1881, Zip 71210–8005; tel. 318/330–7000 **A**1 3 5 9 10 **F**3 11 13 15 25 26 27 31 33 38 40 49 50 53 55 57 58 62 63 64 68 70 72 73 74 75 76 77 79 80 82 84 86 87 88 90 92 96 97 99 100 102 107 119 124 135 **P**1
Primary Contact: H. Aryon McGuire, Administrator
CFO: Linda Lochbrunner, Chief Financial Officer
CMO: LaDonna Ford, M.D., Medical Director
CHR: Jim Hardegree, Assistant Director Human Resource Management
Web address: www.conway.lsuhsc.edu
Control: State–Government, nonfederal **Service:** General Medical and Surgical

Staffed Beds: 158 **Admissions:** 6840 **Census:** 110 **Outpatient Visits:** 145521 **Births:** 1086 **Total Expense ($000):** 83700 **Payroll Expense ($000):** 34500 **Personnel:** 926

GOLDEN AGE SENIOR CARE HOSPITAL (194070), 4310 South Grand Street, Zip 71202; tel. 318/651–0920, (Nonreporting) **A**10
Primary Contact: Walter O. Bigby, Jr., Administrator
Control: Corporation, Investor–owned, for–profit **Service:** Other specialty

Staffed Beds: 12

☐ **MONROE SURGICAL HOSPITAL (190245)**, 2408 Broadmoor Boulevard, Zip 71201, Mailing Address: P.O. Box 4887, Zip 71211–4887; tel. 318/410–0002, (Nonreporting) **A**1 9 10 **S** Hospital Partners of America
Primary Contact: Alan Daugherty, Administrator
Web address: www.monroesurgical.com
Control: Corporation, Investor–owned, for–profit **Service:** Surgical

Staffed Beds: 10

★ **P & S SURGICAL HOSPITAL (190246)**, 312 Grammont Street, Suite 101, Zip 71201; tel. 318/388–4040 **A**9 10 **F**3 12 18 20 25 30 31 32 33 35 37 43 51 56 63 66 77 79 80 81 107 121 124 131 **P**7 8
Primary Contact: Linda S. Holyfield, RN, M.S.N., President and Chief Executive Officer
COO: Terri Hicks, Chief Operating Officer and Chief Financial Officer
CFO: Terri Hicks, Chief Operating Officer and Chief Financial Officer
CMO: Wilson Barham, M.D., Chief of Staff
CIO: Joseph Vicknair, Chief Information Officer
CHR: Kymberli Moris, Manager Human Resources
Web address: www.pssurgery.com
Control: Partnership, Investor–owned, for–profit **Service:** General Medical and Surgical

Staffed Beds: 22 **Admissions:** 650 **Census:** 3 **Outpatient Visits:** 7236 **Births:** 0 **Total Expense ($000):** 21190 **Payroll Expense ($000):** 5304 **Personnel:** 140

★ **PREMIER REHABILITATION HOSPITAL (193082)**, 4310 South Grand Street, Zip 71202; tel. 318/812–1000, (Nonreporting) **A**10
Primary Contact: James A. Joubert, Jr., Chief Executive Officer
CFO: Scott Markstrom, Chief Financial Officer
CIO: Marilyn North, Coordinator Health Information Management
Control: Corporation, Investor–owned, for–profit **Service:** Rehabilitation

Staffed Beds: 32

★ **ST. FRANCIS MEDICAL CENTER (190125)**, 309 Jackson Street, Zip 71201–7407, Mailing Address: P.O. Box 1901, Zip 71210–1901; tel. 318/327–4000, (Includes ST. FRANCIS NORTH HOSPITAL, 3421 Medical Park Drive, Zip 71203–2399; tel. 318/388–1946; Sabrina H. Ramsey, Vice President and Administrator) **A**1 2 9 10 **F**2 3 8 11 12 13 15 17 18 19 20 22 24 25 26 27 28 30 31 33 35 36 38 41 43 46 47 49 50 53 55 57 62 64 67 68 69 70 72 73 74 75 76 77 79 80 82 83 84 85 86 87 88 93 94 95 96 97 99 100 101 102 103 104 105 107 108 109 110 111 116 117 118 119 120 121 124 133 134 135 136 137 **P**6 8 **S** Franciscan Missionaries of Our Lady Health System, Inc.
Primary Contact: Sister Kathleen Cain, Interim President and Chief Executive Officer
CFO: Ronald E. Hogan, Senior Vice President and Chief Financial Officer
CMO: R. Louis Gavioli, M.D., Vice President Medical Affairs
CIO: Thomas H. Hammond, Chief Information Officer
CHR: James Novak, Vice President Human Resources
Web address: www.stfran.com
Control: Church–operated, Nongovernment, not–for profit **Service:** General Medical and Surgical

Staffed Beds: 415 **Admissions:** 19944 **Census:** 285 **Outpatient Visits:** 175949 **Births:** 1828 **Total Expense ($000):** 238529 **Payroll Expense ($000):** 81240 **Personnel:** 2078

Hospital, Medicare Provider Number, Address, Telephone, Approval, Facility, and Physician Codes, Health Care System

★ American Hospital Association (AHA) membership
☐ The Joint Commission accreditation
○ American Osteopathic Association (AOA) accreditation
△ Commission on Accreditation of Rehabilitation Facilities (CARF) accreditation

LA

☒ **ST. FRANCIS SPECIALTY HOSPITAL (192016)**, 309 Jackson Street, Zip 71210, Mailing Address: P.O. Box 1532, Zip 71210–1532; tel. 318/327–4000 **A**1 10 **F**1 3 25 26 27 32 80 96 119 137 **P**8
Primary Contact: George W. Hightower, FACHE, President and Chief Executive Officer
Web address: www.specialtyhospital.com
Control: Church–operated, Nongovernment, not–for profit **Service:** General Medical and Surgical

Staffed Beds: 32 **Admissions:** 368 **Census:** 27 **Outpatient Visits:** 0 **Births:** 0 **Total Expense ($000):** 13882 **Payroll Expense ($000):** 4648 **Personnel:** 93

★ **ST. PATRICK'S PSYCHIATRIC HOSPITAL (194060)**, 3421 Medical Park Drive, Zip 71203–2355; tel. 318/327–4686 **A**10 **F**32 88 93 94 **S** Franciscan Missionaries of Our Lady Health System, Inc.
Primary Contact: Cindy J. Rogers, FACHE, Chief Executive Officer
CFO: Lisa Bradley, Controller
CMO: Alfredo Torres, M.D., Chief of Staff
Web address: www.stpatrickshospital.net
Control: Church–operated, Nongovernment, not–for profit **Service:** Psychiatric

Staffed Beds: 24 **Admissions:** 551 **Census:** 14 **Outpatient Visits:** 14070 **Births:** 0 **Total Expense ($000):** 4376 **Payroll Expense ($000):** 1803 **Personnel:** 57

MORGAN CITY—St. Mary Parish

☒ **TECHE REGIONAL MEDICAL CENTER (190014)**, 1125 Marguerite Street, Zip 70380–1855, Mailing Address: P.O. Box 2308, Zip 70381–2308; tel. 985/384–2200, (Total facility includes 10 beds in nursing home–type unit) (Nonreporting) **A**1 9 10 20 **S** LifePoint Hospitals, Inc.
Primary Contact: Scott M. Smith, Chief Executive Officer
CFO: Michael Mayeux, Chief Financial Officer
CMO: Natalie Dishman, M.D., Chief of Staff
CIO: Cheryl Lipari, Manager Information Systems
CHR: Timothy Hebert, Director Human Resources
Web address: www.techeregional.com
Control: Hospital district or authority, Government, nonfederal **Service:** General Medical and Surgical

Staffed Beds: 127

NAPOLEONVILLE—Assumption Parish

★ **ASSUMPTION COMMUNITY HOSPITAL (191303)**, 135 Highway 402, Zip 70390; tel. 985/369–3600 **A**9 10 18 **F**15 28 38 55 62 63 124 **S** Franciscan Missionaries of Our Lady Health System, Inc.
Primary Contact: Wayne M. Arboneaux, Chief Executive Officer
CHR: Letonia Pierre, Coordinator Human Resources
Web address: www.ololrmc.com
Control: Other not–for–profit (including NFP Corporation) **Service:** General Medical and Surgical

Staffed Beds: 6 **Admissions:** 138 **Census:** 1 **Outpatient Visits:** 23706 **Births:** 0 **Total Expense ($000):** 4955 **Payroll Expense ($000):** 1927 **Personnel:** 41

NATCHITOCHES—Natchitoches Parish

LOUISIANA EXTENDED CARE HOSPITAL OF NATCHITOCHES (192035), 501 Keyser Avenue, Zip 71457; tel. 318/354–2044, (Nonreporting) **A**10
Primary Contact: Kermit Simmons, Administrator
Web address: www.lhcgroup.com
Control: Partnership, Investor–owned, for–profit **Service:** General Medical and Surgical

Staffed Beds: 21

☒ **NATCHITOCHES REGIONAL MEDICAL CENTER (190007)**, 501 Keyser Avenue, Zip 71457–6036, Mailing Address: P.O. Box 2009, Zip 71457–2009; tel. 318/214–4200, (Total facility includes 112 beds in nursing home–type unit) **A**1 9 10 20 **F**1 3 7 11 13 15 25 30 31 33 38 39 55 56 57 65 73 74 75 77 79 80 82 84 86 88 93 94 96 99 102 107 117 119 121 122 124 **P**5 **S** CHRISTUS Health
Primary Contact: Mark E. Marley, CHE, Chief Executive Officer
CFO: Gerard Hebert, Chief Financial Officer
CIO: Major Steve Crowder, Information Technology Manager
CHR: Tammy Broadway, Director Human Resources
Web address: www.natchitocheshospital.org
Control: Hospital district or authority, Government, nonfederal **Service:** General Medical and Surgical

Staffed Beds: 211 **Admissions:** 4171 **Census:** 141 **Outpatient Visits:** 51184 **Births:** 640 **Total Expense ($000):** 43606 **Payroll Expense ($000):** 17503 **Personnel:** 409

NEW IBERIA—Iberia Parish

☒ **DAUTERIVE HOSPITAL (190003)**, 600 North Lewis Street, Zip 70563; tel. 337/365–7311 **A**1 9 10 **F**13 15 17 24 25 32 38 54 68 74 79 81 82 84 85 86 88 93 96 100 107 119 121 135 **S** HCA
Primary Contact: Alan J. Fabian, Chief Executive Officer
CFO: Stephanie Boudreaux, Chief Financial Officer
CMO: Mike Alvarez, M.D., Chief Medical Officer
CIO: Terry Stewart, Director Information Systems
CHR: Michele Broussard, Director Human Resources
Web address: www.dauterivehospital.com
Control: Corporation, Investor–owned, for–profit **Service:** General Medical and Surgical

Staffed Beds: 103 **Admissions:** 3878 **Census:** 51 **Outpatient Visits:** 24849 **Births:** 522 **Total Expense ($000):** 53924 **Payroll Expense ($000):** 15320 **Personnel:** 299

☐ **IBERIA MEDICAL CENTER (190054)**, 2315 East Main Street, Zip 70560–4031, Mailing Address: P.O. Box 13338, Zip 70562–3338; tel. 337/364–0441 **A**1 9 10 **F**3 11 13 15 18 20 24 25 26 27 28 30 31 32 37 38 46 47 48 49 56 57 61 62 63 66 68 70 72 73 74 76 77 79 80 81 82 84 86 87 96 97 103 107 119 133 135 137 **S** Brim Healthcare, Inc.
Primary Contact: John A. Tucker, Chief Executive Officer
COO: Shane P. Myers, R.N., Chief Operating Officer
CFO: Wally Piekarczyk, Chief Financial Officer
CIO: Ross Leleux, Chief Information Officer
CHR: Lori Zachry, Director Human Resources
Web address: www.iberiamedicalcenter.com
Control: Hospital district or authority, Government, nonfederal **Service:** General Medical and Surgical

Staffed Beds: 83 **Admissions:** 5020 **Census:** 48 **Outpatient Visits:** 78254 **Births:** 572 **Total Expense ($000):** 48200 **Payroll Expense ($000):** 19552 **Personnel:** 512

NEW ORLEANS—Orleans Parish

☐ **CHILDREN'S HOSPITAL (193300)**, 200 Henry Clay Avenue, Zip 70118–5799; tel. 504/899–9511 **A**1 2 3 5 9 10 **F**3 8 9 11 16 17 19 21 23 25 26 27 28 32 33 34 37 38 40 43 44 50 53 55 56 57 59 60 62 63 64 69 70 72 73 76 77 78 79 80 81 82 83 84 85 86 87 88 89 90 94 95 96 97 100 103 107 114 118 119 120 121 125 127 128 130 133 135 137 **P**4 8
Primary Contact: Steve Worley, President and Chief Executive Officer
CFO: Greg Feirn, Senior Vice President and Chief Financial Officer
CMO: Alan M. Robson, M.D., Senior Vice President and Medical Director
CIO: Tammy Reites, Assistant Vice President Patient Financial Services
CHR: Doug Mittelstaedt, Vice President Human Resources
Web address: www.chnola.org
Control: Other not–for–profit (including NFP Corporation) **Service:** Children's general

Staffed Beds: 175 **Admissions:** 7225 **Census:** 131 **Outpatient Visits:** 368488 **Births:** 0 **Personnel:** 1460

COMMUNITY CARE HOSPITAL (194056), 1421 General Taylor Street, Zip 70115; tel. 504/899–2500, (Nonreporting) **A**10
Primary Contact: Paul B. Kavanaugh, President and Chief Executive Officer
Web address: www.communitycarehospital.com
Control: State–Government, nonfederal **Service:** Psychiatric

Staffed Beds: 36

☐ **KINDRED HOSPITAL – NEW ORLEANS (192009)**, 3601 Coliseum Street, Zip 70115–3606; tel. 504/899–1555 **A**1 10 **F**1 3 25 26 33 50 54 59 66 68 72 73 75 76 77 82 107 119 124 137 **S** Kindred Healthcare
Primary Contact: Jan Turk, Chief Executive Officer
CFO: Mary Kay Nations, Chief Financial Officer
CMO: Juzar Ali, M.D., Chief of Staff
Web address: www.kindredhealthcare.com
Control: Corporation, Investor–owned, for–profit **Service:** Long–Term Acute Care hospital

Staffed Beds: 55 **Admissions:** 461 **Census:** 42 **Outpatient Visits:** 0 **Births:** 0

☒ **MEDICAL CENTER OF LOUISIANA AT NEW ORLEANS (190005)**, 2021 Perdido Street, Zip 70112–1396; tel. 504/903–3000 **A**1 2 3 5 8 9 10 **F**3 4 8 11 13 15 18 22 25 26 27 31 32 37 38 44 49 50 56 57 58 59 60 62 63 64 66 68 71 72 73 74 75 76 77 79 80 81 82 86 87 96 97 99 100 103 106 107 114 119 121 124 135 **P**1 **S** LSU Health Sciences Center
Primary Contact: Dwayne Thomas, M.D., Administrator
COO: Adler Voltaire, Chief Administrative Officer
CFO: Ed Burke, Chief Financial Officer
CMO: Cathi E. Fontenot, M.D., Medical Director
CIO: Mitch Perlin, Chief Information Officer
CHR: Ronald Broadus, Assistant Administrator Human Resources
Web address: www.mclno.org
Control: State–Government, nonfederal **Service:** General Medical and Surgical

Staffed Beds: 145 **Admissions:** 4808 **Census:** 77 **Outpatient Visits:** 99065 **Births:** 266 **Total Expense ($000):** 233771 **Payroll Expense ($000):** 68441 **Personnel:** 1963

☐ **NEW ORLEANS ADOLESCENT HOSPITAL (194012)**, 210 State Street, Zip 70118–5797; tel. 504/897–3400, (Nonreporting) **A**1 3 5 10 **S** Louisiana State Hospitals
Primary Contact: Shelby Price, Chief Executive Officer
CFO: Ken Portel, Fiscal Director
CMO: Martin Drell, M.D., Clinical Director
CIO: Anita M. Sanders, Chief Information Technology Director
Control: State–Government, nonfederal **Service:** Children's hospital psychiatric

Staffed Beds: 30

★☐ **OCHSNER BAPTIST MEDICAL CENTER (190135)**, (Nonreporting) **A**1 9 10 **S** Ochsner Health System
Primary Contact: Robert Wolterman, Chief Executive Officer
COO: Brad Goodson, Vice President Operations
CFO: Christy Migaud, Controller
CMO: Allen Brown, M.D., Vice President Medical Affairs
CHR: Cindy Mousa, Human Resources Generalist
Web address: www.ochsner.org
Control: Other not–for–profit (including NFP Corporation) **Service:** General Medical and Surgical

Staffed Beds: 10

★☐ △ **OCHSNER MEDICAL CENTER (190036)**, (Formerly Ochsner Clinic Foundation), 1514 Jefferson Highway, Zip 70121–2484; tel. 504/842–3000, (Total facility includes 18 beds in nursing home–type unit) **A**1 2 3 5 7 8 9 10 **F**3 5 8 9 11 12 13 14 15 17 18 19 20 21 22 23 24 25 26 27 28 30 32 33 35 36 38 39 40 41 43 44 45 46 47 48 49 50 51 52 53 54 55 56 57 58 59 60 61 62 63 64 66 68 70 72 73 74 75 76 77 79 80 81 82 83 84 85 86 87 88 89 90 91 92 93 94 95 96 97 100 102 103 104 105 107 108 109 111 112 113 114 116 117 118 119 120 121 123 124 126 127 128 130 131 132 134 135 136 137 **P**6 **S** Ochsner Health System
Primary Contact: Patrick J. Quinlan, M.D., Chief Executive Officer
COO: Warner L. Thomas, President and Chief Operating Officer
CFO: Scott J. Posecai, Executive Vice President and Chief Financial Officer
CMO: Patrick J. Quinlan, M.D., Chief Executive Officer
CIO: Lynn Witherspoon, Vice President and Chief Information Officer
CHR: Joan Mollohan, Vice President Human Resources
Web address: www.ochsner.org
Control: Other not–for–profit (including NFP Corporation) **Service:** General Medical and Surgical

Staffed Beds: 390 **Admissions:** 24636 **Census:** 347 **Outpatient Visits:** 1888722 **Births:** 1779 **Total Expense ($000):** 450459 **Payroll Expense ($000):** 146962 **Personnel:** 3597

RIVER OAKS CHILD AND ADOLESCENT HOSPITAL (194042), 1525 River Oaks Road West, Zip 70123; tel. 504/734–1740, (Nonreporting) **A**10
Primary Contact: Evelyn Nolting, Chief Executive Officer
Web address: www.riveroakshospital.com
Control: Corporation, Investor–owned, for–profit **Service:** Psychiatric

Staffed Beds: 26

☐ **RIVER OAKS HOSPITAL (194031)**, 1525 River Oaks Road West, Zip 70123–2199; tel. 504/734–1740, (Nonreporting) **A**1 10 **S** Universal Health Services, Inc.
Primary Contact: Evelyn Nolting, Chief Executive Officer and Managing Director
COO: Mary Matamores, Chief Operating Officer
CMO: Lincoln Paine, M.D., Medical Director
Web address: www.riveroakshospital.com
Control: Corporation, Investor–owned, for–profit **Service:** Psychiatric

Staffed Beds: 121

★☐ △ **TOURO INFIRMARY (190046)**, 1401 Foucher Street, Zip 70115–3593; tel. 504/897–7011, (Total facility includes 120 beds in nursing home–type unit) **A**1 2 3 5 7 8 9 10 **F**3 8 10 11 13 15 17 18 20 22 24 25 26 27 33 34 35 37 38 40 41 42 43 44 45 50 52 53 55 56 57 59 60 61 62 66 68 70 71 72 73 74 75 76 77 79 80 81 82 85 86 87 96 97 98 99 100 102 103 106 107 109 111 114 115 117 119 120 121 124 132 135 136 137 **P**8
Primary Contact: Michael J. Sniffen, Interim President and Chief Executive Officer
COO: Susan Pitoscia, Chief Operating Officer
CFO: Robert A. Ficken, Vice President Finance
CMO: Kevin Jordan, M.D., Vice President Medical Affairs
CIO: Jeff Lott, Director Information Services
CHR: Joan Williams, Vice President Human Resources
Web address: www.touro.com
Control: Other not–for–profit (including NFP Corporation) **Service:** General Medical and Surgical

Staffed Beds: 395 **Admissions:** 14209 **Census:** 223 **Outpatient Visits:** 197314 **Births:** 2291 **Total Expense ($000):** 244541 **Payroll Expense ($000):** 102478 **Personnel:** 1524

TOURO REHABILITATION CENTER (193034), 1401 Foucher Street, Zip 70115; tel. 504/897–8560, (Nonreporting) **A**10
Primary Contact: Michael J. Sniffen, Interim President and Chief Executive Officer
COO: Susan Pitoscia, Chief Operating Officer
CFO: Robert A. Ficken, Vice President Finance
CMO: Kevin Jordan, M.D., Vice President Medical Affairs
CIO: Jeff Lott, Director Information Services
CHR: Chad Courrege, Vice President Human Resources
Web address: www.touro.com
Control: Corporation, Investor–owned, for–profit **Service:** Rehabilitation

Staffed Beds: 63

★☐ **TULANE UNIVERSITY HOSPITAL AND CLINIC (190176)**, 1415 Tulane Avenue, Zip 70112–2605; tel. 504/988–5263 **A**1 2 3 5 8 9 **F**3 13 15 17 18 20 22 25 26 27 31 32 33 38 39 50 56 57 58 59 66 68 70 72 73 74 76 77 78 79 80 83 84 85 86 87 88 90 92 94 96 97 100 101 102 103 104 105 107 109 116 118 119 120 121 124 125 126 127 128 129 130 131 133 135 136 137 **S** HCA
Primary Contact: Robert Lynch, M.D., Chief Executive Officer
COO: Andre duPlessis, Chief Operating Officer
CFO: Robert Hatcher, Chief Financial Officer
CMO: John Pigott, M.D., Chief Medical Officer
CIO: Sue Rachuig, Director Information Services
CHR: Larry Balyeat, Vice President Human Resources
Web address: www.tuhc.com
Control: Corporation, Investor–owned, for–profit **Service:** General Medical and Surgical

Staffed Beds: 331 **Admissions:** 11303 **Census:** 162 **Outpatient Visits:** 201321 **Births:** 2424 **Total Expense ($000):** 324940 **Payroll Expense ($000):** 112150 **Personnel:** 1591

NEW ROADS—Pointe Coupee Parish

★ **POINTE COUPEE GENERAL HOSPITAL (191316)**, 2202 False River Drive, Zip 70760–2698; tel. 225/638–6331 **A**9 10 18 **F**11 25 31 38 55 56 73 75 79 96 99 100 107 119 122 137
Primary Contact: Chad E. Olinde, Administrator and Chief Executive Officer
CFO: John Cazayoux, Chief Financial Officer
CMO: Paul Rachal, M.D., Chief of Staff
CHR: Lisa Patterson, Director Human Resources
Web address: www.pcgh.org
Control: Hospital district or authority, Government, nonfederal **Service:** General Medical and Surgical

Staffed Beds: 25 **Admissions:** 1146 **Census:** 8 **Outpatient Visits:** 36584 **Births:** 0 **Total Expense ($000):** 10252 **Payroll Expense ($000):** 5331 **Personnel:** 159

OAK GROVE—West Carroll Parish

WEST CARROLL MEMORIAL HOSPITAL (190081), 706 Ross Street, Zip 71263; tel. 318/428–3237, (Nonreporting) **A**9 10
Primary Contact: R. Randall Morris, Administrator
Control: Other not–for–profit (including NFP Corporation) **Service:** General Medical and Surgical

Staffed Beds: 21

OAKDALE—Allen Parish

★☐ **OAKDALE COMMUNITY HOSPITAL (190106)**, 130 North Hospital Drive, Zip 71463, Mailing Address: P.O. Box 629, Zip 71463–0629; tel. 318/335–3700, (Nonreporting) **A**1 9 10 **S** HCA
Primary Contact: John W. Stigall, Chief Executive Officer
CFO: Michael Fontenot, Interim Chief Financial Officer
CMO: Tommy Davis, M.D., Chief of Staff
CIO: Melissa Welch, Health Information Management Director
CHR: Dana Blood, Director Human Resources
Web address: www.oakdalecommunityhospital.com
Control: Partnership, Investor–owned, for–profit **Service:** General Medical and Surgical

Staffed Beds: 59

Hospital, Medicare Provider Number, Address, Telephone, Approval, Facility, and Physician Codes, Health Care System

★ American Hospital Association (AHA) membership
☐ The Joint Commission accreditation
○ American Osteopathic Association (AOA) accreditation
△ Commission on Accreditation of Rehabilitation Facilities (CARF) accreditation

OLLA—La Salle Parish

HARDTNER MEDICAL CENTER (191315), 1102 North Pine Road, Zip 71465; tel. 318/495–3131 **A**9 10 18 **F**7 25 26 31 32 38 54 55 57 62 66 75 79 82 85 86 88 93 94 96 107 117 119 122
Primary Contact: Paul G. Mathews, CPA, Administrator
CIO: Destini Bubrig, Health Information Management Director
Web address: www.hardtnermedical.com
Control: Hospital district or authority, Government, nonfederal **Service:** General Medical and Surgical

Staffed Beds: 35 **Admissions:** 569 **Census:** 10 **Outpatient Visits:** 10006 **Births:** 0 **Total Expense ($000):** 5224 **Payroll Expense ($000):** 3800 **Personnel:** 110

OPELOUSAS—St. Landry Parish

★ **DOCTOR'S HOSPITAL OF OPELOUSAS (190191)**, 3983 I–49 South Service Road, Zip 70570–8975; tel. 337/948–2100, (Nonreporting) **A**1 9 10 **S** LifePoint Hospitals, Inc.
Primary Contact: Phillip Young, FACHE, Chief Executive Officer
CFO: Stephen Downs, Chief Financial Officer
CIO: Jamie D. Miller, Chief Information Officer
Web address: www.doctorshospital.com
Control: Corporation, Investor–owned, for–profit **Service:** General Medical and Surgical

Staffed Beds: 171

★ **OPELOUSAS GENERAL HEALTH SYSTEM (190017)**, 539 East Prudhomme Street, Zip 70570, Mailing Address: P.O. Box 1389, Zip 70571–1389; tel. 337/948–3011 **A**1 2 9 10 19 **F**12 13 15 22 25 26 27 31 32 33 36 38 55 60 68 72 73 74 75 76 77 79 81 82 84 86 96 97 100 104 106 107 108 118 119 135 136 137 **S** QHR
Primary Contact: Gerald A. Fornoff, Chief Executive Officer
CFO: Brian T. Kirk, Vice President Financial Services
CMO: Derek Metoyer, M.D., Chief of Staff
CIO: Jared Lormand, Vice President Information Technology
CHR: Suzanne Kidder, Director Human Resources
Web address: www.opelousasgeneral.com
Control: Hospital district or authority, Government, nonfederal **Service:** General Medical and Surgical

Staffed Beds: 163 **Admissions:** 8276 **Census:** 97 **Outpatient Visits:** 87276 **Births:** 1039 **Total Expense ($000):** 85803 **Payroll Expense ($000):** 33810 **Personnel:** 736

ST. LANDRY EXTENDED CARE HOSPITAL (192034), 539 East Prudhomme Lane, Zip 70570; tel. 337/948–5184, (Nonreporting) **A**10
Primary Contact: Biff David, Administrator
Web address: www.lhcgroup.com
Control: Corporation, Investor–owned, for–profit **Service:** Long–Term Acute Care hospital

Staffed Beds: 23

PINEVILLE—Rapides Parish

☐ **CENTRAL LOUISIANA STATE HOSPITAL (194025)**, 242 West Shamrock Avenue, Zip 71361–5031, Mailing Address: P.O. Box 5031, Zip 71360–5031; tel. 318/484–6200 **A**1 10 **F**26 37 57 66 73 88 89 119 132 **S** Louisiana State Hospitals
Primary Contact: Patrick Kelly, Chief Executive Officer
COO: Paul Benoit, Associate Administrator
CFO: Tina Darbonne, Chief Financial Officer
CMO: L. Lee Tynes, M.D., Ph.D., Medical Director
CIO: William Haynes, Director Information Technology
CHR: Tom Crout, MS, Director Human Resources
Web address: www.dhh.la.gov/omh/inpatient–serv/clsh.htm
Control: State–Government, nonfederal **Service:** Psychiatric

Staffed Beds: 132 **Admissions:** 78 **Census:** 122 **Outpatient Visits:** 0 **Births:** 0 **Total Expense ($000):** 27191 **Payroll Expense ($000):** 14026 **Personnel:** 352

★ **HUEY P. LONG MEDICAL CENTER (190009)**, 352 Hospital Boulevard, Zip 71360, Mailing Address: P.O. Box 5352, Zip 71361–5352; tel. 318/448–0811 **A**1 3 5 9 10 **F**3 8 11 13 15 25 26 27 28 30 31 32 33 36 37 38 40 44 46 50 53 55 57 60 62 68 71 73 74 75 76 79 80 81 82 84 86 87 88 92 96 102 107 119 121 124 **P**6 **S** LSU Health Sciences Center
Primary Contact: Gary L. Crockett, Administrator
CFO: Nita Chambers, Chief Financial Officer
CMO: David Barnard, M.D., Medical Director
CIO: Mickey Roberts, Director Information Systems
CHR: Marsha Crittle, Director Human Resources
Web address: www.lsuhsc.edu/hcsd/hpl
Control: State–Government, nonfederal **Service:** General Medical and Surgical

Staffed Beds: 60 **Admissions:** 2654 **Census:** 42 **Outpatient Visits:** 98487 **Births:** 186 **Total Expense ($000):** 57845 **Payroll Expense ($000):** 20168 **Personnel:** 584

★ **VETERANS AFFAIRS MEDICAL CENTER**, 2495 Shreveport Highway, 71 North, Zip 71360, Mailing Address: P.O. Box 69004, Alexandria, Zip 71306–9004; tel. 318/473–0010, (Total facility includes 154 beds in nursing home–type unit) (Nonreporting) **A**1 2 3 5 9 **S** Department of Veterans Affairs
Primary Contact: Barbara C. Watkins, Director
CFO: Denise Morton, Chief Financial Officer
CMO: Hollis Reed, M.D., Chief of Staff
CIO: Stefan Test, Chief Information Resource Management Service
CHR: Cindy Twilligear, Manager Human Resources
Web address: www.va.gov/sta/guide/home.asp
Control: Veterans Affairs, Government, federal **Service:** General Medical and Surgical

Staffed Beds: 292

PLAQUEMINE—Iberville Parish

☐ **RIVER WEST MEDICAL CENTER (190131)**, 59355 River West Drive, Zip 70764–0737, Mailing Address: P.O. Box 737, Zip 70764–0737; tel. 225/687–9222, (Nonreporting) **A**1 9 10 **S** Shiloh Health Services, Inc.
Primary Contact: James P. Jeansonne, Chief Executive Officer
CFO: Bryan Bogle, Chief Financial Officer
CMO: Michael Green, M.D., Chief of Staff
CHR: Shelly Stafford, Director Human Resources
Web address: www.riverwestmc.com
Control: Corporation, Investor–owned, for–profit **Service:** General Medical and Surgical

Staffed Beds: 75

RACELAND—Lafourche Parish

★ **OCHSNER ST. ANNE GENERAL HOSPITAL (191324)**, 4608 Highway 1, Zip 70394–2623; tel. 985/537–6841, (Nonreporting) **A**9 10 18 **S** Ochsner Health System
Primary Contact: Milton D. Bourgeois, Jr., Chief Executive Officer
CHR: Ann Ritchie, Director Human Resources
Web address: www.stannegeneral.com
Control: Hospital district or authority, Government, nonfederal **Service:** General Medical and Surgical

Staffed Beds: 35

RAYVILLE—Richland Parish

★ **RICHARDSON MEDICAL CENTER (190151)**, 254 Highway 3048 at Christian Drive, Zip 71269–0388, Mailing Address: P.O. Box 388, Zip 71269–0388; tel. 318/728–4181 **A**9 10 **F**30 31 32 38 40 52 53 55 56 57 61 63 64 68 75 79 96 99 100 102 103 107 119 122 124 135 136
Primary Contact: Kerry Dean Goff, Administrator
CFO: Richard Bayland, Chief Financial Officer
CMO: David Thompson, M.D., Chief of Staff
CHR: Rita Brown, Director Human Resources
Web address: www.richardsonmed.org
Control: Other not–for–profit (including NFP Corporation) **Service:** General Medical and Surgical

Staffed Beds: 38 **Admissions:** 1260 **Census:** 16 **Outpatient Visits:** 8158 **Births:** 0 **Total Expense ($000):** 11820 **Payroll Expense ($000):** 5815 **Personnel:** 240

ROSEPINE—Vernon Parish

☐ **TRI PARISH REHABILITATION HOSPITAL (193050)**, 8088 Hawks Road, Zip 70659; tel. 337/462–8880, (Nonreporting) **A**1 10
Primary Contact: Heath Hairgrove, Administrator
Web address: www.triparishrehab.com
Control: Corporation, Investor–owned, for–profit **Service:** Rehabilitation

Staffed Beds: 33

RUSTON—Lincoln Parish

GREEN CLINIC SURGICAL HOSPITAL (190257), 1118 Farmerville Street, Zip 71270; tel. 318/232–7700, (Nonreporting) **A**9 10
Primary Contact: James W. McClurg, Chief Executive Officer
Web address: www.green–clinic.com
Control: Corporation, Investor–owned, for–profit **Service:** Other specialty

Staffed Beds: 13

★ **HEALTHSOUTH SPECIALTY HOSPITAL OF NORTH LOUISIANA (192022)**, 1401 Ezell Street, Zip 71270–7221; tel. 318/251–3126, (Nonreporting) **A**1 10 **S** HEALTHSOUTH Corporation
Primary Contact: Mark J. Rice, Chief Executive Officer
Web address: www.healthsouth.com
Control: Corporation, Investor–owned, for–profit **Service:** Long–Term Acute Care hospital

Staffed Beds: 90

★ **NORTHERN LOUISIANA MEDICAL CENTER (190086)**, (Formerly Lincoln General Hospital), 401 East Vaughn Avenue, Zip 71270–5950, Mailing Address: P.O. Drawer 1368, Zip 71273–1368; tel. 318/254–2100, (Total facility includes 8 beds in nursing home–type unit) (Nonreporting) **A**1 9 10 19 **S** Community Health Systems, Inc.
Primary Contact: Doug Sills, Chief Executive Officer
COO: Tripp Smith, Assistant Chief Executive Officer
CFO: Frank Malek, Chief Financial Officer
CMO: Cynthia Jones, M.D., Chief of Staff
CIO: Robert Clowers, Director Information Services
CHR: Tonya Duggan, Director Human Resources
Web address: www.northernlouisianamedicalcenter.com
Control: Other not–for–profit (including NFP Corporation) **Service:** General Medical and Surgical

Staffed Beds: 99

SAINT FRANCISVILLE—West Feliciana Parish

★ **WEST FELICIANA PARISH HOSPITAL (191306)**, 5266 Commerce Street, Zip 70775–0368, Mailing Address: P.O. Box 368, Zip 70775–0368; tel. 225/635–3811 **A**1 9 10 18 **F**7 25 38 55 96 97 107 117 122 124 132 **P**5
Primary Contact: Mark Chustz, Administrator
CFO: Linda Harvey, Chief Financial Officer
CHR: Neta F. Leake, Administrative Assistant Human Resources
Web address: www.wfph.org
Control: Hospital district or authority, Government, nonfederal **Service:** General Medical and Surgical

Staffed Beds: 22 **Admissions:** 195 **Census:** 2 **Outpatient Visits:** 12948 **Births:** 0 **Total Expense ($000):** 8412 **Payroll Expense ($000):** 3312

SHREVEPORT—Caddo Parish

☐ **BRENTWOOD HOSPITAL (194020)**, 1006 Highland Avenue, Zip 71101–4103; tel. 318/618–7500, (Nonreporting) **A**1 9 10 **S** Psychiatric Solutions
Primary Contact: J. Paul Smith, Chief Executive Officer
COO: J. Paul Smith, Chief Executive Officer
CFO: Tom Mueller, Chief Financial Officer
Web address: www.psysolutions.com
Control: Corporation, Investor–owned, for–profit **Service:** Psychiatric

Staffed Beds: 160

★ **CHRISTUS SCHUMPERT HEALTH SYSTEM (190041)**, One St. Mary Place, Zip 71101–4399; tel. 318/681–4500, (Includes CHRISTUS SCHUMPERT BOSSIER, 2105 Airline Drive, Bossier City, Zip 71111–3190; tel. 318/848–8000; CHRISTUS SCHUMPERT HEALTH SYSTEM, tel. 318/681–4500; CHRISTUS SCHUMPERT HIGHLAND, 1453 East Bert Kouns Industrial Loop, Zip 71105–6050; tel. 318/681–5000) **A**1 2 3 5 9 10 **F**2 3 7 11 12 13 15 18 20 22 24 25 26 27 28 31 32 33 34 37 38 40 42 43 44 46 47 49 52 53 54 55 56 57 58 59 62 63 68 69 70 72 73 74 75 76 77 79 80 82 83 84 85 86 87 88 90 91 92 93 96 97 99 100 103 106 107 108 109 116 118 119 120 121 123 124 132 133 135 136 137 **P**6 **S** CHRISTUS Health
Primary Contact: Charles J. Paine, M.D., President and Chief Executive Officer
CMO: Judy Laviolette, M.D., Vice President Medical Affairs and Chief Medical Officer
CIO: Asha Thakur, Market Information Officer
Web address: www.christusschumpert.org
Control: Church–operated, Nongovernment, not–for profit **Service:** General Medical and Surgical

Staffed Beds: 488 **Admissions:** 17861 **Census:** 247 **Outpatient Visits:** 227368 **Births:** 891 **Total Expense ($000):** 265687 **Payroll Expense ($000):** 102130 **Personnel:** 1587

☐ **DOCTORS' HOSPITAL OF SHREVEPORT (190115)**, 1130 Louisiana Avenue, Zip 71101–3998, Mailing Address: P.O. Box 1526, Zip 71165–1526; tel. 318/227–1211, (Nonreporting) **A**1 9 10
Primary Contact: David J. Holly, Chief Executive Officer
Web address: www.dhshreveport.com
Control: Corporation, Investor–owned, for–profit **Service:** General Medical and Surgical

Staffed Beds: 108

★ **DUBUIS HOSPITAL OF SHREVEPORT (192025)**, One St. Mary Place, 6th Floor, Zip 71101; tel. 318/221–3802 **A**1 10 **F**1 3 25 26 **S** Dubuis Health System
Primary Contact: Berry Gilbert, Administrator
Web address: www.dubuis.org
Control: Church–operated, Nongovernment, not–for profit **Service:** Long–Term Acute Care hospital

Staffed Beds: 36 **Admissions:** 310 **Census:** 23 **Outpatient Visits:** 0 **Births:** 0 **Total Expense ($000):** 9015 **Payroll Expense ($000):** 2974 **Personnel:** 67

☐ **LIFECARE HOSPITALS OF SHREVEPORT (192011)**, 9320 Linwood Avenue, Zip 71106–7003; tel. 318/688–8504, (Nonreporting) **A**1 10 **S** LifeCare Management Services
Primary Contact: Keith Cox, CHE, Chief Executive Officer
CFO: Rick Stockton, Chief Financial Officer
Web address: www.lifecare–hospitals.com
Control: Corporation, Investor–owned, for–profit **Service:** Long–Term Acute Care hospital

Staffed Beds: 130

☐ **LSU MEDICAL CENTER–UNIVERSITY HOSPITAL (190098)**, 1501 Kings Highway, Zip 71130–4299, Mailing Address: P.O. Box 33932, Zip 71130–3932; tel. 318/675–5000 **A**1 2 3 5 9 10 **F**3 8 11 13 15 16 17 18 19 20 21 22 24 25 26 27 28 32 33 34 37 38 40 43 47 49 50 51 53 55 57 59 60 62 64 66 68 70 71 72 73 74 75 76 77 79 80 81 82 83 84 86 87 88 89 90 91 92 93 94 96 97 99 100 102 103 105 106 107 108 109 111 112 118 119 124 125 134 135 136 137 **P**1 4 5 8
Primary Contact: Joseph M. Miciotto, Administrator
COO: Bill Hankins, Associate Administrator
CFO: Harold White, Vice Chancellor
CMO: Roy Clay, M.D., Associate Director Medical Affairs and Clinical Director
CIO: Lee Bairnsfather, Assistant Dean Information Services
CHR: David Fuqua, Director Human Resources Management
Web address: www.lsumc.edu
Control: State–Government, nonfederal **Service:** General Medical and Surgical

Staffed Beds: 459 **Admissions:** 18752 **Census:** 381 **Outpatient Visits:** 458701 **Births:** 1685 **Total Expense ($000):** 320976 **Payroll Expense ($000):** 158599 **Personnel:** 3632

★ **OVERTON BROOKS VETERANS AFFAIRS MEDICAL CENTER**, 510 East Stoner Avenue, Zip 71101–4295; tel. 318/221–8411 **A**1 2 3 5 8 9 **F**5 7 18 20 26 27 30 31 32 33 34 36 37 38 43 44 50 52 53 54 56 57 58 59 60 61 62 63 64 66 68 72 73 75 76 77 79 80 81 82 86 87 88 90 91 92 93 94 95 96 97 100 107 118 119 121 124 132 133 134 135 136 137 **S** Department of Veterans Affairs
Primary Contact: George M. Moore, Jr., Director
CFO: Kim Lane, Chief Fiscal Service
CMO: Virginia Short, M.D., Chief of Staff
CIO: Janey Taylor, Chief Information and Technology
CHR: Michael L. Palmier, Chief Human Resources Management
Web address: www.va.gov/sta/guide/home.asp
Control: Veterans Affairs, Government, federal **Service:** General Medical and Surgical

Staffed Beds: 124 **Admissions:** 5669 **Census:** 97 **Outpatient Visits:** 362391 **Births:** 0 **Personnel:** 1295

☐ **PROMISE SPECIALTY HOSPITAL OF SHREVEPORT (192010)**, 1800 Irving Place, Zip 71101–4608; tel. 318/425–4096, (Nonreporting) **A**1 9 10 **S** Promise Healthcare
Primary Contact: Martin C. Milner, Chief Executive Officer
Web address: www.promise–shreveport.com
Control: Corporation, Investor–owned, for–profit **Service:** Long–Term Acute Care hospital

Staffed Beds: 146

☐ **SHRINERS HOSPITALS FOR CHILDREN, SHREVEPORT**, 3100 Samford Avenue, Zip 71103–4289; tel. 318/222–5704 **A**1 3 5 **F**50 56 57 62 66 77 79 86 107 119 135 **S** Shriners Hospitals for Children
Primary Contact: Garry K. Green, Administrator
CFO: Toni Goodin, Director Fiscal Services
CMO: Richard McCall, M.D., Chief of Staff
CIO: Kim Crockett, Director Management Information Systems
CHR: Fred Krieg, Director Human Resources
Web address: www.shriners.com
Control: Other not–for–profit (including NFP Corporation) **Service:** Children's orthopedic

Staffed Beds: 45 **Admissions:** 968 **Census:** 17 **Personnel:** 163

Hospital, Medicare Provider Number, Address, Telephone, Approval, Facility, and Physician Codes, Health Care System
★ American Hospital Association (AHA) membership
☐ The Joint Commission accreditation
○ American Osteopathic Association (AOA) accreditation
△ Commission on Accreditation of Rehabilitation Facilities (CARF) accreditation

★ △ **WILLIS–KNIGHTON MEDICAL CENTER (190111)**, 2600 Greenwood Road, Zip 71103–2600, Mailing Address: P.O. Box 32600, Zip 71130–2600; tel. 318/212–4600, (Includes WILLIS–KNIGHTON PIERREMONT HEALTH CENTER, 8001 Youree Drive, Zip 71115; tel. 318/212–3000; WILLIS–KNIGHTON SOUTH – THE CENTER FOR WOMEN'S HEALTH, 2510 Bert Kouns Industrial Loop, Zip 71118, Mailing Address: P.O. Box 32600, Zip 71130–2600; tel. 318/212–5000; Keri Elrod, Administrator), (Nonreporting) **A**1 3 5 7 9 10 **S** Willis–Knighton Health System
Primary Contact: Jaf Fielder, Vice President and Administrator
CFO: Robert Huie, Executive Vice President and Chief Financial Officer
CIO: Charles Laster, Director Information Management
CHR: Jaf Fielder, Director Human Resources
Web address: www.wkhs.com
Control: Other not–for–profit (including NFP Corporation) **Service:** General Medical and Surgical

Staffed Beds: 651

SLIDELL—St. Tammany Parish

DOCTORS HOSPITAL OF SLIDELL (190256), 989 Robert Boulevard, Zip 70458; tel. 985/690–8200, (Nonreporting) **A**10
Primary Contact: Jim Bergeron, Administrator
Control: Corporation, Investor–owned, for–profit **Service:** Other specialty

Staffed Beds: 10

★ **NORTHSHORE REGIONAL MEDICAL CENTER (190204)**, 100 Medical Center Drive, Zip 70461–8572; tel. 985/646–5025 **A**1 9 10 **F**3 11 13 15 17 18 20 22 24 25 27 31 32 33 38 43 46 49 51 54 55 56 57 59 62 68 70 72 73 74 75 76 77 79 80 81 82 83 84 85 86 92 96 97 99 100 102 107 112 118 119 121 135 136 137 **S** TENET Healthcare Corporation
Primary Contact: Alan Cason, Chief Executive Officer
COO: Alan Hodges, Chief Operating Officer
CFO: Tony Bonnecarre, Chief Financial Officer
Web address: www.northshoremedctr.com
Control: Corporation, Investor–owned, for–profit **Service:** General Medical and Surgical

Staffed Beds: 165 **Admissions:** 6450 **Census:** 86 **Outpatient Visits:** 53904 **Births:** 719 **Total Expense ($000):** 73547 **Payroll Expense ($000):** 32569 **Personnel:** 532

★ △ **SLIDELL MEMORIAL HOSPITAL (190040)**, 1001 Gause Boulevard, Zip 70458–2987; tel. 985/643–2200 **A**1 2 5 7 9 10 **F**3 8 11 13 15 17 18 19 20 21 22 23 24 25 27 28 30 32 33 38 43 46 49 53 54 55 56 57 62 68 70 72 73 74 76 77 79 80 81 82 84 85 86 87 96 97 98 99 100 102 103 104 106 107 108 109 111 112 118 119 121 133 134 135 136 137 **P**6
Primary Contact: Robert L. Hawley, Jr., FACHE, Chief Executive Officer
CFO: Bill Davis, Chief Financial Officer
CMO: William Williams, M.D., Chief Medical Officer
CIO: Sonya Christian, Chief Information Officer
Web address: www.slidellmemorial.org
Control: Hospital district or authority, Government, nonfederal **Service:** General Medical and Surgical

Staffed Beds: 191 **Admissions:** 8628 **Census:** 115 **Outpatient Visits:** 119098 **Births:** 882 **Total Expense ($000):** 110315 **Payroll Expense ($000):** 47833 **Personnel:** 857

☐ **SOUTHERN SURGICAL HOSPITAL (190270)**, 1700 Lindberg Drive, Zip 70458–8062; tel. 985/641–0600, (Nonreporting) **A**1 9 10
Primary Contact: Michael Pisciotta, Chief Executive Officer
CFO: Michael J. Maurin, Chief Financial Officer
CMO: J. Gosey, M.D., Medical Director
CIO: Buddy Graves, Chief Information Officer
CHR: Lorrie Alfred, Director Human Resources
Control: Corporation, Investor–owned, for–profit **Service:** Surgical

Staffed Beds: 36

SPRINGHILL—Webster Parish

☐ **SPRINGHILL MEDICAL CENTER (190088)**, 2001 Doctors Drive, Zip 71075–4526, Mailing Address: P.O. Box 920, Zip 71075–0920; tel. 318/539–1000, (Nonreporting) **A**1 9 10
Primary Contact: John W. Rainey, Chief Executive Officer
CFO: Tanika Nash, Chief Financial Officer
CMO: Robert Edwards, M.D., Chief Medical Staff
CIO: Brian Griffin, Director Information Services
CHR: Derek Melancon, Director Human Resources and Marketing
Web address: www.sprhill.net/smc
Control: Other not–for–profit (including NFP Corporation) **Service:** General Medical and Surgical

Staffed Beds: 60

STERLINGTON—Ouachita Parish

★ **STERLINGTON REHABILITATION HOSPITAL (193069)**, 111 Highway 2, Zip 71280, Mailing Address: P.O. Box 627, Zip 71280–0627; tel. 318/665–9950, (Nonreporting) **A**10
Primary Contact: Cathy Perot, Administrator
Web address: www.www.sterlingtonrehab.com
Control: Corporation, Investor–owned, for–profit **Service:** Rehabilitation

Staffed Beds: 19

SULPHUR—Calcasieu Parish

☐ **CORNERSTONE HOSPITAL OF SOUTHWEST LOUISIANA (192013)**, 703 Cypress Street, Zip 70663; tel. 337/527–1102, (Nonreporting) **A**1 10 **S** Cornerstone Healthcare Group
Primary Contact: W. Darrell Jean, Chief Executive Officer
CFO: Amy Bryant, Chief Financial Officer
Web address: www.cornerstonehealthcaregroup.com
Control: Partnership, Investor–owned, for–profit **Service:** Long–Term Acute Care hospital

Staffed Beds: 30

☐ **WEST CALCASIEU CAMERON HOSPITAL (190013)**, 701 Cypress Street, Zip 70663–5000, Mailing Address: P.O. Box 2509, Zip 70664–2509; tel. 337/527–4240, (Nonreporting) **A**1 9 10
Primary Contact: J. William Hankins, Chief Executive Officer
COO: Theresa Woods, MSN, FACHE, Chief Operating Officer
CFO: Tammy Broussard, Controller
CIO: Trey Rion, Director Information Systems
CHR: Christi Kingsley, Director Human Resources
Web address: www.wcch.com
Control: Hospital district or authority, Government, nonfederal **Service:** General Medical and Surgical

Staffed Beds: 74

TALLULAH—Madison Parish

MADISON PARISH HOSPITAL (191314), 900 Johnson Street, Zip 71282–4537, Mailing Address: P.O. Box 1559, Zip 71284–1559; tel. 318/574–2374, (Nonreporting) **A**9 10 18
Primary Contact: Wendell Alford, Administrator
CIO: Charles Whitaker, Director Information Technology
CHR: Chasity Whitaker, Administrative Assistant
Web address: www.madisonparishhospital.com
Control: Other not–for–profit (including NFP Corporation) **Service:** General Medical and Surgical

Staffed Beds: 25

THIBODAUX—Lafourche Parish

★ △ **THIBODAUX REGIONAL MEDICAL CENTER (190004)**, 602 North Acadia Road, Zip 70301–4847, Mailing Address: P.O. Box 1118, Zip 70302–1118; tel. 985/447–5500 **A**1 2 7 9 10 **F**3 8 11 12 13 15 18 20 22 24 25 26 27 30 31 32 38 46 49 55 56 57 61 62 68 71 72 73 74 75 76 77 79 80 81 82 85 86 94 95 96 97 99 100 102 103 104 105 107 108 109 111 112 116 118 119 120 121 124 135 136 137 **S** QHR
Primary Contact: Greg K. Stock, Chief Executive Officer
COO: Timothy Allen, Chief Operating Officer
CFO: Steve C. Gaubert, Chief Financial Officer
CMO: Judith Blaise, M.D., Chief Medical Staff
CIO: Terry Evans, Chief Information Officer
CHR: Eric Degravelle, Director Human Resources
Web address: www.thibodaux.com
Control: Hospital district or authority, Government, nonfederal **Service:** General Medical and Surgical

Staffed Beds: 144 **Admissions:** 7610 **Census:** 96 **Outpatient Visits:** 120331 **Births:** 695 **Total Expense ($000):** 90272 **Payroll Expense ($000):** 33808 **Personnel:** 687

VILLE PLATTE—Evangeline Parish

★ **VILLE PLATTE MEDICAL CENTER (190167)**, 800 East Main Street, Zip 70586–4618, Mailing Address: P.O. Box 349, Zip 70586–0349; tel. 337/363–5684 **A**1 9 10 **F**3 11 18 25 27 31 32 33 38 46 52 55 56 57 59 68 73 76 77 79 84 86 87 96 100 102 118 120 122 **S** LifePoint Hospitals, Inc.
Primary Contact: Brian L. Riddle, Sr., Chief Executive Officer
CFO: Lori Petrie, Chief Financial Officer
CMO: Eduardo Alvarez, M.D., Chief of Staff
CIO: Courtney Bieber, Director Information Systems
CHR: Sue Thomas, Director Human Resources
Web address: www.vpmc.com
Control: Corporation, Investor–owned, for–profit **Service:** General Medical and Surgical

Staffed Beds: 60 **Admissions:** 3073 **Census:** 40 **Outpatient Visits:** 37333 **Total Expense ($000):** 26025 **Payroll Expense ($000):** 8957 **Personnel:** 192

Many Facility Codes have changed. Please refer to the AHA Guide Code Chart.

VIVIAN—Caddo Parish

NORTH CADDO MEDICAL CENTER (191304), 1000 South Spruce Street, Zip 71082–3232, Mailing Address: P.O. Box 792, Zip 71082–0792; tel. 318/375–3235 **A**9 10 18 **F**7 13 25 38 52 57 63 74 79 82 84 94 96 100 107 122 135 **P**6
Primary Contact: David C. Jones, Administrator
CFO: Carol Reisz, Chief Financial Officer
CMO: John H. Haynes, M.D., Chief of Medical Staff
CIO: Allyson Allums, Medical Records Director
CHR: Lanell Audirsch, Administrative Assistant
Web address: www.northcaddomedicalcenter.com
Control: Hospital district or authority, Government, nonfederal **Service:** General Medical and Surgical

Staffed Beds: 25 **Admissions:** 1078 **Census:** 10 **Outpatient Visits:** 10422 **Births:** 81 **Total Expense ($000):** 7549 **Payroll Expense ($000):** 3608 **Personnel:** 120

WEST MONROE—Ouachita Parish

☐ **CORNERSTONE HOSPITAL–WEST MONROE (192031)**, 6198 Cypress Street, Zip 71291–9010; tel. 318/396–5600, (Nonreporting) **A**1 10 **S** Cornerstone Healthcare Group
Primary Contact: Chris Simpson, Chief Executive Officer
CFO: Amy Bryant, Chief Financial Officer
Web address: www.cornerstonehealthcaregroup.com
Control: Corporation, Investor–owned, for–profit **Service:** Long–Term Acute Care hospital

Staffed Beds: 40

☐ **GLENWOOD REGIONAL MEDICAL CENTER (190160)**, 503 McMillan Road, Zip 71291–5327, Mailing Address: P.O. Box 35805, Zip 71294–5805; tel. 318/329–4200, (Total facility includes 12 beds in nursing home–type unit) (Nonreporting) **A**1 2 9 10 **S** IASIS Healthcare
Primary Contact: Ronald J. Elder, Chief Executive Officer
CFO: Stephen Thames, Chief Financial Officer
CIO: Ronnie Maxwell, Director Information Systems
CHR: Jan Walker, Director Human Resources
Web address: www.grmc.com
Control: Other not–for–profit (including NFP Corporation) **Service:** General Medical and Surgical

Staffed Beds: 231

☐ **LOUISIANA EXTENDED CARE HOSPITAL WEST MONROE (192055)**, 593 McMillan Road, 3rd Floor, Zip 71291; tel. 318/329–4300 **A**1 10 **F**3 31 32 137 **P**5
Primary Contact: Theresa Marsala, RN, FACHE, Administrator
Control: Individual, Investor–owned, for–profit **Service:** Long–Term Acute Care hospital

Staffed Beds: 18 **Admissions:** 170 **Census:** 12 **Outpatient Visits:** 0 **Births:** 0 **Personnel:** 43

☐ **OUACHITA SURGICAL HOSPITAL (190261)**, 1275 Glenwood Drive, Zip 71291; tel. 318/322–1339, (Nonreporting) **A**1 9 10
Primary Contact: W. Benjamin Patterson, Administrator
Web address: www.ouachitasurgery.com
Control: Corporation, Investor–owned, for–profit **Service:** Other specialty

Staffed Beds: 10

WINNFIELD—Winn Parish

HEALTHSOUTH SPECIALTY HOSPITAL OF WINNFIELD See Specialty Hospital of Winnfield

★☐ **SPECIALTY HOSPITAL OF WINNFIELD (192052)**, (Formerly HEALTHSOUTH Specialty Hospital of Winnfield), 915 First Street, Zip 71483; tel. 318/648–0212, (Nonreporting) **A**1 10
Primary Contact: Kemp Wright, Chief Executive Officer
CFO: Charlie Jurek, Business Office Manager
CIO: Shamada Venzant, Manager Health Information
Web address: www.healthsouth.com
Control: Corporation, Investor–owned, for–profit **Service:** Long–Term Acute Care hospital

Staffed Beds: 20

★☐ **WINN PARISH MEDICAL CENTER (190090)**, 301 West Boundary Street, Zip 71483–3427, Mailing Address: P.O. Box 152, Zip 71483–0152; tel. 318/648–3000 **A**1 9 10 **F**8 15 17 25 30 38 55 68 75 79 80 82 86 96 100 107 117 122 137 **S** HCA
Primary Contact: H. J. Gaspard, Chief Executive Officer
CFO: Jennifer Tarver, Chief Financial Officer
CMO: Eric Dupree, M.D., Chief of Staff
CHR: Kimberly Ingles, Director Human Resources
Web address: www.winnparishmedical.com
Control: Partnership, Investor–owned, for–profit **Service:** General Medical and Surgical

Staffed Beds: 60 **Admissions:** 1577 **Census:** 15 **Outpatient Visits:** 24186 **Births:** 0 **Personnel:** 154

WOODLANDS BEHAVIORAL CENTER (194076), 1400 West Court Street, Zip 71483–1338, Mailing Address: P.O. Box 138, Zip 71483–1338; tel. 318/628–5445, (Nonreporting) **A**10
Primary Contact: Link Martin, Administrator
Control: Corporation, Investor–owned, for–profit **Service:** Psychiatric

Staffed Beds: 19

WINNSBORO—Franklin Parish

★ **FRANKLIN MEDICAL CENTER (190140)**, 2106 Loop Road, Zip 71295–3398, Mailing Address: P.O. Box 1300, Zip 71295–1300; tel. 318/435–9411, (Nonreporting) **A**9 10
Primary Contact: Robert A. Boullion, Chief Executive Officer
CFO: Robert A. Boullion, Chief Executive Officer
CMO: Jay Busby, M.D., President Medical Staff
CIO: Judy Ogden, Director Information Technology
Web address: www.fmc–cares.com
Control: Hospital district or authority, Government, nonfederal **Service:** General Medical and Surgical

Staffed Beds: 43

ZACHARY—East Baton Rouge Parish

★☐ **LANE REGIONAL MEDICAL CENTER (190020)**, 6300 Main Street, Zip 70791–9990; tel. 225/658–4000, (Total facility includes 38 beds in nursing home–type unit) **A**1 9 10 **F**3 11 12 13 15 20 25 33 37 38 46 54 55 56 57 61 62 65 68 71 73 74 75 77 79 80 82 84 85 86 96 97 99 102 107 117 118 119 135 137 **P**6
Primary Contact: Randall M. Olson, Chief Executive Officer
CFO: Michael Zimmerman, Chief Financial Officer
CMO: Brian E. Kozar, M.D., Chief Medical Staff
CHR: David Beck, Chief Administrative Officer and Director Human Resources
Web address: www.lanermc.org
Control: Hospital district or authority, Government, nonfederal **Service:** General Medical and Surgical

Staffed Beds: 162 **Admissions:** 4955 **Census:** 112 **Outpatient Visits:** 60706 **Births:** 300 **Total Expense ($000):** 40506 **Payroll Expense ($000):** 23191 **Personnel:** 515

Hospital, Medicare Provider Number, Address, Telephone, Approval, Facility, and Physician Codes, Health Care System
★ American Hospital Association (AHA) membership
☐ The Joint Commission accreditation
○ American Osteopathic Association (AOA) accreditation
△ Commission on Accreditation of Rehabilitation Facilities (CARF) accreditation

MAINE

ME

AUGUSTA—Kennebec County

MAINEGENERAL MEDICAL CENTER–AUGUSTA CAMPUS See MaineGeneral Medical Center–Waterville Campus, Waterville

☐ **RIVERVIEW PSYCHIATRIC CENTER (204007)**, 250 Arsenal Street, Zip 4330, Mailing Address: P.O. Box 724, Zip 04330–0724; tel. 207/287–7200 **A**1 10 **F**25 26 30 31 32 37 52 56 62 73 81 82 87 88 90 91 92 93 94 119 121 124 **P**6
Primary Contact: David S. Proffitt, Superintendent
COO: Jamie P. Morrill, Director Operations and Administrative Services
CFO: Leon Beaulieu, Financial Analyst
CMO: William Nelson, M.D., Medical Director
CIO: Ron Moores, Director Management Information System
CHR: Lucia Nadeau, Personnel Officer
Web address: www.state.me.us/dhhs/riverview/
Control: State–Government, nonfederal **Service:** Psychiatric

Staffed Beds: 92 **Admissions:** 291 **Census:** 87 **Outpatient Visits:** 0 **Births:** 0 **Total Expense ($000):** 32157 **Payroll Expense ($000):** 13000 **Personnel:** 342

BANGOR—Penobscot County

▣ **ACADIA HOSPITAL (204006)**, 268 Stillwater Avenue, Zip 04401–3945, Mailing Address: P.O. Box 422, Zip 04402–0422; tel. 207/973–6100 **A**1 10 **F**5 25 26 30 31 32 50 62 64 72 73 75 82 88 89 90 91 92 93 94 95 119 121 123 135 **P**6 **S** Eastern Maine Healthcare Systems
Primary Contact: Dorothy E. Hill, Chief Executive Officer
COO: Dorothy E. Hill, Chief Executive Officer
CFO: Marie Suitter, Chief Financial Officer
CMO: Paul W. Tisher, Vice President and Chief Medical Officer
CIO: Jeanne Paradis, Administrator Information Services
CHR: Sally Baughman, Vice President Human Resources
Web address: www.acadiahospital.org
Control: Other not–for–profit (including NFP Corporation) **Service:** Psychiatric

Staffed Beds: 93 **Admissions:** 2415 **Census:** 68 **Outpatient Visits:** 134505 **Births:** 0 **Total Expense ($000):** 39518 **Payroll Expense ($000):** 21781 **Personnel:** 459

☐ **DOROTHEA DIX PSYCHIATRIC CENTER (204004)**, 656 State Street, Zip 4401, Mailing Address: P.O. Box 926, Zip 04402–0926; tel. 207/941–4000 **A**1 10 **F**37 88 94 **P**6
Primary Contact: Mary Louise McEwen, Superintendent
COO: Chip Fussell, Chief Operating Officer
CFO: Steven Thebarge, Director Finance and Outpatient Services
CMO: Marjorie Snyder, M.D., Clinical Director
CIO: Larry Larson, Management Analyst
CHR: Ruth Mullaney, Personnel Officer
Web address: www.maine.gov/dhhs/ddpc
Control: State–Government, nonfederal **Service:** Psychiatric

Staffed Beds: 60 **Admissions:** 269 **Census:** 56 **Outpatient Visits:** 6749 **Births:** 0 **Total Expense ($000):** 26422 **Payroll Expense ($000):** 13529 **Personnel:** 329

▣ **EASTERN MAINE MEDICAL CENTER (200033)**, 489 State Street, Zip 04401–6674, Mailing Address: P.O. Box 404, Zip 04402–0404; tel. 207/973–7000, (Includes ROSS SKILLED NURSING FACILITY) **A**1 2 3 5 9 10 12 13 **F**3 11 12 13 15 17 18 20 22 24 25 26 27 30 31 32 34 35 37 38 40 41 43 44 46 47 48 49 50 51 52 53 55 56 57 58 59 60 62 68 70 72 73 74 75 76 77 79 80 81 82 83 84 85 86 87 92 96 97 99 100 102 103 104 105 106 107 108 109 111 114 116 118 119 120 121 124 133 134 135 136 137 **P**6 **S** Eastern Maine Healthcare Systems
Primary Contact: Deborah Carey Johnson, RN, President and Chief Executive Officer
CFO: Elmer Doucette, Vice President Fiscal Services
CMO: James Raczek, M.D., Vice President and Chief Medical Officer
CIO: Catherine Bruno, Chief Information Officer, Eastern Maine Healthcare System
CHR: Greg Howat, Vice President Human Resources and Education
Web address: www.emh.org
Control: Other not–for–profit (including NFP Corporation) **Service:** General Medical and Surgical

Staffed Beds: 349 **Admissions:** 19656 **Census:** 279 **Outpatient Visits:** 462949 **Births:** 1792 **Total Expense ($000):** 473287 **Payroll Expense ($000):** 190790 **Personnel:** 3108

▣ **ST. JOSEPH HOSPITAL (200001)**, 360 Broadway, Zip 04401–3897, Mailing Address: P.O. Box 403, Zip 04402–0403; tel. 207/262–1000 **A**1 9 10 **F**8 11 15 18 24 25 26 27 30 31 32 33 38 42 43 44 48 49 51 54 55 57 61 62 68 72 73 76 77 79 81 82 96 97 99 102 106 107 118 119 121 124 135 136 137
Primary Contact: Sister Mary Norberta Malinowski, President
COO: Wayne Woodford, Executive Vice President and Chief Operating Officer
CMO: Scott Stern, D.O., Chief of Staff
CHR: TinaMarie Bowlin–Norris, Assistant Vice President Human Resources
Web address: www.sjhhealth.com
Control: Church–operated, Nongovernment, not–for profit **Service:** General Medical and Surgical

Staffed Beds: 84 **Admissions:** 5335 **Census:** 48 **Outpatient Visits:** 112303 **Births:** 0 **Total Expense ($000):** 81650 **Payroll Expense ($000):** 32470 **Personnel:** 668

BAR HARBOR—Hancock County

★ **MOUNT DESERT ISLAND HOSPITAL (201304)**, 10 Wayman Lane, Zip 04609–0008, Mailing Address: P.O. Box 8, Zip 04609–0008; tel. 207/288–5081 **A**9 10 18 **F**3 5 6 10 11 13 15 24 25 27 30 31 32 33 38 53 54 55 56 57 62 63 68 72 73 74 75 76 77 79 80 82 86 87 89 90 91 94 96 97 102 107 115 119 120 121 122 124 134 135 136 **P**6 7
Primary Contact: Arthur J. Blank, President and Chief Executive Officer
CFO: Wendy Fielding, Vice President Finance
CMO: Brian Caine, M.D., President Medical Staff
CIO: Mark White, Director Information Services
CHR: Chris Owen, Director
Web address: www.mdihospital.org
Control: Other not–for–profit (including NFP Corporation) **Service:** General Medical and Surgical

Staffed Beds: 25 **Admissions:** 1159 **Census:** 10 **Outpatient Visits:** 104100 **Births:** 75 **Total Expense ($000):** 39253 **Payroll Expense ($000):** 17703 **Personnel:** 322

BELFAST—Waldo County

WALDO COUNTY GENERAL HOSPITAL (201312), 118 Northport Avenue, Zip 04915–6072, Mailing Address: P.O. Box 287, Zip 04915–0287; tel. 207/338–2500 **A**9 10 18 **F**3 11 13 15 24 25 27 30 31 32 33 38 42 45 46 51 55 57 61 62 63 68 72 73 74 76 77 79 80 86 87 96 97 99 100 102 105 106 107 118 119 121 135
Primary Contact: Mark A. Biscone, Executive Director
COO: Gary Haslam, Director Support Services
CFO: Gordon Tibbetts, Chief Financial Officer
CIO: David Cox, Management Information Systems Director
Web address: www.wchi.com
Control: Other not–for–profit (including NFP Corporation) **Service:** General Medical and Surgical

Staffed Beds: 25 **Admissions:** 1680 **Census:** 15 **Outpatient Visits:** 69424 **Births:** 196 **Total Expense ($000):** 44474 **Payroll Expense ($000):** 21266 **Personnel:** 436

BIDDEFORD—York County

▣ **SOUTHERN MAINE MEDICAL CENTER (200019)**, One Medical Center Drive, Zip 04005–9496, Mailing Address: P.O. Box 626, Zip 04005–0626; tel. 207/283–7000 **A**1 2 9 10 **F**3 5 11 12 13 15 18 20 24 25 26 27 28 30 31 32 33 34 36 38 41 42 44 47 48 49 50 51 53 54 55 56 57 61 62 63 66 68 72 73 74 75 76 77 79 80 81 82 84 86 88 90 91 93 94 95 96 97 100 103 106 107 118 119 121 124 133 135 136 137 **P**5 8
Primary Contact: Edward J. McGeachey, President and Chief Executive Officer
CFO: Ernest G. Enck, Interim Chief Financial Officer
CMO: Frank Lavoie, M.D., Vice President Medical Affairs
CIO: Glenn Stivers, Director Information Systems
CHR: Lorraine Bouchard, Vice President Human Resources
Web address: www.smmc.org
Control: Other not–for–profit (including NFP Corporation) **Service:** General Medical and Surgical

Staffed Beds: 138 **Admissions:** 6000 **Census:** 71 **Outpatient Visits:** 221722 **Births:** 575 **Total Expense ($000):** 100516 **Payroll Expense ($000):** 48725 **Personnel:** 937

BLUE HILL—Hancock County

★ **BLUE HILL MEMORIAL HOSPITAL (201300)**, 57 Water Street, Zip 04614–0823, Mailing Address: P.O. Box 823, Zip 04614–0823; tel. 207/374–3400 **A**9 10 18 **F**10 13 25 26 27 29 30 31 32 33 38 41 44 45 50 53 54 55 57 62 63 66 73 74 75 76 77 79 80 81 84 86 87 90 92 94 96 102 107 115 119 121 122 135 136 **P**6 **S** Eastern Maine Healthcare Systems
Primary Contact: Timothy Garrity, FACHE, President and Chief Executive Officer
CFO: Jeff Provenzano, Chief Financial Officer
CMO: James Raczek, M.D., Chief Medical Officer
CHR: Judy Pendleton, Manager Human Resources
Web address: www.bhmh.org
Control: Other not–for–profit (including NFP Corporation) **Service:** General Medical and Surgical

Staffed Beds: 25 **Admissions:** 976 **Census:** 11 **Outpatient Visits:** 99950 **Births:** 151 **Total Expense ($000):** 27198 **Payroll Expense ($000):** 12876

BOOTHBAY HARBOR—Lincoln County

★ **ST. ANDREWS HOSPITAL AND HEALTHCARE CENTER (201302)**, 6 St. Andrews Lane, Zip 04538–1732, Mailing Address: P.O. Box 417, Zip 04538–0417; tel. 207/633–2121, (Total facility includes 53 beds in nursing home–type unit) **A**9 10 18 **F**2 3 5 6 10 11 15 24 25 26 27 30 33 37 38 43 44 45 50 54 56 57 61 63 65 67 73 75 76 77 79 80 86 87 94 96 102 107 115 117 119 120 121 122 124 135 137 **P**8
Primary Contact: James W. Donovan, President and Chief Executive Officer
CFO: Wayne Printy, Vice President
CMO: Aqui Alamo, M.D., President Medical Staff
CIO: Brooks Betts, Vice President Information Systems
CHR: Lisa Burger, Vice President Human Resources
Web address: www.standrewshealthcare.org
Control: Other not–for–profit (including NFP Corporation) **Service:** General Medical and Surgical

Staffed Beds: 72 **Admissions:** 585 **Census:** 58 **Outpatient Visits:** 42220 **Births:** 0 **Total Expense ($000):** 19508 **Payroll Expense ($000):** 9474 **Personnel:** 155

BRIDGTON—Cumberland County

★ **BRIDGTON HOSPITAL (201310)**, 10 Hospital Drive, Zip 4009; tel. 207/647–6000 **A**9 10 18 **F**3 11 13 15 25 26 27 30 32 33 38 52 53 55 57 68 73 74 76 77 79 80 81 86 87 96 97 107 119 120 121 122 124 135 136 137 **P**4
Primary Contact: John M. Carlson, President and Chief Executive Officer
CMO: Suzanne Dater, M.D., President Medical Staff
CHR: Thomas Reichard, Director Human Resources
Web address: www.bridgtonhospital.org
Control: Other not–for–profit (including NFP Corporation) **Service:** General Medical and Surgical

Staffed Beds: 22 **Admissions:** 1470 **Census:** 14 **Outpatient Visits:** 56975 **Births:** 166 **Total Expense ($000):** 28962 **Payroll Expense ($000):** 13285 **Personnel:** 225

BRUNSWICK—Cumberland County

★□ **MID COAST HOSPITAL (200021)**, 123 Medical Center Drive, Zip 4011; tel. 207/729–0181 **A**1 9 10 **F**3 5 11 13 15 18 24 25 26 30 31 32 33 34 38 43 44 46 47 48 49 51 52 53 55 56 57 58 60 62 68 72 73 74 75 76 77 79 80 81 82 86 87 88 93 95 96 99 100 103 106 107 118 119 121 123 124 135 136 137 **P**6
Primary Contact: Herbert Paris, President
COO: Philip A. Ortolani, Vice President Operations
CFO: Robert N. McCue, Vice President Finance
CMO: Scott Mills, M.D., Vice President Medical Staff Affairs
CIO: Gale Stoy, Manager Information Systems
CHR: George Hunter, Executive Vice President
Web address: www.midcoasthealth.com
Control: Other not–for–profit (including NFP Corporation) **Service:** General Medical and Surgical

Staffed Beds: 74 **Admissions:** 4904 **Census:** 53 **Outpatient Visits:** 162541 **Births:** 729 **Total Expense ($000):** 84555 **Payroll Expense ($000):** 36187 **Personnel:** 720

★ **PARKVIEW ADVENTIST MEDICAL CENTER (200025)**, 329 Maine Street, Zip 04011–3398; tel. 207/373–2000 **A**9 10 **F**11 13 15 25 26 27 30 31 32 33 34 35 36 38 50 54 56 57 60 62 63 64 66 68 73 74 75 76 77 79 80 81 82 84 85 86 87 96 97 99 100 102 104 105 107 118 119 121 124 134 135 136 **P**7 8 **S** QHR
Primary Contact: Theodore M. Lewis, President and Chief Executive Officer
CMO: Jeffrey Maher, M.D., President Medical Staff
CIO: Bill McQuaid, Assistant Vice President and Chief Information Officer
CHR: Robin White, Assistant Vice President Human Resources
Web address: www.parkviewamc.org
Control: Church–operated, Nongovernment, not–for profit **Service:** General Medical and Surgical

Staffed Beds: 55 **Admissions:** 1393 **Census:** 19 **Outpatient Visits:** 79387 **Births:** 95 **Total Expense ($000):** 41414 **Payroll Expense ($000):** 17130 **Personnel:** 331

CALAIS—Washington County

★ **CALAIS REGIONAL HOSPITAL (201305)**, 22 Hospital Lane, Zip 04619–1398; tel. 207/454–7521 **A**9 10 18 **F**3 11 13 15 24 25 27 28 30 31 32 33 38 43 44 45 46 47 50 55 56 57 61 62 63 66 73 74 75 76 77 79 80 81 82 84 85 86 87 96 100 102 106 107 113 119 121 122 124 135 136 **P**6 **S** QHR
Primary Contact: Ray H. Davis, Jr., Chief Executive Officer
CFO: P. Bernard McAdam, Chief Financial Officer
CMO: David Feiner, M.D., Chief of Staff
CIO: Dee Dee Travis, Director Community Relations
CHR: Kristi K. Saunders, Director and Compliance Officer
Web address: www.calaishospital.com
Control: Other not–for–profit (including NFP Corporation) **Service:** General Medical and Surgical

Staffed Beds: 25 **Admissions:** 991 **Census:** 10 **Outpatient Visits:** 32227 **Births:** 111 **Total Expense ($000):** 25978 **Payroll Expense ($000):** 10750 **Personnel:** 234

CARIBOU—Aroostook County

★□ **CARY MEDICAL CENTER (200031)**, 163 Van Buren Road, Suite 1, Zip 04736–2599; tel. 207/498–3111, (Total facility includes 9 beds in nursing home–type unit) **A**1 9 10 **F**3 8 11 13 15 24 25 27 28 30 31 32 33 34 36 38 40 41 43 44 51 52 53 54 55 56 57 60 62 65 66 68 73 74 75 76 77 79 80 81 82 84 85 86 87 96 97 100 103 106 107 109 113 119 120 121 124 133 135 136 137 **S** QHR
Primary Contact: Kris A. Doody, RN, Chief Executive Officer
COO: Shawn Anderson, Chief Operating Officer
CFO: Galen Dickinson, Chief Financial Officer
CMO: Carl Flynn, M.D., Chief of Staff
CIO: Dave Silsbee, Chief Information Officer
CHR: Paula Parent, Director Human Resources
Web address: www.carymedicalcenter.org
Control: City–Government, nonfederal **Service:** General Medical and Surgical

Staffed Beds: 49 **Admissions:** 1716 **Census:** 28 **Outpatient Visits:** 85589 **Births:** 181 **Total Expense ($000):** 41364 **Payroll Expense ($000):** 16720 **Personnel:** 421

DAMARISCOTTA—Lincoln County

★ **MILES MEMORIAL HOSPITAL (200002)**, 35 Miles Street, Zip 04543–9767; tel. 207/563–1234 **A**9 10 20 **F**3 11 13 15 25 26 28 30 31 32 33 38 40 42 50 55 56 57 61 62 63 68 73 74 77 79 80 81 82 86 87 96 97 99 107 118 119 121 122 123 124 135 136 137 **P**6
Primary Contact: Judy McGuire, Interim Chief Executive Officer
CFO: Wayne Printy, Vice President Finance
CMO: Dan Friedland, M.D., Chief of Staff
CIO: Brooks Betts, Vice President Information Technology
CHR: Lisa McIlwain, Vice President Human Resources
Web address: www.mileshealthcare.org
Control: Other not–for–profit (including NFP Corporation) **Service:** General Medical and Surgical

Staffed Beds: 38 **Admissions:** 1840 **Census:** 22 **Outpatient Visits:** 110411 **Births:** 203 **Total Expense ($000):** 48719 **Payroll Expense ($000):** 15463 **Personnel:** 323

ME

Hospital, Medicare Provider Number, Address, Telephone, Approval, Facility, and Physician Codes, Health Care System

★ American Hospital Association (AHA) membership
□ The Joint Commission accreditation
○ American Osteopathic Association (AOA) accreditation
△ Commission on Accreditation of Rehabilitation Facilities (CARF) accreditation

ME

DOVER–FOXCROFT—Piscataquis County

★ **MAYO REGIONAL HOSPITAL (201309)**, 897 West Main Street, Zip 04426–1099; tel. 207/564–8401 **A**9 10 18 **F**3 5 7 8 11 13 15 24 25 26 27 30 31 32 33 38 43 45 50 55 56 57 63 68 73 74 75 76 77 79 80 81 82 86 87 89 90 91 92 93 94 96 97 99 106 107 118 119 122 123 124 135 136 137 **P**7 8
Primary Contact: Ralph Gabarro, Chief Executive Officer
CFO: Dennis Allen, Chief Financial Officer
CMO: Kathleen Thibault, President Medical Staff
CHR: Ken Proctor, Director Human Resources
Web address: www.mayohospital.com
Control: Hospital district or authority, Government, nonfederal **Service:** General Medical and Surgical

Staffed Beds: 25 **Admissions:** 1249 **Census:** 11 **Outpatient Visits:** 106314 **Births:** 171 **Total Expense ($000):** 35263 **Payroll Expense ($000):** 18028 **Personnel:** 394

ELLSWORTH—Hancock County

⊞ **MAINE COAST MEMORIAL HOSPITAL (200050)**, 50 Union Street, Zip 04605–1599; tel. 207/664–5311 **A**1 9 10 **F**3 13 15 25 27 30 31 32 33 38 44 45 53 54 55 56 68 73 74 75 76 77 79 80 81 82 86 87 96 97 99 100 106 107 118 119 122 124 133 135 136
Primary Contact: Douglas T. Jones, Chief Executive Officer
CFO: Kevin Sedgwick, Chief Financial Officer
CMO: Sean Maloney, M.D., President Medical Staff
CIO: Julie Hagle, Director Information Systems
CHR: Lois Macias, Vice President Ancillary Services
Web address: www.mainehospital.org
Control: Other not–for–profit (including NFP Corporation) **Service:** General Medical and Surgical

Staffed Beds: 48 **Admissions:** 2420 **Census:** 23 **Outpatient Visits:** 212405 **Births:** 234 **Total Expense ($000):** 68088 **Payroll Expense ($000):** 32872 **Personnel:** 543

FARMINGTON—Franklin County

⊞ **FRANKLIN MEMORIAL HOSPITAL (200037)**, 111 Franklin Health Commons, Zip 04938–9990; tel. 207/778–6031 **A**1 9 10 20 **F**3 7 8 11 13 15 24 25 26 27 28 30 31 32 33 34 38 45 46 50 51 53 54 55 56 57 60 62 63 68 73 74 75 76 77 79 80 81 82 84 86 87 92 96 97 100 102 103 104 105 106 107 112 117 118 119 120 121 122 124 133 135 136 137 **P**6 8
Primary Contact: Richard A. Batt, President and Chief Executive Officer
COO: Gerald Cayer, Vice President and Chief Operating Officer
CFO: Eric Martinsen, Vice President Finance and Chief Financial Officer
CMO: David Dixon, M.D., Vice President Medical Affairs and Education
CIO: Ralph Johnson, Chief Information Officer
CHR: Tom Hagerstrom, Director Human Resources
Web address: www.fchn.org
Control: Other not–for–profit (including NFP Corporation) **Service:** General Medical and Surgical

Staffed Beds: 48 **Admissions:** 2737 **Census:** 29 **Outpatient Visits:** 131790 **Births:** 384 **Total Expense ($000):** 66906 **Payroll Expense ($000):** 30985 **Personnel:** 630

FORT FAIRFIELD—Aroostook County

COMMUNITY GENERAL HEALTH CENTER See Aroostook Medical Center, Presque Isle

FORT KENT—Aroostook County

⊞ **NORTHERN MAINE MEDICAL CENTER (200052)**, 194 East Main Street, Zip 04743–1497; tel. 207/834–3155, (Total facility includes 45 beds in nursing home–type unit) **A**1 9 10 20 **F**13 15 24 25 27 30 31 32 38 52 53 55 56 57 61 62 65 66 67 68 73 74 75 76 77 79 81 82 86 88 89 90 91 92 93 94 96 97 100 107 117 119 120 121 124 135 136 **P**6
Primary Contact: Martin B. Bernstein, Chief Executive Officer
COO: Peter Sirois, Associate Administrator
CFO: Roger Lagasse, Chief Financial Officer
CMO: Khalid Husain, Chief Medical Staff
CIO: Adam Landry, Coordinator Computer Systems
CHR: Robin Damboise, Director Human Resources
Web address: www.nmmc.org
Control: Other not–for–profit (including NFP Corporation) **Service:** General Medical and Surgical

Staffed Beds: 84 **Admissions:** 1958 **Census:** 68 **Outpatient Visits:** 52266 **Births:** 84 **Total Expense ($000):** 46042 **Payroll Expense ($000):** 24195 **Personnel:** 523

GREENVILLE—Piscataquis County

★ **CHARLES A. DEAN MEMORIAL HOSPITAL AND NURSING HOME (201301)**, 364 Pritham Avenue, Zip 04441–1395, Mailing Address: P.O. Box 1129, Zip 04441–1129; tel. 207/695–5200, (Total facility includes 24 beds in nursing home–type unit) **A**9 10 18 **F**7 11 15 24 25 26 31 33 38 42 52 56 57 62 63 75 77 79 82 86 87 96 102 107 117 119 122 **P**6 **S** Eastern Maine Healthcare Systems
Primary Contact: Geno Murray, President and Chief Executive Officer
CFO: Edward Olivier, Chief Financial Officer
CMO: Darin Peck, M.D., Chief of Staff
CHR: Nancy Pelletier, Director Human Resources
Web address: www.cadean.org
Control: Other not–for–profit (including NFP Corporation) **Service:** General Medical and Surgical

Staffed Beds: 36 **Admissions:** 430 **Census:** 4 **Births:** 0 **Personnel:** 101

HOULTON—Aroostook County

★ **HOULTON REGIONAL HOSPITAL (201308)**, 20 Hartford Street, Zip 04730–9998; tel. 207/532–9471, (Total facility includes 28 beds in nursing home–type unit) **A**9 10 18 **F**1 3 4 11 13 16 17 24 25 30 31 32 38 40 43 51 52 54 55 56 57 63 65 68 70 71 72 73 74 75 76 77 78 79 81 82 83 84 85 86 87 88 96 97 100 102 107 117 118 119 121 135 136 **P**8
Primary Contact: Thomas J. Moakler, Chief Executive Officer
CFO: Cindy Daigle, Chief Financial Officer
CHR: Vicky Moody, Director Human Resources
Web address: www.houlton.net/hrh
Control: Other not–for–profit (including NFP Corporation) **Service:** General Medical and Surgical

Staffed Beds: 53 **Admissions:** 1770 **Census:** 38 **Outpatient Visits:** 102722 **Births:** 203 **Total Expense ($000):** 36991 **Payroll Expense ($000):** 16485 **Personnel:** 373

LEWISTON—Androscoggin County

⊞ **CENTRAL MAINE MEDICAL CENTER (200024)**, 300 Main Street, Zip 04240–0305; tel. 207/795–0111 **A**1 2 3 5 6 9 10 12 13 **F**3 11 12 13 15 18 20 22 24 25 26 27 28 30 31 32 33 34 38 40 41 43 44 47 48 49 50 51 52 55 56 57 58 59 60 62 63 64 65 66 68 69 71 72 73 74 75 76 77 79 80 81 82 84 85 86 87 92 96 97 102 103 106 107 109 111 112 113 114 118 119 120 121 124 133 135 136 137 **P**5 6 8
Primary Contact: Peter E. Chalke, President and Chief Executive Officer
COO: Laird P. Covey, Chief Operating Officer
CFO: Charles T. Orne, Executive Vice President Finance and Chief Financial Officer
CMO: Larry Hopperstead, M.D., Chief Medical Officer
CIO: Cindy Asbury, Interim Chief Information Officer
CHR: Joyce McPhetres, Vice President Human Resources
Web address: www.cmmc.org
Control: Other not–for–profit (including NFP Corporation) **Service:** General Medical and Surgical

Staffed Beds: 190 **Admissions:** 8867 **Census:** 120 **Outpatient Visits:** 397273 **Births:** 821 **Total Expense ($000):** 233294 **Payroll Expense ($000):** 100725 **Personnel:** 1783

⊞ **ST. MARY'S REGIONAL MEDICAL CENTER (200034)**, 330 Sabattus Street, Zip 4240, Mailing Address: P.O. Box 291, Zip 04243–0291; tel. 207/777–8100 **A**1 2 9 10 **F**3 4 5 7 11 13 15 17 18 24 25 26 27 30 31 32 33 37 38 41 42 43 44 46 50 51 55 56 57 58 59 60 62 66 68 72 73 74 75 76 77 79 80 81 82 84 86 88 89 90 91 92 93 94 95 96 97 100 102 104 105 106 107 118 119 121 123 124 135 136 137 **P**6 **S** Covenant Health Systems, Inc.
Primary Contact: Lee T. Myles, Chief Executive Officer
COO: Susan Keiler, Chief Operating Officer
CFO: Carolyn Kasabian, Chief Financial Officer
CMO: Peter Watko, Vice President Medical Affairs and Quality
CIO: Rene Dumont, Vice President Marketing, Planning and Information Systems
CHR: Kevin Healey, Vice President Human Resources
Web address: www.stmarysmaine.com
Control: Other not–for–profit (including NFP Corporation) **Service:** General Medical and Surgical

Staffed Beds: 171 **Admissions:** 6299 **Census:** 94 **Outpatient Visits:** 174132 **Births:** 676 **Total Expense ($000):** 115468 **Payroll Expense ($000):** 33010 **Personnel:** 1411

Many Facility Codes have changed. Please refer to the AHA Guide Code Chart.

LINCOLN—Penobscot County

★ **PENOBSCOT VALLEY HOSPITAL (201303)**, 7 Transalpine Road, Zip 04457–0368, Mailing Address: P.O. Box 368, Zip 04457–0368; tel. 207/794–3321 **A**9 10 18 **F**3 7 8 11 13 15 24 25 26 30 31 32 38 43 44 45 50 54 55 57 66 68 73 74 75 77 79 80 82 84 85 86 96 97 106 107 117 119 122 124 135 137 **P**6 **S** QHR
Primary Contact: David A. Shannon, Chief Executive Officer
CFO: Ann Marie Rush, Chief Financial Officer
CIO: Harry Maynard, Director Information Technology
CHR: David Woodbury, Director Human Resources
Web address: www.pvhhealthcare.org
Control: Other not–for–profit (including NFP Corporation) **Service:** General Medical and Surgical

Staffed Beds: 25 **Admissions:** 1004 **Census:** 7 **Outpatient Visits:** 42353 **Births:** 97 **Total Expense ($000):** 20670 **Payroll Expense ($000):** 8859 **Personnel:** 178

MACHIAS—Washington County

★ **DOWN EAST COMMUNITY HOSPITAL (201311)**, Upper Court Street, Zip 4654, Mailing Address: Rural Route 1, Box 11, Zip 04654–9702; tel. 207/255–3356 **A**9 18 **F**3 13 15 24 25 26 28 30 31 32 33 38 43 44 54 55 56 57 62 63 66 73 74 76 77 79 80 81 84 86 87 96 97 99 107 118 119 121 135 136 **P**6 **S** QHR
Primary Contact: Wayne Dodwell, Chief Executive Officer
CFO: Lynnette Parr, Chief Financial Officer
CMO: David Rioux, D.O., Chief of Staff
CIO: Lynnette Parr, Chief Financial Officer
CHR: Ernie Reisman, Vice President Human Resources
Web address: www.dech.org
Control: Other not–for–profit (including NFP Corporation) **Service:** General Medical and Surgical

Staffed Beds: 25 **Admissions:** 1229 **Census:** 11 **Outpatient Visits:** 35377 **Births:** 132 **Total Expense ($000):** 29890 **Payroll Expense ($000):** 12934 **Personnel:** 216

MARS HILL—Aroostook County

AROOSTOOK HEALTH CENTER See Aroostook Medical Center, Presque Isle

MILLINOCKET—Penobscot County

★ **MILLINOCKET REGIONAL HOSPITAL (201307)**, 200 Somerset Street, Zip 04462–1298; tel. 207/723–5161 **A**9 10 18 **F**3 8 11 15 24 25 26 27 31 32 33 35 38 40 44 50 52 55 56 57 62 63 66 73 77 79 80 81 82 86 87 96 97 117 119 122 124 **P**6 **S** QHR
Primary Contact: Marie E. Vienneau, RN, Chief Executive Officer
CFO: Christine McLaughlin, Chief Financial Officer
CMO: Daniel Herbert, M.D., Medical Administrative Officer
CIO: Joe Grant, Manager Information Systems
CHR: Lisa Arsenault, Director Human Resources
Web address: www.mrhme.org
Control: Other not–for–profit (including NFP Corporation) **Service:** General Medical and Surgical

Staffed Beds: 25 **Admissions:** 1067 **Census:** 13 **Outpatient Visits:** 34895 **Total Expense ($000):** 23483 **Payroll Expense ($000):** 11111 **Personnel:** 190

NORWAY—Oxford County

★ **STEPHENS MEMORIAL HOSPITAL (200032)**, 181 Main Street, Zip 04268–1297; tel. 207/743–5933 **A**2 9 10 **F**3 7 8 13 15 24 25 26 27 30 31 32 33 38 40 44 56 57 62 68 73 74 76 77 79 80 86 96 97 100 103 107 119 121 135 137 **P**8
Primary Contact: Timothy A. Churchill, President
CMO: Kathleen Herlihy, Medical Staff President
CHR: Roberta Metivier, Vice President Human Resources
Web address: www.wmhcc.com
Control: Other not–for–profit (including NFP Corporation) **Service:** General Medical and Surgical

Staffed Beds: 50 **Admissions:** 2303 **Census:** 23 **Outpatient Visits:** 117186 **Births:** 212 **Total Expense ($000):** 37607 **Payroll Expense ($000):** 16515 **Personnel:** 348

PITTSFIELD—Somerset County

★□ **SEBASTICOOK VALLEY HOSPITAL (201313)**, 447 North Main Street, Zip 04967–1199; tel. 207/487–5141 **A**1 9 10 18 **F**7 11 15 24 25 30 31 32 33 37 38 50 51 55 57 62 63 68 73 76 77 79 80 82 86 87 96 97 102 106 107 118 119 121 122 124 132 135 136 137 **P**6 **S** Eastern Maine Healthcare Systems
Primary Contact: John C. May, Chief Executive Officer
COO: Terri Vieira, Vice President Operations
CFO: Randall Clark, Vice President Finance
CMO: James Baldwin, D.O., Chief of Staff
CHR: David Pease, Vice President Human Resources
Web address: www.sebasticookhospital.org
Control: Other not–for–profit (including NFP Corporation) **Service:** General Medical and Surgical

Staffed Beds: 25 **Admissions:** 918 **Census:** 9 **Outpatient Visits:** 58935 **Births:** 0 **Total Expense ($000):** 24338 **Payroll Expense ($000):** 10747 **Personnel:** 287

PORTLAND—Cumberland County

★□ **MAINE MEDICAL CENTER (200009)**, 22 Bramhall Street, Zip 04102–3175; tel. 207/662–0111, (Includes MAINE MEDICAL CENTER, BRIGHTON CAMPUS, 335 Brighton Avenue, Zip 04102–9735; tel. 207/879–8000) **A**1 2 3 5 8 9 10 **F**3 5 8 11 12 13 15 16 17 18 19 20 21 22 23 24 25 26 27 28 30 31 32 33 34 35 36 37 38 40 43 44 46 49 50 51 53 54 55 56 57 58 59 60 62 63 64 66 68 70 72 73 74 75 76 77 79 80 81 82 84 86 87 88 90 91 92 93 94 95 96 97 99 100 102 103 106 107 109 110 111 112 113 114 116 118 119 120 121 123 124 125 127 131 132 133 134 135 136 137 **P**4 6 8
Primary Contact: Richard W. Peterson, Interim President and Chief Executive Officer
CFO: John E. Heye, Chief Financial Officer
CMO: George Higgins, M.D., Vice President Medical Affairs and Chief Medical Officer
CIO: Stephen Rosenfeld, M.D., Chief Information Officer
CHR: Judy West, Vice President Human Resources
Web address: www.mmc.org
Control: Other not–for–profit (including NFP Corporation) **Service:** General Medical and Surgical

Staffed Beds: 557 **Admissions:** 28207 **Census:** 417 **Outpatient Visits:** 283175 **Births:** 2507 **Total Expense ($000):** 539763 **Payroll Expense ($000):** 243202 **Personnel:** 5390

★□ **MERCY HOSPITAL OF PORTLAND (200008)**, 144 State Street, Zip 04101–3795; tel. 207/879–3000 **A**1 2 9 10 **F**4 5 11 13 15 18 25 26 27 30 31 32 33 34 38 41 43 49 50 51 53 54 55 56 57 58 60 62 66 68 72 73 74 75 76 77 79 81 82 86 87 90 92 94 95 96 97 99 100 103 107 119 121 124 132 133 135 136 137 **P**6 **S** Catholic Health East
Primary Contact: Eileen F. Skinner, FACHE, President and Chief Executive Officer
COO: Timothy Prince, Vice President Planning and Ancillary Services
CFO: Russ Gardner, Interim Chief Financial Officer
CMO: Stephen Sears, M.D., Vice President Medical Administration
CIO: Jonathan Roderick, Chief Information Officer
CHR: Robert Nutter, Vice President Human Resources and Support Services
Web address: www.mercyhospital.com
Control: Church–operated, Nongovernment, not–for profit **Service:** General Medical and Surgical

Staffed Beds: 168 **Admissions:** 8933 **Census:** 101 **Outpatient Visits:** 254422 **Births:** 969 **Total Expense ($000):** 154847 **Payroll Expense ($000):** 70286 **Personnel:** 1243

★□ **NEW ENGLAND REHABILITATION HOSPITAL OF PORTLAND (203025)**, 335 Brighton Avenue, Zip 04102–9735; tel. 207/775–4000 **A**1 10 **F**24 25 32 33 43 56 62 66 72 73 75 77 85 86 119 120 121 124 132 135
S HEALTHSOUTH Corporation
Primary Contact: Amy Morse, Chief Executive Officer
CFO: Jeanine Chesley, Controller
CMO: Elissa Charbonneau, D.O., Medical Director
CHR: Leigh Baade, Director Human Resources
Web address: www.healthsouth.com
Control: Partnership, Investor–owned, for–profit **Service:** Rehabilitation

Staffed Beds: 90 **Admissions:** 1591 **Census:** 72 **Outpatient Visits:** 16071 **Births:** 0 **Total Expense ($000):** 20115 **Payroll Expense ($000):** 11162 **Personnel:** 200

Hospital, Medicare Provider Number, Address, Telephone, Approval, Facility, and Physician Codes, Health Care System

★ American Hospital Association (AHA) membership
□ The Joint Commission accreditation
○ American Osteopathic Association (AOA) accreditation
△ Commission on Accreditation of Rehabilitation Facilities (CARF) accreditation

PRESQUE ISLE—Aroostook County

★ **AROOSTOOK MEDICAL CENTER (200018)**, 140 Academy Street, Zip 04769–3171, Mailing Address: P.O. Box 151, Zip 04769–0151; tel. 207/768–4000, (Includes AROOSTOOK HEALTH CENTER, 15 Highland Avenue, Mars Hill, Zip 04758; tel. 207/768–4900; ARTHUR R. GOULD MEMORIAL HOSPITAL; COMMUNITY GENERAL HEALTH CENTER, 3 Green Street, Fort Fairfield, Zip 04742; tel. 207/768–4700), (Total facility includes 72 beds in nursing home–type unit) **A**1 9 10 12 **F**3 5 7 8 12 13 15 18 24 25 26 27 28 30 31 32 33 34 36 37 38 40 42 43 44 45 50 52 53 54 55 56 57 59 60 62 63 65 66 68 72 73 74 75 76 77 78 79 80 81 82 84 85 86 87 89 90 91 93 94 96 97 100 102 103 106 107 109 111 113 114 117 118 119 120 121 123 124 132 135 136 137 **P**6 **S** Eastern Maine Healthcare Systems
Primary Contact: David A. Peterson, President and Chief Executive Officer
COO: Jay Reynolds, M.D., Vice President Medical Affairs
CFO: C. Bruce Sandstrom, Senior Vice President Finance
CMO: Jay Reynolds, M.D., Vice President Medical Affairs
CIO: Catherine Bruno, Chief Information Officer
CHR: Thomas Umphrey, Senior Vice President Human Resources
Web address: www.tamc.org
Control: Other not–for–profit (including NFP Corporation) **Service:** General Medical and Surgical

Staffed Beds: 132 **Admissions:** 2606 **Census:** 82 **Outpatient Visits:** 180471 **Births:** 253 **Total Expense ($000):** 92965 **Payroll Expense ($000):** 46958 **Personnel:** 906

ROCKPORT—Knox County

★ **PENOBSCOT BAY MEDICAL CENTER (200063)**, 6 Glen Cove Drive, Zip 04856–4240; tel. 207/596–8000, (Total facility includes 84 beds in nursing home–type unit) **A**1 2 9 10 20 **F**3 4 5 6 11 13 15 17 24 25 26 27 30 31 32 33 37 38 40 43 51 55 56 57 58 60 62 65 68 72 73 74 75 76 77 79 80 81 82 84 86 87 88 89 90 92 93 94 96 100 102 107 117 118 119 120 121 123 124 133 135 136 137
Primary Contact: Roy A. Hitchings, Jr., FACHE, President and Chief Executive Officer
COO: Eric Waters, Vice President Operations
CFO: Maura Kelly, Vice President Finance
CMO: Dana L. Goldsmith, M.D., Vice President Medical Affairs
CIO: Dennis Puls, Director Information Systems and Chief Information Officer
CHR: Thomas Girard, Vice President Human Resources
Web address: www.penbayhealthcare.org
Control: Other not–for–profit (including NFP Corporation) **Service:** General Medical and Surgical

Staffed Beds: 171 **Admissions:** 4961 **Census:** 140 **Outpatient Visits:** 242060 **Births:** 345 **Total Expense ($000):** 95171 **Payroll Expense ($000):** 43002 **Personnel:** 825

RUMFORD—Oxford County

★ **RUMFORD HOSPITAL (201306)**, 420 Franklin Street, Zip 04276–2145; tel. 207/369–1000 **A**9 10 18 **F**8 11 13 15 24 25 27 30 31 32 33 36 38 43 50 55 56 57 62 68 73 74 75 76 77 79 80 82 86 87 96 100 102 107 117 119 121 122 135 137 **P**6 8
Primary Contact: John H. Welsh, Chief Executive Officer
Web address: www.rumfordhospital.org
Control: Other not–for–profit (including NFP Corporation) **Service:** General Medical and Surgical

Staffed Beds: 20 **Admissions:** 1107 **Census:** 13 **Outpatient Visits:** 45460 **Births:** 79 **Total Expense ($000):** 25747 **Payroll Expense ($000):** 11288 **Personnel:** 229

SANFORD—York County

★ **HENRIETTA D. GOODALL HOSPITAL (200040)**, 25 June Street, Zip 04073–2645; tel. 207/324–4310, (Total facility includes 104 beds in nursing home–type unit) **A**2 9 10 **F**1 2 3 6 8 10 13 15 24 25 27 30 31 32 33 38 43 47 50 52 54 55 56 57 63 65 66 68 71 73 74 75 76 77 79 80 84 85 86 87 96 97 100 102 106 107 115 117 118 119 120 121 123 124 134 135 136 **P**6
Primary Contact: Darlene Stromstad, FACHE, Chief Executive Officer
COO: Patricia Aprile, Vice President Operations
CFO: Ron Bryant, Chief Financial Officer
CMO: Mukesh Bhargava, M.D., Vice President Medical Affairs
CIO: Charles Caruso, Chief Information Officer
CHR: Carolyn Burgess, Director Human Resources
Web address: www.goodallhospital.org
Control: Other not–for–profit (including NFP Corporation) **Service:** General Medical and Surgical

Staffed Beds: 157 **Admissions:** 2238 **Census:** 125 **Outpatient Visits:** 105440 **Births:** 288 **Total Expense ($000):** 63063 **Payroll Expense ($000):** 30101 **Personnel:** 593

SKOWHEGAN—Somerset County

★ **REDINGTON–FAIRVIEW GENERAL HOSPITAL (201314)**, Fairview Avenue, Zip 4976, Mailing Address: P.O. Box 468, Zip 04976–0468; tel. 207/474–5121 **A**2 9 10 18 **F**3 7 11 13 15 24 25 26 27 30 31 32 33 38 43 45 50 52 54 55 56 57 63 66 68 72 73 74 75 76 77 79 80 84 86 87 96 97 102 103 106 107 119 120 121 123 124 135 136 **P**6
Primary Contact: Richard Willett, Chief Executive Officer
CFO: Dana Kempton, Associate Director and Chief Financial Officer
CMO: Roger Renfrew, Medical Director
CHR: Deborah Buckingham, R.N., Director Human Resources
Web address: www.rfgh.net
Control: Other not–for–profit (including NFP Corporation) **Service:** General Medical and Surgical

Staffed Beds: 25 **Admissions:** 1940 **Census:** 20 **Outpatient Visits:** 79970 **Births:** 164 **Total Expense ($000):** 46521 **Payroll Expense ($000):** 19536 **Personnel:** 393

TOGUS—Kennebec County

★ **VETERANS AFFAIRS MEDICAL CENTER**, 1 VA Center, Zip 4330; tel. 207/623–8411, (Total facility includes 100 beds in nursing home–type unit) **A**1 **F**2 3 5 18 25 26 27 29 30 31 32 37 38 42 43 44 45 50 53 54 55 56 57 59 60 61 62 63 66 68 72 73 75 77 79 80 82 86 87 88 90 92 93 94 95 96 100 101 103 107 118 119 121 124 132 135 136 137 **P**6 **S** Department of Veterans Affairs
Primary Contact: Brian Stiller, Director
CFO: Daniel Howard, Chief Financial Officer
CMO: Timothy J. Richardson, M.D., Chief of Staff
CIO: Richard McNaughton, Chief Information Management Service
CHR: Christine Miller, Chief Human Resources Management Services
Web address: www.visn1.med.va.gov/togus/
Control: Veterans Affairs, Government, federal **Service:** General Medical and Surgical

Staffed Beds: 167 **Admissions:** 1708 **Census:** 105 **Outpatient Visits:** 332349 **Births:** 0 **Total Expense ($000):** 188653 **Payroll Expense ($000):** 85055 **Personnel:** 1032

WATERVILLE—Kennebec County

★ ○ **INLAND HOSPITAL (200041)**, 200 Kennedy Memorial Drive, Zip 04901–4595; tel. 207/861–3000 **A**9 10 11 **F**3 13 15 25 26 30 31 32 33 36 38 43 50 55 57 66 68 73 74 77 79 80 81 86 87 96 97 103 106 107 118 121 124 135 136 137 **S** Eastern Maine Healthcare Systems
Primary Contact: John Dalton, President and Chief Executive Officer
COO: Sally Conary, President and Chief Executive Officer
CFO: Dean Bither, Chief Financial Officer
CMO: Michael Palumbo, D.O., Vice President Medical Affairs
CIO: Kevin Dieterich, Director Information Services
CHR: Daniel Booth, Vice President Operations and Chief Human Resources Officer
Web address: www.inlandhospital.org
Control: Other not–for–profit (including NFP Corporation) **Service:** General Medical and Surgical

Staffed Beds: 46 **Admissions:** 1509 **Census:** 16 **Outpatient Visits:** 77143 **Births:** 250 **Total Expense ($000):** 39867 **Payroll Expense ($000):** 17476 **Personnel:** 348

★ **MAINEGENERAL MEDICAL CENTER–WATERVILLE CAMPUS (200039)**, 149 North Street, Zip 04901–4974; tel. 207/872–1000, (Includes MAINEGENERAL MEDICAL CENTER–AUGUSTA CAMPUS, 6 East Chestnut Street, Augusta, Zip 04330–9988; tel. 207/626–1000; Chuck Hays, Chief Executive Officer) **A**1 2 9 10 19 **F**3 4 5 11 12 13 15 18 22 24 25 26 27 30 31 32 33 35 38 41 43 44 50 51 53 57 58 59 60 61 62 63 66 68 72 73 74 75 76 77 79 80 81 82 84 85 86 87 88 89 90 92 93 94 95 96 97 99 100 102 103 104 105 106 107 108 109 111 112 116 118 119 120 124 133 135 137
Primary Contact: Scott B. Bullock, President, MaineGeneral Health
CFO: Norman Belair, Vice President of Finance and Chief Financial Officer
CMO: Steve Diaz, Chief Medical Officer
CIO: Daniel Burgess, Chief Information Officer
CHR: Rebecca Lamey, Vice President Human Resources
Web address: www.mainegeneral.org
Control: Other not–for–profit (including NFP Corporation) **Service:** General Medical and Surgical

Staffed Beds: 278 **Admissions:** 13477 **Census:** 173 **Births:** 1162 **Total Expense ($000):** 271501 **Payroll Expense ($000):** 107119

Many Facility Codes have changed. Please refer to the AHA Guide Code Chart.

WESTBROOK—Cumberland County

★□ **SPRING HARBOR HOSPITAL (204005)**, 123 Andover Road, Zip 04092–3850; tel. 207/761–2200 **A**1 10 **F**4 5 30 31 32 33 41 50 53 62 82 88 89 91 93 94 119 121 124 135
Primary Contact: Dennis P. King, Chief Executive Officer
COO: Richard Hanley, Chief Operating Officer
CFO: Gregory Bowers, Chief Financial Officer
CMO: Girard Robinson, M.D., Chief Medical Officer
CIO: Julie Wooden, Director Project Management, Customer and Information Services
CHR: John Orlowski, Chief Human Resources Officer
Web address: www.springharbor.org
Control: Other not–for–profit (including NFP Corporation) **Service:** Psychiatric

Staffed Beds: 100 **Admissions:** 2184 **Census:** 71 **Outpatient Visits:** 3002 **Births:** 0 **Total Expense ($000):** 29885 **Payroll Expense ($000):** 18749 **Personnel:** 360

YORK—York County

★ **YORK HOSPITAL (200020)**, 15 Hospital Drive, Zip 03909–1099; tel. 207/363–4321 **A**9 10 **F**3 5 11 13 15 18 20 24 25 27 28 30 31 32 33 34 38 42 50 52 53 57 61 62 63 67 68 72 73 74 75 76 77 79 80 82 84 86 90 94 96 97 99 100 102 106 107 112 118 119 120 121 124 132 133 135 137
Primary Contact: Jud Knox, President
COO: Stephen Pelletier, Leader Guest Services
CFO: Robin LaBonte, Leader Financial Care
CMO: Michael Major, M.D., Medical Staff President
CIO: Robin LaBonte, Leader Financial Care
CHR: Olivia Chayer, Lead Human Resources
Web address: www.yorkhospital.com
Control: Other not–for–profit (including NFP Corporation) **Service:** General Medical and Surgical

Staffed Beds: 79 **Admissions:** 5352 **Census:** 55 **Outpatient Visits:** 185426 **Births:** 402 **Total Expense ($000):** 105699 **Payroll Expense ($000):** 43895 **Personnel:** 793

 Many Facility Codes have changed. Please refer to the AHA Guide Code Chart.

MD

MARYLAND

ANDREWS AFB—Prince George's County

★ **MALCOLM GROW MEDICAL CENTER**, 1050 West Perimeter, Zip 20762–6600, Mailing Address: 1050 West Perimeter, Suite A1–19, Zip 20762–6600; tel. 240/857–3001, (Nonreporting) **A**1 2 3 5 9 **S** Department of the Air Force
Primary Contact: Colonel Robert I. Miller, Commanding Officer
COO: Lieutenant Colonel Jaime Rosado, Administrator
CFO: Captain Tonya Brown, Director Medical Resource Management Flight
CMO: Colonel James Bennion, Chief Medical Staff
CIO: Captain Sylvia Kim, Flight Commander Medical Information Management
CHR: Captain Tonya Brown, Director Medical Resource Management Flight
Web address: www.mgmc.af.mil
Control: Air Force, Government, federal **Service:** General Medical and Surgical

Staffed Beds: 60

ANNAPOLIS—Anne Arundel County

★ **ANNE ARUNDEL MEDICAL CENTER (210023)**, 2001 Medical Parkway, Zip 21401–3019; tel. 443/481–1000 **A**1 2 5 9 10 **F**3 4 5 11 13 14 15 18 20 22 24 25 26 27 30 31 32 33 34 36 38 41 42 43 46 49 50 53 54 55 56 57 58 62 64 66 68 70 72 73 74 75 76 77 79 80 81 82 84 86 87 90 92 96 97 99 100 102 104 105 106 107 108 109 111 112 114 116 118 119 121 123 124 134 135 136 137 **P**6 7
Primary Contact: Martin L. Doordan, President and Chief Executive Officer
COO: Victoria Bayless, Chief Operating Officer
CFO: William L. Hughes, Senior Vice President and Chief Financial Officer
CMO: Joseph Moser, M.D., Vice President Medical Staff Affairs
CIO: Douglas A. Abel, Chief Information Officer
CHR: Nancy Luttrell, Interim Vice President Human Resources
Web address: www.aahs.org
Control: Other not–for–profit (including NFP Corporation) **Service:** General Medical and Surgical

Staffed Beds: 348 **Admissions:** 23072 **Census:** 228 **Outpatient Visits:** 403260 **Births:** 5527 **Total Expense ($000):** 316079 **Payroll Expense ($000):** 130822 **Personnel:** 2200

BALTIMORE—Baltimore City County

★ **BON SECOURS BALTIMORE HEALTH SYSTEM (210013)**, 2000 West Baltimore Street, Zip 21223–1597; tel. 410/362–3000 **A**9 10 **F**3 5 15 18 20 22 24 25 26 31 32 33 38 44 46 50 52 55 56 59 60 61 62 68 73 75 77 79 82 88 89 90 92 94 95 96 100 107 119 124 132 135 136 **P**6 **S** Bon Secours Health System, Inc.
Primary Contact: Samuel Lee Ross, M.D., Chief Executive Officer
CFO: Richard Braam, Chief Financial Officer
CMO: Crystal L. Clark, Chief Medical Officer
CIO: Mike King, Director Information Systems
Web address: www.bonsecours.org
Control: Church–operated, Nongovernment, not–for profit **Service:** General Medical and Surgical

Staffed Beds: 141 **Admissions:** 7746 **Census:** 103 **Outpatient Visits:** 155484 **Births:** 0 **Total Expense ($000):** 113987 **Payroll Expense ($000):** 46590 **Personnel:** 893

★ **FRANKLIN SQUARE HOSPITAL CENTER (210015)**, 9000 Franklin Square Drive, Zip 21237–2998; tel. 443/777–7000 **A**1 2 3 5 8 9 10 **F**3 5 8 10 11 12 13 14 15 17 18 20 24 25 26 27 28 30 31 32 33 34 35 36 37 38 41 43 44 46 47 48 49 50 51 54 55 56 57 58 59 60 62 63 64 68 69 70 72 73 74 75 76 77 79 80 81 82 84 86 87 88 89 90 91 92 93 94 95 96 102 103 106 107 113 114 118 119 120 121 123 124 135 136 137 **P**6 **S** MedStar Health
Primary Contact: Carl J. Schindelar, President
CFO: Robert P. Lally, Vice President Finance
CMO: Tony Sclama, M.D., Vice President Medical Affairs
CHR: Karen Robertson–Keck, Vice President Human Resources
Web address: www.franklinsquare.org
Control: Other not–for–profit (including NFP Corporation) **Service:** General Medical and Surgical

Staffed Beds: 347 **Admissions:** 26389 **Census:** 270 **Outpatient Visits:** 220146 **Births:** 2677 **Total Expense ($000):** 339292 **Payroll Expense ($000):** 146639 **Personnel:** 2652

★ △ **GOOD SAMARITAN HOSPITAL OF MARYLAND (210056)**, 5601 Loch Raven Boulevard, Zip 21239–2995; tel. 410/532–8000, (Total facility includes 30 beds in nursing home–type unit) **A**1 2 3 5 7 9 10 **F**3 9 11 14 15 17 18 24 25 26 27 28 30 31 32 33 34 35 36 38 41 43 44 50 51 52 54 55 56 57 58 59 60 62 63 64 65 66 68 69 72 73 75 76 77 78 79 80 81 82 85 86 87 92 96 97 100 102 105 106 107 109 117 118 119 120 121 124 132 135 137 **P**6 **S** MedStar Health
Primary Contact: Lawrence M. Beck, President
CFO: Deanna Stout, Vice President Financial Services
Web address: www.goodsam–md.org
Control: Other not–for–profit (including NFP Corporation) **Service:** General Medical and Surgical

Staffed Beds: 315 **Admissions:** 17708 **Census:** 256 **Outpatient Visits:** 136928 **Births:** 0 **Total Expense ($000):** 250448 **Payroll Expense ($000):** 106475 **Personnel:** 1991

★ **GREATER BALTIMORE MEDICAL CENTER (210044)**, 6701 North Charles Street, Zip 21204–6892; tel. 443/849–2000, (Total facility includes 24 beds in nursing home–type unit) **A**1 2 3 5 8 9 10 **F**3 8 11 12 13 18 20 25 26 27 33 35 38 41 42 43 44 46 47 49 50 51 53 54 55 56 57 59 60 62 66 72 73 75 76 77 79 80 81 82 86 87 92 96 97 102 103 107 108 109 111 112 113 114 116 118 119 121 124 133 134 135 136 137
Primary Contact: Laurence M. Merlis, President and Chief Executive Officer
COO: Keith R. Poisson, Executive Vice President Chief Operating Officer
CFO: Eric L. Melchior, Executive Vice President and Chief Financial Officer
CMO: Rodney W. Williams, M.D., JD, Executive Vice President and Chief Medical Officer
CIO: Tressa Springmann, Chief Information Officer
CHR: Mark R. Thomas, Vice President Human Resources and Organizational Development
Web address: www.gbmc.org
Control: Other not–for–profit (including NFP Corporation) **Service:** General Medical and Surgical

Staffed Beds: 269 **Admissions:** 22048 **Census:** 257 **Births:** 4746 **Total Expense ($000):** 359957 **Payroll Expense ($000):** 162104 **Personnel:** 2363

★ **HARBOR HOSPITAL (210034)**, (Formerly Harbor Hospital Center), 3001 South Hanover Street, Zip 21225–1290; tel. 410/350–3200 **A**1 2 3 5 9 10 **F**2 8 9 11 13 14 15 17 25 26 27 30 31 32 33 34 35 38 40 41 43 50 51 52 53 54 55 56 57 59 60 62 63 64 66 68 72 73 74 75 76 77 79 80 81 82 84 86 87 90 92 96 99 100 102 104 105 107 108 109 114 118 119 120 124 135 136 **S** MedStar Health
Primary Contact: Joseph M. Oddis, President
CHR: Dawn C. Hoffman, Associate Vice President Human Resources
Web address: www.harborhospital.org
Control: Other not–for–profit (including NFP Corporation) **Service:** General Medical and Surgical

Staffed Beds: 240 **Admissions:** 13024 **Census:** 145 **Outpatient Visits:** 76158 **Births:** 1910 **Total Expense ($000):** 151983 **Payroll Expense ($000):** 72958 **Personnel:** 1293

★ △ **JOHNS HOPKINS BAYVIEW MEDICAL CENTER (210029)**, 4940 Eastern Avenue, Zip 21224–2780; tel. 410/550–0100, (Total facility includes 224 beds in nursing home–type unit) **A**1 3 5 7 8 9 10 **F**2 3 4 5 6 8 9 10 12 13 15 16 17 18 20 24 25 26 27 28 30 31 32 33 36 38 40 41 43 44 47 48 49 50 51 54 55 56 57 58 59 60 62 63 64 66 68 69 70 72 73 74 75 76 77 78 79 80 81 82 84 85 86 87 88 89 90 91 92 93 94 95 96 100 102 103 104 106 107 113 114 117 118 119 120 121 123 124 130 132 134 135 136 137 **S** Johns Hopkins Health System
Primary Contact: Gregory F. Schaffer, President
COO: Richard G. Bennett, M.D., Executive Vice President, Chief Operating Officer and Vice President Medical Affairs
CFO: Carl H. Francioli, Vice President Finance
CMO: Richard G. Bennett, M.D., Executive Vice President, Chief Operating Officer and Vice President Medical Affairs
CIO: Sandy Reckert, Director Communications and Public Affairs
CHR: Craig Brodian, Vice President Human Resources
Web address: www.hopkinsbayview.org
Control: Other not–for–profit (including NFP Corporation) **Service:** General Medical and Surgical

Staffed Beds: 560 **Admissions:** 22689 **Census:** 452 **Outpatient Visits:** 395392 **Births:** 1661 **Total Expense ($000):** 328111 **Payroll Expense ($000):** 110396 **Personnel:** 3044

Many Facility Codes have changed. Please refer to the AHA Guide Code Chart.

★ □ △ **JOHNS HOPKINS HOSPITAL (210009)**, 600 North Wolfe Street, Zip 21287–2182; tel. 410/955–5000 **A**1 2 3 5 7 8 9 10 **F**3 5 6 7 9 11 13 14 15 17 18 19 20 21 22 23 24 25 26 27 28 30 31 32 33 34 36 37 38 40 41 43 44 46 47 49 50 53 54 55 56 57 58 59 60 62 63 64 66 68 70 72 73 74 75 76 77 78 79 80 81 82 83 84 85 86 87 88 89 90 91 92 93 94 95 96 97 99 100 101 102 103 104 105 106 107 108 109 111 112 113 114 116 118 119 120 121 123 124 125 126 127 128 129 130 131 132 134 135 136 137 **S** Johns Hopkins Health System
Primary Contact: Ronald R. Peterson, President
COO: Judy A. Reitz, Sc.D., Executive Vice President and Chief Operating Officer
CFO: Ronald J. Werthman, Vice President Finance, Chief Financial Officer and Treasurer
CMO: Beryl Rosenstein, M.D., Vice President Medical Affairs
CIO: Stephanie L. Reel, Vice President Information Services
CHR: Pamela Paulk, Vice President Human Resources
Web address: www.hopkinsmedicine.org
Control: Other not–for–profit (including NFP Corporation) **Service:** General Medical and Surgical

Staffed Beds: 920 **Admissions:** 47031 **Census:** 751 **Outpatient Visits:** 337099 **Births:** 2110 **Total Expense ($000):** 1293410 **Payroll Expense ($000):** 413125 **Personnel:** 7708

□ △ **KENNEDY KRIEGER INSTITUTE (213301)**, 707 North Broadway, Zip 21205–1890; tel. 443/923–9200, (Nonreporting) **A**1 3 5 7 9 10
Primary Contact: Gary W. Goldstein, M.D., President and Chief Executive Officer
COO: James M. Anders, Administrator and Chief Operating Officer
CFO: Michael J. Neuman, Vice President Finance
CMO: Michael V. Johnston, M.D., Chief Medical Officer and Senior Vice President Medical Programs
CIO: Kenneth Davis, Assistant Vice President Information Systems
CHR: Michael Loughran, Vice President Human Resources
Web address: www.kennedykrieger.org
Control: Other not–for–profit (including NFP Corporation) **Service:** Children's other specialty

Staffed Beds: 70

★ □ △ **KERNAN ORTHOPAEDICS AND REHABILITATION (210058)**, 2200 Kernan Drive, Zip 21207–6697; tel. 410/448–2500 **A**1 7 9 10 **F**1 2 9 11 25 30 31 33 34 37 43 52 53 55 56 57 58 62 66 68 72 73 77 79 80 82 85 86 90 96 100 118 119 120 121 135 137 **S** University of Maryland Medical System
Primary Contact: James E. Ross, FACHE, Chief Executive Officer
CFO: W. Walter Augustin, Vice President and Chief Financial Officer
CMO: Michael Jablonover, M.D., Chief Medical Officer
CIO: Allen Tracey, Director Information Systems
CHR: Christine Martin, Director Human Resources
Web address: www.kernan.org
Control: Other not–for–profit (including NFP Corporation) **Service:** Rehabilitation

Staffed Beds: 133 **Admissions:** 3257 **Census:** 114 **Outpatient Visits:** 84759 **Births:** 0 **Total Expense ($000):** 86936 **Payroll Expense ($000):** 37649 **Personnel:** 603

★ □ △ **LEVINDALE HEBREW GERIATRIC CENTER AND HOSPITAL (212005)**, 2434 West Belvedere Avenue, Zip 21215–5299; tel. 410/466–8700, (Total facility includes 323 beds in nursing home–type unit) **A**1 7 9 10 **F**2 6 11 26 31 32 33 37 42 43 44 54 65 66 67 93 94 95 117 119 121 132 135 137 **P**6 **S** LifeBridge Health
Primary Contact: Ronald Rothstein, President and Chief Operating Officer
CFO: Raul Lujan, Vice President Finance
CMO: Susan M. Levy, M.D., Vice President Medical Affairs
CIO: Karen Barker, Vice President and Chief Information Officer
CHR: Elizabeth McMann, Director
Web address: www.sinai–balt.com
Control: Other not–for–profit (including NFP Corporation) **Service:** Long–Term Acute Care hospital

Staffed Beds: 443 **Admissions:** 1252 **Census:** 417 **Outpatient Visits:** 0 **Births:** 0 **Total Expense ($000):** 83159 **Payroll Expense ($000):** 35145

★ □ △ **MARYLAND GENERAL HOSPITAL (210038)**, 827 Linden Avenue, Zip 21201–4681; tel. 410/225–8000 **A**1 3 5 7 9 10 **F**5 11 13 15 17 18 25 26 27 31 32 33 36 38 41 43 49 50 54 55 56 57 59 60 62 63 64 66 68 72 73 74 75 76 77 79 80 82 84 86 87 88 89 90 91 92 93 94 96 97 100 102 106 107 118 119 124 132 133 135 136 137 **S** University of Maryland Medical System
Primary Contact: Sylvia Smith Johnson, President and Chief Executive Officer
CFO: Brian Bailey, Chief Financial Officer
CMO: Roy T. Smoot, M.D., Chief Medical Officer
CHR: David Swift, Senior Vice President Human Resources
Web address: www.marylandgeneral.org
Control: Other not–for–profit (including NFP Corporation) **Service:** General Medical and Surgical

Staffed Beds: 238 **Admissions:** 11544 **Census:** 162 **Outpatient Visits:** 106930 **Births:** 1262 **Total Expense ($000):** 151769 **Payroll Expense ($000):** 72910 **Personnel:** 1258

★ □ **MERCY MEDICAL CENTER (210008)**, 301 St. Paul Place, Zip 21202–2165; tel. 410/332–9000 **A**1 2 3 5 8 9 10 **F**3 4 8 11 13 15 17 18 20 25 26 27 30 31 32 33 37 38 41 46 49 50 51 55 56 57 58 62 64 66 68 70 72 73 74 75 76 77 79 81 82 84 86 90 92 96 97 100 102 104 106 107 109 111 114 117 118 119 121 133 135 136 137 **P**6
Primary Contact: Thomas R. Mullen, President and Chief Executive Officer
COO: Samuel E. Moskowitz, Executive Vice President and Chief Operating Officer
CFO: John E. Topper, Senior Vice President and Chief Financial Officer
CMO: Scott A. Spier, M.D., Senior Vice President Medical Affairs
CIO: James C. Stalder, Senior Vice President and Chief Information Officer
CHR: Jessie Reed, Senior Vice President Human Resources
Web address: www.mercymed.com
Control: Church–operated, Nongovernment, not–for profit **Service:** General Medical and Surgical

Staffed Beds: 285 **Admissions:** 18136 **Census:** 207 **Outpatient Visits:** 183579 **Births:** 2722 **Total Expense ($000):** 282445 **Payroll Expense ($000):** 115788 **Personnel:** 2195

MD

★ □ △ **MT. WASHINGTON PEDIATRIC HOSPITAL (213300)**, (Pediatric Specialty), 1708 West Rogers Avenue, Zip 21209–4537; tel. 410/578–8600 **A**1 5 7 9 10 **F**31 32 53 62 66 73 77 82 84 85 86 89 94 118 119 121 135 137 **P**6 **S** University of Maryland Medical System
Primary Contact: Sheldon J. Stein, President and Chief Executive Officer
CFO: Al Pietsch, CPA, Senior Vice President and Chief Financial Officer
CMO: Richard Katz, M.D., Vice President Medical Affairs
CIO: Tim Brady, Director Information Systems
CHR: Thomas Ellis, Vice President Human Resources
Web address: www.mwph.org
Control: Other not–for–profit (including NFP Corporation) **Service:** Children's other specialty

Staffed Beds: 70 **Admissions:** 674 **Census:** 60 **Outpatient Visits:** 28095 **Births:** 0 **Total Expense ($000):** 37030 **Payroll Expense ($000):** 20595 **Personnel:** 451

□ **SHEPPARD AND ENOCH PRATT HOSPITAL (214000)**, 6501 North Charles Street, Zip 21285, Mailing Address: P.O. Box 6815, Zip 21285–6815; tel. 410/938–3000, (Includes TAYLOR MANOR HOSPITAL, 4100 College Avenue, Ellicott City, Zip 21043–5506, Mailing Address: P.O. Box 396, Zip 21041–0396; tel. 410/465–3322) **A**1 3 5 9 10 **F**10 26 32 33 36 54 55 57 58 73 82 88 89 90 91 93 94 95 119 121 124 132 135 **P**4
Primary Contact: Steven S. Sharfstein, M.D., President and Chief Executive Officer
COO: Diana Ramsay, Executive Vice President and Chief Operating Officer
CFO: Patricia Pinkerton, Chief Financial Officer
CMO: Robert Roca, M.D., Vice President and Medical Director
CIO: Greg Merkle, Director Information Systems
CHR: Cathy Doughty, Vice President, Human Resources
Web address: www.sheppardpratt.org
Control: Other not–for–profit (including NFP Corporation) **Service:** Psychiatric

Staffed Beds: 282 **Admissions:** 7922 **Census:** 225 **Outpatient Visits:** 42780 **Births:** 0 **Total Expense ($000):** 148274 **Payroll Expense ($000):** 73700 **Personnel:** 1647

★ □ △ **SINAI HOSPITAL OF BALTIMORE (210012)**, 2401 West Belvedere Avenue, Zip 21215–5271; tel. 410/601–9000 **A**1 2 3 5 7 8 9 10 **F**3 5 9 11 12 13 15 17 18 20 22 25 26 27 28 30 31 32 33 34 35 36 37 38 40 41 43 46 48 49 50 55 56 57 58 59 60 62 63 64 66 68 70 71 72 73 74 75 76 77 79 80 81 82 83 84 85 86 87 88 89 90 91 92 93 94 96 97 100 102 103 105 106 107 112 114 118 119 121 124 132 135 136 **P**6 **S** LifeBridge Health
Primary Contact: Neil M. Meltzer, President and Chief Operating Officer
COO: Neil M. Meltzer, President and Chief Operating Officer
CFO: Charles Orlando, Senior Vice President and Chief Financial Officer
CIO: Karen Barker, Vice President and Chief Information Officer
CHR: Taylor Foss, Vice President Human Resources
Web address: www.lifebridgehealth.org
Control: Other not–for–profit (including NFP Corporation) **Service:** General Medical and Surgical

Staffed Beds: 439 **Admissions:** 25051 **Census:** 336 **Outpatient Visits:** 146572 **Births:** 2665 **Total Expense ($000):** 525872 **Payroll Expense ($000):** 224949 **Personnel:** 3923

□ **SPRING GROVE HOSPITAL CENTER (214018)**, 55 Wade Avenue, Zip 21228–4689; tel. 410/402–6000 **A**1 3 5 9 10 **F**10 25 26 37 52 56 57 58 66 72 73 88 89 91 93 124
Primary Contact: David S. Helsel, M.D., Chief Executive Officer
CFO: Shawn Hain, Chief Financial Officer
CMO: Barry Rudnick, M.D., Clinical Director and Chief of Staff
Web address: www.springgrove.com
Control: State–Government, nonfederal **Service:** Psychiatric

Staffed Beds: 440 **Admissions:** 720 **Census:** 720 **Outpatient Visits:** 0 **Births:** 0

Hospital, Medicare Provider Number, Address, Telephone, Approval, Facility, and Physician Codes, Health Care System

★ American Hospital Association (AHA) membership
□ The Joint Commission accreditation
○ American Osteopathic Association (AOA) accreditation
△ Commission on Accreditation of Rehabilitation Facilities (CARF) accreditation

ST. AGNES HEALTHCARE (210011), 900 Caton Avenue, Zip 21229–5299; tel. 410/368–6000 **A**1 2 3 5 9 10 **F**3 8 11 12 13 14 15 17 18 20 24 25 26 27 28 30 31 32 33 38 41 42 43 44 46 49 50 51 52 53 54 55 56 57 58 59 60 61 62 63 66 68 70 72 73 74 75 76 77 79 80 81 82 83 84 86 87 92 93 96 97 100 102 103 105 106 107 108 109 111 112 114 118 119 120 121 123 124 133 135 136 137 **P**6 **S** Ascension Health
Primary Contact: Bonnie Phipps, President and Chief Executive Officer
CFO: Rhonda Anderson, Chief Financial Officer
CMO: Adrian Long, Executive Vice President and Chief Medical Officer
CIO: William Greskovich, Chief Information Officer
CHR: James Bobbitt, Vice President Human Resources
Web address: www.stagnes.org
Control: Church–operated, Nongovernment, not–for profit **Service:** General Medical and Surgical

MD

Staffed Beds: 351 **Admissions:** 20576 **Census:** 232 **Outpatient Visits:** 449590 **Births:** 2140 **Total Expense ($000):** 299625 **Payroll Expense ($000):** 140389 **Personnel:** 2108

△ **UNION MEMORIAL HOSPITAL (210024)**, 201 East University Parkway, Zip 21218–2895; tel. 410/554–2000 **A**1 2 3 5 7 9 10 **F**3 5 9 11 14 15 17 18 20 22 24 25 26 27 30 31 32 33 34 35 36 37 38 40 41 42 43 44 46 47 48 49 50 51 52 53 54 55 56 57 58 59 60 62 63 64 66 68 72 73 75 76 77 78 79 80 81 82 84 85 86 87 88 90 91 92 93 94 95 96 97 100 102 103 106 107 108 109 111 112 113 114 118 119 120 121 122 124 132 135 137 **P**6 **S** MedStar Health
Primary Contact: Harrison J. Rider, III, President
COO: Bradley Chambers, Chief Operating Officer
CFO: Joseph B. Smith, Vice President Finance
CMO: Stuart Bell, M.D., Vice President Medical Affairs
CIO: Catherine Szenczy, Senior Vice President and Chief Information Officer
CHR: Holly Phipps–Adams, Vice President Human Resources
Web address: www.unionmemorial.org
Control: Other not–for–profit (including NFP Corporation) **Service:** General Medical and Surgical

Staffed Beds: 273 **Admissions:** 20036 **Census:** 215 **Outpatient Visits:** 171623 **Births:** 0 **Total Expense ($000):** 334509 **Payroll Expense ($000):** 134611 **Personnel:** 2093

UNIVERSITY OF MARYLAND MEDICAL CENTER (210002), 22 South Greene Street, Zip 21201–1595; tel. 410/328–8667 **A**1 2 3 5 8 9 10 **F**3 5 6 7 9 11 12 13 14 15 17 18 19 20 21 22 23 24 25 26 27 28 30 31 32 33 36 37 38 40 41 42 43 44 46 47 48 49 50 51 53 54 55 56 57 58 59 60 62 63 64 66 68 69 70 72 73 74 75 76 77 78 79 80 81 82 83 84 86 87 88 89 90 91 92 93 94 95 96 97 98 99 100 102 103 104 105 106 107 108 109 111 112 113 114 116 118 119 120 121 123 124 125 126 127 128 129 130 131 132 133 134 135 136 137 **P**6 **S** University of Maryland Medical System
Primary Contact: Jeffrey A. Rivest, President and Chief Executive Officer
COO: Herbert Buchanan, Senior Vice President and Chief Operating Officer
CFO: Henry J. Franey, Senior Vice President Finance and Chief Financial Officer
CMO: Timothy J. Babineau, M.D., Chief Medical Officer
CIO: Jon Burns, Chief Information Officer
CHR: R. Keith Allen, Senior Vice President Human Resources
Web address: www.umm.edu
Control: Other not–for–profit (including NFP Corporation) **Service:** General Medical and Surgical

Staffed Beds: 666 **Admissions:** 34780 **Census:** 536 **Outpatient Visits:** 224899 **Births:** 1553 **Total Expense ($000):** 937636 **Payroll Expense ($000):** 351690 **Personnel:** 6515

△ **UNIVERSITY SPECIALTY HOSPITAL (212007)**, 601 South Charles Street, Zip 21230–3898; tel. 410/547–8500 **A**1 7 9 10 **F**1 3 7 12 25 26 30 31 32 33 39 43 56 59 62 63 66 73 75 80 90 118 119 135 137 **P**2 5 **S** University of Maryland Medical System
Primary Contact: James L. Warner, Vice President
COO: James L. Warner, Vice President Operations
CFO: Hank Franey, Chief Financial Officer
CMO: Michael Jablonover, M.D., Chief Medical Officer
CIO: Allen Tracey, Manager
CHR: Diane Posko, Manager Human Resources
Web address: www.umm.edu/ush/
Control: Other not–for–profit (including NFP Corporation) **Service:** Chronic disease

Staffed Beds: 180 **Admissions:** 1094 **Census:** 156 **Outpatient Visits:** 13792 **Births:** 0 **Total Expense ($000):** 53183 **Payroll Expense ($000):** 23194 **Personnel:** 310

△ **VETERANS AFFAIRS MARYLAND HEALTH CARE SYSTEM–BALTIMORE DIVISION**, 10 North Greene Street, Zip 21201–1524; tel. 410/605–7001, (Includes VETERANS AFFAIRS MARYLAND HEALTH CARE SYSTEM–PERRY POINT DIVISION, Circle Drive, Perry Point, Zip 21902; tel. 410/642–2411; Dennis H. Smith, Director), (Total facility includes 275 beds in nursing home–type unit) **A**1 2 3 5 7 8 9 **F**3 4 5 6 7 8 11 12 15 17 18 20 25 26 27 32 33 34 36 37 38 41 42 43 44 45 46 48 49 50 51 52 53 54 55 56 57 58 60 61 62 63 66 68 72 73 75 76 77 79 80 81 82 85 86 87 88 90 91 92 93 94 95 96 97 99 100 102 103 106 107 117 118 119 121 122 124 132 133 134 135 136 137 **S** Department of Veterans Affairs
Primary Contact: Dennis H. Smith, Director
CFO: Major Tom Scheffler, Chief Fiscal Officer
CMO: Dorothy Snow, M.D., Chief of Staff
CIO: Sharon Zielinski, Chief Information Resource Officer
CHR: Jeff Craig, Chief Human Resource Management
Web address: www.va.gov/sta/guide/home.asp
Control: Veterans Affairs, Government, federal **Service:** General Medical and Surgical

Staffed Beds: 727 **Admissions:** 7878 **Census:** 484 **Outpatient Visits:** 614637 **Births:** 0 **Total Expense ($000):** 378330 **Payroll Expense ($000):** 239100 **Personnel:** 2894

BEL AIR—Harford County

UPPER CHESAPEAKE MEDICAL CENTER (210049), 500 Upper Chesapeake Drive, Zip 21014–4324; tel. 443/643–1000 **A**1 9 10 **F**11 12 13 15 24 25 26 31 32 33 34 38 43 44 45 51 53 55 56 57 59 62 68 69 71 72 74 76 77 79 81 82 84 86 92 96 97 100 106 107 119 121 124 135 136 137 **S** Upper Chesapeake Health System
Primary Contact: Lyle Ernest Sheldon, FACHE, President and Chief Executive Officer
COO: Kenneth Kozel, Senior Vice President and Chief Operating Officer
CFO: Joseph E. Hoffman, Senior Vice President and Chief Financial Officer
CMO: Peggy Vaughan, M.D., Senior Vice President Medical Affairs
CIO: Rick Casteel, Vice President Management Information Systems and Chief Information Officer
CHR: Toni Shivery, Vice President Human Resources
Web address: www.uchs.org
Control: Other not–for–profit (including NFP Corporation) **Service:** General Medical and Surgical

Staffed Beds: 168 **Admissions:** 14425 **Census:** 126 **Outpatient Visits:** 129064 **Births:** 1542 **Total Expense ($000):** 145021 **Payroll Expense ($000):** 58426 **Personnel:** 1219

BERLIN—Worcester County

ATLANTIC GENERAL HOSPITAL (210061), 9733 Healthway Drive, Zip 21811–1155; tel. 410/641–1100 **A**1 9 10 **F**3 8 15 17 25 26 30 31 32 33 36 38 39 54 55 56 57 58 62 63 64 65 68 72 73 77 79 80 82 84 87 96 97 98 100 102 107 112 117 118 121 124 135 136 **P**7
Primary Contact: Michael A. Franklin, FACHE, President and Chief Executive Officer
COO: Kim Justice, Vice President Planning and Operations
CFO: Cheryl Nottingham, Chief Financial Officer
CMO: Stephen F. Waters, M.D., Medical Director
CIO: Murray Oltman, Director Information Services
CHR: Jim Brannon, Vice President Human Resources
Web address: www.atlanticgeneral.org
Control: Other not–for–profit (including NFP Corporation) **Service:** General Medical and Surgical

Staffed Beds: 51 **Admissions:** 3675 **Census:** 37 **Outpatient Visits:** 111307 **Births:** 0 **Total Expense ($000):** 51171 **Payroll Expense ($000):** 20925 **Personnel:** 597

BETHESDA—Montgomery County

NATIONAL INSTITUTES OF HEALTH CLINICAL CENTER, (Biomedical research), 9000 Rockville Pike, Building 10, Room 6–2551, Zip 20892–1504; tel. 301/496–4000 **A**1 3 5 8 **F**3 4 5 8 14 26 27 34 37 43 44 46 52 54 58 59 60 62 66 68 73 75 76 79 80 82 84 86 88 89 90 91 93 94 95 96 97 98 99 100 101 104 105 106 107 119 121 125 127 131 132 135 **S** U. S. Indian Health Service
Primary Contact: John I. Gallin, M.D., Director, NIH Clinical Center
COO: Maureen E. Gormley, R.N., M.P.H., Chief Operating Officer
CFO: Maria Joyce, Chief Financial Officer
CMO: David K. Henderson, M.D., Deputy Director Clinical Care
CIO: Jon W. McKeeby, Chief Information Officer
CHR: Bonnie Tuman, Chief Human Resources
Web address: www.clinicalcenter.nih.gov
Control: Public Health Service, Government, federal **Service:** Other specialty

Staffed Beds: 234 **Admissions:** 5825 **Census:** 140 **Outpatient Visits:** 90889 **Births:** 0 **Total Expense ($000):** 344535 **Payroll Expense ($000):** 135805 **Personnel:** 1779

Many Facility Codes have changed. Please refer to the AHA Guide Code Chart.

★ **NATIONAL NAVAL MEDICAL CENTER**, 8901 Wisconsin Avenue, Zip 20889–5600; tel. 301/295–5800, (Nonreporting) **A**1 2 3 5 9 **S** Bureau of Medicine and Surgery, Department of the Navy
Primary Contact: Rear Admiral Richard Jeffries, Commanding Officer
CFO: Joseph Pickel, Director Resource Management
CIO: Lieutenant Colonel Cayetano Thornton, Chief Information Officer
Web address: www.bethesda.med.navy.mil
Control: Navy, Government, federal **Service:** General Medical and Surgical

Staffed Beds: 240

★ **SUBURBAN HOSPITAL HEALTHCARE SYSTEM (210022)**, 8600 Old Georgetown Road, Zip 20814–1497; tel. 301/896–3100 **A**1 2 3 5 9 10 **F**3 4 5 11 15 17 18 20 22 24 25 26 27 30 31 32 33 34 35 36 37 38 40 41 43 44 49 50 51 52 55 56 57 58 60 61 62 66 68 73 75 76 77 78 79 80 81 82 84 86 87 88 89 90 91 92 93 94 95 96 97 100 102 103 107 108 109 111 118 119 121 123 124 135 136 **P**4
Primary Contact: Brian A. Gragnolati, FACHE, President and Chief Executive Officer
COO: Gene A. Corapi, Senior Vice President Operations
CFO: Marty Basso, Senior Vice President Finance and Treasurer
CMO: Eugene R. Passamani, M.D., Senior Vice President Medical Affairs
CIO: Christopher T. Timbers, Vice President Medical Information Systems
CHR: Dennis Parnell, Senior Vice President Human Resources
Web address: www.suburbanhospital.org
Control: Other not–for–profit (including NFP Corporation) **Service:** General Medical and Surgical

Staffed Beds: 227 **Admissions:** 14204 **Census:** 166 **Outpatient Visits:** 130650 **Births:** 0 **Total Expense ($000):** 199415 **Payroll Expense ($000):** 88681 **Personnel:** 1427

CAMBRIDGE—Dorchester County

★ **DORCHESTER GENERAL HOSPITAL**, 300 Byrn Street, Zip 21613–1908; tel. 410/228–5511 **A**1 9 **F**3 11 15 24 25 26 27 30 32 37 38 43 55 57 62 68 72 73 75 76 77 79 80 82 86 88 89 90 92 93 94 95 96 97 100 102 106 107 119 121 **S** Shore Health System
Primary Contact: Joseph P. Ross, President and Chief Executive Officer
COO: Gerard M. Walsh, Senior Vice President and Chief Operating Officer
CFO: Deidra S. Bell, Senior Vice President and Chief Financial Officer
CMO: Michael Tooke, M.D., Vice President Medical Affairs
CIO: Tara Newman–Bell, Chief Information Officer
CHR: Michael Zimmerman, Vice President Human Resources
Web address: www.shorehealth.org
Control: Other not–for–profit (including NFP Corporation) **Service:** General Medical and Surgical

Staffed Beds: 46 **Admissions:** 3388 **Census:** 36 **Outpatient Visits:** 76419 **Births:** 0 **Total Expense ($000):** 37135 **Payroll Expense ($000):** 17606 **Personnel:** 234

□ **EASTERN SHORE HOSPITAL CENTER (214002)**, 5262 Woods Road, Zip 21613, Mailing Address: P.O. Box 800, Zip 21613–0800; tel. 410/221–2525 **A**1 9 10 **F**30 31 32 88 90 91 93 119 135 **P**6
Primary Contact: Mary Kay Noren, Superintendent
COO: Randy L. Bradford, Assistant Superintendent
CMO: David Pytlewski, M.D., Clinical Director
CHR: Cassandra Stanley, Director Personnel
Web address: www.dhmh.state.md.us/eshc
Control: State–Government, nonfederal **Service:** Psychiatric

Staffed Beds: 80 **Admissions:** 107 **Census:** 77 **Total Expense ($000):** 18393 **Payroll Expense ($000):** 9910 **Personnel:** 199

CHESTERTOWN—Kent County

★ **CHESTER RIVER HOSPITAL CENTER (210030)**, 100 Brown Street, Zip 21620–1499; tel. 410/778–3300, (Nonreporting) **A**1 9 10
Primary Contact: William R. Kirk, Jr., President and Chief Executive Officer
COO: Scott D. Burleson, Executive Vice President
CFO: Terry Weaver, Vice President Finance and Chief Financial Officer
CIO: Allison Trumpy, Information Technology Director
CHR: Beverly Churchill, Vice President Human Resources
Web address: www.chesterriverhealth.org
Control: Other not–for–profit (including NFP Corporation) **Service:** General Medical and Surgical

Staffed Beds: 57

□ **UPPER SHORE COMMUNITY MENTAL HEALTH CENTER (214019)**, Scheeler Road, Zip 21620–1031, Mailing Address: P.O. Box 229, Zip 21620–0229; tel. 410/778–6800 **A**1 9 10 **F**11 30 31 32 43 88 90 91 92 119 121 124 135
Primary Contact: Mary Kay Noren, Chief Executive Officer
COO: Randy L. Bradford, Chief Operating Officer
CFO: Randy L. Bradford, Chief Operating Officer
CMO: David Pytlewski, M.D., Clinical Director
CIO: Lisa Jones, Chief Health Information Services
CHR: Cassandra Stanley, Director Personnel
Control: State–Government, nonfederal **Service:** Psychiatric

Staffed Beds: 40 **Admissions:** 210 **Census:** 38 **Outpatient Visits:** 0 **Births:** 0 **Total Expense ($000):** 8663 **Payroll Expense ($000):** 4746 **Personnel:** 91

MD

CHEVERLY—Prince George's County

□ **GLADYS SPELLMAN SPECIALTY HOSPITAL AND NURSING CENTER**, 2900 Mercy Lane, Zip 20785–1157; tel. 301/618–2010, (Nonreporting) **A**1
Primary Contact: Stewart R. Seitz, Chief Executive Officer
CFO: Robert Eiring, Chief Financial Officer
CMO: Paul A. Devore, M.D., Medical Director
CIO: Hank Schonzeit, Chief Information Officer
CHR: Frank Venuto, Vice President Human Resources
Web address: www.dimensionshealth.org
Control: Corporation, Investor–owned, for–profit **Service:** Chronic disease

Staffed Beds: 30

□ **PRINCE GEORGE'S HOSPITAL CENTER (210003)**, 3001 Hospital Drive, Zip 20785–1189; tel. 301/618–2000, (Total facility includes 107 beds in nursing home–type unit) **A**1 3 5 9 10 **F**1 3 11 13 14 15 17 18 20 22 24 25 26 27 30 31 32 33 36 38 39 40 43 44 45 46 49 50 53 54 55 56 57 59 60 62 63 64 66 68 70 72 73 74 75 76 77 79 80 81 82 84 86 87 88 90 91 92 94 95 96 97 106 107 114 117 119 121 123 124 133 135 136 137 **P**6 **S** Dimensions Healthcare System
Primary Contact: John A. O'Brien, FACHE, President
CFO: Neil Moore, Chief Financial Officer
CMO: David Goldman, Vice President Medical Affairs and Education
CIO: Dennis Lilik, Chief Information Officer
CHR: Michael Jacobs, Interim Vice President Human Resources
Web address: www.princegeorgeshospital.org
Control: Other not–for–profit (including NFP Corporation) **Service:** General Medical and Surgical

Staffed Beds: 395 **Admissions:** 14382 **Census:** 278 **Outpatient Visits:** 89423 **Births:** 2728 **Total Expense ($000):** 219638 **Payroll Expense ($000):** 97456 **Personnel:** 1478

CLINTON—Prince George's County

★ **SOUTHERN MARYLAND HOSPITAL CENTER (210054)**, 7503 Surratts Road, Zip 20735–3397; tel. 301/868–8000, (Total facility includes 24 beds in nursing home–type unit) **A**1 2 9 10 **F**3 8 13 17 18 20 24 25 26 27 28 30 31 32 33 34 35 38 43 46 47 48 49 50 55 56 57 58 62 63 66 68 69 71 72 73 74 75 76 77 79 80 81 82 84 86 88 89 90 91 92 93 95 96 97 102 103 106 107 117 118 119 121 124 134 135 137 **P**6
Primary Contact: Francis P. Chiaramonte, M.D., President and Chairman
COO: Patricia I. Christensen, Chief Operating Officer
CFO: Charles R. Stewart, Vice President Business, Finance and Corporate Compliance
CMO: Ronald Bortnick, M.D., Vice President Medical Affairs
CIO: Lou Mavromatis, Vice President Data Processing
CHR: Paul Zeller, Vice President Human Resources
Web address: www.smhchealth.org
Control: Corporation, Investor–owned, for–profit **Service:** General Medical and Surgical

Staffed Beds: 306 **Admissions:** 17782 **Census:** 198 **Outpatient Visits:** 88802 **Births:** 1791 **Total Expense ($000):** 187877 **Payroll Expense ($000):** 69699 **Personnel:** 1374

Hospital, Medicare Provider Number, Address, Telephone, Approval, Facility, and Physician Codes, Health Care System
★ American Hospital Association (AHA) membership
□ The Joint Commission accreditation
○ American Osteopathic Association (AOA) accreditation
△ Commission on Accreditation of Rehabilitation Facilities (CARF) accreditation

COLUMBIA—Howard County

★ **HOWARD COUNTY GENERAL HOSPITAL (210048)**, 5755 Cedar Lane, Zip 21044–2999; tel. 410/740–7890 **A**1 2 5 9 10 **F**3 8 11 13 15 18 20 24 25 26 27 28 31 32 33 37 38 41 46 49 50 51 55 56 57 59 60 62 63 66 68 70 72 73 74 75 76 77 78 79 80 81 82 84 86 88 89 90 91 92 93 96 97 100 102 103 107 114 118 119 120 121 124 135 136 137 **S** Johns Hopkins Health System
Primary Contact: Victor A. Broccolino, President and Chief Executive Officer
COO: Jay H. Blackman, Senior Vice President and Chief Operating Officer
CFO: James Young, Senior Vice President Finance and Chief Financial Officer
CIO: Rick Edwards, Director Information Systems
CHR: Dorothy Brillantes, Senior Vice President Human Resources
Web address: www.hcgh.org
Control: Other not–for–profit (including NFP Corporation) **Service:** General Medical and Surgical

Staffed Beds: 203 **Admissions:** 13799 **Census:** 155 **Outpatient Visits:** 131716 **Births:** 2853 **Total Expense ($000):** 166170 **Payroll Expense ($000):** 62512 **Personnel:** 1211

CRISFIELD—Somerset County

☐ **MCCREADY HEALTH SERVICES FOUNDATION (210045)**, 201 Hall Highway, Zip 21817–1299; tel. 410/968–1200, (Total facility includes 76 beds in nursing home–type unit) **A**1 9 10 **F**11 15 24 28 33 34 36 38 43 46 52 53 54 55 56 57 61 62 66 73 75 77 79 81 86 96 97 100 107 119 120 122 124 132 135 **P**6
Primary Contact: Charles F. Pinkerman, Chief Executive Officer
CFO: David Tawes, Chief Financial Officer
Web address: www.mccreadyfoundation.org
Control: Other not–for–profit (including NFP Corporation) **Service:** General Medical and Surgical

Staffed Beds: 89 **Admissions:** 756 **Census:** 82 **Outpatient Visits:** 30909 **Births:** 0 **Total Expense ($000):** 17973 **Payroll Expense ($000):** 8684 **Personnel:** 239

CUMBERLAND—Allegany County

★ △ **MEMORIAL HOSPITAL AND MEDICAL CENTER OF CUMBERLAND (210025)**, 600 Memorial Avenue, Zip 21502–3797; tel. 301/723–4000 **A**1 2 7 9 10 **F**3 11 13 14 18 25 26 30 31 32 33 36 38 40 41 42 43 44 50 53 54 55 56 57 59 61 62 67 68 71 72 73 74 75 77 78 79 80 81 82 84 85 86 90 92 93 96 97 102 106 107 118 119 121 124 133 135 137 **P**6 **S** Western Maryland Health System
Primary Contact: Thomas C. Dowdell, FACHE, Senior Vice President and Chief Operating Officer
COO: Thomas C. Dowdell, FACHE, Senior Vice President and Chief Operating Officer
CFO: Kimberly S. Repac, Senior Vice President and Chief Financial Officer
CMO: James M. Raver, M.D., Senior Vice President Medical Affairs
CIO: William Byers, Director Information Systems
CHR: Mark J. Sullivan, Vice President Human Resources
Web address: www.wmhs.com
Control: Other not–for–profit (including NFP Corporation) **Service:** General Medical and Surgical

Staffed Beds: 151 **Admissions:** 7744 **Census:** 90 **Outpatient Visits:** 223667 **Births:** 975 **Total Expense ($000):** 98066 **Payroll Expense ($000):** 40100 **Personnel:** 850

☐ **THOMAS B. FINAN CENTER (214012)**, 10102 Country Club Road S.E., Zip 21502–8339, Mailing Address: P.O. Box 1722, Zip 21501–1722; tel. 301/777–2240, (Nonreporting) **A**1 9 10
Primary Contact: Judith Hott, Chief Executive Officer
CFO: Craig Alexander, Fiscal Specialist
CMO: Linda de Hoyos, Clinical Director
Web address: www.dhmh.state.md.us
Control: State–Government, nonfederal **Service:** Psychiatric

Staffed Beds: 80

★ **WMHS BRADDOCK HOSPITAL (210027)**, 900 Seton Drive, Zip 21502–1874; tel. 301/723–4200, (Total facility includes 88 beds in nursing home–type unit) **A**1 2 9 10 **F**2 3 5 11 14 15 17 18 20 22 25 26 27 30 31 32 33 36 38 41 43 44 50 51 53 54 55 56 57 59 62 67 68 72 73 75 76 77 78 79 80 81 82 87 88 90 92 93 94 96 97 99 100 102 103 104 105 106 107 108 109 110 111 117 119 121 133 135 **P**6 **S** Western Maryland Health System
Primary Contact: Thomas C. Dowdell, FACHE, Senior Vice President and Chief Operating Officer
COO: Thomas C. Dowdell, FACHE, Senior Vice President and Chief Operating Officer
CFO: Kimberly S. Repac, Senior Vice President and Chief Financial Officer
CMO: James M. Raver, M.D., Senior Vice President Medical Affairs
CIO: William Byers, Director Information Systems
CHR: Mark J. Sullivan, Vice President Human Resources
Web address: www.wmhs.com
Control: Other not–for–profit (including NFP Corporation) **Service:** General Medical and Surgical

Staffed Beds: 256 **Admissions:** 9915 **Census:** 206 **Outpatient Visits:** 103847 **Births:** 0 **Total Expense ($000):** 134204 **Payroll Expense ($000):** 50657 **Personnel:** 1060

EAST NEW MARKET—Dorchester County

WARWICK MANOR BEHAVIORAL HEALTH, 3680 Warwick Road, Zip 21631–1420; tel. 410/943–8108, (Nonreporting) **A**9
Primary Contact: Marie McBee, Chief Executive Officer
Control: Corporation, Investor–owned, for–profit **Service:** Alcoholism and other chemical dependency

Staffed Beds: 42

EASTON—Talbot County

★ **MEMORIAL HOSPITAL AT EASTON MARYLAND (210037)**, 219 South Washington Street, Zip 21601–2996; tel. 410/822–1000 **A**1 9 10 **F**3 11 13 15 18 24 25 26 27 30 35 37 38 43 44 45 49 53 55 56 57 58 59 61 62 63 68 72 73 74 76 77 79 81 82 84 85 86 90 92 96 97 100 102 104 105 106 107 108 109 111 112 118 119 121 133 136 137 **P**3 **S** Shore Health System
Primary Contact: Joseph P. Ross, President and Chief Executive Officer
COO: Gerard M. Walsh, Senior Vice President and Chief Operating Officer
CFO: Walter Zajac, Senior Vice President and Chief Financial Officer
CMO: Chris Galan, M.D., Chief Medical Staff
CIO: Tara Newman–Bell, Chief Information Officer
CHR: Michael Zimmerman, Vice President Human Resources
Web address: www.shorehealth.org
Control: Other not–for–profit (including NFP Corporation) **Service:** General Medical and Surgical

Staffed Beds: 123 **Admissions:** 9222 **Census:** 90 **Outpatient Visits:** 207114 **Births:** 1124 **Total Expense ($000):** 125644 **Payroll Expense ($000):** 55410 **Personnel:** 1066

ELKTON—Cecil County

★ **UNION HOSPITAL (210032)**, 106 Bow Street, Zip 21921–5596; tel. 410/398–4000 **A**1 2 9 10 **F**2 3 11 13 15 25 26 27 30 31 32 33 38 41 42 43 44 46 49 50 51 53 55 56 57 60 62 67 68 72 73 74 75 76 77 79 80 81 82 84 87 88 92 94 95 96 97 100 102 106 107 118 119 120 121 124 135 136 **P**6
Primary Contact: Kenneth S. Lewis, M.D., J.D., President and Chief Executive Officer
COO: David Gipson, Senior Vice President and Chief Clinical Operations Officer
CFO: Laurie Beyer, Senior Vice President and Chief Financial Officer
CMO: Jose Ma, M.D., Vice President Medical Affairs
CIO: Mary Jane Kamps, Chief Information Officer
CHR: Peter Gloggner, Vice President Human Resources
Web address: www.uhcc.com
Control: Other not–for–profit (including NFP Corporation) **Service:** General Medical and Surgical

Staffed Beds: 118 **Admissions:** 7888 **Census:** 76 **Outpatient Visits:** 145037 **Births:** 706 **Total Expense ($000):** 93912 **Payroll Expense ($000):** 38242 **Personnel:** 790

ELLICOTT CITY—Howard County

TAYLOR MANOR HOSPITAL See Sheppard and Enoch Pratt Hospital, Baltimore

EMMITSBURG—Frederick County

MOUNTAIN MANOR TREATMENT CENTER, Route 15, Zip 21727, Mailing Address: Box 136, Zip 21727; tel. 301/447–2361, (Nonreporting)
Primary Contact: William J. Roby, Executive Vice President
CFO: Susan Liedlich, Director Finance
CHR: Craig Cutter, Corporate Director Human Resources
Control: Corporation, Investor–owned, for–profit **Service:** Alcoholism and other chemical dependency

Staffed Beds: 140

FORT WASHINGTON—Prince George's County

★ **FORT WASHINGTON MEDICAL CENTER (210060)**, 11711 Livingston Road, Zip 20744–5164; tel. 301/292–7000 **A**1 9 10 **F**3 15 25 31 33 38 56 68 75 77 78 79 80 85 97 102 119
Primary Contact: Paul E. Porter, Chief Executive Officer
COO: Donald C. Brown, Vice President, Corporate Operations
CFO: Joseph B. Tucker, Senior Vice President and Chief Financial Officer
CMO: Patrick Daly, President Medical Staff
CIO: Fred Ashby, Director Information Technology
CHR: Jane Tinsley, Corporate Director Human Resources
Web address: www.fortwashingtonmc.org
Control: Other not–for–profit (including NFP Corporation) **Service:** General Medical and Surgical

Staffed Beds: 37 **Admissions:** 2961 **Census:** 30 **Outpatient Visits:** 41639 **Births:** 0 **Total Expense ($000):** 36316 **Payroll Expense ($000):** 16412 **Personnel:** 192

Many Facility Codes have changed. Please refer to the AHA Guide Code Chart.

FREDERICK—Frederick County

★ **FREDERICK MEMORIAL HOSPITAL (210005)**, 400 West Seventh Street, Zip 21701–4593; tel. 240/566–3300, (Total facility includes 20 beds in nursing home–type unit) **A**1 2 9 10 **F**3 7 8 11 13 15 18 24 25 26 27 28 30 31 32 33 34 36 37 38 41 42 44 46 48 49 50 51 52 53 55 56 57 59 60 61 62 66 68 69 71 72 73 74 75 76 77 79 80 81 82 84 86 87 88 90 91 92 93 94 95 96 97 99 100 102 103 104 105 106 107 109 111 112 117 118 119 120 121 124 132 133 135 136 137 **P**6 7
Primary Contact: Thomas A. Kleinhanzl, President and Chief Executive Officer
COO: John R. Verbus, Senior Vice President and Chief Operations Officer
CFO: Michelle K. Mahan, Senior Vice President and Chief Financial Officer
CMO: Manuel Casiano, M.D., Vice President Medical Affairs
CIO: David Quirke, Vice President Information Services
CHR: Terry O'Malley, Vice President Human Resources
Web address: www.fmh.org
Control: Other not–for–profit (including NFP Corporation) **Service:** General Medical and Surgical

Staffed Beds: 219 **Admissions:** 17361 **Census:** 202 **Outpatient Visits:** 381382 **Births:** 2601 **Total Expense ($000):** 251314 **Payroll Expense ($000):** 105851 **Personnel:** 1923

GLEN BURNIE—Anne Arundel County

★ **BALTIMORE WASHINGTON MEDICAL CENTER (210043)**, 301 Hospital Drive, Zip 21061–5899; tel. 410/787–4000 **A**1 2 9 10 **F**3 11 15 17 18 20 24 25 26 27 31 32 33 37 38 48 49 54 55 56 57 59 62 66 68 72 73 75 76 77 79 80 81 84 86 88 90 92 93 94 95 96 100 102 104 105 107 109 111 112 114 118 119 120 121 132 135 136 137 **P**6 **S** University of Maryland Medical System
Primary Contact: James R. Walker, FACHE, President and Chief Executive Officer
COO: Karen Olscamp, Chief Operating Officer
CFO: Al Pietsch, CPA, Vice President Finance
CMO: Lawrence Linder, M.D., Senior Vice President and Chief Medical Officer
CIO: David Peterson, Chief Information Officer
CHR: Patricia Loughlin, Director Human Resources
Web address: www.bwmc.umms.org
Control: Other not–for–profit (including NFP Corporation) **Service:** General Medical and Surgical

Staffed Beds: 277 **Admissions:** 18247 **Census:** 206 **Outpatient Visits:** 101582 **Births:** 15 **Total Expense ($000):** 226351 **Payroll Expense ($000):** 101628 **Personnel:** 2021

HAGERSTOWN—Washington County

BROOK LANE HEALTH SERVICES (214003), 13218 Brook Lane Drive, Zip 21742–1945, Mailing Address: P.O. Box 1945, Zip 21742–1945; tel. 301/733–0330 **A**9 10 **F**5 26 30 31 32 54 66 88 89 90 91 93 94 95 119 135 **P**4 6
Primary Contact: R. Lynn Rushing, Chief Executive Officer
CFO: Floyd Klauka, Chief Financial Officer
CIO: Sharon Gladfelter, Health Information Officer
CHR: Patricia Bourdeau, Director Human Resources
Web address: www.brooklane.org
Control: Other not–for–profit (including NFP Corporation) **Service:** Psychiatric

Staffed Beds: 44 **Admissions:** 1322 **Census:** 28 **Outpatient Visits:** 15743 **Births:** 0 **Total Expense ($000):** 15801 **Payroll Expense ($000):** 10112 **Personnel:** 278

★ △ **WASHINGTON COUNTY HEALTH SYSTEM (210001)**, 251 East Antietam Street, Zip 21740–5771; tel. 301/790–8000 **A**1 2 7 9 10 **F**3 5 11 12 13 15 17 18 24 25 26 27 30 31 32 33 36 38 40 41 43 44 45 49 51 53 54 55 56 57 58 59 60 61 62 63 66 68 72 73 74 75 76 77 79 80 81 82 84 85 86 87 88 89 90 91 92 93 94 95 96 97 100 102 103 106 107 109 111 113 119 120 121 124 132 133 134 135 136 137 **P**6 8
Primary Contact: James P. Hamill, President and Chief Executive Officer
CFO: Raymond A. Grahe, Vice President Finance
CMO: Robert L. Brooks, M.D., Vice President Medical Affairs
CIO: Carey O. Leverett, Vice President Information Services
Web address: www.wchsys.org
Control: Other not–for–profit (including NFP Corporation) **Service:** General Medical and Surgical

Staffed Beds: 300 **Admissions:** 16270 **Census:** 201 **Outpatient Visits:** 207598 **Births:** 2034 **Total Expense ($000):** 203387 **Payroll Expense ($000):** 90076 **Personnel:** 1712

□ **WESTERN MARYLAND CENTER (212002)**, 1500 Pennsylvania Avenue, Zip 21742–3194; tel. 301/791–4400, (Total facility includes 60 beds in nursing home–type unit) (Nonreporting) **A**1 9 10
Primary Contact: Cynthia Miller Pellegrino, Director and Chief Executive Officer
CFO: David Davis, Assistant Superintendent and Chief Financial Officer
CMO: Rose M. Chan–Sri, M.D., Chief of Staff
CIO: Ron Keplinger, Chief Information Officer
Web address: www.wc–link.org/wmhc/caring.htm
Control: State–Government, nonfederal **Service:** Long–Term Acute Care hospital

Staffed Beds: 120

HAVRE DE GRACE—Harford County

★ **HARFORD MEMORIAL HOSPITAL (210006)**, 501 South Union Avenue, Zip 21078–3493; tel. 443/843–5000, (Total facility includes 17 beds in nursing home–type unit) **A**1 9 10 **F**12 15 25 26 31 32 33 34 38 44 45 51 55 57 59 62 68 69 72 73 75 76 77 79 82 86 88 92 96 97 100 107 117 118 119 121 135 137 **S** Upper Chesapeake Health System
Primary Contact: Lyle Ernest Sheldon, FACHE, President and Chief Executive Officer
COO: Kenneth Kozel, Senior Vice President and Chief Operating Officer
CFO: Joseph E. Hoffman, Senior Vice President and Chief Financial Officer
CMO: Peggy Vaughan, M.D., Senior Vice President Medical Affairs
CIO: Rick Casteel, Vice President Management Information Systems and Chief Information Officer
CHR: Toni Shivery, Vice President Human Resources
Web address: www.uchs.org
Control: Other not–for–profit (including NFP Corporation) **Service:** General Medical and Surgical

Staffed Beds: 108 **Admissions:** 7251 **Census:** 85 **Outpatient Visits:** 82993 **Births:** 0 **Total Expense ($000):** 67579 **Payroll Expense ($000):** 30729 **Personnel:** 614

JESSUP—Anne Arundel County

□ **CLIFTON T. PERKINS HOSPITAL CENTER**, 8450 Dorsey Run Road, Zip 20794–9414; tel. 410/724–3000, (Nonreporting) **A**1 3 5
Primary Contact: Sheilah Davenport, J.D., M.S., RN, Chief Executive Officer and Superintendent
COO: Steve Mason, Assistant Superintendent and Chief Operating Officer
CFO: George Parnel, Chief Financial Officer
CMO: Muhammed Ajanah, M.D., Clinical Director
CIO: Chanda Hamilton, Chief Information Officer
CHR: Michael Faulkner, Director Human Resources
Web address: www.dhmh.state.md.us/perkins/
Control: State–Government, nonfederal **Service:** Psychiatric

Staffed Beds: 215

LA PLATA—Charles County

★ **CIVISTA HEALTH (210035)**, 5 Garrett Avenue, Zip 20646–1070, Mailing Address: P.O. Box 1070, Zip 20646–1070; tel. 301/609–4000 **A**1 2 9 10 **F**3 8 11 13 15 17 18 20 24 25 26 27 30 31 32 33 34 38 43 46 49 50 51 53 55 56 57 59 62 68 72 74 75 76 77 79 80 81 82 84 86 87 96 97 98 100 102 103 106 107 119 121 134 135 136 137
Primary Contact: Christine M. Stefanides, FACHE, President and Chief Executive Officer
COO: Gary J. Herbek, Chief Operating Officer
CFO: Mickey Slade, Vice President Finance and Chief Financial Officer
CMO: Sanjeeb Mishra, M.D., Chief of Staff
CIO: Kevin Burbules, Chief Information Officer
CHR: Stacey Cook, Director Human Resources
Web address: www.civista.org
Control: Other not–for–profit (including NFP Corporation) **Service:** General Medical and Surgical

Staffed Beds: 127 **Admissions:** 7666 **Census:** 89 **Outpatient Visits:** 39894 **Births:** 887 **Total Expense ($000):** 85152 **Payroll Expense ($000):** 33501 **Personnel:** 669

MD

Hospital, Medicare Provider Number, Address, Telephone, Approval, Facility, and Physician Codes, Health Care System
★ American Hospital Association (AHA) membership
□ The Joint Commission accreditation
○ American Osteopathic Association (AOA) accreditation
△ Commission on Accreditation of Rehabilitation Facilities (CARF) accreditation

MD

LANHAM—Prince George's County

DOCTORS COMMUNITY HOSPITAL (210051), 8118 Good Luck Road, Zip 20706–3596; tel. 301/552–8118 **A**1 9 10 **F**3 11 17 18 20 24 25 26 27 30 32 33 38 40 43 46 47 49 55 56 57 58 61 68 72 73 75 76 77 79 80 81 86 96 97 100 106 107 112 118 119 121 133 135 136 137
Primary Contact: Philip B. Down, President and Chief Executive Officer
COO: Thomas J. Crowley, Executive Vice President
CFO: Dennis P. Scanlon, Vice President Finance
CMO: Gabriel Jaffe, M.D., Vice President Medical Affairs
CIO: Alan Johnson, Chief Information Officer
CHR: Charlene Lundgren, Vice President
Web address: www.dchweb.org
Control: Other not–for–profit (including NFP Corporation) **Service:** General Medical and Surgical

Staffed Beds: 186 **Admissions:** 11888 **Census:** 138 **Outpatient Visits:** 91431 **Births:** 0 **Total Expense ($000):** 143010 **Payroll Expense ($000):** 59349 **Personnel:** 1055

LAUREL—Prince George's County

□ △ **LAUREL REGIONAL HOSPITAL (210055)**, 7300 Van Dusen Road, Zip 20707–9266; tel. 301/725–4300 **A**1 7 9 10 **F**3 8 11 13 15 25 27 31 33 38 42 50 52 55 57 59 68 72 74 75 77 78 79 80 82 85 86 88 90 92 95 96 97 99 106 107 118 119 121 124 135 **S** Dimensions Healthcare System
Primary Contact: Douglas Shepherd, FACHE, President
CFO: Neil Moore, Chief Financial Officer
CIO: Dennis Lilik, Chief Information Officer
Web address: www.laurelregionalhospital.org
Control: Other not–for–profit (including NFP Corporation) **Service:** General Medical and Surgical

Staffed Beds: 124 **Admissions:** 6590 **Census:** 80 **Outpatient Visits:** 39932 **Births:** 596 **Total Expense ($000):** 79156 **Payroll Expense ($000):** 39558 **Personnel:** 481

LEONARDTOWN—St. Marys County

ST. MARY'S HOSPITAL (210028), 25500 Point Lookout Road, Zip 20650–0527, Mailing Address: P.O. Box 527, Zip 20650–0527; tel. 301/475–6001 **A**1 2 9 10 **F**2 3 5 8 11 13 15 25 26 27 28 30 31 32 33 34 37 38 41 42 43 44 50 51 53 54 55 56 57 59 62 63 66 68 69 72 73 74 75 76 77 79 80 81 82 84 86 88 92 94 95 97 100 102 106 107 118 119 121 124 133 135 136 137 **P**6
Primary Contact: Christine R. Wray, President and Chief Executive Officer
CFO: Paul M. Barber, Vice President Finance
CIO: Donald Sirk, Director Information Systems
CHR: Barbara Hendricks, Director Human Resources
Web address: www.smhwecare.com
Control: Other not–for–profit (including NFP Corporation) **Service:** General Medical and Surgical

Staffed Beds: 110 **Admissions:** 9254 **Census:** 77 **Outpatient Visits:** 145371 **Births:** 1074 **Total Expense ($000):** 91381 **Payroll Expense ($000):** 41923 **Personnel:** 833

OAKLAND—Garrett County

GARRETT COUNTY MEMORIAL HOSPITAL (210017), 251 North Fourth Street, Zip 21550–1398; tel. 301/533–4000, (Total facility includes 10 beds in nursing home–type unit) **A**1 9 10 **F**3 11 13 15 24 25 26 27 28 30 31 32 33 36 38 43 54 55 56 57 63 68 72 73 76 77 79 80 82 92 96 97 98 100 102 106 107 117 119 135 136 **P**8
Primary Contact: Donald P. Battista, President and Chief Executive Officer
CFO: Tracy Lipscomb, Vice President Financial Services and Chief Financial Officer
CIO: Sandy Swanson, Director Information System
CHR: Annette Livengood, Vice President Human Resources
Web address: www.gcmh.com
Control: Other not–for–profit (including NFP Corporation) **Service:** General Medical and Surgical

Staffed Beds: 55 **Admissions:** 2747 **Census:** 25 **Outpatient Visits:** 71657 **Births:** 300 **Total Expense ($000):** 31249 **Payroll Expense ($000):** 13906 **Personnel:** 302

OLNEY—Montgomery County

MONTGOMERY GENERAL HOSPITAL (210018), 18101 Prince Philip Drive, Zip 20832–1512; tel. 301/774–8882 **A**1 2 9 10 **F**3 5 11 13 18 24 25 26 27 30 31 32 33 36 38 44 46 48 49 50 51 54 55 56 57 61 63 68 72 73 74 75 76 77 78 79 80 81 84 86 88 89 90 92 93 94 95 96 97 103 106 107 114 118 119 121 123 124 132 135 **S** MedStar Health
Primary Contact: Peter W. Monge, President
CFO: John F. Hogarty, Chief Financial Officer
CMO: Roger Leonard, M.D., Vice President Medical Affairs
CHR: Kevin Mell, Vice President Human Resources
Web address: www.montgomerygeneral.com
Control: Other not–for–profit (including NFP Corporation) **Service:** General Medical and Surgical

Staffed Beds: 149 **Admissions:** 9635 **Census:** 110 **Outpatient Visits:** 51679 **Births:** 649 **Total Expense ($000):** 102678 **Payroll Expense ($000):** 43851 **Personnel:** 660

PERRY POINT—Cecil County

VETERANS AFFAIRS MARYLAND HEALTH CARE SYSTEM–PERRY POINT DIVISION See Veterans Affairs Maryland Health Care System–Baltimore Division, Baltimore

PRINCE FREDERICK—Calvert County

CALVERT MEMORIAL HOSPITAL (210039), 100 Hospital Road, Zip 20678–9675; tel. 410/535–4000, (Total facility includes 18 beds in nursing home–type unit) **A**1 2 9 10 **F**3 8 11 13 15 18 24 25 26 27 28 29 30 31 32 33 34 36 38 43 44 50 52 53 55 56 57 61 62 66 68 72 73 74 75 76 77 79 80 81 82 84 86 88 89 91 92 95 96 97 100 102 106 107 118 119 120 121 123 124 133 135 137 **P**4
Primary Contact: James J. Xinis, President and Chief Executive Officer
CFO: Kirk Blandford, Vice President Finance
CMO: Emad Albanna, M.D., Chief of Staff
CIO: Ed Grogan, Vice President Information Services and Chief Information Officer
CHR: Carrie Forrest, Vice President Human Resources
Web address: www.calverthospital.com
Control: Other not–for–profit (including NFP Corporation) **Service:** General Medical and Surgical

Staffed Beds: 138 **Admissions:** 8432 **Census:** 89 **Outpatient Visits:** 122711 **Births:** 978 **Total Expense ($000):** 93947 **Payroll Expense ($000):** 41943 **Personnel:** 789

RANDALLSTOWN—Baltimore County

NORTHWEST HOSPITAL CENTER (210040), 5401 Old Court Road, Zip 21133–5185; tel. 410/521–2200, (Total facility includes 24 beds in nursing home–type unit) **A**1 2 9 10 **F**3 11 14 15 18 25 26 27 30 31 32 33 36 38 42 43 44 45 49 50 51 54 55 56 57 58 59 62 63 66 68 72 73 75 76 77 78 79 80 82 86 88 90 92 96 97 99 100 102 103 107 117 118 119 121 124 135 137 **S** LifeBridge Health
Primary Contact: Erik G. Wexler, President and Chief Operating Officer
CFO: David Krajewski, Vice President Finance
CMO: Ronald L. Ginsberg, Vice President Medical Affairs
CIO: Karen Barker, Vice President and Chief Information Officer
CHR: Mark Ostrowski, Director Human Resources
Web address: www.lifebridgehealth.org
Control: Other not–for–profit (including NFP Corporation) **Service:** General Medical and Surgical

Staffed Beds: 230 **Admissions:** 13899 **Census:** 176 **Outpatient Visits:** 84628 **Births:** 0 **Total Expense ($000):** 161166 **Payroll Expense ($000):** 66440 **Personnel:** 1221

ROCKVILLE—Montgomery County

△ **ADVENTIST REHABILITATION HOSPITAL OF MARYLAND (213029)**, 9909 Medical Center Drive, Zip 20850; tel. 240/864–6000 **A**1 7 9 10 **F**3 25 26 30 33 53 56 62 85 86 119 121 124 135 **P**6 **S** Adventist HealthCare
Primary Contact: Doris B. Reinhart, Vice President and Administrator
COO: Doris B. Reinhart, Vice President and Administrator
CFO: Val C. Daniels, Chief Financial Officer
CMO: Terrence P. Sheehan, M.D., Medical Director
CHR: Caroline Lunenfeld, Manager Human Resources
Web address: www.adventisthealthcare.com
Control: Other not–for–profit (including NFP Corporation) **Service:** Rehabilitation

Staffed Beds: 73 **Admissions:** 1570 **Census:** 50 **Outpatient Visits:** 24148 **Births:** 0 **Total Expense ($000):** 23580 **Payroll Expense ($000):** 11601 **Personnel:** 238

★ **POTOMAC RIDGE BEHAVIORAL HEALTH SYSTEM (214013)**, 14901 Broschart Road, Zip 20850–3395; tel. 301/251–4500 **A**9 10 **F**5 25 26 88 89 91 94 95 119 121 **P**5 **S** Adventist HealthCare
Primary Contact: Sako Maki, President
COO: Sako Maki, President
CMO: Steven Israel, M.D., Medical Director
CIO: Edna Bruehl, Vice President and Chief Information Officer
CHR: Mary Cloutier, Director
Web address: www.potomacridge.com
Control: Other not–for–profit (including NFP Corporation) **Service:** Psychiatric

Staffed Beds: 181 **Admissions:** 3070 **Census:** 160 **Outpatient Visits:** 3889 **Births:** 0 **Total Expense ($000):** 34880 **Payroll Expense ($000):** 19802 **Personnel:** 450

Many Facility Codes have changed. Please refer to the AHA Guide Code Chart.

★ **SHADY GROVE ADVENTIST HOSPITAL (210057)**, 9901 Medical Center Drive, Zip 20850–3395; tel. 301/279–6000 **A**1 2 9 10 **F**3 12 13 15 18 20 24 25 26 27 28 30 31 32 33 34 35 37 38 39 41 43 44 46 47 48 49 50 51 54 55 56 57 58 59 60 62 64 66 68 69 70 71 72 73 74 75 76 77 79 80 82 83 84 90 92 96 97 98 100 102 103 104 107 108 109 111 112 118 119 120 121 122 124 135 136 137 **P**3 **S** Adventist HealthCare
Primary Contact: Dennis Hansen, Interim President
COO: Dennis Hansen, President
CFO: Ronald K. Benfield, Vice President and Chief Financial Officer
CMO: Robert Eisdorfer, M.D., President Medical and Affiliate Staff
CIO: Kathleen Dyer, Vice President and Chief Information Officer
CHR: Jeff Jones, Assistant Vice President Human Resources
Web address: www.adventisthealthcare.com
Control: Church–operated, Nongovernment, not–for profit **Service:** General Medical and Surgical

Staffed Beds: 243 **Admissions:** 20330 **Census:** 207 **Outpatient Visits:** 139870 **Births:** 4720 **Total Expense ($000):** 251738 **Payroll Expense ($000):** 95024 **Personnel:** 1402

SALISBURY—Wicomico County

☐ **DEER'S HEAD HOSPITAL CENTER (212003)**, 351 Deer's Head Hospital Road, Zip 21801, Mailing Address: P.O. Box 2018, Zip 21802–2018; tel. 410/543–4000, (Total facility includes 70 beds in nursing home–type unit) **A**1 10 **F**1 3 11 24 25 26 30 31 32 41 43 44 50 54 55 57 59 60 66 73 75 80 81 82 85 86 117 119 121 135 137 **P**6
Primary Contact: Sandra K. Smith, Director and Chief Executive Officer
COO: Richard E. Keefer, Assistant Superintendent
CFO: Steven Nusbaum, Fiscal Administrator
CMO: Richard Schlottman, M.D., Acting Medical Director
CIO: Mac Beattie, Computer Network Specialist
CHR: Michael Dollinger, Personnel Administrator
Web address: www.deershead.org
Control: State–Government, nonfederal **Service:** Chronic disease

Staffed Beds: 90 **Admissions:** 249 **Census:** 81 **Outpatient Visits:** 20043 **Births:** 0 **Total Expense ($000):** 31392 **Payroll Expense ($000):** 12409 **Personnel:** 248

★ △ **HEALTHSOUTH CHESAPEAKE REHABILITATION HOSPITAL (213028)**, 220 Tilghman Road, Zip 21804–1921; tel. 410/546–4600, (Nonreporting) **A**1 7 9 10 **S** HEALTHSOUTH Corporation
Primary Contact: Gary Crowley, Chief Executive Officer
CFO: Karen Rounsley, Controller
CHR: Belinda Thompson, Coordinator Human Resources
Web address: www.healthsouth.com
Control: Corporation, Investor–owned, for–profit **Service:** Rehabilitation

Staffed Beds: 42

★ **PENINSULA REGIONAL HEALTH SYSTEM (210019)**, 100 East Carroll Street, Zip 21801–5422; tel. 410/546–6400, (Total facility includes 30 beds in nursing home–type unit) **A**1 2 9 10 **F**3 11 12 13 15 17 18 20 22 24 25 26 27 30 31 32 33 35 38 40 43 44 50 51 52 53 55 57 59 60 61 62 66 68 72 73 74 75 76 77 79 80 82 84 86 87 88 90 92 96 97 98 100 104 105 106 107 108 109 111 112 114 116 117 118 119 121 132 133 135 136 137
Primary Contact: R. Alan Newberry, President and Chief Executive Officer
COO: Peggy Naleppa, Executive Vice President and Chief Operating Officer
CFO: Bruce Ritchie, Chief Financial Officer
CMO: Conworth Dayton–Jones, M.D., President Medical Staff
CIO: Raymond Adkins, Chief Information Officer
CHR: Scott Peterson, Vice President Human Resources
Web address: www.peninsula.org
Control: Other not–for–profit (including NFP Corporation) **Service:** General Medical and Surgical

Staffed Beds: 401 **Admissions:** 21600 **Census:** 289 **Outpatient Visits:** 441422 **Births:** 2216 **Total Expense ($000):** 291565 **Payroll Expense ($000):** 117148 **Personnel:** 2378

SILVER SPRING—Montgomery County

★ **HOLY CROSS HOSPITAL (210004)**, 1500 Forest Glen Road, Zip 20910–1487; tel. 301/754–7000 **A**1 2 3 5 8 9 10 **F**2 3 11 12 13 15 17 20 25 26 27 28 30 31 32 33 34 35 38 42 43 44 46 49 50 53 54 55 56 57 58 59 61 62 64 66 68 70 72 73 74 75 76 77 79 80 81 82 84 86 87 90 96 97 100 102 103 107 114 118 119 120 121 124 133 135 136 **S** Trinity Health
Primary Contact: Kevin J. Sexton, President and Chief Executive Officer
COO: Brooks Sutton, R.N., Chief Operating Officer
CFO: Gary Vogan, Chief Financial Officer
CMO: Blair Eig, M.D., Senior Vice President Medical Affairs
CIO: Manuel Ocasio, Vice President Information Services
Web address: www.holycrosshealth.org
Control: Church–operated, Nongovernment, not–for profit **Service:** General Medical and Surgical

Staffed Beds: 425 **Admissions:** 28060 **Census:** 287 **Outpatient Visits:** 138262 **Births:** 9169 **Total Expense ($000):** 311646 **Payroll Expense ($000):** 136025 **Personnel:** 2069

SAINT LUKE INSTITUTE, 8901 New Hampshire Avenue, Zip 20903–3611; tel. 301/445–7970, (Nonreporting)
Primary Contact: Father Stephen J. Rossetti, Ph.D., President and Chief Executive Officer
COO: Sister Danile Lynch, Chief Operating Officer
Web address: www.sli.org
Control: Other not–for–profit (including NFP Corporation) **Service:** Psychiatric

Staffed Beds: 24

SYKESVILLE—Carroll County

☐ **SPRINGFIELD HOSPITAL CENTER (214004)**, 6655 Sykesville Road, Zip 21784–7966; tel. 410/970–7000 **A**1 9 10 **F**10 11 30 32 33 41 52 54 55 66 73 75 81 82 88 89 91 93 119 124 135
Primary Contact: Paula A. Langmead, Chief Executive Officer
COO: Janice Bowen, Chief Operating Officer
CFO: Dallas Snyder, Chief Financial Officer
CMO: Jonathan D. Book, M.D., Clinical Director
CIO: Dan Triplett, Director Information Technology
CHR: Gary Compher, Director Human Resources
Web address: www.dhmh.state.md.us/springfield
Control: State–Government, nonfederal **Service:** Psychiatric

Staffed Beds: 375 **Admissions:** 413 **Census:** 327 **Outpatient Visits:** 0 **Births:** 0 **Total Expense ($000):** 72836 **Payroll Expense ($000):** 41223 **Personnel:** 797

TAKOMA PARK—Montgomery County

★ △ **WASHINGTON ADVENTIST HOSPITAL (210016)**, 7600 Carroll Avenue, Zip 20912–6392; tel. 301/891–7600 **A**1 3 5 7 9 10 **F**3 5 13 15 17 18 20 22 24 25 26 27 30 31 32 38 43 44 46 49 50 59 62 63 66 68 69 72 74 75 76 77 79 80 81 82 86 88 89 90 91 92 93 94 95 96 97 100 102 103 106 107 108 109 111 118 119 121 124 135 136 137 **S** Adventist HealthCare
Primary Contact: Jere D. Stocks, President
Web address: www.adventisthealthcare.com
Control: Church–operated, Nongovernment, not–for profit **Service:** General Medical and Surgical

Staffed Beds: 210 **Admissions:** 17771 **Census:** 210 **Outpatient Visits:** 61866 **Births:** 2276 **Total Expense ($000):** 231323 **Payroll Expense ($000):** 85421 **Personnel:** 1245

TOWSON—Baltimore County

★ **ST. JOSEPH MEDICAL CENTER (210007)**, 7601 Osler Drive, Zip 21204–7582; tel. 410/337–1000, (Total facility includes 32 beds in nursing home–type unit) **A**1 2 9 10 **F**3 11 12 13 17 18 19 20 21 22 24 25 26 27 30 31 32 33 34 35 38 41 43 46 47 49 50 54 55 56 57 58 59 60 62 63 64 66 68 69 70 72 73 74 75 76 77 79 80 81 82 84 86 87 88 89 90 91 92 93 94 95 96 97 102 103 106 107 109 114 116 117 118 119 120 121 123 124 133 135 136 137 **P**6 **S** Catholic Health Initiatives
Primary Contact: John Kerr Tolmie, President and Chief Executive Officer
COO: Sylvia Moore, Executive Vice President and Chief Operating Officer
CFO: Ron Wood, Interim Vice President Finance and Chief Financial Officer
CMO: Richard Boehler, M.D., Vice President and Chief Medical Officer
CIO: David Hynson, Director Information Systems
CHR: Carmel Taibi–Lehn, Vice President People
Web address: www.sjmcmd.org
Control: Church–operated, Nongovernment, not–for profit **Service:** General Medical and Surgical

Staffed Beds: 364 **Admissions:** 24398 **Census:** 277 **Outpatient Visits:** 210483 **Births:** 2266 **Total Expense ($000):** 327371 **Payroll Expense ($000):** 130212 **Personnel:** 1787

Hospital, Medicare Provider Number, Address, Telephone, Approval, Facility, and Physician Codes, Health Care System
★ American Hospital Association (AHA) membership
☐ The Joint Commission accreditation
○ American Osteopathic Association (AOA) accreditation
△ Commission on Accreditation of Rehabilitation Facilities (CARF) accreditation

WESTMINSTER—Carroll County

★ **CARROLL HOSPITAL CENTER (210033)**, 200 Memorial Avenue, Zip 21157–5799; tel. 410/848–3000 **A**1 2 9 10 **F**3 5 8 11 13 15 18 24 25 26 27 28 30 31 32 33 34 35 36 38 41 42 43 44 49 50 51 54 55 56 57 61 62 63 68 73 74 76 77 78 79 80 81 82 84 88 89 90 91 92 93 95 96 97 103 107 118 119 121 124 135 136 137 **P**6 8
Primary Contact: John M. Sernulka, President and Chief Executive Officer
COO: Leslie Simmons, Chief Operating Officer
CFO: Kevin Kelbly, Senior Vice President Finance and Corporate Fiscal Affairs
CMO: Kevin Smothers, M.D., Senior Vice President Medical Affairs
CIO: Kim Moreau, Director Information Systems
CHR: Tracey Ellison, Assistant Vice President Human Resources
Web address: www.carrollhospitalcenter.org
Control: Other not–for–profit (including NFP Corporation) **Service:** General Medical and Surgical

Staffed Beds: 210 **Admissions:** 15926 **Census:** 155 **Outpatient Visits:** 264202 **Births:** 1249 **Total Expense ($000):** 188750 **Payroll Expense ($000):** 80040 **Personnel:** 1434

Many Facility Codes have changed. Please refer to the AHA Guide Code Chart.

MASSACHUSETTS

AMHERST—Hampshire County

UNIVERSITY HEALTH SERVICES (220172), University of Massachusetts, Box 34310, Zip 01003–4310; tel. 413/577–5000, (Nonreporting) **A**10
Primary Contact: Bernette A. Melby, Executive Director
Control: State–Government, nonfederal **Service:** Hospital unit of an institution (prison hospital, college infimary, etc.)

Staffed Beds: 6

ANDOVER—Essex County

ISHAM HEALTH CENTER, 180 Main Street, Zip 01810–4161; tel. 978/749–4455, (Nonreporting)
Primary Contact: Catherine Golas, Administrator
Web address: www.andover.edu
Control: Other not–for–profit (including NFP Corporation) **Service:** Children's other specialty

Staffed Beds: 20

ATHOL—Worcester County

□ **ATHOL MEMORIAL HOSPITAL (221303)**, 2033 Main Street, Zip 01331–3598; tel. 978/249–3511 **A**1 9 10 18 **F**11 25 27 31 32 33 38 68 73 75 76 79 86 96 107 118 119 132 135 **P**5
Primary Contact: Steven Penka, President and Chief Executive Officer
CFO: Dean Fleming, Director Finance
CMO: Mohsen Noreldin, M.D., President Medical Staff
CIO: Lorrie Bernard, Manager Patient Accounts and Information Systems
CHR: John G. Kelleher, Manager Human Resources
Web address: www.atholhospital.org
Control: Other not–for–profit (including NFP Corporation) **Service:** General Medical and Surgical

Staffed Beds: 12 **Admissions:** 996 **Census:** 9 **Outpatient Visits:** 53417 **Total Expense ($000):** 19338 **Payroll Expense ($000):** 9320 **Personnel:** 194

ATTLEBORO—Bristol County

□ **ARBOUR–FULLER HOSPITAL (224021)**, 200 May Street, Zip 02703–5515; tel. 508/761–8500, (Nonreporting) **A**1 10 **S** Universal Health Services, Inc.
Primary Contact: Robert Mansfield, Chief Executive Officer
CFO: James Rollins, Chief Financial Officer
CMO: Gregg Etter, M.D., Medical Director
CHR: Brian Jenkins, Director Human Resources
Web address: www.arbourhealth.com
Control: Corporation, Investor–owned, for–profit **Service:** Psychiatric

Staffed Beds: 46

★□ **STURDY MEMORIAL HOSPITAL (220008)**, 211 Park Street, Zip 02703–3137, Mailing Address: P.O. Box 2963, Zip 02703–2963; tel. 508/222–5200 **A**1 2 9 10 **F**3 8 13 15 18 24 25 26 27 28 30 31 32 33 34 37 38 41 43 49 50 53 54 55 56 57 58 60 62 68 72 73 74 75 76 77 79 80 81 82 84 86 87 96 97 99 100 103 106 107 118 119 120 121 123 133 135 136 137 **P**2
Primary Contact: Linda Shyavitz, CHE, President and Chief Executive Officer
CFO: Joseph Casey, Chief Financial Officer
CMO: Daniel Pietro, M.D., Medical Director
CIO: Lisa McCluskie, Director Marketing and Planning
CHR: Cheryl Barrows, Vice President Human Resources
Web address: www.sturdymemorial.org
Control: Other not–for–profit (including NFP Corporation) **Service:** General Medical and Surgical

Staffed Beds: 128 **Admissions:** 6815 **Census:** 72 **Outpatient Visits:** 225690 **Births:** 1019 **Total Expense ($000):** 123225 **Payroll Expense ($000):** 61015 **Personnel:** 1044

AYER—Middlesex County

□ **NASHOBA VALLEY MEDICAL CENTER (220098)**, 200 Groton Road, Zip 01432–3300; tel. 978/784–9000 **A**1 9 10 **F**2 11 15 17 25 28 33 38 53 54 55 56 57 60 62 73 75 76 79 81 82 84 86 87 96 97 100 107 119 121 135 136 **S** Essent Healthcare
Primary Contact: Steven P. Roach, Chief Executive Officer
CFO: Ben Moll, Assistant Chief Financial Officer
CMO: Michael Older, M.D., President Medical Staff
CIO: Armen Arakelian, Chief Information Officer
Web address: www.nashobamed.com
Control: Other not–for–profit (including NFP Corporation) **Service:** General Medical and Surgical

Staffed Beds: 57 **Admissions:** 2288 **Census:** 23 **Outpatient Visits:** 113235 **Births:** 0

MA

BEDFORD—Middlesex County

★□ △ **EDITH NOURSE ROGERS MEMORIAL VETERANS HOSPITAL**, 200 Springs Road, Zip 01730–1198; tel. 781/687–2000, (Total facility includes 306 beds in nursing home–type unit) (Nonreporting) **A**1 3 5 7 **S** Department of Veterans Affairs
Primary Contact: Karen Y. Waghorn, Director
CFO: Warren Berger, Chief Fiscal Service
CIO: Joseph Calabresi, Chief Information Service
Web address: www.va.gov/sta/guide/home.asp
Control: Veterans Affairs, Government, federal **Service:** Psychiatric

Staffed Beds: 453

BELMONT—Middlesex County

★□ **MCLEAN HOSPITAL (224007)**, 115 Mill Street, Zip 02478–9106; tel. 617/855–2000 **A**1 3 5 10 **F**2 4 5 11 50 52 54 57 58 62 66 72 73 75 81 87 88 89 91 93 94 95 100 104 119 124 **P**6 **S** Partners HealthCare System, Inc.
Primary Contact: Scott L. Rauch, M.D., President
COO: Michele L. Gougeon, Executive Vice President and Chief Operating Officer
CFO: David A. Lagasse, Senior Vice President Fiscal Affairs
CIO: Marc DiFabbio, Director Information System
Web address: www.mclean.harvard.edu
Control: Partnership, Investor–owned, for–profit **Service:** Psychiatric

Staffed Beds: 172 **Admissions:** 5426 **Census:** 150 **Outpatient Visits:** 238940 **Births:** 0 **Total Expense ($000):** 144782 **Payroll Expense ($000):** 56847 **Personnel:** 947

BEVERLY—Essex County

□ **BEVERLY HOSPITAL (220033)**, 85 Herrick Street, Zip 01915–1777; tel. 978/922–3000, (Includes ADDISON GILBERT HOSPITAL, 298 Washington Street, Gloucester, Zip 01930–4887; tel. 978/283–4000) **A**1 5 9 10 **F**3 5 8 9 11 12 13 15 18 20 22 24 25 26 27 30 31 32 33 38 40 42 43 44 45 46 48 49 50 51 52 53 54 55 56 57 62 63 66 68 72 73 74 76 77 79 80 81 82 84 86 87 88 90 92 93 94 95 96 97 99 100 102 103 107 118 119 120 121 123 124 135 136 137 **P**1 6
Primary Contact: Stephen R. Laverty, President and Chief Executive Officer
COO: Philip M. Cormier, Chief Operating Officer and Executive Vice President
CFO: Denis Conroy, Chief Financial Officer
CMO: Peter H. Short, M.D., Senior Vice President Medical Affairs
CIO: Michael Hicks, Director Information Systems
CHR: Althea C. Lyons, Vice President Human Resources
Web address: www.nhshealth.org
Control: Other not–for–profit (including NFP Corporation) **Service:** General Medical and Surgical

Staffed Beds: 332 **Admissions:** 18421 **Census:** 244 **Outpatient Visits:** 472676 **Births:** 2127 **Total Expense ($000):** 245041 **Payroll Expense ($000):** 123568 **Personnel:** 1965

BOSTON—Suffolk County

□ **ARBOUR HOSPITAL (224013)**, 49 Robinwood Avenue, Zip 02130–2156, Mailing Address: P.O. Box 9, Zip 2130; tel. 617/522–4400, (Nonreporting) **A**1 10 **S** Universal Health Services, Inc.
Primary Contact: Joseph Murphy, Chief Executive Officer
Web address: www.arbourhealth.com
Control: Other not–for–profit (including NFP Corporation) **Service:** Psychiatric

Staffed Beds: 118

Hospital, Medicare Provider Number, Address, Telephone, Approval, Facility, and Physician Codes, Health Care System

★ American Hospital Association (AHA) membership
□ The Joint Commission accreditation
○ American Osteopathic Association (AOA) accreditation
△ Commission on Accreditation of Rehabilitation Facilities (CARF) accreditation

★ **BETH ISRAEL DEACONESS MEDICAL CENTER (220086)**, 330 Brookline Avenue, Zip 02215–5491; tel. 617/667–7000, (Includes BETH ISRAEL DEACONESS HOSPITAL–NEEDHAM CAMPUS, 148 Chestnut Street, Needham, Zip 02492; tel. 781/453–3000; Jeffrey H. Liebman, President and Chief Executive Officer) **A**1 2 3 5 8 9 10 **F**3 6 9 11 12 13 14 15 17 18 20 22 24 25 26 27 30 31 32 33 34 36 38 39 40 41 42 43 44 46 47 48 49 50 51 52 53 54 55 56 57 58 60 62 63 64 66 68 70 71 72 73 74 75 76 77 79 80 81 82 86 87 88 90 91 92 93 94 96 97 98 99 100 102 103 104 105 106 107 108 109 111 112 119 120 121 123 125 127 128 131 132 134 135 136 137 **P**5 7
Primary Contact: Paul F. Levy, President and Chief Executive Officer
COO: Eric Buehrens, Chief Operating Officer
CFO: Steven P. Fischer, Chief Financial Officer
CIO: John Halamka, M.D., Chief Information Officer
CHR: Lisa Zankman, Senior Vice President Human Resources
Web address: www.bidmc.harvard.edu
Control: Other not–for–profit (including NFP Corporation) **Service:** General Medical and Surgical

Staffed Beds: 585 **Admissions:** 36566 **Census:** 507 **Outpatient Visits:** 542997 **Births:** 4864 **Total Expense ($000):** 1075738 **Payroll Expense ($000):** 439754 **Personnel:** 6864

★ △ **BOSTON MEDICAL CENTER (220031)**, One Boston Medical Center Place, Zip 02118–2393; tel. 617/638–8000 **A**1 2 3 5 7 8 9 10 **F**3 5 8 9 12 13 15 17 18 20 22 24 25 26 27 28 30 31 32 33 34 36 38 40 41 43 44 45 50 51 53 54 55 56 57 58 60 62 63 64 66 68 70 71 72 73 74 75 76 77 79 80 81 82 83 84 85 86 87 89 90 91 92 93 94 96 97 99 100 102 104 105 106 107 108 109 111 112 113 116 118 119 120 121 123 124 127 131 132 133 134 135 136 137 **P**7
Primary Contact: Elaine S. Ullian, President and Chief Executive Officer
CFO: Ronald E. Bartlett, Chief Financial Officer
CMO: Susan Haas, M.D., Chief Medical Officer
Web address: www.bmc.org
Control: Other not–for–profit (including NFP Corporation) **Service:** General Medical and Surgical

Staffed Beds: 520 **Admissions:** 27170 **Census:** 384 **Outpatient Visits:** 985356 **Births:** 2301 **Total Expense ($000):** 884876 **Payroll Expense ($000):** 316292 **Personnel:** 5018

★ **BRIGHAM AND WOMEN'S HOSPITAL (220110)**, 75 Francis Street, Zip 02115–6195; tel. 617/732–5500 **A**1 3 5 8 9 10 **F**3 5 6 7 9 11 12 13 14 15 16 17 18 20 22 24 25 26 27 28 29 30 31 32 33 34 35 36 37 38 40 41 43 44 45 46 47 48 49 50 53 54 55 56 57 58 59 60 62 63 64 66 68 70 72 73 74 75 76 77 79 80 81 82 86 87 89 90 91 92 93 94 96 97 99 100 101 102 103 104 105 106 107 108 109 111 112 113 114 116 118 119 120 121 123 124 125 126 127 129 130 131 132 133 134 135 136 137 **P**6 **S** Partners HealthCare System, Inc.
Primary Contact: Gary L. Gottlieb, M.D., President
COO: Kate Walsh, Chief Operating Officer
CMO: Anthony Whittemore, Chief Medical Officer
CIO: Sue Schade, Chief Information Officer
CHR: Lisa Ponton, Vice President Human Resources
Web address: www.brighamandwomens.org
Control: Other not–for–profit (including NFP Corporation) **Service:** General Medical and Surgical

Staffed Beds: 746 **Admissions:** 45400 **Census:** 665 **Outpatient Visits:** 667076 **Births:** 8399 **Total Expense ($000):** 1640916 **Payroll Expense ($000):** 525412 **Personnel:** 11263

★ **CHILDREN'S HOSPITAL BOSTON (223302)**, 300 Longwood Avenue, Zip 02115–5737; tel. 617/355–6000 **A**1 3 5 8 9 10 **F**3 5 8 12 14 18 19 20 21 22 23 25 26 27 28 30 31 32 33 34 35 36 37 38 40 41 42 43 44 46 48 49 50 51 53 55 56 57 58 59 60 61 62 63 66 70 72 73 75 76 77 79 80 81 82 83 84 86 87 88 89 90 91 92 94 96 97 98 100 101 102 103 104 105 106 107 112 114 116 118 119 120 121 123 125 126 127 128 129 130 131 132 133 135 136 137 **P**3 5
Primary Contact: James Mandell, M.D., President and Chief Executive Officer
COO: Sandra Fenwick, Chief Operating Officer
CFO: David Kirshner, Senior Vice President and Chief Financial Officer
CIO: Daniel Nigrin, M.D., Vice President Information Services and Chief Information Officer
CHR: Inez Stewart, Vice President
Web address: www.childrenshospital.org/
Control: Other not–for–profit (including NFP Corporation) **Service:** Children's general

Staffed Beds: 359 **Admissions:** 17106 **Census:** 282 **Outpatient Visits:** 471641 **Births:** 0 **Total Expense ($000):** 860705 **Payroll Expense ($000):** 364880 **Personnel:** 7043

★ **DANA–FARBER CANCER INSTITUTE (220162)**, 44 Binney Street, Zip 02115–6084; tel. 617/632–3000 **A**1 3 5 9 10 **F**3 11 14 15 25 26 27 28 30 31 32 33 34 41 43 44 50 53 55 56 57 58 62 63 66 69 73 75 76 80 81 82 89 90 91 94 96 97 100 102 104 105 107 108 109 111 114 119 121 123 124 125 135 136 137 **P**6
Primary Contact: Edward J. Benz, Jr., M.D., President and Chief Executive Officer
COO: Janet E. Porter, Ph.D., Executive Vice President and Chief Operating Officer
CFO: Dorothy E. Puhy, Executive Vice President and Chief Financial Officer
CMO: Lawrence N. Shulman, M.D., Senior Vice President Medical Affairs and Chief Medical Officer
CIO: Jeffrey R. Kessler, Vice President Information Services
CHR: Emily Barclay, Vice President Human Resources
Web address: www.dana–farber.org
Control: Other not–for–profit (including NFP Corporation) **Service:** Cancer

Staffed Beds: 27 **Admissions:** 984 **Census:** 23 **Outpatient Visits:** 200988 **Births:** 0 **Total Expense ($000):** 646223 **Payroll Expense ($000):** 213815 **Personnel:** 3143

★ **FAULKNER HOSPITAL (220119)**, Mailing Address: 1153 Centre Sreet, Zip 02130–3400; tel. 617/983–7000, (Nonreporting) **A**1 2 3 5 8 9 10 **S** Partners HealthCare System, Inc.
Primary Contact: David J. Trull, President and Chief Executive Officer
CFO: Michael E. Conklin, Senior Vice President Finance
CMO: Stephen C. Wright, M.D., Chief Medical Officer
CIO: Jim Anzeveno, Chief Information Officer
CHR: Rebecca Blair, Vice President Human Resources and Service Excellence
Web address: www.faulknerhospital.org
Control: Other not–for–profit (including NFP Corporation) **Service:** General Medical and Surgical

Staffed Beds: 104

★ **FRANCISCAN HOSPITAL FOR CHILDREN (223300)**, (Formerly Franciscan Hospital for Children and Rehabilitation Center), 30 Warren Street, Zip 02135–3680; tel. 617/254–3800, (Nonreporting) **A**1 5 9 10
Primary Contact: Paul J. DellaRocco, President and Chief Executive Officer
COO: Donna Pohselli, Chief Operating Officer
CFO: Debra Bruss, Chief Financial Officer
CMO: Jane E. O'Brien, M.D., Medical Director
CHR: Steven Snyder, Vice President Human Resources
Web address: www.franciscanhospital.org
Control: Other not–for–profit (including NFP Corporation) **Service:** Children's rehabilitation

Staffed Beds: 60

△ **HEBREW REHABILITATION CENTER FOR AGED (222007)**, 1200 Centre Street, Zip 02131–1097; tel. 617/325–8000, (Total facility includes 21 beds in nursing home–type unit) (Nonreporting) **A**7 10
Primary Contact: Carl Zack, President and Chief Executive Officer
CFO: Fred Leathers, Chief Financial Officer
CMO: Rob Schreiber, M.D., Physician–in–Chief
CIO: Fran Hinckley, Chief Information Officer
CHR: Alessandra de Vaca, Vice President Human Resources
Web address: www.hebrewseniorlife.org
Control: Other not–for–profit (including NFP Corporation) **Service:** Long–Term Acute Care hospital

Staffed Beds: 721

□ **KINDRED HOSPITAL–BOSTON (222045)**, 1515 Commonwealth Avenue, Zip 02135–3696; tel. 617/254–1100, (Nonreporting) **A**1 10 **S** Kindred Healthcare
Primary Contact: Jacqueline Arocho, Chief Executive Officer
CFO: John Couillard, Chief Financial Officer
CMO: Mark Rohrer, Chief Medical Officer
CHR: Debra Pantoja, Coordinator Human Resources
Web address: www.kindredhealthcare.com
Control: Corporation, Investor–owned, for–profit **Service:** General Medical and Surgical

Staffed Beds: 36

□ **MASSACHUSETTS EYE AND EAR INFIRMARY (220075)**, 243 Charles Street, Zip 02114–3096; tel. 617/523–7900 **A**1 3 5 9 10 **F**3 11 25 26 27 30 31 32 33 34 37 38 40 43 50 54 55 56 57 58 62 66 72 73 75 76 79 80 81 82 84 86 96 100 102 107 110 119 121 124 130 132 133 135 137 **P**6 8
Primary Contact: John R. Fernandez, President and Chief Executive Officer
CFO: Peter J. Chinetti, Chief Financial Officer
CIO: Alec Cheloff, Chief Information Officer
CHR: Christine Regan, Vice President Human Resources
Web address: www.meei.harvard.edu
Control: Other not–for–profit (including NFP Corporation) **Service:** Eye, ear, nose, and throat

Staffed Beds: 42 **Admissions:** 1213 **Census:** 12 **Outpatient Visits:** 254221 **Births:** 0 **Total Expense ($000):** 137479 **Payroll Expense ($000):** 39719 **Personnel:** 1325

 Many Facility Codes have changed. Please refer to the AHA Guide Code Chart.

★ **MASSACHUSETTS GENERAL HOSPITAL (220071)**, 55 Fruit Street, Zip 02114–2696; tel. 617/726–2000 **A**1 3 5 8 9 10 **F**3 5 7 8 9 11 12 13 14 15 16 17 18 19 20 21 22 23 24 25 26 27 28 30 31 32 33 34 35 36 37 38 40 41 42 43 44 46 47 48 49 50 51 52 53 54 55 56 57 58 59 60 61 62 63 64 66 68 70 71 72 73 74 75 76 77 78 79 80 81 82 83 84 86 87 88 89 90 91 92 93 94 95 96 97 99 100 101 102 103 104 105 106 107 108 109 110 111 112 113 114 118 119 120 121 123 124 125 126 127 128 129 130 131 132 133 134 135 136 137 **P**6 **S** Partners HealthCare System, Inc.
Primary Contact: Peter L. Slavin, M.D., President
CFO: Sally Mason Boemer, Senior Vice President Finance
CMO: Britain Nicholson, M.D., Chief Medical Officer
CIO: James W. Noga, Chief Information Officer
CHR: Jeff Davis, Senior Vice President Human Resources
Web address: www.massgeneral.org
Control: Other not–for–profit (including NFP Corporation) **Service:** General Medical and Surgical

Staffed Beds: 907 **Admissions:** 46748 **Census:** 745 **Outpatient Visits:** 827318 **Births:** 3503 **Total Expense ($000):** 2195173 **Payroll Expense ($000):** 724999 **Personnel:** 13966

★ **NEW ENGLAND BAPTIST HOSPITAL (220088)**, 125 Parker Hill Avenue, Zip 02120–3297; tel. 617/754–5800 **A**1 3 5 10 **F**3 8 11 14 18 25 26 27 30 31 32 33 35 41 43 50 51 53 55 56 57 58 59 62 64 66 68 73 75 76 77 79 80 81 82 86 87 90 96 97 100 102 104 106 107 116 119 120 121 132 135 **P**8
Primary Contact: Joseph D. Dionisio, President and Chief Executive Officer
Web address: www.nebh.org
Control: Other not–for–profit (including NFP Corporation) **Service:** Orthopedic

Staffed Beds: 95 **Admissions:** 7128 **Census:** 82 **Outpatient Visits:** 136406 **Births:** 0 **Total Expense ($000):** 164136 **Payroll Expense ($000):** 64403 **Personnel:** 1028

★ **RADIUS SPECIALTY HOSPITAL BOSTON (222010)**, 59 Townsend Street, Zip 02119–9918; tel. 617/442–8760, (Nonreporting) **A**1 10
Primary Contact: William F. Duffy, Chief Executive Officer
CFO: John Shea, Chief Financial Officer
CMO: R. Nicholas Nace, M.D., Chief Medical Officer
CIO: Anthony DiPrizio, Director Information Services
CHR: Christine Bresnahan, Manager Human Resources
Web address: www.radiushospital.com
Control: Other not–for–profit (including NFP Corporation) **Service:** Long–Term Acute Care hospital

Staffed Beds: 153

□ **SHRINERS HOSPITALS FOR CHILDREN–BOSTON**, (Burns), 51 Blossom Street, Zip 2114; tel. 617/722–3000 **A**1 3 5 **F**16 25 26 32 33 55 62 73 75 79 80 81 82 86 89 94 119 121 130 132 135 137 **S** Shriners Hospitals for Children
Primary Contact: C. Thomas D'Esmond, Administrator
CFO: Maria Chung, Director Fiscal Services
CMO: Ronald G. Tompkins, M.D., Sc.D., Chief of Staff
CIO: Solomon Kenea, Director Management Information Services
CHR: Maureen Huffam, Director Human Resources
Web address: www.shrinershospitals.org
Control: Other not–for–profit (including NFP Corporation) **Service:** Children's other specialty

Staffed Beds: 30 **Admissions:** 1115 **Census:** 17 **Outpatient Visits:** 6677 **Births:** 0 **Personnel:** 249

★ △ **SPAULDING REHABILITATION HOSPITAL (223034)**, 125 Nashua Street, Zip 02114–1198; tel. 617/573–7000 **A**1 3 5 7 10 **F**3 7 25 26 30 31 32 33 34 37 50 55 56 57 58 59 62 66 72 73 75 80 81 82 85 86 94 118 119 120 121 132 135 137 **P**8 **S** Partners HealthCare System, Inc.
Primary Contact: Judith C. Waterston, M.S., President
CFO: Mary Shaughnessy, Vice President Finance
CIO: John Campbell, Director Management Information Systems
CHR: Colleen M. Moran, Director Human Resources
Web address: www.spauldingrehab.org
Control: Other not–for–profit (including NFP Corporation) **Service:** Rehabilitation

Staffed Beds: 196 **Admissions:** 2510 **Census:** 166 **Outpatient Visits:** 134846 **Births:** 0 **Total Expense ($000):** 96347 **Payroll Expense ($000):** 47639 **Personnel:** 915

□ △ **TUFTS MEDICAL CENTER (220116)**, (Formerly Tufts–New England Medical Center), 750 Washington Street, Zip 02111–1845; tel. 617/636–5000 **A**1 2 3 5 7 8 9 10 **F**3 12 13 14 15 18 19 20 21 22 23 24 25 26 27 28 30 31 32 33 37 38 40 41 43 50 51 55 56 57 60 62 66 68 69 70 72 73 74 75 76 77 79 80 81 82 83 84 86 87 88 89 90 92 94 96 97 100 102 103 104 105 106 107 109 111 114 118 119 120 121 123 124 125 126 127 128 132 135 136 **P**3 5
Primary Contact: Ellen Zane, CHE, President and Chief Executive Officer
CIO: Glen Johnson, Regional Information Officer
Web address: www.nemc.org
Control: Other not–for–profit (including NFP Corporation) **Service:** General Medical and Surgical

Staffed Beds: 280 **Admissions:** 16302 **Census:** 255 **Outpatient Visits:** 364375 **Births:** 1361 **Total Expense ($000):** 452870 **Payroll Expense ($000):** 195629

★ △ **VETERANS AFFAIRS BOSTON HEALTHCARE SYSTEM**, 1400 VFW Parkway, Zip 2132; tel. 617/232–9500, (Total facility includes 141 beds in nursing home–type unit) **A**1 2 3 5 7 8 **F**3 4 5 12 15 17 18 20 22 24 25 26 27 30 31 32 33 36 37 38 42 43 44 45 46 47 49 50 53 54 55 57 58 59 60 61 62 66 68 72 73 75 76 77 78 79 80 82 85 86 87 88 90 92 93 94 95 96 97 100 103 104 106 107 109 117 118 119 121 124 133 134 135 136 137 **P**6 **S** Department of Veterans Affairs
Primary Contact: Michael M. Lawson, Director
COO: Susan A. MacKenzie, Ph.D., Associate Director
CFO: Joseph R. Costa, Chief Financial Officer
CMO: Brian Hoffman, M.D., Chief Medical Services
CIO: David M. Goodman, Ph.D., Chief Information Officer
CHR: William Warfield, Chief Human Resources Management
Web address: www.va.gov/sta/guide/home.asp
Control: Veterans Affairs, Government, federal **Service:** General Medical and Surgical

Staffed Beds: 502 **Admissions:** 10575 **Census:** 459 **Outpatient Visits:** 795064 **Births:** 0 **Personnel:** 3349

VETERANS AFFAIRS MEDICAL CENTER See Brockton Veterans Affairs Medical Center, Brockton

BRAINTREE—Norfolk County

★ **BRAINTREE REHABILITATION HOSPITAL (223027)**, (Formerly HEALTHSOUTH Braintree Rehabilitation Hospital), 250 Pond Street, Zip 2184; tel. 781/848–5353, (Nonreporting) **A**1 10 **S** Five Star Quality Care
Primary Contact: Randy Doherty, Administrator
CFO: Andrew Rando, Chief Financial Officer
CMO: John Stevenson, M.D., Medical Director
CHR: Tara Spellacy, Director Human Resources
Web address: www.braintreerehabhospital.com
Control: Corporation, Investor–owned, for–profit **Service:** Rehabilitation

Staffed Beds: 187

□ **NORTHEAST SPECIALTY HOSPITAL (222002)**, 2001 Washington Street, Zip 02184–8664; tel. 781/848–2600 **A**1 10 **F**1 3 6 17 18 25 26 29 34 37 38 40 43 50 54 55 59 62 68 72 73 75 76 77 78 80 81 82 85 86 87 96 97 98 100 102 104 106 107 115 119 121 137
Primary Contact: Judyth McTiernan, Chief Executive Officer
COO: Scott Ariel, Administrator and Chief Operating Officer
CFO: Larry Toye, Chief Financial Officer
CMO: Svetlozar Natov, M.D., Medical Director
CIO: Glen Ushrey, Director Information Technology
CHR: Tom Phillips, Director Human Resources
Web address: www.commonwealthcommunity.com
Control: Corporation, Investor–owned, for–profit **Service:** General Medical and Surgical

Staffed Beds: 404 **Admissions:** 20562 **Census:** 266 **Outpatient Visits:** 224909 **Births:** 0

BRIDGEWATER—Plymouth County

BRIDGEWATER STATE HOSPITAL, 20 Administration Road, Zip 02324–3201; tel. 508/279–4521, (Nonreporting) **A**3 5
Primary Contact: Kenneth W. Nelson, Superintendent
CFO: Diane Wholley, Director Fiscal Services
Control: State–Government, nonfederal **Service:** Psychiatric

Staffed Beds: 350

Hospital, Medicare Provider Number, Address, Telephone, Approval, Facility, and Physician Codes, Health Care System
★ American Hospital Association (AHA) membership
□ The Joint Commission accreditation
○ American Osteopathic Association (AOA) accreditation
△ Commission on Accreditation of Rehabilitation Facilities (CARF) accreditation

BRIGHTON—Suffolk County

★ **CARITAS ST. ELIZABETH'S MEDICAL CENTER (220036)**, 736 Cambridge Street, Zip 02135–2997; tel. 617/789–3000 **A**1 2 3 5 8 9 10 **F**3 4 5 8 11 12 13 15 17 18 20 22 24 25 26 27 33 36 38 41 43 44 50 51 52 53 54 55 56 57 59 62 64 66 68 70 72 73 74 75 76 77 79 80 81 82 86 87 88 90 91 92 93 94 95 96 97 100 102 103 106 107 114 117 118 119 120 121 124 132 134 135 136 137 **P**5 **S** Caritas Christi Health Care
Primary Contact: Christopher M. O'Connor, President
CFO: Miles Coverdale, Chief Financial Officer
CMO: Michael Kneeland, Vice President Medical Affairs
CIO: Charles Podesta, Vice President and Chief Information Officer
CHR: Nanette Smith Callihan, Vice President Human Resources
Web address: www.semc.org
Control: Church–operated, Nongovernment, not–for profit **Service:** General Medical and Surgical

Staffed Beds: 338 **Admissions:** 14733 **Census:** 198 **Outpatient Visits:** 141725 **Births:** 1218

MA

BROCKTON—Plymouth County

BROCKTON HOSPITAL See Signature Healthcare Brockton Hospital

★ **BROCKTON VETERANS AFFAIRS MEDICAL CENTER**, 940 Belmont Street, Zip 02401–5596; tel. 508/583–4500, (Includes VETERANS AFFAIRS MEDICAL CENTER, 1400 VFW Parkway, West Roxbury, Boston, Zip 02132, Mailing Address: 1400 VWF Parkway, West Roxbury, Zip 02132; tel. 617/323–7700; William H. Kelleher, Director), (Total facility includes 141 beds in nursing home–type unit) **A**1 3 5 8 **F**3 4 5 12 15 17 18 20 22 24 25 26 27 30 31 32 33 36 37 38 42 43 44 45 46 47 48 49 50 53 54 55 57 58 59 60 61 62 63 66 68 72 73 75 76 77 78 79 81 82 85 86 87 88 90 91 92 93 94 95 96 97 100 103 104 107 108 109 117 118 119 121 124 133 134 135 136 137 **P**6 **S** Department of Veterans Affairs
Primary Contact: Michael E. Lawson, Director
CFO: Joe Costa, Acting Chief Fiscal Officer
Web address: www.va.gov/sta/guide/home.asp
Control: Veterans Affairs, Government, federal **Service:** General Medical and Surgical

Staffed Beds: 502 **Admissions:** 10575 **Census:** 459 **Outpatient Visits:** 795064

★ **CARITAS GOOD SAMARITAN MEDICAL CENTER (220111)**, 235 North Pearl Street, Zip 02301–1794; tel. 508/427–3000, (Includes GOOD SAMARITAN MEDICAL CENTER – CUSHING CAMPUS) **A**1 2 3 5 9 10 **F**3 4 5 8 13 15 17 18 20 24 25 26 27 31 32 33 38 40 42 43 50 53 54 55 57 59 62 63 66 68 73 74 75 76 77 79 80 81 82 84 88 93 96 97 100 102 103 106 107 112 118 119 121 124 132 133 135 136 **P**4 5 **S** Caritas Christi Health Care
Primary Contact: John J. Holiver, President
CFO: Joseph Iannoni, Vice President Finance
CMO: Scott Stewart, M.D., Vice President Medical Management
CIO: Daniel O'Neil, Vice President Information Technology
CHR: Victor Munger, Vice President Human Resources
Web address: www.caritasgoodsam.org
Control: Other not–for–profit (including NFP Corporation) **Service:** General Medical and Surgical

Staffed Beds: 258 **Admissions:** 15692 **Census:** 179 **Outpatient Visits:** 168730 **Births:** 926 **Total Expense ($000):** 155226 **Payroll Expense ($000):** 71819 **Personnel:** 1347

★ **SIGNATURE HEALTHCARE BROCKTON HOSPITAL (220052)**, (Formerly Brockton Hospital), 680 Centre Street, Zip 02302–3395; tel. 508/941–7000, (Total facility includes 29 beds in nursing home–type unit) **A**1 2 3 5 6 9 10 **F**11 13 15 17 18 20 24 25 26 27 28 30 31 32 33 36 38 43 44 49 50 51 53 54 55 56 57 58 59 60 61 62 63 64 66 68 71 72 73 74 75 76 77 79 80 82 84 86 87 88 90 91 92 93 94 95 96 97 100 102 103 105 107 108 109 111 114 117 119 120 121 124 132 133 135 136 137 **P**6 8
Primary Contact: Norman B. Goodman, President and Chief Executive Officer
CFO: Michael Connors, Vice President and Chief Financial Officer
CIO: Craig Fletcher, Chief Information Officer
CHR: Donald Anderson, Vice President Human Resources
Web address: www.signature–healthcare.org
Control: Other not–for–profit (including NFP Corporation) **Service:** General Medical and Surgical

Staffed Beds: 253 **Admissions:** 14415 **Census:** 173 **Outpatient Visits:** 178067 **Births:** 1410 **Total Expense ($000):** 174717 **Payroll Expense ($000):** 105579 **Personnel:** 1422

BROOKLINE—Norfolk County

☐ **ARBOUR H. R. I. HOSPITAL (224018)**, 227 Babcock Street, Zip 02146–6799; tel. 617/731–3200, (Nonreporting) **A**1 10 **S** Universal Health Services, Inc.
Primary Contact: Patrick Moallemian, Chief Executive Officer and Managing Director
CFO: James Rollins, Chief Financial Officer
CMO: Anthony Raynes, M.D., Psychiatrist in Chief
CHR: Kris Munson, Director Human Resources
Web address: www.arbourhealth.com
Control: Corporation, Investor–owned, for–profit **Service:** Psychiatric

Staffed Beds: 68

☐ **BOURNEWOOD HEALTH SYSTEM (224022)**, 300 South Street, Zip 02467–3694; tel. 617/469–0300 **A**1 3 5 10 **F**4 5 30 88 89 94 95 119 121 **P**1
Primary Contact: Nasir A. Khan, M.D., Chief Executive Officer
CFO: Michael Gale, Chief Financial Officer
CMO: Carmel Heinsohn, M.D., Medical Director
CHR: Paula Berardi, Human Resources Manager
Web address: www.bournewood.com
Control: Corporation, Investor–owned, for–profit **Service:** Psychiatric

Staffed Beds: 81 **Admissions:** 3534 **Census:** 73 **Outpatient Visits:** 12114 **Births:** 0 **Total Expense ($000):** 18198 **Payroll Expense ($000):** 10935 **Personnel:** 178

BURLINGTON—Middlesex County

★ **LAHEY CLINIC HOSPITAL (220171)**, 41 Mall Road, Zip 01805–0001; tel. 781/744–5100 **A**1 2 3 5 8 9 10 **F**3 5 6 8 9 11 12 14 15 17 18 20 22 24 25 26 27 30 31 32 33 34 35 36 37 38 39 40 41 42 43 44 45 46 47 48 49 50 51 53 54 55 56 57 58 60 62 63 64 66 68 72 73 75 76 77 79 80 81 82 86 87 89 90 91 92 93 94 96 97 99 100 101 102 103 104 105 106 107 108 109 111 112 114 116 118 119 120 121 123 124 125 127 128 130 131 132 133 134 135 136 137 **P**6
Primary Contact: David M. Barrett, M.D., Chief Executive Officer
COO: Sanford R. Kurtz, M.D., Chief Operating Officer
CFO: Timothy O'Connor, Chief Financial Officer
CMO: Joseph C. Corkery, M.D., Chief Medical Officer
CIO: Nelson R. Gagnon, Chief Information Officer
CHR: Joan M. Robbio, Senior Vice President Human Resources
Web address: www.lahey.org
Control: Other not–for–profit (including NFP Corporation) **Service:** General Medical and Surgical

Staffed Beds: 327 **Admissions:** 20866 **Census:** 271 **Outpatient Visits:** 723212 **Births:** 0 **Total Expense ($000):** 534613 **Payroll Expense ($000):** 226187 **Personnel:** 4740

CAMBRIDGE—Middlesex County

★ **CAMBRIDGE HEALTH ALLIANCE (220011)**, 1493 Cambridge Street, Zip 02139–1099; tel. 617/665–1000, (Includes CAMBRIDGE HOSPITAL, 1493 Cambridge Street; SOMERVILLE HOSPITAL, 230 Highland Avenue, Somerville, Zip 02143; tel. 617/666–4400; WHIDDEN MEMORIAL HOSPITAL, 103 Garland Street, Everett, Zip 02149–5095; tel. 617/389–6270) **A**1 2 3 5 8 9 10 **F**1 2 4 5 7 9 11 13 15 16 17 25 26 27 28 29 30 31 32 33 34 35 36 37 38 40 41 43 46 47 48 49 50 51 53 54 55 56 57 58 60 62 63 64 65 66 68 70 71 72 73 74 75 76 77 78 79 81 82 83 84 85 86 87 88 89 90 91 92 93 94 95 96 97 99 100 102 103 107 112 113 114 117 118 119 120 121 123 124 132 133 135 136 **P**6
Primary Contact: Dennis D. Keefe, Chief Executive Officer
COO: Allison Bayer, Senior Vice President Operations and Chief Operating Officer
CFO: Gordon Boudrow, Chief Financial Officer
CMO: David Bor, M.D., Chief of Medicine
CIO: Judith K. Klickstein, Chief Information Officer
CHR: Joan Bennett, Senior Vice President Human Resources
Web address: www.challiance.org
Control: Hospital district or authority, Government, nonfederal **Service:** General Medical and Surgical

Staffed Beds: 349 **Admissions:** 16415 **Census:** 268 **Outpatient Visits:** 634650 **Births:** 1415 **Total Expense ($000):** 501121 **Payroll Expense ($000):** 279552 **Personnel:** 3354

☐ **M. I. T. MEDICAL DEPARTMENT**, 77 Massachusetts Avenue, Zip 02139–4307; tel. 617/253–4481, (Nonreporting) **A**1
Primary Contact: Arnold N. Weinberg, M.D., Director
Control: Other not–for–profit (including NFP Corporation) **Service:** Hospital unit of an institution (prison hospital, college infimary, etc.)

Staffed Beds: 18

★ **MOUNT AUBURN HOSPITAL (220002)**, 330 Mount Auburn Street, Zip 02138–5597; tel. 617/492–3500 **A**1 2 3 5 8 9 10 **F**3 5 11 13 14 15 17 18 20 22 25 26 27 30 31 32 33 35 38 49 50 51 54 55 56 57 58 59 60 61 62 63 66 68 71 72 73 74 75 76 77 79 81 82 86 87 88 90 91 92 93 94 96 97 99 100 102 103 105 106 107 108 109 111 113 114 118 119 120 121 124 133 134 135 136 **P**5 6 7
Primary Contact: Jeanette G. Clough, President and Chief Executive Officer
COO: Nicholas T. Dileso, R.N., Chief Operating Officer
CFO: Peter Semenza, Vice President Financial Operations
CMO: Anthony Abner, M.D., President Medical Staff
CIO: Bob Todd, Director Information Systems
CHR: Tom Fabiano, Director Human Resources
Web address: www.mtauburn.caregroup.org
Control: Other not–for–profit (including NFP Corporation) **Service:** General Medical and Surgical

Staffed Beds: 196 **Admissions:** 12509 **Census:** 154 **Outpatient Visits:** 194271 **Births:** 2085 **Total Expense ($000):** 232240 **Payroll Expense ($000):** 108822 **Personnel:** 2042

STILLMAN INFIRMARY, HARVARD UNIVERSITY HEALTH SERVICES (220133), 75 Mount Auburn Street, Zip 02138–4960; tel. 617/495–2010, (Nonreporting) **A**10
Primary Contact: David S. Rosenthal, M.D., Director
COO: Kathi Tracy, Chief Operating Officer
CFO: Melanie Green, Chief Financial Officer
CIO: Michael Brown, M.D., Chief Information Officer
CHR: David Kearns, Assistant Director Human Resources
Web address: www.uhs.harvard.edu
Control: Other not–for–profit (including NFP Corporation) **Service:** Hospital unit of an institution (prison hospital, college infimary, etc.)

Staffed Beds: 18

□ **YOUVILLE HOSPITAL AND REHABILITATION CENTER (222000)**, 1575 Cambridge Street, Zip 02138–4398; tel. 617/876–4344, (Nonreporting) **A**1 3 5 10 **S** Covenant Health Systems, Inc.
Primary Contact: Daniel P. Leahey, President and Chief Executive Officer
COO: Timothy Lynch, Vice President Operations
CFO: Michael J. Keller, Vice President Financial Affairs and Chief Financial Officer
CMO: Melvyn L. Hecht, M.D., Medical Director and Chief Medical Officer
CIO: John Wilder, Director Information Systems
CHR: Jack Carroll, Senior Director Human Resources
Web address: www.youville.org
Control: Church–operated, Nongovernment, not–for profit **Service:** General Medical and Surgical

Staffed Beds: 150

CANTON—Norfolk County

★□ **MASSACHUSETTS HOSPITAL SCHOOL (222025)**, 3 Randolph Street, Zip 02021–2397; tel. 781/828–2440 **A**1 5 10 **F**25 31 37 41 53 57 63 73 75 77 80 81 82 86 87 96 107 119 132 135 **S** Massachusetts Department of Public Health
Primary Contact: Katherine Ann Chmiel, RN, M.S., Chief Executive Officer
COO: Brian V. Devin, Chief Operating Officer
CFO: Sharon Porter, Chief Financial Officer
CMO: Aruna Sachdev, M.D., Medical Director
CIO: Robert Lima, Director Information Systems
CHR: Gene Rivers, Manager Employment Services
Web address: www.state.ma.us/dph/hosp/mhs.htm
Control: State–Government, nonfederal **Service:** Children's chronic disease

Staffed Beds: 86 **Admissions:** 158 **Census:** 74 **Outpatient Visits:** 0 **Births:** 0 **Total Expense ($000):** 15932 **Payroll Expense ($000):** 9875 **Personnel:** 231

CHELSEA—Suffolk County

★ **LAWRENCE F. QUIGLEY MEMORIAL HOSPITAL (220154)**, 91 Crest Avenue, Zip 02150–2199; tel. 617/884–5660, (Total facility includes 109 beds in nursing home–type unit) (Nonreporting) **A**10
Primary Contact: Michael Resca, Commandant
CIO: Thomas Rosa, Director Human Resources
Control: State–Government, nonfederal **Service:** Other specialty

Staffed Beds: 156

CLINTON—Worcester County

★□ **CLINTON HOSPITAL (220058)**, 201 Highland Street, Zip 01510–1096; tel. 978/368–3000 **A**1 5 9 10 **F**8 15 25 27 33 38 57 62 66 72 73 77 78 79 80 82 86 88 93 96 97 107 119 120 135 136 **S** UMass Memorial Health Care, Inc.
Primary Contact: Sheila Daly, President and Chief Executive Officer
CFO: Steven McCue, Controller
CHR: Martha Chiarchiaro, Vice President Human Resources
Web address: www.clintonhospital.org
Control: Other not–for–profit (including NFP Corporation) **Service:** General Medical and Surgical

Staffed Beds: 41 **Admissions:** 1436 **Census:** 28 **Outpatient Visits:** 16432 **Births:** 0

CONCORD—Middlesex County

★□ **EMERSON HOSPITAL (220084)**, 133 Old Road to Nine Acre Corner, Zip 01742–9120; tel. 978/369–1400, (Total facility includes 20 beds in nursing home–type unit) **A**1 2 5 9 10 **F**3 5 7 11 12 13 14 15 17 24 25 26 27 30 31 32 33 34 38 40 43 49 50 51 53 55 56 57 59 61 62 63 66 68 69 70 71 72 73 74 76 77 79 80 81 82 84 86 88 90 93 94 95 96 97 99 100 102 103 105 106 107 109 117 118 119 121 133 135 136 137 **P**1 5
Primary Contact: Christine C. Schuster, President and Chief Executive Officer
CFO: John O. Wilhelm, Senior Vice President and Chief Financial Officer
CMO: C. Gregory Martin, M.D., Chief Medical Officer
CIO: Martin Belscher, Chief Information Officer
CHR: Eric Stastny, Vice President Human Resources
Web address: www.emersonhospital.org
Control: Other not–for–profit (including NFP Corporation) **Service:** General Medical and Surgical

Staffed Beds: 186 **Admissions:** 10544 **Census:** 124 **Outpatient Visits:** 328999 **Births:** 1039 **Total Expense ($000):** 152161 **Payroll Expense ($000):** 75113

DORCHESTER—Suffolk County

★□ **CARITAS CARNEY HOSPITAL (220017)**, 2100 Dorchester Avenue, Zip 02124–5666; tel. 617/296–4000 **A**1 2 3 5 9 10 **F**3 5 15 17 18 20 22 24 25 26 27 30 31 32 33 38 43 52 55 56 57 60 62 66 68 72 73 75 76 77 79 80 81 82 84 86 87 88 89 90 91 92 93 94 95 96 102 104 105 106 107 118 119 121 123 135 136 **P**5 **S** Caritas Christi Health Care
Primary Contact: Daniel H. O'Leary, M.D., President
CFO: Nancy Hoffmann, Vice President Finance
CHR: Mary Orlandi, Manager Human Resources
Web address: www.carneyhospital.org
Control: Church–operated, Nongovernment, not–for profit **Service:** General Medical and Surgical

Staffed Beds: 133 **Admissions:** 6761 **Census:** 97 **Outpatient Visits:** 92324 **Births:** 0 **Total Expense ($000):** 113296 **Payroll Expense ($000):** 57403

EAST SANDWICH—Barnstable County

□ △ **REHABILITATION HOSPITAL OF THE CAPE AND ISLANDS (223032)**, 311 Service Road, Zip 2537; tel. 508/833–4000 **A**1 7 10 **F**24 25 26 33 34 54 56 59 62 72 73 77 80 85 86 119 120 135
Primary Contact: Carol Sim, President and Chief Executive Officer
COO: Stephanie Nadolny, Vice President Clinical Services
CFO: Mary Shaughnessy, Vice President Finance
CMO: David Lowell, M.D., Medical Director
CHR: Del Pontremoli, Director Human Resources
Web address: www.rhci.org
Control: Other not–for–profit (including NFP Corporation) **Service:** Rehabilitation

Staffed Beds: 60 **Admissions:** 1241 **Census:** 49 **Outpatient Visits:** 78744 **Births:** 0 **Total Expense ($000):** 29216 **Payroll Expense ($000):** 15746

EVERETT—Middlesex County

WHIDDEN MEMORIAL HOSPITAL See Cambridge Health Alliance, Cambridge

FALL RIVER—Bristol County

CHARLTON MEMORIAL HOSPITAL See Southcoast Hospitals Group

DR. J. CORRIGAN MENTAL HEALTH CENTER (224028), 49 Hillside Street, Zip 02720–5266; tel. 508/235–7200, (Nonreporting) **A**10 **S** Massachusetts Department of Mental Health
Primary Contact: Steve Figueiredo, Interim Director
Control: State–Government, nonfederal **Service:** Psychiatric

Staffed Beds: 16

★□ **SAINT ANNE'S HOSPITAL (220020)**, 795 Middle Street, Zip 02721–1798; tel. 508/674–5741, (Total facility includes 16 beds in nursing home–type unit) **A**1 2 5 9 10 **F**2 3 5 11 15 24 25 26 27 28 30 31 32 33 34 38 43 49 50 55 56 57 60 62 66 68 73 75 76 77 79 80 81 82 84 86 89 92 93 94 95 96 97 99 102 103 106 107 108 109 111 112 117 118 119 121 124 135 136 137 **P**5 6 **S** Caritas Christi Health Care
Primary Contact: Richard L. Cunningham, Interim Chief Executive Officer
COO: Susan Labus, Chief Operating Officer
CFO: Michael Bushell, Vice President Business Development and Finance
CMO: Christopher Sanders, M.D., Vice President Medical Staff Affairs
CIO: Dan O'Neil, Director Management Information Systems
CHR: Sarah Jackson, Director
Web address: www.saintanneshospital.org
Control: Church–operated, Nongovernment, not–for profit **Service:** General Medical and Surgical

Staffed Beds: 108 **Admissions:** 5961 **Census:** 90 **Outpatient Visits:** 173900 **Births:** 0 **Total Expense ($000):** 114652 **Payroll Expense ($000):** 48026 **Personnel:** 939

MA

Hospital, Medicare Provider Number, Address, Telephone, Approval, Facility, and Physician Codes, Health Care System
★ American Hospital Association (AHA) membership
□ The Joint Commission accreditation
○ American Osteopathic Association (AOA) accreditation
△ Commission on Accreditation of Rehabilitation Facilities (CARF) accreditation

★ **SOUTHCOAST HOSPITALS GROUP (220074)**, 363 Highland Avenue, Zip 02720–3703; tel. 508/679–3131, (Includes CHARLTON MEMORIAL HOSPITAL, 363 Highland Avenue, tel. 508/679–3131; ST. LUKE'S HOSPITAL, 101 Page Street, New Bedford, Zip 02740; tel. 508/997–1515; TOBEY HOSPITAL, 43 High Street, Wareham, Zip 02571; tel. 508/295–0880) **A**1 2 9 10 **F**3 8 11 12 13 14 15 17 18 20 22 24 25 26 27 30 31 32 33 34 36 38 41 42 43 44 49 50 53 54 55 56 57 59 60 61 62 64 66 68 71 72 73 74 75 76 77 79 80 81 82 84 85 86 88 90 92 93 95 96 97 100 102 103 106 107 119 120 121 123 135 136 **P**6
Primary Contact: Keith A. Hovan, President and Chief Executive Officer
COO: Linda Bodenmann, Chief Operating Officer
CFO: William Grigg, Chief Financial Officer
CMO: Eugene J. McMahon, M.D., Senior Vice President and Chief Medical Officer
CIO: Christopher Baldwin, Vice President Information Systems
CHR: David DeJesus, Vice President Human Resources
Web address: www.southcoast.org
Control: Other not–for–profit (including NFP Corporation) **Service:** General Medical and Surgical

Staffed Beds: 781 **Admissions:** 35950 **Census:** 551 **Outpatient Visits:** 868892 **Births:** 3651 **Total Expense ($000):** 525551 **Payroll Expense ($000):** 259006 **Personnel:** 4233

FALMOUTH—Barnstable County

★ **FALMOUTH HOSPITAL (220135)**, 100 Ter Heun Drive, Zip 02540–2599; tel. 508/548–5300 **A**1 2 5 9 10 **F**10 11 13 15 18 24 25 26 30 31 32 33 34 35 38 43 46 51 53 54 55 56 57 59 60 62 66 68 72 73 74 75 76 77 79 80 82 84 86 90 96 97 100 102 104 105 106 107 118 119 120 121 132 133 134 135 136 137 **P**5 **S** Cape Cod Healthcare, Inc.
Primary Contact: Susan M. Wing, Chief Operating Officer
COO: Susan M. Wing, Chief Operating Officer
CFO: Stephen J. Guimond, Senior Vice President and Chief Financial Officer
CMO: Richard Adams, M.D., Chief Medical Officer
CIO: John E. Kilroy, Vice President and Chief Information Officer
Web address: www.capecodhealth.org
Control: Other not–for–profit (including NFP Corporation) **Service:** General Medical and Surgical

Staffed Beds: 95 **Admissions:** 5970 **Census:** 64 **Outpatient Visits:** 168514 **Births:** 612 **Total Expense ($000):** 123802 **Payroll Expense ($000):** 50519 **Personnel:** 681

FRAMINGHAM—Middlesex County

★ **METROWEST MEDICAL CENTER (220175)**, 115 Lincoln Street, Zip 01702–6342; tel. 508/383–1000, (Includes FRAMINGHAM UNION HOSPITAL; LEONARD MORSE HOSPITAL, 67 Union Street, Natick, Zip 01760; tel. 508/650–7000) **A**1 2 3 5 9 10 **F**3 5 13 15 17 20 25 26 27 28 33 34 38 41 42 43 50 52 53 54 55 56 57 60 61 62 66 68 71 72 73 74 75 76 77 79 80 81 82 84 86 87 88 89 90 91 92 93 94 95 96 97 102 106 107 117 118 119 120 121 123 124 132 133 135 136 137 **S** Vanguard Health System
Primary Contact: Andrei Soran, Chief Executive Officer
COO: Deborah Bitsoli, Chief Operating Officer
CFO: Thomas Sullivan, Chief Financial Officer
CMO: Michael Gottlieb, M.D., Chief Medical Officer
CIO: Michael Hebert, Director Technology
CHR: Rebecca Heffernan, Director Human Resources
Web address: www.mwmc.com
Control: Corporation, Investor–owned, for–profit **Service:** General Medical and Surgical

Staffed Beds: 407 **Admissions:** 17045 **Census:** 208 **Outpatient Visits:** 144607 **Births:** 1942

GARDNER—Worcester County

★ **HEYWOOD HOSPITAL (220095)**, 242 Green Street, Zip 01440–1373; tel. 978/632–3420, (Total facility includes 19 beds in nursing home–type unit) **A**1 5 9 10 **F**3 9 11 13 15 18 24 25 27 31 32 33 38 40 43 46 50 54 55 56 57 62 66 68 72 73 74 75 76 77 79 80 82 84 86 87 88 92 93 95 96 97 102 106 107 112 113 117 118 119 120 121 124 135 136 **P**8
Primary Contact: Daniel P. Moen, President and Chief Executive Officer
CFO: Kimberly Webb, Interim Chief Financial Officer
CIO: Kevin Irish, Chief Information Officer
CHR: Thomas Cady, Vice President Human Resources
Web address: www.heywood.org
Control: Other not–for–profit (including NFP Corporation) **Service:** General Medical and Surgical

Staffed Beds: 128 **Admissions:** 4844 **Census:** 77 **Outpatient Visits:** 218762 **Births:** 591 **Total Expense ($000):** 76087 **Payroll Expense ($000):** 35430 **Personnel:** 710

GLOUCESTER—Essex County

ADDISON GILBERT HOSPITAL See Beverly Hospital, Beverly

GREAT BARRINGTON—Berkshire County

★ **FAIRVIEW HOSPITAL (221302)**, 29 Lewis Avenue, Zip 01230–1713; tel. 413/528–0790 **A**1 9 10 18 **F**3 13 15 24 25 30 31 32 34 38 50 56 62 66 68 73 77 79 80 82 86 87 96 97 102 107 119 120 121 122 124 135 **P**6 **S** Berkshire Health Systems, Inc.
Primary Contact: Eugene A. Dellea, President
COO: Doreen M. Sylvia–Hutchinson, Vice President Operations and Chief Nurse Executive
CMO: Brian Burke, M.D., Chief Medical Officer
CIO: Joe Diver, Chief Information Officer
CHR: Bertha Holcomb, Director Human Resources
Web address: www.berkshirehealthsystems.com
Control: Other not–for–profit (including NFP Corporation) **Service:** General Medical and Surgical

Staffed Beds: 25 **Admissions:** 1178 **Census:** 12 **Outpatient Visits:** 14880 **Births:** 170 **Total Expense ($000):** 30291 **Payroll Expense ($000):** 12679 **Personnel:** 210

GREENFIELD—Franklin County

★ **BAYSTATE FRANKLIN MEDICAL CENTER (220016)**, 164 High Street, Zip 01301–2613; tel. 413/773–0211 **A**1 2 9 10 **F**3 11 13 15 24 25 26 27 30 31 32 38 43 50 51 54 56 57 62 66 68 72 73 74 75 76 77 79 80 81 82 84 86 88 89 93 95 96 97 100 102 106 107 118 119 121 124 135 136 **S** Baystate Health, Inc.
Primary Contact: Charles Gijanto, President
CFO: Greg Brink, Director Finance
CMO: Jacques Blanchet, M.D., Interim Director Medical Affairs
CHR: John Brady, Director Human Resources
Web address: www.baystatehealth.com
Control: Other not–for–profit (including NFP Corporation) **Service:** General Medical and Surgical

Staffed Beds: 90 **Admissions:** 4293 **Census:** 51 **Outpatient Visits:** 136253 **Births:** 523 **Total Expense ($000):** 77176 **Payroll Expense ($000):** 33538 **Personnel:** 484

HAVERHILL—Essex County

BALDPATE HOSPITAL (224033), 83 Baldpate Road, Zip 01833–2399; tel. 978/352–2131, (Nonreporting) **A**9 10
Primary Contact: Lucille M. Batal, Administrator
Control: Corporation, Investor–owned, for–profit **Service:** Psychiatric

Staffed Beds: 59

☐ **MERRIMACK VALLEY HOSPITAL (220174)**, 140 Lincoln Avenue, Zip 01830–6798; tel. 978/374–2000 **A**1 9 10 **F**3 8 15 25 26 27 33 38 41 43 50 51 55 56 57 62 66 68 73 75 79 81 82 86 88 93 96 97 100 106 107 117 118 119 121 134 135 **S** Essent Healthcare
Primary Contact: Michael F. Collins, M.D., Chief Executive Officer
COO: Diane Lovallo, R.N., Chief Nursing Officer
CMO: George Kwass, M.D., Chief of Staff
CIO: Mark Nightingale, Senior Administrator
CHR: Gina Lagana, Director Human Resources
Web address: www.merrimackvalleyhospital.com
Control: Corporation, Investor–owned, for–profit **Service:** General Medical and Surgical

Staffed Beds: 90 **Admissions:** 4497 **Census:** 64 **Outpatient Visits:** 70368 **Births:** 0

★ △ **WHITTIER REHABILITATION HOSPITAL (223028)**, 76 Summer Street, Zip 01830–5896; tel. 978/372–8000, (Nonreporting) **A**1 7 10
Primary Contact: Alfred J. Arcidi, M.D., Senior Vice President
Web address: www.whittierhealth.com
Control: State–Government, nonfederal **Service:** General Medical and Surgical

Staffed Beds: 60

HOLYOKE—Hampden County

★ **HOLYOKE MEDICAL CENTER (220024)**, 575 Beech Street, Zip 01040–2296; tel. 413/534–2500, (Total facility includes 22 beds in nursing home–type unit) **A**1 2 5 9 10 **F**3 5 9 11 13 14 15 17 18 24 25 27 30 31 32 33 36 37 38 41 46 49 50 51 55 56 57 59 62 63 66 68 72 73 74 75 76 77 79 80 81 82 84 86 88 90 91 92 94 95 96 97 100 102 106 107 108 109 111 117 118 119 121 124 132 134 135 136 137 **P**8
Primary Contact: Hank J. Porten, CHE, President and Chief Executive Officer
CFO: Antonio Correia, Chief Financial Officer
CMO: Karen Ferroni, M.D., Medical Director
CIO: Carl Cameron, Manager Information Systems
CHR: Mary Kelleher, Vice President Human Resources
Web address: www.holyokehealth.com
Control: Other not–for–profit (including NFP Corporation) **Service:** General Medical and Surgical

Staffed Beds: 202 **Admissions:** 7103 **Census:** 108 **Outpatient Visits:** 236497 **Births:** 591 **Total Expense ($000):** 109897 **Payroll Expense ($000):** 56292 **Personnel:** 936

Many Facility Codes have changed. Please refer to the AHA Guide Code Chart.

SOLDIERS' HOME IN HOLYOKE (220153), 110 Cherry Street, Zip 01040–2829; tel. 413/532–9475, (Total facility includes 274 beds in nursing home–type unit) (Nonreporting) **A**10
Primary Contact: Paul A. Morin, Superintendent
COO: Lee Anne St Martin, Director Operations
CFO: Anthony Di Stefano, Director Finance
CMO: John E. McHugh, M.D., Medical Director
CIO: Robert Morissette, Coordinator Management Information Systems
CHR: James M. Black, Director Administration
Web address: www.mass.gov/hly
Control: State–Government, nonfederal **Service:** General Medical and Surgical

Staffed Beds: 286

HYANNIS—Barnstable County

★□ **CAPE COD HOSPITAL (220012)**, 27 Park Street, Zip 02601–5203; tel. 508/771–1800 **A**1 2 5 9 10 20 **F**2 3 5 11 13 15 17 18 20 22 25 26 27 30 31 32 33 34 38 40 41 43 50 51 55 56 57 58 59 60 62 63 66 68 72 73 74 75 76 77 79 80 81 82 84 86 87 88 89 90 92 93 94 95 96 97 100 102 107 111 114 119 120 121 124 135 136 137 **P**5 6 **S** Cape Cod Healthcare, Inc.
Primary Contact: Margaret Hanson, RN, Chief Administrative Officer
COO: Patricia Nadle, R.N., Chief Operating Officer and Chief Nursing Officer
CFO: Stephen J. Guimond, Senior Vice President and Chief Financial Officer
CMO: James D. Butterick, M.D., Chief Medical Officer
CIO: John E. Kilroy, Vice President and Chief Information Officer
Web address: www.capecodhealth.org
Control: Other not–for–profit (including NFP Corporation) **Service:** General Medical and Surgical

Staffed Beds: 268 **Admissions:** 15921 **Census:** 189 **Outpatient Visits:** 89486 **Births:** 1021 **Total Expense ($000):** 335297 **Payroll Expense ($000):** 119805 **Personnel:** 1495

JAMAICA PLAIN—Suffolk County

★□ **LEMUEL SHATTUCK HOSPITAL (222006)**, 170 Morton Street, Zip 02130–3787; tel. 617/522–8110 **A**1 3 5 10 **F**3 5 6 15 25 26 27 30 31 32 33 34 37 41 42 43 44 45 47 48 49 50 53 54 55 56 57 59 60 62 66 68 72 73 75 76 77 78 79 80 81 82 85 86 87 88 90 91 92 93 94 95 96 97 100 103 107 119 121 122 124 132 135 137 **P**6 **S** Massachusetts Department of Public Health
Primary Contact: Paul Romary, Chief Executive Officer
CFO: Mike Donovan, Chief Financial Officer
CMO: Joseph Cohen, M.D., Director Medical Services
CIO: Kathryn Noonan, Vice President Information
CHR: Greg Guba, Director Human Resources
Web address: www.shattuckhospital.org
Control: State–Government, nonfederal **Service:** General Medical and Surgical

Staffed Beds: 260 **Admissions:** 1482 **Census:** 247 **Outpatient Visits:** 39176 **Births:** 0 **Total Expense ($000):** 81577 **Payroll Expense ($000):** 51008 **Personnel:** 789

LAWRENCE—Essex County

□ **LAWRENCE GENERAL HOSPITAL (220010)**, 1 General Street, Zip 01842–0389, Mailing Address: P.O. Box 189, Zip 01842–0389; tel. 978/683–4000 **A**1 2 3 5 9 10 **F**3 11 13 15 17 18 25 26 27 30 31 32 33 38 40 43 46 48 49 50 51 55 56 57 59 60 62 63 66 68 72 73 74 75 76 77 79 80 81 82 84 96 97 99 102 106 107 119 124 133 135 136 137 **P**2 5
Primary Contact: Joseph S. McManus, CHE, President and Chief Executive Officer
COO: Gerard J. Foley, Executive Vice President
CFO: Edward L. Dudley, Vice President Fiscal Affairs
CMO: Norman L. Stein, M.D., Vice President Clinical Affairs
CIO: Peter Cole, Director Information Systems
CHR: Cynthia Phelan, Vice President Human Resources
Web address: www.lawrencegeneral.org
Control: Other not–for–profit (including NFP Corporation) **Service:** General Medical and Surgical

Staffed Beds: 189 **Admissions:** 11246 **Census:** 127 **Outpatient Visits:** 87988 **Births:** 2041 **Total Expense ($000):** 143725 **Payroll Expense ($000):** 73541 **Personnel:** 1028

LEEDS—Hampshire County

★□ △ **VETERANS AFFAIRS MEDICAL CENTER**, 421 North Main Street, Zip 01053–9764; tel. 413/584–4040, (Total facility includes 66 beds in nursing home–type unit) **A**1 7 **F**25 26 30 32 36 37 43 44 45 50 53 54 56 57 60 61 62 63 66 72 73 75 76 77 81 82 86 87 88 91 92 93 94 96 119 121 124 133 135 136 137 **S** Department of Veterans Affairs
Primary Contact: Gary M. De Gasta, Acting Director
CMO: William E. Bouttelle, M.D., Chief of Staff and Service Line Manager Mental Health
CIO: James Como, Chief Information Officer
Web address: www.va.gov/sta/guide/home.asp
Control: Veterans Affairs, Government, federal **Service:** Psychiatric

Staffed Beds: 167 **Admissions:** 1114 **Census:** 87 **Outpatient Visits:** 153138 **Births:** 0 **Personnel:** 591

LEOMINSTER—Worcester County

★□ **HEALTH ALLIANCE HOSPITALS (220001)**, 60 Hospital Road, Zip 01453–8004; tel. 978/466–2000 **A**1 2 5 9 10 **F**3 13 15 24 26 27 30 32 33 34 38 39 44 45 46 47 49 50 51 56 59 62 66 68 73 74 75 76 77 79 80 81 84 85 86 87 88 90 94 95 96 97 102 103 106 107 120 121 124 133 135 136 **P**8 **S** UMass Memorial Health Care, Inc.
Primary Contact: Patrick L. Muldoon, FACHE, President and Chief Executive Officer
CFO: Michael Cofone, Chief Financial Officer
CMO: Val Slayton, M.D., Chief Medical Officer
CIO: Richard Monhk, Chief Information Officer
CHR: Allison Wollen, Vice President Human Resources
Web address: www.healthalliance.com
Control: Other not–for–profit (including NFP Corporation) **Service:** General Medical and Surgical

Staffed Beds: 97 **Admissions:** 7624 **Census:** 87 **Outpatient Visits:** 221480 **Births:** 1119 **Total Expense ($000):** 127567 **Payroll Expense ($000):** 57494 **Personnel:** 1047

LOWELL—Middlesex County

★□ **LOWELL GENERAL HOSPITAL (220063)**, 295 Varnum Avenue, Zip 01854–2195; tel. 978/937–6000 **A**1 2 9 10 **F**3 8 11 12 13 15 18 20 24 25 26 27 28 30 31 32 33 34 36 38 40 41 42 43 44 49 50 53 54 55 56 57 58 60 61 62 64 66 68 71 72 73 74 75 76 77 79 80 81 82 84 86 87 96 97 100 102 103 106 107 109 111 112 113 114 118 119 120 121 123 124 133 135 136 **P**8
Primary Contact: Normand E. Deschene, FACHE, President and Chief Executive Officer
COO: Jody White, Executive Vice President and Chief Operating Officer
CFO: Richard Jeffcote, Chief Financial Officer
CMO: Wayne Pasanen, Vice President Medical Affairs
CHR: Peter Zarrilla, Vice President Human Resources
Web address: www.lowellgeneral.org
Control: Other not–for–profit (including NFP Corporation) **Service:** General Medical and Surgical

Staffed Beds: 186 **Admissions:** 11169 **Census:** 122 **Outpatient Visits:** 237947 **Births:** 1905 **Total Expense ($000):** 166432 **Payroll Expense ($000):** 71586 **Personnel:** 1318

□ **SAINTS MEDICAL CENTER (220082)**, One Hospital Drive, Zip 01852–1389; tel. 978/458–1411, (Nonreporting) **A**1 2 5 9 10
Primary Contact: Michael G. Guley, FACHE, President and Chief Executive Officer
COO: Judith Casagrande, Chief Operating Officer
CFO: Steve O'Connor, Chief Financial Officer
CHR: Deborah Bradshaw, Vice President Human Resources
Web address: www.saints–memorial.org
Control: Other not–for–profit (including NFP Corporation) **Service:** General Medical and Surgical

Staffed Beds: 150

LUDLOW—Hampden County

★□ **HEALTHSOUTH REHABILITATION HOSPITAL OF WESTERN MASSACHUSETTS (223030)**, 14 Chestnut Place, Zip 01056–3460; tel. 413/589–7581 **A**1 10 **F**12 16 25 26 30 31 32 33 34 50 55 56 62 72 73 75 80 81 82 85 86 90 93 119 120 121 124 135 137 **S** HEALTHSOUTH Corporation
Primary Contact: R. David Richer, Chief Executive Officer
CFO: Victoria Healy, Controller
CMO: Adnan Dahdul, M.D., Medical Director
CHR: Mary Mazza, Director Human Resources
Web address: www.healthsouth.com
Control: Corporation, Investor–owned, for–profit **Service:** Rehabilitation

Staffed Beds: 53 **Admissions:** 1037 **Census:** 41 **Outpatient Visits:** 42760 **Births:** 0 **Total Expense ($000):** 14207 **Payroll Expense ($000):** 8596 **Personnel:** 177

MA

Hospital, Medicare Provider Number, Address, Telephone, Approval, Facility, and Physician Codes, Health Care System

★ American Hospital Association (AHA) membership
□ The Joint Commission accreditation
○ American Osteopathic Association (AOA) accreditation
△ Commission on Accreditation of Rehabilitation Facilities (CARF) accreditation

LYNN—Essex County

UNION HOSPITAL See North Shore Medical Center, Salem

MALDEN—Middlesex County

HALLMARK HEALTH SYSTEM See Melrose

MARLBOROUGH—Middlesex County

★ **UMASS MEMORIAL–MARLBOROUGH HOSPITAL (220049)**, 157 Union Street, Zip 01752–1297; tel. 508/481–5000 **A**1 5 9 10 **F**3 11 15 24 25 26 27 33 38 43 46 49 50 51 52 53 55 56 57 59 62 63 66 68 72 73 75 76 77 79 80 81 86 88 92 95 96 99 102 106 107 118 119 121 135 136 **S** UMass Memorial Health Care, Inc.
Primary Contact: John Polanowicz, President and Chief Executive Officer
COO: Candra Szymanski, Chief Operating Officer
CFO: Jeff Dion, Chief Financial Officer
CHR: Suzanne Parsons, Vice President Human Resources
Web address: www.marlboroughhospital.org
Control: Other not–for–profit (including NFP Corporation) **Service:** General Medical and Surgical

Staffed Beds: 67 **Admissions:** 3795 **Census:** 46 **Outpatient Visits:** 57426 **Births:** 0 **Total Expense ($000):** 61574 **Payroll Expense ($000):** 30534

MA

MEDFORD—Middlesex County

LAWRENCE MEMORIAL HOSPITAL OF MEDFORD See Hallmark Health System, Melrose

MELROSE—Middlesex County

★ **HALLMARK HEALTH SYSTEM (220070)**, 585 Lebanon Street, Zip 2176; tel. 781/979–3000, (Includes LAWRENCE MEMORIAL HOSPITAL OF MEDFORD, 170 Governors Avenue, Medford, Zip 02155–1643; tel. 781/306–6000; MELROSE–WAKEFIELD HOSPITAL, 585 Lebanon Street, Zip 02176) **A**1 2 5 10 **F**3 5 11 12 13 15 18 20 24 25 26 27 28 30 31 32 33 38 42 44 46 49 50 51 53 54 55 56 57 60 62 63 68 71 72 73 74 75 76 77 79 80 81 82 86 87 88 90 91 92 93 94 95 96 97 99 100 102 107 109 117 119 120 121 122 124 135 136 137 **P**5 6
Primary Contact: Michael V. Sack, President and Chief Executive Officer
CFO: James A. Nania, System Vice President and Chief Financial Officer
CMO: Mike H. Summerer, M.D., Chief Medical Officer
CIO: Richard A. Pozniak, Director Marketing and Communications
CHR: Richard Kenny, Vice President Human Resources
Web address: www.hallmarkhealth.org
Control: Other not–for–profit (including NFP Corporation) **Service:** General Medical and Surgical

Staffed Beds: 319 **Admissions:** 16330 **Census:** 240 **Outpatient Visits:** 616304 **Births:** 1251 **Total Expense ($000):** 258899 **Payroll Expense ($000):** 133934 **Personnel:** 1901

METHUEN—Essex County

★ **CARITAS HOLY FAMILY HOSPITAL AND MEDICAL CENTER (220080)**, 70 East Street, Zip 01844–4597; tel. 978/687–0151, (Total facility includes 18 beds in nursing home–type unit) **A**1 2 5 9 10 **F**3 11 13 14 15 17 18 24 25 26 27 33 36 37 38 40 41 43 50 51 54 55 56 57 59 60 62 66 68 71 72 73 74 75 76 77 79 80 81 82 84 86 87 88 90 91 92 93 96 97 102 106 107 109 111 112 114 117 118 119 120 121 124 133 135 136 137 **P**5 6 7 **S** Caritas Christi Health Care
Primary Contact: Thomas K. Sager, President and Chief Executive Officer
COO: Martha M. McDrury, R.N., Senior Vice President and Chief Operating Officer
CFO: Robert Kotsonis, Chief Financial Officer
CMO: Robert Karpman, M.D., Vice President Medical Affairs
CIO: Dan O'Neil, Director Management Information Systems
Web address: www.holyfamilyhosp.org
Control: Church–operated, Nongovernment, not–for profit **Service:** General Medical and Surgical

Staffed Beds: 255 **Admissions:** 10303 **Census:** 131 **Outpatient Visits:** 196847 **Births:** 1153 **Total Expense ($000):** 132623 **Payroll Expense ($000):** 60165

MILFORD—Worcester County

★ **MILFORD REGIONAL MEDICAL CENTER (220090)**, 14 Prospect Street, Zip 01757–3090; tel. 508/473–1190, (Includes WHITINSVILLE MEDICAL CENTER, 18 Granite Street, Whitinsville, Zip 01588; tel. 508/234–6311) **A**1 2 5 9 10 **F**3 11 13 15 24 25 26 27 28 30 31 32 33 38 43 46 49 50 51 55 56 57 61 62 66 68 72 73 74 75 76 77 78 79 80 81 82 84 86 96 97 99 102 103 106 107 112 119 121 123 124 135 136 137
Primary Contact: Francis M. Saba, Chief Executive Officer
CFO: Edward Kelly, President
CMO: William Muller, M.D., Vice President Medical Affairs
CIO: Larry Fraize, Director Management Information Systems
CHR: Linda Greasom, Vice President Human Resources
Web address: www.milfordregional.org
Control: Other not–for–profit (including NFP Corporation) **Service:** General Medical and Surgical

Staffed Beds: 121 **Admissions:** 8421 **Census:** 94 **Outpatient Visits:** 372019 **Births:** 1030 **Total Expense ($000):** 143456 **Payroll Expense ($000):** 69037 **Personnel:** 1444

MILTON—Norfolk County

☐ **MILTON HOSPITAL (220108)**, 199 Reedsdale Road, Zip 02186–3807; tel. 617/696–4600 **A**1 9 10 **F**11 15 25 26 27 38 43 55 57 62 66 68 72 75 76 77 79 80 81 82 86 96 97 100 106 107 117 119 120 121 122 124 135
Primary Contact: Joseph V. Morrissey, President
CFO: Jay Holleran, Chief Financial Officer
CMO: Joseph Raduazzo, M.D., Vice President Affairs and Chief Medical Officer
CIO: Jean Fernandez, Chief Information Officer
CHR: Kathleen Harrington, Vice President Human Resources
Web address: www.miltonhospital.org
Control: Other not–for–profit (including NFP Corporation) **Service:** General Medical and Surgical

Staffed Beds: 82 **Admissions:** 4747 **Census:** 64 **Outpatient Visits:** 28398 **Births:** 0

NANTUCKET—Nantucket County

★ **NANTUCKET COTTAGE HOSPITAL (221301)**, 57 Prospect Street, Zip 02554–2799; tel. 508/825–8100 **A**1 9 10 18 **F**13 15 24 27 30 31 32 33 38 42 43 46 50 55 57 59 61 62 63 66 67 68 73 74 75 76 79 80 84 86 90 92 96 100 107 119 121 122 137 **P**5 **S** Partners HealthCare System, Inc.
Primary Contact: Sylvia Getman, President and Chief Executive Officer
CFO: John R. Fitzgerald, Chief Financial Officer
CMO: Timothy J. Lepore, FACS, M.D., Medical Director
CIO: Terry Hughes, Management Information Systems Coordinator
CHR: Kelly John, Manager Human Resources
Web address: www.nantuckethospital.org
Control: Other not–for–profit (including NFP Corporation) **Service:** General Medical and Surgical

Staffed Beds: 19 **Admissions:** 719 **Census:** 5 **Outpatient Visits:** 47307 **Births:** 147 **Total Expense ($000):** 28674 **Payroll Expense ($000):** 10215 **Personnel:** 145

NATICK—Middlesex County

☐ **KINDRED HOSPITAL NORTHEAST–NATICK**, 67 Union Street, 6th Floor, Zip 1760; tel. 508/650–7630, (Nonreporting) **A**1 **S** Kindred Healthcare
Primary Contact: Robert A. Gundersen, Chief Executive Officer
Web address: www.kindredhealthcare.com
Control: Corporation, Investor–owned, for–profit **Service:** Long–Term Acute Care hospital

Staffed Beds: 23

LEONARD MORSE HOSPITAL See MetroWest Medical Center, Framingham

NEEDHAM—Norfolk County

BETH ISRAEL DEACONESS HOSPITAL–NEEDHAM CAMPUS See Beth Israel Deaconess Medical Center, Boston

NEW BEDFORD—Bristol County

☐ **NEW BEDFORD REHABILITATION HOSPITAL (222043)**, 4499 Acushnet Avenue, Zip 2745; tel. 508/995–6900, (Nonreporting) **A**1 **S** Vibra Healthcare
Primary Contact: Edward B. Leary, Chief Executive Officer
Web address: www.newbedfordrehab.com
Control: Corporation, Investor–owned, for–profit **Service:** Long–Term Acute Care hospital

Staffed Beds: 90

ST. LUKE'S HOSPITAL See Southcoast Hospitals Group, Fall River

NEWBURYPORT—Essex County

★ **ANNA JAQUES HOSPITAL (220029)**, 25 Highland Avenue, Zip 01950–3894; tel. 978/463–1000 **A**1 9 10 **F**3 13 14 15 18 24 25 27 30 33 36 38 40 43 44 55 56 62 66 68 73 74 75 76 77 79 80 81 82 84 86 87 88 89 92 95 96 97 99 100 102 106 107 117 118 119 120 121 135 **P**8
Primary Contact: Delia O'Connor, Chief Executive Officer
CFO: Mark L. Goldstein, Chief Financial Officer
CMO: Leslie Sebba, M.D., Medical Director
CIO: Robert Buchanan, M.D., Chief Information Officer
CHR: Stephen Salvo, Vice President Human Resources
Web address: www.ajh.org
Control: Other not–for–profit (including NFP Corporation) **Service:** General Medical and Surgical

Staffed Beds: 143 **Admissions:** 7441 **Census:** 102 **Outpatient Visits:** 215137 **Births:** 717 **Total Expense ($000):** 89380 **Payroll Expense ($000):** 42861 **Personnel:** 627

NEWTON LOWER FALLS—Middlesex County

★ **NEWTON–WELLESLEY HOSPITAL (220101)**, 2014 Washington Street, Zip 02462–1699; tel. 617/243–6000 **A**1 2 3 5 9 10 **F**3 8 11 12 13 15 24 25 26 27 28 29 33 34 36 38 40 41 43 49 50 52 53 54 55 56 57 58 59 62 63 66 68 71 72 73 74 75 76 77 79 80 82 84 86 88 90 91 92 96 99 102 103 104 105 106 107 113 114 118 119 120 121 124 132 133 135 136 137 **P**1 **S** Partners HealthCare System, Inc.
Primary Contact: Michael Jellinek, M.D., President
COO: Patrick Jordan, Senior Vice President Administration
CFO: Daniel Gross, Senior Vice President Finance and Chief Financial Officer
CMO: Leslie Selbovitz, M.D., Senior Vice President Medical Affairs
CIO: Scott T. MacLean, Chief Information Officer
CHR: Beth Taylor, Director Human Resources
Web address: www.nwh.org
Control: Other not–for–profit (including NFP Corporation) **Service:** General Medical and Surgical

Staffed Beds: 226 **Admissions:** 14336 **Census:** 195 **Outpatient Visits:** 531663 **Births:** 3296

NORTH ADAMS—Berkshire County

★ **NORTH ADAMS REGIONAL HOSPITAL (220051)**, 71 Hospital Avenue, Zip 01247–2584; tel. 413/664–5000 **A**1 2 9 10 **F**3 8 13 15 25 26 31 32 33 37 38 50 56 60 62 63 66 68 73 74 79 81 82 84 86 88 96 97 99 100 107 115 119 124 135 136 137 **P**6
Primary Contact: Richard T. Palmisano, II, RN, President and Chief Executive Officer
CFO: Paul Dabrody, Interim Chief Financial Officer
CMO: Paul Donovan, M.D., President Medical Staff
CIO: Dave Delano, Director Information Technology
CHR: Arthur Scott, Vice President Human Resources
Web address: www.nbhealth.org
Control: Other not–for–profit (including NFP Corporation) **Service:** General Medical and Surgical

Staffed Beds: 54 **Admissions:** 3323 **Census:** 38 **Outpatient Visits:** 130690 **Births:** 311 **Total Expense ($000):** 54199 **Payroll Expense ($000):** 23023 **Personnel:** 386

NORTHAMPTON—Hampshire County

★ **COOLEY DICKINSON HOSPITAL (220015)**, 30 Locust Street, Zip 01060–2093, Mailing Address: P.O. Box 5001, Zip 01061–5001; tel. 413/582–2000 **A**1 2 9 10 **F**3 5 11 13 14 15 18 24 25 26 27 30 31 33 34 36 37 38 40 43 49 50 51 53 54 55 56 57 59 60 62 68 72 73 74 76 77 79 81 82 84 86 88 89 90 91 92 93 94 95 96 97 100 102 105 106 107 109 111 112 116 119 120 121 123 124 135 136 137 **P**8
Primary Contact: Carol M. Smith, RN, Acting President and Chief Executive Officer
COO: Carol M. Smith, R.N., Chief Operating Officer, Chief Nursing Officer and Senior Executive Vice President
CFO: Edith S. Peter, Chief Financial Officer and Vice President Finance
CMO: Glenn Focht, M.D., Vice President Medical Affairs
CIO: Wayne Freeberg, Chief Information Officer
CHR: Wilmont Davis, Vice President Human Resources
Web address: www.cooley–dickinson.org
Control: Other not–for–profit (including NFP Corporation) **Service:** General Medical and Surgical

Staffed Beds: 142 **Admissions:** 8326 **Census:** 101 **Outpatient Visits:** 217768 **Births:** 873 **Total Expense ($000):** 140416 **Payroll Expense ($000):** 68516 **Personnel:** 1086

NORWOOD—Norfolk County

★ **CARITAS NORWOOD HOSPITAL (220126)**, 800 Washington Street, Zip 02062–3487; tel. 781/769–4000 **A**1 2 5 9 10 **F**3 7 11 12 13 17 18 24 25 26 31 33 38 41 43 50 52 54 56 57 63 66 68 72 73 74 77 79 82 84 86 88 90 92 93 96 97 100 102 103 104 106 107 110 111 112 114 118 119 120 121 124 135 136 137 **P**5 **S** Caritas Christi Health Care
Primary Contact: John B. Chessare, M.D., M.P.H., President
COO: William P. Fleming, Chief Operating Officer
CFO: Robert Guyon, Vice President Finance and Chief Financial Officer
CMO: Shanker Nesathurai, M.D., Vice President Medical Affairs
CIO: Charles Podesta, Vice President and Chief Information Officer
CHR: Marian Cheevers, Director Human Resources
Web address: www.caritasnorwood.org
Control: Church–operated, Nongovernment, not–for profit **Service:** General Medical and Surgical

Staffed Beds: 264 **Admissions:** 12538 **Census:** 171 **Outpatient Visits:** 132992 **Births:** 533 **Total Expense ($000):** 145322 **Payroll Expense ($000):** 73086 **Personnel:** 1018

OAK BLUFFS—Dukes County

★ **MARTHA'S VINEYARD HOSPITAL (221300)**, One Hospital Road, Zip 2557, Mailing Address: P.O. Box 1477, Zip 02557–1477; tel. 508/693–0410 **A**1 9 10 18 **F**8 13 15 24 25 26 38 50 55 66 68 73 74 75 76 77 79 84 86 87 96 102 107 119 122 133 135 136 **S** Partners HealthCare System, Inc.
Primary Contact: Timothy J. Walsh, Chief Executive Officer
CMO: Pieter Pil, M.D., Chief Medical Staff
CHR: Ken Chisholm, Director Human Resources
Web address: www.marthasvineyardhospital.org
Control: Other not–for–profit (including NFP Corporation) **Service:** General Medical and Surgical

Staffed Beds: 25 **Admissions:** 1231 **Census:** 16 **Outpatient Visits:** 25775 **Births:** 104

PALMER—Hampden County

★ **WING MEMORIAL HOSPITAL AND MEDICAL CENTERS (220030)**, 40 Wright Street, Zip 01069–1138; tel. 413/283–7651 **A**1 5 9 10 **F**3 5 11 15 25 26 27 29 31 32 34 35 38 42 43 49 50 54 55 56 57 60 61 62 63 66 68 72 75 76 77 79 80 84 86 87 88 89 90 91 92 93 94 95 96 97 99 102 106 107 118 119 120 121 135 136 137 **P**6 **S** UMass Memorial Health Care, Inc.
Primary Contact: Charles E. Cavagnaro, III, M.D., President and Chief Executive Officer
COO: Janice A. Kucewicz, Senior Vice President
CFO: Keary T. Allicon, Vice President Finance and Chief Financial Officer
CMO: David L. Maguire, M.D., Vice President Medical Affairs
CIO: Kenneth Riley, Director Information Systems
CHR: Thomas Guilfoil, Director Human Resources
Web address: www.winghealth.org
Control: Other not–for–profit (including NFP Corporation) **Service:** General Medical and Surgical

Staffed Beds: 52 **Admissions:** 2789 **Census:** 32 **Outpatient Visits:** 243386 **Births:** 0 **Total Expense ($000):** 59729 **Payroll Expense ($000):** 29802 **Personnel:** 524

PEABODY—Essex County

□ **KINDRED HOSPITAL BOSTON NORTH SHORE (222044)**, 15 King Street, Zip 01960–4268; tel. 978/531–2900, (Nonreporting) **A**1 10 **S** Kindred Healthcare
Primary Contact: Thomas Dowley, Interim Chief Executive Officer
COO: Rosalind Tryder, Chief Operating Officer
CFO: Thomas Dowley, Chief Financial Officer
Web address: www.kindredbns.com
Control: Corporation, Investor–owned, for–profit **Service:** General Medical and Surgical

Staffed Beds: 50

PEMBROKE—Plymouth County

□ **PEMBROKE HOSPITAL**, 199 Oak Street, Zip 02359–1953; tel. 781/826–8161, (Nonreporting) **A**1 **S** Universal Health Services, Inc.
Primary Contact: Paul Zani, Chief Executive Officer and Managing Director
Control: Partnership, Investor–owned, for–profit **Service:** Psychiatric

Staffed Beds: 80

PITTSFIELD—Berkshire County

★ **BERKSHIRE MEDICAL CENTER (220046)**, 725 North Street, Zip 01201–4124; tel. 413/447–2000, (Includes HILLCREST HOSPITAL, 165 Tor Court, Zip 01201–3099, Mailing Address: Box 1155, Zip 01202–1155; tel. 413/443–4761), (Nonreporting) **A**1 2 3 5 8 9 10 12 13 **S** Berkshire Health Systems, Inc.
Primary Contact: Helen Downey, RN, Chief Operating Officer and Chief Nursing Officer
COO: Helen Downey, R.N., Chief Operating Officer and Chief Nursing Officer
CFO: Darlene Rodowicz, Chief Financial Officer
CMO: Robert Cella, M.D., Vice President Medical Affairs
CIO: Joseph Diver, Chief Information Officer
CHR: Arthur Milano, Vice President Human Resources
Web address: www.berkshirehealthsystems.com
Control: Other not–for–profit (including NFP Corporation) **Service:** General Medical and Surgical

Staffed Beds: 283

MA

Hospital, Medicare Provider Number, Address, Telephone, Approval, Facility, and Physician Codes, Health Care System
★ American Hospital Association (AHA) membership
□ The Joint Commission accreditation
○ American Osteopathic Association (AOA) accreditation
△ Commission on Accreditation of Rehabilitation Facilities (CARF) accreditation

PLYMOUTH—Plymouth County

★ **JORDAN HOSPITAL (220060)**, 275 Sandwich Street, Zip 02360–2196; tel. 508/746–2000 **A**1 2 9 10 **F**3 13 15 17 18 24 25 26 27 30 31 32 33 34 35 38 41 43 49 51 55 56 57 58 60 62 66 68 72 73 74 75 76 77 79 80 81 82 84 86 90 92 96 97 100 102 105 106 107 108 109 111 119 120 121 123 124 132 133 134 135 136 137 **P**6
Primary Contact: Peter J. Holden, President and Chief Executive Officer
CFO: Elliot L. Schwartz, Vice President Finance
CMO: Harvey Kowaloff, M.D., Vice President Medical Affairs
CIO: Dennis Fonseca, Chief Information Officer
CHR: Russell Averna, Vice President Clinical and Support Services
Web address: www.jordanhospital.org
Control: Other not–for–profit (including NFP Corporation) **Service:** General Medical and Surgical

Staffed Beds: 136 **Admissions:** 11026 **Census:** 113 **Outpatient Visits:** 380926 **Births:** 738 **Total Expense ($000):** 166741 **Payroll Expense ($000):** 74557 **Personnel:** 966

QUINCY—Norfolk County

★ **QUINCY MEDICAL CENTER (220067)**, 114 Whitwell Street, Zip 02169–1899; tel. 617/773–6100 **A**1 2 5 9 10 **F**3 8 11 12 15 18 24 25 26 27 30 31 32 33 38 41 42 43 44 46 50 54 55 56 57 60 62 66 68 72 73 75 76 77 79 80 81 82 84 86 87 88 90 91 93 94 95 96 97 102 107 112 118 119 120 121 124 132 133 135 136 137 **P**6
Primary Contact: Gary W. Gibbons, M.D., President and Chief Executive Officer
CFO: Mark O'Neill, Chief Financial Officer
CMO: Tom Barber, M.D., Chief Medical Officer
CIO: Meg Aranow, Chief Information Officer
CHR: David Ryan, Vice President Human Resources
Web address: www.quincymc.org
Control: Other not–for–profit (including NFP Corporation) **Service:** General Medical and Surgical

Staffed Beds: 130 **Admissions:** 7268 **Census:** 111 **Outpatient Visits:** 93757 **Births:** 0 **Total Expense ($000):** 105635 **Payroll Expense ($000):** 51650

ROCHDALE—Worcester County

☐ **KINDRED HOSPITAL PARK VIEW–CENTRAL MASSACHUSETTS (222046)**, 111 Huntoon Memorial Highway, Zip 1542; tel. 508/892–6000, (Nonreporting) **A**1 10 **S** Kindred Healthcare
Primary Contact: Scott MacLean, Administrator
Web address: www.kindredhealthcare.com
Control: Corporation, Investor–owned, for–profit **Service:** Long–Term Acute Care hospital

Staffed Beds: 10

SALEM—Essex County

★ **NORTH SHORE MEDICAL CENTER (220035)**, 81 Highland Avenue, Zip 01970–2768; tel. 978/741–1200, (Includes NORTH SHORE CHILDREN'S HOSPITAL, 57 Highland Avenue, Zip 01970–6508; tel. 978/745–2100; SALEM HOSPITAL, 81 Highland Avenue, Zip 01970; tel. 978/741–1200; UNION HOSPITAL, 500 Lynnfield Street, Lynn, Zip 01904–1487; tel. 781/581–9200) **A**1 2 3 5 9 10 **F**5 12 13 15 17 18 20 22 25 26 27 28 30 31 32 33 34 36 38 40 42 43 50 51 55 56 57 60 62 66 68 71 72 73 74 75 76 77 79 80 81 82 84 86 88 89 90 91 92 93 94 95 96 97 100 102 104 106 107 109 111 113 114 118 119 120 121 132 135 136 137 **P**6 8 **S** Partners HealthCare System, Inc.
Primary Contact: Robert G. Norton, CHE, President and Chief Executive Officer
COO: Louis J. Woolf, Executive Vice President and Chief Operating Officer
CFO: Roger D. Wiseman, Senior Vice President and Chief Financial Officer
CMO: Mitchell S. Rein, M.D., Chief Medical Officer
CIO: Mark Hulse, Vice President Information Services
CHR: Arthur Bowes, Senior Vice President Human Resources
Web address: www.nsmc.partners.org
Control: Other not–for–profit (including NFP Corporation) **Service:** General Medical and Surgical

Staffed Beds: 415 **Admissions:** 22820 **Census:** 304 **Outpatient Visits:** 142041 **Births:** 1915 **Total Expense ($000):** 383114 **Payroll Expense ($000):** 174786

★ △ **SHAUGHNESSY–KAPLAN REHABILITATION HOSPITAL (222026)**, Dove Avenue, Zip 01970–2999; tel. 978/745–9000, (Total facility includes 40 beds in nursing home–type unit) **A**1 7 10 **F**1 24 25 26 32 42 43 44 54 55 56 57 59 66 72 75 77 80 82 86 117 119 120 121 135 136 137 **P**6 **S** Partners HealthCare System, Inc.
Primary Contact: Maureen Banks, President
COO: Joanne Fucile, Vice President Patient Care Services
CFO: Virginia Mirisola, Fiscal Director
CMO: Maurice Greenbaum, M.D., Medical Director
CIO: Robert Sawyer, Senior Project Specialist
CHR: Hugh Burke, Director Human Resources
Web address: www.shaughnessy–kaplan.org
Control: Other not–for–profit (including NFP Corporation) **Service:** Long–Term Acute Care hospital

Staffed Beds: 160 **Admissions:** 1931 **Census:** 121 **Outpatient Visits:** 56426 **Births:** 0 **Total Expense ($000):** 38516 **Payroll Expense ($000):** 22061 **Personnel:** 380

SOMERVILLE—Middlesex County

SOMERVILLE HOSPITAL See Cambridge Health Alliance, Cambridge

SOUTH WEYMOUTH—Norfolk County

★ **SOUTH SHORE HOSPITAL (220100)**, 55 Fogg Road, Zip 02190–2455; tel. 781/340–8000 **A**1 2 5 9 10 **F**7 11 13 15 17 18 20 24 25 26 27 28 30 33 35 38 41 42 43 44 46 50 51 55 56 57 59 61 62 66 68 70 71 72 73 74 76 77 79 80 81 82 84 86 96 97 99 100 102 103 106 107 112 113 114 118 119 121 123 124 132 133 135 136 137 **P**1
Primary Contact: Richard Aubut, President and Chief Executive Officer
COO: Joseph Cahill, Executive Vice President and Chief Operating Officer
CIO: Del Dixon, Chief Information Officer
CHR: Robert Wheeler, Vice President Human Resources
Web address: www.southshorehospital.org
Control: Other not–for–profit (including NFP Corporation) **Service:** General Medical and Surgical

Staffed Beds: 299 **Admissions:** 19842 **Census:** 209 **Outpatient Visits:** 457305 **Births:** 3795 **Total Expense ($000):** 322485 **Payroll Expense ($000):** 157286 **Personnel:** 2360

SOUTHBRIDGE—Worcester County

★ **HARRINGTON MEMORIAL HOSPITAL (220019)**, 100 South Street, Zip 01550–4045; tel. 508/765–9771 **A**1 5 9 10 **F**1 3 4 5 6 8 11 13 15 16 17 24 25 27 28 30 31 32 33 36 38 40 41 42 49 50 53 54 55 56 57 62 65 66 68 70 71 72 73 74 75 76 77 78 79 80 81 82 83 84 85 86 87 88 89 90 91 92 93 94 96 99 100 102 104 107 112 117 118 119 121 123 124 135 **P**1
Primary Contact: Edward H. Moore, President and Chief Executive Officer
COO: Douglas Crapser, Executive Vice President
CFO: Dana P. Diggins, Acting Vice President Fiscal Services
CMO: Vladas Litani, M.D., President Medical Staff
CIO: Mark Forsman, Director Management Information Systems
CHR: Charlene Richard, Director Human Resources
Web address: www.harringtonhospital.org
Control: Other not–for–profit (including NFP Corporation) **Service:** General Medical and Surgical

Staffed Beds: 79 **Admissions:** 2746 **Census:** 36 **Outpatient Visits:** 195080 **Births:** 412 **Total Expense ($000):** 64618 **Payroll Expense ($000):** 34015 **Personnel:** 525

SPRINGFIELD—Hampden County

★ **BAYSTATE MEDICAL CENTER (220077)**, 759 Chestnut Street, Zip 01199–0001; tel. 413/794–0000 **A**1 2 3 5 8 9 10 **F**3 5 8 11 12 13 14 15 17 18 20 22 24 25 26 27 28 30 31 32 33 36 38 40 41 43 46 47 48 49 50 51 52 53 54 55 56 57 58 59 60 62 63 66 68 70 72 73 74 75 76 77 79 80 81 82 83 84 86 87 88 89 90 91 92 93 94 95 96 97 98 99 100 102 103 106 107 108 109 111 112 113 114 116 118 119 120 121 127 130 132 134 135 136 137 **P**1 **S** Baystate Health, Inc.
Primary Contact: Mark R. Tolosky, FACHE, J.D., President and Chief Executive Officer
COO: Trish Hannon, Senior Vice President and Chief Operating Officer
CFO: Keith C McLean Shinaman, Senior Vice President Finance
CMO: Loring S. Flint, M.D., Senior Vice President Medical Affairs
CIO: Mark Gorrell, Vice President Information Services
CHR: Elizabeth B. Simpson, Senior Vice President Human Resources
Web address: www.baystatehealth.com
Control: Other not–for–profit (including NFP Corporation) **Service:** General Medical and Surgical

Staffed Beds: 653 **Admissions:** 35146 **Census:** 498 **Outpatient Visits:** 792897 **Births:** 4250 **Total Expense ($000):** 747799 **Payroll Expense ($000):** 290224 **Personnel:** 5275

☐ **KINDRED HOSPITAL PARK VIEW (222046)**, 1400 State Street, Zip 01109–2589; tel. 413/726–6700, (Total facility includes 172 beds in nursing home–type unit) (Nonreporting) **A**1 10 **S** Kindred Healthcare
Primary Contact: Karen O. Moore, RN, M.S., Chief Executive Officer
CFO: Anna Dyrkacz, Chief Financial Officer
CMO: Kenneth Santiago, M.D., Medical Director
CHR: Donna Ciarefella, Director Human Resources
Web address: www.kindredhealthcare.com
Control: Corporation, Investor–owned, for–profit **Service:** Long–Term Acute Care hospital

Staffed Beds: 284

☒ **MERCY MEDICAL CENTER (220066)**, 271 Carew Street, Zip 01104–2398, Mailing Address: P.O. Box 9012, Zip 01102–9012; tel. 413/748–9000 **A**1 2 9 10 **F**1 4 5 8 11 12 13 15 16 17 18 20 24 25 26 27 30 31 32 33 38 43 46 49 50 51 54 55 57 62 65 66 68 70 71 72 74 75 76 77 78 79 80 83 84 85 86 88 89 92 93 94 95 96 97 99 100 102 103 106 107 108 109 111 112 116 117 118 119 121 124 132 133 135 136 137 **P**6 **S** Catholic Health East
Primary Contact: Vincent J. McCorkle, CHE, President and Chief Executive Officer
CFO: Michael Hammond, Interim Chief Financial Officer
CIO: Joan Methe, Chief Information Officer
CHR: Leonard F. Pansa, Vice President Human Resources
Web address: www.mercycares.com
Control: Other not–for–profit (including NFP Corporation) **Service:** General Medical and Surgical

Staffed Beds: 325 **Admissions:** 14972 **Census:** 260 **Outpatient Visits:** 465846 **Births:** 1237 **Total Expense ($000):** 187829 **Payroll Expense ($000):** 83371 **Personnel:** 1401

☐ **SHRINERS HOSPITALS FOR CHILDREN, SPRINGFIELD**, 516 Carew Street, Zip 01104–2396; tel. 413/787–2000 **A**1 3 5 **F**25 32 33 62 73 77 79 80 84 86 107 119 132 135 **P**6 **S** Shriners Hospitals for Children
Primary Contact: Mark L. Niederpruem, FACHE, Administrator
CFO: Stuart Young, Director Fiscal Services
CMO: David M. Drvaric, M.D., Chief of Staff
CIO: Howard Tuber, Director Information Services
Web address: www.shrinershq.org
Control: Other not–for–profit (including NFP Corporation) **Service:** Children's orthopedic

Staffed Beds: 20 **Admissions:** 723 **Census:** 8 **Outpatient Visits:** 19661 **Births:** 0 **Personnel:** 203

STOCKBRIDGE—Berkshire County

★ **AUSTEN RIGGS CENTER**, 25 Main Street, Zip 01262–0962, Mailing Address: P.O. Box 962, Zip 01262–0962; tel. 413/298–5511, (Nonreporting)
Primary Contact: Chauncey Collins, Director Operations
COO: Edward R. Shapiro, M.D., Medical Director and Chief Executive Officer
CFO: Chauncey Collins, Director Operations
CMO: Edward R. Shapiro, M.D., Medical Director and Chief Executive Officer
CHR: Lisa Scale, Director Human Resources
Web address: www.austenriggs.org
Control: Other not–for–profit (including NFP Corporation) **Service:** Psychiatric

Staffed Beds: 47

STOUGHTON—Norfolk County

☐ **KINDRED HOSPITAL NORTHEAST–STOUGHTON**, 909 Sumner Street, 1st Floor, Zip 2072; tel. 781/297–8200, (Nonreporting) **A**1 **S** Kindred Healthcare
Primary Contact: James MacKenzie, Administrator
Web address: www.kindredhealthcare.com
Control: Corporation, Investor–owned, for–profit **Service:** Long–Term Acute Care hospital

Staffed Beds: 10

☒ △ **NEW ENGLAND SINAI HOSPITAL AND REHABILITATION CENTER (222027)**, 150 York Street, Zip 02072–1881; tel. 781/344–0600 **A**1 3 5 7 10 **F**1 2 3 6 9 11 24 25 26 30 33 43 44 45 50 54 55 56 57 58 60 62 66 73 75 76 80 81 82 85 86 118 119 120 121 132 135 137 **P**6
Primary Contact: Lester P. Schindel, President and Chief Executive Officer
COO: Ronald M. Lombardi, Executive Vice President and Chief Operating Officer
CFO: Charles Champagne, Chief Financial Officer
CMO: Lawrence S. Hotes, M.D., Chief Medical Officer
CIO: Francine Sousa, Director Management Information Service
CHR: David Tedesco, Vice President Human Resources
Web address: www.newenglandsinai.org
Control: Other not–for–profit (including NFP Corporation) **Service:** Long–Term Acute Care hospital

Staffed Beds: 212 **Admissions:** 1843 **Census:** 178 **Outpatient Visits:** 37590 **Births:** 0 **Total Expense ($000):** 70737 **Payroll Expense ($000):** 39778 **Personnel:** 659

TAUNTON—Bristol County

☒ **MORTON HOSPITAL AND MEDICAL CENTER (220073)**, 88 Washington Street, Zip 02780–2499; tel. 508/828–7000, (Total facility includes 21 beds in nursing home–type unit) **A**1 2 9 10 **F**1 3 4 5 8 11 13 15 16 17 25 26 27 31 32 33 38 40 43 50 55 56 57 60 61 62 65 66 68 70 71 72 73 74 75 76 77 78 79 80 82 83 84 85 86 88 89 90 91 92 93 94 96 97 100 102 106 107 112 117 118 119 120 121 133 135 136 137 **P**6 8
Primary Contact: Thomas C. Porter, President
COO: Maureen A. Bryant, Executive Vice President
CFO: Lawrence E. Seck, Senior Vice President
Web address: www.mortonhospital.org
Control: Other not–for–profit (including NFP Corporation) **Service:** General Medical and Surgical

Staffed Beds: 153 **Admissions:** 6730 **Census:** 102 **Outpatient Visits:** 88423 **Births:** 482 **Total Expense ($000):** 106991 **Payroll Expense ($000):** 53638 **Personnel:** 843

MA

☐ **TAUNTON STATE HOSPITAL (224001)**, 60 Hodges Avenue Extension, Zip 02780–3034, Mailing Address: P.O. Box 4007, Zip 02780–4007; tel. 508/977–3000, (Nonreporting) **A**1 10 **S** Massachusetts Department of Mental Health
Primary Contact: Roberta H. Guez, Administrator and Chief Operating Officer
COO: Roberta H. Guez, Administrator and Chief Operating Officer
CMO: Masood Aslam, M.D., Medical Director
CHR: Trish Cobb, Director Human Resources
Control: State–Government, nonfederal **Service:** Psychiatric

Staffed Beds: 185

TEWKSBURY—Middlesex County

☐ **TEWKSBURY HOSPITAL (222003)**, 365 East Street, Zip 01876–1998; tel. 978/851–7321, (Nonreporting) **A**1 10 **S** Massachusetts Department of Public Health
Primary Contact: Sandra Akers, Chief Executive Officer
COO: Debra Tosti, Chief Operating Officer
CFO: Maureen DiPalma, Director Finance
CMO: Val Slayton, M.D., Chief Medical Officer
Web address: www.state.ma.us/dph/hosp/th.htm
Control: State–Government, nonfederal **Service:** Long–Term Acute Care hospital

Staffed Beds: 720

WALTHAM—Middlesex County

☐ **KINDRED HOSPITAL NORTHEAST–WALTHAM**, 9 Hope Avenue, 4th Floor, Zip 2453; tel. 781/647–6600, (Nonreporting) **A**1
Primary Contact: Valerie Gingras, Administrator
Web address: www.kindredhealthcare.com
Control: Corporation, Investor–owned, for–profit **Service:** Long–Term Acute Care hospital

Staffed Beds: 10

WARE—Hampshire County

☒ **BAYSTATE MARY LANE HOSPITAL (220050)**, 85 South Street, Zip 01082–1697; tel. 413/967–6211 **A**1 9 10 **F**2 3 11 13 15 25 26 27 28 30 31 32 33 38 43 50 53 54 55 56 57 62 63 66 68 73 74 75 76 77 79 80 81 82 84 86 87 96 100 107 118 119 120 121 123 132 133 135 136 **S** Baystate Health, Inc.
Primary Contact: Christine Shirtcliff, FACHE, President
CFO: Curtis Davis, Finance Director
CMO: Richard Gerstein, M.D., Director Medical Staff
CHR: Donna Arsenault, Manager Human Resources
Web address: www.baystatehealth.com
Control: Other not–for–profit (including NFP Corporation) **Service:** General Medical and Surgical

Staffed Beds: 31 **Admissions:** 1552 **Census:** 13 **Outpatient Visits:** 74280 **Births:** 180 **Total Expense ($000):** 27604 **Payroll Expense ($000):** 13589 **Personnel:** 285

WAREHAM—Plymouth County

TOBEY HOSPITAL See Southcoast Hospitals Group, Fall River

Hospital, Medicare Provider Number, Address, Telephone, Approval, Facility, and Physician Codes, Health Care System

★ American Hospital Association (AHA) membership
☐ The Joint Commission accreditation
◯ American Osteopathic Association (AOA) accreditation
△ Commission on Accreditation of Rehabilitation Facilities (CARF) accreditation

WEBSTER—Worcester County

★ **HUBBARD REGIONAL HOSPITAL (220025)**, 340 Thompson Road, Zip 01570–0608; tel. 508/943–2600, (Nonreporting) **A**1 5 9 10
Primary Contact: William R. Falkowski, Chief Executive Officer
CFO: William R. Falkowski, Chief Executive Officer
CHR: Lisa Mason, Human Resources Director
Web address: www.hubbardhealth.com
Control: Other not–for–profit (including NFP Corporation) **Service:** General Medical and Surgical

Staffed Beds: 22

WELLESLEY—Norfolk County

SIMPSON INFIRMARY, WELLESLEY COLLEGE, 106 Central Street, Zip 02481–8203; tel. 781/283–2810, (Nonreporting)
Primary Contact: Vanessa M. Britto, M.D., MSC, Director Health Service
CFO: Susan Vogt, Vice President Finance and Treasurer
Control: Other not–for–profit (including NFP Corporation) **Service:** Hospital unit of an institution (prison hospital, college infirmary, etc.)

Staffed Beds: 11

MA

WESTBOROUGH—Worcester County

☐ **WESTBOROUGH STATE HOSPITAL (224026)**, Lyman Street, Zip 01581–0288, Mailing Address: P.O. Box 288, Zip 01581–0288; tel. 508/616–2100, (Nonreporting) **A**1 3 5 10 **S** Massachusetts Department of Mental Health
Primary Contact: Joel Skolnick, Chief Operating Officer
Control: State–Government, nonfederal **Service:** Psychiatric

Staffed Beds: 220

☐ △ **WHITTIER REHABILITATION HOSPITAL (223033)**, 150 Flanders Road, Zip 1581; tel. 508/871–2000, (Nonreporting) **A**1 7 10
Primary Contact: Alfred J. Arcidi, M.D., Senior Vice President
Web address: www.whittierhealth.com
Control: Individual, Investor–owned, for–profit **Service:** Long–Term Acute Care hospital

Staffed Beds: 74

WESTFIELD—Hampden County

★ **NOBLE HOSPITAL (220065)**, 115 West Silver Street, Zip 01086–1634; tel. 413/568–2811 **A**1 2 5 9 10 **F**4 8 14 15 17 24 25 26 27 30 31 32 33 34 36 38 42 43 46 47 48 49 50 55 56 57 59 61 62 63 65 66 68 72 73 75 76 77 79 80 81 82 84 85 86 88 89 90 91 92 93 94 95 96 97 99 100 102 103 104 107 119 120 121 124 133 135 136 137 **P**7 8
Primary Contact: George J. Koller, President and Chief Executive Officer
CFO: Robert Blondin, Vice President Finance
CMO: Francis D. Horrigan, M.D., Medical Director
CHR: Jeff Whorton, Director Human Resources
Web address: www.noblehealth.org
Control: Other not–for–profit (including NFP Corporation) **Service:** General Medical and Surgical

Staffed Beds: 97 **Admissions:** 3440 **Census:** 59 **Outpatient Visits:** 121752 **Births:** 0 **Total Expense ($000):** 47908 **Payroll Expense ($000):** 22363 **Personnel:** 382

☐ **WESTERN MASSACHUSETTS HOSPITAL (222023)**, 91 East Mountain Road, Zip 1085; tel. 413/562–4131, (Nonreporting) **A**1 10 **S** Massachusetts Department of Public Health
Primary Contact: Blake M. Molleur, Chief Executive Officer
CMO: Chabilal Neergheen, M.D., Medical Director
CHR: James E. Duggan, Director Human Resources
Web address: www.mass.gov/dph/hosp/wmh.htm
Control: State–Government, nonfederal **Service:** General Medical and Surgical

Staffed Beds: 80

WESTWOOD—Norfolk County

☐ **WESTWOOD LODGE HOSPITAL (224023)**, 45 Clapboardtree Street, Zip 02090–2930; tel. 781/762–7764, (Nonreporting) **A**1 5 9 10 **S** Universal Health Services, Inc.
Primary Contact: Robert W. Spiegel, Chief Executive Officer and Managing Director
COO: Doris Sinkevich, Chief Nurse Executive and Chief Operating Officer
CFO: Charles Denno, Chief Financial Officer
Web address: www.arbourhealth.com
Control: Other not–for–profit (including NFP Corporation) **Service:** Psychiatric

Staffed Beds: 65

WHITINSVILLE—Worcester County

WHITINSVILLE MEDICAL CENTER See Milford Regional Medical Center, Milford

WINCHESTER—Middlesex County

★ **WINCHESTER HOSPITAL (220105)**, 41 Highland Avenue, Zip 01890–1496; tel. 781/729–9000 **A**1 2 3 5 9 10 **F**8 12 13 15 24 25 26 27 28 29 30 31 32 33 34 36 38 39 43 48 49 50 51 54 55 56 57 61 62 66 68 70 72 73 74 75 76 77 79 80 81 82 84 86 96 97 99 100 106 107 116 118 119 121 133 134 135 136 137 **P**2 5 6 7
Primary Contact: Dale M. Lodge, President and Chief Executive Officer
CFO: Kevin F. Smith, Executive Vice President Finance and Administrator
CMO: Richard Iseke, M.D., Vice President Medical Affairs
CHR: Anne Lang, Vice President Human Resources and Compliance and Privacy Officer
Web address: www.winchesterhospital.org
Control: Other not–for–profit (including NFP Corporation) **Service:** General Medical and Surgical

Staffed Beds: 178 **Admissions:** 12103 **Census:** 130 **Outpatient Visits:** 526961 **Births:** 1976 **Total Expense ($000):** 209198 **Payroll Expense ($000):** 102569 **Personnel:** 1494

WOBURN—Middlesex County

★ **NEW ENGLAND REHABILITATION HOSPITAL (223026)**, Two Rehabilitation Way, Zip 01801–6098; tel. 781/935–5050, (Nonreporting) **A**1 3 5 10 **S** Five Star Quality Care
Primary Contact: Joel Rudin, Chief Executive Officer
CFO: Lester Felege, Controller
CMO: A. Deniz Ozel, M.D., Medical Director
CHR: Annamarie Cronin, Director Human Resources
Web address: www.newenglandrehab.com
Control: Corporation, Investor–owned, for–profit **Service:** Rehabilitation

Staffed Beds: 210

WORCESTER—Worcester County

ADCARE HOSPITAL OF WORCESTER (220062), 107 Lincoln Street, Zip 01605–2499; tel. 508/799–9000, (Nonreporting) **A**3 5 10
Primary Contact: David W. Hillis, President and Chief Executive Officer
CFO: Christine Judycki–Crepeault, Chief Financial Officer
CMO: Ronald F. Pike, M.D., Medical Director
Web address: www.adcare.com
Control: Other not–for–profit (including NFP Corporation) **Service:** Alcoholism and other chemical dependency

Staffed Beds: 114

★ **FAIRLAWN REHABILITATION HOSPITAL (223029)**, 189 May Street, Zip 01602–4399; tel. 508/791–6351 **A**1 5 10 **F**24 25 26 30 31 32 33 43 54 57 62 72 73 75 77 82 85 86 119 135 137 **P**8 **S** HEALTHSOUTH Corporation
Primary Contact: Peter M. Mantegazza, Chief Executive Officer
CFO: John Flaherty, Controller
CMO: Peter Bagley, M.D., Medical Director
CHR: Brandon Hay, Human Resources Director
Web address: www.fairlawnrehab.org
Control: Corporation, Investor–owned, for–profit **Service:** Rehabilitation

Staffed Beds: 110 **Admissions:** 1766 **Census:** 73 **Outpatient Visits:** 15916 **Births:** 0 **Total Expense ($000):** 21501 **Payroll Expense ($000):** 12205 **Personnel:** 257

★ **SAINT VINCENT HOSPITAL AT WORCESTER MEDICAL CENTER (220176)**, 123 Summer Street, Zip 1608; tel. 508/363–5000 **A**1 2 3 5 9 10 12 **F**13 15 17 25 27 36 38 43 50 53 57 59 62 66 67 68 70 72 73 74 75 76 77 79 81 82 84 86 87 88 90 91 92 96 97 100 107 118 119 135 136 **S** Vanguard Health System
Primary Contact: John E. Smithhisler, CHE, President and Chief Executive Officer
COO: Rita J. Wilder, Chief Operating Officer
CFO: Stephen Gilmore, Chief Financial Officer
CMO: Harvey Kowaloff, Chief Medical Officer
CIO: Patricia Chassey, Director Information Services
Web address: www.stvincenthospital.com
Control: Corporation, Investor–owned, for–profit **Service:** General Medical and Surgical

Staffed Beds: 351 **Admissions:** 18359 **Census:** 217 **Outpatient Visits:** 102867 **Births:** 1826

Many Facility Codes have changed. Please refer to the AHA Guide Code Chart.

★ **UMASS MEMORIAL MEDICAL CENTER (220163)**, 119 Belmont Street, Zip 01605–2982; tel. 508/334–1000, (Includes HAHNEMANN CAMPUS, 281 Lincoln Street, Zip 01605; tel. 508/334–1000; MEMORIAL CAMPUS; UNIVERSITY CAMPUS, 55 Lake Avenue North, Zip 01655–0002; tel. 508/334–1000) **A**1 2 3 5 8 9 10 **F**3 6 7 9 12 13 14 15 16 17 18 19 20 21 22 23 24 25 26 27 30 31 32 33 34 38 40 42 43 44 50 52 54 55 56 57 59 60 61 62 66 68 70 71 72 73 74 75 76 77 79 80 81 82 83 84 86 87 88 89 90 91 92 93 94 95 96 97 102 103 104 106 107 109 111 112 113 114 116 118 119 120 121 123 124 125 127 128 131 132 133 135 136 137 **P**6 **S** UMass Memorial Health Care, Inc.
Primary Contact: Walter Ettinger, M.D., President and Chief Executive Officer
COO: Andrew Sussman, M.D., Chief Operating Officer
CFO: Therese Day, Chief Financial Officer
CMO: Stephen Tosi, M.D., Chief Medical Officer
CIO: George Brenkle, Chief Information Officer
CHR: Patricia Webb, Senior Vice President Human Resources
Web address: www.umassmemorial.org
Control: Other not–for–profit (including NFP Corporation) **Service:** General Medical and Surgical

Staffed Beds: 723 **Admissions:** 44241 **Census:** 566 **Outpatient Visits:** 970361 **Births:** 4353 **Total Expense ($000):** 1095761 **Payroll Expense ($000):** 374343 **Personnel:** 8697

☐ **WORCESTER STATE HOSPITAL (224032)**, 305 Belmont Street, Zip 01604–1695; tel. 508/368–3300 **A**1 3 5 10 **F**26 32 33 37 50 66 73 75 81 82 88 93 119 121 124 135 **S** Massachusetts Department of Mental Health
Primary Contact: Anthony Riccitelli, Chief Operating Officer
COO: Anthony Riccitelli, Chief Operating Officer
CMO: Kathleen Whitley, M.D., Director Clinical and Professional Service
CIO: Rod Flakes, Director Applied Information Technology
Control: State–Government, nonfederal **Service:** Psychiatric

Staffed Beds: 126 **Admissions:** 196 **Census:** 123 **Outpatient Visits:** 0 **Births:** 0 **Total Expense ($000):** 39479 **Payroll Expense ($000):** 19912 **Personnel:** 385

MA

Hospital, Medicare Provider Number, Address, Telephone, Approval, Facility, and Physician Codes, Health Care System

★ American Hospital Association (AHA) membership
☐ The Joint Commission accreditation
○ American Osteopathic Association (AOA) accreditation
△ Commission on Accreditation of Rehabilitation Facilities (CARF) accreditation

MICHIGAN

ADRIAN—Lenawee County

★ **BIXBY MEDICAL CENTER (230005)**, 818 Riverside Avenue, Zip 49221–1496; tel. 517/265–0900 **A**1 2 9 10 **F**3 5 8 10 11 13 15 18 24 25 26 27 31 32 33 36 38 40 43 44 46 55 56 61 62 63 66 68 72 73 74 75 76 77 79 80 82 84 86 87 94 96 97 100 102 105 106 107 108 109 111 112 113 118 119 120 121 132 133 135 136 137 **P**6 7 8 **S** ProMedica Health System
Primary Contact: Gregory Corbett, President
CFO: James F. Wheeler, Vice President Finance
CMO: Julie Yaioch, Vice President Medical Affairs
CIO: Carol Boyce, Administrative Director Support Services
CHR: Dennis Wright, Vice President Human Resources
Web address: www.promedica.org
Control: Other not–for–profit (including NFP Corporation) **Service:** General Medical and Surgical

Staffed Beds: 66 **Admissions:** 3937 **Census:** 38 **Outpatient Visits:** 158897 **Births:** 665 **Total Expense ($000):** 62934 **Payroll Expense ($000):** 19832 **Personnel:** 430

ALLEGAN—Allegan County

★ **ALLEGAN GENERAL HOSPITAL (231328)**, 555 Linn Street, Zip 49010–1594; tel. 269/673–8424 **A**9 10 18 **F**3 7 8 13 14 15 25 26 27 29 30 31 32 34 35 38 40 55 56 57 59 61 62 63 68 72 73 74 75 76 77 79 81 82 86 88 92 93 94 96 97 100 101 103 105 107 118 119 124 134 135 137 **P**3 6 **S** QHR
Primary Contact: Gerald J. Barbini, President and Chief Executive Officer
CFO: Richard Harning, Vice President Finance
CMO: Nabil Nouna, M.D., Chief of Staff
CIO: David Federinko, Chief Information Officer
CHR: Joann Gerrish, Director Human Resources
Web address: www.aghosp.org
Control: Other not–for–profit (including NFP Corporation) **Service:** General Medical and Surgical

Staffed Beds: 34 **Admissions:** 1682 **Census:** 18 **Outpatient Visits:** 73485 **Births:** 207 **Total Expense ($000):** 36499 **Payroll Expense ($000):** 14756 **Personnel:** 301

ALMA—Gratiot County

★ △ **GRATIOT MEDICAL CENTER (230030)**, 300 East Warwick Drive, Zip 48801–1096; tel. 989/463–1101 **A**1 7 9 10 19 **F**3 11 12 13 15 18 24 25 26 27 30 31 32 37 38 43 54 55 56 57 59 60 62 63 66 68 73 74 75 76 77 79 80 81 82 84 85 86 88 90 91 92 93 95 96 97 100 102 106 107 118 119 121 133 135 **P**6 **S** MidMichigan Health
Primary Contact: Mark E. Bush, President and Chief Executive Officer
CFO: Scott D. Currie, Vice President Finance
CHR: Michelle McGill, Vice President Human Resources
Web address: www.gratiothealth.com
Control: Other not–for–profit (including NFP Corporation) **Service:** General Medical and Surgical

Staffed Beds: 127 **Admissions:** 5805 **Census:** 69 **Outpatient Visits:** 203780 **Births:** 673 **Total Expense ($000):** 97830 **Payroll Expense ($000):** 43712 **Personnel:** 899

ALPENA—Alpena County

★ **ALPENA REGIONAL MEDICAL CENTER (230036)**, 1501 West Chisholm Street, Zip 49707–1498; tel. 989/356–7390 **A**1 2 9 10 19 20 **F**3 5 11 13 14 15 18 20 24 25 27 30 31 32 33 38 40 41 43 46 47 48 49 50 56 57 61 62 63 68 69 71 72 73 74 75 76 77 79 80 81 82 84 85 86 87 88 89 90 91 92 93 94 96 97 100 102 106 107 118 119 120 121 124 135 136 137 **P**6
Primary Contact: Karmon T. Bjella, Chief Executive Officer
COO: Aldean J. Moe, Chief Operating Officer
CFO: Damone Sorensen, CPA, Chief Financial Officer
CHR: Diane Shields, Chief Human Resources Officer
Web address: www.agh.org
Control: County–Government, nonfederal **Service:** General Medical and Surgical

Staffed Beds: 125 **Admissions:** 5011 **Census:** 66 **Outpatient Visits:** 164813 **Births:** 416 **Total Expense ($000):** 101610 **Payroll Expense ($000):** 42772 **Personnel:** 853

ANN ARBOR—Washtenaw County

★ **UNIVERSITY OF MICHIGAN HOSPITALS AND HEALTH CENTERS (230046)**, 1500 East Medical Center Drive, Zip 48109; tel. 734/936–4000 **A**1 2 3 5 8 9 10 **F**3 5 6 8 9 11 12 13 15 16 17 18 19 20 21 22 23 24 25 26 27 28 30 31 32 33 34 35 36 37 38 40 41 43 44 46 47 48 49 50 51 52 53 54 55 56 57 58 59 60 61 62 63 64 66 67 68 70 71 72 73 74 75 76 77 78 79 80 81 82 83 84 85 86 87 88 89 90 91 92 93 94 96 97 99 100 102 103 104 105 106 107 108 109 111 112 113 114 116 118 119 120 121 123 124 125 126 127 128 129 130 131 135 136 137
Primary Contact: Douglas Strong, Chief Executive Officer
COO: Tony Denton, Chief Operating Officer
CFO: Dave Morlock, Chief Financial Officer
CMO: Darrell Campbell, M.D., Chief Clinical Affairs
CIO: Jocelyn DeWitt, Chief Information Officer
CHR: Deborah Childs, Chief Human Resources Officer
Web address: www.med.umich.edu
Control: Other not–for–profit (including NFP Corporation) **Service:** General Medical and Surgical

Staffed Beds: 849 **Admissions:** 42830 **Census:** 699 **Outpatient Visits:** 1512523 **Births:** 3875 **Total Expense ($000):** 1464667 **Payroll Expense ($000):** 603401 **Personnel:** 13374

★ **VETERANS AFFAIRS ANN ARBOR HEALTHCARE SYSTEM**, 2215 Fuller Road, Zip 48105–2399; tel. 734/769–7100, (Total facility includes 40 beds in nursing home–type unit) **A**1 2 3 5 8 9 **F**3 5 17 18 20 22 24 25 26 27 30 31 32 33 34 36 37 38 42 43 44 45 46 49 50 53 54 55 56 57 58 59 60 61 62 63 66 68 69 72 73 75 76 77 79 80 81 82 86 87 88 90 91 92 93 94 95 96 97 100 102 107 111 117 119 121 124 132 133 135 136 137 **S** Department of Veterans Affairs
Primary Contact: Lou Ann Atkins, Director
COO: Randall Ritter, Associate Director Operations
CFO: Karen Ruedel, Chief Resource Officer
CMO: Eric Young, M.D., Chief of Staff
CIO: Shannon Rhodes, Chief Information Officer
CHR: Paul Serefine, Acting Personnel Officer
Web address: www.va.gov/sta/guide/home.asp
Control: Veterans Affairs, Government, federal **Service:** General Medical and Surgical

Staffed Beds: 136 **Admissions:** 4794 **Census:** 80 **Outpatient Visits:** 307568 **Births:** 0 **Total Expense ($000):** 162480 **Payroll Expense ($000):** 100105 **Personnel:** 1707

AUBURN HILLS—Oakland County

☐ **HAVENWYCK HOSPITAL (234023)**, 1525 University Drive, Zip 48326–2675; tel. 248/373–9200 **A**1 9 10 **F**88 89 92 95 119 **P**8 **S** Psychiatric Solutions
Primary Contact: Robert A. Kercorian, Chief Executive Officer
CFO: Mirhee Chun, Chief Financial Officer
Web address: www.havenwyckhospital.com
Control: Corporation, Investor–owned, for–profit **Service:** Psychiatric

Staffed Beds: 181 **Admissions:** 3763 **Census:** 150 **Outpatient Visits:** 5400 **Births:** 0 **Total Expense ($000):** 20314 **Payroll Expense ($000):** 10588 **Personnel:** 252

BAD AXE—Huron County

★ **HURON MEDICAL CENTER (230118)**, 1100 South Van Dyke Road, Zip 48413–9799; tel. 989/269–8933 **A**9 10 20 **F**3 11 13 14 15 25 28 31 32 38 52 54 55 56 57 62 68 72 73 74 75 79 86 87 96 97 102 107 118 119 121 123 124 133 135 **P**7
COO: Fred Meyer, Chief Operating Officer
CFO: Jeffery Longbrake, Chief Financial Officer
CMO: William Corsini, M.D., Chief of Staff
CHR: Nancy Bouck, Director Human Resources
Web address: www.huronmedicalcenter.org
Control: Other not–for–profit (including NFP Corporation) **Service:** General Medical and Surgical

Staffed Beds: 64 **Admissions:** 1848 **Census:** 15 **Outpatient Visits:** 50253 **Births:** 325 **Total Expense ($000):** 29151 **Payroll Expense ($000):** 10766 **Personnel:** 243

BATTLE CREEK—Calhoun County

★ **BATTLE CREEK HEALTH SYSTEM (230075)**, tel. 269/966–8000, (Includes FIELDSTONE CENTER, 165 North Washington Avenue, Zip 49037; MAIN CAMPUS, 300 North Avenue, Zip 49017) **A**1 2 9 10 **F**10 13 15 18 24 25 26 27 31 32 33 38 40 49 58 59 62 63 66 68 69 72 73 74 75 76 77 79 80 81 82 84 86 87 88 90 91 92 93 94 96 97 99 100 102 103 104 105 106 107 109 111 116 118 119 120 121 124 132 133 135 136 137 **P**8 **S** Trinity Health
Primary Contact: Patrick R. Garrett, President and Chief Executive Officer
CFO: Kenneth Barth, Vice President Finance
CMO: Jeffrey Mitchell, M.D., Vice President Medical Affairs, Quality and Informatics
CIO: Jim Keller, Site Director Information Systems
CHR: Cathy Edwards, Director Human Resources
Web address: www.bchealth.com
Control: Church–operated, Nongovernment, not–for profit **Service:** General Medical and Surgical

Staffed Beds: 211 **Admissions:** 12301 **Census:** 143 **Outpatient Visits:** 168309 **Births:** 1203 **Total Expense ($000):** 192154 **Payroll Expense ($000):** 73540 **Personnel:** 1339

☐ **SELECT SPECIALTY HOSPITAL–BATTLE CREEK (232028)**, 300 North Avenue, 6th Floor, Zip 49016; tel. 269/565–8900, (Nonreporting) **A**1 10 **S** Select Medical Corporation
Primary Contact: Dave Gehringer, Chief Executive Officer
Web address: www.selectmedicalcorp.com
Control: Corporation, Investor–owned, for–profit **Service:** Long–Term Acute Care hospital

Staffed Beds: 32

★ **SOUTHWEST REGIONAL REHABILITATION CENTER (233025)**, 393 East Roosevelt Avenue, Zip 49017–3333; tel. 269/965–3206 **A**1 9 10 **F**2 3 25 52 54 57 62 85 86 119 121 132 **P**6
Primary Contact: Stan Tooley, President and Chief Executive Officer
CFO: Stephen Jessup, Chief Financial Officer
CMO: Mehmet Yilmaz, M.D., Medical Director
CIO: Rick Albaugh, Manager Information Services
CHR: Karol A. Jenney, Director Business Operations
Web address: www.sw–rehab.org
Control: Other not–for–profit (including NFP Corporation) **Service:** Rehabilitation

Staffed Beds: 26 **Admissions:** 573 **Census:** 15 **Outpatient Visits:** 17935 **Births:** 0 **Total Expense ($000):** 11028 **Payroll Expense ($000):** 5382 **Personnel:** 121

★ △ **VETERANS AFFAIRS MEDICAL CENTER**, 5500 Armstrong Road, Zip 49015; tel. 269/966–5600, (Total facility includes 135 beds in nursing home–type unit) (Nonreporting) **A**1 7 9 **S** Department of Veterans Affairs
Primary Contact: Alice L. Wood, Director
COO: Gregory R. Harris, Acting Associate Director
CFO: Mike Rupert, Chief Fiscal Services
CMO: Alan M. Sooho, M.D., Chief of Staff
CIO: Rhys Foulkes, Chief Information Management Service
CHR: Palma Simkins, Chief Human Resources Management Services
Web address: www.va.gov/sta/guide/home.asp
Control: Veterans Affairs, Government, federal **Service:** Psychiatric

Staffed Beds: 368

BAY CITY—Bay County

★ △ **BAY REGIONAL MEDICAL CENTER (230041)**, 1900 Columbus Avenue, Zip 48708–6880; tel. 989/894–3000, (Includes BAY REGIONAL MEDICAL CENTER–WEST CAMPUS, 3250 East Midland Road, Zip 48706; tel. 989/667–6750) **A**1 2 7 9 10 12 13 **F**3 7 11 13 15 17 18 20 22 24 25 26 27 30 31 32 33 36 38 43 46 47 48 49 50 55 57 62 66 68 72 73 74 76 77 79 80 81 82 84 85 86 87 88 96 97 100 102 103 104 105 106 107 108 109 110 112 118 119 121 124 135 137 **S** McLaren Health Care Corporation
Primary Contact: Alice Gerard, President and Chief Executive Officer
CFO: Brian Kay, Chief Financial Officer
CMO: Jay Summer, M.D., Vice President Corporate Medical Affairs
CIO: Curt Valley, Customer Site Manager
CHR: Joseph Lyons, Vice President Human Resources
Web address: www.bayregional.org
Control: Other not–for–profit (including NFP Corporation) **Service:** General Medical and Surgical

Staffed Beds: 320 **Admissions:** 17793 **Census:** 222 **Outpatient Visits:** 339823 **Births:** 901 **Total Expense ($000):** 222263 **Payroll Expense ($000):** 90933 **Personnel:** 1623

BAY SPECIAL CARE HOSPITAL (232020), Mailing Address: 3250 East Midland Road, Suite 1, Zip 48706–2835; tel. 989/667–6802 **A**10 **F**1 3 25 26 27 30 31 77 82 137
Primary Contact: Cheryl A. Burzynski, President
CFO: Brian Kay, Chief Financial Officer
CMO: Janet Sutton, M.D., Medical Director
CHR: Joseph Lyons, Vice President Human Resources
Web address: www.bayspecialcare.org
Control: Other not–for–profit (including NFP Corporation) **Service:** Long–Term Acute Care hospital

Staffed Beds: 26 **Admissions:** 313 **Census:** 24 **Outpatient Visits:** 0 **Births:** 0 **Total Expense ($000):** 7036 **Payroll Expense ($000):** 3348 **Personnel:** 86

BERRIEN CENTER—Berrien County

☐ **LAKELAND SPECIALTY HOSPITAL, BERRIEN CENTER (232025)**, 6418 Dean's Hill Road, Zip 49102–9704; tel. 269/473–3003, (Total facility includes 166 beds in nursing home–type unit) **A**1 **F**1 3 6 11 25 26 30 31 32 43 54 66 73 75 85 88 117 119 135 137 **P**5 **S** Lakeland Healthcare
Primary Contact: Joseph A. Wasserman, President and Chief Executive Officer
Web address: www.lakelandhealth.org
Control: Other not–for–profit (including NFP Corporation) **Service:** Long–Term Acute Care hospital

Staffed Beds: 221 **Admissions:** 537 **Census:** 159 **Outpatient Visits:** 0 **Births:** 0 **Total Expense ($000):** 20724 **Payroll Expense ($000):** 10063 **Personnel:** 241

BIG RAPIDS—Mecosta County

★ **MECOSTA COUNTY MEDICAL CENTER (230093)**, 605 Oak Street, Zip 49307–2099; tel. 231/796–8691 **A**1 9 10 20 **F**3 11 13 15 17 24 30 31 32 38 40 57 61 62 63 67 73 74 75 77 79 80 81 82 84 85 86 96 97 100 107 118 119 121 124 135 137 **P**1 **S** QHR
Primary Contact: Thomas E. Daugherty, Administrator
CFO: Joseph W. Hohenberger, Chief Financial Officer
Web address: www.mcmcbr.com
Control: County–Government, nonfederal **Service:** General Medical and Surgical

Staffed Beds: 64 **Admissions:** 2577 **Census:** 21 **Outpatient Visits:** 122329 **Births:** 667 **Total Expense ($000):** 42076 **Payroll Expense ($000):** 18190 **Personnel:** 331

BRIGHTON—Livingston County

★ **BRIGHTON HOSPITAL (230279)**, 12851 East Grand River Avenue, Zip 48116–8596; tel. 810/227–1211, (Nonreporting) **A**10 **S** Ascension Health
Primary Contact: Denise Bertin–Epp, Chief Executive Officer
CFO: Jackie Hill, Chief Financial Officer
CMO: John Hopper, M.D., Vice President Medical Affairs
CIO: Melissa Whelan, Associate Director Health Information
CHR: Marissa DeLisle, Director Human Resources
Web address: www.stjohn.org/brighton/
Control: Other not–for–profit (including NFP Corporation) **Service:** Alcoholism and other chemical dependency

Staffed Beds: 92

CADILLAC—Wexford County

★ **MERCY HOSPITAL CADILLAC (230081)**, 400 Hobart Street, Zip 49601–9596; tel. 231/876–7200 **A**1 9 10 20 **F**3 11 13 15 22 24 25 26 30 31 32 33 37 38 41 43 50 51 57 62 64 66 68 73 74 75 76 77 79 80 82 84 86 87 96 97 100 102 106 107 118 119 121 135 136 137 **P**8 **S** Trinity Health
Primary Contact: John L. MacLeod, President and Chief Executive Officer
COO: Mary L. Neff, R.N., Chief Operating Officer and Chief Nursing Officer
CFO: Dan Hogan, Vice President Finance
CMO: Elizabeth Adamson, M.D., Chief of Staff
CIO: Randi Oehlers, Site Director Management Information Systems
CHR: Peter Lane, Director Human Resources
Web address: www.munsonhealthcare.org
Control: Church–operated, Nongovernment, not–for profit **Service:** General Medical and Surgical

Staffed Beds: 65 **Admissions:** 4065 **Census:** 32 **Outpatient Visits:** 80666 **Births:** 438 **Total Expense ($000):** 53649 **Payroll Expense ($000):** 20136 **Personnel:** 504

MI

Hospital, Medicare Provider Number, Address, Telephone, Approval, Facility, and Physician Codes, Health Care System

★ American Hospital Association (AHA) membership
☐ The Joint Commission accreditation
○ American Osteopathic Association (AOA) accreditation
△ Commission on Accreditation of Rehabilitation Facilities (CARF) accreditation

CARO—Tuscola County

☐ **CARO CENTER (234025)**, 2000 Chambers Road, Zip 48723–9296; tel. 989/673–3191, (Nonreporting) **A**1 9 10
Primary Contact: Rose Laskowski, RN, Director
COO: Rose Laskowski, R.N., Director
CFO: Maurice Forrest, Administrative Manager
CMO: William Clark, M.D., Chief Clinical Affairs
Control: State–Government, nonfederal **Service:** Psychiatric

Staffed Beds: 193

★ **CARO COMMUNITY HOSPITAL (231329)**, 401 North Hooper Street, Zip 48723–1476, Mailing Address: P.O. Box 435, Zip 48723–0435; tel. 989/673–3141, (Nonreporting) **A**9 10 18
Primary Contact: William P. Miller, President and Chief Executive Officer
COO: Marc Augsburger, Vice President Operations
CFO: James L. Singles, Vice President Finance
Control: Other not–for–profit (including NFP Corporation) **Service:** General Medical and Surgical

Staffed Beds: 25

CARSON CITY—Montcalm County

MI

★ ○ **CARSON CITY HOSPITAL (230208)**, 406 East Elm Street, Zip 48811–0879, Mailing Address: P.O. Box 879, Zip 48811–0879; tel. 989/584–3131 **A**9 10 11 19 **F**11 13 15 24 25 26 27 30 31 33 38 43 46 55 56 57 61 63 66 68 72 74 75 76 77 79 86 87 88 90 91 92 94 96 100 103 107 119 121 124 135 136 **P**8
Primary Contact: Bruce L. Traverse, President
COO: Matt Thompson, Chief Operating Officer
CFO: Duane Miller, Vice President Finance
CMO: Lawrence Brown, D.O., Medical Director
CIO: Richard Terry, Chief Information Officer
CHR: Georgette Russell, Director Human Resources
Web address: www.carsoncityhospital.com
Control: Other not–for–profit (including NFP Corporation) **Service:** General Medical and Surgical

Staffed Beds: 63 **Admissions:** 2144 **Census:** 20 **Outpatient Visits:** 69164 **Births:** 395 **Total Expense ($000):** 36515 **Payroll Expense ($000):** 17828 **Personnel:** 481

CASS CITY—Tuscola County

⊛ **HILLS AND DALES GENERAL HOSPITAL (231316)**, 4675 Hill Street, Zip 48726–1099; tel. 989/872–2121 **A**1 9 10 18 **F**3 11 15 25 26 27 28 30 31 32 33 38 46 52 54 55 56 57 60 61 62 72 73 75 76 77 79 80 81 82 86 87 96 97 98 103 106 107 118 119 120 121 124 133 135 136 137 **P**6
Primary Contact: Michael J. Falatko, FACHE, Chief Executive Officer
COO: Jean Anthony, Chief Operating Officer and Chief Patient Services
CMO: Surrendra Raythatha, M.D., Chief of Staff
CIO: Ashley Patrick, Director Business Development
CHR: Tom Bardwell, Director Human Resources
Web address: www.hillsanddales.com
Control: Other not–for–profit (including NFP Corporation) **Service:** General Medical and Surgical

Staffed Beds: 25 **Admissions:** 680 **Census:** 5 **Outpatient Visits:** 51141 **Births:** 0 **Total Expense ($000):** 18317 **Payroll Expense ($000):** 8740 **Personnel:** 190

CHARLEVOIX—Charlevoix County

⊛ **CHARLEVOIX AREA HOSPITAL (231322)**, 14700 Lake Shore Drive, Zip 49720–1931; tel. 231/547–4024 **A**1 9 10 18 **F**11 13 15 24 30 31 32 38 55 57 68 74 75 76 77 79 84 86 96 97 100 107 118 119 120 122 124 133 135
Primary Contact: William Jackson, President
COO: Christine Wilhelm, Vice President Operations
CFO: Joseph Schodde, Vice President Financial Services
CIO: David Priest, Director Information Systems
CHR: Diane Kidder, Vice President Staff Services
Web address: www.cah.org
Control: Other not–for–profit (including NFP Corporation) **Service:** General Medical and Surgical

Staffed Beds: 25 **Admissions:** 1126 **Census:** 11 **Outpatient Visits:** 31251 **Births:** 214 **Total Expense ($000):** 28420 **Payroll Expense ($000):** 13028 **Personnel:** 256

CHARLOTTE—Eaton County

⊛ **HAYES GREEN BEACH MEMORIAL HOSPITAL (231327)**, 321 East Harris Street, Zip 48813–1697; tel. 517/543–1050 **A**1 9 10 18 **F**3 7 11 13 15 24 25 31 38 43 46 52 55 56 61 62 66 67 73 74 75 77 79 80 84 86 87 96 97 102 106 107 118 119 120 132 133 135 137 **P**6 **S** QHR
Primary Contact: Matthew Rush, President and Chief Executive Officer
CFO: Kim Capps, Chief Financial Officer
CMO: Robert Leeser, M.D., Chief Medical Officer
CIO: Kim Capps, Chief Financial Officer
CHR: Jennifer Bucienski, Director Human Resources
Web address: www.hgbhealth.com
Control: Other not–for–profit (including NFP Corporation) **Service:** General Medical and Surgical

Staffed Beds: 25 **Admissions:** 1344 **Census:** 12 **Outpatient Visits:** 134051 **Births:** 310 **Total Expense ($000):** 39944 **Payroll Expense ($000):** 17026 **Personnel:** 372

CHEBOYGAN—Cheboygan County

⊛ **CHEBOYGAN MEMORIAL HOSPITAL (230034)**, 748 South Main Street, Zip 49721–2299, Mailing Address: P.O. Box 419, Zip 49721–0419; tel. 231/627–5601, (Total facility includes 50 beds in nursing home–type unit) **A**1 9 10 20 **F**11 13 15 24 25 26 30 31 32 33 38 42 53 54 55 56 57 61 62 66 68 73 74 75 77 79 80 86 96 97 102 107 117 121 124 133 135 136 **P**6
Primary Contact: Barbara J. Cliff, President and Chief Executive Officer
COO: Beth Daugherty, Senior Vice President and Chief Operating Officer
CFO: Ted Anderson, Senior Vice President and Chief Financial Officer
CMO: Donald Watson, M.D., President Medical Staff
CIO: Nancy Barr, Director Information Technology
CHR: Beth Walter, Director Human Resources
Web address: www.cheboyganhospital.org
Control: Other not–for–profit (including NFP Corporation) **Service:** General Medical and Surgical

Staffed Beds: 92 **Admissions:** 2243 **Census:** 68 **Outpatient Visits:** 108844 **Births:** 256 **Total Expense ($000):** 44555 **Payroll Expense ($000):** 20203 **Personnel:** 422

CHELSEA—Washtenaw County

⊛ **CHELSEA COMMUNITY HOSPITAL (230259)**, 775 South Main Street, Zip 48118–1399; tel. 734/475–1311 **A**1 3 5 9 10 **F**3 5 8 10 11 15 24 26 30 31 32 33 34 38 42 43 46 51 52 54 56 57 61 62 63 66 68 73 75 77 79 81 82 85 86 87 88 89 90 91 93 94 95 96 97 100 103 106 107 115 118 119 120 121 124 135 136
Primary Contact: Kathleen S. Griffiths, President and Chief Executive Officer
CFO: James Birchler, Vice President Finance
CMO: Larry Handelsman, M.D., Vice President Medical Affairs
CIO: Sherry Brown, Director Information Services
CHR: Cindy Harrison, Vice President Human Resources
Web address: www.cch.org
Control: Other not–for–profit (including NFP Corporation) **Service:** General Medical and Surgical

Staffed Beds: 99 **Admissions:** 4046 **Census:** 57 **Outpatient Visits:** 192158 **Births:** 0 **Total Expense ($000):** 86477 **Payroll Expense ($000):** 39573 **Personnel:** 762

CLARE—Clare County

⊛ **MIDMICHIGAN MEDICAL CENTER–CLARE (230180)**, 703 North McEwan Street, Zip 48617–1409; tel. 989/802–5000 **A**1 9 10 **F**3 11 13 15 24 26 27 30 31 32 33 38 52 55 57 60 62 68 72 73 74 75 77 79 80 82 84 86 96 97 102 106 107 119 121 124 133 137 **S** MidMichigan Health
Primary Contact: Lawrence F. Barco, President
CFO: Victor Morgan, Chief Financial Officer
CHR: Penny Parsons, Assistant Vice President
Web address: www.midmichigan.org
Control: Other not–for–profit (including NFP Corporation) **Service:** General Medical and Surgical

Staffed Beds: 55 **Admissions:** 2278 **Census:** 20 **Outpatient Visits:** 110848 **Births:** 214 **Total Expense ($000):** 33603 **Payroll Expense ($000):** 13863 **Personnel:** 276

CLINTON TOWNSHIP—Macomb County

★ **HENRY FORD MACOMB HOSPITAL (230047)**, (Includes HENRY FORD MACOMB HOSPITAL – MOUNT CLEMENS CAMPUS, 215 North Avenue, Mount Clemens, Zip 48043; tel. 586/466–9300; ST. JOSEPH'S MERCY HOSPITAL–WEST, 15855 19 Mile Road, Zip 48038; tel. 586/263–2707; ST. JOSEPH'S MERCY–NORTH, 80650 North Van Dyke, Romeo, Zip 48065; tel. 810/798–3551) **A**1 9 10 12 13 **F**3 7 8 11 13 15 18 20 22 24 25 26 27 28 30 31 32 33 34 36 38 41 43 44 46 49 50 51 53 55 56 57 58 61 62 63 64 66 68 72 73 74 75 76 77 79 80 81 82 84 85 86 87 88 89 90 91 92 93 94 95 96 97 99 100 102 103 104 105 107 109 116 118 119 121 123 124 132 133 134 135 136 137 **P**5 6 8 **S** Henry Ford Health System
Primary Contact: Barbara Rossmann, President and Chief Executive Officer
COO: Gary Beaulac, Chief Operating Officer
CFO: Steve Hathaway, Vice President Finance and Chief Financial Officer
CIO: Robert Jones, Director Information Systems
CHR: Joel Gibson, Vice President Human Resources
Web address: www.stjoe–macomb.com
Control: Other not–for–profit (including NFP Corporation) **Service:** General Medical and Surgical

Staffed Beds: 419 **Admissions:** 22226 **Census:** 312 **Outpatient Visits:** 276652 **Births:** 1612 **Total Expense ($000):** 292960 **Payroll Expense ($000):** 126505 **Personnel:** 2420

COLDWATER—Branch County

★ **COMMUNITY HEALTH CENTER OF BRANCH COUNTY (230022)**, 274 East Chicago Street, Zip 49036–2088; tel. 517/279–5400 **A**1 9 10 12 13 19 **F**3 5 11 12 13 15 24 26 27 30 31 32 35 38 40 42 46 55 56 57 60 61 62 63 64 68 72 73 74 75 76 77 79 80 82 84 86 87 88 90 91 92 93 94 96 97 100 103 106 107 118 119 121 124 135 137 **P**6 8
Primary Contact: Randy DeGroot, President and Chief Executive Officer
CFO: Richard Trufant, Chief Financial Officer
CMO: John Sennish, M.D., Chief of Staff
CIO: Sheila Preston, Information Systems Director
CHR: Amy Jensen, Director Human Resources
Web address: www.chcbc.com
Control: County–Government, nonfederal **Service:** General Medical and Surgical

Staffed Beds: 96 **Admissions:** 3859 **Census:** 44 **Outpatient Visits:** 119975 **Births:** 431 **Total Expense ($000):** 60922 **Payroll Expense ($000):** 26484 **Personnel:** 541

COMMERCE TOWNSHIP—Oakland County

★ **HURON VALLEY–SINAI HOSPITAL (230277)**, 1 William Carls Drive, Zip 48382–2201; tel. 248/937–3300 **A**1 9 10 12 13 **F**3 6 8 11 12 13 15 18 24 25 26 27 30 31 32 33 35 38 41 42 43 44 46 49 50 51 54 55 56 57 59 60 62 63 66 68 72 73 74 75 76 77 79 80 81 82 84 90 93 96 97 99 100 102 105 106 107 109 111 118 119 120 121 124 133 135 136 **P**6 **S** Detroit Medical Center
Primary Contact: Lynn M. Torossian, President
COO: Lynn M. Torossian, President
CFO: William Lantzy, Vice President Finance
CMO: Marc Bocknek, M.D., Vice President Medical Affairs
CHR: Paul Sturgis, Director Human Resources
Web address: www.hvsh.org
Control: Other not–for–profit (including NFP Corporation) **Service:** General Medical and Surgical

Staffed Beds: 153 **Admissions:** 9194 **Census:** 109 **Outpatient Visits:** 92294 **Births:** 1865 **Total Expense ($000):** 145656 **Payroll Expense ($000):** 52862 **Personnel:** 1010

DEARBORN—Wayne County

★ **OAKWOOD HOSPITAL AND MEDICAL CENTER–DEARBORN (230020)**, 18101 Oakwood Boulevard, Zip 48124–4093, Mailing Address: P.O. Box 2500, Zip 48123–2500; tel. 313/593–7000 **A**1 2 3 5 8 9 10 **F**3 11 12 13 15 17 18 20 22 24 25 26 27 28 30 31 32 33 34 36 37 38 41 42 43 44 46 49 50 54 55 56 57 58 59 60 61 62 63 66 68 70 72 73 74 75 76 77 79 80 81 82 84 86 87 90 96 97 100 102 103 104 105 106 107 108 109 111 112 113 114 116 119 120 121 123 124 125 134 135 136 137 **P**8 **S** Oakwood Healthcare, Inc.
Primary Contact: Michael Geheb, M.D., Division President
COO: J. Joseph Diederich, Executive Vice President and Chief Operating Officer
CFO: Douglas D. Welday, Executive Vice President and Chief Financial Officer
CMO: Malcolm S. Henoch, M.D., Chief Medical Officer
CIO: Paula Smith, Leader Information Services and Chief Information Officer
CHR: John Furman, Executive Vice President Human Resources
Web address: www.oakwood.org
Control: Other not–for–profit (including NFP Corporation) **Service:** General Medical and Surgical

Staffed Beds: 594 **Admissions:** 33357 **Census:** 462 **Outpatient Visits:** 174133 **Births:** 4692 **Total Expense ($000):** 487003 **Payroll Expense ($000):** 193624 **Personnel:** 3530

DECKERVILLE—Sanilac County

DECKERVILLE COMMUNITY HOSPITAL (231311), 3559 Pine Street, Zip 48427–0126, Mailing Address: P.O. Box 126, Zip 48427–0126; tel. 810/376–2835 **A**9 10 18 **F**3 11 15 25 27 30 31 32 33 38 41 50 52 54 55 56 57 62 63 64 73 75 79 82 84 85 86 87 92 96 107 120 124 133 136 **P**6
Primary Contact: Edward L. Gamache, Administrator
CFO: Caren Puvalowski, Business Manager
CMO: Levi Guerrero, M.D., Chief of Staff
CIO: David West, Supervisor Information Technology
CHR: Tina Osantosri, Director Human Resources
Web address: www.deckervillehosp.org
Control: Other not–for–profit (including NFP Corporation) **Service:** General Medical and Surgical

Staffed Beds: 15 **Admissions:** 254 **Census:** 2 **Outpatient Visits:** 12376 **Births:** 0 **Total Expense ($000):** 5766 **Payroll Expense ($000):** 2591 **Personnel:** 67

DETROIT—Wayne County

★ △ **CHILDREN'S HOSPITAL OF MICHIGAN (233300)**, (PEDIATRICS), 3901 Beaubien Boulevard, Zip 48201–9985; tel. 313/745–5437 **A**1 3 5 7 9 10 **F**3 8 11 16 19 21 23 25 26 27 28 30 31 32 33 34 36 37 38 40 41 43 44 46 47 48 49 50 53 55 56 57 58 59 60 62 63 66 69 70 72 73 75 76 77 78 79 80 81 82 83 84 85 86 87 89 90 91 92 94 96 97 100 102 104 105 106 107 108 109 111 114 116 118 119 120 121 123 125 126 127 133 135 137 **P**6 **S** Detroit Medical Center
Primary Contact: Herman B. Gray, M.D., President
COO: Shawn Levitt, Chief Operating Officer
CFO: Joseph Scallen, Chief Financial Officer
CMO: Jefrey Devries, M.D., Vice President Medical Affairs
CIO: Lori Mouton, Director Public Relations and Marketing
CHR: Tarry Paylor, Director Human Resources
Web address: www.chmkids.org
Control: Other not–for–profit (including NFP Corporation) **Service:** Children's other specialty

Staffed Beds: 225 **Admissions:** 13504 **Census:** 158 **Outpatient Visits:** 282670 **Births:** 0 **Total Expense ($000):** 307921 **Payroll Expense ($000):** 111626 **Personnel:** 2035

CIRCLE OF LIFE CENTER (234048), 15000 Gratiot Avenue, Zip 48205; tel. 313/245–0600, (Nonreporting) **A**9 10
Primary Contact: Pam Lamb, Chief Executive Officer
Control: Corporation, Investor–owned, for–profit **Service:** Psychiatric

Staffed Beds: 90

DETROIT HOPE HOSPITAL (230298), 801 Virginia Park Street, Zip 48202; tel. 313/874–0100, (Nonreporting) **A**10
Primary Contact: Ramsay Dass, M.D., Chief Executive Officer
Web address: www.thecityofdetroit.com/hospital
Control: Corporation, Investor–owned, for–profit **Service:** Long–Term Acute Care hospital

Staffed Beds: 116

★ **DETROIT RECEIVING HOSPITAL AND UNIVERSITY HEALTH CENTER (230273)**, 4201 St. Antoine Boulevard, Zip 48201–2194; tel. 313/745–3603 **A**1 3 5 9 10 **F**3 16 17 25 26 30 31 32 33 36 38 40 41 43 44 50 54 55 56 57 62 64 66 68 72 73 75 77 79 80 82 86 87 88 89 90 92 93 94 96 102 105 107 119 120 121 124 130 132 133 135 137 **P**6 **S** Detroit Medical Center
Primary Contact: Iris Taylor, Ph.D., President
CFO: Kathleen Ralston, Vice President and Chief Financial Officer
CMO: Fernando Diaz, M.D., Ph.D., Senior Vice President and Chief Medical Officer
Web address: www.dmc.org
Control: Other not–for–profit (including NFP Corporation) **Service:** General Medical and Surgical

Staffed Beds: 217 **Admissions:** 13765 **Census:** 188 **Outpatient Visits:** 166119 **Births:** 0 **Total Expense ($000):** 304458 **Payroll Expense ($000):** 78712 **Personnel:** 1459

MI

Hospital, Medicare Provider Number, Address, Telephone, Approval, Facility, and Physician Codes, Health Care System

★ American Hospital Association (AHA) membership
□ The Joint Commission accreditation
○ American Osteopathic Association (AOA) accreditation
△ Commission on Accreditation of Rehabilitation Facilities (CARF) accreditation

★ **HARPER UNIVERSITY HOSPITAL (230104)**, 3990 John R. Street, Zip 48201–9027; tel. 313/745–8040, (Includes HUTZEL HOSPITAL; MICHIGAN ORTHOPAEDIC SPECIALTY HOSPITAL, 30671 Stephenson Highway, Madison Heights, Zip 48071–1678; tel. 248/733–2200; Frank P. Iacobell, President) **A**1 3 5 9 10 **F**3 8 11 12 13 15 17 18 20 22 24 25 26 27 30 31 32 33 34 36 38 41 42 43 44 46 47 48 49 50 53 54 55 56 57 58 59 60 62 63 66 68 70 71 72 73 74 75 76 77 78 79 80 81 82 86 87 90 91 92 96 97 98 100 102 103 105 106 107 112 113 114 116 118 119 120 121 123 124 125 127 130 131 132 135 136 137 **P**6 **S** Detroit Medical Center
Primary Contact: Brooks Bock, M.D., President
COO: Mark Harrison, Vice President Operations
CFO: Kevin Smith, Vice President Finance
CMO: Reginald J. Eadie, Vice President Medical Affairs
CIO: Michael LeRoy, Senior Vice President and Chief Information Officer
CHR: Deloris Hunt, Corporate Vice President Human Resources
Web address: www.harperhospital.org
Control: Other not–for–profit (including NFP Corporation) **Service:** General Medical and Surgical

Staffed Beds: 471 **Admissions:** 20350 **Census:** 272 **Outpatient Visits:** 182038 **Births:** 5461 **Total Expense ($000):** 511432 **Payroll Expense ($000):** 140721 **Personnel:** 2355

MI

★ **HENRY FORD HOSPITAL (230053)**, 2799 West Grand Boulevard, Zip 48202–2689; tel. 313/916–2600 **A**1 2 3 5 8 9 10 **F**3 5 6 8 9 11 12 13 15 17 18 20 22 24 25 26 27 28 29 30 31 32 33 34 36 37 38 39 40 41 42 43 44 45 46 47 48 49 50 51 53 54 55 56 57 58 59 60 61 62 63 66 68 69 70 71 72 73 74 75 76 77 78 79 80 81 82 86 87 89 90 91 92 93 94 95 96 97 99 100 102 103 104 105 106 107 108 109 111 112 113 114 116 118 119 120 121 123 124 125 126 127 128 129 130 131 132 133 135 136 137 **P**6 **S** Henry Ford Health System
Primary Contact: Anthony A. Armada, President and Chief Executive Officer
COO: Veronica Hall, Chief Operating Officer
CFO: Joseph Schmitt, Vice President Finance and Chief Financial Officer
CMO: Mark A. Kelley, M.D., Executive Vice President and Chief Medical Officer
CIO: Arther Gross, Chief Information Officer
CHR: Kathy Oswald, Interim Senior Vice President and Chief Human Resources Officer
Web address: www.henryfordhealth.org
Control: Other not–for–profit (including NFP Corporation) **Service:** General Medical and Surgical

Staffed Beds: 768 **Admissions:** 40198 **Census:** 605 **Outpatient Visits:** 2097850 **Births:** 2418 **Total Expense ($000):** 1392149 **Payroll Expense ($000):** 685404 **Personnel:** 9114

★ △ **JOHN D. DINGELL VETERANS AFFAIRS MEDICAL CENTER**, 4646 John R Street, Zip 48201–1932; tel. 313/576–1000, (Total facility includes 109 beds in nursing home–type unit) **A**1 2 3 5 7 8 9 **F**3 4 5 8 9 10 11 12 17 18 20 24 25 26 27 30 31 32 33 34 36 37 38 41 42 43 44 45 49 50 53 54 55 56 57 58 59 60 61 62 63 64 65 66 68 72 73 75 76 77 79 80 81 82 86 87 88 90 91 92 93 94 95 96 97 100 102 106 107 111 117 118 119 121 124 132 133 135 136 137 **P**6 **S** Department of Veterans Affairs
Primary Contact: Pamela Reeves, M.D., Director
COO: Leslie Wiggins, Associate Director
CFO: Patricia Kelly, Chief Fiscal Service
CMO: Basim Dubaybo, M.D., Chief of Staff
CIO: Annette Walker, Secretary to Director
CHR: Kathleen Osinski, Chief Human Resources Officer
Web address: www.va.gov/sta/guide/home.asp
Control: Veterans Affairs, Government, federal **Service:** General Medical and Surgical

Staffed Beds: 217 **Admissions:** 3745 **Census:** 125 **Outpatient Visits:** 358215 **Births:** 0 **Total Expense ($000):** 220717 **Payroll Expense ($000):** 100176 **Personnel:** 1531

★ **KARMANOS CANCER CENTER (230297)**, 4100 John R, Zip 48201; tel. 313/576–8670 **A**1 2 9 10 **F**3 8 11 15 25 26 27 30 31 32 33 34 37 41 42 43 44 45 46 47 48 49 50 53 55 56 57 58 62 63 64 66 72 73 76 77 79 80 81 82 90 96 97 99 100 101 102 103 104 105 106 107 108 109 111 112 114 116 119 121 124 125 132 135 136 137 **P**6
Primary Contact: John C. Ruckdeschel, M.D., President and Chief Executive Officer
CMO: Manuel Valdivieso, M.D., Chief Medical Officer
CIO: George G. Yacoub, Chief Information Officer
CHR: David Jansen, Vice President Human Resources
Web address: www.karmanos.org
Control: Other not–for–profit (including NFP Corporation) **Service:** Cancer

Staffed Beds: 97 **Admissions:** 4669 **Census:** 80 **Outpatient Visits:** 145322 **Births:** 0 **Total Expense ($000):** 178931 **Payroll Expense ($000):** 40623 **Personnel:** 654

★ △ **REHABILITATION INSTITUTE OF MICHIGAN (233027)**, 261 Mack Boulevard, Zip 48201–2495; tel. 313/745–1203 **A**1 3 5 7 9 10 **F**25 26 30 31 32 33 34 41 43 50 52 53 54 55 56 57 58 62 66 73 81 82 85 86 119 120 121 124 132 135 137 **P**6 **S** Detroit Medical Center
Primary Contact: Terry Reiley, President
COO: Mildred Matlock, Ph.D., Chief Operating Officer
CFO: Asad M. Malik, Vice President Finance
CMO: Ali Bitar, M.D., Vice President Medical Affairs
CHR: Paul Sturgis, Vice President Human Resources
Web address: www.rimrehab.org
Control: Other not–for–profit (including NFP Corporation) **Service:** Rehabilitation

Staffed Beds: 62 **Admissions:** 1202 **Census:** 54 **Outpatient Visits:** 175646 **Births:** 0 **Total Expense ($000):** 62010 **Payroll Expense ($000):** 29984 **Personnel:** 560

☐ **SELECT SPECIALTY HOSPITAL–NORTHWEST DETROIT (232032)**, 6071 West Outer Drive, Zip 48235; tel. 313/966–4747, (Nonreporting) **A**1 10 **S** Select Medical Corporation
Primary Contact: Sandra Baumchen, Chief Executive Officer
Web address: www.selectmedicalcorp.com
Control: Corporation, Investor–owned, for–profit **Service:** Long–Term Acute Care hospital

Staffed Beds: 36

★ △ **SINAI–GRACE HOSPITAL (230024)**, 6071 West Outer Drive, Zip 48235–2679; tel. 313/966–3300 **A**1 3 5 7 8 9 10 **F**3 5 7 8 11 13 15 17 18 20 22 24 25 26 27 30 31 32 33 36 38 40 41 42 43 44 46 49 50 51 52 53 54 55 56 57 58 59 60 62 63 64 66 68 70 72 73 74 75 76 77 78 79 80 81 82 85 86 87 88 90 91 92 93 94 95 96 97 99 100 102 105 106 107 108 109 111 112 114 118 119 120 121 123 124 132 133 135 136 137 **P**6 **S** Detroit Medical Center
Primary Contact: Conrad L. Mallett, Jr., President
COO: Vernell Williams, Vice President Operations
CFO: Kenneth Lipan, Vice President Finance
CMO: Melvin L. Hollowell, M.D., Vice President Medical Affairs
Web address: www.sinaigrace.org
Control: Other not–for–profit (including NFP Corporation) **Service:** General Medical and Surgical

Staffed Beds: 380 **Admissions:** 18855 **Census:** 282 **Outpatient Visits:** 98709 **Births:** 1859 **Total Expense ($000):** 352129 **Payroll Expense ($000):** 109640 **Personnel:** 2146

★ **ST. JOHN HOSPITAL AND MEDICAL CENTER (230165)**, 22101 Moross Road, Zip 48236–2172; tel. 313/343–4000 **A**1 2 3 5 8 9 10 12 13 **F**3 8 11 12 13 14 15 17 18 20 22 24 25 26 27 30 31 32 33 34 35 36 37 38 39 40 41 42 43 44 46 47 48 49 50 51 53 55 56 57 58 59 60 62 66 68 70 72 73 74 75 76 77 79 80 81 82 83 84 86 87 88 90 91 92 93 96 97 99 100 102 103 104 105 106 107 109 111 112 116 118 119 120 121 124 127 132 133 135 136 137 **P**8 **S** Ascension Health
Primary Contact: David B. Stephens, President and Chief Executive Officer
COO: Christopher Palazzolo, Chief Operating Officer
CFO: Tomasine Marx, Chief Financial Officer
CMO: Jim Orosz, M.D., Chief Medical Officer
CIO: Claudia Allen, Chief Information Officer
CHR: Debbie Condino, Vice President Customer Service
Web address: www.stjohn.org
Control: Church–operated, Nongovernment, not–for profit **Service:** General Medical and Surgical

Staffed Beds: 612 **Admissions:** 33605 **Census:** 480 **Outpatient Visits:** 498130 **Births:** 3923 **Total Expense ($000):** 525695 **Payroll Expense ($000):** 239129 **Personnel:** 4005

☐ **TRIUMPH HOSPITAL DETROIT (232027)**, 4777 East Outer Drive, Zip 48234; tel. 313/369–5800 **A**1 10 **F**1 3 25 26 43 44 73 75 77 80 81 82 119 137 **S** Triumph HealthCare
Primary Contact: Kim Knight, Chief Executive Officer
CFO: David Mak, Chief Financial Officer
Web address: www.triumph–healthcare.com
Control: Corporation, Investor–owned, for–profit **Service:** Long–Term Acute Care hospital

Staffed Beds: 65 **Admissions:** 701 **Census:** 48 **Outpatient Visits:** 0 **Births:** 0 **Total Expense ($000):** 16754 **Payroll Expense ($000):** 6878 **Personnel:** 115

DOWAGIAC—Cass County

★□ **BORGESS–LEE MEMORIAL HOSPITAL (231315)**, 420 West High Street, Zip 49047–1907; tel. 269/782–8681 **A**1 9 10 18 **F**11 15 25 26 27 30 31 32 33 38 50 53 55 56 57 62 64 66 68 73 75 76 77 79 80 81 82 84 86 87 89 94 96 97 98 99 102 107 121 124 133 135 137 **P**6 **S** Ascension Health
Primary Contact: Joy Strand, Chief Executive Officer
COO: William Daam, Chief Operating Officer
CFO: Ken Holst, Chief Financial Officer
CMO: Mohammad S. Zaman, M.D., Chief of Staff
CIO: Bill Schuur, Director Material Management
CHR: Pete Krueger, Director Human Resources
Web address: www.borgess.com
Control: Church–operated, Nongovernment, not–for profit **Service:** General Medical and Surgical

Staffed Beds: 25 **Admissions:** 848 **Census:** 8 **Outpatient Visits:** 79534 **Births:** 0 **Total Expense ($000):** 22427 **Payroll Expense ($000):** 10115 **Personnel:** 199

EAST CHINA—St. Clair County

★□ **ST. JOHN RIVER DISTRICT HOSPITAL (230241)**, 4100 River Road, Zip 48054–2909; tel. 810/329–7111 **A**1 9 10 **F**11 13 15 25 27 31 32 33 34 38 43 44 54 56 57 62 63 68 73 74 75 76 77 79 80 82 84 86 87 90 92 96 99 102 107 118 119 121 135 136 **P**8 **S** Ascension Health
Primary Contact: Frank W. Poma, President
CFO: Philip Wild, Controller
CMO: H. Lee Bacheldor, D.O., Medical Director
CIO: Linda Osterland, Director Information Services
Web address: www.stjohn.org
Control: Church–operated, Nongovernment, not–for profit **Service:** General Medical and Surgical

Staffed Beds: 68 **Admissions:** 2493 **Census:** 26 **Outpatient Visits:** 65457 **Births:** 427 **Total Expense ($000):** 37820 **Payroll Expense ($000):** 19913 **Personnel:** 375

EATON RAPIDS—Eaton County

★□ **EATON RAPIDS MEDICAL CENTER (231324)**, 1500 South Main Street, Zip 48827–0130, Mailing Address: P.O. Box 130, Zip 48827–0130; tel. 517/663–2671 **A**1 9 10 18 **F**3 11 15 25 26 31 33 38 43 52 55 56 57 58 62 66 73 75 77 79 81 82 84 86 96 102 107 119 121 122 124 133 135
Primary Contact: Jack L. Denton, President and Chief Executive Officer
CFO: Tim Johnson, Chief Operating Officer
CMO: Ashok K. Gupta, M.D., Chief of Staff
CHR: Laurie Field, Director Human Resources
Web address: www.eatonrapidsmedicalcenter.org
Control: Other not–for–profit (including NFP Corporation) **Service:** General Medical and Surgical

Staffed Beds: 20 **Admissions:** 475 **Census:** 4 **Outpatient Visits:** 13924 **Births:** 0 **Total Expense ($000):** 17206 **Payroll Expense ($000):** 6339 **Personnel:** 169

ESCANABA—Delta County

★□ **OSF ST. FRANCIS HOSPITAL (230101)**, 3401 Ludington Street, Zip 49829–1377; tel. 906/786–3311, (Nonreporting) **A**1 9 10 20 **S** OSF Healthcare System
Primary Contact: Peter G. Jennings, Chief Executive Officer
CFO: Jim Wayne, Chief Financial Officer
CIO: Mark Irving, Manager Management Information Systems
CHR: Wayne Seibert, Assistant Administrator
Web address: www.osfstfrancis.org
Control: Church–operated, Nongovernment, not–for profit **Service:** General Medical and Surgical

Staffed Beds: 48

FARMINGTON HILLS—Oakland County

★ ○ **BOTSFORD HOSPITAL (230151)**, 28050 Grand River Avenue, Zip 48336–5933; tel. 248/471–8000 **A**9 10 11 12 13 **F**3 8 9 11 13 15 17 18 20 24 25 26 27 28 30 31 32 33 34 36 37 38 40 41 44 46 47 48 49 50 51 52 53 54 55 56 57 58 59 60 62 63 66 68 71 72 73 74 75 76 77 78 79 80 81 82 84 85 86 87 88 89 90 91 92 93 96 97 102 106 107 118 119 120 121 123 124 135 136 137 **P**5 6
Primary Contact: Paul E. LaCasse, D.O., President and Chief Executive Officer
CFO: David Marcellino, Corporate Vice President and Chief Financial Officer
CMO: David Walters, D.O., Vice President and Chief Medical Officer
CIO: John Czahor, Chief Information Officer
CHR: Barbara Palmer, Corporate Vice President Human Resources
Web address: www.botsford.org
Control: Other not–for–profit (including NFP Corporation) **Service:** General Medical and Surgical

Staffed Beds: 306 **Admissions:** 17192 **Census:** 217 **Outpatient Visits:** 392000 **Births:** 868 **Total Expense ($000):** 244810 **Payroll Expense ($000):** 124759 **Personnel:** 2118

FERNDALE—Oakland County

★□ **HENRY FORD KINGSWOOD HOSPITAL (234011)**, 10300 West Eight Mile Road, Zip 48220–2198; tel. 248/398–3200 **A**1 9 10 **F**2 30 31 32 50 73 75 81 82 88 89 91 93 95 **P**6 8 **S** Henry Ford Health System
Primary Contact: Richard T. Young, FACHE, Chief Operating Officer
COO: Richard T. Young, FACHE, Chief Operating Officer
CFO: Mike Cimino, Chief Financial Officer
CMO: Taft Parson, M.D., Medical Director
Web address: www.henryford.com
Control: Other not–for–profit (including NFP Corporation) **Service:** Psychiatric

Staffed Beds: 80 **Admissions:** 2362 **Census:** 53 **Outpatient Visits:** 1654 **Births:** 0 **Payroll Expense ($000):** 7669 **Personnel:** 151

FLINT—Genesee County

★□ △ **HURLEY MEDICAL CENTER (230132)**, One Hurley Plaza, Zip 48503–5993; tel. 810/257–9000 **A**1 2 3 5 7 8 9 10 **F**1 3 11 12 13 15 16 17 18 20 24 25 26 28 30 31 32 33 35 38 40 43 44 46 49 50 52 53 54 55 57 58 60 62 64 65 68 70 72 73 74 75 76 77 78 79 80 81 82 83 84 85 86 87 88 90 91 92 93 96 97 102 103 105 106 107 108 109 111 112 113 114 117 118 119 120 121 124 127 130 132 133 135 136 137 **P**1 7
Primary Contact: Patrick R. Wardell, President and Chief Executive Officer
COO: Jamal Ghani, Senior Vice President Operations
CFO: Cass Wisniewski, Interim Chief Financial Officer
CMO: Michael Jaggi, D.O., Vice President and Chief Medical Officer
CIO: Gary Townsend, Chief Information Officer
CHR: Jay Kitson, Vice President Human Resources
Web address: www.hurleymc.com
Control: City–Government, nonfederal **Service:** General Medical and Surgical

Staffed Beds: 443 **Admissions:** 27098 **Census:** 294 **Outpatient Visits:** 443882 **Births:** 2839 **Total Expense ($000):** 316820 **Payroll Expense ($000):** 132005 **Personnel:** 2333

★□ **MCLAREN REGIONAL MEDICAL CENTER (230141)**, 401 South Ballenger Highway, Zip 48532–3685; tel. 810/342–2000, (Total facility includes 23 beds in nursing home–type unit) **A**1 2 3 5 8 9 10 **F**3 5 11 12 13 15 17 18 20 22 24 25 26 27 28 30 31 32 33 34 36 37 38 41 43 46 49 50 52 53 54 55 56 57 58 59 60 62 66 68 72 73 74 75 76 77 79 80 81 82 84 85 86 87 88 89 90 91 92 93 94 95 96 97 102 103 106 107 108 109 111 112 113 114 116 118 119 120 121 124 130 133 135 136 137 **P**6 7 **S** McLaren Health Care Corporation
Primary Contact: Donald C. Kooy, President and Chief Executive Officer
COO: Brent Wheeler, Vice President Ancillary and Support Services
CFO: Rick Wyles, Chief Financial Officer
CMO: Edwin H. Gullekson, M.D., Vice President Medical Affairs
CIO: Joan Maten, Vice President Nursing Services
CHR: Timothy Srock, Vice President Human Resources
Web address: www.mclarenregional.org
Control: Other not–for–profit (including NFP Corporation) **Service:** General Medical and Surgical

Staffed Beds: 324 **Admissions:** 20574 **Census:** 272 **Outpatient Visits:** 416832 **Births:** 693 **Total Expense ($000):** 283692 **Payroll Expense ($000):** 117472 **Personnel:** 2083

□ **SELECT SPECIALTY HOSPITAL–FLINT (232012)**, One Hurley Plaza, 11th Floor, Zip 48503; tel. 810/237–6793, (Nonreporting) **A**1 10 **S** Select Medical Corporation
Primary Contact: Lorie Powell, Chief Executive Officer
Web address: www.selectmedicalcorp.com
Control: Corporation, Investor–owned, for–profit **Service:** Long–Term Acute Care hospital

Staffed Beds: 32

MI

Hospital, Medicare Provider Number, Address, Telephone, Approval, Facility, and Physician Codes, Health Care System
★ American Hospital Association (AHA) membership
□ The Joint Commission accreditation
○ American Osteopathic Association (AOA) accreditation
△ Commission on Accreditation of Rehabilitation Facilities (CARF) accreditation

FRANKFORT—Benzie County

★ **PAUL OLIVER MEMORIAL HOSPITAL (231300)**, 224 Park Avenue, Zip 49635–9658; tel. 231/352–2200, (Total facility includes 40 beds in nursing home–type unit) **A**9 10 18 **F**11 15 24 26 31 32 33 38 46 50 55 57 62 75 79 81 86 96 102 107 119 121 122 135 137 **S** Munson Healthcare
Primary Contact: James D. Austin, FACHE, Administrator
COO: Peter Marinoff, Director Operations
CFO: Edward B. Carlson, Vice President and Chief Financial Officer
CMO: Gerard Mahoney, M.D., Chief of Staff
CHR: Julie Banktson, Human Resources Manager
Web address: www.munsonhealthcare.org
Control: Other not–for–profit (including NFP Corporation) **Service:** General Medical and Surgical

Staffed Beds: 48 **Admissions:** 98 **Census:** 40 **Outpatient Visits:** 34383 **Births:** 0 **Total Expense ($000):** 12021 **Payroll Expense ($000):** 4165 **Personnel:** 119

FREMONT—Newaygo County

⊠ **GERBER MEMORIAL HEALTH SERVICES (230106)**, 212 South Sullivan Street, Zip 49412–1596; tel. 231/924–3300 **A**1 9 10 **F**11 13 15 24 26 27 30 31 32 33 34 36 38 40 43 48 52 54 56 57 61 62 63 66 68 73 74 75 76 77 79 81 82 86 88 90 91 92 93 94 96 97 100 102 106 107 112 118 119 120 121 122 124 135 136
Primary Contact: Ned B. Hughes, Jr., President
COO: John Sella, Chief Financial Officer
CFO: John Sella, Chief Financial Officer
CMO: Michael DeWeerd, M.D., Chief of Staff
CIO: Pete Mulford, Director Information Systems
CHR: Ted Britton, Director Human Resources
Web address: www.gerberhospital.org
Control: Other not–for–profit (including NFP Corporation) **Service:** General Medical and Surgical

Staffed Beds: 77 **Admissions:** 2943 **Census:** 30 **Outpatient Visits:** 102778 **Births:** 522 **Total Expense ($000):** 53486 **Payroll Expense ($000):** 23547 **Personnel:** 510

MI

GARDEN CITY—Wayne County

★ ○ **GARDEN CITY HOSPITAL (230244)**, 6245 North Inkster Road, Zip 48135–4001; tel. 734/421–3300 **A**9 10 11 12 13 **F**3 4 11 13 15 17 18 20 24 25 27 30 31 32 33 34 38 40 41 43 46 47 49 50 51 55 56 61 62 63 64 66 68 72 73 74 75 76 77 78 79 80 82 84 85 86 87 96 100 101 102 105 107 118 119 120 121 124 132 135 137 **P**5 6
Primary Contact: Gary R. Ley, President and Chief Executive Officer
COO: Tom Daskalakis, Chief Operating Officer
CFO: Daniel Babb, Chief Financial Officer
CIO: Bill Moncrief, Director Information Systems
CHR: Mitchell Nimmoor, Vice President Human Resources
Web address: www.gchosp.org
Control: Other not–for–profit (including NFP Corporation) **Service:** General Medical and Surgical

Staffed Beds: 222 **Admissions:** 9479 **Census:** 134 **Outpatient Visits:** 105776 **Births:** 862 **Total Expense ($000):** 122195 **Payroll Expense ($000):** 53272 **Personnel:** 1033

GAYLORD—Otsego County

⊠ **OTSEGO MEMORIAL HOSPITAL (230133)**, 825 North Center Avenue, Zip 49735–1560; tel. 989/731–2100, (Includes MCREYNOLDS HALL), (Total facility includes 34 beds in nursing home–type unit) **A**1 9 10 20 **F**3 13 15 24 25 27 28 30 31 32 33 34 35 38 40 43 46 49 50 53 54 55 56 57 59 62 63 68 72 73 74 75 76 77 79 80 81 82 86 87 96 97 100 102 106 107 112 117 118 119 120 121 123 124 133 135 136 137 **P**6
Primary Contact: Thomas R. Lemon, Chief Executive Officer
CFO: Timothy Eckert, Vice President Finance
CMO: Rick Mee, M.D., Chief of Staff
CIO: Timothy Hella, Director Information Management
CHR: Terra Deming, Director Human Resources
Web address: www.otsegomemorialhospital.org
Control: Other not–for–profit (including NFP Corporation) **Service:** General Medical and Surgical

Staffed Beds: 87 **Admissions:** 2005 **Census:** 48 **Outpatient Visits:** 100503 **Births:** 291 **Total Expense ($000):** 55419 **Payroll Expense ($000):** 24862 **Personnel:** 507

GLADWIN—Gladwin County

⊠ **MIDMICHIGAN MEDICAL CENTER–GLADWIN (231325)**, 515 South Quarter Street, Zip 48624–1918; tel. 989/426–9286 **A**1 9 10 18 **F**3 11 15 24 25 26 31 32 38 52 55 56 57 62 66 75 79 80 81 84 86 87 96 97 99 100 102 107 119 121 124 132 135 **S** MidMichigan Health
Primary Contact: Ray Stover, Executive Vice President
Web address: www.midmichigan.org
Control: Other not–for–profit (including NFP Corporation) **Service:** General Medical and Surgical

Staffed Beds: 25 **Admissions:** 1232 **Census:** 11 **Outpatient Visits:** 55503 **Births:** 0 **Total Expense ($000):** 20750 **Payroll Expense ($000):** 8695 **Personnel:** 223

GRAND BLANC—Genesee County

⊠ ○ △ **GENESYS REGIONAL MEDICAL CENTER (230197)**, One Genesys Parkway, Zip 48439–8066; tel. 810/606–5000 **A**1 2 3 5 7 9 10 11 12 13 **F**3 7 8 11 13 15 17 18 20 22 24 25 26 27 30 31 32 33 35 38 39 40 41 43 44 46 48 49 50 51 53 54 55 56 57 58 59 60 62 66 68 72 73 74 75 76 77 79 80 81 82 84 85 86 87 96 99 102 103 106 107 118 119 121 123 124 134 135 136 **P**6 **S** Ascension Health
Primary Contact: Elizabeth Aderholdt, President
COO: Elizabeth Aderholdt, President
CIO: Daniel Stross, Chief Information Officer
CHR: Tammy Saunaitis, Vice President
Web address: www.genesys.org
Control: Church–operated, Nongovernment, not–for profit **Service:** General Medical and Surgical

Staffed Beds: 410 **Admissions:** 27094 **Census:** 331 **Outpatient Visits:** 1043738 **Births:** 2947 **Total Expense ($000):** 402885 **Payroll Expense ($000):** 174567 **Personnel:** 2984

GRAND HAVEN—Ottawa County

⊠ **NORTH OTTAWA COMMUNITY HOSPITAL (230174)**, 1309 Sheldon Road, Zip 49417–2488; tel. 616/842–3600 **A**1 9 10 **F**3 7 11 13 15 24 25 30 32 33 38 50 55 56 57 61 63 66 68 73 74 77 79 80 84 86 87 96 97 100 102 107 118 119 120 121 135 136 137 **P**6
Primary Contact: Shelleye Yaklin, President and Chief Executive Officer
CFO: Donald J. Longpre, Vice President Finance and Chief Financial Officer
CMO: Kay Aardema, M.D., Chief of Staff
CIO: Greg Shunta, Director Information Technology
CHR: Carla Wallis, Director Human Resources
Web address: www.noch.org
Control: Other not–for–profit (including NFP Corporation) **Service:** General Medical and Surgical

Staffed Beds: 40 **Admissions:** 1959 **Census:** 17 **Outpatient Visits:** 129044 **Births:** 422 **Total Expense ($000):** 50217 **Payroll Expense ($000):** 19435 **Personnel:** 379

GRAND RAPIDS—Kent County

☐ **FOREST VIEW PSYCHIATRIC HOSPITAL (234030)**, (Formerly Forest View Hospital), 1055 Medical Park Drive S.E., Zip 49546–8323; tel. 616/942–9610 **A**1 9 10 **F**25 31 82 88 89 91 94 95 119 121 132 **P**5 **S** Universal Health Services, Inc.
Primary Contact: Wayne T. Miller, Chief Executive Officer and Managing Director
CFO: Terry Cross, Controller
CMO: Stan Gunadi, M.D., Medical Director
CHR: Billie Williams, Director Human Resources
Web address: www.forestviewhospital.com
Control: Corporation, Investor–owned, for–profit **Service:** Psychiatric

Staffed Beds: 62 **Admissions:** 2172 **Census:** 53 **Outpatient Visits:** 3685 **Births:** 0 **Total Expense ($000):** 12051 **Payroll Expense ($000):** 5785 **Personnel:** 132

⊠ △ **MARY FREE BED REHABILITATION HOSPITAL (233026)**, 235 Wealthy Street S.E., Zip 49503–5299; tel. 616/242–0300 **A**1 7 9 10 **F**26 30 31 32 43 53 56 62 66 73 75 81 85 86 90 94 119 120 121 132 135
Primary Contact: William H. Blessing, President
CFO: Randall DeNeff, Vice President Finance
CMO: John Butzer, M.D., Medical Director
CHR: Kelli Miller, Vice President Human Resources
Web address: www.maryfreebed.com
Control: Other not–for–profit (including NFP Corporation) **Service:** Rehabilitation

Staffed Beds: 80 **Admissions:** 1067 **Census:** 41 **Outpatient Visits:** 47346 **Births:** 0 **Total Expense ($000):** 30733 **Payroll Expense ($000):** 18295 **Personnel:** 468

⊠ **PINE REST CHRISTIAN MENTAL HEALTH SERVICES (234006)**, 300 68th Street S.E., Zip 49501–0165, Mailing Address: P.O. Box 165, Zip 49501–0165; tel. 616/455–5000 **A**1 5 9 10 **F**4 5 6 25 26 30 31 32 33 36 54 56 57 61 66 73 81 88 89 90 91 92 93 94 95 119 121 123 135 **P**6
Primary Contact: Mark C. Eastburg, Ph.D., President and Chief Executive Officer
COO: Mark C. Eastburg, Ph.D., President and Chief Executive Officer
CFO: Paul H. Karsten, Vice President Finance and Chief Financial Officer
CMO: Denise Gribbin, M.D., Vice President and Chief Medical Officer
Web address: www.pinerest.org
Control: Other not–for–profit (including NFP Corporation) **Service:** Psychiatric

Staffed Beds: 296 **Admissions:** 4812 **Census:** 133 **Outpatient Visits:** 206233 **Births:** 0 **Total Expense ($000):** 66246 **Personnel:** 912

Many Facility Codes have changed. Please refer to the AHA Guide Code Chart.

★ **SAINT MARY'S HEALTH CARE (230059)**, 200 Jefferson Avenue S.E., Zip 49503–4598; tel. 616/685–6090 **A**1 2 3 5 9 10 **F**3 8 13 15 17 20 24 25 26 27 30 31 32 33 34 35 38 39 40 41 42 43 44 45 46 48 49 50 52 53 54 55 56 57 58 59 60 62 64 66 68 69 70 71 72 73 74 75 76 77 79 80 81 82 84 87 88 89 90 92 95 96 97 99 100 102 103 106 107 108 109 111 112 116 118 119 120 121 124 127 133 135 136 137 **P**7 **S** Trinity Health
Primary Contact: Philip H. McCorkle, Jr., President and Chief Executive Officer
COO: Randall J. Wagner, Chief Operating Officer
CFO: Steve Pirog, Vice President Finance
CMO: David Baumgartner, M.D., Vice President Medical Affairs
CIO: William Van Doornik, Site Director Information Services
CHR: Thomas Karel, Vice President Organization and Talent Effectiveness
Web address: www.smhealthcare.org
Control: Church–operated, Nongovernment, not–for profit **Service:** General Medical and Surgical

Staffed Beds: 336 **Admissions:** 18687 **Census:** 262 **Outpatient Visits:** 753410 **Births:** 2505 **Total Expense ($000):** 373502 **Payroll Expense ($000):** 147474 **Personnel:** 2285

★ △ **SPECTRUM HEALTH (230038)**, 100 Michigan Street N.E., Zip 49503; tel. 616/774–7444, (Includes SPECTRUM HEALTH – BLODGETT CAMPUS; SPECTRUM HEALTH – BUTTERWORTH CAMPUS, 100 Michigan Street N.E., Zip 49503–2551; tel. 616/391–1774) **A**1 2 3 5 7 8 9 10 **F**3 7 8 9 11 12 13 15 16 17 18 19 20 21 22 23 24 25 26 27 28 30 31 32 33 35 36 38 40 41 43 49 50 51 52 53 54 55 56 57 58 59 60 61 62 63 64 66 68 69 70 71 72 73 74 75 76 77 79 80 81 82 83 84 86 87 89 96 97 98 99 100 102 103 104 105 106 107 109 112 113 114 116 118 119 120 121 123 124 125 127 132 133 135 136 137 **P**6 8 **S** Spectrum Health
Primary Contact: Matthew Van Vranken, President
COO: Marc Chircop, Senior Vice President
CFO: Joseph J. Fifer, Vice President Finance
CMO: Lowell Bursch, M.D., Executive Vice President Medical Affairs
CIO: Steven Sarros, Vice President Technology and Information Solutions
CHR: Tanja Oquendo, Vice President Human Resources
Web address: www.spectrum–health.org
Control: Other not–for–profit (including NFP Corporation) **Service:** General Medical and Surgical

Staffed Beds: 987 **Admissions:** 58774 **Census:** 696 **Outpatient Visits:** 176849 **Births:** 8122 **Total Expense ($000):** 1014214 **Payroll Expense ($000):** 415026 **Personnel:** 8680

★ △ **SPECTRUM HEALTH–SPECIAL CARE HOSPITAL (232029)**, 750 Fuller Avenue N.E., Zip 49503–1995; tel. 616/486–3000 **A**1 7 10 **F**1 25 26 30 32 41 50 59 66 73 80 119 137 **S** Spectrum Health
Primary Contact: Don Romain, Chief Executive Officer
CFO: James Davidson, Vice President Finance
CMO: Iris Boettcher, M.D., Medical Director
CIO: Frank Thomas, Director Information Systems
CHR: Floyd Wilson, Chief Human Resources Officer
Web address: www.kentcommunity.spectrum–health.org
Control: Other not–for–profit (including NFP Corporation) **Service:** Children's Long–Term Acute Care

Staffed Beds: 36 **Admissions:** 319 **Census:** 21 **Outpatient Visits:** 5480 **Births:** 0 **Total Expense ($000):** 34524 **Payroll Expense ($000):** 14383 **Personnel:** 63

GRAYLING—Crawford County

★ **MERCY HOSPITAL GRAYLING (230058)**, 1100 East Michigan Avenue, Zip 49738–1398; tel. 989/348–5461, (Total facility includes 40 beds in nursing home–type unit) **A**1 9 10 20 **F**3 11 13 15 24 25 26 28 30 31 32 33 34 36 38 41 43 50 51 53 56 57 62 64 68 73 74 75 77 79 80 81 82 86 87 89 90 91 92 94 96 97 100 107 119 120 121 132 135 136 137 **P**6 8 **S** Trinity Health
Primary Contact: Stephanie J. Riemer–Matuzak, Chief Executive Officer
CFO: Dan Hogan, Vice President Finance
CMO: Douglas Slater, M.D., Vice President Medical Affairs
CHR: Kirsten Korth–White, Chief Human Resources Officer
Web address: www.mercygrayling.munsonhealthcare.org
Control: Church–operated, Nongovernment, not–for profit **Service:** General Medical and Surgical

Staffed Beds: 95 **Admissions:** 3991 **Census:** 68 **Outpatient Visits:** 122931 **Births:** 285 **Total Expense ($000):** 60150 **Payroll Expense ($000):** 26955 **Personnel:** 497

GREENVILLE—Montcalm County

★ **SPECTRUM HEALTH–UNITED MEMORIAL (231317)**, 615 South Bower Street, Zip 48838–2628; tel. 616/754–4691, (Includes SPECTRUM HEALTH – KELSEY CAMPUS, 418 Washington Avenue, Lakeview, Zip 48850; tel. 989/352–7211), (Total facility includes 71 beds in nursing home–type unit) **A**1 9 10 **F**3 8 11 13 15 25 28 31 38 40 41 44 46 50 62 68 74 75 79 80 82 84 86 87 96 97 102 107 117 118 119 120 122 135 136 **P**8 **S** Spectrum Health
Primary Contact: Paul Bonis, Chief Executive Officer
COO: Priscillia Mahar, Chief Operating Officer
CFO: Mary Anne Jones, Chief Financial Officer
CMO: Bennett Walstatler, M.D., President
CIO: David Dutmers, Team Leader Information and Technology Management
CHR: Vicki Jensen, Chief Human Resources Officer
Web address: www.umha.org
Control: Other not–for–profit (including NFP Corporation) **Service:** General Medical and Surgical

Staffed Beds: 141 **Admissions:** 3061 **Census:** 96 **Outpatient Visits:** 400103 **Births:** 359 **Total Expense ($000):** 53584 **Payroll Expense ($000):** 20900 **Personnel:** 503

GROSSE POINTE—Wayne County

★ **BEAUMONT HOSPITAL GROSSE POINTE (230089)**, (Formerly Bon Secours Cottage Health Services–Bon Secours Campus), 468 Cadieux Road, Zip 48230–1592; tel. 313/343–1000 **A**1 9 10 **F**3 11 13 15 18 24 25 26 30 31 32 33 34 36 38 40 41 42 43 44 45 46 47 49 50 51 55 56 57 60 61 62 63 64 66 68 69 72 73 74 75 76 77 79 81 82 84 87 90 92 96 97 100 102 103 106 107 119 121 124 135 136 137 **P**6 **S** Beaumont Hospitals
Primary Contact: Richard P. Swaine, Chief Executive Officer
COO: Chris Stesney–Ridenour, Chief Operating Officer
CIO: Tim Chavis, Chief Information Officer
CHR: Ruthann Liagre, Vice President Human Resources
Web address: www.bschealth.com
Control: Other not–for–profit (including NFP Corporation) **Service:** General Medical and Surgical

Staffed Beds: 234 **Admissions:** 9895 **Census:** 132 **Outpatient Visits:** 149594 **Births:** 752 **Total Expense ($000):** 37420 **Payroll Expense ($000):** 16522 **Personnel:** 1107

SELECT SPECIALTY HOSPITAL – GROSSE POINTE (230300), 159 Kercheval Avenue, Zip 48236; tel. 313/640–2220, (Nonreporting) **A**10 **S** Select Medical Corporation
Primary Contact: Linda Steiger, Chief Executive Officer
Control: Corporation, Investor–owned, for–profit **Service:** Long–Term Acute Care hospital

Staffed Beds: 30

GROSSE POINTE FARMS—Wayne County

★ **HENRY FORD COTTAGE HOSPITAL (230135)**, 159 Kercheval Avenue, Zip 48236–3692; tel. 313/640–1000, (Nonreporting) **A**1 9 10 **S** Henry Ford Health System
Primary Contact: Denise Allar, Interim Administrator
COO: Catherine Newhouse, Executive Vice President Operations
CIO: Tim Chavis, Chief Information Officer
CHR: Ruthann Liagre, Vice President Human Resources
Web address: www.bonsecourscottage.org
Control: Church–operated, Nongovernment, not–for profit **Service:** General Medical and Surgical

Staffed Beds: 63

HANCOCK—Houghton County

★ **PORTAGE HEALTH (230108)**, (Formerly Portage Health System), 500 Campus Drive, Zip 49930–1569; tel. 906/483–1000, (Total facility includes 60 beds in nursing home–type unit) **A**1 9 10 20 **F**3 7 8 11 13 15 24 25 26 27 30 31 32 33 38 40 42 43 44 46 50 52 53 54 55 56 57 61 62 63 65 66 67 68 73 74 75 76 77 79 80 81 82 84 85 86 87 96 100 106 107 108 118 119 120 121 122 124 132 133 135 136 137 **P**6
Primary Contact: James Bogan, President and Chief Executive Officer
CFO: Brian Donahue, Chief Financial Officer
CMO: Kirk Lufkin, M.D., Medical Director
CIO: John Steenport, Director Information Technology
CHR: Robbyn Lucier, Chief Human Resources Officer
Web address: www.portagehealth.org
Control: Other not–for–profit (including NFP Corporation) **Service:** General Medical and Surgical

Staffed Beds: 96 **Admissions:** 1998 **Census:** 65 **Outpatient Visits:** 114894 **Births:** 417 **Total Expense ($000):** 60389 **Payroll Expense ($000):** 27504 **Personnel:** 545

MI

Hospital, Medicare Provider Number, Address, Telephone, Approval, Facility, and Physician Codes, Health Care System
★ American Hospital Association (AHA) membership
□ The Joint Commission accreditation
○ American Osteopathic Association (AOA) accreditation
△ Commission on Accreditation of Rehabilitation Facilities (CARF) accreditation

HARBOR BEACH—Huron County

★ **HARBOR BEACH COMMUNITY HOSPITAL (231313)**, 210 South First Street, Zip 48441–1236; tel. 989/479–3201, (Total facility includes 40 beds in nursing home–type unit) **A**9 10 18 **F**2 3 11 15 25 30 31 32 33 38 54 55 57 62 73 79 81 86 96 107 117 119 121 122 135 136 **P**3 6
Primary Contact: Edward L. Gamache, President and Chief Executive Officer
CFO: Jill Wehner, Vice President Financial Services
CMO: Richard Lloyd, D.O., Chief of Staff
CIO: Tami Nickrand, Director Information Technology
Web address: www.hbch.org
Control: Other not–for–profit (including NFP Corporation) **Service:** General Medical and Surgical

Staffed Beds: 55 **Admissions:** 207 **Census:** 39 **Outpatient Visits:** 11042 **Births:** 0 **Total Expense ($000):** 9977 **Payroll Expense ($000):** 4348 **Personnel:** 130

HARRISON TOWNSHIP—Macomb County

☒ **ST. JOHN NORTH SHORES HOSPITAL (230257)**, 26755 Ballard Road, Zip 48045–2458; tel. 586/465–5501 **A**1 9 10 **F**3 8 15 25 26 30 31 32 33 37 38 40 42 51 52 55 57 59 62 66 72 73 75 79 80 85 86 89 96 102 107 119 120 121 132 135 **S** Ascension Health
Primary Contact: David Sessions, Administrator
COO: Dennis Franks, Administrative Director Operations
CFO: Jeffrey Ewald, Director Finance
CMO: Anthony Southall, M.D., Chief of Staff
Web address: www.stjohn.org
Control: Church–operated, Nongovernment, not–for profit **Service:** General Medical and Surgical

Staffed Beds: 60 **Admissions:** 1155 **Census:** 29 **Outpatient Visits:** 24606 **Births:** 1 **Total Expense ($000):** 24615 **Payroll Expense ($000):** 12546 **Personnel:** 219

HASTINGS—Barry County

☒ **PENNOCK HOSPITAL (230040)**, 1009 West Green Street, Zip 49058–1790; tel. 269/945–3451 **A**1 9 10 **F**3 11 13 15 25 26 28 30 31 32 33 37 38 42 43 46 52 53 54 55 56 57 61 62 63 66 68 72 73 74 75 76 77 79 80 81 82 86 87 92 96 97 100 103 106 107 115 118 119 120 121 122 124 133 135 137 **P**1
Primary Contact: Sheryl Lewis Blake, FACHE, Chief Executive Officer
COO: Carla Wilson–Neil, Chief Operating Officer
CFO: Connie Downs, Chief Financial Officer
CHR: Anita Henderson, Director Human Resources
Web address: www.pennockhealth.com
Control: Other not–for–profit (including NFP Corporation) **Service:** General Medical and Surgical

Staffed Beds: 88 **Admissions:** 3264 **Census:** 34 **Outpatient Visits:** 23321 **Births:** 396 **Total Expense ($000):** 47200 **Payroll Expense ($000):** 20335 **Personnel:** 523

HILLSDALE—Hillsdale County

☒ ○ **HILLSDALE COMMUNITY HEALTH CENTER (230037)**, 168 South Howell Street, Zip 49242–2081; tel. 517/437–4451, (Total facility includes 21 beds in nursing home–type unit) **A**1 9 10 11 12 13 19 **F**3 11 12 13 15 24 25 27 31 33 35 36 37 38 43 50 57 61 68 73 74 76 77 79 82 84 86 87 88 90 92 94 96 99 100 102 107 117 118 119 120 121 124 133 135 136 137 **P**6 8
Primary Contact: Duke Anderson, President and Chief Executive Officer
CFO: Valerie Fetters, Chief Financial Officer
CMO: Dan McCance, D.O., Chief of Staff
CIO: Jim Christy, Manager, Information Technology
CHR: Janet Marsh, Director Human Resources
Web address: www.hchc.com
Control: Other not–for–profit (including NFP Corporation) **Service:** General Medical and Surgical

Staffed Beds: 82 **Admissions:** 3231 **Census:** 46 **Outpatient Visits:** 131318 **Births:** 399 **Total Expense ($000):** 50165 **Payroll Expense ($000):** 17082 **Personnel:** 352

HOLLAND—Ottawa County

☒ **HOLLAND HOSPITAL (230072)**, 602 Michigan Avenue, Zip 49423–4999; tel. 616/392–5141, (Nonreporting) **A**1 9 10
Primary Contact: Dale Sowders, President and Chief Executive Officer
CFO: Terry L. Steele, Vice President Finance and Chief Financial Officer
CHR: Chuck Kohlruss, Vice President Human Resources and Operations Support
Web address: www.hollandhospital.org
Control: Other not–for–profit (including NFP Corporation) **Service:** General Medical and Surgical

Staffed Beds: 178

HOWELL—Livingston County

☒ **SAINT JOSEPH MERCY LIVINGSTON HOSPITAL (230069)**, 620 Byron Road, Zip 48843–1093; tel. 517/545–6000 **A**1 3 5 9 10 12 13 **F**3 8 11 13 15 24 25 26 27 28 31 32 33 38 42 43 44 45 50 51 53 56 57 61 62 63 66 68 72 73 74 75 76 77 79 80 81 82 86 87 96 97 100 102 107 118 119 120 121 124 132 133 135 137 **P**5 **S** Trinity Health
Primary Contact: Garry C. Faja, President and Chief Executive Officer
COO: Douglas A. Edema, M.D., Vice President and Chief Operating Officer
CFO: Charles Hoffman, Vice President Financial Services and Chief Financial Officer
CMO: Mark Baumeier, M.D., Chief of Staff
CIO: David Koch, Director Information Systems
CHR: Marcie Wilson, Chief Human Resources Officer
Web address: www.sjmh.com/who/mcphersn.shtml
Control: Church–operated, Nongovernment, not–for profit **Service:** General Medical and Surgical

Staffed Beds: 83 **Admissions:** 4074 **Census:** 31 **Outpatient Visits:** 94481 **Births:** 668 **Total Expense ($000):** 83114 **Payroll Expense ($000):** 32095 **Personnel:** 617

IONIA—Ionia County

☒ **IONIA COUNTY MEMORIAL HOSPITAL (231331)**, 479 Lafayette Street, Zip 48846–1834, Mailing Address: Box 1001, Zip 48846–1899; tel. 616/527–4200, (Nonreporting) **A**1 9 10 18
Primary Contact: William Roeser, Chief Executive Officer
Web address: www.ioniahospital.org
Control: Other not–for–profit (including NFP Corporation) **Service:** General Medical and Surgical

Staffed Beds: 25

IRON MOUNTAIN—Dickinson County

☒ **DICKINSON COUNTY HEALTHCARE SYSTEM (230055)**, 1721 South Stephenson Avenue, Zip 49801–3637; tel. 906/774–1313 **A**1 9 10 20 **F**3 12 13 15 17 24 25 26 27 32 33 38 40 51 52 54 55 56 57 61 62 66 68 73 74 75 76 77 78 79 80 81 82 84 86 87 96 97 100 102 103 106 107 109 111 112 118 119 120 121 122 124 133 134 135 137 **P**6
Primary Contact: John Schon, Administrator and Chief Executive Officer
COO: Jeff Gussert, Director Operations
CFO: John Lee, Director Finance
CMO: Don Kube, Chief of Staff
CIO: Dean Decremer, Chief Information Officer
CHR: James Husing, Manager Human Resources
Web address: www.dchs.org
Control: County–Government, nonfederal **Service:** General Medical and Surgical

Staffed Beds: 96 **Admissions:** 3890 **Census:** 40 **Outpatient Visits:** 202438 **Births:** 482 **Total Expense ($000):** 63798 **Payroll Expense ($000):** 32620 **Personnel:** 579

☒ **VETERANS AFFAIRS MEDICAL CENTER**, 325 East H Street, Zip 49801–4792; tel. 906/774–3300, (Total facility includes 40 beds in nursing home–type unit) **A**1 9 **F**1 5 17 25 26 27 29 30 31 32 33 36 37 42 43 44 50 54 56 57 60 61 62 63 65 66 68 73 74 75 76 77 79 81 82 86 87 88 90 91 92 93 94 96 97 102 107 117 118 119 121 124 135 136 137 **P**6 **S** Department of Veterans Affairs
Primary Contact: Michael Murphy, Director
Web address: www.va.gov/sta/guide/home.asp
Control: Veterans Affairs, Government, federal **Service:** General Medical and Surgical

Staffed Beds: 57 **Admissions:** 1321 **Census:** 51 **Outpatient Visits:** 137631 **Births:** 0 **Personnel:** 585

IRON RIVER—Iron County

☒ **IRON COUNTY COMMUNITY HOSPITAL (231318)**, 1400 West Ice Lake Road, Zip 49935–9594; tel. 906/265–6121 **A**1 9 10 18 **F**11 15 24 25 27 28 31 32 33 38 40 50 52 53 54 55 56 57 59 61 62 68 73 75 76 77 79 81 82 84 86 87 96 100 102 107 117 119 120 121 122 124 133 134 135 136 137
Primary Contact: Bruce E. Rampage, Chief Executive Officer
CFO: Glenn E. Dobson, Chief Financial Officer
CHR: Lindsay Harmon, Director Human Resources
Web address: www.icch.org
Control: Other not–for–profit (including NFP Corporation) **Service:** General Medical and Surgical

Staffed Beds: 25 **Admissions:** 1075 **Census:** 10 **Outpatient Visits:** 64830 **Births:** 0 **Total Expense ($000):** 24057 **Payroll Expense ($000):** 10147 **Personnel:** 233

Many Facility Codes have changed. Please refer to the AHA Guide Code Chart.

IRONWOOD—Gogebic County

★ **GRAND VIEW HOSPITAL (231333)**, N10561 Grand View Lane, Zip 49938–9622; tel. 906/932–2525 **A**1 9 10 18 **F**3 11 13 15 25 26 27 33 38 41 42 50 54 55 56 57 61 62 63 64 66 68 73 74 75 79 80 82 84 96 97 100 102 106 107 113 118 119 121 122 124 136 **P**6
Primary Contact: Carol Goffnett, Chief Executive Officer
COO: Mary Nemetz, Vice President Patient Care Services
CFO: Charmaine Chiantello, Chief Financial Officer
CMO: Jeffery Edwards, M.D., Chief Medical Staff
CIO: Ron Eyer, Chief Management Information Services
Web address: www.gvhs.org
Control: Other not–for–profit (including NFP Corporation) **Service:** General Medical and Surgical

Staffed Beds: 25 **Admissions:** 1103 **Census:** 9 **Outpatient Visits:** 57754 **Births:** 140 **Total Expense ($000):** 26593 **Payroll Expense ($000):** 9730 **Personnel:** 266

ISHPEMING—Marquette County

★ △ **BELL HOSPITAL (231321)**, 101 South Fourth Street, Zip 49849–2151; tel. 906/486–4431 **A**7 9 10 18 **F**5 7 10 11 13 15 30 31 32 33 38 51 52 55 57 68 73 74 75 77 79 82 84 86 96 97 107 118 120 122 133 135 **P**6
Primary Contact: Rick Ament, Chief Executive Officer
COO: John Wodniak, Clinic Administrator
CFO: Greg Perttula, Chief Financial Officer
CMO: Richard Cooley, Chief of Staff
CHR: Tami Ketchen, Director Human Resources
Web address: www.bellmemorial.org
Control: Other not–for–profit (including NFP Corporation) **Service:** General Medical and Surgical

Staffed Beds: 25 **Admissions:** 1309 **Census:** 11 **Outpatient Visits:** 58586 **Births:** 219 **Total Expense ($000):** 27798 **Payroll Expense ($000):** 11601 **Personnel:** 323

JACKSON—Jackson County

★ **ALLEGIANCE HEALTH (230092)**, (Formerly Foote Health System), 205 North East Avenue, Zip 49201–1789; tel. 517/788–4800 **A**1 2 9 10 **F**3 4 5 8 9 11 13 15 17 18 20 24 25 26 27 30 31 32 33 36 38 42 43 44 45 46 47 48 49 51 52 53 54 55 56 57 60 61 62 63 64 66 67 68 71 72 73 74 75 77 79 80 82 84 86 88 89 90 91 92 93 94 95 96 97 100 101 102 103 104 105 106 107 116 117 118 119 120 121 123 124 135 136 137 **P**6
Primary Contact: Georgia R. Fojtasek, President and Chief Executive Officer
COO: Karen Chaprnka, Senior Vice President and Chief Operating Officer
CFO: Jeanne Wickens, Chief Financial Officer
CMO: Ray King, M.D., Chief Medical Officer
CIO: Richard Warren, Vice President Health Information Systems
CHR: Jan Blair, Vice President Human Resources
Web address: www.allegiancehealth.org
Control: Other not–for–profit (including NFP Corporation) **Service:** General Medical and Surgical

Staffed Beds: 411 **Admissions:** 17694 **Census:** 220 **Outpatient Visits:** 415510 **Births:** 1933 **Total Expense ($000):** 278799 **Payroll Expense ($000):** 126440 **Personnel:** 2868

★ **CARELINK OF JACKSON (232036)**, 110 North Elm Avenue, Zip 49202–3595; tel. 517/787–1440 **A**1 10 **F**1 3 25 26 31 32 55 57 59 66 119 135 137 **P**1 **S** Ascension Health
Primary Contact: Victoria Webster, Vice President and Chief Operating Officer
COO: Victoria Webster, Vice President and Chief Operating Officer
CFO: Renae Veldhoven, Controller
CMO: Gregg Patten, M.D., Chief Medical Officer
CIO: Debora Slone, Director Human Resources
CHR: Debora Slone, Director Human Resources
Web address: www.carelinkofjackson.org
Control: Other not–for–profit (including NFP Corporation) **Service:** General Medical and Surgical

Staffed Beds: 30 **Admissions:** 310 **Census:** 22 **Outpatient Visits:** 0 **Births:** 0 **Total Expense ($000):** 9996 **Payroll Expense ($000):** 3709 **Personnel:** 89

DUANE L. WATERS HOSPITAL, 3857 Cooper Street, Zip 49201–7521; tel. 517/780–5600 **F**1 7 26 37 38 42 43 44 57 60 65 86 96 117 119 124 **P**5
Primary Contact: Gerald De Voss, Acting Administrator
Control: State–Government, nonfederal **Service:** Hospital unit of an institution (prison hospital, college infimary, etc.)

Staffed Beds: 120 **Admissions:** 1340 **Census:** 103 **Outpatient Visits:** 6585 **Births:** 0 **Total Expense ($000):** 15780 **Payroll Expense ($000):** 9310

KALAMAZOO—Kalamazoo County

★ △ **BORGESS MEDICAL CENTER (230117)**, 1521 Gull Road, Zip 49048–1640; tel. 269/226–7000 **A**1 3 5 7 9 10 **F**1 3 7 8 9 11 12 13 15 17 18 20 22 24 25 26 27 28 30 31 32 33 34 36 37 38 40 41 42 43 44 49 50 52 53 54 55 56 57 58 59 60 61 62 66 68 72 73 74 75 76 77 79 80 81 82 84 85 86 87 88 89 90 91 92 93 94 95 96 97 99 102 103 106 107 118 119 120 121 123 124 133 135 136 137 **P**3 6 8 **S** Ascension Health
Primary Contact: Paul A. Spaude, FACHE, President and Chief Executive Officer
COO: Lois Van Donselaar, Chief Nursing Officer
CFO: Richard Felbinger, Senior Vice President and Chief Financial Officer
CMO: Terry Baxter, M.D., Chief Medical Officer
CIO: George Dix, Chief Information Officer
CHR: Laura Lentenbrink, Vice President Human Resources
Web address: www.borgess.com
Control: Church–operated, Nongovernment, not–for profit **Service:** General Medical and Surgical

Staffed Beds: 392 **Admissions:** 20458 **Census:** 276 **Outpatient Visits:** 375589 **Births:** 1425 **Total Expense ($000):** 357050 **Payroll Expense ($000):** 136282 **Personnel:** 2549

★ **BRONSON METHODIST HOSPITAL (230017)**, 601 John Street, Zip 49007–5345; tel. 269/341–6000 **A**1 3 5 8 9 10 **F**3 11 12 13 15 16 17 18 20 22 24 25 26 27 28 30 31 32 33 35 37 38 40 43 44 46 49 50 51 54 55 56 57 58 60 61 62 66 68 70 71 72 73 74 75 76 77 79 80 81 82 83 84 85 86 87 92 96 97 99 100 102 103 106 107 114 119 120 121 123 124 135 136 137 **P**6 **S** Bronson Healthcare Group, Inc.
Primary Contact: Frank J. Sardone, President and Chief Executive Officer
COO: Kenneth L. Taft, Executive Vice President and Chief Operating Officer
CFO: Mary Meitz, Vice President Finance
CMO: Scott Larson, M.D., Vice President Medical Affairs and Chief Medical Officer
CHR: John Hayden, Vice President and Chief Human Resources Officer
Web address: www.bronsonhealth.com
Control: Other not–for–profit (including NFP Corporation) **Service:** General Medical and Surgical

Staffed Beds: 356 **Admissions:** 22276 **Census:** 279 **Outpatient Visits:** 408267 **Births:** 3449 **Total Expense ($000):** 420707 **Payroll Expense ($000):** 195569 **Personnel:** 2920

□ **KALAMAZOO PSYCHIATRIC HOSPITAL (234026)**, 1312 Oakland Drive, Zip 49008–1205; tel. 269/337–3000 **A**1 9 10 **F**3 30 31 32 37 50 52 54 63 73 75 81 82 88 91 92 93 119 121 124 132 135 **P**6
Primary Contact: James J. Coleman, Ed.D., Director
CMO: N. Gajare, M.D., Chief Clinical Affairs
CHR: Kerry Bloom, Human Resource Director
Control: State–Government, nonfederal **Service:** Psychiatric

Staffed Beds: 188 **Admissions:** 468 **Census:** 160 **Outpatient Visits:** 0 **Births:** 0 **Total Expense ($000):** 36130 **Payroll Expense ($000):** 20191 **Personnel:** 419

□ **SELECT SPECIALTY HOSPITAL OF KALAMAZOO (232035)**, 601 John Street, Zip 49007; tel. 269/836–1300, (Nonreporting) **A**1 10 **S** Select Medical Corporation
Primary Contact: Robert C. Desotelle, Chief Executive Officer
Web address: www.selectmedicalcorp.com
Control: Corporation, Investor–owned, for–profit **Service:** Long–Term Acute Care hospital

Staffed Beds: 25

KALKASKA—Kalkaska County

★ **KALKASKA MEMORIAL HEALTH CENTER (231301)**, 419 South Coral Street, Zip 49646–2500; tel. 231/258–7500, (Total facility includes 88 beds in nursing home–type unit) **A**9 10 18 **F**2 7 15 24 27 30 31 32 33 38 53 55 56 57 59 62 64 76 86 87 96 107 117 118 119 121 123 132 133 135 136 137 **S** Munson Healthcare
Primary Contact: James D. Austin, FACHE, Administrator
CMO: Jeremy Holmes, D.O., Chief of Staff
CHR: Kimberly Babcock, Administrator Chief Quality Improvement
Web address: www.munsonhealthcare.org
Control: Hospital district or authority, Government, nonfederal **Service:** General Medical and Surgical

Staffed Beds: 96 **Admissions:** 196 **Census:** 85 **Outpatient Visits:** 46526 **Total Expense ($000):** 18715 **Payroll Expense ($000):** 7850 **Personnel:** 240

MI

Hospital, Medicare Provider Number, Address, Telephone, Approval, Facility, and Physician Codes, Health Care System
★ American Hospital Association (AHA) membership
□ The Joint Commission accreditation
○ American Osteopathic Association (AOA) accreditation
△ Commission on Accreditation of Rehabilitation Facilities (CARF) accreditation

L'ANSE—Baraga County

☐ **BARAGA COUNTY MEMORIAL HOSPITAL (231307)**, 770 North Main Street, Zip 49946–1195; tel. 906/524–3300, (Total facility includes 28 beds in nursing home–type unit) **A**1 9 10 18 **F**3 8 11 15 24 27 30 31 38 42 43 44 52 57 61 62 76 77 79 84 86 96 97 102 106 107 117 119 120 121 122 **P**6
Primary Contact: John P. Tembreull, Administrator
CFO: Gail Jestila–Peltola, Chief Financial Officer
CMO: Elizabeth Benyi, D.O., Chief of Staff
CHR: Carol Seppanen, Director Human Resources
Web address: www.bcmh.org
Control: County–Government, nonfederal **Service:** General Medical and Surgical

Staffed Beds: 52 **Admissions:** 730 **Census:** 33 **Outpatient Visits:** 29086 **Births:** 0 **Total Expense ($000):** 18656 **Payroll Expense ($000):** 8657 **Personnel:** 172

LAKEVIEW—Montcalm County

SPECTRUM HEALTH – KELSEY CAMPUS See Spectrum Health–United Memorial, Greenville

LANSING—Ingham County

MI

★ ○ **INGHAM REGIONAL MEDICAL CENTER (230167)**, 401 West Greenlawn Avenue, Zip 48910–2819; tel. 517/334–2121, (Includes INGHAM REGIONAL MEDICAL CENTER, GREENLAWN CAMPUS; INGHAM REGIONAL MEDICAL CENTER, PENNSYLVANIA CAMPUS, 2727 South Pennsylvania Avenue, Zip 48910; tel. 517/372–8220) **A**1 2 3 5 8 9 10 11 12 13 **F**3 10 11 12 13 15 17 18 19 20 21 22 23 24 25 26 30 31 32 33 36 37 38 42 43 44 45 50 51 54 55 56 57 58 59 60 62 63 68 72 73 74 75 76 77 79 80 81 82 84 86 87 88 90 91 92 93 94 96 97 100 106 107 118 119 120 121 124 133 135 136 137 **P**1 **S** McLaren Health Care Corporation
Primary Contact: Robert N. Wright, President and Chief Executive Officer
CFO: Paula Reichle, Vice President Finance and Chief Financial Officer
CMO: Geoffrey Linz, M.D., Chief Medical Officer
CIO: Sally Bender, Director Information Services
CHR: Laiine Brewis, Chief Human Resources Officer
Web address: www.irmc.org
Control: Other not–for–profit (including NFP Corporation) **Service:** General Medical and Surgical

Staffed Beds: 352 **Admissions:** 18856 **Census:** 241 **Outpatient Visits:** 510086 **Births:** 1607 **Total Expense ($000):** 295961 **Payroll Expense ($000):** 120095 **Personnel:** 1801

★ ○ △ **SPARROW HOSPITAL (230230)**, (Formerly Sparrow Health System), 1215 East Michigan Avenue, Zip 48912–1811, Mailing Address: P.O. Box 30480, Zip 48909–7980; tel. 517/364–1000 **A**1 2 3 5 7 9 10 11 12 13 **F**2 3 4 5 7 11 12 13 14 15 17 18 20 24 25 26 27 28 30 31 32 33 34 36 38 40 41 42 43 45 46 49 50 51 52 53 54 55 56 57 58 59 62 63 64 65 66 67 68 70 72 73 74 75 76 77 79 80 81 82 83 84 85 86 87 88 89 90 91 92 93 94 95 96 97 99 100 102 103 105 106 107 108 109 111 112 113 114 116 118 119 120 121 123 124 132 133 135 136 137 **P**1 6 **S** Sparrow Health System
Primary Contact: Dennis A. Swan, President and Chief Executive Officer
COO: Andrea R. Price, Chief Operating Officer
CFO: Chris Bergman, Senior Vice President and Chief Financial Officer
CMO: Larry Rawsthorne, M.D., Senior Vice President Medical Affairs
CIO: Ronald Swenson, M.D., Vice President and Chief Information Officer
CHR: Thomas Ostrander, Vice President Human Resources
Web address: www.sparrow.org
Control: Other not–for–profit (including NFP Corporation) **Service:** General Medical and Surgical

Staffed Beds: 560 **Admissions:** 30714 **Census:** 410 **Outpatient Visits:** 460431 **Births:** 3928 **Total Expense ($000):** 568231 **Payroll Expense ($000):** 266649 **Personnel:** 4962

SPARROW SPECIALTY HOSPITAL (232037), 1210 West Saginaw Street, Zip 48915, Mailing Address: P.O. Box 85201, Zip 48915; tel. 517/364–6800 **A**10 **F**1 3 25 26 27 31 32 34 54 59 60 66 72 73 75 76 77 80 90 91 107 119 135 137 **S** Sparrow Health System
Primary Contact: Kira Carter, President and Chief Executive Officer
CFO: Steven Mackenzie, Controller
CMO: Cynthia Boynton, M.D., Medical Director
CHR: Shawn Williams, Manager Employee Services
Web address: www.sparrowspecialty.org
Control: Other not–for–profit (including NFP Corporation) **Service:** Long–Term Acute Care hospital

Staffed Beds: 36 **Admissions:** 322 **Census:** 27 **Outpatient Visits:** 0 **Births:** 0 **Total Expense ($000):** 11431 **Payroll Expense ($000):** 5755 **Personnel:** 121

LAPEER—Lapeer County

☐ **LAPEER REGIONAL MEDICAL CENTER (230193)**, 1375 North Main Street, Zip 48446–1376; tel. 810/667–5500, (Total facility includes 19 beds in nursing home–type unit) **A**1 9 10 **F**3 4 5 11 13 15 24 25 26 27 30 32 38 40 42 43 46 50 51 53 54 55 56 57 61 62 66 68 73 74 75 76 77 79 80 81 82 86 87 88 92 96 97 99 100 102 103 105 107 108 109 110 111 117 118 119 120 121 124 135 **S** McLaren Health Care Corporation
Primary Contact: Barton Buxton, President and Chief Executive Officer
COO: Brent Wheeler, Associate Administrator
CFO: Mary Beth Callahan, Chief Financial Officer
CHR: Amy Dorr, Director Human Resources
Web address: www.lapeerhospital.org
Control: Other not–for–profit (including NFP Corporation) **Service:** General Medical and Surgical

Staffed Beds: 222 **Admissions:** 6612 **Census:** 74 **Outpatient Visits:** 134028 **Births:** 580 **Total Expense ($000):** 66702 **Payroll Expense ($000):** 31334 **Personnel:** 579

LAURIUM—Houghton County

★ **KEWEENAW MEMORIAL MEDICAL CENTER (231319)**, 205 Osceola Street, Zip 49913–2199; tel. 906/337–6500 **A**1 9 10 18 **F**3 10 11 13 15 17 24 25 26 27 32 33 38 51 52 54 55 57 60 68 74 77 79 82 84 86 96 97 99 102 103 107 113 118 119 120 121 122 124 134 135 136 **P**6
Primary Contact: Charles Nelson, Chief Executive Officer
COO: Michael Hauswirth, Chief Operating Officer
CFO: Michael Hagwell, Chief Financial Officer
CMO: Paul Lyle, M.D., Chief of Staff
CHR: Arthur Wasek, Manager Human Resources
Web address: www.kmmc.org
Control: Other not–for–profit (including NFP Corporation) **Service:** General Medical and Surgical

Staffed Beds: 25 **Admissions:** 1143 **Census:** 11 **Outpatient Visits:** 36664 **Births:** 75 **Total Expense ($000):** 27196 **Payroll Expense ($000):** 14170 **Personnel:** 319

LINCOLN PARK—Wayne County

☐ **KINDRED HOSPITAL–DETROIT (232019)**, 26400 West Outer Drive, Zip 48146; tel. 313/386–2000 **A**1 10 **F**1 3 25 30 32 73 78 80 81 82 119 135 137 **P**6
Primary Contact: Judy Ingala, Interim Chief Executive Officer
Control: Corporation, Investor–owned, for–profit **Service:** Long–Term Acute Care hospital

Staffed Beds: 140 **Admissions:** 309 **Census:** 28 **Outpatient Visits:** 0 **Births:** 0 **Total Expense ($000):** 14031 **Payroll Expense ($000):** 6088 **Personnel:** 110

LIVONIA—Wayne County

★ **ST. MARY MERCY HOSPITAL (230002)**, 36475 West Five Mile Road, Zip 48154–1988; tel. 734/655–4800 **A**1 2 9 10 **F**3 4 5 12 13 15 18 20 25 26 27 30 31 32 33 34 36 38 40 41 42 44 46 47 49 50 51 54 55 56 57 58 62 66 68 72 73 74 76 77 79 80 81 82 85 86 88 90 91 92 93 94 96 97 100 102 103 104 105 106 107 109 118 119 121 124 132 134 135 136 137 **P**5 6 **S** Trinity Health
Primary Contact: David A. Spivey, President and Chief Executive Officer
COO: C. W. Lauderbach, Chief Operating Officer
CFO: Kathy O'Connor, Interim Chief Financial Officer
CMO: Asit Gokli, M.D., Vice President Medical Affairs
CIO: Julie Moran, Director Information Services
CHR: Kenneth Antczak, Vice President Human Resources
Web address: www.stmarymercy.org
Control: Church–operated, Nongovernment, not–for profit **Service:** General Medical and Surgical

Staffed Beds: 293 **Admissions:** 15529 **Census:** 197 **Outpatient Visits:** 167382 **Births:** 1428 **Total Expense ($000):** 176402 **Payroll Expense ($000):** 83811 **Personnel:** 1189

LUDINGTON—Mason County

MEMORIAL MEDICAL CENTER OF WEST MICHIGAN (230110), One Atkinson Drive, Zip 49431–1999; tel. 231/843–2591 **A**9 10 20 **F**8 11 13 15 17 24 27 30 33 38 43 49 51 56 57 61 63 66 72 73 74 75 76 77 79 80 86 87 88 90 92 93 96 97 100 102 106 107 118 119 121 124 135 136 137
Primary Contact: Mark Vipperman, President and Chief Executive Officer
CFO: Bruno Bettin, Vice President Finance
CMO: Richard York, M.D., Chief of Staff
CIO: Daryl Crowley, Director Information Services
CHR: James Wood, Director Human Resources
Web address: www.mmcwm.com
Control: Other not–for–profit (including NFP Corporation) **Service:** General Medical and Surgical

Staffed Beds: 80 **Admissions:** 3271 **Census:** 40 **Outpatient Visits:** 93434 **Births:** 411 **Total Expense ($000):** 47783 **Payroll Expense ($000):** 20553 **Personnel:** 402

Many Facility Codes have changed. Please refer to the AHA Guide Code Chart.

MADISON HEIGHTS—Oakland County

MICHIGAN ORTHOPAEDIC SPECIALTY HOSPITAL See Harper University Hospital, Detroit

★ ○ **ST. JOHN OAKLAND HOSPITAL (230223)**, (Formerly St. John Oakland Hospital), 27351 Dequindre, Zip 48071–3499; tel. 248/967–7000 **A**9 10 11 12 13 **F**3 12 15 18 25 26 27 28 30 31 32 33 34 36 38 41 42 43 46 49 50 51 52 53 54 55 56 57 58 59 60 61 62 63 64 66 68 72 73 75 76 77 79 80 81 82 86 87 88 90 91 92 94 95 96 97 98 100 101 102 103 106 107 118 119 121 124 132 133 135 136 137 **P**5 8 **S** Ascension Health
Primary Contact: Joseph M. Tasse, FACHE, President
COO: Michael Beaubien, Chief Operating Officer
CFO: Randolph H. Kummler, Chief Financial Officer
CMO: Gary L. Berg, D.O., Chief Medical Officer
Web address: www.stjohn.org
Control: Church–operated, Nongovernment, not–for profit **Service:** General Medical and Surgical

Staffed Beds: 159 **Admissions:** 7821 **Census:** 108 **Outpatient Visits:** 101728 **Births:** 0 **Total Expense ($000):** 95601 **Payroll Expense ($000):** 44493 **Personnel:** 877

MANISTEE—Manistee County

WEST SHORE MEDICAL CENTER (230060), 1465 East Parkdale Avenue, Zip 49660–9785; tel. 231/398–1000 **A**9 10 20 **F**3 7 11 13 15 17 24 25 28 30 31 32 37 38 46 49 52 53 55 56 57 62 72 73 74 75 77 79 80 81 84 86 96 97 103 106 107 119 121 122 124 135 136 137 **P**6
Primary Contact: Burton O. Parks, III, President
COO: Suzanne Cleere, Vice President Patient Care Services
CFO: Donn J. Lemmer, Vice President Finance
CIO: Louise Maik, Manager, Information Services
CHR: Jeff Rose, Vice President Human Resources
Web address: www.westshoremedcenter.org
Control: County–Government, nonfederal **Service:** General Medical and Surgical

Staffed Beds: 54 **Admissions:** 1659 **Census:** 19 **Outpatient Visits:** 80847 **Births:** 171 **Total Expense ($000):** 36775 **Payroll Expense ($000):** 16217 **Personnel:** 303

MANISTIQUE—Schoolcraft County

★ **SCHOOLCRAFT MEMORIAL HOSPITAL (231303)**, 500 Main Street, Zip 49854–0000; tel. 906/341–3200 **A**9 10 18 **F**3 10 11 15 24 25 26 27 28 30 31 32 33 34 37 38 41 42 43 44 50 52 54 55 56 57 61 62 63 73 75 76 77 79 80 81 82 84 86 87 95 96 97 100 102 106 107 117 118 119 121 122 124 132 133 135 136 **P**6
Primary Contact: Frederick J. Makowski, Chief Executive Officer
CFO: Tanya Hoar, Chief Financial Officer
CMO: David Schoenow, M.D., Chief Medical Officer
CIO: Sherry Arnold, Risk Manager
CHR: Gina Lindquist, Director Human Resources
Web address: www.scmh.org
Control: County–Government, nonfederal **Service:** General Medical and Surgical

Staffed Beds: 25 **Admissions:** 356 **Census:** 3 **Outpatient Visits:** 40069 **Births:** 0 **Total Expense ($000):** 19543 **Payroll Expense ($000):** 9981 **Personnel:** 189

MARLETTE—Sanilac County

★ △ **MARLETTE REGIONAL HOSPITAL (231330)**, 2770 Main Street, Zip 48453–0307, Mailing Address: P.O. Box 307, Zip 48453–0307; tel. 989/635–4000, (Total facility includes 43 beds in nursing home–type unit) **A**1 7 9 10 18 **F**3 7 10 11 15 25 28 30 31 32 33 36 38 42 43 44 45 46 50 53 54 55 56 57 62 63 66 73 75 77 79 80 81 82 85 86 87 96 97 100 104 106 107 115 117 118 119 120 121 122 123 124 132 135 **P**6 **S** QHR
Primary Contact: Michael A. Kozar, Chief Executive Officer
CFO: Daniel Babcock, Chief Financial Officer
CIO: Daniel Babcock, Chief Financial Officer
CHR: Connie Kennedy, Director Human Resources
Web address: www.marlettecommunityhospital.com
Control: Other not–for–profit (including NFP Corporation) **Service:** General Medical and Surgical

Staffed Beds: 84 **Admissions:** 966 **Census:** 57 **Outpatient Visits:** 42578 **Births:** 0 **Total Expense ($000):** 30500 **Payroll Expense ($000):** 13640 **Personnel:** 364

MARQUETTE—Marquette County

★ **MARQUETTE GENERAL HEALTH SYSTEM (230054)**, 580 West College Avenue, Zip 49855–2794; tel. 906/228–9440 **A**1 2 3 5 9 10 13 19 20 **F**3 4 5 7 8 10 11 12 13 14 15 17 18 20 22 24 25 26 27 28 30 31 32 33 36 37 38 40 43 44 46 49 50 51 53 54 55 56 57 58 59 61 62 63 66 68 70 72 73 74 75 76 77 79 80 81 82 84 85 86 87 88 89 90 91 92 93 94 96 97 100 102 103 104 105 106 107 108 109 111 112 113 118 119 120 121 123 124 132 133 134 135 136 137 **P**6
Primary Contact: A. Gary Muller, FACHE, Chief Executive Officer
CFO: Mike Beckstrom, Chief Financial Officer
CMO: Stanley Russin, M.D., Chief Medical Officer
CIO: Jim Sundberg, Director Information Systems
Web address: www.mgh.org
Control: Other not–for–profit (including NFP Corporation) **Service:** General Medical and Surgical

Staffed Beds: 287 **Admissions:** 12076 **Census:** 155 **Outpatient Visits:** 427922 **Births:** 819 **Total Expense ($000):** 276773 **Payroll Expense ($000):** 113565 **Personnel:** 1812

MARSHALL—Calhoun County

★ **OAKLAWN HOSPITAL (230217)**, 200 North Madison Street, Zip 49068–1199; tel. 269/781–4271 **A**1 9 10 **F**3 11 13 15 25 27 30 31 32 33 38 48 52 55 56 57 61 62 63 68 72 73 74 75 76 77 79 81 82 84 86 87 88 90 91 92 93 94 95 96 97 99 100 102 103 104 105 106 107 116 118 119 120 121 **P**1
Primary Contact: Rob Covert, President and Chief Executive Officer
CFO: Colleen Koppenhaver, Chief Financial Officer
CMO: Ginger Williams, M.D., Chief Medical Officer
CIO: Natalie Spivak, Director Information Services
CHR: Alec Allen, Director Personnel
Web address: www.oaklawnhospital.org
Control: Other not–for–profit (including NFP Corporation) **Service:** General Medical and Surgical

Staffed Beds: 78 **Admissions:** 3913 **Census:** 40 **Outpatient Visits:** 141293 **Births:** 591 **Total Expense ($000):** 76302 **Payroll Expense ($000):** 33785 **Personnel:** 636

MIDLAND—Midland County

★ **MIDMICHIGAN MEDICAL CENTER–MIDLAND (230222)**, 4005 Orchard Drive, Zip 48670–0001; tel. 989/839–3000 **A**1 2 3 5 9 10 20 **F**1 3 4 7 11 13 15 16 17 18 20 22 24 25 26 27 30 31 32 38 43 48 49 50 52 53 55 56 57 58 62 63 65 66 68 70 71 72 73 74 75 76 77 78 79 80 81 82 83 84 85 86 87 88 90 91 92 94 96 97 99 100 102 103 106 107 108 109 111 112 117 118 119 120 121 124 132 134 135 136 137 **S** MidMichigan Health
Primary Contact: Gregory H. Rogers, Senior Vice President and Treasurer
CMO: James Bicknell, M.D., Medical Director
CIO: C. Harlan Goodrich, Vice President and Chief Information Officer
CHR: Lynn Bruchhof, Vice President
Web address: www.midmichigan.org
Control: Other not–for–profit (including NFP Corporation) **Service:** General Medical and Surgical

Staffed Beds: 222 **Admissions:** 11432 **Census:** 116 **Outpatient Visits:** 302848 **Births:** 1187 **Total Expense ($000):** 219744 **Payroll Expense ($000):** 80386 **Personnel:** 1659

MONROE—Monroe County

★ **MERCY MEMORIAL HOSPITAL SYSTEM (230099)**, 718 North Macomb Street, Zip 48162–2930; tel. 734/240–8400 **A**1 9 10 **F**3 5 7 8 11 13 15 24 25 26 30 31 32 33 36 38 39 40 41 42 44 46 50 51 53 54 55 56 57 61 62 63 67 68 73 74 75 77 79 80 81 82 84 86 87 88 90 91 92 93 94 96 97 98 99 100 102 103 104 106 107 112 118 119 120 121 122 124 133 134 135 136
Primary Contact: Annette S. Phillips, President and Chief Executive Officer
CFO: Sam D. Radke, Interim Chief Financial Officer
CMO: Gilbert Burgos, Chief Medical Officer and Senior Vice President Health Care Services
CIO: Teri Boos, Interim Director Information Management
CHR: Maureen Henson, Vice President Human Resources
Web address: www.mercymemorial.org
Control: Other not–for–profit (including NFP Corporation) **Service:** General Medical and Surgical

Staffed Beds: 169 **Admissions:** 9040 **Census:** 99 **Outpatient Visits:** 231632 **Births:** 893 **Total Expense ($000):** 139555 **Payroll Expense ($000):** 58459 **Personnel:** 1340

MOUNT CLEMENS—Macomb County

HENRY FORD MACOMB HOSPITAL – MOUNT CLEMENS CAMPUS See Henry Ford Macomb Hospital, Clinton Township

MI

Hospital, Medicare Provider Number, Address, Telephone, Approval, Facility, and Physician Codes, Health Care System

★ American Hospital Association (AHA) membership
□ The Joint Commission accreditation
○ American Osteopathic Association (AOA) accreditation
△ Commission on Accreditation of Rehabilitation Facilities (CARF) accreditation

★ ○ **MOUNT CLEMENS REGIONAL MEDICAL CENTER (230227)**, 1000 Harrington Boulevard, Zip 48043–2992; tel. 586/493–8000 **A**9 10 11 12 13 **F**3 7 8 11 12 13 15 17 18 20 22 24 25 26 27 30 32 33 34 38 42 43 46 49 50 51 53 54 55 56 57 58 61 62 63 64 66 68 69 72 73 74 75 76 77 79 80 81 82 84 86 87 96 97 99 102 106 107 109 111 116 118 119 120 121 124 130 133 135 137 **P**8 **S** McLaren Health Care Corporation
Primary Contact: Mark S. O'Halla, President and Chief Executive Officer
CFO: Donna Kopinski, Chief Financial Officer
CMO: Michael K. Smith, D.O., Vice President Medical Affairs
CHR: Greg Purtell, Vice President Human Resources
Web address: www.mcrmc.org
Control: Other not–for–profit (including NFP Corporation) **Service:** General Medical and Surgical

Staffed Beds: 288 **Admissions:** 11322 **Census:** 170 **Outpatient Visits:** 130811 **Births:** 815 **Total Expense ($000):** 174313 **Payroll Expense ($000):** 66770 **Personnel:** 1497

☐ **SELECT SPECIALTY HOSPITAL–MACOMB (232023)**, 215 North Avenue, Zip 48043; tel. 586/307–9000, (Nonreporting) **A**1 10 **S** Select Medical Corporation
Primary Contact: Linda Steiger, Chief Executive Officer
Control: Corporation, Investor–owned, for–profit **Service:** Long–Term Acute Care hospital

Staffed Beds: 32

MI

MOUNT PLEASANT—Isabella County

★ ○ **CENTRAL MICHIGAN COMMUNITY HOSPITAL (230080)**, 1221 South Drive, Zip 48858–3234; tel. 989/772–6700 **A**9 10 11 19 **F**3 11 12 13 15 24 25 26 27 28 29 30 31 32 33 34 37 38 44 50 52 53 54 55 56 57 60 61 62 63 66 68 72 73 74 75 76 77 79 80 81 82 84 86 87 92 96 97 99 100 102 106 107 108 109 111 118 119 120 121 133 134 135 136 137 **P**1
Primary Contact: Jeffrey A. Collins, Interim Chief Executive Officer
CFO: Gregg Beeg, Vice President Finance and Operations
CMO: Christian Allan, M.D., Chief Medical Officer
CHR: Julie Ward, Vice President Human Resources
Web address: www.cmch.org
Control: Other not–for–profit (including NFP Corporation) **Service:** General Medical and Surgical

Staffed Beds: 83 **Admissions:** 3671 **Census:** 32 **Outpatient Visits:** 214617 **Births:** 470 **Total Expense ($000):** 68472 **Payroll Expense ($000):** 32468 **Personnel:** 627

MUNISING—Alger County

MUNISING MEMORIAL HOSPITAL (231308), 1500 Sand Point Road, Zip 49862–1406; tel. 906/387–4110 **A**9 10 18 **F**10 11 30 31 33 38 55 56 57 59 62 64 67 73 75 79 84 86 87 96 97 99 107 118 119 120 121 134 **P**6
Primary Contact: Carl J. Velte, Chief Executive Officer
CFO: Lorraine Hawley, Controller
Web address: www.uphcn.org
Control: Other not–for–profit (including NFP Corporation) **Service:** General Medical and Surgical

Staffed Beds: 25 **Admissions:** 176 **Census:** 1 **Outpatient Visits:** 21028 **Births:** 0 **Total Expense ($000):** 6782 **Payroll Expense ($000):** 3505 **Personnel:** 82

MUSKEGON—Muskegon County

☐ **HACKLEY HOSPITAL (230066)**, 1700 Clinton Street, Zip 49443–3302, Mailing Address: P.O. Box 3302, Zip 49443–3302; tel. 231/726–3511 **A**1 2 9 10 **F**3 11 12 13 15 18 25 26 27 31 32 33 37 38 40 43 44 49 50 51 52 53 55 57 60 62 66 68 72 74 75 76 77 79 80 84 85 86 88 92 93 95 96 97 98 100 102 103 105 106 107 109 111 112 114 116 118 119 120 121 122 133 135 136 137 **P**6 8 **S** Hackley Health System
Primary Contact: Gordon A. Mudler, President and Chief Executive Officer
COO: Gayle R. Miller, Vice President and Chief Operating Officer
CFO: David J. Gingras, Vice President and Chief Financial Officer
CIO: Gary Matthews, Director Information Systems
Web address: www.hackley.org
Control: Other not–for–profit (including NFP Corporation) **Service:** General Medical and Surgical

Staffed Beds: 181 **Admissions:** 8706 **Census:** 98 **Outpatient Visits:** 301921 **Births:** 1002 **Total Expense ($000):** 161033 **Payroll Expense ($000):** 64703 **Personnel:** 1183

☐ **LIFECARE HOSPITALS OF WEST MICHIGAN (232026)**, 1700 Oak Avenue, 3rd Floor, Zip 49442; tel. 231/777–6202, (Nonreporting) **A**1 10 **S** LifeCare Management Services
Primary Contact: Jevne Conover, Administrator
Web address: www.lifecare–hospitals.com
Control: Corporation, Investor–owned, for–profit **Service:** Long–Term Acute Care hospital

Staffed Beds: 20

⊠ ○ **MERCY HEALTH PARTNERS (230004)**, (Formerly Mercy General Health Partners), 1500 East Sherman Boulevard, Zip 49443; tel. 231/672–2000, (Includes MERCY HEALTH PARTNERS–MERCY CAMPUS; MERCY HEALTH PARTNERS–MUSKEGON GENERAL CAMPUS, 1700 Oak Avenue, Zip 49442; tel. 231/672–3311) **A**1 2 9 10 11 12 13 **F**3 11 12 13 15 18 20 22 24 25 26 27 30 31 32 33 38 41 43 44 50 51 53 54 55 56 57 58 62 66 68 72 73 74 75 76 77 79 80 81 82 84 85 86 87 96 97 100 104 106 107 118 119 120 121 124 133 135 136 137 **P**6 8 **S** Trinity Health
Primary Contact: Roger Spoelman, President and Chief Executive Officer
COO: Greg Loomis, Chief Operation Officer
CFO: Gary Allore, Chief Financial Officer
CMO: Remington Sprague, M.D., Chief Medical Officer
Web address: www.mghp.com
Control: Other not–for–profit (including NFP Corporation) **Service:** General Medical and Surgical

Staffed Beds: 230 **Admissions:** 11675 **Census:** 127 **Outpatient Visits:** 379274 **Births:** 1474 **Total Expense ($000):** 211820 **Payroll Expense ($000):** 90030 **Personnel:** 1370

☐ **SELECT SPECIALTY HOSPITAL OF WESTERN MICHIGAN (232021)**, 1700 Clinton Street, Suite S2, Zip 49442; tel. 231/728–5811, (Nonreporting) **A**1 10 **S** Select Medical Corporation
Primary Contact: Jonathan Cohee, Interim Chief Executive Officer
Web address: www.selectmedicalcorp.com
Control: Corporation, Investor–owned, for–profit **Service:** Long–Term Acute Care hospital

Staffed Beds: 32

NEW BALTIMORE—Macomb County

HARBOR OAKS HOSPITAL (234021), 35031 23 Mile Road, Zip 48047–2097; tel. 586/725–5777, (Nonreporting) **A**9 10 **S** Pioneer Behavioral Health
Primary Contact: Tina Lesnik, Chief Operating Officer
COO: Tina Lesnik, Chief Operating Officer
CFO: Paula C. Wurts, Chief Financial Officer
CMO: Teymour Sepahbodi, M.D., Medical Director
CHR: Ryan King, Director Human Resources
Web address: www.harboroaks.com
Control: Corporation, Investor–owned, for–profit **Service:** Psychiatric

Staffed Beds: 64

NEWBERRY—Luce County

⊠ **HELEN NEWBERRY JOY HOSPITAL (231304)**, 502 West Harrie Street, Zip 49868–0070; tel. 906/293–9200, (Includes HELEN NEWBERRY JOY HOSPITAL ANNEX), (Total facility includes 48 beds in nursing home–type unit) **A**1 9 10 18 **F**15 24 25 26 27 28 30 31 32 33 34 36 38 41 42 43 52 53 55 56 57 62 63 73 76 79 80 81 82 85 86 87 96 97 102 106 107 117 118 119 120 121 122 123 124 132 133 135 137 **P**6
Primary Contact: Wayne P. Hellerstedt, Chief Executive Officer
CFO: Scott Pillion, Chief Financial Officer
CMO: Raghu Rao, M.D., Chief of Staff
CIO: Michelle Sears, Director Information Systems
CHR: Roger Bergh, Director Human Resources
Web address: www.hnjh.org
Control: County–Government, nonfederal **Service:** General Medical and Surgical

Staffed Beds: 73 **Admissions:** 511 **Census:** 51 **Outpatient Visits:** 59388 **Births:** 0 **Total Expense ($000):** 25345 **Payroll Expense ($000):** 11258 **Personnel:** 262

NORTHVILLE—Wayne County

☐ **HAWTHORN CENTER**, 18471 Haggerty Road, Zip 48167–9575; tel. 248/735–6771 **A**1 3 5 9 **F**37 88 89
Primary Contact: Shobhana Joshi, M.D., Facility Director
CIO: Robert W. Bailey, Chief Information Officer
Control: State–Government, nonfederal **Service:** Children's hospital psychiatric

Staffed Beds: 67 **Admissions:** 530 **Census:** 58 **Outpatient Visits:** 0 **Births:** 0 **Total Expense ($000):** 19623 **Payroll Expense ($000):** 12084 **Personnel:** 192

ONTONAGON—Ontonagon County

⊠ **ASPIRUS ONTONAGON HOSPITAL (231309)**, (Formerly Ontonagon Memorial Hospital), 601 Seventh Street, Zip 49953–1496; tel. 906/884–8000, (Total facility includes 46 beds in nursing home–type unit) **A**1 9 10 18 **F**3 15 24 25 27 30 33 38 42 46 52 54 55 56 57 62 66 77 79 80 86 87 96 97 107 117 119 121 122 **P**6
Primary Contact: Mike Gutsch, Chief Executive Officer
COO: Michael R. Drew, Assistant Administrator and Director Pharmacy
CMO: John Austin, M.D., Director Medical Staff
CIO: Pam Karttunen, Administrative Assistant
CHR: Gina Linna, Administrative Assistant
Web address: www.aspirus–ontonagon.org
Control: Other not–for–profit (including NFP Corporation) **Service:** General Medical and Surgical

Staffed Beds: 64 **Admissions:** 563 **Census:** 50 **Outpatient Visits:** 18100 **Births:** 0 **Total Expense ($000):** 7129 **Payroll Expense ($000):** 6288 **Personnel:** 144

OWOSSO—Shiawassee County

★ **MEMORIAL HEALTHCARE (230121)**, 826 West King Street, Zip 48867–2198; tel. 989/723–5211, (Total facility includes 20 beds in nursing home–type unit) **A**1 2 5 9 10 **F**2 11 12 13 15 24 25 26 27 30 31 32 33 36 38 42 43 44 46 49 50 51 54 55 56 57 58 61 62 63 67 68 72 73 74 75 76 77 79 80 81 82 84 85 86 87 88 90 91 92 93 96 97 100 103 107 117 118 119 120 121 133 135 136 137 **P**1 6 7
Primary Contact: Cheryl Peterson, President and Chief Executive Officer
CFO: Michael Grisdela, Vice President Administration and Chief Financial Officer
CMO: Michael Schmidt, D.O., Chief of Staff
CIO: Frank Fear, Chief Information Officer
CHR: Geoffrey Washburn, Vice President Ancillary and Human Resources
Web address: www.memorialhealthcare.org
Control: Other not–for–profit (including NFP Corporation) **Service:** General Medical and Surgical

Staffed Beds: 131 **Admissions:** 4921 **Census:** 66 **Outpatient Visits:** 268168 **Births:** 542 **Total Expense ($000):** 80789 **Payroll Expense ($000):** 34255 **Personnel:** 880

PAW PAW—Van Buren County

★ **BRONSON LAKEVIEW HOSPITAL (231332)**, (Formerly LakeView Community Hospital), 408 Hazen Street, Zip 49079–0209, Mailing Address: P.O. Box 209, Zip 49079–0209; tel. 269/657–3141, (Total facility includes 120 beds in nursing home–type unit) **A**9 10 18 **F**3 11 15 25 26 30 33 38 43 46 54 56 57 61 62 63 66 72 73 75 77 79 80 81 82 84 86 88 90 91 92 93 94 96 102 107 117 119 121 124 135 136 137 **S** Bronson Healthcare Group, Inc.
Primary Contact: Frank J. Sardone, President and Chief Executive Officer
COO: Sally L. Berglin, Vice President, Bronson Lakeveiw Operations
CMO: Ravinder P. Mediratta, M.D., Chief of Staff
CHR: Jeff Johnson, Director Human Resources and Community Services
Web address: www.bronsonhealth.com/lakeview
Control: Hospital district or authority, Government, nonfederal **Service:** General Medical and Surgical

Staffed Beds: 155 **Admissions:** 1314 **Census:** 130 **Outpatient Visits:** 61649 **Births:** 0 **Total Expense ($000):** 40320 **Payroll Expense ($000):** 18861 **Personnel:** 455

PETOSKEY—Emmet County

☐ **NORTHERN MICHIGAN REGIONAL HOSPITAL (230105)**, (Formerly Northern Michigan Regional Health System), 416 Connable Avenue, Zip 49770–2297; tel. 231/487–4000 **A**1 2 9 10 19 20 **F**3 12 13 15 17 18 20 22 24 25 26 27 30 31 32 33 34 36 38 41 43 49 50 52 55 56 57 58 59 66 68 71 72 73 74 75 76 77 79 80 81 82 84 85 86 88 90 91 92 93 96 97 99 100 102 103 107 108 109 111 118 119 121 124 135 137
Primary Contact: Thomas C. Mroczkowski, President and Chief Executive Officer
COO: Reezie DeVet, R.N., Ph.D., Chief Operating Officer
CFO: Timothy Jodway, Chief Financial Officer
CMO: Andrew Smith, Chief Medical Officer
CIO: Mark Gray, Chief Information Officer
CHR: Eugene Kaminski, Vice President Human Resources Officer
Web address: www.northernhealth.org
Control: Other not–for–profit (including NFP Corporation) **Service:** General Medical and Surgical

Staffed Beds: 214 **Admissions:** 10739 **Census:** 123 **Outpatient Visits:** 111990 **Births:** 798 **Total Expense ($000):** 161295 **Payroll Expense ($000):** 61952 **Personnel:** 1284

PIGEON—Huron County

★ **SCHEURER HOSPITAL (231310)**, 170 North Caseville Road, Zip 48755–9704; tel. 989/453–3223, (Total facility includes 19 beds in nursing home–type unit) **A**1 9 10 18 **F**7 10 11 15 24 26 27 32 34 38 41 52 53 54 55 56 57 62 66 67 73 75 76 77 79 80 81 82 86 87 96 97 102 107 115 119 120 121 122 132 135 **P**6
Primary Contact: Dwight Gascho, President and Chief Executive Officer
CFO: Terry Lutz, Chief Financial Officer
CMO: Ali Khan, M.D., Chief of Staff
CIO: Suzanne LeMaire, Manager Health Information Management Services
CHR: Greg Foy, Human Resources System Leader
Web address: www.scheurer.org
Control: Other not–for–profit (including NFP Corporation) **Service:** General Medical and Surgical

Staffed Beds: 44 **Admissions:** 670 **Census:** 25 **Outpatient Visits:** 49650 **Births:** 0 **Total Expense ($000):** 27014 **Payroll Expense ($000):** 12890 **Personnel:** 294

PLAINWELL—Allegan County

☐ **BORGESS–PIPP HOSPITAL (232034)**, (Formerly Borgess–Pipp Health Center), 411 Naomi Street, Zip 49080–9911; tel. 269/685–6811, (Nonreporting) **A**1 9 10 **S** Ascension Health
Web address: www.borgess.com
Control: Other not–for–profit (including NFP Corporation) **Service:** Long–Term Acute Care hospital

Staffed Beds: 43

PONTIAC—Oakland County

☐ **NORTH OAKLAND MEDICAL CENTERS (230013)**, 461 West Huron Street, Zip 48341–1651; tel. 248/857–7200 **A**1 9 10 **F**3 11 15 17 18 25 26 30 31 32 33 34 36 37 38 39 41 49 50 53 54 55 56 57 60 62 63 64 66 68 72 73 75 76 77 79 80 81 82 85 86 87 88 90 91 92 93 96 97 99 100 106 107 109 112 113 114 119 121 123 132 133 135 136 137
Primary Contact: John R. Graham, President and Chief Executive Officer
CFO: Michael DeRubeis, Chief Financial Officer
CMO: Raouf Seifeldin, M.D., Chief of Staff
CIO: Chuck Laufle, Director Information Systems
Web address: www.nomc.org
Control: Other not–for–profit (including NFP Corporation) **Service:** General Medical and Surgical

Staffed Beds: 137 **Admissions:** 5575 **Census:** 91 **Outpatient Visits:** 75035 **Births:** 542 **Total Expense ($000):** 100454 **Payroll Expense ($000):** 49527 **Personnel:** 958

★ ○ **POH REGIONAL MEDICAL CENTER (230207)**, (Formerly POH Medical Center), 50 North Perry Street, Zip 48342–2253; tel. 248/338–5000, (Total facility includes 120 beds in nursing home–type unit) **A**9 10 11 12 13 **F**3 4 7 8 11 12 14 15 18 22 24 25 26 28 29 30 31 32 33 34 38 39 40 41 42 43 50 52 53 55 56 57 61 62 63 64 66 68 72 73 75 77 79 85 86 88 93 96 97 100 102 106 107 112 117 119 120 121 124 125 126 127 128 129 130 131 132 133 135 137 **P**4 8 **S** McLaren Health Care Corporation
Primary Contact: Patrick Lamberti, Chief Executive Officer
CFO: Thomas Schilling, Chief Financial Officer
CIO: Sharon Lucik, Senior Vice President Marketing and Public Relations
Web address: www.pohmedical.org
Control: Other not–for–profit (including NFP Corporation) **Service:** General Medical and Surgical

Staffed Beds: 268 **Admissions:** 6344 **Census:** 216 **Outpatient Visits:** 205645 **Births:** 0 **Total Expense ($000):** 120631 **Payroll Expense ($000):** 48634 **Personnel:** 1072

☐ **SELECT SPECIALTY HOSPITAL–PONTIAC (232030)**, 44405 Woodward Avenue, 8th Floor, Zip 48341, Mailing Address: 4405 Woodward Avenue, 8th Floor, Zip 48341; tel. 248/452–5206, (Nonreporting) **A**1 10 **S** Select Medical Corporation
Primary Contact: Peggy Kingston, Chief Executive Officer and Administrator
Control: Corporation, Investor–owned, for–profit **Service:** Long–Term Acute Care hospital

Staffed Beds: 32

★ **ST. JOSEPH MERCY OAKLAND (230029)**, 44405 Woodward Avenue, Zip 48341–2985; tel. 248/858–3000 **A**1 2 3 5 9 10 12 13 **F**3 8 11 12 13 15 17 18 20 22 24 25 26 27 28 30 31 32 33 34 36 37 38 40 41 43 44 46 49 50 51 53 55 56 57 58 62 63 64 66 68 70 72 73 74 75 76 77 79 80 81 82 84 85 86 87 88 92 93 95 96 97 98 99 100 102 103 104 105 106 107 112 114 118 119 120 121 124 133 134 135 136 137 **P**6 **S** Trinity Health
Primary Contact: Jack Weiner, President and Chief Executive Officer
COO: Barbara Hertzler, Chief Operating Officer
CFO: Michael Gusho, Chief Financial Officer
CMO: Donald Bignotti, M.D., Vice President Medical Affairs
CIO: Robert Jones, Director Management Information Systems
CHR: Martha Murphy, Vice President Human Resources
Web address: www.stjoesoakland.com
Control: Church–operated, Nongovernment, not–for profit **Service:** General Medical and Surgical

Staffed Beds: 403 **Admissions:** 21406 **Census:** 283 **Outpatient Visits:** 282188 **Births:** 2881 **Total Expense ($000):** 311399 **Payroll Expense ($000):** 128683 **Personnel:** 2198

Hospital, Medicare Provider Number, Address, Telephone, Approval, Facility, and Physician Codes, Health Care System

★ American Hospital Association (AHA) membership
☐ The Joint Commission accreditation
○ American Osteopathic Association (AOA) accreditation
△ Commission on Accreditation of Rehabilitation Facilities (CARF) accreditation

PORT HURON—St. Clair County

★ **MERCY HOSPITAL (230031)**, 2601 Electric Avenue, Zip 48060–6518; tel. 810/985–1500 **A**1 2 9 10 **F**3 11 15 18 25 26 27 30 31 32 33 38 40 43 44 49 50 53 55 57 58 60 62 64 66 68 72 73 75 76 77 79 80 81 82 84 85 86 96 97 102 104 105 106 107 109 111 119 120 121 135 136 137 **P**6 8
S Trinity Health
Primary Contact: Peter Karadjoff, President and Chief Executive Officer
CFO: Deborah Armstrong, Chief Financial Officer
CMO: Gail McIntyre, M.D., Vice President Medical Affairs
CIO: Cathy Geiger, Director Information Services
CHR: Robert Gunn, Vice President Human Resources
Web address: www.mercyporthuron.com
Control: Church–operated, Nongovernment, not–for profit **Service:** General Medical and Surgical

Staffed Beds: 119 **Admissions:** 4976 **Census:** 63 **Outpatient Visits:** 157749 **Births:** 0 **Total Expense ($000):** 82264 **Payroll Expense ($000):** 31259 **Personnel:** 716

★ **PORT HURON HOSPITAL (230216)**, 1221 Pine Grove Avenue, Zip 48061–5011; tel. 810/987–5000 **A**1 2 9 10 **F**2 3 5 11 12 13 15 17 18 20 22 25 26 27 28 30 31 32 33 34 37 38 40 41 43 44 46 48 49 50 51 53 54 55 56 57 58 60 62 63 66 68 70 72 73 74 76 77 79 80 81 82 84 86 87 88 89 90 91 92 93 94 95 96 97 102 103 104 105 106 107 118 119 120 121 123 124 133 135 136 137 **S** Blue Water Health Services Corporation
Primary Contact: Thomas D. DeFauw, FACHE, President and Chief Executive Officer
CFO: John Liston, Chief Financial Officer
CMO: Daniel Angeli, D.O., Vice President Medical Affairs
CIO: Dennis Belter, Director Information Systems
CHR: Dennis L. Hoover, Vice President Human Resources
Web address: www.porthuronhospital.org
Control: Other not–for–profit (including NFP Corporation) **Service:** General Medical and Surgical

Staffed Beds: 186 **Admissions:** 11222 **Census:** 128 **Outpatient Visits:** 165153 **Births:** 1448 **Total Expense ($000):** 131008 **Payroll Expense ($000):** 56732 **Personnel:** 1124

REED CITY—Osceola County

★ **SPECTRUM HEALTH REED CITY HOSPITAL (231323)**, (Formerly Spectrum Health–Reed City Campus), 300 North Patterson Road, Zip 49677–0075, Mailing Address: P.O. Box 75, Zip 49677–0075; tel. 231/832–3271, (Total facility includes 54 beds in nursing home–type unit) **A**1 9 10 18 **F**3 15 25 26 27 30 31 32 38 44 50 51 52 53 54 55 56 57 63 66 68 73 75 76 77 79 80 82 86 87 96 97 100 102 106 107 111 117 118 119 120 122 135 **P**6
S Spectrum Health
Primary Contact: Thomas D. Kaufman, President and Chief Executive Officer
COO: Linda Rubin, Chief Operating Officer
CFO: Thomas Knoerl, Chief Financial Officer
CMO: Marshall Wickens, M.D., Chief of Staff
CHR: Erika Duncan, Chief Human Resources Officer
Web address: www.reedcity.spectrum–health.org
Control: Other not–for–profit (including NFP Corporation) **Service:** General Medical and Surgical

Staffed Beds: 79 **Admissions:** 1093 **Census:** 59 **Outpatient Visits:** 96086 **Births:** 0 **Total Expense ($000):** 38311 **Payroll Expense ($000):** 15648 **Personnel:** 376

ROCHESTER—Oakland County

□ △ **CRITTENTON HOSPITAL MEDICAL CENTER (230254)**, 1101 West University Drive, Zip 48307–1831; tel. 248/652–5000 **A**1 2 7 9 10 **F**3 11 12 13 15 17 18 20 22 24 25 26 27 28 30 32 33 34 37 38 41 42 43 44 46 47 49 50 52 53 55 56 57 58 59 61 62 63 66 68 71 72 73 74 75 76 77 79 80 81 82 84 85 86 87 88 90 91 92 96 97 99 102 103 106 107 114 118 119 120 121 123 124 132 133 135 136 137
Primary Contact: Lynn C. Orfgen, President and Chief Executive Officer
COO: Gregory A. Partamian, Chief Operating Officer
CFO: Cynthia Long, Chief Financial Officer
CMO: Frank Sottile, M.D., Chief Medical Officer
CIO: Tom Ventameglia, Director Information Systems
Web address: www.crittenton.com
Control: Other not–for–profit (including NFP Corporation) **Service:** General Medical and Surgical

Staffed Beds: 256 **Admissions:** 11593 **Census:** 157 **Outpatient Visits:** 187251 **Births:** 994 **Total Expense ($000):** 173299 **Payroll Expense ($000):** 70694 **Personnel:** 1083

ROGERS CITY—Presque Isle County

□ △ **ROGERS CITY REHABILITATION HOSPITAL (233029)**, 555 North Bradley Highway, Suite C., Zip 49779–1599; tel. 989/734–7545 **A**1 7 9 10 **F**30 32 85 132 **P**5
Primary Contact: Bill Ostola, Executive Director
CFO: John Evans, Controller
CMO: Randall Bonfiglio, M.D., Medical Director
Web address: www.rogerscityrehab.com
Control: Individual, Investor–owned, for–profit **Service:** Rehabilitation

Staffed Beds: 15 **Admissions:** 230 **Census:** 8 **Outpatient Visits:** 0 **Births:** 0 **Total Expense ($000):** 4453 **Payroll Expense ($000):** 1639 **Personnel:** 37

ROMEO—Macomb County

ST. JOSEPH'S MERCY–NORTH See Henry Ford Macomb Hospital, Clinton Township

ROYAL OAK—Oakland County

★ **BEAUMONT HOSPITAL – ROYAL OAK (230130)**, 3601 West Thirteen Mile Road, Zip 48073–6769; tel. 248/898–5000 **A**1 2 3 5 8 9 10 **F**2 3 6 8 11 12 13 14 15 17 18 20 22 24 25 26 27 28 30 31 32 33 34 36 38 40 41 42 43 44 45 46 47 48 49 50 51 53 54 55 56 57 58 59 60 61 62 63 64 66 68 69 70 71 72 73 75 76 77 79 80 81 82 83 84 85 86 87 88 89 90 91 92 93 95 96 97 98 99 100 102 103 104 105 106 107 108 109 111 112 113 114 116 118 119 120 121 123 124 127 133 134 135 136 137 **P**6
S Beaumont Hospitals
Primary Contact: John D. Labriola, Senior Vice President and Director
COO: Eugene F. Michalski, Executive Vice President and Chief Operating Officer
CFO: Nickolas A. Vitale, Vice President Finance
CMO: Ananias C. Diokno, M.D., Executive Vice President and Chief Medical Officer
CIO: Paul Peabody, Vice President and Chief Information Officer
CHR: Ronald B. Lilek, Vice President Human Resources
Web address: www.beaumonthospitals.com
Control: Other not–for–profit (including NFP Corporation) **Service:** General Medical and Surgical

Staffed Beds: 1061 **Admissions:** 58212 **Census:** 862 **Outpatient Visits:** 1172580 **Births:** 6120 **Total Expense ($000):** 973917 **Payroll Expense ($000):** 515311 **Personnel:** 8147

SAGINAW—Saginaw County

★ **ALEDA E. LUTZ VETERANS AFFAIRS MEDICAL CENTER**, 1500 Weiss Street, Zip 48602–5298; tel. 989/497–2500 **A**1 9 **F**3 5 8 11 15 17 25 26 27 30 31 32 33 34 36 37 38 41 42 43 44 45 50 52 53 54 55 56 57 58 60 62 66 68 72 73 75 76 79 80 81 82 86 87 90 91 92 93 94 96 97 107 117 119 120 121 122 124 125 126 127 128 129 130 131 132 133 135 136 137 **P**6
S Department of Veterans Affairs
Primary Contact: Gabriel Perez, Medical Director
CFO: Angela Morris, Fiscal Officer
CIO: Stephanie Young, Acting Chief Information Technology
CHR: Shelly Pullen, Chief Human Resources Management Service
Web address: www.va.gov/sta/guide/home.asp
Control: Veterans Affairs, Government, federal **Service:** General Medical and Surgical

Staffed Beds: 114 **Admissions:** 1251 **Census:** 66 **Outpatient Visits:** 198567 **Births:** 0 **Total Expense ($000):** 95554 **Payroll Expense ($000):** 42443 **Personnel:** 827

★ ○ △ **COVENANT MEDICAL CENTER (230070)**, 1447 North Harrison Street, Zip 48602–4785; tel. 989/583–0000, (Includes COVENANT MEDICAL CENTER–COOPER, 700 Cooper Avenue, Zip 48602–5399; tel. 517/583–0000; COVENANT MEDICAL CENTER–HARRISON), (Total facility includes 20 beds in nursing home–type unit) **A**3 5 7 9 10 11 **F**3 8 11 13 15 17 18 20 22 24 25 26 27 30 31 32 33 34 38 39 42 43 44 45 47 48 49 50 53 55 57 58 59 60 61 62 63 68 70 72 73 74 75 76 77 79 81 82 83 84 85 86 87 96 97 100 101 102 103 105 106 107 110 117 118 119 120 121 124 132 133 135 136 137 **P**7 8
Primary Contact: Spencer Maidlow, President and Chief Executive Officer
COO: Edward Bruff, Executive Vice President and Chief Operating Officer
CFO: Mark E. Gronda, Vice President and Chief Financial Officer
CMO: John Kosanovich, M.D., Vice President Medical Affairs
CIO: Keith Grantham, Director Information Technology
CHR: Al Van Arsdal, Director Human Resources
Web address: www.covenanthealthcare.com
Control: Other not–for–profit (including NFP Corporation) **Service:** General Medical and Surgical

Staffed Beds: 521 **Admissions:** 26249 **Census:** 349 **Outpatient Visits:** 522929 **Total Expense ($000):** 388599 **Payroll Expense ($000):** 163906 **Personnel:** 3868

☐ △ **HEALTHSOURCE SAGINAW (230275)**, (LTC Rehabilitation Psychiatric Chemical Dependency), 3340 Hospital Road, Zip 48603, Mailing Address: P.O. Box 6280, Zip 48608–6280; tel. 989/790–7700, (Total facility includes 213 beds in nursing home–type unit) **A**1 7 9 10 **F**4 5 11 43 54 55 60 62 65 73 75 81 82 85 86 88 89 90 91 92 93 94 117 119 121 124 132 135 137 **P**6
Primary Contact: Lester Heyboer, Jr., President and Chief Executive Officer
COO: Richard Firebaugh, Executive Operations Officer
CFO: Jeffrey Engelsman, Chief Financial Officer
CMO: Daniel Duffy, D.O., Chief Medical Director
CHR: Katie Adams, Director Human Resources
Web address: www.healthsourcesaginaw.org
Control: Other not–for–profit (including NFP Corporation) **Service:** Other specialty

Staffed Beds: 319 **Admissions:** 2696 **Census:** 228 **Outpatient Visits:** 2047 **Births:** 0 **Total Expense ($000):** 34204 **Payroll Expense ($000):** 14564 **Personnel:** 423

☐ **SELECT SPECIALTY HOSPITAL–SAGINAW (232033)**, 1447 North Harrison Street, Zip 48602; tel. 989/583–4850, (Nonreporting) **A**1 10 **S** Select Medical Corporation
Primary Contact: Jonathan Cohee, Chief Executive Officer
Web address: www.selectmedicalcorp.com
Control: Corporation, Investor–owned, for–profit **Service:** Long–Term Acute Care hospital

Staffed Beds: 32

★☐ **ST. MARY'S OF MICHIGAN (230077)**, 800 South Washington Avenue, Zip 48601–2594; tel. 989/776–8000 **A**1 2 3 5 9 10 **F**2 3 8 11 15 17 18 20 22 24 25 26 27 30 31 32 33 34 38 39 41 42 49 50 51 53 55 56 57 58 62 66 68 72 73 75 76 77 79 80 81 82 86 87 90 92 96 97 99 100 102 103 105 106 107 108 109 111 112 116 118 119 121 132 133 135 136 137 **P**6 8 **S** Ascension Health
Primary Contact: Andrew W. Allen, Interim President and Chief Executive Officer
COO: Craig Carmichael, Vice President Operations
CFO: Gary W. Chawk, Chief Financial Officer
CIO: Karen Hollingsworth, Chief Information Officer
CHR: Jerry Chiplock, Vice President Human Resources
Web address: www.saintmarys–saginaw.org
Control: Church–operated, Nongovernment, not–for profit **Service:** General Medical and Surgical

Staffed Beds: 268 **Admissions:** 13455 **Census:** 191 **Outpatient Visits:** 176654 **Births:** 0 **Total Expense ($000):** 233301 **Payroll Expense ($000):** 90853 **Personnel:** 1818

SAINT IGNACE—Mackinac County

★ **MACKINAC STRAITS HOSPITAL AND HEALTH CENTER (231306)**, 220 Burdette Street, Zip 49781–1792; tel. 906/643–8585, (Total facility includes 75 beds in nursing home–type unit) **A**9 10 18 **F**11 15 27 28 30 31 32 38 39 53 59 62 63 75 76 81 86 87 96 102 107 117 119 121 122 132 135 136 **P**6
Primary Contact: Rodney M. Nelson, President and Chief Executive Officer
CFO: Jason Anderson, Chief Financial Officer
CMO: John Stephenson, M.D., Chief of Staff
CHR: Karen Cheeseman, Director Human Resources
Web address: www.mshosp.org
Control: Hospital district or authority, Government, nonfederal **Service:** General Medical and Surgical

Staffed Beds: 90 **Admissions:** 260 **Census:** 79 **Outpatient Visits:** 22774 **Births:** 0 **Total Expense ($000):** 17528 **Payroll Expense ($000):** 8077 **Personnel:** 183

SAINT JOHNS—Clinton County

★☐ **CLINTON MEMORIAL HOSPITAL (231326)**, 805 South Oakland Street, Zip 48879–0260; tel. 989/224–6881 **A**1 9 10 18 **F**8 11 15 27 30 33 38 52 55 56 57 68 73 75 76 77 79 80 86 96 100 102 107 118 119 120 122 135 **P**6 **S** Sparrow Health System
Primary Contact: Edward Bruun, President and Chief Executive Officer
COO: Kevin A. Price, Vice President and Chief Operating Officer
CFO: Janice Stitt, Controller
CMO: B. P. Rajesh, M.D., Chief of Staff
CIO: Jami Thering, Manager Information Systems
CHR: Jolene Jacobs, Director Human Resources
Web address: www.clintonmemorial.org
Control: Other not–for–profit (including NFP Corporation) **Service:** General Medical and Surgical

Staffed Beds: 25 **Admissions:** 753 **Census:** 7 **Outpatient Visits:** 52953 **Births:** 0 **Total Expense ($000):** 29122 **Payroll Expense ($000):** 10406 **Personnel:** 207

SAINT JOSEPH—Berrien County

★☐ **LAKELAND REGIONAL MEDICAL CENTER–ST. JOSEPH (230021)**, 1234 Napier Avenue, Zip 49085–2112; tel. 269/983–8300, (Includes LAKELAND COMMUNITY HOSPITAL–NILES, 31 North St. Joseph Avenue, Niles, Zip 49120–2287; tel. 269/683–5510), (Total facility includes 277 beds in nursing home–type unit) **A**1 2 9 10 19 **F**1 3 6 11 12 13 15 18 20 22 24 25 26 27 30 31 32 33 34 35 38 40 41 42 46 49 50 51 52 53 54 55 56 57 59 60 61 62 66 68 72 73 74 75 76 77 79 80 81 84 85 86 88 92 93 96 97 99 100 102 103 105 106 107 108 109 116 117 118 119 120 121 123 124 134 135 136 137 **P**8 **S** Lakeland Healthcare
Primary Contact: Joseph A. Wasserman, President and Chief Executive Officer
CFO: Timothy Calhoun, Vice President Finance and Chief Financial Officer
CMO: Dennis Thompson, M.D., President Medical Staff
CIO: Emily Gallay, Vice President and Chief Information Officer
Web address: www.lakelandhealth.org
Control: Other not–for–profit (including NFP Corporation) **Service:** General Medical and Surgical

Staffed Beds: 671 **Admissions:** 14818 **Census:** 440 **Outpatient Visits:** 323687 **Births:** 2020 **Total Expense ($000):** 271689 **Payroll Expense ($000):** 110575 **Personnel:** 2511

SALINE—Washtenaw County

★☐ **SAINT JOSEPH MERCY SALINE HOSPITAL (230212)**, 400 West Russell Street, Zip 48176–1101; tel. 734/429–1500 **A**1 9 10 **F**11 12 15 25 26 30 31 32 33 34 38 40 41 42 43 44 46 50 51 54 55 56 57 62 64 66 72 73 75 76 77 79 80 81 82 86 87 90 91 92 93 94 96 100 102 103 107 119 120 121 122 123 124 132 133 135 137 **S** Trinity Health
Primary Contact: Kathleen Rhine, Executive Director
COO: Julie MacDonald, R.N., Senior Vice President Patient Care Services and Chief Operating Officer
CFO: Barbara Fielder, Unit Financial Director
CMO: Rolland Mambourg, M.D., Vice President Physician Services
CIO: Joan Hurray, Regional Director Information Services
Web address: www.sjmercyhealth.org
Control: Church–operated, Nongovernment, not–for profit **Service:** General Medical and Surgical

Staffed Beds: 40 **Admissions:** 1239 **Census:** 11 **Outpatient Visits:** 89793 **Births:** 0 **Total Expense ($000):** 28960 **Payroll Expense ($000):** 10292 **Personnel:** 200

SANDUSKY—Sanilac County

MCKENZIE MEMORIAL HOSPITAL (231314), 120 Delaware Street, Zip 48471–1087; tel. 810/648–3770 **A**9 10 18 **F**5 7 15 24 25 31 32 38 54 55 56 62 74 77 79 80 81 82 86 92 96 97 102 106 107 119 122 124 135 **P**6
Primary Contact: Steve Barnett, Chief Executive Officer
COO: Janet Herbert, R.N., Chief Operating Officer
CFO: Ron Srebinski, Chief Financial Officer
Web address: www.mckenziehospital.org
Control: Other not–for–profit (including NFP Corporation) **Service:** General Medical and Surgical

Staffed Beds: 25 **Admissions:** 676 **Census:** 7 **Outpatient Visits:** 25142 **Births:** 114 **Total Expense ($000):** 15031 **Payroll Expense ($000):** 6633 **Personnel:** 181

SAULT STE. MARIE—Chippewa County

★☐ **WAR MEMORIAL HOSPITAL (230239)**, 500 Osborn Boulevard, Zip 49783–4467; tel. 906/635–4460, (Total facility includes 51 beds in nursing home–type unit) **A**1 9 10 20 **F**3 11 13 15 24 25 26 27 30 31 32 33 36 37 38 40 42 43 44 50 52 54 55 57 59 60 61 63 66 68 72 73 74 75 76 77 79 80 82 86 90 92 93 96 97 99 100 102 107 117 118 119 120 121 122 124 132 133 135 136 137
Primary Contact: David B. Jahn, President and Chief Executive Officer
COO: Susan Clow, R.N., Vice President Operations
CFO: Kevin Kalchik, Chief Financial Officer
CIO: Steve Pietrangelo, Director Information Services
CHR: Susan Sliger, Director Human Resources
Web address: www.warmemorialhospital.org
Control: Other not–for–profit (including NFP Corporation) **Service:** General Medical and Surgical

Staffed Beds: 98 **Admissions:** 2617 **Census:** 79 **Outpatient Visits:** 136659 **Births:** 306 **Total Expense ($000):** 59775 **Payroll Expense ($000):** 21847 **Personnel:** 535

MI

Hospital, Medicare Provider Number, Address, Telephone, Approval, Facility, and Physician Codes, Health Care System
★ American Hospital Association (AHA) membership
☐ The Joint Commission accreditation
○ American Osteopathic Association (AOA) accreditation
△ Commission on Accreditation of Rehabilitation Facilities (CARF) accreditation

SHELBY—Oceana County

☐ **HACKLEY LAKESHORE HOSPITAL (231320)**, 72 South State Street, Zip 49455–1299; tel. 231/861–2156, (Nonreporting) **A**1 9 10 18 **S** Hackley Health System
Primary Contact: Jay Bryan, Chief Executive Officer
CFO: Mark Gross, Chief Financial Officer
Web address: www.hackley.org
Control: Other not–for–profit (including NFP Corporation) **Service:** General Medical and Surgical

Staffed Beds: 24

SHERIDAN—Montcalm County

★ ○ **SHERIDAN COMMUNITY HOSPITAL (231312)**, 301 North Main Street, Zip 48884–9220, Mailing Address: P.O. Box 279, Zip 48884–0279; tel. 989/291–3261 **A**9 10 11 18 **F**3 11 15 28 30 31 32 33 38 42 46 55 56 57 62 75 77 79 80 81 82 86 87 96 99 102 107 118 120 121 122 124 133 135 136 137 **P**1
Primary Contact: Kevin Cawley, Chief Executive Officer
COO: Steve Scott, Chief Operating Officer
CMO: Darrell Cunningham, D.O., Chief of Staff
CIO: Jill Wills, Chief Information Officer
CHR: Charlene Cilibraise, Payroll Manager
Web address: www.sheridanhospital.com
Control: Other not–for–profit (including NFP Corporation) **Service:** General Medical and Surgical

Staffed Beds: 18 **Admissions:** 419 **Census:** 4 **Outpatient Visits:** 27711 **Births:** 0 **Total Expense ($000):** 13151 **Payroll Expense ($000):** 6355 **Personnel:** 140

SOUTH HAVEN—Van Buren County

⊠ **SOUTH HAVEN COMMUNITY HOSPITAL (230085)**, 955 South Bailey Avenue, Zip 49090–9797; tel. 269/637–5271 **A**1 9 10 **F**3 11 13 15 24 25 26 27 30 32 33 34 38 52 55 56 57 61 62 63 66 67 73 74 75 76 77 79 80 82 84 86 87 96 97 101 103 106 107 118 119 121 133 135 136 137 **P**4
Primary Contact: Joanne Urbanski, Interim President and Chief Executive Officer
CFO: Brian Long, Vice President and Chief Financial Officer
CIO: John Kirshman, Chief Information Officer
CHR: Charlene Wilson, Interim Director Human Resources
Web address: www.shch.org
Control: Hospital district or authority, Government, nonfederal **Service:** General Medical and Surgical

Staffed Beds: 33 **Admissions:** 1172 **Census:** 8 **Outpatient Visits:** 112421 **Births:** 458 **Total Expense ($000):** 31465 **Payroll Expense ($000):** 13004 **Personnel:** 312

SOUTHFIELD—Oakland County

○ **OAKLAND REGIONAL HOSPITAL (233028)**, 22401 Foster Winter Drive, Zip 48075–3708; tel. 248/423–5100, (Total facility includes 26 beds in nursing home–type unit) **A**9 10 11 **F**8 25 62 77 79 85 86 117
Primary Contact: Raji Kumar, Chief Executive Officer
COO: Andia Jones, Chief Operating Officer
CFO: Earl Romans, Chief Financial Officer
CMO: Robert Barbosa, D.O., Medical Officer
CIO: Daniel Bowen, Director Information Technology
CHR: Gordon Meyer, Director Human Resources
Web address: www.oaklandregionalhospital.com
Control: Corporation, Investor–owned, for–profit **Service:** Rehabilitation

Staffed Beds: 81 **Admissions:** 547 **Census:** 22 **Births:** 0

⊠ **PROVIDENCE HOSPITAL AND MEDICAL CENTER (230019)**, 16001 West Nine Mile Road, Zip 48075–4854, Mailing Address: Box 2043, Zip 48037–2043; tel. 248/424–3000 **A**1 2 3 5 9 10 12 13 **F**2 3 5 8 9 11 13 14 15 17 18 20 22 24 25 26 27 30 31 32 33 34 36 38 41 42 43 44 46 47 48 49 50 53 54 55 56 57 58 59 60 62 63 64 66 68 69 70 72 73 74 75 76 77 79 80 81 82 84 85 86 87 88 89 90 91 92 93 94 95 96 97 99 100 102 103 106 107 109 111 116 118 119 120 121 124 135 136 137 **P**1 6 **S** Ascension Health
Primary Contact: Michael Wiemann, M.D., Senior Vice President and Chief Medical Officer
CFO: William T. Crowe, Vice President Finance and Chief Financial Officer
CMO: Tammy Lundstrom, M.D., Chief Medical Officer
CHR: Therese Bologna, Director Human Resources
Web address: www.providence–stjohnhealth.org
Control: Church–operated, Nongovernment, not–for profit **Service:** General Medical and Surgical

Staffed Beds: 453 **Admissions:** 27102 **Census:** 366 **Outpatient Visits:** 575812 **Births:** 3501 **Total Expense ($000):** 485620 **Payroll Expense ($000):** 210062 **Personnel:** 3530

⊠ **STRAITH HOSPITAL FOR SPECIAL SURGERY (230071)**, 23901 Lahser Road, Zip 48034–3296; tel. 248/357–3360 **A**1 9 10 **F**25 30 77 79 85 119 131 137 **P**5
Primary Contact: Gregory R. Hoose, Chief Executive Officer
CFO: H. Roger Jones, Chief Financial Officer
Control: Other not–for–profit (including NFP Corporation) **Service:** General Medical and Surgical

Staffed Beds: 27 **Admissions:** 850 **Census:** 13 **Outpatient Visits:** 5460 **Births:** 0 **Total Expense ($000):** 13362 **Payroll Expense ($000):** 6074 **Personnel:** 142

STANDISH—Arenac County

⊠ **ST. MARY'S OF MICHIGAN STANDISH HOSPITAL (231305)**, 805 West Cedar Street, Zip 48658–9526; tel. 989/846–4521, (Total facility includes 43 beds in nursing home–type unit) **A**1 9 10 18 **F**3 11 15 17 24 25 26 30 32 33 38 54 55 56 57 62 63 73 75 79 81 82 86 96 97 100 102 106 107 117 119 121 122 135 **S** Ascension Health
Primary Contact: Sheri Leaman–Case, Administrator and Chief Executive Officer
CFO: Tony Doud, Controller
CMO: Rasheed Siddiqui, M.D., Chief of Staff
CIO: David Wanner, Director Information Systems
CHR: Renee Reetz, Director Human Resources
Web address: www.stmarysofmichigan.org/standish
Control: Other not–for–profit (including NFP Corporation) **Service:** General Medical and Surgical

Staffed Beds: 68 **Admissions:** 1002 **Census:** 43 **Outpatient Visits:** 46363 **Births:** 0 **Total Expense ($000):** 18584 **Payroll Expense ($000):** 9139 **Personnel:** 240

STURGIS—St. Joseph County

⊠ **STURGIS HOSPITAL (230096)**, 916 Myrtle, Zip 49091–2001; tel. 269/651–7824 **A**1 9 10 **F**3 11 13 15 24 25 26 27 30 31 32 33 38 42 46 49 50 55 56 57 61 62 63 66 68 72 73 74 75 76 77 79 80 82 84 86 87 92 96 97 103 106 107 118 119 120 121 135 136 137 **P**6 **S** QHR
Primary Contact: Robert J. LaBarge, Chief Executive Officer
CFO: Michael A. Barger, Associate Administrator Finance and Chief Financial Officer
CMO: Edward Griffin, M.D., Medical Staff President
CIO: Rita Denison, Information Systems Manager
CHR: Mary Kay Schultz, Director Human Resources
Web address: www.sturgishospital.com
Control: City–Government, nonfederal **Service:** General Medical and Surgical

Staffed Beds: 49 **Admissions:** 2194 **Census:** 18 **Outpatient Visits:** 100066 **Births:** 422 **Total Expense ($000):** 39667 **Payroll Expense ($000):** 15781 **Personnel:** 289

TAWAS CITY—Iosco County

⊠ **ST. JOSEPH HEALTH SYSTEM (230100)**, 200 Hemlock Street, Zip 48763–9360, Mailing Address: P.O. Box 659, Zip 48764–0659; tel. 989/362–3411, (Nonreporting) **A**1 9 10 20 **S** Ascension Health
Primary Contact: Patrick Murtha, President and Chief Executive Officer
CFO: Linda Stancill, Vice President and Chief Financial Officer
CHR: Georgette Alexander, Director Human Resources
Web address: www.sjhsys.org
Control: Other not–for–profit (including NFP Corporation) **Service:** General Medical and Surgical

Staffed Beds: 20

TAYLOR—Wayne County

⊠ **OAKWOOD HERITAGE HOSPITAL (230270)**, 10000 Telegraph Road, Zip 48180–3349; tel. 313/295–5000 **A**1 9 10 **F**3 11 15 25 26 30 31 32 35 36 37 38 41 42 43 44 46 49 50 54 55 57 59 60 62 63 66 68 72 73 76 77 78 79 80 81 82 85 86 88 90 92 93 94 95 96 97 100 103 106 107 119 121 135 137 **P**8 **S** Oakwood Healthcare, Inc.
Primary Contact: Michael Geheb, M.D., Division President
COO: Eric W. Widner, Chief Operating Officer
CFO: Jackie Porter, Controller
CMO: Vijay Khanna, M.D., Chief of Staff
CIO: Paula Smith, Chief Information Officer
CHR: Sherry Huffman, Administrator Human Resources
Web address: www.oakwood.org
Control: Other not–for–profit (including NFP Corporation) **Service:** General Medical and Surgical

Staffed Beds: 153 **Admissions:** 8804 **Census:** 149 **Outpatient Visits:** 50005 **Births:** 0 **Total Expense ($000):** 93467 **Payroll Expense ($000):** 40555 **Personnel:** 672

☐ **SELECT SPECIALTY HOSPITAL–DOWNRIVER (232031)**, (Formerly Select Specialty Hospital–Wyandotte), 10000 Telegraph Road, Zip 48180; tel. 313/375–7075, (Nonreporting) **A**1 10 **S** Select Medical Corporation
Primary Contact: Robert Padalino, Chief Executive Officer
CMO: Roderick Boyer, M.D., Medical Director
CHR: Barb Wiezbicir, Manager Human Resources
Web address: www.selectmedicalcorp.com
Control: Corporation, Investor–owned, for–profit **Service:** Long–Term Acute Care hospital

Staffed Beds: 32

SELECT SPECIALTY HOSPITAL–WYANDOTTE See Select Specialty Hospital–Downriver

TECUMSEH—Lenawee County

★ **HERRICK MEDICAL CENTER (231334)**, 500 East Pottawatamie Street, Zip 49286–2097; tel. 517/424–3000, (Total facility includes 25 beds in nursing home–type unit) **A**9 10 18 **F**3 5 8 10 11 13 15 24 25 26 31 32 33 36 38 52 55 56 57 61 62 63 66 68 72 73 74 75 77 79 80 82 86 87 88 89 90 91 92 93 94 96 97 102 106 107 113 117 119 120 121 133 135 136 137 **P**6 7 8 **S** ProMedica Health System
Primary Contact: Gregory Corbett, President
CFO: James F. Wheeler, Vice President Finance
CMO: Gordon Guild, D.O., Vice President Medical Affairs
CIO: Carol Boyce, Administrative Director Information Resources
CHR: Dennis Wright, Vice President Human Resources
Web address: www.promedica.org
Control: Other not–for–profit (including NFP Corporation) **Service:** General Medical and Surgical

Staffed Beds: 60 **Admissions:** 1931 **Census:** 43 **Outpatient Visits:** 52809 **Births:** 214 **Total Expense ($000):** 33595 **Payroll Expense ($000):** 11700 **Personnel:** 180

THREE RIVERS—St. Joseph County

⊠ △ **THREE RIVERS HEALTH (230015)**, 701 South Health Parkway, Zip 49093–9362; tel. 269/278–1145 **A**1 7 9 10 **F**3 11 13 15 24 25 27 28 30 31 32 33 38 42 50 52 56 57 61 62 63 64 66 68 73 74 75 76 77 79 80 81 82 84 85 86 87 90 96 97 100 103 106 107 118 119 121 122 124 133 136 **P**6 8 **S** QHR
Primary Contact: Matthew Chambers, President and Chief Executive Officer
COO: Laurie Herbert, Vice President Operations
CFO: Steve Andrews, Chief Financial Officer
CIO: Dave Parks, Chief Information Officer
Web address: www.threeriverhealth.org
Control: Hospital district or authority, Government, nonfederal **Service:** General Medical and Surgical

Staffed Beds: 60 **Admissions:** 1773 **Census:** 19 **Outpatient Visits:** 131892 **Births:** 370 **Total Expense ($000):** 47732 **Payroll Expense ($000):** 17594 **Personnel:** 437

TRAVERSE CITY—Grand Traverse County

⊠ △ **MUNSON MEDICAL CENTER (230097)**, 1105 Sixth Street, Zip 49684–2386; tel. 231/935–5000 **A**1 2 3 5 7 9 10 12 13 19 20 **F**3 5 6 11 12 13 14 15 18 20 22 24 25 26 27 28 30 31 32 33 34 36 38 40 41 42 43 44 46 48 49 50 51 52 53 54 55 56 57 58 59 60 61 62 63 66 68 69 70 72 73 74 75 76 77 79 80 81 82 85 86 87 88 90 91 92 93 94 95 96 97 100 102 106 107 108 109 111 114 118 119 120 121 123 130 131 132 133 135 136 137 **P**6 **S** Munson Healthcare
Primary Contact: Edwin Ness, President and Chief Executive Officer
CFO: Edward B. Carlson, Vice President and Chief Financial Officer
CMO: David S. McGreaham, M.D., Vice President Medical Affairs
CIO: Christopher J. Podges, Vice President and Chief Information Officer
CHR: Sue Peters, Vice President Human Resources
Web address: www.munsonhealthcare.org
Control: Other not–for–profit (including NFP Corporation) **Service:** General Medical and Surgical

Staffed Beds: 391 **Admissions:** 20632 **Census:** 263 **Outpatient Visits:** 439703 **Births:** 2013 **Total Expense ($000):** 324439 **Payroll Expense ($000):** 136455 **Personnel:** 3111

TRENTON—Wayne County

⊠ ○ **OAKWOOD SOUTHSHORE MEDICAL CENTER (230176)**, 5450 Fort Street, Zip 48183–4625; tel. 734/671–3800 **A**1 9 10 11 12 13 **F**3 8 11 13 15 17 18 24 25 26 27 30 31 32 33 37 38 42 43 44 46 49 50 54 55 56 57 58 59 60 62 63 66 68 72 73 74 76 77 78 79 80 81 82 86 96 97 99 100 103 104 105 106 107 119 135 137 **P**8 **S** Oakwood Healthcare, Inc.
Primary Contact: Edith M. Hughes, Division President
COO: J. Joseph Diederich, Executive Vice President and Chief Operating Officer
CFO: Patricia Vannoy, Controller
CMO: Iqbal Nasir, M.D., Chief of Staff
CIO: Paula Smith, Vice President Information Services and Chief Information Officer
CHR: Juliet Hafford, Director Human Resources
Web address: www.oakwood.org
Control: Other not–for–profit (including NFP Corporation) **Service:** General Medical and Surgical

Staffed Beds: 129 **Admissions:** 6465 **Census:** 78 **Outpatient Visits:** 55299 **Births:** 648 **Total Expense ($000):** 87079 **Payroll Expense ($000):** 37958 **Personnel:** 698

TROY—Oakland County

⊠ **BEAUMONT HOSPITAL – TROY (230269)**, 44201 Dequindre Road, Zip 48085; tel. 248/964–5000 **A**1 2 9 10 **F**3 6 8 11 12 13 15 17 18 20 22 24 25 26 27 28 30 31 32 33 34 36 38 40 41 42 43 44 45 46 47 49 50 51 53 54 55 56 57 58 59 60 61 62 63 64 66 68 69 71 72 73 74 75 76 77 79 80 81 82 84 86 87 90 92 96 97 98 99 100 102 103 106 107 108 109 111 116 118 119 120 121 123 124 133 134 135 136 137 **P**6 **S** Beaumont Hospitals
Primary Contact: Thomas Brisse, Senior Vice President and Hospital Director
COO: Heidi Shepard, Vice President Operations
CFO: Mark Leonard, Controller
CMO: Roger Howard, M.D., Senior Vice President and Medical Director
CIO: Paul Peabody, Vice President and Chief Information Officer
CHR: Ronald B. Lilek, Vice President Human Resources
Web address: www.beaumonthospitals.com
Control: Other not–for–profit (including NFP Corporation) **Service:** General Medical and Surgical

Staffed Beds: 346 **Admissions:** 25254 **Census:** 284 **Outpatient Visits:** 558121 **Births:** 3382 **Total Expense ($000):** 387222 **Payroll Expense ($000):** 162420 **Personnel:** 2809

WARREN—Macomb County

★ **BEHAVIORAL CENTER OF MICHIGAN (234039)**, 4050 East 12 Mile Road, Zip 48092; tel. 586/261–2266, (Nonreporting) **A**10
Primary Contact: Ryan Gunabalan, Chief Executive Officer
COO: John Knisely, Director Nursing and Clinical
CFO: Dave Satawa, Controller
CMO: Eleanor Medina, M.D., Chief Medical Officer and Psychiatric
CIO: Karen Apsey, Chief Information Officer and Director Information Health
CHR: Sharon Upshaw, Chief Human Resources Officer
Web address: www.behavioralcenter.com
Control: Corporation, Investor–owned, for–profit **Service:** Psychiatric

Staffed Beds: 42

★ ○ △ **HENRY FORD MACOMB HOSPITAL–WARREN CAMPUS (230204)**, (Formerly Henry Ford Bi–County Hospital), 13355 East Ten Mile Road, Zip 48089–2065; tel. 586/759–7300 **A**7 9 10 11 12 13 **F**3 12 15 24 25 26 27 30 31 32 33 34 38 42 44 47 49 51 52 55 56 57 58 60 62 63 67 68 72 73 75 76 77 79 80 81 82 85 86 96 97 99 100 106 107 113 118 119 120 121 124 132 135 136 137 **P**5 **S** Henry Ford Health System
Primary Contact: Barbara Rossmann, President and Chief Executive Officer
COO: Margaret Dimond, Chief Operating Officer
CMO: Gary L. Moorman, M.D., Chief Medical Officer
Web address: www.bicountyhospital.org
Control: Other not–for–profit (including NFP Corporation) **Service:** General Medical and Surgical

Staffed Beds: 137 **Admissions:** 6017 **Census:** 91 **Outpatient Visits:** 97499 **Births:** 0 **Total Expense ($000):** 97525 **Payroll Expense ($000):** 45163 **Personnel:** 810

☐ **SOUTHEAST MICHIGAN SURGICAL HOSPITAL (230264)**, 21230 Dequindre, Zip 48091–2287; tel. 586/427–1000 **A**1 9 10 **F**25 33 43 56 57 58 59 62 63 73 77 79 107 137 **P**2 **S** National Surgical Hospitals
Primary Contact: John Kolozsvary, Chief Executive Officer
CMO: Benjamin Paolucci, D.O., Chief of Staff
CHR: Dawn Meiers, Coordinator Medical Staff and Personnel Services
Web address: www.nshinc.com
Control: Partnership, Investor–owned, for–profit **Service:** General Medical and Surgical

Staffed Beds: 13 **Admissions:** 202 **Census:** 1 **Outpatient Visits:** 2060 **Births:** 0 **Total Expense ($000):** 9841 **Payroll Expense ($000):** 3474 **Personnel:** 63

MI

Hospital, Medicare Provider Number, Address, Telephone, Approval, Facility, and Physician Codes, Health Care System

★ American Hospital Association (AHA) membership
☐ The Joint Commission accreditation
○ American Osteopathic Association (AOA) accreditation
△ Commission on Accreditation of Rehabilitation Facilities (CARF) accreditation

☒ **ST. JOHN MACOMB HOSPITAL (230195)**, (Formerly St John Macomb Hospital), 11800 East Twelve Mile Road, Zip 48093–3494; tel. 586/573–5000 **A**1 2 9 10 **F**3 11 13 15 18 20 22 24 25 26 27 30 31 32 33 34 36 37 38 40 41 42 43 44 46 48 49 50 55 56 57 59 61 62 66 68 69 72 73 74 75 76 77 78 79 80 81 82 85 86 87 88 90 91 92 93 94 95 96 97 100 102 103 104 105 106 107 109 111 119 120 121 122 124 132 133 135 136 137 **P**6 8 **S** Ascension Health
Primary Contact: Patricia A. Maryland, Dr.P.h., President and Chief Executive Officer
COO: Michael Beaubien, Chief Operating Officer
CFO: Randolph H. Kummler, Vice President Finance
CMO: Roberto Barretto, M.D., Vice President Medical Affairs
CIO: Mary Kay LaChance, Director Information Systems
CHR: Sue Gronbach, Director Worklife Services
Web address: www.stjohn.org
Control: Church–operated, Nongovernment, not–for profit **Service:** General Medical and Surgical

Staffed Beds: 353 **Admissions:** 19995 **Census:** 285 **Outpatient Visits:** 210556 **Births:** 1278 **Total Expense ($000):** 236763 **Payroll Expense ($000):** 110240 **Personnel:** 1912

WATERVLIET—Berrien County

☒ △ **COMMUNITY HOSPITAL (230078)**, 400 Medical Park Drive, Zip 49098–9225; tel. 269/463–3111 **A**1 7 9 10 **F**3 11 15 25 26 31 32 33 35 36 38 50 53 55 56 57 66 68 69 73 75 77 79 80 81 82 85 86 96 107 119 121 124 133 135 **P**6 8 **S** QHR
Primary Contact: Ray Cruse, Interim Chief Executive Officer
CFO: Thomas Bedeck, Chief Financial Officer
CIO: Bill Roberts, Information Systems Director
CHR: Kevin Kalinowski, Director Human Resources
Web address: www.communityhospitalwatervliet.com
Control: Other not–for–profit (including NFP Corporation) **Service:** General Medical and Surgical

Staffed Beds: 46 **Admissions:** 1221 **Census:** 14 **Outpatient Visits:** 51168 **Births:** 0 **Total Expense ($000):** 26649 **Payroll Expense ($000):** 11115 **Personnel:** 234

WAYNE—Wayne County

☒ **OAKWOOD ANNAPOLIS HOSPITAL (230142)**, 33155 Annapolis Avenue, Zip 48184–2493; tel. 734/467–4000 **A**1 9 10 **F**3 11 13 15 18 20 24 25 26 27 30 31 32 33 36 37 38 41 42 43 44 46 49 50 54 55 57 58 59 60 62 63 66 68 72 73 74 76 77 78 79 80 81 82 86 90 96 97 100 102 103 104 105 106 107 119 121 132 135 136 137 **P**8 **S** Oakwood Healthcare, Inc.
Primary Contact: Kathleen Cronin, RN, Interim President
Web address: www.oakwood.org
Control: Other not–for–profit (including NFP Corporation) **Service:** General Medical and Surgical

Staffed Beds: 193 **Admissions:** 9933 **Census:** 119 **Outpatient Visits:** 74551 **Births:** 814 **Total Expense ($000):** 114981 **Payroll Expense ($000):** 50743 **Personnel:** 774

WEST BLOOMFIELD—Oakland County

☒ **HENRY FORD WEST BLOOMFIELD HOSPITAL**, 6777 West Maple Road, Zip 48322; tel. 248/661–4100, (Nonreporting) **A**1 9 **S** Henry Ford Health System
Primary Contact: Gerard van Grinsven, President and Chief Executive Officer
COO: Christine Zambrini, Chief Operating Officer and Chief Nursing Officer
Web address: www.henryford.com
Control: Partnership, Investor–owned, for–profit **Service:** General Medical and Surgical

Staffed Beds: 300

WEST BRANCH—Ogemaw County

☒ **WEST BRANCH REGIONAL MEDICAL CENTER (230095)**, 2463 South M–30, Zip 48661–1199; tel. 989/345–3660 **A**1 9 10 20 **F**11 13 15 17 18 24 26 31 32 38 42 43 44 50 55 56 57 62 73 74 77 79 86 96 100 102 105 106 107 119
Primary Contact: Douglas E. Pattullo, Chief Executive Officer
COO: Edward A. Napierala, Chief Operating Officer
CFO: Robert McGrail, Chief Financial Officer
CMO: Michael Beasley, M.D., President Medical Staff
CIO: Randy Lewis, Director Information Technology
CHR: Janet Norton, Manager Human Resources
Web address: www.wbrmc.com
Control: City–Government, nonfederal **Service:** General Medical and Surgical

Staffed Beds: 88 **Admissions:** 3051 **Census:** 35 **Outpatient Visits:** 84830 **Births:** 326 **Total Expense ($000):** 36258 **Payroll Expense ($000):** 13479 **Personnel:** 348

WESTLAND—Wayne County

☐ **WALTER P. REUTHER PSYCHIATRIC HOSPITAL (234035)**, 30901 Palmer Road, Zip 48186–5389; tel. 734/367–8400 **A**1 9 10 **F**30 31 32 54 73 75 81 82 88 90 91 93 119 124 135 **P**5
Primary Contact: Ron Denstedt, Acting Director
CMO: Venkata Lingam, M.D., Chief Clinical Affairs
CHR: Gerald Gibson, Director Human Resources
Control: State–Government, nonfederal **Service:** Psychiatric

Staffed Beds: 244 **Admissions:** 238 **Census:** 221 **Outpatient Visits:** 0 **Births:** 0 **Total Expense ($000):** 40525 **Payroll Expense ($000):** 22613 **Personnel:** 402

WYANDOTTE—Wayne County

☒ ○ △ **HENRY FORD WYANDOTTE HOSPITAL (230146)**, 2333 Biddle Avenue, Zip 48192–4693; tel. 734/246–6000 **A**1 7 9 10 11 12 13 **F**2 3 5 11 12 13 15 17 18 24 26 27 33 36 38 39 42 43 44 46 47 49 50 51 53 55 56 57 58 59 62 63 64 66 67 68 72 73 74 75 76 77 79 80 82 84 85 86 88 90 91 92 93 96 97 100 102 104 105 106 107 116 118 119 120 121 124 135 137 **P**6 **S** Henry Ford Health System
Primary Contact: James J. Sexton, FACHE, President and Chief Executive Officer
CFO: James J. Miller, Vice President and Chief Financial Officer
CMO: Mohammed Al–Ansari, M.D., Medical Staff President
CIO: Arthur K. Gross, FACHE, Executive Vice President and Chief Information Officer
CHR: Aline Lafferty, Vice President Human Resources
Web address: www.henryfordhealth.org
Control: Other not–for–profit (including NFP Corporation) **Service:** General Medical and Surgical

Staffed Beds: 344 **Admissions:** 18965 **Census:** 264 **Outpatient Visits:** 254387 **Births:** 1796 **Total Expense ($000):** 235748 **Payroll Expense ($000):** 105406 **Personnel:** 2063

WYOMING—Kent County

★ ○ **METRO HEALTH HOSPITAL (230236)**, 5900 Byron Center Avenue S.W., Zip 49519–0916, Mailing Address: P.O. Box 916, Zip 49519–0916; tel. 616/252–7200 **A**9 10 11 12 13 **F**3 12 13 15 18 20 22 23 24 25 26 30 31 32 33 34 38 41 43 46 50 51 53 55 57 58 62 63 66 68 69 72 73 74 75 77 79 81 84 85 86 87 96 97 100 102 105 106 107 118 119 120 121 124 135 137 **P**6 7 8
Primary Contact: Michael D. Faas, President and Chief Executive Officer
COO: Daniel L. Holwerda, Chief Operating Officer
CFO: Robert Smedes, Chief Financial Officer
CMO: William Cunningham, D.O., Chief Medical Officer
CIO: William Lewkowski, Vice President Information Services and Chief Information Officer
CHR: Sandy Sefton, Chief People Officer
Web address: www.metrohealth.net
Control: Other not–for–profit (including NFP Corporation) **Service:** General Medical and Surgical

Staffed Beds: 198 **Admissions:** 7995 **Census:** 114 **Outpatient Visits:** 294449 **Births:** 1513 **Total Expense ($000):** 167555 **Payroll Expense ($000):** 65983 **Personnel:** 1422

YPSILANTI—Washtenaw County

☐ **FOREST HEALTH MEDICAL CENTER (230144)**, 135 South Prospect Street, Zip 48198–7914; tel. 734/547–4700 **A**1 9 10 **F**12 26 46 62 73 79 80 107 119 121
Primary Contact: Trevor J. Dykstehouse, President
COO: Trevor J. Dykstehouse, President
CMO: Steven Poplawski, M.D., FACS, Medical Director
CHR: Karen Pinto, Coordinator Human Resources
Web address: www.barixclinics.com
Control: Corporation, Investor–owned, for–profit **Service:** General Medical and Surgical

Staffed Beds: 24 **Admissions:** 1367 **Census:** 6 **Outpatient Visits:** 1482 **Births:** 0 **Personnel:** 58

☐ **SELECT SPECIALTY HOSPITAL–ANN ARBOR (232024)**, 5301 East Huron River Drive, 5th Floor, Zip 48197; tel. 734/712–0103, (Nonreporting) **A**1 10 **S** Select Medical Corporation
Primary Contact: Carol Littleton, Chief Executive Officer
Control: Corporation, Investor–owned, for–profit **Service:** Long–Term Acute Care hospital

Staffed Beds: 36

★ **ST. JOSEPH MERCY HOSPITAL (230156)**, 5301 McAuley Drive, Zip 48197, Mailing Address: P.O. Box 995, Ann Arbor, Zip 48106–0995; tel. 734/712–3456 **A**2 8 9 10 **F**3 5 6 8 9 11 12 13 15 17 18 20 22 24 25 26 27 28 29 30 31 32 33 34 35 36 37 38 40 41 42 43 44 46 50 51 52 53 54 55 56 57 58 59 60 61 62 63 64 66 68 69 70 71 72 73 74 75 76 77 79 80 81 82 84 85 86 87 88 89 90 91 92 93 94 95 96 97 98 99 100 102 103 104 105 106 107 108 109 111 115 116 118 119 120 121 122 123 124 132 133 134 135 136 137 **P**1 5 **S** Trinity Health
Primary Contact: Garry C. Faja, President and Chief Executive Officer
CFO: Chuck Hoffman, Chief Financial Officer
CMO: Rolland Mambourg, M.D., Vice President Physician Services
CIO: Joan Hurray, Regional Director Information Services
CHR: Kathleen Rhine, Vice President Administrative Services and Chief Operating Officer
Web address: www.sjmercyhealth.org
Control: Church–operated, Nongovernment, not–for profit **Service:** General Medical and Surgical

Staffed Beds: 529 **Admissions:** 32416 **Census:** 421 **Outpatient Visits:** 902630 **Births:** 3919 **Total Expense ($000):** 561148 **Payroll Expense ($000):** 210621 **Personnel:** 4585

ZEELAND—Ottawa County

★☐ **ZEELAND COMMUNITY HOSPITAL (230003)**, 8333 Felch Street, Zip 49464–1619; tel. 616/772–4644 **A**1 9 10 **F**3 13 15 25 30 31 32 33 38 42 45 46 57 62 66 67 68 73 74 77 79 80 86 87 96 102 107 119 121 124 135 **P**4 8
Primary Contact: Henry A. Veenstra, President
CFO: George Smart, Vice President Finance and System Services
CMO: Dale Terpstra, D.O., Medical Director
CIO: Gil Lalo, Information Systems Manager
CHR: Robert W. Dean, Vice President Human Resources and Community Relations
Web address: www.zch.org
Control: Other not–for–profit (including NFP Corporation) **Service:** General Medical and Surgical

Staffed Beds: 52 **Admissions:** 2248 **Census:** 21 **Outpatient Visits:** 69895 **Births:** 521 **Total Expense ($000):** 43524 **Payroll Expense ($000):** 20469 **Personnel:** 422

MI

Hospital, Medicare Provider Number, Address, Telephone, Approval, Facility, and Physician Codes, Health Care System

★ American Hospital Association (AHA) membership
☐ The Joint Commission accreditation
○ American Osteopathic Association (AOA) accreditation
△ Commission on Accreditation of Rehabilitation Facilities (CARF) accreditation

MINNESOTA

ADA—Norman County

★ **BRIDGES MEDICAL CENTER (241313)**, (Formerly Bridges Medical Services), 201 9th Street West, Zip 56510–1243; tel. 218/784–5000, (Nonreporting) **A**9 10 18 **S** Essentia Health
Primary Contact: Dan Rohrbach, Chief Executive Officer
CFO: Ryan Hill, Chief Financial Officer
CMO: Jeff Peterson, M.D., Chief of Staff
CHR: Shaun Crowell, Director Human Resources
Web address: www.bridgesmed.com
Control: City–Government, nonfederal **Service:** General Medical and Surgical

Staffed Beds: 14

AITKIN—Aitkin County

★ **RIVERWOOD HEALTHCARE CENTER (241305)**, 200 Bunker Hill Drive, Zip 56431–1844; tel. 218/927–2121 **A**9 10 18 **F**3 8 11 13 15 24 25 27 28 30 31 32 33 38 40 43 46 53 54 55 56 57 62 63 68 73 74 75 76 77 79 81 82 86 87 96 99 102 107 118 119 120 121 122 124 133 135 136 137 **P**6
Primary Contact: Michael Hagen, Chief Executive Officer
COO: Michael Delfs, Chief Operating Officer
CFO: James West, Chief Financial Officer
CMO: Mark Heggem, M.D., Medical Director
CHR: Teresa Jacobson, Director Human Resources
Web address: www.riverwoodhealthcare.com
Control: Other not–for–profit (including NFP Corporation) **Service:** General Medical and Surgical

Staffed Beds: 24 **Admissions:** 1359 **Census:** 13 **Outpatient Visits:** 65675 **Births:** 79 **Total Expense ($000):** 36131 **Payroll Expense ($000):** 15180 **Personnel:** 241

MN

ALBANY—Stearns County

★ **ALBANY AREA HOSPITAL AND MEDICAL CENTER (241331)**, 300 Third Avenue, Zip 56307–9363; tel. 320/845–2121 **A**9 10 18 **F**13 14 15 26 31 32 33 38 42 50 57 61 62 74 75 79 86 96 102 107 119 122 135 **P**6 **S** Catholic Health Initiatives
Primary Contact: Nicholas R. Brandner, Administrator
CFO: Stephen Plaisance, Vice President Finance
CMO: Heather Swanson, M.D., Chief of Staff
Web address: www.albanyareahospital.com
Control: Church–operated, Nongovernment, not–for profit **Service:** General Medical and Surgical

Staffed Beds: 17 **Admissions:** 315 **Census:** 2 **Outpatient Visits:** 10867 **Births:** 61 **Total Expense ($000):** 8680 **Payroll Expense ($000):** 3464 **Personnel:** 102

ALBERT LEA—Freeborn County

□ △ **ALBERT LEA MEDICAL CENTER (240043)**, 404 West Fountain Street, Zip 56007–2473; tel. 507/373–2384, (Total facility includes 61 beds in nursing home–type unit) (Nonreporting) **A**1 5 7 9 10 **S** Mayo Foundation
Primary Contact: Mark Ciota, M.D., Chief Executive Officer
CFO: Dave Pilot, Chief Financial Officer
CMO: John Grzybowski, M.D., Medical Director
CIO: Daryl Kallevig, Information Technology Director
CHR: Monica Fleegel, Director Human Resources
Web address: www.almedcenter.org
Control: Other not–for–profit (including NFP Corporation) **Service:** General Medical and Surgical

Staffed Beds: 129

ALEXANDRIA—Douglas County

□ **COMMUNITY BEHAVIORAL HEALTH HOSPITAL – ALEXANDRIA**, 1610 8th Avenue East, Zip 55308; tel. 320/335–6201, (Nonreporting) **A**1 **S** Minnesota Deparment of Human Services
Primary Contact: John A. Cosco, Ph.D., FACHE, Administrator
Web address: www.health.state.mn.us
Control: State–Government, nonfederal **Service:** Psychiatric

Staffed Beds: 16

★ ○ **DOUGLAS COUNTY HOSPITAL (240030)**, 111 17th Avenue East, Zip 56308–3798; tel. 320/762–1511 **A**9 10 11 19 20 **F**3 8 11 13 15 24 26 27 30 31 34 38 40 55 56 60 61 62 66 67 68 74 75 76 77 79 80 81 84 86 90 91 92 94 96 97 100 102 105 107 118 119 120 121 124 135
Primary Contact: William G. Flaig, Administrator
Web address: www.dchospital.com
Control: County–Government, nonfederal **Service:** General Medical and Surgical

Staffed Beds: 99 **Admissions:** 4859 **Census:** 47 **Outpatient Visits:** 49211 **Births:** 660 **Total Expense ($000):** 63673 **Payroll Expense ($000):** 24346 **Personnel:** 435

ANOKA—Anoka County

□ **ANOKA–METROPOLITAN REGIONAL TREATMENT CENTER (244002)**, 3301 Seventh Avenue, Zip 55303–1119; tel. 763/712–4000, (Nonreporting) **A**1 10 **S** Minnesota Deparment of Human Services
Primary Contact: David Hartford, Administrator
Web address: www.health.state.mn.us
Control: State–Government, nonfederal **Service:** Psychiatric

Staffed Beds: 227

APPLETON—Swift County

★ **APPLETON MUNICIPAL HOSPITAL AND NURSING HOME (241341)**, 30 South Behl Street, Zip 56208–1699; tel. 320/289–2422, (Total facility includes 84 beds in nursing home–type unit) (Nonreporting) **A**9 10 18
Primary Contact: Daniel J. Swenson, Chief Executive Officer and Administrator
CFO: Mike DeFoe, Chief Financial Officer
Web address: www.appletonareahealth.com
Control: City–Government, nonfederal **Service:** General Medical and Surgical

Staffed Beds: 99

ARLINGTON—Sibley County

★ **SIBLEY MEDICAL CENTER (241311)**, 601 West Chandler Street, Zip 55307–4500; tel. 507/964–2271 **A**9 10 18 **F**11 15 17 24 25 27 31 33 38 55 56 57 61 62 67 75 79 81 82 86 87 96 107 117 119 122 **P**6
Primary Contact: Rhonda Matz, Chief Executive Officer
CFO: Darla Anderson, Chief Financial Officer
CMO: Dean Bergersen, M.D., Chief Medical Officer
CIO: Chris Bulau, Director Information Technology
CHR: Ashleigh Rose, Director Human Resources
Web address: www.sibleymedical.org
Control: City–Government, nonfederal **Service:** General Medical and Surgical

Staffed Beds: 17 **Admissions:** 282 **Census:** 4 **Outpatient Visits:** 6425 **Births:** 0 **Total Expense ($000):** 9270 **Payroll Expense ($000):** 3954 **Personnel:** 93

AURORA—St. Louis County

★ **WHITE COMMUNITY HOSPITAL (241340)**, 5211 Highway 110, Zip 55705–1599; tel. 218/229–2211, (Total facility includes 69 beds in nursing home–type unit) (Nonreporting) **A**9 10 18
Primary Contact: James J. Carroll, Administrator and Chief Executive Officer
CFO: Paula Schaefbauer, Chief Financial Officer
Web address: www.whitech.org
Control: Other not–for–profit (including NFP Corporation) **Service:** General Medical and Surgical

Staffed Beds: 84

AUSTIN—Mower County

□ **AUSTIN MEDICAL CENTER (240117)**, 1000 First Drive N.W., Zip 55912–2904; tel. 507/437–4551 **A**1 5 9 10 **F**3 4 5 11 13 15 24 27 32 38 42 43 56 57 61 62 63 64 66 67 68 74 75 77 79 80 81 82 84 85 86 87 88 89 90 91 92 93 94 96 97 98 100 103 106 107 117 118 119 120 121 122 124 133 134 135 **S** Mayo Foundation
Primary Contact: Timothy Johnson, M.D., President and Chief Executive Officer
Web address: www.austinmedicalcenter.org
Control: Other not–for–profit (including NFP Corporation) **Service:** General Medical and Surgical

Staffed Beds: 82 **Admissions:** 3665 **Census:** 38 **Outpatient Visits:** 293842 **Births:** 459 **Total Expense ($000):** 85916 **Payroll Expense ($000):** 46418

BAGLEY—Clearwater County

★ **CLEARWATER HEALTH SERVICES (241328)**, 203 Fourth Street N.W., Zip 56621–8307; tel. 218/694–6501, (Total facility includes 70 beds in nursing home–type unit) (Nonreporting) **A**9 10 18 **S** MeritCare Health System
Primary Contact: Bonnie Anderson, Interim Chief Executive Officer
CFO: Rachel Rosenbush, Account Manager
CMO: Rudd Thabes, M.D., Chief Medical Staff
CHR: John Nelson, Chairman
Web address: www.clearwaterhs.com
Control: County–Government, nonfederal **Service:** General Medical and Surgical

Staffed Beds: 95

 Many Facility Codes have changed. Please refer to the AHA Guide Code Chart.

BAUDETTE—Lake of the Woods County

★ **LAKEWOOD HEALTH CENTER (241301)**, 600 Main Avenue South, Zip 56623–2855; tel. 218/634–2120, (Total facility includes 46 beds in nursing home–type unit) **A**9 10 18 **F**7 10 13 15 26 27 31 32 33 38 42 52 55 56 57 61 63 74 79 80 86 96 100 107 117 119 124 137 **P**6 **S** Catholic Health Initiatives
Primary Contact: SharRay Feickert, President and Chief Executive Officer
CFO: Lynn Ellis, Chief Financial Officer
Web address: www.lakewoodhealthcenter.org
Control: Church–operated, Nongovernment, not–for profit **Service:** General Medical and Surgical

Staffed Beds: 61 **Admissions:** 279 **Census:** 48 **Outpatient Visits:** 16927 **Births:** 25 **Total Expense ($000):** 12650 **Payroll Expense ($000):** 5720 **Personnel:** 130

BEMIDJI—Beltrami County

★ **NORTH COUNTRY REGIONAL HOSPITAL (240100)**, 1300 Anne Street N.W., Zip 56601; tel. 218/751–5430, (Total facility includes 78 beds in nursing home–type unit) **A**9 10 19 20 **F**3 10 11 13 15 24 25 26 30 31 32 33 38 42 43 50 52 56 57 61 62 68 73 74 75 77 79 80 81 82 85 86 93 96 97 99 100 102 107 115 117 118 119 121 124 135 137 **P**6
Primary Contact: James F. Hanko, President and Chief Executive Officer
CFO: Craig Boyer, Vice President
CMO: Maria Statton, M.D., President Medical Staff
CHR: Robert Verchota, Vice President Ancillary Service and Human Resources
Web address: www.nchs.com
Control: Other not–for–profit (including NFP Corporation) **Service:** General Medical and Surgical

Staffed Beds: 196 **Admissions:** 6014 **Census:** 144 **Outpatient Visits:** 69789 **Births:** 1074 **Total Expense ($000):** 79291 **Payroll Expense ($000):** 33119 **Personnel:** 560

BENSON—Swift County

★ **SWIFT COUNTY–BENSON HOSPITAL (241365)**, 1815 Wisconsin Avenue, Zip 56215–1653; tel. 320/843–4232, (Nonreporting) **A**9 10 18
Primary Contact: Frank Lawatsch, Chief Executive Officer
CFO: Jayne Thielke, Chief Financial Officer
CIO: Jayne Thielke, Chief Financial Officer
CHR: Stella Kalthoff, Quality Improvement Coordinator
Web address: www.scbh.org
Control: Hospital district or authority, Government, nonfederal **Service:** General Medical and Surgical

Staffed Beds: 18

BIGFORK—Itasca County

★ **BIGFORK VALLEY HOSPITAL (241316)**, 258 Pine Tree Drive, Zip 56628, Mailing Address: P.O. Box 258, Zip 56628–0258; tel. 218/743–3177, (Total facility includes 40 beds in nursing home–type unit) (Nonreporting) **A**9 10 18
Primary Contact: Daniel Odegaard, Chief Executive Officer
COO: Ken Westman, Administrator Long Term Care and Chief Operating Officer
CFO: Karen M. Campbell, Controller
CMO: George Rounds, M.D., Chief of Staff
CIO: Sally Sedgwick, Manager Public Relations and Marketing
CHR: Jennifer Drotts, Manager Human Resources
Web address: www.bigforkvalley.org
Control: Hospital district or authority, Government, nonfederal **Service:** General Medical and Surgical

Staffed Beds: 60

BLUE EARTH—Faribault County

★□ **UNITED HOSPITAL DISTRICT (241369)**, 515 South Moore Street, Zip 56013–2158, Mailing Address: P.O. Box 160, Zip 56013–0160; tel. 507/526–3273 **A**1 9 10 18 **F**3 4 7 8 11 12 13 15 17 24 25 26 27 32 33 38 42 43 53 55 56 57 61 62 63 66 67 68 69 73 74 75 77 79 81 82 84 86 87 96 102 107 117 119 122 124 133 135 137 **P**6
Primary Contact: Jeffrey M. Lang, Chief Executive Officer
CFO: Kyle Chase, Chief Financial Officer
Web address: www.uhd.org
Control: Hospital district or authority, Government, nonfederal **Service:** General Medical and Surgical

Staffed Beds: 48 **Admissions:** 710 **Census:** 20 **Outpatient Visits:** 48063 **Births:** 58 **Total Expense ($000):** 18539 **Payroll Expense ($000):** 8614 **Personnel:** 202

BRAINERD—Crow Wing County

□ **BRAINERD REGIONAL HUMAN SERVICES CENTER (244008)**, 11800 State Highway 18, Zip 56401–7300; tel. 218/828–2201, (Nonreporting) **A**1 9 10
Primary Contact: Bill Peters, Acting Director of Psychiatry
Control: State–Government, nonfederal **Service:** Psychiatric

Staffed Beds: 16

□ **ST. JOSEPH'S MEDICAL CENTER (240075)**, 523 North Third Street, Zip 56401–3098; tel. 218/829–2861 **A**1 9 10 19 **F**3 4 5 11 12 13 15 24 25 26 27 30 31 32 33 38 40 41 48 49 55 56 57 62 63 68 73 74 75 76 77 78 79 80 81 82 84 85 86 88 90 91 92 93 94 95 96 97 100 102 104 107 119 120 121 135 137 **P**2 **S** Essentia Health
Primary Contact: Jani Wiebolt, President and Chief Executive Officer
CMO: David Sabir, M.D., Chief of Staff
CIO: Pat DeLong, Information Services Manager
CHR: Dale Benson, Director Human Resources
Web address: www.sjmcmn.org
Control: Church–operated, Nongovernment, not–for profit **Service:** General Medical and Surgical

Staffed Beds: 162 **Admissions:** 7456 **Census:** 78 **Outpatient Visits:** 136530 **Births:** 651 **Total Expense ($000):** 91305 **Payroll Expense ($000):** 39519 **Personnel:** 609

BRECKENRIDGE—Wilkin County

★ **ST. FRANCIS HEALTHCARE CAMPUS (241377)**, 2400 St. Francis Drive, Zip 56520–1298; tel. 218/643–3000, (Total facility includes 120 beds in nursing home–type unit) **A**5 9 10 18 **F**3 5 8 11 13 15 17 24 25 26 28 30 31 32 33 34 36 37 38 40 42 43 44 46 50 52 54 55 56 57 61 62 66 68 73 74 75 79 81 82 84 86 87 89 90 91 92 93 94 96 99 100 102 103 107 117 118 119 121 122 123 124 132 135 136 **S** Catholic Health Initiatives
Primary Contact: David A. Nelson, President and Chief Executive Officer
CFO: Nancy Whitney, Chief Financial Officer
Web address: www.sfcare.org
Control: Church–operated, Nongovernment, not–for profit **Service:** General Medical and Surgical

Staffed Beds: 145 **Admissions:** 1469 **Census:** 127 **Outpatient Visits:** 24327 **Births:** 184 **Total Expense ($000):** 24258 **Payroll Expense ($000):** 10603 **Personnel:** 260

BUFFALO—Wright County

★□ **BUFFALO HOSPITAL (240076)**, 303 Catlin Street, Zip 55313–1947; tel. 763/682–1212 **A**1 9 10 **F**1 3 4 11 13 15 16 17 24 25 27 32 33 38 41 44 55 57 65 68 70 71 73 74 76 77 78 79 80 81 82 83 84 85 86 88 96 100 102 107 117 118 119 120 133 135 **S** Allina Hospitals & Clinics
Primary Contact: Steve Hatkin, President
COO: Bill Priest, Director Operations and Finance
CFO: Joyce Dehmer, Manager Finance
CHR: Nikki Mills, Director Human Resources
Web address: www.buffalohospital.org
Control: Other not–for–profit (including NFP Corporation) **Service:** General Medical and Surgical

Staffed Beds: 40 **Admissions:** 3010 **Census:** 20 **Outpatient Visits:** 62789 **Births:** 611 **Total Expense ($000):** 45136 **Payroll Expense ($000):** 19680 **Personnel:** 298

BURNSVILLE—Dakota County

★□ **FAIRVIEW RIDGES HOSPITAL (240207)**, 201 East Nicollet Boulevard, Zip 55337–5799; tel. 952/892–2000 **A**1 9 10 **F**3 11 13 15 24 25 26 27 30 31 32 33 38 43 44 49 51 62 66 68 71 73 74 75 76 77 79 80 81 82 84 86 96 97 98 99 100 102 106 107 114 119 121 135 **S** Fairview Health Services
Primary Contact: Beth Krehbiel, President and Chief Executive Officer
CFO: Laura DeNeui, Vice President Finance and Quality Performance
CMO: Jamie Peters, M.D., Vice President Medical Services
Web address: www.fairview.org
Control: Other not–for–profit (including NFP Corporation) **Service:** General Medical and Surgical

Staffed Beds: 149 **Admissions:** 12727 **Census:** 104 **Outpatient Visits:** 104620 **Births:** 3062 **Total Expense ($000):** 127348 **Payroll Expense ($000):** 66354 **Personnel:** 933

MN

Hospital, Medicare Provider Number, Address, Telephone, Approval, Facility, and Physician Codes, Health Care System

★ American Hospital Association (AHA) membership
□ The Joint Commission accreditation
○ American Osteopathic Association (AOA) accreditation
△ Commission on Accreditation of Rehabilitation Facilities (CARF) accreditation

CAMBRIDGE—Isanti County

★ **CAMBRIDGE MEDICAL CENTER (240020)**, 701 South Dellwood Street, Zip 55008–1920; tel. 763/689–7700 **A**1 9 10 **F**3 4 5 11 13 14 15 24 25 26 27 28 30 31 32 33 36 38 40 43 50 54 55 56 57 60 62 63 67 68 72 73 74 75 76 77 79 80 81 82 84 86 87 88 89 90 91 92 93 94 96 97 100 102 107 115 118 119 120 121 123 124 133 135 136 137 **P**5 6 **S** Allina Hospitals & Clinics
Primary Contact: Dennis J. Doran, President
CFO: Nancy Treacy, Chief Financial Officer
Web address: www.allina.com/ahs/cambridge.nsf
Control: Other not–for–profit (including NFP Corporation) **Service:** General Medical and Surgical

Staffed Beds: 78 **Admissions:** 4306 **Census:** 48 **Outpatient Visits:** 372641 **Births:** 582 **Total Expense ($000):** 95419 **Payroll Expense ($000):** 48867 **Personnel:** 672

CANBY—Yellow Medicine County

★ **SANFORD CANBY MEDICAL CENTER (241347)**, (Formerly Sioux Valley Canby Campus), 112 St. Olaf Avenue South, Zip 56220–1433; tel. 507/223–7277, (Includes SENIOR HAVEN CONVALESCENT NURSING CENTER), (Total facility includes 75 beds in nursing home–type unit) **A**9 10 18 **F**2 3 6 7 10 11 13 15 24 25 27 31 33 37 38 46 49 52 54 57 59 61 62 63 68 69 74 77 79 84 86 96 102 107 115 117 119 121 122 132 133 135 **P**6 **S** Sanford Health
Primary Contact: Robert J. Salmon, Chief Executive Officer
CFO: Allison Nelson, Chief Financial Officer
CMO: Maritza Lopez, M.D., Chief of Staff
CIO: Cheryl Ferguson, Associate Administrator
Web address: www.sanfordcanby.org
Control: Other not–for–profit (including NFP Corporation) **Service:** General Medical and Surgical

Staffed Beds: 100 **Admissions:** 685 **Census:** 80 **Outpatient Visits:** 20498 **Births:** 57 **Total Expense ($000):** 17624 **Payroll Expense ($000):** 8455 **Personnel:** 247

MN

CANNON FALLS—Goodhue County

★ **CANNON FALLS MEDICAL CENTER (241346)**, 1116 West Mill Street, Zip 55009–1898; tel. 507/263–4221, (Nonreporting) **A**9 10 18 **S** Mayo Foundation
Primary Contact: Glenn Christian, Administrator
Web address: www.cannonhealth.org/
Control: Hospital district or authority, Government, nonfederal **Service:** General Medical and Surgical

Staffed Beds: 21

CASS LAKE—Cass County

★ **U. S. PUBLIC HEALTH SERVICE INDIAN HOSPITAL (241358)**, 7th Street and Grant Utley Avenue N.W., Zip 56633, Mailing Address: Rural Route 3, Box 211, Zip 56633; tel. 218/335–3200, (Nonreporting) **A**5 9 10 18 **S** U. S. Indian Health Service
Primary Contact: Earl Cournoyer, Interim Chief Executive Officer
CFO: Randall Jordan, Budget Analyst
Web address: www.ihs.gov
Control: PHS, Indian Service, Government, federal **Service:** General Medical and Surgical

Staffed Beds: 11

CLOQUET—Carlton County

★ **COMMUNITY MEMORIAL HOSPITAL (241364)**, 512 Skyline Boulevard, Zip 55720–1199; tel. 218/879–4641, (Total facility includes 88 beds in nursing home–type unit) **A**9 10 18 **F**3 13 15 24 25 26 27 32 33 38 43 56 57 62 68 73 74 75 77 79 80 82 86 96 100 102 107 117 119 120 121 122 133 135 136 137 **P**6
Primary Contact: Rick Breuer, Chief Executive Officer and Administrator
CFO: Brad Anderson, Chief Financial Officer
CIO: Jay Knute, Director Management Information Systems
CHR: Denise Frankki, Director Human Resources
Web address: www.cloquethospital.com
Control: Other not–for–profit (including NFP Corporation) **Service:** General Medical and Surgical

Staffed Beds: 113 **Admissions:** 1518 **Census:** 98 **Outpatient Visits:** 49078 **Births:** 97 **Total Expense ($000):** 35439 **Payroll Expense ($000):** 17254 **Personnel:** 321

COOK—St. Louis County

★ **COOK HOSPITAL AND CONVALESCENT NURSING CARE UNIT (241312)**, 10 Fifth Street S.E., Zip 55723–9745; tel. 218/666–5945, (Total facility includes 41 beds in nursing home–type unit) **A**9 10 18 **F**2 3 11 15 24 30 31 32 33 38 52 54 55 62 63 75 86 96 100 107 117 119 120 122 135 137 **P**5
Primary Contact: Allen J. Vogt, Administrator
CFO: Dan McCarthy, Chief Financial Officer
Control: Hospital district or authority, Government, nonfederal **Service:** General Medical and Surgical

Staffed Beds: 55 **Admissions:** 447 **Census:** 44 **Outpatient Visits:** 10403 **Births:** 0 **Total Expense ($000):** 10147 **Payroll Expense ($000):** 4634 **Personnel:** 118

COON RAPIDS—Anoka County

★ **MERCY HOSPITAL (240115)**, 4050 Coon Rapids Boulevard, Zip 55433–2586; tel. 763/236–6000, (Nonreporting) **A**1 5 9 10 **S** Allina Hospitals & Clinics
Primary Contact: Thomas O'Connor, President
COO: Philip Patterson, Vice President Operations
CFO: Earl Beitzel, Vice President Finance
CMO: Dennis O'Hare, M.D., Vice President Medical Affairs
CIO: Robert Plaszcz, Chief Information Officer
CHR: Nancy Watson, Director Human Resources
Web address: www.allinamercy.org
Control: Other not–for–profit (including NFP Corporation) **Service:** General Medical and Surgical

Staffed Beds: 264

CROOKSTON—Polk County

★ **RIVERVIEW HEALTHCARE ASSOCIATION (241320)**, 323 South Minnesota Street, Zip 56716–1600; tel. 218/281–9200, (Total facility includes 125 beds in nursing home–type unit) (Nonreporting) **A**5 9 10 18
Primary Contact: Debra K. Boardman, President and Chief Executive Officer
COO: Vicky Korynta, Chief Nursing Officer
CFO: William Bennett, Chief Financial Officer
CMO: Ron Dorman, M.D., Chief of Staff
CIO: Chris Bruggeman, Chief Information Officer
CHR: Jean Tate, Manager Human Resources
Web address: www.riverviewhealth.org
Control: Other not–for–profit (including NFP Corporation) **Service:** General Medical and Surgical

Staffed Beds: 187

CROSBY—Crow Wing County

★ **CUYUNA REGIONAL MEDICAL CENTER (241353)**, 320 East Main Street, Zip 56441–1690; tel. 218/546–7000, (Total facility includes 115 beds in nursing home–type unit) (Nonreporting) **A**9 10 18
Primary Contact: Thomas F. Reek, Chief Executive Officer
CFO: Kyle Bauer, Chief Financial Officer
CMO: George Kuhlmann, M.D., Chief of Staff
CHR: Theresa Sullivan, Administrator Organizational Support
Web address: www.cuyunamed.org
Control: Hospital district or authority, Government, nonfederal **Service:** General Medical and Surgical

Staffed Beds: 140

DAWSON—Lac Qui Parle County

JOHNSON MEMORIAL HEALTH SERVICES (241314), 1282 Walnut Street, Zip 56232–2333; tel. 320/769–4323 **A**9 10 18 **F**3 7 11 15 24 30 38 55 56 57 61 62 63 66 69 74 75 79 80 84 86 96 99 100 107 117 119 122 124 135 **P**6
Primary Contact: Kathy Johnson, Administrator
CFO: Stacey Lee, Chief Financial Officer
CMO: Ralph Gerbig, M.D., Chief of Staff
CHR: Jody Bjerke, Director Human Resources
Web address: www.jmhsdawson.com
Control: Hospital district or authority, Government, nonfederal **Service:** General Medical and Surgical

Staffed Beds: 18 **Admissions:** 316 **Census:** 5 **Outpatient Visits:** 802 **Births:** 15 **Total Expense ($000):** 5004 **Payroll Expense ($000):** 2588 **Personnel:** 31

DEER RIVER—Itasca County

★ **DEER RIVER HEALTHCARE CENTER (241360)**, 1002 Comstock Drive, Zip 56636–9700; tel. 218/246–2900, (Total facility includes 50 beds in nursing home–type unit) (Nonreporting) **A**9 10 18
Primary Contact: Jeffry Stampohar, Chief Executive Officer
CFO: Steven Larson, Chief Financial Officer
CMO: David Goodall, M.D., Chief Medical Staff
CHR: Amy Lane Myers, Director Human Resources
Web address: www.drhc.org
Control: Other not–for–profit (including NFP Corporation) **Service:** General Medical and Surgical

Staffed Beds: 65

Many Facility Codes have changed. Please refer to the AHA Guide Code Chart.

DETROIT LAKES—Becker County

☒ **ST. MARY'S REGIONAL HEALTH CENTER (240101)**, 1027 Washington Avenue, Zip 56501–3598; tel. 218/847–5611, (Total facility includes 100 beds in nursing home–type unit) **A**1 5 9 10 **F**3 6 7 8 10 11 13 14 24 26 30 31 33 38 40 44 46 47 50 54 55 56 57 61 62 68 73 74 75 77 79 80 84 86 96 97 102 107 115 117 119 121 122 124 132 135 **S** Essentia Health
Primary Contact: Thomas R. Thompson, Chief Executive Officer
CHR: Chad Engstrom, Manager Human Resources
Web address: www.smrhc.com
Control: Church–operated, Nongovernment, not–for profit **Service:** General Medical and Surgical

Staffed Beds: 154 **Admissions:** 3638 **Census:** 122 **Outpatient Visits:** 27132 **Births:** 548 **Total Expense ($000):** 41589 **Payroll Expense ($000):** 19859 **Personnel:** 370

DULUTH—St. Louis County

☒ △ **MILLER–DWAN MEDICAL CENTER (240019)**, 502 East Second Street, Zip 55805–1982; tel. 218/727–8762 **A**1 7 9 10 **F**3 5 11 16 26 30 31 32 33 34 36 43 50 51 54 55 62 68 72 73 75 76 77 79 80 81 82 85 86 88 89 90 91 92 93 94 95 107 108 109 111 112 119 121 123 135 137 **P**6 **S** Essentia Health
Primary Contact: Rocklon B. Chapin, Executive Vice President and Chief Operating Officer
CFO: Robert Norman, Chief Financial Officer
CMO: Jeff Garland, M.D., Vice President Medical Affairs
CIO: Dennis Dassenko, Chief Information Officer
CHR: Diane Davidson, Senior Vice President Human Resources
Web address: www.miller–dwan.com
Control: Other not–for–profit (including NFP Corporation) **Service:** General Medical and Surgical

Staffed Beds: 154 **Admissions:** 4415 **Census:** 78 **Outpatient Visits:** 56023 **Births:** 0 **Total Expense ($000):** 69494 **Payroll Expense ($000):** 32300 **Personnel:** 496

☒ △ **ST. LUKE'S HOSPITAL (240047)**, 915 East First Street, Zip 55805–2193; tel. 218/249–5555 **A**1 2 3 5 7 9 10 **F**3 7 8 9 12 13 15 17 18 20 22 24 25 26 27 30 31 32 33 37 38 40 42 43 44 45 46 47 48 49 51 53 56 57 58 59 60 61 62 63 68 72 73 74 75 76 77 79 80 81 82 84 85 86 87 88 90 91 92 93 94 96 97 99 100 102 103 104 106 107 108 109 111 112 118 119 121 133 135 137 **P**6
Primary Contact: John Strange, President and Chief Executive Officer
CFO: James F. Wuellner, Chief Financial Officer
CMO: Gary Peterson, M.D., Vice President Medical Affairs and Medical Director
CIO: Clark Averill, Director Information Technology
CHR: Marla Halvorson, Director Human Resources
Web address: www.slhduluth.com
Control: Other not–for–profit (including NFP Corporation) **Service:** General Medical and Surgical

Staffed Beds: 267 **Admissions:** 12440 **Census:** 144 **Outpatient Visits:** 143221 **Births:** 1035 **Total Expense ($000):** 271005 **Payroll Expense ($000):** 128689 **Personnel:** 1669

☒ **ST. MARY'S MEDICAL CENTER (240002)**, 407 East Third Street, Zip 55805–1984; tel. 218/786–4000 **A**1 2 3 5 9 10 **F**3 7 11 12 13 17 18 20 22 24 25 26 27 28 30 31 32 33 34 35 36 38 40 41 42 43 44 45 46 48 49 50 55 56 60 61 62 63 65 66 68 70 72 73 74 75 76 77 79 80 82 83 84 86 96 97 100 103 106 107 116 118 119 121 130 134 135 136 137 **P**6 **S** Essentia Health
Primary Contact: Peter E. Person, M.D., President and Chief Executive Officer
COO: MariBeth Olson, Chief Operating Officer
CMO: Hugh Renier, M.D., Vice President Medical Affairs
CIO: Tess Jettergren, Director Clinical Informatics
CHR: Glen Porter, Vice President Human Resources
Web address: www.smdc.org
Control: Other not–for–profit (including NFP Corporation) **Service:** General Medical and Surgical

Staffed Beds: 337 **Admissions:** 18765 **Census:** 222 **Outpatient Visits:** 136896 **Births:** 1423 **Total Expense ($000):** 288865 **Payroll Expense ($000):** 120536 **Personnel:** 1708

EDINA—Hennepin County

☒ **FAIRVIEW SOUTHDALE HOSPITAL (240078)**, 6401 France Avenue South, Zip 55435–2199; tel. 952/924–5000 **A**1 2 9 10 **F**3 5 8 11 12 13 15 17 18 20 22 24 25 26 27 30 31 32 33 36 38 40 43 44 49 50 51 55 56 57 59 62 63 67 68 71 72 73 74 76 77 79 82 86 88 90 92 96 97 98 99 100 102 103 104 107 109 112 114 118 119 120 121 123 124 135 136 137 **P**6 **S** Fairview Health Services
Primary Contact: Bradley Beard, President
CFO: Alan Lem, Vice President Finance
CMO: James Bishop, M.D., Director Medical Affairs
CHR: Jennifer Preston, Director Human Resources
Web address: www.fairview.org
Control: Other not–for–profit (including NFP Corporation) **Service:** General Medical and Surgical

Staffed Beds: 357 **Admissions:** 21824 **Census:** 219 **Outpatient Visits:** 127407 **Births:** 3656 **Total Expense ($000):** 340809 **Payroll Expense ($000):** 142830 **Personnel:** 1786

ELBOW LAKE—Grant County

★ **ELEAH MEDICAL CENTER (241379)**, 930 First Street N.E., Zip 56531–4611; tel. 218/685–4461 **A**9 10 18 **F**7 15 27 30 38 52 57 61 62 68 79 86 106 121 122 **P**4
Primary Contact: Larry Rapp, M.D., Chief Medical and Executive Officer
COO: Larry Rapp, M.D., Chief Medical and Executive Officer
CMO: Larry Rapp, M.D., Chief Medical and Executive Officer
Web address: www.eleahmed.org
Control: Other not–for–profit (including NFP Corporation) **Service:** General Medical and Surgical

Staffed Beds: 20 **Admissions:** 353 **Census:** 3 **Outpatient Visits:** 979 **Births:** 0 **Total Expense ($000):** 6045 **Payroll Expense ($000):** 2273 **Personnel:** 72

MN

ELY—St. Louis County

★ **ELY–BLOOMENSON COMMUNITY HOSPITAL (241318)**, 328 West Conan Street, Zip 55731–1198; tel. 218/365–3271, (Total facility includes 79 beds in nursing home–type unit) **A**9 10 18 **F**7 11 13 15 17 24 27 30 31 33 34 38 61 62 67 74 79 84 86 96 99 107 117 119 121 122 135 **P**6
Primary Contact: John Fossum, Chief Executive Officer and Administrator
CFO: Scott Kellerman, Chief Financial Officer
CHR: Richard Rand, Director Human Resources
Web address: www.ebch.org
Control: Other not–for–profit (including NFP Corporation) **Service:** General Medical and Surgical

Staffed Beds: 104 **Admissions:** 603 **Census:** 79 **Outpatient Visits:** 8861 **Births:** 32 **Total Expense ($000):** 19263 **Payroll Expense ($000):** 7904 **Personnel:** 194

FAIRMONT—Martin County

☒ **FAIRMONT MEDICAL CENTER–MAYO HEALTH SYSTEM (240166)**, 800 Medical Center Drive, Zip 56031–0800; tel. 507/238–8100, (Includes LUTZ WING CONVALESCENT AND NURSING CARE UNIT), (Total facility includes 40 beds in nursing home–type unit) (Nonreporting) **A**1 9 10 **S** Mayo Foundation
Primary Contact: Barbara Allen, M.D., President and Chief Executive Officer
COO: Gayle Hansen, Chief Operating Officer
CFO: Brian Suter, Chief Financial Officer
CMO: Marie Morris, M.D., Medical Director
Web address: www.fairmontmedicalcenter.org
Control: Other not–for–profit (including NFP Corporation) **Service:** General Medical and Surgical

Staffed Beds: 97

FARIBAULT—Rice County

★ **DISTRICT ONE HOSPITAL (240071)**, 200 State Avenue, Zip 55021–6345; tel. 507/334–6451 **A**9 10 **F**3 8 11 13 15 24 27 30 31 33 38 40 42 43 46 55 56 57 66 68 73 74 79 80 81 82 84 96 100 107 119 121 124 135 136
Primary Contact: James N. Wolf, Chief Executive Officer
CFO: Patrick A. Justin, Chief Financial Officer
CIO: Patrick A. Justin, Chief Financial Officer
CHR: Rose Dube, Manager Human Resources
Web address: www.districtonehospital.com
Control: Hospital district or authority, Government, nonfederal **Service:** General Medical and Surgical

Staffed Beds: 42 **Admissions:** 2243 **Census:** 17 **Outpatient Visits:** 33070 **Births:** 467 **Total Expense ($000):** 38484 **Payroll Expense ($000):** 14564 **Personnel:** 253

Hospital, Medicare Provider Number, Address, Telephone, Approval, Facility, and Physician Codes, Health Care System

★ American Hospital Association (AHA) membership
☐ The Joint Commission accreditation
○ American Osteopathic Association (AOA) accreditation
△ Commission on Accreditation of Rehabilitation Facilities (CARF) accreditation

FERGUS FALLS—Otter Tail County

☐ **COMMUNITY BEHAVIORAL HEALTH HOSPITAL – FERGUS FALLS**, 1801 West Alcott Avenue, Zip 56538–0478, Mailing Address: P.O. Box 478, Zip 56538–0478; tel. 218/332–5001, (Nonreporting) **A**1 **S** Minnesota Deparment of Human Services
Primary Contact: Derrick A. Jones, Administrator
Control: State–Government, nonfederal **Service:** Psychiatric

Staffed Beds: 138

★ △ **LAKE REGION HEALTHCARE CORPORATION (240052)**, 712 South Cascade Street, Zip 56537–2900, Mailing Address: P.O. Box 728, Zip 56538–0728; tel. 218/736–8000 **A**1 7 9 10 20 **F**3 10 11 13 15 17 24 25 26 27 30 31 32 33 34 38 41 43 51 52 54 55 56 57 60 62 66 68 73 74 75 76 77 79 80 81 82 84 85 86 88 90 91 92 93 96 97 100 102 105 106 107 118 119 120 121 124 135 136 137 **P**5
Primary Contact: Edward A. Strand, CPA, Interim Administrator
CFO: Edward A. Strand, CPA, Assistant Administrator and Chief Financial Officer
CMO: James E. Andrews, M.D., Chief of Staff
CHR: Cheryl Buck, Manager Human Resources
Web address: www.lrhc.org
Control: Other not–for–profit (including NFP Corporation) **Service:** General Medical and Surgical

Staffed Beds: 108 **Admissions:** 4394 **Census:** 50 **Outpatient Visits:** 57139 **Births:** 365 **Total Expense ($000):** 48371 **Payroll Expense ($000):** 24202 **Personnel:** 486

MN

FOSSTON—Polk County

★ **FIRST CARE MEDICAL SERVICES (241357)**, 900 South Hilligoss Boulevard East, Zip 56542–1599; tel. 218/435–1133, (Total facility includes 50 beds in nursing home–type unit) **A**9 10 18 **F**2 3 7 8 10 13 15 24 27 33 36 38 40 42 43 44 50 52 55 56 57 61 62 63 67 69 73 74 77 78 79 80 82 84 86 87 96 102 107 115 117 119 121 122 124 133 134 135 137
Primary Contact: Patricia Wangler, Chief Executive Officer
CFO: Kim Bodensteiner, Chief Financial Officer
CIO: Kris Dally, Manager Business Office
CHR: Diane Sundrud, Human Resource Director
Web address: www.firstcare.org
Control: Other not–for–profit (including NFP Corporation) **Service:** General Medical and Surgical

Staffed Beds: 72 **Admissions:** 832 **Census:** 56 **Outpatient Visits:** 21239 **Births:** 67

FRIDLEY—Anoka County

★ **UNITY HOSPITAL (240132)**, 550 Osborne Road N.E., Zip 55432–2799; tel. 763/236–5000 **A**1 2 5 9 10 **F**3 4 5 11 12 13 15 17 18 20 22 24 25 26 31 32 33 34 38 43 46 49 54 57 62 63 67 68 70 71 73 74 75 76 79 80 82 84 86 87 88 93 96 97 100 103 107 109 113 114 119 121 124 135 136 137 **P**4 5 **S** Allina Hospitals & Clinics
Primary Contact: Rickie L. Ressler, RN, President
COO: Julie Lapensky, Vice President Operations
CFO: Lisa K. Anderson, Vice President Finance
CMO: John J. Stoltenberg, M.D., Vice President Medical Affairs
CIO: Bob Plaszcz, Executive Vice President Information Services and Chief Information Officer
CHR: Scott Hamman, Director Human Resources
Web address: www.allina.com
Control: Other not–for–profit (including NFP Corporation) **Service:** General Medical and Surgical

Staffed Beds: 237 **Admissions:** 12945 **Census:** 131 **Outpatient Visits:** 94140 **Births:** 1874 **Total Expense ($000):** 164195 **Payroll Expense ($000):** 70051 **Personnel:** 1089

GLENCOE—McLeod County

★ **GLENCOE REGIONAL HEALTH SERVICES (241355)**, 1805 Hennepin Avenue North, Zip 55336–1416; tel. 320/864–3121, (Total facility includes 110 beds in nursing home–type unit) **A**9 10 18 **F**2 3 7 11 13 15 17 25 27 30 31 32 38 40 54 56 62 66 68 73 74 75 79 81 82 84 86 87 96 99 102 107 115 117 119 121 122 124 134 135 **P**6 **S** Park Nicollet Health Services
Primary Contact: Jon D. Braband, President and Chief Executive Officer
CFO: Cheryl Trippel, Director Finance
CMO: John H. Bergseng, D.O., Vice President Medical Affairs
CIO: Michael Sprandel, Administrator Network
CHR: Jill Hatlestad, Vice President Human Resources and Organizational Support
Web address: www.grhsonline.com
Control: Other not–for–profit (including NFP Corporation) **Service:** General Medical and Surgical

Staffed Beds: 135 **Admissions:** 1310 **Census:** 120 **Outpatient Visits:** 25267 **Births:** 196 **Total Expense ($000):** 44330 **Payroll Expense ($000):** 20864 **Personnel:** 425

GLENWOOD—Pope County

★ **GLACIAL RIDGE HEALTH SYSTEM (241376)**, 10 Fourth Avenue S.E., Zip 56334–1898; tel. 320/634–4521 **A**9 10 18 **F**7 11 13 15 17 24 27 30 31 33 38 40 42 52 57 61 62 74 79 96 102 107 119 122 **P**6
Primary Contact: Kirk Stensrud, Chief Executive Officer
CFO: Casey R. Johnson, Chief Financial Officer
CHR: Gordon Paulson, Manager Personnel
Web address: www.glacialridge.org
Control: Hospital district or authority, Government, nonfederal **Service:** General Medical and Surgical

Staffed Beds: 34 **Admissions:** 818 **Census:** 7 **Outpatient Visits:** 11502 **Births:** 48 **Total Expense ($000):** 12749 **Payroll Expense ($000):** 6193 **Personnel:** 134

GOLDEN VALLEY—Hennepin County

★ **REGENCY HOSPITAL OF MINNEAPOLIS (242005)**, 1300 Hidden Lakes Parkway, Zip 55422–4299; tel. 763/588–2750 **A**1 **F**1 3 25 30 55 56 80 119 135 137 **P**8 **S** Regency Hospital Company
Primary Contact: Deborah Graves, RN, Chief Executive Officer
CMO: Norm Yunis, M.D., Medical Director
Web address: www.regencyhospital.com
Control: Corporation, Investor–owned, for–profit **Service:** Long–Term Acute Care hospital

Staffed Beds: 54 **Admissions:** 413 **Census:** 37 **Outpatient Visits:** 0 **Births:** 0 **Total Expense ($000):** 26814 **Payroll Expense ($000):** 11510 **Personnel:** 166

GRACEVILLE—Big Stone County

GRACEVILLE HEALTH CENTER (241321), 115 West Second Street, Zip 56240–0157, Mailing Address: P.O. Box 157, Zip 56240–0157; tel. 320/748–7223, (Total facility includes 50 beds in nursing home–type unit) (Nonreporting) **A**9 10 18 **S** Essentia Health
Primary Contact: A. Todd Howell, Administrator and Chief Executive Officer
CFO: Diane Sullivan, Chief Financial Officer
CMO: Arthur Van Vranken, M.D., Chief of Staff
CHR: Mary Bauer, Director Human Resources
Web address: www.gracevillehealth.com
Control: Other not–for–profit (including NFP Corporation) **Service:** General Medical and Surgical

Staffed Beds: 65

GRAND MARAIS—Cook County

COOK COUNTY NORTH SHORE HOSPITAL (241317), 515 5th Avenue West, Zip 55604–9716, Mailing Address: 515 5th Avenue West, Zip 55604–0010; tel. 218/387–3040, (Total facility includes 47 beds in nursing home–type unit) **A**9 10 18 **F**7 13 15 24 27 30 38 40 61 74 84 86 96 102 117 119 122 137 **P**6
Primary Contact: Diane L. Pearson, Administrator
CFO: Yvonne Gennrich, Controller
Web address: www.boreal.org/nshcf/index.html
Control: Hospital district or authority, Government, nonfederal **Service:** General Medical and Surgical

Staffed Beds: 56 **Admissions:** 387 **Census:** 47 **Outpatient Visits:** 15648 **Births:** 9 **Total Expense ($000):** 11719 **Payroll Expense ($000):** 5717 **Personnel:** 133

GRAND RAPIDS—Itasca County

★ **GRAND ITASCA CLINIC AND HOSPITAL (240064)**, 1601 Golf Course Road, Zip 55744–3698; tel. 218/326–5000 **A**1 10 20 **F**3 11 12 13 15 17 24 25 26 27 29 31 38 40 52 54 61 62 63 68 73 74 75 77 79 85 86 87 96 97 98 99 100 103 106 107 119 120 121 135 136
Primary Contact: John M. Kutch, President and Chief Executive Officer
CFO: Steven Feltman, Senior Vice President Finance, Operations and Chief Financial Officer
CHR: Robert Cocker, Vice President Organizational Effectiveness
Web address: www.granditasca.org
Control: Other not–for–profit (including NFP Corporation) **Service:** General Medical and Surgical

Staffed Beds: 64 **Admissions:** 2924 **Census:** 28 **Outpatient Visits:** 160867 **Births:** 413 **Total Expense ($000):** 64822 **Payroll Expense ($000):** 30673 **Personnel:** 492

GRANITE FALLS—Yellow Medicine County

★ **GRANITE FALLS MUNICIPAL HOSPITAL AND MANOR (241343)**, 345 Tenth Avenue, Zip 56241–1499; tel. 320/564–3111, (Total facility includes 57 beds in nursing home–type unit) **A**9 10 18 **F**3 7 13 15 24 25 32 33 38 54 55 56 57 61 63 66 67 73 74 75 77 79 80 81 82 84 86 96 115 117 118 119 122 132 135
Primary Contact: George Gerlach, Chief Executive Officer
CFO: Larry Lee, Chief Financial Officer
Web address: www.gfmhm.com
Control: City–Government, nonfederal **Service:** General Medical and Surgical

Staffed Beds: 82 **Admissions:** 837 **Census:** 59 **Outpatient Visits:** 24893 **Births:** 49 **Total Expense ($000):** 14985 **Payroll Expense ($000):** 7540 **Personnel:** 116

Many Facility Codes have changed. Please refer to the AHA Guide Code Chart.

HALLOCK—Kittson County

★ **KITTSON MEMORIAL HEALTHCARE CENTER (241336)**, 1010 South Birch Street, Zip 56728–0700, Mailing Address: P.O. Box 700, Zip 56728–0700; tel. 218/843–3612, (Total facility includes 77 beds in nursing home–type unit) (Nonreporting) **A**9 10 18
Primary Contact: Jason Carlson, Chief Executive Officer
CFO: Sandra Gjervold, Chief Financial Officer
Control: Other not–for–profit (including NFP Corporation) **Service:** General Medical and Surgical

Staffed Beds: 92

HASTINGS—Dakota County

☐ **REGINA MEDICAL CENTER (240059)**, 1175 Nininger Road, Zip 55033–1098; tel. 651/480–4100 **A**1 9 10 **F**10 11 13 15 25 26 38 42 55 57 67 68 73 74 75 79 82 86 96 100 102 107 115 117 119 122 132 135
Primary Contact: Mark D. Wilson, President and Chief Executive Officer
CFO: Nate Meyer, Chief Financial Officer
CMO: James Noreen, M.D., Chief Medical Officer
Web address: www.reginamedical.org
Control: Other not–for–profit (including NFP Corporation) **Service:** General Medical and Surgical

Staffed Beds: 44 **Admissions:** 2773 **Census:** 28 **Outpatient Visits:** 42093 **Births:** 405 **Total Expense ($000):** 51408 **Payroll Expense ($000):** 27227 **Personnel:** 403

HENDRICKS—Lincoln County

★ **HENDRICKS COMMUNITY HOSPITAL (241339)**, 503 East Lincoln Street, Zip 56136–0106, Mailing Address: P.O. Box 1016, Zip 56136–0106; tel. 507/275–3134, (Total facility includes 70 beds in nursing home–type unit) **A**9 10 18 **F**2 7 10 11 15 17 24 25 27 30 31 33 38 42 43 44 52 61 68 74 79 84 86 107 115 117 119 122 132 135 137 **P**5
Primary Contact: Jeffrey Gollaher, Chief Executive Officer
CFO: Julie Hogie, Manager Business Office
CMO: Tabb McCluskey, M.D., Chief Medical Officer
CHR: Lynn Olson, Director Human Resources
Web address: www.hendrickshosp.org
Control: Other not–for–profit (including NFP Corporation) **Service:** General Medical and Surgical

Staffed Beds: 80 **Admissions:** 304 **Census:** 70 **Outpatient Visits:** 7273 **Births:** 17 **Total Expense ($000):** 9328 **Payroll Expense ($000):** 3916 **Personnel:** 125

HIBBING—St. Louis County

★ **FAIRVIEW RANGE REGIONAL HEALTH SERVICES (240040)**, 750 East 34th Street, Zip 55746–4600; tel. 218/262–4881 **A**2 9 10 **F**2 3 6 8 10 11 13 15 25 26 27 30 31 32 33 38 42 43 44 46 50 55 56 57 61 62 63 66 67 68 73 74 75 76 77 79 80 81 82 84 86 87 88 96 97 100 103 104 107 108 109 118 119 121 124 132 133 134 135 136 137 **S** Fairview Health Services
Primary Contact: Lawrence W. Pfaff, President and Chief Executive Officer
CFO: John D. Kritz, Senior Vice President and Chief Financial Officer
CMO: Michael Heck, M.D., Chief Medical Officer
CIO: Joe Wivoda, Vice President Information Services and Chief Information Officer
CHR: Mitch Vincent, Vice President Human Resources
Web address: www.range.fairview.org
Control: Other not–for–profit (including NFP Corporation) **Service:** General Medical and Surgical

Staffed Beds: 107 **Admissions:** 4733 **Census:** 54 **Outpatient Visits:** 128808 **Births:** 399 **Total Expense ($000):** 82145 **Payroll Expense ($000):** 39302 **Personnel:** 575

HUTCHINSON—McLeod County

⊠ **HUTCHINSON AREA HEALTH CARE (240187)**, 1095 Highway 15 South, Zip 55350–3182; tel. 320/234–5000, (Total facility includes 120 beds in nursing home–type unit) **A**1 9 10 **F**2 3 5 7 11 13 15 24 25 27 31 32 33 34 36 38 54 55 57 62 67 68 73 74 75 76 77 79 80 82 86 88 89 90 91 92 93 94 96 102 106 107 117 119 120 121 122 135 136 137 **S** Allina Hospitals & Clinics
Primary Contact: Mary Ellen Wells, President
COO: Mary Ellen Wells, President
CFO: Pamela Larson, Chief Financial Officer
CMO: Steven Mulder, M.D., Director Medical Affairs
CIO: Pamela Larson, Chief Financial Officer
CHR: Robyn Erickson, Division Director Human Resources
Web address: www.hahc-hmc.com
Control: City–Government, nonfederal **Service:** General Medical and Surgical

Staffed Beds: 179 **Admissions:** 3078 **Census:** 144 **Outpatient Visits:** 76432 **Births:** 372 **Total Expense ($000):** 59493 **Payroll Expense ($000):** 25716 **Personnel:** 476

INTERNATIONAL FALLS—Koochiching County

⊠ **FALLS MEMORIAL HOSPITAL (241322)**, 1400 Highway 71, Zip 56649–2189; tel. 218/283–4481 **A**1 9 10 18 **F**11 13 15 24 25 27 30 31 32 38 56 66 74 75 79 80 86 96 107 122 133 136 **S** QHR
Primary Contact: Bonnie Erickson, Interim Chief Executive Officer
CFO: Robert Henshaw, Chief Financial Officer
CMO: Douglas A. Johnson, M.D., Chief of Staff
CHR: Mary Phillipe, Vice President Human Resources
Web address: www.fmh–mn.com
Control: Other not–for–profit (including NFP Corporation) **Service:** General Medical and Surgical

Staffed Beds: 25 **Admissions:** 818 **Census:** 8 **Outpatient Visits:** 27864 **Births:** 85 **Total Expense ($000):** 14062 **Payroll Expense ($000):** 6758 **Personnel:** 16

JACKSON—Jackson County

★ **SANFORD JACKSON MEDICAL CENTER (241315)**, 1430 North Highway, Zip 56143–1098; tel. 507/847–2420 **A**9 10 18 **F**3 8 24 25 26 27 30 33 38 46 50 54 55 56 57 62 63 66 69 73 75 76 79 80 81 82 85 86 87 107 121 122 **P**8 **S** Sanford Health
Primary Contact: Mary J. Ruyter, Chief Executive Officer
CFO: Gail Eike, Chief Financial Officer
CHR: Naomi Pederson, Director Human Resources
Web address: www.sanfordjackson.org
Control: Other not–for–profit (including NFP Corporation) **Service:** General Medical and Surgical

Staffed Beds: 20 **Admissions:** 256 **Census:** 2 **Outpatient Visits:** 11255 **Births:** 0 **Total Expense ($000):** 4423 **Payroll Expense ($000):** 2005 **Personnel:** 44

MN

LAKE CITY—Goodhue County

⊠ **LAKE CITY MEDICAL CENTER–MAYO (241338)**, 500 West Grant Street, Zip 55041–1143; tel. 651/345–3321, (Total facility includes 93 beds in nursing home–type unit) **A**1 9 10 18 **F**11 13 15 24 30 31 32 33 38 55 57 63 66 67 69 73 74 75 77 79 80 82 86 96 97 100 103 107 117 118 119 121 122 124 134 135 137 **S** Mayo Foundation
Primary Contact: Thomas J. Witt, M.D., President and Chief Executive Officer
COO: Mark Brown, Chief Operating Officer
CFO: Sue Diercks, Chief Financial Officer
CMO: Dennis Spano, M.D., Medical Director
Web address: www.lakecitymedicalcenter.org
Control: Other not–for–profit (including NFP Corporation) **Service:** General Medical and Surgical

Staffed Beds: 111 **Admissions:** 661 **Census:** 93 **Outpatient Visits:** 14191 **Births:** 80 **Total Expense ($000):** 18004 **Payroll Expense ($000):** 4978 **Personnel:** 91

LE SUEUR—Le Sueur County

MINNESOTA VALLEY HEALTH CENTER (241375), 621 South Fourth Street, Zip 56058–2298; tel. 507/665–3375, (Includes GARDENVIEW NURSING HOME), (Total facility includes 85 beds in nursing home–type unit) (Nonreporting) **A**9 10 18
Primary Contact: Patricia J. Townsdin, Chief Executive Officer and Administrator
CFO: Patricia Schlegel, Director Finance
CMO: Carolyn Stelter, M.D., Chief of Staff
CHR: Jennifer Baron, Director Human Resources
Web address: www.mvhc.org
Control: Other not–for–profit (including NFP Corporation) **Service:** General Medical and Surgical

Staffed Beds: 110

LITCHFIELD—Meeker County

★ **MEEKER COUNTY MEMORIAL HOSPITAL (241366)**, 612 South Sibley Avenue, Zip 55355–3398; tel. 320/693–3242 **A**9 10 18 **F**11 13 15 24 25 27 30 31 32 38 54 55 56 57 66 68 73 74 75 76 79 84 93 96 107 119 121 122 135
Primary Contact: Michael Schramm, Chief Executive Officer
CFO: Gary Sogge, Chief Financial Officer
CMO: Debra G. Peterson, M.D., Chief of Staff
CIO: Connie Liimatta, Director Medical Records and Business Office
CHR: Cindi Twardy, Manager Human Resources
Web address: www.mcmh–litchfield.org
Control: County–Government, nonfederal **Service:** General Medical and Surgical

Staffed Beds: 38 **Admissions:** 1102 **Census:** 14 **Outpatient Visits:** 26145 **Births:** 143 **Total Expense ($000):** 18196 **Payroll Expense ($000):** 6598 **Personnel:** 125

Hospital, Medicare Provider Number, Address, Telephone, Approval, Facility, and Physician Codes, Health Care System
★ American Hospital Association (AHA) membership
☐ The Joint Commission accreditation
○ American Osteopathic Association (AOA) accreditation
△ Commission on Accreditation of Rehabilitation Facilities (CARF) accreditation

LITTLE FALLS—Morrison County

☒ **ST. GABRIEL'S HOSPITAL (241370)**, 815 Second Street S.E., Zip 56345–3596; tel. 320/632–5441, (Total facility includes 118 beds in nursing home–type unit) **A**1 9 10 18 **F**2 3 11 13 15 24 25 26 27 30 31 32 38 42 43 44 57 58 61 62 63 66 68 73 74 75 77 79 80 81 82 86 96 97 102 106 107 117 119 120 121 122 135 **P**5 **S** Catholic Health Initiatives
Primary Contact: Carl P. Vaagenes, President and Chief Executive Officer
CFO: Stephen Plaisance, Vice President Finance
CMO: Mark Moe, Chief of Staff
CHR: Cory Glad, Vice President Human Resources
Web address: www.stgabriels.com
Control: Church–operated, Nongovernment, not–for profit **Service:** General Medical and Surgical

Staffed Beds: 167 **Admissions:** 1678 **Census:** 122 **Outpatient Visits:** 54600 **Births:** 225 **Total Expense ($000):** 40163 **Payroll Expense ($000):** 16272 **Personnel:** 386

LONG PRAIRIE—Todd County

★ **LONG PRAIRIE MEMORIAL HOSPITAL AND HOME (241326)**, 20 Ninth Street S.E., Zip 56347–1404; tel. 320/732–2141, (Total facility includes 95 beds in nursing home–type unit) **A**9 10 18 **F**2 7 8 12 13 15 24 25 27 30 31 32 38 55 57 62 66 74 75 76 79 80 86 87 96 97 99 107 117 118 119 121 122 132 135 137 **S** CentraCare Health System
Primary Contact: Roger B. Oberg, Administrator
CFO: Larry Knutson, Finance Director
CMO: Paul Van Gorp, M.D., Chief of Staff
CHR: Joyce Chan, Manager Human Resources
Web address: www.centracare.com
Control: Other not–for–profit (including NFP Corporation) **Service:** General Medical and Surgical

Staffed Beds: 122 **Admissions:** 785 **Census:** 96 **Outpatient Visits:** 21086 **Births:** 151 **Total Expense ($000):** 18976 **Payroll Expense ($000):** 8055 **Personnel:** 223

LUVERNE—Rock County

★ **SIOUX VALLEY LUVERNE MEDICAL CENTER (241371)**, 1600 North Kniss, Zip 56156–2519; tel. 507/283–2321 **A**9 10 18 **F**3 4 5 7 8 11 13 15 24 25 27 28 30 31 32 33 38 42 43 44 45 54 55 56 57 62 63 66 73 74 75 76 79 80 81 82 84 86 87 96 102 103 107 118 120 121 122 124 135 136 137 **P**5 **S** Sanford Health
Primary Contact: Mark Henke, Chief Executive Officer
COO: Tammy Loosbrock, Chief Operating Officer
CFO: Christopher Brown, Chief Financial Officer
CMO: Joshua Crabtree, M.D., Chief of Staff
Web address: www.sanfordluverne.org
Control: Other not–for–profit (including NFP Corporation) **Service:** General Medical and Surgical

Staffed Beds: 25 **Admissions:** 860 **Census:** 7 **Outpatient Visits:** 19701 **Births:** 140 **Total Expense ($000):** 13944 **Payroll Expense ($000):** 5091 **Personnel:** 157

MADELIA—Watonwan County

☒ **MADELIA COMMUNITY HOSPITAL (241323)**, 121 Drew Avenue S.E., Zip 56062–1899; tel. 507/642–3255 **A**1 9 10 18 **F**11 13 15 30 31 32 33 38 44 55 57 61 62 66 67 73 74 75 79 80 81 85 86 92 96 102 117 119 121 122 134 **P**6
Primary Contact: Candace Fenske, Chief Executive Officer
CFO: Donna M. Klinkner, Chief Financial Officer
CHR: Donna M. Klinkner, Chief Financial Officer
Web address: www.mchospital.org
Control: Other not–for–profit (including NFP Corporation) **Service:** General Medical and Surgical

Staffed Beds: 21 **Admissions:** 427 **Census:** 4 **Outpatient Visits:** 9917 **Births:** 37 **Total Expense ($000):** 6639 **Payroll Expense ($000):** 3026 **Personnel:** 63

MADISON—Lac Qui Parle County

MADISON HOSPITAL (241372), 820 Third Avenue, Zip 56256–1014, Mailing Address: 900 Second Avenue, Zip 56256–1006; tel. 320/598–7556 **A**9 10 18 **F**10 11 15 24 25 26 27 31 32 38 55 57 61 62 63 75 77 79 84 86 87 96 100 107 115 119 122 134 136 **P**5
Primary Contact: Scott Larson, Chief Executive Officer
CIO: Jerry Harberts, Information Technologist
CHR: Sally Fernholz, Director Human Resources
Web address: www.madisonlutheranhome.com
Control: Other not–for–profit (including NFP Corporation) **Service:** General Medical and Surgical

Staffed Beds: 12 **Admissions:** 540 **Census:** 5 **Outpatient Visits:** 22620 **Births:** 12 **Total Expense ($000):** 4202 **Payroll Expense ($000):** 1427 **Personnel:** 56

MAHNOMEN—Mahnomen County

★ **MAHNOMEN HEALTH CENTER (241300)**, 414 West Jefferson Avenue, Zip 56557–4912, Mailing Address: P.O. Box 396, Zip 56557–0396; tel. 218/935–2511, (Total facility includes 48 beds in nursing home–type unit) **A**9 10 18 **F**7 15 26 33 38 42 43 54 55 56 57 61 66 75 86 93 96 117 119 120 121 122 135 137 **S** MeritCare Health System
Primary Contact: Susan Klabo, Administrator
CFO: Mary Pazdernik, Chief Financial Officer
CMO: Sanjit Dutta, M.D., Chief Medical Officer
CHR: Kristi Agnew, Human Resources Generalist
Web address: www.mahnomenhealthcenter.com
Control: City–County, Government, nonfederal **Service:** General Medical and Surgical

Staffed Beds: 66 **Admissions:** 225 **Census:** 48 **Outpatient Visits:** 10666 **Births:** 0 **Total Expense ($000):** 6204 **Payroll Expense ($000):** 2902 **Personnel:** 105

MANKATO—Blue Earth County

☒ **IMMANUEL ST. JOSEPH'S–MAYO HEALTH SYSTEM (240093)**, 1025 Marsh Street, Zip 56002–8673, Mailing Address: P.O. Box 8673, Zip 56002–8673; tel. 507/625–4031 **A**1 3 5 9 10 19 **F**3 5 11 13 15 18 20 24 25 26 27 29 30 31 32 33 34 36 37 38 40 42 43 49 52 53 55 57 58 59 60 61 62 63 64 66 68 72 73 74 75 76 77 79 80 81 82 84 86 87 88 90 92 93 94 96 97 99 100 102 103 106 107 108 109 111 118 119 121 124 133 135 136 137 **P**6 **S** Mayo Foundation
Primary Contact: Greg Kutcher, M.D., President and Chief Executive Officer
CFO: Gregory Burkel, Chief Financial Officer
CMO: Anthony Jaspers, M.D., President Medical Staff
CIO: Thomas Borowski, Chief Information Officer
CHR: Julie Oliver, Chief Human Resources Officer
Web address: www.isj–mhs.org
Control: Other not–for–profit (including NFP Corporation) **Service:** General Medical and Surgical

Staffed Beds: 174 **Admissions:** 10688 **Census:** 105 **Outpatient Visits:** 311239 **Births:** 1638 **Total Expense ($000):** 191550 **Payroll Expense ($000):** 94411 **Personnel:** 1599

MARSHALL—Lyon County

☒ **AVERA MARSHALL REGIONAL MEDICAL CENTER (241359)**, 300 South Bruce Street, Zip 56258–3900; tel. 507/532–9661, (Total facility includes 76 beds in nursing home–type unit) **A**1 9 10 18 **F**2 3 10 11 12 13 15 24 25 27 30 31 32 34 38 41 46 52 56 57 61 68 73 74 75 76 79 80 81 82 86 87 88 90 92 94 95 96 100 103 107 115 117 118 119 121 122 124 132 135 136 **P**3 6 **S** Avera Health
Primary Contact: Mary Maertens, Chief Executive Officer
CFO: Sharon Williams, Vice President Information and Financial Services
CMO: Jane Willett, D.O., Chief of Staff
CIO: Sharon Williams, Vice President Information and Financial Services
CHR: Bonnie Barnhardt, Vice President Human Resources
Web address: www.wmmc.org
Control: City–Government, nonfederal **Service:** General Medical and Surgical

Staffed Beds: 111 **Admissions:** 1202 **Census:** 89 **Outpatient Visits:** 15911 **Births:** 352 **Total Expense ($000):** 17302 **Payroll Expense ($000):** 9559 **Personnel:** 334

MELROSE—Stearns County

★ **MELROSE AREA HOSPITAL – CENTRACARE (241330)**, 11 North Fifth Avenue West, Zip 56352–1098; tel. 320/256–4231, (Total facility includes 75 beds in nursing home–type unit) **A**9 10 18 **F**2 6 13 15 24 26 27 30 31 32 33 38 45 46 54 55 56 57 62 68 73 74 75 76 77 79 80 84 86 96 102 107 109 115 117 118 119 121 122 135 137 **P**5 **S** CentraCare Health System
Primary Contact: Joan D. Jackson, Chief Executive Officer
CFO: Todd Stordahl, Chief Financial Officer
Web address: www.centracare.com
Control: Other not–for–profit (including NFP Corporation) **Service:** General Medical and Surgical

Staffed Beds: 93 **Admissions:** 583 **Census:** 80 **Outpatient Visits:** 14100 **Births:** 81 **Total Expense ($000):** 13457 **Payroll Expense ($000):** 5461 **Personnel:** 149

Many Facility Codes have changed. Please refer to the AHA Guide Code Chart.

MINNEAPOLIS—Hennepin County

⊠ **ABBOTT NORTHWESTERN HOSPITAL (240057)**, 800 East 28th Street, Zip 55407–3799; tel. 612/863–4000, (Includes SISTER KENNY REHABILITATION INSTITUTE) **A**1 2 3 5 8 9 10 **F**3 8 9 12 13 15 17 18 20 22 24 25 26 27 30 31 32 33 34 35 36 38 40 41 43 44 45 46 47 48 49 50 51 52 53 54 55 56 57 58 59 60 62 64 66 68 72 73 74 75 76 77 79 80 81 82 85 86 87 88 89 90 91 92 93 94 95 96 97 98 99 100 101 102 103 104 105 106 107 108 109 110 111 112 114 116 118 119 120 121 124 125 126 127 128 129 130 131 132 134 135 136 137 **P**1 5 **S** Allina Hospitals & Clinics
Primary Contact: Jeffrey D. Peterson, President and Chief Executive Officer
COO: Ken Paulus, Chief Operating Officer
CFO: Brian Weinreis, Vice President Operations and Finance
CMO: Robert Wieland, M.D., Vice President Medical Affairs
Web address: www.abbottnorthwestern.com
Control: Other not–for–profit (including NFP Corporation) **Service:** General Medical and Surgical

Staffed Beds: 637 **Admissions:** 38964 **Census:** 487 **Outpatient Visits:** 332000 **Births:** 4324 **Total Expense ($000):** 757526 **Payroll Expense ($000):** 303790 **Personnel:** 4047

☐ **CHILDREN'S HOSPITALS AND CLINICS OF MINNESOTA (243302)**, (pediatric), 2525 Chicago Avenue South, Zip 55404–9976; tel. 612/813–6100 **A**1 3 5 9 10 **F**3 5 8 9 11 12 17 19 21 23 25 26 27 28 30 33 34 36 38 39 42 43 44 50 52 53 55 56 57 58 60 61 62 63 64 66 70 71 72 73 75 76 77 79 80 81 82 83 84 86 87 89 90 91 92 94 96 97 100 102 103 104 107 108 109 111 112 114 118 119 120 121 122 123 124 135 137 **P**1 5 6 **S** Children's Hospitals and Clinics of Minnesota
Primary Contact: Alan L. Goldbloom, M.D., President and Chief Executive Officer
COO: Julie Morath, Chief Operating Officer
CFO: Jerry Massmann, Chief Financial Officer
CMO: Phillip M. Kibort, M.D., Chief Medical Officer
CIO: Dave S. Overman, Chief Information Officer
CHR: David Brumbaugh, Vice President Human Resources
Web address: www.childrenshc.org
Control: Other not–for–profit (including NFP Corporation) **Service:** Children's other specialty

Staffed Beds: 193 **Admissions:** 7901 **Census:** 150 **Outpatient Visits:** 148589 **Births:** 0 **Total Expense ($000):** 286722 **Payroll Expense ($000):** 142989 **Personnel:** 2215

FAIRVIEW RIVERSIDE HOSPITAL See University of Minnesota Medical Center, Fairview

⊠ **HENNEPIN COUNTY MEDICAL CENTER (240004)**, 701 Park Avenue South, Zip 55415–1829; tel. 612/873–3000 **A**1 2 3 5 8 9 10 **F**3 5 7 11 12 13 15 16 17 18 20 22 24 25 26 27 28 29 30 31 32 33 36 37 38 40 41 43 44 46 49 50 51 53 54 55 56 57 58 60 62 63 64 66 68 70 72 73 74 75 76 77 79 80 81 82 83 84 85 86 87 88 89 90 91 92 93 94 95 96 97 99 100 101 102 103 106 107 109 111 114 118 119 120 121 123 124 127 133 135 136 137
Primary Contact: Lynn M. Abrahamsen, Chief Executive Officer
CFO: Larry Kryzaniak, Chief Financial Officer
CMO: Michael Belzer, Medical Director
CIO: Joanne Sunquist, Chief Information Officer
CHR: Hilary Marden–Resnik, Vice President Human Resources
Web address: www.hcmc.org
Control: County–Government, nonfederal **Service:** General Medical and Surgical

Staffed Beds: 431 **Admissions:** 21191 **Census:** 318 **Outpatient Visits:** 430554 **Births:** 2892 **Total Expense ($000):** 518171 **Payroll Expense ($000):** 264264 **Personnel:** 3915

⊠ **PHILLIPS EYE INSTITUTE (240196)**, 2215 Park Avenue, Zip 55404–3756; tel. 612/775–8800, (Nonreporting) **A**1 9 10 **S** Allina Hospitals & Clinics
Primary Contact: David B. Orbuch, President
CFO: Mark T. Gillen, Director Finance
CMO: Emmett Carpel, M.D., Medical Director and Chief of Staff
Web address: www.allina.com
Control: Other not–for–profit (including NFP Corporation) **Service:** Eye, ear, nose, and throat

Staffed Beds: 10

☐ **SHRINERS HOSPITALS FOR CHILDREN, TWIN CITIES**, 2025 East River Parkway, Zip 55414–3696; tel. 612/596–6100, (Nonreporting) **A**1 **S** Shriners Hospitals for Children
Primary Contact: Charles C. Lobeck, Administrator
CFO: Edward A. Tusa, Director Finance
CMO: Kenneth Guidera, Chief of Staff
CHR: Karen Frigen, Director Human Resources
Web address: www.shrinershq.org
Control: Other not–for–profit (including NFP Corporation) **Service:** Children's orthopedic

Staffed Beds: 40

SISTER KENNY REHABILITATION INSTITUTE See Abbott Northwestern Hospital

ST. MARY'S HOSPITAL AND REHABILITATION CENTER See University of Minnesota Medical Center, Fairview

UNIVERSITY OF MINNESOTA HOSPITAL AND CLINIC See University of Minnesota Medical Center, Fairview

⊠ **UNIVERSITY OF MINNESOTA MEDICAL CENTER, FAIRVIEW (240080)**, 2450 Riverside Avenue, Zip 55454–1400; tel. 612/672–6000, (Includes FAIRVIEW RIVERSIDE HOSPITAL, 2312 South Sixth Street, Zip 55454; ST. MARY'S HOSPITAL AND REHABILITATION CENTER, 2414 South Seventh Street, Zip 55454; tel. 612/338–2229; UNIVERSITY OF MINNESOTA HOSPITAL AND CLINIC, 420 S.E. Delaware Street, Zip 55455–0392; tel. 612/626–3000), (Total facility includes 41 beds in nursing home–type unit) **A**1 3 5 8 9 10 **F**2 3 4 5 6 8 9 11 12 13 14 15 17 18 19 20 21 22 23 24 25 26 27 28 30 31 32 33 34 36 37 38 39 40 41 43 44 45 46 47 48 49 50 51 54 55 56 57 58 59 60 62 66 67 68 69 70 72 73 74 75 76 77 78 79 80 81 82 83 84 85 86 87 88 89 90 91 92 93 94 95 96 97 98 99 100 101 102 103 104 105 106 107 108 109 111 112 113 114 116 117 118 119 120 121 122 123 124 125 126 127 128 129 130 131 132 133 135 136 137 **P**5 **S** Fairview Health Services
Primary Contact: Gordon L. Alexander, President
CFO: Steven Hill, Vice President Finance
CHR: Charles McIntosh, Senior Director Human Resources
Web address: www.fairview.org
Control: Other not–for–profit (including NFP Corporation) **Service:** General Medical and Surgical

Staffed Beds: 819 **Admissions:** 34573 **Census:** 580 **Outpatient Visits:** 516338 **Births:** 2834 **Total Expense ($000):** 898729 **Payroll Expense ($000):** 332662 **Personnel:** 4853

⊠ △ **VETERANS AFFAIRS MEDICAL CENTER**, One Veterans Drive, Zip 55417–2399; tel. 612/725–2000, (Total facility includes 104 beds in nursing home–type unit) (Nonreporting) **A**1 2 3 5 7 8 **S** Department of Veterans Affairs
Primary Contact: Steven P. Kleinglass, Director
CFO: Paul Resel, Chief Financial Officer
CMO: John Drucker, M.D., Chief of Staff
CHR: Rick Erredge, Chief Human Resources Officer
Web address: www.va.gov/sta/guide/home.asp
Control: Veterans Affairs, Government, federal **Service:** General Medical and Surgical

Staffed Beds: 365

MONTEVIDEO—Chippewa County

★ **CHIPPEWA COUNTY–MONTEVIDEO HOSPITAL (241325)**, 824 North 11th Street, Zip 56265–1683; tel. 320/269–8877 **A**9 10 18 **F**3 7 13 15 24 27 30 31 32 33 38 42 54 55 56 57 61 62 66 73 76 77 79 80 86 87 96 99 102 121 122 124 132 135 **P**5
Primary Contact: Mark E. Paulson, Chief Executive Officer
CFO: Darlene Boike, Manager Business Office
CIO: Jane Myhre, MS, Director Health Information
Web address: www.montevideomedical.com
Control: City–County, Government, nonfederal **Service:** General Medical and Surgical

Staffed Beds: 25 **Admissions:** 1110 **Census:** 10 **Outpatient Visits:** 11683 **Births:** 90 **Total Expense ($000):** 23269 **Payroll Expense ($000):** 9383 **Personnel:** 185

MONTICELLO—Wright County

⊠ **MONTICELLO–BIG LAKE HOSPITAL (241362)**, 1013 Hart Boulevard, Zip 55362–8230; tel. 763/295–2945, (Total facility includes 89 beds in nursing home–type unit) **A**1 9 10 18 **F**3 7 11 13 15 17 26 27 30 31 38 41 51 56 62 66 67 68 74 76 77 79 80 84 96 97 100 102 106 107 117 118 119 135 137 **P**5
Primary Contact: Marshall E. Smith, Chief Executive Officer
COO: Lynn Olson, Chief Operations Officer
CFO: Nancy Friesen, Chief Financial Officer
CMO: William Scheig, M.D., Chief of Staff
CHR: Kathy Voss, Organizational Support Officer
Web address: www.mblch.com
Control: Hospital district or authority, Government, nonfederal **Service:** General Medical and Surgical

Staffed Beds: 114 **Admissions:** 2109 **Census:** 97 **Outpatient Visits:** 33354 **Births:** 664 **Total Expense ($000):** 42882 **Payroll Expense ($000):** 20526 **Personnel:** 343

MN

Hospital, Medicare Provider Number, Address, Telephone, Approval, Facility, and Physician Codes, Health Care System
★ American Hospital Association (AHA) membership
☐ The Joint Commission accreditation
○ American Osteopathic Association (AOA) accreditation
△ Commission on Accreditation of Rehabilitation Facilities (CARF) accreditation

MOOSE LAKE—Carlton County

★ **MERCY HOSPITAL AND HEALTH CARE CENTER (241350)**, 710 South Kenwood Avenue, Zip 55767–9405; tel. 218/485–4481, (Total facility includes 84 beds in nursing home–type unit) **A**9 10 18 **F**3 7 8 10 11 13 15 24 25 27 30 31 32 33 38 40 46 52 55 56 57 61 62 66 68 73 74 75 79 80 81 82 84 86 96 100 102 107 117 119 121 122 124 132 133 135 137 **P**5
Primary Contact: Jason T. Douglas, Chief Executive Officer
COO: William Storck, Chief Operating Officer and Director Human Resources
CFO: Gregg Chartrand, Chief Financial Officer
CHR: William Storck, Chief Operating Officer and Director Human Resources
Web address: www.mercymooselake.org
Control: Hospital district or authority, Government, nonfederal **Service:** General Medical and Surgical

Staffed Beds: 109 **Admissions:** 1348 **Census:** 92 **Outpatient Visits:** 30824 **Births:** 156 **Total Expense ($000):** 31828 **Payroll Expense ($000):** 13327

MORA—Kanabec County

▣ **KANABEC HOSPITAL (241367)**, 301 South Highway 65, Zip 55051; tel. 320/679–1212 **A**1 9 10 18 **F**3 7 11 13 15 24 26 27 30 31 32 33 38 40 42 51 52 55 56 68 73 74 75 76 77 79 80 82 86 96 102 119 121 122 124 133 135 137
Primary Contact: Randy Ulseth, Chief Executive Officer
COO: Christine M. Kimbler, R.N., Chief Operating Officer
CFO: Gordy Forbort, Chief Financial Officer
Web address: www.kanabechospital.org
Control: County–Government, nonfederal **Service:** General Medical and Surgical

Staffed Beds: 25 **Admissions:** 1808 **Census:** 13 **Outpatient Visits:** 23869 **Births:** 181 **Total Expense ($000):** 28808 **Payroll Expense ($000):** 11753 **Personnel:** 226

MN

MORRIS—Stevens County

★ **STEVENS COMMUNITY MEDICAL CENTER (241363)**, 400 East First Street, Zip 56267–0660, Mailing Address: P.O. Box 660, Zip 56267–0660; tel. 320/589–1313 **A**9 10 18 **F**11 12 13 15 24 25 27 30 32 33 37 38 55 57 62 68 74 77 79 80 81 82 84 87 96 100 102 107 119 120 121 122 124 133 134 135 137 **P**6
Primary Contact: John Rau, President and Chief Executive Officer
CFO: Kerrie McEvilly, Director Finance and Information Systems
CIO: Kerrie McEvilly, Director Finance and Information Systems
CHR: Karla Larson, Director Human Resources
Web address: www.scmcmorris.com
Control: Other not–for–profit (including NFP Corporation) **Service:** General Medical and Surgical

Staffed Beds: 25 **Admissions:** 1773 **Census:** 15 **Outpatient Visits:** 109936 **Births:** 94 **Total Expense ($000):** 30635 **Payroll Expense ($000):** 15135 **Personnel:** 222

NEW PRAGUE—Scott County

▣ **QUEEN OF PEACE HOSPITAL (241361)**, 301 Second Street N.E., Zip 56071–1799; tel. 952/758–4431 **A**1 9 10 18 **F**8 11 13 15 17 24 25 26 27 32 33 34 37 38 40 42 43 46 52 55 56 57 61 62 66 68 72 73 74 75 76 77 79 80 82 84 85 86 87 96 97 100 102 105 107 115 118 119 120 121 122 124 135 136 **P**6
Primary Contact: Mary Klimp, Chief Executive Officer
CFO: Paula Nelson, Chief Financial Officer
CMO: Dan Berg, M.D., Chief of Staff
CHR: Jes Kennedy, Director Human Resources
Web address: www.queenofpeacehospital.org
Control: Other not–for–profit (including NFP Corporation) **Service:** General Medical and Surgical

Staffed Beds: 25 **Admissions:** 1411 **Census:** 11 **Outpatient Visits:** 38886 **Births:** 154 **Total Expense ($000):** 28728 **Payroll Expense ($000):** 12643 **Personnel:** 205

NEW ULM—Brown County

▣ **NEW ULM MEDICAL CENTER (241378)**, 1324 Fifth Street North, Zip 56073–1553, Mailing Address: P.O. Box 577, Zip 56073–0577; tel. 507/233–1000 **A**1 9 10 18 **F**3 4 5 7 8 11 12 13 15 17 24 25 27 28 30 31 32 38 42 43 44 53 54 55 56 57 61 62 66 68 73 74 75 76 77 79 80 84 86 87 88 89 90 91 92 93 94 95 96 100 102 107 118 119 120 121 122 124 133 135 137 **S** Allina Hospitals & Clinics
Primary Contact: Lori L. Wightman, President
CFO: Toby Freier, Director Operations, Finance and Assistant Administrator
CMO: Joan Krikava, M.D., Director Medical Affairs
CIO: Toby Freier, Director Operations, Finance and Assistant Administrator
CHR: Diane Rasmussen, Director Human Resources
Web address: www.newulmmedicalcenter.com
Control: Other not–for–profit (including NFP Corporation) **Service:** General Medical and Surgical

Staffed Beds: 35 **Admissions:** 2431 **Census:** 22 **Births:** 347 **Total Expense ($000):** 57460 **Payroll Expense ($000):** 20233 **Personnel:** 372

NORTHFIELD—Dakota County

★ **NORTHFIELD HOSPITAL (240014)**, 2000 North Avenue, Zip 55057–1498; tel. 507/646–1000, (Includes LONG TERM CARE CENTER), (Total facility includes 40 beds in nursing home–type unit) **A**9 10 **F**3 7 11 13 15 26 27 31 33 34 38 42 43 54 55 56 57 61 66 67 74 75 76 77 79 80 84 86 96 100 102 107 117 118 119 120 121 122 135 136
Primary Contact: Kendall C. Bank, President
COO: Mary Crow, Chief Operating Officer
CFO: Roger Stapek, Vice President and Chief Financial Officer
CHR: Kirsten Budin, Director Human Resources
Web address: www.northfieldhospital.org
Control: City–Government, nonfederal **Service:** General Medical and Surgical

Staffed Beds: 75 **Admissions:** 2332 **Census:** 53 **Outpatient Visits:** 34466 **Births:** 415 **Total Expense ($000):** 50706 **Payroll Expense ($000):** 20970 **Personnel:** 420

OLIVIA—Renville County

RC HOSPITAL AND CLINICS (241306), (Formerly Renville County Hospital), 611 East Fairview Avenue, Zip 56277–0800; tel. 320/523–1261 **A**9 10 18 **F**2 3 13 15 17 24 38 42 43 44 67 68 73 74 77 79 80 84 96 102 106 107 118 119 121 122
Primary Contact: Glenn Haugo, Chief Executive Officer
CFO: Nate Blad, Chief Financial Officer
CIO: Cherry Weigel, Director Health Information Management
Web address: www.renvillecountyhospital.org
Control: County–Government, nonfederal **Service:** General Medical and Surgical

Staffed Beds: 25 **Admissions:** 540 **Census:** 5 **Outpatient Visits:** 16708 **Births:** 31 **Total Expense ($000):** 10342 **Payroll Expense ($000):** 4332 **Personnel:** 90

ONAMIA—Mille Lacs County

★ **MILLE LACS HEALTH SYSTEM (241356)**, 200 North Elm Street, Zip 56359–7978; tel. 320/532–3154, (Total facility includes 72 beds in nursing home–type unit) **A**9 10 18 **F**6 7 11 13 24 25 26 27 28 29 30 31 32 33 38 40 42 50 54 55 57 61 62 79 80 81 86 87 97 117 118 119 120 121 122 124 133 137 **P**6
Primary Contact: Larry A. Schulz, Interim Chief Executive Officer
CFO: Chris Gross, Chief Financial Officer
CMO: Thomas H. Bracken, Chief of Staff
CHR: Jeffrey S. Mutz, Vice President Human Resources
Web address: www.millelacshealth.com
Control: Other not–for–profit (including NFP Corporation) **Service:** General Medical and Surgical

Staffed Beds: 90 **Admissions:** 968 **Census:** 74 **Outpatient Visits:** 21779 **Births:** 92 **Total Expense ($000):** 30474 **Payroll Expense ($000):** 14182

ORTONVILLE—Big Stone County

★ **ORTONVILLE AREA HEALTH SERVICES (241342)**, 450 Eastvold Avenue, Zip 56278–1133; tel. 320/839–2502, (Total facility includes 64 beds in nursing home–type unit) **A**5 9 10 18 **F**2 3 11 13 15 24 26 27 30 31 32 33 38 41 42 43 44 49 50 54 55 56 57 61 62 66 67 72 73 74 75 76 77 79 80 81 82 84 86 96 100 102 105 107 117 119 120 122 124 135 **P**4 **S** Sanford Health
Primary Contact: Richard M. Ash, Chief Executive Officer
CFO: James Foster, Administrator Finance
CMO: Robert Ross, M.D., Medical Director
CHR: Kim McCrea, Chief Human Resources Officer
Web address: www.ortonvilleareahealth.org
Control: City–Government, nonfederal **Service:** General Medical and Surgical

Staffed Beds: 81 **Admissions:** 588 **Census:** 64 **Outpatient Visits:** 23283 **Births:** 60 **Total Expense ($000):** 12743 **Payroll Expense ($000):** 4881 **Personnel:** 132

OWATONNA—Steele County

▣ **OWATONNA HOSPITAL (240069)**, 903 South Oak Street, Zip 55060–3234; tel. 507/451–3850 **A**1 9 10 **F**11 13 24 25 30 31 32 33 38 43 55 56 67 68 73 74 75 77 79 84 86 88 90 91 92 93 96 97 102 107 118 119 120 134 **S** Allina Hospitals & Clinics
Primary Contact: Dorothy Erdmann, President
CFO: David Albrecht, Director Finance and Operations and Assistant Administrator
CHR: Mark Sevenich, Director Human Resources
Web address: www.owatonnahospital.com
Control: Other not–for–profit (including NFP Corporation) **Service:** General Medical and Surgical

Staffed Beds: 43 **Admissions:** 2653 **Census:** 23 **Outpatient Visits:** 31803 **Births:** 592 **Total Expense ($000):** 32673 **Payroll Expense ($000):** 14042 **Personnel:** 226

PARK RAPIDS—Hubbard County

☒ **ST. JOSEPH'S AREA HEALTH SERVICES (241380)**, 600 Pleasant Avenue, Zip 56470–1432; tel. 218/732–3311 **A**1 5 9 10 18 **F**3 11 12 13 15 24 25 26 28 30 31 32 33 37 38 42 44 47 55 56 57 61 62 63 68 73 74 75 77 79 80 86 96 97 100 102 106 107 110 118 119 120 121 122 123 135 **S** Catholic Health Initiatives
Primary Contact: Benjamin Koppelman, President and Chief Executive Officer
CFO: Brent Schmidt, Chief Financial Officer
Web address: www.sjahs.org
Control: Church–operated, Nongovernment, not–for profit **Service:** General Medical and Surgical

Staffed Beds: 25 **Admissions:** 1556 **Census:** 16 **Outpatient Visits:** 39595 **Births:** 136 **Total Expense ($000):** 32011 **Payroll Expense ($000):** 14192 **Personnel:** 299

PAYNESVILLE—Stearns County

★ **PAYNESVILLE AREA HEALTH CARE SYSTEM (241349)**, 200 West 1st Street, Zip 56362–1496; tel. 320/243–3767, (Total facility includes 107 beds in nursing home–type unit) **A**9 10 18 **F**2 7 10 11 13 15 17 24 27 30 31 32 38 54 62 73 79 96 97 107 115 117 119 121 122 132 134 135 137 **P**8
Primary Contact: Steven T. Moburg, Chief Executive Officer
CFO: Kirk Johnson, Chief Financial Officer
CMO: Robert Gardner, M.D., Chief of Staff
CIO: Gary Smith, Manager Information Technology
CHR: Paulette Hagen, Director Human Resources
Web address: www.pahcs.com
Control: Hospital district or authority, Government, nonfederal **Service:** General Medical and Surgical

Staffed Beds: 132 **Admissions:** 798 **Census:** 112 **Outpatient Visits:** 20079 **Births:** 117 **Total Expense ($000):** 23309 **Payroll Expense ($000):** 10033 **Personnel:** 166

PERHAM—Otter Tail County

☒ **PERHAM MEMORIAL HOSPITAL AND HOME (241373)**, 665 Third Street S.W., Zip 56573–1199; tel. 218/346–4500, (Total facility includes 96 beds in nursing home–type unit) **A**1 9 10 18 **F**15 24 29 30 31 32 33 38 55 56 57 61 67 74 79 80 84 86 96 107 119 121 122 124 135 **S** MeritCare Health System
Primary Contact: Chuck Hofius, Chief Executive Officer and Administrator
CFO: Brad D. Wurgler, Chief Financial Officer
CIO: Jim Rieber, Director Information Systems
CHR: Kathy Johnson, Director Human Resources
Web address: www.pmhh.com
Control: Hospital district or authority, Government, nonfederal **Service:** General Medical and Surgical

Staffed Beds: 115 **Admissions:** 732 **Census:** 102 **Outpatient Visits:** 15701 **Births:** 105 **Total Expense ($000):** 18949 **Payroll Expense ($000):** 8692 **Personnel:** 265

PINE CITY—Pine County

LAKESIDE MEDICAL CENTER (240211), 129 East Sixth Avenue, Zip 55063; tel. 320/629–2542, (Nonreporting) **A**9 10
Primary Contact: Max Blaufuss, Administrator and Chief Executive Officer
Web address: www.lmc–pcac.com
Control: Corporation, Investor–owned, for–profit **Service:** Other specialty

Staffed Beds: 10

PIPESTONE—Pipestone County

★ **PIPESTONE COUNTY MEDICAL CENTER/AVERA HEALTH (241374)**, 916 4th Avenue S.W., Zip 56164–0370; tel. 507/825–6125, (Total facility includes 43 beds in nursing home–type unit) (Nonreporting) **A**9 10 18 **S** Avera Health
Primary Contact: Bradley D. Burris, Chief Executive Officer
CHR: Claudia Krueger, Director Human Resources
Web address: www.pcmchealth.org
Control: County–Government, nonfederal **Service:** General Medical and Surgical

Staffed Beds: 68

PRINCETON—Sherburne County

☒ **FAIRVIEW NORTHLAND MEDICAL CENTER (240141)**, (Formerly Fairview Northland Health Services), 911 Northland Drive, Zip 55371–2173; tel. 763/389–1313 **A**1 9 10 **F**3 11 13 15 24 25 26 27 28 29 30 31 32 33 38 50 54 57 68 73 74 75 79 80 82 84 86 87 96 100 102 107 119 121 136 **P**6 **S** Fairview Health Services
Primary Contact: Michael Youso, President
CFO: Kim Ericson, Vice President Finance
CMO: Greg Schoen, M.D., Regional Medical Director
Web address: www.fairview.org/northland/
Control: Other not–for–profit (including NFP Corporation) **Service:** General Medical and Surgical

Staffed Beds: 54 **Admissions:** 2233 **Census:** 19 **Outpatient Visits:** 83609 **Births:** 533 **Total Expense ($000):** 75086 **Payroll Expense ($000):** 33373 **Personnel:** 482

RED WING—Goodhue County

☒ **FAIRVIEW RED WING MEDICAL CENTER (240018)**, 701 Fairview Boulevard, Zip 55066–2848, Mailing Address: P.O. Box 95, Zip 55066–0095; tel. 651/267–5000, (Total facility includes 85 beds in nursing home–type unit) **A**1 9 10 **F**3 8 11 13 15 17 24 25 26 27 30 31 32 33 38 40 42 44 45 50 53 55 57 61 62 66 67 68 73 74 75 76 77 79 80 81 82 84 86 87 89 94 96 97 100 102 106 107 115 117 118 119 120 121 124 133 135 136 **P**6 **S** Fairview Health Services
Primary Contact: Scott Wordelman, President and Chief Executive Officer
CFO: Mike Larson, Chief Financial Officer
CMO: Jack Alexander, M.D., Chief Medical Officer
CHR: Kim Trittin, Manager Human Resources
Web address: www.fairview.org
Control: Other not–for–profit (including NFP Corporation) **Service:** General Medical and Surgical

Staffed Beds: 135 **Admissions:** 2455 **Census:** 89 **Outpatient Visits:** 29356 **Births:** 380 **Total Expense ($000):** 85971 **Payroll Expense ($000):** 41855 **Personnel:** 605

REDLAKE—Beltrami County

☒ **U.S. PUBLIC HEALTH SERVICE INDIAN HOSPITAL (240206)**, Highway 1, Zip 56671, Mailing Address: P.O. Box 497, Zip 56671–0497; tel. 218/679–3912 **A**1 9 10 **F**3 15 25 26 30 31 32 36 37 38 39 55 56 57 58 62 63 66 82 84 87 89 90 91 92 94 119 121 123 124 133 137 **P**5 **S** U. S. Indian Health Service
Primary Contact: Constance James, Chief Executive Officer
CMO: John Robinson, M.D., Clinical Director
Web address: www.ihs.gov
Control: PHS, Indian Service, Government, federal **Service:** General Medical and Surgical

Staffed Beds: 19 **Admissions:** 350 **Census:** 4 **Outpatient Visits:** 52919 **Births:** 2

REDWOOD FALLS—Redwood County

★ **REDWOOD AREA HOSPITAL (241351)**, 100 Fallwood Road, Zip 56283–1828; tel. 507/637–4500 **A**9 10 18 **F**2 3 11 13 15 24 25 27 30 38 42 43 44 55 56 57 61 62 63 66 68 73 74 75 76 79 81 82 84 86 102 117 118 119 121 122 124 135 **P**5
Primary Contact: James E. Schulte, Administrator
CFO: John Peyerl, Chief Financial Officer
CIO: Tom Balko, Manager Information Systems
CHR: Jody Rindfleisch, Manager Human Resources
Web address: www.redwoodareahospital.org
Control: City–Government, nonfederal **Service:** General Medical and Surgical

Staffed Beds: 25 **Admissions:** 790 **Census:** 9 **Outpatient Visits:** 13584 **Births:** 114 **Total Expense ($000):** 15461 **Payroll Expense ($000):** 6586 **Personnel:** 136

MN

Hospital, Medicare Provider Number, Address, Telephone, Approval, Facility, and Physician Codes, Health Care System
★ American Hospital Association (AHA) membership
□ The Joint Commission accreditation
○ American Osteopathic Association (AOA) accreditation
△ Commission on Accreditation of Rehabilitation Facilities (CARF) accreditation

ROBBINSDALE—Hennepin County

☒ △ **NORTH MEMORIAL HEALTH CARE (240001)**, 3300 Oakdale Avenue North, Zip 55422–2926; tel. 763/520–5200 **A**1 2 3 5 7 9 10 **F**3 7 11 13 15 17 18 20 22 24 25 26 27 28 30 31 32 33 34 35 36 38 40 41 42 43 44 45 50 52 53 54 55 56 57 59 61 62 66 67 68 70 71 72 73 74 75 76 77 78 79 80 81 82 84 85 86 87 88 90 92 95 96 97 100 102 104 105 107 112 114 118 119 121 122 124 132 133 135 136 137 **P**6 8
Primary Contact: David W. Cress, President and Chief Executive Officer
CFO: Patrick Boran, Chief Financial Officer
CMO: Tom Timmons, M.D., Vice President Medical Affairs
CIO: Patrick Taffe, Vice President Information Services
CHR: David Abrams, Vice President Human Resources
Web address: www.northmemorial.com
Control: Other not–for–profit (including NFP Corporation) **Service:** General Medical and Surgical

Staffed Beds: 424 **Admissions:** 27777 **Census:** 308 **Outpatient Visits:** 345647 **Births:** 3214 **Total Expense ($000):** 565899 **Payroll Expense ($000):** 271783 **Personnel:** 3225

ROCHESTER—Olmsted County

☐ **COMMUNITY BEHAVIORAL HEALTH HOSPITAL – ROCHESTER**, 251 Wood Lake Drive S.E., Zip 55904; tel. 507/206–2561, (Nonreporting) **A**1 **S** Minnesota Deparment of Human Services
Primary Contact: Rod Kornrumpf, Regional Administrator
Web address: www.health.state.mn.us
Control: State–Government, nonfederal **Service:** Psychiatric

Staffed Beds: 16

MN

★ **OLMSTED MEDICAL CENTER (240006)**, 1650 Fourth Street S.E., Zip 55904–4717, Mailing Address: 210 Ninth Street S.E., Zip 55904–4717; tel. 507/288–3443, (Nonreporting) **A**9 10
Primary Contact: Roy A. Yawn, M.D., President and Chief Executive Officer
CFO: Kevin A. Higgins, Assistant Administrator Finance
CMO: David E. Westgard, M.D., MS, Chief Medical Officer
CIO: Susan M. Schuett, Assistant Administrator Information Systems
CHR: Lois Till–Tarara, Assistant Administrator Human Resources
Web address: www.olmmed.org
Control: Other not–for–profit (including NFP Corporation) **Service:** General Medical and Surgical

Staffed Beds: 37

☒ **ROCHESTER METHODIST HOSPITAL (240061)**, 201 West Center Street, Zip 55902–3084; tel. 507/266–7890, (Nonreporting) **A**1 3 5 9 10 **S** Mayo Foundation
Primary Contact: Lynn Frederick, Administrator
COO: Jeffrey Korsmo, Chief Administrative Officer
CFO: Brad Schmidt, Chief Financial Officer
CMO: Michael Rock, M.D., Chair Hospital Practice Committee
CIO: Jessica Grosset, Director Information Technology
CHR: Ken Schneider, Chair Human Resources
Web address: www.mayoclinic.org
Control: Other not–for–profit (including NFP Corporation) **Service:** General Medical and Surgical

Staffed Beds: 335

☒ △ **SAINT MARYS HOSPITAL (240010)**, 1216 Second Street S.W., Zip 55902–1970; tel. 507/255–5123, (Nonreporting) **A**1 3 5 7 8 9 10 **S** Mayo Foundation
Primary Contact: Lynn Frederick, Administrator
COO: Jeffrey Korsmo, Chief Administrative Officer
CFO: Brad Schmidt, Chief Financial Officer
CMO: Michael Rock, M.D., Chair Hospital Practice Committee
CIO: Jessica Grosset, Director Information Technology
CHR: Ken Schneider, Chair Human Resources
Web address: www.mayoclinic.org
Control: Other not–for–profit (including NFP Corporation) **Service:** General Medical and Surgical

Staffed Beds: 797

ROSEAU—Roseau County

☒ **LIFECARE MEDICAL CENTER (241344)**, (Formerly Roseau Area Hospital & Homes), 715 Delmore Avenue, Zip 56751–1599; tel. 218/463–2500, (Total facility includes 124 beds in nursing home–type unit) **A**1 5 9 10 18 **F**3 7 11 13 15 24 25 26 27 28 32 33 38 40 42 43 52 54 55 56 57 61 62 63 66 73 74 75 78 79 80 81 82 84 86 89 90 91 93 94 96 100 102 107 117 118 119 120 121 122 124 133 135 137 **P**6
Primary Contact: Keith Okeson, Chief Executive Officer
COO: Susan C. Lisell, Senior Leader Patient Services
CFO: Cathy Huss, Chief Financial Officer
CHR: Carol Klotz, Director Human Resources
Web address: www.lifecaremedicalcenter.org
Control: Other not–for–profit (including NFP Corporation) **Service:** General Medical and Surgical

Staffed Beds: 149 **Admissions:** 965 **Census:** 133 **Outpatient Visits:** 49939 **Births:** 196 **Total Expense ($000):** 27668 **Payroll Expense ($000):** 12845 **Personnel:** 301

SAINT CLOUD—Stearns County

☒ **ST. CLOUD HOSPITAL (240036)**, 1406 Sixth Avenue North, Zip 56303–1901; tel. 320/251–2700 **A**1 2 3 5 9 10 **F**3 5 11 12 13 14 15 17 18 20 22 24 25 26 27 28 30 32 33 35 36 37 38 40 41 42 43 44 48 49 50 51 53 54 55 56 57 58 59 60 61 62 64 66 67 68 70 72 73 74 75 76 77 78 79 80 81 82 83 84 85 86 87 88 89 90 91 92 93 94 95 96 97 100 102 103 105 106 107 108 109 111 112 116 118 119 121 123 124 133 135 136 137 **P**6 **S** CentraCare Health System
Primary Contact: Craig J. Broman, President
COO: Linda Chmielewski, R.N., Vice President Operations
CFO: John Seckinger, Vice President Corporate Services and Chief Financial Officer
CMO: Dan Whitlock, M.D., Vice President Medical Affairs
CIO: Chuck Dooley, Vice President Information Services
CHR: Duane Rasmusson, Vice President Human Resources
Web address: www.centracare.com
Control: Other not–for–profit (including NFP Corporation) **Service:** General Medical and Surgical

Staffed Beds: 447 **Admissions:** 25785 **Census:** 287 **Outpatient Visits:** 403085 **Births:** 2787 **Total Expense ($000):** 422227 **Payroll Expense ($000):** 189973 **Personnel:** 3546

☒ △ **VETERANS AFFAIRS MEDICAL CENTER**, 4801 Veterans Drive, Zip 56303–2099; tel. 320/252–1670, (Total facility includes 225 beds in nursing home–type unit) **A**1 7 **F**2 3 4 5 11 12 15 25 26 30 31 32 33 37 42 44 45 46 50 52 53 54 57 58 60 62 63 66 73 75 76 77 79 82 86 87 88 90 92 93 94 95 107 117 119 121 124 132 133 135 136 137 **P**6 **S** Department of Veterans Affairs
Primary Contact: Barry I. Bahl, Director
COO: Barry I. Bahl, Director
CFO: Mary Clausen, Chief Financial Officer
CMO: Susan Markstrom, M.D., Chief of Staff
CHR: Lisa Rosendahl, Director Human Resources
Web address: www.visn13.med.va.gov
Control: Veterans Affairs, Government, federal **Service:** Psychiatric

Staffed Beds: 388 **Admissions:** 2223 **Census:** 304 **Outpatient Visits:** 199917 **Births:** 0 **Total Expense ($000):** 114499 **Payroll Expense ($000):** 73257 **Personnel:** 1095

SAINT JAMES—Watonwan County

☒ **ST. JAMES MEDICAL CENTER (241333)**, (Formerly St. James Health Services), 1101 Moulton and Parsons Drive, Zip 56081; tel. 507/375–3261 **A**1 9 10 18 **F**3 13 15 30 38 42 46 55 56 57 61 63 74 77 79 87 96 99 100 119 121 122 124 135 **S** Mayo Foundation
Primary Contact: Matthew Grimshaw, Administrator
CFO: Gregory Burkel, Chief Financial Officer
CMO: Lindy C. Eatwell, M.D., Medical Director
CIO: Pam Kunkel, Manager Information Services
CHR: Philip Berg, Manager Human Resources
Web address: www.stjmc–mhs.org
Control: Other not–for–profit (including NFP Corporation) **Service:** General Medical and Surgical

Staffed Beds: 13 **Admissions:** 317 **Census:** 5 **Outpatient Visits:** 31704 **Births:** 23 **Total Expense ($000):** 11364 **Payroll Expense ($000):** 4183 **Personnel:** 91

SAINT LOUIS PARK—Hennepin County

☒ △ **METHODIST HOSPITAL (240053)**, 6500 Excelsior Boulevard, Zip 55426–4702; tel. 952/993–5000, (Nonreporting) **A**1 2 3 5 7 9 10 **S** Park Nicollet Health Services
Primary Contact: David K. Wessner, President and Chief Executive Officer
COO: Michael Kaupa, Executive Vice President and Chief Operating Officer
CFO: David J. Cooke, Senior Vice President and Chief Financial Officer
CMO: Sam Carlson, M.D., Executive Vice President and Chief Medical Officer
CIO: Francis Cheung, Chief Information Officer
CHR: Arthur La Point, Vice President Human Resources
Web address: www.parknicollet.com
Control: Other not–for–profit (including NFP Corporation) **Service:** General Medical and Surgical

Staffed Beds: 426

SAINT PAUL—Ramsey County

★ △ **BETHESDA HOSPITAL (242004)**, 559 Capitol Boulevard, Zip 55103–2101; tel. 651/232–2000 **A**1 5 7 9 10 **F**1 3 6 25 26 30 31 32 36 41 50 52 54 59 60 62 66 72 73 75 77 80 81 82 86 90 91 93 94 95 96 102 107 118 119 121 135 **P**8 **S** HealthEast Care System
Primary Contact: Catherine Barr, Chief Executive Officer
COO: Ann M. Schrader, Chief Operating Officer
CFO: Brian Johnson, Chief Financial Officer
CMO: Robert Beck, M.D., Vice President Medical Affairs
CIO: Ronald Strachan, Chief Information Officer
CHR: Ginny Sullivan, Vice President Human Resources
Web address: www.healtheast.org
Control: Other not–for–profit (including NFP Corporation) **Service:** General Medical and Surgical

Staffed Beds: 140 **Admissions:** 1195 **Census:** 107 **Outpatient Visits:** 7068 **Births:** 0 **Personnel:** 557

★ **CHILDREN'S HOSPITALS AND CLINICS OF MINNESOTA (243301)**, (pediatric), 345 North Smith Avenue, Zip 55102–2392; tel. 651/220–6000 **A**1 3 5 9 10 **F**3 8 11 12 18 19 20 21 22 23 25 26 27 28 30 33 34 36 38 39 41 42 43 44 50 52 55 56 57 58 59 60 61 62 63 64 66 70 72 73 75 76 77 79 80 81 82 83 84 86 87 89 90 91 92 94 96 97 100 102 103 104 107 108 109 111 112 114 118 119 120 121 122 123 124 135 137 **P**1 5 6 **S** Children's Hospitals and Clinics of Minnesota
Primary Contact: Alan L. Goldbloom, M.D., President and Chief Executive Officer
COO: Julie Morath, Chief Operating Officer
CFO: Jerry Massmann, Chief Financial Officer
CMO: Phillip M. Kibort, M.D., Chief Medical Officer
CIO: David S. Overman, Chief Information Officer
CHR: David Brumbaugh, Vice President Human Resources
Web address: www.childrensmn.org
Control: Other not–for–profit (including NFP Corporation) **Service:** Children's other specialty

Staffed Beds: 133 **Admissions:** 6132 **Census:** 95 **Outpatient Visits:** 172137 **Births:** 0 **Total Expense ($000):** 193070 **Payroll Expense ($000):** 99071 **Personnel:** 1006

□ △ **GILLETTE CHILDREN'S SPECIALTY HEALTHCARE (243300)**, (Pediatric Specialty Hospital), 200 East University Avenue, Zip 55101–2598; tel. 651/291–2848 **A**1 3 5 7 9 10 **F**3 9 25 26 30 32 33 34 37 44 50 53 62 66 69 72 77 78 79 80 83 84 85 86 119 135 **P**6
Primary Contact: Margaret E. Perryman, President and Chief Executive Officer
CFO: James Haddican, Vice President Finance
CMO: Steven Koop, M.D., Medical Director
CIO: Vennifer Fall, Chief Information Officer
CHR: Betty Rivard, Vice President Human Resources
Web address: www.gillettechildrens.org
Control: Other not–for–profit (including NFP Corporation) **Service:** Children's other specialty

Staffed Beds: 60 **Admissions:** 1920 **Census:** 28 **Outpatient Visits:** 95246 **Births:** 0 **Total Expense ($000):** 108103 **Payroll Expense ($000):** 48807 **Personnel:** 737

★ △ **REGIONS HOSPITAL (240106)**, 640 Jackson Street, Zip 55101–2595; tel. 651/254–3456, (Nonreporting) **A**1 2 3 5 7 8 9 10 **S** HealthPartners
Primary Contact: Brock D. Nelson, President and Chief Executive Officer
CFO: Heidi Conrad, Vice President and Chief Financial Officer
CMO: George J. Isham, M.D., Chief Health Officer and Medical Director Health Plan
CIO: Kim LaReau, Vice President and Chief Information Officer
CHR: Bruce W. Edison, Director Human Resources
Web address: www.regionshospital.com
Control: Other not–for–profit (including NFP Corporation) **Service:** General Medical and Surgical

Staffed Beds: 416

★ **ST. JOHN'S HOSPITAL (240210)**, 1575 Beam Avenue, Zip 55109–1126; tel. 651/232–7000 **A**2 9 10 **F**3 13 15 24 25 26 27 30 31 32 33 34 35 36 38 41 42 46 49 50 51 53 55 56 57 59 60 62 66 68 70 72 73 74 75 76 77 79 80 81 82 84 86 90 92 94 96 97 99 100 102 103 105 106 107 109 111 114 116 119 120 121 133 135 136 **P**8 **S** HealthEast Care System
Primary Contact: Scott North, Chief Executive Officer
COO: Ann M. Schrader, Chief Operating Officer
CFO: Robert D. Gill, Vice President and Chief Financial Officer
CMO: Thomas Lundsten, M.D., Medical Director
CHR: Ginny Sullivan, Vice President Human Resources
Web address: www.stjohnshospital-mn.org
Control: Other not–for–profit (including NFP Corporation) **Service:** General Medical and Surgical

Staffed Beds: 193 **Admissions:** 16114 **Census:** 150 **Outpatient Visits:** 199351 **Births:** 2793 **Total Expense ($000):** 181346 **Payroll Expense ($000):** 75756 **Personnel:** 1284

★ **ST. JOSEPH'S HOSPITAL (240063)**, 69 West Exchange Street, Zip 55102–1053; tel. 651/232–3000 **A**1 3 5 9 10 **F**3 4 5 11 12 13 15 17 18 20 22 24 25 26 27 30 31 32 33 34 35 36 38 40 41 42 44 45 46 49 50 54 55 56 57 58 59 60 62 66 68 71 72 73 74 75 76 77 79 80 82 86 88 90 91 92 93 94 95 96 97 100 102 107 108 109 112 118 119 121 135 136 137 **P**8 **S** HealthEast Care System
Primary Contact: Sara J. Criger, Chief Executive Officer
COO: Ann M. Schrader, Vice President and Chief Operating Officer
CFO: Robert D. Gill, Vice President and Chief Financial Officer
CMO: Robert Beck, M.D., Vice President Medical Affairs
Web address: www.healtheast.org
Control: Other not–for–profit (including NFP Corporation) **Service:** General Medical and Surgical

Staffed Beds: 258 **Admissions:** 13066 **Census:** 180 **Outpatient Visits:** 91474 **Births:** 1020 **Total Expense ($000):** 203009 **Payroll Expense ($000):** 82734 **Personnel:** 1403

★ △ **UNITED HOSPITAL (240038)**, 333 North Smith Avenue, Zip 55102–2389; tel. 651/241–8000, (Nonreporting) **A**1 2 3 5 7 9 10 **S** Allina Hospitals & Clinics
Primary Contact: Mark G. Mishek, President
COO: Ken Paulus, Chief Operating Officer
CFO: John Bien, Vice President Finance
CMO: Daniel Foley, M.D., Vice President Medical Affairs
CIO: Robert Plaszcz, Chief Information Officer
CHR: James McGlade, Director Human Resources
Web address: www.allina.com
Control: Other not–for–profit (including NFP Corporation) **Service:** General Medical and Surgical

Staffed Beds: 449

MN

SAINT PETER—Nicollet County

□ **COMMUNITY BEHAVIORAL HEALTH HOSPITAL – ST. PETER (244004)**, 2000 Klein Street, Zip 56082–5800; tel. 507/933–5001, (Nonreporting) **A**1 10 **S** Minnesota Deparment of Human Services
Primary Contact: Carol Olson, Administrator
Web address: www.health.state.mn.us
Control: State–Government, nonfederal **Service:** Psychiatric

Staffed Beds: 560

★ **ST. PETER COMMUNITY HOSPITAL (241334)**, 1900 North Sunrise Drive, Zip 56082–1327; tel. 507/931–2200, (Nonreporting) **A**9 10 18
Primary Contact: Colleen A. Spike, Administrator
CFO: Kenneth D. Cornish, Chief Financial Officer
CMO: Benjamin Chaska, M.D., Chief Medical Staff
CIO: Paulette Redman, Manager Health Information Management
CHR: Tammie Hudspith, Director Human Resources
Web address: www.stpeterhealth.org
Control: City–Government, nonfederal **Service:** General Medical and Surgical

Staffed Beds: 17

SANDSTONE—Pine County

★ **PINE MEDICAL CENTER (241309)**, 109 Court Avenue South, Zip 55072–5120; tel. 320/245–2212, (Total facility includes 69 beds in nursing home–type unit) (Nonreporting) **A**9 10 18 **S** Essentia Health
Primary Contact: Timothy E. Zwickey, Administrator and Chief Executive Officer
CFO: Greg Tarnowski, Chief Financial Officer
CMO: Brian Barstad, M.D., Chief of Staff
Web address: www.pinemedical.org
Control: Other not–for–profit (including NFP Corporation) **Service:** General Medical and Surgical

Staffed Beds: 94

SAUK CENTRE—Stearns County

★ **ST. MICHAEL'S HOSPITAL AND NURSING HOME (241368)**, 425 North Elm Street, Zip 56378–1010; tel. 320/352–2221, (Total facility includes 60 beds in nursing home–type unit) (Nonreporting) **A**9 10 18
Primary Contact: Delano Christianson, Administrator
CFO: Delano Christianson, Administrator
Web address: www.stmichaelshospital.org
Control: City–Government, nonfederal **Service:** General Medical and Surgical

Staffed Beds: 85

Hospital, Medicare Provider Number, Address, Telephone, Approval, Facility, and Physician Codes, Health Care System
★ American Hospital Association (AHA) membership
□ The Joint Commission accreditation
○ American Osteopathic Association (AOA) accreditation
△ Commission on Accreditation of Rehabilitation Facilities (CARF) accreditation

SHAKOPEE—Scott County

★ **ST. FRANCIS REGIONAL MEDICAL CENTER (240104)**, 1455 St. Francis Avenue, Zip 55379–3380; tel. 952/403–3000 **A**1 2 9 10 **F**3 11 13 14 15 25 26 27 31 32 33 36 38 43 44 50 55 56 57 66 67 68 71 73 74 75 76 77 79 81 82 84 86 96 100 102 107 118 119 120 121 124 132 133 135 136 **P**5 **S** Allina Hospitals & Clinics
Primary Contact: Michael A. Baumgartner, President
COO: Lori Peterson, Chief Operating Officer and Vice President Patient Care
CFO: Cynthia Vincent, Vice President Finance
CMO: Brian Prokosch, M.D., Vice President Medical Affairs
CIO: Joe Delveaux, Manager Information Services
CHR: Ann Glaves, Vice President Human Resources
Web address: www.stfrancis–shakopee.com
Control: Other not–for–profit (including NFP Corporation) **Service:** General Medical and Surgical

Staffed Beds: 86 **Admissions:** 5934 **Census:** 45 **Outpatient Visits:** 109717 **Births:** 1231 **Total Expense ($000):** 88533 **Payroll Expense ($000):** 36903 **Personnel:** 531

SLAYTON—Murray County

★ **MURRAY COUNTY MEDICAL CENTER (241319)**, 2042 Juniper Avenue, Zip 56172–1016; tel. 507/836–6111 **A**9 10 18 **F**3 7 8 24 25 27 28 33 37 38 40 52 54 55 62 63 68 73 79 80 81 82 86 87 96 102 118 119 120 122 124 137 **P**5 **S** Sanford Health
Primary Contact: Meldon L. Snow, Chief Executive Officer
CFO: Renee Logan, Chief Financial Officer
CMO: Sajjad Rizvi, M.D., Chief Medical Officer
CIO: Paul Pettit, Director Information Technology
CHR: Nancy Andert, Director Human Resources
Web address: www.murraycountymed.org
Control: County–Government, nonfederal **Service:** General Medical and Surgical

Staffed Beds: 25 **Admissions:** 486 **Census:** 4 **Outpatient Visits:** 15751 **Births:** 0 **Total Expense ($000):** 7057 **Payroll Expense ($000):** 3760

SLEEPY EYE—Brown County

SLEEPY EYE MEDICAL CENTER (241327), 400 Fourth Avenue N.W., Zip 56085–1109, Mailing Address: P.O. Box 323, Zip 56085–0323; tel. 507/794–3571 **A**10 18 **F**3 13 15 24 33 38 55 57 67 74 75 79 84 86 96 102 118 119 122 **P**6
Primary Contact: Kevin Sellheim, Chief Executive Officer
Web address: www.semedicalcenter.org
Control: City–Government, nonfederal **Service:** General Medical and Surgical

Staffed Beds: 25 **Admissions:** 388 **Census:** 3 **Outpatient Visits:** 11149 **Births:** 12 **Total Expense ($000):** 6863 **Payroll Expense ($000):** 3137 **Personnel:** 83

SPRINGFIELD—Brown County

☐ **SPRINGFIELD MEDICAL CENTER–MAYO HEALTH SYSTEM (241352)**, 625 North Jackson Avenue, Zip 56087–1714, Mailing Address: P.O. Box 146, Zip 56087–0146; tel. 507/723–6201 **A**1 9 10 18 **F**3 13 15 24 27 30 31 32 34 37 38 55 56 57 63 73 74 79 80 84 86 87 96 102 117 121 122 124 **P**6 **S** Mayo Foundation
Primary Contact: Scott D. Thoreson, Administrator
CHR: Marian Schoper, Manager Human Resources
Web address: www.smc–mhs.org
Control: Other not–for–profit (including NFP Corporation) **Service:** General Medical and Surgical

Staffed Beds: 24 **Admissions:** 557 **Census:** 5 **Outpatient Visits:** 21252 **Births:** 43 **Total Expense ($000):** 11129 **Payroll Expense ($000):** 5659 **Personnel:** 101

STAPLES—Todd County

LAKEWOOD HEALTH SYSTEM (241329), 49725 County 83, Zip 56479–5280; tel. 218/894–1515, (Total facility includes 100 beds in nursing home–type unit) **A**9 10 18 **F**3 6 7 8 10 11 12 13 15 24 25 26 27 31 32 33 34 37 38 42 43 44 50 52 54 55 56 57 61 62 63 66 73 75 76 77 79 80 81 82 86 89 90 91 92 93 94 96 102 107 113 115 117 118 119 120 121 122 124 132 135 136 137 **P**7
Primary Contact: Tim Rice, President
CFO: Jim Dregney, Chief Financial Officer
CMO: John Halfen, M.D., Medical Director
CIO: JoEllen Einerwold, Director Information Services
CHR: Janet Jacobson, Director Human Resources
Web address: www.lakewoodhealthsystem.com
Control: Other not–for–profit (including NFP Corporation) **Service:** General Medical and Surgical

Staffed Beds: 125 **Admissions:** 1298 **Census:** 100 **Outpatient Visits:** 213600 **Births:** 292 **Total Expense ($000):** 55827 **Payroll Expense ($000):** 22534 **Personnel:** 592

STILLWATER—Washington County

★ **LAKEVIEW HOSPITAL (240066)**, 927 West Churchill Street, Zip 55082–5930; tel. 651/439–5330 **A**1 5 9 10 **F**3 7 11 12 13 15 17 24 25 27 28 30 31 32 33 34 38 42 43 44 45 50 52 55 56 57 61 62 68 73 74 76 77 79 80 81 82 84 86 96 97 99 100 102 106 107 118 119 121 123 124 131 134 135 137 **P**6
Primary Contact: Curt Geissler, President
CFO: Doug Johnson, Chief Financial Officer
CMO: Charles Bransford, M.D., Medical Director
CIO: Bill Overby, Manager Information Systems
CHR: Angy Duchesneau, Director Human Resources
Web address: www.lakeview.org
Control: Other not–for–profit (including NFP Corporation) **Service:** General Medical and Surgical

Staffed Beds: 66 **Admissions:** 4741 **Census:** 35 **Outpatient Visits:** 57650 **Births:** 704 **Total Expense ($000):** 80894 **Payroll Expense ($000):** 31337 **Personnel:** 545

THIEF RIVER FALLS—Pennington County

★ **MERITCARE THIEF RIVER FALLS NORTHWEST MEDICAL CENTER (241381)**, (Formerly Northwest Medical Center), 120 LaBree Avenue South, Zip 56701–2819, Mailing Address: P.O. Box 531, Zip 56701–0531; tel. 218/681–4240, (Total facility includes 90 beds in nursing home–type unit) (Nonreporting) **A**9 10 18
Primary Contact: Christine K. Harff, Chief Executive Officer
COO: Rob Lovejoy, Chief Operating Officer
CFO: Thomas Wang, Director Finance
CMO: Janell Hudson, Chief Clinical Officer
CHR: Rob Lovejoy, Chief Operating Officer
Control: Other not–for–profit (including NFP Corporation) **Service:** General Medical and Surgical

Staffed Beds: 125

TRACY—Lyon County

★ **SANFORD TRACY MEDICAL CENTER (241303)**, (Formerly Sanford Tracy), 251 Fifth Street East, Zip 56175–1536; tel. 507/629–3200 **A**9 10 18 **F**3 11 24 27 28 31 32 38 54 55 56 57 61 62 66 69 75 79 80 82 84 86 87 96 97 100 115 118 119 120 121 122 124 132 **S** Sanford Health
Primary Contact: Richard E. Nordahl, Administrator and Chief Executive Officer
CFO: Stacy Barstad, Chief Financial Officer and Director Operations
CMO: M. Fareed, M.D., Chief Medical Officer
CIO: Janet Theisen, Chief Information Officer
CHR: Becky Foster, Manager Human Resources
Web address: www.tracyareamedical.org
Control: Other not–for–profit (including NFP Corporation) **Service:** General Medical and Surgical

Staffed Beds: 25 **Admissions:** 348 **Census:** 4 **Outpatient Visits:** 17349 **Births:** 0 **Total Expense ($000):** 8565 **Payroll Expense ($000):** 3763 **Personnel:** 97

TWO HARBORS—Lake County

LAKE VIEW MEMORIAL HOSPITAL AND HOME (241308), 325 11th Avenue, Zip 55616–1360; tel. 218/834–7300, (Total facility includes 50 beds in nursing home–type unit) **A**9 10 18 **F**5 10 17 24 32 33 38 42 43 44 52 57 62 73 75 79 86 90 100 102 107 117 119 122 133 137 **P**5
Primary Contact: Brian J. Carlson, FACHE, President and Chief Executive Officer
Web address: www.lvmhospital.com
Control: Other not–for–profit (including NFP Corporation) **Service:** General Medical and Surgical

Staffed Beds: 68 **Admissions:** 326 **Census:** 41 **Outpatient Visits:** 12649 **Births:** 0 **Total Expense ($000):** 11263 **Payroll Expense ($000):** 4969 **Personnel:** 108

TYLER—Lincoln County

TYLER HEALTHCARE CENTER/AVERA HEALTH (241348), 240 Willow Street, Zip 56178–0280, Mailing Address: P.O. Box 280, Zip 56178–0280; tel. 507/247–5521, (Total facility includes 38 beds in nursing home–type unit) **A**9 10 18 **F**3 7 12 15 27 29 30 32 33 38 42 52 55 56 57 61 62 63 67 75 79 86 96 117 119 121 122 135 **P**6 **S** Avera Health
Primary Contact: Dale K. Kruger, Chief Executive Officer and Chief Financial Officer
CFO: Dale K. Kruger, Chief Executive Officer and Chief Financial Officer
Web address: www.averamckennan.org/amck/regionalfacilities/tyler/
Control: Other not–for–profit (including NFP Corporation) **Service:** General Medical and Surgical

Staffed Beds: 52 **Admissions:** 236 **Census:** 39 **Outpatient Visits:** 2040 **Births:** 0 **Total Expense ($000):** 8665 **Payroll Expense ($000):** 4508 **Personnel:** 113

MN

Many Facility Codes have changed. Please refer to the AHA Guide Code Chart.

VIRGINIA—St. Louis County

★ △ **VIRGINIA REGIONAL MEDICAL CENTER (240084)**, 901 Ninth Street North, Zip 55792–2398; tel. 218/741–3340, (Total facility includes 116 beds in nursing home–type unit) **A**1 7 9 10 **F**3 7 11 13 15 17 24 25 26 30 31 32 33 38 40 43 44 51 54 55 56 57 62 66 68 72 73 74 78 79 82 84 85 87 96 97 100 102 107 112 117 118 119 121 135 136 137 **P**6
Primary Contact: Keith D. Harvey, Chief Executive Officer
CFO: Daniel J. Rabideaux, Chief Financial Officer
CMO: John Linstromberg, M.D., Chief of Staff
CIO: Barb Johnson, Manager Business and Medical Records
CHR: Stephen Roskoski, Director Human Resources
Web address: www.vrmc.org
Control: City–Government, nonfederal **Service:** General Medical and Surgical

Staffed Beds: 199 **Admissions:** 3087 **Census:** 140 **Outpatient Visits:** 47144 **Births:** 295 **Total Expense ($000):** 47832 **Payroll Expense ($000):** 21996 **Personnel:** 435

WABASHA—Wabasha County

★ **SAINT ELIZABETH'S MEDICAL CENTER (241335)**, 1200 Grant Boulevard West, Zip 55981–1098; tel. 651/565–4531, (Total facility includes 148 beds in nursing home–type unit) **A**9 10 18 **F**2 5 6 10 11 12 13 15 24 25 26 30 31 32 33 38 40 50 52 54 55 57 61 62 63 73 74 75 79 80 82 86 89 90 91 93 94 96 99 102 107 115 117 119 121 122 132 133 134 135 137 **P**6 **S** Marian Health System
Primary Contact: Thomas Crowley, President and Chief Executive Officer
CFO: John Wolfe, Chief Financial Officer
CMO: Rob Taylor, M.D., President Medical Staff
CHR: Jim Root, Director Human Resources
Web address: www.stelizabethswabasha.org
Control: Church–operated, Nongovernment, not–for profit **Service:** General Medical and Surgical

Staffed Beds: 168 **Admissions:** 719 **Census:** 140 **Outpatient Visits:** 24995 **Births:** 87 **Total Expense ($000):** 20081 **Payroll Expense ($000):** 9678 **Personnel:** 249

WACONIA—Carver County

★ **RIDGEVIEW MEDICAL CENTER (240056)**, 500 South Maple Street, Zip 55387–1791; tel. 952/442–2191 **A**1 2 9 10 **F**3 7 13 15 18 20 24 26 27 28 29 30 31 32 33 36 38 42 43 55 56 57 58 61 62 63 68 72 73 74 75 76 77 79 80 81 82 84 86 96 97 100 102 106 107 118 119 120 121 124 135 136 137
Primary Contact: Robert Stevens, President and Chief Executive Officer
CFO: Gordon Gablenz, Vice President Finance
CIO: Marilyn Foss, Director Management Information Systems
CHR: Sarah Hastings, Director Human Resources
Web address: www.ridgeviewmedical.org
Control: Other not–for–profit (including NFP Corporation) **Service:** General Medical and Surgical

Staffed Beds: 91 **Admissions:** 6672 **Census:** 50 **Outpatient Visits:** 118048 **Births:** 1268 **Total Expense ($000):** 99869 **Payroll Expense ($000):** 49758 **Personnel:** 662

WADENA—Wadena County

★ **TRI–COUNTY HOSPITAL (241354)**, 415 North Jefferson Street, Zip 56482–1297; tel. 218/631–3510 **A**1 9 10 18 **F**3 7 10 11 13 15 17 24 27 30 31 32 33 38 42 43 44 50 53 54 55 57 61 62 63 68 73 74 75 76 79 80 81 84 86 96 107 119 120 121 122 124 135 137 **P**5
Primary Contact: Dennis C. Miley, President and Chief Executive Officer
CFO: Joel Beiswenger, Chief Financial Officer and Treasurer
CMO: Tim Schmitt, M.D., Chief Medical Officer
CIO: Bill Blaha, Manager Information Technology
CHR: Kellie Weller, Manager Human Resources
Web address: www.tricountyhospital.org
Control: Other not–for–profit (including NFP Corporation) **Service:** General Medical and Surgical

Staffed Beds: 25 **Admissions:** 1371 **Census:** 15 **Outpatient Visits:** 68965 **Births:** 170 **Total Expense ($000):** 33818 **Payroll Expense ($000):** 14416 **Personnel:** 266

WARREN—Marshall County

★ **NORTH VALLEY HEALTH CENTER (241337)**, 109 South Minnesota Street, Zip 56762–1499; tel. 218/745–4211, (Nonreporting) **A**9 10 18
Primary Contact: Kevin J. Smith, Chief Executive Officer
CFO: Susan Butler, Chief Financial Officer
Web address: www.nvhc.net
Control: Other not–for–profit (including NFP Corporation) **Service:** General Medical and Surgical

Staffed Beds: 20

WASECA—Waseca County

□ **WASECA MEDICAL CENTER (241345)**, 501 North State Street, Zip 56093–2811; tel. 507/835–1210, (Nonreporting) **A**1 5 9 10 12 13 18 **S** Mayo Foundation
Primary Contact: Michael Milbrath, Executive Vice President
CFO: Michael Kubat, Director Finance and Information
Web address: www.wmc–mhs.org
Control: Other not–for–profit (including NFP Corporation) **Service:** General Medical and Surgical

Staffed Beds: 25

WESTBROOK—Cottonwood County

★ **SANFORD WESTBROOK MEDICAL CENTER (241302)**, 920 Bell Avenue, Zip 56183–0188, Mailing Address: P.O. Box 188, Zip 56183–0188; tel. 507/274–6121 **A**9 10 18 **F**3 27 30 31 32 38 54 55 56 57 61 62 66 69 73 75 79 80 84 86 87 89 90 91 92 93 94 96 97 100 115 119 120 121 122 124 132 **P**6 **S** Sanford Health
Primary Contact: Richard E. Nordahl, Administrator and Chief Executive Officer
COO: Gordon Kopperud, Director Operations
CFO: Stacy Barstad, Chief Financial Officer
CIO: Janet Theisen, Chief Information Officer
CHR: Becky Foster, Manager Human Resources
Web address: www.westbrookhealthcenter.org
Control: Other not–for–profit (including NFP Corporation) **Service:** General Medical and Surgical

Staffed Beds: 6 **Admissions:** 170 **Census:** 2 **Outpatient Visits:** 7721 **Births:** 0 **Total Expense ($000):** 4174 **Payroll Expense ($000):** 1686 **Personnel:** 35

WHEATON—Traverse County

★ **WHEATON COMMUNITY HOSPITAL (241304)**, 401 12th Street North, Zip 56296–1099; tel. 320/563–8226 **A**9 10 18 **F**3 7 11 13 15 24 25 27 30 31 32 33 34 38 50 52 54 55 56 57 62 63 68 73 74 75 76 79 80 81 87 92 96 99 102 107 117 121 122 123 124 136 137 **P**6
Primary Contact: Jesse G. Tischer, Administrator
CFO: Shane Ayres, Chief Financial Officer
CHR: Brenda Petersen, Director Human Resources
Web address: www.wheatonhealthcare.org
Control: City–Government, nonfederal **Service:** General Medical and Surgical

Staffed Beds: 15 **Admissions:** 1088 **Census:** 6 **Outpatient Visits:** 10496 **Births:** 17 **Total Expense ($000):** 6664 **Payroll Expense ($000):** 2537 **Personnel:** 57

WILLMAR—Kandiyohi County

★ **RICE MEMORIAL HOSPITAL (240088)**, 301 Becker Avenue S.W., Zip 56201–3395; tel. 320/235–4543, (Total facility includes 74 beds in nursing home–type unit) **A**1 2 9 10 19 **F**7 11 12 13 15 24 25 26 27 30 33 34 37 38 42 43 44 47 48 49 55 56 57 59 62 66 68 71 73 74 75 76 77 79 81 82 86 88 90 91 92 93 94 95 96 97 100 102 106 107 109 117 118 119 120 121 124 132 135 136 137
Primary Contact: Lawrence J. Massa, Chief Executive Officer
COO: Dale Hustedt, Associate Administrator Administrative Services
CFO: Bill Fenske, Chief Financial Officer
CMO: George Gordon, M.D., Chief Medical Officer
CHR: Dale Hustedt, Associate Administrator Administrative Services
Web address: www.ricehospital.com
Control: City–Government, nonfederal **Service:** General Medical and Surgical

Staffed Beds: 183 **Admissions:** 4809 **Census:** 115 **Outpatient Visits:** 23664 **Births:** 866 **Total Expense ($000):** 83073 **Payroll Expense ($000):** 38355 **Personnel:** 688

□ **WILLMAR ADULT MENTAL HEALTH PROGRAM (244005)**, 1550 Highway 71 N.E., Zip 56201; tel. 320/231–5100, (Nonreporting) **A**1 9 10 **S** Minnesota Deparment of Human Services
Primary Contact: Sandra J. Butturff, Site Director
COO: Fran Bly, Chief Operating Officer
CFO: Shirley Jacobson, Chief Financial Officer
CMO: Alan Radke, M.D., Chief Medical Officer
CIO: Tom Meierhofer, Utilization and Performance Management Director
Control: State–Government, nonfederal **Service:** Psychiatric

Staffed Beds: 164

MN

Hospital, Medicare Provider Number, Address, Telephone, Approval, Facility, and Physician Codes, Health Care System

★ American Hospital Association (AHA) membership
□ The Joint Commission accreditation
○ American Osteopathic Association (AOA) accreditation
△ Commission on Accreditation of Rehabilitation Facilities (CARF) accreditation

WINDOM—Cottonwood County

★ **WINDOM AREA HOSPITAL (241332)**, 2150 Hospital Drive, Zip 56101–0339, Mailing Address: P.O. Box 339, Zip 56101–0339; tel. 507/831–2400 **A**9 10 18 **F**11 13 15 24 27 32 33 38 52 55 56 57 74 75 79 86 96 102 107 119 122 **S** Sanford Health
Primary Contact: Geraldine S. Burmeister, Chief Executive Officer
CFO: Kim Armstrong, Chief Financial Officer
CIO: Lori Ling, Information Technician
CHR: Katie Slette, Director Human Resources and Marketing
Web address: www.windomareahospital.com
Control: City–Government, nonfederal **Service:** General Medical and Surgical

Staffed Beds: 25 **Admissions:** 814 **Census:** 6 **Outpatient Visits:** 20500 **Births:** 134 **Total Expense ($000):** 10723 **Payroll Expense ($000):** 4271 **Personnel:** 96

WINONA—Winona County

★ **WINONA HEALTH (240044)**, 855 Mankato Avenue, Zip 55987–5377, Mailing Address: P.O. Box 5600, Zip 55987–0600; tel. 507/454–3650 **A**9 10 20 **F**11 13 15 24 25 26 28 30 32 33 34 36 38 43 48 50 52 54 55 56 57 59 60 62 66 68 72 73 74 75 76 77 79 80 81 82 84 86 88 89 90 91 92 93 94 96 97 99 100 102 106 107 108 112 118 119 120 121 124 133 135 136 137 **P**6
Primary Contact: Rachelle H. Schultz, President and Chief Executive Officer
CFO: Michael Allen, Chief Financial Officer
CMO: Charles Shepard, M.D., Medical Director
CHR: Bill Gould, Chief People Resource Officer
Web address: www.winonahealth.org
Control: Other not–for–profit (including NFP Corporation) **Service:** General Medical and Surgical

Staffed Beds: 68 **Admissions:** 3154 **Census:** 32 **Outpatient Visits:** 66099 **Births:** 408 **Total Expense ($000):** 53380 **Payroll Expense ($000):** 23885 **Personnel:** 743

MN

WOODBURY—Washington County

★ **WOODWINDS HEALTH CAMPUS (240213)**, 1925 Woodwinds Drive, Zip 55125; tel. 651/232–0100 **A**1 5 9 10 **F**3 13 15 24 25 26 27 30 31 32 33 34 35 36 38 41 42 49 50 55 56 57 58 60 62 63 66 68 71 72 73 74 75 76 77 79 80 81 82 86 96 97 100 102 107 118 119 121 124 135 **P**8 **S** HealthEast Care System
Primary Contact: Julie A. Schmidt, Chief Executive Officer
CMO: Lynne Lillie, M.D., Medical Director
CHR: Tammy Arrigoni, Human Resources Lead
Web address: www.woodwinds.org
Control: Other not–for–profit (including NFP Corporation) **Service:** General Medical and Surgical

Staffed Beds: 78 **Admissions:** 6890 **Census:** 57 **Outpatient Visits:** 73868 **Births:** 1590 **Total Expense ($000):** 97819 **Payroll Expense ($000):** 34694 **Personnel:** 562

WORTHINGTON—Nobles County

★ **WORTHINGTON REGIONAL HOSPITAL (240022)**, 1018 Sixth Avenue, Zip 56187–2202, Mailing Address: P.O. Box 997, Zip 56187–0997; tel. 507/372–2941 **A**9 10 20 **F**7 11 13 17 24 27 30 31 32 33 38 40 43 57 59 61 62 66 67 68 70 73 74 75 77 79 80 81 82 84 85 86 87 88 89 90 91 92 93 96 100 102 107 109 111 119 120 121 122 124 135 136 137 **S** Sanford Health
Primary Contact: Melvin J. Platt, Chief Executive Officer
Web address: www.worthingtonhospital.com
Control: City–Government, nonfederal **Service:** General Medical and Surgical

Staffed Beds: 64 **Admissions:** 2025 **Census:** 20 **Outpatient Visits:** 40300 **Births:** 442 **Total Expense ($000):** 23023 **Payroll Expense ($000):** 11041 **Personnel:** 212

WYOMING—Chisago County

★ **FAIRVIEW LAKES REGIONAL HEALTH CARE (240050)**, 5200 Fairview Boulevard, Zip 55092–8013; tel. 651/982–7000 **A**1 9 10 **F**3 5 11 13 15 24 25 26 27 28 30 31 32 33 38 40 42 43 44 45 51 52 53 54 55 56 57 61 62 63 68 73 74 75 76 79 81 82 86 87 96 100 102 107 109 113 118 119 120 121 122 123 132 133 135 136 137 **P**6 **S** Fairview Health Services
Primary Contact: Daniel K. Anderson, President
COO: Dave Dobosenski, Chief Operating Officer
CFO: Mark Bortnem, Vice President Finance
CMO: Terry Martinson, M.D., Medical Director
CHR: Darci Tanberg, Director Human Resources
Web address: www.fairview.org/lakes/flrmc.htm
Control: Other not–for–profit (including NFP Corporation) **Service:** General Medical and Surgical

Staffed Beds: 55 **Admissions:** 4781 **Census:** 38 **Outpatient Visits:** 118831 **Births:** 894 **Total Expense ($000):** 133175 **Payroll Expense ($000):** 63567 **Personnel:** 889

MISSISSIPPI

ABERDEEN—Monroe County

PIONEER COMMUNITY HOSPITAL OF ABERDEEN (251302), 400 South Chestnut Street, Zip 39730–3335, Mailing Address: P.O. Box 548, Zip 39730–0747; tel. 662/369–2455 **A**9 10 18 **F**3 10 11 15 25 30 31 32 33 38 40 46 52 53 54 55 56 57 62 73 79 81 82 86 87 88 90 91 92 93 94 95 96 118 119 120 121 122 **S** Pioneer Health Services
Primary Contact: Steven M. Fontaine, Administrator
CFO: Julie Gieger, Chief Financial Officer
CMO: Kevin Hayes, M.D., Chief of Staff
CHR: Lee Rob, Director Human Resources
Web address: www.pchaberdeen.com
Control: Corporation, Investor–owned, for–profit **Service:** General Medical and Surgical

Staffed Beds: 35 **Admissions:** 407 **Census:** 8 **Outpatient Visits:** 3512 **Births:** 0 **Total Expense ($000):** 12780 **Payroll Expense ($000):** 4839 **Personnel:** 149

ACKERMAN—Choctaw County

CHOCTAW COUNTY MEDICAL CENTER (251310), 148 West Cherry Street, Zip 39735–0417, Mailing Address: P.O. Box 1039, Zip 39735–0417; tel. 662/285–6235, (Total facility includes 60 beds in nursing home–type unit) **A**9 10 18 **F**38 40 84 88 117 119 122 **P**6
Primary Contact: Tami Jones, Administrator
CFO: James L. Miller, Chief Financial Officer
CMO: Ronnie Medlin, M.D., Chief of Staff
CHR: Debra Ward, Executive Administrative Assistant and Manager Human Resources
Control: Corporation, Investor–owned, for–profit **Service:** General Medical and Surgical

Staffed Beds: 83 **Admissions:** 565 **Census:** 62 **Outpatient Visits:** 19374 **Births:** 0 **Personnel:** 145

AMORY—Monroe County

☐ **GILMORE MEMORIAL REGIONAL MEDICAL CENTER (250025)**, 1105 Earl Frye Boulevard, Zip 38821–0459, Mailing Address: P.O. Box 459, Zip 38821–0459; tel. 662/256–7111 **A**1 9 10 **F**13 15 17 25 30 31 32 33 38 40 52 68 70 71 73 74 75 79 81 82 83 84 85 86 97 100 107 119 135 136 **P**6 **S** Health Management Associates
Primary Contact: Dwayne Blaylock, Chief Executive Officer
COO: Paul V. Peiffer, Chief Operating Officer
CFO: Shea Sutherland, Chief Financial Officer
CMO: Dwight McComb, M.D., Chief Medical Officer
CIO: Jeff Wideman, Director Information Systems
CHR: Debbie Carson, Director Human Resources
Web address: www.gilmorehealth.com
Control: Corporation, Investor–owned, for–profit **Service:** General Medical and Surgical

Staffed Beds: 95 **Admissions:** 3464 **Census:** 36 **Outpatient Visits:** 40790 **Births:** 636 **Personnel:** 348

BATESVILLE—Panola County

BATESVILLE SPECIALTY HOSPITAL (252011), 303 Medical Center Drive, Zip 38606; tel. 662/712–2484 **A**10 **F**30 31 32
Primary Contact: Candace Eldib, Administrator
Control: Corporation, Investor–owned, for–profit **Service:** Long–Term Acute Care hospital

Staffed Beds: 12 **Admissions:** 33 **Census:** 2 **Outpatient Visits:** 0 **Births:** 0 **Personnel:** 13

TRI–LAKES MEDICAL CENTER (250128), 303 Medical Center Drive, Zip 38606–8608; tel. 662/563–5611 **A**9 10 **F**3 4 5 11 13 15 17 25 26 28 30 31 32 33 38 50 52 54 56 62 63 66 68 74 79 80 82 84 87 88 90 91 93 94 95 96 97 102 106 119 121 132 135 136 137
Primary Contact: Barry Morrison, Chief Executive Officer
CFO: John Gregory, Chief Financial Officer
CMO: Robert S. Corkern, M.D., Medical Director
CIO: Edward Pipkin, Director Information Technology
CHR: Sarah Dale Ball, JD, Vice President Human Resources and Risk Management
Web address: www.trilakesmedical.com
Control: Other not–for–profit (including NFP Corporation) **Service:** General Medical and Surgical

Staffed Beds: 88 **Admissions:** 3633 **Census:** 60 **Outpatient Visits:** 16571 **Births:** 202 **Total Expense ($000):** 29180 **Payroll Expense ($000):** 16392 **Personnel:** 404

BAY SAINT LOUIS—Hancock County

★☐ **HANCOCK MEDICAL CENTER (250162)**, 149 Drinkwater Boulevard, Zip 39521–2790, Mailing Address: P.O. Box 2790, Zip 39521–2790; tel. 228/467–8600 **A**1 9 10 **F**3 11 13 15 17 24 25 28 30 31 32 33 37 38 40 51 55 56 57 63 64 66 68 73 74 75 77 79 80 81 82 84 85 86 87 96 97 98 99 100 102 107 118 119 120 124 134 135 136 137 **S** QHR
Primary Contact: Hal W. Leftwich, FACHE, Administrator
CHR: Audrey Dunn, Director Human Resources
Web address: www.hmc.org
Control: County–Government, nonfederal **Service:** General Medical and Surgical

Staffed Beds: 41 **Admissions:** 2450 **Census:** 25 **Outpatient Visits:** 25477 **Births:** 294 **Total Expense ($000):** 23538 **Payroll Expense ($000):** 17703 **Personnel:** 347

MS

BAY SPRINGS—Jasper County

★ **JASPER GENERAL HOSPITAL (250018)**, 15 A South Sixth Street, Zip 39422–9738, Mailing Address: P.O. Box 527, Zip 39422–0527; tel. 601/764–2101, (Includes JASPER COUNTY NURSING HOME), (Total facility includes 110 beds in nursing home–type unit) **A**9 10 **F**30 31 42 61 82 117 119 122
Primary Contact: M. Kenneth Posey, FACHE, Administrator
CFO: Steve Green, Comptroller
CMO: A. K. Lay, M.D., Chief Medical Officer
CHR: JoAnn Boyd, Administrative Assistant
Control: County–Government, nonfederal **Service:** General Medical and Surgical

Staffed Beds: 126 **Admissions:** 71 **Census:** 108 **Outpatient Visits:** 0 **Births:** 0 **Personnel:** 56

BELZONI—Humphreys County

HUMPHREYS COUNTY MEMORIAL HOSPITAL (251311), 500 CCC Road, Zip 39038–3806, Mailing Address: P.O. Box 510, Zip 39038–0510; tel. 662/247–3831 **A**9 10 18 **F**2 13 25 30 31 32 38 54 84 85 86 88 93 107 117 122
Primary Contact: Ray Shoemaker, Chief Executive Officer
CFO: Gaye Walker, Controller
Control: County–Government, nonfederal **Service:** General Medical and Surgical

Staffed Beds: 34 **Admissions:** 909 **Census:** 11 **Outpatient Visits:** 7776 **Births:** 0 **Personnel:** 135

BILOXI—Harrison County

☐ **BILOXI REGIONAL MEDICAL CENTER (250007)**, 150 Reynoir Street, Zip 39530–4199, Mailing Address: P.O. Box 128, Zip 39533–0128; tel. 228/432–1571 **A**1 9 10 **F**13 15 17 25 30 31 32 33 38 40 60 68 71 73 74 75 76 78 79 81 82 83 84 85 86 87 90 93 96 97 100 106 107 119 132 135 136 **P**8 **S** Health Management Associates
Primary Contact: Timothy W. Mitchell, Chief Executive Officer
COO: Joan Strayham, Chief Operating Officer
CFO: Brenda Whitwell, Chief Financial Officer
CMO: Stephen Jones, M.D., President Medical Affairs
CHR: Dale Shaw, Director Human Resources
Web address: www.hmamississippi.com
Control: Corporation, Investor–owned, for–profit **Service:** General Medical and Surgical

Staffed Beds: 153 **Admissions:** 6370 **Census:** 78 **Outpatient Visits:** 79813 **Births:** 821 **Personnel:** 535

Hospital, Medicare Provider Number, Address, Telephone, Approval, Facility, and Physician Codes, Health Care System

★ American Hospital Association (AHA) membership
☐ The Joint Commission accreditation
○ American Osteopathic Association (AOA) accreditation
△ Commission on Accreditation of Rehabilitation Facilities (CARF) accreditation

☒ △ **VETERANS AFFAIRS GULF COAST VETERANS HEALTH CARE SYSTEM**, 400 Veterans Avenue, Zip 39531–2410; tel. 228/523–5000, (Total facility includes 160 beds in nursing home–type unit) (Nonreporting) **A**1 3 5 7 **S** Department of Veterans Affairs
Primary Contact: Charles E. Sepich, FACHE, Director
COO: Deborah M. Johnson, Associate Director
CFO: Wayne I. Deal, Chief Financial Officer
CMO: Ana Mello, M.D., Chief of Staff
CIO: David D. Wagner, Chief Information Management Service
CHR: Frank Kehus, Acting Chief Human Resource Management and Workforce Development Service
Web address: www.va.gov/biloxi
Control: Veterans Affairs, Government, federal **Service:** General Medical and Surgical

Staffed Beds: 552

BOONEVILLE—Prentiss County

☒ **BAPTIST MEMORIAL HOSPITAL–BOONEVILLE (250044)**, 100 Hospital Street, Zip 38829–3359; tel. 662/720–5000 **A**1 9 10 **F**3 11 15 17 24 25 26 30 31 32 38 40 52 55 56 57 63 66 68 73 79 81 82 84 87 88 90 93 96 97 100 102 107 118 119 121 122 124 **P**3 **S** Baptist Memorial Health Care Corporation
Primary Contact: Larkin Kennedy, Administrator and Chief Executive Officer
CFO: Diane Wilson, Chief Financial Officer
CMO: Nathan Baldwin, M.D., President Medical Staff
CIO: Linda Chaffin, Director Quality
Web address: www.bmhcc.org
Control: Church–operated, Nongovernment, not–for profit **Service:** General Medical and Surgical

Staffed Beds: 66 **Admissions:** 1472 **Census:** 23 **Outpatient Visits:** 31591 **Births:** 1 **Personnel:** 218

BRANDON—Rankin County

MS

☐ **CROSSGATES RIVER OAKS HOSPITAL (250096)**, (Formerly Rankin Medical Center), 350 Crossgates Boulevard, Zip 39042–2698; tel. 601/825–2811 **A**1 9 10 **F**17 30 31 32 38 40 52 61 68 75 76 79 82 83 84 85 86 87 88 93 96 97 100 106 107 119 **P**8 **S** Health Management Associates
Primary Contact: J. Allen Tyra, Chief Executive Officer
COO: Nathan Howell, Chief Operating Officer
CFO: Brad Sinclair, Chief Financial Officer
CMO: James Jefferson, M.D., Chief of Staff
CIO: Cindy White, Director Health Information Systems
CHR: Mark Cook, Director Human Resources
Web address: www.rankinmedcenter.com
Control: Corporation, Investor–owned, for–profit **Service:** General Medical and Surgical

Staffed Beds: 134 **Admissions:** 4275 **Census:** 61 **Outpatient Visits:** 50753 **Births:** 0 **Personnel:** 418

BROOKHAVEN—Lincoln County

☒ **KING'S DAUGHTERS MEDICAL CENTER (250057)**, 427 Highway 51 North, Zip 39601–2600, Mailing Address: P.O. Box 948, Zip 39602–0948; tel. 601/833–6011 **A**1 9 10 20 **F**13 15 17 25 31 32 33 37 38 40 42 52 60 68 71 73 74 75 78 79 81 83 84 86 87 97 119 120 121 135 136 **S** QHR
Primary Contact: Alvin Hoover, FACHE, Chief Executive Officer
CFO: Dean Snider, Chief Financial Officer
CIO: Carl Smith, Director Information Systems
CHR: Celine Craig, Director Human Resources
Web address: www.kdmc.org
Control: Other not–for–profit (including NFP Corporation) **Service:** General Medical and Surgical

Staffed Beds: 99 **Admissions:** 3945 **Census:** 40 **Outpatient Visits:** 69447 **Births:** 514 **Personnel:** 470

CALHOUN CITY—Calhoun County

★ **CALHOUN HEALTH SERVICES (250112)**, 140 Burke–Calhoun City Road, Zip 38916–9690; tel. 662/628–6611, (Total facility includes 120 beds in nursing home–type unit) **A**9 10 **F**7 31 38 40 66 82 84 86 88 93 96 100 102 107 117 119 122 **S** North Mississippi Health Services, Inc.
Primary Contact: James P. Franklin, Administrator
CFO: Mandy Suber, Controller
CMO: Guy Farmer, M.D., President Medical Staff
Web address: www.nmhs.net/calhoun_city
Control: City–County, Government, nonfederal **Service:** General Medical and Surgical

Staffed Beds: 150 **Admissions:** 722 **Census:** 123 **Outpatient Visits:** 4970 **Births:** 0 **Total Expense ($000):** 12355 **Payroll Expense ($000):** 6677 **Personnel:** 251

CANTON—Madison County

MADISON COUNTY MEDICAL CENTER (250038), Highway 16 East, Zip 39046–8823, Mailing Address: P.O. Box 1607, Zip 39046–1607; tel. 601/859–1331 **A**9 10 **F**15 25 32 33 38 73 74 79 82 84 86 96 107 119 122 135 136 **S** Health Management Associates
Primary Contact: Joseph Weaver, Chief Executive Officer
CFO: Denise Baker, Chief Financial Officer
CMO: Larry Cooper, M.D., Chief of Staff
CIO: Shannon Strong, Director Health Information Management
CHR: Lu Harding, Human Resource Director
Web address: www.madisonregionalmedicalcenter.com
Control: Corporation, Investor–owned, for–profit **Service:** General Medical and Surgical

Staffed Beds: 67 **Admissions:** 2080 **Census:** 22 **Outpatient Visits:** 28149 **Births:** 403 **Personnel:** 141

CARTHAGE—Leake County

LEAKE MEMORIAL HOSPITAL (251315), 310 Ellis Street, Zip 39051, Mailing Address: P.O. Box 909, Zip 39051–0909; tel. 601/267–1100, (Total facility includes 44 beds in nursing home–type unit) **A**9 10 18 **F**25 30 31 32 38 40 82 86 96 107 117 119 122 **P**6
Primary Contact: Robert Faulkner, Administrator
COO: Robert Faulkner, Administrator
CFO: Sandy Goolsby, Accountant
CMO: Manuel Ong, M.D., Chief of Staff
Web address: www.leakemh.org
Control: County–Government, nonfederal **Service:** General Medical and Surgical

Staffed Beds: 69 **Admissions:** 707 **Census:** 49 **Outpatient Visits:** 16254 **Births:** 5 **Personnel:** 157

CENTREVILLE—Wilkinson County

☒ **FIELD MEMORIAL COMMUNITY HOSPITAL (251309)**, 270 West Main Street, Zip 39631, Mailing Address: P.O. Box 639, Zip 39631–0639; tel. 601/645–5221 **A**1 9 10 18 **F**15 25 32 33 37 38 40 60 73 75 79 84 86 96 97 107 119 121 122
Primary Contact: Chao Netterville, Administrator
CFO: Jacquelyn Richoux, Chief Financial Officer
CHR: Debbie Willingham, Administrative Assistant
Web address: www.fmch.org
Control: County–Government, nonfederal **Service:** General Medical and Surgical

Staffed Beds: 25 **Admissions:** 798 **Census:** 8 **Outpatient Visits:** 13320 **Births:** 0 **Personnel:** 159

CHARLESTON—Tallahatchie County

TALLAHATCHIE GENERAL HOSPITAL (251304), 201 South Market, Zip 38921–2236, Mailing Address: P.O. Box 230, Zip 38921–0230; tel. 662/647–5535, (Total facility includes 68 beds in nursing home–type unit) **A**9 10 18 **F**37 38 82 96 117 119 122 **P**6
Primary Contact: Bobby J. Brunson, Jr., Chief Executive Officer
CFO: Sammie Bell, Chief Financial Officer
Control: County–Government, nonfederal **Service:** General Medical and Surgical

Staffed Beds: 77 **Admissions:** 249 **Census:** 67 **Outpatient Visits:** 3216 **Births:** 0 **Personnel:** 161

CLARKSDALE—Coahoma County

☐ **NORTHWEST MISSISSIPPI REGIONAL MEDICAL CENTER (250042)**, 1970 Hospital Drive, Zip 38614–7204, Mailing Address: P.O. Box 1218, Zip 38614–1218; tel. 662/627–3211 **A**1 9 10 19 **F**13 15 16 17 25 30 31 32 33 38 40 60 68 70 71 74 75 76 78 79 81 82 83 84 85 86 96 97 100 106 107 119 120 121 **S** Health Management Associates
Primary Contact: Mark W. Caton, Chief Executive Officer
COO: Jack Hill, Chief Operating Officer
CFO: Steve Marinelli, Chief Financial Officer
CMO: Rodney Baine, M.D., Chief of Staff
CIO: Kayla Carpenter, Health Information Management Systems Officer
CHR: Martha Harthcock, Director Human Resources
Web address: www.nwmsregionalmedcenter.com
Control: Corporation, Investor–owned, for–profit **Service:** General Medical and Surgical

Staffed Beds: 195 **Admissions:** 6471 **Census:** 84 **Outpatient Visits:** 25081 **Births:** 970 **Personnel:** 519

CLEVELAND—Bolivar County

★ **BOLIVAR MEDICAL CENTER (250093)**, 901 East Sunflower Road, Zip 38732–9722, Mailing Address: P.O. Box 1380, Zip 38732–1380; tel. 662/846–0061, (Total facility includes 35 beds in nursing home–type unit) **A**1 10 20 **F**13 15 17 25 32 33 37 38 40 68 71 74 79 82 83 84 86 96 97 100 106 107 117 119 121 **S** LifePoint Hospitals, Inc.
Primary Contact: Stephen Nichols, Chief Executive Officer
CFO: Chad Miller, Chief Financial Officer
CMO: Michael Portrer, Chief Medical Staff
CIO: Dusty Griffith, Director Information Systems
CHR: David Kent, Director Human Resources
Web address: www.bolivarmedical.com
Control: Corporation, Investor–owned, for–profit **Service:** General Medical and Surgical

Staffed Beds: 156 **Admissions:** 5823 **Census:** 97 **Outpatient Visits:** 43288 **Births:** 651 **Personnel:** 364

COLLINS—Covington County

COVINGTON COUNTY HOSPITAL (251325), Gerald McRaney Street, Zip 39428–3899, Mailing Address: P.O. Box 1149, Zip 39428–1149; tel. 601/765–6711 **A**9 10 18 **F**13 15 30 31 32 37 38 40 60 71 74 79 84 85 86 87 88 93 96 107 119 122 **P**6 7
Primary Contact: Thomas Bland, Interim Chief Executive Officer
Control: County–Government, nonfederal **Service:** General Medical and Surgical

Staffed Beds: 35 **Admissions:** 956 **Census:** 16 **Outpatient Visits:** 24445 **Births:** 77 **Personnel:** 187

COLUMBIA—Marion County

MARION GENERAL HOSPITAL (250085), 1560 Sumrall Road, Zip 39429–2654, Mailing Address: P.O. Box 630, Zip 39429–0630; tel. 601/736–6303 **A**9 10 **F**15 17 25 31 33 37 38 60 61 68 79 82 83 84 85 86 87 96 97 100 106 107 119 120 122
Primary Contact: Jerry M. Howell, Chief Executive Officer
Control: County–Government, nonfederal **Service:** General Medical and Surgical

Staffed Beds: 51 **Admissions:** 1450 **Census:** 17 **Outpatient Visits:** 30779 **Births:** 1 **Personnel:** 201

COLUMBUS—Lowndes County

★ **BAPTIST MEMORIAL HOSPITAL–GOLDEN TRIANGLE (250100)**, 2520 Fifth Street North, Zip 39705–2095, Mailing Address: P.O. Box 1307, Zip 39703–1307; tel. 662/244–1000 **A**1 9 10 19 **F**3 4 5 7 13 15 17 18 20 22 24 25 26 27 30 31 32 33 38 40 42 44 49 51 55 56 57 60 62 68 70 71 72 73 74 75 76 78 79 80 81 82 83 84 86 88 90 92 93 94 95 96 97 100 103 104 105 106 107 109 112 116 118 119 120 121 123 135 136 **S** Baptist Memorial Health Care Corporation
Primary Contact: Paul Cade, Interim Administrator and Chief Executive Officer
CFO: Jimmy Robertson, Chief Financial Officer
CIO: Sheila Bardwell, Director Information Systems
CHR: Bob McCallister, Director Human Resources
Web address: www.bmhcc.org
Control: Other not–for–profit (including NFP Corporation) **Service:** General Medical and Surgical

Staffed Beds: 328 **Admissions:** 8588 **Census:** 124 **Outpatient Visits:** 45793 **Births:** 1055 **Total Expense ($000):** 111179 **Payroll Expense ($000):** 37505 **Personnel:** 988

CORINTH—Alcorn County

☐ **MAGNOLIA REGIONAL HEALTH CENTER (250009)**, 611 Alcorn Drive, Zip 38834–9368; tel. 662/293–1000 **A**1 9 10 19 **F**13 15 17 25 30 31 32 33 37 38 40 42 51 52 61 68 73 74 75 76 79 81 82 84 86 88 90 91 92 93 96 97 104 106 107 119 120 121 132 **P**8
Primary Contact: Rick D. Napper, Chief Executive Officer
COO: Jason Boyd, Chief Operating Officer
CFO: Jeff Taylor, Chief Financial Officer
CIO: Hershell Foster, Director Information Technology
CHR: Regenia Brown, Director Human Resources
Web address: www.mrhc.org
Control: City–County, Government, nonfederal **Service:** General Medical and Surgical

Staffed Beds: 164 **Admissions:** 7081 **Census:** 85 **Outpatient Visits:** 104312 **Births:** 603 **Personnel:** 925

ELLISVILLE—Jones County

SOUTH CENTRAL EXTENDED CARE See South Central Regional Medical Center, Laurel

EUPORA—Webster County

★ **NORTH MISSISSIPPI MEDICAL CENTER–EUPORA (250020)**, 70 Medical Plaza, Zip 39744–2215; tel. 662/258–6221, (Total facility includes 35 beds in nursing home–type unit) **A**1 9 10 **F**15 30 31 32 33 38 40 52 81 82 84 96 107 117 119 122 **S** North Mississippi Health Services, Inc.
Primary Contact: John R. Jones, Administrator
CFO: Adonna Mitchell, Manager Business Services
CMO: Sue Simmons, M.D., Chairman Medical Staff
CIO: Shirley Griffin, Manager
CHR: Dorothy Castle, Manager
Web address: www.nmhs.net/eupora
Control: Other not–for–profit (including NFP Corporation) **Service:** General Medical and Surgical

Staffed Beds: 73 **Admissions:** 1654 **Census:** 55 **Outpatient Visits:** 18516 **Births:** 0 **Personnel:** 196

FAYETTE—Jefferson County

JEFFERSON COUNTY HOSPITAL (250060), 870 South Main Street, Zip 39069, Mailing Address: P.O. Box 577, Zip 39069–0577; tel. 601/786–3401 **A**9 10 **F**31 38 93 119
Primary Contact: Jerry Kennedy, Administrator
CFO: Jerry Kennedy, Administrator
CHR: Rochelle McKenzie, R.N., Chief Human Resources
Web address: www.jeffersoncountyhospital@yahoo.com
Control: County–Government, nonfederal **Service:** General Medical and Surgical

Staffed Beds: 30 **Admissions:** 793 **Census:** 19 **Outpatient Visits:** 2285 **Births:** 0 **Personnel:** 61

FOREST—Scott County

S. E. LACKEY MEMORIAL HOSPITAL (251300), 330 Broad Street, Zip 39074–0428, Mailing Address: P.O. Box 428, Zip 39074–0428; tel. 601/469–4151, (Total facility includes 20 beds in nursing home–type unit) **A**10 18 **F**15 25 30 31 32 33 37 38 40 42 46 52 54 55 56 57 62 63 79 81 84 90 94 95 96 97 100 107 117 118 119 120 122 **P**5 **S** Pioneer Health Services
Primary Contact: Donna Riser, Administrator
CIO: Eddie Pope, Chief Information Officer
Web address: www.selackey.com
Control: Other not–for–profit (including NFP Corporation) **Service:** General Medical and Surgical

Staffed Beds: 55 **Admissions:** 1557 **Census:** 40 **Outpatient Visits:** 14962 **Births:** 6 **Total Expense ($000):** 14180 **Payroll Expense ($000):** 4698 **Personnel:** 191

GREENVILLE—Washington County

★ **DELTA REGIONAL MEDICAL CENTER (250082)**, 1400 East Union Street, Zip 38703; tel. 662/334–2099, (Includes THE KING'S DAUGHTERS HOSPITAL, 300 Washington Avenue, Zip 38701–3614, Mailing Address: P.O. Box 1857, Zip 38702–1857; tel. 662/378–2020; L. Ray Humphreys, Chief Executive Officer) **A**1 9 10 19 **F**2 13 15 17 25 30 31 32 33 37 38 40 42 51 52 54 60 61 68 74 76 79 84 86 87 93 94 96 97 100 106 107 119 120 121 133 135 136 **P**6 8
Primary Contact: L. Ray Humphreys, Chief Executive Officer
COO: Allyson Williams, Chief Operating Officer and Chief Nursing Officer
CFO: Courtney Phillips, Chief Financial Officer
CIO: Shane Coleman, Director Information Services
CHR: Alphe Wells, Chief Human Resources Officer
Web address: www.deltaregional.com
Control: County–Government, nonfederal **Service:** General Medical and Surgical

Staffed Beds: 190 **Admissions:** 9655 **Census:** 123 **Outpatient Visits:** 125371 **Births:** 977 **Personnel:** 1254

GREENWOOD—Leflore County

★ △ **GREENWOOD LEFLORE HOSPITAL (250099)**, 1401 River Road, Zip 38930, Mailing Address: Drawer 1410, Zip 38935–1410; tel. 662/459–7000 **A**1 7 9 10 19 **F**13 15 17 30 31 32 33 37 38 40 52 60 68 73 74 79 81 82 84 85 86 88 93 96 97 100 106 107 119 120 121 123 132 135 136 **P**6 8
Primary Contact: Jerry W. Adams, Executive Director
COO: Jeff Curtis, Chief Operating Officer
CFO: James H. Jackson, Chief Financial Officer
CMO: A. Randle White, M.D., Chief Medical Staff
CIO: Mark S. Hutson, Chief Information Officer
CHR: Key Britt, Associate Director
Web address: www.glh.org
Control: City–County, Government, nonfederal **Service:** General Medical and Surgical

Staffed Beds: 198 **Admissions:** 9455 **Census:** 130 **Outpatient Visits:** 252100 **Births:** 859 **Personnel:** 904

MS

Hospital, Medicare Provider Number, Address, Telephone, Approval, Facility, and Physician Codes, Health Care System

★ American Hospital Association (AHA) membership
☐ The Joint Commission accreditation
○ American Osteopathic Association (AOA) accreditation
△ Commission on Accreditation of Rehabilitation Facilities (CARF) accreditation

GREENWOOD SPECIALTY HOSPITAL (252010), 1401 River Road, 2nd Floor, Zip 38935; tel. 662/459–2681 **A**10
Control: Corporation, Investor–owned, for–profit **Service:** Long–Term Acute Care hospital

Staffed Beds: 40 **Admissions:** 441 **Census:** 28 **Outpatient Visits:** 0 **Births:** 0 **Personnel:** 61

GRENADA—Grenada County

★ **GRENADA LAKE MEDICAL CENTER (250015)**, 960 Avent Drive, Zip 38901–5094; tel. 662/227–7000 **A**1 9 10 20 **F**3 7 11 13 15 17 18 20 25 31 32 33 37 38 40 52 55 57 60 61 62 63 66 68 71 72 74 75 77 78 79 80 84 85 86 87 96 97 100 103 106 107 118 119 124 132 136 137
Primary Contact: Charles L. Denton, Chief Executive Officer
CFO: Keith Heartsill, Chief Financial Officer
CIO: Sarah Longest, Chief Information Officer
CHR: Ken Baker, Administrative Director Human Resources
Web address: www.glmc.net
Control: County–Government, nonfederal **Service:** General Medical and Surgical

Staffed Beds: 142 **Admissions:** 3880 **Census:** 52 **Outpatient Visits:** 40077 **Births:** 648 **Total Expense ($000):** 40755 **Payroll Expense ($000):** 17234 **Personnel:** 471

GULFPORT—Harrison County

★ **GARDEN PARK MEDICAL CENTER (250123)**, 15200 Community Road, Zip 39503–3085, Mailing Address: P.O. Box 1240, Zip 39502–1240; tel. 228/575–7000 **A**1 9 10 **F**13 15 17 25 30 31 32 33 38 40 52 68 73 74 75 79 82 84 85 86 87 88 93 96 97 100 104 106 107 119 132 135 136 **P**5 **S** HCA
Primary Contact: William E. Peaks, Chief Executive Officer
CFO: Regina Ramazani, Chief Financial Officer
CHR: Krystyna Jarnado, Director Human Resources
Web address: www.gpmedical.com
Control: Corporation, Investor–owned, for–profit **Service:** General Medical and Surgical

Staffed Beds: 130 **Admissions:** 2698 **Census:** 46 **Outpatient Visits:** 36647 **Births:** 562 **Personnel:** 280

★ △ **MEMORIAL HOSPITAL AT GULFPORT (250019)**, 4500 13th Street, Zip 39501–2569, Mailing Address: P.O. Box 1810, Zip 39502–1810; tel. 228/867–4000, (Includes MEMORIAL BEHAVIORAL HEALTH, 11150 Highway 49 North, Zip 39503–4110; tel. 228/831–1700; Michael A. Zieman, Administrator) **A**1 2 7 9 10 **F**2 4 5 13 15 17 25 31 32 33 38 40 42 51 52 68 70 71 74 75 76 78 79 82 84 85 86 88 89 90 91 92 94 95 96 97 100 104 106 107 119 121 133 **P**3 8
Primary Contact: Gary G. Marchand, President and Chief Executive Officer
COO: Jennifer H. Dumal, Vice President Patient Care Services
CFO: Jeffrey T. Steiner, Vice President Finance
CMO: Nancy Downs, M.D., Vice President Medical Affairs
CIO: Richard Ferrans, M.D., Vice President and Medical Information Officer
CHR: Cathy Wood, Director Human Resources
Web address: www.gulfportmemorial.com
Control: City–County, Government, nonfederal **Service:** General Medical and Surgical

Staffed Beds: 445 **Admissions:** 15708 **Census:** 256 **Outpatient Visits:** 238321 **Births:** 1492 **Personnel:** 2365

☐ **SELECT SPECIALTY HOSPITAL – GULFPORT (252005)**, 1520 Broad Avenue, Suite 300, Zip 39501, Mailing Address: 1521 Broad Avenue, Suite 300, Zip 39501; tel. 228/575–7500 **A**1 10 **F**30 31 32 82 85 119 **S** Select Medical Corporation
Primary Contact: Ray Owens, Chief Executive Officer
Web address: www.selectmedicalcorp.com
Control: Corporation, Investor–owned, for–profit **Service:** Long–Term Acute Care hospital

Staffed Beds: 61 **Admissions:** 314 **Census:** 23 **Outpatient Visits:** 0 **Births:** 0 **Personnel:** 125

HATTIESBURG—Forrest and Lamar County

★ △ **FORREST GENERAL HOSPITAL (250078)**, 6051 U.S. Highway 49, Zip 39401–7243, Mailing Address: P.O. Box 16389, Zip 39404–6389; tel. 601/288–7000 **A**2 5 7 9 10 19 **F**4 5 13 15 17 25 30 31 32 33 38 40 42 52 61 68 70 71 73 74 75 76 79 81 82 84 85 86 88 89 90 92 93 94 96 97 100 106 107 119 120 121 135 136
Primary Contact: William C. Oliver, President
COO: Evan S. Dillard, Vice President and Chief Operating Officer
CFO: Andy Woodward, Chief Financial Officer
CIO: G. Edward Tucker, Vice President Corporate Services
CHR: Robert G. Stultz, Vice President Human Resources
Web address: www.forrestgeneral.com
Control: County–Government, nonfederal **Service:** General Medical and Surgical

Staffed Beds: 512 **Admissions:** 24622 **Census:** 326 **Outpatient Visits:** 126681 **Births:** 2546 **Personnel:** 2724

★ **REGENCY HOSPITAL OF HATTIESBURG (252009)**, 125 South 25th Avenue, Zip 39401; tel. 601/288–8510, (Nonreporting) **A**1 10 **S** Regency Hospital Company
Primary Contact: Douglas L. Johnson, FACHE, Chief Executive Officer
CFO: Lori Baxter, Manager Human Resources
CMO: Steven E. Farrell, M.D., Medical Director
Web address: www.regencyhospital.com/hattiesburg
Control: Partnership, Investor–owned, for–profit **Service:** General Medical and Surgical

Staffed Beds: 33

★ **WESLEY MEDICAL CENTER (250094)**, 5001 Hardy Street, Zip 39402–1366, Mailing Address: P.O. Box 16509, Zip 39404–6509; tel. 601/268–8000 **A**1 9 10 19 **F**13 15 17 25 30 31 32 33 37 38 52 61 68 70 71 73 74 75 76 79 82 84 85 86 87 97 100 106 107 119 121 **S** Community Health Systems, Inc.
Primary Contact: Ronald T. Seal, Chief Executive Officer
COO: Travis Sisson, Chief Operating Officer
CFO: Randy Humphrey, Chief Financial Officer
CMO: John Gaudet, President Medical Staff
CIO: William Toon, Director Information Technology
CHR: Terry Trigg, Director Human Resources
Web address: www.wesley.com
Control: Corporation, Investor–owned, for–profit **Service:** General Medical and Surgical

Staffed Beds: 211 **Admissions:** 10077 **Census:** 131 **Outpatient Visits:** 81063 **Births:** 1700 **Personnel:** 837

HAZLEHURST—Copiah County

★ **HARDY WILSON MEMORIAL HOSPITAL (251327)**, 233 Magnolia Street, Zip 39083–2229, Mailing Address: P.O. Box 889, Zip 39083–0889; tel. 601/894–4541 **A**9 10 18 **F**15 38 74 79 84 86 88 93 96 100 104 107 119 122
Primary Contact: Mike Boleware, Administrator
Control: County–Government, nonfederal **Service:** General Medical and Surgical

Staffed Beds: 35 **Admissions:** 1004 **Census:** 18 **Outpatient Visits:** 10551 **Births:** 0 **Personnel:** 158

HOLLY SPRINGS—Marshall County

★ **ALLIANCE HEALTHCARE SYSTEM (250012)**, 1430 Highway 4 East, Zip 38635, Mailing Address: P.O. Box 6000, Zip 38634–6000; tel. 662/252–1212 **A**9 10 20 **F**15 25 31 32 33 38 40 54 73 79 82 84 88 93 94 96 97 107 119 121 122 132
Primary Contact: Perry E. Williams, Sr., Administrator and Chief Executive Officer
COO: Cecelia Bost, Chief Operating Officer
CFO: Greg G. Underwood, Chief Financial Officer
CMO: Peter Dews, M.D., Medical Director
Web address: www.alliancehealth.us
Control: Corporation, Investor–owned, for–profit **Service:** General Medical and Surgical

Staffed Beds: 40 **Admissions:** 910 **Census:** 13 **Outpatient Visits:** 14409 **Births:** 12 **Personnel:** 120

HOUSTON—Chickasaw County

☐ **TRACE REGIONAL HOSPITAL (250017)**, Highway 8 East, Zip 38851–9396, Mailing Address: P.O. Box 626, Zip 38851–0626; tel. 662/456–3700 **A**1 10 **F**3 15 17 24 30 32 33 38 50 56 57 60 63 64 66 68 73 79 84 85 86 88 93 96 100 102 107 117 119 122 124 137 **P**6 **S** Sunlink Health Systems
Primary Contact: Gary L. Staten, Chief Executive Officer
CFO: Pamela W. Cook, Chief Financial Officer
CMO: J. Ronald Staten, M.D., Chief of Staff
CHR: Carol Colbert, Director Human Resources
Web address: www.traceregional.com
Control: Corporation, Investor–owned, for–profit **Service:** General Medical and Surgical

Staffed Beds: 84 **Admissions:** 1186 **Census:** 16 **Outpatient Visits:** 15402 **Births:** 0 **Total Expense ($000):** 13592 **Payroll Expense ($000):** 6342 **Personnel:** 229

INDIANOLA—Sunflower County

★ **SOUTH SUNFLOWER COUNTY HOSPITAL (250095)**, 121 East Baker Street, Zip 38751–2498; tel. 662/887–5235 **A**1 9 10 20 **F**13 15 17 38 40 68 74 77 79 84 96 100 107 119 **P**8
Primary Contact: Harold J. Blessitt, Administrator
COO: Barbara Prichard, Assistant Administrator
CFO: Meredith Taylor, Comptroller
CMO: Wade Dowell, M.D., Chief of Staff
CIO: Julie Sterling, Information System Manager
Control: County–Government, nonfederal **Service:** General Medical and Surgical

Staffed Beds: 49 **Admissions:** 2569 **Census:** 20 **Outpatient Visits:** 12925 **Births:** 442 **Total Expense ($000):** 13374 **Payroll Expense ($000):** 8017 **Personnel:** 132

Many Facility Codes have changed. Please refer to the AHA Guide Code Chart.

IUKA—Tishomingo County

★ **NORTH MISSISSIPPI MEDICAL CENTER–IUKA (250002)**, 1777 Curtis Drive, Zip 38852–1001, Mailing Address: P.O. Box 860, Zip 38852–0860; tel. 662/423–6051 **A**1 9 10 **F**17 25 30 31 32 33 38 40 52 68 73 79 81 82 84 85 86 96 107 119 121 122 123 **S** North Mississippi Health Services, Inc.
Primary Contact: Fred A. Truesdale, Jr., Administrator
CFO: Betty Moore, Business Manager
CMO: Margaret Glynn, M.D., Chief Medical Staff
CIO: Fred A. Truesdale, Administrator
CHR: Jane Chamblee, Manager Human Resources
Web address: www.nmhs.net
Control: Other not–for–profit (including NFP Corporation) **Service:** General Medical and Surgical

Staffed Beds: 48 **Admissions:** 1671 **Census:** 18 **Outpatient Visits:** 12186 **Births:** 0 **Personnel:** 154

JACKSON—Hinds and Rankin County

☐ **BRENTWOOD BEHAVIORAL HEALTHCARE OF MISSISSIPPI (254007)**, 3531 East Lakeland Drive, Zip 39296–9794; tel. 601/936–2024, (Nonreporting) **A**1 9 10 **S** Psychiatric Solutions
Primary Contact: Michael J. Carney, Chief Executive Officer
Web address: www.psysolutions.com
Control: Corporation, Investor–owned, for–profit **Service:** Psychiatric

Staffed Beds: 107

☐ **CENTRAL MISSISSIPPI MEDICAL CENTER (250072)**, 1850 Chadwick Drive, Zip 39204–3479, Mailing Address: P.O. Box 59001, Zip 39204–9001; tel. 601/376–1000 **A**1 2 10 **F**13 17 30 31 32 33 38 51 60 68 70 71 74 76 78 79 81 82 83 84 85 86 87 88 90 92 93 96 97 100 104 106 107 119 121 135 136 **P**8 **S** Health Management Associates
Primary Contact: Joe D. Pinion, Chief Executive Officer
CFO: Glen Silverman, Chief Financial Officer
CHR: Kevin Korner, Director Human Resources
Web address: www.centralmississippimedicalcenter.com
Control: Corporation, Investor–owned, for–profit **Service:** General Medical and Surgical

Staffed Beds: 429 **Admissions:** 9750 **Census:** 140 **Outpatient Visits:** 35855 **Births:** 1333 **Personnel:** 1067

★ **G.V. MONTGOMERY VETERANS AFFAIRS MEDICAL CENTER**, 1500 East Woodrow Wilson Drive, Zip 39216–5199; tel. 601/364–1201, (Total facility includes 120 beds in nursing home–type unit) (Nonreporting) **A**1 2 3 5 8 **S** Department of Veterans Affairs
Primary Contact: Richard J. Baltz, FACHE, Center Director
COO: Jed Fillingim, Acting Chief Operating Officer and Associate Director
CFO: Joy Willis, Acting Chief Fiscal Service
CMO: Kent Kirchner, M.D., Chief of Staff
CIO: Robert Wolak, Chief Information Resource Management Service
CHR: Sam Evans, Chief Human Resources Management
Web address: www.va.gov
Control: Veterans Affairs, Government, federal **Service:** General Medical and Surgical

Staffed Beds: 443

★ △ **METHODIST REHABILITATION CENTER (250152)**, 1350 Woodrow Wilson Drive, Zip 39216–5198; tel. 601/981–2611, (Total facility includes 60 beds in nursing home–type unit) **A**1 3 5 7 8 9 10 **F**25 30 31 32 33 75 79 81 82 85 86 107 119 121 132
Primary Contact: Mark A. Adams, President and Chief Executive Officer
COO: Joseph M. Morette, Executive Vice President
CFO: Gary Armstrong, Executive Vice President
CIO: Gary Armstrong, Executive Vice President
CHR: Steve Hope, Vice President Corporate Services
Web address: www.methodistrehab.org
Control: Other not–for–profit (including NFP Corporation) **Service:** Rehabilitation

Staffed Beds: 157 **Admissions:** 920 **Census:** 98 **Outpatient Visits:** 38273 **Births:** 0 **Personnel:** 462

★ **MISSISSIPPI BAPTIST MEDICAL CENTER (250102)**, 1225 North State Street, Zip 39202–2002; tel. 601/968–1000 **A**1 2 3 5 9 10 **F**3 4 5 11 13 14 15 17 18 20 22 24 25 26 27 30 31 32 33 35 36 37 38 43 51 55 56 57 58 59 60 62 63 66 68 70 71 72 73 74 76 77 78 79 80 81 84 85 86 88 89 90 93 94 95 96 97 99 100 102 103 104 105 106 107 108 109 112 114 116 119 121 124 133 135 136 137 **P**1 **S** Mississippi Baptist Health System
Primary Contact: C. Gerald Cotton, President
CFO: Russell W. York, Vice President and Chief Financial Officer
CMO: Eric A. McVey, M.D., Vice President and Chief Medical Officer
CIO: Scott C. Groom, Vice President and Chief Information Officer
CHR: Jerry Jones, Vice President Human Resources
Web address: www.mbhs.org
Control: Other not–for–profit (including NFP Corporation) **Service:** General Medical and Surgical

Staffed Beds: 638 **Admissions:** 20423 **Census:** 285 **Outpatient Visits:** 125589 **Births:** 1210 **Total Expense ($000):** 285120 **Payroll Expense ($000):** 98378 **Personnel:** 2672

☐ **MISSISSIPPI HOSPITAL FOR RESTORATIVE CARE (252003)**, 1225 North State Street, Zip 39202–2097, Mailing Address: P.O. Box 23695, Zip 39225–3695; tel. 601/968–1000 **A**1 10 **F**25 30 31 32 54 78 119 **P**7 **S** Mississippi Baptist Health System
Primary Contact: David Jackson, Chief Executive Officer
CFO: Russell W. York, Vice President and Chief Financial Officer
CMO: Holland M. Addison, M.D., Medical Director
CIO: Scott C. Groom, Vice President and Chief Information Officer
CHR: Jerry Jones, Vice President Human Resources
Web address: www.mbhs.org
Control: Other not–for–profit (including NFP Corporation) **Service:** Long–Term Acute Care hospital

Staffed Beds: 25 **Admissions:** 183 **Census:** 18 **Outpatient Visits:** 0 **Births:** 0 **Personnel:** 67

MS

★ **REGENCY HOSPITAL OF JACKSON (250161)**, 971 Lakeland Drive, Zip 39216; tel. 601/364–6200 **F**1 25 38 **S** Regency Hospital Company
Primary Contact: Tommy Jackson, Chief Executive Officer
Web address: www.regencyhospital.com
Control: Partnership, Investor–owned, for–profit **Service:** Long–Term Acute Care hospital

Staffed Beds: 36 **Admissions:** 341 **Census:** 27 **Outpatient Visits:** 0 **Births:** 0 **Personnel:** 117

★ **RIVER OAKS HOSPITAL (250138)**, 1030 River Oaks Drive, Zip 39232, Mailing Address: P.O. Box 5100, Zip 39296–5100; tel. 601/932–1030 **A**1 9 10 **F**3 11 12 13 15 18 25 26 33 37 38 40 41 44 49 50 51 55 56 57 62 66 68 70 71 72 74 76 77 79 80 82 84 85 86 96 97 100 103 106 107 119 124 135 136 **S** Health Management Associates
Primary Contact: Davis A. Richards, III, President and Chief Executive Officer
COO: Cynthia L. Dishongh, Executive Vice President and Chief Operating Officer
CFO: Jeff Bedford, Executive Vice President and Chief Financial Officer
CMO: Peter Neglen, M.D., Chief of Staff
CIO: Pat Jones, Director Information Systems
CHR: Warren Weed, Director Human Resources
Web address: www.riveroakshospital.org
Control: Corporation, Investor–owned, for–profit **Service:** General Medical and Surgical

Staffed Beds: 109 **Admissions:** 7559 **Census:** 79 **Outpatient Visits:** 65098 **Births:** 1829 **Personnel:** 656

☐ **SELECT SPECIALTY HOSPITAL OF JACKSON (252007)**, 5903 Ridgewood Road, Zip 39211; tel. 601/899–3800 **A**1 10 **F**25 30 31 32 75 86 96 119 **S** Select Medical Corporation
Primary Contact: Aaron Anothayanontha, Chief Executive Officer
CFO: Melissa Smith, Controller
CMO: Greg Oden, M.D., Medical Director and Chief of Staff
CIO: Jacqueline Barnes, Manager Health Information
CHR: Vicki Watson, Manager Human Resources
Web address: www.selectmedicalcorp.com
Control: Corporation, Investor–owned, for–profit **Service:** Long–Term Acute Care hospital

Staffed Beds: 53 **Admissions:** 557 **Census:** 40 **Outpatient Visits:** 0 **Births:** 0 **Personnel:** 175

Hospital, Medicare Provider Number, Address, Telephone, Approval, Facility, and Physician Codes, Health Care System

★ American Hospital Association (AHA) membership
☐ The Joint Commission accreditation
○ American Osteopathic Association (AOA) accreditation
△ Commission on Accreditation of Rehabilitation Facilities (CARF) accreditation

★ **ST. DOMINIC–JACKSON MEMORIAL HOSPITAL (250048)**, 969 Lakeland Drive, Zip 39216–4699; tel. 601/200–2000 **A**1 2 3 5 9 10 **F**4 5 13 15 17 25 30 31 32 33 37 38 51 52 60 68 71 73 74 75 76 78 79 81 84 85 86 87 88 89 90 91 92 93 94 95 96 97 100 104 106 107 119 120 135 136 **P**8
Primary Contact: Claude W. Harbarger, President
COO: Lester K. Diamond, Executive Vice President, Operations
CFO: Jennifer Sinclair, Vice President Finance
CMO: Robert L. Mobley, M.D., Executive Vice President Medical Affairs and Quality
CIO: Keith Van Camp, Vice President Information Services
CHR: Lamar Nesbit, Senior Vice President Human Resources and Customer Services
Web address: www.stdom.com
Control: Other not–for–profit (including NFP Corporation) **Service:** General Medical and Surgical

Staffed Beds: 523 **Admissions:** 25523 **Census:** 315 **Outpatient Visits:** 83852 **Births:** 1516 **Personnel:** 2509

★ △ **UNIVERSITY HOSPITALS AND CLINICS, UNIVERSITY OF MISSISSIPPI MEDICAL CENTER (250001)**, 2500 North State Street, Zip 39216–4505; tel. 601/984–1000 **A**1 2 3 5 7 8 9 10 **F**3 7 8 9 11 12 13 15 17 18 19 20 21 22 23 24 25 26 27 30 31 32 33 37 38 40 46 47 48 49 50 51 53 55 56 57 58 60 62 63 64 66 68 69 70 71 72 73 74 75 76 77 78 79 80 81 82 83 84 85 86 87 88 89 90 91 92 94 96 97 99 100 101 102 103 104 106 107 108 109 111 112 113 114 118 119 120 121 123 124 125 126 127 135 136 137 **P**6
Primary Contact: William Ferniany, Ph.D., Chief Executive Officer
COO: David G. Putt, FACHE, Chief Operating Officer
CFO: Dan Janicak, Chief Financial Officer
CMO: Michael Baumann, M.D., Chief Medical Officer
CHR: Paul Trussell, Director Human Resources
Web address: www.umc.edu
Control: State–Government, nonfederal **Service:** General Medical and Surgical

Staffed Beds: 530 **Admissions:** 23560 **Census:** 420 **Outpatient Visits:** 245299 **Births:** 3307 **Total Expense ($000):** 522055 **Payroll Expense ($000):** 194536 **Personnel:** 4246

MS

□ **WOMAN'S HOSPITAL AT RIVER OAKS (250136)**, 1026 North Flowood Drive, Zip 39232, Mailing Address: P.O. Box 4546, Zip 39296–4546; tel. 601/932–1000 **A**1 9 10 **F**13 15 25 26 30 31 32 33 37 55 56 57 70 71 74 79 80 82 107 119 135 136 137 **S** Health Management Associates
Primary Contact: Sherry J. Pitts, Chief Executive Officer
COO: Cynthia L. Dishongh, Executive Vice President and Chief Operating Officer
CFO: Jeff Bedford, Executive Vice President and Chief Financial Officer
CMO: Kim Nichols, M.D., Chief of Staff
CHR: Warren Weed, Director Human Resources
Web address: www.womanshospitalms.com
Control: Corporation, Investor–owned, for–profit **Service:** Obstetrics and gynecology

Staffed Beds: 60 **Admissions:** 2737 **Census:** 26 **Outpatient Visits:** 18673 **Births:** 1588 **Personnel:** 207

KEESLER AFB—Harrison County

★ **U. S. AIR FORCE MEDICAL CENTER KEESLER**, 301 Fisher Street, Suite 1A132, Zip 39534–2519; tel. 228/377–1110, (Nonreporting) **A**1 2 3 5 **S** Department of the Air Force
Primary Contact: Colonel Anthony S. Lonigro, MSC, USAF, Administrator
COO: Brigadier General James Dougherty, Commander
CFO: Major Brenda Yi, Director Medical Resource Management and Chief Financial Officer
CMO: Colonel James Gasque, Chief Hospital Services
CIO: Major Samuel Silverthorne, Chief Information Officer
CHR: Major Brenda Yi, Director Medical Resource Management and Chief Financial Officer
Web address: www.keesler.af.mil
Control: Air Force, Government, federal **Service:** General Medical and Surgical

Staffed Beds: 185

KILMICHAEL—Montgomery County

★ **KILMICHAEL HOSPITAL (250051)**, 301 Lamar Avenue, Zip 39747–0188, Mailing Address: P.O. Box 188, Zip 39747–0188; tel. 662/262–4311 **A**9 10 **F**31 32 84 122 **P**8
Primary Contact: Calvin D. Johnson, Administrator
Control: County–Government, nonfederal **Service:** General Medical and Surgical

Staffed Beds: 19 **Admissions:** 667 **Census:** 6 **Outpatient Visits:** 3335 **Births:** 0 **Personnel:** 50

KOSCIUSKO—Attala County

★ **MONTFORT JONES MEMORIAL HOSPITAL (250059)**, 220 Highway 12 West, Zip 39090–3209, Mailing Address: P.O. Box 887, Zip 39090–0887; tel. 662/289–4311 **A**9 10 **F**3 15 17 31 37 38 40 55 57 68 79 83 84 96 97 99 102 106 107 119 122
Primary Contact: Richard W. Manning, Administrator
CFO: James Thomas, Chief Financial Officer
CHR: Paige Duke, Chief Human Resources and Marketing
Web address: www.mjmh.com
Control: County–Government, nonfederal **Service:** General Medical and Surgical

Staffed Beds: 71 **Admissions:** 2054 **Census:** 27 **Outpatient Visits:** 18129 **Births:** 0 **Total Expense ($000):** 12305 **Payroll Expense ($000):** 7644 **Personnel:** 164

LAUREL—Jones County

★ **SOUTH CENTRAL REGIONAL MEDICAL CENTER (250058)**, 1220 Jefferson Street, Zip 39440–4374, Mailing Address: P.O. Box 607, Zip 39441–0607; tel. 601/426–4000, (Includes SOUTH CENTRAL EXTENDED CARE, Ivy Street, Ellisville, Zip 39437; tel. 601/477–9159), (Total facility includes 248 beds in nursing home–type unit) **A**1 9 10 19 20 **F**4 13 15 17 25 30 31 32 33 37 38 40 42 52 54 61 68 73 74 75 76 79 81 82 84 85 86 87 88 90 93 94 97 100 104 117 119 120 121 123 132 135 136 **P**3
Primary Contact: G. Douglas Higginbotham, Executive Director
CFO: Tom Canizaro, Associate Executive Director
CMO: Michael Weber, M.D., President Medical Staff
CIO: Linda Gavin, Associate Executive Director Marketing and Physician Recruitment
CHR: Janet Staples, Director Human Resources
Web address: www.scrmc.com
Control: County–Government, nonfederal **Service:** General Medical and Surgical

Staffed Beds: 464 **Admissions:** 9864 **Census:** 383 **Outpatient Visits:** 177379 **Births:** 1164 **Personnel:** 1757

LEAKESVILLE—Greene County

★ **GREENE COUNTY HOSPITAL (251329)**, 1017 Jackson Avenue, Zip 39451; tel. 601/394–4139, (Nonreporting) **A**10 18
Primary Contact: Donna Freeman, Administrator
Control: County–Government, nonfederal **Service:** General Medical and Surgical

Staffed Beds: 6

LEXINGTON—Holmes County

★ **HOLMES COUNTY HOSPITAL AND CLINICS (251319)**, (Formerly University Hospital and Clinics –Holmes County), 239 Bowling Green Road, Zip 39095–9332; tel. 662/834–1321 **A**1 9 10 18 **F**15 25 30 31 32 38 40 81 82 84 85 86 87 88 93 96 97 107 119 122
Primary Contact: Phillip L. Grady, Chief Executive Officer
COO: Dewery Montgomery, Chief Operating Officer
CFO: Dan Janicak, Chief Financial Officer
CMO: Mark Smothers, Chief Medical Staff
CIO: Paula Pepper, LAN Administrator
CHR: Gloria Bordelon, Human Resources Generalist
Control: State–Government, nonfederal **Service:** General Medical and Surgical

Staffed Beds: 35 **Admissions:** 891 **Census:** 12 **Outpatient Visits:** 7820 **Births:** 0 **Personnel:** 142

LOUISVILLE—Winston County

WINSTON MEDICAL CENTER (250027), 562 East Main Street, Zip 39339–2742, Mailing Address: P.O. Box 967, Zip 39339–0967; tel. 662/773–6211, (Total facility includes 120 beds in nursing home–type unit) **A**9 10 **F**15 17 38 40 55 68 84 93 96 102 107 117 119 122
Primary Contact: W. Dale Saulters, Administrator
Web address: www.winstonmedical.org
Control: Other not–for–profit (including NFP Corporation) **Service:** General Medical and Surgical

Staffed Beds: 149 **Admissions:** 829 **Census:** 126 **Outpatient Visits:** 21857 **Births:** 0 **Total Expense ($000):** 15363 **Payroll Expense ($000):** 5110 **Personnel:** 174

LUCEDALE—George County

GEORGE COUNTY HOSPITAL (250036), 859 Winter Street, Zip 39452–6603, Mailing Address: P.O. Box 607, Zip 39452–0607; tel. 601/947–3161 **A**9 10 20 **F**13 15 17 30 31 32 33 38 40 52 68 74 79 81 82 86 93 96 97 100 107 119 122 **P**8
Primary Contact: Paul A. Gardner, CPA, Administrator
CFO: Debbie Brannon, Chief Financial Officer
CMO: Michael Huber, M.D., Chief of Staff
CHR: Carla Shows, Payroll Clerk
Web address: www.georgeregional.com
Control: County–Government, nonfederal **Service:** General Medical and Surgical

Staffed Beds: 53 **Admissions:** 2334 **Census:** 25 **Outpatient Visits:** 35942 **Births:** 210 **Personnel:** 307

MACON—Noxubee County

★ **NOXUBEE GENERAL HOSPITAL (251307)**, 606 North Jefferson Street, Zip 39341–2236, Mailing Address: P.O. Box 480, Zip 39341–0480; tel. 662/726–4231, (Total facility includes 60 beds in nursing home–type unit) **A**9 10 18 **F**31 37 38 40 60 84 96 117 119 122
Primary Contact: Danny H. McKay, Administrator
Web address: www.noxubeemedical.com
Control: County–Government, nonfederal **Service:** General Medical and Surgical

Staffed Beds: 85 **Admissions:** 818 **Census:** 62 **Outpatient Visits:** 4952 **Births:** 0 **Personnel:** 139

MAGEE—Simpson County

MAGEE GENERAL HOSPITAL (250124), 300 Third Avenue, S.E., Zip 39111–3698; tel. 601/849–5070 **A**9 10 **F**15 38 74 79 84 93 96 97 100 107 119 122
Primary Contact: Althea H. Crumpton, Administrator
CFO: Missy Hudson, Chief Financial Officer
CIO: Kirby Craft, Chief Information Officer
CHR: Steve Beckham, Director Human Resources
Web address: www.mghosp.org
Control: Other not–for–profit (including NFP Corporation) **Service:** General Medical and Surgical

Staffed Beds: 64 **Admissions:** 2719 **Census:** 31 **Outpatient Visits:** 38444 **Births:** 121 **Personnel:** 293

MAGNOLIA—Pike County

BEACHAM MEMORIAL HOSPITAL (250049), 205 North Cherry Street, Zip 39652–2819, Mailing Address: P.O. Box 351, Zip 39652–0351; tel. 601/783–2351 **A**9 10 **F**31 32 33 96 119 122
Primary Contact: Guy Geller, Administrator and Chief Executive Officer
CMO: Lucius Lampton, M.D., Chief of Staff
CHR: Jackie McKenzie, Director Administrative Services
Web address: www.beachammemhos.com
Control: Other not–for–profit (including NFP Corporation) **Service:** General Medical and Surgical

Staffed Beds: 37 **Admissions:** 1136 **Census:** 17 **Outpatient Visits:** 0 **Births:** 0 **Personnel:** 98

MARKS—Quitman County

QUITMAN COUNTY HOSPITAL (251314), 340 Getwell Drive, Zip 38646–9785; tel. 662/326–8031 **A**9 10 18 **F**38 40 54 84 96 107 117 119 122
Primary Contact: Sean Johnson, Administrator
Control: Corporation, Investor–owned, for–profit **Service:** General Medical and Surgical

Staffed Beds: 33 **Admissions:** 961 **Census:** 13 **Outpatient Visits:** 10705 **Births:** 0 **Total Expense ($000):** 6783 **Payroll Expense ($000):** 2648 **Personnel:** 87

MCCOMB—Pike County

☒ △ **SOUTHWEST MISSISSIPPI REGIONAL MEDICAL CENTER (250097)**, 215 Marion Avenue, Zip 39648–2798, Mailing Address: P.O. Box 1307, Zip 39649–1307; tel. 601/249–5500 **A**1 7 9 10 19 **F**13 15 17 25 30 31 32 37 38 51 52 61 68 70 71 73 74 75 76 79 81 82 84 85 86 96 97 100 106 107 119 120 121 **P**6
Primary Contact: Norman M. Price, FACHE, Chief Executive Officer
CFO: Reece Nunnery, Chief Financial Officer
CMO: Simon Cofrancesco, M.D., Chief of Staff
CIO: Mike Moak, Chief Information Officer
CHR: Balfour Lipscomb, Administrative Director Human Resources
Web address: www.smrmc.com
Control: Hospital district or authority, Government, nonfederal **Service:** General Medical and Surgical

Staffed Beds: 170 **Admissions:** 8511 **Census:** 83 **Outpatient Visits:** 77330 **Births:** 1107 **Personnel:** 1008

MEADVILLE—Franklin County

FRANKLIN COUNTY MEMORIAL HOSPITAL (250035), Hospital Road, Zip 39653–4402, Mailing Address: P.O. Box 636, Zip 39653–0636; tel. 601/384–5801 **A**9 10 20 **F**25 30 33 38 40 54 79 81 84 86 88 93 95 96 107 119 122 132 **P**6
Primary Contact: Lance Moak, Administrator
Web address: www.fcmh.net
Control: County–Government, nonfederal **Service:** General Medical and Surgical

Staffed Beds: 36 **Admissions:** 959 **Census:** 14 **Outpatient Visits:** 6340 **Births:** 0 **Personnel:** 129

MENDENHALL—Simpson County

★ **SIMPSON GENERAL HOSPITAL (251317)**, 1842 Simpson Highway 149, Zip 39114–3592; tel. 601/847–2221 **A**10 18 **F**3 11 31 32 33 38 40 52 54 60 79 81 82 85 88 90 91 92 93 96 107 119 121 122 123 **P**5 7
Primary Contact: Audrey Wedgeworth, Interim Chief Executive Officer
CMO: Teresa Windham, Director Nursing
CIO: David Welch, Director Information Technology
CHR: Stephanie Smith, Manager Human Resources
Web address: www.simpsongeneralhospital.com
Control: Other not–for–profit (including NFP Corporation) **Service:** General Medical and Surgical

Staffed Beds: 25 **Admissions:** 995 **Census:** 13 **Outpatient Visits:** 10564 **Births:** 0 **Total Expense ($000):** 8823 **Payroll Expense ($000):** 4813 **Personnel:** 156

MERIDIAN—Lauderdale County

☐ **ALLIANCE HEALTH CENTER (250151)**, 5000 Highway 39 North, Zip 39301; tel. 601/483–6211 **A**1 9 10 **F**4 5 33 81 82 88 89 90 91 93 119 121 **S** Psychiatric Solutions
Primary Contact: William M. Patterson, Chief Executive Officer
CFO: Robert Jackson, Chief Financial Officer
CMO: Terry Jordan, M.D., Chief of Staff
CIO: John Eakes, Director Financial Services and Management Information Systems
CHR: Major Stephanie Williams, Vice President Human Resources
Web address: www.psysolutions.com
Control: Corporation, Investor–owned, for–profit **Service:** Psychiatric

Staffed Beds: 122 **Admissions:** 2436 **Census:** 92 **Outpatient Visits:** 0 **Births:** 0 **Personnel:** 248

EAST MISSISSIPPI STATE HOSPITAL, 4555 Highland Park Drive, Zip 39307–5498, Mailing Address: Box 4128, West Station, Zip 39304–4128; tel. 601/482–6186 **F**4 25 30 31 32 82 88 89 91 93 117 119 **S** Mississippi State Department of Mental Health
Primary Contact: Charles Carlisle, Director
CFO: Geri Rutledge, Director Business
CMO: Rolando Abangan, M.D., Medical Director
CIO: Susie Broadhead, Director Public Information
CHR: Shearmaine Calaway, Director Human Resources
Web address: www.emsh.state.ms.us
Control: State–Government, nonfederal **Service:** Psychiatric

Staffed Beds: 334 **Admissions:** 898 **Census:** 321 **Outpatient Visits:** 0 **Births:** 0 **Personnel:** 1101

☒ **JEFF ANDERSON REGIONAL MEDICAL CENTER (250104)**, 2124 14th Street, Zip 39301–4093; tel. 601/553–6000 **A**1 2 9 10 19 **F**13 15 17 30 31 32 33 37 38 40 52 68 70 71 73 74 75 76 78 79 81 82 83 84 85 86 88 96 97 104 106 107 119 120 121 **P**7 8
Primary Contact: Mark D. McPhail, President and Chief Executive Officer
CFO: Larry Fortenberry, Controller
CHR: Irby Lang, Vice President Human Resources
Web address: www.jarmc.org
Control: Other not–for–profit (including NFP Corporation) **Service:** General Medical and Surgical

Staffed Beds: 260 **Admissions:** 10764 **Census:** 160 **Outpatient Visits:** 76212 **Births:** 1503 **Personnel:** 1076

☒ **REGENCY HOSPITAL OF MERIDIAN (252006)**, 1102 Constitution Avenue, 2nd Floor, Zip 39301; tel. 601/484–7900 **A**1 10 **F**31 32 100 **S** Regency Hospital Company
Primary Contact: Benny Costello, Chief Executive Officer
Web address: www.regencyhospital.com
Control: Partnership, Investor–owned, for–profit **Service:** Long–Term Acute Care hospital

Staffed Beds: 40 **Admissions:** 460 **Census:** 32 **Outpatient Visits:** 0 **Births:** 0 **Personnel:** 121

☐ △ **RILEY HOSPITAL (250081)**, 1102 21st Avenue, Zip 39301–4096, Mailing Address: P.O. Box 1810, Zip 39301–1810; tel. 601/693–2511 **A**1 7 9 10 19 **F**4 13 15 17 25 30 33 38 40 60 61 68 71 73 74 76 79 81 82 84 85 86 87 88 96 97 106 107 119 120 121 135 136 **S** Health Management Associates
Primary Contact: Kerry Tirman, Chief Executive Officer
COO: Pam Tvarkunas, Chief Operating Officer
CFO: David Grizzard, Chief Financial Officer
CMO: Azhar Pasha, M.D., Chief of Staff
CHR: Amy Boutwell, Director Human Resources
Web address: www.hmamississippi.com
Control: Corporation, Investor–owned, for–profit **Service:** General Medical and Surgical

Staffed Beds: 140 **Admissions:** 3727 **Census:** 53 **Outpatient Visits:** 56849 **Births:** 547 **Personnel:** 398

MS

Hospital, Medicare Provider Number, Address, Telephone, Approval, Facility, and Physician Codes, Health Care System

★ American Hospital Association (AHA) membership
☐ The Joint Commission accreditation
○ American Osteopathic Association (AOA) accreditation
△ Commission on Accreditation of Rehabilitation Facilities (CARF) accreditation

★ **RUSH FOUNDATION HOSPITAL (250069)**, 1314 19th Avenue, Zip 39301–4195; tel. 601/483–0011 **A**1 9 10 19 **F**8 13 15 17 18 20 22 25 26 27 31 33 35 37 38 43 49 50 68 70 71 74 75 76 77 79 80 81 84 86 96 97 100 102 106 107 119 120 135 136 137 **P**3 8 **S** Rush Health Systems
Primary Contact: Wallace Strickland, President and Chief Executive Officer
COO: Morris A. Reece, Executive Vice President and Chief Operating Officer
CFO: Darrell Wildman, Chief Financial Officer
CIO: Angela Sherrill, Corporate Director Information System
CHR: Donnie Smith, Director Human Resources
Web address: www.rushhealthsystems.org
Control: Other not–for–profit (including NFP Corporation) **Service:** General Medical and Surgical

Staffed Beds: 182 **Admissions:** 7174 **Census:** 86 **Outpatient Visits:** 105040 **Births:** 877 **Total Expense ($000):** 116410 **Payroll Expense ($000):** 43155 **Personnel:** 949

★ **SPECIALTY HOSPITAL OF MERIDIAN (252004)**, 1314 19th Avenue, Zip 39301–4116; tel. 601/703–4211 **A**10 **F**76 82 121 122 133 **S** Rush Health Systems
Primary Contact: Wallace Strickland, President and Chief Executive Officer
CFO: Lexie Fuller, Controller
CMO: Richmond Alexander, M.D., President Medical Staff
CIO: Angela Sherrill, Corporate Director Information System
Web address: www.rushhealthsystems.org
Control: Other not–for–profit (including NFP Corporation) **Service:** Long–Term Acute Care hospital

Staffed Beds: 49 **Admissions:** 518 **Census:** 40 **Outpatient Visits:** 0 **Births:** 0 **Personnel:** 203

MONTICELLO—Lawrence County

LAWRENCE COUNTY HOSPITAL (251305), Highway 84 East, Zip 39654–0788, Mailing Address: P.O. Box 788, Zip 39654–0788; tel. 601/587–4051 **A**9 10 18 **F**37 38 40 82 84 96 119 122
Primary Contact: Semmes Ross, Jr., Administrator
CFO: Jennifer Moak, Business Office Manager
Web address: www.smrmc.com
Control: County–Government, nonfederal **Service:** General Medical and Surgical

Staffed Beds: 25 **Admissions:** 678 **Census:** 6 **Outpatient Visits:** 8759 **Births:** 0 **Personnel:** 109

MORTON—Scott County

★ **SCOTT REGIONAL HOSPITAL (251323)**, 317 Highway 13 South, Zip 39117–3353, Mailing Address: P.O. Box 259, Zip 39117–0259; tel. 601/732–6301, (Nonreporting) **A**9 10 18 **S** Rush Health Systems
Primary Contact: Michael R. Edwards, Chief Executive Officer
Control: Other not–for–profit (including NFP Corporation) **Service:** General Medical and Surgical

Staffed Beds: 30

NATCHEZ—Adams County

□ **NATCHEZ COMMUNITY HOSPITAL (250122)**, 129 Jefferson Davis Boulevard, Zip 39120–5100, Mailing Address: P.O. Box 1203, Zip 39121–1203; tel. 601/445–6200 **A**1 9 10 **F**13 15 17 25 30 32 38 40 51 60 68 74 76 79 82 84 93 96 97 107 119 **S** Health Management Associates
Primary Contact: Timothy Trottier, Chief Executive Officer
CFO: Melissa Johnson, Chief Financial Officer
CHR: Hal Harrington, Director Human Resources
Web address: www.hmamississippi.com
Control: Corporation, Investor–owned, for–profit **Service:** General Medical and Surgical

Staffed Beds: 101 **Admissions:** 4031 **Census:** 45 **Outpatient Visits:** 31806 **Births:** 560 **Personnel:** 259

★ △ **NATCHEZ REGIONAL MEDICAL CENTER (250084)**, 54 Seargent S Prentiss Drive, Zip 39120–4726; tel. 601/443–2100 **A**1 7 9 10 **F**13 17 25 31 32 33 38 40 68 71 74 82 83 84 85 88 93 96 97 100 104 107 119 121 **S** QHR
Primary Contact: Scott Phillips, Chief Executive Officer
CMO: Ed Daly, M.D., Chief of Staff
CIO: Walt Roddy, Director Information Management Systems
CHR: Eileen Richardson, Director Human Resources
Web address: www.natchezregional.com
Control: County–Government, nonfederal **Service:** General Medical and Surgical

Staffed Beds: 132 **Admissions:** 4160 **Census:** 61 **Outpatient Visits:** 31089 **Births:** 654 **Personnel:** 440

NEW ALBANY—Union County

★ **BAPTIST MEMORIAL HOSPITAL–UNION COUNTY (250006)**, 200 Highway 30 West, Zip 38652–3197; tel. 662/538–7631 **A**1 9 10 **F**13 15 17 25 31 33 37 38 51 52 68 73 74 75 76 79 81 82 84 85 86 96 97 100 107 117 119 121 135 136 **S** Baptist Memorial Health Care Corporation
Primary Contact: James Huffman, Administrator and Chief Executive Officer
CFO: Kim High, Controller
CMO: Jason Dees, M.D., Chief of Staff
CIO: Missy Coltharp, Director
CHR: Lori Goode, Director Human Resources
Web address: www.bmhcc.org
Control: Other not–for–profit (including NFP Corporation) **Service:** General Medical and Surgical

Staffed Beds: 153 **Admissions:** 4022 **Census:** 42 **Outpatient Visits:** 40686 **Births:** 1102 **Personnel:** 418

NEWTON—Newton County

NEWTON REGIONAL HOSPITAL (250149), (Formerly Rush Hospital–Newton), 9421 Eastside Drive, Zip 39345–0299, Mailing Address: P.O. Box 299, Zip 39345–0299; tel. 601/683–2031 **A**9 10 **F**30 31 33 38 40 79 81 82 84 86 88 93 96 100 107 119
Primary Contact: Bobby Welborn, Administrator/Chief Executive Officer
CHR: Jo Ann Adams, Executive Assistant
Web address: www.newtonregionalhospital.com
Control: Other not–for–profit (including NFP Corporation) **Service:** General Medical and Surgical

Staffed Beds: 30 **Admissions:** 1265 **Census:** 14 **Outpatient Visits:** 12358 **Births:** 0 **Personnel:** 127

OCEAN SPRINGS—Jackson County

OCEAN SPRINGS HOSPITAL See Singing River Hospital System, Pascagoula

OLIVE BRANCH—De Soto County

□ **PARKWOOD BEHAVIORAL HEALTH SYSTEM (254005)**, 8135 Goodman Road, Zip 38654–2199; tel. 662/895–4900 **A**1 9 10 **F**4 5 30 31 32 33 36 39 73 75 81 88 89 90 91 92 94 95 119 **S** Universal Health Services, Inc.
Primary Contact: M. Andrew Mayo, Ph.D., Chief Executive Officer and Managing Director
CFO: Sandra Wallace, Chief Financial Officer
CMO: Paul King, M.D., Medical Director
CHR: Audrey Johnson, Director Human Resources
Web address: www.parkwoodbhs.com
Control: Corporation, Investor–owned, for–profit **Service:** Psychiatric

Staffed Beds: 128 **Admissions:** 2373 **Census:** 104 **Outpatient Visits:** 4151 **Births:** 0 **Personnel:** 163

OXFORD—Lafayette County

★ △ **BAPTIST MEMORIAL HOSPITAL–NORTH MISSISSIPPI (250034)**, 2301 South Lamar Boulevard, Zip 38655–5373, Mailing Address: P.O. Box 946, Zip 38655–0946; tel. 662/232–8100, (Total facility includes 14 beds in nursing home–type unit) **A**1 2 7 9 10 19 **F**7 12 13 15 18 20 22 24 25 26 27 28 30 31 32 33 34 37 38 40 42 43 44 49 50 52 55 56 57 61 62 63 66 68 74 75 76 77 79 80 81 82 84 85 86 94 96 97 100 102 103 104 107 108 117 118 119 120 121 124 134 135 136 137 **S** Baptist Memorial Health Care Corporation
Primary Contact: Jim Ainsworth, Interim Administrator and Chief Executive Officer
CFO: Dana Williams, Assistant Administrator and Chief Financial Officer
CIO: Linda Britt, Director Information Systems
CHR: Roger Brune, Director Human Resources
Web address: www.bmhcc.org
Control: Other not–for–profit (including NFP Corporation) **Service:** General Medical and Surgical

Staffed Beds: 203 **Admissions:** 9209 **Census:** 129 **Outpatient Visits:** 58000 **Births:** 1016 **Personnel:** 1047

PASCAGOULA—Jackson County

★ **SINGING RIVER HOSPITAL SYSTEM (250040)**, 2809 Denny Avenue, Zip 39581–5301; tel. 228/809–5000, (Includes OCEAN SPRINGS HOSPITAL, 3109 Bienville Boulevard, Ocean Springs, Zip 39564–4361; tel. 228/818–1111; SINGING RIVER HOSPITAL, tel. 228/809–5000) **A**1 2 9 10 **F**3 13 15 17 18 20 22 24 25 27 30 31 32 36 37 38 40 41 47 48 49 50 55 56 57 58 60 62 66 68 71 72 74 76 77 78 79 80 81 83 84 85 88 90 91 92 93 94 96 97 100 102 103 106 107 119 124 134 137 **P**8
Primary Contact: Chris Anderson, Chief Executive Officer
CFO: Michael E. Crews, Chief Financial Officer
CMO: Larry D. Shoemaker, M.D., Chief Medical Officer
CIO: Chris Oubre, Director Information Systems
CHR: Nebo Carter, Director Human Resources
Web address: www.srhshealth.com
Control: County–Government, nonfederal **Service:** General Medical and Surgical

Staffed Beds: 369 **Admissions:** 16814 **Census:** 205 **Outpatient Visits:** 348458 **Births:** 1689 **Total Expense ($000):** 266289 **Payroll Expense ($000):** 105078 **Personnel:** 2151

MS

PHILADELPHIA—Neshoba County

☒ **CHOCTAW HEALTH CENTER (250127)**, 210 Hospital Circle, Zip 39350–6781; tel. 601/656–2211, (Nonreporting) **A**1 5 10
Primary Contact: Howard Billie, Acting Administrator
CFO: Donita Stephens, Administrative Assistant Financial Services
CMO: Joann Coates, M.D., Chief of Staff
CHR: Linda McMillan, Patient Relations and Personnel Specialist
Control: Other not–for–profit (including NFP Corporation) **Service:** General Medical and Surgical

Staffed Beds: 35

★ **NESHOBA COUNTY GENERAL HOSPITAL (250043)**, 1001 Holland Avenue, Zip 39350–2161, Mailing Address: P.O. Box 648, Zip 39350–0648; tel. 601/663–1200, (Total facility includes 148 beds in nursing home–type unit) **A**9 10 20 **F**6 7 11 15 25 38 40 54 60 79 80 84 85 93 96 102 107 117 119 122 132 **S** QHR
Primary Contact: Karen A. Fiducia, Interim Chief Executive Officer
CFO: Michael Weeks, Chief Financial Officer
CMO: Walt Willis, M.D., Medical Director
CHR: Hedda Stewart, Director Human Resources
Web address: www.neshobageneral.com
Control: County–Government, nonfederal **Service:** General Medical and Surgical

Staffed Beds: 200 **Admissions:** 2064 **Census:** 180 **Outpatient Visits:** 34350 **Births:** 0 **Total Expense ($000):** 24551 **Payroll Expense ($000):** 14429 **Personnel:** 443

PICAYUNE—Pearl River County

HIGHLAND COMMUNITY HOSPITAL (250117), 801 Goodyear Boulevard, Zip 39466–3221, Mailing Address: P.O. Box 909, Zip 39466–0909; tel. 601/798–4711 **A**9 10 **F**12 13 15 25 30 31 32 38 40 68 73 74 79 81 82 86 96 97 100 107 118 119 120 135 136
Primary Contact: Steve Grimm, FACHE, Administrator
COO: Shirley Bertolasi, Chief Nursing Officer
CFO: Bryan N. Stevens, Chief Financial Officer
CHR: Josh Lowery, Director Human Resources
Web address: www.highlandch.com
Control: County–Government, nonfederal **Service:** General Medical and Surgical

Staffed Beds: 61 **Admissions:** 2398 **Census:** 18 **Outpatient Visits:** 39033 **Births:** 370 **Total Expense ($000):** 11283 **Payroll Expense ($000):** 11325 **Personnel:** 271

PONTOTOC—Pontotoc County

☒ **NORTH MISSISSIPPI MEDICAL CENTER–PONTOTOC HOSPITAL AND NURSING HOME (251308)**, 176 South Main Street, Zip 38863–3311, Mailing Address: P.O. Box 790, Zip 38863–0790; tel. 662/488–7640, (Total facility includes 44 beds in nursing home–type unit) **A**1 9 10 18 **F**15 30 31 32 33 73 81 82 85 86 96 107 117 119 121 122 132 **S** North Mississippi Health Services, Inc.
Primary Contact: Fred B. Hood, FACHE, Administrator
CFO: M. Denise Heard, Director Business Services
Web address: www.nmhs.net
Control: Other not–for–profit (including NFP Corporation) **Service:** General Medical and Surgical

Staffed Beds: 69 **Admissions:** 578 **Census:** 49 **Outpatient Visits:** 17939 **Births:** 0 **Personnel:** 159

POPLARVILLE—Pearl River County

PEARL RIVER COUNTY HOSPITAL (250023), 305 West Moody Street, Zip 39470–7242, Mailing Address: P.O. Box 392, Zip 39470–0392; tel. 601/795–4543, (Total facility includes 126 beds in nursing home–type unit) **A**9 10 **F**30 31 32 75 82 85 86 87 97 107 119 120 121 122 123 132
Primary Contact: Dorothy C. Bilbo, Administrator
Control: County–Government, nonfederal **Service:** General Medical and Surgical

Staffed Beds: 150 **Admissions:** 128 **Census:** 105 **Outpatient Visits:** 0 **Births:** 0 **Personnel:** 200

PORT GIBSON—Claiborne County

CLAIBORNE COUNTY HOSPITAL (251320), 123 McComb Avenue, Zip 39150–2915, Mailing Address: P.O. Box 1004, Zip 39150–1004; tel. 601/437–5141 **A**9 10 18 **F**31 32 40 84 85 88 90 91 92 93 94 107 119 122
Primary Contact: Wanda C. Fleming, Administrator and Chief Executive Officer
CFO: Linda Caho–Mooney, Chief Financial Officer
CIO: Ada Ratliff, Chief Information Officer
Control: County–Government, nonfederal **Service:** General Medical and Surgical

Staffed Beds: 25 **Admissions:** 632 **Census:** 8 **Outpatient Visits:** 13932 **Births:** 0 **Personnel:** 89

PRENTISS—Jefferson Davis County

JEFFERSON DAVIS COMMUNITY HOSPITAL (251326), 1102 Rose Street, Zip 39474, Mailing Address: P.O. Box 1288, Zip 39474; tel. 601/792–4276, (Total facility includes 60 beds in nursing home–type unit) **A**9 10 18 **F**30 31 32 33 38 40 52 54 81 82 85 86 88 90 91 92 93 96 100 107 117 119 122
Primary Contact: Mary R. Curtis, Chief Executive Officer
Control: Other not–for–profit (including NFP Corporation) **Service:** General Medical and Surgical

Staffed Beds: 95 **Admissions:** 710 **Census:** 69 **Outpatient Visits:** 9585 **Births:** 1 **Personnel:** 190

PURVIS—Lamar County

☐ **SOUTH MISSISSIPPI STATE HOSPITAL (254008)**, 823 Highway 589, Zip 39475–4194; tel. 601/794–0100 **A**1 10 **F**3 30 31 32 88 119 **S** Mississippi State Department of Mental Health
Primary Contact: Wynona C. Winfield, Director
Web address: www.smsh.state.ms.us
Control: State–Government, nonfederal **Service:** Psychiatric

Staffed Beds: 50 **Admissions:** 325 **Census:** 31 **Outpatient Visits:** 0 **Births:** 0 **Total Expense ($000):** 9537 **Payroll Expense ($000):** 4601 **Personnel:** 109

QUITMAN—Clarke County

★ **H. C. WATKINS MEMORIAL HOSPITAL (251316)**, 605 South Archusa Avenue, Zip 39355–2398; tel. 601/776–6925 **A**9 10 18 **F**25 31 32 33 38 40 46 78 79 81 84 86 93 94 96 117 118 119 122 **P**8
Primary Contact: Michael Nester, Chief Executive Officer
CFO: Jerry Sims, Vice President Finance
CMO: O. Wayne Byrd, M.D., Chief of Staff
CIO: Melinda Smith, Chief Information Systems
CHR: Leigh Moore, Administrative Assistant Human Resources
Control: Other not–for–profit (including NFP Corporation) **Service:** General Medical and Surgical

Staffed Beds: 25 **Admissions:** 818 **Census:** 14 **Outpatient Visits:** 7126 **Births:** 0 **Total Expense ($000):** 9640 **Payroll Expense ($000):** 3364 **Personnel:** 147

RICHTON—Perry County

PERRY COUNTY GENERAL HOSPITAL (251306), 206 Bay Avenue, Zip 39476; tel. 601/788–6316 **A**9 10 18 **F**30 31 32 38 40 82 86 87 88 93 96 107 119 122
Primary Contact: David Paris, Chief Executive Officer
Control: Partnership, Investor–owned, for–profit **Service:** General Medical and Surgical

Staffed Beds: 30 **Admissions:** 585 **Census:** 10 **Outpatient Visits:** 4166 **Births:** 0 **Personnel:** 88

RIPLEY—Tippah County

☒ **TIPPAH COUNTY HOSPITAL (250010)**, 1005 City Avenue North, Zip 38663–0499, Mailing Address: P.O. Box 499, Zip 38663–0499; tel. 662/837–9221, (Total facility includes 40 beds in nursing home–type unit) **A**1 9 10 20 **F**3 7 15 31 32 38 40 79 96 103 107 117 119 122
Primary Contact: Tom Hood, Administrator
CFO: Stephanie McAlister, Controller
CMO: Charles M. Elliott, M.D., Chief of Staff
CHR: Margaret Weeks, Manager Personnel
Web address: www.tippahcountyhospital.com
Control: County–Government, nonfederal **Service:** General Medical and Surgical

Staffed Beds: 85 **Admissions:** 968 **Census:** 52 **Outpatient Visits:** 18766 **Births:** 0 **Total Expense ($000):** 11602 **Payroll Expense ($000):** 6121 **Personnel:** 176

ROLLING FORK—Sharkey County

SHARKEY–ISSAQUENA COMMUNITY HOSPITAL (250079), 108 South Fourth Street, Zip 39159–2612, Mailing Address: P.O. Box 339, Zip 39159–0339; tel. 662/873–4396 **A**9 10 20 **F**38 52 54 84 93 96 100 107 122
Primary Contact: Jerry Keever, Administrator
Control: County–Government, nonfederal **Service:** General Medical and Surgical

Staffed Beds: 29 **Admissions:** 476 **Census:** 7 **Outpatient Visits:** 2288 **Births:** 0 **Personnel:** 65

MS

Hospital, Medicare Provider Number, Address, Telephone, Approval, Facility, and Physician Codes, Health Care System

★ American Hospital Association (AHA) membership
☐ The Joint Commission accreditation
○ American Osteopathic Association (AOA) accreditation
△ Commission on Accreditation of Rehabilitation Facilities (CARF) accreditation

RULEVILLE—Sunflower County

★ **NORTH SUNFLOWER MEDICAL CENTER (251318)**, 840 North Oak Avenue, Zip 38771–0369, Mailing Address: P.O. Box 369, Zip 38771–0369; tel. 662/756–2711, (Total facility includes 60 beds in nursing home–type unit) **A**9 10 18 **F**25 30 31 32 33 38 40 52 54 61 73 75 79 82 85 86 87 93 96 107 117 119 121 122 123 132 **P**7
Primary Contact: Billy Marlow, Administrator
COO: Sam Miller, Chief Operating Officer
CFO: Charlotte Sherwood, Chief Financial Officer
CMO: Adelo Aquino, M.D., Chief of Staff
CIO: T J Weeks, Director Information Services
CHR: Robbie Taylor, Director Human Resources
Web address: www.northsunflower.com
Control: County–Government, nonfederal **Service:** General Medical and Surgical

Staffed Beds: 95 **Admissions:** 780 **Census:** 73 **Outpatient Visits:** 8821 **Births:** 0 **Personnel:** 285

SENATOBIA—Tate County

☐ **NORTH OAK REGIONAL MEDICAL CENTER (250126)**, 401 Getwell Drive, Zip 38668–2213, Mailing Address: P.O. Box 648, Zip 38668–0648; tel. 662/562–3100 **A**1 9 10 **F**30 31 32 33 38 40 54 79 84 93 96 107 119
Primary Contact: James D. Tesar, Chief Executive Officer
CMO: Pravin Chandra Patel, M.D., Chief Medical Officer
CHR: Vickie Barksdale, Manager Human Resources
Web address: www.normc.org
Control: Corporation, Investor–owned, for–profit **Service:** General Medical and Surgical

Staffed Beds: 41 **Admissions:** 1510 **Census:** 19 **Outpatient Visits:** 12413 **Births:** 0 **Personnel:** 105

SOUTHAVEN—De Soto County

MS

★ △ **BAPTIST MEMORIAL HOSPITAL–DESOTO (250141)**, 7601 Southcrest Parkway, Zip 38671–4742; tel. 662/772–4000 **A**1 7 9 10 **F**3 8 11 13 15 17 18 20 22 24 25 26 27 30 31 32 33 38 40 44 46 47 48 49 51 56 60 62 66 68 71 72 74 75 76 77 78 79 80 81 82 85 86 96 97 100 102 103 104 106 107 109 111 118 119 120 121 124 132 135 136 137 **S** Baptist Memorial Health Care Corporation
Primary Contact: Randy King, Administrator and Chief Executive Officer
CFO: Kimberly Young, Chief Financial Officer
CMO: Jacinto A. Hernandez, M.D., Chief Medical Officer
CHR: Walter Banks, Director Human Resources
Web address: www.bmhcc.org
Control: Other not–for–profit (including NFP Corporation) **Service:** General Medical and Surgical

Staffed Beds: 305 **Admissions:** 13879 **Census:** 187 **Outpatient Visits:** 91651 **Births:** 1933 **Personnel:** 1433

STARKVILLE—Oktibbeha County

★ **OKTIBBEHA COUNTY HOSPITAL (250050)**, 400 Hospital Road, Zip 39759–2163, Mailing Address: Drawer 1506, Zip 39760–1506; tel. 662/323–4320 **A**1 9 10 **F**7 11 13 15 17 24 25 30 31 32 33 37 38 40 51 52 55 56 57 60 62 68 71 74 75 77 79 80 82 83 84 85 86 87 88 96 97 100 103 106 107 118 119 120 121 122 124 134 135 136
Primary Contact: Arthur C. Kelly, Administrator and Chief Executive Officer
COO: Mike Andrews, Assistant Administrator and Chief Operating Officer
CFO: Richard G. Hilton, Associate Administrator and Chief Financial Officer
CIO: Chamath Wijewardane, Director Information Technology
CHR: Mike Andrews, Assistant Administrator and Chief Operating Officer
Web address: www.och.org
Control: County–Government, nonfederal **Service:** General Medical and Surgical

Staffed Beds: 96 **Admissions:** 3552 **Census:** 35 **Outpatient Visits:** 182950 **Births:** 1162 **Total Expense ($000):** 47927 **Payroll Expense ($000):** 27505 **Personnel:** 575

TUPELO—Lee County

★ △ **NORTH MISSISSIPPI MEDICAL CENTER – TUPELO (250004)**, 830 South Gloster Street, Zip 38801–4934; tel. 662/377–3000, (Total facility includes 107 beds in nursing home–type unit) **A**1 2 3 5 7 9 10 19 **F**4 5 13 15 17 25 30 31 32 33 38 40 42 51 52 54 60 61 68 70 71 73 74 75 76 78 79 81 82 83 84 85 86 87 88 90 91 93 94 96 97 100 104 106 107 117 119 120 121 123 135 136 **P**6 **S** North Mississippi Health Services, Inc.
Primary Contact: Charles D. Stokes, FACHE, President
CIO: Tom Bozeman, Chief Information Officer
CHR: Rodger Brown, Vice President Human Resources
Web address: www.nmhs.net
Control: Other not–for–profit (including NFP Corporation) **Service:** General Medical and Surgical

Staffed Beds: 726 **Admissions:** 29300 **Census:** 515 **Outpatient Visits:** 118431 **Births:** 2632 **Personnel:** 3853

☐ **NORTH MISSISSIPPI STATE HOSPITAL (254009)**, 1937 Briar Ridge Road, Zip 38804; tel. 662/690–4200 **A**1 10 **F**3 25 31 32 56 57 63 82 88 91 119 121 124 132 **S** Mississippi State Department of Mental Health
Primary Contact: Paul A. Callens, Ph.D., Director
CFO: Joe Rials, Director Fiscal Services
CMO: Ken Lippincott, M.D., Chief of Staff
CIO: James Wilhite, Director Systems Information
Web address: www.nmsh.state.ms.us
Control: State–Government, nonfederal **Service:** Psychiatric

Staffed Beds: 50 **Admissions:** 341 **Census:** 49 **Outpatient Visits:** 0 **Births:** 0 **Total Expense ($000):** 12861 **Payroll Expense ($000):** 6392 **Personnel:** 116

TYLERTOWN—Walthall County

★ **WALTHALL COUNTY GENERAL HOSPITAL (251324)**, 100 Hospital Drive, Zip 39667–2099; tel. 601/876–2122 **A**9 10 18 **F**3 11 31 38 40 48 62 79 82 84 86 96 107 119 122 137
Primary Contact: Jimmy Graves, Administrator
Web address: www.wcghospital.datastar.net/
Control: County–Government, nonfederal **Service:** General Medical and Surgical

Staffed Beds: 25 **Admissions:** 1142 **Census:** 10 **Outpatient Visits:** 17970 **Births:** 0 **Total Expense ($000):** 8844 **Payroll Expense ($000):** 4535 **Personnel:** 175

UNION—Newton County

★ **LAIRD HOSPITAL (251322)**, 25117 Highway 15, Zip 39365–9099; tel. 601/774–8214 **A**9 10 18 **F**3 11 15 25 30 31 32 33 38 40 44 55 56 57 62 79 82 84 85 86 96 99 100 102 107 119 122
Primary Contact: Thomas G. Bartlett, III, M.D., Administrator
Control: Other not–for–profit (including NFP Corporation) **Service:** General Medical and Surgical

Staffed Beds: 25 **Admissions:** 1070 **Census:** 9 **Outpatient Visits:** 20355 **Births:** 0 **Total Expense ($000):** 13782 **Payroll Expense ($000):** 4255 **Personnel:** 128

VICKSBURG—Warren County

PROMISE HOSPITAL OF VICKSBURG (252008), (Formerly Promise Specialty Hospital of Vicksburg), 1111 North Frontage Road, 2nd Floor, Zip 39180; tel. 601/619–3526 **A**10 **F**30 31 32 85 **S** Promise Healthcare
Primary Contact: Lee Huckaby, Chief Executive Officer
COO: Dawn Posey, Chief Operating Officer
CFO: Christopher A. Stegall, Regional Chief Financial Officer and Chief Operating Officer
CMO: Daniel Edney, M.D., Chief of Staff
CIO: Barbara Whiting, Director Health Information Management
CHR: Roxan Houghton, Director Human Resources
Web address: www.promise–vicksburg.com
Control: Corporation, Investor–owned, for–profit **Service:** Long–Term Acute Care hospital

Staffed Beds: 35 **Admissions:** 351 **Census:** 24 **Outpatient Visits:** 0 **Births:** 0 **Personnel:** 87

★ **RIVER REGION MEDICAL CENTER (250031)**, 2100 Highway 61 North, Zip 39183, Mailing Address: P.O. Box 590, Zip 39181–0590; tel. 601/883–5000, (Includes RIVER REGION WEST CAMPUS, 1111 North Frontage Road, Zip 39180–5102; tel. 601/636–2611), (Total facility includes 16 beds in nursing home–type unit) (Nonreporting) **A**1 2 9 10 19 20 **S** Community Health Systems, Inc.
Primary Contact: Phillip A. Clendenin, Chief Executive Officer
COO: Brad D. Holland, Administrator and Chief Operating Officer
CFO: John Milazzo, Chief Financial Officer
CMO: W. Briggs Hopson, M.D., Clinical Medical Director
CIO: J. B. White, Chief Information Officer
CHR: Wendy Alexander, Director Human Resources
Web address: www.riverregion.com
Control: Corporation, Investor–owned, for–profit **Service:** General Medical and Surgical

Staffed Beds: 324

WATER VALLEY—Yalobusha County

YALOBUSHA GENERAL HOSPITAL (250061), 630 South Main, Zip 38965, Mailing Address: P.O. Box 728, Zip 38965–0728; tel. 662/473–1411, (Total facility includes 120 beds in nursing home–type unit) **A**9 10 **F**3 7 25 26 50 56 57 75 96 101 102 107 117 119 122 132 **P**4
Primary Contact: Terry Varner, Administrator
CMO: Paul Odom, M.D., Chief Medical Staff
CHR: Katie Baggett, Administrative Assistant
Control: County–Government, nonfederal **Service:** General Medical and Surgical

Staffed Beds: 146 **Admissions:** 884 **Census:** 125 **Outpatient Visits:** 18320 **Births:** 0 **Personnel:** 193

WAYNESBORO—Wayne County

☐ **WAYNE GENERAL HOSPITAL (250077)**, 950 Matthew Drive, Zip 39367–2590, Mailing Address: P.O. Box 1249, Zip 39367–1249; tel. 601/735–5151 **A**1 9 10 20 **F**13 15 31 32 33 37 38 40 42 52 60 61 68 73 74 79 81 83 84 85 86 96 97 100 107 119 121 122
Primary Contact: Donald Hemeter, Administrator
Web address: www.waynegeneralhospital.org
Control: County–Government, nonfederal **Service:** General Medical and Surgical

Staffed Beds: 80 **Admissions:** 2796 **Census:** 36 **Outpatient Visits:** 34081 **Births:** 284 **Personnel:** 329

WEST POINT—Clay County

★☐ **NORTH MISSISSIPPI MEDICAL CENTER–WEST POINT (250067)**, 835 Medical Center Drive, Zip 39773–9320; tel. 662/495–2300 **A**1 9 10 **F**3 7 8 11 13 15 17 24 25 26 27 28 30 31 32 33 37 38 39 40 52 55 56 57 62 63 68 71 73 74 76 77 78 79 80 81 82 84 85 87 96 97 98 99 100 102 107 108 118 119 121 122 124 132 134 135 136 137 **S** North Mississippi Health Services, Inc.
Primary Contact: W. Kent Rogers, Administrator
CFO: Athena Adams, Chief Financial Officer
CMO: John Cox, M.D., Chief Medical Staff
CHR: Brenda Johnson, Director Human Resources
Web address: www.nmhs.net
Control: Other not–for–profit (including NFP Corporation) **Service:** General Medical and Surgical

Staffed Beds: 60 **Admissions:** 2646 **Census:** 25 **Outpatient Visits:** 49906 **Births:** 495 **Total Expense ($000):** 26433 **Payroll Expense ($000):** 12520 **Personnel:** 290

WHITFIELD—Rankin County

★☐ **MISSISSIPPI STATE HOSPITAL (254010)**, 3550 Highway 468 West, Zip 39193, Mailing Address: P.O. Box 157–A, Zip 39193–0157; tel. 601/351–8000, (Includes WHITFIELD MEDICAL SURGICAL HOSPITAL, Oak Circle, tel. 601/351–8023), (Total facility includes 454 beds in nursing home–type unit) **A**1 10 **F**4 25 31 32 37 73 82 88 89 90 91 92 93 94 117 119 132 **P**1 **S** Mississippi State Department of Mental Health
Primary Contact: James G. Chastain, CHE, Director
COO: Kelly R. Breland, CPA, Director Support Services
CFO: Warren Williams, CPA, Fiscal Services Director
CMO: Duncan Stone, M.D., Chief Medical Staff
CIO: James Dunaway, Director Information Management
CHR: Stephanie Macraugh, Director Human Resources
Web address: www.msh.state.ms.us
Control: State–Government, nonfederal **Service:** Psychiatric

Staffed Beds: 1119 **Admissions:** 2353 **Census:** 1068 **Births:** 0 **Personnel:** 1382

WIGGINS—Stone County

STONE COUNTY HOSPITAL (251303), 1434 East Central Avenue, Zip 39577; tel. 601/928–6600 **A**9 10 18 **F**25 30 31 32 33 79 82 85 96 97 107 119 122
Primary Contact: Julie Cain, Administrator
Control: Corporation, Investor–owned, for–profit **Service:** General Medical and Surgical

Staffed Beds: 25 **Admissions:** 537 **Census:** 5 **Outpatient Visits:** 5896 **Births:** 0 **Personnel:** 124

WINONA—Montgomery County

TYLER HOLMES MEMORIAL HOSPITAL (251312), 409 Tyler Holmes Drive, Zip 38967–1599; tel. 662/283–4114 **A**9 10 18 **F**3 11 31 32 33 38 40 55 57 62 82 96 100 102 107 119 122 124 **P**8
Primary Contact: Rosamond M. Tyler, Administrator
Control: County–Government, nonfederal **Service:** General Medical and Surgical

Staffed Beds: 25 **Admissions:** 808 **Census:** 9 **Outpatient Visits:** 13306 **Births:** 0 **Total Expense ($000):** 7072 **Payroll Expense ($000):** 3787 **Personnel:** 124

YAZOO CITY—Yazoo County

★ **KING'S DAUGHTERS HOSPITAL (251313)**, 823 Grand Avenue, Zip 39194–3233; tel. 662/746–2261, (Nonreporting) **A**9 10 18
Primary Contact: Daryl W. Weaver, Chief Executive Officer
COO: Marsha Jones, R.N., Director Nursing
CFO: Robert E. Harper, Chief Financial Officer
CMO: Will P. Thompson, M.D., Chief of Staff
CHR: Lauren Henderson, Director Human Resources
Web address: www.kdhyazoo.com
Control: Other not–for–profit (including NFP Corporation) **Service:** General Medical and Surgical

Staffed Beds: 35

MS

Hospital, Medicare Provider Number, Address, Telephone, Approval, Facility, and Physician Codes, Health Care System

★ American Hospital Association (AHA) membership
☐ The Joint Commission accreditation
○ American Osteopathic Association (AOA) accreditation
△ Commission on Accreditation of Rehabilitation Facilities (CARF) accreditation

MISSOURI

ALBANY—Gentry County

★ **NORTHWEST MEDICAL CENTER (261328)**, 705 North College Street, Zip 64402–1433; tel. 660/726–3941 **A**9 10 18 **F**3 11 15 24 25 26 30 31 32 33 37 38 41 50 52 54 55 56 57 61 62 66 72 73 75 76 77 79 80 81 82 85 86 87 96 97 99 100 102 105 106 107 119 120 121 122 124 137 **P**6
Primary Contact: John W. Richmond, President and Chief Executive Officer
CFO: Mark Thorn, Vice President Finance
CMO: Arturo Tenorio, M.D., Chief of Staff
CIO: James Crouch, Vice President Technical Services
CHR: Chuck Davis, Vice President Human Resources and Marketing
Web address: www.northwestmedicalcenter.org
Control: Other not–for–profit (including NFP Corporation) **Service:** General Medical and Surgical

Staffed Beds: 25 **Admissions:** 898 **Census:** 12 **Outpatient Visits:** 27479 **Births:** 0 **Total Expense ($000):** 10765 **Payroll Expense ($000):** 4706 **Personnel:** 135

APPLETON CITY—St. Clair County

★ **ELLETT MEMORIAL HOSPITAL (261301)**, 610 North Ohio Avenue, Zip 64724–1609, Mailing Address: P.O. Box 6, Zip 64724–0006; tel. 660/476–2111 **A**9 10 18 **F**7 26 31 33 38 55 57 79 85 86 96 100 102 107 117 119 122 132 **P**6 **S** Hospital Management Consulting, LLC
Primary Contact: Stephanie Lyon, RN, Administrator
CMO: James Wirkkula, M.D., Chief Medical Officer
Web address: www.ellettmemorial.com
Control: Hospital district or authority, Government, nonfederal **Service:** General Medical and Surgical

Staffed Beds: 25 **Admissions:** 277 **Census:** 5 **Outpatient Visits:** 9554 **Births:** 0 **Total Expense ($000):** 4367 **Payroll Expense ($000):** 2475 **Personnel:** 66

AURORA—Lawrence County

MO

★ **ST. JOHN'S HOSPITAL – AURORA (261316)**, 500 Porter Street, Zip 65605–2365; tel. 417/678–2122 **A**1 10 18 **F**3 11 13 15 24 25 26 32 33 38 50 55 57 62 66 73 74 75 78 79 80 81 82 84 86 96 97 100 107 118 119 121 122 124 137 **P**6 **S** Sisters of Mercy Health System
Primary Contact: Gary W. Jordan, President
CFO: Sherry Clouse Day, CPA, Chief Financial Officer
Web address: www.stjohns.com/aboutus/aurora.aspx
Control: Church–operated, Nongovernment, not–for profit **Service:** General Medical and Surgical

Staffed Beds: 25 **Admissions:** 1268 **Census:** 10 **Outpatient Visits:** 28169 **Births:** 276 **Total Expense ($000):** 14209 **Payroll Expense ($000):** 7765 **Personnel:** 191

BELTON—Cass County

★ **RESEARCH BELTON HOSPITAL (260214)**, 17065 South 71 Highway, Zip 64012–4631; tel. 816/348–1200 **A**1 9 10 **F**3 15 25 26 30 31 32 33 35 38 43 55 57 62 63 66 68 72 73 75 77 79 80 82 85 86 96 97 100 102 107 118 119 121 124 135 **P**5 **S** HCA
Primary Contact: Todd Krass, Chief Executive Officer
COO: Nicole Smith Hendricks, Vice President Operations
CFO: Susan Shreeve, Chief Financial Officer
CMO: Douglas Bradley, Vice President Medical Affairs
CIO: Paul Klehn, Director Information Systems
CHR: Yvonne Brewington, Director Human Resources
Web address: www.researchbeltonhospital.com
Control: Corporation, Investor–owned, for–profit **Service:** General Medical and Surgical

Staffed Beds: 38 **Admissions:** 1250 **Census:** 10 **Outpatient Visits:** 76143 **Births:** 0 **Total Expense ($000):** 27787 **Payroll Expense ($000):** 8851 **Personnel:** 141

BETHANY—Harrison County

★ **HARRISON COUNTY COMMUNITY HOSPITAL (261312)**, 2600 Miller Street, Zip 64424–2701, Mailing Address: P.O. Box 428, Zip 64424–0428; tel. 660/425–2211 **A**5 9 10 18 **F**3 11 15 24 25 30 31 32 33 38 41 43 52 55 56 57 61 62 63 65 68 73 75 77 79 82 84 85 86 96 97 100 102 106 107 117 118 119 122 132 134 135 137 **P**5
Primary Contact: Richard C. Hamilton, Administrator
CFO: Christina Gillespie, Chief Financial Officer
Web address: www.hcchospital.org
Control: Hospital district or authority, Government, nonfederal **Service:** General Medical and Surgical

Staffed Beds: 20 **Admissions:** 465 **Census:** 5 **Outpatient Visits:** 28289 **Births:** 0 **Total Expense ($000):** 10697 **Payroll Expense ($000):** 4881 **Personnel:** 154

BLUE SPRINGS—Jackson County

★ **ST. MARY'S MEDICAL CENTER (260193)**, 201 West R. D. Mize Road, Zip 64014–2518; tel. 816/228–5900 **A**1 9 10 12 13 **F**3 8 11 13 15 18 24 25 26 27 30 31 32 33 38 43 44 49 50 60 62 66 68 70 72 73 74 75 76 77 79 80 82 85 96 97 99 100 102 106 107 109 111 118 119 121 124 135 137 **S** Ascension Health
Primary Contact: Robin M. Schluter, Chief Executive Officer
CFO: Steven R. Cleary, Vice President Finance
CMO: Michael Feder, M.D., Chief Medical Officer
CHR: Dawn Bryant, Vice President Organizational Development
Web address: www.carondelethealth.org
Control: Other not–for–profit (including NFP Corporation) **Service:** General Medical and Surgical

Staffed Beds: 139 **Admissions:** 6404 **Census:** 75 **Outpatient Visits:** 84223 **Births:** 1147 **Total Expense ($000):** 72684 **Payroll Expense ($000):** 27187 **Personnel:** 459

BOLIVAR—Polk County

★ **CITIZENS MEMORIAL HOSPITAL (260195)**, 1500 North Oakland Avenue, Zip 65613–3011; tel. 417/326–6000 **A**1 9 10 20 **F**3 7 11 13 15 18 24 25 26 27 30 31 32 33 34 36 37 38 40 41 42 43 50 54 55 56 57 61 62 66 68 72 73 74 75 76 77 78 79 80 81 82 84 85 86 88 90 92 93 94 96 97 100 102 107 118 119 120 121 122 124 132 135 136 137 **P**6
Primary Contact: Donald J. Babb, Chief Executive Officer
COO: Allen Waldo, FACHE, Chief Operating Officer
CFO: Gary D. Fullbright, Comptroller
CMO: Steven Butcher, D.O., Director Medical Affairs
CIO: Denni McColm, Chief Information Officer
CHR: Jeremy MacLaughlin, Director Human Resources
Web address: www.citizensmemorial.com
Control: Hospital district or authority, Government, nonfederal **Service:** General Medical and Surgical

Staffed Beds: 76 **Admissions:** 3439 **Census:** 38 **Outpatient Visits:** 242597 **Births:** 524 **Total Expense ($000):** 71539 **Payroll Expense ($000):** 33660 **Personnel:** 771

BONNE TERRE—St. Francois County

★ **PARKLAND HEALTH CENTER–BONNE TERRE (261315)**, 7245 Raider Road, Zip 63628–3767; tel. 573/358–1400 **A**1 9 10 18 **F**3 11 15 25 26 27 30 31 32 33 38 50 52 55 56 57 62 63 73 75 76 81 82 84 85 86 118 119 124 135 **S** BJC HealthCare
Primary Contact: Richard L. Conklin, President
CFO: Thomas P. Karl, Assistant Administrator Operations
CMO: Patrick W. O'Hara, M.D., Chief of Staff
CHR: Sheri S. Graham, Director Human Resources and Administrative Services
Web address: www.parklandhealthcenter.org
Control: Other not–for–profit (including NFP Corporation) **Service:** General Medical and Surgical

Staffed Beds: 3 **Admissions:** 3916 **Census:** 40 **Outpatient Visits:** 18862 **Births:** 0 **Personnel:** 51

BOONVILLE—Cooper County

★ **COOPER COUNTY MEMORIAL HOSPITAL (260004)**, 17651 B Highway, Zip 65233–2839, Mailing Address: P.O. Box 88, Zip 65233–0088; tel. 660/882–7461, (Total facility includes 24 beds in nursing home–type unit) **A**5 9 10 20 **F**2 3 7 24 25 30 31 32 33 38 52 55 57 61 62 66 73 77 79 84 86 90 96 100 102 107 117 118 119 121 122 124 135 137 **S** University of Missouri Health Care
Primary Contact: Jeffrey L. Durham, Interim Chief Executive Officer
COO: Larry D. Kay, Chief Operating Officer
CFO: Brenda Campbell, Controller
Control: County–Government, nonfederal **Service:** General Medical and Surgical

Staffed Beds: 49 **Admissions:** 740 **Census:** 35 **Outpatient Visits:** 39856 **Births:** 0 **Total Expense ($000):** 13762 **Payroll Expense ($000):** 5446 **Personnel:** 190

Many Facility Codes have changed. Please refer to the AHA Guide Code Chart.

BRANSON—Taney County

☒ **SKAGGS COMMUNITY HEALTH CENTER (260094)**, Business Highway 65 and Skaggs Road, Zip 65616–2035, Mailing Address: P.O. Box 650, Zip 65615–0650; tel. 417/335–7000, (Total facility includes 16 beds in nursing home–type unit) **A**1 5 9 10 20 **F**3 11 13 15 17 18 20 22 24 25 26 27 30 31 32 33 36 38 42 43 44 50 51 52 54 55 56 57 59 60 61 62 63 65 66 68 72 73 74 75 76 77 78 79 80 81 82 84 85 86 87 90 96 97 100 102 105 106 107 117 118 119 120 121 124 132 133 135 137 **P**6 8
Primary Contact: Stephen M. Erixon, Chief Executive Officer
CFO: Robert C. Tyk, Chief Financial Officer
CMO: Peter R. Marcellus, M.D., Vice President Medical Services and Chief Medical Officer
CIO: Crystal Stallings, Chief Information Officer
CHR: Royce W. Allen, Vice President Human Resources
Web address: www.skaggs.net
Control: Other not–for–profit (including NFP Corporation) **Service:** General Medical and Surgical

Staffed Beds: 116 **Admissions:** 6512 **Census:** 79 **Outpatient Visits:** 292758 **Births:** 640 **Total Expense ($000):** 122425 **Payroll Expense ($000):** 45888 **Personnel:** 994

BRIDGETON—St. Louis County

☒ **SSM DEPAUL HEALTH CENTER (260104)**, 12303 DePaul Drive, Zip 63044–2588; tel. 314/344–6000, (Total facility includes 54 beds in nursing home–type unit) **A**1 9 10 **F**3 5 8 11 12 13 15 17 18 20 22 24 25 26 27 30 31 32 33 34 36 38 40 41 43 44 50 52 54 55 56 57 59 60 62 67 68 71 72 73 74 76 77 79 80 81 82 84 88 89 90 91 92 93 94 95 96 97 100 102 107 108 109 111 112 114 117 119 121 124 132 135 136 137 **P**6 8 **S** SSM Health Care
Primary Contact: Patrice L. Komoroski, M.S.N., RN, President
COO: Sean Hogan, Vice President and Chief Operating Officer
CFO: Hal Holder, Director Finance
CMO: Andrew Karanas, M.D., Vice President Medical Affairs
CIO: Matt Woodall, Director Information Management
CHR: Ken Clark, Human Resources Leader
Web address: www.ssmdepaul.com
Control: Church–operated, Nongovernment, not–for profit **Service:** General Medical and Surgical

Staffed Beds: 457 **Admissions:** 23185 **Census:** 351 **Outpatient Visits:** 156750 **Births:** 1755 **Total Expense ($000):** 253615 **Payroll Expense ($000):** 97563 **Personnel:** 1538

BROOKFIELD—Linn County

GENERAL JOHN J. PERSHING MEMORIAL HOSPITAL (261307), 130 East Lockling Avenue, Zip 64628–0130, Mailing Address: P.O. Box 408, Zip 64628–0408; tel. 660/258–2222 **A**9 10 18 **F**11 15 24 25 30 31 32 34 38 41 42 53 55 57 61 62 73 79 82 86 87 96 100 102 107 119 122 135 **P**6
Primary Contact: Phil Hamilton, RN, Chief Executive Officer
CFO: Gary R. Tandy, Chief Financial Officer
CMO: P. C. Rivera, M.D., Chief of Staff
CIO: Elaine Sutton, Director Perform Improvement and Privacy Officer
CHR: Amy Sayre, Director Human Resources
Web address: www.pershinghealthsystem.com
Control: Other not–for–profit (including NFP Corporation) **Service:** General Medical and Surgical

Staffed Beds: 25 **Admissions:** 660 **Census:** 8 **Outpatient Visits:** 56793 **Births:** 0 **Total Expense ($000):** 11251 **Payroll Expense ($000):** 4810 **Personnel:** 132

BUTLER—Bates County

★ **BATES COUNTY MEMORIAL HOSPITAL (260034)**, 615 West Nursery Street, Zip 64730–0370, Mailing Address: P.O. Box 370, Zip 64730–0370; tel. 660/200–7000 **A**9 10 **F**3 7 11 13 15 24 25 26 38 50 53 55 56 57 61 62 66 68 74 75 77 79 82 86 96 97 99 100 103 106 107 118 119 121 122 132 **P**6
Primary Contact: Wendell R. Harris, CPA, Ph.D., Chief Executive Officer
CFO: Wendell R. Harris, CPA, Ph.D., Chief Executive Officer
CMO: James L. Miller, M.D., Chief of Staff
CHR: Melinda Jackson, Director Human Resources
Web address: www.bcmhospital.com
Control: County–Government, nonfederal **Service:** General Medical and Surgical

Staffed Beds: 60 **Admissions:** 2062 **Census:** 25 **Outpatient Visits:** 43561 **Births:** 49 **Total Expense ($000):** 29943 **Payroll Expense ($000):** 10692 **Personnel:** 243

CAMERON—Clinton County

CAMERON REGIONAL MEDICAL CENTER (260057), 1600 East Evergreen, Zip 64429–1498, Mailing Address: P.O. Box 557, Zip 64429–0557; tel. 816/632–2101 **A**9 10 **F**3 11 13 15 17 24 25 27 31 32 33 34 37 38 42 43 44 46 47 49 54 55 56 57 60 61 62 65 68 72 73 74 75 76 77 79 80 82 84 85 86 88 90 93 94 96 100 102 105 107 117 118 119 120 122 132 135 137 **P**6
Primary Contact: Joseph F. Abrutz, Jr., Administrator
CFO: Rosa Patti, Chief Financial Officer
CIO: Bill Walser, Coordinator Technology
CHR: Pat Bestgen, Manager Human Resources
Web address: www.cameronregional.org
Control: Other not–for–profit (including NFP Corporation) **Service:** General Medical and Surgical

Staffed Beds: 58 **Admissions:** 1469 **Census:** 39 **Outpatient Visits:** 197295 **Births:** 163 **Total Expense ($000):** 34711 **Payroll Expense ($000):** 13705 **Personnel:** 352

CAPE GIRARDEAU—Cape Girardeau County

☐ **LANDMARK HOSPITAL (260220)**, 3255 Independence Street, Zip 63701–4904; tel. 573/335–1091 **A**1 9 10 **F**1 25 73 107 119 **S** Landmark Hospitals
Primary Contact: Deborah Sabella, Chief Executive Officer
COO: Michael L. Norman, CHE, Executive Vice President and Chief Operating Officer
CFO: Richard H. Hogan, CPA, Chief Financial Officer
CMO: Khalid I. Khan, M.D., Chief of Staff and Medical Director
CIO: Renee Hesselrode, Director Health Information Management
CHR: Angela Kisner, Director Human Resources and Coordinator Medical Staff
Web address: www.landmarkhospitals.com
Control: Partnership, Investor–owned, for–profit **Service:** Long–Term Acute Care hospital

Staffed Beds: 25 **Admissions:** 256 **Census:** 18 **Outpatient Visits:** 0 **Births:** 0 **Total Expense ($000):** 8081 **Payroll Expense ($000):** 2912 **Personnel:** 91

MO

☒ **SAINT FRANCIS MEDICAL CENTER (260183)**, 211 St. Francis Drive, Zip 63703–5049; tel. 573/331–3000 **A**1 2 5 9 10 19 **F**3 9 11 12 13 15 17 18 20 22 24 25 26 27 28 30 31 32 33 37 38 40 41 43 44 50 52 53 55 56 57 59 60 61 62 66 68 70 71 72 73 74 75 76 77 78 79 80 81 82 84 85 86 96 97 99 100 102 103 106 107 112 118 119 120 121 124 130 131 132 133 135 136 137 **P**6
Primary Contact: Steven C. Bjelich, President and Chief Executive Officer
CFO: Tony Balsano, Vice President Finance
CMO: James Schell, M.D., Vice President Medical Affairs
CIO: Diane Gammon, Director Information Systems
CHR: Teri Kreitzer, Director Human Resources
Web address: www.sfmc.net
Control: Church–operated, Nongovernment, not–for profit **Service:** General Medical and Surgical

Staffed Beds: 254 **Admissions:** 11110 **Census:** 160 **Outpatient Visits:** 185497 **Births:** 634 **Total Expense ($000):** 231414 **Payroll Expense ($000):** 90135 **Personnel:** 1534

☒ **SOUTHEAST MISSOURI HOSPITAL (260110)**, 1701 Lacey Street, Zip 63701–5230; tel. 573/334–4822 **A**1 2 5 9 10 19 **F**3 11 12 13 15 17 18 20 22 24 25 26 27 28 30 31 33 38 42 43 44 49 50 51 52 55 56 57 59 60 61 62 63 66 67 68 70 71 72 73 74 75 76 77 78 79 80 81 82 83 84 85 86 87 88 90 91 92 93 96 97 99 100 102 103 104 106 107 108 109 111 112 116 118 119 121 123 124 132 133 135 136 137
Primary Contact: James W. Wente, CPA, CHE, President and Chief Executive Officer
CFO: David Strong, Vice President
CMO: Lee Taylor, M.D., Vice President
CIO: Jay McGuire, Director Information Systems
Web address: www.southeastmissourihospital.com
Control: Other not–for–profit (including NFP Corporation) **Service:** General Medical and Surgical

Staffed Beds: 229 **Admissions:** 10237 **Census:** 127 **Outpatient Visits:** 165367 **Births:** 1273 **Total Expense ($000):** 217645 **Payroll Expense ($000):** 79702 **Personnel:** 1702

Hospital, Medicare Provider Number, Address, Telephone, Approval, Facility, and Physician Codes, Health Care System

★ American Hospital Association (AHA) membership
☐ The Joint Commission accreditation
○ American Osteopathic Association (AOA) accreditation
△ Commission on Accreditation of Rehabilitation Facilities (CARF) accreditation

CARROLLTON—Carroll County

CARROLL COUNTY MEMORIAL HOSPITAL (261332), 1502 North Jefferson Street, Zip 64633–1948; tel. 660/542–1695, (Total facility includes 15 beds in nursing home–type unit) **A**5 9 10 18 **F**2 3 10 15 24 25 26 31 33 34 38 52 54 55 57 58 61 62 63 65 73 75 77 79 85 86 96 97 100 102 105 107 115 117 118 119 122 **P**6
Primary Contact: Jerry Dover, Administrator and Chief Executive Officer
COO: Jeff Tindle, Associate Administrator and Chief Financial Officer
CFO: Jeff Tindle, Associate Administrator and Chief Financial Officer
CMO: Alex Dymek, M.D., Medical Director
CIO: Jeff Tindle, Associate Administrator and Chief Financial Officer
CHR: Karen Pfaff, Director Human Resources
Web address: www.carrollcountyhospital.org
Control: Other not–for–profit (including NFP Corporation) **Service:** General Medical and Surgical

Staffed Beds: 40 **Admissions:** 1337 **Census:** 20 **Outpatient Visits:** 39880 **Births:** 0 **Total Expense ($000):** 9384 **Payroll Expense ($000):** 4341 **Personnel:** 125

CARTHAGE—Jasper County

★ **MCCUNE–BROOKS REGIONAL HOSPITAL (261326)**, (Formerly McCune–Brooks Hospital), 3125 Drive Russell Smith Way, Zip 64836–7402; tel. 417/358–8121 **A**9 10 18 **F**3 7 11 15 24 25 26 33 38 44 50 51 52 55 57 61 62 66 67 68 73 77 79 82 84 88 93 96 100 102 107 118 119 120 121 122 124 135
Primary Contact: Robert Y. Copeland, Jr., FACHE, Chief Executive Officer
CFO: Tony Wright, Chief Financial Officer
CIO: Ken Masters, Director Information Systems
CHR: Brenda Kaiser, Director Human Resources
Web address: www.mccune–brooks.org
Control: City–Government, nonfederal **Service:** General Medical and Surgical

Staffed Beds: 35 **Admissions:** 1595 **Census:** 21 **Outpatient Visits:** 40769 **Births:** 0 **Total Expense ($000):** 21066 **Payroll Expense ($000):** 10286 **Personnel:** 279

CASSVILLE—Barry County

MO

▣ **ST. JOHN'S HOSPITAL – CASSVILLE (261317)**, 94 Main Street, Zip 65625–1610; tel. 417/847–6000 **A**1 10 18 **F**11 15 24 25 26 32 38 50 52 55 57 62 66 73 75 79 80 81 82 86 96 97 100 107 119 121 122 124 137 **P**6 **S** Sisters of Mercy Health System
Primary Contact: Gary W. Jordan, President
CFO: Douglas M. Hoban, Chief Financial Officer
Web address: www.southbarrycountyhospital.com
Control: Church–operated, Nongovernment, not–for profit **Service:** General Medical and Surgical

Staffed Beds: 18 **Admissions:** 218 **Census:** 2 **Outpatient Visits:** 18714 **Births:** 0 **Total Expense ($000):** 8529 **Payroll Expense ($000):** 4187 **Personnel:** 100

CHESTERFIELD—St. Louis County

▣ **DUBUIS HOSPITAL OF ST. LOUIS (262012)**, 13190 South Outer Forty Road, Zip 63017–5917; tel. 314/392–6380 **A**1 9 10 **F**1 3 25 26 31 43 119 137 **S** Dubuis Health System
Primary Contact: John F. Brothers, Interim Administrator
CMO: Anthony Masi, M.D., Medical Director
Web address: www.dubuis.org
Control: Other not–for–profit (including NFP Corporation) **Service:** Long–Term Acute Care hospital

Staffed Beds: 54 **Admissions:** 345 **Census:** 31 **Outpatient Visits:** 0 **Births:** 0 **Total Expense ($000):** 16105 **Payroll Expense ($000):** 6911 **Personnel:** 78

▣ **ST. LUKE'S HOSPITAL (260179)**, 232 South Woods Mill Road, Zip 63017–3417; tel. 314/434–1500, (Total facility includes 140 beds in nursing home–type unit) **A**1 2 9 10 **F**10 11 12 13 15 17 18 20 22 24 25 26 27 28 30 31 32 33 34 37 38 39 41 43 44 45 49 50 52 53 54 55 56 57 59 60 62 63 64 66 67 68 69 71 72 73 74 75 76 77 79 80 81 82 84 85 86 87 96 97 100 102 107 108 109 111 112 113 114 115 117 119 120 121 124 133 134 135 136 137 **P**6 8
Primary Contact: Gary R. Olson, President and Chief Executive Officer
CFO: Brian Spillers, Chief Financial Officer
CIO: William Meyers, Chief Information Officer
CHR: Janette Taaffe, Administrator Human Resources
Web address: www.stlukes–stl.com
Control: Church–operated, Nongovernment, not–for profit **Service:** General Medical and Surgical

Staffed Beds: 521 **Admissions:** 19750 **Census:** 372 **Outpatient Visits:** 684699 **Births:** 2192 **Total Expense ($000):** 343660 **Payroll Expense ($000):** 161174 **Personnel:** 2929

CHILLICOTHE—Livingston County

▣ **HEDRICK MEDICAL CENTER (261321)**, 100 Central Avenue, Zip 64601–1554; tel. 660/646–1480 **A**1 5 9 10 18 **F**3 11 13 15 24 25 26 27 30 31 32 33 38 41 42 43 50 55 57 61 62 63 67 68 72 73 74 75 76 77 79 80 81 82 84 85 86 87 94 96 97 100 102 106 107 117 118 119 120 121 122 124 132 133 135 136 137 **P**6 **S** Saint Luke's Health System
Primary Contact: Brian J. Johnston, FACHE, Chief Executive Officer
CFO: Dana Hoover, Chief Financial Officer
CMO: George A. Pagels, M.D., President and Chief Executive Officer
CIO: Matthew Wenzel, Senior Information System Site Analyst
CHR: Lisa Hecker, Director Human Resources
Web address: www.saintlukeshealthsystem.org
Control: Other not–for–profit (including NFP Corporation) **Service:** General Medical and Surgical

Staffed Beds: 25 **Admissions:** 948 **Census:** 9 **Outpatient Visits:** 64099 **Births:** 222 **Total Expense ($000):** 27769 **Payroll Expense ($000):** 11900 **Personnel:** 264

CLINTON—Henry County

▣ ○ **GOLDEN VALLEY MEMORIAL HOSPITAL (260175)**, 1600 North Second Street, Zip 64735–1192; tel. 660/885–5511 **A**1 9 10 11 19 20 **F**3 7 11 13 15 24 26 27 30 31 32 33 34 38 43 44 46 48 49 52 55 57 60 61 62 66 68 73 74 75 76 77 79 80 81 82 85 86 96 97 99 100 102 105 106 107 117 118 119 120 121 122 124 135 136 137
Primary Contact: Randy S. Wertz, Chief Executive Officer
CFO: Gordon Glass, Assistant Administrator Finance
CIO: James Begin, Director Information Technology
CHR: Roger Cook, Assistant Administrator Human Resources
Web address: www.gvmh.org
Control: Hospital district or authority, Government, nonfederal **Service:** General Medical and Surgical

Staffed Beds: 84 **Admissions:** 3387 **Census:** 43 **Outpatient Visits:** 238174 **Births:** 361 **Total Expense ($000):** 52492 **Payroll Expense ($000):** 25837 **Personnel:** 548

COLUMBIA—Boone County

▣ **BOONE HOSPITAL CENTER (260068)**, 1600 East Broadway, Zip 65201–5844; tel. 573/815–8000 **A**1 2 3 5 9 10 **F**3 7 11 12 13 15 17 18 20 22 24 25 26 27 30 31 32 33 34 38 43 44 46 48 49 50 51 52 54 55 56 57 59 60 62 63 66 68 70 71 72 73 74 75 76 77 78 79 80 81 82 84 85 86 87 88 90 91 92 93 94 95 96 97 99 100 102 103 104 106 107 118 119 120 121 124 134 135 136 137 **S** BJC HealthCare
Primary Contact: Daniel J. Rothery, President
COO: Randy Morrow, Vice President and Chief Operating Officer
CFO: Randy Morrow, Vice President and Chief Operating Officer
CMO: Carol Danuser, M.D., Chief Medical Officer
Web address: www.boone.org
Control: Other not–for–profit (including NFP Corporation) **Service:** General Medical and Surgical

Staffed Beds: 349 **Admissions:** 17628 **Census:** 231 **Outpatient Visits:** 146024 **Births:** 2125 **Total Expense ($000):** 239234 **Payroll Expense ($000):** 71550 **Personnel:** 1690

▣ **COLUMBIA REGIONAL HOSPITAL (260178)**, 404 Keene Street, Zip 65201–6626; tel. 573/875–9000 **A**1 3 5 9 10 **F**3 11 13 15 18 20 25 26 30 32 38 50 51 52 54 58 59 62 63 66 68 70 71 72 73 74 76 77 79 80 81 82 85 86 96 97 100 101 107 110 113 114 118 119 120 133 135 136 **P**6 **S** University of Missouri Health Care
Primary Contact: Keri Simon, Executive Director
CMO: Steven Dresner, M.D., Chief of Staff
CIO: Mark Bollinger, Manager Data Processing
Web address: www.columbiaregional.org
Control: State–Government, nonfederal **Service:** General Medical and Surgical

Staffed Beds: 176 **Admissions:** 5792 **Census:** 77 **Outpatient Visits:** 111827 **Births:** 1708 **Total Expense ($000):** 115045 **Payroll Expense ($000):** 37413 **Personnel:** 887

ELLIS FISCHEL CANCER CENTER See University of Missouri Hospitals and Clinics

▣ **HARRY S. TRUMAN MEMORIAL VETERANS HOSPITAL**, 800 Hospital Drive, Zip 65201–5275; tel. 573/814–6000, (Total facility includes 41 beds in nursing home–type unit) **A**1 3 5 **F**3 4 5 17 18 20 22 24 25 26 27 30 32 33 37 38 41 42 43 44 45 49 53 54 56 57 58 60 61 62 65 68 72 73 76 77 79 80 81 82 85 86 87 88 90 91 92 93 94 95 96 97 100 103 104 106 107 117 118 119 121 124 135 136 **P**6 **S** Department of Veterans Affairs
Primary Contact: Sallie Houser–Hanfelder, FACHE, Director
CFO: Curtis R. Russell, Chief Financial Officer
CMO: William Patterson, M.D., Chief of Staff
CIO: Rex Toles, Director Information Management Service Line
CHR: Thomas J. Patterson, Manager Human Resources
Web address: www.va.gov/cmo
Control: Veterans Affairs, Government, federal **Service:** General Medical and Surgical

Staffed Beds: 118 **Admissions:** 3518 **Census:** 83 **Outpatient Visits:** 416910 **Births:** 0 **Total Expense ($000):** 171425 **Payroll Expense ($000):** 64113 **Personnel:** 1048

★ △ **HOWARD A. RUSK REHABILITATION CENTER (263027)**, 315 Business Loop 70 West, Zip 65203–3248; tel. 573/817–2703 **A**1 5 7 9 10 **F**25 30 55 81 85 132 **S** HEALTHSOUTH Corporation
Primary Contact: Gary Payne, Chief Executive Officer
CFO: Scott Garrett, Controller
CMO: Gregory Worsowicz, M.D., Medical Director
CHR: Robin Prater, Director Human Resources
Web address: www.healthsouth.com
Control: Partnership, Investor–owned, for–profit **Service:** Rehabilitation

Staffed Beds: 60 **Admissions:** 909 **Census:** 44 **Outpatient Visits:** 11867 **Births:** 0 **Total Expense ($000):** 16751 **Payroll Expense ($000):** 6754 **Personnel:** 186

□ **MID–MISSOURI MENTAL HEALTH CENTER (264011)**, 3 Hospital Drive, Zip 65201–5296; tel. 573/884–1300 **A**1 3 5 10 **F**4 31 32 56 88 89 90 91 92 93 95 119
Primary Contact: Robert Reitz, Ph.D., Chief Executive Officer
COO: Marla Smith, Chief Operating Officer
CFO: Ken Lyle, Chief Financial Officer
CMO: Ronald Lacey, M.D., Medical Director
CHR: Lori Hollinger, Manager Human Resources
Web address: www.dmh.missouri.gov/mid_mo
Control: State–Government, nonfederal **Service:** Psychiatric

Staffed Beds: 69 **Admissions:** 1587 **Census:** 68 **Outpatient Visits:** 0 **Births:** 0 **Total Expense ($000):** 17742 **Payroll Expense ($000):** 8161 **Personnel:** 261

★ **UNIVERSITY OF MISSOURI HOSPITALS AND CLINICS (260141)**, One Hospital Drive, Zip 65212–0001; tel. 573/882–4141, (Includes ELLIS FISCHEL CANCER CENTER, 115 Business Loop 70 West, Zip 65203; tel. 573/882–5460) **A**1 2 3 5 8 9 10 **F**3 7 9 11 12 15 16 17 18 19 20 21 22 23 24 25 26 27 28 30 32 33 36 37 38 40 43 44 46 47 48 49 50 51 52 54 55 56 57 58 59 60 62 63 66 68 69 72 73 75 76 77 79 80 81 82 83 84 86 87 90 91 92 94 96 97 100 101 102 104 107 108 109 110 111 113 114 118 119 120 121 123 124 127 131 133 135 137 **P**1 **S** University of Missouri Health Care
Primary Contact: James H. Ross, Chief Executive Officer
COO: Anita Larsen, R.N., Interim Chief Operating Officer
CFO: Kevin Necas, Chief Financial Officer
CMO: Les Hall, M.D., Chief Medical Officer
CIO: George Carr, Chief Information Officer
CHR: Sue Kopfle, Chief Human Resources Officer
Web address: www.muhealth.org
Control: State–Government, nonfederal **Service:** General Medical and Surgical

Staffed Beds: 282 **Admissions:** 14319 **Census:** 201 **Outpatient Visits:** 575338 **Births:** 0 **Total Expense ($000):** 389579 **Payroll Expense ($000):** 150971 **Personnel:** 2844

CRYSTAL CITY—Jefferson County

○ **JEFFERSON MEMORIAL HOSPITAL (260023)**, Highway 61 South, Zip 63019, Mailing Address: P.O. Box 350, Zip 63019–0350; tel. 636/933–1000, (Total facility includes 10 beds in nursing home–type unit) **A**9 10 11 **F**3 4 5 7 8 11 13 15 18 20 22 24 25 26 30 31 32 33 35 38 41 42 43 44 49 50 51 52 53 54 55 56 57 61 62 68 72 73 74 75 77 79 80 81 82 84 85 86 87 88 89 90 91 92 93 94 96 97 100 102 104 105 106 107 117 118 119 120 121 124 132 135 136 137
Primary Contact: Lloyd F. Ford, Jr., Ph.D., FACHE, President and Chief Executive Officer
CFO: Jim Muehlhauser, Chief Financial Officer
CHR: Jeff Buck, Executive Director Human Resources
Web address: www.jeffersonmemorial.org
Control: Other not–for–profit (including NFP Corporation) **Service:** General Medical and Surgical

Staffed Beds: 188 **Admissions:** 10588 **Census:** 123 **Outpatient Visits:** 124235 **Births:** 749 **Total Expense ($000):** 95526 **Payroll Expense ($000):** 42228 **Personnel:** 1062

DEXTER—Stoddard County

MISSOURI SOUTHERN HEALTHCARE (260160), 1200 North One Mile Road, Zip 63841–1000; tel. 573/624–5566 **A**9 10 **F**3 11 15 17 25 31 32 37 38 55 61 62 66 68 73 75 78 79 80 84 85 86 87 96 97 100 102 107 117 118 119 121 122 124 137 **P**6 **S** Sunlink Health Systems
Primary Contact: James P. Crawford, Jr., Chief Executive Officer
Web address: www.msh-hospital.com
Control: Corporation, Investor–owned, for–profit **Service:** General Medical and Surgical

Staffed Beds: 45 **Admissions:** 1513 **Census:** 16 **Outpatient Visits:** 89867 **Births:** 0 **Total Expense ($000):** 11795 **Payroll Expense ($000):** 5612 **Personnel:** 116

DONIPHAN—Ripley County

★ **RIPLEY COUNTY MEMORIAL HOSPITAL (260080)**, 109 Plum Street, Zip 63935–1299; tel. 573/996–2141 **A**9 10 **F**11 25 30 31 38 57 61 82 86 87 96 100 119 122 124
Primary Contact: Robert E. Garrison, Chief Executive Officer
CFO: Monya York, Chief Financial Officer
CIO: Tony Hahn, Manager Information Technology
Web address: www.rcmhospital.net
Control: County–Government, nonfederal **Service:** General Medical and Surgical

Staffed Beds: 27 **Admissions:** 778 **Census:** 8 **Outpatient Visits:** 28123 **Births:** 0 **Total Expense ($000):** 7986 **Payroll Expense ($000):** 4627 **Personnel:** 140

EL DORADO SPRINGS—Cedar County

CEDAR COUNTY MEMORIAL HOSPITAL (261323), 1401 South Park Street, Zip 64744–2037; tel. 417/876–2511 **A**9 10 18 **F**11 15 24 25 26 28 30 31 32 33 38 50 52 54 55 56 57 61 62 63 73 74 75 79 80 81 82 84 86 92 96 100 106 107 119 121 122 123 124 135 136 **P**6
Primary Contact: Jackie Boyles, Administrator
CFO: Carla Gilbert, Controller
CHR: Diana Pyle, Director Human Resources
Web address: www.cedarcountyhospital.org
Control: County–Government, nonfederal **Service:** General Medical and Surgical

Staffed Beds: 25 **Admissions:** 809 **Census:** 7 **Outpatient Visits:** 36711 **Births:** 90 **Total Expense ($000):** 9618 **Payroll Expense ($000):** 4290 **Personnel:** 132

SOUTHWEST MISSOURI PSYCHIATRIC REHABILITATION CENTER (264027), 1301 Industrial Parkway East, Zip 64744–6263; tel. 417/876–1000 **A**10 **F**30 31 32 88 91 92
Primary Contact: Denise Norbury, Regional Executive Officer
Control: State–Government, nonfederal **Service:** Psychiatric

Staffed Beds: 24 **Admissions:** 120 **Census:** 22 **Outpatient Visits:** 0 **Births:** 0 **Total Expense ($000):** 3187 **Payroll Expense ($000):** 2463 **Personnel:** 15

ELLINGTON—Reynolds County

ADVANCED HEALTHCARE MEDICAL CENTER (261304), Highway 21 South, Zip 63638–7427, Mailing Address: Rural Route 4, Box 4269, Zip 63638–4269; tel. 573/663–2511 **A**9 10 18 **F**3 7 30 31 32 38 61 62 75 77 79 80 82 86 96 100 102 107 118 119 122 **P**6
Primary Contact: Paula Harris, Chief Executive Officer
COO: Steve Myers, Assistant Administrator
CFO: Katie Caudel, Controller
CIO: Thomas Barker, Director Information
Control: Partnership, Investor–owned, for–profit **Service:** General Medical and Surgical

Staffed Beds: 25 **Admissions:** 478 **Census:** 5 **Outpatient Visits:** 98600 **Births:** 1 **Total Expense ($000):** 21552 **Payroll Expense ($000):** 10237 **Personnel:** 174

EXCELSIOR SPRINGS—Clay County

★ **EXCELSIOR SPRINGS MEDICAL CENTER (261322)**, 1700 Rainbow Boulevard, Zip 64024–1190; tel. 816/630–6081, (Total facility includes 80 beds in nursing home–type unit) **A**1 9 10 18 **F**3 8 10 11 15 25 26 27 28 30 31 32 33 37 38 42 43 44 54 55 56 57 61 62 65 66 68 72 73 75 76 77 79 80 81 82 86 96 97 100 102 104 105 106 107 115 117 118 119 121 122 124 132 135 136
Primary Contact: Sally S. Nance, Chief Executive Officer
CFO: Dennis Hartman, Chief Financial Officer
CMO: Manoch Kuangparichat, M.D., President Medical Staff
CIO: Alicia Harrison, Data Management Officer
CHR: Joni Schwan, Human Resources Director
Web address: www.esmc.org
Control: City–Government, nonfederal **Service:** General Medical and Surgical

Staffed Beds: 105 **Admissions:** 697 **Census:** 77 **Outpatient Visits:** 30438 **Births:** 0 **Total Expense ($000):** 17789 **Payroll Expense ($000):** 8391 **Personnel:** 225

MO

Hospital, Medicare Provider Number, Address, Telephone, Approval, Facility, and Physician Codes, Health Care System

★ American Hospital Association (AHA) membership
□ The Joint Commission accreditation
○ American Osteopathic Association (AOA) accreditation
△ Commission on Accreditation of Rehabilitation Facilities (CARF) accreditation

FAIRFAX—Atchison County

★ **COMMUNITY HOSPITAL ASSOCIATION (261303)**, 405 East Main, Zip 64446–0107, Mailing Address: P.O. Box 107, Zip 64446–0107; tel. 660/686–2211 **A**5 9 10 18 **F**11 13 15 24 30 38 57 61 62 65 74 79 80 82 84 86 96 107 117 122
Primary Contact: Myra L. Evans, Chief Executive Officer
COO: Myra L. Evans, Chief Executive Officer
CFO: Suzanne Southard, Director Finance
CMO: Aron Burke, M.D., Chief Medical Officer
CIO: Toni Ray, Information Systems Supervisor
CHR: Myra L. Evans, Chief Executive Officer
Web address: www.chafx.org
Control: Other not–for–profit (including NFP Corporation) **Service:** General Medical and Surgical

Staffed Beds: 25 **Admissions:** 651 **Census:** 7 **Outpatient Visits:** 19094 **Births:** 63 **Total Expense ($000):** 8261 **Payroll Expense ($000):** 3718 **Personnel:** 93

FARMINGTON—St. Francois County

★ ○ **MINERAL AREA REGIONAL MEDICAL CENTER (260116)**, 1212 Weber Road, Zip 63640–3325; tel. 573/756–4581 **A**9 10 11 19 **F**3 13 15 24 25 26 32 38 55 57 61 62 68 74 75 77 79 80 84 85 86 90 94 96 100 102 106 107 118 119 121 122 136 **S** Capella Healthcare
Primary Contact: Philip H. Walkley, Jr., FACHE, Chief Executive Officer
CFO: Rick Jenkins, Chief Financial Officer
CMO: Russel Deidiker, M.D., Chief of Staff
CIO: Jim Smith, Director Information Systems
Web address: www.marmc.org
Control: Corporation, Investor–owned, for–profit **Service:** General Medical and Surgical

Staffed Beds: 98 **Admissions:** 3233 **Census:** 32 **Outpatient Visits:** 110776 **Births:** 353 **Total Expense ($000):** 45887 **Payroll Expense ($000):** 17968 **Personnel:** 393

⊠ ○ **PARKLAND HEALTH CENTER (260163)**, 1101 West Liberty Street, Zip 63640–1921; tel. 573/756–6451 **A**1 5 9 10 11 **F**3 11 13 15 24 25 26 27 30 31 32 33 34 37 38 41 43 46 49 50 51 52 55 56 57 59 60 62 63 66 67 68 72 73 74 75 76 77 79 80 81 82 84 86 88 93 96 97 100 102 106 107 119 120 121 124 135 137 **S** BJC HealthCare
Primary Contact: Richard L. Conklin, President
CFO: Thomas P. Karl, Assistant Administrator Operations
CMO: Patrick W. O'Hara, M.D., Chief of Staff
CHR: Sheri S. Graham, Director Human Resources and Administrative Services
Web address: www.parklandhealthcenter.org
Control: Other not–for–profit (including NFP Corporation) **Service:** General Medical and Surgical

Staffed Beds: 94 **Admissions:** 3916 **Census:** 40 **Outpatient Visits:** 65303 **Births:** 745 **Total Expense ($000):** 55949 **Payroll Expense ($000):** 20518 **Personnel:** 466

☐ **SOUTHEAST MISSOURI MENTAL HEALTH CENTER (264005)**, 1010 West Columbia Street, Zip 63640–2997; tel. 573/218–6701 **A**1 9 10 **F**4 26 30 31 32 38 52 81 88 91 92 93 119
Primary Contact: Karen L. Adams, Chief Executive Officer
COO: Melissa Ring, Ph.D., Chief Operating Officer
CFO: Julie Inman, Chief Financial Officer
CMO: Jay Englehart, M.D., Medical Director
CIO: Julie Inman, Chief Financial Officer
CHR: Mark Remspecher, Director Human Resources
Web address: www.dmh.missouri.gov/southeast/
Control: State–Government, nonfederal **Service:** Psychiatric

Staffed Beds: 172 **Admissions:** 1761 **Census:** 157 **Outpatient Visits:** 2188 **Births:** 0 **Total Expense ($000):** 29308 **Payroll Expense ($000):** 12811 **Personnel:** 536

FORT LEONARD WOOD—Pulaski County

⊠ **GENERAL LEONARD WOOD ARMY COMMUNITY HOSPITAL**, 126 Missouri Avenue, Zip 65473–8952; tel. 573/596–0414 **A**1 5 **F**3 4 7 13 14 15 25 26 29 30 31 32 33 37 38 50 55 56 57 63 66 68 72 73 74 75 77 79 80 81 82 84 85 86 87 88 89 90 92 96 99 100 107 119 121 124 135 136 **S** Department of the Army, Office of the Surgeon General
Primary Contact: Lieutenant Colonel Margaret Toillion, Interim Deputy Commander
CFO: Major Michael Hogan, Chief Resource Management
CMO: Lieutenant Colonel John Lowery, Deputy Commander Clinical Services
CIO: Major Frederick White, Chief Information Management
CHR: Major Sandra Roper, Chief Human Resources
Web address: www.amedd.army.mil
Control: Army, Government, federal **Service:** General Medical and Surgical

Staffed Beds: 42 **Admissions:** 2111 **Census:** 20 **Outpatient Visits:** 382952 **Births:** 469 **Total Expense ($000):** 80188 **Personnel:** 956

FREDERICKTOWN—Madison County

MADISON MEDICAL CENTER (261302), 611 West Main, Zip 63645–1111, Mailing Address: P.O. Box 431, Zip 63645–0431; tel. 573/783–3341, (Total facility includes 102 beds in nursing home–type unit) **A**9 10 18 **F**6 7 11 15 30 31 33 38 57 61 62 65 68 75 77 79 82 86 87 93 96 100 107 117 119 122 135
Primary Contact: Rodney D. Gross, Ph.D., Administrator
CFO: Lisa Twidwell, Chief Financial Officer
CMO: P. A. George, M.D., Chief of Staff
CHR: Jennifer Penuel, Director Human Resources
Web address: www.madisonmedicalcenter.net
Control: County–Government, nonfederal **Service:** General Medical and Surgical

Staffed Beds: 119 **Admissions:** 441 **Census:** 90 **Outpatient Visits:** 52304 **Births:** 0 **Total Expense ($000):** 14653 **Payroll Expense ($000):** 7766 **Personnel:** 275

FULTON—Callaway County

☐ **CALLAWAY COMMUNITY HOSPITAL (260209)**, 10 South Hospital Drive, Zip 65251–2510; tel. 573/642–3376 **A**1 5 9 10 **F**3 8 11 13 15 25 26 27 30 31 32 38 57 61 62 65 68 74 76 77 79 80 81 84 87 96 97 100 102 107 117 119 122 135 **S** Sunlink Health Systems
Primary Contact: John T. Graves, CHE, Chief Executive Officer
CFO: William Akers, Chief Financial Officer
CHR: Martie Jeney, Director Human Resources
Web address: www.sunlinkhealth.com/callaway.html
Control: Corporation, Investor–owned, for–profit **Service:** General Medical and Surgical

Staffed Beds: 35 **Admissions:** 1267 **Census:** 11 **Outpatient Visits:** 40033 **Births:** 142 **Total Expense ($000):** 14749 **Payroll Expense ($000):** 6774 **Personnel:** 166

☐ **FULTON STATE HOSPITAL (264004)**, 600 East Fifth Street, Zip 65251–1798; tel. 573/592–4100 **A**1 5 10 **F**3 11 25 26 30 37 41 43 50 52 54 55 57 58 63 73 75 81 82 88 90 91 92 93 119 121 124 132 135 **P**6
Primary Contact: Robert Reitz, Ph.D., Chief Executive Officer
COO: Marty Ann Martin, Chief Operating Officer
CFO: J. Kenneth Lyle, Chief Financial Officer
CMO: Judith Fisher, D.O., Clinical Director
CIO: Robert Smith, Chief Information Officer
CHR: Lori Hollinger, Manager Human Resources
Web address: www.dmh.missouri.gov/fulton
Control: State–Government, nonfederal **Service:** Psychiatric

Staffed Beds: 496 **Admissions:** 273 **Census:** 509 **Outpatient Visits:** 0 **Births:** 0 **Total Expense ($000):** 75389 **Payroll Expense ($000):** 41469 **Personnel:** 1295

HANNIBAL—Marion County

⊠ **HANNIBAL REGIONAL HOSPITAL (260025)**, 6000 Hospital Drive, Zip 63401–6749, Mailing Address: P.O. Box 551, Zip 63401–0551; tel. 573/248–1300 **A**1 2 5 9 10 19 20 **F**3 11 13 15 18 20 24 26 27 30 32 33 36 37 38 43 44 46 49 54 55 56 57 59 60 61 62 68 72 73 74 75 76 77 78 79 80 81 82 84 85 86 87 88 89 90 91 92 93 94 96 97 100 106 107 108 109 118 119 120 121 124 132 133 135 136 137 **P**1
Primary Contact: John C. Grossmeier, President and Chief Executive Officer
CFO: Roger J. Dix, Senior Vice President and Chief Financial Officer
CMO: John Bennett, M.D., President Medical Staff
CIO: Phyllis Paris, Director
CHR: Penny Nunley, Vice President Human Resources
Web address: www.hrhonline.org
Control: Other not–for–profit (including NFP Corporation) **Service:** General Medical and Surgical

Staffed Beds: 105 **Admissions:** 5663 **Census:** 63 **Outpatient Visits:** 89540 **Births:** 677 **Total Expense ($000):** 77514 **Payroll Expense ($000):** 34470 **Personnel:** 770

HARRISONVILLE—Cass County

★ **CASS MEDICAL CENTER (261324)**, 1800 East Mechanic Street, Zip 64701–2017; tel. 816/380–3474 **A**9 10 18 **F**3 11 15 24 25 26 27 28 30 31 32 33 37 38 49 50 53 54 55 57 62 64 66 68 72 73 75 76 77 79 80 81 82 84 87 88 96 100 102 107 118 119 121 122 124 135 137 **P**6
Primary Contact: John Christopher Lang, Chief Executive Officer
CFO: Steve Klein, Chief Financial Officer
CIO: Cynthia Miltenberger, Director Organizational Effectiveness
CHR: Carla Wallen, Manager Human Resources
Web address: www.cassmedicalcenter.com
Control: County–Government, nonfederal **Service:** General Medical and Surgical

Staffed Beds: 35 **Admissions:** 1726 **Census:** 20 **Outpatient Visits:** 84088 **Births:** 2 **Total Expense ($000):** 31159 **Payroll Expense ($000):** 12522 **Personnel:** 274

Many Facility Codes have changed. Please refer to the AHA Guide Code Chart.

HAYTI—Pemiscot County

PEMISCOT MEMORIAL HEALTH SYSTEM (260070), Highway 61 and Reed, Zip 63851–1245, Mailing Address: P.O. Box 489, Zip 63851–0489; tel. 573/359–1372, (Total facility includes 120 beds in nursing home–type unit) **A**9 10 **F**3 7 11 13 15 17 24 25 26 30 31 32 37 38 50 55 56 57 62 65 66 68 73 74 75 77 79 80 82 84 85 86 87 96 100 107 117 118 119 122 132 133 135 136 137 **P**6
Primary Contact: Kerry L. Noble, Administrator
Control: County–Government, nonfederal **Service:** General Medical and Surgical

Staffed Beds: 169 **Admissions:** 3210 **Census:** 95 **Outpatient Visits:** 85455 **Total Expense ($000):** 31637 **Payroll Expense ($000):** 13526 **Personnel:** 417

HERMANN—Gasconade County

★ **HERMANN AREA DISTRICT HOSPITAL (261314)**, Mailing Address: P.O. Box 470, Zip 65041–0470; tel. 573/486–2191 **A**9 10 18 **F**11 15 24 25 26 30 31 32 33 38 52 55 57 61 62 65 67 73 75 76 77 79 82 84 86 87 93 94 96 107 117 119 121 122 124 135 **P**6
Primary Contact: Dan McKinney, Administrator
COO: Dan McKinney, Administrator
CFO: Denise Witthaus, Accountant
CMO: Jaya Appal, M.D., Chief of Staff
CIO: Darrell D. Jung, Assistant Administrator
CHR: Carol Schaefer, Director Human Resources
Web address: www.hadh.org
Control: Hospital district or authority, Government, nonfederal **Service:** General Medical and Surgical

Staffed Beds: 25 **Admissions:** 470 **Census:** 12 **Outpatient Visits:** 51292 **Births:** 0 **Total Expense ($000):** 14223 **Payroll Expense ($000):** 6664 **Personnel:** 161

HOUSTON—Texas County

TEXAS COUNTY MEMORIAL HOSPITAL (260024), 1333 South Sam Houston Boulevard, Zip 65483–2046; tel. 417/967–3311 **A**9 10 20 **F**3 7 13 15 24 25 32 38 42 52 57 61 62 68 73 74 75 79 80 81 82 84 86 87 96 100 102 107 119 122 132 137 **P**6
Primary Contact: Wesley E. Murray, Chief Executive Officer
CFO: Linda Pamperien, Chief Financial Officer
CMO: Charles Mueller, M.D., Chief Medical Officer
CHR: Anita Kuhn, Coordinator Human Resources
Web address: www.tcmh.org
Control: County–Government, nonfederal **Service:** General Medical and Surgical

Staffed Beds: 47 **Admissions:** 1731 **Census:** 18 **Outpatient Visits:** 159043 **Births:** 291 **Total Expense ($000):** 25229 **Payroll Expense ($000):** 11476 **Personnel:** 308

INDEPENDENCE—Jackson County

☒ ○ **CENTERPOINT MEDICAL CENTER (260095)**, 19600 East 39th Street, Zip 64057; tel. 816/698–7000 **A**1 2 5 9 10 11 12 13 **F**3 8 13 15 17 18 20 22 24 25 26 27 30 31 32 33 36 38 40 53 54 55 56 57 59 62 68 69 70 71 72 73 74 75 76 77 78 79 80 81 82 86 96 97 100 103 107 118 119 120 121 124 134 135 136 137 **P**5 6 **S** HCA
Primary Contact: Carolyn W. Caldwell, President and Chief Executive Officer
COO: Natalie Mussi, Chief Operating Officer
CFO: James H. Brown, Chief Financial Officer
CMO: Paul Chu, M.D., President Medical Staff
CIO: Shannan Pfeiffer, Director Information Technology and System Services
CHR: Nancy Hill, Vice President Human Resources
Control: Corporation, Investor–owned, for–profit **Service:** General Medical and Surgical

Staffed Beds: 221 **Admissions:** 10211 **Census:** 113 **Outpatient Visits:** 97907 **Births:** 1062 **Total Expense ($000):** 107642 **Payroll Expense ($000):** 47961 **Personnel:** 843

JEFFERSON CITY—Cole County

☒ ○ **CAPITAL REGION MEDICAL CENTER (260047)**, 1125 Madison Street, Zip 65101–5227, Mailing Address: P.O. Box 1128, Zip 65102–1128; tel. 573/632–5000 **A**1 5 9 10 11 12 13 19 **F**3 5 7 11 13 15 18 20 22 24 25 26 27 28 30 31 32 33 34 36 38 46 47 48 49 52 53 54 55 56 57 60 61 62 64 68 72 73 74 75 76 77 78 79 80 82 84 85 86 87 89 90 92 94 96 97 99 102 106 107 108 109 118 119 120 121 124 133 135 136 **P**6 **S** University of Missouri Health Care
Primary Contact: Edward F. Farnsworth, FACHE, President
CFO: James McMillan, Vice President Finance
CMO: Lisa Kolb, M.D., Chief of Staff
CIO: Cerise Seifert, Interim Chief Information Officer
CHR: Bob Mazur, Vice President Human Resources
Web address: www.crmc.org
Control: Other not–for–profit (including NFP Corporation) **Service:** General Medical and Surgical

Staffed Beds: 114 **Admissions:** 7898 **Census:** 92 **Outpatient Visits:** 305585 **Births:** 923 **Total Expense ($000):** 132000 **Payroll Expense ($000):** 51911 **Personnel:** 1152

☒ **ST. MARYS HEALTH CENTER (260011)**, 100 St. Marys Medical Plaza, Zip 65101–1602; tel. 573/761–7000 **A**1 6 9 10 19 **F**3 8 11 13 15 18 20 22 24 25 26 27 30 31 32 33 36 37 38 43 44 45 49 50 51 55 56 57 58 59 60 62 68 72 73 74 75 76 77 78 79 80 81 82 84 86 87 88 90 91 92 93 94 95 96 97 100 102 104 105 106 107 109 111 118 119 120 121 124 133 135 136 137 **P**6 **S** SSM Health Care
Primary Contact: R. Brent VanConia, President
CFO: Tom Luebbering, Vice President Finance
CMO: John Lucio, D.O., President Medical Staff
CHR: Susan Mankoski, Vice President Human Resources
Web address: www.stmarys–jeffcity.com
Control: Church–operated, Nongovernment, not–for profit **Service:** General Medical and Surgical

Staffed Beds: 167 **Admissions:** 10634 **Census:** 101 **Outpatient Visits:** 252025 **Births:** 584 **Total Expense ($000):** 146367 **Payroll Expense ($000):** 51992 **Personnel:** 923

JOPLIN—Newton County

★ ○ **FREEMAN HEALTH SYSTEM (260137)**, 1102 West 32nd Street, Zip 64804–3503; tel. 417/347–1111, (Includes FREEMAN HOSPITAL EAST, 932 East 34th Street, Zip 64804–3999; FREEMAN HOSPITAL WEST, Mailing Address: 1102 West 32nd Street, Zip 64804–3599), (Total facility includes 32 beds in nursing home–type unit) **A**2 9 10 11 12 13 **F**3 11 13 15 17 18 20 22 24 25 26 27 28 30 31 32 33 34 37 38 39 40 41 43 44 45 46 47 49 50 53 54 55 56 57 58 59 60 61 62 63 66 68 69 70 72 73 74 75 76 77 79 80 81 82 84 85 86 87 88 90 92 93 96 97 100 102 103 105 107 112 114 117 118 119 120 121 124 133 134 135 136 137 **P**1 6 **S** Freeman Health System
Primary Contact: Gary D. Duncan, President and Chief Executive Officer
COO: Joe L. Kirk, Executive Vice President
CFO: Steve W. Graddy, Chief Financial Officer
CMO: Richard D. Schooler, M.D., Chief Medical Officer
CIO: Sue Annesser, Director Information Technology
CHR: Deborah Chiodo, Director Human Resources
Web address: www.freemanhealth.com
Control: Other not–for–profit (including NFP Corporation) **Service:** General Medical and Surgical

Staffed Beds: 326 **Admissions:** 17269 **Census:** 244 **Outpatient Visits:** 662250 **Births:** 2615 **Total Expense ($000):** 339661 **Payroll Expense ($000):** 162969 **Personnel:** 2821

★ △ **ST. JOHN'S REGIONAL MEDICAL CENTER (260001)**, 2727 McClelland Boulevard, Zip 64804–1626; tel. 417/781–2727, (Includes ST. JOHN'S REHABILITATION CENTER, 2727 McClelland Boulevard, Zip 64804; tel. 417/659–6716), (Total facility includes 10 beds in nursing home–type unit) **A**2 7 9 10 **F**3 5 7 11 12 13 15 17 18 20 22 24 25 26 27 30 31 32 33 35 36 37 38 40 41 42 43 44 45 50 51 53 55 56 57 58 59 60 61 62 63 64 66 67 68 72 73 74 75 76 77 79 80 81 82 84 85 86 87 88 89 90 91 92 93 94 95 96 97 100 102 103 104 107 108 109 111 117 118 119 120 121 123 124 133 135 136 137 **P**1 6 **S** Catholic Health Initiatives
Primary Contact: George P. Caralis, President and Chief Executive Officer
COO: John Mentgen, Chief Operating Officer
CFO: Dennis G. Wilson, Interim Chief Financial Officer
CMO: Stephen Nesbit, M.D., Vice President Medical Affairs
CIO: Robert Honeywell, Vice President Information Systems
CHR: Pete Pzeminski, Interim Vice President Human Resources
Web address: www.stj.com
Control: Church–operated, Nongovernment, not–for profit **Service:** General Medical and Surgical

Staffed Beds: 367 **Admissions:** 16405 **Census:** 214 **Outpatient Visits:** 212065 **Births:** 906 **Total Expense ($000):** 218362 **Payroll Expense ($000):** 75864 **Personnel:** 1919

MO

Hospital, Medicare Provider Number, Address, Telephone, Approval, Facility, and Physician Codes, Health Care System

★ American Hospital Association (AHA) membership
□ The Joint Commission accreditation
○ American Osteopathic Association (AOA) accreditation
△ Commission on Accreditation of Rehabilitation Facilities (CARF) accreditation

KANSAS CITY—Jackson County

★ **CHILDREN'S MERCY HOSPITALS AND CLINICS (263302)**, 2401 Gillham Road, Zip 64108–4619; tel. 816/234–3000 **A**1 2 3 5 8 9 10 **F**3 7 8 9 11 12 16 18 19 20 21 22 23 25 26 27 28 31 32 33 34 37 38 40 41 43 44 48 49 50 53 55 56 57 58 59 60 61 62 63 66 70 71 72 73 75 76 77 79 80 81 82 83 84 85 86 87 89 90 94 96 97 100 102 106 107 114 119 120 121 123 125 127 128 131 133 135 137 **P**6 8
Primary Contact: Randall L. O'Donnell, Ph.D., President and Chief Executive Officer
COO: Jo Stueve, Co Chief Operating Officer
CFO: Sandra A J Lawrence, Executive Vice President and Chief Financial Officer
CMO: V. Fred Burry, M.D., Executive Medical Director
CIO: Jean Ann Breedlove, Chief Information Officer
CHR: Dan Wright, Vice President Human Resources
Web address: www.childrens–mercy.org
Control: Other not–for–profit (including NFP Corporation) **Service:** Children's general

Staffed Beds: 260 **Admissions:** 12485 **Census:** 185 **Outpatient Visits:** 307802 **Births:** 0 **Total Expense ($000):** 447374 **Payroll Expense ($000):** 221647 **Personnel:** 3636

☐ **CRITTENTON CHILDREN'S CENTER (264018)**, 10918 Elm Avenue, Zip 64134–4108; tel. 816/765–6600 **A**1 10 **F**5 25 26 28 30 31 32 33 56 73 75 81 82 88 89 90 91 92 94 119 121 135 **P**6 **S** Saint Luke's Health System
Primary Contact: Stephen W. Churchill, M.D., Chief Executive Officer and Medical Director
COO: JoAnn McDonough, Director Operations and Chief Nursing Officer
CFO: Willard Staron, Chief Financial Officer
CIO: John Wade, Vice President and Chief Information Officer
Web address: www.saintlukeshealthsystem.org/app/hpcrittenton.asp
Control: Other not–for–profit (including NFP Corporation) **Service:** Children's hospital psychiatric

Staffed Beds: 46 **Admissions:** 1509 **Census:** 33 **Outpatient Visits:** 16785 **Births:** 0 **Total Expense ($000):** 19987 **Payroll Expense ($000):** 11911 **Personnel:** 78

☐ **KINDRED HOSPITAL KANSAS CITY (262011)**, 8701 Troost Avenue, Zip 64131–2767; tel. 816/995–2000 **A**1 9 10 **F**1 3 25 56 59 62 68 73 75 82 85 90 96 119 137 **S** Kindred Healthcare
Primary Contact: Cindy Mostaffa, Chief Executive Officer
CFO: Mike Delaney, Chief Financial Officer
Web address: www.kindredhospitalkc.com
Control: Corporation, Investor–owned, for–profit **Service:** Long–Term Acute Care hospital

Staffed Beds: 130 **Admissions:** 739 **Census:** 72 **Outpatient Visits:** 799 **Births:** 0 **Total Expense ($000):** 31408 **Payroll Expense ($000):** 10700 **Personnel:** 199

NORTH KANSAS CITY HOSPITAL See North Kansas City

★ **RESEARCH MEDICAL CENTER (260027)**, 2316 East Meyer Boulevard, Zip 64132–1136; tel. 816/276–4000 **A**1 2 3 5 9 10 **F**3 8 11 13 15 17 18 20 22 24 25 26 27 30 31 32 33 36 37 38 39 40 43 44 49 50 51 52 55 56 57 58 59 60 62 66 68 70 71 72 73 74 75 76 77 78 79 80 81 82 85 86 87 88 90 96 97 100 103 104 106 107 109 111 112 113 114 118 119 121 123 124 127 130 131 135 136 137 **P**5 6 **S** HCA
Primary Contact: Kevin J. Hicks, President and Chief Executive Officer
COO: Jacqueline DeSouza, Chief Operating Officer
CFO: Susan Shreeve, Chief Financial Officer
CIO: Tressy McKinney, Director Information Services
CHR: Dennis K. Johnson, Director Human Resources
Web address: www.researchmedicalcenter.com
Control: Corporation, Investor–owned, for–profit **Service:** General Medical and Surgical

Staffed Beds: 383 **Admissions:** 13922 **Census:** 213 **Outpatient Visits:** 117219 **Births:** 1200 **Total Expense ($000):** 300664 **Payroll Expense ($000):** 87297 **Personnel:** 1611

★ **RESEARCH MEDICAL CENTER – BROOKSIDE CAMPUS**, 6601 Rockhill Road, Zip 64131–1197; tel. 816/276–7000, (Total facility includes 23 beds in nursing home–type unit) (Nonreporting) **A**1 2 **S** HCA
Primary Contact: Kevin J. Hicks, President and Chief Executive Officer
COO: Troy DeDecker, Vice President Operations
CFO: Susan Shreeve, Chief Financial Officer
CHR: Dennis K. Johnson, Director Human Resources
Web address: www.b–lmc.com
Control: Corporation, Investor–owned, for–profit **Service:** General Medical and Surgical

Staffed Beds: 265

★ **RESEARCH PSYCHIATRIC CENTER (264016)**, 2323 East 63rd Street, Zip 64130–3462; tel. 816/444–8161 **A**1 10 **F**5 25 30 31 32 33 82 88 89 90 91 92 93 94 95 119 **S** HCA
Primary Contact: Todd Krass, President and Chief Executive Officer
CFO: Susan Shreeve, Chief Financial Officer
CMO: M. David Brown, M.D., Medical Director
CIO: Dan Fehr, Controller
CHR: Peggy Tyson, Director Human Resources
Web address: www.researchpsychiatriccenter.com
Control: Corporation, Investor–owned, for–profit **Service:** Psychiatric

Staffed Beds: 100 **Admissions:** 3063 **Census:** 57 **Outpatient Visits:** 6623 **Births:** 0 **Total Expense ($000):** 19277 **Payroll Expense ($000):** 8317 **Personnel:** 146

SAINT LUKE'S CANCER INSTITUTE (260211), 4323 Wornall Road, Zip 64111–3214; tel. 816/932–2823 **A**9 10 **F**3 12 15 27 31 32 33 55 57 62 69 76 80 96 97 99 102 104 105 107 109 111 119 121 125 135 **P**6 **S** Saint Luke's Health System
Primary Contact: Jeffrey Wieman, M.D., Chief Executive Officer
Web address: www.saint–lukes.org
Control: Other not–for–profit (including NFP Corporation) **Service:** Cancer

Staffed Beds: 30 **Admissions:** 1023 **Census:** 12 **Outpatient Visits:** 52277 **Births:** 0 **Total Expense ($000):** 50663 **Payroll Expense ($000):** 21595 **Personnel:** 222

★ **SAINT LUKE'S HOSPITAL OF KANSAS CITY (260138)**, 4401 Wornall Road, Zip 64111–3238; tel. 816/932–2000 **A**1 2 3 5 8 9 10 **F**3 9 11 12 13 15 17 18 20 22 23 24 25 26 27 30 31 32 33 38 40 41 43 44 47 49 50 52 53 54 55 56 57 58 59 60 61 62 64 66 68 70 72 73 74 75 76 77 79 80 81 82 84 85 86 87 90 91 92 94 96 97 99 100 102 106 107 109 111 112 114 116 118 119 120 121 124 126 127 130 134 135 136 137 **S** Saint Luke's Health System
Primary Contact: G. Richard Hastings, Chief Executive Officer
CFO: Jama Johnson, Chief Financial Officer
CMO: John Yeast, M.D., Director Medical Affairs
CIO: Deborah Gash, Chief Information Officer
CHR: Doris Rogers, Vice President Human Resources
Web address: www.saint–lukes.org
Control: Church–operated, Nongovernment, not–for profit **Service:** General Medical and Surgical

Staffed Beds: 404 **Admissions:** 19069 **Census:** 274 **Outpatient Visits:** 220618 **Births:** 2444 **Total Expense ($000):** 401323 **Payroll Expense ($000):** 161064 **Personnel:** 2861

☐ **SAINT LUKE'S NORTHLAND HOSPITAL (260062)**, 5830 N.W. Barry Road, Zip 64154–2778; tel. 816/891–6000 **A**1 9 10 **F**3 11 13 15 20 24 25 26 27 28 30 31 32 33 34 36 38 41 43 44 50 52 54 55 56 57 59 62 67 68 69 71 72 73 74 75 79 80 81 85 86 87 88 89 90 91 92 93 94 95 96 97 100 102 107 114 118 119 120 121 123 124 132 133 135 136 137 **S** Saint Luke's Health System
Primary Contact: N. Gary Wages, FACHE, President and Chief Executive Officer
COO: Kevin Trimble, R.N., Chief Operating Officer and Chief Nursing Officer
CFO: Julie Murphy, Chief Financial Officer
CIO: Carolyn Masoner, Director Information Services
CHR: Alan Abramovitz, Director Human Resources
Web address: www.saint–lukes.org
Control: Church–operated, Nongovernment, not–for profit **Service:** General Medical and Surgical

Staffed Beds: 134 **Admissions:** 6517 **Census:** 76 **Outpatient Visits:** 83321 **Births:** 1025 **Total Expense ($000):** 83037 **Payroll Expense ($000):** 34759 **Personnel:** 718

☐ **SELECT SPECIALTY HOSPITAL – WESTERN MISSOURI (262014)**, 2316 East Meyer Boulevard, 3 West, Zip 64132; tel. 816/276–9444 **A**1 9 10 **F**1 3 25 32 75 80 81 119 137 **S** Select Medical Corporation
Primary Contact: Larry Brown, Chief Executive Officer
Web address: www.selectmedicalcorp.com
Control: Corporation, Investor–owned, for–profit **Service:** Long–Term Acute Care hospital

Staffed Beds: 34 **Admissions:** 362 **Census:** 27 **Outpatient Visits:** 0 **Births:** 0 **Total Expense ($000):** 14916 **Payroll Expense ($000):** 5833 **Personnel:** 66

★ **ST. JOSEPH MEDICAL CENTER (260085)**, 1000 Carondelet Drive, Zip 64114–4673; tel. 816/942–4400 **A**1 2 5 9 10 **F**3 5 11 13 15 18 20 22 24 25 26 27 30 31 32 33 34 38 43 44 49 50 54 55 56 57 62 66 68 70 71 72 73 74 75 76 77 78 79 80 81 82 85 96 97 99 100 103 106 107 118 119 121 124 135 136 **S** Ascension Health
Primary Contact: Scott Kashman, Chief Executive Officer
CFO: Steven R. Cleary, Vice President Finance
CMO: Michael Feder, M.D., Chief Medical Officer
CIO: Thomas Pagano, Vice President and Chief Information Officer
CHR: Dawn Bryant, Vice President Organizational Development
Web address: www.carondelethealth.org
Control: Other not–for–profit (including NFP Corporation) **Service:** General Medical and Surgical

Staffed Beds: 242 **Admissions:** 12136 **Census:** 162 **Outpatient Visits:** 127765 **Births:** 1225 **Total Expense ($000):** 156435 **Payroll Expense ($000):** 50971 **Personnel:** 975

 Many Facility Codes have changed. Please refer to the AHA Guide Code Chart.

★ **TRUMAN MEDICAL CENTER–HOSPITAL HILL (260048)**, 2301 Holmes Street, Zip 64108–2640; tel. 816/404–1000 **A**1 2 3 5 8 9 10 **F**3 5 11 12 13 15 17 18 20 25 26 27 30 31 32 33 36 37 38 40 41 43 44 50 54 55 56 57 58 60 61 62 63 64 66 68 70 72 73 74 75 76 77 79 81 82 86 87 88 89 90 91 92 93 94 96 97 99 100 102 106 107 113 114 118 119 121 123 124 132 135 136 137 **P**5 6 **S** Truman Medical Centers
Primary Contact: John W. Bluford, President and Chief Executive Officer
COO: Catherine D. Disch, Executive Vice President and Chief Operating Officer
CFO: Allen Johnson, Chief Financial Officer
CMO: Mark Steele, M.D., Chief Medical Officer
CIO: Mitzi Cardenas, Chief Information Officer
CHR: Valerie Fulbright, Vice President Human Resources
Web address: www.trumed.org
Control: Other not–for–profit (including NFP Corporation) **Service:** General Medical and Surgical

Staffed Beds: 229 **Admissions:** 13220 **Census:** 175 **Outpatient Visits:** 389111 **Births:** 2668 **Total Expense ($000):** 270323 **Payroll Expense ($000):** 119122 **Personnel:** 2259

★ **TRUMAN MEDICAL CENTER–LAKEWOOD (260102)**, 7900 Lee's Summit Road, Zip 64139–1236; tel. 816/404–7000, (Total facility includes 212 beds in nursing home–type unit) **A**1 3 5 9 10 **F**3 4 5 6 11 13 15 25 26 28 30 31 32 33 34 36 37 38 41 43 50 53 54 55 56 57 60 62 63 64 65 66 68 71 72 73 74 75 76 77 79 80 81 82 84 85 86 87 88 89 90 91 92 93 94 96 102 107 117 119 120 121 124 132 135 136 **P**5 6 **S** Truman Medical Centers
Primary Contact: John W. Bluford, President and Chief Executive Officer
COO: Harold L. Siglar, Chief Operating Officer
CFO: Daniel J. Williams, Chief Financial Officer
CMO: Mark Steele, M.D., Chief Medical Officer
CIO: Mitzi Cardenas, Chief Information Officer
CHR: Valerie Fulbright, Vice President Human Resources
Web address: www.trumanmed.org
Control: Other not–for–profit (including NFP Corporation) **Service:** General Medical and Surgical

Staffed Beds: 301 **Admissions:** 5198 **Census:** 240 **Outpatient Visits:** 431540 **Births:** 975 **Total Expense ($000):** 91366 **Payroll Expense ($000):** 40262 **Personnel:** 815

★ **TWO RIVERS PSYCHIATRIC HOSPITAL (264017)**, 5121 Raytown Road, Zip 64133–2141; tel. 816/382–6300 **A**1 10 **F**4 5 6 25 26 30 31 32 33 36 56 73 81 82 88 89 91 92 93 94 95 119 121 123 132 **S** Universal Health Services, Inc.
Primary Contact: Norma Ferris, Chief Executive Officer and Managing Director
CFO: Kevin Walker, Chief Financial Officer
CMO: John Schmitz, M.D., Medical Director
CHR: Troy Angell, Director Human Resources
Web address: www.tworivershospital.com
Control: Corporation, Investor–owned, for–profit **Service:** Psychiatric

Staffed Beds: 105 **Admissions:** 3714 **Census:** 75 **Outpatient Visits:** 7280 **Births:** 0 **Total Expense ($000):** 17512 **Payroll Expense ($000):** 8263 **Personnel:** 223

★ **VETERANS AFFAIRS MEDICAL CENTER**, 4801 East Linwood Boulevard, Zip 64128–2226; tel. 816/861–4700 **A**1 2 3 5 **F**4 5 8 18 20 26 27 29 37 38 46 47 49 54 58 59 64 68 73 75 76 78 85 86 87 88 90 91 92 93 94 95 96 98 100 102 105 106 107 119 121 124 136 **S** Department of Veterans Affairs
Primary Contact: Kent D. Hill, Director
CFO: Charles Henning, Program Director Business
Web address: www.va.gov/sta/guide/home.asp
Control: Veterans Affairs, Government, federal **Service:** General Medical and Surgical

Staffed Beds: 157 **Admissions:** 5964 **Census:** 121 **Outpatient Visits:** 480025 **Births:** 0 **Total Expense ($000):** 194357 **Payroll Expense ($000):** 88392 **Personnel:** 683

□ **WESTERN MISSOURI MENTAL HEALTH CENTER (264008)**, 1000 East 24th Street, Zip 64108–2776; tel. 816/512–7000 **A**1 3 5 10 **F**4 5 25 26 33 34 36 38 50 52 66 81 82 88 89 90 91 92
Primary Contact: Dick Gregory, Ph.D., Chief Executive Officer
COO: Mark D. Miller, Chief Operating Officer
CFO: Scott Carter, Chief Financial Officer
CMO: Rob Hornstra, M.D., Clinical Director
CIO: Eduardo Abaricia, Director Information Technology
CHR: Silva Ward, Director Human Resources
Web address: www.dmhonline.dmh.state.mo.us
Control: State–Government, nonfederal **Service:** Psychiatric

Staffed Beds: 165 **Admissions:** 1261 **Census:** 131 **Outpatient Visits:** 6154 **Births:** 0 **Total Expense ($000):** 27374 **Payroll Expense ($000):** 15828 **Personnel:** 514

KENNETT—Dunklin County

★ **TWIN RIVERS REGIONAL MEDICAL CENTER (260015)**, 1301 First Street, Zip 63857–2508, Mailing Address: P.O. Box 728, Zip 63857–0728; tel. 573/888–4522 **A**1 9 10 **F**3 13 15 17 25 26 27 30 31 32 33 38 43 50 54 55 57 59 62 66 68 74 75 76 77 79 80 84 85 88 96 100 102 107 118 119 124 133 135 136 **S** Health Management Associates
Primary Contact: John W. McClellan, Chief Executive Officer
CFO: Curtis Herrin, Chief Financial Officer
CHR: Sherry Malone, Director Human Resources
Web address: www.twinriversmedctr.com
Control: Corporation, Investor–owned, for–profit **Service:** General Medical and Surgical

Staffed Beds: 116 **Admissions:** 5181 **Census:** 54 **Outpatient Visits:** 45461 **Births:** 493 **Total Expense ($000):** 35929 **Payroll Expense ($000):** 12360 **Personnel:** 340

KIRKSVILLE—Adair County

★ ○ **NORTHEAST REGIONAL MEDICAL CENTER (260022)**, 315 South Osteopathy, Zip 63501–8599, Mailing Address: P.O. Box C8502, Zip 63501–8599; tel. 660/785–1000 **A**9 10 11 12 13 19 20 **F**3 13 15 18 20 24 25 26 31 32 33 38 40 43 46 49 51 52 55 56 57 59 61 62 66 68 72 73 74 75 77 79 80 81 82 85 86 96 97 100 107 118 119 121 122 124 135 136 137 **S** Community Health Systems, Inc.
Primary Contact: Bob Moore, FACHE, Chief Executive Officer
COO: Ranee C. Brayton, R.N., MSN, Associate Chief Executive Officer
CFO: Loren Rials, Chief Financial Officer
CMO: E. Glenn Browning, D.O., Chief of Staff
CIO: Chad Tatro, Supervisor Information Systems
CHR: Bruce Canan, Director Human Resources
Web address: www.nermc.com
Control: Corporation, Investor–owned, for–profit **Service:** General Medical and Surgical

Staffed Beds: 115 **Admissions:** 4187 **Census:** 42 **Outpatient Visits:** 75171 **Births:** 508 **Total Expense ($000):** 55094 **Payroll Expense ($000):** 18423 **Personnel:** 432

MO

LAKE SAINT LOUIS—St. Charles County

★ **SSM ST. JOSEPH HOSPITAL WEST (260200)**, 100 Medical Plaza, Zip 63367–1366; tel. 636/625–5200 **A**1 9 10 **F**3 11 13 15 17 24 25 26 27 30 31 32 33 34 36 38 40 41 43 49 50 52 53 54 55 56 57 60 62 68 71 72 73 74 76 77 80 81 82 84 92 96 97 100 102 106 107 114 119 121 124 135 136 137 **P**6 8 **S** SSM Health Care
Primary Contact: Verna Meacham, Interim President
COO: Verna Meacham, Executive Vice President and Chief Operating Officer
CFO: Carole Campbell, Director Finance
CMO: Michael Handler, M.D., Chief Medical Officer
CIO: Sharon Gardner, Manager Information Systems
CHR: H. Layne Ebers, Director Human Resources
Web address: www.ssmstjoseph.com
Control: Church–operated, Nongovernment, not–for profit **Service:** General Medical and Surgical

Staffed Beds: 129 **Admissions:** 8081 **Census:** 74 **Outpatient Visits:** 105302 **Births:** 1257 **Total Expense ($000):** 92341 **Payroll Expense ($000):** 39818 **Personnel:** 541

LAMAR—Barton County

★ **BARTON COUNTY MEMORIAL HOSPITAL (261325)**, 29 N.W. First Lane, Zip 64759–8105; tel. 417/681–5100 **A**9 10 18 **F**3 11 15 24 27 30 31 32 37 38 43 55 57 62 66 73 75 79 80 82 84 85 86 87 96 97 100 102 107 117 118 119 120 121 122 137
Primary Contact: Rudy C. Snedigar, Administrator and Chief Executive Officer
COO: Virginia Rutledge, Assistant Administrator
CFO: Wendy Duvall, Chief Financial Officer
CIO: Brad Butler, Network Administrator
CHR: Sheila Boice, Director Human Resources
Web address: www.bcmh.net
Control: County–Government, nonfederal **Service:** General Medical and Surgical

Staffed Beds: 25 **Admissions:** 1322 **Census:** 15 **Outpatient Visits:** 54440 **Births:** 0 **Total Expense ($000):** 13820 **Payroll Expense ($000):** 5507 **Personnel:** 167

Hospital, Medicare Provider Number, Address, Telephone, Approval, Facility, and Physician Codes, Health Care System

★ American Hospital Association (AHA) membership
□ The Joint Commission accreditation
○ American Osteopathic Association (AOA) accreditation
△ Commission on Accreditation of Rehabilitation Facilities (CARF) accreditation

LEBANON—Laclede County

★ **ST. JOHN'S HOSPITAL – LEBANON (260059)**, 100 Hospital Drive, Zip 65536–9210; tel. 417/533–6100 **A**1 10 20 **F**3 11 13 15 24 25 26 27 28 31 32 33 34 35 43 50 52 55 57 62 63 66 68 69 73 74 75 76 77 78 79 80 81 82 84 85 86 96 97 100 107 112 118 119 120 121 122 124 133 135 136 137 **P**6 **S** Sisters of Mercy Health System
Primary Contact: Michael J. Gillen, President
CFO: Douglas M. Hoban, Vice President and Chief Financial Officer
CHR: Gary Moor, Director Human Resources
Web address: www.stjohnslebanon.com
Control: Church–operated, Nongovernment, not–for profit **Service:** General Medical and Surgical

Staffed Beds: 48 **Admissions:** 2904 **Census:** 27 **Outpatient Visits:** 46508 **Births:** 453 **Total Expense ($000):** 41769 **Payroll Expense ($000):** 20144 **Personnel:** 459

LEE'S SUMMIT—Jackson County

★ **LEE'S SUMMIT MEDICAL CENTER (260190)**, (Formerly Lee's Summit Hospital), 2100 S.E. Blue Parkway, Zip 64063; tel. 816/282–5000 **A**1 9 10 **F**3 13 15 18 20 24 25 26 27 30 31 32 38 39 44 49 55 57 59 62 63 66 67 68 72 73 74 75 76 77 79 80 82 86 96 97 100 102 107 108 109 118 119 120 121 124 134 **P**5 **S** HCA
Primary Contact: Damond Boatright, Chief Executive Officer
COO: Don King, Chief Operating Officer
CFO: Matthew Leary, Chief Financial Officer
CIO: Evan Kenney, Manager Information Technology Systems
CHR: DeeDee Hawman, Director Human Resources
Web address: www.leessummitmedicalcenter.com
Control: Corporation, Investor–owned, for–profit **Service:** General Medical and Surgical

Staffed Beds: 64 **Admissions:** 3974 **Census:** 46 **Outpatient Visits:** 43988 **Births:** 74 **Total Expense ($000):** 52958 **Payroll Expense ($000):** 24558 **Personnel:** 318

☐ **SAINT LUKE'S EAST–LEE'S SUMMIT (260216)**, 100 N.E. Saint Luke's Boulevard, Zip 64086–6000; tel. 816/347–5000 **A**1 5 9 10 **F**3 13 15 18 20 24 25 26 27 30 31 32 33 36 38 43 44 46 49 50 54 55 56 57 59 66 68 71 72 73 74 76 77 79 80 81 82 85 86 87 96 97 99 100 102 107 118 119 121 132 135 136 137 **S** Saint Luke's Health System
Primary Contact: George A. Pagels, M.D., President and Chief Executive Officer
COO: Gloria Solis, R.N., MSN, Chief Operating Officer and Chief Nursing Officer
Web address: www.saint–lukes.org
Control: Church–operated, Nongovernment, not–for profit **Service:** General Medical and Surgical

Staffed Beds: 57 **Admissions:** 4245 **Census:** 41 **Outpatient Visits:** 63755 **Births:** 998 **Total Expense ($000):** 63608 **Payroll Expense ($000):** 23119 **Personnel:** 413

LEXINGTON—Lafayette County

★ **LAFAYETTE REGIONAL HEALTH CENTER (261320)**, 1500 State Street, Zip 64067–1107; tel. 660/259–2203 **A**1 9 10 18 **F**11 15 25 27 30 31 32 38 57 62 66 68 73 76 77 79 80 82 86 96 100 102 107 118 119 122 **P**6 **S** HCA
Primary Contact: Bret Kolman, CPA, Chief Executive Officer
CFO: Teri James, Chief Financial Officer
CHR: Lee Tagai, Director Human Resources
Web address: www.lafayetteregionalhealthcenter.com
Control: Corporation, Investor–owned, for–profit **Service:** General Medical and Surgical

Staffed Beds: 25 **Admissions:** 1172 **Census:** 12 **Outpatient Visits:** 68025 **Births:** 0 **Total Expense ($000):** 24401 **Payroll Expense ($000):** 9401 **Personnel:** 176

LIBERTY—Clay County

★ **LIBERTY HOSPITAL (260177)**, 2525 Glenn Hendren Drive, Zip 64068–9600, Mailing Address: P.O. Box 1002, Zip 64069–1002; tel. 816/781–7200, (Total facility includes 12 beds in nursing home–type unit) **A**1 2 3 5 9 10 **F**3 9 11 13 15 18 20 24 26 27 30 31 33 38 40 41 42 43 44 49 54 55 56 57 59 61 62 66 67 68 70 72 73 74 75 76 77 79 80 81 84 86 92 96 97 100 102 103 104 107 116 117 118 119 121 132 135 137
Primary Contact: Joseph W. Crossett, Administrator
CFO: Erin Parde, Chief Financial Officer
CIO: David Feess, Assistant Administrator
CHR: Patti Downey, Assistant Administrator
Web address: www.Libertyhospital.org
Control: Hospital district or authority, Government, nonfederal **Service:** General Medical and Surgical

Staffed Beds: 245 **Admissions:** 13732 **Census:** 164 **Outpatient Visits:** 128600 **Births:** 1168 **Total Expense ($000):** 142921 **Payroll Expense ($000):** 59973 **Personnel:** 1145

LOUISIANA—Pike County

★ **PIKE COUNTY MEMORIAL HOSPITAL (261333)**, 2305 West Georgia Street, Zip 63353–2559; tel. 573/754–5531 **A**1 9 10 18 **F**3 7 11 15 24 25 26 30 31 32 33 38 50 53 55 57 62 63 73 77 79 80 84 86 96 102 119 122 132
Primary Contact: Lorraine L. Harness, Administrator
CFO: Ann Perry, Chief Financial Officer
CIO: Jeremy Gruen, Director Information Systems
CHR: Brad Hufty, Director Human Resources
Web address: www.pcmh–mo.org
Control: County–Government, nonfederal **Service:** General Medical and Surgical

Staffed Beds: 24 **Admissions:** 725 **Census:** 5 **Outpatient Visits:** 38122 **Births:** 0 **Total Expense ($000):** 11707 **Payroll Expense ($000):** 5717 **Personnel:** 143

MACON—Macon County

★ **SAMARITAN MEMORIAL HOSPITAL (261313)**, 1205 North Missouri Street, Zip 63552–2095; tel. 660/385–8700 **A**9 10 18 **F**3 7 8 11 14 15 25 26 30 31 32 33 34 38 42 43 44 50 52 55 56 57 59 60 61 62 63 66 73 75 77 79 80 81 82 86 87 96 100 102 107 117 118 119 120 121 122 124 132 135 **P**3 5
Primary Contact: Bernard A. Orman, Jr., Administrator
CFO: Susan Spencer, Chief Financial Officer
CHR: Suzanne Britt, Director Human Resources
Web address: www.samaritanhospital.net
Control: County–Government, nonfederal **Service:** General Medical and Surgical

Staffed Beds: 25 **Admissions:** 881 **Census:** 12 **Outpatient Visits:** 59856 **Births:** 0 **Total Expense ($000):** 15744 **Payroll Expense ($000):** 6535 **Personnel:** 176

MARSHALL—Saline County

★ **FITZGIBBON HOSPITAL (260142)**, 2305 South 65 Highway, Zip 65340–0250, Mailing Address: P.O. Box 250, Zip 65340–0250; tel. 660/886–7431 **A**3 5 9 10 20 **F**3 11 13 15 29 30 31 32 33 38 42 43 52 55 57 61 62 66 68 72 73 74 75 77 79 80 82 86 88 93 96 100 102 106 107 117 118 119 120 121 122 132 135 136
Primary Contact: Ronald A. Ott, Chief Executive Officer
CFO: Nancy Harris, Chief Financial Officer
CHR: Kevin Hart, Director Human Resources
Web address: www.fitzgibbon.org
Control: Other not–for–profit (including NFP Corporation) **Service:** General Medical and Surgical

Staffed Beds: 52 **Admissions:** 2630 **Census:** 31 **Outpatient Visits:** 103611 **Births:** 388 **Total Expense ($000):** 34396 **Payroll Expense ($000):** 14623 **Personnel:** 358

MARYLAND HEIGHTS—St. Louis County

★ **RANKEN JORDAN – A PEDIATRIC SPECIALTY HOSPITAL (263303)**, (Pediatric Specialty Hospital), 11365 Dorsett Road, Zip 63043–3411; tel. 314/872–6400 **A**10 **F**12 16 25 28 30 33 41 50 62 78 81 82 84 85 86 119 121 132 135 137 **P**6
Primary Contact: Laureen K. Tanner, RN, M.S.N., Chief Executive Officer
COO: Brett Moorehouse, Vice President and Chief Operating Officer
CFO: Jean Bardwell, Vice President and Chief Financial Officer
CMO: Nicholas Holekamp, M.D., Medical Director
CIO: Jean Bardwell, Vice President and Chief Financial Officer
Web address: www.rankenjordan.org
Control: Other not–for–profit (including NFP Corporation) **Service:** Children's other specialty

Staffed Beds: 30 **Admissions:** 246 **Census:** 24 **Outpatient Visits:** 2181 **Births:** 0 **Total Expense ($000):** 16822 **Payroll Expense ($000):** 6459 **Personnel:** 178

MARYVILLE—Nodaway County

★ **ST. FRANCIS HOSPITAL AND HEALTH SERVICES (260050)**, 2016 South Main Street, Zip 64468–2655; tel. 660/562–2600 **A**1 5 9 10 20 **F**3 11 13 15 24 25 26 30 31 32 33 36 38 55 57 62 68 73 74 77 79 80 84 86 88 89 90 91 92 93 94 95 96 100 102 107 119 120 122 124 130 131 135 **P**6 **S** SSM Health Care
Primary Contact: Gray Cox, President
COO: Cathy New, Vice President Clinical Services
CFO: Jocelyn Skidmore, Director Finance
CMO: James Bradley, M.D., President Medical Staff
CIO: Dave Lewis, Director Information Services
CHR: Martha Archer, Director Human Resources
Web address: www.stfrancismaryville.com
Control: Church–operated, Nongovernment, not–for profit **Service:** General Medical and Surgical

Staffed Beds: 57 **Admissions:** 2008 **Census:** 23 **Outpatient Visits:** 71004 **Births:** 279 **Total Expense ($000):** 51170 **Payroll Expense ($000):** 23031 **Personnel:** 426

Many Facility Codes have changed. Please refer to the AHA Guide Code Chart.

MEMPHIS—Scotland County

★ **SCOTLAND COUNTY MEMORIAL HOSPITAL (261310)**, Sigler Avenue, Zip 63555–9767, Mailing Address: Rural Route 1, Box 53, Zip 63555–9767; tel. 660/465–8511 **A**9 10 18 **F**7 9 11 13 15 24 25 26 28 30 31 32 33 34 38 43 51 54 55 56 57 62 65 66 68 73 74 75 79 80 81 82 84 85 86 87 96 100 107 117 119 120 121 122 124 135 136 137 **P**6
Primary Contact: Marcia R. Dial, Administrator and Chief Executive Officer
CFO: Sheryl Templeton, Chief Financial Officer
CMO: William Dixon, M.D., Chief of Staff
CIO: Angela Schmitter, Director Health Information Management
Web address: www.scotlandcountyhospital.com
Control: Hospital district or authority, Government, nonfederal **Service:** General Medical and Surgical

Staffed Beds: 25 **Admissions:** 742 **Census:** 9 **Outpatient Visits:** 77228
Births: 98 **Total Expense ($000):** 12383 **Payroll Expense ($000):** 6244
Personnel: 154

MEXICO—Audrain County

□ **AUDRAIN MEDICAL CENTER (260064)**, 620 East Monroe Street, Zip 65265–2919; tel. 573/582–5000 **A**1 2 9 10 19 20 **F**3 7 11 13 15 18 20 24 25 26 27 30 31 32 43 44 51 52 53 55 56 57 62 63 68 72 73 74 75 76 77 79 80 81 82 84 85 86 87 88 90 92 93 94 96 97 100 102 106 107 111 118 119 120 121 124 135 136 **P**6
Primary Contact: David A. Neuendorf, FACHE, President and Chief Executive Officer
COO: David A. Neuendorf, FACHE, President and Chief Executive Officer
CFO: Greg Shaw, Vice President and Chief Financial Officer
CMO: Patricia Burke, M.D., Chief of Staff
CIO: Dawn Evans, Manager Information Technology
CHR: Christy Smiley, Director Human Resources
Web address: www.audrainmedicalcenter.com
Control: Other not–for–profit (including NFP Corporation) **Service:** General Medical and Surgical

Staffed Beds: 107 **Admissions:** 4136 **Census:** 42 **Outpatient Visits:** 172260
Births: 257 **Total Expense ($000):** 67426 **Payroll Expense ($000):** 26186
Personnel: 604

MILAN—Sullivan County

★ **SULLIVAN COUNTY MEMORIAL HOSPITAL (261306)**, 630 West Third Street, Zip 63556–1076; tel. 660/265–4212, (Total facility includes 14 beds in nursing home–type unit) **A**9 10 18 **F**24 25 28 31 32 33 38 52 55 56 57 62 63 65 66 73 75 79 82 87 96 100 102 107 117 118 119 122 124 135 137 **P**5 6
Primary Contact: Amy J. Michael, Chief Executive Officer
CFO: Mary Tredway, Director Finance
CMO: Anthony Mattaline, Chief of Staff
CIO: Kimberly Ray, Director Risk Management and Health Information
CHR: Billie Ryals, Director Human Resources
Control: County–Government, nonfederal **Service:** General Medical and Surgical

Staffed Beds: 39 **Admissions:** 346 **Census:** 26 **Outpatient Visits:** 17040
Births: 0 **Total Expense ($000):** 5271 **Payroll Expense ($000):** 2786
Personnel: 89

MOBERLY—Randolph County

★□ **MOBERLY REGIONAL MEDICAL CENTER (260074)**, 1515 Union Avenue, Zip 65270–9449; tel. 660/263–8400, (Total facility includes 21 beds in nursing home–type unit) **A**1 9 10 12 13 **F**3 13 15 18 24 25 26 30 31 32 33 36 37 38 41 43 47 48 49 50 54 55 56 57 62 68 72 73 74 75 77 78 79 80 81 82 84 86 88 90 93 96 97 100 102 106 107 117 118 119 120 121 122 124 135 136 137 **S** Community Health Systems, Inc.
Primary Contact: Kevin Clement, Chief Executive Officer
CFO: Tracey Bradley, Interim Chief Financial Officer
CMO: Ahmad Habib, M.D., Chief Medical Officer
CIO: Doris Whelan, Chief Information Officer
Web address: www.moberlyhospital.com
Control: Corporation, Investor–owned, for–profit **Service:** General Medical and Surgical

Staffed Beds: 100 **Admissions:** 2756 **Census:** 42 **Outpatient Visits:** 60978
Births: 263 **Total Expense ($000):** 45899 **Payroll Expense ($000):** 15540
Personnel: 341

MONETT—Barry County

□ **COX MONETT HOSPITAL (261329)**, 801 Lincoln Avenue, Zip 65708–1641; tel. 417/235–3144 **A**1 9 10 18 **F**3 8 11 13 15 24 25 27 28 31 32 33 38 50 52 53 54 55 56 57 61 62 63 66 73 74 75 77 79 80 81 86 96 97 100 102 107 118 119 120 121 122 124 134 135 136 **P**6 **S** CoxHealth
Primary Contact: Gregory D. Johnson, Administrator and Chief Executive Officer
CFO: R. Martin Williams, Director Financial Services
CMO: Allison Heider, M.D., Chief of Staff
CHR: Pamela Foland, Director Human Resources
Web address: www.coxhealth.com
Control: Other not–for–profit (including NFP Corporation) **Service:** General Medical and Surgical

Staffed Beds: 25 **Admissions:** 1257 **Census:** 11 **Outpatient Visits:** 69533
Births: 447 **Total Expense ($000):** 27606 **Payroll Expense ($000):** 13404
Personnel: 280

MOUNT VERNON—Lawrence County

★□ △ **MISSOURI REHABILITATION CENTER (262001)**, 600 North Main Street, Zip 65712–1004; tel. 417/466–3711 **A**1 7 9 10 **F**1 3 11 24 26 30 50 52 55 57 62 68 75 85 86 107 118 119 132 135 **P**6 **S** University of Missouri Health Care
Primary Contact: Steve Patterson, Executive Director
CFO: Amy Baker, Manager Finance
CMO: Najdat Atallah, M.D., Co–Medical Director
CIO: Gary Mackie, Manager Information Systems
CHR: David Thiessen, Associate Director Support Services
Web address: www.muhealth.org/~MOrehab
Control: State–Government, nonfederal **Service:** Long–Term Acute Care hospital

Staffed Beds: 115 **Admissions:** 463 **Census:** 52 **Outpatient Visits:** 53634
Births: 0 **Total Expense ($000):** 36049 **Payroll Expense ($000):** 18366
Personnel: 471

MOUNTAIN VIEW—Howell County

★□ **ST. JOHN'S ST. FRANCIS HOSPITAL (261335)**, 100 West Highway 60, Zip 65548–7125; tel. 417/934–7000 **A**1 10 18 **F**3 11 15 24 25 26 30 31 32 38 55 62 73 79 84 85 86 96 107 121 122 135 **P**6 **S** Sisters of Mercy Health System
Primary Contact: Douglas R. Trembath, President
CMO: Barry Spoon, M.D., Chief of Staff
CIO: Joyce Grogan, Manager Medical Records
CHR: Linda Divine, Manager Human Resources
Web address: www.stjohns.com/aboutus/stfrancis.aspx
Control: Church–operated, Nongovernment, not–for profit **Service:** General Medical and Surgical

Staffed Beds: 20 **Admissions:** 512 **Census:** 5 **Outpatient Visits:** 23018
Births: 0 **Total Expense ($000):** 9388 **Payroll Expense ($000):** 4784
Personnel: 132

NEOSHO—Newton County

★ **FREEMAN NEOSHO HOSPITAL (261331)**, 113 West Hickory Street, Zip 64850–1705; tel. 417/455–4352 **A**2 9 10 18 **F**3 7 11 15 17 24 25 26 27 30 31 32 33 38 40 41 54 55 56 57 62 68 73 75 76 77 79 80 81 82 84 85 86 87 96 100 102 106 107 117 119 120 121 122 135 137 **S** Freeman Health System
Primary Contact: Daxton Holcomb, Chief Executive Officer
CFO: Steve W. Graddy, Chief Financial Officer
CMO: Rodney McFarland, M.D., Medical Director
CIO: Sue Annesser, Director Information Systems
CHR: Deborah Chiodo, Director Human Resources
Web address: www.freemanhealth.com
Control: Other not–for–profit (including NFP Corporation) **Service:** General Medical and Surgical

Staffed Beds: 25 **Admissions:** 2017 **Census:** 20 **Outpatient Visits:** 83861
Births: 0 **Total Expense ($000):** 22891 **Payroll Expense ($000):** 9784
Personnel: 198

MO

Hospital, Medicare Provider Number, Address, Telephone, Approval, Facility, and Physician Codes, Health Care System
★ American Hospital Association (AHA) membership
□ The Joint Commission accreditation
○ American Osteopathic Association (AOA) accreditation
△ Commission on Accreditation of Rehabilitation Facilities (CARF) accreditation

NEVADA—Vernon County

☐ **HEARTLAND BEHAVIORAL HEALTH SERVICES**, 1500 West Ashland Street, Zip 64772–1710; tel. 417/667–2666, (Total facility includes 122 beds in nursing home–type unit) **A**1 **F**25 30 31 32 63 88 89 90 91 92 119
S Psychiatric Solutions
Primary Contact: Michael D. Ham, Chief Executive Officer
CFO: Tara Stevens, Chief Financial Officer
CMO: Ahmad Tarar, M.D., Medical Director
CHR: Joe Hardin, Director Human Resources
Web address: www.psysolutions.com/heartland/site/index.html
Control: Corporation, Investor–owned, for–profit **Service:** Psychiatric

Staffed Beds: 159 **Admissions:** 844 **Census:** 78 **Outpatient Visits:** 0 **Births:** 0 **Total Expense ($000):** 10929 **Payroll Expense ($000):** 6052 **Personnel:** 161

★ **NEVADA REGIONAL MEDICAL CENTER (260061)**, 800 South Ash Street, Zip 64772–3223; tel. 417/667–3355 **A**1 9 10 **F**3 11 13 15 24 25 26 28 30 31 32 33 38 42 43 44 49 50 51 53 55 56 57 61 62 63 67 68 73 74 75 77 79 80 81 82 84 85 86 88 90 92 94 96 99 100 102 107 118 119 120 121 122 124 132 135 137 **S** QHR
Primary Contact: Judith K. Feuquay, Chief Executive Officer
CFO: Cindy D. Buck, Vice President Financial Services and Chief Financial Officer
CMO: Scott Compton, D.O., Chief of Staff
CIO: Carrie Compton–Ogle, Chief Information Officer
CHR: Pam Sweger, Administrative Officer and Director Human Resources
Web address: www.nrmchealth.com
Control: City–Government, nonfederal **Service:** General Medical and Surgical

Staffed Beds: 63 **Admissions:** 2211 **Census:** 26 **Outpatient Visits:** 48743 **Births:** 361 **Total Expense ($000):** 29605 **Payroll Expense ($000):** 10565 **Personnel:** 286

NORTH KANSAS CITY—Clay County

★ **NORTH KANSAS CITY HOSPITAL (260096)**, 2800 Clay Edwards Drive, Zip 64116–3220; tel. 816/691–2000, (Total facility includes 18 beds in nursing home–type unit) **A**1 2 9 10 **F**3 11 13 15 17 18 20 22 24 25 26 27 30 31 32 33 35 36 37 38 40 41 42 43 44 45 49 50 52 55 56 57 61 62 67 68 71 72 73 74 75 76 77 78 79 80 81 82 84 85 86 96 97 99 100 102 103 106 107 109 111 112 116 117 118 119 121 124 135 **P**6
Primary Contact: David R. Carpenter, FACHE, President and Chief Executive Officer
COO: Jody Abbott, Senior Vice President and Chief Operating Officer
CFO: Jim McNey, Vice President Finance and Chief Financial Officer
CIO: Art Fisk, Chief Information Officer
CHR: Beverly Johnson, Vice President Human Resources
Web address: www.nkch.org
Control: City–Government, nonfederal **Service:** General Medical and Surgical

Staffed Beds: 411 **Admissions:** 22514 **Census:** 312 **Outpatient Visits:** 202729 **Births:** 1882 **Total Expense ($000):** 322515 **Payroll Expense ($000):** 120003 **Personnel:** 2442

OSAGE BEACH—Camden County

★ **LAKE REGIONAL HEALTH SYSTEM (260186)**, 54 Hospital Drive, Zip 65065–3050; tel. 573/348–8000, (Total facility includes 16 beds in nursing home–type unit) **A**1 5 9 10 19 **F**3 11 13 15 17 18 20 22 24 25 26 27 30 31 32 33 37 38 40 41 43 48 49 50 51 52 55 56 57 59 61 62 63 66 68 72 73 74 75 76 77 79 80 81 82 84 86 96 97 100 102 103 104 106 107 109 117 118 119 120 121 124 134 135 **P**6
Primary Contact: Michael E. Henze, Chief Executive Officer
COO: Vicki L. Franklin, Senior Vice President and Chief Operating Officer
CFO: Dan Probstfield, Senior Vice President and Chief Financial Officer
CMO: Robert Hyatt, M.D., Chief of Staff
CIO: Cindy Otradovec, Chief Information Officer
CHR: Tom Williams, Director Human Resources
Web address: www.lakeregional.com
Control: Other not–for–profit (including NFP Corporation) **Service:** General Medical and Surgical

Staffed Beds: 116 **Admissions:** 7009 **Census:** 76 **Outpatient Visits:** 214952 **Births:** 829 **Total Expense ($000):** 136689 **Payroll Expense ($000):** 50689 **Personnel:** 1079

OSCEOLA—St. Clair County

★ **SAC–OSAGE HOSPITAL (260147)**, Junction Highways 13 & Business 13, Zip 64776–0426, Mailing Address: P.O. Box 426, Zip 64776–0426; tel. 417/646–8181 **A**9 10 20 **F**3 7 8 15 26 27 30 31 32 38 42 55 56 57 60 62 68 73 75 76 79 81 82 84 85 86 96 100 107 117 119 122 135
Primary Contact: Jeffrey T. Speaks, Chief Executive Officer
Web address: www.sac–osagehospital.com
Control: Hospital district or authority, Government, nonfederal **Service:** General Medical and Surgical

Staffed Beds: 47 **Admissions:** 733 **Census:** 9 **Outpatient Visits:** 15305 **Births:** 0 **Total Expense ($000):** 8896 **Payroll Expense ($000):** 3995 **Personnel:** 92

PERRYVILLE—Perry County

★ **PERRY COUNTY MEMORIAL HOSPITAL (261311)**, 434 North West Street, Zip 63775–1398; tel. 573/547–2536 **A**1 9 10 18 **F**3 7 8 11 13 15 25 26 27 30 31 32 33 38 41 48 51 52 53 54 55 56 57 59 61 62 64 66 73 74 75 76 77 79 80 82 84 85 86 89 90 91 92 93 94 96 97 100 102 105 107 118 119 120 121 122 124 132 133 134 135 136
Primary Contact: Patrick E. Carron, CHE, President and Chief Executive Officer
CFO: Randall Wolf, Vice President Finance
CMO: Mohammad Moaddabi, M.D., Chief of Staff
CIO: Ron Heuring, Director Information Systems
CHR: Linda Todaro, Director Human Resources
Web address: www.pchmo.org
Control: Other not–for–profit (including NFP Corporation) **Service:** General Medical and Surgical

Staffed Beds: 25 **Admissions:** 805 **Census:** 13 **Outpatient Visits:** 46350 **Births:** 158 **Total Expense ($000):** 21144 **Payroll Expense ($000):** 9051 **Personnel:** 292

POPLAR BLUFF—Butler County

★ **JOHN J. PERSHING VETERANS AFFAIRS MEDICAL CENTER**, 1500 North Westwood Boulevard, Zip 63901–3318; tel. 573/686–4151, (Total facility includes 40 beds in nursing home–type unit) **A**1 **F**3 5 11 25 26 32 36 37 38 44 52 53 54 57 61 62 63 73 75 77 79 81 82 85 86 87 90 94 96 100 102 107 117 119 124 132 133 135 136 137 **S** Department of Veterans Affairs
Primary Contact: Nancy Arnold, RN, Director
COO: Stan Skorniak, MS, FACHE, Associate Medical Center Director
CFO: Kristy Eagle, Manager Finance
CMO: Vijayachandran Nair, M.D., Chief of Staff
CIO: Janice Vernon, Supervisory Information Technology Specialist
CHR: Kay Riggs, Manager Human Resources
Web address: www.va.gov/sta/guide/home.asp
Control: Veterans Affairs, Government, federal **Service:** General Medical and Surgical

Staffed Beds: 58 **Admissions:** 1446 **Census:** 44 **Outpatient Visits:** 70881 **Births:** 0 **Total Expense ($000):** 78124 **Payroll Expense ($000):** 25057 **Personnel:** 430

★ △ **POPLAR BLUFF REGIONAL MEDICAL CENTER (260119)**, 2620 North Westwood Boulevard, Zip 63901–3396, Mailing Address: P.O. Box 88, Zip 63901–0088; tel. 573/686–5311, (Includes POPLAR BLUFF REGIONAL MEDICAL CENTER–NORTH CAMPUS; POPLAR BLUFF REGIONAL MEDICAL CENTER–SOUTH CAMPUS, 621 Pine Boulevard, Zip 63901; tel. 573/785–7721) **A**1 2 7 9 10 19 **F**3 11 13 15 18 20 22 24 25 27 31 32 33 37 38 43 46 49 50 51 52 55 57 59 60 61 62 63 66 68 72 73 74 75 76 77 79 80 81 82 84 85 86 88 90 92 96 97 100 102 107 109 118 119 120 121 135 137 **P**6
S Health Management Associates
Primary Contact: Bruce Eady, Chief Executive Officer
CFO: Richard Ervin, Chief Financial Officer
CMO: Austin Tinsley, M.D., Chief Medical Officer
CIO: Gary Dollins, Director Management Information Systems
CHR: Denise Dye, Director Human Resources
Web address: www.poplarbluffregional.com
Control: Corporation, Investor–owned, for–profit **Service:** General Medical and Surgical

Staffed Beds: 255 **Admissions:** 12668 **Census:** 141 **Outpatient Visits:** 229337 **Births:** 1402 **Total Expense ($000):** 117160 **Payroll Expense ($000):** 38666 **Personnel:** 934

POTOSI—Washington County

★ **WASHINGTON COUNTY MEMORIAL HOSPITAL (261308)**, 300 Health Way, Zip 63664–1420; tel. 573/438–5451 **A**9 10 18 **F**3 11 15 24 25 30 33 38 55 56 57 61 62 79 82 85 86 87 96 97 100 102 107 118 119 122 135 136
Primary Contact: Leah Osbahr, Administrator
COO: Leah Osbahr, Administrator
CFO: Allan Sucharski, Chief Financial Officer
CMO: J. Paul Tindall, D.O., Chief of Staff
CIO: Greg Riddle, Director Information Systems
CHR: Hopie Jenkins, Director Personnel
Web address: www.wcmhosp.org
Control: County–Government, nonfederal **Service:** General Medical and Surgical

Staffed Beds: 25 **Admissions:** 437 **Census:** 5 **Outpatient Visits:** 56789 **Births:** 0 **Total Expense ($000):** 14861 **Payroll Expense ($000):** 5859 **Personnel:** 166

RICHMOND—Ray County

RAY COUNTY MEMORIAL HOSPITAL (261327), 904 Wollard Boulevard, Zip 64085–2229; tel. 816/470–5432 **A**9 10 18 **F**3 11 15 24 25 27 30 38 42 43 61 62 66 72 73 76 77 79 80 82 86 96 100 102 104 107 119 122 135
Primary Contact: Tommy L. Hicks, Administrator
CFO: Donald Harr, Controller
Control: County–Government, nonfederal **Service:** General Medical and Surgical

Staffed Beds: 25 **Admissions:** 1061 **Census:** 14 **Outpatient Visits:** 12707 **Births:** 0 **Total Expense ($000):** 16848 **Payroll Expense ($000):** 7027 **Personnel:** 207

 Many Facility Codes have changed. Please refer to the AHA Guide Code Chart.

ROLLA—Phelps County

★ △ **PHELPS COUNTY REGIONAL MEDICAL CENTER (260017)**, 1000 West Tenth Street, Zip 65401–2905; tel. 573/458–8899, (Total facility includes 20 beds in nursing home–type unit) **A**1 2 7 9 10 19 20 **F**3 7 8 11 13 15 17 18 24 25 26 27 30 31 32 33 37 38 40 42 47 48 49 51 55 56 57 59 66 68 71 72 73 74 75 76 77 79 80 81 82 84 85 86 88 89 90 91 92 93 94 98 100 102 106 107 109 111 112 117 118 119 120 121 124 132 133 135 137
Primary Contact: John Denbo, Chief Executive Officer
COO: Gerald Paule, Vice President, Chief Operating Officer and Chief Financial Officer
CFO: Gerald Paule, Vice President, Chief Operating Officer and Chief Financial Officer
CMO: Jay Crump, M.D., Director Medical Staff
CIO: David Dawdy, Director Information Technology
CHR: Frank A. Lazzaro, Chief Human Resources Officer
Web address: www.pcrmc.com
Control: County–Government, nonfederal **Service:** General Medical and Surgical

Staffed Beds: 204 **Admissions:** 8944 **Census:** 116 **Outpatient Visits:** 169222 **Births:** 992 **Total Expense ($000):** 125390 **Payroll Expense ($000):** 46683 **Personnel:** 847

SAINT CHARLES—St. Charles County

★ **CENTERPOINTE HOSPITAL (264012)**, 5931 Highway 94 South, Zip 63304–5611; tel. 636/441–7300 **A**1 10 **F**4 5 31 32 33 53 56 58 88 89 90 91 92 93 94 95 119 121 132
Primary Contact: Azfar Malik, M.D., Chief Executive Officer
COO: Susan Mathis, Chief Operating Officer
CFO: Tariq F. Malik, CPA, Acting Chief Financial Officer
CMO: Azfar Malik, M.D., Chief Executive Officer and Chief Medical Officer
CIO: Jennifer Bourn, Coordinator Health Information Systems
CHR: Jan Mullenix, Director Human Resources
Web address: www.centerpointehospital.com
Control: Corporation, Investor–owned, for–profit **Service:** Psychiatric

Staffed Beds: 72 **Admissions:** 2555 **Census:** 58 **Outpatient Visits:** 26408 **Births:** 0 **Total Expense ($000):** 21765 **Payroll Expense ($000):** 11764 **Personnel:** 275

★ **PROGRESS WEST HEALTHCARE CENTER (260219)**, Two Progress Point, Zip 63368–2208; tel. 636/344–2273 **A**10 **F**3 13 15 25 32 38 51 55 57 59 68 74 77 79 84 96 100 103 106 107 119 124 **S** BJC HealthCare
Primary Contact: John Antes, President
Web address: www.progresswesthealthcare.org
Control: Other not–for–profit (including NFP Corporation) **Service:** General Medical and Surgical

Staffed Beds: 34 **Admissions:** 1559 **Census:** 16 **Outpatient Visits:** 17971 **Births:** 229 **Total Expense ($000):** 40108 **Payroll Expense ($000):** 12517 **Personnel:** 262

★ **SSM ST. JOSEPH HEALTH CENTER (260005)**, 300 First Capitol Drive, Zip 63301–2844; tel. 636/947–5000, (Includes SSM ST. JOSEPH HEALTH CENTER – WENTZVILLE, 500 Medical Drive, Wentzville, Zip 63385–3421; tel. 636/327–1000) **A**1 2 9 10 **F**2 3 4 5 8 11 13 15 17 18 20 22 24 25 26 27 30 31 32 33 34 36 37 38 40 41 43 47 49 50 52 54 55 56 57 60 62 68 71 72 73 74 76 77 79 80 81 82 87 88 89 90 91 92 93 94 95 96 97 100 102 106 107 108 109 111 114 118 119 120 121 123 124 132 135 136 137 **P**6 8 **S** SSM Health Care
Primary Contact: Gaspare Calvaruso, President
CFO: Hal Holder, Director Finance
CMO: Filippo Ferrigni, M.D., Vice President Clinical Affairs and Medical Director
CIO: Margaret Feilner, Director Information Services
CHR: Jana Mayfield, Director President Human Resources
Web address: www.ssmstjoseph.com
Control: Church–operated, Nongovernment, not–for profit **Service:** General Medical and Surgical

Staffed Beds: 297 **Admissions:** 14773 **Census:** 198 **Outpatient Visits:** 162813 **Births:** 729 **Total Expense ($000):** 178567 **Payroll Expense ($000):** 75163 **Personnel:** 1164

SAINT JOSEPH—Buchanan County

★ **HEARTLAND REGIONAL MEDICAL CENTER (260006)**, 5325 Faraon Street, Zip 64506–3488; tel. 816/271–6000 **A**1 2 5 9 10 20 **F**3 8 9 11 13 15 17 18 20 22 24 25 26 28 29 30 31 32 33 34 37 38 40 42 43 44 49 50 52 53 55 56 57 58 59 60 61 62 63 64 68 69 72 74 75 77 78 79 80 81 82 84 85 86 87 88 90 92 93 96 97 100 102 103 105 107 109 111 118 119 120 133 135 136 137 **P**6
Primary Contact: Lowell C. Kruse, President and Chief Executive Officer
COO: Curt Kretzinger, Chief Operating Officer
CFO: John P. Wilson, Chief Financial Officer
CMO: Robert Permut, M.D., Chief Medical Officer
CIO: Helen Thompson, Chief Information Officer
CHR: Michael Pulido, Process Leader Human Resources
Web address: www.heartland–health.com
Control: Other not–for–profit (including NFP Corporation) **Service:** General Medical and Surgical

Staffed Beds: 350 **Admissions:** 19124 **Census:** 235 **Outpatient Visits:** 651961 **Births:** 1832 **Total Expense ($000):** 360748 **Payroll Expense ($000):** 157441 **Personnel:** 2569

□ **NORTHWEST MISSOURI PSYCHIATRIC REHABILITATION CENTER (264007)**, 3505 Frederick Avenue, Zip 64506–2914; tel. 816/387–2300 **A**1 10 **F**4 25 36 50 56 57 58 63 73 75 81 82 87 88 91 92 93 119 124 135 **P**6
Primary Contact: Dick Gregory, Ph.D., Chief Executive Officer
COO: Mary Attebury, Chief Operating Officer
CFO: Randy Riley, Fiscal and Administrative Manager
CMO: James B. Reynolds, M.D., Medical Director
CIO: Eduardo Abaricia, Director Information Technology
CHR: Mary Blakey Gorman, Human Resources Director
Web address: www.dmh.missouri.gov/hr/faclist.htm
Control: State–Government, nonfederal **Service:** Psychiatric

Staffed Beds: 108 **Admissions:** 54 **Census:** 110 **Outpatient Visits:** 33 **Births:** 0 **Total Expense ($000):** 18412 **Payroll Expense ($000):** 10514 **Personnel:** 313

SAINT LOUIS—St. Louis County

★ **BARNES–JEWISH HOSPITAL (260032)**, One Barnes–Jewish Hospital Plaza, Zip 63110–1003; tel. 314/747–3000, (Total facility includes 120 beds in nursing home–type unit) **A**1 2 3 5 8 9 10 **F**1 3 4 5 6 7 8 9 11 12 13 14 15 16 17 18 19 20 21 22 23 24 25 26 27 30 31 32 33 34 35 36 37 38 40 41 43 44 46 47 48 49 50 51 52 53 54 55 56 57 58 59 60 62 63 64 65 66 68 69 71 72 73 74 75 76 77 78 79 80 81 82 84 85 86 87 88 90 91 92 93 94 95 96 97 98 99 100 101 102 103 104 105 106 107 108 109 110 111 112 113 114 116 117 118 119 120 121 123 124 125 126 127 128 129 130 131 132 133 134 135 136 137 **P**5 6 7 **S** BJC HealthCare
Primary Contact: Andrew A. Ziskind, M.D., President
COO: Sharon O'Keefe, R.N., Chief Operating Officer
CFO: Mark Krieger, Vice President and Chief Financial Officer
CMO: Jonathan Gottlieb, M.D., Chief Medical Officer
CIO: Jerry Vuchak, Vice President Information Systems
CHR: John Beatty, Vice President Human Resources
Web address: www.barnesjewish.org
Control: Other not–for–profit (including NFP Corporation) **Service:** General Medical and Surgical

Staffed Beds: 1207 **Admissions:** 54656 **Census:** 884 **Outpatient Visits:** 514768 **Births:** 3932 **Total Expense ($000):** 1265523 **Payroll Expense ($000):** 403127 **Personnel:** 8884

★ **BARNES–JEWISH WEST COUNTY HOSPITAL (260162)**, 12634 Olive Boulevard, Zip 63141–6337; tel. 314/996–8000, (Total facility includes 10 beds in nursing home–type unit) **A**1 3 5 9 10 **F**3 12 14 15 25 26 30 31 32 33 38 43 46 49 50 51 52 55 57 62 63 68 72 75 77 79 80 81 82 85 86 96 97 100 102 105 106 107 117 118 119 120 121 135 **S** BJC HealthCare
Primary Contact: Larry Tracy, Vice President and Chief Operating Officer
COO: Larry Tracy, Vice President and Chief Operating Officer
CFO: Mark Krieger, Vice President and Chief Financial Officer
CMO: Alan Londe, M.D., Chief of Staff
CIO: Jerry Vuchak, Vice President Information Systems
CHR: John Beatty, Vice President Human Resources
Web address: www.barnesjewishwestcounty.org
Control: Other not–for–profit (including NFP Corporation) **Service:** General Medical and Surgical

Staffed Beds: 79 **Admissions:** 3591 **Census:** 43 **Outpatient Visits:** 75447 **Births:** 0 **Total Expense ($000):** 79125 **Payroll Expense ($000):** 24854 **Personnel:** 455

MO

Hospital, Medicare Provider Number, Address, Telephone, Approval, Facility, and Physician Codes, Health Care System

★ American Hospital Association (AHA) membership
□ The Joint Commission accreditation
○ American Osteopathic Association (AOA) accreditation
△ Commission on Accreditation of Rehabilitation Facilities (CARF) accreditation

[★] **CHRISTIAN HOSPITAL (260180)**, 11133 Dunn Road, Zip 63136–6119; tel. 314/653–5000, (Total facility includes 24 beds in nursing home–type unit) **A**1 2 9 10 **F**2 3 7 11 15 18 20 22 24 25 26 27 30 32 33 38 39 43 47 49 50 51 52 54 55 57 59 67 68 69 72 73 75 76 77 78 79 80 81 82 85 86 88 91 93 94 95 96 100 102 103 104 105 106 107 108 109 111 117 118 119 121 124 135 137 **S** BJC HealthCare
Primary Contact: Ronald B. McMullen, President
CFO: John Katsianis, Chief Financial Officer
CMO: Melanie Mueth, M.D., Vice President Medical Affairs and Clinical Effectiveness
CIO: Diane Tattich, Group Manager
CHR: Bryan Hartwick, Vice President Human Resources
Web address: www.bjc.org
Control: Other not–for–profit (including NFP Corporation) **Service:** General Medical and Surgical

Staffed Beds: 244 **Admissions:** 14820 **Census:** 247 **Outpatient Visits:** 177668 **Births:** 0 **Total Expense ($000):** 259488 **Payroll Expense ($000):** 87926 **Personnel:** 1713

★ ○ **DES PERES HOSPITAL (260176)**, 2345 Dougherty Ferry Road, Zip 63122–3313; tel. 314/966–9100 **A**3 5 9 10 11 12 13 **F**3 6 9 11 12 15 17 18 20 22 25 26 30 31 32 33 34 38 41 43 44 49 50 54 55 56 57 59 62 66 67 68 72 73 75 77 79 80 81 82 86 87 90 91 92 93 96 100 102 107 119 120 121 124 132 135 136 137 **S** TENET Healthcare Corporation
Primary Contact: Michele C. Meyer, Chief Executive Officer
COO: Michael Kendrick, Chief Operating Officer
CFO: David Byrd, Chief Financial Officer
CMO: Karen Webb, M.D., Chief Medical Officer
CIO: Kay Hannon, Director Information Systems
CHR: Ron Birlew, Director Human Resources
Web address: www.despereshospital.com
Control: Corporation, Investor–owned, for–profit **Service:** General Medical and Surgical

Staffed Beds: 143 **Admissions:** 9256 **Census:** 109 **Outpatient Visits:** 35253 **Births:** 0 **Total Expense ($000):** 122389 **Payroll Expense ($000):** 33911 **Personnel:** 731

MO

□ △ **FOREST PARK COMMUNITY HOSPITAL (260021)**, 6150 Oakland Avenue, Zip 63139–3215; tel. 314/768–3000 **A**1 3 5 7 9 10 **F**3 8 15 17 18 25 26 27 30 31 32 38 41 46 50 51 54 55 56 57 62 66 68 72 73 75 76 77 78 79 80 85 86 87 88 90 91 92 93 94 96 100 102 106 107 109 111 119 120 121 132 135 137 **P**6 **S** Envision Hospital Corporation
Primary Contact: Jordan Tenenbaum, Chief Executive Officer
CFO: Lawrence Tyrrell, Chief Financial Officer
CHR: Kathaleen Clutts, Director Human Resources
Web address: www.forestparkhospital.com
Control: Corporation, Investor–owned, for–profit **Service:** General Medical and Surgical

Staffed Beds: 178 **Admissions:** 4461 **Census:** 76 **Outpatient Visits:** 57572 **Births:** 0 **Total Expense ($000):** 67745 **Payroll Expense ($000):** 28350 **Personnel:** 634

□ **HAWTHORN CHILDREN PSYCHIATRIC HOSPITAL**, 1901 Pennsylvania, Zip 63133; tel. 314/512–7800 **A**1 3 5 **F**30 31 32 88 89 **P**6
Primary Contact: Laurent D. Javois, Regional Executive Officer
Web address: www.dmh.missouri.gov\hcph\
Control: State–Government, nonfederal **Service:** Children's hospital psychiatric

Staffed Beds: 52 **Admissions:** 223 **Census:** 45 **Outpatient Visits:** 0 **Births:** 0 **Total Expense ($000):** 12416 **Payroll Expense ($000):** 6833 **Personnel:** 209

[★] **KINDRED HOSPITAL–ST. LOUIS (262010)**, 4930 Lindell Boulevard, Zip 63108–1510; tel. 314/361–8700, (Includes KINDRED HOSPITAL ST. LOUIS–ST. ANTHONY'S, 10018 Kennerly Road, 3rd Floor, Zip 63128; tel. 314/525–8100) **A**1 9 10 **F**1 3 25 30 32 43 59 75 80 107 119 137 **S** Kindred Healthcare
Primary Contact: Peter Miller, FACHE, Chief Executive Officer
COO: Wendi Lakeman, Chief Clinical Officer
CFO: Mary Berry, Senior Chief Financial Officer
CMO: Neil Ettinger, M.D., Medical Director
CHR: Tiana Taylor, Human Resources Recruiter
Web address: www.kindredhealthcare.com
Control: Corporation, Investor–owned, for–profit **Service:** Long–Term Acute Care hospital

Staffed Beds: 98 **Admissions:** 869 **Census:** 60 **Outpatient Visits:** 0 **Births:** 0 **Total Expense ($000):** 28346 **Payroll Expense ($000):** 10238 **Personnel:** 181

□ **METROPOLITAN ST. LOUIS PSYCHIATRIC CENTER (264025)**, 5351 Delmar, Zip 63112–3198; tel. 314/877–0500 **A**1 3 5 10 **F**4 11 26 30 31 32 38 88 92 135 **P**6
Primary Contact: Laurent D. Javois, Regional Executive Officer
COO: Anthony J. Cuneo, Chief Operating Officer
CFO: Laura Wayer, Chief Financial Officer
CMO: Rakhshanda Hassan, M.D., Medical Director
Web address: www.dmh.missouri.gov/mpc
Control: State–Government, nonfederal **Service:** Psychiatric

Staffed Beds: 112 **Admissions:** 2219 **Census:** 72 **Outpatient Visits:** 3544 **Births:** 0 **Total Expense ($000):** 20154 **Payroll Expense ($000):** 11112 **Personnel:** 299

[★] **MISSOURI BAPTIST MEDICAL CENTER (260108)**, 3015 North Ballas Road, Zip 63131–2329; tel. 314/996–5000 **A**1 2 5 9 10 **F**3 11 13 14 15 17 18 20 22 24 25 26 27 30 31 32 33 38 44 45 46 48 49 50 51 53 55 56 57 58 59 60 62 63 66 68 69 71 72 73 74 75 76 77 78 79 80 81 82 84 85 86 96 97 99 100 102 103 104 107 109 111 113 114 116 119 120 121 134 135 136 137 **P**6 **S** BJC HealthCare
Primary Contact: Joan Magruder, President
CFO: Anthony A. Noronha, Vice President Finance and Chief Financial Officer
CMO: John Krettek, M.D., Vice President Medical Affairs and Chief Medical Officer
CIO: Jane Schaefer, Director Information Systems
CHR: Rhonda Brandon, Vice President Human Resources
Web address: www.missouribaptistmedicalcenter.org
Control: Other not–for–profit (including NFP Corporation) **Service:** General Medical and Surgical

Staffed Beds: 418 **Admissions:** 21835 **Census:** 286 **Outpatient Visits:** 207179 **Births:** 4099 **Total Expense ($000):** 356447 **Payroll Expense ($000):** 122901 **Personnel:** 2426

[★] **SAINT LOUIS UNIVERSITY HOSPITAL (260105)**, 3635 Vista at Grand Boulevard, Zip 63110–0250, Mailing Address: P.O. Box 15250, Zip 63110–0250; tel. 314/577–8000 **A**1 2 3 5 8 9 10 **F**3 6 8 9 11 14 15 17 18 20 22 25 26 27 30 31 32 33 34 35 36 37 38 40 41 43 44 46 47 48 49 50 51 54 56 57 58 59 60 62 63 66 68 72 73 75 76 77 79 80 81 82 85 86 87 88 90 91 92 93 94 96 97 100 101 102 103 104 105 106 107 109 111 112 116 119 120 121 124 125 127 128 129 130 131 135 136 137 **P**1 **S** TENET Healthcare Corporation
Primary Contact: Crystal L. Haynes, Chief Executive Officer
COO: Dawn Anuszkiewicz, Chief Operating Officer
CFO: Raymond Alvey, Chief Financial Officer
CMO: Karen Webb, M.D., Chief Medical Officer
CIO: Beckie Patrick, Director Information System Technology
CHR: Ann Relling, Chief Human Resources Officer
Web address: www.sluhospital.com
Control: Corporation, Investor–owned, for–profit **Service:** General Medical and Surgical

Staffed Beds: 332 **Admissions:** 14233 **Census:** 229 **Outpatient Visits:** 110531 **Births:** 0 **Total Expense ($000):** 326426 **Payroll Expense ($000):** 77920 **Personnel:** 1308

□ **SELECT SPECIALTY HOSPITAL (262013)**, 6150 Oakland Avenue, 5th Floor, Zip 63139–3297; tel. 314/768–3513 **A**1 9 10 **F**1 25 26 30 59 72 75 82 119 137 **S** Select Medical Corporation
Primary Contact: Megan Schmidt, Chief Executive Officer
Web address: www.selectmedicalcorp.com
Control: Corporation, Investor–owned, for–profit **Service:** Long–Term Acute Care hospital

Staffed Beds: 33 **Admissions:** 254 **Census:** 21 **Outpatient Visits:** 0 **Births:** 0 **Total Expense ($000):** 11227 **Payroll Expense ($000):** 4047 **Personnel:** 66

□ **SHRINERS HOSPITALS FOR CHILDREN, ST. LOUIS**, 2001 South Lindbergh Boulevard, Zip 63131–3597; tel. 314/432–3600 **A**1 3 5 **F**3 25 30 31 55 56 57 62 63 66 72 73 77 78 80 81 82 84 86 87 119 120 121 135 137 **S** Shriners Hospitals for Children
Primary Contact: John W. O'Shaughnessy, FACHE, Administrator
CMO: Perry L. Schoenecker, M.D., Chief of Staff
CIO: Jeanne Hall, Director Management Information Systems
CHR: Christina Devine, Director Human Resources
Web address: www.shrinershq.org
Control: Other not–for–profit (including NFP Corporation) **Service:** Children's orthopedic

Staffed Beds: 42 **Admissions:** 1537 **Census:** 13 **Outpatient Visits:** 12804 **Births:** 0 **Total Expense ($000):** 0 **Payroll Expense ($000):** 0 **Personnel:** 223

★ **SSM CARDINAL GLENNON CHILDREN'S MEDICAL CENTER**, 1465 South Grand Boulevard, Zip 63104–1095; tel. 314/577–5600 **A**1 3 5 9 **F**3 8 11 19 21 23 25 26 27 28 30 31 32 33 34 36 37 38 40 41 43 44 45 46 47 48 49 50 53 55 56 57 59 60 62 63 64 70 71 72 73 75 76 77 78 79 81 82 83 84 85 86 87 89 90 91 92 94 96 100 101 106 107 114 118 119 120 121 123 125 126 127 128 129 130 131 133 135 137 **P**6 7 8 **S** SSM Health Care
Primary Contact: Douglas A. Ries, FACHE, President
COO: Sherlyn Hailstone, MSN, CHE, Chief Operating Officer
CMO: Susan Heaney, M.D., Vice President Medical Affairs
CIO: Joe Provaznik, Manager Information Systems
CHR: Mary Pat Campbell, Director Human Resources
Web address: www.cardinalglennon.com
Control: Church–operated, Nongovernment, not–for profit **Service:** Children's general

Staffed Beds: 176 **Admissions:** 6767 **Census:** 128 **Outpatient Visits:** 215017 **Births:** 0 **Total Expense ($000):** 204115 **Payroll Expense ($000):** 72800 **Personnel:** 1412

★ **SSM ST. JOSEPH HOSPITAL OF KIRKWOOD (260081)**, 525 Couch Avenue, Zip 63122–5536; tel. 314/966–1500 **A**1 9 10 **F**3 11 13 14 15 17 18 20 22 24 25 26 27 30 31 32 33 37 38 41 42 43 44 49 50 51 54 55 57 59 60 62 63 66 68 71 72 73 74 76 77 79 80 81 82 90 96 97 99 100 102 104 105 106 107 108 109 111 118 119 121 124 132 135 136 137 **P**6 8 **S** SSM Health Care
Primary Contact: Sherry Hausmann, President
COO: Lee Bernstein, Executive Vice President and Chief Operating Officer
CFO: Alita Prosser, Director Finance
CMO: Timothy J. Pratt, M.D., President Medical Staff
CIO: Leighton Wassilak, Director Information Systems
CHR: Kurt Delabar, Director Human Resources
Web address: www.st josephkirkwood.com
Control: Church–operated, Nongovernment, not–for profit **Service:** General Medical and Surgical

Staffed Beds: 187 **Admissions:** 7597 **Census:** 81 **Outpatient Visits:** 78500 **Births:** 993 **Total Expense ($000):** 96752 **Payroll Expense ($000):** 38693 **Personnel:** 571

★ **SSM ST. MARY'S HEALTH CENTER (260091)**, 6420 Clayton Road, Zip 63117–1811; tel. 314/768–8000 **A**1 2 3 5 8 9 10 **F**3 8 11 13 15 17 18 20 22 24 25 26 27 30 31 32 33 35 36 38 41 43 44 49 54 55 56 57 58 59 62 64 68 70 71 72 73 74 76 77 79 80 81 82 87 88 90 91 92 93 94 95 96 97 100 102 104 105 106 107 108 109 111 113 114 119 121 124 132 135 136 137 **S** SSM Health Care
Primary Contact: William M. Jennings, President
COO: Sharon R. Dudley, R.N., Executive Vice President and Chief Operating Officer
CFO: Jo Bertram, Vice President Finance
CMO: Darren E. Wethers, M.D., President Medical Staff
CIO: Bob Curran, Director Health Information Management
CHR: Robert F. Scott, Director Human Resources
Web address: www.stmarys–stlouis.com
Control: Church–operated, Nongovernment, not–for profit **Service:** General Medical and Surgical

Staffed Beds: 293 **Admissions:** 19388 **Census:** 262 **Outpatient Visits:** 181218 **Births:** 3207 **Total Expense ($000):** 247637 **Payroll Expense ($000):** 97765 **Personnel:** 1592

□ **ST. ALEXIUS HOSPITAL (260210)**, 3933 South Broadway, Zip 63118–4601; tel. 314/865–3333, (Includes SOUTHPOINTE HOSPITAL, 2639 Miami Street, Zip 63118–3929; tel. 314/772–1456) **A**1 6 9 10 **F**3 12 15 18 25 26 32 33 36 37 38 54 55 57 59 66 68 72 75 76 77 79 81 82 88 91 92 93 94 96 97 100 106 107 119 132 135 **S** Envision Hospital Corporation
Primary Contact: Robert S. Adcock, Chief Executive Officer
CFO: Johnny Watkins, Chief Financial Officer
CIO: Jennifer Schempp, Manager Information Systems
Web address: www.stalexiushospital.com
Control: Corporation, Investor–owned, for–profit **Service:** General Medical and Surgical

Staffed Beds: 169 **Admissions:** 7309 **Census:** 121 **Outpatient Visits:** 36972 **Births:** 0 **Total Expense ($000):** 75567 **Payroll Expense ($000):** 32465 **Personnel:** 697

★ △ **ST. ANTHONY'S MEDICAL CENTER (260077)**, 10010 Kennerly Road, Zip 63128–2106; tel. 314/525–1000 **A**1 7 9 10 **F**3 4 5 8 11 12 13 15 17 18 20 22 24 25 26 27 28 30 32 33 36 38 39 40 42 43 44 47 49 50 52 53 54 55 56 57 59 60 61 62 63 66 67 68 71 72 73 74 75 76 77 78 79 80 81 82 84 85 86 87 88 89 90 91 92 93 94 95 96 97 99 100 102 106 107 108 109 111 112 118 119 120 121 124 132 133 135 136 137 **P**6
Primary Contact: Thomas H. Rockers, President and Chief Executive Officer
COO: Michalene D. Maringer, R.N., Executive Vice President and Chief Hospital Officer
CFO: John McGuire, Executive Vice President and Chief Financial Officer
CMO: Robert V. Griesbaum, M.D., Vice President Patient Care Quality
CIO: Gordon Lashmett, Chief Information Officer
CHR: Ann Bollone, Vice President Human Resources
Web address: www.stanthonysmedcenter.com
Control: Other not–for–profit (including NFP Corporation) **Service:** General Medical and Surgical

Staffed Beds: 602 **Admissions:** 29108 **Census:** 398 **Outpatient Visits:** 454218 **Births:** 1750 **Total Expense ($000):** 359230 **Payroll Expense ($000):** 161744 **Personnel:** 3728

★ △ **ST. JOHN'S MERCY MEDICAL CENTER (260020)**, 615 South New Ballas Road, Zip 63141–8277; tel. 314/569–6000 **A**1 2 3 5 7 8 9 10 **F**3 5 8 9 11 13 14 15 16 17 18 20 22 23 24 25 26 27 28 29 30 31 32 33 34 36 37 38 40 44 46 47 49 51 52 53 54 55 56 57 58 59 60 62 64 66 67 68 69 70 71 72 73 74 76 77 78 79 80 81 82 83 84 85 86 87 88 89 90 91 92 93 94 95 96 97 99 100 102 104 105 106 107 108 109 111 113 114 116 118 119 120 121 123 124 132 133 135 136 137 **P**6 8 **S** Sisters of Mercy Health System
Primary Contact: Margaret DeNarvaez, President and Chief Executive Officer
CFO: Randy Combs, Chief Financial Officer
CMO: Paul Hintze, M.D., Vice President Medical Affairs
CIO: Eugene Roth, Vice President Information Services
CHR: Rocky Ruello, Vice President Human Resources
Web address: www.stjohnsmercy.org
Control: Other not–for–profit (including NFP Corporation) **Service:** General Medical and Surgical

Staffed Beds: 822 **Admissions:** 42554 **Census:** 620 **Outpatient Visits:** 666157 **Births:** 7915 **Total Expense ($000):** 620454 **Payroll Expense ($000):** 252425 **Personnel:** 4912

★ △ **ST. LOUIS CHILDREN'S HOSPITAL (263301)**, One Children's Place, Zip 63110–1002; tel. 314/454–6000 **A**1 3 5 7 8 9 10 **F**3 5 7 11 16 17 18 19 20 21 23 25 26 27 28 30 31 32 33 36 37 38 39 40 41 42 43 44 45 49 50 53 55 56 57 58 59 60 61 62 63 66 69 70 72 73 75 76 77 79 80 81 82 83 84 85 86 89 90 91 92 94 96 97 98 100 102 107 118 119 120 121 123 124 125 126 127 128 129 130 131 132 133 134 135 137 **S** BJC HealthCare
Primary Contact: Lee F. Fetter, President and Senior Executive Officer
CFO: Doug Vanderslice, Vice President and Chief Financial Officer
CMO: F. Sessions Cole, M.D., Chief Medical Officer
CHR: David Cook, Vice President Human Resources
Web address: www.stlouischildrens.org
Control: Other not–for–profit (including NFP Corporation) **Service:** Children's general

Staffed Beds: 250 **Admissions:** 10986 **Census:** 180 **Outpatient Visits:** 156449 **Births:** 0 **Total Expense ($000):** 366061 **Payroll Expense ($000):** 111393 **Personnel:** 2725

□ **ST. LOUIS PSYCHIATRIC REHABILITATION CENTER (264010)**, 5300 Arsenal Street, Zip 63139–1494; tel. 314/877–6500 **A**1 10 **F**11 26 32 37 50 52 63 73 81 82 88 90 91 119 121 132 135 **P**6
Primary Contact: Laurent D. Javois, Regional Executive Officer
COO: Curtis L. Trager, Chief Operating Officer
CFO: Laura Wayer, Chief Operations
CMO: Lori DeRosear, D.O., Medical Director
CIO: Richard Moore, Director Information Technology
CHR: Ronald Moore, Manager Human Resources
Web address: www.dmh.missouri.gov
Control: State–Government, nonfederal **Service:** Psychiatric

Staffed Beds: 196 **Admissions:** 83 **Census:** 189 **Outpatient Visits:** 0 **Births:** 0 **Total Expense ($000):** 29952 **Payroll Expense ($000):** 16035 **Personnel:** 466

★ **THE REHABILITATION INSTITUTE OF ST. LOUIS (263028)**, 4455 Duncan Avenue, Zip 63110–1111; tel. 314/658–3800 **A**1 10 **F**2 25 26 30 41 43 53 58 62 72 73 77 82 85 86 119 120 121 132 135 137
S HEALTHSOUTH Corporation
Primary Contact: Barbara Jacobsmeyer, Chief Executive Officer
Web address: www.healthsouth.com
Control: Partnership, Investor–owned, for–profit **Service:** Rehabilitation

Staffed Beds: 80 **Admissions:** 1693 **Census:** 65 **Outpatient Visits:** 37356 **Births:** 0 **Total Expense ($000):** 24906 **Payroll Expense ($000):** 12333 **Personnel:** 247

MO

Hospital, Medicare Provider Number, Address, Telephone, Approval, Facility, and Physician Codes, Health Care System

★ American Hospital Association (AHA) membership
□ The Joint Commission accreditation
○ American Osteopathic Association (AOA) accreditation
△ Commission on Accreditation of Rehabilitation Facilities (CARF) accreditation

★ △ **VETERANS AFFAIRS MEDICAL CENTER**, 915 North Grand, Zip 63106–1621; tel. 314/652–4100, (Total facility includes 71 beds in nursing home–type unit) **A**1 3 5 7 **F**1 3 4 5 15 18 20 24 25 26 27 29 30 31 32 33 37 38 42 43 44 49 50 53 54 55 56 59 60 61 62 64 65 68 72 73 75 76 77 79 80 82 85 86 87 88 90 92 93 94 95 96 97 99 100 102 103 106 107 109 111 117 118 119 121 124 132 133 134 135 136 137 **S** Department of Veterans Affairs
Primary Contact: Glen E. Struchtemeyer, Director
CFO: Karen Westerheide, Chief Financial Officer
CMO: Nathan Ravi, M.D., Chief of Staff
CIO: Steve Warmbold, Director Information Management Service Line
CHR: Marie Lewis, Human Resources Liaison
Web address: www.va.gov/sta/guide/home.asp
Control: Veterans Affairs, Government, federal **Service:** General Medical and Surgical

Staffed Beds: 339 **Admissions:** 9235 **Census:** 257 **Outpatient Visits:** 536881 **Births:** 0 **Total Expense ($000):** 284899 **Payroll Expense ($000):** 159032 **Personnel:** 2009

SAINT PETERS—St. Charles County

★ **BARNES–JEWISH ST. PETERS HOSPITAL (260191)**, 10 Hospital Drive, Zip 63376–1659; tel. 636/916–9000, (Total facility includes 8 beds in nursing home–type unit) **A**1 5 9 10 **F**3 8 11 13 15 18 20 24 25 26 27 30 31 32 33 38 55 56 57 62 68 73 74 75 76 77 79 80 81 82 85 86 96 97 100 102 107 109 117 118 119 121 124 135 136 **S** BJC HealthCare
Primary Contact: David Ross, President
CFO: Cindy Gross, Assistant Administrator Finance
CHR: Keith Bolton, Manager
Web address: www.bjsph.org/
Control: Other not–for–profit (including NFP Corporation) **Service:** General Medical and Surgical

Staffed Beds: 101 **Admissions:** 6652 **Census:** 80 **Outpatient Visits:** 112664 **Births:** 720 **Total Expense ($000):** 100810 **Payroll Expense ($000):** 34943 **Personnel:** 711

SALEM—Dent County

★ **SALEM MEMORIAL DISTRICT HOSPITAL (261318)**, Highway 72 North, Zip 65560–0774, Mailing Address: P.O. Box 774, Zip 65560–0774; tel. 573/729–6626, (Total facility includes 18 beds in nursing home–type unit) **A**9 10 18 **F**3 7 11 25 26 30 31 32 38 55 57 59 61 65 73 78 79 80 82 84 96 107 117 119 122 124 135
Primary Contact: Dennis P. Pryor, Administrator
CFO: Stephanie Wofford, Controller
Web address: www.smdh.net
Control: Hospital district or authority, Government, nonfederal **Service:** General Medical and Surgical

Staffed Beds: 43 **Admissions:** 917 **Census:** 27 **Outpatient Visits:** 32891 **Births:** 0 **Total Expense ($000):** 13674 **Payroll Expense ($000):** 5690 **Personnel:** 134

MO

SEDALIA—Pettis County

★ **BOTHWELL REGIONAL HEALTH CENTER (260009)**, 601 East 14th Street, Zip 65301–1706, Mailing Address: P.O. Box 1706, Zip 65302–1706; tel. 660/826–8833, (Total facility includes 10 beds in nursing home–type unit) **A**1 9 10 20 **F**3 11 12 13 14 15 18 20 24 25 26 27 30 31 32 33 37 38 42 43 44 53 54 55 57 59 61 62 63 66 68 71 72 73 74 75 76 77 78 79 81 82 84 85 86 96 97 99 100 102 104 105 106 107 111 112 117 118 119 120 121 124 133 135 136 137
Primary Contact: John M. Dawes, FACHE, Chief Executive Officer
COO: Mark I. Hirshberg, Chief Operating Officer
CFO: David Halsell, Chief Financial Officer
CIO: Greg Collins, Information Systems Director
CHR: Deb Clemmer, Vice President Human Resources
Web address: www.brhc.org
Control: City–Government, nonfederal **Service:** General Medical and Surgical

Staffed Beds: 152 **Admissions:** 6650 **Census:** 79 **Outpatient Visits:** 122134 **Births:** 634 **Total Expense ($000):** 80667 **Payroll Expense ($000):** 35008 **Personnel:** 734

SIKESTON—Scott County

☐ △ **MISSOURI DELTA MEDICAL CENTER (260113)**, 1008 North Main Street, Zip 63801–5044; tel. 573/471–1600 **A**1 5 7 9 10 19 20 **F**3 11 13 15 18 19 20 24 25 26 27 28 30 31 32 33 37 38 41 43 44 50 51 52 53 54 55 56 57 59 61 62 66 68 72 73 74 75 76 77 79 80 81 82 84 85 86 87 88 89 90 91 92 93 94 96 97 98 100 103 104 107 118 119 120 121 133 135
Primary Contact: Charles D. Ancell, President
CFO: Jon Branstetter, Vice President Finance
Web address: www.missouridelta.com
Control: Other not–for–profit (including NFP Corporation) **Service:** General Medical and Surgical

Staffed Beds: 160 **Admissions:** 5422 **Census:** 70 **Outpatient Visits:** 205854 **Births:** 586 **Total Expense ($000):** 76872 **Payroll Expense ($000):** 32961 **Personnel:** 690

SMITHVILLE—Clay County

★ △ **SAINT LUKE'S NORTHLAND HOSPITAL–SMITHVILLE CAMPUS (260062)**, 601 South 169 Highway, Zip 64089–9317; tel. 816/532–3700, (Total facility includes 11 beds in nursing home–type unit) (Nonreporting) **A**1 7 9 10 **S** Saint Luke's Health System
Primary Contact: Don Sipes, Chief Executive Officer
COO: Kevin Trimble, R.N., Chief Operating Officer and Chief Nursing Officer
CFO: Julie Murphy, Chief Financial Officer
CMO: George A. Pagels, M.D., Senior Vice President and Chief Medical Officer
CIO: Deborah Gash, Chief Information Officer
CHR: Alan Abramovitz, Senior Director Human Resources
Web address: www.saintlukeshealthsystem.org
Control: Other not–for–profit (including NFP Corporation) **Service:** General Medical and Surgical

Staffed Beds: 51

SPRINGFIELD—Greene County

☐ **LAKELAND REGIONAL HOSPITAL (264024)**, 440 South Market Street, Zip 65806–2026; tel. 417/865–5581 **A**1 9 10 **F**38 88 89 91 119 135 **P**6 **S** Youth and Family Centered Services
Primary Contact: Rick Crump, Chief Executive Officer
CMO: Richard Aiken, M.D., Vice President and Medical Director
CHR: Kay Hill, Director Human Resources
Web address: www.yfcs.com/facilities/lakeland/index.html
Control: Corporation, Investor–owned, for–profit **Service:** Children's hospital psychiatric

Staffed Beds: 60 **Admissions:** 1560 **Census:** 53 **Outpatient Visits:** 0 **Births:** 0 **Total Expense ($000):** 8553 **Payroll Expense ($000):** 4750 **Personnel:** 233

★ **LESTER E. COX MEDICAL CENTERS (260040)**, 1423 North Jefferson Street, Zip 65802–1988; tel. 417/269–3000, (Includes LESTER E. COX MEDICAL CENTER NORTH; LESTER E. COX MEDICAL CENTER SOUTH, 3801 South National Avenue, Zip 65807; tel. 417/269–6000), (Total facility includes 34 beds in nursing home–type unit) **A**1 2 9 10 **F**3 4 5 7 11 12 13 15 17 18 20 22 24 25 26 27 28 30 31 32 33 36 37 38 39 40 41 43 44 47 49 50 51 52 53 54 55 56 57 59 60 61 62 63 66 67 68 69 70 72 73 74 75 76 77 78 79 80 81 82 83 84 85 86 87 88 89 90 91 92 93 94 96 97 99 100 103 104 105 106 107 108 109 111 112 113 114 117 118 119 120 121 124 132 133 135 136 137 **P**3 6 **S** CoxHealth
Primary Contact: Robert H. Bezanson, President and Chief Executive Officer
COO: Steven Edwards, Executive Vice President and Chief Operating Officer
CFO: Jacob McWay, Senior Vice President and Chief Financial Officer
CMO: Wolfe Gerecht, M.D., Vice President Medical Affairs
CIO: Bruce Robison, Executive Director Information Technology
CHR: John Hursh, Vice President Human Resources
Web address: www.coxhealth.com
Control: Other not–for–profit (including NFP Corporation) **Service:** General Medical and Surgical

Staffed Beds: 623 **Admissions:** 29902 **Census:** 423 **Outpatient Visits:** 1316524 **Births:** 3945 **Total Expense ($000):** 778918 **Payroll Expense ($000):** 273278 **Personnel:** 6016

○ **OZARKS COMMUNITY HOSPITAL (260207)**, (Formerly Doctors Hospital of Springfield), 2828 North National, Zip 65803–4306; tel. 417/837–4000 **A**9 10 11 **F**3 25 30 31 32 37 38 39 43 53 54 55 57 63 66 72 73 75 77 79 80 81 82 85 86 87 88 90 93 94 96 97 100 102 107 118 119 124 132 133 136 137 **P**6
Primary Contact: Paul Taylor, Administrator
CFO: Janet Taylor, CPA, Chief Financial Officer
Control: Corporation, Investor–owned, for–profit **Service:** General Medical and Surgical

Staffed Beds: 35 **Admissions:** 1252 **Census:** 21 **Outpatient Visits:** 167831 **Births:** 0 **Total Expense ($000):** 42271 **Payroll Expense ($000):** 13329 **Personnel:** 453

SELECT SPECIALTY HOSPITAL – SPRINGFIELD (260221), 1630 East Primrose Street, Zip 65804; tel. 417/885–4700, (Nonreporting) **A**10
Primary Contact: Cynthia Whitten, RN, Chief Executive Officer
Control: Corporation, Investor–owned, for–profit **Service:** Long–Term Acute Care hospital

Staffed Beds: 44

Many Facility Codes have changed. Please refer to the AHA Guide Code Chart.

▣ △ **ST. JOHN'S HOSPITAL (260065)**, 1235 East Cherokee Street, Zip 65804–2263; tel. 417/820–2000, (Total facility includes 21 beds in nursing home–type unit) **A**1 2 7 10 **F**3 5 6 7 8 9 11 12 13 15 16 17 18 20 22 24 25 26 27 29 30 31 32 33 34 36 37 38 40 41 43 44 49 50 51 53 54 55 56 57 59 60 61 62 63 66 68 69 70 71 72 73 74 75 76 77 79 80 81 82 83 84 85 86 87 88 90 91 92 93 94 96 97 100 102 104 105 106 107 109 111 114 117 118 119 120 121 123 124 132 133 135 136 137 **P**6 8 **S** Sisters of Mercy Health System
Primary Contact: Jon Swope, President
COO: Michele Schaefer, Senior Vice President and Chief Operating Officer
CFO: Jim Budzinski, Chief Financial Officer
CMO: Allan Allphin, M.D., Chief of Staff
CIO: Mark Pasquale, Vice President Information Systems
CHR: Trisha Holbert, Vice President Human Resources
Web address: www.stjohns.com
Control: Church–operated, Nongovernment, not–for profit **Service:** General Medical and Surgical

Staffed Beds: 623 **Admissions:** 32985 **Census:** 434 **Outpatient Visits:** 596471 **Births:** 2654 **Total Expense ($000):** 634027 **Payroll Expense ($000):** 220814 **Personnel:** 5168

STE. GENEVIEVE—Ste. Genevieve County

★ **STE. GENEVIEVE COUNTY MEMORIAL HOSPITAL (261330)**, 800 Suite Genevieve Drive, Zip 63670–0468; tel. 573/883–2751 **A**9 10 18 **F**3 11 13 15 24 25 27 30 32 33 36 37 38 50 52 54 55 56 57 61 62 63 66 72 73 74 75 76 77 79 80 81 82 84 86 96 100 107 118 119 120 121 122 135 136 137 **P**6
Primary Contact: Thomas Keim, Chief Executive Officer
CFO: Susan Eckenfels, Chief Financial Officer
CMO: Bhargau Kanani, M.D., Chief of Staff
CIO: Marsha Norris, Director Information Systems
CHR: Sarah Glueck, Director Human Resources
Web address: www.stegenevievehospital.org
Control: County–Government, nonfederal **Service:** General Medical and Surgical

Staffed Beds: 25 **Admissions:** 1355 **Census:** 12 **Outpatient Visits:** 96854 **Births:** 108 **Total Expense ($000):** 23544 **Payroll Expense ($000):** 10655 **Personnel:** 250

SULLIVAN—Crawford County

★ **MISSOURI BAPTIST HOSPITAL–SULLIVAN (260115)**, 751 Sappington Bridge Road, Zip 63080–2354; tel. 573/468–4186 **A**9 10 **F**3 7 11 13 15 24 25 26 27 30 31 32 33 38 42 43 45 52 54 55 57 62 63 66 68 73 74 75 76 77 79 80 81 82 84 85 86 87 88 92 93 96 100 102 107 118 119 120 122 124 135 **P**5 7 **S** BJC HealthCare
Primary Contact: Tony Schwarm, President
CFO: Tonya Cottrell, Senior Financial Analyst
CMO: Barbara Dixon–Scott, M.D., Chief of Staff
CHR: Lisa Lochner, Assistant Administrator
Web address: www.missouribaptistsullivan.org
Control: Other not–for–profit (including NFP Corporation) **Service:** General Medical and Surgical

Staffed Beds: 55 **Admissions:** 1734 **Census:** 20 **Outpatient Visits:** 70453 **Births:** 204 **Total Expense ($000):** 33469 **Payroll Expense ($000):** 12553 **Personnel:** 322

SWEET SPRINGS—Saline County

I–70 MEDICAL CENTER (261334), 105 Hospital Drive, Zip 65351–2229; tel. 660/335–4700 **A**9 10 18 **F**3 11 25 31 32 33 38 54 55 57 62 63 66 77 80 82 84 85 86 96 117 119 122 **P**6 **S** Hospital Management Consulting, LLC
Primary Contact: Ronald D. Baker, Chief Executive Officer
CFO: Gary Clifton, Chief Financial Officer
CMO: Charles E. Lea, Chief of Staff
CHR: Diane Steinkuhler, Administrative Assistant Human Resources
Web address: www.i70medcenter.com
Control: Other not–for–profit (including NFP Corporation) **Service:** General Medical and Surgical

Staffed Beds: 15 **Admissions:** 167 **Census:** 4 **Outpatient Visits:** 8652 **Births:** 0 **Total Expense ($000):** 5861 **Payroll Expense ($000):** 1909 **Personnel:** 44

TRENTON—Grundy County

WRIGHT MEMORIAL HOSPITAL (261309), 701 East First Street, Zip 64683–2402, Mailing Address: P.O. Box 628, Zip 64683–0628; tel. 660/359–5621 **A**9 10 18 **F**11 13 15 24 26 27 30 31 32 33 38 42 43 55 56 57 61 62 66 72 73 74 75 76 77 78 79 80 84 85 86 87 94 96 97 100 102 107 118 119 122 124 132 135 **P**1 **S** Saint Luke's Health System
Primary Contact: Karen S. Cole, FACHE, Chief Executive Officer
CFO: Leslie Reed, Chief Financial Officer
CHR: Gail Ledesma, Director Human Resources
Web address: www.saintlukeshealthsystem.org
Control: Other not–for–profit (including NFP Corporation) **Service:** General Medical and Surgical

Staffed Beds: 25 **Admissions:** 1076 **Census:** 11 **Outpatient Visits:** 65978 **Births:** 230 **Total Expense ($000):** 18628 **Payroll Expense ($000):** 8440 **Personnel:** 196

TROY—Lincoln County

□ **LINCOLN COUNTY MEDICAL CENTER (261319)**, 1000 East Cherry Street, Zip 63379–1513; tel. 636/528–8551 **A**1 9 10 18 **F**3 11 15 17 24 25 26 30 31 32 33 38 41 50 51 55 56 57 61 62 63 66 68 73 75 77 79 80 81 82 84 86 96 100 107 118 119 120 121 122 124 135
Primary Contact: Floyd B. Dowell, Jr., Administrator
CFO: Albert Wiss, Chief Financial Officer
CMO: Dale Reinker, M.D., Medical Director
CIO: Travis Boyd, Manager Information Technology
CHR: Toni Price, Director Human Resources
Web address: www.lcmctroy.com
Control: County–Government, nonfederal **Service:** General Medical and Surgical

Staffed Beds: 25 **Admissions:** 1067 **Census:** 13 **Outpatient Visits:** 67926 **Births:** 0 **Total Expense ($000):** 27015 **Payroll Expense ($000):** 11767 **Personnel:** 263

UNIONVILLE—Putnam County

★ **PUTNAM COUNTY MEMORIAL HOSPITAL (261305)**, 1926 Oak Street, Zip 63565–1100, Mailing Address: P.O. Box 389, Zip 63565–0389; tel. 660/947–2411 **A**9 10 18 **F**3 24 30 31 32 33 38 50 55 57 62 63 79 80 82 84 87 100 102 107 119 122 124 **P**6
Primary Contact: Ray Magers, Chief Executive Officer
COO: Katherine Smith, Chief Operating Officer
CFO: Jan Slayton, Chief Financial Officer
CMO: W. Stephen Casady, M.D., Chief of Staff
CIO: Ray Magers, Chief Executive Officer
CHR: Judy Green, Director Human Resources
Web address: www.pcmhosp.com
Control: County–Government, nonfederal **Service:** General Medical and Surgical

Staffed Beds: 25 **Admissions:** 365 **Census:** 4 **Outpatient Visits:** 50609 **Births:** 0 **Total Expense ($000):** 7052 **Payroll Expense ($000):** 3787 **Personnel:** 102

WARRENSBURG—Johnson County

▣ **WESTERN MISSOURI MEDICAL CENTER (260097)**, 403 Burkarth Road, Zip 64093–3101; tel. 660/747–2500 **A**1 9 10 20 **F**3 8 11 13 15 17 24 25 26 27 28 30 31 32 38 43 47 55 56 57 60 62 63 66 68 73 74 75 76 77 79 80 84 85 86 92 96 97 100 106 107 117 118 119 120 121 122 124 135 136 137 **P**6
Primary Contact: Craig J. Marks, President and Chief Executive Officer
COO: John Smolen, Vice President Clinical Services and Chief Operating Officer
CFO: Roberta Nienhueser, Vice President Financial Services and Chief Financial Officer
CMO: David Pulliam, D.O., President Medical Staff
CIO: Carol McKinney, Director Information Services
CHR: Dennis Long, Director Human Resources
Web address: www.wmmconline.org
Control: County–Government, nonfederal **Service:** General Medical and Surgical

Staffed Beds: 77 **Admissions:** 3319 **Census:** 32 **Outpatient Visits:** 76211 **Births:** 870 **Total Expense ($000):** 53555 **Payroll Expense ($000):** 24323 **Personnel:** 499

MO

Hospital, Medicare Provider Number, Address, Telephone, Approval, Facility, and Physician Codes, Health Care System
★ American Hospital Association (AHA) membership
□ The Joint Commission accreditation
○ American Osteopathic Association (AOA) accreditation
△ Commission on Accreditation of Rehabilitation Facilities (CARF) accreditation

WASHINGTON—Franklin County

★ **ST. JOHN'S MERCY HOSPITAL (260052)**, 901 East Fifth Street, Zip 63090–3127; tel. 636/239–8000 **A**1 9 10 **F**3 8 11 12 13 14 15 17 18 24 25 26 28 30 31 32 33 38 40 43 44 46 48 49 50 55 57 60 62 64 68 71 73 74 75 76 77 78 79 80 84 85 86 87 94 96 97 99 100 102 106 107 113 118 119 120 121 123 124 135 136 **P**8 **S** Sisters of Mercy Health System
Primary Contact: Terri L. McLain, FACHE, President
CFO: Cheryl Matejka, Vice President Finance
CMO: Thomas Riechers, M.D., Chief Medical Staff
CIO: Eugene Roth, Vice President Information Services
CHR: Sheila Shortt, Manager Human Resources
Web address: www.stjohnsmercy.org
Control: Church–operated, Nongovernment, not–for profit **Service:** General Medical and Surgical

Staffed Beds: 169 **Admissions:** 6449 **Census:** 61 **Outpatient Visits:** 135225 **Births:** 990 **Total Expense ($000):** 81842 **Payroll Expense ($000):** 34068 **Personnel:** 713

WENTZVILLE—St. Charles County

SSM ST. JOSEPH HEALTH CENTER – WENTZVILLE See SSM St. Joseph Health Center, Saint Charles

WEST PLAINS—Howell County

★ **OZARKS MEDICAL CENTER (260078)**, 1100 Kentucky Avenue, Zip 65775–1100, Mailing Address: P.O. Box 1100, Zip 65775–1100; tel. 417/256–9111 **A**1 5 9 10 20 **F**2 3 5 7 11 13 15 17 18 20 22 24 25 26 27 30 31 32 36 38 41 42 43 44 55 57 60 61 62 66 68 72 73 74 75 76 77 79 80 81 82 84 86 88 89 90 91 92 93 94 96 97 99 100 103 106 107 109 118 119 120 121 124 133 135 136 137 **P**8
Primary Contact: David Zechman, President and Chief Executive Officer
COO: Edward R. Henegar, D.O., Vice President
CFO: Michael Gross, Vice President Finance
CIO: Edward Boys, Director Information Services
CHR: Greg Shannon, Director Human Resources
Web address: www.ozarksmedicalcenter.com
Control: Other not–for–profit (including NFP Corporation) **Service:** General Medical and Surgical

Staffed Beds: 114 **Admissions:** 5053 **Census:** 51 **Outpatient Visits:** 528820 **Births:** 743 **Total Expense ($000):** 96702 **Payroll Expense ($000):** 45840 **Personnel:** 954

MO

WINDSOR—Henry County

☐ **ROYAL OAKS HOSPITAL (264020)**, 307 North Main, Zip 65360–1449; tel. 660/647–2182 **A**1 3 5 10 **F**88 89 90 91 92 93 94 95 119
Primary Contact: Jon L. Bair, Administrator
Web address: www.royal–oaks–hospital.org
Control: Other not–for–profit (including NFP Corporation) **Service:** Psychiatric

Staffed Beds: 41 **Admissions:** 1384 **Census:** 31 **Outpatient Visits:** 1783 **Births:** 0 **Total Expense ($000):** 11225 **Payroll Expense ($000):** 6397 **Personnel:** 170

MONTANA

ANACONDA—Deer Lodge County

★ **COMMUNITY HOSPITAL OF ANACONDA (271335)**, 401 West Pennsylvania Street, Zip 59711–1931; tel. 406/563–8500, (Total facility includes 62 beds in nursing home–type unit) **A**9 10 18 **F**1 3 6 8 11 13 15 18 25 26 27 31 32 38 42 51 55 57 61 62 68 73 74 75 77 79 82 86 96 100 107 117 119 122 132 133 135 **P**6 **S** Providence Health & Services
Primary Contact: Steve McNeece, Chief Executive Officer
CFO: Laura Austin, Chief Financial Officer
CIO: Laura Austin, Chief Financial Officer
CHR: Meg Hickey–Boynton, Director Human Resources and Marketing
Control: Other not–for–profit (including NFP Corporation) **Service:** General Medical and Surgical

Staffed Beds: 87 **Admissions:** 1062 **Census:** 70 **Outpatient Visits:** 22285 **Births:** 31 **Total Expense ($000):** 17195 **Payroll Expense ($000):** 7751 **Personnel:** 195

BAKER—Fallon County

FALLON MEDICAL COMPLEX (271301), 202 South 4th Street West, Zip 59313–0820, Mailing Address: P.O. Box 820, Zip 59313–0820; tel. 406/778–3331, (Total facility includes 27 beds in nursing home–type unit) **A**9 10 18 **F**11 15 24 27 28 30 31 32 34 38 54 55 56 57 61 63 67 73 79 86 87 96 107 117 119 120 121 122 **P**6
Primary Contact: David Espeland, Chief Executive Officer
CFO: Selena Nelson, Chief Financial Officer
CMO: Darryl Espeland, D.O., Chief Medical Staff
Control: Other not–for–profit (including NFP Corporation) **Service:** General Medical and Surgical

Staffed Beds: 52 **Admissions:** 258 **Census:** 38 **Outpatient Visits:** 16053 **Births:** 0 **Total Expense ($000):** 6140 **Payroll Expense ($000):** 2077 **Personnel:** 85

BIG SANDY—Chouteau County

★ **BIG SANDY MEDICAL CENTER (271311)**, Mailing Address: P.O. Box 530, Zip 59520–0530; tel. 406/378–2188, (Total facility includes 22 beds in nursing home–type unit) **A**9 10 18 **F**30 31 38 61 62 86 117
Primary Contact: Harry Bold, Administrator
Web address: www.bsmc.org
Control: Other not–for–profit (including NFP Corporation) **Service:** General Medical and Surgical

Staffed Beds: 30 **Admissions:** 111 **Census:** 19 **Outpatient Visits:** 6347 **Births:** 0 **Total Expense ($000):** 2499 **Payroll Expense ($000):** 1340 **Personnel:** 34

BIG TIMBER—Sweet Grass County

★ **PIONEER MEDICAL CENTER (271313)**, 301 West Seventh Avenue, Zip 59011–1228, Mailing Address: P.O. Box 1228, Zip 59011–1228; tel. 406/932–4603, (Total facility includes 35 beds in nursing home–type unit) **A**9 10 18 **F**2 7 10 24 38 42 46 55 57 62 65 67 75 79 86 87 92 117 119 120 121 122 **P**3 6
Primary Contact: Bren Lowe, Chief Executive Officer
CFO: Kyle Gee, Chief Financial Officer
CMO: Wallace C. Walker, M.D., Chief of Staff
CHR: Miki Gregorich, Director Human Resources
Web address: www.billingsclinic.com/body.cfm?id=152
Control: County–Government, nonfederal **Service:** General Medical and Surgical

Staffed Beds: 60 **Admissions:** 220 **Census:** 49 **Outpatient Visits:** 8022 **Births:** 0 **Personnel:** 100

BILLINGS—Yellowstone County

★ **BILLINGS CLINIC (270004)**, 2800 10th Avenue North, Zip 59101, Mailing Address: P.O. Box 37000, Zip 59107–7000; tel. 406/657–4000, (Total facility includes 125 beds in nursing home–type unit) **A**1 2 3 5 9 10 **F**3 7 9 10 11 13 15 17 18 20 22 24 25 26 27 28 30 31 32 33 34 36 38 40 41 42 43 44 48 49 50 51 53 54 55 56 57 58 59 60 62 63 64 66 68 69 70 72 73 74 75 76 77 79 80 81 82 86 87 88 89 90 91 92 93 94 95 96 97 102 103 106 107 113 117 118 119 120 121 123 124 132 133 135 136 137 **P**6
Primary Contact: Nicholas Wolter, M.D., Chief Executive Officer
COO: Jon D. Ness, Chief Operating Officer
CFO: Robert E. Wilson, Chief Financial Officer
CMO: Mark C. Rumans, M.D., Physician in Chief
CIO: Chris E. Stevens, Chief Information Officer
CHR: Kellee J. Fisk, Vice President People Resources
Web address: www.billingsclinic.com
Control: Other not–for–profit (including NFP Corporation) **Service:** General Medical and Surgical

Staffed Beds: 344 **Admissions:** 14300 **Census:** 289 **Outpatient Visits:** 890859 **Births:** 1294 **Total Expense ($000):** 361167 **Payroll Expense ($000):** 175119 **Personnel:** 2843

★ △ **ST. VINCENT HEALTHCARE (270049)**, 1233 North 30th Street, Zip 59101–0165, Mailing Address: P.O. Box 35200, Zip 59107–5200; tel. 406/237–7000, (Total facility includes 21 beds in nursing home–type unit) **A**1 2 3 5 7 9 10 **F**3 8 11 12 13 15 17 18 20 22 24 25 26 28 30 31 32 33 34 35 36 37 38 40 41 43 44 45 47 49 50 51 54 55 56 57 59 60 62 66 68 69 70 71 72 73 74 75 76 77 79 80 81 82 83 84 85 86 87 89 90 91 93 94 96 97 102 106 107 117 118 119 120 121 123 124 132 133 135 136 **P**6 **S** Sisters of Charity of Leavenworth Health System
Primary Contact: James T. Paquette, President and Chief Executive Officer
COO: Jack E. Bell, Executive Vice President and Chief Operating Officer
CFO: Steve Ballock, Chief Financial Officer
CIO: Jay McKiernan, Director Information Systems
CHR: Harold Anderson, Vice President Human Resources
Web address: www.svh–mt.org
Control: Church–operated, Nongovernment, not–for profit **Service:** General Medical and Surgical

Staffed Beds: 234 **Admissions:** 13943 **Census:** 182 **Outpatient Visits:** 438938 **Births:** 1296 **Total Expense ($000):** 250084 **Payroll Expense ($000):** 107529 **Personnel:** 1929

BOZEMAN—Gallatin County

★ **BOZEMAN DEACONESS HOSPITAL (270057)**, 915 Highland Boulevard, Zip 59715–6902; tel. 406/585–5000, (Nonreporting) **A**9 10 20
Primary Contact: John A. Nordwick, President and Chief Executive Officer
Web address: www.bozemandeaconess.org
Control: Other not–for–profit (including NFP Corporation) **Service:** General Medical and Surgical

Staffed Beds: 70

BUTTE—Silver Bow County

★ **ST. JAMES HEALTHCARE (270017)**, 400 South Clark Street, Zip 59702–3300, Mailing Address: P.O. Box 3300, Zip 59702–3300; tel. 406/723–2500 **A**1 9 10 19 20 **F**3 11 13 18 20 24 25 26 31 32 33 35 38 43 44 45 47 48 49 50 51 52 55 56 60 62 68 70 72 73 74 75 76 77 79 80 82 84 86 92 96 97 100 102 105 106 107 109 111 117 119 120 134 135 **P**8 **S** Sisters of Charity of Leavenworth Health System
Primary Contact: James Kiser, II, President and Chief Executive Officer
CFO: Bruce Whitfield, Chief Financial Officer
CMO: Keith Popovich, M.D., Medical Staff President
CHR: Patrick Dudley, Director
Web address: www.stjameshealthcare.org
Control: Other not–for–profit (including NFP Corporation) **Service:** General Medical and Surgical

Staffed Beds: 65 **Admissions:** 4893 **Census:** 50 **Outpatient Visits:** 56534 **Births:** 491 **Total Expense ($000):** 61633 **Payroll Expense ($000):** 24245 **Personnel:** 475

MT

Hospital, Medicare Provider Number, Address, Telephone, Approval, Facility, and Physician Codes, Health Care System
★ American Hospital Association (AHA) membership
□ The Joint Commission accreditation
○ American Osteopathic Association (AOA) accreditation
△ Commission on Accreditation of Rehabilitation Facilities (CARF) accreditation

CHESTER—Liberty County

★ **LIBERTY COUNTY HOSPITAL AND NURSING HOME (271334)**, 315 West Madison Avenue, Zip 59522, Mailing Address: P.O. Box 705, Zip 59522–0705; tel. 406/759–5181, (Total facility includes 40 beds in nursing home–type unit) **A**9 10 18 **F**2 3 10 11 15 25 28 33 34 38 40 46 50 54 55 57 62 73 79 81 82 84 86 87 96 107 117 118 119 122
Primary Contact: Ronald M. Gleason, Chief Executive Officer
CFO: Shari Meissner, Chief Financial Officer
CMO: Anna Earl, M.D., Chief of Staff
CIO: Mark Burnham, System Analyst
CHR: Jane Allen, Director Human Resources and Payroll
Web address: www.lchnh.org
Control: Other not–for–profit (including NFP Corporation) **Service:** General Medical and Surgical

Staffed Beds: 51 **Admissions:** 168 **Census:** 12 **Outpatient Visits:** 6169 **Births:** 0 **Total Expense ($000):** 6204 **Payroll Expense ($000):** 3145 **Personnel:** 88

CHOTEAU—Teton County

★ **TETON MEDICAL CENTER (271307)**, 915 Fourth Street N.W., Zip 59422–9123; tel. 406/466–5763, (Total facility includes 34 beds in nursing home–type unit) **A**9 10 18 **F**2 15 30 31 32 33 38 42 52 53 54 55 56 57 61 62 66 82 86 96 117 119 120 122 132 135
Primary Contact: H. Ray Gibbons, FACHE, Administrator
Web address: www.tetonmedicalcenter.net
Control: Hospital district or authority, Government, nonfederal **Service:** General Medical and Surgical

Staffed Beds: 46 **Admissions:** 342 **Census:** 29 **Outpatient Visits:** 6971 **Births:** 0 **Total Expense ($000):** 4866 **Payroll Expense ($000):** 3129 **Personnel:** 75

CIRCLE—McCone County

★ **MCCONE COUNTY HEALTH CENTER (271305)**, Mailing Address: P.O. Box 48, Zip 59215–0048; tel. 406/485–3381, (Total facility includes 30 beds in nursing home–type unit) **A**9 10 18 **F**2 11 38 63 65 117 122 124 132 135
Primary Contact: Nancy Hansen, Administrator
Control: Other not–for–profit (including NFP Corporation) **Service:** General Medical and Surgical

Staffed Beds: 38 **Admissions:** 116 **Census:** 24 **Outpatient Visits:** 2879 **Births:** 0 **Total Expense ($000):** 2669 **Payroll Expense ($000):** 1170 **Personnel:** 38

COLUMBUS—Stillwater County

MT

STILLWATER COMMUNITY HOSPITAL (271330), 44 West Fourth Avenue North, Zip 59019–7126, Mailing Address: P.O. Box 959, Zip 59019–0959; tel. 406/322–5316 **A**9 10 18 **F**10 15 24 25 28 33 38 46 54 57 61 63 73 86 117 119 122 134 **P**1 3
Primary Contact: Tim Russell, Administrator
Control: Other not–for–profit (including NFP Corporation) **Service:** General Medical and Surgical

Staffed Beds: 23 **Admissions:** 241 **Census:** 9 **Outpatient Visits:** 8055 **Births:** 0 **Total Expense ($000):** 4072 **Payroll Expense ($000):** 1750 **Personnel:** 51

CONRAD—Pondera County

PONDERA MEDICAL CENTER (271324), 805 Sunset Boulevard, Zip 59425–1717, Mailing Address: P.O. Box 758, Zip 59425–0757; tel. 406/271–3211, (Total facility includes 59 beds in nursing home–type unit) **A**9 10 18 **F**1 2 3 6 7 11 13 15 24 25 31 32 33 38 52 55 57 61 63 74 75 79 82 86 87 92 96 97 102 107 117 119 122 133 135 **P**6
Primary Contact: Richard L. Palagi, Interim Chief Executive Officer
CFO: Mack N. Simpson, Chief Financial Officer
CMO: Jay Taylor, M.D., Chief of Staff
CIO: Jill Swanson, Supervisor Information Technology and Information Systems
CHR: Laura Elliot, Director Human Resources
Web address: www.ourpmc.com
Control: Other not–for–profit (including NFP Corporation) **Service:** General Medical and Surgical

Staffed Beds: 79 **Admissions:** 409 **Census:** 60 **Outpatient Visits:** 13201 **Births:** 45 **Total Expense ($000):** 10256 **Payroll Expense ($000):** 5679 **Personnel:** 154

CROW AGENCY—Big Horn County

★ **CROW/NORTHERN CHEYENNE HOSPITAL (271339)**, Mailing Address: P.O. Box 9, Zip 59022–0009; tel. 406/638–2626, (Nonreporting) **A**10 18 **S** U. S. Indian Health Service
Primary Contact: Charlene Johnson, Service Unit Director
COO: Curtis Brien, Administrative Officer
CFO: Dan Gunshews, Administrative Officer
CMO: David Mark, Chief Medical Officer
CIO: Melanie Falls Down, Site Manager
Control: Public Health Service, Government, federal **Service:** General Medical and Surgical

Staffed Beds: 24

CULBERTSON—Roosevelt County

★ **ROOSEVELT MEDICAL CENTER (271308)**, 818 Second Avenue East, Zip 59218, Mailing Address: P.O. Box 419, Zip 59218–0419; tel. 406/787–6401, (Total facility includes 34 beds in nursing home–type unit) **A**9 10 18 **F**2 3 7 11 28 33 38 50 54 57 62 67 78 82 84 86 87 117 119 122 124 132 **P**6
Primary Contact: Audrey Stromberg, Administrator
CFO: Carolyn Casterline, Financial Director
Web address: www.roosmem.org
Control: Other not–for–profit (including NFP Corporation) **Service:** General Medical and Surgical

Staffed Beds: 41 **Admissions:** 102 **Census:** 28 **Outpatient Visits:** 7867 **Births:** 0 **Total Expense ($000):** 3526 **Payroll Expense ($000):** 2100 **Personnel:** 63

CUT BANK—Glacier County

★ **NORTHERN ROCKIES MEDICAL CENTER (271337)**, 802 Second Street S.E., Zip 59427–3329; tel. 406/873–2251 **A**9 10 18 **F**8 11 25 30 32 38 50 55 56 57 62 73 74 75 79 84 86 87 96 97 107 119 122 135 **P**4 6
Primary Contact: Thane Bedwell, Chief Executive Officer
CFO: Dave Doran, Chief Financial Officer
CMO: Randy Webb, M.D., Chief Medical Staff
CHR: Kandie Lemieux, Administrative Assistant and Director Human Resources
Web address: www.nrmciac.org
Control: Other not–for–profit (including NFP Corporation) **Service:** General Medical and Surgical

Staffed Beds: 20 **Admissions:** 466 **Census:** 4 **Outpatient Visits:** 11885 **Births:** 43 **Total Expense ($000):** 6300 **Payroll Expense ($000):** 3070 **Personnel:** 77

DEER LODGE—Powell County

POWELL COUNTY MEDICAL CENTER (271314), 1101 Texas Avenue, Zip 59722–1828; tel. 406/846–2212, (Total facility includes 16 beds in nursing home–type unit) (Nonreporting) **A**9 10 18 **S** Cypress Health Systems
Primary Contact: Mike Walsh, Chief Executive Officer
CFO: Jaena Richards, Chief Financial Officer
CMO: Michelle Corbin, M.D., Chief of Staff
CIO: Chris Foster, Director Health Information Management
Web address: www.pcmh.org
Control: Other not–for–profit (including NFP Corporation) **Service:** General Medical and Surgical

Staffed Beds: 35

DILLON—Beaverhead County

★ **BARRETT HOSPITAL & HEALTHCARE (271318)**, 90 Highway 91 South, Zip 59725–3597; tel. 406/683–3000 **A**9 10 18 **F**3 13 15 22 25 28 30 31 32 33 35 36 38 41 42 43 44 45 50 55 56 57 61 62 66 68 73 74 75 77 79 80 81 82 86 87 96 97 102 106 107 117 119 120 121 122 124 135 136 137 **P**5 6 8 **S** Brim Healthcare, Inc.
Primary Contact: Steve Hannah, Chief Executive Officer
CFO: Dick Achter, Chief Financial Officer
CIO: Dick Achter, Chief Financial Officer
CHR: Judy Marshall, Human Resource Officer
Web address: www.barretthospital.org
Control: Hospital district or authority, Government, nonfederal **Service:** General Medical and Surgical

Staffed Beds: 20 **Admissions:** 736 **Census:** 7 **Outpatient Visits:** 18880 **Births:** 82 **Total Expense ($000):** 14100 **Payroll Expense ($000):** 5989 **Personnel:** 135

EKALAKA—Carter County

DAHL MEMORIAL HEALTHCARE ASSOCIATION (271302), (Formerly Dahl Memorial Medical Assistance Facility), 215 Sandy Street, Zip 59324, Mailing Address: P.O. Box 46, Zip 59324–0046; tel. 406/775–8730, (Total facility includes 23 beds in nursing home–type unit) **A**9 10 18 **F**2 7 30 31 32 38 55 57 67 84 117 119 120 122 132 135 **P**6
Primary Contact: Nadine Elmore, Chief Executive Officer
Control: Other not–for–profit (including NFP Corporation) **Service:** General Medical and Surgical

Staffed Beds: 31 **Admissions:** 35 **Census:** 19 **Outpatient Visits:** 1192 **Births:** 0 **Total Expense ($000):** 1730 **Payroll Expense ($000):** 801 **Personnel:** 36

ENNIS—Madison County

MADISON VALLEY HOSPITAL (271329), 217 North Main Street, Zip 59729–0397, Mailing Address: P.O. Box 397, Zip 59729–0397; tel. 406/682–4222 **A**9 10 18 **F**38 55 57 87 96 119 122 124 **P**6
Primary Contact: Pete Brekhus, Chief Executive Officer
CMO: Jeff Bern, M.D., Chief Medical Officer
Web address: www.mvhospital–clinic.com
Control: Hospital district or authority, Government, nonfederal **Service:** General Medical and Surgical

Staffed Beds: 8 **Admissions:** 109 **Census:** 2 **Outpatient Visits:** 14593 **Births:** 0 **Total Expense ($000):** 3670 **Payroll Expense ($000):** 1522 **Personnel:** 38

FORSYTH—Rosebud County

★ **ROSEBUD HEALTH CARE CENTER (271327)**, 383 North 17th Avenue, Zip 59327–0268, Mailing Address: P.O. Box 268, Zip 59327–0268; tel. 406/346–2161, (Total facility includes 41 beds in nursing home–type unit) **A**9 10 18 **F**15 17 31 38 55 56 86 96 117 119 120 122 132 134 137 **P**5
Primary Contact: James E. Ferguson, Chief Executive Officer
CFO: Ryan Tooke, Manager Business Office
CMO: William Anderson, M.D., Chief of Staff
CHR: Karla Allies, Director Human Resources
Web address: www.billingsclinic.com
Control: Other not–for–profit (including NFP Corporation) **Service:** General Medical and Surgical

Staffed Beds: 66 **Admissions:** 493 **Census:** 44 **Outpatient Visits:** 1635 **Births:** 0

FORT BENTON—Chouteau County

★ **MISSOURI RIVER MEDICAL CENTER (271304)**, 1501 St. Charles Street, Zip 59442–0249, Mailing Address: P.O. Box 249, Zip 59442–0249; tel. 406/622–3331, (Total facility includes 41 beds in nursing home–type unit) **A**9 10 18 **F**2 3 10 15 38 42 44 55 57 61 62 65 75 86 117 119 122 124 132 135 **P**5
Primary Contact: Jay Pottenger, Administrator
CFO: Lynn Asbeck, Manager Business Office
CHR: Carolyn Johnsrud, Manager Human Resources
Web address: www.mrmcfb.org
Control: Hospital district or authority, Government, nonfederal **Service:** Long–Term Acute Care hospital

Staffed Beds: 52 **Admissions:** 210 **Census:** 36 **Outpatient Visits:** 6390 **Births:** 0 **Total Expense ($000):** 4812 **Payroll Expense ($000):** 2802 **Personnel:** 79

FORT HARRISON—Lewis and Clark County

★ **VETERANS AFFAIRS MONTANA HEALTH CARE SYSTEM**, 1892 Williams Street, Zip 59636; tel. 406/442–6410, (Total facility includes 30 beds in nursing home–type unit) **A**1 **F**1 3 4 5 11 17 18 20 25 26 27 29 30 31 32 33 36 37 38 41 42 43 44 46 50 51 53 54 55 56 57 60 62 63 64 68 72 73 75 76 77 79 80 81 82 86 87 88 90 92 93 94 96 97 100 102 107 117 118 119 121 124 132 133 135 136 137 **P**6 **S** Department of Veterans Affairs
Primary Contact: Joseph Underkofler, Director
CFO: Brian Gustafson, Chief Financial Officer
CMO: Faust M. Alvarez, M.D., Chief of Staff
CIO: Paul Gauthier, Chief Information Resources Management
CHR: Aggie Hamilton, Chief Human Resources
Web address: www.va.gov/sta/guide/home.asp
Control: Veterans Affairs, Government, federal **Service:** General Medical and Surgical

Staffed Beds: 80 **Admissions:** 2214 **Census:** 28 **Outpatient Visits:** 246130 **Births:** 0 **Total Expense ($000):** 130698 **Payroll Expense ($000):** 43205 **Personnel:** 685

GLASGOW—Valley County

★ **FRANCES MAHON DEACONESS HOSPITAL (271316)**, 621 Third Street South, Zip 59230–2699; tel. 406/228–3500 **A**1 9 10 18 **F**1 3 4 7 11 13 15 16 17 24 25 26 27 30 31 32 33 38 40 43 52 54 55 56 57 60 62 65 68 70 71 73 74 76 77 78 79 81 82 83 84 85 86 88 90 92 95 96 97 100 102 106 107 117 118 119 122 124 134 135 **P**6 7
Primary Contact: Randall G. Holom, Chief Executive Officer
COO: Ellen Guttenberg, Chief Operating Officer
CFO: Del Gienger, Director Financial Services
CMO: Martin Kurland, M.D., Chief of Staff
CHR: Shelly Van Buren, Director Human Resources
Web address: www.fmdh.org
Control: Other not–for–profit (including NFP Corporation) **Service:** General Medical and Surgical

Staffed Beds: 25 **Admissions:** 766 **Census:** 6 **Outpatient Visits:** 35431 **Births:** 187 **Total Expense ($000):** 15650 **Payroll Expense ($000):** 7130 **Personnel:** 158

GLENDIVE—Dawson County

★ **GLENDIVE MEDICAL CENTER (271332)**, 202 Prospect Drive, Zip 59330–1999; tel. 406/345–3306, (Total facility includes 75 beds in nursing home–type unit) **A**9 10 18 **F**3 10 11 13 15 24 25 26 27 30 31 33 36 38 40 42 43 54 55 57 60 61 62 65 67 68 73 74 75 76 77 79 82 84 86 88 92 96 97 100 102 107 117 119 120 121 122 132 133 135 136 137 **P**6 7 8
Primary Contact: Scott Duke, Chief Executive Officer
CFO: Barbara Markham, Chief Financial Officer
CIO: Mike Janeway, M.D., Director Information Systems
CHR: Sandra McGovern, Director Human Resources
Web address: www.gmc.org
Control: Other not–for–profit (including NFP Corporation) **Service:** General Medical and Surgical

Staffed Beds: 100 **Admissions:** 1126 **Census:** 76 **Outpatient Visits:** 33046 **Births:** 100 **Total Expense ($000):** 20706 **Payroll Expense ($000):** 9691 **Personnel:** 255

GREAT FALLS—Cascade County

★ △ **BENEFIS HEALTHCARE SYSTEM (270012)**, 1101 26th Street South, Zip 59405–5104; tel. 406/455–5000, (Includes BENEFIS HEALTH CARE–EAST CAMPUS, 1101 26th Street, Zip 59405; BENEFIS HEALTH CARE–WEST CAMPUS, 500 15th Avenue South, Zip 59405), (Total facility includes 146 beds in nursing home–type unit) **A**1 2 7 9 10 20 **F**3 4 5 6 8 11 12 13 15 17 18 20 22 24 25 26 27 30 31 32 33 35 36 38 40 42 43 44 45 46 48 49 50 53 54 55 56 57 58 59 60 61 62 63 68 69 70 71 72 73 74 75 76 77 78 79 80 81 82 83 84 85 86 87 88 90 91 92 93 94 95 96 97 99 100 102 103 107 108 109 111 112 114 117 118 119 120 121 123 124 125 130 132 133 135 136 **P**4 5 6 8
Primary Contact: John H. Goodnow, Chief Executive Officer
COO: Laura Goldhahn, Senior Vice President
CFO: Wayne Dunn, Vice President Finance
CMO: Paul Dolan, M.D., Chief Medical Affairs Officer
CIO: Wayne Thompson, Manager Information Systems
CHR: Terry Olinger, Chief Human Resources Officer
Web address: www.benefis.org
Control: Other not–for–profit (including NFP Corporation) **Service:** General Medical and Surgical

Staffed Beds: 465 **Admissions:** 13528 **Census:** 316 **Outpatient Visits:** 124381 **Births:** 1406 **Total Expense ($000):** 192216 **Payroll Expense ($000):** 78986 **Personnel:** 1637

CENTRAL MONTANA HOSPITAL (270086), (Formerly Central Montana Surgical Hospital), 1411 9th Street South, Zip 59405; tel. 406/216–8000, (Nonreporting) **A**9 10 **S** Essentia Health
Primary Contact: Jane Drolet, Administrator
CFO: Brian Chandler, Chief Financial Officer
CMO: Tamim Khaliqi, M.D., Medical Director
Control: Corporation, Investor–owned, for–profit **Service:** Surgical

Staffed Beds: 20

MT

Hospital, Medicare Provider Number, Address, Telephone, Approval, Facility, and Physician Codes, Health Care System

★ American Hospital Association (AHA) membership
□ The Joint Commission accreditation
○ American Osteopathic Association (AOA) accreditation
△ Commission on Accreditation of Rehabilitation Facilities (CARF) accreditation

HAMILTON—Ravalli County

★ **MARCUS DALY MEMORIAL HOSPITAL (271340)**, 1200 Westwood Drive, Zip 59840–2395; tel. 406/363–2211 **A**9 10 18 **F**7 8 11 13 15 24 26 30 31 32 33 38 40 42 44 46 55 56 57 61 62 68 73 74 75 77 79 80 81 82 84 86 87 92 96 99 100 103 107 117 119 120 121 122 133 134 135 136 137
Primary Contact: John M. Bartos, Chief Executive Officer
CFO: Donja Erdman, Chief Financial Officer
CMO: Mark Jergens, M.D., Chief Medical Officer
CIO: Pamela Chaplin, Director Data Processing
CHR: Debbie Morris, Director Human Resources
Web address: www.mdmh.org
Control: Other not–for–profit (including NFP Corporation) **Service:** General Medical and Surgical

Staffed Beds: 31 **Admissions:** 2017 **Census:** 15 **Outpatient Visits:** 27238 **Births:** 120 **Total Expense ($000):** 26790 **Payroll Expense ($000):** 15021 **Personnel:** 360

HARDIN—Big Horn County

★ **BIG HORN COUNTY MEMORIAL HOSPITAL (271338)**, 17 North Miles Avenue, Zip 59034–0430; tel. 406/665–2310, (Total facility includes 36 beds in nursing home–type unit) **A**9 10 18 **F**10 11 13 15 24 31 32 38 50 55 57 62 63 66 73 74 75 79 80 81 82 85 86 96 102 107 115 117 119 121 122 132 135
Primary Contact: Gary W. Robertson, Chief Executive Officer
CFO: Roxie Cain, Chief Financial Officer
Web address: www.bighornhospital.org
Control: Other not–for–profit (including NFP Corporation) **Service:** General Medical and Surgical

Staffed Beds: 61 **Admissions:** 325 **Census:** 40 **Outpatient Visits:** 5928 **Births:** 29 **Total Expense ($000):** 7893 **Payroll Expense ($000):** 3852 **Personnel:** 130

HARLEM—Blaine County

★ **FORT BELKNAP U. S. PUBLIC HEALTH SERVICE INDIAN HOSPITAL (271315)**, Rural Route 1, Box 67, Zip 59526; tel. 406/353–3100, (Nonreporting) **A**10 18 **S** U. S. Indian Health Service
Primary Contact: Daryl A. Brockie, Director
CMO: Robert B. Andrews, M.D., Chief Medical Officer
CIO: Mikki Grant, Chief Information Officer
CHR: Mary H. Mount, Administrative Officer
Web address: www.ihs.gov
Control: PHS, Indian Service, Government, federal **Service:** General Medical and Surgical

Staffed Beds: 6

MT

HARLOWTON—Wheatland County

★ **WHEATLAND MEMORIAL HEALTHCARE (271321)**, 530 Third Street North West, Zip 59036, Mailing Address: P.O. Box 287, Zip 59036–0287; tel. 406/632–4351 **A**9 10 18 **F**15 26 28 31 32 33 38 54 55 56 57 60 62 63 75 77 80 82 86 87 96 107 119 121 122 132 135 136 **P**6
Primary Contact: Scot Mitchell, FACHE, Chief Executive Officer
CFO: Jerry Wright, Chief Financial Officer
CHR: Peggy Hiner, Executive Secretary and Manager Human Resources
Web address: www.wheatlandmemorial.org
Control: Other not–for–profit (including NFP Corporation) **Service:** General Medical and Surgical

Staffed Beds: 25 **Admissions:** 104 **Census:** 23 **Outpatient Visits:** 4943 **Births:** 0 **Total Expense ($000):** 4466 **Payroll Expense ($000):** 2530 **Personnel:** 60

HAVRE—Hill County

★ **NORTHERN MONTANA HOSPITAL (270032)**, 30 13th Street, Zip 59501–5222, Mailing Address: P.O. Box 1231, Zip 59501–1231; tel. 406/265–2211, (Total facility includes 114 beds in nursing home–type unit) **A**9 10 20 **F**10 11 13 15 24 27 30 31 32 33 36 38 42 43 44 50 54 55 56 57 59 61 62 66 68 73 74 75 76 77 79 80 84 86 87 88 89 91 92 93 94 95 96 97 99 100 102 106 107 117 118 119 121 122 124 135 137 **P**6
Primary Contact: David Henry, President and Chief Executive Officer
CFO: Kim Lucke, Director Finance
CHR: Joe Schmier, Vice President Human Resources
Web address: www.nmhcare.org
Control: Other not–for–profit (including NFP Corporation) **Service:** General Medical and Surgical

Staffed Beds: 141 **Admissions:** 2926 **Census:** 140 **Outpatient Visits:** 77852 **Births:** 388 **Total Expense ($000):** 47197 **Payroll Expense ($000):** 23895 **Personnel:** 534

HELENA—Lewis and Clark County

★ **SHODAIR CHILDREN'S HOSPITAL (274004)**, 2755 Colonial Drive, Zip 59601–4926, Mailing Address: P.O. Box 5539, Zip 59604–5539; tel. 406/444–7500 **A**9 10 **F**31 32 88 89 91 92 94 114 119 **P**6
Primary Contact: John P. Casey, Administrator
COO: John P. Casey, Administrator
CFO: Ron Wiens, Chief Financial Officer
CMO: James Reynolds, M.D., President Medical Staff
CIO: Judy Jackson, Director Health Information Management and Privacy Officer
CHR: Gary Willis, Director Human Resources
Web address: www.shodairhospital.org
Control: Other not–for–profit (including NFP Corporation) **Service:** Children's hospital psychiatric

Staffed Beds: 88 **Admissions:** 552 **Census:** 54 **Outpatient Visits:** 4169 **Births:** 0 **Total Expense ($000):** 14330 **Payroll Expense ($000):** 8013 **Personnel:** 187

⊠ **ST. PETER'S HOSPITAL (270003)**, 2475 Broadway, Zip 59601–4999; tel. 406/442–2480 **A**1 2 9 10 20 **F**3 7 8 13 15 18 20 24 25 26 27 30 31 32 33 34 36 38 40 42 43 44 48 50 51 54 55 56 57 59 61 62 68 72 73 74 75 76 77 79 80 81 82 84 86 87 90 92 96 97 99 100 102 103 105 106 107 111 117 118 119 120 121 122 132 135 136 137 **P**6
Primary Contact: John H. Solheim, President and Chief Executive Officer
CFO: John Green, Vice President Finance
CMO: James Haley, M.D., Vice President Medical Affairs
CHR: Thomas Gregg, Vice President Human Resources
Web address: www.stpetes.org
Control: Other not–for–profit (including NFP Corporation) **Service:** General Medical and Surgical

Staffed Beds: 99 **Admissions:** 5164 **Census:** 50 **Outpatient Visits:** 24658 **Births:** 781 **Total Expense ($000):** 96318 **Payroll Expense ($000):** 40044 **Personnel:** 757

JORDAN—Garfield County

GARFIELD COUNTY HEALTH CENTER (271310), 332 Leavitt Avenue, Zip 59337; tel. 406/557–2500, (Total facility includes 24 beds in nursing home–type unit) (Nonreporting) **A**9 10 18
Primary Contact: Wanda Hageman, Administrator
COO: Wanda Hageman, Administrator
CFO: Sandi Williams, Manager Business Officer
CMO: Daniel Muniak, Chief Medical Officer
CIO: Sandi Williams, Manager Business Officer
Control: County–Government, nonfederal **Service:** General Medical and Surgical

Staffed Beds: 28

KALISPELL—Flathead County

★ **HEALTHCENTER NORTHWEST (270087)**, 320 Sunnyview Lane, Zip 59901; tel. 406/751–7500 **A**9 10 **F**3 8 15 27 30 37 42 43 62 66 69 72 76 77 79 80 82 90 96 99 100 102 103 107 112 **P**2
Primary Contact: Velinda Stevens, President and Chief Executive Officer
COO: Tate J. Kreitinger, Chief Operating Officer and Chief Financial Officer
CFO: Tate J. Kreitinger, Chief Operating Officer and Chief Financial Officer
CHR: Susan Stevens, Director Human Resources
Web address: www.krmc.org
Control: Corporation, Investor–owned, for–profit **Service:** General Medical and Surgical

Staffed Beds: 12 **Admissions:** 955 **Census:** 6 **Outpatient Visits:** 47107 **Births:** 0 **Total Expense ($000):** 24085 **Payroll Expense ($000):** 4269 **Personnel:** 112

⊠ △ **KALISPELL REGIONAL MEDICAL CENTER (270051)**, 310 Sunnyview Lane, Zip 59901–3199; tel. 406/752–5111, (Includes PATHWAYS TREATMENT CENTER, 200 Heritage Way, Zip 59901; tel. 406/756–3950) **A**1 7 9 10 19 20 **F**3 4 5 8 13 14 15 18 20 22 24 25 26 27 30 31 32 33 34 37 38 40 42 46 49 50 54 55 56 57 61 62 68 70 71 72 73 74 76 77 78 79 80 82 85 86 88 89 90 91 92 93 94 95 96 97 98 100 102 103 107 108 109 111 112 119 121 124 133 135 137
Primary Contact: Velinda Stevens, President
COO: Ted W. Hirsch, Chief Executive Officer
CFO: Charles T. Pearce, Chief Financial and Information Officer
CHR: Pat Wilson, Director Human Resources
Web address: www.krmc.org
Control: Other not–for–profit (including NFP Corporation) **Service:** General Medical and Surgical

Staffed Beds: 163 **Admissions:** 7952 **Census:** 85 **Outpatient Visits:** 160267 **Births:** 880 **Total Expense ($000):** 113373 **Payroll Expense ($000):** 43210 **Personnel:** 1130

LEWISTOWN—Fergus County

★ **CENTRAL MONTANA MEDICAL CENTER (270011)**, 408 Wendell Avenue, Zip 59457–2261; tel. 406/538–7711, (Total facility includes 85 beds in nursing home–type unit) **A**9 10 **F**2 3 7 11 13 15 24 25 26 27 30 31 32 33 38 42 43 46 50 52 54 55 56 57 61 62 63 68 73 74 75 76 77 79 80 81 82 86 90 92 95 96 97 100 106 107 112 117 118 119 120 121 122 124 132 135 137 **P**6 **S** QHR
Primary Contact: David M. Faulkner, Chief Executive Officer
COO: Dianne Scotten, Chief Clinical Officer
CFO: Alan Aldrich, Chief Financial Officer
Web address: www.cmmccares.com
Control: Other not–for–profit (including NFP Corporation) **Service:** General Medical and Surgical

Staffed Beds: 124 **Admissions:** 1447 **Census:** 75 **Outpatient Visits:** 38523 **Births:** 96 **Total Expense ($000):** 22491 **Payroll Expense ($000):** 10967 **Personnel:** 292

LIBBY—Lincoln County

★ **ST. JOHN'S LUTHERAN HOSPITAL (271320)**, 350 Louisiana Avenue, Zip 59923–2130; tel. 406/293–0100 **A**9 10 18 **F**3 11 13 15 17 24 25 26 27 33 38 42 43 44 54 55 57 61 62 66 68 73 74 75 77 79 80 81 82 84 86 87 92 96 100 102 107 117 118 119 120 121 122 124 133 135 136 137 **P**6
Primary Contact: William Patten, Administrator and Chief Executive Officer
CFO: Steve Chavez, Chief Financial Officer
CMO: Gregory Rice, M.D., Chief of Staff
CHR: Jeanie Gentry, Director Support Services
Web address: www.sjlh.com
Control: Other not–for–profit (including NFP Corporation) **Service:** General Medical and Surgical

Staffed Beds: 25 **Admissions:** 1010 **Census:** 10 **Outpatient Visits:** 30819 **Births:** 87 **Total Expense ($000):** 17189 **Payroll Expense ($000):** 8118 **Personnel:** 189

LIVINGSTON—Park County

★ **LIVINGSTON MEMORIAL HOSPITAL (271317)**, 504 South 13th Street, Zip 59047–3727; tel. 406/222–3541 **A**9 10 18 **F**8 13 15 17 24 25 27 30 31 32 33 38 42 43 50 61 62 64 66 68 75 76 77 79 80 81 82 86 96 97 100 102 107 112 118 120 122 **P**3
Primary Contact: Samuel G. Pleshar, Chief Executive Officer
CFO: William Vanderhoff, Director Finance
CMO: Michelle Donaldson, M.D., President Medical Staff
CIO: Sandra Marlowe, Director Community Development
CHR: Connie Dunn, Director Human Resources
Web address: www.livingstonhealthcare.org
Control: Other not–for–profit (including NFP Corporation) **Service:** General Medical and Surgical

Staffed Beds: 25 **Admissions:** 1231 **Census:** 11 **Outpatient Visits:** 31690 **Births:** 138 **Total Expense ($000):** 29123 **Payroll Expense ($000):** 13935 **Personnel:** 292

MALTA—Phillips County

★ **PHILLIPS COUNTY HOSPITAL (271312)**, 417 South Fourth East, Zip 59538, Mailing Address: P.O. Box 640, Zip 59538–0640; tel. 406/654–1100 **A**9 10 18 **F**3 25 26 27 28 30 31 32 33 38 46 54 57 58 61 62 72 76 77 86 87 107 117 122 136 **P**4
Primary Contact: Ward C. VanWichen, Chief Executive Officer
CFO: Stephanie Denham, Chief Financial Officer and Human Resources Officer
CMO: Ed Medina, M.D., Medical Director
CHR: Stephanie Denham, Chief Financial Officer and Human Resources Officer
Web address: www.phillipscountyhospital.com
Control: Other not–for–profit (including NFP Corporation) **Service:** General Medical and Surgical

Staffed Beds: 12 **Admissions:** 222 **Census:** 2 **Outpatient Visits:** 6029 **Births:** 0 **Total Expense ($000):** 3848 **Payroll Expense ($000):** 1366 **Personnel:** 66

MILES CITY—Custer County

★□ **HOLY ROSARY HEALTHCARE (270002)**, 2600 Wilson Street, Zip 59301–5094; tel. 406/233–2600, (Total facility includes 55 beds in nursing home–type unit) **A**1 9 10 20 **F**3 13 15 24 25 26 27 30 31 32 33 38 42 55 56 57 62 68 74 75 76 77 79 80 81 82 84 86 87 92 96 97 98 100 103 107 118 119 120 122 132 133 135 137 **P**6 **S** Sisters of Charity of Leavenworth Health System
Primary Contact: Greg A. Nielsen, Chief Executive Officer
CIO: Jana Anderson, Director Information Services
CHR: Cathy Rodenbaugh, Human Resource Director
Web address: www.holyrosaryhealthcare.org
Control: Church–operated, Nongovernment, not–for profit **Service:** General Medical and Surgical

Staffed Beds: 99 **Admissions:** 2241 **Census:** 82 **Outpatient Visits:** 42467 **Births:** 285 **Total Expense ($000):** 27853 **Payroll Expense ($000):** 13732 **Personnel:** 305

MISSOULA—Missoula County

★□ △ **COMMUNITY MEDICAL CENTER (270023)**, 2827 Fort Missoula Road, Zip 59804–7408; tel. 406/728–4100 **A**1 5 7 9 10 19 20 **F**3 13 15 17 24 25 26 27 30 33 34 38 39 40 43 44 45 46 49 50 55 56 57 63 68 70 71 72 73 74 75 76 77 79 80 83 84 85 86 96 97 101 102 103 107 119 121 124 132 133 134 135 136 137 **P**6
Primary Contact: Stephen G. Carlson, President and Chief Executive Officer
CFO: David Richhart, Vice President Fiscal Services
CMO: Thomas Randall, M.D., Vice President Medical Affairs
CIO: Leigh Thurston, Vice President Information Systems
CHR: Larry Fagerhaug, Vice President Organizational Development
Web address: www.communitymed.org
Control: Other not–for–profit (including NFP Corporation) **Service:** General Medical and Surgical

Staffed Beds: 146 **Admissions:** 6671 **Census:** 64 **Outpatient Visits:** 160821 **Births:** 1671 **Total Expense ($000):** 122048 **Payroll Expense ($000):** 50268 **Personnel:** 944

★□ **ST. PATRICK HOSPITAL (270014)**, 500 West Broadway, Zip 59802–4096, Mailing Address: P.O. Box 4587, Zip 59806–4587; tel. 406/543–7271 **A**1 2 5 9 10 19 **F**3 5 8 11 12 15 18 19 20 21 22 23 24 25 26 27 30 31 32 33 34 36 38 40 43 44 49 50 51 52 55 56 57 58 59 60 62 63 66 68 72 73 75 76 77 78 79 80 81 83 84 85 86 87 88 89 90 91 92 93 94 95 96 97 98 99 100 102 103 104 105 106 107 108 109 110 111 112 117 118 119 120 121 124 130 135 136 137 **P**1 6 7 **S** Providence Health & Services
Primary Contact: Jeff Fee, Chief Executive Officer
CFO: Bruce Whitfield, Vice President and Chief Financial Officer
CIO: Rita Spear, Director Information Services
CHR: Barbara Blanchard, Vice President Human Resources
Web address: www.saintpatrick.org
Control: Church–operated, Nongovernment, not–for profit **Service:** General Medical and Surgical

Staffed Beds: 185 **Admissions:** 8587 **Census:** 126 **Outpatient Visits:** 145438 **Births:** 0 **Total Expense ($000):** 176990 **Payroll Expense ($000):** 65419 **Personnel:** 1279

PHILIPSBURG—Granite County

GRANITE COUNTY MEDICAL CENTER (271303), 310 Sansome Street, Zip 59858–0729, Mailing Address: P.O. Box 729, Zip 59858–0729; tel. 406/859–3271, (Total facility includes 30 beds in nursing home–type unit) (Nonreporting) **A**9 10 18
Primary Contact: Amy Edwards Webb, Administrator
CFO: Susan Ossello, Chief Financial Officer
CMO: John Moore, M.D., Medical Director
Control: County–Government, nonfederal **Service:** General Medical and Surgical

Staffed Beds: 35

PLAINS—Sanders County

★ **CLARK FORK VALLEY HOSPITAL (271323)**, 10 Kruger Road, Zip 59859–0768, Mailing Address: P.O. Box 768, Zip 59859–0768; tel. 406/826–4800, (Total facility includes 28 beds in nursing home–type unit) **A**9 10 18 **F**3 13 15 38 40 41 42 44 45 50 55 56 57 58 61 62 63 68 73 74 79 84 86 96 102 107 117 119 122 **P**6
Primary Contact: Gregory S. Hanson, M.D., Chief Executive Officer
CFO: Carla Neiman, Chief Financial Officer
CIO: Carla Neiman, Chief Financial Officer
CHR: Barry Fowler, Director Human and System Resources
Web address: www.cfvh.org
Control: Other not–for–profit (including NFP Corporation) **Service:** General Medical and Surgical

Staffed Beds: 44 **Admissions:** 527 **Census:** 32 **Outpatient Visits:** 17186 **Births:** 50 **Total Expense ($000):** 14077 **Payroll Expense ($000):** 6380 **Personnel:** 160

MT

Hospital, Medicare Provider Number, Address, Telephone, Approval, Facility, and Physician Codes, Health Care System

★ American Hospital Association (AHA) membership
□ The Joint Commission accreditation
○ American Osteopathic Association (AOA) accreditation
△ Commission on Accreditation of Rehabilitation Facilities (CARF) accreditation

PLENTYWOOD—Sheridan County

SHERIDAN MEMORIAL HOSPITAL (271322), 440 West Laurel Avenue, Zip 59254–1596; tel. 406/765–1420, (Total facility includes 78 beds in nursing home–type unit) **A**9 10 18 **F**1 3 7 11 13 15 17 26 33 38 42 55 57 61 65 75 78 79 85 86 96 102 107 117 119 122 134 135 **P**5
Primary Contact: Wayne Nelson, Chief Executive Officer
Web address: www.sheridanhospital.org
Control: Other not–for–profit (including NFP Corporation) **Service:** General Medical and Surgical

Staffed Beds: 97 **Admissions:** 503 **Census:** 65 **Outpatient Visits:** 8947 **Births:** 21 **Total Expense ($000):** 5285 **Payroll Expense ($000):** 3888 **Personnel:** 136

POLSON—Lake County

ST. JOSEPH HOSPITAL (271343), 6 Thirteenth Avenue East, Zip 59860–5316, Mailing Address: P.O. Box 1010, Zip 59860–1010; tel. 406/883–5377 **A**1 9 10 18 **F**3 10 11 13 15 24 25 26 30 31 32 33 38 43 44 46 50 52 55 56 57 61 62 66 73 74 75 77 79 80 84 86 87 90 96 100 102 107 119 120 122 124 135 136 137 **P**5 6 **S** Providence Health & Services
Primary Contact: John W. Glueckert, President
CFO: Kirk Bodlovic, Vice President and Chief Financial Officer
CMO: R. Stephen Irwin, M.D., Chief of Staff
Web address: www.saintjoes.org
Control: Church–operated, Nongovernment, not–for profit **Service:** General Medical and Surgical

Staffed Beds: 22 **Admissions:** 626 **Census:** 5 **Outpatient Visits:** 76006 **Births:** 153 **Total Expense ($000):** 18986 **Payroll Expense ($000):** 8866 **Personnel:** 219

POPLAR—Roosevelt County

★ **POPLAR COMMUNITY HOSPITAL (271300)**, H and Court Avenue, Zip 59255, Mailing Address: P.O. Box 38, Zip 59255; tel. 406/768–3452 **A**9 10 18 **F**7 32 38 50 67 73 85 86 102 119 122 132 **P**6
Primary Contact: Margaret B. Norgaard, Chief Executive Officer
CHR: Annie Block, Director Human Resources
Web address: www.nemhs.net
Control: Other not–for–profit (including NFP Corporation) **Service:** General Medical and Surgical

Staffed Beds: 20 **Admissions:** 335 **Census:** 8 **Outpatient Visits:** 7473 **Births:** 4 **Total Expense ($000):** 4037 **Payroll Expense ($000):** 2193 **Personnel:** 69

RED LODGE—Carbon County

★ **BEARTOOTH HOSPITAL AND HEALTH CENTER (271326)**, 600 West 20th Street, Zip 59068, Mailing Address: P.O. Box 590, Zip 59068–0590; tel. 406/446–2345, (Total facility includes 30 beds in nursing home–type unit) **A**9 10 18 **F**11 15 24 27 30 33 38 42 43 44 50 52 54 55 56 57 58 61 63 66 68 75 79 80 81 82 86 87 96 99 107 117 119 120 122 124 132 135 137 **P**3 5
Primary Contact: Kelley Evans, Administrator
CFO: Kyle Gee, Chief Financial Officer
CMO: Billy Oley, M.D., Chief of Staff
CIO: Susan Scott, Director Medical Records
CHR: Katie Nordstrom, Director Human Resources
Web address: www.beartoothhospital.org
Control: Other not–for–profit (including NFP Corporation) **Service:** General Medical and Surgical

Staffed Beds: 52 **Admissions:** 312 **Census:** 28 **Outpatient Visits:** 21207 **Births:** 0 **Total Expense ($000):** 5986 **Payroll Expense ($000):** 3021 **Personnel:** 98

RONAN—Lake County

★ **ST. LUKE COMMUNITY HOSPITAL (271325)**, 107 Sixth Avenue S.W., Zip 59864–2634; tel. 406/676–4441, (Total facility includes 75 beds in nursing home–type unit) **A**9 10 18 **F**2 13 15 30 31 32 38 40 46 52 55 57 60 62 63 73 74 75 79 80 86 87 96 97 100 103 107 117 120 122 124 **P**6
Primary Contact: Shane H. Roberts, Chief Executive Officer
COO: Steve J. Todd, Chief Operating Officer
CFO: Paul Soukup, Chief Financial Officer
CMO: Paul D. Gochis, M.D., Chief of Staff
CHR: Theresa Jones, Manager Human Resources
Web address: www.stlukehealthnet.org
Control: Other not–for–profit (including NFP Corporation) **Service:** General Medical and Surgical

Staffed Beds: 104 **Admissions:** 1068 **Census:** 68 **Outpatient Visits:** 68920 **Births:** 169 **Total Expense ($000):** 22814 **Payroll Expense ($000):** 11364 **Personnel:** 262

ROUNDUP—Musselshell County

★ **ROUNDUP MEMORIAL HEALTHCARE (271346)**, 1202 Third Street West, Zip 59072–1816, Mailing Address: P.O. Box 40, Zip 59072–0040; tel. 406/323–2302, (Total facility includes 37 beds in nursing home–type unit) **A**9 10 18 **F**2 11 30 33 38 55 63 87 96 107 117 119 122 135 **P**6 **S** Brim Healthcare, Inc.
Primary Contact: Lee Rhodes, Chief Executive Officer
CFO: Gary Bostrom, Chief Financial Officer
CMO: Tony Ham, M.D., Chief Medical Officer
CHR: Rochelle Hatter, Chief Human Resources Officer
Control: Other not–for–profit (including NFP Corporation) **Service:** General Medical and Surgical

Staffed Beds: 48 **Admissions:** 303 **Census:** 27 **Outpatient Visits:** 8997 **Total Expense ($000):** 3805 **Payroll Expense ($000):** 2545 **Personnel:** 82

SAINT MARY—Glacier County

U. S. PUBLIC HEALTH SERVICE BLACKFEET COMMUNITY HOSPITAL (270074), Mailing Address: P.O. Box 760, Browning, Zip 59417–0760; tel. 406/338–6100, (Nonreporting) **A**1 5 10 **S** U. S. Indian Health Service
Primary Contact: James Kennedy, Chief Executive Officer
Web address: www.phs.ihs.gov
Control: PHS, Indian Service, Government, federal **Service:** General Medical and Surgical

Staffed Beds: 25

SCOBEY—Daniels County

DANIELS MEMORIAL HEALTHCARE CENTER (271342), 105 Fifth Avenue East, Zip 59263, Mailing Address: P.O. Box 400, Zip 59263–0400; tel. 406/487–2296, (Total facility includes 30 beds in nursing home–type unit) **A**9 10 18 **F**2 25 27 30 31 32 33 38 54 55 57 61 62 63 80 81 82 86 87 92 93 107 117 119 120 121 122 **P**6
Primary Contact: Steve Hubbard, Interim Chief Executive Officer
CMO: Darrel Stock, M.D., Medical Director
CHR: Edith Huda, Director Human Resources
Control: Hospital district or authority, Government, nonfederal **Service:** General Medical and Surgical

Staffed Beds: 54 **Admissions:** 124 **Census:** 30 **Outpatient Visits:** 4319 **Births:** 0 **Total Expense ($000):** 4298 **Payroll Expense ($000):** 2090

SHELBY—Toole County

★ **MARIAS MEDICAL CENTER (271328)**, 640 Park Drive, Zip 59474–1663, Mailing Address: P.O. Box 915, Zip 59474–0915; tel. 406/434–3200, (Total facility includes 63 beds in nursing home–type unit) **A**9 10 18 **F**7 10 11 13 14 15 17 31 38 42 50 54 55 56 57 61 62 63 68 73 74 75 76 79 81 96 97 100 107 115 117 119 121 122 132 135 137 **P**6
Primary Contact: Mark A. Cross, Chief Executive Officer
CMO: George A. Biancarelli, M.D., Chief of Staff
CIO: Jayce Yarn, Director Information Technology
CHR: Cindy Lamb, Director Human Resources
Web address: www.mmcmt.org
Control: County–Government, nonfederal **Service:** General Medical and Surgical

Staffed Beds: 88 **Admissions:** 582 **Census:** 38 **Outpatient Visits:** 51024 **Births:** 28 **Total Expense ($000):** 11812 **Payroll Expense ($000):** 4421 **Personnel:** 210

SHERIDAN—Madison County

★ **RUBY VALLEY HOSPITAL (271319)**, 220 East Crofoot Street, Zip 59749, Mailing Address: P.O. Box 336, Zip 59749–0336; tel. 406/842–5453 **A**9 10 12 13 18 **F**11 31 33 38 42 55 57 64 75 86 122 **P**5
Primary Contact: John H. Semingson, Chief Executive Officer
CFO: Dennis Holschbuch, Chief Financial Officer and Director Human Resources
CMO: Sara Googe, M.D., Medical Director
CHR: Dennis Holschbuch, Chief Financial Officer and Director Human Resources
Control: Hospital district or authority, Government, nonfederal **Service:** General Medical and Surgical

Staffed Beds: 10 **Admissions:** 240 **Census:** 2 **Outpatient Visits:** 4979 **Personnel:** 36

SIDNEY—Richland County

★ **SIDNEY HEALTH CENTER (271344)**, 216 14th Avenue S.W., Zip 59270–3586; tel. 406/488–2100, (Total facility includes 93 beds in nursing home–type unit) **A**9 10 18 **F**2 3 7 10 13 15 17 24 25 26 27 30 31 32 33 38 42 43 50 54 55 56 57 61 62 67 68 73 74 75 76 77 79 80 81 82 84 86 87 96 97 103 107 112 113 114 115 117 118 119 120 121 122 124 135 136 137 **P**5 6 7
Primary Contact: Richard Haraldson, Chief Executive Officer
CFO: Tina Montgomery, Chief Financial Officer
CIO: Brian Fay, Information Systems Director
Web address: www.sidneyhealth.org
Control: Other not–for–profit (including NFP Corporation) **Service:** General Medical and Surgical

Staffed Beds: 118 **Admissions:** 1226 **Census:** 106 **Outpatient Visits:** 41851 **Births:** 88 **Total Expense ($000):** 30738 **Payroll Expense ($000):** 13580 **Personnel:** 427

Many Facility Codes have changed. Please refer to the AHA Guide Code Chart.

SUPERIOR—Mineral County

★ **MINERAL COMMUNITY HOSPITAL (271331)**, 1208 6th Avenue East, Zip 59872–9603, Mailing Address: P.O. Box 66, Zip 59872–0066; tel. 406/822–4841 **A**9 10 18 **F**3 10 11 15 25 26 28 30 31 32 33 38 50 54 55 56 57 62 63 69 72 73 75 79 81 82 86 87 96 99 107 115 118 119 121 122 132 133 137 **P**6 **S** Brim Healthcare, Inc.
Primary Contact: Barry Kenfield, Interim Chief Executive Officer
CFO: Cliff Case, Chief Financial Officer
CMO: Patrick Tufts, M.D., Medical Director
Control: Other not–for–profit (including NFP Corporation) **Service:** General Medical and Surgical

Staffed Beds: 25 **Admissions:** 208 **Census:** 17 **Outpatient Visits:** 7057 **Births:** 0 **Total Expense ($000):** 4909 **Payroll Expense ($000):** 2270 **Personnel:** 76

TERRY—Prairie County

★ **PRAIRIE COMMUNITY HEALTH CENTER (271309)**, 312 South Adams Avenue, Zip 59349–0156, Mailing Address: P.O. Box 156, Zip 59349–0156; tel. 406/635–5511 **A**9 10 18 **F**1 2 3 11 28 30 31 32 38 55 57 63 65 67 73 87 117 119 122 132 135 136 **P**6
Primary Contact: Reed Reyman, Administrator
CFO: Reed Reyman, Administrator
CMO: Joseph M. Leal, M.D., Medical Director
CIO: Laurie Chandler, Chairman
Control: Hospital district or authority, Government, nonfederal **Service:** General Medical and Surgical

Staffed Beds: 21 **Admissions:** 125 **Census:** 19 **Outpatient Visits:** 4939 **Births:** 0 **Total Expense ($000):** 1584 **Payroll Expense ($000):** 791 **Personnel:** 37

TOWNSEND—Broadwater County

BROADWATER HEALTH CENTER (271333), 110 North Oak Street, Zip 59644–2306; tel. 406/266–3186 **A**9 10 18 **F**3 7 11 38 55 56 57 62 65 86 117 119 122 132 **P**7
Primary Contact: Sam J. Allen, Administrator
CFO: Lorrie Vennes, Chief Financial Officer
Web address: www.broadwaterhealthcenter.com
Control: Other not–for–profit (including NFP Corporation) **Service:** General Medical and Surgical

Staffed Beds: 44 **Admissions:** 100 **Census:** 2 **Births:** 0

WARM SPRINGS—Deer Lodge County

MONTANA STATE HOSPITAL (274086), 300 Garnet Way, Zip 59756–0300, Mailing Address: P.O. Box 300, Zip 59756–0300; tel. 406/693–7000 **A**10 **F**25 30 36 37 50 57 64 66 72 73 75 81 87 88 90 93 119 121 124 **P**6
Primary Contact: Edward Amberg, Administrator
CFO: Tracey Sweeney, Director Business and Support Services
CMO: Thomas Gray, M.D., Medical Director
CIO: Billie Holmlund, Director Information Services
CHR: Todd Thun, Director Human Resources
Web address: www.msh.mt.gov
Control: State–Government, nonfederal **Service:** Psychiatric

Staffed Beds: 214 **Admissions:** 699 **Census:** 198 **Outpatient Visits:** 0 **Births:** 0 **Total Expense ($000):** 27226 **Payroll Expense ($000):** 15089 **Personnel:** 401

WHITE SULPHUR SPRINGS—Meagher County

★ **MOUNTAINVIEW MEDICAL CENTER (271306)**, 16 West Main Street, Zip 59645, Mailing Address: P.O. Box Q, Zip 59645; tel. 406/547–3321 **A**9 10 18 **F**38 57 62 65 82 85 86 87 96 117 122 137 **P**6
Primary Contact: Denzel Davis, Interim Chief Executive Officer
CMO: Ben Bullington, M.D., Chief Medical Officer
Web address: www.mvmc.org
Control: Other not–for–profit (including NFP Corporation) **Service:** General Medical and Surgical

Staffed Beds: 25 **Admissions:** 99 **Census:** 15 **Outpatient Visits:** 6552 **Births:** 0 **Total Expense ($000):** 4243 **Payroll Expense ($000):** 2216 **Personnel:** 62

WHITEFISH—Flathead County

★ **NORTH VALLEY HOSPITAL (271336)**, 1600 Hospital Way, Zip 59937–2958; tel. 406/863–3500 **A**9 10 18 **F**3 11 13 15 24 25 26 27 33 38 43 50 54 55 56 57 62 66 68 73 74 77 79 80 81 82 84 87 96 100 103 107 117 118 119 120 121 122 135 **P**5 **S** QHR
Primary Contact: Craig E. Aasved, Chief Executive Officer
CFO: Marilyn Hays, Chief Financial Officer
CIO: Jay Adams, Chief Information Officer
CHR: Susan Catt, Director Human Resources
Web address: www.nvhosp.org
Control: Other not–for–profit (including NFP Corporation) **Service:** General Medical and Surgical

Staffed Beds: 25 **Admissions:** 1651 **Census:** 14 **Outpatient Visits:** 44386 **Births:** 351 **Total Expense ($000):** 23622 **Payroll Expense ($000):** 8935 **Personnel:** 148

WOLF POINT—Roosevelt County

★ **TRINITY HOSPITAL (271341)**, (Total facility includes 60 beds in nursing home–type unit) **A**9 10 18 **F**2 3 6 7 13 15 25 27 30 31 32 38 50 54 55 56 57 62 67 68 73 74 76 79 84 99 107 108 115 117 119 122 132 134 **P**3 6
Primary Contact: Margaret B. Norgaard, Chief Executive Officer
Web address: www.nemhs.net
Control: Other not–for–profit (including NFP Corporation) **Service:** General Medical and Surgical

Staffed Beds: 82 **Admissions:** 501 **Census:** 57 **Outpatient Visits:** 14376 **Births:** 80 **Total Expense ($000):** 7823 **Payroll Expense ($000):** 4295 **Personnel:** 151

MT

Hospital, Medicare Provider Number, Address, Telephone, Approval, Facility, and Physician Codes, Health Care System

★ American Hospital Association (AHA) membership
□ The Joint Commission accreditation
○ American Osteopathic Association (AOA) accreditation
△ Commission on Accreditation of Rehabilitation Facilities (CARF) accreditation

NEBRASKA

AINSWORTH—Brown County

BROWN COUNTY HOSPITAL (281325), 945 East Zero Street, Zip 69210–1547; tel. 402/387–2800, (Nonreporting) **A**9 10 18
Primary Contact: Neil Hilton, Chief Executive Officer
CMO: Melvin Campbell, M.D., Medical Staff Chairman
CHR: Lisa Fischer, Director Human Resources
Web address: www.browncountyhospital.org
Control: County–Government, nonfederal **Service:** General Medical and Surgical

Staffed Beds: 25

ALBION—Boone County

★ **BOONE COUNTY HEALTH CENTER (281334)**, 723 West Fairview Street, Zip 68620–1725, Mailing Address: P.O. Box 151, Zip 68620–0151; tel. 402/395–2191 **A**9 10 18 **F**3 11 13 15 24 25 27 28 30 31 32 33 36 38 43 52 55 56 57 61 62 63 73 74 75 76 77 79 80 81 82 86 94 107 113 117 119 120 121 122 123 124 135 136 137 **P**5 6
Primary Contact: Victor N. Lee, FACHE, President and Chief Executive Officer
CFO: Mandy Price, Vice President Fiscal Services
CIO: Larry Zoucha, Chief Information Officer
CHR: Jennifer Beierman, Director Human Resources
Web address: www.boonecohealth.org
Control: County–Government, nonfederal **Service:** General Medical and Surgical

Staffed Beds: 25 **Admissions:** 859 **Census:** 7 **Outpatient Visits:** 33832 **Births:** 77 **Total Expense ($000):** 15172 **Payroll Expense ($000):** 7338 **Personnel:** 179

ALLIANCE—Box Butte County

☒ **BOX BUTTE GENERAL HOSPITAL (281360)**, 2101 Box Butte Avenue, Zip 69301–0810, Mailing Address: P.O. Box 810, Zip 69301–0810; tel. 308/762–6660 **A**1 9 10 18 **F**3 5 11 13 15 24 25 27 28 30 31 32 33 34 36 38 40 43 50 52 55 56 57 59 62 66 67 73 75 76 77 79 80 81 82 86 87 90 91 92 94 96 97 100 102 104 106 107 118 119 120 121 122 123 124 133 135 137
Primary Contact: Dan Griess, Chief Executive Officer
COO: Jim Parks, Chief Operating Officer
CFO: Tracy E. Jatczak, CPA, Chief Financial Officer
CMO: Raymond Carlson, D.O., Chief of Staff
CIO: Jim Parks, Chief Operating Officer
CHR: Rebecca Sisler, Director Human Resources
Web address: www.bbgh.org
Control: County–Government, nonfederal **Service:** General Medical and Surgical

Staffed Beds: 25 **Admissions:** 1112 **Census:** 11 **Outpatient Visits:** 33891 **Births:** 70 **Total Expense ($000):** 17204 **Payroll Expense ($000):** 7558 **Personnel:** 195

NE

ALMA—Harlan County

★ **HARLAN COUNTY HEALTH SYSTEM (281300)**, 717 North Brown Street, Zip 68920–0836, Mailing Address: P.O. Box 836, Zip 68920–0836; tel. 308/928–2151 **A**9 10 18 **F**3 11 25 26 27 30 31 32 38 40 50 62 73 79 80 81 86 96 102 107 117 119 121 122 **S** Great Plains Health Alliance, Inc.
Primary Contact: Allen Van Driel, CHE, Administrator
CFO: Rebekah Mussman, Chief Financial Officer
Web address: www.gpha.com
Control: County–Government, nonfederal **Service:** General Medical and Surgical

Staffed Beds: 25 **Admissions:** 277 **Census:** 4 **Outpatient Visits:** 7465 **Births:** 0 **Total Expense ($000):** 4498 **Payroll Expense ($000):** 1730 **Personnel:** 51

ATKINSON—Holt County

WEST HOLT MEMORIAL HOSPITAL (281343), 406 West Neely Street, Zip 68713–0200; tel. 402/925–2811 **A**9 10 18 **F**3 24 30 31 38 55 56 57 73 74 79 86 96 107 119 122 **P**4 **S** Sanford Health
Primary Contact: John N. Olson, Chief Executive Officer
CFO: Karen Nollette, Chief Financial Officer
CMO: John Tubbs, M.D., Chief of Staff
CHR: Margaret Linse, Administrative Secretary and Director Human Resources
Web address: www.westholtmed.org
Control: Other not–for–profit (including NFP Corporation) **Service:** General Medical and Surgical

Staffed Beds: 18 **Admissions:** 419 **Census:** 5 **Outpatient Visits:** 13727 **Births:** 32 **Total Expense ($000):** 5939 **Payroll Expense ($000):** 2858 **Personnel:** 70

AUBURN—Nemaha County

★ **NEMAHA COUNTY HOSPITAL (281324)**, 2022 13th Street, Zip 68305–1799; tel. 402/274–4366 **A**9 10 18 **F**3 7 11 12 13 15 24 25 26 27 30 33 38 40 43 61 62 65 72 73 75 76 77 79 80 82 84 86 96 100 105 107 117 118 122 124 130 135 136
Primary Contact: Marty Fattig, Administrator and Chief Executive Officer
COO: Kermit Moore, Chief Operating Officer and Chief Nursing Officer
CFO: Stacy Taylor, Chief Financial Officer
CHR: Susie Shupp, Director Human Resources
Web address: www.nchnet.org
Control: County–Government, nonfederal **Service:** General Medical and Surgical

Staffed Beds: 20 **Admissions:** 287 **Census:** 3 **Outpatient Visits:** 14359 **Births:** 0 **Total Expense ($000):** 7479 **Payroll Expense ($000):** 3008 **Personnel:** 69

AURORA—Hamilton County

★ **MEMORIAL HOSPITAL (281320)**, 1423 Seventh Street, Zip 68818–1197; tel. 402/694–3171, (Total facility includes 49 beds in nursing home–type unit) (Nonreporting) **A**9 10 18
Primary Contact: Diane R. Keller, Chief Executive Officer
CFO: Phil Fendt, Chief Financial Officer
CMO: Mark Jobman, M.D., Chief of Staff
CHR: Laurie Andrews, Chief Human Resources Officer
Web address: www.memorialcommunityhealth.org
Control: Other not–for–profit (including NFP Corporation) **Service:** General Medical and Surgical

Staffed Beds: 74

BASSETT—Rock County

ROCK COUNTY HOSPITAL (281333), 102 East South Street, Zip 68714; tel. 402/684–3366, (Total facility includes 28 beds in nursing home–type unit) **A**9 10 18 **F**7 11 24 38 44 55 79 117 122
Primary Contact: Stacey A. Knox, Administrator
CMO: John I. Cherry, M.D., Chief of Staff
CHR: Jackie Carpenter, Office Manager
Web address: www.rockcountyhospital.com
Control: County–Government, nonfederal **Service:** General Medical and Surgical

Staffed Beds: 45 **Admissions:** 255 **Census:** 27 **Outpatient Visits:** 3911 **Births:** 0 **Total Expense ($000):** 3754 **Payroll Expense ($000):** 2046 **Personnel:** 68

BEATRICE—Gage County

☒ **BEATRICE COMMUNITY HOSPITAL AND HEALTH CENTER (281364)**, 1110 North Tenth Street, Zip 68310–2039, Mailing Address: P.O. Box 278, Zip 68310–0278; tel. 402/228–3344, (Total facility includes 71 beds in nursing home–type unit) **A**1 9 10 18 **F**2 13 15 24 25 26 27 30 31 32 33 38 42 43 52 55 57 61 62 63 65 66 67 68 73 74 76 77 79 80 82 86 87 96 97 100 102 106 107 117 118 119 121 122 124 135 136 137
Primary Contact: Thomas W. Sommers, President and Chief Executive Officer
CFO: James A. Garbarino, Chief Financial Officer
CMO: James Van Brocklin, M.D., Chief of Staff
CHR: Charlotte Campbell, Director Human Resources
Web address: www.beatricecommunityhospital.com
Control: Other not–for–profit (including NFP Corporation) **Service:** General Medical and Surgical

Staffed Beds: 96 **Admissions:** 1155 **Census:** 68 **Outpatient Visits:** 97394 **Births:** 121 **Total Expense ($000):** 32491 **Payroll Expense ($000):** 15136 **Personnel:** 354

BENKELMAN—Dundy County

★ **DUNDY COUNTY HOSPITAL (281340)**, 1313 North Cheyenne Street, Zip 69021, Mailing Address: P.O. Box 626, Zip 69021–0626; tel. 308/423–2204 **A**9 10 18 **F**3 13 15 24 25 26 27 30 31 32 38 40 50 54 55 57 73 74 76 77 79 80 81 82 86 87 96 117 120 121 122 136 137 **P**6
Primary Contact: Rita A. Jones, Chief Executive Officer
COO: Wendy Elkins, Director Operations
CFO: Dwana Roschewski, Director Administration
CMO: Shiuvaun Jaeger, M.D., Chief Medical Staff
CIO: Anna Elliot, Head Information Technology
CHR: Sandy Noffsinger, Executive Assistant
Web address: www.bwtelcom.net/dch
Control: County–Government, nonfederal **Service:** General Medical and Surgical

Staffed Beds: 14 **Admissions:** 274 **Census:** 3 **Outpatient Visits:** 9700 **Births:** 20 **Personnel:** 73

BLAIR—Washington County

MEMORIAL COMMUNITY HOSPITAL AND HEALTH SYSTEM (281359), 810 North 22nd Street, Zip 68008–1199, Mailing Address: P.O. Box 250, Zip 68008–0250; tel. 402/426–2182, (Nonreporting) **A**9 10 18 **S** Alegent Health
Primary Contact: Sally Harvey, RN, Regional Administrator
COO: Pam Reynolds, Chief Operating Officer
CFO: Dan Schonlau, Chief Financial Officer
CMO: Brad Sawtelle, M.D., President Medical Staff
CIO: Deann Rosenau, Operations Director Information Technology and Revenue Cycle
CHR: Carol Bartholct, Human Resources Generalist
Web address: www.mchhs.org
Control: Other not–for–profit (including NFP Corporation) **Service:** General Medical and Surgical

Staffed Beds: 25

BRIDGEPORT—Morrill County

MORRILL COUNTY COMMUNITY HOSPITAL (281318), 1313 S Street, Zip 69336–0579, Mailing Address: P.O. Box 579, Zip 69336–0579; tel. 308/262–1616, (Nonreporting) **A**9 10 18
Primary Contact: Julia Morrow, Administrator
Web address: www.morrillcountyhospital.org
Control: County–Government, nonfederal **Service:** General Medical and Surgical

Staffed Beds: 20

BROKEN BOW—Custer County

JENNIE M. MELHAM MEMORIAL MEDICAL CENTER (281365), 145 Memorial Drive, Zip 68822–1378, Mailing Address: P.O. Box 250, Zip 68822–0250; tel. 308/872–4100, (Total facility includes 65 beds in nursing home–type unit) (Nonreporting) **A**9 10 18
Primary Contact: Michael J. Steckler, President and Chief Executive Officer
CFO: Tim Schuckman, Chief Financial Officer
CIO: Tim Schuckman, Chief Financial Officer
Web address: www.brokenbow-ne.com/community/healthcare/melham.htm
Control: Other not–for–profit (including NFP Corporation) **Service:** General Medical and Surgical

Staffed Beds: 90

CALLAWAY—Custer County

★ **CALLAWAY DISTRICT HOSPITAL (281335)**, 211 Kimball, Zip 68825–0100, Mailing Address: P.O. Box 100, Zip 68825–0100; tel. 308/836–2228, (Nonreporting) **A**9 10 18
Primary Contact: Marvin Neth, Administrator
Web address: www.callaway-ne.com/hospital/
Control: Hospital district or authority, Government, nonfederal **Service:** General Medical and Surgical

Staffed Beds: 12

CAMBRIDGE—Furnas County

★ **TRI–VALLEY HEALTH SYSTEM (281348)**, 1305 West Highway 6 and 34, Zip 69022–0488, Mailing Address: P.O. Box 488, Zip 69022–0488; tel. 308/697–3329, (Total facility includes 34 beds in nursing home–type unit) (Nonreporting) **A**9 10 18 **S** Brim Healthcare, Inc.
Primary Contact: Carol H. Hanes, Chief Executive Officer
COO: Carol H. Hanes, Chief Executive Officer
CFO: Diana Rippe, Financial Services Executive
CMO: Shelly Kasper–Cope, M.D., Chief of Staff
CIO: Doug Hall, Director Information Systems
CHR: Leanne Miller, Employee Services Executive
Web address: www.trivalleyhealth.com
Control: Other not–for–profit (including NFP Corporation) **Service:** General Medical and Surgical

Staffed Beds: 51

CENTRAL CITY—Merrick County

★ **LITZENBERG MEMORIAL COUNTY HOSPITAL (281328)**, 1715 26th Street, Zip 68826–9620, Mailing Address: Route 2, Box 1, Zip 68826–0001; tel. 308/946–3015, (Total facility includes 46 beds in nursing home–type unit) (Nonreporting) **A**9 10 18
Primary Contact: Michael R. Bowman, Administrator
Web address: www.lmchealth.com
Control: County–Government, nonfederal **Service:** General Medical and Surgical

Staffed Beds: 71

CHADRON—Dawes County

★ **CHADRON COMMUNITY HOSPITAL AND HEALTH SERVICES (281341)**, 821 Morehead Street, Zip 69337–2599; tel. 308/432–5586, (Nonreporting) **A**9 10 18
Primary Contact: Harold L. Krueger, Jr., Chief Executive Officer
CFO: Russ Bohnenkamp, Director Finance
Web address: www.chadronhospital.com
Control: Other not–for–profit (including NFP Corporation) **Service:** General Medical and Surgical

Staffed Beds: 25

COLUMBUS—Platte County

★☐ **COLUMBUS COMMUNITY HOSPITAL (280111)**, 4600 38th Street, Zip 68601, Mailing Address: P.O. Box 1800, Zip 68602–1800; tel. 402/564–7118, (Total facility includes 4 beds in nursing home–type unit) **A**1 9 10 20 **F**3 8 11 13 15 17 24 25 30 31 32 33 35 36 37 38 40 42 43 44 55 57 61 62 63 66 67 68 73 74 75 77 79 80 81 82 86 96 97 99 100 103 105 106 107 112 117 118 119 120 121 122 124 135 **P**8
Primary Contact: Claude Chatterton, President and Chief Executive Officer
COO: James P. Goulet, Vice President Operations
CFO: J. Joseph Barbaglia, Vice President Financial Services
CMO: Deborah Anderson, M.D., President Medical Staff
CIO: Cheryl Tira, Director Information Systems
CHR: Scott E. Messersmith, Director Human Resources
Web address: www.columbushosp.org
Control: Other not–for–profit (including NFP Corporation) **Service:** General Medical and Surgical

Staffed Beds: 51 **Admissions:** 2749 **Census:** 26 **Outpatient Visits:** 55944 **Births:** 505 **Total Expense ($000):** 44729 **Payroll Expense ($000):** 19624 **Personnel:** 391

COZAD—Dawson County

★ **COZAD COMMUNITY HOSPITAL (281327)**, 300 East 12th Street, Zip 69130–1505, Mailing Address: P.O. Box 108, Zip 69130–0108; tel. 308/784–2261 **A**5 9 10 18 **F**3 10 13 15 24 26 27 30 31 33 38 40 42 43 44 50 52 54 56 57 61 68 73 74 75 79 81 86 87 96 107 117 119 120 121 122 124 135 137 **P**6
Primary Contact: Lyle E. Davis, Administrator
Web address: www.cozadhealthcare.com
Control: Hospital district or authority, Government, nonfederal **Service:** General Medical and Surgical

Staffed Beds: 21 **Admissions:** 426 **Census:** 5 **Outpatient Visits:** 8159 **Births:** 48 **Total Expense ($000):** 7776 **Payroll Expense ($000):** 4266 **Personnel:** 118

CREIGHTON—Knox County

CREIGHTON AREA HEALTH SERVICES (281331), 1503 Main Street, Zip 68729–0186, Mailing Address: P.O. Box 186, Zip 68729–0186; tel. 402/358–5700, (Total facility includes 47 beds in nursing home–type unit) **A**9 10 18 **F**2 11 12 24 25 27 30 31 32 33 38 41 50 52 54 55 56 57 61 62 65 73 75 76 77 79 81 84 85 86 87 96 102 117 119 120 121 122 124 132 135 137 **P**6
Primary Contact: Jeff Lingerfelt, Chief Executive Officer
CFO: Kim Hixson, Chief Financial Officer
CHR: June Kotrous, Director Human Resources
Web address: www.cahs-ne.org
Control: City–Government, nonfederal **Service:** General Medical and Surgical

Staffed Beds: 70 **Admissions:** 509 **Census:** 47 **Outpatient Visits:** 9693 **Births:** 0 **Total Expense ($000):** 7462 **Payroll Expense ($000):** 3698 **Personnel:** 110

CRETE—Saline County

★ **CRETE AREA MEDICAL CENTER (281354)**, 2910 Betten Drive, Zip 68333–0220, Mailing Address: P.O. Box 220, Zip 68333–0220; tel. 402/826–2102, (Total facility includes 1 beds in nursing home–type unit) **A**9 10 18 **F**13 15 25 27 30 31 32 38 55 56 62 63 66 76 77 79 86 87 96 100 102 107 122 **P**6 **S** BryanLGH Health System
Primary Contact: Carol Friesen, Chief Executive Officer
CFO: Bryce Betke, Chief Financial Officer
CIO: Sheri Thompson, Director Information Technology
CHR: Bobbie Wilson, Director Human Resources
Web address: www.creteareamedicalcenter.com
Control: Other not–for–profit (including NFP Corporation) **Service:** General Medical and Surgical

Staffed Beds: 25 **Admissions:** 506 **Census:** 15 **Outpatient Visits:** 41891 **Births:** 115 **Total Expense ($000):** 15979 **Payroll Expense ($000):** 6311 **Personnel:** 143

NE

Hospital, Medicare Provider Number, Address, Telephone, Approval, Facility, and Physician Codes, Health Care System
★ American Hospital Association (AHA) membership
☐ The Joint Commission accreditation
○ American Osteopathic Association (AOA) accreditation
△ Commission on Accreditation of Rehabilitation Facilities (CARF) accreditation

DAVID CITY—Butler County

★ **BUTLER COUNTY HEALTH CARE CENTER (281332)**, 372 South Ninth Street, Zip 68632–2199; tel. 402/367–1200 **A**9 10 18 **F**7 11 13 15 24 25 30 31 32 38 43 51 52 55 56 57 58 59 62 63 73 74 76 77 79 81 84 86 96 97 100 107 117 118 119 120 122 124 132 134 135 **P**6
Primary Contact: Donald T. Naiberk, Administrator
CFO: Ron Jones, Chief Financial Officer
CMO: Victor Thoendel, M.D., Chief Medical Officer
CHR: Andra Vandenberg, Director Human Resources
Web address: www.bchccnet.org
Control: County–Government, nonfederal **Service:** General Medical and Surgical

Staffed Beds: 25 **Admissions:** 446 **Census:** 4 **Outpatient Visits:** 14110
Births: 68 **Total Expense ($000):** 7912 **Payroll Expense ($000):** 3408
Personnel: 82

FAIRBURY—Jefferson County

★ **JEFFERSON COMMUNITY HEALTH CENTER (281319)**, 2200 H Street, Zip 68352–1119, Mailing Address: P.O. Box 277, Zip 68352–0277; tel. 402/729–3351, (Total facility includes 39 beds in nursing home–type unit) **A**9 10 18 **F**3 10 11 12 13 15 24 25 26 27 28 30 31 32 33 38 43 50 52 55 56 57 61 63 73 74 75 76 77 79 80 81 82 86 96 107 119 120 121 122 124 135 **P**5
Primary Contact: William L. Welch, FACHE, Chief Executive Officer
CFO: Chad Jurgens, Chief Financial Officer
CHR: Sandy Bauer, Director Human Resources
Web address: www.jchc.us
Control: Other not–for–profit (including NFP Corporation) **Service:** General Medical and Surgical

Staffed Beds: 64 **Admissions:** 598 **Census:** 42 **Outpatient Visits:** 16693
Births: 66 **Total Expense ($000):** 12299 **Payroll Expense ($000):** 5297
Personnel: 146

FALLS CITY—Richardson County

★ **COMMUNITY MEDICAL CENTER (281352)**, 2307 Barada Street, Zip 68355–1599, Mailing Address: P.O. Box 399, Zip 68355–0399; tel. 402/245–2428 **A**9 10 18 **F**3 7 13 15 24 27 30 33 38 55 56 57 68 74 75 76 79 80 84 96 100 105 107 119 122
Primary Contact: Ryan C. Larsen, Chief Executive Officer
CFO: Scott Sawyer, Chief Financial Officer
CIO: Karen Brown, Director Health Information
CHR: Amy Olberding, Director Human Resources
Web address: www.cmcfc.org
Control: Other not–for–profit (including NFP Corporation) **Service:** General Medical and Surgical

Staffed Beds: 25 **Admissions:** 901 **Census:** 11 **Outpatient Visits:** 27000
Births: 47 **Total Expense ($000):** 13217 **Payroll Expense ($000):** 5724
Personnel: 164

NE

FRANKLIN—Franklin County

★ **FRANKLIN COUNTY MEMORIAL HOSPITAL (281311)**, 1406 Q Street, Zip 68939–0315, Mailing Address: P.O. Box 315, Zip 68939–0315; tel. 308/425–6221 **A**9 10 18 **F**3 11 17 24 26 27 30 31 32 33 38 40 42 50 55 56 57 62 73 75 77 79 86 87 119 121 122 **P**6
Primary Contact: Jerrell F. Gerdes, FACHE, Administrator
COO: Linda Bush, Chief Operating Officer
CMO: Linda Mazour, M.D., President
CIO: Cathy Webber, Chief Information Officer
Web address: www.fcmh.com
Control: County–Government, nonfederal **Service:** General Medical and Surgical

Staffed Beds: 12 **Admissions:** 211 **Census:** 1 **Outpatient Visits:** 6560
Births: 0 **Total Expense ($000):** 4107 **Payroll Expense ($000):** 2081
Personnel: 57

FREMONT—Dodge County

⊠ **FREMONT AREA MEDICAL CENTER (280077)**, 450 East 23rd Street, Zip 68025–2387; tel. 402/721–1610, (Total facility includes 162 beds in nursing home–type unit) **A**1 2 9 10 **F**3 11 13 15 17 18 20 24 25 26 27 30 31 32 33 35 38 42 43 44 52 54 55 56 57 61 62 66 68 71 73 74 75 76 77 79 80 81 82 84 86 96 97 100 102 107 108 109 111 116 117 118 119 120 121 124 132 135 **P**8
Primary Contact: Patrick M. Booth, Chief Executive Officer
COO: Peggy S. Kennedy, R.N., Vice President, Chief Operating Officer and Chief Nursing Officer
CFO: David G. Hanen, Vice President Fiscal Services and Chief Financial Officer
Web address: www.famc.org
Control: County–Government, nonfederal **Service:** General Medical and Surgical

Staffed Beds: 252 **Admissions:** 4920 **Census:** 190 **Outpatient Visits:** 67526
Births: 431 **Total Expense ($000):** 75534 **Payroll Expense ($000):** 34770
Personnel: 712

FRIEND—Saline County

WARREN MEMORIAL HOSPITAL (281330), 905 Second Street, Zip 68359–1198; tel. 402/947–2541, (Total facility includes 50 beds in nursing home–type unit) **A**9 10 18 **F**11 31 32 33 38 43 55 56 62 65 67 79 119 121 122
Primary Contact: John W. Wilson, Chief Executive Officer
CFO: Don Williamson, Chief Financial Officer
CMO: Roger Meyer, M.D., Chief of Staff
CIO: Colleen Classen, Director Health Information Systems
CHR: Jamie Tuttle, Coordinator Human Resources
Web address: www.warrenmemorialhospital.org
Control: City–Government, nonfederal **Service:** General Medical and Surgical

Staffed Beds: 61 **Admissions:** 82 **Census:** 39 **Outpatient Visits:** 8219
Births: 0

GENEVA—Fillmore County

FILLMORE COUNTY HOSPITAL (281301), 1325 H Street, Zip 68361–1325, Mailing Address: P.O. Box 193, Zip 68361–0193; tel. 402/759–3167, (Nonreporting) **A**9 10 18
Primary Contact: Paul Utemark, Chief Executive Officer
CFO: Gary Kudlacek, Chief Financial Officer
CMO: C. L. Verhage, M.D., Chief of Staff
CIO: Tyler Gewecke, Information Technology Technician
CHR: Ranee Hoarty, Business Manager Human Resources
Web address: www.fhsofgeneva.org
Control: County–Government, nonfederal **Service:** General Medical and Surgical

Staffed Beds: 25

GENOA—Nance County

GENOA COMMUNITY HOSPITAL (281312), 706 Ewing Avenue, Zip 68640, Mailing Address: P.O. Box 310, Zip 68640–0310; tel. 402/993–2283, (Total facility includes 45 beds in nursing home–type unit) (Nonreporting) **A**9 10 18
Primary Contact: Shelli Cornwell, Chief Executive Officer
CFO: Jennifer Wieck, Business Manager
CMO: Brian Buhlke, M.D., Medical Director
CHR: Kathy Kruse, Manager Human Resources
Control: City–County, Government, nonfederal **Service:** General Medical and Surgical

Staffed Beds: 65

GORDON—Sheridan County

★ **GORDON MEMORIAL HOSPITAL (281358)**, 300 East Eighth Street, Zip 69343–9990; tel. 308/282–0401, (Total facility includes 40 beds in nursing home–type unit) (Nonreporting) **A**9 10 18
Primary Contact: Kay Garcia, Chief Executive Officer
CMO: S. K. Shrestha, M.D., Chief of Staff
CIO: Tony Hindman, Director Information Technology
CHR: Tina Mills, Director Personnel and Administrative Assistant
Web address: www.gordonhospital.org
Control: Hospital district or authority, Government, nonfederal **Service:** General Medical and Surgical

Staffed Beds: 65

GOTHENBURG—Dawson County

★ **GOTHENBURG MEMORIAL HOSPITAL (281313)**, 910 20th Street, Zip 69138–1237, Mailing Address: P.O. Box 469, Zip 69138–0469; tel. 308/537–3661, (Total facility includes 35 beds in nursing home–type unit) **A**9 10 18 **F**3 13 15 24 25 28 31 33 38 52 55 56 62 63 74 75 77 79 86 96 102 107 117 119 120 122 **P**5
Primary Contact: John H. Johnson, Chief Executive Officer
CFO: Taci Bartlett, Chief Financial Officer
CMO: Craig Bartruff, M.D., Medical Director
CIO: John H. Johnson, Chief Executive Officer
CHR: Lisa Gieken, Director Human Resources
Web address: www.ghospital.org
Control: Hospital district or authority, Government, nonfederal **Service:** General Medical and Surgical

Staffed Beds: 47 **Admissions:** 295 **Census:** 25 **Outpatient Visits:** 13846
Births: 16 **Total Expense ($000):** 5648 **Payroll Expense ($000):** 3886
Personnel: 98

GRAND ISLAND—Hall County

☒ **SAINT FRANCIS MEDICAL CENTER (280023)**, 2620 West Faidley Avenue, Zip 68803–4297, Mailing Address: P.O. Box 9804, Zip 68802–9804; tel. 308/384–4600, (Includes SAINT FRANCIS MEMORIAL HEALTH CENTER, 2116 West Faidley Avenue, Zip 68803), (Total facility includes 34 beds in nursing home–type unit) **A**1 2 3 5 9 10 19 **F**3 4 5 11 12 13 17 18 20 24 26 27 30 31 32 33 35 36 38 40 42 43 44 50 52 55 56 57 59 61 62 66 68 70 71 72 73 74 75 76 77 79 80 81 84 86 94 108 109 111 117 118 119 121 132 135 137 **S** Catholic Health Initiatives
Primary Contact: Daniel P. McElligott, FACHE, President and Chief Executive Officer
CFO: Lisa Webb, Vice President Finance and Chief Financial Officer
CMO: Mike Horn, M.D., Vice President Medical Affairs
CIO: Tammy Williams, Director Information Systems
CHR: Lee Elliott, Vice President Human Resources and Fund Development
Web address: www.saintfrancisgi.org
Control: Church–operated, Nongovernment, not–for profit **Service:** General Medical and Surgical

Staffed Beds: 179 **Admissions:** 7473 **Census:** 94 **Outpatient Visits:** 224615 **Births:** 1009 **Total Expense ($000):** 114557 **Payroll Expense ($000):** 49537 **Personnel:** 1010

GRANT—Perkins County

★ **PERKINS COUNTY HEALTH SERVICES (281356)**, 900 Lincoln Avenue, Zip 69140–9799; tel. 308/352–7200, (Includes GOLDEN OURS CONVALESCENT HOME), (Total facility includes 64 beds in nursing home–type unit) (Nonreporting) **A**9 10 18
Primary Contact: Pam Holm, RN, Administrator
CFO: Tiffany Weber, Chief Financial Officer
CIO: Jennifer Baumgartner, Chief Information Officer
CHR: Candace Frickey, Chief Human Resources and Payroll
Web address: www.pchsgrant.com
Control: Hospital district or authority, Government, nonfederal **Service:** General Medical and Surgical

Staffed Beds: 84

HASTINGS—Adams County

HASTINGS REGIONAL CENTER (284002), 4200 West Second Street, Zip 68901–9700, Mailing Address: P.O. Box 579, Zip 68902–0579; tel. 402/462–1971, (Nonreporting) **A**9 10
Primary Contact: William R. Gibson, Chief Executive Officer
COO: Marj A. Colburn, Facility Operating Officer, Risk Manager and Performance Improvement Coordinator
CMO: Gene Wyse, D.O., Medical Director
CIO: Nancy Kinyoun, Director Health Information Management
CHR: LaDene Madson, Director Human Resources
Web address: www.dhhs.ne.gov
Control: State–Government, nonfederal **Service:** Other specialty

Staffed Beds: 156

☒ **MARY LANNING MEMORIAL HOSPITAL (280032)**, 715 North St. Joseph Avenue, Zip 68901–4497; tel. 402/463–4521 **A**1 2 9 10 19 **F**11 13 15 17 24 26 27 30 31 32 33 35 38 42 43 44 46 52 53 61 62 64 66 68 70 72 73 74 75 76 77 79 80 81 82 84 85 86 87 88 90 91 92 93 94 95 96 97 100 102 103 105 107 109 110 111 117 118 119 120 121 124 135 136 137
Primary Contact: W. Michael Kearney, President and Chief Executive Officer
CFO: Timothy L. Gronseth, Senior Vice President and Chief Financial Officer
CMO: Joe Davis, M.D., Vice President Medical Affairs
CIO: George Sullivan, Director Management Information Systems
CHR: Bruce Cutright, Vice President Human Resources
Web address: www.mlmh.org
Control: Other not–for–profit (including NFP Corporation) **Service:** General Medical and Surgical

Staffed Beds: 161 **Admissions:** 5745 **Census:** 73 **Outpatient Visits:** 148225 **Births:** 708 **Total Expense ($000):** 82400 **Payroll Expense ($000):** 36805 **Personnel:** 835

HEBRON—Thayer County

★ **THAYER COUNTY HEALTH SERVICES (281304)**, 120 Park Avenue, Zip 68370–2019, Mailing Address: P.O. Box 49, Zip 68370–0049; tel. 402/768–6041 **A**9 10 18 **F**27 30 31 32 38 55 56 57 61 63 74 75 76 77 79 81 86 96 107 117 119 122 124
Primary Contact: Joyce Beck, Administrator
COO: Susan L. Moore, R.N., Director Nursing
CFO: Michael Pracheil, Chief Financial Officer
CMO: Michelle Kuhlmann, M.D., Director Medical Staff
Web address: www.thayercountyhealth.com
Control: County–Government, nonfederal **Service:** General Medical and Surgical

Staffed Beds: 19 **Admissions:** 667 **Census:** 5 **Outpatient Visits:** 25240 **Births:** 47 **Total Expense ($000):** 12013 **Payroll Expense ($000):** 5600 **Personnel:** 99

HENDERSON—York County

HENDERSON HEALTH CARE SERVICES (281308), 1621 Front Street, Zip 68371; tel. 402/723–4512, (Total facility includes 40 beds in nursing home–type unit) (Nonreporting) **A**9 10 18
Primary Contact: Marianna Harris, Administrator
COO: Marianna Harris, Administrator
CMO: James M. Ohrt, M.D., Director Medical Staff
CHR: Lynette Friesen, Manager Human Resources
Web address: www.telcoweb.net/health
Control: Other not–for–profit (including NFP Corporation) **Service:** General Medical and Surgical

Staffed Beds: 56

HOLDREGE—Phelps County

☒ **PHELPS MEMORIAL HEALTH CENTER (281362)**, 1215 Tibbals Street, Zip 68949–1280; tel. 308/995–2211 **A**1 9 10 18 **F**3 7 13 15 24 25 26 27 30 31 32 33 38 40 43 55 56 57 61 62 68 73 74 75 77 79 80 81 82 86 93 96 97 100 102 107 118 119 120 121 122 124 135 **P**5 **S** QHR
Primary Contact: Mark Harrel, Chief Executive Officer
CFO: Loren D. Schroder, Chief Financial Officer
CMO: Stuart Embury, M.D., Chief Medical Officer
CIO: Leora Smith, Information System and Health Information Management Team Leader
CHR: Cindy Jackson, Director Human Resources
Web address: www.phelpsmemorial.com
Control: Other not–for–profit (including NFP Corporation) **Service:** General Medical and Surgical

Staffed Beds: 25 **Admissions:** 1211 **Census:** 13 **Outpatient Visits:** 30778 **Births:** 122 **Total Expense ($000):** 18138 **Payroll Expense ($000):** 7211 **Personnel:** 187

IMPERIAL—Chase County

CHASE COUNTY COMMUNITY HOSPITAL (281351), 600 West 12th Street, Zip 69033–0819, Mailing Address: P.O. Box 819, Zip 69033–0819; tel. 308/882–7111 **A**9 10 18 **F**11 13 15 24 27 31 32 38 40 55 57 74 79 84 86 96 102 117 122 137 **P**6
Primary Contact: Lola Jones, RN, Administrator
CFO: Renee Fink, CPA, Chief Financial Officer
CMO: Jonathan Richman, M.D., Chief of Staff
CHR: Julie Sharp, Supervisor Human Resources
Web address: www.chasecountyhospital.com
Control: County–Government, nonfederal **Service:** General Medical and Surgical

Staffed Beds: 25 **Admissions:** 336 **Census:** 4 **Outpatient Visits:** 13325 **Births:** 31 **Total Expense ($000):** 6972 **Payroll Expense ($000):** 2082 **Personnel:** 71

Hospital, Medicare Provider Number, Address, Telephone, Approval, Facility, and Physician Codes, Health Care System

★ American Hospital Association (AHA) membership
□ The Joint Commission accreditation
○ American Osteopathic Association (AOA) accreditation
△ Commission on Accreditation of Rehabilitation Facilities (CARF) accreditation

KEARNEY—Buffalo County

★ **GOOD SAMARITAN HEALTH SYSTEMS (280009)**, 10 East 31st Street, Zip 68847–2926, Mailing Address: P.O. Box 1990, Zip 68848–1990; tel. 308/865–7100, (Total facility includes 40 beds in nursing home–type unit) **A**1 2 3 5 9 10 19 **F**3 7 9 13 15 18 20 22 24 25 26 27 30 31 32 33 36 37 38 40 41 42 43 50 52 55 56 57 59 61 62 66 67 68 69 70 72 73 74 75 76 77 78 79 80 81 82 84 85 86 88 89 91 92 93 94 96 97 100 102 106 107 108 109 111 112 117 118 119 121 123 124 135 137 **P**6 8 **S** Catholic Health Initiatives
Primary Contact: John Allen, President and Chief Executive Officer
CFO: George Harms, Chief Financial Officer
CMO: Timothy Ranney, M.D., Vice President Medical Affairs
CIO: Tanya Arthur, Chief Information Officer
CHR: Robert Cunningham, Vice President Human Resources
Web address: www.gshs.org
Control: Church–operated, Nongovernment, not–for profit **Service:** General Medical and Surgical

Staffed Beds: 238 **Admissions:** 9192 **Census:** 165 **Outpatient Visits:** 65266 **Births:** 1071 **Total Expense ($000):** 156849 **Payroll Expense ($000):** 59684 **Personnel:** 1215

★ **RICHARD H. YOUNG HOSPITAL (284007)**, 1755 Prairie View Place, Zip 68848; tel. 308/865–2000, (Nonreporting) **A**1 9 **S** Catholic Health Initiatives
CFO: George Harms, Chief Financial Officer
CMO: Timothy Ranney, M.D., Vice President Medical Affairs
CIO: Tanya Arthur, Regional Chief Information Officer
CHR: Robert Cunningham, Vice President Human Resources
Web address: www.gshs.org
Control: Church–operated, Nongovernment, not–for profit **Service:** Psychiatric

Staffed Beds: 67

KIMBALL—Kimball County

★ **KIMBALL HEALTH SERVICES (281305)**, 505 South Burg Street, Zip 69145–1398; tel. 308/235–1952 **A**9 10 18 **F**1 3 15 32 38 40 55 63 65 79 80 84 85 86 87 96 117 119 122 135 137 **P**6
Primary Contact: Julie Schnell, Chief Executive Officer
CMO: Richard Jay, M.D., Chief of Staff
CIO: Nicole Nielan, Director Information Technology
CHR: James R. Imler, Director Human Resources
Web address: www.kimballhealth.org
Control: County–Government, nonfederal **Service:** General Medical and Surgical

Staffed Beds: 10 **Admissions:** 326 **Census:** 3 **Outpatient Visits:** 21399 **Births:** 0 **Total Expense ($000):** 6233 **Payroll Expense ($000):** 3015 **Personnel:** 73

LEXINGTON—Dawson County

★ **TRI–COUNTY AREA HOSPITAL (281361)**, 1201 North Erie Street, Zip 68850–0980, Mailing Address: P.O. Box 980, Zip 68850–0980; tel. 308/324–5651 **A**9 10 18 **F**3 11 13 15 24 27 30 38 42 44 45 47 49 52 55 57 61 62 65 66 73 74 77 79 80 81 86 96 102 107 115 117 119 122 124
Primary Contact: Calvin A. Hiner, Jr., Administrator
CFO: Gretchin Heckenlively, Director Financial Services
CMO: Edward M. Ford, Chief of Staff
CHR: Carolyn Malzahn, Director Human Resources
Web address: www.tricountyhospital.com
Control: Hospital district or authority, Government, nonfederal **Service:** General Medical and Surgical

Staffed Beds: 25 **Admissions:** 1155 **Census:** 12 **Outpatient Visits:** 22812 **Births:** 207 **Total Expense ($000):** 14718 **Payroll Expense ($000):** 6697 **Personnel:** 167

LINCOLN—Lancaster County

★ △ **BRYANLGH MEDICAL CENTER (280003)**, 1600 South 48th Street, Zip 68506–1299; tel. 402/489–0200, (Includes BRYANLGH MEDICAL CENTER–EAST; BRYANLGH MEDICAL CENTER–WEST, 2300 South 16th Street, Zip 68502–3781; tel. 402/475–1011) **A**1 6 7 9 10 **F**3 4 5 8 13 15 17 18 20 22 24 25 26 27 30 31 32 35 36 38 40 43 46 49 52 55 56 57 58 60 61 62 66 68 69 72 73 74 76 77 79 80 81 82 84 85 86 88 89 90 91 92 93 94 95 96 97 98 99 100 102 103 106 107 108 109 111 112 116 118 119 120 121 123 124 126 134 135 **S** BryanLGH Health System
Primary Contact: Craig M. Ames, President and Chief Operating Officer
CFO: Jennifer Lesoing–Lucs, Vice President and Chief Financial Officer
CMO: Carolyn Cody, M.D., Vice President Medical Affairs
CIO: Richard Marreel, Chief Information Officer
CHR: Gary Moore, Vice President Human Resources
Web address: www.bryanlgh.org
Control: Other not–for–profit (including NFP Corporation) **Service:** General Medical and Surgical

Staffed Beds: 349 **Admissions:** 22212 **Census:** 280 **Outpatient Visits:** 227201 **Births:** 1955 **Total Expense ($000):** 373497 **Payroll Expense ($000):** 146715 **Personnel:** 2882

LINCOLN DIVISION See Veterans Affairs Nebraska–Western Iowa Health Care System

□ **LINCOLN REGIONAL CENTER (284003)**, West Prospector Place and South Folsom, Zip 68522–2299, Mailing Address: P.O. Box 94949, Zip 68509–4949; tel. 402/471–4444, (Nonreporting) **A**1 9 10
Primary Contact: William R. Gibson, Chief Executive Officer
COO: Stacey Werth–Sweeney, Facility Operating Officer
CFO: Marion Schmidt, Business Manager
CMO: Vijay Dewan, M.D., Clinical Director
CHR: Scott Rasmussen, Director Human Resources
Control: State–Government, nonfederal **Service:** Psychiatric

Staffed Beds: 253

LINCOLN SURGICAL HOSPITAL (280127), 1710 South 70th Street, Suite 200, Zip 68506; tel. 402/484–9090, (Nonreporting) **A**9 10
Primary Contact: Robb Linafelter, Chief Executive Officer
Web address: www.lincolnsurgery.com
Control: Corporation, Investor–owned, for–profit **Service:** Other specialty

Staffed Beds: 7

★ △ **MADONNA REHABILITATION HOSPITAL (282000)**, 5401 South Street, Zip 68506–2134; tel. 402/489–7102, (Total facility includes 141 beds in nursing home–type unit) **A**7 9 10 **F**1 2 6 10 12 24 25 26 28 30 33 34 42 43 44 50 52 53 54 55 56 57 58 62 72 73 75 81 82 85 86 117 119 120 121 132 135 137 **P**4 6
Primary Contact: Marsha Lommel, FACHE, President and Chief Executive Officer
COO: Paul Dongilli, Ph.D., FACHE, Executive Vice President and Chief Operating Officer
CFO: Victor J. Witkowicz, Senior Vice President and Chief Financial Officer
CMO: Andrew Bohart, Vice President Medical Affairs
CIO: David Rolfe, Chief Information Officer
CHR: Lou Ann Manske, Director Human Resources
Web address: www.madonna.org
Control: Other not–for–profit (including NFP Corporation) **Service:** Rehabilitation

Staffed Beds: 303 **Admissions:** 2227 **Census:** 232 **Outpatient Visits:** 48006 **Births:** 0 **Total Expense ($000):** 74728 **Payroll Expense ($000):** 47364 **Personnel:** 1065

NEBRASKA HEART HOSPITAL (280128), 7500 South 91st Street, Zip 68526; tel. 402/327–2700, (Nonreporting) **A**9 10
Primary Contact: Thomas Burnell, Chief Executive Officer
CFO: Mark Smith, Chief Financial Officer
CIO: Doug Colburn, Chief Information Officer
Web address: www.neheart.com
Control: Corporation, Investor–owned, for–profit **Service:** General Medical and Surgical

Staffed Beds: 52

★ **SAINT ELIZABETH REGIONAL MEDICAL CENTER (280020)**, 555 South 70th Street, Zip 68510–2494; tel. 402/219–8000 **A**1 2 3 5 9 10 **F**11 12 13 15 16 17 18 20 22 24 25 26 27 30 31 32 33 35 37 38 41 42 43 44 45 49 50 51 52 55 56 57 58 59 60 61 62 66 68 70 72 73 74 75 76 77 78 79 80 81 82 84 86 90 96 97 99 100 102 103 105 106 107 108 109 111 116 118 119 120 121 124 133 134 135 136 137 **P**6 **S** Catholic Health Initiatives
Primary Contact: Robert J. Lanik, President and Chief Executive Officer
CFO: Jeanette Wojtalewicz, Vice President Finance
CMO: Cary Ward, M.D., Chief Medical Officer
CIO: Tanya Arthur, Chief Information Officer
CHR: John Dumonceaux, Vice President Human Resources
Web address: www.saintelizabethonline.com
Control: Other not–for–profit (including NFP Corporation) **Service:** General Medical and Surgical

Staffed Beds: 257 **Admissions:** 13471 **Census:** 171 **Outpatient Visits:** 124180 **Births:** 3087 **Total Expense ($000):** 204071 **Payroll Expense ($000):** 73731 **Personnel:** 1941

★ **VETERANS AFFAIRS NEBRASKA–WESTERN IOWA HEALTH CARE SYSTEM**, 600 South 70th Street, Zip 68510–2493; tel. 402/489–3802, (Includes LINCOLN DIVISION), (Nonreporting) **A**9 **S** Department of Veterans Affairs
Primary Contact: Denise Harrison, Site Manager
CFO: Russell Lloyd, Chief Financial Officer
CMO: Rowen K. Zetterman, M.D., Chief of Staff
CIO: David Daiker, Chief Information Resource Management
CHR: David Peters, Chief Human Resources Officer
Web address: www.va.gov/sta/guide/home.asp
Control: Veterans Affairs, Government, federal **Service:** General Medical and Surgical

Staffed Beds: 186

NE

Many Facility Codes have changed. Please refer to the AHA Guide Code Chart.

LYNCH—Boyd County

NIOBRARA VALLEY HOSPITAL (281303), 401 South Fifth Street, Zip 68746–0118, Mailing Address: P.O. Box 118, Zip 68746–0118; tel. 402/569–2451, (Total facility includes 5 beds in nursing home–type unit) **A**9 10 18 **F**2 3 11 38 52 55 57 79 80 86 96 117 122 132 **P**5 6 **S** Sanford Health
Primary Contact: Kelly Kalkowski, Chief Executive Officer
CFO: Martha Nelson, Chief Financial Officer
Web address: www.ci.lynch.ne.us/health.htm
Control: Other not–for–profit (including NFP Corporation) **Service:** General Medical and Surgical

Staffed Beds: 20 **Admissions:** 63 **Census:** 9 **Outpatient Visits:** 2052 **Births:** 0 **Total Expense ($000):** 1748 **Payroll Expense ($000):** 805 **Personnel:** 23

MCCOOK—Red Willow County

☒ **COMMUNITY HOSPITAL (281363)**, 1301 East H Street, Zip 69001–1328, Mailing Address: P.O. Box 1328, Zip 69001–1328; tel. 308/344–2650 **A**1 5 9 10 18 **F**3 11 13 15 24 30 31 32 33 35 38 40 42 43 44 55 56 57 61 62 66 73 75 77 79 80 81 82 96 102 107 118 119 121 122 135 136 137
Primary Contact: James P. Ulrich, Jr., President and Chief Executive Officer
CFO: Troy Bruntz, Vice President Finance and Chief Financial Officer
CIO: Lori Beeby, Director Information Systems
Web address: www.chmccook.org
Control: Other not–for–profit (including NFP Corporation) **Service:** General Medical and Surgical

Staffed Beds: 25 **Admissions:** 1399 **Census:** 13 **Outpatient Visits:** 42444 **Births:** 127 **Total Expense ($000):** 24184 **Payroll Expense ($000):** 8592 **Personnel:** 210

MINDEN—Kearney County

★ **KEARNEY COUNTY HEALTH SERVICES (281306)**, 727 East First Street, Zip 68959–1700; tel. 308/832–3400, (Total facility includes 50 beds in nursing home–type unit) (Nonreporting) **A**9 10 18
Primary Contact: Connie Jorgensen, Interim Chief Executive Officer
CFO: Mike Clymer, Chief Financial Officer
CMO: John Grove, M.D., Chief Medical Staff
CHR: Donna Dyke, Human Resources Officer
Web address: www.kchs.org
Control: County–Government, nonfederal **Service:** General Medical and Surgical

Staffed Beds: 75

NEBRASKA CITY—Otoe County

★ **ST. MARY'S COMMUNITY HOSPITAL (281342)**, 1314 Third Avenue, Zip 68410–1999; tel. 402/873–3321 **A**9 10 18 **F**3 13 15 17 24 31 32 33 38 55 62 65 66 67 68 74 76 79 80 82 84 96 100 102 106 107 117 118 121 122 **S** Catholic Health Initiatives
Primary Contact: Daniel J. Kelly, President and Chief Executive Officer
CFO: Shawn Closner, Chief Financial Officer
CMO: Dean R. Thomson, M.D., Chief of Staff
Web address: www.stmaryshospitalnecity.org
Control: Church–operated, Nongovernment, not–for profit **Service:** General Medical and Surgical

Staffed Beds: 18 **Admissions:** 573 **Census:** 5 **Outpatient Visits:** 30526 **Births:** 154 **Total Expense ($000):** 11219 **Payroll Expense ($000):** 4331 **Personnel:** 118

NELIGH—Antelope County

★ **ANTELOPE MEMORIAL HOSPITAL (281326)**, 102 West Ninth Street, Zip 68756–0229, Mailing Address: P.O. Box 229, Zip 68756–0229; tel. 402/887–4151 **A**9 10 18 **F**7 11 13 33 34 38 42 52 54 61 62 66 74 79 84 86 96 107 117 119 120 122 136 **P**6
Primary Contact: Jack W. Green, Administrator
CFO: Martha Nelson, Chief Financial Officer
CIO: Jack W. Green, Administrator
Web address: www.amhne.org/
Control: Other not–for–profit (including NFP Corporation) **Service:** General Medical and Surgical

Staffed Beds: 25 **Admissions:** 491 **Census:** 7 **Outpatient Visits:** 32468 **Births:** 24 **Total Expense ($000):** 9294 **Payroll Expense ($000):** 3791 **Personnel:** 105

NORFOLK—Madison County

☒ **FAITH REGIONAL HEALTH SERVICES (280125)**, 2700 West Norfolk Avenue, Zip 68701, Mailing Address: P.O. Box 869, Zip 68702–0869; tel. 402/644–7201, (Includes EAST CAMPUS, 1500 Koenigstein Avenue; WEST CAMPUS), (Total facility includes 99 beds in nursing home–type unit) **A**1 3 5 9 10 19 20 **F**3 5 8 10 13 15 18 20 22 24 25 26 27 28 30 31 32 33 37 38 40 41 42 43 44 45 46 48 49 50 51 52 53 54 55 56 57 59 60 61 62 65 66 68 72 73 74 75 76 77 79 80 81 82 84 85 86 87 88 89 90 91 92 93 94 95 96 97 100 102 103 104 105 106 107 108 109 111 117 118 119 120 121 124 132 135 136 137 **P**6 7 **S** Missionary Benedictine Sisters American Province
Primary Contact: Michael Hammond, Interim Chief Executive Officer
CFO: Dale Pohlman, Chief Financial Officer
CMO: Dean O. French, M.D., Chief of Staff
CIO: Donald Cope, Director Information Systems
CHR: Janet Pinkelman, Director Human Resources
Web address: www.frhs.org
Control: Other not–for–profit (including NFP Corporation) **Service:** General Medical and Surgical

Staffed Beds: 245 **Admissions:** 6531 **Census:** 168 **Outpatient Visits:** 72740 **Births:** 904 **Total Expense ($000):** 105715 **Payroll Expense ($000):** 47876 **Personnel:** 1071

NORFOLK REGIONAL CENTER (284004), 1700 North Victory Road, Zip 68701–6859, Mailing Address: P.O. Box 1209, Zip 68702–1209; tel. 402/370–3400, (Nonreporting) **A**9 10
Primary Contact: William R. Gibson, Chief Executive Officer
CFO: Sharon Broders, Business Manager
CIO: Marilyn Blunck, Director Health Information Management
CHR: Don Dammast, Manager Human Resources
Web address: www.hhss.ne.gov/beh/rc/nrcserv.htm
Control: State–Government, nonfederal **Service:** Psychiatric

Staffed Beds: 179

NORTH PLATTE—Lincoln County

☒ **GREAT PLAINS REGIONAL MEDICAL CENTER (280065)**, 601 West Leota Street, Zip 69101–6598, Mailing Address: P.O. Box 1167, Zip 69103–1167; tel. 308/696–8000 **A**1 2 3 5 9 10 20 **F**3 5 11 13 15 24 25 26 27 30 33 38 40 42 43 50 51 55 56 57 61 62 68 71 72 73 74 75 76 77 79 80 81 82 84 86 88 89 90 92 93 94 95 96 97 100 102 103 104 106 107 108 109 111 115 118 119 120 121 124 135 137 **P**8 **S** QHR
Primary Contact: Lucinda A. Bradley, Chief Executive Officer
COO: Mel McNea, Vice President Operations
CFO: Lana J. Webster, Vice President Finance
CIO: Jim Anderson, Chief Information Officer
Web address: www.gprmc.com
Control: Other not–for–profit (including NFP Corporation) **Service:** General Medical and Surgical

Staffed Beds: 96 **Admissions:** 4768 **Census:** 49 **Outpatient Visits:** 195757 **Births:** 623 **Total Expense ($000):** 84852 **Payroll Expense ($000):** 37302 **Personnel:** 674

O'NEILL—Holt County

★ **AVERA ST. ANTHONY'S HOSPITAL (281329)**, 300 North 2nd Street, Zip 68763–1569; tel. 402/336–2611 **A**9 10 18 **F**3 8 13 15 24 25 26 27 28 30 31 32 33 36 37 38 43 46 48 54 55 56 57 59 60 61 62 63 66 72 73 74 75 76 77 79 81 82 86 96 97 100 101 102 107 108 112 113 118 119 120 122 124 132 135 137 **P**6 **S** Avera Health
Primary Contact: Ronald J. Cork, President and Chief Executive Officer
CFO: Michael Garman, Chief Financial Officer
CMO: Mark Ptacek, M.D., President Medical Staff
CIO: Michael Garman, Chief Financial Officer
CHR: Crystal Kahle, Director Human Resources and Marketing
Web address: www.avera–sta.org
Control: Church–operated, Nongovernment, not–for profit **Service:** General Medical and Surgical

Staffed Beds: 27 **Admissions:** 1068 **Census:** 10 **Outpatient Visits:** 29949 **Births:** 95 **Total Expense ($000):** 18077 **Payroll Expense ($000):** 6402 **Personnel:** 162

OAKLAND—Burt County

★ **OAKLAND MERCY HOSPITAL (281321)**, 601 East Second Street, Zip 68045–1499; tel. 402/685–5601, (Nonreporting) **A**9 10 18 **S** Trinity Health
Primary Contact: Timothy Fischer, Administrator and Chief Executive Officer
CFO: Mike Clymer, Chief Financial Officer
CHR: Karolyn McEnroy, Business Office Manager
Web address: www.oaklandhospital.org
Control: Hospital district or authority, Government, nonfederal **Service:** General Medical and Surgical

Staffed Beds: 18

NE

Hospital, Medicare Provider Number, Address, Telephone, Approval, Facility, and Physician Codes, Health Care System
★ American Hospital Association (AHA) membership
□ The Joint Commission accreditation
○ American Osteopathic Association (AOA) accreditation
△ Commission on Accreditation of Rehabilitation Facilities (CARF) accreditation

OGALLALA—Keith County

★ **OGALLALA COMMUNITY HOSPITAL (281355)**, 2601 North Spruce Street, Zip 69153–2465; tel. 308/284–4011 **A**9 10 18 **F**3 13 15 25 26 27 30 33 38 40 46 55 57 74 75 76 77 79 80 82 84 86 87 96 102 107 118 122 137 **P**6 **S** Banner Health
Primary Contact: Bob S. Edwards, Jr., Chief Executive Officer
CFO: Dena Klockman, Chief Financial Officer
CMO: Kurt Johnson, M.D., Chief of Staff
CHR: Bethany Childers, Manager People Resources
Web address: www.bannerhealth.com
Control: Other not–for–profit (including NFP Corporation) **Service:** General Medical and Surgical

Staffed Beds: 18 **Admissions:** 778 **Census:** 8 **Outpatient Visits:** 64975 **Births:** 95 **Total Expense ($000):** 14472 **Payroll Expense ($000):** 6604 **Personnel:** 113

OMAHA—Douglas County

🞵 **ALEGENT HEALTH BERGAN MERCY MEDICAL CENTER (280060)**, 7500 Mercy Road, Zip 68124–2319; tel. 402/398–6060 **A**1 2 3 5 9 10 **F**3 8 11 13 15 17 18 20 22 24 25 26 27 28 30 31 32 33 36 37 38 39 40 41 42 43 44 45 50 51 53 54 55 56 57 59 60 61 62 63 66 68 70 73 74 75 76 77 78 79 80 81 82 84 87 90 92 95 97 98 99 100 103 105 106 107 108 109 111 112 114 119 120 121 123 132 134 135 136 137 **P**6 8 **S** Alegent Health
Primary Contact: David Tew, Chief Operating Officer
COO: David Tew, Chief Operating Officer
CIO: Dan Connolly, Chief Information Officer
Web address: www.alegent.com/bergan
Control: Church–operated, Nongovernment, not–for profit **Service:** General Medical and Surgical

Staffed Beds: 304 **Admissions:** 14311 **Census:** 166 **Outpatient Visits:** 170567 **Births:** 2826 **Total Expense ($000):** 219245 **Payroll Expense ($000):** 88801 **Personnel:** 1737

🞵 △ **ALEGENT HEALTH IMMANUEL MEDICAL CENTER (280081)**, 6901 North 72nd Street, Zip 68122–1799; tel. 402/572–2121, (Total facility includes 175 beds in nursing home–type unit) **A**1 2 3 5 7 9 10 **F**3 4 5 6 11 12 13 15 17 18 20 22 24 25 26 27 28 30 31 32 33 35 36 37 38 40 41 42 43 44 45 49 50 52 53 54 55 56 57 58 61 66 68 71 72 73 74 75 76 77 78 79 80 81 82 85 86 87 88 89 90 91 92 93 94 95 97 100 102 105 106 107 108 109 111 117 118 119 120 121 123 125 131 132 133 135 136 **P**6 8 **S** Alegent Health
Primary Contact: Ann Schumacher, Vice President and Chief Operating Officer
CIO: Kenneth Lawonn, Senior Vice President and Chief Information Officer
Web address: www.alegent.com/immanuel
Control: Church–operated, Nongovernment, not–for profit **Service:** General Medical and Surgical

Staffed Beds: 471 **Admissions:** 11925 **Census:** 356 **Outpatient Visits:** 67451 **Births:** 756 **Total Expense ($000):** 159130 **Payroll Expense ($000):** 75409 **Personnel:** 1664

🞵 **ALEGENT HEALTH LAKESIDE HOSPITAL (280130)**, 16901 Lakeside Hills Court, Zip 68130–2318; tel. 402/717–8000 **A**1 2 9 10 **F**3 8 11 13 15 18 20 24 25 26 27 28 30 31 32 33 34 36 37 38 40 41 43 44 46 52 53 54 55 56 57 59 61 62 63 66 68 72 73 74 75 76 77 78 79 80 81 82 86 92 94 96 97 99 100 103 106 107 108 109 112 118 119 120 121 123 124 132 133 134 135 136 **P**6 8 **S** Alegent Health
Primary Contact: Cindy Alloway, RN, Vice President and Chief Operating Officer
Web address: www.alegent.org
Control: Church–operated, Nongovernment, not–for profit **Service:** General Medical and Surgical

Staffed Beds: 83 **Admissions:** 4371 **Census:** 46 **Outpatient Visits:** 47830 **Births:** 987 **Total Expense ($000):** 62282 **Payroll Expense ($000):** 27278 **Personnel:** 563

☐ **BOYS TOWN NATIONAL RESEARCH HOSPITAL (283300)**, 555 North 30th Street, Zip 68131–2198; tel. 402/498–6511 **A**1 3 5 9 10 **F**30 31 32 33 58 63 66 77 79 81 82 87 89 94 96 97 120 **P**6
Primary Contact: John K. Arch, Administrator
CFO: Leigh Jean Koinzan, Director Finance
CMO: Patrick E. Brookhouser, M.D., Director and Chief Medical Officer
CIO: Ann Ducey, Chief Information Officer
CHR: Michael Gell, Director Human Resources
Web address: www.boystownhospital.org
Control: Other not–for–profit (including NFP Corporation) **Service:** Children's general

Staffed Beds: 149 **Admissions:** 62 **Census:** 1 **Outpatient Visits:** 168860 **Births:** 0 **Payroll Expense ($000):** 26846 **Personnel:** 668

🞵 **CHILDREN'S HOSPITAL (283301)**, 8200 Dodge Street, Zip 68114–4113; tel. 402/955–5400 **A**1 3 5 9 10 **F**3 11 19 21 23 25 26 27 28 30 31 32 33 38 43 44 46 48 49 50 55 56 57 58 61 62 66 70 72 73 76 79 80 81 82 83 84 86 89 91 94 95 96 97 100 103 107 112 118 119 121 124 132 133 135 **P**8
Primary Contact: Gary A. Perkins, President and Chief Executive Officer
COO: Kathy L. English, R.N., Executive Vice President and Chief Operating Officer
CFO: Michael Brown, Senior Vice President Finance and Chief Financial Officer
CMO: David Christensen, M.D., Senior Vice President Medical Affairs and Chief Medical Officer
CIO: Allana Cummings, Vice President and Chief Information Officer
CHR: Corliss Lovstad, Vice President Human Resources
Web address: www.childrensomaha.org
Control: Other not–for–profit (including NFP Corporation) **Service:** Children's general

Staffed Beds: 142 **Admissions:** 4913 **Census:** 113 **Outpatient Visits:** 149027 **Births:** 0 **Total Expense ($000):** 214622 **Payroll Expense ($000):** 103867 **Personnel:** 1522

🞵 **CREIGHTON UNIVERSITY MEDICAL CENTER (280030)**, 601 North 30th Street, Zip 68131–2197; tel. 402/449–5021, (Nonreporting) **A**1 3 5 8 9 10 **S** TENET Healthcare Corporation
Primary Contact: Linda Neu Ollis, FACHE, Administrator and Chief Operating Officer
CMO: Stephen Lanspa, M.D., Vice President Medical Affairs
Web address: www.saintjosephhospital.com
Control: Corporation, Investor–owned, for–profit **Service:** General Medical and Surgical

Staffed Beds: 334

○ **DOUGLAS COUNTY HEALTH CENTER (284009)**, 4102 Woolworth Avenue, Zip 68105–1899; tel. 402/444–7000, (Total facility includes 254 beds in nursing home–type unit) (Nonreporting) **A**9 10 11
Primary Contact: James C. Tourville, Administrator
CFO: Dee Maine, Director Finance
CMO: Blaine Roffman, M.D., Medical Director
Web address: www.co.douglas.ne.us
Control: County–Government, nonfederal **Service:** Psychiatric

Staffed Beds: 284

🞵 **NEBRASKA MEDICAL CENTER (280013)**, 987400 Nebraska Medical Center, Zip 68198–7400; tel. 402/552–2000 **A**1 2 3 5 8 9 10 **F**3 8 11 12 13 15 16 17 18 20 22 24 25 26 27 30 31 32 33 35 37 38 39 40 41 43 44 45 46 48 49 50 51 52 53 54 55 56 57 58 59 60 62 64 66 68 69 70 72 73 74 76 77 78 79 80 81 82 83 84 86 87 88 90 91 92 93 96 97 99 100 102 103 104 105 106 107 108 109 111 112 116 118 119 120 121 124 125 126 127 128 130 131 134 135 136 137 **P**8
Primary Contact: Glenn A. Fosdick, FACHE, President and Chief Executive Officer
COO: Joe B. Graham, Chief Operating Officer
CFO: William S. Dinsmoor, Chief Financial Officer
CMO: Stephen B. Smith, M.D., Chief Medical Officer
CIO: Lianne Stevens, Vice President Information Technology
CHR: Nat Ponticello, Vice President Human Resources
Web address: www.nebraskamed.com
Control: Other not–for–profit (including NFP Corporation) **Service:** General Medical and Surgical

Staffed Beds: 518 **Admissions:** 25771 **Census:** 385 **Outpatient Visits:** 446967 **Births:** 2709 **Total Expense ($000):** 559614 **Payroll Expense ($000):** 205259 **Personnel:** 4101

🞵 △ **NEBRASKA METHODIST HOSPITAL (280040)**, 8303 Dodge Street, Zip 68114–4199; tel. 402/354–4000, (Total facility includes 22 beds in nursing home–type unit) **A**1 2 3 5 7 9 10 **F**3 8 11 12 13 15 17 18 20 22 24 25 26 27 30 31 32 33 38 40 42 43 44 45 46 51 54 55 56 57 59 61 62 63 65 66 68 72 73 74 75 76 77 79 81 82 85 86 87 90 96 97 98 99 100 102 103 104 105 106 107 108 109 111 112 113 114 116 118 119 120 121 123 124 125 133 134 135 136 137 **P**8 **S** Nebraska Methodist Health System, Inc.
Primary Contact: Stephen L. Goeser, President and Chief Executive Officer
CFO: Linda K. Burt, Corporate Vice President Finance
CMO: William Shiffermiller, M.D., Vice President Medical Affairs
CIO: Roger Hertz, Vice President Information Technology
CHR: Holly Huerter, Vice President Human Resources
Web address: www.bestcare.org
Control: Other not–for–profit (including NFP Corporation) **Service:** General Medical and Surgical

Staffed Beds: 334 **Admissions:** 18901 **Census:** 235 **Births:** 3776 **Total Expense ($000):** 306359 **Payroll Expense ($000):** 120885 **Personnel:** 1875

Many Facility Codes have changed. Please refer to the AHA Guide Code Chart.

☐ **NEBRASKA ORTHOPAEDIC HOSPITAL (280129)**, 2808 South 143rd Plaza, Zip 68144; tel. 402/637–0600 **A**1 5 9 10 **F**3 25 30 31 35 43 62 75 77 79 80 81 82 86 100 120
Primary Contact: Tom Macy, FACHE, Chief Executive Officer
COO: Mark Longacre, Director Operations
CFO: Anna McCaslin, Chief Financial Officer
CMO: Ian Crabb, M.D., Medical Director
CIO: Tim Pugsley, Manager Information Technology
CHR: Kathleen Kelley–Robinson, Manager Human Resources
Web address: www.neorthohospital.com
Control: Partnership, Investor–owned, for–profit **Service:** Orthopedic

Staffed Beds: 24 **Admissions:** 2046 **Census:** 10 **Outpatient Visits:** 43983 **Births:** 0 **Total Expense ($000):** 34007 **Payroll Expense ($000):** 9729 **Personnel:** 214

☐ **SELECT SPECIALTY HOSPITAL – OMAHA NORTH**, 6901 North 72nd Street, 7th Floor West, Zip 68122; tel. 402/572–2714, (Nonreporting) **A**1 **S** Select Medical Corporation
Primary Contact: Thomas N. Theroult, Administrator
Web address: www.selectmedicalcorp.com
Control: Corporation, Investor–owned, for–profit **Service:** Other specialty

Staffed Beds: 36

⊠ **VETERANS AFFAIRS MEDICAL CENTER**, 4101 Woolworth Avenue, Zip 68105–1873; tel. 402/346–8800, (Total facility includes 76 beds in nursing home–type unit) (Nonreporting) **A**1 3 5 8 9 **S** Department of Veterans Affairs
Primary Contact: Albert B. Washko, Director
COO: Nancy Gregory, Associate Director
CFO: Kirk Kay, Chief Financial Officer
CMO: Rowen K. Zetterman, M.D., Chief of Staff
CIO: James Dank, Manager Business Office
CHR: Dave Peters, Chief Human Resources Officer
Web address: www.va.gov/sta/guide/home.asp
Control: Veterans Affairs, Government, federal **Service:** General Medical and Surgical

Staffed Beds: 202

ORD—Valley County

★ **VALLEY COUNTY HEALTH SYSTEM (281353)**, 217 Westridge Drive, Zip 68862–1675; tel. 308/728–3211, (Total facility includes 60 beds in nursing home–type unit) **A**9 10 18 **F**7 13 15 18 24 27 30 31 32 38 40 42 52 54 55 56 57 61 62 69 73 75 76 77 79 86 93 96 99 100 107 108 118 119 120 121 122 132 134 137 **P**6
Primary Contact: Larry Schrage, Chief Executive Officer
CFO: Ashley Woodward, Director Financial Services
CMO: Jennifer Bengston, M.D., Chief Medical Officer
CIO: Josh Dieckmann, Manager Information Technology
CHR: Karlie Koinzan, Director Human Resources
Web address: www.valleycountyhospital.org
Control: County–Government, nonfederal **Service:** General Medical and Surgical

Staffed Beds: 85 **Admissions:** 543 **Census:** 49 **Outpatient Visits:** 20489 **Births:** 6 **Total Expense ($000):** 13535 **Payroll Expense ($000):** 7106 **Personnel:** 217

OSCEOLA—Polk County

ANNIE JEFFREY MEMORIAL COUNTY HEALTH CENTER (281314), 531 Beebe Street, Zip 68651, Mailing Address: P.O. Box 428, Zip 68651–0428; tel. 402/747–2031, (Nonreporting) **A**9 10 18
Primary Contact: Joseph W. Lohrman, Chief Executive Officer
CFO: Joseph W. Lohrman, Chief Executive Officer
CMO: David Jameson, M.D., Chief of Staff
CIO: Frank Vrba, Chief Information Officer
CHR: Sue Leif, R.N., Director Human Resources
Web address: www.ajhc.org
Control: County–Government, nonfederal **Service:** General Medical and Surgical

Staffed Beds: 21

OSHKOSH—Garden County

GARDEN COUNTY HEALTH SERVICES (281310), (Formerly Garden County Hospital), (Nursing Home), 1100 West Second Street, Zip 69154, Mailing Address: P.O. Box 320, Zip 69154–0320; tel. 308/772–3283, (Total facility includes 63 beds in nursing home–type unit) **A**9 10 18 **F**7 10 38 62 63 75 93 94 96 100 107 122
Primary Contact: Carol A. Kraus, Chief Executive Officer
CFO: Jennifer Moffat, Staff Accountant
CMO: Harold Keenan, M.D., Chief Medical Officer
CIO: DeeDee Waltman, Information Officer
CHR: Dodi Moffat, Human Resources Supervisor
Web address: www.gchealth.org
Control: County–Government, nonfederal **Service:** Other specialty

Staffed Beds: 73 **Admissions:** 248 **Census:** 2 **Births:** 0 **Total Expense ($000):** 4857 **Payroll Expense ($000):** 1286 **Personnel:** 52

OSMOND—Pierce County

★ **OSMOND GENERAL HOSPITAL (281347)**, 402 North Maple Street, Zip 68765–0429, Mailing Address: P.O. Box 429, Zip 68765–0429; tel. 402/748–3393 **A**9 10 18 **F**2 11 24 31 38 55 57 67 77 79 96 122 132 **P**6
Primary Contact: Celine M. Mlady, Chief Executive Officer
CFO: Jodi Aschoff, Chief Financial Officer
CMO: Gilberto Collazo, M.D., Chief of Staff
Web address: www.osmondhospital.com
Control: Other not–for–profit (including NFP Corporation) **Service:** General Medical and Surgical

Staffed Beds: 25 **Admissions:** 241 **Census:** 2 **Outpatient Visits:** 4957 **Births:** 0 **Total Expense ($000):** 5566 **Payroll Expense ($000):** 2863 **Personnel:** 71

PAPILLION—Sarpy County

⊠ **ALEGENT–HEALTH MIDLANDS HOSPITAL (280105)**, (Formerly Alegent Health Midlands Community Hospital), 11111 South 84th Street, Zip 68046–4157; tel. 402/593–3000 **A**1 2 3 5 9 10 **F**3 11 13 15 18 20 25 26 30 31 32 33 36 37 38 41 43 44 50 54 55 56 57 60 61 62 63 66 68 74 75 76 77 79 80 81 82 87 88 89 96 99 100 102 103 105 106 107 118 119 120 121 124 132 135 136 **P**6 8 **S** Alegent Health
Primary Contact: Kevin Nokels, Vice President and Chief Operating Officer
COO: Kevin Nokels, Vice President and Chief Operating Officer
CFO: Tim Meier, Chief Financial Officer
CMO: Fred Hosler, M.D., Senior Vice President and Chief Medical Officer
CIO: Kenneth Lawonn, Senior Vice President and Chief Information Officer
CHR: Margaret Breen, Senior Vice President Human Resources
Web address: www.alegent.org/midlands
Control: Church–operated, Nongovernment, not–for profit **Service:** General Medical and Surgical

Staffed Beds: 121 **Admissions:** 2950 **Census:** 35 **Outpatient Visits:** 45451 **Births:** 377 **Total Expense ($000):** 43169 **Payroll Expense ($000):** 22976 **Personnel:** 478

☐ **SELECT SPECIALTY HOSPITAL–OMAHA (282001)**, 11111 South 84th Street, 6th Floor, Zip 68046; tel. 402/898–2700, (Nonreporting) **A**1 9 10 **S** Select Medical Corporation
Primary Contact: Thomas N. Theroult, Chief Executive Officer
COO: Cynde McCall, Chief Operating Officer
CMO: Bill Huerta, M.D., Medical Director
Web address: www.selectmedicalcorp.com
Control: Corporation, Investor–owned, for–profit **Service:** Long–Term Acute Care hospital

Staffed Beds: 30

PAWNEE CITY—Pawnee County

★ **PAWNEE COUNTY MEMORIAL HOSPITAL (281302)**, 600 I Street, Zip 68420–3001, Mailing Address: P.O. Box 313, Zip 68420–0313; tel. 402/852–2231, (Nonreporting) **A**9 10 18
Primary Contact: James A. Kubik, Administrator
Control: County–Government, nonfederal **Service:** General Medical and Surgical

Staffed Beds: 17

NE

Hospital, Medicare Provider Number, Address, Telephone, Approval, Facility, and Physician Codes, Health Care System

★ American Hospital Association (AHA) membership
☐ The Joint Commission accreditation
○ American Osteopathic Association (AOA) accreditation
△ Commission on Accreditation of Rehabilitation Facilities (CARF) accreditation

PENDER—Thurston County

★ **PENDER COMMUNITY HOSPITAL (281349)**, 603 Earl Street, Zip 68047–0100, Mailing Address: P.O. Box 100, Zip 68047–0100; tel. 402/385–3083, (Total facility includes 42 beds in nursing home–type unit) (Nonreporting) **A**9 10 18 **S** Trinity Health
Primary Contact: Michael Hansen, FACHE, Administrator and Chief Executive Officer
CFO: Melissa Kelly, Controller
CMO: Matt Felber, M.D., Medical Director
CIO: Teresa Heise, Coordinator Management Information Systems
CHR: Nancy Suhr, Manager Human Resources and Patient Accounts
Web address: www.pendercommunityhospital.com
Control: Hospital district or authority, Government, nonfederal **Service:** General Medical and Surgical

Staffed Beds: 137

PLAINVIEW—Pierce County

PLAINVIEW AREA HEALTH SYSTEM (281346), 704 North Third Street, Zip 68769, Mailing Address: P.O. Box 489, Zip 68769–0489; tel. 402/582–4245, (Nonreporting) **A**9 10 18
Primary Contact: Becky Lambrecht, Administrator
CFO: Tiffany Guenther, Manager Business Office and Chief Financial Officer
CMO: Richard Bell, M.D., Chief of Staff
CHR: Diane Blair, Director Human Resources and Admissions
Web address: www.plainviewhealth.org
Control: City–Government, nonfederal **Service:** General Medical and Surgical

Staffed Beds: 18

RED CLOUD—Webster County

★ **WEBSTER COUNTY COMMUNITY HOSPITAL (281316)**, Sixth Avenue and Franklin Street, Zip 68970–0465; tel. 402/746–2291, (Nonreporting) **A**9 10 18
Primary Contact: Robert L. Sheckler, Administrator
COO: Robert L. Sheckler, Administrator
Web address: www.websterhospital.org
Control: County–Government, nonfederal **Service:** General Medical and Surgical

Staffed Beds: 16

SAINT PAUL—Howard County

★ **HOWARD COUNTY COMMUNITY HOSPITAL (281338)**, 1113 Sherman Street, Zip 68873–1536, Mailing Address: P.O. Box 406, Zip 68873–0406; tel. 308/754–4421 **A**9 10 18 **F**3 11 13 24 25 30 32 38 55 57 74 79 80 86 96 102 107 119 122 124 135 **P**6
Primary Contact: Arthur H. Frable, Chief Executive Officer
CFO: Jeanine Soneson, Chief Financial Officer
CMO: Christopher Tomhave, M.D., Chief of Staff
CIO: Kari Pierson, Manager
CHR: Shauna Birchard, Director Human Resources
Web address: www.hcchmc.org
Control: County–Government, nonfederal **Service:** General Medical and Surgical

Staffed Beds: 25 **Admissions:** 541 **Census:** 14 **Outpatient Visits:** 38834 **Births:** 48 **Total Expense ($000):** 9293 **Payroll Expense ($000):** 4893 **Personnel:** 131

SCHUYLER—Colfax County

★ **ALEGENT HEALTH–MEMORIAL HOSPITAL (281323)**, 104 West 17th Street, Zip 68661–1396; tel. 402/352–2441 **A**9 10 18 **F**3 11 13 15 24 27 31 38 55 57 61 62 66 69 74 76 77 79 80 82 84 86 87 96 103 107 119 122 124 **P**5 **S** Alegent Health
Primary Contact: Connie Peters, RN, Regional Health Administrator
CFO: Tim H. Schnack, Chief Financial Officer
Web address: www.alegent.org
Control: Other not–for–profit (including NFP Corporation) **Service:** General Medical and Surgical

Staffed Beds: 25 **Admissions:** 505 **Census:** 3 **Outpatient Visits:** 6555 **Births:** 78 **Total Expense ($000):** 9552 **Payroll Expense ($000):** 3324 **Personnel:** 72

SCOTTSBLUFF—Scotts Bluff County

★ △ **REGIONAL WEST MEDICAL CENTER (280061)**, 4021 Avenue B, Zip 69361–4695; tel. 308/635–3711, (Total facility includes 13 beds in nursing home–type unit) (Nonreporting) **A**1 2 3 5 7 9 10 19 20
Primary Contact: Todd Sorensen, M.D., Chief Executive Officer
CFO: David Griffiths, Vice President and Chief Financial Officer
CIO: Lisa Bewley, Vice President and Chief Information Officer
CHR: Steve Hodges, Vice President Human Resources
Web address: www.rwhs.org
Control: Other not–for–profit (including NFP Corporation) **Service:** General Medical and Surgical

Staffed Beds: 89

SEWARD—Seward County

★ **MEMORIAL HEALTH CARE SYSTEMS (281339)**, 300 North Columbia Avenue, Zip 68434–9907; tel. 402/643–2971, (Total facility includes 115 beds in nursing home–type unit) **A**9 10 18 **F**8 10 13 15 24 31 32 38 46 62 73 79 96 104 105 107 117 122
Primary Contact: Roger J. Reamer, Chief Executive Officer
CFO: Greg Jerger, Chief Financial Officer
CMO: Jason Summa, M.D., Medical Director
CIO: Carol Carlson, Director Marketing
Web address: www.mhcs–seward.org
Control: Other not–for–profit (including NFP Corporation) **Service:** General Medical and Surgical

Staffed Beds: 152 **Admissions:** 1001 **Census:** 81 **Outpatient Visits:** 25817 **Births:** 80 **Total Expense ($000):** 23762 **Payroll Expense ($000):** 11739 **Personnel:** 272

SIDNEY—Cheyenne County

★ **MEMORIAL HEALTH CENTER (281357)**, 645 Osage Street, Zip 69162–1799; tel. 308/254–5825, (Total facility includes 63 beds in nursing home–type unit) **A**9 10 18 **F**17 31 32 79 **S** QHR
Primary Contact: Danielle Gearhart, Chief Executive Officer
COO: Jim Hansel, Chief Operating Officer and Chief Human Resources Officer
CFO: Kelly Utley, Chief Financial Officer
CMO: James D. Thayer, M.D., Chief of Staff
CHR: Jim Hansel, Chief Operating Officer and Chief Human Resources Officer
Web address: www.memorialhealthcenter.org
Control: Other not–for–profit (including NFP Corporation) **Service:** General Medical and Surgical

Staffed Beds: 88 **Admissions:** 1025 **Census:** 60 **Outpatient Visits:** 51542 **Births:** 99 **Total Expense ($000):** 62348 **Payroll Expense ($000):** 8834 **Personnel:** 218

SUPERIOR—Nuckolls County

★ **BRODSTONE MEMORIAL HOSPITAL (281315)**, 520 East Tenth Street, Zip 68978–1225, Mailing Address: P.O. Box 187, Zip 68978–0187; tel. 402/879–3281, (Nonreporting) **A**9 10 18
Primary Contact: John E. Keelan, Administrator and Chief Executive Officer
CFO: Sandy Borden, Chief Financial Officer
CMO: Timothy Blecha, M.D., Medical Director
CIO: Gary Keeling, Chief Information Officer
CHR: Jeremy Littrell, Director Human Resources
Web address: www.brodstonehospital.org
Control: Other not–for–profit (including NFP Corporation) **Service:** General Medical and Surgical

Staffed Beds: 25

SYRACUSE—Otoe County

★ **COMMUNITY MEMORIAL HOSPITAL (281309)**, 1579 Midland Street, Zip 68446–9732, Mailing Address: P.O. Box N, Zip 68446; tel. 402/269–2011 **A**9 10 18 **F**11 13 15 24 25 30 31 33 38 43 52 57 61 62 73 77 79 87 107 122 124 **P**6
Primary Contact: Michael Harvey, Chief Executive Officer
COO: Julie Werner, Chief Operating Officer
CFO: Michael Harvey, Chief Executive Officer
CMO: Zak Tempelmeyer, M.D., Chief Medical Staff
CIO: Matthew Steinblock, Systems Administrator
CHR: Karrie Beach, Director Human Resources
Web address: www.syracusecmh.org
Control: Hospital district or authority, Government, nonfederal **Service:** General Medical and Surgical

Staffed Beds: 18 **Admissions:** 177 **Census:** 1 **Outpatient Visits:** 15617 **Births:** 7 **Total Expense ($000):** 6091 **Payroll Expense ($000):** 2935 **Personnel:** 69

TECUMSEH—Johnson County

★ **JOHNSON COUNTY HOSPITAL (281350)**, 202 High Street, Zip 68450–0599, Mailing Address: P.O. Box 599, Zip 68450–0599; tel. 402/335–3361, (Nonreporting) **A**9 10 18
Primary Contact: Diane Newman, Administrator
COO: Diane Newman, Administrator
CFO: Janice Oehm, Manager Business Officer
CMO: Stacey Goodrich, M.D., Chief Medical Staff
CIO: Fred Pooch, Supervisor Information Technology
CHR: Susan Hessheimer, Director Human Resources
Control: County–Government, nonfederal **Service:** General Medical and Surgical

Staffed Beds: 25

NE

TILDEN—Antelope County

TILDEN COMMUNITY HOSPITAL (281317), 308 West 2nd Street, Zip 68781–0340, Mailing Address: P.O. Box 340, Zip 68781–0340; tel. 402/368–5343 **A**9 10 18 **F**17 30 31 38 46 54 55 56 57 82 86 87 122 135
Primary Contact: Julie Roemhildt, Chief Executive Officer
CFO: Sarah Mitchell, Chief Financial Officer
CMO: Thomas Fennessy, M.D., Chief Medical Officer
CIO: Sarah Mitchell, Chief Financial Officer
CHR: Lon Knievel, Assistant Administrator
Web address: www.tildenhospital.org
Control: City–Government, nonfederal **Service:** General Medical and Surgical

Staffed Beds: 21 **Admissions:** 220 **Census:** 4 **Outpatient Visits:** 7659 **Births:** 0 **Total Expense ($000):** 2950 **Payroll Expense ($000):** 1741 **Personnel:** 50

VALENTINE—Cherry County

★ **CHERRY COUNTY HOSPITAL (281344)**, Highway 12 and Green Street, Zip 69201–0410; tel. 402/376–2525 **A**9 10 18 **F**3 7 11 15 17 24 27 30 31 32 33 38 40 55 59 61 62 68 74 79 82 84 86 87 96 107 122 132 135 **P**6
Primary Contact: Brent A. Peterson, Administrator
CFO: Peggy Snell, Chief Finance Officer
Control: County–Government, nonfederal **Service:** General Medical and Surgical

Staffed Beds: 25 **Admissions:** 684 **Census:** 6 **Outpatient Visits:** 14328 **Births:** 112 **Total Expense ($000):** 10189 **Payroll Expense ($000):** 4528 **Personnel:** 116

WAHOO—Saunders County

★ **SAUNDERS MEDICAL CENTER (281307)**, 1760 County Road J., Zip 68066–4152; tel. 402/443–4191, (Total facility includes 59 beds in nursing home–type unit) (Nonreporting) **A**9 10 18
Primary Contact: Earl N. Sheehy, President and Chief Executive Officer
CFO: Annette Stanton, Chief Financial Officer
CMO: Bradley Freidel, D.O., Chief Medical Officer
CIO: Carrie Stephens, Information Systems Coordinator
CHR: Karen Leise, Coordinator Human Resources
Web address: www.saunders–health.org
Control: County–Government, nonfederal **Service:** General Medical and Surgical

Staffed Beds: 82

WAYNE—Wayne County

★ **PROVIDENCE MEDICAL CENTER (281345)**, 1200 Providence Road, Zip 68787–1299; tel. 402/375–3800, (Nonreporting) **A**9 10 18 **S** Missionary Benedictine Sisters American Province
Primary Contact: Marcile Thomas, Administrator
Web address: www.providencemedical.com
Control: Church–operated, Nongovernment, not–for profit **Service:** General Medical and Surgical

Staffed Beds: 25

WEST POINT—Cuming County

★ **ST. FRANCIS MEMORIAL HOSPITAL (281322)**, 430 North Monitor Street, Zip 68788–1595; tel. 402/372–2404, (Total facility includes 67 beds in nursing home–type unit) **A**9 10 18 **F**3 6 11 13 15 24 25 26 27 31 32 33 38 42 43 52 55 56 57 61 62 66 73 74 75 76 77 79 80 81 85 86 89 90 93 96 100 102 107 117 119 120 121 122 124 135 136 137 **P**6 **S** Franciscan Sisters of Christian Charity HealthCare Ministry, Inc
Primary Contact: Ronald O. Briggs, FACHE, President and Chief Executive Officer
CFO: Dennis Dinslage, Vice President Finance and Chief Financial Officer
CMO: Rhett Eckmann, M.D., Chief of Staff
CIO: Jean Meiergerd, Chief Information Officer
CHR: Terri Ridder, Director Human Resources
Web address: www.fcswp.org
Control: Church–operated, Nongovernment, not–for profit **Service:** General Medical and Surgical

Staffed Beds: 92 **Admissions:** 560 **Census:** 62 **Outpatient Visits:** 64247 **Births:** 82 **Total Expense ($000):** 17629 **Payroll Expense ($000):** 9111 **Personnel:** 198

WINNEBAGO—Thurston County

☒ **U. S. PUBLIC HEALTH SERVICE INDIAN HOSPITAL (280119)**, Highway 7577, Zip 68071; tel. 402/878–2231, (Nonreporting) **A**1 9 10 **S** U. S. Indian Health Service
Primary Contact: Sheriann Moore, Service Unit Director
CFO: Audrey Parker, Budget Analyst
Web address: www.ihs.gov
Control: PHS, Indian Service, Government, federal **Service:** General Medical and Surgical

Staffed Beds: 30

YORK—York County

★ **YORK GENERAL HOSPITAL (281336)**, (Formerly York General Health Care Services), 2222 North Lincoln Avenue, Zip 68467–1095; tel. 402/362–6671, (Total facility includes 129 beds in nursing home–type unit) **A**5 9 10 18 **F**3 10 11 13 15 24 25 27 33 38 43 52 54 55 56 57 59 61 62 66 68 73 74 75 76 77 79 80 81 82 86 96 97 99 100 102 105 106 107 115 117 118 119 120 121 122 135 137
Primary Contact: Charles K. Schulz, Chief Executive Officer
COO: Jane Thompson, Administrator and Chief Operating Officer
CFO: Bob McQuistan, Vice President Finance
CIO: John Temple, Director Information Systems
CHR: Barb Koester, Director Human Resources
Web address: www.yorkgeneral.org
Control: Other not–for–profit (including NFP Corporation) **Service:** General Medical and Surgical

Staffed Beds: 154 **Admissions:** 1161 **Census:** 128 **Outpatient Visits:** 40743 **Births:** 161 **Total Expense ($000):** 29926 **Payroll Expense ($000):** 13695 **Personnel:** 351

NE

Hospital, Medicare Provider Number, Address, Telephone, Approval, Facility, and Physician Codes, Health Care System

★ American Hospital Association (AHA) membership
□ The Joint Commission accreditation
○ American Osteopathic Association (AOA) accreditation
△ Commission on Accreditation of Rehabilitation Facilities (CARF) accreditation

NEVADA

BATTLE MOUNTAIN—Lander County

BATTLE MOUNTAIN GENERAL HOSPITAL (291303), 535 South Humboldt Street, Zip 89820–1988; tel. 775/635–2550, (Nonreporting) **A**9 10 18
Primary Contact: Kathy Ancho, Administrator
CFO: Cindy Fagg, Fiscal Officer
CIO: Judi Benvenuto, R.N., Risk Manager and Staff Educator
Web address: www.bmgh.org
Control: Hospital district or authority, Government, nonfederal **Service:** General Medical and Surgical

Staffed Beds: 7

BOULDER CITY—Clark County

BOULDER CITY HOSPITAL (291309), 901 Adams Boulevard, Zip 89005–2213; tel. 702/293–4111, (Total facility includes 47 beds in nursing home–type unit) (Nonreporting) **A**9 10 18
Primary Contact: Tom Maher, Chief Executive Officer and Administrator
COO: Charles Harrison, Chief Operating Officer
CFO: Yvonne Waggener, Chief Financial Officer
CMO: Craig Jorgenson, M.D., Chief of Staff
CHR: Carol Davenport, Director Human Resources
Web address: www.bouldercityhospital.org
Control: Other not–for–profit (including NFP Corporation) **Service:** General Medical and Surgical

Staffed Beds: 67

CALIENTE—Lincoln County

GROVER C. DILS MEDICAL CENTER (290027), Highway 93 North, Zip 89008, Mailing Address: P.O. Box 1010, Zip 89008–1010; tel. 775/726–3171, (Nonreporting) **A**9 10 20
Primary Contact: Jason Bleak, Administrator
Web address: www.dilsmedicalcenter.org
Control: Other not–for–profit (including NFP Corporation) **Service:** Other specialty

Staffed Beds: 20

CARSON CITY—Carson City County

★ **CARSON TAHOE REGIONAL HEALTHCARE (290019)**, 1600 Medical Parkway, Zip 89703, Mailing Address: P.O. Box 2168, Zip 89702–2168; tel. 775/882–1361, (Includes CARSON REHABILITATION CENTER, 900 East Long Street, Zip 89706; tel. 775/881–7000; Edward L. Epperson, Chief Executive Officer) **A**1 2 9 10 19 20 **F**3 4 5 8 11 12 13 15 17 18 20 22 24 25 26 27 31 33 36 38 39 48 49 55 56 57 62 66 68 73 74 75 76 77 79 81 82 84 85 86 88 89 90 91 92 93 94 95 96 97 100 107 119 121 124 133 135 137 **P**5
Primary Contact: Edward L. Epperson, Chief Executive Officer
CFO: Ann Beck, Vice President Finance
CMO: Andrea Weed, D.O., Chief of Staff
CIO: Cheri Glockner, Director Development
CHR: Richard Lawley, Vice President Human Resources
Web address: www.carsontahoe.com
Control: Other not–for–profit (including NFP Corporation) **Service:** General Medical and Surgical

Staffed Beds: 172 **Admissions:** 10122 **Census:** 105 **Outpatient Visits:** 161026 **Births:** 1031 **Total Expense ($000):** 151141 **Payroll Expense ($000):** 57678 **Personnel:** 989

NV

☐ **SIERRA SURGERY HOSPITAL (290051)**, 1400 Medical Parkway, Zip 89703; tel. 775/883–1700, (Nonreporting) **A**1 9 10
Primary Contact: Joan Lapham, Chief Executive Officer
CFO: Sheryl Hayden, Chief Financial Officer
Web address: www.sierrasurgery.com
Control: Corporation, Investor–owned, for–profit **Service:** Surgical

Staffed Beds: 15

ELKO—Elko County

★ **NORTHEASTERN NEVADA REGIONAL HOSPITAL (290008)**, 2001 Errecart Boulevard, Zip 89801–3499; tel. 775/738–5151 **A**1 9 10 20 **F**3 8 11 13 15 18 25 26 27 38 55 57 62 63 66 72 73 74 76 77 79 80 81 82 86 96 97 100 107 118 121 124 137 **S** LifePoint Hospitals, Inc.
Primary Contact: David L. Henson, Chief Executive Officer
COO: Ann Cariker, Chief Operating Officer
CFO: James P. Barbuat, Chief Financial Officer
CIO: Jeff Morgan, Information Systems Director
CHR: Janie Wadford, Director Human Resources
Web address: www.nnrhospital.com
Control: Corporation, Investor–owned, for–profit **Service:** General Medical and Surgical

Staffed Beds: 50 **Admissions:** 2360 **Census:** 18 **Outpatient Visits:** 50418 **Births:** 669 **Total Expense ($000):** 27735 **Payroll Expense ($000):** 13409 **Personnel:** 214

ELY—White Pine County

☐ **WILLIAM BEE RIRIE HOSPITAL (291302)**, 1500 Avenue H, Zip 89301–2699; tel. 775/289–3001 **A**1 9 10 18 **F**11 13 15 25 29 31 32 38 43 55 57 62 63 73 74 75 79 96 100 107 118 135 **P**6
Primary Contact: Richard L. Kilburn, Chief Executive Officer and Administrator
CMO: Steven MacArthur, M.D., Physician
Web address: www.elynevadahospital.org
Control: Hospital district or authority, Government, nonfederal **Service:** General Medical and Surgical

Staffed Beds: 25 **Admissions:** 752 **Census:** 6 **Outpatient Visits:** 74767 **Births:** 73 **Total Expense ($000):** 17328 **Payroll Expense ($000):** 12015 **Personnel:** 152

FALLON—Churchill County

★ **BANNER CHURCHILL COMMUNITY HOSPITAL (290006)**, 801 East Williams Avenue, Zip 89406–3052; tel. 775/423–3151 **A**1 3 5 9 10 20 **F**3 7 11 13 15 25 26 27 30 31 33 38 40 55 56 57 63 66 68 73 74 75 76 77 79 80 81 82 84 86 87 96 97 99 100 103 107 112 135 137 **S** Banner Health
Primary Contact: Charles Myers, Chief Executive Officer
COO: Skip Reeves, Assistant Administrator Operations
CFO: Steven Fraker, Chief Financial Officer
Web address: www.bannerhealth.com
Control: Other not–for–profit (including NFP Corporation) **Service:** General Medical and Surgical

Staffed Beds: 40 **Admissions:** 1898 **Census:** 16 **Outpatient Visits:** 159198 **Births:** 423 **Total Expense ($000):** 43670 **Payroll Expense ($000):** 22093 **Personnel:** 320

GARDNERVILLE—Douglas County

★ **CARSON VALLEY MEDICAL CENTER (291306)**, 1107 Highway 395, Zip 89410; tel. 775/782–1600 **A**9 10 18 **F**8 15 25 27 30 32 38 55 56 57 62 68 73 75 79 81 86 96 99 100 102 107 118 119 135
Primary Contact: William R. Hale, Administrator
CFO: Steve Geidl, Chief Financial Officer
Web address: www.carsonvalleymedicalcenter.com
Control: Other not–for–profit (including NFP Corporation) **Service:** General Medical and Surgical

Staffed Beds: 23 **Admissions:** 705 **Census:** 7 **Outpatient Visits:** 68246 **Births:** 0 **Total Expense ($000):** 28029 **Payroll Expense ($000):** 9157 **Personnel:** 172

HAWTHORNE—Mineral County

MOUNT GRANT GENERAL HOSPITAL (291300), First and A Street, Zip 89415, Mailing Address: P.O. Box 1510, Zip 89415–1510; tel. 775/945–2461, (Nonreporting) **A**9 10 18
Primary Contact: Richard Munger, Administrator
Control: Other not–for–profit (including NFP Corporation) **Service:** General Medical and Surgical

Staffed Beds: 11

HENDERSON—Clark County

★ **HEALTHSOUTH REHABILITATION HOSPITAL – HENDERSON (293032)**, 10301 Jeffreys Street, Zip 89052; tel. 702/939–9400, (Nonreporting) **A**1 9 10 **S** HEALTHSOUTH Corporation
Primary Contact: William Schoonmaker, Chief Executive Officer
CFO: Robert Bollard, Chief Financial Officer
Web address: www.healthsouth.com
Control: Corporation, Investor–owned, for–profit **Service:** Rehabilitation

Staffed Beds: 60

★ **ST. ROSE DOMINICAN HOSPITALS – ROSE DE LIMA CAMPUS (290012)**, 102 East Lake Mead Parkway, Zip 89015–5524; tel. 702/616–5000 **A**1 9 10 **F**3 12 13 15 18 25 26 28 31 32 33 36 38 41 42 43 44 49 50 51 55 56 57 60 61 62 63 66 68 70 72 73 74 75 76 77 79 80 81 82 85 86 87 96 97 100 102 106 107 119 120 121 123 124 134 135 136 137 **S** Catholic Healthcare West
Primary Contact: Renato V. Baciarelli, President
COO: Teressa Conley, Vice President and Chief Operating Officer
CFO: Kevin Walters, Chief Financial Officer
CMO: Stephen K. Jones, M.D., Vice President Medical Staff Affairs
CIO: Sharon Hester, Information Technology Site Manager
Web address: www.strosecares.com
Control: Church–operated, Nongovernment, not–for profit **Service:** General Medical and Surgical

Staffed Beds: 145 **Admissions:** 8795 **Census:** 98 **Outpatient Visits:** 36154 **Births:** 1153 **Total Expense ($000):** 107573 **Payroll Expense ($000):** 49107 **Personnel:** 667

Many Facility Codes have changed. Please refer to the AHA Guide Code Chart.

☒ **ST. ROSE DOMINICAN HOSPITALS – SIENA CAMPUS (290045)**, 3001 St. Rose Parkway, Zip 89052; tel. 702/616–5000 **A**1 3 5 9 10 **F**3 13 15 17 18 19 20 21 22 25 26 27 28 31 32 33 36 38 40 41 43 44 49 50 51 52 55 56 57 60 61 62 63 66 68 70 72 73 74 75 76 77 79 80 81 82 83 84 86 87 96 97 99 100 102 103 106 107 116 119 120 121 123 124 134 135 136 **S** Catholic Healthcare West
Primary Contact: Rod A. Davis, President and Chief Executive Officer
COO: Teressa Conley, Chief Operating Officer
CFO: Kevin Walters, Chief Financial Officer
CMO: Stephen K. Jones, M.D., Vice President Medical Staff Affairs
CIO: Sharon Hester, Site Manager Information Technology
CHR: LeRoy Walker, Vice President Human Resources
Web address: www.strosehospitals.com
Control: Church–operated, Nongovernment, not–for profit **Service:** General Medical and Surgical

Staffed Beds: 245 **Admissions:** 17976 **Census:** 192 **Outpatient Visits:** 56664 **Births:** 2451 **Total Expense ($000):** 216438 **Payroll Expense ($000):** 89892 **Personnel:** 1297

INCLINE VILLAGE—Washoe County

★ ○ **INCLINE VILLAGE COMMUNITY HOSPITAL (291301)**, 880 Alder Avenue, Zip 89450; tel. 775/833–4100 **A**9 10 11 18 **F**3 8 11 15 25 26 27 31 32 33 34 38 42 43 44 52 55 56 57 61 63 64 66 73 75 76 77 79 80 81 82 86 87 96 99 100 102 107 118 119 120 122 124 132 134 135 136 137 **S** Tahoe Forest Health System
Primary Contact: Peter A. Basler, Chief Executive Officer
CFO: Crystal Betts, Chief Financial Officer
CIO: Jay O'Hanlon, Director Management Information Systems
CHR: Marcie Mortenson, Director Human Resources
Web address: www.tfhd.com
Control: Hospital district or authority, Government, nonfederal **Service:** General Medical and Surgical

Staffed Beds: 4 **Admissions:** 20 **Census:** 1 **Outpatient Visits:** 11329 **Births:** 0 **Total Expense ($000):** 7621 **Payroll Expense ($000):** 2347 **Personnel:** 52

LAS VEGAS—Clark County

☐ **DESERT SPRINGS HOSPITAL MEDICAL CENTER (290022)**, 2075 East Flamingo Road, Zip 89119–5121; tel. 702/733–8800, (Nonreporting) **A**1 9 10 **S** Universal Health Services, Inc.
Primary Contact: Samuel Kaufman, Chief Executive Officer and Managing Director
CFO: Lynn Kennington, Chief Financial Officer
CMO: Adel R. Shehata, M.D., Medical Director
CIO: Tom Schoenig, System Director Information Services
CHR: J. Mason Hudson, Administrator Human Resources
Web address: www.desertspringshospital.net
Control: Corporation, Investor–owned, for–profit **Service:** General Medical and Surgical

Staffed Beds: 346

HARMON MEDICAL AND REHABILITATION HOSPITAL (290042), 2170 East Harmon Avenue, Zip 89119; tel. 702/794–0100, (Nonreporting) **A**10 **S** Fundamental Long Term Care Holdings, LLC
Primary Contact: Darrin Cook, Administrator
Control: Corporation, Investor–owned, for–profit **Service:** Rehabilitation

Staffed Beds: 118

☒ **HEALTHSOUTH HOSPITAL OF TENAYA (292006)**, 2500 North Tenaya, Zip 89128; tel. 702/562–2021 **A**1 10 **F**1 3 25 26 43 44 72 73 75 82 119 137 **P**8 **S** HEALTHSOUTH Corporation
Primary Contact: Kenneth D'Amico, Chief Executive Officer
CFO: Marciano Patricio, Chief Financial Officer
CMO: C. Dean Milne, D.O., Medical Director
CIO: Rose Mary Danuloff, Manager Medical Records
CHR: Barbara Staresinc, Human Resources Director
Web address: www.healthsouth.com
Control: Corporation, Investor–owned, for–profit **Service:** Long–Term Acute Care hospital

Staffed Beds: 70 **Admissions:** 716 **Census:** 55 **Outpatient Visits:** 0 **Births:** 0 **Total Expense ($000):** 23999 **Payroll Expense ($000):** 11651 **Personnel:** 212

☒ **HEALTHSOUTH REHABILITATION HOSPITAL–LAS VEGAS (293026)**, (Formerly Rehabilitation Hospital), 1250 South Valley View Boulevard, Zip 89102–1861; tel. 702/877–8898 **A**1 10 **F**3 24 25 53 55 66 72 73 75 77 85 86 137 **S** HEALTHSOUTH Corporation
Primary Contact: Cheryl Williams, Chief Executive Officer
CFO: Ashley Rushford, Chief Financial Officer
CMO: David Oliveri, M.D., Medical Director
CHR: Donna Webster, Director Human Resources
Web address: www.healthsouth.com
Control: Corporation, Investor–owned, for–profit **Service:** Rehabilitation

Staffed Beds: 79 **Admissions:** 1908 **Census:** 70 **Outpatient Visits:** 5591 **Births:** 0 **Total Expense ($000):** 19169 **Payroll Expense ($000):** 10424

☐ **HORIZON SPECIALTY HOSPITAL (292003)**, 640 Desert Lane, Zip 89106; tel. 702/382–3155, (Nonreporting) **A**1 9 10 **S** Fundamental Long Term Care Holdings, LLC
Primary Contact: Frank Bellinger, Chief Executive Officer and Administrator
CFO: Christopher Morrow, Manager Business Office
CMO: Alok Saxena, M.D., Chief of Staff
CIO: Lynn Muserelle, Director Health Information Management
CHR: Danna Botwick, Director Human Resources
Control: Corporation, Investor–owned, for–profit **Service:** Long–Term Acute Care hospital

Staffed Beds: 25

☐ **KINDRED HOSPITAL LAS VEGAS–SAHARA (292002)**, 5110 West Sahara Avenue, Zip 89146–3406; tel. 702/871–1418, (Includes KINDRED HOSPITAL LAS VEGAS, DESERT SPRINGS CAMPUS, 2075 East Flamingo Road, Suite 114, Zip 89119; tel. 702/894–5728; Dianne Chartier, Administrator; KINDRED HOSPITAL–FLAMINGO, 2250 East Flamingo Road, Zip 89119; tel. 702/871–1418; Michael A. Fenello, Chief Executive Officer), (Nonreporting) **A**1 9 10 **S** Kindred Healthcare
Primary Contact: Jennifer Schomburg, Administrator
CFO: Mark Hall, Chief Financial Officer
CMO: Paeel Stewart, M.D., Medical Director
CHR: Fred Herrera, Regional Director Human Resources
Web address: www.kindredhealthcare.com
Control: Corporation, Investor–owned, for–profit **Service:** Long–Term Acute Care hospital

Staffed Beds: 144

☐ **MONTEVISTA HOSPITAL (294009)**, 5900 West Rochelle Avenue, Zip 89103–3327; tel. 702/364–1111 **A**1 9 10 **F**5 88 89 92 93 94 95 119 **S** Psychiatric Solutions
Primary Contact: Ingrid L. Whipple, Chief Executive Officer
CFO: Dana Calhoun, Chief Financial Officer
CMO: William Bauer, M.D., Medical Director
CHR: Dianna Todd, Director Human Resources
Web address: www.montevistahospital.com
Control: Corporation, Investor–owned, for–profit **Service:** Psychiatric

Staffed Beds: 80 **Admissions:** 3588 **Census:** 68 **Births:** 0

☒ **MOUNTAINVIEW HOSPITAL (290039)**, 3100 North Tenaya Way, Zip 89128–0436; tel. 702/255–5000 **A**1 9 10 **F**3 11 12 13 18 20 22 24 25 27 30 31 32 33 38 46 47 48 49 50 57 68 71 73 74 75 76 77 79 80 81 86 96 97 100 102 103 107 119 135 136 **P**1 **S** HCA
Primary Contact: William Wagnon, Chief Executive Officer
COO: J. D. Melchiode, Chief Operating Officer
CFO: Lana Arad, Chief Financial Officer
CMO: Jack Collier, M.D., Chief of Staff
CIO: Gary Sharp, Director Information Services
CHR: Robert Nettles, Director Human Resources
Web address: www.mountainview–hospital.com
Control: Corporation, Investor–owned, for–profit **Service:** General Medical and Surgical

Staffed Beds: 235 **Admissions:** 15358 **Census:** 181 **Outpatient Visits:** 67590 **Births:** 2335 **Total Expense ($000):** 178054 **Payroll Expense ($000):** 62939 **Personnel:** 834

PROGRESSIVE HOSPITAL (292007), 4015 South McLeod Drive, Zip 89121; tel. 702/433–2200, (Nonreporting) **A**10
Primary Contact: Rosemary Thiele, Chief Executive Officer
Control: Corporation, Investor–owned, for–profit **Service:** Long–Term Acute Care hospital

Staffed Beds: 24

REHABILITATION HOSPITAL See HEALTHSOUTH Rehabilitation Hospital–Las Vegas

Hospital, Medicare Provider Number, Address, Telephone, Approval, Facility, and Physician Codes, Health Care System

★ American Hospital Association (AHA) membership
☐ The Joint Commission accreditation
○ American Osteopathic Association (AOA) accreditation
△ Commission on Accreditation of Rehabilitation Facilities (CARF) accreditation

★ **SOUTHERN HILLS HOSPITAL AND MEDICAL CENTER (290047)**, 9300 West Sunset Road, Zip 89148; tel. 702/880–2100 **A**1 9 10 **F**3 15 18 20 25 26 27 30 31 32 33 35 38 41 46 49 50 55 56 57 59 66 68 70 72 73 74 75 76 77 79 80 82 86 96 99 100 102 107 119 135 **S** HCA
Primary Contact: Stephen E. Dixon, Chief Executive Officer
COO: Jen Sweeney, Chief Operating Officer
CFO: Steve Killian, Chief Financial Officer
CIO: Cameron Bellamy, Director Information Technology and Systems
CHR: Robert Brown, Director Human Resources
Web address: www.southernhillshospital.com
Control: Corporation, Investor–owned, for–profit **Service:** General Medical and Surgical

Staffed Beds: 139 **Admissions:** 5753 **Census:** 70 **Outpatient Visits:** 27159 **Births:** 1206 **Total Expense ($000):** 68218 **Payroll Expense ($000):** 29694 **Personnel:** 592

☐ **SOUTHERN NEVADA ADULT MENTAL HEALTH SERVICES (294002)**, 6161 West Charleston Boulevard, Zip 89146; tel. 702/486–6000 **A**1 5 10 **F**5 30 32 63 69 88 90 91 92 93 94 119 121
Primary Contact: James Northrop, Director
Web address: www.mhds.state.nv.us
Control: State–Government, nonfederal **Service:** Psychiatric

Staffed Beds: 293 **Admissions:** 5973 **Census:** 191 **Outpatient Visits:** 146545 **Births:** 0 **Total Expense ($000):** 107473 **Payroll Expense ($000):** 33226 **Personnel:** 492

☐ **SPRING MOUNTAIN SAHARA (294010)**, 5460 West Sahara, Zip 89146; tel. 702/216–8900, (Nonreporting) **A**1 10 **S** Universal Health Services, Inc.
Web address: www.springmountainsahara.com
Control: Corporation, Investor–owned, for–profit **Service:** Psychiatric

Staffed Beds: 30

☐ **SPRING VALLEY HOSPITAL MEDICAL CENTER (290046)**, 5400 South Rainbow Boulevard, Zip 89118; tel. 702/853–3000, (Nonreporting) **A**1 9 10 **S** Universal Health Services, Inc.
Primary Contact: Leonard Freehof, Chief Executive Officer and Managing Director
COO: Jason M. Adams, Chief Operating Officer
CFO: Leanne Shields, Chief Financial Officer
CMO: Dan McBride, M.D., Chief of Staff
Web address: www.springvalleyhospital.com
Control: Corporation, Investor–owned, for–profit **Service:** General Medical and Surgical

Staffed Beds: 210

★ **ST. ROSE DOMINCIAN HOSPITALS – SAN MARTIN CAMPUS (290053)**, 8280 West Warm Springs Road, Zip 89113; tel. 702/492–8000 **A**1 9 10 **F**3 13 15 18 20 22 25 26 28 30 31 32 33 36 38 41 43 44 49 50 51 55 56 57 60 62 63 66 68 70 72 73 74 75 76 77 79 80 81 82 84 86 87 96 97 99 100 102 106 107 119 120 121 123 124 134 135 136 **S** Catholic Healthcare West
Primary Contact: Victoria J. VanMeetren, President
COO: Teressa Conley, Vice President and Chief Operating Officer
CFO: Kevin Walters, Chief Financial Officer
CMO: Stephen K. Jones, M.D., Chief Medical Officer
CIO: Sharon Hester, Information Technology Site Manager
CHR: LeRoy Walker, Vice President Human Resources
Web address: www.strosehospitals.org
Control: Church–operated, Nongovernment, not–for profit **Service:** General Medical and Surgical

Staffed Beds: 147 **Admissions:** 2940 **Census:** 44 **Outpatient Visits:** 9898 **Births:** 223 **Total Expense ($000):** 62859 **Payroll Expense ($000):** 23217 **Personnel:** 473

☐ **SUMMERLIN HOSPITAL MEDICAL CENTER (290041)**, 657 Town Center Drive, Zip 89144; tel. 702/233–7000, (Nonreporting) **A**1 9 10 **S** Universal Health Services, Inc.
Primary Contact: Tim Hingtgen, Chief Executive Officer and Managing Director
COO: Alex Villa, Chief Operating Officer
CFO: Vanessa Kochevar, Chief Financial Officer
Web address: www.summerlinhospital.org
Control: Corporation, Investor–owned, for–profit **Service:** General Medical and Surgical

Staffed Beds: 148

★ △ **SUNRISE HOSPITAL AND MEDICAL CENTER (290003)**, 3186 Maryland Parkway, Zip 89109–2306, Mailing Address: P.O. Box 98530, Zip 89193–8530; tel. 702/731–8000, (Includes SUNRISE CHILDREN'S HOSPITAL) **A**1 2 3 5 7 9 10 **F**3 8 13 15 17 18 19 20 21 22 23 25 26 27 28 30 31 32 33 38 40 46 47 49 50 53 55 56 57 58 59 62 63 65 66 68 70 72 73 74 75 76 77 78 79 80 81 82 83 84 85 86 87 90 96 97 99 100 101 102 103 104 105 106 107 112 116 118 119 121 124 125 127 131 132 135 136 137 **S** HCA
Primary Contact: Sylvia Young, Chief Executive Officer
COO: Steve Otto, Chief Operating Officer
CFO: Daniel Perritt, Chief Financial Officer
CMO: Katherine Keeley, M.D., Chief of Staff
CIO: Alan Burt, Director Information Services
CHR: Stuart Thompson, Vice President
Web address: www.sunrisehospital.com
Control: Corporation, Investor–owned, for–profit **Service:** General Medical and Surgical

Staffed Beds: 645 **Admissions:** 31661 **Census:** 484 **Outpatient Visits:** 100595 **Births:** 4620 **Total Expense ($000):** 431948 **Payroll Expense ($000):** 174119 **Personnel:** 2480

★ **UNIVERSITY MEDICAL CENTER (290007)**, 1800 West Charleston Boulevard, Zip 89102–2386; tel. 702/383–2000 **A**1 2 3 5 9 10 **F**3 8 11 12 13 15 16 17 18 20 22 24 25 26 27 30 32 33 38 40 49 50 51 53 54 55 56 57 58 59 60 62 64 66 68 70 71 72 73 74 75 76 77 78 79 80 82 83 84 85 86 87 96 97 100 102 103 107 118 119 121 127 133 135 136 137
Primary Contact: Kathy Silver, Interim Chief Executive Officer
CFO: George Stevens, Acting Chief Administrative Officer and Acting Chief Financial Officer
CMO: John Ellerton, M.D., Chief of Staff
CIO: Doug Northcutt, Chief Information Officer
CHR: John Espinoza, Chief Human Resources Officer
Web address: www.umc-cares.org
Control: County–Government, nonfederal **Service:** General Medical and Surgical

Staffed Beds: 575 **Admissions:** 30767 **Census:** 485 **Outpatient Visits:** 665544 **Births:** 5104 **Total Expense ($000):** 148821 **Payroll Expense ($000):** 212916 **Personnel:** 3626

☐ **UNIVERSITY MEDICAL CENTER–RANCHO REHAB**, 4333 North Rancho Drive, Zip 89130; tel. 702/656–0467, (Nonreporting) **A**1
Primary Contact: Kathy Silver, Interim Chief Executive Officer
Control: County–Government, nonfederal **Service:** Rehabilitation

Staffed Beds: 34

☐ **VALLEY HOSPITAL MEDICAL CENTER (290021)**, 620 Shadow Lane, Zip 89106–4119; tel. 702/388–4000, (Nonreporting) **A**1 9 10 12 13 **S** Universal Health Services, Inc.
Primary Contact: Gregory E. Boyer, Chief Executive Officer and Managing Director
CFO: Betsy A. Sponsler, Chief Financial Officer
CMO: R. M. Vennart, M.D., Chief of Staff
CIO: Mary Siero, Information Services Regional Director
CHR: Dana Thorne, Administrator Human Resources
Web address: www.valleyhospital.net
Control: Corporation, Investor–owned, for–profit **Service:** General Medical and Surgical

Staffed Beds: 365

LOVELOCK—Pershing County

★ **PERSHING GENERAL HOSPITAL (291304)**, 855 Sixth Street, Zip 89419, Mailing Address: P.O. Box 661, Zip 89419–0661; tel. 775/273–2621, (Total facility includes 25 beds in nursing home–type unit) **A**9 10 18 **F**24 25 30 31 38 54 55 56 57 62 63 66 73 75 81 82 86 90 96 100 107 117 119 122 124 132 135 137
Primary Contact: Matt Rees, Chief Executive Officer and Administrator
COO: Matt Rees, Chief Executive Officer and Administrator
CFO: Marjorie Skinner, Director Finance
CMO: Yousri Gadallah, M.D., Chief Medical Officer
CHR: Cynthia Hixenbaugh, Director Human Resources
Web address: www.pershinggenhospital.org
Control: Hospital district or authority, Government, nonfederal **Service:** General Medical and Surgical

Staffed Beds: 47 **Admissions:** 280 **Census:** 25 **Outpatient Visits:** 12779 **Births:** 0 **Total Expense ($000):** 10858 **Payroll Expense ($000):** 4525 **Personnel:** 98

Many Facility Codes have changed. Please refer to the AHA Guide Code Chart.

MESQUITE—Clark County

☒ **MESA VIEW REGIONAL HOSPITAL (291307)**, 1299 Bertha Howe Avenue, Zip 89027; tel. 702/346–8040 **A**1 9 10 18 **F**3 13 15 25 31 32 33 38 43 50 51 55 56 57 62 68 73 74 75 77 79 80 86 87 96 97 100 102 107 117 119 135 136 **S** Community Health Systems, Inc.
Primary Contact: Sue Conley, Chief Executive Officer
CFO: Jorge Latibeaudiere, Chief Financial Officer
CHR: Matthew Anderson, Director Human Resources
Web address: www.mesaviewhospital.com
Control: Corporation, Investor–owned, for–profit **Service:** General Medical and Surgical

Staffed Beds: 25 **Admissions:** 936 **Census:** 7 **Outpatient Visits:** 17192 **Births:** 214 **Total Expense ($000):** 19956 **Payroll Expense ($000):** 9031 **Personnel:** 141

NELLIS AFB—Clark County

☒ **MIKE O'CALLAGHAN FEDERAL HOSPITAL**, 4700 Las Vegas Boulevard North, Suite 2419, Zip 89191–6601; tel. 702/653–2000 **A**1 **F**7 8 13 14 15 25 26 28 31 32 37 38 46 50 52 53 55 56 57 62 63 68 72 73 74 75 76 77 79 81 82 86 87 88 89 90 91 92 94 96 97 100 102 103 107 124 134 135 136 137 **S** Department of the Air Force
Primary Contact: Colonel Christian Benjamin, USAF, MC, Commander
COO: Colonel Linnes L. Chester, USAF, MSC, Administrator
CFO: Major Kari Turkal–Barrett, Flight Commander Resource Management Officer
CMO: Lieutenant Colonel Markham Brown, Chief Medical Staff
CIO: Major Kevin Seeley, Chief Information Officer
Control: Air Force, Government, federal **Service:** General Medical and Surgical

Staffed Beds: 102 **Admissions:** 2724 **Census:** 11 **Outpatient Visits:** 224880 **Births:** 672 **Total Expense ($000):** 101000 **Personnel:** 1056

NORTH LAS VEGAS—Clark County

☐ **NORTH VISTA HOSPITAL (290005)**, 1409 East Lake Mead Boulevard, Zip 89030–7197; tel. 702/649–7711, (Nonreporting) **A**1 9 10 **S** IASIS Healthcare
Primary Contact: Anthony Marinello, Chief Executive Officer
COO: Michael Heindel, Chief Operating Officer
CFO: Kim Forbes–Daniels, Chief Financial Officer
Web address: www.northvistahospital.com
Control: Corporation, Investor–owned, for–profit **Service:** General Medical and Surgical

Staffed Beds: 198

★ **VETERANS AFFAIRS SOUTHERN NEVADA HEALTHCARE SYSTEM**, Mailing Address: P.O. Box 360001, Zip 89036; tel. 702/636–3000, (Nonreporting) **A**3 5 **S** Department of Veterans Affairs
Primary Contact: John Bright, Director
CFO: Richard O. Hays, Chief Fiscal Service
CMO: Ramanujam Komanduri, M.D., Chief of Staff
Web address: www.va.gov/sta/guide/home.asp
Control: Veterans Affairs, Government, federal **Service:** General Medical and Surgical

Staffed Beds: 52

PAHRUMP—Nye County

★ **DESERT VIEW REGIONAL MEDICAL CENTER**, 360 South Lola Lane, Zip 89048; tel. 775/751–7500, (Nonreporting) **A**9 18 **S** Rural Health Group
Primary Contact: Susan Davila, Administrator and Chief Executive Officer
CFO: Alan Barnes, Chief Financial Officer
CHR: Alecia Stoddard, Manager Human Resources
Web address: www.dvrmc.org
Control: Other not–for–profit (including NFP Corporation) **Service:** General Medical and Surgical

Staffed Beds: 24

RENO—Washoe County

☒ **RENOWN REGIONAL MEDICAL CENTER (290001)**, 1155 Mill Street, Zip 89502; tel. 775/982–4100 **A**1 2 3 5 9 10 **F**3 5 11 13 15 17 18 19 20 21 22 23 24 25 26 27 30 31 32 33 38 40 43 53 54 55 56 57 59 60 61 62 64 66 68 70 72 73 74 75 76 77 79 80 81 82 83 84 86 89 90 91 92 93 94 95 96 97 98 99 100 102 103 106 107 108 109 111 112 119 120 121 124 132 133 135 136 137 **P**6 **S** Renown Health
Primary Contact: James I. Miller, President and Chief Executive Officer
CMO: David Fiore, M.D., Chief of Staff
CIO: Charles Scully, Chief Information Officer
CHR: Kris Gaw, Vice President Human Resources
Web address: www.renown.org
Control: Other not–for–profit (including NFP Corporation) **Service:** General Medical and Surgical

Staffed Beds: 517 **Admissions:** 25475 **Census:** 347 **Outpatient Visits:** 205615 **Births:** 4960 **Total Expense ($000):** 396529 **Payroll Expense ($000):** 137505 **Personnel:** 2143

RENOWN REHABILITATION HOSPITAL, 1495 Mill Street, Zip 89502–1449; tel. 775/982–3500 **F**25 30 31 32 85 86 132 137 **P**5 **S** Renown Health
Primary Contact: Troy Smith, Interim Administrator
Web address: www.renown.org
Control: Other not–for–profit (including NFP Corporation) **Service:** Rehabilitation

Staffed Beds: 62 **Admissions:** 660 **Census:** 30 **Outpatient Visits:** 59512 **Births:** 0 **Total Expense ($000):** 18250 **Payroll Expense ($000):** 9203 **Personnel:** 160

☒ **RENOWN SOUTH MEADOWS MEDICAL CENTER (290049)**, 10101 Double R Boulevard, Zip 89521; tel. 775/982–7000 **A**1 9 10 **F**10 11 15 25 26 30 31 32 33 38 46 49 66 68 72 73 77 79 80 82 87 96 97 100 107 119 120 135 **S** Renown Health
Primary Contact: Alan C. Olive, Chief Executive Officer
CFO: Jane Postin, Chief Financial Officer
CMO: Max Jackson, M.D., Chief Medical Officer
CIO: Charles Scully, Chief Information Officer
CHR: Kris Gaw, Vice President Human Resources
Web address: www.renown.org
Control: Other not–for–profit (including NFP Corporation) **Service:** General Medical and Surgical

Staffed Beds: 76 **Admissions:** 2598 **Census:** 30 **Outpatient Visits:** 55141 **Births:** 0 **Total Expense ($000):** 56782 **Payroll Expense ($000):** 21420 **Personnel:** 323

☒ △ **SAINT MARY'S REGIONAL MEDICAL CENTER (290009)**, 235 West Sixth Street, Zip 89503; tel. 775/770–3000 **A**1 5 7 10 **F**3 11 12 13 15 17 18 19 20 22 24 25 26 27 28 31 32 33 37 38 42 43 44 45 49 50 51 52 54 55 56 57 61 62 63 66 68 69 70 72 73 74 75 76 77 79 80 81 82 84 85 86 96 97 98 99 100 102 103 106 107 109 111 119 120 121 124 135 136 137 **S** Catholic Healthcare West
Primary Contact: Michael J. Uboldi, President
COO: Helen Lidholm, Chief Operating Officer
CFO: Sam King, Chief Financial Officer
CIO: Roy Hagerman, Site Leader
CHR: David Milovich, Vice President Human Resources
Web address: www.saintmarysreno.com
Control: Church–operated, Nongovernment, not–for profit **Service:** General Medical and Surgical

Staffed Beds: 269 **Admissions:** 15203 **Census:** 178 **Outpatient Visits:** 324194 **Births:** 2433 **Total Expense ($000):** 251730 **Payroll Expense ($000):** 93419 **Personnel:** 1635

☐ **TAHOE PACIFIC HOSPITALS (292004)**, 10405 Double R Boulevard, Zip 89512; tel. 775/355–5970 **A**1 9 10 **F**1 3 25 26 31 32 43 44 85 117 119 137 **S** LifeCare Management Services
Primary Contact: Phil Greenhill, Chief Executive Officer
COO: Theresa Fegan, Chief Clinical Officer
CFO: Nena Swenson, Financial Manager
CMO: T. Brian Callister, M.D., Chief Medical Officer
CIO: Kaylene Reeves, Director
CHR: Nelson Coy, Director Human Resources
Web address: www.lifecare–hospitals.com
Control: Corporation, Investor–owned, for–profit **Service:** Long–Term Acute Care hospital

Staffed Beds: 50 **Admissions:** 387 **Census:** 38 **Outpatient Visits:** 0 **Births:** 0 **Total Expense ($000):** 20332 **Payroll Expense ($000):** 8486 **Personnel:** 105

NV

Hospital, Medicare Provider Number, Address, Telephone, Approval, Facility, and Physician Codes, Health Care System

★ American Hospital Association (AHA) membership
☐ The Joint Commission accreditation
○ American Osteopathic Association (AOA) accreditation
△ Commission on Accreditation of Rehabilitation Facilities (CARF) accreditation

★ **VETERANS AFFAIRS SIERRA NEVADA HEALTH CARE SYSTEM**, 1000 Locust Street, Zip 89502–2597; tel. 775/786–7200, (Total facility includes 60 beds in nursing home–type unit) **A**1 3 5 **F**3 5 8 9 11 18 25 26 27 30 31 32 33 34 36 37 38 41 42 43 44 45 46 50 52 53 54 55 56 57 58 60 61 62 63 64 66 68 72 73 75 76 77 79 80 81 82 86 87 88 90 91 92 93 94 95 96 97 100 102 107 117 118 119 121 124 132 133 135 136 137 **P**6 **S** Department of Veterans Affairs
Primary Contact: Kurt W. Schlegelmilch, M.D., FACHE, Director
COO: Peggy W. Kearns, MS, FACHE, Associate Director
CFO: Kathy Munday, Chief Business Service
CMO: Steven Brilliant, M.D., Chief of Staff
CIO: Tony Steverson, Chief Information Resources Management Service
CHR: Debbie Jenkins, Chief Human Resources Management Service
Web address: www.va.gov/sta/guide/home.asp
Control: Veterans Affairs, Government, federal **Service:** General Medical and Surgical

Staffed Beds: 116 **Admissions:** 3465 **Census:** 96 **Outpatient Visits:** 255544 **Births:** 0 **Total Expense ($000):** 147983 **Payroll Expense ($000):** 60944 **Personnel:** 810

☐ **WEST HILLS HOSPITAL (294003)**, 1240 East Ninth Street, Zip 89512–2997, Mailing Address: P.O. Box 30012, Zip 89520–3012; tel. 775/323–0478, (Nonreporting) **A**1 3 5 9 10 **S** Psychiatric Solutions
Primary Contact: Jeffrey Rice, Chief Executive Officer
CFO: Sabrina Patton, Chief Financial Officer
CMO: Philip Malinas, M.D., Chief Medical Officer
Web address: www.psysolutions.com/facilities/westhills/
Control: Corporation, Investor–owned, for–profit **Service:** Psychiatric

Staffed Beds: 95

WILLOW SPRINGS CENTER, 690 Edison Way, Zip 89502–4135; tel. 775/858–3303, (Nonreporting) **S** Psychiatric Solutions
Primary Contact: Jim Serratt, Chief Executive Officer
CFO: Sabrina Pahon, Chief Financial Officer
CMO: Philip Malinas, M.D., Chief Medical Officer
Web address: www.psysolutions.com/facilities/willowsprings/index.html
Control: Corporation, Investor–owned, for–profit **Service:** Children's hospital psychiatric

Staffed Beds: 76

SPARKS—Washoe County

☐ **NORTHERN NEVADA ADULT MENTAL HEALTH SERVICES (294000)**, 480 Galletti Way, Zip 89431–5574; tel. 775/688–2001, (Nonreporting) **A**1 3 5 10
Primary Contact: Rosalyne Reynolds, Acting Agency Director
CFO: Elizabeth O'Brien, Chief Financial Officer
CMO: Lorrie Oksenholt, D.O., Chief of Staff
Web address: www.mhds.state.nv.us/nn
Control: State–Government, nonfederal **Service:** Psychiatric

Staffed Beds: 50

NV

☐ **NORTHERN NEVADA MEDICAL CENTER (290032)**, 2375 East Prater Way, Zip 89434–9900; tel. 775/331–7000, (Nonreporting) **A**1 9 10 **S** Universal Health Services, Inc.
Primary Contact: Mark W. Crawford, Interim Chief Executive Officer
CFO: Gina Anderson, Chief Financial Officer
CHR: Patricia Downs, Director Human Resources
Web address: www.nnmc.com
Control: Corporation, Investor–owned, for–profit **Service:** General Medical and Surgical

Staffed Beds: 80

TONOPAH—Nye County

NYE REGIONAL MEDICAL CENTER (290020), 825 South Main Street, Zip 89049, Mailing Address: P.O. Box 391, Zip 89049–0391; tel. 775/482–6233, (Nonreporting) **A**9 10 20
COO: Jennifer McMillan, Assistant Administrator
CFO: Karin Richardson, Chief Financial Officer
CMO: Vincent Scoccia, D.O., Chief Medical Staff
CHR: Karla Snider, Executive Assistant Payroll and Supervisor Human Resources
Web address: www.nyeregional.org
Control: Corporation, Investor–owned, for–profit **Service:** General Medical and Surgical

Staffed Beds: 44

WINNEMUCCA—Humboldt County

★ **HUMBOLDT GENERAL HOSPITAL (291308)**, 118 East Haskell Street, Zip 89445–3299; tel. 775/623–5222, (Total facility includes 30 beds in nursing home–type unit) (Nonreporting) **A**10 18
Primary Contact: James G. Parrish, FACHE, Chief Executive Officer
COO: Bill Barsanti, Operations Services Director
CFO: Eddy D. Davis, Chief Financial Officer and Administrative Service Director
CMO: Richard M. Ingle, M.D., Chief of Staff
CIO: Eddy D. Davis, Chief Financial Officer and Administrative Service Director
CHR: Rose Marie Green, Director Human Resources
Web address: www.hghospital.ws
Control: Hospital district or authority, Government, nonfederal **Service:** General Medical and Surgical

Staffed Beds: 52

YERINGTON—Lyon County

SOUTH LYON MEDICAL CENTER (290002), 213 South Whitacre, Zip 89447, Mailing Address: P.O. Box 940, Zip 89447–0940; tel. 775/463–2301, (Total facility includes 49 beds in nursing home–type unit) (Nonreporting) **A**9 10 20
Primary Contact: Joan S. Hall, RN, Administrator
Web address: www.southlyonmedicalcenter.org
Control: Other not–for–profit (including NFP Corporation) **Service:** General Medical and Surgical

Staffed Beds: 63

Many Facility Codes have changed. Please refer to the AHA Guide Code Chart.

NEW HAMPSHIRE

BERLIN—Coos County

ANDROSCOGGIN VALLEY HOSPITAL (301310), 59 Page Hill Road, Zip 03570–3531; tel. 603/752–2200 **A**10 18 **F**3 8 11 13 15 17 24 25 26 30 31 32 38 40 42 43 55 56 57 60 61 62 68 73 74 75 77 79 80 83 84 86 92 96 97 102 107 118 119 120 121 122 135 136 **P**6
Primary Contact: Russell G. Keene, Chief Executive Officer
CFO: James R. Brannen, Senior Vice President Finance
CMO: Keith M. Shute, M.D., Senior Vice President Medical Affairs and Clinical Services
CIO: Linda M. Laperle, Vice President Administrative Services
CHR: James R. Brannen, Senior Vice President Finance
Web address: www.avhnh.org
Control: Other not–for–profit (including NFP Corporation) **Service:** General Medical and Surgical

> **Staffed Beds:** 25 **Admissions:** 1857 **Census:** 22 **Outpatient Visits:** 68029 **Births:** 111 **Total Expense ($000):** 41404 **Payroll Expense ($000):** 17974 **Personnel:** 318

CLAREMONT—Sullivan County

★ **VALLEY REGIONAL HOSPITAL (301308)**, 243 Elm Street, Zip 03743–2099; tel. 603/542–7771 **A**9 10 18 **F**2 3 11 13 14 15 24 25 30 31 32 33 36 38 42 43 46 49 50 51 52 53 55 56 57 61 62 66 68 72 73 74 75 76 77 79 80 82 86 87 94 96 97 102 107 119 121 122 124 135 136 **P**6
Primary Contact: Claire L. Bowen, Chief Executive Officer
CFO: Steven Monette, Chief Financial Officer
CMO: Ellen M. Joyce, M.D., President Medical Staff
CIO: Patricia Witthaus, Director Information Services
CHR: Gregg Burdett, Vice President Administration and Physician Services
Web address: www.vrh.org
Control: Other not–for–profit (including NFP Corporation) **Service:** General Medical and Surgical

> **Staffed Beds:** 25 **Admissions:** 1666 **Census:** 17 **Outpatient Visits:** 57979 **Births:** 210 **Total Expense ($000):** 35202 **Payroll Expense ($000):** 16147 **Personnel:** 395

COLEBROOK—Coos County

★ **UPPER CONNECTICUT VALLEY HOSPITAL (301300)**, 181 Corliss Lane, Zip 03576–9533; tel. 603/237–4971 **A**9 10 18 **F**3 7 15 24 25 26 27 30 31 32 33 38 42 50 54 55 56 57 61 62 65 66 68 73 76 77 79 80 84 86 92 96 99 102 107 117 119 122 123 124 135 136 137
Primary Contact: Louise A. McCleery, Chief Executive Officer
COO: Kimberlee H. Daley, R.N., Chief Operating Officer
CFO: Lori Gambrell, Controller
CMO: Gerald Westover, Medical Director
Web address: www.dartmouth–hitchcock.org/ucvh/
Control: Other not–for–profit (including NFP Corporation) **Service:** General Medical and Surgical

> **Staffed Beds:** 16 **Admissions:** 599 **Census:** 6 **Outpatient Visits:** 20317 **Births:** 0 **Total Expense ($000):** 12537 **Payroll Expense ($000):** 6253 **Personnel:** 120

CONCORD—Merrimack County

[★] **CONCORD HOSPITAL (300001)**, 250 Pleasant Street, Zip 03301–2598; tel. 603/225–2711 **A**1 2 3 5 9 10 **F**3 8 13 14 15 17 18 20 22 24 25 26 27 29 30 31 32 33 34 35 36 37 38 39 40 41 43 44 46 49 50 51 52 53 54 55 56 57 58 60 62 63 64 66 67 68 69 72 73 74 75 76 77 78 79 80 81 82 84 86 87 88 89 90 91 92 93 94 95 96 97 100 102 103 104 105 106 107 109 113 114 116 118 119 120 121 123 124 133 135 136 137 **P**6
Primary Contact: Michael B. Green, President and Chief Executive Officer
COO: Joseph M. Conley, Chief Operating Officer
CFO: Bruce R. Burns, Chief Financial Officer
CMO: David F. Green, M.D., Chief Medical Officer
CIO: Deane Morrison, Chief Information Officer
CHR: Robin A. Moore, Vice President Human Resources
Web address: www.concordhospital.org
Control: Other not–for–profit (including NFP Corporation) **Service:** General Medical and Surgical

> **Staffed Beds:** 220 **Admissions:** 11180 **Census:** 148 **Outpatient Visits:** 531240 **Births:** 1394 **Total Expense ($000):** 263514 **Payroll Expense ($000):** 123643 **Personnel:** 2389

[★] **HEALTHSOUTH REHABILITATION HOSPITAL (303027)**, 254 Pleasant Street, Zip 03301–2508; tel. 603/226–9800 **A**1 10 **F**24 25 31 32 54 56 62 72 73 77 81 82 85 86 119 **S** HEALTHSOUTH Corporation
Primary Contact: Catherine Devaney, Chief Executive Officer
CFO: Jeanine Chesley, Controller
CMO: Shanmugam Uthamalingam, M.D., Medical Director
CHR: Erika Pouliot, Manager Human Resources
Web address: www.healthsouth.com
Control: Corporation, Investor–owned, for–profit **Service:** Rehabilitation

> **Staffed Beds:** 50 **Admissions:** 737 **Census:** 28 **Outpatient Visits:** 5394 **Births:** 0

☐ **NEW HAMPSHIRE HOSPITAL (304000)**, 36 Clinton Street, Zip 03301–3861; tel. 603/271–5200 **A**1 10 **F**3 25 26 30 31 32 37 54 60 66 72 73 75 81 82 88 89 91 93 119 124 135 **P**4 6
Primary Contact: Chester G. Batchelder, Superintendent
CFO: Jamie Dall, Director Finance and Support Operations
CMO: Alexander de Nesherea, M.D., Medical Director
CHR: Kimberly Saucier, Administrator Human Resources
Web address: www.dhhs.state.nh.us./dhhs/default.htm
Control: State–Government, nonfederal **Service:** Psychiatric

> **Staffed Beds:** 224 **Admissions:** 2123 **Census:** 204 **Outpatient Visits:** 0 **Births:** 0 **Total Expense ($000):** 59598 **Payroll Expense ($000):** 32989 **Personnel:** 815

DERRY—Rockingham County

[★] **PARKLAND MEDICAL CENTER (300017)**, One Parkland Drive, Zip 03038–2750; tel. 603/432–1500 **A**1 2 9 10 **F**3 8 12 13 15 18 20 24 25 27 30 31 32 33 34 36 38 40 43 46 49 51 55 56 57 62 65 68 72 73 74 76 77 79 80 82 84 86 96 97 99 100 103 104 105 106 107 113 118 119 121 132 133 135 **S** HCA
Primary Contact: Anne Jamieson, Chief Executive Officer
COO: Jeff Scionti, Chief Operating Officer
CFO: Dean Carucci, Chief Financial Officer
CIO: Brad George, Director Information Systems
CHR: Molly Lahti, Director Human Resources
Web address: www.parklandmedicalcenter.com
Control: Corporation, Investor–owned, for–profit **Service:** General Medical and Surgical

> **Staffed Beds:** 82 **Admissions:** 3514 **Census:** 39 **Outpatient Visits:** 110088 **Births:** 357 **Total Expense ($000):** 57311 **Payroll Expense ($000):** 25967 **Personnel:** 424

DOVER—Strafford County

[★] **WENTWORTH–DOUGLASS HOSPITAL (300018)**, 789 Central Avenue, Zip 03820–2589; tel. 603/742–5252 **A**1 2 9 10 **F**3 11 12 13 17 18 20 24 25 26 27 28 30 31 32 33 34 37 38 40 41 43 44 46 49 50 51 52 53 54 55 56 57 58 59 60 62 66 68 71 72 73 74 75 76 77 79 80 81 82 84 86 87 96 97 100 102 103 104 105 106 107 109 111 114 116 118 119 120 121 124 132 133 134 135 136 137 **P**5 7 8
Primary Contact: Gregory J. Walker, Chief Executive Officer
COO: Daniel N. Dunn, Vice President Operations
CFO: Peter Walcek, Vice President Finance
CMO: Paul Cass, M.D., Vice President Medical Affairs
CIO: Jeffrey Pollock, Chief Information Officer
CHR: Erin Flanigan, Vice President Human Resources
Web address: www.wdhospital.com
Control: Other not–for–profit (including NFP Corporation) **Service:** General Medical and Surgical

> **Staffed Beds:** 134 **Admissions:** 6552 **Census:** 69 **Outpatient Visits:** 147464 **Births:** 934 **Total Expense ($000):** 161106 **Payroll Expense ($000):** 68251 **Personnel:** 1104

Hospital, Medicare Provider Number, Address, Telephone, Approval, Facility, and Physician Codes, Health Care System

★ American Hospital Association (AHA) membership
☐ The Joint Commission accreditation
○ American Osteopathic Association (AOA) accreditation
△ Commission on Accreditation of Rehabilitation Facilities (CARF) accreditation

EXETER—Rockingham County

★ **EXETER HOSPITAL (300023)**, 5 Alumni Drive, Zip 3833; tel. 603/778-7311 **A**1 2 9 10 **F**3 11 13 14 15 18 20 24 25 26 27 28 29 30 31 32 33 34 35 36 37 38 41 42 43 44 46 47 49 50 51 53 55 56 57 59 60 62 63 64 66 68 69 72 73 74 75 76 77 78 79 80 81 82 84 86 96 97 99 100 102 106 107 109 111 113 114 118 119 120 121 124 132 133 135 136 137
Primary Contact: Kevin J. Callahan, President and Chief Executive Officer
CFO: Kevin J. O'Leary, Senior Vice President and Chief Financial Officer
CIO: David Briden, Chief Information Officer
Web address: www.ehr.org
Control: Other not-for-profit (including NFP Corporation) **Service:** General Medical and Surgical

Staffed Beds: 97 **Admissions:** 5265 **Census:** 59 **Outpatient Visits:** 153643 **Births:** 777 **Total Expense ($000):** 148523 **Payroll Expense ($000):** 60013 **Personnel:** 1149

FRANKLIN—Merrimack County

★ **FRANKLIN REGIONAL HOSPITAL (301306)**, 15 Aiken Avenue, Zip 03235-1299; tel. 603/934-2060 **A**9 10 18 **F**11 15 25 26 27 30 31 32 33 34 38 41 43 44 45 46 47 48 49 50 55 56 57 58 60 62 64 66 68 72 73 75 76 77 78 79 80 81 82 86 87 89 90 91 92 93 96 104 107 117 118 119 120 121 122 124 133 135 136 137 **P**4 6 8 **S** LRGHealthcare
Primary Contact: Thomas Clairmont, President
CFO: Henry D. Lipman, Executive Vice President and Chief Financial Officer
CMO: Peter Walkley, M.D., Chief of Staff
Web address: www.lrgh.org
Control: Other not-for-profit (including NFP Corporation) **Service:** General Medical and Surgical

Staffed Beds: 31 **Admissions:** 1399 **Census:** 17 **Outpatient Visits:** 53162 **Births:** 0 **Total Expense ($000):** 30713 **Payroll Expense ($000):** 15841 **Personnel:** 255

GREENFIELD—Hillsborough County

CROTCHED MOUNTAIN REHABILITATION CENTER, 1 Verney Drive, Zip 03047-5000; tel. 603/547-3311, (Total facility includes 62 beds in nursing home-type unit) **F**2 10 25 31 32 33 34 36 37 50 52 53 55 73 81 82 85 86 89 90 94 119 121 124 132 135 137 **P**6
Primary Contact: Donald L. Shumway, Chief Executive Officer
CFO: Randal Loubier, Vice President Finance
CMO: W. Carl Cooley, M.D., Medical Director
Web address: www.cmf.org
Control: Other not-for-profit (including NFP Corporation) **Service:** Rehabilitation

Staffed Beds: 181 **Admissions:** 52 **Census:** 151 **Outpatient Visits:** 5875 **Births:** 0 **Total Expense ($000):** 44494 **Payroll Expense ($000):** 23845 **Personnel:** 656

HAMPSTEAD—Rockingham County

☐ **HAMPSTEAD HOSPITAL (304001)**, 218 East Road, Zip 03841-2228; tel. 603/329-5311 **A**1 9 10 **F**88
Primary Contact: Phillip J. Kubiak, President
COO: Cynthia A. Gove, Chief Operating Officer
CFO: John J. Whittier, Vice President Finance
CMO: Kenneth S. Brown, M.D., Medical Director
CIO: Sandra J. Lucia, Director Health Information and Corporate Compliance Officer
CHR: Lisa M. Ryan, Coordinator Human Resources
Web address: www.hampsteadhospital.com
Control: Corporation, Investor-owned, for-profit **Service:** Psychiatric

Staffed Beds: 60 **Admissions:** 967 **Census:** 45 **Births:** 0 **Total Expense ($000):** 14060 **Payroll Expense ($000):** 8544 **Personnel:** 164

KEENE—Cheshire County

★ △ **CHESHIRE MEDICAL CENTER (300019)**, 580 Court Street, Zip 03431-1718; tel. 603/354-5400 **A**1 2 7 10 19 **F**3 13 15 17 18 24 25 26 27 30 31 32 33 34 36 38 40 41 43 44 46 49 51 52 54 55 56 57 60 62 63 66 68 72 73 74 75 76 77 79 80 81 82 84 85 86 87 88 89 90 91 92 93 94 95 96 97 100 102 106 107 109 118 119 120 121 122 124 135 136 137
Primary Contact: Arthur W. Nichols, President and Chief Executive Officer
CFO: Jill I. Batty, Chief Financial Officer
CMO: John Schlegelmilch, M.D., Medical Director Healthcare Improvement Services
CIO: Peter Malloy, Director Information Services
CHR: Julie Green, Vice President Human Resources
Web address: www.cheshire-med.com
Control: Other not-for-profit (including NFP Corporation) **Service:** General Medical and Surgical

Staffed Beds: 146 **Admissions:** 4796 **Census:** 70 **Outpatient Visits:** 125351 **Births:** 504 **Total Expense ($000):** 117249 **Payroll Expense ($000):** 38028 **Personnel:** 1054

LACONIA—Belknap County

★ **LAKES REGION GENERAL HOSPITAL (300005)**, 80 Highland Street, Zip 03246-3298; tel. 603/524-3211 **A**9 10 19 **F**3 5 7 8 11 13 15 18 24 25 26 27 28 30 31 32 33 34 37 38 40 41 43 44 45 46 47 48 49 50 52 54 55 56 57 58 59 60 62 64 66 68 72 73 74 75 76 77 79 80 81 82 84 86 87 88 89 90 91 92 93 96 102 106 107 118 119 120 121 122 124 133 135 136 137 **P**4 6 8 **S** LRGHealthcare
Primary Contact: Thomas Clairmont, President
CFO: Henry D. Lipman, Executive Vice President and Chief Financial Officer
CMO: Peter Walkley, M.D., Chief of Staff
Web address: www.lrgh.org
Control: Other not-for-profit (including NFP Corporation) **Service:** General Medical and Surgical

Staffed Beds: 113 **Admissions:** 5360 **Census:** 80 **Outpatient Visits:** 46667 **Births:** 513 **Total Expense ($000):** 125951 **Payroll Expense ($000):** 59553 **Personnel:** 884

LANCASTER—Coos County

★ **WEEKS MEDICAL CENTER (301303)**, 173 Middle Street, Zip 03584-3561; tel. 603/788-4911 **A**9 10 18 **F**3 11 13 15 24 25 26 27 28 30 31 32 33 34 38 42 50 51 54 55 56 57 60 61 62 63 64 66 68 69 73 74 75 76 77 79 80 82 84 86 87 90 94 96 97 99 100 102 106 107 119 120 121 122 123 124 135 136 137 **P**6
Primary Contact: Scott W. Howe, Chief Executive Officer
CFO: Celeste Pitts, Controller
CMO: Lars Nielson, M.D., Chief Medical Officer
CIO: Eric Livingstone, Director Information
CHR: Linda Rexford, Director Human Resources
Web address: www.weeks.hitchcock.org
Control: Other not-for-profit (including NFP Corporation) **Service:** General Medical and Surgical

Staffed Beds: 25 **Admissions:** 1185 **Census:** 14 **Outpatient Visits:** 78053 **Births:** 124 **Total Expense ($000):** 33760 **Payroll Expense ($000):** 18290 **Personnel:** 329

LEBANON—Grafton County

★ **ALICE PECK DAY MEMORIAL HOSPITAL (301305)**, 125 Mascoma Street, Zip 03766-2650; tel. 603/448-3121, (Total facility includes 50 beds in nursing home-type unit) **A**9 10 18 **F**3 11 13 15 30 31 33 35 37 38 42 44 47 51 53 54 55 56 57 62 63 64 65 73 74 75 77 79 80 86 87 90 96 102 103 107 117 118 119 122 124 133 134 135 136 137 **P**5 6 8
Primary Contact: Harry G. Dorman, III, President and Chief Executive Officer
COO: Harry G. Dorman, President and Chief Executive Officer
CFO: Theresa M. Koehler, Vice President Finance
CMO: Susan E. Mooney, M.D., Medical Director
CIO: Lorraine Nichols, Director Information Services
CHR: Brenda Blair, Director Human Resources
Web address: www.alicepeckday.org
Control: Other not-for-profit (including NFP Corporation) **Service:** General Medical and Surgical

Staffed Beds: 75 **Admissions:** 840 **Census:** 52 **Outpatient Visits:** 47823 **Births:** 280 **Total Expense ($000):** 33703 **Payroll Expense ($000):** 16996 **Personnel:** 363

★ **DARTMOUTH-HITCHCOCK MEDICAL CENTER (300003)**, One Medical Center Drive, Zip 03756-0001; tel. 603/650-5000 **A**1 3 5 8 9 10 19 **F**3 5 6 7 9 11 12 13 14 15 17 18 19 20 21 22 23 24 25 26 27 28 30 31 32 33 34 35 36 37 38 40 41 42 43 44 45 46 47 48 49 50 51 52 53 54 55 56 57 58 59 60 62 63 64 66 68 69 70 72 73 74 75 76 77 78 79 80 81 82 83 84 86 87 88 89 90 91 92 93 94 95 96 97 99 100 102 103 104 105 106 107 108 109 111 112 113 114 116 118 119 120 121 123 124 125 127 130 131 132 135 136 137 **P**8
Primary Contact: Nancy A. Formella, President
COO: Steve LeBlanc, Chief Operating Officer
CFO: Daniel Jantzen, Chief Financial Officer
CMO: John R. Butterly, Medical Director
CIO: Peter A. Johnson, Vice President Information Services
CHR: Richard B. Davis, Chief Human Resources Officer
Web address: www.hitchcock.org
Control: Other not-for-profit (including NFP Corporation) **Service:** General Medical and Surgical

Staffed Beds: 361 **Admissions:** 18485 **Census:** 281 **Outpatient Visits:** 732819 **Births:** 1131 **Total Expense ($000):** 758299 **Payroll Expense ($000):** 364311 **Personnel:** 5325

NH

Many Facility Codes have changed. Please refer to the AHA Guide Code Chart.

LITTLETON—Grafton County

★ **LITTLETON REGIONAL HOSPITAL (301302)**, 600 Saint Johnsbury Road, Zip 03561–3436; tel. 603/444–9000 **A**9 10 18 **F**3 11 13 15 25 26 27 30 31 32 33 38 40 43 44 50 51 55 56 57 62 63 65 66 68 71 72 73 74 75 76 77 79 80 82 84 86 87 96 97 106 107 112 117 119 121 122 124 132 135 137 **P**6
Primary Contact: Warren K. West, Administrator
COO: Peter J. Wright, Senior Director Planning Development and Medical Group Operations
CIO: Peg Buckley, Information Services Coordinator
CHR: Georgene Novak, Director Human Resources
Web address: www.littletonhospital.org
Control: Other not–for–profit (including NFP Corporation) **Service:** General Medical and Surgical

Staffed Beds: 25 **Admissions:** 1359 **Census:** 14 **Outpatient Visits:** 68082 **Births:** 237 **Total Expense ($000):** 45825 **Payroll Expense ($000):** 21137 **Personnel:** 325

MANCHESTER—Hillsborough County

★ **CATHOLIC MEDICAL CENTER (300034)**, 100 McGregor Street, Zip 03102–3770; tel. 603/668–3545 **A**1 2 9 10 **F**1 3 4 9 11 12 13 15 16 17 18 20 22 24 25 26 27 28 30 31 32 33 34 35 36 37 38 41 42 43 44 47 48 49 50 52 55 56 57 58 59 60 62 63 64 65 68 69 70 71 72 73 74 75 76 77 78 79 80 81 82 83 84 85 86 88 90 92 93 94 95 96 97 99 100 102 103 106 107 112 116 117 118 119 120 121 123 124 132 133 135 136 137 **P**6
Primary Contact: Alyson Pitman Giles, President and Chief Executive Officer
COO: Raymond J. Bonito, Senior Vice President and Chief Operating Officer
CFO: Kevin Kilday, Chief Financial Officer
CMO: Joseph Pepe, M.D., Medical Director
CIO: Brian Tew, Vice President and Chief Information Officer
CHR: Margo Compagna, Vice President Human Resources
Web address: www.catholicmedicalcenter.org
Control: Other not–for–profit (including NFP Corporation) **Service:** General Medical and Surgical

Staffed Beds: 224 **Admissions:** 9056 **Census:** 130 **Outpatient Visits:** 148846 **Births:** 909 **Total Expense ($000):** 182970 **Payroll Expense ($000):** 75712 **Personnel:** 1373

★ △ **ELLIOT HOSPITAL (300012)**, One Elliot Way, Zip 03103–3599; tel. 603/669–5300 **A**1 2 7 9 10 **F**2 3 8 11 12 13 15 18 20 24 25 26 27 28 30 31 32 33 34 35 36 37 38 40 41 43 44 45 46 47 48 49 50 51 52 53 54 55 56 57 62 63 66 68 70 72 73 74 75 76 77 79 80 81 82 84 86 87 88 90 91 92 93 95 96 97 99 100 102 103 106 107 108 109 111 112 114 118 119 120 121 123 124 132 133 135 136 137 **P**6
Primary Contact: Douglas F. Dean, Jr., President and Chief Executive Officer
CFO: Richard Elwell, Senior Vice President, Chief Financial Officer and Administrative Services
CMO: Rick Phelps, M.D., Executive Vice President, Chief Clinical Operations & Chief Medical Officer
CIO: Denise Purington, Vice President and Chief Information Officer
CHR: Sabrina M. Granville, Vice President Human Resources
Web address: www.elliothospital.org
Control: Other not–for–profit (including NFP Corporation) **Service:** General Medical and Surgical

Staffed Beds: 264 **Admissions:** 12551 **Census:** 159 **Outpatient Visits:** 363947 **Births:** 2470 **Total Expense ($000):** 225317 **Payroll Expense ($000):** 90553 **Personnel:** 1743

★ **VETERANS AFFAIRS MEDICAL CENTER**, 718 Smyth Road, Zip 03104–4098; tel. 603/624–4366, (Total facility includes 90 beds in nursing home–type unit) (Nonreporting) **A**5 **S** Department of Veterans Affairs
Primary Contact: Marc Levenson, Administrator
COO: Susan Kimmey, Associate Director
CFO: Frank Ryan, Chief Financial Officer
CMO: Andrew Breuder, M.D., Chief of Staff
CIO: Cynthia Obermiller, Chief Information Officer
CHR: Mary Ellen Kenney, Chief Human Services
Web address: www.va.gov/sta/guide/home.asp
Control: Veterans Affairs, Government, federal **Service:** Rehabilitation

Staffed Beds: 90

NASHUA—Hillsborough County

★ **SOUTHERN NEW HAMPSHIRE MEDICAL CENTER (300020)**, 8 Prospect Street, Zip 03060–3925, Mailing Address: P.O. Box 2014, Zip 03061–2014; tel. 603/577–2000 **A**1 2 3 5 9 10 **F**2 3 11 13 15 18 20 24 25 26 27 30 31 32 33 36 38 40 49 50 51 55 56 57 60 63 68 70 73 74 75 76 79 80 81 82 84 86 87 88 90 92 93 94 95 96 99 100 102 103 104 105 106 107 112 113 118 119 120 121 124 133 134 135 136 137 **P**6 8
Primary Contact: Thomas E. Wilhelmsen, Jr., President and Chief Executive Officer
CFO: Michael S. Rose, Senior Vice President Finance and Chief Financial Officer
CMO: Stephanie Wolf–Rosenblum, M.D., Vice President Medical Affairs
CIO: Dwight Muller, Vice President Information Systems and Chief Information Officer
CHR: Merryll Rosenfeld, Vice President Human Resources
Web address: www.snhmc.org
Control: Other not–for–profit (including NFP Corporation) **Service:** General Medical and Surgical

Staffed Beds: 179 **Admissions:** 9763 **Census:** 116 **Outpatient Visits:** 216381 **Births:** 1440 **Total Expense ($000):** 142343 **Payroll Expense ($000):** 71254 **Personnel:** 1333

★ △ **ST. JOSEPH HOSPITAL (300011)**, 172 Kinsley Street, Zip 03060–3688; tel. 603/882–3000 **A**1 2 7 9 10 **F**2 3 7 8 11 13 15 18 24 25 26 27 28 30 31 32 33 34 38 39 40 41 42 43 44 45 49 50 51 53 54 55 56 57 60 61 62 63 66 68 72 73 74 75 76 77 79 80 81 82 84 85 86 88 93 94 96 97 99 100 103 104 105 107 118 119 121 124 132 135 136 137 **P**6 8 **S** Covenant Health Systems, Inc.
Primary Contact: Peter B. Davis, President and Chief Executive Officer
COO: Pam Duchene, R.N., Vice President Patient Care Services
CFO: Richard Plamondon, Vice President Finance
CMO: William Stephan, M.D., Vice President Medical Affairs
CIO: Keith A. Choinka, Vice President Information Systems and Chief Information Officer
CHR: Jacqueline Woolley, Vice President Human Resources
Web address: www.stjosephhealthcare.com
Control: Church–operated, Nongovernment, not–for profit **Service:** General Medical and Surgical

Staffed Beds: 144 **Admissions:** 5104 **Census:** 85 **Outpatient Visits:** 206438 **Births:** 538 **Total Expense ($000):** 133548 **Payroll Expense ($000):** 58609 **Personnel:** 1154

NEW LONDON—Merrimack County

★ **NEW LONDON HOSPITAL (301304)**, 273 County Road, Zip 03257–4570; tel. 603/526–2911, (Total facility includes 58 beds in nursing home–type unit) **A**9 10 18 **F**3 7 11 15 25 27 28 30 31 32 38 43 50 51 53 54 55 56 57 62 65 68 73 75 76 77 79 80 82 84 86 87 96 99 100 102 107 117 118 119 120 122 123 135 136 **P**6
Primary Contact: Bruce King, President and Chief Executive Officer
CFO: Tina Naimie, Chief Financial Officer and Vice President Fiscal Services
CMO: Timothy Wolfe, M.D., President Medical Staff
Web address: www.newlondonhospital.org
Control: Other not–for–profit (including NFP Corporation) **Service:** General Medical and Surgical

Staffed Beds: 83 **Admissions:** 1014 **Census:** 61 **Outpatient Visits:** 166188 **Births:** 0 **Total Expense ($000):** 42327 **Payroll Expense ($000):** 20859 **Personnel:** 360

NORTH CONWAY—Carroll County

MEMORIAL HOSPITAL (301307), 3073 White Mountain Highway, Zip 03860–5001, Mailing Address: P.O. Box 5001, Zip 03860–5001; tel. 603/356–5461, (Total facility includes 45 beds in nursing home–type unit) **A**9 10 18 **F**2 3 8 11 13 15 24 25 26 30 31 32 33 38 40 51 55 57 62 65 66 68 73 74 75 76 77 79 80 81 82 85 86 95 96 97 99 100 102 106 107 117 119 120 121 122 123 124 135 136 137 **P**3
Primary Contact: Gary R. Poquette, FACHE, Executive Director
CFO: John Newton, Assistant Director Financial and Support Services
CIO: David Fitch, Director Information and Facility Services
CHR: Beverly Holmes, Assistant Administrator Human Resources
Web address: www.thememorialhospital.org
Control: Other not–for–profit (including NFP Corporation) **Service:** General Medical and Surgical

Staffed Beds: 80 **Admissions:** 1588 **Census:** 60 **Outpatient Visits:** 48501 **Births:** 251 **Total Expense ($000):** 46238 **Payroll Expense ($000):** 15536 **Personnel:** 406

NH

Hospital, Medicare Provider Number, Address, Telephone, Approval, Facility, and Physician Codes, Health Care System

★ American Hospital Association (AHA) membership
□ The Joint Commission accreditation
○ American Osteopathic Association (AOA) accreditation
△ Commission on Accreditation of Rehabilitation Facilities (CARF) accreditation

PETERBOROUGH—Hillsborough County

★ **MONADNOCK COMMUNITY HOSPITAL (301309)**, 452 Old Street Road, Zip 03458–1295; tel. 603/924–7191 **A**5 9 10 18 **F**3 9 13 15 24 25 26 27 30 31 32 33 34 36 37 38 41 43 50 52 54 55 56 57 62 63 68 72 73 74 75 76 77 79 80 81 82 84 86 87 89 90 91 92 93 94 96 97 103 106 107 119 120 121 122 123 124 135 136 137 **P**6
Primary Contact: Peter L. Gosline, Chief Executive Officer
COO: Sarah K. Taylor, Vice President Physician Practices
CFO: Richard Scheinblum, Chief Financial Officer
CMO: Peter L. Forssell, Medical Director
CIO: Carol Roosa, Chief Information Officer
CHR: Michael Blood, Director Human Resources
Web address: www.monadnockhospital.org
Control: Other not–for–profit (including NFP Corporation) **Service:** General Medical and Surgical

Staffed Beds: 25 **Admissions:** 1549 **Census:** 17 **Outpatient Visits:** 160449 **Births:** 357 **Total Expense ($000):** 55107 **Payroll Expense ($000):** 26058 **Personnel:** 686

PLYMOUTH—Grafton County

★ **SPEARE MEMORIAL HOSPITAL (301311)**, 16 Hospital Road, Zip 03264–1199; tel. 603/536–1120 **A**9 10 18 **F**3 8 13 15 24 25 27 28 30 31 32 33 37 38 44 55 56 57 62 68 73 74 75 76 77 79 80 86 87 96 102 107 119 121 122 133 135 136 **P**8
Primary Contact: Michelle McEwen, President and Chief Executive Officer
CFO: Peter Kritikos, Chief Financial Officer
CMO: Joseph Ebner, M.D., Chief Medical Officer
CIO: Jerry Coffey, Director Information Technology
CHR: Lauri Bolognani, Human Resources Officer
Web address: www.spearehospital.com
Control: Other not–for–profit (including NFP Corporation) **Service:** General Medical and Surgical

Staffed Beds: 25 **Admissions:** 1373 **Census:** 12 **Outpatient Visits:** 73977 **Births:** 178 **Total Expense ($000):** 32262 **Payroll Expense ($000):** 15385 **Personnel:** 274

PORTSMOUTH—Rockingham County

⊠ **PORTSMOUTH REGIONAL HOSPITAL (300029)**, 333 Borthwick Avenue, Zip 03801–7004; tel. 603/436–5110 **A**1 9 10 **F**3 8 12 13 15 18 20 22 24 25 26 27 28 33 34 36 38 39 40 43 44 50 51 54 55 56 57 59 60 62 66 68 72 73 74 75 76 77 79 81 82 84 86 87 88 89 90 91 92 93 94 95 96 97 99 100 103 105 106 107 113 118 119 120 121 124 135 136 137 **P**1 **S** HCA
Primary Contact: William J. Schuler, Chief Executive Officer
COO: Stuart Hemming, Chief Operating Officer
CFO: Richard Senger, Chief Financial Officer
CIO: Ed Sovetskhy, Director Information Services
CHR: Jackie Brayton, Vice President Human Resources
Web address: www.portsmouthhospital.com
Control: Corporation, Investor–owned, for–profit **Service:** General Medical and Surgical

Staffed Beds: 165 **Admissions:** 6809 **Census:** 97 **Outpatient Visits:** 139817 **Births:** 699 **Personnel:** 761

ROCHESTER—Strafford County

★ **FRISBIE MEMORIAL HOSPITAL (300014)**, 11 Whitehall Road, Zip 03867–3297; tel. 603/332–5211 **A**9 10 **F**3 7 11 13 17 18 19 24 25 27 28 30 31 32 33 38 43 46 49 50 54 55 56 57 62 66 68 73 74 75 76 77 79 81 82 84 86 87 88 93 94 95 96 100 103 104 106 107 118 119 121 124 133 135 136 **P**5 8
Primary Contact: Alvin D. Felgar, President and Chief Executive Officer
CFO: John A. Marzinzik, Vice President Finance
CMO: Sara Stacey, D.O., Vice President Medical Affairs
CHR: Carol Themelis, Vice President Human Resources
Web address: www.frisbiehospital.com
Control: Other not–for–profit (including NFP Corporation) **Service:** General Medical and Surgical

Staffed Beds: 70 **Admissions:** 3906 **Census:** 47 **Outpatient Visits:** 103432 **Births:** 378 **Total Expense ($000):** 98435 **Payroll Expense ($000):** 37548 **Personnel:** 821

SALEM—Rockingham County

☐ **NORTHEAST REHABILITATION HOSPITAL (303026)**, 70 Butler Street, Zip 03079–3925; tel. 603/893–2900 **A**1 9 10 **F**25 30 31 32 33 43 52 53 55 56 57 61 62 66 72 73 75 77 80 81 82 85 86 119 120 121 124 135
Primary Contact: John F. Prochilo, Chief Executive Officer and Administrator
CFO: James E. Murphy, Chief Financial Officer
CMO: James A. Whitlock, M.D., Medical Director
CIO: Kathleen Blaine, Director Information Systems
CHR: Thomas A. Prince, Vice President Operations and Human Resources
Web address: www.northeastrehab.com
Control: Corporation, Investor–owned, for–profit **Service:** Rehabilitation

Staffed Beds: 80 **Admissions:** 1506 **Census:** 64 **Outpatient Visits:** 163461 **Births:** 0 **Total Expense ($000):** 41223 **Payroll Expense ($000):** 22141 **Personnel:** 365

WOLFEBORO—Carroll County

★ **HUGGINS HOSPITAL (301312)**, 240 South Main Street, Zip 03894–4455, Mailing Address: P.O. Box 912, Zip 03894–0912; tel. 603/569–7500, (Total facility includes 27 beds in nursing home–type unit) **A**9 10 18 **F**2 10 11 13 15 24 30 31 32 38 50 54 55 56 57 62 63 68 72 73 74 75 77 79 80 81 82 86 87 96 107 112 115 117 119 121 122 124 135 136 **P**6
Primary Contact: David W. Tower, FACHE, President
CFO: Daniel R. O'Neill, Vice President Finance
CMO: John Boornazian, M.D., Chief Medical Officer
CHR: Angela Closson, Director Human Resources
Web address: www.hugginshospital.org
Control: Other not–for–profit (including NFP Corporation) **Service:** General Medical and Surgical

Staffed Beds: 52 **Admissions:** 1942 **Census:** 35 **Outpatient Visits:** 106771 **Births:** 102 **Total Expense ($000):** 34778 **Payroll Expense ($000):** 15582 **Personnel:** 311

WOODSVILLE—Grafton County

★ **COTTAGE HOSPITAL (301301)**, Swiftwater Road, Zip 03785–2001, Mailing Address: P.O. Box 2001, Zip 03785–2001; tel. 603/747–2761 **A**9 10 18 **F**3 11 13 15 24 25 26 27 30 31 32 33 38 40 43 46 49 50 56 57 62 63 65 66 68 72 73 74 75 76 77 79 80 82 84 86 87 96 100 102 107 117 119 121 122 124 135 136 137 **P**8
Primary Contact: Reginald J. Lavoie, Administrator
CFO: Steven L. Plant, Chief Financial Officer
CHR: Helen Torrey, Director Human Resources
Web address: www.cottagehospital.org
Control: Other not–for–profit (including NFP Corporation) **Service:** General Medical and Surgical

Staffed Beds: 25 **Admissions:** 792 **Census:** 7 **Outpatient Visits:** 43219 **Births:** 101 **Total Expense ($000):** 23497 **Payroll Expense ($000):** 10290 **Personnel:** 192

Many Facility Codes have changed. Please refer to the AHA Guide Code Chart.

NEW JERSEY

ANCORA—Camden County

☐ **ANCORA PSYCHIATRIC HOSPITAL (314005)**, 301 Spring Garden Road, Zip 08037–9699; tel. 609/561–1700, (Nonreporting) **A**1 10 **S** Division of Mental Health Services, Department of Human Services, State of New Jersey
Primary Contact: LaTanya Wood El, Chief Executive Officer
COO: Joseph Canale, Assistant Business Manager
CFO: John Holmes, Business Manager
CMO: Marie Hasson, M.D., Acting Medical Director
CIO: Debbie Bensel, Director Information Technology Development
CHR: Terry O'Lone, Manager Human Resources
Web address: www.peoplefirstnurses.nj.gov/ancora.htm
Control: State–Government, nonfederal **Service:** Psychiatric

Staffed Beds: 709

ATLANTIC CITY—Atlantic County

★☐ **ATLANTICARE REGIONAL MEDICAL CENTER (310064)**, 1925 Pacific Avenue, Zip 08401–6713; tel. 609/345–4000, (Includes ATLANTIC CITY MEDICAL CENTER–MAINLAND DIVISION, Jimmie Leeds Road, Pomona, Zip 08240; tel. 609/652–1000) **A**1 2 10 **F**1 3 4 7 11 12 13 15 16 17 18 20 22 25 26 27 30 31 32 33 38 40 42 43 44 45 46 47 48 49 57 58 59 60 62 65 66 68 70 71 72 73 74 76 77 78 79 80 81 82 83 84 85 87 88 92 93 96 97 98 99 100 101 102 103 106 107 108 109 111 112 114 117 119 121 123 124 132 134 135 136 **P**6 **S** AtlantiCare
Primary Contact: David P. Tilton, President and Chief Executive Officer
COO: Lori Herndon, Vice President and Chief Operating Officer
CFO: Walter Greiner, Chief Financial Officer
CMO: Marilouise Venditti, M.D., Chief Medical Officer
CIO: Daniel Morreale, Chief Information Officer
CHR: Richard Lovering, Corporate Vice President Human Resources and Organizational Development
Web address: www.atlanticare.org
Control: Other not–for–profit (including NFP Corporation) **Service:** General Medical and Surgical

Staffed Beds: 494 **Admissions:** 28133 **Census:** 380 **Outpatient Visits:** 264652 **Births:** 2380 **Total Expense ($000):** 448431 **Payroll Expense ($000):** 202108 **Personnel:** 3924

BAYONNE—Hudson County

★☐ **BAYONNE MEDICAL CENTER (310025)**, 29 East 29th Street, Zip 07002–4699; tel. 201/858–5000 **A**1 2 6 9 10 **F**3 18 20 24 25 27 28 37 38 41 46 49 50 56 57 59 63 64 68 72 73 74 76 77 79 80 82 84 87 88 92 96 97 99 100 102 106 107 108 109 111 119 121 135 136 137 **S** Bridge Regional Health System
Primary Contact: Daniel A. Kane, Dr.P.h., President and Chief Executive Officer
COO: Marvin Apsel, Acting Chief Operating Officer and Senior Vice President
CFO: Gary G. Terrinoni, Chief Financial Officer
CMO: John Dedousis, M.D., President Medical Staff
CIO: Richard T. Pery, Chief Information Officer
CHR: Jennifer Dobin, Vice President Human Resources
Web address: www.bayonnemedicalcenter.org
Control: Other not–for–profit (including NFP Corporation) **Service:** General Medical and Surgical

Staffed Beds: 206 **Admissions:** 7010 **Census:** 129 **Births:** 0 **Payroll Expense ($000):** 48492

BELLE MEAD—Somerset County

★ **CARRIER CLINIC (314012)**, 252 County Route 601, Zip 08502–0147, Mailing Address: P.O. Box 147, Zip 08502–0147; tel. 908/281–1000 **A**3 5 10 **F**4 5 30 31 32 88 89 90 91 92 93 **P**6
Primary Contact: C. Richard Sarle, CPA, FACHE, President and Chief Executive Officer
COO: Mary Pawlikowski, Chief Operating Officer
CFO: Randolph Jacobson, Chief Financial Officer
CMO: David Greenspan, M.D., Medical Director
CIO: Peter Schwartz, Manager Information Services
Web address: www.carrier.org
Control: Other not–for–profit (including NFP Corporation) **Service:** Psychiatric

Staffed Beds: 260 **Admissions:** 4235 **Census:** 188 **Outpatient Visits:** 0 **Births:** 0 **Total Expense ($000):** 46776 **Payroll Expense ($000):** 27272 **Personnel:** 461

EAST MOUNTAIN HOSPITAL (314026), 40 East Mountain Road, Zip 8502; tel. 908/281–1545, (Nonreporting) **A**10
Primary Contact: Peter Casey, Acting Director
Control: Corporation, Investor–owned, for–profit **Service:** Other specialty

Staffed Beds: 16

BELLEVILLE—Essex County

★☐ **CLARA MAASS MEDICAL CENTER (310009)**, One Clara Maass Drive, Zip 07109–3557; tel. 973/450–2000 **A**1 2 9 10 **F**1 3 4 8 11 13 15 16 17 18 24 25 26 27 30 31 32 33 38 39 40 43 47 49 50 54 55 56 57 58 59 61 62 64 65 66 68 70 71 72 73 74 76 77 78 79 80 81 82 83 84 85 86 88 90 91 92 93 96 97 100 102 105 106 107 108 109 111 114 117 118 119 121 132 135 136 137 **P**5 **S** Saint Barnabas Health Care System
Primary Contact: Thomas A. Biga, Executive Director
CMO: Frank Mazzarella, M.D., Vice President Medical Affairs
CIO: Michael McTigue, Chief Information Officer
Web address: www.sbhcs.com
Control: Other not–for–profit (including NFP Corporation) **Service:** General Medical and Surgical

Staffed Beds: 426 **Admissions:** 15988 **Census:** 204 **Outpatient Visits:** 322878 **Births:** 1463 **Total Expense ($000):** 171645 **Payroll Expense ($000):** 75775 **Personnel:** 1338

SELECT SPECIALTY HOSPITAL–BELLEVILLE See Select Specialty Hospital of Northeast, Rochelle Park

BERKELEY HEIGHTS—Union County

★ **RUNNELLS SPECIALIZED HOSPITAL OF UNION COUNTY (312002)**, (Long Term Care Nursing Home), 40 Watchung Way, Zip 07922–2618; tel. 908/771–5700, (Total facility includes 300 beds in nursing home–type unit) **A**10 **F**3 6 11 12 25 26 29 31 32 33 34 36 41 43 44 50 54 55 56 57 62 63 66 69 81 82 85 86 88 93 117 119 132 135 137 **P**6
Primary Contact: Joseph W. Sharp, Administrator
COO: Joan Wheeler, MSN, R.N., Associate Administrator
CFO: Michael Drummond, Chief Financial Officer
CMO: Raymond Lanza, D.O., Medical Director
CIO: Margaret A. Salisbury, Director Marketing
Web address: www.ucnj.org/runnells
Control: County–Government, nonfederal **Service:** Other specialty

Staffed Beds: 369 **Admissions:** 1232 **Census:** 343 **Outpatient Visits:** 1253 **Births:** 0 **Total Expense ($000):** 45006 **Payroll Expense ($000):** 30321 **Personnel:** 594

BERLIN—Camden County

★☐ **VIRTUA WEST JERSEY HOSPITAL–BERLIN (310022)**, 100 Townsend Avenue, Zip 08009–9035; tel. 856/322–3000, (Nonreporting) **A**1 10 **S** Virtua Health
Primary Contact: Christopher A. Chekouras, Vice President and Chief Operating Officer
COO: Christopher A. Chekouras, Vice President and Chief Operating Officer
CFO: Robert Segin, Chief Financial Officer
CMO: Joseph Reichman, M.D., Vice President Clinical Outcomes and Medical Affairs
CIO: John Bloomer, Vice President and Chief Information Officer
CHR: AnneMarie Horan, Director Human Resources
Web address: www.virtua.org
Control: Other not–for–profit (including NFP Corporation) **Service:** General Medical and Surgical

Staffed Beds: 84

NJ

Hospital, Medicare Provider Number, Address, Telephone, Approval, Facility, and Physician Codes, Health Care System

★ American Hospital Association (AHA) membership
☐ The Joint Commission accreditation
○ American Osteopathic Association (AOA) accreditation
△ Commission on Accreditation of Rehabilitation Facilities (CARF) accreditation

BLACKWOOD—Camden County

★ **CAMDEN COUNTY HEALTH SERVICES CENTER (314018)**, 20 North Woodbury Turnersville Road, Zip 08012–2799; tel. 856/374–6600, (Total facility includes 300 beds in nursing home–type unit) **A**1 10 **F**4 30 31 32 44 54 63 82 88 91 93 117 119 135 137
Primary Contact: Kevin G. Halpern, Chief Executive Officer
COO: Gene Lynam, Chief Operating Officer and Treasurer
CFO: Gene Lynam, Chief Operating Officer and Treasurer
CMO: Michael S. DeShields, M.D., Director Medical Affairs
CIO: Frank Maestrale, Director Information Technology
CHR: Brian Eisen, Director Human Resources
Web address: www.cchsc.com
Control: County–Government, nonfederal **Service:** Psychiatric

Staffed Beds: 458 **Admissions:** 1409 **Census:** 440 **Outpatient Visits:** 42 **Births:** 0 **Total Expense ($000):** 64498 **Payroll Expense ($000):** 28502 **Personnel:** 541

BOONTON TOWNSHIP—Morris County

SAINT CLARE'S HOSPITAL/BOONTON TOWNSHIP See Saint Clare's Hospital, Dover

BRICK TOWNSHIP—Ocean County

★ **OCEAN MEDICAL CENTER (310052)**, 425 Jack Martin Boulevard, Zip 8724; tel. 732/840–2200 **A**1 2 9 10 **F**3 6 11 13 15 17 18 20 24 25 26 27 28 30 31 32 33 34 38 39 41 43 44 46 49 51 52 54 55 57 58 59 62 64 66 67 68 71 72 73 74 75 76 77 78 79 80 81 82 84 86 87 90 91 92 93 96 97 100 102 107 109 111 114 118 119 121 123 124 133 135 136 **P**7 **S** Meridian Health
Primary Contact: W. Peter Daniels, President
COO: Richard Epstein, Vice President Operations
CFO: William Phillips, Senior Vice President Finance and Chief Financial Officer
CIO: Rebecca Weber, Vice President Information System and Chief Information Officer
CHR: John E. Sindoni, Senior Vice President Human Resources
Web address: www.meridianhealth.com
Control: Other not–for–profit (including NFP Corporation) **Service:** General Medical and Surgical

Staffed Beds: 229 **Admissions:** 14530 **Census:** 190 **Outpatient Visits:** 137954 **Births:** 1082 **Total Expense ($000):** 173427 **Payroll Expense ($000):** 74895 **Personnel:** 999

BRIDGETON—Cumberland County

BRIDGETON HEALTH CENTER See South Jersey Healthcare – Regional Medical Center, Vineland

BROWNS MILLS—Burlington County

☐ **DEBORAH HEART AND LUNG CENTER (310031)**, 200 Trenton Road, Zip 08015–1799; tel. 609/893–6611, (Nonreporting) **A**1 3 5 9 10 13
Primary Contact: John R. Ernst, President and Chief Executive Officer
CFO: R. Grant Leidy, Vice President Finance
CMO: Lynn McGrath, M.D., Vice President Medical Affairs
CHR: James Carlino, Director Human Resources
Web address: www.deborah.org
Control: Other not–for–profit (including NFP Corporation) **Service:** Other specialty

Staffed Beds: 161

CAMDEN—Camden County

★ **COOPER HEALTH SYSTEM (310014)**, One Cooper Plaza, Zip 08103–1489; tel. 856/342–2000 **A**1 2 3 5 8 9 10 **F**3 5 8 9 11 12 13 15 17 18 20 22 25 26 27 28 30 31 32 33 34 35 36 37 38 40 41 43 46 47 48 49 50 51 53 54 55 56 57 58 60 62 63 64 66 68 70 71 72 73 74 76 77 79 80 81 82 83 84 86 87 88 89 90 91 92 93 94 96 97 99 100 102 103 104 105 106 107 109 111 112 113 114 116 118 119 120 121 123 124 135 136 137 **P**6
Primary Contact: John P. Sheridan, Jr., President and Chief Executive Officer
COO: Jeffrey N. Yarmel, Senior Executive Vice President and Chief Operating Officer
CFO: John Gates, Chief Financial Officer
CMO: Simon J. Samaha, M.D., Senior Executive Vice President and Chief Medical Officer
CIO: Karen Graham, Chief Information Officer
CHR: Douglas Allen, Vice President Human Resources
Web address: www.cooperhealth.org
Control: Other not–for–profit (including NFP Corporation) **Service:** General Medical and Surgical

Staffed Beds: 438 **Admissions:** 23523 **Census:** 312 **Outpatient Visits:** 231602 **Births:** 2352 **Total Expense ($000):** 455333 **Payroll Expense ($000):** 182103 **Personnel:** 4642

★ △ **OUR LADY OF LOURDES MEDICAL CENTER (310029)**, 1600 Haddon Avenue, Zip 08103–3117; tel. 856/757–3500 **A**1 2 6 7 9 10 **F**3 11 12 13 15 17 18 20 22 24 25 26 27 28 31 32 33 34 36 38 41 43 44 47 49 50 54 55 56 57 58 59 60 62 63 64 66 68 69 70 72 73 74 76 77 79 80 81 82 84 85 86 87 90 92 96 97 100 102 103 106 107 114 116 119 121 123 124 127 128 131 135 136 **P**7 **S** Catholic Health East
Primary Contact: Mark T. Bateman, Chief Administrative Officer
CFO: Andrew Guarni, Vice President Finance and Chief Financial Officer
CMO: John P. Capelli, M.D., Vice President Medical Affairs
CIO: Maureen Hetu, Chief Information Officer
CHR: Janet Moran, Vice President Human Resources
Web address: www.lourdesnet.org
Control: Other not–for–profit (including NFP Corporation) **Service:** General Medical and Surgical

Staffed Beds: 391 **Admissions:** 17416 **Census:** 279 **Outpatient Visits:** 178090 **Births:** 1440 **Total Expense ($000):** 267786 **Payroll Expense ($000):** 108736 **Personnel:** 1903

CAPE MAY COURT HOUSE—Cape May County

★ **CAPE REGIONAL MEDICAL CENTER (310011)**, Two Stone Harbor Boulevard, Zip 08210–9990; tel. 609/463–2000 **A**1 2 9 10 **F**3 8 11 13 15 18 24 25 26 27 30 31 32 33 38 41 43 44 46 49 50 52 55 56 57 62 68 72 73 74 75 76 77 79 80 81 82 84 86 87 96 106 107 109 111 119 121 124 132 135 137
Primary Contact: Joanne Carrocino, FACHE, President and Chief Executive Officer
CFO: Mark Gill, Vice President Finance and Chief Financial Officer
CMO: Richard Falivena, D.O., M.P.H., Vice President Medical Affairs
CIO: Mike Cordi, Director Information Systems
CHR: Byron Hunter, Vice President Human Resources
Web address: www.caperegional.com
Control: Other not–for–profit (including NFP Corporation) **Service:** General Medical and Surgical

Staffed Beds: 208 **Admissions:** 10301 **Census:** 122 **Outpatient Visits:** 142801 **Births:** 570 **Total Expense ($000):** 106879 **Payroll Expense ($000):** 42048 **Personnel:** 867

CEDAR GROVE—Essex County

☐ **ESSEX COUNTY HOSPITAL CENTER (314020)**, 204 Grove Avenue, Zip 07009–1436; tel. 973/571–2800 **A**1 10 **F**26 31 32 37 56 58 73 82 88 91 93 119 121 132
Primary Contact: Lucia A. Guarini, Administrator
CFO: Teodora Kasper, Comptroller
CMO: N. Elangovan, M.D., Medical Director
CHR: BettyAnn Jannuzzi, Supervisor Personnel
Web address: www.essexcountynj.org
Control: Hospital district or authority, Government, nonfederal **Service:** Psychiatric

Staffed Beds: 180 **Admissions:** 357 **Census:** 149 **Outpatient Visits:** 0 **Births:** 0 **Total Expense ($000):** 42025 **Payroll Expense ($000):** 20350 **Personnel:** 361

CHERRY HILL—Camden County

★ ○ **KENNEDY MEMORIAL HOSPITALS–UNIVERSITY MEDICAL CENTER (310086)**, 2201 Chapel Avenue West, Zip 08002–2048; tel. 856/488–6500, (Includes KENNEDY MEMORIAL HOSPITAL, 18 East Laurel Road, Stratford, Zip 08084; tel. 609/346–6000; KENNEDY MEMORIAL HOSPITAL, 435 Hurffville–Cross Keys Road, Turnersville, Zip 08012; tel. 609/582–2500) **A**1 9 10 11 12 **F**3 4 5 7 11 12 13 15 18 20 25 26 27 28 30 31 32 33 36 37 38 41 43 44 46 49 50 54 55 56 57 59 60 61 62 63 64 66 68 70 71 72 73 74 76 77 78 79 80 81 82 84 86 87 88 89 90 91 92 93 94 95 96 97 100 102 106 107 109 111 114 118 119 120 121 123 132 135 136 137
Primary Contact: Richard E. Murray, President and Chief Executive Officer
COO: Martin A. Bieber, Senior Vice President Operations
CFO: Joseph Lario, Senior Vice President and Chief Financial Officer
CMO: Daniel L. Herriman, M.D., JD, Senior Vice President Medical Affairs and Chief Medical Officer
CIO: Thomas Balcavage, Vice President Information Systems and Chief Information Officer
CHR: Annaliese McMenamin, Vice President Human Resources
Web address: www.kennedyhealth.org
Control: Other not–for–profit (including NFP Corporation) **Service:** General Medical and Surgical

Staffed Beds: 482 **Admissions:** 28191 **Census:** 324 **Outpatient Visits:** 368056 **Births:** 1604 **Total Expense ($000):** 320203 **Payroll Expense ($000):** 139308 **Personnel:** 2307

DENVILLE—Morris County

SAINT CLARE'S HOSPITAL/DENVILLE See Saint Clare's Hospital, Dover

NJ

Many Facility Codes have changed. Please refer to the AHA Guide Code Chart.

DOVER—Morris County

☐ **KINDRED HOSPITAL–NEW JERSEY MORRIS COUNTY (312020)**, 400 West Blackwell Street, Zip 7801; tel. 973/537–3818, (Nonreporting) **A**1 10
Primary Contact: Beth Cullum, Administrator
CFO: Rishab Punjabi, Chief Financial Officer
CMO: Edward J. McManus, M.D., President Medical Staff and Medical Director
CHR: Neil Rosner, Area Director Human Resources
Web address: www.kindredhealthcare.com
Control: Corporation, Investor–owned, for–profit **Service:** Long–Term Acute Care hospital

Staffed Beds: 45

★☐ **SAINT CLARE'S HOSPITAL (310050)**, 400 West Blackwell Street, Zip 7801; tel. 973/625–6000, (Includes SAINT CLARE'S HOSPITAL/BOONTON TOWNSHIP, 130 Powerville Road, Boonton Township, Zip 07005; tel. 973/316–1800; SAINT CLARE'S HOSPITAL/DENVILLE, 25 Pocono Road, Denville, Zip 07834; tel. 973/625–6000; SAINT CLARE'S HOSPITAL/SUSSEX, 20 Walnut Street, Sussex, Zip 07461; tel. 973/702–2200), (Total facility includes 137 beds in nursing home–type unit) (Nonreporting) **A**1 9 10 **S** Catholic Health Initiatives
Primary Contact: Leslie D. Hirsch, FACHE, President and Chief Executive Officer
COO: David Lundquist, Chief Operating Officer
CFO: Dennis Pignato, Executive Vice President and Chief Financial Officer
CMO: Alma Ratcliffe, M.D., Executive Vice President Medical Staff and Business Development
CIO: Richard Temple, Chief Information Officer
CHR: Joseph Marsicovete, Vice President Administrative and Regulatory Services
Web address: www.saintclares.org
Control: Other not–for–profit (including NFP Corporation) **Service:** General Medical and Surgical

Staffed Beds: 607

EAST ORANGE—Essex County

★☐ **EAST ORANGE GENERAL HOSPITAL (310083)**, 300 Central Avenue, Zip 07019–2897; tel. 973/672–8400 **A**1 9 10 **F**5 11 15 25 26 27 29 30 31 32 33 36 38 43 46 54 55 56 57 59 60 62 63 64 66 68 69 73 75 76 77 78 79 82 86 87 88 89 90 91 92 93 94 95 96 97 99 107 119 120 121 123 135 136 **P**6
Primary Contact: Kevin Slavin, President and Chief Executive Officer
CFO: Robert C. Hood, Chief Financial Officer
CMO: Gnana Sunderam, M.D., Chief Medical Officer
CIO: Thomas Ciccarelli, Chief Information Officer
CHR: Chester Banks, Director Human Resources
Web address: www.evh.org
Control: Other not–for–profit (including NFP Corporation) **Service:** General Medical and Surgical

Staffed Beds: 211 **Admissions:** 7246 **Census:** 149 **Outpatient Visits:** 120341 **Births:** 0 **Total Expense ($000):** 87251 **Payroll Expense ($000):** 47896 **Personnel:** 885

★☐ △ **VETERANS AFFAIRS NEW JERSEY HEALTH CARE SYSTEM**, 385 Tremont Avenue, Zip 07018–1095; tel. 973/676–1000, (Includes EAST ORANGE DIVISION; LYONS DIVISION, 151 Knollcroft Road, Lyons, Zip 07939–9998; tel. 908/647–0180), (Total facility includes 270 beds in nursing home–type unit) (Nonreporting) **A**1 2 3 5 7 8 **S** Department of Veterans Affairs
Primary Contact: Kenneth H. Mizrach, Director
COO: Kenneth H. Mizrach, Director
CFO: Tyrone Taylor, Chief Financial Officer
CMO: Steven L. Lieberman, M.D., Chief of Staff
CIO: Marsha Evens, Acting Chief Information Resource Management
CHR: Joseph Capodiferro, Chief Human and Learning Resources
Web address: www.va.gov/sta/guide/home.asp
Control: Veterans Affairs, Government, federal **Service:** Other specialty

Staffed Beds: 684

EATONTOWN—Monmouth County

REHABILITATION HOSPITAL OF TINTON FALLS See Tinton Falls

EDISON—Middlesex County

★ △ **JFK JOHNSON REHABILITATION INSTITUTE**, 65 James Street, Zip 08818–3059; tel. 732/321–7050, (Nonreporting) **A**7 **S** Solaris Health System
Primary Contact: Anthony Cuzzola, Vice President Rehabilitation Services
CFO: Raymond F. Fredericks, Senior Vice President and Chief Financial Officer
CIO: Louis H. Hermans, Vice President Information Systems
Web address: www.solarishs.org
Control: Other not–for–profit (including NFP Corporation) **Service:** Rehabilitation

Staffed Beds: 92

★☐ **JFK MEDICAL CENTER (310108)**, 65 James Street, Zip 08818–3059; tel. 732/321–7000, (Nonreporting) **A**1 2 3 5 9 10 **S** Solaris Health System
Primary Contact: Scott Gebhard, Executive Vice President and Chief Operating Officer
COO: Scott Gebhard, Executive Vice President and Chief Operating Officer
CFO: Richard C. Smith, Senior Vice President and Chief Financial Officer
CMO: William F. Oser, M.D., JD, Senior Vice President and Chief Medical Officer
CIO: Louis H. Hermans, Vice President Information Systems
CHR: Shirley Higgins–Bowers, Vice President Human Resources
Web address: www.solarishs.org
Control: Other not–for–profit (including NFP Corporation) **Service:** General Medical and Surgical

Staffed Beds: 325

ELIZABETH—Union County

★☐ **TRINITAS HOSPITAL–WILLIAMSON STREET CAMPUS (310027)**, 225 Williamson Street, Zip 7202; tel. 908/994–5000, (Includes TRINITAS HOSPITAL; TRINITAS HOSPITAL – NEW POINT CAMPUS, 655 East Jersey Street, Zip 07206), (Total facility includes 157 beds in nursing home–type unit) **A**1 2 6 9 10 **F**3 5 7 11 13 15 18 20 24 25 26 27 28 30 31 32 33 36 38 41 43 44 49 50 52 53 54 55 56 57 59 60 62 64 65 68 71 72 73 74 75 76 77 79 80 82 84 86 87 88 89 90 91 92 93 94 95 96 97 100 102 105 106 107 108 109 111 116 117 118 119 121 123 124 135 136 137
Primary Contact: Gary S. Horan, FACHE, President and Chief Executive Officer
CFO: Karen Lumpp, Senior Vice President and Chief Financial Officer
CMO: William McHugh, M.D., Chief Medical Officer
CIO: Judy Comitto, Vice President Information Services and Chief Information Officer
CHR: Glenn Nacion, Vice President Human Resources
Web address: www.trinitashospital.com
Control: Other not–for–profit (including NFP Corporation) **Service:** General Medical and Surgical

Staffed Beds: 493 **Admissions:** 15163 **Census:** 410 **Outpatient Visits:** 402127 **Births:** 1963 **Total Expense ($000):** 277880 **Payroll Expense ($000):** 118548 **Personnel:** 2105

ELMER—Salem County

☐ **SOUTH JERSEY HEALTHCARE – ELMER HOSPITAL (310069)**, (Formerly Elmer Hospital), 501 West Front Street, Zip 08318–1090; tel. 856/363–1000, (Nonreporting) **A**1 9 10 **S** South Jersey Healthcare
Primary Contact: Chester B. Kaletkowski, President and Chief Executive Officer
COO: John Bickings, Chief Operating Officer
CFO: John A. DiAngelo, Senior Vice President Finance and Chief Financial Officer
CMO: Steven C. Linn, M.D., Chief Medical Officer
CIO: Thomas Pacek, Vice President Information Systems and Chief Information Officer
CHR: Erich Florentine, Chief People Officer
Web address: www.sjhealthcare.net
Control: Other not–for–profit (including NFP Corporation) **Service:** General Medical and Surgical

Staffed Beds: 91

ENGLEWOOD—Bergen County

★☐ **ENGLEWOOD HOSPITAL AND MEDICAL CENTER (310045)**, 350 Engle Street, Zip 07631–1898; tel. 201/894–3000 **A**1 2 3 5 9 10 **F**3 7 8 11 12 13 15 17 18 20 22 24 25 26 27 28 30 31 32 33 34 35 36 38 41 42 43 44 46 47 48 49 50 51 54 55 56 57 58 59 60 61 62 63 64 66 68 70 71 72 73 74 75 76 77 79 80 81 82 84 86 87 88 91 92 93 95 96 97 99 100 102 103 104 105 106 107 109 111 112 114 118 119 120 121 124 134 135 136 137
Primary Contact: Douglas A. Duchak, President and Chief Executive Officer
CFO: Anthony T. Orlando, Senior Vice President Finance
CMO: Joseph Willner, M.D., President Medical Staff
CIO: Diane Caesar, Director
CHR: Patricia Wilson, Vice President Human Resources
Web address: www.englewoodhospital.com
Control: Other not–for–profit (including NFP Corporation) **Service:** General Medical and Surgical

Staffed Beds: 283 **Admissions:** 16411 **Census:** 220 **Outpatient Visits:** 306782 **Births:** 2134 **Total Expense ($000):** 282487 **Payroll Expense ($000):** 115113 **Personnel:** 2081

NJ

Hospital, Medicare Provider Number, Address, Telephone, Approval, Facility, and Physician Codes, Health Care System

★ American Hospital Association (AHA) membership
☐ The Joint Commission accreditation
○ American Osteopathic Association (AOA) accreditation
△ Commission on Accreditation of Rehabilitation Facilities (CARF) accreditation

FLEMINGTON—Hunterdon County

★ **HUNTERDON MEDICAL CENTER (310005)**, 2100 Wescott Drive, Zip 08822–4604; tel. 908/788–6100 **A**1 2 3 5 9 10 **F**3 5 11 13 14 15 18 20 24 25 26 27 28 30 31 32 33 36 38 43 44 45 46 47 48 49 51 52 53 54 55 56 57 58 59 60 61 62 63 68 69 71 72 73 74 75 76 77 79 80 81 82 84 86 87 88 89 90 91 92 93 94 95 96 97 102 106 107 109 111 118 119 120 121 123 124 135 136 137 **P**1 5
Primary Contact: Robert P. Wise, President and Chief Executive Officer
COO: Lawrence N. Grand, Executive Vice President and Chief Operating Officer
CFO: Daniel J. Deets, Chief Financial Officer
CMO: Robert M. Pickoff, M.D., Chief Medical Officer
CIO: Glenn Mamary, Chief Information Officer
CHR: Violet Kocsis, Vice President Human Resources and Development
Web address: www.hunterdonhealthcare.org
Control: Other not–for–profit (including NFP Corporation) **Service:** General Medical and Surgical

Staffed Beds: 178 **Admissions:** 8671 **Census:** 112 **Outpatient Visits:** 479927 **Births:** 1241 **Total Expense ($000):** 190523 **Payroll Expense ($000):** 96278 **Personnel:** 1807

FREEHOLD—Monmouth County

★ **CENTRASTATE HEALTHCARE SYSTEM (310111)**, 901 West Main Street, Zip 07728–2549; tel. 732/431–2000 **A**1 2 3 5 9 10 **F**3 11 12 13 15 17 18 24 25 26 27 28 30 31 32 33 34 35 36 38 43 44 49 54 55 56 57 58 60 62 63 68 71 72 73 74 75 76 77 79 81 82 84 86 87 88 90 91 92 96 97 102 104 105 106 107 108 109 112 118 119 120 121 123 124 133 135 136 137 **P**1 5
Primary Contact: John T. Gribbin, President and Chief Executive Officer
COO: Daniel J. Messina, Senior Vice President and Chief Operating Officer
CFO: John Dellocono, Senior Vice President and Chief Financial Officer
CMO: Benjamin Weinstein, M.D., Senior Vice President and Medical Director
CIO: Indranil Ganguly, Vice President and Chief Information Officer
CHR: Fran Keane, Vice President Human Resources
Web address: www.centrastate.com
Control: Other not–for–profit (including NFP Corporation) **Service:** General Medical and Surgical

Staffed Beds: 260 **Admissions:** 16816 **Census:** 200 **Outpatient Visits:** 221365 **Births:** 2026 **Total Expense ($000):** 191612 **Payroll Expense ($000):** 81699 **Personnel:** 1452

GLEN GARDNER—Hunterdon County

☐ **SENATOR GARRETT W. HAGEDORN PSYCHIATRIC HOSPITAL (314017)**, 200 Sanatorium Road, Zip 08826–3291; tel. 908/537–2141 **A**1 10 **F**26 37 41 43 54 62 63 66 72 73 75 81 82 88 89 91 93 119 124 135 137 **P**7 **S** Division of Mental Health Services, Department of Human Services, State of New Jersey
Primary Contact: Debra A. Smith, Chief Executive Officer
CFO: Mercedes Ayala, Business Manager
CMO: Ahmad Mur, M.D., Acting Medical Director
CHR: Janice Decker, Manager Human Resources
Control: State–Government, nonfederal **Service:** Psychiatric

Staffed Beds: 288 **Admissions:** 465 **Census:** 288 **Outpatient Visits:** 0 **Births:** 0 **Personnel:** 632

HACKENSACK—Bergen County

★ **HACKENSACK UNIVERSITY MEDICAL CENTER (310001)**, 30 Prospect Avenue, Zip 07601–1991; tel. 201/996–2000 **A**1 2 3 5 8 9 10 **F**2 3 4 5 6 7 8 9 10 11 12 13 14 15 16 17 18 20 22 24 25 26 27 28 30 31 32 33 34 36 37 38 40 41 42 43 44 46 47 48 49 50 51 52 53 54 55 56 57 58 59 60 61 62 63 64 66 67 68 69 70 71 72 73 74 75 76 77 79 80 81 82 83 84 85 86 87 88 89 90 91 92 93 94 96 97 98 99 100 102 103 104 105 106 107 109 111 112 113 114 116 118 119 120 121 123 124 125 127 130 131 132 133 134 135 136 137 **P**4 5 6 8
Primary Contact: John P. Ferguson, FACHE, President and Chief Executive Officer
COO: Robert C. Garrett, Executive Vice President and Chief Operating Officer
CFO: Robert Glenning, Executive Vice President Finance and Chief Financial Officer
CMO: Peter A. Gross, M.D., Senior Vice President and Chief Medical Officer
CIO: Lex Ferrauiola, Vice President Information Technology and Chief Information Officer
CHR: Nancy R. Corcoran, Senior Vice President Human Resources and Service Quality
Web address: www.humed.com
Control: Other not–for–profit (including NFP Corporation) **Service:** General Medical and Surgical

Staffed Beds: 679 **Admissions:** 69727 **Census:** 679 **Outpatient Visits:** 2543319 **Births:** 5870 **Total Expense ($000):** 1048976 **Payroll Expense ($000):** 472023 **Personnel:** 7288

HACKETTSTOWN—Warren County

★ **HACKETTSTOWN REGIONAL MEDICAL CENTER (310115)**, 651 Willow Grove Street, Zip 07840–1792; tel. 908/852–5100, (Nonreporting) **A**1 9 10 **S** Adventist HealthCare
Primary Contact: Gene C. Milton, President and Chief Executive Officer
COO: Jason Coe, Chief Operating Officer
CFO: Stella Visaggio, Chief Financial Officer
CMO: Kenneth Janowski, M.D., Chief Medical Officer
CIO: Dorothy Cox, Manager Information Systems
CHR: Jeanne Jepson, Director Human Resources
Web address: www.hrmcnj.org
Control: Church–operated, Nongovernment, not–for profit **Service:** General Medical and Surgical

Staffed Beds: 99

HAMILTON—Mercer County

★ **ROBERT WOOD JOHNSON UNIVERSITY HOSPITAL AT HAMILTON (310110)**, One Hamilton Health Place, Zip 08690–3599; tel. 609/586–7900 **A**1 2 3 5 9 10 **F**3 8 9 11 12 13 15 17 18 20 24 25 26 27 28 30 31 32 33 34 37 38 41 42 43 44 46 47 48 49 50 51 52 53 54 55 56 57 58 59 60 62 63 64 66 67 68 69 71 72 73 74 75 76 77 79 80 81 82 86 87 90 92 93 96 97 99 100 102 104 105 106 107 108 109 111 112 114 118 119 120 121 123 124 132 133 134 135 136 137 **P**6 **S** Robert Wood Johnson Health System & Network
Primary Contact: Ellen Guarnieri, President and Chief Executive Officer
CFO: Paul Pernice, Vice President Finance and Chief Financial Officer
CMO: Mahmoud Ghusson, M.D., Chief of Staff
CIO: Paul Pernice, Vice President Finance and Chief Financial Officer
Web address: www.rwjhamilton.org
Control: Other not–for–profit (including NFP Corporation) **Service:** General Medical and Surgical

Staffed Beds: 270 **Admissions:** 15496 **Census:** 213 **Outpatient Visits:** 295247 **Births:** 1386 **Total Expense ($000):** 202358 **Payroll Expense ($000):** 89085 **Personnel:** 1689

HAMMONTON—Atlantic County

☐ **WILLIAM B. KESSLER MEMORIAL HOSPITAL (310088)**, 600 South White Horse Pike, Zip 08037–2099; tel. 609/561–6700, (Nonreporting) **A**1 9 10
Primary Contact: Sharon Rosetti, RN, Administrator
Web address: www.kesslerhospital.org
Control: Other not–for–profit (including NFP Corporation) **Service:** General Medical and Surgical

Staffed Beds: 84

HOBOKEN—Hudson County

★ **HOBOKEN UNIVERSITY MEDICAL CENTER (310040)**, 308 Willow Avenue, Zip 07030–3889; tel. 201/418–1000 **A**1 3 5 8 9 10 **F**3 5 8 10 11 13 15 17 18 24 25 26 27 28 30 31 32 33 34 36 37 38 43 44 45 49 50 52 53 54 55 56 57 59 60 62 63 64 66 68 71 73 74 75 76 77 79 80 81 82 84 85 86 87 88 89 90 91 92 93 94 95 96 99 100 103 107 112 114 118 119 121 123 124 132 135 136 137
Primary Contact: Harvey A. Holzberg, Chief Executive Officer
CFO: Ronald F. DiVito, Chief Financial Officer
CMO: Joseph Kozel, M.D., President Medical Staff
CIO: Lior Blik, Chief Information Officer
CHR: Yleana Contrera, Executive Director Human Resources
Web address: www.hobokenumc.com
Control: Hospital district or authority, Government, nonfederal **Service:** General Medical and Surgical

Staffed Beds: 364 **Admissions:** 10515 **Census:** 132 **Outpatient Visits:** 113632 **Births:** 1372 **Total Expense ($000):** 130301 **Payroll Expense ($000):** 60328 **Personnel:** 1503

HOLMDEL—Monmouth County

★ **BAYSHORE COMMUNITY HOSPITAL (310112)**, 727 North Beers Street, Zip 07733–1598; tel. 732/739–5900, (Total facility includes 13 beds in nursing home–type unit) **A**1 2 9 10 **F**3 12 15 17 18 24 25 26 27 30 31 32 33 35 38 40 42 43 46 49 50 51 54 55 56 57 59 62 64 66 67 68 72 73 75 76 77 79 80 81 82 84 86 90 96 97 100 102 106 107 118 119 120 121 124 135 137 **P**6 7
Primary Contact: Raimonda Clark, President and Chief Executive Officer
CFO: Jane Kaye, Vice President Finance
CMO: Gerald Costa, M.D., Vice President Medical Affairs
CIO: Linda Woods, Vice President Information Services
CHR: Emro Krasovec, Vice President Human Resources
Web address: www.bchs.com
Control: Other not–for–profit (including NFP Corporation) **Service:** General Medical and Surgical

Staffed Beds: 161 **Admissions:** 7764 **Census:** 124 **Outpatient Visits:** 103020 **Births:** 0 **Total Expense ($000):** 96880 **Payroll Expense ($000):** 43924 **Personnel:** 973

NJ

Many Facility Codes have changed. Please refer to the AHA Guide Code Chart.

JERSEY CITY—Hudson County

★ **CHRIST HOSPITAL (310016)**, 176 Palisade Avenue, Zip 07306–1196, Mailing Address: P.O. Box J–1, Zip 07306–1196; tel. 201/795–8200 **A**1 5 6 9 10 12 13 **F**3 4 5 11 13 15 18 20 24 25 26 27 28 30 31 32 33 35 36 37 38 42 43 44 46 48 50 54 55 56 57 59 60 61 62 63 66 68 72 73 74 75 76 77 79 80 81 82 84 86 87 88 89 90 91 92 93 94 95 96 97 98 99 100 101 102 103 106 107 109 111 112 114 117 118 119 120 121 122 123 124 132 135 136 137
Primary Contact: Peter A. Kelly, President and Chief Executive Officer
CFO: George A. Popko, Senior Vice President and Chief Financial Officer
CMO: Bhavani P. Mekala, M.D., President Medical Staff
CIO: Marty Grossman, Director Information Technology
CHR: Eileen Clyne, Director Human Resources
Web address: www.christhospital.org
Control: Other not–for–profit (including NFP Corporation) **Service:** General Medical and Surgical

Staffed Beds: 381 **Admissions:** 13974 **Census:** 219 **Outpatient Visits:** 79552 **Births:** 1230 **Total Expense ($000):** 138005 **Payroll Expense ($000):** 79494 **Personnel:** 1300

□ **LIBERTYHEALTH–JERSEY CITY MEDICAL CENTER (310074)**, 355 Grand Street, Zip 7302; tel. 201/915–2000 **A**1 3 5 9 10 **F**3 7 11 12 13 17 18 20 22 25 26 27 28 30 31 32 33 36 37 38 40 41 43 44 46 48 49 50 53 54 55 56 57 58 59 60 61 62 64 66 68 70 71 72 73 74 75 76 77 79 80 81 82 84 86 87 88 89 90 91 92 93 94 95 96 97 100 101 102 106 107 113 114 119 121 123 132 133 135 136 137 **S** LibertyHealth
Primary Contact: E. Stephen Kirby, Interim Chief Executive Officer
COO: Timothy P. Selz, Interim Chief Operating Officer
CFO: Donald Parseghian, Chief Financial Officer
CMO: Robert P. Jacobs, M.D., Senior Vice President Medical Affairs
CIO: James Yost, Vice President Management Information Systems
CHR: Mary Cataudella, Corporate Director Human Resources
Web address: www.libertyhcs.org
Control: Other not–for–profit (including NFP Corporation) **Service:** General Medical and Surgical

Staffed Beds: 324 **Admissions:** 14621 **Census:** 199 **Outpatient Visits:** 184251 **Births:** 1637 **Total Expense ($000):** 247450 **Payroll Expense ($000):** 107549 **Personnel:** 1513

LAKEWOOD—Ocean County

★ **KIMBALL MEDICAL CENTER (310084)**, 600 River Avenue, Zip 08701–4281; tel. 732/363–1900, (Nonreporting) **A**1 2 9 10 **S** Saint Barnabas Health Care System
Primary Contact: Joe Hicks, Executive Director
CFO: Gerald Tofani, Chief Financial Officer
CMO: Tony Lombardino, Vice President Medical Affairs
CIO: Richard Wheatley, Vice President Information Services
CHR: Michele Schweers, Vice President Human Resources
Web address: www.sbhcs.com
Control: Other not–for–profit (including NFP Corporation) **Service:** General Medical and Surgical

Staffed Beds: 302

LIVINGSTON—Essex County

★ **SAINT BARNABAS MEDICAL CENTER (310076)**, 94 Old Short Hills Road, Zip 07039–5668; tel. 973/322–5000 **A**1 2 3 5 8 9 10 12 13 **F**3 11 12 13 16 17 18 20 22 24 25 26 27 28 31 32 33 38 40 42 43 44 46 49 55 56 57 58 59 62 64 66 68 70 71 72 73 74 75 76 77 78 79 80 81 82 83 84 86 87 96 97 100 102 103 106 107 108 109 111 112 113 114 116 118 119 121 124 127 131 135 136 137 **P**5 **S** Saint Barnabas Health Care System
Primary Contact: John F. Bonamo, M.D., Executive Director
COO: Patricia Carroll, Chief Operating Officer
CFO: Patrick Ahearn, Senior Vice President Finance and Administrative Services
CMO: Gregory Rokosz, D.O., Senior Vice President Medical and Academic Affairs
CIO: Michael McTigue, Chief Information Officer
CHR: Arnie Manzo, Vice President Human Resources
Web address: www.sbhcs.com
Control: Other not–for–profit (including NFP Corporation) **Service:** General Medical and Surgical

Staffed Beds: 601 **Admissions:** 32019 **Census:** 443 **Outpatient Visits:** 215341 **Births:** 6357 **Total Expense ($000):** 496512 **Payroll Expense ($000):** 194128 **Personnel:** 2841

LONG BRANCH—Monmouth County

★ **MONMOUTH MEDICAL CENTER (310075)**, 300 Second Avenue, Zip 07740–6303; tel. 732/222–5200 **A**1 2 3 5 8 9 10 **F**1 3 5 8 9 11 12 13 14 15 18 20 24 25 26 27 28 30 31 32 33 34 36 37 38 42 43 44 46 47 48 49 50 51 52 53 54 55 56 57 58 60 62 63 64 66 67 68 70 71 72 73 74 75 76 77 79 80 81 82 83 84 87 88 89 90 91 92 93 94 95 96 97 98 99 100 102 104 107 108 109 111 112 113 114 116 118 119 120 121 122 123 124 132 133 134 135 136 137 **P**5 6 7 8 **S** Saint Barnabas Health Care System
Primary Contact: Frank J. Vozos, M.D., FACS, Executive Director
COO: Bill Arnold, Chief Operating Officer
CFO: Gerald Tofani, Chief Financial Officer
CMO: Eric Burkett, M.D., Vice President Medical Affairs
CHR: Glenn Oppito, Vice President Human Resources
Web address: www.sbhcs.com
Control: Other not–for–profit (including NFP Corporation) **Service:** General Medical and Surgical

Staffed Beds: 324 **Admissions:** 17681 **Census:** 230 **Outpatient Visits:** 53354 **Births:** 4104 **Total Expense ($000):** 262347 **Payroll Expense ($000):** 103852 **Personnel:** 1665

SPECIALTY HOSPITAL AT MONMOUTH (312017), 300 Second Avenue, Zip 7740; tel. 732/923–5037, (Nonreporting) **A**10
Primary Contact: Violeta Peters, Chief Executive Officer
CMO: Howard Lebowitz, M.D., Chief Medical Officer
CHR: Mary Pat Napolitano, Director Human Resources
Web address: www.acutecarehs.com
Control: Corporation, Investor–owned, for–profit **Service:** Long–Term Acute Care hospital

Staffed Beds: 25

LYONS—Somerset County

LYONS DIVISION See Veterans Affairs New Jersey Health Care System, East Orange

MANAHAWKIN—Ocean County

★ **SOUTHERN OCEAN COUNTY HOSPITAL (310113)**, 1140 Route 72 West, Zip 08050–2499; tel. 609/978–8900 **A**1 2 9 10 **F**3 8 11 13 15 18 24 25 26 27 28 30 31 32 33 38 41 43 44 46 50 51 52 53 54 55 56 57 62 63 64 66 68 72 73 74 75 76 77 79 80 81 82 86 96 97 100 102 106 107 117 118 119 121 123 124 135 136 137 **P**7 8
Primary Contact: Joseph P. Coyle, President and Chief Executive Officer
COO: E. Joseph Hummel, Chief Strategy Officer
CFO: Richard A. Hand, Vice President Information and Chief Financial Officer
CMO: Edward Niewiadomski, M.D., Vice President Medical Affairs and Chief Medical Officer
CIO: Kevin Bryant, Vice President Information
CHR: Raymond Green, Vice President Human Resources
Web address: www.soch.com
Control: Other not–for–profit (including NFP Corporation) **Service:** General Medical and Surgical

Staffed Beds: 176 **Admissions:** 8362 **Census:** 110 **Outpatient Visits:** 169377 **Births:** 329 **Total Expense ($000):** 116704 **Payroll Expense ($000):** 46331 **Personnel:** 863

MARLTON—Burlington County

□ △ **MARLTON REHABILITATION HOSPITAL (313032)**, 92 Brick Road, Zip 08053–2177; tel. 856/988–8778 **A**1 7 10 **F**3 25 26 33 41 50 56 57 62 66 72 73 75 77 81 82 85 86 90 119 120 121 **S** Vibra Healthcare
Primary Contact: David T. Shannon, Chief Executive Officer
CFO: Stuart Moss, Chief Financial Officer
CMO: Kenneth Wu, M.D., Medical Director
CHR: Joanne Cornava, Director Human Resources
Web address: www.marltonrehab.com
Control: Corporation, Investor–owned, for–profit **Service:** Rehabilitation

Staffed Beds: 46 **Admissions:** 1414 **Census:** 44 **Outpatient Visits:** 15350 **Births:** 0

★ **VIRTUA WEST JERSEY HOSPITAL–MARLTON (313032)**, 90 Brick Road, Zip 08053–9697; tel. 856/355–6000, (Nonreporting) **A**1 9 10 **S** Virtua Health
Primary Contact: Gary L. Long, Vice President and Chief Operating Officer
CFO: Brian Malone, Director Finance
Web address: www.virtua.org
Control: Other not–for–profit (including NFP Corporation) **Service:** General Medical and Surgical

Staffed Beds: 165

Hospital, Medicare Provider Number, Address, Telephone, Approval, Facility, and Physician Codes, Health Care System

★ American Hospital Association (AHA) membership
□ The Joint Commission accreditation
○ American Osteopathic Association (AOA) accreditation
△ Commission on Accreditation of Rehabilitation Facilities (CARF) accreditation

☐ **WEISMAN CHILDREN'S REHABILITATION HOSPITAL (313034),** 92 Brick Road, 3rd Floor, Zip 8053; tel. 856/589–4520 **A**1 10 **F**3 25 31 32 33 41 50 55 56 66 75 81 82 85 86 119 120 121 135
Primary Contact: Richard W. Shepherd, Chief Executive Officer
CMO: Connie Domingo, Medical Director
CIO: Darren Pedersen, Coordinator Information Technology
CHR: Eileen Dumsha, Manager Employee Relations
Web address: www.weismanchildrens.com
Control: Corporation, Investor–owned, for–profit **Service:** Children's rehabilitation

Staffed Beds: 24 **Admissions:** 119 **Census:** 10 **Outpatient Visits:** 14670 **Births:** 0 **Personnel:** 70

MONTCLAIR—Essex County

★ **MOUNTAINSIDE HOSPITAL (310054),** 1 Bay Avenue, Zip 07042–4898; tel. 973/429–6000 **A**1 2 3 5 6 9 10 **F**3 11 12 13 14 15 18 20 24 25 26 27 28 30 31 32 33 34 36 37 38 41 43 44 46 49 50 51 52 53 54 55 56 57 58 59 60 62 63 64 66 72 73 75 76 77 79 80 81 82 84 86 87 89 90 91 92 93 94 95 96 97 98 99 100 101 102 103 104 105 106 107 108 109 110 111 112 118 119 120 121 124 132 133 135 136 137 **P**5 **S** Merit Health Systems
Primary Contact: C. Barry Dykes, President and Chief Executive Officer
COO: Ed Devaney, Vice President and Chief Operating Officer
CFO: Al Aboud, Vice President Finance and Chief Financial Officer
CMO: Craig Hersh, M.D., Vice President and Chief Medical Officer
CIO: Jay Sharon, Director Information Technology and Telecommunications
CHR: Fran Corridon, Vice President Human Resources and Shared Services
Web address: www.mountainsidenow.com
Control: Corporation, Investor–owned, for–profit **Service:** General Medical and Surgical

Staffed Beds: 233 **Admissions:** 11892 **Census:** 174 **Outpatient Visits:** 105847 **Births:** 773 **Total Expense ($000):** 100607 **Payroll Expense ($000):** 45019 **Personnel:** 1385

MORRIS PLAINS—Morris County

☐ **GREYSTONE PARK PSYCHIATRIC HOSPITAL (314016),** 99 Central Avenue, Zip 07950–1005, Mailing Address: P.O. Box A, Zip 07950–1005; tel. 973/538–1800 **A**1 10 **F**26 37 63 73 82 88 119 124 132 135 **P**6 **S** Division of Mental Health Services, Department of Human Services, State of New Jersey
Primary Contact: Janet Monroe, Chief Executive Officer
COO: John Whitenack, Chief Operating Officer
CFO: Jack Frey, Business Manager
CMO: Milton Luria, M.D., Chief of Medicine
CIO: Louise Perugini, Assistant to Chief Executive Officer
CHR: Jerri Casazza, Manager Human Resources
Web address: www.state.nj.us/humanservices/pfnurse/greystone.htm
Control: State–Government, nonfederal **Service:** Psychiatric

Staffed Beds: 557 **Admissions:** 338 **Census:** 585 **Outpatient Visits:** 0 **Births:** 0

MORRISTOWN—Morris County

★ △ **MORRISTOWN MEMORIAL HOSPITAL (310015),** 100 Madison Avenue, Zip 07962–1956; tel. 973/971–5000, (Includes REHABILITATION INSTITUTE AT THE MOUNT KEMBLE DIVISION), (Total facility includes 40 beds in nursing home–type unit) **A**1 2 3 5 7 8 9 10 **F**3 5 7 8 9 11 12 13 14 15 17 18 20 22 24 25 26 27 28 29 30 31 32 33 34 35 36 37 38 40 41 42 43 44 45 46 48 49 50 51 52 53 54 55 56 57 58 59 60 61 62 63 64 66 67 68 69 70 71 72 73 74 75 76 77 79 80 81 82 83 84 85 86 87 88 89 90 91 92 93 94 95 96 97 99 100 102 103 104 105 106 107 108 109 111 114 116 117 118 119 120 121 123 124 130 132 133 134 135 136 137 **P**6 **S** Atlantic Health
Primary Contact: Joseph A. Trunfio, Ph.D., President and Chief Executive Officer
COO: Joanne M. Conroy, M.D., Chief Operating Officer
CFO: Kevin Shanley, Vice President Finance and Chief Financial Officer
CMO: Joanne M. Conroy, M.D., Executive Vice President and Chief Operating Officer
CIO: Linda Reed, Vice President and Chief Information Officer
CHR: Andrew Kovach, Vice President Human Resources and Shared Services
Web address: www.atlantichealth.org/cons/hospitals/at_MMH
Control: Other not–for–profit (including NFP Corporation) **Service:** General Medical and Surgical

Staffed Beds: 626 **Admissions:** 34253 **Census:** 513 **Outpatient Visits:** 363752 **Births:** 3646 **Total Expense ($000):** 595519 **Payroll Expense ($000):** 280919 **Personnel:** 5029

MOUNT HOLLY—Burlington County

★ **VIRTUA MEMORIAL HOSPITAL BURLINGTON COUNTY (310057),** 175 Madison Avenue, Zip 08060–2099; tel. 609/267–0700 **A**1 3 5 9 10 **F**3 5 8 11 13 15 17 18 20 25 26 27 30 31 32 38 42 43 46 48 49 54 55 57 59 68 71 72 73 74 75 76 79 80 81 82 84 86 88 89 90 96 97 100 106 107 109 111 118 119 132 135 136 137 **S** Virtua Health
Primary Contact: Stephen Kolesk, M.D., Vice President and Chief Operating Officer
CFO: Robert Segin, Chief Financial Officer
CMO: James P. Dwyer, D.O., Executive Vice President and Chief Medical Officer
CIO: Maria Foschi, Acting Chief Information Officer
CHR: E. D. Dunn, Vice President Human Resources
Web address: www.virtua.org
Control: Other not–for–profit (including NFP Corporation) **Service:** General Medical and Surgical

Staffed Beds: 326 **Admissions:** 18182 **Census:** 226 **Outpatient Visits:** 178023 **Births:** 2319 **Total Expense ($000):** 234459 **Payroll Expense ($000):** 82859 **Personnel:** 5463

NEPTUNE—Monmouth County

★ **JERSEY SHORE UNIVERSITY MEDICAL CENTER (310073),** 1945 Route 33, Zip 07754–0397; tel. 732/775–5500 **A**1 2 3 5 8 9 10 **F**3 5 8 11 13 15 17 18 20 22 24 25 26 27 28 30 31 32 34 37 38 40 42 43 44 45 46 47 48 49 50 51 53 55 57 58 59 60 62 64 66 68 70 71 72 73 74 76 77 78 79 80 81 82 83 84 86 87 88 89 90 91 92 93 94 95 96 97 100 102 103 105 106 107 109 111 114 118 119 120 121 124 133 134 135 136 137 **S** Meridian Health
Primary Contact: Steven G. Littleson, President
COO: Jill Ostrem, Vice President Operations
CFO: William Phillips, Senior Vice President Finance and Chief Financial Officer
CMO: Carl M. Marchetti, M.D., Senior Vice President Medical Affairs
CIO: Rebecca Weber, Vice President Information Technology
CHR: John Sinnoni, Senior Vice President Human Resources
Web address: www.meridianhealth.com
Control: Other not–for–profit (including NFP Corporation) **Service:** General Medical and Surgical

Staffed Beds: 453 **Admissions:** 28838 **Census:** 374 **Outpatient Visits:** 187088 **Births:** 1728 **Total Expense ($000):** 411621 **Payroll Expense ($000):** 165970 **Personnel:** 2275

NEW BRUNSWICK—Middlesex County

☐ △ **CHILDREN'S SPECIALIZED HOSPITAL (313300),** 200 Somerset Street, Zip 08901; tel. 732/258–7000, (Includes CHILDREN'S SPECIALIZED HOSPITAL, 150 New Providence Road, Mountainside, Zip 07092–2590; tel. 908/233–3720; CHILDREN'S SPECIALIZED HOSPITAL–TOM'S RIVER, 94 Stevens Road, Mountainside, Zip 08755–1237; tel. 732/914–1100), (Total facility includes 66 beds in nursing home–type unit) **A**1 3 5 7 10 **F**3 25 26 28 32 33 37 56 61 62 66 72 73 77 81 85 86 87 89 90 94 132 135 **P**6 **S** Robert Wood Johnson Health System & Network
Primary Contact: Amy B. Mansue, President and Chief Executive Officer
COO: Warren E. Moore, Executive Vice President and Chief Operating Officer
CFO: Joseph J. Dobosh, Vice President and Chief Financial Officer
CMO: Frank V. Castello, M.D., Medical Director
CIO: Pat DeMartino, Chief Information Officer
CHR: William Dwyer, Vice President Human Resources
Web address: www.childrens–specialized.org
Control: Other not–for–profit (including NFP Corporation) **Service:** Children's rehabilitation

Staffed Beds: 126 **Admissions:** 388 **Census:** 106 **Outpatient Visits:** 141483 **Births:** 0 **Total Expense ($000):** 86516 **Payroll Expense ($000):** 52659 **Personnel:** 865

★ **ROBERT WOOD JOHNSON UNIVERSITY HOSPITAL (310038),** 1 Robert Wood Johnson Place, Zip 08903–2601; tel. 732/828–3000 **A**1 2 3 5 8 9 10 **F**3 6 7 8 9 11 13 14 15 17 18 19 20 21 22 23 24 25 26 27 28 30 31 32 33 34 35 36 37 38 40 41 43 44 46 47 48 49 50 51 52 53 54 55 56 57 58 59 60 61 62 63 64 66 68 69 70 71 72 73 74 75 76 77 79 80 81 82 83 84 86 87 89 90 92 94 96 97 98 99 100 101 102 103 104 105 106 107 108 109 111 112 113 114 116 118 119 120 121 123 124 125 126 127 130 131 132 135 136 137 **P**5 **S** Robert Wood Johnson Health System & Network
Primary Contact: Stephen K. Jones, President and Chief Executive Officer
COO: Vincent D. Joseph, Executive Vice President and Chief Operating Officer
CFO: Carl O'Brien, Senior Vice President Finance and Chief Financial Officer
CMO: Joshua M. Bershad, M.D., Acting Vice President Medical Affairs
CIO: Robert G. Irwin, Vice President Information Systems
CHR: John Regina, Senior Vice President Human Resources
Web address: www.rwjuh.edu
Control: Other not–for–profit (including NFP Corporation) **Service:** General Medical and Surgical

Staffed Beds: 610 **Admissions:** 30738 **Census:** 523 **Outpatient Visits:** 251000 **Births:** 2492 **Total Expense ($000):** 315768 **Payroll Expense ($000):** 258920 **Personnel:** 3976

NJ

★ **SAINT PETER'S UNIVERSITY HOSPITAL (310070)**, 254 Easton Avenue, Zip 08901–1780, Mailing Address: P.O. Box 591, Zip 08903–0591; tel. 732/745–8600 **A**1 2 3 5 8 9 10 **F**2 3 8 11 13 15 17 18 20 25 26 27 28 30 31 32 33 35 37 38 41 43 44 45 46 47 49 50 51 53 54 55 56 57 58 59 60 62 63 64 66 68 69 70 71 72 73 74 76 77 79 80 81 82 83 84 86 87 96 97 100 102 106 107 109 111 114 116 117 118 119 120 121 123 124 132 135 136 137 **P**3 6
Primary Contact: Alfred Glover, President and Chief Executive Officer
COO: Alfred Glover, President and Chief Executive Officer
CFO: Garrick J. Stoldt, Chief Financial Officer
CMO: John D'Anna, M.D., Chief Medical Officer
CIO: Frank DiSanzo, Chief Information Officer
CHR: Susan Ballestero, Senior Vice President Human Resources
Web address: www.saintpetersuh.com
Control: Church–operated, Nongovernment, not–for profit **Service:** General Medical and Surgical

Staffed Beds: 438 **Admissions:** 23733 **Census:** 303 **Outpatient Visits:** 351376 **Births:** 5958 **Total Expense ($000):** 356249 **Payroll Expense ($000):** 174802 **Personnel:** 2351

NEWARK—Essex County

□ **COLUMBUS HOSPITAL (310093)**, 495 North 13th Street, Zip 07107–1397; tel. 973/268–1400, (Nonreporting) **A**1 2 5 9 10 **S** Cathedral Healthcare System, Inc.
Primary Contact: Patricia Fehring White, Administrator
COO: Robert H. Evans, Chief Operating Officer
CFO: John S. Grywalski, CPA, Executive Vice President Financial Services
CMO: Bart De Gregorio, M.D., President Medical Staff
CIO: Angelo Schittone, Vice President and Chief Information Officer
CHR: Robert Lawrence, Vice President Human Resources and Educational Development
Web address: www.cathedralhealth.org
Control: Other not–for–profit (including NFP Corporation) **Service:** General Medical and Surgical

Staffed Beds: 206

MT. CARMEL BEHAVIORAL HEALTHCARE SYSTEM (314010), 1160 Raymond Boulevard, Zip 7102; tel. 973/596–4100, (Nonreporting) **A**9 10
Primary Contact: Ronald A. Finch, Ed.D., Director Healthcare
Control: Church–operated, Nongovernment, not–for profit **Service:** Psychiatric

Staffed Beds: 20

★ **NEWARK BETH ISRAEL MEDICAL CENTER (310002)**, 201 Lyons Avenue, Zip 07112–2027; tel. 973/926–7000 **A**1 2 3 5 8 9 10 12 13 **F**2 3 5 9 11 12 13 15 17 18 19 20 21 22 23 24 25 26 27 28 30 31 32 33 34 36 37 38 40 41 42 43 44 45 46 50 53 54 55 56 57 58 59 60 62 63 64 66 68 69 70 71 72 73 74 75 76 77 79 80 81 82 83 84 86 87 88 89 90 91 92 93 94 95 96 97 100 102 103 104 105 106 107 108 109 111 112 114 116 119 120 121 122 123 124 126 127 131 132 135 136 137 **P**5 8 **S** Saint Barnabas Health Care System
Primary Contact: John A. Brennan, M.D., Executive Director
COO: Kenneth L. Tyson, Senior Vice President Operations
CFO: Veronica Zeichner, Chief Financial Officer
CIO: Thomas Gregorio, Chief Information Officer
CHR: Zach Lipner, Vice President Human Resources
Web address: www.sbhcs.com
Control: Other not–for–profit (including NFP Corporation) **Service:** General Medical and Surgical

Staffed Beds: 407 **Admissions:** 22905 **Census:** 394 **Outpatient Visits:** 312447 **Births:** 3327 **Total Expense ($000):** 475216 **Payroll Expense ($000):** 226346 **Personnel:** 2945

★ **SAINT MICHAEL'S MEDICAL CENTER (310096)**, 268 Dr. Martin Luther King Jr. Boulevard, Zip 07102–2094; tel. 973/877–5000 **A**1 2 3 5 10 12 13 **F**3 4 5 11 12 15 17 18 20 22 24 25 26 27 30 32 33 36 38 43 46 48 49 50 55 56 57 59 60 62 64 66 68 72 73 76 77 79 80 81 82 84 86 87 88 90 91 92 94 95 96 97 99 100 101 102 107 109 111 112 116 118 119 121 135 136 137 **S** Cathedral Healthcare System, Inc.
Primary Contact: Felicia Karsos, Administrator
COO: Robert H. Evans, Chief Operating Officer
CFO: John S. Grywalski, CPA, Chief Financial Officer
CIO: Angelo Schittone, Chief Information Officer
CHR: Brendan Farrelly, Vice President Human Resources
Web address: www.cathedralhealthcare.org
Control: Church–operated, Nongovernment, not–for profit **Service:** General Medical and Surgical

Staffed Beds: 223 **Admissions:** 11257 **Census:** 170 **Outpatient Visits:** 69083 **Births:** 0 **Total Expense ($000):** 193373 **Payroll Expense ($000):** 86436 **Personnel:** 1305

★ **UNIVERSITY OF MEDICINE AND DENTISTRY OF NEW JERSEY–UNIVERSITY HOSPITAL (310119)**, 150 Bergen Street, Zip 07103–2496; tel. 973/972–4300 **A**1 2 3 5 8 9 10 **F**3 7 11 12 15 17 18 20 22 24 25 26 27 28 31 32 33 34 35 36 37 38 40 41 43 44 46 47 48 49 50 54 55 56 57 58 59 60 62 63 64 66 68 69 70 71 72 73 74 75 76 77 79 80 82 83 84 86 87 88 90 92 93 96 97 98 99 100 101 103 105 106 107 108 109 111 112 113 114 116 119 120 121 122 123 124 128 131 132 133 134 135 136 137
Primary Contact: Darlene L. Cox, President and Chief Executive Officer
CFO: Edward C. Burke, Chief Financial Officer and Special Advisor
CMO: Suzanne Atkin, M.D., Chief of Staff and Associate Dean Clinical Affairs
CIO: Richard Tunnell, Director Information Systems Technology and Health Management Information Systems
CHR: Gerard Garcia, Acting Vice President Human Resources
Web address: www.umdnj.edu
Control: State–Government, nonfederal **Service:** General Medical and Surgical

Staffed Beds: 444 **Admissions:** 20611 **Census:** 360 **Outpatient Visits:** 307064 **Births:** 1926 **Total Expense ($000):** 481456 **Payroll Expense ($000):** 284366 **Personnel:** 3363

NEWTON—Sussex County

★ **NEWTON MEMORIAL HOSPITAL (310028)**, 175 High Street, Zip 07860–1004; tel. 973/383–2121 **A**1 2 9 10 **F**1 3 4 5 8 11 12 13 15 16 17 18 20 24 25 26 27 28 30 31 32 33 36 37 38 43 46 55 56 57 59 60 61 62 63 64 65 66 68 70 71 72 73 74 75 76 77 78 79 80 81 82 83 84 85 86 87 88 89 90 91 92 93 94 95 96 97 102 106 107 117 118 119 120 121 124 132 133 135 137
Primary Contact: Thomas J. Senker, President and Chief Executive Officer
COO: Sean O'Rourke, Senior Vice President and Chief Operating Officer
CFO: David Rikkola, Vice President Finance and Chief Financial Officer
CMO: David Lazarus, M.D., Vice President Medical Affairs
CIO: Michael Zegar, Vice President Information Technology
CHR: Eva Goldenberg, Vice President Human Resources
Web address: www.nmhnj.org
Control: Other not–for–profit (including NFP Corporation) **Service:** General Medical and Surgical

Staffed Beds: 146 **Admissions:** 11581 **Census:** 102 **Outpatient Visits:** 243226 **Births:** 686 **Total Expense ($000):** 121597 **Payroll Expense ($000):** 58601 **Personnel:** 778

NORTH BERGEN—Hudson County

★ **PALISADES MEDICAL CENTER (310003)**, 7600 River Road, Zip 07047–6217; tel. 201/854–5000 **A**1 10 **F**11 13 15 18 24 25 26 27 30 32 33 36 38 42 46 52 54 55 56 57 62 66 68 71 72 73 74 75 76 77 79 80 81 82 84 86 92 94 96 99 100 103 107 118 119 120 121 124 132 135 136 137 **P**6
Primary Contact: Bruce J. Markowitz, President and Chief Executive Officer
COO: David J. Berkowitz, Vice President and Chief Operating Officer
CFO: John Calandriello, Vice President and Chief Financial Officer
CMO: Maria E. Bornia, M.D., Vice President Medical Staff
CIO: Maria Nunes, Director Management Information Systems
CHR: Donna Cahill, Vice President Human Resources
Web address: www.palisadesmedical.org
Control: Other not–for–profit (including NFP Corporation) **Service:** General Medical and Surgical

Staffed Beds: 194 **Admissions:** 9873 **Census:** 149 **Outpatient Visits:** 45359 **Births:** 1466 **Total Expense ($000):** 117347 **Payroll Expense ($000):** 53360 **Personnel:** 817

NORTH PLAINFIELD—Somerset County

★ **MUHLENBERG REGIONAL MEDICAL CENTER (310063)**, Park Avenue and Randolph Road, Zip 7060; tel. 908/668–2000 **A**1 2 3 5 6 10 **F**2 4 7 8 11 12 13 14 15 17 18 20 24 25 26 27 30 31 32 33 38 42 46 47 49 50 51 59 61 62 66 68 71 73 74 76 77 79 80 82 85 86 88 92 95 96 97 98 99 100 101 102 103 104 105 106 107 108 109 110 111 112 118 119 121 132 134 135 136 137 **S** Solaris Health System
Primary Contact: Nancy A. Fiamingo, Senior Vice President and Chief Operating Officer
COO: Nancy A. Fiamingo, Senior Vice President and Chief Operating Officer
CFO: Richard C. Smith, Senior Vice President and Chief Financial Officer
CMO: Robert Bayly, M.D., Vice President Medical Affairs
CIO: Louis H. Hermans, Vice President Information Systems and Chief Information Officer
CHR: Shirley Higgins–Bowers, Vice President Human Resources
Web address: www.solarishs.org
Control: Other not–for–profit (including NFP Corporation) **Service:** General Medical and Surgical

Staffed Beds: 184 **Admissions:** 9267 **Census:** 135 **Outpatient Visits:** 117620 **Births:** 2475 **Total Expense ($000):** 143003 **Payroll Expense ($000):** 71796 **Personnel:** 1193

NJ

Hospital, Medicare Provider Number, Address, Telephone, Approval, Facility, and Physician Codes, Health Care System
★ American Hospital Association (AHA) membership
□ The Joint Commission accreditation
○ American Osteopathic Association (AOA) accreditation
△ Commission on Accreditation of Rehabilitation Facilities (CARF) accreditation

OLD BRIDGE—Middlesex County

OLD BRIDGE DIVISION See Raritan Bay Medical Center, Perth Amboy

PARAMUS—Bergen County

☐ **BERGEN REGIONAL MEDICAL CENTER (310058)**, 230 East Ridgewood Avenue, Zip 07652–4131; tel. 201/967–4000, (Total facility includes 574 beds in nursing home–type unit) **A**1 9 10 **F**3 4 5 6 11 15 26 27 30 31 32 33 36 38 41 42 43 44 45 50 54 55 56 57 59 60 64 66 68 72 73 75 76 77 79 80 81 86 87 88 89 91 92 93 94 95 96 100 103 107 117 118 119 121 134 135 137 **P**6
Primary Contact: Heather Aaron, President and Chairperson
COO: Susan Mendelowitz, Executive Vice President and Chief Operating Officer
CFO: James Alund, Executive Vice President and Chief Financial Officer
CMO: Robert M. Harris, M.D., President Medical and Dental Staff
CIO: Ronald Li, Vice President Management Information Systems
CHR: Guy Mennonna, Senior Vice President Human Resources
Web address: www.bergenregional.com
Control: County–Government, nonfederal **Service:** Psychiatric

Staffed Beds: 993 **Admissions:** 10730 **Census:** 993 **Outpatient Visits:** 68299 **Births:** 0 **Total Expense ($000):** 180287 **Payroll Expense ($000):** 79445 **Personnel:** 1635

PASSAIC—Passaic County

PBI REGIONAL MEDICAL CENTER (310020), 70 Parker Avenue, Zip 07055–7000; tel. 973/365–5000, (Nonreporting) **A**9 10
Primary Contact: Hank Wells, Interim President and Chief Executive Officer
CFO: Joe Aquilante, Vice President Finance
Web address: www.pbih.org
Control: Other not–for–profit (including NFP Corporation) **Service:** General Medical and Surgical

Staffed Beds: 210

⊠ **ST. MARY'S HOSPITAL (310006)**, 350 Boulevard, Zip 7055; tel. 973/365–4300 **A**1 9 10 **F**8 13 15 18 20 22 24 25 26 27 33 36 38 43 46 48 56 59 60 63 66 68 71 73 74 76 77 79 84 86 87 88 89 90 91 92 94 95 96 97 100 101 107 108 118 119 123 124 133 135 136 137 **P**5 8
Primary Contact: Colene Y. Daniel, M.S., M.P.H., FACHE, President and Chief Executive Officer
COO: Robert C. Iannaccone, Executive Vice President and Chief Operating Officer
CFO: Brian McIndoe, Vice President Finance and Chief Financial Officer
CMO: Charles Herbstman, M.D., President Medical and Dental Staff
CHR: Ronald Brooks, Vice President Human Resources
Web address: www.smh–passaic.org
Control: Other not–for–profit (including NFP Corporation) **Service:** General Medical and Surgical

Staffed Beds: 289 **Admissions:** 11516 **Census:** 170 **Outpatient Visits:** 193332 **Births:** 1457 **Total Expense ($000):** 159400 **Payroll Expense ($000):** 68222 **Personnel:** 1406

PATERSON—Passaic County

★ ○ **ST. JOSEPH'S REGIONAL MEDICAL CENTER (310019)**, 703 Main Street, Zip 07503–2691; tel. 973/754–2000, (Total facility includes 151 beds in nursing home–type unit) **A**2 3 5 9 10 11 12 13 **F**3 5 13 14 15 17 18 19 20 21 22 23 24 25 26 27 28 31 32 33 36 37 38 40 41 42 43 44 46 47 48 49 50 53 54 55 56 57 58 59 60 61 62 63 64 66 68 69 70 71 72 73 74 75 76 77 79 80 81 82 83 84 86 87 88 89 90 91 92 93 94 95 96 97 98 100 102 103 104 105 106 107 108 109 111 114 119 120 121 122 123 124 133 134 135 136 137 **P**5 **S** St. Joseph's Healthcare System
Primary Contact: William A. McDonald, President and Chief Executive Officer
COO: Gloria A. Kunze, R.N., Vice President Operations
CFO: Jack Robinson, Chief Financial Officer
CMO: James Labagnara, M.D., Vice President Medical Affairs
CIO: James Cavanagh, Chief Information Officer
CHR: John Bruno, Vice President Human Resources
Web address: www.stjosephshealth.org
Control: Church–operated, Nongovernment, not–for profit **Service:** General Medical and Surgical

Staffed Beds: 651 **Admissions:** 26360 **Census:** 388 **Outpatient Visits:** 2399445 **Births:** 3392 **Total Expense ($000):** 433820 **Payroll Expense ($000):** 216448 **Personnel:** 3463

PEAPACK—Somerset County

☐ **MATHENY MEDICAL AND EDUCATIONAL CENTER (312014)**, 65 Highland Avenue, Zip 7977, Mailing Address: P.O. Box 339, Zip 07977–0339; tel. 908/234–0011 **A**1 5 10 **F**2 25 26 31 32 33 37 53 62 69 72 75 77 86 87 94 119 133 135 136 137 **P**1 6
Primary Contact: Steven M. Proctor, President
COO: Christopher King, Director Operations and Administrative Services
CFO: Wayne Guberman, Director Finance
CMO: Gary E. Eddey, M.D., Medical Director
CIO: Ron Daniel, Manager Information Systems
CHR: Nancy Petrillo, Director Human Resources
Web address: www.matheny.org
Control: Other not–for–profit (including NFP Corporation) **Service:** Chronic disease

Staffed Beds: 101 **Admissions:** 7 **Census:** 97 **Outpatient Visits:** 1600 **Births:** 0 **Total Expense ($000):** 33167 **Payroll Expense ($000):** 20024 **Personnel:** 455

PERTH AMBOY—Middlesex County

☐ **CARE ONE REHABILITATION HOSPITAL (312018)**, 530 New Brunswick Avenue, Zip 8861; tel. 732/324–6090, (Nonreporting) **A**1 10
Primary Contact: Michael Burns, Chief Executive Officer
CFO: Richard Burguillos, Chief Financial Officer
Control: Corporation, Investor–owned, for–profit **Service:** Long–Term Acute Care hospital

Staffed Beds: 30

⊠ **RARITAN BAY MEDICAL CENTER (310039)**, 530 New Brunswick Avenue, Zip 8861; tel. 732/442–3700, (Includes OLD BRIDGE DIVISION, One Hospital Plaza, Old Bridge, Zip 08857; tel. 732/360–1000; PERTH AMBOY DIVISION) **A**1 2 3 5 6 9 10 **F**7 11 12 13 15 25 26 27 30 31 32 33 34 36 38 42 43 44 46 53 54 55 57 60 62 63 68 72 73 74 76 77 79 84 88 90 92 93 94 96 97 100 102 105 107 118 121 132 135 136 137 **P**5
Primary Contact: Michael R. D'Agnes, President and Chief Executive Officer
COO: Vincent Costantino, Vice President Operations and Human Resources
CFO: Thomas Shanahan, Chief Financial Officer and Senior Vice President
CMO: Michael Ciencewicki, M.D., Vice President Medical Affairs
CHR: Vincent Costantino, Vice President Operations and Human Resources
Web address: www.rbmc.org
Control: Other not–for–profit (including NFP Corporation) **Service:** General Medical and Surgical

Staffed Beds: 396 **Admissions:** 17275 **Census:** 249 **Outpatient Visits:** 139995 **Births:** 1100 **Total Expense ($000):** 223064 **Payroll Expense ($000):** 107281 **Personnel:** 1781

PHILLIPSBURG—Warren County

⊠ **WARREN HOSPITAL (310060)**, 185 Roseberry Street, Zip 08865–9955; tel. 908/859–6700 **A**1 2 3 5 9 10 12 13 **F**3 5 8 11 13 15 18 24 25 26 27 30 31 32 33 37 38 43 49 52 53 54 56 57 60 62 63 64 66 68 73 74 75 76 79 81 82 86 87 88 90 92 93 96 97 100 102 106 107 118 119 120 121 123 135 137 **P**7
Primary Contact: Jeffrey C. Goodwin, President and Chief Executive Officer
COO: Jeffrey W. Kelly, Senior Vice President Administration and Chief Operating Officer
CFO: Carl M. Alberto, Vice President Finance and Chief Financial Officer
CMO: Frank Gilly, M.D., Vice President Medical Affairs
CIO: Debbie Bowlby, Director Information Systems
CHR: William Durett, Director Human Resources
Web address: www.warrenhospital.org
Control: Other not–for–profit (including NFP Corporation) **Service:** General Medical and Surgical

Staffed Beds: 150 **Admissions:** 6839 **Census:** 86 **Outpatient Visits:** 141948 **Births:** 354 **Total Expense ($000):** 110725 **Payroll Expense ($000):** 44405 **Personnel:** 996

PISCATAWAY—Middlesex County

UNIVERSITY OF MEDICINE AND DENTISTRY OF NEW JERSEY, UNIVERSITY BEHAVIORAL HEALTHCARE (314011), 671 Hoes Lane, Zip 8855, Mailing Address: P.O. Box 1392, Zip 08855–1392; tel. 732/235–5900, (Nonreporting) **A**9 10
Primary Contact: Christopher O. Kosseff, President and Chief Executive Officer
COO: Susan Furrer, PsyD, Acting Chief Operating Officer and Executive Director Behavioral Research and Training Institute
CFO: Alan Weinkrantz, Chief Financial Officer
CMO: Theresa Miskimen, M.D., Vice President Medical Services
CIO: Bruce Blakeslee, Director Information Services
Web address: www.umdnj.edu
Control: State–Government, nonfederal **Service:** Psychiatric

Staffed Beds: 64

POMONA—Atlantic County

ATLANTIC CITY MEDICAL CENTER–MAINLAND DIVISION See Atlanticare Regional Medical Center, Atlantic City

 Many Facility Codes have changed. Please refer to the AHA Guide Code Chart.

★ △ **BACHARACH INSTITUTE FOR REHABILITATION (313030)**, 61 West Jimmie Leeds Road, Zip 08240–0723, Mailing Address: P.O. Box 723, Zip 08240–0723; tel. 609/652–7000, (Nonreporting) **A**1 7 10
Primary Contact: Richard J. Kathrins, President and Chief Executive Officer
CFO: Janet Turso, Vice President Finance
CMO: Craig Anmuth, M.D., Medical Director
CIO: Jeff Rees, Director Information Systems
CHR: Diane Croshaw, Vice President Human Resources
Web address: www.bacharach.org
Control: Other not–for–profit (including NFP Corporation) **Service:** Rehabilitation

Staffed Beds: 80

POMPTON PLAINS—Morris County

★ **CHILTON MEMORIAL HOSPITAL (310017)**, 97 West Parkway, Zip 07444–1696; tel. 973/831–5000 **A**1 2 9 10 **F**3 7 11 12 13 15 17 18 20 24 25 26 27 28 30 31 32 33 38 41 43 44 47 49 50 53 55 56 57 62 63 64 66 68 70 71 72 73 74 75 76 77 79 80 81 82 84 86 87 88 89 90 92 93 96 97 98 99 100 102 104 105 106 107 109 111 118 119 120 121 124 135 137
Primary Contact: Deborah K. Zastocki, FACHE, President and Chief Executive Officer
COO: Thomas Scott, Chief Operating Officer
CFO: Michael Richetti, Chief Financial Officer
CMO: Charles Ross, M.D., Vice President Medical Affairs
CIO: Karen S. Smith, Director Information Services
CHR: Julia McGovern, Vice President Human Resources
Web address: www.chiltonmemorial.org
Control: Other not–for–profit (including NFP Corporation) **Service:** General Medical and Surgical

Staffed Beds: 260 **Admissions:** 11768 **Census:** 151 **Outpatient Visits:** 135803 **Births:** 1011 **Total Expense ($000):** 137547 **Payroll Expense ($000):** 65060 **Personnel:** 1168

PRINCETON—Mercer County

★ △ **UNIVERSITY MEDICAL CENTER AT PRINCETON (310010)**, 253 Witherspoon Street, Zip 08540–3213; tel. 609/497–4000, (Includes ACUTE GENERAL HOSPITAL, MERWICK UNIT–EXTENDED CARE AND REHABILITATION, PRINCETON HOUSE UNIT–COMMUNITY MENTAL HEALTH AND SUBSTANCE ABUSE), (Total facility includes 93 beds in nursing home–type unit) (Nonreporting) **A**1 2 3 5 7 8 9 10
Primary Contact: Vincent D. Joseph, President
CFO: Bruce Traub, Chief Financial Officer
CMO: Melissa Schori, M.D., Vice President Medical Affairs
CIO: Steve Locke, Vice President and Chief Information Officer
CHR: Lucille Mason, Vice President Human Resources
Web address: www.princetonhcs.org
Control: Other not–for–profit (including NFP Corporation) **Service:** General Medical and Surgical

Staffed Beds: 392

RAHWAY—Union County

☐ **KINDRED HOSPITAL NEW JERSEY – RAHWAY**, 865 Stone Street, Zip 7065; tel. 732/453–2950, (Nonreporting) **A**1 **S** Kindred Healthcare
Primary Contact: Janet Biedron, Chief Executive Officer
Control: Corporation, Investor–owned, for–profit **Service:** Other specialty

Staffed Beds: 28

★ **ROBERT WOOD JOHNSON UNIVERSITY HOSPITAL AT RAHWAY (310024)**, 865 Stone Street, Zip 07065–2797; tel. 732/381–4200, (Total facility includes 24 beds in nursing home–type unit) **A**1 10 **F**3 11 15 17 18 25 26 27 30 31 32 33 36 38 42 43 46 47 49 50 54 55 56 57 62 63 66 68 72 73 75 76 77 79 81 82 86 87 90 91 92 96 97 100 105 106 107 117 119 121 123 132 135 136 137 **S** Robert Wood Johnson Health System & Network
Primary Contact: Kirk C. Tice, President and Chief Executive Officer
CFO: Peter Bihuniak, Vice President Finance
CMO: Howard Pecker, M.D., President Medical Staff
CIO: Denine Izzi, Site Manager Information Systems
CHR: Kathryn Tarantino, Vice President Human Resources
Web address: www.rahwayhospital.com
Control: Other not–for–profit (including NFP Corporation) **Service:** General Medical and Surgical

Staffed Beds: 165 **Admissions:** 8181 **Census:** 131 **Outpatient Visits:** 64562 **Births:** 0 **Total Expense ($000):** 106639 **Payroll Expense ($000):** 46607 **Personnel:** 824

RED BANK—Monmouth County

★ △ **RIVERVIEW MEDICAL CENTER (310034)**, 1 Riverview Plaza, Zip 07701–9982; tel. 732/741–2700 **A**1 2 7 9 10 **F**3 5 11 13 15 17 18 20 24 25 26 27 30 31 32 33 36 38 41 43 46 47 49 51 54 55 57 59 60 62 64 66 68 71 72 73 74 76 77 78 79 80 81 82 84 85 86 87 88 89 90 91 92 93 94 95 96 97 99 100 102 103 105 107 108 109 111 112 114 118 119 121 122 124 133 134 135 136 137 **S** Meridian Health
Primary Contact: Timothy J. Hogan, President
CFO: Chitra Kasinathan, Site Manager Finance
CMO: Richard Scott, M.D., Vice President Medical Affairs and Clinical Effectiveness
CIO: Donna Sellmann, Manager Communications and Marketing
CHR: Sheila Hintze, Manager
Web address: www.meridianhealth.com
Control: Other not–for–profit (including NFP Corporation) **Service:** General Medical and Surgical

Staffed Beds: 278 **Admissions:** 15363 **Census:** 200 **Outpatient Visits:** 124377 **Births:** 1663 **Total Expense ($000):** 172880 **Payroll Expense ($000):** 76571 **Personnel:** 985

RIDGEWOOD—Bergen County

★ **VALLEY HOSPITAL (310012)**, 223 North Van Dien Avenue, Zip 07450–9982; tel. 201/447–8000 **A**1 2 5 9 10 **F**3 8 11 12 13 15 17 18 20 22 24 25 26 27 28 30 31 32 33 34 35 36 38 43 44 46 47 49 50 51 52 53 54 55 56 57 58 59 60 62 63 64 66 67 68 70 71 72 73 74 75 76 77 78 79 80 81 82 83 84 86 87 90 91 92 93 96 97 98 100 102 104 106 107 108 109 111 112 113 114 116 118 119 120 121 123 124 132 135 136 137 **P**6
Primary Contact: Audrey Meyers, President and Chief Executive Officer
CFO: Richard Keenan, Senior Vice President Finance and Chief Financial Officer
CMO: Mitchell Rubinstein, M.D., Vice President Medical Affairs
CIO: Peter Schwartz, Vice President Information Systems and Chief Information Officer
CHR: Anne Raftery, Vice President Human Resources
Web address: www.valleyhealth.com
Control: Other not–for–profit (including NFP Corporation) **Service:** General Medical and Surgical

Staffed Beds: 437 **Admissions:** 27040 **Census:** 343 **Outpatient Visits:** 286340 **Births:** 3286 **Total Expense ($000):** 429536 **Payroll Expense ($000):** 206811 **Personnel:** 3058

ROCHELLE PARK—Bergen County

SELECT SPECIALTY HOSPITAL OF NORTHEAST (312019), (Formerly Select Specialty Hospital–Belleville), 96 Parkway, Zip 7662; tel. 201/221–2351, (Nonreporting) **A**10 **S** Select Medical Corporation
Primary Contact: Barbara E. Hannan, Chief Executive Officer
Web address: www.selectmedicalcorp.com
Control: Corporation, Investor–owned, for–profit **Service:** Other specialty

Staffed Beds: 25

SALEM—Salem County

★ **MEMORIAL HOSPITAL OF SALEM COUNTY (310091)**, 310 Woodstown Road, Zip 08079–2080; tel. 856/935–1000 **A**1 9 10 **F**13 15 18 24 25 26 30 31 32 38 42 50 55 56 61 62 63 68 72 73 74 79 81 82 84 86 96 100 102 107 135 **P**7 **S** Community Health Systems, Inc.
Primary Contact: James L. Angle, Chief Executive Officer
CFO: James Waschecka, Chief Financial Officer
CIO: Brian McCarthy, Information Systems Director
Web address: www.salemhospitalnj.org
Control: Corporation, Investor–owned, for–profit **Service:** General Medical and Surgical

Staffed Beds: 110 **Admissions:** 5405 **Census:** 53 **Outpatient Visits:** 59972 **Births:** 378 **Total Expense ($000):** 52025 **Payroll Expense ($000):** 21073 **Personnel:** 410

NJ

Hospital, Medicare Provider Number, Address, Telephone, Approval, Facility, and Physician Codes, Health Care System
★ American Hospital Association (AHA) membership
☐ The Joint Commission accreditation
○ American Osteopathic Association (AOA) accreditation
△ Commission on Accreditation of Rehabilitation Facilities (CARF) accreditation

SECAUCUS—Hudson County

☐ **LIBERTYHEALTH–MEADOWLANDS HOSPITAL MEDICAL CENTER (310118)**, 55 Meadowland Parkway, Zip 07094–1580; tel. 201/392–3100, (Total facility includes 8 beds in nursing home–type unit) **A**1 9 10 **F**3 4 5 11 13 15 17 18 20 24 25 26 27 29 30 31 32 33 34 36 38 40 41 43 44 46 49 50 52 54 55 57 59 62 63 66 68 71 72 73 74 77 78 79 80 81 82 83 84 85 86 90 96 97 102 106 107 113 117 118 119 120 121 124 132 135 136 137 **S** LibertyHealth
Primary Contact: Joseph F. Scott, Chief Executive Officer
COO: Martin W. Baicker, CHE, Senior Vice President and Administrator
CFO: Donald Parseghian, Chief Financial Officer
CMO: Kenneth Garay, M.D., Chief Medical Officer
CIO: James Yost, Director Management Information Systems
CHR: Mary Cataudella, Corporate Director Human Resources
Web address: www.libertyhcs.com
Control: Other not–for–profit (including NFP Corporation) **Service:** General Medical and Surgical

Staffed Beds: 163 **Admissions:** 6023 **Census:** 96 **Outpatient Visits:** 28563 **Births:** 784 **Total Expense ($000):** 67905 **Payroll Expense ($000):** 30973 **Personnel:** 442

SOMERS POINT—Atlantic County

★ **SHORE MEMORIAL HOSPITAL (310047)**, 1 East New York Avenue, Zip 08244–2387; tel. 609/653–3500 **A**1 2 9 10 **F**3 11 13 15 17 18 24 25 26 27 30 31 32 33 35 38 41 43 44 49 50 53 55 56 57 59 60 62 64 66 68 71 72 73 74 75 76 77 79 80 81 82 84 86 96 97 99 100 102 106 107 108 109 111 118 119 121 124 132 135 136 137
Primary Contact: Albert Gutierrez, President and Chief Executive Officer
COO: Ronald Johnson, Vice President Operations and Chief Operating Officer
CFO: James T. Foley, Vice President and Chief Financial Officer
CMO: Peter R. Jungblut, M.D., Vice President Medical Affairs and Chief Medical Officer
CIO: Ronald Johnson, Vice President Operations and Chief Operating Officer
CHR: Alan Beatty, Vice President Human Resources
Web address: www.shorememorial.org
Control: Other not–for–profit (including NFP Corporation) **Service:** General Medical and Surgical

Staffed Beds: 208 **Admissions:** 12076 **Census:** 151 **Outpatient Visits:** 102991 **Births:** 1470 **Total Expense ($000):** 173740 **Payroll Expense ($000):** 77062 **Personnel:** 1336

SOMERVILLE—Somerset County

★ **SOMERSET MEDICAL CENTER (310048)**, 110 Rehill Avenue, Zip 08876–2598; tel. 908/685–2200 **A**1 2 3 5 9 10 **F**7 12 13 14 15 18 20 24 25 26 27 33 38 43 46 52 54 55 56 57 58 59 60 62 63 65 66 68 72 73 74 75 76 79 82 84 86 87 89 90 91 92 93 94 95 96 97 99 100 104 105 106 107 109 118 119 120 121 124 135 136
Primary Contact: Kenneth Bateman, President and Chief Executive Officer
COO: Maureen Schneider, Vice President Patient Care Services and Chief Operating Officer
CFO: James De Rosa, Assistant Vice President Finance
CMO: Richard Paris, M.D., Chief Medical Officer
CIO: Dave Dyer, Vice President and Chief Information Officer
CHR: Mary Ann Bross, Vice President Human Resources
Web address: www.smchealthwise.com
Control: State–Government, nonfederal **Service:** General Medical and Surgical

Staffed Beds: 308 **Admissions:** 15868 **Census:** 224 **Births:** 1471 **Total Expense ($000):** 220959 **Payroll Expense ($000):** 96087

STRATFORD—Camden County

KENNEDY MEMORIAL HOSPITAL See Kennedy Memorial Hospitals–University Medical Center, Cherry Hill

SUMMIT—Union County

★ **OVERLOOK HOSPITAL (310051)**, 99 Beauvoir Avenue, Zip 07902–0220; tel. 908/522–2000 **A**1 2 3 5 9 10 12 13 **F**3 7 11 12 13 14 15 17 18 20 24 25 26 27 28 30 31 32 33 34 35 36 37 38 39 41 42 43 44 45 46 48 49 50 51 52 53 54 55 56 57 58 59 60 61 62 63 64 66 67 68 69 70 71 72 73 74 75 76 77 79 80 81 82 84 86 87 88 89 90 91 92 93 94 95 96 97 98 99 100 102 103 104 105 106 107 108 109 111 112 113 114 118 119 120 121 123 124 130 132 133 134 135 136 137 **P**6 **S** Atlantic Health
Primary Contact: Alan R. Lieber, Chief Operating Officer
COO: Alan R. Lieber, Chief Operating Officer
CFO: Kevin Shanley, Vice President Finance and Chief Financial Officer
CMO: Joanne M. Conroy, M.D., Executive Vice President and Chief Operating Officer
CIO: Linda Reed, Vice President and Chief Information Officer
CHR: Andrew Kovach, Vice President Human Resources and Shared Services
Web address: www.atlantichealth.org/cons/hospitals/at_OH
Control: Other not–for–profit (including NFP Corporation) **Service:** General Medical and Surgical

Staffed Beds: 373 **Admissions:** 18586 **Census:** 278 **Outpatient Visits:** 319955 **Births:** 2341 **Total Expense ($000):** 312008 **Payroll Expense ($000):** 157825 **Personnel:** 2843

☐ **SUMMIT OAKS HOSPITAL (314001)**, 19 Prospect Street, Zip 07902–0100; tel. 908/522–7000, (Nonreporting) **A**1 9 10 **S** Psychiatric Solutions
Primary Contact: James P. Gallagher, Chief Executive Officer
Control: Corporation, Investor–owned, for–profit **Service:** Psychiatric

Staffed Beds: 90

SUSSEX—Sussex County

SAINT CLARE'S HOSPITAL/SUSSEX See Saint Clare's Hospital, Dover

TEANECK—Bergen County

★ **HOLY NAME HOSPITAL (310008)**, 718 Teaneck Road, Zip 07666–4281; tel. 201/833–3000 **A**1 2 6 9 10 **F**2 3 7 11 12 13 15 18 20 24 25 26 27 28 31 32 33 34 37 38 42 43 45 46 47 49 50 51 52 53 54 55 56 57 58 59 61 62 63 64 66 68 71 72 73 74 75 76 77 79 80 81 82 84 86 87 88 90 92 93 96 97 99 100 102 103 104 105 106 107 108 109 111 112 114 118 119 121 122 124 132 133 135 136 137 **P**5
Primary Contact: Michael Maron, President and Chief Executive Officer
CFO: Gregory Adams, Senior Vice President and Chief Financial Officer
CMO: Paul Mendelowitz, M.D., Senior Vice President Medical Affairs
CIO: Michael Skuarenina, Assistant Vice President Information Systems
CHR: Anthony Pellicano, Vice President Human Resources
Web address: www.holyname.org
Control: Other not–for–profit (including NFP Corporation) **Service:** General Medical and Surgical

Staffed Beds: 318 **Admissions:** 17599 **Census:** 213 **Outpatient Visits:** 259916 **Births:** 1183 **Total Expense ($000):** 208506 **Payroll Expense ($000):** 97719 **Personnel:** 1813

TINTON FALLS—Monmouth County

★ **REHABILITATION HOSPITAL OF TINTON FALLS (313035)**, 2 Centre Plaza, Zip 7724; tel. 732/460–5320 **A**1 10 **F**24 25 31 32 53 54 55 56 57 72 77 85 86 119 120 121 137 **S** HEALTHSOUTH Corporation
Primary Contact: Linda A. Savino, Chief Executive Officer
CFO: Lynne Freel, Controller
CMO: Todd Cooperman, M.D., Medical Director
CHR: Anita Saum, Manager Human Resources
Web address: www.rehabnj.com
Control: Corporation, Investor–owned, for–profit **Service:** Rehabilitation

Staffed Beds: 60 **Admissions:** 1197 **Census:** 43 **Outpatient Visits:** 9785 **Births:** 0 **Total Expense ($000):** 13196 **Payroll Expense ($000):** 8576 **Personnel:** 164

TOMS RIVER—Ocean County

★ **COMMUNITY MEDICAL CENTER (310041)**, 99 Route 37 West, Zip 08755–6423; tel. 732/557–8000 **A**1 2 9 10 **F**2 3 11 12 13 14 15 17 18 24 25 26 27 28 31 32 33 34 36 38 40 41 42 43 44 49 50 51 52 54 55 56 57 58 59 60 61 62 66 67 68 71 72 73 74 75 76 77 79 80 81 82 84 86 87 90 96 97 98 100 102 103 106 107 108 109 111 112 116 117 118 119 120 121 122 123 124 135 136 137 **P**5 **S** Saint Barnabas Health Care System
Primary Contact: Mark D. Pilla, Executive Director
COO: Frank Gelormini, Vice President Support Services
CFO: Thomas Percello, Vice President Financial Services
CMO: John Crisanti, M.D., Vice President Medical Affairs
CIO: Richard Wheatley, Vice President Information Services
CHR: Jane Palaia, Vice President Human Resources
Web address: www.sbhcs.com
Control: Other not–for–profit (including NFP Corporation) **Service:** General Medical and Surgical

Staffed Beds: 495 **Admissions:** 27769 **Census:** 383 **Outpatient Visits:** 311277 **Births:** 1736 **Total Expense ($000):** 313080 **Payroll Expense ($000):** 135874 **Personnel:** 2156

★ **HEALTHSOUTH REHABILITATION HOSPITAL OF NEW JERSEY (313029)**, 14 Hospital Drive, Zip 08755–6470; tel. 732/244–3100, (Total facility includes 33 beds in nursing home–type unit) (Nonreporting) **A**1 10 **S** HEALTHSOUTH Corporation
Primary Contact: Patricia Ostaszewski, Chief Executive Officer
CFO: David Totaro, Controller
CMO: Joseph Stillo, M.D., Medical Director
CIO: Lori Munyan, Director Quality Services
Web address: www.healthsouth.com
Control: Corporation, Investor–owned, for–profit **Service:** Rehabilitation

Staffed Beds: 131

NJ

 Many Facility Codes have changed. Please refer to the AHA Guide Code Chart.

TRENTON—Mercer County

★ **CAPITAL HEALTH SYSTEM AT FULD (310092)**, 750 Brunswick Avenue, Zip 08638–4174; tel. 609/394–6000 **A**1 3 5 6 10 **F**3 5 11 15 17 24 25 26 27 30 31 32 33 34 36 38 40 41 43 44 49 50 51 53 54 56 58 59 60 62 64 66 68 72 73 76 77 79 80 82 84 86 87 88 89 90 91 92 93 94 95 96 97 100 102 107 111 118 119 121 134 **P**6 **S** Capital Health System
Primary Contact: Al Maghazehe, Chief Executive Officer
COO: Larry DiSanto, Executive Vice President and Chief Operating Officer
CFO: Ronald J. Guy, Chief Financial Officer
CMO: Robert Remstein, D.O., Vice President Medical Affairs
CIO: Gene Grochala, Vice President Information Systems
CHR: Scott Clemmensen, Vice President Human Resources and Leadership Enhancement
Web address: www.capitalhealth.org
Control: Other not–for–profit (including NFP Corporation) **Service:** General Medical and Surgical

Staffed Beds: 195 **Admissions:** 7846 **Census:** 131 **Outpatient Visits:** 126071 **Births:** 0 **Total Expense ($000):** 170710 **Payroll Expense ($000):** 80372 **Personnel:** 1370

★ **CAPITAL HEALTH SYSTEM AT MERCER (310044)**, 446 Bellevue Avenue, Zip 08618–4597, Mailing Address: P.O. Box 1658, Zip 08607–1658; tel. 609/394–4000 **A**1 2 3 5 6 9 10 **F**3 11 13 15 17 18 20 24 25 26 27 28 30 31 32 33 34 38 41 42 43 44 49 50 51 53 54 56 58 59 62 64 66 68 70 71 72 73 74 76 77 79 80 82 84 86 87 90 96 97 98 102 104 107 109 111 112 114 118 119 121 134 135 136 137 **P**6 **S** Capital Health System
Primary Contact: Al Maghazehe, Chief Executive Officer
COO: Larry DiSanto, Executive Vice President and Chief Operating Officer
CFO: Ronald J. Guy, Chief Financial Officer
CMO: Norman Coopersmith, M.D., Vice President Medical Affairs
CIO: Gene Grochala, Vice President Information Systems
CHR: Scott Clemmensen, Vice President Human Resources and Leadership Enhancement
Web address: www.capitalhealth.org
Control: Other not–for–profit (including NFP Corporation) **Service:** General Medical and Surgical

Staffed Beds: 235 **Admissions:** 10576 **Census:** 130 **Outpatient Visits:** 160540 **Births:** 2515 **Total Expense ($000):** 183743 **Payroll Expense ($000):** 88028 **Personnel:** 1278

★ **ST. FRANCIS MEDICAL CENTER (310021)**, 601 Hamilton Avenue, Zip 08629–1986; tel. 609/599–5000 **A**1 2 6 9 10 **F**3 11 12 15 17 18 20 22 24 25 26 27 30 31 32 33 38 42 43 46 48 49 50 54 55 56 57 58 59 60 61 62 63 64 66 67 68 69 72 73 75 76 77 79 80 81 82 86 87 88 89 90 91 92 93 94 95 96 97 99 100 102 103 106 107 109 112 118 119 121 123 124 132 133 135 136 137 **P**5 6 **S** Catholic Health East
Primary Contact: Gerard J. Jablonowski, President and Chief Executive Officer
COO: Joseph Flamini, Vice President Operations
CFO: Gail Kosyla, Executive Vice President and Chief Financial Officer
CMO: C. James Romano, M.D., President Medical Staff
CIO: Richard Dowgun, Chief Information Officer
CHR: Laura James, Director Human Resources
Web address: www.stfrancismedical.org
Control: Church–operated, Nongovernment, not–for profit **Service:** General Medical and Surgical

Staffed Beds: 165 **Admissions:** 6713 **Census:** 100 **Outpatient Visits:** 88332 **Births:** 0 **Total Expense ($000):** 115831 **Payroll Expense ($000):** 46760 **Personnel:** 846

★ **ST. LAWRENCE REHABILITATION CENTER (313027)**, 2381 Lawrenceville Road, Zip 08648–2024; tel. 609/896–9500, (Total facility includes 30 beds in nursing home–type unit) (Nonreporting) **A**1 10
Primary Contact: Charles L. Brennan, President and Chief Executive Officer
CFO: Thomas W. Boyle, Chief Financial Officer
CIO: Jane Millner, Director Community Relations and Development
Web address: www.slrc.org
Control: Church–operated, Nongovernment, not–for profit **Service:** Rehabilitation

Staffed Beds: 116

★ **TRENTON PSYCHIATRIC HOSPITAL (314013)**, Route 29 and Sullivan Way, Zip 08628–3425, Mailing Address: P.O. Box 7500, West Trenton, Zip 08628–7500; tel. 609/633–1500, (Nonreporting) **A**1 10 **S** Division of Mental Health Services, Department of Human Services, State of New Jersey
Primary Contact: Teresa A. McQuaide, Chief Executive Officer
COO: Christopher Morrison, Deputy Chief Executive Officer
CFO: Joseph Canale, Business Manager
CMO: Lawrence Rossi, M.D., Chief Medicine
CIO: Christopher Morrison, Director Information Technology
Control: State–Government, nonfederal **Service:** Psychiatric

Staffed Beds: 436

TURNERSVILLE—Camden County

KENNEDY MEMORIAL HOSPITAL See Kennedy Memorial Hospitals–University Medical Center, Cherry Hill

VINELAND—Cumberland County

□ **REHABILITATION HOSPITAL OF SOUTH JERSEY (313036)**, 1237 West Sherman Avenue, Zip 8360; tel. 856/696–7100 **A**1 10 **F**32 85 86 **P**5
Primary Contact: Frank Bonner, M.D., Chief Executive Officer and Medical Director
Web address: www.rhsj.com
Control: State–Government, nonfederal **Service:** Rehabilitation

Staffed Beds: 34 **Admissions:** 753 **Census:** 24 **Outpatient Visits:** 5040 **Births:** 0

★ **SOUTH JERSEY HEALTHCARE – REGIONAL MEDICAL CENTER (310032)**, 1505 West Sherman Avenue, Zip 8360; tel. 856/641–8000, (Includes BRIDGETON HEALTH CENTER, 333 Irving Avenue, Bridgeton, Zip 08302–2100; tel. 856/575–4500) **A**1 2 9 10 **F**3 11 12 13 15 17 18 24 25 26 30 31 32 33 36 38 39 41 43 50 55 56 57 59 62 66 68 71 72 73 74 75 76 77 79 80 81 82 84 86 88 89 90 91 92 93 94 95 96 97 99 100 102 103 106 107 108 109 111 119 120 121 123 135 136 137 **P**6 **S** South Jersey Healthcare
Primary Contact: Chester B. Kaletkowski, President and Chief Executive Officer
COO: Elizabeth Sheridan, Chief Operating Officer
CFO: John A. DiAngelo, Senior Vice President Finance and Chief Financial Officer
CMO: Steven C. Linn, M.D., Chief Medical Officer
CIO: Thomas Pacek, Vice President Information Systems and Chief Information Officer
CHR: Erich Florentine, Chief People Officer
Web address: www.sjhealthcare.net
Control: Other not–for–profit (including NFP Corporation) **Service:** General Medical and Surgical

Staffed Beds: 421 **Admissions:** 19563 **Census:** 284 **Outpatient Visits:** 249372 **Births:** 2622 **Total Expense ($000):** 286561 **Payroll Expense ($000):** 124268 **Personnel:** 2309

VOORHEES—Camden County

★ **VIRTUA WEST JERSEY HOSPITAL–VOORHEES (310022)**, 101 Carnie Boulevard, Zip 08043–1597; tel. 856/325–3000, (Nonreporting) **A**1 3 5 10 **S** Virtua Health
Primary Contact: Michael S. Kotzen, Vice President and Chief Operating Officer
COO: Michael S. Kotzen, Vice President and Chief Operating Officer
CFO: Peter J. Powell, Director Finance
CMO: James P. Dwyer, D.O., Executive Vice President and Chief Medical Officer
CHR: Edward J. Dunn, Vice President Human Resources
Web address: www.virtua.org
Control: Other not–for–profit (including NFP Corporation) **Service:** General Medical and Surgical

Staffed Beds: 258

WAYNE—Passaic County

□ **KINDRED HOSPITAL NEW JERSEY – WAYNE**, 224 Hamburg Turnpike, Zip 7470; tel. 973/636–7200, (Nonreporting) **A**1 **S** Kindred Healthcare
Primary Contact: Robert Meyers, Chief Executive Officer
Web address: www.kindredhealthcare.com
Control: Corporation, Investor–owned, for–profit **Service:** Other specialty

Staffed Beds: 38

★ **ST. JOSEPH'S WAYNE HOSPITAL (310116)**, 224 Hamburg Turnpike, Zip 07470–2100; tel. 973/942–6900 **A**1 9 10 **F**3 7 8 11 15 17 18 20 24 25 26 27 31 32 33 38 41 42 43 44 45 46 47 48 49 50 54 55 56 57 60 61 62 68 73 75 76 77 79 80 81 82 85 86 96 97 100 101 106 107 118 119 121 124 135 137 **P**5 **S** St. Joseph's Healthcare System
Primary Contact: William A. McDonald, President and Chief Executive Officer
COO: Gloria A. Kunze, R.N., Vice President Operations
CFO: Jack Robinson, Chief Financial Officer
CMO: James Labagnara, M.D., Vice President Medical Affairs
CIO: Jim Kavanagh, Vice President and Chief Information Officer
CHR: John Bruno, Vice President Human Resources
Web address: www.sjwh.net
Control: Church–operated, Nongovernment, not–for profit **Service:** General Medical and Surgical

Staffed Beds: 136 **Admissions:** 6080 **Census:** 111 **Outpatient Visits:** 51350 **Births:** 0 **Total Expense ($000):** 69883 **Payroll Expense ($000):** 31899 **Personnel:** 640

NJ

Hospital, Medicare Provider Number, Address, Telephone, Approval, Facility, and Physician Codes, Health Care System
★ American Hospital Association (AHA) membership
□ The Joint Commission accreditation
○ American Osteopathic Association (AOA) accreditation
△ Commission on Accreditation of Rehabilitation Facilities (CARF) accreditation

WEST ORANGE—Essex County

★ △ **KESSLER INSTITUTE FOR REHABILITATION (313025)**, 1199 Pleasant Valley Way, Zip 07052–1419; tel. 973/731–3600, (Includes EAST ORANGE FACILITY, WEST ORANGE FACILITY, SADDLE BROOK FACILITY AND CHESTER FACILITY), (Nonreporting) **A**1 3 5 7 10 **S** Select Medical Corporation
Primary Contact: Robert Brehm, President
CFO: Ted Bolcavage, Regional Controller
CMO: Bruce M. Gans, M.D., Executive Vice President and Chief Medical Officer
CIO: James Talalai, Chief Information Officer
CHR: Frank Fritsch, Chief Human Resources Officer
Web address: www.kessler–rehab.com
Control: Corporation, Investor–owned, for–profit **Service:** Rehabilitation

Staffed Beds: 322

WESTAMPTON TOWNSHIP—Burlington County

☐ **HAMPTON BEHAVIORAL HEALTH CENTER (314021)**, 650 Rancocas Road, Zip 08060–5613; tel. 609/267–7000 **A**1 9 10 **F**5 30 31 32 62 88 89 93 94 95 **P**6 **S** Universal Health Services, Inc.
Primary Contact: Craig Hilton, Chief Executive Officer
COO: Joanne Wijaya, Chief Operating Officer
CFO: Art Randall, CPA, Chief Financial Officer
CHR: Polly Costantini, Director Human Resources
Web address: www.hamptonhospital.com
Control: Corporation, Investor–owned, for–profit **Service:** Psychiatric

Staffed Beds: 100 **Admissions:** 3014 **Census:** 83 **Outpatient Visits:** 15481 **Births:** 0 **Total Expense ($000):** 16779 **Payroll Expense ($000):** 9271 **Personnel:** 102

WILLINGBORO—Burlington County

★ **LOURDES MEDICAL CENTER OF BURLINGTON COUNTY (310061)**, 218–A Sunset Road, Zip 08046–1162; tel. 609/835–2900 **A**1 2 9 10 **F**3 5 11 12 13 15 17 18 25 26 27 31 32 33 34 36 38 41 43 47 48 49 50 54 55 56 57 59 60 62 64 66 68 71 72 73 74 76 77 79 80 81 82 86 87 88 90 92 94 95 96 97 98 100 102 106 107 114 118 119 121 124 135 136 137 **S** Catholic Health East
Primary Contact: Eugene Johnson, Chief Administrative Officer
COO: Robert Ruggero, Senior Vice President Operations
CFO: Andrew Guarni, Chief Financial Officer
CIO: Mike Elfert, Director Information Services
CHR: Janet Moran, Vice President Human Resources
Web address: www.lourdesnet.org
Control: Other not–for–profit (including NFP Corporation) **Service:** General Medical and Surgical

Staffed Beds: 188 **Admissions:** 8925 **Census:** 129 **Outpatient Visits:** 98464 **Births:** 965 **Total Expense ($000):** 101388 **Payroll Expense ($000):** 43809 **Personnel:** 642

WOODBRIDGE—Middlesex County

WOODBRIDGE DEVELOPMENT CENTER, Rahway Avenue, Zip 07095–3697, Mailing Address: P.O. Box 189, Zip 07095–0189; tel. 732/499–5951, (Nonreporting)
Primary Contact: Amy R. Bailon, M.D., Medical Director
Control: State–Government, nonfederal **Service:** Hospital unit within an institution for the mentally retarded

Staffed Beds: 125

WOODBURY—Gloucester County

★ **UNDERWOOD–MEMORIAL HOSPITAL (310081)**, 509 North Broad Street, Zip 08096–1697, Mailing Address: P.O. Box 359, Zip 08096–7359; tel. 856/845–0100 **A**1 3 5 9 10 **F**3 11 13 15 17 18 24 25 26 27 31 32 33 36 37 38 43 49 50 54 55 56 57 58 60 61 62 64 65 68 71 72 73 74 75 76 77 78 79 80 82 84 86 87 88 89 90 92 94 95 96 102 103 106 107 118 119 121 124 132 135 136 137 **P**6
Primary Contact: Eileen K. Cardile, President and Chief Executive Officer
COO: John W. Graham, Executive Vice President and Chief Operating Officer
CFO: James R. Brant, Senior Vice President Finance and Chief Financial Officer
CIO: Robert Mizia, Director Information Systems and Chief Information Officer
CHR: Robert Manestrina, Director Human Resources
Web address: www.umhospital.org
Control: Other not–for–profit (including NFP Corporation) **Service:** General Medical and Surgical

Staffed Beds: 240 **Admissions:** 13600 **Census:** 181 **Outpatient Visits:** 102645 **Births:** 1217 **Total Expense ($000):** 154785 **Payroll Expense ($000):** 75483 **Personnel:** 1406

WYCKOFF—Bergen County

★ **CHRISTIAN HEALTH CARE CENTER (314019)**, 301 Sicomac Avenue, Zip 07481–2194; tel. 201/848–5200, (Total facility includes 252 beds in nursing home–type unit) **A**1 9 10 **F**2 10 11 25 26 30 32 33 42 43 44 54 62 66 67 73 75 88 89 90 91 93 94 95 115 117 135 137 **P**6
Primary Contact: Douglas A. Struyk, President and Chief Executive Officer
COO: Denise Ratcliffe, Executive Vice President and Chief Operating Officer
CFO: Kevin Stagg, Vice President Finance and Chief Financial Officer
CMO: Howard Gilman, M.D., Medical Executive
CHR: Bob Zierold, Vice President Human Resources
Web address: www.chccnj.org
Control: Other not–for–profit (including NFP Corporation) **Service:** Psychiatric

Staffed Beds: 514 **Admissions:** 1367 **Census:** 509 **Outpatient Visits:** 35865 **Births:** 0 **Total Expense ($000):** 55648 **Payroll Expense ($000):** 33742 **Personnel:** 687

Many Facility Codes have changed. Please refer to the AHA Guide Code Chart.

NEW MEXICO

ALAMOGORDO—Otero County

☒ **GERALD CHAMPION REGIONAL MEDICAL CENTER (320004)**, 2669 North Scenic Drive, Zip 88310–8799; tel. 575/439–6100, (Nonreporting) **A**1 9 10 20 **S** QHR
Primary Contact: Robert J. Heckert, Jr., Chief Executive Officer
CFO: Jim Childers, Chief Financial Officer
CMO: Arthur Austin, M.D., Senior Vice President Medical Staff Affairs
CHR: Karen O'Brien, Director President Human Resources
Web address: www.gcrmc.org
Control: Other not–for–profit (including NFP Corporation) **Service:** General Medical and Surgical

Staffed Beds: 99

ALBUQUERQUE—Bernalillo County

DESERT HILLS, 5310 Sequoia Road N.W., Zip 87120–1249; tel. 505/836–7330, (Nonreporting)
Primary Contact: Carol Bickelman, President and Chief Executive Officer
CFO: Melissa Doggett, Chief Financial Officer
Web address: www.yfcs.com
Control: Corporation, Investor–owned, for–profit **Service:** Psychiatric

Staffed Beds: 88

☒ **HEALTHSOUTH REHABILITATION HOSPITAL (323027)**, 7000 Jefferson N.E., Zip 87109–4357; tel. 505/344–9478, (Nonreporting) **A**1 10 **S** HEALTHSOUTH Corporation
Primary Contact: Sylvia K. Kelly, Chief Executive Officer
CFO: Byron Aten, Controller
CMO: Patrick Schmitt, M.D., Medical Director
CHR: Eliza Marquez, Director Human Resources
Web address: www.healthsouth.com
Control: Corporation, Investor–owned, for–profit **Service:** Rehabilitation

Staffed Beds: 60

☒ **HEART HOSPITAL OF NEW MEXICO (320083)**, 504 Elm Street, Zip 87102; tel. 505/724–2000 **A**1 9 10 **F**3 17 18 20 22 25 26 30 33 38 50 56 57 66 73 79 80 81 82 96 97 107 122 135 **S** MedCath, Inc.
Primary Contact: Ronald C. Winger, President
COO: Terry Odom, Vice President Clinical Services
CFO: Duane Scholer, Chief Financial Officer
CMO: Harvey White, M.D., Medical Director
Web address: www.hearthospitalnm.com
Control: Corporation, Investor–owned, for–profit **Service:** Heart

Staffed Beds: 55 **Admissions:** 2768 **Census:** 30 **Outpatient Visits:** 4611 **Births:** 0 **Total Expense ($000):** 54084 **Payroll Expense ($000):** 16336 **Personnel:** 244

☐ **KINDRED HOSPITAL – ALBUQUERQUE (322002)**, 700 High Street N.E., Zip 87102–2565; tel. 505/242–4444, (Nonreporting) **A**1 9 10 **S** Kindred Healthcare
Primary Contact: Charles Tozer, Interim Chief Executive Officer
CFO: Margaret Wantland, Chief Financial Officer
CMO: Jeffrey Dorf, M.D., Medical Director
CHR: Donald Whitney, Director Human Resources
Web address: www.kindredhealthcare.com
Control: Corporation, Investor–owned, for–profit **Service:** Long–Term Acute Care hospital

Staffed Beds: 61

☒ **LOVELACE MEDICAL CENTER–DOWNTOWN (320009)**, 601 Martin Luther King Jr. Avenue N.E., Zip 87102–3670, Mailing Address: P.O. Box 25555, Zip 87125–0555; tel. 505/727–8000, (Nonreporting) **A**1 9 10 **S** Ardent Health Services
Primary Contact: Clay Holderman, Chief Executive Officer
CFO: Brian Vaughan, Chief Financial Officer
CMO: William J. Mitchell, M.D., Chief Medical Officer
CIO: Lance Henderson, Technology Director
CHR: Randy Royster, Vice President Human Resources
Web address: www.albuquerquehospital.com
Control: Corporation, Investor–owned, for–profit **Service:** General Medical and Surgical

Staffed Beds: 128

★ △ **LOVELACE REHABILITATION HOSPITAL (323028)**, 505 Elm Street N.E., Zip 87102–2500; tel. 505/727–4700, (Total facility includes 17 beds in nursing home–type unit) (Nonreporting) **A**7 9 10 **S** Ardent Health Services
Primary Contact: Ulrike Berzau, Chief Executive Officer
CFO: Tyler Felt, Chief Financial Officer
CHR: Becky Falance, Director Human Resources
Web address: www.lovelace.com
Control: Corporation, Investor–owned, for–profit **Service:** Rehabilitation

Staffed Beds: 62

☒ **LOVELACE WESTSIDE HOSPITAL (320074)**, 10501 Golf Course Road N.W., Zip 87114–5000, Mailing Address: P.O. Box 25555, Zip 87125–0555; tel. 505/727–2000, (Total facility includes 22 beds in nursing home–type unit) (Nonreporting) **A**1 9 10 **S** Ardent Health Services
Primary Contact: Troy Greer, Chief Executive Officer
COO: Karrie Brazaski, Chief Operating Officer and Chief Nursing Officer
CFO: Leonard Tapia, Chief Financial Officer
CMO: William J. Mitchell, M.D., Chief Medical Officer
Web address: www.lovelacesandia.com
Control: Corporation, Investor–owned, for–profit **Service:** General Medical and Surgical

Staffed Beds: 48

☒ **LOVELACE WOMEN'S HOSPITAL (320017)**, 4701 Montgomery Boulevard N.E., Zip 87109–1251, Mailing Address: P.O. Box 25555, Zip 87125–0555; tel. 505/727–7800, (Nonreporting) **A**1 9 10 **S** Ardent Health Services
Primary Contact: Sheri Milone, Chief Executive Officer and Administrator
COO: Lynn Arnold, Chief Operating Officer
CFO: Cindy Miller, Chief Financial Officer
CHR: Carol Shelton, Director Human Resources
Web address: www.lovelacesandia.com
Control: Corporation, Investor–owned, for–profit **Service:** General Medical and Surgical

Staffed Beds: 84

☒ **PRESBYTERIAN HOSPITAL (320021)**, 1100 Central Avenue S.E., Zip 87106–4934, Mailing Address: P.O. Box 26666, Zip 87125–6666; tel. 505/841–1234 **A**1 2 3 5 9 10 **F**3 7 8 11 13 14 17 18 19 20 21 22 23 25 26 27 31 32 33 36 38 39 46 47 49 55 57 59 66 68 70 71 72 73 74 75 76 77 79 80 81 82 83 84 86 87 96 97 100 102 106 107 112 119 120 121 127 131 133 135 136 137 **P**6 **S** Presbyterian Healthcare Services
Primary Contact: Lauren Cates, Vice President Central New Mexico Operations
COO: David Scrase, M.D., Executive Senior Vice President and Chief Operating Officer
CFO: Paul Briggs, Senior Vice President and Chief Financial Officer
CMO: Eddie Benge, M.D., Vice President Medical Staff Affairs
CIO: Donna Agnew, Chief Information Officer
Web address: www.phs.org
Control: Other not–for–profit (including NFP Corporation) **Service:** General Medical and Surgical

Staffed Beds: 552 **Admissions:** 31776 **Census:** 401 **Outpatient Visits:** 1260411 **Births:** 6146 **Total Expense ($000):** 623034 **Payroll Expense ($000):** 332128 **Personnel:** 3911

☒ **PRESBYTERIAN KASEMAN HOSPITAL (320079)**, 8300 Constitution Avenue N.E., Zip 87110–7624, Mailing Address: P.O. Box 26666, Zip 87125–6666; tel. 505/291–2000 **A**1 9 10 **F**3 5 15 25 26 27 30 31 32 38 39 42 43 44 50 52 54 62 63 66 73 76 79 80 81 82 86 87 88 89 90 91 92 93 94 95 96 97 100 102 103 104 105 107 108 109 111 117 118 119 121 123 135 137 **S** Presbyterian Healthcare Services
Primary Contact: Matt Pehrson, Administrative Director
COO: David Scrase, M.D., Executive Senior Vice President and Chief Operating Officer
CFO: Paul Briggs, Senior Vice President Finance
CMO: Eddie Benge, M.D., Vice President Medical Staff Affairs
CIO: Donna Agnew, Chief Information Officer
CHR: Margaret Eaton, Vice President Human Resources
Web address: www.phs.org
Control: Other not–for–profit (including NFP Corporation) **Service:** General Medical and Surgical

Staffed Beds: 124 **Admissions:** 4155 **Census:** 74 **Outpatient Visits:** 145976 **Births:** 0 **Total Expense ($000):** 79299 **Payroll Expense ($000):** 41054 **Personnel:** 546

NM

Hospital, Medicare Provider Number, Address, Telephone, Approval, Facility, and Physician Codes, Health Care System

★ American Hospital Association (AHA) membership
☐ The Joint Commission accreditation
○ American Osteopathic Association (AOA) accreditation
△ Commission on Accreditation of Rehabilitation Facilities (CARF) accreditation

☐ **SPECIALTY HOSPITAL OF ALBUQUERQUE (322003)**, 235 Elm Street N.E., Zip 87102; tel. 505/842–5550, (Nonreporting) **A**1 9 10 **S** Fundamental Long Term Care Holdings, LLC
Primary Contact: Kathi Gleim, Chief Executive Officer
Control: Corporation, Investor–owned, for–profit **Service:** Long–Term Acute Care hospital

Staffed Beds: 25

▣ **UNIVERSITY OF NEW MEXICO HOSPITALS (320001)**, 2211 Lomas Boulevard N.E., Zip 87106–2745; tel. 505/272–2111, (Includes CARRIE TINGLEY HOSPITAL, 1127 University Boulevard N.E., Zip 87102–1715; tel. 505/272–5200; Crystal Frantz, Executive Director; MENTAL HEALTH CENTER, 2600 Marble N.E., Zip 87131–2600; tel. 505/272–2800; UNIVERSITY OF NEW MEXICO CHILDREN'S PSYCHIATRIC HOSPITAL, 1001 Yale Boulevard N.E., Zip 87131–3830; tel. 505/272–2890) **A**1 2 3 5 8 9 10 12 13 **F**3 9 11 13 15 16 17 18 19 20 21 22 24 25 26 27 28 30 32 33 36 37 38 40 41 42 43 46 47 48 49 50 51 53 54 55 56 57 59 60 62 63 66 68 70 71 72 73 74 75 76 77 79 80 81 82 83 84 85 86 87 90 96 97 100 102 103 104 105 107 108 109 111 113 114 118 119 120 121 124 125 127 135 136 137
Primary Contact: Stephen W. McKernan, Chief Executive Officer
CFO: Ella Watt, Chief Financial Officer
CMO: Robert Katz, M.D., Vice President Clinical Affairs
CIO: Ron Margolis, Chief Information Officer
CHR: Jim Pendergast, Administrator Human Resources
Web address: www.unm.edu
Control: State–Government, nonfederal **Service:** General Medical and Surgical

Staffed Beds: 501 **Admissions:** 24690 **Census:** 321 **Outpatient Visits:** 570271 **Births:** 3760 **Total Expense ($000):** 480195 **Payroll Expense ($000):** 196371 **Personnel:** 3883

▣ △ **VETERANS AFFAIRS MEDICAL CENTER**, 1501 San Pedro S.E., Zip 87108–5138; tel. 505/265–1711 **A**1 2 3 5 7 8 **F**1 3 4 5 8 11 12 15 16 17 18 20 22 25 26 27 29 32 33 36 37 38 41 43 44 45 50 51 54 55 56 57 58 59 60 61 62 63 65 66 68 70 71 72 73 74 75 76 77 78 79 80 81 82 83 84 85 86 87 88 90 91 92 93 94 95 96 97 98 100 102 105 106 107 117 119 121 124 132 135 136 137 **P**6 **S** Department of Veterans Affairs
Primary Contact: George Marnell, Director
CFO: Michael McNeill, Chief Financial Management
CMO: Meghan Gerety, M.D., Chief of Staff
CIO: Ronald Ferrell, Facility Chief Information Officer
CHR: Melvin Hooker, Chief Human Resources
Web address: www.southwest.va.gov/albuquerque/
Control: Veterans Affairs, Government, federal **Service:** General Medical and Surgical

Staffed Beds: 307 **Admissions:** 6171 **Census:** 208 **Outpatient Visits:** 534988 **Births:** 0 **Total Expense ($000):** 318121 **Payroll Expense ($000):** 120809 **Personnel:** 1937

ARTESIA—Eddy County

★ **ARTESIA GENERAL HOSPITAL (320030)**, 702 North 13th Street, Zip 88210–1199; tel. 505/748–3333 **A**9 10 20 **F**3 11 25 26 32 33 37 38 51 55 57 62 63 73 74 79 87 96 97 100 107 118 119 122 **P**6
Primary Contact: Kenneth W. Randall, Chief Executive Officer
CFO: Jerry Pickett, Chief Financial Officer
CMO: Joe Salgado, M.D., Chief of Staff
CIO: Paul Groh, Coordinator Information Systems
CHR: Donnie Lambert, Director Human Resources
Web address: www.artesiageneral.com
Control: Other not–for–profit (including NFP Corporation) **Service:** General Medical and Surgical

Staffed Beds: 34 **Admissions:** 911 **Census:** 7 **Outpatient Visits:** 21592 **Births:** 58 **Total Expense ($000):** 17795 **Payroll Expense ($000):** 7334 **Personnel:** 110

CARLSBAD—Eddy County

▣ **CARLSBAD MEDICAL CENTER (320063)**, 2430 West Pierce Street, Zip 88220–3597; tel. 505/887–4100 **A**1 9 10 19 20 **F**1 4 8 15 16 17 18 20 25 26 30 31 32 33 37 38 41 46 51 55 56 57 62 65 66 68 70 71 72 73 74 75 76 78 79 80 81 82 83 84 85 86 88 96 97 100 102 103 107 117 118 119 124 136 137 **S** Community Health Systems, Inc.
Primary Contact: Janet Carbary, Interim Chief Executive Officer
CFO: Janet Carbary, Chief Financial Officer
CIO: Kenneth Kemp, Director Information Systems
CHR: Tonk Chester, Director Human Resources
Web address: www.carlsbadmedicalcenter.com
Control: Corporation, Investor–owned, for–profit **Service:** General Medical and Surgical

Staffed Beds: 127 **Admissions:** 4214 **Census:** 40 **Outpatient Visits:** 76404 **Births:** 548 **Total Expense ($000):** 52267 **Payroll Expense ($000):** 16267 **Personnel:** 549

CLAYTON—Union County

★ **UNION COUNTY GENERAL HOSPITAL (321304)**, 301 Harding Street, Zip 88415–3321, Mailing Address: P.O. Box 489, Zip 88415–0489; tel. 575/374–2585 **A**9 10 18 **F**3 11 13 15 25 27 30 31 32 33 38 50 55 57 61 62 63 64 68 74 79 80 82 84 86 87 92 96 102 107 119 122 133 134 137 **S** Brim Healthcare, Inc.
Primary Contact: Stephen J. Campbell, Administrator
CFO: Texas Davis, Controller
CHR: Jill Swagerty, Director Human Resources
Web address: www.unioncountygeneral.com
Control: Other not–for–profit (including NFP Corporation) **Service:** General Medical and Surgical

Staffed Beds: 21 **Admissions:** 457 **Census:** 4 **Outpatient Visits:** 9661 **Births:** 19 **Total Expense ($000):** 7236 **Payroll Expense ($000):** 2914 **Personnel:** 74

CLOVIS—Curry County

▣ **PLAINS REGIONAL MEDICAL CENTER (320022)**, 2100 Martin Luther King, Jr. Boulevard, Zip 88101–9412, Mailing Address: P.O. Box 1688, Zip 88101–1688; tel. 505/769–2141 **A**1 9 10 20 **F**3 11 13 15 18 20 22 25 26 27 30 31 32 33 38 42 43 44 50 51 52 57 59 61 62 66 67 68 73 75 76 77 79 80 82 86 87 96 97 100 102 106 107 109 111 118 119 124 135 136 137 **S** Presbyterian Healthcare Services
Primary Contact: Hoyt Skabelund, Administrator
Web address: www.phs.org
Control: Other not–for–profit (including NFP Corporation) **Service:** General Medical and Surgical

Staffed Beds: 106 **Admissions:** 5026 **Census:** 44 **Births:** 1317 **Total Expense ($000):** 74186 **Payroll Expense ($000):** 28164 **Personnel:** 517

CROWNPOINT—McKinley County

★ **U. S. PUBLIC HEALTH SERVICE INDIAN HOSPITAL (320062)**, Mailing Address: P.O. Box 358, Zip 87313–0358; tel. 505/786–5291 **A**10 **F**3 7 13 15 25 31 32 33 37 38 50 55 56 57 62 63 66 69 73 74 81 82 84 86 87 89 92 93 94 99 102 119 123 136 **P**5 **S** U. S. Indian Health Service
Primary Contact: Fannessa Comer, Acting Chief Executive Officer
COO: Mary Ann O'Neal, Administrative Officer
CFO: Darlene Kirk, Finance Manager
CMO: Harry Goldenberg, Director Clinical
CIO: Mary Ann O'Neal, Administrative Officer
CHR: Victoria Pablo, Human Resource Specialist
Web address: www.ihs.gov
Control: PHS, Indian Service, Government, federal **Service:** General Medical and Surgical

Staffed Beds: 12 **Admissions:** 674 **Census:** 5 **Outpatient Visits:** 84277 **Births:** 70 **Total Expense ($000):** 26044 **Payroll Expense ($000):** 11816 **Personnel:** 331

DEMING—Luna County

▣ **MIMBRES MEMORIAL HOSPITAL (320014)**, 900 West Ash Street, Zip 88030–4098, Mailing Address: P.O. Box 710, Zip 88031–0710; tel. 505/546–2761, (Total facility includes 70 beds in nursing home–type unit) (Nonreporting) **A**1 9 10 20 **S** Community Health Systems, Inc.
Primary Contact: John M. Gallagher, Chief Executive Officer
CFO: Brian Ebright, Chief Financial Officer
CHR: Kevin Driver, Human Resource Director
Web address: www.mimbresmemorial.com
Control: Corporation, Investor–owned, for–profit **Service:** General Medical and Surgical

Staffed Beds: 119

ESPANOLA—Rio Arriba County

▣ **ESPANOLA HOSPITAL (320011)**, 1010 Spruce Street, Zip 87532–2746; tel. 505/753–7111 **A**1 9 10 20 **F**7 8 11 13 15 25 26 30 31 32 33 38 55 56 61 62 64 66 68 73 74 75 77 79 86 87 96 97 100 102 103 106 107 118 119 121 124 133 135 136 137 **P**3 8 **S** Presbyterian Healthcare Services
Primary Contact: Derrick Yu, Administrator
Web address: www.phs.org
Control: Other not–for–profit (including NFP Corporation) **Service:** General Medical and Surgical

Staffed Beds: 80 **Admissions:** 1987 **Census:** 18 **Outpatient Visits:** 101261 **Births:** 348 **Total Expense ($000):** 41608 **Payroll Expense ($000):** 16690 **Personnel:** 326

FARMINGTON—San Juan County

★ **SAN JUAN REGIONAL MEDICAL CENTER (320005)**, 801 West Maple Street, Zip 87401–5698; tel. 505/609–2000, (Includes SAN JUAN REGIONAL MEDICAL CENTER REHABILITATION HOSPITAL, 525 South Schwartz, Zip 87401; tel. 505/609–2625) **A**1 2 5 9 10 19 20 **F**7 8 11 13 15 18 24 25 26 27 28 30 31 32 33 38 40 47 48 49 52 53 55 56 57 59 62 63 66 68 72 73 74 76 77 79 80 82 84 85 86 87 88 89 90 92 96 97 100 101 102 106 107 109 119 124 132 133 135 137 **P**5
Primary Contact: Steve Altmiller, President and Chief Executive Officer
COO: John Buffington, Chief Operating Officer
CFO: J. Michael Philips, Chief Strategy Officer
CMO: Robert Fabrey, M.D., Chief Medical Officer
CIO: Steve Franken, Chief Information Officer
CHR: Elizabeth Volkerding, Director Human Resources
Web address: www.sanjuanregional.com
Control: Other not–for–profit (including NFP Corporation) **Service:** General Medical and Surgical

Staffed Beds: 205 **Admissions:** 9996 **Census:** 115 **Outpatient Visits:** 186683 **Births:** 1375 **Total Expense ($000):** 161669 **Payroll Expense ($000):** 70962 **Personnel:** 1317

GALLUP—McKinley County

★ **GALLUP INDIAN MEDICAL CENTER (320061)**, 516 East Nizhoni Boulevard, Zip 87301–5748, Mailing Address: P.O. Box 1337, Zip 87305–1337; tel. 505/722–1000 **A**1 10 **F**3 4 13 15 25 28 33 36 37 38 42 43 50 54 55 57 60 61 62 63 65 66 68 71 73 74 75 77 79 80 82 84 85 86 87 89 90 91 92 93 94 95 96 100 102 107 117 119 121 132 133 136 137 **S** U. S. Indian Health Service
Primary Contact: Bennie C. Yazzie, Interim Chief Executive Officer
COO: Bennie C. Yazzie, Administrative Officer
CFO: Alva R. Tom, Manager Finance
CMO: Douglas G. Peter, M.D., Chief Medical Officer
CIO: Adrian C. Haven, Site Manager
CHR: Karen Lee, Director Human Resources
Web address: www.ihs.gov/facilitiesservices/areaoffices/navajo/naihs–hcc–gallup.asp
Control: Public Health Service, Government, federal **Service:** General Medical and Surgical

Staffed Beds: 65 **Admissions:** 3439 **Census:** 38 **Births:** 684

★ **REHOBOTH MCKINLEY CHRISTIAN HEALTH CARE SERVICES (320038)**, (Formerly Rehoboth McKinley Christain Hospital), 1901 Red Rock Drive, Zip 87301–1901; tel. 505/863–7000 **A**1 5 9 10 20 **F**3 4 5 11 13 15 24 25 26 31 33 35 38 42 44 50 53 54 55 56 57 59 61 62 63 66 68 72 73 74 77 79 80 82 84 86 87 90 91 93 94 96 97 100 102 103 107 118 119 121 124 135 136 **P**6
Primary Contact: Chuck Wright, Chief Executive Officer
CFO: Deb Mohesky, Chief Financial Officer
CMO: Mary L. Poel, M.D., Chief Medical Officer
CHR: Theresa Padilla, Director Human Resources
Web address: www.rmch.org
Control: Other not–for–profit (including NFP Corporation) **Service:** General Medical and Surgical

Staffed Beds: 80 **Admissions:** 3315 **Census:** 38 **Outpatient Visits:** 132606 **Births:** 475 **Total Expense ($000):** 63318 **Payroll Expense ($000):** 33606 **Personnel:** 558

GRANTS—Cibola County

★ **CIBOLA GENERAL HOSPITAL (320037)**, 1016 Roosevelt Avenue, Zip 87020–2104; tel. 505/287–4446 **A**1 9 10 20 **F**3 11 13 15 25 26 33 37 38 46 55 56 57 62 66 68 73 74 79 80 84 86 96 102 107 118 119 120 121 135 136 137 **P**8 **S** QHR
Primary Contact: Kenneth Cochran, RN, FACHE, Chief Executive Officer
CFO: Jeff Rimel, Chief Financial Officer
CIO: Norman Wilder, Director Information Services
CHR: Sheila Cox, Director Human Resources
Web address: www.cibolahospital.com
Control: County–Government, nonfederal **Service:** General Medical and Surgical

Staffed Beds: 25 **Admissions:** 895 **Census:** 8 **Outpatient Visits:** 21970 **Births:** 221 **Total Expense ($000):** 15740 **Payroll Expense ($000):** 6261 **Personnel:** 136

HOBBS—Lea County

★ **LEA REGIONAL MEDICAL CENTER (320065)**, 5419 North Lovington Highway, Zip 88240–9125, Mailing Address: P.O. Box 3000, Zip 88240–3000; tel. 505/492–5000, (Nonreporting) **A**1 9 10 19 20 **S** Community Health Systems, Inc.
Primary Contact: Larry W. Payton, Chief Executive Officer
CFO: Steven Smith, Chief Financial Officer
CMO: Al Jecius, M.D., Chief of Staff
CIO: Tom Motejzik, Director Information Services
CHR: Kim Smith, Director Human Resources
Web address: www.learegional.com
Control: Corporation, Investor–owned, for–profit **Service:** General Medical and Surgical

Staffed Beds: 214

LAS CRUCES—Dona Ana County

★ **MEMORIAL MEDICAL CENTER (320018)**, 2450 South Telshor Boulevard, Zip 88011–5076; tel. 575/522–8641 **A**1 9 10 **F**3 8 11 13 15 18 20 22 24 25 26 27 30 31 32 33 37 38 41 49 50 51 53 55 57 59 60 61 62 63 66 68 71 72 73 74 76 77 79 80 84 86 87 88 92 93 95 96 97 100 102 103 106 107 109 110 111 112 119 121 123 124 136 137 **S** LifePoint Hospitals, Inc.
Primary Contact: Paul F. Herzog, Chief Executive Officer
COO: Steve O. Hyde, Chief Operating Officer
CFO: Randolph F. Harrison, Chief Financial Officer
CMO: Bruce San Filippo, M.D., Chief Medical Officer
CIO: Berton Stevens, Director Information Systems
CHR: Laura Pierce, Human Resources Director
Web address: www.mmclc.org
Control: Corporation, Investor–owned, for–profit **Service:** General Medical and Surgical

Staffed Beds: 198 **Admissions:** 11117 **Census:** 134 **Outpatient Visits:** 152237 **Births:** 2136 **Total Expense ($000):** 122361 **Payroll Expense ($000):** 59813 **Personnel:** 920

☐ **MESILLA VALLEY HOSPITAL (324010)**, 3751 Del Rey Boulevard, Zip 88012–8526; tel. 505/382–3500 **A**1 9 10 **F**4 5 25 31 32 82 88 89 90 91 92 93 94 **S** Psychiatric Solutions
Primary Contact: Margaret McCowen, Chief Executive Officer
CFO: Douglas Smith, Chief Financial Officer
CMO: Georgina Herrera, M.D., Medical Director
CHR: Linda Moya, Director Human Resources
Web address: www.mesillavalleyhospital.com
Control: Corporation, Investor–owned, for–profit **Service:** Psychiatric

Staffed Beds: 121 **Admissions:** 1665 **Census:** 91 **Outpatient Visits:** 33190 **Births:** 0 **Total Expense ($000):** 17020 **Payroll Expense ($000):** 9591 **Personnel:** 205

★ **MOUNTAINVIEW REGIONAL MEDICAL CENTER (320085)**, 4311 East Lohman Avenue, Zip 88011; tel. 505/556–7600 **A**1 9 10 **F**3 8 13 15 18 20 22 24 25 26 30 32 33 38 55 56 57 62 68 71 73 74 75 77 79 80 81 82 84 86 96 97 100 102 107 119 120 121 132 135 136 137 **P**5 **S** Community Health Systems, Inc.
Primary Contact: Randall Hempling, Chief Executive Officer
CFO: Gene Alexander, Chief Financial Officer
Web address: www.mountainviewregional.com
Control: Corporation, Investor–owned, for–profit **Service:** General Medical and Surgical

Staffed Beds: 131 **Admissions:** 6968 **Census:** 86 **Outpatient Visits:** 69382 **Births:** 833 **Total Expense ($000):** 80260 **Payroll Expense ($000):** 26460 **Personnel:** 661

★ **REHABILITATION HOSPITAL OF SOUTHERN NEW MEXICO (323032)**, 4441 East Lohman Avenue, Zip 88011; tel. 575/521–6400, (Nonreporting) **A**1 9 10 **S** Ernest Health, Inc.
Primary Contact: Tony Hernandez, Chief Executive Officer
COO: Beverly Munoz, Director Quality, Risk Management and Chief Operating Officer
CFO: Jared Udall, Chief Financial Officer
CMO: Kevin F. Brown, D.O., Medical Director
CHR: Yolanda Mendoza, Director Human Resources
Web address: www.rhsnm.ernesthealth.com
Control: Corporation, Investor–owned, for–profit **Service:** Rehabilitation

Staffed Beds: 40

NM

Hospital, Medicare Provider Number, Address, Telephone, Approval, Facility, and Physician Codes, Health Care System
★ American Hospital Association (AHA) membership
☐ The Joint Commission accreditation
○ American Osteopathic Association (AOA) accreditation
△ Commission on Accreditation of Rehabilitation Facilities (CARF) accreditation

LAS VEGAS—San Miguel County

ALTA VISTA REGIONAL HOSPITAL (320003), 104 Legion Drive, Zip 87701; tel. 505/426–3500, (Nonreporting) **A**1 9 10 20 **S** Community Health Systems, Inc.
Primary Contact: Richard Grogan, Chief Executive Officer
CMO: Michael Lopez, M.D., Chief Medical Staff
CIO: Samuel Lujan, Director Information Systems
CHR: Beth Irizarry, Director Human Resources
Web address: www.altavistaregionalhospital.com
Control: Corporation, Investor–owned, for–profit **Service:** General Medical and Surgical

Staffed Beds: 42

NEW MEXICO BEHAVIORAL HEALTH INSTITUTE AT LAS VEGAS, 3695 Hot Springs Boulevard, Zip 87701–9575; tel. 505/454–2100, (Total facility includes 167 beds in nursing home–type unit) (Nonreporting) **A**9
Primary Contact: Steve Martinez, Executive Director and Administrator
CFO: Albino Martinez, Director Finance and Budget
Web address: www.health.state.nm.us
Control: State–Government, nonfederal **Service:** Psychiatric

Staffed Beds: 357

LOS ALAMOS—Los Alamos County

LOS ALAMOS MEDICAL CENTER (320033), 3917 West Road, Zip 87544–2293; tel. 505/662–4201, (Nonreporting) **A**1 9 10 20 **S** LifePoint Hospitals, Inc.
Primary Contact: Sandra C. Podley, Chief Executive Officer
CFO: Heather Teter, Chief Financial Officer
CMO: Jeffrey Sauer, DPM, Chief of Staff
CIO: Kevin Vigil, Director Information Systems
CHR: Jacqueline Carroll, Director Human Resources
Web address: www.losalamosmedicalcenter.com
Control: Other not–for–profit (including NFP Corporation) **Service:** General Medical and Surgical

Staffed Beds: 47

LOVINGTON—Lea County

★ **NOR–LEA GENERAL HOSPITAL (321305)**, 1600 North Main Avenue, Zip 88260–2871; tel. 505/396–6611 **A**9 10 18 **F**3 9 11 15 24 25 26 27 28 30 31 32 33 38 42 50 51 53 55 56 57 61 62 64 66 73 76 79 87 89 93 96 100 102 107 118 119 121 122 124 136 **P**6 **S** Covenant Health System
Primary Contact: David B. Shaw, Chief Executive Officer and Administrator
CFO: Allyson Roberts, CPA, Chief Financial Officer
CMO: Chad Carver, M.D., Chief of Staff
CHR: Carol Dearment, Director Human Resources
Web address: www.nlgh.org
Control: Hospital district or authority, Government, nonfederal **Service:** General Medical and Surgical

Staffed Beds: 12 **Admissions:** 572 **Census:** 5 **Outpatient Visits:** 108112 **Births:** 0 **Total Expense ($000):** 23285 **Payroll Expense ($000):** 9522 **Personnel:** 204

MESCALERO—Otero County

MESCALERO PUBLIC HEALTH SERVICE INDIAN HOSPITAL (320058), (Formerly PHS Indian Hospital), Mailing Address: Box 210, Zip 88340–0210; tel. 505/671–4441 **A**1 10 **F**25 28 30 31 32 33 34 37 41 43 44 50 55 56 57 61 62 63 64 66 73 82 84 87 107 119 133 135 136 137 **P**6 **S** U. S. Indian Health Service
Primary Contact: Dorlynn Simmons, Chief Executive Officer
CFO: Rainey Enjady, Administrative Officer
CIO: Kathy Murphy, Site Manager
Web address: www.ihs.gov
Control: PHS, Indian Service, Government, federal **Service:** General Medical and Surgical

Staffed Beds: 13 **Admissions:** 147 **Census:** 1 **Outpatient Visits:** 38387 **Births:** 0 **Total Expense ($000):** 6882 **Payroll Expense ($000):** 3299 **Personnel:** 68

NM

PORTALES—Roosevelt County

ROOSEVELT GENERAL HOSPITAL (320084), 14121 U.S. Highway 70, Zip 88130, Mailing Address: P.O. Box 868, Zip 88130–0868; tel. 575/359–1800, (Nonreporting) **A**9 10 **S** Covenant Health System
Primary Contact: James P. D'Agostino, Chief Executive Officer
CFO: Eva Steven, Chief Financial Officer
CMO: Les Donaldson, M.D., Chief of Staff
CHR: Cindy Duncan, Director Human Resources
Control: Hospital district or authority, Government, nonfederal **Service:** General Medical and Surgical

Staffed Beds: 22

RATON—Colfax County

★ **MINERS' COLFAX MEDICAL CENTER (320069)**, 200 Hospital Drive, Zip 87740–2099; tel. 505/445–3661, (Includes MINERS' HOSPITAL OF NEW MEXICO), (Total facility includes 47 beds in nursing home–type unit) **A**9 10 20 **F**3 8 11 12 13 15 24 25 27 30 31 33 38 43 46 52 54 55 56 57 58 62 64 65 66 68 69 73 74 76 79 81 82 96 99 102 107 118 119 122 **P**6
Primary Contact: Donald R. Holl, Chief Executive Officer
CFO: Albino Martinez, Director Budget and Finance
CIO: Richard Laner, Manager Information Systems
CHR: Jamie Johnson, Director Human Resources
Web address: www.minershosp.com
Control: State–Government, nonfederal **Service:** General Medical and Surgical

Staffed Beds: 80 **Admissions:** 1157 **Census:** 39 **Outpatient Visits:** 20379 **Births:** 24 **Total Expense ($000):** 16069 **Payroll Expense ($000):** 7811 **Personnel:** 149

ROSWELL—Chaves County

EASTERN NEW MEXICO MEDICAL CENTER (320006), 405 West Country Club Road, Zip 88201–9981; tel. 505/622–8170 **A**1 3 5 9 10 19 20 **F**3 8 11 13 15 18 20 25 26 27 30 38 40 43 46 49 51 55 56 59 66 68 73 74 75 76 77 79 80 82 84 86 88 90 91 92 96 97 99 100 102 107 108 118 119 135 136 137 **P**7 **S** Community Health Systems, Inc.
Primary Contact: Bradley McGrath, Chief Executive Officer
CFO: Leanne Hacker, Chief Financial Officer
CMO: Jan Hobbs, M.D., Chief Medical Officer
CIO: Deepak Surl, Chief Information Officer
CHR: Barry Nateman, Chief Human Resources Officer
Web address: www.enmmc.com
Control: Corporation, Investor–owned, for–profit **Service:** General Medical and Surgical

Staffed Beds: 162 **Admissions:** 7343 **Census:** 73 **Outpatient Visits:** 232984 **Births:** 722 **Total Expense ($000):** 109894 **Payroll Expense ($000):** 44499 **Personnel:** 573

☐ **NEW MEXICO REHABILITATION CENTER (323026)**, 31 Gail Harris Avenue, Zip 88203–8134; tel. 505/347–3400, (Includes PECOS VALLEY LODGE) **A**1 10 **F**4 5 25 30 31 32 45 63 66 81 85 86 124 **P**6
Primary Contact: Thomas Tutor, Administrator
COO: Thomas Tutor, Administrator
CFO: Janie Banda, Chief Financial Officer
CMO: Soofia Khan, M.D., Medical Director
CHR: Dorie Isler, Director Human Resources
Control: State–Government, nonfederal **Service:** Rehabilitation

Staffed Beds: 41 **Admissions:** 513 **Census:** 23 **Outpatient Visits:** 379 **Births:** 0 **Total Expense ($000):** 3249 **Payroll Expense ($000):** 3775 **Personnel:** 118

RUIDOSO—Lincoln County

LINCOLN COUNTY MEDICAL CENTER (321306), 211 Sudderth Drive, Zip 88345–6043, Mailing Address: P.O. Box 8000, Zip 88345–8000; tel. 505/257–7381 **A**1 9 10 18 **F**7 11 13 15 25 30 31 32 33 37 38 46 52 54 55 57 62 68 74 75 76 79 86 93 96 100 103 107 109 121 135 **P**6 **S** Presbyterian Healthcare Services
Primary Contact: James P. Gibson, Administrator
COO: James P. Gibson, Administrator
CFO: Dudley McCauley, Controller
CMO: Tim Harkins, M.D., Chief of Staff
CHR: Deana Moses, Manager Human Resources
Web address: www.phs.org
Control: Other not–for–profit (including NFP Corporation) **Service:** General Medical and Surgical

Staffed Beds: 25 **Admissions:** 1172 **Census:** 9 **Outpatient Visits:** 84134 **Births:** 333 **Total Expense ($000):** 28384 **Payroll Expense ($000):** 11915 **Personnel:** 229

SAN FIDEL—Cibola County

ACOMA–CANONCITO–LAGUNA HOSPITAL (320070), Mailing Address: P.O. Box 130, Zip 87049–0130; tel. 505/552–5300 **A**1 10 **F**3 7 25 28 30 32 36 37 38 50 53 62 63 66 73 86 87 89 94 107 119 121 123 132 133 136 137 **P**1 6 **S** U. S. Indian Health Service
Primary Contact: William Thorne, Jr., Chief Executive Officer
Control: PHS, Indian Service, Government, federal **Service:** General Medical and Surgical

Staffed Beds: 7 **Admissions:** 251 **Census:** 4 **Outpatient Visits:** 65881 **Births:** 3 **Total Expense ($000):** 22273 **Payroll Expense ($000):** 10861 **Personnel:** 139

Many Facility Codes have changed. Please refer to the AHA Guide Code Chart.

SANTA FE—Santa Fe County

☒ **PHS SANTA FE INDIAN HOSPITAL (320057)**, 1700 Cerrillos Road, Zip 87505–3554; tel. 505/988–9821, (Nonreporting) **A**1 10 **S** U. S. Indian Health Service
Primary Contact: Robert J. Lyon, Chief Executive Officer
CMO: Bret Smoker, M.D., Clinical Director
CIO: Vernita Jones, Site Manager
Control: Public Health Service, Government, federal **Service:** General Medical and Surgical

Staffed Beds: 39

☒ **ST. VINCENT REGIONAL MEDICAL CENTER (320002)**, 455 St. Michael's Drive, Zip 87505–7663, Mailing Address: P.O. Box 2107, Zip 87504–2107; tel. 505/983–3361, (Nonreporting) **A**1 2 3 5 9 10 20
Primary Contact: J. Alex Valdez, J.D., Chief Executive Officer
COO: Rick Crabtree, Chief Operating Officer
CFO: Rick Doxtator, Chief Financial Officer
CMO: Kevin Garrett, M.D., Chief Medical Officer
CHR: Barbara Roe, Vice President and Director Human Resources
Web address: www.stvin.org
Control: Other not–for–profit (including NFP Corporation) **Service:** General Medical and Surgical

Staffed Beds: 180

SANTA ROSA—Guadalupe County

GUADALUPE COUNTY HOSPITAL (320067), 535 Lake Drive, Zip 88435–2542, Mailing Address: P.O. Box 500, Zip 88435–0500; tel. 505/472–3246 **A**9 10 20 **F**31 32 33 38 55 57 96 106 107 119 137 **P**5
Primary Contact: Christina Campos, Administrator
COO: Christina Campos, Administrator
CFO: Bret Goebel, Finance Officer
CMO: Randal Brown, M.D., Chief of Staff
CHR: Colleen Galligos, Director Human Resources
Control: County–Government, nonfederal **Service:** General Medical and Surgical

Staffed Beds: 10 **Admissions:** 255 **Census:** 2 **Outpatient Visits:** 6279 **Births:** 0 **Total Expense ($000):** 3515 **Payroll Expense ($000):** 969 **Personnel:** 29

SANTA TERESA—Dona Ana County

☒ **PEAK BEHAVIORAL HEALTH SERVICES (324012)**, 5065 McNut Road, Zip 88008; tel. 505/589–3000, (Nonreporting) **A**1 9 10 **S** Psychiatric Solutions
Primary Contact: Bruce Waldo, Chief Executive Officer
COO: Katie Cosper, R.N., Director of Nursing
CFO: Shirley Milligan, Chief Financial Officer
CHR: Sonia Rodriguez, Director Human Resources
Web address: www.psysolutions.com/facilities/peak/index.html
Control: Corporation, Investor–owned, for–profit **Service:** Psychiatric

Staffed Beds: 36

SHIPROCK—San Juan County

☒ **NORTHERN NAVAJO MEDICAL CENTER (320059)**, Mailing Address: P.O. Box 160, Zip 87420–0160; tel. 505/368–6001, (Nonreporting) **A**1 10 **S** U. S. Indian Health Service
Primary Contact: George C. Baacke, II, M.D., Acting Chief Executive Officer
CFO: Dorothy Smith, Finance Officer
CMO: Stephen Bowers, M.D., Clinical Director
CIO: Roland Chapman, Chief Information Officer
CHR: Cecelia A. Anderson, Director Human Resources
Web address: www.home.nnmc.ihs.gov/
Control: Public Health Service, Government, federal **Service:** General Medical and Surgical

Staffed Beds: 64

SILVER CITY—Grant County

☒ **GILA REGIONAL MEDICAL CENTER (320016)**, 1313 East 32nd Street, Zip 88061; tel. 505/538–4000 **A**1 9 10 20 **F**3 7 11 13 15 26 27 30 31 32 33 35 38 40 42 50 52 55 57 61 62 68 73 74 75 76 77 79 80 82 86 88 90 92 93 96 97 100 102 107 118 119 137 **P**5
Primary Contact: Brian S. Bentley, Chief Executive Officer
CFO: Craig Stewart, Chief Financial Officer
CMO: Jean Remillard, M.D., Chief Medical Officer
CIO: David Furnas, Chief Information Officer
CHR: Barbara Barela, Director Human Resources
Web address: www.grmc.org
Control: County–Government, nonfederal **Service:** General Medical and Surgical

Staffed Beds: 68 **Admissions:** 3778 **Census:** 32 **Outpatient Visits:** 89296 **Births:** 512 **Total Expense ($000):** 55392 **Payroll Expense ($000):** 24018 **Personnel:** 569

SOCORRO—Socorro County

☒ **SOCORRO GENERAL HOSPITAL (321301)**, 1202 Highway 60 West, Zip 87801, Mailing Address: P.O. Box 1009, Zip 87801–1009; tel. 505/835–1140 **A**1 9 10 18 **F**3 11 13 14 25 26 31 32 38 42 52 55 61 62 66 79 86 90 93 96 119 122 123 132 **S** Presbyterian Healthcare Services
Primary Contact: Bo Beames, Administrator
CHR: Pam Miller–Balfour, Director Human Resources
Web address: www.phs.org/facilities/facsocorro.htm
Control: Other not–for–profit (including NFP Corporation) **Service:** General Medical and Surgical

Staffed Beds: 24 **Admissions:** 892 **Census:** 7 **Outpatient Visits:** 61111 **Births:** 188 **Total Expense ($000):** 20109 **Payroll Expense ($000):** 9664 **Personnel:** 169

TAOS—Taos County

★ **HOLY CROSS HOSPITAL (320013)**, 1397 Weimer Road, Zip 87571–6284, Mailing Address: P.O. Box DD, Zip 87571–6284; tel. 575/758–8883 **A**9 10 20 **F**8 11 13 15 25 26 31 32 33 38 40 46 51 55 56 57 62 68 73 74 75 79 81 84 96 100 102 107 121 124 136 137 **P**8 **S** QHR
Primary Contact: Warren K. Spellman, Chief Executive Officer
CFO: Richard Eisenring, Chief Financial Officer
CMO: Jack Garland, M.D., Chief of Staff
CIO: Ed Flores, Director Information System
CHR: James Arkens, Director Human Resources
Web address: www.taoshospital.org
Control: Other not–for–profit (including NFP Corporation) **Service:** General Medical and Surgical

Staffed Beds: 47 **Admissions:** 2805 **Census:** 27 **Outpatient Visits:** 59696 **Births:** 292 **Total Expense ($000):** 42496 **Payroll Expense ($000):** 17186 **Personnel:** 361

TRUTH OR CONSEQUENCES—Sierra County

★ **SIERRA VISTA HOSPITAL (321300)**, 800 East Ninth Avenue, Zip 87901–1961; tel. 505/894–2111 **A**9 10 18 **F**5 7 11 14 25 26 30 31 32 33 36 38 41 43 57 62 64 66 79 80 82 86 87 89 90 92 93 94 96 117 119 121 122 124 137 **P**6
Primary Contact: Jeff White, Chief Executive Officer
CFO: Bret Gobel, Interim Chief Financial Officer
CMO: James F. Malcolmson, M.D., Chief of Staff
CIO: Dan Morrell, Manager Information Systems
CHR: Lana Dillon, Chief Human Resources Officer
Control: City–County, Government, nonfederal **Service:** General Medical and Surgical

Staffed Beds: 16 **Admissions:** 391 **Census:** 4 **Outpatient Visits:** 32083 **Births:** 1 **Total Expense ($000):** 7612 **Payroll Expense ($000):** 4974 **Personnel:** 115

TUCUMCARI—Quay County

★ **DR. DAN C. TRIGG MEMORIAL HOSPITAL (321302)**, 301 East Miel De Luna Avenue, Zip 88401–3810, Mailing Address: P.O. Box 608, Zip 88401–0608; tel. 505/461–7003 **A**9 10 18 **F**3 11 15 25 31 32 33 38 40 57 61 65 66 79 80 82 85 86 96 102 107 117 118 122 124 135 **P**5 **S** Presbyterian Healthcare Services
Primary Contact: Hoyt Skabelund, Administrator
Web address: www.phs.org
Control: Other not–for–profit (including NFP Corporation) **Service:** General Medical and Surgical

Staffed Beds: 25 **Admissions:** 575 **Census:** 6 **Outpatient Visits:** 25934 **Births:** 2 **Total Expense ($000):** 11585 **Payroll Expense ($000):** 4378 **Personnel:** 98

ZUNI—McKinley County

☒ **U. S. PUBLIC HEALTH SERVICE INDIAN HOSPITAL (320060)**, Route 301 North B. Street, Zip 87327, Mailing Address: P.O. Box 467, Zip 87327–0467; tel. 505/782–4431 **A**1 10 **F**13 15 37 38 57 74 84 99 107 **S** U. S. Indian Health Service
Primary Contact: Jean Othole, Chief Executive Officer
CFO: Clyde Yatsattie, Administrative Officer
CMO: David Kessler, M.D., Clinical Director
CHR: Cynthia Tsalate, Human Resource Specialist
Web address: www.ihs.gov
Control: PHS, Indian Service, Government, federal **Service:** General Medical and Surgical

Staffed Beds: 32 **Admissions:** 706 **Census:** 7 **Outpatient Visits:** 86783 **Births:** 87

NM

Hospital, Medicare Provider Number, Address, Telephone, Approval, Facility, and Physician Codes, Health Care System

★ American Hospital Association (AHA) membership
☐ The Joint Commission accreditation
○ American Osteopathic Association (AOA) accreditation
△ Commission on Accreditation of Rehabilitation Facilities (CARF) accreditation

NEW YORK

ALBANY—Albany County

★ **ALBANY MEDICAL CENTER (330013)**, 43 New Scotland Avenue, Zip 12208–3478; tel. 518/262–3125, (Includes ALBANY MEDICAL CENTER SOUTH–CLINICAL CAMPUS, 25 Hackett Boulevard, Zip 12208–3499; tel. 518/242–1200; Timothy W. Duffy, General Director) **A**1 2 3 5 8 9 10 12 13 **F**6 11 12 13 15 17 18 19 20 21 22 23 24 25 26 27 28 30 31 32 33 38 40 46 49 50 54 55 56 59 60 62 66 68 70 71 72 73 74 75 76 77 79 80 81 82 83 84 85 86 87 88 90 92 93 94 95 96 97 98 99 100 102 103 104 105 106 107 108 109 111 112 113 114 116 119 126 127 131 135
Primary Contact: James J. Barba, President and Chief Executive Officer
COO: Bernadette R. Pedlow, Senior Vice President Hospital Business and Hospital Chief Operating Officer
CFO: William C. Hasselbarth, Chief Financial Officer
CMO: Robert A. Catalano, M.D., Medical Director
CIO: George Hickman, Senior Vice President and Chief Information Officer
CHR: Cathy Halakan, Senior Vice President
Web address: www.amc.edu
Control: Other not–for–profit (including NFP Corporation) **Service:** General Medical and Surgical

Staffed Beds: 600 **Admissions:** 29019 **Census:** 509 **Outpatient Visits:** 286894 **Births:** 2341 **Total Expense ($000):** 507532 **Payroll Expense ($000):** 184514 **Personnel:** 4322

ALBANY MEMORIAL HOSPITAL (330003), 600 Northern Boulevard, Zip 12204–1083; tel. 518/471–3221, (Nonreporting) **A**5 6 9 10
Primary Contact: Norman E. Dascher, Jr., Chief Executive Officer
COO: Karen Tassey, Chief Operating Officer
CFO: Lori Santos, Vice President Finance
CMO: Daniel Kopp, M.D., Senior Vice President Medical Affairs
CIO: Robert J. Duthe, Vice President Corporate Management Information Systems
CHR: Barbara McCandless, Corporate Vice President Human Resources
Web address: www.nehealth.com
Control: Other not–for–profit (including NFP Corporation) **Service:** General Medical and Surgical

Staffed Beds: 165

□ **CAPITAL DISTRICT PSYCHIATRIC CENTER (334046)**, 75 New Scotland Avenue, Zip 12208–3474; tel. 518/447–9611, (Nonreporting) **A**1 3 5 10 **S** New York State Office of Mental Health
Primary Contact: Lewis Campbell, Executive Director
CFO: Bonnie Erickson, Director Business Office
Web address: www.omh.state.ny.us/omhweb/facilities/cdpc/facility.htm
Control: State–Government, nonfederal **Service:** Psychiatric

Staffed Beds: 200

★ **ST. PETER'S HOSPITAL (330057)**, 315 South Manning Boulevard, Zip 12208–1789; tel. 518/525–1550, (Total facility includes 320 beds in nursing home–type unit) **A**1 2 3 5 9 10 **F**4 5 11 12 13 14 15 17 18 20 22 24 25 26 27 30 31 32 33 34 35 36 37 38 42 43 44 50 51 52 53 54 55 56 57 59 60 61 62 64 66 68 69 70 71 72 73 74 75 76 77 79 80 81 82 83 84 85 86 87 90 91 92 93 96 97 98 99 100 102 103 104 105 106 107 108 109 111 112 114 116 117 118 119 121 122 123 124 132 134 135 136 137 **S** Catholic Health East
Primary Contact: Steven P. Boyle, President and Chief Executive Officer
CFO: James M. Gavin, Chief Financial Officer
CMO: Robert Cella, M.D., Vice President Medical Affairs
CIO: Jonathan Goldberg, Chief Information Officer
CHR: Judy Gray, Vice President Human Resources
Web address: www.stpetershealthcare.org
Control: Church–operated, Nongovernment, not–for profit **Service:** General Medical and Surgical

Staffed Beds: 762 **Admissions:** 26774 **Census:** 404 **Outpatient Visits:** 515768 **Births:** 2824 **Total Expense ($000):** 318283 **Payroll Expense ($000):** 140225 **Personnel:** 4106

★ △ **VETERANS AFFAIRS MEDICAL CENTER**, 113 Holland Avenue, Zip 12208–3473; tel. 518/626–5000, (Total facility includes 40 beds in nursing home–type unit) **A**1 2 3 5 7 8 9 **F**2 3 4 5 12 15 17 18 20 24 25 26 27 30 31 32 33 37 38 42 43 44 45 46 47 50 52 54 55 56 57 58 59 60 61 62 63 66 68 72 73 75 76 77 79 80 81 82 86 87 88 90 92 93 94 96 97 100 106 107 109 110 117 118 119 121 124 132 135 136 137 **S** Department of Veterans Affairs
Primary Contact: Mary–Ellen Piche, Director
COO: Douglas Erickson, Associate Director
CMO: Lourdes Irizarry, M.D., Chief Medical Officer
CIO: Mike Mullahey, Manager Operations
Web address: www.va.gov/sta/guide/home.asp
Control: Veterans Affairs, Government, federal **Service:** General Medical and Surgical

Staffed Beds: 177 **Admissions:** 2548 **Census:** 50 **Outpatient Visits:** 295592 **Births:** 0 **Total Expense ($000):** 160989 **Payroll Expense ($000):** 102562 **Personnel:** 1192

ALEXANDRIA BAY—Jefferson County

★ **RIVER HOSPITAL (331309)**, 4 Fuller Street, Zip 13607; tel. 315/482–2511, (Total facility includes 27 beds in nursing home–type unit) (Nonreporting) **A**9 10 18
Primary Contact: Ben Moore, III, President and Chief Executive Officer
COO: William Connor, Assistant Administrator and Director Human Resources
CFO: Traci Mintonye, Interim Chief Financial Officer
CMO: Harriet Burris, M.D., Medical Director
CIO: Phillip Edie, Director Information and Communication Systems
CHR: William Connor, Assistant Administrator and Director Human Resources
Web address: www.riverhospital.org
Control: Other not–for–profit (including NFP Corporation) **Service:** General Medical and Surgical

Staffed Beds: 51

AMITYVILLE—Suffolk County

□ **BRUNSWICK PHYSICAL MEDICINE AND REHABILITATION HOSPITAL (334026)**, 366 Broadway, Zip 11701–9820; tel. 631/789–7000, (Includes BRUNSWICK HALL, 80 Louden Avenue, Zip 11701–2735; tel. 516/789–7100), (Nonreporting) **A**1 9 10
Primary Contact: Amar Jit Singh, M.D., Chief Executive Officer
CFO: Harry Fruhman, Chief Financial Officer
Web address: www.brunswickhospital.com
Control: Corporation, Investor–owned, for–profit **Service:** Rehabilitation

Staffed Beds: 36

□ **SOUTH OAKS HOSPITAL (334027)**, 400 Sunrise Highway, Zip 11701–2508; tel. 631/264–4000, (Total facility includes 320 beds in nursing home–type unit) (Nonreporting) **A**1 9 10
Primary Contact: Robert E. Detor, Chief Executive Officer
CFO: Patricia Porter, Chief Financial Officer
CMO: Yogendra Upadhyay, M.D., Senior Vice President Medical Affairs
CHR: Pam Quiroga, Vice President Human Resources
Web address: www.longislandhome.org
Control: Other not–for–profit (including NFP Corporation) **Service:** Psychiatric

Staffed Beds: 554

AMSTERDAM—Montgomery County

★ ○ △ **AMSTERDAM MEMORIAL HOSPITAL (330010)**, 4988 State Highway 30, Zip 12010–1699; tel. 518/842–3100, (Total facility includes 160 beds in nursing home–type unit) **A**7 9 10 11 **F**2 3 8 11 15 25 26 33 49 50 52 54 56 57 60 62 66 72 73 75 79 82 85 87 96 99 102 107 117 119 120 121 122 124 133 134 135 136 137 **P**6
Primary Contact: Donald W. Massey, President and Chief Executive Officer
CFO: Richard G. Braun, CPA, Chief Financial Officer
CMO: Kevin P. Cope, M.D., Chief Medical Officer
CIO: Ivan Antonyuk, Director Information Technology
CHR: Martin Patrick, Chief Human Resources Officer
Web address: www.amsterdammemorial.org
Control: Other not–for–profit (including NFP Corporation) **Service:** General Medical and Surgical

Staffed Beds: 199 **Admissions:** 636 **Census:** 167 **Outpatient Visits:** 74159 **Births:** 0 **Total Expense ($000):** 31143 **Payroll Expense ($000):** 15193 **Personnel:** 360

★ **ST. MARY'S HOSPITAL (330047)**, 427 Guy Park Avenue, Zip 12010–1095; tel. 518/842–1900 **A**1 9 10 **F**3 4 11 13 15 17 24 25 26 27 30 31 32 33 34 38 42 43 44 45 50 55 56 57 59 62 66 68 69 74 75 76 79 80 81 82 86 87 88 89 90 91 92 93 94 95 96 99 100 103 107 119 121 123 124 135 136 **S** Ascension Health
Primary Contact: Victor Giulianelli, FACHE, President and Chief Executive Officer
COO: Scott Bruce, Vice President Operations
CFO: John Sagan, Vice President Finance
CMO: Timothy Shoen, M.D., Vice President Medical Staff Services
CIO: James DeGroff, Director Technology and Network Services
CHR: Beth Case, Vice President Human Resources
Web address: www.smha.org
Control: Other not–for–profit (including NFP Corporation) **Service:** General Medical and Surgical

Staffed Beds: 143 **Admissions:** 6520 **Census:** 100 **Outpatient Visits:** 263614 **Births:** 512 **Total Expense ($000):** 85312 **Payroll Expense ($000):** 43542 **Personnel:** 878

NY

Many Facility Codes have changed. Please refer to the AHA Guide Code Chart.

AUBURN—Cayuga County

★ **AUBURN MEMORIAL HOSPITAL (330235)**, 17 Lansing Street, Zip 13021–1943; tel. 315/255–7011, (Total facility includes 80 beds in nursing home–type unit) **A**9 10 **F**3 11 12 13 15 17 24 25 27 33 38 42 44 53 62 66 73 74 77 79 84 85 86 88 90 92 96 98 106 107 117 118 119 121 133 135 137
Primary Contact: Scott A. Berlucchi, President and Chief Executive Officer
CFO: John Baran, Interim Chief Financial Officer
CHR: Chad Hoffman, Director Employee Relations
Web address: www.auburnhospital.org
Control: Other not–for–profit (including NFP Corporation) **Service:** General Medical and Surgical

Staffed Beds: 131 **Admissions:** 4750 **Census:** 131 **Outpatient Visits:** 147667 **Births:** 250 **Total Expense ($000):** 69961 **Payroll Expense ($000):** 31711 **Personnel:** 672

BATAVIA—Genesee County

☒ **UNITED MEMORIAL MEDICAL CENTER (330073)**, 127 North Street, Zip 14020–2260; tel. 585/343–6030, (Includes UNITED MEMORIAL MEDICAL CENTER–BANK STREET; UNITED MEMORIAL MEDICAL CENTER–NORTH STREET, 16 Banks Street, Zip 14020–1697; tel. 585/343–6030) **A**1 9 10 **F**3 4 8 13 15 17 24 25 26 27 30 31 32 33 38 40 43 49 55 56 57 62 68 73 74 75 77 79 80 84 86 87 96 97 100 102 103 107 119
Primary Contact: Mark C. Schoell, Chief Executive Officer
CFO: Robert Chiavetta, Vice President Finance
CMO: Michael Merrill, M.D., Interim Vice President Medical Affairs
CIO: Daniel O'Connor, Chief Information Officer
CHR: Sonja Gonyea, Director Human Resources
Web address: www.ummc.org
Control: Other not–for–profit (including NFP Corporation) **Service:** General Medical and Surgical

Staffed Beds: 131 **Admissions:** 4901 **Census:** 71 **Outpatient Visits:** 185158 **Births:** 573 **Total Expense ($000):** 55225 **Payroll Expense ($000):** 24198 **Personnel:** 670

★ **VETERANS AFFAIRS WESTERN NEW YORK HEALTHCARE SYSTEM–BATAVIA DIVISION**, 222 Richmond Avenue, Zip 14020–1288; tel. 585/297–1000, (Total facility includes 70 beds in nursing home–type unit) (Nonreporting) **A**5 9 **S** Department of Veterans Affairs
Primary Contact: Michael S. Finegan, Director
Web address: www.va.gov/visns/visn02
Control: Veterans Affairs, Government, federal **Service:** General Medical and Surgical

Staffed Beds: 158

BATH—Steuben County

☒ **IRA DAVENPORT MEMORIAL HOSPITAL (330144)**, 7571 State Route 54, Zip 14810–9590; tel. 607/776–8500, (Total facility includes 120 beds in nursing home–type unit) (Nonreporting) **A**1 9 10
Primary Contact: James B. Watson, Chief Executive Officer
CFO: James L. Smith, Chief Financial Officer
CMO: Dennis O'Connor, M.D., Medical Director
CIO: Hendrik Van der Horst, Chief Information Officer
CHR: Marybess Hazlett, Director Human Resources
Web address: www.davenportandtaylor.org
Control: Other not–for–profit (including NFP Corporation) **Service:** General Medical and Surgical

Staffed Beds: 156

☒ **VETERANS AFFAIRS MEDICAL CENTER**, 76 Veterans Avenue, Zip 14810–0842; tel. 607/664–4000, (Total facility includes 124 beds in nursing home–type unit) **A**1 9 **F**3 5 7 11 15 24 25 26 29 30 31 32 33 34 37 38 42 43 44 52 54 55 56 57 61 62 72 73 75 81 82 86 87 90 91 93 94 96 102 107 117 119 121 124 132 135 136 137 **S** Department of Veterans Affairs
Primary Contact: David J. West, Director
CFO: Jill Haynes, Financial Coach
CMO: Alan Fantuzzo, D.O., Chief of Staff
CIO: Karen Clancy, Manager, Information Systems Operations
CHR: Edward Yankowski, Manager Human Resources
Web address: www.va.gov/sta/guide/home.asp
Control: Veterans Affairs, Government, federal **Service:** General Medical and Surgical

Staffed Beds: 344 **Admissions:** 2293 **Census:** 277 **Outpatient Visits:** 150973 **Births:** 0 **Total Expense ($000):** 64956 **Payroll Expense ($000):** 46818 **Personnel:** 590

BAY SHORE—Suffolk County

☒ **SOUTHSIDE HOSPITAL (330043)**, 301 East Main Street, Zip 11706–8458; tel. 631/968–3000 **A**1 2 3 5 9 10 **F**3 4 11 12 13 15 17 18 20 25 26 27 30 31 32 33 34 36 38 40 41 42 43 44 50 53 54 55 56 57 58 59 60 62 63 64 66 68 71 72 73 74 75 76 77 79 80 81 82 84 85 86 87 88 89 90 91 92 93 96 97 100 102 106 107 108 109 111 113 114 119 120 121 123 124 135 136 137 **S** North Shore–LIJ Health System
Primary Contact: Winifred Mack, Executive Director
CFO: Robert Power, Associate Executive Director Finance
CMO: Jay Enden, Medical Director
CIO: Lowney Mincy, Director Information Services
CHR: Anne Barrett, Associate Executive Director Human Resources
Web address: www.southsidehospital.org
Control: Other not–for–profit (including NFP Corporation) **Service:** General Medical and Surgical

Staffed Beds: 296 **Admissions:** 16104 **Census:** 225 **Outpatient Visits:** 130142 **Births:** 2837 **Total Expense ($000):** 233177 **Payroll Expense ($000):** 109271 **Personnel:** 1755

BEACON—Dutchess County

SAINT FRANCIS HOSPITAL See Saint Francis Hospital and Health Centers, Poughkeepsie

BELLEROSE—Queens County, See New York City

BETHPAGE—Nassau County

☐ **NEW ISLAND HOSPITAL (330332)**, 4295 Hempstead Turnpike, Zip 11714–5769; tel. 516/579–6000, (Nonreporting) **A**1 9 10
Primary Contact: Aaron Glatt, M.D., President and Chief Executive Officer
CFO: Drew Pallas, Vice President Finance
CMO: Lawrence A. Reduto, M.D., President and Chief Medical Officer
CIO: Blake Benz, Director Management Information Systems
CHR: Peter Chiacchiaro, Vice President Human Resources
Web address: www.newislandhospital.org
Control: Other not–for–profit (including NFP Corporation) **Service:** General Medical and Surgical

Staffed Beds: 140

BINGHAMTON—Broome County

BINGHAMTON GENERAL HOSPITAL See United Health Services Hospitals–Binghamton

☐ **GREATER BINGHAMTON HEALTH CENTER (334012)**, 425 Robinson Street, Zip 13901–4198; tel. 607/724–1391 **A**1 10 **F**25 26 33 37 58 73 88 89 93 94 95 119 121 135 **P**1 **S** New York State Office of Mental Health
Primary Contact: Margaret R. Dugan, Executive Director
Web address: www.omh.state.ny.us
Control: State–Government, nonfederal **Service:** Psychiatric

Staffed Beds: 168 **Admissions:** 233 **Census:** 163 **Outpatient Visits:** 45788 **Births:** 0 **Total Expense ($000):** 42747 **Payroll Expense ($000):** 23324 **Personnel:** 436

☒ **OUR LADY OF LOURDES MEMORIAL HOSPITAL (330011)**, 169 Riverside Drive, Zip 13905–4198; tel. 607/798–5111 **A**1 2 9 10 **F**3 11 13 15 24 25 26 30 31 32 33 34 37 38 42 43 44 46 47 49 50 51 52 53 54 55 56 57 59 61 62 63 66 68 69 72 73 74 75 76 77 79 80 81 82 84 86 87 96 97 99 100 102 103 106 107 108 109 112 118 119 120 121 123 124 133 135 136 137 **P**7 **S** Ascension Health
Primary Contact: John D. O'Neil, President and Chief Executive Officer
CFO: Gregg Hayton, Vice President Finance
CMO: Robert Taylor, M.D., Vice President Medical Affairs
CIO: John Laliberte, Director Information Services
CHR: Dan Bonsick, Assistant Vice President Human Resources
Web address: www.lourdes.com
Control: Church–operated, Nongovernment, not–for profit **Service:** General Medical and Surgical

Staffed Beds: 169 **Admissions:** 8887 **Census:** 112 **Outpatient Visits:** 1270279 **Births:** 1177 **Total Expense ($000):** 194542 **Payroll Expense ($000):** 81067 **Personnel:** 1736

Hospital, Medicare Provider Number, Address, Telephone, Approval, Facility, and Physician Codes, Health Care System

★ American Hospital Association (AHA) membership
☐ The Joint Commission accreditation
○ American Osteopathic Association (AOA) accreditation
△ Commission on Accreditation of Rehabilitation Facilities (CARF) accreditation

★ **UNITED HEALTH SERVICES HOSPITALS–BINGHAMTON (330394)**, 10–42 Mitchell Avenue, Zip 13903–1678; tel. 607/763–6000, (Includes BINGHAMTON GENERAL HOSPITAL, 10–42 Mitchell Avenue, Zip 13903; MEDICENTER, 600 High Avenue, Endicott, Zip 13760; tel. 607/754–7171; WILSON MEMORIAL REGIONAL MEDICAL CENTER, 33–57 Harrison Street, Johnson City, Zip 13790) **A**1 8 9 10 **F**1 3 4 5 11 12 13 15 17 18 20 22 24 25 26 27 28 30 31 32 33 35 36 37 38 40 44 46 47 49 50 51 56 57 58 59 60 62 63 66 68 70 72 73 74 75 76 77 79 80 81 82 84 85 86 87 88 90 91 92 93 94 96 97 99 102 103 106 107 112 113 116 119 120 121 124 134 135 136 137 **P**6 **S** United Health Services
Primary Contact: Matthew J. Salanger, President and Chief Executive Officer
Web address: www.uhs.net
Control: Other not–for–profit (including NFP Corporation) **Service:** General Medical and Surgical

Staffed Beds: 465 **Admissions:** 16961 **Census:** 314 **Outpatient Visits:** 313358 **Births:** 1592 **Total Expense ($000):** 338204 **Payroll Expense ($000):** 133396 **Personnel:** 2579

BRENTWOOD—Suffolk County

☐ **PILGRIM PSYCHIATRIC CENTER (334013)**, 998 Crooked Hill Road, Zip 11717–1087; tel. 631/761–3500, (Includes KINGS PARK PSYCHIATRIC CENTER), (Nonreporting) **A**1 10 **S** New York State Office of Mental Health
Primary Contact: Dean R. Weinstock, RN, Executive Director
CFO: Carole Isasi, Director for Administration
Web address: www.omh.state.ny.us/omhweb/facilities/pgpc/facility.htm
Control: State–Government, nonfederal **Service:** Psychiatric

Staffed Beds: 569

BROCKPORT—Monroe County

★ **LAKESIDE MEMORIAL HOSPITAL (330037)**, 156 West Avenue, Zip 14420–1286; tel. 585/395–6095, (Total facility includes 120 beds in nursing home–type unit) **A**1 9 10 **F**3 8 13 25 28 38 42 43 53 56 62 64 66 68 73 74 75 77 79 80 86 87 96 97 100 102 107 113 119 121 124 135 **P**6
Primary Contact: Kevin C. Nacy, Chief Executive Officer
COO: Michael Stapleton, Chief Operating Officer
CFO: Michelle Kingdollar, Controller
CMO: James E. Szalados, M.D., Vice President Medical Affairs
CIO: John Schrenker, Chief Information Officer
CHR: James Cummings, Vice President Human Resources
Web address: www.lakesidehealth.com
Control: Other not–for–profit (including NFP Corporation) **Service:** General Medical and Surgical

Staffed Beds: 181 **Admissions:** 2251 **Census:** 34 **Births:** 215

BRONX—Bronx County, See New York City

BRONXVILLE—Westchester County

★ **LAWRENCE HOSPITAL CENTER (330061)**, 55 Palmer Avenue, Zip 10708–3491; tel. 914/787–1000 **A**1 2 5 9 10 **F**3 12 13 15 24 25 26 27 33 38 41 42 43 44 46 51 56 57 61 63 66 67 68 70 74 76 77 79 80 82 84 86 90 96 97 99 100 102 107 114 119 120 121 124 135 136
Primary Contact: Edward M. Dinan, President and Chief Executive Officer
COO: James Y. Lee, Executive Vice President and Chief Operating Officer
CFO: Murray Askinazi, Vice President Finance
CMO: Werner Roeder, M.D., Vice President Medical Affairs
CHR: Tom Mastroianni, Vice President Human Resources
Web address: www.lawrencehealth.org
Control: Other not–for–profit (including NFP Corporation) **Service:** General Medical and Surgical

Staffed Beds: 164 **Admissions:** 10800 **Census:** 140 **Outpatient Visits:** 171635 **Births:** 1740 **Total Expense ($000):** 128880 **Payroll Expense ($000):** 60789 **Personnel:** 891

BROOKLYN—Kings County, See New York City

BUFFALO—Erie County

BRYLIN HOSPITALS (334022), 1263 Delaware Avenue, Zip 14209–2497; tel. 716/886–8200, (Nonreporting) **A**9 10
Primary Contact: Eric D. Pleskow, President and Chief Executive Officer
CFO: E. Paul Hettich, Chief Financial Officer
CMO: Balvinder Kang, M.D., Medical Director
CIO: Pawel Wieczorek, Director Information Technology
CHR: Jacquelyn Bixler, Vice President Human Resources
Web address: www.brylin.com
Control: Individual, Investor–owned, for–profit **Service:** Psychiatric

Staffed Beds: 88

☐ **BUFFALO PSYCHIATRIC CENTER (334052)**, 400 Forest Avenue, Zip 14213–1298; tel. 716/885–2261, (Nonreporting) **A**1 3 5 10 **S** New York State Office of Mental Health
Primary Contact: Thomas Dodson, Executive Director
COO: Celia Spacone, M.D., Director Operations
CFO: Pamela Esposito, Interim Director Facility Administration
CMO: Norma Panahon, M.D., President Medical Staff
CIO: Anne Buchheit, Coordinator Mental Health Local Information Systems
CHR: Charles Siewert, Director Human Resources
Web address: www.omh.state.ny.us
Control: State–Government, nonfederal **Service:** Psychiatric

Staffed Beds: 240

☐ **ERIE COUNTY MEDICAL CENTER (330219)**, 462 Grider Street, Zip 14215–3098; tel. 716/898–3000, (Total facility includes 794 beds in nursing home–type unit) (Nonreporting) **A**1 3 5 9 10
Primary Contact: Michael A. Young, FACHE, Chief Executive Officer
COO: Mark C. Barabas, Chief Operating Officer
CFO: Sue McCarthy, Chief Financial Officer
CMO: John Fudyma, M.D., Medical Director
CIO: Debbie Cancilla, Director Information Systems
CHR: Kathleen O'Hara, Vice President Human Resources
Web address: www.ecmc.edu
Control: County–Government, nonfederal **Service:** General Medical and Surgical

Staffed Beds: 1200

☐ **KALEIDA HEALTH (330005)**, 100 High Street, Zip 14203–1154; tel. 716/859–5600, (Includes DE GRAFF MEMORIAL HOSPITAL, 445 Tremont Street, North Tonawanda, Zip 14120–0750, Mailing Address: P.O. Box 0750, Zip 14120–0750; tel. 716/694–4500; Tamara Owen, President; MILLARD FILLMORE GATES CIRCLE HOSPITAL, 3 Gates Circle, Zip 14209–9986; tel. 716/887–4600; Don Boyd, Interim President; MILLARD FILLMORE SUBURBAN HOSPITAL, 1540 Maple Road, Williamsville, Zip 14221; tel. 716/688–3100; WOMEN AND CHILDREN'S HOSPITAL, 219 Bryant Street, Zip 14222–2099; tel. 716/878–7000; Cheryl Klass, President), (Total facility includes 397 beds in nursing home–type unit) **A**1 3 5 8 9 10 **F**2 5 8 11 12 13 15 17 18 19 20 21 22 23 24 25 26 27 28 30 31 32 33 34 37 38 40 41 42 43 44 45 46 49 50 51 53 54 55 56 57 58 59 60 61 62 63 64 66 68 70 71 72 73 74 75 76 77 79 80 81 82 83 84 85 86 87 88 89 90 91 92 93 94 95 96 97 98 99 100 101 102 103 104 105 106 107 117 119 120 121 124 125 127 131 132 133 134 135 136 137 **P**6
Primary Contact: James R. Kaskie, President and Chief Executive Officer
COO: Connie Vari, Executive Vice President and Chief Operating Officer
CFO: Joseph Kessler, Executive Vice President and Chief Financial Officer
CMO: Margaret Paroski, M.D., Executive Vice President and Chief Medical Officer
CIO: Francis Meyer, Vice President Information Systems Technology
Web address: www.kaleidahealth.org
Control: State–Government, nonfederal **Service:** General Medical and Surgical

Staffed Beds: 1558 **Admissions:** 58462 **Census:** 1465 **Outpatient Visits:** 400023 **Births:** 5853 **Total Expense ($000):** 987042 **Payroll Expense ($000):** 418052 **Personnel:** 8381

★ **MERCY HOSPITAL (330279)**, 565 Abbott Road, Zip 14220–2095; tel. 716/826–7000, (Total facility includes 74 beds in nursing home–type unit) **A**1 3 5 9 10 **F**3 8 13 14 15 17 18 20 22 24 26 27 31 32 33 38 39 42 43 44 45 46 48 49 50 51 53 54 55 57 58 59 62 64 66 68 70 71 72 73 74 76 77 79 80 82 84 85 87 90 96 97 100 102 103 106 107 116 117 118 119 135 **P**5 **S** Catholic Health System
Primary Contact: Charles J. Urlaub, President and Chief Executive Officer
COO: Nils Gunnersen, Chief Operating Officer
CFO: James Dunlop, Senior Vice President and Chief Financial Officer
CMO: Timothy Gabryel, M.D., Vice President Medical Affairs and Medical Director
CHR: Joseph A. Scrivo, Director Human Resources
Web address: www.chsbuffalo.org
Control: Other not–for–profit (including NFP Corporation) **Service:** General Medical and Surgical

Staffed Beds: 420 **Admissions:** 18126 **Census:** 320 **Outpatient Visits:** 464102 **Births:** 2485 **Total Expense ($000):** 226660 **Payroll Expense ($000):** 96383 **Personnel:** 1791

☐ **ROSWELL PARK CANCER INSTITUTE (330354)**, Elm and Carlton Streets, Zip 14263–0001; tel. 716/845–2300 **A**1 2 3 5 8 9 10 **F**3 8 11 14 15 18 25 26 27 28 30 31 32 33 34 36 37 41 42 43 44 46 47 49 50 53 55 56 57 58 60 62 63 64 66 68 72 73 75 76 77 78 79 80 81 82 83 84 85 86 87 88 90 94 96 97 99 100 101 102 103 104 105 106 107 108 109 111 112 113 114 116 119 121 124 125 130 133 134 135 136 137 **P**6
Primary Contact: Donald L. Trump, M.D., President and Chief Executive Officer
COO: Rochelle L. Krowinski, Chief Clinical Operations Officer
CFO: Gregory McDonald, Vice President Finance and Chief Financial Officer
CMO: Judy Smith, M.D., Medical Director
CIO: JoAnne Ruh, Vice President Information Technology
CHR: Rick Paris, Vice President Human Resources
Web address: www.roswellpark.org
Control: Hospital district or authority, Government, nonfederal **Service:** Cancer

Staffed Beds: 106 **Admissions:** 4215 **Census:** 82 **Outpatient Visits:** 161869 **Births:** 0 **Total Expense ($000):** 420130 **Payroll Expense ($000):** 159825 **Personnel:** 3034

NY

SHEEHAN MEMORIAL HOSPITAL (330029), 425 Michigan Avenue, Zip 14203–2297; tel. 716/848–2000 **A**9 10 **F**3 4 5 8 30 31 32 56 81 87 97 99 107 124 **P**3 8
Primary Contact: Sheila Kee, President and Chief Executive Officer
COO: Althea Morgan Smith, Ph.D., Chief Operating Officer
CFO: Norman Dow, Controller
CMO: Kenton Forte, M.D., Medical Director
CIO: Dale Spellman, Manager Information Systems
CHR: Darlene Thomas, Director Human Resources
Web address: www.smhhealth.org
Control: Other not–for–profit (including NFP Corporation) **Service:** Rehabilitation

Staffed Beds: 40 **Admissions:** 1514 **Census:** 38 **Outpatient Visits:** 9404 **Births:** 0 **Payroll Expense ($000):** 3617 **Personnel:** 132

★ □ **SISTERS OF CHARITY HOSPITAL OF BUFFALO (330078)**, 2157 Main Street, Zip 14214–2692; tel. 716/862–1000, (Total facility includes 80 beds in nursing home–type unit) **A**1 2 3 5 9 10 12 13 **F**3 5 8 12 13 15 24 25 26 27 30 31 32 33 34 37 38 42 43 44 47 49 50 52 53 55 56 57 59 61 62 63 66 68 70 71 72 73 74 76 77 79 80 82 84 85 86 87 96 97 100 103 106 107 113 117 119 120 121 135 136 **P**5 **S** Catholic Health System
Primary Contact: Peter U. Bergmann, President and Chief Executive Officer
COO: Matthew Hamp, Chief Operating Officer
CFO: James Dunlop, Chief Financial Officer
CMO: Nady Shehata, M.D., Vice President Medical Affairs
CIO: Doug Torre, Director Information Technology
CHR: David DeLorenzo, Director Human Resources
Web address: www.chsbuffalo.org
Control: Other not–for–profit (including NFP Corporation) **Service:** General Medical and Surgical

Staffed Beds: 325 **Admissions:** 12643 **Census:** 218 **Outpatient Visits:** 253256 **Births:** 2832 **Total Expense ($000):** 164779 **Payroll Expense ($000):** 74082 **Personnel:** 1422

★ □ △ **VETERANS AFFAIRS WESTERN NEW YORK HEALTHCARE SYSTEM–BUFFALO DIVISION**, 3495 Bailey Avenue, Zip 14215–1129; tel. 716/834–9200, (Total facility includes 120 beds in nursing home–type unit) (Nonreporting) **A**1 2 7 8 9 **S** Department of Veterans Affairs
Primary Contact: Michael S. Finegan, Director
CFO: Royce Calhoun, Business Manager
CMO: Miguel Rainstein, M.D., Acting Chief of Staff
CIO: Margaret Owczarzak, Facility Chief Information Officer
Web address: www.va.gov/visns/visn02
Control: Veterans Affairs, Government, federal **Service:** General Medical and Surgical

Staffed Beds: 233

WESTERN NEW YORK CHILDREN'S PSYCHIATRIC CENTER See West Seneca

CALLICOON—Sullivan County

□ **CATSKILL REGIONAL MEDICAL CENTER (331303)**, 8881 Route 97, Zip 12723; tel. 845/887–5530, (Nonreporting) **A**1 9 10
Primary Contact: Chris L. White, Administrator
Web address: www.catskillregional.com
Control: Other not–for–profit (including NFP Corporation) **Service:** General Medical and Surgical

Staffed Beds: 25

CANANDAIGUA—Ontario County

★ □ **THOMPSON HEALTH (330074)**, 350 Parrish Street, Zip 14424–1793; tel. 585/396–6000, (Total facility includes 188 beds in nursing home–type unit) **A**1 9 10 **F**3 11 13 15 24 25 26 27 28 29 30 31 32 33 34 38 43 44 45 49 51 55 56 57 66 68 72 73 74 75 76 77 79 80 81 84 86 87 96 97 102 107 118 119 120 121 124 133 134 135 136 137
Primary Contact: Linda M. Janczak, President and Chief Executive Officer
COO: Deborah Weymouth, Senior Vice President Operations and Chief Financial Officer
CFO: Deborah Weymouth, Senior Vice President Operations and Chief Financial Officer
CMO: Carlos Ortiz, M.D., Senior Vice President Medical Services
CIO: Mark Halladay, Director Information Services
CHR: Jennifer DeVault, Director Associate Services
Web address: www.thompsonhealth.com
Control: Other not–for–profit (including NFP Corporation) **Service:** General Medical and Surgical

Staffed Beds: 301 **Admissions:** 4610 **Census:** 234 **Outpatient Visits:** 895320 **Births:** 694 **Total Expense ($000):** 79499 **Payroll Expense ($000):** 40940 **Personnel:** 823

★ □ **VETERANS AFFAIRS MEDICAL CENTER**, (Nursing Home), 400 Fort Hill Avenue, Zip 14424–1197; tel. 585/394–2000, (Total facility includes 138 beds in nursing home–type unit) **A**1 5 **F**2 4 5 6 10 25 26 30 31 32 33 34 36 37 42 43 44 45 50 52 53 54 55 56 57 60 61 62 63 66 72 73 75 81 82 86 87 90 91 93 94 95 96 107 117 119 121 124 132 135 136 **P**6 **S** Department of Veterans Affairs
Primary Contact: Craig Howard, Acting Director
CMO: Robert Babcock, M.D., Chief of Staff
CIO: Patricia Simon, Manager Information Systems
Web address: www.va.gov/sta/guide/home.asp
Control: Veterans Affairs, Government, federal **Service:** Other specialty

Staffed Beds: 218 **Admissions:** 745 **Census:** 174 **Outpatient Visits:** 196430 **Births:** 0 **Total Expense ($000):** 83942 **Payroll Expense ($000):** 58429 **Personnel:** 765

CARMEL—Putnam County

ARMS ACRES, 75 Seminary Hill Road, Zip 10512–1921; tel. 845/225–3400, (Nonreporting)
Primary Contact: Patrice Wallace–Moore, Executive Director
CFO: Lena Jiggetts, Controller
CMO: Frederick Hesse, M.D., Medical Director
CIO: Michelle Clark, Director Health Information Management
Web address: www.armsacres.com
Control: Corporation, Investor–owned, for–profit **Service:** Alcoholism and other chemical dependency

Staffed Beds: 129

★ □ **PUTNAM HOSPITAL CENTER (330273)**, 670 Stoneleigh Avenue, Zip 10512–9948; tel. 845/279–5711 **A**1 2 9 10 **F**3 11 13 15 24 25 26 28 29 31 32 33 36 38 42 43 49 51 52 53 54 55 56 57 59 61 62 66 68 72 73 74 75 76 77 79 80 81 82 84 86 88 89 90 91 92 93 94 95 96 97 100 102 104 105 107 112 114 118 119 120 121 124 135 136 137 **S** Health Quest Systems, Inc.
Primary Contact: Donna McGregor, President and Chief Executive Officer
COO: Maureen Zipparo, Senior Vice President Patient Care Services and Chief Operating Officer
CFO: Anthony Mirdita, Assistant Vice President Financial Operations and Chief Financial Officer
CMO: Arun Agarwal, M.D., Senior Vice President Medical Affairs
CHR: Clifford Gibberman, Vice President Human Resources
Web address: www.putnamhospital.org
Control: Other not–for–profit (including NFP Corporation) **Service:** General Medical and Surgical

Staffed Beds: 144 **Admissions:** 7714 **Census:** 106 **Outpatient Visits:** 180265 **Births:** 504 **Total Expense ($000):** 113958 **Payroll Expense ($000):** 48774 **Personnel:** 817

CARTHAGE—Jefferson County

□ **CARTHAGE AREA HOSPITAL (330263)**, 1001 West Street, Zip 13619–9703; tel. 315/493–1000, (Total facility includes 30 beds in nursing home–type unit) **A**1 9 10 20 **F**11 13 15 24 25 26 28 30 31 32 33 34 36 37 38 42 43 44 50 52 53 54 55 56 57 62 64 66 69 73 74 75 77 79 80 81 82 84 85 86 87 90 94 96 107 114 117 119 120 121 122 123 124 132 135 136
Primary Contact: Walter S. Becker, Chief Executive Officer
CFO: Mark Hills, CPA, Chief Financial Officer
CMO: Mirza Ashraf, M.D., Medical Director
CIO: Glenn Clark, Director Data Processing
CHR: Beckey Kamguia, Director Human Resources
Web address: www.carthagehospital.com
Control: Other not–for–profit (including NFP Corporation) **Service:** General Medical and Surgical

Staffed Beds: 78 **Admissions:** 1471 **Census:** 49 **Outpatient Visits:** 125191 **Births:** 202 **Total Expense ($000):** 28363 **Payroll Expense ($000):** 14207 **Personnel:** 308

CASTLE POINT—Dutchess County

VETERAN AFFAIRS HUDSON VALLEY HEALTH CARE SYSTEM–CASTLE POINT DIVISION See Veterans Affairs Hudson Valley Health Care System–F.D. Roosevelt Hospital, Montrose

CATSKILL—Columbia County

KAATERSKILL CARE See Columbia Memorial Hospital, Hudson

Hospital, Medicare Provider Number, Address, Telephone, Approval, Facility, and Physician Codes, Health Care System
★ American Hospital Association (AHA) membership
□ The Joint Commission accreditation
○ American Osteopathic Association (AOA) accreditation
△ Commission on Accreditation of Rehabilitation Facilities (CARF) accreditation

CHEEKTOWAGA—Erie County

★ **ST. JOSEPH HOSPITAL (330091)**, 2605 Harlem Road, Zip 14225–4097; tel. 716/891–2400 **A**1 9 10 **F**15 17 25 26 30 31 32 38 43 44 45 46 48 49 50 52 53 57 58 62 63 66 68 73 77 79 80 81 82 86 87 96 97 107 118 119 121 125 130 135 **P**5 **S** Catholic Health System
Primary Contact: James M. Millard, President and Senior Administrative Officer
COO: James M. Millard, President and Senior Administrative Officer
CMO: Jagdeep Singh, M.D., Vice President Medical Affairs
CIO: Doug Torre, Vice President Information Technology
CHR: Kimberly Juzdowski, Manager Human Resources
Web address: www.chsbuffalo.org
Control: Other not–for–profit (including NFP Corporation) **Service:** General Medical and Surgical

Staffed Beds: 127 **Admissions:** 6280 **Census:** 99 **Outpatient Visits:** 101830 **Births:** 0 **Total Expense ($000):** 74048 **Payroll Expense ($000):** 33891 **Personnel:** 637

CLIFTON SPRINGS—Ontario County

★ **CLIFTON SPRINGS HOSPITAL AND CLINIC (330265)**, 2 Coulter Road, Zip 14432–1189; tel. 315/462–1311, (Total facility includes 108 beds in nursing home–type unit) (Nonreporting) **A**1 9 10
Primary Contact: John P. Galati, President and Chief Executive Officer
COO: Arthur Dehey, Senior Vice President and Chief Financial Officer
CFO: Jim Cullen, Director Finance
CIO: David Markant, Director Information Systems
Web address: www.cliftonspringshospital.org
Control: Other not–for–profit (including NFP Corporation) **Service:** General Medical and Surgical

Staffed Beds: 204

COBLESKILL—Schoharie County

□ **COBLESKILL REGIONAL HOSPITAL (330268)**, 178 Grandview Drive, Zip 12043; tel. 518/254–3456, (Nonreporting) **A**1 9 10
Primary Contact: Eric H. Stein, FACHE, President and Chief Executive Officer
COO: Gayle Jones, Senior Vice President Operations
CFO: Leanna Jensen, Vice President Finance and Chief Financial Officer
CMO: Roy Korn, M.D., Medical Director
CIO: William Mackey, Director Information Systems
CHR: Terri Ann Montanye, Vice President Human Resources
Web address: www.cobleskillhospital.org
Control: Other not–for–profit (including NFP Corporation) **Service:** General Medical and Surgical

Staffed Beds: 40

COHOES—Albany County

EDDY COHOES REHABILITATION CENTER (333029), 421 West Columbia Street, Zip 12047; tel. 518/237–5630, (Nonreporting) **A**10
Primary Contact: Laurie Mante, Administrator and Vice President
Web address: www.nehealth.com/Medical_Care/Eddy_Cohoes_Rehabilitation_Center/
Control: Other not–for–profit (including NFP Corporation) **Service:** Rehabilitation

Staffed Beds: 37

COOPERSTOWN—Otsego County

★ **MARY IMOGENE BASSETT HOSPITAL (330136)**, One Atwell Road, Zip 13326–1394; tel. 607/547–3100 **A**1 2 3 5 8 9 10 12 19 20 **F**12 13 15 18 20 22 24 25 26 27 28 31 32 33 36 37 38 40 41 46 51 53 54 55 56 57 58 59 60 62 63 66 68 69 72 73 74 75 76 77 79 80 81 82 84 86 87 88 90 91 92 93 94 96 97 100 102 103 104 105 106 107 108 109 111 118 119 120 121 123 124 131 132 133 135 136 137 **P**6
Primary Contact: William F. Streck, M.D., President and Chief Executive Officer
COO: Bertine C. McKenna, Ph.D., Executive Vice President and Chief Operating Officer
CFO: Nicholas Nicoletta, Vice President Finance and Chief Financial Officer
CMO: Gerald D. Groff, M.D., Vice President Medical Affairs
CIO: Kenneth R. Deans, Vice President Information Services and Chief Information Officer
CHR: Robin A. Moore, Vice President Human Resources
Web address: www.bassetthealthcare.org
Control: Other not–for–profit (including NFP Corporation) **Service:** General Medical and Surgical

Staffed Beds: 154 **Admissions:** 8864 **Census:** 115 **Outpatient Visits:** 607331 **Births:** 780 **Total Expense ($000):** 300964 **Payroll Expense ($000):** 155479 **Personnel:** 2528

CORNING—Steuben County

★ **CORNING HOSPITAL (330277)**, 176 Denison Parkway East, Zip 14830–2899; tel. 607/937–7200 **A**1 9 10 **F**3 8 11 13 15 24 25 26 27 30 31 33 35 36 38 41 43 49 50 52 55 56 57 62 68 73 74 75 76 77 79 82 84 86 90 96 97 100 102 107 108 109 112 118 119 120 121 124 134 135 136 **S** Guthrie Healthcare System
Primary Contact: Shirley P. Magana, President and Chief Operating Officer
CFO: Francis M. Macafee, Vice President Finance, Corning Hospital Chief Financial Officer
CMO: William Sorber, M.D., Medical Director
CIO: Trish Colabine, Director Community Relations
CHR: Laura Manning, Administrative Director
Web address: www.corninghospital.com
Control: Other not–for–profit (including NFP Corporation) **Service:** General Medical and Surgical

Staffed Beds: 82 **Admissions:** 3895 **Census:** 37 **Outpatient Visits:** 127925 **Births:** 410 **Total Expense ($000):** 60614 **Payroll Expense ($000):** 21401 **Personnel:** 527

CORNWALL—Orange County

ST. LUKE'S CORNWALL HOSPITAL – CORNWALL CAMPUS See St. Luke's Cornwall Hospital – Newburgh Campus, Newburgh

CORTLAND—Cortland County

★ **CORTLAND REGIONAL MEDICAL CENTER (330175)**, 134 Homer Avenue, Zip 13045–0960; tel. 607/756–3500, (Total facility includes 82 beds in nursing home–type unit) **A**1 9 10 20 **F**2 3 11 13 15 24 25 26 30 31 32 33 38 43 49 50 53 54 55 57 61 62 66 68 74 75 77 79 80 81 82 84 86 88 90 92 96 97 99 100 102 103 106 107 117 118 119 120 121 122 124 133 135 136 137
Primary Contact: Brian R. Mitteer, Chief Executive Officer
CFO: David Hardy, Senior Vice President Operations and Chief Financial Officer
CMO: Richard Rohr, M.D., Vice President Medical Affairs
CIO: Thomas Hallisey, Vice President Information Management
Web address: www.cortlandregional.org
Control: Other not–for–profit (including NFP Corporation) **Service:** General Medical and Surgical

Staffed Beds: 217 **Admissions:** 5327 **Census:** 167 **Outpatient Visits:** 128134 **Births:** 554 **Total Expense ($000):** 70793 **Payroll Expense ($000):** 32519 **Personnel:** 753

CORTLANDT MANOR—Westchester County

★ **HUDSON VALLEY HOSPITAL CENTER (330267)**, 1980 Crompond Road, Zip 10567–4182; tel. 914/737–9000 **A**1 9 10 **F**3 9 11 13 15 24 25 26 27 30 31 32 33 38 43 52 55 57 65 68 70 74 75 76 77 79 80 81 82 84 86 96 97 100 102 104 107 119 121 134 135 136 137
Primary Contact: John C. Federspiel, President and Chief Executive Officer
CFO: Mark Webster, Vice President Finance
CIO: Chryl Pynn, Director Management Information Systems
Web address: www.hvhc.org
Control: Other not–for–profit (including NFP Corporation) **Service:** General Medical and Surgical

Staffed Beds: 128 **Admissions:** 6393 **Census:** 81 **Outpatient Visits:** 150906 **Total Expense ($000):** 94814 **Payroll Expense ($000):** 46089 **Personnel:** 789

CUBA—Allegany County

CUBA MEMORIAL HOSPITAL (331301), 140 West Main Street, Zip 14727–1398; tel. 585/968–2000, (Total facility includes 61 beds in nursing home–type unit) (Nonreporting) **A**9 10 18
Primary Contact: Andrew Boser, Chief Executive Officer
CFO: Jack Ormond, Chief Financial Officer
Web address: www.cubamemorialhospital.com
Control: Other not–for–profit (including NFP Corporation) **Service:** General Medical and Surgical

Staffed Beds: 81

DANSVILLE—Livingston County

★ **NICHOLAS H. NOYES MEMORIAL HOSPITAL (330238)**, 111 Clara Barton Street, Zip 14437–9527; tel. 585/335–6001, (Nonreporting) **A**1 9 10
Primary Contact: James Wissler, President and Chief Executive Officer
CFO: Jay T. Maslyn, Chief Financial Officer
CMO: Douglas Mayhle, M.D., Medical Director
CIO: Ernest Lehmann, Chief Information Officer
CHR: Denise Morley, Director Human Resources
Web address: www.noyes–health.org
Control: Other not–for–profit (including NFP Corporation) **Service:** General Medical and Surgical

Staffed Beds: 54

DELHI—Delaware County

★ **O'CONNOR HOSPITAL (331305)**, 460 Andes Road, State Route 28, Zip 13753; tel. 607/746–0300 **A**1 9 10 18 **F**15 25 31 32 33 38 55 56 57 62 73 77 79 80 81 82 86 96 107 113 119 121 122 134 136
CFO: Nicolas Nicoletta, Chief Financial Officer and Vice President
CMO: Alberto Gaitan, M.D., Medical Director
CHR: Barbara Green, Director Human Resources
Web address: www.oconnorhosp.org
Control: Other not–for–profit (including NFP Corporation) **Service:** General Medical and Surgical

Staffed Beds: 16 **Admissions:** 400 **Census:** 6 **Outpatient Visits:** 31804 **Births:** 0 **Total Expense ($000):** 13932 **Payroll Expense ($000):** 4443 **Personnel:** 124

DIX HILLS—Suffolk County

☐ **SAGAMORE CHILDREN'S PSYCHIATRIC CENTER**, 197 Half Hollow Road, Zip 11746–5861; tel. 631/370–1700, (Nonreporting) **A**1 **S** New York State Office of Mental Health
Primary Contact: Dennis Dubey, Ph.D., Executive Director
Web address: www.omh.state.ny.us/ombweb/facilities/scpc/facility.htm
Control: State–Government, nonfederal **Service:** Children's hospital psychiatric

Staffed Beds: 69

DOBBS FERRY—Westchester County

☐ **COMMUNITY HOSPITAL AT DOBBS FERRY (330036)**, 128 Ashford Avenue, Zip 10522–1896; tel. 914/693–0700, (Nonreporting) **A**1 9 10
Primary Contact: Ronald Corti, President and Chief Executive Officer
CFO: Dennis M. Keane, Vice President Finance and Chief Financial Officer
CMO: Francis C. Golier, M.D., Chief of Staff
CIO: Peter Weidner, Director Management Information Systems
CHR: Pam La France, Vice President Human Resources
Web address: www.riversidehealth.org
Control: Other not–for–profit (including NFP Corporation) **Service:** General Medical and Surgical

Staffed Beds: 50

DUNKIRK—Chautauqua County

★ **BROOKS MEMORIAL HOSPITAL (330229)**, 529 Central Avenue, Zip 14048–2599; tel. 716/366–1111 **A**1 9 10 **F**1 3 4 11 13 15 16 17 24 25 30 32 33 38 46 54 55 56 57 59 62 63 65 66 67 68 70 71 72 73 74 76 77 78 79 80 81 82 83 84 85 86 88 96 97 100 102 106 107 109 111 117 118 119 120 121 124 134 135 136 **P**5
Primary Contact: Richard H. Ketcham, President
CFO: Ralph Webdale, Vice President Finance
CIO: Kathy Kucharski, Director Management Information Systems
CHR: Joan VanDette, Vice President Human Resources
Web address: www.brookshospital.org
Control: Other not–for–profit (including NFP Corporation) **Service:** General Medical and Surgical

Staffed Beds: 65 **Admissions:** 2631 **Census:** 32 **Outpatient Visits:** 109238 **Births:** 512 **Total Expense ($000):** 33191 **Payroll Expense ($000):** 15189 **Personnel:** 381

EAST MEADOW—Nassau County

★ **NASSAU UNIVERSITY MEDICAL CENTER (330027)**, 2201 Hempstead Turnpike, Zip 11554–1854; tel. 516/572–0123, (Nonreporting) **A**1 2 3 5 9 10 12 13
Primary Contact: Arthur Gianelli, President and Chief Executive Officer
COO: Paul J. Rowland, Senior Vice President and Chief Operating Officer
CFO: Gary Bie, Senior Vice President Finance, Administration and Chief Financial Officer
CMO: Steven Walerstein, M.D., Medical Director
CIO: Christine Forman, Vice President and Chief Information Officer
CHR: George Boerum, Vice President Human Resources
Web address: www.numc.edu
Control: Hospital district or authority, Government, nonfederal **Service:** General Medical and Surgical

Staffed Beds: 481

ELIZABETHTOWN—Essex County

★ **ELIZABETHTOWN COMMUNITY HOSPITAL (331302)**, Park Street, Zip 12932–0277, Mailing Address: P.O. Box 277, Zip 12932–0277; tel. 518/873–6377, (Nonreporting) **A**1 9 10 18
Primary Contact: Rodney C. Boula, Administrator and Chief Executive Officer
CFO: John Anderson, Chief Financial Officer
CMO: Rob DeMuro, M.D., Medical Staff President
CHR: Michelle Meachem, Director Human Resources
Web address: www.ech.org
Control: Other not–for–profit (including NFP Corporation) **Service:** General Medical and Surgical

Staffed Beds: 15

ELLENVILLE—Ulster County

ELLENVILLE REGIONAL HOSPITAL (331310), Route 209, Zip 12428–0668, Mailing Address: P.O. Box 668, Zip 12428–0668; tel. 845/647–6400, (Nonreporting) **A**9 10 18
Primary Contact: Steven L. Kelley, President and Chief Executive Officer
CFO: Patricia Gavis, Chief Financial Officer
CMO: Helen Robinson, Chief Clinical Officer
CIO: Robert Rue, Controller
CHR: Debbie Briggs, Director Human Resources
Web address: www.ellenvilleregional.org
Control: Other not–for–profit (including NFP Corporation) **Service:** General Medical and Surgical

Staffed Beds: 25

ELMHURST—Queens County, See New York City

ELMIRA—Chemung County

★ **ARNOT OGDEN MEDICAL CENTER (330090)**, 600 Roe Avenue, Zip 14905–1629; tel. 607/737–4100, (Total facility includes 40 beds in nursing home–type unit) **A**1 2 6 9 10 19 **F**1 3 4 8 11 12 13 14 15 16 17 18 20 22 24 25 26 27 28 30 31 32 33 34 38 40 41 43 46 49 50 52 53 54 55 56 57 59 60 62 63 65 66 68 69 70 71 72 73 74 75 76 77 78 79 80 81 82 83 84 85 86 87 88 90 96 97 98 99 100 102 103 104 105 106 107 108 109 111 112 114 117 118 119 120 121 123 124 132 133 134 135 136 137 **P**6
Primary Contact: Anthony J. Cooper, FACHE, President and Chief Executive Officer
COO: H. Fred Farley, FACHE, Ph.D., Chief Operating Officer
CFO: Ronald J. Kintz, Vice President and Treasurer
CMO: William Huffner, M.D., Vice President Medical Affairs
CIO: Gregg Martin, Manager Management Information Systems
CHR: Brian Forrest, Director Human Resources
Web address: www.aomc.org
Control: Other not–for–profit (including NFP Corporation) **Service:** General Medical and Surgical

Staffed Beds: 256 **Admissions:** 10219 **Census:** 186 **Outpatient Visits:** 325000 **Births:** 1523 **Total Expense ($000):** 180131 **Payroll Expense ($000):** 82707 **Personnel:** 1582

☐ **ELMIRA PSYCHIATRIC CENTER (334045)**, 100 Washington Street, Zip 14901–2898; tel. 607/737–4739, (Nonreporting) **A**1 10 **S** New York State Office of Mental Health
Primary Contact: William Benedict, Executive Director
CFO: Timothy J. Lamitie, Assistant Business Officer
CIO: Smith B. Paulison, Director Operations
Web address: www.omh.state.ny.us/omhweb/facilities/elpc/facility.htm
Control: State–Government, nonfederal **Service:** Psychiatric

Staffed Beds: 93

★ **ST. JOSEPH'S HOSPITAL (330108)**, 555 East Market Street, Zip 14902–1512; tel. 607/733–6541, (Includes TWIN TIERS REHABILITATION CENTER), (Total facility includes 71 beds in nursing home–type unit) (Nonreporting) **A**1 9 10
Primary Contact: Sister Marie Castagnaro, President and Chief Executive Officer
COO: Albert A. Barto, Chief Operating Officer
CFO: Robert McNamara, Vice President Finance
CMO: Kimberly Panosian, M.D., Vice President Medical Services
CIO: Len Kaner, Director Information Services
CHR: Roger Rockwell, Director Human Resources
Web address: www.stjosephs.org
Control: Church–operated, Nongovernment, not–for profit **Service:** General Medical and Surgical

Staffed Beds: 240

ENDICOTT—Broome County

MEDICENTER See United Health Services Hospitals–Binghamton, Binghamton

NY

Hospital, Medicare Provider Number, Address, Telephone, Approval, Facility, and Physician Codes, Health Care System
★ American Hospital Association (AHA) membership
☐ The Joint Commission accreditation
○ American Osteopathic Association (AOA) accreditation
△ Commission on Accreditation of Rehabilitation Facilities (CARF) accreditation

FAR ROCKAWAY—Queens County, See New York City

FLUSHING—Queens County, See New York City

FOREST HILLS—Queens County

★ **FOREST HILLS HOSPITAL (330353)**, Mailing Address: 102–01 66th Road, Zip 11375–2029; tel. 718/830–4000 **A**1 9 10 **F**3 11 12 13 15 25 26 27 30 31 32 33 36 37 38 40 41 43 44 46 50 51 53 55 56 57 58 59 62 63 64 66 68 71 72 74 76 77 79 80 81 82 87 90 96 100 102 107 113 119 121 124 132 135 136 **P**6 **S** North Shore–LIJ Health System
Primary Contact: Robert T. Hettenbach, Executive Director
COO: Mark J. Solazzo, Senior Vice President and Chief Operating Officer
CFO: Robert S. Shapiro, Senior Vice President and Chief Financial Officer
CMO: Lawrence Smith, M.D., Senior Vice President and Chief Medical Officer
CIO: John Bosco, Vice President Chief Information Officer
CHR: Joseph Cabral, Vice President Chief Human Resources Officer
Web address: www.northshorelij.com
Control: Other not–for–profit (including NFP Corporation) **Service:** General Medical and Surgical

Staffed Beds: 199 **Admissions:** 13483 **Census:** 192 **Outpatient Visits:** 58506 **Births:** 2085 **Total Expense ($000):** 145805 **Payroll Expense ($000):** 66110 **Personnel:** 1047

☐ **PARKWAY HOSPITAL (330041)**, 70–35 113th Street, Zip 11375–4699; tel. 718/990–4100, (Nonreporting) **A**1 9 10
Primary Contact: Robert Aquino, M.D., President and Chief Executive Officer
COO: Jeanine Aquino, Chief Operating Officer
CFO: Jeffrey Bayer, Chief Financial Officer
CMO: Girish Desai, M.D., Chief Medical Officer
CIO: Ray Young, Director Management Information Systems
CHR: Mother Superior Joseph Fiorentino, Vice President Human Resources
Web address: www.parkwayhospital.org
Control: Corporation, Investor–owned, for–profit **Service:** General Medical and Surgical

Staffed Beds: 251

FULTON—Oswego County

★ **ALBERT LINDLEY LEE MEMORIAL HOSPITAL (330075)**, 510 South Fourth Street, Zip 13069–2994; tel. 315/591–9400, (Nonreporting) **A**1 9 10
Primary Contact: Dennis A. Casey, Executive Director
CFO: Richard T. Lang, Chief Financial Officer
CMO: Anurag Sahai, M.D., Medical Director
CHR: M. Rita Tickle, Director Human Resources
Web address: www.allee.org
Control: Other not–for–profit (including NFP Corporation) **Service:** General Medical and Surgical

Staffed Beds: 55

GENEVA—Ontario County

★ △ **GENEVA GENERAL HOSPITAL (330058)**, 196 North Street, Zip 14456–1694; tel. 315/787–4000 **A**1 6 7 9 10 **F**3 4 8 11 13 15 17 24 25 26 27 28 30 31 32 33 38 49 50 53 55 56 57 59 60 62 64 66 67 68 72 73 74 75 77 79 80 81 82 85 86 87 96 97 102 107 118 119 121 124 135 136 137 **S** Finger Lakes Health
Primary Contact: James J. Dooley, President and Chief Executive Officer
COO: Mary Ann Eldred, Executive Vice President and Chief Operating Officer
CFO: Lawrence J. Farnand, Treasurer and Chief Financial Officer
CMO: Jose Acevedo, M.D., Vice President Medical Affairs and Chief Medical Officer
CIO: Daniel Pletcher, Director Management Information System
CHR: Patrick Boyle, Vice President Human Resources
Web address: www.flhealth.org
Control: Other not–for–profit (including NFP Corporation) **Service:** General Medical and Surgical

Staffed Beds: 119 **Admissions:** 5132 **Census:** 56 **Outpatient Visits:** 460998 **Births:** 656 **Total Expense ($000):** 65262 **Payroll Expense ($000):** 35508 **Personnel:** 774

GLEN COVE—Nassau County

★ **GLEN COVE HOSPITAL (330181)**, 101 St. Andrews Lane, Zip 11542–2254; tel. 516/674–7300 **A**1 2 3 5 9 10 **F**3 5 9 11 12 14 15 17 24 25 26 27 28 29 30 31 32 33 34 36 37 38 40 41 42 43 44 46 47 48 49 50 53 54 55 56 57 58 59 60 62 63 66 67 68 72 73 75 76 77 79 80 81 82 85 86 87 88 90 91 92 93 94 96 97 100 102 106 107 111 114 119 120 121 123 124 132 134 135 136 137 **P**6 **S** North Shore–LIJ Health System
Primary Contact: Dennis Connors, Executive Director
CFO: Jon Sendach, Associate Executive Director Finance
CMO: George Dunn, M.D., Senior Vice President Medical Affairs
Web address: www.northshorelij.com
Control: Other not–for–profit (including NFP Corporation) **Service:** General Medical and Surgical

Staffed Beds: 265 **Admissions:** 9527 **Census:** 196 **Outpatient Visits:** 88607 **Births:** 0 **Total Expense ($000):** 147572 **Payroll Expense ($000):** 69466 **Personnel:** 935

GLEN OAKS—Queens County, See New York City

GLENS FALLS—Warren County

★ **GLENS FALLS HOSPITAL (330191)**, 100 Park Street, Zip 12801; tel. 518/926–1000, (Nonreporting) **A**1 2 5 9 10
Primary Contact: David G. Kruczlnicki, President and Chief Executive Officer
COO: Dianne Shugrue, Executive Vice President Operations and Chief Operating Officer
CFO: D. Michael Niles, Vice President Finance
CMO: John Bulova, Vice President Medical Affairs and Medical Director
CHR: Marcy Dreimiller, Vice President Human Resources and Support Services
Web address: www.glensfallshospital.org
Control: Other not–for–profit (including NFP Corporation) **Service:** General Medical and Surgical

Staffed Beds: 335

GLENVILLE—Schenectady County

CONIFER PARK, 79 Glenridge Road, Zip 12302–4523; tel. 518/399–6446, (Nonreporting)
Primary Contact: Patrick Carrese, Executive Director
COO: Jeanne Gluchowski, Executive Director
CFO: Jason Burczeuski, Controller
CMO: John Melbourne, M.D., Medical Director
CIO: Amy Kentera, Chief Information Officer
CHR: Jenna Bongermino, Chief Human Resource Officer
Web address: www.libertymgt.com
Control: Corporation, Investor–owned, for–profit **Service:** Alcoholism and other chemical dependency

Staffed Beds: 190

GLOVERSVILLE—Fulton County

★ **NATHAN LITTAUER HOSPITAL AND NURSING HOME (330276)**, 99 East State Street, Zip 12078–1293; tel. 518/725–8621, (Total facility includes 84 beds in nursing home–type unit) **A**1 5 9 10 **F**3 8 11 13 15 24 25 26 27 28 30 31 32 33 34 35 38 50 52 53 55 56 57 60 62 63 68 72 73 75 76 77 79 80 81 82 86 87 96 97 99 103 106 107 112 117 119 121 124 135 136 **P**6
Primary Contact: Laurence E. Kelly, President and Chief Executive Officer
CFO: Henry Legendziewicz, Senior Vice President and Chief Financial Officer
CMO: Brian Cannon, M.D., Vice President Medical Affairs
CIO: Martin Brown, Vice President Information Services and Chief Information Officer
CHR: Lana Wydra, Vice President Human Resources
Web address: www.nlh.org
Control: Other not–for–profit (including NFP Corporation) **Service:** General Medical and Surgical

Staffed Beds: 158 **Admissions:** 3791 **Census:** 127 **Outpatient Visits:** 194228 **Births:** 400 **Total Expense ($000):** 66076 **Payroll Expense ($000):** 35408 **Personnel:** 719

GOSHEN—Orange County

ORANGE REGIONAL MEDICAL CENTER–ARDEN HILL CAMPUS See Orange Regional Medical Center, Middletown

GOUVERNEUR—St. Lawrence County

☐ **EDWARD JOHN NOBLE HOSPITAL OF GOUVERNEUR (330177)**, 77 West Barney Street, Zip 13642–1090; tel. 315/287–1000, (Total facility includes 40 beds in nursing home–type unit) **A**1 9 10 20 **F**3 8 11 13 15 25 26 28 30 31 32 33 34 36 37 38 40 43 53 54 55 56 57 62 63 68 69 73 74 75 77 79 80 81 82 84 86 87 96 97 102 107 114 117 119 120 121 122 124 132 135 136 137 **P**6
Primary Contact: Charles P. Conole, FACHE, Chief Executive Officer
COO: Charles P. Conole, FACHE, Chief Executive Officer
CFO: Joseph B. Vaganek, Chief Financial Officer
CMO: Donald Schuessler, M.D., Medical Director
CIO: Linda Fishel, Manager Information Services
CHR: Cathy Chirico, Director Human Resources
Web address: www.ejnoble.com
Control: Other not–for–profit (including NFP Corporation) **Service:** General Medical and Surgical

Staffed Beds: 87 **Admissions:** 1216 **Census:** 54 **Outpatient Visits:** 61101 **Births:** 107 **Total Expense ($000):** 18231 **Payroll Expense ($000):** 8544 **Personnel:** 222

GOWANDA—Cattaraugus County

○ **TRI–COUNTY MEMORIAL HOSPITAL (330132)**, 100 Memorial Drive, Zip 14070–1194; tel. 716/532–3377, (Total facility includes 120 beds in nursing home–type unit) (Nonreporting) **A**9 10 11 **S** TLC Health Network
Primary Contact: Louis J. Frascella, President and Chief Executive Officer
CFO: John Salerno, Director Finance
Web address: www.tlchealth.org
Control: Other not–for–profit (including NFP Corporation) **Service:** General Medical and Surgical

Staffed Beds: 576

 Many Facility Codes have changed. Please refer to the AHA Guide Code Chart.

GREENPORT—Suffolk County

★ **EASTERN LONG ISLAND HOSPITAL (330088)**, 201 Manor Place, Zip 11944–1298; tel. 631/477–1000, (Nonreporting) **A**1 9 10
Primary Contact: Paul J. Connor, III, President and Chief Executive Officer
CFO: Robert A. Ragona, Vice President Finance
CIO: Dan Scotto, Director Data Processing
CHR: August F. Menchini, Director Human Resources
Web address: www.elih.org
Control: Other not–for–profit (including NFP Corporation) **Service:** General Medical and Surgical

Staffed Beds: 80

HAMILTON—Madison County

★ **COMMUNITY MEMORIAL HOSPITAL (330249)**, 150 Broad Street, Zip 13346–9518; tel. 315/824–1100, (Total facility includes 40 beds in nursing home–type unit) (Nonreporting) **A**1 9 10
Primary Contact: David Felton, President and Chief Executive Officer
CFO: Richard S. Kirby, Executive Vice President and Chief Financial Officer
CMO: Michael S. Jastremski, M.D., Vice President Medical Affairs and Director Emergency Services
Web address: www.communitymemorial.org
Control: Other not–for–profit (including NFP Corporation) **Service:** General Medical and Surgical

Staffed Beds: 84

HARRIS—Sullivan County

★ **CATSKILL REGIONAL MEDICAL CENTER (330386)**, 68 Harris Bushville Road, Zip 12742–5030, Mailing Address: P.O. Box 800, Zip 12742–0800; tel. 845/794–3300, (Total facility includes 64 beds in nursing home–type unit) (Nonreporting) **A**1 2 9 10 19 20
Primary Contact: Steven T. Ruwoldt, Chief Executive Officer
CFO: Nicholas Lanza, Vice President and Chief Financial Officer
CMO: Peter J. Panzarino, M.D., Director Medical Affairs
CIO: Ruth Ann Lange, Director Information Services
CHR: Jennifer DeFrank, Director Human Resources
Web address: www.catskillregional.org
Control: Other not–for–profit (including NFP Corporation) **Service:** General Medical and Surgical

Staffed Beds: 211

HOLLISWOOD—Queens County, See New York City

HORNELL—Steuben County

★ **ST. JAMES MERCY HOSPITAL (330151)**, 411 Canisteo Street, Zip 14843–2197; tel. 607/324–8000, (Total facility includes 120 beds in nursing home–type unit) **A**1 9 10 20 **F**3 4 13 14 15 24 25 26 30 31 32 38 40 55 56 57 67 68 69 72 73 74 75 76 77 79 80 82 84 85 86 88 89 96 97 102 107 117 118 119 121 124 133 135 **P**1 **S** Catholic Health East
Primary Contact: Mary E. LaRowe, FACHE, President and Chief Executive Officer
COO: Pamela Urban, Senior Vice President Operations and Chief Operating Officer
CFO: Jennifer Sullivan, Senior Vice President Finance and Chief Financial Officer
CMO: Sue Wesley, M.D., Senior Vice President Medical Staff Affairs
CHR: Brenda Sobeck, Vice President Human Resources
Web address: www.stjamesmercy.org
Control: Other not–for–profit (including NFP Corporation) **Service:** General Medical and Surgical

Staffed Beds: 212 **Admissions:** 4030 **Census:** 174 **Outpatient Visits:** 216714 **Births:** 325 **Total Expense ($000):** 62143 **Payroll Expense ($000):** 28098 **Personnel:** 767

HUDSON—Columbia County

☐ **COLUMBIA MEMORIAL HOSPITAL (330094)**, 71 Prospect Avenue, Zip 12534–2900; tel. 518/828–7601, (Includes KAATERSKILL CARE, 161 Jefferson Heights, Catskill, Zip 12414; tel. 518/943–6363), (Total facility includes 120 beds in nursing home–type unit) **A**1 9 10 19 **F**8 11 12 13 15 25 26 30 31 32 33 38 42 46 48 49 53 54 55 56 57 59 62 66 68 72 74 75 77 79 80 81 82 84 86 87 88 92 95 96 97 99 100 103 107 117 119 124 133 135 136 137 **P**1
Primary Contact: Jane Ehrlich, President and Chief Executive Officer
COO: Jay P. Cahalan, Chief Operating Officer
CFO: Vincent Dingman, Chief Financial Officer
CMO: Norman Chapin, M.D., Medical Director
CHR: Ray Jones, Vice President
Web address: www.columbiamemorial.com
Control: Other not–for–profit (including NFP Corporation) **Service:** General Medical and Surgical

Staffed Beds: 232 **Admissions:** 6124 **Census:** 202 **Outpatient Visits:** 242607 **Births:** 505 **Total Expense ($000):** 90415 **Payroll Expense ($000):** 45098 **Personnel:** 953

HUNTINGTON—Suffolk County

★ **HUNTINGTON HOSPITAL (330045)**, 270 Park Avenue, Zip 11743–2799; tel. 631/351–2200 **A**1 2 9 10 **F**3 11 12 13 15 17 18 20 25 26 27 30 31 32 33 34 36 38 40 42 43 44 53 55 56 57 58 59 60 62 63 66 67 68 71 72 73 74 76 77 79 80 81 84 86 87 88 90 91 92 93 94 96 97 100 102 107 111 119 120 121 124 135 136 **S** North Shore–LIJ Health System
Primary Contact: Kevin F. Lawlor, President and Chief Executive Officer
CMO: Michael Grosso, M.D., Senior Vice President Medical Affairs
CIO: Linda Fisher, Director Information Services
CHR: Michael J. Quartier, Vice President Administrative Services
Web address: www.hunthosp.org
Control: Other not–for–profit (including NFP Corporation) **Service:** General Medical and Surgical

Staffed Beds: 303 **Admissions:** 15452 **Census:** 232 **Outpatient Visits:** 127354 **Births:** 1736 **Total Expense ($000):** 214978 **Payroll Expense ($000):** 103434 **Personnel:** 1626

HUNTINGTON STATION—Suffolk County

SAGAMORE CHILDREN'S PSYCHIATRIC CENTER See Dix Hills

IRVING—Chautauqua County

○ **LAKE SHORE HEALTH CARE CENTER**, 845 Route 5 and 20, Zip 14081–9716; tel. 716/951–7000, (Total facility includes 160 beds in nursing home–type unit) (Nonreporting) **A**9 11 **S** TLC Health Network
Primary Contact: Louis J. Frascella, President and Chief Executive Officer
CFO: John Schreier, Chief Financial Officer
CMO: James Wild, M.D., Medical Director
CIO: Louis Di Rienzo, Chief Information Officer
CHR: Tracie Luther, Vice President Human Resources
Web address: www.tlchealth.org
Control: Other not–for–profit (including NFP Corporation) **Service:** General Medical and Surgical

Staffed Beds: 576

ITHACA—Tompkins County

★ **CAYUGA MEDICAL CENTER AT ITHACA (330307)**, 101 Dates Drive, Zip 14850–1383; tel. 607/274–4011 **A**1 2 3 5 9 10 **F**3 8 11 12 13 15 18 25 26 27 30 31 32 36 38 43 44 49 51 52 53 55 56 57 60 62 66 68 70 72 73 74 75 76 77 79 80 81 82 85 86 88 89 90 92 93 96 97 99 100 102 104 106 107 109 118 119 120 121 122 124 133 134 135 136 137 **P**6
Primary Contact: D. Robert Mackenzie, M.D., President and Chief Executive Officer
COO: D. Robert Mackenzie, M.D., President and Chief Executive Officer
CFO: John Rudd, Chief Financial Officer
CMO: David M. Evelyn, M.D., Vice President Medical Affairs
CIO: Anthony Votaw, Chief Information Officer
CHR: Alan Pedersen, Vice President Human Resources
Web address: www.cayugamed.org
Control: Other not–for–profit (including NFP Corporation) **Service:** General Medical and Surgical

Staffed Beds: 209 **Admissions:** 7108 **Census:** 98 **Outpatient Visits:** 207684 **Births:** 904 **Total Expense ($000):** 112449 **Payroll Expense ($000):** 41074 **Personnel:** 901

JACKSON HEIGHTS—Queens County, See New York City

JAMAICA—Queens County, See New York City

JAMESTOWN—Chautauqua County

★ **WOMAN'S CHRISTIAN ASSOCIATION HOSPITAL (330239)**, 207 Foote Avenue, Zip 14702–9975, Mailing Address: P.O. Box 840, Zip 14702–0840; tel. 716/487–0141 **A**1 2 9 10 **F**4 5 8 11 13 15 18 24 25 27 30 31 32 33 38 43 44 45 46 53 55 56 57 59 60 62 66 68 72 73 74 75 79 80 81 82 85 86 87 88 89 90 91 92 93 94 96 97 100 102 105 107 118 119 120 121 123 124 132 135 136 137
Primary Contact: Betsy T. Wright, President and Chief Executive Officer
CFO: Charles Iverson, Vice President Finance and Chief Financial Officer
CMO: Marlene Garone, M.D., Vice President Medical Affairs and Medical Director
CIO: Keith Robison, Chief Information Officer
CHR: Karen Bohall, Interim Director Human Resources
Web address: www.wcahospital.org
Control: Other not–for–profit (including NFP Corporation) **Service:** General Medical and Surgical

Staffed Beds: 230 **Admissions:** 8434 **Census:** 128 **Outpatient Visits:** 243699 **Births:** 729 **Total Expense ($000):** 97018 **Payroll Expense ($000):** 45209 **Personnel:** 1122

Hospital, Medicare Provider Number, Address, Telephone, Approval, Facility, and Physician Codes, Health Care System

★ American Hospital Association (AHA) membership
☐ The Joint Commission accreditation
○ American Osteopathic Association (AOA) accreditation
△ Commission on Accreditation of Rehabilitation Facilities (CARF) accreditation

JOHNSON CITY—Broome County

WILSON MEMORIAL REGIONAL MEDICAL CENTER See United Health Services Hospitals–Binghamton, Binghamton

KATONAH—Westchester County

☐ **FOUR WINDS HOSPITAL (334002)**, 800 Cross River Road, Zip 10536–3549; tel. 914/763–8151 **A**1 9 10 **F**25 26 31 32 33 66 73 88 89 91 95 119 121 132 135
Primary Contact: Martin A. Buccolo, Ph.D., Chief Executive Officer
CFO: Barry S. Weinstein, Chief Financial Officer
CMO: Jonathan Bauman, M.D., Chief Medical Officer
CIO: Barry S. Weinstein, Chief Financial Officer
CHR: Susan Cusano, Director Human Resources
Web address: www.fourwindshospital.com
Control: Corporation, Investor–owned, for–profit **Service:** Psychiatric

Staffed Beds: 175 **Admissions:** 3300 **Census:** 170 **Outpatient Visits:** 0 **Births:** 0

KENMORE—Erie County

★ **KENMORE MERCY HOSPITAL (330102)**, 2950 Elmwood Avenue, Zip 14217–1390; tel. 716/447–6100, (Total facility includes 160 beds in nursing home–type unit) **A**1 9 10 **F**3 14 15 17 25 26 27 30 31 32 33 38 42 43 49 52 53 55 57 58 59 62 63 66 67 68 72 73 75 76 77 79 81 82 85 86 87 96 97 103 106 107 116 117 119 120 121 124 135 137 **P**5 **S** Catholic Health System
Primary Contact: Mary Hoffman, President and Chief Executive Officer
COO: John J. Herman, Chief Operating Officer
CFO: James Dunlop, Senior Vice President and Chief Financial Officer
CMO: James Fitzpatrick, M.D., Vice President Medical Affairs
CHR: Pam Nicastro, Director Human Resources
Web address: www.chsbuffalo.org
Control: Other not–for–profit (including NFP Corporation) **Service:** General Medical and Surgical

Staffed Beds: 313 **Admissions:** 8422 **Census:** 264 **Outpatient Visits:** 148808 **Births:** 0 **Total Expense ($000):** 108622 **Payroll Expense ($000):** 47197 **Personnel:** 970

KINGSTON—Ulster County

★ **BENEDICTINE HOSPITAL (330224)**, 105 Marys Avenue, Zip 12401–5894; tel. 845/338–2500 **A**1 2 9 10 19 **F**3 7 11 13 15 18 20 25 26 27 30 31 32 33 34 35 38 42 43 44 45 46 47 50 53 54 55 56 57 58 59 64 66 68 72 73 74 76 77 79 80 82 84 85 86 88 89 92 94 95 96 99 100 101 104 107 108 109 111 118 119 120 121 124 132 135 136 137 **P**7
Primary Contact: Thomas A. Dee, President and Chief Executive Officer
CFO: David Scarpino, Senior Vice President and Chief Financial Officer
CMO: Rafael Olazagasti, M.D., Vice President Medical Affairs and Network Development
CIO: John Finch, Vice President Corporate Development
CHR: Heidi Rosborough, Manager Human Resources
Web address: www.benedictine.org
Control: Church–operated, Nongovernment, not–for profit **Service:** General Medical and Surgical

Staffed Beds: 169 **Admissions:** 6992 **Census:** 127 **Outpatient Visits:** 97149 **Births:** 359 **Total Expense ($000):** 77464 **Payroll Expense ($000):** 36114 **Personnel:** 739

★ **KINGSTON HOSPITAL (330004)**, 396 Broadway, Zip 12401–4692; tel. 845/331–3131 **A**1 9 10 **F**3 4 5 8 11 13 15 18 24 25 26 27 30 31 32 33 35 38 42 43 49 50 53 54 55 57 59 62 66 68 72 73 74 75 76 77 79 80 81 82 84 85 86 96 97 99 100 102 107 118 119 120 121 124 135 136 137
Primary Contact: Michael S. Kaminski, President and Chief Executive Officer
CFO: David Scarpino, Senior Vice President Finance and Chief Financial Officer
CMO: Alfred Frontera, M.D., Vice President Medical Services
CIO: John Finch, Vice President Information Services
CHR: Greg Howard, Vice President Human Resources, Corporate Compliance and Communications
Web address: www.kingstonregionalhealth.org
Control: Other not–for–profit (including NFP Corporation) **Service:** General Medical and Surgical

Staffed Beds: 160 **Admissions:** 6374 **Census:** 93 **Outpatient Visits:** 142134 **Births:** 469 **Total Expense ($000):** 79704 **Payroll Expense ($000):** 35333 **Personnel:** 687

LEWISTON—Niagara County

★ **MOUNT ST. MARY'S HOSPITAL AND HEALTH CENTER (330188)**, 5300 Military Road, Zip 14092–1997; tel. 716/297–4800, (Total facility includes 250 beds in nursing home–type unit) **A**1 9 10 **F**3 4 11 13 15 17 24 25 26 27 31 33 38 49 55 56 57 60 62 66 68 72 73 74 75 76 77 79 80 82 86 87 95 96 97 99 100 102 106 107 114 117 118 119 120 121 124 132 135 136 137 **P**5 **S** Ascension Health
Primary Contact: Judith A. Maness, FACHE, President and Chief Executive Officer
COO: Gary Tucker, Senior Vice President Operations
CFO: Michael F. Ickowski, Vice President Finance and Chief Financial Officer
CMO: Domonic F. Falsetti, M.D., Chief of Staff and Medical Director
CIO: Richard J. Witkowski, Director Management Information Systems
CHR: Deborah Serafin, Vice President Human Resources
Web address: www.msmh.org
Control: Church–operated, Nongovernment, not–for profit **Service:** General Medical and Surgical

Staffed Beds: 373 **Admissions:** 7357 **Census:** 341 **Outpatient Visits:** 137899 **Births:** 383 **Total Expense ($000):** 92906 **Payroll Expense ($000):** 42156 **Personnel:** 880

LITTLE FALLS—Herkimer County

★ **LITTLE FALLS HOSPITAL (331311)**, 140 Burwell Street, Zip 13365–1725; tel. 315/823–1000, (Total facility includes 34 beds in nursing home–type unit) (Nonreporting) **A**9 10 18
Primary Contact: Jonathan I. Lawrence, President and Chief Executive Officer
CFO: James Vielkind, Chief Financial Officer
CMO: Laurance C. Lee, M.D., Medical Director
CIO: Duane Merry, Chief Information Officer
CHR: Jack Fredericks, Vice President Human Resources
Web address: www.lfhny.org
Control: Other not–for–profit (including NFP Corporation) **Service:** General Medical and Surgical

Staffed Beds: 59

LITTLE NECK—Queens County, See New York City

LOCKPORT—Niagara County

LOCKPORT MEMORIAL HOSPITAL (330163), 521 East Avenue, Zip 14094–3299; tel. 716/514–5700, (Nonreporting) **A**9 10
Primary Contact: Clare A. Haar, Chief Executive Officer
COO: David J. Di Bacco, Chief Operating Officer
CFO: Donald L. Kepner, Chief Financial Officer
CMO: Bruce J. Cusenz, M.D., Medical Director
CHR: Joseph J. DeFazio, Director Human Resources
Control: Other not–for–profit (including NFP Corporation) **Service:** General Medical and Surgical

Staffed Beds: 100

LONG BEACH—Nassau County

★ **LONG BEACH MEDICAL CENTER (330225)**, 455 East Bay Drive, Zip 11561–2300, Mailing Address: P.O. Box 300, Zip 11561–2300; tel. 516/897–1000, (Total facility includes 200 beds in nursing home–type unit) **A**1 9 10 12 13 **F**3 4 5 8 9 11 15 17 25 26 27 30 31 32 33 34 36 37 38 43 46 49 50 52 54 55 56 57 59 60 61 62 63 64 66 68 72 73 76 77 79 80 81 82 84 85 86 87 88 89 90 91 92 93 94 96 97 100 102 106 107 117 118 119 120 121 123 124 132 134 135 137
Primary Contact: Douglas L. Melzer, Chief Executive Officer
CFO: Barry Stern, Chief Financial Officer
CMO: Harish Sood, M.D., Medical Director
CIO: Peter Genova, Chief Information Officer
CHR: Michelle Levine, Director Human Resources
Web address: www.lbmc.org
Control: Other not–for–profit (including NFP Corporation) **Service:** General Medical and Surgical

Staffed Beds: 334 **Admissions:** 4592 **Census:** 97 **Outpatient Visits:** 118673 **Births:** 0 **Total Expense ($000):** 66384 **Payroll Expense ($000):** 33709 **Personnel:** 741

LONG ISLAND CITY—Queens County, See New York City

LOWVILLE—Lewis County

★ **LEWIS COUNTY GENERAL HOSPITAL (330213)**, 7785 North State Street, Zip 13367–1297; tel. 315/376–5200, (Total facility includes 160 beds in nursing home–type unit) **A**1 9 10 20 **F**2 3 6 11 13 15 25 26 31 32 33 38 43 53 54 55 56 57 68 73 74 75 77 79 80 81 82 86 96 97 99 100 107 112 119 120 121 122 132 135 136 **P**1 5 6
Primary Contact: Eric Burch, Chief Executive Officer
CMO: Catherine Williams, M.D., Medical Director
CIO: Rob Uttendorfsky, Director Information Management
CHR: Timothy Ryan, Director Human Resources
Web address: www.lcgh.net
Control: County–Government, nonfederal **Service:** General Medical and Surgical

Staffed Beds: 214 **Admissions:** 1868 **Census:** 168 **Outpatient Visits:** 86589 **Births:** 213 **Total Expense ($000):** 38333 **Payroll Expense ($000):** 15939 **Personnel:** 410

MALONE—Franklin County

★ **ALICE HYDE MEDICAL CENTER (330084)**, 133 Park Street, Zip 12953–0729, Mailing Address: P.O. Box 729, Zip 12953–0729; tel. 518/483–3000, (Total facility includes 75 beds in nursing home–type unit) **A**1 9 10 20 **F**3 11 13 15 24 25 27 30 31 32 33 37 38 42 43 44 50 51 55 56 57 59 62 66 68 73 74 76 77 79 80 81 82 86 87 96 100 102 105 106 107 112 117 118 119 120 121 124 132 135 137
Primary Contact: John W. Johnson, President and Chief Executive Officer
CFO: Sandra MacDonald, Vice President Finance
CMO: Jan Close, M.D., Chief Medical Officer
CIO: Joel Benware, Chief Information Officer
CHR: Emily Campbell, Director Human Resources
Web address: www.alicehyde.com
Control: Other not–for–profit (including NFP Corporation) **Service:** General Medical and Surgical

Staffed Beds: 129 **Admissions:** 2659 **Census:** 103 **Outpatient Visits:** 106825 **Births:** 284 **Total Expense ($000):** 54853 **Payroll Expense ($000):** 27500 **Personnel:** 644

MANHASSET—Nassau County

MANHASSET AMBULATORY CARE PAVILION See Long Island Jewish Medical Center, New York

★ **NORTH SHORE UNIVERSITY HOSPITAL (330106)**, 300 Community Drive, Zip 11030–3876; tel. 516/562–0100 **A**1 2 3 5 8 9 10 **F**2 3 5 7 8 9 11 12 13 14 15 17 18 19 20 21 22 23 25 26 27 28 30 31 32 33 34 35 36 37 38 40 41 42 43 44 45 46 47 48 49 50 51 53 54 55 56 57 58 59 60 61 62 63 64 66 67 68 69 70 71 72 73 74 75 76 77 78 79 80 81 82 83 84 86 87 88 89 90 91 92 93 94 95 96 97 98 99 100 101 102 103 104 105 106 107 108 109 111 112 113 114 116 118 119 120 121 123 124 125 127 130 131 132 134 135 136 137 **P**6 **S** North Shore–LIJ Health System
Primary Contact: Susan Somerville, RN, Executive Director
COO: Mark J. Solazzo, Senior Vice President and Chief Operating Officer
CFO: Michael DiTaranto, Deputy Executive Director and Vice President Tertiary Financial Services
CMO: Vicki LoPachin, M.D., Medical Director
CIO: Robin Slone–Marx, Vice President and Chief Information Officer
CHR: Ronald Stone, Regional Chief Human Resource Officer
Web address: www.northshorelij.com
Control: Other not–for–profit (including NFP Corporation) **Service:** General Medical and Surgical

Staffed Beds: 798 **Admissions:** 49053 **Census:** 780 **Outpatient Visits:** 638458 **Births:** 5513 **Total Expense ($000):** 1181565 **Payroll Expense ($000):** 570583 **Personnel:** 6345

MANHATTAN—New York County, See New York City

MARCY—Oneida County

☐ **CENTRAL NEW YORK PSYCHIATRIC CENTER**, Mailing Address: P.O. Box 300, Zip 13403–0300; tel. 315/736–3620, (Nonreporting) **A**1 5 **S** New York State Office of Mental Health
Primary Contact: Donald Sawyer, Ph.D., Executive Director
Web address: www.omh.state.ny.us/
Control: State–Government, nonfederal **Service:** Psychiatric

Staffed Beds: 206

MARGARETVILLE—Delaware County

☐ **MARGARETVILLE HOSPITAL (331304)**, (Formerly Margaretville Memorial Hospital), 42084 State Highway 28, Zip 12455–0200; tel. 845/586–2631, (Nonreporting) **A**1 9 10 18
Primary Contact: Edmond Morache, Chief Executive Officer
CFO: David Scarpino, Chief Financial Officer
CHR: Linda Mead, Director Human Resources
Web address: www.margaretvillehospital.org
Control: Other not–for–profit (including NFP Corporation) **Service:** General Medical and Surgical

Staffed Beds: 15

MASSENA—St. Lawrence County

★ **MASSENA MEMORIAL HOSPITAL (330223)**, One Hospital Drive, Zip 13662–1097; tel. 315/764–1711 **A**1 9 10 20 **F**3 8 11 13 15 17 18 25 27 30 31 32 33 38 43 51 54 55 57 59 62 68 74 76 78 79 80 81 82 84 86 87 96 97 98 99 100 102 104 105 106 107 114 119 121 124 135 136 **P**3
Primary Contact: Charles F. Fahd, II, Chief Executive Officer
CFO: Kelley Tiernan, Chief Financial Officer
CMO: Nimesh Desai, M.D., Medical Director
CIO: Jana Grose, Director Management Information Systems
Web address: www.massenahospital.org
Control: City–Government, nonfederal **Service:** General Medical and Surgical

Staffed Beds: 50 **Admissions:** 3559 **Census:** 37 **Outpatient Visits:** 123766 **Births:** 273 **Total Expense ($000):** 40988 **Payroll Expense ($000):** 17624 **Personnel:** 340

MEDINA—Orleans County

★ △ **MEDINA MEMORIAL HOSPITAL (330053)**, 200 Ohio Street, Zip 14103–1095; tel. 585/798–2000, (Total facility includes 30 beds in nursing home–type unit) **A**1 7 9 10 **F**3 8 11 13 15 24 25 27 31 32 33 34 38 49 53 56 57 59 61 62 65 66 68 73 74 75 77 79 80 81 82 84 85 86 87 88 90 92 93 96 97 102 104 105 107 113 117 119 121 122 124 134 135 136 **P**6
Primary Contact: James E. Sinner, President and Chief Executive Officer
COO: Mary Kargbo, Chief Operating Officer
CFO: Raj Mehta, Chief Financial Officer
CMO: Mohammed Khalaf, M.D., President Medical Staff
CHR: Mary Williams, Director Human Resources
Web address: www.medinamemorial.org
Control: Other not–for–profit (including NFP Corporation) **Service:** General Medical and Surgical

Staffed Beds: 101 **Admissions:** 2849 **Census:** 68

MIDDLETOWN—Orange County

★ △ **ORANGE REGIONAL MEDICAL CENTER (330126)**, 60 Prospect Avenue, Zip 10940–4133; tel. 845/343–2424, (Includes ORANGE REGIONAL MEDICAL CENTER–ARDEN HILL CAMPUS, 4 Harriman Drive, Goshen, Zip 10924–2499; tel. 845/294–5441) **A**1 2 7 9 10 **F**3 5 7 8 11 12 13 15 17 18 24 25 26 27 30 31 32 33 38 43 44 49 51 53 55 56 57 59 62 65 66 68 72 73 74 75 76 77 78 79 80 81 82 84 85 86 88 89 90 91 92 93 94 95 96 97 99 100 102 103 105 106 107 108 109 111 112 114 118 119 121 124 133 135 136 137
Primary Contact: Scott Batulis, Chief Executive Officer
COO: Robert G. Wolleben, Vice President Horton Campus
CFO: Mitch Amodo, Vice President and Chief Financial Officer
CMO: James Oxley, D.O., Vice President Medical Affairs
CIO: Shafiq Rab, Chief Information Officer
CHR: Deborah Carr, Vice President Human Resources
Web address: www.ormc.org
Control: Other not–for–profit (including NFP Corporation) **Service:** General Medical and Surgical

Staffed Beds: 343 **Admissions:** 19858 **Census:** 298 **Outpatient Visits:** 208354 **Births:** 1985 **Total Expense ($000):** 260230 **Payroll Expense ($000):** 122892 **Personnel:** 1998

MINEOLA—Nassau County

★ **WINTHROP–UNIVERSITY HOSPITAL (330167)**, 259 First Street, Zip 11501–3987; tel. 516/663–0333 **A**1 2 3 5 8 9 10 **F**3 5 8 11 12 13 14 15 17 18 20 22 24 25 26 27 28 30 31 32 33 36 38 40 41 42 43 44 46 47 49 50 51 54 55 56 57 58 59 60 61 62 66 67 68 69 70 71 72 73 74 75 76 77 79 80 81 82 83 84 86 90 96 97 100 102 103 104 106 107 108 109 111 112 114 118 119 120 121 123 124 125 134 135 136 137 **P**5
Primary Contact: Daniel P. Walsh, President and Chief Executive Officer
COO: John F. Collins, Chief Operating Officer and Chief Financial Officer
CFO: John F. Collins, Chief Operating Officer and Chief Financial Officer
CMO: Joseph Greensher, M.D., Medical Director
CIO: Nicholas Casabona, Director Management Information Services
CHR: George Rainer, Vice President Human Resources
Web address: www.winthrop.org
Control: Other not–for–profit (including NFP Corporation) **Service:** General Medical and Surgical

Staffed Beds: 512 **Admissions:** 30663 **Census:** 469 **Outpatient Visits:** 281802 **Births:** 4588 **Total Expense ($000):** 625016 **Payroll Expense ($000):** 242828 **Personnel:** 4342

Hospital, Medicare Provider Number, Address, Telephone, Approval, Facility, and Physician Codes, Health Care System

★ American Hospital Association (AHA) membership
☐ The Joint Commission accreditation
○ American Osteopathic Association (AOA) accreditation
△ Commission on Accreditation of Rehabilitation Facilities (CARF) accreditation

MONTOUR FALLS—Schuyler County

★ **SCHUYLER HOSPITAL (331313)**, 220 Steuben Street, Zip 14865–9709; tel. 607/535–7121, (Total facility includes 120 beds in nursing home–type unit) (Nonreporting) **A**1 9 10 18 **S** Brim Healthcare, Inc.
Primary Contact: V. Richard Stelzer, Jr., FACHE, President and Chief Executive Officer
CFO: Tracy Gates, Vice President and Chief Financial Officer
CMO: Ashraf Sabahat, M.D., Medical Director
CHR: Troy Preston, Director Human Resources
Web address: www.schuylerhospital.org
Control: Other not–for–profit (including NFP Corporation) **Service:** General Medical and Surgical

Staffed Beds: 145

MONTROSE—Westchester County

★ **VETERANS AFFAIRS HUDSON VALLEY HEALTH CARE SYSTEM–F.D. ROOSEVELT HOSPITAL**, Mailing Address: P.O. Box 100, Zip 10548–0110; tel. 914/737–4400, (Includes VETERAN AFFAIRS HUDSON VALLEY HEALTH CARE SYSTEM–CASTLE POINT DIVISION, Castle Point, Zip 12511–9999; tel. 914/831–2000; VETERANS AFFAIRS HUDSON VALLEY HEALTH CARE SYSTEM–MONTROSE DIVISION, Zip 10548) **A**1 3 5 **F**3 4 5 8 11 12 25 26 27 30 32 33 34 36 37 40 41 42 43 44 50 52 54 55 56 57 60 61 62 63 64 72 73 75 76 77 78 79 81 82 86 87 88 90 91 93 94 96 97 107 108 117 119 121 122 124 132 133 135 136 137 **P**6 **S** Department of Veterans Affairs
Primary Contact: Robert Walton, Acting Director
COO: John M. Grady, Associate Director
CFO: John Walsh, Chief Fiscal Services
CMO: Joanne J. Malina, M.D., Chief of Staff
CIO: Thomas Rooney, Chief Information Resource Management
CHR: Dale Kutzbach, Chief Human Resources Management Service
Web address: www.va.gov/sta/guide/home.asp
Control: Veterans Affairs, Government, federal **Service:** Psychiatric

Staffed Beds: 383 **Admissions:** 1744 **Census:** 325 **Outpatient Visits:** 307406 **Births:** 0 **Total Expense ($000):** 185900 **Payroll Expense ($000):** 98126 **Personnel:** 1499

MOUNT KISCO—Westchester County

★ **NORTHERN WESTCHESTER HOSPITAL (330162)**, 400 East Main Street, Zip 10549–3477; tel. 914/666–1200 **A**1 2 9 10 **F**3 8 12 13 15 17 25 26 27 28 30 31 32 33 34 38 43 44 46 47 48 49 50 53 54 55 56 57 59 60 62 63 66 68 70 71 72 73 74 76 77 79 80 81 82 84 86 87 88 89 90 91 92 93 96 97 100 102 103 106 107 108 109 111 112 114 118 119 120 121 124 135 136 137
Primary Contact: Joel Seligman, President and Chief Executive Officer
COO: Warren Geller, Senior Vice President Administration
CFO: John Partenza, Vice President and Treasurer
CMO: Marla Koroly, M.D., Chief Medical Officer and Senior Vice President Medical Affairs
CIO: Sue Prince, Director Information Systems
CHR: Kerry Flynn Barrett, Vice President Human Resources
Web address: www.nwhc.net
Control: Other not–for–profit (including NFP Corporation) **Service:** General Medical and Surgical

Staffed Beds: 163 **Admissions:** 9616 **Census:** 122 **Outpatient Visits:** 100020 **Births:** 1821 **Total Expense ($000):** 156105 **Payroll Expense ($000):** 63794 **Personnel:** 1003

MOUNT VERNON—Westchester County

☐ **MOUNT VERNON HOSPITAL (330086)**, 12 North Seventh Avenue, Zip 10550–2098; tel. 914/664–8000, (Nonreporting) **A**1 3 5 9 10 **S** Sound Shore Health System
Primary Contact: John R. Spicer, President and Chief Executive Officer
COO: George Haskins, Senior Vice President and Chief Operating Officer
CFO: Thomas M. Daly, Chief Financial Officer
CMO: Paul Tucci, M.D., Vice President Medical Affairs
CIO: Barbara Cooke, Director Health Information Systems
CHR: Dennis Ashley, Vice President Human Resources
Web address: www.sshsw.org
Control: Other not–for–profit (including NFP Corporation) **Service:** General Medical and Surgical

Staffed Beds: 132

NEW HAMPTON—Orange County

☐ **MID–HUDSON FORENSIC PSYCHIATRIC CENTER (334061)**, Route 17M, Zip 10958, Mailing Address: P.O. Box 158, Zip 10958–0158; tel. 845/374–8700, (Nonreporting) **A**1 10 **S** New York State Office of Mental Health
Primary Contact: Howard Holanchock, Executive Director
Web address: www.omh.state.ny.us
Control: State–Government, nonfederal **Service:** Psychiatric

Staffed Beds: 268

NEW HYDE PARK—Queens County, See New York City

NEW ROCHELLE—Westchester County

★ **SOUND SHORE MEDICAL CENTER OF WESTCHESTER (330184)**, 16 Guion Place, Zip 10801–5500; tel. 914/632–5000, (Total facility includes 150 beds in nursing home–type unit) (Nonreporting) **A**1 2 3 5 8 9 10 **S** Sound Shore Health System
Primary Contact: John R. Spicer, President and Chief Executive Officer
COO: Douglas O. Landy, Executive Vice President and Chief Operating Officer
CFO: Thomas M. Daly, Senior Vice President and Chief Financial Officer
CMO: Jeffrey Stier, M.D., Medical Director
CIO: Barbara Cooke, Director Health Information Systems
CHR: Dennis Ashley, Vice President Human Resources
Web address: www.sshsw.org
Control: Other not–for–profit (including NFP Corporation) **Service:** General Medical and Surgical

Staffed Beds: 356

NEW YORK (Includes all hospitals located within the five boroughs)
BRONX - Bronx County (Mailing Address - Bronx)
BROOKLYN - Kings County (Mailing Address - Brooklyn)
MANHATTAN - New York County (Mailing Address - New York)
QUEENS - Queens County (Mailing Addresses - Bellerose, Elmhurst, Far Rockaway, Flushing, Forest Hills, Glen Oaks, Holliswood, Jackson Heights, Jamaica, Little Neck, Long Island City, New Hyde Park, and Queens Village)
RICHMOND VALLEY - Richmond County (Mailing Address - Staten Island)

★ **BELLEVUE HOSPITAL CENTER (330204)**, 462 First Avenue, Zip 10016–9198; tel. 212/562–4141 **A**1 3 5 8 9 10 **F**2 3 4 5 8 13 14 15 17 18 22 25 26 27 28 30 31 32 33 36 37 38 50 55 56 57 58 59 60 62 63 64 66 68 70 71 72 74 76 79 82 83 84 85 88 89 90 92 94 95 96 97 100 118 119 123 124 132 133 135 **S** New York City Health and Hospitals Corporation
Primary Contact: Lynda D. Curtis, Senior Vice President and Executive Director
COO: Terry Miles, Chief Operating Officer
CFO: Aaron Cohen, Chief Financial Officer
CMO: Eric Manheimer, M.D., Medical Director
CIO: Mary McKenna, Chief Information Officer
CHR: Brenda Chapman, Director Human Resources
Web address: www.nyc.gov/bellevue
Control: Public Health Service, Government, federal **Service:** General Medical and Surgical

Staffed Beds: 788 **Admissions:** 25675 **Census:** 643 **Outpatient Visits:** 587722 **Births:** 1863 **Total Expense ($000):** 629059 **Payroll Expense ($000):** 261849

★ **BETH ISRAEL MEDICAL CENTER (330169)**, First Avenue and 16th Street, Zip 10003–3803; tel. 212/420–2000, (Includes BETH ISRAEL MEDICAL CENTER–KINGS HIGHWAY DIVISION, 3201 Kings Highway, Zip 11234; tel. 718/252–3000), (Total facility includes 28 beds in nursing home–type unit) **A**1 3 5 8 9 10 12 13 **F**3 4 5 7 8 9 11 12 13 14 15 17 18 20 22 24 25 26 27 28 29 30 31 32 33 34 36 37 38 40 41 42 43 44 45 46 49 50 51 53 54 55 56 57 58 59 60 62 63 64 66 68 70 71 72 73 74 75 76 77 78 79 80 81 82 83 84 85 86 87 88 89 90 91 92 93 94 96 97 99 100 102 103 104 105 106 107 109 111 113 114 116 118 119 120 121 124 134 135 136 137 **P**6 **S** Continuum Health Partners
Primary Contact: David J. Shulkin, M.D., President and Chief Executive Officer
CFO: John Collura, Executive Vice President Financial Services and Chief Financial Officer
CMO: David Bernard, M.D., Chief Medical Officer
CIO: Bonnie Sessa, Vice President and Chief Information Officer
CHR: Marvin Russell, Corporate Senior Vice President Human Resources
Web address: www.bethisraelny.org
Control: Other not–for–profit (including NFP Corporation) **Service:** General Medical and Surgical

Staffed Beds: 1077 **Admissions:** 48349 **Census:** 749 **Outpatient Visits:** 613443 **Births:** 3673 **Total Expense ($000):** 1168471 **Payroll Expense ($000):** 555694 **Personnel:** 7517

☐ **BRONX CHILDREN'S PSYCHIATRIC CENTER**, 1000 Waters Place, Bronx, Zip 10461–2799; tel. 718/239–3600, (Nonreporting) **A**1 **S** New York State Office of Mental Health
Primary Contact: Mark D. Bienstock, Executive Director
Web address: www.omh.state.ny.us
Control: State–Government, nonfederal **Service:** Children's hospital psychiatric

Staffed Beds: 75

☐ **BRONX PSYCHIATRIC CENTER (334053)**, 1500 Waters Place, Bronx, Zip 10461–2796; tel. 718/931–0600, (Nonreporting) **A**1 3 5 10 **S** New York State Office of Mental Health
Primary Contact: Pamela Turner, Interim Executive Director
CFO: Robert Erway, Director for Administration
Web address: www.omh.state.ny.us
Control: State–Government, nonfederal **Service:** Psychiatric

Staffed Beds: 450

NY

★ **BRONX–LEBANON HOSPITAL CENTER (330009)**, 1276 Fulton Avenue, Bronx, Zip 10456–3499; tel. 718/590–1800, (Includes CONCOURSE DIVISION, 1650 Grand Concourse, Zip 10457; tel. 718/590–1800; FULTON DIVISION), (Total facility includes 240 beds in nursing home–type unit) (Nonreporting) **A**1 3 5 8 9 10
Primary Contact: Miguel A. Fuentes, Jr., President and Chief Executive Officer
COO: Steven Anderman, Senior Vice President and Chief Operating Officer
CFO: Victor DeMarco, Senior Vice President and Chief Financial Officer
CMO: Milton A. Gumbs, M.D., Vice President Medical Affairs and Medical Director
CIO: Steven Anderman, Senior Vice President and Chief Operating Officer
CHR: Sheldon Ortsman, Vice President Operations and Human Resources
Web address: www.bronxcare.org
Control: Other not–for–profit (including NFP Corporation) **Service:** General Medical and Surgical

Staffed Beds: 784

☐ **BROOKDALE HOSPITAL MEDICAL CENTER (330233)**, Linden Boulevard at Brookdale Plaza, Brooklyn, Zip 11212–3198; tel. 718/240–5000, (Total facility includes 448 beds in nursing home–type unit) **A**1 3 5 9 10 12 **F**2 5 8 10 12 13 14 15 17 18 19 20 24 25 26 27 28 30 31 32 33 36 37 38 40 42 43 44 46 50 51 53 54 55 56 57 58 59 60 61 62 63 64 66 67 68 69 70 71 72 73 74 75 76 77 78 79 80 81 82 83 84 86 87 88 89 90 91 92 93 94 95 96 97 99 100 107 113 114 117 119 120 121 123 124 134 135 136 137 **P**5 7
Primary Contact: David P. Rosen, President and Chief Executive Officer
COO: Bruce J. Flanz, Executive Vice President and Chief Operating Officer
CFO: Mounir F. Doss, Executive Vice President and Chief Financial Officer
CMO: Richard Fogler, M.D., Senior Vice President and Chief Medical Officer
CIO: Douglas Thompson, Director Information Systems
CHR: Max Sclair, Vice President Human Resources
Web address: www.brookdalehospital.com
Control: Other not–for–profit (including NFP Corporation) **Service:** General Medical and Surgical

Staffed Beds: 934 **Admissions:** 21486 **Census:** 826 **Outpatient Visits:** 284537 **Births:** 1449 **Total Expense ($000):** 545470 **Payroll Expense ($000):** 245629 **Personnel:** 3974

☐ **BROOKLYN CHILDREN'S PSYCHIATRIC CENTER**, 1819 Bergen Street, Brooklyn, Zip 11233–4513; tel. 718/221–4500, (Nonreporting) **A**1 **S** New York State Office of Mental Health
Primary Contact: Diane Aman, Acting Executive Director
Control: State–Government, nonfederal **Service:** Psychiatric

Staffed Beds: 36

☐ **BROOKLYN HOSPITAL CENTER (330056)**, 121 DeKalb Avenue, Brooklyn, Zip 11201–5493; tel. 718/250–8000, (Nonreporting) **A**1 2 3 5 8 9 10 **S** New York Presbyterian Healthcare System
Primary Contact: Richard B. Becker, M.D., President and Chief Executive Officer
COO: Paul Albertson, Senior Vice President Operations and Ambulatory Care
CFO: Joseph Guarracino, Senior Vice President and Chief Financial Officer
CMO: John Carroll, M.D., Chief Medical Officer
CIO: Irene Farrelly, Vice President Information Systems
Web address: www.tbh.org
Control: Other not–for–profit (including NFP Corporation) **Service:** General Medical and Surgical

Staffed Beds: 653

★ **CALVARY HOSPITAL (332006)**, 1740 Eastchester Road, Bronx, Zip 10461–2392; tel. 718/863–6900, (Nonreporting) **A**1 9 10
Primary Contact: Frank A. Calamari, President and Chief Executive Officer
COO: Richard J. Kutilek, Chief Operating Officer
CFO: Frank J. Locaparra, Chief Financial Officer
CMO: Michael J. Brescia, M.D., Executive Medical Director
CIO: Patrick Martin, Director Information Systems
CHR: Mary Kelly, Director Human Resources
Web address: www.calvaryhospital.org
Control: Church–operated, Nongovernment, not–for profit **Service:** General Medical and Surgical

Staffed Beds: 225

★ △ **COLER–GOLDWATER SPECIALTY HOSPITAL AND NURSING FACILITY (332008)**, One Main Street, Zip 10044; tel. 212/318–8000, (Includes COLER MEMORIAL HOSPITAL, Roosevelt Island, tel. 212/848–6000; GOLDWATER MEMORIAL HOSPITAL, Franklin D. Roosevelt Island, tel. 212/318–8000), (Total facility includes 1389 beds in nursing home–type unit) (Nonreporting) **A**1 3 5 7 10 **S** New York City Health and Hospitals Corporation
Primary Contact: Claude Ritman, Executive Director
COO: Robert Hughes, Chief Operating Officer
CFO: Gloria Ranghelli, Deputy Chief Financial Officer
CMO: Yolanda Bruno, M.D., Medical Director
CHR: Howard Kritz, Director
Web address: www.coler–goldwater.org
Control: City–Government, nonfederal **Service:** Long–Term Acute Care hospital

Staffed Beds: 2013

CONCOURSE DIVISION See Bronx–Lebanon Hospital Center

★ **CONEY ISLAND HOSPITAL (330196)**, 2601 Ocean Parkway, Brooklyn, Zip 11235–7795; tel. 718/616–3000 **A**1 3 5 8 9 10 12 13 **F**4 5 8 11 12 13 14 15 17 18 24 25 26 27 28 30 31 32 33 34 36 37 38 43 44 45 49 50 51 53 54 55 56 57 58 59 60 61 62 63 64 66 68 69 72 73 74 75 76 77 79 82 84 85 86 87 88 89 90 92 93 94 96 97 100 102 103 106 107 113 114 119 120 121 123 124 **S** New York City Health and Hospitals Corporation
Primary Contact: Peter Wolf, Senior Vice President and Executive Director
CFO: Paul Pandolfini, Chief Financial Officer
CMO: Edmund Giegerich, M.D., Medical Director
CIO: Silvana DeSimone, Chief Information Officer
CHR: Irma Suarez, Associate Executive Director
Web address: www.ci.nyc.ny.us/html/hhc/html/coneyisland.html
Control: City–Government, nonfederal **Service:** General Medical and Surgical

Staffed Beds: 351 **Admissions:** 17447 **Census:** 283 **Outpatient Visits:** 328720 **Births:** 1208 **Total Expense ($000):** 328152 **Payroll Expense ($000):** 139678 **Personnel:** 2611

CORNERSTONE OF MEDICAL ARTS CENTER HOSPITAL, 57 West 57th Street, Zip 10019–2802; tel. 212/755–0200, (Nonreporting)
Primary Contact: Norman J. Sokolow, Chairman and Chief Executive Officer
COO: Thomas C. Puzo, President and Chief Operating Officer
CFO: Jeff OniFather, Chief Financial Officer
CMO: Sami Kaddouri, M.D., Medical Director
CHR: Gloria Burtch, Director Human Resources
Web address: www.cornerstoneny.com
Control: Corporation, Investor–owned, for–profit **Service:** Alcoholism and other chemical dependency

Staffed Beds: 162

☐ **CREEDMOOR PSYCHIATRIC CENTER (334004)**, Jamaica, Mailing Address: 80–45 Winchester Boulevard, Queens Village, Zip 11427–2199; tel. 718/264–3600 **A**1 10 **F**25 26 33 37 53 88 94 119 **S** New York State Office of Mental Health
Primary Contact: Kathleen Iverson, Executive Director
CFO: Viodelda Ho–Shing, Deputy Director Administration
CIO: Connie Mitchell, Ph.D., Chief Information Officer
CHR: Rhonda Cicha, Director Human Resources
Web address: www.omh.state.ny.us
Control: State–Government, nonfederal **Service:** Psychiatric

Staffed Beds: 420 **Admissions:** 292 **Census:** 414 **Personnel:** 1097

★ **ELMHURST HOSPITAL CENTER (330128)**, 79–01 Broadway, Flushing, Zip 11373–1368; tel. 718/334–4000 **A**1 2 3 5 8 9 10 **F**5 8 9 13 15 17 18 19 20 21 25 26 27 28 30 31 32 33 36 38 40 50 51 52 54 55 56 57 59 60 62 66 68 70 71 72 73 74 75 76 77 79 81 82 83 84 85 87 88 89 90 91 92 93 94 95 96 97 100 107 109 119 120 121 123 132 135 **P**6 **S** New York City Health and Hospitals Corporation
Primary Contact: Chris D. Constantino, Executive Director
COO: Wayne Zimmermann, Chief Operating Officer
CFO: Julius Wool, Chief Financial Officer
CMO: Jasmin Moshirpur, M.D., Dean and Medical Director
CIO: Alfred Marino, Chief Information Officer
CHR: Carol White, Associate Executive Director
Web address: www.elmhursthospitalcenter.org
Control: City–Government, nonfederal **Service:** General Medical and Surgical

Staffed Beds: 527 **Admissions:** 24852 **Census:** 482 **Outpatient Visits:** 719642 **Births:** 4236 **Total Expense ($000):** 472731 **Payroll Expense ($000):** 198227 **Personnel:** 3527

NY

Hospital, Medicare Provider Number, Address, Telephone, Approval, Facility, and Physician Codes, Health Care System
★ American Hospital Association (AHA) membership
☐ The Joint Commission accreditation
○ American Osteopathic Association (AOA) accreditation
△ Commission on Accreditation of Rehabilitation Facilities (CARF) accreditation

☐ **FLUSHING HOSPITAL MEDICAL CENTER (330193)**, 45th Avenue at Parsons Boulevard, Flushing, Zip 11355–2100; tel. 718/670–5000 **A**1 9 10 **F**3 4 5 7 8 11 13 15 17 25 26 27 28 30 31 32 33 34 37 38 43 44 45 50 53 54 55 57 59 60 62 63 66 68 69 70 72 73 74 75 76 77 79 80 82 84 86 87 88 90 91 92 93 94 96 97 107 119 121 124 135 136 137 **P**5 7
Primary Contact: David P. Rosen, President and Chief Executive Officer
COO: Bruce J. Flanz, Executive Vice President and Chief Operating Officer
CFO: Mounir F. Doss, Executive Vice President and Chief Financial Officer
CMO: Peter Barra, M.D., Chief Medical Officer
CIO: Tony Gatto, Chief Information Officer
CHR: Max Sclair, Vice President Human Resources
Web address: www.flushinghospital.org
Control: Other not–for–profit (including NFP Corporation) **Service:** General Medical and Surgical

Staffed Beds: 293 **Admissions:** 14905 **Census:** 232 **Outpatient Visits:** 153068 **Births:** 2163 **Total Expense ($000):** 204770 **Payroll Expense ($000):** 97082 **Personnel:** 1572

FULTON DIVISION See Bronx–Lebanon Hospital Center

GOLDWATER MEMORIAL HOSPITAL See Coler–Goldwater Specialty Hospital and Nursing Facility

☐ **GRACIE SQUARE HOSPITAL (334048)**, 420 East 76th Street, Zip 10021–3104; tel. 212/988–4400, (Nonreporting) **A**1 9 10 **S** New York Presbyterian Healthcare System
Primary Contact: Frank Bruno, Chief Executive Officer
Web address: www.nygsh.org
Control: Other not–for–profit (including NFP Corporation) **Service:** Psychiatric

Staffed Beds: 157

★ △ **HARLEM HOSPITAL CENTER (330240)**, 506 Lenox Avenue, Zip 10037–1894; tel. 212/939–1000, (Includes HARLEM GENERAL CARE UNIT AND HARLEM PSYCHIATRIC UNIT) **A**1 3 5 7 8 9 10 **F**2 3 4 5 8 11 12 13 15 16 17 18 19 20 21 25 26 27 28 31 32 33 36 37 38 40 41 43 44 46 47 50 54 55 56 57 58 59 60 62 63 64 66 68 69 70 71 72 73 74 75 76 77 79 80 81 82 84 85 86 87 88 89 90 91 92 93 94 95 96 97 100 106 107 113 114 119 121 123 124 135 136 137 **S** New York City Health and Hospitals Corporation
Primary Contact: John M. Palmer, Ph.D., Executive Director
Web address: www.nyclink.org/hhc
Control: City–Government, nonfederal **Service:** General Medical and Surgical

Staffed Beds: 286 **Admissions:** 12125 **Census:** 209 **Personnel:** 2328

☐ **HOLLISWOOD HOSPITAL (334055)**, 87–37 Palermo Street, Jamaica, Zip 11423–1209; tel. 718/776–8181 **A**1 9 10 **F**25 32 54 88 89 90 91 93 95 119 121 **S** Liberty Management Group, Inc.
Primary Contact: Jeffrey Borenstein, M.D., Chief Executive Officer and Medical Director
CMO: Jeffrey Borenstein, M.D., Chief Executive Officer and Medical Director
CHR: Dorothy Muller, Director Human Resources
Web address: www.holliswoodhospital.com
Control: Corporation, Investor–owned, for–profit **Service:** Psychiatric

Staffed Beds: 110 **Admissions:** 2438 **Census:** 105 **Outpatient Visits:** 0 **Births:** 0 **Total Expense ($000):** 23515 **Payroll Expense ($000):** 11211 **Personnel:** 197

★ **HOSPITAL FOR SPECIAL SURGERY (330270)**, 535 East 70th Street, Zip 10021–4898; tel. 212/606–1000 **A**1 3 5 8 9 10 **F**3 8 9 25 26 28 29 30 31 32 33 34 35 36 40 41 42 43 44 50 52 53 54 55 56 57 58 62 64 66 72 73 75 77 78 79 80 81 82 84 86 87 90 96 97 98 100 102 103 104 105 106 107 109 111 116 119 120 121 123 130 131 135 136 **P**8 **S** New York Presbyterian Healthcare System
Primary Contact: Louis A. Shapiro, President and Chief Executive Officer
COO: Lisa Goldstein, Executive Vice President and Chief Operating Officer
CFO: Stacey Malakoff, Executive Vice President and Chief Financial Officer
CMO: Thomas P. Sculco, M.D., Surgeon–in–Chief and Medical Director
CIO: John Cox, Vice President and Chief Information Officer
CHR: Stephen A. Reday, Vice President Human Resources
Web address: www.hss.edu
Control: Other not–for–profit (including NFP Corporation) **Service:** Orthopedic

Staffed Beds: 162 **Admissions:** 11255 **Census:** 131 **Outpatient Visits:** 251032 **Births:** 0 **Total Expense ($000):** 422115 **Payroll Expense ($000):** 177278 **Personnel:** 2662

☐ **INTERFAITH MEDICAL CENTER (330397)**, 1545 Atlantic Avenue, Brooklyn, Zip 11213; tel. 718/613–4000 **A**1 3 5 9 10 **F**4 5 8 15 25 26 27 37 38 39 68 84 88 96 97 100 102 107
Primary Contact: Edward J. Glicksman, FACHE, President and Chief Executive Officer
CFO: Gregory Dixon, Chief Financial Officer
CMO: Jochanan Weisenfreund, M.D., Senior Vice President Academic and Medical Affairs
CIO: Mark Lederman, Chief Information Officer
CHR: Venra Mathurin, Vice President Human Resources
Web address: www.interfaithmedical.com
Control: Other not–for–profit (including NFP Corporation) **Service:** General Medical and Surgical

Staffed Beds: 277 **Admissions:** 10688 **Census:** 274 **Outpatient Visits:** 232971

JACK D WEILER HOSPITAL OF ALBERT EINSTEIN COLLEGE OF MEDICINE See Montefiore Medical Center

★ **JACOBI MEDICAL CENTER (330127)**, Pelham Parkway South and Eastchester Road, Bronx, Zip 10461–1197; tel. 718/918–5000 **A**1 3 5 8 9 10 **F**3 4 5 7 8 11 12 13 15 16 17 18 25 26 27 28 30 31 32 33 34 36 37 38 40 43 44 46 47 49 51 52 53 54 55 56 57 59 60 61 62 63 64 66 68 69 70 71 72 73 74 75 76 77 79 80 81 82 83 84 85 86 87 88 89 90 91 92 93 94 96 97 99 100 102 106 107 114 119 120 121 123 124 131 132 133 135 136 137 **P**6 **S** New York City Health and Hospitals Corporation
Primary Contact: William P. Walsh, Senior Vice President and Executive Director
COO: Arthur Wagner, Chief Operating Officer
CFO: Kathy Garramone, Chief Financial Officer
CMO: Joseph Skarzynski, M.D., Medical Director
CIO: Diane Carr, Chief Information Officer
CHR: Dolores Leite, Chief Human Resource Executive
Web address: www.nyc.gov/html/hhc/jacobi/home.html
Control: City–Government, nonfederal **Service:** General Medical and Surgical

Staffed Beds: 457 **Admissions:** 20057 **Census:** 377 **Outpatient Visits:** 511905 **Births:** 2263 **Total Expense ($000):** 547099 **Payroll Expense ($000):** 219989

★ **JAMAICA HOSPITAL MEDICAL CENTER (330014)**, 8900 Van Wyck Expressway, Jamaica, Zip 11418–2832; tel. 718/206–6000, (Total facility includes 204 beds in nursing home–type unit) **A**1 3 5 9 10 12 13 **F**3 7 11 13 15 17 18 20 25 26 27 31 32 33 34 37 38 40 41 43 44 50 52 53 54 55 56 57 58 59 60 61 62 63 66 68 69 70 71 72 73 74 75 76 77 78 79 80 81 82 83 84 85 86 87 88 90 91 92 93 94 96 97 100 102 106 107 113 114 117 119 120 121 123 124 132 133 135 136 **P**5 7
Primary Contact: David P. Rosen, President and Chief Executive Officer
CFO: Mounir F. Doss, Executive Vice President and Chief Financial Officer
CMO: Anthony Di Maria, M.D., Chief Medical Officer
CIO: Richard Hlavenka, Director Management Information Systems
CHR: Max Sclair, Vice President Human Resources
Web address: www.Jamaicahospital.org
Control: Other not–for–profit (including NFP Corporation) **Service:** General Medical and Surgical

Staffed Beds: 588 **Admissions:** 21904 **Census:** 524 **Outpatient Visits:** 445212 **Births:** 2952 **Personnel:** 2784

★ **KINGS COUNTY HOSPITAL CENTER (330202)**, 451 Clarkson Avenue, Brooklyn, Zip 11203–2097; tel. 718/245–3131 **A**1 2 3 5 8 9 10 **F**3 4 5 8 11 13 15 17 18 25 26 27 28 30 31 32 33 36 37 38 40 43 44 45 50 51 52 54 55 56 57 58 59 60 61 62 63 64 66 68 69 70 71 72 73 74 75 76 77 78 79 80 81 82 83 84 85 86 87 88 89 90 91 92 93 94 95 96 97 99 100 102 104 106 107 108 109 111 114 118 119 121 122 124 133 135 136 137 **P**6 **S** New York City Health and Hospitals Corporation
Primary Contact: Jean G. Leon, RN, Senior Vice President and Executive Director
COO: George M. Proctor, Chief Operating Officer
CFO: Julian John, Chief Financial Officer
CMO: Kathie Rones, M.D., M.P.H., Medical Director
CIO: Al Porco, Chief Information Officer
CHR: Stephen Small Warner, Deputy Executive Director Network and Human Resources
Web address: www.ci.nyc.ny.us/html/hhc/html/kings.html
Control: City–Government, nonfederal **Service:** General Medical and Surgical

Staffed Beds: 616 **Admissions:** 23060 **Census:** 521 **Outpatient Visits:** 686427 **Births:** 2423 **Total Expense ($000):** 608562 **Payroll Expense ($000):** 298620 **Personnel:** 4482

☐ **KINGSBORO PSYCHIATRIC CENTER (334058)**, 681 Clarkson Avenue, Brooklyn, Zip 11203–2199; tel. 718/221–7395 **A**1 3 5 10 **F**25 33 37 75 88 94 119 **S** New York State Office of Mental Health
Primary Contact: Martin Darcy, Executive Director
CFO: Ralph Lopez, Business Officer
CMO: Mark Lerman, D.O., Clinical Director
CIO: George Gavora, Director Program Evaluation
CHR: Mahendra Jorawar, Director Human Resources
Web address: www.omh.state.ny.us/omhweb/facilities/kbpc/facility/htm
Control: State–Government, nonfederal **Service:** Psychiatric

Staffed Beds: 290 **Admissions:** 340 **Census:** 283 **Outpatient Visits:** 16050 **Births:** 0 **Total Expense ($000):** 72353 **Personnel:** 695

★ △ **KINGSBROOK JEWISH MEDICAL CENTER (330201)**, 585 Schenectady Avenue, Brooklyn, Zip 11203–1891; tel. 718/604–5000, (Total facility includes 538 beds in nursing home–type unit) (Nonreporting) **A**1 3 5 7 9 10
Primary Contact: Linda Brady, M.D., President and Chief Executive Officer
COO: Kevin Molloy, Executive Vice President Operations and Chief Operating Officer
CFO: John Schmitt, Vice President Finance and Chief Financial Officer
CMO: Sibte Burney, M.D., Senior Vice President Medical Affairs
CIO: Nympha Meindel, R.N., Vice President and Chief Information Officer
CHR: John McKeon, Vice President Human Resources
Web address: www.kingsbrook.org
Control: Other not–for–profit (including NFP Corporation) **Service:** General Medical and Surgical

Staffed Beds: 864

★ **LENOX HILL HOSPITAL (330119)**, 100 East 77th Street, Zip 10021–1883; tel. 212/434–2000, (Nonreporting) **A**1 3 5 8 9 10
Primary Contact: Gladys George, President and Chief Executive Officer
COO: Terence M. O'Brien, Executive Vice President and Chief Operating Officer
CIO: Louis Ajamy, Vice President and Chief Information Officer
Web address: www.lenoxhillhospital.org
Control: Other not–for–profit (including NFP Corporation) **Service:** General Medical and Surgical

Staffed Beds: 515

★ **LINCOLN MEDICAL AND MENTAL HEALTH CENTER (330080)**, 234 East 149th Street, Bronx, Zip 10451–9998; tel. 718/579–5700 **A**1 2 3 5 8 9 10 **F**3 5 8 11 13 15 25 26 27 28 30 31 32 33 36 37 38 40 43 50 54 55 57 59 60 62 63 64 66 68 69 70 71 72 73 74 75 76 77 79 81 82 83 84 86 87 88 89 90 91 92 93 94 95 96 97 99 100 107 119 121 123 124 133 135 136 137 **P**4 **S** New York City Health and Hospitals Corporation
Primary Contact: Jose R. Sanchez, Senior Vice President and Executive Director
COO: Lauren Johnston, Deputy Executive Director
CFO: Victor Bekker, Chief Financial Officer
CMO: Anita Soni, M.D., Medical Director
CIO: Maricar Barrameda, Chief Information Officer
CHR: Herman Smith, Senior Associate Executive Director
Control: City–Government, nonfederal **Service:** General Medical and Surgical

Staffed Beds: 332 **Admissions:** 22409 **Census:** 264 **Outpatient Visits:** 550799 **Births:** 2350 **Total Expense ($000):** 412956 **Payroll Expense ($000):** 164552

LOEB CENTER NURSING REHABILITATION See Montefiore Medical Center

★ **LONG ISLAND COLLEGE HOSPITAL (330152)**, 339 Hicks Street, Brooklyn, Zip 11201–5509; tel. 718/780–1000 **A**1 2 3 5 6 8 9 10 **F**1 3 4 7 8 11 12 13 15 16 17 18 20 22 25 26 27 28 30 31 32 33 36 37 38 40 41 42 43 44 49 50 51 54 55 56 57 58 59 60 62 63 64 65 66 68 70 71 72 73 74 75 76 77 78 79 80 81 82 83 84 85 86 87 88 89 90 92 93 94 96 97 100 102 106 107 109 111 113 114 117 119 121 123 124 135 136 137 **P**6 **S** Continuum Health Partners
Primary Contact: Rita Battles, President and Chief Executive Officer
CFO: Tomas Del Rio, Vice President Finance
CIO: Hal Wachter, Director Information Systems
Web address: www.wehealny.org
Control: Other not–for–profit (including NFP Corporation) **Service:** General Medical and Surgical

Staffed Beds: 352 **Admissions:** 20601 **Census:** 290 **Outpatient Visits:** 294973 **Births:** 2653 **Total Expense ($000):** 310932 **Payroll Expense ($000):** 154765 **Personnel:** 2415

★ **LONG ISLAND JEWISH MEDICAL CENTER (330195)**, 270–05 76th Avenue, New Hyde Park, Zip 11040–1496; tel. 718/470–7000, (Includes MANHASSET AMBULATORY CARE PAVILION, 1554 Northern Boulevard, Manhasset, Zip 11030; tel. 516/365–2070; SCHNEIDER CHILDREN'S HOSPITAL, 270–05 76th Avenue, Zip 11040; tel. 718/470–3000; ZUCKER HILLSIDE HOSPITAL, 75–59 263rd Street, Glen Oaks, Zip 11004; tel. 718/470–8000) **A**1 2 3 5 8 9 10 12 13 **F**2 3 5 6 7 8 9 11 12 13 15 17 18 19 20 21 22 23 25 26 27 28 30 31 32 33 34 35 36 37 38 40 41 42 43 44 46 47 48 49 50 51 53 54 55 56 57 58 59 60 61 62 63 64 66 68 69 70 71 72 73 74 75 76 77 79 80 81 82 83 84 86 87 88 89 90 91 92 93 94 95 96 97 98 99 100 102 103 104 105 106 107 108 109 111 112 113 114 116 118 119 120 121 123 124 125 130 131 132 133 134 135 136 137 **P**6 **S** North Shore–LIJ Health System
Primary Contact: John Steel, Executive Director
COO: John Steel, Executive Director
CFO: Michael DiTaranto, Deputy Executive Director and Vice President Tertiary Financial Services
CMO: Jeremy Boal, M.D., Medical Director
CIO: Jim Bosco, Chief Information Officer
CHR: Ronald Stone, Regional Chief Human Resource Officer
Web address: www.lij.edu
Control: Other not–for–profit (including NFP Corporation) **Service:** General Medical and Surgical

Staffed Beds: 840 **Admissions:** 42833 **Census:** 786 **Outpatient Visits:** 559627 **Births:** 5504 **Total Expense ($000):** 1028597 **Payroll Expense ($000):** 507579 **Personnel:** 6671

★ **LUTHERAN MEDICAL CENTER (330306)**, 150 55th Street, Brooklyn, Zip 11220–2570; tel. 718/630–7000 **A**1 3 5 9 10 12 13 **F**3 4 5 11 12 13 14 15 17 20 25 26 27 28 30 31 32 33 34 36 37 38 40 43 46 47 48 49 50 51 53 54 55 56 57 58 59 60 61 62 63 64 66 67 68 70 71 72 73 74 75 76 77 79 80 81 82 84 85 86 87 88 90 91 92 93 94 96 97 100 102 107 108 109 111 112 115 118 119 120 121 132 135 136 137 **P**8
Primary Contact: Wendy Z. Goldstein, President and Chief Executive Officer
COO: Claudia Caine, Executive Vice President and Chief Operating Officer
CFO: Richard Langfelder, Executive Vice President and Chief Financial Officer
CMO: Beth Raucher, M.D., Senior Vice President and Chief Medical Officer
CIO: Steve Art, Senior Vice President and Chief Information Officer
CHR: Frank Scheets, Senior Vice President
Web address: www.lmcmc.com
Control: Church–operated, Nongovernment, not–for profit **Service:** General Medical and Surgical

Staffed Beds: 476 **Admissions:** 22682 **Census:** 360 **Total Expense ($000):** 413779 **Payroll Expense ($000):** 197760

★ **MAIMONIDES MEDICAL CENTER (330194)**, 4802 Tenth Avenue, Brooklyn, Zip 11219–2916; tel. 718/283–6000 **A**1 3 5 8 9 10 12 13 **F**2 3 7 8 9 11 12 13 14 15 17 18 20 22 24 25 26 27 28 30 31 32 33 36 37 38 41 43 44 46 47 48 49 50 51 53 54 55 56 57 58 59 60 62 63 64 66 68 70 71 72 73 74 75 76 77 79 80 82 84 86 87 88 89 90 91 92 93 94 95 96 97 99 100 102 103 106 107 108 109 111 112 113 114 116 118 119 120 121 123 124 134 135 136 137 **P**5 6 8
Primary Contact: Pamela S. Brier, President and Chief Executive Officer
COO: Mark McDougle, Executive Vice President and Chief Operating Officer
CFO: Robert Naldi, Chief Financial Officer
CMO: Samuel Kopel, M.D., Medical Director
CIO: Walter Fahey, Chief Information Officer
CHR: Marc Leff, Vice President Human Resources
Web address: www.maimonidesmed.org
Control: Other not–for–profit (including NFP Corporation) **Service:** General Medical and Surgical

Staffed Beds: 610 **Admissions:** 35670 **Census:** 580 **Outpatient Visits:** 366776 **Births:** 7207 **Total Expense ($000):** 800890 **Payroll Expense ($000):** 398321 **Personnel:** 5023

★ **MANHATTAN EYE, EAR AND THROAT HOSPITAL (330247)**, 210 East 64th Street, Zip 10021–9885; tel. 212/838–9200, (Nonreporting) **A**1 3 5 9 10
Primary Contact: Philip Rosenthal, Executive Director
COO: Terence M. O'Brien, Executive Vice President and Chief Operating Officer
CFO: Michael Breslin, Chief Financial Officer
CMO: Marc Napp, M.D., Vice President Medical Affairs
CIO: Louis Ajamy, Vice President and Chief Information Officer
CHR: Glen Courounis, Vice President Human Resources
Control: Other not–for–profit (including NFP Corporation) **Service:** Eye, ear, nose, and throat

Staffed Beds: 30

☐ **MANHATTAN PSYCHIATRIC CENTER–WARD'S ISLAND (334054)**, 600 East 125th Street, Zip 10035–9998; tel. 646/672–6767, (Nonreporting) **A**1 3 5 10 **S** New York State Office of Mental Health
Primary Contact: Stephen Rabinowitz, Acting Executive Director
CFO: James Collins, Business Officer
Control: State–Government, nonfederal **Service:** Psychiatric

Staffed Beds: 745

★ **MARY IMMACULATE HOSPITAL (330357)**, 88–25 153rd Street, Jamaica, Zip 11432–3731; tel. 718/558–2000, (Includes HOLY FAMILY HOME, 1740 84th Street, Brooklyn, Zip 11214; tel. 718/232–3666; MONSIGNOR JAMES H FITZPATRICK PAVILION FOR SKILLED NURSING CARE, 152–11 89th Avenue, Zip 11432; tel. 718/558–2800), (Nonreporting) **A**8 10
Primary Contact: Rose Britt, Executive Director
CFO: Richard Sarli, Chief Financial Officer
CIO: Malcolm Murray, Vice President Information Services
Control: Church–operated, Nongovernment, not–for profit **Service:** General Medical and Surgical

Staffed Beds: 261

Hospital, Medicare Provider Number, Address, Telephone, Approval, Facility, and Physician Codes, Health Care System
★ American Hospital Association (AHA) membership
☐ The Joint Commission accreditation
○ American Osteopathic Association (AOA) accreditation
△ Commission on Accreditation of Rehabilitation Facilities (CARF) accreditation

★ **MEMORIAL SLOAN–KETTERING CANCER CENTER (330154)**, 1275 York Avenue, Zip 10021–6094; tel. 212/639–2000 **A**1 2 3 5 8 9 10 **F**3 11 14 15 25 26 27 28 30 31 32 33 34 35 37 41 43 44 46 47 49 50 53 54 55 56 57 58 59 60 62 66 68 72 73 75 76 77 79 80 81 82 84 86 89 90 94 96 97 99 100 101 102 103 104 105 106 107 108 109 111 112 114 116 119 121 124 125 131 132 133 134 135 136 **P**1
Primary Contact: Harold Varmus, M.D., President and Chief Executive Officer
COO: John R. Gunn, Executive Vice President and Chief Operating Officer
CFO: Michael Gutnick, Senior Vice President Finance
CMO: Robert E. Wittes, M.D., Physician in Chief
CIO: Patricia Skarulis, Vice President Information Systems
CHR: Dennis Dowdell, Vice President Human Resources
Web address: www.mskcc.org
Control: Other not–for–profit (including NFP Corporation) **Service:** Cancer

Staffed Beds: 432 **Admissions:** 21869 **Census:** 378 **Outpatient Visits:** 979136 **Births:** 0 **Total Expense ($000):** 1499165 **Payroll Expense ($000):** 593750 **Personnel:** 8431

★ **METROPOLITAN HOSPITAL CENTER (330199)**, 1901 First Avenue, Zip 10029–7496; tel. 212/423–6262, (Includes METROPOLITAN GENERAL CARE UNIT, METROPOLITAN DRUG DETOXIFICATION AND METROPOLITAN PSYCHIATRIC UNIT) **A**1 3 5 8 9 10 **F**4 5 7 8 11 13 15 17 25 26 27 28 30 31 32 37 38 43 50 54 55 59 60 62 63 64 66 69 70 71 72 73 74 75 76 77 79 81 82 83 84 85 86 87 88 89 90 91 92 93 94 95 96 97 99 100 107 119 121 123 124 133 135 136 **S** New York City Health and Hospitals Corporation
Primary Contact: Meryl Weinberg, Executive Director
CFO: Todd Hixson, Chief Financial Officer
CMO: Richard Stone, M.D., Medical Director
CIO: Maricar Barrameda, Chief Information Officer
Web address: www.nyc.gov/html/hhc/metropolitan.html
Control: City–Government, nonfederal **Service:** General Medical and Surgical

Staffed Beds: 333 **Admissions:** 14265 **Census:** 291 **Outpatient Visits:** 413369 **Births:** 1854 **Total Expense ($000):** 314898 **Payroll Expense ($000):** 127224

MONSIGNOR JAMES H FITZPATRICK PAVILION FOR SKILLED NURSING CARE See Mary Immaculate Hospital

★ **MONTEFIORE MEDICAL CENTER (330059)**, 111 East 210th Street, Bronx, Zip 10467–2490; tel. 718/920–4321, (Includes JACK D WEILER HOSPITAL OF ALBERT EINSTEIN COLLEGE OF MEDICINE, 1825 Eastchester Road, Zip 10461–2373; tel. 718/904–2000; LOEB CENTER NURSING REHABILITATION) **A**1 3 5 8 9 10 **F**2 3 5 12 13 14 15 17 18 19 20 21 22 23 24 25 26 27 28 30 31 32 33 37 38 41 42 43 44 45 46 47 48 49 50 51 53 54 55 56 57 58 59 60 61 62 63 64 66 68 69 70 72 73 74 75 76 77 78 79 80 81 82 83 84 85 86 87 88 89 90 91 92 93 94 96 97 99 100 102 103 106 107 108 109 111 112 113 114 116 118 119 120 121 123 124 125 126 127 133 134 135 136 137 **P**5 **S** Montefiore Health System
Primary Contact: Steven M. Safyer, M.D., President and Chief Executive Officer
COO: Robert B. Conaty, Executive Vice President Operations
CFO: Joel A. Perlman, Executive Vice President Finance
CMO: Gary Kalkut, M.D., Senior Vice President – Chief Medical Officer
CIO: Jack Wolf, Vice President Management Information Systems
CHR: Milton C. Anderson, Senior Vice President Human Resources
Web address: www.montefiore.org
Control: Other not–for–profit (including NFP Corporation) **Service:** General Medical and Surgical

Staffed Beds: 1094 **Admissions:** 65908 **Census:** 1000 **Outpatient Visits:** 1546797 **Births:** 5203 **Total Expense ($000):** 2130668 **Payroll Expense ($000):** 946384 **Personnel:** 12120

MORGAN STANLEY CHILDREN'S HOSPITAL OF NEW YORK–PRESBYTERIAN See New York–Presbyterian Hospital

★ △ **MOUNT SINAI HOSPITAL (330024)**, One Gustave L. Levy Place, Zip 10029–6574; tel. 212/241–6500 **A**1 3 5 7 8 9 10 **F**2 3 5 6 7 9 11 12 13 14 15 16 17 18 19 20 21 22 23 24 25 26 27 28 30 31 32 33 34 35 36 37 38 39 40 41 42 43 44 45 46 47 48 49 50 51 53 54 55 56 57 58 59 60 61 62 63 64 66 68 69 70 71 72 73 74 75 76 77 79 80 81 82 83 84 85 86 87 88 89 90 91 92 93 94 95 96 97 98 99 100 101 102 103 104 105 106 107 108 109 110 111 112 113 114 116 118 119 120 121 123 124 125 126 127 128 129 130 131 132 133 134 135 136 137 **P**5
Primary Contact: Burton P. Drayer, M.D., President
COO: Wayne Keathley, M.P.H., Chief Operating Officer
CFO: Donald Scanlon, Chief Financial Officer
CMO: Derborah Marin, M.D., Chief Medical Officer
CIO: Jack Nelson, Senior Vice President and Chief Information Officer
CHR: Jane Maksoud, Director Human Resources
Web address: www.mountsinai.org
Control: Other not–for–profit (including NFP Corporation) **Service:** General Medical and Surgical

Staffed Beds: 1016 **Admissions:** 51469 **Census:** 888 **Outpatient Visits:** 514490 **Births:** 5717 **Total Expense ($000):** 1165183 **Payroll Expense ($000):** 469714 **Personnel:** 6800

☐ **NEW YORK COMMUNITY HOSPITAL (330019)**, 2525 Kings Highway, Brooklyn, Zip 11229–1798, Mailing Address: 2513 Avenue O, Zip 11210; tel. 718/692–5300, (Nonreporting) **A**1 5 9 10 **S** New York Presbyterian Healthcare System
Primary Contact: Lin H. Mo, President and Chief Executive Officer
COO: Una E. Morrissey, Senior Vice President, Chief Nursing Officer and Chief Operating Officer
CFO: Rich Ortiz, Divisional Chief Financial Officer
CMO: Herbert Rader, Senior Vice President and Medical Director
CIO: Steve Meyers, Director Management Information Systems
CHR: Steve Meyers, Director Management Information Systems
Web address: www.nych.com
Control: Other not–for–profit (including NFP Corporation) **Service:** General Medical and Surgical

Staffed Beds: 125

★ **NEW YORK DOWNTOWN HOSPITAL (330064)**, 170 William Street, Zip 10038–2649; tel. 212/312–5000 **A**1 3 5 9 10 **F**7 8 13 15 17 24 25 26 27 30 31 32 33 38 45 46 49 53 54 55 56 57 58 59 60 62 63 64 66 68 71 72 73 74 75 76 77 79 80 82 85 86 87 92 96 97 102 103 107 112 113 114 119 132 133 135 136 137 **P**3 5 8
Primary Contact: Jeffrey Menkes, President and Chief Executive Officer
CFO: Frank A. Vutrano, Senior Vice President Finance and Chief Financial Officer
CMO: Warren Licht, M.D., Chief Medical Officer
CIO: Kathleen Parker, Director Information Systems
CHR: Anthony Alfano, Senior Vice President Human Resources
Web address: www.downtownhospital.org
Control: Other not–for–profit (including NFP Corporation) **Service:** General Medical and Surgical

Staffed Beds: 180 **Admissions:** 9396 **Census:** 112 **Outpatient Visits:** 146686 **Births:** 2708 **Total Expense ($000):** 155243 **Payroll Expense ($000):** 75433 **Personnel:** 1051

★ **NEW YORK EYE AND EAR INFIRMARY (330100)**, 310 East 14th Street, Zip 10003–4201; tel. 212/979–4000 **A**1 3 5 9 10 **F**11 25 26 30 31 32 33 40 41 43 50 53 55 56 57 58 62 63 64 66 72 79 80 81 86 96 102 107 118 119 121 131 135 **P**8 **S** Continuum Health Partners
Primary Contact: D. McWilliams Kessler, President and Chief Executive Officer
COO: Allan Fine, Vice President Strategy and Business Development
CFO: Charles Figliozzi, CPA, Vice President and Chief Financial Officer
CMO: J. Robert Rosenthal, M.D., Senior Vice President Medical Affairs
CIO: Don Ushak, Director Information Systems
CHR: Susan Singer, Director Human Resources
Web address: www.nyee.edu
Control: Other not–for–profit (including NFP Corporation) **Service:** Eye, ear, nose, and throat

Staffed Beds: 32 **Admissions:** 1458 **Census:** 10 **Outpatient Visits:** 183094 **Births:** 0 **Total Expense ($000):** 95428 **Payroll Expense ($000):** 43512 **Personnel:** 729

☐ **NEW YORK HOSPITAL QUEENS (330055)**, 56–45 Main Street, Flushing, Zip 11355–5000; tel. 718/670–1231, (Nonreporting) **A**1 2 3 5 9 10 **S** New York Presbyterian Healthcare System
Primary Contact: Stephen S. Mills, President and Chief Executive Officer
COO: John E. Sciortino, Senior Vice President and Chief Operating Officer
CFO: Kevin J. Ward, Vice President and Chief Financial Officer
CMO: Stephen Rimar, M.D., Senior Vice President Medical Affairs
CIO: Thomas Kemp, Chief Information Officer
CHR: Lorraine Orlando, Vice President Human Resources
Web address: www.nyhq.org
Control: Other not–for–profit (including NFP Corporation) **Service:** General Medical and Surgical

Staffed Beds: 439

★ **NEW YORK METHODIST HOSPITAL (330236)**, 506 Sixth Street, Brooklyn, Zip 11215–3645; tel. 718/780–3000 **A**1 2 3 5 8 9 10 **F**8 13 14 15 17 18 20 22 25 26 27 33 37 38 43 46 49 51 53 55 56 57 59 62 63 66 68 70 72 73 74 75 76 77 79 80 81 82 84 85 86 88 94 96 97 100 107 109 112 113 114 118 119 134 135 136 **P**6 **S** New York Presbyterian Healthcare System
Primary Contact: Mark J. Mundy, President and Chief Executive Officer
CFO: Edward A. Zaidberg, Senior Vice President Finance
CMO: Stanley Sherbell, M.D., Executive Vice President Medical Affairs
CIO: Robert Dulak, Director Management Information Systems
CHR: Dennis Buchanan, Vice President Human Resources
Web address: www.nym.org
Control: Other not–for–profit (including NFP Corporation) **Service:** General Medical and Surgical

Staffed Beds: 576 **Admissions:** 29657 **Census:** 507 **Outpatient Visits:** 268955 **Births:** 5044 **Total Expense ($000):** 537860 **Payroll Expense ($000):** 209942 **Personnel:** 3572

Many Facility Codes have changed. Please refer to the AHA Guide Code Chart.

☐ **NEW YORK STATE PSYCHIATRIC INSTITUTE (334009)**, 1051 Riverside Drive, Zip 10032–2695; tel. 212/543–5000, (Nonreporting) **A**1 3 5 10 **S** New York State Office of Mental Health
Primary Contact: Jeffrey A. Lieberman, M.D., Executive Director
CFO: Jonathan Segal, Chief Financial Officer
CIO: Joseph Grun, Chief Information Officer
Web address: www.nyspi.org
Control: State–Government, nonfederal **Service:** Psychiatric

Staffed Beds: 58

★ **NEW YORK UNIVERSITY MEDICAL CENTER (330214)**, 550 First Avenue, Zip 10016–4576; tel. 212/263–7300, (Includes RUSK INSTITUTE) **A**1 3 5 8 9 10 **F**3 5 6 7 8 9 11 12 13 14 15 17 18 19 20 21 22 23 24 25 26 27 28 30 31 32 33 34 35 36 37 38 40 41 43 44 46 47 48 49 50 52 53 54 55 56 57 58 59 60 62 63 64 66 68 70 71 72 73 74 75 76 77 78 79 80 81 82 83 84 85 86 87 88 89 90 91 92 93 94 96 97 99 100 102 103 104 105 106 107 108 109 111 112 113 114 116 118 119 120 121 123 124 125 127 128 130 131 133 134 135 136 137 **P**5 6 7
Primary Contact: Robert I. Grossman, M.D., Chief Executive Officer
COO: John Harney, Executive Vice President and Chief Operating Officer
CMO: Max M. Cohen, M.D., Chief Medical Officer
CIO: Paul Conocenti, Senior Vice President and Chief Information Officer
CHR: Ira Warm, Senior Vice President Human Resources
Web address: www.nyumedicalcenter.org
Control: Other not–for–profit (including NFP Corporation) **Service:** General Medical and Surgical

Staffed Beds: 812 **Admissions:** 37962 **Census:** 628 **Outpatient Visits:** 562405 **Births:** 4680 **Total Expense ($000):** 1055913 **Payroll Expense ($000):** 450148 **Personnel:** 7497

☐ **NEW YORK WESTCHESTER SQUARE MEDICAL CENTER (330316)**, 2475 St. Raymond Avenue, Bronx, Zip 10461–3198; tel. 718/430–7300 **A**1 5 9 10 **F**3 7 8 15 17 25 27 33 38 50 55 56 59 62 66 68 72 73 76 77 79 82 86 87 92 96 97 100 107 119 135 **S** New York Presbyterian Healthcare System
Primary Contact: Alan Kopman, President and Chief Executive Officer
CFO: Elliott Gamberg, Vice President Finance
CMO: Rudolph Nisi, M.D., Vice President Medical Affairs
CIO: Mary O'Brien, Director Information Systems and Telecommunications
CHR: Barbara DeAngelo, Manager Human Resources
Web address: www.nywsmc.org
Control: Other not–for–profit (including NFP Corporation) **Service:** General Medical and Surgical

Staffed Beds: 169 **Admissions:** 7437 **Census:** 130 **Outpatient Visits:** 41478 **Births:** 0 **Total Expense ($000):** 75110 **Payroll Expense ($000):** 33488 **Personnel:** 592

★ △ **NEW YORK–PRESBYTERIAN HOSPITAL (330101)**, 525 East 68th Street, Zip 10021–4885; tel. 212/746–5454, (Includes MORGAN STANLEY CHILDREN'S HOSPITAL OF NEW YORK–PRESBYTERIAN, 3959 Broadway, Zip 10032–3784; tel. 212/305–2500; NEW YORK–PRESBYTERIAN HOSPITAL, WESTCHESTER DIVISION, Zip 10605; NEW YORK–PRESBYTERIAN HOSPITAL/WEILL CORNELL MEDICAL CENTER; NEW YORK–PRESBYTERIAN/COLUMBIA UNIVERSITY MEDICAL CENTER, 161 Fort Washington Avenue, Zip 10032; tel. 212/305–2500; PAYNE WHITNEY PSYCHIATRIC CLINIC; THE ALLEN PAVILION, 5141 Broadway, Zip 10032; tel. 212/932–5000) **A**1 2 3 5 7 8 9 10 **F**2 3 4 5 6 7 8 9 10 11 12 13 14 15 16 17 18 19 20 21 22 23 24 25 26 27 28 30 31 32 33 34 36 37 38 39 40 41 43 44 46 47 48 49 50 51 52 53 54 55 56 57 58 59 60 62 63 66 68 70 71 72 73 74 75 76 77 78 79 80 81 82 83 84 85 86 87 88 89 90 91 92 93 94 95 96 97 99 100 101 102 103 104 105 106 107 108 109 111 112 113 114 116 118 119 120 121 122 123 124 125 126 127 128 129 130 131 132 133 134 135 136 137 **S** New York Presbyterian Healthcare System
Primary Contact: Herbert Pardes, M.D., President and Chief Executive Officer
COO: Robert Kelly, M.D., Senior Vice President, Chief Medical Officer and Chief Operating Officer
CFO: Phyllis R. Lantos, Executive Vice President, Chief Financial Officer and Treasurer
CMO: Laura Forese, M.D., M.P.H., Senior Vice President, Chief Medical Officer and Chief Operating Officer
CIO: Aurelia Boyer, Senior Vice President and Chief Information Officer
CHR: G. Thomas Ferguson, Senior Vice President and Chief Human Resources Officer
Web address: www.nyp.org
Control: Other not–for–profit (including NFP Corporation) **Service:** General Medical and Surgical

Staffed Beds: 2207 **Admissions:** 99367 **Census:** 1863 **Outpatient Visits:** 1860878 **Births:** 12345 **Total Expense ($000):** 2785024 **Payroll Expense ($000):** 1321723 **Personnel:** 17243

NEW YORK–PRESBYTERIAN HOSPITAL/WEILL CORNELL MEDICAL CENTER See New York–Presbyterian Hospital

NEW YORK–PRESBYTERIAN/COLUMBIA UNIVERSITY MEDICAL CENTER See New York–Presbyterian Hospital

★ **NORTH CENTRAL BRONX HOSPITAL (330385)**, 3424 Kossuth Avenue, Bronx, Zip 10467–2489; tel. 718/519–3500 **A**1 8 9 10 **F**3 5 7 8 11 15 25 26 27 30 31 32 33 34 36 37 38 46 53 54 55 56 57 59 60 62 63 64 66 68 70 71 73 74 75 76 77 79 81 82 84 86 87 88 89 90 91 92 93 94 95 96 97 99 100 106 107 118 119 120 121 123 124 132 135 **P**6 **S** New York City Health and Hospitals Corporation
Primary Contact: Arthur Wagner, Executive Director
COO: Arthur Wagner, Executive Director
CIO: Diane Carr, Chief Information Officer
CHR: Dolores Leite, Chief Human Resource Executive
Web address: www.ci.nyc.ny.us/html/hhc/html/northcentralbronx.html
Control: City–Government, nonfederal **Service:** General Medical and Surgical

Staffed Beds: 213 **Admissions:** 8063 **Census:** 148 **Outpatient Visits:** 262544 **Births:** 1769 **Total Expense ($000):** 177534 **Payroll Expense ($000):** 75811 **Personnel:** 1343

★ **NORTH GENERAL HOSPITAL (330390)**, 1879 Madison Avenue, Zip 10035–2745; tel. 212/423–4000, (Nonreporting) **A**1 3 5 6 9 10
Primary Contact: Samuel J. Daniel, M.D., President and Chief Executive Officer
COO: John P. Maher, Chief Operating Officer
CFO: John P. Maher, Chief Financial Officer
CMO: Abraham Warshaw, M.D., Medical Director
CIO: Michele Prisco, Director
CHR: Marchene Noel, Director Human Resources
Web address: www.northgeneral.org
Control: Other not–for–profit (including NFP Corporation) **Service:** General Medical and Surgical

Staffed Beds: 200

★ △ **NYU HOSPITAL FOR JOINT DISEASES (330389)**, 301 East 17th Street, Zip 10003–3890; tel. 212/598–6000, (Nonreporting) **A**1 3 5 7 8 9 10
Primary Contact: David A. Dibner, FACHE, Senior Vice President Operations
CFO: Gerald R. Ferlisi, Senior Director Finance
CMO: H. Michael Belmont, M.D., Medical Director
CIO: Paul Conocenti, Senior Vice President, Vice Dean and Chief Information Officer
CHR: Austin Bender, Director Human Resources
Web address: www.nyuhjd.org
Control: Other not–for–profit (including NFP Corporation) **Service:** Orthopedic

Staffed Beds: 157

☐ **OUR LADY OF MERCY MEDICAL CENTER (330072)**, 600 East 233rd Street, Bronx, Zip 10466–2697; tel. 718/920–9000 **A**1 2 3 5 8 9 10 **F**3 5 7 11 13 15 25 26 27 28 32 33 36 37 38 43 46 47 48 49 50 53 54 55 57 59 61 62 63 64 66 68 70 72 73 74 75 76 77 79 80 82 84 86 87 88 89 90 91 92 93 94 96 97 98 100 103 107 111 112 119 121 135 137 **P**5 6 8 **S** Montefiore Health System
Primary Contact: Richard Celiberti, President and Chief Executive Officer
COO: Gerard Villucci, Senior Vice President Operations
CFO: Alex Mirdita, Acting Chief Financial Officer
CMO: Maguid Megalli, Executive Vice President Medical Affairs
CIO: Donna Farago, Chief Technology Officer
CHR: Eileen Montalto, Director Human Resources
Web address: www.ourladyofmercy.com
Control: Other not–for–profit (including NFP Corporation) **Service:** General Medical and Surgical

Staffed Beds: 341 **Admissions:** 15517 **Census:** 250 **Outpatient Visits:** 124795 **Births:** 1646 **Total Expense ($000):** 225921 **Payroll Expense ($000):** 112370 **Personnel:** 1633

PAYNE WHITNEY PSYCHIATRIC CLINIC See New York–Presbyterian Hospital

☐ **PENINSULA HOSPITAL CENTER (330002)**, 51–15 Beach Channel Drive, Far Rockaway, Zip 11691–1074; tel. 718/734–2000, (Nonreporting) **A**1 9 10 12 13
Primary Contact: Robert V. Levine, President and Chief Executive Officer
CFO: Mark Skulnick, Chief Financial Officer
CMO: Peter A. Galvin, M.D., Director Medical Affairs
CIO: Peter Ribolla, Director Management Information Systems
Control: Other not–for–profit (including NFP Corporation) **Service:** General Medical and Surgical

Staffed Beds: 190

☐ **QUEENS CHILDREN'S PSYCHIATRIC CENTER**, 74–03 Commonwealth Boulevard, Jamaica, Zip 11426–1890; tel. 718/264–4506, (Nonreporting) **A**1 **S** New York State Office of Mental Health
Primary Contact: Keith Little, Acting Executive Director
CMO: David M. Rube, M.D., Clinical Director
Web address: www.omh.state.ny.us
Control: State–Government, nonfederal **Service:** Children's hospital psychiatric

Staffed Beds: 84

NY

Hospital, Medicare Provider Number, Address, Telephone, Approval, Facility, and Physician Codes, Health Care System

★ American Hospital Association (AHA) membership
☐ The Joint Commission accreditation
○ American Osteopathic Association (AOA) accreditation
△ Commission on Accreditation of Rehabilitation Facilities (CARF) accreditation

★ **QUEENS HOSPITAL CENTER (330231)**, 82–68 164th Street, Jamaica, Zip 11432–1104; tel. 718/883–3000 **A**1 2 3 5 8 9 10 **F**4 5 8 11 15 26 27 28 30 31 32 33 36 37 38 50 52 53 54 55 56 62 66 68 70 74 75 76 79 84 85 86 87 88 89 90 92 93 94 95 96 100 118 119 123 135 136 **P**6 **S** New York City Health and Hospitals Corporation
Primary Contact: Antonio D. Martin, Executive Director
CFO: Julius Wool, Chief Financial Officer
CIO: Alfred Marino, Chief Information Officer
Web address: www.ci.nyc.ny.us/html/hhc/html/facilities/queens.shtml
Control: City–Government, nonfederal **Service:** General Medical and Surgical

Staffed Beds: 261 **Admissions:** 15096 **Census:** 232 **Outpatient Visits:** 426863 **Births:** 1959 **Total Expense ($000):** 285391 **Payroll Expense ($000):** 116428 **Personnel:** 2063

★ **RICHMOND UNIVERSITY MEDICAL CENTER (330028)**, 355 Bard Avenue, Staten Island, Zip 10310–1699; tel. 718/818–1234, (Nonreporting) **A**1 2 3 5 9 10 **S** Bridge Regional Health System
Primary Contact: Richard J. Murphy, President and Chief Executive Officer
COO: Richard Salhany, Chief Operating Officer
CFO: Robert Zupa, Vice President Finance
CMO: Edward Arsura, M.D., Chief Medical Officer
CIO: Richard Perry, Chief Information Officer
CHR: Patricia Caldari, Vice President
Web address: www.svcmc.org/statenisland/
Control: Church–operated, Nongovernment, not–for profit **Service:** General Medical and Surgical

Staffed Beds: 449

□ **ROCKEFELLER UNIVERSITY HOSPITAL (330387)**, 1230 York Avenue, Zip 10021–6399; tel. 212/327–8000, (Nonreporting) **A**1 10
Primary Contact: Barbara O'Sullivan, M.D., M.P.H., Chief Executive Officer
Web address: www.rucares.org
Control: Other not–for–profit (including NFP Corporation) **Service:** Other specialty

Staffed Beds: 40

ROOSEVELT HOSPITAL See St. Luke's–Roosevelt Hospital Center

RUSK INSTITUTE See New York University Medical Center

★ **SAINT VINCENT'S HOSPITAL – MANHATTAN (330290)**, 170 West 12th Street, Zip 10011–8397; tel. 212/604–7000 **A**1 2 3 5 9 10 **F**3 4 5 7 8 11 13 14 17 18 19 20 21 22 23 24 25 26 27 28 30 31 32 33 34 35 36 37 38 40 43 44 45 46 47 48 49 50 53 54 55 56 57 58 59 60 62 63 64 66 68 69 70 71 72 73 74 75 76 77 79 80 81 82 83 84 85 86 87 88 89 90 91 93 94 95 96 97 102 103 107 113 114 118 119 120 121 123 124 132 133 134 135 136 137 **P**8
Primary Contact: Henry J. Amoroso, Chief Executive Officer
COO: Michael Greene, Chief Operating Officer
CFO: Domenic Segalla, Senior Vice President and Chief Financial Officer
CMO: George Neuman, M.D., Chief Medical Officer
CIO: John McDaniel, Chief Information Officer
CHR: Bart Metzger, Chief Human Resources Officer
Web address: www.svcmcny.org
Control: Other not–for–profit (including NFP Corporation) **Service:** General Medical and Surgical

Staffed Beds: 440 **Admissions:** 17743 **Census:** 272 **Outpatient Visits:** 408922 **Births:** 1382 **Personnel:** 3682

SCHNEIDER CHILDREN'S HOSPITAL See Long Island Jewish Medical Center

□ **SOUTH BEACH PSYCHIATRIC CENTER (334043)**, 777 Seaview Avenue, Staten Island, Zip 10305–3499; tel. 718/667–2300, (Nonreporting) **A**1 10 **S** New York State Office of Mental Health
Primary Contact: William Henri, Executive Director
COO: Eileen Klein, Ph.D., Deputy Director Operations
CFO: Jeffrey Einbond, Director Facility Administration
CIO: Thomas Uttaro, Chief Information Officer
Web address: www.omh.state.ny.us
Control: State–Government, nonfederal **Service:** Psychiatric

Staffed Beds: 316

★ **ST. BARNABAS HOSPITAL (330399)**, 183rd Street & Third Avenue, Bronx, Zip 10457–9998; tel. 718/960–9000, (Includes UNION HOSPITAL OF THE BRONX, 260 East 188th Street, Zip 10458; tel. 718/220–2020), (Total facility includes 199 beds in nursing home–type unit) **A**1 9 10 12 13 **F**2 3 4 5 7 8 11 13 15 18 25 26 27 28 30 31 32 33 34 36 37 38 40 41 43 46 47 48 49 50 51 53 54 55 56 57 58 59 60 62 63 64 66 68 69 70 72 73 74 75 76 77 79 80 81 82 84 86 87 88 89 90 92 93 94 96 97 98 100 102 106 107 108 109 110 111 112 114 119 120 121 123 124 134 135 136 137 **P**6
Primary Contact: Scott Cooper, Chief Executive Officer
COO: Len Walsh, Executive Vice President and Chief Executive Officer
CFO: Richard Rank, Chief Financial Officer
CMO: Jerry Balentine, D.O., Senior Vice President and Chief Medical Director
CIO: Noah Caldwell, Senior Vice President and Chief Information Officer
CHR: Marc Wolf, Director Human Resources
Web address: www.stbarnabashospital.org
Control: Other not–for–profit (including NFP Corporation) **Service:** General Medical and Surgical

Staffed Beds: 660 **Admissions:** 24673 **Census:** 530 **Outpatient Visits:** 306550 **Births:** 1171 **Total Expense ($000):** 306771 **Payroll Expense ($000):** 125603 **Personnel:** 2088

□ ○ **ST. JOHN'S EPISCOPAL HOSPITAL–SOUTH SHORE (330395)**, 327 Beach 19th Street, Far Rockaway, Zip 11691–4424; tel. 718/869–7000 **A**1 3 5 9 10 11 12 13 **F**3 4 8 11 15 17 26 27 30 32 33 38 42 49 50 51 54 55 56 57 59 60 62 63 66 68 71 72 73 74 75 76 77 79 80 81 82 84 86 87 88 90 92 93 94 95 96 97 100 102 107 119 121 135 137 **P**6
Primary Contact: John Gupta, Chief Executive Officer
COO: Patrick Sullivan, Chief Operating Officer
CFO: Kathleen Garcia, Controller
CMO: Raymond Pastore, M.D., Chief Medical Officer
CIO: Ronald A. Tomo, Chief Information Officer
CHR: Dorette Norris, Director Human Resources
Web address: www.ehs.org
Control: Church–operated, Nongovernment, not–for profit **Service:** General Medical and Surgical

Staffed Beds: 251 **Admissions:** 9927 **Census:** 217 **Outpatient Visits:** 127575 **Births:** 785 **Total Expense ($000):** 178337 **Payroll Expense ($000):** 78753 **Personnel:** 1145

★ **ST. LUKE'S–ROOSEVELT HOSPITAL CENTER (330046)**, 1111 Amsterdam Avenue, Zip 10025; tel. 212/523–4000, (Includes ROOSEVELT HOSPITAL, 1000 Tenth Avenue, Zip 10019; tel. 212/523–5700; ST. LUKE'S HOSPITAL CENTER) **A**1 2 3 5 8 9 10 **F**3 4 5 7 8 11 12 13 14 15 17 18 20 22 25 26 27 28 30 31 32 33 36 37 38 40 41 42 43 44 46 49 50 53 54 55 56 57 58 59 60 62 63 64 66 68 70 72 73 74 75 76 77 79 80 81 82 84 85 86 87 88 89 90 91 92 93 94 95 96 97 99 100 102 106 107 109 111 112 113 114 116 118 119 120 121 123 124 127 134 135 136 137 **P**6 **S** Continuum Health Partners
Primary Contact: Frank J. Cracolici, President and Chief Executive Officer
CFO: John Collura, Executive Vice President and Chief Financial Officer
CMO: Carl W. Braun, M.D., Interim Chief Medical Officer
CIO: Bonnie Sessa, Interim Vice President and Chief Information Officer
CHR: Marvin Russell, Senior Vice President Human Resources
Web address: www.slrhc.org
Control: Other not–for–profit (including NFP Corporation) **Service:** General Medical and Surgical

Staffed Beds: 702 **Admissions:** 44765 **Census:** 702 **Outpatient Visits:** 608459 **Births:** 5963 **Total Expense ($000):** 991435 **Payroll Expense ($000):** 469960 **Personnel:** 5746

□ **ST. VINCENT'S MIDTOWN HOSPITAL (330230)**, 415 West 51st Street, Zip 10019–6394; tel. 212/459–8000, (Nonreporting) **A**1 9 10 12
Primary Contact: Sister Jane Iannucelli, President and Chief Executive Officer
COO: Regina Zuvich, Senior Vice President Operations
CFO: John Mertens, Chief Financial Officer
CMO: Paul Marino, M.D., Medical Director
CIO: Harry Volin, Chief Information Officer
Web address: www.svcmc.org
Control: Church–operated, Nongovernment, not–for profit **Service:** General Medical and Surgical

Staffed Beds: 143

★ △ **STATEN ISLAND UNIVERSITY HOSPITAL (330160)**, 475 Seaview Avenue, Staten Island, Zip 10305–9998; tel. 718/226–9000 **A**1 2 3 5 7 8 9 10 **F**3 4 5 7 8 11 12 13 14 15 16 17 18 20 22 25 26 27 28 30 31 32 33 34 36 37 38 40 41 42 43 44 49 50 51 53 54 55 56 57 58 59 60 62 63 64 66 68 70 71 72 73 74 75 76 77 78 79 80 81 82 83 84 85 86 87 88 90 91 92 93 94 95 96 97 99 100 102 103 104 105 106 107 109 111 112 113 114 118 119 121 123 124 135 136 137 **P**6 **S** North Shore–LIJ Health System
Primary Contact: Anthony C. Ferreri, President and Chief Executive Officer
COO: Donna Proske, Executive Vice President and Chief Nursing Executive
CFO: Thomas Reca, Senior Vice President Finance and Chief Financial Officer
CMO: Mark Jarrett, M.D., Chief Medical Officer
CIO: Kathy Kania, Chief Information Officer
CHR: Margaret Dialto, Vice President Human Resources
Web address: www.siuh.edu
Control: Other not–for–profit (including NFP Corporation) **Service:** General Medical and Surgical

Staffed Beds: 672 **Admissions:** 39014 **Census:** 620 **Outpatient Visits:** 352114 **Births:** 3282 **Total Expense ($000):** 596286 **Payroll Expense ($000):** 283199 **Personnel:** 4550

★ **SUNY DOWNSTATE MEDICAL CENTER UNIVERSITY HOSPITAL OF BROOKLYN (330350)**, 445 Lenox Road, Brooklyn, Zip 11203–2098; tel. 718/270–1000 **A**1 2 3 5 8 9 10 **F**7 8 13 15 17 18 19 20 21 22 23 24 25 26 27 28 30 31 32 33 36 37 38 43 46 51 52 53 54 55 56 57 58 59 60 62 64 68 70 72 73 74 75 76 77 79 81 82 83 84 86 87 88 89 90 91 92 93 94 95 96 97 99 100 101 103 104 105 106 107 112 116 118 119 120 121 122 127 132 133 134 135 136 **P**5
Primary Contact: Debra D. Carey, Chief Executive Officer
COO: David Conley, Chief Administrative Officer
CFO: Gerry Dantis, Assistant Vice President Finance
CMO: Michael Lucchesi, M.D., Interim Chief Medical Officer
CIO: Bert Robles, Chief Information Officer
CHR: Hendrina Goeloe–Alston, Assistant Vice President Personnel
Web address: www.downstate.edu
Control: State–Government, nonfederal **Service:** General Medical and Surgical

Staffed Beds: 332 **Admissions:** 16777 **Census:** 291 **Outpatient Visits:** 306859 **Births:** 1709 **Total Expense ($000):** 441061 **Payroll Expense ($000):** 230419 **Personnel:** 3051

THE ALLEN PAVILION See New York–Presbyterian Hospital

□ **THE MOUNT SINAI HOSPITAL OF QUEENS (330258)**, 25–10 30th Avenue, Long Island City, Zip 11102–2495; tel. 718/932–1000 **A**1 10 **F**3 8 15 17 25 26 27 30 31 32 33 38 43 44 45 46 48 49 50 51 53 54 55 56 57 59 62 63 66 68 72 73 75 76 77 78 79 80 81 82 86 90 93 96 97 100 102 103 107 119 120 124 135 **P**6
Primary Contact: Caryn A. Schwab, Executive Director
COO: Judy Trilivas, Vice President and Chief Operating Officer
CFO: Salvatore Morello, Vice President Finance
CMO: David M. Nierman, M.D., Vice President and Chief Medical Officer
CIO: Jack Abuin, Director Management Information Systems
CHR: Norma Calame, Director Human Resources
Web address: www.mshq.org
Control: Other not–for–profit (including NFP Corporation) **Service:** General Medical and Surgical

Staffed Beds: 192 **Admissions:** 10269 **Census:** 162 **Outpatient Visits:** 80388 **Births:** 0 **Total Expense ($000):** 112273 **Payroll Expense ($000):** 60033 **Personnel:** 989

UNION HOSPITAL OF THE BRONX See St. Barnabas Hospital

★□ △ **VETERANS ADMINISTRATION NEW YORK HARBOR HEALTHCARE SYSTEM**, 800 Poly Place, Brooklyn, Zip 11209–7104; tel. 718/630–3500, (Includes VETERANS AFFAIRS MEDICAL CENTER, 423 East 23rd Street, New York, Zip 10010–5050; tel. 212/686–7500), (Total facility includes 229 beds in nursing home–type unit) **A**1 2 3 5 7 8 **F**2 3 4 5 7 8 9 15 17 18 20 22 24 25 26 27 32 33 36 37 38 42 43 44 45 46 48 49 52 53 54 55 56 57 58 59 60 61 62 63 66 68 72 73 75 76 77 79 80 81 82 85 86 87 88 90 91 92 93 94 95 96 97 100 102 106 107 109 117 119 120 121 124 132 135 136 137 **P**6 **S** Department of Veterans Affairs
Primary Contact: John J. Donnellan, Jr., Director
CFO: Daniel Downey, Chief Fiscal Service
CIO: Maria Schay, Chief Information Officer
Web address: www.va.gov/sta/guide/home.asp
Control: Veterans Affairs, Government, federal **Service:** General Medical and Surgical

Staffed Beds: 547 **Admissions:** 10292 **Census:** 438 **Outpatient Visits:** 687957 **Births:** 0 **Total Expense ($000):** 531380 **Payroll Expense ($000):** 251230 **Personnel:** 3617

★□ △ **VETERANS AFFAIRS MEDICAL CENTER**, 130 West Kingsbridge Road, Bronx, Zip 10468–3992; tel. 718/584–9000, (Total facility includes 112 beds in nursing home–type unit) **A**1 2 3 5 7 8 **F**3 5 6 8 11 14 15 17 18 20 24 25 26 27 29 30 31 32 33 34 35 36 37 38 41 42 43 44 45 46 49 50 51 52 53 54 55 56 57 58 59 60 61 62 63 65 66 68 72 73 75 76 77 78 79 80 81 82 85 86 87 88 90 91 92 93 94 96 97 100 102 103 106 107 111 117 119 121 124 132 135 136 137 **S** Department of Veterans Affairs
Primary Contact: Maryann Musumeci, Director
COO: Robert Walton, Associate Director
CFO: Gregory Angelo, Chief Fiscal Program
CMO: Clive Rosendorff, M.D., Chief Medical Program
CIO: Linda Bund, Chief Information Officer and Director Education
CHR: Peter Tinker, Chief Human Resources Officer
Web address: www.va.gov/sta/guide/home.asp
Control: Veterans Affairs, Government, federal **Service:** General Medical and Surgical

Staffed Beds: 330 **Admissions:** 4710 **Census:** 158 **Outpatient Visits:** 301925 **Births:** 0 **Total Expense ($000):** 227469 **Payroll Expense ($000):** 122118 **Personnel:** 2054

□ **VICTORY MEMORIAL HOSPITAL (330242)**, 9036 Seventh Avenue, Brooklyn, Zip 11228–3625; tel. 718/567–1234, (Nonreporting) **A**1 9 10
Primary Contact: Krishin L. Bhatia, Administrator
CFO: Joe Mazzella, Interim Chief Financial Officer
CMO: John Reilly, Medical Director
CIO: Cynthia Naglio, Director Public Relations
CHR: August Manzini, Director Human Resources
Web address: www.vmhny.org
Control: Other not–for–profit (including NFP Corporation) **Service:** General Medical and Surgical

Staffed Beds: 346

★□ **WOODHULL MEDICAL AND MENTAL HEALTH CENTER (330396)**, 760 Broadway Street, Brooklyn, Zip 11206–5383; tel. 718/963–8000, (Nonreporting) **A**1 8 9 10 **S** New York City Health and Hospitals Corporation
Primary Contact: Iris Jimenez–Hernandez, Senior Vice President and Executive Director
CFO: Milton Nunez, Chief Financial Officer
CMO: Edward Fishkin, M.D., Medical Director
CIO: Cynthia Bianchi, Chief Information Officer
CHR: Yvette Villanueva, Senior Associate Executive Director
Web address: www.nyc.gov/html/hhc
Control: City–Government, nonfederal **Service:** General Medical and Surgical

Staffed Beds: 406

★□ ○ **WYCKOFF HEIGHTS MEDICAL CENTER (330221)**, 374 Stockholm Street, Brooklyn, Zip 11237–4099; tel. 718/963–7272, (Nonreporting) **A**1 3 5 9 10 11 12 13
Primary Contact: Nirmal K. Mattoo, M.D., Interim President and Chief Executive Officer
COO: Harold E. McDonald, Executive Vice President and Chief Operating Officer
CFO: Wah Chung Hsu, Vice President and Chief Financial Officer
CMO: Bushan Khashu, Chief Medical Officer
CIO: Cletis Earle, Chief Information Officer
CHR: Fred Eisgrub, Vice President Human Resources
Web address: www.wyckoffhospital.org
Control: Other not–for–profit (including NFP Corporation) **Service:** General Medical and Surgical

Staffed Beds: 279

ZUCKER HILLSIDE HOSPITAL See Long Island Jewish Medical Center

NEWARK—Wayne County

□ **NEWARK–WAYNE COMMUNITY HOSPITAL (330030)**, Driving Park Avenue, Zip 14513, Mailing Address: P.O. Box 111, Zip 14513–0111; tel. 315/332–2022, (Total facility includes 180 beds in nursing home–type unit) **A**1 9 10 **F**2 3 8 11 13 15 24 25 26 30 31 32 33 36 38 40 41 50 54 55 56 57 66 68 72 73 74 75 77 79 80 81 82 86 87 88 90 92 93 96 100 107 117 119 120 121 124 135 136 137 **P**5 7 **S** ViaHealth
Primary Contact: Annette B. Leahy, President and Chief Executive Officer
COO: Brad Smith, Senior Vice President and Chief Operating Officer
CFO: Richard Hogg, Senior Vice President and Chief Financial Officer
CIO: David Kamowski, Senior Vice President and Chief Information Officer
CHR: Cheryl Henke, Senior Vice President Human Resources
Web address: www.viahealth.org
Control: Other not–for–profit (including NFP Corporation) **Service:** General Medical and Surgical

Staffed Beds: 263 **Admissions:** 3235 **Census:** 224 **Outpatient Visits:** 45431 **Births:** 395 **Total Expense ($000):** 54147 **Payroll Expense ($000):** 26180 **Personnel:** 582

NEWBURGH—Orange County

★□ **ST. LUKE'S CORNWALL HOSPITAL – NEWBURGH CAMPUS (330264)**, 70 Dubois Street, Zip 12550–4898; tel. 845/561–4400, (Includes ST LUKE'S CAMPUS; ST. LUKE'S CORNWALL HOSPITAL – CORNWALL CAMPUS, 19 Laurel Avenue, Cornwall, Zip 12518–1499; tel. 845/534–7711) **A**1 2 9 10 **F**3 8 11 13 15 17 18 24 25 27 30 32 33 34 35 38 43 46 49 50 51 53 55 56 57 59 62 66 68 71 72 73 74 75 76 77 79 80 81 82 84 86 88 90 92 96 97 106 107 116 119 121 124 132 135 137
Primary Contact: Allan E. Atzrott, President and Chief Executive Officer
COO: Robert Ross, Senior Vice President Operations
CFO: Mary Elizabeth Duffy, Senior Vice President and Chief Financial Officer
CMO: Christine Jelalian, M.D., Medical Director
CIO: Jane Lake, Director Information Technology
CHR: Deborah Turner, Vice President Human Resources
Web address: www.stlukescornwallhospital.org
Control: Other not–for–profit (including NFP Corporation) **Service:** General Medical and Surgical

Staffed Beds: 270 **Admissions:** 13079 **Census:** 174 **Outpatient Visits:** 182577 **Births:** 1116 **Total Expense ($000):** 153459 **Payroll Expense ($000):** 73498 **Personnel:** 1256

NEWFANE—Niagara County

★ **INTER–COMMUNITY MEMORIAL HOSPITAL (330025)**, 2600 William Street, Zip 14108–1093; tel. 716/778–5111, (Nonreporting) **A**9 10
Primary Contact: Clare A. Haar, Chief Executive Officer
COO: David J. Di Bacco, Chief Operating Officer
CFO: Donald L. Kepner, Chief Financial Officer
CMO: Bruce J. Cusenz, M.D., Medical Director
CHR: Joseph J. DeFazio, Director Human Resources
Control: Other not–for–profit (including NFP Corporation) **Service:** General Medical and Surgical

Staffed Beds: 71

Hospital, Medicare Provider Number, Address, Telephone, Approval, Facility, and Physician Codes, Health Care System

★ American Hospital Association (AHA) membership
□ The Joint Commission accreditation
○ American Osteopathic Association (AOA) accreditation
△ Commission on Accreditation of Rehabilitation Facilities (CARF) accreditation

NIAGARA FALLS—Niagara County

NIAGARA FALLS MEMORIAL MEDICAL CENTER (330065), 621 Tenth Street, Zip 14302–0708, Mailing Address: P.O. Box 708, Zip 14302–0708; tel. 716/278–4000, (Nonreporting) **A**3 5 9 10
Primary Contact: Joseph A. Ruffolo, President and Chief Executive Officer
CFO: Philip Johnson, Chief Financial Officer
CMO: Fatma Patel, M.D., Vice President Medical Affairs
CIO: Diane Martin–Pratt, Director Information Systems
Web address: www.nfmmc.org
Control: Other not–for–profit (including NFP Corporation) **Service:** General Medical and Surgical

Staffed Beds: 288

NORTH TONAWANDA—Niagara County

DE GRAFF MEMORIAL HOSPITAL See KALEIDA Health, Buffalo

NORTHPORT—Suffolk County

★ △ **VETERANS AFFAIRS MEDICAL CENTER**, 79 Middleville Road, Zip 11768–2293; tel. 631/261–4400, (Total facility includes 170 beds in nursing home–type unit) (Nonreporting) **A**1 2 3 5 7 8 **S** Department of Veterans Affairs
Primary Contact: Robert Schuster, Director
CFO: Mary Pat Hessman, Chief Fiscal
CMO: Edward Mack, M.D., Chief of Staff
CIO: Robert Ziskin, Chief Information Officer
Web address: www.va.gov/sta/guide/home.asp
Control: Veterans Affairs, Government, federal **Service:** General Medical and Surgical

Staffed Beds: 331

NORWICH—Chenango County

★ ○ **CHENANGO MEMORIAL HOSPITAL (330033)**, 179 North Broad Street, Zip 13815–1097; tel. 607/337–4111, (Total facility includes 80 beds in nursing home–type unit) **A**9 10 11 **F**3 8 11 13 15 17 25 28 30 31 32 33 36 37 38 43 44 50 53 54 55 56 57 60 62 63 66 68 73 74 75 77 79 80 81 82 84 86 87 96 97 102 106 107 117 119 121 122 135 136 **P**6 **S** United Health Services
Primary Contact: Drake M. Lamen, M.D., President and Chief Executive Officer
COO: Drake M. Lamen, M.D., President and Chief Executive Officer
CFO: Robert R. McCarthy, Vice President Finance and Chief Financial Officer
CMO: Michael F. Trevisani, M.D., Vice President Medical Affairs and Chief Medical Officer
CIO: Tracy McCumber, Manager Information Systems
CHR: Anne L. English, Director Human Resources
Web address: www.chenangomemorial.com
Control: Other not–for–profit (including NFP Corporation) **Service:** General Medical and Surgical

Staffed Beds: 138 **Admissions:** 2121 **Census:** 100 **Outpatient Visits:** 194778 **Births:** 275 **Total Expense ($000):** 47285 **Payroll Expense ($000):** 20031 **Personnel:** 374

NYACK—Rockland County

☐ **NYACK HOSPITAL (330104)**, 160 North Midland Avenue, Zip 10960–1998; tel. 845/348–2000 **A**1 2 5 9 10 **F**4 5 8 11 13 14 15 17 25 26 27 31 32 38 40 43 46 68 71 73 74 75 76 77 79 83 84 96 97 100 106 107 109 112 118 119 124 **S** New York Presbyterian Healthcare System
Primary Contact: David H. Freed, President and Chief Executive Officer
CFO: John Burke, Chief Financial Officer
CMO: Michael E. Rader, M.D., Vice President and Medical Director
CIO: John Volanto, Vice President and Chief Information Officer
CHR: Mary K. Shinick, Vice President Human Resources
Web address: www.nyackhospital.org
Control: Other not–for–profit (including NFP Corporation) **Service:** General Medical and Surgical

Staffed Beds: 267 **Admissions:** 13684 **Census:** 176 **Outpatient Visits:** 152139 **Births:** 2135 **Total Expense ($000):** 147559 **Payroll Expense ($000):** 70522 **Personnel:** 1392

OCEANSIDE—Nassau County

★ **SOUTH NASSAU COMMUNITIES HOSPITAL (330198)**, One Healthy Way, Zip 11572–1500; tel. 516/632–3000 **A**1 2 3 5 9 10 **F**3 5 11 12 13 15 17 18 20 24 25 26 27 30 31 32 33 35 36 38 40 41 43 46 49 50 53 54 55 56 57 58 59 61 62 64 66 67 68 71 72 73 74 75 76 77 79 80 82 84 86 87 88 89 90 92 93 94 95 96 97 98 99 100 102 106 107 108 109 111 112 114 116 118 119 120 121 124 134 135 137
Primary Contact: Joseph A. Quagliata, President and Chief Executive Officer
COO: Joseph Lamantia, Executive Vice President and Chief Operating Officer
CFO: Gerard Haas, Senior Vice President and Chief Financial Officer
CMO: Joshua Kugler, M.D., Medical Director
CIO: John Mertz, Chief Information Officer
CHR: Paul Giordano, Vice President Human Resources
Web address: www.southnassau.org
Control: Other not–for–profit (including NFP Corporation) **Service:** General Medical and Surgical

Staffed Beds: 392 **Admissions:** 18963 **Census:** 356 **Outpatient Visits:** 353251 **Births:** 1797 **Total Expense ($000):** 279010 **Payroll Expense ($000):** 129567 **Personnel:** 1994

OGDENSBURG—St. Lawrence County

★ **CLAXTON–HEPBURN MEDICAL CENTER (330211)**, 214 King Street, Zip 13669–1192; tel. 315/393–3600, (Total facility includes 29 beds in nursing home–type unit) **A**1 2 9 10 20 **F**3 11 13 15 24 25 26 27 30 31 32 33 34 36 38 41 43 50 51 52 53 54 55 56 57 59 60 62 68 72 73 74 75 76 77 79 80 81 82 85 86 87 88 90 91 92 93 96 97 100 104 106 107 109 111 117 118 119 121 122 123 124 134 135 136 **P**7
Primary Contact: Mark Webster, President and Chief Executive Officer
CFO: Frederick Morey, Chief Financial Officer
CMO: Adam Jarrett, M.D., Chief Medical Officer
CIO: Christiana Navan, Manager Management Information Systems
CHR: John Ziegler, Director Human Resources
Web address: www.chmed.org
Control: Other not–for–profit (including NFP Corporation) **Service:** General Medical and Surgical

Staffed Beds: 159 **Admissions:** 4488 **Census:** 88 **Outpatient Visits:** 162686 **Births:** 444 **Total Expense ($000):** 71968 **Payroll Expense ($000):** 31720 **Personnel:** 619

☐ **ST. LAWRENCE PSYCHIATRIC CENTER (334003)**, 1 Chimney Point Drive, Zip 13669–2291; tel. 315/541–2001, (Nonreporting) **A**1 5 10 **S** New York State Office of Mental Health
Primary Contact: Samua A. Bastien, IV, Ph.D., Executive Director
CFO: Timothy J. Lamitie, Deputy Director Administration
CMO: Harishankar Sangni, M.D., Clinical Director
CIO: Christopher Ashwood, Coordinator Information Systems
Web address: www.omh.state.ny.us/omhweb/facilities/slpc/facility.htm
Control: State–Government, nonfederal **Service:** Psychiatric

Staffed Beds: 114

OLEAN—Cattaraugus County

★ **OLEAN GENERAL HOSPITAL (330103)**, 515 Main Street, Zip 14760–9912; tel. 716/373–2600 **A**1 3 5 9 10 19 20 **F**3 8 11 13 15 17 24 25 26 27 30 31 32 33 36 37 38 43 46 47 48 49 50 51 52 53 55 56 57 58 59 60 61 62 63 68 72 73 74 75 76 77 79 80 81 82 84 86 87 88 90 91 92 93 96 97 100 103 104 106 107 109 112 118 119 120 121 122 123 124 132 133 134 135 137 **P**2
Primary Contact: Timothy J. Finan, FACHE, President and Chief Executive Officer
COO: David Kobis, Vice President Operations
CFO: John Eichner, Vice President and Chief Financial Officer
CMO: William Mills, M.D., Vice President Medical Affairs
CIO: Jason Yaworsky, Director Information Systems
Web address: www.ogh.org
Control: Other not–for–profit (including NFP Corporation) **Service:** General Medical and Surgical

Staffed Beds: 156 **Admissions:** 8138 **Census:** 111 **Outpatient Visits:** 143056 **Births:** 738 **Total Expense ($000):** 74255 **Payroll Expense ($000):** 31843 **Personnel:** 809

ONEIDA—Madison County

★ **ONEIDA HEALTHCARE CENTER (330115)**, 321 Genesee Street, Zip 13421–0321; tel. 315/363–6000, (Total facility includes 160 beds in nursing home–type unit) **A**1 9 10 **F**3 13 15 30 31 32 38 49 55 56 68 73 74 75 77 79 81 82 84 86 96 97 100 103 106 107 117 118 119 124 135 **P**1
Primary Contact: Gene Morreale, Chief Executive Officer
COO: Paul A. Scopac, Chief Operating Officer
CFO: Vincent S. Maneen, Chief Financial Officer
CMO: John Wight, M.D., Chief of Staff
CIO: Mary Fox, Director Information Systems
CHR: John G. Margo, Director Human Resources
Web address: www.oneidahealthcare.org
Control: Other not–for–profit (including NFP Corporation) **Service:** General Medical and Surgical

Staffed Beds: 237 **Admissions:** 3519 **Census:** 191 **Outpatient Visits:** 154205 **Births:** 567 **Total Expense ($000):** 60271 **Payroll Expense ($000):** 29042 **Personnel:** 701

ONEONTA—Otsego County

★ **AURELIA OSBORN FOX MEMORIAL HOSPITAL (330085)**, 1 Norton Avenue, Zip 13820–2697; tel. 607/432–2000, (Total facility includes 131 beds in nursing home–type unit) **A**1 9 10 19 20 **F**2 3 11 13 15 17 24 25 26 27 30 31 32 33 37 38 43 46 48 50 52 53 54 55 56 57 62 63 66 68 72 73 74 75 76 77 79 80 81 82 84 86 87 96 97 99 100 103 106 107 108 109 111 117 119 120 133 135 136 137 **P**6
Primary Contact: John R. Remillard, President
CFO: Mark J. Wright, Vice President Finance
CMO: Carlton Rule, M.D., Executive Vice President Medical Affairs
CIO: Joseph Phillips, Director Information Systems
CHR: Keith Valk, Vice President Human Resources
Web address: www.foxcarenetwork.com
Control: Other not–for–profit (including NFP Corporation) **Service:** General Medical and Surgical

Staffed Beds: 231 **Admissions:** 4675 **Census:** 191 **Outpatient Visits:** 232628 **Births:** 409 **Total Expense ($000):** 76603 **Payroll Expense ($000):** 35591 **Personnel:** 682

ORANGEBURG—Rockland County

☐ **ROCKLAND CHILDREN'S PSYCHIATRIC CENTER (334015)**, 599 Convent Road, Zip 10962; tel. 845/359–7400, (Nonreporting) **A**1 **S** New York State Office of Mental Health
Primary Contact: Raul Silva, M.D., Executive Director
COO: Kenneth Perrotte, Director Operations
CFO: Peter Gorey, Administrative Coordinator
CMO: Sadhana Sardana, M.D., Clinical Director
CIO: Mary Pivonka, Director Quality Management
Control: State–Government, nonfederal **Service:** Children's hospital psychiatric

Staffed Beds: 54

☐ **ROCKLAND PSYCHIATRIC CENTER (334015)**, 140 Old Orangeburg Road, Zip 10962–0071; tel. 845/359–1000, (Nonreporting) **A**1 3 5 10 **S** New York State Office of Mental Health
Primary Contact: James H. Bopp, Executive Director
Control: State–Government, nonfederal **Service:** Psychiatric

Staffed Beds: 525

OSSINING—Westchester County

OSSINING CORRECTIONAL FACILITIES HOSPITAL, 354 Hunter Street, Zip 10562–5498; tel. 914/941–0108, (Nonreporting)
Primary Contact: John Perilli, M.D., Health Services Director
Control: State–Government, nonfederal **Service:** Hospital unit of an institution (prison hospital, college infimary, etc.)

Staffed Beds: 25

STONY LODGE HOSPITAL (334059), 40 Croton Dam Road, Zip 10562–2644, Mailing Address: P.O. Box 1250, Briarcliff Manor, Zip 10510–1250; tel. 914/941–7400 **A**9 10 **F**88 89 **P**6
Primary Contact: Kevin F. Czipo, Executive Director and Chief Executive Officer
CMO: Fady Hajal, M.D., Medical Director
CHR: Anne Alley, Director Human Resources
Web address: www.stonylodge.com
Control: Corporation, Investor–owned, for–profit **Service:** Children's hospital psychiatric

Staffed Beds: 61 **Admissions:** 625 **Census:** 58 **Births:** 0 **Total Expense ($000):** 14327 **Payroll Expense ($000):** 8127 **Personnel:** 200

OSWEGO—Oswego County

★ **OSWEGO HOSPITAL (330218)**, 110 West Sixth Street, Zip 13126–9985; tel. 315/349–5511 **A**1 9 10 **F**3 5 11 13 15 17 24 25 30 31 32 36 38 43 44 49 50 53 55 56 57 61 62 66 68 72 73 74 75 76 77 79 80 81 82 84 86 87 88 89 90 91 92 93 94 95 96 97 98 100 102 106 107 119 120 121 124 135 137 **P**6
Primary Contact: Ann C. Gilpin, President and Chief Executive Officer
COO: Gail Greenwood, Executive Vice President and Chief Operating Officer
CFO: Paul Snyder, Vice President and Chief Financial Officer
CMO: Patsy Iannolo, M.D., Vice President Medical Affairs
CIO: Craig Dumas, Vice President and Chief Information Officer
CHR: Michael Russell, Vice President Human Resources
Web address: www.oswegohealth.org
Control: Other not–for–profit (including NFP Corporation) **Service:** General Medical and Surgical

Staffed Beds: 89 **Admissions:** 5285 **Census:** 66 **Outpatient Visits:** 275240 **Births:** 687 **Total Expense ($000):** 61002 **Payroll Expense ($000):** 28586 **Personnel:** 653

PATCHOGUE—Suffolk County

★ **BROOKHAVEN MEMORIAL HOSPITAL MEDICAL CENTER (330141)**, 101 Hospital Road, Zip 11772–4897; tel. 631/654–7100, (Nonreporting) **A**1 9 10
Primary Contact: Thomas Ockers, President and Chief Executive Officer
COO: Richard T. Margulis, Senior Vice President and Chief Operating Officer
CFO: Ronald A. Giraulo, Senior Vice President and Chief Financial Officer
CMO: Ronald Klen, M.D., Interim Chief Medical Officer
CIO: Donald Fleming, Vice President and Chief Information Officer
CHR: Virginia Raffaele, Vice President Human Resources
Web address: www.bmhmc.org
Control: Other not–for–profit (including NFP Corporation) **Service:** General Medical and Surgical

Staffed Beds: 345

PENN YAN—Yates County

★ **SOLDIERS AND SAILORS MEMORIAL HOSPITAL OF YATES COUNTY (331314)**, 418 North Main Street, Zip 14527–1085; tel. 315/531–2000, (Total facility includes 151 beds in nursing home–type unit) **A**9 10 18 **F**2 3 11 15 24 25 30 31 32 33 38 46 53 54 55 57 62 63 64 66 68 73 75 77 79 82 86 87 88 89 90 91 92 93 94 96 107 117 119 121 122 124 132 135 136 **S** Finger Lakes Health
Primary Contact: James J. Dooley, President and Chief Executive Officer
COO: Mary Ann Eldred, Executive Vice President and Chief Operating Officer
CFO: Lawrence J. Farnand, Treasurer and Chief Financial Officer
CMO: Jose Acevedo, M.D., Vice President Medical Affairs and Chief Medical Officer
CIO: Daniel Pletcher, Director Management Information System
CHR: Patrick Boyle, Vice President Human Resources
Web address: www.flhealth.org
Control: Other not–for–profit (including NFP Corporation) **Service:** General Medical and Surgical

Staffed Beds: 186 **Admissions:** 1487 **Census:** 162 **Outpatient Visits:** 80849 **Births:** 0 **Total Expense ($000):** 28142 **Payroll Expense ($000):** 14990 **Personnel:** 391

PLAINVIEW—Nassau County

★ **NORTH SHORE UNIVERSITY HOSPITAL AT PLAINVIEW (330331)**, 888 Old Country Road, Zip 11803–4978; tel. 516/719–3000 **A**1 2 9 10 12 13 **F**3 9 13 15 17 25 26 27 30 31 32 33 34 36 38 40 41 44 46 49 50 55 56 57 58 59 62 63 66 67 68 69 71 72 73 74 76 77 79 80 81 82 87 91 92 96 97 99 100 105 107 119 121 124 135 **P**6 **S** North Shore–LIJ Health System
Primary Contact: Deborah Tascone, RN, M.S., Executive Director
CFO: Michael Fener, Associate Executive Director Finance
CMO: Abdallah Mishrick, M.D., Senior Vice President Medical Affairs
CIO: Nicholas O'Connor, Vice President and Chief Information Officer
Web address: www.northshorelij.com
Control: Other not–for–profit (including NFP Corporation) **Service:** General Medical and Surgical

Staffed Beds: 211 **Admissions:** 14178 **Census:** 206 **Outpatient Visits:** 55911 **Births:** 1409 **Total Expense ($000):** 155001 **Payroll Expense ($000):** 74466 **Personnel:** 1068

PLATTSBURGH—Clinton County

★ **CHAMPLAIN VALLEY PHYSICIANS HOSPITAL MEDICAL CENTER (330250)**, 75 Beekman Street, Zip 12901–1493; tel. 518/561–2000, (Total facility includes 90 beds in nursing home–type unit) **A**1 2 9 10 19 20 **F**7 8 11 13 14 15 17 18 20 22 24 25 26 27 28 31 32 33 34 35 36 37 38 40 41 43 46 49 51 52 53 55 56 57 59 60 62 63 64 68 72 73 74 75 76 77 79 80 81 82 84 86 87 88 89 90 91 92 94 96 97 100 102 105 107 109 117 118 119 120 121 124 133 135 136 137 **P**1
Primary Contact: Stephens M. Mundy, President and Chief Executive Officer
CFO: Joyce Rafferty, Vice President Finance
CMO: Wouter Rietsema, M.D., Medical Director
CIO: Rosemary Miller, Associate Vice President Information Systems Services
CHR: Noreen Brady, Vice President Human Resources
Web address: www.cvph.org
Control: Other not–for–profit (including NFP Corporation) **Service:** General Medical and Surgical

Staffed Beds: 322 **Admissions:** 10532 **Census:** 186 **Outpatient Visits:** 288678 **Births:** 790 **Total Expense ($000):** 197920 **Payroll Expense ($000):** 94026 **Personnel:** 2305

POMONA—Rockland County

☐ **SUMMIT PARK HOSPITAL AND NURSING CARE CENTER (332014)**, 50 Sanatorium Road, Building A., Zip 10970; tel. 845/364–2700, (Total facility includes 300 beds in nursing home–type unit) (Nonreporting) **A**1 10
Primary Contact: Aldo A. Troiani, Acting Commissioner
CFO: Chris Kopf, Chief Fiscal Officer
CMO: Paul M. Adler, M.D., Medical Director
CHR: Anita Caminez, Director Human Resources
Web address: www.co.rockland.ny.us
Control: County–Government, nonfederal **Service:** Long–Term Acute Care hospital

Staffed Beds: 408

Hospital, Medicare Provider Number, Address, Telephone, Approval, Facility, and Physician Codes, Health Care System

★ American Hospital Association (AHA) membership
☐ The Joint Commission accreditation
○ American Osteopathic Association (AOA) accreditation
△ Commission on Accreditation of Rehabilitation Facilities (CARF) accreditation

PORT JEFFERSON—Suffolk County

★ **JOHN T. MATHER MEMORIAL HOSPITAL (330185)**, 75 North Country Road, Zip 11777–2190; tel. 631/473–1320 **A**1 2 9 10 **F**5 8 12 14 15 17 25 27 30 31 32 33 34 35 36 38 41 43 49 51 54 55 56 57 59 62 63 67 68 73 75 76 77 79 80 82 88 89 90 92 93 94 95 96 97 99 100 102 103 106 107 108 113 114 118 119 121 135 136 137
Primary Contact: Kenneth D. Roberts, President
CFO: Joseph Wisnoski, Vice President Finance and Chief Financial Officer
CMO: Joan Faro, M.D., Chief Medical Officer
CIO: Thomas Heiman, Assistant Vice President Information Services
CHR: Diane Marotta, Vice President Human Resources
Web address: www.matherhospital.com
Control: Other not–for–profit (including NFP Corporation) **Service:** General Medical and Surgical

Staffed Beds: 248 **Admissions:** 12149 **Census:** 216 **Outpatient Visits:** 132757 **Births:** 0 **Total Expense ($000):** 190725 **Payroll Expense ($000):** 93781 **Personnel:** 1640

☐ **ST. CHARLES HOSPITAL (330246)**, 200 Belle Terre Road, Zip 11777–1928; tel. 631/474–6000, (Nonreporting) **A**1 2 9 10 **S** Catholic Health Services of Long Island
Primary Contact: James O'Connor, President and Chief Executive Officer
COO: Ronald Weingartner, Chief Operating Officer
CFO: John Pohlman, Interim Vice President and Chief Financial Officer
CMO: Craig Smestad, M.D., Chief Medical Officer
CIO: Felix Pabon–Ramirez, Chief Information Officer
CHR: Mark Boehrer, Director Human Resources
Web address: www.stcharleshospital.chsli.org
Control: Church–operated, Nongovernment, not–for profit **Service:** General Medical and Surgical

Staffed Beds: 289

PORT JERVIS—Orange County

★ **BON SECOURS COMMUNITY HOSPITAL (330135)**, 160 East Main Street, Zip 12771–2245, Mailing Address: P.O. Box 1014, Zip 12771–1014; tel. 845/858–7000 **A**1 2 9 10 **F**4 8 12 13 15 17 25 26 27 30 31 32 37 38 43 44 45 46 54 55 56 57 59 60 63 64 66 68 73 74 75 76 77 79 82 84 85 86 87 88 91 92 93 96 97 107 117 119 121 124 136 137 **S** Bon Secours Health System, Inc.
Primary Contact: Leah Cerkvenik, Executive Vice President, Administrator and Chief Executive Officer
COO: Gaynor Rosenstein, Vice President Operations
CFO: Stephen D. Majetich, CPA, Senior Vice President and Chief Financial Officer
CMO: Jeffrey Auerbach, D.O., Medical Director
CHR: Kim Hirkaler, Director Human Resources
Web address: www.bonsecourscommunityhosp.org
Control: Other not–for–profit (including NFP Corporation) **Service:** General Medical and Surgical

Staffed Beds: 187 **Admissions:** 4979 **Census:** 78 **Outpatient Visits:** 76137 **Births:** 304

POTSDAM—St. Lawrence County

★ **CANTON–POTSDAM HOSPITAL (330197)**, 50 Leroy Street, Zip 13676–1799; tel. 315/265–3300, (Nonreporting) **A**1 9 10 20
Primary Contact: David B. Acker, FACHE, President and Chief Executive Officer
CFO: Richard Jacobs, Vice President Finance and Chief Financial Officer
CMO: Robert T. Rogers, M.D., Medical Director
CIO: Corey Zeigler, Chief Information Officer
Web address: www.cphospital.org
Control: Other not–for–profit (including NFP Corporation) **Service:** General Medical and Surgical

Staffed Beds: 94

POUGHKEEPSIE—Dutchess County

☐ **HUDSON RIVER PSYCHIATRIC CENTER (334010)**, 10 Ross Circle, Zip 12601–1078; tel. 845/452–8000, (Nonreporting) **A**1 10 **S** New York State Office of Mental Health
Primary Contact: Jean L. Wolfersteig, Acting Executive Director
COO: Claire Newquist, Director Program Operations
CFO: Naomi Garrell, Business Officer
CMO: Kren K. Shriver, M.P.H., M.D., Director Clinical Services
CIO: Roger Christenfeld, Ph.D., Director Public Relations
CHR: Alexander Walsh, Director Human Resources Management
Web address: www.omh.state.ny.us
Control: State–Government, nonfederal **Service:** Psychiatric

Staffed Beds: 460

☐ △ **SAINT FRANCIS HOSPITAL AND HEALTH CENTERS (330067)**, 241 North Road, Zip 12601–1399; tel. 845/483–5000, (Includes SAINT FRANCIS HOSPITAL, 11 Hastings Drive, Beacon, Zip 12508; tel. 845/838–4500) **A**1 2 7 9 10 **F**3 4 5 8 11 12 15 17 18 25 26 27 28 30 31 32 33 34 35 38 40 43 46 49 50 54 55 56 57 59 60 61 62 63 64 66 68 72 73 75 76 77 78 79 80 81 82 84 85 86 88 89 90 91 92 93 94 96 97 100 102 106 107 118 119 120 121 122 123 124 133 135 137
Primary Contact: Robert L. Savage, President and Chief Executive Officer
COO: Suzanne McLaughlin, Chief Operating Officer and Chief Nursing Officer
CFO: Will de la Pena, Chief Financial Officer
CMO: J. Keith Festa, M.D., Vice President Medical Affairs
CIO: Robert Wagner, Director Information Systems
CHR: Helen Rinaudo, Vice President Human Resources
Web address: www.sfhhc.org
Control: Church–operated, Nongovernment, not–for profit **Service:** General Medical and Surgical

Staffed Beds: 322 **Admissions:** 9974 **Census:** 198 **Outpatient Visits:** 188595 **Births:** 0 **Total Expense ($000):** 142765 **Payroll Expense ($000):** 67442

★ **VASSAR BROTHERS MEDICAL CENTER (330023)**, 45 Reade Place, Zip 12601–3990; tel. 845/454–8500 **A**1 2 9 10 **F**3 8 11 13 14 15 17 18 20 22 25 26 27 28 30 31 32 33 34 36 37 38 42 43 44 46 49 50 51 53 54 55 56 57 59 60 62 64 66 68 70 72 73 74 76 77 79 80 81 82 84 86 87 96 97 99 100 102 105 107 108 109 112 114 118 119 121 123 124 135 136 137 **S** Health Quest Systems, Inc.
Primary Contact: Daniel Z. Aronzon, M.D., President and Chief Executive Officer
COO: Janet L. Ready, Senior Vice President Operations and Chief Operating Officer
CFO: Jeffrey Kruger, Chief Financial Officer
CMO: Stephen A. Katz, M.D., Chief Medical Officer and Senior Vice President Medical Affairs
CIO: Robert Diamond, Chief Information Officer
CHR: Patrick Borek, Vice President Human Resources
Web address: www.vassarbrothers.org
Control: Other not–for–profit (including NFP Corporation) **Service:** General Medical and Surgical

Staffed Beds: 355 **Admissions:** 19660 **Census:** 277 **Outpatient Visits:** 245654 **Births:** 2469 **Total Expense ($000):** 290173 **Payroll Expense ($000):** 109646 **Personnel:** 1762

QUEENS—Queens County, See New York City

QUEENS VILLAGE—Queens County, See New York City

RHINEBECK—Dutchess County

★ △ **NORTHERN DUTCHESS HOSPITAL (330049)**, 6511 Springbrook Avenue, Zip 12572–5002, Mailing Address: P.O. Box 5002, Zip 12572–5002; tel. 845/876–3001 **A**1 7 9 10 **F**3 9 11 13 15 24 25 26 33 34 35 38 43 52 53 54 55 56 57 62 66 68 72 73 74 75 77 79 80 85 86 96 97 100 102 107 118 119 120 121 124 135 136 **S** Health Quest Systems, Inc.
Primary Contact: Denise George, RN, President and Chief Executive Officer
CFO: Maryann Kepple, Interim Chief Financial Officer
CMO: John Sabia, M.D., Medical Director
CIO: Catherine Schuster, Chief Information Officer
CHR: Eileen Miller, Director Human Resources
Web address: www.ndhosp.com
Control: Other not–for–profit (including NFP Corporation) **Service:** General Medical and Surgical

Staffed Beds: 68 **Admissions:** 3290 **Census:** 41 **Outpatient Visits:** 66217 **Births:** 777 **Total Expense ($000):** 50494 **Payroll Expense ($000):** 18712 **Personnel:** 374

RICHMOND VALLEY—Richmond County, See New York City

RIVERHEAD—Suffolk County

☐ **PECONIC BAY MEDICAL CENTER (330107)**, 1300 Roanoke Avenue, Zip 11901–2028; tel. 631/548–6000, (Total facility includes 60 beds in nursing home–type unit) (Nonreporting) **A**1 9 10
Primary Contact: Andrew J. Mitchell, President and Chief Executive Officer
COO: Ronald McManus, Vice President Operations and Continuum of Care
CFO: Michael O'Donnell, Chief Financial Officer
CMO: Saul Rosenstreich, Vice President Medical Affairs
CIO: Thomas Chiasera, Director Information Systems
CHR: Peter Chiacchiaro, Director Human Resources
Web address: www.peconicbaymedicalcenter.org
Control: Other not–for–profit (including NFP Corporation) **Service:** General Medical and Surgical

Staffed Beds: 100

 Many Facility Codes have changed. Please refer to the AHA Guide Code Chart.

ROCHESTER—Monroe County

★ **HIGHLAND HOSPITAL OF ROCHESTER (330164)**, 1000 South Avenue, Zip 14620–2782; tel. 585/473–2200 **A**1 3 5 9 10 **F**5 10 12 13 15 18 20 22 25 26 27 28 30 31 32 33 34 35 36 37 38 42 43 46 49 50 54 57 59 60 62 63 66 68 72 73 74 76 77 79 81 82 87 96 97 98 99 104 105 107 108 109 110 111 112 116 119 120 132 134 135 136 **S** Strong Memorial Hospital
Primary Contact: Steven I. Goldstein, President and Chief Executive Officer
COO: Cindy Becker, Vice President and Chief Operating Officer
CFO: Leonard J. Shute, Chief Financial Officer
CMO: Raymond Mayewski, M.D., Chief Medical Officer
CIO: Jerry Powell, Chief Information Officer
Web address: www.stronghealth.com
Control: Hospital district or authority, Government, nonfederal **Service:** General Medical and Surgical

Staffed Beds: 261 **Admissions:** 15225 **Census:** 213 **Outpatient Visits:** 33691 **Births:** 3308 **Total Expense ($000):** 218680 **Payroll Expense ($000):** 90587 **Personnel:** 1892

□ **ROCHESTER GENERAL HOSPITAL (330125)**, 1425 Portland Avenue, Zip 14621–3099; tel. 585/922–4000 **A**1 2 3 5 6 9 10 **F**3 5 8 11 12 13 14 15 17 18 20 22 24 25 26 27 28 30 31 32 33 34 36 37 38 40 41 43 49 50 53 54 55 56 57 58 59 62 64 66 68 71 72 73 74 75 76 77 78 79 80 81 82 84 85 86 87 88 89 90 91 92 93 94 95 96 97 100 102 103 106 107 109 111 112 116 119 120 121 123 124 132 135 136 137 **P**5 7 **S** ViaHealth
Primary Contact: Mark C. Clement, President and Chief Executive Officer
COO: Bill Horner, Senior Vice President Operations
CFO: Robert Nesselbush, Senior Vice President Finance and Chief Financial Officer
CMO: Richard Gangemi, M.D., Senior Vice President Academic and Medical Affairs
CIO: David Kamowski, Interim Chief Information Officer
CHR: Cheryl Henke, Senior Vice President Human Resources
Web address: www.viahealth.org/
Control: Other not–for–profit (including NFP Corporation) **Service:** General Medical and Surgical

Staffed Beds: 494 **Admissions:** 27345 **Census:** 423 **Outpatient Visits:** 1313552 **Births:** 2524 **Total Expense ($000):** 513217 **Payroll Expense ($000):** 245712 **Personnel:** 4614

□ **ROCHESTER PSYCHIATRIC CENTER (334020)**, 1111 Elmwood Avenue, Zip 14620–3005; tel. 585/241–1200, (Nonreporting) **A**1 3 5 9 10 **S** New York State Office of Mental Health
Primary Contact: Michael P. Zuber, Ph.D., Executive Director
COO: Joseph Coffey, Director Facility Administration
CFO: Ned Miller, Business Officer
CMO: Laurence Guttmacher, M.D., Clinical Director
CIO: Stephen Font, Information Systems Coordinator
CHR: Christine Hally, Director Human Resources
Web address: www.omh.state.ny.us/omhweb/facilities/ropc/facility.htm
Control: State–Government, nonfederal **Service:** Psychiatric

Staffed Beds: 180

★ △ **STRONG MEMORIAL HOSPITAL OF THE UNIVERSITY OF ROCHESTER (330285)**, 601 Elmwood Avenue, Zip 14642–0002; tel. 585/275–2100, (Total facility includes 267 beds in nursing home–type unit) **A**1 3 5 7 8 9 10 **F**2 3 5 6 8 9 10 11 12 13 14 15 16 17 18 19 20 21 22 23 24 25 26 27 28 29 30 31 32 33 34 35 36 37 38 40 41 42 43 44 45 46 47 48 49 50 51 52 53 54 55 56 57 58 59 60 61 62 63 64 66 67 68 69 70 71 72 73 74 75 76 77 78 79 80 81 82 83 84 85 86 87 88 89 90 91 92 93 94 95 96 97 99 100 102 103 104 105 106 107 108 109 111 112 113 114 115 116 117 118 119 120 121 123 124 125 126 127 128 130 131 132 133 134 135 136 137 **P**5 6 **S** Strong Memorial Hospital
Primary Contact: Steven I. Goldstein, President and Chief Executive Officer
COO: Kathleen M. Parrinello, Ph.D., Chief Operating Officer
CFO: Leonard J. Shute, Chief Financial Officer
CMO: Raymond Mayewski, M.D., Chief Medical Officer
CIO: D. Jerome Powell, Chief Information Officer
CHR: Charles J. Murphy, Associate Vice President Human Resources
Web address: www.urmc.rochester.edu
Control: Other not–for–profit (including NFP Corporation) **Service:** General Medical and Surgical

Staffed Beds: 1006 **Admissions:** 37830 **Census:** 947 **Outpatient Visits:** 1229835 **Births:** 2999 **Total Expense ($000):** 827258 **Payroll Expense ($000):** 346020 **Personnel:** 7307

★ **UNITY HOSPITAL (330226)**, 1555 Long Pond Road, Zip 14626–4182; tel. 585/723–7000 **A**1 2 3 5 9 10 **F**4 5 8 11 12 13 15 18 20 22 24 25 26 27 28 33 36 37 38 39 43 46 47 49 50 54 55 56 57 58 59 60 62 63 64 68 74 85 88 96 102 107 117 118 119 120 121 122 123 124 133 135 136 137
Primary Contact: Timothy McCormick, President and Chief Executive Officer
COO: Stewart C. Putnam, Executive Vice President and Chief Operating Officer
CFO: Warren Hern, Executive Vice President and Chief Financial Officer
CMO: Joseph Salipante, M.D., Vice President Medical Affairs
CIO: John Glynn, Vice President and Chief Information Officer
CHR: James Rancourt, Vice President Human Resources
Web address: www.unityhealth.org
Control: State–Government, nonfederal **Service:** General Medical and Surgical

Staffed Beds: 441 **Admissions:** 12622 **Census:** 181 **Outpatient Visits:** 965587 **Births:** 1194

ROCKVILLE CENTRE—Nassau County

□ **MERCY MEDICAL CENTER (330259)**, 1000 North Village Avenue, Zip 11570–1098; tel. 516/705–2525, (Nonreporting) **A**1 2 9 10 **S** Catholic Health Services of Long Island
Primary Contact: Alan D. Guerci, M.D., Chief Executive Officer
CIO: Beth Hammerman, Director Community Relations and Planning
Web address: www.mercymedicalcenter.chsli.org
Control: Church–operated, Nongovernment, not–for profit **Service:** General Medical and Surgical

Staffed Beds: 387

ROME—Oneida County

★ △ **ROME MEMORIAL HOSPITAL (330215)**, 1500 North James Street, Zip 13440–2898; tel. 315/338–7000, (Total facility includes 82 beds in nursing home–type unit) **A**1 7 9 10 **F**3 5 8 13 15 25 27 28 30 31 32 33 38 43 46 49 54 55 56 57 58 60 62 63 64 68 72 73 74 75 76 77 78 79 80 81 82 84 85 86 87 88 93 96 97 103 106 107 108 109 111 117 118 119 120 121 123 124 132 135 136 **P**6
Primary Contact: Darlene A. Burns, RN, President and Chief Executive Officer
COO: Basil Ariglio, Senior Vice President and Chief Operating Officer
CFO: Nick Mayhew, Vice President and Chief Financial Officer
CMO: Walled Albert, M.D., Chief Medical Officer
CIO: Maryann Dubai, Chief Information Officer
CHR: Gina Chambers, Assistant Vice President Human Resource
Web address: www.romehospital.org
Control: Other not–for–profit (including NFP Corporation) **Service:** General Medical and Surgical

Staffed Beds: 195 **Admissions:** 5339 **Census:** 148 **Outpatient Visits:** 142542 **Births:** 623 **Total Expense ($000):** 69452 **Payroll Expense ($000):** 33607 **Personnel:** 784

ROSLYN—Nassau County

★ **ST. FRANCIS HOSPITAL (330182)**, 100 Port Washington Boulevard, Zip 11576–1348; tel. 516/562–6000 **A**1 9 10 **F**3 15 17 18 19 20 21 22 24 25 26 27 30 31 32 33 34 35 37 38 40 42 43 44 45 46 48 49 50 52 53 54 55 56 57 58 62 63 66 67 68 69 72 76 77 79 80 81 82 86 87 90 92 96 97 98 99 100 102 103 106 107 112 116 119 120 121 123 124 135 136 **S** Catholic Health Services of Long Island
Primary Contact: Alan D. Guerci, M.D., Chief Executive Officer
COO: Ruth Hennessey, Senior Vice President and Chief Operating Officer
CFO: William C. Armstrong, Vice President and Chief Financial Officer
CMO: Jack Soterakis, M.D., Executive Vice President Medical Affairs
Web address: www.stfrancisheartcenter.chsli.org
Control: Church–operated, Nongovernment, not–for profit **Service:** General Medical and Surgical

Staffed Beds: 311 **Admissions:** 17338 **Census:** 267 **Outpatient Visits:** 85785 **Births:** 0 **Total Expense ($000):** 323640 **Payroll Expense ($000):** 140858 **Personnel:** 2014

RYE—Westchester County

★ **RYE HOSPITAL CENTER (334033)**, 754 Boston Post Road, Zip 10580–2724; tel. 914/967–4567 **A**1 10 **F**88 89 93 119 135
Primary Contact: Jack C. Schoenholtz, M.D., Medical Director, Administrator, President and Chief Executive Officer
CFO: John Marcogliese, Vice President Financial Operations
Web address: www.ryehospitalcenter.org
Control: Corporation, Investor–owned, for–profit **Service:** Psychiatric

Staffed Beds: 34 **Admissions:** 258 **Census:** 24 **Total Expense ($000):** 5705 **Payroll Expense ($000):** 2809 **Personnel:** 61

NY

Hospital, Medicare Provider Number, Address, Telephone, Approval, Facility, and Physician Codes, Health Care System
★ American Hospital Association (AHA) membership
□ The Joint Commission accreditation
○ American Osteopathic Association (AOA) accreditation
△ Commission on Accreditation of Rehabilitation Facilities (CARF) accreditation

SARANAC LAKE—Franklin County

★ ○ **ADIRONDACK MEDICAL CENTER (330079)**, 2233 State Route 86, Zip 12983, Mailing Address: P.O. Box 471, Zip 12983–0471; tel. 518/891–4141, (Total facility includes 186 beds in nursing home–type unit) **A**1 9 10 11 19 20 **F**3 8 11 12 13 15 24 25 26 27 30 31 33 37 38 39 40 43 53 54 55 56 57 59 62 68 72 73 74 75 76 77 79 80 81 84 86 87 88 92 93 96 97 100 102 104 106 107 117 118 119 120 121 122 124 135 136 **P**1 5 **S** Brim Healthcare, Inc.
Primary Contact: Chandler M. Ralph, President and Chief Executive Officer
CFO: Patrick M. Facteau, Vice President Finance
CMO: William Viscardo, M.D., Vice President Medical Affairs
CIO: William Kelly, Director Information Systems
CHR: Michael Lee, Vice President Human Resources
Web address: www.amccares.org
Control: Other not–for–profit (including NFP Corporation) **Service:** General Medical and Surgical

Staffed Beds: 263 **Admissions:** 2979 **Census:** 43 **Outpatient Visits:** 111012 **Births:** 208 **Total Expense ($000):** 73296 **Payroll Expense ($000):** 33532 **Personnel:** 564

SARATOGA SPRINGS—Saratoga County

□ **FOUR WINDS HOSPITAL (334049)**, 30 Crescent Avenue, Zip 12866; tel. 518/584–3600, (Nonreporting) **A**1 10
Primary Contact: Michael O'Neil, Administrator
Web address: www.fourwindshospital.com
Control: Corporation, Investor–owned, for–profit **Service:** Children's hospital psychiatric

Staffed Beds: 83

★ **SARATOGA HOSPITAL (330222)**, 211 Church Street, Zip 12866–1003; tel. 518/587–3222, (Total facility includes 72 beds in nursing home–type unit) **A**1 9 10 **F**3 8 13 15 17 18 25 26 27 32 33 35 36 38 42 43 49 53 54 55 56 57 62 66 68 72 73 74 75 76 77 79 80 82 86 88 89 90 91 92 93 96 97 99 100 102 103 104 105 107 116 117 119 120 121 124 133 134 135 136
Primary Contact: Angelo G. Calbone, President and Chief Executive Officer
CFO: Gary Foster, Vice President and Chief Financial Officer
CMO: Joyce Peabody, M.D., Vice President and Chief Medical Officer
CIO: John Mangona, Chief Information Officer and Compliance Officer
CHR: Jeffrey M. Methven, Vice President and Chief Human Resources Officer
Web address: www.saratogacare.org
Control: Other not–for–profit (including NFP Corporation) **Service:** General Medical and Surgical

Staffed Beds: 213 **Admissions:** 8339 **Census:** 183 **Outpatient Visits:** 188267 **Births:** 888 **Total Expense ($000):** 129277 **Payroll Expense ($000):** 58613 **Personnel:** 1384

SCHENECTADY—Schenectady County

CONIFER PARK See Glenville

★ **ELLIS HOSPITAL (330153)**, 1101 Nott Street, Zip 12308–2487; tel. 518/243–4000, (Includes BELLEVUE WOMAN'S CARE CENTER, 2210 Troy Road, Zip 12309–4797; tel. 518/346–9400), (Total facility includes 82 beds in nursing home–type unit) (Nonreporting) **A**1 3 5 6 9 10
Primary Contact: James W. Connolly, President and Chief Executive Officer
COO: Paul A. Milton, Executive Vice President and Chief Operating Officer
CFO: Daniel Rinaldi, Chief Financial Officer
CMO: David Liebers, M.D., Chief Medical Officer and Vice President Medical Affairs
CIO: William Young, Chief Information Officer and Vice President Information Technology
CHR: Joseph Giansante, Vice President Human Resources
Web address: www.ellishospital.org
Control: Other not–for–profit (including NFP Corporation) **Service:** General Medical and Surgical

Staffed Beds: 351

□ **ST. CLARE'S HOSPITAL OF SCHENECTADY (330066)**, 600 McClellan Street, Zip 12304–1090; tel. 518/382–2000 **A**1 3 5 9 10 12 **F**3 8 11 13 15 25 26 27 30 31 32 33 37 38 41 46 49 50 51 54 55 57 58 59 60 62 63 64 66 68 72 73 74 75 76 77 79 80 81 82 84 86 87 96 97 99 100 102 107 118 119 120 121 124 132 133 134 135 137
Primary Contact: Robert P. Perry, President and Chief Executive Officer
CFO: Edward Gasparovic, Vice President Finance
CMO: Richard Gullot, M.D., Vice President Medical Affairs
CIO: James DeGroff, Director Technology and Network Services
CHR: Randy Stark, Vice President Human Resources
Web address: www.stclares.org
Control: Other not–for–profit (including NFP Corporation) **Service:** General Medical and Surgical

Staffed Beds: 136 **Admissions:** 5680 **Census:** 79 **Outpatient Visits:** 192268 **Total Expense ($000):** 87580 **Payroll Expense ($000):** 44307 **Personnel:** 796

★ △ **SUNNYVIEW REHABILITATION HOSPITAL (330406)**, 1270 Belmont Avenue, Zip 12308–2104; tel. 518/382–4500 **A**1 3 5 7 9 10 **F**3 11 12 24 25 31 32 52 54 55 57 62 72 77 85 86 96 107 119 121 124 135 **P**5
Primary Contact: Edward Eisenman, Chief Executive Officer
CFO: Juanita Wheeler, Director Finance
CMO: Lynne T. Nicolson, M.D., Medical Director
CIO: Patrick Clark, Manager Information Technology
CHR: Meghan Glowa, Director Human Resources
Web address: www.sunnyview.org
Control: Other not–for–profit (including NFP Corporation) **Service:** Rehabilitation

Staffed Beds: 104 **Admissions:** 1582 **Census:** 68 **Outpatient Visits:** 49522 **Births:** 0 **Total Expense ($000):** 38717 **Payroll Expense ($000):** 22126 **Personnel:** 500

SLEEPY HOLLOW—Westchester County

★ **PHELPS MEMORIAL HOSPITAL CENTER (330261)**, 701 North Broadway, Zip 10591–1096; tel. 914/366–3000 **A**1 9 10 **F**3 4 5 8 9 11 13 14 15 17 24 25 26 27 28 30 31 32 33 36 37 38 40 42 43 44 46 47 48 49 50 52 54 55 56 57 59 60 61 62 63 66 67 68 72 73 74 75 76 77 79 80 81 82 84 85 86 87 88 91 92 93 94 96 97 99 102 106 107 113 114 118 119 120 121 124 132 133 134 135 136 137 **P**1 5 8
Primary Contact: Keith F. Safian, President and Chief Executive Officer
COO: Bruce B. Davidow, Senior Vice President and Chief Operating Officer
CFO: Vincent DeSantis, Vice President Finance
CMO: Lawrence L. Faltz, M.D., Senior Vice President Medical Affairs and Medical Director
CHR: Kevin T. Byrne, Vice President Human Resources
Web address: www.phelpshospital.org
Control: Other not–for–profit (including NFP Corporation) **Service:** General Medical and Surgical

Staffed Beds: 235 **Admissions:** 7866 **Census:** 146 **Outpatient Visits:** 239534 **Births:** 1061 **Total Expense ($000):** 143509 **Payroll Expense ($000):** 72531 **Personnel:** 1048

SMITHTOWN—Suffolk County

□ **ST. CATHERINE OF SIENA MEDICAL CENTER (330401)**, 50 Route 25–A, Zip 11787–1398; tel. 631/862–3000, (Total facility includes 240 beds in nursing home–type unit) (Nonreporting) **A**1 9 10 **S** Catholic Health Services of Long Island
Primary Contact: Sharon A. Kennish, Executive Director and Administrative Officer
COO: Nancy B. Simmons, Senior Vice President and Chief Operating Officer
CFO: Ronald Steimel, Director Financial Operations
CMO: Augustus Mantia, M.D., Vice President Medical Affairs
Web address: www.stcatherinemedicalcenter.org
Control: Church–operated, Nongovernment, not–for profit **Service:** General Medical and Surgical

Staffed Beds: 503

SOUTHAMPTON—Suffolk County

□ **SOUTHAMPTON HOSPITAL (330340)**, 240 Meeting House Lane, Zip 11968–5090; tel. 631/726–8200 **A**1 9 10 **F**3 8 11 12 13 15 25 27 30 31 32 33 35 38 42 43 46 49 53 54 55 56 57 59 60 62 63 66 68 72 73 74 75 76 77 79 80 81 82 84 86 87 90 96 97 99 100 106 107 112 119 120 121 124 132 133 134 135 136 137 **P**5 6
Primary Contact: Robert S. Chaloner, President and Chief Executive Officer
CFO: Chris Schulteis, Chief Financial Officer
CMO: Frederic Weinbaum, M.D., Executive Vice President Operations and Chief Medical Officer
CIO: William Bifulco, Chief Information Officer
CHR: Paul Davin, Vice President Human Resources
Web address: www.southamptonhospital.org
Control: Other not–for–profit (including NFP Corporation) **Service:** General Medical and Surgical

Staffed Beds: 80 **Admissions:** 5807 **Census:** 57 **Outpatient Visits:** 520370 **Births:** 844 **Total Expense ($000):** 81521 **Payroll Expense ($000):** 36030 **Personnel:** 712

SPRINGVILLE—Erie County

BERTRAND CHAFFEE HOSPITAL (330111), 224 East Main Street, Zip 14141–1497; tel. 716/592–2871, (Total facility includes 80 beds in nursing home–type unit) **A**9 10 **F**3 15 17 24 38 42 56 62 67 73 75 77 79 80 86 96 97 100 107 117 119 136
Primary Contact: Paul A. DeSantis, Chief Executive Officer
COO: Paul A. DeSantis, Chief Executive Officer
CFO: George Vasiliouskas, Interim Chief Financial Officer
CMO: Priscilla Dale, M.D., President Medical Staff
CHR: Mary Beth Brown, Director Human Resources
Web address: www.chaffeehospitalandhome.com
Control: Other not–for–profit (including NFP Corporation) **Service:** General Medical and Surgical

Staffed Beds: 104 **Admissions:** 1359 **Census:** 91 **Outpatient Visits:** 38000 **Births:** 0 **Total Expense ($000):** 12001 **Payroll Expense ($000):** 6270 **Personnel:** 175

STAR LAKE—St. Lawrence County

★ **CLIFTON–FINE HOSPITAL (331307)**, Oswegatchie Trail, Zip 13690, Mailing Address: P.O. Box 10, Zip 13690–0010; tel. 315/848–3351, (Total facility includes 11 beds in nursing home–type unit) (Nonreporting) **A**9 10 18
Primary Contact: Roger A. Masse, FACHE, Chief Executive Officer
COO: Roger A. Masse, FACHE, Chief Executive Officer
CFO: Nancy Russell, Chief Accounting
CMO: David Welch, M.D., Medical Director
CIO: Nancy Russell, Chief Accounting
Web address: www.northnet.org
Control: Other not–for–profit (including NFP Corporation) **Service:** General Medical and Surgical

Staffed Beds: 20

STATEN ISLAND—Richmond County, See New York City

STONY BROOK—Suffolk County

★ □ **STONY BROOK UNIVERSITY HOSPITAL (330393)**, State University of New York, Zip 11794–8410; tel. 631/689–8333 **A**1 2 3 5 8 9 10 **F**3 6 7 8 11 13 14 15 16 17 18 20 22 24 25 26 27 28 30 31 32 33 34 35 37 38 40 43 44 46 48 49 50 51 53 54 55 56 57 58 59 60 62 63 64 66 68 70 71 72 73 74 75 76 77 78 79 80 81 82 83 84 86 87 88 89 90 91 92 93 94 95 96 97 99 100 102 103 105 106 107 108 109 111 112 113 114 116 118 119 120 121 124 125 127 130 132 134 135 136 137
Primary Contact: Steven Strongwater, M.D., President and Chief Executive Officer
COO: Fred S. Sganga, CHE, Chief Operating Officer
CFO: Dennis Mitchell, Chief Financial Officer
CMO: Thomas Biancaniello, Chief Medical Officer
CIO: Dennis Proul, Chief Information Officer
Web address: www.stonybrookmedicalcenter.org
Control: State–Government, nonfederal **Service:** General Medical and Surgical

Staffed Beds: 536 **Admissions:** 28891 **Census:** 446 **Outpatient Visits:** 268609 **Births:** 3363 **Total Expense ($000):** 685494 **Payroll Expense ($000):** 301078 **Personnel:** 4990

SUFFERN—Rockland County

★ □ **GOOD SAMARITAN HOSPITAL (330158)**, 255 Lafayette Avenue, Zip 10901–4869; tel. 845/368–5000, (Nonreporting) **A**1 2 9 10 **S** Bon Secours Health System, Inc.
Primary Contact: Dominick M. Stanzione, Chief Executive Officer
COO: Joseph J. Cassidy, Vice President Operations
CFO: Stephen D. Majetich, CPA, Chief Financial Officer
CMO: William K. Cors, M.D., Vice President Medical Affairs
CHR: Elizabeth Savage, Senior Vice President Human Resources
Web address: www.goodsamhosp.org
Control: Church–operated, Nongovernment, not–for profit **Service:** General Medical and Surgical

Staffed Beds: 308

SYOSSET—Nassau County

★ □ **NORTH SHORE UNIVERSITY HOSPITAL AT SYOSSET**, 221 Jericho Turnpike, Zip 11791–4567; tel. 516/496–6400 **A**1 9 **F**3 12 15 25 26 30 31 32 33 34 36 38 40 41 43 44 50 55 56 57 58 62 63 66 68 72 73 77 79 80 82 87 88 90 91 92 96 97 107 119 121 124 135 **P**6 **S** North Shore–LIJ Health System
Primary Contact: Deborah Tascone, RN, M.S., Executive Director
COO: Mark J. Solazzo, Regional Chief Operating Officer
CFO: Richard Reilly, Assistant Administrator Finance
CMO: Randolph DiLorenzo, M.D., Medical Director
CIO: Charles M. Trunz, Chief Information Officer and Chief Administrative Officer
CHR: Rosemarie Milano, Chief Human Resources Director
Web address: www.northshorelij.com
Control: Other not–for–profit (including NFP Corporation) **Service:** General Medical and Surgical

Staffed Beds: 79 **Admissions:** 4577 **Census:** 64 **Outpatient Visits:** 37605 **Births:** 0 **Total Expense ($000):** 88575 **Payroll Expense ($000):** 41818 **Personnel:** 522

SYRACUSE—Onondaga County

★ □ **COMMUNITY–GENERAL HOSPITAL OF GREATER SYRACUSE (330159)**, 4900 Broad Road, Zip 13215–2293; tel. 315/492–5011, (Total facility includes 50 beds in nursing home–type unit) **A**1 3 5 9 10 **F**1 3 11 12 13 15 18 25 26 27 30 31 32 38 47 49 50 55 56 57 62 66 68 72 73 74 75 76 77 79 80 81 85 86 88 95 96 97 102 106 107 117 118 119 124 135 137
Primary Contact: Thomas P. Quinn, President and Chief Executive Officer
CFO: Pamela Johnson, Corporate Vice President and Chief Financial Officer
CMO: Andrew Merritt, M.D., Acting Senior Vice President Medical Affairs
CIO: Mitchell P. Rozonkiewiecz, Corporate Vice President Information Systems
CHR: Lisa Dittrich, Director Human Resources
Web address: www.cgh.org
Control: Other not–for–profit (including NFP Corporation) **Service:** General Medical and Surgical

Staffed Beds: 252 **Admissions:** 9460 **Census:** 174 **Outpatient Visits:** 76249 **Births:** 1296 **Total Expense ($000):** 117262 **Payroll Expense ($000):** 51618 **Personnel:** 923

★ □ **CROUSE HOSPITAL (330203)**, 736 Irving Avenue, Zip 13210–1690; tel. 315/470–7111, (Nonreporting) **A**1 3 5 6 9 10
Primary Contact: Paul J. Kronenberg, M.D., President and Chief Executive Officer
CFO: Kimberly Boynton, Chief Financial Officer
CMO: Ronald Stahl, M.D., Chief Medical Officer
CIO: Marc Gibbs, Chief Information Officer
Web address: www.crouse.org
Control: Other not–for–profit (including NFP Corporation) **Service:** General Medical and Surgical

Staffed Beds: 576

□ **RICHARD H. HUTCHINGS PSYCHIATRIC CENTER (334001)**, 620 Madison Street, Zip 13210–2319; tel. 315/426–3632, (Nonreporting) **A**1 3 5 10 **S** New York State Office of Mental Health
Primary Contact: Colleen Sawyer, Executive Director
COO: David Peppel, Director Operations
CMO: David K. Frey, M.D., Clinical Director
CIO: Don Fredericks, Administrator Facility Information Center
CHR: Katherine Herron, Director Human Resources
Web address: www.omh.state.ny.us
Control: State–Government, nonfederal **Service:** Psychiatric

Staffed Beds: 131

□ **ST. JOSEPH'S HOSPITAL HEALTH CENTER (330140)**, 301 Prospect Avenue, Zip 13203–1895; tel. 315/448–5111, (Nonreporting) **A**1 3 5 9 10 **S** Sisters of Saint Francis
Primary Contact: Theodore M. Pasinski, President
CFO: Michael Shaffer, Vice President Fiscal Services
CMO: Dennis Ehrich, M.D., Vice President Medical Affairs
CIO: Charles Fennell, Vice President Information Management
CHR: Frank Panzetta, Director Human Resources
Web address: www.sjhsyr.org
Control: Other not–for–profit (including NFP Corporation) **Service:** General Medical and Surgical

Staffed Beds: 431

★ □ **UPSTATE MEDICAL UNIVERSITY (330241)**, 750 East Adams Street, Zip 13210–2399; tel. 315/464–5540 **A**1 2 8 9 10 **F**3 9 11 12 15 16 17 18 19 20 21 22 23 24 25 26 27 28 31 32 33 36 37 38 40 41 43 44 46 47 48 49 50 51 53 54 55 56 57 58 59 60 62 64 66 68 72 73 75 76 77 79 80 81 82 83 84 85 86 87 88 89 90 91 92 93 94 96 97 99 100 102 103 105 106 107 108 109 111 112 113 114 116 119 120 121 123 124 125 127 131 135 136 137 **P**7
Primary Contact: Phillip S. Schaengold, J.D., Chief Executive Officer and Senior Vice President for Hospital Affairs
COO: Paul E. Seale, FACHE, Chief Operating Officer
CFO: Stuart M. Wright, CPA, Chief Financial Officer
CMO: Colleen O'Leary, M.D., Medical Director
CIO: Terry Wagner, Chief Information Officer
CHR: Eric Frost, Associate Vice President Human Resources
Web address: www.universityhospital.org/
Control: State–Government, nonfederal **Service:** General Medical and Surgical

Staffed Beds: 347 **Admissions:** 16213 **Census:** 297 **Outpatient Visits:** 391056 **Births:** 0 **Total Expense ($000):** 472423 **Payroll Expense ($000):** 189226 **Personnel:** 3571

NY

Hospital, Medicare Provider Number, Address, Telephone, Approval, Facility, and Physician Codes, Health Care System
★ American Hospital Association (AHA) membership
□ The Joint Commission accreditation
○ American Osteopathic Association (AOA) accreditation
△ Commission on Accreditation of Rehabilitation Facilities (CARF) accreditation

★ △ **VETERANS AFFAIRS MEDICAL CENTER**, 800 Irving Avenue, Zip 13210–2796; tel. 315/425–4400, (Total facility includes 48 beds in nursing home–type unit) **A**1 3 5 7 8 9 **F**2 3 5 17 18 24 26 27 30 33 34 36 37 38 41 42 43 44 45 46 49 50 51 53 54 55 57 59 60 61 62 68 72 73 75 76 77 79 80 81 82 85 86 87 88 90 91 92 93 94 96 97 100 101 102 106 107 118 119 121 124 132 135 136 137 **P**6 **S** Department of Veterans Affairs
Primary Contact: James Cody, Director
COO: Michael J. Swartz, Associate Medical Center Director
CFO: Marcia Wadsworth, Chief Financial Officer
CMO: William Marx, M.D., Chief of Staff
CIO: James Nichols, Chief Information Officer
CHR: Mark Antinelli, Human Resources Manager
Web address: www.va.gov/sta/guide/home.asp
Control: Veterans Affairs, Government, federal **Service:** General Medical and Surgical

Staffed Beds: 167 **Admissions:** 4118 **Census:** 85 **Outpatient Visits:** 314375 **Births:** 0 **Total Expense ($000):** 179157 **Payroll Expense ($000):** 105780 **Personnel:** 1470

TICONDEROGA—Essex County

★ **MOSES LUDINGTON HOSPITAL (331306)**, 1019 Wicker Street, Zip 12883–1097; tel. 518/585–2831 **A**9 10 18 **F**8 24 30 31 32 37 38 42 55 62 75 79 86 96 107 118 119 122 132 134
Primary Contact: Kevin Haughney, Chief Executive Officer
COO: Kevin Haughney, Chief Executive Officer and Chief Financial Officer
CFO: Kevin Haughney, Chief Executive Officer and Chief Financial Officer
CMO: Robert Holterman, M.D., Medical Director
CIO: Lisa Busby, Manager Information Systems
Web address: www.mosesludington.com
Control: Other not–for–profit (including NFP Corporation) **Service:** General Medical and Surgical

Staffed Beds: 15 **Admissions:** 310 **Census:** 6 **Outpatient Visits:** 7574 **Births:** 0 **Total Expense ($000):** 11501 **Payroll Expense ($000):** 5593 **Personnel:** 136

TROY—Rensselaer County

SAMARITAN HOSPITAL (330180), 2215 Burdett Avenue, Zip 12180–2475; tel. 518/271–3300, (Nonreporting) **A**5 9 10
Primary Contact: Norman E. Dascher, Jr., Chief Executive Officer
COO: Karen Tassey, Chief Operating Officer
CFO: Lori Santos, Vice President Finance
CMO: Daniel Kopp, M.D., Senior Vice President Medical Affairs
CIO: Robert J. Duthe, Vice President Corporate Management Information Systems
CHR: Barbara McCandless, Corporate Vice President Human Resources
Web address: www.nehealth.com
Control: Other not–for–profit (including NFP Corporation) **Service:** General Medical and Surgical

Staffed Beds: 238

SETON HEALTH SYSTEM See St. Mary's Hospital

★ **ST. MARY'S HOSPITAL (330232)**, (Formerly Seton Health System), 1300 Massachusetts Avenue, Zip 12180–1695; tel. 518/268–5000 **A**1 9 10 **F**2 4 5 8 11 13 15 17 18 24 25 26 27 30 31 32 33 34 36 37 38 42 43 44 50 51 53 54 60 62 66 68 72 73 74 75 76 77 78 79 80 81 82 84 96 97 99 100 102 103 107 117 118 119 121 134 135 136 **P**6 **S** Ascension Health
Primary Contact: Gino J. Pazzaglini, FACHE, President and Chief Executive Officer
COO: Frederick H. Kuriger, Executive Vice President and Chief Operating Officer
CFO: Scott St George, Senior Vice President and Chief Financial Officer
CMO: Richard Rubin, M.D., Chief Medical Officer
CIO: Robert Charbonneau, Senior Vice President Operations
CHR: Kathleen Occhiogrosso, Vice President Human Resources
Web address: www.setonhealth.org
Control: Other not–for–profit (including NFP Corporation) **Service:** General Medical and Surgical

Staffed Beds: 177 **Admissions:** 8372 **Census:** 114 **Outpatient Visits:** 457813 **Births:** 656 **Total Expense ($000):** 119363 **Payroll Expense ($000):** 60875 **Personnel:** 1301

UTICA—Oneida County

★ △ **FAXTON–ST. LUKE'S HEALTHCARE (330044)**, 1676 Sunset Avenue, Zip 13502–5475, Mailing Address: P.O. Box 479, Zip 13503–0479; tel. 315/624–6000, (Includes FAXTON CAMPUS; ST. LUKE'S CAMPUS, Mailing Address: P.O. Box 479, Zip 13503–0479; tel. 315/624–6000) **A**1 2 7 9 10 **F**3 12 13 15 17 18 20 24 25 26 27 28 31 32 33 37 38 43 44 45 49 50 55 56 57 59 62 63 65 66 68 71 73 74 75 76 77 79 80 84 85 86 87 88 92 96 97 99 100 102 104 106 107 108 109 111 112 119 121 124 133 135 136
Primary Contact: Keith A. Fenstemacher, President and Chief Executive Officer
COO: Scott H. Perra, Executive Vice President and Chief Operating Officer
CFO: Michael Haile, Senior Vice President Finance
CMO: Daniel Kopp, M.D., Senior Vice President and Medical Director
CIO: Kevin Mahoney, Vice President and Chief Information Officer
CHR: Tony Scibelli, Vice President Human Resources
Web address: www.mvnhealth.com
Control: Other not–for–profit (including NFP Corporation) **Service:** General Medical and Surgical

Staffed Beds: 319 **Admissions:** 16228 **Census:** 236 **Outpatient Visits:** 305874 **Births:** 2186 **Total Expense ($000):** 221811 **Payroll Expense ($000):** 97762 **Personnel:** 2174

☐ **MOHAWK VALLEY PSYCHIATRIC CENTER (334021)**, 1400 Noyes Street, Zip 13502–3803; tel. 315/738–3800, (Nonreporting) **A**1 10 **S** New York State Office of Mental Health
Primary Contact: Collen A. Sawyer, RN, M.S.N., Executive Director
Web address: www.omh.state.ny.us/omhweb/facilities/mvpc/facility.htm
Control: State–Government, nonfederal **Service:** Psychiatric

Staffed Beds: 614

★ **ST. ELIZABETH MEDICAL CENTER (330245)**, 2209 Genesee Street, Zip 13501–5999; tel. 315/798–8100 **A**1 6 9 10 12 13 **F**3 11 12 15 17 18 20 22 24 25 26 27 28 30 31 32 34 35 38 40 49 50 55 57 60 61 62 63 64 66 68 72 73 75 76 77 79 80 82 84 86 87 88 89 90 92 93 96 97 99 102 106 107 118 119 120 121 135 136 137 **P**6 **S** Sisters of Saint Francis
Primary Contact: Sister M. Johanna DeLelys, President and Chief Executive Officer
COO: Matthew D. Babcock, Chief Operating Officer
CFO: Louis Aiello, Chief Financial Officer
CMO: Albert D'Accurzio, Medical Director
CIO: Robert Gillette, Chief Information Officer
CHR: Patrick Buckley, Vice President Human Resources
Web address: www.stemc.org
Control: Church–operated, Nongovernment, not–for profit **Service:** General Medical and Surgical

Staffed Beds: 190 **Admissions:** 11469 **Census:** 167 **Outpatient Visits:** 426514 **Births:** 0 **Total Expense ($000):** 173900 **Payroll Expense ($000):** 80145 **Personnel:** 1695

ST. LUKE'S CAMPUS See Faxton–St. Luke's Healthcare

VALHALLA—Westchester County

★ **BLYTHEDALE CHILDREN'S HOSPITAL (333301)**, 95 Bradhurst Avenue, Zip 10595–1697; tel. 914/592–7555, (Nonreporting) **A**1 10
Primary Contact: Larry L. Levine, President and Chief Executive Officer
COO: Maureen Desimone, Chief Operating Officer
CFO: John Canning, Chief Financial Officer
CMO: Joelle Mast, Ph.D., M.D., Chief Medical Officer
CHR: Ronald Gallo, Director Human Resources
Web address: www.blythedale.org
Control: Other not–for–profit (including NFP Corporation) **Service:** Children's rehabilitation

Staffed Beds: 92

☐ **WESTCHESTER MEDICAL CENTER (330234)**, Valhalla Campus, Zip 10595–1696; tel. 914/493–7000, (Total facility includes 275 beds in nursing home–type unit) (Nonreporting) **A**1 3 5 8 9 10
Primary Contact: Michael D. Israel, President and Chief Executive Officer
COO: Gary F. Brudnicki, Executive Vice President, Chief Operating Officer and Chief Financial Officer
CFO: Gary F. Brudnicki, Executive Vice President, Chief Operating Officer and Chief Financial Officer
CMO: Renee Garrick, M.D., Chief Medical Officer
CHR: Thomas Fentner, Acting Director Human Resources
Web address: www.wcmc.com
Control: Hospital district or authority, Government, nonfederal **Service:** General Medical and Surgical

Staffed Beds: 910

VALLEY STREAM—Nassau County

☒ **FRANKLIN HOSPITAL (330372)**, 900 Franklin Avenue, Zip 11580–2190; tel. 516/256–6000, (Total facility includes 120 beds in nursing home–type unit) **A**1 2 9 10 **F**2 3 11 15 17 25 26 27 30 31 32 38 40 42 43 45 49 50 54 55 57 58 59 61 62 63 66 68 72 73 75 76 77 79 80 81 82 84 87 88 89 90 92 93 96 97 100 102 106 107 117 119 124 132 135 136 137 **P**6 **S** North Shore–LIJ Health System
Primary Contact: Deborah Tascone, RN, M.S., Executive Director
CFO: Elizabeth Zubko, Associate Executive Director Finance
CMO: Jack Rubenstein, M.D., Medical Director
CIO: Nicholas O'Connor, Chief Information Officer
CHR: Stacie Caplan, Director Human Resources
Web address: www.fhmc.org
Control: Other not–for–profit (including NFP Corporation) **Service:** General Medical and Surgical

Staffed Beds: 356 **Admissions:** 11824 **Census:** 305 **Outpatient Visits:** 233346 **Births:** 0 **Total Expense ($000):** 159885 **Payroll Expense ($000):** 76732 **Personnel:** 1099

WALTON—Delaware County

★ **DELAWARE VALLEY HOSPITAL (331312)**, 1 Titus Place, Zip 13856–1498; tel. 607/865–2100 **A**9 10 18 **F**4 8 11 15 24 25 26 30 31 32 33 38 46 53 63 73 75 79 82 86 87 96 107 119 120 122 124 132 134 135 136 137 **P**6 **S** United Health Services
Primary Contact: David J. Polge, President and Chief Executive Officer
CFO: Paul Summers, Chief Financial Officer
CHR: David J. Polge, President and Chief Executive Officer
Web address: www.uhs.net
Control: Other not–for–profit (including NFP Corporation) **Service:** General Medical and Surgical

Staffed Beds: 25 **Admissions:** 884 **Census:** 15 **Outpatient Visits:** 90099 **Births:** 0 **Total Expense ($000):** 13084 **Payroll Expense ($000):** 7526 **Personnel:** 153

WARSAW—Wyoming County

☐ **WYOMING COUNTY COMMUNITY HOSPITAL (330008)**, 400 North Main Street, Zip 14569–1025; tel. 585/786–2233, (Total facility includes 160 beds in nursing home–type unit) **A**1 9 10 20 **F**13 24 25 31 32 38 49 55 57 62 66 74 75 77 79 80 82 84 86 88 92 96 100 107 117 119 121 122 124 135
Primary Contact: Ronald J. Krawiec, Administrator and Chief Executive Officer
CFO: Paul H. Brozyna, Chief Financial Officer
CIO: Jane Beechler, Director Healthcare Information Systems
Web address: www.wcchs.net
Control: County–Government, nonfederal **Service:** General Medical and Surgical

Staffed Beds: 235 **Admissions:** 2841 **Census:** 184 **Outpatient Visits:** 46564 **Births:** 331 **Total Expense ($000):** 36602 **Payroll Expense ($000):** 19317 **Personnel:** 499

WARWICK—Orange County

☒ **ST. ANTHONY COMMUNITY HOSPITAL (330205)**, 15 Maple Avenue, Zip 10990–5180; tel. 845/987–5173, (Nonreporting) **A**1 9 10 **S** Bon Secours Health System, Inc.
Primary Contact: Thomas R. Brunelle, Executive Vice President and Administrator
CFO: John Whitesel, Senior Vice President and Chief Financial Officer
Web address: www.stanthonycommunityhosp.org
Control: Church–operated, Nongovernment, not–for profit **Service:** General Medical and Surgical

Staffed Beds: 73

WATERTOWN—Jefferson County

☒ **SAMARITAN MEDICAL CENTER (330157)**, 830 Washington Street, Zip 13601–4066; tel. 315/785–4000 **A**1 3 5 9 10 12 13 **F**5 8 13 15 18 25 26 27 31 32 33 38 49 51 55 59 62 66 68 71 72 73 74 75 76 77 79 82 84 85 86 87 88 89 90 92 93 94 96 97 100 102 104 107 108 109 118 119 124 135 136 137 **P**6
Primary Contact: Thomas H. Carman, President and Chief Executive Officer
CFO: Paul Kraeger, Vice President Finance and Chief Financial Officer
CMO: Spencer P. Falcon, M.D., Vice President Medical Affairs
CIO: Edward Ricks, Vice President Information Services
CHR: Lynda Goldman, Vice President Human Resources
Web address: www.samaritanhealth.com
Control: Other not–for–profit (including NFP Corporation) **Service:** General Medical and Surgical

Staffed Beds: 228 **Admissions:** 7681 **Census:** 141 **Outpatient Visits:** 221784 **Births:** 1615 **Total Expense ($000):** 131136 **Payroll Expense ($000):** 61731 **Personnel:** 1185

WELLSVILLE—Allegany County

☒ **JONES MEMORIAL HOSPITAL (330096)**, 191 North Main Street, Zip 14895–1197, Mailing Address: P.O. Box 72, Zip 14895–0072; tel. 585/593–1100 **A**1 9 10 20 **F**8 11 13 15 17 24 25 26 27 30 31 32 33 38 40 43 60 62 68 73 74 75 76 77 79 80 81 84 86 87 96 102 107 120 121 122 135
Primary Contact: Eva Benedict, President and Chief Executive Officer
CFO: Robert Bruckner, Chief Financial Officer
Web address: www.jmhny.org
Control: Other not–for–profit (including NFP Corporation) **Service:** General Medical and Surgical

Staffed Beds: 70 **Admissions:** 2469 **Census:** 25 **Outpatient Visits:** 111278 **Births:** 368 **Total Expense ($000):** 30810 **Payroll Expense ($000):** 15054 **Personnel:** 332

WEST HAVERSTRAW—Rockland County

☐ △ **HELEN HAYES HOSPITAL (330405)**, Route 9W, Zip 10993–1195; tel. 845/786–4000, (Total facility includes 25 beds in nursing home–type unit) **A**1 5 7 10 **F**9 24 25 26 31 32 33 37 41 52 55 56 57 58 62 63 72 75 77 79 81 82 85 86 90 107 117 119 121 135 136 137 **P**6
Primary Contact: Magdalena Ramirez, Chief Executive Officer
COO: Edmund Coletti, Chief Operating Officer
CFO: Richard Buhowski, Chief Financial Officer
CMO: John T. Pellicone, M.D., Medical Director
CIO: Virgil Ennis, Chief Information Officer
CHR: Kathleen Martucci, Director Human Resources
Web address: www.helenhayeshospital.org
Control: State–Government, nonfederal **Service:** Rehabilitation

Staffed Beds: 155 **Admissions:** 2591 **Census:** 110 **Outpatient Visits:** 67784 **Births:** 0 **Total Expense ($000):** 68130 **Payroll Expense ($000):** 30213 **Personnel:** 638

WEST ISLIP—Suffolk County

☒ **GOOD SAMARITAN HOSPITAL MEDICAL CENTER (330286)**, 1000 Montauk Highway, Zip 11795–4958; tel. 631/376–3000, (Total facility includes 100 beds in nursing home–type unit) (Nonreporting) **A**1 2 9 10 12 13 **S** Catholic Health Services of Long Island
Primary Contact: William Allison, President and Chief Executive Officer
COO: Charles Bove, Chief Administrative Officer
CFO: John Pohlman, Interim Vice President and Chief Financial Officer
CMO: M. Abul Fazal, M.D., Senior Vice President Medical Affairs
CIO: Marcy Dunn, Vice President and Chief Information Officer
CHR: Lori Spina, Vice President Human Resources
Web address: www.good–samaritan–hospital.org
Control: Church–operated, Nongovernment, not–for profit **Service:** General Medical and Surgical

Staffed Beds: 531

WEST POINT—Orange County

☒ **KELLER ARMY COMMUNITY HOSPITAL**, 900 Washington Road, Zip 10996–1197; tel. 845/938–5169, (Nonreporting) **A**1 **S** Department of the Army, Office of the Surgeon General
Primary Contact: Colonel Van Coots, Commanding Officer
COO: Lieutenant Colonel Scott F. Cass, Deputy Commander Administration
CMO: Lieutenant Colonel Italo Bastianelli, Deputy Commander for Clinical Services
CIO: Patrick McGuinness, Chief Information Management
CHR: Captain Alex L. Hayman, Chief Human Resources
Web address: www.usma.edu/meddac/
Control: Army, Government, federal **Service:** General Medical and Surgical

Staffed Beds: 31

WEST SENECA—Erie County

☐ **WESTERN NEW YORK CHILDREN'S PSYCHIATRIC CENTER**, 1010 East and West Road, Zip 14224–3698; tel. 716/677–7000, (Nonreporting) **A**1 3 5 **S** New York State Office of Mental Health
Primary Contact: Kathe Hayes, Executive Director
COO: David Privett, Deputy Director
CFO: Steven Cobb, Business Officer
CMO: Patrick Stein, M.D., Clinical Director
CIO: Dan Hrubiak, Associate Computer Program Analyst
CHR: Charles Siewert, Director Human Resources
Web address: www.omh.state.ny.us
Control: State–Government, nonfederal **Service:** Children's hospital psychiatric

Staffed Beds: 46

Hospital, Medicare Provider Number, Address, Telephone, Approval, Facility, and Physician Codes, Health Care System

★ American Hospital Association (AHA) membership
☐ The Joint Commission accreditation
○ American Osteopathic Association (AOA) accreditation
△ Commission on Accreditation of Rehabilitation Facilities (CARF) accreditation

WESTFIELD—Chautauqua County

★ **WESTFIELD MEMORIAL HOSPITAL (330166)**, 189 East Main Street, Zip 14787–1195; tel. 716/326–4921, (Nonreporting) **A**9 10 **S** St. Vincent Health System
Primary Contact: C. Angela Bontempo, President and Chief Executive Officer
CFO: Henry J. Ward, Vice President and Chief Financial Officer
CMO: Russell Elwell, M.D., Medical Director
CIO: Cindy Harper, Director Information Systems
CHR: Christine Schuyler, Vice President Administration and Director Human Resources
Web address: www.wmhinc.org
Control: Other not–for–profit (including NFP Corporation) **Service:** General Medical and Surgical

Staffed Beds: 19

WHITE PLAINS—Westchester County

★ △ **BURKE REHABILITATION HOSPITAL (330404)**, 785 Mamaroneck Avenue, Zip 10605–2593; tel. 914/597–2500, (Nonreporting) **A**1 5 7 10
Primary Contact: Mary Beth Walsh, M.D., Chief Executive Officer
COO: Brian Swift, Senior Administrator Plant Operations
CFO: John Stewart, Director Finance
CMO: Mary Beth Walsh, M.D., Chief Executive Officer
CIO: Ken Kupetsky, Senior Administrator Information Systems
CHR: Marlo Asencio, Senior Administrator Human Resources
Web address: www.burke.org
Control: Other not–for–profit (including NFP Corporation) **Service:** Rehabilitation

Staffed Beds: 150

NEW YORK–PRESBYTERIAN HOSPITAL, WESTCHESTER DIVISION See New York–Presbyterian Hospital, New York

★ **WHITE PLAINS HOSPITAL CENTER (330304)**, Davis Avenue and Post Road, Zip 10601–4699; tel. 914/681–0600 **A**1 2 9 10 **F**3 11 12 13 14 15 17 25 26 27 30 31 32 33 34 38 43 44 46 47 48 49 50 54 55 56 57 58 59 60 61 62 63 66 68 70 71 72 73 74 75 76 77 79 80 81 82 84 86 87 89 90 92 94 96 97 99 100 101 102 103 104 105 106 107 109 116 118 119 121 134 135 137 **P**2 5 8
Primary Contact: Jon B. Schandler, President and Chief Executive Officer
CFO: John Sciurba, Vice President and Chief Financial Officer
CMO: Lawrence J. Kadish, M.D., Executive Vice President and Medical Director
CHR: John Sanchez, Acting Director Human Resources
Web address: www.wphospital.org
Control: Other not–for–profit (including NFP Corporation) **Service:** General Medical and Surgical

Staffed Beds: 292 **Admissions:** 13974 **Census:** 218 **Outpatient Visits:** 155713 **Births:** 2105 **Total Expense ($000):** 235392 **Payroll Expense ($000):** 113320 **Personnel:** 1662

WILLIAMSVILLE—Erie County

MILLARD FILLMORE SUBURBAN HOSPITAL See KALEIDA Health, Buffalo

YONKERS—Westchester County

ANDRUS PAVILION See St. John's Riverside Hospital

PARKCARE PAVILION See St. John's Riverside Hospital

☐ **ST. JOHN'S RIVERSIDE HOSPITAL (330208)**, 967 North Broadway, Zip 10701–1399; tel. 914/964–4444, (Includes ANDRUS PAVILION, 967 North Broadway, tel. 914/964–4444; PARKCARE PAVILION, Two Park Avenue, Zip 10703–3497; tel. 914/964–7300), (Total facility includes 120 beds in nursing home–type unit) (Nonreporting) **A**1 9 10
Primary Contact: James Foy, President and Chief Executive Officer
COO: Lynn M. Nelson, R.N., Chief Operating Officer
CFO: Dennis M. Keane, Vice President Finance and Chief Financial Officer
CMO: Paul Antonecchia, M.D., Vice President Medical Affairs
CIO: Peter Weidner, Director Management Information Systems
CHR: Pam LaFrance, Vice President Human Resources
Web address: www.riversidehealth.org
Control: Other not–for–profit (including NFP Corporation) **Service:** General Medical and Surgical

Staffed Beds: 504

★ **ST. JOSEPH'S MEDICAL CENTER (330006)**, 127 South Broadway, Zip 10701–4080; tel. 914/378–7000, (Total facility includes 200 beds in nursing home–type unit) **A**1 3 5 9 10 **F**2 3 5 8 11 12 15 25 26 27 28 30 31 32 33 37 38 46 47 48 49 51 53 54 55 56 57 59 60 61 62 63 64 66 68 72 73 75 76 77 78 79 80 82 84 86 87 88 90 91 93 94 95 96 97 99 100 102 103 107 115 117 119 132 133 135 136 **P**8
Primary Contact: Michael J. Spicer, President and Chief Executive Officer
CFO: James J. Curcuruto, Senior Vice President Finance
CMO: Nicholas De Robertis, M.D., Medical Director
CIO: Deborah Di Bernardo, Chief Information Officer
CHR: Dean Civitello, Vice President Human Resources
Web address: www.saintjosephs.org
Control: Other not–for–profit (including NFP Corporation) **Service:** General Medical and Surgical

Staffed Beds: 386 **Admissions:** 7779 **Census:** 337 **Outpatient Visits:** 330545 **Births:** 0 **Total Expense ($000):** 143849 **Payroll Expense ($000):** 65485 **Personnel:** 1401

NORTH CAROLINA

AHOSKIE—Hertford County

★ **ROANOKE–CHOWAN HOSPITAL (340099)**, 500 South Academy Street, Zip 27910–3261, Mailing Address: P.O. Box 1385, Zip 27910–1385; tel. 252/209–3000 **A**1 9 10 20 **F**3 11 13 15 24 25 26 27 28 30 31 32 33 38 43 46 52 54 55 56 57 62 68 72 74 75 76 77 79 80 82 84 86 87 88 90 92 93 94 96 97 99 100 102 107 118 119 121 124 133 135 136 **P**6 7 **S** University Health Systems of Eastern Carolina
Primary Contact: Susan S. Lassiter, President
CFO: Jon Graham, Chief Financial Officer
CHR: John Rankins, Director Human Resources
Web address: www.uhseast.com
Control: Other not–for–profit (including NFP Corporation) **Service:** General Medical and Surgical

Staffed Beds: 102 **Admissions:** 5373 **Census:** 59 **Outpatient Visits:** 65183 **Births:** 464 **Total Expense ($000):** 51857 **Payroll Expense ($000):** 21716 **Personnel:** 628

ALBEMARLE—Stanly County

★ **STANLY REGIONAL MEDICAL CENTER (340119)**, 301 Yadkin Street, Zip 28001–3448, Mailing Address: P.O. Box 1489, Zip 28002–1489; tel. 704/984–4000 **A**1 9 10 **F**3 11 13 17 18 24 25 26 27 31 32 33 37 38 49 55 56 57 59 60 61 62 66 68 72 73 74 75 76 77 79 80 81 84 85 86 88 90 91 92 93 94 96 97 100 102 107 111 118 119 120 121 124 135 137 **P**6
Primary Contact: Alfred P. Taylor, Chief Executive Officer
COO: Debra B. Smith, Senior Vice President and Chief Operating Officer
CFO: Nick Samilo, Vice President Fiscal Services and Chief Financial Officer
CMO: Leonard D. Saltzman, Chief of Staff
CIO: Brian Freeman, Vice President Ambulatory Services and Information Systems
CHR: Paul Morlock, Vice President Human Resources
Web address: www.stanly.org
Control: Other not–for–profit (including NFP Corporation) **Service:** General Medical and Surgical

Staffed Beds: 119 **Admissions:** 5046 **Census:** 52 **Outpatient Visits:** 80184 **Births:** 736 **Total Expense ($000):** 76808 **Payroll Expense ($000):** 28590 **Personnel:** 715

ASHEBORO—Randolph County

★ **RANDOLPH HOSPITAL (340123)**, 364 White Oak Street, Zip 27203–5400, Mailing Address: P.O. Box 1048, Zip 27204–1048; tel. 336/625–5151 **A**1 2 9 10 **F**3 13 15 18 24 25 26 28 31 32 33 37 38 41 44 48 49 50 55 56 57 60 61 62 63 66 68 69 72 73 74 75 76 77 78 79 80 81 82 84 86 87 96 98 100 102 103 106 107 118 119 121 124 135 137 **P**6
Primary Contact: Robert E. Morrison, President
CMO: Francisco Hodges, M.D., Chief of Staff
CIO: Angela Burgess, Chief Information Officer
Web address: www.randolphhospital.org
Control: Other not–for–profit (including NFP Corporation) **Service:** General Medical and Surgical

Staffed Beds: 136 **Admissions:** 6493 **Census:** 67 **Outpatient Visits:** 138739 **Births:** 923 **Total Expense ($000):** 83129 **Payroll Expense ($000):** 37608 **Personnel:** 912

ASHEVILLE—Buncombe County

ASHEVILLE SPECIALTY HOSPITAL (342017), 428 Biltmore Avenue, 4th Floor, Zip 28802; tel. 828/213–5400, (Nonreporting) **A**10
Primary Contact: Jay Cutspec, President and Chief Executive Officer
Web address: www.ashevillespecialtyhospital.org
Control: Corporation, Investor–owned, for–profit **Service:** Long–Term Acute Care hospital

Staffed Beds: 32

★ △ **CAREPARTNERS REHABILITATION HOSPITAL (343025)**, 68 Sweeten Creek Road, Zip 28803–1599, Mailing Address: P.O. Box 5779, Zip 28813–5779; tel. 828/277–4800 **A**1 7 10 **F**2 25 26 30 31 32 34 41 42 43 44 50 54 55 56 57 61 62 66 69 72 73 75 76 77 81 82 85 86 108 119 120 121 132 135 137 **P**5
Primary Contact: Charles D. Norvell, President and Chief Executive Officer
COO: Tracy Buchanan, Chief Operating Officer
CFO: Diann Bolick, Chief Financial Officer
CIO: Drake Thomas, Chief Information Officer
CHR: Karen Vernon–Young, Vice President Human Resources and Communications
Web address: www.thoms.org
Control: Other not–for–profit (including NFP Corporation) **Service:** Rehabilitation

Staffed Beds: 107 **Admissions:** 1727 **Census:** 68 **Outpatient Visits:** 289731 **Births:** 0 **Total Expense ($000):** 61244 **Payroll Expense ($000):** 36991 **Personnel:** 772

★ **MISSION HOSPITAL (340002)**, 509 Biltmore Avenue, Zip 28801–4690; tel. 828/213–1111, (Includes MEMORIAL MISSION HOSPITAL; ST. JOSEPH'S HOSPITAL, 428 Biltmore Avenue, Zip 28801–9839) **A**1 2 9 10 **F**3 7 8 11 12 13 15 17 18 20 22 24 25 26 27 28 30 31 32 33 34 35 37 38 40 41 43 44 46 47 48 49 50 51 52 53 54 55 56 57 58 59 60 61 62 63 64 66 68 69 70 71 72 73 74 75 76 77 78 79 80 81 82 83 84 86 87 88 89 90 91 92 93 94 95 96 97 99 100 102 103 104 105 106 107 108 109 111 112 114 116 118 119 120 121 123 124 131 132 133 135 136 137 **P**6
Primary Contact: Joseph F. Damore, President and Chief Executive Officer
COO: Brian W. Aston, Chief Operating Officer
CFO: Charles F. Ayscue, Senior Vice President Finance and Chief Financial Officer
CMO: George M. Bilbrey, M.D., Chief of Staff
CIO: D. Arlo Jennings, Ph.D., Chief Information Officer
CHR: Maria Roloff, Vice President Human Resources
Web address: www.missionhospitals.org
Control: Other not–for–profit (including NFP Corporation) **Service:** General Medical and Surgical

Staffed Beds: 730 **Admissions:** 38592 **Census:** 547 **Outpatient Visits:** 337380 **Births:** 4062 **Total Expense ($000):** 622207 **Payroll Expense ($000):** 261337 **Personnel:** 4818

★ **VETERANS AFFAIRS MEDICAL CENTER**, 1100 Tunnel Road, Zip 28805–2087; tel. 828/298–7911, (Total facility includes 80 beds in nursing home–type unit) **A**1 3 5 **F**3 4 5 8 17 18 20 22 24 25 26 27 33 34 36 37 38 41 42 43 44 46 49 50 53 54 55 56 57 58 60 61 62 63 64 66 68 72 73 75 76 77 78 79 81 82 86 87 88 89 90 91 92 93 94 95 96 97 100 101 102 103 107 108 119 121 122 124 135 136 137 **S** Department of Veterans Affairs
Primary Contact: Susan Pendergrass, Director
CMO: Mary Ann Curl, M.D., Interim Chief of Staff
CIO: Carla McLendon, Director Information Resource Management Services
CHR: Melissa Bragg, Chief Human Resources Management
Web address: www.va.gov/sta/guide/home.asp
Control: Veterans Affairs, Government, federal **Service:** General Medical and Surgical

Staffed Beds: 196 **Admissions:** 4100 **Census:** 164 **Outpatient Visits:** 32000 **Births:** 0

BELHAVEN—Beaufort County

PUNGO DISTRICT HOSPITAL (341310), 202 East Water Street, Zip 27810–9998; tel. 252/943–2111, (Total facility includes 10 beds in nursing home–type unit) **A**9 10 18 **F**11 13 15 25 26 30 31 32 38 46 50 55 56 57 62 63 68 73 75 79 82 86 94 96 102 107 117 118 119 122 132 135 137
Primary Contact: Kenneth E. Ragland, Chief Executive Officer
COO: Kenneth E. Ragland, Chief Executive Officer
CFO: Gerald Hardison, Director Finance
CMO: Mark Beamer, M.D., Chief of Staff
CIO: Jenny Brown, Director Human Resources
CHR: Jenny Brown, Director Human Resources
Control: Other not–for–profit (including NFP Corporation) **Service:** General Medical and Surgical

Staffed Beds: 35 **Admissions:** 942 **Census:** 16 **Outpatient Visits:** 13578 **Births:** 0 **Total Expense ($000):** 10534 **Payroll Expense ($000):** 5321 **Personnel:** 141

Hospital, Medicare Provider Number, Address, Telephone, Approval, Facility, and Physician Codes, Health Care System
★ American Hospital Association (AHA) membership
□ The Joint Commission accreditation
○ American Osteopathic Association (AOA) accreditation
△ Commission on Accreditation of Rehabilitation Facilities (CARF) accreditation

BLACK MOUNTAIN—Buncombe County

JULIAN F. KEITH ALCOHOL AND DRUG ABUSE TREATMENT CENTER (344023), 201 Tabernacle Road, Zip 28711–2599; tel. 828/669–3400, (Nonreporting) **A**10
Primary Contact: W. Douglas Baker, Director
CFO: Jackie Maurer, Fiscal Officer
CMO: Anthony Burnett, M.D., Medical Director
CHR: Faye Hamlin, Manager Human Resources
Web address: www.jfkadatc.net
Control: State–Government, nonfederal **Service:** Alcoholism and other chemical dependency

Staffed Beds: 110

BLOWING ROCK—Watauga County

★ **BLOWING ROCK HOSPITAL (341321)**, Chestnut Street, Zip 28605–0148, Mailing Address: Box 148, Zip 28605–0148; tel. 828/295–3136, (Includes DAVANT REHABILITATION AND EXTENDED CARE CENTER), (Total facility includes 72 beds in nursing home–type unit) **A**1 9 10 18 **F**2 37 38 55 57 61 62 82 86 96 117 119 122 133 135
Primary Contact: Timothy R. Ford, Chief Executive Officer
CMO: Charles Davant, M.D., Chief Medical Officer
CHR: Charles Lentz, Coordinator Human Resources
Web address: www.blowingrockhospital.org
Control: Other not–for–profit (including NFP Corporation) **Service:** General Medical and Surgical

Staffed Beds: 100 **Admissions:** 350 **Census:** 67 **Outpatient Visits:** 8960 **Births:** 0 **Total Expense ($000):** 9510 **Payroll Expense ($000):** 4850 **Personnel:** 124

BOILING SPRINGS—Cleveland County

CRAWLEY MEMORIAL HOSPITAL (340104), 315 West College Avenue, Zip 28017, Mailing Address: P.O. Box 996, Zip 28017–0996; tel. 704/434–9466, (Total facility includes 10 beds in nursing home–type unit) **A**9 10 **F**30 31 117 122 137 **S** Carolinas HealthCare System
Primary Contact: Angela M. Orsky, President
CFO: Elizabeth Presnell, Accountant
CMO: Julia Roos, M.D., Chief of Staff
Web address: www.carolinas.org
Control: Hospital district or authority, Government, nonfederal **Service:** Rehabilitation

Staffed Beds: 60 **Admissions:** 287 **Census:** 54 **Outpatient Visits:** 175 **Births:** 0 **Total Expense ($000):** 5374 **Payroll Expense ($000):** 2098 **Personnel:** 71

BOONE—Watauga County

★ **WATAUGA MEDICAL CENTER (340051)**, Deerfield Road, Zip 28607–2600, Mailing Address: P.O. Box 2600, Zip 28607–2600; tel. 828/262–4100 **A**1 2 9 10 19 **F**3 5 13 15 16 17 18 20 24 25 26 27 28 30 31 32 33 36 38 41 43 46 47 48 49 50 52 53 55 56 57 59 61 62 68 70 71 72 73 74 75 76 77 79 80 81 82 83 84 85 86 89 90 92 93 94 96 97 100 102 103 106 107 110 111 112 117 118 119 120 121 124 134 135 136 137 **P**6 7 8
Primary Contact: Richard G. Sparks, President
COO: John E. Barrett, Chief Operating Officer
CFO: Kevin May, Senior Vice President Finance
CMO: Herman A. Godwin, M.D., Senior Vice President and Medical Director
CIO: Mike Quinto, Chief Information Officer
CHR: Amy Crabbe, Vice President Human Resources
Web address: www.wataugamc.org
Control: Other not–for–profit (including NFP Corporation) **Service:** General Medical and Surgical

Staffed Beds: 101 **Admissions:** 5226 **Census:** 62 **Outpatient Visits:** 89419 **Births:** 615 **Total Expense ($000):** 87996 **Payroll Expense ($000):** 35797 **Personnel:** 807

BREVARD—Transylvania County

★ **TRANSYLVANIA COMMUNITY HOSPITAL (341319)**, Hospital Drive, Zip 28712–1116, Mailing Address: Box 1116, Zip 28712–1116; tel. 828/884–9111, (Total facility includes 10 beds in nursing home–type unit) **A**1 9 10 18 **F**2 3 11 13 15 24 25 26 31 32 33 38 42 46 49 52 54 55 56 57 61 62 63 68 71 74 75 77 78 79 80 87 96 97 100 102 107 112 117 119 121 122 124 135 **P**5 6 8
Primary Contact: Robert J. Bednarek, President and Chief Executive Officer
COO: Rebecca W. Carter, MSN, Chief Operating Officer
CFO: Theresa Parker, Chief Financial Officer
CMO: Carmelo Hernandez, M.D., Chief of Staff
CIO: Pat Perry, Manager Information Systems
CHR: Mark L. Emory, Vice President Human Resources and Support Services
Web address: www.tchospital.org
Control: Other not–for–profit (including NFP Corporation) **Service:** General Medical and Surgical

Staffed Beds: 54 **Admissions:** 1705 **Census:** 24 **Outpatient Visits:** 47756 **Births:** 204 **Total Expense ($000):** 40829 **Payroll Expense ($000):** 16600 **Personnel:** 472

BRYSON CITY—Swain County

★ **SWAIN COUNTY HOSPITAL (341305)**, 45 Plateau Street, Zip 28713–6784; tel. 828/488–4013 **A**1 9 10 18 **F**8 11 15 25 26 30 31 32 33 38 41 42 43 44 55 57 61 66 73 75 77 79 80 86 96 107 118 119 122 135 137 **S** WestCare Health System
Primary Contact: Ronald A. Sloan, Administrator
COO: Mark T. Leonard, Chief Executive Officer
CFO: Steve Heatherly, Executive Vice President Finance and Operations
CMO: Martha Anderson, M.D., Chief of Staff
CIO: Dale Chernich, Chief Information Officer
CHR: Janet Millsaps, Vice President Staff Services
Web address: www.westcare.org
Control: Other not–for–profit (including NFP Corporation) **Service:** General Medical and Surgical

Staffed Beds: 25 **Admissions:** 840 **Census:** 5 **Outpatient Visits:** 23131 **Births:** 0 **Total Expense ($000):** 12382 **Payroll Expense ($000):** 3883 **Personnel:** 83

BURGAW—Pender County

★ **PENDER MEMORIAL HOSPITAL (341307)**, 507 Freemont Street, Zip 28425–5131; tel. 910/259–5451, (Total facility includes 43 beds in nursing home–type unit) **A**1 9 10 18 **F**3 11 15 25 31 33 38 46 54 55 57 61 62 63 66 75 79 86 96 102 107 117 119 121 122 124 135 **S** New Hanover Health Network
Primary Contact: David Long, Administrator
CMO: Michael G. Rallis, M.D., Chief of Staff
CIO: Michael Jones, Manager Information Systems
CHR: Holly Horton, Director Human Resources
Web address: www.pendermemorial.org
Control: County–Government, nonfederal **Service:** General Medical and Surgical

Staffed Beds: 68 **Admissions:** 995 **Census:** 44 **Outpatient Visits:** 26959 **Births:** 0 **Total Expense ($000):** 16519 **Payroll Expense ($000):** 8470 **Personnel:** 243

BURLINGTON—Alamance County

★ **ALAMANCE REGIONAL MEDICAL CENTER (340070)**, 1240 Huffman Mill Road, Zip 27216–0202, Mailing Address: P.O. Box 202, Zip 27216–0202; tel. 336/538–7000 **A**1 2 9 10 **F**3 5 11 12 13 15 18 20 24 25 26 27 28 30 31 32 33 34 35 36 37 38 41 43 44 46 49 50 52 53 54 55 56 57 60 62 66 68 71 72 73 74 75 76 77 79 80 81 82 84 86 88 90 91 92 93 94 95 96 97 99 100 102 103 106 107 108 109 111 119 120 121 123 124 130 132 135 136 137 **P**6
Primary Contact: John G. Currin, Jr., President
COO: John G. Currin, President
CFO: Rex Street, Senior Vice President and Chief Financial Officer
CMO: Connie Kincius, M.D., Chief of Staff
CIO: Jesse Long, Director Information Technology
CHR: Dick Donahey, Senior Vice President Human Resources
Web address: www.armc.com
Control: Other not–for–profit (including NFP Corporation) **Service:** General Medical and Surgical

Staffed Beds: 210 **Admissions:** 11214 **Census:** 139 **Outpatient Visits:** 177075 **Births:** 1365 **Total Expense ($000):** 167263 **Payroll Expense ($000):** 64031 **Personnel:** 1494

BURNSVILLE—Yancey County

YANCEY COMMUNITY MEDICAL CENTER (341301), 800 Medical Campus Drive, Zip 28714–9010; tel. 828/682–6136, (Nonreporting) **A**9 10
Primary Contact: Dena Hensley, Administrator
Control: Other not–for–profit (including NFP Corporation) **Service:** General Medical and Surgical

Staffed Beds: 6

BUTNER—Granville County

☐ **JOHN UMSTEAD HOSPITAL (344004)**, 1003 12th Street, Zip 27509–1626; tel. 919/575–7211, (Includes ALCOHOL AND DRUG ABUSE TREATMENT CENTER, 205 West East Street, Zip 27509; tel. 919/575–7928; Cliff Hood, Director), (Nonreporting) **A**1 3 5 10
Primary Contact: Patricia L. Christian, Ph.D., RN, Chief Executive Officer
Web address: www.juh.dhhs.state.nc.us
Control: State–Government, nonfederal **Service:** Psychiatric

Staffed Beds: 514

CAMP LEJEUNE—Onslow County

★ **NAVAL HOSPITAL**, Mailing Address: P.O. Box 10100, Zip 28547–0100; tel. 910/450–4300, (Nonreporting) **A**1 **S** Bureau of Medicine and Surgery, Department of the Navy
Primary Contact: Captain Mark C. Olesen, Commanding Officer
Web address: www.lej–www.med.navy.mil
Control: Navy, Government, federal **Service:** General Medical and Surgical

Staffed Beds: 117

CARY—Wake County

★ △ **WAKEMED CARY HOSPITAL (340173)**, 1900 Kildaire Farm Road, Zip 27511; tel. 919/350–2300, (Includes WAKE MED FUQUAY–VARINA OUTPATIENT AND SKILLED NURSING FACILITY, 400 West Ranson Street, Fuquay–Varina, Zip 27526; tel. 919/350–4600), (Total facility includes 36 beds in nursing home–type unit) **A**1 7 9 10 **F**3 7 11 13 15 18 20 22 25 26 27 30 31 32 33 38 41 43 48 49 50 55 56 57 60 62 66 68 70 71 72 73 74 75 76 77 79 80 81 86 96 97 100 102 103 106 107 117 118 119 121 134 135 136 **S** WakeMed
COO: Deborah G. Friberg, Senior Vice President and Chief Operating Officer
CFO: Michael D. DeVaughn, Senior Vice President and Chief Financial Officer
CMO: West Lawson, M.D., Chief Medical Officer
CIO: Denton Arledge, Vice President and Chief Information Officer
CHR: Jeanene R. Martin, Senior Vice President Human Resources
Web address: www.wakemed.org
Control: Other not–for–profit (including NFP Corporation) **Service:** General Medical and Surgical

Staffed Beds: 150 **Admissions:** 9192 **Census:** 128 **Outpatient Visits:** 230331 **Births:** 2519 **Total Expense ($000):** 124913 **Payroll Expense ($000):** 52166 **Personnel:** 1065

CHAPEL HILL—Orange County

★ △ **UNIVERSITY OF NORTH CAROLINA HOSPITALS (340061)**, 101 Manning Drive, Zip 27514–4220; tel. 919/966–4131, (Includes NORTH CAROLINA CHILDREN'S AND WOMEN'S HOSPITAL ; NORTH CAROLINA NEUROSCIENCES HOSPITAL) **A**1 2 3 5 7 8 9 10 **F**3 4 5 7 8 9 11 12 13 14 15 16 17 18 19 20 21 22 23 24 25 26 27 28 30 31 32 33 34 36 37 38 40 41 42 43 44 46 47 48 49 50 52 53 54 55 56 57 58 59 60 61 62 63 64 66 68 70 71 72 73 74 75 76 77 78 79 80 81 82 83 84 85 86 87 88 89 90 91 92 93 94 95 96 97 99 100 102 103 104 105 106 107 108 109 111 112 113 114 116 118 119 120 121 123 124 125 126 127 128 129 130 131 132 133 134 135 136 137
Primary Contact: Gary L. Park, President
COO: Todd L. Peterson, Executive Vice President and Chief Operating Officer
CFO: John P. Lewis, Vice President Finance and Chief Financial Officer
CMO: Brian Goldstein, M.D., Chief of Staff
CIO: J. P. Kichak, Vice President Information Services
CHR: William Rotella, Vice President Human Resources
Web address: www.unchealthcare.org
Control: State–Government, nonfederal **Service:** General Medical and Surgical

Staffed Beds: 711 **Admissions:** 35015 **Census:** 597 **Outpatient Visits:** 1247748 **Births:** 3678 **Total Expense ($000):** 741151 **Payroll Expense ($000):** 326865 **Personnel:** 6188

CHARLOTTE—Mecklenburg County

★ **CAROLINAS MEDICAL CENTER (340113)**, 1000 Blythe Boulevard, Zip 28203–5871, Mailing Address: P.O. Box 32861, Zip 28232–2861; tel. 704/355–2000 **A**1 2 3 5 6 8 9 10 **F**3 7 8 13 15 17 18 19 20 21 22 23 24 25 26 27 28 31 33 35 36 37 38 40 41 43 44 46 47 48 49 50 53 54 55 56 57 58 59 60 61 62 63 64 66 68 70 71 72 73 74 75 76 77 78 79 80 81 82 83 84 85 86 87 88 89 90 91 92 93 94 95 96 97 100 102 103 104 105 106 107 108 109 111 112 113 114 116 118 119 120 121 123 124 125 126 127 128 130 131 132 134 135 136 137 **P**2 6 **S** Carolinas HealthCare System
Primary Contact: Suzanne H. Freeman, RN, President
CFO: Greg A. Gombar, Chief Financial Officer
CMO: Roger A. Ray, M.D., Chief Medical Officer
CIO: Craig Richardville, Senior Vice President and Chief Information Officer
CHR: F. Traylor Renfro, Senior Vice President Human Resources
Web address: www.carolinasmedicalcenter.org
Control: Hospital district or authority, Government, nonfederal **Service:** General Medical and Surgical

Staffed Beds: 874 **Admissions:** 45316 **Census:** 702 **Outpatient Visits:** 888063 **Births:** 6951 **Total Expense ($000):** 1298818 **Payroll Expense ($000):** 476671 **Personnel:** 8913

★ △ **CAROLINAS MEDICAL CENTER–MERCY (340098)**, 2001 Vail Avenue, Zip 28207–1289; tel. 704/304–5000, (Includes CAROLINAS MEDICAL CENTER–PINEVILLE, 10628 Park Road, Zip 28210; tel. 704/543–2025; Christopher R. Hummer, Administrator) **A**1 2 7 9 10 **F**4 12 18 20 22 25 26 27 31 38 41 43 44 49 50 55 56 57 59 62 63 66 68 72 73 76 77 79 81 82 86 96 97 100 102 103 106 107 118 119 135 137 **S** Carolinas HealthCare System
Primary Contact: Phyllis Wingate–Jones, Administrator
CFO: David Thomas, Chief Financial Officer
CMO: William Bock, M.D., President Medical Staff
CHR: Stephanie McGary, Regional Director Human Resources
Web address: www.carolinashealthcare.org
Control: Hospital district or authority, Government, nonfederal **Service:** General Medical and Surgical

Staffed Beds: 157 **Admissions:** 6533 **Census:** 94 **Outpatient Visits:** 61277 **Births:** 0 **Total Expense ($000):** 114451 **Payroll Expense ($000):** 40094 **Personnel:** 702

★ **CAROLINAS MEDICAL CENTER–PINEVILLE**, 10628 Park Road, Zip 28210; tel. 704/543–2000 **A**1 2 9 10 **F**13 18 25 26 31 38 41 43 44 49 50 55 56 57 62 63 66 68 70 72 73 74 77 79 81 82 86 96 100 102 103 106 107 118 119 135 137 **S** Carolinas HealthCare System
Primary Contact: Christopher R. Hummer, Administrator
Web address: www.carolinashealthcare.org
Control: Hospital district or authority, Government, nonfederal **Service:** General Medical and Surgical

Staffed Beds: 109 **Admissions:** 7257 **Census:** 76 **Outpatient Visits:** 90197 **Births:** 2149 **Total Expense ($000):** 84042 **Payroll Expense ($000):** 34836 **Personnel:** 615

★ **CAROLINAS MEDICAL CENTER–UNIVERSITY (340166)**, 8800 North Tryon Street, Zip 28262–8415, Mailing Address: P.O. Box 560727, Zip 28256–0727; tel. 704/863–6000 **A**1 2 9 10 **F**8 13 18 25 26 27 31 38 41 43 44 49 50 55 56 57 62 63 66 68 70 72 73 74 76 77 79 81 82 86 96 100 102 103 106 107 116 118 119 134 135 137 **S** Carolinas HealthCare System
Primary Contact: W. Spencer Lilly, Vice President and Administrator
CFO: Greg A. Gombar, Chief Financial Officer
CIO: John J. Knox, Senior Vice President and Chief Information Officer
Web address: www.carolinashealthcare.org
Control: Hospital district or authority, Government, nonfederal **Service:** General Medical and Surgical

Staffed Beds: 130 **Admissions:** 5675 **Census:** 61 **Outpatient Visits:** 118321 **Births:** 1677 **Total Expense ($000):** 96581 **Payroll Expense ($000):** 38976 **Personnel:** 647

★ △ **CAROLINAS REHABILITATION (343026)**, 1100 Blythe Boulevard, Zip 28203–5864; tel. 704/355–4300 **A**1 7 10 **F**25 26 30 31 32 62 66 80 85 86 88 119 132 135 137 **P**1 **S** Carolinas HealthCare System
Primary Contact: C. Curtis Copenhaver, Vice President and Administrator
CFO: William Hopkins, Director Finance
CMO: William Bockenek, M.D., Chief Medical Staff
Web address: www.carolinashealthcare.org
Control: Other not–for–profit (including NFP Corporation) **Service:** Rehabilitation

Staffed Beds: 159 **Admissions:** 2833 **Census:** 108 **Outpatient Visits:** 48974 **Births:** 0 **Total Expense ($000):** 49124 **Payroll Expense ($000):** 25222 **Personnel:** 464

CAROLINAS SPECIALTY HOSPITAL (342015), 2001 Vail Avenue, 7th Floor, Zip 28207; tel. 704/379–6450, (Nonreporting) **A**10
Web address: www.carolinashealthcare.org
Control: Corporation, Investor–owned, for–profit **Service:** Long–Term Acute Care hospital

Staffed Beds: 38

★ **PRESBYTERIAN HOSPITAL (340053)**, 200 Hawthorne Lane, Zip 28204–2528, Mailing Address: P.O. Box 33549, Zip 28233–3549; tel. 704/384–4000 **A**1 2 9 10 **F**3 5 7 8 11 12 13 15 17 18 20 22 24 25 26 27 28 30 31 32 33 34 36 38 42 43 44 47 48 49 52 53 54 55 56 57 58 59 60 61 62 66 68 69 70 71 72 73 74 76 77 79 80 81 82 83 84 86 88 89 90 91 92 93 94 95 96 97 99 100 102 103 104 105 106 107 108 109 114 116 118 119 121 124 131 132 135 136 137 **P**6 **S** Novant Health
Primary Contact: Carl S. Armato, President and Chief Executive Officer
COO: Lynn Ingram Boggs, Executive Vice President and Chief Operating Officer
CFO: Mark Moyer, Vice President and Chief Financial Officer
CMO: Stephen Wallenhaupt, M.D., Executive Vice President Medical Affairs
CIO: Rich B. McKnight, Senior Vice President Information Technology
Web address: www.presbyterian.org
Control: Other not–for–profit (including NFP Corporation) **Service:** General Medical and Surgical

Staffed Beds: 529 **Admissions:** 30862 **Census:** 488 **Outpatient Visits:** 361245 **Births:** 5198 **Total Expense ($000):** 466274 **Payroll Expense ($000):** 175483 **Personnel:** 3352

★ **PRESBYTERIAN–ORTHOPAEDIC HOSPITAL (340153)**, 1901 Randolph Road, Zip 28207–1195; tel. 704/316–2000 **A**1 9 10 **F**3 11 25 26 30 31 32 35 41 43 50 62 66 73 77 79 81 82 96 100 102 107 117 119 120 121 135 **S** Novant Health
Primary Contact: Tanya S. Blackmon, Vice President and Administrator
CFO: Tammy Geist, Chief Financial Officer
CIO: Shelia Cook, Director Information Systems
Web address: www.novanthealth.org
Control: Other not–for–profit (including NFP Corporation) **Service:** Orthopedic

Staffed Beds: 80 **Admissions:** 4158 **Census:** 46 **Outpatient Visits:** 40246 **Births:** 0 **Total Expense ($000):** 74512 **Payroll Expense ($000):** 20693 **Personnel:** 333

Hospital, Medicare Provider Number, Address, Telephone, Approval, Facility, and Physician Codes, Health Care System

★ American Hospital Association (AHA) membership
□ The Joint Commission accreditation
○ American Osteopathic Association (AOA) accreditation
△ Commission on Accreditation of Rehabilitation Facilities (CARF) accreditation

CHEROKEE—Swain County

☒ **CHEROKEE INDIAN HOSPITAL AUTHORITY (340156)**, Hospital Road, Zip 28719, Mailing Address: Caller Box C–268, Zip 28719; tel. 828/497–9163, (Nonreporting) **A**1 10
Primary Contact: Casey Cooper, Chief Executive Officer
CFO: Shirley Hilton, Budget Analyst
Control: Other not–for–profit (including NFP Corporation) **Service:** General Medical and Surgical

Staffed Beds: 28

CLINTON—Sampson County

☒ **SAMPSON REGIONAL MEDICAL CENTER (340024)**, 607 Beaman Street, Zip 28328–2697, Mailing Address: P.O. Box 260, Zip 28329–0260; tel. 910/592–8511, (Total facility includes 30 beds in nursing home–type unit) **A**1 9 10 **F**3 7 8 11 13 14 15 18 24 25 27 28 30 31 32 33 37 38 43 44 50 52 53 54 55 56 57 61 62 66 68 73 74 75 76 77 79 80 81 82 84 86 96 97 100 102 103 107 109 111 117 119 120 121 124 132 135 136 137
Primary Contact: Lee Pridgen, Jr., Chief Executive Officer
COO: Wanda L. Boyette, R.N., Senior Vice President and Chief Operating Officer
CFO: Jerry Heinzman, Senior Vice President and Chief Financial Officer
CMO: Ted Bavman, M.D., President Medical Staff
CIO: David Ziolkowski, Chief Information Officer
CHR: Patricia Britt–Boyette, Vice President Human Resources
Web address: www.sampsonrmc.org
Control: County–Government, nonfederal **Service:** General Medical and Surgical

Staffed Beds: 132 **Admissions:** 4585 **Census:** 74 **Outpatient Visits:** 66715 **Births:** 520 **Total Expense ($000):** 55382 **Payroll Expense ($000):** 25080 **Personnel:** 588

CLYDE—Haywood County

☒ **HAYWOOD REGIONAL MEDICAL CENTER (340025)**, 262 Leroy George Drive, Zip 28721–9434; tel. 828/456–7311, (Total facility includes 20 beds in nursing home–type unit) **A**1 9 10 **F**3 11 13 15 18 24 25 26 27 30 31 32 33 38 42 44 46 50 51 52 55 56 57 61 62 63 68 69 72 73 74 75 76 77 79 80 81 86 90 96 97 100 102 106 107 117 118 119 120 121 133 135 136 137 **P**8
Primary Contact: Alton T. Byers, Chief Executive Officer
CFO: Gwen Evans, Chief Financial Officer
CMO: Robert Reible, M.D., Chief Medical Officer
Web address: www.haymed.org
Control: Hospital district or authority, Government, nonfederal **Service:** General Medical and Surgical

Staffed Beds: 125 **Admissions:** 5588 **Census:** 59 **Outpatient Visits:** 185355 **Births:** 387 **Total Expense ($000):** 68415 **Payroll Expense ($000):** 34170 **Personnel:** 806

COLUMBUS—Polk County

☐ **ST. LUKE'S HOSPITAL (341322)**, 101 Hospital Drive, Zip 28722–9473; tel. 828/894–3311 **A**1 9 10 18 **F**3 11 15 25 26 30 31 32 33 38 46 54 55 56 57 61 62 68 73 75 77 79 80 86 88 93 96 97 102 107 119 122 124 135 137
Primary Contact: C. Cameron Highsmith, President and Chief Executive Officer
CFO: Robert D. Cress, Chief Financial Officer
CMO: James Holleman, M.D., Chief of Staff
CHR: Amy Arledge, Coordinator Support Services
Web address: www.saintlukeshospital.com
Control: Other not–for–profit (including NFP Corporation) **Service:** General Medical and Surgical

Staffed Beds: 35 **Admissions:** 1263 **Census:** 23 **Outpatient Visits:** 25431 **Births:** 0 **Total Expense ($000):** 23068 **Payroll Expense ($000):** 10092 **Personnel:** 308

CONCORD—Cabarrus County

☒ **CAROLINAS MEDICAL CENTER–NORTHEAST (340001)**, (Formerly NorthEast Medical Center), 920 Church Street North, Zip 28025–2983; tel. 704/403–3000 **A**1 2 9 10 **F**3 5 7 8 9 11 12 13 14 15 17 18 20 22 24 25 26 27 28 31 32 33 34 35 36 38 41 42 43 44 46 47 49 50 51 52 53 54 55 56 57 58 59 60 62 63 64 66 67 68 69 70 71 72 73 74 75 76 77 78 79 80 81 82 83 84 86 87 88 89 90 92 93 94 95 96 97 99 100 101 102 103 104 105 106 107 109 111 112 114 116 118 119 120 121 124 132 134 135 136 137 **P**6 **S** Carolinas HealthCare System
Primary Contact: Mark Nantz, President and Chief Executive Officer
CFO: James Ramsey, Vice President Finance
CMO: Karim Nazer, M.D., Chief Medical Officer
CIO: Keith McNeice, Vice President and Chief Information Officer
CHR: Paula Beaver, Vice President Human Resources
Web address: www.northeastmedical.org
Control: Other not–for–profit (including NFP Corporation) **Service:** General Medical and Surgical

Staffed Beds: 418 **Admissions:** 22323 **Census:** 281 **Outpatient Visits:** 853821 **Births:** 2933 **Total Expense ($000):** 409162 **Payroll Expense ($000):** 193669 **Personnel:** 3538

DANBURY—Stokes County

★ **STOKES–REYNOLDS MEMORIAL HOSPITAL (341317)**, 1570 Highway 8 and 89 North, Zip 27016, Mailing Address: P.O. Box 10, Zip 27016–0010; tel. 336/593–2831, (Total facility includes 40 beds in nursing home–type unit) **A**9 10 18 **F**3 8 15 31 32 33 38 39 42 53 55 56 57 62 73 79 80 86 87 94 96 102 107 117 119 122 132 133 135 **P**6 **S** North Carolina Baptist Hospital
Primary Contact: Lance C. Labine, President
CFO: James McDonnell, Chief Financial Officer
CMO: Samuel C. Newsome, M.D., President Medical Staff
Web address: www.wfubmc.edu/stokes
Control: Other not–for–profit (including NFP Corporation) **Service:** General Medical and Surgical

Staffed Beds: 65 **Admissions:** 409 **Census:** 43 **Outpatient Visits:** 45060 **Births:** 0 **Total Expense ($000):** 14815 **Payroll Expense ($000):** 6722 **Personnel:** 213

DUNN—Harnett County

☒ **BETSY JOHNSON REGIONAL HOSPITAL (340071)**, 800 Tilghman Drive, Zip 28334–5599, Mailing Address: Drawer 1706, Zip 28335–1706; tel. 910/892–7161 **A**1 9 10 **F**3 11 13 15 24 25 26 31 32 33 37 38 43 46 54 55 57 66 68 71 73 74 75 77 79 80 81 84 86 87 96 97 99 100 102 106 107 118 119 121 124 135 137 **S** WakeMed
Primary Contact: Kenneth E. Bryan, President and Chief Executive Officer
COO: Kenneth E. Bryan, President and Chief Executive Officer
CFO: Eric L. Young, Chief Financial Officer
CMO: Patrick Gray, M.D., Chief Medical Staff
CIO: Demetrius Hagins, Director Information Systems
CHR: Sondra Davis, Vice President Human Resources
Web address: www.bjrh.org
Control: Hospital district or authority, Government, nonfederal **Service:** General Medical and Surgical

Staffed Beds: 101 **Admissions:** 6417 **Census:** 76 **Outpatient Visits:** 98485 **Births:** 849 **Total Expense ($000):** 72416 **Payroll Expense ($000):** 33062 **Personnel:** 700

DURHAM—Durham County

☒ **DUKE UNIVERSITY HOSPITAL (340030)**, 2301 Erwin Road, Zip 27710–0001, Mailing Address: P.O. Box 3708, Zip 27710–3708; tel. 919/684–8111 **A**1 2 8 9 10 **F**3 5 6 7 8 11 12 13 15 16 17 18 19 20 21 22 23 24 25 26 27 28 30 31 32 33 34 35 36 37 38 40 41 43 44 46 47 48 49 50 52 53 54 55 56 57 58 59 60 62 64 66 68 70 71 72 73 74 75 76 77 78 79 80 81 82 83 84 86 87 88 90 91 92 93 94 96 97 98 99 100 102 103 104 105 106 107 108 109 111 112 113 114 116 118 119 120 121 123 124 125 126 127 128 129 130 131 134 135 136 137 **P**1 **S** Duke University Health System
Primary Contact: William J. Fulkerson, M.D., Chief Executive Officer
COO: Kevin W. Sowers, R.N., MSN, Chief Operating Officer
CFO: Mark F. Miller, Chief Financial Officer
CMO: Steven Olson, M.D., Chief Medical Officer
CIO: Asif Ahmad, Chief Information Officer
CHR: Deborah Page, Chief Human Resources Officer
Web address: www.dukehealth.org
Control: Other not–for–profit (including NFP Corporation) **Service:** General Medical and Surgical

Staffed Beds: 784 **Admissions:** 37864 **Census:** 656 **Outpatient Visits:** 863038 **Births:** 3202 **Total Expense ($000):** 1058887 **Payroll Expense ($000):** 425317 **Personnel:** 7660

☒ **DURHAM REGIONAL HOSPITAL (340155)**, 3643 North Roxboro Road, Zip 27704–2763; tel. 919/470–4000 **A**1 3 5 6 9 10 **F**3 8 11 12 13 15 17 18 20 22 24 25 26 27 30 31 32 33 38 41 43 44 46 47 50 51 55 56 57 59 62 64 66 68 71 72 73 74 75 76 77 78 79 80 82 85 86 88 90 92 93 95 96 97 100 102 106 107 116 119 120 121 135 136 137 **P**6 **S** Duke University Health System
Primary Contact: Kerry Watson, Chief Executive Officer
CFO: Mark F. Miller, Chief Financial Officer
CMO: Edward N. LaMay, M.D., Chief Medical Officer
CIO: Terry Mears, Director Information Systems
CHR: Richard J. Walsh, Ph.D., Chief Human Resources Officer
Web address: www.durhamregional.org
Control: Other not–for–profit (including NFP Corporation) **Service:** General Medical and Surgical

Staffed Beds: 201 **Admissions:** 16024 **Census:** 201 **Outpatient Visits:** 121034 **Births:** 2043 **Total Expense ($000):** 209378 **Payroll Expense ($000):** 105720 **Personnel:** 1882

☒ **DURHAM VETERANS AFFAIRS MEDICAL CENTER**, 508 Fulton Street, Zip 27705–3897; tel. 919/286–0411, (Total facility includes 90 beds in nursing home–type unit) (Nonreporting) **A**1 3 5 8 **S** Department of Veterans Affairs
Primary Contact: Ralph T. Gigliotti, Director
CMO: John D. Shelburne, M.D., Chief of Staff
CIO: Conrad Raber, Chief Information Resources Management Service
Web address: www.va.gov/sta/guide/facility.asp?id=43
Control: Veterans Affairs, Government, federal **Service:** General Medical and Surgical

Staffed Beds: 232

□ **NORTH CAROLINA SPECIALTY HOSPITAL (340049)**, 3916 Ben Franklin Boulevard, Zip 27704; tel. 919/956–9300 **A**1 9 10 **F**3 25 30 31 32 43 50 57 62 66 73 77 79 80 81 82 84 107 119 120 **S** National Surgical Hospitals
Primary Contact: Randi L. Pisko, Chief Executive Officer
CFO: Bill Wilson, Chief Financial Officer
CMO: Thomas Dimmig, M.D., Medical Director
CHR: Deborah Wheeler, Director Human Resources
Web address: www.ncspecialty.com
Control: Partnership, Investor–owned, for–profit **Service:** General Medical and Surgical

Staffed Beds: 14 **Admissions:** 1049 **Census:** 8 **Outpatient Visits:** 8594 **Births:** 0 **Total Expense ($000):** 22652 **Payroll Expense ($000):** 8179 **Personnel:** 116

□ **SELECT SPECIALTY HOSPITAL OF DURHAM (342018)**, 3643 North Roxboro Road, 6th Floor, Zip 27704; tel. 919/470–9000, (Nonreporting) **A**1 10 **S** Select Medical Corporation
Primary Contact: Matthew Womble, Chief Executive Officer
Web address: www.selectmedicalcorp.com
Control: Corporation, Investor–owned, for–profit **Service:** Long–Term Acute Care hospital

Staffed Beds: 30

EDEN—Rockingham County

★ **MOREHEAD MEMORIAL HOSPITAL (340060)**, 117 East King's Highway, Zip 27288–5299; tel. 336/623–9711, (Total facility includes 121 beds in nursing home–type unit) **A**1 2 9 10 **F**3 11 13 15 24 25 26 27 31 32 33 38 43 44 49 50 53 54 55 56 57 61 62 63 65 68 72 73 74 75 76 77 79 80 82 84 86 87 96 97 100 102 106 107 109 113 117 118 119 120 121 123 124 135 136 137 **P**6 8 **S** QHR
Primary Contact: Robert Enders, President
CFO: Dan Elmer, Vice President Finance
CHR: Tom Stevens, Director Personnel
Web address: www.morehead.org
Control: Other not–for–profit (including NFP Corporation) **Service:** General Medical and Surgical

Staffed Beds: 224 **Admissions:** 6588 **Census:** 184 **Outpatient Visits:** 170143 **Births:** 699 **Total Expense ($000):** 81952 **Payroll Expense ($000):** 36119 **Personnel:** 830

EDENTON—Chowan County

★ **CHOWAN HOSPITAL (341318)**, 211 Virginia Road, Zip 27932–0629, Mailing Address: P.O. Box 629, Zip 27932–0629; tel. 252/482–8451, (Total facility includes 32 beds in nursing home–type unit) **A**1 9 10 18 **F**3 11 13 15 24 25 26 27 30 31 32 33 38 43 54 55 57 61 62 68 73 74 75 76 77 79 80 84 86 96 97 102 107 117 119 121 122 124 135 136 **P**6 **S** University Health Systems of Eastern Carolina
Primary Contact: Jeffrey N. Sackrison, FACHE, President
CFO: Michael Dacus, Vice President Financial Services
CHR: Debbie Swicegood, Director Human Resources
Web address: www.uhseast.com
Control: Other not–for–profit (including NFP Corporation) **Service:** General Medical and Surgical

Staffed Beds: 67 **Admissions:** 1904 **Census:** 46 **Outpatient Visits:** 34205 **Births:** 398 **Total Expense ($000):** 40061 **Payroll Expense ($000):** 17567 **Personnel:** 445

ELIZABETH CITY—Pasquotank County

★ **ALBEMARLE HEALTH (340109)**, 1144 North Road Street, Zip 27909, Mailing Address: P.O. Box 1587, Zip 27906–1587; tel. 252/335–0531 **A**1 9 10 19 20 **F**3 13 15 17 18 24 25 26 27 30 31 32 33 37 38 44 46 52 55 56 57 62 66 68 72 73 74 75 76 77 79 81 82 86 96 97 100 106 107 109 118 119 121 132 135 136 137
Primary Contact: Sharon M. Tanner, President and Chief Executive Officer
CFO: Raymond Owings, Chief Financial Officer
CMO: Jasvinder Singh, M.D., Chief of Staff
CIO: Steve Clark, Chief Information Officer
CHR: Jan King Robinson, Vice President Human Resources and Organizational Development
Web address: www.albemarlehealth.org
Control: Hospital district or authority, Government, nonfederal **Service:** General Medical and Surgical

Staffed Beds: 140 **Admissions:** 7246 **Census:** 84 **Outpatient Visits:** 139781 **Births:** 828 **Total Expense ($000):** 94033 **Payroll Expense ($000):** 41686 **Personnel:** 869

ELIZABETHTOWN—Bladen County

★ **BLADEN COUNTY HOSPITAL (341315)**, 501 South Poplar Street, Zip 28337–0398, Mailing Address: P.O. Box 398, Zip 28337–0398; tel. 910/862–5100 **A**1 9 10 18 **F**11 13 15 25 26 31 32 38 57 62 68 74 75 79 80 82 86 87 96 102 107 122 124 133 135 136 **P**6
Primary Contact: David J. Masterson, Chief Executive Officer
COO: Beverly Grayman–Rice, Vice President Patient Care Services
CFO: Jay Leatherman, Chief Financial Officer
CMO: Anthony Clary, M.D., President Medical Staff
CIO: Richard Bryan, Director Management Information Systems
CHR: Ginger Parks, Director Human Resources
Web address: www.bchn.org
Control: County–Government, nonfederal **Service:** General Medical and Surgical

Staffed Beds: 25 **Admissions:** 1376 **Census:** 12 **Outpatient Visits:** 20937 **Births:** 260 **Total Expense ($000):** 23617 **Payroll Expense ($000):** 9769 **Personnel:** 219

ELKIN—Surry County

★ **HUGH CHATHAM MEMORIAL HOSPITAL (340097)**, 180 Parkwood Drive, Zip 28621–0560, Mailing Address: P.O. Box 560, Zip 28621–0560; tel. 336/527–7000, (Total facility includes 127 beds in nursing home–type unit) **A**1 9 10 **F**1 3 4 6 8 10 11 12 13 15 16 17 24 25 26 30 31 33 38 42 44 49 50 55 56 57 61 62 63 65 66 67 68 69 70 71 73 74 75 78 79 80 82 83 85 86 87 88 96 97 99 100 102 103 106 107 115 117 118 119 121 122 124 135 **P**6 7
Primary Contact: Stephen Pennington, Chief Executive Officer
CFO: Donald E. Trippel, Chief Financial Officer
CMO: Tony Canupp, M.D., Chief of Staff
CHR: Jeff Seaford, Director Human Resources
Web address: www.hughchatham.org
Control: Other not–for–profit (including NFP Corporation) **Service:** General Medical and Surgical

Staffed Beds: 220 **Admissions:** 4993 **Census:** 170 **Outpatient Visits:** 55477 **Births:** 436 **Total Expense ($000):** 58609 **Payroll Expense ($000):** 22844 **Personnel:** 639

FAYETTEVILLE—Cumberland County

★ △ **CAPE FEAR VALLEY HEALTH SYSTEM (340028)**, 1638 Owen Drive, Zip 28304–3431, Mailing Address: P.O. Box 2000, Zip 28302–2000; tel. 910/609–4000, (Includes SOUTHEASTERN REGIONAL REHABILITATION CENTER ; BEHAVIORAL HEALTH CARE OF CAPE FEAR VALLEY HEALTH SYSTEM, 3425 Melrose Road, Zip 28304–1695; tel. 910/609–3000; Stanley D. Dodson, Director for Psychiatric Services; HIGHSMITH–RAINEY MEMORIAL HOSPITAL, 150 Robeson Street, Zip 28301–5570; tel. 910/609–1000; Walt Rose, Vice President; SOUTHEASTERN REGIONAL REHABILITATION CENTER) **A**1 2 7 9 10 **F**1 5 7 12 13 14 15 17 18 20 22 24 25 26 27 30 31 32 33 34 36 37 38 42 43 44 45 46 49 50 51 52 53 54 55 56 57 58 59 60 61 62 63 66 68 70 71 72 73 74 75 76 77 78 79 80 81 82 83 84 85 86 87 88 89 90 91 92 93 94 95 96 97 98 100 102 104 107 108 109 118 119 120 121 124 132 133 135 136 137 **P**5 6
Primary Contact: Joyce P. Korzen, RN, Interim Chief Executive Officer
COO: Joyce P. Korzen, R.N., Senior Vice President and Chief Operating Officer
CFO: Torrey M. Johnson, Senior Vice President and Chief Financial Officer
CIO: William Avenel, Vice President Information Systems and Chief Information Officer
CHR: Steve Thomas, Vice President Human Resources
Web address: www.capefearvalley.com
Control: Other not–for–profit (including NFP Corporation) **Service:** General Medical and Surgical

Staffed Beds: 581 **Admissions:** 30491 **Census:** 504 **Outpatient Visits:** 575762 **Births:** 4481 **Total Expense ($000):** 502497 **Payroll Expense ($000):** 234102 **Personnel:** 4183

★ **VETERANS AFFAIRS MEDICAL CENTER**, 2300 Ramsey Street, Zip 28301–3899; tel. 910/822–7059, (Total facility includes 39 beds in nursing home–type unit) (Nonreporting) **A**1 **S** Department of Veterans Affairs
Primary Contact: Janet S. Stout, Director
CIO: Clint Nordan, Chief Information Resource Management
Web address: www.va.gov/sta/guide/home.asp
Control: Veterans Affairs, Government, federal **Service:** General Medical and Surgical

Staffed Beds: 159

Hospital, Medicare Provider Number, Address, Telephone, Approval, Facility, and Physician Codes, Health Care System

★ American Hospital Association (AHA) membership
□ The Joint Commission accreditation
○ American Osteopathic Association (AOA) accreditation
△ Commission on Accreditation of Rehabilitation Facilities (CARF) accreditation

NC

FLETCHER—Henderson County

★ ○ **PARK RIDGE HOSPITAL (340023)**, Naples Road, Zip 28732, Mailing Address: P.O. Box 1569, Zip 28732–1569; tel. 828/684–8501 **A**1 9 10 11 19 **F**3 11 13 15 24 25 26 27 28 30 31 32 33 38 44 45 46 47 48 49 50 56 57 61 63 66 68 73 74 76 77 78 79 84 86 88 92 93 95 96 97 100 103 107 118 119 120 121 122 124 131 133 134 135 136 137 **P**6 **S** Adventist Health System Sunbelt Health Care Corporation
Primary Contact: Jimm Bunch, President and Chief Executive Officer
CFO: Kelly J. Pettijohn, Vice President Finance
CMO: Martin Black, M.D., Chief of Staff
CHR: Charlotte Lyda, Director Human Resources
Web address: www.parkridgehospital.org
Control: Other not–for–profit (including NFP Corporation) **Service:** General Medical and Surgical

Staffed Beds: 98 **Admissions:** 4466 **Census:** 68 **Outpatient Visits:** 225490 **Births:** 458 **Total Expense ($000):** 92555 **Payroll Expense ($000):** 39453 **Personnel:** 782

FORT BRAGG—Cumberland County

★ **WOMACK ARMY MEDICAL CENTER**, Normandy Drive, Zip 28307–5000; tel. 910/907–6000, (Nonreporting) **A**1 3 5 **S** Department of the Army, Office of the Surgeon General
Primary Contact: Colonel Terry Walters, Commander
Web address: www.wamc.amedd.army.mil/
Control: Army, Government, federal **Service:** General Medical and Surgical

Staffed Beds: 156

FRANKLIN—Macon County

★ **ANGEL MEDICAL CENTER (340012)**, 120 Riverview Street, Zip 28734, Mailing Address: P.O. Box 1209, Zip 28744; tel. 828/524–8411 **A**1 9 10 **F**3 8 11 13 15 25 26 27 30 31 32 33 34 38 42 43 44 45 51 55 56 57 61 62 63 68 73 74 75 76 77 79 80 82 86 96 97 100 102 106 107 112 118 121 122 133 135 136 137
Primary Contact: Donald D. Sandoval, FACHE, Chief Executive Officer
COO: Martin Wadewitz, Chief Operating Officer
CFO: Tracy Gihl, Interim Chief Financial Officer
CIO: Gary Hanold, Director Management Information Systems
CHR: Mark Garber, Chief Human Resources Officer
Web address: www.angelmed.org
Control: Other not–for–profit (including NFP Corporation) **Service:** General Medical and Surgical

Staffed Beds: 50 **Admissions:** 1665 **Census:** 18 **Outpatient Visits:** 97572 **Births:** 310 **Total Expense ($000):** 35697 **Payroll Expense ($000):** 13319 **Personnel:** 357

FUQUAY–VARINA—Wake County

WAKE MED FUQUAY–VARINA OUTPATIENT AND SKILLED NURSING FACILITY See WakeMed Cary Hospital, Cary

GASTONIA—Gaston County

★ **GASTON MEMORIAL HOSPITAL (340032)**, 2525 Court Drive, Zip 28054–2142, Mailing Address: P.O. Box 1747, Zip 28053–1747; tel. 704/834–2000 **A**1 2 9 10 **F**3 13 15 17 18 20 22 24 25 26 27 31 32 38 42 43 44 46 48 49 52 53 59 68 70 71 72 73 74 75 76 77 78 79 80 82 84 88 89 90 92 96 97 99 100 102 103 104 105 106 107 108 109 111 118 119 124 135 136 137 **P**6
Primary Contact: Wayne F. Shovelin, President and Chief Executive Officer
COO: Terry L. Jones, Executive Vice President and Chief Operating Officer
CFO: David O'Connor, Chief Financial Officer
CMO: J. David Huber, Vice President Medical Services Division
CIO: Mike Johnson, Director Information Systems
CHR: Elizabeth McCraw, Director Human Resources
Web address: www.caromont.org
Control: Other not–for–profit (including NFP Corporation) **Service:** General Medical and Surgical

Staffed Beds: 395 **Admissions:** 22314 **Census:** 276 **Outpatient Visits:** 315890 **Births:** 2934 **Total Expense ($000):** 280360 **Payroll Expense ($000):** 116771 **Personnel:** 2173

GOLDSBORO—Wayne County

☐ **CHERRY HOSPITAL (344003)**, 201 Stevens Mill Road, Zip 27530–1057; tel. 919/731–3200 **A**1 10 **F**3 26 30 31 32 37 66 73 75 81 82 88 89 91 93 119 121 124 135 **P**6
Primary Contact: Jack St. Clair, Ed.D., Director
COO: Richard Courliss, Chief Support Services
CFO: Susie Sherrod Sanders, Budget Officer
CMO: Kimberly Johnson, M.D., Clinical Director
CIO: Lisa Pettus, Manager Information Systems
CHR: Angela Crawford, Director Human Resources
Web address: www.cherryhospital.org
Control: State–Government, nonfederal **Service:** Psychiatric

Staffed Beds: 284 **Admissions:** 3996 **Census:** 260 **Outpatient Visits:** 0 **Births:** 0 **Total Expense ($000):** 68320 **Payroll Expense ($000):** 42790 **Personnel:** 1000

★ **WAYNE MEMORIAL HOSPITAL (340010)**, 2700 Wayne Memorial Drive, Zip 27534, Mailing Address: P.O. Box 8001, Zip 27533; tel. 919/736–1110 **A**1 9 10 19 **F**3 8 13 15 18 24 25 26 27 28 31 32 33 37 38 43 49 59 66 68 69 72 74 75 76 77 79 80 81 84 86 88 89 92 94 96 97 99 100 102 106 107 118 119 121 123 124 135 137
Primary Contact: J. William Paugh, President and Chief Executive Officer
COO: Thomas A. Bradshaw, Vice President Operations
CFO: Rebecca W. Craig, Vice President and Chief Financial Officer
CIO: Lori Cole, Director Information Management
CHR: Richard K. Rogers, Vice President Human Resources
Web address: www.waynehealth.org
Control: Other not–for–profit (including NFP Corporation) **Service:** General Medical and Surgical

Staffed Beds: 267 **Admissions:** 13375 **Census:** 178 **Outpatient Visits:** 143309 **Births:** 1455 **Total Expense ($000):** 159442 **Payroll Expense ($000):** 70184 **Personnel:** 1447

GREENSBORO—Guilford County

☐ **KINDRED HOSPITAL–GREENSBORO (342012)**, 2401 Southside Boulevard, Zip 27406–3311; tel. 336/271–2800, (Total facility includes 23 beds in nursing home–type unit) **A**1 9 10 **F**1 3 4 17 25 26 31 32 33 36 43 44 54 57 59 60 63 65 68 73 75 76 77 78 79 85 88 96 117 119 135 137 **P**5 **S** Kindred Healthcare
Primary Contact: David M. Polunas, Chief Executive Officer
COO: Deana Knight, MSN, Chief Clinical Officer
CFO: Michael Nelson, Chief Financial Officer
CMO: Percy E. Jones, M.D., Chief of Staff
CIO: Little Shuford, Medical Information Manager
CHR: Michele Roberts, Hospital Recruiter
Web address: www.kindredhealthcare.com
Control: Corporation, Investor–owned, for–profit **Service:** Long–Term Acute Care hospital

Staffed Beds: 124 **Admissions:** 645 **Census:** 73 **Outpatient Visits:** 82 **Births:** 0 **Total Expense ($000):** 32835 **Payroll Expense ($000):** 14467 **Personnel:** 331

★ △ **MOSES CONE HEALTH SYSTEM (340091)**, 1200 North Elm Street, Zip 27401–1020; tel. 336/832–7000, (Includes ANNIE PENN HOSPITAL, 618 South Main Street, Reidsville, Zip 27320–5094; tel. 336/951–4000; Susan H. Fitzgibbon, President and Executive Vice President; BEHAVIORAL HEALTH CENTER, 700 Walter Reed Drive, Zip 27403–1129; tel. 336/832–9600; Troy Chisolm, Vice President and Administrator; MOSES H. CONE MEMORIAL HOSPITAL; WESLEY LONG COMMUNITY HOSPITAL, 501 North Elam Avenue, Zip 27403; tel. 336/832–1000; Paul A. Jeffrey, Vice President and Administrator; WOMEN'S HOSPITAL OF GREENSBORO, 801 Green Valley Road, Zip 27408; tel. 336/832–6500), (Total facility includes 92 beds in nursing home–type unit) **A**1 2 3 5 7 9 10 **F**3 5 7 8 11 12 13 15 17 18 20 22 24 25 26 27 28 30 31 32 33 35 37 38 40 41 42 43 44 45 46 49 50 53 54 55 56 57 58 59 60 62 64 66 68 70 72 73 74 75 76 77 78 79 80 81 82 83 84 85 86 87 88 89 90 91 92 93 94 96 97 99 100 102 103 105 106 107 108 109 111 116 117 118 119 120 121 123 124 133 134 135 136 137 **P**6 8
Primary Contact: R. Timothy Rice, President and Chief Executive Officer
COO: Glenn D. Waters, Chief Operating Officer
CFO: Beth Ward, Vice President and Chief Financial Officer
CMO: William Bowman, M.D., Vice President Medical Affairs
CIO: John Jenkins, Vice President and Chief Information Officer
CHR: Noel Burt, Ph.D., Vice President Human Resources
Web address: www.mosescone.com
Control: Other not–for–profit (including NFP Corporation) **Service:** General Medical and Surgical

Staffed Beds: 997 **Admissions:** 46784 **Census:** 744 **Outpatient Visits:** 661484 **Births:** 6184 **Total Expense ($000):** 704924 **Payroll Expense ($000):** 298269 **Personnel:** 6171

GREENVILLE—Pitt County

★ △ **PITT COUNTY MEMORIAL HOSPITAL (340040)**, 2100 Stantonsburg Road, Zip 27834, Mailing Address: P.O. Box 6028, Zip 27835–6028; tel. 252/847–4100 **A**1 2 3 5 7 8 9 10 **F**3 7 8 12 13 14 15 17 18 19 20 21 22 23 24 25 26 27 28 30 31 32 33 36 37 38 39 40 41 43 44 45 46 47 48 49 50 51 53 54 55 56 57 58 59 60 62 63 64 66 68 70 71 72 73 74 75 76 77 78 79 80 81 82 83 84 85 86 87 88 90 91 92 93 94 96 97 100 102 103 104 105 106 107 108 112 113 114 116 118 119 120 121 123 124 127 132 133 134 135 136 137 **S** University Health Systems of Eastern Carolina
Primary Contact: Stephen J. Lawler, President
CFO: Jack W. Holsten, Chief Financial Officer
CMO: Ernest Larkin, M.D., Chief Medical Officer
CIO: Stuart James, Chief Information Officer
CHR: Tyree Walker, Chief Human Resources Officer
Web address: www.uhseast.com
Control: Other not–for–profit (including NFP Corporation) **Service:** General Medical and Surgical

Staffed Beds: 737 **Admissions:** 34374 **Census:** 608 **Outpatient Visits:** 284438 **Births:** 3659 **Total Expense ($000):** 702102 **Payroll Expense ($000):** 287496 **Personnel:** 5621

Many Facility Codes have changed. Please refer to the AHA Guide Code Chart.

WALTER B. JONES ALCOHOL AND DRUG ABUSE TREATMENT CENTER (344024), 2577 West Fifth Street, Zip 27834–7813; tel. 252/830–3426 **A**10 **F**4 25 43 52 66 81 82 119 124 **P**6
Primary Contact: Theresa Edmondson, Director
CFO: Tom Basnight, Chief Financial Officer
CMO: Gary Leonhardt, M.D., Clinical Director
Control: State–Government, nonfederal **Service:** Alcoholism and other chemical dependency

Staffed Beds: 80 **Admissions:** 974 **Census:** 46 **Outpatient Visits:** 0 **Births:** 0 **Total Expense ($000):** 7825 **Payroll Expense ($000):** 5056 **Personnel:** 175

HAMLET—Richmond County

□ **SANDHILLS REGIONAL MEDICAL CENTER (340106)**, 1000 West Hamlet Avenue, Zip 28345–4522, Mailing Address: P.O. Box 1109, Zip 28345–1109; tel. 910/205–8000 **A**1 9 10 **F**3 15 18 25 26 30 31 32 38 43 50 55 59 63 66 68 73 77 79 80 86 88 92 94 95 96 97 100 102 107 118 119 135 137 **P**6 **S** Health Management Associates
Primary Contact: Andrew L. Davis, Chief Executive Officer
CFO: Kyle Johnson, Chief Financial Officer
CHR: Kathy Shapiro, Director
Web address: www.hma–corp.com
Control: Corporation, Investor–owned, for–profit **Service:** General Medical and Surgical

Staffed Beds: 64 **Admissions:** 3380 **Census:** 44 **Outpatient Visits:** 34113 **Births:** 0 **Total Expense ($000):** 23615 **Payroll Expense ($000):** 10371 **Personnel:** 298

HENDERSON—Vance County

★ △ **MARIA PARHAM MEDICAL CENTER (340132)**, 566 Ruin Creek Road, Zip 27536–2957; tel. 252/438–4143 **A**1 7 9 10 **F**3 11 13 15 18 24 25 26 27 31 32 33 34 38 41 43 46 50 51 53 55 56 57 60 61 62 66 68 72 73 74 76 77 78 79 80 81 82 85 86 87 96 97 100 102 107 109 112 118 119 120 121 124 135 136 137 **P**3 8
Primary Contact: Robert G. Singletary, President and Chief Executive Officer
CFO: Jim Chatman, Chief Financial Officer
CIO: Randy Williams, Director Management Information Systems
CHR: Tonya Jones, Vice President Human Resources
Web address: www.mphosp.org
Control: Other not–for–profit (including NFP Corporation) **Service:** General Medical and Surgical

Staffed Beds: 102 **Admissions:** 5203 **Census:** 63 **Outpatient Visits:** 159451 **Births:** 842 **Total Expense ($000):** 65733 **Payroll Expense ($000):** 25255 **Personnel:** 625

HENDERSONVILLE—Henderson County

□ **MARGARET R. PARDEE MEMORIAL HOSPITAL (340017)**, 800 North Justice Street, Zip 28791–2563; tel. 828/696–1000, (Total facility includes 130 beds in nursing home–type unit) (Nonreporting) **A**1 2 9 10
Primary Contact: Kris Hoce, Chief Executive Officer
CFO: Alan House, Vice President Finance
CIO: Sherman Moore, Director Information Systems
Web address: www.pardeehospital.org
Control: County–Government, nonfederal **Service:** General Medical and Surgical

Staffed Beds: 300

HICKORY—Catawba County

★ △ **CATAWBA VALLEY MEDICAL CENTER (340143)**, 810 Fairgrove Church Road S.E., Zip 28602–9643; tel. 828/326–3000 **A**1 2 5 7 9 10 **F**3 5 11 12 13 15 18 20 24 25 26 27 30 31 32 33 34 35 37 38 41 43 44 46 47 48 49 50 51 52 53 54 55 56 57 60 62 63 64 66 68 69 71 72 73 74 75 76 77 79 80 81 82 84 85 86 87 88 90 91 92 93 94 96 97 98 99 100 102 103 105 106 107 109 110 111 112 116 118 119 120 121 124 132 133 134 135 136 137
Primary Contact: J. Anthony Rose, President and Chief Executive Officer
COO: Scott Echelberger, Vice President Operations
CFO: David J. Boone, Vice President Finance
CIO: Jerry Reardon, Director Information Systems
CHR: Phyllis Johnston, Director
Web address: www.catawbavalleymc.org
Control: County–Government, nonfederal **Service:** General Medical and Surgical

Staffed Beds: 213 **Admissions:** 8439 **Census:** 136 **Outpatient Visits:** 272694 **Births:** 1674 **Total Expense ($000):** 161370 **Payroll Expense ($000):** 68353 **Personnel:** 1286

★ **FRYE REGIONAL MEDICAL CENTER (340116)**, 420 North Center Street, Zip 28601–5049; tel. 828/322–6070, (Includes FRYE REGIONAL MEDICAL CENTER–SOUTH CAMPUS, tel. 704/315–5777) **A**1 2 9 10 **F**11 12 13 15 17 18 20 22 24 25 26 27 30 31 32 33 38 42 43 44 50 51 53 55 56 57 62 66 70 71 72 73 74 75 76 77 79 80 81 82 85 86 88 89 91 93 96 97 99 100 102 103 104 106 107 117 118 119 120 121 122 124 133 135 136 137 **S** TENET Healthcare Corporation
Primary Contact: Michael R. Blackburn, Chief Executive Officer
COO: Craig P. Hume, Senior Vice President and Chief Operating Officer
CFO: Sherry Henderson, Vice President Financial Services and Chief Financial Officer
CMO: Frank C. Smeeks, M.D., Chief Medical Officer
CIO: Nathan White, Administrative Director Information Systems
CHR: Liz Elich, Vice President Human Resources
Web address: www.fryemedctr.com
Control: Corporation, Investor–owned, for–profit **Service:** General Medical and Surgical

Staffed Beds: 322 **Admissions:** 13585 **Census:** 209 **Outpatient Visits:** 136065 **Births:** 744 **Personnel:** 1332

HIGH POINT—Guilford County

★ △ **HIGH POINT REGIONAL HEALTH SYSTEM (340004)**, 601 North Elm Street, Zip 27262–4398, Mailing Address: P.O. Box HP–5, Zip 27261; tel. 336/878–6000, (Total facility includes 18 beds in nursing home–type unit) **A**1 2 7 9 10 **F**3 4 5 7 8 9 11 12 13 15 17 18 20 22 24 25 26 27 30 31 32 33 34 37 38 40 41 43 44 49 50 51 52 53 55 56 57 58 59 60 62 64 66 68 69 71 72 73 74 75 76 77 78 79 80 81 82 84 85 86 88 90 91 92 93 94 96 97 98 100 102 103 104 105 106 107 108 109 113 116 117 118 119 121 124 133 135 136 137 **P**6
Primary Contact: Jeffrey S. Miller, President and Chief Executive Officer
COO: Martha Barham, Vice President and Chief Operating Officer
CMO: Gregory W. Taylor, M.D., Senior Vice President and Chief Medical Director
CIO: Diana Sharkey, Chief Information Officer
CHR: Katherine Burns, Vice President Human Resources
Web address: www.highpointregional.com
Control: Other not–for–profit (including NFP Corporation) **Service:** General Medical and Surgical

Staffed Beds: 353 **Admissions:** 17897 **Census:** 246 **Outpatient Visits:** 193715 **Births:** 1986 **Total Expense ($000):** 229455 **Payroll Expense ($000):** 94413 **Personnel:** 1790

HIGHLANDS—Macon County

★ **HIGHLANDS–CASHIERS HOSPITAL (341316)**, 190 Hospital Drive, Zip 28741–7600, Mailing Address: P.O. Drawer 190, Zip 28741–0190; tel. 828/526–1200, (Total facility includes 84 beds in nursing home–type unit) **A**1 9 10 18 **F**3 11 15 24 25 26 30 31 38 42 43 52 55 56 57 65 67 73 75 77 79 82 86 93 96 100 107 117 119 122 124 135 136 **P**6
Primary Contact: Kenneth A. Shull, FACHE, President and Chief Executive Officer
COO: Frank Leslie, Vice President Operations
CFO: Michael E. Daiken, Chief Financial Officer
Web address: www.hchospital.org
Control: Other not–for–profit (including NFP Corporation) **Service:** General Medical and Surgical

Staffed Beds: 108 **Admissions:** 455 **Census:** 92 **Outpatient Visits:** 14573 **Births:** 0 **Total Expense ($000):** 19640 **Payroll Expense ($000):** 8444 **Personnel:** 198

HUNTERSVILLE—Mecklenburg County

★ **PRESBYTERIAN HOSPITAL HUNTERSVILLE (340183)**, 10030 Gilead Road, Zip 28078, Mailing Address: P.O. Box 3508, Zip 28070–3508; tel. 704/316–4000 **A**1 9 10 **F**3 11 13 25 26 27 30 31 32 33 38 43 50 55 56 62 66 68 71 73 74 75 76 77 79 80 81 82 86 92 96 97 100 102 106 107 118 119 121 124 135 136 **S** Novant Health
Primary Contact: Jeffrey T. Lindsay, Vice President and Administrator
COO: Melissa Robson, Chief Operating Officer
CFO: Jason Yanni, Senior Financial Analyst
CMO: David Cook, M.D., Chief Medical Officer
CIO: Rich B. McKnight, Senior Vice President Chief Information Officer
CHR: Tracy Craig, Director Human Resources
Web address: www.novanthealth.org
Control: Other not–for–profit (including NFP Corporation) **Service:** General Medical and Surgical

Staffed Beds: 50 **Admissions:** 5187 **Census:** 47 **Outpatient Visits:** 128716 **Births:** 1030 **Total Expense ($000):** 66195 **Payroll Expense ($000):** 24751 **Personnel:** 424

Hospital, Medicare Provider Number, Address, Telephone, Approval, Facility, and Physician Codes, Health Care System
★ American Hospital Association (AHA) membership
□ The Joint Commission accreditation
○ American Osteopathic Association (AOA) accreditation
△ Commission on Accreditation of Rehabilitation Facilities (CARF) accreditation

JACKSONVILLE—Onslow County

☐ **BRYNN MARR HOSPITAL (344016)**, 192 Village Drive, Zip 28546–7299; tel. 910/577–1400 **A**1 10 **F**30 36 88 89 91 92 93 119 **P**6
S Psychiatric Solutions
Primary Contact: Sarah Wiltgen, Chief Executive Officer
COO: Nancy Mumma, Chief Operating Officer
CFO: David Warmerdam, Chief Financial Officer
CMO: Rayna Rogers, Medical Director
CIO: Sue Jackson, Director Performance Improvement, Regulatory Preparedness and Risk Management
CHR: Richard Walker, Director Human Resources
Web address: www.brynnmarr.org
Control: Corporation, Investor–owned, for–profit **Service:** Psychiatric

Staffed Beds: 87 **Admissions:** 1465 **Census:** 69 **Outpatient Visits:** 0 **Births:** 0 **Total Expense ($000):** 10803 **Payroll Expense ($000):** 7499 **Personnel:** 227

★ **ONSLOW MEMORIAL HOSPITAL (340042)**, 317 Western Boulevard, Zip 28540–6379, Mailing Address: P.O. Box 1358, Zip 28541–1358; tel. 910/577–2345 **A**9 10 20 **F**1 3 4 8 11 13 15 16 17 18 24 25 30 31 32 38 43 44 53 55 56 57 59 62 65 66 68 70 71 73 74 75 77 78 79 80 81 82 83 84 85 86 88 96 97 100 102 107 117 118 119 120 121 124 135 136 137 **P**8
Primary Contact: Ed Piper, Chief Executive Officer
CFO: Roy Smith, Chief Financial Officer
CMO: Lennox Williams, Chief of Staff
CHR: Sue Keyley, Director Human Resources
Web address: www.onslowmemorial.org
Control: Hospital district or authority, Government, nonfederal **Service:** General Medical and Surgical

Staffed Beds: 133 **Admissions:** 8326 **Census:** 90 **Outpatient Visits:** 156080 **Births:** 1683 **Total Expense ($000):** 71483 **Payroll Expense ($000):** 39053 **Personnel:** 1000

JEFFERSON—Ashe County

★ **ASHE MEMORIAL HOSPITAL (341325)**, 200 Hospital Avenue, Zip 28640–9244; tel. 336/846–7101, (Total facility includes 60 beds in nursing home–type unit) **A**1 9 10 18 **F**3 8 11 13 15 24 26 30 31 32 33 38 46 52 55 56 57 62 73 74 77 78 79 80 81 84 86 96 97 102 106 107 117 119 121 122 124 130 131 133 135 **S** QHR
Primary Contact: R. D. Williams, Administrator and Chief Executive Officer
COO: Joe Thore, Chief Operating Officer
CFO: Joy McClure, Chief Financial Officer
CMO: Kevin Kurtz, M.D., Chief of Staff
CIO: William Baldwin, Chief Information Officer
CHR: Sherry Cox, Chief Human Resources Officer
Web address: www.ashememorial.org
Control: Other not–for–profit (including NFP Corporation) **Service:** General Medical and Surgical

Staffed Beds: 85 **Admissions:** 1676 **Census:** 71 **Outpatient Visits:** 44903 **Births:** 110 **Total Expense ($000):** 25081 **Payroll Expense ($000):** 10991 **Personnel:** 290

KENANSVILLE—Duplin County

★ **DUPLIN GENERAL HOSPITAL (340120)**, 401 North Main Street, Zip 28349–9989, Mailing Address: P.O. Box 278, Zip 28349–0278; tel. 910/296–0941, (Total facility includes 20 beds in nursing home–type unit) **A**1 9 10 **F**11 13 15 25 26 31 32 37 38 54 55 60 66 68 73 74 77 79 86 87 88 91 92 93 96 97 100 102 107 117 118 119 124 135 136
Primary Contact: Harvey Case, Chief Executive Officer
CFO: Lucinda Maready, Vice President Financial Services
CMO: Danny Pate, M.D., Chief Medical Staff
CIO: Lucinda Maready, Vice President Financial Services
CHR: Panry Chase, Interim Director Human Resources
Web address: www.uhseast.org
Control: County–Government, nonfederal **Service:** General Medical and Surgical

Staffed Beds: 89 **Admissions:** 3581 **Census:** 60 **Outpatient Visits:** 47621 **Births:** 777 **Total Expense ($000):** 22944 **Payroll Expense ($000):** 13726 **Personnel:** 369

KINGS MOUNTAIN—Cleveland County

★ **KINGS MOUNTAIN HOSPITAL (340037)**, 706 West King Street, Zip 28086–2708; tel. 704/739–3601, (Total facility includes 10 beds in nursing home–type unit) **A**1 9 10 **F**3 4 15 17 25 26 30 31 32 38 43 46 49 65 68 77 79 80 84 86 88 96 100 102 107 117 119 122 135 137 **S** Carolinas HealthCare System
Primary Contact: John E. Young, President and Chief Executive Officer
COO: Sheri Deshazo, Chief Operating Officer and Chief Nursing Executive
CFO: Terry Edwards, Controller
CMO: David Johnson, M.D., Chief of Staff
CHR: Debra Kale, Director Human Resources
Web address: www.carolinas.org
Control: County–Government, nonfederal **Service:** General Medical and Surgical

Staffed Beds: 72 **Admissions:** 2911 **Census:** 38 **Outpatient Visits:** 43442 **Births:** 0 **Total Expense ($000):** 29912 **Payroll Expense ($000):** 11456 **Personnel:** 255

KINSTON—Lenoir County

CASWELL CENTER, 2415 West Vernon Avenue, Zip 28504–3321; tel. 252/208–4000 **F**26 37 55 57 66 73 75 132 135 137
Primary Contact: Beverly Vinson, Director
COO: Tim Russell, Director Administrative Services
CFO: Jim Hall, Budget Officer
CMO: Tony Bright, M.D., Administrator Medical Services
CIO: Danny Rice, Director Specialized Services
CHR: Ken Lafone, Director Human Resources
Web address: www.caswellcenter.org
Control: State–Government, nonfederal **Service:** Institution for mental retardation

Staffed Beds: 825 **Admissions:** 20 **Census:** 423 **Outpatient Visits:** 0 **Total Expense ($000):** 83082 **Payroll Expense ($000):** 52255 **Personnel:** 1552

☐ **LENOIR MEMORIAL HOSPITAL (340027)**, 100 Airport Road, Zip 28501–1634, Mailing Address: P.O. Box 1678, Zip 28503–1678; tel. 252/522–7000, (Total facility includes 26 beds in nursing home–type unit) **A**1 2 9 10 19 20 **F**3 8 11 12 13 18 24 25 26 27 31 32 33 36 38 40 43 47 48 49 50 52 54 55 56 57 59 60 62 63 66 68 72 73 74 75 76 77 78 79 80 81 82 84 85 86 92 96 97 100 102 106 107 109 111 117 118 119 121 123 124 132 134 135 137
Primary Contact: Gary E. Black, President and Chief Executive Officer
CFO: Sarah Mayo, Vice President Financial and Information Services
CMO: Laddie Crisp, M.D., President Medical Staff
CIO: Mary Jo Nimmo, Director Management Information Systems
CHR: Jim Dobbins, Vice President Human Resources
Web address: www.lenoirmemorial.org
Control: Other not–for–profit (including NFP Corporation) **Service:** General Medical and Surgical

Staffed Beds: 219 **Admissions:** 10062 **Census:** 150 **Outpatient Visits:** 91652 **Births:** 670 **Total Expense ($000):** 98964 **Payroll Expense ($000):** 43257 **Personnel:** 889

LAURINBURG—Scotland County

★ **SCOTLAND MEMORIAL HOSPITAL (340008)**, 500 Lauchwood Drive, Zip 28352–5599; tel. 910/291–7000, (Total facility includes 50 beds in nursing home–type unit) **A**1 9 10 **F**3 11 13 15 24 25 27 30 31 35 38 43 53 55 56 57 62 64 68 69 71 72 73 74 75 76 77 79 80 82 84 85 86 87 96 100 102 107 112 117 119 121 124 132 133 134 135 136 137 **P**8
Primary Contact: Gregory C. Wood, Chief Executive Officer
COO: Ruth Glaser, Senior Vice President Operations
CFO: Matthew Pracht, Vice President Finance
CMO: Glenn Harris, M.D., Chief of Staff
CIO: Larry Pergerson, Chief Information Systems
CHR: Ann Locklear, Director Human Resources
Web address: www.scotlandhealth.org
Control: Other not–for–profit (including NFP Corporation) **Service:** General Medical and Surgical

Staffed Beds: 152 **Admissions:** 6341 **Census:** 127 **Outpatient Visits:** 136018 **Births:** 887 **Total Expense ($000):** 92704 **Payroll Expense ($000):** 39995 **Personnel:** 864

LENOIR—Caldwell County

★ **CALDWELL MEMORIAL HOSPITAL (340041)**, 321 Mulberry Street S.W., Zip 28645–5720, Mailing Address: P.O. Box 1890, Zip 28645–1890; tel. 828/757–5100 **A**1 2 9 10 **F**3 8 11 13 15 18 20 22 24 25 33 35 38 43 46 51 52 54 55 56 57 58 62 63 64 66 68 69 72 73 74 75 76 77 79 80 82 84 86 87 96 99 100 102 107 108 109 110 111 112 119 121 124 135 136 137 **P**6
Primary Contact: Laura J. Easton, President and Chief Executive Officer
CFO: Donald F. Gardner, Vice President Fiscal Services
CMO: Mark Batts, M.D., Chief of Staff
CIO: Adam Sears, Director Information Systems
CHR: Rebecca Smith, Vice President
Web address: www.caldwell-mem.org
Control: Other not–for–profit (including NFP Corporation) **Service:** General Medical and Surgical

Staffed Beds: 110 **Admissions:** 4355 **Census:** 42 **Outpatient Visits:** 104856 **Births:** 680 **Total Expense ($000):** 74801 **Payroll Expense ($000):** 33937 **Personnel:** 764

LEXINGTON—Davidson County

★ **LEXINGTON MEMORIAL HOSPITAL (340096)**, 250 Hospital Drive, Zip 27292–6728, Mailing Address: P.O. Box 1817, Zip 27293–1817; tel. 336/248–5161 **A**1 9 10 **F**11 13 15 17 25 26 32 56 57 60 62 68 73 74 75 76 77 79 80 81 82 84 85 86 96 97 100 106 107 118 119 121 124 133 135
Primary Contact: John A. Cashion, FACHE, President
CFO: Danny Squires, Vice President and Chief Financial Officer
CMO: Martin Allen, M.D., Chief of Staff
CIO: Kevin Buchanan, Director Management Information Systems
CHR: Dolly Mayerchak, Director Human Resources
Web address: www.lexingtonmemorial.com
Control: Other not–for–profit (including NFP Corporation) **Service:** General Medical and Surgical

Staffed Beds: 85 **Admissions:** 3721 **Census:** 32 **Outpatient Visits:** 91969 **Births:** 781 **Total Expense ($000):** 51948 **Payroll Expense ($000):** 23494 **Personnel:** 587

LINCOLNTON—Lincoln County

★ **CAROLINAS MEDICAL CENTER–LINCOLN (340145)**, 200 Gamble Drive, Zip 28092–4421, Mailing Address: P.O. Box 677, Zip 28093–0677; tel. 704/735–3071 **A**1 9 10 **F**8 9 11 12 13 14 15 25 26 28 30 32 33 38 40 41 43 46 50 51 55 56 57 62 63 66 67 68 69 72 73 74 75 77 79 81 82 84 86 96 102 103 104 105 107 118 119 120 121 124 135 137 **S** Carolinas HealthCare System
Primary Contact: Peter W. Acker, President and Chief Executive Officer
COO: Jarrett Morris, Vice President Finance
CIO: Jarrett Morris, Vice President Finance
CHR: Lesley Chambless, Assistant Vice President Human Resources
Web address: www.cmc–lincoln.org
Control: Hospital district or authority, Government, nonfederal **Service:** General Medical and Surgical

Staffed Beds: 92 **Admissions:** 3733 **Census:** 42 **Outpatient Visits:** 89063 **Births:** 500 **Total Expense ($000):** 51969 **Payroll Expense ($000):** 22183 **Personnel:** 554

LINVILLE—Avery County

★ **CHARLES A. CANNON JR. MEMORIAL HOSPITAL (341323)**, (Critical Access Hospital), 434 Hospital Drive, Zip 28646, Mailing Address: P.O. Box 767, Zip 28646; tel. 828/737–7000 **A**1 9 10 18 **F**3 13 15 24 25 26 27 38 68 74 79 80 85 86 94 96 107 117 119 122 124 135 **P**8
Primary Contact: Chuck Mantooth, Chief Executive Officer
CFO: Jodi O'Leary, System Director Finance
CMO: Thomas M. Haizlip, M.D., Chief of Staff
CHR: Amy Crabbe, Vice President Human Resources
Web address: www.apprhs.org
Control: Other not–for–profit (including NFP Corporation) **Service:** Other specialty

Staffed Beds: 25 **Admissions:** 1570 **Census:** 21 **Outpatient Visits:** 10430 **Births:** 124 **Total Expense ($000):** 22987 **Payroll Expense ($000):** 9552

LOUISBURG—Franklin County

□ **FRANKLIN REGIONAL MEDICAL CENTER (340036)**, 100 Hospital Drive, Zip 27549–2256, Mailing Address: P.O. Box 609, Zip 27549–0609; tel. 919/497–8401 **A**1 9 10 **F**8 11 12 15 25 26 33 38 43 46 48 51 55 56 57 59 62 66 72 73 75 76 77 79 80 82 86 90 96 97 100 107 118 119 135 **S** Health Management Associates
Primary Contact: Michael H. McNair, Chief Executive Officer
CFO: Julie Do, Chief Financial Officer
CMO: Steve Schwam, M.D., Chief of Staff
CIO: Kim Webster, Information Systems Manager
CHR: Chuck Gavazzi, Director Human Resources
Web address: www.franklinregionalmedicalctr.com
Control: Individual, Investor–owned, for–profit **Service:** General Medical and Surgical

Staffed Beds: 59 **Admissions:** 2903 **Census:** 37 **Outpatient Visits:** 52708 **Births:** 0 **Total Expense ($000):** 36464 **Payroll Expense ($000):** 13702

LUMBERTON—Robeson County

★ **SOUTHEASTERN REGIONAL MEDICAL CENTER (340050)**, 300 West 27th Street, Zip 28358–3017, Mailing Address: P.O. Box 1408, Zip 28359–1408; tel. 910/671–5000, (Total facility includes 115 beds in nursing home–type unit) **A**1 9 10 19 20 **F**3 5 7 9 13 17 18 20 22 24 25 26 27 30 31 32 33 38 42 43 45 49 50 52 55 56 57 59 60 61 65 66 68 70 71 74 75 76 77 78 79 80 82 84 86 87 88 92 93 96 97 100 102 103 106 107 109 117 118 119 120 121 135 137 **P**8
Primary Contact: Joann Anderson, President and Chief Executive Officer
CFO: C. Thomas Johnson, Vice President Finance
CMO: Ricky Johnson, M.D., President Medical Staff
CIO: Nancy Waters, Chief Information Officer
CHR: Joseph W. Glezen, Director Human Resources
Web address: www.srmc.org
Control: Other not–for–profit (including NFP Corporation) **Service:** General Medical and Surgical

Staffed Beds: 400 **Admissions:** 15050 **Census:** 299 **Outpatient Visits:** 263776 **Births:** 1633 **Total Expense ($000):** 193963 **Payroll Expense ($000):** 81566 **Personnel:** 1839

MARION—McDowell County

★ **MCDOWELL HOSPITAL (340087)**, 430 Rankin Drive, Zip 28752–4989, Mailing Address: P.O. Box 730, Zip 28752–0730; tel. 828/659–5000 **A**1 9 10 **F**3 11 13 15 24 25 26 27 31 33 38 40 43 46 53 55 57 62 66 68 73 74 76 77 79 80 81 82 86 96 97 100 102 106 107 119 121 122 135 **P**6
Primary Contact: Edward J. Hannon, Chief Executive Officer
COO: Jason Clapsaddle, Vice President Operations
CFO: Katrina McDevitt, Controller
CMO: Terry McCall, M.D., Chief of Staff
CIO: Martha Stepp, Director Information Services
CHR: Cathy Gallett, Director Human Resources
Web address: www.mcdhospital.org
Control: Other not–for–profit (including NFP Corporation) **Service:** General Medical and Surgical

Staffed Beds: 49 **Admissions:** 2142 **Census:** 21 **Outpatient Visits:** 74487 **Births:** 314 **Total Expense ($000):** 25187 **Payroll Expense ($000):** 11836 **Personnel:** 332

MATTHEWS—Mecklenburg County

★ **PRESBYTERIAN HOSPITAL–MATTHEWS (340171)**, 1500 Matthews Township Parkway, Zip 28105–4656, Mailing Address: P.O. Box 3310, Zip 28106–3310; tel. 704/384–6500 **A**1 9 10 **F**3 11 13 15 18 25 26 27 28 30 31 32 33 34 38 43 44 49 54 55 56 57 62 66 68 71 73 74 75 76 77 79 80 81 82 84 86 96 97 99 100 102 103 107 118 119 121 135 136 137 **S** Novant Health
Primary Contact: Derrick Mark Billings, President
COO: Lynn Ingram Boggs, Executive Vice President and Chief Operating Officer
CFO: Greg Klein, Senior Director Finance
CMO: Thomas Zweng, M.D., Senior Vice President Medical Affairs
CIO: Rich B. McKnight, Chief Information Officer
CHR: Susan Kennedy, Manager Human Resources
Web address: www.presbyterian.org
Control: Other not–for–profit (including NFP Corporation) **Service:** General Medical and Surgical

Staffed Beds: 102 **Admissions:** 7561 **Census:** 80 **Outpatient Visits:** 207326 **Births:** 1484 **Total Expense ($000):** 90682 **Payroll Expense ($000):** 35023 **Personnel:** 607

MOCKSVILLE—Davie County

★ **DAVIE COUNTY HOSPITAL (341313)**, 223 Hospital Street, Zip 27028–2038, Mailing Address: P.O. Box 1209, Zip 27028–1209; tel. 336/751–8100 **A**1 9 10 18 **F**3 11 15 26 31 32 33 38 55 57 62 75 77 79 80 87 96 102 107 119 122 133
Primary Contact: Lynne T. Doss, Administrator
CFO: Terry R. Bowman, Chief Financial Officer
CMO: Larry Pearce, M.D., President Medical Staff
CHR: Linda Pate, Director Human Resources
Web address: www.daviehospital.org
Control: Other not–for–profit (including NFP Corporation) **Service:** General Medical and Surgical

Staffed Beds: 25 **Admissions:** 443 **Census:** 4 **Outpatient Visits:** 20829 **Births:** 0 **Total Expense ($000):** 10391 **Payroll Expense ($000):** 4462 **Personnel:** 126

Hospital, Medicare Provider Number, Address, Telephone, Approval, Facility, and Physician Codes, Health Care System
★ American Hospital Association (AHA) membership
□ The Joint Commission accreditation
○ American Osteopathic Association (AOA) accreditation
△ Commission on Accreditation of Rehabilitation Facilities (CARF) accreditation

MONROE—Union County

★ **CAROLINAS MEDICAL CENTER–UNION (340130)**, 600 Hospital Drive, Zip 28112–6000, Mailing Address: P.O. Box 5003, Zip 28111–5003; tel. 704/283–3100, (Total facility includes 70 beds in nursing home–type unit) **A**1 2 9 10 **F**3 4 5 11 13 15 18 24 25 26 27 30 31 33 37 38 43 49 54 55 56 57 61 62 64 65 68 71 72 73 74 75 76 77 79 80 81 82 84 86 96 97 100 102 106 107 108 109 111 117 118 119 121 124 133 135 136 137 **S** Carolinas HealthCare System
Primary Contact: Michael Lutes, President
COO: Dave Anderson, FACHE, Vice President Operations
CFO: John Moore, Vice President Services
CMO: Dan Hagler, M.D., Vice President and Chief Medical Officer
CIO: Lisa Sykes, Director Information Services
CHR: Annette Myers, Director Human Resources
Web address: www.cmc–union.org
Control: Hospital district or authority, Government, nonfederal **Service:** General Medical and Surgical

Staffed Beds: 241 **Admissions:** 9661 **Census:** 175 **Outpatient Visits:** 155965 **Births:** 1593 **Total Expense ($000):** 131809 **Payroll Expense ($000):** 53228 **Personnel:** 1223

MOORESVILLE—Iredell County

☐ **LAKE NORMAN REGIONAL MEDICAL CENTER (340129)**, 171 Fairview Road, Zip 28117–9500, Mailing Address: P.O. Box 3250, Zip 28117–3250; tel. 704/660–4000, (Nonreporting) **A**1 9 10 19 **S** Health Management Associates
Primary Contact: J. Michael Cowling, Chief Executive Officer
CFO: James Stoner, Chief Financial Officer
CHR: Gae Elliot, Director Human Resources
Web address: www.lnrmc.com
Control: Corporation, Investor–owned, for–profit **Service:** General Medical and Surgical

Staffed Beds: 129

MOREHEAD CITY—Carteret County

★ **CARTERET GENERAL HOSPITAL (340142)**, 3500 Arendell Street, Zip 28557–1619, Mailing Address: P.O. Box 1619, Zip 28557–1619; tel. 252/808–6000, (Total facility includes 104 beds in nursing home–type unit) **A**1 9 10 19 20 **F**7 11 13 15 24 25 26 27 30 31 32 33 38 42 43 44 45 46 47 49 53 55 56 57 61 62 63 66 69 73 74 75 76 77 79 80 81 82 84 87 96 97 100 102 107 111 117 118 119 121 124 132 134 135 137 **P**5
Primary Contact: Frederick A. Odell, III, FACHE, President
CFO: Riley Gray, Vice President Fiscal Services
CIO: Robert Walker, Manager Information Services
CHR: Elizabeth Beswick, Vice President Human Resources and Public Relations
Web address: www.ccgh.org
Control: County–Government, nonfederal **Service:** General Medical and Surgical

Staffed Beds: 239 **Admissions:** 7126 **Census:** 145 **Outpatient Visits:** 137240 **Births:** 678 **Total Expense ($000):** 95622 **Payroll Expense ($000):** 39532 **Personnel:** 874

MORGANTON—Burke County

☐ **BROUGHTON HOSPITAL (344002)**, 1000 South Sterling Street, Zip 28655–3999; tel. 828/433–2111, (Nonreporting) **A**1 5 10
Primary Contact: Seth P. Hunt, Jr., Director and Chief Executive Officer
COO: John Esse, Ph.D., Deputy Director and Chief Operating Officer
CFO: Jonathan Berry, Chief Support Services and Chief Financial Officer
CMO: George Krebs, M.D., Acting Chief Medical Officer
CIO: Phil Shirley, Director Information Resource Management
CHR: Mary Ragsdale, Director Human Resources
Web address: www.broughtonhospital.org
Control: State–Government, nonfederal **Service:** Psychiatric

Staffed Beds: 370

★ **GRACE HOSPITAL (340075)**, 2201 South Sterling Street, Zip 28655–4058; tel. 828/580–5000, (Total facility includes 120 beds in nursing home–type unit) **A**1 2 9 10 **F**3 11 13 15 18 24 25 26 27 30 31 32 33 34 38 43 44 45 46 52 54 55 56 57 61 62 66 67 68 71 73 74 75 76 77 79 80 81 82 86 87 88 90 91 92 93 94 95 96 97 98 99 100 102 104 106 107 112 117 119 120 121 122 124 132 133 135 136 **S** Carolinas HealthCare System
Primary Contact: Kenneth W. Wood, President and Chief Executive Officer
CFO: Robert Fritts, Chief Financial Officer
CMO: Lee Rogers, M.D., Senior Vice President Medical Affairs
CHR: Phil Satey, Vice President Human Resources
Web address: www.gracehcs.org
Control: Other not–for–profit (including NFP Corporation) **Service:** General Medical and Surgical

Staffed Beds: 269 **Admissions:** 6387 **Census:** 178 **Outpatient Visits:** 144926 **Births:** 1051 **Total Expense ($000):** 89678 **Payroll Expense ($000):** 35757 **Personnel:** 774

MOUNT AIRY—Surry County

★ **NORTHERN HOSPITAL OF SURRY COUNTY (340003)**, 830 Rockford Street, Zip 27030–5365, Mailing Address: P.O. Box 1101, Zip 27030–1101; tel. 336/719–7000, (Total facility includes 33 beds in nursing home–type unit) **A**1 9 10 **F**3 11 13 15 18 25 26 27 30 31 32 33 37 38 42 43 44 46 49 50 51 54 55 56 57 61 62 63 66 68 72 73 74 75 77 78 79 80 81 82 86 92 96 97 100 102 103 105 106 107 117 118 119 120 121 122 134 135 136 137 **S** QHR
Primary Contact: William B. James, Chief Executive Officer
CFO: Robert G. Hetrick, Chief Financial Officer
CMO: Bruce Middleton, M.D., Chief of Staff
CHR: Jeannie Moore, Director Human Resources
Web address: www.northernhospital.com
Control: Hospital district or authority, Government, nonfederal **Service:** General Medical and Surgical

Staffed Beds: 120 **Admissions:** 5294 **Census:** 87 **Outpatient Visits:** 159242 **Births:** 653 **Total Expense ($000):** 68198 **Payroll Expense ($000):** 30249 **Personnel:** 678

MURPHY—Cherokee County

★ **MURPHY MEDICAL CENTER (340160)**, 4130 U.S. Highway 64 East, Zip 28906–7917; tel. 828/837–8161, (Total facility includes 134 beds in nursing home–type unit) **A**1 9 10 **F**3 6 13 15 26 27 31 32 33 38 41 42 44 51 52 53 55 57 61 62 65 66 68 73 74 75 76 77 79 80 86 96 100 102 107 117 119 133 135 137
Primary Contact: Mike Stevenson, Administrator
CFO: Steve Gilgen, Assistant Administrator Fiscal Services
CHR: Russ Paine, Human Resources Officer
Web address: www.murphymedical.org
Control: Other not–for–profit (including NFP Corporation) **Service:** General Medical and Surgical

Staffed Beds: 191 **Admissions:** 2438 **Census:** 149 **Outpatient Visits:** 60114 **Births:** 156 **Total Expense ($000):** 48657 **Payroll Expense ($000):** 24146 **Personnel:** 701

NAGS HEAD—Dare County

★ **THE OUTER BANKS HOSPITAL (341324)**, 4800 South Croatan Highway, Zip 27959–9704; tel. 252/449–4500 **A**1 9 10 18 **F**3 13 15 25 26 31 32 33 38 50 54 55 56 57 62 63 66 71 73 74 75 77 79 80 86 100 106 107 119 122 135 **S** University Health Systems of Eastern Carolina
Primary Contact: D. Van Smith, Jr., President
CFO: Todd Warlitner, Vice President Business Operations
CMO: Michael Russell, M.D., President Medical Staff
CHR: Mary Kelley, Director Human Resources
Web address: www.theouterbankshospital.com
Control: Other not–for–profit (including NFP Corporation) **Service:** General Medical and Surgical

Staffed Beds: 19 **Admissions:** 1511 **Census:** 10 **Outpatient Visits:** 38191 **Births:** 422 **Total Expense ($000):** 29484 **Payroll Expense ($000):** 10922 **Personnel:** 183

NEW BERN—Craven County

★ △ **CRAVEN REGIONAL MEDICAL CENTER (340131)**, 2000 Neuse Boulevard, Zip 28560–3499, Mailing Address: P.O. Box 12157, Zip 28561–2157; tel. 252/633–8111 **A**1 2 7 9 10 19 20 **F**3 7 11 13 15 17 18 20 22 24 25 26 27 30 31 32 33 38 46 47 48 49 55 56 57 59 60 61 62 65 66 68 72 73 74 75 76 77 79 80 82 84 85 86 87 88 90 91 92 93 94 95 96 97 99 100 102 103 104 105 106 107 108 109 111 116 118 119 121 124 132 135 137
Primary Contact: Raymond Budrys, President and Chief Executive Officer
COO: Rosanne Leahy, Vice President Nursing Services
CFO: David Cauble, Chief Financial Officer
CMO: Ronald B. May, M.D., Vice President Medical Affairs
CIO: G. Raymond Leggett, Vice President Administration
CHR: Bruce A. Martin, Vice President Human Resources
Web address: www.cravenhealthcare.org
Control: Hospital district or authority, Government, nonfederal **Service:** General Medical and Surgical

Staffed Beds: 313 **Admissions:** 16377 **Census:** 243 **Outpatient Visits:** 160653 **Births:** 1159 **Total Expense ($000):** 201775 **Payroll Expense ($000):** 77335 **Personnel:** 1528

NORTH WILKESBORO—Wilkes County

★ □ **WILKES REGIONAL MEDICAL CENTER (340064)**, 1370 West D Street, Zip 28659–3506, Mailing Address: P.O. Box 609, Zip 28659–0609; tel. 336/651–8100, (Total facility includes 10 beds in nursing home–type unit) **A**1 9 10 **F**3 11 13 15 17 25 26 31 37 38 42 46 47 49 50 51 52 53 55 57 59 61 62 66 68 72 74 75 77 79 80 82 84 86 92 96 97 99 100 102 103 106 107 112 117 118 119 120 134 137
Primary Contact: Ted G. Chapin, Chief Executive Officer
CFO: Anthony C. Rispoli, Chief Financial Officer
CMO: Zbiqniew Cichon, M.D., Chief Medical Officer
CIO: Mark Cullison, Director Facility Services
CHR: Vanya Baker, Director
Web address: www.wilkesregional.org
Control: City–Government, nonfederal **Service:** General Medical and Surgical

Staffed Beds: 93 **Admissions:** 4998 **Census:** 48 **Outpatient Visits:** 62937 **Births:** 409

OXFORD—Granville County

★ □ **GRANVILLE MEDICAL CENTER (340127)**, 1010 College Street, Zip 27565–2507, Mailing Address: P.O. Box 947, Zip 27565–0947; tel. 919/690–3000, (Total facility includes 80 beds in nursing home–type unit) **A**1 9 10 **F**2 3 11 13 15 25 26 27 31 33 36 37 38 43 50 53 54 55 56 57 62 68 73 74 75 76 77 79 80 81 86 90 91 93 94 96 97 100 106 107 114 117 118 119 121 122 132 133 135 136 137 **P**1
Primary Contact: L. Lee Isley, Chief Executive Officer
CFO: Bruce Brooks, Chief Financial Officer
CMO: Steven Winters, M.D., Chief Medical Staff
Web address: www.granvillemedical.com
Control: County–Government, nonfederal **Service:** General Medical and Surgical

Staffed Beds: 142 **Admissions:** 2482 **Census:** 89 **Outpatient Visits:** 43306 **Births:** 400 **Total Expense ($000):** 35317 **Payroll Expense ($000):** 15912 **Personnel:** 405

PINEHURST—Moore County

★ □ △ **FIRSTHEALTH MOORE REGIONAL HOSPITAL (340115)**, 155 Memorial Drive, Zip 28374–8710, Mailing Address: P.O. Box 3000, Zip 28374–3000; tel. 910/715–1000 **A**1 2 7 9 10 19 **F**3 4 5 11 12 13 15 17 18 20 22 24 25 26 27 30 31 32 33 34 38 41 43 46 48 50 51 52 53 54 55 56 57 58 59 62 63 66 68 70 72 73 74 75 76 77 79 81 82 84 85 86 88 89 90 91 92 93 94 95 96 97 100 102 103 106 107 108 109 116 118 119 121 123 124 132 133 135 136 137 **S** FirstHealth of the Carolinas
Primary Contact: Stuart Voelpel, President and Chief Operating Officer
COO: Stuart Voelpel, President and Chief Operating Officer
CFO: Lynn S. DeJaco, Chief Financial Officer
CMO: George Bussey, M.D., Chief Medical Officer
CIO: David B. Dillehunt, Chief Information Officer
CHR: Dan Biediger, Vice President Human Resources
Web address: www.firsthealth.org
Control: Other not–for–profit (including NFP Corporation) **Service:** General Medical and Surgical

Staffed Beds: 356 **Admissions:** 21585 **Census:** 262 **Outpatient Visits:** 164069 **Births:** 1650 **Total Expense ($000):** 271810 **Payroll Expense ($000):** 108158 **Personnel:** 2350

PLYMOUTH—Washington County

★ □ **WASHINGTON COUNTY HOSPITAL (341314)**, 958 U.S. Highway 64 East, Zip 27962–9591; tel. 252/793–4135 **A**1 9 10 18 **F**3 8 11 15 25 26 27 30 31 32 38 41 62 66 73 79 81 82 87 96 107 122 135
Primary Contact: Jeffrey M. Judd, Chief Executive Officer
COO: Betty Bowen, Chief Operating Officer
CFO: Al Arrowood, Chief Financial Officer
CMO: Robert Venable, M.D., Chief Medical Staff
CHR: Christina Craft, Director Human Resources
Web address: www.wchonline.com
Control: County–Government, nonfederal **Service:** General Medical and Surgical

Staffed Beds: 25 **Admissions:** 689 **Census:** 6 **Outpatient Visits:** 27181 **Births:** 0 **Total Expense ($000):** 11365 **Payroll Expense ($000):** 5140 **Personnel:** 151

RAEFORD—Hoke County

MCCAIN CORRECTIONAL HOSPITAL, 855 Old Highway 211, Zip 28376; tel. 910/944–2351, (Nonreporting)
Primary Contact: F. David Hubbard, Superintendent
Web address: www.doc.state.nc.us/DOP/prisons/mccain.htm
Control: State–Government, nonfederal **Service:** Hospital unit of an institution (prison hospital, college infimary, etc.)

Staffed Beds: 81

RALEIGH—Wake County

CENTRAL PRISON HOSPITAL, 1300 Western Boulevard, Zip 27606–2148; tel. 919/733–0800, (Nonreporting)
Primary Contact: Thomas J. Hawkins, Administrator
CFO: Annette Goforth, Administrative Services Manager
CMO: Olushola Metiko, M.D., Medical Director
Web address: www.doc.state.nc.us/dop/prisons/central.htm/
Control: State–Government, nonfederal **Service:** Hospital unit of an institution (prison hospital, college infimary, etc.)

Staffed Beds: 230

□ **DOROTHEA DIX HOSPITAL (344001)**, 3601 Mail Service Center, Zip 27699–3601; tel. 919/733–5540, (Nonreporting) **A**1 3 5 10
Primary Contact: James Osberg, III, Ph.D., Director
CMO: Susan Saik, M.D., Medical Director
CHR: Terry Johnston, Director Human Resources
Control: State–Government, nonfederal **Service:** Psychiatric

Staffed Beds: 443

★ □ **DUKE RALEIGH HOSPITAL (340073)**, (Formerly Duke Health Raleigh Hospital), 3400 Wake Forest Road, Zip 27609–7373, Mailing Address: P.O. Box 28280, Zip 27611–8280; tel. 919/954–3000 **A**1 2 9 10 **F**3 11 15 18 20 24 25 26 27 30 31 32 33 38 43 44 46 47 49 52 55 56 57 58 59 62 68 72 73 75 76 77 79 80 82 86 96 97 100 102 104 107 109 111 118 119 120 121 124 135 137 **S** Duke University Health System
Primary Contact: Douglas B. Vinsel, Chief Executive Officer
COO: Richard Gannotta, Chief Operating Officer
CFO: Terri Newsom, Divisional Chief Financial Officer
CMO: Ted Kunstling, M.D., Chief Medical Officer
CIO: Billie Kennedy–Hutchinson, Director Information Technology
CHR: Don Barnes, Chief Human Resources Officer
Web address: www.dukehealthraleigh.org
Control: Other not–for–profit (including NFP Corporation) **Service:** General Medical and Surgical

Staffed Beds: 146 **Admissions:** 4959 **Census:** 62 **Outpatient Visits:** 85418 **Births:** 0 **Total Expense ($000):** 141341 **Payroll Expense ($000):** 57164 **Personnel:** 973

□ **HOLLY HILL HOSPITAL (344014)**, 3019 Falstaff Road, Zip 27610–1812; tel. 919/250–7000 **A**1 10 **F**4 88 89 92 93 94 95 **P**6 **S** Psychiatric Solutions
Primary Contact: Robert L. Turner, Ph.D., Chief Executive Officer
CFO: Ron Howard, Chief Financial Officer
CMO: Thomas Cornwall, M.D., Medical Director
CHR: Teresa Sulit, Director Human Resources
Web address: www.hollyhillhospital.com
Control: Corporation, Investor–owned, for–profit **Service:** Psychiatric

Staffed Beds: 108 **Admissions:** 3360 **Census:** 85 **Outpatient Visits:** 2513 **Total Expense ($000):** 15626 **Payroll Expense ($000):** 9134

LARRY B. ZIEVERINK, SR. ALCOHOLISM TREATMENT CENTER, 3000 Falstaff Road, Zip 27610–1897; tel. 919/250–1500 **F**4 5 32 94 121 124 132 **P**5
Primary Contact: Martin D. Woodward, Director Acute Care Services
COO: Martin D. Woodward, Director Acute Care Services
CFO: Robert Sorrells, Director Operations
CMO: Enrique Lopez, M.D., Medical Director
CIO: Jane Martin, Communications Director
Web address: www.wakegov.com/county/family/atc
Control: County–Government, nonfederal **Service:** Alcoholism and other chemical dependency

Staffed Beds: 34 **Admissions:** 808 **Census:** 24 **Outpatient Visits:** 10000 **Births:** 0 **Total Expense ($000):** 3682 **Payroll Expense ($000):** 3105 **Personnel:** 81

★ □ △ **REX HEALTHCARE (340114)**, 4420 Lake Boone Trail, Zip 27607–6599; tel. 919/784–3100, (Total facility includes 227 beds in nursing home–type unit) **A**1 2 7 9 10 **F**3 7 8 11 12 13 14 15 17 18 20 22 24 25 26 27 30 31 32 33 34 38 41 42 43 44 46 47 48 49 50 52 53 55 56 57 58 59 61 62 64 66 68 69 71 72 73 74 75 76 77 79 80 81 82 84 86 92 96 97 99 100 102 103 104 105 107 108 109 111 116 117 118 119 120 133 134 135 136 137 **P**6
Primary Contact: David W. Strong, President
CFO: Bernadette Spong, Chief Financial Officer
CMO: Timothy Carter, M.D., Medical Director Patient Safety
CIO: Novlet Bradshaw, Vice President Information Technology and Chief Information Officer
CHR: Sylvia D. Hackett, Vice President Human Resources
Web address: www.rexhealth.com
Control: Other not–for–profit (including NFP Corporation) **Service:** General Medical and Surgical

Staffed Beds: 621 **Admissions:** 27324 **Census:** 489 **Outpatient Visits:** 233857 **Births:** 6085 **Total Expense ($000):** 399816 **Payroll Expense ($000):** 172824 **Personnel:** 3483

Hospital, Medicare Provider Number, Address, Telephone, Approval, Facility, and Physician Codes, Health Care System

★ American Hospital Association (AHA) membership
□ The Joint Commission accreditation
○ American Osteopathic Association (AOA) accreditation
△ Commission on Accreditation of Rehabilitation Facilities (CARF) accreditation

NC

★ △ **WAKEMED RALEIGH CAMPUS (340069)**, 3000 New Bern Avenue, Zip 27610–1295; tel. 919/350–8000, (Total facility includes 19 beds in nursing home–type unit) **A**1 3 5 7 9 10 **F**3 7 9 11 12 13 15 17 18 20 22 24 25 26 27 28 30 31 32 33 35 36 37 38 39 40 41 42 43 44 48 49 50 52 53 54 55 56 57 58 59 60 61 62 63 64 66 68 69 70 71 72 73 74 75 76 77 79 80 81 82 83 84 85 86 87 94 96 97 99 100 102 103 106 107 116 117 118 119 120 121 124 132 134 135 136 137 **P**6 **S** WakeMed
Primary Contact: William K. Atkinson, II, President and Chief Executive Officer
COO: Deborah G. Friberg, Senior Vice President and Chief Operating Officer
CFO: Michael D. DeVaughn, Senior Vice President Finance and Chief Financial Officer
CMO: West Lawson, M.D., Chief Medical Officer
CIO: Denton Arledge, Vice President and Chief Information Officer
CHR: Jeanene R. Martin, Senior Vice President Human Resources
Web address: www.wakemed.org
Control: Other not–for–profit (including NFP Corporation) **Service:** General Medical and Surgical

Staffed Beds: 612 **Admissions:** 37131 **Census:** 554 **Outpatient Visits:** 870230 **Births:** 5319 **Total Expense ($000):** 640703 **Payroll Expense ($000):** 324779 **Personnel:** 5559

REIDSVILLE—Rockingham County

ANNIE PENN HOSPITAL See Moses Cone Health System, Greensboro

ROANOKE RAPIDS—Halifax County

★ **HALIFAX REGIONAL MEDICAL CENTER (340151)**, 250 Smith Church Road, Zip 27870, Mailing Address: P.O. Box 1089, Zip 27870; tel. 252/535–8011 **A**1 9 10 20 **F**3 11 13 15 18 25 30 31 32 33 36 38 44 49 50 52 53 55 56 57 58 59 60 62 63 64 66 67 68 73 74 75 76 77 79 80 81 86 87 88 91 92 93 94 96 97 98 100 107 118 119 121 124 135 **P**6
Primary Contact: William Mahone, V, President and Chief Executive Officer
CFO: Sherry Jensen, Chief Financial Officer
CIO: Robert Gordon, Manager Information Systems
CHR: Susan Hayes, Manager Human Resources
Web address: www.halifaxmedicalcenter.org
Control: Other not–for–profit (including NFP Corporation) **Service:** General Medical and Surgical

Staffed Beds: 142 **Admissions:** 7855 **Census:** 108 **Outpatient Visits:** 87156 **Births:** 844 **Total Expense ($000):** 77126 **Payroll Expense ($000):** 32133 **Personnel:** 785

ROCKINGHAM—Richmond County

★ **FIRSTHEALTH RICHMOND MEMORIAL HOSPITAL (340035)**, 925 Long Drive, Zip 28379–4815; tel. 910/417–3000, (Total facility includes 51 beds in nursing home–type unit) **A**1 9 10 **F**13 15 18 25 26 28 30 31 32 33 38 43 46 49 51 54 55 56 57 58 62 66 68 73 74 77 79 81 82 84 86 96 99 100 103 107 117 118 119 121 124 133 135 136 137 **S** FirstHealth of the Carolinas
Primary Contact: John J. Jackson, President
COO: Allison Duckworth, Chief Operating Officer and Chief Nursing Officer
CFO: John D. Price, Chief Financial Officer
CMO: Len Newton, M.D., Chief Medical Officer
Web address: www.firsthealth.org
Control: Other not–for–profit (including NFP Corporation) **Service:** General Medical and Surgical

Staffed Beds: 141 **Admissions:** 4078 **Census:** 78 **Outpatient Visits:** 48289 **Births:** 615 **Total Expense ($000):** 37368 **Payroll Expense ($000):** 18878 **Personnel:** 415

ROCKY MOUNT—Nash County

☐ **LIFECARE HOSPITALS OF NORTH CAROLINA (342013)**, 1051 Noell Lane, Zip 27804–1761; tel. 252/451–2300 **A**1 10 **F**1 3 25 26 80 137 **S** LifeCare Management Services
Primary Contact: Kevin S. Cooper, RN, Chief Executive Officer and Administrator
COO: Robyn Perkerson, Clinical Operations Officer
CMO: Daniel Crocker, Chief Medical Officer
CHR: Vicky Goode, Manager Human Resources
Web address: www.lifecare–hospitals.com
Control: Corporation, Investor–owned, for–profit **Service:** Long–Term Acute Care hospital

Staffed Beds: 50 **Admissions:** 452 **Census:** 37 **Outpatient Visits:** 0 **Births:** 0 **Total Expense ($000):** 16615 **Payroll Expense ($000):** 5850 **Personnel:** 135

★ **NASH HEALTH CARE SYSTEMS (340147)**, 2460 Curtis Ellis Drive, Zip 27804–2297; tel. 252/443–8000 **A**1 2 9 10 **F**3 4 5 11 12 13 15 18 24 25 26 27 30 32 33 36 38 39 42 43 44 46 47 48 49 50 52 55 56 57 59 62 68 72 73 74 75 76 77 78 79 80 81 82 84 85 86 88 90 91 92 93 94 96 97 100 102 106 107 109 111 118 119 120 121 124 133 135 136 137
Primary Contact: Larry H. Chewning, III, President and Chief Executive Officer
COO: Brad Weisner, Executive Vice President and Chief Operating Officer
CFO: Al Hooks, Senior Vice President and Chief Financial Officer
CMO: Rick Guarino, M.D., Senior Vice President and Chief Medical Officer
CIO: David Hinkle, Vice President and Chief Information Officer
CHR: Cam Blalock, Senior Vice President Corporate Services
Web address: www.nhcs.org
Control: Hospital district or authority, Government, nonfederal **Service:** General Medical and Surgical

Staffed Beds: 310 **Admissions:** 14341 **Census:** 204 **Outpatient Visits:** 197417 **Births:** 1298 **Total Expense ($000):** 183018 **Payroll Expense ($000):** 83828 **Personnel:** 1659

ROXBORO—Person County

★ **PERSON MEMORIAL HOSPITAL (340159)**, 615 Ridge Road, Zip 27573–4630; tel. 336/599–2121, (Total facility includes 60 beds in nursing home–type unit) **A**1 9 10 **F**11 13 15 24 25 27 30 31 32 33 38 43 44 55 57 62 68 73 75 76 77 79 80 81 86 93 94 96 97 102 106 107 117 118 119 121 135 **S** Duke University Health System
Primary Contact: Jamie W. Guin, Jr., Chief Executive Officer
CFO: James L. Leis, Chief Financial Officer
CMO: Kenneth Flowe, M.D., Chief Medical Officer
CIO: Kelly Lucas, Manager Information Systems
CHR: Mary Paylor, Director Human Resources
Web address: www.personhospital.com
Control: Other not–for–profit (including NFP Corporation) **Service:** General Medical and Surgical

Staffed Beds: 110 **Admissions:** 2467 **Census:** 85 **Outpatient Visits:** 51301 **Births:** 150 **Total Expense ($000):** 33820 **Payroll Expense ($000):** 13193 **Personnel:** 329

RUTHERFORDTON—Rutherford County

★ **RUTHERFORD HOSPITAL (340013)**, 288 South Ridgecrest Avenue, Zip 28139–3097; tel. 828/286–5000 **A**1 2 9 10 19 **F**3 11 13 15 18 24 25 26 27 30 31 32 33 38 43 44 50 52 53 54 55 56 57 61 62 68 72 73 75 76 77 79 80 81 82 86 87 88 90 91 92 94 96 97 100 103 104 105 106 107 112 119 120 121 124 133 135 136 137 **S** QHR
Primary Contact: David Bixler, President
CFO: James B. Bross, Vice President and Chief Financial Officer
CMO: Dean Backstrom, M.D., Vice President Medical Affairs
CIO: Tommy Finley, Chief Information Officer
CHR: James Rowell, Vice President Human Resources
Web address: www.rutherfordhosp.org
Control: Other not–for–profit (including NFP Corporation) **Service:** General Medical and Surgical

Staffed Beds: 116 **Admissions:** 6119 **Census:** 62 **Outpatient Visits:** 85312 **Births:** 700 **Total Expense ($000):** 69050 **Payroll Expense ($000):** 32786 **Personnel:** 779

SALISBURY—Rowan County

★ **ROWAN REGIONAL MEDICAL CENTER (340015)**, 612 Mocksville Avenue, Zip 28144–2799; tel. 704/210–5000 **A**1 9 10 **F**3 4 6 8 11 13 15 17 18 20 24 25 26 27 30 33 35 38 42 43 44 46 48 49 50 51 52 53 55 56 57 59 60 61 62 66 68 71 72 73 74 75 76 77 79 80 81 82 85 86 88 90 92 96 100 102 107 109 112 119 120 121 124 135 136 137 **P**2 **S** Novant Health
Primary Contact: Charles W. Elliott, Jr., Chief Executive Officer
COO: Lee Roy Kirk, Senior Vice President and Chief Operating Officer
CFO: Marlin Markham, Senior Vice President and Chief Financial Officer
CMO: David N. Smith, M.D., Vice President Medical Affairs
CIO: Jerry Reardon, Director Information Systems
CHR: Jerry Clevenger, Vice President Human Resources
Web address: www.rowan.org
Control: Other not–for–profit (including NFP Corporation) **Service:** General Medical and Surgical

Staffed Beds: 180 **Admissions:** 8977 **Census:** 112 **Outpatient Visits:** 204597 **Births:** 898 **Total Expense ($000):** 162159 **Payroll Expense ($000):** 62339 **Personnel:** 1191

★ △ **VETERANS AFFAIRS MEDICAL CENTER**, 1601 Brenner Avenue, Zip 28144–2559; tel. 704/638–9000, (Total facility includes 300 beds in nursing home–type unit) (Nonreporting) **A**1 5 7 **S** Department of Veterans Affairs
Primary Contact: Carolyn L. Adams, Director
COO: Sheila Womack, Interim Associate Director
CFO: Steve Patil, Chief Financial Officer
CIO: Deborah Gunn, Director
CHR: Sandra Fischer, Director
Web address: www.va.gov/sta/guide/home.asp
Control: Veterans Affairs, Government, federal **Service:** Psychiatric

Staffed Beds: 533

 Many Facility Codes have changed. Please refer to the AHA Guide Code Chart.

SANFORD—Lee County

★ **CENTRAL CAROLINA HOSPITAL (340020)**, 1135 Carthage Street, Zip 27330–4111; tel. 919/774–2100, (Nonreporting) **A**1 9 10 **S** TENET Healthcare Corporation
Primary Contact: Doug Doris, Chief Executive Officer
COO: Kevin Zachary, Chief Operating Officer
CFO: Sharon Dickens, Chief Financial Officer
CMO: Richard Ebken, M.D., Chief Medical Officer
CIO: Jimmy Whitaker, Director Information Systems
CHR: Tom Macklin, Director Human Resources
Web address: www.centralcarolinahosp.com
Control: Corporation, Investor–owned, for–profit **Service:** General Medical and Surgical

Staffed Beds: 129

SCOTLAND NECK—Halifax County

OUR COMMUNITY HOSPITAL (341302), 921 Junior High Road, Zip 27874–0405, Mailing Address: Box 405, Zip 27874–0405; tel. 252/826–4144, (Total facility includes 60 beds in nursing home–type unit) **A**9 10 18 **F**38 52 54 56 57 67 86 87 93 96 117 118 122 137
Primary Contact: Thomas K. Majure, Administrator
COO: Rob Calhoun, Chief Operating Officer
CFO: Angela Hicks, Controller
Web address: www.och–bltc.org
Control: Other not–for–profit (including NFP Corporation) **Service:** General Medical and Surgical

Staffed Beds: 100 **Admissions:** 108 **Census:** 4 **Outpatient Visits:** 6322 **Births:** 0 **Total Expense ($000):** 3732 **Payroll Expense ($000):** 2291 **Personnel:** 37

SHELBY—Cleveland County

★ **CLEVELAND REGIONAL MEDICAL CENTER (340021)**, 201 East Grover Street, Zip 28150; tel. 704/487–3000, (Total facility includes 120 beds in nursing home–type unit) **A**1 2 9 10 19 **F**3 5 8 11 13 15 18 24 25 26 27 28 30 31 32 33 36 37 38 40 41 43 47 48 49 50 51 54 55 56 57 60 62 63 65 68 72 73 74 75 76 77 78 79 80 81 82 84 86 92 94 96 97 100 102 106 107 109 111 117 119 121 124 132 135 136 137 **S** Carolinas HealthCare System
Primary Contact: John E. Young, President and Chief Executive Officer
COO: Veronica Poole–Adams, Vice President, Chief Operating Officer and Chief Nursing Executive
CFO: Rose Coyne, Vice President and Chief Financial Officer
CIO: Craig Richardville, Chief Information Officer
CHR: Debbie Kale, Vice President Human Resources
Web address: www.clevelandregional.org
Control: Hospital district or authority, Government, nonfederal **Service:** General Medical and Surgical

Staffed Beds: 309 **Admissions:** 9321 **Census:** 218 **Outpatient Visits:** 116626 **Births:** 1032 **Total Expense ($000):** 136255 **Payroll Expense ($000):** 56466 **Personnel:** 1231

SILER CITY—Chatham County

★ **CHATHAM HOSPITAL (341311)**, West Third Street and Ivy Avenue, Zip 27344–2343, Mailing Address: P.O. Box 649, Zip 27344; tel. 919/663–2113 **A**1 9 10 18 **F**3 11 15 17 24 25 26 33 38 55 56 57 66 73 79 86 96 100 107 118 119 122 124 135 **P**5
Primary Contact: Carol Straight, Chief Executive Officer
CFO: Bert Barnette, Chief Financial Officer
CIO: Mike McCoy, Coordinator Information Technology
CHR: Kathy Thomas, Director Human Resources
Web address: www.chathamhospital.org
Control: Other not–for–profit (including NFP Corporation) **Service:** General Medical and Surgical

Staffed Beds: 25 **Admissions:** 774 **Census:** 8 **Outpatient Visits:** 22395 **Births:** 3 **Total Expense ($000):** 14787 **Payroll Expense ($000):** 6284 **Personnel:** 180

SMITHFIELD—Johnston County

★ **JOHNSTON MEMORIAL HOSPITAL (340090)**, 509 North Bright Leaf Boulevard, Zip 27577–1376, Mailing Address: P.O. Box 1376, Zip 27577–1376; tel. 919/934–8171 **A**1 9 10 **F**3 8 11 13 15 17 18 24 25 26 27 28 30 31 32 33 38 39 42 43 46 47 48 49 50 52 53 54 55 56 57 59 61 62 63 64 66 68 72 73 74 75 77 79 80 81 82 84 86 87 88 89 90 92 93 96 97 100 102 106 107 118 119 120 121 124 132 133 135 136 **P**6 **S** QHR
Primary Contact: Kevin L. Rogols, CHE, President and Chief Executive Officer
COO: Jackie Ring, Chief Operating Officer and Chief Nursing Executive
CFO: Stephen Sawyer, Chief Financial Officer
CMO: Eric Gloss, M.D., Vice President Medical Affairs
CHR: Timothy A. Hays, Vice President Human Resources
Web address: www.johnstonmemorial.org
Control: Hospital district or authority, Government, nonfederal **Service:** General Medical and Surgical

Staffed Beds: 167 **Admissions:** 8651 **Census:** 124 **Outpatient Visits:** 198431 **Births:** 1358 **Total Expense ($000):** 123519 **Payroll Expense ($000):** 48544 **Personnel:** 1126

SOUTHPORT—Brunswick County

★ **J. ARTHUR DOSHER MEMORIAL HOSPITAL (340121)**, 924 North Howe Street, Zip 28461–3099; tel. 910/457–3800, (Total facility includes 64 beds in nursing home–type unit) **A**1 9 10 **F**3 15 24 26 30 31 32 33 38 41 43 44 45 46 52 55 56 57 63 65 66 69 73 75 77 79 80 86 96 100 102 107 117 119 121 122 124 132 135
Primary Contact: Edgar Haywood, III, Administrator
COO: Lynda Stanley, Senior Vice President and Chief Operating Officer
CFO: Dennis J. Coffey, CPA, Chief Financial Officer and Senior Vice President
CMO: Brad L. Hilaman, M.D., Chief of Staff
CIO: Susan Shomaker, Director Information Management Systems
CHR: Kelley Richards, Director Human Resources
Web address: www.dosher.org
Control: Other not–for–profit (including NFP Corporation) **Service:** General Medical and Surgical

Staffed Beds: 100 **Admissions:** 1589 **Census:** 65 **Outpatient Visits:** 178109 **Births:** 0 **Total Expense ($000):** 27578 **Payroll Expense ($000):** 10710 **Personnel:** 300

SPARTA—Alleghany County

★ **ALLEGHANY MEMORIAL HOSPITAL (341320)**, 233 Doctors Street, Zip 28675–0009, Mailing Address: P.O. Box 9, Zip 28675–0009; tel. 336/372–5511 **A**1 9 10 18 **F**3 15 25 26 30 31 32 33 38 40 43 55 57 62 65 75 79 82 85 86 87 96 100 107 117 118 119 122 124 135 **P**5 **S** QHR
Primary Contact: Ralph Castillo, Chief Executive Officer
CFO: Katie Myers, Chief Financial Officer
CMO: Mary Emma Beres, Chief Medical Staff
CIO: Darlene Keith, Chief Information Systems
CHR: John Spencer, Director Human Resources
Web address: www.amhsparta.org
Control: Other not–for–profit (including NFP Corporation) **Service:** General Medical and Surgical

Staffed Beds: 25 **Admissions:** 842 **Census:** 8 **Outpatient Visits:** 25350 **Births:** 0 **Total Expense ($000):** 9473 **Payroll Expense ($000):** 4143 **Personnel:** 133

SPRUCE PINE—Mitchell County

□ **BLUE RIDGE REGIONAL HOSPITAL (340011)**, 125 Hospital Drive, Zip 28777, Mailing Address: P.O. Drawer 9, Zip 28777; tel. 828/765–4201 **A**1 9 10 20 **F**1 3 4 13 15 16 17 24 25 26 27 28 30 31 32 33 37 38 40 43 52 53 55 57 62 64 65 68 70 71 73 74 75 76 77 78 79 80 82 83 84 85 86 87 88 96 100 102 107 117 118 119 120 121 122 124 133 134 135 137
Primary Contact: Keith S. Holtsclaw, Chief Executive Officer
CFO: Jonathan Smith, Chief Financial Officer
CMO: Steven Hill, M.D., Chief of Staff
CIO: Kathy Calhoun, Director Management Information System Services
CHR: Fonda Harris, R.N., Director Human Resources
Web address: www.spchospital.org
Control: Other not–for–profit (including NFP Corporation) **Service:** General Medical and Surgical

Staffed Beds: 40 **Admissions:** 2251 **Census:** 19 **Outpatient Visits:** 50573 **Births:** 180 **Total Expense ($000):** 30548 **Payroll Expense ($000):** 15484 **Personnel:** 370

Hospital, Medicare Provider Number, Address, Telephone, Approval, Facility, and Physician Codes, Health Care System
★ American Hospital Association (AHA) membership
□ The Joint Commission accreditation
○ American Osteopathic Association (AOA) accreditation
△ Commission on Accreditation of Rehabilitation Facilities (CARF) accreditation

STATESVILLE—Iredell County

☐ **DAVIS REGIONAL MEDICAL CENTER (340144)**, 218 Old Mocksville Road, Zip 28625–1930, Mailing Address: P.O. Box 1823, Zip 28687–1823; tel. 704/873–0281, (Total facility includes 13 beds in nursing home–type unit) **A**1 9 10 19 **F**3 11 12 13 15 17 18 24 25 26 30 31 32 33 38 42 43 44 50 52 54 55 57 59 62 68 72 73 74 75 77 79 80 82 84 86 88 90 91 92 94 95 96 100 102 107 117 118 119 120 121 124 135 136 137 **P**4 6 **S** Health Management Associates
Primary Contact: Karen Metz, Chief Executive Officer
COO: John Phillips, Chief Operating Officer
CFO: Rodney Ball, Chief Financial Officer
CMO: Lisa Fair, M.D., Chief of Staff
CIO: Janie Stikeleather, Director Marketing and Community Relations
CHR: Alison Kay, Director Human Resources
Web address: www.davisregional.com
Control: Corporation, Investor–owned, for–profit **Service:** General Medical and Surgical

Staffed Beds: 149 **Admissions:** 5369 **Census:** 56 **Outpatient Visits:** 45403 **Births:** 476 **Total Expense ($000):** 47192 **Payroll Expense ($000):** 19574 **Personnel:** 386

★ **IREDELL MEMORIAL HOSPITAL (340039)**, 557 Brookdale Drive, Zip 28677–1828, Mailing Address: P.O. Box 1828, Zip 28687–1828; tel. 704/873–5661, (Total facility includes 48 beds in nursing home–type unit) **A**1 2 9 10 **F**3 11 13 15 17 18 24 25 26 27 28 30 31 32 33 38 43 48 49 50 54 55 56 57 59 61 62 66 68 72 73 74 75 76 77 79 80 81 82 84 86 87 96 97 100 102 103 105 106 107 109 111 117 118 119 121 124 135 136 137 **P**6
Primary Contact: Ed Rush, President and Chief Executive Officer
CFO: Fred W. Karnap, Vice President Finance
CMO: Anthony Meluch, M.D., President Medical Staff
CIO: Myers M. David, Chief Information Officer
CHR: Elaine Allison, Vice President Human Resources
Web address: www.iredellmemorial.org
Control: Other not–for–profit (including NFP Corporation) **Service:** General Medical and Surgical

Staffed Beds: 203 **Admissions:** 9587 **Census:** 155 **Outpatient Visits:** 152953 **Births:** 854 **Total Expense ($000):** 131110 **Payroll Expense ($000):** 62299 **Personnel:** 1239

SUPPLY—Brunswick County

★ **BRUNSWICK COMMUNITY HOSPITAL (340158)**, 1 Medical Center Drive, Zip 28462–3350, Mailing Address: P.O. Box 139, Zip 28462–0139; tel. 910/755–8121 **A**1 9 10 **F**13 15 24 25 26 30 31 32 33 38 54 55 56 57 62 68 73 74 77 79 82 86 96 97 100 106 107 119 124 135 **P**6 **S** Novant Health
Primary Contact: Denise B. Mihal, RN, President
CFO: Joan Thomas, Chief Financial Officer
CMO: Robert Hassler, M.D., Director Medical Affairs
CIO: Pamela Parrish, Information Systems Director
Web address: www.brunswickcommunityhospital.com
Control: Other not–for–profit (including NFP Corporation) **Service:** General Medical and Surgical

Staffed Beds: 60 **Admissions:** 3382 **Census:** 30 **Outpatient Visits:** 91900 **Births:** 341 **Total Expense ($000):** 44954 **Payroll Expense ($000):** 19098 **Personnel:** 413

SYLVA—Jackson County

★ **HARRIS REGIONAL HOSPITAL (340016)**, 68 Hospital Road, Zip 28779–2795; tel. 828/586–7000, (Total facility includes 114 beds in nursing home–type unit) **A**1 9 10 **F**3 7 8 11 13 15 24 25 26 27 30 31 33 38 42 43 44 46 50 53 56 61 62 66 68 70 73 74 75 76 77 79 80 81 82 84 85 86 96 97 100 102 107 108 109 117 118 119 120 124 132 135 136 137 **S** WestCare Health System
Primary Contact: Mark T. Leonard, Chief Executive Officer
CFO: Pam Buchanan, Chief Financial Officer
CMO: Randy Savell, M.D., Chief of Staff
CIO: Shawn Remacle, Chief Information Officer
CHR: Janet Millsaps, Vice President Staff Services
Web address: www.westcare.org
Control: Other not–for–profit (including NFP Corporation) **Service:** General Medical and Surgical

Staffed Beds: 200 **Admissions:** 5631 **Census:** 157 **Outpatient Visits:** 68513 **Births:** 721 **Total Expense ($000):** 72253 **Payroll Expense ($000):** 30616 **Personnel:** 744

TARBORO—Edgecombe County

★ **HERITAGE HOSPITAL (340107)**, 111 Hospital Drive, Zip 27886–2011; tel. 252/641–7700 **A**1 9 10 **F**3 8 11 13 15 25 26 27 30 31 32 37 38 43 50 55 57 67 68 71 73 74 76 77 79 80 82 84 85 86 96 107 119 120 121 122 124 135 **S** University Health Systems of Eastern Carolina
Primary Contact: Wendell H. Baker, Jr., President
CFO: Charles Alford, Vice President Financial Services
CMO: Barry Bunn, M.D., Chief of Staff
CHR: Arenda Battle, Director Human Resources
Web address: www.heritage.uhseast.com
Control: Other not–for–profit (including NFP Corporation) **Service:** General Medical and Surgical

Staffed Beds: 117 **Admissions:** 4996 **Census:** 49 **Outpatient Visits:** 51568 **Births:** 633 **Total Expense ($000):** 50097 **Payroll Expense ($000):** 20896 **Personnel:** 517

THOMASVILLE—Davidson County

★ **THOMASVILLE MEDICAL CENTER (340085)**, 207 Old Lexington Road, Zip 27360–3428, Mailing Address: P.O. Box 789, Zip 27361–0789; tel. 336/472–2000 **A**1 2 9 10 **F**13 15 24 25 26 30 31 32 33 38 46 47 48 54 55 56 57 63 68 72 73 74 75 77 79 80 81 82 84 86 88 93 94 96 97 100 102 106 107 118 121 124 135 136 **P**6 **S** Novant Health
Primary Contact: Gabrielle K. Causby, President
CFO: Tom Pogue, Vice President
CHR: Andrea West, Manager Human Resources
Web address: www.thomasvillemedicalcenter.org
Control: Other not–for–profit (including NFP Corporation) **Service:** General Medical and Surgical

Staffed Beds: 94 **Admissions:** 4116 **Census:** 54 **Outpatient Visits:** 111685 **Births:** 550 **Total Expense ($000):** 47870 **Payroll Expense ($000):** 20418 **Personnel:** 443

TROY—Montgomery County

★ **FIRSTHEALTH MONTGOMERY MEMORIAL HOSPITAL (341303)**, 520 Allen Street, Zip 27371–2802, Mailing Address: P.O. Box 486, Zip 27371–0486; tel. 910/572–1301 **A**1 9 10 18 **F**3 11 15 25 26 30 31 32 38 46 54 57 62 77 79 80 82 86 87 96 102 107 118 122 135 137 **S** FirstHealth of the Carolinas
Primary Contact: Kerry A. Hensley, RN, President
COO: Beth Walker, Chief Operating Officer and Chief Nursing Officer
CFO: Bryan Hawkins, Controller
CHR: Ellie Wiles, Director Human Resources
Web address: www.firsthealth.org
Control: Other not–for–profit (including NFP Corporation) **Service:** General Medical and Surgical

Staffed Beds: 25 **Admissions:** 527 **Census:** 7 **Outpatient Visits:** 23212 **Total Expense ($000):** 12305 **Payroll Expense ($000):** 6132 **Personnel:** 129

VALDESE—Burke County

★ **VALDESE GENERAL HOSPITAL (340055)**, 720 Malcolm Boulevard, Zip 28690, Mailing Address: P.O. Box 700, Zip 28690–0700; tel. 828/874–2251, (Total facility includes 108 beds in nursing home–type unit) **A**1 2 9 10 **F**3 11 12 15 18 21 24 25 26 27 30 31 32 33 38 43 44 45 46 54 55 57 62 66 68 73 75 76 77 79 80 81 82 86 96 97 98 99 100 103 104 106 107 109 115 117 119 121 124 132 135 136 137 **S** Carolinas HealthCare System
Primary Contact: Kenneth W. Wood, President and Chief Executive Officer
COO: Kathy C. Bailey, Ph.D., FACHE, Vice President
CFO: Robert Fritts, Chief Financial Officer
CMO: Dorwyn Croon, President Medical Staff
CHR: Phil Satey, Vice President Human Resources
Web address: www.blueridgehealth.org
Control: Hospital district or authority, Government, nonfederal **Service:** General Medical and Surgical

Staffed Beds: 163 **Admissions:** 3027 **Census:** 134 **Outpatient Visits:** 107819 **Births:** 0 **Total Expense ($000):** 54382 **Payroll Expense ($000):** 19716 **Personnel:** 362

WADESBORO—Anson County

★ **ANSON COMMUNITY HOSPITAL (340084)**, 500 Morven Road, Zip 28170–2745; tel. 704/694–5131, (Total facility includes 95 beds in nursing home–type unit) **A**1 9 10 **F**11 15 24 25 26 30 31 32 33 38 43 54 55 56 57 58 61 62 63 69 75 79 81 82 86 96 99 102 106 107 117 119 121 122 124 134 135 **P**5 **S** Carolinas HealthCare System
Primary Contact: Frederick G. Thompson, Ph.D., Administrator and Chief Executive Officer
CFO: Dale Spencer, Chief Financial Officer
CHR: Sherri McRorie, Director Human Resources
Web address: www.carolinashealthcare.org
Control: Hospital district or authority, Government, nonfederal **Service:** General Medical and Surgical

Staffed Beds: 125 **Admissions:** 1445 **Census:** 105 **Outpatient Visits:** 30822 **Births:** 0 **Total Expense ($000):** 24397 **Payroll Expense ($000):** 10900 **Personnel:** 346

WASHINGTON—Beaufort County

★ **BEAUFORT COUNTY HOSPITAL (340038)**, 628 East 12th Street, Zip 27889–3498; tel. 252/975–4100 **A**1 9 10 **F**3 7 13 15 24 25 26 27 30 31 32 33 34 38 52 55 56 57 61 62 68 73 74 76 77 79 80 81 82 86 87 88 89 90 91 92 94 96 97 100 102 106 107 118 119 121 132 133 134 135
Primary Contact: Bill R. Bedsole, Chief Executive Officer
COO: Susan Gerard, Assistant Administrator
CFO: Chris Riggs, Chief Financial Officer
CMO: Russel Cook, M.D., Chief of Staff
CIO: Amy Boyd, Manager Information Systems
CHR: Penny Leggett, Manager Human Resources
Web address: www.beaufortcountyhospital.org
Control: Hospital district or authority, Government, nonfederal **Service:** General Medical and Surgical

Staffed Beds: 95 **Admissions:** 3681 **Census:** 43 **Outpatient Visits:** 163387 **Births:** 435 **Total Expense ($000):** 53729 **Payroll Expense ($000):** 25344 **Personnel:** 708

WHITEVILLE—Columbus County

★ **COLUMBUS REGIONAL HEALTHCARE SYSTEM (340068)**, 500 Jefferson Street, Zip 28472–9987; tel. 910/642–8011 **A**1 9 10 19 **F**3 8 11 13 15 18 24 25 26 27 30 31 32 33 35 38 46 50 51 53 55 56 57 58 59 66 68 72 73 74 75 76 77 79 80 81 82 84 86 96 100 102 107 112 118 119 121 124 134 135 136 137 **S** Carolinas HealthCare System
Primary Contact: Henry Hawthorne, III, President and Chief Executive Officer
COO: Ann Johnston, Vice President Operations
CFO: Carl Biber, Chief Financial Officer
CMO: Erik Kenyon, D.O., Chief of Staff
CIO: Lisa Ward, Director Management Information Systems
CHR: Ginger Scott, Vice President Human Resources
Web address: www.crhealthcare.org
Control: Other not–for–profit (including NFP Corporation) **Service:** General Medical and Surgical

Staffed Beds: 151 **Admissions:** 5908 **Census:** 78 **Outpatient Visits:** 90599 **Births:** 509 **Total Expense ($000):** 62656 **Payroll Expense ($000):** 26527 **Personnel:** 593

WILLIAMSTON—Martin County

★ **MARTIN GENERAL HOSPITAL (340133)**, 310 South McCaskey Road, Zip 27892–2150, Mailing Address: P.O. Box 1128, Zip 27892–1128; tel. 252/809–6179, (Nonreporting) **A**1 9 10 **S** Community Health Systems, Inc.
Primary Contact: Glenn Carney, Chief Executive Officer
CFO: Kevin Randall, Chief Financial Officer
CIO: James Griffin, Manager Information Systems
CHR: Vickie Coleman, Director Human Resources
Web address: www.martingeneral.com
Control: County–Government, nonfederal **Service:** General Medical and Surgical

Staffed Beds: 49

WILMINGTON—New Hanover County

CAPE FEAR HOSPITAL See New Hanover Regional Medical Center

★ △ **NEW HANOVER REGIONAL MEDICAL CENTER (340141)**, 2131 South 17th Street, Zip 28401–7483, Mailing Address: P.O. Box 9000, Zip 28402–9000; tel. 910/343–7000, (Includes CAPE FEAR HOSPITAL, 5301 Wrightsville Avenue, Zip 28403–6599; tel. 910/452–8100; Donna Bost, RN, Administrator) **A**1 2 7 9 10 12 13 **F**3 7 8 11 12 13 15 17 18 20 22 24 25 26 27 30 31 32 33 34 37 38 40 43 44 46 49 50 54 55 56 57 58 59 60 62 64 66 68 69 70 71 72 73 74 75 76 77 78 79 80 81 82 84 85 86 87 88 90 91 92 93 94 95 96 97 100 102 103 104 105 106 107 109 111 118 119 120 121 124 135 136 137 **P**6 **S** New Hanover Health Network
Primary Contact: John K. Barto, Jr., President and Chief Executive Officer
COO: Matthew Heywood, Chief Operating Officer
CFO: Edwin J. Ollie, Executive Vice President and Chief Financial Officer
CMO: Sam Spicer, M.D., Vice President Medical Affairs
CIO: Avery Cloud, Vice President and Chief Information Officer
CHR: Keith Strawn, Vice President Human Resources
Web address: www.nhhn.org
Control: County–Government, nonfederal **Service:** General Medical and Surgical

Staffed Beds: 646 **Admissions:** 30133 **Census:** 470 **Outpatient Visits:** 416605 **Births:** 4128 **Total Expense ($000):** 520380 **Payroll Expense ($000):** 206011 **Personnel:** 3919

WILMINGTON TREATMENT CENTER (340168), 2520 Troy Drive, Zip 28401–7643; tel. 910/762–2727, (Nonreporting) **A**10
Primary Contact: Charles S. Sharp, Chief Executive Officer
COO: Paige Bottom, Director Operations
CFO: Virginia Powell, Director Finance
CMO: Patrick Martin, M.D., Medical Director
Web address: www.wilmtreatment.com
Control: Corporation, Investor–owned, for–profit **Service:** Alcoholism and other chemical dependency

Staffed Beds: 94

WILSON—Wilson County

★ **WILSON MEDICAL CENTER (340126)**, 1705 Tarboro Street, S.W., Zip 27893–3428; tel. 252/399–8040 **A**1 2 9 10 19 **F**3 11 13 15 18 24 25 26 27 30 31 37 38 44 45 47 48 49 55 56 59 62 72 73 74 75 76 77 78 79 80 81 82 84 86 87 88 91 92 93 96 97 99 100 102 103 107 108 109 111 118 119 121 124 135 137 **P**6
Primary Contact: Richard E. Hudson, FACHE, President and Chief Executive Officer
CMO: Linda Christmann, M.D., Vice President Medical Affairs
CIO: Rex Burnworth, Director Information Systems
CHR: Lynne Gallimore, Vice President Human Resources
Web address: www.wilmed.org
Control: Other not–for–profit (including NFP Corporation) **Service:** General Medical and Surgical

Staffed Beds: 220 **Admissions:** 9174 **Census:** 98 **Outpatient Visits:** 146736 **Births:** 1602 **Total Expense ($000):** 120234 **Payroll Expense ($000):** 51448 **Personnel:** 1057

WINDSOR—Bertie County

★ **BERTIE MEMORIAL HOSPITAL (341304)**, 1403 South King Street, Zip 27983–1726, Mailing Address: P.O. Box 40, Zip 27983–1726; tel. 252/794–6600 **A**1 9 10 18 **F**15 30 31 38 55 62 75 79 96 103 135 136 **S** University Health Systems of Eastern Carolina
Primary Contact: Jeffrey N. Sackrison, FACHE, President
CFO: Michael Dacus, Vice President Financial Services
Web address: www.bertie.uhseast.com
Control: Other not–for–profit (including NFP Corporation) **Service:** General Medical and Surgical

Staffed Beds: 6 **Admissions:** 444 **Census:** 4 **Outpatient Visits:** 19959 **Births:** 0 **Total Expense ($000):** 13358 **Payroll Expense ($000):** 5350 **Personnel:** 120

WINSTON–SALEM—Forsyth County

★ **FORSYTH MEDICAL CENTER (340014)**, 3333 Silas Creek Parkway, Zip 27103–3090; tel. 336/718–5000, (Total facility includes 10 beds in nursing home–type unit) **A**1 2 3 5 9 10 **F**3 5 7 9 10 13 14 17 18 20 22 24 25 26 27 28 30 31 32 33 35 36 38 41 43 44 45 46 49 50 52 53 54 55 56 57 58 59 60 62 63 64 65 66 68 69 70 72 73 74 75 76 77 78 79 80 81 82 84 85 86 88 90 91 92 93 94 95 96 97 98 100 101 102 103 104 105 106 107 108 109 111 112 117 119 120 121 124 132 135 136 137 **P**6 **S** Novant Health
Primary Contact: Gregory J. Beier, President and Chief Executive Officer
COO: Sallye A. Liner, Executive Vice President and Chief Operating Officer
CFO: Dean Swindle, Chief Financial Officer
CMO: Elms Allen, M.D., Senior Vice President Medical Affairs
CIO: Rich B. McKnight, Chief Information Officer
Web address: www.novanthealth.org
Control: Other not–for–profit (including NFP Corporation) **Service:** General Medical and Surgical

Staffed Beds: 852 **Admissions:** 40172 **Census:** 654 **Outpatient Visits:** 345039 **Births:** 7103 **Total Expense ($000):** 513514 **Payroll Expense ($000):** 204956 **Personnel:** 3991

★ **MEDICAL PARK HOSPITAL (340148)**, 1950 South Hawthorne Road, Zip 27103–3993, Mailing Address: P.O. Box 24728, Zip 27114–4728; tel. 336/718–0600 **A**1 2 9 10 **F**3 25 30 31 32 33 56 62 66 72 73 76 77 79 80 82 116 118 119 124 132 135 **S** Novant Health
Primary Contact: Timothy S. Shelton, Administrator
COO: Sallye A. Liner, Executive Vice President and Chief Operating Officer
CFO: Dean Swindle, Executive Vice President and Chief Financial Officer Novant Health
CMO: Elms Allen, M.D., Senior Vice President Medical Affairs
CIO: Richard McKnight, Senior Vice President Chief Information Officer
CHR: Jason Carter, Vice President Human Resources
Web address: www.novanthealth.org
Control: Other not–for–profit (including NFP Corporation) **Service:** General Medical and Surgical

Staffed Beds: 22 **Admissions:** 1501 **Census:** 16 **Outpatient Visits:** 41849 **Births:** 0 **Total Expense ($000):** 41682 **Payroll Expense ($000):** 13482 **Personnel:** 268

Hospital, Medicare Provider Number, Address, Telephone, Approval, Facility, and Physician Codes, Health Care System

★ American Hospital Association (AHA) membership
□ The Joint Commission accreditation
○ American Osteopathic Association (AOA) accreditation
△ Commission on Accreditation of Rehabilitation Facilities (CARF) accreditation

NC

★ △ **NORTH CAROLINA BAPTIST HOSPITAL (WAKE FOREST UNIVERSITY BAPTIST MEDICAL CENTER) (340047)**, Medical Center Boulevard, Zip 27157–0001; tel. 336/716–2011, (Total facility includes 170 beds in nursing home–type unit) **A**1 7 8 9 10 **F**3 7 8 11 12 15 16 17 18 19 20 21 22 23 24 25 26 27 28 29 30 31 32 33 34 35 36 38 40 41 43 44 45 46 48 49 50 52 53 54 55 56 57 58 59 60 61 62 63 64 66 68 70 71 72 73 75 76 77 78 79 80 81 82 83 84 85 86 87 88 89 90 91 92 93 96 97 99 100 102 103 104 105 106 107 108 109 111 112 114 116 117 118 119 120 121 122 123 124 125 126 127 130 131 132 134 135 136 137 **P**1 6 **S** North Carolina Baptist Hospital
Primary Contact: Donny C. Lambeth, Interim President
COO: Donny C. Lambeth, Interim President and Chief Operating Officer
CFO: Gina B. Ramsey, Vice President Financial Services and Chief Financial Officer
CMO: Patricia L. Adams, M.D., Chief Professional Services
CIO: Paul M. LoRusso, Vice President Information Services and Chief Information Officer
CHR: Steven C. Snelgrove, Interim Vice President Human Resources
Web address: www.wfubmc.edu
Control: Other not–for–profit (including NFP Corporation) **Service:** General Medical and Surgical

Staffed Beds: 965 **Admissions:** 35136 **Census:** 773 **Outpatient Visits:** 198928 **Births:** 0 **Total Expense ($000):** 796758 **Payroll Expense ($000):** 339918 **Personnel:** 7403

OLD VINEYARD BEHAVIORAL HEALTH SERVICES (344007), (Formerly Old Vineyard Youth Services), 3637 Old Vineyard Road, Zip 27104–4835; tel. 336/794–3550 **A**10 **F**25 30 31 32 82 88 89 91 92 95 119 **P**5 **S** Universal Health Services, Inc.
Primary Contact: Wesley E. Mason, III, Chief Executive Officer
COO: Andrew Hotaling, Chief Operating Officer
CMO: Raj Thotakura, M.D., Medical Director
CHR: Cheryl McKinney, Director Human Resources
Web address: www.oldvineyard.net
Control: Corporation, Investor–owned, for–profit **Service:** Psychiatric

Staffed Beds: 108 **Admissions:** 1335 **Census:** 60 **Outpatient Visits:** 82 **Births:** 0 **Total Expense ($000):** 12824 **Payroll Expense ($000):** 6818 **Personnel:** 216

☐ **SELECT SPECIALTY HOSPITAL OF WINSTON–SALEM (342016)**, 3333 Silas Creek Parkway, 6th Floor, Zip 27103; tel. 336/718–6300 **A**1 10 **F**1 25 30 32 119 137 **P**2 **S** Select Medical Corporation
Primary Contact: Marion Reef, Chief Executive Officer
Web address: www.selectmedicalcorp.com
Control: Corporation, Investor–owned, for–profit **Service:** Long–Term Acute Care hospital

Staffed Beds: 25 **Admissions:** 245 **Census:** 20 **Outpatient Visits:** 0 **Births:** 0 **Total Expense ($000):** 12468 **Payroll Expense ($000):** 4908 **Personnel:** 73

☐ **WAKE FOREST UNIVERSITY HEALTH SERVICE**, Medical Center Boulevard, Zip 27109, Mailing Address: P.O. Box 7386, Winston Salem, Zip 27109–7386; tel. 336/758–5937, (Nonreporting) **A**1 2
Primary Contact: Cecil Price, Director
Web address: www.wfu.edu
Control: Other not–for–profit (including NFP Corporation) **Service:** Hospital unit of an institution (prison hospital, college infimary, etc.)

Staffed Beds: 6

YADKINVILLE—Yadkin County

★ **HOOTS MEMORIAL HOSPITAL (341308)**, 624 West Main Street, Zip 27055–7804, Mailing Address: P.O. Box 68, Zip 27055–0068; tel. 336/679–2041 **A**1 9 10 18 **F**3 11 15 25 26 31 32 33 38 44 45 50 52 54 57 62 63 79 80 84 85 86 87 96 107 119 122 135 **P**6 **S** North Carolina Baptist Hospital
Primary Contact: Lance C. Labine, President
CFO: James McDonnell, Chief Financial Officer
CHR: Bruce Niemeyer, Director Human Resources
Web address: www.bgsm.edu/hoots/
Control: Other not–for–profit (including NFP Corporation) **Service:** General Medical and Surgical

Staffed Beds: 22 **Admissions:** 266 **Census:** 5 **Outpatient Visits:** 15857 **Births:** 0 **Total Expense ($000):** 9572 **Payroll Expense ($000):** 3844 **Personnel:** 119

NORTH DAKOTA

ASHLEY—McIntosh County

★ **ASHLEY MEDICAL CENTER (351322)**, 612 North Center Avenue, Zip 58413–0556, Mailing Address: P.O. Box 450, Zip 58413–0450; tel. 701/288–3433, (Total facility includes 44 beds in nursing home–type unit) **A**9 10 18 **F**3 11 15 24 27 28 31 32 33 38 40 42 43 44 50 52 54 55 57 61 62 63 66 68 73 79 80 81 82 86 87 96 102 115 117 119 120 121 122 132 134 135 136 137 **P**6
Primary Contact: Kathleen Hoeft, Administrator and Chief Executive Officer
CFO: Jerry Lepp, Chief Financial Officer
CMO: Udom Tinsa, M.D., Medical Director
Web address: www.amctoday.org
Control: Other not–for–profit (including NFP Corporation) **Service:** General Medical and Surgical

Staffed Beds: 64 **Admissions:** 225 **Census:** 41 **Outpatient Visits:** 5161 **Births:** 0 **Total Expense ($000):** 5307 **Payroll Expense ($000):** 2940 **Personnel:** 117

BELCOURT—Rolette County

★☐ **PUBLIC HEALTH SERVICE INDIAN HOSPITAL – QUENTIN N. BURDICK MEMORIAL HEALTH FACILITY (350063)**, 2 Blocks North of Highway 5, Zip 58316, Mailing Address: P.O. Box 160, Zip 58316–0160; tel. 701/477–6111 **A**1 5 10 **F**7 15 25 31 32 33 37 38 40 50 55 56 57 62 63 74 79 84 86 89 92 94 96 107 119 124 132 136 **S** U. S. Indian Health Service
Primary Contact: David L. Quincy, Chief Executive Officer
CFO: Lynn Davis, Chief Financial Officer
Web address: www.ihs.gov
Control: PHS, Indian Service, Government, federal **Service:** General Medical and Surgical

Staffed Beds: 27 **Admissions:** 1045 **Census:** 8 **Outpatient Visits:** 111942 **Births:** 231 **Personnel:** 243

BISMARCK—Burleigh County

★☐ △ **MEDCENTER ONE (350015)**, 300 North Seventh Street, Zip 58501–4439, Mailing Address: P.O. Box 5525, Zip 58506–5525; tel. 701/323–6000, (Total facility includes 19 beds in nursing home–type unit) **A**1 2 3 5 7 9 10 **F**3 9 11 12 13 15 17 18 20 22 24 25 26 27 28 32 33 34 35 38 40 41 42 43 44 47 49 51 52 54 55 56 57 58 59 60 61 62 63 67 68 70 71 72 73 74 75 76 77 79 80 81 82 83 84 85 86 87 88 89 90 91 92 93 94 95 96 97 100 102 105 106 107 113 117 118 119 120 121 123 127 133 135 136 137 **P**6
Primary Contact: James C. Cooper, President and Chief Executive Officer
CFO: Paul Morth, Vice President Finance
CMO: Craig Lambrecht, M.D., Medical Director
CIO: John Miller, Vice President Information Services
CHR: Scott Boehm, Vice President Human Resources
Web address: www.medcenterone.com
Control: Other not–for–profit (including NFP Corporation) **Service:** General Medical and Surgical

Staffed Beds: 223 **Admissions:** 9276 **Census:** 113 **Outpatient Visits:** 393455 **Births:** 692 **Total Expense ($000):** 224591 **Payroll Expense ($000):** 117289 **Personnel:** 1927

★☐ △ **ST. ALEXIUS MEDICAL CENTER (350002)**, 900 East Broadway, Zip 58501–4586, Mailing Address: P.O. Box 5510, Zip 58506–5510; tel. 701/530–7000, (Total facility includes 19 beds in nursing home–type unit) **A**1 2 3 5 7 9 10 **F**3 8 9 11 12 13 15 17 18 20 22 23 24 25 26 27 28 30 31 32 33 34 36 38 40 42 43 52 54 55 56 57 59 61 62 66 68 70 71 72 73 74 76 77 79 83 84 85 86 88 89 90 91 92 93 94 95 96 100 102 104 105 107 117 118 119 120 121 122 124 134 135 136 137 **P**8 **S** Benedictine Sisters of the Annunciation
Primary Contact: Andrew L. Wilson, President and Chief Executive Officer
CFO: Gary Miller, Senior Vice President and Chief Financial Officer
CMO: Shiraz Hyder, M.D., Director Medical Affairs
CIO: Ron Hindt, Chief Information Officer
CHR: Wanda Pfaff, Vice President Human Resources
Web address: www.st.alexius.org
Control: Church–operated, Nongovernment, not–for profit **Service:** General Medical and Surgical

Staffed Beds: 280 **Admissions:** 9938 **Census:** 126 **Outpatient Visits:** 181066 **Births:** 1251 **Total Expense ($000):** 171666 **Payroll Expense ($000):** 69783 **Personnel:** 1666

BOTTINEAU—Bottineau County

ST. ANDREW'S HEALTH CENTER (351307), 316 Ohmer Street, Zip 58318–1018; tel. 701/228–9300 **A**5 9 10 18 **F**8 15 24 26 27 30 38 40 50 55 57 62 79 86 87 96 115 119 121 122 135 **P**1 **S** Sisters of Mary of the Presentation Health System
Primary Contact: Jodi Atkinson, President and Chief Executive Officer
CFO: Kerri Christenson, Chief Financial Officer
CHR: Brenda Arneson, Administrative Assistant
Web address: www.standrewshealth.com
Control: Other not–for–profit (including NFP Corporation) **Service:** General Medical and Surgical

Staffed Beds: 25 **Admissions:** 163 **Census:** 1 **Outpatient Visits:** 8400 **Births:** 0 **Total Expense ($000):** 4924 **Payroll Expense ($000):** 1852 **Personnel:** 76

BOWMAN—Bowman County

SOUTHWEST HEALTHCARE SERVICES (351313), 202 Sixth Avenue S.W., Zip 58623–0009, Mailing Address: P.O. Drawer C, Zip 58623; tel. 701/523–5265, (Total facility includes 67 beds in nursing home–type unit) (Nonreporting) **A**9 10 18
Primary Contact: Darrold Bertsch, Administrator
CFO: Becky Hansen, Chief Financial Officer
Web address: www.swhealthcare.net
Control: Other not–for–profit (including NFP Corporation) **Service:** General Medical and Surgical

Staffed Beds: 90

CANDO—Towner County

★ **TOWNER COUNTY MEDICAL CENTER (351331)**, Mailing Address: P.O. Box 688, Zip 58324–0688; tel. 701/968–4411, (Total facility includes 60 beds in nursing home–type unit) (Nonreporting) **A**5 9 10 18
Primary Contact: Jac McTaggart, Chief Executive Officer
CFO: Tammy Larson, Chief Financial Officer
CMO: Greg Culver, M.D., Chief of Staff
CHR: Pat Klingenberg, Director Human Resources
Web address: www.tcmedcenter.com
Control: Other not–for–profit (including NFP Corporation) **Service:** General Medical and Surgical

Staffed Beds: 80

CARRINGTON—Foster County

★ **CARRINGTON HEALTH CENTER (351318)**, 800 North Fourth Street, Zip 58421–1217, Mailing Address: P.O. Box 461, Zip 58421–0461; tel. 701/652–3141, (Total facility includes 24 beds in nursing home–type unit) **A**5 9 10 18 **F**3 7 10 11 15 24 25 26 27 30 31 32 38 40 42 50 54 55 56 57 62 66 73 77 79 80 86 87 96 97 100 102 107 117 119 120 121 122 133 135 136 137 **P**6 **S** Catholic Health Initiatives
Primary Contact: Mariann Doeling, RN, Executive Vice President
CFO: Jeff Durham, Interim Chief Financial Officer
CMO: Todd Schaffer, M.D., Chief Medical Officer
CHR: Sarah Aberle, Generalist
Web address: www.carringtonhealthcenter.net
Control: Church–operated, Nongovernment, not–for profit **Service:** General Medical and Surgical

Staffed Beds: 49 **Admissions:** 509 **Census:** 29 **Outpatient Visits:** 20717 **Births:** 0 **Total Expense ($000):** 10892 **Payroll Expense ($000):** 5363 **Personnel:** 119

Hospital, Medicare Provider Number, Address, Telephone, Approval, Facility, and Physician Codes, Health Care System
★ American Hospital Association (AHA) membership
☐ The Joint Commission accreditation
○ American Osteopathic Association (AOA) accreditation
△ Commission on Accreditation of Rehabilitation Facilities (CARF) accreditation

CAVALIER—Pembina County

★ **PEMBINA COUNTY MEMORIAL HOSPITAL AND WEDGEWOOD MANOR (351319)**, 301 Mountain Street East, Zip 58220–4015, Mailing Address: P.O. Box 380, Zip 58220–0380; tel. 701/265–8461, (Total facility includes 60 beds in nursing home–type unit) **A**5 9 10 18 **F**3 11 24 25 27 31 38 40 43 44 54 57 63 66 76 79 80 81 82 84 86 87 96 102 107 117 119 120 121 122 124 135 **P**5
Primary Contact: Everett A. Butler, Chief Executive Officer
CFO: Jeni Schwenzfeier, Director Finance
CMO: K. S. Sumra, M.D., Chief of Staff
CIO: Robert Heidt, Director Information Systems
Web address: www.cavalierhospital.com
Control: Other not–for–profit (including NFP Corporation) **Service:** General Medical and Surgical

Staffed Beds: 85 **Admissions:** 709 **Census:** 59 **Outpatient Visits:** 18316 **Births:** 0 **Total Expense ($000):** 9844 **Payroll Expense ($000):** 5337 **Personnel:** 130

COOPERSTOWN—Griggs County

COOPERSTOWN MEDICAL CENTER (351306), 1200 Roberts Avenue, Zip 58425; tel. 701/797–2221, (Nonreporting) **A**9 10 18
Primary Contact: Gregory Stomp, Chief Executive Officer
CFO: Jill Anderson, CPA, Chief Financial Officer
CMO: Rohini Becherl, M.D., Medical Director
CHR: Kristi Halvorson, Chief Human Resources Officer
Web address: www.cooperstownnd.com/index.php
Control: Other not–for–profit (including NFP Corporation) **Service:** General Medical and Surgical

Staffed Beds: 10

CROSBY—Divide County

ST. LUKE'S HOSPITAL (351325), 702 First Street Southwest, Zip 58730–0010; tel. 701/965–6384 **A**5 9 10 18 **F**3 11 17 30 38 56 57 67 75 79 81 82 84 86 122 **P**6
Primary Contact: Leslie O. Urvand, Administrator
Control: Other not–for–profit (including NFP Corporation) **Service:** General Medical and Surgical

Staffed Beds: 12 **Admissions:** 104 **Census:** 1 **Outpatient Visits:** 4071 **Births:** 0 **Total Expense ($000):** 3030 **Payroll Expense ($000):** 1572 **Personnel:** 47

DEVILS LAKE—Ramsey County

⊞ **MERCY HOSPITAL (350030)**, 1031 Seventh Street N.E., Zip 58301–2798; tel. 701/662–2131 **A**1 5 9 10 20 **F**3 11 13 17 24 26 30 31 32 33 38 40 42 43 50 55 56 57 63 68 73 74 79 81 82 84 86 96 97 100 102 107 119 120 121 122 124 **S** Catholic Health Initiatives
Primary Contact: Marlene J. Krein, President and Chief Executive Officer
CHR: Tanya Knutson, Director Human Resources
Web address: www.mercyhospitaldl.com
Control: Other not–for–profit (including NFP Corporation) **Service:** General Medical and Surgical

Staffed Beds: 35 **Admissions:** 1363 **Census:** 13 **Outpatient Visits:** 20513 **Births:** 294 **Total Expense ($000):** 14750 **Payroll Expense ($000):** 6670 **Personnel:** 186

DICKINSON—Stark County

⊞ **ST. JOSEPH'S HOSPITAL AND HEALTH CENTER (350003)**, 30 Seventh Street West, Zip 58601–4399; tel. 701/456–4000 **A**1 5 9 10 20 **F**3 8 11 13 15 24 25 26 31 32 33 38 40 42 44 52 55 56 57 61 62 68 73 74 75 77 79 80 82 84 86 87 96 97 100 102 105 107 118 119 121 122 135 **S** Catholic Health Initiatives
Primary Contact: Claudia Ann Eisenmann, President and Chief Executive Officer
CFO: Stephen O'Grady, Chief Financial Officer
Web address: www.stjoeshospital.org
Control: Church–operated, Nongovernment, not–for profit **Service:** General Medical and Surgical

Staffed Beds: 49 **Admissions:** 2991 **Census:** 41 **Outpatient Visits:** 40768 **Births:** 326 **Total Expense ($000):** 51285 **Payroll Expense ($000):** 16491 **Personnel:** 363

ELGIN—Grant County

JACOBSON MEMORIAL HOSPITAL CARE CENTER (351314), 601 East Street North, Zip 58533–0376; tel. 701/584–2792, (Total facility includes 25 beds in nursing home–type unit) (Nonreporting) **A**9 10 18
Primary Contact: Jim Opdahl, Administrator
COO: Jim Opdahl, Administrator
CFO: Brandon Vaughan, Accountant
CMO: S. K. Patel, M.D., Chief of Staff
CHR: Paula Rivinius, Manager Human Resources
Web address: www.jacobsonhospital.org
Control: Other not–for–profit (including NFP Corporation) **Service:** General Medical and Surgical

Staffed Beds: 46

FARGO—Cass County

HEARTLAND HEALTH SYSTEM See MeritCare South University

⊞ **INNOVIS HEALTH (350070)**, 3000 32nd Avenue South, Zip 58103; tel. 701/364–8000 **A**1 2 3 5 9 10 **F**3 13 15 17 18 20 22 24 25 26 27 30 31 32 33 38 40 41 43 44 50 68 70 71 72 73 74 75 76 77 79 80 81 82 84 86 119 121 135 136 137 **S** Essentia Health
Primary Contact: Greg Glasner, M.D., Chief Executive Officer
COO: Kevin M. Pitzer, Chief Administrative Officer
CFO: Dennis Fuhrman, Vice President Finance
CMO: Michael Briggs, M.D., Chief Medical Officer
CIO: Ken Gilles, Chief Information Officer
CHR: Keith Wahlund, Vice President Human Resources
Web address: www.innovishealth.com
Control: Other not–for–profit (including NFP Corporation) **Service:** General Medical and Surgical

Staffed Beds: 96 **Admissions:** 6543 **Census:** 67 **Outpatient Visits:** 18254 **Births:** 1108 **Total Expense ($000):** 78200 **Payroll Expense ($000):** 24489 **Personnel:** 594

⊞ △ **MERITCARE MEDICAL CENTER (350011)**, 720 Fourth Street North, Zip 58122; tel. 701/234–6000, (Includes MERITCARE SOUTH UNIVERSITY, 1720 South University Drive, Zip 58103–4994; tel. 701/280–4100; Jeff Hoss, Executive Partner), (Total facility includes 33 beds in nursing home–type unit) **A**1 2 3 5 7 8 9 10 **F**1 3 4 5 9 11 12 13 16 17 18 19 20 21 22 23 24 25 26 27 30 31 32 33 37 38 40 41 42 43 44 45 46 47 49 50 51 52 53 54 58 59 60 61 62 63 65 66 68 70 71 72 73 74 76 77 78 79 80 82 83 84 85 86 88 89 91 92 94 95 96 97 100 101 102 103 104 106 107 108 109 111 112 116 117 118 119 120 124 127 131 135 137 **P**6 **S** MeritCare Health System
Primary Contact: Roger L. Gilbertson, M.D., President and Chief Executive Officer
COO: Bruce Pitts, M.D., Executive Vice President Clinical Services
CFO: Lisa Carlson, Chief Financial Officer
CMO: Rhonda L. Ketterling, M.D., Chief Medical Officer
CIO: Craig Hewit, Executive Partner Information Technology
CHR: Harriette McCaul, Executive Partner Human Resources
Web address: www.meritcare.com
Control: Other not–for–profit (including NFP Corporation) **Service:** General Medical and Surgical

Staffed Beds: 447 **Admissions:** 21039 **Census:** 296 **Outpatient Visits:** 278627 **Births:** 2142 **Total Expense ($000):** 348752 **Payroll Expense ($000):** 133040 **Personnel:** 2318

☐ **PRAIRIE ST. JOHN'S (354004)**, 510 4th Street South, Zip 58103–1914; tel. 701/476–7200, (Nonreporting) **A**1 9 10
Primary Contact: Emmet M. Kenney, Jr., M.D., Chief Executive Officer
COO: Diana Ketterling, Chief Operating Officer
CMO: Neil Venard, M.D., Medical Director
CHR: Karen Frigen, Director Human Resources
Web address: www.prairie–stjohns.com
Control: Corporation, Investor–owned, for–profit **Service:** Other specialty

Staffed Beds: 25

☐ **TRIUMPH HOSPITAL – FARGO (352004)**, 1720 University Drive South, Zip 58103; tel. 701/241–9099, (Nonreporting) **A**1 9 10 **S** Triumph HealthCare
Primary Contact: Custer Huseby, Chief Executive Officer
Web address: www.triumph–healthcare.com
Control: Corporation, Investor–owned, for–profit **Service:** Long–Term Acute Care hospital

Staffed Beds: 31

⊞ **VETERANS AFFAIRS MEDICAL CENTER**, 2101 Elm Street, Zip 58102–2498; tel. 701/232–3241, (Total facility includes 35 beds in nursing home–type unit) (Nonreporting) **A**1 2 3 5 **S** Department of Veterans Affairs
Primary Contact: Robert P. McDivitt, FACHE, Director
CFO: Roger Sayler, Finance Officer
CMO: William K. Becker, M.D., Chief of Staff
CHR: Jason Wells, Chief Human Resources Management Service
Web address: www.va.gov/sta/guide/home.asp
Control: Veterans Affairs, Government, federal **Service:** General Medical and Surgical

Staffed Beds: 77

FORT YATES—Sioux County

★ **U. S. PUBLIC HEALTH SERVICE INDIAN HOSPITAL (350064)**, N 10 North River Road, Zip 58538, Mailing Address: P.O. Box J, Zip 58538; tel. 701/854–3831, (Nonreporting) **A**5 9 10 **S** U. S. Indian Health Service
Primary Contact: Tim Yellow, Director
CFO: William Condon, Deputy Administrative Officer
Web address: www.ihs.gov
Control: PHS, Indian Service, Government, federal **Service:** General Medical and Surgical

Staffed Beds: 14

Many Facility Codes have changed. Please refer to the AHA Guide Code Chart.

GARRISON—McLean County

★ **GARRISON MEMORIAL HOSPITAL (351303)**, 407 Third Avenue S.E., Zip 58540–0039; tel. 701/463–2275, (Total facility includes 28 beds in nursing home–type unit) **A**5 9 10 18 **F**2 15 24 26 38 39 40 50 54 55 57 65 85 86 96 102 117 119 120 121 122 132 136 **S** Benedictine Sisters of the Annunciation
Primary Contact: Dean Mattern, President and Chief Executive Officer
CFO: Tod Graeber, Controller
Web address: www.garrisonmh.com
Control: Other not–for–profit (including NFP Corporation) **Service:** General Medical and Surgical

Staffed Beds: 50 **Admissions:** 209 **Census:** 43 **Outpatient Visits:** 9418 **Births:** 0 **Total Expense ($000):** 5457 **Payroll Expense ($000):** 2809 **Personnel:** 132

GRAFTON—Walsh County

★ **UNITY MEDICAL CENTER (351320)**, 164 West 13th Street, Zip 58237–1896; tel. 701/352–1620, (Nonreporting) **A**5 9 10 18
Primary Contact: Everett A. Butler, Chief Executive Officer
CFO: Rachel Ray, Chief Financial Officer
Web address: www.unitymedcenter.com
Control: Other not–for–profit (including NFP Corporation) **Service:** General Medical and Surgical

Staffed Beds: 17

GRAND FORKS—Grand Forks County

★ △ **ALTRU HEALTH SYSTEM (350019)**, 1000 South Columbia Road, Zip 58201–4032; tel. 701/780–5000, (Includes ALTRU HOSPITAL, 1200 South Columbia Road, Zip 58201; tel. 701/780–5000; ALTRU REHABILITATION CENTER, 1300 South Columbia Road, Zip 58201; tel. 701/780–2311) **A**1 2 3 5 7 9 10 20 **F**3 5 7 8 10 11 12 13 14 15 18 20 22 24 25 26 27 28 30 31 32 33 34 35 36 38 40 41 42 43 44 48 49 50 52 54 55 56 57 58 59 60 61 62 64 66 67 68 69 70 72 73 75 76 77 79 80 81 82 85 86 87 88 89 90 91 92 93 94 95 96 97 98 100 102 104 105 106 107 109 111 113 115 118 119 120 121 124 132 133 135 136 137 **P**6
Primary Contact: David R. Molmen, Chief Executive Officer
COO: Timothy Sayler, Chief Operating Officer
CFO: Dwight Thompson, Chief Financial Officer
CMO: James Van Looy, M.D., Chief Medical Executive
CIO: Mark Waind, Administrative Director Information Services
CHR: Lee Lindquist, Administrative Director Human Services
Web address: www.altru.org
Control: Other not–for–profit (including NFP Corporation) **Service:** General Medical and Surgical

Staffed Beds: 263 **Admissions:** 12921 **Census:** 159 **Outpatient Visits:** 116215 **Births:** 1515 **Total Expense ($000):** 342024 **Payroll Expense ($000):** 176862 **Personnel:** 2917

RICHARD P. STADTER PSYCHIATRIC CENTER (354005), 1451 44th Avenue South, Zip 58201; tel. 701/772–2500, (Nonreporting) **A**9 10
Primary Contact: Thomas Peterson, Chief Executive Officer
COO: Bonnie Peterson, Chief Operating Officer and Vice President Clinical Services
CFO: Darin Ohe, Chief Financial Officer
CMO: Thomas Peterson, Chief Executive Officer
CHR: Dan Bjerknes, Director Human Resources
Web address: www.stadtercenter.com
Control: Corporation, Investor–owned, for–profit **Service:** Psychiatric

Staffed Beds: 34

HARVEY—Wells County

★ **ST. ALOISIUS MEDICAL CENTER (351327)**, 325 East Brewster Street, Zip 58341–1605; tel. 701/324–4651, (Total facility includes 106 beds in nursing home–type unit) **A**5 9 10 18 **F**13 15 24 26 27 38 40 52 54 55 57 68 75 76 79 86 115 117 119 120 121 122 135 136 **S** Sisters of Mary of the Presentation Health System
Primary Contact: Rockford Zastoupil, President and Chief Executive Officer
CFO: Sandra Teubner, Chief Financial Officer
Web address: www.staloisius.com
Control: Church–operated, Nongovernment, not–for profit **Service:** General Medical and Surgical

Staffed Beds: 131 **Admissions:** 457 **Census:** 109 **Outpatient Visits:** 8155 **Births:** 6 **Total Expense ($000):** 10849 **Payroll Expense ($000):** 5294 **Personnel:** 235

HAZEN—Mercer County

SAKAKAWEA MEDICAL CENTER (351310), 510 Eighth Avenue N.E., Zip 58545–4637; tel. 701/748–2225, (Nonreporting) **A**5 9 10 18 **S** Cypress Health Systems
Primary Contact: James L. Marshall, Chief Executive Officer
CFO: Renae Snyder, Manager Business Office
CHR: Cheryl Axtman, Administrative Assistant
Web address: www.sakmedcenter.com
Control: Other not–for–profit (including NFP Corporation) **Service:** General Medical and Surgical

Staffed Beds: 25

HETTINGER—Adams County

WEST RIVER REGIONAL MEDICAL CENTER (351330), 1000 Highway 12, Zip 58639–7530; tel. 701/567–4561, (Nonreporting) **A**5 9 10 18
Primary Contact: James K. Long, CPA, Administrator and Chief Executive Officer
CFO: Karan Ehlers, Chief Financial Officer
CMO: Brian Willoughby, M.D., Chief of Staff
CIO: Julia Gochenour, Information Systems Manager
CHR: Christi Miller, Manager Human Resources
Web address: www.wrhs.com
Control: Other not–for–profit (including NFP Corporation) **Service:** General Medical and Surgical

Staffed Beds: 25

HILLSBORO—Traill County

★ **HILLSBORO MEDICAL CENTER (351329)**, 12 Third Street S.E., Zip 58045, Mailing Address: P.O. Box 609, Zip 58045–0609; tel. 701/636–4501, (Total facility includes 42 beds in nursing home–type unit) **A**5 9 10 18 **F**1 7 30 31 32 38 119 122 **P**7 **S** MeritCare Health System
Primary Contact: Patricia Dirk, Administrator
COO: Patricia Dirk, Administrator
CFO: Darlene Swanson, Business Manager
CMO: Charles J. Breen, M.D., Medical Director
CIO: Darlene Swanson, Business Manager
CHR: Jenny Jacobson, Manager Human Resources
Web address: www.hillsboromedicalcenter.com
Control: Corporation, Investor–owned, for–profit **Service:** Long–Term Acute Care hospital

Staffed Beds: 62 **Admissions:** 302 **Census:** 40 **Outpatient Visits:** 19007 **Births:** 0 **Total Expense ($000):** 4327 **Payroll Expense ($000):** 3018 **Personnel:** 79

JAMESTOWN—Stutsman County

★ **JAMESTOWN HOSPITAL (350009)**, 419 Fifth Street N.E., Zip 58401–3360; tel. 701/252–1050 **A**1 5 9 10 20 **F**3 11 13 15 17 24 27 33 34 38 40 42 43 44 50 52 55 56 57 61 62 68 73 74 75 79 80 81 82 86 96 97 99 100 102 106 107 118 119 121 122 124 135
Primary Contact: Martin I. Richman, President and Chief Executive Officer
CFO: Wes Smith, Chief Financial Officer
CIO: Jeremey Schiele, Chief Information Officer
CHR: Ricki Ramlo, Vice President Human Resources
Web address: www.jamestownhospital.com
Control: Other not–for–profit (including NFP Corporation) **Service:** General Medical and Surgical

Staffed Beds: 56 **Admissions:** 1635 **Census:** 13 **Outpatient Visits:** 25419 **Births:** 302 **Total Expense ($000):** 19453 **Payroll Expense ($000):** 8653 **Personnel:** 220

□ **NORTH DAKOTA STATE HOSPITAL (354003)**, 2605 Circle Drive, Zip 58401–6905; tel. 701/253–3964, (Nonreporting) **A**1 5 9 10
Primary Contact: Alex Schweitzer, Superintendent and Chief Executive Officer
CFO: Gene O. Wahl, Chief Financial Officer
Control: State–Government, nonfederal **Service:** Psychiatric

Staffed Beds: 140

Hospital, Medicare Provider Number, Address, Telephone, Approval, Facility, and Physician Codes, Health Care System

★ American Hospital Association (AHA) membership
□ The Joint Commission accreditation
○ American Osteopathic Association (AOA) accreditation
△ Commission on Accreditation of Rehabilitation Facilities (CARF) accreditation

KENMARE—Ward County

★ **KENMARE COMMUNITY HOSPITAL (351305)**, 317 First Avenue N.W., Zip 58746–7104, Mailing Address: P.O. Box 697, Zip 58746–0697; tel. 701/385–4296, (Nonreporting) **A**9 10 18
Primary Contact: Margaret Shawn Smothers, Administrator
COO: Bev Heninger, Director Nursing
CFO: Kevin Seehafer, Chief Financial Officer
CMO: Jesse Sabitti, M.D., Chief Medical Officer
CIO: Alan Okerson, Director Information Technology
CHR: Ranae Ehlke, Administrative Secretary and Coordinator Risk Management and Human Resources
Web address: www.kenmarend.net/hospital.htm
Control: Other not–for–profit (including NFP Corporation) **Service:** General Medical and Surgical

Staffed Beds: 25

LANGDON—Cavalier County

★ **CAVALIER COUNTY MEMORIAL HOSPITAL (351323)**, 909 Second Street, Zip 58249–2499; tel. 701/256–6100 **A**5 9 10 18 **F**3 7 8 15 25 26 37 38 46 55 56 57 62 63 64 66 68 73 75 79 80 81 82 86 87 96 119 122 **P**6
Primary Contact: Lawrence Blue, Administrator and Chief Executive Officer
COO: Lawrence Blue, Administrator and Chief Executive Officer
CFO: Julie Feil, Accountant
CMO: John Baugh, M.D., Medical Director
CHR: Christie Sauer, Human Resources Officer
Web address: www.cavaliercountyhospital.com
Control: Other not–for–profit (including NFP Corporation) **Service:** General Medical and Surgical

Staffed Beds: 24 **Admissions:** 378 **Census:** 4 **Outpatient Visits:** 13000 **Births:** 0 **Total Expense ($000):** 6076 **Payroll Expense ($000):** 3185 **Personnel:** 76

LINTON—Emmons County

★ **LINTON HOSPITAL (351328)**, 518 North Broadway, Zip 58552–7308, Mailing Address: P.O. Box 850, Zip 58552–0850; tel. 701/254–4511 **A**5 9 10 18 **F**3 7 8 10 15 24 25 30 31 32 38 40 55 56 57 62 73 79 80 81 86 87 96 100 107 118 119 122 124 133 137 **P**6
Primary Contact: Roger R. Unger, Administrator
CFO: Beverly Vilhauer, Chief Operating Officer and Chief Financial Officer
CMO: Edgar Oliveira, M.D., Chief Medical Staff
CHR: Sue Meidinger, Manager Business Office
Web address: www.lintonhospital.com
Control: Other not–for–profit (including NFP Corporation) **Service:** General Medical and Surgical

Staffed Beds: 14 **Admissions:** 299 **Census:** 4 **Births:** 0

LISBON—Ransom County

★ **LISBON AREA HEALTH SERVICES (351311)**, 905 Main Street, Zip 58054–0353, Mailing Address: P.O. Box 353, Zip 58054–0353; tel. 701/683–5241, (Nonreporting) **A**5 9 10 18 **S** Catholic Health Initiatives
Primary Contact: Jeffrey S. Drop, Senior Vice President and Division Executive Officer
COO: Diane Weispfenning, Chief Operating Officer
Control: Church–operated, Nongovernment, not–for profit **Service:** General Medical and Surgical

Staffed Beds: 25

MANDAN—Morton County

☐ **TRIUMPH HOSPITAL – CENTRAL DAKOTAS (352005)**, 1000 18th Street N.W., Zip 58554; tel. 701/667–2000, (Nonreporting) **A**1 9 10
S Triumph HealthCare
Primary Contact: Cora Pifer, Chief Executive Officer
Web address: www.triumph-healthcare.com
Control: Corporation, Investor–owned, for–profit **Service:** Long–Term Acute Care hospital

Staffed Beds: 41

MAYVILLE—Traill County

★ **UNION HOSPITAL (351309)**, 42 Sixth Avenue S.E., Zip 58257–1598; tel. 701/786–3800 **A**5 9 10 18 **F**24 27 31 32 38 73 79 96 100 107 119 122 135
Primary Contact: Roger Baier, Chief Executive Officer
CMO: Jeremiah Penn, M.D., Chief of Staff
Web address: www.unionhospital.com
Control: Other not–for–profit (including NFP Corporation) **Service:** General Medical and Surgical

Staffed Beds: 18 **Admissions:** 298 **Census:** 4 **Outpatient Visits:** 8321 **Total Expense ($000):** 3720 **Payroll Expense ($000):** 1637 **Personnel:** 48

MCVILLE—Nelson County

NELSON COUNTY HEALTH SYSTEM (351308), 200 Main Street, Zip 58254–4002, Mailing Address: P.O. Box 367, Zip 58254–0367; tel. 701/322–4328, (Total facility includes 39 beds in nursing home–type unit) (Nonreporting) **A**9 10 18
Primary Contact: Cathy Swenson, Chief Executive Officer
CFO: Steve Forde, Chief Financial Officer
CMO: Erling Martinson, M.D., Medical Director
Control: Other not–for–profit (including NFP Corporation) **Service:** General Medical and Surgical

Staffed Beds: 58

MINOT—Ward County

⊠ △ **TRINITY HEALTH (350006)**, One Burdick Expressway West, Zip 58701, Mailing Address: P.O. Box 5020, Zip 58702–5020; tel. 701/857–5000, (Includes TRINITY HOSPITAL–ST. JOSEPH'S), (Total facility includes 294 beds in nursing home–type unit) **A**1 2 3 5 7 9 10 20 **F**3 4 5 7 8 11 12 13 15 17 18 20 22 24 26 27 30 31 32 33 34 38 40 41 42 43 44 46 49 50 51 53 54 55 56 57 59 61 62 65 68 69 70 71 72 73 74 75 76 77 78 79 80 81 82 84 85 86 87 88 89 90 91 92 93 94 95 96 97 99 100 102 103 104 105 106 107 108 109 111 113 114 115 117 118 119 120 121 123 124 132 134 135 136 137 **P**3 6
Primary Contact: Terry G. Hoff, President
CFO: Kevin Seehafer, Chief Financial Officer
CHR: Paul Simonson, Vice President
Web address: www.trinityhealth.org
Control: Other not–for–profit (including NFP Corporation) **Service:** General Medical and Surgical

Staffed Beds: 586 **Admissions:** 9594 **Census:** 395 **Outpatient Visits:** 152733 **Births:** 1315 **Total Expense ($000):** 241880 **Payroll Expense ($000):** 117319 **Personnel:** 2253

NORTHWOOD—Grand Forks County

★ **NORTHWOOD DEACONESS HEALTH CENTER (351312)**, 4 North Park Street, Zip 58267–0190; tel. 701/587–6060, (Total facility includes 61 beds in nursing home–type unit) **A**5 9 10 18 **F**2 3 7 11 12 15 24 26 31 32 33 38 43 44 52 54 55 56 57 62 67 73 75 86 87 107 115 117 119 122 132 135 136 **P**5
Primary Contact: Pete Antonson, Chief Executive Officer
CMO: Jon Berg, M.D., Chief of Staff
CIO: Chad Peterson, Chief Information Officer
Web address: www.ndhc.net
Control: Church–operated, Nongovernment, not–for profit **Service:** General Medical and Surgical

Staffed Beds: 73 **Admissions:** 276 **Census:** 66 **Outpatient Visits:** 2713 **Births:** 0 **Total Expense ($000):** 7916 **Payroll Expense ($000):** 3906 **Personnel:** 124

OAKES—Dickey County

★ **OAKES COMMUNITY HOSPITAL (351315)**, 1200 North Seventh Street, Zip 58474–2502; tel. 701/742–3291 **A**5 9 10 18 **F**3 11 13 25 26 27 30 31 32 33 38 40 41 44 50 61 62 66 68 73 74 76 79 80 81 82 84 96 102 107 119 122 124 **P**5 **S** Catholic Health Initiatives
Primary Contact: Major James Gabriel, Administrator
CMO: Vani Nagala, M.D., Chief Medical Officer
CIO: Terry Engel, Information Technology Manager
CHR: Julie Entzminger, Manager Human Resources
Web address: www.oakeshospital.com
Control: Other not–for–profit (including NFP Corporation) **Service:** General Medical and Surgical

Staffed Beds: 20 **Admissions:** 623 **Census:** 6 **Outpatient Visits:** 9555 **Births:** 39 **Total Expense ($000):** 7470 **Payroll Expense ($000):** 3333 **Personnel:** 64

PARK RIVER—Walsh County

★ **FIRST CARE HEALTH CENTER (351326)**, 115 Vivian Street, Zip 58270–0708; tel. 701/284–7500 **A**5 9 10 18 **F**11 13 15 24 25 26 27 31 33 38 50 57 62 63 66 74 75 79 84 86 94 96 100 102 107 119 122 **P**6
Primary Contact: Louise Dryburgh, Administrator
CFO: Layne Ensrude, Chief Financial Officer
CMO: K. J. Midgarden, M.D., Chief Medical Staff
Web address: www.firstcarehc.org
Control: Other not–for–profit (including NFP Corporation) **Service:** General Medical and Surgical

Staffed Beds: 14 **Admissions:** 391 **Census:** 8 **Outpatient Visits:** 28285 **Births:** 34 **Total Expense ($000):** 6478 **Payroll Expense ($000):** 2575 **Personnel:** 67

Many Facility Codes have changed. Please refer to the AHA Guide Code Chart.

RICHARDTON—Stark County

RICHARDTON HEALTH CENTER (351317), 212 Third Avenue West, Zip 58652–7103, Mailing Address: P.O. Box H, Zip 58652; tel. 701/974–3304, (Nonreporting) **A**9 10 18
Primary Contact: Jim Opdahl, Interim Administrator
CFO: Niki Mitchell, Director Administrative Services
CMO: Shelley Selph, M.D., Chief Medical Officer
CHR: Niki Mitchell, Director Administrative Services
Web address: www.richardtonhospital.org
Control: Other not–for–profit (including NFP Corporation) **Service:** General Medical and Surgical

Staffed Beds: 25

ROLLA—Rolette County

PRESENTATION MEDICAL CENTER (351316), 213 Second Avenue N.E., Zip 58367–7153, Mailing Address: P.O. Box 759, Zip 58367–0759; tel. 701/477–3161 **A**5 9 10 18 **F**8 11 13 15 24 25 26 27 30 33 38 50 55 56 57 62 74 76 77 79 80 82 84 86 87 96 100 107 117 119 120 122 124 136 **P**6 **S** Sisters of Mary of the Presentation Health System
Primary Contact: Kimber Wraalstad, President and Chief Executive Officer
CFO: Paula Wilkie, Chief Financial Officer
CMO: Norman Gordner, M.D., President Medical Staff
CHR: Holly Cahill, Director Human Resources
Web address: www.pmc–rolla.com
Control: Church–operated, Nongovernment, not–for profit **Service:** General Medical and Surgical

Staffed Beds: 25 **Admissions:** 400 **Census:** 8 **Outpatient Visits:** 8473 **Births:** 32 **Total Expense ($000):** 7764 **Payroll Expense ($000):** 3578 **Personnel:** 98

RUGBY—Pierce County

★ **HEART OF AMERICA MEDICAL CENTER (351332)**, 800 Main Avenue South, Zip 58368–2198; tel. 701/776–5261, (Total facility includes 148 beds in nursing home–type unit) **A**5 9 10 **F**3 7 11 13 15 24 26 27 38 42 44 52 54 62 68 73 74 75 79 84 86 96 102 107 115 117 119 120 121 122 135 **P**2 6
Primary Contact: Jerry E. Jurena, Executive Director
CFO: Bonnie Kuehnemund, Comptroller
Web address: www.hamc.com
Control: Other not–for–profit (including NFP Corporation) **Service:** General Medical and Surgical

Staffed Beds: 168 **Admissions:** 795 **Census:** 147 **Outpatient Visits:** 32290 **Births:** 25 **Total Expense ($000):** 15054 **Payroll Expense ($000):** 7652 **Personnel:** 254

STANLEY—Mountrail County

★ **MOUNTRAIL COUNTY MEDICAL CENTER (351301)**, 615 6th Street S.E., Zip 58784–4323, Mailing Address: P.O. Box 399, Zip 58784–0399; tel. 701/628–2424 **A**9 10 18 **F**11 24 28 38 55 56 57 62 64 66 75 79 86 87 119 122 **P**6
Primary Contact: Mitch Leupp, Administrator
CFO: Ramona Edwards, Assistant Administrator
CMO: Robert Heninger, M.D., Chief Medical Officer
CIO: Stacey Ramburg, Director Medical Records
CHR: Linda Halvorson, Director Human Resources
Web address: www.stanleyhealth.org
Control: Other not–for–profit (including NFP Corporation) **Service:** General Medical and Surgical

Staffed Beds: 11 **Admissions:** 146 **Census:** 4 **Outpatient Visits:** 7301 **Births:** 0 **Total Expense ($000):** 2899 **Payroll Expense ($000):** 526 **Personnel:** 14

TIOGA—Williams County

★ **TIOGA MEDICAL CENTER (351300)**, 810 North Welo Street, Zip 58852–0159, Mailing Address: P.O. Box 159, Zip 58852–0159; tel. 701/664–3305, (Total facility includes 30 beds in nursing home–type unit) (Nonreporting) **A**5 9 10 18
Primary Contact: Randall K. Pederson, Chief Executive Officer
CFO: Brian A. Lovdahl, Vice President and Chief Financial Officer
Web address: www.tiogahealth.org
Control: Other not–for–profit (including NFP Corporation) **Service:** General Medical and Surgical

Staffed Beds: 55

TURTLE LAKE—McLean County

COMMUNITY MEMORIAL HOSPITAL (351304), 220 Fifth Avenue, Zip 58575–4005, Mailing Address: P.O. Box 280, Zip 58575–0280; tel. 701/448–2331, (Nonreporting) **A**9 10 18
Primary Contact: Dean Mattern, President and Chief Executive Officer
CFO: Karen Aafedt, Assistant Administrator and Controller
Web address: www.wrtc.com/cullum/hospital
Control: Church–operated, Nongovernment, not–for profit **Service:** General Medical and Surgical

Staffed Beds: 25

VALLEY CITY—Barnes County

★ **MERCY HOSPITAL (351324)**, 570 Chautauqua Boulevard, Zip 58072–3199; tel. 701/845–6400 **A**5 9 10 18 **F**3 11 13 17 24 25 26 27 28 32 38 40 61 62 68 73 74 75 79 80 81 84 86 96 119 120 121 122 135 137 **S** Catholic Health Initiatives
CHR: Kathy Buck, Human Resources Generalist
Web address: www.mercyhospital.biz
Control: Church–operated, Nongovernment, not–for profit **Service:** General Medical and Surgical

Staffed Beds: 25 **Admissions:** 810 **Census:** 10 **Outpatient Visits:** 17226 **Births:** 70 **Total Expense ($000):** 10834 **Payroll Expense ($000):** 5619 **Personnel:** 113

WATFORD CITY—McKenzie County

★ **MCKENZIE COUNTY HEALTHCARE SYSTEM (351302)**, 516 North Main Street, Zip 58854–0548; tel. 701/842–3000 **A**9 10 18 **F**11 24 31 38 40 50 52 55 56 57 63 65 73 75 79 86 87 96 102 117 122 **P**8
Primary Contact: Daniel R. Kelly, Chief Executive Officer
CFO: Colette Anderson, Manager Finance
CMO: Gary Ramage, M.D., Chief Medical Officer
CHR: Colette Anderson, Manager Human Resources
Web address: www.mckenziehealth.com
Control: Other not–for–profit (including NFP Corporation) **Service:** General Medical and Surgical

Staffed Beds: 24 **Admissions:** 231 **Census:** 7 **Outpatient Visits:** 10155 **Births:** 0 **Total Expense ($000):** 3425 **Payroll Expense ($000):** 1525 **Personnel:** 25

WILLISTON—Williams County

★□ **MERCY MEDICAL CENTER (350017)**, 1301 15th Avenue West, Zip 58801–3896; tel. 701/774–7400 **A**1 5 9 10 20 **F**3 4 5 8 11 13 15 24 25 26 27 28 30 31 32 33 36 38 40 42 43 44 50 51 52 54 55 56 57 59 60 61 62 63 66 68 73 74 75 76 77 78 79 80 81 82 84 85 86 87 88 89 90 91 92 93 94 95 96 97 98 100 102 106 107 108 109 111 117 118 119 120 121 122 124 132 135 137 **P**6 **S** Catholic Health Initiatives
Primary Contact: Dennis Goebel, President and Chief Executive Officer
CFO: Kerry Monson, Vice President Finance and Chief Financial Officer
CMO: A. Marc Nielsen, M.D., Chief of Staff
CIO: Sean Key, Director Information Technology
CHR: Mary Banta, Director Human Resources
Web address: www.mercy–williston.org
Control: Church–operated, Nongovernment, not–for profit **Service:** General Medical and Surgical

Staffed Beds: 86 **Admissions:** 2119 **Census:** 33 **Outpatient Visits:** 56793 **Births:** 391 **Total Expense ($000):** 36448 **Payroll Expense ($000):** 16746 **Personnel:** 383

WISHEK—McIntosh County

★ **WISHEK COMMUNITY HOSPITAL AND CLINICS (351321)**, 1007 Fourth Avenue South, Zip 58495–7527, Mailing Address: P.O. Box 647, Zip 58495–0647; tel. 701/452–2326 **A**5 9 10 18 **F**3 7 11 15 17 24 25 26 28 31 32 33 34 38 41 42 45 50 52 54 55 56 57 59 61 62 63 65 66 73 79 82 85 86 87 96 102 117 119 120 122 132 135 136 **P**3 8
Primary Contact: Trina Schilling, Chief Executive Officer
CFO: Sahlenia Braun, Chief Financial Officer
CMO: Rogelio Cruz, M.D., Chief of Staff
CIO: Kari Buchholz, Director Health Information Management
CHR: Shar Bauer, Executive Secretary
Web address: www.wishekhospital.com
Control: Other not–for–profit (including NFP Corporation) **Service:** General Medical and Surgical

Staffed Beds: 17 **Admissions:** 336 **Census:** 4 **Outpatient Visits:** 30972 **Births:** 1 **Total Expense ($000):** 4782 **Payroll Expense ($000):** 2247 **Personnel:** 73

Hospital, Medicare Provider Number, Address, Telephone, Approval, Facility, and Physician Codes, Health Care System

★ American Hospital Association (AHA) membership
□ The Joint Commission accreditation
○ American Osteopathic Association (AOA) accreditation
△ Commission on Accreditation of Rehabilitation Facilities (CARF) accreditation

OH

OHIO

AKRON—Summit County

★ **AKRON CHILDREN'S HOSPITAL (363303)**, One Perkins Square, Zip 44308–1062; tel. 330/543–1000 **A**1 2 3 5 8 9 10 **F**3 7 11 16 19 21 23 24 25 26 27 28 29 30 31 32 33 34 36 37 38 39 40 41 42 43 44 50 53 55 56 57 58 59 60 61 62 63 64 66 70 72 73 75 76 77 78 79 80 81 82 83 84 86 87 88 89 90 91 92 94 95 96 97 100 101 102 105 106 107 114 118 119 120 121 123 124 125 130 132 133 135 137 **P**6
Primary Contact: William H. Considine, President
COO: Mark Watson, Chief Operating Officer
CFO: Dennis P. Jancsy, Chief Financial Officer
CMO: Michael Bird, M.D., Vice President Medical Services
CIO: Chuck Kozak, Chief Information Officer
CHR: Walter Schwoeble, Vice President Human Resources
Web address: www.akronchildrens.org
Control: Other not–for–profit (including NFP Corporation) **Service:** Children's general

Staffed Beds: 253 **Admissions:** 8594 **Census:** 138 **Outpatient Visits:** 478254 **Births:** 0 **Total Expense ($000):** 326086 **Payroll Expense ($000):** 160055 **Personnel:** 2681

AKRON CITY HOSPITAL See Summa Health System

★ **AKRON GENERAL MEDICAL CENTER (360027)**, 400 Wabash Avenue, Zip 44307–2433; tel. 330/344–6000 **A**1 2 3 5 8 9 10 **F**3 5 7 8 11 12 13 14 15 17 18 20 22 24 25 26 27 28 30 31 32 33 34 36 37 38 39 40 41 42 43 44 48 49 50 51 52 53 54 55 56 57 58 59 60 61 62 63 64 66 68 69 71 72 73 74 75 76 77 79 80 81 82 86 87 88 90 91 92 93 94 95 96 97 98 99 100 102 103 104 105 106 107 109 113 114 116 118 119 120 121 123 124 132 134 135 136 137 **P**1 6 **S** Akron General Health System
Primary Contact: Alan J. Bleyer, President and Chief Executive Officer
COO: Cathy M. Ceccio, MSN, Executive Vice President and Chief Operating Officer
CMO: Thomas L. Stover, M.D., Senior Vice President Medical Affairs
CIO: Nancy Jones, Chief Information Officer
CHR: Maureen Van Duser, Vice President Human Resources
Web address: www.akrongeneral.org
Control: Other not–for–profit (including NFP Corporation) **Service:** General Medical and Surgical

Staffed Beds: 473 **Admissions:** 24828 **Census:** 328 **Outpatient Visits:** 433870 **Births:** 3156 **Total Expense ($000):** 367557 **Payroll Expense ($000):** 164162 **Personnel:** 3665

☐ △ **EDWIN SHAW REHAB (360241)**, 1621 Flickinger Road, Zip 44312–4495; tel. 330/784–1271, (Total facility includes 49 beds in nursing home–type unit) (Nonreporting) **A**1 5 7 9 10 12 13 **S** Akron General Health System
Primary Contact: Cathy M. Ceccio, M.S.N., President
CFO: Debbie Gorbach, Vice President and Treasurer
CMO: Michael J. Delahanty, D.O., Medical Director
Web address: www.edwinshaw.com
Control: County–Government, nonfederal **Service:** Rehabilitation

Staffed Beds: 161

SAINT THOMAS HOSPITAL See Summa Health System

☐ **SELECT SPECIALTY HOSPITAL–AKRON (362027)**, 525 East Market Street, Zip 44309–3617; tel. 330/375–4390, (Nonreporting) **A**1 10 **S** Select Medical Corporation
Primary Contact: Gregory T. Storer, Chief Executive Officer
Web address: www.selectmedicalcorp.com
Control: Corporation, Investor–owned, for–profit **Service:** Long–Term Acute Care hospital

Staffed Beds: 34

☐ **SELECT SPECIALTY HOSPITAL–NORTHEAST OHIO (362016)**, 400 Wabash Avenue, 9th Floor, Zip 44307; tel. 330/344–6910, (Nonreporting) **A**1 10 **S** Select Medical Corporation
Primary Contact: Pat Mahovich, Chief Executive Officer
Web address: www.selectmedicalcorp.com
Control: Corporation, Investor–owned, for–profit **Service:** Long–Term Acute Care hospital

Staffed Beds: 31

★ **SUMMA HEALTH SYSTEM (360020)**, (Includes AKRON CITY HOSPITAL, 525 East Market Street, Zip 44309–2090, Mailing Address: P.O. Box 2090, Zip 44309–2090; tel. 330/375–3000; SAINT THOMAS HOSPITAL, 444 North Main Street, Zip 44310; tel. 330/375–3000), (Total facility includes 12 beds in nursing home–type unit) **A**1 2 3 5 8 9 10 **F**1 2 3 4 5 6 7 8 9 11 12 13 15 17 18 20 22 24 25 26 27 29 30 31 32 33 34 35 36 37 38 40 41 42 43 44 45 46 47 48 49 50 51 52 53 54 55 56 57 58 59 60 61 62 63 64 66 67 68 69 70 72 73 74 75 76 77 78 79 80 81 82 85 86 87 88 89 90 91 92 93 94 95 96 97 98 99 100 102 103 104 105 106 107 108 109 111 112 113 114 116 117 118 119 120 121 122 123 124 127 132 133 134 135 136 137 **P**6 8 **S** Summa Health System
Primary Contact: Thomas J. Strauss, President and Chief Executive Officer
COO: Robert Harrigan, Vice President and Chief Operating Officer
CFO: Michael Rutherford, Chief Financial Officer
CMO: Dale Murphy, M.D., Vice President Medical Affairs
CIO: Greg Kall, Chief Information Officer
CHR: Kyle Klawitter, Vice President Human Resources
Web address: www.summahealth.org
Control: Other not–for–profit (including NFP Corporation) **Service:** General Medical and Surgical

Staffed Beds: 481 **Admissions:** 36737 **Census:** 473 **Outpatient Visits:** 394381 **Births:** 3159 **Total Expense ($000):** 517311 **Payroll Expense ($000):** 212154 **Personnel:** 4447

ALLIANCE—Stark County

☐ **ALLIANCE COMMUNITY HOSPITAL (360131)**, 200 East State Street, Zip 44601–4399; tel. 330/596–6000, (Total facility includes 78 beds in nursing home–type unit) **A**1 2 5 9 10 **F**3 8 11 13 15 24 25 26 27 30 32 33 34 38 42 43 49 50 54 55 56 57 59 61 62 67 68 72 73 74 75 77 79 80 81 82 86 88 93 96 97 100 103 106 107 117 118 119 121 124 132 135 136 **P**5 8
Primary Contact: Stanley W. Jonas, Chief Executive Officer
COO: Kerry Swanson, Chief Operating Officer and Chief Nursing Officer
CFO: Dale Wells, Chief Financial Officer
CMO: Ashraf Ahmed, M.D., Chief Medical Officer
CIO: David W. Shroades, Chief Technology Officer
CHR: Sam Donohoe, Director Executive Management and Colleague
Web address: www.achosp.org
Control: Other not–for–profit (including NFP Corporation) **Service:** General Medical and Surgical

Staffed Beds: 194 **Admissions:** 5106 **Census:** 118 **Outpatient Visits:** 146516 **Births:** 523 **Total Expense ($000):** 79196 **Payroll Expense ($000):** 34824 **Personnel:** 801

AMHERST—Lorain County

☐ **AMHERST HOSPITAL (360130)**, (Formerly Hospital for Orthopaedic and Specialty Services), 254 Cleveland Avenue, Zip 44001–1620; tel. 440/988–6000 **A**1 9 10 **F**17 25 30 38 39 41 50 55 56 57 62 68 75 77 79 81 86 96 102 107 118 119
Primary Contact: Kevin C. Martin, President and Chief Executive Officer
CFO: James M. Simone, Vice President and Chief Financial Officer
CMO: Donald Sheldon, M.D., Vice President Medical Affairs
CIO: Edward E. Duryee, Vice President and Chief Information Officer
CHR: Daniel Miller, Vice President Human Resources
Web address: www.emh–healthcare.org
Control: Other not–for–profit (including NFP Corporation) **Service:** General Medical and Surgical

Staffed Beds: 34 **Admissions:** 941 **Census:** 10 **Outpatient Visits:** 22449 **Births:** 0 **Total Expense ($000):** 16314 **Payroll Expense ($000):** 6176 **Personnel:** 126

★ **SPECIALTY HOSPITAL OF LORAIN (362025)**, 205 West 20th Street, Suite 200, Zip 44001; tel. 440/988–6260, (Nonreporting) **A**1 10 **S** Catholic Healthcare Partners
Primary Contact: Julia M. Meeks, President and Chief Executive Officer
CFO: Shelly Newson, Chief Financial Officer
Web address: www.specialtyhospitaloflorain.com
Control: Corporation, Investor–owned, for–profit **Service:** Long–Term Acute Care hospital

Staffed Beds: 30

ARCHBOLD—Fulton County

ARCHBOLD HOSPITAL See Community Hospitals and Wellness Centers, Bryan

Many Facility Codes have changed. Please refer to the AHA Guide Code Chart.

ASHLAND—Ashland County

★ **SAMARITAN REGIONAL HEALTH SYSTEM (360002)**, 1025 Center Street, Zip 44805–4011; tel. 419/289–0491 **A**1 5 9 10 **F**11 13 15 18 24 26 27 30 31 32 33 38 43 50 51 53 55 56 57 61 62 66 68 73 74 75 76 77 79 81 82 86 96 97 100 106 107 118 119 120 121 122 124 135 136
Primary Contact: Danny L. Boggs, President and Chief Executive Officer
CFO: Mary Griest, Vice President Finance and Chief Financial Officer
CHR: Alyce Legg, Vice President Human Resources
Web address: www.samaritanhospital.org
Control: Other not–for–profit (including NFP Corporation) **Service:** General Medical and Surgical

Staffed Beds: 55 **Admissions:** 2678 **Census:** 23 **Outpatient Visits:** 136919 **Births:** 507

ASHTABULA—Ashtabula County

□ **ASHTABULA COUNTY MEDICAL CENTER (360125)**, 2420 Lake Avenue, Zip 44004–4954; tel. 440/997–2262, (Total facility includes 16 beds in nursing home–type unit) **A**1 5 9 10 19 20 **F**3 4 5 11 13 15 17 25 26 30 31 32 33 36 38 42 43 49 55 56 57 60 61 62 66 68 72 73 74 75 77 79 80 82 84 85 86 87 88 92 93 96 97 100 102 104 105 107 117 118 119 120 121 124 132 133 135 **P**4 8
Primary Contact: Kevin J. Miller, FACHE, President and Chief Executive Officer
CFO: Jason Kopczak, Vice President Finance and Chief Financial Officer
CMO: David L. Parker, M.D., Chief of Staff
CIO: David Jacobs, Director Information Systems
CHR: Robert Sincich, Vice President Human Resources
Web address: www.acmchealth.org
Control: Other not–for–profit (including NFP Corporation) **Service:** General Medical and Surgical

Staffed Beds: 174 **Admissions:** 6184 **Census:** 81 **Outpatient Visits:** 142310 **Births:** 600 **Total Expense ($000):** 77078 **Payroll Expense ($000):** 32711 **Personnel:** 627

ATHENS—Athens County

★ **O'BLENESS MEMORIAL HOSPITAL (360014)**, 55 Hospital Drive, Zip 45701–2302; tel. 740/593–5551, (Nonreporting) **A**1 9 10 12 13 19
Primary Contact: Richard F. Castrop, President
COO: Ward E. Howe, CPA, Executive Vice President
CFO: Kim Dettwiller, Vice President Finance
CIO: Kristine Barr, Vice President Communication Services
CHR: Sandie Leasure, Senior Vice President Human Resources
Web address: www.obleness.org
Control: Other not–for–profit (including NFP Corporation) **Service:** General Medical and Surgical

Staffed Beds: 77

BARBERTON—Summit County

★ **REGENCY HOSPITAL OF AKRON (362029)**, 155 Fifth Street N.E., Zip 44203; tel. 330/861–2065, (Nonreporting) **A**1 10 **S** Regency Hospital Company
Primary Contact: Andrew Escamilla, Chief Executive Officer
CFO: Gene Winters, Chief Financial Officer
CMO: Akram Dar, M.D., Medical Director
Web address: www.regencyhospital.com
Control: Corporation, Investor–owned, for–profit **Service:** Long–Term Acute Care hospital

Staffed Beds: 36

★ **SUMMA BARBERTON CITIZENS HOSPITAL (360019)**, (Formerly Barberton Citizens Hospital), 155 Fifth Street N.E., Zip 44203–3332; tel. 330/615–3000, (Total facility includes 20 beds in nursing home–type unit) **A**1 2 3 5 9 10 **F**3 8 13 14 15 17 18 20 22 24 25 26 27 30 31 32 33 37 38 43 46 47 48 49 50 51 52 53 54 55 56 57 58 59 60 62 66 68 72 73 74 75 76 77 79 80 81 82 85 86 87 88 90 92 93 96 97 99 100 102 105 106 107 108 109 111 117 118 119 120 121 124 135 136 137 **P**4 6 **S** Summa Health System
Primary Contact: Willard P. Roderick, Chief Executive Officer
COO: Thomas DeBord, Chief Operating Officer
CFO: David Nosacka, Chief Financial Officer
CMO: Mark Parker, M.D., Medical Director
CIO: David Lynch, Director Information Systems
Web address: www.barbhosp.com
Control: Other not–for–profit (including NFP Corporation) **Service:** General Medical and Surgical

Staffed Beds: 245 **Admissions:** 8210 **Census:** 127 **Outpatient Visits:** 355309 **Births:** 673 **Total Expense ($000):** 123941 **Payroll Expense ($000):** 50433 **Personnel:** 989

BARNESVILLE—Belmont County

★ **BARNESVILLE HOSPITAL ASSOCIATION (361321)**, 639 West Main Street, Zip 43713–0309, Mailing Address: P.O. Box 309, Zip 43713–0309; tel. 740/425–3941 **A**1 9 10 18 **F**3 11 15 17 24 25 26 27 30 32 33 37 38 50 55 56 57 61 62 63 67 68 72 73 75 76 77 79 80 81 82 84 86 96 97 100 102 107 117 118 119 122 124 134 135 **P**6
Primary Contact: Richard L. Doan, CHE, Chief Executive Officer
CFO: Willie Cooper–Lohr, Chief Financial Officer
CMO: David J. Hilliard, D.O., Chief of Staff
CIO: Tiffany Gramby, Director Health Information Management and Privacy Officer
CHR: Beth Brill, Director Human Resources
Web address: www.barnesvillehospital.com
Control: Other not–for–profit (including NFP Corporation) **Service:** General Medical and Surgical

Staffed Beds: 25 **Admissions:** 1729 **Census:** 18 **Outpatient Visits:** 47237 **Births:** 0 **Total Expense ($000):** 19183 **Payroll Expense ($000):** 8824 **Personnel:** 236

BATAVIA—Clermont County

★ **MERCY HOSPITAL CLERMONT (360236)**, 3000 Hospital Drive, Zip 45103–1921; tel. 513/732–8200, (Nonreporting) **A**1 2 9 10 **S** Catholic Healthcare Partners
Primary Contact: Gayle M. Heintzelman, President and Chief Executive Officer
COO: Brad Bertke, Vice President Support Services
CMO: Richard Cardella, M.D., Chief of Staff
CHR: Sandie Ferrigno, Director Human Resources
Web address: www.e–mercy.com
Control: Church–operated, Nongovernment, not–for profit **Service:** General Medical and Surgical

Staffed Beds: 114

BELLAIRE—Belmont County

★ **BELMONT COMMUNITY HOSPITAL (360153)**, 4697 Harrison Street, Zip 43906–1338, Mailing Address: P.O. Box 653, Zip 43906–0653; tel. 740/671–1200 **A**1 9 10 **F**11 15 27 32 33 38 40 53 62 68 77 79 85 86 88 92 95 96 100 105 106 107 119 135 **P**6
Primary Contact: Gary R. Gould, FACHE, Administrator and Chief Executive Officer
CFO: James Holden, Chief Financial Officer
CMO: F. Brian Brautigan, M.D., Chief of Staff
CHR: Donna Moore, Director Human Resources
Web address: www.wheelinghospital.org/facilities/bch/
Control: Other not–for–profit (including NFP Corporation) **Service:** General Medical and Surgical

Staffed Beds: 72 **Admissions:** 1933 **Census:** 29 **Outpatient Visits:** 57708 **Births:** 0 **Total Expense ($000):** 20608 **Payroll Expense ($000):** 8869 **Personnel:** 253

BELLEFONTAINE—Logan County

★ **MARY RUTAN HOSPITAL (360197)**, 205 Palmer Avenue, Zip 43311–2281; tel. 937/592–4015 **A**1 3 5 9 10 **F**3 11 13 14 15 18 24 25 26 27 28 31 32 38 43 53 55 57 62 64 66 68 73 74 75 76 79 80 81 82 84 86 96 97 100 102 106 107 118 119 121 124 135 136
Primary Contact: Mandy C. Goble, President and Chief Executive Officer
CFO: Ron Carmin, Vice President Fiscal Affairs
CMO: Grant Varian, M.D., Medical Director
CIO: Robert Reynolds, Director Information Systems
CHR: Tim Froebe, Vice President Human Resources
Web address: www.maryrutan.org
Control: Other not–for–profit (including NFP Corporation) **Service:** General Medical and Surgical

Staffed Beds: 110 **Admissions:** 3193 **Census:** 33 **Outpatient Visits:** 116436 **Births:** 478 **Total Expense ($000):** 64409 **Payroll Expense ($000):** 25721 **Personnel:** 559

Hospital, Medicare Provider Number, Address, Telephone, Approval, Facility, and Physician Codes, Health Care System

★ American Hospital Association (AHA) membership
□ The Joint Commission accreditation
○ American Osteopathic Association (AOA) accreditation
△ Commission on Accreditation of Rehabilitation Facilities (CARF) accreditation

BELLEVUE—Sandusky County

▣ **BELLEVUE HOSPITAL (360107)**, 1400 West Main Street, Zip 44811–1028, Mailing Address: P.O. Box 8004, Zip 44811–8004; tel. 419/483–4040 **A**1 2 5 9 10 **F**3 11 13 15 24 27 30 31 32 33 34 38 43 46 50 54 55 56 57 60 61 66 68 72 73 74 75 77 79 80 84 86 96 97 100 102 106 107 118 119 120 121 122 124 132 135 **P**8
Primary Contact: Michael K. Winthrop, President
CFO: Alan Ganci, Executive Vice President
CMO: Patrick Waters, M.D., President Medical Staff
CIO: Laura Collier, Coordinator Data Processing
CHR: Deborah Ganci, Vice President Human Resources
Web address: www.bellevuehospital.com
Control: Other not–for–profit (including NFP Corporation) **Service:** General Medical and Surgical

Staffed Beds: 50 **Admissions:** 2943 **Census:** 26 **Outpatient Visits:** 86669 **Births:** 421 **Total Expense ($000):** 46920 **Payroll Expense ($000):** 17070 **Personnel:** 394

BOARDMAN—Mahoning County

☐ **GREENBRIAR REHABILITATION HOSPITAL (363032)**, 8064 South Avenue, Suite One, Zip 44512; tel. 330/726–3700, (Nonreporting) **A**1 10
Primary Contact: Daphne Bonner, Administrator
Control: Corporation, Investor–owned, for–profit **Service:** Rehabilitation

Staffed Beds: 29

★ **ST. ELIZABETH BOARDMAN HEALTH CENTER (360276)**, 8401 Market Street, Zip 44512–6777; tel. 330/729–2929, (Nonreporting) **A**9 10 **S** Catholic Healthcare Partners
Primary Contact: Eugenia Aubel, President
Web address: www.ehealthconnection.com/regions/youngstown/content/show_facility.asp?facility_id=190
Control: Church–operated, Nongovernment, not–for profit **Service:** General Medical and Surgical

Staffed Beds: 108

BOWLING GREEN—Wood County

▣ **WOOD COUNTY HOSPITAL (360029)**, 950 West Wooster Street, Zip 43402–2603; tel. 419/354–8900 **A**1 5 9 10 **F**3 11 12 13 15 17 24 25 28 30 31 32 33 38 41 43 46 50 53 55 56 57 66 67 68 73 74 75 77 79 80 84 86 96 97 99 100 102 103 107 112 118 119 120 121 123 124 133 135 136 137 **P**7 8
Primary Contact: Stanley R. Korducki, President
COO: Carole Matthews, Vice President Patient Care
CFO: Karol Bortel, Vice President Financial Services
CIO: Joanne White, Chief Information Officer
CHR: Frank Day, Vice President Patient Services
Web address: www.wch.net
Control: Other not–for–profit (including NFP Corporation) **Service:** General Medical and Surgical

Staffed Beds: 92 **Admissions:** 3693 **Census:** 36 **Outpatient Visits:** 122017 **Births:** 407 **Total Expense ($000):** 54977 **Payroll Expense ($000):** 23650 **Personnel:** 539

BRYAN—Williams County

☐ **COMMUNITY HOSPITALS AND WELLNESS CENTERS (360121)**, 433 West High Street, Zip 43506–1679; tel. 419/636–1131, (Includes ARCHBOLD HOSPITAL, 121 Westfield Drive, Archbold, Zip 43502; tel. 419/445–4415; BRYAN HOSPITAL; MONTPELIER HOSPITAL, 909 East Snyder Avenue, Montpelier, Zip 43543; tel. 419/485–3154), (Nonreporting) **A**1 2 5 9 10 19
Primary Contact: Philip L. Ennen, Vice President and Chief Executive Officer
CFO: Leroy P. Feather, Vice President Finance
CIO: Greg Slattery, Vice President Information
CHR: Mary Ann Potts, Director Personnel
Web address: www.chwchospital.com
Control: Other not–for–profit (including NFP Corporation) **Service:** General Medical and Surgical

Staffed Beds: 113

BUCYRUS—Crawford County

▣ **BUCYRUS COMMUNITY HOSPITAL (361316)**, 629 North Sandusky Avenue, Zip 44820–1821; tel. 419/562–4677 **A**1 5 9 10 18 **F**3 8 11 14 15 24 25 27 31 32 33 38 43 44 54 55 56 57 68 73 75 76 77 79 80 81 86 96 97 102 106 107 118 120 121 122 124 135 136 **P**6
Primary Contact: Gerard D. Klein, President and Chief Executive Officer
CFO: Lori Falter, Vice President Finance
CMO: Ron Frazier, M.D., Chief of Staff
CIO: Cathy Brown, Manager Information Systems
CHR: Jaime Hatlay, Manager Human Resources
Web address: www.bchonline.org
Control: Other not–for–profit (including NFP Corporation) **Service:** General Medical and Surgical

Staffed Beds: 25 **Admissions:** 864 **Census:** 9 **Outpatient Visits:** 53060 **Births:** 0 **Total Expense ($000):** 25035 **Payroll Expense ($000):** 9460 **Personnel:** 231

CADIZ—Harrison County

▣ **HARRISON COMMUNITY HOSPITAL (361311)**, 951 East Market Street, Zip 43907–9799; tel. 740/942–4631 **A**1 9 10 18 **F**7 11 15 24 25 26 28 31 32 33 37 38 43 50 52 55 56 57 61 62 66 72 73 77 79 80 81 82 86 87 96 97 99 102 107 119 121 122 124 132 135 136 137
Primary Contact: Terry M. Carson, Chief Executive Officer
CFO: Sally Huff, Controller
CMO: Isam Tabbah, M.D., Chief of Staff
CHR: Marcella Evans, Director Human Resources
Web address: www.harrisoncommunity.com
Control: Other not–for–profit (including NFP Corporation) **Service:** General Medical and Surgical

Staffed Beds: 25 **Admissions:** 595 **Census:** 9 **Outpatient Visits:** 30586 **Births:** 0 **Total Expense ($000):** 12938 **Payroll Expense ($000):** 5860 **Personnel:** 168

CAMBRIDGE—Guernsey County

☐ **APPALACHIAN BEHAVIORAL HEALTHCARE (364027)**, 66737 Old 21 Road North, Zip 43725–9298; tel. 740/439–1371, (Nonreporting) **A**1 9 10
Primary Contact: Jane E. Krason, RN, Chief Executive Officer
COO: Kelly D. Markins, Chief Operating Officer
CMO: Mark F. McGee, M.D., Chief Clinical Officer
CIO: Kevin Waller, Regional Director Management Information Systems
Web address: www.mh.state.oh.us
Control: State–Government, nonfederal **Service:** Psychiatric

Staffed Beds: 224

▣ **SOUTHEASTERN OHIO REGIONAL MEDICAL CENTER (360203)**, 1341 North Clark Street, Zip 43725–9614, Mailing Address: P.O. Box 610, Zip 43725–0610; tel. 740/439–3561 **A**1 2 5 9 10 **F**3 7 11 13 15 18 24 25 26 27 28 30 31 32 33 38 40 42 43 44 45 46 49 51 55 56 57 59 61 62 63 64 68 73 74 75 76 77 79 80 81 82 86 87 96 97 99 100 102 104 106 107 118 119 120 121 124 133 135 136 137 **P**6 8
Primary Contact: Raymond M. Chorey, President and Chief Executive Officer
CFO: Donald P. Huelskamp, Vice President Finance and Chief Financial Officer
CMO: Andrew D. Eddy, M.D., Vice President Medical Affairs and Chief Medical Officer
CIO: Michael Price, Director Information Systems
CHR: Patricia Grubbs, Director Human Resources
Web address: www.seormc.org
Control: Other not–for–profit (including NFP Corporation) **Service:** General Medical and Surgical

Staffed Beds: 120 **Admissions:** 4535 **Census:** 43 **Outpatient Visits:** 133312 **Births:** 538 **Total Expense ($000):** 65764 **Payroll Expense ($000):** 27460 **Personnel:** 648

CANTON—Stark County

ACUTE CARE SPECIALTY HOSPITAL OF AULTMAN (362032), 2600 Sixth Street, S.W., Zip 44710; tel. 330/363–4000, (Nonreporting) **A**10
Primary Contact: Jackie Toth, Administrator
Control: Corporation, Investor–owned, for–profit **Service:** Long–Term Acute Care hospital

Staffed Beds: 30

▣ △ **AULTMAN HOSPITAL (360084)**, 2600 Sixth Street S.W., Zip 44710–1702; tel. 330/452–9911, (Total facility includes 60 beds in nursing home–type unit) **A**1 2 3 5 6 7 8 9 10 12 13 **F**3 7 8 11 12 13 14 15 17 18 20 22 24 25 26 27 30 31 32 33 37 38 40 41 42 43 44 49 50 51 52 53 54 55 56 57 58 59 60 61 62 66 68 70 72 73 74 75 76 77 79 80 81 82 84 85 86 87 88 92 93 95 96 97 98 99 100 102 106 107 108 109 111 114 117 118 119 120 121 122 123 124 132 133 135 136 137 **P**3 6 7
Primary Contact: Edward J. Roth, III, President and Chief Executive Officer
COO: Christopher Remark, Chief Operating Officer
CFO: Mark Wright, Vice President
CIO: Martin Tursky, Vice President Information Systems
CHR: Sue Olivera, Vice President
Web address: www.aultman.com
Control: Other not–for–profit (including NFP Corporation) **Service:** General Medical and Surgical

Staffed Beds: 577 **Admissions:** 31187 **Census:** 429 **Outpatient Visits:** 478601 **Births:** 2738 **Total Expense ($000):** 324921 **Payroll Expense ($000):** 151832 **Personnel:** 4135

★ △ **MERCY MEDICAL CENTER (360070)**, 1320 Mercy Drive N.W., Zip 44708–2641; tel. 330/489–1000 **A**1 2 3 5 7 9 10 **F**3 5 11 13 15 17 18 20 22 24 25 26 27 30 31 32 33 37 38 40 41 42 43 46 49 50 51 52 53 54 55 56 57 59 61 62 64 66 68 70 72 73 74 75 76 77 79 80 81 82 84 85 86 87 88 90 91 92 93 94 96 97 100 102 103 104 105 106 107 108 109 111 112 118 119 120 121 124 132 133 135 136 137 **P**6 7 **S** Sisters of Charity Health System
Primary Contact: Thomas E. Cecconi, President and Chief Executive
COO: Jeffrey Smith, Senior Vice President and Chief Operating Officer
CFO: Michael S. Rieger, Vice President and Chief Financial Officer
CMO: David Gormsen, D.O., Chief Medical Officer
CIO: James H. Carroll, Chief Information Officer
CHR: Lorraine Washington, Vice President Human Resources
Web address: www.cantonmercy.com
Control: Other not–for–profit (including NFP Corporation) **Service:** General Medical and Surgical

Staffed Beds: 345 **Admissions:** 15743 **Census:** 208 **Outpatient Visits:** 536349 **Births:** 1738 **Total Expense ($000):** 218062 **Payroll Expense ($000):** 93914 **Personnel:** 1931

CHARDON—Geauga County

☐ **UNIVERSITY HOSPITALS EXTENDED CARE CAMPUS (362014)**, 12340 Bass Lake Road, Zip 44024–8327; tel. 440/285–4040, (Total facility includes 62 beds in nursing home–type unit) **A**1 9 10 **F**1 2 6 10 25 26 30 31 32 37 54 55 56 57 62 63 66 72 73 75 76 77 80 86 93 107 117 119 120 132 135 137 **S** University Hospitals
Primary Contact: Susan V. Juris, President and Chief Executive Officer
COO: Linton Sharpnack, R.N., Director Nursing
CFO: Rebecca Ivcic, Chief Financial Officer
CMO: Donald Goddard, M.D., Chief Medical Officer
CIO: Edward Marx, Vice President and Chief Information Officer
CHR: Danialle Lynce, Manager Human Resources
Web address: www.heatherhill.com
Control: Other not–for–profit (including NFP Corporation) **Service:** Long–Term Acute Care hospital

Staffed Beds: 215 **Admissions:** 1284 **Census:** 215 **Outpatient Visits:** 8205 **Births:** 0 **Total Expense ($000):** 37571 **Payroll Expense ($000):** 18255 **Personnel:** 314

★ **UNIVERSITY HOSPITALS GEAUGA REGIONAL HOSPITAL (360192)**, 13207 Ravenna Road, Zip 44024–7032; tel. 440/269–6000 **A**1 2 9 10 **F**3 11 12 13 15 17 18 20 24 25 26 27 30 31 32 33 35 37 38 40 41 43 45 46 48 49 50 51 54 55 56 57 58 59 60 62 63 66 68 72 73 74 75 76 77 79 80 81 82 84 86 87 88 90 91 92 93 96 97 100 104 106 107 112 117 119 120 121 124 132 135 136 137 **S** University Hospitals
Primary Contact: Richard J. Frenchie, President and Chief Executive Officer
COO: M. Steven Jones, Vice President and Chief Operating Officer
CMO: Martin Macklin, M.D., Ph.D., Vice President Medical Affairs
CIO: Lou Ciraldo, Community Hospitals Representative Information Services
Web address: www.uhhsgrh.com
Control: Other not–for–profit (including NFP Corporation) **Service:** General Medical and Surgical

Staffed Beds: 137 **Admissions:** 6542 **Census:** 65 **Outpatient Visits:** 226701 **Births:** 1131 **Total Expense ($000):** 67792 **Payroll Expense ($000):** 28135 **Personnel:** 525

CHILLICOTHE—Ross County

★ **ADENA HEALTH SYSTEM (360159)**, 272 Hospital Road, Zip 45601–9031; tel. 740/779–7500 **A**1 2 5 9 10 19 **F**3 5 8 11 13 15 17 18 20 22 24 25 26 27 30 31 32 33 36 38 42 43 54 55 56 60 61 62 66 68 72 73 74 75 76 77 78 79 80 82 86 87 88 89 90 92 94 96 97 107 109 114 118 119 120 121 124 133 134 135 136 137 **P**6
Primary Contact: Mark H. Shuter, President and Chief Executive Officer
COO: Jeff Graham, Chief Operating Officer
CFO: Keith T. Coleman, Chief Financial Officer
CMO: John Fortney, M.D., Medical Director
CIO: Marcus Bost, Director Information Services and Chief Information Officer
Web address: www.adena.org
Control: Other not–for–profit (including NFP Corporation) **Service:** General Medical and Surgical

Staffed Beds: 170 **Admissions:** 14751 **Census:** 120 **Outpatient Visits:** 49455 **Personnel:** 1833

★ **VETERANS AFFAIRS MEDICAL CENTER**, 17273 State Route 104, Zip 45601–8608; tel. 740/773–1141, (Total facility includes 162 beds in nursing home–type unit) **A**1 5 **F**3 11 25 26 32 33 36 37 41 42 43 44 46 50 53 54 55 56 57 60 61 62 63 65 72 73 75 77 78 79 81 82 86 87 88 90 92 93 94 95 96 97 100 102 107 117 118 119 121 124 132 133 135 136 **P**6 **S** Department of Veterans Affairs
Primary Contact: Jeffrey T. Gering, Medical Center Director
COO: Keith Sullivan, Acting Associate Director
CFO: Rick Deckard, Chief Fiscal Service
CIO: Joseph Enderle, Chief Information Officer
CHR: Angela Young, Human Resources Officer
Web address: www.va.gov/sta/guide/home.asp
Control: Veterans Affairs, Government, federal **Service:** Psychiatric

Staffed Beds: 297 **Admissions:** 3965 **Census:** 250 **Outpatient Visits:** 254766 **Births:** 0 **Total Expense ($000):** 131348 **Payroll Expense ($000):** 65075 **Personnel:** 1128

CINCINNATI—Hamilton County

☐ **BETHESDA NORTH HOSPITAL (360179)**, 10500 Montgomery Road, Zip 45242–4402; tel. 513/745–1111 **A**1 3 5 9 10 **F**3 11 13 15 17 18 20 22 24 25 26 27 30 31 32 33 34 35 37 38 39 40 41 43 44 45 46 49 50 52 53 54 55 56 57 58 60 62 64 66 68 71 72 73 74 75 76 77 79 80 81 82 85 86 87 90 92 96 97 100 102 103 106 107 114 116 118 119 120 121 123 124 132 134 135 136 137 **P**6
Primary Contact: John S. Prout, President and Chief Executive Officer
COO: Gerald P. Oliphant, Executive Vice President and Chief Operating Officer
CFO: Frank Skala, Interim Chief Financial Officer
CIO: Rick Moore, Vice President and Chief Information Officer
CHR: Walter McLarty, Vice President Human Resources
Web address: www.trihealth.com
Control: Other not–for–profit (including NFP Corporation) **Service:** General Medical and Surgical

Staffed Beds: 330 **Admissions:** 24218 **Census:** 259 **Outpatient Visits:** 257647 **Births:** 4430 **Total Expense ($000):** 317071 **Payroll Expense ($000):** 118428 **Personnel:** 1792

★ △ **CHRIST HOSPITAL (360163)**, 2139 Auburn Avenue, Zip 45219–2906; tel. 513/585–2000 **A**1 2 3 5 6 7 9 10 **F**3 5 8 11 12 13 15 17 18 20 22 24 25 26 27 30 31 32 33 34 35 36 37 38 41 43 44 46 49 50 52 53 54 55 56 57 58 59 60 62 64 66 68 71 72 73 74 75 76 77 78 79 80 81 82 85 86 87 88 89 90 92 93 94 95 96 97 99 100 102 103 104 105 106 107 108 109 111 113 114 116 119 120 121 123 124 127 130 132 134 135 136 137
Primary Contact: Susan Croushore, Executive Director and Senior Vice President
COO: Victor DiPilla, Vice President
CFO: John K. Renner, Vice President Finance
CMO: Bernard B. Gawne, M.D., Vice President Medical Affairs
CIO: Chester Maze, Chief Information Officer
CHR: Rick Tolson, Vice President Human Resources
Web address: www.health–alliance.com
Control: Other not–for–profit (including NFP Corporation) **Service:** General Medical and Surgical

Staffed Beds: 511 **Admissions:** 24600 **Census:** 301 **Outpatient Visits:** 182750 **Births:** 3224 **Total Expense ($000):** 392335 **Payroll Expense ($000):** 135177 **Personnel:** 2622

★ △ **CINCINNATI CHILDREN'S HOSPITAL MEDICAL CENTER (363300)**, (Formerly Children's Hospital Medical Center), (Pediatric medical and surgical), 3333 Burnet Avenue, Zip 45229–3039; tel. 513/636–4200, (Includes DIVISION OF ADOLESCENT MEDICINE, CINCINNATI CENTER FOR DEVELOPMENTAL DISORDERS, AND CONVALESCENT HOSPITAL FOR CHILDREN ; CHILDREN'S HOSPITAL) **A**1 2 3 5 7 8 9 10 **F**3 5 7 9 11 12 17 19 21 23 25 26 27 28 30 31 32 33 34 35 36 37 38 40 41 42 43 44 48 49 50 51 53 55 56 57 58 59 60 61 62 63 64 66 70 72 73 75 76 77 79 80 81 82 83 84 85 86 87 88 89 90 91 92 94 95 96 97 100 101 102 103 104 105 106 107 114 118 119 120 121 123 124 125 126 127 128 130 131 133 135 137 **P**1
Primary Contact: James M. Anderson, President and Chief Executive Officer
CFO: Scott J. Hamlin, Chief Financial Officer
CIO: Marianne Speight, Vice President Information System and Chief Information Officer
CHR: Ronald McKinley, Ph.D., Vice President Human Resources
Web address: www.cincinnatichildrens.org
Control: Other not–for–profit (including NFP Corporation) **Service:** Children's other specialty

Staffed Beds: 452 **Admissions:** 16645 **Census:** 305 **Outpatient Visits:** 900559 **Births:** 8 **Total Expense ($000):** 863506 **Payroll Expense ($000):** 302697 **Personnel:** 9120

Hospital, Medicare Provider Number, Address, Telephone, Approval, Facility, and Physician Codes, Health Care System
★ American Hospital Association (AHA) membership
☐ The Joint Commission accreditation
○ American Osteopathic Association (AOA) accreditation
△ Commission on Accreditation of Rehabilitation Facilities (CARF) accreditation

☐ △ **DEACONESS HOSPITAL (360038)**, 311 Straight Street, Zip 45219–1018; tel. 513/559–2100 **A**1 7 9 10 **F**3 9 11 12 15 17 18 20 22 24 25 26 27 30 31 32 33 38 43 46 52 54 55 56 57 59 62 63 66 68 72 73 75 76 77 79 80 81 82 85 86 87 88 90 91 92 93 94 96 97 100 101 107 117 119 120 121 132 135 137
Primary Contact: E. Anthony Woods, President
COO: David A. Ferrell, Chief Operating Officer
CFO: David McAdmas, Vice President Finance
CMO: Emmett O'Neal, M.D., President Medical Staff
CIO: Ted Averbeck, Director Information Systems
CHR: Jeff Beckman, Vice President Human Resources
Web address: www.Deaconess–healthcare.com
Control: Other not–for–profit (including NFP Corporation) **Service:** General Medical and Surgical

Staffed Beds: 167 **Admissions:** 3764 **Census:** 59 **Outpatient Visits:** 27298 **Births:** 0 **Total Expense ($000):** 59479 **Payroll Expense ($000):** 21368 **Personnel:** 541

★ △ **DRAKE CENTER (362004)**, 151 West Galbraith Road, Zip 45216–1015; tel. 513/418–2500, (Total facility includes 110 beds in nursing home–type unit) **A**1 3 5 7 9 10 **F**1 3 10 11 24 25 26 30 31 32 33 34 41 50 55 56 57 58 62 66 73 75 80 81 82 86 90 94 96 102 115 117 119 121 124 135 137 **P**6 **S** Health Alliance of Greater Cincinnati
Primary Contact: Karen Bankston, Ph.D., Senior Vice President
CFO: Nancy Binder, Director Financial Services
CHR: Alan Jones, Director Human Resources
Web address: www.drakecenter.com
Control: Other not–for–profit (including NFP Corporation) **Service:** Long–Term Acute Care hospital

Staffed Beds: 278 **Admissions:** 1642 **Census:** 164 **Outpatient Visits:** 21572 **Births:** 0 **Total Expense ($000):** 68404 **Payroll Expense ($000):** 35018 **Personnel:** 624

★ △ **GOOD SAMARITAN HOSPITAL (360134)**, 375 Dixmyth Avenue, Zip 45220–2489; tel. 513/872–1400 **A**1 2 3 5 6 7 8 9 10 **F**3 5 11 12 13 15 17 18 20 22 24 25 26 27 30 31 32 33 34 35 37 38 41 42 43 44 45 46 49 50 52 53 54 55 56 57 58 59 60 62 64 66 68 70 72 73 74 75 76 77 79 80 81 82 85 86 87 88 89 90 91 92 93 94 95 96 97 100 102 103 106 107 109 111 114 116 118 119 120 121 124 132 134 135 136 137 **P**6 **S** Catholic Health Initiatives
Primary Contact: John S. Prout, President and Chief Executive Officer
COO: Gerald P. Oliphant, Executive Vice President and Chief Operating Officer
CFO: Frank Skala, Interim Chief Financial Officer
CIO: Rick Moore, Vice President and Chief Information Officer
CHR: Walter McLarty, Vice President Human Resources
Web address: www.trihealth.com
Control: Church–operated, Nongovernment, not–for profit **Service:** General Medical and Surgical

Staffed Beds: 499 **Admissions:** 26698 **Census:** 343 **Outpatient Visits:** 185939 **Births:** 7120 **Total Expense ($000):** 359079 **Payroll Expense ($000):** 130090 **Personnel:** 2312

★ **JEWISH HOSPITAL (360016)**, 4777 East Galbraith Road, Zip 45236–2725; tel. 513/686–3000 **A**1 2 3 5 9 10 **F**3 11 12 15 17 18 20 22 24 26 27 29 30 31 32 33 35 37 38 43 46 49 50 54 59 62 64 66 68 72 73 76 77 78 79 80 82 85 86 87 90 96 97 99 100 103 106 107 108 111 112 119 120 121 125 135 **P**6 **S** Health Alliance of Greater Cincinnati
Primary Contact: M. Aurora Lambert, Senior Vice President
Web address: www.health–alliance.com/jewish.html
Control: Other not–for–profit (including NFP Corporation) **Service:** General Medical and Surgical

Staffed Beds: 209 **Admissions:** 13205 **Census:** 169 **Outpatient Visits:** 38251 **Births:** 0 **Total Expense ($000):** 182901 **Payroll Expense ($000):** 69314 **Personnel:** 1321

★ **MERCY HOSPITAL ANDERSON (360001)**, 7500 State Road, Zip 45255–2492; tel. 513/624–4500, (Nonreporting) **A**1 2 9 10 **S** Catholic Healthcare Partners
Primary Contact: Patricia A. Schroer, President and Chief Executive Officer
CFO: Deborah Bloomfield, Chief Financial Officer
CMO: Leonard M. Randolph, M.D., Senior Vice President and Chief Medical Officer
CIO: Yousuf Ahmad, Regional Vice President Information Services
CHR: Sandie Ferrigno, Director Human Resources
Web address: www.e–mercy.com
Control: Church–operated, Nongovernment, not–for profit **Service:** General Medical and Surgical

Staffed Beds: 160

★ **MERCY HOSPITAL MOUNT AIRY (360234)**, 2446 Kipling Avenue, Zip 45239–6650; tel. 513/853–5000 **A**1 2 9 10 **F**3 11 15 18 24 25 26 27 28 30 31 32 33 38 41 42 43 44 47 50 55 57 59 62 66 72 76 77 79 80 85 87 88 89 96 97 100 102 104 106 107 119 135 137 **S** Catholic Healthcare Partners
Primary Contact: Paul C. Hiltz, President and Chief Executive Officer
CMO: Leonard M. Randolph, M.D., Senior Vice President and Chief Medical Officer
CIO: Yousuf Ahmad, Regional Vice President Information Services
CHR: Chris Browning, Regional Vice President Human Resources
Web address: www.e–mercy.com
Control: Other not–for–profit (including NFP Corporation) **Service:** General Medical and Surgical

Staffed Beds: 184 **Admissions:** 6723 **Census:** 184 **Births:** 0 **Total Expense ($000):** 88221 **Payroll Expense ($000):** 37347

★ **MERCY HOSPITAL WESTERN HILLS (360113)**, 3131 Queen City Avenue, Zip 45238–2396; tel. 513/389–5000 **A**1 2 9 10 **F**8 11 15 18 20 24 25 26 27 30 31 32 33 34 35 38 39 42 43 44 45 46 49 52 55 59 62 63 66 68 72 73 75 76 77 79 80 82 85 86 88 93 96 100 102 104 107 117 119 121 124 135 136 137 **S** Catholic Healthcare Partners
Primary Contact: Patrick A. Kowalski, President and Chief Executive Officer
COO: Patrick A. Kowalski, Chief Financial Officer
Web address: www.e–mercy.com
Control: Other not–for–profit (including NFP Corporation) **Service:** General Medical and Surgical

Staffed Beds: 181 **Admissions:** 7541 **Census:** 96 **Outpatient Visits:** 131719 **Births:** 0 **Total Expense ($000):** 79885 **Payroll Expense ($000):** 36756 **Personnel:** 736

★ **REGENCY HOSPITAL OF CINCINNATI (362034)**, 311 Straight Street, 8th Floor, Zip 45219; tel. 513/559–5900, (Nonreporting) **A**1 10 **S** Regency Hospital Company
Primary Contact: Russell Dean, Chief Executive Officer
Web address: www.regencyhospital.com
Control: Corporation, Investor–owned, for–profit **Service:** Long–Term Acute Care hospital

Staffed Beds: 15

☐ **SELECT SPECIALTY HOSPITAL (362019)**, 375 Dixmyth Avenue, Zip 45220; tel. 513/487–4105 **A**1 9 10 **F**1 3 24 25 30 31 55 63 80 119 137 **S** Select Medical Corporation
Primary Contact: Damian Jones, Administrator and Chief Executive
Web address: www.selectmedicalcorp.com
Control: Corporation, Investor–owned, for–profit **Service:** Long–Term Acute Care hospital

Staffed Beds: 36 **Admissions:** 326 **Census:** 22 **Outpatient Visits:** 0 **Births:** 0 **Total Expense ($000):** 10342 **Payroll Expense ($000):** 4635 **Personnel:** 74

☐ **SHRINERS HOSPITALS FOR CHILDREN, SHRINERS BURNS HOSPITAL, CINCINNATI**, 3229 Burnet Avenue, Zip 45229–3095; tel. 513/872–6000, (Nonreporting) **A**1 **S** Shriners Hospitals for Children
Primary Contact: Ronald R. Hitzler, Administrator
CFO: James Lester, Director Fiscal Services
CMO: Richard J. Kagan, M.D., Chief of Staff
CIO: Mark Washam, Chief Information Officer
CHR: Sally Skillman, Director Human Resources
Web address: www.shrinershq.org
Control: Other not–for–profit (including NFP Corporation) **Service:** Children's other specialty

Staffed Beds: 30

★ **SUMMIT BEHAVIORAL HEALTHCARE (364035)**, 1101 Summit Road, Zip 45237–2652; tel. 513/948–3600 **A**1 9 10 **F**4 25 26 37 52 73 75 88 91 94 119 124 135 **P**5
Primary Contact: Elizabeth Banks, Chief Executive Officer
CFO: Steven Burns, Director Fiscal Services
CMO: Lawrence Ostrowski, M.D., Chief Clinical Officer
CIO: Eric Bradley, Director Computer Information Services
CHR: Rhonda Milton, Director Human Resources
Web address: www.prime/prime.htm
Control: State–Government, nonfederal **Service:** Psychiatric

Staffed Beds: 258 **Admissions:** 400 **Census:** 242 **Outpatient Visits:** 0 **Births:** 0 **Total Expense ($000):** 31261 **Payroll Expense ($000):** 20864 **Personnel:** 313

 Many Facility Codes have changed. Please refer to the AHA Guide Code Chart.

★ **UNIVERSITY HOSPITAL (360003)**, 234 Goodman Street, Zip 45219–2316; tel. 513/584–1000 **A**1 2 3 5 8 9 10 **F**3 7 9 11 12 13 15 16 17 18 20 22 24 25 26 27 30 31 32 33 34 35 36 37 38 40 41 42 43 44 46 47 48 49 50 52 53 54 55 56 57 58 59 60 62 64 66 68 69 70 72 73 74 76 77 78 79 80 81 82 86 87 88 90 91 92 93 94 96 97 99 100 101 102 103 104 105 106 107 109 111 112 114 116 119 120 121 123 124 126 127 128 130 131 132 133 135 136 137 **S** Health Alliance of Greater Cincinnati
Primary Contact: Lee Ann Liska, Executive Director and Senior Vice President
CFO: Rick Hinds, Vice President and Chief Financial Officer
CMO: Michael Archdeacon, M.D., Chief of Staff
CHR: Clarence Pauley, Vice President Human Resources
Web address: www.health-alliance.com/Univ_control.html
Control: Other not–for–profit (including NFP Corporation) **Service:** General Medical and Surgical

Staffed Beds: 438 **Admissions:** 27766 **Census:** 354 **Outpatient Visits:** 384307 **Births:** 2661 **Total Expense ($000):** 434610 **Payroll Expense ($000):** 195342 **Personnel:** 3826

★ **VETERANS AFFAIRS MEDICAL CENTER**, 3200 Vine Street, Zip 45220–2288; tel. 513/861–3100, (Total facility includes 64 beds in nursing home–type unit) **A**1 3 5 8 **F**1 3 4 5 8 18 20 25 26 27 30 31 32 33 35 36 37 38 39 41 43 44 46 48 50 53 54 55 56 57 58 59 60 61 62 63 68 69 72 73 75 76 77 79 80 81 82 86 87 88 90 91 93 94 95 96 97 100 102 103 104 105 106 107 117 118 119 121 124 132 133 134 135 136 137 **S** Department of Veterans Affairs
Primary Contact: Linda Smith, Director
COO: David Ninneman, Associate Director
CFO: Sandra Selvidge, Chief Fiscal Service
CMO: Sidney Steinberg, M.D., Chief of Staff
CIO: Debra Luttjohann, Chief Information Officer
CHR: Iola Dews, Chief Human Resources
Web address: www.va.gov/sta/guide/home.asp
Control: Veterans Affairs, Government, federal **Service:** General Medical and Surgical

Staffed Beds: 277 **Admissions:** 5472 **Census:** 91 **Outpatient Visits:** 366444 **Total Expense ($000):** 173604 **Payroll Expense ($000):** 112514 **Personnel:** 1566

CIRCLEVILLE—Pickaway County

★ **BERGER HEALTH SYSTEM (360170)**, 600 North Pickaway Street, Zip 43113–1447; tel. 740/474–2126 **A**1 5 9 10 **F**3 11 13 15 20 24 25 26 27 30 31 32 33 34 38 41 42 43 50 53 55 56 57 62 66 68 72 73 74 75 76 77 79 80 81 82 84 85 86 96 97 100 102 104 105 107 112 118 119 120 121 124 132 134 135 136 137
Primary Contact: Larry Willard, Interim Chief Executive Officer
COO: Sandra Rudawsky, Corporate Senior Vice President and Chief Operating Officer
CFO: Tim Colburn, Corporate Vice President Finance
CMO: Yadwinder Singh, M.D., Chief of Staff
CIO: Andy Chileski, Corporate Vice President Management Information Systems
CHR: Suzanne Welker, Corporate Vice President Human Resources
Web address: www.bergerhealth.com
Control: City–County, Government, nonfederal **Service:** General Medical and Surgical

Staffed Beds: 80 **Admissions:** 3133 **Census:** 32 **Outpatient Visits:** 90034 **Total Expense ($000):** 52702 **Payroll Expense ($000):** 20691 **Personnel:** 470

CLEVELAND—Cuyahoga County

CLEVELAND CAMPUS See Northcoast Behavioral Healthcare System, Northfield

□ △ **CLEVELAND CLINIC CHILDREN'S HOSPITAL FOR REHABILITATION (363304)**, Mailing Address: 2801 Martin Luther King Jr. Drive, Zip 44104–3865; tel. 216/721–5400 **A**1 7 9 10 **F**25 26 28 30 31 32 33 43 50 53 59 62 73 80 81 82 85 86 119 121 132 135 **S** Cleveland Clinic Health System
Primary Contact: David Kenagny, M.D., Medical Director
COO: Loretta C. Pierce, R.N., MSN, Director Operations
CFO: Debra Nyikes, Chief Financial Officer and Director Finance
CMO: Nancy Roizen, M.D., Chair Medical Staff
CHR: Jan Hlahol, Manager Human Resources
Web address: www.clevelandclinic.org/childrenshospital
Control: Other not–for–profit (including NFP Corporation) **Service:** Children's rehabilitation

Staffed Beds: 25 **Admissions:** 243 **Census:** 15 **Outpatient Visits:** 36366 **Total Expense ($000):** 21035 **Payroll Expense ($000):** 13437 **Personnel:** 300

★ △ **CLEVELAND CLINIC FOUNDATION (360180)**, 9500 Euclid Avenue, Zip 44195–5108; tel. 216/444–2200 **A**1 3 5 7 8 9 10 **F**3 4 5 6 7 8 9 11 12 14 15 17 18 19 20 21 22 23 24 25 26 27 28 30 31 32 33 34 35 36 37 38 41 42 43 44 45 46 47 48 49 50 51 52 53 54 55 56 57 58 59 60 61 62 63 64 66 68 69 70 72 73 75 76 77 78 79 80 81 82 83 84 86 87 88 89 90 91 92 93 94 95 96 97 99 100 101 102 103 104 105 106 107 108 109 111 112 113 114 116 118 119 120 121 123 124 125 126 127 128 129 131 132 133 134 135 136 137 **P**1 3 **S** Cleveland Clinic Health System
Primary Contact: Delos Cosgrove, M.D., President and Chief Executive Officer
COO: Michael P. O'Boyle, Chief Operating Officer
CFO: Steven Glass, Chief Financial Officer
CMO: Joseph Hahn, M.D., Chief of Staff
CIO: C. Martin Harris, M.D., Chief Information Officer
CHR: Joseph Patrnchak, Chief Human Resources Officer
Web address: www.clevelandclinic.org
Control: Other not–for–profit (including NFP Corporation) **Service:** General Medical and Surgical

Staffed Beds: 1080 **Admissions:** 52561 **Census:** 922 **Outpatient Visits:** 3282510 **Births:** 0 **Total Expense ($000):** 2837967 **Payroll Expense ($000):** 1337706 **Personnel:** 18715

□ **FAIRVIEW HOSPITAL (360077)**, 18101 Lorain Avenue, Zip 44111–5656; tel. 216/476–7000, (Total facility includes 20 beds in nursing home–type unit) **A**1 2 3 5 9 10 **F**2 8 13 15 17 18 20 22 24 25 26 27 28 30 31 32 33 38 40 42 43 46 49 51 52 54 55 56 57 58 59 62 63 66 67 68 70 72 73 74 75 76 77 79 80 81 82 84 85 86 87 90 92 96 97 100 105 106 107 108 109 111 117 119 121 135 136 **S** Cleveland Clinic Health System
Primary Contact: Fred M. DeGrandis, Chief Executive Officer
COO: John C. Mills, Senior Vice President Operations
CFO: Mary Ann Freas, Vice President and Chief Financial Officer
CMO: Neal Chadwick, M.D., Chief Medical Officer
CIO: Pam Piar, Chief Information Officer
CHR: Joanne Zeroske, Regional Vice President Human Resources
Web address: www.fairviewhospital.org
Control: Other not–for–profit (including NFP Corporation) **Service:** General Medical and Surgical

Staffed Beds: 410 **Admissions:** 19440 **Census:** 280 **Outpatient Visits:** 332310 **Births:** 4247 **Total Expense ($000):** 296217 **Payroll Expense ($000):** 129940 **Personnel:** 2605

□ **GRACE HOSPITAL (362015)**, 2307 West 14th Street, Zip 44113–3698; tel. 216/687–1500, (Nonreporting) **A**1 10
Primary Contact: Rajive Khanna, Chief Executive Officer
COO: Rajive Khanna, Chief Executive Officer
CMO: John Nickels, M.D., President Medical Staff
CIO: Mary Zimpfer, Vice President Quality Management
Web address: www.gracehospital.org
Control: Other not–for–profit (including NFP Corporation) **Service:** Long–Term Acute Care hospital

Staffed Beds: 87

HANNA HOUSE SKILLED NURSING FACILITY See University Hospitals Case Medical Center

□ **HILLCREST HOSPITAL (360230)**, 6780 Mayfield Road, Zip 44124–2202; tel. 440/449–4500 **A**1 2 9 10 **F**11 13 15 17 18 20 21 22 24 25 26 27 30 31 32 33 36 38 40 43 44 46 49 55 56 57 59 62 63 66 67 68 70 72 73 74 75 76 77 79 81 82 84 86 87 90 96 97 99 100 102 103 104 105 107 109 111 118 119 121 124 132 133 135 136 137 **S** Cleveland Clinic Health System
Primary Contact: Jeffrey A. Leimgruber, President
Web address: www.hillcresthospital.org
Control: Other not–for–profit (including NFP Corporation) **Service:** General Medical and Surgical

Staffed Beds: 361 **Admissions:** 20474 **Census:** 260 **Outpatient Visits:** 293418 **Births:** 3810 **Total Expense ($000):** 260687 **Payroll Expense ($000):** 109276 **Personnel:** 2224

□ **HURON HOSPITAL (360101)**, 13951 Terrace Road, Zip 44112–4399; tel. 216/761–3300 **A**1 6 9 10 **F**4 5 13 15 25 26 28 30 31 32 33 38 40 43 44 46 49 50 51 54 55 56 57 58 59 60 62 68 70 73 74 75 76 77 79 80 82 86 87 88 96 100 102 107 119 132 133 135 136 137 **S** Cleveland Clinic Health System
Primary Contact: A. Gus Kious, M.D., Chief Administrative Officer
CFO: Joseph Beatty, Finance Director
Web address: www.meridia.org
Control: Other not–for–profit (including NFP Corporation) **Service:** General Medical and Surgical

Staffed Beds: 197 **Admissions:** 9525 **Census:** 118 **Outpatient Visits:** 95171 **Births:** 935 **Total Expense ($000):** 104848 **Payroll Expense ($000):** 56723 **Personnel:** 1105

Hospital, Medicare Provider Number, Address, Telephone, Approval, Facility, and Physician Codes, Health Care System

★ American Hospital Association (AHA) membership
□ The Joint Commission accreditation
○ American Osteopathic Association (AOA) accreditation
△ Commission on Accreditation of Rehabilitation Facilities (CARF) accreditation

☐ **KINDRED HOSPITAL CLEVELAND – GATEWAY (362026)**, 2351 East 22nd Street, 7th Floor, Zip 44115; tel. 216/363–2671, (Nonreporting) **A**1
Primary Contact: Janice Hanna, Chief Executive Officer
Web address: www.kindredhealthcare.com
Control: Corporation, Investor–owned, for–profit **Service:** Long–Term Acute Care hospital

Staffed Beds: 75

★ **LUTHERAN HOSPITAL (360087)**, 1730 West 25th Street, Zip 44113–3170; tel. 216/696–4300, (Total facility includes 10 beds in nursing home–type unit) **A**1 9 10 **F**9 25 27 29 30 31 32 33 38 43 46 54 55 56 57 58 59 62 63 68 73 75 77 79 81 82 85 86 87 88 90 91 93 94 96 97 100 107 117 118 119 120 121 124 132 133 135 137 **S** Cleveland Clinic Health System
Primary Contact: David Perse, M.D., President
COO: Hugh Pearson, Vice President
CFO: Thomas P. O'Neill, Vice President and Director Finance
Web address: www.lutheranhospital.org
Control: Other not–for–profit (including NFP Corporation) **Service:** General Medical and Surgical

Staffed Beds: 191 **Admissions:** 7057 **Census:** 113 **Outpatient Visits:** 84755 **Total Expense ($000):** 86096 **Payroll Expense ($000):** 40669 **Personnel:** 786

★ △ **METROHEALTH MEDICAL CENTER (360059)**, 2500 MetroHealth Drive, Zip 44109–1998; tel. 216/778–7800, (Total facility includes 294 beds in nursing home–type unit) **A**1 2 3 5 7 8 9 10 12 13 **F**3 5 6 7 8 9 11 12 13 15 16 17 18 20 22 24 25 26 27 28 30 31 32 33 34 36 37 38 40 41 42 43 44 46 47 49 50 51 52 53 54 55 56 57 58 59 60 62 63 64 66 68 69 70 72 73 74 75 76 77 78 79 80 81 82 83 84 85 86 87 88 89 90 91 92 93 94 95 96 97 100 102 103 104 105 106 107 109 111 113 114 117 118 119 120 121 123 124 132 133 135 136 137 **P**6
Primary Contact: Mark J. Moran, Interim President and Chief Executive Officer
CFO: Nancy Fisher Crum, Chief Financial Officer
CMO: Ben H. Brouhard, M.D., Executive Vice President Medical Affairs and Chief Medical Officer
CIO: Vince Miller, Vice President and Chief Information Officer
CHR: Daniel Lewis, Vice President Human Resources
Web address: www.metrohealth.org
Control: County–Government, nonfederal **Service:** General Medical and Surgical

Staffed Beds: 868 **Admissions:** 27869 **Census:** 696 **Outpatient Visits:** 813880 **Births:** 3598 **Total Expense ($000):** 641390 **Payroll Expense ($000):** 357612 **Personnel:** 5918

RAINBOW BABIES AND CHILDREN'S HOSPITAL See University Hospitals Case Medical Center

SAINT LUKE'S MEDICAL CENTER See St. Vincent Charity Hospital

☐ ○ **ST. JOHN WEST SHORE HOSPITAL (360123)**, 29000 Center Ridge Road, Zip 44145–5219; tel. 440/835–8000, (Total facility includes 11 beds in nursing home–type unit) **A**1 2 9 10 11 12 13 **F**3 8 13 15 17 18 20 22 24 25 26 27 30 31 32 33 37 38 39 40 41 43 44 49 50 51 54 55 56 57 59 62 66 68 69 72 73 74 76 77 78 79 80 81 82 84 86 96 97 100 102 107 117 118 119 121 132 133 135 136 137 **P**4 **S** Sisters of Charity Health System
Primary Contact: Cliff J. Coker, President
CFO: Allen R. Tracy, Senior Vice President and Chief Financial Officer
CMO: Michael Dobrovich, M.D., Chief Medical Officer
CIO: James H. Carroll, Chief Information Officer
CHR: Gary Lazroff, Vice President Human Resources
Web address: www.sjws.net
Control: Other not–for–profit (including NFP Corporation) **Service:** General Medical and Surgical

Staffed Beds: 183 **Admissions:** 10867 **Census:** 114 **Outpatient Visits:** 192892 **Births:** 630 **Total Expense ($000):** 108873 **Payroll Expense ($000):** 46412 **Personnel:** 1033

☐ **ST. VINCENT CHARITY HOSPITAL (360037)**, 2351 East 22nd Street, Zip 44115–3111; tel. 216/861–6200, (Includes SAINT LUKE'S MEDICAL CENTER, 11311 Shaker Boulevard, Zip 44104–3805; tel. 216/368–7000) **A**1 2 3 5 9 10 **F**3 4 5 6 9 12 15 17 18 20 22 24 25 26 27 29 30 31 32 33 34 35 36 37 38 39 41 42 43 44 49 50 53 54 55 56 57 59 60 62 63 64 66 68 72 73 75 76 77 79 80 81 82 86 87 88 89 90 91 92 93 94 95 96 97 100 102 106 107 114 117 118 119 120 121 123 124 132 133 135 136 137 **P**4 **S** Sisters of Charity Health System
Primary Contact: Jeffrey S. Jeney, President and Chief Executive Officer
COO: Beverly Lozar, Vice President Professional and Support Services
CFO: Allen R. Tracy, Senior Vice President and Chief Financial Officer
CMO: Adnan Tahir, M.D., Chief Medical Officer
CIO: James H. Carroll, Chief Information Officer
CHR: Gary Lazroff, Vice President Human Resources
Web address: www.svch.net
Control: Other not–for–profit (including NFP Corporation) **Service:** General Medical and Surgical

Staffed Beds: 182 **Admissions:** 9153 **Census:** 125 **Outpatient Visits:** 169519 **Births:** 0 **Total Expense ($000):** 122489 **Payroll Expense ($000):** 53589 **Personnel:** 1077

★ **UNIVERSITY HOSPITALS BEDFORD MEDICAL CENTER (360115)**, 44 Blaine Avenue, Zip 44146–2709; tel. 440/735–3900 **A**1 2 9 10 **F**8 14 15 18 20 22 24 25 26 27 29 30 31 32 33 34 35 38 43 46 50 51 53 55 56 57 58 59 61 62 63 67 68 69 72 73 75 76 77 79 81 82 85 86 87 96 97 98 99 100 102 103 104 105 107 118 119 121 122 132 134 135 136 **S** University Hospitals
Primary Contact: Sean McKibben, President
COO: Michelle Giltner, Director Professional and Support Staff Services
CFO: Scott Platz, Director Finance
CMO: Marwan Hilal, M.D., Chief Medical Officer
CHR: Donna Kwiecien, Manager Human Resources
Web address: www.uhhsbmc.com
Control: Other not–for–profit (including NFP Corporation) **Service:** General Medical and Surgical

Staffed Beds: 77 **Admissions:** 3947 **Census:** 57 **Outpatient Visits:** 163853 **Births:** 0 **Total Expense ($000):** 44965 **Payroll Expense ($000):** 21860 **Personnel:** 428

★ **UNIVERSITY HOSPITALS CASE MEDICAL CENTER (360137)**, 11100 Euclid Avenue, Zip 44106–2602; tel. 216/844–1000, (Includes ALFRED AND NORMA LERNER TOWER, BOLWELL HEALTH CENTER, HANNA PAVILION, LAKESIDE HOSPITAL, SAMUEL MATHER PAVILION ; HANNA HOUSE SKILLED NURSING FACILITY; RAINBOW BABIES AND CHILDREN'S HOSPITAL; UNIVERSITY MACDONALD WOMEN'S HOSPITAL), (Total facility includes 33 beds in nursing home–type unit) **A**1 2 3 5 8 9 10 12 13 **F**3 5 6 7 8 9 11 12 13 14 15 16 17 18 19 20 21 22 23 24 25 26 27 28 30 31 32 33 34 35 36 37 38 39 40 41 42 43 44 46 47 48 49 50 51 53 54 55 56 57 58 59 60 61 62 63 64 66 67 68 69 70 71 72 73 74 75 76 77 79 80 81 82 83 84 85 86 87 88 89 90 91 92 93 94 95 96 97 98 99 100 101 102 103 104 105 106 107 108 109 111 112 113 114 116 117 118 119 120 121 123 124 125 126 127 128 129 130 131 132 133 134 135 136 137 **P**6 **S** University Hospitals
Primary Contact: Fred C. Rothstein, M.D., President
COO: Ron Dziedzicki, Senior Vice President and General Manager Operations
CFO: Matt Love, Vice President Financial Services
CMO: Nathan Levitan, M.D., Chief Medical Officer and Senior Vice President Academic Affairs
CIO: Mike Kelly, Vice President and Chief Information Officer
CHR: Julie Chester, Director Human Resources
Web address: www.UHhospitals.org
Control: Other not–for–profit (including NFP Corporation) **Service:** General Medical and Surgical

Staffed Beds: 649 **Admissions:** 43478 **Census:** 589 **Outpatient Visits:** 1187813 **Births:** 3880 **Total Expense ($000):** 787101 **Payroll Expense ($000):** 296810 **Personnel:** 6297

★ ○ **UNIVERSITY HOSPITALS RICHMOND MEDICAL CENTER (360075)**, 27100 Chardon Road, Zip 44143–1116; tel. 440/585–6500 **A**9 10 11 12 13 **F**8 15 18 25 31 32 33 38 43 46 48 49 50 51 56 57 62 64 65 66 68 72 73 75 77 79 80 82 85 86 90 96 100 104 107 118 119 135 137
S University Hospitals
Primary Contact: Michael Szubski, Interim President
CFO: Kris Bennett, Director Finance
CMO: Michael Devereaux, M.D., Medical Director and Vice President Clinical Integration
Web address: www.uhhsrh.org
Control: Other not–for–profit (including NFP Corporation) **Service:** General Medical and Surgical

Staffed Beds: 80 **Admissions:** 4026 **Census:** 46 **Outpatient Visits:** 176556 **Births:** 0 **Total Expense ($000):** 49003 **Payroll Expense ($000):** 20862 **Personnel:** 446

★ △ **VETERANS AFFAIRS MEDICAL CENTER**, 10701 East Boulevard, Zip 44106–1702; tel. 216/791–3800, (Total facility includes 190 beds in nursing home–type unit) **A**1 3 5 7 8 **F**2 3 4 5 6 7 8 9 10 11 12 15 17 18 20 22 24 25 26 27 30 31 32 33 34 35 36 37 38 41 42 43 44 45 46 47 48 49 50 53 54 55 56 57 58 59 60 61 62 63 64 66 68 69 72 73 75 76 77 78 79 80 81 82 85 86 87 88 90 91 92 93 94 95 96 97 100 101 102 103 104 105 107 108 109 111 117 118 119 121 124 132 133 135 136 137 **S** Department of Veterans Affairs
Primary Contact: William D. Montague, Director
CFO: Gene DeAngelis, Chief Fiscal Service
CIO: Michael Hickman, Chief Information Resource Management
Web address: www.va.gov/sta/guide/home.asp
Control: Veterans Affairs, Government, federal **Service:** General Medical and Surgical

Staffed Beds: 671 **Admissions:** 11270 **Census:** 575 **Outpatient Visits:** 1004926 **Births:** 0 **Total Expense ($000):** 582409 **Payroll Expense ($000):** 229749 **Personnel:** 3550

 Many Facility Codes have changed. Please refer to the AHA Guide Code Chart.

COLDWATER—Mercer County

★ **MERCER COUNTY JOINT TOWNSHIP COMMUNITY HOSPITAL (360058)**, 800 West Main Street, Zip 45828–1698; tel. 419/678–2341 **A**1 9 10 **F**3 7 11 13 15 24 25 26 27 31 32 33 34 38 51 53 55 57 61 62 64 66 68 73 74 75 76 77 79 80 82 86 96 97 99 100 102 106 107 118 119 120 121 122 124 133 135 137 **P**3
Primary Contact: James A. Wermert, Chief Executive Officer
CFO: Cindy Berning, Chief Financial Officer
CMO: Venkatarao Neelati, M.D., Chief of Staff
CIO: Rich Branch, Director Information Systems
CHR: Peggy Schultz, Director Human Resources
Web address: www.mercerhospital.com
Control: Hospital district or authority, Government, nonfederal **Service:** General Medical and Surgical

Staffed Beds: 60 **Admissions:** 2103 **Census:** 17 **Outpatient Visits:** 62808 **Births:** 328 **Total Expense ($000):** 36661 **Payroll Expense ($000):** 14438 **Personnel:** 380

COLUMBUS—Franklin County

CHILDREN'S HOSPITAL See Nationwide Children's Hospital

★ ○ **DOCTORS HOSPITAL (360152)**, 5100 West Broad Street, Zip 43228–1607; tel. 614/544–1000 **A**1 2 9 10 11 12 13 **F**3 11 13 15 17 18 20 22 24 25 26 27 30 31 32 33 38 43 45 49 53 55 56 57 58 59 60 62 63 64 66 68 70 71 72 73 74 75 76 77 79 80 81 82 86 87 96 97 99 100 102 103 104 105 106 107 111 112 119 121 124 132 133 135 136 137 **S** OhioHealth
Primary Contact: Michael L. Reichfield, President
CFO: Nathan Van Laningham, Vice President and Chief Financial Officer
CMO: Dean Colwell, D.O., Vice President Medical Affairs
CIO: Michael Krouse, Chief Information Officer
CHR: Barbara Otey, Vice President Human Resources
Web address: www.ohiohealth.com
Control: Church–operated, Nongovernment, not–for profit **Service:** General Medical and Surgical

Staffed Beds: 193 **Admissions:** 8847 **Census:** 109 **Outpatient Visits:** 149711 **Births:** 1124 **Total Expense ($000):** 156355 **Payroll Expense ($000):** 73826 **Personnel:** 1297

★ **GRANT MEDICAL CENTER (360017)**, 111 South Grant Avenue, Zip 43215–1898; tel. 614/566–9000 **A**1 2 8 9 10 **F**3 7 8 11 13 14 15 17 18 20 22 24 25 26 27 30 31 32 33 34 35 36 37 38 40 42 43 44 45 46 47 48 49 50 52 53 54 55 56 57 58 59 60 61 62 63 64 65 66 67 68 69 70 72 73 74 75 76 77 79 80 81 82 86 87 90 92 94 95 96 97 98 99 100 101 102 103 104 105 106 107 108 109 111 112 114 118 119 120 121 122 123 124 132 133 135 136 137 **S** OhioHealth
Primary Contact: Karen H. Connors, President
COO: Tom Chickerella, Senior Vice President Operations
CFO: Vinson Yates, Vice President Finance
CMO: Sean Gleason, M.D., Chief Medical Officer
CIO: Michael Krouse, Chief Information Officer
CHR: John Boswell, Vice President Human Resources
Web address: www.ohiohealth.com
Control: Church–operated, Nongovernment, not–for profit **Service:** General Medical and Surgical

Staffed Beds: 404 **Admissions:** 22186 **Census:** 258 **Outpatient Visits:** 209674 **Births:** 2157 **Total Expense ($000):** 349885 **Payroll Expense ($000):** 142032 **Personnel:** 2461

★ **JAMES CANCER HOSPITAL AND SOLOVE RESEARCH INSTITUTE (360242)**, 300 West Tenth Avenue, Zip 43210–1240; tel. 614/293–3300 **A**1 2 3 5 8 9 10 **F**3 7 9 11 12 13 14 15 17 18 20 22 24 25 26 27 28 29 30 31 32 33 34 35 36 37 38 39 40 41 42 43 44 45 46 47 48 49 50 51 52 53 54 55 56 57 58 59 60 62 64 66 68 69 72 73 75 76 77 79 80 81 82 85 86 87 90 92 93 94 96 97 99 100 101 102 103 104 105 106 107 108 109 111 112 113 114 116 119 121 123 124 125 130 132 133 134 135 136 137 **P**2 **S** Ohio State University Health System
Primary Contact: Dennis J. Smith, Chief Operating Officer
CFO: Bell Julian, Associate Executive Director and Chief Financial Officer
CIO: Twyla Pohar, Manager Business Relations
CHR: Jill Hannah, Director Human Resources
Web address: www.jamesline.com
Control: State–Government, nonfederal **Service:** Cancer

Staffed Beds: 163 **Admissions:** 8307 **Census:** 151 **Outpatient Visits:** 182014 **Births:** 0 **Total Expense ($000):** 301141 **Payroll Expense ($000):** 72667 **Personnel:** 2485

★ △ **MOUNT CARMEL (360035)**, Mailing Address: 793 West State Street, Zip 43222–1551; tel. 614/234–5000, (Includes MOUNT CARMEL EAST HOSPITAL, 6001 East Broad Street, Zip 43213; tel. 614/234–6000; MOUNT CARMEL WEST HOSPITAL) **A**1 2 3 5 7 9 10 **F**3 11 12 13 15 17 18 20 22 24 25 26 27 28 30 31 32 33 34 35 38 40 41 42 43 44 45 46 47 48 49 50 56 57 58 60 61 62 63 64 66 68 69 70 71 72 73 74 76 77 79 80 81 82 85 86 87 88 90 91 92 93 94 96 97 98 99 100 102 103 104 106 107 109 111 114 116 119 120 121 122 124 135 136 137 **S** Trinity Health
Primary Contact: Claus von Zychlin, President and Chief Executive Officer
COO: Mary R. Trimmer, Interim Chief Operating Officer
CFO: Russell W. Gardner, Chief Financial Officer
CIO: Cindy Sheets, Chief Information Officer
Web address: www.mountcarmelhealth.com
Control: Church–operated, Nongovernment, not–for profit **Service:** General Medical and Surgical

Staffed Beds: 760 **Admissions:** 40754 **Census:** 502 **Outpatient Visits:** 438492 **Births:** 4912 **Total Expense ($000):** 546904 **Payroll Expense ($000):** 190540 **Personnel:** 3832

★ △ **NATIONWIDE CHILDREN'S HOSPITAL (363305)**, (Formerly Children's Hospital), (Pediatric Medical–Surgical), 700 Children's Drive, Zip 43205–2696; tel. 614/722–2000 **A**1 3 5 7 8 9 10 **F**3 7 8 12 16 17 18 19 20 21 22 23 24 25 26 27 28 30 31 32 33 37 38 40 41 42 43 44 48 50 52 53 55 56 57 58 59 60 61 62 63 64 66 69 70 72 73 75 76 77 79 80 81 82 83 84 85 86 87 89 90 91 92 94 96 97 100 102 103 106 107 114 118 119 120 121 122 123 124 125 126 127 129 132 133 135 137 **P**6 8
Primary Contact: Steve Allen, M.D., Chief Executive Officer
COO: Rick Miller, President and Chief Operating Officer
CFO: Tim Robinson, Chief Financial Officer and Treasurer
CMO: Terry Davis, M.D., Interim Medical Director
CIO: Denise Zabawski, Vice President Information Services and Chief Information Officer
CHR: Jose Balderrama, Vice President Human Resources
Web address: www.nationwidechildrens.org
Control: Other not–for–profit (including NFP Corporation) **Service:** Children's other specialty

Staffed Beds: 404 **Admissions:** 15444 **Census:** 289 **Outpatient Visits:** 743660 **Births:** 0 **Total Expense ($000):** 502790 **Payroll Expense ($000):** 236362 **Personnel:** 4591

★ **OHIO STATE UNIVERSITY HOSPITALS EAST (360062)**, 1492 East Broad Street, Zip 43205–1546; tel. 614/257–3000 **A**1 3 5 9 10 **F**3 4 5 7 15 18 24 25 26 30 31 32 33 35 38 41 43 46 48 49 50 52 55 56 57 58 59 62 63 66 68 72 73 75 76 77 79 80 81 82 86 87 90 96 97 100 102 107 118 119 120 121 124 135 137 **S** Ohio State University Health System
Primary Contact: Elizabeth Seely, Executive Director
CFO: Patrick Robertson, Chief Financial Officer
CMO: Joel Lucas, M.D., Medical Director
Web address: www.medicalcenter.osu.edu
Control: State–Government, nonfederal **Service:** General Medical and Surgical

Staffed Beds: 172 **Admissions:** 10221 **Census:** 140 **Outpatient Visits:** 160846 **Births:** 0 **Total Expense ($000):** 147856 **Payroll Expense ($000):** 57170 **Personnel:** 2212

★ △ **OHIO STATE UNIVERSITY MEDICAL CENTER (360085)**, 370 West 9th Avenue, Zip 43210–1240; tel. 614/293–8000 **A**1 3 5 7 8 9 10 **F**3 5 7 9 11 12 13 15 16 17 18 20 22 24 25 26 27 29 30 31 32 33 34 35 36 37 38 40 41 43 44 46 47 48 49 50 51 52 53 54 55 56 57 58 59 60 62 63 64 66 68 70 71 72 73 74 75 77 78 79 80 81 82 85 86 87 88 89 90 91 92 93 94 95 96 97 100 101 102 103 106 107 113 116 118 119 121 123 124 126 127 128 129 130 131 133 134 135 136 137 **P**6 **S** Ohio State University Health System
Primary Contact: Peter E. Geier, Chief Operating Officer
COO: Jay D. Kasey, Chief Operating Officer
CFO: John B. Stone, Chief Financial Officer
CMO: Hagop Mekhjian, M.D., Medical Director
CIO: Herb Smaltz, Chief Information Officer
CHR: Les Ridout, Human Resources Officer
Web address: www.osumedcenter.edu
Control: State–Government, nonfederal **Service:** General Medical and Surgical

Staffed Beds: 732 **Admissions:** 33851 **Census:** 534 **Outpatient Visits:** 577027 **Births:** 4440 **Total Expense ($000):** 808293 **Payroll Expense ($000):** 251259 **Personnel:** 7093

Hospital, Medicare Provider Number, Address, Telephone, Approval, Facility, and Physician Codes, Health Care System

★ American Hospital Association (AHA) membership
□ The Joint Commission accreditation
○ American Osteopathic Association (AOA) accreditation
△ Commission on Accreditation of Rehabilitation Facilities (CARF) accreditation

★ △ **RIVERSIDE METHODIST HOSPITAL (360006)**, 3535 Olentangy River Road, Zip 43214–3998; tel. 614/566–5000 **A**1 2 7 8 9 10 **F**2 3 4 5 6 7 8 9 11 12 13 14 15 17 18 20 22 24 25 26 27 28 29 30 31 32 33 34 35 36 37 38 40 41 42 43 44 45 46 47 48 49 50 51 52 53 54 55 56 57 58 59 60 61 62 63 64 66 68 69 70 71 72 73 74 75 76 77 78 79 80 81 82 84 85 86 87 88 90 91 92 93 94 95 96 97 99 100 102 103 104 105 106 107 108 109 111 112 113 114 116 118 119 120 121 122 124 130 132 133 134 135 136 137 **S** OhioHealth
Primary Contact: Bruce P. Hagen, President
COO: Stephen Markovich, M.D., Senior Vice President Operations
CFO: John Lindaman, Interim Vice President Finance
CMO: Leonard J. Lozada, M.D., Vice President Medical Affairs
CIO: Michael Krouse, Chief Information Officer
CHR: Paul N. Patton, Vice President Human Resources
Web address: www.ohiohealth.com
Control: Church–operated, Nongovernment, not–for profit **Service:** General Medical and Surgical

Staffed Beds: 826 **Admissions:** 50230 **Census:** 572 **Outpatient Visits:** 740297 **Births:** 6734 **Total Expense ($000):** 694009 **Payroll Expense ($000):** 288880 **Personnel:** 5091

☐ **SELECT SPECIALTY HOSPITAL–COLUMBUS**, 410 West 10th Avenue, 11th Floor, Zip 43210; tel. 614/293–6931, (Nonreporting) **A**1 **S** Select Medical Corporation
Primary Contact: Dan West, Chief Executive Officer
Web address: www.selectmedicalcorp.com
Control: Corporation, Investor–owned, for–profit **Service:** Long–Term Acute Care hospital

Staffed Beds: 50

☐ **SELECT SPECIALTY HOSPITAL–COLUMBUS (362022)**, 111 South Grant Avenue, 5th Floor, Zip 43215; tel. 614/566–8211, (Nonreporting) **A**1 10 **S** Select Medical Corporation
Primary Contact: Mary Burkett, Interim Chief Executive Officer
Web address: www.selectmedicalcorp.com
Control: Corporation, Investor–owned, for–profit **Service:** Long–Term Acute Care hospital

Staffed Beds: 37

☐ **SELECT SPECIALTY HOSPITAL–COLUMBUS (362017)**, 1492 East Broad Street, 8th Floor, Zip 43205; tel. 614/252–4440, (Nonreporting) **A**1 10 **S** Select Medical Corporation
Primary Contact: Craig A. Hoover, Chief Executive Officer
Web address: www.selectmedicalcorp.com
Control: Corporation, Investor–owned, for–profit **Service:** Long–Term Acute Care hospital

Staffed Beds: 44

★ **TWIN VALLEY BEHAVIORAL HEALTHCARE–COLUMBUS CAMPUS (364007)**, 2200 West Broad Street, Zip 43223–1295; tel. 614/752–0333 **A**1 9 10 **F**25 26 30 31 32 37 66 82 88 90 95 119 121 124 135
Primary Contact: Robert Short, Chief Executive Officer
COO: David Blahnik, Chief Operating Officer
CFO: John Eardley, Chief Financial Officer
CMO: Marion E. Sherman, M.D., Chief Clinical Officer
CIO: Missy McGarvey, Director Computer Information Systems
CHR: Gilbert Murphy, Director Human Services
Web address: www.mh.state.oh.us/ibhs/bhos/tvbh.html
Control: State–Government, nonfederal **Service:** Psychiatric

Staffed Beds: 317 **Admissions:** 1121 **Census:** 299 **Outpatient Visits:** 54545 **Births:** 0 **Total Expense ($000):** 49254 **Payroll Expense ($000):** 37587 **Personnel:** 504

CONNEAUT—Ashtabula County

★ **UNIVERSITY HOSPITALS CONNEAUT MEDICAL CENTER (361308)**, 158 West Main Road, Zip 44030–2039; tel. 440/593–1131 **A**1 9 10 18 **F**3 7 11 15 24 25 30 31 32 33 38 43 51 55 56 57 62 66 68 73 76 79 81 82 86 96 107 119 121 122 124 132 135 136 **S** University Hospitals
Primary Contact: Laurie Delgado, President and Chief Executive Officer
CFO: Rob David, Director Finance Services
CMO: Gary Huston, D.O., Director Medical Affairs
CIO: Alnita B. Russell, Director Medical Care Evaluation
Web address: www.uhhs.com
Control: Other not–for–profit (including NFP Corporation) **Service:** General Medical and Surgical

Staffed Beds: 25 **Admissions:** 997 **Census:** 11 **Outpatient Visits:** 138666 **Births:** 0 **Total Expense ($000):** 22562 **Payroll Expense ($000):** 8845 **Personnel:** 166

COSHOCTON—Coshocton County

☐ **COSHOCTON COUNTY MEMORIAL HOSPITAL (360109)**, 1460 Orange Street, Zip 43812–6330, Mailing Address: P.O. Box 1330, Zip 43812–6330; tel. 740/622–6411, (Total facility includes 61 beds in nursing home–type unit) **A**1 5 9 10 20 **F**13 24 25 27 30 31 32 38 40 55 68 73 75 76 77 79 86 96 97 100 102 103 107 108 117 118 119 121 132 133 135 136 137 **P**7
Primary Contact: Gregory M. Nowak, Administrator and Chief Executive Officer
CFO: Robert Miller, Chief Financial Officer
CMO: David Lozowski, M.D., Chief of Staff
CIO: Rob Rizk, Director Information Services
CHR: Rick Davis, Senior Director Human Resources
Web address: www.ccmh.com
Control: Other not–for–profit (including NFP Corporation) **Service:** General Medical and Surgical

Staffed Beds: 135 **Admissions:** 3725 **Census:** 87 **Outpatient Visits:** 67418 **Births:** 351 **Total Expense ($000):** 51906 **Payroll Expense ($000):** 18616 **Personnel:** 435

CUYAHOGA FALLS—Summit County

○ **CUYAHOGA FALLS GENERAL HOSPITAL (360150)**, 1900 23rd Street, Zip 44223–1499; tel. 330/971–7000 **A**9 10 11 12 13 **F**2 3 13 25 26 27 30 31 32 33 38 42 43 55 57 59 62 63 64 66 68 72 73 74 75 76 77 79 80 86 87 96 97 100 102 107 118 119 132 135 136 137 **P**1 6 **S** Summa Health System
Primary Contact: Kathleen A. Rice, President and Chief Operating Officer
CFO: John Brockettі, Vice President and Chief Financial Officer
CMO: Rob Kent, M.D., Vice President Medical Affairs
Web address: www.summahealth.org
Control: Other not–for–profit (including NFP Corporation) **Service:** General Medical and Surgical

Staffed Beds: 105 **Admissions:** 3738 **Census:** 41 **Outpatient Visits:** 105837 **Births:** 436 **Total Expense ($000):** 76378 **Payroll Expense ($000):** 29403 **Personnel:** 577

DAYTON—Montgomery County

☐ **CHILDREN'S MEDICAL CENTER (363306)**, One Children's Plaza, Zip 45404–1815; tel. 937/641–3000 **A**1 2 3 5 8 9 10 **F**3 7 11 19 25 26 27 28 30 31 32 33 37 38 40 41 42 43 44 50 53 55 56 57 58 59 60 61 62 63 64 70 72 73 75 76 77 79 80 81 82 83 84 86 87 96 100 102 107 114 118 119 121 123 124 133 135 **P**6
Primary Contact: David Kinsaul, President and Chief Executive Officer
CFO: David T. Miller, Vice President and Chief Financial Officer
CMO: Thomas Murphy, M.D., Vice President Medical Affairs
CIO: Beth Fredette, Chief Information Officer
Web address: www.childrensdayton.org
Control: Other not–for–profit (including NFP Corporation) **Service:** Children's general

Staffed Beds: 123 **Admissions:** 6111 **Census:** 81 **Outpatient Visits:** 250162 **Births:** 0 **Total Expense ($000):** 149859 **Payroll Expense ($000):** 65089 **Personnel:** 1374

☐ **DAYTON HEART HOSPITAL (360253)**, 707 South Edwin C. Moses Boulevard, Zip 45408; tel. 937/221–8000, (Nonreporting) **A**1 9 10 **S** MedCath, Inc.
Web address: www.daytonhearthospital.com
Control: Corporation, Investor–owned, for–profit **Service:** General Medical and Surgical

Staffed Beds: 47

★ **GOOD SAMARITAN HOSPITAL (360052)**, 2222 Philadelphia Drive, Zip 45406–1813; tel. 937/278–2612 **A**1 2 3 5 9 10 **F**3 5 6 8 10 11 12 13 15 17 18 20 22 24 25 26 27 30 31 32 33 34 35 36 37 38 40 41 43 44 45 47 49 50 53 54 55 56 57 58 59 60 62 64 66 68 71 72 73 74 76 77 79 80 81 82 86 87 88 89 90 91 92 93 94 95 96 97 99 100 102 103 105 106 107 115 118 119 120 121 123 124 130 133 135 136 137 **S** Catholic Health Initiatives
Primary Contact: James R. Pancoast, President and Chief Executive Officer
COO: Mark S. Shaker, Executive Vice President and Chief Operating Officer
CFO: Thomas Duncan, Vice President and Chief Financial Officer
CMO: Daniel L. Schoulties, M.D., Vice President Medical Affairs
CIO: Mikki Clancy, Vice President and Chief Information Officer
CHR: William Linesch, Vice President Human Resources
Web address: www.goodsamdayton.com
Control: Church–operated, Nongovernment, not–for profit **Service:** General Medical and Surgical

Staffed Beds: 353 **Admissions:** 19133 **Census:** 231 **Outpatient Visits:** 243591 **Births:** 1273 **Total Expense ($000):** 309278 **Payroll Expense ($000):** 132117 **Personnel:** 2687

★ ○ △ **GRANDVIEW HOSPITAL AND MEDICAL CENTER (360133)**, 405 Grand Avenue, Zip 45405–4796; tel. 937/226–3200, (Includes SOUTHVIEW HOSPITAL AND FAMILY HEALTH CENTER, 1997 Miamisburg–Centerville Road, Zip 45459–3800; tel. 937/439–6000; Gregory Henderson, Vice President Operations and Senior Executive Officer) **A**2 7 9 10 11 12 13 **F**3 4 5 8 11 12 13 15 17 18 20 22 24 25 26 27 28 30 31 32 33 34 35 36 37 38 39 41 42 43 47 48 49 50 52 53 55 56 57 58 59 60 61 62 63 64 66 68 70 71 72 73 74 75 76 77 78 79 80 81 82 84 85 86 87 88 90 91 92 93 94 95 96 97 100 102 103 106 107 118 119 120 121 124 130 133 134 135 136 137 **P**7 8 **S** Kettering Health Network
Primary Contact: Roy G. Chew, Ph.D., President
COO: Peter J. King, Senior Vice President and Chief Financial Officer
CFO: Peter J. King, Senior Vice President and Chief Financial Officer
CMO: Tom Hardy, D.O., Vice President Medical Affairs
Web address: www.kmcnetwork.org
Control: Church–operated, Nongovernment, not–for profit **Service:** General Medical and Surgical

Staffed Beds: 318 **Admissions:** 13285 **Census:** 174 **Outpatient Visits:** 234156 **Births:** 1988 **Total Expense ($000):** 218873 **Payroll Expense ($000):** 92053 **Personnel:** 1701

KETTERING YOUTH SERVICES See Kettering Medical Center–Sycamore, Miamisburg

□ **KINDRED HOSPITAL–DAYTON (362033)**, One Elizabeth Place, 5th Floor, Zip 45408; tel. 937/222–5963, (Nonreporting) **A**1 9 10
Primary Contact: Christina Stover, Chief Executive Officer
CMO: Felipe Rubio, M.D., Medical Director
Web address: www.khdayton.com
Control: Corporation, Investor–owned, for–profit **Service:** Long–Term Acute Care hospital

Staffed Beds: 67

★□ △ **MIAMI VALLEY HOSPITAL (360051)**, One Wyoming Street, Zip 45409–2793; tel. 937/208–8000 **A**1 2 3 5 7 8 9 10 **F**2 3 5 12 13 15 16 17 18 20 22 24 25 26 27 30 31 32 33 35 36 37 38 39 40 41 43 44 46 47 48 49 50 52 53 54 55 56 57 58 59 60 62 64 65 66 68 70 72 73 74 76 77 78 79 80 81 82 85 86 88 90 91 92 93 94 95 96 97 99 100 101 102 103 104 105 106 107 114 116 118 119 120 121 122 123 124 125 127 130 132 135 136 137 **P**6
Primary Contact: Mary H. Boosalis, President and Chief Executive Officer
COO: Bobbie Gerhart, Executive Vice President and Chief Operating Officer
CFO: Scott Shelton, Executive Vice President and Chief Financial Officer
CMO: Gary Collier, M.D., Vice President Medical Affairs and Chief Medical Officer
CIO: Mikki Clancy, Vice President and Chief Information Officer
CHR: William Linesch, Vice President Human Resources
Web address: www.miamivalleyhospital.org
Control: Other not–for–profit (including NFP Corporation) **Service:** General Medical and Surgical

Staffed Beds: 712 **Admissions:** 32369 **Census:** 525 **Outpatient Visits:** 392197 **Births:** 5108 **Total Expense ($000):** 588570 **Payroll Expense ($000):** 254264 **Personnel:** 5047

SOUTHVIEW HOSPITAL AND FAMILY HEALTH CENTER See Grandview Hospital and Medical Center

★□ **VETERANS AFFAIRS MEDICAL CENTER**, 4100 West Third Street, Zip 45428–1002; tel. 937/268–6511, (Total facility includes 265 beds in nursing home–type unit) (Nonreporting) **A**1 2 3 5 8 **S** Department of Veterans Affairs
Primary Contact: Guy B. Richardson, Director
COO: Terry Taylor, Associate Director
CFO: Lawrence Andrews, Chief Fiscal Services
CMO: Steven M. Cohen, M.D., Chief of Staff
CIO: Susan Sherer, Chief Information Resource Management
CHR: Theresa Webb, Chief Human Resources Management Service
Web address: www.va.gov/sta/guide/home.asp
Control: Veterans Affairs, Government, federal **Service:** General Medical and Surgical

Staffed Beds: 500

DEFIANCE—Defiance County

★□ **DEFIANCE REGIONAL MEDICAL CENTER (361328)**, 1200 Ralston Avenue, Zip 43512–1396; tel. 419/783–6955 **A**1 5 9 10 18 **F**3 11 13 15 18 24 27 28 30 31 32 38 40 55 56 57 62 66 68 73 74 75 76 77 79 80 81 82 86 88 90 91 92 93 94 95 96 97 100 102 106 107 118 119 121 124 133 135 136 **S** ProMedica Health System
Primary Contact: Timothy Jakacki, President and Chief Executive Officer
CFO: Bernie Nawrocki, Vice President Finance
CMO: Kermit Erwin, M.D., Medical Director
CIO: Kevin Wietrzykowski, Director Information Management Systems
CHR: Linda Shaffer, Director Human Resources
Web address: www.promedica.org
Control: Other not–for–profit (including NFP Corporation) **Service:** General Medical and Surgical

Staffed Beds: 35 **Admissions:** 2500 **Census:** 20 **Outpatient Visits:** 16300 **Births:** 680 **Total Expense ($000):** 39489 **Payroll Expense ($000):** 12461 **Personnel:** 235

★□ **MERCY HOSPITAL OF DEFIANCE (360270)**, 1404 East Second Street, Zip 43512; tel. 419/782–8444 **A**1 9 10 **F**3 8 25 26 30 31 32 38 43 46 55 56 62 63 66 72 73 77 79 80 82 87 124 **P**8 **S** Catholic Healthcare Partners
Primary Contact: William A. Sutton, Administrator
CFO: Samantha M. Platzke, Senior Vice President Finance and Chief Financial Officer
CMO: John Racciato, M.D., Chief of Staff
CIO: James Albin, Regional Vice President and Chief Information Officer
CHR: Marilyn Reineke, Director Human Resources
Web address: www.ehealthconnection.com/regions/toledo/
Control: Partnership, Investor–owned, for–profit **Service:** General Medical and Surgical

Staffed Beds: 23 **Admissions:** 1361 **Census:** 13 **Outpatient Visits:** 10212 **Births:** 0 **Personnel:** 102

DELAWARE—Delaware County

★□ △ **GRADY MEMORIAL HOSPITAL (360210)**, 561 West Central Avenue, Zip 43015–1485; tel. 740/369–8711 **A**1 2 5 7 9 10 **F**3 13 15 18 24 25 26 27 30 31 32 33 38 42 55 56 57 58 61 62 64 66 68 72 73 74 75 76 77 79 81 86 96 99 100 102 106 107 112 118 119 120 121 124 135 136 **P**3 7 **S** OhioHealth
Primary Contact: Steven J. Garlock, President
CFO: Eric Draime, Director Finance
CMO: Thomas Hubbell, M.D., Chief of Staff
CHR: Beth Crow, Associate Relations Representative
Web address: www.ohiohealth.com
Control: Church–operated, Nongovernment, not–for profit **Service:** General Medical and Surgical

Staffed Beds: 61 **Admissions:** 2700 **Census:** 23 **Outpatient Visits:** 187756 **Births:** 407 **Total Expense ($000):** 61346 **Payroll Expense ($000):** 25853 **Personnel:** 453

DENNISON—Tuscarawas County

★□ **TWIN CITY HOSPITAL (361302)**, 819 North First Street, Zip 44621–1098; tel. 740/922–2800, (Nonreporting) **A**1 9 10 18
Primary Contact: Marge Jentes, Chief Executive Officer
CFO: Halli Sell, Director Accounting
CMO: Galen Durose, M.D., Chief of Staff
CHR: Dawn Furniss, Director Human Resources
Web address: www.twincityhospital.org
Control: Other not–for–profit (including NFP Corporation) **Service:** General Medical and Surgical

Staffed Beds: 25

DOVER—Tuscarawas County

★□ **UNION HOSPITAL (360010)**, 659 Boulevard, Zip 44622–2077; tel. 330/343–3311 **A**1 9 10 19 **F**3 8 11 13 14 15 24 25 30 31 32 33 38 43 50 52 55 56 57 61 62 68 73 74 75 76 77 78 79 80 81 84 86 96 97 99 106 107 118 119 120 121 135 137 **P**8
Primary Contact: William W. Harding, President and Chief Executive Officer
CFO: Eugene A. Thorn, Vice President Finance and Chief Financial Officer
CMO: Thomas J. Kelly, M.P.H., D.O., Vice President Medical Affairs
CIO: David Baumgardner, Director Information Management
CHR: Darwin K. Smith, Vice President Human Resources
Web address: www.unionhospital.org
Control: Other not–for–profit (including NFP Corporation) **Service:** General Medical and Surgical

Staffed Beds: 144 **Admissions:** 6809 **Census:** 74 **Outpatient Visits:** 290506 **Births:** 760 **Total Expense ($000):** 93855 **Payroll Expense ($000):** 37973 **Personnel:** 857

Hospital, Medicare Provider Number, Address, Telephone, Approval, Facility, and Physician Codes, Health Care System
★ American Hospital Association (AHA) membership
□ The Joint Commission accreditation
○ American Osteopathic Association (AOA) accreditation
△ Commission on Accreditation of Rehabilitation Facilities (CARF) accreditation

OH

EAST LIVERPOOL—Columbiana County

★ **EAST LIVERPOOL CITY HOSPITAL (360096)**, 425 West Fifth Street, Zip 43920–2498; tel. 330/385–7200, (Total facility includes 20 beds in nursing home–type unit) **A**1 9 10 **F**3 11 13 15 18 24 25 26 27 28 30 31 32 33 37 38 41 46 49 50 51 52 55 56 57 59 61 62 68 72 73 74 75 76 77 79 80 81 82 84 86 87 96 97 100 103 106 107 117 119 121 124 135 137 **P**1
Primary Contact: Melvin R. Creeley, President
CFO: Michael H. Winiarski, Vice President Finance
CMO: Vern Orlang, M.D., Medical Director
CIO: Frank Mader, Director Information Services
CHR: Pam Amos, Director Human Resources
Web address: www.elch.org
Control: Other not–for–profit (including NFP Corporation) **Service:** General Medical and Surgical

Staffed Beds: 158 **Admissions:** 6566 **Census:** 80 **Outpatient Visits:** 101856 **Births:** 220 **Total Expense ($000):** 54668 **Payroll Expense ($000):** 22762 **Personnel:** 535

ELYRIA—Lorain County

★ **EMH REGIONAL MEDICAL CENTER (360145)**, 630 East River Street, Zip 44035–5902; tel. 440/329–7500 **A**1 2 9 10 **F**3 11 12 13 15 17 18 20 22 24 25 26 30 32 33 38 39 43 50 52 55 56 57 61 62 68 71 72 73 74 75 76 77 79 80 81 82 84 86 88 96 97 100 102 106 107 118 119 120 124 135 **P**6 7
Primary Contact: Kevin C. Martin, President and Chief Executive Officer
CFO: Dave Cook, Vice President and Chief Financial Officer
CMO: Donald Sheldon, M.D., Vice President Medical Affairs
CIO: Scott Smith, Director Information Systems
CHR: Daniel Miller, Vice President Human Resources
Web address: www.emh–healthcare.org
Control: Other not–for–profit (including NFP Corporation) **Service:** General Medical and Surgical

Staffed Beds: 285 **Admissions:** 13754 **Census:** 153 **Outpatient Visits:** 175330 **Births:** 1066 **Total Expense ($000):** 168164 **Payroll Expense ($000):** 65294 **Personnel:** 1302

EUCLID—Cuyahoga County

□ △ **EUCLID HOSPITAL (360082)**, 18901 Lake Shore Boulevard, Zip 44119–1090; tel. 216/531–9000, (Total facility includes 40 beds in nursing home–type unit) **A**1 2 7 9 10 **F**11 15 17 18 20 24 25 27 30 31 32 33 37 38 43 46 47 49 54 57 68 72 73 75 76 77 79 85 88 93 94 95 100 107 117 119 120 135 137 **S** Cleveland Clinic Health System
Primary Contact: Robert Stall, President
CFO: Shirley Lawson, Manager Finance
CHR: Gloria Donnelly, Director Human Resources
Web address: www.euclidhospital.org
Control: Other not–for–profit (including NFP Corporation) **Service:** General Medical and Surgical

Staffed Beds: 190 **Admissions:** 8505 **Census:** 150 **Outpatient Visits:** 81169 **Total Expense ($000):** 90008 **Payroll Expense ($000):** 41989 **Personnel:** 886

FAIRFIELD—Butler County

★ **MERCY HOSPITAL FAIRFIELD (360056)**, 3000 Mack Road, Zip 45014; tel. 513/870–7000 **A**1 2 9 10 **F**3 8 11 13 15 17 22 24 25 26 27 30 31 32 33 38 41 43 44 46 49 50 53 55 56 57 62 63 66 68 71 72 73 74 75 76 77 79 80 82 86 96 97 99 100 102 103 106 107 119 121 124 135 136 137 **S** Catholic Healthcare Partners
Primary Contact: Thomas S. Urban, President and Chief Executive Officer
COO: Roland Cruickshank, Vice President Operations
CMO: Leonard M. Randolph, M.D., Chief Medical Officer
CIO: Yousuf Ahmad, Regional Vice President Information Services
CHR: Christine Browning, Regional Vice President Human Resources
Web address: www.e–mercy.com
Control: Church–operated, Nongovernment, not–for profit **Service:** General Medical and Surgical

Staffed Beds: 207 **Admissions:** 11707 **Census:** 148 **Outpatient Visits:** 61782 **Births:** 2130 **Total Expense ($000):** 154382 **Payroll Expense ($000):** 50145 **Personnel:** 1095

FINDLAY—Hancock County

★ **BLANCHARD VALLEY HEALTH SYSTEM (361322)**, 1900 South Main Street, Zip 45840; tel. 419/423–4500, (Includes BLANCHARD VALLEY HOSPITAL, John L. Bookmyer, Executive Vice President and Chief Operating Officer; BLUFFTON HOSPITAL, 139 Garau Street, Bluffton, Zip 45817–0048; tel. 419/358–9010; William Watkins, Chief Administrative Officer) **A**1 2 5 9 10 18 19 **F**3 11 12 13 15 17 18 20 22 24 25 26 27 30 31 32 33 38 40 43 44 46 48 49 54 56 57 59 62 68 70 72 74 75 76 77 79 80 81 82 86 87 88 93 96 97 100 102 104 105 106 107 108 112 118 119 120 121 123 124 135 136 137 **P**5
Primary Contact: Scott C. Malaney, President and Chief Executive Officer
COO: John L. Bookmyer, Executive Vice President and Chief Operating Officer
CFO: John L. Bookmyer, Executive Vice President and Chief Operating Officer
CMO: Bill Kose, M.D., Senior Vice President Medical Affairs
CIO: Annette Elchert, Director Information Services
CHR: Doug DeFrain, Director Human Resources
Web address: www.bvhealthsystem.org
Control: Other not–for–profit (including NFP Corporation) **Service:** General Medical and Surgical

Staffed Beds: 174 **Admissions:** 9067 **Census:** 87 **Outpatient Visits:** 238344 **Births:** 1402 **Total Expense ($000):** 159064 **Payroll Expense ($000):** 65892 **Personnel:** 1222

FOSTORIA—Hancock County

★ **FOSTORIA COMMUNITY HOSPITAL (361318)**, 501 Van Buren Street, Zip 44830–0907, Mailing Address: P.O. Box 907, Zip 44830–0907; tel. 419/435–7734 **A**1 5 9 10 18 **F**3 11 13 15 24 27 28 30 31 32 33 38 42 55 56 57 59 61 62 64 66 67 68 73 74 75 76 77 79 80 81 84 86 87 96 97 99 100 103 106 107 117 118 119 120 121 122 124 132 135 **P**7 **S** ProMedica Health System
Primary Contact: Timothy Jakacki, President and Chief Executive Officer
COO: Dan Schwanke, Senior Vice President Operations
CFO: Ken Swint, Vice President Finance and Chief Financial Officer
CMO: Terrence Fondessy, M.D., Vice President Medical Affairs
CIO: David G. Selman, Corporate Vice President Information Resources
CHR: Charles McDowell, Corporate Vice President Human Resources
Web address: www.promedica.org
Control: Other not–for–profit (including NFP Corporation) **Service:** General Medical and Surgical

Staffed Beds: 25 **Admissions:** 1244 **Census:** 11 **Outpatient Visits:** 50546 **Births:** 187 **Total Expense ($000):** 33204 **Payroll Expense ($000):** 10966 **Personnel:** 229

FRANKLIN—Warren County

□ **ATRIUM MEDICAL CENTER (360076)**, (Formerly Middletown Regional Hospital), One Medical Center Drive, Zip 45005–1066; tel. 513/424–2111 **A**1 10 **F**3 6 10 11 12 13 15 17 18 24 25 26 27 28 30 31 32 33 35 38 40 42 43 46 49 50 51 53 54 55 56 57 59 61 62 63 64 66 67 68 72 73 74 75 76 77 79 80 81 82 85 86 88 89 90 91 92 93 94 95 96 97 100 102 105 106 107 112 116 119 120 121 124 133 135 136 **P**8
Primary Contact: Douglas W. McNeill, FACHE, President and Chief Executive Officer
COO: Carol Turner, Chief Operating Officer and Executive Vice President
CFO: Tom Maloney, Chief Financial Officer
CHR: Ted Ripperger, Administrative Director Human Resources
Web address: www.atriummedcenter.org
Control: Other not–for–profit (including NFP Corporation) **Service:** General Medical and Surgical

Staffed Beds: 200 **Admissions:** 11293 **Census:** 141 **Outpatient Visits:** 252535 **Births:** 984 **Total Expense ($000):** 181418 **Payroll Expense ($000):** 71065 **Personnel:** 1272

FREMONT—Sandusky County

★ **MEMORIAL HOSPITAL (360156)**, 715 South Taft Avenue, Zip 43420–3200; tel. 419/332–7321 **A**1 2 5 9 10 **F**3 8 11 13 14 15 24 25 26 28 30 31 32 33 36 38 42 43 44 45 46 49 51 54 55 56 57 61 62 63 66 67 68 72 73 74 75 76 77 78 79 80 81 82 84 86 89 90 94 96 97 100 103 106 107 112 118 119 121 123 124 132 135 136 137 **P**1 5 **S** QHR
Primary Contact: John A. Gorman, Chief Executive Officer
COO: Sandra J. Foster, Chief Operating Officer
CFO: Rick Ruppel, Chief Financial Officer
CIO: John Allen, Chief Information Officer
Web address: www.fremontmemorial.org
Control: Other not–for–profit (including NFP Corporation) **Service:** General Medical and Surgical

Staffed Beds: 102 **Admissions:** 2853 **Census:** 26 **Outpatient Visits:** 91336 **Births:** 443 **Total Expense ($000):** 57525 **Payroll Expense ($000):** 21811 **Personnel:** 482

Many Facility Codes have changed. Please refer to the AHA Guide Code Chart.

GALION—Crawford County

★ **GALION COMMUNITY HOSPITAL (361325)**, 269 Portland Way South, Zip 44833–2399; tel. 419/468–4841, (Total facility includes 33 beds in nursing home–type unit) (Nonreporting) **A**1 9 10 18
Primary Contact: LaMar L. Wyse, President and Chief Executive Officer
CFO: Robert V. Melaragno, Vice President and Chief Financial Officer
CHR: Traci Oswald, Vice President Human Resources
Web address: www.galionhospital.org
Control: Other not–for–profit (including NFP Corporation) **Service:** General Medical and Surgical

Staffed Beds: 68

GALLIPOLIS—Gallia County

☐ △ **HOLZER MEDICAL CENTER (360054)**, 100 Jackson Pike, Zip 45631–1563; tel. 740/446–5000 **A**1 2 5 7 9 10 19 **F**3 12 13 17 20 22 25 26 27 28 30 32 33 38 42 49 52 55 56 57 59 61 62 68 74 75 76 77 79 80 82 84 85 86 96 97 102 103 105 106 107 119 121 124 135 137 **P**6
Primary Contact: James R. Phillipe, President
CFO: Kevin Yeager, Vice President Fiscal Services
CMO: Jamal Haddad, D.O., President Medical Staff
CIO: Kevin Yeager, Vice President Fiscal Services
CHR: Lisa Halley, Vice President Human Resources
Web address: www.holzer.org
Control: Other not–for–profit (including NFP Corporation) **Service:** General Medical and Surgical

Staffed Beds: 181 **Admissions:** 8140 **Census:** 93 **Outpatient Visits:** 57246 **Births:** 807 **Total Expense ($000):** 100748 **Payroll Expense ($000):** 35975 **Personnel:** 948

GARFIELD HEIGHTS—Cuyahoga County

☐ △ **MARYMOUNT HOSPITAL (360143)**, 12300 McCracken Road, Zip 44125–2975; tel. 216/581–0500, (Total facility includes 1 beds in nursing home–type unit) **A**1 2 7 9 10 **F**3 8 11 13 15 18 24 25 26 27 30 31 32 33 36 37 38 39 41 42 43 46 47 48 49 50 51 52 53 54 55 56 57 58 59 60 62 63 66 67 68 72 73 74 75 76 77 79 80 81 82 86 87 88 89 90 91 92 93 94 95 96 97 100 102 104 105 106 107 112 118 119 120 121 124 132 133 135 136 137 **S** Cleveland Clinic Health System
Primary Contact: David J. Kilarski, President and Chief Executive Officer
COO: William D. Keckan, Chief Operating Officer
CMO: George V. Topalsky, M.D., Vice President Medical Affairs
CIO: Ralph A. Cagna, Director Information Technology
CHR: Christina Webb, Director Human Resources
Web address: www.marymount.org
Control: Other not–for–profit (including NFP Corporation) **Service:** General Medical and Surgical

Staffed Beds: 282 **Admissions:** 13861 **Census:** 194 **Outpatient Visits:** 140806 **Births:** 898 **Total Expense ($000):** 151235 **Payroll Expense ($000):** 68742 **Personnel:** 1437

GENEVA—Ashtabula County

★ **UNIVERSITY HOSPITALS GENEVA MEDICAL CENTER (361307)**, 870 West Main Street, Zip 44041–1295; tel. 440/466–1141 **A**1 9 10 18 **F**3 7 11 15 25 30 31 32 33 38 43 46 51 55 56 57 62 66 68 73 75 79 81 82 86 96 100 104 118 119 121 122 124 132 135 **S** University Hospitals
Primary Contact: Laurie Delgado, President and Chief Executive Officer
COO: Laurie Delgado, President and Chief Executive Officer
CFO: Rob David, Director Finance Services
Web address: www.uhhs.com
Control: Other not–for–profit (including NFP Corporation) **Service:** General Medical and Surgical

Staffed Beds: 25 **Admissions:** 1499 **Census:** 16 **Outpatient Visits:** 193146 **Births:** 0 **Total Expense ($000):** 28970 **Payroll Expense ($000):** 11099 **Personnel:** 200

GEORGETOWN—Brown County

★ **BROWN COUNTY GENERAL HOSPITAL (360116)**, 425 Home Street, Zip 45121–1407; tel. 937/378–7500 **A**1 9 10 **F**8 11 13 15 24 25 27 30 31 32 38 43 55 57 61 62 68 71 73 74 75 76 77 79 81 82 84 85 86 87 96 97 98 100 101 102 104 106 107 108 109 118 119 120 133 135 **P**6
Primary Contact: Michael C. Patterson, Chief Executive Officer
CHR: Matt Hess, Director Human Resources
Web address: www.browncountygeneralhospital.org
Control: County–Government, nonfederal **Service:** General Medical and Surgical

Staffed Beds: 59 **Admissions:** 2289 **Census:** 15 **Outpatient Visits:** 62315 **Births:** 452 **Total Expense ($000):** 35790 **Payroll Expense ($000):** 16624 **Personnel:** 396

GREEN SPRINGS—Sandusky County

★ **ST. FRANCIS HEALTH CARE CENTRE (362007)**, 401 North Broadway, Zip 44836–9653; tel. 419/639–2626, (Total facility includes 150 beds in nursing home–type unit) (Nonreporting) **A**1 9 10 **S** Vibra Healthcare
Primary Contact: Kim D. Eicher, Chief Executive Officer
CFO: Douglas Morris, Chief Financial Officer
CMO: John Yuhas, D.O., Medical Director
CHR: Joan E. Schmidt, Director Human Resources
Web address: www.sfhcc.org
Control: Church–operated, Nongovernment, not–for profit **Service:** General Medical and Surgical

Staffed Beds: 186

GREENFIELD—Highland County

☐ △ **GREENFIELD AREA MEDICAL CENTER (361304)**, 550 Mirabeau Street, Zip 45123–1617; tel. 937/981–9400 **A**1 7 9 10 18 **F**3 15 30 38 75 79 82 86 87 96 107 117 119 122 137
Primary Contact: Daniel J. Schaetzle, Administrator
COO: Jeff Graham, Chief Operating Officer
CFO: Ralph W. Sorrell, Chief Financial Officer
CIO: Marcus Bost, Director Information Services and Chief Information Officer
CHR: Brandt Lippert, Vice President Human Resources
Web address: www.adena.org
Control: Other not–for–profit (including NFP Corporation) **Service:** General Medical and Surgical

Staffed Beds: 25 **Admissions:** 707 **Census:** 12 **Outpatient Visits:** 32999 **Births:** 0 **Total Expense ($000):** 9042 **Payroll Expense ($000):** 4800 **Personnel:** 105

GREENVILLE—Darke County

★ **WAYNE HOSPITAL (360044)**, 835 Sweitzer Street, Zip 45331–1077; tel. 937/548–1141 **A**1 9 10 **F**3 8 11 13 15 25 26 30 31 32 33 37 38 42 44 54 55 56 57 62 66 67 68 73 74 75 76 77 79 81 82 84 86 96 97 100 102 106 107 118 119 121 122 124 135 137 **P**1
Primary Contact: Wayne G. Deschambeau, President and Chief Executive Officer
CFO: Marvella Fletcher, Vice President Fiscal Services
CMO: M. Lynn Hawley, M.D., President Medical Staff
CHR: Jim Stamcoff, Vice President Human Resources
Web address: www.waynehospital.com
Control: Other not–for–profit (including NFP Corporation) **Service:** General Medical and Surgical

Staffed Beds: 73 **Admissions:** 2715 **Census:** 25 **Outpatient Visits:** 101114 **Births:** 367 **Total Expense ($000):** 41560 **Payroll Expense ($000):** 18111 **Personnel:** 367

GROVEPORT—Franklin County

☐ **BARIX CLINICS OF OHIO (360258)**, 3964 Hamilton Square Boulevard, Zip 43125–9119; tel. 614/834–6800, (Nonreporting) **A**1 10
Primary Contact: David Globig, President
Web address: www.barixclinics.com/contact_us/ohio.jsp
Control: Individual, Investor–owned, for–profit **Service:** Surgical

Staffed Beds: 24

HAMILTON—Butler County

☐ **BUTLER COUNTY MEDICAL CENTER (360269)**, 3125 Hamilton Mason Road, Zip 45011; tel. 513/894–8888, (Nonreporting) **A**1 9
Primary Contact: Ajay Mangal, M.D., Chief Executive Officer
COO: Mary Ann Gellenbeck, Chief Operating Officer
CFO: Michael L. Griffin, Chief Financial Officer
CHR: Amy Turner, Director Human Resources
Web address: www.bcsurg.com
Control: Corporation, Investor–owned, for–profit **Service:** Surgical

Staffed Beds: 8

★ **FORT HAMILTON HOSPITAL (360132)**, 630 Eaton Avenue, Zip 45013–2770; tel. 513/867–2000 **A**1 2 9 10 **F**3 11 13 15 18 24 25 26 27 28 30 31 32 33 38 41 42 43 47 49 50 52 53 54 55 56 57 58 62 66 68 71 72 73 74 76 77 79 80 81 82 84 85 86 88 90 92 93 95 96 97 100 102 103 107 116 118 119 120 121 123 124 135 136 137 **S** Health Alliance of Greater Cincinnati
Primary Contact: Lynn M. Oswald, FACHE, Senior Vice President
CFO: Leslie Snyder, Director Finance
CHR: Joseph Geigle, Director Human Resources
Web address: www.forthamiltonhospital.com
Control: Other not–for–profit (including NFP Corporation) **Service:** General Medical and Surgical

Staffed Beds: 185 **Admissions:** 9189 **Census:** 117 **Outpatient Visits:** 112243 **Births:** 1146 **Total Expense ($000):** 95397 **Payroll Expense ($000):** 41443 **Personnel:** 891

Hospital, Medicare Provider Number, Address, Telephone, Approval, Facility, and Physician Codes, Health Care System

★ American Hospital Association (AHA) membership
☐ The Joint Commission accreditation
○ American Osteopathic Association (AOA) accreditation
△ Commission on Accreditation of Rehabilitation Facilities (CARF) accreditation

HICKSVILLE—Defiance County

☒ **COMMUNITY MEMORIAL HOSPITAL (361301)**, 208 North Columbus Street, Zip 43526–1299; tel. 419/542–6692 **A**1 9 10 18 **F**3 8 11 13 15 24 25 26 30 31 33 35 38 43 52 55 56 57 64 66 74 75 77 79 80 82 84 86 87 96 107 118 119 120 122 132 133 135 **P**6
Primary Contact: Melvin H. Fahs, Chief Executive Officer
COO: Michelle Waggoner, Chief Operating Officer
CFO: Sharon McGowan, Chief Financial Officer
CIO: Pete Rife, Chief Information Officer
CHR: Pam Franklin, Director Administrative Services
Web address: www.cmhosp.com
Control: Hospital district or authority, Government, nonfederal **Service:** General Medical and Surgical

Staffed Beds: 25 **Admissions:** 637 **Census:** 7 **Outpatient Visits:** 23180 **Births:** 96 **Total Expense ($000):** 15629 **Payroll Expense ($000):** 6017 **Personnel:** 161

HILLSBORO—Highland County

☒ **HIGHLAND DISTRICT HOSPITAL (361332)**, 1275 North High Street, Zip 45133–8571; tel. 937/393–6100 **A**1 9 10 18 **F**3 11 13 15 25 26 27 30 31 32 33 38 47 49 55 56 57 61 62 66 72 74 75 76 77 79 80 81 82 86 88 93 96 100 107 119 120 121 124 135 137 **P**3
Primary Contact: Paula J. Detterman, President and Chief Executive Officer
CFO: Thomas Degen, Chief Financial Officer
CMO: Ramesh Shivani, M.D., Chief of Staff
CIO: Steve Lemaster, Director Information Technology
Web address: www.hdh.org
Control: Hospital district or authority, Government, nonfederal **Service:** General Medical and Surgical

Staffed Beds: 25 **Admissions:** 2112 **Census:** 21 **Outpatient Visits:** 86082 **Births:** 361 **Total Expense ($000):** 34374 **Payroll Expense ($000):** 15707 **Personnel:** 339

JACKSON—Jackson County

☐ **HOLZER MEDICAL CENTER – JACKSON (361320)**, 500 Burlington Road, Zip 45640–9360; tel. 740/395–8500, (Nonreporting) **A**1 9 10 18
Primary Contact: Ross A. Matlack, FACHE, President and Chief Executive Officer
CFO: Kevin Yeager, Vice President Fiscal Services
CMO: Nimal Dutla, M.D., Chief Medical Staff
CHR: Sandy Carlisle, Manager Human Resources
Web address: www.holzer.org
Control: Other not–for–profit (including NFP Corporation) **Service:** General Medical and Surgical

Staffed Beds: 24

KENTON—Hardin County

☒ **HARDIN MEMORIAL HOSPITAL (361315)**, 921 East Franklin Street, Zip 43326–2099, Mailing Address: P.O. Box 710, Zip 43326–0710; tel. 419/673–0761 **A**1 9 10 18 **F**11 15 25 26 30 31 32 38 55 56 57 60 73 75 76 77 79 81 82 86 87 92 96 97 99 100 102 104 107 118 119 120 121 122 135 136 **S** OhioHealth
Primary Contact: Mark R. Seckinger, Administrator and Chief Executive Officer
CFO: Ron Snyder, Chief Financial Officer
Web address: www.hardinmemorial.org
Control: Other not–for–profit (including NFP Corporation) **Service:** General Medical and Surgical

Staffed Beds: 25 **Admissions:** 1204 **Census:** 13 **Outpatient Visits:** 56638 **Births:** 0 **Total Expense ($000):** 18312 **Payroll Expense ($000):** 8641 **Personnel:** 210

KETTERING—Montgomery County

☒ △ **CHARLES F. KETTERING MEMORIAL HOSPITAL (360079)**, 3535 Southern Boulevard, Zip 45429; tel. 937/298–4331, (Total facility includes 100 beds in nursing home–type unit) **A**1 2 3 5 7 8 10 **F**3 4 5 6 8 10 11 12 13 15 17 18 20 22 24 25 26 27 28 30 31 32 33 34 35 36 37 38 41 42 43 47 48 49 50 51 52 53 54 55 56 57 58 59 60 61 62 63 64 65 66 68 69 70 71 72 73 74 75 76 77 78 79 80 81 82 84 85 86 87 88 89 90 91 92 93 94 96 97 99 100 102 103 104 105 106 107 108 109 111 112 113 115 116 117 118 119 120 121 123 124 130 132 134 135 136 137 **P**7 8 **S** Kettering Health Network
Primary Contact: Fred M. Manchur, President
CMO: Gregory Wise, M.D., Vice President Medical Affairs
CHR: Beverly Morris, Vice President Human Resources
Web address: www.kmcnetwork.org
Control: Church–operated, Nongovernment, not–for profit **Service:** General Medical and Surgical

Staffed Beds: 507 **Admissions:** 24126 **Census:** 339 **Outpatient Visits:** 224164 **Births:** 2386 **Total Expense ($000):** 354072 **Payroll Expense ($000):** 150330 **Personnel:** 1149

LAKEWOOD—Cuyahoga County

☐ △ **LAKEWOOD HOSPITAL (360212)**, 14519 Detroit Avenue, Zip 44107–4383; tel. 216/521–4200, (Total facility includes 45 beds in nursing home–type unit) **A**1 2 7 9 10 **F**2 8 13 15 17 18 20 22 25 26 28 30 31 32 33 38 39 40 46 49 51 53 54 55 56 57 58 59 60 61 62 63 66 67 68 72 73 74 75 77 79 81 82 84 85 86 87 88 89 90 91 92 93 94 95 96 97 100 106 107 117 119 121 123 124 133 135 136 **S** Cleveland Clinic Health System
Primary Contact: Jack D. Gustin, President
COO: William Baddour, Chief Operating Officer
CFO: Jeff Dyibec, Director Finance
CMO: A. Mary Walborn, M.D., Vice President Medical Operations
CIO: Pam Piar, Chief Information Officer
CHR: Suzanne Rogachuk, Director Human Resources
Web address: www.lakewoodhospital.org
Control: Other not–for–profit (including NFP Corporation) **Service:** General Medical and Surgical

Staffed Beds: 271 **Admissions:** 12328 **Census:** 179 **Outpatient Visits:** 184771 **Births:** 880 **Total Expense ($000):** 135697 **Payroll Expense ($000):** 64554 **Personnel:** 1200

LANCASTER—Fairfield County

☒ △ **FAIRFIELD MEDICAL CENTER (360072)**, 401 North Ewing Street, Zip 43130–3371; tel. 740/687–8000 **A**1 2 5 7 9 10 **F**3 8 9 11 13 15 18 20 22 24 25 26 30 31 32 33 34 36 38 41 43 44 45 47 48 49 50 52 53 55 56 57 61 62 68 72 73 74 75 76 77 79 80 82 84 86 87 88 92 94 96 97 100 102 103 106 107 119 120 121 124 134 135 136 137 **P**4
Primary Contact: Mina H. Ubbing, President and Chief Executive Officer
COO: Howard Sniderman, Vice President Professional and Support Services
CFO: Sky Gettys, Vice President Finance
CMO: Jerome J. Roche, Chief Medical Officer
CHR: Dominic Prunte, Director Human Resources
Web address: www.fmchealth.org
Control: Other not–for–profit (including NFP Corporation) **Service:** General Medical and Surgical

Staffed Beds: 222 **Admissions:** 11354 **Census:** 129 **Outpatient Visits:** 218441 **Births:** 1125 **Total Expense ($000):** 163831 **Payroll Expense ($000):** 70581 **Personnel:** 1428

LIMA—Allen County

☒ **INSTITUTE FOR ORTHOPAEDIC SURGERY (360263)**, 801 Medical Drive, Suite B., Zip 45804; tel. 419/224–7586, (Nonreporting) **A**1 9 10 **S** Catholic Healthcare Partners
Primary Contact: Mark McDonald, M.D., President
COO: Brian Smith, Executive Vice President and Chief Operating Officer
CFO: Jaime Welsch, Manager Accounts Payable and Finance
CMO: Mark McDonald, M.D., President
CHR: Pat Farmer, Coordinator Human Resources and Safety Officer
Web address: www.ioshospital.com
Control: Partnership, Investor–owned, for–profit **Service:** Orthopedic

Staffed Beds: 3

☒ △ **LIMA MEMORIAL HEALTH SYSTEM (360009)**, 1001 Bellefontaine Avenue, Zip 45804–2899; tel. 419/228–3335, (Total facility includes 17 beds in nursing home–type unit) **A**1 2 7 9 10 **F**3 11 13 14 15 17 18 20 22 24 25 26 27 30 31 32 33 38 40 43 44 46 47 49 50 53 55 56 57 58 59 61 62 63 66 67 68 72 73 75 76 77 78 79 80 81 85 86 96 97 99 100 103 106 107 108 109 114 117 118 119 120 121 135 136 137 **P**8
Primary Contact: Michael D. Swick, President and Chief Executive Officer
COO: Robert Armstrong, Senior Vice President and Chief Operating Officer
CFO: Eric Pohjala, Vice President and Chief Financial Officer
CMO: C. Lynn Thompson, M.D., Vice President Medical Affairs
CIO: Cheryl Homan, Administrative Director
CHR: Theresa Bowen, Administrative Director
Web address: www.limamemorial.org
Control: Other not–for–profit (including NFP Corporation) **Service:** General Medical and Surgical

Staffed Beds: 257 **Admissions:** 8850 **Census:** 117 **Outpatient Visits:** 231505 **Births:** 707 **Total Expense ($000):** 131999 **Payroll Expense ($000):** 53616 **Personnel:** 949

☐ **OAKWOOD CORRECTIONAL FACILITY**, 3200 North West Street, Zip 45801–2000; tel. 419/225–8052 **A**1 **F**25 26 30 32 54 55 56 57 60 66 73 81 82 88 89 90 91 92 93 94 95 119 121 124 132 135 136 **P**5
Primary Contact: Christopher Yanai, Warden and Chief Executive Officer
CFO: Thomas Ferry, Business Administrator
CHR: Glenda Turner, Director Personnel
Web address: www.drc.state.oh.us/public/ocf.htm
Control: State–Government, nonfederal **Service:** Psychiatric

Staffed Beds: 61 **Admissions:** 209 **Census:** 42 **Outpatient Visits:** 12 **Births:** 0 **Total Expense ($000):** 23361 **Payroll Expense ($000):** 19913 **Personnel:** 286

 Many Facility Codes have changed. Please refer to the AHA Guide Code Chart.

★ △ **ST. RITA'S MEDICAL CENTER (360066)**, 730 West Market Street, Zip 45801–4670; tel. 419/227–3361 **A**1 2 7 9 10 **F**3 4 5 9 11 13 15 17 18 20 22 24 25 26 27 28 30 31 32 33 34 37 38 39 40 42 43 44 46 49 50 52 53 54 55 56 57 58 59 60 61 62 64 66 68 70 71 72 73 74 76 77 79 80 81 82 84 85 86 87 88 90 91 93 96 97 99 100 102 103 104 105 106 107 108 109 117 118 119 120 121 124 133 135 136 137 **P**8 **S** Catholic Healthcare Partners
Primary Contact: James P. Reber, President and Chief Executive Officer
COO: Brian Smith, Executive Vice President and Chief Operating Officer
CFO: William Roe, Chief Financial Officer
CMO: Herbert Schumm, M.D., Vice President Medical Affairs
CHR: Will Cason, Vice President Human Resources
Web address: www.stritas.org
Control: Church–operated, Nongovernment, not–for profit **Service:** General Medical and Surgical

Staffed Beds: 413 **Admissions:** 19872 **Census:** 221 **Outpatient Visits:** 380192 **Births:** 1837 **Total Expense ($000):** 286646 **Payroll Expense ($000):** 116955 **Personnel:** 2571

★ **TRIUMPH HOSPITAL LIMA (362020)**, 730 West Market Street, 6th Floor, Zip 45801; tel. 419/224–1888 **A**1 9 10 **F**1 3 25 30 32 68 73 80 85 119 137 **P**5 **S** Triumph HealthCare
Primary Contact: Kimberly Thomas, Chief Executive Officer
Web address: www.triumph–healthcare.com
Control: Corporation, Investor–owned, for–profit **Service:** Long–Term Acute Care hospital

Staffed Beds: 26 **Admissions:** 276 **Census:** 19 **Outpatient Visits:** 0 **Births:** 0 **Total Expense ($000):** 9917 **Payroll Expense ($000):** 3234 **Personnel:** 48

LODI—Medina County

☐ **LODI COMMUNITY HOSPITAL (361303)**, 225 Elyria Street, Zip 44254–1096; tel. 330/948–1222 **A**1 9 10 18 **F**3 11 15 25 26 30 31 32 33 38 43 56 57 62 67 73 75 77 79 86 87 96 103 107 118 119 121 122 135 **S** Akron General Health System
Primary Contact: Thomas Whelan, President
CFO: Cindy Dennison, Senior Director Fiscal and Support Services
CIO: Robb Baldauf, Coordinator Information Systems
CHR: Christine Harris, Coordinator Human Resources
Web address: www.lodihospital.com
Control: Other not–for–profit (including NFP Corporation) **Service:** General Medical and Surgical

Staffed Beds: 25 **Admissions:** 467 **Census:** 8 **Outpatient Visits:** 26377 **Births:** 1 **Total Expense ($000):** 13408 **Payroll Expense ($000):** 6030 **Personnel:** 104

LOGAN—Hocking County

★ **HOCKING VALLEY COMMUNITY HOSPITAL (361330)**, 601 State Route 664 North, Zip 43138–0966, Mailing Address: P.O. Box 966, Zip 43138–0966; tel. 740/380–8000, (Total facility includes 30 beds in nursing home–type unit) **A**1 9 10 18 **F**3 8 11 13 15 24 25 27 30 31 32 38 54 55 56 57 62 68 73 74 75 76 77 79 80 81 86 88 93 96 100 103 106 107 117 118 119 122 124 133 135 136 137 **P**1 3
Primary Contact: LeeAnn Lucas–Helber, President
CMO: Duane Mast, M.D., Medical Director
CHR: Robert Schmidt, Director Human Resources
Web address: www.hvch.org
Control: County–Government, nonfederal **Service:** General Medical and Surgical

Staffed Beds: 65 **Admissions:** 1639 **Census:** 41 **Outpatient Visits:** 58885 **Births:** 178 **Total Expense ($000):** 29754 **Payroll Expense ($000):** 12783 **Personnel:** 314

LONDON—Madison County

★ **MADISON COUNTY HOSPITAL (360189)**, 210 North Main Street, Zip 43140–1115; tel. 740/845–7000 **A**1 9 10 **F**11 13 15 24 25 27 30 31 32 33 36 38 42 43 44 52 53 55 56 57 61 62 68 73 74 75 76 77 79 80 81 82 85 86 96 97 100 102 106 107 117 118 119 120 121 124 133 135 136
Primary Contact: Fred L. Kolb, Chief Executive Officer
CFO: Michael Browning, Chief Financial Officer
CMO: Mitchell Spahn, M.D., Chief Medical Staff
CIO: Dennis Vogt, Director Information Technology
CHR: Becky Rozell, Director Human Resources
Web address: www.madisoncountyhospital.org
Control: Other not–for–profit (including NFP Corporation) **Service:** General Medical and Surgical

Staffed Beds: 75 **Admissions:** 1674 **Census:** 23 **Outpatient Visits:** 38198 **Births:** 271 **Total Expense ($000):** 31733 **Payroll Expense ($000):** 12653 **Personnel:** 243

LORAIN—Lorain County

★ △ **COMMUNITY HEALTH PARTNERS REGIONAL MEDICAL CENTER (360172)**, (Formerly Community Health Partners Hospital and Surgical Center), 3700 Kolbe Road, Zip 44053–1697; tel. 440/960–4000 **A**1 2 7 9 10 **F**3 8 13 15 18 20 22 24 25 26 27 30 31 32 33 34 35 37 38 41 42 43 44 50 52 53 54 55 56 57 61 62 63 64 66 68 71 72 73 74 75 76 77 79 80 81 82 84 85 86 87 88 89 90 91 92 93 95 96 97 98 100 102 107 108 109 111 118 119 120 121 124 132 135 136 137 **P**5 **S** Catholic Healthcare Partners
Primary Contact: Edwin M. Oley, President and Chief Executive Officer
CFO: Gary Wengerd, Vice President Finance and Chief Financial Officer
CMO: Donald Blanford, M.D., Chief Medical Officer
CHR: Sarah Nickell, Vice President Human Resources
Web address: www.community–health–partners.com
Control: Church–operated, Nongovernment, not–for profit **Service:** General Medical and Surgical

Staffed Beds: 291 **Admissions:** 14345 **Census:** 178 **Births:** 1115 **Total Expense ($000):** 168739 **Payroll Expense ($000):** 67339 **Personnel:** 1413

SPECIALTY HOSPITAL OF LORAIN See Amherst

MANSFIELD—Richland County

★ **MEDCENTRAL – MANSFIELD HOSPITAL (360118)**, 335 Glessner Avenue, Zip 44903–2265; tel. 419/526–8000, (Includes MANSFIELD HOSPITAL) **A**1 2 5 6 9 10 **F**3 17 31 32 68 74 79 84 85 88 **S** MedCentral Health System
Primary Contact: James E. Meyer, President and Chief Executive Officer
CMO: Terry Weston, M.D., Vice President Physician Services
CIO: Mike Mistretta, Vice President Information Systems and Chief Information Officer
CHR: Beth Hildreth, Vice President Human Resources
Web address: www.medcentral.org
Control: Other not–for–profit (including NFP Corporation) **Service:** General Medical and Surgical

Staffed Beds: 308 **Admissions:** 17774 **Census:** 219 **Outpatient Visits:** 360295 **Births:** 1408 **Total Expense ($000):** 243634 **Payroll Expense ($000):** 104595 **Personnel:** 2121

☐ **TRIUMPH HOSPITAL MANSFIELD (362021)**, 335 Glessner Avenue, 5th Floor, Zip 44903; tel. 419/526–0777, (Nonreporting) **A**1 10 **S** Triumph HealthCare
Primary Contact: Kimberly Thomas, Chief Executive Officer
Web address: www.triumph–healthcare.com
Control: Corporation, Investor–owned, for–profit **Service:** Long–Term Acute Care hospital

Staffed Beds: 17

MARIETTA—Washington County

★ △ **MARIETTA MEMORIAL HOSPITAL (360147)**, 401 Matthew Street, Zip 45750–1699; tel. 740/374–1400 **A**1 2 5 7 9 10 **F**3 4 5 8 11 13 14 15 18 24 25 26 27 30 31 32 33 38 42 43 44 49 51 52 53 54 55 56 57 61 62 66 68 72 73 74 75 76 77 78 79 80 81 82 84 85 86 88 90 91 92 93 95 96 97 100 102 104 106 107 109 111 112 118 119 121 135 136 137 **P**7 8
Primary Contact: Larry J. Unroe, President
COO: J. Scott Cantley, Senior Vice President and Chief Operating Officer
CFO: Orvie E. Fischer, Senior Vice President and Chief Financial Officer
CMO: Richard Cain, M.D., Chief of Staff
CIO: Charles Morgan, Director Information Technology
CHR: Dee Ann Gehlauf, Administrative Director Human Resources
Web address: www.mmhospital.org
Control: Other not–for–profit (including NFP Corporation) **Service:** General Medical and Surgical

Staffed Beds: 150 **Admissions:** 7855 **Census:** 92 **Outpatient Visits:** 40619 **Births:** 611 **Total Expense ($000):** 136080 **Payroll Expense ($000):** 55860 **Personnel:** 1035

★ ○ **SELBY GENERAL HOSPITAL (361319)**, 1106 Colegate Drive, Zip 45750–1323; tel. 740/568–2000 **A**9 10 11 18 **F**3 11 15 25 26 28 30 31 32 33 38 43 50 53 54 55 56 57 62 68 73 76 77 79 80 82 87 88 93 96 97 99 106 107 120 121 122 123 124 135 **P**6 **S** QHR
Primary Contact: Robert M. Peterson, Chief Executive Officer
CFO: Steven Hall, Chief Financial Officer
CMO: Deborah Harris, M.D., Chief of Staff
CHR: Cindy Hall, Coordinator Human Resources
Web address: www.selbygeneralhospital.com
Control: Other not–for–profit (including NFP Corporation) **Service:** General Medical and Surgical

Staffed Beds: 35 **Admissions:** 1316 **Census:** 18 **Outpatient Visits:** 27689 **Births:** 0 **Total Expense ($000):** 21524 **Payroll Expense ($000):** 8879 **Personnel:** 228

Hospital, Medicare Provider Number, Address, Telephone, Approval, Facility, and Physician Codes, Health Care System

★ American Hospital Association (AHA) membership
☐ The Joint Commission accreditation
○ American Osteopathic Association (AOA) accreditation
△ Commission on Accreditation of Rehabilitation Facilities (CARF) accreditation

MARION—Marion County

☒ △ **MARION GENERAL HOSPITAL (360011)**, 1000 McKinley Park Drive, Zip 43302–6397; tel. 740/383–8400 **A**1 2 5 7 9 10 19 **F**3 13 15 18 20 22 24 25 26 27 30 31 33 38 42 52 55 57 59 61 66 68 70 71 72 73 74 76 77 79 82 84 88 94 95 96 100 102 107 119 121 124 135 **S** OhioHealth
Primary Contact: Ronald J. Bachman, President and Chief Executive Officer
CFO: Jerry G. Feyh, Vice President Finance
CMO: Carol M. Solie, M.D., Vice President Medical Affairs
CIO: Chuck Tudor, Director Information Services
CHR: Debra K. Rapert, Director Human Resources
Web address: www.mariongeneral.com
Control: Other not–for–profit (including NFP Corporation) **Service:** General Medical and Surgical

Staffed Beds: 204 **Admissions:** 10676 **Census:** 105 **Outpatient Visits:** 82417 **Births:** 1053 **Total Expense ($000):** 114582 **Payroll Expense ($000):** 49051 **Personnel:** 938

MARTINS FERRY—Belmont County

☐ **EAST OHIO REGIONAL HOSPITAL (360080)**, 90 North Fourth Street, Zip 43935–1648; tel. 740/633–1100, (Total facility includes 94 beds in nursing home–type unit) **A**1 9 10 **F**3 11 13 15 18 24 25 27 30 31 32 33 38 40 41 50 52 55 56 57 61 62 66 68 72 73 74 75 77 79 80 82 86 96 97 103 106 107 118 119 120 121 124 133 135 137 **P**5 **S** Ohio Valley Health Services and Education Corporation
Primary Contact: Brian K. Felici, President and Chief Executive Officer
COO: Anne Hellstern, Associate Administrator and Chief Operating Officer
CFO: David T. Baranik, Senior Vice President and Chief Financial Officer
CIO: Robert Panichi, Chief Information Officer
CHR: James R. Stultz, Senior Vice President Human Resources
Web address: www.eorh–online.com
Control: Other not–for–profit (including NFP Corporation) **Service:** General Medical and Surgical

Staffed Beds: 172 **Admissions:** 5393 **Census:** 138 **Outpatient Visits:** 171051 **Births:** 477 **Total Expense ($000):** 67914 **Payroll Expense ($000):** 29557 **Personnel:** 731

MARYSVILLE—Union County

☐ **MEMORIAL HOSPITAL OF UNION COUNTY (360092)**, 500 London Avenue, Zip 43040–1594; tel. 937/644–6115 **A**1 5 9 10 **F**3 11 13 15 24 25 26 27 30 31 32 33 36 38 42 43 46 50 52 54 55 56 57 61 62 63 64 66 67 68 72 73 74 75 76 77 79 80 82 86 88 90 91 92 93 94 96 97 100 102 103 105 107 118 119 121 124 133 134 135 136 137 **P**6
Primary Contact: Olas A. Hubbs, III, FACHE, President and Chief Executive Officer
COO: Laurie A. Whittington, Chief Operating Officer
CFO: Jeffrey Ehlers, Vice President Finance and Information Services
CMO: Brian Seifferth, M.D., Chief of Staff
CIO: Carl Zani, Director Information Systems
CHR: Carman Wirtz, Vice President Human Resources
Web address: www.memorialhosp.org
Control: County–Government, nonfederal **Service:** General Medical and Surgical

Staffed Beds: 66 **Admissions:** 2711 **Census:** 23 **Outpatient Visits:** 125587 **Births:** 663 **Total Expense ($000):** 55014 **Payroll Expense ($000):** 23952 **Personnel:** 484

MASSILLON—Stark County

★ ○ △ **AFFINITY MEDICAL CENTER, DOCTORS CAMPUS (360151)**, 400 Austin Avenue N.W., Zip 44646–3554; tel. 330/837–7200, (Nonreporting) **A**7 9 10 11 12 13 **S** Community Health Systems, Inc.
Primary Contact: Ronald L. Bierman, Chief Executive Officer
CFO: Gay Huff, Interim Chief Financial Officer
CMO: Brian E. Wind, D.O., Chief of Staff
CIO: William J. Mars, Vice President and Chief Information Officer
CHR: Angie Boyle, Director Human Resources
Web address: www.drshospital.com
Control: Corporation, Investor–owned, for–profit **Service:** General Medical and Surgical

Staffed Beds: 166

★ △ **AFFINITY MEDICAL CENTER, MASSILLON CAMPUS (360100)**, 875 Eighth Street N.E., Zip 44646–8503, Mailing Address: P.O. Box 805, Zip 44648–8503; tel. 330/832–8761, (Total facility includes 16 beds in nursing home–type unit) (Nonreporting) **A**7 9 10 **S** Community Health Systems, Inc.
Primary Contact: Ronald L. Bierman, Chief Executive Officer
COO: Beverly Bokowitz, Chief Operating Officer
CFO: James Miltner, System Chief Financial Officer
CIO: Stacy Malcolm, Director Information Systems
Web address: www.mchosp.org
Control: Corporation, Investor–owned, for–profit **Service:** General Medical and Surgical

Staffed Beds: 128

☐ **HEARTLAND BEHAVIORAL HEALTHCARE (364031)**, 3000 Erie Street, Zip 44646–7993, Mailing Address: Box 540, Zip 44648–0540; tel. 330/833–3135, (Nonreporting) **A**1 5 9 10
Primary Contact: Helen L. Stevens, Chief Executive Officer
COO: Kelly D. Markins, Regional Operations Director
CFO: Patricia Eddleman, Fiscal Officer
CMO: Steven Thomson, M.D., Medical Director
CIO: Kevin Waller, Regional Director Management Information Systems
CHR: Michele Szantay, Administrator Human Resources
Web address: www.mh.state.oh.us/ibhs/bhos/hoh.html
Control: State–Government, nonfederal **Service:** Psychiatric

Staffed Beds: 184

MAUMEE—Lucas County

☐ **FOCUS HEALTHCARE OF OHIO (364036)**, 1725 Timber Line Road, Zip 43537–4015; tel. 419/891–9333, (Nonreporting) **A**1 9 10 **S** Horizon Health Corporation
Primary Contact: Gene Riegle, Chief Executive Officer
CFO: Tammy Bowen, Business Office Manager and Accounting
CMO: Nancy Carroll, M.D., Medical Director
CIO: Lynette Box, Director Medical Records
Web address: www.focushealthcare.com
Control: Corporation, Investor–owned, for–profit **Service:** Other specialty

Staffed Beds: 42

☒ **ST. LUKE'S HOSPITAL (360090)**, 5901 Monclova Road, Zip 43537–1899; tel. 419/893–5911 **A**1 2 3 5 9 10 **F**3 11 12 13 15 17 18 20 22 24 25 26 27 30 31 32 33 38 43 46 49 55 56 57 62 66 68 72 74 75 76 77 79 80 81 82 84 85 86 90 96 97 100 102 106 107 116 118 119 120 121 123 124 132 135 136 137 **P**8
Primary Contact: Daniel L. Wakeman, President and Chief Executive Officer
CFO: David M. Oppenlander, Vice President and Treasurer
CIO: Eric Perron, Director Computer Information Services
CHR: Debra A. Ball, Vice President Human Resources
Web address: www.stlukeshospital.com
Control: Other not–for–profit (including NFP Corporation) **Service:** General Medical and Surgical

Staffed Beds: 201 **Admissions:** 9657 **Census:** 109 **Outpatient Visits:** 170834 **Births:** 621 **Total Expense ($000):** 131879 **Payroll Expense ($000):** 54886

MEDINA—Medina County

☐ **MEDINA GENERAL HOSPITAL (360091)**, 1000 East Washington Street, Zip 44256–2170; tel. 330/725–1000, (Nonreporting) **A**1 2 5 9 10
Primary Contact: Gary D. Hallman, President and Chief Executive Officer
CFO: Timothy Buit, Vice President Finance
CMO: Kenneth Weiner, M.D., Vice President Medical Affairs
CHR: Ronald Robinson, Vice President Human Resources
Web address: www.medinahospital.org
Control: Other not–for–profit (including NFP Corporation) **Service:** General Medical and Surgical

Staffed Beds: 118

MIAMISBURG—Montgomery County

☒ **KETTERING MEDICAL CENTER–SYCAMORE (360239)**, 2150 Leiter Road, Zip 45342; tel. 937/866–0551, (Includes KETTERING YOUTH SERVICES, 5350 Lamme Road, Dayton, Zip 45439; tel. 513/299–9511) **A**1 9 10 **F**3 4 5 8 11 12 17 24 25 26 28 30 31 32 33 34 35 36 37 38 41 42 43 47 48 49 50 52 53 54 55 56 57 58 59 60 61 62 63 64 65 66 68 72 73 75 76 77 78 79 80 81 82 84 86 87 88 89 90 91 92 94 95 96 97 99 100 102 103 106 107 115 119 120 121 123 124 130 135 136 137 **P**7 8 **S** Kettering Health Network
Primary Contact: Richard Haas, Senior Executive Officer
COO: Richard Haas, Senior Executive Officer
CMO: Gregory Wise, M.D., Vice President Medical Affairs
CIO: Nyle Morgan, Director Information Systems
CHR: Beverly Morris, Vice President Human Resources
Web address: www.kmcnetwork.org
Control: Church–operated, Nongovernment, not–for profit **Service:** General Medical and Surgical

Staffed Beds: 136 **Admissions:** 6301 **Census:** 82 **Outpatient Visits:** 87278 **Births:** 0 **Total Expense ($000):** 87641 **Payroll Expense ($000):** 30894 **Personnel:** 239

☐ **LIFECARE HOSPITAL OF DAYTON (362028)**, 4000 Miamisburg–Centerville Road, Zip 45342; tel. 937/384–8300, (Nonreporting) **A**1 9 10 **S** LifeCare Management Services
Primary Contact: Brent Martin, Chief Executive Officer
CMO: Richard Gregg, M.D., Medical Director
CHR: Pam Fannin, Coordinator Human Resources
Web address: www.lifecare–hospitals.com
Control: Corporation, Investor–owned, for–profit **Service:** Long–Term Acute Care hospital

Staffed Beds: 42

MIDDLEBURG HEIGHTS—Cuyahoga County

☐ **SOUTHWEST GENERAL HEALTH CENTER (360155)**, 18697 Bagley Road, Zip 44130–3497; tel. 440/816–8000 **A**1 2 10 **F**3 5 7 11 13 15 17 18 20 22 24 25 26 27 28 30 31 32 33 34 35 36 37 38 40 41 42 43 50 51 52 53 54 55 56 57 59 61 62 63 64 66 68 72 73 74 75 76 77 79 80 81 82 84 85 86 87 88 89 90 91 92 93 94 95 96 97 100 102 103 104 105 106 107 109 111 112 116 117 118 119 120 121 123 124 132 133 135 136 137 **P**6 **S** University Hospitals
Primary Contact: Thomas A. Selden, President and Chief Executive Officer
CFO: Janice Dunn, Vice President and Chief Financial Officer
CMO: Marilyn McNamara, M.D., Vice President Medical Affairs
CIO: Teresa Rini Barber, Chief Information Officer
CHR: Judy Murphy, Director Human Resources
Web address: www.swgeneral.com
Control: Other not–for–profit (including NFP Corporation) **Service:** General Medical and Surgical

Staffed Beds: 300 **Admissions:** 16175 **Census:** 199 **Outpatient Visits:** 371349 **Births:** 1205 **Total Expense ($000):** 225014 **Payroll Expense ($000):** 87743 **Personnel:** 1934

MIDDLETOWN—Warren County

MIDDLETOWN REGIONAL HOSPITAL See Atrium Medical Center, Franklin

MILLERSBURG—Holmes County

☐ **POMERENE HOSPITAL (360148)**, 981 Wooster Road, Zip 44654–1094; tel. 330/674–1015 **A**1 9 10 **F**3 11 13 15 25 26 30 31 32 33 38 52 55 56 57 66 68 72 73 74 75 77 79 80 84 86 96 97 102 107 118 119 120 121 124 132 135 136 137 **P**1
Primary Contact: Tony Snyder, Administrator and Chief Executive Officer
CFO: Robert Molnar, Chief Financial Officer
CMO: Yasser Omran, M.D., President Medical Staff
CIO: Randy Millard, Director Information Services
CHR: Connie Poulton, Vice President Human Resources and Support Services
Web address: www.pomerenehospital.org
Control: County–Government, nonfederal **Service:** General Medical and Surgical

Staffed Beds: 40 **Admissions:** 1964 **Census:** 18 **Outpatient Visits:** 13480 **Births:** 509 **Total Expense ($000):** 24419 **Payroll Expense ($000):** 10425 **Personnel:** 244

MONTPELIER—Williams County

☐ △ **COMMUNITY HOSPITAL (361327)**, 909 East Snyder Avenue, Zip 43543; tel. 419/636–1131, (Nonreporting) **A**1 7 9 10 18
Primary Contact: Rusty O. Brunicardi, President
Web address: www.chwchospital.com
Control: Corporation, Investor–owned, for–profit **Service:** General Medical and Surgical

Staffed Beds: 35

MONTPELIER HOSPITAL See Community Hospitals and Wellness Centers, Bryan

MOUNT GILEAD—Morrow County

★☐ **MORROW COUNTY HOSPITAL (361313)**, 651 West Marion Road, Zip 43338–1027; tel. 419/946–5015, (Total facility includes 38 beds in nursing home–type unit) **A**1 5 9 10 18 **F**3 11 15 24 25 26 33 38 55 57 61 62 68 77 79 80 96 102 105 107 117 118 119 135 **S** OhioHealth
Primary Contact: Diana D. Fisher, President and Chief Executive Officer
CFO: Joe Schueler, Chief Financial Officer
Web address: www.morrowcountyhospital.com
Control: County–Government, nonfederal **Service:** General Medical and Surgical

Staffed Beds: 53 **Admissions:** 965 **Census:** 42 **Outpatient Visits:** 57949 **Births:** 0

MOUNT VERNON—Knox County

★☐ **KNOX COMMUNITY HOSPITAL (360040)**, 1330 Coshocton Road, Zip 43050–1495; tel. 740/393–9000 **A**1 5 9 10 20 **F**3 11 13 15 18 20 24 25 26 27 32 33 38 40 41 43 44 51 52 55 56 57 62 66 67 68 71 73 74 75 76 77 79 80 81 82 86 96 97 100 102 107 111 118 119 124 135 136 137 **P**6 **S** QHR
Primary Contact: Bruce D. White, Chief Executive Officer
CMO: Eric J. Glose, D.O., Vice President Medical Affairs
CIO: Kwi Holland, Director Information Services
CHR: Betty Lucci, Vice President Human Resources
Web address: www.knoxcommhosp.org
Control: Other not–for–profit (including NFP Corporation) **Service:** General Medical and Surgical

Staffed Beds: 96 **Admissions:** 3886 **Census:** 39 **Outpatient Visits:** 83972 **Births:** 432 **Total Expense ($000):** 74368 **Payroll Expense ($000):** 34077 **Personnel:** 585

NAPOLEON—Henry County

★☐ **HENRY COUNTY HOSPITAL (361309)**, 11600 State Route 424, Zip 43545–9399; tel. 419/592–4015 **A**1 5 9 10 18 **F**3 5 11 13 15 24 25 27 31 32 33 34 38 43 52 55 57 62 66 68 73 74 75 76 77 79 80 81 82 86 89 90 91 94 96 97 100 106 107 112 118 119 120 121 122 124 135
Primary Contact: Kimberly Bordenkircher, Chief Executive Officer
COO: Michelle Burkholder, Chief Operating Officer
CFO: Mary Clapp, Controller
CHR: Jennifer Fisher, Manager Human Resources
Web address: www.henrycountyhospital.org
Control: Other not–for–profit (including NFP Corporation) **Service:** General Medical and Surgical

Staffed Beds: 25 **Admissions:** 866 **Census:** 9 **Outpatient Visits:** 31319 **Births:** 140 **Total Expense ($000):** 20983 **Payroll Expense ($000):** 8583 **Personnel:** 202

NELSONVILLE—Athens County

★ ○ **DOCTORS HOSPITAL NELSONVILLE (361305)**, 1950 Mount Saint Mary Drive, Zip 45764–1193; tel. 740/753–1931, (Total facility includes 45 beds in nursing home–type unit) **A**9 10 11 18 **F**3 15 25 27 31 32 33 38 55 57 73 77 79 80 96 97 102 106 117 119 122 137 **P**6 **S** OhioHealth
Primary Contact: Steve Swart, Administrator
CFO: Lewis Newberry, Chief Financial Officer
CMO: James Foglesong, D.O., Chief Medical Officer
CHR: Terry Wilson, Director Human Resources and Compliance
Web address: www.ohiohealth.com
Control: Other not–for–profit (including NFP Corporation) **Service:** General Medical and Surgical

Staffed Beds: 70 **Admissions:** 560 **Census:** 40 **Outpatient Visits:** 24255 **Births:** 0 **Total Expense ($000):** 16010 **Payroll Expense ($000):** 8406 **Personnel:** 201

NEW ALBANY—Franklin County

☐ **MOUNT CARMEL NEW ALBANY SURGICAL HOSPITAL (360266)**, 7333 Smith's Mill Road, Zip 43054; tel. 614/775–6600 **A**1 9 10 **F**25 30 31 32 34 35 56 58 62 72 77 79 80 81 82 96 100 102 107 120 124 135 **S** Trinity Health
Primary Contact: Richard D'Enbeau, Chief Operating Officer
Web address: www.newalbanysurgicalhospital.com
Control: Church–operated, Nongovernment, not–for profit **Service:** General Medical and Surgical

Staffed Beds: 42 **Admissions:** 3856 **Census:** 22 **Outpatient Visits:** 9495 **Births:** 0 **Total Expense ($000):** 59625 **Payroll Expense ($000):** 11022 **Personnel:** 193

NEWARK—Licking County

☐ **LICKING MEMORIAL HOSPITAL (360218)**, 1320 West Main Street, Zip 43055–3699; tel. 740/348–4000 **A**1 2 9 10 **F**3 4 5 13 15 18 20 24 25 26 27 28 30 31 32 33 38 43 50 52 55 56 57 61 62 63 66 68 73 74 75 76 79 80 81 82 84 86 87 88 90 91 92 94 95 96 97 100 102 106 107 118 119 121 124 133 135 137 **P**6
Primary Contact: Robert A. Montagnese, President and Chief Executive Officer
CFO: Thomas Poulson, Vice President Financial Services
CMO: Craig Cairns, M.D., Vice President Medical Affairs
CIO: Sallie Arnett, Vice President Information Systems
CHR: Anne Peterson, Vice President Human Resources
Web address: www.lmhealth.org
Control: Other not–for–profit (including NFP Corporation) **Service:** General Medical and Surgical

Staffed Beds: 197 **Admissions:** 7648 **Census:** 67 **Outpatient Visits:** 264543 **Births:** 1060 **Total Expense ($000):** 116956 **Payroll Expense ($000):** 49503 **Personnel:** 1213

NORTHFIELD—Summit County

☐ **NORTHCOAST BEHAVIORAL HEALTHCARE SYSTEM (364011)**, 1756 Sagamore Road, Zip 44067–1086; tel. 330/467–7131, (Includes CLEVELAND CAMPUS, 1708 Southpoint Drive, Cleveland, Zip 44109–1999; tel. 216/787–0500; NORTHFIELD CAMPUS; TOLEDO CAMPUS, 930 South Detroit Avenue, Toledo, Zip 43614–2701; tel. 419/381–1881), (Nonreporting) **A**1 3 5 10
Primary Contact: Thomas M. Cheek, Chief Executive Officer
CFO: Jeff Comfort, Vice President Administration
CIO: Karl Donenwirth, Vice President Information Services
Control: State–Government, nonfederal **Service:** Psychiatric

Staffed Beds: 376

Hospital, Medicare Provider Number, Address, Telephone, Approval, Facility, and Physician Codes, Health Care System

★ American Hospital Association (AHA) membership
☐ The Joint Commission accreditation
○ American Osteopathic Association (AOA) accreditation
△ Commission on Accreditation of Rehabilitation Facilities (CARF) accreditation

NORWALK—Huron County

★ ○ **FISHER–TITUS MEDICAL CENTER (360065)**, 272 Benedict Avenue, Zip 44857–2374; tel. 419/668–8101, (Total facility includes 69 beds in nursing home–type unit) **A**1 2 9 10 11 19 **F**3 10 11 13 15 18 24 25 27 30 31 32 33 34 37 38 43 49 50 51 54 55 56 57 58 61 62 68 72 73 74 75 76 77 79 80 81 82 86 96 97 100 103 104 105 107 112 115 117 118 119 120 121 124 134 135 136 **P**2 7
Primary Contact: Patrick J. Martin, President and Chief Executive Officer
COO: Margaret Baird, Executive Vice President Administrative Services
CFO: Duane L. Woods, Chief Financial Officer
CIO: John Britton, Director Information Services
CHR: Stan Hire, Vice President Human Resources
Web address: www.fisher-titus.com
Control: Other not–for–profit (including NFP Corporation) **Service:** General Medical and Surgical

Staffed Beds: 173 **Admissions:** 4527 **Census:** 173 **Outpatient Visits:** 137207 **Births:** 741 **Total Expense ($000):** 83480 **Payroll Expense ($000):** 34402 **Personnel:** 741

OBERLIN—Lorain County

★ **ALLEN COMMUNITY HOSPITAL (361306)**, (Formerly Allen Medical Center), 200 West Lorain Street, Zip 44074–1077; tel. 440/775–1211, (Total facility includes 8 beds in nursing home–type unit) **A**1 9 10 18 **F**7 8 11 30 31 38 50 54 57 62 67 68 73 75 76 77 79 80 81 84 86 96 97 107 117 119 120 121 122 124 135 136 **S** Catholic Healthcare Partners
Primary Contact: Susan Bowers, RN, President
CFO: Dave Richards, Chief Financial Officer
CMO: Georgia Newman, M.D., Chief of Staff
CIO: David Noll, Director Information Services
Web address: www.ehealthconnection.com/lorain
Control: Other not–for–profit (including NFP Corporation) **Service:** General Medical and Surgical

Staffed Beds: 25 **Admissions:** 934 **Census:** 9 **Outpatient Visits:** 21701 **Births:** 0 **Total Expense ($000):** 15557 **Payroll Expense ($000):** 8109 **Personnel:** 152

OREGON—Lucas County

★ **BAY PARK COMMUNITY HOSPITAL (360259)**, 2801 Bay Park Drive, Zip 43616; tel. 419/690–7900 **A**1 9 10 **F**3 11 13 15 18 25 26 27 30 31 32 33 38 41 43 49 50 51 55 56 57 62 66 68 72 73 74 75 76 77 79 80 81 82 86 96 97 99 100 102 106 107 118 119 120 121 124 135 136 137 **S** ProMedica Health System
Primary Contact: Bill Mueller, President
CFO: Darrin Arquette, Vice President Finance, Diagnostics and Support Services
CMO: David Lindstrom, M.D., Vice President Medical Affairs
CIO: David G. Selman, Corporate Vice President Information Resources
CHR: Charles McDowell, Corporate Vice President Human Resources
Web address: www.promedica.org
Control: Other not–for–profit (including NFP Corporation) **Service:** General Medical and Surgical

Staffed Beds: 70 **Admissions:** 3191 **Census:** 37 **Outpatient Visits:** 93426 **Births:** 644 **Total Expense ($000):** 56787 **Payroll Expense ($000):** 18812 **Personnel:** 389

★ △ **ST. CHARLES MERCY HOSPITAL (360081)**, 2600 Navarre Avenue, Zip 43616–3297; tel. 419/696–7200 **A**1 2 7 9 10 **F**5 7 11 12 13 15 25 26 27 30 31 32 33 34 38 40 43 46 48 49 52 53 54 55 57 58 60 62 63 66 68 71 74 75 76 77 79 80 84 85 86 87 88 89 90 91 92 93 94 95 96 97 98 99 100 102 103 104 106 107 109 111 118 119 120 121 122 132 135 136 137 **P**8 **S** Catholic Healthcare Partners
Primary Contact: Carol A. Whittaker, President and Chief Executive Officer
CFO: Todd Warner, Interim Chief Financial Officer
CMO: Surendra Kumar, M.D., Chief of Staff
CIO: James Albin, Regional Vice President and Chief Information Officer
CHR: Gary George, Regional Vice President Human Resources
Web address: www.mercyweb.org
Control: Church–operated, Nongovernment, not–for profit **Service:** General Medical and Surgical

Staffed Beds: 294 **Admissions:** 10942 **Census:** 161 **Outpatient Visits:** 181343 **Births:** 700 **Personnel:** 1132

ORRVILLE—Wayne County

★ **DUNLAP COMMUNITY HOSPITAL (361323)**, (Formerly Dunlap Memorial Hospital), 832 South Main Street, Zip 44667–2208; tel. 330/682–3010 **A**1 9 10 18 **F**3 11 13 15 24 25 26 30 31 32 33 38 43 47 50 51 52 55 56 57 66 68 73 74 75 77 79 80 81 82 84 86 96 97 100 102 106 107 117 118 119 120 121 122 124 132 135
Primary Contact: Rod Steiger, President and Chief Executive Officer
CFO: Steve Knox, Vice President Finance
CMO: Marchelle Suppan, M.D., Senior Vice President Medical Affairs and Chief Medical Officer
CHR: Kathy Loede, Vice President Human Resources
Web address: www.dunlaphospital.org
Control: Other not–for–profit (including NFP Corporation) **Service:** General Medical and Surgical

Staffed Beds: 25 **Admissions:** 884 **Census:** 7 **Outpatient Visits:** 48573 **Births:** 304 **Total Expense ($000):** 22477 **Payroll Expense ($000):** 8459 **Personnel:** 205

OXFORD—Butler County

○ **MCCULLOUGH–HYDE MEMORIAL HOSPITAL (360046)**, 110 North Poplar Street, Zip 45056–1292; tel. 513/523–2111 **A**9 10 11 **F**3 11 13 15 24 25 26 27 28 30 33 38 49 53 55 56 57 62 63 67 68 73 74 75 76 77 79 80 84 86 96 100 102 106 107 118 119 120 121 124 132 135 136
Primary Contact: Richard A. Daniels, President and Chief Executive Officer
COO: Tammy B. Wood, Vice President and Chief Administrative Officer
CFO: Christopher Lauer, Vice President and Chief Financial Officer
CHR: Dennis Johnson, Director Human Resources
Web address: www.mhmh.org
Control: Other not–for–profit (including NFP Corporation) **Service:** General Medical and Surgical

Staffed Beds: 45 **Admissions:** 2588 **Census:** 22 **Outpatient Visits:** 105202 **Births:** 499 **Total Expense ($000):** 45696 **Payroll Expense ($000):** 19105 **Personnel:** 393

PAINESVILLE—Lake County

★ △ **LAKE HOSPITAL SYSTEM (360098)**, 10 East Washington, Zip 44077–3472; tel. 440/354–2400 **A**1 2 7 9 10 **F**3 8 11 13 15 18 20 22 24 25 26 30 31 32 33 38 41 42 43 49 50 51 53 54 55 56 57 58 59 61 62 66 67 68 71 72 73 74 75 77 79 80 81 82 85 86 87 88 93 96 97 99 100 102 104 107 117 118 119 120 121 124 132 133 134 135 136 **P**1
Primary Contact: Cynthia Ann Moore–Hardy, President and Chief Executive Officer
CFO: Robert Tracz, Chief Financial Officer
CMO: Theodore Nichols, M.D., Senior Vice President Medical Affairs
Web address: www.lhs.net
Control: Other not–for–profit (including NFP Corporation) **Service:** General Medical and Surgical

Staffed Beds: 360 **Admissions:** 16429 **Census:** 204 **Outpatient Visits:** 228310 **Births:** 2017 **Total Expense ($000):** 239417 **Payroll Expense ($000):** 92749 **Personnel:** 1789

PARMA—Cuyahoga County

★ △ **PARMA COMMUNITY GENERAL HOSPITAL (360041)**, 7007 Powers Boulevard, Zip 44129–5495; tel. 440/743–3000, (Total facility includes 27 beds in nursing home–type unit) (Nonreporting) **A**1 2 7 9 10
Primary Contact: Patricia A. Ruflin, President and Chief Executive Officer
COO: Terrence G. Deis, Executive Vice President and Chief Operating Officer
CFO: Barry L. Franklin, Executive Vice President and Chief Financial Officer
CMO: Donn Wolfson, M.D., Vice President Medical Affairs
CIO: Terrence G. Deis, Executive Vice President and Chief Operating Officer
CHR: Larry Jeffries, Senior Director Human Resources
Web address: www.parmahospital.org
Control: Other not–for–profit (including NFP Corporation) **Service:** General Medical and Surgical

Staffed Beds: 325

PAULDING—Paulding County

□ **PAULDING COUNTY HOSPITAL (361300)**, 1035 West Wayne Street, Zip 45879–9220; tel. 419/399–4080 **A**1 9 10 18 **F**3 11 15 24 25 27 30 31 32 38 52 55 57 61 62 66 67 75 76 77 79 80 86 96 97 100 107 117 118 122 132 135 137
Primary Contact: Gary W. Adkins, Chief Executive Officer
COO: Randy Ruge, Chief Operating Officer
CFO: Rob Goshia, Chief Financial Officer
CMO: William H. Strawter, M.D., Chief of Staff
CIO: Dan Kaufman, Director Information Services
CHR: Amy Lieb, Director Human Resources
Web address: www.pauldingcountyhospital.com
Control: County–Government, nonfederal **Service:** General Medical and Surgical

Staffed Beds: 25 **Admissions:** 544 **Census:** 4 **Outpatient Visits:** 49058 **Births:** 39 **Total Expense ($000):** 17965 **Payroll Expense ($000):** 7999 **Personnel:** 178

 Many Facility Codes have changed. Please refer to the AHA Guide Code Chart.

PORT CLINTON—Ottawa County

★ **H. B. MAGRUDER MEMORIAL HOSPITAL (361314)**, 615 Fulton Street, Zip 43452–2034; tel. 419/734–3131, (Nonreporting) **A**1 5 9 10 18
Primary Contact: Clifford K. Harmon, Chief Executive Officer
COO: Michael E. Long, Senior Vice President
CFO: J. Todd Almendinger, Vice President Finance
CMO: Sean P. Callahan, M.D., President Medical Staff
CHR: Jennifer Capizzi, Vice President Human Resources
Web address: www.magruderhospital.com
Control: Other not–for–profit (including NFP Corporation) **Service:** General Medical and Surgical

Staffed Beds: 15

PORTSMOUTH—Scioto County

★ △ **SOUTHERN OHIO MEDICAL CENTER (360008)**, 1805 27th Street, Zip 45662–2400; tel. 740/354–5000 **A**1 5 7 9 10 12 13 19 **F**3 11 13 15 18 20 24 25 26 27 30 31 32 33 36 37 38 39 42 44 46 49 50 52 55 56 57 61 62 63 66 68 72 73 74 75 76 77 79 80 81 82 84 85 87 90 92 94 96 98 99 100 102 103 104 105 106 107 108 109 110 111 112 114 115 118 119 120 121 124 133 134 135 **P**3
Primary Contact: Randal M. Arnett, President and Chief Executive Officer
COO: Claudia Burchett, Vice President Patient Services
CFO: Dean Wray, Vice President Finance
CMO: Kendall Stewart, M.D., Medical Director
CIO: Brent Richard, Director Information Systems
CHR: Vicki Noel, Vice President Human Resources
Web address: www.somc.org
Control: Other not–for–profit (including NFP Corporation) **Service:** General Medical and Surgical

Staffed Beds: 230 **Admissions:** 11705 **Census:** 142 **Outpatient Visits:** 300875 **Births:** 1339 **Total Expense ($000):** 188893 **Payroll Expense ($000):** 76545 **Personnel:** 1947

RAVENNA—Portage County

★ **REGENCY HOSPITAL OF RAVENNA**, 6847 North Chestnut Street, Zip 44266; tel. 330/296–2350, (Nonreporting) **A**1 **S** Regency Hospital Company
Primary Contact: Andrew Escamilla, Chief Executive Officer
Web address: www.regencyhospital.com
Control: Corporation, Investor–owned, for–profit **Service:** Long–Term Acute Care hospital

Staffed Beds: 19

□ **ROBINSON MEMORIAL HOSPITAL (360078)**, 6847 North Chestnut Street, Zip 44266–1204, Mailing Address: P.O. Box 1204, Zip 44266–1204; tel. 330/297–0811 **A**1 2 3 5 9 10 **F**3 8 11 13 15 17 18 20 24 25 26 27 28 30 31 32 33 38 40 41 42 43 44 47 49 50 51 53 54 55 56 57 58 60 61 62 68 72 73 74 75 76 77 79 80 81 82 86 87 90 96 97 100 102 104 106 107 109 111 118 119 120 121 133 134 135 136 137 **P**6 8 **S** Summa Health System
Primary Contact: Stephen Colecchi, President and Chief Executive Officer
CFO: Carl Ebner, Vice President Finance
CIO: David Baldwin, Chief Information Officer
CHR: Pamela Mackintosh, Vice President Human Resources
Web address: www.robinsonmemorial.org
Control: County–Government, nonfederal **Service:** General Medical and Surgical

Staffed Beds: 115 **Admissions:** 8714 **Census:** 101 **Outpatient Visits:** 131706 **Births:** 835 **Total Expense ($000):** 140088 **Payroll Expense ($000):** 55135 **Personnel:** 1202

ROCK CREEK—Ashtabula County

GLENBEIGH HOSPITAL AND OUTPATIENT CENTERS (360245), Route 45, Zip 44084, Mailing Address: P.O. Box 298, Zip 44084–0298; tel. 440/563–3400 **A**9 10 **F**4 5 25 52 55 73 81 82 90 119 121 **P**5
Primary Contact: Patricia Weston–Hall, Chief Executive Officer
CFO: Dave Erra, Accountant
CIO: Linda Advey, Manager Information Systems
CHR: Shirley Deary, Director Human Resources
Web address: www.glenbeigh.com
Control: Other not–for–profit (including NFP Corporation) **Service:** Alcoholism and other chemical dependency

Staffed Beds: 112 **Admissions:** 2560 **Census:** 51 **Outpatient Visits:** 45709 **Births:** 0 **Total Expense ($000):** 11259 **Payroll Expense ($000):** 5813 **Personnel:** 169

SAINT MARYS—Auglaize County

★ **JOINT TOWNSHIP DISTRICT MEMORIAL HOSPITAL (360032)**, 200 St. Clair Street, Zip 45885–2400; tel. 419/394–3335, (Total facility includes 15 beds in nursing home–type unit) **A**1 9 10 **F**3 7 8 11 13 15 18 24 25 26 27 28 30 31 32 33 34 38 40 42 43 44 51 52 55 56 57 61 62 68 72 73 74 75 76 77 79 80 82 84 85 86 87 96 97 99 103 107 117 119 120 121 124 132 133 135 136 137
Primary Contact: Kevin W. Harlan, President
CFO: Jeffrey W. Vossler, Vice President Financial Services
CIO: DeWayne Marsee, Director Information Systems
CHR: Art Swain, Vice President Support Services
Web address: www.grandlakehealth.org
Control: Other not–for–profit (including NFP Corporation) **Service:** General Medical and Surgical

Staffed Beds: 90 **Admissions:** 3387 **Census:** 29 **Outpatient Visits:** 95990 **Births:** 297 **Total Expense ($000):** 55030 **Payroll Expense ($000):** 20013 **Personnel:** 450

SALEM—Columbiana County

★ **SALEM COMMUNITY HOSPITAL (360185)**, 1995 East State Street, Zip 44460–0121; tel. 330/332–1551, (Total facility includes 15 beds in nursing home–type unit) **A**1 5 9 10 **F**11 13 15 18 20 24 25 26 27 30 31 32 38 43 49 51 55 57 62 68 72 73 74 75 76 77 79 80 84 86 96 97 100 102 105 106 107 117 118 119 121 124 135 137
Primary Contact: Howard E. Rohleder, President and Chief Executive Officer
CFO: Mike Giangardella, Vice President Finance and Administration
CMO: Anita Hackstedde, M.D., Vice President Medical Affairs
CIO: Mark L'Italien, Director Information Services
CHR: Barb Hirst, Vice President Human Resources
Web address: www.salemhosp.com
Control: Other not–for–profit (including NFP Corporation) **Service:** General Medical and Surgical

Staffed Beds: 140 **Admissions:** 6041 **Census:** 77 **Outpatient Visits:** 149757 **Births:** 611 **Total Expense ($000):** 89354 **Payroll Expense ($000):** 38693 **Personnel:** 833

SANDUSKY—Erie County

□ ○ **FIRELANDS REGIONAL HEALTH SYSTEM (360025)**, 1111 Hayes Avenue, Zip 44870; tel. 419/557–7400, (Includes FIRELANDS REGIONAL MEDICAL CENTER – MAIN CAMPUS, Zip 44870–8005; FIRELANDS REGIONAL MEDICAL CENTER SOUTH CAMPUS, 1912 Hayes Avenue, Zip 44870–4736; tel. 419/557–7000; Charles A. Stark, FACHE, President and Chief Executive Officer) **A**1 2 5 6 9 10 11 12 13 19 **F**2 3 5 8 9 11 12 13 15 17 18 20 22 24 25 26 27 28 29 31 32 33 34 35 36 37 38 40 41 42 43 44 50 51 54 55 56 57 59 60 61 62 64 66 67 68 72 73 74 75 76 77 79 80 81 82 84 85 86 87 88 89 90 91 92 93 94 95 96 97 98 99 100 102 103 104 105 106 107 108 109 111 118 119 120 121 122 123 124 132 135 136 137 **P**1
Primary Contact: Charles A. Stark, FACHE, President and Chief Executive Officer
COO: Tam Jackson, R.N., MSN, Senior Vice President and Chief Nursing Officer
CFO: Daniel J. Moncher, Vice President and Chief Financial Officer
CIO: Robert Ayres, Director Information Systems
CHR: James Sennish, Vice President Human Resources
Web address: www.firelands.com
Control: Other not–for–profit (including NFP Corporation) **Service:** General Medical and Surgical

Staffed Beds: 219 **Admissions:** 9951 **Census:** 141 **Outpatient Visits:** 287246 **Births:** 709 **Total Expense ($000):** 163527 **Payroll Expense ($000):** 68575 **Personnel:** 1346

SHELBY—Richland County

□ **MEDCENTRAL – SHELBY HOSPITAL (361324)**, (Formerly Shelby Hospital), 20 Morris Road, Zip 44875; tel. 419/342–5015, (Nonreporting) **A**1 9 10 18 **S** MedCentral Health System
Primary Contact: Ron Distl, Chief Executive Officer
Web address: www.medcentral.org/body.cfm?id=153
Control: Other not–for–profit (including NFP Corporation) **Service:** General Medical and Surgical

Staffed Beds: 25

Hospital, Medicare Provider Number, Address, Telephone, Approval, Facility, and Physician Codes, Health Care System

★ American Hospital Association (AHA) membership
□ The Joint Commission accreditation
○ American Osteopathic Association (AOA) accreditation
△ Commission on Accreditation of Rehabilitation Facilities (CARF) accreditation

OH

SIDNEY—Shelby County

★ **WILSON MEMORIAL HOSPITAL (360013)**, 915 West Michigan Street, Zip 45365–2491; tel. 937/498–2311 **A**1 9 10 **F**3 7 11 13 15 24 25 26 27 30 31 32 38 42 46 49 54 55 57 61 62 66 68 73 74 75 76 77 79 80 81 82 84 86 88 93 96 97 100 106 107 112 118 119 121 124 135 136 **P**6
Primary Contact: Thomas J. Boecker, President and Chief Executive Officer
CFO: Douglas Bomba, Vice President Finance
CMO: Paul Thorpe, M.D., Chief of Staff
CIO: Jeff Partee, Chief Information Officer
CHR: Bill McCaskey, Director Human Resources
Web address: www.wilsonhospital.com
Control: Other not–for–profit (including NFP Corporation) **Service:** General Medical and Surgical

Staffed Beds: 71 **Admissions:** 3523 **Census:** 41 **Outpatient Visits:** 187067 **Births:** 861 **Total Expense ($000):** 63613 **Payroll Expense ($000):** 24262 **Personnel:** 582

SPRINGFIELD—Clark County

★ **SPRINGFIELD REGIONAL MEDICAL CENTER – FOUNTAIN CAMPUS (360086)**, (Formerly Mercy Medical Center), 1343 North Fountain Boulevard, Zip 45501–1380; tel. 937/390–5000 **A**1 2 5 9 10 **F**3 5 11 15 17 18 20 22 25 26 28 30 31 32 33 36 38 42 43 44 54 55 57 60 62 63 66 67 68 72 73 75 77 79 81 82 84 86 96 97 100 102 106 107 112 118 119 121 123 124 133 134 135 136 137 **S** Catholic Healthcare Partners
Primary Contact: George N. Miller, Jr., President and Chief Executive Officer
CMO: Donald Johnson, M.D., Chief Medical Officer
Web address: www.mercy–health.org
Control: Church–operated, Nongovernment, not–for profit **Service:** General Medical and Surgical

Staffed Beds: 154 **Admissions:** 7626 **Census:** 95 **Outpatient Visits:** 109203 **Births:** 0 **Total Expense ($000):** 109154 **Payroll Expense ($000):** 39176 **Personnel:** 860

★ **SPRINGFIELD REGIONAL MEDICAL CENTER – HIGH STREET CAMPUS (360187)**, (Formerly Community Hospital of Springfield), 2615 East High Street, Zip 45505–1422, Mailing Address: P.O. Box 1228, Zip 45501–1228; tel. 937/325–0531 **A**1 6 9 10 **F**3 11 12 13 17 18 20 22 25 26 30 31 32 38 51 56 57 60 62 66 68 70 71 72 73 74 77 79 80 81 82 85 86 96 97 99 100 106 107 119 121 124 134 135 137 **S** Catholic Healthcare Partners
Primary Contact: George N. Miller, Jr., Regional President and Chief Executive Officer
COO: Mark S. Wiener, Chief Operating Officer
CFO: Renato Suntay, Vice President and Chief Financial Officer
CMO: Kamel Abraham, M.D., Chief of Staff
CIO: Yousuf Ahmad, Chief Information Officer
CHR: Cherie Lamborn, Interim Vice President Human Resources
Web address: www.communityhospital.com
Control: Church–operated, Nongovernment, not–for profit **Service:** General Medical and Surgical

Staffed Beds: 215 **Admissions:** 9976 **Census:** 129 **Outpatient Visits:** 142409 **Births:** 1687 **Total Expense ($000):** 116933 **Payroll Expense ($000):** 45214 **Personnel:** 957

STEUBENVILLE—Jefferson County

☐ **ACUITY SPECIALTY HOSPITAL – OHIO VALLEY (362035)**, 380 Summit Avenue, 3rd Floor, Zip 43952; tel. 740/283–7497, (Nonreporting) **A**1 10
Primary Contact: Leanne Fiorentino, Chief Executive Officer
Web address: www.acuityhealthcare.net
Control: Corporation, Investor–owned, for–profit **Service:** Long–Term Acute Care hospital

Staffed Beds: 40

★ **TRINITY HEALTH SYSTEM (360211)**, 380 Summit Avenue, Zip 43952–2699; tel. 740/283–7000, (Includes TRINITY MEDICAL CENTER EAST; TRINITY MEDICAL CENTER WEST, 4000 Johnson Road, Zip 43952–2393; tel. 740/264–8000) **A**1 2 6 9 10 **F**3 4 5 11 13 15 17 18 20 22 24 25 26 27 28 30 31 32 33 36 38 49 52 53 54 55 56 57 59 61 62 63 66 68 72 73 74 75 76 77 79 80 81 82 84 85 86 87 88 89 90 91 92 93 94 95 96 97 100 102 106 107 109 111 117 118 119 120 121 124 133 135 136 137 **P**6 **S** Franciscan Services Corporation
Primary Contact: Fred B. Brower, President and Chief Executive Officer
COO: JoAnn M. Mulrooney, R.N., Vice President Nursing
CFO: Elizabeth Allen, Vice President Finance
CMO: Ivan Wright, M.D., Vice President Medical Affairs
CIO: Tom Kiger, Director Information Systems
CHR: Lewis C. Musso, Vice President Human Resources
Web address: www.trinityhealth.com
Control: Other not–for–profit (including NFP Corporation) **Service:** General Medical and Surgical

Staffed Beds: 308 **Admissions:** 11400 **Census:** 183 **Outpatient Visits:** 233723 **Births:** 635 **Total Expense ($000):** 143212 **Payroll Expense ($000):** 59745 **Personnel:** 1409

SYLVANIA—Lucas County

★ **FLOWER HOSPITAL (360074)**, 5200 Harroun Road, Zip 43560–2196; tel. 419/824–1444 **A**1 2 9 10 **F**3 11 12 13 15 18 20 22 24 25 26 27 30 31 32 33 34 36 38 40 43 44 48 49 50 54 55 56 57 58 62 63 66 68 73 74 75 76 77 79 80 81 82 85 86 87 88 90 91 92 93 96 97 98 100 102 105 106 107 108 109 111 112 118 119 120 121 124 132 135 136 **S** ProMedica Health System
Primary Contact: Kevin C. Webb, FACHE, President
CFO: Alan Sattler, Senior Vice President Finance
CMO: John D. Meier, M.D., Vice President Medical Affairs
CIO: David G. Selman, Vice President Information
Web address: www.promedica.org
Control: Other not–for–profit (including NFP Corporation) **Service:** General Medical and Surgical

Staffed Beds: 225 **Admissions:** 10764 **Census:** 156 **Outpatient Visits:** 186734 **Births:** 1066 **Total Expense ($000):** 135032 **Payroll Expense ($000):** 54984 **Personnel:** 1210

TIFFIN—Seneca County

★ **MERCY HOSPITAL OF TIFFIN (360089)**, 45 St. Lawrence Drive, Zip 44883–0727; tel. 419/447–3130 **A**1 5 9 10 **F**3 11 12 13 15 24 25 26 27 30 31 32 33 34 38 43 44 45 49 50 54 55 56 57 61 62 64 66 68 72 73 74 75 76 77 79 80 81 82 84 87 96 97 102 106 107 108 109 111 117 118 119 121 123 124 132 134 135 136 137 **S** Catholic Healthcare Partners
Primary Contact: Dale E. Thornton, M.P.H., CHE, President and Chief Executive Officer
CFO: Lynn Detterman, Chief Financial Officer
CMO: Wesley Hedges, M.D., President Medical Staff
CHR: Diana Olson, Chief Human Resources Officer
Web address: www.mercyweb.org
Control: Church–operated, Nongovernment, not–for profit **Service:** General Medical and Surgical

Staffed Beds: 70 **Admissions:** 2343 **Census:** 31 **Outpatient Visits:** 106715 **Births:** 403 **Total Expense ($000):** 44949 **Payroll Expense ($000):** 18165 **Personnel:** 400

TOLEDO—Lucas County

★ ○ **ST. ANNE MERCY HOSPITAL (360262)**, 3404 West Sylvania Avenue, Zip 43623; tel. 419/407–2663 **A**1 2 9 10 11 **F**3 13 15 25 26 27 30 31 32 33 34 36 38 40 44 46 53 54 55 56 57 62 63 66 68 72 73 76 77 79 80 81 86 87 96 97 100 102 106 107 119 120 121 135 136 **P**8 **S** Catholic Healthcare Partners
Primary Contact: Richard R. Evens, President and Chief Executive Officer
CFO: Samantha Platyke, Chief Financial Officer
CIO: James Albin, Regional Vice President and Chief Information Officer
CHR: Gary George, Regional Vice President Human Resources
Web address: www.mercyweb.org
Control: Church–operated, Nongovernment, not–for profit **Service:** General Medical and Surgical

Staffed Beds: 128 **Admissions:** 5377 **Census:** 63 **Outpatient Visits:** 191451 **Births:** 0 **Personnel:** 629

★ ○ **ST. VINCENT MERCY MEDICAL CENTER (360112)**, 2213 Cherry Street, Zip 43608–2691; tel. 419/251–3232, (Includes MERCY CHILDREN'S HOSPITAL, tel. 419/251–8000) **A**1 2 3 5 9 10 11 12 13 **F**3 7 8 11 12 13 15 16 17 18 19 20 21 22 23 24 25 26 27 28 30 31 32 33 34 35 36 38 40 41 43 44 45 46 48 49 50 51 53 54 55 56 57 58 59 60 62 63 64 65 66 68 70 71 72 73 74 75 76 77 79 80 81 83 84 85 86 87 88 90 91 92 93 94 95 96 97 98 99 100 102 104 106 107 108 111 116 118 119 120 121 123 124 130 135 136 137 **P**8 **S** Catholic Healthcare Partners
Primary Contact: Michael L. McEachern, President and Chief Executive Officer
CFO: Samantha M. Platzke, Senior Vice President Finance and Chief Financial Officer
CMO: David R. Franzblau, M.D., Chief Medical Officer
CIO: James Albin, Regional Vice President and Chief Information Officer
CHR: Gary George, Regional Vice President Human Resources
Web address: www.mercyweb.org
Control: Church–operated, Nongovernment, not–for profit **Service:** General Medical and Surgical

Staffed Beds: 462 **Admissions:** 20922 **Census:** 296 **Outpatient Visits:** 274195 **Births:** 1423 **Personnel:** 2434

Many Facility Codes have changed. Please refer to the AHA Guide Code Chart.

★ **THE TOLEDO HOSPITAL (360068)**, 2142 North Cove Boulevard, Zip 43606–3896; tel. 419/291–4000, (Includes TOLEDO CHILDREN'S HOSPITAL, Kathy Carlson, M.D., President), (Total facility includes 25 beds in nursing home–type unit) **A**1 3 5 9 10 12 13 **F**3 4 5 7 8 9 11 12 13 15 17 18 19 20 21 22 23 25 26 27 28 30 31 32 33 34 36 37 38 40 43 44 48 49 50 51 52 53 55 56 57 58 59 62 63 66 68 69 70 72 73 74 75 76 77 79 80 81 82 83 84 86 87 88 89 90 91 92 94 95 96 97 98 99 100 102 103 106 107 111 113 114 117 118 119 120 121 123 124 132 133 135 136 137 **S** ProMedica Health System
Primary Contact: Barbara Steele, Chief Executive Officer
CFO: Alan Sattler, Senior Vice President Finance
CMO: Rob Fredrick, M.D., Vice President Medical Affairs
CIO: David G. Selman, Chief Information Officer
CHR: Randy Schimmoeller, Vice President Human Resources
Web address: www.promedica.org
Control: Other not–for–profit (including NFP Corporation) **Service:** General Medical and Surgical

Staffed Beds: 587 **Admissions:** 29648 **Census:** 418 **Outpatient Visits:** 649644 **Births:** 4141 **Total Expense ($000):** 505260 **Payroll Expense ($000):** 187448 **Personnel:** 4609

★ △ **THE UNIVERSITY OF TOLEDO MEDICAL CENTER (360048)**, 3000 Arlington Avenue, Zip 43614–5805; tel. 419/383–4000 **A**1 2 3 5 7 8 9 10 **F**3 8 9 11 12 15 18 20 22 24 25 26 27 28 30 31 32 33 35 37 38 40 41 43 44 46 47 49 50 51 52 53 54 55 56 57 58 59 60 62 63 64 65 66 68 72 73 75 76 77 79 80 81 82 85 86 87 88 89 90 91 92 93 94 95 96 97 98 99 100 102 103 104 105 106 107 108 109 111 112 114 119 120 121 123 124 127 135 136 137 **P**4
Primary Contact: Mark J. Chastang, Executive Director
COO: Mark J. Chastang, Executive Director
CFO: Daniel Morissette, Senior Vice President Finance and Administration
CMO: Ronald McGinnis, M.D., Medical Director
CIO: Lawrence Burns, Vice President Institutional Advancement
CHR: William Logie, Vice President Human Resources
Web address: www.utoledo.edu
Control: State–Government, nonfederal **Service:** General Medical and Surgical

Staffed Beds: 228 **Admissions:** 11839 **Census:** 167 **Outpatient Visits:** 222368 **Births:** 0 **Total Expense ($000):** 219637 **Payroll Expense ($000):** 91205 **Personnel:** 2025

TOLEDO CAMPUS See Northcoast Behavioral Healthcare System, Northfield

TROY—Miami County

□ △ **UPPER VALLEY MEDICAL CENTER (360174)**, 3130 North Dixie Highway, Zip 45373–1309; tel. 937/440–4000, (Includes DETTMER HOSPITAL, tel. 937/440–7500), (Nonreporting) **A**1 2 3 5 7 9 10
Primary Contact: David J. Meckstroth, President and Chief Executive Officer
COO: Michael J. Maiberger, Executive Vice President and Chief Operating Officer
CFO: Randal Lennartz, Senior Vice President and Chief Financial Officer
CMO: Barbara Evert, M.D., Vice President Medical Services and Chief Medical Officer
CIO: William Watercutter, Director Management Information System
CHR: Tracy Moser, Director Human Resources
Web address: www.uvmc.com
Control: Other not–for–profit (including NFP Corporation) **Service:** General Medical and Surgical

Staffed Beds: 168

UPPER SANDUSKY—Wyandot County

★ **WYANDOT MEMORIAL HOSPITAL (361329)**, 885 North Sandusky Avenue, Zip 43351–1098; tel. 419/294–4991 **A**9 10 18 **F**3 11 13 15 17 24 25 27 31 32 38 46 55 57 62 63 72 73 74 75 76 77 79 80 81 82 84 86 87 96 97 103 106 107 118 122 124 135 137 **P**6
Primary Contact: Joseph A. D'Ettorre, Chief Executive Officer
COO: Ty Shaull, Chief Operating Officer
CFO: Alan H. Yeates, Vice President Fiscal Services
CMO: Eric M. Stemmer, D.O., Chief of Staff
CHR: Vickie Underwood, Director Human Resources
Web address: www.wyandotmemorial.com
Control: Hospital district or authority, Government, nonfederal **Service:** General Medical and Surgical

Staffed Beds: 25 **Admissions:** 786 **Census:** 7 **Outpatient Visits:** 47380 **Births:** 128 **Total Expense ($000):** 21077 **Payroll Expense ($000):** 8833 **Personnel:** 181

URBANA—Champaign County

★ **MERCY MEMORIAL HOSPITAL (361312)**, 904 Scioto Street, Zip 43078–2200; tel. 937/653–5231 **A**1 9 10 18 **F**11 30 31 32 38 66 68 73 75 77 79 80 82 86 96 107 119 122 123 124 135 **S** Catholic Healthcare Partners
Primary Contact: Jeanne Bowman, Administrator and Chief Nursing Officer
Web address: www.mercy–health.org
Control: Church–operated, Nongovernment, not–for profit **Service:** General Medical and Surgical

Staffed Beds: 25 **Admissions:** 1014 **Census:** 9 **Outpatient Visits:** 57008 **Births:** 0 **Total Expense ($000):** 17018 **Payroll Expense ($000):** 6359 **Personnel:** 116

VAN WERT—Van Wert County

★ **VAN WERT COUNTY HOSPITAL (360071)**, 1250 South Washington Street, Zip 45891–2599; tel. 419/238–2390 **A**1 5 9 10 **F**8 13 24 27 32 33 37 38 52 53 55 56 57 62 68 71 74 77 79 80 84 86 96 97 102 107 118 119 120 121 135 **P**7 8
Primary Contact: Mark J. Minick, President and Chief Executive Officer
CFO: Michael T. Holliday, Vice President Fiscal and Administrative Services
CMO: Scott Jarvis, M.D., President Medical Staff
CIO: Jerry Borton, Manager Information
CHR: Joyce Pothast, Vice President Human and Environmental Services
Web address: www.vanwerthospital.org
Control: Other not–for–profit (including NFP Corporation) **Service:** General Medical and Surgical

Staffed Beds: 79 **Admissions:** 1955 **Census:** 19 **Outpatient Visits:** 63566 **Births:** 309 **Total Expense ($000):** 36107 **Payroll Expense ($000):** 12182 **Personnel:** 270

WADSWORTH—Medina County

□ **WADSWORTH–RITTMAN HOSPITAL (360195)**, 195 Wadsworth Road, Zip 44281–9505; tel. 330/334–1504, (Nonreporting) **A**1 5 9 10 **S** Summa Health System
Primary Contact: James W. Pope, FACHE, President and Chief Executive Officer
COO: Carolyn Laughlin, Chief Operating Officer
CFO: Charles Alderson, Chief Financial Officer
CMO: Jeffrey Morris, M.D., Vice President Medical Affairs
CIO: Gina Rood, Director Information Services
CHR: Marilyn Haskins, Senior Director Human Resources
Web address: www.wrhhs.org
Control: Other not–for–profit (including NFP Corporation) **Service:** General Medical and Surgical

Staffed Beds: 67

WARREN—Trumbull County

□ **FORUM HEALTH TRUMBULL MEMORIAL HOSPITAL (360055)**, 1350 East Market Street, Zip 44482–6628; tel. 330/841–9011, (Nonreporting) **A**1 2 3 5 9 10 **S** Forum Health
Primary Contact: Todd Hickey, CHE, Interim Chief Executive Officer
COO: Todd Hickey, CHE, Vice President Operations
CFO: Doug Wermer, Senior Vice President and Chief Financial Officer
CMO: Thomas L. James, M.D., Senior Vice President and Chief Medical Officer
CIO: Timothy Roe, Chief Information Officer
CHR: David Swift, Senior Vice President Human Resources
Web address: www.forumhealth.org
Control: Other not–for–profit (including NFP Corporation) **Service:** General Medical and Surgical

Staffed Beds: 292

□ △ **FORUM HILLSIDE REHABILITATION HOSPITAL (363026)**, 8747 Squires Lane N.E., Zip 44484–1649; tel. 330/841–3700, (Nonreporting) **A**1 5 7 9 10 **S** Forum Health
Primary Contact: Marilyn Titus, Vice President and Chief Operating Officer
COO: Marilyn Titus, Vice President and Chief Operating Officer
CFO: Truman Esmond, Senior Vice President and Chief Financial Officer
CMO: Terry Puet, M.D., Medical Director
CIO: Timothy Roe, Chief Information Officer
CHR: David Swift, Senior Vice President Human Resources
Web address: www.forumhealth.org
Control: County–Government, nonfederal **Service:** Rehabilitation

Staffed Beds: 47

Hospital, Medicare Provider Number, Address, Telephone, Approval, Facility, and Physician Codes, Health Care System

★ American Hospital Association (AHA) membership
□ The Joint Commission accreditation
○ American Osteopathic Association (AOA) accreditation
△ Commission on Accreditation of Rehabilitation Facilities (CARF) accreditation

★ ○ **ST. JOSEPH HEALTH CENTER (360161)**, 667 Eastland Avenue S.E., Zip 44484–4531; tel. 330/841–4000 **A**1 2 9 10 11 12 13 **F**3 5 8 11 12 13 15 24 25 26 27 30 32 33 38 39 40 41 43 44 46 50 51 52 53 54 55 57 59 60 62 64 67 68 73 74 75 76 77 79 80 81 82 84 86 87 88 89 90 91 92 93 94 96 97 98 100 102 104 105 106 107 109 111 118 119 121 132 133 135 136 137 **S** Catholic Healthcare Partners
Primary Contact: Robert W. Shroder, President and Chief Executive Officer
COO: John Finizio, President
CFO: Donald E. Kline, Senior Vice President Finance
CMO: Nicholas Kreatsoulas, M.D., Senior Vice President and Chief Medical Officer
CIO: Charles Folkwein, Vice President Ancillary Services and Information Technology
CHR: Molly Seals, Senior Vice President Human Resources and Organizational Development
Web address: www.hmpartners.org
Control: Church–operated, Nongovernment, not–for profit **Service:** General Medical and Surgical

Staffed Beds: 162 **Admissions:** 8536 **Census:** 104 **Outpatient Visits:** 164237 **Births:** 772 **Total Expense ($000):** 98372 **Payroll Expense ($000):** 35845 **Personnel:** 586

WARRENSVILLE HEIGHTS—Morgan County

□ ○ **SOUTH POINTE HOSPITAL (360144)**, 20000 Harvard Road, Zip 44122–7099; tel. 216/491–6000, (Total facility includes 29 beds in nursing home–type unit) **A**1 2 9 10 11 12 13 **F**11 15 18 24 25 26 27 28 30 31 32 33 34 36 37 38 39 41 43 44 46 49 50 51 52 53 55 56 57 58 59 60 62 64 67 68 69 75 76 77 79 80 82 86 87 88 89 90 91 92 93 94 95 96 97 100 102 104 105 106 107 113 117 119 120 121 123 124 132 133 135 136 137 **S** Cleveland Clinic Health System
Primary Contact: David J. Kilarski, President and Chief Executive Officer
COO: William A. Young, Chief Operating Officer
CFO: Georgianna Umbel, Director Finance
CMO: Charles Webb, M.D., Chief of Staff
CIO: Ralph A. Cagna, Director Information Technology
CHR: Doris Zajec, Director
Web address: www.southpointehospital.org
Control: Other not–for–profit (including NFP Corporation) **Service:** General Medical and Surgical

Staffed Beds: 259 **Admissions:** 10575 **Census:** 187 **Outpatient Visits:** 173321 **Total Expense ($000):** 134986 **Payroll Expense ($000):** 63813 **Personnel:** 1383

WASHINGTON COURT HOUSE—Lucas County

★ **FAYETTE COUNTY MEMORIAL HOSPITAL (361331)**, 1430 Columbus Avenue, Zip 43160–1791; tel. 740/335–1210 **A**9 10 18 **F**3 11 13 15 25 31 33 37 38 43 55 56 57 61 62 66 67 68 72 73 75 76 77 79 80 81 82 86 87 92 96 97 99 100 107 118 120 121 124 135 136 137 **P**4 **S** Trinity Health
Primary Contact: Lyndon J. Christman, Administrator
CFO: Chris Peters, Vice President Finance
CMO: Greg Schall, D.O., Chief of Staff
CIO: Bruce Denen, Manager Data Processing
CHR: Earlene Christensen, Director Human Resources
Web address: www.fcmh.org
Control: County–Government, nonfederal **Service:** General Medical and Surgical

Staffed Beds: 25 **Admissions:** 1337 **Census:** 11 **Outpatient Visits:** 78219 **Births:** 330 **Total Expense ($000):** 32875 **Payroll Expense ($000):** 13737 **Personnel:** 303

WAUSEON—Fulton County

★ **FULTON COUNTY HEALTH CENTER (361333)**, 725 South Shoop Avenue, Zip 43567–1701; tel. 419/335–2015, (Total facility includes 71 beds in nursing home–type unit) **A**1 2 9 10 18 **F**8 11 13 15 24 25 27 30 31 32 38 52 55 56 57 65 67 68 73 74 75 76 77 79 82 86 88 91 92 93 94 95 96 97 100 103 106 107 115 117 118 119 120 121 124 135 137
Primary Contact: E. Dean Beck, Administrator
COO: Patti Finn, Assistant Administrator
CFO: Darrell Topmiller, Director Finance
CIO: Larry Hefflinger, Director Information Systems
CHR: Kristy Snyder, Director Human Resources
Web address: www.fultoncountyhealthcenter.org
Control: Other not–for–profit (including NFP Corporation) **Service:** General Medical and Surgical

Staffed Beds: 121 **Admissions:** 2317 **Census:** 89 **Outpatient Visits:** 155154 **Births:** 365 **Total Expense ($000):** 64156 **Payroll Expense ($000):** 26257 **Personnel:** 677

WAVERLY—Pike County

○ **PIKE COMMUNITY HOSPITAL (361334)**, 100 Dawn Lane, Zip 45690–9664; tel. 740/947–2186 **A**9 10 11 18 **F**11 15 33 53 56 68 79 86 96 100 102 107 119 122 135 **P**6
Primary Contact: Craig E. Solle, President and Chief Executive Officer
COO: Craig E. Solle, President and Chief Executive Officer
CFO: Sharon Novak, CPA, Vice President
CMO: David Roddy, M.D., Medical Director and Chief of Staff
CHR: Wanda Guggisberg, Vice President Human Resources
Web address: www.pikecommunityhospital.org
Control: Other not–for–profit (including NFP Corporation) **Service:** General Medical and Surgical

Staffed Beds: 25 **Admissions:** 1200 **Census:** 10 **Outpatient Visits:** 47400 **Births:** 0 **Personnel:** 303

WEST CHESTER—Butler County

□ **UNIVERSITY POINTE SURGICAL HOSPITAL (360271)**, 7750 University Court, Zip 45069; tel. 513/475–8300 **A**1 9 10 **F**3 15 30 43 46 47 48 49 55 62 79 80 96 100 103 107
Primary Contact: Carol King, Executive Director
COO: Sara Deem, Director Operations
CFO: Tom Ducro, Chief Financial Officer
CMO: Lesley Gilbertson, M.D., Medical Director
CHR: Penny Elder, Manager Human Resources
Web address: www.upsurgicalhospital.com
Control: Other not–for–profit (including NFP Corporation) **Service:** Surgical

Staffed Beds: 8 **Admissions:** 25 **Census:** 1 **Outpatient Visits:** 15587 **Births:** 0 **Personnel:** 50

WEST UNION—Adams County

★ **ADAMS COUNTY HOSPITAL (361326)**, 210 North Wilson Drive, Zip 45693–1574; tel. 937/544–5571, (Nonreporting) **A**1 9 10 18
Primary Contact: Linda Niles, Chief Executive Officer
CFO: Dewey Applegate, Chief Financial Officer
CHR: Joyce Porter, Chief Human Resources Officer
Web address: www.bright.net/~ach
Control: County–Government, nonfederal **Service:** General Medical and Surgical

Staffed Beds: 25

WESTERVILLE—Franklin County

★ **MOUNT CARMEL ST. ANN'S (360012)**, 500 South Cleveland Avenue, Zip 43081–8998; tel. 614/898–4000 **A**1 2 3 5 9 10 **F**3 6 11 13 15 18 25 26 27 30 31 32 33 34 35 38 41 42 43 44 45 46 47 48 49 50 56 57 58 60 61 62 63 64 66 68 69 70 71 72 73 74 76 77 79 80 81 82 86 87 90 91 92 93 94 96 97 98 100 102 103 104 106 107 109 111 114 119 120 121 122 124 135 136 137 **S** Trinity Health
Primary Contact: Claus von Zychlin, Executive Vice President and Chief Operating Officer
Web address: www.mountcarmelhealth.com
Control: Church–operated, Nongovernment, not–for profit **Service:** General Medical and Surgical

Staffed Beds: 273 **Admissions:** 17470 **Census:** 183 **Outpatient Visits:** 187195 **Births:** 4882 **Total Expense ($000):** 178406 **Payroll Expense ($000):** 68668 **Personnel:** 1291

WILLARD—Huron County

★ **MERCY HOSPITAL OF WILLARD (361310)**, 110 East Howard Street, Zip 44890–1611; tel. 419/964–5000 **A**1 5 9 10 18 **F**3 5 13 15 24 26 30 31 32 33 38 44 46 55 56 57 68 73 74 75 77 79 80 82 84 86 94 96 100 102 105 107 119 121 122 132 135 136 **S** Catholic Healthcare Partners
Primary Contact: Robert E. Gospodarek, President and Chief Executive Officer
CFO: Lynn Detterman, Chief Financial Officer
CMO: Christopher Bohach, DPM, Chief of Staff
CHR: Diana Olson, Chief Human Resources Officer
Web address: www.mercyweb.org
Control: Church–operated, Nongovernment, not–for profit **Service:** General Medical and Surgical

Staffed Beds: 25 **Admissions:** 703 **Census:** 10 **Outpatient Visits:** 42707 **Births:** 131 **Total Expense ($000):** 20441 **Payroll Expense ($000):** 8704 **Personnel:** 188

WILLOUGHBY—Lake County

□ **WINDSOR–LAURELWOOD CENTER FOR BEHAVIORAL MEDICINE (364029)**, (Formerly Laurelwood Hospital), 35900 Euclid Avenue, Zip 44094–4648; tel. 440/953–3000, (Nonreporting) **A**1 9 10 **S** Horizon Health Corporation
Primary Contact: David Fletcher–Janzen, Chief Executive Officer
CMO: Leonard Barley, M.D., Chief Medical Officer
CHR: Nicole Ostrosky, Director Human Resources
Web address: www.laurelwoodhospital.com
Control: Individual, Investor–owned, for–profit **Service:** Psychiatric

Staffed Beds: 160

WILMINGTON—Clinton County

★ △ **CLINTON MEMORIAL HOSPITAL (360175)**, 610 West Main Street, Zip 45177–0600; tel. 937/382–6611 **A**1 2 3 5 7 9 10 **F**11 13 15 18 25 26 27 30 31 32 33 37 38 50 51 52 53 54 56 57 61 62 66 67 68 69 72 73 74 75 76 77 79 81 82 85 86 87 96 97 100 102 105 107 109 118 119 120 121 124 133 135 136 137 **P**1
Primary Contact: Andrew J. Riddell, President and Chief Executive Officer
CFO: Karen Shadowens, Vice President and Chief Financial Officer
CMO: Michael C. Choo, M.D., Chief of Staff
CHR: Mary Ann Foland, Manager Human Resources
Web address: www.cmhregional.com
Control: County–Government, nonfederal **Service:** General Medical and Surgical

Staffed Beds: 93 **Admissions:** 4220 **Census:** 45 **Outpatient Visits:** 133888 **Births:** 699 **Total Expense ($000):** 98238 **Payroll Expense ($000):** 39136 **Personnel:** 788

WOOSTER—Wayne County

☐ **WOOSTER COMMUNITY HOSPITAL (360036)**, 1761 Beall Avenue, Zip 44691–2342; tel. 330/263–8100 **A**1 2 5 9 10 19 **F**3 11 13 14 15 18 24 25 26 27 28 30 31 32 33 38 49 51 52 55 57 60 61 62 68 72 73 74 75 76 77 79 80 81 82 84 85 86 96 97 99 100 102 103 106 107 118 119 121 124 132 135 136 137 **P**8 **S** QHR
Primary Contact: William E. Sheron, Chief Executive Officer
Web address: www.woosterhospital.org
Control: City–Government, nonfederal **Service:** General Medical and Surgical

Staffed Beds: 150 **Admissions:** 5700 **Census:** 58 **Outpatient Visits:** 184362 **Births:** 1080 **Total Expense ($000):** 73141 **Payroll Expense ($000):** 32691 **Personnel:** 705

WRIGHT–PATTERSON AFB—Greene County

★ **WRIGHT PATTERSON MEDICAL CENTER**, 4881 Sugar Maple Drive, Zip 45433–5529; tel. 937/257–9133, (Nonreporting) **A**1 2 3 5 **S** Department of the Air Force
Primary Contact: Colonel Mark S. White, Administrator
COO: Colonel Mark S. White, Administrator
CFO: Levi Braswell, Flight Commander Resource Management
CMO: Colonel Brantley Baynes, M.D., Chief Medical Officer
CIO: Matt Osborne, Medical Information Systems Flight Chief
CHR: Rhonda Buie, Chief Civilian Personnel
Web address: www.wpmc1.wpafb.af.mil
Control: Air Force, Government, federal **Service:** General Medical and Surgical

Staffed Beds: 70

XENIA—Greene County

★ △ **GREENE MEMORIAL HOSPITAL (360026)**, 1141 North Monroe Drive, Zip 45385–1600; tel. 937/352–2000, (Total facility includes 90 beds in nursing home–type unit) **A**1 2 5 7 9 10 **F**3 5 6 8 9 10 11 12 13 15 18 24 25 26 27 30 31 33 38 40 41 42 43 44 46 50 53 54 55 56 57 59 60 61 62 63 66 67 68 69 72 73 74 75 76 77 78 79 80 81 85 86 87 88 89 90 91 92 93 94 95 96 97 100 102 106 107 109 115 116 117 118 119 120 121 124 133 135 136 137 **P**4 8 **S** Kettering Health Network
Primary Contact: Michael R. Stephens, President
COO: Timothy Ols, Vice President and Chief Operating Officer
CFO: Timothy J. Pollard, Chief Financial Officer
CMO: David Goldberg, M.D., Medical Director
CIO: Ellen M. Predaina, Director Management Information Systems
CHR: Barbara Coalter, Director Human Resources
Web address: www.greenehealth.org
Control: Other not–for–profit (including NFP Corporation) **Service:** General Medical and Surgical

Staffed Beds: 204 **Admissions:** 4600 **Census:** 47 **Outpatient Visits:** 28467 **Births:** 214 **Total Expense ($000):** 81106 **Payroll Expense ($000):** 31188 **Personnel:** 752

YOUNGSTOWN—Mahoning County

☐ **BELMONT PINES HOSPITAL (364038)**, 615 Churchill–Hubbard Road, Zip 44505–1379; tel. 330/759–2700, (Nonreporting) **A**1 9 10 **S** Psychiatric Solutions
Primary Contact: George H. Perry, Ph.D., Chief Executive Officer
CFO: Robin Stough, Chief Financial Officer
CMO: Phillip Maiden, M.D., Medical Director
Web address: www.belmontpines.com
Control: Corporation, Investor–owned, for–profit **Service:** Psychiatric

Staffed Beds: 46

☐ **MAHONING VALLEY HOSPITAL (362023)**, 345 Oak Hill Avenue, Suite 210, Zip 44502; tel. 330/480–1250, (Nonreporting) **A**1 10
Primary Contact: Michael S. Senchak, President and Chief Executive Officer
Control: Corporation, Investor–owned, for–profit **Service:** Long–Term Acute Care hospital

Staffed Beds: 45

NORTHSIDE MEDICAL CENTER See Western Reserve Care System

☐ **SELECT SPECIALTY HOSPITAL–YOUNGSTOWN (362024)**, 1044 Belmont Avenue, Zip 44501; tel. 330/480–2349, (Nonreporting) **A**1 10 **S** Select Medical Corporation
Primary Contact: MaryJo Shuntich, Chief Executive Officer
Web address: www.selectmedicalcorp.com
Control: Corporation, Investor–owned, for–profit **Service:** Long–Term Acute Care hospital

Staffed Beds: 31

★ △ **ST. ELIZABETH HEALTH CENTER (360064)**, 1044 Belmont Avenue, Zip 44504–1096, Mailing Address: P.O. Box 1790, Zip 44501–1790; tel. 330/746–7211 **A**1 2 3 5 7 8 9 10 **F**3 7 8 11 12 13 14 15 18 20 22 24 25 26 27 28 30 32 33 37 38 39 40 41 43 44 46 50 51 52 53 54 55 56 57 58 59 60 62 64 66 67 68 69 70 72 73 74 75 76 77 79 80 81 82 84 85 86 87 88 90 91 92 93 94 96 97 98 99 100 102 103 104 105 106 107 111 112 116 118 119 120 121 124 132 135 136 137 **S** Catholic Healthcare Partners
Primary Contact: Robert W. Shroder, President and Chief Executive Officer
COO: James R. Davis, Executive Vice President and Chief Operating Officer
CFO: Donald E. Kline, Senior Vice President Finance
CMO: Nicholas Kreatsoulas, M.D., Senior Vice President and Chief Medical Officer
CIO: Charles Folkwein, Senior Vice President Ancillary Services and Information Technology
CHR: Molly Seals, Senior Vice President Human Resources
Web address: www.hmpartners.org
Control: Church–operated, Nongovernment, not–for profit **Service:** General Medical and Surgical

Staffed Beds: 418 **Admissions:** 24858 **Census:** 331 **Outpatient Visits:** 349344 **Births:** 1201 **Total Expense ($000):** 280244 **Payroll Expense ($000):** 99173 **Personnel:** 1712

TOD CHILDREN'S HOSPITAL See Western Reserve Care System

☐ **WESTERN RESERVE CARE SYSTEM (360141)**, 500 Gypsy Lane, Zip 44501–0240, Mailing Address: P.O. Box 990, Zip 44501–0990; tel. 330/747–1444, (Includes NORTHSIDE MEDICAL CENTER, tel. 330/747–1444; TOD CHILDREN'S HOSPITAL, tel. 330/747–6700), (Nonreporting) **A**1 3 5 8 9 10 **S** Forum Health
Primary Contact: Keith T. Ghezzi, M.D., President and Chief Executive Officer
COO: Roxia B. Boykin, R.N., Interim Chief Operating Officer
CFO: Henry Seybold, Senior Vice President and Chief Financial Officer
CMO: Robert Sinsheimer, M.D., Senior Vice President Medical Affairs
CIO: Timothy Roe, Chief Information Officer
Web address: www.forumhealth.org
Control: Other not–for–profit (including NFP Corporation) **Service:** General Medical and Surgical

Staffed Beds: 373

ZANESVILLE—Muskingum County

★ △ **GENESIS HEALTHCARE SYSTEM (360039)**, 2951 Maple Avenue, Zip 43701–2881; tel. 740/454–5000, (Includes BETHESDA HOSPITAL, 2951 Maple Avenue, Zip 43701–1465; tel. 614/454–4000; GOOD SAMARITAN MEDICAL AND REHABILITATION CENTER, 800 Forest Avenue), (Total facility includes 17 beds in nursing home–type unit) **A**1 2 5 7 9 10 19 **F**3 5 11 13 15 17 18 20 22 24 25 26 27 28 30 31 32 33 34 38 41 42 43 44 45 50 51 53 54 55 56 57 58 59 62 63 66 68 72 73 74 75 76 77 78 79 80 81 82 84 85 86 87 88 89 90 91 92 93 94 95 96 97 99 100 102 104 105 106 107 109 110 111 112 117 118 119 121 124 133 135 136 **P**8 **S** Franciscan Sisters of Christian Charity HealthCare Ministry, Inc
Primary Contact: Matthew J. Perry, President and Chief Executive Officer
CFO: Paul Masterson, Chief Financial Officer
CIO: Ed Romito, Director Information Systems
Web address: www.genesishcs.org
Control: Other not–for–profit (including NFP Corporation) **Service:** General Medical and Surgical

Staffed Beds: 395 **Admissions:** 16114 **Census:** 191 **Outpatient Visits:** 266870 **Births:** 1445 **Total Expense ($000):** 207594 **Payroll Expense ($000):** 84063 **Personnel:** 2182

Hospital, Medicare Provider Number, Address, Telephone, Approval, Facility, and Physician Codes, Health Care System

★ American Hospital Association (AHA) membership
☐ The Joint Commission accreditation
○ American Osteopathic Association (AOA) accreditation
△ Commission on Accreditation of Rehabilitation Facilities (CARF) accreditation

☐ **SELECT SPECIALTY HOSPITAL–ZANESVILLE (362031)**, 800 Forest Avenue, 6th Floor, Zip 43701; tel. 740/588–7888 **A**1 10 **F**1 55 56 57 63 80 137
S Select Medical Corporation
Primary Contact: Linda Supplee, Chief Executive Officer
Web address: www.selectmedicalcorp.com
Control: Corporation, Investor–owned, for–profit **Service:** Long–Term Acute Care hospital

Staffed Beds: 35 **Admissions:** 257 **Census:** 17 **Outpatient Visits:** 0 **Births:** 0 **Personnel:** 59

 Many Facility Codes have changed. Please refer to the AHA Guide Code Chart.

OKLAHOMA

ADA—Pontotoc County

★□ **CHICKASAW NATION HEALTH SYSTEM (370180)**, 1001 North Country Club Road, Zip 74820–2847; tel. 580/436–3980, (Nonreporting) **A**1 10
Primary Contact: Bill Lance, Administrator
COO: Sandi Sanders, Chief Operating Officer
CFO: Jenny Trett, Chief Financial Officer
CMO: Tina Cooper, M.D., Medical Director
CIO: Terry Clark, Chief Information Officer
CHR: Jalinda Kelley, Director
Web address: www.ihs.gov
Control: Other not–for–profit (including NFP Corporation) **Service:** General Medical and Surgical

Staffed Beds: 51

□ **ROLLING HILLS HOSPITAL (374016)**, 1000 Rolling Hills Lane, Zip 74820–9415; tel. 580/436–3600 **A**1 9 10 **F**4 31 32 88 91 92 93 119 **S** Liberty Management Group, Inc.
Primary Contact: Brian Beutin, M.S., Chief Executive Officer
CFO: Ted McKinney, Chief Financial Officer
CMO: Robert Morton, M.D., Medical Director
CIO: Sherry Barnes, Director Health Information Management and Quality Management
CHR: Timothy Blackwell, Manager Human Resources
Web address: www.rollinghillshospital.com
Control: Corporation, Investor–owned, for–profit **Service:** Psychiatric

Staffed Beds: 40 **Admissions:** 974 **Census:** 37 **Births:** 0 **Total Expense ($000):** 6686 **Payroll Expense ($000):** 3524 **Personnel:** 166

★□ △ **VALLEY VIEW REGIONAL HOSPITAL (370020)**, 430 North Monta Vista, Zip 74820–4610; tel. 580/332–2323 **A**1 2 7 9 10 19 20 **F**3 7 8 15 18 25 26 27 32 38 51 61 67 68 72 73 74 76 77 79 84 85 97 100 105 107 118 119 122 124 133 135 137 **P**8
Primary Contact: Ronald W. Webb, President and Chief Executive Officer
CFO: Rory Ward, Chief Financial Officer
CIO: Dennis Jackson, Director Management Information Systems
CHR: David Jordan, Vice President Human Resources
Web address: www.valleyviewregional.com
Control: Other not–for–profit (including NFP Corporation) **Service:** General Medical and Surgical

Staffed Beds: 131 **Admissions:** 5244 **Census:** 61 **Outpatient Visits:** 56070 **Births:** 605 **Total Expense ($000):** 68098 **Payroll Expense ($000):** 25449 **Personnel:** 606

ALTUS—Jackson County

★□ **JACKSON COUNTY MEMORIAL HOSPITAL (370022)**, 1200 East Pecan Street, Zip 73521–6192, Mailing Address: Box 8190, Zip 73522–8190; tel. 580/482–4781, (Total facility includes 16 beds in nursing home–type unit) **A**1 5 9 10 19 20 **F**3 10 11 13 15 25 26 27 31 33 38 40 42 55 57 59 61 62 63 66 68 73 74 75 76 77 79 80 81 82 85 86 90 91 93 94 96 97 100 102 107 117 118 119 121 124 134 135 136 137
Primary Contact: William G. Wilson, President and Chief Executive Officer
COO: Jim King, Executive Vice President and Chief Operating Officer
CFO: Nancy Davidson, Senior Vice President and Chief Financial Officer
CMO: M. George Zakhary, M.D., Chief of Staff
CIO: David Parker, Director Information Systems
CHR: Tom Graham, Vice President Human Resources
Web address: www.jcmh.com
Control: Hospital district or authority, Government, nonfederal **Service:** General Medical and Surgical

Staffed Beds: 85 **Admissions:** 5608 **Census:** 54 **Births:** 543 **Total Expense ($000):** 58423 **Payroll Expense ($000):** 26634 **Personnel:** 675

ALVA—Woods County

★ **SHARE MEDICAL CENTER (370080)**, 800 Share Drive, Zip 73717–3699, Mailing Address: P.O. Box 727, Zip 73717–0727; tel. 580/327–2800, (Total facility includes 65 beds in nursing home–type unit) **A**9 10 20 **F**15 30 31 38 42 55 61 65 67 79 85 96 100 107 122 137 **S** QHR
Primary Contact: Barbara Oestmann, Chief Executive Officer
CFO: Denise Reed, Chief Financial Officer
CMO: Kirt Bierig, D.O., Chief of Staff
CHR: Kristi Moorman, Supervisor Human Resources
Web address: www.smcok.com
Control: Hospital district or authority, Government, nonfederal **Service:** General Medical and Surgical

Staffed Beds: 102 **Admissions:** 691 **Census:** 67 **Outpatient Visits:** 14827 **Births:** 0 **Total Expense ($000):** 9262 **Payroll Expense ($000):** 4756 **Personnel:** 161

ANADARKO—Caddo County

PHYSICIANS' HOSPITAL IN ANADARKO (371314), 1002 Central Boulevard East, Zip 73005–4496; tel. 405/247–2551, (Nonreporting) **A**9 10 18 **S** The Schuster Group
Primary Contact: Joe Swart, Administrator
Control: Partnership, Investor–owned, for–profit **Service:** General Medical and Surgical

Staffed Beds: 25

ANTLERS—Pushmataha County

PUSHMATAHA COUNTY–TOWN OF ANTLERS HOSPITAL AUTHORITY (370083), 510 East Main Street, Zip 74523–3262, Mailing Address: P.O. Box 518, Zip 74523–3262; tel. 580/298–3342, (Nonreporting) **A**9 10
Primary Contact: Mark Rogers, Chief Executive Officer
CFO: Stephen Poe, Chief Financial Officer
CMO: Herbert Rowland, M.D., Chief of Staff
CHR: Pat McCarty, Director Human Resources
Web address: www.pushhospital.com
Control: City–County, Government, nonfederal **Service:** General Medical and Surgical

Staffed Beds: 33

ARDMORE—Carter County

★□ **MERCY MEMORIAL HEALTH CENTER (370047)**, 1011 14th Avenue N.W., Zip 73401–1889; tel. 580/223–5400 **A**1 9 10 19 20 **F**3 11 13 15 18 20 25 26 30 31 32 33 37 38 40 52 54 55 56 57 60 61 62 68 74 75 76 79 81 82 85 96 100 107 118 119 133 135 137 **P**6 8 **S** Sisters of Mercy Health System
Primary Contact: Bobby G. Thompson, President and Chief Executive Officer
COO: Jay Johnson, Chief Operating Officer
CMO: William Parsons, D.O., Vice President Medical Affairs
Web address: www.mercyok.net
Control: Church–operated, Nongovernment, not–for profit **Service:** General Medical and Surgical

Staffed Beds: 159 **Admissions:** 10081 **Census:** 115 **Outpatient Visits:** 70201 **Births:** 1009 **Total Expense ($000):** 85771 **Payroll Expense ($000):** 33906 **Personnel:** 719

ATOKA—Atoka County

★ **ATOKA MEMORIAL HOSPITAL (371300)**, 1501 South Virginia Avenue, Zip 74525–3298; tel. 580/889–3333 **A**9 10 18 **F**3 11 24 25 32 33 38 55 56 57 62 79 80 86 92 96 102 107 122 135 137 **P**5 6
Primary Contact: Charles E. Young, Ph.D., Chief Executive Officer
CFO: Jamie McGaugh, Controller
CMO: Bruce Rumbaugh, M.D., Director Patient Care
CHR: Naomi Farris, Director Human Resources
Web address: www.atoka–hosp.otnnet.net
Control: County–Government, nonfederal **Service:** General Medical and Surgical

Staffed Beds: 25 **Admissions:** 432 **Census:** 4 **Outpatient Visits:** 10097 **Births:** 0 **Total Expense ($000):** 6052 **Payroll Expense ($000):** 3438 **Personnel:** 85

Hospital, Medicare Provider Number, Address, Telephone, Approval, Facility, and Physician Codes, Health Care System

★ American Hospital Association (AHA) membership
□ The Joint Commission accreditation
○ American Osteopathic Association (AOA) accreditation
△ Commission on Accreditation of Rehabilitation Facilities (CARF) accreditation

BARTLESVILLE—Washington County

CONTINUOUS CARE CENTERS OF BARTLESVILLE (372014), 3500 East Frank Phillips Boulevard, 4 Tower, Zip 74006; tel. 918/331–1452 **A**9 10 **F**1 25 38 43 44 75 119 137 **P**8
Primary Contact: John Kerlin, Administrator
COO: Mike Harris, Vice President and Chief Operating Officer
CFO: Basil Wyatt, Vice President and Chief Financial Officer
CMO: Mark Myers, M.D., Chief Medical Officer
CIO: Dana Jetton, Director Information Technology
CHR: Sunny Benjamin, Director Human Resources
Web address: www.cccok.com
Control: Other not–for–profit (including NFP Corporation) **Service:** Long–Term Acute Care hospital

Staffed Beds: 16 **Admissions:** 171 **Census:** 13 **Outpatient Visits:** 0 **Births:** 0 **Total Expense ($000):** 5152 **Payroll Expense ($000):** 1916 **Personnel:** 44

☒ **JANE PHILLIPS MEDICAL CENTER (370018)**, 3500 East Frank Phillips Boulevard, Zip 74006–2409; tel. 918/333–7200 **A**1 2 3 5 9 10 19 **F**3 11 13 15 17 18 20 22 24 25 26 27 30 31 32 33 38 40 43 50 51 52 55 56 57 58 59 60 61 66 69 72 73 74 75 76 77 79 80 81 82 85 86 88 93 96 100 102 103 104 105 106 107 111 118 119 120 124 132 133 135 136 137 **P**4
S Marian Health System
Primary Contact: David R. Stire, President and Chief Executive Officer
CFO: Mike Moore, Chief Financial Officer
CIO: Rob Poole, Director
CHR: Jennifer Workman, Director Human Resources
Web address: www.jpmc.org
Control: Church–operated, Nongovernment, not–for profit **Service:** General Medical and Surgical

Staffed Beds: 137 **Admissions:** 6663 **Census:** 80 **Outpatient Visits:** 67717 **Births:** 789 **Total Expense ($000):** 85275 **Payroll Expense ($000):** 32907 **Personnel:** 725

BEAVER—Beaver County

BEAVER COUNTY MEMORIAL HOSPITAL (371322), 212 East Eighth Street, Zip 73932, Mailing Address: P.O. Box 640, Zip 73932–0640; tel. 580/625–4551 **A**9 10 18 **F**31 38 57 122 **P**6
Primary Contact: Brent Meyers, Administrator
Control: Hospital district or authority, Government, nonfederal **Service:** General Medical and Surgical

Staffed Beds: 15 **Admissions:** 154 **Census:** 1 **Outpatient Visits:** 1047 **Births:** 0 **Total Expense ($000):** 4237 **Payroll Expense ($000):** 1627 **Personnel:** 43

BLACKWELL—Kay County

☒ **INTEGRIS BLACKWELL REGIONAL HOSPITAL (370030)**, 710 South 13th Street, Zip 74631–3700; tel. 580/363–2311, (Nonreporting) **A**1 9 10
S INTEGRIS Health
Primary Contact: Rex Van Meter, President
CMO: Paul Briggs, M.D., Chief of Staff
Web address: www.integris–health.com
Control: Other not–for–profit (including NFP Corporation) **Service:** General Medical and Surgical

Staffed Beds: 34

BOISE CITY—Cimarron County

CIMARRON MEMORIAL HOSPITAL (371307), 100 South Ellis Street, Zip 73933; tel. 580/544–2501, (Nonreporting) **A**9 10 18
Primary Contact: David M. Peyok, Chief Executive Officer
Control: County–Government, nonfederal **Service:** General Medical and Surgical

Staffed Beds: 20

BRISTOW—Creek County

★ **BRISTOW MEDICAL CENTER (370041)**, 700 West 7th Street, Suite 6, Zip 74010; tel. 918/367–2215 **A**9 10 **F**3 11 25 33 38 55 56 61 77 79 84 86 96 107 122 135 **P**1 7
Primary Contact: David Jamin, Chief Executive Officer
CFO: Robin Van Vickle, Chief Financial Officer
Control: Corporation, Investor–owned, for–profit **Service:** General Medical and Surgical

Staffed Beds: 17 **Admissions:** 514 **Census:** 5 **Outpatient Visits:** 10067 **Births:** 0 **Total Expense ($000):** 6372 **Payroll Expense ($000):** 3265 **Personnel:** 63

BUFFALO—Harper County

★ **HARPER COUNTY COMMUNITY HOSPITAL (371324)**, Highway 64 North, Zip 73834, Mailing Address: P.O. Box 60, Zip 73834–0060; tel. 580/735–2555 **A**9 10 18 **F**31 38 67 73 74 79 82 84 86 96 107 117 122 **P**5
Primary Contact: Karen Ives, Interim Administrator
CIO: Kim Hudson, Chief Information Officer
Control: County–Government, nonfederal **Service:** General Medical and Surgical

Staffed Beds: 20 **Admissions:** 274 **Census:** 2 **Outpatient Visits:** 1061 **Births:** 15 **Total Expense ($000):** 2224 **Payroll Expense ($000):** 1089 **Personnel:** 41

CARNEGIE—Caddo County

★ **CARNEGIE TRI–COUNTY MUNICIPAL HOSPITAL (371334)**, 102 North Broadway, Zip 73015, Mailing Address: P.O. Box 97, Zip 73015–0097; tel. 580/654–1050 **A**9 10 18 **F**3 7 31 38 56 57 63 87 96
Primary Contact: Shane Dunning, Administrator
Control: Hospital district or authority, Government, nonfederal **Service:** General Medical and Surgical

Staffed Beds: 19 **Admissions:** 483 **Census:** 4 **Outpatient Visits:** 4655 **Births:** 0 **Total Expense ($000):** 3638 **Payroll Expense ($000):** 1686

CHEYENNE—Roger Mills County

★ **ROGER MILLS MEMORIAL HOSPITAL (371303)**, Fifth and L. L Males Avenue, Zip 73628, Mailing Address: P.O. Box 219, Zip 73628–0219; tel. 580/497–3336 **A**9 10 18 **F**31 32 38 55 57 122
Primary Contact: Marilyn Bryan, Administrator
CFO: Lois Wilson, Controller
Control: County–Government, nonfederal **Service:** General Medical and Surgical

Staffed Beds: 15 **Admissions:** 110 **Census:** 1 **Outpatient Visits:** 867 **Births:** 0 **Personnel:** 64

CHICKASHA—Grady County

★ **GRADY MEMORIAL HOSPITAL (370054)**, 2220 West Iowa Avenue, Zip 73018–2738; tel. 405/224–2300 **A**5 9 10 19 20 **F**3 11 13 15 17 25 26 32 33 38 40 55 56 64 66 67 68 73 74 77 79 80 86 87 96 97 99 100 102 107 118 119 121 122 124 134 135 **P**6
Primary Contact: Michael Nunamaker, Chief Executive Officer
CFO: Linda Hart, Vice President Finance
CMO: Laura Black–Wickes, M.D., Chief of Staff
CIO: Sylvia Ho, Director Information Services
CHR: Steve Hutchens, Vice President General Services
Web address: www.gradymem.org
Control: Hospital district or authority, Government, nonfederal **Service:** General Medical and Surgical

Staffed Beds: 55 **Admissions:** 2700 **Census:** 26 **Outpatient Visits:** 101297 **Births:** 361 **Total Expense ($000):** 38038 **Payroll Expense ($000):** 18618 **Personnel:** 347

CLAREMORE—Rogers County

☒ **CLAREMORE INDIAN HOSPITAL (370173)**, 101 South Moore Avenue, Zip 74017–5091; tel. 918/342–6200 **A**1 5 10 **F**3 15 32 37 38 43 62 68 74 79 84 96 107 **P**6 **S** U. S. Indian Health Service
Primary Contact: Marty Smith, Interim Chief Executive Officer
CFO: Toni Loneman, Supervisor Accounting
CMO: Paul Mobley, D.O., Clinical Director
CIO: David Ponder, Information Technology Officer
CHR: Jamelle King, Director Human Resources
Web address: www.ihs.gov
Control: PHS, Indian Service, Government, federal **Service:** General Medical and Surgical

Staffed Beds: 46 **Admissions:** 1543 **Census:** 17 **Outpatient Visits:** 119241 **Births:** 309 **Total Expense ($000):** 33968 **Payroll Expense ($000):** 18526 **Personnel:** 350

☒ **CLAREMORE REGIONAL HOSPITAL (370039)**, 1202 North Muskogee Place, Zip 74017–3036; tel. 918/341–2556 **A**1 9 10 **F**12 15 17 18 24 25 26 30 31 32 33 38 51 72 74 75 77 79 80 81 86 88 93 96 97 100 107 117 118 119 120 122 124 134 135 136 137 **P**6 **S** Community Health Systems, Inc.
Primary Contact: David Chaussard, Chief Executive Officer
CFO: Jay Johnson, Chief Operating Officer
CIO: Misty Jones, Chief Information Officer
CHR: Pat Goad, Director Human Resources
Web address: www.claremoreregho spital.com
Control: Corporation, Investor–owned, for–profit **Service:** General Medical and Surgical

Staffed Beds: 71 **Admissions:** 3795 **Census:** 42 **Outpatient Visits:** 46742 **Births:** 644 **Total Expense ($000):** 36843 **Payroll Expense ($000):** 13824 **Personnel:** 390

CLEVELAND—Pawnee County

★ **CLEVELAND AREA HOSPITAL (371320)**, 1401 West Pawnee Street, Zip 74020–3019; tel. 918/358–2501 **A**9 10 18 **F**25 38 52 54 55 57 62 75 79 82 84 85 86 93 94 96 102 107 117 119 122 124 132 137
Primary Contact: James Klough, Interim Chief Executive Officer
CFO: David Ward, Business Manager
Web address: www.hillcrest.com
Control: Corporation, Investor–owned, for–profit **Service:** General Medical and Surgical

Staffed Beds: 14 **Admissions:** 230 **Census:** 4 **Outpatient Visits:** 7428 **Births:** 0 **Total Expense ($000):** 7435 **Payroll Expense ($000):** 3424 **Personnel:** 93

CLINTON—Custer County

☒ **INTEGRIS CLINTON REGIONAL HOSPITAL (370029)**, 100 North 30th Street, Zip 73601–3117, Mailing Address: P.O. Box 1569, Zip 73601–1569; tel. 580/323–2363 **A**1 9 10 **F**3 11 13 15 25 26 27 30 31 32 38 42 55 56 57 61 62 66 68 73 74 75 76 79 81 85 86 96 97 102 107 111 118 119 120 121 122 135 136 137 **S** INTEGRIS Health
Primary Contact: Jerry Jones, President
CFO: Richard Foster, CHE, Chief Financial Officer
CHR: Karen Hunter, Director Human Resources
Web address: www.integris–health.com
Control: Other not–for–profit (including NFP Corporation) **Service:** General Medical and Surgical

Staffed Beds: 49 **Admissions:** 1576 **Census:** 16 **Outpatient Visits:** 18580 **Births:** 235 **Total Expense ($000):** 21489 **Payroll Expense ($000):** 8517 **Personnel:** 169

COALGATE—Coal County

★ **COAL COUNTY GENERAL HOSPITAL (371319)**, 6 North Covington Street, Zip 74538–2002, Mailing Address: P.O. Box 326, Zip 74538; tel. 580/927–2327, (Nonreporting) **A**9 10 18
Primary Contact: Dan A. Clements, Chief Executive Officer
CFO: Jamie Massie, Chief Financial Officer
Web address: www.hillcrest.com
Control: Other not–for–profit (including NFP Corporation) **Service:** General Medical and Surgical

Staffed Beds: 20

CORDELL—Washita County

★ **CORDELL MEMORIAL HOSPITAL (371325)**, 1220 North Glenn English Street, Zip 73632–2099; tel. 580/832–3339 **A**9 10 18 **F**7 30 38 55 57 63 79 84 117 122
Primary Contact: Charles H. Greene, Jr., Administrator
CFO: Sue Kelley, Chief Financial Officer
Control: City–Government, nonfederal **Service:** General Medical and Surgical

Staffed Beds: 25 **Admissions:** 363 **Census:** 3 **Outpatient Visits:** 4379 **Births:** 0 **Total Expense ($000):** 3037 **Payroll Expense ($000):** 1339 **Personnel:** 42

CUSHING—Payne County

☒ **CUSHING REGIONAL HOSPITAL (370099)**, 1027 East Cherry Street, Zip 74023–4101, Mailing Address: P.O. Box 1409, Zip 74023–1409; tel. 918/225–2915 **A**1 9 10 **F**3 11 13 15 25 26 30 32 33 38 40 43 50 51 55 56 57 61 62 66 67 68 73 74 77 79 80 82 86 88 90 91 93 94 96 97 100 102 107 117 118 119 121 122 132 136 137 **S** Ardent Health Services
Primary Contact: Ron Cackler, President and Chief Executive Officer
Web address: www.hillcrest.com
Control: Corporation, Investor–owned, for–profit **Service:** General Medical and Surgical

Staffed Beds: 88 **Admissions:** 3736 **Census:** 44 **Outpatient Visits:** 35447 **Births:** 498 **Total Expense ($000):** 28105 **Payroll Expense ($000):** 11390 **Personnel:** 216

DRUMRIGHT—Creek County

DRUMRIGHT REGIONAL HOSPITAL (371331), 610 West Bypass Street, Zip 74030; tel. 918/382–2300 **A**9 10 18 **F**3 11 31 38 55 56 77 79 81 96 100 107 118 119 122 **S** Hospital Management Consulting, LLC
Primary Contact: Darrel Morris, Chief Executive Officer
CFO: Jeremy Clingenpeel, Chief Financial Officer
Control: City–Government, nonfederal **Service:** General Medical and Surgical

Staffed Beds: 15 **Admissions:** 640 **Census:** 10 **Outpatient Visits:** 7975 **Total Expense ($000):** 7470 **Payroll Expense ($000):** 3056 **Personnel:** 62

DUNCAN—Stephens County

☒ **DUNCAN REGIONAL HOSPITAL (370023)**, 1407 North Whisenant Drive, Zip 73533–1650, Mailing Address: P.O. Box 2000, Zip 73534–2000; tel. 580/252–5300, (Total facility includes 16 beds in nursing home–type unit) **A**1 5 9 10 20 **F**3 11 13 15 17 24 25 26 30 33 38 40 42 50 51 52 55 56 57 61 63 66 68 73 74 75 77 79 82 85 86 96 100 102 103 104 107 117 118 119 120 121 124 133 135 **P**6 8
Primary Contact: Scott Street, President and Chief Executive Officer
CFO: Melissa Walker, Vice President and Chief Financial Officer
CIO: Roger Neal, Assistant Vice President Chief Information Officer
CHR: Mark Rhoades, Vice President Human Resources
Web address: www.duncanregional.com
Control: Other not–for–profit (including NFP Corporation) **Service:** General Medical and Surgical

Staffed Beds: 108 **Admissions:** 4906 **Census:** 60 **Outpatient Visits:** 96684 **Births:** 507 **Total Expense ($000):** 56522 **Payroll Expense ($000):** 22795 **Personnel:** 659

DURANT—Bryan County

☒ **MEDICAL CENTER OF SOUTHEASTERN OKLAHOMA (370014)**, 1800 University Boulevard, Zip 74701–3006, Mailing Address: P.O. Box 1207, Zip 74702–1207; tel. 580/924–3080 **A**1 9 10 12 13 19 **F**8 11 12 13 15 17 18 24 25 30 37 38 51 52 54 57 61 68 72 73 74 77 79 80 81 82 84 86 96 97 100 103 106 107 118 121 124 134 135 136 137 **P**8 **S** Health Management Associates
Primary Contact: Jacquelyn Harms, RN, Chief Executive Officer
COO: Dave Wallace, Chief Operating Officer
CFO: Dale Maddox, Chief Financial Officer
CMO: Peter Hedberg, M.D., Chief of Staff
CIO: Katy Stinson, Director Information Services
Web address: www.mcso.com
Control: Corporation, Investor–owned, for–profit **Service:** General Medical and Surgical

Staffed Beds: 120 **Admissions:** 8296 **Census:** 86 **Outpatient Visits:** 30767 **Births:** 1089 **Personnel:** 536

EDMOND—Oklahoma County

☒ **EDMOND MEDICAL CENTER (370148)**, 1 South Bryant Street, Zip 73034–4798; tel. 405/341–6100 **A**1 3 5 9 10 **F**3 8 11 15 18 20 25 27 32 33 37 38 40 43 54 55 56 66 68 72 73 75 76 77 79 80 82 88 92 93 96 100 103 107 119 120 121 124 135 136 137 **P**5 **S** HCA
Primary Contact: Tayo Fichtl, Chief Executive Officer
CFO: Lavaughn Carey, Chief Financial Officer
CMO: Michael Olay, M.D., Chief of Staff
CIO: Michael Upton, Director Information Systems
CHR: Leslie Buford, Director Marketing and Public Relations
Web address: www.edmondhospital.com
Control: Corporation, Investor–owned, for–profit **Service:** General Medical and Surgical

Staffed Beds: 92 **Admissions:** 3494 **Census:** 50 **Outpatient Visits:** 57169 **Births:** 0 **Total Expense ($000):** 60890 **Payroll Expense ($000):** 19650 **Personnel:** 401

□ **EDMOND SPECIALTY HOSPITAL (372005)**, 1100 East Ninth Street, Zip 73034–5755; tel. 405/341–8150 **A**1 9 10 **F**25 30 **S** Fundamental Long Term Care Holdings, LLC
Primary Contact: Phyllis Williams, Chief Executive Officer
CFO: Rowena Davidson, Business Office Manager
CMO: Brian Levy, Medical Director
CHR: Pam Grimes, Director Human Resources
Web address: www.thicare.com/EdmondSpecialty/
Control: Corporation, Investor–owned, for–profit **Service:** Long–Term Acute Care hospital

Staffed Beds: 37 **Admissions:** 271 **Census:** 20 **Outpatient Visits:** 0 **Births:** 0

FOUNDATION BARIATRIC HOSPITAL OF OKLAHOMA (370225), (Bariatrics), 1800 South Renaissance Boulevard, Zip 73013–3023; tel. 405/359–2400 **A**10 **F**68
Primary Contact: Curtis Summers, Chief Executive Officer
Control: Corporation, Investor–owned, for–profit **Service:** Other specialty

Staffed Beds: 15 **Admissions:** 157 **Census:** 1 **Births:** 0

Hospital, Medicare Provider Number, Address, Telephone, Approval, Facility, and Physician Codes, Health Care System

★ American Hospital Association (AHA) membership
□ The Joint Commission accreditation
○ American Osteopathic Association (AOA) accreditation
△ Commission on Accreditation of Rehabilitation Facilities (CARF) accreditation

EL RENO—Canadian County

★ **PARKVIEW HOSPITAL (370011)**, 2115 Parkview Drive, Zip 73036–2199, Mailing Address: P.O. Box 129, Zip 73036–0129; tel. 405/262–2640 **A**9 10 **F**3 7 11 13 25 26 29 31 32 33 37 38 43 55 56 57 61 62 68 73 74 77 79 81 86 92 96 97 100 107 119 121 135 136 137
Primary Contact: Lex Smith, Chief Executive Officer
CFO: Rod Shook, Chief Financial Officer
CMO: Michael Dean Sullivan, M.D., Chief of Staff
CIO: Karen Heldreth, Director Data Processing
CHR: Wendy Ward, Director Human Resources
Web address: www.parkview–hospital.com
Control: Hospital district or authority, Government, nonfederal **Service:** General Medical and Surgical

Staffed Beds: 48 **Admissions:** 1403 **Census:** 14 **Outpatient Visits:** 9505 **Births:** 141 **Total Expense ($000):** 16397 **Payroll Expense ($000):** 8106 **Personnel:** 206

ELK CITY—Beckham County

☒ **GREAT PLAINS REGIONAL MEDICAL CENTER (370019)**, 1705 West Second Street, Zip 73644–4496, Mailing Address: P.O. Box 2339, Zip 73648–2339; tel. 580/225–2511 **A**1 9 10 **F**3 11 13 15 18 20 25 26 27 30 31 32 33 38 40 41 43 50 51 54 55 56 57 61 62 63 66 68 72 73 74 75 76 77 79 80 81 82 86 88 90 91 92 93 96 97 100 103 106 107 111 118 119 120 121 122 124 132 135 136 137 **P**7 8
Primary Contact: Robin E. Lake, Chief Executive Officer
COO: Don Ikner, Senior Vice President and Chief Operating Officer
CFO: Richard McBryde, Vice President Finance
CMO: David Bank, M.D., Chief of Staff
CIO: Terry Davis, Chief Information Officer
CHR: Bill Barrett, Vice President Human Resources
Web address: www.gprmc–ok.com
Control: Other not–for–profit (including NFP Corporation) **Service:** General Medical and Surgical

Staffed Beds: 71 **Admissions:** 3281 **Census:** 34 **Outpatient Visits:** 62550 **Births:** 399 **Total Expense ($000):** 33514 **Payroll Expense ($000):** 14534 **Personnel:** 352

ENID—Garfield County

☒ **INTEGRIS BASS BAPTIST HEALTH CENTER (370016)**, 600 South Monroe Street, Zip 73701–7211, Mailing Address: P.O. Box 3168, Zip 73702–3168; tel. 580/233–2300, (Includes INTEGRIS BASS BEHAVIORAL HEALTH SYSTEM, 2216 South Van Buren Street, Zip 73703–8299; tel. 580/234–2220) **A**1 3 5 9 10 19 **F**3 11 13 15 17 18 19 20 22 24 25 26 27 32 38 40 53 54 55 56 57 61 62 66 67 68 73 74 75 76 77 79 81 82 87 88 90 93 94 96 97 100 102 105 106 107 111 117 120 121 133 135 136 137 **S** INTEGRIS Health
Primary Contact: Jeffrey S. Tarrant, FACHE, President
CMO: Edward Herrman, Assistant Administrator, Patient Care Services
CHR: Jeryl Gates, Director Human Resources
Web address: www.integris–health.com
Control: Other not–for–profit (including NFP Corporation) **Service:** General Medical and Surgical

Staffed Beds: 151 **Admissions:** 5364 **Census:** 107 **Outpatient Visits:** 50533 **Births:** 961 **Total Expense ($000):** 81273 **Payroll Expense ($000):** 34372 **Personnel:** 745

☐ **INTEGRIS BASS PAVILION (372016)**, 401 South Third, Zip 73701; tel. 580/249–4260 **A**1 9 10 **F**1 11 24 25 26 32 38 40 43 55 61 66 67 73 75 80 81 82 86 120 121 135 137 **S** INTEGRIS Health
Primary Contact: Jeffrey S. Tarrant, FACHE, President
CMO: Edward Herrman, Assistant Administrator, Patient Care Services
CHR: Jeryl Gates, Director Human Resources
Web address: www.integris–health.com/integris/en–us/locations/bass–enid
Control: Other not–for–profit (including NFP Corporation) **Service:** General Medical and Surgical

Staffed Beds: 24 **Admissions:** 205 **Census:** 15 **Outpatient Visits:** 1297 **Births:** 0 **Total Expense ($000):** 7985 **Payroll Expense ($000):** 3071 **Personnel:** 70

☐ △ **ST. MARY'S REGIONAL MEDICAL CENTER (370026)**, 305 South Fifth Street, Zip 73701–5899, Mailing Address: Box 232, Zip 73702–0232; tel. 580/233–6100 **A**1 2 3 5 7 9 10 **F**3 11 13 15 17 18 20 22 24 25 26 27 30 31 32 33 37 38 40 51 55 56 57 59 60 66 67 68 70 72 74 75 76 77 79 80 81 84 85 86 96 97 98 99 100 102 103 105 106 107 117 121 135 136 **P**4 **S** Universal Health Services, Inc.
Primary Contact: Rick Wallace, FACHE, Chief Executive Officer and Managing Director
COO: Nicholas Crafts, Chief Operating Officer
CFO: Ralph Mercuri, Chief Financial Officer
CMO: Dan Washburn, M.D., Chief of Staff
CHR: Linda Hoag, Director Human Resources
Web address: www.stmarysregional.com
Control: Corporation, Investor–owned, for–profit **Service:** General Medical and Surgical

Staffed Beds: 176 **Admissions:** 6735 **Census:** 103 **Outpatient Visits:** 58394 **Births:** 322 **Total Expense ($000):** 78266 **Payroll Expense ($000):** 27105

EUFAULA—Mcintosh County

COMMUNITY HOSPITAL–LAKEVIEW (370169), 1 Hospital Drive, Zip 74432–4010, Mailing Address: P.O. Box 629, Zip 74432–0629; tel. 918/689–2535, (Nonreporting) **A**9 10
Primary Contact: Chris A. Larkin, Administrator
CFO: Phyllis Eakle, Chief Financial Officer
CMO: Ed Farrow, M.D., Chief Medical Staff
Web address: www.swnd@cwis.com
Control: Other not–for–profit (including NFP Corporation) **Service:** General Medical and Surgical

Staffed Beds: 33

FAIRFAX—Osage County

★ **FAIRFAX MEMORIAL HOSPITAL (371318)**, Taft Avenue and Highway 18, Zip 74637–4028, Mailing Address: P.O. Box 219, Zip 74637–0219; tel. 918/642–3291 **A**9 10 18 **F**3 11 25 31 32 33 38 54 55 61 62 75 79 86 93 96 107 118 122 135
Primary Contact: Emery Brautigan, Chief Executive Officer
CFO: Emery Brautigan, Chief Executive Officer
Web address: www.hillcrest.com
Control: Partnership, Investor–owned, for–profit **Service:** General Medical and Surgical

Staffed Beds: 15 **Admissions:** 281 **Census:** 4 **Outpatient Visits:** 4093 **Births:** 0 **Total Expense ($000):** 3597 **Payroll Expense ($000):** 1835 **Personnel:** 45

FAIRVIEW—Major County

FAIRVIEW REGIONAL MEDICAL CENTER (371329), 523 East State Road, Zip 73737–1498, Mailing Address: P.O. Box 548, Zip 73737–0548; tel. 580/227–3721 **A**9 10 18 **F**24 30 31 38 43 55 56 57 62 73 75 79 80 86 96 102 117 122 135 **P**6 **S** Cypress Health Systems
Primary Contact: Roger Knak, Administrator
CFO: Jamie Eitzen, Director Finance
CMO: Solomon Ali, M.D., Chief of Staff
CHR: Macky Martin, Director Human Resources
Web address: www.fairviewhospital.net
Control: City–Government, nonfederal **Service:** General Medical and Surgical

Staffed Beds: 25 **Admissions:** 517 **Census:** 5 **Outpatient Visits:** 9282 **Births:** 0 **Total Expense ($000):** 4913 **Payroll Expense ($000):** 2712 **Personnel:** 63

FORT SILL—Comanche County

☒ **REYNOLDS ARMY COMMUNITY HOSPITAL**, 4301 Mow Way Road, Zip 73503–6300; tel. 580/458–3000 **A**1 5 **F**3 5 7 12 13 15 25 26 28 29 30 31 32 33 36 37 38 40 41 43 50 53 54 55 56 57 62 63 66 68 72 73 74 75 77 79 80 82 84 86 87 90 91 92 94 96 97 100 103 106 107 112 113 114 118 119 120 121 123 124 132 133 134 135 136 **S** Department of the Army, Office of the Surgeon General
Primary Contact: Colonel Ellen E. Forster, Commander
COO: Lieutenant Colonel Paul Roberts, Chief of Staff and Deputy Commander for Administration
CFO: Captain Shelley Mizelle, Chief Resource Management Division
CMO: Colonel Donald Mondragon, M.D., Deputy Commander Clinical Services
CIO: Major Eric McClung, Chief Information Management Division
CHR: Homer Williams, Chief Civilian Personnel Branch
Web address: www.rach.sill.amedd.army.mil
Control: Army, Government, federal **Service:** General Medical and Surgical

Staffed Beds: 46 **Admissions:** 2587 **Census:** 16 **Outpatient Visits:** 524517 **Births:** 612 **Total Expense ($000):** 47455 **Personnel:** 1229

FREDERICK—Tillman County

★ **MEMORIAL HOSPITAL AND PHYSICIAN GROUP (370051)**, 319 East Josephine, Zip 73542–2200; tel. 580/335–7565, (Total facility includes 30 beds in nursing home–type unit) **A**9 10 20 **F**11 25 33 38 57 61 62 65 79 84 86 96 102 107 122 **P**6
Primary Contact: Al Allee, Chief Executive Officer
Control: Hospital district or authority, Government, nonfederal **Service:** General Medical and Surgical

Staffed Beds: 55 **Admissions:** 752 **Census:** 36 **Outpatient Visits:** 31698 **Births:** 0 **Total Expense ($000):** 6808 **Payroll Expense ($000):** 3021 **Personnel:** 116

Many Facility Codes have changed. Please refer to the AHA Guide Code Chart.

GROVE—Delaware County

☒ **INTEGRIS GROVE GENERAL HOSPITAL (370113)**, 1310 South Main Street, Zip 74344–1310; tel. 918/786–2243, (Total facility includes 30 beds in nursing home–type unit) **A**1 9 10 20 **F**3 7 11 13 25 26 31 32 38 53 55 61 62 68 74 75 77 79 80 96 99 100 102 107 115 118 135 136 **S** INTEGRIS Health
Primary Contact: Greg Martin, President
CFO: David Zych, Chief Financial Officer
CMO: James Rutter, M.D., Chief of Staff
CHR: Vicki Cossairt, Director Human Resources
Web address: www.integris–health.com
Control: Other not–for–profit (including NFP Corporation) **Service:** General Medical and Surgical

Staffed Beds: 50 **Admissions:** 3323 **Census:** 26 **Outpatient Visits:** 80536 **Births:** 353 **Total Expense ($000):** 36869 **Payroll Expense ($000):** 14715 **Personnel:** 320

GUTHRIE—Logan County

★ **LOGAN MEDICAL CENTER (371317)**, Highway 33 West at Academy Road, Zip 73044–3700, Mailing Address: P.O. Box 1017, Zip 73044–1017; tel. 405/282–6700 **A**9 10 18 **F**3 11 15 25 26 37 38 55 61 62 73 75 77 79 86 87 96 100 103 107 117 118 119 122 **S** QHR
Primary Contact: K. Steven Rowley, CHE, Chief Executive Officer
COO: Abe Sims, Chief Operating Officer
CFO: Jane Bissel, Chief Financial Officer
CMO: Laurie Orme, M.D., Chief of Staff
CHR: Mary Jo Messelt, Director Human Resources
Web address: www.loganhosp.com
Control: County–Government, nonfederal **Service:** General Medical and Surgical

Staffed Beds: 25 **Admissions:** 872 **Census:** 11 **Outpatient Visits:** 23983 **Births:** 0 **Total Expense ($000):** 14158 **Payroll Expense ($000):** 7565 **Personnel:** 172

GUYMON—Texas County

★ **MEMORIAL HOSPITAL OF TEXAS COUNTY (370138)**, 520 Medical Drive, Zip 73942–4438; tel. 580/338–6515 **A**9 10 20 **F**3 11 13 15 25 26 30 31 33 38 40 42 43 55 56 57 61 63 66 67 73 74 77 79 80 86 96 100 102 107 120 122 135 136 137 **P**6
Primary Contact: James F. Grocholski, Chief Executive Officer
CFO: Jim Ellickson, Chief Financial Officer
Web address: www.mhtcguymon.org
Control: County–Government, nonfederal **Service:** General Medical and Surgical

Staffed Beds: 28 **Admissions:** 1703 **Census:** 13 **Outpatient Visits:** 29551 **Births:** 368 **Total Expense ($000):** 16324 **Payroll Expense ($000):** 6837 **Personnel:** 160

HEALDTON—Carter County

★ **HEALDTON MUNICIPAL HOSPITAL (371310)**, 918 S.W. Eighth Street, Zip 73438, Mailing Address: P.O. Box 928, Zip 73438; tel. 580/229–0701 **A**9 10 18 **F**11 25 31 38 62 75 86 96 107 118 122 **P**5
Primary Contact: Ricklin Pack, Administrator and Chief Executive Officer
Control: City–Government, nonfederal **Service:** General Medical and Surgical

Staffed Beds: 22 **Admissions:** 342 **Census:** 5 **Outpatient Visits:** 6437 **Births:** 0 **Total Expense ($000):** 2922 **Payroll Expense ($000):** 1440 **Personnel:** 34

HENRYETTA—Okmulgee County

☒ **HENRYETTA MEDICAL CENTER (370183)**, Dewey Bartlett and Main Streets, Zip 74437–6820, Mailing Address: P.O. Box 1269, Zip 74437–1269; tel. 918/652–4463 **A**1 9 10 **F**3 7 11 15 25 31 32 33 38 54 55 77 79 82 88 93 96 107 118 122 **S** Ardent Health Services
Primary Contact: Eric N. Looper, Chief Executive Officer
CFO: Becky Speight, Chief Financial Officer
Web address: www.hillcrest.com/henryetta
Control: Corporation, Investor–owned, for–profit **Service:** General Medical and Surgical

Staffed Beds: 41 **Admissions:** 1586 **Census:** 22 **Births:** 0

HOBART—Kiowa County

★ **ELKVIEW GENERAL HOSPITAL (370153)**, 429 West Elm Street, Zip 73651–1699; tel. 580/726–3324 **A**9 10 20 **F**3 11 13 15 25 27 38 43 54 56 57 61 62 63 66 76 77 79 80 86 92 96 97 103 106 107 122 135 137
Primary Contact: J. W. Finch, Jr., Chief Executive Officer
COO: Harold Moad, Chief Operating Officer
CFO: Lisa Hart, Chief Financial Officer
CMO: Samatha Lewellen, M.D., Chief of Staff
Control: Hospital district or authority, Government, nonfederal **Service:** General Medical and Surgical

Staffed Beds: 38 **Admissions:** 1369 **Census:** 15 **Outpatient Visits:** 11590 **Births:** 50 **Total Expense ($000):** 9177 **Payroll Expense ($000):** 5994 **Personnel:** 190

HOLDENVILLE—Hughes County

★ **HOLDENVILLE GENERAL HOSPITAL (371321)**, 100 McDougal Drive, Zip 74848–9700; tel. 405/379–4200 **A**9 10 18 **F**3 11 25 26 31 38 55 61 62 73 79 82 86 96 122 **S** Brim Healthcare, Inc.
Primary Contact: Alden M. Vandeveer, Jr., CHE, Chief Executive Officer
CFO: Bridget Cosby, Chief Financial Officer
CHR: Heather Heard, Director Human Resources
Web address: www.holdenvillegeneral.org
Control: City–Government, nonfederal **Service:** General Medical and Surgical

Staffed Beds: 25 **Admissions:** 622 **Census:** 6 **Outpatient Visits:** 21683 **Births:** 0 **Total Expense ($000):** 8193 **Payroll Expense ($000):** 3745 **Personnel:** 106

HOLLIS—Harmon County

★ **HARMON MEMORIAL HOSPITAL (370036)**, 400 East Chestnut Street, Zip 73550–2030, Mailing Address: P.O. Box 791, Zip 73550–0791; tel. 580/688–3363 **A**9 10 20 **F**11 30 31 38 61 84 117 122 **P**5
Primary Contact: Billy Burge, Chief Executive Officer
CFO: Ruthie Matheson, Chief Financial Officer
CHR: Marti Taylor, Director Human Resources
Control: Hospital district or authority, Government, nonfederal **Service:** General Medical and Surgical

Staffed Beds: 22 **Admissions:** 1019 **Census:** 8 **Outpatient Visits:** 6511 **Births:** 0 **Total Expense ($000):** 4644 **Payroll Expense ($000):** 2395 **Personnel:** 50

HUGO—Choctaw County

★ **CHOCTAW MEMORIAL HOSPITAL (370100)**, 1405 East Kirk Road, Zip 74743–3603; tel. 580/317–9500, (Nonreporting) **A**9 10 **S** QHR
Primary Contact: Davie Lloyd, Chief Executive Officer
CFO: Mary Stinson, Chief Financial Officer
CHR: Darlene Galyon, Administrator Human Resources
Control: Hospital district or authority, Government, nonfederal **Service:** General Medical and Surgical

Staffed Beds: 34

LANE FROST HEALTH AND REHABILITATION CENTER (372017), 2815 East Jackson Street, Zip 74743; tel. 580/326–9200 **A**10 **F**1 25 26 32 33 43 56 62 86 132 137 **P**1
Primary Contact: Marla Beatty, Chief Executive Officer
Control: Other not–for–profit (including NFP Corporation) **Service:** Long–Term Acute Care hospital

Staffed Beds: 30 **Admissions:** 285 **Census:** 22 **Outpatient Visits:** 100 **Births:** 0 **Total Expense ($000):** 7648 **Payroll Expense ($000):** 2226 **Personnel:** 66

IDABEL—Mccurtain County

★ **MCCURTAIN MEMORIAL HOSPITAL (370048)**, 1301 Lincoln Road, Zip 74745–7341; tel. 580/286–7623 **A**9 10 20 **F**3 11 13 15 24 25 26 30 38 55 61 68 74 79 86 88 93 96 100 102 107 119 122 **P**8
Primary Contact: Bristol Messer, Chief Executive Officer
CFO: Ray B. Whitmore, Chief Financial Officer
CMO: Michael C. West, M.D., Chief of Staff
CIO: Dana A. Stowell, Chief Information Officer
CHR: Frank Drobil, Director Human Resources
Web address: www.mmhok.com
Control: Other not–for–profit (including NFP Corporation) **Service:** General Medical and Surgical

Staffed Beds: 71 **Admissions:** 2512 **Census:** 24 **Outpatient Visits:** 43461 **Births:** 357 **Total Expense ($000):** 19541 **Payroll Expense ($000):** 8663 **Personnel:** 231

Hospital, Medicare Provider Number, Address, Telephone, Approval, Facility, and Physician Codes, Health Care System

★ American Hospital Association (AHA) membership
□ The Joint Commission accreditation
○ American Osteopathic Association (AOA) accreditation
△ Commission on Accreditation of Rehabilitation Facilities (CARF) accreditation

OK

KINGFISHER—Kingfisher County

★ **KINGFISHER REGIONAL HOSPITAL (371313)**, 500 South Ninth Street, Zip 73750–3528, Mailing Address: P.O. Box 59, Zip 73750–0059; tel. 405/375–3141 **A**9 10 18 **F**13 15 25 31 32 33 38 57 69 74 79 86 135 **S** QHR
Primary Contact: Damon Benson, Chief Executive Officer and Administrator
CFO: Doran Hammett, Chief Financial Officer
CMO: Brett Krablin, M.D., Chief of Staff
CIO: Rose Sherwood, Information Technology Specialist
CHR: Carolyn Bjerke, Director Human Resources
Web address: www.kingfisherhospital.com
Control: Other not–for–profit (including NFP Corporation) **Service:** General Medical and Surgical

Staffed Beds: 25 **Admissions:** 1378 **Census:** 15 **Outpatient Visits:** 8544 **Births:** 120 **Total Expense ($000):** 10374 **Payroll Expense ($000):** 4079 **Personnel:** 119

LAWTON—Comanche County

☒ △ **COMANCHE COUNTY MEMORIAL HOSPITAL (370056)**, 3401 West Gore Boulevard, Zip 73505–0129, Mailing Address: P.O. Box 129, Zip 73502–0129; tel. 580/355–8620, (Total facility includes 135 beds in nursing home–type unit) **A**1 2 3 5 7 9 10 **F**3 7 8 11 13 15 17 18 20 22 24 25 26 27 28 30 32 33 35 37 38 40 43 51 54 55 56 57 59 60 61 62 66 68 72 73 74 75 76 77 79 80 81 82 85 86 87 88 90 92 93 94 96 97 99 100 102 103 106 107 111 117 118 119 120 121 124 133 135 136 137 **P**6
Primary Contact: Randall K. Segler, Chief Executive Officer
COO: Douglas K. Weaver, Chief Operating Officer
CFO: David Blackmon, Chief Financial Officer
CMO: Scott Michener, M.D., Medical Staff President
CIO: Kent Lewis, Director Information Services
CHR: Donna Wade, Division Director Human Resources
Web address: www.memorialhealthsource.com
Control: Hospital district or authority, Government, nonfederal **Service:** General Medical and Surgical

Staffed Beds: 220 **Admissions:** 10344 **Census:** 137 **Outpatient Visits:** 97702 **Births:** 1318 **Total Expense ($000):** 172713 **Payroll Expense ($000):** 75319 **Personnel:** 1543

JIM TALIAFERRO COMMUNITY MENTAL HEALTH (374008), 602 S.W. 37th Street, Zip 73505; tel. 580/248–5780, (Nonreporting) **A**9 10
Primary Contact: Jim Regan, Interim Executive Director
Control: State–Government, nonfederal **Service:** Psychiatric

Staffed Beds: 26

☒ **LAWTON INDIAN HOSPITAL (370170)**, 1515 Lawrie Tatum Road, Zip 73507–3099; tel. 580/353–0350 **A**1 10 **F**8 37 38 43 56 57 63 73 79 87 94 96 102 107 119 124 135 136 **S** U. S. Indian Health Service
Primary Contact: Greg Ketcher, Acting Chief Executive Officer
CFO: Sarabeth Sahmaunt, Supervisory Accountant
CMO: Bryce Poolaw, Clinical Director
CIO: Steve Barse, Chief Information Officer
CHR: Twylla Jimboy, Supervisor Human Resources
Web address: www.ihs.gov
Control: Public Health Service, Government, federal **Service:** General Medical and Surgical

Staffed Beds: 26 **Admissions:** 560 **Census:** 6 **Births:** 0 **Personnel:** 113

☐ △ **SOUTHWESTERN MEDICAL CENTER (370097)**, 5602 S.W. Lee Boulevard, Zip 73505–9635, Mailing Address: P.O. Box 7290, Zip 73506–7290; tel. 580/531–4700 **A**1 2 3 5 7 9 10 **F**3 11 13 25 26 27 32 33 38 40 54 55 57 58 62 68 72 74 75 76 77 78 79 84 85 87 88 92 93 94 96 97 100 102 106 107 108 111 118 119 121 122 135 136 137 **P**8 **S** Capella Healthcare
Primary Contact: Jon C. O'Shaughnessy, Chief Executive Officer
COO: Steven Henderson, Chief Operating Officer
CFO: George Kruger, CPA, Chief Financial Officer
CMO: Dan Criswell, M.D., Chief of Staff
CIO: Ashish Sharma, Director Information Services
CHR: Helen Hooper, Director Human Resources
Web address: www.swmconline.com
Control: Corporation, Investor–owned, for–profit **Service:** General Medical and Surgical

Staffed Beds: 166 **Admissions:** 4877 **Census:** 97 **Outpatient Visits:** 37832 **Births:** 382 **Total Expense ($000):** 56605 **Payroll Expense ($000):** 19963 **Personnel:** 570

LINDSAY—Garvin County

LINDSAY MUNICIPAL HOSPITAL (370214), Highway 19 West, Zip 73052, Mailing Address: P.O. Box 888, Zip 73052–0888; tel. 405/756–1404 **A**9 10 **F**3 31 32 38 79 96 107 122
Primary Contact: Norma N. Howard, Chief Executive Officer
Control: City–Government, nonfederal **Service:** General Medical and Surgical

Staffed Beds: 26 **Admissions:** 989 **Census:** 17 **Outpatient Visits:** 4885 **Births:** 0 **Total Expense ($000):** 6431 **Payroll Expense ($000):** 2871 **Personnel:** 79

MADILL—Marshall County

☒ **INTEGRIS MARSHALL COUNTY MEDICAL CENTER (371326)**, 1 Hospital Drive, Zip 73446, Mailing Address: P.O. Box 827, Zip 73446–0827; tel. 580/795–3384 **A**1 9 10 18 **F**3 11 25 26 31 38 42 43 44 51 55 57 61 62 73 77 79 86 96 100 107 119 122 124 135 137 **P**1 **S** INTEGRIS Health
Primary Contact: Karen Reynolds, Administrator
CFO: Thomas Briggs, Chief Financial Officer
CMO: Shannon G. Chambers, M.D., Chief of Staff
CHR: Shenita Jones, Director Human Resources
Web address: www.integris–health.com
Control: Other not–for–profit (including NFP Corporation) **Service:** General Medical and Surgical

Staffed Beds: 21 **Admissions:** 1052 **Census:** 9 **Outpatient Visits:** 14472 **Births:** 0 **Total Expense ($000):** 9498 **Payroll Expense ($000):** 4156 **Personnel:** 115

MANGUM—Greer County

MANGUM COMMUNITY HOSPITAL (371330), One Wickersham Drive, Zip 73554–9116, Mailing Address: P.O. Box 280, Zip 73554–0280; tel. 580/782–3353, (Nonreporting) **A**9 10 18 **S** Blackhawk Healthcare
Primary Contact: Brian Roland, Chief Executive Officer
COO: Danny Avery, Chief Financial Officer and Chief Operating Officer
CIO: Gregg Burnam, Chief Information Officer and Business Office Manager
Web address: www.mangumhealth.com
Control: City–Government, nonfederal **Service:** General Medical and Surgical

Staffed Beds: 21

MARIETTA—Love County

★ **MERCY HEALTH LOVE COUNTY (371306)**, 300 Wanda Street, Zip 73448–1200; tel. 580/276–3347 **A**9 10 18 **F**3 7 31 38 55 96 107 117 122 133
Primary Contact: Richard Barker, Administrator
Control: County–Government, nonfederal **Service:** General Medical and Surgical

Staffed Beds: 26 **Admissions:** 368 **Census:** 3 **Outpatient Visits:** 10154 **Births:** 0 **Total Expense ($000):** 6595 **Payroll Expense ($000):** 4148 **Personnel:** 97

MCALESTER—Pittsburg County

CARL ALBERT COMMUNITY MENTAL HEALTH CENTER (374006), 1101 East Monroe Avenue, Zip 74501–4826; tel. 918/426–7800 **A**9 10 **F**5 25 30 31 32 33 36 88 90 91 92 93 94 119 121
Primary Contact: Debbie Smith, Director
CFO: Konnie Taylor, Chief Financial Officer
CMO: Eric Broadway, M.D., Medical Director
CHR: Judy Allen, Human Resource Specialist
Web address: www.odmhsas.org
Control: State–Government, nonfederal **Service:** Psychiatric

Staffed Beds: 15 **Admissions:** 712 **Census:** 11 **Births:** 0 **Total Expense ($000):** 9730 **Payroll Expense ($000):** 5418 **Personnel:** 160

☒ △ **MCALESTER REGIONAL HEALTH CENTER (370034)**, One Clark Bass Boulevard, Zip 74501–4267, Mailing Address: P.O. Box 1228, Zip 74502–1228; tel. 918/426–1800 **A**1 7 9 10 19 20 **F**3 10 11 13 15 18 25 26 30 33 38 40 43 51 52 55 56 57 60 61 62 66 67 68 72 73 74 75 77 79 80 81 85 86 96 99 100 103 107 112 117 118 119 121 123 124 135 136 137 **P**7
Primary Contact: Shaun Beggs, Chief Executive Officer
CFO: Ben Scott, Vice President Finances and Chief Financial Officer
CMO: Elliott Metcalfe, M.D., Vice President Medical Affairs
CIO: Chris Ossenbeck, Vice President Information Systems and Chief Information Officer
CHR: Emily Mouser, Vice President Human Resources and Organizational Development
Web address: www.mrhcok.com
Control: Hospital district or authority, Government, nonfederal **Service:** General Medical and Surgical

Staffed Beds: 163 **Admissions:** 6410 **Census:** 93 **Outpatient Visits:** 70706 **Births:** 712 **Total Expense ($000):** 56925 **Payroll Expense ($000):** 30441 **Personnel:** 816

MIAMI—Ottawa County

★ **INTEGRIS BAPTIST REGIONAL HEALTH CENTER (370004)**, 200 Second Street S.W., Zip 74354–6830, Mailing Address: P.O. Box 1207, Zip 74355–1207; tel. 918/542–6611 **A**9 10 20 **F**3 5 7 11 13 15 24 25 26 27 28 30 31 32 33 38 40 42 50 51 54 55 56 57 58 61 62 63 64 66 67 68 72 73 74 75 76 77 79 80 81 82 84 85 86 88 90 91 92 93 94 96 97 100 102 107 115 118 119 120 121 122 124 135 136 137 **P**5 7 **S** INTEGRIS Health
Primary Contact: Joel A. Hart, FACHE, President
CFO: Kevin Cox, Assistant Administrator Finance and Operations
CMO: James Pletcher, D.O., Chief of Staff
CHR: Ginger Ratliff, Director Human Resources
Web address: www.integris–health.com
Control: Other not–for–profit (including NFP Corporation) **Service:** General Medical and Surgical

Staffed Beds: 99 **Admissions:** 4483 **Census:** 47 **Outpatient Visits:** 68457 **Births:** 443 **Total Expense ($000):** 38607 **Payroll Expense ($000):** 16267 **Personnel:** 394

★ **WILLOW CREST HOSPITAL (374017)**, 130 A Street S.W., Zip 74354–6800; tel. 918/542–1836 **A**9 10 **F**25 88 91 92 **P**6
Primary Contact: Anne G. Anthony, President and Chief Executive Officer
COO: Steven Goodman, Chief Operating Officer
CFO: Cindy Bell, Director Finance
CMO: Mark Elkington, M.D., Chief Medical Officer
CIO: Steven Goodman, Chief Operating Officer
CHR: Kathy Henderson, Director Human Resources, Media and Public Relations
Web address: www.willowcresthospital.com
Control: Corporation, Investor–owned, for–profit **Service:** Children's hospital psychiatric

Staffed Beds: 75 **Admissions:** 434 **Census:** 69 **Births:** 0 **Total Expense ($000):** 8172 **Payroll Expense ($000):** 5344 **Personnel:** 138

MIDWEST CITY—Oklahoma County

★ **MIDWEST REGIONAL MEDICAL CENTER (370094)**, 2825 Parklawn Drive, Zip 73110–4258; tel. 405/610–4411 **A**1 5 9 10 **F**3 7 8 11 13 14 15 17 18 20 22 24 25 26 27 30 31 32 38 40 50 55 56 57 59 61 68 72 73 74 75 76 77 79 80 81 82 86 88 90 91 92 94 95 96 97 99 100 102 103 106 107 116 118 119 121 135 136 137 **P**6 **S** Health Management Associates
Primary Contact: Douglas Arnold, Chief Executive Officer
COO: Charles Nasem, Chief Operating Officer and Administrator
CFO: Reed Hurley, Chief Financial Officer
CMO: Don Wilber, M.D., Chief of Staff
CHR: Richard Baranek, Director Human Resources
Web address: www.midwestregional.com
Control: Corporation, Investor–owned, for–profit **Service:** General Medical and Surgical

Staffed Beds: 255 **Admissions:** 16830 **Census:** 181 **Outpatient Visits:** 111058 **Births:** 957 **Total Expense ($000):** 133554 **Payroll Expense ($000):** 55360 **Personnel:** 1144

☐ **SPECIALTY HOSPITAL OF MIDWEST CITY (372012)**, 8210 National Avenue, Zip 73110; tel. 405/739–0800 **A**1 9 10 **F**1
Primary Contact: Diana McMiller, Chief Executive Officer
CFO: Kathi Loftin, Manager Business Office
Control: Corporation, Investor–owned, for–profit **Service:** General Medical and Surgical

Staffed Beds: 31 **Admissions:** 273 **Census:** 20

MOORE—Cleveland County

MOORE MEDICAL CENTER See Norman Regional Health System, Norman

MUSKOGEE—Muskogee County

★ **JACK C. MONTGOMERY VETERANS AFFAIRS MEDICAL CENTER**, 1011 Honor Heights Drive, Zip 74401–1399; tel. 918/683–3261 **A**1 5 **F**3 5 15 25 26 27 31 32 33 37 38 42 43 44 50 52 53 54 57 58 62 63 68 73 76 77 79 80 82 85 86 87 88 90 92 93 94 96 107 119 121 124 132 135 136 137 **P**1 **S** Department of Veterans Affairs
Primary Contact: Adam C. Walmus, Director
COO: Rudy Klopfer, Associate Director
CFO: Robert Wood, Chief Fiscal Services
CMO: Karen Gribbin, M.D., Chief of Staff
CIO: Gary Duvall, Chief Information Resource Management
CHR: Kay DeCamp, Chief Human Resources Officer
Web address: www.visn16.med.va.gov/muskogee.asp
Control: Veterans Affairs, Government, federal **Service:** General Medical and Surgical

Staffed Beds: 88 **Admissions:** 4441 **Census:** 63 **Outpatient Visits:** 256770 **Births:** 0 **Total Expense ($000):** 86195 **Payroll Expense ($000):** 51726 **Personnel:** 850

☐ **MUSKOGEE REGIONAL MEDICAL CENTER (370025)**, 300 Rockefeller Drive, Zip 74401–5081; tel. 918/682–5501 **A**1 2 9 10 19 **F**3 8 11 13 15 18 25 26 27 33 37 38 40 43 50 51 53 54 55 57 58 59 61 62 66 68 72 73 74 75 76 77 79 80 81 82 84 85 86 88 90 92 93 94 95 96 97 100 102 103 107 108 111 118 119 120 121 133 135 136 137 **S** Capella Healthcare
Primary Contact: Stephen W. Mahan, Chief Executive Officer
COO: Chris Whybrew, Chief Operating Officer
CFO: David N. Pennington, FACHE, Chief Financial Officer
CHR: Elmo Vinas, Director Human Resources
Web address: www.muskogeehealth.com
Control: Other not–for–profit (including NFP Corporation) **Service:** General Medical and Surgical

Staffed Beds: 245 **Admissions:** 10064 **Census:** 134 **Outpatient Visits:** 93451 **Births:** 771 **Total Expense ($000):** 85041 **Payroll Expense ($000):** 35142 **Personnel:** 800

SOLARA HOSPITAL OF MUSKOGEE (372022), 351 South 40th Street, Zip 74401; tel. 918/682–6161, (Nonreporting) **A**9 10
Primary Contact: Craig Koele, Chief Executive Officer
Control: Other not–for–profit (including NFP Corporation) **Service:** Long–Term Acute Care hospital

Staffed Beds: 41

NORMAN—Cleveland County

☐ **GRIFFIN MEMORIAL HOSPITAL (374000)**, 900 East Main Street, Zip 73071–5305, Mailing Address: P.O. Box 151, Zip 73070–0151; tel. 405/321–4880 **A**1 9 10 **F**88 92 93 **P**1 **S** Oklahoma State Department of Mental Health and Substance Abuse Services
Primary Contact: Don Bowen, Executive Director
CFO: Bob Mathew, Director Finance
CMO: Stan Ardoin, M.D., State Medical Director
Web address: www.odmhsas.org
Control: State–Government, nonfederal **Service:** Psychiatric

Staffed Beds: 132 **Admissions:** 2436 **Census:** 153 **Outpatient Visits:** 0 **Births:** 0 **Total Expense ($000):** 28756 **Payroll Expense ($000):** 15666 **Personnel:** 425

J. D. MCCARTY CENTER FOR CHILDREN WITH DEVELOPMENTAL DISABILITIES (373300), 2002 East Robinson, Zip 73071–5264, Mailing Address: PO Box 490, Zip 73070–0490; tel. 405/307–2800 **A**10 **F**37 62 73 75 85 86 119 135
Primary Contact: Curtis A. Peters, Chief Executive Officer
COO: Vicki Kuestersteffen, Director Rehabilitation Services
CFO: Ken Younkin, Comptroller
CMO: Thomas Thurston, M.D., Medical Director
CIO: Joel Mann, Administrator Information Systems
CHR: Debbie Barrett, Director Human Resources
Web address: www.jdmc.org
Control: State–Government, nonfederal **Service:** Children's rehabilitation

Staffed Beds: 36 **Admissions:** 198 **Census:** 33 **Outpatient Visits:** 4047 **Births:** 0 **Total Expense ($000):** 12808 **Payroll Expense ($000):** 7024 **Personnel:** 203

★ △ **NORMAN REGIONAL HEALTH SYSTEM (370008)**, 901 North Porter Street, Zip 73071–6482, Mailing Address: P.O. Box 1308, Zip 73070–1308; tel. 405/307–1000, (Includes MOORE MEDICAL CENTER, 700 South Telephone Road, Moore, Zip 73160; tel. 405/793–9355; Ryan Gehris, Chief Administrative Officer; NORMAN REGIONAL HOSPITAL, 901 North Porter Street, Mailing Address: P.O. Box 1308, Zip 73070–1308; tel. 405/307–1000) **A**1 2 7 9 10 **F**3 7 8 11 12 13 15 17 18 20 22 24 25 26 27 30 31 32 35 38 40 43 50 52 53 55 56 57 59 62 65 66 67 68 72 73 74 75 76 77 79 80 81 82 84 85 86 88 90 92 93 96 97 99 100 102 103 107 111 118 119 120 124 130 **P**1 7
Primary Contact: David D. Whitaker, FACHE, President and Chief Executive Officer
COO: Greg Terrell, Senior Vice President and Chief Operating Officer
CFO: Melvin Alexander, Senior Vice President Administrative Services and Chief Financial Officer
CMO: William McMillan, M.D., Vice President Medical Affairs
CIO: Edward L. Fisher, Vice President
CHR: Carolyn Shockey, Director Human Resources
Web address: www.normanregional.com
Control: Hospital district or authority, Government, nonfederal **Service:** General Medical and Surgical

Staffed Beds: 377 **Admissions:** 16894 **Census:** 228 **Outpatient Visits:** 253916 **Births:** 2158 **Total Expense ($000):** 171871 **Payroll Expense ($000):** 98078 **Personnel:** 2320

Hospital, Medicare Provider Number, Address, Telephone, Approval, Facility, and Physician Codes, Health Care System

★ American Hospital Association (AHA) membership
☐ The Joint Commission accreditation
○ American Osteopathic Association (AOA) accreditation
△ Commission on Accreditation of Rehabilitation Facilities (CARF) accreditation

★ **NORMAN SPECIALTY HOSPITAL (372021)**, 1210 West Robinson Street, Zip 73069; tel. 405/321–8824 **A**10 **F**1 **P**8
Primary Contact: Talitha Glosemeyer, Administrator
CFO: Stephanie Wortham, Director Financial Services
CHR: Stephanie Bloomer, Director Human Resources
Web address: www.normanspecialtyhospital.com
Control: Corporation, Investor–owned, for–profit **Service:** Long–Term Acute Care hospital

Staffed Beds: 50 **Admissions:** 433 **Census:** 30 **Outpatient Visits:** 0 **Births:** 0 **Total Expense ($000):** 19608 **Payroll Expense ($000):** 4760 **Personnel:** 171

NOWATA—Nowata County

JANE PHILLIPS NOWATA HEALTH CENTER (371305), 237 South Locust Street, Zip 74048–0426, Mailing Address: P.O. Box 426, Zip 74048–0426; tel. 918/273–3102 **A**9 10 18 **F**38 40 107 117 122
Primary Contact: Maggie Blevins, Administrator
CMO: David Caughell, M.D., Chief of Staff
Web address: www.jpmc.org
Control: Other not–for–profit (including NFP Corporation) **Service:** General Medical and Surgical

Staffed Beds: 15 **Admissions:** 283 **Census:** 5 **Outpatient Visits:** 2998 **Births:** 0 **Total Expense ($000):** 2547 **Payroll Expense ($000):** 1255 **Personnel:** 32

OKEENE—Blaine County

★ **OKEENE MUNICIPAL HOSPITAL (371327)**, 207 East F Street, Zip 73763, Mailing Address: P.O. Box 489, Zip 73763–0489; tel. 580/822–4417, (Total facility includes 20 beds in nursing home–type unit) **A**9 10 18 **F**3 10 25 30 38 55 57 63 67 73 75 79 80 81 82 86 87 96 120 122 135 **P**6
Primary Contact: Shelly Dunham, Chief Executive Officer
COO: Pat Lorenz, Chief Operating Officer
CFO: Sandra Lamle, Chief Financial Officer
CIO: Marsha Price, Supervisor Medical Records
Web address: www.okeenehospital.com
Control: Hospital district or authority, Government, nonfederal **Service:** General Medical and Surgical

Staffed Beds: 37 **Admissions:** 298 **Census:** 19 **Outpatient Visits:** 6833 **Births:** 0 **Total Expense ($000):** 4552 **Payroll Expense ($000):** 2294 **Personnel:** 67

OKEMAH—Okfuskee County

★ **CREEK NATION COMMUNITY HOSPITAL (371333)**, 309 North 14th Street, Zip 74859–2099; tel. 918/623–1424 **A**9 10 18 **F**3 5 7 8 15 25 31 38 55 56 79 84 107 122 137 **P**6
Primary Contact: Tyler McIntosh, Administrator
COO: Jodi Boyd, Administrative Officer
CFO: Rodney Ramsey, Chief Financial Officer
CMO: Lawrence Vark, Chief Medical Officer
CHR: Russell Torbett, Manager
Control: PHS, Indian Service, Government, federal **Service:** General Medical and Surgical

Staffed Beds: 18 **Admissions:** 386 **Census:** 3 **Outpatient Visits:** 16401 **Births:** 0 **Total Expense ($000):** 13502 **Payroll Expense ($000):** 5178 **Personnel:** 110

OKLAHOMA CITY—Oklahoma County

🞸 **BONE AND JOINT HOSPITAL (370105)**, 1111 North Dewey Avenue, Zip 73103–2615; tel. 405/552–9100 **A**1 3 5 9 10 **F**3 11 25 38 40 43 62 64 66 73 77 79 80 120 135 137 **S** SSM Health Care
Primary Contact: Chad Aduddell, President
CFO: Eric Ericson, Director Finance
CMO: William Herndon, M.D., Chief of Staff
CIO: Kevin Olson, Director Information Systems
CHR: Cheryl McConnell, Director Human Resources
Web address: www.boneandjoint.com
Control: Partnership, Investor–owned, for–profit **Service:** Orthopedic

Staffed Beds: 11 **Admissions:** 1072 **Census:** 8 **Outpatient Visits:** 4821 **Births:** 0 **Total Expense ($000):** 31545 **Payroll Expense ($000):** 8006 **Personnel:** 154

CEDAR RIDGE HOSPITAL (374023), 6501 N.E. 50th Street, Zip 73141; tel. 405/605–6111, (Nonreporting) **A**10 **S** Universal Health Services, Inc.
Primary Contact: John A. Holter, Chief Executive Officer
Control: Other not–for–profit (including NFP Corporation) **Service:** Psychiatric

Staffed Beds: 36

CHILDREN'S HOSPITAL OF OKLAHOMA See OU Medical Center

☐ **COMMUNITY HOSPITAL (370203)**, 3100 S.W. 89th Street, Zip 73159–7900; tel. 405/378–3755 **A**1 9 10 **F**3 38 68 79 80 85 96 102 107 118 119 121 124
Primary Contact: Thomas R. Rice, FACHE, President and Chief Operating Officer
Control: Partnership, Investor–owned, for–profit **Service:** General Medical and Surgical

Staffed Beds: 49 **Admissions:** 1814 **Census:** 15 **Outpatient Visits:** 20113 **Births:** 0 **Total Expense ($000):** 42490 **Payroll Expense ($000):** 9367

🞸 △ **DEACONESS HOSPITAL (370032)**, 5501 North Portland Avenue, Zip 73112–2099; tel. 405/604–6000 **A**1 2 7 9 10 **F**3 8 11 13 15 17 18 20 22 25 26 27 30 31 32 33 38 40 43 50 55 56 57 68 70 71 72 73 74 76 77 79 80 81 82 85 86 87 88 90 91 92 93 94 96 97 98 99 100 102 107 108 112 117 118 119 120 121 122 124 135 136 137 **P**8 **S** Community Health Systems, Inc.
Primary Contact: Cathryn A. Hibbs, Chief Executive Officer
COO: R. Andrew Wachtel, Vice President Operations
CFO: Cully Chapman, Vice President Finance
CMO: Kenneth W. Whittington, M.D., Vice President Medical Affairs
CIO: Rex Vaughn, Director Information Technology
CHR: M. L. Wood, Vice President Human Resources and Education
Web address: www.deaconessokc.com
Control: Partnership, Investor–owned, for–profit **Service:** General Medical and Surgical

Staffed Beds: 273 **Admissions:** 10957 **Census:** 167 **Outpatient Visits:** 108106 **Births:** 1374 **Total Expense ($000):** 127123 **Payroll Expense ($000):** 50917 **Personnel:** 1234

EVERETT TOWER See OU Medical Center

🞸 △ **INTEGRIS BAPTIST MEDICAL CENTER (370028)**, 3300 N.W. Expressway, Zip 73112–4481; tel. 405/949–3011, (Includes INTEGRIS MENTAL HEALTH SYSTEM–SPENCER, 2601 North Spencer Road, Spencer, Mailing Address: P.O. Box 11137, Zip 73136–0137; tel. 405/717–9800) **A**1 2 3 5 7 9 10 **F**3 8 11 12 13 15 16 17 18 20 22 24 25 26 27 30 31 32 33 34 37 38 40 42 43 50 52 53 54 55 56 57 58 59 61 62 64 66 68 69 70 71 72 73 74 75 76 77 78 79 81 82 83 84 86 87 88 90 91 92 94 96 97 98 99 102 103 106 107 113 114 118 119 121 122 126 127 128 129 130 131 135 136 137 **P**7 8 **S** INTEGRIS Health
Primary Contact: Chris Hammes, President
COO: C. Bruce Lawrence, Executive Vice President and Chief Operating Officer Integris Health
CFO: Wentz J. Miller, Managing Director and Chief Financial Officer
CMO: James P. White, M.D., Chief Medical Officer
CIO: John Delano, Vice President Chief Information Officer
CHR: Robert Quiring, Vice President Human Resources
Web address: www.integris–health.com
Control: Other not–for–profit (including NFP Corporation) **Service:** General Medical and Surgical

Staffed Beds: 570 **Admissions:** 23276 **Census:** 417 **Outpatient Visits:** 131311 **Births:** 2181 **Total Expense ($000):** 408051 **Payroll Expense ($000):** 154777 **Personnel:** 2408

🞸 △ **INTEGRIS SOUTHWEST MEDICAL CENTER (370106)**, 4401 South Western, Zip 73109–3441; tel. 405/636–7000 **A**1 2 7 9 10 12 13 **F**3 11 13 15 18 20 22 24 25 26 27 28 30 31 32 33 36 37 38 40 43 55 56 57 58 59 61 62 65 66 68 72 73 74 75 76 77 79 80 81 82 85 86 87 96 97 99 100 102 107 108 111 112 118 119 121 123 132 135 136 137 **P**7 8 **S** INTEGRIS Health
Primary Contact: Patricia Dorris, President
COO: Patricia Dorris, President
CFO: Errol Mitchell, Vice President
CIO: John Delano, Vice President and Chief Information Officer
Web address: www.integris–health.com
Control: Other not–for–profit (including NFP Corporation) **Service:** General Medical and Surgical

Staffed Beds: 358 **Admissions:** 14412 **Census:** 222 **Outpatient Visits:** 133778 **Births:** 1525 **Total Expense ($000):** 197744 **Payroll Expense ($000):** 81598 **Personnel:** 1422

☐ **KINDRED HOSPITAL– OKLAHOMA CITY (372004)**, 1407 North Robinson Avenue, Zip 73103; tel. 405/232–8000, (Includes KINDRED HOSPITAL–OKLAHOMA CITY SOUTH, 2129 S.W. 59th Street, Zip 73119; tel. 405/713–5955; Martha J. Heubach, Chief Executive Officer) **A**1 3 5 10 **F**1 25 31 38 59 66 68 80 82 107 119 134 137 **S** Kindred Healthcare
Primary Contact: Gayla Campbell, Chief Executive Officer
Web address: www.kindredoklahoma.com
Control: Corporation, Investor–owned, for–profit **Service:** Long–Term Acute Care hospital

Staffed Beds: 93 **Admissions:** 769 **Census:** 57 **Births:** 0 **Payroll Expense ($000):** 9190 **Personnel:** 118

 Many Facility Codes have changed. Please refer to the AHA Guide Code Chart.

☐ **LAKESIDE WOMEN'S HOSPITAL (370199)**, 11200 North Portland Avenue, Zip 73120; tel. 405/936–1500 **A**1 9 10 **F**3 13 15 26 30 32 33 38 57 62 71 74 79 80 82 99 107 118 121 136 **P**6
Primary Contact: Kelley Brewer, Chief Executive Officer
CFO: Darla McCallister, Chief Financial Officer
CMO: Dana Stone, M.D., Chief Medical Officer
CHR: Renee Beene, Manager Human Resources
Web address: www.lakeside-wh.net
Control: Corporation, Investor–owned, for–profit **Service:** Obstetrics and gynecology

Staffed Beds: 23 **Admissions:** 1535 **Census:** 10 **Births:** 1240 **Total Expense ($000):** 15068 **Payroll Expense ($000):** 5372 **Personnel:** 129

MCBRIDE CLINIC ORTHOPEDIC HOSPITAL (370222), 9600 North Broadway Extension, Zip 73114; tel. 405/478–1717 **A**10 **F**3 25 26 31 38 43 55 57 62 66 75 77 79 80 81 82 85 96 102 107 119 120
Primary Contact: Troy Hensarling, Chief Executive Officer
COO: Christine Weigel, Clinical Operations Officer
CFO: Annie Bassett, Director Finance
CMO: David Holden, M.D., Chief of Staff
CIO: Ronnie Green, Director Information Systems
CHR: Cathy Withiam, Vice President Human Resources
Web address: www.mcbrideclinicorthopedichospital.com
Control: Corporation, Investor–owned, for–profit **Service:** Orthopedic

Staffed Beds: 78 **Admissions:** 2820 **Census:** 24 **Outpatient Visits:** 3036 **Births:** 0 **Total Expense ($000):** 34526 **Payroll Expense ($000):** 10938 **Personnel:** 228

★ △ **MERCY HEALTH CENTER (370013)**, 4300 West Memorial Road, Zip 73120–8362; tel. 405/755–1515 **A**1 2 7 9 10 **F**3 11 13 15 17 18 20 22 24 25 26 27 30 31 32 33 34 38 39 40 42 43 44 50 52 53 55 56 57 59 61 62 66 68 70 72 73 74 75 76 77 79 80 81 82 84 85 96 97 99 100 102 103 104 107 111 112 114 118 119 121 124 133 135 136 137 **S** Sisters of Mercy Health System
Primary Contact: Diana Smalley, President
COO: Jeff Johnston, Chief Operating Officer
CFO: James Newman, Senior Vice President and Chief Financial Officer
CMO: Mark Johnson, M.D., Chief Medical Officer
CIO: Ron Fovargue, Vice President Information Services
CHR: Cathy Withiam, Vice President Human Resources
Web address: www.mercyok.net
Control: Church–operated, Nongovernment, not–for profit **Service:** General Medical and Surgical

Staffed Beds: 338 **Admissions:** 15535 **Census:** 237 **Outpatient Visits:** 199501 **Births:** 3019 **Total Expense ($000):** 220357 **Payroll Expense ($000):** 91671 **Personnel:** 2301

☐ **NORTHWEST SURGICAL HOSPITAL (370192)**, 9204 North May Avenue, Zip 73120–4419; tel. 405/848–1918 **A**1 9 10 **F**30 32 38 43 77 79 80 96 100 104 107 119
Primary Contact: Debbie Foster, RN, Chief Executive Officer
CFO: Cindy Thompson, Chief Financial Officer
CMO: Jimmy Conway, M.D., President Medical Staff
Control: Partnership, Investor–owned, for–profit **Service:** Surgical

Staffed Beds: 9 **Admissions:** 474 **Census:** 3 **Outpatient Visits:** 12281 **Births:** 0 **Total Expense ($000):** 19852 **Payroll Expense ($000):** 2889 **Personnel:** 79

☐ **OKLAHOMA CENTER FOR ORTHOPEDIC AND MULTI–SPECIALTY SURGERY (370212)**, 8100 South Walker, Suite C., Zip 73139, Mailing Address: P.O. Box 890609, Zip 73189; tel. 405/602–6500, (Nonreporting) **A**1 9 10 **S** United Surgical Partners International
Primary Contact: Teri Philbrick, Chief Executive Officer
CFO: Donna Avant, Chief Financial Officer
CHR: Sherry Wagner, Director Human Resources
Control: Corporation, Investor–owned, for–profit **Service:** Orthopedic

Staffed Beds: 10

☐ **OKLAHOMA HEART HOSPITAL (370215)**, 4050 West Memorial Road, Zip 73120; tel. 405/608–3200 **A**1 9 10 **F**3 17 18 20 22 24 25 26 30 31 32 33 38 55 56 57 59 73 75 78 79 80 82 96 102 103 107 116 119 126 135
Primary Contact: John Harvey, M.D., Chief Executive Officer
COO: Peggy Tipton, Chief Operating Officer and Chief Nursing
CFO: Carol Walker, Chief Financial Officer
CMO: John Harvey, M.D., Chief Executive Officer
CIO: Steve Miller, Chief Information Officer
CHR: Katherine Wynn, Director Human Resource
Web address: www.okheart.com
Control: Partnership, Investor–owned, for–profit **Service:** Heart

Staffed Beds: 78 **Admissions:** 9195 **Census:** 54 **Outpatient Visits:** 33673 **Births:** 0 **Total Expense ($000):** 111902 **Payroll Expense ($000):** 38373 **Personnel:** 751

☐ **OKLAHOMA SPINE HOSPITAL (370206)**, 14101 Parkway Commons Drive, Zip 73134; tel. 405/749–2700, (Nonreporting) **A**1 10
Primary Contact: Kevin Blaylock, Chief Executive Officer
Web address: www.oklahomaspine.com
Control: Corporation, Investor–owned, for–profit **Service:** Other specialty

Staffed Beds: 12

ORTHOPEDIC HOSPITAL (370220), 1044 S.W. 44th Street, Suite 620, Zip 73109–3609; tel. 405/631–3085 **A**10
Primary Contact: Denny Oreb, Administrator
Control: Corporation, Investor–owned, for–profit **Service:** Orthopedic

Staffed Beds: 8 **Admissions:** 228 **Census:** 3 **Outpatient Visits:** 772 **Births:** 0 **Total Expense ($000):** 6360 **Payroll Expense ($000):** 1601

★ **OU MEDICAL CENTER (370093)**, 1200 Everett Drive, Zip 73104–5047, Mailing Address: P.O. Box 26307, Zip 73126; tel. 405/271–5911, (Includes CHILDREN'S HOSPITAL OF OKLAHOMA; EVERETT TOWER; PRESBYTERIAN TOWER) **A**1 2 3 5 8 9 10 **F**3 7 11 13 15 17 18 19 20 21 22 23 24 25 26 27 28 30 31 32 33 36 37 38 40 43 44 52 54 55 56 57 58 59 60 62 64 66 68 70 72 73 74 76 77 79 80 83 84 86 88 90 91 92 96 97 100 102 103 105 107 112 113 114 118 119 121 124 125 127 135 136 137 **S** HCA
Primary Contact: Cole C. Eslyn, FACHE, President and Chief Executive Officer
COO: Rebecca Benoit, Chief Operating Officer Adult Services
CFO: Jim Watson, Chief Financial Officer
CIO: Larry Forsyth, Director Information Services
CHR: Laura Land, Chief Human Resources Officer
Web address: www.oumedcenter.com
Control: Corporation, Investor–owned, for–profit **Service:** General Medical and Surgical

Staffed Beds: 587 **Admissions:** 26451 **Census:** 427 **Outpatient Visits:** 213906 **Births:** 4490 **Total Expense ($000):** 449506 **Payroll Expense ($000):** 140148 **Personnel:** 2592

PRESBYTERIAN TOWER See OU Medical Center

☐ **SELECT SPECIALTY HOSPITAL–OKLAHOMA CITY (372009)**, 3524 N.W. 56th Stret, Zip 73112–4510; tel. 405/606–6700 **A**1 9 10 **F**1 3 12 25 38 72 73 77 80 82 96 107 119 137 **S** Select Medical Corporation
Primary Contact: Connie Strickland, Administrator
Web address: www.selectmedicalcorp.com
Control: Corporation, Investor–owned, for–profit **Service:** Long–Term Acute Care hospital

Staffed Beds: 72 **Admissions:** 751 **Census:** 58 **Outpatient Visits:** 0 **Births:** 0 **Total Expense ($000):** 26224 **Payroll Expense ($000):** 10164 **Personnel:** 228

★ △ **ST. ANTHONY HOSPITAL (370037)**, 1000 North Lee Street, Zip 73102–1080, Mailing Address: P.O. Box 205, Zip 73101–0205; tel. 405/272–7000, (Includes ST. ANTHONY SOUTH, 2129 S.W. 59th Street, Zip 73119–7001; tel. 405/713–5700) **A**1 2 3 5 7 9 10 12 13 **F**3 4 5 8 12 13 15 17 18 20 22 23 24 25 26 27 30 31 32 33 37 38 40 43 44 51 54 55 56 57 62 63 64 65 68 72 74 75 76 77 79 80 81 82 85 86 87 88 90 91 92 93 94 95 96 97 99 100 101 102 103 105 106 107 108 118 119 120 121 124 127 135 137 **P**4 7 **S** SSM Health Care
Primary Contact: Joe Hodges, President
COO: Marti Jourden, FACHE, Vice President Operations
CFO: Greg Simia, Vice President Finance
CMO: Kersey Winfree, M.D., Chief Medical Officer
CIO: Kevin Olson, Director Information Systems
CHR: Cynthia Brundise, Vice President Human Resources
Web address: www.saintsok.com
Control: Church–operated, Nongovernment, not–for profit **Service:** General Medical and Surgical

Staffed Beds: 499 **Admissions:** 17548 **Census:** 366 **Outpatient Visits:** 92767 **Births:** 1254 **Total Expense ($000):** 224361 **Payroll Expense ($000):** 83355 **Personnel:** 1761

ST. ANTHONY SOUTH See St. Anthony Hospital

☐ **SURGICAL HOSPITAL OF OKLAHOMA (370201)**, 100 S.E. 59th Street, Zip 73129; tel. 405/634–9300 **A**1 10 **F**3 32 38 79
Primary Contact: Phil Ross, Chief Executive Officer
Control: Partnership, Investor–owned, for–profit **Service:** Surgical

Staffed Beds: 12 **Admissions:** 356 **Census:** 2 **Outpatient Visits:** 5488 **Births:** 0 **Total Expense ($000):** 12868 **Payroll Expense ($000):** 3789 **Personnel:** 90

Hospital, Medicare Provider Number, Address, Telephone, Approval, Facility, and Physician Codes, Health Care System

★ American Hospital Association (AHA) membership
☐ The Joint Commission accreditation
○ American Osteopathic Association (AOA) accreditation
△ Commission on Accreditation of Rehabilitation Facilities (CARF) accreditation

☒ **VALIR REHABILITATION HOSPITAL (373025)**, 700 N.W. Seventh Street, Zip 73102–1295; tel. 405/236–3131 **A**1 10 **F**24 25 26 30 32 33 38 43 54 57 62 64 73 81 82 85 86 119 120 124
Primary Contact: Stacy Smith, Chief Executive Officer
COO: Ginger Castleberry, Chief Operating Officer
CFO: Scott Brown, Chief Financial Officer
CMO: Tonya Washburn, M.D., Medical Director
CIO: Mark Dickey, Director Business Development
CHR: Judy Rutledge, Manager Human Resources
Web address: www.valir.com
Control: Corporation, Investor–owned, for–profit **Service:** Rehabilitation

Staffed Beds: 81 **Admissions:** 940 **Census:** 32 **Outpatient Visits:** 6938 **Births:** 0 **Personnel:** 162

☒ △ **VETERANS AFFAIRS MEDICAL CENTER**, 921 N.E. 13th Street, Zip 73104–5028; tel. 405/270–0501 **A**1 3 5 7 8 **F**1 2 3 4 5 7 8 17 18 20 22 24 25 26 27 37 38 40 43 44 53 54 55 57 58 60 61 62 65 68 72 73 75 76 77 79 80 81 82 86 87 88 90 91 92 93 94 95 96 99 100 102 103 104 105 107 117 118 119 121 124 132 133 135 136 137 **S** Department of Veterans Affairs
Primary Contact: David P. Wood, Medical Center Director
CFO: Haze McDougal, Chief Fiscal Service
CMO: Robert McCaffree, M.D., Chief of Staff
CIO: Jerry Melvin, Chief Information Management Services
CHR: Kyle Inhofe, Chief Human Resources Officer
Web address: www.va.gov/sta/guide/home.asp
Control: Veterans Affairs, Government, federal **Service:** General Medical and Surgical

Staffed Beds: 205 **Admissions:** 6719 **Census:** 160 **Births:** 0 **Total Expense ($000):** 305000 **Payroll Expense ($000):** 124000 **Personnel:** 1607

OKMULGEE—Okmulgee County

GEORGE NIGH REHABILITATION CENTER (373026), 900 East Airport Road, Zip 74447–9762, Mailing Address: P.O. Box 1118, Zip 74447–1118; tel. 918/756–9211, (Total facility includes 13 beds in nursing home–type unit) (Nonreporting) **A**10
Primary Contact: Gala McBee, Administrator
CFO: Djogan Djogan, Chief Financial Officer
CHR: Denaye Atwell, Manager Human Resources
Web address: www.gnrc.ouhsc.edu
Control: State–Government, nonfederal **Service:** Rehabilitation

Staffed Beds: 20

★ **OKMULGEE MEMORIAL HOSPITAL (370057)**, 1401 Morris Drive, Zip 74447–6419, Mailing Address: P.O. Box 1038, Zip 74447–1038; tel. 918/756–4233 **A**9 10 **F**3 11 15 25 31 38 61 79 82 85 88 93 96 106 107 119 122 135 **S** QHR
Primary Contact: Rex Jones, Chief Executive Officer
CMO: Tim Sanford, D.O., Chief of Staff
CIO: Sharon Riker, Data Processing Manager
CHR: Ron Mathis, Director Human Resources
Web address: www.okmulgeehospital.com
Control: Other not–for–profit (including NFP Corporation) **Service:** General Medical and Surgical

Staffed Beds: 66 **Admissions:** 1616 **Census:** 18 **Outpatient Visits:** 29368 **Total Expense ($000):** 12394 **Payroll Expense ($000):** 6976 **Personnel:** 214

OWASSO—Tulsa County

★ **BAILEY MEDICAL CENTER (370228)**, 10502 North 110th East Avenue, Zip 74055; tel. 918/376–8000 **A**9 10 **F**3 11 12 13 15 25 26 30 31 32 33 35 38 55 56 57 63 68 73 74 75 77 79 80 85 96 99 100 103 107 118 119 120 121 135 **P**5 **S** Ardent Health Services
Primary Contact: Dee Renshaw, Chief Executive Officer
COO: Keith Mason, R.N., Chief Operating Officer and Chief Nursing Officer
CFO: Rhonda McCabe, Chief Financial Officer
CHR: Rachel Steward, Manager Human Resources
Web address: www.baileymedicalcenter.com
Control: Corporation, Investor–owned, for–profit **Service:** General Medical and Surgical

Staffed Beds: 67 **Admissions:** 1176 **Census:** 9 **Outpatient Visits:** 8172 **Births:** 37 **Total Expense ($000):** 32100 **Payroll Expense ($000):** 7441 **Personnel:** 166

★ **ST. JOHN OWASSO (370227)**, 12451 East 100th Street North, Zip 74055; tel. 918/274–5000 **A**9 10 **F**38 74 77 79 86 100 103 107 136 **P**7 **S** Marian Health System
Primary Contact: David Phillips, President and Chief Executive Officer
CFO: Lex S. Anderson, Chief Financial Officer
CMO: Tim Hepner, M.D., Medical Director
CIO: Mike Reeves, Chief Information Officer
Web address: www.stjohnowasso.com
Control: Church–operated, Nongovernment, not–for profit **Service:** General Medical and Surgical

Staffed Beds: 24 **Admissions:** 2110 **Census:** 6 **Outpatient Visits:** 16156 **Births:** 128

PAULS VALLEY—Garvin County

★ **PAULS VALLEY GENERAL HOSPITAL (370156)**, 100 Valley Drive, Zip 73075–6613, Mailing Address: Box 368, Zip 73075–0368; tel. 405/238–5501, (Total facility includes 8 beds in nursing home–type unit) **A**9 10 20 **F**7 10 11 13 15 25 38 42 43 44 54 55 61 62 74 75 79 80 96 102 107 117 119 121 122
Primary Contact: Charles Johnston, Chief Executive Officer
CFO: Brent Mynhier, Chief Financial Officer
Web address: www.pvgh.net
Control: Hospital district or authority, Government, nonfederal **Service:** General Medical and Surgical

Staffed Beds: 50 **Admissions:** 1806 **Census:** 23 **Outpatient Visits:** 24709 **Births:** 63 **Total Expense ($000):** 12363 **Payroll Expense ($000):** 7951

PAWHUSKA—Osage County

PAWHUSKA HOSPITAL (371309), 1101 East 15th Street, Zip 74056–1920; tel. 918/287–3232 **A**9 10 18 **F**3 11 25 30 38 117 122
Primary Contact: Ron Dunkle, Administrator
CMO: Mike Priest, M.D., Chief of Staff
CHR: Karen Arrowsmith, Assistant Administrator and Human Resource Director
Control: City–Government, nonfederal **Service:** General Medical and Surgical

Staffed Beds: 25 **Admissions:** 168 **Census:** 3 **Outpatient Visits:** 4533 **Births:** 0 **Total Expense ($000):** 2464 **Payroll Expense ($000):** 1499 **Personnel:** 23

PERRY—Noble County

★ **PERRY MEMORIAL HOSPITAL (370139)**, 501 14th Street, Zip 73077–5099; tel. 580/336–3541 **A**9 10 20 **F**3 11 15 25 26 30 31 32 37 38 55 57 61 62 77 79 80 86 96 97 100 107 119 122 135 137 **S** QHR
Primary Contact: Joe Duerr, Chief Executive Officer
CFO: Milena Davis, Chief Financial Officer
CIO: Chelsie Kinkade, Director Health Information Management
CHR: Robin Webb, Director Human Resources
Web address: www.pmh–ok.org
Control: Hospital district or authority, Government, nonfederal **Service:** General Medical and Surgical

Staffed Beds: 26 **Admissions:** 756 **Census:** 11 **Outpatient Visits:** 16247 **Births:** 1 **Total Expense ($000):** 6643 **Payroll Expense ($000):** 3126 **Personnel:** 77

PONCA CITY—Kay County

☒ **PONCA CITY MEDICAL CENTER (370006)**, 1900 North 14th Street, Zip 74601–2035; tel. 580/765–3321 **A**1 9 10 19 **F**3 8 13 15 18 25 26 30 31 32 33 35 38 40 43 51 52 54 55 56 57 63 64 66 67 68 70 72 73 74 77 79 80 86 87 88 93 96 100 103 104 105 107 112 118 119 121 122 134 135 137 **S** Community Health Systems, Inc.
Primary Contact: Dennis Barts, Chief Executive Officer
CFO: Dennis T. Bynum, Interim Chief Financial Officer
CIO: David Williams, Director Information Systems
CHR: Lisa Zaloudek, Chief Human Resources Officer
Web address: www.poncamedcenter.com
Control: Corporation, Investor–owned, for–profit **Service:** General Medical and Surgical

Staffed Beds: 85 **Admissions:** 3906 **Census:** 40 **Outpatient Visits:** 55504 **Births:** 569 **Total Expense ($000):** 47075 **Payroll Expense ($000):** 15345 **Personnel:** 390

POTEAU—Le Flore County

☒ **EASTERN OKLAHOMA MEDICAL CENTER (370040)**, 105 Wall Street, Zip 74953–4428, Mailing Address: P.O. Box 1148, Zip 74953–1148; tel. 918/647–8161 **A**1 9 10 20 **F**3 11 15 25 30 38 43 55 61 62 68 74 79 86 96 99 100 103 107 135 136 **P**5
Primary Contact: Terry Buckner, Chief Executive Officer
CFO: Nancy Frier, Chief Financial Officer
CMO: Dennis Carter, M.D., Chief of Staff
CIO: Michael C. Huggins, Network System Administrator
CHR: Michele Oglesby, Human Resources Manager
Control: County–Government, nonfederal **Service:** General Medical and Surgical

Staffed Beds: 84 **Admissions:** 2866 **Census:** 28 **Outpatient Visits:** 25625 **Births:** 472 **Total Expense ($000):** 10672 **Payroll Expense ($000):** 6760 **Personnel:** 239

PRAGUE—Lincoln County

★ **PRAGUE MUNICIPAL HOSPITAL (371301)**, 1322 Klabzuba Avenue, Zip 74864–9005, Mailing Address: P.O. Drawer S, Zip 74864–9005; tel. 405/567–4922 **A**9 10 18 **F**25 38 40 55 56 57 62 66 79 86 96 107 119 121 122 **P**6 **S** The Schuster Group
Primary Contact: Joan Walters, RN, M.S.N., Administrator
CFO: Doug Erickson, Chief Financial Officer
CMO: Darryl Jackson, D.O., Chief of Staff
CIO: Krista Grooms, Director Health Improvement Management
CHR: Angie Brezny, Director Human Resources
Web address: www.praguehospital.com
Control: Corporation, Investor–owned, for–profit **Service:** General Medical and Surgical

Staffed Beds: 19 **Admissions:** 298 **Census:** 3 **Outpatient Visits:** 6902 **Births:** 0 **Total Expense ($000):** 2427 **Payroll Expense ($000):** 1136 **Personnel:** 44

PRYOR—Mayes County

☒ **INTEGRIS MAYES COUNTY MEDICAL CENTER (370015)**, 111 North Bailey Street, Zip 74361–4211, Mailing Address: P.O. Box 278, Zip 74362–0278; tel. 918/825–1600 **A**1 9 10 **F**3 11 13 14 15 25 26 30 31 32 33 38 42 55 56 57 61 62 66 73 74 75 79 80 82 86 96 97 107 119 121 122 124 135 136 **S** INTEGRIS Health
Primary Contact: W. Charles Jordan, President
CFO: Kristy McCollough, Assistant Administrator and Chief Financial Officer
CMO: Lora Collier, M.D., Chief Medical Staff
CHR: Jamil Haynes, Director Human Resources
Web address: www.integris–health.com
Control: Other not–for–profit (including NFP Corporation) **Service:** General Medical and Surgical

Staffed Beds: 39 **Admissions:** 1432 **Census:** 11 **Outpatient Visits:** 36706 **Births:** 277 **Total Expense ($000):** 19023 **Payroll Expense ($000):** 8104 **Personnel:** 205

PURCELL—McClain County

★ **PURCELL MUNICIPAL HOSPITAL (370158)**, 1500 North Green Avenue, Zip 73080–1699, Mailing Address: P.O. Box 511, Zip 73080–0511; tel. 405/527–6524 **A**9 10 **F**3 11 13 25 26 30 33 38 55 57 62 63 73 74 75 77 79 81 82 84 86 102 107 119 121 122 **P**8 **S** QHR
COO: Mark Alfonso, Interim Chief Operating Officer
CFO: Jennifer Warren, Chief Financial Officer
CMO: Bryan Dye, Chief of Staff
CIO: Jennifer Coates, Coordinator Information Technology
CHR: Fran Ray, Manager Human Resources
Web address: www.purcellhospital.com
Control: City–Government, nonfederal **Service:** General Medical and Surgical

Staffed Beds: 30 **Admissions:** 1451 **Census:** 15 **Outpatient Visits:** 41155 **Births:** 60 **Total Expense ($000):** 11241 **Payroll Expense ($000):** 5096 **Personnel:** 150

SALLISAW—Sequoyah County

SEQUOYAH MEMORIAL HOSPITAL (370112), 213 East Redwood Street, Zip 74955–2811, Mailing Address: P.O. Box 505, Zip 74955–0505; tel. 918/774–1100 **A**9 10 **F**31 32 38 40 42 43 44 57 61 62 79 86 96 100 102 107 118
Primary Contact: Charles Wade, Interim Administrator
CFO: Glenn Click, Chief Financial Officer
CMO: James D. Campbell, M.D., Chief of Staff
Web address: www.smhok.com
Control: Hospital district or authority, Government, nonfederal **Service:** General Medical and Surgical

Staffed Beds: 26 **Admissions:** 914 **Census:** 8 **Outpatient Visits:** 47449 **Births:** 3 **Total Expense ($000):** 11005 **Payroll Expense ($000):** 5763 **Personnel:** 303

SAPULPA—Creek County

★ **ST. JOHN SAPULPA (371312)**, 519 South Division Street, Zip 74066–4501, Mailing Address: P.O. Box 1368, Zip 74067–1368; tel. 918/224–4280 **A**9 10 18 **F**3 15 25 26 32 38 62 77 79 86 96 107 122 124 135 **P**5 **S** Marian Health System
Primary Contact: Raymond L. Replogle, President and Chief Executive Officer
CFO: Donna Nagel, Senior Director Operations
CMO: Roger D. Wilson, M.D., Medical Director
Web address: www.sjmc.org
Control: Church–operated, Nongovernment, not–for profit **Service:** General Medical and Surgical

Staffed Beds: 25 **Admissions:** 1493 **Census:** 14 **Outpatient Visits:** 46427 **Births:** 0 **Total Expense ($000):** 19935 **Payroll Expense ($000):** 5324 **Personnel:** 157

SAYRE—Beckham County

★ **SAYRE MEMORIAL HOSPITAL (370103)**, 501 East Washington Street, Zip 73662–1337; tel. 580/928–5541 **A**9 10 **F**3 32 38 57 61 82 86 96 107 117 119 122 **S** QHR
Primary Contact: Jason Anglin, Chief Executive Officer
CFO: Monica Scott, Chief Financial Officer
CHR: Misty Carter, Director Human Resources and Marketing
Web address: www.sayrehospital.org
Control: Other not–for–profit (including NFP Corporation) **Service:** General Medical and Surgical

Staffed Beds: 35 **Admissions:** 958 **Census:** 22 **Births:** 0

SEILING—Dewey County

★ **SEILING HOSPITAL (371332)**, Highway 60 N.E., Zip 73663, Mailing Address: P.O. Box 720, Zip 73663–0720; tel. 580/922–7361 **A**9 18 **F**38 40 96 107 122 **P**5
Primary Contact: Jennifer Jones, Chief Executive Officer
CFO: Nancy Freed, Chief Financial Officer
CMO: Porter Leslie, M.D., Medical Director
CHR: Roy Jones, Director Human Resources
Control: City–Government, nonfederal **Service:** General Medical and Surgical

Staffed Beds: 18 **Admissions:** 312 **Census:** 4 **Outpatient Visits:** 4788 **Births:** 0 **Personnel:** 35

SEMINOLE—Seminole County

★ **INTEGRIS SEMINOLE MEDICAL CENTER (370200)**, (Formerly Seminole Medical Center), 2401 Wrangler Boulevard, Zip 74868–1917; tel. 405/303–4000 **A**9 10 **F**3 11 15 25 26 31 33 38 56 57 66 77 79 82 86 87 96 107 118 119 **S** INTEGRIS Health
Primary Contact: C. David Hill, President
CFO: Sarah Edwards, Chief Financial Officer
CMO: Randall Kemp, M.D., Medical Director
CHR: Sherri Kemp, Director Human Resources
Web address: www.seminolemedicalcenter.com
Control: Other not–for–profit (including NFP Corporation) **Service:** General Medical and Surgical

Staffed Beds: 32 **Admissions:** 603 **Census:** 5 **Outpatient Visits:** 17284 **Births:** 0

SHATTUCK—Ellis County

★ **NEWMAN MEMORIAL HOSPITAL (370007)**, 905 South Main Street, Zip 73858–9802; tel. 580/938–2551 **A**9 10 20 **F**3 11 13 15 25 26 31 32 33 37 38 52 55 57 61 62 63 67 74 79 82 86 96 100 102 107 118 122 135 **P**6
Primary Contact: Gary W. Mitchell, Chief Executive Officer
COO: Kevin O'Brien, Chief Operating Officer
Web address: www.newmanmemorialhospital.org
Control: Other not–for–profit (including NFP Corporation) **Service:** General Medical and Surgical

Staffed Beds: 27 **Admissions:** 897 **Census:** 8 **Outpatient Visits:** 42270 **Births:** 162 **Total Expense ($000):** 8798 **Payroll Expense ($000):** 3210 **Personnel:** 83

SHAWNEE—Pottawatomie County

SOLARA HOSPITAL OF SHAWNEE (372019), 1900 Gordan Cooper Drive, 2nd Floor, Zip 74801; tel. 405/395–5800 **A**10
Primary Contact: David M. Peyok, Chief Executive Officer
Web address: www.solarahc.com
Control: Corporation, Investor–owned, for–profit **Service:** General Medical and Surgical

Staffed Beds: 30 **Admissions:** 281 **Census:** 21

☒ **UNITY HEALTH CENTER (370149)**, 1102 West MacArthur Street, Zip 74804–1744; tel. 405/273–2270 **A**1 2 9 10 19 **F**3 11 13 15 18 25 26 27 30 31 32 33 38 40 43 50 55 56 57 62 63 67 68 73 74 75 76 77 79 82 85 86 96 97 100 106 107 108 112 118 119 120 121 124 133 135 136 137 **P**5
Primary Contact: Charles E. Skillings, President and Chief Executive Officer
COO: Thomas Keller, Executive Vice President and Chief Operating Officer
CFO: Vicky Fine, Vice President and Chief Financial Officer
CMO: David Hadley, M.D., Medical Director
CIO: Linda E. Brown, R.N., Vice President Clinical Support
CHR: Michael Spears, Vice President Workforce Development
Web address: www.unityhealthcenter.com
Control: Other not–for–profit (including NFP Corporation) **Service:** General Medical and Surgical

Staffed Beds: 95 **Admissions:** 5209 **Census:** 53 **Outpatient Visits:** 97887 **Births:** 1023 **Total Expense ($000):** 77669 **Payroll Expense ($000):** 22373 **Personnel:** 582

Hospital, Medicare Provider Number, Address, Telephone, Approval, Facility, and Physician Codes, Health Care System
★ American Hospital Association (AHA) membership
□ The Joint Commission accreditation
○ American Osteopathic Association (AOA) accreditation
△ Commission on Accreditation of Rehabilitation Facilities (CARF) accreditation

SPENCER—Oklahoma County

INTEGRIS MENTAL HEALTH SYSTEM–SPENCER See Integris Baptist Medical Center, Oklahoma City

STIGLER—Haskell County

OK

★ **HASKELL COUNTY HEALTHCARE SYSTEM (370084)**, 401 N.W. H Street, Zip 74462–1625, Mailing Address: P.O. Box 728, Zip 74462; tel. 918/967–4682 **A**9 10 20 **F**15 25 38 42 55 79 96 107 122 137
Primary Contact: Nathan Speer, Interim Chief Executive Officer
COO: Ben Helm, Interim Chief Financial Officer
CFO: Jeff Burns, Chief Financial Officer
CMO: Thomas Conklin, M.D., Chief of Staff
CIO: Larry Gregg, Information Technology Specialist
CHR: Stephanie Kroth, Director Human Resources
Web address: www.hchs.otnnet.net
Control: City–County, Government, nonfederal **Service:** General Medical and Surgical

Staffed Beds: 30 **Admissions:** 1057 **Census:** 12 **Outpatient Visits:** 12627 **Births:** 0 **Total Expense ($000):** 9574 **Payroll Expense ($000):** 5157

STILLWATER—Payne County

★ △ **STILLWATER MEDICAL CENTER (370049)**, 1323 West Sixth Avenue, Zip 74074–4399, Mailing Address: P.O. Box 2408, Zip 74076–2408; tel. 405/372–1480 **A**1 7 9 10 19 20 **F**3 11 13 15 18 32 33 38 40 43 52 61 67 68 72 73 74 77 79 80 82 85 86 95 96 97 100 103 104 107 117 118 119 120 124 135 **P**7
Primary Contact: Jerry G. Moeller, President and Chief Executive Officer
COO: Karen Hendren, Chief Operating Officer
CIO: Chris Roark, Chief Information Officer
CHR: Keith Hufnagel, Director Human Resources
Web address: www.stillwater–medical.org
Control: Hospital district or authority, Government, nonfederal **Service:** General Medical and Surgical

Staffed Beds: 87 **Admissions:** 4789 **Census:** 52 **Outpatient Visits:** 90514 **Births:** 913 **Total Expense ($000):** 74773 **Payroll Expense ($000):** 29736 **Personnel:** 702

STILWELL—Adair County

★ **MEMORIAL HOSPITAL (370178)**, 1401 West Locust, Zip 74960, Mailing Address: P.O. Box 272, Zip 74960; tel. 918/696–3101 **A**9 10 20 **F**11 13 15 25 26 32 38 56 57 74 77 84 85 86 94 96 100 107 135 **P**4
Primary Contact: Alan L. Adams, President
Control: Other not–for–profit (including NFP Corporation) **Service:** General Medical and Surgical

Staffed Beds: 30 **Admissions:** 2070 **Census:** 15 **Outpatient Visits:** 51311 **Births:** 78 **Total Expense ($000):** 11338 **Payroll Expense ($000):** 6258 **Personnel:** 167

STROUD—Lincoln County

STROUD REGIONAL MEDICAL CENTER (371316), Highway 66 West, Zip 74079, Mailing Address: P.O. Box 530, Zip 74079–0530; tel. 918/968–3571, (Nonreporting) **A**9 10 18 **S** The Schuster Group
Primary Contact: Beverly Ash, Chief Executive Officer
Control: Other not–for–profit (including NFP Corporation) **Service:** General Medical and Surgical

Staffed Beds: 22

SULPHUR—Murray County

ARBUCKLE MEMORIAL HOSPITAL (371328), 2011 West Broadway Street, Zip 73086–4221; tel. 580/622–2161 **A**9 10 18 **F**30 32 38 55 62 79 96 107 122 135 **P**4 **S** Preferred Management Corporation
Primary Contact: Darin Farrell, Chief Executive Officer
CFO: Chris Bottoms, Chief Financial Officer
Web address: www.arbucklehospital.com/
Control: County–Government, nonfederal **Service:** General Medical and Surgical

Staffed Beds: 25 **Admissions:** 575 **Census:** 13 **Outpatient Visits:** 17967 **Births:** 0 **Total Expense ($000):** 6296 **Payroll Expense ($000):** 3376 **Personnel:** 91

TAHLEQUAH—Cherokee County

TAHLEQUAH CITY HOSPITAL (370089), 1400 East Downing Street, Zip 74464–3324, Mailing Address: P.O. Box 1008, Zip 74465–1008; tel. 918/456–0641 **A**9 10 20 **F**3 7 11 15 17 18 20 22 24 25 26 30 31 32 33 38 40 43 55 57 68 73 74 75 77 79 80 82 84 85 86 88 93 96 100 102 107 118 119 122 124 135
Primary Contact: Brian K. Woodliff, President and Chief Executive Officer
COO: David McClain, Executive Vice President Operations
CFO: Julie Newman, Chief Financial Officer
CIO: Julie Newman, Vice President Finance
CHR: Phyllis Smith, Vice President Human Resources
Web address: www.tch–ok.org
Control: City–Government, nonfederal **Service:** General Medical and Surgical

Staffed Beds: 78 **Admissions:** 3766 **Census:** 49 **Outpatient Visits:** 65536 **Births:** 452 **Total Expense ($000):** 42139 **Payroll Expense ($000):** 14664 **Personnel:** 441

★ **WILLIAM W. HASTINGS INDIAN HOSPITAL (370171)**, 100 South Bliss Avenue, Zip 74464–3399; tel. 918/458–3100, (Nonreporting) **A**1 10 **S** U. S. Indian Health Service
Primary Contact: Edwin McLemore, Chief Executive Officer
Control: PHS, Indian Service, Government, federal **Service:** General Medical and Surgical

Staffed Beds: 60

TALIHINA—La Flore County

★ **CHOCTAW NATION HEALTH CARE CENTER (370172)**, One Choctaw Way, Zip 74571–9517; tel. 918/567–7000 **A**1 10 **F**3 5 6 13 15 25 28 30 31 32 33 37 38 41 43 52 53 54 55 56 57 58 62 63 73 74 77 79 80 81 82 84 85 86 87 88 91 92 94 96 107 113 119 124 132 133 136 137 **P**6
Primary Contact: Teresa Jackson, Chief Executive Officer
COO: Todd Hallmark, Chief Operating Officer
CFO: Teresa Jackson, Chief Executive Officer
CMO: Jason Hill, M.D., Chief Medical Officer
CIO: Skip Leader, Chief Information Officer
CHR: Evelyn Jones, Director Human Resources
Web address: www.choctawnationhealth.com
Control: PHS, Indian Service, Government, federal **Service:** General Medical and Surgical

Staffed Beds: 37 **Admissions:** 1663 **Census:** 14 **Outpatient Visits:** 135124 **Births:** 498 **Personnel:** 575

TISHOMINGO—Johnston County

JOHNSTON MEMORIAL HOSPITAL (371304), 1000 South Byrd Street, Zip 73460–3299; tel. 580/371–2327 **A**9 10 18 **F**3 31 38 56 96 122 **S** The Schuster Group
Primary Contact: Mary Owen, RN, Administrator
CFO: Lisa Dowling, Manager Finance
CHR: Arlita Hummelke, Manager Human Resources
Control: Corporation, Investor–owned, for–profit **Service:** General Medical and Surgical

Staffed Beds: 21 **Admissions:** 524 **Census:** 5 **Outpatient Visits:** 3256 **Births:** 0 **Personnel:** 49

TULSA—Tulsa County

BROOKHAVEN HOSPITAL (374012), 201 South Garnett Road, Zip 74128–1800; tel. 918/438–4257, (Nonreporting) **A**10
Primary Contact: Rolf B. Gainer, Chief Executive Officer and Administrator
CFO: Kenneth Pierce, Chief Financial Officer
CMO: Stephen Marish, M.D., Medical Director
CHR: Betsy Davis, Director Administrative Services
Web address: www.brookhavenhospital.com
Control: Corporation, Investor–owned, for–profit **Service:** Psychiatric

Staffed Beds: 40

★ **CONTINUOUS CARE CENTER OF TULSA (372011)**, 1924 South Utica Avenue, Zip 74105–6510; tel. 918/749–8930 **A**9 10 **F**1 25 38 43 44 75 119 137 **P**8
Primary Contact: Raymond L. Replogle, President and Chief Executive Officer
CFO: Basil Wyatt, Chief Financial Officer
CMO: Gordon Lantz, M.D., Medical Director
CIO: Dana Jetton, Chief Information Officer
CHR: Sunny Benjamin, Director Human Resources
Web address: www.cccok.com
Control: Other not–for–profit (including NFP Corporation) **Service:** Long–Term Acute Care hospital

Staffed Beds: 46 **Admissions:** 452 **Census:** 39 **Outpatient Visits:** 0 **Births:** 0 **Total Expense ($000):** 18260 **Payroll Expense ($000):** 7104 **Personnel:** 131

★ **HILLCREST MEDICAL CENTER (370001)**, 1120 South Utica, Zip 74104–4090; tel. 918/579–1000 **A**1 3 5 9 10 **F**3 8 11 13 15 16 17 18 20 22 24 25 26 27 28 30 32 33 35 37 38 40 42 43 50 51 52 54 55 56 57 58 59 60 61 62 66 68 69 70 72 73 74 75 76 77 79 80 81 82 84 85 86 88 90 91 92 95 96 97 98 99 100 101 102 103 104 105 106 107 108 111 112 118 119 120 121 124 133 134 135 136 137 **S** Ardent Health Services
Primary Contact: Steve Dobbs, Chief Executive Officer
COO: Sandra S. Jackson, Ed.D., R.N., Chief Operating Officer
CFO: Donald Baker, Chief Financial Officer
CMO: Steven Landgarten, M.D., Chief Medical Officer
CHR: Claudia Underwood, Vice President Human Resources
Web address: www.hillcrest.com
Control: Other not–for–profit (including NFP Corporation) **Service:** General Medical and Surgical

Staffed Beds: 418 **Admissions:** 20975 **Census:** 274 **Outpatient Visits:** 98512 **Births:** 3722 **Total Expense ($000):** 218354 **Payroll Expense ($000):** 67651 **Personnel:** 1548

★ **HILLCREST SPECIALTY HOSPITAL (372007)**, 1145 South Utica Avenue, Suite 1200, Zip 74104; tel. 918/579–7260 **A**1 9 10 **F**1 25 26 30 31 38 56 63 73 119 137 **P**5 **S** Ardent Health Services
Primary Contact: Tracy Ferlet, Chief Executive Officer
CFO: Bryon Briggs, Assistant Chief Financial Officer
Web address: www.hillcrestspecialty.com
Control: Corporation, Investor–owned, for–profit **Service:** Long–Term Acute Care hospital

Staffed Beds: 84 **Admissions:** 715 **Census:** 55 **Births:** 0 **Total Expense ($000):** 28443 **Payroll Expense ($000):** 7055 **Personnel:** 128

★ **LAUREATE PSYCHIATRIC CLINIC AND HOSPITAL (374020)**, 6655 South Yale Avenue, Zip 74136–3329; tel. 918/481–4000 **A**1 3 5 9 10 **F**4 5 32 88 90 91 92 93 94 95 **P**6 **S** Saint Francis Health System
Primary Contact: John M. Robson, Executive Director
COO: John M. Robson, Executive Director
CFO: Barry L. Steichen, Executive Vice President and Chief Financial Officer
CMO: David B. Thomas, M.D., Senior Vice President and Chief Medical Officer
CIO: Mark Stastny, Vice President Information Technology
CHR: Amy Adams, Executive Director Human Resources
Web address: www.laureate.com
Control: Other not–for–profit (including NFP Corporation) **Service:** Psychiatric

Staffed Beds: 75 **Admissions:** 3633 **Census:** 62 **Outpatient Visits:** 76802 **Births:** 0 **Personnel:** 247

□ ○ **OKLAHOMA STATE UNIVERSITY MEDICAL CENTER (370078)**, 744 West Ninth Street, Zip 74127–9990; tel. 918/587–2561 **A**1 9 10 11 12 13 **F**3 8 11 13 15 18 20 22 24 25 26 27 30 31 32 33 34 38 40 50 54 55 56 57 60 62 68 70 72 73 74 75 76 77 79 80 81 84 86 87 88 90 91 92 93 94 95 96 97 100 107 118 119 120 121 123 124 132 133 135 137 **P**5 **S** Ardent Health Services
Primary Contact: Earl Denning, Chief Executive Officer
COO: Eric Burch, Chief Operating Officer
CFO: Shasta Manuel, Chief Financial Officer
CMO: Damon Baker, D.O., Chief Medical Officer
Web address: www.osu–medcenter.com
Control: Corporation, Investor–owned, for–profit **Service:** General Medical and Surgical

Staffed Beds: 331 **Admissions:** 11509 **Census:** 193 **Outpatient Visits:** 73515 **Births:** 982 **Total Expense ($000):** 181220 **Payroll Expense ($000):** 56185 **Personnel:** 1186

OKLAHOMA SURGICAL HOSPITAL (370210), (Formerly Orthopedic Surgical Hospital), 2408 East 81st Street, Suite 300, Zip 74137; tel. 918/477–5000 **A**10 **F**12 25 30 31 32 33 38 55 62 72 77 79 80 81 82 86 96 100 102 107 119 120 **P**2
Primary Contact: Rick Ferguson, Interim Chief Executive Officer
Web address: www.oklahomasurgicalhospital.com
Control: Partnership, Investor–owned, for–profit **Service:** Orthopedic

Staffed Beds: 41 **Admissions:** 2505 **Census:** 16 **Outpatient Visits:** 27645 **Births:** 0 **Total Expense ($000):** 46144 **Payroll Expense ($000):** 10928 **Personnel:** 239

PARKSIDE HOSPITAL (374021), 1620 East 12th Street, Zip 74120–5499; tel. 918/582–2131 **A**3 5 10 **F**5 30 88 90 92 94 95 119
Primary Contact: Debra Moore, Chief Executive Officer
CFO: Jim White, Chief Financial Officer
CMO: Virginia Heller, M.D., Medical Director
CIO: Nita Gould, Director Information Services
CHR: Jack Giordano, Director Human Resources
Web address: www.parksideinc.org
Control: Other not–for–profit (including NFP Corporation) **Service:** Psychiatric

Staffed Beds: 52 **Admissions:** 1586 **Census:** 44 **Outpatient Visits:** 25854 **Births:** 0 **Total Expense ($000):** 9560 **Payroll Expense ($000):** 5329 **Personnel:** 112

□ **SAINT FRANCIS HEART HOSPITAL (370218)**, 10501 East 91st Street South, Zip 74133; tel. 918/307–6000, (Nonreporting) **A**1 9 10 **S** Saint Francis Health System
Primary Contact: Joseph H. Neely, Senior Vice President and Administrator
Web address: www.saintfrancisheart.com
Control: Partnership, Investor–owned, for–profit **Service:** Heart

Staffed Beds: 40

★ △ **SAINT FRANCIS HOSPITAL (370091)**, 6161 South Yale Avenue, Zip 74136–1902; tel. 918/494–2200 **A**1 2 3 5 7 9 10 **F**3 7 8 11 12 13 15 17 18 19 20 21 22 23 24 25 26 27 28 31 32 33 37 38 40 41 43 44 50 51 52 55 56 57 58 59 60 62 64 66 67 68 69 70 72 73 74 75 76 77 78 79 80 81 82 83 84 86 97 99 100 101 102 104 106 107 108 111 114 118 119 120 124 125 126 127 130 132 135 137 **P**4 **S** Saint Francis Health System
Primary Contact: Lynn Sund, Administrator
COO: Lynn Sund, Administrator
CFO: Barry L. Steichen, Executive Vice President and Chief Financial Officer
CMO: Thomas David, M.D., Senior Vice President and Chief Medical Officer
CIO: Mark Stastny, Vice President Information Technology
CHR: Amy Adams, Executive Director Human Resources
Web address: www.saintfrancis.com
Control: Other not–for–profit (including NFP Corporation) **Service:** General Medical and Surgical

Staffed Beds: 682 **Admissions:** 38747 **Census:** 518 **Outpatient Visits:** 368778 **Births:** 3929 **Total Expense ($000):** 449332 **Payroll Expense ($000):** 175741 **Personnel:** 4492

SELECT SPECIALTY HOSPITAL – TULSA (372006), 744 West Ninth Street, Zip 74127–9096; tel. 918/502–1400 **A**9 10 **F**1 3 25 30 32 56 59 80 137 **P**8 **S** Select Medical Corporation
Primary Contact: David Bennett, Chief Executive Officer
Control: Corporation, Investor–owned, for–profit **Service:** Long–Term Acute Care hospital

Staffed Beds: 30 **Admissions:** 291 **Census:** 20 **Births:** 0 **Total Expense ($000):** 10133 **Payroll Expense ($000):** 4368

□ **SHADOW MOUNTAIN BEHAVIORAL HEALTH SYSTEM**, 6262 South Sheridan Road, Zip 74133–4099; tel. 918/492–8200, (Nonreporting) **A**1 9 **S** Psychiatric Solutions
Primary Contact: Kevin A. Burgess, Chief Executive Officer
COO: Selena Stockley, Chief Operating Officer
CFO: Kirt Penrod, Chief Financial Officer
CMO: Dean Martin, M.D., Medical Director
CHR: Duane Harris, Director Human Resources
Web address: www.psysolutions.com
Control: Corporation, Investor–owned, for–profit **Service:** Children's hospital psychiatric

Staffed Beds: 100

★ **SOUTHCREST HOSPITAL (370202)**, 8801 South 101st East Avenue, Zip 74133; tel. 918/294–4000 **A**1 9 10 **F**3 13 15 18 20 22 24 25 26 30 31 32 38 40 51 53 55 56 57 68 73 74 77 79 80 81 82 86 87 96 97 99 100 102 103 106 107 119 120 135 136 137 **S** Community Health Systems, Inc.
Primary Contact: Anthony R. Young, Chief Executive Officer
COO: Nikia Beene, Assistant Administrator
CFO: Matt Romero, Vice President Finance and Chief Financial Officer
CMO: Adam Myers, M.D., Chief of Staff
CIO: Frank Evans, Director Information Services
CHR: Shelia Nelson, Director Human Resources
Web address: www.southcresthospital.com
Control: Corporation, Investor–owned, for–profit **Service:** General Medical and Surgical

Staffed Beds: 148 **Admissions:** 9759 **Census:** 103 **Outpatient Visits:** 77187 **Births:** 2476 **Total Expense ($000):** 111206 **Payroll Expense ($000):** 31519 **Personnel:** 716

Hospital, Medicare Provider Number, Address, Telephone, Approval, Facility, and Physician Codes, Health Care System

★ American Hospital Association (AHA) membership
□ The Joint Commission accreditation
○ American Osteopathic Association (AOA) accreditation
△ Commission on Accreditation of Rehabilitation Facilities (CARF) accreditation

OK

☐ **SOUTHWESTERN REGIONAL MEDICAL CENTER (370190)**, 10109 East 79th Street, Zip 74133; tel. 918/286–5000, (Nonreporting) **A**1 2 10 **S** Cancer Treatment Centers of America
Primary Contact: Steve Mackin, President and Chief Executive Officer
CFO: David Hedges, Chief Financial Officer
CMO: James P. Flynn, M.D., President Medical Staff
Web address: www.cancercenter.com
Control: Corporation, Investor–owned, for–profit **Service:** General Medical and Surgical

Staffed Beds: 42

☒ **ST. JOHN MEDICAL CENTER (370114)**, 1923 South Utica Avenue, Zip 74104–6502; tel. 918/744–2345 **A**1 2 3 5 9 10 **F**3 7 8 9 11 13 15 17 18 20 22 24 25 26 27 30 31 32 33 35 38 40 42 43 44 50 51 52 53 54 55 56 57 58 59 60 61 62 63 64 66 68 69 70 71 72 73 74 76 77 78 79 80 81 82 83 84 85 86 87 88 90 94 96 97 98 99 100 102 103 104 105 106 107 108 111 112 116 117 118 119 120 121 124 125 127 130 134 135 136 137 **P**6 8 **S** Marian Health System
Primary Contact: S. Charles Anderson, President and Chief Executive Officer
CFO: Lex S. Anderson, Chief Financial Officer
CMO: William Allred, M.D., Vice President Medical Affairs
CIO: Mike Reeves, Vice President
CHR: Page Bachman, Corporate Vice President
Web address: www.sjmc.org
Control: Church–operated, Nongovernment, not–for profit **Service:** General Medical and Surgical

Staffed Beds: 560 **Admissions:** 30195 **Census:** 417 **Outpatient Visits:** 299369 **Births:** 1978 **Total Expense ($000):** 421881 **Payroll Expense ($000):** 152284 **Personnel:** 3116

☒ **TULSA SPECIALTY HOSPITAL (372018)**, 3219 South 79th East Avenue, Zip 74145–1312; tel. 918/663–8183 **A**1 10 **F**1 3 25 31 38 43 132 137 **P**5 **S** RehabCare Group, Inc.
Primary Contact: Ginger Creech, Chief Executive Officer
Web address: www.mbhealth.com
Control: Corporation, Investor–owned, for–profit **Service:** Long–Term Acute Care hospital

Staffed Beds: 60 **Admissions:** 476 **Census:** 33 **Outpatient Visits:** 0 **Births:** 0 **Personnel:** 157

☒ **TULSA SPINE AND SPECIALTY HOSPITAL (370216)**, 6901 South Olympia Avenue, Zip 74132; tel. 918/388–5701 **A**1 10 **F**25 26 38 43 63 72 77 79 80 82 84 96 100 101 102 119 124
Primary Contact: Terry L. Woodbeck, Administrator
COO: Beverly Pickett, R.N., MSN, Chief Operating Officer and Chief Nursing Officer
CFO: Thom Biby, Chief Financial Officer
CMO: David Fell, M.D., Chief Medical Officer
Web address: www.tulsaspinehospital.com
Control: Corporation, Investor–owned, for–profit **Service:** General Medical and Surgical

Staffed Beds: 21 **Admissions:** 1678 **Census:** 12 **Outpatient Visits:** 14264 **Births:** 0 **Total Expense ($000):** 39321 **Payroll Expense ($000):** 7591 **Personnel:** 171

VINITA—Craig County

★ **CRAIG GENERAL HOSPITAL (370065)**, 735 North Foreman Street, Zip 74301–1418, Mailing Address: Box 326, Zip 74301–0326; tel. 918/256–7551 **A**9 10 20 **F**11 13 25 26 27 30 31 32 33 38 50 55 56 57 61 62 63 67 73 74 75 79 80 84 85 86 88 90 93 94 96 97 100 103 105 107 118 119 122 124 135 137 **P**6
Primary Contact: B. Joe Gunn, Ed.D., FACHE, Chief Executive Officer
COO: Terry W. Shambles, Chief Administrative Officer
CFO: James Brasel, Chief Financial Officer
CMO: Ed Allensworth, M.D., Medical Director
CIO: Terry W. Shambles, Chief Administrative Officer
CHR: Marsha Emerson, Chief Support Officer
Web address: www.craiggeneralhospital.com
Control: Hospital district or authority, Government, nonfederal **Service:** General Medical and Surgical

Staffed Beds: 47 **Admissions:** 2143 **Census:** 29 **Outpatient Visits:** 32872 **Births:** 84 **Total Expense ($000):** 20255 **Payroll Expense ($000):** 7697 **Personnel:** 237

OKLAHOMA FORENSIC CENTER, Mailing Address: P.O. Box 69, Zip 74301–0069; tel. 918/256–7841, (Nonreporting) **S** Oklahoma State Department of Mental Health and Substance Abuse Services
Primary Contact: William T. Burkett, Chief Executive Officer
CFO: Glenda Gray, Director Finance
Control: State–Government, nonfederal **Service:** Psychiatric

Staffed Beds: 221

WAGONER—Wagoner County

WAGONER COMMUNITY HOSPITAL (370166), 1200 West Cherokee, Zip 74467–4681, Mailing Address: P.O. Box 407, Zip 74477–0407; tel. 918/485–5514 **A**9 10 **F**11 15 25 38 40 52 55 56 63 66 68 72 73 75 77 79 80 82 84 86 88 90 92 93 94 96 97 100 102 106 107 118 119 121 **P**8
Primary Contact: Jimmy Leopard, Chief Executive Officer
COO: Louise Easter, R.N., Chief Nursing Officer
CFO: Kathy Frost, Chief Financial Officer
CMO: Casey Hanna, M.D., Chief of Staff
CHR: Barnetta Webb, Director
Control: Hospital district or authority, Government, nonfederal **Service:** General Medical and Surgical

Staffed Beds: 100 **Admissions:** 2017 **Census:** 31 **Outpatient Visits:** 16606 **Births:** 2 **Total Expense ($000):** 12312 **Payroll Expense ($000):** 6303 **Personnel:** 147

WATONGA—Blaine County

★ **WATONGA MUNICIPAL HOSPITAL (371302)**, 500 North Nash Boulevard, Zip 73772–0370, Mailing Address: Box 370, Zip 73772–0370; tel. 580/623–7211 **A**9 10 18 **F**3 7 11 25 31 32 38 55 56 57 62 66 86 96 97 100 107 119 122 134 137
Primary Contact: Brenda K. Doyel, Chief Executive Officer
CFO: LeAnn Darst, Controller
CIO: Alisha Glazier, Compliance Officer and Director Health Information Management
CHR: LeAnn Darst, Controller
Web address: www.watongahospital.com
Control: Hospital district or authority, Government, nonfederal **Service:** General Medical and Surgical

Staffed Beds: 22 **Admissions:** 490 **Census:** 4 **Outpatient Visits:** 9015 **Births:** 2 **Total Expense ($000):** 3951 **Payroll Expense ($000):** 1813 **Personnel:** 65

WAURIKA—Jefferson County

★ **JEFFERSON COUNTY HOSPITAL (371311)**, Highway 70 and 81, Zip 73573–3075, Mailing Address: P.O. Box 90, Zip 73573–0090; tel. 580/228–2344 **A**9 10 18 **F**11 38 96 107 122
Primary Contact: Jane McDowell, Administrator
CFO: Richard Tallon, Chief Financial Officer
CMO: Rob Linzman, D.O., Chief of Staff
CIO: Nikki McGahey, Information Officer
Web address: www.jeffersoncountyhospital.net
Control: County–Government, nonfederal **Service:** General Medical and Surgical

Staffed Beds: 25 **Admissions:** 279 **Census:** 4 **Outpatient Visits:** 10755 **Births:** 0 **Total Expense ($000):** 2571 **Payroll Expense ($000):** 1423 **Personnel:** 39

WEATHERFORD—Custer County

★ **WEATHERFORD REGIONAL HOSPITAL (371323)**, 3701 East Main Street, Zip 73096; tel. 580/772–5551 **A**9 10 18 **F**3 11 13 15 25 32 38 56 62 66 73 74 75 79 81 82 86 96 97 100 103 107 122 135 136 137
Primary Contact: Debbie Howe, Chief Executive Officer
CFO: Stephanie Helton, Chief Financial Officer
CMO: Gary Lawrence, M.D., Chief of Staff
CIO: Cassie Matlock, Director Health Information Management
CHR: Tawnya Paden, Director Human Resources
Web address: www.weatherfordhospital.com
Control: Hospital district or authority, Government, nonfederal **Service:** General Medical and Surgical

Staffed Beds: 25 **Admissions:** 1074 **Census:** 7 **Outpatient Visits:** 26694 **Births:** 238 **Total Expense ($000):** 8533 **Payroll Expense ($000):** 4271 **Personnel:** 123

WILBURTON—Latimer County

LATIMER COUNTY GENERAL HOSPITAL (370072), 806 Highway 2 North, Zip 74578–3698; tel. 918/465–2391 **A**9 10 **F**3 31 32 38 40 61 96 107 135 **P**5
Primary Contact: M. Sue Mings, Administrator
COO: M. Sue Mings, Administrator
CMO: Richard Valbuena, M.D., Medical Director
Control: County–Government, nonfederal **Service:** General Medical and Surgical

Staffed Beds: 24 **Admissions:** 774 **Census:** 6 **Outpatient Visits:** 35100 **Births:** 0 **Total Expense ($000):** 6507 **Payroll Expense ($000):** 3129 **Personnel:** 91

Many Facility Codes have changed. Please refer to the AHA Guide Code Chart.

WOODWARD—Woodward County

NORTHWESTERN CENTER FOR BEHAVIORAL HEALTH (374001), 1222 10th Street, Suite 211, Zip 73801; tel. 580/571–3233 **A**10 **F**4 5 88 92 94 **P**6 **S** Oklahoma State Department of Mental Health and Substance Abuse Services
Primary Contact: Trudy Hoffman, Executive Director
CFO: Mike Terry, Director Fiscal Services
Control: State–Government, nonfederal **Service:** Psychiatric

Staffed Beds: 28 **Admissions:** 743 **Census:** 20 **Outpatient Visits:** 41125 **Births:** 0 **Total Expense ($000):** 17256 **Payroll Expense ($000):** 7642 **Personnel:** 210

★□ **WOODWARD REGIONAL HOSPITAL (370002)**, 900 17th Street, Zip 73801–2423; tel. 580/256–5511 **A**1 9 10 20 **F**13 15 25 26 27 30 31 32 33 38 40 42 57 61 62 67 68 73 74 75 80 88 93 96 97 100 102 107 118 119 120 122 135 **S** Community Health Systems, Inc.
Primary Contact: Lavah Lowe, Interim Chief Executive Officer
CFO: Bonnie Sorensen, Chief Financial Officer
Web address: www.woodwardhospital.com
Control: Corporation, Investor–owned, for–profit **Service:** General Medical and Surgical

Staffed Beds: 68 **Admissions:** 2207 **Census:** 28 **Outpatient Visits:** 37352 **Births:** 267 **Total Expense ($000):** 25673 **Payroll Expense ($000):** 9739 **Personnel:** 359

YUKON—Canadian County

★□ **INTEGRIS CANADIAN VALLEY REGIONAL HOSPITAL (370211)**, 1201 Health Center Parkway, Zip 73099; tel. 405/717–6800 **A**1 9 10 **F**3 13 15 25 26 30 31 32 38 57 62 68 74 77 79 86 96 97 100 107 135 **S** INTEGRIS Health
Primary Contact: James D. Moore, FACHE, President
CFO: Cindy White, CPA, Chief Financial Officer
CMO: James D. Lackey, M.D., Chief of Staff
CHR: Lynn Ketch, Director Human Resources and Volunteer Services
Web address: www.integris–health.com
Control: Other not–for–profit (including NFP Corporation) **Service:** General Medical and Surgical

Staffed Beds: 44 **Admissions:** 2683 **Census:** 24 **Outpatient Visits:** 40817 **Births:** 697 **Total Expense ($000):** 32875 **Payroll Expense ($000):** 13521 **Personnel:** 249

Hospital, Medicare Provider Number, Address, Telephone, Approval, Facility, and Physician Codes, Health Care System
★ American Hospital Association (AHA) membership
□ The Joint Commission accreditation
○ American Osteopathic Association (AOA) accreditation
△ Commission on Accreditation of Rehabilitation Facilities (CARF) accreditation

OREGON

OR

ALBANY—Linn County

★ **SAMARITAN ALBANY GENERAL HOSPITAL (380022)**, 1046 West Sixth Avenue, Zip 97321–1999; tel. 541/812–4000 **A**1 9 10 **F**3 11 12 13 15 24 25 26 30 31 32 33 38 40 42 44 45 47 49 55 56 57 62 68 73 74 77 79 80 82 84 86 96 100 102 107 121 124 134 135 136 137 **S** Samaritan Health Services
Primary Contact: David G. Triebes, Chief Executive Officer
CFO: Daniel B. Smith, Vice President Finance
Web address: www.samhealth.org
Control: Other not–for–profit (including NFP Corporation) **Service:** General Medical and Surgical

Staffed Beds: 67 **Admissions:** 3630 **Census:** 31 **Outpatient Visits:** 123421 **Births:** 689 **Total Expense ($000):** 71668 **Payroll Expense ($000):** 30745 **Personnel:** 480

ASHLAND—Jackson County

★ **ASHLAND COMMUNITY HOSPITAL (380005)**, 280 Maple Street, Zip 97520–1593; tel. 541/201–4000 **A**1 9 10 **F**2 3 6 8 11 13 15 25 26 30 31 32 33 34 38 40 42 43 44 46 48 49 53 54 55 56 57 61 62 63 64 66 67 68 72 73 74 75 77 79 80 81 82 84 86 87 96 102 106 107 108 119 120 121 133 134 135 136 137 **P**6
Primary Contact: Mark E. Marchetti, President and Chief Executive Officer
CFO: Thomas Birmingham, Chief Financial Officer
CMO: Craig Mather, M.D., Chief Medical Staff
CHR: Karen Herwig, Director Human Resources
Web address: www.ashlandhospital.org
Control: City–Government, nonfederal **Service:** General Medical and Surgical

Staffed Beds: 39 **Admissions:** 1720 **Census:** 17 **Outpatient Visits:** 70315 **Births:** 337 **Total Expense ($000):** 45136 **Payroll Expense ($000):** 18164 **Personnel:** 328

ASTORIA—Clatsop County

★ **COLUMBIA MEMORIAL HOSPITAL (381320)**, 2111 Exchange Street, Zip 97103–3329; tel. 503/325–4321 **A**1 9 10 18 **F**3 11 13 15 25 26 27 31 32 33 34 38 40 42 47 51 55 56 57 61 66 68 73 74 75 77 79 80 81 82 86 87 96 97 100 102 107 119 121 123 124 132 135 136 **P**6
Primary Contact: Terry O. Finklein, Chief Executive Officer
COO: Bill Thorn, Chief Operating Officer
CFO: Erik Thorsen, Chief Financial Officer
CMO: Angela Hairn, M.D., Chief of Staff
CHR: Cheryl Martin, Director Human Resources
Web address: www.columbiamemorial.org
Control: Other not–for–profit (including NFP Corporation) **Service:** General Medical and Surgical

Staffed Beds: 25 **Admissions:** 2041 **Census:** 17 **Outpatient Visits:** 72634 **Births:** 343 **Total Expense ($000):** 37958 **Payroll Expense ($000):** 16950 **Personnel:** 332

BAKER CITY—Baker County

★ **ST. ELIZABETH HEALTH SERVICES (381315)**, 3325 Pocahontas Road, Zip 97814–1464; tel. 541/523–6461, (Total facility includes 50 beds in nursing home–type unit) **A**1 9 10 18 **F**3 11 13 15 26 30 31 32 33 35 38 40 55 56 57 62 65 68 73 74 75 77 79 80 84 86 96 102 107 118 119 120 122 132 134 135 136 137 **S** Catholic Health Initiatives
Primary Contact: George Winn, President and Chief Executive Officer
CFO: Scott Spears, Vice President Finance and Chief Financial Officer
CHR: Jerry Nickell, Vice President Human Resource and Mission
Web address: www.stelizabethhealth.com
Control: Other not–for–profit (including NFP Corporation) **Service:** General Medical and Surgical

Staffed Beds: 75 **Admissions:** 1179 **Census:** 51 **Outpatient Visits:** 32021 **Births:** 145 **Total Expense ($000):** 23245 **Payroll Expense ($000):** 9566 **Personnel:** 152

BANDON—Coos County

★ **SOUTHERN COOS HOSPITAL AND HEALTH CENTER (381304)**, 900 11th Street S.E., Zip 97411–9114; tel. 541/347–2426 **A**9 10 18 **F**3 11 15 25 26 30 31 33 38 44 45 46 47 48 49 50 54 55 56 60 62 63 66 75 79 80 81 82 96 102 107 118 119 121 122 123 124 132 137 **P**6
Primary Contact: James A. Wathen, Chief Executive Officer
CFO: David Rollins, Chief Financial Officer
CMO: Sandra Wilson, M.D., Chief Medical Officer
CHR: Monica Reisner, Director Human Resources
Web address: www.southerncoos.com
Control: Hospital district or authority, Government, nonfederal **Service:** General Medical and Surgical

Staffed Beds: 19 **Admissions:** 739 **Census:** 7 **Outpatient Visits:** 11784 **Births:** 0 **Total Expense ($000):** 13314 **Payroll Expense ($000):** 6020 **Personnel:** 113

BEND—Deschutes County

★ **CASCADE HEALTHCARE COMMUNITY ST. CHARLES MEDICAL CENTER – BEND (380047)**, (Formerly St. Charles Medical Center – Bend), 2500 N.E. Neff Road, Zip 97701–6015; tel. 541/382–4321 **A**1 2 3 5 9 10 19 **F**3 8 11 12 13 17 18 20 22 24 25 26 27 30 33 34 35 36 38 40 42 43 44 46 49 50 51 55 56 57 59 61 62 63 65 66 68 70 71 72 73 74 75 76 77 78 79 80 81 83 84 85 86 88 90 91 92 94 96 97 100 102 103 104 105 106 107 109 111 112 118 119 121 124 134 135 137 **P**6 7 **S** Cascade Healthcare Community
Primary Contact: James A. Diegel, FACHE, President and Chief Executive Officer
COO: Tim Bricker, Executive Vice President
CFO: Michael E. McGinnis, Interim Senior Vice President Finance
CMO: Alan Ertle, M.D., Senior Vice President Medical Affairs
CIO: Marilynn Black, Senior Vice President and Chief Information Officer
CHR: Katy Vitcovich, Vice President Human Resources
Web address: www.scmc.org
Control: Other not–for–profit (including NFP Corporation) **Service:** General Medical and Surgical

Staffed Beds: 261 **Admissions:** 14125 **Census:** 160 **Outpatient Visits:** 158805 **Births:** 2042 **Total Expense ($000):** 307879 **Payroll Expense ($000):** 117080 **Personnel:** 1843

BURNS—Harney County

★ **HARNEY DISTRICT HOSPITAL (381307)**, 557 West Washington Street, Zip 97720–1497; tel. 541/573–7281 **A**9 10 18 **F**3 7 13 15 25 32 33 38 40 43 55 57 62 68 69 73 74 79 80 86 96 102 107 121 122 124 135 **P**5
Primary Contact: Jim Bishop, Chief Executive Officer
CMO: Kevin Johnston, M.D., Chief Medical Staff
CHR: Sammie Masterson, Chief Human Resources Officer
Web address: www.harneydh.com
Control: Hospital district or authority, Government, nonfederal **Service:** General Medical and Surgical

Staffed Beds: 25 **Admissions:** 565 **Census:** 6 **Outpatient Visits:** 18271 **Births:** 63 **Total Expense ($000):** 12741 **Payroll Expense ($000):** 5427 **Personnel:** 108

CLACKAMAS—Clackamas County

★ **KAISER SUNNYSIDE MEDICAL CENTER (380091)**, 10180 S.E. Sunnyside Road, Zip 97015–9303; tel. 503/652–2880 **A**1 2 10 **F**3 11 12 13 15 18 26 27 30 38 44 47 56 59 60 62 66 68 71 72 73 74 75 76 77 79 80 81 82 86 87 92 96 97 100 106 107 119 135 136 137 **P**6 **S** Kaiser Foundation Hospitals
Primary Contact: William Butcher, Administrator and Chief Executive Officer
CFO: Dennis Reese, Chief Financial Officer
CMO: Rick Olson, M.D., Chief of Staff
CIO: Larry Wheeler, Vice President Communications and External Affairs
CHR: Tricia Peters, Vice President Human Resources
Web address: www.kaiserpermanente.org
Control: Other not–for–profit (including NFP Corporation) **Service:** General Medical and Surgical

Staffed Beds: 233 **Admissions:** 14350 **Census:** 155 **Outpatient Visits:** 55140 **Births:** 1601 **Personnel:** 1945

COOS BAY—Coos County

★ **BAY AREA HOSPITAL (380090)**, 1775 Thompson Road, Zip 97420–2198; tel. 541/269–8111 **A**2 9 10 19 20 **F**3 8 11 12 13 15 24 27 30 31 32 38 40 44 46 49 50 51 55 56 57 61 66 68 71 72 73 74 75 76 77 79 80 84 86 88 89 91 92 94 96 97 100 105 106 107 108 109 111 118 119 121 124 135 137
Primary Contact: Daniel L. Smith, President and Chief Executive Officer
CFO: Tim Salisbury, Vice President Finance
CMO: Terry Bach, M.D., Director Medical Affairs
CIO: Bob Adams, Information Services Manager
CHR: Tom Shine, Vice President Human Resources
Web address: www.bayareahospital.org
Control: Hospital district or authority, Government, nonfederal **Service:** General Medical and Surgical

Staffed Beds: 134 **Admissions:** 7545 **Census:** 77 **Outpatient Visits:** 69477 **Births:** 656 **Total Expense ($000):** 96857 **Payroll Expense ($000):** 49228 **Personnel:** 808

COQUILLE—Coos County

★ **COQUILLE VALLEY HOSPITAL (381312)**, 940 East Fifth Street, Zip 97423–1699; tel. 541/396–3101 **A**9 10 18 **F**1 3 4 11 13 15 16 17 25 30 31 32 33 38 40 46 50 55 56 57 61 65 68 70 71 73 74 77 78 79 80 81 84 85 88 96 100 102 106 107 117 121 122 134 137 **P**6
Primary Contact: Dennis G. Zielinski, Chief Executive Officer and Administrator
CFO: Gail Ludington, Chief Financial Officer
CMO: James Sinnott, M.D., Chief Medical Staff
CIO: Charlotte Barrett, Manager Marketing and Community Relations
CHR: Monte Johnston, Manager Human Resources
Web address: www.cvhospital.org
Control: Hospital district or authority, Government, nonfederal **Service:** General Medical and Surgical

Staffed Beds: 25 **Admissions:** 588 **Census:** 4 **Outpatient Visits:** 16906 **Births:** 33 **Total Expense ($000):** 10588 **Payroll Expense ($000):** 4790 **Personnel:** 93

CORVALLIS—Benton County

☒ **GOOD SAMARITAN REGIONAL MEDICAL CENTER (380014)**, 3600 N.W. Samaritan Drive, Zip 97330–3737, Mailing Address: P.O. Box 1068, Zip 97339–1068; tel. 541/768–5111 **A**1 2 9 10 19 **F**3 5 8 11 12 13 15 18 20 22 24 25 26 27 30 31 32 34 38 40 43 46 51 55 57 59 61 62 66 68 71 72 73 74 75 76 77 79 80 81 82 86 87 88 90 91 92 93 94 96 97 99 100 102 103 106 107 108 109 111 112 118 119 120 121 124 134 135 136 137 **P**1 6 7 8 **S** Samaritan Health Services
Primary Contact: Steven W. Jasperson, Chief Executive Officer
CFO: Daniel B. Smith, Vice President Finance
CIO: Robert French, Vice President Information Services
CHR: Sheryl Helms, Vice President Human Resources
Web address: www.samhealth.org
Control: Other not–for–profit (including NFP Corporation) **Service:** General Medical and Surgical

Staffed Beds: 185 **Admissions:** 8633 **Census:** 106 **Outpatient Visits:** 241974 **Births:** 1125 **Total Expense ($000):** 209345 **Payroll Expense ($000):** 87484 **Personnel:** 1160

COTTAGE GROVE—Lane County

★ **COTTAGE GROVE COMMUNITY HOSPITAL (381301)**, 1515 Village Drive, Zip 97424; tel. 541/942–0511 **A**9 10 18 **F**3 11 15 25 26 30 31 32 33 38 44 50 54 62 63 66 73 86 87 96 99 102 107 119 121 136 137 **S** PeaceHealth
Primary Contact: Randall L. Mee, RN, Chief Executive Officer
Web address: www.peacehealth.org
Control: Other not–for–profit (including NFP Corporation) **Service:** General Medical and Surgical

Staffed Beds: 14 **Admissions:** 508 **Census:** 4 **Outpatient Visits:** 35165 **Births:** 0 **Total Expense ($000):** 10037 **Payroll Expense ($000):** 4585 **Personnel:** 62

DALLAS—Polk County

WEST VALLEY HOSPITAL (381308), 525 S.E. Washington Street, Zip 97338–2899, Mailing Address: P.O. Box 378, Zip 97338–0378; tel. 503/623–8301 **A**9 10 18 **F**3 11 15 32 33 38 40 50 57 62 73 77 79 80 84 86 96 107 120 121 122 132 135 137 **P**6 **S** Salem Health
Primary Contact: Eric Buckland, CHE, Site Administrator
CFO: Eric Buckland, CHE, Site Administrator
Web address: www.westvalleyhospital.org
Control: Other not–for–profit (including NFP Corporation) **Service:** General Medical and Surgical

Staffed Beds: 6 **Admissions:** 125 **Census:** 1 **Outpatient Visits:** 54033 **Births:** 0 **Total Expense ($000):** 13699 **Payroll Expense ($000):** 6296 **Personnel:** 109

ENTERPRISE—Wallowa County

★ **WALLOWA MEMORIAL HOSPITAL (381306)**, 601 Medical Parkway, Zip 97828–1167; tel. 541/426–3111, (Total facility includes 32 beds in nursing home–type unit) **A**5 9 10 18 **F**3 7 11 13 15 24 26 27 30 31 32 33 38 40 42 44 46 54 57 61 65 66 73 74 76 77 79 80 82 86 92 96 102 107 117 120 121 122 124 132 135
Primary Contact: David L. Harman, Chief Executive Officer
CFO: Lexi M. Fields, Chief Financial Officer
CMO: Kirsten Caine, M.D., Chief Medical Staff
CHR: Linda Childers, Director Human Resources
Web address: www.wchcd.org
Control: Hospital district or authority, Government, nonfederal **Service:** General Medical and Surgical

Staffed Beds: 57 **Admissions:** 756 **Census:** 37 **Outpatient Visits:** 19839 **Births:** 49 **Total Expense ($000):** 12297 **Payroll Expense ($000):** 5322 **Personnel:** 117

EUGENE—Lane County

☒ △ **SACRED HEART MEDICAL CENTER (380033)**, 1255 Hilyard Street, Zip 97401–3700, Mailing Address: P.O. Box 10905, Zip 97440–0905; tel. 541/686–7300 **A**1 7 9 10 **F**3 8 11 12 13 18 20 22 24 25 26 27 30 31 32 33 38 40 42 43 44 45 50 51 55 56 57 58 59 62 66 68 70 72 73 74 76 77 79 80 81 84 85 86 88 89 90 91 92 93 94 96 97 101 102 103 107 108 118 119 121 135 136 137 **P**6 **S** PeaceHealth
Primary Contact: Jill Hoggard Green, RN, Ph.D., Administrator and Chief Executive Officer
COO: Jill Hoggard Green, R.N., Ph.D., Administrator and Chief Operating Officer
CFO: Karen Shepard, Vice President Finance and Chief Financial Officer
CMO: Bill Moshofsky, M.D., Chief of Staff
CIO: Don McMillan, Chief Information Officer
CHR: Craig Mills, Vice President Human Resources
Web address: www.peacehealth.org
Control: Church–operated, Nongovernment, not–for profit **Service:** General Medical and Surgical

Staffed Beds: 476 **Admissions:** 26664 **Census:** 319 **Outpatient Visits:** 110299 **Births:** 2857 **Total Expense ($000):** 405540 **Payroll Expense ($000):** 165836 **Personnel:** 2870

SERENITY LANE, 616 East 16th, Zip 97401–4357; tel. 541/687–1110, (Nonreporting)
Primary Contact: Peter J. Asmuth, Executive Director and Administrator
CMO: Ron Schwerzler, M.D., Director Medical Services
CIO: Josh Bolton, Chief Information Officer
Web address: www.serenitylane.org
Control: Other not–for–profit (including NFP Corporation) **Service:** Alcoholism and other chemical dependency

Staffed Beds: 55

FLORENCE—Lane County

☒ **PEACE HARBOR HOSPITAL (381316)**, 400 Ninth Street, Zip 97439–7398; tel. 541/997–8412 **A**1 9 10 18 **F**11 13 15 24 25 26 30 31 32 33 38 40 42 43 44 50 55 56 57 61 62 66 68 74 75 77 79 86 87 96 97 100 102 107 121 122 136 137 **P**6 **S** PeaceHealth
Primary Contact: James R. Barnhart, Chief Executive Officer
CFO: Rick Yecny, Vice President and Chief Financial Officer
CMO: Sharon F. Catlin, D.O., Regional Medical Director
CIO: Ginni Boughal, Manager Health Information
CHR: Don Bourland, Vice President Human Resources
Web address: www.peacehealth.org
Control: Church–operated, Nongovernment, not–for profit **Service:** General Medical and Surgical

Staffed Beds: 21 **Admissions:** 1500 **Census:** 13 **Outpatient Visits:** 27272 **Births:** 41 **Total Expense ($000):** 43863 **Payroll Expense ($000):** 22646 **Personnel:** 422

FOREST GROVE—Washington County

TUALITY FOREST GROVE HOSPITAL See Tuality Healthcare, Hillsboro

OR

Hospital, Medicare Provider Number, Address, Telephone, Approval, Facility, and Physician Codes, Health Care System

★ American Hospital Association (AHA) membership
□ The Joint Commission accreditation
○ American Osteopathic Association (AOA) accreditation
△ Commission on Accreditation of Rehabilitation Facilities (CARF) accreditation

GOLD BEACH—Curry County

★ **CURRY GENERAL HOSPITAL (381322)**, 94220 Fourth Street, Zip 97444–9990; tel. 541/247–6621 **A**9 10 18 **F**3 10 13 15 24 25 30 31 32 38 54 55 56 57 62 63 68 73 74 79 96 102 107 115 122 133
Primary Contact: William I. McMillan, FACHE, Chief Executive Officer
CFO: Mark Sayler, Chief Financial Officer
CIO: Kwang Veloso, Director Information Systems
CHR: Terri Tomberlin, Manager Human Resources
Web address: www.currygeneralhospital.com
Control: Hospital district or authority, Government, nonfederal **Service:** General Medical and Surgical

Staffed Beds: 21 **Admissions:** 793 **Census:** 6 **Outpatient Visits:** 47161 **Births:** 53 **Total Expense ($000):** 14727 **Payroll Expense ($000):** 6359 **Personnel:** 136

OR

GRANTS PASS—Josephine County

★ **THREE RIVERS COMMUNITY HOSPITAL AND HEALTH CENTER (380002)**, 500 S.W. Ramsey Avenue, Zip 97527; tel. 541/472–7000 **A**1 9 10 **F**11 13 15 24 25 26 30 31 32 33 34 38 40 41 46 50 53 55 56 57 61 62 63 68 73 74 76 79 82 86 92 96 97 100 101 102 106 107 110 111 119 121 132 135 136 137 **P**6 **S** Asante Health System
Primary Contact: Paul Janke, FACHE, Chief Executive Officer
CFO: Marvin Haas, Chief Administration and Finance Officer
CMO: Thomas Turek, M.D., Interim Vice President Medical Affairs
CIO: Mark Hetz, Chief Information Officer
CHR: Gregg Edwards, Chief People Officer
Web address: www.asante.org
Control: Other not–for–profit (including NFP Corporation) **Service:** General Medical and Surgical

Staffed Beds: 115 **Admissions:** 7489 **Census:** 69 **Outpatient Visits:** 200999 **Births:** 821 **Total Expense ($000):** 97767 **Payroll Expense ($000):** 37649 **Personnel:** 675

GRESHAM—Multnomah County

★ **LEGACY MOUNT HOOD MEDICAL CENTER (380025)**, 24800 S.E. Stark, Zip 97030–0154; tel. 503/667–1122 **A**1 2 9 10 **F**3 11 13 15 18 25 26 27 28 30 31 32 33 36 38 41 46 49 50 54 55 57 59 62 66 68 72 73 74 75 76 77 79 80 81 82 86 90 91 92 96 97 99 100 102 106 107 108 109 119 121 135 136 **P**8 **S** Legacy Health System
Primary Contact: Bryce R. Helgerson, Chief Administrative Officer
CFO: Pamela S. Vukovich, Senior Vice President and Chief Financial Officer
CMO: Jack Cioffi, M.D., Senior Vice President and Chief Medical Officer
CIO: Richard Gibson, M.D., Senior Vice President and Chief Information Officer
CHR: Sonja Steves, Vice President Human Resources and Marketing
Web address: www.legacyhealth.org
Control: Other not–for–profit (including NFP Corporation) **Service:** General Medical and Surgical

Staffed Beds: 81 **Admissions:** 5293 **Census:** 49 **Outpatient Visits:** 90410 **Births:** 979 **Total Expense ($000):** 61746 **Payroll Expense ($000):** 26377 **Personnel:** 401

HEPPNER—Morrow County

PIONEER MEMORIAL HOSPITAL (381310), 564 East Pioneer Drive, Zip 97836, Mailing Address: P.O. Box 9, Zip 97836; tel. 541/676–9133 **A**9 10 18 **F**3 7 17 33 38 42 57 61 62 64 66 67 73 87 96 107 122 132 137 **P**6
Primary Contact: Victor Vander Does, Administrator
CFO: Nicole Mahoney, Chief Financial Officer
CIO: Ray Greenlaw, Information Systems Officer
CHR: Patti Allstott, Administrative Coordinator Human Resources and Grant Writer
Web address: www.morrowcountyhealthdistrict.org
Control: Hospital district or authority, Government, nonfederal **Service:** General Medical and Surgical

Staffed Beds: 12 **Admissions:** 88 **Census:** 1 **Outpatient Visits:** 5365 **Births:** 0 **Total Expense ($000):** 5444 **Payroll Expense ($000):** 2698 **Personnel:** 49

HERMISTON—Umatilla County

★ **GOOD SHEPHERD HEALTHCARE SYSTEM (381325)**, 610 N.W. 11th Street, Zip 97838–9696; tel. 541/667–3400 **A**1 9 10 18 **F**3 8 11 13 15 25 26 30 31 32 33 38 40 42 43 50 52 55 56 57 61 62 63 66 68 73 74 75 77 79 80 81 82 84 86 87 96 97 99 100 102 107 119 121 122 123 124 130 132 135 137 **P**3 7
Primary Contact: Dennis E. Burke, President
COO: David T. Hughes, FACHE, Senior Vice President Operations
CFO: William H. Alsdurf, Vice President Fiscal Services
CMO: Thomas Farney, M.D., President Medical Staff
CHR: Kelly Sanders, Vice President Human Resources
Web address: www.gshealth.org
Control: Other not–for–profit (including NFP Corporation) **Service:** General Medical and Surgical

Staffed Beds: 25 **Admissions:** 2035 **Census:** 17 **Outpatient Visits:** 55006 **Births:** 603 **Total Expense ($000):** 38155 **Payroll Expense ($000):** 17023 **Personnel:** 348

HILLSBORO—Washington County

★ **TUALITY HEALTHCARE (380021)**, 335 S.E. Eighth Avenue, Zip 97123–4246; tel. 503/681–1111, (Includes TUALITY COMMUNITY HOSPITAL, Mailing Address: P.O. Box 309, Zip 97123; TUALITY FOREST GROVE HOSPITAL, 1809 Maple Street, Forest Grove, Zip 97116–1995; tel. 503/357–2173) **A**1 9 10 **F**3 11 13 15 17 18 20 22 24 25 26 27 28 30 31 32 33 34 35 38 41 49 50 52 53 54 55 56 57 61 62 66 68 69 72 73 74 75 76 77 78 79 80 81 82 86 87 88 90 93 94 96 97 100 102 106 107 119 120 121 124 132 133 134 135 136 137 **P**1 6
Primary Contact: Richard Stenson, President and Chief Executive Officer
COO: Manuel S. Berman, Administrator and Chief Operating Officer
CFO: Tim Fleischmann, Chief Financial Officer
CMO: Darell Lumaco, M.D., Chief of Staff
CIO: John Stoneburg, Chief Information Officer
CHR: Kathy Ratliffe, Director Human Resources
Web address: www.tuality.com
Control: Other not–for–profit (including NFP Corporation) **Service:** General Medical and Surgical

Staffed Beds: 149 **Admissions:** 6635 **Census:** 82 **Outpatient Visits:** 221545 **Births:** 1449 **Total Expense ($000):** 147699 **Payroll Expense ($000):** 65581 **Personnel:** 1173

HOOD RIVER—Hood River County

★ **PROVIDENCE HOOD RIVER MEMORIAL HOSPITAL (381318)**, 811 13th Street, Zip 97031–1204, Mailing Address: P.O. Box 149, Zip 97031–0149; tel. 541/386–3911 **A**1 9 10 18 **F**2 3 5 8 9 10 11 12 13 15 24 25 26 27 31 32 33 34 38 40 47 48 52 53 54 55 56 57 59 62 63 66 68 69 73 74 75 77 79 80 81 87 89 90 91 92 94 96 97 100 102 107 115 118 121 123 124 132 133 135 136 137 **S** Providence Health & Services
Primary Contact: Ty W. Erickson, Chief Executive Officer
CFO: Ron Guth, Chief Financial Officer
CHR: Catherine Bourgault, Director Human Resources
Web address: www.providence.org/hoodriver
Control: Church–operated, Nongovernment, not–for profit **Service:** General Medical and Surgical

Staffed Beds: 25 **Admissions:** 1705 **Census:** 13 **Outpatient Visits:** 120091 **Births:** 367 **Total Expense ($000):** 44159 **Payroll Expense ($000):** 18004 **Personnel:** 342

JOHN DAY—Grant County

★ **BLUE MOUNTAIN HOSPITAL (381305)**, 170 Ford Road, Zip 97845–2009; tel. 541/575–1311, (Total facility includes 52 beds in nursing home–type unit) **A**5 9 10 18 **F**2 3 7 8 11 13 15 17 25 26 27 31 33 34 38 40 42 43 54 55 56 57 61 62 65 66 68 73 74 79 81 82 84 86 96 100 102 103 107 117 119 120 121 122 132 134 137 **P**6 **S** Brim Healthcare, Inc.
Primary Contact: Robert Houser, FACHE, Chief Executive Officer
CFO: Sam Grant, Chief Financial Officer
CMO: Keith Thomas, M.D., Chief of Staff
CHR: Verlene Davis, Director Human Resources
Web address: www.bluemountainhospital.org
Control: Hospital district or authority, Government, nonfederal **Service:** General Medical and Surgical

Staffed Beds: 68 **Admissions:** 409 **Census:** 30 **Outpatient Visits:** 20197 **Births:** 49 **Total Expense ($000):** 13478 **Payroll Expense ($000):** 6479 **Personnel:** 157

KLAMATH FALLS—Klamath County

★ **SKY LAKES MEDICAL CENTER (380050)**, 2865 Daggett Avenue, Zip 97601–1180; tel. 541/882–6311 **A**1 2 3 5 9 10 19 20 **F**3 8 11 12 13 15 18 20 24 25 27 30 31 32 33 38 40 41 46 47 48 50 52 53 55 56 57 58 59 60 61 62 66 68 69 72 73 74 75 76 77 79 80 81 82 86 87 90 92 96 97 99 100 102 103 104 106 107 108 109 111 119 121 124 132 135 137 **P**6
Primary Contact: Paul R. Stewart, Chief Executive Officer
CFO: Joe Chamberlain, Vice President and Chief Financial Officer
CMO: Rick Zwartverwer, M.D., Vice President Medical Affairs
CIO: David Chabner, Director Information Services
CHR: Don York, Vice President Human Resources
Web address: www.skylakes.org
Control: Other not–for–profit (including NFP Corporation) **Service:** General Medical and Surgical

Staffed Beds: 100 **Admissions:** 6517 **Census:** 67 **Outpatient Visits:** 229830 **Births:** 865 **Total Expense ($000):** 136263 **Payroll Expense ($000):** 54066 **Personnel:** 1028

Many Facility Codes have changed. Please refer to the AHA Guide Code Chart.

LA GRANDE—Union County

★ **GRANDE RONDE HOSPITAL (381321)**, 900 Sunset Drive, Zip 97850–1362, Mailing Address: P.O. Box 3290, Zip 97850–3290; tel. 541/963–8421 **A**9 10 18 **F**3 8 11 13 14 15 17 25 26 27 30 35 37 38 40 41 42 46 50 52 55 56 57 61 62 64 68 73 74 75 76 77 79 80 81 82 84 86 87 90 96 97 99 100 102 107 114 119 120 121 122 124 135 136 137
Primary Contact: James A. Mattes, President and Chief Executive Officer
CFO: Wade Weis, Director Finance
CIO: Parhez Sattar, Senior Director Information Technology
CHR: Kristi Puckett, Director Human Resources
Web address: www.grh.org
Control: Other not–for–profit (including NFP Corporation) **Service:** General Medical and Surgical

Staffed Beds: 25 **Admissions:** 1983 **Census:** 17 **Outpatient Visits:** 52140 **Births:** 320 **Total Expense ($000):** 36141 **Payroll Expense ($000):** 18224 **Personnel:** 309

LAKEVIEW—Lake County

★ **LAKE DISTRICT HOSPITAL (381309)**, 700 South J Street, Zip 97630–1679; tel. 541/947–2114, (Total facility includes 47 beds in nursing home–type unit) **A**5 9 10 18 **F**3 4 11 13 15 17 30 32 38 40 42 46 55 57 61 62 66 68 74 79 84 86 92 96 107 117 119 121 122 124 135 137 **P**4
Primary Contact: Gordon Ensley, Chief Executive Officer
CFO: Ken Landau, Chief Financial Officer
CMO: Stephen Hussey, M.D., Chief of Staff
CHR: Linda Michaelson, Director Human Resources
Web address: www.lake–health.com
Control: Hospital district or authority, Government, nonfederal **Service:** General Medical and Surgical

Staffed Beds: 68 **Admissions:** 682 **Census:** 37 **Outpatient Visits:** 28971 **Births:** 59 **Total Expense ($000):** 11935 **Payroll Expense ($000):** 5691 **Personnel:** 138

LEBANON—Linn County

★☐ **SAMARITAN LEBANON COMMUNITY HOSPITAL (381323)**, 525 North Santiam Highway, Zip 97355–4363, Mailing Address: P.O. Box 739, Zip 97355–0739; tel. 541/258–2101 **A**1 9 10 18 **F**3 11 13 15 24 25 26 27 30 31 32 33 38 40 41 42 46 47 50 52 56 57 62 66 73 74 76 77 79 80 81 82 84 86 87 96 97 99 100 103 106 107 112 119 120 121 124 133 135 136 137 **P**5 6 **S** Samaritan Health Services
Primary Contact: Becky A. Pape, RN, Chief Executive Officer
CFO: Daniel B. Smith, Vice President Finance
CMO: Alden Forrester, M.D., President Medical Staff
CIO: Robert French, Vice President Information Services
CHR: Connie Erwin, Manager
Web address: www.samhealth.org
Control: Other not–for–profit (including NFP Corporation) **Service:** General Medical and Surgical

Staffed Beds: 25 **Admissions:** 1900 **Census:** 17 **Outpatient Visits:** 102894 **Births:** 302 **Total Expense ($000):** 55917 **Payroll Expense ($000):** 25986 **Personnel:** 417

LINCOLN CITY—Lincoln County

★☐ **SAMARITAN NORTH LINCOLN HOSPITAL (381302)**, 3043 N.E. 28th Street, Zip 97367–4523, Mailing Address: P.O. Box 767, Zip 97367–0767; tel. 541/994–3661 **A**1 9 10 18 **F**3 8 11 13 15 25 26 30 31 32 33 38 40 42 50 55 56 57 61 62 66 73 74 79 81 82 86 87 96 97 102 106 107 119 121 122 124 133 135 137 **S** Samaritan Health Services
Primary Contact: Sue Massart, Chief Executive Officer
CFO: Matthew M. Sherwood, Chief Financial Officer
CMO: Darrel Prins, DPM, President Medical Staff
CIO: Robert French, Director Information Services
CHR: Lauri Bolton, Director Human Resources
Web address: www.samhealth.org
Control: Other not–for–profit (including NFP Corporation) **Service:** General Medical and Surgical

Staffed Beds: 25 **Admissions:** 1705 **Census:** 13 **Outpatient Visits:** 53438 **Births:** 177 **Total Expense ($000):** 39014 **Payroll Expense ($000):** 19775 **Personnel:** 294

MADRAS—Jefferson County

★ **MOUNTAIN VIEW HOSPITAL DISTRICT (381324)**, 470 N.E. A Street, Zip 97741–1844; tel. 541/475–3882, (Total facility includes 34 beds in nursing home–type unit) **A**9 10 18 **F**1 3 8 13 15 25 26 30 31 32 33 38 40 42 44 45 52 55 57 60 61 62 65 66 68 73 74 75 77 79 80 82 84 85 86 88 96 102 107 117 119 121 122 124 133 135 136 **P**7
Primary Contact: Jay Henry, Chief Executive Officer
COO: Bob Krickbaum, Vice President Support Services
CFO: Shawn Whalen, Chief Financial Officer
CIO: Phil MacTaggart, Project Manager HealthSync
CHR: Janet Morgan, Director Talent
Web address: www.mvhd.org
Control: Hospital district or authority, Government, nonfederal **Service:** General Medical and Surgical

Staffed Beds: 59 **Admissions:** 1065 **Census:** 30 **Outpatient Visits:** 31547 **Births:** 229 **Total Expense ($000):** 19891 **Payroll Expense ($000):** 9025 **Personnel:** 207

MCMINNVILLE—Yamhill County

★☐ **WILLAMETTE VALLEY MEDICAL CENTER (380071)**, 2700 S.E. Stratus Avenue, Zip 97128–6498; tel. 503/472–6131 **A**1 2 9 10 **F**3 11 13 15 18 24 25 26 27 30 31 32 33 38 40 43 54 55 57 59 62 68 72 73 74 75 76 77 79 82 85 86 96 97 100 102 103 106 107 111 112 118 119 121 124 135 136 137 **P**5 6 **S** Capella Healthcare
Primary Contact: Rosemari Davis, Chief Executive Officer
COO: Daniel Ordyna, Chief Operating Officer
CFO: Cory Rhoades, Chief Financial Officer
CHR: Cheryl Gebhart, Director Human Resources
Web address: www.wvmcweb.com
Control: Corporation, Investor–owned, for–profit **Service:** General Medical and Surgical

Staffed Beds: 88 **Admissions:** 4287 **Census:** 46 **Outpatient Visits:** 107522 **Births:** 749 **Total Expense ($000):** 65656 **Payroll Expense ($000):** 24218 **Personnel:** 488

MEDFORD—Jackson County

★☐ △ **PROVIDENCE MEDFORD MEDICAL CENTER (380075)**, 1111 Crater Lake Avenue, Zip 97504–6241; tel. 541/732–5000 **A**1 2 7 9 10 **F**3 11 13 15 18 20 22 25 26 27 28 30 31 32 33 38 40 42 43 44 49 50 51 54 55 56 57 60 61 62 66 68 72 73 74 75 76 77 79 80 81 82 85 86 87 92 96 99 102 103 106 107 108 109 111 112 114 116 119 121 132 135 136 137 **S** Providence Health & Services
Primary Contact: Thomas S. Hanenburg, Chief Executive
CFO: Michael Strasser, Assistant Administrator Fiscal Services
CHR: Todd Tangeman, Director Human Resources
Web address: www.providence.org
Control: Church–operated, Nongovernment, not–for profit **Service:** General Medical and Surgical

Staffed Beds: 135 **Admissions:** 6467 **Census:** 78 **Outpatient Visits:** 247567 **Births:** 625 **Total Expense ($000):** 126086 **Payroll Expense ($000):** 53276 **Personnel:** 887

★☐ **ROGUE VALLEY MEDICAL CENTER (380018)**, 2825 East Barnett Road, Zip 97504–8332; tel. 541/789–7000 **A**1 2 9 10 **F**11 12 13 15 17 18 19 20 21 22 23 24 25 26 27 28 30 31 32 33 34 35 36 38 40 42 43 46 50 51 55 56 57 61 62 63 68 70 72 73 74 76 77 79 81 82 84 85 86 88 90 92 96 97 99 107 108 109 110 119 121 132 135 136 137 **P**6 **S** Asante Health System
Primary Contact: Kent L. Brown, FACHE, Chief Executive Officer
CFO: Marvin Haas, Chief Administrative and Finance Officer
CIO: Mark Hetz, Chief Information Officer
CHR: Gregg Edwards, Chief People Officer
Web address: www.asante.org
Control: Other not–for–profit (including NFP Corporation) **Service:** General Medical and Surgical

Staffed Beds: 312 **Admissions:** 14515 **Census:** 183 **Outpatient Visits:** 337347 **Births:** 1465 **Total Expense ($000):** 261374 **Payroll Expense ($000):** 91974 **Personnel:** 1745

Hospital, Medicare Provider Number, Address, Telephone, Approval, Facility, and Physician Codes, Health Care System

★ American Hospital Association (AHA) membership
☐ The Joint Commission accreditation
○ American Osteopathic Association (AOA) accreditation
△ Commission on Accreditation of Rehabilitation Facilities (CARF) accreditation

OR

MILWAUKIE—Clackamas County

★ **PROVIDENCE MILWAUKIE HOSPITAL (380082)**, 10150 S.E. 32nd Avenue, Zip 97222–6593; tel. 503/513–8300 **A**1 2 3 5 9 10 **F**3 13 15 25 26 30 31 32 33 34 38 41 42 43 44 46 50 52 53 55 56 57 62 66 68 72 73 74 75 77 79 80 82 86 87 90 95 96 97 100 102 103 107 118 119 120 121 122 124 135 136 137 **S** Providence Health & Services
Primary Contact: Theron Park, Administrator
CFO: Dale Hiserote, Chief Financial Officer
CHR: Laurie Ayers Pino, Director Human Resources
Web address: www.providence.org
Control: Church–operated, Nongovernment, not–for profit **Service:** General Medical and Surgical

Staffed Beds: 66 **Admissions:** 3123 **Census:** 27 **Outpatient Visits:** 202166 **Births:** 634 **Total Expense ($000):** 67085 **Payroll Expense ($000):** 26139 **Personnel:** 386

NEWBERG—Yamhill County

★ **PROVIDENCE NEWBERG MEDICAL CENTER (380037)**, 1001 Providence Drive, Zip 97132–7485; tel. 503/537–1555 **A**1 9 10 **F**3 11 13 15 18 25 26 30 31 32 33 38 40 46 50 55 56 57 61 62 66 68 73 74 75 77 79 80 82 86 90 96 97 99 100 102 106 107 118 119 121 124 135 136 137 **S** Providence Health & Services
Primary Contact: Larry Bowe, Chief Executive, Yamhill Service Area
CFO: Jack R. Sumner, Assistant Administrator Finance
CIO: Laureen O'Brien, Chief Information Officer
CHR: Jeannie Mikulic, Director Human Resources
Web address: www.phsor.org
Control: Church–operated, Nongovernment, not–for profit **Service:** General Medical and Surgical

Staffed Beds: 40 **Admissions:** 1856 **Census:** 15 **Outpatient Visits:** 178844 **Births:** 575 **Total Expense ($000):** 59161 **Payroll Expense ($000):** 23048 **Personnel:** 368

NEWPORT—Lincoln County

★ **SAMARITAN PACIFIC COMMUNITIES HOSPITAL (381314)**, 930 S.W. Abbey Street, Zip 97365–4820, Mailing Address: P.O. Box 945, Zip 97365–4820; tel. 541/265–2244 **A**1 9 10 18 **F**8 11 15 17 24 25 26 27 31 38 40 41 42 50 61 62 68 73 74 75 76 77 79 82 86 87 96 97 99 102 103 107 118 119 121 122 135 136 137 **P**6 **S** Samaritan Health Services
Primary Contact: David C. Bigelow, Chief Executive Officer
CHR: Penny Dunne, R.N., Director Human Resources
Web address: www.samhealth.org
Control: Church–operated, Nongovernment, not–for profit **Service:** General Medical and Surgical

Staffed Beds: 42 **Admissions:** 1236 **Census:** 10 **Outpatient Visits:** 71268 **Births:** 185 **Total Expense ($000):** 49372 **Payroll Expense ($000):** 22083 **Personnel:** 402

ONTARIO—Malheur County

★ **HOLY ROSARY MEDICAL CENTER (380052)**, 351 S.W. Ninth Street, Zip 97914–2693; tel. 541/881–7000 **A**1 5 9 10 **F**3 11 12 13 15 25 26 30 31 32 33 38 41 42 43 50 51 53 54 55 56 57 61 62 63 64 66 68 73 74 75 77 79 82 86 87 96 97 102 107 118 119 120 121 122 124 133 135 137 **P**6 **S** Catholic Health Initiatives
Primary Contact: Mark F. Dalley, Administrator and Chief Executive Officer
CFO: Matthew Cox, Chief Financial Officer
CHR: Karen Kosowan, Vice President Human Resources
Web address: www.holyrosary–ontario.org
Control: Church–operated, Nongovernment, not–for profit **Service:** General Medical and Surgical

Staffed Beds: 49 **Admissions:** 2666 **Census:** 23 **Outpatient Visits:** 72037 **Births:** 712 **Total Expense ($000):** 49849 **Payroll Expense ($000):** 18518 **Personnel:** 421

OREGON CITY—Clackamas County

★ **WILLAMETTE FALLS HOSPITAL (380038)**, 1500 Division Street, Zip 97045–1597; tel. 503/656–1631 **A**1 2 9 10 **F**11 13 15 24 30 37 38 42 49 53 55 56 57 62 66 68 73 74 75 76 77 79 80 81 86 87 96 97 99 100 102 106 107 119 120 121 133 135 136
Primary Contact: Russ Reinhard, Chief Executive Officer
CFO: Tim Blanchard, Vice President Finance and Chief Financial Officer
CHR: Barb Applebee, Director Human Resources
Web address: www.willamettefallshospital.org
Control: Other not–for–profit (including NFP Corporation) **Service:** General Medical and Surgical

Staffed Beds: 91 **Admissions:** 5485 **Census:** 41 **Outpatient Visits:** 82000 **Births:** 1164 **Total Expense ($000):** 81832 **Payroll Expense ($000):** 35675 **Personnel:** 603

PENDLETON—Umatilla County

EASTERN OREGON PSYCHIATRIC CENTER (384011), 2575 Westgate, Zip 97801–9613; tel. 541/276–4511, (Nonreporting) **A**10
Primary Contact: Maxine Stone, Superintendent
CMO: Satua Chandragiri, M.D., Chief Medical Officer
Control: State–Government, nonfederal **Service:** Psychiatric

Staffed Beds: 60

★ **ST. ANTHONY HOSPITAL (381319)**, 1601 S.E. Court Avenue, Zip 97801–3297; tel. 541/276–5121 **A**1 2 5 9 10 18 **F**3 13 15 25 26 27 30 31 32 33 37 38 40 42 51 52 53 55 57 61 62 63 66 73 74 75 76 77 79 80 81 82 86 87 96 97 99 100 102 106 107 119 120 121 122 123 124 135 **S** Catholic Health Initiatives
Primary Contact: Theodore P. Fox, President and Chief Executive Officer
CFO: Steven Taylor, Vice President and Chief Financial Officer
CMO: Malcolm Townsley, M.D., Chief of Staff
CHR: Jon Oravec, Vice President Human Resources
Web address: www.sahpendleton.org
Control: Church–operated, Nongovernment, not–for profit **Service:** General Medical and Surgical

Staffed Beds: 25 **Admissions:** 1725 **Census:** 15 **Outpatient Visits:** 45651 **Births:** 351 **Total Expense ($000):** 32685 **Payroll Expense ($000):** 12794 **Personnel:** 254

PORTLAND—Multnomah County

★ **ADVENTIST MEDICAL CENTER (380060)**, 10123 S.E. Market Street, Zip 97216–2599; tel. 503/257–2500 **A**1 2 9 10 **F**3 4 5 11 13 15 18 20 24 25 26 27 30 31 32 33 38 41 42 43 44 49 50 52 53 55 56 57 61 62 68 69 72 73 74 75 76 77 79 81 82 86 87 88 92 96 97 99 100 102 106 107 109 118 119 120 121 124 133 135 136 137 **P**6 7 **S** Adventist Health
Primary Contact: Deryl L. Jones, President
CFO: V. Mark Perry, Chief Financial Officer
CMO: Wesley E. Rippey, M.D., Chief Medical Officer
CIO: Jon Russell, Regional Chief Information Officer
CHR: Herbert Hill, Director Human Resources
Web address: www.adventisthealthnw.com
Control: Church–operated, Nongovernment, not–for profit **Service:** General Medical and Surgical

Staffed Beds: 252 **Admissions:** 11483 **Census:** 140 **Outpatient Visits:** 449377 **Births:** 1253 **Total Expense ($000):** 221180 **Payroll Expense ($000):** 100839 **Personnel:** 1916

DOERNBECHER CHILDREN'S HOSPITAL See OHSU Hospital

GOOD SAMARITAN HOSPITAL AND MEDICAL CENTER See Legacy Good Samaritan Hospital and Medical Center

★ △ **LEGACY EMANUEL HOSPITAL AND HEALTH CENTER (380007)**, 2801 North Gantenbein Avenue, Zip 97227–1674; tel. 503/413–2200 **A**1 2 3 5 7 9 10 **F**3 11 13 15 16 18 19 20 21 22 23 25 26 27 28 30 31 32 33 36 38 40 41 44 45 46 47 49 50 51 52 53 54 55 56 57 59 60 62 63 66 68 70 72 73 74 75 76 77 78 79 80 81 82 83 84 86 87 88 89 90 91 92 95 96 97 99 100 102 106 107 108 109 111 112 119 121 135 136 137 **P**8 **S** Legacy Health System
Primary Contact: April Whitworth, Chief Administrative Officer
CFO: Pamela S. Vukovich, Senior Vice President and Chief Financial Officer
CIO: Matthew Calais, Senior Vice President and Chief Information Officer
Web address: www.legacyhealth.org
Control: Other not–for–profit (including NFP Corporation) **Service:** General Medical and Surgical

Staffed Beds: 401 **Admissions:** 18179 **Census:** 279 **Outpatient Visits:** 188543 **Births:** 1636 **Total Expense ($000):** 425946 **Payroll Expense ($000):** 187957 **Personnel:** 2735

★ **LEGACY GOOD SAMARITAN HOSPITAL AND MEDICAL CENTER (380017)**, 1015 N.W. 22nd Avenue, Zip 97210–3099; tel. 503/413–7711, (Includes GOOD SAMARITAN HOSPITAL AND MEDICAL CENTER; REHABILITATION INSTITUTE OF OREGON) **A**1 2 3 5 9 10 **F**3 8 12 13 15 18 19 20 22 24 25 26 27 28 30 31 32 33 36 38 41 43 44 45 46 47 49 50 52 53 54 55 56 57 59 60 62 63 64 68 72 73 74 75 76 77 78 79 80 81 82 85 86 87 88 90 91 92 93 96 97 99 100 102 106 107 109 116 118 119 121 125 127 131 135 136 **P**8 **S** Legacy Health System
Primary Contact: Tony Melaragno, M.D., Chief Administrative Officer
CFO: Pamela S. Vukovich, Vice President Financial Services
CIO: C. Matthew Calais, Senior Vice President and Chief Information Officer
CHR: Sonja Steves, Vice President Marketing
Web address: www.legacyhealth.org
Control: Other not–for–profit (including NFP Corporation) **Service:** General Medical and Surgical

Staffed Beds: 263 **Admissions:** 13331 **Census:** 171 **Outpatient Visits:** 172285 **Births:** 1236 **Total Expense ($000):** 229114 **Payroll Expense ($000):** 89244 **Personnel:** 1449

Many Facility Codes have changed. Please refer to the AHA Guide Code Chart.

★ **OHSU HOSPITAL (380009)**, 3181 S.W. Sam Jackson Park Road, Zip 97201–3098; tel. 503/494–8311, (Includes DOERNBECHER CHILDREN'S HOSPITAL) **A**1 2 3 5 8 9 10 **F**3 5 8 9 11 12 13 15 17 18 19 20 21 22 23 24 25 26 27 28 29 30 31 32 33 34 36 37 38 40 41 43 44 46 49 50 52 53 54 55 56 57 58 60 62 63 64 66 68 70 72 73 74 75 76 77 79 80 81 82 83 84 86 87 88 89 90 91 92 93 94 95 96 97 99 100 101 102 103 104 105 106 107 108 109 111 112 113 114 116 118 119 120 121 123 124 125 126 127 128 130 133 134 135 136 137 **P**1
Primary Contact: Peter F. Rapp, Vice President and Executive Director
COO: Cynthia M. Grueber, Chief Operating Officer
CFO: Brad King, Vice President and Chief Financial Officer
CMO: A. Roy Magnusson, M.D., Chief Medical Officer
CIO: Bridget Haggerty, Interim Chief Information Officer
CHR: Rick Bentzinger, Vice President Human Resources
Web address: www.ohsu.edu
Control: Hospital district or authority, Government, nonfederal **Service:** General Medical and Surgical

Staffed Beds: 503 **Admissions:** 26759 **Census:** 395 **Outpatient Visits:** 367676 **Births:** 2645 **Total Expense ($000):** 758755 **Payroll Expense ($000):** 283766 **Personnel:** 4509

★ **PROVIDENCE PORTLAND MEDICAL CENTER (380061)**, 4805 N.E. Glisan Street, Zip 97213–2967; tel. 503/215–1111 **A**1 2 3 5 9 10 **F**3 4 5 9 13 15 17 18 20 22 25 26 27 30 31 32 33 34 35 36 38 41 42 43 44 46 49 50 51 52 53 54 55 56 57 58 59 60 61 62 63 64 66 68 71 72 73 74 75 76 77 79 80 81 82 85 86 87 88 89 90 92 93 94 95 96 97 98 99 100 102 104 105 106 107 109 111 112 118 119 120 121 122 124 125 126 134 135 136 137 **S** Providence Health & Services
Primary Contact: Lisa Vance, Administrator
COO: James Arp, Associate Administrator
CFO: Eric Olson, Chief Financial Officer
CIO: Laureen O'Brien, Chief Information Officer
Web address: www.providence.org
Control: Church–operated, Nongovernment, not–for profit **Service:** General Medical and Surgical

Staffed Beds: 409 **Admissions:** 21483 **Census:** 278 **Outpatient Visits:** 994360 **Births:** 2606 **Total Expense ($000):** 466568 **Payroll Expense ($000):** 163703 **Personnel:** 2575

★ **PROVIDENCE ST. VINCENT MEDICAL CENTER (380004)**, 9205 S.W. Barnes Road, Zip 97225–6661; tel. 503/216–1234 **A**1 2 3 5 9 10 **F**3 5 13 15 17 18 20 22 25 26 27 30 31 32 33 34 35 36 38 41 42 43 44 46 47 48 49 50 51 52 53 54 55 56 57 58 59 60 61 62 63 66 68 70 72 73 74 75 76 77 79 80 81 82 84 86 87 88 90 93 94 95 96 97 98 99 100 102 103 104 105 106 107 109 111 116 118 119 120 121 122 124 126 135 136 137 **S** Providence Health & Services
Primary Contact: Janice Burger, Administrator
CFO: William Olson, Director Finance
CIO: Kate Chester, Senior Public Relations Coordinator
Web address: www.providence.org/portland/hospitals
Control: Church–operated, Nongovernment, not–for profit **Service:** General Medical and Surgical

Staffed Beds: 523 **Admissions:** 33211 **Census:** 395 **Outpatient Visits:** 769773 **Births:** 6425 **Total Expense ($000):** 578630 **Payroll Expense ($000):** 197575 **Personnel:** 3099

REHABILITATION INSTITUTE OF OREGON See Legacy Good Samaritan Hospital and Medical Center

□ **SHRINERS HOSPITALS FOR CHILDREN, PORTLAND**, 3101 S.W. Sam Jackson Park Road, Zip 97239; tel. 503/241–5090 **A**1 3 5 **F**31 79 84 **P**6 **S** Shriners Hospitals for Children
Primary Contact: Gayle Littlejohn, Interim Administrator
CFO: Mark Knudsen, Director Fiscal Services
CMO: Ivan Krajbich, M.D., Chief of Staff
CHR: Patricia Sussman, Director Human Resources
Web address: www.shcc.org
Control: Other not–for–profit (including NFP Corporation) **Service:** Children's orthopedic

Staffed Beds: 22 **Admissions:** 1450 **Census:** 11 **Outpatient Visits:** 15340 **Births:** 0 **Payroll Expense ($000):** 14194 **Personnel:** 235

★ **VETERANS AFFAIRS MEDICAL CENTER**, 3710 S.W. U.S. Veterans Hospital Road, Zip 97239; tel. 503/220–8262, (Total facility includes 72 beds in nursing home–type unit) (Nonreporting) **A**1 2 3 5 8 **S** Department of Veterans Affairs
Primary Contact: James Tuchschmidt, M.D., Director
CFO: Susan P. Heublein, Chief Financial Officer
CMO: John Dryden, M.D., Chief of Staff
CIO: David M. Douglas, M.D., Chief Information Officer
CHR: Linda Condich, Chief Human Resources Management
Web address: www.va.gov/sta/guide/home.asp
Control: Veterans Affairs, Government, federal **Service:** General Medical and Surgical

Staffed Beds: 221

OR

PRINEVILLE—Crook County

PIONEER MEMORIAL HOSPITAL (381313), 1201 N.E. Elm Street, Zip 97754–1206; tel. 541/447–6254 **A**9 10 18 **F**3 11 13 15 25 31 33 38 40 42 44 50 56 57 61 62 66 68 73 74 77 79 82 96 102 107 119 121 122 124 135 **S** Cascade Healthcare Community
Primary Contact: Donald J. Wee, Executive Director
CHR: Laurie Romine, Manager Human Resources
Web address: www.cascadehealthcare.org
Control: Other not–for–profit (including NFP Corporation) **Service:** General Medical and Surgical

Staffed Beds: 25 **Admissions:** 944 **Census:** 9 **Outpatient Visits:** 100805 **Births:** 172 **Total Expense ($000):** 21053 **Payroll Expense ($000):** 8848 **Personnel:** 157

REDMOND—Deschutes County

★ **CASCADE HEALTHCARE COMMUNITY ST. CHARLES MEDICAL CENTER – REDMOND (380040)**, (Formerly St. Charles Medical Center – Redmond), 1253 North Canal Boulevard, Zip 97756–1395; tel. 541/548–8131 **A**1 9 10 20 **F**3 11 13 15 25 26 30 31 32 38 40 43 47 51 55 56 57 61 62 68 73 74 79 80 86 92 96 97 107 119 124 135 137 **P**7 **S** Cascade Healthcare Community
Primary Contact: James A. Diegel, FACHE, President and Chief Executive Officer
COO: Tim Bricker, Executive Vice President
CFO: Michael E. McGinnis, Interim Senior Vice President Finance
CMO: Alan Ertle, M.D., Senior Vice President Medical Affairs
CIO: Marilynn Black, Senior Vice President and Chief Information Officer
CHR: Katy Vitcovich, Vice President Human Resources
Web address: www.cascadehealthcare.org
Control: Other not–for–profit (including NFP Corporation) **Service:** General Medical and Surgical

Staffed Beds: 48 **Admissions:** 1837 **Census:** 16 **Outpatient Visits:** 48738 **Births:** 261 **Total Expense ($000):** 33893 **Payroll Expense ($000):** 14335 **Personnel:** 325

REEDSPORT—Douglas County

LOWER UMPQUA HOSPITAL DISTRICT (381311), 600 Ranch Road, Zip 97467–1795; tel. 541/271–2171, (Total facility includes 29 beds in nursing home–type unit) **A**9 10 18 **F**3 7 11 15 27 33 38 40 46 65 68 73 75 77 79 82 86 96 99 103 107 119 121 122 124 132 135 137 **P**6
Primary Contact: Sandra Reese, Administrator
CFO: John Chivers, Chief Financial Officer
CMO: Ronald Vail, M.D., Chief of Staff
CIO: Timothy Picou, Manager Information Technology
Web address: www.lowerumpquahospital.com
Control: Hospital district or authority, Government, nonfederal **Service:** General Medical and Surgical

Staffed Beds: 53 **Admissions:** 829 **Census:** 35 **Outpatient Visits:** 19020 **Births:** 0 **Total Expense ($000):** 16749 **Payroll Expense ($000):** 7652 **Personnel:** 166

Hospital, Medicare Provider Number, Address, Telephone, Approval, Facility, and Physician Codes, Health Care System
★ American Hospital Association (AHA) membership
□ The Joint Commission accreditation
○ American Osteopathic Association (AOA) accreditation
△ Commission on Accreditation of Rehabilitation Facilities (CARF) accreditation

ROSEBURG—Douglas County

★ **MERCY MEDICAL CENTER (380027)**, 2700 Stewart Parkway, Zip 97470–1297; tel. 541/673–0611 **A**1 2 9 10 19 20 **F**3 11 13 15 17 18 20 24 25 26 27 30 31 32 33 36 38 40 41 42 43 44 47 49 50 51 53 54 55 57 59 60 61 62 63 66 68 72 73 74 75 76 77 79 80 81 82 84 85 86 88 89 90 91 92 93 94 96 97 99 100 102 103 106 107 115 118 119 121 124 132 135 136 137 **P**6 **S** Catholic Health Initiatives
Primary Contact: Kelly C. Morgan, President and Chief Executive Officer
COO: Debbie Boswell, Chief Operating Officer and Chief Nursing Officer
CFO: John Kasberger, Vice President, Chief Financial Officer and Corporate Responsibility Officer
CIO: Kathleen Nickel, Director Communications
CHR: Deb Lightcap, Director Human Resources
Web address: www.mercyrose.org
Control: Church–operated, Nongovernment, not–for profit **Service:** General Medical and Surgical

Staffed Beds: 163 **Admissions:** 10220 **Census:** 109 **Outpatient Visits:** 230599 **Births:** 985 **Total Expense ($000):** 132210 **Payroll Expense ($000):** 53059 **Personnel:** 938

★ **VETERANS AFFAIRS ROSEBURG HEALTHCARE SYSTEM**, 913 N.W. Garden Valley Boulevard, Zip 97470–6513; tel. 541/440–1000, (Total facility includes 69 beds in nursing home–type unit) (Nonreporting) **A**1 **S** Department of Veterans Affairs
Primary Contact: Susan Yeager, Director
Web address: www.va.gov/sta/guide/home.asp
Control: Veterans Affairs, Government, federal **Service:** General Medical and Surgical

Staffed Beds: 157

SALEM—Marion County

☐ **OREGON STATE HOSPITAL (384008)**, 2600 Center Street N.E., Zip 97301–2682; tel. 503/945–2870, (Nonreporting) **A**1 3 5 10
Primary Contact: Marvin D. Fickle, M.D., Superintendent
CFO: Maynard Hammer, Deputy Superintendent
Web address: www.oregon.gov/dhs/mentalhealth/osh/main.shtml
Control: State–Government, nonfederal **Service:** Psychiatric

Staffed Beds: 679

★ **SALEM HOSPITAL (380051)**, 665 Winter Street S.E., Zip 97301–3959, Mailing Address: P.O. Box 14001, Zip 97309–5014; tel. 503/561–5200, (Includes PSYCHIATRIC MEDICINE CENTER, 1127 Oak Street S.E., Zip 97301; REGIONAL REHABILITATION CENTER, 2561 Center Street N.E., Zip 97301; tel. 503/370–5986) **A**1 2 9 10 **F**3 8 11 12 13 15 17 18 20 22 24 25 26 27 30 32 35 38 40 43 44 46 52 53 55 56 57 61 62 64 66 68 70 71 72 73 74 75 76 77 78 79 80 82 84 85 86 88 89 90 92 93 94 95 96 97 98 99 100 102 103 106 107 109 111 118 119 120 121 124 133 134 135 137 **P**6 **S** Salem Health
Primary Contact: Norman F. Gruber, President and Chief Executive Officer
COO: Cheryl Nester–Bowers, Senior Vice President Operations and Chief Nursing Officer
CFO: Aaron Crane, Chief Financial Officer
CMO: W. David Holloway, M.D., Chief Medical Officer
CIO: Ken Kudla, Chief Information Officer
CHR: Beverly Bow, Vice President Human Resources
Web address: www.salemhospital.org
Control: Other not–for–profit (including NFP Corporation) **Service:** General Medical and Surgical

Staffed Beds: 417 **Admissions:** 19722 **Census:** 246 **Outpatient Visits:** 506042 **Births:** 3699 **Total Expense ($000):** 364667 **Payroll Expense ($000):** 165421 **Personnel:** 2600

SEASIDE—Clatsop County

★ **PROVIDENCE SEASIDE HOSPITAL (381303)**, 725 South Wahanna Road, Zip 97138–7735; tel. 503/717–7000, (Total facility includes 20 beds in nursing home–type unit) **A**1 9 10 18 **F**3 8 11 12 13 15 17 26 27 28 30 31 32 33 38 43 46 53 55 56 57 61 62 64 65 68 73 74 75 77 79 80 81 82 84 86 87 94 96 107 117 119 121 122 124 135 136 137 **P**6 **S** Providence Health & Services
Primary Contact: William P. Sexton, Chief Executive
CFO: Pamela Cooper, Director Finance
CMO: Lisa Huddleston, M.D., Chief of Staff
CHR: Martie Teske, Human Resources Director
Web address: www.providence.org
Control: Church–operated, Nongovernment, not–for profit **Service:** General Medical and Surgical

Staffed Beds: 47 **Admissions:** 1176 **Census:** 30 **Outpatient Visits:** 97474 **Births:** 147 **Total Expense ($000):** 34119 **Payroll Expense ($000):** 18718 **Personnel:** 289

SILVERTON—Marion County

★ **SILVERTON HOSPITAL (380029)**, 342 Fairview Street, Zip 97381–1993; tel. 503/873–1500 **A**1 9 10 **F**3 11 13 15 25 26 30 32 33 38 40 50 52 53 55 56 57 62 63 64 66 68 73 74 75 77 79 80 81 82 84 96 100 103 107 112 118 119 121 122 124 132 133 135 136 137
Primary Contact: Gary W. Pulsipher, Vice President and Chief Executive Officer
COO: Jeffrey D. Lorenz, Vice President Corporate Services
CFO: Jeff Fritsche, Chief Financial Officer
CMO: John Gilliam, M.D., President Medical Staff
CIO: Lentz Farrell, Information Services Specialist
CHR: Jim Washam, Director Human Resources
Web address: www.silvertonhospital.org
Control: Other not–for–profit (including NFP Corporation) **Service:** General Medical and Surgical

Staffed Beds: 48 **Admissions:** 3225 **Census:** 23 **Outpatient Visits:** 111152 **Births:** 1737 **Total Expense ($000):** 67715 **Payroll Expense ($000):** 33641 **Personnel:** 600

SPRINGFIELD—Lane County

★ **MCKENZIE–WILLAMETTE MEDICAL CENTER (380020)**, 1460 G Street, Zip 97477–4197; tel. 541/726–4400 **A**1 9 10 **F**3 11 13 17 18 20 22 24 25 26 27 30 31 32 33 37 38 40 46 49 60 68 70 71 74 76 77 79 80 82 84 86 96 97 100 102 103 107 116 118 119 121 124 135 136 137 **P**6 **S** Community Health Systems, Inc.
Primary Contact: Maurine Cate, Chief Executive Officer
COO: Elmer Hyde, Chief Operating Officer
CFO: Richard Rico, Chief Financial Officer
CIO: Randy Burrows, Director Information Technology
CHR: Cathy Starkey, Vice President Human Resources
Web address: www.mckweb.com
Control: Corporation, Investor–owned, for–profit **Service:** General Medical and Surgical

Staffed Beds: 112 **Admissions:** 6758 **Census:** 60 **Outpatient Visits:** 70188 **Births:** 908 **Total Expense ($000):** 91105 **Payroll Expense ($000):** 40299 **Personnel:** 571

STAYTON—Marion County

★ **SANTIAM MEMORIAL HOSPITAL (380056)**, 1401 North 10th Avenue, Zip 97383–1399; tel. 503/769–2175 **A**1 9 10 **F**1 3 4 7 11 13 15 16 17 25 26 30 32 38 40 50 63 65 68 70 71 74 78 79 80 82 83 84 85 88 96 100 103 107 117 119 122 124 132 **P**8
Primary Contact: Terry L. Fletchall, Administrator
COO: Maggie Hudson, Director Operations and Financial Services
CFO: Rachael Seeder, Controller
CMO: Thomas VanVeen, M.D., Chief Medical Officer
Web address: www.santiamhospital.com
Control: Other not–for–profit (including NFP Corporation) **Service:** General Medical and Surgical

Staffed Beds: 40 **Admissions:** 1098 **Census:** 9 **Outpatient Visits:** 32452 **Births:** 162 **Total Expense ($000):** 19439 **Payroll Expense ($000):** 8574 **Personnel:** 186

THE DALLES—Wasco County

★ **MID–COLUMBIA MEDICAL CENTER (380001)**, 1700 East 19th Street, Zip 97058–3316; tel. 541/296–1111 **A**1 2 9 10 19 20 **F**11 12 13 15 17 24 25 26 27 28 31 32 33 34 38 40 43 44 45 46 47 50 51 52 53 54 55 56 57 61 62 63 66 68 73 74 75 76 77 79 81 82 84 85 86 87 96 97 100 106 107 108 109 111 113 118 119 121 122 124 135 136 **P**4
Primary Contact: Duane Francis, President
COO: Randy Skov, Vice President
CFO: Don Arbon, Vice President Finance
CMO: Jeffrey Mathisen, M.D., President Medical Staff
CIO: Erick Larson, Vice President and Chief Information Officer
CHR: Linda Miller, Director Human Resources
Web address: www.mcmc.net
Control: Other not–for–profit (including NFP Corporation) **Service:** General Medical and Surgical

Staffed Beds: 49 **Admissions:** 2216 **Census:** 22 **Outpatient Visits:** 115411 **Births:** 314 **Total Expense ($000):** 61958 **Payroll Expense ($000):** 27496 **Personnel:** 611

TILLAMOOK—Tillamook County

★ **TILLAMOOK COUNTY GENERAL HOSPITAL (381317)**, 1000 Third Street, Zip 97141–3430; tel. 503/842–4444 **A**1 9 10 18 **F**2 3 7 13 15 17 25 26 27 30 31 32 33 38 40 50 55 56 57 62 66 73 74 75 77 79 80 82 86 92 96 97 99 100 103 105 107 119 121 122 134 135 137 **S** Adventist Health
Primary Contact: Larry Davy, President and Chief Executive Officer
CFO: Walt Larson, Vice President Finance
Web address: www.tcgh.com
Control: Church–operated, Nongovernment, not–for profit **Service:** General Medical and Surgical

Staffed Beds: 25 **Admissions:** 1372 **Census:** 12 **Outpatient Visits:** 38069 **Births:** 162 **Total Expense ($000):** 39685 **Payroll Expense ($000):** 15701 **Personnel:** 280

TUALATIN—Clackamas County

★☐ **LEGACY MERIDIAN PARK HOSPITAL (380089)**, 19300 S.W. 65th Avenue, Zip 97062–9741; tel. 503/692–1212 **A**1 2 9 10 **F**2 3 11 13 15 18 20 25 26 27 28 30 31 32 33 36 38 41 46 49 50 54 55 56 57 59 62 66 68 72 73 74 75 76 77 78 79 80 81 82 86 90 91 92 96 97 99 100 102 103 104 105 106 107 108 109 119 121 135 136 **P**8 **S** Legacy Health System
Primary Contact: Allyson Anderson, Chief Administrative Officer
CFO: Pamela S. Vukovich, Senior Vice President and Chief Financial Officer
CIO: C. Matthew Calais, Senior Vice President and Chief Information Officer
CHR: Sonja Steves, Vice President Human Resources and Marketing
Web address: www.legacyhealth.org
Control: Other not–for–profit (including NFP Corporation) **Service:** General Medical and Surgical

Staffed Beds: 133 **Admissions:** 7469 **Census:** 75 **Outpatient Visits:** 130789 **Births:** 1168 **Total Expense ($000):** 102165 **Payroll Expense ($000):** 38402 **Personnel:** 628

Hospital, Medicare Provider Number, Address, Telephone, Approval, Facility, and Physician Codes, Health Care System

★ American Hospital Association (AHA) membership
☐ The Joint Commission accreditation
○ American Osteopathic Association (AOA) accreditation
△ Commission on Accreditation of Rehabilitation Facilities (CARF) accreditation

PENNSYLVANIA

ABINGTON—Montgomery County

★ **ABINGTON MEMORIAL HOSPITAL (390231)**, 1200 Old York Road, Zip 19001–3720; tel. 215/481–2000 **A**1 2 3 5 6 9 10 12 13 **F**2 3 11 12 13 14 15 17 18 20 22 24 25 26 27 28 29 30 31 32 33 34 35 36 37 38 40 41 42 43 44 45 47 49 50 52 53 54 55 56 57 58 59 60 61 62 63 64 65 66 67 68 70 72 73 74 75 76 77 79 80 81 82 84 85 86 87 88 89 90 91 92 93 94 95 96 97 100 102 103 104 105 106 107 108 109 111 112 113 114 116 118 119 120 121 123 124 132 135 136 137 **P**6 7
Primary Contact: Richard L. Jones, Jr., FACHE, President and Chief Executive Officer
COO: Margaret M. McGoldrick, Executive Vice President and Administrator
CFO: Michael Walsh, Senior Vice President Finance and Chief Financial Officer
CMO: John J. Kelly, M.D., Chief of Staff
CIO: Alison Ferren, Vice President Information Technology and Chief Information Officer
CHR: Meghan Patton, Vice President Human Resources
Web address: www.amh.org
Control: Other not–for–profit (including NFP Corporation) **Service:** General Medical and Surgical

Staffed Beds: 606 **Admissions:** 36781 **Census:** 465 **Outpatient Visits:** 534526 **Births:** 4925 **Total Expense ($000):** 517833 **Payroll Expense ($000):** 228560 **Personnel:** 4321

ALIQUIPPA—Beaver County

COMMONWEALTH MEDICAL CENTER (390176), (Formerly Aliquippa Community Hospital), 2500 Hospital Drive, Zip 15001–2191; tel. 724/857–1212, (Nonreporting) **A**9 10
Primary Contact: Willie E. Wilson, Chief Executive Officer
CIO: James Stafford, Director Information Systems
CHR: Jamie Malloy, Director Human Resources
Web address: www.achonline.org
Control: Church–operated, Nongovernment, not–for profit **Service:** General Medical and Surgical

Staffed Beds: 208

ALLENTOWN—Lehigh County

☐ **ALLENTOWN STATE HOSPITAL (394011)**, 1600 Hanover Avenue, Zip 18103–2408; tel. 610/740–3200, (Nonreporting) **A**1 10
Primary Contact: Gregory M. Smith, Chief Executive Officer
COO: Carol Eliashevsky, Chief Operating Officer
CMO: Dung P. Tran, Chief Medical Officer
Web address: www.dpw.state.paus/family/mentalhealthserv/statementalhospa
Control: State–Government, nonfederal **Service:** Psychiatric

Staffed Beds: 181

☐ △ **GOOD SHEPHERD REHABILITATION NETWORK (393035)**, 850 South 5th Street, Zip 18103–3231; tel. 610/776–3299, (Nonreporting) **A**1 7 9 10
Primary Contact: Sally Gammon, President and Chief Executive Officer
CFO: Daniel Confalone, Chief Financial Officer
CMO: Phillip Bryant, D.O., Chief Medical Officer
CIO: John Kravitz, Chief Information Officer
CHR: Anthony Bongiovanni, Senior Vice President Human Resources and Corporate Performance
Web address: www.goodshepherdrehab.org
Control: Other not–for–profit (including NFP Corporation) **Service:** Rehabilitation

Staffed Beds: 82

★ **LEHIGH VALLEY HOSPITAL (390133)**, 1200 South Cedar Crest Boulevard, Zip 18105–6248, Mailing Address: P.O. Box 689, Zip 18105–0689; tel. 610/402–8000, (Total facility includes 52 beds in nursing home–type unit) **A**1 2 3 5 8 9 10 12 13 **F**3 6 7 9 11 12 13 15 16 17 18 20 22 24 25 26 27 28 30 31 32 33 34 36 37 38 40 41 42 43 44 45 46 48 49 50 51 52 53 54 55 56 57 58 59 60 61 62 63 64 66 68 69 70 71 72 73 74 75 76 77 78 79 80 81 82 83 84 85 86 87 88 89 90 91 92 93 94 95 96 97 99 100 102 103 104 105 106 107 108 109 111 112 113 114 116 117 118 119 120 121 123 124 125 127 131 132 133 135 136 137 **P**4 5 6 7 8 **S** Lehigh Valley Hospital and Health Network
Primary Contact: Elliot J. Sussman, M.D., President and Chief Executive Officer
COO: Stuart S. Paxton, Chief Operating Officer
CFO: Vaughn C. Gower, Senior Vice President and Chief Financial Officer
CMO: Ronald W. Swinfard, M.D., Chief Medical Officer
CIO: Harry Lukens, Senior Vice President and Chief Information Officer
CHR: Mary Kay Grim, Senior Vice President Human Resources
Web address: www.lvhhn.org
Control: Other not–for–profit (including NFP Corporation) **Service:** General Medical and Surgical

Staffed Beds: 701 **Admissions:** 40375 **Census:** 604 **Outpatient Visits:** 305852 **Births:** 3418 **Total Expense ($000):** 666947 **Payroll Expense ($000):** 238485 **Personnel:** 5534

☐ △ **SACRED HEART HOSPITAL (390197)**, 421 Chew Street, Zip 18102–3490; tel. 610/776–4500, (Total facility includes 20 beds in nursing home–type unit) **A**1 2 3 5 7 9 10 12 13 **F**3 11 12 13 15 18 20 22 24 25 26 27 28 30 32 33 36 37 38 40 42 43 44 46 47 49 50 52 53 54 55 56 57 60 61 62 64 66 71 72 73 74 75 76 77 78 79 80 82 86 87 88 90 91 92 93 96 97 100 102 107 109 111 117 118 119 121 124 132 135 136 137 **P**8
Primary Contact: Leo J. Connors, Interim Chief Executive Officer
CFO: Laurie H. Gombert, Vice President Finance
CMO: Frank Sparandero, M.D., M.P.H., President and Chief Executive Officer
CIO: Tracy Burkhart, Vice President Information Services
CHR: Joseph Mikitka, Vice President Human Resources
Web address: www.shh.org
Control: Other not–for–profit (including NFP Corporation) **Service:** General Medical and Surgical

Staffed Beds: 224 **Admissions:** 7969 **Census:** 126 **Outpatient Visits:** 184401 **Births:** 444 **Total Expense ($000):** 112734 **Payroll Expense ($000):** 48753 **Personnel:** 1178

ST LUKE'S HOSPITAL–ALLENTOWN CAMPUS See St. Luke's Hospital – Bethlehem Campus, Bethlehem

ALTOONA—Blair County

ALTOONA CENTER, 1515 Fourth Street, Zip 16601–4595; tel. 814/946–6900, (Nonreporting)
Primary Contact: Barry C. Benford, Director
Web address: www.altoonacenter.com/
Control: State–Government, nonfederal **Service:** Institution for mental retardation

Staffed Beds: 138

★ ○ **ALTOONA REGIONAL HEALTH SYSTEM (390073)**, 620 Howard Avenue, Zip 16601–4899; tel. 814/889–2011, (Includes ALTOONA HOSPITAL CAMPUS, 620 Howard Avenue, tel. 814/889–2011; BON SECOURS HOSPITAL CAMPUS, 2500 Seventh Avenue, Zip 16602–2099; tel. 814/944–1681) **A**1 2 9 10 11 12 13 **F**3 4 5 8 11 12 13 15 18 20 22 24 25 26 27 28 30 31 32 33 36 38 40 43 44 45 46 47 48 49 50 51 53 54 55 57 59 62 63 64 66 68 71 72 73 74 75 76 77 79 80 81 82 84 85 86 88 89 90 91 92 93 94 96 97 100 102 103 104 105 106 107 108 109 111 114 117 118 119 120 121 124 134 135 136 137 **P**8
Primary Contact: James W. Barner, President and Chief Executive Officer
COO: Ron McConnell, Chief Operating Officer
CFO: Charles Zorger, Senior Vice President Finance
CMO: Anthony J. Maniglia, M.D., President Medical Staff
CIO: Ron McConnell, Chief Operating Officer
CHR: Gary Naugle, Vice President Human Resources
Web address: www.altoonaregional.org
Control: Other not–for–profit (including NFP Corporation) **Service:** General Medical and Surgical

Staffed Beds: 450 **Admissions:** 20755 **Census:** 272 **Outpatient Visits:** 448481 **Births:** 1275 **Total Expense ($000):** 284278 **Payroll Expense ($000):** 106935 **Personnel:** 2116

★ **HEALTHSOUTH REHABILITATION HOSPITAL OF ALTOONA (393040)**, 2005 Valley View Boulevard, Zip 16602–4598; tel. 814/944–3535 **A**1 10 **F**2 24 25 30 31 32 50 54 55 57 59 73 77 85 86 120 121 132 **S** HEALTHSOUTH Corporation
Primary Contact: Scott Filler, Chief Executive Officer
CFO: Michael Zenone, Controller
CMO: Rakesh Patel, D.O., Medical Director
CHR: Christine Filer, Director Human Resources
Web address: www.healthsouthaltoona.com
Control: Corporation, Investor–owned, for–profit **Service:** Rehabilitation

Staffed Beds: 70 **Admissions:** 1407 **Census:** 57 **Outpatient Visits:** 44582 **Births:** 0 **Total Expense ($000):** 18531 **Payroll Expense ($000):** 11153 **Personnel:** 259

★ **JAMES E. VAN ZANDT VETERANS AFFAIRS MEDICAL CENTER**, 2907 Pleasant Valley Boulevard, Zip 16602–4377; tel. 814/943–8164, (Total facility includes 40 beds in nursing home–type unit) **A**1 9 **F**5 15 25 26 33 37 38 41 42 43 53 54 56 57 60 61 62 63 66 68 72 73 75 77 79 81 82 86 87 90 94 96 102 107 119 121 124 132 135 136 137 **P**6 **S** Department of Veterans Affairs
Primary Contact: Anthony Bennett, Director
Web address: www.va.gov/sta/guide/home.asp
Control: Veterans Affairs, Government, federal **Service:** General Medical and Surgical

Staffed Beds: 68 **Admissions:** 954 **Census:** 33 **Outpatient Visits:** 151538 **Births:** 0 **Total Expense ($000):** 78909 **Payroll Expense ($000):** 27739 **Personnel:** 511

AMBLER—Montgomery County

☐ **HORSHAM CLINIC (394034)**, 722 East Butler Pike, Zip 19002–2310; tel. 215/643–7800, (Nonreporting) **A**1 5 9 10 **S** Universal Health Services, Inc.
Primary Contact: Phyllis Weisfield, Chief Executive Officer and Managing Director
CFO: Robert Chavez, Chief Financial Officer
CMO: Susan Au, M.D., Medical Director
CIO: Suzanne Scholz, Director Medical Records
CHR: Kathleen Nichelson, Director Human Resources
Web address: www.horshamclinic.com
Control: Individual, Investor–owned, for–profit **Service:** Psychiatric

Staffed Beds: 138

ASHLAND—Schuylkill County

☐ **SAINT CATHERINE MEDICAL CENTER FOUNTAIN SPRINGS (390313)**, 101 Broad Street, Zip 17921–0000; tel. 570/875–2000, (Total facility includes 40 beds in nursing home–type unit) **A**1 9 10 **F**3 8 11 15 25 26 38 42 43 49 50 56 57 66 68 72 77 79 82 86 90 96 100 107 117 119 135 **P**6 **S** Saint Catherine Healthcare, LLC
Primary Contact: Robert C. Marquardt, FACHE, President and Chief Executive Officer
CFO: Jeffrey Chilson, Chief Financial Officer
CMO: Yasser Khoudeir, M.D., Medical Staff President
CHR: Laura LaBuda, Director Human Resources
Control: Corporation, Investor–owned, for–profit **Service:** General Medical and Surgical

Staffed Beds: 79 **Admissions:** 1503 **Census:** 49 **Outpatient Visits:** 258757 **Births:** 0 **Total Expense ($000):** 18710 **Payroll Expense ($000):** 8040 **Personnel:** 205

BEAVER—Beaver County

☐ **HERITAGE VALLEY BEAVER (390036)**, (Formerly The Medical Center, Beaver), 1000 Dutch Ridge Road, Zip 15009–9727; tel. 724/728–7000, (Nonreporting) **A**1 9 10 12 13 **S** Heritage Valley Health System
Primary Contact: Norman F. Mitry, President and Chief Executive Officer
COO: Rosemary Nolan, Chief Operating Officer and Chief Nursing Officer
CFO: Bryan J. Randall, Vice President Finance and Chief Financial Officer
CMO: Oliver Hayes, D.O., Chief Medical Officer
CIO: David Carleton, Chief Information Officer
CHR: Bruce Edwards, Vice President Human Resources
Web address: www.heritagevalley.org
Control: Other not–for–profit (including NFP Corporation) **Service:** General Medical and Surgical

Staffed Beds: 300

☐ **KINDRED HOSPITAL–HERITAGE VALLEY (392043)**, 1000 Dutch Ridge Road, Zip 15009; tel. 724/773–8210, (Nonreporting) **A**1 10 **S** Kindred Healthcare
Primary Contact: Timothy Bugin, Administrator
CFO: Kevin Varley, Chief Financial Officer
CMO: Jeffrey Erukhimou, M.D., Medical Director
Web address: www.kindredhealthcare.com
Control: Corporation, Investor–owned, for–profit **Service:** Long–Term Acute Care hospital

Staffed Beds: 35

BENSALEM—Bucks County

LIVENGRIN FOUNDATION, 4833 Hulmeville Road, Zip 19020–3099; tel. 215/638–5200, (Nonreporting) **A**9
Primary Contact: Richard M. Pine, President and Chief Executive Officer
CFO: James D. Flis, Chief Financial Officer
CMO: William J. Lorman, Ph.D., Clinical Director
CIO: William Miller, Coordinator Management Information Systems
Web address: www.livengrin.org
Control: Other not–for–profit (including NFP Corporation) **Service:** Alcoholism and other chemical dependency

Staffed Beds: 76

BERWICK—Columbia County

★☐ **BERWICK HOSPITAL CENTER (390072)**, 701 East 16th Street, Zip 18603–2397; tel. 570/759–5000, (Total facility includes 240 beds in nursing home–type unit) **A**1 9 10 **F**3 13 15 18 24 25 27 30 31 32 37 38 42 43 46 54 55 56 57 61 62 68 72 73 74 75 76 77 79 80 86 88 90 91 92 93 96 97 100 102 106 107 117 118 119 121 122 135 136 137 **P**6 **S** Community Health Systems, Inc.
Primary Contact: John Kristel, Chief Executive Officer
CFO: Mike Stephens, Chief Financial Officer
CMO: Frank Giugliano, M.D., Chief of Staff
CHR: Jackie Ridall, Director Human Resources
Web address: www.berwick–hospital.com
Control: Corporation, Investor–owned, for–profit **Service:** General Medical and Surgical

Staffed Beds: 341 **Admissions:** 4109 **Census:** 240 **Outpatient Visits:** 89422 **Births:** 138 **Personnel:** 500

PA

BETHLEHEM—Lehigh County

☐ **GOOD SHEPHERD SPECIALTY HOSPITAL (392033)**, 2545 Schoenersville Road, 3rd Floor, Zip 18017; tel. 484/884–5051, (Nonreporting) **A**1 10
Primary Contact: Pam Miles, Administrator
Web address: www.goodshepherdrehab.org
Control: Corporation, Investor–owned, for–profit **Service:** Long–Term Acute Care hospital

Staffed Beds: 32

★☐ **LEHIGH VALLEY HOSPITAL–MUHLENBERG (390263)**, 2545 Schoenersville Road, Zip 18017–7384; tel. 484/884–2201 **A**1 2 9 10 12 13 **F**3 11 15 17 18 20 22 24 25 26 27 30 31 32 33 34 36 37 38 41 42 43 44 49 50 51 52 53 55 56 57 58 59 61 62 63 66 68 72 73 75 76 77 78 79 80 81 82 85 86 87 92 96 97 99 100 102 103 106 107 108 109 111 112 113 114 118 119 120 121 123 124 132 135 137 **P**4 5 6 7 8 **S** Lehigh Valley Hospital and Health Network
Primary Contact: Elliot J. Sussman, M.D., President and Chief Executive Officer
COO: James F. Geiger, Senior Vice President Operations
CFO: Vaughn C. Gower, Senior Vice President Finance and Chief Financial Officer
CMO: Ronald W. Swinfard, M.D., Chief Medical Officer
CIO: Harry Lukens, Senior Vice President and Chief Information Officer
CHR: Mary Kay Grim, Senior Vice President Human Resources
Web address: www.lvhhn.org
Control: Other not–for–profit (including NFP Corporation) **Service:** General Medical and Surgical

Staffed Beds: 156 **Admissions:** 9030 **Census:** 115 **Outpatient Visits:** 163212 **Births:** 0 **Total Expense ($000):** 150247 **Payroll Expense ($000):** 55363 **Personnel:** 1231

☐ **ST. LUKE'S HOSPITAL – BETHLEHEM CAMPUS (390049)**, 801 Ostrum Street, Zip 18015–1065; tel. 610/954–4000, (Includes ST LUKE'S HOSPITAL–ALLENTOWN CAMPUS, 1736 Hamilton Street, Allentown, Zip 18104–5656; tel. 610/770–8300) **A**1 2 3 5 6 8 9 10 12 13 **F**3 7 9 11 12 13 15 17 18 20 22 24 25 26 27 28 30 31 32 33 34 35 36 37 38 39 40 41 42 43 44 46 49 50 51 52 53 54 55 56 57 58 59 60 62 63 64 66 68 69 70 71 72 73 74 75 76 77 79 80 81 82 84 85 86 87 88 89 90 91 92 93 94 95 96 97 99 100 102 103 104 105 106 107 108 109 111 112 113 114 116 118 119 120 121 123 124 133 134 135 136 137 **P**6 8
Primary Contact: Richard A. Anderson, President and Chief Executive Officer
COO: Joel Fagerstrom, Executive Vice President and Chief Operating Officer
CFO: Tom Lichtenwalner, Interim Vice President Finance
CMO: Jeffrey Jahre, M.D., Vice President Medical and Academic Affairs
CIO: Albert Sinisi, Chief Information Officer
CHR: Robert Zimmel, Senior Vice President Human Resources
Web address: www.slhn–lehighvalley.org
Control: Other not–for–profit (including NFP Corporation) **Service:** General Medical and Surgical

Staffed Beds: 579 **Admissions:** 34410 **Census:** 416 **Outpatient Visits:** 693513 **Births:** 4205 **Total Expense ($000):** 456834 **Payroll Expense ($000):** 190601 **Personnel:** 3882

Hospital, Medicare Provider Number, Address, Telephone, Approval, Facility, and Physician Codes, Health Care System

★ American Hospital Association (AHA) membership
☐ The Joint Commission accreditation
○ American Osteopathic Association (AOA) accreditation
△ Commission on Accreditation of Rehabilitation Facilities (CARF) accreditation

BLOOMSBURG—Columbia County

★ **BLOOMSBURG HOSPITAL (390003)**, 549 Fair Street, Zip 17815–0340; tel. 570/387–2100 **A**9 10 **F**3 11 13 15 24 25 26 27 30 31 33 34 38 41 43 50 51 54 55 56 57 62 63 66 68 73 74 75 76 77 79 80 82 88 89 91 92 93 96 97 100 103 106 107 112 118 119 121 124
Primary Contact: Regis Cabonor, President and Chief Executive Officer
COO: Joseph M. DeVito, Chief Operating Officer
CFO: Joseph M. DeVito, Chief Financial Officer
CMO: Paul Salory, M.D., President Medical Staff
CIO: Robert Theiss, Chief Information Officer
CHR: Mary Lenzini Howe, Vice President Human Resources
Web address: www.bloomhealth.net
Control: Other not–for–profit (including NFP Corporation) **Service:** General Medical and Surgical

Staffed Beds: 72 **Admissions:** 2799 **Census:** 29 **Outpatient Visits:** 63301 **Births:** 260 **Total Expense ($000):** 32728 **Payroll Expense ($000):** 12763 **Personnel:** 305

PA

BRADDOCK—Allegheny County

☐ **UPMC BRADDOCK (390128)**, 400 Holland Avenue, Zip 15104–1598; tel. 412/636–5000, (Total facility includes 30 beds in nursing home–type unit) **A**1 9 10 **F**3 4 8 15 25 26 28 30 31 32 33 36 37 38 50 55 56 57 60 65 67 68 73 76 77 79 80 88 90 91 92 93 96 102 106 107 117 119 121 123 124 135 **P**5 **S** UPMC
Primary Contact: Cynthia M. Dorundo, President
COO: Rodney B. Jones, Vice President Operations
CFO: Charles LaClair, Chief Financial Officer
CIO: Toni McKeever, Director Information Systems
CHR: Helene Brown, Director Human Resources
Web address: www.upmc.edu
Control: Other not–for–profit (including NFP Corporation) **Service:** General Medical and Surgical

Staffed Beds: 176 **Admissions:** 7827 **Census:** 130 **Outpatient Visits:** 75355 **Births:** 0 **Total Expense ($000):** 55077 **Payroll Expense ($000):** 25211 **Personnel:** 515

BRADFORD—McKean County

★ **BRADFORD REGIONAL MEDICAL CENTER (390118)**, 116 Interstate Parkway, Zip 16701–0218; tel. 814/368–4143, (Total facility includes 95 beds in nursing home–type unit) **A**9 10 **F**11 13 15 18 24 25 27 30 31 32 33 37 38 42 43 49 50 52 54 55 57 61 62 68 72 74 75 76 77 79 80 81 82 86 87 88 90 91 92 93 94 95 96 97 100 102 106 107 117 118 119 120 121 124 135 136 137 **P**8
Primary Contact: George E. Leonhardt, CHE, President and Chief Executive Officer
CFO: James Tarasovitch, Senior Vice President and Chief Financial Officer
CIO: Terry Palmer, Chief Information Officer
CHR: Dennis Geitner, Vice President Human Resources
Web address: www.brmc.com
Control: Other not–for–profit (including NFP Corporation) **Service:** General Medical and Surgical

Staffed Beds: 191 **Admissions:** 4190 **Census:** 141 **Outpatient Visits:** 116787 **Births:** 296 **Total Expense ($000):** 71084 **Payroll Expense ($000):** 28960 **Personnel:** 605

BRIDGEVILLE—Allegheny County

☐ **MAYVIEW STATE HOSPITAL (394018)**, 1601 Mayview Road, Zip 15017–1547; tel. 412/257–6500, (Nonreporting) **A**1 5 10
Primary Contact: Richard Kuppelweiser, Chief Executive Officer
Control: State–Government, nonfederal **Service:** Psychiatric

Staffed Beds: 438

BRISTOL—Bucks County

☐ **LOWER BUCKS HOSPITAL (390070)**, 501 Bath Road, Zip 19007–3190; tel. 215/785–9200 **A**1 5 9 10 **F**8 11 13 15 17 18 20 22 24 25 26 30 31 32 36 38 43 52 53 55 56 57 61 62 68 70 73 74 75 76 77 79 81 82 84 86 88 90 91 92 96 97 100 106 107 118 119 120 121 135 136 137
Primary Contact: Austin B. Cleveland, President and Chief Executive Officer
CFO: Michael Drabot, Chief Financial Officer
CMO: Vincent LaRosa, M.D., President Medical Staff
CIO: John McHale, Vice President Management Information Systems
CHR: Kellie Pearson, Director Human Resources
Web address: www.lowerbuckshospital.org
Control: Other not–for–profit (including NFP Corporation) **Service:** General Medical and Surgical

Staffed Beds: 159 **Admissions:** 8360 **Census:** 100 **Outpatient Visits:** 124941 **Births:** 998 **Personnel:** 867

BROOKVILLE—Jefferson County

BROOKVILLE HOSPITAL (391312), 100 Hospital Road, Zip 15825–1367; tel. 814/849–2312 **A**9 10 18 **F**3 11 15 17 24 25 26 30 31 32 33 37 38 55 56 57 61 73 75 77 79 80 81 86 88 93 96 97 102 106 107 118 119 120 122 135 **P**5
Primary Contact: John Sutika, President and Chief Executive Officer
CFO: Julie Peer, Vice President Finance
CMO: Susan A. Connor, M.D., President Medical Staff
CIO: Fred Terwilliger, Director Information Systems
Web address: www.brookvillehospital.org
Control: Other not–for–profit (including NFP Corporation) **Service:** General Medical and Surgical

Staffed Beds: 34 **Admissions:** 1733 **Census:** 20 **Outpatient Visits:** 78800 **Births:** 0 **Total Expense ($000):** 23995 **Payroll Expense ($000):** 9700 **Personnel:** 236

BRYN MAWR—Montgomery County

☐ **BRYN MAWR HOSPITAL (390139)**, 130 South Bryn Mawr Avenue, Zip 19010–3160; tel. 610/526–3000 **A**1 2 3 5 9 10 **F**3 11 13 15 17 18 20 22 24 25 26 27 30 31 32 33 38 43 44 46 48 49 52 53 55 56 57 58 62 68 70 72 73 74 76 77 79 80 81 82 84 86 88 89 90 92 93 96 97 99 102 103 106 107 108 109 111 112 114 116 118 119 120 121 124 135 136 137
S Jefferson Health System
Primary Contact: Andrea F. Gilbert, CHE, President
COO: Andrea F. Gilbert, CHE, President
CFO: Michael J. Buongiorno, Senior Vice President Finance
CMO: Donald C. Arthur, M.D., Chief Medical Officer
CIO: Karen A. Thomas, R.N., Chief Information Officer
CHR: Terry Dougherty, Director Human Resources
Web address: www.brynmawrhospital.org
Control: Other not–for–profit (including NFP Corporation) **Service:** General Medical and Surgical

Staffed Beds: 311 **Admissions:** 17643 **Census:** 210 **Outpatient Visits:** 194129 **Births:** 1749 **Total Expense ($000):** 212997 **Payroll Expense ($000):** 83639 **Personnel:** 1540

BUTLER—Butler County

☒ **BUTLER HEALTH SYSTEM (390168)**, 911 East Brady Street, Zip 16001–4697; tel. 724/283–6666, (Total facility includes 23 beds in nursing home–type unit) **A**1 9 10 **F**4 5 13 15 17 18 20 22 24 25 27 28 30 31 32 33 38 43 55 57 68 72 74 77 79 80 82 86 88 90 93 96 97 100 102 106 107 117 118 119 121 124 135 136 137
Primary Contact: Ken DeFurio, President and Chief Executive Officer
CFO: Anne Krebs, Chief Financial Officer
CMO: John C. Reefer, M.D., Director
CIO: Chuck Oleson, Chief Information Officer
CHR: Mike Swank, Interim Vice President Human Resources
Web address: www.butlerhealthsystem.org
Control: Other not–for–profit (including NFP Corporation) **Service:** General Medical and Surgical

Staffed Beds: 258 **Admissions:** 13400 **Census:** 189 **Outpatient Visits:** 436284 **Births:** 789 **Total Expense ($000):** 147829 **Payroll Expense ($000):** 62639 **Personnel:** 1377

★ △ **VETERANS AFFAIRS MEDICAL CENTER**, (VA Outpatient, Nursing Home), 325 New Castle Road, Zip 16001–2480; tel. 724/287–4781, (Total facility includes 60 beds in nursing home–type unit) **A**7 9 **F**1 2 3 4 5 11 12 25 26 29 30 31 32 33 36 37 42 43 44 45 50 52 54 55 56 57 61 62 63 65 72 73 75 78 81 82 85 86 87 88 94 96 102 103 107 117 119 121 124 132 135 **P**6
S Department of Veterans Affairs
Primary Contact: Patricia Nealon, Director
COO: Richard W. Cotter, Chief Operating Officer
CFO: Doug George, Financial Manager
CMO: Varsha Mehta, M.D., Chief of Staff
CIO: Jupe Fowkes, Chief Information Officer
CHR: David Cord, Human Resources Officer
Web address: www.va.gov/sta/guide/home.asp
Control: Veterans Affairs, Government, federal **Service:** Other specialty

Staffed Beds: 126 **Admissions:** 536 **Census:** 111 **Outpatient Visits:** 126947 **Births:** 0 **Total Expense ($000):** 81358 **Payroll Expense ($000):** 35232 **Personnel:** 512

Many Facility Codes have changed. Please refer to the AHA Guide Code Chart.

CAMP HILL—Cumberland County

★ **HOLY SPIRIT HOSPITAL (390004)**, 503 North 21st Street, Zip 17011–2288; tel. 717/763–2100 **A**1 5 9 10 **F**3 8 11 13 14 15 17 18 20 22 24 25 26 27 30 32 33 36 38 41 42 43 44 50 53 55 56 57 58 60 62 63 68 70 71 72 73 74 75 76 77 78 79 80 81 82 86 88 89 90 91 92 93 94 95 96 97 99 100 102 103 106 107 118 119 121 123 124 133 135 136 137
Primary Contact: Sister Romaine Niemeyer, President and Chief Executive Officer
COO: Richard Schaffner, Chief Operating Officer
CFO: Manuel J. Evans, Chief Financial Officer
CMO: Joseph Torchia, M.D., Vice President Clinical Resource Management
CIO: Edith Hunter, Chief Information Officer
CHR: William Shartle, Senior Vice President Human Resources
Web address: www.hsh.org
Control: Church–operated, Nongovernment, not–for profit **Service:** General Medical and Surgical

Staffed Beds: 298 **Admissions:** 15012 **Census:** 204 **Outpatient Visits:** 182438 **Births:** 1033 **Total Expense ($000):** 195163 **Payroll Expense ($000):** 86499 **Personnel:** 1821

□ **SELECT SPECIALTY HOSPITAL–CAMP HILL (392039)**, 503 North 21st Street, 5th Floor, Zip 17011; tel. 717/972–4560, (Nonreporting) **A**1 10 **S** Select Medical Corporation
Primary Contact: Marcia Medlin, Chief Executive Officer
Web address: www.selectmedicalcorp.com
Control: Corporation, Investor–owned, for–profit **Service:** Long–Term Acute Care hospital

Staffed Beds: 31

STATE CORRECTIONAL INSTITUTION AT CAMP HILL, 2500 Lisbon Road, Zip 17011, Mailing Address: P.O. Box 200, Zip 17011–0200; tel. 717/737–4531, (Nonreporting)
Primary Contact: Kathy Montag, Administrator Health Care
Control: State–Government, nonfederal **Service:** Other specialty

Staffed Beds: 34

CANONSBURG—Washington County

★ **CANONSBURG GENERAL HOSPITAL (390160)**, 100 Medical Boulevard, Zip 15317–9762; tel. 724/745–6100 **A**1 9 10 **F**3 7 11 15 25 26 27 28 30 31 32 33 38 49 55 56 57 62 63 66 68 73 75 76 77 79 80 85 96 102 106 107 118 119 132 135 **P**6 **S** West Penn Allegheny Health System
Primary Contact: Kim Malinky, President and Chief Executive Officer
COO: Terry Wiltrout, Vice President Operations
CFO: Gene Trout, Chief Financial Officer
CMO: Jeffrey Gretz, D.O., President Medical Staff
CIO: David Vincent, Director Information Systems
CHR: Martha L. Clister, Director Human Resources
Web address: www.wpahs.org
Control: Other not–for–profit (including NFP Corporation) **Service:** General Medical and Surgical

Staffed Beds: 104 **Admissions:** 4429 **Census:** 63 **Outpatient Visits:** 85202 **Births:** 0 **Total Expense ($000):** 49118 **Payroll Expense ($000):** 21111 **Personnel:** 445

CARBONDALE—Lackawanna County

★ **MARIAN COMMUNITY HOSPITAL (390095)**, 100 Lincoln Avenue, Zip 18407–2198; tel. 570/281–1000 **A**1 9 10 **F**3 8 15 24 25 26 27 30 31 32 38 53 56 57 62 68 72 73 76 77 79 84 86 88 96 97 100 107 119 121 132 135 **S** Catholic Health East
Primary Contact: Mary Theresa Vautrinot, President and Chief Executive Officer
CFO: Richard J. Hager, Chief Financial Officer
CMO: Jeffrey Mogerman, M.D., President Medical Staff
CIO: Doug Tippins, Director Information Services
CHR: Ronald Boldt, Vice President Human Resources
Web address: www.marianhospital.org
Control: Church–operated, Nongovernment, not–for profit **Service:** General Medical and Surgical

Staffed Beds: 80 **Admissions:** 3130 **Census:** 42 **Outpatient Visits:** 70059 **Births:** 0 **Total Expense ($000):** 34864 **Payroll Expense ($000):** 14269 **Personnel:** 309

CARLISLE—Cumberland County

□ **CARLISLE REGIONAL MEDICAL CENTER (390058)**, 361 Alexander Spring Road, Zip 17013–3661; tel. 717/249–1212, (Nonreporting) **A**1 9 10 **S** Health Management Associates
Primary Contact: Nathan Staggs, Chief Executive Officer
CFO: Jeffrey Morgan, Associate Executive Director and Chief Financial Officer
CMO: Howard Alster, M.D., President, Medical Staff
CIO: Kemp Beatty, Director Information Management
Web address: www.chhs.org/home/default.asp
Control: Corporation, Investor–owned, for–profit **Service:** General Medical and Surgical

Staffed Beds: 103

CENTRE HALL—Centre County

□ **MEADOWS PSYCHIATRIC CENTER (394040)**, 132 The Meadows Drive, Zip 16828–9798; tel. 814/364–2161 **A**1 9 10 **F**30 88 89 92 93 94 95 **P**6 **S** Universal Health Services, Inc.
Primary Contact: Larry Grimes, Chief Executive Officer
CFO: Ernest C. Priddy, Chief Financial Officer
CMO: Nalin Patel, M.D., Medical Director
CHR: Kimberly J. Tate, Director Human Resources
Web address: www.themeadows.net
Control: Corporation, Investor–owned, for–profit **Service:** Psychiatric

Staffed Beds: 101 **Admissions:** 2525 **Census:** 77 **Outpatient Visits:** 28662 **Births:** 0 **Total Expense ($000):** 12551 **Payroll Expense ($000):** 6461 **Personnel:** 177

CHAMBERSBURG—Franklin County

★ **CHAMBERSBURG HOSPITAL (390151)**, 112 North Seventh Street, Zip 17201–0187; tel. 717/267–3000 **A**1 2 9 10 19 **F**3 11 12 13 15 17 20 24 25 26 27 30 31 32 33 34 36 38 43 44 48 49 50 52 53 54 55 56 57 60 62 63 66 68 72 73 74 75 76 77 79 80 81 82 84 85 86 87 88 89 90 91 92 93 94 96 97 99 100 102 105 106 107 108 111 118 119 120 121 124 133 135 136 **P**6 7 8 **S** Summit Health
Primary Contact: Norman B. Epstein, FACHE, President
COO: John P. Massimilla, FACHE, Vice President Administration
CFO: Patrick W. O'Donnell, CPA, Senior Vice President and Chief Operating Officer
CMO: Thomas Anderson, M.D., Vice President Medical Affairs
CIO: Michael Zeigler, Vice President and Chief Information Officer
CHR: Lou Gregorio, Vice President Human Resources
Web address: www.summithealth.org
Control: Other not–for–profit (including NFP Corporation) **Service:** General Medical and Surgical

Staffed Beds: 240 **Admissions:** 13249 **Census:** 159 **Outpatient Visits:** 349411 **Births:** 1442 **Total Expense ($000):** 180467 **Payroll Expense ($000):** 79727 **Personnel:** 1439

CHESTER—Delaware County

KEYSTONE CENTER, 2001 Providence Avenue, Zip 19013–5504; tel. 610/876–9000, (Nonreporting) **S** Universal Health Services, Inc.
Primary Contact: Michael Salazar, XPsyD, Chief Executive Officer and Managing Director
CFO: Delia Gonzalez, Director Accounting
CMO: Michael Glacken, M.D., Medical Director
CHR: Kevin Williams, Director Human Resources
Web address: www.keystonecenter.net
Control: Corporation, Investor–owned, for–profit **Service:** Alcoholism and other chemical dependency

Staffed Beds: 119

CLAIRTON—Allegheny County

□ **JEFFERSON REGIONAL MEDICAL CENTER (390265)**, 565 Coal Valley Road, Zip 15025, Mailing Address: Box 18119, Pittsburgh, Zip 15236–0119; tel. 412/469–5000 **A**1 9 10 **F**17 68 85 88
Primary Contact: Thomas P. Timcho, President and Chief Executive Officer
COO: Robert A. Frank, Executive Vice President and Chief Operating Officer
CFO: Joanne A. Hahey, Vice President and Chief Financial Officer
CMO: Richard F. Collins, M.D., Vice President Medical Affairs
CIO: James Witenske, Chief Information Officer and Director Information Systems
CHR: Rosanne Sanders, Vice President Human Resources
Web address: www.jeffersonregional.com
Control: Other not–for–profit (including NFP Corporation) **Service:** General Medical and Surgical

Staffed Beds: 373 **Admissions:** 18453 **Census:** 280 **Outpatient Visits:** 290182 **Births:** 0 **Payroll Expense ($000):** 79

PA

Hospital, Medicare Provider Number, Address, Telephone, Approval, Facility, and Physician Codes, Health Care System

★ American Hospital Association (AHA) membership
□ The Joint Commission accreditation
○ American Osteopathic Association (AOA) accreditation
△ Commission on Accreditation of Rehabilitation Facilities (CARF) accreditation

PA

CLARION—Clarion County

★ ○ **CLARION HOSPITAL (390093)**, One Hospital Drive, Zip 16214–8599; tel. 814/226–9500 **A**9 10 11 12 13 19 **F**3 7 11 13 15 25 26 27 38 40 43 44 55 57 62 68 74 75 76 77 79 80 96 97 100 107 117 118 119 134 135 137 **S** QHR
Primary Contact: Byron Quinton, Chief Executive Officer
CFO: Vincent M. Lamorella, Chief Financial Officer
CHR: Michael Wienand, Manager Human Resources
Web address: www.clarionhospital.org
Control: Other not–for–profit (including NFP Corporation) **Service:** General Medical and Surgical

Staffed Beds: 83 **Admissions:** 3007 **Census:** 36 **Outpatient Visits:** 107166 **Births:** 329 **Total Expense ($000):** 40150 **Payroll Expense ($000):** 15360 **Personnel:** 449

□ **CLARION PSYCHIATRIC CENTER (394043)**, 2 Hospital Drive, Zip 16214; tel. 814/226–9545 **A**1 9 10 **F**25 32 54 57 66 69 73 82 88 89 90 93 95 119 **P**6 **S** Universal Health Services, Inc.
Primary Contact: Curtis J. Dyer, Chief Executive Officer
CFO: Shelly Rhoades, Chief Financial Officer
CMO: Gerald M. Streets, M.D., Medical Director
CHR: Dianne C. Bilunka, Director Human Resources
Web address: www.clarioncenter.com
Control: Corporation, Investor–owned, for–profit **Service:** Psychiatric

Staffed Beds: 74 **Admissions:** 1844 **Census:** 41 **Outpatient Visits:** 2152 **Births:** 0 **Total Expense ($000):** 7499 **Payroll Expense ($000):** 3540 **Personnel:** 101

CLARKS SUMMIT—Lackawanna County

□ **CLARKS SUMMIT STATE HOSPITAL (394012)**, 1451 Hillside Drive, Zip 18411–9504; tel. 570/586–2011 **A**1 10 **F**25 26 30 32 33 34 36 37 43 44 50 52 54 55 56 57 58 60 63 66 72 73 75 81 82 86 87 88 90 91 92 93 119 121 124 132 135 **P**6
Primary Contact: Thomas P. Comerford, Jr., Superintendent
COO: Gordon Weber, Chief Operating Officer
CMO: David Waibel, M.D., Medical Director
CHR: William Abda, Chief Human Resources Officer
Web address: www.dpw.state.pa.us/
Control: State–Government, nonfederal **Service:** Psychiatric

Staffed Beds: 245 **Admissions:** 136 **Census:** 221 **Outpatient Visits:** 0 **Total Expense ($000):** 42677 **Payroll Expense ($000):** 23580 **Personnel:** 508

CLEARFIELD—Clearfield County

★ **CLEARFIELD HOSPITAL (390052)**, 809 Turnpike Avenue, Zip 16830–1232, Mailing Address: P.O. Box 992, Zip 16830–0992; tel. 814/765–5341, (Nonreporting) **A**9 10
Primary Contact: David J. McConnell, President and Chief Executive Officer
CFO: Robert Locke, Chief Financial Officer
CMO: Gregory Sheffo, M.D., President Medical Staff
CIO: Linda Dunworth, Director Management Information Systems
CHR: Jon Steen, Vice President Support Services
Web address: www.clearfieldhosp.org
Control: Other not–for–profit (including NFP Corporation) **Service:** General Medical and Surgical

Staffed Beds: 96

COAL TOWNSHIP—Northumberland County

★ **SHAMOKIN AREA COMMUNITY HOSPITAL (390189)**, 4200 Hospital Road, Zip 17866–9697; tel. 570/644–4200, (Total facility includes 15 beds in nursing home–type unit) **A**9 10 **F**3 8 11 15 24 25 26 30 31 32 33 34 38 43 49 50 51 54 55 56 57 62 63 66 68 73 75 77 79 80 82 86 88 92 93 96 97 99 100 102 107 117 119 121 124 135 136
Primary Contact: Thomas R. Harlow, FACHE, President and Chief Executive Officer
CFO: Randy B. Morris, Vice President and Chief Financial Officer
CMO: Duane R. Donmoyer, M.D., Chief of Staff
CIO: Kimberly Chaundy, Manager Information Systems
CHR: Rick Flynn, Vice President Human Resources
Web address: www.shamokinhospital.org
Control: Other not–for–profit (including NFP Corporation) **Service:** General Medical and Surgical

Staffed Beds: 70 **Admissions:** 3314 **Census:** 47 **Outpatient Visits:** 84219 **Births:** 1 **Total Expense ($000):** 30034 **Payroll Expense ($000):** 12914 **Personnel:** 294

COALDALE—Schuylkill County

□ **ST. LUKE'S MINER'S MEMORIAL HOSPITAL (390183)**, 360 West Ruddle Street, Zip 18218–1099; tel. 570/645–2131, (Total facility includes 48 beds in nursing home–type unit) **A**1 9 10 **F**3 7 15 24 25 27 30 31 32 38 49 52 53 54 55 56 57 61 62 63 66 68 73 75 76 77 79 80 81 86 96 97 100 103 106 107 112 117 118 119 120 121 135 137 **P**6 8
Primary Contact: William J. Crossin, President
CFO: Michele Levitz, Director Finance
CMO: Robert De Joseph, M.D., Medical Director
CHR: Stephen Peters, Director Human Resources
Web address: www.slhhn.org
Control: Other not–for–profit (including NFP Corporation) **Service:** General Medical and Surgical

Staffed Beds: 93 **Admissions:** 2270 **Census:** 71 **Outpatient Visits:** 80491 **Births:** 0 **Total Expense ($000):** 37909 **Payroll Expense ($000):** 14915 **Personnel:** 326

COATESVILLE—Chester County

☒ **BRANDYWINE HOSPITAL (390076)**, 201 Reeceville Road, Zip 19320–1536; tel. 610/383–8000, (Nonreporting) **A**1 2 6 9 10 **S** Community Health Systems, Inc.
Primary Contact: Mark A. Benz, Chief Executive Officer
COO: Jill Tillman, Assistant Chief Executive Officer
CFO: Anthony Esposito, Chief Financial Officer
CHR: Amy Linsin, Director Human Resources
Web address: www.brandywinehospital.com
Control: Corporation, Investor–owned, for–profit **Service:** General Medical and Surgical

Staffed Beds: 164

☒ △ **VETERANS AFFAIRS MEDICAL CENTER**, 1400 Black Horse Hill Road, Zip 19320–2040; tel. 610/384–7711, (Total facility includes 164 beds in nursing home–type unit) (Nonreporting) **A**1 7 9 **S** Department of Veterans Affairs
Primary Contact: Gary W. Devansky, Director
CFO: Thomas Robinson, Chief Financial Officer
CMO: James F. Tischler, M.D., Chief of Staff
CIO: Eugene Doria, Chief Information Officer
CHR: George Pearson, Director Human Resources Management Service
Web address: www.va.gov/sta/guide/home.asp
Control: Veterans Affairs, Government, federal **Service:** Alcoholism and other chemical dependency

Staffed Beds: 472

CONNELLSVILLE—Fayette County

HIGHLANDS HOSPITAL (390184), 401 East Murphy Avenue, Zip 15425–2700; tel. 724/628–1500 **A**9 10 **F**3 11 12 15 24 25 26 31 32 33 34 37 38 41 46 49 50 51 52 54 55 56 57 60 62 63 68 73 75 77 79 80 82 84 86 88 89 90 91 92 93 96 97 102 107 118 119 121 122 132 135
Primary Contact: Michelle P. Cunningham, Chief Executive Officer
CFO: John Andursky, Chief Financial Officer
CMO: Paul Means, M.D., Medical Staff President
CIO: John Andursky, Chief Financial Officer
CHR: Mary June Krosoff, Chief Human Resources Officer
Web address: www.highlandshospital.org
Control: Other not–for–profit (including NFP Corporation) **Service:** General Medical and Surgical

Staffed Beds: 71 **Admissions:** 2787 **Census:** 37 **Outpatient Visits:** 57106 **Births:** 0 **Total Expense ($000):** 23622 **Payroll Expense ($000):** 9901 **Personnel:** 301

CORRY—Erie County

CORRY MEMORIAL HOSPITAL (391308), 612 West Smith Street, Zip 16407–1196; tel. 814/664–4641, (Nonreporting) **A**9 10 18
Primary Contact: Barbara Nichols, RN, President and Chief Executive Officer
COO: Barbara Moore, Chief Operating Officer
CFO: Michael Heller, Chief Financial Officer
CIO: Ryan Merrow, Supervisor Information Systems
CHR: Gary Webb, Director Human Resources
Web address: www.corryhospital.com
Control: Other not–for–profit (including NFP Corporation) **Service:** General Medical and Surgical

Staffed Beds: 35

COUDERSPORT—Potter County

★ **CHARLES COLE MEMORIAL HOSPITAL (391313)**, 1001 East Second Street, Zip 16915–9762; tel. 814/274–9300, (Total facility includes 49 beds in nursing home–type unit) **A**1 9 10 **F**3 10 11 13 15 24 25 26 27 30 32 33 38 42 48 49 52 55 57 61 62 68 74 75 76 77 79 82 85 86 88 93 96 100 102 107 109 117 119 120 121 122 124 134 135 136 137
Primary Contact: Edward C. Pitchford, President and Chief Executive Officer
CMO: Michael E. Callahan, M.D., President Medical Staff
CIO: Thomas Lamb, Chief Information Officer
CHR: J. Thomas Noe, Director Human Resources
Web address: www.charlescolehospital.com
Control: Other not–for–profit (including NFP Corporation) **Service:** General Medical and Surgical

Staffed Beds: 94 **Admissions:** 2641 **Census:** 80 **Outpatient Visits:** 175066 **Births:** 309 **Total Expense ($000):** 55723 **Payroll Expense ($000):** 20355 **Personnel:** 494

CRANBERRY—Butler County

UPMC PASSAVANT CRANBERRY See UPMC Passavant, Pittsburgh

DANVILLE—Montour County

☐ **DANVILLE STATE HOSPITAL (394004)**, 200 State Hospital Drive, Zip 17821–9198; tel. 570/271–4500 **A**1 10 **F**26 30 37 63 73 75 82 88 119 124 135 **P**6
Primary Contact: Donna M. Ashbridge, Chief Executive Officer
COO: Thomas J. Burk, Chief Operating Officer
CFO: Dennis Frazier, Director Fiscal Services
CMO: Anthony Montecalvo, M.D., Chief Medical Officer
CHR: Deborah Lenig, Director Human Resources
Control: State–Government, nonfederal **Service:** Psychiatric

Staffed Beds: 184 **Admissions:** 104 **Census:** 172 **Outpatient Visits:** 0 **Births:** 0 **Total Expense ($000):** 37312 **Payroll Expense ($000):** 19425 **Personnel:** 371

★ **GEISINGER HEALTHSOUTH REHABILITATION HOSPITAL (393047)**, 2 Rehab Lane, Zip 17821; tel. 570/271–6733 **A**1 9 10 **F**12 25 26 30 31 33 57 62 66 72 73 77 85 86 90 120 121 132 136 137 **P**1 **S** HEALTHSOUTH Corporation
Primary Contact: Lorie Dillon, Chief Executive Officer
COO: Thomas Hoy, Chief Operating Officer
CFO: Sally Shipierski, Controller
CMO: Greg Burke, M.D., Medical Director
CHR: Christian Shirley, Director Human Resources
Web address: www.healthsouth.com
Control: Partnership, Investor–owned, for–profit **Service:** Rehabilitation

Staffed Beds: 40 **Admissions:** 755 **Census:** 29 **Outpatient Visits:** 39720 **Births:** 0 **Total Expense ($000):** 12522 **Payroll Expense ($000):** 8091 **Personnel:** 164

★ **GEISINGER MEDICAL CENTER (390006)**, 100 North Academy Avenue, Zip 17822–2201; tel. 570/271–6211 **A**1 2 3 5 8 9 10 12 13 19 **F**1 3 7 8 9 11 12 13 15 17 18 19 20 21 22 23 24 25 26 27 28 30 32 33 34 35 36 37 38 40 41 43 44 46 47 48 49 50 51 52 53 54 55 56 57 58 59 60 62 63 66 68 69 70 72 73 74 76 77 78 79 80 81 82 83 84 85 86 87 88 89 90 91 92 93 94 95 96 97 100 102 103 104 105 106 107 108 109 111 112 113 114 116 118 119 120 121 124 125 127 128 130 131 134 135 136 137 **P**6 **S** Geisinger Health System
Primary Contact: E. Lynn Miller, Chief Administrative Officer
COO: Frank J. Trembulak, Executive Vice President and Chief Operating Officer
CFO: Kevin F. Brennan, CPA, Executive Vice President and Chief Financial Officer
CMO: Howard R. Grant, M.D., Executive Vice President and Chief Medical Officer
CIO: Frank Richards, Chief Information Officer
CHR: Richard E. Merkle, Chief Human Resources Officer
Web address: www.geisinger.org
Control: Other not–for–profit (including NFP Corporation) **Service:** General Medical and Surgical

Staffed Beds: 392 **Admissions:** 22813 **Census:** 318 **Outpatient Visits:** 673091 **Births:** 1656 **Total Expense ($000):** 567708 **Payroll Expense ($000):** 156136 **Personnel:** 3896

☐ **SELECT SPECIALTY HOSPITAL–DANVILLE (392047)**, 100 North Academy Avenue, 3rd Floor, Zip 17822–3050; tel. 570/214–9657, (Nonreporting) **A**1 9 10 **S** Select Medical Corporation
Primary Contact: Brian Mann, Chief Executive Officer
Web address: www.selectmedicalcorp.com
Control: Corporation, Investor–owned, for–profit **Service:** Long–Term Acute Care hospital

Staffed Beds: 30

DARBY—Delaware County

☐ **KINDRED HOSPITAL – DELAWARE COUNTY (392032)**, 1500 Landsdowne Avenue, 6th Floor, Zip 19023, Mailing Address: 1500 Lansdowne Avenue, 6th Floor, Zip 19023; tel. 610/237–5780, (Nonreporting) **A**1 9 10 **S** Kindred Healthcare
Primary Contact: Garrett Arneson, Chief Executive Officer
COO: Susan Ferguson, Chief Operating Officer
CFO: Thomas A. McMullen, Chief Financial Officer
CMO: Joanne Connaughton, M.D., Chief Medical Officer
CHR: Neil Rosner, Area Director Human Resources
Web address: www.kindredhealthcare.com
Control: Corporation, Investor–owned, for–profit **Service:** Long–Term Acute Care hospital

Staffed Beds: 43

★ △ **MERCY FITZGERALD HOSPITAL (390156)**, (Formerly Mercy Catholic Medical Center), 1500 South Lansdowe Avenue, Zip 19023; tel. 610/237–4000, (Includes MERCY HOSPITAL OF PHILADELPHIA, 501 South 54th Street, Philadelphia, Zip 19143; tel. 215/748–9000) **A**1 2 3 5 7 9 10 12 13 **F**3 4 5 11 12 15 17 18 20 22 24 25 26 27 30 31 32 33 36 38 43 46 49 50 51 52 53 55 56 57 58 60 62 64 67 68 73 75 76 77 79 80 81 82 85 86 87 88 89 90 91 92 94 96 97 99 100 102 103 107 109 111 119 121 124 134 135 136 137 **S** Catholic Health East
Primary Contact: Brian Finestein, Executive Director
COO: Ruth Thomas, Chief Operating Officer
CFO: Don Snenk, Chief Financial Officer
CMO: Jeff Komins, M.D., Chief Medical Officer
CIO: Jeff Byda, Vice President Information Technology
Web address: www.mercyhealth.org
Control: Church–operated, Nongovernment, not–for profit **Service:** General Medical and Surgical

Staffed Beds: 413 **Admissions:** 22401 **Census:** 310 **Outpatient Visits:** 239051 **Births:** 0 **Total Expense ($000):** 285658 **Payroll Expense ($000):** 114849 **Personnel:** 1527

DOWNINGTOWN—Chester County

ST. JOHN VIANNEY HOSPITAL, 151 Woodbine Road, Zip 19335–3057; tel. 610/269–2600, (Nonreporting) **A**9
Primary Contact: Edward Maguire, Administrator
Web address: www.sjvcenter.org
Control: Church–operated, Nongovernment, not–for profit **Service:** Psychiatric

Staffed Beds: 42

DOYLESTOWN—Bucks County

★ △ **DOYLESTOWN HOSPITAL (390203)**, 595 West State Street, Zip 18901–2597; tel. 215/345–2200, (Total facility includes 119 beds in nursing home–type unit) **A**1 2 7 9 10 **F**2 3 8 10 11 12 13 15 17 18 20 22 24 25 26 27 28 30 31 32 33 34 37 38 42 43 44 47 49 50 53 54 55 56 57 58 60 61 62 63 66 68 71 72 73 74 75 76 77 79 80 81 82 86 96 97 99 100 106 107 112 115 117 119 121 123 124 132 135 136 **P**5 8
Primary Contact: Richard A. Reif, President and Chief Executive Officer
COO: James C. Brownlow, Vice President Administration and Chief Operating Officer
CFO: Douglas Boyle, Vice President and Chief Financial Officer
CMO: Scott S. Levy, M.D., Vice President and Chief Medical Officer
CIO: Richard Lang, Ph.D., Chief Information Officer
CHR: Barbara Hebel, Director Human Resources
Web address: www.dh.org
Control: Other not–for–profit (including NFP Corporation) **Service:** General Medical and Surgical

Staffed Beds: 306 **Admissions:** 13540 **Census:** 240 **Outpatient Visits:** 308255 **Births:** 1408 **Total Expense ($000):** 199341 **Payroll Expense ($000):** 81518 **Personnel:** 2255

☐ **FOUNDATIONS BEHAVIORAL HEALTH (394038)**, 833 East Butler Avenue, Zip 18901–2280; tel. 215/345–0444, (Total facility includes 40 beds in nursing home–type unit) (Nonreporting) **A**1 9 10 **S** Universal Health Services, Inc.
Primary Contact: Robert Weinhold, Chief Executive Officer
Web address: www.fbh.com
Control: Other not–for–profit (including NFP Corporation) **Service:** Children's hospital psychiatric

Staffed Beds: 94

PA

Hospital, Medicare Provider Number, Address, Telephone, Approval, Facility, and Physician Codes, Health Care System
★ American Hospital Association (AHA) membership
☐ The Joint Commission accreditation
○ American Osteopathic Association (AOA) accreditation
△ Commission on Accreditation of Rehabilitation Facilities (CARF) accreditation

DREXEL HILL—Delaware County

★ ○ △ **DELAWARE COUNTY MEMORIAL HOSPITAL (390081)**, 501 North Lansdowne Avenue, Zip 19026–1114; tel. 610/284–8100 **A**1 2 3 5 7 9 10 11 **F**3 7 11 13 15 17 24 25 26 27 30 31 32 33 34 38 41 42 46 50 51 54 55 57 60 61 62 66 70 72 73 74 75 76 77 79 80 81 82 85 86 87 90 96 97 98 99 100 102 103 104 105 106 107 108 109 111 113 114 118 119 120 121 122 123 132 135 136 137 **P**6 **S** Crozer–Keystone Health System
Primary Contact: William McCune, President
CFO: Richard I. Bennett, Senior Vice President and Chief Financial Officer
CMO: Seth Malin, M.D., President Medical and Dental Staff
CIO: Robert E. Wilson, Vice President and Chief Information Officer
CHR: Eugene Zegar, Vice President Human Resources
Web address: www.crozer.org
Control: Other not–for–profit (including NFP Corporation) **Service:** General Medical and Surgical

Staffed Beds: 214 **Admissions:** 11520 **Census:** 170 **Outpatient Visits:** 106716 **Births:** 1617 **Total Expense ($000):** 154111 **Payroll Expense ($000):** 68623 **Personnel:** 1070

DU BOIS—Clearfield County

★ **DUBOIS REGIONAL MEDICAL CENTER (390086)**, 100 Hospital Avenue, Zip 15801–1440, Mailing Address: P.O. Box 447, Zip 15801–0447; tel. 814/371–2200, (Nonreporting) **A**1 2 9 10 19
Primary Contact: Raymond A. Graeca, President and Chief Executive Officer
CMO: Daniel J. Ahearn, M.D., Vice President Medical Affairs
CIO: Thomas Johnson, Manager Information Systems Manager
CHR: Susan Grady, Vice President Human Resources
Web address: www.drmc.org
Control: Other not–for–profit (including NFP Corporation) **Service:** General Medical and Surgical

Staffed Beds: 203

EAGLEVILLE—Montgomery County

★ **EAGLEVILLE HOSPITAL (390278)**, 100 Eagleville Road, Zip 19408–0045, Mailing Address: P.O. Box 45, Zip 19408–0045; tel. 610/539–6000 **A**5 9 10 **F**4 25 30 31 32 33 50 56 60 66 73 81 88 90 91 93 119 121 123 132 135 136 **P**6
Primary Contact: Maureen King Pollock, Interim Chief Executive Officer
COO: Maureen King Pollock, Chief Operating Officer
CFO: Hon–Chung Tong, Chief Financial Officer
CMO: Robert Wilson, D.O., Director Medical Services
CIO: Richard R. Mitchell, Network Administrator
CHR: Edward Powell, Co–Director Human Resources
Web address: www.eaglevillehospital.org
Control: Other not–for–profit (including NFP Corporation) **Service:** Alcoholism and other chemical dependency

Staffed Beds: 270 **Admissions:** 4657 **Census:** 204 **Outpatient Visits:** 0 **Births:** 0 **Total Expense ($000):** 26740 **Payroll Expense ($000):** 14295 **Personnel:** 333

EAST STROUDSBURG—Monroe County

★ △ **POCONO MEDICAL CENTER (390201)**, 206 East Brown Street, Zip 18301–3006; tel. 570/421–4000 **A**1 2 7 9 10 19 20 **F**3 11 13 14 15 17 18 20 22 24 25 26 27 28 30 31 32 33 34 36 37 38 43 46 48 49 50 53 54 55 56 57 60 62 63 64 68 72 73 74 75 76 77 79 80 81 82 84 86 87 88 90 91 92 93 96 97 99 100 102 106 107 108 109 111 112 119 121 124 135 137
Primary Contact: Kathleen E. Kuck, Interim Chief Operating Officer
CFO: Michael Wilk, Vice President Financial Services
CMO: Howard Z. Davis, M.D., Senior Vice President Medical Affairs
CIO: Nicholas Christiano, Vice President and Chief Information Officer
CHR: Lynn M. Lansdowne, Vice President Human Resources
Web address: www.pmchealthsystem.org
Control: Other not–for–profit (including NFP Corporation) **Service:** General Medical and Surgical

Staffed Beds: 231 **Admissions:** 12131 **Census:** 138 **Outpatient Visits:** 217142 **Births:** 779 **Total Expense ($000):** 156167 **Payroll Expense ($000):** 65003 **Personnel:** 1370

EASTON—Northampton County

★ **EASTON HOSPITAL (390162)**, 250 South 21st Street, Zip 18042–3892; tel. 610/250–4000 **A**1 2 3 5 9 10 12 13 **F**11 12 13 15 17 18 20 22 24 25 26 27 30 31 32 33 38 46 48 49 50 51 55 56 57 58 59 60 61 62 63 64 66 68 70 73 74 76 77 79 80 81 82 86 87 96 97 99 100 102 106 107 108 109 111 112 118 119 121 124 135 136 137 **P**6 **S** Community Health Systems, Inc.
Primary Contact: Angela M. Marchi, FACHE, President and Chief Executive Officer
COO: Peter Wozniak, Chief Operating Officer
CFO: Roy Boyd, Chief Financial Officer
CMO: David Lyon, M.D., Chief Medical Officer
CIO: Kenneth Castle, Chief Information Officer
CHR: Lori Ofner, Vice President Human Resources
Web address: www.easton–hospital.com
Control: Corporation, Investor–owned, for–profit **Service:** General Medical and Surgical

Staffed Beds: 221 **Admissions:** 11487 **Census:** 151 **Outpatient Visits:** 148569 **Births:** 526 **Total Expense ($000):** 157478 **Payroll Expense ($000):** 48129 **Personnel:** 949

☐ **TRIUMPH HOSPITAL EASTON (392034)**, 250 South 21st Street, 3rd Floor, Zip 18042; tel. 610/250–4724, (Nonreporting) **A**1 9 10 **S** Triumph HealthCare
Primary Contact: Linda Luther, Chief Executive Officer
Web address: www.triumph–healthcare.com
Control: Corporation, Investor–owned, for–profit **Service:** Long–Term Acute Care hospital

Staffed Beds: 31

ELKINS PARK—Montgomery County

☐ △ **MOSS REHAB, EINSTEIN AT ELKINS PARK**, 60 East Township Line Road, Zip 19027–2220; tel. 215/663–6000, (Nonreporting) **A**1 7 9 **S** Albert Einstein Healthcare Network
Primary Contact: Ruth Lefton, Chief Operating Officer
COO: Jack Jensen, Chief Operating Officer
CFO: Chuck Hoover, Chief Financial Officer
Web address: www.einstein.edu
Control: Other not–for–profit (including NFP Corporation) **Service:** Rehabilitation

Staffed Beds: 158

ELLWOOD CITY—Lawrence County

ELLWOOD CITY HOSPITAL (390008), 724 Pershing Street, Zip 16117–1474; tel. 724/752–0081, (Total facility includes 23 beds in nursing home–type unit) (Nonreporting) **A**9 10
Primary Contact: Raymond J. Beck, President and Chief Executive Officer
CFO: Christopher M. Little, Vice President and Chief Financial Officer
Control: Other not–for–profit (including NFP Corporation) **Service:** General Medical and Surgical

Staffed Beds: 118

EPHRATA—Lancaster County

☐ **EPHRATA COMMUNITY HOSPITAL (390225)**, 169 Martin Avenue, Zip 17522–1002, Mailing Address: P.O. Box 1002, Zip 17522–1002; tel. 717/733–0311 **A**1 2 9 10 **F**11 13 15 18 24 25 26 27 30 31 32 33 34 38 43 49 51 53 55 56 57 60 61 62 67 68 70 72 73 74 75 76 77 78 79 80 81 82 84 85 87 88 89 90 91 92 93 94 96 97 100 102 105 106 107 118 119 121 124 135 136 137 **P**6 8
Primary Contact: John M. Porter, Jr., President and Chief Executive Officer
COO: Robert Graupensperger, Executive Vice President
CFO: John A. Holmes, Chief Financial Officer
CMO: Vincent D. Glielmi, M.D., Vice President Medical Affairs
CIO: William Johnson, Chief Information Officer
CHR: Barbara Mumma, Vice President Human Resources
Web address: www.ephratahospital.org
Control: Other not–for–profit (including NFP Corporation) **Service:** General Medical and Surgical

Staffed Beds: 138 **Admissions:** 8272 **Census:** 85 **Outpatient Visits:** 384991 **Births:** 787 **Total Expense ($000):** 158063 **Payroll Expense ($000):** 71760 **Personnel:** 1466

PA

ERIE—Erie County

☐ **HAMOT MEDICAL CENTER (390063)**, 201 State Street, Zip 16550–0002; tel. 814/877–6000 **A**1 2 3 5 8 9 10 12 13 **F**3 11 12 13 17 18 20 22 25 26 27 30 31 32 33 34 36 38 40 41 43 44 49 50 51 55 56 57 58 59 60 62 63 66 68 70 72 73 74 75 76 77 78 79 80 81 82 84 86 92 96 97 100 102 103 106 107 112 114 116 118 119 120 121 124 135 136 137 **P**6 8
Primary Contact: John T. Malone, President and Chief Executive Officer
COO: V. James Fiorenzo, Executive Vice President and Chief Operating Officer
CFO: Stephen M. Danch, Chief Financial Officer
CMO: Richard Long, M.D., Chief Medical Officer
CIO: Joseph Butler, Vice President and Chief Information Officer
CHR: Joseph Butler, Vice President and Chief Information Officer
Web address: www.hamot.org
Control: Other not–for–profit (including NFP Corporation) **Service:** General Medical and Surgical

Staffed Beds: 340 **Admissions:** 16995 **Census:** 220 **Outpatient Visits:** 239179 **Births:** 1227 **Total Expense ($000):** 247246 **Payroll Expense ($000):** 92549 **Personnel:** 2263

★ **HEALTHSOUTH REHABILITATION HOSPITAL OF ERIE (393046)**, 143 East Second Street, Zip 16507–1501; tel. 814/878–1200, (Nonreporting) **A**1 10 **S** HEALTHSOUTH Corporation
Primary Contact: John Ferritto, Chief Executive Officer
CFO: Lori Gibbens, Controller
CMO: Douglas Grisier, D.O., Medical Director
CIO: Marybeth Hamm, Manager Health Information
CHR: William Robinson, Director Human Resources
Web address: www.healthsouth.com
Control: Corporation, Investor–owned, for–profit **Service:** Rehabilitation

Staffed Beds: 108

○ **MILLCREEK COMMUNITY HOSPITAL (390198)**, 5515 Peach Street, Zip 16509–2695; tel. 814/864–4031 **A**9 10 11 12 13 **F**3 4 13 14 15 18 20 29 30 31 32 36 37 38 50 62 63 66 68 72 73 74 77 79 80 82 84 87 88 89 90 91 92 93 95 96 97 100 102 107 118 119 124 132 133 135 137
Primary Contact: Mary L. Eckert, President and Chief Executive Officer
CFO: Richard P. Olinger, Chief Financial Officer
CMO: Armando Ricci, D.O., Chief of Staff
CIO: Cheryl Girardier, Director Information Technology
CHR: Ed Pietkiewicz, Manager Human Resources
Web address: www.millcreekcommunityhospital.com
Control: Other not–for–profit (including NFP Corporation) **Service:** General Medical and Surgical

Staffed Beds: 145 **Admissions:** 4331 **Census:** 56 **Outpatient Visits:** 24977 **Births:** 216 **Total Expense ($000):** 29521 **Payroll Expense ($000):** 12378 **Personnel:** 302

★ **SAINT VINCENT HEALTH CENTER (390009)**, 232 West 25th Street, Zip 16544–0002; tel. 814/452–5000, (Total facility includes 14 beds in nursing home–type unit) **A**1 2 9 10 12 13 **F**3 5 8 9 11 13 15 17 18 20 22 24 25 26 27 28 29 30 31 32 33 34 36 37 38 41 42 43 44 45 46 49 50 51 52 53 54 55 56 57 58 59 60 61 62 63 66 68 70 71 72 73 74 75 76 77 78 79 80 81 82 84 85 86 87 88 89 90 91 92 93 94 96 97 100 102 103 104 105 106 107 112 117 118 119 120 121 122 124 133 135 136 137 **S** St. Vincent Health System
Primary Contact: C. Angela Bontempo, President and Chief Executive Officer
COO: Joseph Cacchione, M.D., Executive Vice President
CFO: Steve Gary, Senior Vice President and Chief Financial Officer
CMO: Richard Cogley, M.D., Senior Vice President Medical Affairs
CIO: Robin Stursa, Vice President Information Technology
CHR: John Mashinski, Senior Vice President Human Resources
Web address: www.svhs.org
Control: Other not–for–profit (including NFP Corporation) **Service:** General Medical and Surgical

Staffed Beds: 456 **Admissions:** 15848 **Census:** 225 **Outpatient Visits:** 170951 **Births:** 2145 **Total Expense ($000):** 222138 **Payroll Expense ($000):** 81991 **Personnel:** 1873

☐ **SELECT SPECIALTY HOSPITAL–ERIE (392037)**, 201 State Street, Zip 16550; tel. 814/877–2774, (Nonreporting) **A**1 10 **S** Select Medical Corporation
Primary Contact: Anne Frew, Chief Executive Officer
Web address: www.selectmedicalcorp.com
Control: Corporation, Investor–owned, for–profit **Service:** Long–Term Acute Care hospital

Staffed Beds: 35

☐ **SHRINERS HOSPITALS FOR CHILDREN, ERIE**, 1645 West 8th Street, Zip 16505–5007; tel. 814/875–8700, (Nonreporting) **A**1 **S** Shriners Hospitals for Children
Primary Contact: Richard W. Brzuz, FACHE, Administrator
CFO: Karen L. Wagner, CPA, Director Fiscal Services
CMO: James O. Sanders, M.D., Chief of Staff
CIO: Robert Howden, Director Public Relations
Web address: www.shrinershq.org
Control: Other not–for–profit (including NFP Corporation) **Service:** Children's orthopedic

Staffed Beds: 30

★ **VETERANS AFFAIRS MEDICAL CENTER**, 135 East 38th Street, Zip 16504–1596; tel. 814/860–2576, (Total facility includes 52 beds in nursing home–type unit) (Nonreporting) **A**1 9 **S** Department of Veterans Affairs
Primary Contact: Michael Adelman, M.D., Director
CFO: Joann Pritchard, Chief Financial Officer
CMO: Anthony Behm, D.O., Chief of Staff
CIO: Michael Downey, Chief Information Officer
CHR: Lynn Nies, Human Resources Officer
Web address: www.va.gov/sta/guide/home.asp
Control: Veterans Affairs, Government, federal **Service:** General Medical and Surgical

Staffed Beds: 78

EVERETT—Bedford County

☐ **UPMC BEDFORD MEMORIAL (390117)**, 10455 Lincoln Highway, Zip 15537–7046; tel. 814/623–6161 **A**1 9 10 20 **F**3 8 11 13 15 18 24 25 26 30 31 32 33 37 38 50 51 54 55 56 57 60 62 63 66 68 69 72 73 74 75 76 77 79 80 81 82 84 86 87 92 94 96 97 100 102 107 112 118 119 120 121 122 124 135 136 137 **S** UPMC
Primary Contact: Roger P. Winn, President
CFO: William J. Obert, Vice President Administration
CIO: Mark Wiley, Manager Information Systems Development
CHR: Michelle A. Speck, Vice President Human Resources
Web address: www.bedford.org
Control: Other not–for–profit (including NFP Corporation) **Service:** General Medical and Surgical

Staffed Beds: 27 **Admissions:** 2445 **Census:** 20 **Outpatient Visits:** 113401 **Births:** 238 **Total Expense ($000):** 34070 **Payroll Expense ($000):** 14350 **Personnel:** 352

FARRELL—Mercer County

SHENANGO VALLEY CAMPUS See UPMC Horizon, Greenville

FORT WASHINGTON—Montgomery County

☐ **BROOKE GLEN BEHAVIORAL HOSPITAL (394049)**, 7170 Lafayette Avenue, Zip 19034–0209; tel. 215/641–5300, (Nonreporting) **A**1 9 10 **S** Psychiatric Solutions
Primary Contact: Mark Schor, Chief Executive Officer
COO: William R. Mason, Chief Operating Officer
CFO: Robert Zagerman, Chief Financial Officer
CMO: Chand Nair, M.D., Medical Director
CHR: Dawn Kownacki, Director Human Resources
Web address: www.brookeglenbehavioral.com
Control: Corporation, Investor–owned, for–profit **Service:** Psychiatric

Staffed Beds: 146

GETTYSBURG—Adams County

★ **GETTYSBURG HOSPITAL (390065)**, 147 Gettys Street, Zip 17325–2534; tel. 717/334–2121, (Total facility includes 19 beds in nursing home–type unit) **A**1 9 10 **F**3 11 13 15 17 18 24 25 26 27 28 30 31 32 33 34 38 42 43 46 48 50 51 52 53 55 56 57 59 62 63 66 68 71 73 74 75 76 77 79 80 81 82 86 90 92 96 97 100 102 103 106 107 108 117 118 119 120 121 123 124 135 136 **P**8 **S** WellSpan Health
Primary Contact: Kevin H. Mosser, M.D., Chief Executive Officer
COO: Joseph H. Edgar, Senior Vice President Operations
CMO: Charles Marley, D.O., Vice President Medical Affairs
CIO: Robin Kimple, Director Information Services
CHR: Kim Brister, Director Human Resources
Web address: www.wellspan.org
Control: Other not–for–profit (including NFP Corporation) **Service:** General Medical and Surgical

Staffed Beds: 95 **Admissions:** 4418 **Census:** 50 **Outpatient Visits:** 151786 **Births:** 611 **Total Expense ($000):** 75345 **Payroll Expense ($000):** 34133 **Personnel:** 728

Hospital, Medicare Provider Number, Address, Telephone, Approval, Facility, and Physician Codes, Health Care System

★ American Hospital Association (AHA) membership
☐ The Joint Commission accreditation
○ American Osteopathic Association (AOA) accreditation
△ Commission on Accreditation of Rehabilitation Facilities (CARF) accreditation

PA

GLENSIDE—Montgomery County

☐ △ **CHESTNUT HILL REHABILITATION HOSPITAL (393032)**, 8601 Stenton Avenue, Zip 19038–8395; tel. 215/233–6200, (Nonreporting) **A**1 7 10
Primary Contact: Brooks Turkel, Chief Executive Officer
CMO: Matthew Schwartz, M.D., Medical Director
CIO: Jack Nash, Vice President and Chief Information Officer
CHR: Paul Cavanaugh, Director Human Resources
Web address: www.chh.org
Control: Other not–for–profit (including NFP Corporation) **Service:** Rehabilitation

Staffed Beds: 48

GREENSBURG—Westmoreland County

☐ **EXCELA WESTMORELAND REGIONAL HOSPITAL (390145)**, 532 West Pittsburgh Street, Zip 15601–2282; tel. 724/832–4000, (Total facility includes 25 beds in nursing home–type unit) **A**1 9 10 **F**3 5 8 9 11 12 13 15 17 18 20 22 24 25 26 28 30 31 32 33 34 36 37 38 41 43 44 47 48 49 50 51 54 55 56 57 60 62 63 66 68 71 72 73 74 75 76 77 79 80 81 82 84 85 86 87 88 90 91 92 93 94 95 96 97 100 102 106 107 117 118 119 120 121 123 124 132 135 136 137 **S** Excela Health
Primary Contact: David S. Gallatin, Chief Executive Officer
COO: Samuel Raneri, Senior Vice President Operations and Business Development
CFO: Jeffrey T. Curry, Executive Vice President and Chief Financial Officer
CMO: Ralph Capone, M.D., Chief Medical Officer
CIO: Otto Salguero, Chief Information Officer
CHR: John Caverno, Chief Human Resources Officer
Web address: www.excelahealth.org
Control: Other not–for–profit (including NFP Corporation) **Service:** General Medical and Surgical

Staffed Beds: 299 **Admissions:** 15988 **Census:** 219 **Outpatient Visits:** 302855 **Births:** 1205 **Total Expense ($000):** 155648 **Payroll Expense ($000):** 63455 **Personnel:** 1572

☐ **SELECT SPECIALTY HOSPITAL OF GREENSBURG (392036)**, 532 West Pittsburgh Street, Zip 15601; tel. 724/832–4210, (Nonreporting) **A**1 10 **S** Select Medical Corporation
Primary Contact: Anthony Martino, Chief Executive Officer
Web address: www.selectmedicalcorp.com
Control: Corporation, Investor–owned, for–profit **Service:** Long–Term Acute Care hospital

Staffed Beds: 31

GREENVILLE—Mercer County

☐ ○ **UPMC HORIZON (390178)**, (Includes GREENVILLE CAMPUS, 110 North Main Street, Zip 16125–1795; tel. 724/588–2100; SHENANGO VALLEY CAMPUS, 2200 Memorial Drive, Farrell, Zip 16121–1398; tel. 724/981–3500), (Total facility includes 36 beds in nursing home–type unit) **A**1 2 9 10 11 12 13 **F**3 9 11 12 13 15 18 24 25 26 27 28 30 31 32 33 37 38 41 43 47 49 50 52 53 54 55 56 57 62 66 68 72 73 74 75 76 77 79 81 82 85 86 87 96 97 100 102 103 104 105 106 107 117 118 119 120 121 124 135 136 137 **P**8 **S** UPMC
Primary Contact: Neil Yuhas, President
CFO: David Shulik, Vice President and Chief Financial Officer
CMO: Samuel Daisley, D.O., Vice President Medical Affairs
CHR: Connie Mayle, Vice President Administrative Services
Web address: www.horizon.upmc.com
Control: Other not–for–profit (including NFP Corporation) **Service:** General Medical and Surgical

Staffed Beds: 187 **Admissions:** 8358 **Census:** 113 **Outpatient Visits:** 228771 **Births:** 758 **Total Expense ($000):** 108357 **Payroll Expense ($000):** 40266 **Personnel:** 1009

GROVE CITY—Mercer County

○ **GROVE CITY MEDICAL CENTER (390266)**, 631 North Broad Street Extension, Zip 16127–9703; tel. 724/450–7000, (Total facility includes 20 beds in nursing home–type unit) **A**9 10 11 **F**3 8 13 15 18 24 27 30 31 32 33 38 43 46 49 50 53 57 59 61 62 68 73 74 76 77 79 82 84 86 97 100 102 106 107 117 118 119 121 124 135 136 137 **P**6
Primary Contact: Robert Jackson, Jr., Chief Executive Officer
CFO: Jennifer Davis, Vice President Finance
CMO: Matthew Glenn, D.O., Chief of Staff
CIO: Philip Swartwood, Director Information
CHR: Donald Henley, Vice President Human Resources and Social Services
Web address: www.gcmcpa.org
Control: Other not–for–profit (including NFP Corporation) **Service:** General Medical and Surgical

Staffed Beds: 101 **Admissions:** 2854 **Census:** 41 **Outpatient Visits:** 91409 **Births:** 244 **Total Expense ($000):** 36946 **Payroll Expense ($000):** 15454 **Personnel:** 418

HANOVER—York County

☐ **HANOVER HOSPITAL (390233)**, 300 Highland Avenue, Zip 17331–2297; tel. 717/637–3711 **A**1 9 10 **F**3 11 13 15 18 24 25 26 27 28 30 31 32 33 37 38 44 49 50 51 52 53 54 55 56 57 60 62 63 66 68 72 73 74 75 76 77 79 80 81 82 84 85 86 96 97 100 102 103 106 107 118 119 120 121 123 124 132 135 136 137
Primary Contact: George Kyriacou, President and Chief Executive Officer
COO: Michael A. Hockenberry, Vice President Operations
CFO: Marilyn A. Olejnik, Senior Vice President and Chief Financial Officer
CMO: Carol V. Freer, M.D., Vice President Medical Affairs
CIO: Pamela Owens, Director Health Information Management
CHR: Peter P. Krech, Vice President Human Resources
Web address: www.hanoverhospital.org
Control: Other not–for–profit (including NFP Corporation) **Service:** General Medical and Surgical

Staffed Beds: 116 **Admissions:** 5764 **Census:** 69 **Outpatient Visits:** 230150 **Births:** 708 **Total Expense ($000):** 100949 **Payroll Expense ($000):** 43595 **Personnel:** 1011

HARRISBURG—Dauphin County

COMMUNITY HOSPITAL See PinnacleHealth System

☐ **PINNACLEHEALTH SYSTEM (390067)**, 111 South Front Street, Zip 17101, Mailing Address: P.O. Box 8700, Zip 17105–8700; tel. 717/782–3131, (Includes COMMUNITY HOSPITAL, 4300 Londonderry Road, Zip 17109–5397; tel. 717/652–3000; HARRISBURG HOSPITAL; POLYCLINIC HOSPITAL, 2501 North Third Street, Zip 17110–2098; tel. 717/782–4141), (Total facility includes 35 beds in nursing home–type unit) **A**1 2 3 5 8 9 10 12 13 **F**3 7 11 12 13 14 15 17 18 20 22 24 25 26 27 28 30 31 32 33 34 35 38 41 42 43 44 48 49 50 53 54 55 56 57 58 59 60 61 62 64 66 68 70 72 73 74 75 76 77 78 79 80 81 82 84 85 86 87 88 89 90 91 93 94 95 96 97 99 100 102 106 107 109 111 116 117 118 119 121 123 124 127 131 133 135 136 137
Primary Contact: Roger Longenderfer, M.D., President and Chief Executive Officer
COO: Philip Guarneschelli, Senior Vice President and Chief Operating Officer
CFO: William H. Pugh, Senior Vice President Corporate Finance and Chief Financial Officer
CMO: Dana Kellis, M.D., Senior Vice President Medical Affairs and Chief Medical Officer
CIO: Steven Roth, Vice President Informatics and Chief Information Officer
CHR: Thomas Kess, Vice President Human Resources
Web address: www.pinnaclehealth.org
Control: Other not–for–profit (including NFP Corporation) **Service:** General Medical and Surgical

Staffed Beds: 678 **Admissions:** 33080 **Census:** 476 **Outpatient Visits:** 493550 **Births:** 4594 **Total Expense ($000):** 441517 **Payroll Expense ($000):** 180180 **Personnel:** 4038

POLYCLINIC HOSPITAL See PinnacleHealth System

HASTINGS—Cambria County

MINERS MEDICAL CENTER (390130), 290 Haida Avenue, Zip 16646, Mailing Address: P.O. Box 689, Zip 16646–0689; tel. 814/247–3100 **A**9 10 20 **F**3 15 25 26 27 30 31 32 33 34 38 46 48 54 55 57 62 68 73 76 77 79 81 87 92 96 97 99 107 118 119 120 122 133 135 **P**8 **S** Conemaugh Health System
Primary Contact: William R. Crowe, President
CFO: Kimberly Semelsberger, Vice President Financial Operations
CIO: James Homerski, Director Information Services
CHR: John Fresh, Vice President Human Resources
Web address: www.minersmedicalcenter.org
Control: Other not–for–profit (including NFP Corporation) **Service:** General Medical and Surgical

Staffed Beds: 30 **Admissions:** 813 **Census:** 10 **Outpatient Visits:** 52087 **Births:** 0 **Total Expense ($000):** 16035 **Payroll Expense ($000):** 4943 **Personnel:** 148

HAZLETON—Luzerne County

★ ○ △ **HAZLETON GENERAL HOSPITAL (390185)**, 700 East Broad Street, Zip 18201–6897; tel. 570/501–4000 **A**7 9 10 11 19 **F**3 8 11 12 13 15 24 25 26 27 30 31 32 33 38 43 50 51 52 53 55 56 57 58 59 61 62 66 67 68 72 73 74 75 76 77 79 80 81 82 84 85 86 96 97 99 100 102 106 107 112 118 119 120 121 124 132 135 136 137 **P**7
Primary Contact: James Edwards, President
COO: John R. Fletcher, Senior Vice President and Chief Operating Officer
CFO: William Bauer, Vice President Finance and Chief Financial Officer
CMO: Anthony Valente, M.D., Vice President Medical Affairs
CIO: Carl Shoener, Chief Information Officer
CHR: Timothy Farley, Vice President Human Resources
Web address: www.ghha.org
Control: Other not–for–profit (including NFP Corporation) **Service:** General Medical and Surgical

Staffed Beds: 141 **Admissions:** 7673 **Census:** 99 **Outpatient Visits:** 118102 **Births:** 636 **Total Expense ($000):** 85576 **Payroll Expense ($000):** 31582 **Personnel:** 923

Many Facility Codes have changed. Please refer to the AHA Guide Code Chart.

HERSHEY—Dauphin County

⊠ △ **PENN STATE MILTON S. HERSHEY MEDICAL CENTER (390256)**, 500 University Drive, Zip 17033–0850, Mailing Address: P.O. Box 850, Zip 17033–0850; tel. 717/531–8521 **A**1 2 3 5 7 8 9 10 **F**3 5 7 9 12 13 14 15 17 18 19 20 21 22 23 24 25 26 27 28 30 31 32 33 34 37 38 40 41 43 44 46 47 48 49 50 51 52 53 54 55 56 57 58 59 60 62 63 64 65 66 68 70 71 72 73 74 75 76 77 79 80 81 82 83 84 85 86 87 88 89 90 91 92 93 94 95 96 97 98 99 100 101 102 103 104 105 106 107 108 109 111 112 113 114 118 119 120 121 123 124 125 126 127 128 130 131 132 134 135 136 137 **P**6
Primary Contact: Alan L. Brechbill, Executive Director
COO: Alan L. Brechbill, Executive Director
CFO: Kevin Haley, Chief Financial Officer
CMO: Michael Weitekamp, M.D., Chief Medical Officer
CIO: Thomas Abendroth, M.D., Chief Information Officer
CHR: Charles Wilson, Chief Human Resources Officer
Web address: www.pennstatehershey.org/web/guest/home
Control: Other not–for–profit (including NFP Corporation) **Service:** General Medical and Surgical

Staffed Beds: 477 **Admissions:** 25991 **Census:** 420 **Outpatient Visits:** 518786 **Births:** 1596 **Total Expense ($000):** 591681 **Payroll Expense ($000):** 263746 **Personnel:** 6405

HONESDALE—Wayne County

★ **WAYNE MEMORIAL HOSPITAL (390125)**, 601 Park Street, Zip 18431–1498; tel. 570/253–8100 **A**2 9 10 **F**3 11 13 15 24 27 30 31 32 33 34 37 38 42 46 48 49 50 51 52 53 54 55 56 57 60 61 62 63 73 74 75 76 77 79 81 84 85 86 89 90 91 92 93 94 96 97 100 103 107 112 118 119 120 121 122 123 124 135 136 137 **P**8
Primary Contact: David L. Hoff, Chief Executive Officer
COO: John Conte, Director Facility Services
CFO: Michael J. Clifford, Director Finance
CMO: George Tietjen, M.D., Chief of Staff
CIO: Tom Hoffman, Manager Information Systems
CHR: Elizabeth McDonald, Director Human Resources
Web address: www.wmh.org
Control: Other not–for–profit (including NFP Corporation) **Service:** General Medical and Surgical

Staffed Beds: 104 **Admissions:** 4602 **Census:** 59 **Outpatient Visits:** 127769 **Births:** 402 **Total Expense ($000):** 57990 **Payroll Expense ($000):** 22008 **Personnel:** 540

HUNTINGDON—Huntingdon County

⊠ **J. C. BLAIR MEMORIAL HOSPITAL (390056)**, 1225 Warm Springs Avenue, Zip 16652–2398; tel. 814/643–2290 **A**1 9 10 20 **F**3 11 13 15 25 30 31 33 38 49 55 56 57 62 66 68 74 79 80 81 82 84 88 96 97 99 102 106 107 118 119 121 122 124 135 **P**6 **S** QHR
Primary Contact: Kevin P. Calhoun, Chief Executive Officer
CFO: Nancy Glidden, Chief Financial Officer
CMO: Christopher Patitsas, M.D., Chief of Staff
CIO: Steve Gildea, Director Management Information Systems
CHR: Michael Hubert, Vice President Human Resources
Web address: www.jcblair.org
Control: Other not–for–profit (including NFP Corporation) **Service:** General Medical and Surgical

Staffed Beds: 73 **Admissions:** 2935 **Census:** 34 **Outpatient Visits:** 110553 **Births:** 347 **Total Expense ($000):** 34986 **Payroll Expense ($000):** 14618 **Personnel:** 312

INDIANA—Indiana County

★ **INDIANA REGIONAL MEDICAL CENTER (390173)**, 835 Hospital Road, Zip 15701–0788, Mailing Address: P.O. Box 788, Zip 15701–0788; tel. 724/357–7000 **A**2 9 10 20 **F**3 11 15 18 24 25 26 27 30 31 32 33 37 38 41 43 44 47 49 52 54 55 57 62 63 68 69 72 73 74 75 76 77 79 80 82 84 85 86 88 93 96 97 100 103 106 107 108 109 111 112 118 119 121 135 136 137
Primary Contact: Stephen A. Wolfe, President and Chief Executive Officer
COO: Dominic Paccapaniccia, Chief Operating Officer
CFO: Larry J. Marshall, CPA, Senior Vice President Finance
CMO: Bruce A. Bush, M.D., Senior Vice President Medical Affairs
CIO: Gene Burd, Director Information Services
CHR: Matt Reading, Director Human Resources
Web address: www.indianarmc.org
Control: Other not–for–profit (including NFP Corporation) **Service:** General Medical and Surgical

Staffed Beds: 162 **Admissions:** 8022 **Census:** 99 **Outpatient Visits:** 257977 **Births:** 673 **Total Expense ($000):** 101574 **Payroll Expense ($000):** 47803 **Personnel:** 956

JEANNETTE—Westmoreland County

⊠ **EXCELA HEALTH WESTMORELAND HOSPITAL AT JEANNETTE (390010)**, (Formerly Mercy Jeannette Hospital), 600 Jefferson Avenue, Zip 15644–2599; tel. 724/527–3551, (Total facility includes 11 beds in nursing home–type unit) (Nonreporting) **A**1 9 10 **S** Excela Health
Primary Contact: Julie A. Hester, Administrator
CFO: Kevin B. May, Executive Director Finance
CMO: S. Annamkaju, M.D., Chief Medical Officer
CIO: Laurel Bistko, Director Information Systems
CHR: Jennifer Hornyak, Manager Human Resources
Control: Other not–for–profit (including NFP Corporation) **Service:** General Medical and Surgical

Staffed Beds: 149

JENKINTOWN—Montgomery County

☐ **HOLY REDEEMER HOSPITAL AND MEDICAL CENTER (390097)**, 1648 Huntingdon Pike, Zip 19046–8001; tel. 215/947–3000, (Total facility includes 21 beds in nursing home–type unit) **A**1 2 5 9 10 **F**3 10 11 13 14 15 17 18 20 25 26 27 28 30 31 32 33 37 38 41 42 43 44 46 49 50 52 53 54 55 56 57 58 60 61 62 67 68 70 72 73 74 75 76 77 79 80 81 82 84 86 87 88 90 93 96 97 98 102 103 106 107 108 109 111 117 118 119 120 121 123 124 130 132 135 136 137
Primary Contact: Michael B. Laign, President and Chief Executive Officer
COO: Mark T. Jones, Executive Vice President and System Chief Operating Officer
CFO: Russell R. Wagner, Senior Vice President and Chief Financial Officer
CMO: Charles I. Wagner, M.D., Senior Vice President and Chief Medical Officer
CIO: Anne Searle, Senior Vice President and Chief Information Officer
CHR: Joseph J. Cassidy, Vice President
Web address: www.holyredeemer.com
Control: Other not–for–profit (including NFP Corporation) **Service:** General Medical and Surgical

Staffed Beds: 262 **Admissions:** 15337 **Census:** 187 **Outpatient Visits:** 324251 **Births:** 2298 **Total Expense ($000):** 166403 **Payroll Expense ($000):** 68102 **Personnel:** 1425

JERSEY SHORE—Lycoming County

⊠ **JERSEY SHORE HOSPITAL (391300)**, 1020 Thompson Street, Zip 17740–1794; tel. 570/398–0100, (Nonreporting) **A**1 9 10 18 **S** QHR
Primary Contact: Carey W. Plummer, President and Chief Executive Officer
COO: Kurt Williams, Senior Vice President and Chief Financial Officer
CFO: Kurt Williams, Senior Vice President and Chief Financial Officer
CMO: Carmen E. Spinney, M.D., President Medical and Dental Staff
CHR: Trudi Alexander, Director Human Resources
Web address: www.jsh.org
Control: Other not–for–profit (including NFP Corporation) **Service:** General Medical and Surgical

Staffed Beds: 25

JOHNSTOWN—Cambria County

☐ **MEMORIAL MEDICAL CENTER (390110)**, 1086 Franklin Street, Zip 15905–4398; tel. 814/534–9000, (Includes GOOD SAMARITAN MEDICAL CENTER, 1020 Franklin Street, Zip 15905–4186) **A**1 2 3 5 6 9 10 **F**3 5 8 11 12 13 14 15 17 18 20 22 24 25 26 27 28 30 31 32 33 38 40 41 42 43 44 45 46 49 50 51 52 53 54 55 56 57 60 61 62 66 68 70 72 73 74 75 76 77 79 80 81 82 84 85 86 87 88 89 90 91 93 94 96 97 100 102 104 106 107 114 118 119 120 121 123 124 134 135 136 137 **P**5 8 **S** Conemaugh Health System
Primary Contact: Steven E. Tucker, President
CFO: Edward De Pasquale, Chief Financial Officer
CMO: David J. Carlson, D.O., Chief Medical Officer
CIO: Joseph Dado, Chief Information Officer
CHR: Susan Benya, Vice President Human Resources
Web address: www.conemaugh.org
Control: Other not–for–profit (including NFP Corporation) **Service:** General Medical and Surgical

Staffed Beds: 538 **Admissions:** 23034 **Census:** 327 **Outpatient Visits:** 313339 **Births:** 1357 **Total Expense ($000):** 324288 **Payroll Expense ($000):** 123120 **Personnel:** 3322

PA

Hospital, Medicare Provider Number, Address, Telephone, Approval, Facility, and Physician Codes, Health Care System

★ American Hospital Association (AHA) membership
☐ The Joint Commission accreditation
○ American Osteopathic Association (AOA) accreditation
△ Commission on Accreditation of Rehabilitation Facilities (CARF) accreditation

☐ **MEMORIAL MEDICAL CENTER – LEE CAMPUS**, 320 Main Street, Zip 15901–1694; tel. 814/533–0123, (Total facility includes 18 beds in nursing home–type unit) (Nonreporting) **A**1 9 **S** Conemaugh Health System
Primary Contact: Steven E. Tucker, President
CFO: Edward De Pasquale, Chief Financial Officer
CMO: Michael Tatarko, M.D., Chief Medical Officer
CIO: Joseph Dado, Chief Information Officer
CHR: Susan Benya, Vice President Human Resources
Web address: www.conemaugh.org
Control: Other not–for–profit (including NFP Corporation) **Service:** General Medical and Surgical

Staffed Beds: 212

☐ **SELECT SPECIALTY HOSPITAL – JOHNSTOWN (392031)**, 320 Main Street, Zip 15901; tel. 814/534–7300, (Nonreporting) **A**1 10 **S** Select Medical Corporation
Primary Contact: Marylee Dadey, Chief Executive Officer
CMO: Gary Davidson, M.D., Medical Director
Web address: www.selectmedicalcorp.com
Control: Corporation, Investor–owned, for–profit **Service:** Long–Term Acute Care hospital

Staffed Beds: 38

PA

KANE—McKean County

KANE COMMUNITY HOSPITAL (390104), 4372 Route 6, Zip 16735–9654; tel. 814/837–8585 **A**9 10 20 **F**3 11 12 15 17 24 25 26 31 33 38 46 50 52 55 56 57 61 62 68 73 75 77 79 80 82 96 97 100 102 105 106 107 117 119 120 121 122 124 134 135 136 **P**4 6
Primary Contact: J. Gary Rhodes, FACHE, Chief Executive Officer
CFO: Phyllis A. Fitch, Director Finance
CIO: Margaret Twidale, Manager Information Systems
CHR: Marsha Keller, Director Human Resources
Web address: www.kanehosp.com
Control: Other not–for–profit (including NFP Corporation) **Service:** General Medical and Surgical

Staffed Beds: 31 **Admissions:** 1180 **Census:** 14 **Outpatient Visits:** 29077 **Births:** 0 **Total Expense ($000):** 19433 **Payroll Expense ($000):** 8528 **Personnel:** 171

KITTANNING—Armstrong County

ACMH (390163), (Formerly Armstrong County Memorial Hospital), One Nolte Drive, Zip 16201–8808; tel. 724/543–8500, (Total facility includes 13 beds in nursing home–type unit) (Nonreporting) **A**2 9 10 19
Primary Contact: John I. Lewis, Chief Executive Officer
CFO: Patrick Burns, Vice President Finance
CMO: Harold Altman, M.D., Medical Director and Vice President Medical Affairs
CIO: Dianne Emminger, Vice President Information Services
CHR: Anne Remaley, Vice President Human Resources
Web address: www.acmh.org
Control: Other not–for–profit (including NFP Corporation) **Service:** General Medical and Surgical

Staffed Beds: 170

LANCASTER—Lancaster County

★ **LANCASTER GENERAL HOSPITAL (390100)**, 555 North Duke Street, Zip 17604–3555, Mailing Address: P.O. Box 3555, Zip 17604–3555; tel. 717/544–5511 **A**1 2 3 5 6 9 10 **F**3 7 8 11 12 13 14 15 18 20 22 24 25 26 27 28 30 31 32 33 34 35 37 38 40 41 42 43 44 46 47 48 49 50 52 53 54 55 56 57 58 59 60 62 63 64 66 68 69 70 71 72 73 74 75 76 77 78 79 80 81 82 84 85 86 87 88 89 90 91 92 93 94 96 97 98 99 100 101 102 103 104 105 106 107 108 109 110 111 112 113 114 116 118 119 120 121 123 124 134 135 136 137 **P**6
Primary Contact: Thomas E. Beeman, President and Chief Executive Officer
COO: Marion A. McGowan, Executive Vice President and Chief Operating Officer
CFO: F. Joseph Byorick, Senior Vice President Finance and Chief Financial Officer
CMO: Lee M. Duke, M.D., Senior Vice President and Chief Physician Executive
CIO: Leo Gilmore, Senior Vice President and Chief Information Officer
CHR: Regina Mingle, Senior Vice President and Chief Leadership Officer
Web address: www.lancastergeneral.org
Control: Other not–for–profit (including NFP Corporation) **Service:** General Medical and Surgical

Staffed Beds: 568 **Admissions:** 35055 **Census:** 481 **Outpatient Visits:** 1336666 **Births:** 5184 **Total Expense ($000):** 571717 **Payroll Expense ($000):** 243248 **Personnel:** 4812

☐ **LANCASTER REGIONAL MEDICAL CENTER (390061)**, 250 College Avenue, Zip 17603, Mailing Address: P.O. Box 3434, Zip 17604–3434; tel. 717/291–8211, (Total facility includes 21 beds in nursing home–type unit) (Nonreporting) **A**1 9 10 **S** Health Management Associates
Primary Contact: Rebecca T. Brewer, FACHE, Interim Chief Executive Officer
COO: Deborah Willwerth, Chief Operating Officer
CFO: Lynne Rudisill, Chief Financial Officer
CMO: Mark C. Regan, M.D., Medical Director
CHR: Brian Hoffman, Director Human Resources
Web address: www.lancasterregional.com
Control: Other not–for–profit (including NFP Corporation) **Service:** General Medical and Surgical

Staffed Beds: 226

LANGHORNE—Bucks County

BUCKS COUNTY CAMPUS See Frankford Hospital of the City of Philadelphia, Philadelphia

★ **ST. MARY MEDICAL CENTER (390258)**, Langhorne–Newtown Road, Zip 19047–1295; tel. 215/710–2000 **A**1 2 9 10 **F**15 17 18 20 22 24 25 26 27 28 30 31 32 33 38 40 43 44 52 54 55 56 57 62 68 70 72 73 74 75 76 77 79 81 82 84 85 86 87 96 97 99 102 103 104 105 106 107 109 111 114 118 119 121 124 135 136 137 **S** Catholic Health East
Primary Contact: Gregory T. Wozniak, President and Chief Executive Officer
CFO: Edward Maher, Chief Financial Officer and Vice President Finance
CMO: Joseph Conroy, M.D., Vice President Medical Affairs
CIO: Marian Moran, Chief Information Officer
CHR: Peter LaChance, Vice President Human Resources and Chief Learning Officer
Web address: www.stmaryhealthcare.org
Control: Church–operated, Nongovernment, not–for profit **Service:** General Medical and Surgical

Staffed Beds: 294 **Admissions:** 21819 **Census:** 270 **Outpatient Visits:** 220164 **Births:** 1603 **Total Expense ($000):** 261472 **Payroll Expense ($000):** 110134 **Personnel:** 1866

LANSDALE—Montgomery County

☐ **CENTRAL MONTGOMERY MEDICAL CENTER (390012)**, 100 Medical Campus Drive, Zip 19446–1200; tel. 215/368–2100 **A**1 2 9 10 **F**1 3 4 11 13 15 16 17 24 25 26 27 30 31 32 33 37 38 43 49 55 57 63 65 68 70 71 72 74 75 76 77 78 79 83 84 85 86 88 96 97 100 106 107 112 117 118 119 121 135 137 **P**6 **S** Universal Health Services, Inc.
Primary Contact: James D. Wilson, Chief Executive Officer
CFO: Michael Olivieri, Chief Financial Officer
CMO: Clifford Ehrlich, M.D., President Medical Staff
CIO: Peter Funch, Director Management Information Systems
CHR: John Coker, Director Human Resource
Web address: www.cmmc–uhs.com
Control: Individual, Investor–owned, for–profit **Service:** General Medical and Surgical

Staffed Beds: 125 **Admissions:** 5503 **Census:** 66 **Outpatient Visits:** 71380 **Births:** 417 **Total Expense ($000):** 61668 **Payroll Expense ($000):** 28123 **Personnel:** 587

LATROBE—Westmoreland County

★ **EXCELA LATROBE AREA HOSPITAL (390219)**, 121 West Second Avenue, Zip 15650–1096; tel. 724/537–1000, (Total facility includes 20 beds in nursing home–type unit) **A**1 2 3 5 9 10 12 13 **F**3 8 11 12 13 15 25 26 30 31 32 33 36 38 41 43 48 49 50 51 52 54 55 56 57 59 62 63 66 68 71 72 73 74 75 76 77 79 80 81 82 84 86 87 88 89 90 91 94 96 97 100 102 106 107 117 118 119 121 123 124 132 135 136 137 **P**6 **S** Excela Health
Primary Contact: Kim N. Hollon, FACHE, Chief Executive Officer
COO: Samuel Raneri, Senior Vice President Operations and Business Development
CFO: Jeffrey T. Curry, Executive Vice President and Chief Financial Officer
CMO: Ralph Capone, M.D., Chief Medical Officer
CIO: Otto Salguero, Chief Information Officer
CHR: Jill Clements, Vice President Human Resources
Web address: www.excelahealth.org
Control: Other not–for–profit (including NFP Corporation) **Service:** General Medical and Surgical

Staffed Beds: 164 **Admissions:** 10845 **Census:** 126 **Outpatient Visits:** 239416 **Births:** 570 **Total Expense ($000):** 109917 **Payroll Expense ($000):** 52786 **Personnel:** 1006

LEBANON—Lebanon County

★□ **THE GOOD SAMARITAN HOSPITAL (390066)**, Fourth and Walnut Streets, Zip 17042–1281, Mailing Address: P.O. Box 1281, Zip 17042–1281; tel. 717/270–7500, (Total facility includes 19 beds in nursing home–type unit) **A**1 3 5 9 10 **F**3 8 11 13 14 15 17 18 20 22 24 25 26 27 30 31 32 33 37 38 39 42 43 50 51 52 53 55 57 59 61 62 66 68 73 74 75 76 77 78 79 80 82 84 85 86 96 97 100 102 106 107 117 118 119 121 124 133 135 137 **P**8
Primary Contact: Robert J. Longo, FACHE, President and Chief Executive Officer
COO: William Hendrick, Senior Vice President and Chief Operating Officer
CFO: Robert J. Richards, Vice President Finance and Chief Financial Officer
CMO: Robert D. Sharer, M.D., Vice President Medical Affairs
CIO: Louis Eaglehouse, Site Director and Chief Information Officer
CHR: Kimberly Feeman, Vice President Human Resources
Web address: www.gshleb.org
Control: Other not–for–profit (including NFP Corporation) **Service:** General Medical and Surgical

Staffed Beds: 180 **Admissions:** 10314 **Census:** 135 **Outpatient Visits:** 244007 **Births:** 1013 **Total Expense ($000):** 136114 **Payroll Expense ($000):** 50803 **Personnel:** 1131

★□ △ **VETERANS AFFAIRS MEDICAL CENTER**, 1700 South Lincoln Avenue, Zip 17042–7529; tel. 717/272–6621, (Total facility includes 101 beds in nursing home–type unit) **A**1 3 5 7 9 **F**3 4 5 8 25 26 27 30 31 32 33 36 37 38 41 42 43 44 45 50 52 53 54 55 56 57 58 60 61 62 63 64 66 68 72 73 75 76 77 79 81 82 86 87 88 90 91 92 93 94 95 96 100 102 107 117 119 121 124 132 133 134 135 136 137 **P**6 **S** Department of Veterans Affairs
Primary Contact: Robert W. Callahan, Jr., Director
COO: William H. Mills, Associate Director
CFO: Jeffrey Beiler, Financial Manager
CMO: Rick Hartman, D.O., Chief of Staff
CIO: Ray Bush, Chief Information Officer
CHR: Raymer Kent, Manager Human Resources
Web address: www.va.gov/sta/guide/home.asp
Control: Veterans Affairs, Government, federal **Service:** General Medical and Surgical

Staffed Beds: 213 **Admissions:** 1995 **Census:** 142 **Outpatient Visits:** 353605 **Births:** 0 **Total Expense ($000):** 173520 **Payroll Expense ($000):** 64985 **Personnel:** 1088

LEHIGHTON—Carbon County

★□ △ **GNADEN HUETTEN MEMORIAL HOSPITAL (390194)**, 211 North 12th Street, Zip 18235–1138; tel. 610/377–1300, (Total facility includes 91 beds in nursing home–type unit) **A**1 7 9 10 **F**11 13 15 17 24 25 26 27 30 31 32 33 38 41 52 55 57 61 62 66 67 68 72 73 74 75 77 79 80 84 85 86 87 92 96 100 102 107 117 119 124 **S** Blue Mountain Health System
Primary Contact: Andrew E. Harris, Chief Executive Officer
CFO: David J. Plaviak, Chief Financial Officer
CIO: Ron Freed, Interim Chief Information Officer
CHR: Terry Purcell, Vice President Support Services and Ambulatory Care
Web address: www.bluemountainhealthsystem.org
Control: Other not–for–profit (including NFP Corporation) **Service:** General Medical and Surgical

Staffed Beds: 182 **Admissions:** 3258 **Census:** 128 **Outpatient Visits:** 79198 **Births:** 473 **Total Expense ($000):** 47322 **Payroll Expense ($000):** 20057 **Personnel:** 535

LEWISBURG—Union County

EVANGELICAL COMMUNITY HOSPITAL (390013), One Hospital Drive, Zip 17837–9314; tel. 570/522–2000 **A**9 10 19 **F**3 11 12 13 15 18 20 24 25 26 32 33 38 42 43 46 50 52 53 55 56 57 61 62 63 72 73 74 75 77 79 80 81 82 84 85 86 96 99 100 101 102 103 104 105 106 107 118 119 121 124 135 137 **P**7 8
Primary Contact: Michael N. O'Keefe, President and Chief Executive Officer
COO: Richard E. Smith, Chief Operating Officer
CFO: Christine M. Martin, Vice President Finance and Treasurer
CMO: J. Lawrence Ginsburg, M.D., Vice President Medical Affairs
CIO: Scott Peterson, Vice President Information Management
CHR: Michael Pierce, Vice President Human Resources
Web address: www.evanhospital.com
Control: Other not–for–profit (including NFP Corporation) **Service:** General Medical and Surgical

Staffed Beds: 123 **Admissions:** 6354 **Census:** 56 **Outpatient Visits:** 220344 **Births:** 1003 **Total Expense ($000):** 96800 **Payroll Expense ($000):** 41345 **Personnel:** 1125

U. S. PENITENTIARY INFIRMARY, Route 7, Zip 17837–9303; tel. 570/523–1251, (Nonreporting)
Primary Contact: Arnold Reyes, Administrator
Control: Department of Justice, Government, federal **Service:** Hospital unit of an institution (prison hospital, college infimary, etc.)

Staffed Beds: 17

LEWISTOWN—Mifflin County

★□ **LEWISTOWN HOSPITAL (390048)**, 400 Highland Avenue, Zip 17044–1198; tel. 717/248–5411 **A**1 2 5 9 10 19 **F**3 11 12 13 15 17 24 25 26 27 30 31 32 33 38 42 43 50 51 54 55 56 57 61 62 66 68 69 72 73 74 75 76 77 79 80 81 82 87 88 89 90 91 92 93 94 96 97 100 102 105 106 107 109 112 118 119 121 124 135 136 137 **P**6
Primary Contact: Kay A. Hamilton, RN, M.S., President and Chief Executive Officer
COO: Kirk E. Thomas, Vice President Operations
CFO: Randy E. Tewksbury, Vice President Finance
CMO: Gurpreet Bhalla, M.D., President Medical and Dental Staff
CIO: Ronald M. Cowan, Vice President Information Systems
CHR: N. Sue Reinke, Vice President Human Resources
Web address: www.lewistownhospital.org
Control: Other not–for–profit (including NFP Corporation) **Service:** General Medical and Surgical

Staffed Beds: 123 **Admissions:** 7100 **Census:** 84 **Outpatient Visits:** 30000 **Births:** 600

LITITZ—Lancaster County

□ **HEART OF LANCASTER REGIONAL MEDICAL CENTER (390068)**, 1500 Highlands Avenue, Zip 17543; tel. 717/625–5000, (Nonreporting) **A**1 9 10 12 13 **S** Health Management Associates
Primary Contact: Rebecca T. Brewer, FACHE, Interim Chief Executive Officer
CIO: David Fisher, Director Information Systems
Web address: www.chol.org
Control: Corporation, Investor–owned, for–profit **Service:** General Medical and Surgical

Staffed Beds: 139

LOCK HAVEN—Clinton County

★□ **LOCK HAVEN HOSPITAL (390071)**, 24 Cree Drive, Zip 17745–2699; tel. 570/893–5000, (Total facility includes 112 beds in nursing home–type unit) (Nonreporting) **A**1 9 10 **S** Community Health Systems, Inc.
Primary Contact: Cindy Segar–Gorr, RN, M.S., Chief Executive Officer
CFO: Joanna Zimmerman, Chief Financial Officer
CMO: Frank Parker, M.D., Chief of Staff
CIO: Jackie Haines, Director Information Systems
CHR: Lynn Moon, Director Human Resources
Web address: www.lockhavenhospital.com
Control: Corporation, Investor–owned, for–profit **Service:** General Medical and Surgical

Staffed Beds: 171

MALVERN—Chester County

□ △ **BRYN MAWR REHABILITATION HOSPITAL (393025)**, 414 Paoli Pike, Zip 19355–3300, Mailing Address: P.O. Box 3007, Zip 19355–3300; tel. 610/251–5400 **A**1 7 10 **F**25 30 31 32 33 43 53 54 62 72 75 76 77 81 82 85 86 119 121 135 137 **P**5 **S** Jefferson Health System
Primary Contact: Donna Phillips, President
CFO: Michael J. Buongiorno, Vice President Finance and Treasurer
CMO: John Kraus, M.D., Chief Medical Officer
CIO: Karen A. Thomas, R.N., Chief Information Officer
Web address: www.mainlinehealth.org
Control: Other not–for–profit (including NFP Corporation) **Service:** Rehabilitation

Staffed Beds: 148 **Admissions:** 3018 **Census:** 131 **Outpatient Visits:** 29315 **Births:** 0 **Total Expense ($000):** 48724 **Payroll Expense ($000):** 26299 **Personnel:** 503

DEVEREUX CHILDREN'S BEHAVIORAL HEALTH CENTER, 655 Sugartown Road, Zip 19355–0275, Mailing Address: P.O. Box 275, Zip 19355–0275; tel. 484/595–6777, (Nonreporting) **S** Devereux
Primary Contact: Walter J. Grono, Executive Director
COO: Howard Jarden, Ph.D., Assistant Executive Director
CFO: David Schultheis, Chief Financial Officer
CMO: Jacquelyn Zavodnick, M.D., Medical Director
CIO: MaryLou Hettinger, Director Quality Management
CHR: Sean Maher, Director Human Resources
Web address: www.devereux.org
Control: Other not–for–profit (including NFP Corporation) **Service:** Psychiatric

Staffed Beds: 13

MALVERN INSTITUTE, 940 King Road, Zip 19355–3167; tel. 610/647–0330, (Nonreporting) **A**9
Primary Contact: Richard Mangano, Administrator and Chief Executive Officer
CFO: Janet Corley, Accountant
Web address: www.malverninstitute.com
Control: Corporation, Investor–owned, for–profit **Service:** Alcoholism and other chemical dependency

Staffed Beds: 40

Hospital, Medicare Provider Number, Address, Telephone, Approval, Facility, and Physician Codes, Health Care System
★ American Hospital Association (AHA) membership
□ The Joint Commission accreditation
○ American Osteopathic Association (AOA) accreditation
△ Commission on Accreditation of Rehabilitation Facilities (CARF) accreditation

PA

MCCONNELLSBURG—Fulton County

★ **FULTON COUNTY MEDICAL CENTER (391303)**, 214 Peach Orchard Road, Zip 17233–1399; tel. 717/485–3155, (Total facility includes 57 beds in nursing home–type unit) **A**9 10 18 **F**3 11 15 24 25 30 31 32 38 46 50 55 56 57 61 62 66 68 73 75 79 82 86 96 100 102 107 117 119 121 122 135 137
Primary Contact: Jason F. Hawkins, President and Chief Executive Officer
COO: William Buterbaugh, Director Support Services
CFO: Shana K. Wolfe, Vice President and Chief Financial Officer
CMO: Sharon E. Martin, M.D., Ph.D., President Medical Staff
CIO: Harold M. Gress, Manager Management Information Systems
CHR: Cheryl Rose, Manager Human Resources
Web address: www.fcmc–pa.org
Control: Other not–for–profit (including NFP Corporation) **Service:** General Medical and Surgical

Staffed Beds: 82 **Admissions:** 967 **Census:** 67 **Outpatient Visits:** 43818 **Births:** 0 **Total Expense ($000):** 21758 **Payroll Expense ($000):** 10247 **Personnel:** 269

MCKEES ROCKS—Allegheny County

★ **OHIO VALLEY GENERAL HOSPITAL (390157)**, 25 Heckel Road, Zip 15136–1694; tel. 412/777–6161 **A**6 9 10 **F**3 10 13 18 24 25 38 43 51 57 68 73 74 75 77 79 80 85 86 96 100 104 107 115 118 119 135 137 **P**6
Primary Contact: William F. Provenzano, President and Chief Executive Officer
COO: David W. Scott, Chief Operating Officer
CFO: William J. Day, Vice President Finance
CIO: Joyce Polovich, Director Information Management
CHR: Vicki Mell, Vice President Human Resources
Web address: www.ohiovalleyhospital.org
Control: Other not–for–profit (including NFP Corporation) **Service:** General Medical and Surgical

Staffed Beds: 92 **Admissions:** 4833 **Census:** 65 **Outpatient Visits:** 127703 **Births:** 345 **Total Expense ($000):** 59232 **Payroll Expense ($000):** 21421 **Personnel:** 470

MCKEESPORT—Allegheny County

☐ **SELECT SPECIALTY HOSPITAL OF MCKEESPORT (392045)**, 1500 Fifth Avenue, Zip 15132; tel. 412/664–2900, (Nonreporting) **A**1 10 **S** Select Medical Corporation
Primary Contact: Tina Ruskewicz, Chief Executive Officer
Web address: www.selectmedicalcorp.com
Control: Corporation, Investor–owned, for–profit **Service:** Long–Term Acute Care hospital

Staffed Beds: 30

☐ **UPMC MCKEESPORT (390002)**, 1500 Fifth Avenue, Zip 15132–2482; tel. 412/664–2000, (Total facility includes 19 beds in nursing home–type unit) **A**1 3 5 9 10 12 13 **F**3 8 11 15 17 18 24 25 26 27 28 30 31 32 33 35 38 44 49 50 53 54 55 56 57 59 60 61 62 63 64 66 68 72 73 75 76 77 79 80 81 82 85 86 87 88 91 92 93 96 100 102 103 106 107 109 117 118 119 120 121 123 124 132 135 136 137 **S** UPMC
Primary Contact: Ronald H. Ott, President
CFO: Susan Mammarella, Chief Financial Officer
CIO: Joyce Krut, Senior Director Information Services
CHR: Mark P. Frick, Vice President Human Resources
Web address: www.mckeesport.upmc.com
Control: Other not–for–profit (including NFP Corporation) **Service:** General Medical and Surgical

Staffed Beds: 209 **Admissions:** 10589 **Census:** 167 **Outpatient Visits:** 43888 **Births:** 0 **Total Expense ($000):** 108718 **Payroll Expense ($000):** 54560 **Personnel:** 971

MEADVILLE—Crawford County

⊠ **MEADVILLE MEDICAL CENTER (390113)**, 751 Liberty Street, Zip 16335–2555; tel. 814/333–5000, (Total facility includes 32 beds in nursing home–type unit) **A**1 2 9 10 12 13 19 20 **F**3 4 5 11 13 15 18 24 25 26 27 30 31 32 33 34 36 38 42 43 46 49 52 55 57 61 62 68 72 73 74 75 76 77 79 80 81 82 84 85 86 88 90 92 93 96 100 102 106 107 112 117 118 119 120 121 124 132 135 137 **P**6
Primary Contact: Anthony J. DeFail, FACHE, President and Chief Executive Officer
COO: Philip Pandolph, Chief Operating Officer
CFO: Dave Poland, Chief Financial Officer
CMO: James McLamb, M.D., Medical Director
CIO: Mark Mahoney, Manager Information Systems
CHR: James Privitera, Vice President Human Resources
Web address: www.mmchs.org
Control: Other not–for–profit (including NFP Corporation) **Service:** General Medical and Surgical

Staffed Beds: 236 **Admissions:** 8309 **Census:** 126 **Outpatient Visits:** 204280 **Births:** 572 **Total Expense ($000):** 99437 **Payroll Expense ($000):** 40299 **Personnel:** 1018

MECHANICSBURG—Cumberland County

⊠ **HEALTHSOUTH REGIONAL SPECIALTY HOSPITAL (392038)**, 4950 Wilson Lane, Zip 17055; tel. 717/697–7706, (Nonreporting) **A**1 9 10
S HEALTHSOUTH Corporation
Primary Contact: Brent Burger, Chief Executive Officer
CFO: Jay Shoen, Controller
CHR: David Staskin, Director Human Resources
Web address: www.healthsouth.com
Control: Corporation, Investor–owned, for–profit **Service:** Long–Term Acute Care hospital

Staffed Beds: 46

⊠ **HEALTHSOUTH REHABILITATION HOSPITAL OF MECHANICSBURG (393031)**, 175 Lancaster Boulevard, Zip 17055–0736, Mailing Address: P.O. Box 2016, Zip 17055–2016; tel. 717/691–3700, (Nonreporting) **A**1 9 10
S HEALTHSOUTH Corporation
Primary Contact: Gregory P. Toot, Chief Executive Officer
CFO: Jay Shoen, Controller
CMO: Michael Lupinacci, M.D., Medical Director
CHR: David Staskin, Director Human Resources
Web address: www.healthsouth.com
Control: Corporation, Investor–owned, for–profit **Service:** Rehabilitation

Staffed Beds: 103

MEDIA—Delaware County

⊠ **RIDDLE MEMORIAL HOSPITAL (390222)**, 1068 West Baltimore Pike, Zip 19063–5177; tel. 610/566–9400, (Total facility includes 23 beds in nursing home–type unit) **A**1 2 9 10 **F**3 5 7 11 12 13 15 18 20 24 25 26 27 28 30 31 32 33 34 37 38 41 43 46 50 52 53 54 55 56 57 60 62 63 66 68 70 72 73 74 75 76 77 78 79 80 81 82 86 87 90 96 97 100 102 103 106 107 117 118 119 120 121 123 124 132 135 136 137
Primary Contact: Daniel E. Kennedy, President and Chief Executive Officer
CMO: Ken Boyd, M.D., President Medical Executive Committee
CIO: Denis Tucker, Director Information Services
CHR: Mary Louise Ciciretti, Director Human Resources
Web address: www.riddlehospital.org
Control: Other not–for–profit (including NFP Corporation) **Service:** General Medical and Surgical

Staffed Beds: 205 **Admissions:** 12146 **Census:** 164 **Outpatient Visits:** 103146 **Births:** 1113 **Total Expense ($000):** 127622 **Payroll Expense ($000):** 59452 **Personnel:** 1280

MEYERSDALE—Somerset County

MEYERSDALE MEDICAL CENTER (391302), 200 Hospital Drive, Zip 15552–1249; tel. 814/634–5911 **A**9 10 18 **F**15 24 25 30 38 46 50 55 56 57 62 75 79 96 102 107 119 121 122 **S** Conemaugh Health System
Primary Contact: Mary L. Libengood, President
CFO: Heather Smith, Director Finance
CMO: Nathan Thomas, M.D., President Medical Staff
CHR: Michael Lowry, Director Human Resources and Social Services
Web address: www.conemaugh.org
Control: Other not–for–profit (including NFP Corporation) **Service:** General Medical and Surgical

Staffed Beds: 20 **Admissions:** 497 **Census:** 7 **Outpatient Visits:** 26345 **Births:** 0 **Total Expense ($000):** 8361 **Payroll Expense ($000):** 3233 **Personnel:** 81

MONONGAHELA—Washington County

⊠ **MONONGAHELA VALLEY HOSPITAL (390147)**, 1163 Country Club Road, Rt 88, Zip 15063–1095; tel. 724/258–1000 **A**1 2 9 10 **F**3 9 11 12 15 17 18 20 24 25 26 27 28 30 31 32 33 37 38 43 48 49 50 51 53 54 55 56 57 60 62 66 68 72 73 74 75 76 77 78 79 80 81 82 84 85 86 88 90 91 92 93 96 97 102 106 107 108 109 111 118 119 120 121 123 124 135 136 137 **P**8
Primary Contact: Louis J. Panza, Jr., President and Chief Executive Officer
COO: Patrick J. Alberts, Senior Vice President and Chief Operating Officer
CFO: Daniel F. Simmons, Senior Vice President and Treasurer
CIO: Sandra Osborne, Director Information Systems
CHR: David Clark, Vice President Human Resources
Web address: www.monvalleyhospital.com
Control: Other not–for–profit (including NFP Corporation) **Service:** General Medical and Surgical

Staffed Beds: 226 **Admissions:** 10169 **Census:** 149 **Outpatient Visits:** 252843 **Births:** 463 **Total Expense ($000):** 102529 **Payroll Expense ($000):** 45322 **Personnel:** 1092

MONROEVILLE—Allegheny County

★ **HEALTHSOUTH HOSPITAL OF PITTSBURGH (392041)**, 2380 McGinley Road, Zip 15146–4400; tel. 412/856–2400, (Nonreporting) **A**1 10
S HEALTHSOUTH Corporation
Primary Contact: Cynthia Eiseman, Chief Executive Officer
COO: Cynthia Eiseman, Chief Operating Officer
CFO: Bill Bauer, Controller
CMO: Robert Crossey, D.O., Chief Medical Officer
CIO: Justin Armstrong, Chief Information Officer
CHR: Chelsea Webber, Director Human Resources
Web address: www.healthsouth.com
Control: Corporation, Investor–owned, for–profit **Service:** Long–Term Acute Care hospital

Staffed Beds: 89

★ **WESTERN PENNSYLVANIA HOSPITAL – FORBES REGIONAL CAMPUS (390267)**, 2570 Haymaker Road, Zip 15146–3592; tel. 412/858–2000 **A**1 3 5 9 10 **F**3 11 12 13 15 18 24 25 26 27 30 31 32 33 34 35 38 41 42 43 44 49 50 51 52 55 57 62 63 66 67 68 71 72 73 74 75 76 77 79 80 81 82 85 86 88 92 93 94 96 97 100 102 104 105 106 107 119 121 124 131 132 135
S West Penn Allegheny Health System
Primary Contact: Dawn M. Gideon, President and Chief Executive Officer
COO: Thomas B. Moser, Chief Operating Officer
CFO: James A. Kanuch, Chief Financial Officer
CIO: Sharon Lewis, Manager Client Service
CHR: Rebecca Trumble, Director Human Resources
Web address: www.wpahs.org
Control: Other not–for–profit (including NFP Corporation) **Service:** General Medical and Surgical

Staffed Beds: 264 **Admissions:** 14232 **Census:** 191 **Outpatient Visits:** 164918 **Births:** 748 **Total Expense ($000):** 68293 **Payroll Expense ($000):** 53378 **Personnel:** 1069

MONTROSE—Susquehanna County

ENDLESS MOUNTAIN HEALTH SYSTEMS (391306), 1 Grow Avenue, Zip 18801–1199; tel. 570/278–3801 **A**9 10 18 **F**25 33 38 52 54 55 57 63 68 73 75 77 79 86 96 107 119 121 122 124 **P**4
Primary Contact: Rexford Catlin, Chief Executive Officer
CFO: David Taylor, Manager Finance
CIO: Gary Passmore, Chief Information Officer
CHR: Paula Anderson, Administrative Director Human Resources
Web address: www.endlesscare.org
Control: Other not–for–profit (including NFP Corporation) **Service:** General Medical and Surgical

Staffed Beds: 21 **Admissions:** 1008 **Census:** 9 **Outpatient Visits:** 61170 **Births:** 0 **Total Expense ($000):** 13262 **Payroll Expense ($000):** 4784 **Personnel:** 152

MOUNT GRETNA—Lebanon County

☐ **PHILHAVEN (394020)**, 283 South Butler Road, Zip 17064–0550, Mailing Address: P.O. Box 550, Zip 17064–0550; tel. 717/273–8871 **A**1 9 10 **F**26 30 31 88 89 90 91 92 93 94 95 119 135 **P**6
Primary Contact: Phil Hess, Interim Chief Executive Officer
COO: Phil Hess, Chief Operating Officer
CFO: James Hess, Chief Financial Officer
CMO: Francis D. Sparrow, M.D., Medical Director
CIO: Lori Nolt, Director Information Technology
CHR: Marilynn Brubaker, Director Human Resources
Web address: www.philhaven.org
Control: Church–operated, Nongovernment, not–for profit **Service:** Psychiatric

Staffed Beds: 83 **Admissions:** 1839 **Census:** 69 **Outpatient Visits:** 75836 **Births:** 0 **Total Expense ($000):** 46899 **Payroll Expense ($000):** 29249 **Personnel:** 882

MOUNT PLEASANT—Westmoreland County

☐ **EXCELA FRICK HOSPITAL (390217)**, 508 South Church Street, Zip 15666–1790; tel. 724/547–1500, (Total facility includes 18 beds in nursing home–type unit) **A**1 9 10 **F**3 8 12 15 24 25 26 30 31 32 33 38 49 55 56 57 62 63 66 68 72 73 75 76 77 79 80 81 82 86 92 96 97 100 106 107 117 118 119 121 124 132 135 137 **S** Excela Health
Primary Contact: David S. Gallatin, Chief Executive Officer
COO: Samuel Raneri, Senior Vice President Operations and Business Development
CFO: Jeffrey T. Curry, Executive Vice President and Chief Financial Officer
CMO: Ralph Capone, M.D., Chief Medical Officer
CIO: Otto Salguero, Chief Information Officer
CHR: John Caverno, Chief Human Resources Officer
Web address: www.frickhospital.org
Control: Other not–for–profit (including NFP Corporation) **Service:** General Medical and Surgical

Staffed Beds: 83 **Admissions:** 4471 **Census:** 64 **Outpatient Visits:** 106138 **Births:** 0 **Total Expense ($000):** 42507 **Payroll Expense ($000):** 18608 **Personnel:** 431

PA

MUNCY—Lycoming County

MUNCY VALLEY HOSPITAL (391301), 215 East Water Street, Zip 17756–8700; tel. 570/546–4242, (Total facility includes 69 beds in nursing home–type unit) (Nonreporting) **A**9 10 18
Primary Contact: Steven P. Johnson, President and Chief Executive Officer
Control: Other not–for–profit (including NFP Corporation) **Service:** General Medical and Surgical

Staffed Beds: 94

NANTICOKE—Luzerne County

★ **MERCY SPECIAL CARE HOSPITAL (392025)**, 128 West Washington Street, Zip 18634–3113; tel. 570/735–5000, (Nonreporting) **A**9 10 **S** Catholic Healthcare Partners
Primary Contact: Robert D. Williams, Administrator
CFO: Stephen Franko, Chief Financial Officer
Web address: www.mercyhealthpartners.com
Control: Other not–for–profit (including NFP Corporation) **Service:** Long–Term Acute Care hospital

Staffed Beds: 68

NATRONA HEIGHTS—Allegheny County

★ **ALLE–KISKI MEDICAL CENTER (390032)**, 1301 Carlisle Street, Zip 15065–1192; tel. 724/224–5100 **A**1 2 6 9 10 **F**3 8 11 14 15 17 18 22 24 25 26 27 30 31 32 33 36 37 38 42 43 46 49 51 53 54 55 56 57 62 63 66 68 72 73 75 76 77 79 80 81 82 86 88 90 91 92 93 96 97 100 102 105 106 107 109 111 118 119 120 121 122 124 132 133 135 136 137 **S** West Penn Allegheny Health System
Primary Contact: Michael Harlovic, RN, Interim President and Chief Executive Officer
CFO: George Sandora, Director Finance
CMO: Radha Kambhampati, M.D., Vice President Medical Affairs
CIO: Linda Fergus, Director Information Systems
Web address: www.wpahs.org
Control: Other not–for–profit (including NFP Corporation) **Service:** General Medical and Surgical

Staffed Beds: 250 **Admissions:** 11514 **Census:** 164 **Outpatient Visits:** 222680 **Births:** 0 **Total Expense ($000):** 110367 **Payroll Expense ($000):** 47166 **Personnel:** 1075

NEW CASTLE—Lawrence County

★ **JAMESON HOSPITAL (390016)**, 1211 Wilmington Avenue, Zip 16105–2595; tel. 724/658–9001, (Total facility includes 32 beds in nursing home–type unit) **A**1 2 6 9 10 **F**3 4 8 11 13 15 18 20 24 25 26 27 28 30 31 32 33 36 38 42 46 49 51 53 54 55 56 57 61 62 63 66 68 73 74 75 77 79 80 81 82 85 86 88 89 91 92 93 95 96 97 100 102 103 106 107 108 117 118 119 121 124 135 137
Primary Contact: Thomas White, President and Chief Executive Officer
COO: Douglas Danko, Chief Operating Officer
CFO: James Aubel, Chief Financial Officer
CMO: David Shober, D.O., Medical Staff President
CIO: James Aubel, Chief Financial Officer
CHR: Neil A. Chessin, Vice President
Web address: www.jamesonhealth.org
Control: Other not–for–profit (including NFP Corporation) **Service:** General Medical and Surgical

Staffed Beds: 259 **Admissions:** 11414 **Census:** 166 **Outpatient Visits:** 255923 **Births:** 450 **Total Expense ($000):** 103485 **Payroll Expense ($000):** 46320 **Personnel:** 1375

Hospital, Medicare Provider Number, Address, Telephone, Approval, Facility, and Physician Codes, Health Care System
★ American Hospital Association (AHA) membership
☐ The Joint Commission accreditation
○ American Osteopathic Association (AOA) accreditation
△ Commission on Accreditation of Rehabilitation Facilities (CARF) accreditation

NORRISTOWN—Montgomery County

★ ○ **MERCY SUBURBAN HOSPITAL (390116)**, 2701 DeKalb Pike, Zip 19401–1820; tel. 610/278–2000, (Nonreporting) **A**1 2 9 10 11 12 13 **S** Catholic Health East
Primary Contact: Lisa Mallon, Chief Executive Officer
CFO: Peter B. Kenniff, CPA, Chief Financial Officer
Web address: www.mercyhealth.org
Control: Church–operated, Nongovernment, not–for profit **Service:** General Medical and Surgical

Staffed Beds: 141

☐ **MONTGOMERY COUNTY EMERGENCY SERVICE (394033)**, 50 Beech Drive, Zip 19403–5421; tel. 610/279–6100 **A**1 9 10 **F**4 5 7 25 31 33 36 50 62 88 89 90 91 92 93 94 119 **P**6
Primary Contact: William S. Leopold, Chief Administrative Officer
COO: William S. Leopold, Administrator and Chief Administrative Officer
CFO: William Myers, Chief Financial Officer
CHR: Karen Mossop, Director Human Resources
Web address: www.mces.org
Control: Other not–for–profit (including NFP Corporation) **Service:** Psychiatric

Staffed Beds: 81 **Admissions:** 2496 **Census:** 72 **Outpatient Visits:** 3281 **Births:** 0 **Total Expense ($000):** 14959 **Payroll Expense ($000):** 9737 **Personnel:** 200

★ **MONTGOMERY HOSPITAL MEDICAL CENTER (390108)**, 1301 Powell Street, Zip 19401–3377, Mailing Address: P.O. Box 992, Zip 19404–0992; tel. 610/270–2000 **A**1 2 3 5 9 10 **F**3 11 13 14 15 17 18 20 24 25 26 27 28 30 31 32 33 35 38 42 43 44 45 50 54 55 56 57 61 66 68 70 72 73 74 75 76 77 79 80 82 86 87 88 90 91 92 93 95 96 97 99 100 103 106 107 109 111 118 119 121 124 132 135 136 137 **P**6
Primary Contact: Timothy M. Casey, President and Chief Executive Officer
CFO: Edward Ladely, Senior Vice President and Chief Financial Officer
CIO: Ed Hemschoot, Director Information Systems
CHR: Murray Swim, Chief Human Resources Officer
Web address: www.montgomeryhospital.org
Control: Other not–for–profit (including NFP Corporation) **Service:** General Medical and Surgical

Staffed Beds: 166 **Admissions:** 7945 **Census:** 90 **Outpatient Visits:** 158296 **Births:** 656 **Total Expense ($000):** 91318 **Payroll Expense ($000):** 43573 **Personnel:** 971

☐ **NORRISTOWN STATE HOSPITAL (394001)**, 1001 Sterigere Street, Zip 19401–5300; tel. 610/270–1000 **A**1 9 10 **F**4 5 30 32 37 73 75 82 88 90 91 119 135 **P**1
Primary Contact: Gerald P. Kent, Chief Executive Officer
COO: Gary Raisner, Chief Operating Officer
CMO: Mia Marcovici, M.D., Chief Medical Officer
CHR: Richard Szczurowski, Director Human Resources
Control: State–Government, nonfederal **Service:** Psychiatric

Staffed Beds: 442 **Admissions:** 262 **Census:** 394 **Outpatient Visits:** 186 **Births:** 0 **Total Expense ($000):** 83321 **Payroll Expense ($000):** 36617 **Personnel:** 807

★ **VALLEY FORGE MEDICAL CENTER AND HOSPITAL (390272)**, 1033 West Germantown Pike, Zip 19403–3998; tel. 610/539–8500 **A**1 10 **F**3 4 25 31 32 43 60 66 73 90 119 121 **P**6
Primary Contact: Marian W. Colcher, President
CFO: Gregg Y. Slocum, Chief Financial Officer
CMO: Robert E. Colcher, M.D., Medical Director
CHR: Frederick D. Jackes, Assistant Administrator and Director Human Resources
Web address: www.vfmc.net
Control: Corporation, Investor–owned, for–profit **Service:** Alcoholism and other chemical dependency

Staffed Beds: 86 **Admissions:** 1970 **Census:** 68 **Outpatient Visits:** 0 **Births:** 0 **Total Expense ($000):** 10286 **Payroll Expense ($000):** 6303 **Personnel:** 124

OAKDALE—Allegheny County

☐ **KINDRED HOSPITAL–PITTSBURGH (392028)**, 7777 Steubenville Pike, Zip 15071–3409; tel. 412/494–5500, (Nonreporting) **A**1 10 **S** Kindred Healthcare
Primary Contact: Susan Colpo, Chief Executive Officer
CFO: Kevin Varley, Chief Financial Officer
CMO: Ravi Alagar, M.D., Medical Director
CIO: Kurt Segeleon, Director Health Information Management
CHR: Nancy Smocynski, Director Payroll, Personnel and Human Resources
Web address: www.kindredhealthcare.com
Control: Corporation, Investor–owned, for–profit **Service:** Long–Term Acute Care hospital

Staffed Beds: 63

OREFIELD—Lehigh County

KIDSPEACE CHILDREN'S HOSPITAL (394047), 5300 Kids Peace Drive, Zip 18069–9101; tel. 610/799–8800 **A**9 10 **F**25 30 36 72 88 89 90 91 92 119 **P**6
Primary Contact: Charles Thomas O'Donnell, President and Chief Executive Officer
COO: Lorrie Henderson, M.D., Chief Operating Officer
Web address: www.kidspeace.org
Control: Other not–for–profit (including NFP Corporation) **Service:** Children's hospital psychiatric

Staffed Beds: 56 **Admissions:** 1183 **Census:** 45 **Outpatient Visits:** 0 **Births:** 0 **Total Expense ($000):** 8908 **Payroll Expense ($000):** 6064 **Personnel:** 138

PALMERTON—Carbon County

☐ **PALMERTON HOSPITAL (390019)**, 135 Lafayette Avenue, Zip 18071–1596; tel. 610/826–3141 **A**1 9 10 **F**2 3 11 15 24 25 30 31 32 33 38 46 47 49 50 52 54 55 56 57 63 66 67 68 72 73 75 77 79 80 81 82 86 87 88 92 93 96 99 100 104 107 118 119 121 124 135 **S** Blue Mountain Health System
Primary Contact: Andrew E. Harris, Chief Executive Officer
CFO: David J. Plaviak, Chief Financial Officer
CMO: Clement McGinley, M.D., Vice President Medical Affairs
CHR: Terry Purcell, Vice President Ambulatory Care and Support Services
Web address: www.palmertonhospital.com
Control: Other not–for–profit (including NFP Corporation) **Service:** General Medical and Surgical

Staffed Beds: 59 **Admissions:** 1724 **Census:** 21 **Outpatient Visits:** 41399 **Births:** 0 **Total Expense ($000):** 23416 **Payroll Expense ($000):** 9779 **Personnel:** 281

PAOLI—Chester County

☐ **PAOLI HOSPITAL (390153)**, 255 West Lancaster Avenue, Zip 19301–1792; tel. 610/648–1000 **A**1 2 9 10 **F**3 13 15 17 18 20 22 24 25 26 27 30 31 32 33 34 35 36 37 38 43 44 46 50 51 53 54 55 56 57 62 63 70 72 73 74 75 76 77 79 80 81 82 86 90 94 95 96 97 102 106 107 109 111 112 114 118 119 120 121 123 124 125 130 131 132 135 136 137 **S** Jefferson Health System
Primary Contact: Barbara J. Tachovsky, President
CFO: John Doyle, Vice President Finance
CMO: Thomas G. McCarter, M.D., Chief Medical Officer
CIO: Karen A. Thomas, R.N., Vice President and Chief Information Officer
CHR: Deborah Fedora, Director Human Resources
Web address: www.mainlinehealth.org
Control: Other not–for–profit (including NFP Corporation) **Service:** General Medical and Surgical

Staffed Beds: 157 **Admissions:** 12720 **Census:** 124 **Outpatient Visits:** 205287 **Births:** 2252 **Total Expense ($000):** 146330 **Payroll Expense ($000):** 55944 **Personnel:** 920

PECKVILLE—Lackawanna County

MID–VALLEY HOSPITAL (391311), 1400 Main Street, Zip 18452–2098; tel. 570/383–5500 **A**9 10 18 **F**3 11 15 24 25 30 31 32 33 37 38 41 42 49 50 55 57 62 66 73 75 77 79 81 82 86 96 97 102 107 119 122 124 132 135
Primary Contact: Ann Marie Stevens, Director Operations
CFO: James G. Brittain, Chief Financial Officer
CMO: Rajan Mulloth, M.D., President Medical Staff
CIO: Edward Roman, Chief Information Officer and Chief Privacy Officer
CHR: Paul Gionfriddo, Vice President Human Resources
Web address: www.mth.org
Control: Other not–for–profit (including NFP Corporation) **Service:** General Medical and Surgical

Staffed Beds: 25 **Admissions:** 816 **Census:** 8 **Outpatient Visits:** 38177 **Births:** 0 **Total Expense ($000):** 10785 **Payroll Expense ($000):** 4824 **Personnel:** 116

PHILADELPHIA—Philadelphia County

☐ **ALBERT EINSTEIN MEDICAL CENTER (390142)**, 5501 Old York Road, Zip 19141–3098; tel. 215/456–7890, (Total facility includes 102 beds in nursing home–type unit) (Nonreporting) **A**1 2 3 5 8 9 10 12 13 **S** Albert Einstein Healthcare Network
Primary Contact: A. Susan Bernini, Chief Operating Officer
COO: A. Susan Bernini, Chief Operating Officer
CFO: Brian Derrick, Chief Financial Officer
CIO: Kenneth Levitan, Vice President Information Systems
CHR: Lynne R. Kornblatt, Vice President Human Resources
Web address: www.einstein.edu
Control: Other not–for–profit (including NFP Corporation) **Service:** General Medical and Surgical

Staffed Beds: 701

PA

□ **BELMONT CENTER FOR COMPREHENSIVE TREATMENT (394023)**, 4200 Monument Road, Zip 19131–1625; tel. 215/877–2000, (Nonreporting) **A**1 9 10 **S** Albert Einstein Healthcare Network
Primary Contact: Sharon A. Bergen, Chief Operating Officer
COO: Sharon A. Bergen, Chief Operating Officer
CFO: Guy Romaniello, Director Fiscal Services
CMO: Lawrence A. Real, M.D., Medical Director
CHR: Kymm Steliga, Human Resources Specialist
Web address: www.einstein.edu
Control: Other not–for–profit (including NFP Corporation) **Service:** Psychiatric

Staffed Beds: 146

★□ **CHESTNUT HILL HEALTH SYSTEM (390026)**, 8835 Germantown Avenue, Zip 19118–2765; tel. 215/248–8200, (Nonreporting) **A**1 2 3 5 9 10 **S** Community Health Systems, Inc.
Primary Contact: M. Brooks Turkel, Chief Executive Officer
CMO: Robert J. Gillesby, M.D., Executive Vice President Clinical Services and Chief Medical Officer
CIO: Jack Nash, Interim Director Information Systems
CHR: Rita Guzewski, Director Human Resources
Web address: www.chh.org
Control: Other not–for–profit (including NFP Corporation) **Service:** General Medical and Surgical

Staffed Beds: 212

★□ **CHILDREN'S HOSPITAL OF PHILADELPHIA (393303)**, 34th Street and Civic Center Boulevard, Zip 19104–4304; tel. 215/590–1000 **A**1 3 5 8 9 10 **F**3 7 8 11 17 18 19 21 22 23 24 25 26 27 28 30 32 33 36 37 38 40 41 43 44 45 46 48 50 53 55 56 57 58 59 60 61 62 63 64 66 69 70 71 72 73 75 76 77 79 80 81 82 83 84 85 86 87 89 90 91 92 94 96 97 100 102 103 104 105 106 107 114 116 118 119 120 121 123 125 126 127 128 129 130 133 135 137 **P**6
Primary Contact: Steven M. Altschuler, President and Chief Executive Officer
COO: Madeline Bell, Executive Vice President and Chief Operating Officer
CFO: Thomas Todorow, Chief Financial Officer
CMO: James Steven, M.D., Chief Medical Officer
CHR: Meg Jones, Vice President Human Resources
Web address: www.chop.edu
Control: Other not–for–profit (including NFP Corporation) **Service:** Children's general

Staffed Beds: 422 **Admissions:** 24661 **Census:** 334 **Outpatient Visits:** 1064390 **Births:** 0 **Total Expense ($000):** 834151 **Payroll Expense ($000):** 400133 **Personnel:** 8162

□ **FAIRMOUNT BEHAVIORAL HEALTH SYSTEM (394027)**, 561 Fairthorne Avenue, Zip 19128–2499; tel. 215/487–4000 **A**1 9 10 **F**4 32 38 88 89 92 95 119 **P**6 **S** Universal Health Services, Inc.
Primary Contact: Geoff Botak, Chief Executive Officer and Managing Director
COO: Elizabeth Dean, Assistant Administrator
CFO: Robert Gregor, Chief Financial Officer
CMO: T. Sureshkumar, M.D., President Medical Staff
CIO: Robert Gregor, Chief Financial Officer
CHR: Jenita Lunsford, Interim Director Human Resources
Web address: www.fairmountbhs.com
Control: Corporation, Investor–owned, for–profit **Service:** Psychiatric

Staffed Beds: 182 **Admissions:** 4261 **Census:** 170 **Outpatient Visits:** 6575 **Births:** 0 **Total Expense ($000):** 27701 **Payroll Expense ($000):** 15102 **Personnel:** 345

★□ **FOX CHASE CANCER CENTER–AMERICAN ONCOLOGIC HOSPITAL (390196)**, 333 Cottman Avenue, Zip 19111; tel. 215/728–6900 **A**1 2 3 5 8 9 10 **F**3 8 11 15 25 26 27 30 31 32 33 34 42 43 44 46 47 49 50 52 55 56 57 58 59 60 61 62 66 68 69 72 73 75 76 77 79 80 81 82 86 90 96 97 98 99 100 102 103 104 105 106 107 108 109 111 112 114 116 119 121 135 136 **P**6
Primary Contact: Michael V. Seiden, President and Chief Executive Officer
COO: R. Donald Leedy, Chief Operating Officer
CFO: Theresa Larivee, Vice President Finance and Chief Financial Officer
CMO: Robert F. Ozols, Ph.D., Senior Vice President Medical Sciences
CIO: J. Robert Beck, M.D., Vice President Information Services and Chief Information Officer
CHR: Gary Weyhmuller, Vice President Human Resources
Web address: www.fccc.edu
Control: Other not–for–profit (including NFP Corporation) **Service:** General Medical and Surgical

Staffed Beds: 84 **Admissions:** 4208 **Census:** 59 **Outpatient Visits:** 71508 **Births:** 0 **Total Expense ($000):** 167328 **Payroll Expense ($000):** 45682 **Personnel:** 939

□ △ **FRANKFORD HOSPITAL OF THE CITY OF PHILADELPHIA (390115)**, Knights and Red Lion Roads, Zip 19114–4208; tel. 215/612–4000, (Includes BUCKS COUNTY CAMPUS, 380 North Oxford Valley Road, Langhorne, Zip 19047–8399; tel. 215/949–5000; FRANKFORD CAMPUS, Frankford Avenue and Wakeling Street, Zip 19124; tel. 215/831–2000) **A**1 3 5 6 7 9 10 12 13 **F**3 5 11 14 15 18 20 22 24 25 26 27 28 30 31 32 33 34 37 38 40 41 43 49 52 53 55 56 57 60 61 62 63 64 66 67 68 72 73 75 76 77 78 79 80 81 82 86 87 88 90 91 92 93 94 96 97 102 103 104 105 106 107 108 109 111 112 118 119 120 121 124 132 133 134 135 136 137 **P**6 **S** Jefferson Health System
Primary Contact: Roy A. Powell, President
COO: Eugene R. Johnson, Senior Vice President
CFO: Robert J. Crossin, Vice President Finance
CMO: Howard L. Elefant, M.D., Medical Director
CIO: Joseph Olszewski, Director Information Services
CHR: John R. Osgood, Vice President Human Resources
Web address: www.frankfordhospitals.org
Control: Other not–for–profit (including NFP Corporation) **Service:** General Medical and Surgical

Staffed Beds: 486 **Admissions:** 29700 **Census:** 440 **Outpatient Visits:** 329827 **Births:** 0 **Total Expense ($000):** 354875 **Payroll Expense ($000):** 161655

PA

★□ **FRIENDS BEHAVIORAL HEALTH SYSTEM (394008)**, 4641 Roosevelt Boulevard, Zip 19124–2399; tel. 215/831–4600 **A**1 3 5 9 10 **F**25 26 30 31 36 43 54 66 73 75 88 89 90 91 92 93 119 121 **P**6 **S** Horizon Health Corporation
Primary Contact: Arris S. Veronie, Chief Executive Officer
COO: Diane Carugati, Chief Operating Officer
CFO: Alfred P. Salvitti, Chief Financial Officer
CMO: Marc Rothman, M.D., Medical Director
CIO: John Healy, Manager Information Technology
CHR: Paul Cavanaugh, Director Human Resources
Web address: www.fbhs.org
Control: Partnership, Investor–owned, for–profit **Service:** Psychiatric

Staffed Beds: 219 **Admissions:** 5139 **Census:** 172 **Outpatient Visits:** 14000 **Births:** 0 **Total Expense ($000):** 37731 **Payroll Expense ($000):** 21625 **Personnel:** 430

GIRARD MEDICAL CENTER See North Philadelphia Health System

★□ **HAHNEMANN UNIVERSITY HOSPITAL (390290)**, Broad and Vine Streets, Zip 19102–1192; tel. 215/762–7000 **A**1 2 3 5 8 9 10 **F**3 6 12 13 14 15 17 18 20 22 25 27 30 31 32 33 38 40 43 46 48 49 50 51 55 57 58 59 60 62 63 66 68 70 72 74 75 76 77 79 80 82 87 88 90 92 93 95 96 97 98 100 102 104 105 106 107 109 111 112 113 114 116 118 119 120 121 125 126 127 128 131 133 135 136 137 **P**6 **S** TENET Healthcare Corporation
Primary Contact: Michael P. Halter, Chief Executive Officer
COO: James B. Burke, Chief Operating Officer
CFO: Brian Reilly, Chief Financial Officer
CMO: George Amrom, M.D., Vice President Medical Affairs
CIO: Tom Nataloni, Senior Director Information Technology
CHR: Steven Simmons, Chief Human Resources Officer
Web address: www.hahnemannhospital.com
Control: Corporation, Investor–owned, for–profit **Service:** General Medical and Surgical

Staffed Beds: 483 **Admissions:** 19559 **Census:** 326 **Outpatient Visits:** 92104 **Births:** 2146 **Personnel:** 2496

★□ △ **HOSPITAL OF THE UNIVERSITY OF PENNSYLVANIA (390111)**, 3400 Spruce Street, Zip 19104–4283; tel. 215/662–4000 **A**1 7 8 9 10 **F**3 4 7 9 11 12 13 14 15 16 17 18 19 20 21 22 23 24 25 26 27 30 31 32 33 34 36 37 38 40 41 42 43 44 45 46 47 48 49 50 51 53 54 55 56 57 58 59 60 61 62 63 64 66 68 70 71 72 73 74 75 76 77 79 80 81 82 84 85 86 87 88 89 90 91 92 93 94 96 97 98 99 100 102 103 104 105 106 107 108 109 111 112 113 114 116 117 118 119 120 121 123 124 125 126 127 128 129 130 131 132 134 135 136 137 **P**6 **S** University of Pennsylvania Health System
Primary Contact: Garry L. Scheib, Executive Director
COO: Albert P. Black, Chief Operating Officer
CFO: Keith Kasper, Chief Financial Officer
CMO: Bernett L. Johnson, M.D., Chief Medical Officer
CIO: Michael Restuccia, Chief Information Officer
CHR: Terri Woodruff, Chief Human Resources Officer
Web address: www.pennhealth.com
Control: Other not–for–profit (including NFP Corporation) **Service:** General Medical and Surgical

Staffed Beds: 694 **Admissions:** 38213 **Census:** 616 **Outpatient Visits:** 856749 **Births:** 3739 **Total Expense ($000):** 1294929 **Payroll Expense ($000):** 554488 **Personnel:** 7253

Hospital, Medicare Provider Number, Address, Telephone, Approval, Facility, and Physician Codes, Health Care System

★ American Hospital Association (AHA) membership
□ The Joint Commission accreditation
○ American Osteopathic Association (AOA) accreditation
△ Commission on Accreditation of Rehabilitation Facilities (CARF) accreditation

PA

★ **JEANES HOSPITAL (390080)**, 7600 Central Avenue, Zip 19111–2499; tel. 215/728–2000 **A**1 5 9 10 **F**3 11 12 13 15 18 20 22 24 25 26 27 30 31 32 33 38 40 41 43 54 55 57 59 61 62 63 66 68 70 72 73 74 75 76 77 79 80 82 85 86 96 97 100 102 103 104 107 108 118 119 121 124 134 135 137 **P**6 **S** Temple University Health System
Primary Contact: Linda J. Grass, Executive Director and Chief Executive Officer
CFO: Gerald P. Oetzel, Chief Financial Officer
CMO: Andrea C. McCoy, M.D., Chief Medical Officer
CHR: Elisabeth Donahue, Associate Director Human Resources
Web address: www.jeanes.com
Control: Other not–for–profit (including NFP Corporation) **Service:** General Medical and Surgical

Staffed Beds: 198 **Admissions:** 10701 **Census:** 134 **Outpatient Visits:** 118068 **Births:** 1414 **Total Expense ($000):** 131772 **Payroll Expense ($000):** 54432 **Personnel:** 1044

☐ **KENSINGTON HOSPITAL (390025)**, 136 West Diamond Street, Zip 19122–1721; tel. 215/426–8100, (Nonreporting) **A**1 9 10
Primary Contact: Eileen Hause, Chief Executive Officer
CFO: Kenneth Biddle, Controller
CMO: Luis F. Vera, M.D., Medical Director
CHR: Maria Dimichele, Administrative Assistant
Control: State–Government, nonfederal **Service:** General Medical and Surgical

Staffed Beds: 45

☐ **KINDRED HOSPITAL–PHILADELPHIA (392027)**, 6129 Palmetto Street, Zip 19111–5729; tel. 215/722–8555, (Nonreporting) **A**1 9 10 **S** Kindred Healthcare
Primary Contact: Margaret M. Murphy, Chief Executive Officer
COO: Deborah Karn, Chief Clinical Officer
CFO: Thomas A. McMullen, Chief Financial Officer
Web address: www.kindredhealthcare.com
Control: Corporation, Investor–owned, for–profit **Service:** Long–Term Acute Care hospital

Staffed Beds: 52

★ △ **MAGEE REHABILITATION HOSPITAL (393038)**, 1513 Race Street, Zip 19102–1177; tel. 215/587–3000 **A**1 3 5 7 10 **F**11 25 26 30 33 43 53 55 58 66 73 75 81 85 86 119 121 135 137 **P**6 **S** Jefferson Health System
Primary Contact: Jack A. Carroll, Ph.D., President and Chief Executive Officer
CFO: Patricia A. Underwood, Chief Financial Officer
CMO: Guy Fried, M.D., Chief Medical Officer
CIO: Steven Peterson, Director
CHR: Ed Petka, Director
Web address: www.mageerehab.org
Control: Other not–for–profit (including NFP Corporation) **Service:** Rehabilitation

Staffed Beds: 96 **Admissions:** 1376 **Census:** 77 **Outpatient Visits:** 23360 **Births:** 0 **Total Expense ($000):** 55017 **Payroll Expense ($000):** 28235 **Personnel:** 493

MERCY HOSPITAL OF PHILADELPHIA See Mercy Fitzgerald Hospital, Darby

METHODIST HOSPITAL See Thomas Jefferson University Hospital

★ △ **NAZARETH HOSPITAL (390204)**, 2601 Holme Avenue, Zip 19152–2096; tel. 215/335–6672, (Total facility includes 28 beds in nursing home–type unit) **A**1 7 9 10 **F**3 11 15 17 18 25 26 27 31 32 33 35 37 38 43 44 49 50 52 54 55 56 57 58 62 63 66 68 72 73 75 76 77 79 80 81 82 85 86 87 90 96 97 100 102 103 106 107 110 117 119 120 121 124 132 135 137 **P**7 **S** Catholic Health East
Primary Contact: Christina Fitz–Patrick, RN, President and Chief Executive Officer
COO: Christina Fitz–Patrick, R.N., President and Chief Executive Officer
CFO: David Wajda, Chief Financial Officer
CMO: Patrick Waters, D.O., Chief Medical Officer
CIO: Jeff Buda, Chief Information Technology
CHR: Mary Ellen Cockerham, Vice President Human Resources
Web address: www.nazarethhospital.org
Control: Other not–for–profit (including NFP Corporation) **Service:** General Medical and Surgical

Staffed Beds: 233 **Admissions:** 11568 **Census:** 177 **Outpatient Visits:** 156924 **Births:** 0 **Total Expense ($000):** 120067 **Payroll Expense ($000):** 52988 **Personnel:** 865

☐ **NORTH PHILADELPHIA HEALTH SYSTEM (390132)**, 1524 West Girard Avenue, Zip 19130–1615; tel. 215/787–9000, (Includes GIRARD MEDICAL CENTER, Girard Avenue at Eighth Street, Zip 19122; tel. 215/787–2000; Marlene Walsh, Vice President and Administrator; ST. JOSEPH'S HOSPITAL, Girard Avenue at Sixteenth Street, Zip 19130; tel. 215/787–9000; Catherine Kutzler, RN, Vice President and Administrator), (Nonreporting) **A**1 9 10
Primary Contact: George J. Walmsley, III, CPA, President and Chief Executive Officer
CFO: Ronald Kaplan, Chief Financial Officer
CIO: Tony Iero, Director Management Information Systems
CHR: James Gloner, Senior Vice President
Web address: www.nphs.com
Control: Other not–for–profit (including NFP Corporation) **Service:** General Medical and Surgical

Staffed Beds: 315

★ **PENNSYLVANIA HOSPITAL (390226)**, 800 Spruce Street, Zip 19107–6192; tel. 215/829–3000 **A**1 3 5 9 10 **F**3 9 11 12 13 14 15 17 18 20 22 25 26 27 30 31 32 33 34 35 36 38 41 42 43 44 46 50 52 53 54 55 56 57 59 60 62 64 66 68 70 72 73 74 75 76 77 78 79 80 81 82 85 86 87 88 89 90 91 92 94 96 97 100 102 104 105 106 107 109 111 112 113 114 117 118 119 120 121 123 124 125 130 135 136 137 **P**6 **S** University of Pennsylvania Health System
Primary Contact: Kathleen Kinslow, Ed.D., Executive Director
COO: Ron Kumor, Chief Operating Officer
CFO: Frank Anastasi, Chief Financial Officer
CMO: R. Michael Buckley, M.D., Chief Medical Officer
CIO: Tod Simons, Entity Information Officer
CHR: Dorinda Carolina, Chief Human Resources Officer
Web address: www.pahosp.com
Control: Other not–for–profit (including NFP Corporation) **Service:** General Medical and Surgical

Staffed Beds: 434 **Admissions:** 23257 **Census:** 301 **Outpatient Visits:** 169789 **Births:** 5207 **Total Expense ($000):** 356298 **Payroll Expense ($000):** 137290 **Personnel:** 2399

★ **PRESBYTERIAN MEDICAL CENTER OF THE UNIVERSITY OF PENNSYLVANIA HEALTH SYSTEM (390223)**, 39th and Market Street, Zip 19104–2699; tel. 215/662–8000, (Total facility includes 23 beds in nursing home–type unit) **A**1 3 5 9 10 **F**3 4 5 7 9 11 12 15 17 18 20 22 25 26 27 28 30 31 32 33 34 35 37 38 41 42 43 44 46 50 53 54 55 56 57 58 59 60 61 62 63 64 66 68 72 73 75 76 77 78 79 80 81 82 86 87 88 90 96 97 98 100 102 103 106 107 116 117 119 120 121 123 124 130 131 132 135 137 **P**6 **S** University of Pennsylvania Health System
Primary Contact: Michele M. Volpe, Executive Director and Chief Executive Officer
COO: Robert J. Russell, Associate Vice President Operations
CFO: Stephen Muravsky, Chief Financial Officer
CMO: Ana Pujols–McKee, M.D., Chief Medical Officer and Associate Executive Director
CIO: Theresa Hiltunen, Entity Information Officer
CHR: Gail Kimble, Chief Human Resource Officer
Web address: www.health.upenn.edu/pmc
Control: Other not–for–profit (including NFP Corporation) **Service:** General Medical and Surgical

Staffed Beds: 279 **Admissions:** 15419 **Census:** 221 **Outpatient Visits:** 150006 **Births:** 0 **Total Expense ($000):** 332391 **Payroll Expense ($000):** 118340 **Personnel:** 1550

★ **ROXBOROUGH MEMORIAL HOSPITAL (390304)**, 5800 Ridge Avenue, Zip 19128–1737; tel. 215/483–9900, (Nonreporting) **A**1 6 9 10
Primary Contact: John J. Donnelly, Jr., Chief Executive Officer
CFO: Michael Metts, Chief Financial Officer
Web address: www.roxboroughmemorial.com
Control: Corporation, Investor–owned, for–profit **Service:** General Medical and Surgical

Staffed Beds: 137

☐ **SHRINERS HOSPITALS FOR CHILDREN, PHILADELPHIA**, 3551 North Broad Street, Zip 19140–4131; tel. 215/430–4000, (Nonreporting) **A**1 3 5 **S** Shriners Hospitals for Children
Primary Contact: Ernest N. Perilli, Administrator
CFO: Mario Salvati, Director Fiscal Services
CMO: Randal Betz, M.D., Chief of Staff
CIO: Mark Morrison, Director Support Services
CHR: Wanda Amaro, Director Human Resources
Web address: www.shrinershq.org
Control: Other not–for–profit (including NFP Corporation) **Service:** Children's orthopedic

Staffed Beds: 80

☐ **ST. AGNES CONTINUING CARE CENTER (392046)**, 1900 South Broad Street, Zip 19145–2304; tel. 215/339–4100, (Total facility includes 38 beds in nursing home–type unit) **A**1 9 10 **F**1 2 3 25 26 30 32 33 56 66 72 73 75 80 81 82 90 117 119 132 135 137 **S** Catholic Health East
Primary Contact: Mary Ann Papa, Vice President and General Manager Long Term Care Hospital
CFO: Teresa A. Gresko, Chief Financial Officer
CIO: Charles Schechterly, Director Information Systems
CHR: Maryann Kenkelen, Vice President Human Resources and Tenant Services
Web address: www.stagnesccc.org
Control: Church–operated, Nongovernment, not–for profit **Service:** Long–Term Acute Care hospital

Staffed Beds: 96 **Admissions:** 1278 **Census:** 78 **Outpatient Visits:** 0 **Births:** 0 **Total Expense ($000):** 50373 **Payroll Expense ($000):** 19115 **Personnel:** 320

★ **ST. CHRISTOPHER'S HOSPITAL FOR CHILDREN (393307)**, (Pediatrics), Erie Avenue at Front Street, Zip 19134–1095; tel. 215/427–5000 **A**1 3 5 8 9 10 **F**3 12 16 17 19 21 23 25 26 27 28 30 31 32 37 38 39 40 50 53 55 56 57 59 60 62 63 66 69 70 72 73 75 76 77 78 79 81 83 86 87 89 96 97 98 100 101 102 103 107 114 118 119 120 121 123 125 127 131 132 135 **S** TENET Healthcare Corporation
Primary Contact: Bernadette M. Mangan, Chief Executive Officer
COO: Jeff Snyder, Chief Operating Officer
CFO: Gil Cottle, Chief Financial Officer
CMO: Maureen Fee, M.D., Chief Medical Officer
CIO: Steve Landis, Director Information Services
CHR: Lisa Coulter, Director Human Resources
Web address: www.stchristophershospital.com
Control: Corporation, Investor–owned, for–profit **Service:** Children's other specialty

Staffed Beds: 124 **Admissions:** 9309 **Census:** 114 **Outpatient Visits:** 95585 **Births:** 0 **Total Expense ($000):** 143876 **Payroll Expense ($000):** 63183 **Personnel:** 1170

ST. JOSEPH'S HOSPITAL See North Philadelphia Health System

★ **TEMPLE EAST, NORTHEASTERN HOSPITAL (390023)**, 2301 East Allegheny Avenue, Zip 19134–4497; tel. 215/291–3000 **A**1 3 5 6 9 10 **F**3 8 13 15 25 26 27 30 31 32 33 38 50 53 54 57 62 63 66 68 73 74 75 76 77 78 79 80 82 86 96 100 103 106 107 118 119 121 135 136 **S** Temple University Health System
Primary Contact: John J. Buckley, Executive Director and Chief Executive Officer
COO: Eugene Ott, Associate Director Operations
CFO: Thomas A. Bielecki, Chief Financial Officer
CMO: Marc P. Hurowitz, D.O., Chief Medical Officer
CIO: Andrew J. Cymerman, Chief Information Officer
CHR: David Brodar, Associate Director Human Resources
Web address: www.health.temple.edu/northeastern.html
Control: Other not–for–profit (including NFP Corporation) **Service:** General Medical and Surgical

Staffed Beds: 187 **Admissions:** 10804 **Census:** 127 **Outpatient Visits:** 97430 **Births:** 1542 **Total Expense ($000):** 105762 **Payroll Expense ($000):** 45696 **Personnel:** 722

★ **TEMPLE UNIVERSITY HOSPITAL (390027)**, 3401 North Broad Street, Zip 19140–5192; tel. 215/707–2000, (Includes TEMPLE UNIVERSITY HOSPITAL – EPISCOPAL DIVISION, 100 East Lehigh Avenue, Zip 19125–1098; tel. 215/427–7000) **A**1 2 3 5 6 8 9 10 **F**3 11 12 13 15 16 17 18 20 22 24 25 26 27 30 31 32 33 35 36 38 40 41 43 44 46 47 48 49 50 54 55 56 57 58 59 60 62 66 68 70 72 73 74 75 76 77 78 79 80 81 82 85 86 87 88 89 90 91 92 94 96 97 100 102 103 106 107 108 109 111 112 114 118 119 120 121 124 125 126 127 129 131 134 135 136 137 **P**4 **S** Temple University Health System
Primary Contact: Robert E. Pezzoli, Interim Chief Executive Officer
CFO: Edward Chabalowski, Chief Financial Officer
CIO: Arthur Papacostas, M.D., Vice President and Chief Information Officer
Web address: www.health.temple.edu/tuh/
Control: Other not–for–profit (including NFP Corporation) **Service:** General Medical and Surgical

Staffed Beds: 678 **Admissions:** 34273 **Census:** 571 **Outpatient Visits:** 250937 **Births:** 2449 **Total Expense ($000):** 600041 **Payroll Expense ($000):** 231347 **Personnel:** 4006

□ △ **THOMAS JEFFERSON UNIVERSITY HOSPITAL (390174)**, 111 South 11th Street, Zip 19107–5096; tel. 215/955–6000, (Includes METHODIST HOSPITAL, 2301 South Broad Street, Zip 19148; tel. 215/952–9000) **A**1 2 3 5 6 7 8 9 10 **F**3 5 6 7 8 9 11 12 13 14 15 17 18 20 22 24 25 26 27 28 30 31 32 33 34 35 36 37 38 40 41 43 44 46 47 49 50 51 53 54 55 56 57 58 60 62 63 64 66 68 70 71 72 73 74 75 76 77 78 79 80 81 82 84 85 86 87 88 89 90 92 93 94 96 97 98 99 100 102 103 104 105 106 107 108 109 111 112 113 114 116 118 119 120 121 123 124 125 126 127 128 130 131 132 134 135 136 137 **P**2 8 **S** Jefferson Health System
Primary Contact: Thomas J. Lewis, CHE, President and Chief Executive Officer
COO: David P. McQuaid, Executive Vice President and Chief Operating Officer
CFO: Neil Lubarsky, Senior Vice President Finance
CMO: Geno Merli, M.D., Chief Medical Officer
CIO: Stephen Tranquillo, Chief Information Officer
Web address: www.jeffersonhospital.org
Control: Other not–for–profit (including NFP Corporation) **Service:** General Medical and Surgical

Staffed Beds: 933 **Admissions:** 45050 **Census:** 751 **Outpatient Visits:** 481659 **Births:** 2200 **Total Expense ($000):** 952361 **Payroll Expense ($000):** 385281 **Personnel:** 6793

★ △ **VETERANS AFFAIRS MEDICAL CENTER**, University and Woodland Avenues, Zip 19104–4594; tel. 215/823–5800, (Total facility includes 240 beds in nursing home–type unit) (Nonreporting) **A**1 3 5 7 8 9 **S** Department of Veterans Affairs
Primary Contact: Michael J. Sullivan, Director
COO: Margaret Caplan, Chief Operating Officer
CFO: Vinh Tran, Chief Financial Officer
CMO: Martin F. Heyworth, M.D., Chief of Staff
CIO: Adrienne Ficchi, Vice President Information Management
CHR: Gerald Morelli, Director Human Resources
Control: Veterans Affairs, Government, federal **Service:** General Medical and Surgical

Staffed Beds: 389

□ **WILLS EYE HOSPITAL**, 840 Walnut Street, Zip 19107–5109; tel. 215/928–3000, (Nonreporting) **A**1 3 5 9
Primary Contact: James J. Mulvihill, Chief Executive Officer
CFO: Jeri Mogle, Assistant Executive Director Finance
CMO: William Tasman, M.D., Ophthalmologist in Chief
CIO: William Romano, Director Information Systems and Privacy
CHR: Cynthia Farano, Director Human Resources and Compliance Officer
Web address: www.willseye.org
Control: Other not–for–profit (including NFP Corporation) **Service:** Other specialty

Staffed Beds: 40

PA

PHOENIXVILLE—Chester County

★ **PHOENIXVILLE HOSPITAL (390127)**, 140 Nutt Road, Zip 19460–3900, Mailing Address: P.O. Box 3001, Zip 19460–3001; tel. 610/983–1000 **A**1 9 10 **F**3 8 11 13 15 17 18 20 22 24 25 27 28 30 31 32 33 34 36 37 38 43 49 51 54 55 57 60 62 67 68 70 72 73 74 75 76 77 79 80 81 82 86 90 92 96 97 106 107 119 121 123 124 135 136 137 **S** Community Health Systems, Inc.
Primary Contact: Stephen M. Tullman, Chief Executive Officer
CFO: Richard Haun, Chief Financial Officer
CMO: David Stepansky, M.D., Chief Medical Officer
CIO: Terry Murphy, Director Information Services
CHR: Grant Hoffman, Director Human Resources
Web address: www.phoenixvillehospital.com
Control: Corporation, Investor–owned, for–profit **Service:** General Medical and Surgical

Staffed Beds: 136 **Admissions:** 8744 **Census:** 91 **Outpatient Visits:** 132884 **Births:** 967 **Total Expense ($000):** 125336 **Payroll Expense ($000):** 40513 **Personnel:** 714

PITTSBURGH—Allegheny County

★ **ALLEGHENY GENERAL HOSPITAL (390050)**, 320 East North Avenue, Zip 15212–4756; tel. 412/359–3131, (Includes SUBURBAN GENERAL HOSPITAL, 100 South Jackson Avenue, Zip 15202–3499; tel. 412/734–6000; Kim Sperring, Chief Executive Officer) **A**1 2 3 5 8 9 10 **F**3 7 8 9 11 12 13 15 17 18 20 22 24 25 26 27 28 30 31 32 33 34 36 37 38 40 41 42 43 46 47 48 49 50 51 52 53 55 56 57 58 59 60 61 62 63 64 66 68 70 72 73 74 75 76 77 78 79 80 81 82 83 84 86 87 88 89 90 91 92 93 94 95 96 97 98 99 100 101 102 104 106 107 108 109 110 111 112 113 114 118 119 120 121 123 124 126 127 128 129 131 132 134 135 136 137 **P**6 **S** West Penn Allegheny Health System
Primary Contact: Connie M. Cibrone, President and Chief Executive Officer
COO: Edward D. Banos, Chief Operating Officer
CFO: Dawn Javersack, Vice President and Chief Financial Officer
CMO: Parviz Baghai, M.D., President Medical Staff
CIO: Nicholas J. Valadja, Vice President Information Systems
Web address: www.wpahs.org
Control: Other not–for–profit (including NFP Corporation) **Service:** General Medical and Surgical

Staffed Beds: 473 **Admissions:** 29034 **Census:** 441 **Outpatient Visits:** 436840 **Births:** 1353 **Total Expense ($000):** 575972 **Payroll Expense ($000):** 208269 **Personnel:** 4103

□ **CHILDREN'S HOSPITAL OF PITTSBURGH OF UPMC (393302)**, 3705 Fifth Avenue at De Soto Street, Zip 15213–2583; tel. 412/692–5325, (Nonreporting) **A**1 3 5 9 10 **S** UPMC
Primary Contact: Roger A. Oxendale, President
COO: Christopher Gessner, Chief Operating Officer
Web address: www.chp.edu
Control: Other not–for–profit (including NFP Corporation) **Service:** Children's general

Staffed Beds: 260

EYE AND EAR HOSPITAL OF PITTSBURGH See UPMC Presbyterian

Hospital, Medicare Provider Number, Address, Telephone, Approval, Facility, and Physician Codes, Health Care System
★ American Hospital Association (AHA) membership
□ The Joint Commission accreditation
○ American Osteopathic Association (AOA) accreditation
△ Commission on Accreditation of Rehabilitation Facilities (CARF) accreditation

★ **HEALTHSOUTH HARMARVILLE REHABILITATION HOSPITAL (393027)**, Guys Run Road, Zip 15238–0460, Mailing Address: P.O. Box 11460, Zip 15238–0460; tel. 412/828–1300, (Nonreporting) **A**1 10 **S** HEALTHSOUTH Corporation
Primary Contact: Kenneth J. Anthony, Chief Executive Officer
CFO: Jim Steinkirchner, Regional Controller
CMO: Thomas Franz, M.D., Medical Director
CHR: Ethel Black, Director Human Resources
Web address: www.healthsouth.com
Control: Corporation, Investor–owned, for–profit **Service:** Rehabilitation

Staffed Beds: 202

★ **LIFECARE HOSPITALS OF PITTSBURGH (392024)**, 225 Penn Avenue, Zip 15221–2173; tel. 412/247–2424 **A**1 10 **F**1 3 25 26 54 72 73 79 81 82 88 93 96 107 119 121 137 **P**6 **S** LifeCare Management Services
Primary Contact: Richard Pletz, Chief Executive Officer
CFO: Harry Peterson, Chief Financial Officer
CMO: Steven Sotos, M.D., President of the Medical Staff
CIO: George Fitzgerald, Regional Director Information Systems
CHR: Robin Arslanpay, Director Human Resources
Web address: www.lifecare–hospitals.com
Control: Corporation, Investor–owned, for–profit **Service:** Long–Term Acute Care hospital

Staffed Beds: 159 **Admissions:** 1557 **Census:** 113 **Outpatient Visits:** 0 **Births:** 0 **Total Expense ($000):** 44555 **Payroll Expense ($000):** 19344 **Personnel:** 417

★ **MAGEE–WOMENS HOSPITAL OF UPMC (390114)**, 300 Halket Street, Zip 15213–3180; tel. 412/641–1000 **A**1 2 3 5 8 9 10 **F**3 11 12 13 15 25 26 27 30 31 32 33 38 41 43 44 47 49 53 55 56 57 58 62 63 64 66 68 70 72 73 74 76 77 79 80 81 82 87 96 97 99 100 102 105 107 108 109 113 114 119 120 121 123 124 135 136 137 **P**7 **S** UPMC
Primary Contact: Leslie C. Davis, President
COO: Maribeth McLaughlin, Vice President Patient Care Services
CFO: Eileen Simmons, Chief Financial Officer
CMO: Dennis English, M.D., Vice President Medical Affairs
CIO: Lou Bauerso, Chief Information Officer
CHR: Kelli Reale, Vice President Human Resources
Web address: www.magee.edu
Control: Other not–for–profit (including NFP Corporation) **Service:** Obstetrics and gynecology

Staffed Beds: 278 **Admissions:** 18297 **Census:** 204 **Outpatient Visits:** 407229 **Births:** 9468 **Total Expense ($000):** 253821 **Payroll Expense ($000):** 114312 **Personnel:** 2166

MERCY HOSPITAL OF PITTSBURGH See UPMC Mercy

MONTEFIORE HOSPITAL See UPMC Presbyterian

□ **SELECT SPECIALTY HOSPITAL (392044)**, 200 Lothrop Street, E824, Zip 15213; tel. 412/586–9819, (Nonreporting) **A**1 10 **S** Select Medical Corporation
Primary Contact: Keith J. Weinhold, Chief Executive Officer
Web address: www.selectmedicalcorp.com
Control: Corporation, Investor–owned, for–profit **Service:** Long–Term Acute Care hospital

Staffed Beds: 32

□ **SOUTHWOOD PSYCHIATRIC HOSPITAL**, 2575 Boyce Plaza Road, Zip 15241–3925; tel. 412/257–2290 **A**1 9 **F**88 89 **P**6 **S** Youth and Family Centered Services
Primary Contact: Barbara L. Callaghan, Chief Executive Officer
CFO: Harry Peterson, Chief Financial Officer
CMO: Robert J. Edelman, D.O., Medical Director
CHR: Jenifer Fetcko, Director Human Resources
Web address: www.southwoodhospital.com
Control: Corporation, Investor–owned, for–profit **Service:** Children's hospital psychiatric

Staffed Beds: 174 **Admissions:** 789 **Census:** 114 **Outpatient Visits:** 20630 **Births:** 0 **Total Expense ($000):** 12889 **Payroll Expense ($000):** 8117 **Personnel:** 230

★ **ST. CLAIR MEMORIAL HOSPITAL (390228)**, 1000 Bower Hill Road, Zip 15243–1873; tel. 412/942–4000 **A**1 2 9 10 **F**3 8 11 12 13 15 17 18 20 22 24 25 26 27 28 30 31 32 33 36 38 41 44 49 50 51 52 53 54 55 56 57 59 60 62 63 65 68 71 72 73 74 75 76 77 79 80 81 82 84 85 86 88 90 91 92 93 95 96 97 99 100 102 106 107 111 112 118 119 121 123 124 132 135 136 137
Primary Contact: James M. Collins, President and Chief Executive Officer
COO: Michael J. Flanagan, Senior Vice President and Chief Operating Officer
CFO: Richard C. Chesnos, Senior Vice President Finance and Chief Financial Officer
CMO: G. Alan Yeasted, M.D., Senior Vice President and Chief Medical Officer
CIO: Richard Schaeffer, Vice President Information Systems and Chief Information Officer
CHR: Andrea Kalina, Vice President Human Resources and Organizational Advancement
Web address: www.stclair.org
Control: Other not–for–profit (including NFP Corporation) **Service:** General Medical and Surgical

Staffed Beds: 303 **Admissions:** 15587 **Census:** 203 **Outpatient Visits:** 319595 **Births:** 1153 **Total Expense ($000):** 171298 **Payroll Expense ($000):** 70762 **Personnel:** 1607

★ **THE CHILDREN'S HOME OF PITTSBURGH (393304)**, 5324 Penn Avenue, Zip 15224; tel. 412/441–4884 **A**9 10 **F**3 25 58 81 84 135
Primary Contact: Pamela R. Schanwald, Chief Executive Officer
COO: Karen Schneider, Chief Operating Officer
CFO: Kimberly A. Phillips, Director Finance
CMO: Debrah Flowers, Chief Clinical Officer
Web address: www.childrenshomepgh.org
Control: Other not–for–profit (including NFP Corporation) **Service:** Children's general

Staffed Beds: 28 **Admissions:** 140 **Census:** 8 **Outpatient Visits:** 0 **Total Expense ($000):** 6063 **Payroll Expense ($000):** 3064 **Personnel:** 40

★ △ **THE CHILDREN'S INSTITUTE OF PITTSBURGH (393308)**, 1405 Shady Avenue, Zip 15217–1396; tel. 412/420–2400 **A**1 7 10 **F**3 25 26 30 31 32 33 53 56 62 72 73 77 80 81 82 85 86 89 90 96 119 121 135 **P**6
Primary Contact: David K. Miles, President and Chief Executive Officer
COO: Jane T. Keim, Vice President Operations
CFO: Jody Mulvihill, Vice President Finance
CMO: Maryanne Henderson, Medical Director
CIO: Sharon Dorogy, Director Information Systems
CHR: Bob Brown, Director Human Resources
Web address: www.amazingkids.org
Control: Other not–for–profit (including NFP Corporation) **Service:** Children's rehabilitation

Staffed Beds: 48 **Admissions:** 400 **Census:** 32 **Outpatient Visits:** 34191 **Births:** 0 **Total Expense ($000):** 23473 **Payroll Expense ($000):** 11363 **Personnel:** 275

★ △ **UPMC MERCY (390028)**, (Formerly Mercy Hospital of Pittsburgh), 1400 Locust Street, Zip 15219–5166; tel. 412/232–8111 **A**1 3 5 6 7 8 9 10 12 13 **F**3 4 13 15 16 18 20 22 24 25 26 27 28 30 31 32 33 34 35 38 40 41 43 44 49 50 51 53 54 55 56 57 59 60 61 62 63 64 68 70 72 73 74 75 76 77 79 80 81 82 84 85 86 87 88 92 94 96 97 100 102 104 106 107 108 109 111 112 114 116 118 119 120 121 123 133 135 136 137 **S** UPMC
Primary Contact: Kenneth A. Eshak, President and Chief Executive Officer
CFO: Jack Gaenzle, Senior Vice President Finance and Administration
CIO: Stephen D. Adams, Executive Vice President and Chief Executive Officer
CHR: Kristen Bell, Director Human Resources
Web address: www.upmc.com/HospitalsFacilities/HFHome/Hospitals/Mercy/
Control: Other not–for–profit (including NFP Corporation) **Service:** General Medical and Surgical

Staffed Beds: 413 **Admissions:** 18215 **Census:** 258 **Outpatient Visits:** 201492 **Births:** 1574 **Total Expense ($000):** 258259 **Payroll Expense ($000):** 94991 **Personnel:** 2161

□ **UPMC PASSAVANT (390107)**, 9100 Babcock Boulevard, Zip 15237–5815; tel. 412/367–6700, (Includes UPMC PASSAVANT CRANBERRY, One St. Francis Way, Cranberry, Zip 16066; tel. 724/772–5300; Teresa A. Petrick, President) **A**1 9 10 **F**3 11 15 17 18 20 22 24 25 26 27 30 31 32 33 38 42 43 44 45 46 47 48 49 51 54 55 56 57 61 62 63 66 68 72 73 75 76 77 79 80 81 82 85 86 90 96 100 102 103 104 105 106 107 109 118 119 121 122 124 132 135 137 **S** UPMC
Primary Contact: Teresa A. Petrick, President
COO: Marcie S. Caplan, Vice President
CFO: Dennis Tomassetti, Chief Financial Officer
CMO: James W. Boyle, M.D., Chief Medical Officer
CIO: Karen Borosky, Vice President and Chief Information Officer
CHR: Gary Mignosna, Vice President Human Resources
Web address: www.upmc.edu/passavant
Control: Other not–for–profit (including NFP Corporation) **Service:** General Medical and Surgical

Staffed Beds: 346 **Admissions:** 16052 **Census:** 225 **Outpatient Visits:** 366023 **Births:** 0 **Total Expense ($000):** 207416 **Payroll Expense ($000):** 78454 **Personnel:** 2404

Many Facility Codes have changed. Please refer to the AHA Guide Code Chart.

□ **UPMC PRESBYTERIAN (390164)**, 200 Lothrop Street, Zip 15213–2585; tel. 412/647–2345, (Includes EYE AND EAR HOSPITAL OF PITTSBURGH; MONTEFIORE HOSPITAL; UPMC PRESBYTERIAN HOSPITAL; UPMC SHADYSIDE, 5230 Centre Avenue, Zip 15232–1381; tel. 412/623–2121; WESTERN PSYCHIATRIC INSTITUTE AND CLINIC, 3811 O'Hara Street, Zip 15213–2593; tel. 412/624–2100), (Total facility includes 30 beds in nursing home–type unit) **A**1 3 5 6 8 9 10 13 **F**2 3 5 6 7 8 9 10 11 12 14 15 17 18 20 22 24 25 26 27 28 29 30 31 32 33 34 35 36 37 38 40 41 42 43 44 45 46 47 48 49 50 51 52 53 54 55 56 57 58 59 60 61 62 63 64 66 67 68 69 72 73 75 76 77 79 80 81 82 85 86 87 88 89 90 91 92 93 94 95 96 97 98 99 100 102 103 104 105 106 107 108 109 111 112 113 114 116 117 118 119 120 121 123 124 125 126 127 128 129 130 131 132 134 135 136 137 **P**6 **S** UPMC
Primary Contact: John Innocenti, President and Chief Executive Officer
COO: James Terwilliger, Vice President Operations
CFO: Paul Castillo, Chief Financial Officer
CMO: Margaret Reidy, Vice President Medical Affairs
CIO: James Venturella, Chief Information Officer
CHR: Louis Goodman, Vice President Human Resources
Web address: www.upmc.edu
Control: Other not–for–profit (including NFP Corporation) **Service:** General Medical and Surgical

Staffed Beds: 1501 **Admissions:** 65199 **Census:** 1264 **Outpatient Visits:** 1131058 **Births:** 0 **Total Expense ($000):** 1473446 **Payroll Expense ($000):** 447138 **Personnel:** 13067

□ △ **UPMC SOUTH SIDE (390131)**, 2000 Mary Street, Zip 15203–2095; tel. 412/488–5550 **A**1 5 7 9 10 **F**3 8 15 25 30 31 32 38 43 46 47 49 59 61 63 68 73 77 78 79 80 81 82 86 87 96 97 100 102 106 107 118 119 121 124 135 136 137 **S** UPMC
Primary Contact: Nancy Magee, President
COO: Nancy Magee, President
CFO: William Miller, Vice President Finance
CMO: Jalit Tuchinda, M.D., Medical Staff President
CIO: Lisa Khorey, Chief Information Officer
CHR: Jonathan Forbes, Director Human Resources
Web address: www.upmc.com
Control: Other not–for–profit (including NFP Corporation) **Service:** General Medical and Surgical

Staffed Beds: 150 **Admissions:** 5701 **Census:** 118 **Outpatient Visits:** 68288 **Births:** 0 **Total Expense ($000):** 76176 **Payroll Expense ($000):** 28391 **Personnel:** 609

□ **UPMC ST. MARGARET (390102)**, 815 Freeport Road, Zip 15215–3399; tel. 412/784–4000 **A**1 2 3 5 6 9 10 12 13 **F**3 6 8 9 11 12 15 18 24 25 26 27 30 31 32 33 35 38 41 42 43 44 49 50 51 52 53 54 55 56 57 59 60 62 63 66 68 72 73 75 76 77 79 80 81 82 85 86 87 92 93 94 96 97 100 102 103 106 107 109 111 118 119 120 121 123 124 135 **S** UPMC
Primary Contact: David T. Martin, President
CFO: Thomas M. Newman, Vice President Finance
CMO: Vincent J. Silvaggio, M.D., Medical Staff President
CIO: Charles M. Rudek, Chief Information Officer
CHR: Leeann Cerimele, Vice President Human Resources
Web address: www.horizon.upmc.com
Control: Other not–for–profit (including NFP Corporation) **Service:** General Medical and Surgical

Staffed Beds: 240 **Admissions:** 14021 **Census:** 186 **Outpatient Visits:** 248272 **Births:** 0 **Total Expense ($000):** 188199 **Payroll Expense ($000):** 67194 **Personnel:** 1563

★ **VETERANS AFFAIRS PITTSBURGH HEALTHCARE SYSTEM**, Delafield Road, Zip 15240–1001; tel. 412/688–6000, (Includes VETERANS AFFAIRS MEDICAL CENTER, 7180 Highland Drive, Zip 15206–1297; tel. 412/365–4900; VETERANS AFFAIRS MEDICAL CENTER, University Drive C., tel. 412/688–6000), (Total facility includes 336 beds in nursing home–type unit) **A**1 2 8 **F**1 2 3 4 5 6 7 8 10 11 12 18 20 21 22 24 25 26 27 30 31 32 33 36 37 38 41 42 43 44 45 46 47 49 50 52 53 54 55 56 57 58 59 60 61 62 63 64 65 66 68 69 72 73 75 76 77 79 80 81 82 85 86 87 88 90 91 92 93 94 95 96 100 101 103 107 116 117 118 119 121 122 124 127 128 132 133 134 135 136 137 **P**1 **S** Department of Veterans Affairs
Primary Contact: Terry Gerigk Wolf, Director
CFO: James Baker, Vice President Business Support Services
CMO: Rajiv Jain, M.D., Chief of Staff
CIO: Dewaine Beard, Chief Information Officer
CHR: Michelle Dominski, Acting Human Resources Officer
Web address: www.va.gov/pittsburgh
Control: Veterans Affairs, Government, federal **Service:** General Medical and Surgical

Staffed Beds: 692 **Admissions:** 9047 **Census:** 489 **Outpatient Visits:** 489814 **Total Expense ($000):** 434326 **Payroll Expense ($000):** 147561 **Personnel:** 2680

★ **WESTERN PENNSYLVANIA HOSPITAL (390090)**, 4800 Friendship Avenue, Zip 15224–1722; tel. 412/578–5000 **A**1 2 3 5 6 8 9 10 12 13 **F**3 12 13 15 16 17 18 20 22 24 25 26 27 33 35 38 43 44 45 46 49 51 55 56 57 58 59 61 62 66 68 70 72 73 74 75 76 77 78 79 80 81 82 84 85 86 87 92 96 97 98 99 100 102 103 104 105 106 107 108 109 111 112 114 116 118 119 121 124 125 134 135 136 137 **P**6 **S** West Penn Allegheny Health System
Primary Contact: Dawn M. Gideon, President and Chief Executive Officer
COO: Sherry Zisk, R.N., Chief Operating Officer
CFO: Augustine Lopez, Chief Financial Officer
CMO: Mark Rubino, M.D., President Medical Staff
CIO: Christine B. Middlemiss, Senior Director Information Services
CHR: Tanya Ulrich, Director Human Resources
Web address: www.wpahs.org
Control: Other not–for–profit (including NFP Corporation) **Service:** General Medical and Surgical

Staffed Beds: 448 **Admissions:** 19177 **Census:** 268 **Outpatient Visits:** 138951 **Births:** 2443 **Total Expense ($000):** 272084 **Payroll Expense ($000):** 116640 **Personnel:** 2603

WESTERN PSYCHIATRIC INSTITUTE AND CLINIC See UPMC Presbyterian

PA

PLEASANT GAP—Centre County

★ **HEALTHSOUTH NITTANY VALLEY REHABILITATION HOSPITAL (393039)**, 550 West College Avenue, Zip 16823–7416; tel. 814/359–3421, (Nonreporting) **A**1 9 10 **S** HEALTHSOUTH Corporation
Primary Contact: Susan Hartman, Chief Executive Officer
CFO: Steven Alwine, Controller
CMO: Richard Allatt, M.D., Medical Director
CHR: Jody Hay, Director Human Resources
Web address: www.nittanyvalleyrehab.com
Control: Corporation, Investor–owned, for–profit **Service:** Rehabilitation

Staffed Beds: 85

POTTSTOWN—Montgomery County

★ **POTTSTOWN MEMORIAL MEDICAL CENTER (390123)**, 1600 East High Street, Zip 19464–5093; tel. 610/327–7000 **A**1 2 9 10 **F**10 13 15 18 25 26 27 31 32 33 36 37 38 49 50 52 53 54 55 57 59 61 62 66 68 72 73 74 75 76 77 79 80 82 84 85 86 88 92 93 96 106 107 118 121 124 136 137 **P**6 **S** Community Health Systems, Inc.
Primary Contact: Steven MacLauchlan, Chief Executive Officer
CFO: Neal R. Fegely, Vice President Finance and Chief Financial Officer
CMO: Richard F. Saylor, M.D., Vice President Medical Affairs
CIO: Ron Peterson, Chief Information Officer
Web address: www.pottstownmemorial.com
Control: Corporation, Investor–owned, for–profit **Service:** General Medical and Surgical

Staffed Beds: 226 **Admissions:** 10466 **Census:** 124 **Outpatient Visits:** 139409 **Births:** 756 **Total Expense ($000):** 112769 **Payroll Expense ($000):** 46814 **Personnel:** 827

POTTSVILLE—Schuylkill County

★ △ **GOOD SAMARITAN REGIONAL MEDICAL CENTER (390031)**, 700 East Norwegian Street, Zip 17901–2798; tel. 570/621–4000 **A**1 2 7 9 10 **F**5 11 15 26 27 30 31 32 37 38 40 43 49 54 55 56 57 60 62 68 72 73 75 76 77 79 80 81 82 84 85 86 88 90 93 96 97 99 100 103 107 118 119 121 124 135 136 137 **P**6 **S** Ascension Health
Primary Contact: Bernard G. Koval, President and Chief Executive Officer
CFO: Daniel A. Kochie, CPA, Senior Vice President and Chief Financial Officer
CMO: Thomas McLaughlin, M.D., Chief Medical Officer
CIO: David Schneck, Director Health Information Management and Technology
CHR: Denis Orthaus, Director Human Resources
Web address: www.gsrmc.com
Control: Church–operated, Nongovernment, not–for profit **Service:** General Medical and Surgical

Staffed Beds: 136 **Admissions:** 6672 **Census:** 101 **Outpatient Visits:** 150200 **Births:** 0 **Total Expense ($000):** 67812 **Payroll Expense ($000):** 27778 **Personnel:** 661

Hospital, Medicare Provider Number, Address, Telephone, Approval, Facility, and Physician Codes, Health Care System
★ American Hospital Association (AHA) membership
□ The Joint Commission accreditation
○ American Osteopathic Association (AOA) accreditation
△ Commission on Accreditation of Rehabilitation Facilities (CARF) accreditation

★ △ **POTTSVILLE HOSPITAL AND WARNE CLINIC (390030)**, 420 South Jackson Street, Zip 17901–3692; tel. 570/621–5000 **A**1 2 6 7 9 10 19 **F**3 11 13 15 24 26 28 30 31 32 33 36 37 38 43 46 49 50 51 53 54 55 56 57 60 61 62 66 68 72 73 74 75 76 77 79 80 81 84 85 86 88 89 90 91 92 93 94 95 96 97 99 100 102 104 106 107 118 119 120 124 135 136 137
Primary Contact: John E. Simodejka, President and Chief Executive Officer
CFO: Craig P. Hunt, Vice President Operations and Finance
CIO: Carla Ambrosius, Interim Director Health Information Management
CHR: Martin Treasure, Director Human Resources
Web address: www.pottsvillehospital.com
Control: Other not–for–profit (including NFP Corporation) **Service:** General Medical and Surgical

Staffed Beds: 200 **Admissions:** 8932 **Census:** 123 **Outpatient Visits:** 110304 **Births:** 1158 **Total Expense ($000):** 79357 **Payroll Expense ($000):** 34341 **Personnel:** 768

PUNXSUTAWNEY—Jefferson County

PUNXSUTAWNEY AREA HOSPITAL (390199), 81 Hillcrest Drive, Zip 15767–2616; tel. 814/938–1800, (Nonreporting) **A**9 10
Primary Contact: Daniel D. Blough, Jr., Chief Executive Officer
CFO: Jack Sisk, Chief Financial Officer
CMO: Dajani Zuhd, M.D., President Medical Staff
CIO: Chuck States, Director Information Systems
CHR: Barbara Kostok, Manager Human Resources
Web address: www.pah.org
Control: Other not–for–profit (including NFP Corporation) **Service:** General Medical and Surgical

Staffed Beds: 44

QUAKERTOWN—Bucks County

□ **ST. LUKE'S QUAKERTOWN HOSPITAL (390035)**, 1021 Park Avenue, Zip 18951–9003; tel. 215/538–4510 **A**1 2 9 10 **F**3 7 11 15 24 25 26 30 31 32 33 36 38 41 42 43 49 50 51 52 53 54 55 56 57 58 59 62 66 67 68 72 73 75 76 77 79 80 81 82 86 88 89 90 92 93 96 97 99 100 103 106 107 118 119 121 122 123 124 132 134 135 136 137 **P**6 8
Primary Contact: Edward Nawrocki, President
CFO: Theresa Corrado, Director Finance
CMO: Thomas Filipowicz, Medical Director
CIO: Albert Sinisi, Chief Information Officer
CHR: Shelley Maley, Director
Web address: www.slhhn.org
Control: Other not–for–profit (including NFP Corporation) **Service:** General Medical and Surgical

Staffed Beds: 57 **Admissions:** 3378 **Census:** 38 **Outpatient Visits:** 74097 **Births:** 0 **Total Expense ($000):** 37693 **Payroll Expense ($000):** 14075 **Personnel:** 289

READING—Berks County

★ **HEALTHSOUTH READING REHABILITATION HOSPITAL (393026)**, 1623 Morgantown Road, Zip 19607–9455; tel. 610/796–6000, (Nonreporting) **A**1 9 10 **S** HEALTHSOUTH Corporation
Primary Contact: Richard Kruczek, Chief Executive Officer
CFO: Jason Pulaski, Controller
CMO: Patti Brown, Medical Director
CHR: Steve Walas, Director Human Resources
Web address: www.healthsouthreading.com
Control: Corporation, Investor–owned, for–profit **Service:** Rehabilitation

Staffed Beds: 95

★ **ST. JOSEPH MEDICAL CENTER (390096)**, 2500 Bernville Road, Zip 19605, Mailing Address: P.O. Box 316, Zip 19603–0316; tel. 610/378–2000, (Includes ST. JOSEPH MEDICAL CENTER–DOWNTOWN READING, 145 North Sixth Street, Zip 19601; tel. 610/376–2100), (Total facility includes 24 beds in nursing home–type unit) **A**1 2 9 10 12 13 **F**2 3 8 11 12 13 15 18 20 22 24 25 26 27 28 30 31 32 33 34 36 37 38 41 43 44 49 50 51 52 53 54 55 56 57 60 62 63 64 66 68 70 72 73 74 75 76 77 79 80 81 82 84 86 87 88 89 90 91 92 93 94 95 96 97 100 104 105 106 107 108 109 117 119 120 121 124 133 135 136 137 **P**6 **S** Catholic Health Initiatives
Primary Contact: John R. Morahan, President and Chief Executive Officer
CFO: Lim David, Vice President Finance and Chief Financial Officer
CMO: Samuel Alfano, M.D., Vice President Medical Affairs
CIO: Mary Babb, Director Information Technology
CHR: Scott Mengle, Vice President Human Resources
Web address: www.thefutureofhealthcare.org
Control: Church–operated, Nongovernment, not–for profit **Service:** General Medical and Surgical

Staffed Beds: 232 **Admissions:** 10198 **Census:** 142 **Outpatient Visits:** 287977 **Births:** 737 **Total Expense ($000):** 160061 **Payroll Expense ($000):** 59270 **Personnel:** 1132

RENOVO—Clinton County

BUCKTAIL MEDICAL CENTER (391304), 1001 Pine Street, Zip 17764–1620; tel. 570/923–1000, (Total facility includes 45 beds in nursing home–type unit) **A**9 10 18 **F**31 38 67 96 117 119 122 **P**5
Primary Contact: Anita L. Rathgeber, Administrator
CFO: Kimberly Rossell, Manager Accounting
CMO: David Lennon, M.D., Medical Director
Control: Other not–for–profit (including NFP Corporation) **Service:** General Medical and Surgical

Staffed Beds: 62 **Admissions:** 101 **Census:** 42 **Outpatient Visits:** 10498 **Births:** 0 **Total Expense ($000):** 5877 **Payroll Expense ($000):** 2439 **Personnel:** 77

RIDLEY PARK—Delaware County

TAYLOR HOSPITAL See Crozer–Chester Medical Center, Upland

ROARING SPRING—Blair County

★ **NASON HOSPITAL (390062)**, 105 Nason Drive, Zip 16673–1202; tel. 814/224–2141, (Nonreporting) **A**1 9 10
Primary Contact: Garrett W. Hoover, CHE, President and Chief Executive Officer
CFO: Raymond C. Askey, Vice President Fiscal Services
CIO: Brian Lilly, Director Information Systems
CHR: Patricia McGraw, Director Human Resources
Web address: www.nasonhospital.org
Control: Other not–for–profit (including NFP Corporation) **Service:** General Medical and Surgical

Staffed Beds: 42

SAINT MARYS—Elk County

★ **ELK REGIONAL HEALTH CENTER (390154)**, 763 Johnsonburg Road, Zip 15857–3498; tel. 814/788–8000, (Total facility includes 138 beds in nursing home–type unit) **A**9 10 20 **F**3 6 11 13 15 18 24 25 26 30 31 32 33 38 41 43 55 56 57 68 72 74 75 77 79 80 81 82 84 86 88 93 96 97 100 102 107 117 118 119 120 122 124 133 135 136 137
Primary Contact: Gregory Bauer, President and Chief Executive Officer
CFO: Laurie MacDonald, Chief Financial Officer
CMO: Dean Stokes, M.D., President Medical Staff
CHR: James Chiesa, Director Human Resources
Web address: www.elkregional.org
Control: Other not–for–profit (including NFP Corporation) **Service:** General Medical and Surgical

Staffed Beds: 218 **Admissions:** 3663 **Census:** 157 **Outpatient Visits:** 138546 **Births:** 236 **Total Expense ($000):** 54614 **Payroll Expense ($000):** 24870 **Personnel:** 765

SAYRE—Bradford County

★ **ROBERT PACKER HOSPITAL (390079)**, 1 Guthrie Square, Zip 18840–1698; tel. 570/888–6666 **A**1 2 3 5 9 10 12 13 19 **F**3 11 13 15 17 18 20 22 24 25 26 27 30 31 32 35 36 38 40 43 47 49 50 51 55 56 57 58 59 60 62 66 68 71 72 73 74 75 76 77 79 80 81 82 84 86 88 89 90 91 92 93 95 96 97 100 102 103 106 107 109 118 119 121 130 131 134 135 137 **S** Guthrie Healthcare System
Primary Contact: Marie T. Droege, President and Chief Operating Officer
CFO: Minh Dang, Vice President Finance
CMO: Anthony Oliva, D.O., Chief Medical Officer
CIO: Dale Swingle, Vice President Information Services
CHR: Frank Pinkosky, Senior Vice President
Web address: www.guthrie.org
Control: Other not–for–profit (including NFP Corporation) **Service:** General Medical and Surgical

Staffed Beds: 224 **Admissions:** 12196 **Census:** 144 **Outpatient Visits:** 158077 **Births:** 791 **Total Expense ($000):** 178936 **Payroll Expense ($000):** 51297 **Personnel:** 1144

SCRANTON—Lackawanna County

★ △ **ALLIED SERVICES REHABILITATION HOSPITAL (393030)**, 475 Morgan Highway, Zip 18501–1103, Mailing Address: P.O. Box 1103, Zip 18501–1103; tel. 570/348–1300 **A**1 7 10 **F**11 25 33 43 52 54 56 57 62 72 73 75 76 77 81 82 85 86 119 132 135
Primary Contact: James L. Brady, President
COO: Jackie Brozena, Senior Vice President
CFO: Michael Avvisato, Vice President and Chief Financial Officer
CMO: Gregory Basting, M.D., Vice President Medical Affairs
CIO: John Regula, Chief Information Officer
CHR: Susan D. Montross, Vice President Human Resources
Web address: www.allied–services.org
Control: Other not–for–profit (including NFP Corporation) **Service:** Rehabilitation

Staffed Beds: 117 **Admissions:** 2343 **Census:** 68 **Outpatient Visits:** 102869 **Births:** 0 **Total Expense ($000):** 35787 **Payroll Expense ($000):** 16977 **Personnel:** 424

 Many Facility Codes have changed. Please refer to the AHA Guide Code Chart.

★ **COMMUNITY MEDICAL CENTER (390001)**, 1800 Mulberry Street, Zip 18510–2523, Mailing Address: P.O. Box 2037, Zip 18501–2037; tel. 570/969–8000 **A**1 9 10 **F**3 11 12 13 15 17 18 20 22 24 25 26 27 30 31 32 33 38 40 41 43 47 49 50 54 55 56 57 58 60 62 66 68 70 71 72 73 74 75 76 77 79 80 81 82 84 86 87 88 90 92 93 95 96 97 100 102 103 106 107 114 119 121 124 130 131 135 136 137
Primary Contact: John Nilsson, Interim President and Chief Executive Officer
COO: Barbara Bossi, Senior Vice President Patient Care Services and Operations
CFO: Thomas Kelly, Interim Chief Financial Officer
CIO: Joseph Fisne, Chief Information Officer
CHR: Lois Wolfe, Director Human Resources
Web address: www.cmchealthsys.org
Control: Other not–for–profit (including NFP Corporation) **Service:** General Medical and Surgical

Staffed Beds: 253 **Admissions:** 13688 **Census:** 178 **Outpatient Visits:** 97863 **Births:** 640 **Total Expense ($000):** 141714 **Payroll Expense ($000):** 56350 **Personnel:** 1054

★ △ **MERCY HOSPITAL OF SCRANTON (390237)**, 746 Jefferson Avenue, Zip 18501–1697; tel. 570/348–7100 **A**1 2 3 5 7 9 10 **F**8 11 13 15 17 18 20 22 24 25 26 27 28 30 31 32 33 37 38 41 42 44 45 46 47 48 49 50 51 52 53 55 56 57 58 60 61 62 63 64 66 68 72 73 74 75 76 77 79 80 81 82 84 86 87 96 97 98 99 100 101 102 103 104 105 106 107 108 109 110 111 112 117 118 119 121 132 133 134 135 136 137 **P**6 **S** Catholic Healthcare Partners
Primary Contact: John M. Starcher, Interim President and Chief Executive Officer
COO: Jacquelyn Gaines, President and Chief Executive Officer
CFO: Stephen Franko, Vice President Finance and Chief Financial Officer
CMO: E. Donald Kotchick, M.D., Vice President Medical Affairs
CIO: John Howells, Chief Information Officer
CHR: Maggie Lund, Vice President Human Resources
Web address: www.mhs–nepa.com
Control: Church–operated, Nongovernment, not–for profit **Service:** General Medical and Surgical

Staffed Beds: 230 **Admissions:** 10760 **Census:** 132 **Outpatient Visits:** 177015 **Births:** 239 **Total Expense ($000):** 134784 **Payroll Expense ($000):** 50220 **Personnel:** 1069

★ △ **MOSES TAYLOR HOSPITAL (390119)**, 700 Quincy Avenue, Zip 18510–1798, Mailing Address: P.O. Box 1270, Zip 18501–1270; tel. 570/340–2100, (Total facility includes 32 beds in nursing home–type unit) **A**1 3 5 7 9 10 **F**3 11 13 15 24 25 26 27 30 31 32 38 43 46 49 51 54 55 56 57 60 61 62 63 64 66 68 70 72 73 74 75 76 77 79 80 81 82 84 86 88 93 96 97 100 102 103 107 117 118 119 121 124 135 136 137 **P**6
Primary Contact: Harold E. Anderson, Chief Executive Officer
CFO: James G. Brittain, Acting Chief Financial Officer
CMO: Carmen A. Brutico, M.D., Chief Medical Officer
CIO: Edward Roman, Chief Information Officer and Chief Privacy Officer
CHR: Paul Gionfriddo, Vice President Human Resources
Web address: www.mth.org
Control: Other not–for–profit (including NFP Corporation) **Service:** General Medical and Surgical

Staffed Beds: 227 **Admissions:** 10573 **Census:** 174 **Outpatient Visits:** 149653 **Births:** 2064 **Total Expense ($000):** 117290 **Payroll Expense ($000):** 46852 **Personnel:** 1154

SELLERSVILLE—Bucks County

★ **GRAND VIEW HOSPITAL (390057)**, 700 Lawn Avenue, Zip 18960–1576, Mailing Address: P.O. Box 902, Zip 18960–0902; tel. 215/453–4000 **A**1 2 5 9 10 **F**3 7 11 13 15 24 25 26 27 28 30 31 32 33 35 38 41 42 43 46 49 50 53 54 55 56 57 60 61 62 63 66 68 71 72 74 75 76 77 79 80 81 82 84 85 86 88 96 97 99 100 102 103 106 107 109 111 119 120 121 124 134 135 136 137 **P**6
Primary Contact: Stuart H. Fine, Chief Executive Officer
CFO: Gregory Wuerstle, Vice President Finance
CMO: Jane Ferry, M.D., Vice President Medical Affairs
CIO: Jane Doll Loveless, Vice President Information Services
Web address: www.gvh.org
Control: Other not–for–profit (including NFP Corporation) **Service:** General Medical and Surgical

Staffed Beds: 197 **Admissions:** 10421 **Census:** 123 **Outpatient Visits:** 279330 **Births:** 1445 **Total Expense ($000):** 145733 **Payroll Expense ($000):** 70877 **Personnel:** 1234

SENECA—Venango County

□ **UPMC NORTHWEST (390091)**, 100 Fairfield Drive, Zip 16346; tel. 814/676–7600, (Total facility includes 16 beds in nursing home–type unit) **A**1 2 9 10 19 **F**3 11 13 15 18 24 25 26 27 30 31 32 33 38 41 46 49 50 55 56 57 66 67 68 72 73 74 75 76 77 79 80 81 82 84 85 86 87 88 89 90 93 96 97 100 102 105 107 109 111 117 118 119 120 121 124 134 135 137 **S** UPMC
Primary Contact: Neil E. Todhunter, President
CFO: W. Roger McCauley, Senior Vice President Administration and Chief Financial Officer
CMO: John Shonnard, M.D., Medical Director
CIO: Melinda Remley, Vice Patient Medical and Information Services
CHR: Courtney Cox, Vice President Human Resources
Web address: www.northwest.upmc.com
Control: Other not–for–profit (including NFP Corporation) **Service:** General Medical and Surgical

Staffed Beds: 159 **Admissions:** 8158 **Census:** 101 **Outpatient Visits:** 179951 **Births:** 500 **Total Expense ($000):** 83530 **Payroll Expense ($000):** 30873 **Personnel:** 794

SEWICKLEY—Allegheny County

★ **HEALTHSOUTH REHABILITATION HOSPITAL (393045)**, 303 Camp Meeting Road, Zip 15143–8322; tel. 412/741–9500, (Nonreporting) **A**1 10 **S** HEALTHSOUTH Corporation
Primary Contact: Marlene Hughes, Chief Executive Officer
CFO: Jim Steinkirchner, Regional Controller
CMO: Shelana Gibbs–McElvy, Medical Director
CIO: Daryl Ault, Director Information Services
CHR: Kathy Mischler, Director Human Resources
Web address: www.healthsouth.com
Control: Corporation, Investor–owned, for–profit **Service:** Rehabilitation

Staffed Beds: 31

SEWICKLEY VALLEY HOSPITAL See Sewickley Valley Hospital, (A Division of Valley Medical Facilities)

□ **SEWICKLEY VALLEY HOSPITAL, (A DIVISION OF VALLEY MEDICAL FACILITIES) (390037)**, (Formerly Sewickley Valley Hospital), 720 Blackburn Road, Zip 15143–1459; tel. 412/741–6600, (Nonreporting) **A**1 6 9 10 **S** Heritage Valley Health System
Primary Contact: Norman F. Mitry, President and Chief Executive Officer
COO: Rosemary Nolan, Chief Operating Officer and Chief Nursing Officer
CFO: Bryan J. Randall, Vice President Finance and Chief Financial Officer
CMO: Oliver Hayes, D.O., Chief Medical Officer
CIO: David Carleton, Chief Information Officer
CHR: Bruce Edwards, Vice President Human Resources
Web address: www.heritagevalley.org
Control: Other not–for–profit (including NFP Corporation) **Service:** General Medical and Surgical

Staffed Beds: 175

SHARON—Mercer County

★ **SHARON REGIONAL HEALTH SYSTEM (390211)**, 740 East State Street, Zip 16146–3395; tel. 724/983–3911, (Total facility includes 38 beds in nursing home–type unit) **A**1 2 6 9 10 **F**3 5 11 13 15 17 18 20 22 24 25 26 27 28 30 31 32 33 36 37 38 41 42 43 44 46 47 49 50 51 53 54 55 56 57 58 59 61 62 68 71 72 73 74 75 76 77 78 79 80 81 82 84 85 86 88 89 90 91 92 93 94 95 96 97 99 100 102 103 106 107 109 111 117 118 119 120 121 123 124 135 136 137 **P**6 8
Primary Contact: John A. Zidansek, President and Chief Executive Officer
CFO: Jeffrey Chrosak, Vice President Finance and Chief Financial Officer
CMO: Larry Baling, M.D., Chief Medical Officer
CIO: Jack Janoso, Chief Information Officer
CHR: John Davidson, Vice President Human Resources
Web address: www.sharonregional.com
Control: Other not–for–profit (including NFP Corporation) **Service:** General Medical and Surgical

Staffed Beds: 236 **Admissions:** 10390 **Census:** 156 **Outpatient Visits:** 312444 **Births:** 346 **Total Expense ($000):** 136099 **Payroll Expense ($000):** 54966 **Personnel:** 1424

SHICKSHINNY—Luzerne County

CLEAR BROOK LODGE, 890 Bethel Road, Zip 18655; tel. 570/864–3116, (Nonreporting)
Primary Contact: Nicholas Colangelo, Chief Executive Officer
Web address: www.clearbrookinc.com
Control: Other not–for–profit (including NFP Corporation) **Service:** Alcoholism and other chemical dependency

Staffed Beds: 65

PA

Hospital, Medicare Provider Number, Address, Telephone, Approval, Facility, and Physician Codes, Health Care System

★ American Hospital Association (AHA) membership
□ The Joint Commission accreditation
○ American Osteopathic Association (AOA) accreditation
△ Commission on Accreditation of Rehabilitation Facilities (CARF) accreditation

SOMERSET—Somerset County

★ **SOMERSET HOSPITAL (390039)**, 225 South Center Avenue, Zip 15501–2088; tel. 814/443–5000, (Total facility includes 15 beds in nursing home–type unit) **A**9 10 20 **F**3 5 8 11 12 13 15 17 18 20 24 25 26 28 30 31 32 33 36 38 42 43 44 49 51 52 54 55 56 57 59 60 61 62 63 64 65 66 68 69 72 73 74 75 76 77 79 80 81 82 84 86 87 88 89 90 91 92 93 94 96 97 98 100 102 106 107 117 118 119 120 121 122 123 124 135 136 137 **P**6
Primary Contact: Michael J. Farrell, FACHE, Chief Executive Officer
COO: Cheryl Brill, FACHE, Vice President, Chief Nursing Officer and Chief Operating Officer
CFO: Ron Park, Chief Financial Officer
CIO: Jonathan Bauer, Director Information Services
CHR: Sharon Glover, Director Human Resources
Web address: www.somersethospital.com
Control: Other not–for–profit (including NFP Corporation) **Service:** General Medical and Surgical

Staffed Beds: 134 **Admissions:** 5085 **Census:** 67 **Outpatient Visits:** 163493 **Births:** 422 **Total Expense ($000):** 55208 **Payroll Expense ($000):** 21470 **Personnel:** 578

PA

SPRINGFIELD—Delaware County

SPRINGFIELD HOSPITAL See Crozer–Chester Medical Center, Upland

STATE COLLEGE—Centre County

★ **MOUNT NITTANY MEDICAL CENTER (390268)**, 1800 Park Avenue, Zip 16803–6797; tel. 814/231–7000, (Nonreporting) **A**1 2 5 9 10
Primary Contact: Thomas J. Murray, FACHE, President and Chief Executive Officer
COO: David B. Peterson, Executive Vice President and Chief Operating Officer
CFO: Richard Wisniewski, Senior Vice President Finance and Chief Financial Officer
CMO: Francis X. Speidel, M.D., Senior Vice President Medical Affairs and Chief Quality Officer
CIO: Kenneth Bixel, Senior Vice President and Chief Information Officer
CHR: Jerry Dittmann, Vice President Human Resources
Web address: www.mountnittany.org
Control: Other not–for–profit (including NFP Corporation) **Service:** General Medical and Surgical

Staffed Beds: 199

SUNBURY—Northumberland County

★ **SUNBURY COMMUNITY HOSPITAL (390084)**, 350 North Eleventh Street, Zip 17801–0737; tel. 570/286–3333, (Total facility includes 29 beds in nursing home–type unit) **A**9 10 **F**3 15 17 24 25 26 30 32 38 49 56 57 67 68 73 75 76 77 79 80 84 85 86 88 96 100 107 112 117 119 122 135 **S** Community Health Systems, Inc.
Primary Contact: Cornelio R. Catena, Interim Chief Executive Officer
CFO: Anthony Tortella, Chief Financial Officer
CHR: Talia Beatty, Director Human Resources
Web address: www.schopc.org
Control: Corporation, Investor–owned, for–profit **Service:** General Medical and Surgical

Staffed Beds: 121 **Admissions:** 2620 **Census:** 50 **Outpatient Visits:** 68718 **Births:** 0 **Total Expense ($000):** 25406 **Payroll Expense ($000):** 10097 **Personnel:** 291

SUSQUEHANNA—Susquehanna County

BARNES–KASSON COUNTY HOSPITAL (391309), 400 Turnpike Street, Zip 18847–1638; tel. 570/853–3135, (Total facility includes 58 beds in nursing home–type unit) (Nonreporting) **A**9 10 18
Primary Contact: Sara C. Iveson, Executive Director
COO: Sara C. Iveson, Executive Director
CFO: Sara F. Iveson, Director Finance
CMO: Pravin Chandra Patel, M.D., Chief Medical Officer
CHR: William D. Iveson, Assistant Administrator and Director Human Resources
Web address: www.barnes-kasson.org
Control: Other not–for–profit (including NFP Corporation) **Service:** General Medical and Surgical

Staffed Beds: 83

TITUSVILLE—Crawford County

★ **TITUSVILLE AREA HOSPITAL (390122)**, 406 West Oak Street, Zip 16354–1404; tel. 814/827–1851 **A**9 10 **F**11 13 15 24 26 27 31 32 37 38 43 55 57 61 68 73 74 75 76 77 79 81 82 86 96 97 99 100 102 106 107 119 121 122 124 134 **P**6
Primary Contact: Anthony J. Nasralla, FACHE, President and Chief Executive Officer
CFO: Paul Mattis, Vice President Finance
CMO: William Sonnenberg, M.D., Medical Staff President
CIO: Deanna Callahan, Director Information Systems
CHR: Jeffrey Saintz, Vice President Human Resources
Web address: www.titusvillehospital.org
Control: Other not–for–profit (including NFP Corporation) **Service:** General Medical and Surgical

Staffed Beds: 50 **Admissions:** 2327 **Census:** 26 **Outpatient Visits:** 73059 **Births:** 241 **Total Expense ($000):** 28724 **Payroll Expense ($000):** 11814 **Personnel:** 288

TORRANCE—Westmoreland County

□ **TORRANCE STATE HOSPITAL (394026)**, Torrance Road, Zip 15779–0111, Mailing Address: P.O. Box 111, Zip 15779–0111; tel. 724/459–8000, (Nonreporting) **A**1 10
Primary Contact: Edna I. McCutcheon, Chief Executive Officer
COO: Ronald Stypula, Chief Operating Officer
CFO: Michael Yahner, Chief Financial Officer
CMO: Lisa Issac, M.D., Chief Medical Services
Control: State–Government, nonfederal **Service:** Psychiatric

Staffed Beds: 242

TOWANDA—Bradford County

□ **MEMORIAL HOSPITAL (390236)**, One Hospital Drive, Zip 18848–9702; tel. 570/265–2191, (Total facility includes 118 beds in nursing home–type unit) **A**1 9 10 **F**3 7 10 11 13 15 24 25 31 33 34 38 42 43 44 50 51 55 56 57 61 62 68 73 74 75 79 80 81 82 86 96 97 100 102 107 117 118 119 120 122 124 132 135 137 **S** QHR
Primary Contact: Gary A. Baker, President
CFO: William K. Rohrbach, Vice President Fiscal Affairs
CMO: Constance Sweet, M.D., President Medical Staff
CHR: Linda Berry, Vice President Human Resources
Web address: www.memorialhospital.org
Control: Other not–for–profit (including NFP Corporation) **Service:** General Medical and Surgical

Staffed Beds: 161 **Admissions:** 1759 **Census:** 128 **Outpatient Visits:** 57553 **Births:** 226 **Total Expense ($000):** 30078 **Payroll Expense ($000):** 14186 **Personnel:** 419

TRANSFER—Mercer County

EDGEWOOD SURGICAL HOSPITAL (390307), 239 Edgewood Drive Extension, Zip 16154; tel. 724/646–0400, (Nonreporting) **A**10
Primary Contact: Kurt Gramley, Chief Executive Officer
Web address: www.edgewoodsurgical.com
Control: Corporation, Investor–owned, for–profit **Service:** Surgical

Staffed Beds: 10

TROY—Bradford County

★ ○ **TROY COMMUNITY HOSPITAL (391305)**, 100 John Street, Zip 16947–0036; tel. 570/297–2121 **A**9 10 11 18 **F**3 8 11 15 24 25 26 30 31 38 46 50 56 62 65 66 79 80 82 85 86 96 100 107 117 118 119 122 135 **P**8 **S** Guthrie Healthcare System
Primary Contact: Staci Covey, Administrator
CFO: Bernie Smith, Chief Financial Officer
CMO: Vance A. Good, M.D., Chief Medical Staff
Web address: www.guthrie.org
Control: Other not–for–profit (including NFP Corporation) **Service:** General Medical and Surgical

Staffed Beds: 25 **Admissions:** 740 **Census:** 18 **Outpatient Visits:** 24192 **Births:** 0 **Total Expense ($000):** 9796 **Payroll Expense ($000):** 4194 **Personnel:** 107

TUNKHANNOCK—Wyoming County

★ **TYLER MEMORIAL HOSPITAL (390192)**, 880 State Road 6 West, Zip 18657–6149; tel. 570/836–2161 **A**1 9 10 **F**11 24 25 26 27 30 31 32 38 56 57 62 66 68 73 74 75 76 79 82 84 86 96 121 122 124 135
Primary Contact: Denise S. Gieski, RN, President and Chief Executive Officer
CFO: Thomas Dougherty, Vice President and Chief Financial Officer
CMO: Christopher Andres, M.D., Chief of Staff
CIO: Dan Diljak, Chief Information Officer
CHR: Jill Smith, Director Human Resources
Web address: www.tylerhospital.com
Control: Other not–for–profit (including NFP Corporation) **Service:** General Medical and Surgical

Staffed Beds: 58 **Admissions:** 2486 **Census:** 25 **Outpatient Visits:** 47667 **Births:** 260 **Total Expense ($000):** 26043 **Payroll Expense ($000):** 10212 **Personnel:** 280

TYRONE—Blair County

★ **TYRONE HOSPITAL (391307)**, One Hospital Drive, Zip 16686–1810; tel. 814/684–1255 **A**9 10 18 **F**3 15 38 73 75 77 79 86 96 107 119 122 135
Primary Contact: Walter S. Van Dyke, Chief Executive Officer
CFO: George Berger, Chief Financial Officer
CMO: Jerome DeJulia, M.D., Chief Medical Officer
CIO: Steve Gildea, Director Management Information Systems
CHR: Leeann Price, Director Human Resources
Web address: www.tyronehospital.org
Control: Other not–for–profit (including NFP Corporation) **Service:** General Medical and Surgical

Staffed Beds: 25 **Admissions:** 1129 **Census:** 11 **Outpatient Visits:** 7647 **Total Expense ($000):** 13730 **Payroll Expense ($000):** 7308 **Personnel:** 154

 Many Facility Codes have changed. Please refer to the AHA Guide Code Chart.

UNIONTOWN—Fayette County

★□ **UNIONTOWN HOSPITAL (390041)**, 500 West Berkeley Street, Zip 15401–5596; tel. 724/430–5000, (Total facility includes 19 beds in nursing home–type unit) **A**1 9 10 **F**11 13 15 18 20 24 25 30 31 32 33 38 44 49 51 53 57 62 68 71 72 73 74 76 77 79 84 85 86 96 97 99 100 102 106 107 117 118 119 121 124 135
Primary Contact: Paul Bacharach, President and Chief Executive Officer
CFO: Steven P. Handy, CPA, Senior Vice President, Chief Financial Officer and Chief Information Officer
CIO: Steven P. Handy, CPA, Senior Vice President, Chief Financial Officer and Chief Information Officer
CHR: James Proud, Vice President Human Resources and Marketing
Web address: www.uniontownhospital.com
Control: Other not–for–profit (including NFP Corporation) **Service:** General Medical and Surgical

Staffed Beds: 209 **Admissions:** 11009 **Census:** 143 **Outpatient Visits:** 233691 **Births:** 956 **Total Expense ($000):** 106886 **Payroll Expense ($000):** 41068 **Personnel:** 1155

UPLAND—Delaware County

★□ ○ △ **CROZER–CHESTER MEDICAL CENTER (390180)**, One Medical Center Boulevard, Zip 19013–3995; tel. 610/447–2000, (Includes SPRINGFIELD HOSPITAL, 190 West Sproul Road, Springfield, Zip 19064–2097; tel. 610/328–8700; TAYLOR HOSPITAL, 175 East Chester Pike, Ridley Park, Zip 19078–2212; tel. 610/595–6000) **A**1 2 3 5 7 8 9 10 11 12 13 **F**2 3 6 7 11 12 13 15 16 17 18 20 22 24 25 26 27 28 30 31 32 33 34 35 36 38 40 41 42 43 44 45 46 48 49 50 51 53 54 55 57 58 60 61 62 63 64 66 68 70 72 73 74 75 76 77 79 80 81 82 84 85 86 87 88 89 90 91 92 93 94 95 96 97 98 100 102 103 104 105 106 107 108 109 111 113 114 116 117 118 119 120 121 122 123 127 132 135 136 137 **P**6 **S** Crozer–Keystone Health System
Primary Contact: Joseph Saunders, President
CMO: Sat Arora, M.D., President Medical and Dental Staff
CIO: Robert E. Wilson, Vice President and Chief Information Officer
CHR: Eugene Zegar, Vice President Human Resources
Web address: www.crozer.org
Control: Other not–for–profit (including NFP Corporation) **Service:** General Medical and Surgical

Staffed Beds: 554 **Admissions:** 30640 **Census:** 435 **Outpatient Visits:** 516631 **Births:** 1986 **Total Expense ($000):** 511430 **Payroll Expense ($000):** 214448 **Personnel:** 3735

WARREN—Warren County

WARREN GENERAL HOSPITAL (390146), Two Crescent Park West, Zip 16365–0068, Mailing Address: P.O. Box 68, Zip 16365–0068; tel. 814/723–4973, (Total facility includes 16 beds in nursing home–type unit) **A**9 10 **F**11 13 15 24 25 26 27 31 32 37 38 42 43 44 53 55 57 61 62 66 68 73 74 75 76 77 79 80 82 84 86 87 88 89 92 93 95 96 97 102 106 107 109 111 117 119 120 121 124 135 **P**6
Primary Contact: John P. Papalia, CHE, Chief Executive Officer
COO: Randy California, Assistant Director
CFO: Murray S. Marsh, Vice President Finance
CIO: Rick Setili, Manager Information Systems
CHR: Alice Pedersen, Corporate Director Human Resources
Web address: www.wgh.org
Control: Other not–for–profit (including NFP Corporation) **Service:** General Medical and Surgical

Staffed Beds: 105 **Admissions:** 3522 **Census:** 55 **Outpatient Visits:** 135348 **Births:** 316 **Total Expense ($000):** 59081 **Payroll Expense ($000):** 27507 **Personnel:** 569

□ **WARREN STATE HOSPITAL (394016)**, 33 Main Drive, Zip 16365–5001; tel. 814/723–5500, (Nonreporting) **A**1 10
Primary Contact: David A. Kucherawy, Acting Chief Executive Officer
COO: Jeff Dahlgren, Chief Operating Officer
CFO: Terry Crambes, Manager Finance
CMO: Reynaldo Puesan, M.D., Chief Medical Officer
CIO: Karen Byler, Information Technician
CHR: Nancy Saullo, Director
Web address: www.dpw.state.pa.us
Control: State–Government, nonfederal **Service:** Psychiatric

Staffed Beds: 250

WASHINGTON—Washington County

★□ **WASHINGTON HOSPITAL (390042)**, 155 Wilson Avenue, Zip 15301–3398; tel. 724/225–7000 **A**1 2 3 5 6 9 10 12 13 **F**3 5 11 13 15 18 20 22 24 25 26 27 28 30 31 32 33 34 36 37 38 42 43 44 45 46 49 50 52 53 54 55 56 57 59 60 62 63 68 72 73 74 75 76 77 79 80 81 84 85 86 87 88 89 90 91 92 93 96 97 100 102 103 104 106 107 117 118 119 121 123 124 133 135 136 137 **P**1 7
Primary Contact: Telford W. Thomas, President and Chief Executive Officer
COO: Gary B. Weinstein, Executive Vice President
CFO: Michael J. Roney, Vice President Finance and Chief Financial Officer
CMO: William P. Pearson, M.D., Vice President Medical Affairs
CIO: Rodney Louk, Vice President Information Systems
CHR: William H. Cline, Vice President Human Resources
Web address: www.washingtonhospital.org
Control: Other not–for–profit (including NFP Corporation) **Service:** General Medical and Surgical

Staffed Beds: 265 **Admissions:** 15859 **Census:** 190 **Outpatient Visits:** 702623 **Births:** 1124 **Total Expense ($000):** 200160 **Payroll Expense ($000):** 90438 **Personnel:** 1733

WAYNESBORO—Franklin County

★□ **WAYNESBORO HOSPITAL (390138)**, 501 East Main Street, Zip 17268–2394; tel. 717/765–4000 **A**1 9 10 19 **F**3 11 13 15 24 25 26 27 30 31 32 38 49 53 55 56 57 62 63 66 72 73 74 75 76 77 79 80 81 82 86 97 100 103 106 107 118 119 120 121 122 124 135 136 137 **P**8 **S** Summit Health
Primary Contact: Kenneth L. Shur, FACHE, Vice President and Chief Operating Officer
CFO: Patrick W. O'Donnell, CPA, Vice President Finance
CMO: Thomas Anderson, M.D., Vice President Medical Affairs
Web address: www.summithealth.org
Control: Other not–for–profit (including NFP Corporation) **Service:** General Medical and Surgical

Staffed Beds: 64 **Admissions:** 3585 **Census:** 39 **Outpatient Visits:** 112951 **Births:** 518 **Total Expense ($000):** 47261 **Payroll Expense ($000):** 23824 **Personnel:** 485

WAYNESBURG—Greene County

★ **SOUTHWEST REGIONAL MEDICAL CENTER (390150)**, Seventh Street and Bonar Avenue, Zip 15370–1697; tel. 724/627–3101, (Total facility includes 20 beds in nursing home–type unit) (Nonreporting) **A**9 10 **S** Essent Healthcare
Primary Contact: Cynthia Cowie, Chief Executive Officer
CFO: James C. Rutkowski, Chief Financial Officer
CMO: Jamie Boris, M.D., Medical Staff President
CIO: Chris Zaglama, Director Information Services
CHR: Matt D'Accione, Director Human Resources
Web address: www.sw–rmc.com
Control: Corporation, Investor–owned, for–profit **Service:** General Medical and Surgical

Staffed Beds: 45

WELLSBORO—Tioga County

★□ **SOLDIERS AND SAILORS MEMORIAL HOSPITAL (390043)**, 32–36 Central Avenue, Zip 16901–1899; tel. 570/724–1631 **A**1 9 10 20 **F**3 11 13 15 17 24 30 31 32 38 48 49 62 63 68 73 74 77 79 80 86 88 92 93 94 96 97 100 106 107 118 119 135 **P**7
Primary Contact: Jan E. Fisher, President and Chief Executive Officer
CFO: Ronald Gilbert, Chief Financial Officer
CMO: F. Ardell Thomas, M.D., Chief Medical Officer
CIO: Joe Bubacz, Chief Information Officer
CHR: Gene Yajko, Director Human Resources
Web address: www.laurelhs.org
Control: Other not–for–profit (including NFP Corporation) **Service:** General Medical and Surgical

Staffed Beds: 83 **Admissions:** 2502 **Census:** 28 **Outpatient Visits:** 101021 **Births:** 295 **Total Expense ($000):** 35076 **Payroll Expense ($000):** 14423 **Personnel:** 415

WERNERSVILLE—Berks County

□ **WERNERSVILLE STATE HOSPITAL (394014)**, Route 422, Zip 19565–0300, Mailing Address: P.O. Box 300, Zip 19565–0300; tel. 610/678–3411, (Nonreporting) **A**1 10
Primary Contact: Andrea Kepler, Chief Executive Officer
COO: Cheryl Benson, Chief Operating Officer
CFO: Thomas Parise, Financial Officer
CMO: Dale K. Adair, M.D., Chief Medical Officer
CIO: William Edwards, Information Technology Generalist
CHR: Melvin McMinn, Director Human Resources
Control: State–Government, nonfederal **Service:** Psychiatric

Staffed Beds: 232

Hospital, Medicare Provider Number, Address, Telephone, Approval, Facility, and Physician Codes, Health Care System

★ American Hospital Association (AHA) membership
□ The Joint Commission accreditation
○ American Osteopathic Association (AOA) accreditation
△ Commission on Accreditation of Rehabilitation Facilities (CARF) accreditation

PA

WEST CHESTER—Chester County

★ **CHESTER COUNTY HOSPITAL (390179)**, 701 East Marshall Street, Zip 19380–4412; tel. 610/431–5000 **A**1 2 5 9 10 **F**3 11 13 15 17 18 20 22 24 25 27 28 30 31 32 33 38 42 43 44 49 50 52 54 55 56 57 61 62 63 66 67 68 70 73 74 75 76 77 79 80 81 82 84 86 87 96 97 99 100 102 106 107 109 111 114 119 120 121 123 124 135 136 137 **P**3 6
Primary Contact: H. L. Perry Pepper, FACHE, President and Chief Executive Officer
COO: Michael Barber, Chief Operating Officer
CFO: Kenneth E. Flickinger, Corporate Vice President Finance
CMO: Richard D. Donze, D.O., Senior Vice President Medical Affairs
CIO: Mary Buckley, Vice President Information Technology
CHR: Jacqueline Felicetti, Director Human Resources
Web address: www.cchosp.com
Control: Other not–for–profit (including NFP Corporation) **Service:** General Medical and Surgical

Staffed Beds: 220 **Admissions:** 14941 **Census:** 169 **Outpatient Visits:** 406244 **Births:** 2447 **Total Expense ($000):** 168265 **Payroll Expense ($000):** 72637 **Personnel:** 1447

☐ **LIFECARE HOSPITALS OF CHESTER COUNTY (392048)**, 400 East Marshall Street, Zip 19380; tel. 484/826–0400, (Nonreporting) **A**1 9 10 **S** LifeCare Management Services
Primary Contact: Rosalie Cox, Chief Executive Officer
Web address: www.lifecare–hospitals.com
Control: Corporation, Investor–owned, for–profit **Service:** Long–Term Acute Care hospital

Staffed Beds: 39

WEST GROVE—Chester County

★ **JENNERSVILLE REGIONAL HOSPITAL (390220)**, 1015 West Baltimore Pike, Zip 19390–9499; tel. 610/869–1000 **A**1 2 9 10 **F**3 11 13 15 25 27 31 32 38 42 49 50 51 55 57 61 68 72 73 74 76 77 79 82 86 96 97 99 100 102 107 118 119 120 121 122 134 135 136 **P**6 **S** Community Health Systems, Inc.
Primary Contact: Charles A. Davis, Chief Executive Officer
CFO: Robert Ehinger, Chief Financial Officer
CIO: Joanne Sciotti, Director Information Technology
Web address: www.jennersville.com
Control: Corporation, Investor–owned, for–profit **Service:** General Medical and Surgical

Staffed Beds: 59 **Admissions:** 3713 **Census:** 38 **Outpatient Visits:** 16629 **Births:** 415 **Total Expense ($000):** 42274 **Payroll Expense ($000):** 15757 **Personnel:** 296

WEST READING—Berks County

★ △ **READING HOSPITAL AND MEDICAL CENTER (390044)**, Sixth Avenue and Spruce Street, Zip 19611–1428, Mailing Address: P.O. Box 16052, Zip 19612–6052; tel. 610/988–8000 **A**1 2 3 5 6 7 8 9 10 12 **F**3 5 8 11 12 13 14 15 18 20 22 24 25 26 27 30 31 32 33 35 38 39 40 42 43 44 46 47 48 49 52 53 54 55 56 57 59 60 61 62 63 64 66 68 70 72 73 74 75 76 77 79 80 81 82 84 85 86 87 88 89 90 91 92 93 94 95 96 97 99 100 102 103 104 106 107 108 109 111 112 113 114 117 118 119 120 121 123 124 135 136 137 **P**6 8
Primary Contact: Scott R. Wolfe, CPA, President and Chief Executive Officer
CFO: Steven Finkel, Vice President and Treasurer
CMO: Gerald Malick, M.D., Vice President and Medical Director
CIO: Jayashree Raman, Vice President and Chief Information Officer
Web address: www.readinghospital.org
Control: Other not–for–profit (including NFP Corporation) **Service:** General Medical and Surgical

Staffed Beds: 570 **Admissions:** 28716 **Census:** 437 **Outpatient Visits:** 886394 **Births:** 3600 **Total Expense ($000):** 515986 **Payroll Expense ($000):** 213844 **Personnel:** 4704

WILKES–BARRE—Luzerne County

CLEAR BROOK MANOR, 1100 East Northampton Street, Zip 18702–9803; tel. 570/823–1171, (Nonreporting)
Primary Contact: Robert Piccone, President
Web address: www.clearbrookinc.com
Control: Other not–for–profit (including NFP Corporation) **Service:** Alcoholism and other chemical dependency

Staffed Beds: 50

☐ **FIRST HOSPITAL WYOMING VALLEY (394039)**, 562 Wyoming Avenue, Zip 18704–3721; tel. 570/552–3900 **A**1 9 10 **F**30 31 32 88 89 93 94 95 **P**6
Primary Contact: Joseph H. Knecht, President and Chief Executive Officer
COO: Richard Sapolis, Director Clinical Operations
CMO: Steven R. Kafrissen, M.D., Medical Director
Web address: www.wvhcs.org
Control: Other not–for–profit (including NFP Corporation) **Service:** Psychiatric

Staffed Beds: 103 **Admissions:** 2900 **Census:** 80 **Outpatient Visits:** 0 **Births:** 0 **Personnel:** 100

★ **GEISINGER SOUTH WILKES–BARRE (390169)**, 25 Church Street, Zip 18765–0999; tel. 570/826–3100 **A**1 9 10 **F**11 15 17 18 20 22 24 25 26 27 30 31 32 35 38 41 46 47 49 51 54 55 56 57 59 62 64 66 68 72 73 76 77 79 81 82 86 88 89 90 92 96 97 100 102 106 107 117 118 119 133 135 136 **P**6 8 **S** Geisinger Health System
Primary Contact: Cynthia Brylinsky, Vice President, Administration
COO: Cynthia Brylinsky, Vice President, Administration
CFO: Kathleen Chapman, Chief Financial Officer
CMO: Eric Bieber, M.D., Medical Director
CIO: Mary Rosen, Vice President Information Technology
CHR: Nancy Pearson, Manager Human Resources
Web address: www.geisinger.org
Control: Other not–for–profit (including NFP Corporation) **Service:** General Medical and Surgical

Staffed Beds: 112 **Admissions:** 6615 **Census:** 104 **Outpatient Visits:** 83986 **Births:** 0 **Total Expense ($000):** 86635 **Payroll Expense ($000):** 34262 **Personnel:** 747

★ **GEISINGER WYOMING VALLEY MEDICAL CENTER (390270)**, 1000 East Mountain Drive, Zip 18711–0027; tel. 570/826–7300 **A**1 2 9 10 **F**7 8 11 12 13 15 17 18 20 22 24 25 27 30 31 32 35 37 38 41 43 49 50 55 56 57 62 63 66 72 73 74 75 76 77 79 80 81 82 84 85 86 90 94 96 97 100 102 104 105 107 108 109 111 113 118 119 120 121 124 127 132 133 135 137 **P**6 **S** Geisinger Health System
Primary Contact: Lissa Bryan–Smith, Chief Administrative Officer
CFO: Jeffrey T. Wright, Chief Financial Officer
CMO: Eric Bieber, M.D., Medical Director
CIO: Frank Richards, Chief Information Officer
CHR: Margaret Heffers, Assistant Vice President Human Resources
Web address: www.geisinger.org
Control: Other not–for–profit (including NFP Corporation) **Service:** General Medical and Surgical

Staffed Beds: 148 **Admissions:** 9160 **Census:** 118 **Outpatient Visits:** 341762 **Births:** 949 **Total Expense ($000):** 157077 **Payroll Expense ($000):** 43404 **Personnel:** 870

★ △ **JOHN HEINZ INSTITUTE OF REHABILITATION MEDICINE (393036)**, 150 Mundy Street, Zip 18702; tel. 570/826–3800, (Total facility includes 19 beds in nursing home–type unit) **A**1 7 10 **F**3 11 25 26 28 30 31 32 33 43 53 55 57 61 62 66 73 75 81 85 86 119 120 121 132 135 137
Primary Contact: Thomas E. Pugh, Chief Executive Officer
CFO: Mike Avvisato, Vice President and Chief Financial Officer
CMO: Gregory Basting, M.D., Vice President Medical Affairs
CIO: John Regula, Chief Information Officer
CHR: Susan D. Montross, Vice President Human Resources
Web address: www.allied–services.org
Control: Other not–for–profit (including NFP Corporation) **Service:** Rehabilitation

Staffed Beds: 71 **Admissions:** 1977 **Census:** 63 **Outpatient Visits:** 104106 **Births:** 0 **Total Expense ($000):** 31215 **Payroll Expense ($000):** 16191 **Personnel:** 406

☐ **KINDRED HOSPITAL–WOMING VALLEY (392042)**, 575 North River Street, 7th Floor, Zip 18764; tel. 570/552–7620, (Nonreporting) **A**1 10 **S** Kindred Healthcare
Primary Contact: Erin Pica, Chief Executive Officer
Web address: www.kindredhealthcare.com
Control: Corporation, Investor–owned, for–profit **Service:** Long–Term Acute Care hospital

Staffed Beds: 36

★ △ **VETERANS AFFAIRS MEDICAL CENTER**, 1111 East End Boulevard, Zip 18711–0026; tel. 570/824–3521, (Total facility includes 105 beds in nursing home–type unit) **A**1 2 3 5 7 9 **F**2 3 4 5 8 10 11 12 24 25 26 27 30 31 32 33 36 37 38 41 42 43 44 45 50 52 53 54 55 56 57 58 59 60 61 62 63 66 68 69 72 73 75 76 77 78 79 81 82 86 87 88 89 90 91 92 93 94 96 102 103 106 107 117 118 119 121 124 132 135 136 137 **P**6 **S** Department of Veterans Affairs
Primary Contact: C. Gene Molino, Acting Director
COO: C. Gene Molino, Associate Director
CFO: Donald E. Foote, Fiscal Officer
CMO: Mirza Z. Ali, M.D., Acting Chief of Staff
CIO: David Longmore, Chief Information Officer
CHR: Dawn P. DeMorrow, Chief Human Resources Service
Web address: www.va.gov/vamcwb
Control: Veterans Affairs, Government, federal **Service:** General Medical and Surgical

Staffed Beds: 174 **Admissions:** 2506 **Census:** 152 **Outpatient Visits:** 249316 **Births:** 0 **Total Expense ($000):** 172416 **Payroll Expense ($000):** 60115 **Personnel:** 881

Many Facility Codes have changed. Please refer to the AHA Guide Code Chart.

★ **WYOMING VALLEY HEALTH CARE SYSTEM (390137)**, 575 North River Street, Zip 18764–0001; tel. 570/829–8111, (Includes WILKES–BARRE GENERAL HOSPITAL), (Total facility includes 26 beds in nursing home–type unit) **A**2 3 5 9 10 **F**3 4 11 13 15 17 18 20 22 24 25 26 27 30 32 35 38 41 49 50 52 53 54 55 56 57 60 62 64 68 71 72 73 74 76 77 79 80 81 82 84 86 96 97 99 100 101 102 103 105 106 107 109 111 112 117 119 121 134 135 136 137
Primary Contact: William R. Host, M.D., President and Chief Executive Officer
COO: Robert P. Hoffman, Vice President Direct Patient Care Services
CFO: Maggie Koehler, Senior Vice President and Chief Financial Officer
CMO: Ragupathy Veluswamy, M.D., Vice President Medical Affairs
CIO: Chris Galanda, Chief Information Officer
CHR: James Carmody, Vice President Human Resources
Web address: www.wvhc.org
Control: Other not–for–profit (including NFP Corporation) **Service:** General Medical and Surgical

Staffed Beds: 368 **Admissions:** 18207 **Census:** 266 **Outpatient Visits:** 558789 **Births:** 1484 **Total Expense ($000):** 223744 **Payroll Expense ($000):** 84715 **Personnel:** 1912

WILLIAMSBURG—Blair County

COVE FORGE BEHAVIORAL HEALTH SYSTEM, New Beginnings Road, P.O. Box B, Zip 16693; tel. 814/832–2121, (Nonreporting)
Primary Contact: Mark Sarneso, Chief Executive Officer
CFO: Tom Stoltz, Chief Financial Officer
CIO: Tom Ashburn, Director Information Services
Web address: www.whitedeerrun.com
Control: Corporation, Investor–owned, for–profit **Service:** Alcoholism and other chemical dependency

Staffed Beds: 100

WILLIAMSPORT—Lycoming County

★ △ **SUSQUEHANNA HEALTH (390045)**, 777 Rural Avenue, Zip 17701–3198; tel. 570/321–1000, (Includes DIVINE PROVIDENCE HOSPITAL, 1100 Grampian Boulevard, Zip 17701–1995; tel. 570/326–8000; WILLIAMSPORT HOSPITAL AND MEDICAL CENTER, 777 Rural Avenue, tel. 570/321–1000), (Total facility includes 138 beds in nursing home–type unit) **A**2 7 9 10 **F**6 7 9 11 12 13 15 17 18 20 22 24 25 26 27 28 30 31 32 33 36 37 38 41 42 43 44 45 49 50 51 52 53 54 55 56 57 59 60 61 62 63 64 66 68 72 73 74 75 76 77 79 80 81 82 84 85 86 87 88 89 90 93 96 97 99 100 103 104 107 109 113 117 118 119 120 121 122 123 124 132 133 135 136 137 **P**7 8
Primary Contact: Steven P. Johnson, President and Chief Executive Officer
COO: Neil G. Armstrong, Executive Vice President and Chief Operating Officer
CFO: Charles J. Santangelo, CPA, Executive Vice President and Chief Financial Officer
CMO: George Manchester, M.D., Senior Vice President Medical Affairs
CIO: Karen M. Armstrong, Senior Vice President and Chief Information Officer
CHR: Glenn C. Mechling, Senior Vice President Human Resources
Web address: www.susquehannahealth.org
Control: Other not–for–profit (including NFP Corporation) **Service:** General Medical and Surgical

Staffed Beds: 408 **Admissions:** 13154 **Census:** 292 **Outpatient Visits:** 407253 **Births:** 1221 **Total Expense ($000):** 242755 **Payroll Expense ($000):** 101363 **Personnel:** 2394

WINDBER—Somerset County

☒ **WINDBER MEDICAL CENTER (390112)**, 600 Somerset Avenue, Zip 15963–1331; tel. 814/467–3000 **A**1 9 10 **F**3 12 13 15 24 26 30 32 33 34 38 42 44 45 52 56 57 58 61 66 68 73 74 75 77 79 80 81 86 96 97 99 100 102 105 106 107 112 114 118 119 120 121 124 135 136
Primary Contact: Nicholas Jacobs, FACHE, President
COO: James Eckenrode, M.D., Chief Operating Officer and Chief Medical Officer
CFO: Linda Fanale, Chief Financial Officer
CMO: James Eckenrode, M.D., Chief Operating Officer and Chief Medical Officer
CIO: Cindy Bacon, MS, Director Information Technology and Services
CHR: Jamie Curtis, Director Human Resources
Web address: www.windbercare.com
Control: Other not–for–profit (including NFP Corporation) **Service:** General Medical and Surgical

Staffed Beds: 52 **Admissions:** 2073 **Census:** 20 **Outpatient Visits:** 124972 **Births:** 239 **Total Expense ($000):** 44268 **Payroll Expense ($000):** 17887 **Personnel:** 401

WYNNEWOOD—Montgomery County

LANKENAU HOSPITAL (390195), 100 Lancaster Avenue West, Zip 19096–3411; tel. 610/645–2000 **A**2 3 5 8 9 10 12 13 **F**3 13 15 17 18 20 22 24 25 26 27 28 30 31 32 33 37 38 43 44 46 47 48 49 50 53 54 55 56 57 62 63 64 66 68 70 71 72 73 74 76 77 79 80 81 82 86 87 96 97 99 100 102 106 107 108 109 111 112 114 116 118 119 121 124 126 127 135 137 **P**7 **S** Jefferson Health System
Primary Contact: Elaine Thompson, Ph.D., President
CFO: Michael J. Buongiorno, Vice President Finance
CMO: Thomas G. McCarter, M.D., Chief Medical Officer
CIO: Karen A. Thomas, R.N., Acting Vice President and Chief Information Officer
CHR: Eileen McAnally, Senior Vice President Human Resources
Web address: www.mainlinehealth.org
Control: Other not–for–profit (including NFP Corporation) **Service:** General Medical and Surgical

Staffed Beds: 331 **Admissions:** 20203 **Census:** 274 **Outpatient Visits:** 202360 **Births:** 2294 **Total Expense ($000):** 299045 **Payroll Expense ($000):** 106152 **Personnel:** 2382

YORK—York County

PA

☒ **HEALTHSOUTH REHABILITATION HOSPITAL OF YORK (393037)**, 1850 Normandie Drive, Zip 17408; tel. 717/767–6941, (Nonreporting) **A**1 9 10 **S** HEALTHSOUTH Corporation
Primary Contact: Mark Freeburn, Chief Executive Officer
CFO: Tracey Claxton, Controller
CMO: Bruce Sicilia, M.D., Medical Director
CIO: Cheryl Kuhn, Director Marketing Operations
CHR: Sarah Arthur, Director Human Resources
Web address: www.healthsouth.com
Control: Corporation, Investor–owned, for–profit **Service:** Chronic disease

Staffed Beds: 88

★ ○ **MEMORIAL HOSPITAL (390101)**, 325 South Belmont Street, Zip 17403–2609, Mailing Address: P.O. Box 15118, Zip 17405–7118; tel. 717/843–8623 **A**9 10 11 12 13 **F**3 7 11 13 15 18 25 26 27 30 31 32 33 35 36 38 42 43 48 50 53 54 55 56 57 59 60 61 62 64 66 68 73 74 75 76 77 79 80 81 82 84 86 94 97 99 106 107 112 118 119 120 121 124 135 137 **P**6
Primary Contact: Sally J. Dixon, President and Chief Executive Officer
COO: Rick Lillo, Chief Operating Officer
CFO: Richard Imbimbo, Chief Financial Officer
CMO: Anthony Minissale, M.D., Vice President Medical Affairs
CIO: James Mahoney, Director Management Information Systems
CHR: Corey Hudak, Manager Human Resources
Web address: www.mhyork.org
Control: Other not–for–profit (including NFP Corporation) **Service:** General Medical and Surgical

Staffed Beds: 100 **Admissions:** 6095 **Census:** 65 **Outpatient Visits:** 181203 **Births:** 833 **Total Expense ($000):** 82888 **Payroll Expense ($000):** 37985 **Personnel:** 760

☐ **SELECT SPECIALTY HOSPITAL – YORK**, 1001 South George Street, Zip 17403–3676; tel. 717/851–2661, (Nonreporting) **A**1 9 **S** Select Medical Corporation
Primary Contact: Marcia Medlin, Chief Executive Officer
Web address: www.selectmedicalcorp.com
Control: Corporation, Investor–owned, for–profit **Service:** Long–Term Acute Care hospital

Staffed Beds: 23

☒ **YORK HOSPITAL (390046)**, 1001 South George Street, Zip 17405–3645; tel. 717/851–2345 **A**1 2 3 5 8 9 10 12 13 **F**3 7 11 12 13 14 15 17 18 20 22 24 25 26 27 30 31 32 33 37 38 40 41 43 44 46 48 49 50 53 54 55 56 57 58 59 60 62 63 64 66 68 70 72 73 74 75 76 77 79 80 81 82 84 86 87 88 89 90 91 92 93 94 95 96 97 99 100 102 103 106 107 108 109 111 112 114 118 119 120 121 123 124 134 135 136 137 **S** WellSpan Health
Primary Contact: Richard L. Seim, President and Chief Executive Officer
COO: Raymond Rosen, Vice President Operations
CFO: Michael F. O'Connor, Senior Vice President Finance
CMO: Peter M. Hartmann, M.D., Vice President Medical Affairs
CIO: William J. Gillespie, Vice President and Chief Information Officer
CHR: Robert J. Batory, Vice President Human Resources
Web address: www.wellspan.org
Control: Other not–for–profit (including NFP Corporation) **Service:** General Medical and Surgical

Staffed Beds: 517 **Admissions:** 28679 **Census:** 384 **Outpatient Visits:** 790000 **Births:** 2870 **Total Expense ($000):** 504608 **Payroll Expense ($000):** 194634 **Personnel:** 3702

Hospital, Medicare Provider Number, Address, Telephone, Approval, Facility, and Physician Codes, Health Care System

★ American Hospital Association (AHA) membership
☐ The Joint Commission accreditation
○ American Osteopathic Association (AOA) accreditation
△ Commission on Accreditation of Rehabilitation Facilities (CARF) accreditation

RHODE ISLAND

CRANSTON—Providence County

☐ **ELEANOR SLATER HOSPITAL (412001)**, John O. Pastore Center, 111 Howard Avenue, Zip 02920–0269, Mailing Address: P.O. Box 8269, Zip 02920–8269; tel. 401/462–3085, (Nonreporting) **A**1 10
Primary Contact: Paul G. Despres, Acting Chief Executive Officer
COO: James P. Benedict, Chief Operating Officer
CFO: Michel C. Manosh, Executive Director Office of Operations
CMO: Edward W. Martin, M.D., Chief Medical Staff and Clinical Services
CHR: Lois M. Hayes, Acting Associate Director Human Resource Management
Web address: www.mhrh.state.ri.us
Control: State–Government, nonfederal **Service:** General Medical and Surgical

Staffed Beds: 360

EAST PROVIDENCE—Providence County

☐ **EMMA PENDLETON BRADLEY HOSPITAL (414003)**, 1011 Veterans Memorial Parkway, Zip 02915–5099; tel. 401/432–1000, (Nonreporting) **A**1 3 5 9 10 **S** Lifespan Corporation
Primary Contact: Daniel J. Wall, President and Chief Executive Officer
CFO: Mamie Wakefield, Vice President Finance
CMO: Gregory K. Fritz, M.D., Medical Director
Web address: www.lifespan.org
Control: Other not–for–profit (including NFP Corporation) **Service:** Children's hospital psychiatric

Staffed Beds: 51

NEWPORT—Newport County

☐ △ **NEWPORT HOSPITAL (410006)**, 11 Friendship Street, Zip 02840–2299; tel. 401/846–6400 **A**1 2 7 9 10 **F**8 11 13 15 24 25 26 27 31 32 33 38 49 51 52 54 55 56 57 59 62 66 68 72 73 74 75 76 77 79 80 81 84 85 86 87 88 90 92 95 96 97 99 100 102 106 107 118 119 121 124 135 136 **S** Lifespan Corporation
Primary Contact: Arthur J. Sampson, President and Chief Executive Officer
CFO: Frank J. Byrne, Director Finance and Treasurer
CMO: Terrence R. McWilliams, M.D., Vice President Medical Affairs
CHR: Barbara J. Arcangeli, Vice President Human Resources
Web address: www.newporthospital.org
Control: Other not–for–profit (including NFP Corporation) **Service:** General Medical and Surgical

Staffed Beds: 119 **Admissions:** 5568 **Census:** 76 **Outpatient Visits:** 105614 **Births:** 730 **Total Expense ($000):** 95586 **Payroll Expense ($000):** 37196 **Personnel:** 564

NORTH PROVIDENCE—Providence County

ST. JOSEPH HEALTH SERVICES OF RHODE ISLAND (410005), 200 High Service Avenue, Zip 02904–5199; tel. 401/456–3000, (Includes OUR LADY OF FATIMA HOSPITAL, 200 High Service Avenue, Zip 02904; ST. JOSEPH HOSPITAL FOR SPECIALTY CARE, 21 Peace Street, Providence, Zip 02907; tel. 401/456–3000), (Total facility includes 24 beds in nursing home–type unit) **A**2 6 9 10 **F**8 10 11 15 25 26 27 28 30 31 32 33 37 38 49 50 51 53 54 55 56 57 59 62 63 64 66 68 72 73 75 76 77 79 81 82 85 86 87 88 90 91 92 93 94 95 96 97 100 102 103 107 115 117 118 119 121 132 133 135 136 137 **P**5
Primary Contact: John M. Fogarty, Interim President and Chief Executive Officer
COO: John M. Fogarty, Executive Vice President and Chief Operations Officer
CFO: Kathleen Kenny, Senior Vice President Finance
CIO: Crystal Pilon, Chief Information Officer
CHR: Christopher Callahan, Vice President
Web address: www.saintjosephri.com
Control: Church–operated, Nongovernment, not–for profit **Service:** General Medical and Surgical

Staffed Beds: 295 **Admissions:** 11093 **Census:** 227 **Outpatient Visits:** 224528 **Births:** 0 **Total Expense ($000):** 167015 **Payroll Expense ($000):** 83336 **Personnel:** 1505

NORTH SMITHFIELD—Providence County

LANDMARK MEDICAL CENTER–FOGARTY UNIT See Landmark Medical Center, Woonsocket

☐ **REHABILITATION HOSPITAL OF RHODE ISLAND (413025)**, 116 Eddie Dowling Highway, Zip 2896; tel. 401/766–0800, (Nonreporting) **A**1 9 10
Primary Contact: Richard Charest, Chief Executive Officer
Web address: www.rhri.net
Control: Partnership, Investor–owned, for–profit **Service:** Rehabilitation

Staffed Beds: 70

PAWTUCKET—Providence County

★ △ **MEMORIAL HOSPITAL OF RHODE ISLAND (410001)**, 111 Brewster Street, Zip 02860–4499; tel. 401/729–2000 **A**1 2 3 5 7 8 9 10 **F**3 8 11 13 15 17 18 24 25 27 28 30 31 32 33 37 38 40 43 44 46 49 53 54 55 56 57 58 61 62 63 64 66 67 68 72 73 74 75 76 77 79 80 81 84 85 86 87 92 96 98 99 100 102 103 106 107 118 119 120 121 124 132 133 135 136 137 **P**6 8
Primary Contact: Francis R. Dietz, President
COO: Shelley MacDonald, R.N., Senior Vice President Operations
CFO: Michael Ryan, Senior Vice President Finance
CMO: Andrew Artenstein, M.D., Physician in Chief Medicine
CIO: Lisa Mahar, Director Information Systems
CHR: Lisa Pratt, Vice President Human Resources
Web address: www.mhri.org
Control: Other not–for–profit (including NFP Corporation) **Service:** General Medical and Surgical

Staffed Beds: 159 **Admissions:** 6850 **Census:** 104 **Outpatient Visits:** 333391 **Births:** 414 **Total Expense ($000):** 158719 **Payroll Expense ($000):** 81970 **Personnel:** 1415

PROVIDENCE—Providence County

★ **BUTLER HOSPITAL (414000)**, 345 Blackstone Boulevard, Zip 02906–4829; tel. 401/455–6200 **A**1 3 5 9 10 **F**4 5 26 30 31 33 36 38 41 50 54 55 56 57 66 72 79 81 88 89 91 92 93 94 95 119 121 124 135 **P**6 **S** Care New England Health System
Primary Contact: Patricia R. Recupero, J.D., M.D., President and Chief Executive Officer
COO: Walter Dias, Vice President and Chief Operating Officer
CFO: Bonnie Baker, Vice President Finance and Chief Financial Officer
CMO: Steven Rasmussen, M.D., Medical Director
CIO: Bruce A. Reirden, Vice President and Chief Information Officer
CHR: Timothy Bigelow, Director Human Resources
Web address: www.butler.org
Control: Other not–for–profit (including NFP Corporation) **Service:** Psychiatric

Staffed Beds: 117 **Admissions:** 4429 **Census:** 108 **Outpatient Visits:** 34896 **Births:** 0 **Total Expense ($000):** 64360 **Payroll Expense ($000):** 40291 **Personnel:** 671

☐ **MIRIAM HOSPITAL (410012)**, 164 Summit Avenue, Zip 02906–2895; tel. 401/793–2500 **A**1 2 3 5 8 9 10 **F**8 12 15 17 18 20 22 24 25 26 27 31 32 33 38 46 49 53 54 55 56 57 58 60 62 63 64 66 68 72 73 75 76 77 79 82 86 87 94 96 97 100 103 106 107 116 118 119 121 124 135 136 **P**3 5 6 **S** Lifespan Corporation
Primary Contact: Kathleen C. Hittner, M.D., President and Chief Executive Officer
COO: Sandra L. Coletta, Chief Operating Officer
CFO: Mamie Wakefield, Chief Financial Officer
CMO: Boyd P. King, M.D., Chief Medical Officer
CIO: Carole Cotter, Vice President and Chief Information Officer
CHR: Nancy McMahon, Vice President
Web address: www.lifespan.org
Control: Other not–for–profit (including NFP Corporation) **Service:** General Medical and Surgical

Staffed Beds: 247 **Admissions:** 14036 **Census:** 190 **Outpatient Visits:** 98852 **Births:** 0 **Total Expense ($000):** 292240 **Payroll Expense ($000):** 123348 **Personnel:** 1733

☐ **RHODE ISLAND HOSPITAL (410007)**, 593 Eddy Street, Zip 02903–4900; tel. 401/444–4000 **A**1 2 3 5 8 9 10 **F**3 8 12 15 17 18 19 20 21 22 25 26 27 28 31 32 33 36 37 38 40 43 44 46 47 49 51 52 53 55 56 57 58 59 62 64 66 68 72 73 75 76 77 79 80 81 82 83 84 86 88 90 91 92 93 94 95 96 97 99 100 102 103 105 107 108 109 111 112 114 118 119 120 121 123 124 127 131 133 135 137 **P**3 5 6 **S** Lifespan Corporation
Primary Contact: George A. Vecchione, Interim Chief Executive Officer
COO: Fredrick Macri, Executive Vice President
CFO: Mamie Wakefield, Senior Vice President and Chief Financial Officer
CMO: John B. Murphy, M.D., Vice President Medical Affairs and Chief Medical Officer
CIO: Carole Cotter, Senior Vice President and Chief Information Officer
CHR: Louis Sperling, Vice President Human Resources
Web address: www.lifespan.org
Control: Other not–for–profit (including NFP Corporation) **Service:** General Medical and Surgical

Staffed Beds: 632 **Admissions:** 35151 **Census:** 505 **Outpatient Visits:** 345894 **Births:** 0 **Total Expense ($000):** 826881 **Payroll Expense ($000):** 377953 **Personnel:** 5085

Many Facility Codes have changed. Please refer to the AHA Guide Code Chart.

★□ **ROGER WILLIAMS MEDICAL CENTER (410004)**, 825 Chalkstone Avenue, Zip 02908–4735; tel. 401/456–2000 **A**1 2 3 5 8 9 10 **F**4 5 7 8 12 15 18 20 25 26 27 30 31 32 33 38 44 46 49 51 54 55 56 57 60 61 62 63 66 68 72 73 75 76 77 79 81 82 87 88 90 91 93 94 95 96 97 100 102 103 104 106 107 118 119 121 124 125 135 136 137 **P**3 5 8
Primary Contact: Kenneth H. Belcher, President and Chief Executive Officer
CFO: Addy Kane, Interim Chief Financial Officer
CMO: Michael Bonitati, M.D., President Medical Staff
CIO: Susan Cerrone Abely, Vice President and Chief Information Officer
CHR: Cheryl Perry, Chief Human Resources Officer
Web address: www.rwmc.com
Control: Other not–for–profit (including NFP Corporation) **Service:** General Medical and Surgical

Staffed Beds: 169 **Admissions:** 8630 **Census:** 121 **Outpatient Visits:** 193005 **Births:** 0 **Total Expense ($000):** 141291 **Payroll Expense ($000):** 62373 **Personnel:** 1255

ST. JOSEPH HOSPITAL FOR SPECIALTY CARE See St. Joseph Health Services of Rhode Island, North Providence

★□ **VETERANS AFFAIRS MEDICAL CENTER**, 830 Chalkstone Avenue, Zip 02908–4799; tel. 401/457–3042 **A**1 3 5 **F**3 5 24 25 26 27 36 37 38 49 50 54 57 58 59 60 61 62 65 68 72 73 75 76 77 79 80 81 82 86 87 88 90 91 92 93 94 96 97 106 107 119 121 124 132 135 136 137 **S** Department of Veterans Affairs
Primary Contact: Vincent Ng, Director
Web address: www.va.gov/sta/guide/home.asp
Control: Veterans Affairs, Government, federal **Service:** General Medical and Surgical

Staffed Beds: 73 **Admissions:** 3106 **Census:** 56 **Outpatient Visits:** 294983 **Births:** 0 **Total Expense ($000):** 70189 **Payroll Expense ($000):** 52683 **Personnel:** 896

★□ **WOMEN & INFANTS HOSPITAL OF RHODE ISLAND (410010)**, 101 Dudley Street, Zip 02905–2499; tel. 401/274–1100 **A**1 2 3 5 8 9 10 **F**3 5 11 13 15 25 26 27 30 31 32 33 34 38 41 42 43 44 50 55 56 57 58 62 64 66 69 70 73 74 76 79 80 81 82 87 90 91 94 95 96 99 100 107 112 113 114 119 121 123 124 132 135 136 **P**5 6 8 **S** Care New England Health System
Primary Contact: Constance A. Howes, President and Chief Executive Officer
COO: Dick Argys, Executive Vice President and Chief Operating Officer
CFO: Debra M. Paul, Vice President Finance
CMO: Raymond Powrie, M.D., Senior Vice President Quality and Clinical Effectiveness
CIO: Cedric Priebe, M.D., Vice President Information Services
CHR: Daniel Michaud, Vice President Human Resources
Web address: www.womenandinfants.org
Control: Other not–for–profit (including NFP Corporation) **Service:** Obstetrics and gynecology

Staffed Beds: 197 **Admissions:** 14536 **Census:** 184 **Outpatient Visits:** 167772 **Births:** 9625 **Total Expense ($000):** 319928 **Payroll Expense ($000):** 149099 **Personnel:** 2230

WAKEFIELD—Washington County

★□ **SOUTH COUNTY HOSPITAL (410008)**, 100 Kenyon Avenue, Zip 02879–4299; tel. 401/782–8000 **A**1 2 9 10 **F**3 11 12 13 15 24 25 26 27 30 31 32 35 36 38 46 49 51 52 54 55 56 57 59 62 63 64 68 72 73 74 75 76 77 79 80 81 82 84 86 96 97 100 102 107 118 119 120 121 122 124 132 133 135 136 137 **P**8
Primary Contact: Louis R. Giancola, President and Chief Executive Officer
CFO: Michael J. Koziol, Vice President and Chief Financial Officer
CMO: Joseph J. O'Neill, M.D., Vice President Medical Affairs
CIO: Gary Croteau, Assistant Vice President and Chief Information Officer
CHR: Maggie Thomas, Vice President and Chief Human Resources Officer
Web address: www.schospital.com
Control: Other not–for–profit (including NFP Corporation) **Service:** General Medical and Surgical

Staffed Beds: 78 **Admissions:** 5336 **Census:** 54 **Outpatient Visits:** 194039 **Births:** 408 **Total Expense ($000):** 88449 **Payroll Expense ($000):** 35230 **Personnel:** 533

WARWICK—Kent County

★□ △ **KENT COUNTY MEMORIAL HOSPITAL (410009)**, 455 Tollgate Road, Zip 02886–2770; tel. 401/737–7000 **A**1 2 7 9 10 **F**1 3 11 13 15 17 18 24 25 26 27 28 30 31 32 34 37 38 42 43 44 50 51 54 55 56 57 59 60 62 65 66 68 70 71 72 73 74 75 76 77 79 80 81 82 84 85 86 87 88 90 92 93 96 97 100 102 106 107 117 118 119 120 121 132 135 136 137 **P**6 8 **S** Care New England Health System
Primary Contact: Mark E. Crevier, President and Chief Executive Officer
CFO: Paul Beaudoin, Senior Vice President Finance and Chief Financial Officer
CMO: John R. Audett, M.D., Senior Vice President and Medical Director
CIO: Cedric Priebe, M.D., Senior Vice President and Chief Information Officer
CHR: Marilyn J. Walsh, Vice President Human Resources
Web address: www.kentri.org
Control: Other not–for–profit (including NFP Corporation) **Service:** General Medical and Surgical

Staffed Beds: 320 **Admissions:** 16234 **Census:** 246 **Outpatient Visits:** 229411 **Births:** 1185 **Total Expense ($000):** 223941 **Payroll Expense ($000):** 108430 **Personnel:** 1568

WESTERLY—Washington County

★□ **WESTERLY HOSPITAL (410013)**, 25 Wells Street, Zip 02891–2934; tel. 401/596–6000 **A**1 9 10 **F**3 11 13 15 18 24 25 26 27 30 31 32 33 38 42 43 48 51 54 55 56 57 59 60 62 68 72 73 74 75 76 77 79 81 82 84 86 87 90 92 96 97 99 100 102 106 107 119 120 121 123 124 135 136 137 **P**1
Primary Contact: Charles S. Kinney, President and Chief Executive Officer
CFO: Jeanne LaChance, Vice President Finance and Chief Financial Officer
CIO: Nancy Barisano, Chief Information Officer
CHR: Jodie Arthur, Director Human Resources
Web address: www.westerlyhospital.org
Control: Other not–for–profit (including NFP Corporation) **Service:** General Medical and Surgical

Staffed Beds: 100 **Admissions:** 4199 **Census:** 45 **Outpatient Visits:** 506140 **Births:** 444 **Total Expense ($000):** 74509 **Payroll Expense ($000):** 34754 **Personnel:** 463

WOONSOCKET—Providence County

□ **LANDMARK MEDICAL CENTER (410011)**, 115 Cass Avenue, Zip 02895–4731; tel. 401/769–4100, (Includes LANDMARK MEDICAL CENTER–FOGARTY UNIT, Eddie Dowling Highway, North Smithfield, Zip 02896; tel. 401/766–0800; LANDMARK MEDICAL CENTER–WOONSOCKET UNIT), (Nonreporting) **A**1 2 9 10
Primary Contact: Gary J. Gaube, President
CFO: Mary MacIntosh, Chief Financial Officer
CMO: Fadi Al–Bilbeisi, M.D., President Medical Staff
CIO: Colleen Ryan, Director Management Information Systems
CHR: Mona Willis, Director Human Resources
Web address: www.landmarkmedical.org
Control: Other not–for–profit (including NFP Corporation) **Service:** General Medical and Surgical

Staffed Beds: 133

RI

Hospital, Medicare Provider Number, Address, Telephone, Approval, Facility, and Physician Codes, Health Care System

★ American Hospital Association (AHA) membership
□ The Joint Commission accreditation
○ American Osteopathic Association (AOA) accreditation
△ Commission on Accreditation of Rehabilitation Facilities (CARF) accreditation

SOUTH CAROLINA

ABBEVILLE—Abbeville County

★ **ABBEVILLE AREA MEDICAL CENTER (421301)**, 901 West Greenwood Street, Zip 29620–0887, Mailing Address: P.O. Box 887, Zip 29620–0887; tel. 864/366–5011 **A**1 9 10 18 **F**3 13 15 17 24 25 26 30 31 32 33 38 51 52 54 55 57 61 62 65 68 72 73 74 75 77 79 80 82 84 85 86 96 97 99 102 107 117 118 119 121 122 124 135 136 **S** QHR
Primary Contact: Richard D. Osmus, Chief Executive Officer
CFO: Timothy Wren, Chief Financial Officer
CIO: Tim Stewart, Chief Information Officer
CHR: Alice Rigney, Chief Human Resources Officer
Web address: www.abbevilleareamc.com
Control: County–Government, nonfederal **Service:** General Medical and Surgical

Staffed Beds: 25 **Admissions:** 1059 **Census:** 9 **Births:** 115 **Total Expense ($000):** 24869 **Payroll Expense ($000):** 10311 **Personnel:** 265

AIKEN—Aiken County

☐ **AIKEN REGIONAL MEDICAL CENTERS (420082)**, 302 University Parkway, Zip 29801–2757; tel. 803/641–5000, (Includes AURORA PAVILION, 655 Medical Park Drive, Zip 29801; tel. 803/641–5900) **A**1 5 9 10 **F**3 4 5 11 15 18 20 22 25 26 27 30 31 32 33 38 49 54 55 56 57 58 62 68 71 72 74 76 77 79 80 81 82 84 88 89 90 91 92 93 94 95 96 97 100 102 103 107 109 111 118 119 120 121 124 135 136 137 **P**6 **S** Universal Health Services, Inc.
Primary Contact: Kathryn D. Justyn, Chief Executive Officer and Managing Director
COO: Carlos Milanes, Chief Operating Officer
CFO: Mark A. Tierney, Chief Financial Officer
CMO: Jonathan Anderson, Chief of Staff
Web address: www.aikenregional.com
Control: Corporation, Investor–owned, for–profit **Service:** General Medical and Surgical

Staffed Beds: 230 **Admissions:** 11718 **Census:** 157 **Outpatient Visits:** 133097 **Births:** 1267 **Total Expense ($000):** 138671 **Payroll Expense ($000):** 43308 **Personnel:** 760

SC

ANDERSON—Anderson County

★ **ANMED HEALTH MEDICAL CENTER (420027)**, 800 North Fant Street, Zip 29621–5793; tel. 864/512–1000, (Includes ANMED HEALTH WOMEN'S AND CHILDREN'S HOSPITAL, 2000 East Greenville Street, Zip 29621; tel. 864/512–1000) **A**1 2 3 5 9 10 **F**3 11 12 13 14 15 17 18 20 22 24 25 26 27 30 31 32 33 35 37 38 40 43 44 46 48 49 50 51 52 53 54 55 56 57 58 59 60 61 62 63 66 68 72 73 74 75 76 77 78 79 80 81 82 84 85 86 87 88 89 90 91 92 93 94 96 97 99 100 102 105 106 107 109 111 118 119 120 121 124 133 135 136 137 **P**7 8 **S** AnMed Health
Primary Contact: John A. Miller, Jr., FACHE, President
COO: William T. Manson, Executive Vice President
CFO: Jerry A. Parrish, Vice President
CMO: Mike Tillirson, D.O., Executive Vice President and Chief Medical Officer
CIO: Darrell Hickman, Director Information Services
CHR: Doug Douglas, Vice President Human Resources
Web address: www.anmedhealth.org
Control: Other not–for–profit (including NFP Corporation) **Service:** General Medical and Surgical

Staffed Beds: 369 **Admissions:** 18395 **Census:** 257 **Births:** 2092 **Total Expense ($000):** 349906 **Payroll Expense ($000):** 128018 **Personnel:** 2734

★ **ANMED HEALTH REHABILITATION HOSPITAL (423029)**, 1 Spring Back Way, Zip 29621; tel. 864/716–2600 **A**1 10 **F**3 25 26 30 31 32 54 72 73 77 85 86 **S** HEALTHSOUTH Corporation
Primary Contact: Michele M. Skripps, Chief Executive Officer
CFO: Julie Saylors, Controller
CMO: William Vogentiz, Medical Director
CHR: Tara Myers, Director Human Resources
Web address: www.anmedhealth.org
Control: Corporation, Investor–owned, for–profit **Service:** Rehabilitation

Staffed Beds: 37 **Admissions:** 882 **Census:** 35 **Total Expense ($000):** 8472 **Payroll Expense ($000):** 4716 **Personnel:** 120

☐ **PATRICK B. HARRIS PSYCHIATRIC HOSPITAL (424011)**, 130 Highway 252, Zip 29622; tel. 864/231–2600 **A**1 10 **F**30 31 32 33 55 81 82 88 90 91 92 93 119 132 135
Primary Contact: John Fletcher, Chief Executive Officer
Web address: www.patrickbharrispsychiatrichospital.com/index.htm
Control: State–Government, nonfederal **Service:** Psychiatric

Staffed Beds: 174 **Admissions:** 1329 **Census:** 146 **Total Expense ($000):** 20687 **Payroll Expense ($000):** 10004 **Personnel:** 335

BAMBERG—Bamberg County

★ **BAMBERG COUNTY MEMORIAL HOSPITAL AND NURSING CENTER (420056)**, 509 North Street, Zip 29003–0507, Mailing Address: P.O. Box 507, Zip 29003–0507; tel. 803/245–4321, (Total facility includes 88 beds in nursing home–type unit) **A**1 9 10 **F**3 8 11 13 15 25 26 30 31 32 33 38 44 50 55 56 57 59 62 63 65 66 73 74 75 79 80 82 84 85 86 96 102 107 117 119 121 122 132 135 137
Primary Contact: Warren E. Hammett, Administrator
CFO: Robert A. McVicker, Chief Financial Officer
CMO: Maggie Shatilla, M.D., Chief of Staff
CHR: Susan Hiers, Director Human Resources
Web address: www.bambergcountyhospital.com
Control: County–Government, nonfederal **Service:** General Medical and Surgical

Staffed Beds: 126 **Admissions:** 1530 **Census:** 100 **Outpatient Visits:** 15536 **Births:** 95 **Total Expense ($000):** 31068 **Payroll Expense ($000):** 12909 **Personnel:** 321

BARNWELL—Barnwell County

★ **BARNWELL COUNTY HOSPITAL (420016)**, 811 Reynolds Road, Zip 29812–1555; tel. 803/259–1000 **A**1 9 10 20 **F**3 15 25 31 32 38 49 55 56 57 68 75 79 84 86 96 107 117 119 122
Primary Contact: Robert E. Waters, Chief Executive Officer
CFO: Al Altman, Chief Financial Officer
CMO: Richard E. Boyles, M.D., Chief Medical Staff
CIO: Randal Padgett, Manager Information Systems
CHR: Sherry Donaldson, Director Human Resources
Web address: www.barnwellcountysc.com/healthcare.htm
Control: County–Government, nonfederal **Service:** General Medical and Surgical

Staffed Beds: 33 **Admissions:** 1170 **Census:** 10 **Outpatient Visits:** 13352 **Total Expense ($000):** 13031 **Payroll Expense ($000):** 5716 **Personnel:** 150

BEAUFORT—Beaufort County

★ **BEAUFORT MEMORIAL HOSPITAL (420067)**, 955 Ribaut Road, Zip 29902–5441; tel. 843/522–5200 **A**1 9 10 19 20 **F**3 11 12 13 14 15 18 24 25 26 27 30 31 32 33 38 40 50 51 52 55 56 57 59 62 63 66 67 68 69 71 72 73 74 75 76 77 79 80 81 82 84 85 86 87 88 90 91 92 93 94 96 97 100 102 104 107 116 119 121 123 124 134 135 136 137
Primary Contact: Richard Kirk Toomey, FACHE, President and Chief Executive Officer
CFO: Jeffrey L. White, Chief Financial Officer
CMO: H. Tim Pearce, M.D., Chief of Staff
Web address: www.bmhsc.org
Control: County–Government, nonfederal **Service:** General Medical and Surgical

Staffed Beds: 200 **Admissions:** 10081 **Census:** 127 **Outpatient Visits:** 38879 **Births:** 1987 **Total Expense ($000):** 122016 **Payroll Expense ($000):** 49917 **Personnel:** 1080

★ **NAVAL HOSPITAL**, 1 Pinckney Boulevard, Zip 29902–6148; tel. 843/228–5301, (Nonreporting) **A**1 5 **S** Bureau of Medicine and Surgery, Department of the Navy
Primary Contact: Captain James Hoffower, Commanding Officer
CIO: Lieutenant Dallas Jones, Head Management Information
Control: Navy, Government, federal **Service:** General Medical and Surgical

Staffed Beds: 20

BENNETTSVILLE—Marlboro County

★ **MARLBORO PARK HOSPITAL (420054)**, 1138 Cheraw Highway, Zip 29512–0738, Mailing Address: P.O. Box 738, Zip 29512–0738; tel. 843/479–2881 **A**1 9 10 **F**3 13 15 17 24 25 33 38 55 57 60 68 73 74 75 77 79 81 82 84 85 86 88 91 93 96 97 107 117 118 119 122 135 136 **S** Community Health Systems, Inc.
Primary Contact: Todd Blanchard, Chief Executive Officer
CFO: Troy Pickens, Chief Financial Officer
CMO: Shaukat Iftikhar, M.D., Chief of Staff
CHR: Christi Meggs, Director Human Resources
Web address: www.marlboroparkhospital.com
Control: Partnership, Investor–owned, for–profit **Service:** General Medical and Surgical

Staffed Beds: 102 **Admissions:** 1883 **Census:** 18 **Outpatient Visits:** 14463 **Births:** 126 **Total Expense ($000):** 23277 **Payroll Expense ($000):** 9081 **Personnel:** 155

Many Facility Codes have changed. Please refer to the AHA Guide Code Chart.

CAMDEN—Kershaw County

★ **KERSHAW COUNTY MEDICAL CENTER (420048)**, 1315 Roberts Street, Zip 29020–7003, Mailing Address: P.O. Box 7003, Zip 29021–7003; tel. 803/432–4311, (Total facility includes 88 beds in nursing home–type unit) **A**1 9 10 **F**1 3 7 11 13 15 18 22 24 25 26 27 28 30 31 33 37 38 41 42 49 50 51 52 53 54 55 56 57 60 61 62 65 66 68 73 74 75 76 77 79 80 81 82 84 85 86 87 90 96 97 100 102 103 107 117 118 119 121 132 135 136
Primary Contact: Donnie J. Weeks, FACHE, President and Chief Executive Officer
COO: Mike Bunch, Vice President and Chief Operating Officer
CFO: Rick Humphrey, Vice President and Chief Financial Officer
CHR: Angela Nettles, Director Human Resources
Web address: www.kcmc.org
Control: County–Government, nonfederal **Service:** General Medical and Surgical

Staffed Beds: 191 **Admissions:** 5796 **Census:** 157 **Births:** 443 **Total Expense ($000):** 81988 **Payroll Expense ($000):** 34388 **Personnel:** 853

CHARLESTON—Charleston County

★ **BON SECOURS–ST. FRANCIS XAVIER HOSPITAL (420065)**, 2095 Henry Tecklenburg Drive, Zip 29414–0001; tel. 843/402–1000 **A**1 9 10 **F**1 3 7 13 14 15 18 24 25 26 30 31 32 33 38 40 43 44 46 47 48 49 50 51 54 55 56 57 59 62 66 68 71 72 73 74 75 76 77 78 79 80 81 82 84 86 90 96 97 99 100 102 106 107 117 119 120 121 134 135 136 137 **P**6 **S** Carolinas HealthCare System
Primary Contact: Allen P. Carroll, Administrator
CFO: Bret Johnson, Chief Financial Officer
CMO: Michael Spandorter, M.D., Chief Medical Officer
CIO: Michael Taylor, Chief Information Officer
CHR: Doug Harrison, Vice President Human Resources
Web address: www.ropersaintfrancis.com
Control: Other not–for–profit (including NFP Corporation) **Service:** General Medical and Surgical

Staffed Beds: 145 **Admissions:** 8854 **Census:** 104 **Outpatient Visits:** 126245 **Births:** 1418 **Total Expense ($000):** 104254 **Payroll Expense ($000):** 39660 **Personnel:** 810

★ **CHARLESTON MEMORIAL HOSPITAL (420006)**, 326 Calhoun Street, Zip 29401–1189; tel. 843/792–2300 **A**1 9 10 **F**1 3 15 26 31 32 38 96 107 119 **S** MUSC Medical Center of Medical University of South Carolina
Primary Contact: John Franklin, Director
COO: W. Stuart Smith, Vice President Clinical Operations
CFO: Todd Nimmich, Manager Fiscal Services
CMO: Patrick J. Cawley, M.D., Executive Medical Director
CHR: Helena G. Bastian, Director Human Resource Services
Web address: www.musc.edu
Control: State–Government, nonfederal **Service:** General Medical and Surgical

Staffed Beds: 20 **Admissions:** 118 **Census:** 18 **Outpatient Visits:** 13947 **Births:** 0 **Total Expense ($000):** 17518 **Payroll Expense ($000):** 6840 **Personnel:** 147

★ **HEALTHSOUTH REHABILITATION HOSPITAL OF CHARLESTON (423027)**, 9181 Medcom Street, Zip 29406–9168; tel. 843/820–7777 **A**1 10 **F**1 9 25 32 33 43 52 53 54 55 58 62 63 75 77 81 85 86 121 132 135 137 **S** HEALTHSOUTH Corporation
Primary Contact: Troy Powell, Chief Executive Officer
CFO: Beckye Lariviere, Chief Financial Officer
CMO: Ruth Hoover, M.D., Medical Director
CHR: Donna White, Director Human Resources
Web address: www.healthsouthcharleston.com
Control: Corporation, Investor–owned, for–profit **Service:** Rehabilitation

Staffed Beds: 46 **Admissions:** 929 **Census:** 37 **Outpatient Visits:** 0 **Births:** 0 **Total Expense ($000):** 11004 **Payroll Expense ($000):** 5673 **Personnel:** 118

□ **KINDRED HOSPITAL–CHARLESTON (422005)**, 326 Calhoun Street, 3rd Floor, Zip 29401; tel. 843/876–8670 **A**1 10 **F**1 3 12 16 25 33 44 54 59 73 78 85 137
Primary Contact: Bradley Talbert, Chief Executive Officer
COO: Katherine LaPorte, Chief Operating Officer
CFO: Julia Smith, Chief Financial Officer
CMO: Athena Beldecos, M.D., Medical Director
CHR: Darren Coffing, Area Director Human Resources
Web address: www.khcharleston.com
Control: Corporation, Investor–owned, for–profit **Service:** Long–Term Acute Care hospital

Staffed Beds: 55 **Admissions:** 359 **Census:** 30 **Outpatient Visits:** 0 **Births:** 0 **Total Expense ($000):** 13692 **Payroll Expense ($000):** 4852 **Personnel:** 102

★ **MUSC MEDICAL CENTER OF MEDICAL UNIVERSITY OF SOUTH CAROLINA (420004)**, 169 Ashley Avenue, Zip 29425; tel. 843/792–2300 **A**1 2 3 5 8 9 10 **F**1 3 4 5 6 7 9 11 12 13 15 16 17 18 19 20 21 22 23 24 25 26 27 28 30 31 32 33 35 36 37 38 40 41 43 44 45 46 47 48 49 50 52 54 55 56 57 59 60 62 64 66 68 69 70 71 72 73 74 75 76 77 78 79 80 81 82 83 84 86 87 88 89 90 91 92 93 94 95 96 97 99 100 102 103 104 105 107 108 109 111 112 113 114 117 118 119 120 121 123 124 125 126 127 128 130 131 133 134 135 136 137 **S** MUSC Medical Center of Medical University of South Carolina
Primary Contact: Stuart Smith, Vice President Clinical Operations and Executive Director
CFO: Lisa P. Montgomery, Administrator Finance and Support Services
CMO: Patrick J. Cawley, M.D., Medical Director
CIO: Frank Clark, Chief Information Officer
CHR: Betts Ellis, Administrator Institutional Relations
Web address: www.muschealth.com
Control: State–Government, nonfederal **Service:** General Medical and Surgical

Staffed Beds: 596 **Admissions:** 31546 **Census:** 494 **Outpatient Visits:** 791909 **Births:** 2685 **Total Expense ($000):** 739479 **Payroll Expense ($000):** 265449 **Personnel:** 5270

□ **PALMETTO LOWCOUNTRY BEHAVIORAL HEALTH (424006)**, 2777 Speissegger Drive, Zip 29405–8299; tel. 843/747–5830 **A**1 9 10 **F**4 5 25 62 88 89 91 92 94 95 119 121 **S** Psychiatric Solutions
Primary Contact: Cherie Tolley, Chief Executive Officer
COO: Susan Weinstein, Chief Operating Officer
CMO: Ric Fermo, M.D., Chief Medical Officer
Web address: www.plbhs.com
Control: Corporation, Investor–owned, for–profit **Service:** Psychiatric

Staffed Beds: 70 **Admissions:** 3265 **Census:** 55 **Total Expense ($000):** 14557 **Payroll Expense ($000):** 7490 **Personnel:** 231

★ **RALPH H. JOHNSON VETERANS AFFAIRS MEDICAL CENTER**, 109 Bee Street, Zip 29401–5799; tel. 843/577–5011 **A**1 2 3 5 8 **F**1 3 4 5 8 17 18 20 22 25 26 27 32 37 38 42 43 44 45 46 50 53 54 55 57 59 60 61 62 63 66 68 69 72 73 75 76 77 79 80 81 85 86 87 88 90 91 92 94 96 97 100 103 106 107 117 118 119 124 135 136 137 **P**6 **S** Department of Veterans Affairs
Primary Contact: John E. Barilich, Director
CFO: Michael Holland, Chief Financial Officer
CMO: Florence N. Hutchison, M.D., Chief of Staff
CIO: Michael Cortright, Chief Information Officer
Web address: www.va.gov/sta/guide/home.asp
Control: Veterans Affairs, Government, federal **Service:** General Medical and Surgical

Staffed Beds: 98 **Admissions:** 3932 **Census:** 64 **Outpatient Visits:** 443850 **Total Expense ($000):** 173693 **Payroll Expense ($000):** 106611 **Personnel:** 1237

★ **ROPER HOSPITAL (420087)**, 316 Calhoun Street, Zip 29401–1125; tel. 843/724–2000 **A**1 2 3 5 9 10 **F**1 3 7 8 11 13 15 17 18 20 22 24 25 26 27 30 31 32 33 38 39 40 44 49 50 51 53 54 55 56 57 58 59 60 61 62 66 67 68 71 72 73 74 75 76 77 78 79 80 81 82 85 86 90 96 97 99 100 102 105 106 107 108 109 111 112 114 116 117 118 119 120 121 124 125 132 133 135 136 137 **P**6 **S** Carolinas HealthCare System
Primary Contact: Matthew J. Severance, Chief Executive Officer
CFO: Bret Johnson, Chief Financial Officer
CMO: Steven D. Shapiro, M.D., Vice President Medical Affairs
CIO: Michael Taylor, Chief Information Officer
CHR: Douglas Harrison, Vice President Human Resources
Web address: www.ropersaintfrancis.com
Control: Other not–for–profit (including NFP Corporation) **Service:** General Medical and Surgical

Staffed Beds: 342 **Admissions:** 17196 **Census:** 270 **Outpatient Visits:** 270404 **Births:** 973 **Total Expense ($000):** 305541 **Payroll Expense ($000):** 104998 **Personnel:** 2102

★ **TRIDENT MEDICAL CENTER (420079)**, 9330 Medical Plaza Drive, Zip 29406–9195; tel. 843/797–7000 **A**1 2 3 5 9 10 **F**1 3 13 15 16 18 20 22 24 25 26 27 30 31 32 33 38 39 40 44 48 49 53 54 55 56 57 58 59 60 62 68 70 71 72 73 74 76 77 78 79 80 81 82 84 85 86 96 97 100 102 103 106 107 109 111 117 119 120 121 124 134 135 136 137 **S** HCA
Primary Contact: Terry J. Gunn, President and Chief Executive Officer
COO: Mark Robinson, Chief Operating Officer
CFO: Karl E. Gorrell, Chief Financial Officer
CIO: Susan Murray, Director Information Services
CHR: Joe B. Hill, Vice President Human Resources
Web address: www.tridenthealthsystem.com
Control: Corporation, Investor–owned, for–profit **Service:** General Medical and Surgical

Staffed Beds: 281 **Admissions:** 16261 **Census:** 214 **Outpatient Visits:** 64260 **Births:** 2469 **Total Expense ($000):** 166192 **Personnel:** 1255

Hospital, Medicare Provider Number, Address, Telephone, Approval, Facility, and Physician Codes, Health Care System

★ American Hospital Association (AHA) membership
□ The Joint Commission accreditation
○ American Osteopathic Association (AOA) accreditation
△ Commission on Accreditation of Rehabilitation Facilities (CARF) accreditation

CHERAW—Chesterfield County

★ **CHESTERFIELD GENERAL HOSPITAL (420062)**, 711 Chesterfield Highway, Zip 29520; tel. 843/537–7881 **A**1 9 10 **F**3 11 13 15 24 25 26 30 31 32 33 38 55 56 57 62 63 68 69 72 73 74 75 77 79 80 81 82 84 85 86 92 96 97 102 107 113 119 121 122 124 135 137 **S** Community Health Systems, Inc.
Primary Contact: Vance Reynolds, Chief Executive Officer
CFO: Nathan Crabdree, Chief Financial Officer
CMO: David Bersinger, M.D., Chief of Staff
CHR: Donna Damico, Director Human Resources
Web address: www.chesterfieldgeneral.com
Control: Corporation, Investor–owned, for–profit **Service:** General Medical and Surgical

Staffed Beds: 59 **Admissions:** 2894 **Census:** 28 **Outpatient Visits:** 33946 **Births:** 172 **Total Expense ($000):** 27329 **Payroll Expense ($000):** 10553 **Personnel:** 214

CHESTER—Chester County

☐ **CHESTER REGIONAL MEDICAL CENTER (420019)**, 1 Medical Park Drive, Zip 29706–9799; tel. 803/581–3151, (Total facility includes 100 beds in nursing home–type unit) **A**1 9 10 **F**1 15 18 24 25 32 33 38 54 55 56 61 62 68 73 77 79 80 81 82 84 86 96 97 102 107 118 119 120 121 135 **S** Health Management Associates
Primary Contact: Patrice L. Tavernier, Chief Executive Officer
CIO: Rick Lewis, Chief Information Officer
Web address: www.chospital.org
Control: Corporation, Investor–owned, for–profit **Service:** General Medical and Surgical

Staffed Beds: 156 **Admissions:** 2121 **Census:** 20 **Outpatient Visits:** 15440 **Total Expense ($000):** 27321 **Payroll Expense ($000):** 10642 **Personnel:** 203

CLINTON—Laurens County

★ **LAURENS COUNTY HEALTHCARE SYSTEM (420038)**, Highway 76 East, Zip 29325–2331, Mailing Address: P.O. Box 976, Zip 29325–0976; tel. 864/833–9100, (Includes LAURENS COUNTY HOSPITAL, Mailing Address: P.O. Box 976, Zip 29325; tel. 803/833–9100), (Total facility includes 14 beds in nursing home–type unit) **A**1 9 10 **F**1 3 11 13 15 17 24 25 26 28 30 32 33 38 55 57 60 62 68 73 74 75 77 78 79 80 82 84 85 86 96 97 100 107 117 118 119 121 124 136 137 **P**8
Primary Contact: James Boote, Chief Executive Officer
COO: Kay Swisher, Vice President Patient Care Services
CFO: William Grant, Vice President Fiscal and Support Services
CMO: Mike Wiggins, M.D., Chief of Staff
CIO: Wade Williams, Director Information Systems
CHR: Robin Callas, Director Human Resources
Web address: www.lchcs.org
Control: Hospital district or authority, Government, nonfederal **Service:** General Medical and Surgical

Staffed Beds: 87 **Admissions:** 3068 **Census:** 41 **Outpatient Visits:** 33868 **Births:** 408 **Total Expense ($000):** 47586 **Payroll Expense ($000):** 17636 **Personnel:** 401

WHITTEN CENTER, Highway 76 East, Zip 29325, Mailing Address: P.O. Box 239, Zip 29325; tel. 864/833–2733, (Nonreporting)
Primary Contact: William Killion, Chief Executive Officer
Control: State–Government, nonfederal **Service:** Institution for mental retardation

Staffed Beds: 22

COLUMBIA—Richland County

☐ **G. WERBER BRYAN PSYCHIATRIC HOSPITAL (424005)**, 220 Faison Drive, Zip 29203–3295; tel. 803/935–7146 **A**1 10 **F**4 26 30 31 32 73 87 88 91 93 119 121 124 135
Primary Contact: Ronald Prier, Director
COO: Jaclyn Upfield, Director Operating Officer
CIO: Sam Livingston, Information Resource Consultant
CHR: Kim Church, Manager Human Resources
Web address: www.scdmh.org
Control: State–Government, nonfederal **Service:** Psychiatric

Staffed Beds: 251 **Admissions:** 999 **Census:** 234 **Total Expense ($000):** 28573 **Payroll Expense ($000):** 16230 **Personnel:** 429

★ **HEALTHSOUTH REHABILITATION HOSPITAL (423025)**, 2935 Colonial Drive, Zip 29203–6811; tel. 803/254–7777 **A**1 10 **F**2 25 30 31 32 33 53 54 55 56 57 58 62 72 73 75 77 81 82 85 86 119 120 121 132
S HEALTHSOUTH Corporation
Primary Contact: James H. Rogers, FACHE, Chief Executive Officer
CFO: Jessica Burriss, Chief Financial Officer
CMO: Devin Troyer, M.D., Medical Director
CHR: Luanne Burton, Director Human Resources
Web address: www.healthsouth.com
Control: Corporation, Investor–owned, for–profit **Service:** Rehabilitation

Staffed Beds: 96 **Admissions:** 1248 **Census:** 60 **Outpatient Visits:** 20282 **Births:** 0 **Total Expense ($000):** 17827 **Payroll Expense ($000):** 9220 **Personnel:** 241

INTERMEDICAL HOSPITAL OF SOUTH CAROLINA (422006), Taylor at Marion Street, Zip 29220; tel. 803/296–3097 **A**9 10 **F**1 3 25 30 55 58 119
Primary Contact: Armando Columbo, Chief Executive Officer
Web address: www.intermedicalhospital.com
Control: Other not–for–profit (including NFP Corporation) **Service:** Long–Term Acute Care hospital

Staffed Beds: 35 **Admissions:** 275 **Census:** 26 **Total Expense ($000):** 10772 **Payroll Expense ($000):** 2768 **Personnel:** 64

★ **PALMETTO HEALTH BAPTIST/COLUMBIA (420086)**, Taylor at Marion Street, Zip 29220–0001; tel. 803/296–5010, (Total facility includes 22 beds in nursing home–type unit) **A**1 2 3 5 9 10 **F**1 3 11 12 13 15 17 18 25 26 27 30 31 32 33 38 42 43 44 47 48 49 51 53 55 56 57 60 61 62 64 66 68 69 70 71 72 73 74 75 76 77 79 80 81 82 84 86 88 89 90 91 92 93 94 95 96 97 99 100 101 102 104 105 106 107 117 119 121 135 136 137 **S** Palmetto Health
Primary Contact: James M. Bridges, Executive Vice President and Chief Operating Officer
COO: James M. Bridges, Executive Vice President and Chief Operating Officer
CFO: Paul K. Duane, Executive Vice President and Chief Financial Officer
CMO: Mark J. Mayson, M.D., Chief of Staff
CIO: David Garrett, Executive Vice President Information Technology
CHR: Trip Gregory, Senior Vice President Human Resources
Web address: www.palmettohealth.org
Control: Other not–for–profit (including NFP Corporation) **Service:** General Medical and Surgical

Staffed Beds: 441 **Admissions:** 19732 **Census:** 319 **Outpatient Visits:** 43462 **Births:** 3948 **Total Expense ($000):** 311362 **Payroll Expense ($000):** 127042 **Personnel:** 2305

★ **PALMETTO HEALTH RICHLAND (420018)**, Five Richland Medical Park Drive, Zip 29203–6897, Mailing Address: P.O. Box 2266, Zip 29203–2266; tel. 803/434–7000 **A**1 2 3 5 8 9 10 **F**1 2 3 4 5 6 11 13 15 17 18 20 22 24 25 26 27 28 30 31 32 33 37 38 40 53 54 55 56 57 58 59 60 62 66 68 70 71 73 74 75 76 77 79 81 82 83 84 85 86 87 88 89 90 91 92 93 94 95 96 97 99 100 102 106 107 109 114 116 117 118 119 120 121 123 124 132 135 136 137 **S** Palmetto Health
Primary Contact: John Singerling, Executive Vice President and Chief Operating Officer
CFO: Paul K. Duane, Executive Vice President and Chief Financial Officer
CMO: Edward Catalano, M.D., Chief of Staff
CIO: David Garrett, Executive Vice President Information Technology
CHR: Trip Gregory, Senior Vice President Human Resources
Web address: www.palmettohealth.org
Control: Other not–for–profit (including NFP Corporation) **Service:** General Medical and Surgical

Staffed Beds: 643 **Admissions:** 35291 **Census:** 520 **Outpatient Visits:** 434718 **Births:** 2717 **Total Expense ($000):** 542091 **Payroll Expense ($000):** 204146 **Personnel:** 4050

★ **SISTERS OF CHARITY PROVIDENCE HOSPITALS (420026)**, 2435 Forest Drive, Zip 29204–2098; tel. 803/865–4500, (Includes PROVIDENCE HOSPITAL NORTHEAST, 120 Gateway Corporate Boulevard, Zip 29203–9611; tel. 803/865–4500; Ryan Hall, Vice President) **A**1 9 10 **F**1 3 8 11 17 18 20 22 24 25 26 30 31 32 33 38 49 50 53 55 56 57 58 60 62 66 68 72 77 78 79 80 81 82 85 86 90 96 97 100 102 106 107 119 121 130 135 136 **P**5
S Sisters of Charity Health System
Primary Contact: George A. Zara, President and Chief Executive Officer
CFO: David K. Stewart, Senior Vice President and Chief Financial Officer
CIO: Lib Cumbee, Director Information Systems
CHR: Richard W. Grooms, Vice President Human Resources
Web address: www.provhosp.com
Control: Church–operated, Nongovernment, not–for profit **Service:** General Medical and Surgical

Staffed Beds: 258 **Admissions:** 11853 **Census:** 167 **Births:** 0 **Total Expense ($000):** 181920 **Payroll Expense ($000):** 54465 **Personnel:** 1200

☐ **WILLIAM S. HALL PSYCHIATRIC INSTITUTE (424003)**, 1800 Colonial Drive, Zip 29203–6827, Mailing Address: P.O. Box 119, Zip 29202–0119; tel. 803/898–1693 **A**1 3 5 10 **F**4 26 31 32 72 73 88 89 94 119 135
Primary Contact: Ronald Prier, Director
COO: Jaclyn Upfield, Director Operating Officer
CMO: Timothy Kowalski, Director Medical Services
CIO: Keith Loner, Director Information Technology
CHR: Kim Church, Manager Human Resources
Web address: www.scdmh.org
Control: State–Government, nonfederal **Service:** Psychiatric

Staffed Beds: 81 **Admissions:** 391 **Census:** 37 **Total Expense ($000):** 33596 **Payroll Expense ($000):** 3829 **Personnel:** 214

Many Facility Codes have changed. Please refer to the AHA Guide Code Chart.

★ **WM. JENNINGS BRYAN DORN VETERANS AFFAIRS MEDICAL CENTER**, 6439 Garners Ferry Road, Zip 29209–1639; tel. 803/776–4000, (Nonreporting) **A**1 2 3 5 9 **S** Department of Veterans Affairs
Primary Contact: Brian Heckert, Medical Center Director
COO: Thomas Wisnieski, Associate Director
CFO: James Cavanaugh, Chief Finance Officer
CMO: Alfred Boykin, M.D., Chief of Staff
CIO: David C. Owings, Director Information Management Service Line
Web address: www.va.gov/sta/guide/home.asp
Control: Veterans Affairs, Government, federal **Service:** General Medical and Surgical

Staffed Beds: 109

CONWAY—Horry County

★ **CONWAY MEDICAL CENTER (420049)**, 300 Singleton Ridge Road, Zip 29526–9175, Mailing Address: P.O. Box 829, Zip 29528–0829; tel. 843/347–7111, (Total facility includes 88 beds in nursing home–type unit) **A**1 9 10 **F**1 3 8 11 12 13 15 18 24 25 26 30 31 32 33 38 40 44 46 51 52 55 56 57 59 60 68 71 73 74 75 77 78 79 80 81 82 84 85 86 96 97 100 102 104 105 106 107 117 118 119 121 124 135 136
Primary Contact: Philip A. Clayton, President and Chief Executive Officer
CFO: Bret Barr, Vice President Fiscal Services
CMO: Russell L. Derrick, M.D., Chief of Staff
CIO: Mickey Waters, Director Information Technology
CHR: Craig Hyman, Vice President Human Resources
Web address: www.conwaymedicalcenter.com
Control: Other not–for–profit (including NFP Corporation) **Service:** General Medical and Surgical

Staffed Beds: 254 **Admissions:** 10269 **Census:** 191 **Births:** 1596 **Personnel:** 1024

LIGHTHOUSE CARE CENTER OF CONWAY (424002), 152 Waccamaw Medical Park Drive, Zip 29520; tel. 843/347–8871 **A**9 10 **F**88 **S** Horizon Health Corporation
Primary Contact: Fran Sauvageau, Chief Executive Officer
CFO: Alan Moore, Chief Financial Officer
CMO: Jim Graham, M.D., Medical Director
CHR: Sherry Hetherington, Director Human Resources
Control: Corporation, Investor–owned, for–profit **Service:** Psychiatric

Staffed Beds: 44 **Admissions:** 1229 **Census:** 27 **Total Expense ($000):** 4580 **Payroll Expense ($000):** 2246 **Personnel:** 185

DARLINGTON—Darlington County

MCLEOD MEDICAL CENTER–DARLINGTON See McLeod Health, Florence

DILLON—Dillon County

★ **MCLEOD MEDICAL CENTER–DILLON (420005)**, 301 East Jackson Street, Zip 29536–2509, Mailing Address: P.O. Box 1327, Zip 29536–1327; tel. 843/774–4111 **A**1 9 10 **F**1 3 11 13 15 24 25 26 28 30 31 32 33 38 43 50 55 56 57 62 66 68 73 74 75 79 80 82 84 85 86 96 97 100 107 117 119 121 123 124 135 136 **P**6
Primary Contact: Deborah Locklair, FACHE, Administrator
CFO: Fulton Ervin, Chief Financial Officer
CMO: Robin Shealy, M.D., Chief of Staff
CIO: Jenean Blackmon, Vice President Information System
CHR: Cynthia Causey, Associate Administrator Human and Mission Services
Web address: www.mcleodhealth.org
Control: Other not–for–profit (including NFP Corporation) **Service:** General Medical and Surgical

Staffed Beds: 66 **Admissions:** 3508 **Census:** 33 **Outpatient Visits:** 26699 **Births:** 362 **Total Expense ($000):** 32233 **Payroll Expense ($000):** 13496 **Personnel:** 301

EASLEY—Pickens County

★ **PALMETTO HEALTH BAPTIST EASLEY (420015)**, 200 Fleetwood Drive, Zip 29640–2076, Mailing Address: P.O. Box 2129, Zip 29641–2129; tel. 864/442–7200 **A**1 9 10 **F**3 11 13 15 18 24 25 26 30 31 32 33 37 38 54 55 57 58 62 68 73 74 77 79 80 81 82 84 96 97 107 119 121 123 135 136 **P**8 **S** Palmetto Health
Primary Contact: Roddey E. Gettys, III, Executive Vice President and Chief Operating Officer
COO: Roddey E. Gettys, Executive Vice President and Chief Operating Officer
CFO: J. Larry Pope, Vice President Finance
CMO: Karen Ardis, M.D., President Medical Staff
CHR: Elizabeth Parsons, Human Resources Business Partner
Web address: www.palmettohealth.org
Control: Other not–for–profit (including NFP Corporation) **Service:** General Medical and Surgical

Staffed Beds: 88 **Admissions:** 4911 **Census:** 52 **Outpatient Visits:** 43354 **Births:** 722 **Total Expense ($000):** 68802 **Payroll Expense ($000):** 27602 **Personnel:** 669

EDGEFIELD—Edgefield County

★ **EDGEFIELD COUNTY HOSPITAL (421304)**, 300 Ridge Medical Plaza, Zip 29824; tel. 803/637–3174 **A**1 9 10 18 **F**3 11 33 38 54 55 57 66 73 75 77 79 84 85 86 87 96 100 107 117 119 121 122
Primary Contact: Ray J. Price, Chief Executive Officer
CFO: Diane Robinson, Director Finance
CMO: Tami Massey, M.D., Chief Medical Staff
CIO: Faye Burton, Chief Health Information Management
CHR: Leslie Seigler, Coordinator Human Resources
Web address: www.myech.org
Control: Hospital district or authority, Government, nonfederal **Service:** General Medical and Surgical

Staffed Beds: 25 **Admissions:** 643 **Census:** 6 **Outpatient Visits:** 13066 **Total Expense ($000):** 9313 **Payroll Expense ($000):** 4518 **Personnel:** 120

FAIRFAX—Allendale County

★ **ALLENDALE COUNTY HOSPITAL (421300)**, 1787 Allendale Fairfax Highway, Zip 29827–0278, Mailing Address: P.O. Box 218, Zip 29827–0218; tel. 803/632–3311, (Total facility includes 44 beds in nursing home–type unit) **A**9 10 18 **F**1 3 15 30 31 33 38 42 55 57 60 62 65 82 85 86 87 96 107 117 119 122 136
Primary Contact: M. K. Hiatt, Administrator
Web address: www.allendalecountyhospital.com/
Control: County–Government, nonfederal **Service:** General Medical and Surgical

Staffed Beds: 69 **Admissions:** 297 **Census:** 42 **Births:** 5 **Total Expense ($000):** 10020 **Payroll Expense ($000):** 4495 **Personnel:** 137

FLORENCE—Florence County

★ △ **CAROLINAS HOSPITAL SYSTEM (420091)**, 805 Pamplico Highway, Zip 29505–6050, Mailing Address: P.O. Box 100550, Zip 29501–0550; tel. 843/674–5000, (Total facility includes 24 beds in nursing home–type unit) **A**1 7 9 10 **F**8 15 17 18 20 22 24 25 26 27 28 30 33 37 38 40 42 43 52 54 55 56 57 59 60 61 62 66 68 72 73 75 76 77 78 79 81 82 83 84 85 86 87 88 93 94 96 97 100 102 103 104 105 106 107 109 111 114 116 118 119 120 121 124 133 134 135 136 137 **S** Community Health Systems, Inc.
Primary Contact: James O'Laughlin, Chief Executive Officer
COO: Jodi Beauregard, Chief Operating Officer
CFO: Dennis Eith, Chief Financial Officer
CMO: Kevin Shea, M.D., Chief of Staff
CIO: Marty Parker, Chief Information Officer
CHR: Tammy Dickerson, Director Human Resources
Web address: www.carolinashospital.com
Control: Corporation, Investor–owned, for–profit **Service:** General Medical and Surgical

Staffed Beds: 334 **Admissions:** 13312 **Census:** 206 **Outpatient Visits:** 49057 **Personnel:** 1237

★ **HEALTHSOUTH REHABILITATION HOSPITAL (423026)**, 900 East Cheves Street, Zip 29506–2704; tel. 843/679–9000 **A**1 10 **F**9 25 31 32 33 43 54 55 56 57 62 73 75 81 82 85 86 119 120 121 132 137 **S** HEALTHSOUTH Corporation
Primary Contact: Jeanette Filpi, Chief Executive Officer
CFO: Robert Wheeler, Controller
CMO: Adora Matthews, M.D., Medical Director
CHR: Susan Trantham, Director Human Resources
Web address: www.healthsouth.com
Control: Corporation, Investor–owned, for–profit **Service:** Rehabilitation

Staffed Beds: 88 **Admissions:** 1234 **Census:** 54 **Total Expense ($000):** 13669 **Payroll Expense ($000):** 7623 **Personnel:** 199

SC

Hospital, Medicare Provider Number, Address, Telephone, Approval, Facility, and Physician Codes, Health Care System
★ American Hospital Association (AHA) membership
□ The Joint Commission accreditation
○ American Osteopathic Association (AOA) accreditation
△ Commission on Accreditation of Rehabilitation Facilities (CARF) accreditation

★ **MCLEOD HEALTH (420051)**, 555 East Cheves Street, Zip 29502–2617, Mailing Address: P.O. Box 100551, Zip 29502–0551; tel. 843/777–2000, (Includes MCLEOD MEDICAL CENTER–DARLINGTON, 701 Cashua Ferry Road, Darlington, Zip 29532, Mailing Address: P.O. Box 1859, Zip 29540; tel. 843/395–1100; Pat Godbold, Administrator) **A**1 3 5 9 10 **F**3 7 8 11 13 15 17 18 20 22 24 25 26 27 28 30 31 32 33 38 40 42 43 44 49 50 52 53 54 55 56 57 58 59 60 61 62 64 66 68 69 70 71 72 73 74 75 76 77 78 79 80 81 82 83 84 85 86 87 90 92 96 97 98 100 102 103 104 106 107 108 109 111 112 117 118 119 120 121 124 132 133 134 135 136 137 **P**6
Primary Contact: Robert L. Colones, President and Chief Executive Officer
CFO: Fulton Ervin, Chief Financial Officer
CMO: Alva W. Whitehead, M.D., Vice President Medical Services
CIO: Jenean Blackmon, Associate Vice President and Chief Information Officer
CHR: Jeannette Glenn, Vice President Human Resources, Education and Training
Web address: www.mcleodhealth.org
Control: Other not–for–profit (including NFP Corporation) **Service:** General Medical and Surgical

Staffed Beds: 493 **Admissions:** 22789 **Census:** 342 **Outpatient Visits:** 78108 **Births:** 2188 **Total Expense ($000):** 386420 **Payroll Expense ($000):** 131769 **Personnel:** 3257

★ **REGENCY HOSPITAL OF FLORENCE (422007)**, 121 East Cedar Street, Zip 29506; tel. 843/661–3499 **A**1 9 10 **F**1 3 25 33 43 50 54 55 56 73 75 81 82 107 119 137 **S** Regency Hospital Company
Primary Contact: Timothy T. Poore, Interim Chief Executive Officer
CFO: Timothy T. Poore, Interim Chief Executive Officer
CIO: Linda Morehouse, Manager Health Information
CHR: Jeanette Jackson, Manager Human Resources
Web address: www.regencyhospital.com
Control: Corporation, Investor–owned, for–profit **Service:** Long–Term Acute Care hospital

Staffed Beds: 40 **Admissions:** 371 **Census:** 28 **Outpatient Visits:** 0 **Births:** 0 **Total Expense ($000):** 13899 **Payroll Expense ($000):** 6076 **Personnel:** 111

SC

FORT JACKSON—Richland County

★ **MONCRIEF ARMY COMMUNITY HOSPITAL**, 4500 Stuart Street, Zip 29207–5720; tel. 803/751–2284, (Nonreporting) **A**1 5 **S** Department of the Army, Office of the Surgeon General
Primary Contact: Colonel James A. Mundy, Commander
CFO: Major Jeffery Rimmer, Chief Resource Management Division
CMO: Lieutenant Colonel Larry Andrew, M.D., Deputy Commander Clinical Services
CIO: Captain Jason Roberts, Deputy Commander Information Management
CHR: Major Jeffery Rimmer, Chief Resource Management Division
Web address: www.moncrief.amedd.army.mil
Control: Army, Government, federal **Service:** General Medical and Surgical

Staffed Beds: 60

GAFFNEY—Cherokee County

☐ **UPSTATE CAROLINA MEDICAL CENTER (420043)**, 1530 North Limestone Street, Zip 29340–4738; tel. 864/487–4271 **A**1 9 10 **F**1 3 7 11 13 15 25 26 32 33 38 46 51 55 57 62 68 73 74 75 77 79 81 82 84 96 97 99 100 102 107 117 118 119 120 135 136 137 **S** Health Management Associates
Primary Contact: Joe D. Howell, Executive Director
COO: Thom King, Chief Operating Officer
CFO: Michael Cherry, Chief Financial Officer
CMO: Richard Cutchin, M.D., Chief of Staff
CIO: Richard Bledsoe, Director Information Systems
CHR: Connie Gibson, R.N., Director Human Resources
Web address: www.upstatecarolina.org
Control: Corporation, Investor–owned, for–profit **Service:** General Medical and Surgical

Staffed Beds: 125 **Admissions:** 4223 **Census:** 47 **Births:** 466 **Total Expense ($000):** 33015 **Payroll Expense ($000):** 14339 **Personnel:** 361

GEORGETOWN—Georgetown County

★ **GEORGETOWN MEMORIAL HOSPITAL (420020)**, 606 Black River Road, Zip 29440–3368, Mailing Address: Drawer 421718, Zip 29442–1718; tel. 843/527–7000 **A**1 2 9 10 19 **F**3 11 12 13 15 17 18 20 25 26 27 28 30 31 32 33 37 38 43 44 50 51 52 53 54 55 56 57 59 60 62 63 66 68 71 72 73 74 75 76 77 79 81 82 84 85 86 87 90 92 96 97 98 100 102 105 106 107 109 111 119 120 121 124 135 136 137 **S** QHR
Primary Contact: Bruce P. Bailey, Chief Executive Officer
COO: Gayle L. Resetar, Chief Operating Officer
CFO: Terry L. Kiser, Chief Financial Officer
CMO: Steven B. Vallery, M.D., Chief of Staff
CHR: James F. Harper, Vice President and Chief Human Resources Officer
Web address: www.gmhsc.com
Control: Other not–for–profit (including NFP Corporation) **Service:** General Medical and Surgical

Staffed Beds: 136 **Admissions:** 6277 **Census:** 81 **Outpatient Visits:** 101911 **Births:** 488 **Total Expense ($000):** 100826 **Payroll Expense ($000):** 37796 **Personnel:** 750

GREENVILLE—Greenville County

★ △ **BON SECOURS ST. FRANCIS HEALTH SYSTEM (420023)**, One St. Francis Drive, Zip 29601–3207; tel. 864/255–1000 **A**1 2 7 9 10 **F**3 15 17 18 20 22 24 25 26 27 30 31 32 33 35 38 42 43 44 51 55 56 57 59 61 62 66 68 72 73 75 76 77 78 79 80 81 82 85 86 96 97 100 102 103 106 107 117 119 120 121 124 125 134 135 136 137 **P**1 **S** Bon Secours Health System, Inc.
Primary Contact: Valinda Rutledge, Chief Executive Officer
CFO: Ronnie Hyatt, Senior Vice President Finance
CMO: Mary Jo Cagle, M.D., Chief Medical Officer
CIO: Rita Hooker, Director Information Services
CHR: Lisa C. Slayton, Senior Vice President Human Resources
Web address: www.stfrancishealth.org
Control: Other not–for–profit (including NFP Corporation) **Service:** General Medical and Surgical

Staffed Beds: 245 **Admissions:** 10914 **Census:** 174 **Births:** 0 **Total Expense ($000):** 169516 **Payroll Expense ($000):** 57078 **Personnel:** 1757

★ △ **GREENVILLE MEMORIAL HOSPITAL (420078)**, 701 Grove Road, Zip 29605–4295; tel. 864/455–7000, (Includes MARSHALL I. PICKENS HOSPITAL; ROGER C. PEACE REHABILITATION HOSPITAL), (Total facility includes 15 beds in nursing home–type unit) **A**1 2 3 5 7 8 9 10 **F**3 5 11 13 15 17 18 20 22 24 25 26 27 30 31 32 33 34 36 37 38 40 41 44 46 49 50 52 53 54 55 56 57 58 60 62 63 64 65 66 68 70 71 72 73 74 75 76 77 78 79 80 81 82 83 84 85 86 87 88 89 90 91 92 93 94 95 96 99 100 102 103 106 107 113 118 119 120 121 123 124 135 136 137 **P**6 **S** Greenville Hospital System
Primary Contact: Greg Rusnak, Chief Operating Officer
Web address: www.ghs.org
Control: Other not–for–profit (including NFP Corporation) **Service:** General Medical and Surgical

Staffed Beds: 777 **Admissions:** 38897 **Census:** 644 **Outpatient Visits:** 453949 **Births:** 5645 **Total Expense ($000):** 676426 **Payroll Expense ($000):** 210077 **Personnel:** 4366

★ **PATEWOOD MEMORIAL HOSPITAL (420102)**, 175 Patewood Drive, Zip 29605; tel. 864/797–0112, (Nonreporting) **A**10 **S** Greenville Hospital System
Primary Contact: Scott R. Jones, Administrator
Control: Other not–for–profit (including NFP Corporation) **Service:** General Medical and Surgical

Staffed Beds: 72

★ **REGENCY HOSPITAL OF GREENVILLE (422009)**, One St. Francis Drive, 4th Floor, Zip 29601; tel. 864/255–1438 **A**1 9 10 **F**1 25 32 43 54 55 56 73 75 80 81 82 85 107 119 137 **P**5 **S** Regency Hospital Company
Primary Contact: Stephanie James, Chief Executive Officer
Web address: www.regencyhospital.com
Control: Corporation, Investor–owned, for–profit **Service:** Long–Term Acute Care hospital

Staffed Beds: 32 **Admissions:** 309 **Census:** 25 **Outpatient Visits:** 0 **Total Expense ($000):** 14707 **Payroll Expense ($000):** 6643 **Personnel:** 92

☐ **SHRINERS HOSPITALS FOR CHILDREN, GREENVILLE**, 950 West Faris Road, Zip 29605–4277; tel. 864/271–3444 **A**1 3 5 **F**43 55 62 66 73 77 79 80 81 84 85 86 117 119 135 137 **S** Shriners Hospitals for Children
Primary Contact: Gary F. Fraley, Administrator
CFO: Don Craig, Director Finance
CMO: Jon Davids, Chief of Staff
CHR: Willis Tisdale, Director Human Resources
Web address: www.shrinershq.org
Control: Other not–for–profit (including NFP Corporation) **Service:** Children's orthopedic

Staffed Beds: 50 **Admissions:** 991 **Census:** 10 **Births:** 0 **Personnel:** 221

GREENWOOD—Greenwood County

★ **SELF REGIONAL HEALTHCARE (420071)**, 1325 Spring Street, Zip 29646–3860; tel. 864/725–4111, (Total facility includes 27 beds in nursing home–type unit) **A**1 2 3 5 9 10 19 20 **F**3 8 11 12 13 15 17 18 20 22 24 26 27 28 30 31 32 33 36 37 38 40 43 49 50 52 53 55 56 57 59 61 62 66 68 70 71 72 73 74 75 76 77 78 79 81 82 84 85 86 87 88 89 90 91 92 93 94 95 96 97 99 100 102 103 105 106 107 108 109 111 112 117 118 119 120 121 123 124 133 135 136 137 **P**8
Primary Contact: M. John Heydel, President and Chief Executive Officer
COO: Fred L. Latham, Executive Vice President and Chief Operating Officer
CFO: Camie Patterson, Vice President and Chief Financial Officer
CMO: F. Gregory Mappin, M.D., Vice President Medical Affairs
CIO: Patrick Stewart, Vice President Information Systems
CHR: Susan Jones, Vice President Human Resources
Web address: www.selfregional.org
Control: County–Government, nonfederal **Service:** General Medical and Surgical

Staffed Beds: 382 **Admissions:** 14209 **Census:** 190 **Outpatient Visits:** 47337 **Births:** 1622 **Total Expense ($000):** 265668 **Payroll Expense ($000):** 102323 **Personnel:** 2121

Many Facility Codes have changed. Please refer to the AHA Guide Code Chart.

GREER—Greenville County

★ **ALLEN BENNETT MEMORIAL HOSPITAL (420033)**, (Formerly Allen Bennett Hospital), 313 Memorial Drive, Zip 29650–1521; tel. 864/848–8200, (Includes ROGER HUNTINGTON NURSING CENTER), (Total facility includes 88 beds in nursing home–type unit) **A**1 9 10 **F**1 3 11 13 15 24 25 26 30 31 32 33 38 40 41 49 50 55 56 57 60 62 63 66 68 74 77 79 80 81 82 84 86 96 100 102 107 117 118 119 135 136 **P**6 **S** Greenville Hospital System
Primary Contact: Phil Feisal, Administrator
Web address: www.ghs.org
Control: Other not–for–profit (including NFP Corporation) **Service:** General Medical and Surgical

Staffed Beds: 146 **Admissions:** 3269 **Census:** 121 **Outpatient Visits:** 94188 **Births:** 509 **Total Expense ($000):** 44525 **Payroll Expense ($000):** 18833 **Personnel:** 407

☐ **CAROLINA CENTER FOR BEHAVIORAL HEALTH (424010)**, 2700 East Phillips Road, Zip 29650–4816; tel. 864/235–2335 **A**1 9 10 **F**4 5 30 31 32 54 88 89 90 91 92 93 94 95 **S** Universal Health Services, Inc.
Primary Contact: John Willingham, Chief Executive Officer and Managing Director
COO: Keith Jackson, Director Business Development
CFO: Jeff Skelton, Chief Financial Officer
CMO: Ralph Castriotta, M.D., Medical Director
CHR: George Hammett, Director Human Resources
Web address: www.thecarolinacenter.com
Control: Corporation, Investor–owned, for–profit **Service:** Psychiatric

Staffed Beds: 89 **Admissions:** 2920 **Census:** 76 **Outpatient Visits:** 0 **Total Expense ($000):** 13365 **Payroll Expense ($000):** 7390 **Personnel:** 183

HARDEEVILLE—Jasper County

★ **COASTAL CAROLINA HOSPITAL (420101)**, (Formerly Coastal Carolina Medical Center), 1000 Medical Center Drive, Zip 29927; tel. 843/784–8000 **A**1 9 10 **F**3 15 25 31 33 38 55 57 62 68 72 73 75 77 79 80 84 85 86 96 97 100 102 107 119 120 135 137 **S** TENET Healthcare Corporation
Primary Contact: Teresa C. Urquhart, Chief Executive Officer
CFO: Gerard Diviney, Interim Chief Financial Officer
CIO: Carnel Aiken, Director Information Systems
Web address: www.coastalcarolinamedicalcenter.com
Control: Corporation, Investor–owned, for–profit **Service:** General Medical and Surgical

Staffed Beds: 41 **Admissions:** 1497 **Census:** 19 **Outpatient Visits:** 15796 **Births:** 0 **Total Expense ($000):** 27686 **Payroll Expense ($000):** 10156 **Personnel:** 188

HARTSVILLE—Darlington County

☐ **CAROLINA PINES REGIONAL MEDICAL CENTER (420010)**, 1304 West BoBo Newsom Highway, Zip 29550–4710; tel. 843/339–2100 **A**1 9 10 **F**3 13 15 18 24 25 26 32 33 38 40 46 49 55 57 62 67 68 71 72 73 74 77 79 80 81 82 84 85 86 96 97 100 103 106 107 118 119 121 124 135 136 137 **S** Health Management Associates
Primary Contact: David L. Castleberry, Chief Executive Officer
COO: Michael Kosor, Chief Operating Officer
CFO: James Young, Chief Financial Officer
CMO: Gary A. Barker, M.D., Chief of Staff
CIO: Denise Barefoot, Director Health Information Systems
CHR: Charlotte Adams, Director Human Resources
Web address: www.cprmc.com
Control: Corporation, Investor–owned, for–profit **Service:** General Medical and Surgical

Staffed Beds: 120 **Admissions:** 8283 **Census:** 94 **Births:** 656 **Total Expense ($000):** 57907 **Payroll Expense ($000):** 23282 **Personnel:** 479

HILTON HEAD ISLAND—Beaufort County

★ △ **HILTON HEAD HOSPITAL (420080)**, (Formerly Hilton Head Regional Medical Center), 25 Hospital Center Boulevard, Zip 29926–2738, Mailing Address: P.O. Box 21117, Zip 29925–1117; tel. 843/681–6122 **A**1 7 9 10 20 **F**3 8 11 12 13 15 17 18 20 22 24 25 26 27 28 30 31 32 33 38 44 48 49 50 53 54 55 56 57 59 60 62 63 66 68 72 73 74 75 76 77 79 80 81 82 84 85 86 87 89 90 91 92 93 96 97 99 100 102 107 108 119 120 121 124 133 135 136 137 **S** TENET Healthcare Corporation
Primary Contact: Elizabeth Lamkin, President and Chief Executive Officer
CFO: Todd Lockcuff, Chief Financial Officer
CMO: Glenn Neil Love, M.D., Medical Director
CIO: Stephen Brendler, Director Information Systems
CHR: Darlene Nester, Chief Human Resources Officer
Web address: www.hiltonheadregional.com
Control: Partnership, Investor–owned, for–profit **Service:** General Medical and Surgical

Staffed Beds: 93 **Admissions:** 4717 **Census:** 51 **Outpatient Visits:** 88675 **Births:** 708 **Total Expense ($000):** 81761 **Payroll Expense ($000):** 23130 **Personnel:** 502

KINGSTREE—Williamsburg County

★ **WILLIAMSBURG REGIONAL HOSPITAL (421303)**, 500 Nelson Boulevard, Zip 29556–4027; tel. 843/355–8888 **A**1 9 10 18 **F**1 3 7 11 15 25 26 31 32 33 38 41 50 54 55 57 62 66 75 79 81 82 84 85 86 96 107 119 122 124 135
Primary Contact: John C. Hales, Jr., FACHE, Chief Executive Officer
COO: Dan Harrington, Chief Operating Officer and Human Resources Director
CMO: Raymond K. Allen, M.D., Chief of Medical Staff
CIO: Jamie Newsom, Director Information Systems
Web address: www.wmbgrh.com/
Control: Other not–for–profit (including NFP Corporation) **Service:** General Medical and Surgical

Staffed Beds: 25 **Admissions:** 731 **Census:** 6 **Outpatient Visits:** 28694 **Births:** 0 **Total Expense ($000):** 14011 **Payroll Expense ($000):** 6077 **Personnel:** 167

LAKE CITY—Florence County

★ **LAKE CITY COMMUNITY HOSPITAL (420066)**, 258 North Ron McNair Boulevard, Zip 29560–1029, Mailing Address: P.O. Box 1479, Zip 29560–1479; tel. 843/374–2036 **A**1 9 10 **F**11 15 24 25 26 30 31 32 33 38 50 54 55 57 60 62 67 73 75 77 79 81 86 96 100 107 117 118 119 122 135
Primary Contact: Clarence W. Bowman, Chief Executive Officer
CMO: Wade Lamb, M.D., Chief of Staff
CIO: Kimberly Glover, Director Information Systems
CHR: Anne Poston, Human Resources Officer
Web address: www.lcchospital.org
Control: Hospital district or authority, Government, nonfederal **Service:** General Medical and Surgical

Staffed Beds: 18 **Admissions:** 1351 **Census:** 14 **Outpatient Visits:** 19073 **Total Expense ($000):** 21300 **Payroll Expense ($000):** 10359 **Personnel:** 190

SC

LANCASTER—Lancaster County

★ **SPRINGS MEMORIAL HOSPITAL (420036)**, 800 West Meeting Street, Zip 29720–2298; tel. 803/286–1481, (Total facility includes 14 beds in nursing home–type unit) **A**1 5 9 10 19 20 **F**3 4 8 11 13 15 17 18 25 27 30 32 33 38 40 42 47 49 55 61 62 66 68 71 72 73 74 76 77 79 80 84 85 86 92 96 97 100 102 103 106 107 117 118 121 135 136 **S** Community Health Systems, Inc.
Primary Contact: Tom R. McDougal, Chief Executive Officer
CFO: Julie Soekoro, Chief Financial Officer
CMO: Todd A. Scott, M.D., Chief of Staff
CIO: Chrys Steele, Director Information Systems
Web address: www.springsmemorial.com
Control: Corporation, Investor–owned, for–profit **Service:** General Medical and Surgical

Staffed Beds: 204 **Admissions:** 7173 **Census:** 101 **Outpatient Visits:** 36055 **Births:** 749 **Total Expense ($000):** 90183 **Payroll Expense ($000):** 27849 **Personnel:** 598

LORIS—Horry County

★ **LORIS COMMUNITY HOSPITAL (420064)**, 3655 Mitchell Street, Box 690001, Zip 29569–9601; tel. 843/716–7000, (Total facility includes 88 beds in nursing home–type unit) **A**1 9 10 **F**1 3 8 11 13 15 17 18 24 25 26 28 30 31 32 33 38 40 43 50 52 53 55 56 57 59 60 62 63 65 66 68 72 73 74 75 77 79 80 81 82 84 85 86 96 97 100 106 107 117 118 119 120 121 123 124 135 136 137
Primary Contact: J. Timothy Browne, President and Chief Executive Officer
COO: Arnold Green, Senior Vice President and Chief Operating Officer
CFO: Fred O. Todd, Senior Vice President Finance
CMO: James N. Craigie, M.D., Vice President Medical Affairs
CHR: Teresa Pougnaud, Vice President Human Resources
Web address: www.lorishealth.org
Control: Hospital district or authority, Government, nonfederal **Service:** General Medical and Surgical

Staffed Beds: 193 **Admissions:** 4425 **Census:** 128 **Outpatient Visits:** 116385 **Births:** 427 **Total Expense ($000):** 81115 **Payroll Expense ($000):** 31958 **Personnel:** 586

Hospital, Medicare Provider Number, Address, Telephone, Approval, Facility, and Physician Codes, Health Care System
★ American Hospital Association (AHA) membership
☐ The Joint Commission accreditation
○ American Osteopathic Association (AOA) accreditation
△ Commission on Accreditation of Rehabilitation Facilities (CARF) accreditation

MANNING—Clarendon County

★ **CLARENDON MEMORIAL HOSPITAL (420069)**, 10 Hospital Street, Zip 29102–3153, Mailing Address: P.O. Box 550, Zip 29102–0550; tel. 803/435–8463 **A**1 9 10 **F**1 3 7 11 13 15 24 25 26 30 31 32 33 37 38 43 50 52 53 54 55 57 60 61 62 65 68 73 74 75 77 79 80 84 85 86 96 97 100 102 107 117 118 119 121 124 132 135 136
Primary Contact: Edward R. Frye, Jr., Chief Executive Officer
COO: Eleyce Winn, Assistant Administrator
CFO: Richard Stokes, CPA, Chief Financial Officer
CMO: D. Maxwell Egbonim, M.D., Chief of Staff
CIO: Alicia Bullard, Manager Information Technology
CHR: Gail Duke, Director Human Resources
Web address: www.clarendonhealth.com
Control: Hospital district or authority, Government, nonfederal **Service:** General Medical and Surgical

Staffed Beds: 56 **Admissions:** 3041 **Census:** 40 **Outpatient Visits:** 109289 **Births:** 828 **Total Expense ($000):** 42458 **Payroll Expense ($000):** 17293 **Personnel:** 454

MOUNT PLEASANT—Charleston County

★ **EAST COOPER REGIONAL MEDICAL CENTER (420089)**, 1200 Johnnie Dodds Boulevard, Zip 29464–3294; tel. 843/881–0100 **A**1 5 9 10 **F**1 3 13 15 25 27 30 31 33 38 43 44 55 57 58 62 66 68 71 72 73 74 75 76 77 78 79 80 81 85 86 96 97 106 107 117 118 119 120 124 135 136 137 **S** TENET Healthcare Corporation
Primary Contact: Andrea L. Wozniak, RN, FACHE, Chief Executive Officer
COO: T. William Cone, Executive Vice President
CFO: Steve Woodford, Chief Financial Officer
CMO: W. John Langley, M.D., Chairman
CIO: Jack Goynes, Director Information Resources
CHR: Mike Gilpen, Director Human Resources
Web address: www.eastcoopermedctr.com
Control: Corporation, Investor–owned, for–profit **Service:** General Medical and Surgical

Staffed Beds: 106 **Admissions:** 5384 **Census:** 50 **Outpatient Visits:** 63448 **Births:** 1693 **Total Expense ($000):** 78482 **Payroll Expense ($000):** 26623 **Personnel:** 516

MULLINS—Marion County

★ **MARION COUNTY MEDICAL CENTER (420055)**, 2829 East Highway 76, Zip 29574–6035, Mailing Address: P.O. Drawer 1150, Marion, Zip 29571–1150; tel. 843/431–2000, (Total facility includes 92 beds in nursing home–type unit) **A**1 9 10 20 **F**1 3 11 13 15 24 25 26 28 30 31 32 33 38 43 51 52 54 55 56 57 60 62 63 64 65 68 73 74 75 79 80 81 84 85 87 96 97 100 103 107 117 118 119 120 121 124 135 136 **P**6
Primary Contact: Gene Tucker, Chief Executive Officer
CFO: Alta DuBose, Chief Financial Officer
CMO: Marc Bahan, M.D., Chief Medical Staff
CIO: Pat Strickland, Information Systems Manager
CHR: Kay White, Human Resources and Public Relations
Web address: www.marioncountymedical.com
Control: Corporation, Investor–owned, for–profit **Service:** General Medical and Surgical

Staffed Beds: 216 **Admissions:** 5543 **Census:** 151 **Outpatient Visits:** 25139 **Births:** 489 **Total Expense ($000):** 55425 **Payroll Expense ($000):** 22502 **Personnel:** 611

MURRELLS INLET—Georgetown County

★ **WACCAMAW COMMUNITY HOSPITAL (420098)**, 4070 Highway 17 Bypass, Zip 29576, Mailing Address: P.O. Drawer 3350, Zip 29576; tel. 843/652–1000 **A**1 9 10 **F**3 11 13 15 17 24 25 26 27 28 30 31 33 37 38 43 44 50 51 54 59 60 63 66 68 72 73 74 75 76 77 79 80 81 82 84 85 87 90 92 96 97 98 100 102 106 107 119 135 136 137 **S** QHR
Primary Contact: Gayle L. Resetar, Chief Operating Officer
CFO: Terry L. Kiser, Chief Financial Officer
CMO: Robert Fabrey, M.D., Chief Medical Officer
CIO: Gary Praznik, Chief Information Officer
Web address: www.gmhsc.com
Control: Other not–for–profit (including NFP Corporation) **Service:** General Medical and Surgical

Staffed Beds: 111 **Admissions:** 6791 **Census:** 95 **Outpatient Visits:** 66419 **Births:** 567 **Total Expense ($000):** 88049 **Payroll Expense ($000):** 24990 **Personnel:** 543

MYRTLE BEACH—Horry County

★ **GRAND STRAND REGIONAL MEDICAL CENTER (420085)**, 809 82nd Parkway, Zip 29572–1413; tel. 843/692–1000 **A**1 2 9 10 19 **F**1 3 11 13 15 17 18 20 22 24 25 26 27 30 31 32 33 35 37 38 39 40 43 46 47 49 50 53 54 55 56 57 59 62 68 71 72 73 74 75 76 77 79 80 81 82 84 85 86 96 97 100 102 103 106 107 117 119 121 124 135 136 **P**6 **S** HCA
Primary Contact: Doug White, Chief Executive Officer
CFO: Turner Wortham, Chief Financial Officer
Web address: www.grandstrandmed.com
Control: Corporation, Investor–owned, for–profit **Service:** General Medical and Surgical

Staffed Beds: 221 **Admissions:** 12395 **Census:** 158 **Births:** 1043 **Total Expense ($000):** 138897 **Personnel:** 932

NEWBERRY—Newberry County

★ **NEWBERRY COUNTY MEMORIAL HOSPITAL (420053)**, 2669 Kinard Street, Zip 29108–0497, Mailing Address: P.O. Box 497, Zip 29108–0497; tel. 803/276–7570, (Total facility includes 9 beds in nursing home–type unit) **A**1 9 10 20 **F**1 3 7 11 13 15 17 24 25 26 27 28 30 32 33 38 43 47 52 54 55 56 57 62 66 68 73 74 75 76 77 79 80 81 82 84 85 86 94 95 96 97 98 100 102 107 117 118 119 124 132 135 136 **S** QHR
Primary Contact: Lynn W. Beasley, President and Chief Executive Officer
CFO: Steve Sawyer, Chief Financial Officer
CHR: Shannon Iriel, Director Human Resources
Web address: www.newberryhospital.org
Control: County–Government, nonfederal **Service:** General Medical and Surgical

Staffed Beds: 48 **Admissions:** 2979 **Census:** 34 **Outpatient Visits:** 59154 **Births:** 444 **Total Expense ($000):** 38200 **Payroll Expense ($000):** 15792 **Personnel:** 355

ORANGEBURG—Orangeburg County

★ **REGIONAL MEDICAL CENTER OF ORANGEBURG AND CALHOUN COUNTIES (420068)**, 3000 St. Matthews Road, Zip 29118–1470; tel. 803/395–2200 **A**1 2 9 10 19 **F**3 11 13 14 15 17 18 24 25 26 27 28 33 38 40 41 42 43 44 52 55 56 57 59 60 61 66 68 71 72 73 74 75 76 77 79 80 81 82 84 85 86 88 90 91 92 93 96 97 98 100 102 106 107 109 118 119 120 121 123 124 135 136 137 **S** QHR
Primary Contact: Thomas C. Dandridge, President and Chief Executive Officer
COO: Lisa Goodlett, Chief Operating Officer
CFO: Dean R. Turner, Chief Financial Officer
CIO: Marilyn Tremblay, Director Information
CHR: Howard Harris, Vice President Human Resources
Web address: www.trmchealth.org
Control: County–Government, nonfederal **Service:** General Medical and Surgical

Staffed Beds: 266 **Admissions:** 10842 **Census:** 153 **Outpatient Visits:** 61477 **Births:** 1409 **Total Expense ($000):** 152076 **Payroll Expense ($000):** 66411 **Personnel:** 1225

PICKENS—Pickens County

★ **CANNON MEMORIAL HOSPITAL (420011)**, 123 West G. Acker Drive, Zip 29671–2739, Mailing Address: P.O. Box 188, Zip 29671–0188; tel. 864/878–4791 **A**1 9 10 **F**1 3 11 15 17 25 28 30 31 33 38 49 51 52 54 55 56 57 60 62 63 68 73 77 79 80 81 86 87 96 97 107 117 119 124 135 **P**8
Primary Contact: Norman G. Rentz, President and Chief Executive Officer
CFO: Mary F. Arnette, Chief Financial Officer
CMO: Daniel J. Dahlhausen, M.D., Chief of Staff
CIO: Amanda R. Dow, Director Community Relations
CHR: Lisa G. Bryant, Director Human Resources
Web address: www.cannonhospital.org
Control: Other not–for–profit (including NFP Corporation) **Service:** General Medical and Surgical

Staffed Beds: 42 **Admissions:** 1066 **Census:** 12 **Outpatient Visits:** 41819 **Births:** 0 **Total Expense ($000):** 17145 **Payroll Expense ($000):** 7180 **Personnel:** 251

ROCK HILL—York County

★ **HEALTHSOUTH REHABILITATION HOSPITAL (423028)**, 1795 Frank Gaston Boulevard, Zip 29732; tel. 803/362–3500 **A**1 10 **F**25 32 54 58 73 81 82 85 86 117 119 137 **S** HEALTHSOUTH Corporation
Primary Contact: Anthony W. Jackson, Chief Executive Officer
Web address: www.healthsouth.com
Control: Corporation, Investor–owned, for–profit **Service:** Rehabilitation

Staffed Beds: 40 **Admissions:** 922 **Census:** 32 **Outpatient Visits:** 10091 **Total Expense ($000):** 9424 **Payroll Expense ($000):** 5297 **Personnel:** 96

SC

★ **PIEDMONT MEDICAL CENTER (420002)**, 222 Herlong Avenue, Zip 29732–1952; tel. 803/329–1234 **A**1 2 9 10 **F**3 7 11 12 13 15 17 18 20 22 24 25 26 27 30 32 33 38 40 43 44 49 50 52 55 56 57 59 60 62 68 71 72 73 74 75 76 77 79 80 81 84 85 86 88 90 92 96 97 99 100 102 103 106 107 119 121 124 135 136 137 **S** TENET Healthcare Corporation
Primary Contact: Charles F. Miller, President and Chief Executive Officer
CFO: Neal Saul, Vice President Finance
Web address: www.piedmonthealth.com
Control: Corporation, Investor–owned, for–profit **Service:** General Medical and Surgical

Staffed Beds: 266 **Admissions:** 15205 **Census:** 186 **Outpatient Visits:** 145685 **Births:** 2453 **Total Expense ($000):** 204999 **Payroll Expense ($000):** 66856 **Personnel:** 1399

SENECA—Oconee County

★ **OCONEE MEMORIAL HOSPITAL (420009)**, 298 Memorial Drive, Zip 29672–9499; tel. 864/882–3351, (Includes LILA DOYLE NURSING CARE FACILITY), (Total facility includes 120 beds in nursing home–type unit) **A**1 9 10 **F**3 7 11 13 15 18 24 25 26 27 28 30 31 32 33 38 42 43 53 54 55 56 57 60 61 62 64 65 68 69 72 73 74 75 76 77 78 79 80 81 82 84 85 86 87 90 92 96 97 102 107 117 118 119 120 121 124 132 135 137 **P**8
Primary Contact: Jeanne L. Ward, President
COO: Jeanne L. Ward, President and Chief Executive Officer
CFO: Greg Scarbrough, Vice President Finance and Chief Financial Officer
CMO: Conrad K. Shuler, M.D., Chief Medical Officer
CIO: Jay Hansen, Director Information Services
CHR: Thomas C. Conley, Senior Director Human Resources
Web address: www.oconeemed.org
Control: Other not–for–profit (including NFP Corporation) **Service:** General Medical and Surgical

Staffed Beds: 242 **Admissions:** 7136 **Census:** 197 **Outpatient Visits:** 51121 **Births:** 556 **Total Expense ($000):** 122227 **Payroll Expense ($000):** 47679 **Personnel:** 1048

SIMPSONVILLE—Greenville County

★ **HILLCREST HOSPITAL (420037)**, 729 S.E. Main Street, Zip 29681–3280; tel. 864/967–6100 **A**1 9 10 **F**1 3 11 12 15 25 26 30 31 32 33 38 41 50 52 55 57 60 62 66 68 77 79 80 81 85 96 99 100 102 107 117 118 119 121 135 137 **P**6 **S** Greenville Hospital System
Primary Contact: Dennis R. Burns, FACHE, Administrator
CFO: Pam DeVore, Financial Manager
Web address: www.ghs.org
Control: Other not–for–profit (including NFP Corporation) **Service:** General Medical and Surgical

Staffed Beds: 43 **Admissions:** 1772 **Census:** 24 **Outpatient Visits:** 71486 **Births:** 0 **Total Expense ($000):** 37420 **Payroll Expense ($000):** 12268 **Personnel:** 226

SPARTANBURG—Spartanburg County

★ △ **MARY BLACK MEMORIAL HOSPITAL (420083)**, 1700 Skylyn Drive, Zip 29307–1061, Mailing Address: P.O. Box 3217, Zip 29304–3217; tel. 864/573–3000 **A**1 7 9 10 **F**3 11 13 15 18 25 27 31 33 38 46 47 49 50 53 55 56 57 58 62 68 71 73 74 75 76 77 79 80 81 82 84 85 86 88 93 96 97 100 102 103 106 107 112 119 120 131 133 135 136 137 **P**8 **S** Community Health Systems, Inc.
Primary Contact: Phillip L. Wright, FACHE, Chief Executive Officer
COO: Michael Davis, FACHE, Chief Operating Officer
CFO: Richard A. Meyer, Chief Financial Officer
Web address: www.maryblack.org
Control: Corporation, Investor–owned, for–profit **Service:** General Medical and Surgical

Staffed Beds: 182 **Admissions:** 7718 **Census:** 111 **Births:** 1245 **Total Expense ($000):** 111552 **Payroll Expense ($000):** 37109 **Personnel:** 736

★ **SPARTANBURG HOSPITAL FOR RESTORATIVE CARE (422004)**, 389 Serpentine Drive, Zip 29303–3026; tel. 864/560–3280, (Nonreporting) **A**1 9 10 **S** Spartanburg Regional Healthcare System
Primary Contact: Anita M. Butler, Chief Executive Officer
Web address: www.srhs.com
Control: Hospital district or authority, Government, nonfederal **Service:** Long–Term Acute Care hospital

Staffed Beds: 82

★ **SPARTANBURG REGIONAL MEDICAL CENTER (420007)**, 101 East Wood Street, Zip 29303–3016; tel. 864/560–6000 **A**1 2 3 5 9 10 12 13 **F**3 4 7 11 12 13 15 17 18 20 22 24 25 26 27 30 32 33 34 35 36 37 38 40 42 43 44 45 46 48 49 50 51 53 54 55 56 57 58 59 60 61 62 63 64 66 68 70 71 72 73 74 75 76 77 79 80 81 82 83 84 86 87 88 89 90 91 92 93 94 95 96 97 99 100 102 103 104 105 107 108 109 111 116 118 119 120 121 124 132 133 134 135 136 137 **P**5 **S** Spartanburg Regional Healthcare System
Primary Contact: Ingo Angermeier, FACHE, President and Chief Executive Officer
COO: Randall G. Nyp, Senior Vice President and Chief Operating Officer
CFO: Larry Barnette, Senior Vice President Finance
CMO: Robert Riehle, M.D., Vice President and Chief Medical Officer
CIO: Raymond Shingler, Vice President Information System
CHR: James R. Walker, Vice President Human Resources
Web address: www.srhs.com
Control: County–Government, nonfederal **Service:** General Medical and Surgical

Staffed Beds: 518 **Admissions:** 23407 **Census:** 410 **Outpatient Visits:** 364469 **Births:** 2792 **Total Expense ($000):** 470608 **Payroll Expense ($000):** 193829 **Personnel:** 4504

SUMMERVILLE—Dorchester County

★ **SUMMERVILLE MEDICAL CENTER**, 295 Midland Parkway, Zip 29485–8104; tel. 843/832–5000 **A**1 9 **F**3 13 15 24 25 26 30 31 32 33 38 44 48 49 54 55 56 57 58 62 68 73 74 77 79 80 81 82 84 85 86 96 97 100 102 106 107 118 119 121 124 135 136 137
Primary Contact: Patricia J. Johnson, Chief Executive Officer
COO: Court LeMaistre, Vice President Operations
CFO: Karl E. Gorrell, Chief Financial Officer
CIO: Susan Murray, Director Information Services
CHR: Catherine Johnston, Director Human Resources
Web address: www.tridenthealthsystem.com
Control: Corporation, Investor–owned, for–profit **Service:** General Medical and Surgical

Staffed Beds: 94 **Admissions:** 5763 **Census:** 65 **Outpatient Visits:** 39557 **Births:** 1146 **Total Expense ($000):** 52319 **Personnel:** 312

SUMTER—Sumter County

★ **TUOMEY HEALTHCARE SYSTEM (420070)**, 129 North Washington Street, Zip 29150–4983; tel. 803/774–9000, (Total facility includes 18 beds in nursing home–type unit) **A**1 9 10 **F**1 3 13 15 18 24 25 26 27 28 30 33 38 42 48 49 50 51 53 54 56 57 59 61 62 66 68 71 73 74 75 76 77 79 80 81 82 84 85 86 92 96 97 99 100 102 104 107 109 117 118 119 120 121 124 135 136 137
Primary Contact: Jay Cox, FACHE, President and Chief Executive Officer
COO: Gregg Martin, Vice President and Chief Operating Officer
CFO: William Johnson, Vice President and Chief Financial Officer
CMO: Gene Dickerson, M.D., Vice President Medical Affairs
CIO: Cheryl Martin, Chief Information Officer
CHR: Letitia Pringle, Administrative Director
Web address: www.tuomey.com
Control: Other not–for–profit (including NFP Corporation) **Service:** General Medical and Surgical

Staffed Beds: 281 **Admissions:** 10018 **Census:** 201 **Outpatient Visits:** 146121 **Births:** 1418 **Total Expense ($000):** 170386 **Payroll Expense ($000):** 60173 **Personnel:** 1511

TRAVELERS REST—Greenville County

★ **NORTH GREENVILLE HOSPITAL (422008)**, 807 North Main Street, Zip 29690–0628; tel. 864/834–5132 **A**1 10 **F**1 3 25 26 28 30 31 32 33 38 41 43 50 53 55 56 57 58 62 66 73 77 80 81 82 87 96 117 119 135 137 **P**6
Primary Contact: Michael Batchelor, Administrator
Web address: www.ghs.org
Control: Other not–for–profit (including NFP Corporation) **Service:** Long–Term Acute Care hospital

Staffed Beds: 28 **Admissions:** 280 **Census:** 22 **Outpatient Visits:** 45566 **Births:** 0 **Total Expense ($000):** 17870 **Payroll Expense ($000):** 6683 **Personnel:** 132

□ **SPRINGBROOK BEHAVIORAL HEALTH SYSTEM (424007)**, One Havenwood Lane, Zip 29690, Mailing Address: P.O. Box 1005, Zip 29690–1005; tel. 864/834–8013 **A**1 9 10 **F**31 81 88 89 91 92 93 119
Primary Contact: William A. Touchstone, Chief Executive Officer
CFO: James P. Boynton, Comptroller
CMO: Gretchen Enright, M.D., Medical Director
CHR: Adrienne Carter, Director Human Resources
Web address: www.springbrookbehavioral.com
Control: Corporation, Investor–owned, for–profit **Service:** Psychiatric

Staffed Beds: 88 **Admissions:** 433 **Census:** 13 **Total Expense ($000):** 8228 **Payroll Expense ($000):** 3612 **Personnel:** 128

SC

Hospital, Medicare Provider Number, Address, Telephone, Approval, Facility, and Physician Codes, Health Care System

★ American Hospital Association (AHA) membership
□ The Joint Commission accreditation
○ American Osteopathic Association (AOA) accreditation
△ Commission on Accreditation of Rehabilitation Facilities (CARF) accreditation

UNION—Union County

☒ **WALLACE THOMSON HOSPITAL (420039)**, 322 West South Street, Zip 29379–2857, Mailing Address: P.O. Box 789, Zip 29379–0789; tel. 864/427–0351, (Total facility includes 113 beds in nursing home–type unit) **A**1 9 10 **F**1 3 7 13 15 25 30 31 33 38 43 55 57 62 67 68 73 74 77 79 81 82 84 96 100 107 118 119 135 136 **S** Carolinas HealthCare System
Primary Contact: William H. Leonard, Chief Executive Officer
CFO: Jeff W. Rush, Chief Financial Officer
CIO: Billy Helmandollar, Director Information Services
CHR: Michelle Helton, Director Human Resources
Web address: www.wallacethomson.com
Control: Hospital district or authority, Government, nonfederal **Service:** General Medical and Surgical

Staffed Beds: 220 **Admissions:** 2789 **Census:** 141 **Outpatient Visits:** 35411 **Births:** 0 **Personnel:** 362

VARNVILLE—Hampton County

★ **HAMPTON REGIONAL MEDICAL CENTER (420072)**, 503 Carolina Avenue West, Zip 29944, Mailing Address: P.O. Box 338, Zip 29944–0338; tel. 803/943–2771 **A**9 10 20 **F**15 22 25 33 38 55 57 62 65 68 75 77 79 85 86 96 97 99 102 107 119 135
Primary Contact: Dave H. Hamill, President and Chief Executive Officer
Control: Other not–for–profit (including NFP Corporation) **Service:** General Medical and Surgical

Staffed Beds: 27 **Admissions:** 834 **Census:** 9 **Outpatient Visits:** 11086 **Births:** 3 **Total Expense ($000):** 12643 **Payroll Expense ($000):** 5855 **Personnel:** 166

SC

WALTERBORO—Colleton County

☒ **COLLETON MEDICAL CENTER (420030)**, 501 Robertson Boulevard, Zip 29488–5714; tel. 843/782–2000 **A**1 9 10 20 **F**1 3 11 13 15 25 26 28 31 32 33 34 38 54 55 57 59 62 68 73 74 75 77 79 80 81 82 84 85 86 96 97 100 102 107 117 118 119 120 121 135 136 137 **S** HCA
Primary Contact: Mitchell P. Mongell, Chief Executive Officer
COO: Tony Taylor, Vice President Operations
CFO: Tom Thompson, Chief Financial Officer
CMO: Jeffrey Holman, M.D., Chief Medical Staff
CHR: Patricia Hendrick, Director Human Resources
Web address: www.colletonmedical.com
Control: Corporation, Investor–owned, for–profit **Service:** General Medical and Surgical

Staffed Beds: 131 **Admissions:** 4207 **Census:** 64 **Births:** 543 **Total Expense ($000):** 56301 **Payroll Expense ($000):** 21020 **Personnel:** 392

WEST COLUMBIA—Lexington County

☒ **LEXINGTON MEDICAL CENTER (420073)**, 2720 Sunset Boulevard, Zip 29169–4816; tel. 803/791–2000 **A**1 2 9 10 **F**3 11 12 13 15 18 24 25 26 27 28 31 32 33 35 36 37 38 40 43 49 52 54 55 56 57 59 60 62 66 68 71 72 73 74 75 76 77 79 80 81 82 84 85 86 96 97 100 102 106 107 108 109 119 120 121 124 134 135 136 137 **P**6
Primary Contact: Michael J. Biediger, President and Chief Executive Officer
COO: Tod Augsburger, Senior Vice President and Chief Operating Officer
CFO: Melinda Kruzner, Chief Financial Officer
CMO: Gwendolyn Galphin, M.D., Chief of Staff
CHR: Kathy Howell, Vice President Human Resources
Web address: www.lexmed.com
Control: Hospital district or authority, Government, nonfederal **Service:** General Medical and Surgical

Staffed Beds: 362 **Admissions:** 19623 **Census:** 271 **Births:** 2887 **Total Expense ($000):** 303808 **Payroll Expense ($000):** 114665 **Personnel:** 2254

☐ **THREE RIVERS BEHAVIORAL HEALTH (424008)**, (Formerly Three Rivers Center for Behavioral Health), 2900 Sunset Boulevard, Zip 29169–3422; tel. 803/796–9911 **A**1 9 10 **F**4 5 33 54 55 81 88 89 90 91 92 93 94 95 **S** Psychiatric Solutions
Primary Contact: R. Andy Hanner, Chief Executive Officer
Web address: www.psysolutions.com/facilities/threerivers/site/
Control: Corporation, Investor–owned, for–profit **Service:** Psychiatric

Staffed Beds: 86 **Admissions:** 1766 **Census:** 50 **Outpatient Visits:** 2296 **Total Expense ($000):** 11703 **Payroll Expense ($000):** 5308 **Personnel:** 165

WINNSBORO—Fairfield County

☒ **FAIRFIELD MEMORIAL HOSPITAL (421302)**, 102 U.S. Highway 321 By–Pass North, Zip 29180–9251, Mailing Address: P.O. Box 620, Zip 29180–0620; tel. 803/635–5548 **A**1 5 9 10 18 **F**3 11 15 24 27 33 38 54 55 57 61 62 73 75 76 77 79 80 81 82 85 86 96 97 102 107 117 119 121 122 135
Primary Contact: Michael Williams, Interim Administrator
CFO: David Kline, Chief Financial Officer
CMO: Fred Ferguson, M.D., Chief Medical Officer
CIO: Reynolds Searle, Director
CHR: Shawna Martin Lyde, Director
Web address: www.fairfieldmemorial.com
Control: County–Government, nonfederal **Service:** General Medical and Surgical

Staffed Beds: 25 **Admissions:** 700 **Census:** 7 **Outpatient Visits:** 10531 **Total Expense ($000):** 13648 **Payroll Expense ($000):** 5743 **Personnel:** 136

SOUTH DAKOTA

ABERDEEN—Brown County

★ △ **AVERA ST. LUKE'S (430014)**, 305 South State Street, Zip 57402–4450; tel. 605/622–5000, (Total facility includes 135 beds in nursing home–type unit) **A**2 7 9 10 19 20 **F**2 3 5 7 10 11 13 15 17 18 24 25 26 27 28 30 31 32 33 34 37 38 42 43 44 46 48 54 55 57 59 60 61 62 63 66 68 69 72 73 74 75 76 77 79 80 81 82 84 85 86 87 88 89 90 91 92 93 94 95 96 97 99 100 102 106 107 108 109 111 112 115 117 118 119 120 121 122 124 135 136 137 **S** Avera Health
Primary Contact: Ronald L. Jacobson, Regional President
COO: K. C. DeBoer, Vice President
CFO: Geoff Durst, Vice President Finance
CMO: John Fritz, D.O., Vice President Medical Affairs
CIO: Julie Kusler, Manager Information Services
CHR: Mary Davis, Vice President
Web address: www.averastlukes.org
Control: Church–operated, Nongovernment, not–for profit **Service:** General Medical and Surgical

Staffed Beds: 265 **Admissions:** 5629 **Census:** 197 **Outpatient Visits:** 215276 **Births:** 743 **Total Expense ($000):** 107669 **Payroll Expense ($000):** 47766 **Personnel:** 1088

DAKOTA PLAINS SURGICAL CENTER (430092), 701 8th Avenue N.W., Suite C., Zip 57401; tel. 605/225–3300, (Nonreporting) **A**9 10
Primary Contact: Charles Livingston, Administrator
Control: Corporation, Investor–owned, for–profit **Service:** Surgical

Staffed Beds: 8

ARMOUR—Douglas County

DOUGLAS COUNTY MEMORIAL HOSPITAL (431305), 708 Eighth Street, Zip 57313–2102; tel. 605/724–2159 **A**9 10 18 **F**3 7 10 13 15 24 30 31 32 33 38 42 52 55 57 61 62 63 67 74 75 76 77 79 86 96 100 107 122
Primary Contact: Heath Brouwer, Administrator
CFO: Dorothy Spease, Business Office Manager
Web address: www.dcmhsd.org
Control: Other not–for–profit (including NFP Corporation) **Service:** General Medical and Surgical

Staffed Beds: 11 **Admissions:** 322 **Census:** 3 **Outpatient Visits:** 6689 **Births:** 19 **Total Expense ($000):** 5549 **Payroll Expense ($000):** 2470 **Personnel:** 60

BOWDLE—Edmunds County

BOWDLE HOSPITAL (431318), 8001 West Fifth Street, Zip 57428–0566; tel. 605/285–6146, (Total facility includes 30 beds in nursing home–type unit) **A**9 10 18 **F**2 7 10 11 24 38 52 57 63 117 122
Primary Contact: Jon Kosiak, Chief Executive Officer
CFO: Jeff Poppen, Chief Financial Officer
CMO: Janice Lumnitz, M.D., Chief of Staff
CIO: Kim Miller, Chief Information Officer
Web address: www.bowdlehealthcarecenter.com
Control: City–Government, nonfederal **Service:** General Medical and Surgical

Staffed Beds: 42 **Admissions:** 169 **Census:** 29 **Outpatient Visits:** 4293 **Births:** 0 **Total Expense ($000):** 3840 **Payroll Expense ($000):** 1975 **Personnel:** 74

BRITTON—Marshall County

★ **MARSHALL COUNTY HEALTHCARE CENTER/AVERA HEALTH (431312)**, 413 Ninth Street, Zip 57430; tel. 605/448–2253 **A**9 10 18 **F**1 4 10 11 16 17 25 30 31 32 33 38 52 55 56 57 58 61 62 63 65 68 70 71 75 78 81 82 83 84 85 88 117 122 **P**5 **S** Avera Health
Primary Contact: Stephanie Reasy, Administrator
Web address: www.avera.org
Control: Other not–for–profit (including NFP Corporation) **Service:** General Medical and Surgical

Staffed Beds: 18 **Admissions:** 332 **Census:** 5 **Outpatient Visits:** 8634 **Births:** 0 **Total Expense ($000):** 4475 **Payroll Expense ($000):** 1955 **Personnel:** 62

BROOKINGS—Brookings County

★ **BROOKINGS HEALTH SYSTEM (430008)**, 300 22nd Avenue, Zip 57006–2496; tel. 605/696–9000, (Total facility includes 79 beds in nursing home–type unit) **A**9 10 20 **F**3 7 11 13 25 27 30 31 33 38 42 54 55 56 57 61 67 68 73 74 79 81 82 100 102 107 115 117 118 119 121 122 132 135 136 137 **P**6
Primary Contact: Vern Carda, Administrator and Chief Executive Officer
CFO: Kevin Coffey, Chief Financial Officer
CHR: Donald McCoy, Administrative Services Division Director
Web address: www.brookingshealth.org
Control: City–Government, nonfederal **Service:** General Medical and Surgical

Staffed Beds: 128 **Admissions:** 1336 **Census:** 87 **Outpatient Visits:** 46196 **Births:** 289 **Total Expense ($000):** 20624 **Payroll Expense ($000):** 10117 **Personnel:** 300

BURKE—Gregory County

★ **COMMUNITY MEMORIAL HOSPITAL (431309)**, 809 Jackson Street, Zip 57523, Mailing Address: P.O. Box 319, Zip 57523–0319; tel. 605/775–2621 **A**9 10 18 **F**3 11 24 27 30 31 32 38 55 56 57 63 65 82 87 117 122 **P**5 **S** Sanford Health
Primary Contact: Jim Frank, Chief Executive Officer
CMO: Teresa Marts, M.D., Chief of Medical Staff
CHR: Becky Jacobson, Manager Business Office and Human Resources
Control: Other not–for–profit (including NFP Corporation) **Service:** General Medical and Surgical

Staffed Beds: 16 **Admissions:** 249 **Census:** 6 **Outpatient Visits:** 1720 **Births:** 0 **Total Expense ($000):** 3028 **Payroll Expense ($000):** 1562 **Personnel:** 44

SD

CANTON—Lincoln County

★ **CANTON–INWOOD MEMORIAL HOSPITAL (431333)**, 440 North Hiawatha Drive, Zip 57013–9404; tel. 605/987–2621 **A**9 10 18 **F**10 24 31 32 38 57 62 69 75 79 86 96 119 122 **S** Sanford Health
Primary Contact: Eric C. Hilmoe, Chief Executive Officer
CFO: Paul Gerhart, Chief Financial Officer
Web address: www.cantoninwoodhospital.org
Control: Other not–for–profit (including NFP Corporation) **Service:** General Medical and Surgical

Staffed Beds: 18 **Admissions:** 230 **Census:** 3 **Outpatient Visits:** 16629 **Births:** 1 **Total Expense ($000):** 4871 **Payroll Expense ($000):** 2385 **Personnel:** 75

CHAMBERLAIN—Brule County

★ **SANFORD MID DAKOTA MEDICAL CENTER (431329)**, 300 South Byron Boulevard, Zip 57325–9741; tel. 605/234–5511, (Total facility includes 47 beds in nursing home–type unit) **A**9 10 18 **F**3 8 13 15 24 25 27 30 31 32 33 38 40 55 57 66 68 73 74 75 79 80 81 84 86 96 102 107 119 120 122 135 **P**6 **S** Sanford Health
Primary Contact: Maureen K. Cadwell, Chief Executive Officer
CFO: Erica Peterson, Chief Financial Officer
CMO: Travis Sanger, M.D., Chief Medical Staff
CHR: Dotty Hieb, Director Human Resource
Web address: www.sanfordmiddakota.org
Control: Other not–for–profit (including NFP Corporation) **Service:** General Medical and Surgical

Staffed Beds: 72 **Admissions:** 706 **Census:** 48 **Outpatient Visits:** 10556 **Births:** 65 **Total Expense ($000):** 10874 **Payroll Expense ($000):** 5318 **Personnel:** 155

Hospital, Medicare Provider Number, Address, Telephone, Approval, Facility, and Physician Codes, Health Care System

★ American Hospital Association (AHA) membership
□ The Joint Commission accreditation
○ American Osteopathic Association (AOA) accreditation
△ Commission on Accreditation of Rehabilitation Facilities (CARF) accreditation

CLEAR LAKE—Deuel County

★ **SANFORD DEUEL COUNTY MEDICAL CENTER (431307)**, 701 Third Avenue South, Zip 57226–2016; tel. 605/874–2141 **A**9 10 18 **F**11 24 25 27 28 30 31 32 33 38 43 50 52 55 56 57 61 62 63 65 66 79 81 82 87 117 122 124 133 136 137 **P**6 **S** Sanford Health
Primary Contact: Robert J. Salmon, Chief Executive Officer
CFO: Allison Nelson, Chief Financial Officer
CMO: Terrance Smith, M.D., Chairman Medical Staff
Web address: www.deuelcountymemorial.org
Control: Other not–for–profit (including NFP Corporation) **Service:** General Medical and Surgical

Staffed Beds: 20 **Admissions:** 250 **Census:** 2 **Outpatient Visits:** 17395 **Births:** 0 **Total Expense ($000):** 4518 **Payroll Expense ($000):** 2186 **Personnel:** 53

CUSTER—Custer County

★ **CUSTER REGIONAL HOSPITAL (431323)**, 1039 Montgomery Street, Zip 57730–1397; tel. 605/673–2229, (Total facility includes 76 beds in nursing home–type unit) **A**9 10 18 **F**2 10 11 25 30 31 33 38 50 54 55 57 62 66 73 74 75 84 86 87 92 96 102 107 117 119 120 121 122 137 **P**8 **S** Regional Health
Primary Contact: Jason Petik, Chief Executive Officer
Web address: www.custerhospital.org
Control: Other not–for–profit (including NFP Corporation) **Service:** General Medical and Surgical

Staffed Beds: 87 **Admissions:** 238 **Census:** 65 **Outpatient Visits:** 9776 **Births:** 0 **Total Expense ($000):** 9298 **Payroll Expense ($000):** 4609 **Personnel:** 145

DAKOTA DUNES—Union County

SIOUXLAND SURGERY CENTER (430089), 600 North Sioux Point Road, Zip 57049–5000; tel. 605/232–3332, (Nonreporting) **A**9 10
Primary Contact: Greg Miner, Administrator
Control: Corporation, Investor–owned, for–profit **Service:** Other specialty

Staffed Beds: 10

DE SMET—Kingsbury County

DE SMET MEMORIAL HOSPITAL (431332), 306 Prairie Avenue S.W., Zip 57231–9499; tel. 605/854–3329 **A**9 10 18 **F**15 24 30 31 32 33 38 55 57 62 86 107 122
Primary Contact: John L. Single, Chief Executive Officer and Administrator
Web address: www.desmetmemorial.org
Control: City–Government, nonfederal **Service:** General Medical and Surgical

Staffed Beds: 14 **Admissions:** 192 **Census:** 2 **Outpatient Visits:** 7922 **Births:** 0 **Total Expense ($000):** 2252 **Payroll Expense ($000):** 1135 **Personnel:** 23

DEADWOOD—Lawrence County

★ **LEAD–DEADWOOD REGIONAL HOSPITAL (431320)**, 61 Charles Street, Zip 57732–1303; tel. 605/722–6101 **A**9 10 18 **F**3 7 10 15 25 26 38 41 55 57 65 67 68 73 75 79 80 82 84 85 86 87 96 107 115 117 122 137 **P**6 **S** Regional Health
Primary Contact: Sherry Bea Smith, RN, Chief Executive Officer
CMO: James Holloway, M.D., President Medical Staff
CHR: Kathryn L. Shockey, Director Human Resources
Web address: www.rcrh.org
Control: Other not–for–profit (including NFP Corporation) **Service:** General Medical and Surgical

Staffed Beds: 18 **Admissions:** 391 **Census:** 4 **Outpatient Visits:** 10749 **Births:** 0 **Total Expense ($000):** 8882 **Payroll Expense ($000):** 4212 **Personnel:** 104

DELL RAPIDS—Minnehaha County

★ **AVERA DELLS AREA HEALTH CENTER (431331)**, 909 North Iowa Avenue, Zip 57022–1231; tel. 605/428–5431 **A**9 10 18 **F**11 13 15 24 38 52 57 79 86 122 **P**5 **S** Avera Health
Primary Contact: James A. Faulwell, Chief Executive Officer and Administrator
CFO: Jamie Schafer, Controller
CMO: Matt Herber, Chief of Staff
CHR: Dawn Ingalls, Regional Representative Human Resources
Web address: www.avera.org
Control: Church–operated, Nongovernment, not–for profit **Service:** General Medical and Surgical

Staffed Beds: 20 **Admissions:** 339 **Census:** 3 **Outpatient Visits:** 11650 **Births:** 15 **Total Expense ($000):** 3945 **Personnel:** 36

EAGLE BUTTE—Dewey County

★ **U. S. PUBLIC HEALTH SERVICE INDIAN HOSPITAL (430083)**, 317 Main Street, Zip 57625–1012, Mailing Address: P.O. Box 1012, Zip 57625–1012; tel. 605/964–7724, (Nonreporting) **A**10 **S** U. S. Indian Health Service
Primary Contact: Charlene Red Thunder, Chief Executive Officer
CFO: Lisa Deal, Budget Analyst
Web address: www.ihs.gov
Control: Public Health Service, Government, federal **Service:** General Medical and Surgical

Staffed Beds: 11

EUREKA—McPherson County

★ **EUREKA COMMUNITY HEALTH SERVICES/AVERA (431308)**, 410 Ninth Street, Zip 57437–0517, Mailing Address: P.O. Box 517, Zip 57437–0517; tel. 605/284–2661 **A**9 10 18 **F**10 24 30 31 32 33 38 57 61 63 75 79 86 122 **S** Avera Health
Primary Contact: Robert A. Dockter, Administrator
CFO: Joyce Schwingler, Finance Officer
Control: Other not–for–profit (including NFP Corporation) **Service:** General Medical and Surgical

Staffed Beds: 6 **Admissions:** 176 **Census:** 2 **Outpatient Visits:** 6601 **Births:** 0 **Total Expense ($000):** 1924 **Payroll Expense ($000):** 754 **Personnel:** 37

FAULKTON—Faulk County

FAULKTON AREA MEDICAL CENTER (431301), (Formerly Faulk County Memorial Hospital), 1300 Oak Street, Zip 57438, Mailing Address: P.O. Box 100, Zip 57438–0100; tel. 605/598–6263 **A**9 10 18 **F**17 24 25 32 38 57 75 86 87 122 **P**5
Primary Contact: Jay A. Jahnig, Chief Executive Officer
COO: Jay A. Jahnig, Chief Executive Officer
CFO: Susan Miller, Financial Administrator
CMO: K. A. Bartholomew, M.D., Medical Director
CIO: Cheryl Arthurs, Transcriptionist Health Information
CHR: Susan Miller, Financial Administrator
Web address: www.faulktonmedical.org
Control: County–Government, nonfederal **Service:** General Medical and Surgical

Staffed Beds: 12 **Admissions:** 228 **Census:** 3 **Outpatient Visits:** 8895 **Births:** 0 **Total Expense ($000):** 2916 **Payroll Expense ($000):** 1430 **Personnel:** 40

FLANDREAU—Moody County

★ **FLANDREAU MEDICAL CENTER/AVERA HEALTH (431310)**, 214 North Prairie Avenue, Zip 57028–1243; tel. 605/997–2433 **A**9 10 18 **F**3 11 24 25 27 30 31 32 33 38 42 43 44 55 56 57 61 62 66 73 75 76 79 81 86 87 107 121 122 133 137 **P**8 **S** Avera Health
Primary Contact: Paul Lewis, Administrator and Chief Executive Officer
COO: Marie Myers, Director Patient Care Services
CIO: Melissa Jones, Director Health Information
Web address: www.flandreaumedical.org
Control: Other not–for–profit (including NFP Corporation) **Service:** General Medical and Surgical

Staffed Beds: 18 **Admissions:** 334 **Census:** 3 **Outpatient Visits:** 13797 **Births:** 1 **Total Expense ($000):** 3493 **Payroll Expense ($000):** 1532 **Personnel:** 37

FORT MEADE—Meade County

☒ **VETERANS AFFAIRS BLACK HILLS HEALTH CARE SYSTEM**, 113 Comanche Road, Zip 57741–1099; tel. 605/347–2511, (Includes VETERANS AFFAIRS MEDICAL CENTER, 500 North Fifth Street, Hot Springs, Zip 57747; tel. 605/745–2052), (Total facility includes 104 beds in nursing home–type unit) (Nonreporting) **A**1 5 9 **S** Department of Veterans Affairs
Primary Contact: Peter P. Henry, FACHE, Director
COO: Stephen R. DiStasio, Associate Director Operations
CFO: Bill Gambill, Chief Financial Officer
CHR: Marg McCaleb, Chief Human Resources Management
Web address: www.va.gov/sta/guide/home.asp
Control: Veterans Affairs, Government, federal **Service:** General Medical and Surgical

Staffed Beds: 322

FREEMAN—Hutchinson County

★ **FREEMAN REGIONAL HEALTH SERVICES (431313)**, 510 East Eighth Street, Zip 57029–0370, Mailing Address: P.O. Box 370, Zip 57029–0370; tel. 605/925–4000, (Total facility includes 51 beds in nursing home–type unit) **A**9 10 18 **F**2 3 6 11 15 24 26 27 31 32 33 38 43 50 54 55 56 57 62 63 66 67 68 73 75 76 77 79 81 84 85 96 107 115 117 119 121 122 132 135
Primary Contact: Daniel Gran, Chief Executive Officer
CFO: Mark Miller, Chief Financial Officer
Web address: www.freemanregional.com
Control: Other not–for–profit (including NFP Corporation) **Service:** General Medical and Surgical

Staffed Beds: 70 **Admissions:** 274 **Census:** 46 **Outpatient Visits:** 7716 **Births:** 0 **Total Expense ($000):** 5816 **Payroll Expense ($000):** 2896 **Personnel:** 103

SD

GETTYSBURG—Potter County

★ **GETTYSBURG MEMORIAL HOSPITAL (431302)**, 606 East Garfield Avenue, Zip 57442–1398; tel. 605/765–2480, (Total facility includes 50 beds in nursing home–type unit) **A**9 10 18 **F**3 6 11 24 25 26 33 34 38 43 50 56 57 62 65 75 77 79 81 82 86 96 115 117 119 121 122 135 **S** Catholic Health Initiatives
Primary Contact: Mark Schmidt, Executive Director
Web address: www.st–marys.com
Control: Church–operated, Nongovernment, not–for profit **Service:** General Medical and Surgical

Staffed Beds: 60 **Admissions:** 194 **Census:** 50 **Outpatient Visits:** 5543 **Births:** 0 **Total Expense ($000):** 4628 **Payroll Expense ($000):** 2297 **Personnel:** 62

GREGORY—Gregory County

★ **AVERA GREGORY HEALTHCARE CENTER (431338)**, 400 Park Avenue, Zip 57533–0400, Mailing Address: P.O. Box 408, Zip 57533–0408; tel. 605/835–8394, (Total facility includes 55 beds in nursing home–type unit) **A**9 10 18 **F**2 6 13 15 17 24 25 26 27 30 31 32 33 38 40 43 54 55 56 57 59 61 66 68 73 74 75 76 77 79 81 82 84 96 117 118 119 120 121 122 132 136 **S** Avera Health
Primary Contact: Jack Williams, Jr., Chief Executive Officer
CFO: Trish Keiser, Comptroller
CIO: Justin Keegan, Director Support Services
CHR: Carol Postulka, Executive Assistant
Web address: www.gregoryhealthcare.org
Control: Church–operated, Nongovernment, not–for profit **Service:** General Medical and Surgical

Staffed Beds: 80 **Admissions:** 834 **Census:** 60 **Outpatient Visits:** 19299 **Births:** 34 **Total Expense ($000):** 10262 **Payroll Expense ($000):** 4940 **Personnel:** 136

HOT SPRINGS—Fall River County

★ **FALL RIVER HOSPITAL (431322)**, 209 North 16th Street, Zip 57747–1375; tel. 605/745–3159, (Includes CASTLE MANOR), (Total facility includes 48 beds in nursing home–type unit) **A**9 10 18 **F**24 31 32 38 62 79 86 96 97 107 119 122 134 135 137 **P**6
Primary Contact: John B. Miller, Administrator
CMO: Arthur Raymond, M.D., Medical Director
CIO: Dwayne Heafner, Chief Information Officer
Web address: www.fallriverhealthservices.com
Control: Other not–for–profit (including NFP Corporation) **Service:** General Medical and Surgical

Staffed Beds: 59 **Admissions:** 233 **Census:** 52 **Outpatient Visits:** 14172 **Births:** 0 **Total Expense ($000):** 8016 **Payroll Expense ($000):** 4184 **Personnel:** 106

VETERANS AFFAIRS MEDICAL CENTER See Veterans Affairs Black Hills Health Care System, Fort Meade

HOVEN—Potter County

HOLY INFANT HOSPITAL (430060), Main Street, Zip 57450–0158, Mailing Address: P.O. Box 158, Zip 57450–0158; tel. 605/948–2262, (Nonreporting) **A**9 10 20
Primary Contact: Jay Duenwald, Interim Administrator
COO: Becky Haar, Business Manager
CFO: Becky Haar, Business Manager
CMO: Dion Ramirez, M.D., Chief Medical Officer
CIO: Becky Haar, Business Manager
CHR: Becky Haar, Business Manager
Control: Other not–for–profit (including NFP Corporation) **Service:** General Medical and Surgical

Staffed Beds: 27

HURON—Beadle County

★ **HURON REGIONAL MEDICAL CENTER (431335)**, 172 Fourth Street S.E., Zip 57350–2590; tel. 605/353–6200 **A**9 10 18 **F**3 11 13 14 15 24 25 26 27 30 31 32 33 38 40 42 55 57 59 61 62 66 68 73 74 75 77 79 80 81 86 92 96 97 99 100 103 106 107 119 121 122 135 137 **P**6 **S** QHR
Primary Contact: John L. Single, Chief Executive Officer
COO: Gaea Blue, Vice President Patient Services
CFO: Marcia Zwanziger, Vice President Finance
CMO: Jeff Wheeler, M.D., Chief of Staff
CHR: Rhonda Hanson, Director Human Resources
Web address: www.huronregional.org
Control: Other not–for–profit (including NFP Corporation) **Service:** General Medical and Surgical

Staffed Beds: 25 **Admissions:** 1307 **Census:** 13 **Outpatient Visits:** 52728 **Births:** 245 **Total Expense ($000):** 26296 **Payroll Expense ($000):** 11256 **Personnel:** 227

LEMMON—Perkins County

FIVE COUNTIES HOSPITAL (431303), 405 Sixth Avenue West, Zip 57638–1318, Mailing Address: P.O. Box 479, Zip 57638–0479; tel. 605/374–3871, (Total facility includes 43 beds in nursing home–type unit) (Nonreporting) **A**9 10 18
Primary Contact: Jannette Van Beek, Administrator and Chief Executive Officer
CFO: Linda Ham, Business Office Manager
CMO: Kent Hocrauf, M.D., Medical Director
CHR: Jim Krebs, Director Personnel
Web address: www.rcrh.org/facilities/hospitals/fivecounties.asp
Control: Other not–for–profit (including NFP Corporation) **Service:** General Medical and Surgical

Staffed Beds: 47

MADISON—Lake County

★ **MADISON COMMUNITY HOSPITAL (431300)**, 917 North Washington Avenue, Zip 57042–1696; tel. 605/256–6551 **A**9 10 18 **F**7 11 13 15 24 27 30 31 32 33 38 55 56 57 61 62 68 73 74 75 79 80 86 96 97 102 107 122 124 132 134 135
Primary Contact: Tamara Miller, Administrator
Web address: www.madisonhospital.com
Control: Other not–for–profit (including NFP Corporation) **Service:** General Medical and Surgical

Staffed Beds: 25 **Admissions:** 703 **Census:** 9 **Outpatient Visits:** 23729 **Births:** 43 **Total Expense ($000):** 9530 **Payroll Expense ($000):** 4942 **Personnel:** 133

MARTIN—Bennett County

BENNETT COUNTY HOSPITAL AND NURSING HOME (431314), 102 Major Allen Street, Zip 57551, Mailing Address: P.O. Box 70, Zip 57551; tel. 605/685–6622, (Total facility includes 38 beds in nursing home–type unit) **A**9 10 18 **F**1 2 7 10 30 38 55 57 61 63 122 132 **P**8
Primary Contact: Joseph Caldwell, Administrator
CFO: Jean Kirk, Chief Financial Officer
CMO: Prakash Shrestha, M.D., Medical Director
CIO: Jean Kirk, Chief Financial Officer
CHR: T J Porter, Director Human Resources
Web address: www.bchospital.com
Control: Other not–for–profit (including NFP Corporation) **Service:** General Medical and Surgical

Staffed Beds: 53 **Admissions:** 160 **Census:** 46 **Outpatient Visits:** 2392 **Births:** 2 **Total Expense ($000):** 3704 **Payroll Expense ($000):** 1988 **Personnel:** 73

SD

MILBANK—Grant County

★ **MILBANK AREA HOSPITAL/AVERA HEALTH (431326)**, 901 East Virgil Avenue, Zip 57252; tel. 605/432–4538, (Includes ST. WILLIAM HOME FOR THE AGED) **A**9 10 18 **F**13 15 24 26 27 30 31 32 38 42 61 66 74 75 79 86 96 107 118 119 122 133 136 137 **S** Avera Health
Primary Contact: Marc Lemon, Administrator
CFO: Jamie Shafer, Chief Financial Officer
CMO: Kevin Bjordahl, M.D., Chief Medical Officer
CHR: Mona Schafer, Regional Manager Human Resources
Control: Other not–for–profit (including NFP Corporation) **Service:** General Medical and Surgical

Staffed Beds: 25 **Admissions:** 454 **Census:** 6 **Outpatient Visits:** 14164 **Births:** 47 **Total Expense ($000):** 6604 **Payroll Expense ($000):** 2340 **Personnel:** 52

MILLER—Hand County

★ **AVERA HAND COUNTY MEMORIAL HOSPITAL & CLINIC (431337)**, (Formerly Hand County Memorial Hospital), 300 West Fifth Street, Zip 57362–1238; tel. 605/853–2421, (Total facility includes 23 beds in nursing home–type unit) **A**9 10 18 **F**7 10 11 17 24 25 28 30 31 32 33 38 40 46 50 52 54 55 56 57 61 62 63 67 72 73 75 79 81 82 86 96 102 107 115 117 118 121 122 134 135 136 137 **P**5 **S** Avera Health
Primary Contact: Bryan Breitling, Administrator
CFO: Debbie Pullman, Director Finance
CMO: Joel Huber, M.D., Chief of Staff
CIO: Jessie Ford, Coordinator Medical Records
Web address: www.avera.org
Control: Other not–for–profit (including NFP Corporation) **Service:** General Medical and Surgical

Staffed Beds: 42 **Admissions:** 427 **Census:** 25 **Outpatient Visits:** 8028 **Births:** 0 **Total Expense ($000):** 4233 **Payroll Expense ($000):** 1934 **Personnel:** 68

Hospital, Medicare Provider Number, Address, Telephone, Approval, Facility, and Physician Codes, Health Care System

★ American Hospital Association (AHA) membership
□ The Joint Commission accreditation
○ American Osteopathic Association (AOA) accreditation
△ Commission on Accreditation of Rehabilitation Facilities (CARF) accreditation

MITCHELL—Davison County

★ **AVERA QUEEN OF PEACE (430013)**, 525 North Foster, Zip 57301–2999; tel. 605/995–2000, (Total facility includes 114 beds in nursing home–type unit) **A**1 2 9 10 **F**3 10 12 13 15 24 25 26 27 30 31 32 33 37 38 40 42 43 50 51 52 54 55 56 57 61 62 63 67 68 69 73 74 75 76 77 79 80 81 84 86 92 96 100 102 106 107 109 111 115 117 118 119 120 121 122 124 135 136 137 **P**6 **S** Avera Health
Primary Contact: Thomas P. Rasmusson, Regional President
CFO: Patrick Clark, Senior Vice President Finance and Support Services
CMO: Trevor Meaney, M.D., President Medical Staff
CIO: Patti Brooks, Director Information Systems
CHR: Rita Lemon, Director Human Resources
Web address: www.averaqueenofpeace.org
Control: Church–operated, Nongovernment, not–for profit **Service:** General Medical and Surgical

Staffed Beds: 199 **Admissions:** 3376 **Census:** 143 **Outpatient Visits:** 102695 **Births:** 564 **Total Expense ($000):** 60142 **Payroll Expense ($000):** 28277 **Personnel:** 403

MOBRIDGE—Walworth County

★ **MOBRIDGE REGIONAL HOSPITAL (431325)**, 1401 Tenth Avenue West, Zip 57601–1199, Mailing Address: P.O. Box 580, Zip 57601–0580; tel. 605/845–3693 **A**9 10 18 **F**3 7 8 10 11 13 15 24 27 30 32 33 38 53 54 55 57 61 62 63 68 73 74 79 86 87 96 99 102 107 115 117 118 119 122 **P**6
Primary Contact: Angelia K. Svihovec, Chief Executive Officer
CFO: Renae Tisdall, Chief Financial Officer
CHR: Jodi Lemke, Director Human Resources
Web address: www.mobridgehospital.org
Control: Other not–for–profit (including NFP Corporation) **Service:** General Medical and Surgical

Staffed Beds: 25 **Admissions:** 672 **Census:** 6 **Outpatient Visits:** 24534 **Births:** 83 **Total Expense ($000):** 7095 **Payroll Expense ($000):** 3402 **Personnel:** 128

SD

PARKSTON—Hutchinson County

★ **AVERA ST. BENEDICT HEALTH CENTER (431330)**, 401 Glynn Drive, Zip 57366–2031; tel. 605/928–3311, (Total facility includes 75 beds in nursing home–type unit) **A**9 10 18 **F**2 3 8 10 13 15 24 25 26 27 28 30 31 32 33 38 42 43 45 46 52 54 55 56 57 61 62 63 67 68 74 76 79 81 82 84 92 96 100 102 104 107 117 118 119 120 121 122 124 135 137 **P**6 **S** Avera Health
Primary Contact: Gale Walker, President and Chief Executive Officer
CFO: Rita Blasius, Assistant Administrator and Chief Financial Officer
CMO: Antoinette VanderPol, M.D., Chief of Staff
CIO: Adam Popp, Director Information Systems
CHR: Phyllis Ehler, Director Human Resource
Web address: www.averastbenedict.org
Control: Church–operated, Nongovernment, not–for profit **Service:** General Medical and Surgical

Staffed Beds: 100 **Admissions:** 655 **Census:** 77 **Outpatient Visits:** 23139 **Births:** 46 **Total Expense ($000):** 12922 **Payroll Expense ($000):** 6406 **Personnel:** 192

PHILIP—Haakon County

★ **HANS P. PETERSON MEMORIAL HOSPITAL (431319)**, 503 West Pine Street, Zip 57567, Mailing Address: P.O. Box 790, Zip 57567–0790; tel. 605/859–2511, (Total facility includes 30 beds in nursing home–type unit) **A**10 18 **F**10 11 24 31 32 38 55 61 86 96 117 120 122 **P**6 **S** Regional Health
Primary Contact: Kent Olson, Administrator and Chief Executive Officer
Web address: www.rcrh.org/Facilities/Hospitals/HPPMemorial.asp
Control: Other not–for–profit (including NFP Corporation) **Service:** General Medical and Surgical

Staffed Beds: 48 **Admissions:** 229 **Census:** 43 **Outpatient Visits:** 11787 **Births:** 0 **Total Expense ($000):** 5657 **Payroll Expense ($000):** 2946 **Personnel:** 86

PIERRE—Hughes County

★ **ST. MARY'S HEALTHCARE CENTER (430015)**, 800 East Dakota Avenue, Zip 57501–3313; tel. 605/224–3100, (Total facility includes 105 beds in nursing home–type unit) **A**1 9 10 20 **F**3 11 13 15 24 25 26 27 30 31 32 36 38 42 43 44 45 56 57 59 61 62 66 68 69 74 75 76 79 80 81 84 86 96 100 102 107 115 117 118 119 120 122 124 135 137 **P**5 **S** Catholic Health Initiatives
Primary Contact: Chad Cooper, Chief Executive Officer
CFO: Adam Paul, Vice President Finance
CMO: Joe Villa, M.D., Chief of Staff
CIO: Chris Harrison, Director Information Services
CHR: Paul Marso, Vice President Human Resources
Web address: www.st–marys.com
Control: Other not–for–profit (including NFP Corporation) **Service:** General Medical and Surgical

Staffed Beds: 165 **Admissions:** 2718 **Census:** 114 **Outpatient Visits:** 26906 **Births:** 508 **Total Expense ($000):** 35863 **Payroll Expense ($000):** 16249 **Personnel:** 387

PINE RIDGE—Shannon County

★ **U. S. PUBLIC HEALTH SERVICE INDIAN HOSPITAL (430081)**, Mailing Address: P.O. Box 1201, Zip 57770–1201; tel. 605/867–5131, (Nonreporting) **A**1 10 **S** U. S. Indian Health Service
Primary Contact: William Pourier, Service Unit Director
Web address: www.ihs.gov
Control: Public Health Service, Government, federal **Service:** General Medical and Surgical

Staffed Beds: 45

PLATTE—Charles Mix County

★ **PLATTE HEALTH CENTER/AVERA HEALTH (431306)**, 601 East Seventh, Zip 57369–2123, Mailing Address: P.O. Box 200, Zip 57369–0200; tel. 605/337–3364, (Total facility includes 48 beds in nursing home–type unit) **A**9 10 18 **F**1 2 27 30 31 32 38 56 57 79 86 96 107 117 122 **P**6 **S** Avera Health
Primary Contact: Mark Burket, Chief Executive Officer
CFO: Jerry Hoffman, Chief Financial Officer
Web address: www.phcavera.org
Control: Other not–for–profit (including NFP Corporation) **Service:** General Medical and Surgical

Staffed Beds: 63 **Admissions:** 304 **Census:** 46 **Outpatient Visits:** 10375 **Births:** 11 **Total Expense ($000):** 5464 **Payroll Expense ($000):** 2990 **Personnel:** 71

RAPID CITY—Pennington County

BLACK HILLS SURGERY CENTER (430091), 216 Anamaria Drive, Zip 57701, Mailing Address: 1868 Lombardy Drive, Zip 57701; tel. 605/721–4900 **A**9 10 **F**57 62 72 77 79 80 96 100 103
Primary Contact: Franklin Shobe, Administrator and Chief Executive Officer
Web address: www.bhsc.com
Control: Partnership, Investor–owned, for–profit **Service:** Surgical

Staffed Beds: 26 **Admissions:** 1250 **Census:** 10 **Outpatient Visits:** 14579 **Births:** 0 **Total Expense ($000):** 32395 **Payroll Expense ($000):** 11944 **Personnel:** 239

★ **INDIAN HEALTH SERVICE HOSPITAL (430082)**, 3200 Canyon Lake Drive, Zip 57702–8197; tel. 605/355–2280 **A**1 10 **F**3 5 15 28 30 31 32 33 37 38 41 52 55 56 57 82 84 87 88 90 94 107 119 121 124 **P**6 **S** U. S. Indian Health Service
Primary Contact: Lorraine Jewett, Administrator
CFO: Helen Thompson, Administrative Officer
Web address: www.ihs.gov
Control: PHS, Indian Service, Government, federal **Service:** General Medical and Surgical

Staffed Beds: 19 **Admissions:** 203 **Census:** 3 **Outpatient Visits:** 98383 **Births:** 0 **Payroll Expense ($000):** 8045 **Personnel:** 178

★ **RAPID CITY REGIONAL HOSPITAL (430077)**, 353 Fairmont Boulevard, Zip 57701–7393, Mailing Address: P.O. Box 6000, Zip 57709–6000; tel. 605/719–1000 **A**1 3 5 9 10 19 20 **F**3 5 11 12 13 15 17 18 20 22 24 25 26 27 30 31 32 33 34 36 38 41 42 43 46 48 49 51 54 55 56 57 58 59 61 62 63 64 66 68 70 71 72 73 74 75 76 77 78 79 80 81 82 83 84 85 86 88 89 90 91 92 94 96 97 100 102 105 106 107 108 109 111 118 119 120 121 124 130 132 135 137 **P**1 **S** Regional Health
Primary Contact: Timothy H. Sughrue, Chief Executive Officer
CFO: Mark Thompson, Vice President Financial Services
CMO: Robert Allen, M.D., Vice President Medical Affairs
CIO: Richard Latuchie, Vice President Business Development
CHR: Robert McGlone, Vice President Human Resources
Web address: www.rcrh.org
Control: Other not–for–profit (including NFP Corporation) **Service:** General Medical and Surgical

Staffed Beds: 372 **Admissions:** 14679 **Census:** 220 **Outpatient Visits:** 185543 **Births:** 2344 **Total Expense ($000):** 276640 **Payroll Expense ($000):** 119359 **Personnel:** 2116

SAME DAY SURGERY CENTER (430093), 651 Cathedral Drive, Zip 57701; tel. 605/719–5000, (Nonreporting) **A**9 10
Primary Contact: Doris Fritts, RN, Executive Director
Web address: www.samedaysurgerycenter.org
Control: Corporation, Investor–owned, for–profit **Service:** Surgical

Staffed Beds: 8

Many Facility Codes have changed. Please refer to the AHA Guide Code Chart.

REDFIELD—Spink County

COMMUNITY MEMORIAL HOSPITAL (431316), 110 West Tenth Avenue, Zip 57469–0420, Mailing Address: P.O. Box 420, Zip 57469–0420; tel. 605/472–1110 **A**9 10 18 **F**3 7 8 10 11 17 24 31 32 33 38 44 52 54 55 57 61 62 63 67 73 75 79 80 86 87 96 102 103 107 117 119 120 122 135 **P**6
Primary Contact: Terry DeJong, Chief Executive Officer
CFO: Lynn Moller, Chief Financial Officer
Web address: www.redfield–sd.com/hospital.html
Control: City–Government, nonfederal **Service:** General Medical and Surgical

Staffed Beds: 25 **Admissions:** 475 **Census:** 6 **Outpatient Visits:** 19457 **Births:** 0 **Total Expense ($000):** 7544 **Payroll Expense ($000):** 4130 **Personnel:** 101

ROSEBUD—Todd County

★ **U. S. PUBLIC HEALTH SERVICE INDIAN HOSPITAL (430084)**, Highway 18, Soldier Creek Road, Zip 57570; tel. 605/747–2231 **A**10 **F**3 8 13 15 25 30 31 32 33 36 37 38 50 55 56 57 60 62 63 66 73 74 79 80 81 82 84 86 87 90 96 107 119 120 121 124 135 136 **P**6 **S** U. S. Indian Health Service
Primary Contact: Shelly Harris, Chief Executive Officer
COO: Romeo Vivit, Chief Surgeon
CMO: Valerie Parker, M.D., Clinical Director
CHR: Michelle Zephier, Human Resource Specialist
Web address: www.ihs.gov
Control: PHS, Indian Service, Government, federal **Service:** General Medical and Surgical

Staffed Beds: 35 **Admissions:** 1527 **Census:** 9 **Outpatient Visits:** 81245 **Births:** 200 **Total Expense ($000):** 25677 **Payroll Expense ($000):** 12039 **Personnel:** 230

SCOTLAND—Bon Homme County

★ **LANDMANN–JUNGMAN MEMORIAL HOSPITAL (431317)**, 600 Billars Street, Zip 57059–2026; tel. 605/583–2226 **A**9 10 18 **F**11 24 27 30 32 33 37 38 42 52 55 56 57 61 62 63 79 82 86 96 107 115 121 122 135 **S** Avera Health
Primary Contact: Jay Plucker, Administrator
CFO: Darcy Kepplinger, Manager Business Office
CMO: Melissa Bartling, M.D., Chief of Staff
CHR: Christa Henderson, Chief Human Resources Officer
Web address: www.ljmh.org
Control: Other not–for–profit (including NFP Corporation) **Service:** General Medical and Surgical

Staffed Beds: 19 **Admissions:** 189 **Census:** 3 **Outpatient Visits:** 3754 **Births:** 0 **Total Expense ($000):** 1737 **Payroll Expense ($000):** 1206 **Personnel:** 37

SIOUX FALLS—Minnehaha County

★□ **AVERA HEART HOSPITAL OF SOUTH DAKOTA (430095)**, 4500 West 69th Street, Zip 57108–8148; tel. 605/977–7000 **A**1 9 10 **F**3 11 18 20 22 25 26 30 31 32 33 38 48 55 56 57 59 62 63 69 73 79 80 81 82 96 97 103 106 107 119 124 135 **P**2 8 **S** MedCath, Inc.
Primary Contact: Jon Soderholm, President
CFO: Jean White, Vice President Finance
Web address: www.southdakotaheart.com
Control: Partnership, Investor–owned, for–profit **Service:** General Medical and Surgical

Staffed Beds: 55 **Admissions:** 3669 **Census:** 39 **Outpatient Visits:** 5830 **Births:** 0 **Total Expense ($000):** 47142 **Payroll Expense ($000):** 15928 **Personnel:** 351

★ △ **AVERA MCKENNAN HOSPITAL AND UNIVERSITY HEALTH CENTER (430016)**, (Formerly Avera McKennan Hospital), 800 East 21st Street, Zip 57105–1096, Mailing Address: P.O. Box 5045, Zip 57117–5045; tel. 605/322–8000, (Total facility includes 90 beds in nursing home–type unit) **A**2 3 5 7 8 9 10 **F**3 5 7 10 11 12 13 15 18 19 20 21 22 24 25 26 27 28 30 31 32 33 34 36 37 38 40 41 42 43 44 46 49 50 52 53 54 55 56 57 58 59 60 61 62 63 64 65 66 68 69 70 72 73 74 75 76 77 78 79 80 81 82 83 84 85 86 87 88 89 90 91 92 93 94 95 96 97 99 100 102 103 106 107 109 114 115 117 118 119 120 121 123 124 125 127 130 131 132 135 136 137 **P**1 6 **S** Avera Health
Primary Contact: Fredrick Slunecka, Regional President
CFO: Ron Farr, Senior Vice President Finance
CMO: David Kapaska, D.O., Chief Medical Officer
CIO: Kristin Gross, Director Information Technology Center
CHR: Bill McLean, Senior Vice President Human Resources
Web address: www.averamckennan.org
Control: Church–operated, Nongovernment, not–for profit **Service:** General Medical and Surgical

Staffed Beds: 531 **Admissions:** 18919 **Census:** 350 **Outpatient Visits:** 174236 **Births:** 1487 **Total Expense ($000):** 423113 **Payroll Expense ($000):** 201831 **Personnel:** 3890

CHILDRENS CARE HOSPITAL AND SCHOOL (433300), 2501 West 26th Street, Zip 57105–2498; tel. 605/782–2300 **A**9 10 **F**11 25 30 31 32 53 62 73 85 86 89 119 132 135
Primary Contact: Dianna Rajski, President and Chief Executive Officer
CFO: John Clark, Chief Financial Officer
CMO: Douglas DeHaan, M.D., Chief of Staff
CHR: Tiffany Reilly, Director Human Resources
Web address: www.cchs.org
Control: Other not–for–profit (including NFP Corporation) **Service:** Children's rehabilitation

Staffed Beds: 114 **Admissions:** 41 **Census:** 80 **Outpatient Visits:** 20446 **Births:** 0 **Total Expense ($000):** 21060 **Payroll Expense ($000):** 12185 **Personnel:** 324

★□ **ROYAL C. JOHNSON VETERANS MEMORIAL MEDICAL CENTER**, 2501 West 22nd Street, Zip 57105–9920, Mailing Address: P.O. Box 5046, Zip 57117–5046; tel. 605/336–3230, (Total facility includes 58 beds in nursing home–type unit) **A**1 3 5 **F**1 5 25 26 27 29 32 37 38 41 42 44 50 54 57 58 59 60 61 62 68 72 73 75 76 77 79 80 81 82 86 87 88 90 92 93 94 95 96 97 107 118 119 124 132 135 136 **P**6 **S** Department of Veterans Affairs
Primary Contact: Paul Bockelman, Director
CFO: Richard Jamison, Chief Financial Officer
CMO: Steven Julius, M.D., Chief of Staff
CIO: Eric Heiser, Chief Information Resource Management
CHR: Teri Nyhaug, Chief Human Resources Officer
Web address: www.visn23.med.va.gov
Control: Veterans Affairs, Government, federal **Service:** General Medical and Surgical

Staffed Beds: 103 **Admissions:** 2759 **Census:** 89 **Outpatient Visits:** 199208 **Births:** 0 **Total Expense ($000):** 50733 **Payroll Expense ($000):** 37947 **Personnel:** 804

★□ △ **SANFORD UNIVERSITY OF SOUTH DAKOTA MEDICAL CENTER (430027)**, 1305 West 18th Street, Zip 57105–0496, Mailing Address: P.O. Box 5039, Zip 57117–5039; tel. 605/333–1000 **A**1 2 3 5 7 8 9 10 **F**3 7 8 9 11 12 13 14 15 17 18 19 20 21 22 23 24 25 26 27 28 30 31 32 33 37 38 40 41 42 43 44 48 49 50 51 52 54 55 56 57 58 59 60 62 66 68 69 70 71 72 73 74 75 76 77 78 79 80 81 82 83 84 85 86 96 97 100 102 103 104 105 106 107 108 109 111 112 114 116 118 119 120 121 123 124 127 130 132 135 136 137 **P**6 **S** Sanford Health
Primary Contact: Charles O'Brien, M.D., President
CFO: Jeff Sandene, Chief Finance
CMO: Ken Aspaas, M.D., Chief Medical Officer
CIO: Arlyn Broekhuis, Vice President and Chief Information Officer
CHR: Evan Burkett, Chief Human Resource Officer
Web address: www.sanfordhealth.org
Control: Other not–for–profit (including NFP Corporation) **Service:** General Medical and Surgical

Staffed Beds: 451 **Admissions:** 22659 **Census:** 292 **Outpatient Visits:** 306778 **Births:** 3209 **Total Expense ($000):** 367112 **Payroll Expense ($000):** 156161 **Personnel:** 3481

□ **SELECT SPECIALTY HOSPITAL–SIOUX FALLS (432002)**, 800 East 21st Street, Suite 3300, Zip 57105; tel. 605/322–3500, (Nonreporting) **A**1 9 10 **S** Select Medical Corporation
Primary Contact: Carol Ulmer, Chief Executive Officer
Web address: www.selectmedicalcorp.com
Control: Corporation, Investor–owned, for–profit **Service:** Long–Term Acute Care hospital

Staffed Beds: 24

★ **SIOUX FALLS SURGICAL CENTER (430090)**, 910 East 20th Street, Zip 57105; tel. 605/334–6730, (Nonreporting) **A**9 10
Primary Contact: Douglas V. Johnson, Executive Director
CFO: Kyle Goldammer, Chief Financial Officer
CMO: Donald A. Schellpfeffer, M.D., Medical Director
Web address: www.sfsurgical.com
Control: Partnership, Investor–owned, for–profit **Service:** General Medical and Surgical

Staffed Beds: 13

SISSETON—Roberts County

★ **COTEAU DES PRAIRIES HOSPITAL (430064)**, 205 Orchard Drive, Zip 57262–2398; tel. 605/698–7647 **A**9 10 20 **F**13 24 27 30 33 38 52 55 56 57 61 62 68 73 74 75 79 81 84 85 86 107 122 **P**6
Primary Contact: Paul F. Lavallee, Chief Executive Officer
Web address: www.cdphospital.com
Control: Other not–for–profit (including NFP Corporation) **Service:** General Medical and Surgical

Staffed Beds: 27 **Admissions:** 619 **Census:** 5 **Outpatient Visits:** 23520 **Births:** 163 **Total Expense ($000):** 8561 **Payroll Expense ($000):** 3487 **Personnel:** 95

SD

Hospital, Medicare Provider Number, Address, Telephone, Approval, Facility, and Physician Codes, Health Care System

★ American Hospital Association (AHA) membership
□ The Joint Commission accreditation
○ American Osteopathic Association (AOA) accreditation
△ Commission on Accreditation of Rehabilitation Facilities (CARF) accreditation

★ **U. S. PUBLIC HEALTH SERVICE INDIAN HOSPITAL (430085)**, Chestnut Street, Zip 57262, Mailing Address: P.O. Box 189, Zip 57262–0189; tel. 605/698–7606, (Nonreporting) **A**10 **S** U. S. Indian Health Service
Primary Contact: Richard Huff, Administrator
CFO: Gail Williams, Administrative Officer
CMO: Sandeep Patel, M.D., Clinical Director
CIO: Guy Canku, Information Technology Specialist
CHR: Leslie Hewitt, Administrative Assistant
Web address: www.ihs.gov
Control: PHS, Indian Service, Government, federal **Service:** General Medical and Surgical

Staffed Beds: 18

SPEARFISH—Lawrence County

★ **SPEARFISH REGIONAL HOSPITAL (430048)**, 1440 North Main Street, Zip 57783–1504; tel. 605/644–4000 **A**10 20 **F**3 11 13 15 24 25 27 30 32 38 42 44 55 56 57 61 68 73 74 77 79 80 86 87 96 97 100 102 107 117 118 119 121 122 124 135 136 137 **P**6 **S** Regional Health
Primary Contact: Larry W. Veitz, Chief Executive Officer
Web address: www.rcrh.org
Control: Other not–for–profit (including NFP Corporation) **Service:** General Medical and Surgical

Staffed Beds: 32 **Admissions:** 1462 **Census:** 12 **Outpatient Visits:** 42045 **Births:** 556 **Total Expense ($000):** 21667 **Payroll Expense ($000):** 9455 **Personnel:** 202

SPEARFISH SURGERY CENTER (430094), 1316 10th Street, Zip 57783; tel. 605/642–3113, (Nonreporting) **A**9 10
Primary Contact: Michael DeLano, Director of Patient Services
Control: Corporation, Investor–owned, for–profit **Service:** Other specialty

Staffed Beds: 4

SD

STURGIS—Meade County

★ **STURGIS REGIONAL HOSPITAL (431321)**, 949 Harmon Street, Zip 57785–2452; tel. 605/720–2400, (Total facility includes 84 beds in nursing home–type unit) **A**9 10 18 **F**7 11 15 24 25 30 31 32 38 42 43 45 46 75 79 86 96 107 117 119 121 122 **S** Regional Health
Primary Contact: Van Hyde, Chief Executive Officer
CFO: Jodie Mitchell, Facility Financial Director
CMO: Seann Atkinson, M.D., Chief of Staff
CHR: Ginger Chord, Human Resources Coordinator
Web address: www.rcrh.org/Facilities/Hospitals/SCHCC/Default.asp
Control: Other not–for–profit (including NFP Corporation) **Service:** General Medical and Surgical

Staffed Beds: 108 **Admissions:** 854 **Census:** 87 **Outpatient Visits:** 11363 **Births:** 53 **Total Expense ($000):** 12872 **Payroll Expense ($000):** 6396 **Personnel:** 149

TYNDALL—Bon Homme County

★ **ST. MICHAEL'S HOSPITAL (431327)**, 410 West 16th Avenue, Zip 57066, Mailing Address: P.O. Box 27, Zip 57066–0027; tel. 605/589–3341, (Total facility includes 9 beds in nursing home–type unit) **A**9 10 18 **F**15 24 30 31 32 38 52 57 61 65 68 79 81 84 96 100 107 117 120 122 **P**6 **S** Avera Health
Primary Contact: Carol Deurmier, Chief Executive Officer
CFO: Lisa Ronke, Director Finance
CMO: Herbert A. Saloum, M.D., Medical Director
Control: Church–operated, Nongovernment, not–for profit **Service:** General Medical and Surgical

Staffed Beds: 25 **Admissions:** 293 **Census:** 11 **Outpatient Visits:** 8653 **Births:** 0 **Total Expense ($000):** 6286 **Payroll Expense ($000):** 2552 **Personnel:** 65

VERMILLION—Clay County

★ **SANFORD VERMILLION MEDICAL CENTER (431336)**, (Formerly Sioux Valley Vermillion Medical Center), 20 South Plum Street, Zip 57069–3346; tel. 605/624–2611, (Total facility includes 66 beds in nursing home–type unit) **A**9 10 18 **F**15 25 27 30 33 38 57 65 74 79 86 87 96 104 107 118 119 120 121 122 124 **P**8 **S** Sanford Health
Primary Contact: Timothy J. Tracy, Chief Executive Officer
CFO: Valerie Osterberg, Chief Financial Officer
CMO: Mary Jo Olson, M.D., Chief of Staff
Control: Other not–for–profit (including NFP Corporation) **Service:** General Medical and Surgical

Staffed Beds: 114 **Admissions:** 496 **Census:** 68 **Outpatient Visits:** 21370 **Births:** 107 **Total Expense ($000):** 15571 **Payroll Expense ($000):** 7302 **Personnel:** 189

VIBORG—Turner County

★ **PIONEER MEMORIAL HOSPITAL AND HEALTH SERVICES (431328)**, 315 North Washington Street, Zip 57070–2002, Mailing Address: P.O. Box 368, Zip 57070–0368; tel. 605/326–5161, (Total facility includes 52 beds in nursing home–type unit) **A**9 10 18 **F**6 10 15 24 26 30 31 32 38 42 46 52 54 55 57 63 67 73 77 79 87 96 100 107 115 117 119 121 122 **P**6 **S** Sanford Health
Primary Contact: Georgia C. Pokorney, Chief Executive Officer
CFO: Anne Christiansen, Chief Financial Officer
CMO: Yuya Hagiwara, M.D., Chief Medical Officer
Web address: www.pioneermemorial.org
Control: Other not–for–profit (including NFP Corporation) **Service:** General Medical and Surgical

Staffed Beds: 64 **Admissions:** 319 **Census:** 52 **Outpatient Visits:** 35166 **Births:** 0 **Total Expense ($000):** 11217 **Payroll Expense ($000):** 5534 **Personnel:** 151

WAGNER—Charles Mix County

★ **WAGNER COMMUNITY MEMORIAL HOSPITAL – AVERA (431315)**, 513 Third Street S.W., Zip 57380, Mailing Address: P.O. Box 280, Zip 57380–0280; tel. 605/384–3611 **A**9 10 18 **F**3 11 17 24 31 32 38 40 52 55 57 62 65 68 79 86 87 96 102 107 115 117 119 122 137 **P**6 **S** Avera Health
Primary Contact: Bryan Slaba, Chief Executive Officer
CFO: Lisa Weisser, Finance Supervisor
CIO: Bernadette Koupal, Business Office Supervisor, Information Systems Coordinator and Administrative Assistant
CHR: Marcia Podzimek, Quality Assurance, Risk Management and Corporate Compliance Officer
Web address: www.avera.org
Control: Other not–for–profit (including NFP Corporation) **Service:** General Medical and Surgical

Staffed Beds: 20 **Admissions:** 507 **Census:** 6 **Outpatient Visits:** 7764 **Births:** 0 **Total Expense ($000):** 4457 **Payroll Expense ($000):** 1681 **Personnel:** 49

WATERTOWN—Codington County

★ **PRAIRIE LAKES HEALTHCARE SYSTEM (430005)**, 401 9th Avenue N.W., Zip 57201–6210, Mailing Address: P.O. Box 1210, Zip 57201–1210; tel. 605/882–7000, (Total facility includes 51 beds in nursing home–type unit) **A**2 9 10 20 **F**3 11 12 13 15 18 20 24 25 26 27 30 32 33 36 38 40 42 43 44 55 56 57 59 61 62 63 66 68 73 74 75 76 77 79 80 81 82 86 96 97 100 102 103 104 105 106 107 109 117 118 119 120 121 122 124 132 135 136 137 **P**5
Primary Contact: Paul A. Hanson, Chief Executive Officer
COO: Paige Gors, Chief Development Officer
CFO: Michael Anderson, Chief Financial Officer
CMO: Gerald Rieber, Chief Medical Staff
CIO: Grant Tillett, Director Information Technologies
Web address: www.prairielakes.com
Control: Other not–for–profit (including NFP Corporation) **Service:** General Medical and Surgical

Staffed Beds: 121 **Admissions:** 3542 **Census:** 80 **Outpatient Visits:** 73382 **Births:** 695 **Total Expense ($000):** 54402 **Payroll Expense ($000):** 21351 **Personnel:** 406

WEBSTER—Day County

★ **SANFORD WEBSTER MEDICAL CENTER (431311)**, 1401 West 1st Street, Zip 57274–1816, Mailing Address: P.O. Box 489, Zip 57274–0489; tel. 605/345–3336 **A**9 10 18 **F**15 24 25 31 33 38 42 55 57 60 62 68 69 75 79 81 82 86 87 96 97 100 107 117 119 120 122 137 **P**6 **S** Sanford Health
Primary Contact: Kyle Richards, Chief Executive Officer
CFO: Sheryl Pappas, Chief Financial Officer
Web address: www.sanfordhealth.org
Control: Other not–for–profit (including NFP Corporation) **Service:** General Medical and Surgical

Staffed Beds: 25 **Admissions:** 179 **Census:** 3 **Outpatient Visits:** 8588 **Births:** 0 **Total Expense ($000):** 5171 **Payroll Expense ($000):** 2349 **Personnel:** 50

WESSINGTON SPRINGS—Jerauld County

★ **AVERA WESKOTA MEMORIAL MEDICAL CENTER (431324)**, 604 First Street N.E., Zip 57382; tel. 605/539–1201 **A**9 10 18 **F**3 15 24 27 30 31 32 33 38 52 55 57 62 73 75 79 80 86 107 117 119 120 121 122 **P**5 **S** Avera Health
Primary Contact: Kayleen R. Lee, Chief Executive Officer
COO: Kayleen R. Lee, Chief Executive Officer
CFO: Linda Jager, Director Finance and Reimbursement
CMO: Thomas Dean, M.D., Chief of Staff
Web address: www.averaweskota.org
Control: Other not–for–profit (including NFP Corporation) **Service:** General Medical and Surgical

Staffed Beds: 14 **Admissions:** 141 **Census:** 1 **Outpatient Visits:** 3582 **Births:** 0 **Total Expense ($000):** 2721 **Payroll Expense ($000):** 1408 **Personnel:** 29

 Many Facility Codes have changed. Please refer to the AHA Guide Code Chart.

WINNER—Tripp County

★ **WINNER REGIONAL HEALTHCARE CENTER (431334)**, 745 East Eighth Street, Zip 57580–2677; tel. 605/842–7100, (Total facility includes 81 beds in nursing home–type unit) **A**9 10 18 **F**11 13 15 17 24 27 31 32 33 38 43 54 55 56 57 61 62 63 73 74 76 77 79 96 97 100 102 107 117 120 121 122 124 **P**3 5 **S** Sanford Health
Primary Contact: Michael L. Hall, Chief Executive Officer
CFO: Phil Husher, Chief Financial Officer
CMO: Thomas Kosina, M.D., Chief of Staff
CHR: Karleen Flakus, Director Human Resources
Web address: www.winnerregional.org
Control: Other not–for–profit (including NFP Corporation) **Service:** General Medical and Surgical

Staffed Beds: 106 **Admissions:** 865 **Census:** 84 **Outpatient Visits:** 7481 **Births:** 172 **Total Expense ($000):** 13894 **Payroll Expense ($000):** 5938 **Personnel:** 195

YANKTON—Yankton County

☒ △ **AVERA SACRED HEART HOSPITAL (430012)**, 501 Summit Avenue, Zip 57078–3899; tel. 605/668–8000, (Total facility includes 187 beds in nursing home–type unit) **A**1 2 5 7 9 10 19 20 **F**2 3 8 10 11 13 15 18 20 24 25 26 27 30 31 32 33 38 42 43 44 51 52 54 55 57 59 61 62 63 66 67 68 73 74 75 76 77 79 80 82 84 85 86 87 96 97 100 103 104 105 106 107 109 111 115 117 118 119 120 121 122 124 135 **S** Avera Health
Primary Contact: Pamela J. Rezac, Regional President
COO: Douglas R. Ekeren, Vice President Planning and Development
CFO: Michael Healy, Vice President Finance
CIO: Kathy Quinlivan, Director Management Information Systems
CHR: Kim Jensen, Vice President Human Resources
Web address: www.averasacredheart.com
Control: Church–operated, Nongovernment, not–for profit **Service:** General Medical and Surgical

Staffed Beds: 293 **Admissions:** 4524 **Census:** 230 **Outpatient Visits:** 82150 **Births:** 623 **Total Expense ($000):** 63203 **Payroll Expense ($000):** 26840 **Personnel:** 649

LEWIS AND CLARK SPECIALTY HOSPITAL (430096), 2601 Fox Run Parkway, Zip 57078; tel. 605/665–5100 **A**9 10 **F**51 79 100
Primary Contact: Michelle J. Jordan, Administrator
Web address: www.lewisandclarkspecialty.com
Control: Corporation, Investor–owned, for–profit **Service:** Surgical

Staffed Beds: 6 **Admissions:** 208 **Census:** 2 **Outpatient Visits:** 5180 **Births:** 0 **Total Expense ($000):** 4932 **Payroll Expense ($000):** 1383 **Personnel:** 35

SD

Hospital, Medicare Provider Number, Address, Telephone, Approval, Facility, and Physician Codes, Health Care System

★ American Hospital Association (AHA) membership
□ The Joint Commission accreditation
○ American Osteopathic Association (AOA) accreditation
△ Commission on Accreditation of Rehabilitation Facilities (CARF) accreditation

TENNESSEE

ASHLAND CITY—Cheatham County

★ **CENTENNIAL MEDICAL CENTER AT ASHLAND CITY (441311)**, 313 North Main Street, Zip 37015–1358; tel. 615/792–3030 **A**1 9 10 18 **F**3 25 30 31 32 38 79 86 96 100 107 119 122 **S** HCA
Primary Contact: Renaye Smith, Administrator
CIO: David Archer, Director Information Systems
Web address: www.centennialmedicalcenter.com
Control: Corporation, Investor–owned, for–profit **Service:** General Medical and Surgical

Staffed Beds: 8 **Admissions:** 166 **Census:** 5 **Outpatient Visits:** 17813

ATHENS—McMinn County

★ **ATHENS REGIONAL MEDICAL CENTER (440068)**, 1114 West Madison Avenue, Zip 37303–4150, Mailing Address: P.O. Box 250, Zip 37371–0250; tel. 423/745–1411 **A**1 9 10 **F**3 11 13 15 24 25 26 27 30 31 32 33 35 38 40 44 46 48 50 51 53 55 56 57 60 62 63 66 68 71 73 74 75 76 77 79 80 81 84 85 86 92 96 97 100 102 103 104 105 106 107 118 119 121 122 124 135 136 137 **P**7 **S** LifePoint Hospitals, Inc.
Primary Contact: John R. Workman, Chief Executive Officer
COO: Margie Brusseau, R.N., Chief Nursing Officer
CFO: David Alley, Chief Financial Officer
Web address: www.athensrmc.com
Control: Corporation, Investor–owned, for–profit **Service:** General Medical and Surgical

Staffed Beds: 97 **Admissions:** 2585 **Census:** 26 **Outpatient Visits:** 78206 **Births:** 454 **Total Expense ($000):** 26115 **Payroll Expense ($000):** 12017 **Personnel:** 290

BARTLETT—Shelby County

★ **SAINT FRANCIS HOSPITAL–BARTLETT (440228)**, 2986 Kate Bond Road, Zip 38133–4003; tel. 901/820–7000 **A**1 9 10 **F**3 13 15 18 25 26 27 30 31 32 33 38 41 49 50 55 56 57 59 66 71 72 73 74 76 77 79 80 81 82 86 87 96 97 100 102 107 119 120 135 136 137 **P**5 8 **S** TENET Healthcare Corporation
Primary Contact: Kem Mullins, Chief Executive Officer
COO: Gwen Bonner, Chief Operating Officer
CFO: Theresa Holbrook, Chief Financial Officer
CMO: Syed Shirazee, M.D., President Medical Staff
CIO: Mike Hadley, Director Information Systems
CHR: Deb Lollar, Director Human Resources
Web address: www.saintfrancisbartlett.com
Control: Corporation, Investor–owned, for–profit **Service:** General Medical and Surgical

Staffed Beds: 100 **Admissions:** 4630 **Census:** 64 **Outpatient Visits:** 41828 **Births:** 753 **Total Expense ($000):** 50850 **Payroll Expense ($000):** 20494 **Personnel:** 368

BOLIVAR—Hardeman County

★ **BOLIVAR GENERAL HOSPITAL (440181)**, 650 Nuckolls Road, Zip 38008–1532, Mailing Address: P.O. Box 509, Zip 38008–0509; tel. 731/658–3100 **A**1 9 10 **F**3 15 25 26 30 31 32 33 38 55 57 62 73 79 82 86 96 107 119 121 122 135 **S** West Tennessee Healthcare
Primary Contact: Ruby Kirby, Administrator
CFO: Terry Swindell, Controller
CMO: Sylvester Nicol, M.D., Chief Medical Staff
Web address: www.wth.net
Control: Hospital district or authority, Government, nonfederal **Service:** General Medical and Surgical

Staffed Beds: 23 **Admissions:** 960 **Census:** 7 **Outpatient Visits:** 19343 **Births:** 1 **Total Expense ($000):** 6467 **Payroll Expense ($000):** 2839 **Personnel:** 83

□ **WESTERN MENTAL HEALTH INSTITUTE (444008)**, 11100 Old Highway 64, West, Zip 38008–1554; tel. 731/228–2000, (Nonreporting) **A**1 10
Primary Contact: Roger Pursley, Chief Executive Officer
CFO: Richard Taylor, Chief Financial Officer
CMO: Doug King, M.D., Director Clinical Services
CIO: Earl Bates, Director Information Technology
CHR: Barry Young, Director Human Resources
Control: State–Government, nonfederal **Service:** Psychiatric

Staffed Beds: 247

BRISTOL—Sullivan County

□ **SELECT SPECIALTY HOSPITAL–TRICITIES (442016)**, One Medical Park Boulevard, 5th Floor, Zip 37620–8964; tel. 423/844–5900, (Nonreporting) **A**1 10 **S** Select Medical Corporation
Primary Contact: Christopher E. Anderson, Chief Executive Officer
Web address: www.selectmedicalcorp.com
Control: Individual, Investor–owned, for–profit **Service:** General Medical and Surgical

Staffed Beds: 33

★ **WELLMONT BRISTOL REGIONAL MEDICAL CENTER (440012)**, 1 Medical Park Boulevard, Zip 37620–7434; tel. 423/844–1121, (Total facility includes 30 beds in nursing home–type unit) **A**1 2 3 5 9 10 **F**3 11 12 13 14 15 17 18 20 22 24 25 26 27 30 31 32 33 36 37 38 40 42 43 44 45 46 47 48 49 50 51 52 53 54 55 56 57 58 59 60 61 62 65 68 71 72 73 74 75 76 77 78 79 80 81 82 84 86 87 88 89 90 91 92 93 94 95 96 97 99 100 103 106 107 108 109 111 112 117 118 119 120 121 124 133 134 135 136 137 **P**5 **S** Wellmont Health System
Primary Contact: Barton A. Hove, President
COO: Barton A. Hove, President
CFO: Brad H. Price, Vice President Finance and Operations
CIO: Bill Moran, Chief Information Officer
CHR: Hamlin J. Wilson, Senior Vice President Human Resources
Web address: www.wellmont.org
Control: Other not–for–profit (including NFP Corporation) **Service:** General Medical and Surgical

Staffed Beds: 348 **Admissions:** 16123 **Census:** 207 **Outpatient Visits:** 138031 **Births:** 849 **Total Expense ($000):** 183098 **Payroll Expense ($000):** 66678 **Personnel:** 1519

BROWNSVILLE—Haywood County

★ **HAYWOOD PARK COMMUNITY HOSPITAL (440174)**, 2545 North Washington Avenue, Zip 38012–1697; tel. 731/772–4110, (Nonreporting) **A**1 9 10 **S** Community Health Systems, Inc.
Primary Contact: Kim Anthony, Chief Executive Officer
CFO: Joy Fergie, Chief Financial Officer
CMO: Daniel Cofie, M.D., Chief of Staff
CHR: Phyllis Cozart, Director Human Resources
Web address: www.haywoodparkcommunity.com
Control: Corporation, Investor–owned, for–profit **Service:** General Medical and Surgical

Staffed Beds: 44

CAMDEN—Benton County

★ **CAMDEN GENERAL HOSPITAL (441316)**, 175 Hospital Drive, Zip 38320–1617; tel. 731/584–6135 **A**1 9 10 18 **F**3 15 25 26 30 31 32 33 38 55 57 62 73 77 79 80 82 86 96 107 119 121 122 135 **S** West Tennessee Healthcare
Primary Contact: Denny R. Smith, Administrator
Web address: www.wth.net
Control: Hospital district or authority, Government, nonfederal **Service:** General Medical and Surgical

Staffed Beds: 25 **Admissions:** 385 **Census:** 6 **Outpatient Visits:** 17834 **Births:** 0 **Total Expense ($000):** 6220 **Payroll Expense ($000):** 2518 **Personnel:** 71

CARTHAGE—Smith County

★ **RIVERVIEW REGIONAL MEDICAL CENTER NORTH (440186)**, 158 Hospital Drive, Zip 37030–1096; tel. 615/735–1560 **A**1 9 10 **F**3 15 25 26 30 31 32 38 54 55 62 68 79 80 86 88 92 93 96 97 100 107 117 118 119 121 122 124 135 137 **S** Sumner Regional Health Systems
Primary Contact: Edward J. Sanford, Chief Executive Officer
CFO: Danny Warren, Chief Financial Officer
CIO: Valerie Upchurch, Chief Physician Relations
Control: Other not–for–profit (including NFP Corporation) **Service:** General Medical and Surgical

Staffed Beds: 63 **Admissions:** 1679 **Census:** 21 **Outpatient Visits:** 21833 **Births:** 0 **Total Expense ($000):** 15726 **Payroll Expense ($000):** 6113 **Personnel:** 162

★ **RIVERVIEW REGIONAL MEDICAL CENTER SOUTH (441307)**, 130 Lebanon Highway, Zip 37030–2955, Mailing Address: P.O. Box 319, Zip 37030–0319; tel. 615/735–9815 **A**1 9 10 18 **F**1 4 15 16 17 31 32 38 61 65 68 70 71 73 74 75 78 79 81 82 83 84 85 86 88 96 100 106 107 117 119 120 121 122 123 **S** Sumner Regional Health Systems
Primary Contact: Edward J. Sanford, Chief Executive Officer
COO: Scott Tongate, Assistant Administrator
CIO: David Young, Chief Information Officer
CHR: Amy Overstreet, Human Resources Director
Web address: www.sumner.org
Control: Other not–for–profit (including NFP Corporation) **Service:** General Medical and Surgical

Staffed Beds: 25 **Admissions:** 507 **Census:** 5 **Outpatient Visits:** 33723 **Births:** 92 **Total Expense ($000):** 10011 **Payroll Expense ($000):** 3991 **Personnel:** 95

CELINA—Clay County

☐ **CUMBERLAND RIVER HOSPITAL (440141)**, 100 Old Jefferson Street, Zip 38551–4040, Mailing Address: P. O. Box 427, Zip 38551–0427; tel. 931/243–3581, (Nonreporting) **A**1 9 10
Primary Contact: Andrea Rich–McLerran, Chief Executive Officer
CFO: Tricia Strong, Chief Financial Officer
CMO: Stephen T. Moore, M.D., Chief of Staff
CHR: Susan Renodin Deaton, Chief Human Resources Officer
Web address: www.associatedhospitals.com
Control: Corporation, Investor–owned, for–profit **Service:** General Medical and Surgical

Staffed Beds: 75

CENTERVILLE—Hickman County

★ **HICKMAN COMMUNITY HOSPITAL (441300)**, 135 East Swan Street, Zip 37033–1446; tel. 931/729–4271, (Total facility includes 40 beds in nursing home–type unit) **A**1 9 10 18 **F**8 15 25 26 30 31 32 33 38 54 55 56 57 61 62 63 65 79 81 82 86 94 96 100 102 107 117 118 119 122 124 **P**6 **S** Ascension Health
Primary Contact: Jack M. Keller, Administrator
Web address: www.hickmanhospital.com
Control: Other not–for–profit (including NFP Corporation) **Service:** General Medical and Surgical

Staffed Beds: 65 **Admissions:** 410 **Census:** 29 **Outpatient Visits:** 11611 **Births:** 0 **Total Expense ($000):** 13046 **Payroll Expense ($000):** 5943 **Personnel:** 103

CHATTANOOGA—Hamilton County

CUMBERLAND HALL PSYCHIATRIC HOSPITAL (444016), 7351 Standifer Gap Road, Zip 37421; tel. 423/499–9007, (Nonreporting) **A**10 **S** Psychiatric Solutions
Primary Contact: Stephanie Austin, Chief Executive Officer
CFO: Kathy Boyer, Chief Financial Officer
CMO: Michael Schmits, M.D., Medical Director
CHR: Patrick England, Director Human Resources
Web address: www.psysolutions.com
Control: Corporation, Investor–owned, for–profit **Service:** Psychiatric

Staffed Beds: 64

★ **ERLANGER MEDICAL CENTER (440104)**, 975 East Third Street, Zip 37403–2112; tel. 423/778–7000, (Includes ERLANGER NORTH HOSPITAL, 632 Morrison Springs Road, Zip 37415; tel. 615/778–3300; T. C. THOMPSON CHILDREN'S HOSPITAL, 910 Blackford Street, Zip 37403; tel. 615/778–6011; WILLIE D. MILLER EYE CENTER) **A**1 2 3 5 8 9 10 **F**3 7 8 11 12 13 14 15 16 17 18 19 20 21 22 23 24 25 26 27 28 32 33 36 37 38 40 41 42 43 47 49 50 53 55 56 57 59 60 61 62 66 68 69 70 72 73 74 75 76 77 79 80 81 82 83 84 86 87 88 93 96 97 99 100 102 103 106 107 109 112 114 116 118 119 121 127 133 135 136 137 **S** Erlanger Health System
Primary Contact: James L. Brexler, President and Chief Executive Officer
COO: Charlesetta Woodard–Thompson, Executive Vice President and Chief Operating Officer
CFO: Britt Tabor, Senior Vice President and Chief Financial Officer
CMO: Cy Huffman, M.D., Chief Medical Officer
CIO: Laurene Vamprine, Interim Senior Vice President Information Systems
CHR: Gregg Gentry, Senior Vice President Human Resources
Web address: www.erlanger.org
Control: Hospital district or authority, Government, nonfederal **Service:** General Medical and Surgical

Staffed Beds: 551 **Admissions:** 29047 **Census:** 411 **Outpatient Visits:** 265323 **Births:** 4801 **Total Expense ($000):** 412934 **Payroll Expense ($000):** 187244 **Personnel:** 4012

★ **HEALTHSOUTH CHATTANOOGA REHABILITATION HOSPITAL (440162)**, 2412 McCallie Avenue, Zip 37404–3398; tel. 423/698–0221 **A**1 10 **F**24 25 30 32 56 57 73 75 85 86 121 132 137 **S** HEALTHSOUTH Corporation
Primary Contact: Scott Rowe, Chief Executive Officer
COO: Scott Rowe, Chief Executive Officer
CFO: Karen Klassen, Controller
CMO: Sai Oh, M.D., Medical Director
CIO: Denise Smith, Director Health Information
CHR: Deborah Hersom, Director Human Resources
Web address: www.healthsouth.com
Control: Corporation, Investor–owned, for–profit **Service:** Rehabilitation

Staffed Beds: 46 **Admissions:** 772 **Census:** 37 **Outpatient Visits:** 4601 **Births:** 0 **Total Expense ($000):** 10153 **Payroll Expense ($000):** 5539 **Personnel:** 115

☐ **KINDRED HOSPITAL–CHATTANOOGA (442007)**, 709 Walnut Street, Zip 37402–1961; tel. 423/266–7721, (Nonreporting) **A**1 9 10 **S** Kindred Healthcare
Primary Contact: William J. Bryant, Chief Executive Officer
COO: Rick Rheinheimer, Chief Clinical Officer
CFO: Julia Smith, Chief Financial Officer
CMO: Robert Magill, M.D., President Medical Staff
CHR: Kellie McCampbell, Human Resource Coordinator
Web address: www.kindredhealthcare.com
Control: Corporation, Investor–owned, for–profit **Service:** Long–Term Acute Care hospital

Staffed Beds: 44

★ **MEMORIAL HEALTH CARE SYSTEM (440091)**, 2525 De Sales Avenue, Zip 37404–3322; tel. 423/495–8656, (Includes MEMORIAL NORTH PARK HOSPITAL, 2051 Hamill Road, Zip 37343–4096; tel. 423/495–7100) **A**1 2 9 10 **F**3 7 11 12 15 17 18 20 22 24 25 26 27 30 31 32 33 35 38 41 43 46 47 48 49 50 52 53 54 55 56 57 58 59 60 61 62 66 68 69 72 73 75 76 77 79 80 81 82 85 86 96 97 99 100 102 103 105 106 107 109 111 112 114 116 118 119 120 121 124 132 135 136 137 **P**1 3 7 **S** Catholic Health Initiatives
Primary Contact: Debra L. Moore, Interim Chief Executive Officer
COO: Debra L. Moore, Vice President Operations and Chief Operating Officer
CFO: Carol Newton, Chief Financial Officer
CMO: S. Gale Fellowes, M.D., Chief Medical Officer
CIO: Tommye Billing, Regional Chief Information Officer
CHR: Brad Pope, Vice President Human Resources
Web address: www.memorial.org
Control: Church–operated, Nongovernment, not–for profit **Service:** General Medical and Surgical

Staffed Beds: 405 **Admissions:** 22818 **Census:** 289 **Outpatient Visits:** 369520 **Births:** 0 **Total Expense ($000):** 339548 **Payroll Expense ($000):** 122183 **Personnel:** 2480

☐ **MOCCASIN BEND MENTAL HEALTH INSTITUTE (444002)**, 100 Moccasin Bend Road, Zip 37405–4496; tel. 423/785–3400 **A**1 10 **F**26 30 31 32 37 50 56 57 73 81 82 88 90 91 92 93 94 119 124 135
Primary Contact: William L. Ventress, Chief Executive Officer
COO: Patricia Alverson, Assistant Superintendent Program Services
CFO: Jane Lovell, Director Financial Services
CMO: Terry R. Holmes, M.D., Clinical Director
CHR: Cynthia Honeycutt, Director Human Resources
Web address: www.state.tn.us/mental/mhs/mbhmhi/moc.htm
Control: State–Government, nonfederal **Service:** Psychiatric

Staffed Beds: 172 **Admissions:** 2512 **Census:** 124 **Outpatient Visits:** 0 **Births:** 0 **Total Expense ($000):** 26514 **Payroll Expense ($000):** 15483 **Personnel:** 426

★ **PARKRIDGE MEDICAL CENTER (440156)**, 2333 McCallie Avenue, Zip 37404–3285; tel. 423/698–6061, (Includes EAST RIDGE HOSPITAL, 941 Spring Creek Road, East Ridge, Zip 37412; tel. 423/855–3500; Mark E. Sims, Chief Executive Officer; PARKRIDGE VALLEY HOSPTIAL, 2200 Morris Hill Road, Zip 37421; tel. 423/894–4220; Mark E. Sims, Chief Executive Officer) **A**1 9 10 **F**3 11 15 18 20 22 24 25 26 27 30 31 32 33 35 38 43 46 49 51 54 55 57 59 62 66 68 72 73 75 76 77 79 80 81 82 85 86 87 88 93 96 97 100 102 103 107 109 116 118 119 120 121 134 135 **S** HCA
Primary Contact: Darrell W. Moore, CHE, Chief Executive Officer
CFO: Jim Leamon, Chief Financial Officer
CIO: Paul Marsh, Director Information Systems
CHR: Carole Hoffman, Vice President
Web address: www.parkridgemedicalcenter.com
Control: Corporation, Investor–owned, for–profit **Service:** General Medical and Surgical

Staffed Beds: 185 **Admissions:** 7916 **Census:** 116 **Outpatient Visits:** 59750 **Births:** 0 **Total Expense ($000):** 106586 **Payroll Expense ($000):** 38754 **Personnel:** 646

TN

Hospital, Medicare Provider Number, Address, Telephone, Approval, Facility, and Physician Codes, Health Care System
★ American Hospital Association (AHA) membership
☐ The Joint Commission accreditation
○ American Osteopathic Association (AOA) accreditation
△ Commission on Accreditation of Rehabilitation Facilities (CARF) accreditation

★ △ **SISKIN HOSPITAL FOR PHYSICAL REHABILITATION (443025)**, One Siskin Plaza, Zip 37403–1306; tel. 423/634–1200, (Total facility includes 29 beds in nursing home–type unit) **A**1 7 10 **F**25 26 30 32 33 52 57 62 73 85 86 117 119 121 132 135 137
Primary Contact: Robert P. Main, President and Chief Executive Officer
COO: Linda Knudson–Lind, Senior Vice President and Chief Operating Officer
CFO: Linda A. Knight, Vice President Finance and Chief Financial Officer
CMO: David N. Bowers, M.D., Medical Director
CHR: C. Duaine Long, Director Human Resources
Web address: www.siskinrehab.org
Control: Other not–for–profit (including NFP Corporation) **Service:** Rehabilitation

Staffed Beds: 109 **Admissions:** 1753 **Census:** 55 **Outpatient Visits:** 35282 **Births:** 0 **Total Expense ($000):** 29049 **Payroll Expense ($000):** 14415 **Personnel:** 306

T. C. THOMPSON CHILDREN'S HOSPITAL See Erlanger Medical Center

WILLIE D. MILLER EYE CENTER See Erlanger Medical Center

CLARKSVILLE—Montgomery County

★ **GATEWAY MEDICAL CENTER (440035)**, (Formerly Gateway Health System), 651 Dunlop Lane, Zip 37040–5015, Mailing Address: P.O. Box 31629, Zip 37043–0028; tel. 931/502–1000 **A**1 2 9 10 **F**3 11 12 13 15 17 18 20 22 24 25 26 28 30 31 32 33 38 41 42 49 50 51 55 56 57 58 60 61 62 68 70 73 74 75 77 78 79 80 81 82 84 85 86 96 97 100 103 104 106 107 118 119 121 124 135 136 137 **S** Community Health Systems, Inc.
Primary Contact: Michael L. Mullins, Chief Executive Officer
COO: Russell Pigg, Chief Operating Officer
CFO: Scott Pfister, Chief Financial Officer
CMO: Thomas L. Ely, D.O., Chief Medical Officer
CIO: Frank Rvotolo, Chief Information Officer
CHR: Dianne McGregor, Director Human Resources
Web address: www.ghsystem.com
Control: Partnership, Investor–owned, for–profit **Service:** General Medical and Surgical

Staffed Beds: 198 **Admissions:** 10319 **Census:** 106 **Outpatient Visits:** 133798 **Births:** 1830 **Total Expense ($000):** 93446 **Payroll Expense ($000):** 40696 **Personnel:** 999

CLEVELAND—Bradley County

★ **SKYRIDGE MEDICAL CENTER (440024)**, 2305 Chambliss Avenue N.W., Zip 37311–3847, Mailing Address: P.O. Box 3060, Zip 37320–3060; tel. 423/559–6000, (Includes SKYRIDGE MEDICAL CENTER – WESTSIDE CAMPUS, 2800 Westside Drive N.W., Zip 37312–3599; tel. 423/339–4100; R. Coleman Foss, Chief Executive Officer) **A**1 9 10 **F**5 13 15 18 20 22 24 25 26 27 30 31 32 33 37 38 39 42 43 49 51 55 56 57 59 61 62 66 68 74 76 77 79 80 82 84 86 88 94 96 97 100 102 103 106 107 118 124 135 137 **S** Community Health Systems, Inc.
Primary Contact: R. Coleman Foss, Chief Executive Officer
CFO: Bill Ziesmer, Chief Financial Officer
CMO: Felicito Fernando, M.D., Chief of Staff
CHR: Kristine Godfrey, Director Human Resources
Web address: www.skyridgemedicalcenter.net
Control: Corporation, Investor–owned, for–profit **Service:** General Medical and Surgical

Staffed Beds: 209 **Admissions:** 10212 **Census:** 108 **Outpatient Visits:** 215523 **Births:** 1137 **Total Expense ($000):** 83898 **Payroll Expense ($000):** 36954 **Personnel:** 825

COLLIERVILLE—Shelby County

★ **BAPTIST MEMORIAL HOSPITAL–COLLIERVILLE (440217)**, 1500 West Poplar Avenue, Zip 38017–0601; tel. 901/861–9400 **A**1 9 10 **F**3 15 25 26 27 30 31 32 33 38 52 55 57 59 68 73 75 77 79 80 86 96 97 99 100 102 106 107 118 121 124 134 135 136 **S** Baptist Memorial Health Care Corporation
Primary Contact: Glenn Baker, Administrator and Chief Executive Officer
CFO: Terri Seago, Chief Financial Officer
CIO: Jerry Brantley, Vice President and Chief Information Officer
CHR: Karen Swanson, Director Human Resources
Web address: www.bmhcc.org
Control: Other not–for–profit (including NFP Corporation) **Service:** General Medical and Surgical

Staffed Beds: 61 **Admissions:** 2348 **Census:** 28 **Outpatient Visits:** 31383 **Births:** 0 **Total Expense ($000):** 45569 **Payroll Expense ($000):** 15229 **Personnel:** 258

COLUMBIA—Maury County

★ **MAURY REGIONAL HOSPITAL (440073)**, 1224 Trotwood Avenue, Zip 38401–4802; tel. 931/381–1111, (Total facility includes 20 beds in nursing home–type unit) **A**1 2 9 10 19 **F**7 8 11 13 15 17 18 20 22 24 25 26 27 32 33 38 43 46 48 50 51 53 55 56 57 59 61 62 66 68 70 72 73 74 75 76 77 78 79 80 81 82 84 86 87 96 97 100 102 104 105 106 107 109 111 117 118 119 120 121 124 133 135 136 137
Primary Contact: Robert Otwell, Chief Executive Officer
COO: C. Ron Pope, Vice President Administrative and Ancillary Services
CFO: Larry E. Moore, Chief Financial Officer
CMO: Charles A. Ball, M.D., Chief Medical Officer
CIO: Doug Turner, Chief Information Officer
CHR: Kaye Brewer, Director Human Resources
Web address: www.mauryregional.com
Control: County–Government, nonfederal **Service:** General Medical and Surgical

Staffed Beds: 172 **Admissions:** 12741 **Census:** 143 **Outpatient Visits:** 224255 **Births:** 1668 **Total Expense ($000):** 162437 **Payroll Expense ($000):** 77232 **Personnel:** 1600

COOKEVILLE—Putnam County

★ **COOKEVILLE REGIONAL MEDICAL CENTER (440059)**, 142 West Fifth Street, Zip 38501–1795, Mailing Address: P.O. Box 340, Zip 38503–0340; tel. 931/646–2541 **A**1 2 9 10 19 **F**3 8 11 13 15 17 18 20 22 24 25 26 27 30 31 32 33 38 41 47 49 50 51 53 55 56 57 61 62 63 66 68 72 73 74 75 76 77 79 80 81 82 84 85 86 96 97 99 100 102 103 105 106 107 108 109 111 116 118 119 120 121 124 135 136 **P**7
Primary Contact: Bernard L. Mattingly, Chief Executive Officer
COO: Bill Little, Chief Operating Officer
CFO: Paul Korth, Chief Financial Officer
CIO: Les Bernstein, Director Information Systems
CHR: Angel Lewis, Executive Director Human Resources
Web address: www.crmchealth.org
Control: City–Government, nonfederal **Service:** General Medical and Surgical

Staffed Beds: 217 **Admissions:** 11136 **Census:** 144 **Outpatient Visits:** 66453 **Births:** 1375 **Total Expense ($000):** 154844 **Payroll Expense ($000):** 59677 **Personnel:** 1399

COPPERHILL—Polk County

★ **COPPER BASIN MEDICAL CENTER (441315)**, 144 Medical Center Drive, Zip 37317, Mailing Address: P.O. Box 990, Zip 37317–0990; tel. 423/496–5511, (Nonreporting) **A**9 10 18
Primary Contact: David Hyatt, Interim Chief Executive Officer
CFO: Jaime Pittman, Chief Financial Officer
CMO: Allen Uhlik, M.D., Chief of Staff
CIO: Rick Demers, Director Maintenance
Web address: www.copperbasin.org
Control: Other not–for–profit (including NFP Corporation) **Service:** General Medical and Surgical

Staffed Beds: 25

COVINGTON—Tipton County

★ **BAPTIST MEMORIAL HOSPITAL–TIPTON (440131)**, 1995 Highway 51 South, Zip 38019–3635; tel. 901/476–2621 **A**1 9 10 **F**3 7 11 15 25 26 30 31 32 33 38 55 56 57 68 73 74 75 77 79 80 82 86 90 96 97 100 102 107 118 119 121 124 135 137 **S** Baptist Memorial Health Care Corporation
Primary Contact: Barry Bondurant, Administrator and Chief Executive Officer
CFO: Monique Hart, Chief Financial Officer
CMO: Jimmy Beasley, M.D., Chief of Staff
CHR: Myra Cousar, Director Human Resources
Web address: www.bmhcc.org
Control: Other not–for–profit (including NFP Corporation) **Service:** General Medical and Surgical

Staffed Beds: 50 **Admissions:** 2228 **Census:** 21 **Outpatient Visits:** 44239 **Births:** 466 **Total Expense ($000):** 25024 **Payroll Expense ($000):** 9896 **Personnel:** 255

CROSSVILLE—Cumberland County

★ **CUMBERLAND MEDICAL CENTER (440009)**, 421 South Main Street, Zip 38555–5031; tel. 931/484–9511, (Total facility includes 20 beds in nursing home–type unit) **A**1 9 10 20 **F**3 13 15 24 25 27 31 32 33 38 51 52 55 57 59 61 66 68 72 73 74 75 76 77 78 79 80 82 84 86 87 96 97 100 102 105 106 107 108 109 111 117 118 119 120 121 124 135 136
Primary Contact: Edwin S. Anderson, Interim President and Chief Executive Officer
CFO: Kenneth R. Stephens, Executive Vice President
CMO: Barry Wagner, D.O., Chief Medical Officer
CIO: Joe Lowe, Director Management Information Systems
CHR: Pat Whittenburg, Director Human Resources and Corporate Compliance Officer
Web address: www.cmchealthcare.org
Control: Other not–for–profit (including NFP Corporation) **Service:** General Medical and Surgical

Staffed Beds: 175 **Admissions:** 7816 **Census:** 105 **Outpatient Visits:** 148550 **Births:** 734 **Total Expense ($000):** 84126 **Payroll Expense ($000):** 43891 **Personnel:** 944

TN

 Many Facility Codes have changed. Please refer to the AHA Guide Code Chart.

DAYTON—Rhea County

★ **RHEA MEDICAL CENTER (441310)**, 9400 Rhea County Highway, Zip 37321–7922; tel. 423/775–1121, (Total facility includes 89 beds in nursing home–type unit) **A**1 9 10 18 **F**3 15 24 25 30 31 33 38 55 57 65 68 73 79 96 97 102 107 119 121 122 135 **S** QHR
Primary Contact: Kennedy L. Croom, Jr., Administrator and Chief Executive Officer
CFO: Harv Sanders, Chief Financial Officer
CMO: William T. Bate, M.D., Chief of Staff
CHR: Peri Meadows, Director Human Resources
Web address: www.rheamedical.org
Control: County–Government, nonfederal **Service:** General Medical and Surgical

Staffed Beds: 114 **Admissions:** 1311 **Census:** 92 **Outpatient Visits:** 39215 **Births:** 3 **Total Expense ($000):** 17063 **Payroll Expense ($000):** 7596 **Personnel:** 233

DICKSON—Dickson County

★ **HORIZON MEDICAL CENTER (440046)**, 111 Highway 70 East, Zip 37055–2033; tel. 615/446–0446 **A**1 9 10 **F**11 12 13 15 18 20 24 25 26 27 30 31 32 33 36 37 38 43 46 50 51 54 55 57 59 62 68 72 73 74 75 76 77 79 80 81 82 85 88 93 96 97 99 100 102 107 109 118 119 124 135 136 **S** HCA
Primary Contact: John A. Marshall, Chief Executive Officer
CFO: Clarence Gray, Chief Financial Officer
CIO: Rick Stoker, Director Management Information Systems
CHR: Robbie Tatum, Director Human Resources
Web address: www.horizonmedicalcenter.com
Control: Corporation, Investor–owned, for–profit **Service:** General Medical and Surgical

Staffed Beds: 116 **Admissions:** 4536 **Census:** 56 **Outpatient Visits:** 58681 **Births:** 533 **Total Expense ($000):** 64766 **Payroll Expense ($000):** 21738 **Personnel:** 404

DYERSBURG—Dyer County

★ **DYERSBURG REGIONAL MEDICAL CENTER (440072)**, 400 Tickle Street, Zip 38024–3182; tel. 731/285–2410 **A**1 9 10 20 **F**7 11 13 15 25 26 30 31 32 37 38 50 55 56 57 59 61 74 77 79 81 82 84 96 100 107 118 122 135 **S** Community Health Systems, Inc.
Primary Contact: Greg Lowe, Chief Executive Officer
COO: Tripp Smith, Assistant Chief Executive Officer
CFO: Terri Warren, Chief Financial Officer
CMO: Pankaj Srivastava, M.D., Chief of Staff
CIO: Russ Shephard, Senior Systems Analyst
CHR: Beverly Ray, Director of Human Resources
Web address: www.dyersburgregionalmc.com
Control: Corporation, Investor–owned, for–profit **Service:** General Medical and Surgical

Staffed Beds: 105 **Admissions:** 5704 **Census:** 50 **Outpatient Visits:** 43407 **Births:** 662 **Total Expense ($000):** 51201 **Payroll Expense ($000):** 20081 **Personnel:** 529

EAST RIDGE—Hamilton County

EAST RIDGE HOSPITAL See Parkridge Medical Center, Chattanooga

ELIZABETHTON—Carter County

□ **SYCAMORE SHOALS HOSPITAL (440018)**, 1501 West Elk Avenue, Zip 37643–2874; tel. 423/542–1300 **A**1 9 10 **F**3 11 13 15 25 26 30 31 32 33 38 41 50 52 54 55 57 61 62 66 68 72 74 75 76 77 79 81 82 84 86 88 93 96 97 100 102 118 119 121 124 135 136 **S** Mountain States Health Alliance
Primary Contact: Dwayne Taylor, Chief Executive Officer
COO: Melanie Stanton, Assistant Administrator and Chief Nursing Officer
CFO: Charles Dugger, Chief Financial Officer
CMO: Bomar Herrin, M.D., Medical Director
CIO: Richard Eshbach, Chief Information Officer
CHR: Sharon Sheppard, Manager Human Resources
Web address: www.msha.com
Control: Other not–for–profit (including NFP Corporation) **Service:** General Medical and Surgical

Staffed Beds: 121 **Admissions:** 4210 **Census:** 45 **Outpatient Visits:** 67410 **Births:** 452 **Total Expense ($000):** 33825 **Payroll Expense ($000):** 15456 **Personnel:** 345

ERIN—Houston County

□ **TRINITY HOSPITAL (441312)**, 5001 East Main Street, Zip 37061–0489, Mailing Address: P.O. Box 489, Zip 37061–0489; tel. 931/289–4211 **A**1 9 10 18 **F**15 25 31 32 38 52 57 75 77 79 80 82 86 96 100 107 118 122 **S** Associated Healthcare Systems, Inc.
Primary Contact: Yvette Gillespie, Chief Executive Officer
CFO: Shannon Allison, Chief Financial Officer
CMO: Erin Chambers, M.D., Chief Medical Officer
CHR: Reta Brady, Administrative Assistant and Manager Human Resources
Web address: www.trinityhospitaltn.com
Control: Corporation, Investor–owned, for–profit **Service:** General Medical and Surgical

Staffed Beds: 25 **Admissions:** 1029 **Census:** 10 **Outpatient Visits:** 8504 **Births:** 0 **Total Expense ($000):** 6731 **Payroll Expense ($000):** 3278 **Personnel:** 92

ERWIN—Unicoi County

★ **UNICOI COUNTY MEMORIAL HOSPITAL (440001)**, 100 Greenway Circle, Zip 37650–2196, Mailing Address: P.O. Box 802, Zip 37650–0802; tel. 423/743–3141, (Total facility includes 46 beds in nursing home–type unit) **A**1 9 10 **F**11 15 25 26 30 31 32 33 38 53 55 56 57 61 62 63 66 68 73 75 77 79 80 86 96 100 102 107 117 118 119 135 **P**6
Primary Contact: Jim S. Pate, President and Chief Executive Officer
CFO: Toni Buchanan, Chief Financial Officer
CMO: Frank T. Wegman, M.D., Chief of Staff
CIO: Spencer Levleit, Director Information Technology
CHR: Susan Broyles, Director Human Resources and Safety
Web address: www.ucmhnet.org
Control: Other not–for–profit (including NFP Corporation) **Service:** General Medical and Surgical

Staffed Beds: 83 **Admissions:** 1272 **Census:** 58 **Outpatient Visits:** 36355 **Births:** 0 **Total Expense ($000):** 14624 **Payroll Expense ($000):** 6993 **Personnel:** 224

ETOWAH—McMinn County

★ **WOODS MEMORIAL HOSPITAL (440054)**, (Formerly Woods Memorial Hospital District), 886 Highway 411 North, Zip 37331–1912; tel. 423/263–3600, (Nonreporting) **A**1 9 10
Primary Contact: Steve Clapp, Chief Executive Officer
CFO: Tim S. Brown, Chief Financial Officer
CMO: Brandon Watters, Chief of Staff
CHR: Angela Chaffin, Director Human Resources and Compliance Officer
Web address: www.woodshospital.org
Control: Partnership, Investor–owned, for–profit **Service:** General Medical and Surgical

Staffed Beds: 72

FAYETTEVILLE—Lincoln County

★ **LINCOLN COUNTY HEALTH SYSTEM (440102)**, 106 Medical Center Boulevard, Zip 37334–2684; tel. 931/438–1100, (Total facility includes 278 beds in nursing home–type unit) **A**1 9 10 **F**7 10 11 13 15 25 26 30 31 32 33 38 42 52 54 55 61 62 65 68 73 74 75 79 86 93 96 97 100 102 107 117 118 121 132 135 137 **S** QHR
Primary Contact: Gary G. Kendrick, Chief Executive Officer
CFO: David Groce, Associate Administrator and Chief Financial Officer
CMO: John Leslie, M.D., Chief of Staff
CHR: Pat Marty, Director
Web address: www.lchealthsystem.com
Control: County–Government, nonfederal **Service:** General Medical and Surgical

Staffed Beds: 327 **Admissions:** 2350 **Census:** 263 **Outpatient Visits:** 41569 **Births:** 335 **Personnel:** 507

FRANKLIN—Williamson County

★ **WILLIAMSON MEDICAL CENTER (440029)**, 4321 Carothers Parkway, Zip 37067–8542; tel. 615/435–5000 **A**1 9 10 **F**3 7 8 11 13 15 18 20 24 25 26 27 30 31 32 33 38 40 49 55 56 57 62 68 70 71 73 74 75 76 77 78 79 80 81 82 86 87 92 96 97 100 102 103 106 107 112 116 119 120 121 124 135 137 **P**3 8
Primary Contact: Dennis E. Miller, FACHE, Chief Executive Officer
COO: Rodger G. Klein, Chief Operating Officer
CFO: Donald Webb, Chief Financial Officer
CMO: Starling C. Evins, M.D., Chief of Staff
CIO: Laura Bustetter, Director Marketing and Public Relations
CHR: Debra Foster, Director Human Resources
Web address: www.williamsonmedicalcenter.org
Control: County–Government, nonfederal **Service:** General Medical and Surgical

Staffed Beds: 193 **Admissions:** 9022 **Census:** 96 **Outpatient Visits:** 142341 **Births:** 1109 **Total Expense ($000):** 121688 **Payroll Expense ($000):** 51737 **Personnel:** 1219

Hospital, Medicare Provider Number, Address, Telephone, Approval, Facility, and Physician Codes, Health Care System

★ American Hospital Association (AHA) membership
□ The Joint Commission accreditation
○ American Osteopathic Association (AOA) accreditation
△ Commission on Accreditation of Rehabilitation Facilities (CARF) accreditation

GALLATIN—Sumner County

★ △ **SUMNER REGIONAL MEDICAL CENTER (440003)**, 555 Hartsville Pike, Zip 37066–2449, Mailing Address: P.O. Box 1558, Zip 37066–1558; tel. 615/452–4210 **A**1 2 7 9 10 **F**3 11 13 15 18 20 24 25 26 27 30 31 32 33 35 38 41 43 50 51 52 55 56 57 59 62 68 72 73 74 75 76 77 79 80 81 82 84 85 86 92 96 97 100 102 107 109 111 112 117 118 119 120 121 124 132 135 136 137 **S** Sumner Regional Health Systems
Primary Contact: Bruce James, Administrator
CFO: Lynn Norvell, Senior Vice President Finance and Chief Financial Officer
CIO: David Young, Senior Vice President Planning and Technology
CHR: Jan Hallmark, Senior Vice President Human Development and Community Outreach
Web address: www.sumner.org
Control: Other not–for–profit (including NFP Corporation) **Service:** General Medical and Surgical

Staffed Beds: 155 **Admissions:** 5939 **Census:** 71 **Outpatient Visits:** 97707 **Births:** 823 **Total Expense ($000):** 97901 **Payroll Expense ($000):** 35546 **Personnel:** 726

GERMANTOWN—Shelby County

★ △ **BAPTIST REHABILITATION–GERMANTOWN (440147)**, 2100 Exeter Road, Zip 38138–3978; tel. 901/757–1350, (Nonreporting) **A**1 7 9 10 **S** Baptist Memorial Health Care Corporation
Primary Contact: Susan Stralka, Administrator and Chief Executive Officer
CFO: Chetan Parekh, Chief Financial Officer
CMO: Sunita Jain, M.D., Chief Medical Officer
Web address: www.bmhcc.org
Control: Other not–for–profit (including NFP Corporation) **Service:** Rehabilitation

Staffed Beds: 51

METHODIST LE BONHEUR GERMANTOWN HOSPITAL See Methodist University Hospital, Memphis

GREENEVILLE—Greene County

★ **LAUGHLIN MEMORIAL HOSPITAL (440025)**, 1420 Tusculum Boulevard, Zip 37745–5825; tel. 423/787–5000, (Total facility includes 90 beds in nursing home–type unit) **A**1 9 10 19 **F**3 11 13 15 18 24 27 30 31 32 33 38 46 49 50 51 54 55 56 57 61 62 66 68 71 72 73 74 75 76 77 79 80 81 82 84 86 96 97 100 102 103 105 106 107 109 111 117 118 119 120 121 135 136
Primary Contact: Charles H. Whitfield, Jr., President and Chief Executive Officer
CFO: Mark Compton, Chief Financial Officer
CIO: Mary Crouch, Director Information Technologies
CHR: Robert Roark, Director Human Resources
Web address: www.laughlinmemorial.org
Control: Other not–for–profit (including NFP Corporation) **Service:** General Medical and Surgical

Staffed Beds: 230 **Admissions:** 5140 **Census:** 143 **Outpatient Visits:** 106662 **Births:** 364 **Total Expense ($000):** 60482 **Payroll Expense ($000):** 25306 **Personnel:** 734

★ **TAKOMA REGIONAL HOSPITAL (440050)**, 401 Takoma Avenue, Zip 37743–4647; tel. 423/639–3151 **A**1 9 10 **F**3 11 13 15 25 26 38 55 61 68 85 88 **S** Adventist Health System Sunbelt Health Care Corporation
Primary Contact: Carlyle L. E. Walton, President
CFO: Tom VandenHoven, Chief Financial Officer
CMO: Michael Menz, M.D., Chief of Staff
CHR: Jack Lister, Director Human Resources
Web address: www.takoma.org
Control: Church–operated, Nongovernment, not–for profit **Service:** General Medical and Surgical

Staffed Beds: 100 **Admissions:** 1808 **Census:** 23 **Outpatient Visits:** 104022 **Births:** 493 **Payroll Expense ($000):** 12141 **Personnel:** 382

HARRIMAN—Roane County

★ **ROANE MEDICAL CENTER (440031)**, 412 Devonia Street, Zip 37748–0489, Mailing Address: P.O. Box 489, Zip 37748–0489; tel. 865/882–1323 **A**1 9 10 **F**3 11 15 18 24 25 26 30 32 33 38 39 55 57 68 77 79 88 93 96 100 107 118 119 122 135 136 137 **P**8
Primary Contact: Jim Gann, Administrator
CFO: Janice Bardill, Chief Financial Officer
CIO: Janice Bardill, Chief Financial Officer
CHR: Joyce Marsalis, Human Resource Manager
Web address: www.roanemedical.com
Control: Hospital district or authority, Government, nonfederal **Service:** General Medical and Surgical

Staffed Beds: 56 **Admissions:** 2973 **Census:** 35 **Outpatient Visits:** 64730 **Total Expense ($000):** 30945 **Payroll Expense ($000):** 14001 **Personnel:** 379

HARTSVILLE—Trousdale County

☐ **TROUSDALE MEDICAL CENTER (441301)**, 500 Church Street, Zip 37074–2936, Mailing Address: P.O. Box 319, Carthage, Zip 37030–0319; tel. 615/374–2221, (Nonreporting) **A**1 9 10 18 **S** Sumner Regional Health Systems
Primary Contact: William D. Mize, Administrator
CFO: Lynn Norvell, Senior Vice President Finance and Chief Financial Officer
CIO: David Young, Senior Vice President Planning and Technology
CHR: Amy Overstreet, Director Human Resources
Web address: www.trousdale.org
Control: Other not–for–profit (including NFP Corporation) **Service:** General Medical and Surgical

Staffed Beds: 25

HENDERSONVILLE—Sumner County

★ **HENDERSONVILLE MEDICAL CENTER (440194)**, 355 New Shackle Island Road, Zip 37075–2393; tel. 615/338–1000, (Includes PORTLAND MEDICAL CENTER, 105 Redbud Drive, Portland, Zip 37148; tel. 615/325–7301), (Nonreporting) **A**1 9 10 **S** HCA
Primary Contact: Regina Bartlett, Chief Executive Officer
COO: Brian Cook, Chief Operating Officer
CFO: Michael Morrison, Chief Financial Officer
CIO: Hal Schultheis, Director Information Systems
CHR: Kreg Arnold, Director Human Resources
Web address: www.hendersonvillemedicalcenter.com
Control: Corporation, Investor–owned, for–profit **Service:** General Medical and Surgical

Staffed Beds: 70

HERMITAGE—Davidson County

★ **SUMMIT MEDICAL CENTER (440150)**, 5655 Frist Boulevard, Zip 37076–2053; tel. 615/316–3000 **A**1 2 9 10 **F**3 11 13 15 17 18 20 24 25 26 27 30 31 32 33 35 36 37 38 43 46 47 48 49 50 52 53 54 55 56 57 60 62 68 71 72 73 74 75 76 77 78 79 80 82 84 86 88 90 92 96 97 99 100 102 103 106 107 109 111 112 118 119 120 124 134 135 136 137 **P**6 **S** HCA
Primary Contact: Jeffrey T. Whitehorn, Chief Executive Officer
COO: Melissa Waddey, Chief Operating Officer
CFO: Timothy Stanfill, Chief Financial Officer
Web address: www.summitmedctr.com
Control: Corporation, Investor–owned, for–profit **Service:** General Medical and Surgical

Staffed Beds: 188 **Admissions:** 9895 **Census:** 116 **Outpatient Visits:** 104329 **Births:** 1660 **Total Expense ($000):** 103368 **Payroll Expense ($000):** 41103 **Personnel:** 790

HUMBOLDT—Gibson County

★ **HUMBOLDT GENERAL HOSPITAL (440115)**, 3525 Chere Carol Road, Zip 38343–3699; tel. 731/784–2321 **A**1 9 10 **F**3 15 25 26 30 31 32 33 38 55 57 62 66 73 79 80 82 86 96 107 119 121 122 135 **S** West Tennessee Healthcare
Primary Contact: Bill Kail, Administrator
CFO: Terry Swindell, Chief Financial Officer
CMO: Keith Kirby, Chief of Staff
Web address: www.wth.net
Control: Hospital district or authority, Government, nonfederal **Service:** General Medical and Surgical

Staffed Beds: 35 **Admissions:** 1156 **Census:** 14 **Outpatient Visits:** 19392 **Births:** 0 **Total Expense ($000):** 6582 **Payroll Expense ($000):** 3757 **Personnel:** 120

HUNTINGDON—Carroll County

★ **BAPTIST MEMORIAL HOSPITAL–HUNTINGDON (440016)**, 631 R. B. Wilson Drive, Zip 38344–1675; tel. 731/986–4461, (Nonreporting) **A**9 10 **S** Baptist Memorial Health Care Corporation
Primary Contact: Susan M. Breeden, Administrator and Chief Executive Officer
CFO: Sharron Holland, Chief Financial Officer
CHR: Kim King, Director Human Resources and Public Relations
Web address: www.bmhcc.org
Control: Other not–for–profit (including NFP Corporation) **Service:** General Medical and Surgical

Staffed Beds: 45

TN

 Many Facility Codes have changed. Please refer to the AHA Guide Code Chart.

JACKSON—Madison County

☒ △ **JACKSON–MADISON COUNTY GENERAL HOSPITAL (440002)**, 708 West Forest Avenue, Zip 38301–3956; tel. 731/541–5000, (Total facility includes 50 beds in nursing home–type unit) **A**1 2 3 5 7 9 10 **F**3 7 8 11 13 15 17 18 20 22 24 25 26 27 30 31 32 33 38 42 43 44 45 46 47 48 49 51 54 55 57 58 59 62 63 66 68 70 72 73 74 75 76 77 78 79 80 81 82 83 84 85 86 87 96 99 100 101 103 104 105 106 107 108 112 117 118 119 120 121 124 134 135 136 137 **P**5 8 **S** West Tennessee Healthcare
Primary Contact: Richard H. Parks, FACHE, President and Chief Executive Officer
COO: Bradford J. Baucom, Vice President and Chief Operating Officer
CFO: Bobby Arnold, Vice President and Chief Financial Officer
CMO: Charles Mertz, Chief of Staff
CIO: Jeff Frieling, Chief Information Officer
CHR: Jan Boud, Vice President Communications and Human Resources
Web address: www.wth.org
Control: Hospital district or authority, Government, nonfederal **Service:** General Medical and Surgical

Staffed Beds: 644 **Admissions:** 28141 **Census:** 473 **Outpatient Visits:** 183832 **Births:** 3065 **Total Expense ($000):** 377234 **Payroll Expense ($000):** 164544 **Personnel:** 3972

★ **PATHWAYS OF TENNESSEE (444010)**, 238 Summar Drive, Zip 38301–3982; tel. 731/541–8200 **A**10 **F**5 25 30 31 32 33 36 55 57 88 89 90 91 92 93 94 121 123 124 **S** West Tennessee Healthcare
Primary Contact: Pam Henson, Executive Director
CFO: Bobby Arnold, Vice President and Chief Financial Officer
CMO: Donna McKenzie, Medical Director
CIO: Jeff Frieling, Chief Information Officer
CHR: Barry Phillips, Director Human Resources
Web address: www.wth.net
Control: Hospital district or authority, Government, nonfederal **Service:** Psychiatric

Staffed Beds: 25 **Admissions:** 961 **Census:** 9 **Outpatient Visits:** 137487 **Births:** 0 **Total Expense ($000):** 14755 **Payroll Expense ($000):** 8433 **Personnel:** 250

☒ **REGIONAL HOSPITAL OF JACKSON (440189)**, 367 Hospital Boulevard, Zip 38305–2081; tel. 731/661–2000, (Nonreporting) **A**1 9 10 **S** Community Health Systems, Inc.
Primary Contact: Stephen Grubbs, Chief Executive Officer
CFO: Cully Chapman, Chief Financial Officer
CHR: Debbie Yeager, Director Human Resource
Web address: www.regionalhospital.com
Control: Corporation, Investor–owned, for–profit **Service:** General Medical and Surgical

Staffed Beds: 127

JAMESTOWN—Fentress County

☐ **JAMESTOWN REGIONAL MEDICAL CENTER (440083)**, 436 Central Avenue West, Zip 38556–3031, Mailing Address: P.O. Box 1500, Zip 38556–1500; tel. 931/879–8171, (Total facility includes 14 beds in nursing home–type unit) (Nonreporting) **A**1 9 10 20 **S** Health Management Associates
Primary Contact: John Lee, Chief Executive Officer
CFO: Walter Turner, Chief Financial Officer
CMO: Mark Clapp, M.D., Chief of Staff
CIO: Rick Smith, Director Information Systems
CHR: Shelia Russell, Interim Director Human Resources
Web address: www.jamestownregional.org
Control: Corporation, Investor–owned, for–profit **Service:** General Medical and Surgical

Staffed Beds: 85

JASPER—Marion County

☐ **GRANDVIEW MEDICAL CENTER (440064)**, 1000 Highway 28, Zip 37347–3638; tel. 423/837–9500, (Nonreporting) **A**1 9 10 **S** Capella Healthcare
Primary Contact: Daniel Aranda, Chief Executive Officer
CFO: Debbie Hennessee, Chief Financial Officer
Web address: www.grandviewhospital.com
Control: Corporation, Investor–owned, for–profit **Service:** General Medical and Surgical

Staffed Beds: 68

JEFFERSON CITY—Jefferson County

☒ **ST. MARY'S JEFFERSON MEMORIAL HOSPITAL (440056)**, 110 Hospital Drive, Zip 37760–5281; tel. 865/471–2500 **A**1 9 10 **F**3 11 13 15 24 25 26 30 31 32 38 44 55 57 66 68 73 74 77 79 82 86 96 97 100 102 106 107 118 119 122 124 134 135 **S** Catholic Healthcare Partners
Primary Contact: Michael C. Hicks, Administrator
COO: Carol Wolfenbarger, Chief Operating Officer and Chief Nursing Executive
Web address: www.jeffersonhealthinc.com
Control: Church–operated, Nongovernment, not–for profit **Service:** General Medical and Surgical

Staffed Beds: 30 **Admissions:** 2402 **Census:** 24 **Outpatient Visits:** 56348 **Births:** 134 **Total Expense ($000):** 30335 **Payroll Expense ($000):** 11327 **Personnel:** 228

JELLICO—Campbell County

☒ **JELLICO COMMUNITY HOSPITAL (440180)**, 188 Hospital Lane, Zip 37762–4400; tel. 423/784–7252 **A**1 9 10 20 **F**3 7 11 13 15 25 26 30 31 32 33 38 40 41 43 44 48 50 52 53 55 56 57 58 60 61 62 63 66 68 73 74 75 77 79 80 81 82 86 87 96 97 100 102 107 119 120 121 122 123 124 132 134 135 137 **P**6 **S** Adventist Health System Sunbelt Health Care Corporation
Primary Contact: David A. Butler, President and Chief Executive Officer
COO: Pamela Hodge, Chief Nursing Officer
CFO: Randy Reimer, Chief Financial Officer
CMO: Darryl J. Wilkens, M.D., Chief of Staff
CIO: Richard Helm, Chief Information Officer
CHR: Vince Vannett, Director Human Resources
Web address: www.jellicohospital.com
Control: Other not–for–profit (including NFP Corporation) **Service:** General Medical and Surgical

Staffed Beds: 39 **Admissions:** 1832 **Census:** 16 **Outpatient Visits:** 39302 **Births:** 247 **Total Expense ($000):** 27634 **Payroll Expense ($000):** 10518 **Personnel:** 294

JOHNSON CITY—Washington County

☒ **JOHNSON CITY MEDICAL CENTER (440063)**, 400 North State of Franklin Road, Zip 37604–6094; tel. 423/431–6111 **A**1 2 3 5 8 9 10 **F**3 7 8 11 12 13 15 17 18 19 20 21 22 23 24 25 26 27 28 30 31 32 33 37 38 40 41 42 43 44 46 47 48 49 50 51 52 53 54 55 56 57 58 59 60 61 62 66 68 70 72 73 74 75 76 77 78 79 80 81 82 83 84 86 87 90 92 96 97 100 102 103 105 106 107 109 111 112 114 118 119 120 121 123 124 127 130 131 132 135 136 137 **P**7 **S** Mountain States Health Alliance
Primary Contact: John W. Melton, Senior Vice President Operations and Chief Executive Officer
COO: Candace Jennings, Vice President and Chief Operating Officer
CFO: Kerry Vermillion, Chief Financial Officer
CMO: Ken Marshall, M.D., Senior Vice President and Chief Medical Officer
CIO: Richard Eshbach, Chief Information Officer
CHR: Jamie Parsons, Vice President Human Resources
Web address: www.msha.com
Control: Other not–for–profit (including NFP Corporation) **Service:** General Medical and Surgical

Staffed Beds: 443 **Admissions:** 26214 **Census:** 365 **Outpatient Visits:** 217677 **Births:** 1138 **Total Expense ($000):** 354130 **Payroll Expense ($000):** 110522 **Personnel:** 2232

☐ **JOHNSON CITY SPECIALTY HOSPITAL (440105)**, 203 East Watauga Avenue, Zip 37601–4651; tel. 423/434–1400 **A**1 9 10 **F**3 13 15 25 26 30 31 32 33 41 50 55 57 66 73 74 79 81 107 119 121 136 **S** Mountain States Health Alliance
Primary Contact: Rhonda Mann, Director Nursing and Operations
CFO: Kerry Vermillion, Chief Financial Officer
CIO: Richard Eshbach, Chief Information Officer
Web address: www.jcmc.com
Control: Other not–for–profit (including NFP Corporation) **Service:** Obstetrics and gynecology

Staffed Beds: 36 **Admissions:** 1471 **Census:** 9 **Outpatient Visits:** 13117 **Births:** 1064 **Total Expense ($000):** 11276 **Payroll Expense ($000):** 5436 **Personnel:** 112

☒ **NORTH SIDE HOSPITAL (440184)**, 401 Princeton Road, Zip 37601–2097; tel. 423/854–5600, (Total facility includes 34 beds in nursing home–type unit) **A**1 9 10 **F**3 25 26 30 31 32 38 41 54 66 68 72 75 77 81 86 96 97 100 102 106 107 117 119 132 135 **S** Mountain States Health Alliance
Primary Contact: Rhonda Mann, Administrator, Director and Chief Nursing Officer
Web address: www.msha.com
Control: Other not–for–profit (including NFP Corporation) **Service:** General Medical and Surgical

Staffed Beds: 88 **Admissions:** 2067 **Census:** 49 **Outpatient Visits:** 47704 **Births:** 0 **Total Expense ($000):** 22792 **Payroll Expense ($000):** 10574 **Personnel:** 233

TN

Hospital, Medicare Provider Number, Address, Telephone, Approval, Facility, and Physician Codes, Health Care System
★ American Hospital Association (AHA) membership
☐ The Joint Commission accreditation
○ American Osteopathic Association (AOA) accreditation
△ Commission on Accreditation of Rehabilitation Facilities (CARF) accreditation

☐ △ **QUILLEN REHABILITATION HOSPITAL**, 2511 Wesley Street, Zip 37601–1723; tel. 423/283–0700, (Total facility includes 13 beds in nursing home–type unit) **A**1 7 10 **F**3 25 26 30 31 32 66 72 77 81 85 86 117 119 121 **S** Mountain States Health Alliance
Primary Contact: John W. Melton, Senior Vice President Operations and Chief Executive Officer
Web address: www.msha.com
Control: Other not–for–profit (including NFP Corporation) **Service:** Rehabilitation

Staffed Beds: 60 **Admissions:** 923 **Census:** 33 **Outpatient Visits:** 16853 **Births:** 0 **Total Expense ($000):** 12974 **Payroll Expense ($000):** 4060 **Personnel:** 103

☐ **WOODRIDGE HOSPITAL**, 403 State of Franklin Road, Zip 37604–6034; tel. 423/431–7060, (Nonreporting) **A**1 3 5 **S** Mountain States Health Alliance
Primary Contact: Jeffrey N. Dice, Assistant Vice President
COO: Kim Moore, Director Behavioral Health Operations
CFO: John Doyle, Chief Financial Officer
CMO: Terry Borei, Medical Director
CIO: Edward C. Herbert, Vice President Marketing and Communications
Web address: www.msha.com
Control: Other not–for–profit (including NFP Corporation) **Service:** Psychiatric

Staffed Beds: 75

KINGSPORT—Sullivan County

☒ **HEALTHSOUTH REHABILITATION HOSPITAL (443027)**, 113 Cassel Drive, Zip 37660–3775; tel. 423/246–7240, (Nonreporting) **A**1 10 **S** HEALTHSOUTH Corporation
Primary Contact: Terri Alsbrook, Chief Executive Officer
COO: Robert Ley, Director Marketing
CFO: Natalie Tilson, Controller
CMO: James P. Little, M.D., Medical Director
CIO: Natalie Tilson, Controller
CHR: Joyce Jones, Coordinator Human Resources
Web address: www.healthsouth.com
Control: Corporation, Investor–owned, for–profit **Service:** Rehabilitation

Staffed Beds: 50

☐ **INDIAN PATH MEDICAL CENTER (440176)**, 2000 Brookside Drive, Zip 37660–4682; tel. 423/857–7000, (Includes INDIAN PATH PAVILION, 2300 Pavilion Drive, Zip 37660–4672; tel. 423/857–5500), (Total facility includes 22 beds in nursing home–type unit) **A**1 9 10 **F**3 4 5 8 11 13 15 18 25 26 30 31 32 33 36 38 49 50 51 54 55 57 59 62 66 68 71 72 73 74 75 76 77 79 81 82 84 86 87 88 90 91 92 93 94 95 96 97 100 102 106 107 111 117 118 119 120 121 135 136 137 **S** Mountain States Health Alliance
Primary Contact: Monty E. McLaurin, President and Chief Executive Officer
CFO: John Doyle, Chief Financial Officer
CIO: David Phelps, Manager Information System
CHR: Rachel Bishop, Director Human Resources
Web address: www.msha.com
Control: Other not–for–profit (including NFP Corporation) **Service:** General Medical and Surgical

Staffed Beds: 216 **Admissions:** 5709 **Census:** 75 **Outpatient Visits:** 149706 **Births:** 988 **Total Expense ($000):** 72151 **Payroll Expense ($000):** 27389 **Personnel:** 594

☒ **WELLMONT HOLSTON VALLEY MEDICAL CENTER (440017)**, 130 West Ravine Street, Zip 37660, Mailing Address: P.O. Box 238, Zip 37662–0238; tel. 423/224–4000 **A**1 2 3 5 9 10 **F**3 8 11 12 13 14 15 17 18 20 22 24 25 26 27 30 31 32 33 34 35 38 40 41 43 45 46 49 50 51 53 54 55 56 57 58 59 60 61 62 63 64 66 68 70 72 73 74 75 76 77 79 80 82 83 84 86 96 97 99 100 102 103 104 105 106 107 108 109 111 117 118 119 120 121 135 136 137 **P**8 **S** Wellmont Health System
Primary Contact: Blaine L. Douglas, Chief Executive Officer
COO: Michael Bundy, Chief Operating Officer
CFO: Alice H. Pope, Vice President Finance and Operations
CMO: James Bowden, Chief Medical Officer
CIO: Bill Moran, Chief Information Officer
CHR: Hamlin J. Wilson, Senior Vice President Human Resources
Web address: www.wellmont.org
Control: Other not–for–profit (including NFP Corporation) **Service:** General Medical and Surgical

Staffed Beds: 317 **Admissions:** 18137 **Census:** 241 **Outpatient Visits:** 145034 **Births:** 981 **Total Expense ($000):** 254496 **Payroll Expense ($000):** 87999 **Personnel:** 1732

KNOXVILLE—Knox County

★ **BAPTIST HOSPITAL FOR WOMEN (440225)**, 10820 Parkside Drive, Zip 37922–1956; tel. 865/218–7090, (Nonreporting) **A**9 10 **S** Catholic Healthcare Partners
Primary Contact: David E. Loving, Chief Administrative Officer
Web address: www.baptistoneword.org/women
Control: Other not–for–profit (including NFP Corporation) **Service:** Obstetrics and gynecology

Staffed Beds: 16

★ △ **BAPTIST HOSPITAL OF EAST TENNESSEE (440019)**, 137 Blount Avenue S.E., Zip 37920–1643, Mailing Address: P.O. Box 1788, Zip 37901–1788; tel. 865/632–5011, (Total facility includes 20 beds in nursing home–type unit) **A**2 7 9 **F**3 5 8 11 15 17 18 20 22 24 25 26 27 31 32 33 36 37 38 42 43 44 49 51 54 55 56 57 59 60 61 62 63 66 68 72 73 75 76 77 79 80 82 85 86 87 88 90 91 92 93 94 95 96 97 99 100 106 107 108 109 111 112 117 118 119 121 124 130 135 136 137 **P**6 **S** Catholic Healthcare Partners
Primary Contact: Jeffrey A. Ashin, Chief Executive Officer
CFO: David Nowiski, Regional Chief Financial Officer
CMO: Jerry Sanders, M.D., Vice President Medical Affairs
CIO: Scott Burke, Chief Information Officer
CHR: Marty Margetts, Regional Senior Vice President Human Resource Development
Web address: www.baptistoneword.org
Control: Church–operated, Nongovernment, not–for profit **Service:** General Medical and Surgical

Staffed Beds: 212 **Admissions:** 10646 **Census:** 167 **Outpatient Visits:** 141150 **Births:** 0 **Total Expense ($000):** 138417 **Payroll Expense ($000):** 60392 **Personnel:** 1977

☒ **BAPTIST HOSPITAL WEST (440226)**, 10820 Parkside Drive, Zip 37922–1956; tel. 865/218–7011, (Nonreporting) **A**1 9 10 **S** Catholic Healthcare Partners
Primary Contact: David E. Loving, Chief Administrative Officer
Web address: www.baptistoneword.org/west
Control: Other not–for–profit (including NFP Corporation) **Service:** Other specialty

Staffed Beds: 75

☐ **EAST TENNESSEE CHILDREN'S HOSPITAL (443303)**, (Pediatric Medical–Surgical), 2018 Clinch Avenue, Zip 37916–2393, Mailing Address: P.O. Box 15010, Zip 37901–5010; tel. 865/541–8000 **A**1 9 10 **F**3 9 11 25 26 27 28 31 32 33 37 38 40 41 43 53 55 57 58 61 62 66 70 72 73 75 76 77 79 80 81 82 83 84 86 87 96 100 107 118 119 121 135 **P**8
Primary Contact: Keith D. Goodwin, President and Chief Executive Officer
COO: Rudolph McKinley, Vice President Operations and Chief Operating Officer
CMO: Joe Childs, M.D., Vice President Medical Services
CHR: Paul Bates, Vice President Human Resources
Web address: www.etch.com
Control: Other not–for–profit (including NFP Corporation) **Service:** Children's other specialty

Staffed Beds: 152 **Admissions:** 6813 **Census:** 104 **Outpatient Visits:** 159606 **Births:** 0 **Total Expense ($000):** 115806 **Payroll Expense ($000):** 55074 **Personnel:** 1173

☒ △ **FORT SANDERS REGIONAL MEDICAL CENTER (440125)**, 1901 Clinch Avenue S.W., Zip 37916–2394; tel. 865/541–1111, (Total facility includes 24 beds in nursing home–type unit) **A**1 2 7 9 10 **F**3 11 13 17 18 20 22 24 25 26 27 30 31 32 33 38 42 43 44 46 47 48 49 50 51 53 54 56 57 58 59 60 62 66 68 72 73 74 75 76 77 79 80 81 82 85 86 96 97 100 102 103 106 107 114 116 117 118 119 120 121 125 130 135 136 137 **S** Covenant Health
Primary Contact: Keith Altshuler, President and Chief Administrative Officer
CFO: David McReynolds, Chief Financial Officer
Web address: www.covenanthealth.com
Control: Other not–for–profit (including NFP Corporation) **Service:** General Medical and Surgical

Staffed Beds: 351 **Admissions:** 15382 **Census:** 244 **Outpatient Visits:** 193075 **Births:** 3047 **Total Expense ($000):** 192982 **Payroll Expense ($000):** 69719 **Personnel:** 2145

☐ **LAKESHORE MENTAL HEALTH INSTITUTE (444000)**, 5908 Lyons View Drive, Zip 37919–7598; tel. 865/450–5200, (Nonreporting) **A**1 10
Primary Contact: Richard Lee Thomas, Superintendent
CFO: Diane Matthews, Fiscal Services Director
CMO: Bert Simpson, M.D., Assistant Superintendent Clinical Services
CIO: Thomas Dobbins, Director Management Information Systems
CHR: Laura Morton, Personnel Director
Control: State–Government, nonfederal **Service:** Psychiatric

Staffed Beds: 185

☒ **PARKWEST MEDICAL CENTER (440173)**, 9352 Park West Boulevard, Zip 37923–4325, Mailing Address: P.O. Box 22993, Zip 37933–0993; tel. 865/373–1000 **A**1 2 9 10 **F**3 12 13 15 17 18 20 22 24 25 26 27 30 31 32 38 49 51 54 59 62 66 68 72 73 74 75 76 79 80 82 86 88 93 96 99 100 103 107 118 119 120 124 135 136 **S** Covenant Health
Primary Contact: Rick Lassiter, President and Chief Administrative Officer
COO: Emlyn Cobble, Vice President and Chief Support Officer
CFO: Scott Hamilton, Vice President and Chief Financial Officer
CHR: Randall Carr, Director Human Resources
Web address: www.yesparkwest.com
Control: Other not–for–profit (including NFP Corporation) **Service:** General Medical and Surgical

Staffed Beds: 274 **Admissions:** 14558 **Census:** 185 **Outpatient Visits:** 152091 **Births:** 1403 **Total Expense ($000):** 177018 **Payroll Expense ($000):** 64058 **Personnel:** 1925

☐ **SELECT SPECIALTY HOSPITAL–KNOXVILLE (442012)**, 1901 Clinch Avenue, Suite 404, Zip 37916; tel. 865/541–2615 **A**1 10 **F**1 3 25 30 31 43 54 80 82 119 132 137 **S** Select Medical Corporation
Primary Contact: Vanda Scott, Chief Executive Officer
COO: Steve Plumlee, Chief Operating Officer
CFO: Mike Gillis, Controller
CMO: Walt Zibas, M.D., Medical Director
CHR: Shara Johnson, Coordinator Human Resources
Web address: www.selectmedicalcorp.com
Control: Corporation, Investor–owned, for–profit **Service:** Long–Term Acute Care hospital

Staffed Beds: 35 **Admissions:** 324 **Census:** 23 **Outpatient Visits:** 0 **Births:** 0 **Total Expense ($000):** 9301 **Payroll Expense ($000):** 2899 **Personnel:** 77

☐ **SELECT SPECIALTY HOSPITAL–NORTH KNOXVILLE (442015)**, 900 East Oak Hill Avenue, Zip 37917; tel. 865/541–2615 **A**1 10 **F**1 3 25 30 31 43 54 80 82 119 132 137 **S** Select Medical Corporation
Primary Contact: Vanda Scott, Chief Executive Officer
Web address: www.selectmedicalcorp.com
Control: Corporation, Investor–owned, for–profit **Service:** Long–Term Acute Care hospital

Staffed Beds: 33 **Admissions:** 310 **Census:** 21 **Outpatient Visits:** 0 **Births:** 0 **Total Expense ($000):** 8929 **Payroll Expense ($000):** 2910 **Personnel:** 69

★ △ **ST. MARY'S MEDICAL CENTER (440120)**, 900 East Oak Hill Avenue, Zip 37917–4556; tel. 865/545–8000, (Includes ST MARY'S MEDICAL CENTER NORTH, 7565 Dannaher Way, Powell, Zip 37849–4029; tel. 865/859–7000; Jeremy Biggs, Administrator), (Total facility includes 25 beds in nursing home–type unit) **A**1 2 7 9 10 **F**3 11 13 15 17 18 20 22 24 25 26 27 30 31 32 33 36 38 39 41 42 43 44 45 49 50 51 53 55 57 61 62 66 68 69 70 72 73 74 76 77 79 80 82 85 86 88 90 91 92 93 94 95 96 97 99 100 102 103 104 105 106 107 108 109 111 112 117 118 119 132 135 136 137 **S** Catholic Healthcare Partners
Primary Contact: Debra K. London, President and Chief Executive Officer
COO: Jeffrey A. Ashin, Chief Executive Officer
CFO: David Nowiski, Chief Financial Officer
CMO: Greg Phelps, M.D., Medical Director
CIO: Scott Burke, Chief Information Officer
CHR: Marty Margetts, Senior Vice President Human Resource Development
Web address: www.mercy.com
Control: Church–operated, Nongovernment, not–for profit **Service:** General Medical and Surgical

Staffed Beds: 407 **Admissions:** 19248 **Census:** 286 **Outpatient Visits:** 295801 **Births:** 2024 **Total Expense ($000):** 241072 **Payroll Expense ($000):** 83413 **Personnel:** 2231

☐ **UNIVERSITY OF TENNESSEE MEDICAL CENTER (440015)**, 1924 Alcoa Highway, Box 81, Zip 37920–6900; tel. 865/544–9000 **A**1 2 3 5 8 9 10 **F**3 7 8 11 12 13 14 15 17 18 19 20 21 22 23 24 25 26 27 32 33 38 40 42 43 46 47 48 49 50 51 52 55 56 57 58 59 60 61 62 66 68 69 70 72 73 74 75 76 77 79 80 82 83 84 86 87 96 97 98 99 100 101 102 103 104 105 106 107 108 109 110 111 112 118 119 120 121 127 130 131 133 135 136 **P**6
Primary Contact: Joseph Landsman, President and Chief Executive Officer
COO: David Hall, Senior Vice President and Chief Operating Officer
CFO: Thomas Fisher, Senior Vice President and Chief Financial Officer
CMO: John W. Lacey, M.D., Senior Vice President and Chief Medical Officer
CIO: Douglas Fain, Director Computer Services
CHR: Betty Gissel, Vice President Human Resources
Web address: www.utmedicalcenter.org
Control: Other not–for–profit (including NFP Corporation) **Service:** General Medical and Surgical

Staffed Beds: 485 **Admissions:** 23116 **Census:** 375 **Outpatient Visits:** 159528 **Births:** 2319 **Total Expense ($000):** 405580 **Payroll Expense ($000):** 151077 **Personnel:** 2863

LA FOLLETTE—Campbell County

★ **ST. MARY'S MEDICAL CENTER OF CAMPBELL COUNTY (440033)**, 923 East Central Avenue, Zip 37766–3106, Mailing Address: P.O. Box 1301, Zip 37766–1301; tel. 423/907–1200, (Total facility includes 98 beds in nursing home–type unit) **A**1 9 10 20 **F**3 15 24 25 26 31 32 33 38 44 55 56 57 62 68 73 75 79 80 82 86 87 88 92 93 96 100 107 117 118 119 121 122 135 136 137 **S** Catholic Healthcare Partners
Primary Contact: H. Alan Watson, FACHE, Chief Executive Officer
COO: Sara Heatherly–Lloyd, Chief Operating Officer
CFO: Glenn McGuire, Chief Financial Officer
CMO: Errol Britto, M.D., Chief of Staff
CIO: Doug Kibler, Management Information Systems Specialist
CHR: Bess Stout, Director Human Resources
Web address: www.stmaryshealth.com
Control: Other not–for–profit (including NFP Corporation) **Service:** General Medical and Surgical

Staffed Beds: 164 **Admissions:** 3273 **Census:** 130 **Outpatient Visits:** 109501 **Births:** 0 **Total Expense ($000):** 30296 **Payroll Expense ($000):** 13819 **Personnel:** 388

LAFAYETTE—Macon County

★ **MACON COUNTY GENERAL HOSPITAL (441305)**, 204 Medical Drive, Zip 37083–1799, Mailing Address: P.O. Box 378, Zip 37083–0378; tel. 615/666–2147 **A**1 9 10 18 **F**3 15 25 26 30 31 32 33 38 55 57 63 79 86 96 107 117 119 122 135 **S** QHR
Primary Contact: Dennis A. Wolford, FACHE, Chief Executive Officer
CFO: Thomas J. Kidd, Assistant Administrator and Chief Financial Officer
Web address: www.mcgh.net
Control: Other not–for–profit (including NFP Corporation) **Service:** General Medical and Surgical

Staffed Beds: 25 **Admissions:** 756 **Census:** 7 **Outpatient Visits:** 17779 **Births:** 1 **Total Expense ($000):** 8997 **Payroll Expense ($000):** 3854 **Personnel:** 138

LAWRENCEBURG—Lawrence County

★ **CROCKETT HOSPITAL (440175)**, U.S. Highway 43 South, Zip 38464–0847, Mailing Address: P.O. Box 847, Zip 38464–0847; tel. 931/762–6571, (Nonreporting) **A**1 9 10 **S** LifePoint Hospitals, Inc.
Primary Contact: Jack S. Buck, Chief Executive Officer
CFO: John W. Copeland, Chief Financial Officer
CHR: Robert Augustin, Director Human Resources
Web address: www.crocketthospital.com
Control: Corporation, Investor–owned, for–profit **Service:** General Medical and Surgical

Staffed Beds: 98

TN

LEBANON—Wilson County

☐ **UNIVERSITY MEDICAL CENTER (440193)**, 1411 Baddour Parkway, Zip 37087–2595; tel. 615/444–8262, (Includes MCFARLAND SPECIALTY HOSPITAL, 500 Park Avenue, Zip 37087–3720; tel. 615/449–0500) **A**1 5 9 10 **F**3 13 15 18 24 25 27 31 32 38 40 43 47 48 49 51 54 55 57 62 66 68 72 73 74 75 76 77 79 80 82 84 85 86 88 90 91 92 93 95 96 97 99 100 102 103 107 118 119 120 121 124 133 134 135 136 137 **P**5 **S** Health Management Associates
Primary Contact: Vincent T. Cherry, Jr., Chief Executive Director
COO: Michael G. Morrical, Chief Operating Officer
CFO: Rhonda Maynard, Chief Financial Officer
CMO: Andrew Jordan, M.D., Chief of Staff
CIO: Adrian Fung, Director Information Systems
Web address: www.universitymedicalcenter.com
Control: Corporation, Investor–owned, for–profit **Service:** General Medical and Surgical

Staffed Beds: 245 **Admissions:** 7787 **Census:** 108 **Outpatient Visits:** 71052 **Births:** 760 **Total Expense ($000):** 75936 **Payroll Expense ($000):** 32047 **Personnel:** 675

LENOIR CITY—Loudon County

★ **FORT LOUDOUN MEDICAL CENTER (440110)**, 550 Fort Loudoun Medical Center Drive, Zip 37772–5673; tel. 865/271–6000 **A**1 9 10 **F**3 11 15 24 25 26 31 32 33 38 46 55 56 57 63 66 68 75 77 79 80 86 96 97 99 100 106 107 114 118 121 124 135 137 **S** Covenant Health
Primary Contact: Jeffrey Feike, President and Chief Administrative Officer
Web address: www.covenanthealth.com
Control: Other not–for–profit (including NFP Corporation) **Service:** General Medical and Surgical

Staffed Beds: 32 **Admissions:** 1622 **Census:** 17 **Outpatient Visits:** 70566 **Births:** 0 **Total Expense ($000):** 19043 **Payroll Expense ($000):** 8583 **Personnel:** 264

Hospital, Medicare Provider Number, Address, Telephone, Approval, Facility, and Physician Codes, Health Care System

★ American Hospital Association (AHA) membership
☐ The Joint Commission accreditation
○ American Osteopathic Association (AOA) accreditation
△ Commission on Accreditation of Rehabilitation Facilities (CARF) accreditation

LEWISBURG—Marshall County

☐ **MARSHALL MEDICAL CENTER (441309)**, 1080 North Ellington Parkway, Zip 37091–2227, Mailing Address: P.O. Box 1609, Zip 37091–1609; tel. 931/359–6241 **A**1 9 10 18 **F**3 11 15 25 26 30 31 32 38 50 55 56 57 66 73 75 79 82 86 96 97 100 102 107 118 120 122 135
Primary Contact: Phyllis Brown, Chief Executive Officer
CFO: Kyle Jones, Controller
CMO: Tim Nash, M.D., Chief of Staff
CHR: Mary Wiles, Human Resource Benefits Specialist
Web address: www.mauryregional.com
Control: County–Government, nonfederal **Service:** General Medical and Surgical

Staffed Beds: 12 **Admissions:** 579 **Census:** 5 **Outpatient Visits:** 39323 **Births:** 1 **Total Expense ($000):** 10880 **Payroll Expense ($000):** 6006 **Personnel:** 144

LEXINGTON—Henderson County

★ **HENDERSON COUNTY COMMUNITY HOSPITAL (440008)**, 200 West Church Street, Zip 38351–2014; tel. 731/968–3646, (Nonreporting) **A**1 9 10 **S** Community Health Systems, Inc.
Primary Contact: Holly Clark, Chief Executive Officer
CFO: Roseann M. Devault, Chief Financial Officer
CHR: Patsy Waddle, Director Human Resources
Web address: www.hendersoncchospital.com
Control: Corporation, Investor–owned, for–profit **Service:** General Medical and Surgical

Staffed Beds: 45

LINDEN—Perry County

PERRY COMMUNITY HOSPITAL (440040), 2718 Squirrel Hollow Drive, Zip 37096–9100; tel. 931/589–2121, (Nonreporting) **A**9 10
Primary Contact: John B. Avery, III, Administrator
Control: Other not–for–profit (including NFP Corporation) **Service:** General Medical and Surgical

Staffed Beds: 53

LIVINGSTON—Overton County

★ **LIVINGSTON REGIONAL HOSPITAL (440187)**, 315 Oak Street, Zip 38570, Mailing Address: P.O. Box 550, Zip 38570–0550; tel. 931/823–5611 **A**1 9 10 **F**3 13 15 17 25 26 27 33 37 38 46 54 55 56 57 68 73 74 75 76 77 79 82 84 85 86 88 93 96 100 102 107 118 119 120 122 134 135 136 137 **S** LifePoint Hospitals, Inc.
Primary Contact: Timothy W. McGill, Chief Executive Officer
COO: Michelle Watson, Chief Nursing Officer and Chief Operating Officer
CFO: Joseph Ross, Chief Financial Officer
CMO: Mark Langenberg, M.D., Chief Medical Officer
CIO: Joseph Ross, Chief Financial Officer
CHR: Paula Rainer, Director Human Resources
Web address: www.livingston–hospital.com
Control: Corporation, Investor–owned, for–profit **Service:** General Medical and Surgical

Staffed Beds: 72 **Admissions:** 3363 **Census:** 45 **Outpatient Visits:** 36820 **Births:** 337 **Total Expense ($000):** 19696 **Payroll Expense ($000):** 10304 **Personnel:** 270

LOUISVILLE—Blount County

☐ **PENINSULA HOSPITAL**, 2347 Jones Bend Road, Zip 37777–5213, Mailing Address: P.O. Box 2000, Zip 37777–2000; tel. 865/970–9800 **A**1 **F**4 5 25 26 30 31 32 33 36 62 66 69 82 88 89 91 92 93 94 95 119 121 132 **P**6
Primary Contact: Glenda Sublett, Vice President and Administrator
CFO: Sonja Jones, Chief Financial Officer
CMO: Kris Houser, M.D., Medical Director
CIO: Roger Ricker, Director Marketing and Public Relations
CHR: Angie Montgomery, Director Human Resources
Web address: www.peninsula–hospital.org
Control: Other not–for–profit (including NFP Corporation) **Service:** Psychiatric

Staffed Beds: 239 **Admissions:** 5372 **Census:** 168 **Outpatient Visits:** 124768 **Births:** 0 **Total Expense ($000):** 37671 **Payroll Expense ($000):** 21170 **Personnel:** 633

MADISON—Davidson County

★ **SKYLINE MADISON CAMPUS (440135)**, 500 Hospital Drive, Zip 37115–5032; tel. 615/865–2373, (Nonreporting) **A**1 9 10 **S** HCA
Primary Contact: Michael W. Garfield, Chief Executive Officer
COO: Kay DeLage, Chief Operating Officer
CFO: Bradley Schultz, Chief Financial Officer
CMO: Matthew Speyer, M.D., Chief Medical Officer
CHR: Andy Hooper, Director Human Resources
Web address: www.skylinemadison.com
Control: Corporation, Investor–owned, for–profit **Service:** General Medical and Surgical

Staffed Beds: 284

MANCHESTER—Coffee County

★ ○ **MEDICAL CENTER OF MANCHESTER (441308)**, 481 Interstate Drive, Zip 37355–3108, Mailing Address: P.O. Box 1409, Zip 37349–1409; tel. 931/728–6354, (Nonreporting) **A**9 10 11 18
Primary Contact: Robert J. Couch, Chief Executive Officer
CFO: James Barnes, Chief Financial Officer
CMO: Bill B. Hollins, D.O., Chief of Staff
Control: Corporation, Investor–owned, for–profit **Service:** General Medical and Surgical

Staffed Beds: 25

UNITED REGIONAL MEDICAL CENTER (440007), 1001 McArthur Drive, Zip 37355–2455, Mailing Address: P.O. Box 1079, Zip 37349–1079; tel. 931/728–3586, (Total facility includes 72 beds in nursing home–type unit) **A**9 10 **F**3 15 25 31 32 37 38 43 55 56 57 63 73 75 79 80 82 84 87 90 96 97 100 102 105 107 117 118 119 122
Primary Contact: Robert George, Chief Executive Officer and Chief Financial Officer
COO: Martha Logan, Chief Operating Officer
CFO: Robert George, Chief Executive Officer and Chief Financial Officer
CMO: Glenn A. Davis, M.D., Chief of Staff
CIO: Matt Burks, Director Information Technology
CHR: Doris Bramblett, Director Human Resources
Web address: www.urmchealthcare.com
Control: Corporation, Investor–owned, for–profit **Service:** General Medical and Surgical

Staffed Beds: 108 **Admissions:** 1533 **Census:** 75 **Outpatient Visits:** 22159 **Births:** 0 **Total Expense ($000):** 14313 **Payroll Expense ($000):** 6242 **Personnel:** 178

MARTIN—Weakley County

★ **HEALTHSOUTH CANE CREEK REHABILITATION HOSPITAL (443030)**, 180 Mt Pelia Road, Zip 38237–3812; tel. 731/587–4231, (Nonreporting) **A**1 10 **S** HEALTHSOUTH Corporation
Primary Contact: William P. Macri, Chief Executive Officer
CFO: Cindy Hazlewood, Controller
CMO: William Eason, M.D., Medical Director
CIO: Jan Gill, Health Information Management Systems Director
CHR: Sharon Shihady, Director Human Resources
Web address: www.healthsouth.com
Control: Corporation, Investor–owned, for–profit **Service:** Rehabilitation

Staffed Beds: 40

★ **VOLUNTEER COMMUNITY HOSPITAL (440061)**, 161 Mount Pelia Road, Zip 38237–0967; tel. 731/587–4261 **A**9 10 **F**3 13 15 25 30 33 38 49 50 51 52 56 57 62 63 68 71 72 73 74 75 77 79 80 86 96 100 102 107 121 122 135 136 137 **S** Community Health Systems, Inc.
Primary Contact: Steve Westenhofer, Chief Executive Officer
CFO: John Conti, Chief Financial Officer
CMO: Susan Lowry, Chief of Staff
CHR: Tammie Bell, Director Human Resources
Web address: www.volunteercommunityhospital.com
Control: Corporation, Investor–owned, for–profit **Service:** General Medical and Surgical

Staffed Beds: 65 **Admissions:** 2609 **Census:** 25 **Outpatient Visits:** 23051 **Births:** 352 **Total Expense ($000):** 23464 **Payroll Expense ($000):** 8620 **Personnel:** 206

MARYVILLE—Blount County

★ **BLOUNT MEMORIAL HOSPITAL (440011)**, 907 East Lamar Alexander Parkway, Zip 37804–5016; tel. 865/983–7211, (Total facility includes 76 beds in nursing home–type unit) **A**1 2 9 10 **F**3 4 5 10 11 12 13 15 17 18 20 24 25 26 27 28 32 33 36 38 40 42 43 44 46 49 52 53 54 55 57 61 62 64 65 66 67 68 73 74 75 76 77 78 79 80 81 82 86 87 88 89 90 91 92 93 94 95 96 97 99 100 102 104 105 106 107 109 110 111 115 117 119 120 121 123 124 135 136 137 **P**1 6 7
Primary Contact: Joseph M. Dawson, Administrator
COO: Don Heinemann, Associate Administrator and Chief Operating Officer
CFO: David E. Arriett, Assistant Administrator
CMO: Samuel D. Evans, M.D., Medical Director
CIO: Jason Mashburn, Director Information Systems
CHR: Chris Wilkes, Director Human Resources
Web address: www.blountmemorial.org
Control: County–Government, nonfederal **Service:** General Medical and Surgical

Staffed Beds: 295 **Admissions:** 12763 **Census:** 213 **Outpatient Visits:** 171893 **Births:** 911 **Total Expense ($000):** 153319 **Payroll Expense ($000):** 70605 **Personnel:** 2120

TN

Many Facility Codes have changed. Please refer to the AHA Guide Code Chart.

MCKENZIE—Carroll County

★ **MCKENZIE REGIONAL HOSPITAL (440182)**, 161 Hospital Drive, Zip 38201–1636; tel. 731/352–5344 **A**1 9 10 **F**3 13 15 25 30 31 38 52 55 74 79 80 84 86 96 107 122 135 **S** Community Health Systems, Inc.
Primary Contact: David D. Rasmussen, Chief Executive Officer
CFO: Kevin Harvey, Chief Financial Officer
CHR: Joyce Hamilton, Director Human Resources
Web address: www.mckenzieregionalhospital.com
Control: Corporation, Investor–owned, for–profit **Service:** General Medical and Surgical

Staffed Beds: 31 **Admissions:** 1829 **Census:** 14 **Outpatient Visits:** 24848 **Births:** 503 **Total Expense ($000):** 13606 **Payroll Expense ($000):** 5923 **Personnel:** 137

MCMINNVILLE—Warren County

□ **RIVER PARK HOSPITAL (440151)**, 1559 Sparta Road, Zip 37110–1399; tel. 931/815–4000, (Nonreporting) **A**1 9 10 **S** Capella Healthcare
Primary Contact: John R. McLain, Chief Executive Officer
CFO: Christina Patterson, Chief Financial Officer
CMO: Randal D. Rampp, M.D., Chief Medical Officer
CIO: Jeff Johnson, Director Information Systems
CHR: Clair Cochran, Director Human Resources
Web address: www.riverparkhospital.com
Control: Corporation, Investor–owned, for–profit **Service:** General Medical and Surgical

Staffed Beds: 125

MEMPHIS—Shelby County

★□ **BAPTIST MEMORIAL HOSPITAL – MEMPHIS (440048)**, 6019 Walnut Grove Road, Zip 38120–2173; tel. 901/226–5000, (Total facility includes 30 beds in nursing home–type unit) (Nonreporting) **A**1 2 3 5 9 10 **S** Baptist Memorial Health Care Corporation
Primary Contact: Jason Little, Administrator and Chief Executive Officer
CFO: Cyndi Pittman, Chief Financial Officer
CMO: Richard Drewry, M.D., Vice President and Chief Medical Officer
CIO: Jerry Brantley, Vice President and Chief Information Officer
CHR: Jerry Barbaree, Director Human Resources
Web address: www.baptistonline.org
Control: Other not–for–profit (including NFP Corporation) **Service:** General Medical and Surgical

Staffed Beds: 633

★□ **BAPTIST MEMORIAL HOSPITAL FOR WOMEN (440222)**, 6225 Humphreys Boulevard, Zip 38120–2373; tel. 901/227–9000 **A**1 9 10 **F**3 12 13 15 25 26 30 31 32 33 38 43 46 55 56 57 62 66 68 69 70 71 79 81 82 96 97 99 107 112 119 121 124 135 136 **S** Baptist Memorial Health Care Corporation
Primary Contact: Anita Vaughn, Administrator and Chief Executive Officer
CFO: Margaret Williams, Chief Financial Officer
CMO: Tom Greenwell, M.D., President Medical Staff
CHR: Kristie Brown, Director Human Resources
Web address: www.bmhcc.org
Control: Other not–for–profit (including NFP Corporation) **Service:** Obstetrics and gynecology

Staffed Beds: 140 **Admissions:** 7604 **Census:** 82 **Outpatient Visits:** 42961 **Births:** 4830 **Total Expense ($000):** 61495 **Payroll Expense ($000):** 28084 **Personnel:** 490

★□ **BAPTIST MEMORIAL RESTORATIVE CARE HOSPITAL (442010)**, 6019 Walnut Grove Road, Zip 38120; tel. 901/226–1400, (Nonreporting) **A**1 9 10 **S** Baptist Memorial Health Care Corporation
Primary Contact: Janice Hill, Administrator
CFO: Chetan Parekh, Chief Financial Officer
Web address: www.baptistonline.org/facilities/restorativecare
Control: Other not–for–profit (including NFP Corporation) **Service:** Long–Term Acute Care hospital

Staffed Beds: 30

BAPTIST REHABILITATION–GERMANTOWN See Germantown

□ **DELTA MEDICAL CENTER (440159)**, 3000 Getwell Road, Zip 38118–2299; tel. 901/369–8500 **A**1 9 10 **F**3 15 22 25 26 27 30 31 32 33 38 50 54 59 68 79 80 86 88 93 95 96 100 102 107 118 119 132 137
Primary Contact: J. Gene Faile, Chief Executive Officer
COO: Mary Hammons, Chief Operating Officer
CMO: Michael Agapos, M.D., Chief of Staff
CHR: Karyn Erickson, Director Human Resources
Web address: www.deltamedcenter.com
Control: Corporation, Investor–owned, for–profit **Service:** General Medical and Surgical

Staffed Beds: 170 **Admissions:** 4419 **Census:** 95 **Outpatient Visits:** 29617 **Births:** 0 **Total Expense ($000):** 38872 **Payroll Expense ($000):** 18037 **Personnel:** 465

★□ **HEALTHSOUTH REHABILITATION HOSPITAL (443029)**, 1282 Union Avenue, Zip 38104–3414; tel. 901/722–2000 **A**1 10 **F**3 24 25 26 32 57 59 85 86 121 132 **S** HEALTHSOUTH Corporation
Primary Contact: Traci Willis, Chief Executive Officer
CFO: Phylis Buck, Chief Financial Officer
CMO: Dale Cunningham, M.D., Medical Director
CHR: Sandra Milburn, Director Human Resources
Web address: www.healthsouth.com
Control: Partnership, Investor–owned, for–profit **Service:** Rehabilitation

Staffed Beds: 80 **Admissions:** 1548 **Census:** 56 **Outpatient Visits:** 8891 **Births:** 0 **Total Expense ($000):** 15810 **Payroll Expense ($000):** 8244 **Personnel:** 210

★□ **HEALTHSOUTH REHABILITATION HOSPITAL (443031)**, 4100 Austin Peay Highway, Zip 38128–2503; tel. 901/213–5400 **A**1 10 **F**30 31 32 85 86 **S** HEALTHSOUTH Corporation
Primary Contact: John R. Borden, Chief Executive Officer
Web address: www.healthsouth.com
Control: Corporation, Investor–owned, for–profit **Service:** Rehabilitation

Staffed Beds: 40 **Admissions:** 934 **Census:** 33 **Outpatient Visits:** 4347 **Births:** 0 **Total Expense ($000):** 7997 **Payroll Expense ($000):** 5658 **Personnel:** 96

□ **LAKESIDE BEHAVIORAL HEALTH SYSTEM (444004)**, 2911 Brunswick Road, Zip 38133–4199; tel. 901/377–4700, (Nonreporting) **A**1 10 **S** Universal Health Services, Inc.
Primary Contact: Shelley A. Nowak, Chief Executive Officer
CFO: Felicia Swauncy, Chief Financial Officer
CMO: C. Hal Brunt, Medical Director
CIO: Kevin Pendleton, Chief Information Technology
CHR: James Miller, Human Resource Director
Web address: www.lakesidebhs.com
Control: Corporation, Investor–owned, for–profit **Service:** Psychiatric

Staffed Beds: 295

LE BONHEUR CHILDREN'S MEDICAL CENTER See Methodist University Hospital

□ **MEMPHIS MENTAL HEALTH INSTITUTE (444001)**, 865 Poplar Avenue, Zip 38105–4626, Mailing Address: P.O. Box 40966, Zip 38174–0966; tel. 901/524–1201 **A**1 3 5 10 **F**50 81 82 88 91 93 119 135 **P**6
Primary Contact: Lawrence Ventura, Chief Executive Officer
COO: Clyde Slate, Assistant Superintendent Administrative Services
CFO: Linda White, Director Fiscal Services
CMO: Kayla Fisher, M.D., Medical Director
CHR: Randy Durham, Director Personnel
Control: State–Government, nonfederal **Service:** Psychiatric

Staffed Beds: 98 **Admissions:** 1816 **Census:** 63 **Outpatient Visits:** 0 **Births:** 0 **Total Expense ($000):** 22147 **Payroll Expense ($000):** 13853 **Personnel:** 323

□ **METHODIST EXTENDED CARE HOSPITAL (442013)**, 225 South Claybrook Street, Zip 38104–3537; tel. 901/516–2152, (Nonreporting) **A**1 10 **S** Methodist Le Bonheur Healthcare
Primary Contact: Sandra Bailey, Administrator
COO: Sandra Hugueley, Chief Nursing Officer and Assistant Administrator
CFO: Kris Sanders, Chief Financial Officer
CMO: Hany Mounir Habashy, M.D., Chief Medical Director
CHR: Marty Keith, Director Human Resources
Web address: www.methodisthealth.org
Control: Other not–for–profit (including NFP Corporation) **Service:** General Medical and Surgical

Staffed Beds: 36

TN

Hospital, Medicare Provider Number, Address, Telephone, Approval, Facility, and Physician Codes, Health Care System

★ American Hospital Association (AHA) membership
□ The Joint Commission accreditation
○ American Osteopathic Association (AOA) accreditation
△ Commission on Accreditation of Rehabilitation Facilities (CARF) accreditation

METHODIST UNIVERSITY HOSPITAL (440049), 1265 Union Avenue, Zip 38104; tel. 901/516–7000, (Includes LE BONHEUR CHILDREN'S MEDICAL CENTER, 50 North Dunlap Street, Zip 38103; tel. 901/287–5437; Meri Armour, Chief Executive Officer; METHODIST HEALTHCARE–NORTH HOSPITAL, 3960 New Covington Pike, Zip 38128; tel. 901/384–5389; William A. Kenley, Chief Executive Officer and Administrator; METHODIST HEALTHCARE–SOUTH HOSPITAL, 1300 Wesley Drive, Zip 38116; tel. 901/516–3081; Michael O. Ugwueke, Administrator; METHODIST LE BONHEUR GERMANTOWN HOSPITAL, 7691 Poplar Avenue, Germantown, Zip 38138; tel. 901/516–6000; David G. Baytos, Chief Executive Officer and Administrator), (Total facility includes 44 beds in nursing home–type unit) (Nonreporting) **A**2 3 5 6 8 9 10 **S** Methodist Le Bonheur Healthcare
Primary Contact: Kevin M. Spiegel, FACHE, Chief Executive Officer
COO: Peggy N. Troy, Chief Operating Officer
CFO: Chris J. McLean, Chief Financial Officer
CMO: Robin Womeodu, M.D., Chief Medical Officer
CIO: Andy Fowler, Senior Vice President Information Systems
CHR: Carol Ross–Spang, Senior Vice President
Web address: www.methodisthealth.org
Control: Other not–for–profit (including NFP Corporation) **Service:** General Medical and Surgical

Staffed Beds: 1359

★ **REGIONAL MEDICAL CENTER AT MEMPHIS (440152)**, 877 Jefferson Avenue, Zip 38103–2897; tel. 901/545–7100, (Nonreporting) **A**1 3 5 8 9 10
Primary Contact: Sylvester L. Reeder, III, Chief Executive Officer
COO: Christine A. Pappas, R.N., Chief Operating Officer
CFO: Peggy Allen, Chief Financial Officer
CMO: Stuart Polly, M.D., Medical Director
CIO: Jim Leonard, Chief Information Officer
CHR: Gloria Thomas, Vice President Human Resources
Web address: www.the–med.org
Control: Other not–for–profit (including NFP Corporation) **Service:** General Medical and Surgical

Staffed Beds: 370

TN

★ **SAINT FRANCIS HOSPITAL (440183)**, 5959 Park Avenue, Zip 38119–5198, Mailing Address: P.O. Box 171808, Zip 38187–1808; tel. 901/765–1000, (Nonreporting) **A**1 2 3 5 9 10 **S** TENET Healthcare Corporation
Primary Contact: David L. Archer, Chief Executive Officer
COO: Donald E. Laughlin, Chief Operating Officer
CFO: Edwin J. Bode, Chief Financial Officer
CMO: Michael Lachina, M.D., Chief Medical Officer
CIO: Mike Hadley, Chief Information Officer
CHR: Laura Adler, Senior Vice President Human Relations
Web address: www.saintfrancishosp.com
Control: Corporation, Investor–owned, for–profit **Service:** General Medical and Surgical

Staffed Beds: 533

□ **SELECT SPECIALTY HOSPITAL–MEMPHIS (442014)**, 5959 Park Avenue, 12th Floor, Zip 38119–5200; tel. 901/684–4110, (Nonreporting) **A**1 10 **S** Select Medical Corporation
Primary Contact: David Key, Chief Executive Officer
Web address: www.selectmedicalcorp.com
Control: Corporation, Investor–owned, for–profit **Service:** Long–Term Acute Care hospital

Staffed Beds: 30

★ **ST. JUDE CHILDREN'S RESEARCH HOSPITAL (443302)**, 332 North Lauderdale Street, Zip 38105–2794; tel. 901/495–3300, (Nonreporting) **A**1 3 5 9 10
Primary Contact: William E. Evans, Pharm.D, Director
COO: Mark Barnes, Chief Administrative Officer
CFO: Mike Canarios, Vice President and Chief Financial Officer
CMO: Joseph J. Mirro, M.D., Executive Vice President and Chief Medical Officer
CIO: Sharon Christian, Vice President and Chief Information Officer
CHR: Mary Anna Quinn, Vice President
Web address: www.stjude.org
Control: Other not–for–profit (including NFP Corporation) **Service:** Children's other specialty

Staffed Beds: 56

★ △ **VETERANS AFFAIRS MEDICAL CENTER**, 1030 Jefferson Avenue, Zip 38104–2193; tel. 901/523–8990 **A**1 2 3 5 7 8 **F**3 4 5 8 9 17 18 20 22 24 25 26 27 30 31 32 33 37 38 43 44 50 51 52 53 54 55 57 58 59 60 61 62 63 68 72 73 75 76 77 78 79 82 85 86 87 88 90 91 92 93 94 95 96 97 100 102 106 107 109 118 119 121 124 135 136 137 **P**6 **S** Department of Veterans Affairs
Primary Contact: Patricia O. Pittman, Director
COO: William R. Delamater, Associate Director
CFO: Brian P. Fuchs, Chief Fiscal Service
CMO: Howard R. Bromley, M.D., Chief of Staff
CIO: Charles D. Sternberg, Chief Information Resources Management Service
CHR: Bonnie J. Eareckson, Chief, Human Resource Management Services
Web address: www.va.gov/sta/guide/home.asp
Control: Veterans Affairs, Government, federal **Service:** General Medical and Surgical

Staffed Beds: 280 **Admissions:** 6172 **Census:** 186 **Outpatient Visits:** 498098 **Births:** 0 **Total Expense ($000):** 289203 **Payroll Expense ($000):** 147193 **Personnel:** 1883

MILAN—Gibson County

★ **MILAN GENERAL HOSPITAL (440060)**, 4039 South Highland, Zip 38358–3167; tel. 731/686–1591 **A**1 9 10 **F**3 12 15 25 26 30 31 32 33 38 55 57 62 66 68 79 80 82 86 96 107 119 121 122 135 **S** West Tennessee Healthcare
Primary Contact: John M. Carruth, Administrator
CFO: Terry Swindell, Chief Financial Officer
Web address: www.wth.net
Control: Hospital district or authority, Government, nonfederal **Service:** General Medical and Surgical

Staffed Beds: 28 **Admissions:** 537 **Census:** 9 **Outpatient Visits:** 15522 **Births:** 1 **Total Expense ($000):** 6892 **Payroll Expense ($000):** 3436 **Personnel:** 93

MORRISTOWN—Hamblen County

★ △ **LAKEWAY REGIONAL HOSPITAL (440067)**, 726 McFarland Street, Zip 37814–3990; tel. 423/586–2302 **A**1 7 9 10 19 **F**8 13 15 25 26 30 32 33 35 37 38 49 55 56 57 59 68 72 74 75 77 78 79 80 85 86 96 97 100 102 106 107 112 117 118 119 122 135 136 **S** Community Health Systems, Inc.
Primary Contact: Priscilla Millis, Chief Executive Officer
CFO: Frank Shiffer, Chief Financial Officer
CMO: Paul Cardali, Chief of Staff
CHR: Deirdre Helton, Director Human Resources
Web address: www.lakewayregionalhospital.com
Control: Corporation, Investor–owned, for–profit **Service:** General Medical and Surgical

Staffed Beds: 100 **Admissions:** 3855 **Census:** 40 **Outpatient Visits:** 34214 **Births:** 489 **Total Expense ($000):** 34993 **Payroll Expense ($000):** 12249 **Personnel:** 308

□ **MORRISTOWN–HAMBLEN HOSPITAL (440030)**, 908 West Fourth North Street, Zip 37814–3894, Mailing Address: P.O. Box 1178, Zip 37816–1178; tel. 423/586–4231, (Nonreporting) **A**1 9 10
Primary Contact: Richard L. Clark, President and Chief Executive Officer
CFO: Mark Thompson, Chief Financial Officer
CIO: James Meister, Director Information Systems
CHR: Derek Winkle, Director Human Resources
Web address: www.mhhs1.org
Control: Other not–for–profit (including NFP Corporation) **Service:** General Medical and Surgical

Staffed Beds: 143

MOUNTAIN CITY—Johnson County

★ **JOHNSON COUNTY COMMUNITY HOSPITAL (441304)**, 1901 South Shady Street, Zip 37683–2271; tel. 423/727–1100 **A**9 10 18 **F**3 15 24 26 30 31 32 33 38 41 50 66 81 86 87 96 **S** Mountain States Health Alliance
Primary Contact: Lisa Heaton, Administrator and Chief Nursing Officer
Web address: www.msha.com
Control: Other not–for–profit (including NFP Corporation) **Service:** General Medical and Surgical

Staffed Beds: 2 **Admissions:** 36 **Census:** 1 **Outpatient Visits:** 36010 **Births:** 0 **Total Expense ($000):** 6485 **Payroll Expense ($000):** 3295 **Personnel:** 65

 Many Facility Codes have changed. Please refer to the AHA Guide Code Chart.

MOUNTAIN HOME—Washington County

★ **JAMES H. QUILLEN VETERANS AFFAIRS MEDICAL CENTER**, Mailing Address: P.O. Box 4000, Zip 37684–4000; tel. 423/926–1171, (Total facility includes 120 beds in nursing home–type unit) (Nonreporting) **A**1 2 3 5 8 **S** Department of Veterans Affairs
Primary Contact: John W. McFadden, Interim Director
COO: Rachel Mitchell, Chief Financial Officer
CMO: David Reagan, M.D., Ph.D., Chief of Staff
CIO: Karen Perry, Chief Information Resource Management Services
CHR: Patsy Fish, Chief, Human Resources Management
Web address: www.va.gov
Control: Veterans Affairs, Government, federal **Service:** General Medical and Surgical

Staffed Beds: 603

MURFREESBORO—Rutherford County

ALVIN C. YORK VETERANS AFFAIRS MEDICAL CENTER See Veterans Affairs Tennessee Valley Healthcare System, Nashville

★ **MIDDLE TENNESSEE MEDICAL CENTER (440053)**, 400 North Highland Avenue, Zip 37130–3854, Mailing Address: P.O. Box 1178, Zip 37133–1178; tel. 615/396–4100, (Nonreporting) **A**1 2 3 5 9 10 **S** Ascension Health
Primary Contact: Gordon B. Ferguson, CHE, President and Chief Executive Officer
COO: Gordon B. Ferguson, CHE, President and Chief Executive Officer
CFO: Martha L. Rowland, Vice President Finance
CMO: Andy Brown, M.D., Vice President Medical Affairs
CIO: Chris Young, Vice President and Chief Information Officer
CHR: Carol Bragdon, Director Human Resources
Web address: www.mtmc.org
Control: Church–operated, Nongovernment, not–for profit **Service:** General Medical and Surgical

Staffed Beds: 199

NASHVILLE—Davidson County

★ **BAPTIST HOSPITAL (440133)**, 2000 Church Street, Zip 37236–0002; tel. 615/284–5555, (Nonreporting) **A**1 2 3 5 9 10 **S** Ascension Health
Primary Contact: Bernard Sherry, President and Chief Executive Officer
COO: Renee A. Kessler, Chief Operating Officer
CFO: Carrie Teaford, Vice President Finance
CMO: William Thompson, M.D., Chief Medical Officer
CIO: Jim Drew, Chief Information Officer
CHR: Martha Underwood, Chief Human Resources Officer
Web address: www.baptisthospital.com
Control: Other not–for–profit (including NFP Corporation) **Service:** General Medical and Surgical

Staffed Beds: 425

★ **CENTENNIAL MEDICAL CENTER AND PARTHENON PAVILION (440161)**, 2300 Patterson Street, Zip 37203–1528; tel. 615/342–1000 **A**1 2 3 5 9 10 **F**3 12 13 15 17 18 20 22 24 25 26 27 30 31 32 33 38 51 52 54 57 59 68 69 70 71 72 73 74 75 76 77 79 80 85 86 88 93 96 97 99 100 102 103 104 106 107 109 116 118 119 121 125 127 135 136 **S** HCA
Primary Contact: Thomas L. Herron, FACHE, Chief Executive Officer
COO: Micki J. Slingerland, Chief Operating Officer
CFO: David A. Summers, Chief Financial Officer
CMO: Robert Alford, M.D., Chief Medical Officer
CHR: Patricia Knight, Vice President Human Resources
Web address: www.centennialmedicalcenter.com
Control: Corporation, Investor–owned, for–profit **Service:** General Medical and Surgical

Staffed Beds: 572 **Admissions:** 24677 **Census:** 396 **Outpatient Visits:** 156954 **Births:** 3221 **Total Expense ($000):** 309194 **Payroll Expense ($000):** 118269 **Personnel:** 1981

☐ **KINDRED HOSPITAL – NASHVILLE (442006)**, 1412 County Hospital Road, Zip 37218; tel. 615/687–2600, (Nonreporting) **A**1 10 **S** Kindred Healthcare
Primary Contact: Michael L. Moody, Chief Executive Officer
COO: Connie Long, Chief Clinical Officer
CFO: Philip L. Jones, Chief Financial Officer
CMO: Wayne E. Moore, M.D., Chief Medical Officer
CHR: Darren Coffing, Area Director Human Resources
Web address: www.kindredhealthcare.com
Control: Corporation, Investor–owned, for–profit **Service:** Long–Term Acute Care hospital

Staffed Beds: 60

☐ **MIDDLE TENNESSEE MENTAL HEALTH INSTITUTE (444014)**, 221 Stewarts Ferry Pike, Zip 37214–3325; tel. 615/902–7535, (Nonreporting) **A**1 3 5 10
Primary Contact: Lynn McDonald, Chief Executive Officer
COO: Walter Wilson, Assistant Superintendent Program Services
CFO: Mark Stanley, Director Fiscal Services
CMO: Mohammad S. Jahan, M.D., Clinical Director
CHR: Margie Dunn, Director Human Resources
Control: State–Government, nonfederal **Service:** Psychiatric

Staffed Beds: 245

MONROE CARELL JR. CHILDREN'S HOSPITAL AT VANDERBILT See Vanderbilt University Medical Center

★ **NASHVILLE GENERAL HOSPITAL (440111)**, 1818 Albion Street, Zip 37208–2918; tel. 615/341–4000, (Nonreporting) **A**1 2 3 5 9 10
Primary Contact: Reginald W. Coopwood, M.D., Chief Executive Officer
CFO: Robert Stillwell, Chief Financial Officer
CIO: Dean Gambill, Chief Information Officer
CHR: Diana Wohlfardt, Director Human Resources
Web address: www.nashville.org/hosp/general_hospital
Control: City–County, Government, nonfederal **Service:** General Medical and Surgical

Staffed Beds: 127

☐ **NASHVILLE REHABILITATION HOSPITAL (440026)**, 1034 West Eastland Avenue, Zip 37206–3238; tel. 615/226–4330 **A**1 10 **F**82 85 88 93 **S** Psychiatric Solutions
Primary Contact: B. Touby Witzky, Chief Executive Officer
CFO: Mark Swatzell, Chief Financial Officer
CMO: Catherine Stallworth, M.D., Medical Director
CHR: Sharon Justice, Manager Human Resource and Payroll
Web address: www.nrhcares.com
Control: Corporation, Investor–owned, for–profit **Service:** Rehabilitation

Staffed Beds: 37 **Admissions:** 959 **Census:** 27 **Outpatient Visits:** 0 **Total Expense ($000):** 9197 **Payroll Expense ($000):** 5397 **Personnel:** 105

PSYCHIATRIC HOSPITAL AT VANDERBILT See Vanderbilt University Medical Center

★ **SAINT THOMAS HOSPITAL (440082)**, 4220 Harding Road, Zip 37205–2095, Mailing Address: P.O. Box 380, Zip 37202–0380; tel. 615/222–2111, (Nonreporting) **A**1 2 3 5 9 10 **S** Ascension Health
Primary Contact: Les A. Donahue, Chief Executive Officer
CFO: Mark J. McGinnis, Vice President Operations and Finance
CMO: Dale Batchelor, M.D., Chief Medical Officer
CIO: Chris Young, Vice President and Chief Information Officer
CHR: Angelle Rosata, Chief Human Resources Officer
Web address: www.stthomas.org
Control: Church–operated, Nongovernment, not–for profit **Service:** General Medical and Surgical

Staffed Beds: 420

☐ **SELECT SPECIALTY HOSPITAL OF NASHVILLE (442011)**, 2021 Church Street, Zip 37203–2016; tel. 615/284–4599, (Nonreporting) **A**1 9 10 **S** Select Medical Corporation
Primary Contact: Edward T. Stinson, Chief Executive Officer
Web address: www.selectmedicalcorp.com
Control: Corporation, Investor–owned, for–profit **Service:** Long–Term Acute Care hospital

Staffed Beds: 37

★ **SKYLINE MEDICAL CENTER (440006)**, 3441 Dickerson Pike, Zip 37207–2539; tel. 615/769–2000 **A**1 2 9 10 **F**3 4 5 11 15 18 20 24 25 26 27 36 38 43 49 51 52 54 55 57 66 68 72 75 76 77 79 80 82 85 86 88 89 90 92 93 94 95 96 97 100 102 103 106 107 109 111 118 119 121 124 135 137 **P**6 **S** HCA
Primary Contact: Michael W. Garfield, Chief Executive Officer
COO: Michael Ehrat, Chief Operating Officer
CFO: Bradley Schultz, Chief Financial Officer
CMO: Matthew Speyer, M.D., Chief Medical Officer
CHR: Andy Hooper, Director Human Resources
Web address: www.skylinemedicalcenter.com
Control: Corporation, Investor–owned, for–profit **Service:** General Medical and Surgical

Staffed Beds: 288 **Admissions:** 12860 **Census:** 184 **Outpatient Visits:** 168676 **Births:** 2 **Total Expense ($000):** 140671 **Payroll Expense ($000):** 51671 **Personnel:** 1157

TN

Hospital, Medicare Provider Number, Address, Telephone, Approval, Facility, and Physician Codes, Health Care System
★ American Hospital Association (AHA) membership
☐ The Joint Commission accreditation
○ American Osteopathic Association (AOA) accreditation
△ Commission on Accreditation of Rehabilitation Facilities (CARF) accreditation

★ **SOUTHERN HILLS MEDICAL CENTER (440197)**, 391 Wallace Road, Zip 37211–4859; tel. 615/781–4000 **A**1 2 9 10 **F**3 5 7 8 13 14 15 18 20 24 25 26 30 31 32 33 38 41 50 53 55 56 57 58 62 63 66 67 68 71 72 73 74 75 76 77 78 79 80 82 86 87 96 97 100 102 107 118 119 122 124 135 136 137 **P**5 **S** HCA
Primary Contact: Thomas H. Ozburn, Chief Executive Officer
COO: Travis Capers, Chief Operating Officer
CFO: Mike Reynolds, Chief Financial Officer
CIO: Ronnie Gannon, Director Information Services
CHR: Dale Beaudoin, Director Human Resources
Web address: www.southernhills.com
Control: Corporation, Investor–owned, for–profit **Service:** General Medical and Surgical

Staffed Beds: 120 **Admissions:** 5391 **Census:** 59 **Outpatient Visits:** 77680 **Births:** 659 **Total Expense ($000):** 62913 **Payroll Expense ($000):** 26826 **Personnel:** 507

THE CENTER FOR SPINAL SURGERY (440218), 2011 Murphy Avenue, Zip 37203; tel. 615/284–2970, (Nonreporting) **A**9 10
Primary Contact: Elissa Christiansen, Administrator
Control: Partnership, Investor–owned, for–profit **Service:** General Medical and Surgical

Staffed Beds: 18

★ **VANDERBILT STALLWORTH REHABILITATION HOSPITAL (443028)**, 2201 Childrens Way, Zip 37212–3165; tel. 615/320–7600, (Nonreporting) **A**1 5 10 **S** HEALTHSOUTH Corporation
Primary Contact: Susan Heath, Chief Executive Officer
CFO: Peggy Belyeu, Controller
CMO: Bob Coxe, M.D., Medical Director
CHR: Ruth Beasley, Director Human Resources
Web address: www.healthsouth.com
Control: Corporation, Investor–owned, for–profit **Service:** Rehabilitation

Staffed Beds: 80

TN

★ **VANDERBILT UNIVERSITY MEDICAL CENTER (440039)**, 1211 22nd Avenue South, Zip 37232–2102; tel. 615/322–5000, (Includes MONROE CARELL JR. CHILDREN'S HOSPITAL AT VANDERBILT, 2200 Children's Way, Zip 37232; tel. 615/936–1000; Kevin B. Churchwell, M.D., Chief Executive Officer; PSYCHIATRIC HOSPITAL AT VANDERBILT, 1601 23rd Avenue South, Zip 37212–3198; tel. 615/320–7770), (Total facility includes 1 beds in nursing home–type unit) **A**1 2 3 5 8 9 10 **F**3 4 5 7 9 11 12 13 15 16 17 18 19 20 21 22 23 24 25 26 27 28 30 31 32 33 34 36 37 38 39 40 41 43 44 46 47 48 49 50 51 52 53 54 55 56 57 58 59 60 61 62 63 66 68 70 71 72 73 74 75 76 77 78 79 80 81 82 83 84 86 87 88 89 90 91 92 93 94 95 96 97 98 99 100 102 103 104 105 106 107 108 109 111 112 113 114 116 117 118 119 120 121 123 124 125 126 127 128 129 130 131 132 133 135 136 137 **P**1 7 **S** Vanderbilt Healthcare
Primary Contact: Larry Goldberg, Executive Director and Chief Executive Officer
CFO: Rick Wagers, Chief Financial Officer
CMO: C. Wright Pinson, M.D., Chief Medical Officer
CIO: William Stead, M.D., Director Informatics Center
Web address: www.vanderbilt.edu
Control: Other not–for–profit (including NFP Corporation) **Service:** General Medical and Surgical

Staffed Beds: 833 **Admissions:** 50629 **Census:** 697 **Outpatient Visits:** 1193788 **Births:** 2561 **Total Expense ($000):** 1170575 **Payroll Expense ($000):** 423869 **Personnel:** 8048

★ **VETERANS AFFAIRS TENNESSEE VALLEY HEALTHCARE SYSTEM**, 1310 24th Avenue South, Zip 37212–2637; tel. 615/327–4751, (Includes ALVIN C. YORK VETERANS AFFAIRS MEDICAL CENTER, 3400 Lebanon Pike, Murfreesboro, Zip 37129–1236; tel. 615/867–6100; VETERANS AFFAIRS MEDICAL CENTER, 1310 24th Avenue South, tel. 615/327–4751), (Total facility includes 245 beds in nursing home–type unit) (Nonreporting) **A**1 2 3 5 8 **S** Department of Veterans Affairs
Primary Contact: Juan A. Morales, Interim Director
COO: Kenyon Dupre, Acting Associate Director
CFO: Terry Simmons, Chief Fiscal
CMO: Samuel Pieper, M.D., Interim Chief of Staff
CHR: William Hardwick, Chief Human Resources Officer
Web address: www.tennesseevalley.va.gov
Control: Veterans Affairs, Government, federal **Service:** General Medical and Surgical

Staffed Beds: 498

NEWPORT—Cocke County

★ **BAPTIST HOSPITAL OF COCKE COUNTY (440153)**, 435 Second Street, Zip 37821–3799; tel. 423/625–2200, (Total facility includes 56 beds in nursing home–type unit) **A**1 9 10 **F**8 13 17 25 26 30 31 32 38 42 44 45 46 50 65 66 73 74 75 79 86 96 97 100 102 107 119 136 **S** Catholic Healthcare Partners
Primary Contact: Patricia Ketterman, RN, Interim Administrator
CFO: Jackie Hounshell, Director Fiscal Services
CMO: James Williams, M.D., Chief of Staff
CHR: Scott Shaffer, Vice President Human Resources
Web address: www.baptistoneword.org/
Control: Church–operated, Nongovernment, not–for profit **Service:** General Medical and Surgical

Staffed Beds: 103 **Admissions:** 1968 **Census:** 69 **Outpatient Visits:** 72793 **Births:** 305 **Total Expense ($000):** 24210 **Payroll Expense ($000):** 10773 **Personnel:** 238

OAK RIDGE—Anderson County

★ **METHODIST MEDICAL CENTER OF OAK RIDGE (440034)**, 990 Oak Ridge Turnpike, Zip 37830–6976, Mailing Address: P.O. Box 2529, Zip 37831–2529; tel. 865/835–1000 **A**1 2 9 10 **F**11 13 15 18 20 22 24 25 26 27 30 31 32 33 38 43 44 45 49 51 55 56 57 59 60 62 63 66 68 72 73 74 75 76 77 79 80 81 86 90 96 97 99 100 102 106 107 108 109 110 111 116 118 135 137 **S** Covenant Health
Primary Contact: Michael Belbeck, President and Chief Administrative Officer
COO: Suzanne Koehler, Vice President and Chief Support Officer
CFO: Julie Utterback, Vice President and Chief Financial Officer
CHR: Rick Akens, Director Human Resources
Web address: www.mmcoakridge.com
Control: Other not–for–profit (including NFP Corporation) **Service:** General Medical and Surgical

Staffed Beds: 225 **Admissions:** 11383 **Census:** 145 **Outpatient Visits:** 135709 **Births:** 913 **Total Expense ($000):** 134816 **Payroll Expense ($000):** 49782 **Personnel:** 1298

RIDGEVIEW PSYCHIATRIC HOSPITAL AND CENTER (444003), 240 West Tyrone Road, Zip 37830–6571; tel. 865/482–1076, (Nonreporting) **A**10
Primary Contact: Robert J. Benning, Chief Executive Officer
COO: Brian Buuck, Chief Operating Officer
CFO: Mary Claire Duff, CPA, Chief Financial Officer
CMO: Renu Bhateja, M.D., President Medical Staff
CHR: Sharla Gerrish, Director Human Resources
Web address: www.ridgeviewresources.com
Control: Other not–for–profit (including NFP Corporation) **Service:** Psychiatric

Staffed Beds: 20

ONEIDA—Scott County

☐ **ST. MARY'S MEDICAL CENTER OF SCOTT COUNTY (440052)**, (Formerly Scott County Hospital), 18797 Alberta Avenue, Zip 37841–2127, Mailing Address: P.O. Box 4939, Zip 37841–4939; tel. 423/569–8521, (Nonreporting) **A**1 9 10 20 **S** Catholic Healthcare Partners
Primary Contact: H. Alan Watson, FACHE, Interim Chief Executive Officer
CFO: Bill Duncan, Chief Financial Officer
CMO: Jan Robbins, M.D., Chief of Staff
CIO: Dillon Ward, Director Information Systems
CHR: Charles Sexton, Director Human Resources and Marketing
Web address: www.stmaryshealth.com
Control: Other not–for–profit (including NFP Corporation) **Service:** General Medical and Surgical

Staffed Beds: 54

PARIS—Henry County

★ **HENRY COUNTY MEDICAL CENTER (440132)**, 301 Tyson Avenue, Zip 38242–4544, Mailing Address: P.O. Box 1030, Zip 38242–1030; tel. 731/642–1220, (Total facility includes 174 beds in nursing home–type unit) **A**1 9 10 **F**3 7 11 12 13 15 17 24 25 26 27 28 30 31 32 33 37 38 42 43 51 52 55 57 61 62 65 66 68 74 75 76 77 79 80 81 82 84 86 88 92 93 96 100 106 107 109 117 119 120 121 122 124 135 137
Primary Contact: Thomas H. Gee, Administrator
CFO: Lisa Casteel, Chief Financial Officer
CIO: Pam Ridley, Director Information Systems
CHR: Edwin L. Ledden, Assistant Administrator
Web address: www.hcmc-tn.org
Control: Hospital district or authority, Government, nonfederal **Service:** General Medical and Surgical

Staffed Beds: 275 **Admissions:** 5120 **Census:** 201 **Outpatient Visits:** 56681 **Births:** 344 **Total Expense ($000):** 59064 **Payroll Expense ($000):** 24700 **Personnel:** 725

PARSONS—Decatur County

☐ **DECATUR COUNTY GENERAL HOSPITAL (440070)**, 969 Tennessee Avenue South, Zip 38363–1649, Mailing Address: P.O. Box 250, Zip 38363–0250; tel. 731/847–3031, (Nonreporting) **A**1 9 10
Primary Contact: Norene Pumphrey, Chief Executive Officer
CFO: Donna Hayes, Controller
CMO: Tom Hamilton, M.D., Chief of Staff
CIO: Sue Ringger, R.N., Director Quality Assurance
CHR: Shelley Bartholomew, Director Human Resources
Web address: www.dcgh.org
Control: County–Government, nonfederal **Service:** General Medical and Surgical

Staffed Beds: 40

PIKEVILLE—Bledsoe County

☐ **ERLANGER BLEDSOE HOSPITAL (441306)**, 71 Wheeler Avenue, Zip 37367, Mailing Address: P.O. Box 699, Zip 37367–0699; tel. 423/447–2112 **A**1 9 10 18 **F**3 15 25 31 32 38 44 53 54 55 57 62 80 86 87 90 96 107 117 122 **P**5 **S** Erlanger Health System
Primary Contact: Stephanie Boynton, Administrator
CMO: Arturo L. Quito, M.D., Chief of Staff
CIO: Debbie Rains, Health Information Management Satellite Coordinator
CHR: Patsy Brown, Human Resources Site Coordinator
Web address: www.erlanger.org
Control: Hospital district or authority, Government, nonfederal **Service:** General Medical and Surgical

Staffed Beds: 29 **Admissions:** 356 **Census:** 6 **Outpatient Visits:** 11146 **Births:** 0 **Total Expense ($000):** 7414 **Payroll Expense ($000):** 2661 **Personnel:** 66

PORTLAND—Sumner County

PORTLAND MEDICAL CENTER See Hendersonville Medical Center, Hendersonville

PULASKI—Giles County

★ **HILLSIDE HOSPITAL (440020)**, 1265 East College Street, Zip 38478–4500; tel. 931/363–7531 **A**1 9 10 **F**3 11 13 15 17 25 26 31 32 38 54 55 56 57 66 68 73 74 77 79 80 86 88 93 96 97 99 100 102 107 118 119 120 121 122 132 135 136 137 **P**6 **S** LifePoint Hospitals, Inc.
Primary Contact: James H. Edmondson, Chief Executive Officer
CFO: Donald Gavin, Chief Financial Officer
CHR: Jane Petty, Director Human Resources
Web address: www.hillsidehospital.com
Control: Corporation, Investor–owned, for–profit **Service:** General Medical and Surgical

Staffed Beds: 50 **Admissions:** 2305 **Census:** 27 **Outpatient Visits:** 21732 **Births:** 273 **Total Expense ($000):** 18893 **Payroll Expense ($000):** 8302 **Personnel:** 167

RIPLEY—Lauderdale County

★ **BAPTIST MEMORIAL HOSPITAL–LAUDERDALE (441314)**, 326 Asbury Avenue, Zip 38063–9701; tel. 731/221–2200 **A**1 9 10 18 **F**1 3 11 15 25 26 30 31 32 33 38 54 55 56 57 68 73 75 77 79 80 82 84 86 88 90 93 96 100 107 119 122 124 135 **S** Baptist Memorial Health Care Corporation
Primary Contact: Daryl Blalack, Administrator and Chief Executive Officer
CFO: Monique Hart, Chief Financial Officer
CMO: Syed Zaidi, Chief Medical Staff
CHR: Gail Henderson, Manager Human Resources
Web address: www.lauderdale.baptistonline.org
Control: Other not–for–profit (including NFP Corporation) **Service:** General Medical and Surgical

Staffed Beds: 35 **Admissions:** 1073 **Census:** 16 **Outpatient Visits:** 19887 **Births:** 0 **Total Expense ($000):** 13499 **Payroll Expense ($000):** 5782 **Personnel:** 157

ROGERSVILLE—Hawkins County

★ **WELLMONT HAWKINS COUNTY MEMORIAL HOSPITAL (440032)**, 851 Locust Street, Zip 37857–2407, Mailing Address: P.O. Box 130, Zip 37857–0130; tel. 423/921–7000, (Nonreporting) **A**1 5 9 10 **S** Wellmont Health System
Primary Contact: Fred L. Pelle, FACHE, President
CFO: Troy Clark, Chief Executive Officer
CHR: Robin Poteete, Human Resources Manager
Web address: www.wellmont.org
Control: Other not–for–profit (including NFP Corporation) **Service:** General Medical and Surgical

Staffed Beds: 50

SAVANNAH—Hardin County

★ **HARDIN MEDICAL CENTER (440109)**, 935 Wayne Road, Zip 38372–1937; tel. 731/926–8000, (Total facility includes 73 beds in nursing home–type unit) **A**1 9 10 **F**7 11 13 15 25 26 27 31 38 55 57 61 62 63 65 66 73 74 75 76 77 79 80 81 82 86 96 97 100 102 107 117 119 122 135 137 **P**8
Primary Contact: Charlotte Burns, Administrator and Chief Executive Officer
CFO: Mike Harbor, Chief Financial Officer
CMO: Barry Hennessey, M.D., Chief Medical Staff
CIO: Jacob Bomar, Information Technology
CHR: Jimmy Davis, Director Human Resources
Web address: www.hardinmedicalcenter.org
Control: County–Government, nonfederal **Service:** General Medical and Surgical

Staffed Beds: 106 **Admissions:** 2425 **Census:** 21 **Outpatient Visits:** 67042 **Births:** 397 **Total Expense ($000):** 18144 **Payroll Expense ($000):** 9902

SELMER—McNairy County

★ **MCNAIRY REGIONAL HOSPITAL (440051)**, 705 East Poplar Avenue, Zip 38375–1828; tel. 731/645–3221 **A**1 9 10 **F**3 7 11 13 15 25 26 31 33 37 44 55 56 57 61 73 74 75 79 80 81 84 85 86 96 97 107 122 134 135 136 137 **S** Community Health Systems, Inc.
Primary Contact: Pamela W. Roberts, Chief Executive Officer
CFO: Meredith Jones, Chief Financial Officer
CMO: Daniel Baxter, Chief of Staff
CHR: Linda Durham, Director Human Resources
Web address: www.mcnairyregionalhospital.com
Control: Corporation, Investor–owned, for–profit **Service:** General Medical and Surgical

Staffed Beds: 41 **Admissions:** 1700 **Census:** 15 **Outpatient Visits:** 23059 **Births:** 160 **Total Expense ($000):** 17435 **Payroll Expense ($000):** 7507 **Personnel:** 189

SEVIERVILLE—Sevier County

★ **FORT SANDERS–SEVIER MEDICAL CENTER (440081)**, 709 Middle Creek Road, Zip 37862–5016, Mailing Address: P.O. Box 8005, Zip 37864–8005; tel. 865/429–6100, (Total facility includes 54 beds in nursing home–type unit) **A**1 9 10 **F**3 11 13 15 18 24 25 26 30 31 32 33 34 38 50 51 52 55 56 57 60 62 63 65 66 68 73 74 77 79 80 81 82 86 87 96 97 99 100 102 106 107 117 118 119 120 121 122 124 135 136 137 **S** Covenant Health
Primary Contact: Ellen Wilhoit, President and Chief Administrative Officer
COO: Jeff Friedman, Vice President Support Services
CFO: Rick Carringer, Chief Financial Officer
CMO: Don Parnell, Chief of Staff
CIO: Amanda Brabson, Director Marketing and Public Relations
CHR: Steve Bramble, Director Human Resources
Web address: www.covenanthealth.com
Control: Other not–for–profit (including NFP Corporation) **Service:** General Medical and Surgical

Staffed Beds: 108 **Admissions:** 3563 **Census:** 75 **Outpatient Visits:** 105991 **Births:** 1053 **Total Expense ($000):** 31023 **Payroll Expense ($000):** 16236 **Personnel:** 544

SEWANEE—Franklin County

EMERALD–HODGSON HOSPITAL See Southern Tennessee Medical Center, Winchester

SHELBYVILLE—Bedford County

★ **BEDFORD COUNTY MEDICAL CENTER (440137)**, 845 Union Street, Zip 37160–2609; tel. 931/685–5433, (Total facility includes 107 beds in nursing home–type unit) (Nonreporting) **A**1 9 10 **S** Community Health Systems, Inc.
Primary Contact: Daniel Buckner, Interim Chief Executive Officer
CIO: Debbie Sudduth, Director Information Services
Web address: www.bcmctn.com
Control: County–Government, nonfederal **Service:** General Medical and Surgical

Staffed Beds: 177

SMITHVILLE—DeKalb County

★ **DEKALB COMMUNITY HOSPITAL (440148)**, 520 West Main Street, Zip 37166–0640, Mailing Address: P.O. Box 640, Zip 37166–0640; tel. 615/215–5000, (Nonreporting) **A**1 9 10
Primary Contact: Robert M. Luther, Chief Executive Officer
CFO: Dennis Smock, Chief Financial Officer
CMO: Denise Dingle, M.D., Chief of Staff
CHR: Gingie Braswell, Human Resources Director
Control: Corporation, Investor–owned, for–profit **Service:** General Medical and Surgical

Staffed Beds: 57

TN

Hospital, Medicare Provider Number, Address, Telephone, Approval, Facility, and Physician Codes, Health Care System

★ American Hospital Association (AHA) membership
☐ The Joint Commission accreditation
○ American Osteopathic Association (AOA) accreditation
△ Commission on Accreditation of Rehabilitation Facilities (CARF) accreditation

SMYRNA—Rutherford County

★ **STONECREST MEDICAL CENTER (440227)**, 200 StoneCrest Boulevard, Zip 37167–6810; tel. 615/768–2000, (Nonreporting) **A**1 9 10 **S** HCA
Primary Contact: Neil A. Heatherly, CHE, Chief Executive Officer
CFO: Joe E. Bowman, Chief Financial Officer
CMO: Mark Dickinson, M.D., Chief of Staff
CHR: Joe Hill, Director Human Resources
Web address: www.stonecrestmedical.com
Control: Corporation, Investor–owned, for–profit **Service:** Other specialty

Staffed Beds: 75

SNEEDVILLE—Hancock County

WELLMONT HANCOCK COUNTY HOSPITAL (441313), 1517 Main Street, Highway 33, Zip 37869; tel. 423/921–7023, (Nonreporting) **A**9 18 **S** Wellmont Health System
Primary Contact: Troy Clark, Chief Executive Officer
Web address: www.wellmont.org
Control: Other not–for–profit (including NFP Corporation) **Service:** General Medical and Surgical

Staffed Beds: 10

SOMERVILLE—Fayette County

☐ **METHODIST HEALTHCARE–FAYETTE HOSPITAL (440168)**, 214 Lakeview Drive, Zip 38068–9737; tel. 901/516–4000, (Total facility includes 20 beds in nursing home–type unit) **A**1 9 10 **F**1 3 8 11 12 13 15 17 18 19 20 21 22 23 24 25 26 27 28 30 31 32 33 35 36 37 38 40 41 42 43 44 46 48 49 50 53 54 55 56 57 58 59 60 61 62 63 64 66 68 69 70 71 72 73 74 75 76 77 78 79 80 81 82 83 84 86 87 88 89 90 91 92 93 94 95 96 97 99 100 101 102 103 106 107 108 109 111 112 116 117 118 119 120 121 122 123 124 125 127 128 130 131 132 133 134 135 136 137 **P**5 6 8 **S** Methodist Le Bonheur Healthcare
Primary Contact: David Crislip, Administrator
CFO: Kevin Todd, Controller
Web address: www.methodisthealth.org
Control: Other not–for–profit (including NFP Corporation) **Service:** General Medical and Surgical

Staffed Beds: 1336 **Admissions:** 60273 **Census:** 979 **Outpatient Visits:** 508974 **Births:** 5725 **Total Expense ($000):** 1066946 **Payroll Expense ($000):** 466133 **Personnel:** 10788

TN

SPARTA—White County

★ **WHITE COUNTY COMMUNITY HOSPITAL (440192)**, 401 Sewell Road, Zip 38583–1299; tel. 931/738–9211, (Nonreporting) **A**1 9 10 **S** Capella Healthcare
Primary Contact: Joel Taylor, Chief Executive Officer
CFO: John Langlois, Chief Financial Officer
CMO: Mann Anbart, M.D., Chief of Staff
CIO: Phillip Austin, Director Information Systems
CHR: Stephanie Williams, Director Human Resources
Web address: www.whitecountyhospital.com
Control: Corporation, Investor–owned, for–profit **Service:** General Medical and Surgical

Staffed Beds: 24

SPRINGFIELD—Robertson County

★ **NORTHCREST MEDICAL CENTER (440065)**, 100 North Crest Drive, Zip 37172–3961; tel. 615/384–2411 **A**1 9 10 **F**3 11 13 15 18 20 24 25 26 30 31 32 36 38 40 42 43 46 53 54 55 56 57 62 66 68 73 74 75 77 79 81 82 84 86 96 97 100 102 107 118 119 120 121 124 133 135 136 137 **P**6
Primary Contact: Scott Raynes, President and Chief Executive Officer
COO: Randy Mills, Vice President Operations and Business Development
CFO: James A. Schmidt, Chief Financial Officer
CMO: Jeffrey Brannick, M.D., Chief of Staff
CIO: Jeff Dorris, Chief Information Officer
CHR: Amber King, Vice President Human Resources and Director Compliance
Web address: www.northcrest.com
Control: Other not–for–profit (including NFP Corporation) **Service:** General Medical and Surgical

Staffed Beds: 81 **Admissions:** 4644 **Census:** 51 **Outpatient Visits:** 72790 **Births:** 817 **Total Expense ($000):** 52968 **Payroll Expense ($000):** 22715 **Personnel:** 565

SWEETWATER—Monroe County

★ **SWEETWATER HOSPITAL (440084)**, 304 Wright Street, Zip 37874–2897; tel. 865/213–8200, (Nonreporting) **A**1 9 10
Primary Contact: Scott Bowman, Administrator
Web address: www.sweetwaterhospital.org
Control: Other not–for–profit (including NFP Corporation) **Service:** General Medical and Surgical

Staffed Beds: 59

TAZEWELL—Claiborne County

★ **CLAIBORNE COUNTY HOSPITAL (440057)**, 1850 Old Knoxville Road, Zip 37879–3625, Mailing Address: P.O. Box 219, Zip 37879–0219; tel. 423/626–4211, (Total facility includes 100 beds in nursing home–type unit) **A**1 9 10 20 **F**7 15 25 32 33 38 42 56 57 61 62 68 75 79 81 82 86 96 100 107 118 119 132 135
Primary Contact: Daniel A. Colon, Chief Executive Officer
CFO: Jessica L. Justice, Controller
CIO: Joe Martin, Director Information Systems
CHR: Susan Stone, Director Human Resources
Web address: www.clibornehospital.org
Control: County–Government, nonfederal **Service:** General Medical and Surgical

Staffed Beds: 162 **Admissions:** 2436 **Census:** 24 **Births:** 0

TRENTON—Gibson County

★ **GIBSON GENERAL HOSPITAL (440047)**, 200 Hospital Drive, Zip 38382–3313; tel. 731/855–7900 **A**1 9 10 **F**3 15 25 26 30 31 32 33 38 55 57 62 66 73 79 82 86 96 107 119 122 135 **S** West Tennessee Healthcare
Primary Contact: Sherry Scruggs, Administrator
CFO: Terry Swindell, Controller
CMO: Tom Nelson, M.D., Family Practice
CHR: Nancy Riggs, Director Human Resources
Web address: www.wth.net
Control: Hospital district or authority, Government, nonfederal **Service:** General Medical and Surgical

Staffed Beds: 34 **Admissions:** 704 **Census:** 7 **Outpatient Visits:** 17184 **Births:** 0 **Total Expense ($000):** 7068 **Payroll Expense ($000):** 3122 **Personnel:** 82

TULLAHOMA—Coffee County

☐ **HARTON REGIONAL MEDICAL CENTER (440144)**, 1801 North Jackson Street, Zip 37388–2201; tel. 931/393–3000, (Nonreporting) **A**1 9 10 19 **S** Health Management Associates
Primary Contact: Kenneth Ward, Interim Chief Executive Officer
CFO: Kenneth Ward, Chief Financial Officer
CMO: Dennis Crabtree, M.D., Chief of Staff
Web address: www.hartonmedicalcenter.com
Control: Corporation, Investor–owned, for–profit **Service:** Rehabilitation

Staffed Beds: 104

UNION CITY—Obion County

★ **BAPTIST MEMORIAL HOSPITAL–UNION CITY (440130)**, 1201 Bishop Street, Zip 38261–5403, Mailing Address: P.O. Box 310, Zip 38281–0310; tel. 731/884–8601, (Nonreporting) **A**1 9 10 **S** Baptist Memorial Health Care Corporation
Primary Contact: Donald Hutson, Administrator and Chief Executive Officer
CFO: Mike Perryman, Chief Financial Officer
CMO: Bruce Brown, President Medical Staff
CIO: David Mercer, Coordinator Information Systems
CHR: Tammy Hall, Director Human Resources
Web address: www.bmhcc.org
Control: Other not–for–profit (including NFP Corporation) **Service:** General Medical and Surgical

Staffed Beds: 85

WAVERLY—Humphreys County

☐ **THREE RIVERS HOSPITAL (441303)**, 451 Highway 13 South, Zip 37185–2149, Mailing Address: P.O. Box 437, Zip 37185–2149; tel. 931/296–4203 **A**1 9 10 18 **F**3 15 25 30 31 32 38 66 79 86 96 102 107 119 122 124 **S** Associated Healthcare Systems, Inc.
Primary Contact: R. Kent Koster, Chief Executive Officer
CFO: Sandra Patrick, Chief Financial Officer
CMO: Nestor A. Ojeda, M.D., Chief of Staff
CHR: Linda Rawlings, Director Human Resources and Personnel
Web address: www.threeriversshospital.org
Control: Partnership, Investor–owned, for–profit **Service:** General Medical and Surgical

Staffed Beds: 25 **Admissions:** 705 **Census:** 8 **Outpatient Visits:** 24034 **Births:** 1 **Total Expense ($000):** 7522 **Payroll Expense ($000):** 3345 **Personnel:** 83

WAYNESBORO—Wayne County

☐ **WAYNE MEDICAL CENTER (440010)**, 103 J. V. Mangubat Drive, Zip 38485, Mailing Address: P.O. Box 580, Zip 38485–0580; tel. 931/722–5411, (Total facility includes 46 beds in nursing home–type unit) (Nonreporting) **A**1 9 10 20
Primary Contact: Michael A. Sears, Interim Administrator
CFO: Michael A. Sears, Chief Financial Officer
CHR: Wendy Inman, Manager Human Resources
Web address: www.mauryregional.com
Control: Other not–for–profit (including NFP Corporation) **Service:** General Medical and Surgical

Staffed Beds: 78

Many Facility Codes have changed. Please refer to the AHA Guide Code Chart.

WINCHESTER—Franklin County

★□ **SOUTHERN TENNESSEE MEDICAL CENTER (440058)**, 185 Hospital Road, Zip 37398–9504; tel. 931/967–8200, (Includes EMERALD–HODGSON HOSPITAL, 1260 University Avenue, Sewanee, Zip 37375–2303; tel. 931/598–5691; Ralph Underwood, Administrator), (Total facility includes 46 beds in nursing home–type unit) **A**1 9 10 **F**3 13 15 25 36 38 39 43 46 48 54 55 56 57 68 72 73 74 75 76 77 79 80 81 82 85 86 88 93 96 97 98 100 102 107 117 118 119 135 136 **S** LifePoint Hospitals, Inc.
Primary Contact: William Russell Spray, Chief Executive Officer
COO: Wes Sigler, Chief Operating Officer
CFO: Steve Moore, Chief Financial Officer
CIO: James Payne, Director Information Systems
CHR: Linda Tipps, Director Human Resources
Web address: www.southerntennessee.com
Control: Corporation, Investor–owned, for–profit **Service:** General Medical and Surgical

Staffed Beds: 153 **Admissions:** 5732 **Census:** 92 **Outpatient Visits:** 66195 **Births:** 481 **Total Expense ($000):** 45347 **Payroll Expense ($000):** 19817 **Personnel:** 445

WOODBURY—Cannon County

□ **STONES RIVER HOSPITAL (440200)**, 324 Doolittle Road, Zip 37190–1140; tel. 615/563–4001, (Nonreporting) **A**1 9 10
Primary Contact: Robert M. Luther, Chief Executive Officer
CMO: J C Wall, Chief of Staff
CHR: Brian Woods, Director Human Resources
Web address: www.stonesriverhospital.com
Control: Corporation, Investor–owned, for–profit **Service:** General Medical and Surgical

Staffed Beds: 55

TN

Hospital, Medicare Provider Number, Address, Telephone, Approval, Facility, and Physician Codes, Health Care System

★ American Hospital Association (AHA) membership
□ The Joint Commission accreditation
○ American Osteopathic Association (AOA) accreditation
△ Commission on Accreditation of Rehabilitation Facilities (CARF) accreditation

TEXAS

ABILENE—Taylor County

☐ **ABILENE PSYCHIATRIC HOSPITAL (454098)**, 4225 Woods Place, Zip 79608; tel. 325/698–6600 **A**1 9 10 **F**5 25 31 32 82 88 89 91 92 93 95 107 24 4 5 79 80 81 82 83 84 86 **P**4
Primary Contact: Christopher Kearney, Chief Executive Officer
Web address: www.abilenepsychiatriccenter.onsmartpages.com/home/
Control: Other not–for–profit (including NFP Corporation) **Service:** Psychiatric

Staffed Beds: 28 **Admissions:** 729 **Census:** 19 **Outpatient Visits:** 65 **Births:** 0 **Total Expense ($000):** 3889299 **Payroll Expense ($000):** 2116323 **Personnel:** 69

★ **ABILENE REGIONAL MEDICAL CENTER (450558)**, 6250 Highway 83–84 at Antilley Road, Zip 79606–5299; tel. 325/695–9900, (Total facility includes 25 beds in nursing home–type unit) **A**1 2 9 10 **F**8 11 12 13 15 17 18 20 22 24 25 26 27 30 32 33 36 38 40 46 51 52 54 55 56 57 62 66 68 70 73 74 75 76 77 79 80 81 82 84 86 96 97 100 102 103 106 107 117 119 121 122 135 136 137 **P**3 **S** Community Health Systems, Inc.
Primary Contact: Michael D. Murphy, Chief Executive Officer
CFO: Ron Bennett, Chief Financial Officer
CIO: Dennis Newquist, Director Information Systems
CHR: Emmett Craig, Director Human Resources
Web address: www.abileneregional.com
Control: Corporation, Investor–owned, for–profit **Service:** General Medical and Surgical

Staffed Beds: 205 **Admissions:** 7875 **Census:** 98 **Outpatient Visits:** 56498 **Births:** 1490 **Total Expense ($000):** 80549 **Payroll Expense ($000):** 28714 **Personnel:** 648

HENDRICK CENTER FOR EXTENDED CARE (452029), 1242 North 19th Street, Zip 79601; tel. 325/670–5151 **A**10 **F**1 25 27 30 31 32 66 80 119
Primary Contact: Patty Esposito, Director
Control: Church–operated, Nongovernment, not–for profit **Service:** Long–Term Acute Care hospital

Staffed Beds: 19 **Admissions:** 247 **Census:** 18 **Outpatient Visits:** 0 **Births:** 0 **Total Expense ($000):** 5226 **Payroll Expense ($000):** 1549 **Personnel:** 31

TX

★ **HENDRICK HEALTH SYSTEM (450229)**, 1900 Pine Street, Zip 79601–2432; tel. 325/670–2000, (Total facility includes 26 beds in nursing home–type unit) **A**1 3 5 9 10 **F**3 11 12 13 14 15 17 18 20 22 24 25 26 27 28 30 31 32 33 37 38 40 41 43 44 48 49 50 51 52 54 55 56 57 59 60 61 62 66 68 71 72 73 74 75 76 77 78 79 80 81 82 83 84 85 86 87 92 96 97 99 100 102 103 106 107 111 117 118 119 120 121 124 132 135 136 137
Primary Contact: Tim Lancaster, FACHE, President and Chief Executive Officer
CFO: Stephen Kimmel, Senior Vice President and Chief Financial Officer
CHR: Mike McBroom, Vice President
Web address: www.ehendrick.org
Control: Church–operated, Nongovernment, not–for profit **Service:** General Medical and Surgical

Staffed Beds: 377 **Admissions:** 15624 **Census:** 238 **Outpatient Visits:** 264051 **Births:** 1346 **Total Expense ($000):** 192022 **Payroll Expense ($000):** 79130 **Personnel:** 2109

ALICE—Jim Wells County

★ **CHRISTUS SPOHN HOSPITAL ALICE (450828)**, 2500 East Main Street, Zip 78332–4794; tel. 361/661–8000, (Total facility includes 12 beds in nursing home–type unit) **A**1 9 10 20 **F**3 11 13 15 18 20 25 26 30 31 32 33 37 38 40 46 49 50 51 54 55 57 62 66 68 73 74 75 77 79 81 82 84 85 86 87 88 90 91 92 93 96 97 100 102 107 117 119 135 137 **P**8 **S** CHRISTUS Health
Primary Contact: Mark Casanova, Chief Operating Officer
COO: Mark Casanova, Chief Operating Officer
CFO: Michael Guajardo, Director Finance
CMO: Jerry Liles, Chief of Staff
CIO: Jean Deanoglis, Director Management Information Systems
CHR: Emily Diaz–Lopez, Director Human Resources
Web address: www.christusspohn.org/locations_alice.htm
Control: Church–operated, Nongovernment, not–for profit **Service:** General Medical and Surgical

Staffed Beds: 152 **Admissions:** 5921 **Census:** 63 **Outpatient Visits:** 53823 **Births:** 569 **Total Expense ($000):** 48822 **Payroll Expense ($000):** 21489 **Personnel:** 367

ALLEN—Collin County

★ **TEXAS HEALTH PRESBYTERIAN HOSPITAL OF ALLEN (450840)**, (Formerly Presbyterian Hospital of Allen), 1105 Central Expressway North, Zip 75013; tel. 972/747–1000 **A**1 9 10 **F**3 13 15 25 26 30 31 32 33 36 38 55 56 57 62 68 71 72 73 74 77 79 96 99 100 106 107 118 119 121 124 135 136 **S** Texas Health Resources
Primary Contact: Sheila A. McKinney, President
CFO: Dan Rich, Director Finance
CMO: Todd Pollack, President
CHR: Sharon Chisholm, Director Human Resources
Web address: www.texashealth.org
Control: Other not–for–profit (including NFP Corporation) **Service:** General Medical and Surgical

Staffed Beds: 62 **Admissions:** 3612 **Census:** 34 **Outpatient Visits:** 44194 **Births:** 1207 **Total Expense ($000):** 50519 **Payroll Expense ($000):** 19923 **Personnel:** 269

ALPINE—Brewster County

★ **BIG BEND REGIONAL MEDICAL CENTER (450830)**, 2600 Highway 118 North, Zip 79830–2002; tel. 432/837–3447 **A**1 9 10 20 **F**3 11 13 25 30 31 32 33 38 40 55 56 57 61 62 73 74 79 80 86 96 102 107 119 132 135 136 **P**6 **S** Community Health Systems, Inc.
Primary Contact: Michael J. Ellis, Chief Executive Officer
Web address: www.bigbendhealthcare.com
Control: Corporation, Investor–owned, for–profit **Service:** General Medical and Surgical

Staffed Beds: 25 **Admissions:** 1182 **Census:** 8 **Outpatient Visits:** 22541 **Births:** 221 **Total Expense ($000):** 18788 **Payroll Expense ($000):** 6833 **Personnel:** 121

ALVIN—Brazoria County

ALVIN DIAGNOSTIC AND URGENT CARE CENTER See Clear Lake Regional Medical Center, Webster

AMARILLO—Potter County

★ **AMARILLO VETERANS AFFAIRS HEALTH CARE SYSTEM**, 6010 Amarillo Boulevard West, Zip 79106–1992; tel. 806/355–9703, (Total facility includes 120 beds in nursing home–type unit) (Nonreporting) **A**1 2 3 5 9 **S** Department of Veterans Affairs
Primary Contact: Gracie Specks, Acting Director
CFO: Alton McKinley, Chief Fiscal Services
CMO: Andrew C. Stenhouse, M.D., Chief of Staff
CIO: Toby Dickerson, Acting Chief Information Resource Management
CHR: Ken Creamer, Chief Human Resource
Web address: www.va.gov/sta/guide/home.asp
Control: Veterans Affairs, Government, federal **Service:** General Medical and Surgical

Staffed Beds: 189

★ **BAPTIST ST. ANTHONY HEALTH SYSTEM (450231)**, 1600 Wallace Boulevard, Zip 79106–1799; tel. 806/212–2000 **A**2 3 5 9 10 **F**3 7 8 11 13 15 17 18 20 22 24 25 26 27 30 31 32 33 38 42 43 44 46 49 51 52 53 54 55 57 61 62 68 70 72 73 74 75 76 77 79 80 81 82 83 84 85 86 87 96 97 100 102 103 105 107 116 118 119 120 133 134 135 136 **P**3
Primary Contact: John D. Hicks, FACHE, President and Chief Executive Officer
COO: Michael Cruz, Vice President Operations
CFO: Elizabeth Pulliam, Vice President and Chief Financial Officer
CMO: Kenneth Johnston, M.D., Vice President Medical Affairs
CIO: Ronald Coots, Chief Information Officer
CHR: Iris Hicks, Director Human Resources and Education
Web address: www.bsahs.org
Control: Church–operated, Nongovernment, not–for profit **Service:** General Medical and Surgical

Staffed Beds: 443 **Admissions:** 22390 **Census:** 273 **Outpatient Visits:** 68994 **Births:** 2530 **Total Expense ($000):** 256624 **Payroll Expense ($000):** 104926 **Personnel:** 2607

Many Facility Codes have changed. Please refer to the AHA Guide Code Chart.

NORTHWEST TEXAS HEALTHCARE SYSTEM (450209), 1501 South Coulter Avenue, Zip 79106–1790, Mailing Address: P.O. Box 1110, Zip 79175–1110; tel. 806/354–1000, (Includes PSYCHIATRIC PAVILION, 7201 Evans, Zip 79106) **A**1 2 3 5 9 10 **F**3 4 5 7 11 12 13 17 18 20 22 23 24 25 26 27 28 30 31 32 33 35 36 37 38 40 41 46 48 49 50 53 54 55 56 57 59 60 62 64 66 68 70 72 73 74 75 76 77 79 80 81 82 83 84 86 87 88 89 90 91 92 93 94 95 96 97 100 102 106 107 112 118 119 121 124 135 136 137 **P**6 **S** Universal Health Services, Inc.
Primary Contact: Frank Lopez, FACHE, Chief Executive Officer and Managing Director
COO: Kyle Sanders, Chief Operating Officer
CMO: Nathan Goldstein, M.D., Chief Medical Officer
CIO: Sam Mason, Director Management Information Systems
CHR: Charlyn Snow, Director Human Resources
Web address: www.nwtexashealthcare.com
Control: Corporation, Investor–owned, for–profit **Service:** General Medical and Surgical

Staffed Beds: 419 **Admissions:** 18809 **Census:** 247 **Outpatient Visits:** 249691 **Births:** 2229 **Total Expense ($000):** 250487 **Payroll Expense ($000):** 79100 **Personnel:** 1569

NORTHWEST TEXAS REHABILITATION HOSPITAL (453096), 7200 West 9th Avenue, Zip 79106; tel. 806/468–2900 **A**1 9 10 **F**3 25 41 43 54 73 75 82 85 119 132 137 **S** RehabCare Group, Inc.
Primary Contact: Mark A. Kelly, Chief Executive Officer and Administrator
Web address: www.rehabcare.com
Control: Partnership, Investor–owned, for–profit **Service:** Rehabilitation

Staffed Beds: 42 **Admissions:** 679 **Census:** 23 **Outpatient Visits:** 0 **Births:** 0 **Total Expense ($000):** 8117 **Payroll Expense ($000):** 3787 **Personnel:** 84

NORTHWEST TEXAS SURGERY CENTER (450796), 3501 Soncy Road, Suite 118, Zip 79109; tel. 805/359–7999 **A**10 **F**30 31 38 79 80 108 120 126 137 30 37 70 71
Primary Contact: Dave Clark, M.D., Administrator
Control: Corporation, Investor–owned, for–profit **Service:** Surgical

Staffed Beds: 6 **Admissions:** 5228 **Census:** 1 **Outpatient Visits:** 5164 **Births:** 0 **Total Expense ($000):** 8994600 **Payroll Expense ($000):** 2762651 **Personnel:** 44

PHYSICIANS SURGICAL HOSPITAL OF QUAIL CREEK (450875), 6819 Plum Creek, Zip 79124; tel. 806/354–6100 **A**9 10 **F**25 26 38 41 50 66 73 77 79 80 84 119 124
Primary Contact: Debbie Inman, Chief Executive Officer
Web address: www.foundationsurgery.com
Control: Corporation, Investor–owned, for–profit **Service:** Surgical

Staffed Beds: 37 **Admissions:** 744 **Census:** 5 **Outpatient Visits:** 9116 **Births:** 0 **Total Expense ($000):** 22778 **Payroll Expense ($000):** 1453 **Personnel:** 121

□ **SPECIALTY HOSPITAL AT PLUM CREEK (452066)**, 5601 Plum Creek Drive, Zip 79124–1801; tel. 806/351–1000 **A**1 9 10 **F**1 3 25 31 32 73 75 80 81 119 132 137 **S** Fundamental Long Term Care Holdings, LLC
Primary Contact: Thomas P. Harlan, Chief Executive Officer
Control: Corporation, Investor–owned, for–profit **Service:** Long–Term Acute Care hospital

Staffed Beds: 47 **Admissions:** 369 **Census:** 27 **Outpatient Visits:** 0 **Births:** 0 **Total Expense ($000):** 9516 **Payroll Expense ($000):** 3518 **Personnel:** 81

□ **TRIUMPH HOSPITAL AMARILLO (452060)**, 2828 West 27th Avenue, Zip 79109; tel. 806/351–1600 **A**1 9 10 **F**1 3 25 32 33 57 68 75 96 137 **S** Triumph HealthCare
Primary Contact: Ronda L. Crow, RN, Chief Executive Officer
Web address: www.triumph–healthcare.com
Control: Corporation, Investor–owned, for–profit **Service:** Long–Term Acute Care hospital

Staffed Beds: 97 **Admissions:** 538 **Census:** 37 **Outpatient Visits:** 0 **Births:** 0 **Total Expense ($000):** 17162 **Payroll Expense ($000):** 6098 **Personnel:** 133

ANAHUAC—Chambers County

★ **BAYSIDE COMMUNITY HOSPITAL (451320)**, 200 Hospital Drive, Zip 77514, Mailing Address: P.O. Box 398, Zip 77514; tel. 409/267–3143 **A**9 10 18 **F**3 8 11 25 31 33 38 40 50 53 54 55 56 57 62 64 66 68 69 75 78 79 81 82 83 84 87 96 102 107 117 119 122 135 136 137 **P**3 7
Primary Contact: Robert Pascasio, FACHE, Chief Executive Officer
COO: Robert Pascasio, FACHE, Chief Executive Officer
CFO: Rick Jacobus, Chief Financial Officer
CMO: Leonidas Andres, M.D., Chief of Staff
Web address: www.baysidehospital.org
Control: Hospital district or authority, Government, nonfederal **Service:** General Medical and Surgical

Staffed Beds: 14 **Admissions:** 395 **Census:** 3 **Outpatient Visits:** 21970 **Births:** 0 **Total Expense ($000):** 6050 **Payroll Expense ($000):** 2717 **Personnel:** 68

ANDREWS—Andrews County

★ **PERMIAN REGIONAL MEDICAL CENTER (450144)**, Northeast By–Pass, Zip 79714, Mailing Address: P.O. Box 2108, Zip 79714–2108; tel. 432/523–2200 **A**9 10 20 **F**3 11 13 15 25 30 31 32 33 34 36 37 38 40 41 43 44 50 52 54 55 56 57 61 62 66 68 71 73 74 75 79 80 81 82 84 86 87 96 97 100 107 118 119 120 121 122 124 133 135 137 **P**6 7
Primary Contact: Randy R. Richards, Chief Executive Officer
CFO: Cleo Cagle, Chief Financial Officer
CIO: Dan Smart, Chief Information Management Off
CHR: Pam McCormick, Director Human Resources
Web address: www.permianregional.com
Control: Hospital district or authority, Government, nonfederal **Service:** General Medical and Surgical

Staffed Beds: 44 **Admissions:** 1244 **Census:** 10 **Outpatient Visits:** 54473 **Births:** 272 **Total Expense ($000):** 22623 **Payroll Expense ($000):** 9646 **Personnel:** 213

ANGLETON—Brazoria County

ANGLETON DANBURY MEDICAL CENTER (450591), 132 East Hospital Drive, Zip 77515–4197; tel. 979/849–7721 **A**1 9 10 **F**3 11 13 15 24 25 26 30 31 32 33 34 38 40 43 46 49 52 55 56 57 62 63 66 68 72 73 74 75 77 79 80 81 82 86 96 97 100 102 107 119 121 124 135 **P**1
Primary Contact: David A. Bleakney, Administrator
CFO: William D. Garwood, Associate Administrator and Chief Financial Officer
CHR: Beverly Dahlem, Associate Administrator
Web address: www.admc.org
Control: Hospital district or authority, Government, nonfederal **Service:** General Medical and Surgical

Staffed Beds: 51 **Admissions:** 3353 **Census:** 24 **Outpatient Visits:** 48051 **Births:** 385 **Total Expense ($000):** 29050 **Payroll Expense ($000):** 9621 **Personnel:** 219

ANSON—Jones County

★ **ANSON GENERAL HOSPITAL (450078)**, 101 Avenue J, Zip 79501–2198; tel. 325/823–3231, (Nonreporting) **A**9 10
Primary Contact: Ted D. Matthews, Chief Executive Officer
COO: Lynna B. Cox, Director Health Services
CFO: Pamela Gonzales, Chief Financial Officer
Control: City–Government, nonfederal **Service:** General Medical and Surgical

Staffed Beds: 31

ARANSAS PASS—San Patricio County

NORTH BAY HOSPITAL (450605), 1711 West Wheeler Avenue, Zip 78336–4536; tel. 361/758–8585 **A**9 10 **F**1 3 4 11 15 16 17 25 30 31 32 38 40 50 54 55 57 62 65 68 70 71 73 76 77 78 79 80 81 82 83 84 85 87 88 92 93 96 107 117 118 119 121 122 135 **P**5 7
Primary Contact: Sean L. Marshall, Chief Executive Officer
CFO: Belinda Vera, Chief Financial Officer
CHR: Sherry Gwynn, Administrative Director Human Resources
Web address: www.nbhtx.com
Control: Corporation, Investor–owned, for–profit **Service:** General Medical and Surgical

Staffed Beds: 58 **Admissions:** 1471 **Census:** 17 **Outpatient Visits:** 25725 **Births:** 0 **Total Expense ($000):** 12279 **Payroll Expense ($000):** 4607 **Personnel:** 160

ARLINGTON—Tarrant County

ARLINGTON MEMORIAL HOSPITAL See Texas Health Arlington Memorial Hospital

TX

Hospital, Medicare Provider Number, Address, Telephone, Approval, Facility, and Physician Codes, Health Care System

★ American Hospital Association (AHA) membership
□ The Joint Commission accreditation
○ American Osteopathic Association (AOA) accreditation
△ Commission on Accreditation of Rehabilitation Facilities (CARF) accreditation

★ **HEALTHSOUTH REHABILITATION HOSPITAL OF ARLINGTON (453040),** 3200 Matlock Road, Zip 76015–2911; tel. 817/468–4000 **A**1 9 10 **F**25 30 43 59 62 73 75 77 85 86 118 119 120 121 **S** HEALTHSOUTH Corporation
Primary Contact: Jessica Knox, Chief Executive Officer
CMO: Rizwan Shah, M.D., Medical Director
CHR: Kelly Harris, Director Marketing Operations
Web address: www.healthsouth.com
Control: Corporation, Investor–owned, for–profit **Service:** Rehabilitation

Staffed Beds: 65 **Admissions:** 702 **Census:** 27 **Outpatient Visits:** 15358 **Births:** 0 **Total Expense ($000):** 10773 **Payroll Expense ($000):** 6545 **Personnel:** 90

☐ **KINDRED HOSPITAL TARRANT COUNTY–ARLINGTON (452028),** 1000 North Cooper Street, Zip 76011–5540; tel. 817/548–3400 **A**1 9 10 **F**3 25 26 30 32 38 43 54 55 68 75 86 118 119 137 **S** Kindred Healthcare
Primary Contact: Christina Richard, Administrator
CFO: Jennifer Penland, Controller
CMO: Bernard A. McGowen, M.D., Medical Director
Web address: www.kindredhealthcare.com
Control: Corporation, Investor–owned, for–profit **Service:** Long–Term Acute Care hospital

Staffed Beds: 79 **Admissions:** 689 **Census:** 60 **Outpatient Visits:** 174 **Births:** 0 **Total Expense ($000):** 22282 **Payroll Expense ($000):** 8885 **Personnel:** 165

★ △ **MEDICAL CENTER OF ARLINGTON (450675),** 3301 Matlock Road, Zip 76015–2998; tel. 817/465–3241 **A**1 7 9 10 **F**3 11 12 13 17 18 20 22 24 25 27 30 31 32 33 37 38 40 43 49 50 52 54 55 56 57 59 62 68 70 71 72 73 74 75 76 77 79 80 81 82 84 85 86 96 97 98 100 102 106 107 119 120 121 124 132 133 134 135 136 137 **S** HCA
Primary Contact: Patrick D. Brilliant, Chief Executive Officer
COO: Scott Schmidly, Chief Operating Officer
CFO: Marshall Allen, Chief Financial Officer
CMO: Bruce Railey, M.D., Chief of Staff
CIO: James Lee, Director Information Services
CHR: Donna Coleman, Vice President Human Resources
Web address: www.medicalcenterarlington.com
Control: Corporation, Investor–owned, for–profit **Service:** General Medical and Surgical

Staffed Beds: 266 **Admissions:** 14292 **Census:** 195 **Outpatient Visits:** 115434 **Total Expense ($000):** 167578 **Payroll Expense ($000):** 61113 **Personnel:** 957

☐ **MILLWOOD HOSPITAL (454012),** 1011 North Cooper Street, Zip 76011–5517; tel. 817/261–3121 **A**1 9 10 **F**4 5 25 26 53 54 61 69 82 88 89 90 91 92 93 94 95 119 121 **S** Psychiatric Solutions
Primary Contact: John Baker, Chief Executive Officer
COO: Sammie Sikes, Chief Operating Officer
CFO: Jeff Epperson, Chief Financial Officer
CMO: Ernest Brownlee, M.D., Medical Director
CHR: Shirley Spurlock, Director Human Resources
Web address: www.millwoodhospital.com
Control: Corporation, Investor–owned, for–profit **Service:** Psychiatric

Staffed Beds: 120 **Admissions:** 3914 **Census:** 85 **Outpatient Visits:** 23622 **Births:** 0 **Total Expense ($000):** 17684 **Payroll Expense ($000):** 9460 **Personnel:** 267

★ △ **REHABCARE OF ARLINGTON (453094),** 2601 West Randol Mill Road, Zip 76012; tel. 817/804–4400 **A**1 7 9 10 **F**3 25 30 32 55 57 72 73 81 82 85 119 121 135 137 **S** RehabCare Group, Inc.
Primary Contact: Susan Schaetti, Chief Executive Officer
Web address: www.rehabcare.com/portfolio/long_term_acute_care/Arlington.htm
Control: Corporation, Investor–owned, for–profit **Service:** Rehabilitation

Staffed Beds: 24 **Admissions:** 600 **Census:** 19 **Outpatient Visits:** 0 **Births:** 0 **Total Expense ($000):** 5882 **Payroll Expense ($000):** 3001 **Personnel:** 52

★ **TEXAS HEALTH ARLINGTON MEMORIAL HOSPITAL (450064),** (Formerly Arlington Memorial Hospital), 800 West Randol Mill Road, Zip 76012–2503; tel. 817/548–6100 **A**1 9 10 **F**3 11 12 13 15 17 18 20 22 24 25 26 27 30 31 32 33 35 38 42 51 52 53 55 56 57 59 62 66 68 70 72 73 74 75 76 77 79 80 81 82 84 86 96 97 100 102 106 107 119 121 124 125 135 136 137 **S** Texas Health Resources
Primary Contact: Kirk King, CHE, President
COO: Sandra L. Harris, Senior Vice President and Chief Operating Officer
CFO: Joe Tallon, Director Finance
CMO: Robert N. Cluck, M.D., Vice President and Medical Director
CHR: Yvonne Kyler, Director Human Resources
Web address: www.arlingtonmemorial.org
Control: Other not–for–profit (including NFP Corporation) **Service:** General Medical and Surgical

Staffed Beds: 344 **Admissions:** 17101 **Census:** 247 **Outpatient Visits:** 138150 **Births:** 2635 **Total Expense ($000):** 224485 **Payroll Expense ($000):** 97777 **Personnel:** 1758

☐ **USMD HOSPITAL AT ARLINGTON (450872),** 801 West Interstate 20, Zip 76017; tel. 817/472–3400 **A**1 9 10 **F**3 12 15 25 26 27 32 37 38 43 51 55 57 63 66 73 77 79 80 82 84 92 96 97 100 102 107 112 116 121 135
Primary Contact: Carlos Acosta, M.D., President
Web address: www.usmdhospital.com
Control: Partnership, Investor–owned, for–profit **Service:** General Medical and Surgical

Staffed Beds: 34 **Admissions:** 1665 **Census:** 8 **Outpatient Visits:** 54495 **Births:** 2 **Total Expense ($000):** 64657 **Payroll Expense ($000):** 11405 **Personnel:** 251

ASPERMONT—Stonewall County

STONEWALL MEMORIAL HOSPITAL (451318), 821 North Broadway, Zip 79502–2913, Mailing Address: P.O. Box C, Zip 79502–2913; tel. 940/989–3551, (Total facility includes 60 beds in nursing home–type unit) **A**9 10 18 **F**25 30 31 32 38 55 57 62 87 117 122 **P**6
Primary Contact: Helen Orr, Administrator
COO: Helen Orr, Administrator
CFO: Debra Meador, Assistant Administrator
CMO: Fahed M. Hamadeh, M.D., Chief of Staff
CIO: Debbie Whitman, Administrative Specialist
Control: Hospital district or authority, Government, nonfederal **Service:** General Medical and Surgical

Staffed Beds: 72 **Admissions:** 93 **Census:** 26 **Outpatient Visits:** 3433 **Births:** 0 **Total Expense ($000):** 4406 **Payroll Expense ($000):** 2247 **Personnel:** 110

ATHENS—Henderson County

★ **EAST TEXAS MEDICAL CENTER ATHENS (450389),** 2000 South Palestine Street, Zip 75751–5610; tel. 903/676–1000 **A**1 9 10 **F**3 11 15 18 19 20 21 25 38 39 40 43 46 51 55 62 63 64 68 72 73 74 75 77 79 80 81 84 96 97 100 102 103 107 119 121 134 **P**7 **S** East Texas Medical Center Regional Healthcare System
Primary Contact: Patrick L. Wallace, Administrator
CFO: David A. Travis, Chief Financial Officer
CHR: Jennifer Rummell, Director Human Resources
Web address: www.etmc.org
Control: Other not–for–profit (including NFP Corporation) **Service:** General Medical and Surgical

Staffed Beds: 117 **Admissions:** 7994 **Census:** 78 **Outpatient Visits:** 87670 **Births:** 893 **Total Expense ($000):** 56886 **Payroll Expense ($000):** 21155 **Personnel:** 502

ATLANTA—Cass County

★ **ATLANTA MEMORIAL HOSPITAL (450615),** Highway 77 at South William, Zip 75551, Mailing Address: P.O. Box 1049, Zip 75551–1049; tel. 903/799–3000 **A**9 10 **F**3 11 15 25 26 28 30 32 33 38 40 52 55 56 57 61 62 66 68 73 75 79 82 86 88 90 93 96 100 102 107 118 119 121 122 135 137 **P**8
Primary Contact: Tom Crow, Administrator
COO: Barbara Weems, Assistant Administrator
CIO: Rodney Bynum, Director Information Services
CHR: Debra Embry, Associate Administrator Employee Services
Web address: www.atlantamemorial.com
Control: Hospital district or authority, Government, nonfederal **Service:** General Medical and Surgical

Staffed Beds: 56 **Admissions:** 2134 **Census:** 28 **Outpatient Visits:** 31433 **Births:** 0 **Total Expense ($000):** 19331 **Payroll Expense ($000):** 8737 **Personnel:** 260

AUSTIN—Travis County

☐ **AUSTIN STATE HOSPITAL (454084),** 4110 Guadalupe Street, Zip 78751–4296; tel. 512/452–0381 **A**1 10 **F**25 26 30 32 37 50 54 57 63 66 73 81 88 89 91 93 119 132 135 **P**1 **S** Texas Department of State Health Services
Primary Contact: Carl Schock, Superintendent
CFO: Larry Shanahan, Chief Financial Officer
CMO: Clifford Moy, M.D., Clinical Director
CIO: Wendy Biro–Pollard, Director Community Relations
Web address: www.mhmr.state.tx.us
Control: State–Government, nonfederal **Service:** Psychiatric

Staffed Beds: 299 **Admissions:** 4598 **Census:** 279 **Outpatient Visits:** 0 **Births:** 0 **Total Expense ($000):** 55316 **Payroll Expense ($000):** 30271 **Personnel:** 872

Many Facility Codes have changed. Please refer to the AHA Guide Code Chart.

☐ **AUSTIN SURGICAL HOSPITAL (450871)**, 3003 Bee Caves Road, Zip 78746; tel. 512/314–3800 **A**1 9 10 **F**3 12 25 26 31 35 38 43 51 57 63 66 68 75 77 79 80 96 100 107 118 119 **P**2 **S** Hospital Partners of America
Primary Contact: Todd Mann, Chief Executive Officer
CFO: Lawrence Oldham, Chief Financial Officer
CMO: Barbara Bergin, M.D., Medical Director
CHR: Marilyn Jennings, Director Human Resources
Web address: www.austinsurgicalhospital.com
Control: Partnership, Investor–owned, for–profit **Service:** Orthopedic

Staffed Beds: 23 **Admissions:** 1310 **Census:** 9 **Outpatient Visits:** 4042 **Births:** 0 **Total Expense ($000):** 29874 **Personnel:** 148

CHILDREN'S HOSPITAL OF AUSTIN See Dell Children's Medical Center of Central Texas

CHRISTOPHER HOUSE, 2820 East Martin Luther King, Zip 78702–1544; tel. 512/322–0747, (Nonreporting)
Primary Contact: Marjorie Mulanax, Executive Director
Web address: www.hospiceaustin.org
Control: Other not–for–profit (including NFP Corporation) **Service:** Other specialty

Staffed Beds: 15

☐ **CORNERSTONE HOSPITAL OF AUSTIN (452034)**, 4207 Burnet Road, Zip 78756–3396; tel. 512/706–1900, (Includes CORNERSTONE HOSPITAL OF AUSTIN, 1005 East 32nd Street, Zip 78705; tel. 512/867–5822; Edward J. Sherwood, M.D., Chief Executive Officer; CORNERSTONE HOSPITAL OF AUSTIN, 12221 North Mopac Expressway, Zip 78758; tel. 512/901–6431; Edward J. Sherwood, M.D., Chief Executive Officer) **A**1 9 10 **F**1 3 25 26 73 75 93 110 119 132 **S** Cornerstone Healthcare Group
Primary Contact: Mary Ann Lee, Chief Executive Officer
CFO: Gregory Taylor, Chief Financial Officer
CMO: David Pohl, M.D., Chief of Staff
Web address: www.cornerstonehealthcaregroup.com
Control: Corporation, Investor–owned, for–profit **Service:** Long–Term Acute Care hospital

Staffed Beds: 95 **Admissions:** 966 **Census:** 70 **Outpatient Visits:** 0 **Births:** 0 **Total Expense ($000):** 33056 **Payroll Expense ($000):** 11446 **Personnel:** 199

★ **DELL CHILDREN'S MEDICAL CENTER OF CENTRAL TEXAS (453310)**, (Formerly Children's Hospital of Austin), (Pediatric), 4900 Mueller Boulevard, Zip 78723; tel. 512/324–0000 **A**1 2 3 5 9 10 **F**3 11 19 21 23 25 26 27 28 30 31 32 33 37 38 41 43 44 49 50 53 56 57 58 60 62 63 65 66 69 70 72 73 75 76 77 79 80 81 82 83 84 86 92 96 100 102 103 107 118 119 120 124 132 133 135 137 **P**8 **S** Ascension Health
Primary Contact: Robert I. Bonar, Jr., President and Chief Executive Officer
Web address: www.dellchildrens.net
Control: Church–operated, Nongovernment, not–for profit **Service:** Children's other specialty

Staffed Beds: 168 **Admissions:** 6 **Census:** 118 **Outpatient Visits:** 49 **Births:** 0 **Total Expense ($000):** 7664 **Payroll Expense ($000):** 1461 **Personnel:** 993

★ **HEALTHSOUTH REHABILITATION HOSPITAL OF AUSTIN (453044)**, 1215 Red River Street, Zip 78701–1921; tel. 512/474–5700 **A**1 9 10 **F**25 26 30 31 32 54 61 62 72 73 75 77 81 82 85 86 121 132 137 **S** HEALTHSOUTH Corporation
Primary Contact: Robert A. Prehn, Ph.D., Chief Executive Officer
COO: Lisa Kunz, Chief Operating Officer and Chief Nursing Officer
CFO: Pamela McLaughlin, Chief Financial Officer
CMO: Elena Arizmendez, Executive Medical Director
CHR: Denise Spear, Interim Director Human Resources
Web address: www.healthsouthaustin.com
Control: Corporation, Investor–owned, for–profit **Service:** Rehabilitation

Staffed Beds: 50 **Admissions:** 1256 **Census:** 48 **Outpatient Visits:** 22284 **Births:** 0 **Total Expense ($000):** 16853 **Payroll Expense ($000):** 9660 **Personnel:** 205

☐ **HEART HOSPITAL OF AUSTIN (450824)**, 3801 North Lamar Boulevard, Zip 78756; tel. 512/407–7000 **A**1 9 10 **F**3 17 18 20 22 25 26 30 31 32 33 38 56 79 81 82 96 97 98 103 107 118 119 121 124 135 137 **S** MedCath, Inc.
Primary Contact: David Laird, President
COO: Monica A. Figun, Vice President Clinical Services
CFO: Michelle Hays, Chief Financial Officer
CHR: Amy Reeves, Human Resources Team Leader
Web address: www.hearthospitalofaustin.com
Control: Partnership, Investor–owned, for–profit **Service:** General Medical and Surgical

Staffed Beds: 58 **Admissions:** 3054 **Census:** 30 **Outpatient Visits:** 13664 **Births:** 0 **Total Expense ($000):** 67678 **Payroll Expense ($000):** 18299 **Personnel:** 296

★ **SETON MEDICAL CENTER (450056)**, 1201 West 38th Street, Zip 78705–1056; tel. 512/324–1000, (Total facility includes 26 beds in nursing home–type unit) **A**1 2 9 10 **F**3 11 12 13 15 18 20 22 24 25 26 27 30 31 32 33 35 38 40 41 43 44 46 50 52 53 55 57 58 60 62 66 68 70 72 73 74 75 76 77 79 80 81 82 86 92 96 97 100 102 103 107 117 118 119 120 121 124 126 133 135 137 **P**8 **S** Ascension Health
Primary Contact: John C. Brindley, President and Chief Executive Officer
Primary Contact: Charlotte ThrasherChief Operating Officer and Administrator
COO: Charlotte Thrasher, Chief Operating Officer and Administrator
CFO: Douglas D. Waite, Chief Financial Officer
CMO: Frank Mazza, M.D., Vice President Medical Affairs
CIO: Gerry Lewis, Chief Information Officer
CHR: Trennis Jones, Vice President Human Resources
Web address: www.seton.net
Control: Church–operated, Nongovernment, not–for profit **Service:** General Medical and Surgical

Staffed Beds: 455 **Admissions:** 24288 **Census:** 330 **Outpatient Visits:** 196958 **Births:** 4687 **Total Expense ($000):** 482271 **Payroll Expense ($000):** 188028 **Personnel:** 3301

★ **SETON NORTHWEST HOSPITAL (450867)**, 11113 Research Boulevard, Zip 78759–7513; tel. 512/324–6000 **A**1 2 9 **F**3 11 13 15 25 26 30 31 32 33 34 35 38 41 50 55 56 57 62 66 68 71 72 73 74 75 76 77 79 80 81 82 86 92 96 100 102 107 118 119 120 121 124 135 137 **P**8 **S** Ascension Health
Primary Contact: Charles E. Durant, Jr., FACHE, Administrator
Web address: www.seton.net
Control: Church–operated, Nongovernment, not–for profit **Service:** General Medical and Surgical

Staffed Beds: 124 **Admissions:** 6936 **Census:** 60 **Outpatient Visits:** 74362 **Births:** 1939 **Total Expense ($000):** 71549 **Payroll Expense ($000):** 27346 **Personnel:** 484

★ **SETON SHOAL CREEK HOSPITAL (454029)**, 3501 Mills Avenue, Zip 78731–6391; tel. 512/324–2000 **A**1 9 10 **F**4 5 25 26 30 31 32 56 66 81 82 88 89 90 91 93 94 119 121 124 **P**8 **S** Ascension Health
Primary Contact: Alan Isaacson, Vice President and Chief Operating Officer
COO: Alan Isaacson, Vice President and Chief Operating Officer
CFO: Douglas D. Waite, Chief Financial Officer
CMO: Paul Whitelock, M.D., Medical Director
CIO: Gerry Lewis, Chief Information Officer
CHR: Tom Wilken, Vice President Human Resources
Web address: www.seton.net
Control: Church–operated, Nongovernment, not–for profit **Service:** Psychiatric

Staffed Beds: 89 **Admissions:** 3575 **Census:** 49 **Outpatient Visits:** 21417 **Births:** 0 **Total Expense ($000):** 16733 **Payroll Expense ($000):** 8494 **Personnel:** 177

★ **SETON SOUTHWEST HEALTHCARE CENTER (450865)**, 7900 F. M. 1826, Zip 78737; tel. 512/324–9000 **A**1 9 10 **F**3 11 13 15 25 26 30 31 32 33 34 38 50 55 57 62 66 69 73 74 75 77 79 80 81 82 86 92 96 102 107 118 119 120 121 124 135 **P**8 **S** Ascension Health
Primary Contact: Maria Faria, FACHE, Administrator
Web address: www.seton.net
Control: Church–operated, Nongovernment, not–for profit **Service:** General Medical and Surgical

Staffed Beds: 17 **Admissions:** 1368 **Census:** 9 **Outpatient Visits:** 34804 **Births:** 754 **Total Expense ($000):** 23217 **Payroll Expense ($000):** 9727 **Personnel:** 176

★ **ST. DAVID'S MEDICAL CENTER (450431)**, 919 East 32nd Street, Zip 78705–2709, Mailing Address: P.O. Box 4039, Zip 78765–4039; tel. 512/476–7111 **A**1 2 9 10 **F**3 8 11 12 13 15 17 18 20 22 24 25 26 27 30 31 32 33 35 37 38 40 52 54 55 56 57 60 62 68 70 71 72 73 74 75 76 77 79 80 81 82 84 85 86 96 97 99 100 102 103 107 112 116 118 119 121 134 135 136 137 **S** HCA
Primary Contact: C. David Huffstutler, President
COO: Jeanne Nagy, Chief Operating Officer
CFO: Cindy Brouillette, Chief Financial Officer
CMO: John Marietta, M.D., Chief Medical Officer
CIO: Debi Castelberry, Director Information System
CHR: De De Juel, Director Human Resources
Web address: www.stdavids.com
Control: Other not–for–profit (including NFP Corporation) **Service:** General Medical and Surgical

Staffed Beds: 326 **Admissions:** 15853 **Census:** 240 **Outpatient Visits:** 101831 **Births:** 4834 **Total Expense ($000):** 207329 **Payroll Expense ($000):** 76995 **Personnel:** 1243

TX

Hospital, Medicare Provider Number, Address, Telephone, Approval, Facility, and Physician Codes, Health Care System

★ American Hospital Association (AHA) membership
☐ The Joint Commission accreditation
○ American Osteopathic Association (AOA) accreditation
△ Commission on Accreditation of Rehabilitation Facilities (CARF) accreditation

★ **ST. DAVID'S NORTH AUSTIN MEDICAL CENTER (450809)**, 12221 MoPac Expressway North, Zip 78758–2496; tel. 512/901–1000 **A**1 9 10 **F**3 11 13 15 17 18 20 22 24 25 26 27 30 31 32 33 35 37 38 43 47 49 52 53 54 55 56 57 62 68 70 71 72 73 74 75 76 77 79 80 81 82 84 85 86 96 97 100 102 106 107 116 118 119 120 121 127 134 135 136 137 **P**7 **S** HCA
Primary Contact: Donald H. Wilkerson, Chief Executive Officer
COO: Sheri Dube, Chief Operating Officer
CFO: Cindy Sexton, Chief Financial Officer
CMO: Kenneth W. Mitchell, M.D., Medical Director
CIO: Marshall Pearson, Director Management Information Systems
Web address: www.northaustin.com
Control: Other not–for–profit (including NFP Corporation) **Service:** General Medical and Surgical

Staffed Beds: 228 **Admissions:** 12665 **Census:** 176 **Outpatient Visits:** 96830 **Births:** 3595 **Total Expense ($000):** 155263 **Payroll Expense ($000):** 54479 **Personnel:** 1034

★ **ST. DAVID'S REHABILITATION CENTER (453038)**, 1005 East 32nd Street, Zip 78705–2705, Mailing Address: P.O. Box 4270, Zip 78765–4270; tel. 512/867–5100 **A**1 9 10 **F**25 26 30 31 32 33 34 85 86 **S** HCA
Primary Contact: Diane Owens, Administrator
COO: Richard A. Hammett, Chief Operating Officer
CFO: Cindy Brouillette, Chief Financial Officer
CMO: John Marietta, M.D., Chief Medical Officer
CIO: Debi Castelberry, Director Information System
CHR: De De Juel, Director Human Resources
Web address: www.stdavids.com
Control: Other not–for–profit (including NFP Corporation) **Service:** Rehabilitation

Staffed Beds: 62 **Admissions:** 1313 **Census:** 52 **Outpatient Visits:** 42749 **Births:** 0 **Total Expense ($000):** 19688 **Payroll Expense ($000):** 10999 **Personnel:** 175

★ **ST. DAVID'S SOUTH AUSTIN HOSPITAL (450713)**, (Formerly South Austin Hospital), 901 West Ben White Boulevard, Zip 78704–6903; tel. 512/447–2211 **A**1 2 9 10 **F**3 11 13 15 17 18 20 22 24 25 26 27 30 31 32 33 36 38 43 49 53 54 55 56 57 62 67 68 71 72 73 74 75 76 77 79 80 82 86 96 97 100 102 103 106 107 118 119 121 135 136 137 **S** HCA
Primary Contact: Erol R. Akdamar, Chief Executive Officer
COO: Brett Matens, Chief Operating Officer
CFO: Wesley D. Fountain, Chief Financial Officer
CMO: Albert Goros, Chief Medical Officer
CIO: Richard Lear, Director
CHR: Lisa Talbot, Director Human Resources
Web address: www.southaustinhospital.com
Control: Other not–for–profit (including NFP Corporation) **Service:** General Medical and Surgical

Staffed Beds: 222 **Admissions:** 12853 **Census:** 168 **Outpatient Visits:** 94021 **Births:** 1406 **Total Expense ($000):** 131291 **Payroll Expense ($000):** 46600 **Personnel:** 930

TX

★ **SURGICAL HOSPITAL OF AUSTIN (450808)**, (Formerly HEALTHSOUTH Surgical Hospital of Austin), 6818 Austin Center Boulevard, Zip 78731–3165; tel. 512/346–1994 **A**1 9 10 **F**38 62 77 79
Primary Contact: Shane Schweda, Administrator
Web address: www.healthsouth.com
Control: Partnership, Investor–owned, for–profit **Service:** General Medical and Surgical

Staffed Beds: 8 **Admissions:** 566 **Census:** 2 **Outpatient Visits:** 4960 **Births:** 0 **Total Expense ($000):** 12837 **Payroll Expense ($000):** 2917 **Personnel:** 62

☐ △ **TEXAS NEUROREHAB CENTER (452038)**, 1106 West Dittmar, Zip 78745–6388, Mailing Address: P.O. Box 150459, Zip 78715–0459; tel. 512/444–4835 **A**1 7 9 10 **F**1 10 25 40 72 73 77 97 119 137 **P**5 **S** Psychiatric Solutions
Primary Contact: Edgar E. Prettyman, XPsyD, Chief Executive Officer
CFO: Omar Correa, Chief Financial Officer
CMO: Nancy Childs, M.D., Executive Medical Director
CHR: Peggy Mason, Director Human Resources
Web address: www.psysolutions.com
Control: Partnership, Investor–owned, for–profit **Service:** Long–Term Acute Care hospital

Staffed Beds: 47 **Admissions:** 454 **Census:** 39 **Outpatient Visits:** 0 **Births:** 0 **Total Expense ($000):** 12154 **Payroll Expense ($000):** 6981 **Personnel:** 290

THE HOSPITAL AT WESTLAKE MEDICAL CENTER (670006), 5656 Bee Caves Road, Zip 78746; tel. 512/327–0000 **A**10 **F**3 18 20 22 24 25 37 38 43 52 58 62 66 68 73 75 77 79 80 86 96 100 102 107 116 118 119 120 137
Primary Contact: Rip Miller, Chief Executive Officer
CFO: Julie Churchill, Director Financial Services
CMO: Tom Burns, Chief of Staff
CHR: Kellie Bryson, Director Human Resources
Web address: www.westlakemedical.com
Control: Partnership, Investor–owned, for–profit **Service:** General Medical and Surgical

Staffed Beds: 23 **Admissions:** 1550 **Census:** 10 **Outpatient Visits:** 8319 **Births:** 0 **Total Expense ($000):** 28396 **Payroll Expense ($000):** 9627 **Personnel:** 146

★ **UNIVERSITY MEDICAL CENTER AT BRACKENRIDGE (450124)**, (Formerly Brackenridge Hospital), 601 East 15th Street, Zip 78701–1996; tel. 512/324–7000 **A**1 2 9 10 **F**3 11 13 15 18 19 20 21 22 23 25 26 27 28 30 31 32 33 37 38 40 41 43 44 49 50 55 56 57 58 60 62 63 64 66 68 69 70 72 73 74 75 76 77 79 80 81 82 83 84 86 87 90 92 94 96 97 100 102 103 107 114 118 119 121 124 133 135 137 **P**8 **S** Ascension Health
Primary Contact: Jesus Garza, President and Chief Executive Officer
COO: Bruce Broslat, Vice President and Chief Operating Officer
CFO: Douglas D. Waite, Chief Financial Officer
CMO: Jim Lindsey, M.D., Senior Vice President Medical Affairs
CIO: Gerry Lewis, Chief Information Officer
CHR: Trennis Jones, Vice President Human Resources
Web address: www.seton.net
Control: Church–operated, Nongovernment, not–for profit **Service:** General Medical and Surgical

Staffed Beds: 372 **Admissions:** 21193 **Census:** 262 **Outpatient Visits:** 303075 **Births:** 2649 **Total Expense ($000):** 402977 **Payroll Expense ($000):** 143139 **Personnel:** 1904

AZLE—Tarrant County

★ **TEXAS HEALTH HARRIS METHODIST NORTHWEST (450419)**, (Formerly Harris Methodist Northwest), 108 Denver Trail, Zip 76020–3697; tel. 817/444–8600 **A**1 9 10 **F**3 11 15 25 26 30 31 32 33 38 42 43 55 56 57 62 63 68 73 75 77 79 80 86 96 99 102 107 119 120 124 135 136 137 **S** Texas Health Resources
Primary Contact: Winjie Tang Miao, President
CFO: Brian Blessing, Chief Financial Officer
CMO: Shawn Davis, Chief of Staff
CIO: Edward Marx, Vice President and Chief Information Officer
CHR: Jan Flavin, Manager Human Resources
Web address: www.harrismethodisthospitals.org
Control: Other not–for–profit (including NFP Corporation) **Service:** General Medical and Surgical

Staffed Beds: 31 **Admissions:** 1375 **Census:** 13 **Outpatient Visits:** 29921 **Births:** 0 **Total Expense ($000):** 22810 **Payroll Expense ($000):** 10175 **Personnel:** 170

BALLINGER—Runnels County

BALLINGER MEMORIAL HOSPITAL (451310), 608 Avenue B, Zip 76821–2499, Mailing Address: P.O. Box 617, Zip 76821–0617; tel. 325/365–2531 **A**9 10 18 **F**3 7 11 24 30 31 32 38 40 52 53 54 55 57 60 62 63 66 73 75 82 86 91 93 94 96 119 122 132 137 **P**5
Primary Contact: Lance W. Keilers, Administrator
Web address: www.ballingerhospital.org
Control: Hospital district or authority, Government, nonfederal **Service:** General Medical and Surgical

Staffed Beds: 16 **Admissions:** 221 **Census:** 3 **Outpatient Visits:** 18611 **Births:** 0 **Total Expense ($000):** 4800 **Payroll Expense ($000):** 2087 **Personnel:** 67

BASTROP—Bastrop County

☐ **LAKESIDE HOSPITAL AT BASTROP (670011)**, 3201 Highway 71 East, Zip 78602; tel. 512/321–8200 **A**1 9 **F**3 25 30 31 32 38 43 79 80 96 102 107 135 **P**5
Primary Contact: Johnny L. Burns, Interim Chief Executive Officer
CFO: Richard Barnes, Chief Financial Officer
CHR: Carole Richards, Director Human Resources
Web address: www.lakesidehospital.net
Control: Partnership, Investor–owned, for–profit **Service:** General Medical and Surgical

Staffed Beds: 15 **Admissions:** 813 **Census:** 7 **Outpatient Visits:** 12254 **Births:** 0 **Total Expense ($000):** 11917 **Payroll Expense ($000):** 3816 **Personnel:** 76

BAY CITY—Matagorda County

★ **MATAGORDA COUNTY HOSPITAL DISTRICT (450465)**, (Formerly Matagorda General Hospital), 1115 Avenue G, Zip 77414–3544; tel. 979/245–6383 **A**1 9 10 20 **F**3 11 13 15 24 25 26 28 30 31 32 34 36 37 38 40 43 45 52 54 55 57 62 63 64 68 73 74 75 77 79 80 81 84 86 88 93 96 97 100 102 103 107 111 119 121 124 135 136 137 **S** QHR
Primary Contact: Daryle Voss, Chief Executive Officer
CFO: Bryan Prochnow, Chief Financial Officer
CMO: Moses E. Wilcox, Chief of Staff
CIO: Mary Ann Cervantes, District Director Management Information Systems
CHR: Cindy Krebs, District Director Human Resources
Web address: www.matagordageneral.org
Control: Hospital district or authority, Government, nonfederal **Service:** General Medical and Surgical

Staffed Beds: 60 **Admissions:** 2224 **Census:** 25 **Outpatient Visits:** 31772 **Births:** 311 **Total Expense ($000):** 32759 **Payroll Expense ($000):** 13577 **Personnel:** 236

Many Facility Codes have changed. Please refer to the AHA Guide Code Chart.

BAYTOWN—Harris County

▣ **SAN JACINTO METHODIST HOSPITAL (450424)**, 4401 Garth Road, Zip 77521–3160; tel. 281/420–8600, (Includes SAN JACINTO METHODIST HOSPITAL – ALEXANDER, 1700 James Bowie Drive, Zip 77520–3386; tel. 281/420–6100), (Total facility includes 30 beds in nursing home–type unit) **A**1 2 9 10 **F**3 8 12 13 15 18 20 24 25 26 27 30 31 32 33 36 37 38 41 43 48 49 54 55 56 57 60 62 63 68 71 72 73 74 75 76 77 79 80 81 82 85 86 87 88 91 92 93 95 96 97 100 102 107 109 111 117 119 121 134 135 137 **P**3 **S** The Methodist Hospital System
Primary Contact: Donna Gares, RN, Interim President and Chief Executive Officer
CFO: Jonathan Sturgis, Chief Financial Officer
CMO: Bruce Kennedy, M.D., Chief Medical Officer
CHR: Sherri Davis–Sampson, Director Human Resources
Web address: www.methodisthealth.com
Control: Other not–for–profit (including NFP Corporation) **Service:** General Medical and Surgical

Staffed Beds: 268 **Admissions:** 14684 **Census:** 190 **Outpatient Visits:** 162212 **Births:** 1738 **Total Expense ($000):** 172593 **Payroll Expense ($000):** 82445 **Personnel:** 1602

BEAUMONT—Jefferson County

BEAUMONT BONE AND JOINT INSTITUTE (670007), 3650 Laurel Street, Zip 77707; tel. 409/838–0346 **A**9 10 **F**3 38 77 79 119 120 125 130
Primary Contact: Duane N. Hill, Chief Executive Officer
Web address: www.orthodoc.aaos.org/bbji/
Control: Partnership, Investor–owned, for–profit **Service:** General Medical and Surgical

Staffed Beds: 6 **Admissions:** 10 **Census:** 1 **Outpatient Visits:** 4951 **Births:** 0 **Personnel:** 42

▣ **CHRISTUS HOSPITAL–ST. ELIZABETH (450034)**, 2830 Calder Avenue, Zip 77702–1809, Mailing Address: P.O. Box 5405, Zip 77726–5405; tel. 409/892–7171 **A**1 2 9 10 **F**3 11 13 15 17 18 20 22 24 25 26 30 31 32 33 34 36 38 40 41 43 45 49 50 51 52 53 55 56 57 59 62 68 70 72 73 74 75 77 79 80 81 82 83 84 86 96 97 100 102 106 107 112 118 119 121 133 135 136 137 **P**8 **S** CHRISTUS Health
Primary Contact: Ellen M. Jones, President and Chief Executive Officer
COO: Mario A. Mudano, Administrator
CFO: Bill Hecht, Chief Financial Officer
CMO: Rick Tyler, M.D., Vice President Medical Affairs
CIO: Robert Jacobs, Regional Director Information Management
CHR: Charles Foster, Regional Director Human Resources
Web address: www.christushospital.org
Control: Church–operated, Nongovernment, not–for profit **Service:** General Medical and Surgical

Staffed Beds: 610 **Admissions:** 24172 **Census:** 306 **Outpatient Visits:** 294650 **Births:** 2267 **Total Expense ($000):** 282476 **Payroll Expense ($000):** 118073 **Personnel:** 2164

▣ **DUBUIS HOSPITAL OF BEAUMONT (452042)**, 2830 Calder Avenue, 4th Floor, Zip 77702; tel. 409/899–8154 **A**1 9 10 **F**1 3 25 26 27 30 31 32 119 137 **P**5 **S** Dubuis Health System
Primary Contact: Barbara Flournoy, Administrator
Web address: www.dubuis.org
Control: Church–operated, Nongovernment, not–for profit **Service:** Long–Term Acute Care hospital

Staffed Beds: 51 **Admissions:** 508 **Census:** 36 **Outpatient Visits:** 0 **Births:** 0 **Total Expense ($000):** 15413 **Payroll Expense ($000):** 5292 **Personnel:** 143

▣ **HEALTHSOUTH REHABILITATION HOSPITAL OF BEAUMONT (453048)**, 3340 Plaza 10 Boulevard, Zip 77707–2551; tel. 409/835–0835 **A**1 9 10 **F**3 24 25 26 30 31 32 61 62 72 73 75 77 82 85 86 118 119 120 121 135 137 **S** HEALTHSOUTH Corporation
Primary Contact: Bill Klamforth, Chief Executive Officer
CFO: Lynn Webb, Chief Financial Officer
Web address: www.healthsouth.com
Control: Corporation, Investor–owned, for–profit **Service:** Rehabilitation

Staffed Beds: 61 **Admissions:** 910 **Census:** 33 **Outpatient Visits:** 9839 **Births:** 0 **Total Expense ($000):** 20081 **Payroll Expense ($000):** 5273 **Personnel:** 108

▣ **MEMORIAL HERMANN BAPTIST BEAUMONT HOSPITAL (450346)**, 3080 College Street, Zip 77701–4689, Mailing Address: P.O. Box 1591, Zip 77704–1591; tel. 409/212–5000, (Includes MEMORIAL HERMANN BAPTIST FANNIN BEHAVIORAL HEALTH CENTER, 3250 Fannin Street, Zip 77701; tel. 409/212–7000) **A**1 9 10 **F**3 4 5 11 13 15 17 18 20 22 24 25 26 27 31 32 33 37 38 46 49 55 57 59 62 68 70 71 72 73 74 76 77 79 80 81 82 83 84 85 86 88 89 91 92 93 94 95 96 97 99 100 102 106 107 109 111 119 121 124 133 135 136 **S** Community Hospital Corporation
Primary Contact: David N. Parmer, President and Chief Executive Officer
COO: Guy Giesecke, Chief Operating Officer
CFO: Gary Troutman, CPA, Chief Financial Officer
CIO: Mark Henderson, Chief Information Officer
CHR: April Seymour, Manager Human Resources
Web address: www.mhbh.org
Control: Other not–for–profit (including NFP Corporation) **Service:** General Medical and Surgical

Staffed Beds: 408 **Admissions:** 16301 **Census:** 223 **Outpatient Visits:** 107993 **Births:** 1497 **Total Expense ($000):** 154035 **Payroll Expense ($000):** 59671 **Personnel:** 1237

BEDFORD—Tarrant County

▣ **TEXAS HEALTH HARRIS METHODIST–HEB (450639)**, (Formerly Harris Methodist–HEB), 1600 Hospital Parkway, Zip 76022–6913, Mailing Address: P.O. Box 669, Zip 76095–0669; tel. 817/685–4000, (Includes HARRIS METHODIST–SPRINGWOOD, 1608 Hospital Parkway, Zip 76022; tel. 817/355–7700) **A**1 9 10 **F**11 12 13 15 18 20 22 24 25 26 30 31 32 33 38 43 44 45 47 49 52 59 62 68 69 70 73 74 75 76 78 79 81 82 85 86 96 97 102 106 107 118 119 120 121 124 135 136 137 **S** Texas Health Resources
Primary Contact: Deborah Paganelli, CHE, President
COO: Alice Landers, Administrative Director Operations
CFO: Shelly Miland, Chief Financial Officer and Vice President Finance
CMO: Bob Nowland, M.D., Chief of Staff
CHR: Dale Smith, Director Human Resources
Web address: www.texashealth.org
Control: Other not–for–profit (including NFP Corporation) **Service:** General Medical and Surgical

Staffed Beds: 228 **Admissions:** 12779 **Census:** 154 **Outpatient Visits:** 100209 **Births:** 1989 **Total Expense ($000):** 178274 **Payroll Expense ($000):** 77313 **Personnel:** 1195

BEEVILLE—Bee County

▣ **CHRISTUS SPOHN HOSPITAL BEEVILLE (450082)**, 1500 East Houston Street, Zip 78102–5312; tel. 361/354–2000 **A**1 9 10 20 **F**3 11 13 15 25 26 30 31 32 33 38 40 46 50 52 55 56 57 62 68 73 74 75 77 79 80 81 82 86 87 96 97 100 102 107 119 135 136 137 **P**7 8 **S** CHRISTUS Health
Primary Contact: Jerry Rodriguez, Vice President and Chief Operating Officer
COO: Jerry Rodriguez, Vice President and Chief Operating Officer
Web address: www.christusspohn.org
Control: Church–operated, Nongovernment, not–for profit **Service:** General Medical and Surgical

Staffed Beds: 63 **Admissions:** 2583 **Census:** 21 **Outpatient Visits:** 36345 **Births:** 390 **Total Expense ($000):** 23888 **Payroll Expense ($000):** 11338 **Personnel:** 196

BELLAIRE—Harris County

FOUNDATION SURGICAL HOSPITAL (670012), 5410 West Loop South, Zip 77401; tel. 713/314–4500 **A**10 **F**3 8 25 30 31 32 35 38 55 57 58 62 63 72 75 77 79 80 81 82 86 96 100 102 119 120 **P**2
Primary Contact: Louisa F. Adelung, Chief Executive Officer
CMO: L V Ansell, Medical Director
Web address: www.foundationsurgicalhospital.com
Control: Partnership, Investor–owned, for–profit **Service:** General Medical and Surgical

Staffed Beds: 64 **Admissions:** 2365 **Census:** 14 **Outpatient Visits:** 2008 **Births:** 0 **Total Expense ($000):** 49665 **Payroll Expense ($000):** 10175 **Personnel:** 161

TX

Hospital, Medicare Provider Number, Address, Telephone, Approval, Facility, and Physician Codes, Health Care System

★ American Hospital Association (AHA) membership
□ The Joint Commission accreditation
○ American Osteopathic Association (AOA) accreditation
△ Commission on Accreditation of Rehabilitation Facilities (CARF) accreditation

BELLVILLE—Austin County

★ **BELLVILLE GENERAL HOSPITAL (450253)**, 44 North Cummings Street, Zip 77418–1347; tel. 979/865–3141 **A**1 9 10 **F**3 11 15 25 30 31 32 38 40 50 55 57 62 63 66 73 78 79 96 100 102 107 122 135
Primary Contact: Michael Morris, Administrator
CFO: Stacy Muehlbrad, Chief Financial Officer
CMO: Christophe Gay, M.D., Chief of Staff
CHR: Jacquiline McEwen, Coordinator Human Resources
Web address: www.bellvillehospital.com
Control: Hospital district or authority, Government, nonfederal **Service:** General Medical and Surgical

Staffed Beds: 25 **Admissions:** 728 **Census:** 8 **Outpatient Visits:** 62746 **Births:** 0 **Total Expense ($000):** 7649 **Payroll Expense ($000):** 3809 **Personnel:** 94

BIG LAKE—Reagan County

★ **REAGAN MEMORIAL HOSPITAL (451301)**, 805 North Main Street, Zip 76932–3999; tel. 325/884–2561 **A**9 10 18 **F**3 38 40 52 55 86 122 **P**5
Primary Contact: Sidney Tucker, Administrator
CMO: Joseph Sudolcan, Medical Director
Control: Hospital district or authority, Government, nonfederal **Service:** General Medical and Surgical

Staffed Beds: 14 **Admissions:** 21 **Census:** 1 **Outpatient Visits:** 3310 **Births:** 1 **Total Expense ($000):** 2357 **Payroll Expense ($000):** 701 **Personnel:** 30

BIG SPRING—Howard County

☐ **BIG SPRING STATE HOSPITAL (454000)**, 1901 North Highway 87, Zip 79720; tel. 432/267–8216 **A**1 10 **F**26 30 31 32 38 54 66 73 75 81 82 87 88 91 92 93 119 124 135 **P**6 **S** Texas Department of State Health Services
Primary Contact: Edward Moughon, Superintendent
CFO: Adrienne Suazo, Assistant Chief Financial Officer and Budget Analyst
CIO: Connie Edgemon, Director Information Management
CHR: Jok Simons, Assistant Superintendent
Web address: www.dshs.state.tx.us/mhhospitals/bigspringSH/bigspringsh.html
Control: State–Government, nonfederal **Service:** Psychiatric

Staffed Beds: 200 **Admissions:** 1098 **Census:** 187 **Outpatient Visits:** 1136 **Births:** 0 **Total Expense ($000):** 35329 **Payroll Expense ($000):** 19780 **Personnel:** 569

★ **SCENIC MOUNTAIN MEDICAL CENTER (450653)**, 1601 West 11th Place, Zip 79720–4198; tel. 432/263–1211 **A**1 9 10 20 **F**11 13 15 18 25 26 31 32 38 40 54 55 56 57 62 63 67 68 73 74 75 77 79 82 84 86 88 93 96 100 102 107 119 122 135 136 137 **P**6 **S** Community Health Systems, Inc.
Primary Contact: George N. Parsley, Chief Executive Officer
Web address: www.smmccares.com
Control: Corporation, Investor–owned, for–profit **Service:** General Medical and Surgical

Staffed Beds: 122 **Admissions:** 3435 **Census:** 33 **Outpatient Visits:** 36261 **Births:** 311 **Total Expense ($000):** 38781 **Payroll Expense ($000):** 14451 **Personnel:** 259

★ **WEST TEXAS VA HEALTH CARE SYSTEM**, 300 Veterans Boulevard, Zip 79720–5500; tel. 432/263–7361, (Total facility includes 40 beds in nursing home–type unit) (Nonreporting) **A**1 3 5 9 **S** Department of Veterans Affairs
Primary Contact: Michael L. Bell, Director
CFO: Billy Sullivan, Chief Fiscal Service
CMO: Wilfredo Rodriguez, M.D., Chief of Staff
CIO: Mike McKinley, Information Security Officer
CHR: Patricia Frausto, Chief Human Resources Management Service
Web address: www.va.gov/sta/guide/home.asp
Control: Veterans Affairs, Government, federal **Service:** General Medical and Surgical

Staffed Beds: 189

BONHAM—Fannin County

☐ **RED RIVER REGIONAL HOSPITAL (451370)**, 504 Lipscomb Boulevard, Zip 75418–4096, Mailing Address: P.O. Drawer C, Zip 75418–4096; tel. 903/583–8585 **A**1 9 10 18 **F**3 11 15 17 24 25 26 30 31 32 33 38 46 50 55 56 57 62 63 73 79 82 86 96 97 99 100 106 107 119 122 124 135
Primary Contact: David Conejo, Chief Executive Officer
CFO: Jerry Panter, Chief Financial Officer
CHR: Brenda Bagley, Director Human Resources
Control: Partnership, Investor–owned, for–profit **Service:** General Medical and Surgical

Staffed Beds: 25 **Admissions:** 1247 **Census:** 12 **Outpatient Visits:** 11654 **Births:** 0 **Total Expense ($000):** 13371 **Payroll Expense ($000):** 5615 **Personnel:** 129

SAM RAYBURN MEMORIAL VETERANS CENTER See Veterans Affairs North Texas Health Care System, Dallas

BORGER—Hutchinson County

★ **GOLDEN PLAINS COMMUNITY HOSPITAL (451369)**, 200 South McGee Street, Zip 79007–0495; tel. 806/273–1100 **A**1 9 10 18 **F**7 11 13 15 25 26 28 30 31 32 33 38 40 43 50 53 55 56 61 62 63 64 66 68 73 74 75 77 79 80 81 82 84 86 96 97 102 107 119 120 122 135 136 137
Primary Contact: Charles R. Slaton, President and Chief Operating Officer
COO: Melody Henderson, R.N., Ph.D., CHE, Chief Operating Officer and Chief Nursing Officer
CMO: Wallace Mann, M.D., Chief of Staff
CHR: Kelly McDonald, Human Resource Director
Web address: www.goldenplains.org
Control: Hospital district or authority, Government, nonfederal **Service:** General Medical and Surgical

Staffed Beds: 25 **Admissions:** 1100 **Census:** 8 **Outpatient Visits:** 32787 **Births:** 211 **Total Expense ($000):** 11140 **Payroll Expense ($000):** 6553 **Personnel:** 187

BOWIE—Montague County

★ **BOWIE MEMORIAL HOSPITAL (450497)**, 705 East Greenwood Avenue, Zip 76230–3199; tel. 940/872–1126 **A**9 10 **F**3 10 11 15 24 25 30 31 32 38 40 42 43 44 52 55 61 62 68 73 75 79 86 93 96 103 107 118 119 120 121 122 137 **P**4
Primary Contact: Joyce Crumpler, RN, Administrator and Chief Executive Officer
CFO: T. Kim Lee, CPA, Chief Financial Officer
CMO: Mark Jenkins, Chief of Staff
CIO: Tiffany Egenbacher, Director Data Processing
CHR: Mary Bates, Director Human Resources
Control: Hospital district or authority, Government, nonfederal **Service:** General Medical and Surgical

Staffed Beds: 44 **Admissions:** 1356 **Census:** 15 **Outpatient Visits:** 32510 **Births:** 0 **Total Expense ($000):** 12792 **Payroll Expense ($000):** 6278 **Personnel:** 186

BRADY—McCulloch County

HEART OF TEXAS MEMORIAL HOSPITAL (451348), 2008 Nine Road, Zip 76825–1150, Mailing Address: P.O. Box 1150, Zip 76825–1150; tel. 325/597–2901 **A**9 10 18 **F**11 15 24 38 40 52 55 79 86 95 102 107 118 122 **P**4
Primary Contact: Tim Jones, Interim Chief Executive Officer
CFO: Brad Burnett, Chief Financial Officer
CMO: Pete Castro, D.O., Chief of Staff
Control: Hospital district or authority, Government, nonfederal **Service:** General Medical and Surgical

Staffed Beds: 25 **Admissions:** 432 **Census:** 5 **Outpatient Visits:** 27665 **Births:** 4 **Total Expense ($000):** 5380 **Payroll Expense ($000):** 2515 **Personnel:** 84

BRECKENRIDGE—Stephens County

STEPHENS MEMORIAL HOSPITAL (450498), 200 South Geneva Street, Zip 76424–4799; tel. 254/559–2241 **A**9 10 20 **F**3 7 8 11 15 24 26 30 31 32 34 38 40 42 43 50 52 54 55 56 57 62 66 67 72 75 76 77 79 80 82 84 86 87 96 100 102 107 118 119 122 124 134 135
Primary Contact: Robbie Dewberry, Administrator and Chief Executive Officer
CFO: Stacy T. Williams, Chief Financial Officer and Director Human Resources
CMO: Ryan Ford, Chief of Staff
CIO: Bobby Thompson, Director Information Technology
CHR: Michelle Funderburg, Director Human Resources
Web address: www.smhtx.com
Control: County–Government, nonfederal **Service:** General Medical and Surgical

Staffed Beds: 33 **Admissions:** 714 **Census:** 10 **Outpatient Visits:** 20295 **Births:** 1 **Total Expense ($000):** 7451 **Payroll Expense ($000):** 3652 **Personnel:** 107

BRENHAM—Washington County

★ **TRINITY COMMUNITY MEDICAL CENTER OF BRENHAM (450187)**, 700 Medical Parkway, Zip 77833–5498; tel. 979/836–6173 **A**1 9 10 **F**3 11 13 25 26 28 30 31 32 33 38 40 41 50 51 52 54 55 56 57 62 63 68 73 74 75 77 79 80 81 82 86 96 97 102 107 118 119 121 122 135 **P**6 **S** Franciscan Services Corporation
Primary Contact: John L. Simms, President and Chief Executive Officer
COO: John L. Simms, President and Chief Executive Officer
CFO: Hank Fender, Chief Financial Officer
CMO: Barry Linden, M.D., Chief of Staff
CIO: Cory Alexander, Director Medical Records and Information Systems
CHR: Debra Makowsky, Director Human Resources
Web address: www.trinitymed.org
Control: Church–operated, Nongovernment, not–for profit **Service:** General Medical and Surgical

Staffed Beds: 60 **Admissions:** 2327 **Census:** 22 **Outpatient Visits:** 51095 **Births:** 415 **Total Expense ($000):** 28920 **Payroll Expense ($000):** 11297 **Personnel:** 252

 Many Facility Codes have changed. Please refer to the AHA Guide Code Chart.

BROWNFIELD—Terry County

★ **BROWNFIELD REGIONAL MEDICAL CENTER (450399)**, 705 East Felt, Zip 79316–3439; tel. 806/637–3551 **A**9 10 20 **F**3 7 13 24 25 26 30 31 32 38 40 50 52 55 56 57 61 62 63 66 73 74 78 79 80 81 82 84 85 86 87 96 107 119 124 137 **P**4
Primary Contact: Mike Click, Administrator
CFO: Cherie Parkhill, Chief Financial Officer
CHR: Avis DePoyster, Director Human Resources
Web address: www.brownfield–rmc.org
Control: Hospital district or authority, Government, nonfederal **Service:** General Medical and Surgical

Staffed Beds: 26 **Admissions:** 1139 **Census:** 9 **Outpatient Visits:** 48387 **Births:** 150 **Total Expense ($000):** 10466 **Payroll Expense ($000):** 4895 **Personnel:** 177

BROWNSVILLE—Cameron County

□ **BROWNSVILLE DOCTORS HOSPITAL (450841)**, 4750 North Expressway, Zip 78526; tel. 956/554–2000 **A**1 10 **F**3 8 15 25 30 31 32 37 38 43 51 55 59 62 66 72 77 79 81 82 84 87 96 99 100 102 103 107 109 112 119 121 123 126 132 134 137 14 24 29 3 30 31 36 37 42 49 52 55 57 65 68 70 72 73 78 87 90 91 92 93 97 **P**2
Primary Contact: Joe Jimenez, Ph.D., Chief Executive Officer
CFO: Jorge Ramirez, Chief Financial Officer
CMO: Manuel G. Guajardo, M.D., Medical Director
CIO: Jorge Ramirez, Chief Financial Officer
CHR: Marcela Mejia, Director Human Resources
Web address: www.brownsvilledoctorshospital.com
Control: Partnership, Investor–owned, for–profit **Service:** Surgical

Staffed Beds: 8 **Admissions:** 567 **Census:** 4 **Outpatient Visits:** 13574 **Births:** 109 **Total Expense ($000):** 16053632 **Payroll Expense ($000):** 7368278 **Personnel:** 147

□ **SOUTH TEXAS REHABILITATION HOSPITAL (453092)**, 425 East Alton Gloor Boulevard, Zip 78526; tel. 956/554–6000 **A**1 9 10 **F**3 25 33 57 62 73 75 81 82 85 86 119 121 **P**6 **S** Ernest Health, Inc.
Primary Contact: Jessie Eason Gonzales, Chief Executive Officer
Web address: www.strh.ernesthealth.com
Control: Partnership, Investor–owned, for–profit **Service:** Rehabilitation

Staffed Beds: 40 **Admissions:** 690 **Census:** 31 **Outpatient Visits:** 3178 **Births:** 0 **Total Expense ($000):** 10405 **Payroll Expense ($000):** 5365 **Personnel:** 120

★□ **VALLEY BAPTIST MEDICAL CENTER–BROWNSVILLE (450028)**, 1040 West Jefferson Street, Zip 78520–5829, Mailing Address: P.O. Box 3590, Zip 78523–3590; tel. 956/698–5400 **A**1 9 10 **F**3 11 13 15 18 20 22 25 26 30 31 32 33 38 40 49 55 57 61 62 68 70 71 72 73 74 75 76 77 79 80 81 82 84 86 90 91 92 93 94 96 97 100 102 106 107 119 135 136 137 **P**8 **S** Valley Baptist Health System
Primary Contact: Leslie Bingham, Senior Vice President and Chief Executive Officer
CFO: Glen Boles, Chief Financial Officer
CIO: Carlos Morales, Data Processing Manager
Web address: www.valleybaptist.net/brownsville/
Control: Other not–for–profit (including NFP Corporation) **Service:** General Medical and Surgical

Staffed Beds: 243 **Admissions:** 10165 **Census:** 140 **Outpatient Visits:** 47761 **Births:** 2382 **Total Expense ($000):** 92843 **Payroll Expense ($000):** 37716 **Personnel:** 741

★□ **VALLEY REGIONAL MEDICAL CENTER (450662)**, 100A Alton Gloor Boulevard, Zip 78526–3346, Mailing Address: P.O. Box 3710, Zip 78521–3710; tel. 956/350–7101 **A**1 9 10 **F**3 11 13 15 18 20 22 23 25 26 28 30 31 32 33 37 38 40 41 43 44 47 49 50 52 55 56 57 59 60 62 63 66 68 70 72 73 74 75 77 79 80 81 82 84 86 96 97 99 100 103 107 119 121 124 132 135 136 137 **P**7 **S** HCA
Primary Contact: David Handley, Chief Executive Officer
COO: Matthew Caldwell, Chief Operating Officer and Chief Nursing Officer
CFO: Marcia Patterson, Chief Financial Officer
CHR: Margie Salazar, Director Human Resources
Web address: www.valleyregionalmedicalcenter.com
Control: Partnership, Investor–owned, for–profit **Service:** General Medical and Surgical

Staffed Beds: 214 **Admissions:** 10512 **Census:** 138 **Outpatient Visits:** 47146 **Births:** 2834 **Total Expense ($000):** 106739 **Payroll Expense ($000):** 42940 **Personnel:** 709

BROWNWOOD—Brown County

★□ **BROWNWOOD REGIONAL MEDICAL CENTER (450587)**, 1501 Burnet Drive, Zip 76801–5933, Mailing Address: P.O. Box 760, Zip 76804–0760; tel. 325/646–8541, (Total facility includes 20 beds in nursing home–type unit) **A**1 9 10 20 **F**3 11 13 15 18 24 25 26 27 30 31 32 33 37 38 43 48 49 50 51 52 53 54 55 57 62 66 68 72 73 74 75 76 77 79 80 81 82 86 87 96 97 100 102 107 109 111 117 118 119 121 135 136 137 **P**3 8 **S** Community Health Systems, Inc.
Primary Contact: Matt T. Maxfield, FACHE, Chief Executive Officer
CFO: John K. Sharp, Chief Financial Officer
CMO: Michael Neel, Chief of Staff
CIO: Paul Ferguson, Director Information Systems
CHR: Mikeana Bailey, Director Human Resources
Web address: www.brmc–cares.com
Control: Partnership, Investor–owned, for–profit **Service:** General Medical and Surgical

Staffed Beds: 168 **Admissions:** 6240 **Census:** 88 **Outpatient Visits:** 65837 **Births:** 721 **Total Expense ($000):** 68096 **Payroll Expense ($000):** 24515 **Personnel:** 480

BRYAN—Brazos County

★□ **ST. JOSEPH REGIONAL HEALTH CENTER (450011)**, 2801 Franciscan Drive, Zip 77802–2599; tel. 979/776–3777, (Total facility includes 15 beds in nursing home–type unit) **A**1 2 3 5 9 10 **F**3 7 11 12 13 15 17 18 20 22 24 25 26 27 28 30 31 32 33 35 38 40 41 46 48 49 50 52 53 55 56 57 62 63 66 68 72 73 74 75 76 77 78 79 80 81 82 84 85 86 88 90 91 93 94 95 96 100 102 106 107 109 111 112 117 118 119 120 121 124 132 135 137 **S** Franciscan Services Corporation
Primary Contact: Anthony D. Pfitzer, FACHE, Chief Executive Officer
CFO: Lisa McNair, Senior Vice President and Chief Financial Officer
CMO: Mark Montgomery, M.D., Vice President Quality and Medical Affairs
CIO: John Phillips, Vice President Information Services
CHR: Michael Costa, Vice President Human Resources
Web address: www.st–joseph.org
Control: Church–operated, Nongovernment, not–for profit **Service:** General Medical and Surgical

Staffed Beds: 253 **Admissions:** 16405 **Census:** 204 **Outpatient Visits:** 266390 **Births:** 2341 **Total Expense ($000):** 200414 **Payroll Expense ($000):** 78678 **Personnel:** 1739

□ **THE PHYSICIANS CENTRE (450834)**, 3131 University Drive East, Zip 77802; tel. 979/731–3100 **A**1 10 **F**3 12 15 32 33 36 38 41 43 48 50 51 55 56 57 62 66 72 73 77 79 80 81 82 84 96 98 100 101 107 108 11 110 120 121 14 3 31 32 35 37 40 42 44 45 49 50 51 55 57 63 64 68 70 71 72 73 87 89 91 97 **P**8
Primary Contact: Michelle Fortune, RN, Chief Executive Officer
CFO: Michelle Brost, Chief Financial Officer
CIO: Michelle Brost, Chief Financial Officer
CHR: LeeAnn Ford, Director Human Resources
Web address: www.thephysicianscentre.com
Control: Partnership, Investor–owned, for–profit **Service:** General Medical and Surgical

Staffed Beds: 16 **Admissions:** 547 **Census:** 4 **Outpatient Visits:** 13043 **Births:** 0 **Total Expense ($000):** 15145953 **Payroll Expense ($000):** 4442482 **Personnel:** 109

BURNET—Burnet County

★□ **SETON HIGHLAND LAKES (451365)**, 3201 South Water Street, Zip 78611–7219, Mailing Address: P.O. Box 1219, Zip 78611–7219; tel. 512/715–3000 **A**1 9 10 18 **F**3 11 15 25 26 30 31 32 33 38 41 42 43 44 50 55 57 60 61 62 66 68 69 73 75 76 79 80 81 82 86 87 92 96 99 100 102 107 118 119 121 122 124 133 135 137 **P**8 **S** Ascension Health
Primary Contact: Scott O. Fuller, Vice President and Administrator
CFO: Douglas D. Waite, Senior Vice President and Chief Financial Officer
CIO: Gerry Lewis, Chief Information Officer
Web address: www.seton.net
Control: Church–operated, Nongovernment, not–for profit **Service:** General Medical and Surgical

Staffed Beds: 25 **Admissions:** 1305 **Census:** 13 **Outpatient Visits:** 50171 **Births:** 0 **Total Expense ($000):** 25670 **Payroll Expense ($000):** 9575 **Personnel:** 227

TX

Hospital, Medicare Provider Number, Address, Telephone, Approval, Facility, and Physician Codes, Health Care System

★ American Hospital Association (AHA) membership
□ The Joint Commission accreditation
○ American Osteopathic Association (AOA) accreditation
△ Commission on Accreditation of Rehabilitation Facilities (CARF) accreditation

CALDWELL—Burleson County

★ **BURLESON ST. JOSEPH HEALTH CENTER (451305)**, 1101 Woodson Drive, Zip 77836–1052, Mailing Address: P.O. Drawer 360, Zip 77836–0360; tel. 979/567–3245 **A**9 10 18 **F**7 11 14 25 30 31 32 33 38 40 42 54 55 56 57 62 81 86 96 97 100 102 107 119 122 132 **P**6 **S** Franciscan Services Corporation
Primary Contact: Reed Edmundson, Administrator
CFO: Lisa McNair, Senior Vice President and Chief Financial Officer
CHR: Mary Lou Alford, Director Professional Services
Web address: www.st-joseph.org/
Control: Church–operated, Nongovernment, not–for profit **Service:** General Medical and Surgical

Staffed Beds: 25 **Admissions:** 349 **Census:** 5 **Outpatient Visits:** 16177 **Births:** 0 **Total Expense ($000):** 7307 **Payroll Expense ($000):** 3591 **Personnel:** 67

CAMERON—Milam County

CENTRAL TEXAS HOSPITAL (450770), 806 North Crockett Avenue, Zip 76520–2599; tel. 254/697–6591 **A**9 10 **F**3 11 25 38 53 55 57 62 63 84 86 96 97 102 107 117 118 122 133 135 **P**8
Primary Contact: Tariq Mahmood, Chief Executive Officer
CFO: Joe White, Chief Financial Officer
Web address: www.centexhospital.com
Control: Corporation, Investor–owned, for–profit **Service:** General Medical and Surgical

Staffed Beds: 34 **Admissions:** 1729 **Census:** 16 **Outpatient Visits:** 7647 **Births:** 0 **Total Expense ($000):** 7095 **Payroll Expense ($000):** 2555 **Personnel:** 80

CANADIAN—Hemphill County

HEMPHILL COUNTY HOSPITAL (450578), 1020 South Fourth Street, Zip 79014–3315; tel. 806/323–6422 **A**9 10 20 **F**2 7 24 25 33 38 42 54 55 61 62 66 67 75 82 84 86 87 92 96 97 119 122 135 137
Primary Contact: Robert Ezzell, Administrator
Web address: www.hch.dst.tx.us
Control: Hospital district or authority, Government, nonfederal **Service:** General Medical and Surgical

Staffed Beds: 19 **Admissions:** 210 **Census:** 2 **Outpatient Visits:** 11165 **Births:** 0 **Total Expense ($000):** 4690 **Payroll Expense ($000):** 1972 **Personnel:** 61

CARRIZO SPRINGS—Dimmit County

DIMMIT COUNTY MEMORIAL HOSPITAL (450620), 704 Hospital Drive, Zip 78834–3836; tel. 830/876–2424 **A**9 10 20 **F**11 13 30 31 32 38 40 55 61 62 68 74 79 82 84 86 96 107
Primary Contact: Ernest Flores, Jr., Administrator
CFO: Alma Melendez, Controller
Control: County–Government, nonfederal **Service:** General Medical and Surgical

Staffed Beds: 35 **Admissions:** 1506 **Census:** 16 **Outpatient Visits:** 24260 **Births:** 244 **Total Expense ($000):** 9106 **Payroll Expense ($000):** 4077 **Personnel:** 138

CARROLLTON—Denton County

⊠ **REGENCY HOSPITAL OF NORTH DALLAS (670013)**, 2225 Parker Road, Zip 75010; tel. 972/236–6800 **A**1 9 10 **F**1 3 25 30 72 73 75 80 81 82 119 124 137 **P**5 **S** Regency Hospital Company
Primary Contact: Judith Schiros, Chief Executive Officer
CMO: Vivek Sastry, Medical Director
Web address: www.regencyhospital.com
Control: Corporation, Investor–owned, for–profit **Service:** Long–Term Acute Care hospital

Staffed Beds: 41 **Admissions:** 418 **Census:** 29 **Outpatient Visits:** 576 **Births:** 0 **Total Expense ($000):** 15143 **Payroll Expense ($000):** 7559 **Personnel:** 144

☐ **TRINITY MEDICAL CENTER (450730)**, 4343 North Josey Lane, Zip 75010–4691; tel. 972/492–1010 **A**1 9 10 **F**3 11 12 13 15 18 25 26 27 30 31 32 33 38 43 48 49 50 53 54 55 57 62 68 70 71 72 73 74 75 76 77 79 81 82 84 96 97 98 100 102 106 107 113 114 118 119 120 121 135 136 **S** Hospital Partners of America
Primary Contact: Spencer Turner, Chief Executive Officer
CFO: Norma Ramos, Chief Financial Officer
CIO: Paul Ratcliff, Director Information Services
CHR: Sheila Richards, Director Human Resources
Web address: www.trinitymedicalcenter.com
Control: Corporation, Investor–owned, for–profit **Service:** General Medical and Surgical

Staffed Beds: 149 **Admissions:** 7115 **Census:** 77 **Outpatient Visits:** 74400 **Births:** 1940 **Total Expense ($000):** 79039 **Payroll Expense ($000):** 33722 **Personnel:** 727

CARTHAGE—Panola County

⊠ **EAST TEXAS MEDICAL CENTER CARTHAGE (450210)**, 409 Cottage Road, Zip 75633–1466, Mailing Address: P.O. Box 549, Zip 75633–0549; tel. 903/693–3841 **A**1 9 10 20 **F**3 11 13 15 24 25 26 27 28 30 31 32 33 37 38 40 41 50 55 57 62 66 68 73 74 79 80 81 84 87 96 97 100 103 107 118 119 124 134 135 136 **S** East Texas Medical Center Regional Healthcare System
Primary Contact: Gary Mikeal Hudson, Administrator
COO: Gary Mikeal Hudson, Administrator
CFO: Kathy Conway, Chief Financial Officer
CMO: A R Barrett, Chief of Staff
CIO: Renee Lawhorn, Director Medical Records
CHR: Crystal Mauritzen, Director Human Resources
Web address: www.etmc.org
Control: Other not–for–profit (including NFP Corporation) **Service:** General Medical and Surgical

Staffed Beds: 37 **Admissions:** 1458 **Census:** 11 **Outpatient Visits:** 58413 **Births:** 108 **Total Expense ($000):** 16757 **Payroll Expense ($000):** 6302 **Personnel:** 157

CEDAR PARK—Williamson County

⊠ **CEDAR PARK REGIONAL MEDICAL CENTER**, 1490 East Whitestone Boulevard, Zip 78613–2274; tel. 512/528–7000, (Nonreporting) **A**1 **S** Community Health Systems, Inc.
Primary Contact: David G. Klein, M.D., Chief Executive Officer
Web address: www.cedarparkregional.com
Control: Partnership, Investor–owned, for–profit **Service:** General Medical and Surgical

Staffed Beds: 75

CENTER—Shelby County

⊠ **SHELBY REGIONAL MEDICAL CENTER (450839)**, 602 Hurst Street, Zip 75935–3414, Mailing Address: P.O. Box 1749, Zip 75935–1749; tel. 936/598–2781, (Nonreporting) **A**1 9 10
Primary Contact: Gary L. Stokes, Chief Executive Officer
Web address: www.shelbyregional.com
Control: Partnership, Investor–owned, for–profit **Service:** General Medical and Surgical

Staffed Beds: 46

CHANNELVIEW—Harris County

☐ **TRIUMPH HOSPITAL EAST HOUSTON (452075)**, 15101 East Freeway, Zip 77530; tel. 832/200–5500, (Includes TRIUMPH HOSPITAL BAYTOWN, 1700 James Bowie Drive, 3rd Floor, Baytown, Zip 77520; tel. 281/420–7800; Michael Higginbotham, Chief Executive Officer; TRIUMPH HOSPITAL CLEAR LAKE, 350 Blossom Street, Webster, Zip 77598; tel. 281/316–7800; Ronald J. Castagno, FACHE, President and Chief Executive Officer) **A**1 9 10 **F**1 3 25 59 62 66 73 75 79 80 96 107 137 **S** Triumph HealthCare
Primary Contact: Mike Files, Chief Executive Officer
Web address: www.triumph–healthcare.com
Control: Partnership, Investor–owned, for–profit **Service:** Long–Term Acute Care hospital

Staffed Beds: 230 **Admissions:** 2405 **Census:** 169 **Outpatient Visits:** 2788 **Births:** 0 **Total Expense ($000):** 79806 **Payroll Expense ($000):** 27179 **Personnel:** 557

CHILDRESS—Childress County

★ **CHILDRESS REGIONAL MEDICAL CENTER (450369)**, Highway 83 North, Zip 79201–5800, Mailing Address: P.O. Box 1030, Zip 79201–1030; tel. 940/937–6371 **A**9 10 20 **F**7 8 13 15 25 28 30 31 32 33 38 40 42 50 54 55 56 57 60 61 62 64 74 79 80 81 82 84 86 96 103 107 118 119 122
Primary Contact: John Henderson, Administrator
COO: Holly Holcomb, Compliance and Privacy Officer
CFO: Kathy McLain, Chief Financial Officer
CIO: Callie Saunders, Administrator Network
CHR: Gayle Cannon, Director Human Resources
Web address: www.childresshospital.com
Control: Hospital district or authority, Government, nonfederal **Service:** General Medical and Surgical

Staffed Beds: 39 **Admissions:** 1418 **Census:** 13 **Outpatient Visits:** 37493 **Births:** 271 **Total Expense ($000):** 15919 **Payroll Expense ($000):** 7130 **Personnel:** 259

TX

CHILLICOTHE—Hardeman County

★ **CHILLICOTHE HOSPITAL DISTRICT (451326)**, 303 Avenue I, Zip 79225, Mailing Address: P.O. Box 370, Zip 79225–0370; tel. 940/852–5131 **A**9 10 18 **F**25 38 40 55 56 57 79 122 **P**5
Primary Contact: Linda Hall, Administrator
CFO: Linda Hall, Administrator
CMO: Weldon Glidden, M.D., Chief of Staff
CIO: Kathy Busby, Medical Record Technician
CHR: Linda Hall, Administrator
Web address: www.chillicothehospital.org
Control: Hospital district or authority, Government, nonfederal **Service:** General Medical and Surgical

Staffed Beds: 21 **Admissions:** 59 **Census:** 1 **Outpatient Visits:** 3142 **Births:** 0 **Total Expense ($000):** 1621 **Payroll Expense ($000):** 762 **Personnel:** 23

CLARKSVILLE—Red River County

★☐ **EAST TEXAS MEDICAL CENTER CLARKSVILLE (450188)**, 3000 West Main Street, Zip 75426, Mailing Address: P.O. Box 1270, Zip 75426–1270; tel. 903/427–6400 **A**1 9 10 **F**11 17 25 31 37 38 40 41 53 54 55 56 57 62 66 73 79 80 81 82 96 97 102 106 107 118 119 124 135 **P**8 **S** East Texas Medical Center Regional Healthcare System
Primary Contact: John S. Hart, Administrator
CFO: James Hines, Chief Financial Officer
CMO: Devabrata Ganguly, M.D., Chief of Staff
CIO: James Hines, Chief Financial Officer
CHR: Susan Hill, Director Human Resources
Web address: www.etmc.org
Control: Other not–for–profit (including NFP Corporation) **Service:** General Medical and Surgical

Staffed Beds: 36 **Admissions:** 1714 **Census:** 17 **Outpatient Visits:** 20416 **Births:** 0 **Total Expense ($000):** 10915 **Payroll Expense ($000):** 4492 **Personnel:** 128

CLEBURNE—Johnson County

★☐ **WALLS REGIONAL HOSPITAL (450148)**, 201 Walls Drive, Zip 76033–4008; tel. 817/641–2551 **A**1 9 10 **F**3 11 13 15 25 28 32 33 38 40 41 46 50 51 54 55 56 57 62 63 66 68 73 74 75 77 79 80 84 86 96 97 100 105 106 107 112 118 119 135 137 **S** Texas Health Resources
Primary Contact: Blake Kretz, President
CFO: James E. Frosch, Director Finance
CHR: Dianne Mayfield, Director
Web address: www.texashealth.org
Control: Other not–for–profit (including NFP Corporation) **Service:** General Medical and Surgical

Staffed Beds: 48 **Admissions:** 3643 **Census:** 32 **Outpatient Visits:** 39530 **Births:** 667 **Total Expense ($000):** 42283 **Payroll Expense ($000):** 17868 **Personnel:** 350

CLEVELAND—Liberty County

★☐ **CLEVELAND REGIONAL MEDICAL CENTER (450296)**, 300 East Crockett Street, Zip 77327–4062, Mailing Address: P.O. Box 1688, Zip 77328–1688; tel. 281/593–1811 **A**1 9 10 **F**3 11 13 15 25 26 30 31 32 33 38 40 50 55 57 61 62 66 68 72 73 74 75 77 79 80 82 86 96 97 102 107 119 121 122 135 **P**6 **S** Community Health Systems, Inc.
Primary Contact: Jude Torchia, Chief Executive Officer
Web address: www.clevelandregionalmedicalcenter.com
Control: Partnership, Investor–owned, for–profit **Service:** General Medical and Surgical

Staffed Beds: 98 **Admissions:** 3795 **Census:** 39 **Outpatient Visits:** 47017 **Births:** 480 **Total Expense ($000):** 46258 **Payroll Expense ($000):** 14889 **Personnel:** 289

☐ **DOCTORS DIAGNOSTIC HOSPITAL (670018)**, 1017 South Travis Street, Zip 77327–5152; tel. 281/622–2900 **A**1 10 **F**1 3 4 9 16 17 38 45 46 62 65 66 68 70 71 73 74 77 78 79 80 81 82 83 84 85 88 96 100 107 117 133
Primary Contact: Tracy Allen, Chief Executive Officer
Control: Partnership, Investor–owned, for–profit **Service:** General Medical and Surgical

Staffed Beds: 4 **Admissions:** 272 **Census:** 2 **Births:** 0

CLIFTON—Bosque County

★ **GOODALL–WITCHER HEALTHCARE (450052)**, 101 South Avenue T, Zip 76634–1897, Mailing Address: P.O. Box 549, Zip 76634–0549; tel. 254/675–8322 **A**9 10 20 **F**3 11 13 15 25 26 30 31 32 33 34 38 40 43 44 55 56 57 61 62 63 66 68 74 75 79 86 96 97 107 119 122 135 136 **P**3
Primary Contact: Clarence Fields, Jr., President and Chief Executive Officer
CFO: Vickie Gloff, Accountant
Web address: www.gwhf.org
Control: Other not–for–profit (including NFP Corporation) **Service:** General Medical and Surgical

Staffed Beds: 40 **Admissions:** 1530 **Census:** 17 **Outpatient Visits:** 48400 **Births:** 148 **Total Expense ($000):** 15842 **Payroll Expense ($000):** 7373 **Personnel:** 225

COLEMAN—Coleman County

★ **COLEMAN COUNTY MEDICAL CENTER (451347)**, 310 South Pecos Street, Zip 76834–4159; tel. 325/625–2135 **A**9 10 18 **F**7 11 24 25 30 31 32 38 46 57 63 73 75 76 79 82 86 96 100 107 122 135
Primary Contact: Douglas Langley, Chief Executive Officer
CHR: Judy Espitia, Director Human Resources
Control: Hospital district or authority, Government, nonfederal **Service:** General Medical and Surgical

Staffed Beds: 25 **Admissions:** 668 **Census:** 6 **Outpatient Visits:** 4393 **Births:** 41 **Total Expense ($000):** 6366 **Payroll Expense ($000):** 3333 **Personnel:** 99

COLLEGE STATION—Brazos County

★☐ **COLLEGE STATION MEDICAL CENTER (450299)**, 1604 Rock Prairie Road, Zip 77845–8345, Mailing Address: P.O. Box 10000, Zip 77842–3500; tel. 979/764–5100 **A**1 2 3 5 9 10 **F**3 11 12 13 15 18 20 22 25 26 27 30 31 32 33 38 40 43 46 48 49 51 52 55 56 57 60 62 65 68 70 72 74 75 76 77 79 80 82 84 85 86 96 97 100 102 104 107 116 118 119 120 121 124 135 136 137 **P**7 **S** Community Health Systems, Inc.
Primary Contact: Thomas W. Jackson, Chief Executive Officer
CFO: Wayne Colson, Chief Financial Officer
CHR: Sharon Bond, Director Human Resources
Web address: www.csmedcenter.com
Control: Partnership, Investor–owned, for–profit **Service:** General Medical and Surgical

Staffed Beds: 150 **Admissions:** 6096 **Census:** 70 **Outpatient Visits:** 60483 **Births:** 1547 **Total Expense ($000):** 70003 **Payroll Expense ($000):** 26349 **Personnel:** 432

TX

COLORADO CITY—Mitchell County

★ **MITCHELL COUNTY HOSPITAL (451342)**, 997 West Interstate 20, Zip 79512–2685; tel. 325/728–3431 **A**9 10 18 **F**3 7 11 24 25 30 31 32 38 40 41 50 57 61 62 66 79 86 96 107 119 122 135 **P**6
Primary Contact: Linda G. Mize, Chief Executive Officer
CFO: Shirley McMahan, Chief Financial Officer
CMO: Dee A. Roach, M.D., Chief of Staff
CIO: Lu Lu Boyd, Information Technology Director
CHR: Sandra Sullivan, Director Human Resources and Payroll
Web address: www.mitchellcountyhospital.com
Control: Hospital district or authority, Government, nonfederal **Service:** General Medical and Surgical

Staffed Beds: 25 **Admissions:** 617 **Census:** 8 **Outpatient Visits:** 41599 **Births:** 0 **Total Expense ($000):** 12882 **Payroll Expense ($000):** 6915 **Personnel:** 163

COLUMBUS—Colorado County

★ **COLUMBUS COMMUNITY HOSPITAL (450370)**, 110 Shult Drive, Zip 78934–3010, Mailing Address: P.O. Box 865, Zip 78934–0865; tel. 979/732–2371 **A**3 5 9 10 **F**11 13 15 25 27 31 32 38 40 54 55 61 66 74 77 79 84 96 97 102 107 119 122
Primary Contact: Robert Thomas, Administrator
Web address: www.columbusch.com
Control: Other not–for–profit (including NFP Corporation) **Service:** General Medical and Surgical

Staffed Beds: 40 **Admissions:** 1173 **Census:** 12 **Outpatient Visits:** 36295 **Births:** 230 **Total Expense ($000):** 17140 **Payroll Expense ($000):** 6062 **Personnel:** 129

Hospital, Medicare Provider Number, Address, Telephone, Approval, Facility, and Physician Codes, Health Care System

★ American Hospital Association (AHA) membership
☐ The Joint Commission accreditation
○ American Osteopathic Association (AOA) accreditation
△ Commission on Accreditation of Rehabilitation Facilities (CARF) accreditation

COMANCHE—Comanche County

★ **COMANCHE COUNTY MEDICAL CENTER (450234)**, 10201 Highway 16 North, Zip 76442–4462; tel. 254/879–4900 **A**9 10 20 **F**7 8 11 24 25 26 38 42 43 44 50 55 61 62 66 68 73 75 77 79 80 82 86 92 96 102 107 119 121 122 124 135 137 **P**4
Primary Contact: Kevin Storey, Chief Executive Officer
CFO: Tom Letz, Chief Financial Officer
CMO: Howard Dickey, D.O., Chief of Staff
CIO: David Cisneroz, Director Information Systems
CHR: Peggy Jordan, Director Human Resources
Web address: www.comanchecmc.org
Control: Hospital district or authority, Government, nonfederal **Service:** General Medical and Surgical

Staffed Beds: 38 **Admissions:** 1742 **Census:** 20 **Outpatient Visits:** 26228 **Births:** 0 **Total Expense ($000):** 15038 **Payroll Expense ($000):** 6703 **Personnel:** 201

COMMERCE—Hunt County

⊠ **PRESBYTERIAN HOSPITAL OF COMMERCE (451321)**, 2900 Sterling Hart Drive, Zip 75428; tel. 903/886–3161 **A**1 9 10 18 **F**3 11 25 26 30 31 38 55 73 80 82 86 96 102 107 119 122 135
Primary Contact: Michael R. Klepin, Administrator
CFO: Jeri Rich, Assistant Administrator and Chief Financial Officer
CMO: Richard Selvaggi, M.D., Chief of Staff
CIO: Joe Hartley, Director Information Systems
CHR: John Heatherly, Assistant Administrator Human and Support Services Director
Web address: www.hmhd.org
Control: Hospital district or authority, Government, nonfederal **Service:** General Medical and Surgical

Staffed Beds: 24 **Admissions:** 503 **Census:** 6 **Outpatient Visits:** 8212 **Births:** 0 **Total Expense ($000):** 6610 **Payroll Expense ($000):** 2459 **Personnel:** 35

CONROE—Montgomery County

⊠ **CONROE REGIONAL MEDICAL CENTER (450222)**, 504 Medical Boulevard, Zip 77304, Mailing Address: P.O. Box 1538, Zip 77305–1538; tel. 936/539–1111 **A**1 9 10 **F**3 11 12 13 15 17 18 20 22 24 25 27 30 31 32 33 38 43 52 53 55 56 57 62 66 68 70 71 72 73 74 76 77 79 80 81 84 86 96 97 100 102 103 106 107 109 112 118 119 121 124 135 136 137 **P**7 **S** HCA
Primary Contact: Jerry A. Nash, Chief Executive Officer
COO: Eric Becker, Chief Operating Officer
CFO: Thomas A. Holt, Chief Financial Officer
CIO: Daniel Andresen, Director Information Services
CHR: Diana Howell, Director Human Resources
Web address: www.conroeregional.com
Control: Corporation, Investor–owned, for–profit **Service:** General Medical and Surgical

Staffed Beds: 267 **Admissions:** 13576 **Census:** 195 **Outpatient Visits:** 99943 **Births:** 1138 **Total Expense ($000):** 174520 **Payroll Expense ($000):** 55874 **Personnel:** 950

⊠ **HEALTHSOUTH REHABILITATION HOSPITAL OF NORTH HOUSTON (453059)**, 18550 I 45 South, Zip 77384; tel. 281/364–2000 **A**1 9 10 **F**3 25 26 30 31 32 33 41 43 54 55 57 61 62 66 73 75 77 81 82 85 86 119 121 137 **S** HEALTHSOUTH Corporation
Primary Contact: Russell Bailey, Chief Executive Officer
CMO: Ben Agana, M.D., Medical Director
CHR: Valerie Wells, Manager Human Resources
Web address: www.healthsouth.com
Control: Corporation, Investor–owned, for–profit **Service:** Rehabilitation

Staffed Beds: 84 **Admissions:** 1307 **Census:** 48 **Outpatient Visits:** 15610 **Births:** 0 **Total Expense ($000):** 12903 **Payroll Expense ($000):** 7391 **Personnel:** 188

☐ **SELECT SPECIALTY HOSPITAL–CONROE (452089)**, 506 Medical Center Boulevard, Zip 77304; tel. 936/538–3154 **A**1 9 10 **F**1 3 25 27 31 32 38 80 81 82 119 137 **S** Select Medical Corporation
Primary Contact: Sandra Stephens, RN, Administrator and Chief Executive Officer
CMO: John Griffin, M.D., Medical Director
CIO: DeAngela Fordjour, Manager Health Information Management
CHR: Sharon Nail, Coordinator Human Resources
Web address: www.selectmedicalcorp.com
Control: Corporation, Investor–owned, for–profit **Service:** Long–Term Acute Care hospital

Staffed Beds: 46 **Admissions:** 490 **Census:** 36 **Outpatient Visits:** 0 **Births:** 0 **Total Expense ($000):** 14128 **Payroll Expense ($000):** 5802 **Personnel:** 107

CORPUS CHRISTI—Nueces County

⊠ △ **CHRISTUS SPOHN HOSPITAL CORPUS CHRISTI MEMORIAL (450046)**, 2606 Hospital Boulevard, Zip 78405–1818, Mailing Address: P.O. Box 5280, Zip 78465–5280; tel. 361/902–4000, (Includes CHRISTUS SPOHN HOSPITAL CORPUS CHRISTI SHORELINE, 600 Elizabeth Street, Zip 78404–2235; tel. 361/881–3000; CHRISTUS SPOHN HOSPITAL CORPUS CHRISTUS SOUTH, 5950 Saratoga, Zip 78414–4100; tel. 361/985–5000; Steven G. Daniel, Chief Operating Officer), (Total facility includes 24 beds in nursing home–type unit) **A**1 2 3 5 7 9 10 **F**3 5 11 13 15 16 17 18 20 22 24 25 26 27 30 31 32 33 35 36 37 38 40 45 46 49 50 51 52 53 54 56 58 59 62 64 66 68 70 72 73 74 75 76 77 79 80 81 82 85 86 87 88 89 90 91 92 93 94 95 96 97 99 100 101 102 103 106 107 117 119 121 131 135 136 137 **P**7 8 **S** CHRISTUS Health
Primary Contact: Estela Chapa, FACHE, Vice President and Chief Operating Officer
COO: Estela Chapa, FACHE, Vice President and Chief Operating Officer
CMO: Richard Davis, M.D., Regional Chief Medical Officer
CIO: Jeanne DeAngelis, Director Information Management
CHR: Mary LaFrancois, Vice President Human Resources
Web address: www.christusspohn.org
Control: Church–operated, Nongovernment, not–for profit **Service:** General Medical and Surgical

Staffed Beds: 809 **Admissions:** 35070 **Census:** 556 **Outpatient Visits:** 350021 **Births:** 3805 **Total Expense ($000):** 392537 **Payroll Expense ($000):** 178347 **Personnel:** 3271

⊠ **CORPUS CHRISTI MEDICAL CENTER (450788)**, 3315 South Alameda Street, Zip 78411–1883, Mailing Address: P.O. Box 8991, Zip 78468–8991; tel. 361/761–1400, (Includes CORPUS CHRISTI MEDICAL CENTER BAY AREA, 7101 South Padre Island Drive, Zip 78412–4999; tel. 361/985–1200), (Total facility includes 26 beds in nursing home–type unit) **A**1 9 10 12 13 **F**3 11 12 13 15 17 18 20 22 24 25 26 27 30 31 32 35 37 38 39 41 49 50 52 55 56 57 62 66 68 70 71 72 73 74 75 76 77 79 80 81 82 84 86 87 96 97 100 102 106 107 117 118 119 135 136 137 **P**8 **S** HCA
Primary Contact: James T. Montgomery, CHE, Chief Executive Officer
CFO: Chris Nicosia, Chief Financial Officer
CMO: Deborah Carver, M.D., Chief of Staff
CIO: Sharon Orton, Director Information Services and Technology
CHR: Michael Conwill, Director Human Resources
Web address: www.ccmedicalcenter.com
Control: Partnership, Investor–owned, for–profit **Service:** General Medical and Surgical

Staffed Beds: 362 **Admissions:** 15077 **Census:** 195 **Outpatient Visits:** 84554 **Births:** 3682 **Total Expense ($000):** 160206 **Payroll Expense ($000):** 56862 **Personnel:** 1168

☐ **CORPUS CHRISTI SPECIALTY HOSPITAL (452036)**, 1310 Third Street, Zip 78404–2208; tel. 361/888–4323 **A**1 9 10 **F**1 3 25 30 31 32 119 137
Primary Contact: Diana Schultz, Chief Executive Officer
CFO: Cynthia Barron, Manager Business Office
CMO: Raymond Acebo, M.D., Director Medical Staff
CHR: Carmen Newton, Manager Human Resources
Control: Corporation, Investor–owned, for–profit **Service:** General Medical and Surgical

Staffed Beds: 31 **Admissions:** 268 **Census:** 19 **Outpatient Visits:** 0 **Births:** 0 **Total Expense ($000):** 6491 **Payroll Expense ($000):** 2758 **Personnel:** 62

⊠ **DRISCOLL CHILDREN'S HOSPITAL (453301)**, 3533 South Alameda Street, Zip 78411–1785, Mailing Address: P.O. Box 6530, Zip 78466–6530; tel. 361/694–5000 **A**1 3 5 9 10 **F**3 7 11 19 21 23 25 26 27 28 30 31 32 33 36 37 38 39 43 49 50 52 53 55 56 57 58 59 60 62 63 66 69 70 72 73 75 76 77 79 80 81 82 83 84 86 87 96 97 100 103 106 107 114 118 119 120 121 123 125 127 132 133 135 137 **P**3 5
Primary Contact: Steve Woerner, Chief Executive Officer
COO: Donna Quinn, Vice President Operations and Quality
CFO: Eric Hamon, Chief Financial Officer
CIO: Miguel Perez, Director Information Systems
CHR: Bill Larsen, Vice President Human Resources
Web address: www.driscollchildrens.org
Control: Other not–for–profit (including NFP Corporation) **Service:** Children's general

Staffed Beds: 162 **Admissions:** 6462 **Census:** 93 **Outpatient Visits:** 127457 **Births:** 0 **Total Expense ($000):** 163529 **Payroll Expense ($000):** 66757 **Personnel:** 1442

⊠ **DUBUIS HOSPITAL OF CORPUS CHRISTI (452086)**, 600 Elizabeth Street, 5rd Floor, Zip 78404, Mailing Address: 600 Elizabeth Street, 3rd Floor, Zip 78404; tel. 361/881–3223 **A**1 9 10 **F**1 3 18 20 22 25 26 27 30 44 59 66 72 73 76 77 80 96 97 100 104 107 119 137 **S** Dubuis Health System
Primary Contact: Diane Kaiser, Administrator
Web address: www.dubuis.org
Control: Church–operated, Nongovernment, not–for profit **Service:** Long–Term Acute Care hospital

Staffed Beds: 22 **Admissions:** 266 **Census:** 20 **Outpatient Visits:** 0 **Births:** 0 **Total Expense ($000):** 8510 **Payroll Expense ($000):** 2963 **Personnel:** 60

Many Facility Codes have changed. Please refer to the AHA Guide Code Chart.

□ **KINDRED HOSPITAL–CORPUS CHRISTI (452092)**, 6226 Saratoga Boulevard, Zip 78414; tel. 361/986–1600 **A**1 9 10 **F**1 3 25 26 27 30 31 32 33 43 55 56 57 59 60 62 68 72 73 75 77 80 81 82 86 87 90 96 119 135 137
Primary Contact: Brian L. Pugh, Interim Chief Executive Officer
CFO: Eva De La Paz, Chief Financial Officer
CMO: Salim Surani, M.D., Medical Director
CIO: Lisa Morgan, Coordinator Health Information Management
CHR: Nancy Matthews, Manager Human Resources
Web address: www.kindredhealthcare.com
Control: Corporation, Investor–owned, for–profit **Service:** General Medical and Surgical

Staffed Beds: 65 **Admissions:** 712 **Census:** 50 **Outpatient Visits:** 1606 **Births:** 0 **Total Expense ($000):** 18716 **Payroll Expense ($000):** 6950 **Personnel:** 149

□ **PADRE BEHAVIORAL HOSPITAL (454096)**, 6629 Wooldridge Road, Zip 78414; tel. 361/986–9444 **A**1 9 10 **F**1 4 5 25 33 73 81 82 88 89 90 91 93 94 95 119 121
Primary Contact: Jeff Parsons, Interim Administrator
Control: Corporation, Investor–owned, for–profit **Service:** Psychiatric

Staffed Beds: 68 **Admissions:** 1813 **Census:** 47 **Outpatient Visits:** 5167 **Births:** 0 **Total Expense ($000):** 10308 **Payroll Expense ($000):** 4323 **Personnel:** 143

CORSICANA—Navarro County

★□ **NAVARRO REGIONAL HOSPITAL (450447)**, 3201 West State Highway 22, Zip 75110–2469; tel. 903/654–6800, (Total facility includes 19 beds in nursing home–type unit) **A**1 9 10 19 **F**3 11 13 14 15 25 26 30 31 32 38 47 49 51 55 57 59 62 66 68 73 74 77 79 80 84 85 86 96 97 99 100 102 107 117 118 119 121 124 135 137 **P**7 8 **S** Community Health Systems, Inc.
Primary Contact: Xavier Villarreal, Chief Executive Officer
CFO: Marco Rodriguez, Chief Financial Officer
CIO: Marco Rodriguez, Chief Financial Officer
CHR: Sarah Covert, Director Human Resources
Web address: www.navarrohospital.com
Control: Partnership, Investor–owned, for–profit **Service:** General Medical and Surgical

Staffed Beds: 148 **Admissions:** 3030 **Census:** 34 **Outpatient Visits:** 38156 **Births:** 479 **Total Expense ($000):** 37995 **Payroll Expense ($000):** 14098 **Personnel:** 299

CRANE—Crane County

★ **CRANE MEMORIAL HOSPITAL (451353)**, 1310 South Alford Street, Zip 79731–3899; tel. 432/558–3555 **A**9 10 18 **F**3 25 28 30 32 38 55 56 57 62 63 66 73 79 81 87 96 107 134 136 137 **P**6
Primary Contact: Dianne Yeager, Chief Executive Officer
CMO: Jay Sigel, M.D., Chief Medical Staff
Web address: www.cranememorial.org
Control: County–Government, nonfederal **Service:** General Medical and Surgical

Staffed Beds: 25 **Admissions:** 198 **Census:** 1 **Outpatient Visits:** 14357 **Births:** 0 **Total Expense ($000):** 3855 **Payroll Expense ($000):** 1533 **Personnel:** 37

CROCKETT—Houston County

★□ **EAST TEXAS MEDICAL CENTER CROCKETT (450580)**, 1100 Loop 304 East, Zip 75835–1810; tel. 936/546–3862 **A**1 9 10 20 **F**3 11 13 15 18 20 24 25 28 30 31 32 33 38 40 46 50 53 55 57 58 60 62 68 73 74 79 82 87 96 97 100 102 106 107 119 121 122 133 135 **P**5 7 **S** East Texas Medical Center Regional Healthcare System
Primary Contact: Terry Cutler, Administrator and Chief Operating Officer
Web address: www.etmc.org
Control: Other not–for–profit (including NFP Corporation) **Service:** General Medical and Surgical

Staffed Beds: 49 **Admissions:** 2311 **Census:** 22 **Outpatient Visits:** 50366 **Births:** 218 **Total Expense ($000):** 17669 **Payroll Expense ($000):** 7198 **Personnel:** 178

CROSBYTON—Crosby County

CROSBYTON CLINIC HOSPITAL (451345), 710 West Main Street, Zip 79322–2143; tel. 806/675–2382 **A**9 10 18 **F**7 25 31 33 34 38 42 44 50 55 56 57 62 66 75 82 86 100 107 115 119 122 137 **P**6 **S** Covenant Health System
Primary Contact: Steve Beck, Chief Executive Officer
COO: Debra Miller, Chief Operating Officer
CFO: Ed Watson, Chief Financial Officer
CMO: Steve B. Alley, M.D., Chief of Staff
CIO: Jane Wheeless, Administrative Assistant
CHR: Debbie Hill, Director Human Resources
Control: Other not–for–profit (including NFP Corporation) **Service:** General Medical and Surgical

Staffed Beds: 25 **Admissions:** 641 **Census:** 8 **Outpatient Visits:** 13750 **Births:** 0 **Total Expense ($000):** 6406 **Payroll Expense ($000):** 2164 **Personnel:** 78

CUERO—De Witt County

★ **CUERO COMMUNITY HOSPITAL (450597)**, 2550 North Esplanade Street, Zip 77954–4716; tel. 361/275–6191 **A**5 9 10 **F**3 7 11 13 15 25 26 31 32 38 40 55 57 61 62 68 73 74 75 77 79 80 81 86 93 96 97 100 103 106 107 118 119 120
Primary Contact: Darryl Stefka, Administrator
COO: Dick L. Stout, Chief Operating Officer
CFO: Greg Pritchett, Controller
CIO: Arthur Mueller, Director Management Information Systems
CHR: Wanda Kolodziejcyk, Director Human Resources
Web address: www.cuerohosp.org
Control: Hospital district or authority, Government, nonfederal **Service:** General Medical and Surgical

Staffed Beds: 49 **Admissions:** 2780 **Census:** 27 **Outpatient Visits:** 130177 **Births:** 205 **Total Expense ($000):** 26704 **Payroll Expense ($000):** 11616 **Personnel:** 344

CYPRESS—Harris County

□ **NORTH CYPRESS MEDICAL CENTER (670024)**, 21214 Northwest Freeway, Zip 77429–3373; tel. 832/912–3500 **A**1 10 **F**3 8 12 15 18 20 22 24 25 27 33 35 37 38 43 49 50 51 56 62 68 72 73 76 77 79 80 81 82 86 96 97 98 99 100 102 103 104 105 106 107 108 109 111 112 118 119 121 135 136 137
Primary Contact: Robert Behar, M.D., Chief Executive Officer
Web address: www.ncmc–hospital.com
Control: Partnership, Investor–owned, for–profit **Service:** General Medical and Surgical

Staffed Beds: 91 **Admissions:** 4707 **Census:** 51 **Outpatient Visits:** 64940 **Births:** 0 **Total Expense ($000):** 76316 **Payroll Expense ($000):** 27734 **Personnel:** 669

DALHART—Dallam County

★ **COON MEMORIAL HOSPITAL AND HOME (451331)**, 1411 Denver Avenue, Zip 79022–4809, Mailing Address: P.O. Box 2014, Zip 79022–6014; tel. 806/244–4571 **A**9 10 18 **F**3 7 10 11 13 26 31 32 33 38 40 42 43 45 50 52 55 57 61 62 63 66 67 69 74 75 77 79 80 82 84 85 86 87 96 102 107 120 122 132 133 135 137 **P**5
Primary Contact: Leroy Schaffner, Chief Executive Officer
CFO: Donny Pettit, Chief Financial Officer
CMO: Randy Herring, M.D., Chief of Staff
CIO: Joshua Gray, Director Information Technology
CHR: Dee Dawn McCormick, Director Personnel and Human Resources
Web address: www.coonmemorial.org
Control: Hospital district or authority, Government, nonfederal **Service:** General Medical and Surgical

Staffed Beds: 21 **Admissions:** 555 **Census:** 5 **Outpatient Visits:** 11918 **Births:** 109 **Total Expense ($000):** 17122 **Payroll Expense ($000):** 6447 **Personnel:** 162

DALLAS—Dallas County

A. WEBB ROBERTS HOSPITAL See Baylor University Medical Center

TX

Hospital, Medicare Provider Number, Address, Telephone, Approval, Facility, and Physician Codes, Health Care System

★ American Hospital Association (AHA) membership
□ The Joint Commission accreditation
○ American Osteopathic Association (AOA) accreditation
△ Commission on Accreditation of Rehabilitation Facilities (CARF) accreditation

★ △ **BAYLOR INSTITUTE FOR REHABILITATION (453036)**, 909 North Washington Avenue, Zip 75246–2018; tel. 214/820–9300 **A**1 7 9 10 **F**25 26 30 31 32 33 41 61 62 63 66 72 75 80 81 82 85 86 119 120 121 124 132 137 **S** Baylor Health Care System
Primary Contact: Jon C. Skinner, President
CFO: Cheryl McMullan, Vice President Financial Services and Controller
CMO: Amy Wilson, Medical Director
CHR: Cheri Gibson, Director Human Resources
Web address: www.bhcs.com
Control: Other not–for–profit (including NFP Corporation) **Service:** Rehabilitation

Staffed Beds: 100 **Admissions:** 1733 **Census:** 92 **Outpatient Visits:** 37746 **Births:** 0 **Total Expense ($000):** 45323 **Payroll Expense ($000):** 22053 **Personnel:** 404

□ **BAYLOR JACK AND JANE HAMILTON HEART AND VASCULAR HOSPITAL (450851)**, 621 North Hall Street, Zip 75226–1337; tel. 214/820–0600 **A**1 9 10 **F**3 11 18 19 20 24 25 26 30 31 32 33 50 55 56 57 58 62 66 73 79 80 81 82 86 90 96 103 107 119 121 124
Primary Contact: Nancy Vish, Ph.D., President
Web address: www.baylorhealth.com
Control: Partnership, Investor–owned, for–profit **Service:** Heart

Staffed Beds: 65 **Admissions:** 2690 **Census:** 14 **Outpatient Visits:** 18896 **Births:** 0 **Total Expense ($000):** 68950 **Payroll Expense ($000):** 16019 **Personnel:** 253

★ **BAYLOR SPECIALTY HOSPITAL (452017)**, 3504 Swiss Avenue, Zip 75204–6224; tel. 214/820–9700 **A**1 9 10 **F**1 25 26 30 31 43 50 58 62 119 137 **S** Baylor Health Care System
Primary Contact: Scott Peek, President
CFO: Julius Wicke, Vice President
CMO: Michael Highbaugh, M.D., Medical Director
CHR: Karen Hill, Coordinator Human Resources
Web address: www.bhcs.com
Control: Other not–for–profit (including NFP Corporation) **Service:** General Medical and Surgical

Staffed Beds: 98 **Admissions:** 1182 **Census:** 84 **Outpatient Visits:** 1417 **Births:** 0 **Total Expense ($000):** 39437 **Payroll Expense ($000):** 16093 **Personnel:** 270

TX

★ **BAYLOR UNIVERSITY MEDICAL CENTER (450021)**, 3500 Gaston Avenue, Zip 75246–2088; tel. 214/820–0111, (Includes A. WEBB ROBERTS HOSPITAL; ERIK AND MARGARET JONSSON HOSPITAL; GEORGE W. TRUETT MEMORIAL HOSPITAL; KARL AND ESTHER HOBLITZELLE MEMORIAL HOSPITAL) **A**1 2 3 5 8 9 10 **F**3 4 5 7 11 12 13 14 15 17 18 20 22 24 25 26 27 28 30 31 32 33 34 35 36 37 38 40 41 42 43 44 46 47 48 49 50 51 53 54 55 56 57 58 59 60 62 63 64 66 68 69 70 71 72 73 74 76 77 78 79 80 81 82 84 85 86 87 88 90 91 92 93 94 95 96 97 99 100 102 103 104 105 106 107 108 109 111 112 114 116 118 119 120 121 124 125 126 127 128 129 130 131 132 134 135 136 137 **S** Baylor Health Care System
Primary Contact: John B. McWhorter, III, President
CFO: Janie Wade, Chief Financial Officer
CMO: Irving Prengler, M.D., Vice President Medical Staff Affairs
CIO: David S. Muntz, Senior Vice President and Chief Information Officer
CHR: Queen Greene, Director
Web address: www.baylorhealth.com
Control: Other not–for–profit (including NFP Corporation) **Service:** General Medical and Surgical

Staffed Beds: 923 **Admissions:** 37497 **Census:** 641 **Outpatient Visits:** 316222 **Births:** 3730 **Total Expense ($000):** 772999 **Payroll Expense ($000):** 266256 **Personnel:** 4820

★ **CHILDREN'S MEDICAL CENTER OF DALLAS (453302)**, 1935 Medical District Drive, Zip 75235–7794; tel. 214/456–7000 **A**1 3 5 8 9 10 **F**3 7 8 11 12 17 19 21 23 25 26 27 28 30 31 32 33 36 37 38 40 41 43 44 46 48 49 50 53 55 56 57 58 59 60 62 63 66 70 72 73 75 76 77 79 80 81 82 83 84 86 87 88 89 90 91 92 94 95 96 97 100 102 104 105 106 107 114 118 119 120 121 123 125 126 127 128 131 132 133 135 137
Primary Contact: Christopher J. Durovich, President and Chief Executive Officer
CFO: Ray R. Dziesinski, Senior Vice President and Chief Financial Officer
CMO: Thomas Zellers, M.D., Interim Chief Medical Officer
CIO: Pamela Arora, Vice President Information Systems
CHR: Jim Herring, Senior Vice President
Web address: www.childrens.com
Control: Other not–for–profit (including NFP Corporation) **Service:** Children's general

Staffed Beds: 314 **Admissions:** 17778 **Census:** 241 **Outpatient Visits:** 359070 **Births:** 0 **Total Expense ($000):** 546124 **Payroll Expense ($000):** 226571 **Personnel:** 4131

★ **DOCTORS HOSPITAL AT WHITE ROCK LAKE (450678)**, (Formerly Doctors Hospital of Dallas), 9440 Poppy Drive, Zip 75218–3694; tel. 214/324–6100 **A**1 5 9 10 **F**3 8 11 12 13 15 17 18 20 22 24 25 26 27 32 33 35 38 43 46 49 50 55 56 57 62 68 71 72 73 74 77 79 80 86 96 97 100 102 107 118 119 134 135 136 137 **S** TENET Healthcare Corporation
Primary Contact: Mitch Edgeworth, Chief Executive Officer
COO: Chakilla Robinson–White, Chief Operating Officer
CFO: Roger D. Hutchins, Chief Financial Officer
CMO: Ruben Sandoval, Chief Medical Officer
CIO: Dianne Yarborough, Director Information Systems
CHR: Marlene Urbach, Director Human Resources
Web address: www.doctorshospitaldallas.com
Control: Partnership, Investor–owned, for–profit **Service:** General Medical and Surgical

Staffed Beds: 156 **Admissions:** 7312 **Census:** 91 **Outpatient Visits:** 65202 **Births:** 940 **Total Expense ($000):** 81784 **Payroll Expense ($000):** 33453 **Personnel:** 583

ERIK AND MARGARET JONSSON HOSPITAL See Baylor University Medical Center

GEORGE W. TRUETT MEMORIAL HOSPITAL See Baylor University Medical Center

★ **GREEN OAKS HOSPITAL (454094)**, 7808 Clodus Fields Drive, Zip 75251–2206; tel. 972/991–9504 **A**1 9 10 **F**4 5 25 30 31 32 53 82 88 89 92 93 94 95 119 121 **P**5 **S** HCA
Primary Contact: Thomas M. Collins, Chief Executive Officer
COO: Pam Whitley, R.N., Chief Operating Officer and Chief Nursing Officer
CFO: Jason Tillman, Chief Financial Officer
CMO: Joel Holiner, M.D., Executive Medical Director
CIO: Chebon Bravo, Director Information Systems
CHR: Kevin Adkins, Director Human Resources
Web address: www.greenoakspsych.com
Control: Corporation, Investor–owned, for–profit **Service:** Psychiatric

Staffed Beds: 105 **Admissions:** 6405 **Census:** 100 **Outpatient Visits:** 24946 **Births:** 0 **Total Expense ($000):** 35309 **Payroll Expense ($000):** 13885 **Personnel:** 305

★ **HEALTHSOUTH MEDICAL CENTER (450758)**, 2124 Research Row, Zip 75235–2504; tel. 214/904–6100 **A**1 5 9 10 **F**3 25 32 52 61 62 72 75 77 85 86 132 **S** HEALTHSOUTH Corporation
Primary Contact: Daniel L. Gideon, CHE, Chief Executive Officer
CFO: Patti Ross, Controller
CMO: Hooman Sedighi, M.D., Medical Director
CHR: Tara Kleas, Manager Human Resources
Web address: www.healthsouth.com
Control: Corporation, Investor–owned, for–profit **Service:** Rehabilitation

Staffed Beds: 73 **Admissions:** 744 **Census:** 34 **Outpatient Visits:** 9496 **Births:** 0 **Total Expense ($000):** 14191 **Payroll Expense ($000):** 6388 **Personnel:** 141

KARL AND ESTHER HOBLITZELLE MEMORIAL HOSPITAL See Baylor University Medical Center

□ **KINDRED HOSPITAL – DALLAS (452015)**, 9525 Greenville Avenue, Zip 75243–4116; tel. 214/355–2600, (Includes KINDRED HOSPITAL DALLAS–WALNUT HILL, 8200 Walnut Hill Lane, Zip 75231; tel. 214/345–6500; Rhonda Y. Williams, Chief Executive Officer) **A**1 9 10 **F**1 3 25 38 68 79 86 96 119 137 **P**5 **S** Kindred Healthcare
Primary Contact: Robert M. Smart, Chief Executive Officer
CFO: Jean McDowell, Chief Financial Officer
Web address: www.kindredhealthcare.com
Control: Partnership, Investor–owned, for–profit **Service:** Long–Term Acute Care hospital

Staffed Beds: 130 **Admissions:** 930 **Census:** 71 **Outpatient Visits:** 278 **Births:** 0 **Total Expense ($000):** 32178 **Payroll Expense ($000):** 12645 **Personnel:** 240

□ **KINDRED HOSPITAL–WHITE ROCK (452071)**, 9440 Poppy Drive, 5th Floor, Zip 75218; tel. 214/324–6562 **A**1 9 10 **F**1 25 80 81 82 1 107 119 126 137 24 71 72 73 **P**5
Primary Contact: Judy Wolfe, Chief Executive Officer
COO: Lynn Coutre, Director Nursing and Clinical Services
CFO: Mary Mwaniki, Chief Financial Officer
CMO: Mark Ferris, M.D., Medical Director
Web address: www.khwhiterock.com
Control: Partnership, Investor–owned, for–profit **Service:** Long–Term Acute Care hospital

Staffed Beds: 23 **Admissions:** 321 **Census:** 21 **Outpatient Visits:** 0 **Births:** 0 **Total Expense ($000):** 9750099 **Payroll Expense ($000):** 3602528 **Personnel:** 65

 Many Facility Codes have changed. Please refer to the AHA Guide Code Chart.

□ **LIFECARE HOSPITALS OF NORTH TEXAS–DALLAS (452044)**, 6161 Harry Hines Boulevard, Suite 100, Zip 75235–5306; tel. 214/525–6300 **A**1 9 10 **F**1 3 25 26 32 96 137 **S** LifeCare Management Services
Primary Contact: Edward Downs, Chief Executive Officer
Web address: www.lifecare–hospitals.com
Control: Partnership, Investor–owned, for–profit **Service:** Long–Term Acute Care hospital

Staffed Beds: 64 **Admissions:** 628 **Census:** 44 **Outpatient Visits:** 0 **Births:** 0 **Total Expense ($000):** 20512 **Payroll Expense ($000):** 8947 **Personnel:** 219

★□ **MARY SHIELS HOSPITAL (450422)**, 3515 Howell Street, Zip 75204–2895; tel. 214/443–3000 **A**1 9 10 **F**38 62 66 79 80 96 100 **S** United Surgical Partners International
Primary Contact: Suzanne Greever, Chief Executive Officer
Web address: www.maryshiels.com
Control: Partnership, Investor–owned, for–profit **Service:** General Medical and Surgical

Staffed Beds: 14 **Admissions:** 19 **Census:** 1 **Outpatient Visits:** 4266 **Births:** 0 **Total Expense ($000):** 14283 **Payroll Expense ($000):** 3980 **Personnel:** 56

★□ **MEDICAL CITY DALLAS HOSPITAL (450647)**, 7777 Forest Lane, Zip 75230–2598; tel. 972/566–7000 **A**1 2 9 10 **F**3 11 12 13 15 17 18 19 20 21 22 23 24 25 26 27 32 33 38 43 47 49 50 51 54 55 56 57 58 59 62 63 66 68 70 71 72 73 74 75 76 77 79 80 81 82 83 84 85 86 96 97 100 102 104 105 107 109 114 118 119 121 124 125 126 127 128 131 135 136 137 **P**6 **S** HCA
Primary Contact: Britt Berrett, President and Chief Executive Officer
COO: Scott Schmidly, Chief Operating Officer
CFO: Tim Burroughs, Vice President and Chief Financial Officer
CMO: Leslie Walters, Chief of Staff
CHR: Virginia Rose, Vice President Human Resources
Web address: www.medicalcityhospital.com
Control: Corporation, Investor–owned, for–profit **Service:** General Medical and Surgical

Staffed Beds: 542 **Admissions:** 22652 **Census:** 355 **Outpatient Visits:** 153019 **Births:** 2973 **Total Expense ($000):** 336763 **Payroll Expense ($000):** 135064 **Personnel:** 1798

★□ **METHODIST CHARLTON MEDICAL CENTER (450723)**, 3500 West Wheatland Road, Zip 75237–3460, Mailing Address: Box 225357, Zip 75222–5357; tel. 214/947–7777 **A**1 9 10 12 13 **F**3 11 13 15 18 20 24 25 26 27 30 31 32 33 38 43 44 46 47 49 50 52 56 57 58 59 62 66 68 71 72 76 77 79 80 81 82 87 96 97 100 102 106 107 113 119 120 121 135 137 **P**1 7 **S** Methodist Health System
Primary Contact: Zachary Chandler, President
CFO: Michael J. Schaefer, Executive Vice President and Chief Financial Officer
CMO: Nick Bellos, President Medical Staff
CIO: Pamela McNutt, Vice President Information Systems
CHR: John S. Lacy, Senior Vice President Human Resources
Web address: www.mhs.com
Control: Other not–for–profit (including NFP Corporation) **Service:** General Medical and Surgical

Staffed Beds: 240 **Admissions:** 13044 **Census:** 154 **Outpatient Visits:** 148142 **Births:** 2151 **Total Expense ($000):** 149143 **Payroll Expense ($000):** 67691 **Personnel:** 1316

★□ **METHODIST DALLAS MEDICAL CENTER (450051)**, 1441 North Beckley Avenue, Zip 75203–1201, Mailing Address: Box 655999, Zip 75265–5999; tel. 214/947–8181 **A**1 2 3 5 8 9 10 **F**3 11 12 13 15 17 18 20 22 24 25 26 27 31 32 33 35 38 40 43 44 46 47 48 49 50 52 53 56 57 58 59 62 66 68 70 72 74 76 77 79 80 82 85 86 87 96 97 100 102 106 107 119 121 127 128 131 135 137 **P**1 7 **S** Methodist Health System
Primary Contact: Michael A. Mayo, FACHE, President
CFO: Randy Walker, Vice President
Web address: www.mhd.com
Control: Other not–for–profit (including NFP Corporation) **Service:** General Medical and Surgical

Staffed Beds: 488 **Admissions:** 17739 **Census:** 296 **Outpatient Visits:** 164832 **Births:** 3324 **Total Expense ($000):** 295917 **Payroll Expense ($000):** 130397 **Personnel:** 2442

NORTH DALLAS REHABILITATION HOSPITAL (453032), 8383 Meadow Road, Zip 75231–3798; tel. 214/369–7811, (Nonreporting) **A**10
Primary Contact: Pam Duhon, Administrator and Chief Executive Officer
COO: Pam Duhon, Administrator and Chief Executive Officer
CFO: Hank Barber, Regional Controller
CMO: Bobby Huynh, Chief Medical Officer
CIO: Suzie Gable, Director Health Information Management
CHR: Kathy Edmonds, Director Human Resources
Control: Corporation, Investor–owned, for–profit **Service:** Rehabilitation

Staffed Beds: 34

★ **OUR CHILDREN'S HOUSE AT BAYLOR (453308)**, 3504 Swiss Avenue, Zip 75204–6219; tel. 214/820–9838 **A**9 10 **F**3 25 26 28 30 31 32 33 43 44 50 62 73 79 80 81 82 84 85 86 119 135 137 **S** Baylor Health Care System
Primary Contact: Scott Peek, President
CFO: Julius Wicke, Vice President Finance
CMO: Andrew Gelfand, M.D., Medical Director
CHR: Karen Hill, Coordinator Human Resources
Web address: www.bhcs.com
Control: Other not–for–profit (including NFP Corporation) **Service:** Children's other specialty

Staffed Beds: 54 **Admissions:** 317 **Census:** 24 **Outpatient Visits:** 79084 **Births:** 0 **Total Expense ($000):** 22574 **Payroll Expense ($000):** 11451 **Personnel:** 233

★□ **PARKLAND HEALTH & HOSPITAL SYSTEM (450015)**, 5201 Harry Hines Boulevard, Zip 75235–7731; tel. 214/590–8000 **A**1 2 3 5 8 9 10 **F**3 9 11 12 13 15 16 17 18 20 22 24 25 26 27 30 31 32 33 36 37 38 40 43 44 45 46 47 48 49 50 51 52 53 54 55 56 57 58 59 60 62 63 66 68 69 70 72 73 74 75 76 77 79 80 81 82 85 86 87 88 89 90 91 92 93 94 96 97 100 101 102 103 106 107 112 113 114 118 119 121 123 124 127 130 131 132 133 135 136 137 **P**1
Primary Contact: Ron J. Anderson, M.D., President and Chief Executive Officer
COO: John M. Haupert, Chief Operating Officer
CFO: John Dragovits, Executive Vice President and Chief Financial Officer
CMO: John Jay Shannon, Chief Medical Officer
CIO: Jack Kowitt, Senior Vice President and Chief Information Officer
Web address: www.parklandhospital.com
Control: Hospital district or authority, Government, nonfederal **Service:** General Medical and Surgical

Staffed Beds: 814 **Admissions:** 42788 **Census:** 609 **Outpatient Visits:** 1056765 **Births:** 16252 **Total Expense ($000):** 922282 **Payroll Expense ($000):** 441367 **Personnel:** 8550

TX

PINE CREEK MEDICAL CENTER (450894), 9032 Harry Hines Boulevard, Zip 75235; tel. 214/231–2273 **A**10 **F**3 12 32 38 56 62 77 79 80 86 96 100 102
Primary Contact: Katherine Lower, Administrator
COO: Corazon Rameriz, M.D., Chief Operating Officer
CFO: Michael Conroy, Chief Financial Officer
CIO: Kevin Carney, Senior Information Systems Analyst
CHR: Rory Money, Human Resources Generalist
Web address: www.pinecreekmedicalcenter.com
Control: Partnership, Investor–owned, for–profit **Service:** General Medical and Surgical

Staffed Beds: 18 **Admissions:** 766 **Census:** 4 **Outpatient Visits:** 2570 **Births:** 0 **Total Expense ($000):** 23179 **Payroll Expense ($000):** 4170 **Personnel:** 103

PRESBYTERIAN HOSPITAL OF DALLAS See Texas Health Presbyterian Hospital of Dallas

RENAISSANCE HOSPITAL OF DALLAS (670002), 2929 South Hampton Road, Zip 75224; tel. 214/623–4400 **A**9 10 **F**3 12 13 15 25 38 40 47 55 68 72 73 74 75 77 79 80 84 86 96 100 103 107 118 119 132 136 137 **P**8 **S** Renaissance Healthcare Systems
Primary Contact: Sammy E. Davis, Chief Executive Officer
Web address: www.dallas.renhealthcare.org
Control: Corporation, Investor–owned, for–profit **Service:** General Medical and Surgical

Staffed Beds: 108 **Admissions:** 3234 **Census:** 35 **Outpatient Visits:** 21791 **Births:** 153 **Total Expense ($000):** 45758 **Payroll Expense ($000):** 18113 **Personnel:** 380

Hospital, Medicare Provider Number, Address, Telephone, Approval, Facility, and Physician Codes, Health Care System

★ American Hospital Association (AHA) membership
□ The Joint Commission accreditation
○ American Osteopathic Association (AOA) accreditation
△ Commission on Accreditation of Rehabilitation Facilities (CARF) accreditation

☐ **RHD MEMORIAL MEDICAL CENTER (450379)**, Seven Medical Parkway, Zip 75234, Mailing Address: P.O. Box 819094, Zip 75381–9094; tel. 972/247–1000 **A**1 9 10 **F**3 11 12 13 15 17 18 22 24 25 27 30 31 32 33 37 38 41 43 50 53 54 55 56 57 62 68 72 74 75 76 77 79 80 81 82 85 86 96 97 100 102 107 119 120 121 135 136 137 **P**5 **S** Hospital Partners of America
Primary Contact: Kenneth Howell, Chief Executive Officer
CFO: Karen Bomersbach, Chief Financial Officer
CIO: Mary Jo Tallant–Ball, Director Health Information Systems
CHR: Stephanie Talley, Associate Administrator and Director Human Resources
Web address: www.rhdmemorial.com
Control: Corporation, Investor–owned, for–profit **Service:** General Medical and Surgical

Staffed Beds: 118 **Admissions:** 3616 **Census:** 54 **Outpatient Visits:** 47696 **Births:** 620 **Total Expense ($000):** 41149 **Payroll Expense ($000):** 24837 **Personnel:** 334

SELECT SPECIALTY HOSPITAL – DALLAS (452022), 10 Medical Parkway, Suite 205, Zip 75234–7845; tel. 972/488–9167 **A**10 **F**1 3 25 31 32 38 54 72 73 75 80 96 102 119 137 **P**4 5 **S** Select Medical Corporation
Primary Contact: Joy Dier, RN, M.S., Administrator and Chief Executive Officer
Web address: www.selectmedicalcorp.com
Control: Corporation, Investor–owned, for–profit **Service:** Long–Term Acute Care hospital

Staffed Beds: 60 **Admissions:** 480 **Census:** 34 **Outpatient Visits:** 0 **Births:** 0 **Total Expense ($000):** 17310 **Payroll Expense ($000):** 6251 **Personnel:** 139

★ △ **TEXAS HEALTH PRESBYTERIAN HOSPITAL OF DALLAS (450462)**, (Formerly Presbyterian Hospital of Dallas), 8200 Walnut Hill Lane, Zip 75231–4402; tel. 214/345–6789 **A**1 2 3 5 7 9 10 **F**3 5 9 11 12 13 15 17 18 20 22 24 25 26 27 28 30 31 32 33 34 35 36 38 39 41 42 43 46 47 49 50 51 52 53 54 55 56 57 58 59 60 61 62 64 66 68 70 72 73 74 75 76 77 79 80 81 82 84 85 86 87 88 90 91 92 93 94 95 96 97 99 100 101 102 103 106 107 108 109 111 112 113 114 118 119 120 121 124 132 135 136 137 **P**6 **S** Texas Health Resources
Primary Contact: Mark H. Merrill, President
COO: Jeffrey Canose, M.D., Senior Vice President and Chief Operating Officer
Web address: www.texashealth.org
Control: Other not–for–profit (including NFP Corporation) **Service:** General Medical and Surgical

Staffed Beds: 655 **Admissions:** 27739 **Census:** 419 **Outpatient Visits:** 414642 **Births:** 5992 **Total Expense ($000):** 493102 **Payroll Expense ($000):** 196518 **Personnel:** 3305

☐ **TEXAS INSTITUTE FOR SURGERY AT PRESBYTERIAN HOSPITAL OF DALLAS (450889)**, 7115 Greenville Avenue, Suite 215, Zip 75231–5101; tel. 214/647–5300 **A**1 9 10 **F**38 51 62 77 79 80 96
Primary Contact: Debbie Hay, RN, Chief Executive Officer
CFO: Andrew Summers, Vice President Finance
CMO: Presley Mock, Chief of Staff
CHR: Jack Martin, Administrative Services Manager
Web address: www.texasinstituteforsurgery.org
Control: Partnership, Investor–owned, for–profit **Service:** General Medical and Surgical

Staffed Beds: 9 **Admissions:** 71 **Census:** 1 **Outpatient Visits:** 12569 **Births:** 0 **Total Expense ($000):** 31370 **Payroll Expense ($000):** 6851 **Personnel:** 123

★ **TEXAS SCOTTISH RITE HOSPITAL FOR CHILDREN**, 2222 Welborn Street, Zip 75219–9982, Mailing Address: P.O. Box 190567, Zip 75219–0567; tel. 214/559–5000 **A**1 3 5 **F**3 9 11 25 26 33 37 41 50 52 56 58 62 64 66 72 73 75 77 79 80 81 82 84 96 100 107 119 121 132 135 137 **P**6
Primary Contact: J. C. Montgomery, Jr., President
COO: Robert L. Walker, Executive Vice President and Administrator
CFO: John T. Schoonmaker, Senior Vice President and Chief Financial Officer
CMO: John A. Herring, M.D., Chief of Staff
CIO: Hunt Gregg, Director Information Systems
CHR: James D. Sturgis, Director
Web address: www.tsrhc.org
Control: Other not–for–profit (including NFP Corporation) **Service:** Children's orthopedic

Staffed Beds: 52 **Admissions:** 2032 **Census:** 26 **Outpatient Visits:** 36925 **Births:** 0 **Total Expense ($000):** 86495 **Payroll Expense ($000):** 42502 **Personnel:** 705

☐ **TEXAS SPECIALTY HOSPITAL AT DALLAS (452067)**, 7955 Harry Hines Boulevard, Zip 75235–3395; tel. 214/637–0000 **A**1 9 10 **F**1 3 **S** Fundamental Long Term Care Holdings, LLC
Primary Contact: Cathy Campbell, Chief Executive Officer
CFO: Diana B. Smith, Chief Financial Officer
CMO: Juan Herrera, M.D., Medical Director
CHR: Tim Lozier, Director Human Resources
Web address: www.thicare.com
Control: Corporation, Investor–owned, for–profit **Service:** General Medical and Surgical

Staffed Beds: 66 **Admissions:** 484 **Census:** 33 **Outpatient Visits:** 1439 **Births:** 0 **Total Expense ($000):** 13755 **Payroll Expense ($000):** 5931 **Personnel:** 139

☐ **TIMBERLAWN MENTAL HEALTH SYSTEM (454081)**, 4600 Samuell Boulevard, Zip 75228–6800; tel. 214/381–7181 **A**1 9 10 **F**4 5 31 32 53 54 57 62 82 88 89 90 91 92 93 94 95 119 121 132 **S** Universal Health Services, Inc.
Primary Contact: Craig Nuckles, Chief Executive Officer, Managing and Regional Vice President
CMO: John Pascoe, M.D., Executive Medical Director
CIO: Jill Dorjee, Director Health Information Management & Quality Improvement
Web address: www.timberlawn.com
Control: Corporation, Investor–owned, for–profit **Service:** Psychiatric

Staffed Beds: 144 **Admissions:** 4906 **Census:** 108 **Outpatient Visits:** 18772 **Births:** 0 **Total Expense ($000):** 18203 **Payroll Expense ($000):** 8793 **Personnel:** 221

★ △ **UNIVERSITY OF TEXAS SOUTHWESTERN MEDICAL CENTER**, 5323 Harry Hines Boulevard, Zip 75390–9265; tel. 214/645–5555, (Includes UNIVERSITY OF TEXAS SOUTHWESTERN MEDICAL CENTER – ST. PAUL, 5909 Harry Hines Boulevard, Zip 75390–9200; UNIVERSITY OF TEXAS SOUTHWESTERN MEDICAL CENTER – ZALE LIPSHY, 5151 Harry Hines Boulevard, Sharon L. Riley, Chief Executive Officer) **A**2 3 5 7 8 9 10 **F**3 5 6 7 8 9 11 12 13 15 17 18 20 22 24 25 26 27 30 31 32 33 36 37 38 41 43 44 45 46 47 49 50 51 52 53 54 55 56 57 58 59 61 62 63 64 66 68 69 70 72 73 74 75 76 77 78 79 80 81 82 85 86 87 88 90 91 92 93 94 96 97 99 10 100 101 102 103 104 105 106 107 108 109 11 110 111 112 113 114 115 116 118 119 12 120 121 123 124 125 126 127 128 129 130 131 132 134 135 136 137 14 16 17 19 21 23 24 25 26 29 3 30 31 32 35 36 37 40 42 44 45 46 47 48 49 5 51 52 54 55 57 59 6 60 61 63 64 65 66 67 68 69 7 70 71 72 73 76 77 78 79 8 81 82 83 84 85 87 88 90 91 92 94 95 96 97 98 99 **P**5 6
Primary Contact: Sharon L. Riley, Chief Executive Officer
CFO: Jim Wentz, Associate Vice President and Chief Financial Officer
CMO: Patricia Bergen, M.D., Chief Medical Officer
CIO: Suresh Gunasekaran, Assistant Vice President Information Resources
CHR: William Behrendt, Ph.D., Vice President Human Resources
Web address: www.utsouthwestern.edu
Control: State–Government, nonfederal **Service:** General Medical and Surgical

Staffed Beds: 424 **Admissions:** 12688 **Census:** 313 **Outpatient Visits:** 70783 **Births:** 1143 **Total Expense ($000):** 184117884 **Payroll Expense ($000):** 74639392 **Personnel:** 1848

★ △ **VETERANS AFFAIRS NORTH TEXAS HEALTH CARE SYSTEM**, 4500 South Lancaster Road, Zip 75216–7167; tel. 214/742–8387, (Includes SAM RAYBURN MEMORIAL VETERANS CENTER, 1201 East Ninth Street, Bonham, Zip 75418–4091; tel. 903/583–2111), (Nonreporting) **A**1 2 3 5 7 8 9 **S** Department of Veterans Affairs
Primary Contact: Betty Bolin Brown, Ed.D., Director
CFO: Garry Martin, Chief Fiscal
CIO: Lucy Rogers, Chief Information Resource Management Systems
Web address: www.va.gov/sta/guide/home.asp
Control: Veterans Affairs, Government, federal **Service:** General Medical and Surgical

Staffed Beds: 875

☐ **VIBRA SPECIALTY HOSPITAL OF DALLAS (670022)**, 1950 Record Crossing Road, Zip 75235–6223; tel. 214/638–1500 **A**1 9 10 **F**1 3 25 73 75 82 119 137 **S** Vibra Healthcare
Primary Contact: Paul P. Hall, Jr., Chief Executive Officer
COO: Staci Jones, Chief Clinical Officer
CFO: Guy Lindholm, Chief Financial Officer
CMO: John Herrera, Medical Director
CHR: Tim Lozier, Director Human Resources
Web address: www.vshdallas.com
Control: Corporation, Investor–owned, for–profit **Service:** Long–Term Acute Care hospital

Staffed Beds: 60 **Admissions:** 153 **Census:** 9 **Outpatient Visits:** 0 **Births:** 0 **Total Expense ($000):** 6244 **Payroll Expense ($000):** 4837 **Personnel:** 84

DE SOTO—Dallas County

☐ **HICKORY TRAIL HOSPITAL (454065)**, 2000 North Old Hickory Trail, Zip 75115–2242; tel. 972/298–7323 **A**1 9 10 **F**4 5 25 31 32 36 66 82 88 89 93 94 95 119 **S** Psychiatric Solutions
Primary Contact: Shanti Carter, Chief Executive Officer
CFO: Terri Logsdon, Chief Financial Officer
CMO: Manoochehr Khatami, M.D., Medical Director
CHR: Sarah Warren, Coordinator Human Resources
Web address: www.cedarshospital.com
Control: Corporation, Investor–owned, for–profit **Service:** Psychiatric

Staffed Beds: 86 **Admissions:** 1632 **Census:** 42 **Outpatient Visits:** 5080 **Births:** 0 **Total Expense ($000):** 7802 **Payroll Expense ($000):** 4171 **Personnel:** 136

TX

☐ **SELECT SPECIALTY HOSPITAL–SOUTH DALLAS (452078)**, 800 Kirkwood Drive, Zip 75115; tel. 972/780–6500 **A**1 9 10 **F**1 25 31 32 38 80 119 137 **P**8 **S** Select Medical Corporation
Primary Contact: James Camp, Chief Executive Officer
Web address: www.selectmedicalcorp.com
Control: Corporation, Investor–owned, for–profit **Service:** Long–Term Acute Care hospital

Staffed Beds: 100 **Admissions:** 775 **Census:** 55 **Outpatient Visits:** 0 **Births:** 0 **Total Expense ($000):** 25521 **Payroll Expense ($000):** 10849 **Personnel:** 183

DECATUR—Wise County

★ **WISE REGIONAL HEALTH SYSTEM (450271)**, 2000 South FM 51, Zip 76234–9295; tel. 940/627–5921 **A**1 9 10 20 **F**3 11 12 13 15 17 18 20 22 24 25 26 27 30 31 32 38 40 43 52 54 55 56 57 59 62 68 72 73 74 75 76 77 79 84 85 86 88 89 93 94 96 97 100 102 103 106 107 119 120 121 124 137 **P**7
Primary Contact: Stephen M. Summers, CPA, FACHE, Chief Executive Officer
COO: Leon Fuqua, Assistant Administrator
CFO: Jim Eaton, Chief Financial Officer
CMO: Jon Walker, Chief of Staff
CIO: Joe Arispie, Director Information Systems
CHR: Mike McQuiston, Director Human Resources
Web address: www.wiseregional.com
Control: Hospital district or authority, Government, nonfederal **Service:** General Medical and Surgical

Staffed Beds: 131 **Admissions:** 4659 **Census:** 51 **Outpatient Visits:** 148712 **Births:** 804 **Total Expense ($000):** 84585 **Payroll Expense ($000):** 28772 **Personnel:** 790

DEL RIO—Val Verde County

★ **VAL VERDE REGIONAL MEDICAL CENTER (450154)**, 801 Bedell Avenue, Zip 78840–4185, Mailing Address: P.O. Box 1527, Zip 78840–1527; tel. 830/775–8566 **A**1 9 10 20 **F**3 7 11 13 15 18 25 26 31 32 33 35 38 40 42 46 50 51 55 56 70 71 74 75 77 79 81 82 84 86 93 96 97 99 100 103 106 107 118 119 122 135 136 **P**5 **S** Community Hospital Corporation
Primary Contact: Jack F. Houghton, Chief Executive Officer
Web address: www.vvrmc.org
Control: Hospital district or authority, Government, nonfederal **Service:** General Medical and Surgical

Staffed Beds: 86 **Admissions:** 3175 **Census:** 31 **Outpatient Visits:** 45600 **Births:** 968 **Total Expense ($000):** 36006 **Payroll Expense ($000):** 15061 **Personnel:** 333

DENISON—Grayson County

CARRUS SPECIALTY HOSPITAL (452041), (Formerly Texoma Medical Center Restorative Care Hospital), 1000 Memorial Drive, 4th Floor, Zip 75020–2035; tel. 903/415–4007, (Total facility includes 13 beds in nursing home–type unit) **A**9 10 **F**1 3 25 26 27 30 31 32 43 50 54 56 63 72 73 75 76 77 80 117 119 137 **P**8
Primary Contact: Verlinda Cobb, Administrator
Web address: www.thcs.org
Control: Other not–for–profit (including NFP Corporation) **Service:** General Medical and Surgical

Staffed Beds: 29 **Admissions:** 153 **Census:** 11 **Outpatient Visits:** 0 **Births:** 0 **Total Expense ($000):** 1309 **Payroll Expense ($000):** 970 **Personnel:** 38

☐ **TEXOMA MEDICAL CENTER (450324)**, 1000 Memorial Drive, Zip 75020–2035, Mailing Address: P.O. Box 890, Zip 75021–9988; tel. 903/416–4000 **A**1 9 10 **F**3 4 5 8 11 13 15 18 20 22 24 25 26 27 30 31 32 38 40 43 46 47 49 50 53 56 57 61 62 66 68 69 72 73 74 75 77 79 81 82 84 85 86 88 90 92 93 94 95 96 97 100 102 107 109 118 119 120 121 133 135 136 **P**3 5 **S** Universal Health Services, Inc.
Primary Contact: W. Mackey Watkins, M.D., President and Chief Executive Officer
CFO: Bobby Pruiett, Chief Financial Officer
CMO: Robert Sanders, M.D., Executive Vice President Medical Staff Affairs
CIO: Ty Sweeney, Vice President and Chief Information Officer
CHR: Minnie Burkhardt, Vice President and General Counsel
Web address: www.texomamedicalcenter.net
Control: Other not–for–profit (including NFP Corporation) **Service:** General Medical and Surgical

Staffed Beds: 205 **Admissions:** 5270 **Census:** 151 **Outpatient Visits:** 31519 **Births:** 295 **Total Expense ($000):** 58429 **Payroll Expense ($000):** 25575 **Personnel:** 1273

DENTON—Denton County

★ △ **DENTON REGIONAL MEDICAL CENTER (450634)**, 3535 South 1–35 East, Zip 76210; tel. 940/384–3535 **A**1 2 7 9 10 **F**3 12 13 18 20 22 24 25 26 27 30 31 32 33 38 43 44 49 50 55 56 57 62 64 66 67 68 72 73 74 75 76 77 79 80 81 82 84 85 86 96 97 100 102 106 107 116 119 121 124 135 136 137 **S** HCA
Primary Contact: Caleb F. O'Rear, Chief Executive Officer
COO: Jeffrey T. Lawrence, Chief Operating Officer
CFO: Elia Stokes, Chief Financial Officer
CMO: Filippo Masciarelli, Chief of Staff
CIO: Jason Sims, Manager Information Technology and Technical Services
CHR: Jenna Sutherland, Manager Human Resources
Web address: www.dentonregional.com
Control: Partnership, Investor–owned, for–profit **Service:** General Medical and Surgical

Staffed Beds: 208 **Admissions:** 9702 **Census:** 136 **Outpatient Visits:** 99804 **Births:** 978 **Total Expense ($000):** 107865 **Payroll Expense ($000):** 42954 **Personnel:** 773

MAYHILL HOSPITAL (670010), (Psych & Physical Rehab), 2809 South Mayhill Road, Zip 76208–5910; tel. 940/239–3000 **A**9 10 **F**38 85 88 92 93 94 119 **P**8 **S** SeniorHealth Incorporated
Primary Contact: William W. Brattvet, Administrator
Web address: www.mayhillhospital.com
Control: Partnership, Investor–owned, for–profit **Service:** Other specialty

Staffed Beds: 57 **Admissions:** 1109 **Census:** 32 **Outpatient Visits:** 2386 **Births:** 0 **Total Expense ($000):** 10854 **Payroll Expense ($000):** 4145 **Personnel:** 83

NORTH TEXAS HOSPITAL (450893), 2801 South Mayhill Road, Zip 76208; tel. 940/220–0600 **A**9 10 **F**3 12 32 38 49 51 77 79 80 84 96 100 102 107 116 137 **S** Cirrus Health
Primary Contact: Randy B. Bacus, FACHE, Chief Executive Officer and Administrator
Web address: www.northtexashospital.com
Control: Partnership, Investor–owned, for–profit **Service:** General Medical and Surgical

Staffed Beds: 16 **Admissions:** 508 **Census:** 2 **Outpatient Visits:** 11848 **Births:** 0 **Total Expense ($000):** 24069 **Payroll Expense ($000):** 4810 **Personnel:** 87

TX

★ **PRESBYTERIAN HOSPITAL OF DENTON (450743)**, 3000 I. 35 North, Zip 76201–3798; tel. 940/898–7000 **A**1 9 10 **F**3 8 11 12 13 15 18 20 22 24 25 26 27 30 31 32 33 38 43 46 48 49 55 56 57 68 70 72 73 74 76 77 79 80 81 84 86 96 97 100 102 103 106 107 118 119 120 121 124 134 135 136 137 **S** Community Health Systems, Inc.
Primary Contact: Stan C. Morton, Chief Executive Officer
COO: Jeff Reecer, Chief Operating Officer
CFO: David B. Meltzer, Chief Financial Officer
CIO: Ellen Painter, Director Marketing
CHR: Linda Bryan, Director Human Resources
Web address: www.dentonhospital.com
Control: Partnership, Investor–owned, for–profit **Service:** General Medical and Surgical

Staffed Beds: 208 **Admissions:** 9928 **Census:** 120 **Outpatient Visits:** 64312 **Births:** 2093 **Total Expense ($000):** 109219 **Payroll Expense ($000):** 35762 **Personnel:** 714

☐ **UNIVERSITY BEHAVIORAL HEALTH OF DENTON (454104)**, 2026 University Drive, Zip 76201; tel. 940/320–8100 **A**1 9 10 **F**4 5 31 78 88 89 93 94 95
Primary Contact: Susan M. Young, Chief Executive Officer
CFO: Cathi Spencer, Chief Financial Officer
CMO: Atique Khan, M.D., Medical Director
CHR: Henry In, Director Human Resources
Web address: www.ubhdenton.net
Control: Partnership, Investor–owned, for–profit **Service:** Psychiatric

Staffed Beds: 76 **Admissions:** 2578 **Census:** 57 **Outpatient Visits:** 13979 **Births:** 0 **Total Expense ($000):** 13342 **Payroll Expense ($000):** 6237 **Personnel:** 186

Hospital, Medicare Provider Number, Address, Telephone, Approval, Facility, and Physician Codes, Health Care System
★ American Hospital Association (AHA) membership
☐ The Joint Commission accreditation
○ American Osteopathic Association (AOA) accreditation
△ Commission on Accreditation of Rehabilitation Facilities (CARF) accreditation

DENVER CITY—Yoakum County

★ **YOAKUM COUNTY HOSPITAL (451308)**, 412 Mustang Avenue, Zip 79323–2750, Mailing Address: P.O. Drawer 1130, Zip 79323–1130; tel. 806/592–2121 **A**9 10 18 **F**3 11 13 24 25 30 31 32 33 38 40 50 52 55 56 57 59 61 62 73 74 79 82 84 86 96 107 119 122 135 **P**6 **S** Covenant Health System
Primary Contact: Clay Taylor, Chief Executive Officer
CFO: Suann Parrish, Chief Financial Officer
CMO: Christopher Cotton, M.D., Chief Medical Officer
CHR: Teresa Howard, Manager Human Resources
Web address: www.ych.us
Control: County–Government, nonfederal **Service:** General Medical and Surgical

Staffed Beds: 22 **Admissions:** 644 **Census:** 7 **Outpatient Visits:** 70808 **Births:** 100 **Total Expense ($000):** 16408 **Payroll Expense ($000):** 5326 **Personnel:** 154

DILLEY—Frio County

☐ **COMMUNITY GENERAL HOSPITAL (450813)**, 230 West Miller, Zip 78017; tel. 830/965–2003, (Nonreporting) **A**1 9 10
Primary Contact: Syed Parvez, M.D., Administrator
Control: Corporation, Investor–owned, for–profit **Service:** General Medical and Surgical

Staffed Beds: 18

DIMMITT—Castro County

★ **PLAINS MEMORIAL HOSPITAL (451350)**, 310 West Halsell Street, Zip 79027–1846, Mailing Address: P.O. Box 278, Zip 79027–0278; tel. 806/647–2191 **A**9 10 18 **F**7 11 31 32 33 38 40 42 46 50 52 55 56 57 61 62 64 66 67 75 79 80 81 84 86 87 96 102 107 119 122 124 137 **P**1 6
Primary Contact: Linda Rasor, RN, Chief Executive Officer
COO: Peggy A. Bradley, Chief Operating Officer
CFO: Milton Wilhite, Chief Financial Officer
CMO: Skylar Bizzell, Medical Director
CIO: Milton Wilhite, Chief Financial Officer
CHR: Debbie Underwood, Manager Human Resources
Web address: www.plainsmemorial.com
Control: Hospital district or authority, Government, nonfederal **Service:** General Medical and Surgical

Staffed Beds: 25 **Admissions:** 816 **Census:** 8 **Outpatient Visits:** 32722 **Births:** 0 **Total Expense ($000):** 7449 **Payroll Expense ($000):** 3646 **Personnel:** 131

TX

DUMAS—Moore County

☒ **MOORE COUNTY HOSPITAL DISTRICT (450221)**, 224 East Second Street, Zip 79029–3808; tel. 806/935–7171, (Total facility includes 60 beds in nursing home–type unit) **A**1 9 10 20 **F**3 7 11 13 15 24 30 31 32 33 37 38 40 42 46 50 51 55 56 57 61 68 73 74 75 77 79 80 81 84 86 96 100 103 107 117 119 120 121 122 135 136 137
Primary Contact: Jeff Turner, FACHE, Chief Executive Officer
COO: Yvonne Blue, Chief Operations Officer
CMO: Berta Kaemmerling, Chief Nursing Officer
CIO: Christopher Killion, Director Information Services
CHR: Eric Bleak, Director Human Resources
Web address: www.mchd.net
Control: Hospital district or authority, Government, nonfederal **Service:** General Medical and Surgical

Staffed Beds: 107 **Admissions:** 1532 **Census:** 72 **Outpatient Visits:** 29148 **Births:** 364 **Total Expense ($000):** 20698 **Payroll Expense ($000):** 9018 **Personnel:** 259

EAGLE LAKE—Colorado County

★ **RICE MEDICAL CENTER (451312)**, 600 South Austin Road, Zip 77434–3298, Mailing Address: P.O. Box 277, Zip 77434–0277; tel. 979/234–5571 **A**9 10 18 **F**11 13 15 25 30 31 38 40 55 57 62 63 68 74 77 79 96 100 107 122 **P**6 **S** CHRISTUS Health
Primary Contact: Susan Hernandez, RN, Interim Administrator
COO: Susan Hernandez, R.N., Director Nursing
CFO: Noble Anderson, Director Financial Services
CMO: Larry Penick, Chief of Staff
CHR: Erica Wilkerson, Administrative Secretary
Web address: www.ricemedicalcenter.org
Control: Hospital district or authority, Government, nonfederal **Service:** General Medical and Surgical

Staffed Beds: 25 **Admissions:** 554 **Census:** 6 **Outpatient Visits:** 17314 **Births:** 70 **Total Expense ($000):** 7318 **Payroll Expense ($000):** 2590 **Personnel:** 81

EAGLE PASS—Maverick County

☐ **FORT DUNCAN REGIONAL MEDICAL CENTER (450092)**, 3333 North Foster Maldonado Boulevard, Zip 78852; tel. 830/773–5321 **A**1 9 10 20 **F**3 13 15 25 31 32 33 38 40 46 55 57 59 62 63 66 68 73 74 75 79 81 82 84 85 86 96 100 102 107 118 119 135 136 137 **S** Universal Health Services, Inc.
Primary Contact: Rene Lopez, Chief Executive Officer
COO: Richard Prati, Chief Operating Officer
CFO: Joel Morales, Chief Financial Officer
CMO: Hector Trevino, Chief Medical Staff
CHR: Daisy Rodriquez, Director Human Resources
Web address: www.fortduncanmedicalcenter.com
Control: Corporation, Investor–owned, for–profit **Service:** General Medical and Surgical

Staffed Beds: 101 **Admissions:** 5088 **Census:** 57 **Outpatient Visits:** 33458 **Births:** 1127 **Total Expense ($000):** 45720 **Payroll Expense ($000):** 17987 **Personnel:** 318

EASTLAND—Eastland County

★ **EASTLAND MEMORIAL HOSPITAL (450411)**, 304 South Daugherty Street, Zip 76448–2609, Mailing Address: P.O. Box 897, Zip 76448–0897; tel. 254/629–2601 **A**9 10 20 **F**7 15 24 30 32 38 40 46 49 52 54 55 56 57 62 63 73 75 77 79 80 81 82 86 96 100 102 107 119 120 135 137
Primary Contact: Rick J. Montelongo, Chief Executive Officer
CFO: Shane Kernell, Chief Financial Officer
Web address: www.eastlandmemorial.com
Control: Hospital district or authority, Government, nonfederal **Service:** General Medical and Surgical

Staffed Beds: 36 **Admissions:** 1372 **Census:** 14 **Outpatient Visits:** 25642 **Births:** 61 **Total Expense ($000):** 9595 **Payroll Expense ($000):** 5276 **Personnel:** 154

EDEN—Concho County

CONCHO COUNTY HOSPITAL (451325), 614 Eaker Street, Zip 76837–0359, Mailing Address: P.O. Box 987, Zip 76837–0359; tel. 325/869–5911 **A**9 10 18 **F**3 31 32 38 40 53 55 57 63 66 75 82 122 135
Primary Contact: Dudley R. White, Administrator and Chief Executive Officer
CFO: Melanie Escamilla, Chief Financial Officer
CIO: Mary Castanuela, Associate Administrator
CHR: Melanie Escamilla, Chief Financial Officer
Web address: www.conchocountyhospital.com
Control: Hospital district or authority, Government, nonfederal **Service:** General Medical and Surgical

Staffed Beds: 16 **Admissions:** 95 **Census:** 1 **Outpatient Visits:** 10730 **Births:** 0 **Total Expense ($000):** 2527 **Payroll Expense ($000):** 1128 **Personnel:** 32

EDINBURG—Hidalgo County

☒ **CORNERSTONE REGIONAL HOSPITAL (450825)**, 2302 Cornerstone Boulevard, Zip 78539–8471; tel. 956/618–4444 **A**1 10 **F**3 25 30 31 32 35 37 38 43 46 51 55 62 72 77 79 80 82 107 **P**8 **S** Universal Health Services, Inc.
Primary Contact: Alma Medina, RN, Interim Chief Executive Officer
CFO: Chris Garza, Billing Coordinator
CMO: John G. Orfanos, M.D., Chief of Staff
CIO: Rene Villareal, Compliance Officer
CHR: Erika Betancourt, Coordinator Human Resources
Control: Partnership, Investor–owned, for–profit **Service:** General Medical and Surgical

Staffed Beds: 14 **Admissions:** 558 **Census:** 5 **Outpatient Visits:** 6528 **Births:** 0 **Total Expense ($000):** 12407 **Payroll Expense ($000):** 3441 **Personnel:** 82

☐ **DOCTOR'S HOSPITAL AT RENAISSANCE (450869)**, 5501 South McColl Road, Zip 78539; tel. 956/664–0036 **A**1 9 10 **F**3 12 13 15 17 18 20 22 25 26 27 30 31 32 33 37 38 43 50 51 55 56 57 59 62 66 68 70 72 73 74 76 77 79 80 82 84 85 87 88 89 90 91 92 93 94 95 96 97 99 100 101 102 103 104 105 106 107 109 119 121 132 135 136 137 **P**3
Primary Contact: Laurence Gelman, M.D., Chief Executive Officer
COO: Marissa Castaneda, Chief Operating Officer and Director Marketing
CFO: Susan S. Turley, Chief Financial Officer
CIO: Les Clonch, Chief Information Officer
Web address: www.doctorshospitalatrenaissance.com
Control: Partnership, Investor–owned, for–profit **Service:** General Medical and Surgical

Staffed Beds: 403 **Admissions:** 16453 **Census:** 175 **Outpatient Visits:** 133923 **Births:** 1708 **Total Expense ($000):** 215090 **Payroll Expense ($000):** 75098 **Personnel:** 2298

Many Facility Codes have changed. Please refer to the AHA Guide Code Chart.

☐ △ **EDINBURG REGIONAL MEDICAL CENTER (450119)**, 1102 West Trenton Road, Zip 78539–6199; tel. 956/388–6000, (Includes EDINBURG CHILDREN'S HOSPITAL, 1400 West Trenton Road, Zip 78539; tel. 956/388–8000), (Total facility includes 8 beds in nursing home–type unit) **A**1 7 10 **F**3 7 11 12 13 15 17 18 20 22 25 26 30 31 32 38 40 41 43 44 46 49 50 55 56 57 59 62 65 68 70 72 73 74 75 76 77 79 80 81 82 83 84 85 86 88 89 90 91 92 93 94 95 96 97 100 102 103 106 107 109 117 119 121 127 135 136 137 **P**1 **S** Universal Health Services, Inc.
Primary Contact: Linda Resendez, RN, Chief Executive Officer
COO: Mike Adams, Chief Operating Officer
CMO: Humberto Hidalgo, M.D., Chief of Staff
CIO: Rosie L. Mendiola, Director Information Systems
CHR: Cindi Mistrot, Associate Administrator
Web address: www.edinburgregional.com
Control: Partnership, Investor–owned, for–profit **Service:** General Medical and Surgical

Staffed Beds: 848 **Admissions:** 15910 **Census:** 199 **Outpatient Visits:** 49468 **Births:** 721 **Total Expense ($000):** 155715 **Payroll Expense ($000):** 53355 **Personnel:** 2334

LIFECARE HOSPITALS OF SOUTH TEXAS (452063), 333 West Freddy Gonzalez Drive, Zip 78539–6132; tel. 956/388–1800 **A**9 10 **F**1 3 24 25 44 55 59 66 73 75 80 137 **S** LifeCare Management Services
Primary Contact: David L. Tupper, Chief Executive Officer
CHR: Blanca Sierra, Human Resources Director
Web address: www.lifecare–hospitals.com
Control: Corporation, Investor–owned, for–profit **Service:** Long–Term Acute Care hospital

Staffed Beds: 94 **Admissions:** 971 **Census:** 67 **Outpatient Visits:** 0 **Births:** 0 **Total Expense ($000):** 29632 **Payroll Expense ($000):** 12225 **Personnel:** 216

EDNA—Jackson County

JACKSON COUNTY HOSPITAL DISTRICT (451363), 1013 South Wells Street, Zip 77957–4098; tel. 361/782–5241, (Total facility includes 37 beds in nursing home–type unit) **A**9 10 18 **F**11 15 24 25 28 30 32 33 38 40 50 54 55 56 57 61 62 63 64 66 73 75 79 80 82 86 93 94 96 100 107 118 119 122 135 137 **P**8
Primary Contact: Asa B. Wilson, Ph.D., Administrator and Chief Executive Officer
COO: Asa B. Wilson, Ph.D., Administrator and Chief Executive Officer
CFO: Diana Williams, Chief Financial Officer
CMO: Eugene Hernandez, Chief of Staff
CIO: Jackie Venuto, Director Health Improvement Management
CHR: Jan Clinkscales, Director Human Resources
Web address: www.jchd.org
Control: Hospital district or authority, Government, nonfederal **Service:** General Medical and Surgical

Staffed Beds: 62 **Admissions:** 394 **Census:** 37 **Outpatient Visits:** 4160 **Births:** 0 **Total Expense ($000):** 8958 **Payroll Expense ($000):** 3193 **Personnel:** 103

EL CAMPO—Wharton County

EL CAMPO MEMORIAL HOSPITAL (450694), 303 Sandy Corner Road, Zip 77437–9535; tel. 979/543–6251 **A**9 10 **F**3 11 15 25 31 32 33 38 46 54 55 56 57 61 62 66 68 73 75 77 79 81 86 87 96 97 100 107 118 119 121 122 137 **P**6
Primary Contact: Steve Gularte, Administrator
CFO: Tisha Zalman, Chief Financial Officer
CMO: Ted Scott, Chief of Staff
Web address: www.ecmh.org
Control: Hospital district or authority, Government, nonfederal **Service:** General Medical and Surgical

Staffed Beds: 30 **Admissions:** 834 **Census:** 9 **Outpatient Visits:** 59733 **Births:** 1 **Total Expense ($000):** 13662 **Payroll Expense ($000):** 5314 **Personnel:** 131

EL PASO—El Paso County

★ △ **DEL SOL MEDICAL CENTER (450646)**, 10301 Gateway West, Zip 79925–7798; tel. 915/595–9000 **A**1 2 7 9 10 **F**11 12 13 15 17 18 20 22 24 25 26 27 30 31 32 33 34 38 40 43 46 50 51 52 53 54 55 56 57 60 62 66 68 70 72 73 74 75 76 77 79 80 81 82 84 85 86 96 97 98 100 102 106 107 118 119 120 121 123 124 135 136 137 **S** HCA
Primary Contact: Jacob Cintron, Chief Executive Officer
COO: Chris Mowan, Chief Operating Officer
CFO: Julie Hayes, Chief Financial Officer
CMO: Manuel Feliberti, M.D., Medical Director
CIO: Barbara Nelson, Chief Information Officer
Web address: www.delsolmedicalcenter.com
Control: Partnership, Investor–owned, for–profit **Service:** General Medical and Surgical

Staffed Beds: 289 **Admissions:** 15604 **Census:** 218 **Outpatient Visits:** 137692 **Births:** 2606 **Total Expense ($000):** 138363 **Payroll Expense ($000):** 54523 **Personnel:** 1082

☐ **EL PASO PSYCHIATRIC CENTER (454100)**, 4615 Alameda Avenue, Zip 79905–2702; tel. 915/532–2202 **A**1 3 5 9 10 **F**25 30 32 88 89 93 119 **P**6 **S** Texas Department of State Health Services
Primary Contact: Zulema Carrillo, Chief Executive Officer
CMO: Nicolas Baida–Fragoso, Director Clinical
Control: State–Government, nonfederal **Service:** Psychiatric

Staffed Beds: 74 **Admissions:** 1058 **Census:** 68 **Outpatient Visits:** 0 **Births:** 0 **Total Expense ($000):** 16148 **Personnel:** 234

☐ **EL PASO SPECIALTY HOSPITAL (450845)**, 1755 Curie Drive, Zip 79902; tel. 915/533–7465 **A**1 9 10 **F**3 25 30 38 43 55 57 66 73 77 79 82 119 120 **S** National Surgical Hospitals
Primary Contact: Paul Gallagher, Chief Executive Officer
COO: Fred Arellano, Chief Operating Officer
CFO: Pauline Motts, Chief Financial Officer
Web address: www.elpasospecialtyhospital.com
Control: Partnership, Investor–owned, for–profit **Service:** Orthopedic

Staffed Beds: 31 **Admissions:** 830 **Census:** 8 **Outpatient Visits:** 11380 **Births:** 0 **Total Expense ($000):** 20078 **Payroll Expense ($000):** 5306 **Personnel:** 162

☐ △ **HIGHLANDS REGIONAL REHABILITATION HOSPITAL (453086)**, 1395 George Dieter Drive, Zip 79936; tel. 915/298–7222 **A**1 7 9 10 **F**3 25 32 55 56 57 62 72 73 77 81 82 85 86 90 107 119 121 132 135 137 **S** United Rehab Corporation
Primary Contact: William G. Collins, Chief Executive Officer
Control: Partnership, Investor–owned, for–profit **Service:** Rehabilitation

Staffed Beds: 41 **Admissions:** 793 **Census:** 26 **Outpatient Visits:** 6150 **Births:** 0 **Total Expense ($000):** 11845 **Payroll Expense ($000):** 4982 **Personnel:** 120

★ **LAS PALMAS MEDICAL CENTER (450107)**, 1801 North Oregon Street, Zip 79902–3591; tel. 915/521–1200, (Includes LAS PALMAS REHABILITATION HOSPITAL, 300 Waymore Drive, Zip 79902–1628; tel. 915/577–2600) **A**1 2 5 9 10 **F**11 12 13 15 18 20 22 24 25 26 27 30 31 32 33 34 38 40 46 50 51 52 53 54 55 56 57 60 62 63 66 68 70 71 72 73 74 75 76 77 79 81 82 83 84 85 86 96 97 100 103 106 107 109 119 120 121 135 136 137 **S** HCA
Primary Contact: Hank Hernandez, Chief Executive Officer
COO: Don Karl, Chief Operating Officer
Web address: www.laspalmashealth.com
Control: Partnership, Investor–owned, for–profit **Service:** General Medical and Surgical

Staffed Beds: 261 **Admissions:** 11248 **Census:** 160 **Outpatient Visits:** 92022 **Births:** 1935 **Total Expense ($000):** 151742 **Payroll Expense ($000):** 47175 **Personnel:** 887

☐ **MESA HILL SPECIALTY HOSPITAL (452035)**, 2311 North Oregon Street, Zip 79902–3216; tel. 915/545–1823 **A**1 9 10 **F**1 8 25 30 31 32 43 44 45 53 54 55 56 57 58 60 62 63 72 73 75 80 81 82 119 132 137
Primary Contact: JoAnn Beatty, Chief Executive Officer
COO: Elena Pino, Chief Nursing Officer and Chief Operating Officer
CFO: Priscilla Carter, Chief Financial Officer
Web address: www.ihs–inc.com
Control: Corporation, Investor–owned, for–profit **Service:** Long–Term Acute Care hospital

Staffed Beds: 32 **Admissions:** 330 **Census:** 22 **Outpatient Visits:** 1198 **Births:** 0 **Total Expense ($000):** 7029 **Payroll Expense ($000):** 2892 **Personnel:** 61

TX

Hospital, Medicare Provider Number, Address, Telephone, Approval, Facility, and Physician Codes, Health Care System

★ American Hospital Association (AHA) membership
☐ The Joint Commission accreditation
○ American Osteopathic Association (AOA) accreditation
△ Commission on Accreditation of Rehabilitation Facilities (CARF) accreditation

☐ **PHYSICIANS HOSPITAL (450877)**, 1416 George Dieter Drive, Zip 79936–7601; tel. 915/598–4240 **A**1 10 **F**3 18 20 22 25 26 30 38 46 49 50 55 62 66 77 79 80 82 96 97 100 102 107 119
Primary Contact: Gregory Padilla, Chief Executive Officer
CFO: Melissa Campa, Interim Chief Financial Officer
CIO: Jaime Gonzalez, Director Information Technology
CHR: Glen Hinton, Director Human Resources
Web address: www.physicianshospital.net
Control: Partnership, Investor–owned, for–profit **Service:** General Medical and Surgical

Staffed Beds: 40 **Admissions:** 2132 **Census:** 23 **Outpatient Visits:** 31536 **Births:** 0 **Total Expense ($000):** 41279 **Payroll Expense ($000):** 10580 **Personnel:** 266

★ **PROVIDENCE MEMORIAL HOSPITAL (450002)**, 2001 North Oregon Street, Zip 79902–3368; tel. 915/577–6011 **A**1 2 9 10 **F**3 11 12 13 14 15 17 18 19 20 21 22 23 25 26 27 28 31 32 33 38 40 41 42 43 46 49 50 51 53 55 56 57 62 63 68 70 71 72 73 74 75 76 77 79 80 81 82 83 84 86 96 97 99 100 102 106 107 116 118 119 121 123 124 135 136 137 **P**8 **S** TENET Healthcare Corporation
Primary Contact: Irene Chavez, Chief Executive Officer
CFO: Charles Hondley, Chief Financial Officer
CIO: Ray Davis, Administrative Director
CHR: Mark Thomasson, Vice President Human Resources
Web address: www.sphn.com
Control: Partnership, Investor–owned, for–profit **Service:** General Medical and Surgical

Staffed Beds: 359 **Admissions:** 19260 **Census:** 236 **Outpatient Visits:** 164566 **Births:** 4330 **Total Expense ($000):** 208155 **Payroll Expense ($000):** 70438 **Personnel:** 1376

★ **R. E. THOMASON GENERAL HOSPITAL (450024)**, 4815 Alameda Avenue, Zip 79905–2794, Mailing Address: P.O. Box 20009, Zip 79998–0009; tel. 915/544–1200 **A**1 2 3 5 9 10 **F**3 8 11 13 15 18 20 22 24 25 26 27 30 31 32 33 35 37 38 40 46 47 48 49 50 51 52 53 55 57 59 60 62 63 66 68 70 71 72 73 74 75 77 79 80 81 82 84 86 87 90 96 99 100 102 106 107 119 123 132 133 134 135 136 137 **P**6
Primary Contact: James N. Valenti, FACHE, President and Chief Executive Officer
COO: James N. Valenti, FACHE, President and Chief Executive Officer
CFO: Philip Rivera, Chief Financial Officer
CMO: Alan Tyroch, Chief of Staff
CIO: Janina Prada, Director
CHR: Gilbert Blancas, Director Human Resources
Web address: www.thomasoncares.org
Control: Hospital district or authority, Government, nonfederal **Service:** General Medical and Surgical

Staffed Beds: 282 **Admissions:** 15353 **Census:** 183 **Outpatient Visits:** 504257 **Births:** 4952 **Total Expense ($000):** 269445 **Payroll Expense ($000):** 81448 **Personnel:** 1809

TX

★ **SIERRA MEDICAL CENTER (450668)**, 1625 Medical Center Drive, Zip 79902–5044; tel. 915/747–4000 **A**1 2 9 10 **F**3 11 13 15 17 18 20 22 24 25 26 27 31 32 33 38 41 43 44 46 47 48 49 50 53 55 56 57 60 62 63 66 68 70 72 73 74 75 76 77 79 80 81 96 97 99 100 102 103 106 107 112 119 121 123 127 134 135 136 137 **P**8 **S** TENET Healthcare Corporation
Primary Contact: Edmundo Castaneda, Chief Executive Officer
CFO: Lynne Mitchell, Chief Financial Officer
Web address: www.sphn.com
Control: Partnership, Investor–owned, for–profit **Service:** General Medical and Surgical

Staffed Beds: 334 **Admissions:** 12498 **Census:** 164 **Outpatient Visits:** 87049 **Births:** 2058 **Total Expense ($000):** 140863 **Payroll Expense ($000):** 44673 **Personnel:** 887

★ △ **SIERRA PROVIDENCE PHYSICAL REHABILITATION HOSPITAL (453033)**, 1740 Curie Drive, Zip 79902–2900; tel. 915/544–3399 **A**1 7 9 10 **F**3 24 25 26 30 31 32 53 62 72 75 77 85 86 119 121 124 132 **S** TENET Healthcare Corporation
Primary Contact: John Harris, President
COO: Gene Miller, Senior Vice President and Chief Operating Officer
CFO: Paul Hymel, Chief Financial Officer
CHR: Mark Thomasson, Vice President Human Resources
Web address: www.sphn.com
Control: Corporation, Investor–owned, for–profit **Service:** Rehabilitation

Staffed Beds: 42 **Admissions:** 1072 **Census:** 35 **Outpatient Visits:** 26474 **Total Expense ($000):** 14144 **Payroll Expense ($000):** 7197 **Personnel:** 182

☐ **SOUTHWESTERN GENERAL HOSPITAL (450760)**, 1221 North Cotton, Zip 79902–3096; tel. 915/496–9600, (Nonreporting) **A**1 9 10
Primary Contact: Joseph Wright, Chief Executive Officer
CFO: Eddie Martinez, Chief Financial Officer
CMO: Perry W. Reding, M.D., Chief of Staff
CIO: Peter Zenker, Director Information Technology
CHR: Arlene E. Contreras, Director Human Resources
Web address: www.pachosp.com
Control: Corporation, Investor–owned, for–profit **Service:** General Medical and Surgical

Staffed Beds: 23

☐ **TRIUMPH HOSPITAL EL PASO (452079)**, 1740 Curie Drive, Zip 79902; tel. 915/351–9044 **A**1 9 10 **F**1 3 25 30 31 32 56 75 82 119 133 137 **P**5 **S** Triumph HealthCare
Primary Contact: Jay Quintana, Chief Executive Officer
CFO: Glen Powers, Chief Financial Officer
CMO: Mauricio Jimenez, M.D., Chief Medical Officer
CHR: Laura Anchondo, Administrator Human Resources
Web address: www.triumph–healthcare.com
Control: Corporation, Investor–owned, for–profit **Service:** Long–Term Acute Care hospital

Staffed Beds: 29 **Admissions:** 246 **Census:** 23 **Outpatient Visits:** 0 **Births:** 0 **Total Expense ($000):** 10388 **Payroll Expense ($000):** 3885 **Personnel:** 73

★ **WILLIAM BEAUMONT ARMY MEDICAL CENTER**, 5005 North Piedras Street, Zip 79920–5001; tel. 915/569–2121, (Nonreporting) **A**1 2 3 5 **S** Department of the Army, Office of the Surgeon General
Primary Contact: Colonel John A. Powell, Commanding Officer
COO: Colonel James J. Leech, Commander
CMO: Colonel Homer Lemar, M.D., Deputy Commander Clinical Services
CIO: Major Rion Koon, Chief Information Management Division
Web address: www.wbamc.amedd.army.mil
Control: Army, Government, federal **Service:** General Medical and Surgical

Staffed Beds: 209

ELDORADO—Schleicher County

SCHLEICHER COUNTY MEDICAL CENTER (451304), 400 West Murchison, Zip 76936, Mailing Address: Box V, Zip 76936; tel. 325/853–2507 **A**9 10 18 **F**11 30 31 32 33 38 40 43 44 45 55 57 64 66 82 86 96 102 107 119 122 **P**6 **S** Preferred Management Corporation
Primary Contact: Sharon Dietz, Administrator
CFO: Beverly Minor, Assistant Administrator and Chief Financial Officer
Control: Corporation, Investor–owned, for–profit **Service:** General Medical and Surgical

Staffed Beds: 14 **Admissions:** 108 **Census:** 1 **Outpatient Visits:** 2969 **Births:** 0 **Total Expense ($000):** 1690 **Payroll Expense ($000):** 893 **Personnel:** 33

ELECTRA—Wichita County

★ **ELECTRA MEMORIAL HOSPITAL (451343)**, 1207 South Bailey Street, Zip 76360–3221, Mailing Address: P.O. Box 1112, Zip 76360–1112; tel. 940/495–3981 **A**9 10 18 **F**3 7 11 28 31 34 38 40 50 52 54 55 57 61 62 63 64 75 79 86 87 96 102 118 120 122 135 136 137
Primary Contact: Jan A. Reed, CPA, Administrator and Chief Executive Officer
CFO: Rebecca McCain, Chief Financial Officer and Assistant Administrator
Web address: www.electrahospital.com
Control: Hospital district or authority, Government, nonfederal **Service:** General Medical and Surgical

Staffed Beds: 23 **Admissions:** 448 **Census:** 6 **Outpatient Visits:** 16557 **Births:** 0 **Total Expense ($000):** 6856 **Payroll Expense ($000):** 3676 **Personnel:** 114

ENNIS—Ellis County

★ **ENNIS REGIONAL MEDICAL CENTER (450833)**, 2201 West Lampasas Street, Zip 75119; tel. 972/875–0900 **A**1 9 10 **F**3 11 13 15 25 30 31 32 38 40 50 51 55 56 57 66 68 74 75 77 79 80 84 86 96 100 103 107 135 **S** LifePoint Hospitals, Inc.
Primary Contact: David Anderson, Chief Executive Officer
CFO: Jack Wilcox, Chief Financial Officer
CMO: Basem Jassin, M.D., Chief of Staff
CHR: Judy Laister, Director Human Resources
Web address: www.ennisregional.com
Control: Partnership, Investor–owned, for–profit **Service:** General Medical and Surgical

Staffed Beds: 56 **Admissions:** 2121 **Census:** 14 **Outpatient Visits:** 29648 **Births:** 447 **Total Expense ($000):** 26730 **Payroll Expense ($000):** 9250 **Personnel:** 196

FAIRFIELD—Freestone County

★ **EAST TEXAS MEDICAL CENTER FAIRFIELD (450658)**, 125 Newman Street, Zip 75840–1499; tel. 903/389–2121 **A**9 10 20 **F**15 24 31 32 38 43 55 57 73 79 96 107 119 121 122 **P**7 **S** East Texas Medical Center Regional Healthcare System
Primary Contact: Ruth Cook, Administrator
CFO: David A. Travis, Chief Financial Officer
CMO: J. Michael Orms, M.D., Chief of Staff
CHR: Jennifer Rummell, Director Human Resources
Web address: www.etmc.org
Control: Other not–for–profit (including NFP Corporation) **Service:** General Medical and Surgical

Staffed Beds: 20 **Admissions:** 728 **Census:** 8 **Outpatient Visits:** 33368 **Births:** 0 **Total Expense ($000):** 9511 **Payroll Expense ($000):** 3388 **Personnel:** 96

Many Facility Codes have changed. Please refer to the AHA Guide Code Chart.

FLORESVILLE—Wilson County

CONNALLY MEDICAL CENTER (450108), 499 10th Street, Zip 78114–2798; tel. 830/393–1300 **A**9 10 **F**3 15 25 33 38 40 55 57 61 62 68 73 79 81 96 97 100 107 119 121 122 124 135
Primary Contact: Frances L. Chilek, RN, Administrator
CFO: Martin Tanneberger, Chief Financial Officer
CMO: Harry Chavez, M.D., Chief of Staff
CIO: Melvin Albert, Manager Information
CHR: Dan Hernandez, Director Human Resources
Web address: www.connally.com
Control: Hospital district or authority, Government, nonfederal **Service:** General Medical and Surgical

Staffed Beds: 44 **Admissions:** 1607 **Census:** 14 **Outpatient Visits:** 36395 **Births:** 0 **Total Expense ($000):** 18561 **Payroll Expense ($000):** 7746 **Personnel:** 210

FORT HOOD—Bell County

★ **CARL R. DARNALL ARMY MEDICAL CENTER**, 36000 Darnall Loop, Zip 76544–4752; tel. 254/288–8000, (Nonreporting) **A**1 2 3 5 9 **S** Department of the Army, Office of the Surgeon General
Primary Contact: Colonel Casper P. Jones, III, Commander
CFO: Lieutenant Colonel Patrick Grady, Chief Resource Management
CMO: Lieutenant Colonel Wilma Larsen, Deputy Commander Clinical Services
CIO: Major David Bowen, Chief Information Management
CHR: Lieutenant Colonel Paul Anderson, Chief Human Resources
Web address: www.hood–meddac.army.mil
Control: Army, Government, federal **Service:** General Medical and Surgical

Staffed Beds: 109

FORT SAM HOUSTON—Bexar County

★ **BROOKE ARMY MEDICAL CENTER**, 3851 Roger Brookes Drive, Zip 78234–6200; tel. 210/916–4141, (Nonreporting) **A**1 2 3 5 9 **S** Department of the Army, Office of the Surgeon General
Primary Contact: Brigadier General James K. Gilman, Commander
COO: Colonel John Shero, M.D., Deputy Commander for Administration
CFO: Lieutenant Colonel Talford Mindingal, Chief Resource Management Division
CMO: Colonel Carlos Angueira, Deputy Commander Clinical Services
CIO: Lieutenant Colonel Hailey Windham, Chief Information Management
CHR: Rose Juarez, Chief Civilian Personnel Branch
Web address: www.bamc.amedd.army.mil
Control: Army, Government, federal **Service:** General Medical and Surgical

Staffed Beds: 226

FORT STOCKTON—Pecos County

★ **PECOS COUNTY MEMORIAL HOSPITAL (450178)**, 387 West I. H–10, Zip 79735–8912, Mailing Address: P.O. Box 1648, Zip 79735–1648; tel. 432/336–2241 **A**9 10 20 **F**3 11 13 25 30 31 32 33 38 40 52 55 57 61 63 73 74 79 86 96 100 107 118 119 **P**5 6
Primary Contact: Russell Tippin, Administrator and Chief Executive Officer
CFO: Leticia Fox, Chief Financial Officer
CMO: Subodh Mallik, M.D., Chief of Staff
CHR: Diana Mesa, Director Human Resources
Web address: www.pcmhfs.com
Control: County–Government, nonfederal **Service:** General Medical and Surgical

Staffed Beds: 27 **Admissions:** 1315 **Census:** 11 **Outpatient Visits:** 35287 **Births:** 190 **Total Expense ($000):** 16874 **Payroll Expense ($000):** 6753 **Personnel:** 216

FORT WORTH—Tarrant County

★ **BAYLOR ALL SAINTS MEDICAL CENTER AT FORT WORTH (450137)**, 1400 Eighth Avenue, Zip 76104–4192; tel. 817/926–2544, (Includes BAYLOR MEDICAL CENTER AT SOUTHWEST FORT WORTH, 7100 Oakmont Boulevard, Zip 76132–3999; tel. 817/346–5700) **A**1 9 10 **F**3 11 13 15 17 18 20 22 24 25 26 27 30 31 32 33 34 36 38 47 49 52 53 57 61 62 66 68 70 71 72 73 74 75 76 77 78 79 81 82 85 86 87 88 90 91 92 93 94 95 96 97 100 102 107 119 120 121 124 127 128 131 135 136 137 **P**5 6 **S** Baylor Health Care System
Primary Contact: Steven R. Newton, President and Chief Executive Officer
COO: Sandra Aaron, Chief Operating Officer
CFO: Jay Whitfield, Vice President Finance
CIO: Sandy Vaughn, Director Information Services
CHR: Julie Strittmatter, Director Human Resources
Web address: www.baylorhealth.com
Control: Other not–for–profit (including NFP Corporation) **Service:** General Medical and Surgical

Staffed Beds: 393 **Admissions:** 16807 **Census:** 226 **Outpatient Visits:** 142252 **Births:** 2643 **Total Expense ($000):** 264764 **Payroll Expense ($000):** 97481 **Personnel:** 1702

□ **BAYLOR SURGICAL HOSPITAL AT FORT WORTH (450880)**, 750 12th Avenue, Zip 76104; tel. 817/334–5050 **A**1 10 **F**3 25 30 31 38 51 56 62 73 75 77 79 80 81 82 96 100 102 107 130
Primary Contact: Jeff Andrews, Chief Executive Officer
Web address: www.mcsh–hospital.com
Control: Partnership, Investor–owned, for–profit **Service:** General Medical and Surgical

Staffed Beds: 22 **Admissions:** 887 **Census:** 5 **Outpatient Visits:** 12901 **Births:** 0 **Total Expense ($000):** 32716 **Payroll Expense ($000):** 6688 **Personnel:** 134

★ **COOK CHILDREN'S MEDICAL CENTER (453300)**, 801 Seventh Avenue, Zip 76104–2796; tel. 682/885–4000 **A**1 9 10 **F**3 7 8 19 21 23 25 26 27 28 31 32 33 36 37 38 41 43 44 50 53 55 56 57 58 59 60 62 66 70 72 73 75 76 77 78 79 80 81 82 83 84 85 86 87 88 89 90 91 92 94 95 96 97 100 101 102 106 107 114 118 119 120 121 123 125 127 132 133 135 **P**6
Primary Contact: Rick W. Merrill, President and Chief Executive Officer
CMO: James C. Cunningham, M.D., Chief Medical Officer
CIO: Matthew Murray, M.D., Interim Senior Vice President Information Systems
CHR: Frank J. Rossi, Senior Vice President Human Resources
Web address: www.cookchildrens.org
Control: Other not–for–profit (including NFP Corporation) **Service:** Children's general

Staffed Beds: 240 **Admissions:** 10852 **Census:** 192 **Outpatient Visits:** 251260 **Births:** 0 **Total Expense ($000):** 345100 **Payroll Expense ($000):** 127835 **Personnel:** 2289

★ △ **HARRIS CONTINUED CARE HOSPITAL (452018)**, 1301 Pennsylvania Avenue, 4th Floor, Zip 76104–2190; tel. 817/250–5500 **A**1 7 9 10 **F**1 3 30 31 32 41 82 119 137 **S** Texas Health Resources
Primary Contact: Susan Louise Baldwin, RN, FACHE, President and Chief Nursing Officer
CFO: Lynn Gipson, Chief Financial Officer
CMO: John Pender, M.D., Medical Director
CHR: Mary Braddock, Human Resources Generalist
Web address: www.texashealth.org
Control: Church–operated, Nongovernment, not–for profit **Service:** Long–Term Acute Care hospital

Staffed Beds: 10 **Admissions:** 123 **Census:** 9 **Outpatient Visits:** 0 **Births:** 0 **Total Expense ($000):** 6382 **Payroll Expense ($000):** 2433 **Personnel:** 43

HARRIS METHODIST FORT WORTH See Texas Health Harris Methodist Fort Worth

HARRIS METHODIST SOUTHWEST See Texas Health Harris Methodist Southwest

★ **HEALTHSOUTH REHABILITATION HOSPITAL (453041)**, 1212 West Lancaster Avenue, Zip 76102–4510; tel. 817/870–2336 **A**1 9 10 **F**3 25 43 62 72 73 77 81 85 86 90 118 119 120 132 137 **S** HEALTHSOUTH Corporation
Primary Contact: Jon McPike, Chief Executive Officer
CFO: Sherry Hapney, Chief Financial Officer
CMO: Patrick Donovan, M.D., Director Medical Staff
CHR: Dori Woods, Director Human Resources
Web address: www.healthsouth.com
Control: Corporation, Investor–owned, for–profit **Service:** Rehabilitation

Staffed Beds: 60 **Admissions:** 803 **Census:** 30 **Outpatient Visits:** 10485 **Births:** 0 **Total Expense ($000):** 10447 **Payroll Expense ($000):** 5817 **Personnel:** 138

★ **HEALTHSOUTH REHABILITATION HOSPITAL–CITYVIEW (453042)**, 6701 Oakmont Boulevard, Zip 76132–2957; tel. 817/370–4700 **A**1 9 10 **F**3 25 32 43 53 61 62 75 85 86 118 119 120 121 132 137 **S** HEALTHSOUTH Corporation
Primary Contact: Barbara Mobley, Chief Executive Officer
Web address: www.healthsouth.com
Control: Corporation, Investor–owned, for–profit **Service:** Rehabilitation

Staffed Beds: 62 **Admissions:** 989 **Census:** 39 **Outpatient Visits:** 28302 **Births:** 0 **Total Expense ($000):** 13906 **Payroll Expense ($000):** 7966 **Personnel:** 197

TX

Hospital, Medicare Provider Number, Address, Telephone, Approval, Facility, and Physician Codes, Health Care System
★ American Hospital Association (AHA) membership
□ The Joint Commission accreditation
○ American Osteopathic Association (AOA) accreditation
△ Commission on Accreditation of Rehabilitation Facilities (CARF) accreditation

★ **HUGULEY MEMORIAL MEDICAL CENTER (450677)**, 11801 South Freeway, Zip 76134, Mailing Address: P.O. Box 6337, Zip 76115–6337; tel. 817/293–9110 **A**1 9 10 **F**3 5 13 15 17 18 20 22 24 25 26 27 28 30 31 32 33 36 38 41 49 51 52 53 54 55 56 57 59 61 62 66 68 69 73 74 75 76 77 78 79 80 81 82 84 86 88 90 91 92 93 94 95 96 97 99 100 102 106 107 108 109 119 121 124 135 136 137 **S** Adventist Health System Sunbelt Health Care Corporation
Primary Contact: Peter M. Weber, President and Chief Executive Officer
CFO: Dan Enderson, Chief Financial Officer
CMO: Edward Laue, M.D., Chief Medical Officer
CIO: David Smith, Manager Data Center
CHR: Leah Foley, Director Human Resources
Web address: www.huguley.org
Control: Church–operated, Nongovernment, not–for profit **Service:** General Medical and Surgical

Staffed Beds: 207 **Admissions:** 10275 **Census:** 117 **Outpatient Visits:** 104331 **Births:** 923 **Total Expense ($000):** 119403 **Payroll Expense ($000):** 44371 **Personnel:** 1111

JOHN PETER SMITH HOSPITAL See JPS Health Network

★ **JPS HEALTH NETWORK (450039)**, 1500 South Main Street, Zip 76104–4941; tel. 817/921–3431, (Includes JOHN PETER SMITH HOSPITAL; TRINITY SPRINGS PAVILION, 1500 South Main Street, Zip 76104–4917; tel. 817/927–3636; Lily Wong, Director Psychiatry), (Total facility includes 15 beds in nursing home–type unit) **A**3 5 8 9 10 12 13 **F**3 11 12 13 15 18 20 25 26 27 28 30 31 32 33 34 35 36 37 38 40 41 43 49 50 53 54 55 57 58 59 60 62 63 66 68 70 72 73 74 75 76 77 78 79 80 81 82 84 86 87 88 89 90 91 92 93 94 96 97 99 100 102 106 107 109 111 114 117 119 120 121 123 124 131 132 133 135 136 137 **P**3
Primary Contact: David M. Cecero, President and Chief Executive Officer
COO: David M. Cecero, President and Chief Executive Officer
CFO: Gale S. Pileggi, Chief Financial Officer
CMO: Jay Haynes, M.D., Chief Medical Officer
CHR: Althea Williams, Vice President Human Resources
Web address: www.jpshealthnet.org
Control: Hospital district or authority, Government, nonfederal **Service:** General Medical and Surgical

Staffed Beds: 451 **Admissions:** 25495 **Census:** 372 **Outpatient Visits:** 822421 **Births:** 6614 **Total Expense ($000):** 498079 **Payroll Expense ($000):** 175560 **Personnel:** 3250

□ **KINDRED HOSPITAL TARRANT COUNTY–FORT WORTH SOUTHWEST (452088)**, 7800 Oakmont Boulevard, Zip 76132–4299; tel. 817/346–0094 **A**1 9 10 **F**1 3 24 25 31 32 78 96 119 137 **S** Kindred Healthcare
Primary Contact: Audra Early, Chief Executive Officer
COO: Anna Rojas, Chief Operating Officer
CFO: Tom Spencer, Chief Financial Officer
CMO: Henry Cunningham, M.D., President Medical Staff
CHR: Joy Raines, Coordinator Human Resources and Administrative Assistant
Web address: www.kindredhealthcare.com
Control: Corporation, Investor–owned, for–profit **Service:** General Medical and Surgical

Staffed Beds: 57 **Admissions:** 730 **Census:** 58 **Outpatient Visits:** 820 **Births:** 0 **Total Expense ($000):** 23981 **Payroll Expense ($000):** 9606 **Personnel:** 163

□ **KINDRED HOSPITAL–FORT WORTH (452088)**, 715 Eighth Avenue, Zip 76104; tel. 817/332–4812 **A**1 9 10 **F**3 12 25 46 48 59 68 75 77 79 80 96 102 107 119 137
Primary Contact: Peggy Cliffe, Administrator
Control: Corporation, Investor–owned, for–profit **Service:** Long–Term Acute Care hospital

Staffed Beds: 64 **Admissions:** 751 **Census:** 55 **Outpatient Visits:** 88 **Births:** 0 **Total Expense ($000):** 23238 **Payroll Expense ($000):** 8810 **Personnel:** 184

□ **LIFECARE HOSPITALS OF FORT WORTH (452044)**, 6201 Overton Ridge Boulevard, Zip 76132; tel. 817/370–6078 **A**1 9 10 **F**1 3 24 25 43 44 60 68 73 75 96 102 119 137 **S** LifeCare Management Services
Primary Contact: Barbara Schmidt, Chief Executive Officer
COO: Barbara Schmidt, Chief Executive Officer
CFO: Chris Pate, Director Finance
CMO: Ladi Haroona, Director Medical Staff
CIO: Patricia Spear, Director Health Information Management
CHR: Donna O'Connor, Director Human Resources
Web address: www.lifecare–hospitals.com
Control: Partnership, Investor–owned, for–profit **Service:** Long–Term Acute Care hospital

Staffed Beds: 80 **Admissions:** 741 **Census:** 54 **Outpatient Visits:** 0 **Births:** 0 **Total Expense ($000):** 21739 **Payroll Expense ($000):** 11691 **Personnel:** 216

★ **PLAZA MEDICAL CENTER OF FORT WORTH (450672)**, 900 Eighth Avenue, Zip 76104–3986; tel. 817/336–2100 **A**1 9 10 12 13 **F**3 9 11 12 17 18 20 22 24 25 26 27 30 31 32 33 34 37 38 43 46 47 49 50 51 52 53 54 55 56 57 58 62 66 68 72 73 75 76 77 78 79 81 86 87 96 97 100 102 103 106 107 119 121 124 135 137 **P**8 **S** HCA
Primary Contact: Troy Villarreal, Chief Executive Officer
COO: Greg Haralson, Chief Operating Officer
CFO: Wayne Gordon, Chief Financial Officer
CIO: Tom Dawson, Director Information Services
Web address: www.plazamedicalcenter.com
Control: Partnership, Investor–owned, for–profit **Service:** General Medical and Surgical

Staffed Beds: 211 **Admissions:** 10677 **Census:** 159 **Outpatient Visits:** 54052 **Births:** 0 **Total Expense ($000):** 165976 **Payroll Expense ($000):** 53812 **Personnel:** 891

★ **REGENCY HOSPITAL OF FORT WORTH (670015)**, 6801 Oakmont Boulevard, Zip 76132; tel. 817/840–2500 **A**9 10 **F**1 25 73 75 80 81 82 86 119 137 **P**5 **S** Regency Hospital Company
Primary Contact: Denise Scurlock, Chief Executive Officer
Web address: www.regencyhospital.com
Control: Corporation, Investor–owned, for–profit **Service:** Long–Term Acute Care hospital

Staffed Beds: 41 **Admissions:** 368 **Census:** 25 **Outpatient Visits:** 0 **Births:** 0 **Total Expense ($000):** 12271 **Payroll Expense ($000):** 5767 **Personnel:** 111

★ △ **TEXAS HEALTH HARRIS METHODIST FORT WORTH (450135)**, (Formerly Harris Methodist Fort Worth), 1301 Pennsylvania Avenue, Zip 76104–2895; tel. 817/250–2000 **A**1 2 7 9 10 **F**3 8 11 12 13 15 17 18 20 22 24 25 26 27 30 31 32 33 34 38 40 43 44 46 49 50 51 52 53 55 56 57 59 62 66 68 69 70 71 72 73 74 75 76 77 79 80 81 82 85 86 90 96 97 100 102 103 107 112 113 116 119 120 121 127 134 135 136 137 **P**3 **S** Texas Health Resources
Primary Contact: Oscar Amparan, President
COO: Terrence Akin, Senior Vice President and Chief Operating Officer
CFO: Lynn Gipson, Chief Financial Officer
CMO: Harold Berenzweig, M.D., Vice President Medical Information Management
CHR: Kathy Hardcastle, Manager Employee Relations
Web address: www.texashealth.org
Control: Other not–for–profit (including NFP Corporation) **Service:** General Medical and Surgical

Staffed Beds: 603 **Admissions:** 36982 **Census:** 520 **Outpatient Visits:** 148232 **Births:** 7024 **Total Expense ($000):** 510103 **Payroll Expense ($000):** 200382 **Personnel:** 3786

★ **TEXAS HEALTH HARRIS METHODIST SOUTHWEST (450779)**, (Formerly Harris Methodist Southwest), 6100 Harris Parkway, Zip 76132–4199; tel. 817/433–6550 **A**1 9 10 **F**3 11 13 15 18 25 26 27 30 31 32 33 38 43 44 49 50 51 54 55 56 57 62 66 68 70 73 74 75 76 77 79 80 81 86 92 96 97 99 100 102 106 107 118 119 134 135 136 **S** Texas Health Resources
Primary Contact: Brett McClung, President
COO: Allen Tseng, Administrative Director
CFO: Vicki L. Galati, Chief Financial Officer and Director Finance
CMO: Curtis Evans, Chief of Staff
CHR: Robert Stansel, Director Human Resources
Web address: www.texashealth.org
Control: Church–operated, Nongovernment, not–for profit **Service:** General Medical and Surgical

Staffed Beds: 156 **Admissions:** 8344 **Census:** 85 **Outpatient Visits:** 83096 **Births:** 2363 **Total Expense ($000):** 96589 **Payroll Expense ($000):** 39912 **Personnel:** 796

FREDERICKSBURG—Gillespie County

★ **HILL COUNTRY MEMORIAL HOSPITAL (450604)**, 1020 Highway 16 South, Zip 78624, Mailing Address: P.O. Box 835, Zip 78624–0835; tel. 830/997–4353 **A**1 9 10 20 **F**3 11 13 15 18 24 25 26 27 31 32 33 35 38 40 43 46 48 49 62 66 68 72 73 74 75 76 77 79 80 81 82 86 96 97 100 102 106 107 111 118 119 120 121 122 135 137 **P**8
Primary Contact: Michael R. Williams, D.O., Interim Chief Executive Officer
CFO: Robert W. Smelser, Chief Financial Officer
CMO: Leo C. Tynan, M.D., Chief of Staff
CIO: Fred Evans, Chief Information Officer
CHR: Erin Cates, Director Human Resources
Web address: www.hcmhs.org
Control: Other not–for–profit (including NFP Corporation) **Service:** General Medical and Surgical

Staffed Beds: 78 **Admissions:** 3889 **Census:** 40 **Outpatient Visits:** 59488 **Births:** 543 **Total Expense ($000):** 47935 **Payroll Expense ($000):** 20477 **Personnel:** 426

Many Facility Codes have changed. Please refer to the AHA Guide Code Chart.

FRIONA—Parmer County

PARMER COUNTY COMMUNITY HOSPITAL (451300), 1307 Cleveland Street, Zip 79035–1121; tel. 806/250–2754 **A**9 10 18 **F**38 40 62 67 73 84 86 96 107 117 122 **P**5 **S** Preferred Management Corporation
Primary Contact: Brandon L. Gatlin, Administrator
Control: Other not–for–profit (including NFP Corporation) **Service:** General Medical and Surgical

Staffed Beds: 15 **Admissions:** 282 **Census:** 3 **Outpatient Visits:** 9502 **Births:** 0 **Total Expense ($000):** 4056 **Payroll Expense ($000):** 1629 **Personnel:** 55

FRISCO—Collin County

□ **BAYLOR MEDICAL CENTER AT FRISCO (450853)**, 5601 Warren Parkway, Zip 75034; tel. 214/618–2000 **A**1 9 10 **F**3 13 25 31 32 37 38 51 55 56 62 66 70 72 73 74 77 79 80 82 96 100 102 107 133 136 **S** United Surgical Partners International
Primary Contact: William A. Keaton, Chief Executive Officer
CFO: Kevin Coots, Chief Financial Officer
CIO: Domingo Garcia, Director Information Systems
Web address: www.bmcf.com
Control: Partnership, Investor–owned, for–profit **Service:** General Medical and Surgical

Staffed Beds: 68 **Admissions:** 1927 **Census:** 13 **Outpatient Visits:** 34538 **Births:** 411 **Total Expense ($000):** 56771 **Payroll Expense ($000):** 20617 **Personnel:** 373

★□ **CENTENNIAL MEDICAL CENTER (450885)**, 12505 Lebanon Road, Zip 75035–8298; tel. 972/963–3333 **A**1 9 10 **F**3 13 15 18 20 22 25 27 38 50 51 55 56 57 59 68 70 74 79 80 82 84 96 97 99 100 102 103 107 119 135 136 **S** TENET Healthcare Corporation
Primary Contact: William C. Henning, Chief Executive Officer
COO: Paul Abraham, Chief Operating Officer
CFO: Blaise Bondi, Chief Financial Officer
CHR: Terry LaCombe, Interim Director Human Resources
Web address: www.centennialmedcenter.com
Control: Corporation, Investor–owned, for–profit **Service:** General Medical and Surgical

Staffed Beds: 108 **Admissions:** 4117 **Census:** 49 **Outpatient Visits:** 37562 **Births:** 1102 **Total Expense ($000):** 62387 **Payroll Expense ($000):** 22950 **Personnel:** 430

GAINESVILLE—Cooke County

★ **NORTH TEXAS MEDICAL CENTER (450090)**, 1900 Hospital Boulevard, Zip 76240–3539; tel. 940/665–1751 **A**9 10 20 **F**3 11 13 15 24 25 26 30 32 33 38 40 50 57 59 61 62 66 68 73 74 75 77 79 80 82 86 96 97 100 102 106 107 119 121 122 124 135 136 137
Primary Contact: Steven D. Porter, FACHE, Chief Executive Officer
CFO: Kelly Hayes, Chief Financial Officer
Web address: www.ntmconline.net
Control: Hospital district or authority, Government, nonfederal **Service:** General Medical and Surgical

Staffed Beds: 60 **Admissions:** 2639 **Census:** 28 **Outpatient Visits:** 45653 **Births:** 477 **Total Expense ($000):** 21738 **Payroll Expense ($000):** 12219 **Personnel:** 304

GALVESTON—Galveston County

□ **SHRINERS HOSPITALS FOR CHILDREN, GALVESTON BURNS HOSPITAL**, (Burn Care), 815 Market Street, Zip 77550–2725; tel. 409/770–6600 **A**1 3 5 **F**11 16 25 62 79 81 90 119 135 **S** Shriners Hospitals for Children
Primary Contact: John A. Swartwout, Administrator
CFO: M. K. Joseph, Controller
CMO: David N. Herndon, M.D., Chief of Staff
CIO: Brian Clarke, Director Information Systems
CHR: Lynn Clements, Director Human Resources
Web address: www.shrinershq.org
Control: Other not–for–profit (including NFP Corporation) **Service:** Children's other specialty

Staffed Beds: 30 **Admissions:** 1557 **Census:** 13 **Outpatient Visits:** 12523 **Births:** 0 **Total Expense ($000):** 31041 **Payroll Expense ($000):** 15356 **Personnel:** 353

★□ **UNIVERSITY OF TEXAS MEDICAL BRANCH HOSPITALS (450018)**, 301 University Boulevard, Zip 77555–0518; tel. 409/772–1011 **A**1 2 8 9 10 12 13 **F**1 3 4 5 11 12 13 14 15 16 17 18 19 20 21 22 23 24 25 26 27 28 30 31 32 33 36 38 40 43 46 49 50 51 52 53 54 55 56 57 58 59 60 62 63 65 66 68 69 70 71 72 73 74 75 76 77 78 79 80 81 82 83 84 85 86 87 88 89 90 91 92 93 94 96 97 99 100 101 105 106 107 108 109 110 113 114 116 117 118 119 120 121 123 126 127 129 130 131 132 133 135 136 137 **P**6 **S** University of Texas System
Primary Contact: Karen H. Sexton, RN, Ph.D., Vice President and Chief Executive Officer
COO: David Marshall, Chief Operating Officer
CFO: Larry Revill, Chief Financial Officer
CMO: Peter Hoffmann, M.D., Chief Medical Officer
CIO: Ralph Farr, Chief Information Officer
CHR: Kathy Shingleton, Chief Human Resources Officer
Web address: www.utmb.edu
Control: State–Government, nonfederal **Service:** General Medical and Surgical

Staffed Beds: 679 **Admissions:** 32935 **Census:** 444 **Outpatient Visits:** 752560 **Births:** 8519 **Total Expense ($000):** 622362 **Payroll Expense ($000):** 245932 **Personnel:** 4414

GARLAND—Dallas County

★□ **BAYLOR MEDICAL CENTER AT GARLAND (450280)**, 2300 Marie Curie Boulevard, Zip 75042–5706; tel. 972/487–5000 **A**1 9 10 **F**3 11 12 13 15 18 20 22 25 26 27 30 31 32 33 38 40 42 43 45 49 50 54 55 57 59 62 63 68 70 72 73 74 75 76 77 79 82 85 86 96 97 100 102 104 105 106 107 112 114 118 119 121 124 134 135 136 137 **S** Baylor Health Care System
Primary Contact: James D. Thaxton, President
CFO: Rhonda McCabe, Vice President and Chief Financial Officer
CMO: Mark Bailey, M.D., Chief of Staff
CIO: Michael Larsen, Director Information Systems
Web address: www.baylorhealth.com
Control: Other not–for–profit (including NFP Corporation) **Service:** General Medical and Surgical

Staffed Beds: 214 **Admissions:** 12778 **Census:** 155 **Outpatient Visits:** 127108 **Births:** 1842 **Total Expense ($000):** 165014 **Payroll Expense ($000):** 62411 **Personnel:** 1021

VISTA HOSPITAL OF DALLAS (450315), 2696 West Walnut Street, Zip 75042–6499; tel. 972/665–3000 **A**10 **F**3 12 38 66 68 73 77 79 80 96 107 121 132 **P**8 **S** Dynacq Healthcare, Inc.
Primary Contact: Alan A. Beauchamp, Chief Executive Officer
COO: Alan A. Beauchamp, Chief Executive Officer
CMO: Steve Thompson, M.D., Chief of Staff
CIO: David Way, Director Information Services
Web address: www.vista-hospital-dallas.com
Control: Partnership, Investor–owned, for–profit **Service:** General Medical and Surgical

Staffed Beds: 29 **Admissions:** 500 **Census:** 3 **Outpatient Visits:** 1624 **Births:** 0 **Total Expense ($000):** 17345 **Payroll Expense ($000):** 4190 **Personnel:** 104

GATESVILLE—Coryell County

□ **CORYELL MEMORIAL HOSPITAL (450239)**, 1507 West Main Street, Zip 76528–1098; tel. 254/865–8251, (Total facility includes 90 beds in nursing home–type unit) **A**1 9 10 **F**3 7 10 11 15 18 24 31 32 38 40 50 52 55 61 63 68 79 82 86 87 96 100 107 115 117 119 122 **P**4 6
Primary Contact: David Byrom, Chief Executive Officer
COO: David Byrom, Chief Executive Officer
CFO: Carol Jones, Controller and Manager Business Office
CMO: Jill Clay, President Medical Staff
CIO: Mike Huckabee, Network Administrator
CHR: Paula Smithhart, Director Human Resources
Web address: www.cmhos.org
Control: Hospital district or authority, Government, nonfederal **Service:** General Medical and Surgical

Staffed Beds: 138 **Admissions:** 1414 **Census:** 98 **Outpatient Visits:** 50718 **Births:** 0 **Total Expense ($000):** 19057 **Payroll Expense ($000):** 9086 **Personnel:** 333

TX

Hospital, Medicare Provider Number, Address, Telephone, Approval, Facility, and Physician Codes, Health Care System
★ American Hospital Association (AHA) membership
□ The Joint Commission accreditation
○ American Osteopathic Association (AOA) accreditation
△ Commission on Accreditation of Rehabilitation Facilities (CARF) accreditation

GEORGETOWN—Williamson County

★ **ST. DAVID'S GEORGETOWN HOSPITAL (450191)**, 2000 Scenic Drive, Zip 78626–7793; tel. 512/943–3000 **A**1 9 10 **F**3 11 13 15 24 25 26 27 30 31 33 38 43 49 50 52 55 57 62 68 73 74 75 76 77 79 80 81 82 85 86 96 97 100 102 107 111 119 121 135 **S** HCA
Primary Contact: Hugh Brown, Chief Executive Officer
COO: Court LeMaistre, Chief Operating Officer
CFO: Laura Wiess, Chief Financial Officer
CMO: David Martin, Vice President, Medical Staff Affairs
Web address: www.stdavidsgeorgetown.com
Control: Other not–for–profit (including NFP Corporation) **Service:** General Medical and Surgical

Staffed Beds: 96 **Admissions:** 4551 **Census:** 45 **Outpatient Visits:** 66289 **Births:** 1286 **Total Expense ($000):** 54679 **Payroll Expense ($000):** 22449 **Personnel:** 370

GILMER—Upshur County

★ **EAST TEXAS MEDICAL CENTER–GILMER (450884)**, 712 North Wood Street, Zip 75644; tel. 903/841–7100 **A**9 10 **F**11 25 26 32 38 40 43 50 55 77 79 87 96 97 100 107 **P**6 7 **S** East Texas Medical Center Regional Healthcare System
Primary Contact: Michael W. Pruitt, Chief Executive Officer
CFO: Michael Choate, Chief Financial Officer
CHR: William Henry, Director Human Resources
Web address: www.etmc.org
Control: Other not–for–profit (including NFP Corporation) **Service:** General Medical and Surgical

Staffed Beds: 37 **Admissions:** 1344 **Census:** 11 **Outpatient Visits:** 27606 **Total Expense ($000):** 12803 **Payroll Expense ($000):** 5057 **Personnel:** 105

GLEN ROSE—Somervell County

★ **GLEN ROSE MEDICAL CENTER (450451)**, 1021 Holden Street, Zip 76043–4937, Mailing Address: P.O. Box 2099, Zip 76043–2099; tel. 254/897–2215 **A**1 9 10 **F**15 25 30 31 32 38 40 54 55 57 63 79 86 96 100 107 119 121 122 132 **P**7
Primary Contact: Gary A. Marks, Executive Director
COO: Mo S. Sheldon, Chief Operating Officer
CFO: Hal Mayo, Chief Financial Officer
CHR: Janice Nickell, Administrative Assistant
Web address: www.glenrosemedicalcenter.com
Control: Other not–for–profit (including NFP Corporation) **Service:** General Medical and Surgical

Staffed Beds: 16 **Admissions:** 717 **Census:** 8 **Outpatient Visits:** 143803 **Births:** 0 **Total Expense ($000):** 13604 **Payroll Expense ($000):** 5243 **Personnel:** 116

GONZALES—Gonzales County

★ **MEMORIAL HOSPITAL (450235)**, 1110 Sarah Dewitt Drive, Zip 78629–2021, Mailing Address: P.O. Box 587, Zip 78629–0587; tel. 830/672–7581 **A**9 10 **F**3 11 13 15 25 30 31 32 33 36 38 40 52 55 56 57 61 62 63 66 68 73 74 75 79 82 86 87 96 100 103 107 118 119 121 122 **S** QHR
Primary Contact: Charles Norris, Chief Executive Officer
CFO: Patty Stewart, Chief Financial Officer
CMO: Commie Hisey, D.O., Chief of Staff
CHR: Joni Leland, Director Human Resources
Web address: www.gonzaleshealthcare.com
Control: Hospital district or authority, Government, nonfederal **Service:** General Medical and Surgical

Staffed Beds: 34 **Admissions:** 1161 **Census:** 11 **Outpatient Visits:** 56268 **Births:** 215 **Total Expense ($000):** 17971 **Payroll Expense ($000):** 7141 **Personnel:** 209

GRAHAM—Young County

★ **GRAHAM REGIONAL MEDICAL CENTER (450085)**, 1301 Montgomery Road, Zip 76450–4224, Mailing Address: P.O. Box 1390, Zip 76450–1390; tel. 940/549–3400 **A**9 10 20 **F**7 11 13 15 24 25 30 38 40 42 46 52 55 57 61 68 73 74 75 76 77 79 80 86 94 96 100 103 106 107 119 122 124 **P**5
Primary Contact: Steve Hartgraves, Chief Executive Officer
CFO: Bonnie Blevins, Chief Financial Officer
CIO: Jeff Clark, Director Information Systems
CHR: Judy Guinn, Chief Human Resources Officer
Web address: www.grahamrmc.com
Control: City–Government, nonfederal **Service:** General Medical and Surgical

Staffed Beds: 35 **Admissions:** 1420 **Census:** 13 **Outpatient Visits:** 68381 **Births:** 284 **Total Expense ($000):** 15410 **Payroll Expense ($000):** 7556 **Personnel:** 216

GRANBURY—Hood County

★ **LAKE GRANBURY MEDICAL CENTER (450596)**, 1310 Paluxy Road, Zip 76048–5699; tel. 817/573–2273 **A**1 9 10 **F**3 8 11 13 15 24 25 26 30 31 32 38 40 43 55 56 57 68 73 74 75 77 79 80 81 86 96 97 100 102 106 107 112 122 135 136 **P**5 **S** Community Health Systems, Inc.
Primary Contact: David Orcutt, Chief Executive Officer
COO: Patrick Trammell, Assistant Chief Executive Officer
CFO: Erich Wallschlaeger, Chief Financial Officer
CIO: Kevin Myers, Director Information Systems
CHR: Carol Langley, Director Human Resources
Web address: www.lakegranburymedicalcenter.com
Control: Corporation, Investor–owned, for–profit **Service:** General Medical and Surgical

Staffed Beds: 59 **Admissions:** 2612 **Census:** 20 **Outpatient Visits:** 34063 **Births:** 555 **Total Expense ($000):** 30169 **Payroll Expense ($000):** 12105 **Personnel:** 241

GRAND SALINE—Van Zandt County

★ **COZBY–GERMANY HOSPITAL (450283)**, 707 North Waldrip Street, Zip 75140–1555; tel. 903/962–4242 **A**9 10 20 **F**24 38 40 54 62 79 94 95 96 107 119 122
Primary Contact: Ronald J. Ensor, Chief Executive Officer
CFO: Laura Preston, Controller
CMO: Richard L. Ingrim, M.D., Chief of Staff
CIO: Becky Champion, Manager Business Office
Web address: www.cozbygermanyhospital.com
Control: Other not–for–profit (including NFP Corporation) **Service:** General Medical and Surgical

Staffed Beds: 24 **Admissions:** 604 **Census:** 7 **Outpatient Visits:** 9191 **Births:** 0 **Total Expense ($000):** 6222 **Payroll Expense ($000):** 3251 **Personnel:** 87

GRAPEVINE—Tarrant County

★ **BAYLOR REGIONAL MEDICAL CENTER AT GRAPEVINE (450563)**, 1650 West College Street, Zip 76051–1650; tel. 817/481–1588 **A**1 9 10 **F**3 11 13 15 18 20 22 24 25 26 27 30 31 32 33 38 43 51 54 55 56 57 60 62 63 66 68 70 72 73 74 75 76 78 79 81 82 86 96 97 99 100 102 103 107 113 114 118 119 120 121 124 133 134 135 136 **S** Baylor Health Care System
Primary Contact: Doug Lawson, President
CFO: Preshie Wilson, Vice President Finance Services
CMO: Thomas Purgett, M.D., Chief Medical Staff
CIO: David Krzjci, Director Information Systems
CHR: Donna Stark, Director Human Resources
Web address: www.bhcs.com
Control: Other not–for–profit (including NFP Corporation) **Service:** General Medical and Surgical

Staffed Beds: 233 **Admissions:** 12292 **Census:** 138 **Outpatient Visits:** 83751 **Births:** 3166 **Total Expense ($000):** 146655 **Payroll Expense ($000):** 54781 **Personnel:** 1003

GREENVILLE—Hunt County

☐ **GLEN OAKS HOSPITAL (454050)**, 301 East Division, Zip 75402–4199; tel. 903/454–6000 **A**1 9 10 **F**4 5 25 38 56 66 88 89 90 91 92 93 94 95 **S** Universal Health Services, Inc.
Primary Contact: Joel Klein, Chief Executive Officer and Managing Director
CFO: Lowell K. Hudson, Chief Financial Officer
CMO: Paul Lee, M.D., Medical Director
CHR: Joe Carson, Director Human Resources
Web address: www.glenoakshospital.com
Control: Corporation, Investor–owned, for–profit **Service:** Psychiatric

Staffed Beds: 54 **Admissions:** 1858 **Census:** 37 **Outpatient Visits:** 4878 **Births:** 0 **Total Expense ($000):** 6874 **Payroll Expense ($000):** 3603 **Personnel:** 92

★ **HUNT MEMORIAL HOSPITAL DISTRICT (450352)**, 4215 Joe Ramsey Boulevard, Zip 75401–7899, Mailing Address: P.O. Drawer 1059, Zip 75403–1059; tel. 903/408–5000, (Includes PRESBYTERIAN HOSPITAL OF GREENVILLE), (Total facility includes 7 beds in nursing home–type unit) **A**1 9 10 **F**3 8 11 13 15 24 25 26 27 30 31 38 40 43 46 49 52 55 56 57 61 68 71 72 73 74 75 76 77 79 80 81 82 86 94 96 97 100 102 103 106 107 117 118 119 121 122 135 137
Primary Contact: Richard Carter, District Chief Executive Officer
COO: Michael R. Klepin, Administrator
CFO: Jeri Rich, Assistant Administrator and Chief Financial Officer
CMO: Moushira Ebrahim, Chief of Staff
CIO: Joe Hartley, Director Information Systems
CHR: John Heatherly, Assistant Administrator Support Services
Web address: www.hmhd.org
Control: Hospital district or authority, Government, nonfederal **Service:** General Medical and Surgical

Staffed Beds: 162 **Admissions:** 8646 **Census:** 95 **Outpatient Visits:** 108475 **Births:** 1213 **Total Expense ($000):** 83095 **Payroll Expense ($000):** 34607 **Personnel:** 672

TX

Many Facility Codes have changed. Please refer to the AHA Guide Code Chart.

☐ **REHABILITATION HOSPITAL OF GREENVILLE (453093)**, 4215 Joe Ramsey Boulevard, 7th Floor, Zip 75401; tel. 903/408–1770, (Nonreporting) **A**1 9 10 **S** SeniorHealth Incorporated
Primary Contact: Lorraine Cook, Administrator
Web address: www.seniorhealthrehab.com
Control: Corporation, Investor–owned, for–profit **Service:** Rehabilitation

Staffed Beds: 16

GROESBECK—Limestone County

LIMESTONE MEDICAL CENTER (451303), 701 McClintic Street, Zip 76642–2105; tel. 254/729–3281 **A**9 10 18 **F**3 7 11 28 30 31 32 33 38 40 46 55 56 62 63 73 75 79 80 86 87 94 96 102 118 119 122 124 135
Primary Contact: Penny Gray, Administrator and Chief Executive Officer
COO: Larry Price, Assistant Administrator
CIO: Sherald Wood, Director Marketing and Public Relations
CHR: Jean Koester, Manager Human Resources
Control: Hospital district or authority, Government, nonfederal **Service:** General Medical and Surgical

Staffed Beds: 16 **Admissions:** 325 **Census:** 5 **Outpatient Visits:** 10488 **Births:** 0 **Total Expense ($000):** 6372 **Payroll Expense ($000):** 3916 **Personnel:** 131

GROVES—Jefferson County

○ **RENAISSANCE HOSPITAL (450123)**, 5500 39th Street, Zip 77619–9805; tel. 409/962–5733 **A**9 10 11 **F**12 15 17 18 22 25 31 38 62 68 73 75 79 82 86 96 97 100 107 119 **P**8 **S** Renaissance Healthcare Systems
Primary Contact: Chris McMahon, Administrator
CFO: John Murphy, Chief Financial Officer
Web address: www.renhealthcare.org
Control: Corporation, Investor–owned, for–profit **Service:** General Medical and Surgical

Staffed Beds: 72 **Admissions:** 2371 **Census:** 30 **Outpatient Visits:** 26558 **Births:** 0 **Total Expense ($000):** 33489 **Payroll Expense ($000):** 13730 **Personnel:** 325

HALLETTSVILLE—Lavaca County

LAVACA MEDICAL CENTER (451376), 1400 North Texana Street, Zip 77964–2099; tel. 361/798–3671 **A**9 10 18 **F**11 15 25 30 31 32 38 40 52 54 55 56 57 62 63 66 75 78 79 80 81 82 86 87 96 100 102 107 122 124 135 137
Primary Contact: James Vanek, Chief Executive Officer
Control: Hospital district or authority, Government, nonfederal **Service:** General Medical and Surgical

Staffed Beds: 25 **Admissions:** 818 **Census:** 8 **Outpatient Visits:** 20646 **Births:** 0 **Total Expense ($000):** 12200 **Payroll Expense ($000):** 3866 **Personnel:** 125

HAMILTON—Hamilton County

★ **HAMILTON GENERAL HOSPITAL (450754)**, 400 North Brown Street, Zip 76531–1518; tel. 254/386–1600 **A**9 10 20 **F**3 7 11 24 30 31 38 40 41 43 46 50 52 54 55 56 57 62 63 75 77 78 79 80 87 93 94 96 102 119 121 **P**4 5
Primary Contact: James R. Shafer, Administrator
CFO: Michele Cathey, Chief Financial Officer
Web address: www.hamiltonhospital.org
Control: Hospital district or authority, Government, nonfederal **Service:** General Medical and Surgical

Staffed Beds: 34 **Admissions:** 1980 **Census:** 17 **Outpatient Visits:** 60954 **Births:** 1 **Total Expense ($000):** 13143 **Payroll Expense ($000):** 5647 **Personnel:** 153

HAMLIN—Jones County

HAMLIN MEMORIAL HOSPITAL (450243), 632 Northwest Second Street, Zip 79520–3831, Mailing Address: P.O. Box 400, Zip 79520–0400; tel. 325/576–3646 **A**9 10 **F**3 7 11 24 31 32 38 40 62 66 67 86 122 124 135 137 **P**5
Primary Contact: James L. Barnett, Administrator
Web address: www.hamlinedc.org
Control: Hospital district or authority, Government, nonfederal **Service:** General Medical and Surgical

Staffed Beds: 23 **Admissions:** 293 **Census:** 5 **Outpatient Visits:** 7055 **Births:** 0 **Total Expense ($000):** 2962 **Personnel:** 75

HARLINGEN—Cameron County

☐ **HARLINGEN MEDICAL CENTER (450855)**, 5501 South Expressway 77, Zip 78550; tel. 956/365–1000 **A**1 9 **F**3 13 15 17 18 20 22 25 26 30 31 32 38 49 50 51 55 57 59 62 66 68 72 73 74 77 79 80 81 96 97 99 100 102 103 106 107 119 135 136 137 **P**2 **S** MedCath, Inc.
Primary Contact: Daniel P. McLean, President and Chief Executive Officer
CFO: Jo Beth Vance, Vice President Finance and Chief Financial Officer
CMO: Hugo Blake, M.D., Chief Medical Staff
CHR: Yvonne Alsbury, Director Human Resources
Web address: www.harlingenmedicalcenter.com
Control: Partnership, Investor–owned, for–profit **Service:** General Medical and Surgical

Staffed Beds: 88 **Admissions:** 6148 **Census:** 49 **Outpatient Visits:** 28500 **Births:** 1274 **Total Expense ($000):** 56716 **Payroll Expense ($000):** 20569 **Personnel:** 397

☐ **RIO GRANDE STATE CENTER/SOUTH TEXAS HEALTH CARE SYSTEM (454088)**, 1401 South Rangerville Road, Zip 78552–7638; tel. 956/364–8000, (Includes RIO GRANDE STATE CENTER; SOUTH TEXAS HEALTH CARE SYSTEM, 1401 Rangerville Road, Zip 78552–7609) **A**1 5 10 **F**15 26 31 32 52 53 55 64 66 73 82 87 88 91 96 107 119 121 124 132 135 136 **P**6 **S** Texas Department of State Health Services
Primary Contact: Sonia Hernandez–Keeble, Superintendent
CFO: Tom Garza, Director Fiscal and Support
CMO: David Moron, M.D., Clinical Director
CIO: Blas Ortiz, Assistant Superintendent and Public Information Officer
CHR: Irma Garcia, Job Coordinator
Web address: www.dshs.state.tx.us/mhospital/riograndesc/default.shtm
Control: State–Government, nonfederal **Service:** Psychiatric

Staffed Beds: 132 **Admissions:** 1171 **Census:** 46 **Outpatient Visits:** 52756 **Births:** 0 **Total Expense ($000):** 14006 **Payroll Expense ($000):** 7184 **Personnel:** 495

SOLARA HOSPITAL HARLINGEN (670020), 508 Victoria Lane, Zip 78550–3225; tel. 956/425–9600 **A**9 10 **F**1 3 25 26 33 56 73 80 81 119 137
Primary Contact: Joanne Saltzman, Chief Executive Officer
Control: Partnership, Investor–owned, for–profit **Service:** Long–Term Acute Care hospital

Staffed Beds: 41 **Admissions:** 170 **Census:** 11 **Outpatient Visits:** 0 **Births:** 0 **Total Expense ($000):** 7346 **Payroll Expense ($000):** 2722 **Personnel:** 68

★☐ **VALLEY BAPTIST MEDICAL CENTER–HARLINGEN (450033)**, (Formerly Valley Baptist Health System), 2101 Pease Street, Zip 78550–8307, Mailing Address: P.O. Drawer 2588, Zip 78551–2588; tel. 956/389–1100 **A**1 3 5 9 10 **F**3 8 11 12 13 15 17 18 20 22 24 25 26 27 30 31 32 33 34 37 38 40 41 42 43 44 50 52 53 54 55 57 59 61 62 68 69 70 71 72 73 74 75 76 77 79 81 82 83 84 85 86 87 90 91 93 94 96 97 99 100 101 102 106 107 119 120 132 133 135 136 137 **P**6 8 **S** Valley Baptist Health System
Primary Contact: Jim D. Wesson, Senior Vice President and Chief Executive Officer
CFO: Joe Beck, Chief Financial Officer
CMO: E. Chandler Deal, Vice President Medical Affairs and Chief Medical Officer
CIO: Jim Barbaglia, Chief Information Officer
CHR: Irma Pye, Senior Vice President and Chief Human Resource Officer
Web address: www.valleybaptist.net
Control: Other not–for–profit (including NFP Corporation) **Service:** General Medical and Surgical

Staffed Beds: 481 **Admissions:** 22124 **Census:** 271 **Outpatient Visits:** 104824 **Births:** 2919 **Total Expense ($000):** 266261 **Payroll Expense ($000):** 97602 **Personnel:** 1556

HASKELL—Haskell County

HASKELL MEMORIAL HOSPITAL (451341), 1 North Avenue N, Zip 79521–5499, Mailing Address: P.O. Box 1117, Zip 79521–1117; tel. 940/864–2621 **A**9 10 18 **F**11 24 25 30 31 32 33 38 43 52 53 55 56 57 66 73 75 76 81 82 86 107 119 120 122 124 **P**1
Primary Contact: Bill Nemir, Administrator
Control: Hospital district or authority, Government, nonfederal **Service:** General Medical and Surgical

Staffed Beds: 25 **Admissions:** 197 **Census:** 4 **Outpatient Visits:** 1538 **Births:** 0 **Total Expense ($000):** 3024 **Payroll Expense ($000):** 1524 **Personnel:** 53

TX

Hospital, Medicare Provider Number, Address, Telephone, Approval, Facility, and Physician Codes, Health Care System

★ American Hospital Association (AHA) membership
☐ The Joint Commission accreditation
○ American Osteopathic Association (AOA) accreditation
△ Commission on Accreditation of Rehabilitation Facilities (CARF) accreditation

HEMPHILL—Sabine County

★ **SABINE COUNTY HOSPITAL (451361)**, Highway 83 West, Zip 75948, Mailing Address: P.O. Box 750, Zip 75948–0750; tel. 409/787–3300 **A**9 10 18 **F**32 38 40 55 96 102 107 **P**5 **S** Preferred Management Corporation
Primary Contact: Deanna Lathrop, Interim Chief Executive Officer
CFO: Cindy Erickson, Chief Financial Officer
CMO: Peter Forrest, Chief of Staff
CIO: Margaret Moore, Business Office Manager
CHR: Cindy Erickson, Chief Financial Officer
Control: Hospital district or authority, Government, nonfederal **Service:** General Medical and Surgical

Staffed Beds: 25 **Admissions:** 275 **Census:** 3 **Outpatient Visits:** 7009 **Births:** 0 **Total Expense ($000):** 5599 **Payroll Expense ($000):** 1696 **Personnel:** 50

HENDERSON—Rusk County

☒ **HENDERSON MEMORIAL HOSPITAL (450475)**, 300 Wilson Street, Zip 75652–5956; tel. 903/657–7541 **A**1 9 10 **F**3 11 13 15 17 24 25 30 31 32 33 38 40 43 50 55 56 57 62 68 73 74 77 79 80 81 82 83 84 86 96 97 100 103 107 117 118 119 121 122 124 134 135 136 137 **P**6 8
Primary Contact: Mark Leitner, Chief Executive Officer
COO: Carla Degges, Chief Clinical Officer
CFO: Gary Gunder, Chief Financial Officer
CHR: Anita Hays, Assistant Director Human Resources
Web address: www.hmhtx.org
Control: Other not–for–profit (including NFP Corporation) **Service:** General Medical and Surgical

Staffed Beds: 76 **Admissions:** 2666 **Census:** 25 **Outpatient Visits:** 48325 **Births:** 652 **Total Expense ($000):** 24825 **Payroll Expense ($000):** 11460 **Personnel:** 254

HENRIETTA—Clay County

CLAY COUNTY MEMORIAL HOSPITAL (451362), 310 West South Street, Zip 76365–3346; tel. 940/538–5621 **A**9 10 18 **F**7 8 11 31 32 38 40 52 55 61 78 79 85 86 96 100 105 107 122 **P**5
Primary Contact: Jeff Huskey, Chief Executive Officer and Administrator
COO: Larry Evangelista, Supervisor Information Technology
CFO: Debra Haehn, Chief Financial Officer
CMO: Mitchell Wolfe, M.D., Chief of Staff
CIO: Michael Clark, Director Operations
CHR: Linda Burleson, Administrative Secretary
Web address: www.ccmhospital.com
Control: County–Government, nonfederal **Service:** General Medical and Surgical

Staffed Beds: 25 **Admissions:** 447 **Census:** 6 **Outpatient Visits:** 10209 **Births:** 0 **Total Expense ($000):** 5264 **Payroll Expense ($000):** 2163 **Personnel:** 74

HEREFORD—Deaf Smith County

HEREFORD REGIONAL MEDICAL CENTER (450155), 801 East Third Street, Zip 79045–5727; tel. 806/364–2141 **A**9 10 **F**3 7 11 17 24 25 30 31 33 38 40 50 55 57 61 62 68 74 75 79 80 84 85 86 96 102 107 117 119 122 136 **P**5
Primary Contact: Nathan A. Flood, Chief Executive Officer
COO: Meri Killingsworth, Chief Operating Officer
CFO: Greg Reinart, Chief Financial Officer
Control: Hospital district or authority, Government, nonfederal **Service:** General Medical and Surgical

Staffed Beds: 35 **Admissions:** 836 **Census:** 8 **Outpatient Visits:** 77373 **Births:** 342 **Total Expense ($000):** 9982 **Payroll Expense ($000):** 6124 **Personnel:** 155

HILLSBORO—Hill County

☒ **HILL REGIONAL HOSPITAL (450192)**, 101 Circle Drive, Zip 76645–2670; tel. 254/580–8950 **A**1 9 10 **F**3 13 15 17 25 31 32 38 50 55 56 57 62 63 66 68 73 74 75 79 81 82 83 84 86 96 106 107 122 135 136 **S** Community Health Systems, Inc.
Primary Contact: Jan McClure, Chief Executive Officer
CFO: Bill Beauchamp, Chief Financial Officer
CHR: Glenn Gray, Director Human Resources
Web address: www.chs.net
Control: Corporation, Investor–owned, for–profit **Service:** General Medical and Surgical

Staffed Beds: 84 **Admissions:** 2416 **Census:** 22 **Outpatient Visits:** 22650 **Births:** 346 **Total Expense ($000):** 22124 **Payroll Expense ($000):** 8018 **Personnel:** 192

HONDO—Medina County

MEDINA COMMUNITY HOSPITAL (451330), 3100 Avenue E., Zip 78861–3599; tel. 830/426–7838 **A**9 10 18 **F**3 11 13 15 25 26 30 31 33 38 40 50 55 57 62 74 79 82 85 86 87 96 102 107 117 122 135 **P**4
Primary Contact: Beverly Gruber, Administrator
CFO: Dale Semar, Chief Financial Officer
CMO: John Meyer, M.D., Chief of Staff
CIO: Michael Smith, Director Support Services and Information Technology
CHR: Tarik Esquerra, Director Human Resources
Web address: www.medinahospital.net
Control: Hospital district or authority, Government, nonfederal **Service:** General Medical and Surgical

Staffed Beds: 25 **Admissions:** 1127 **Census:** 10 **Outpatient Visits:** 82436 **Births:** 162 **Total Expense ($000):** 13239 **Payroll Expense ($000):** 5410 **Personnel:** 177

HOUSTON—Harris County

BEN TAUB GENERAL HOSPITAL See Harris County Hospital District

CHILDREN'S MEMORIAL HERMANN HOSPITAL See Memorial Hermann Hospital

CHRISTUS ST. JOHN HOSPITAL See Nassau Bay

☐ **CORNERSTONE HOSPITAL OF HOUSTON – BELLAIRE (452032)**, 5314 Dashwood, Zip 77081; tel. 713/295–5300, (Includes CORNERSTONE HOSPITAL OF HOUSTON AT CLEARLAKE, 709 Medical Center Boulevard, Webster, Zip 77598; tel. 281/332–3322; Steve Flaherty, Chief Executive Officer) **A**1 9 10 **F**1 3 25 30 31 32 54 73 80 81 82 119 137
Primary Contact: Brenda Hingle, Chief Executive Officer
COO: Ken McGee, Vice President Hospital Operations
CFO: Shane Wells, Chief Financial Officer
CMO: Mark Barlow, President Medical Staff
CIO: Kent Chambless, Chief Information Officer
CHR: Margaret Blunt, Director Human Resources
Web address: www.chghospitals.com
Control: Partnership, Investor–owned, for–profit **Service:** General Medical and Surgical

Staffed Beds: 148 **Admissions:** 1081 **Census:** 81 **Outpatient Visits:** 502 **Births:** 0 **Total Expense ($000):** 44295 **Payroll Expense ($000):** 15177 **Personnel:** 252

☐ **CYPRESS CREEK HOSPITAL (454063)**, 17750 Cali Drive, Zip 77090–2700; tel. 281/586–7600 **A**1 9 10 **F**4 5 25 26 30 31 32 54 62 69 82 88 89 90 91 92 93 94 95 119 121 **S** Psychiatric Solutions
Primary Contact: Diane P. Reidy, Chief Executive Officer
CFO: Tom Ball, Chief Financial Officer
CMO: Marshall Lucas, M.D., Medical Director
CHR: Brenda Dominguez, Director Human Resources
Web address: www.psysolutions.com
Control: Corporation, Investor–owned, for–profit **Service:** Psychiatric

Staffed Beds: 64 **Admissions:** 2940 **Census:** 51 **Outpatient Visits:** 8334 **Births:** 0 **Total Expense ($000):** 12919 **Payroll Expense ($000):** 6833 **Personnel:** 89

☒ **CYPRESS FAIRBANKS MEDICAL CENTER (450716)**, 10655 Steepletop Drive, Zip 77065–4297; tel. 281/890–4285 **A**1 9 10 **F**3 11 12 13 15 18 20 22 24 25 26 27 30 31 32 38 43 46 47 49 52 55 56 57 62 68 70 72 73 74 75 77 78 79 82 84 86 96 97 99 100 101 102 103 106 107 112 119 120 121 133 134 135 136 137 **P**8 **S** TENET Healthcare Corporation
Primary Contact: Terry J. Wheeler, Chief Executive Officer
COO: Bobby Bluford, Chief Operating Officer
CFO: James Wright, Chief Financial Officer
CMO: Magdy Tadros, Chief of Staff
CHR: Lorinnsa Bridges Kee, Director Human Resource
Web address: www.cyfairhospital.com
Control: Corporation, Investor–owned, for–profit **Service:** General Medical and Surgical

Staffed Beds: 170 **Admissions:** 9156 **Census:** 108 **Outpatient Visits:** 82269 **Births:** 2185 **Total Expense ($000):** 95321 **Payroll Expense ($000):** 39983 **Personnel:** 733

☐ **DOCTOR'S HOSPITAL – TIDWELL (450803)**, 510 West Tidwell Road, Zip 77091–4399; tel. 713/691–1111, (Includes DOCTORS HOSPITAL PARKWAY, 233 West Parker Road, Zip 77076–2999; tel. 281/765–2600; Max L. Ludeke, Chief Executive Officer), (Nonreporting) **A**1 9 10
Primary Contact: Max L. Ludeke, Chief Executive Officer
CIO: Richard Barlow, Director Information Systems
Control: Partnership, Investor–owned, for–profit **Service:** General Medical and Surgical

Staffed Beds: 200

TX

★ **DUBUIS HOSPITAL OF HOUSTON (452055)**, 1919 Labranch 7GWS Street, Zip 77002; tel. 713/756–8660 **A**1 9 10 **F**1 3 25 26 27 30 31 32 66 72 75 76 80 81 82 119 124 137 **P**5 **S** Dubuis Health System
Primary Contact: Marissa Henry, Administrator
COO: Sam D. Barkman, Vice President Operations
Web address: www.dubuis.org
Control: Church–operated, Nongovernment, not–for profit **Service:** Long–Term Acute Care hospital

Staffed Beds: 30 **Admissions:** 215 **Census:** 14 **Outpatient Visits:** 0 **Births:** 0 **Total Expense ($000):** 6674 **Payroll Expense ($000):** 2660 **Personnel:** 59

★ **EAST HOUSTON REGIONAL MEDICAL CENTER (450126)**, 13111 East Freeway, Zip 77015–5820; tel. 713/393–2000 **A**1 9 10 **F**3 11 13 15 25 26 31 32 33 38 40 43 55 56 57 59 68 71 72 74 75 77 79 82 84 86 96 97 100 103 106 107 118 119 121 133 135 **S** HCA
Primary Contact: Clay Franklin, Chief Executive Officer
COO: Michael Roussos, Chief Operating Officer
CFO: Claudia Leal, Chief Financial Officer
CMO: Steven Levy, Chief Medical Officer
Web address: www.easthoustonrmc.com
Control: Partnership, Investor–owned, for–profit **Service:** General Medical and Surgical

Staffed Beds: 131 **Admissions:** 8280 **Census:** 88 **Outpatient Visits:** 70813 **Births:** 1587 **Total Expense ($000):** 67125 **Payroll Expense ($000):** 30795 **Personnel:** 471

★ △ **HARRIS COUNTY HOSPITAL DISTRICT (450289)**, 2525 Holly Hall Street, Zip 77054–4108, Mailing Address: P.O. Box 66769, Zip 77266–6769; tel. 713/566–6403, (Includes BEN TAUB GENERAL HOSPITAL, 1504 Taub Loop, Zip 77030; tel. 713/873–2300; LYNDON B JOHNSON GENERAL HOSPITAL, 5656 Kelley, Zip 77026; tel. 713/566–5000; Lester Martinez–Lopez, M.D., Administrator; QUENTIN MEASE HOSPITAL, 3601 North MacGregor, Zip 77004; tel. 713/873–3700; Jeffrey Webster, Administrator), (Total facility includes 24 beds in nursing home–type unit) **A**2 3 5 7 8 9 10 **F**3 5 7 13 15 17 18 20 22 25 26 27 28 31 32 33 37 38 40 43 44 46 49 50 51 53 54 55 56 57 58 59 60 62 63 66 68 69 70 71 72 73 74 75 76 77 79 80 82 83 84 85 86 87 88 89 90 91 92 93 94 96 97 99 100 102 106 107 112 114 117 118 119 121 123 124 132 133 134 135 136 137
Primary Contact: David S. Lopez, FACHE, President and Chief Executive Officer
COO: George V. Masi, Chief Operating Officer
CFO: Ferdinand Gaenzel, Chief Financial Officer
CMO: Fred Sutton, Chief Medical Officer
CIO: Tim Tindle, Chief Information Officer
CHR: Lou Gould, Administrator People and Organizational Development
Web address: www.hchdonline.com
Control: Hospital district or authority, Government, nonfederal **Service:** General Medical and Surgical

Staffed Beds: 875 **Admissions:** 44892 **Census:** 698 **Outpatient Visits:** 1464389 **Births:** 11205 **Personnel:** 6381

□ **HEALTHBRIDGE CHILDREN'S HOSPITAL OF HOUSTON (453309)**, (Specialty Pediatric), 2929 Woodland Park Drive, Zip 77082; tel. 281/293–7774 **A**1 9 10 **F**3 25 32 72 73 77 80 84 90 119 135 137 **S** Nexus Health Systems
Primary Contact: Geoffrey Swaby, Administrator
CHR: Leta Shideler, Director Human Resources
Web address: www.nhsltd.com/HealthBridge–Houston/Default.htm
Control: Partnership, Investor–owned, for–profit **Service:** Children's other specialty

Staffed Beds: 24 **Admissions:** 223 **Census:** 20 **Outpatient Visits:** 0 **Births:** 0 **Total Expense ($000):** 7681 **Payroll Expense ($000):** 3841 **Personnel:** 101

□ **HEALTHSOUTH HOSPITAL FOR SPECIALIZED SURGERY (450797)**, 5400 La Branch Street, Zip 77004–6836; tel. 713/528–6800 **A**1 9 10 **F**3 8 38 43 46 47 49 77 79 **S** HEALTHSOUTH Corporation
Primary Contact: Trent Gastineau, Chief Executive Officer
Web address: www.healthsouth.com
Control: Partnership, Investor–owned, for–profit **Service:** General Medical and Surgical

Staffed Beds: 7 **Admissions:** 66 **Census:** 1 **Outpatient Visits:** 2700 **Births:** 0 **Total Expense ($000):** 6105 **Payroll Expense ($000):** 1633 **Personnel:** 40

★ **HEALTHSOUTH HOSPITAL OF HOUSTON (452077)**, 17506 Red Oak Drive, Zip 77090–7721; tel. 281/580–1212 **A**1 9 10 **F**1 3 9 25 30 31 32 43 54 62 72 73 75 77 81 86 119 120 121 132 135 137 **S** HEALTHSOUTH Corporation
Primary Contact: Aleen D. Arabit, Chief Executive Officer
CFO: Shantra Wayne, Controller
Web address: www.healthsouth.com
Control: Partnership, Investor–owned, for–profit **Service:** General Medical and Surgical

Staffed Beds: 74 **Admissions:** 477 **Census:** 32 **Outpatient Visits:** 5011 **Births:** 0 **Total Expense ($000):** 13801 **Payroll Expense ($000):** 6810 **Personnel:** 131

★ **HOUSTON NORTHWEST MEDICAL CENTER (450638)**, 710 FM 1960 West, Zip 77090–3496; tel. 281/440–1000 **A**1 2 3 5 9 10 **F**3 8 11 12 13 15 18 20 22 24 25 26 27 31 32 38 46 49 56 57 62 63 68 70 72 73 75 76 77 79 80 81 84 86 96 97 98 99 100 101 102 104 105 107 118 119 121 134 135 136 137 **S** TENET Healthcare Corporation
Primary Contact: Drew Kahn, Chief Executive Officer
COO: Linda Mercier, Chief Operating Officer
CFO: Sean B. Gallagher, Chief Financial Officer
CMO: Terry Kirk, Chief Nursing Officer
CIO: Steve Peacock, Director Information Systems
CHR: Judy White House, Director Human Resources
Web address: www.hnmc.com
Control: Partnership, Investor–owned, for–profit **Service:** General Medical and Surgical

Staffed Beds: 369 **Admissions:** 16522 **Census:** 225 **Outpatient Visits:** 127779 **Births:** 2418 **Total Expense ($000):** 215432 **Payroll Expense ($000):** 81923 **Personnel:** 1390

□ **INTRACARE MEDICAL CENTER HOSPITAL (454089)**, 7601 Fannin Street, Zip 77054–1905; tel. 713/790–0949 **A**1 9 10 **F**5 30 31 32 88 89 90 91 92 93 94 95 **P**6 **S** Cambridge Health Foundation
Primary Contact: Terry Scovill, Chief Executive Officer
CFO: Victor Cuffee, Chief Financial Officer
Web address: www.intracarehospital.com
Control: Other not–for–profit (including NFP Corporation) **Service:** Psychiatric

Staffed Beds: 120 **Admissions:** 3597 **Census:** 81 **Outpatient Visits:** 4250 **Births:** 0 **Total Expense ($000):** 16671 **Payroll Expense ($000):** 7836 **Personnel:** 238

□ **INTRACARE NORTH HOSPITAL (454083)**, 1120 Cypress Station Drive, Zip 77090–3031; tel. 281/893–7200 **A**1 9 10 **F**5 31 32 88 89 90 91 92 93 94 95 **P**6 **S** Cambridge Health Foundation
Primary Contact: Teisha York, Chief Executive Officer
CFO: Fred Chan, Chief Financial Officer
CMO: Javier Ruiz, M.D., Medical Director
Web address: www.intracare.org
Control: Other not–for–profit (including NFP Corporation) **Service:** Psychiatric

Staffed Beds: 68 **Admissions:** 2192 **Census:** 41 **Outpatient Visits:** 925 **Births:** 0 **Total Expense ($000):** 7848 **Payroll Expense ($000):** 3993 **Personnel:** 143

□ **KINDRED HOSPITAL–HOUSTON (452023)**, 6441 Main Street, Zip 77030–1596; tel. 713/790–0500 **A**1 5 9 10 **F**1 3 25 26 27 32 38 62 72 73 75 76 77 80 82 96 119 137 **S** Kindred Healthcare
Primary Contact: Randy E. Johnson, Chief Executive Officer
CFO: Nancy Richardson, Chief Financial Officer
Web address: www.kindredhealthcare.com
Control: Corporation, Investor–owned, for–profit **Service:** General Medical and Surgical

Staffed Beds: 92 **Admissions:** 773 **Census:** 66 **Outpatient Visits:** 122 **Births:** 0 **Total Expense ($000):** 31507 **Payroll Expense ($000):** 11700 **Personnel:** 273

□ **KINDRED HOSPITAL–HOUSTON NORTHWEST (452039)**, 11297 Fallbrook Drive, Zip 77065–4292; tel. 281/897–8114 **A**1 9 10 **F**1 3 25 30 32 55 62 68 75 82 86 96 102 118 119 137 **P**5 **S** Kindred Healthcare
Primary Contact: Mary Anne Craig, Chief Executive Officer
Web address: www.kindredhealthcare.com
Control: Corporation, Investor–owned, for–profit **Service:** Long–Term Acute Care hospital

Staffed Beds: 84 **Admissions:** 876 **Census:** 59 **Outpatient Visits:** 43 **Births:** 0 **Total Expense ($000):** 20772 **Payroll Expense ($000):** 9498 **Personnel:** 184

LYNDON B JOHNSON GENERAL HOSPITAL See Harris County Hospital District

Hospital, Medicare Provider Number, Address, Telephone, Approval, Facility, and Physician Codes, Health Care System

★ American Hospital Association (AHA) membership
□ The Joint Commission accreditation
○ American Osteopathic Association (AOA) accreditation
△ Commission on Accreditation of Rehabilitation Facilities (CARF) accreditation

☒ △ **MEMORIAL HERMANN – THE INSTITUTE FOR REHABILITATION AND RESEARCH (453025)**, 1333 Moursund, Zip 77030–3405; tel. 713/797–5278 **A**1 3 5 7 9 10 **F**3 11 25 26 32 37 41 43 50 56 58 62 72 73 75 77 81 82 85 86 113 119 120 121 135 137 **S** Memorial Hermann Healthcare System
Primary Contact: Carl E. Josehart, Chief Executive Officer
CFO: Barrie Strickland, Chief Financial Officer
CMO: William Donovan, M.D., Medical Director
CIO: Mother Superior Andy Draper, Director Hospital Systems
CHR: Vivian Kardow, Chief Human Resources Officer
Web address: www.memorialhermann.org/locations/tirr.html
Control: Other not–for–profit (including NFP Corporation) **Service:** Rehabilitation

Staffed Beds: 98 **Admissions:** 1198 **Census:** 83 **Outpatient Visits:** 34493 **Births:** 0 **Total Expense ($000):** 54884 **Payroll Expense ($000):** 26634 **Personnel:** 506

★ **MEMORIAL HERMANN CONTINUING CARE HOSPITAL (452072)**, 3043 Gessner Drive, Zip 77080–2597; tel. 713/462–2515, (Nonreporting) **A**2 9 10 **S** Triumph HealthCare
Primary Contact: Joe G. Baldwin, Chief Executive Officer
Web address: www.memorialhermann.org
Control: Other not–for–profit (including NFP Corporation) **Service:** General Medical and Surgical

Staffed Beds: 191

☒ **MEMORIAL HERMANN HOSPITAL (450068)**, 6411 Fannin, Zip 77030–1501; tel. 713/704–4000, (Includes CHILDREN'S MEMORIAL HERMANN HOSPITAL, tel. 713/704–5437; Craig Cordola, Chief Executive Officer), (Total facility includes 9 beds in nursing home–type unit) **A**1 3 5 8 9 10 **F**3 7 12 13 15 16 17 18 19 20 21 22 23 24 25 26 27 28 30 31 32 33 34 35 37 38 40 41 43 44 45 46 47 48 49 50 51 54 55 56 57 58 59 60 61 62 66 68 70 71 72 73 74 75 76 77 79 81 82 83 84 85 86 87 90 96 97 98 100 102 103 104 105 106 107 112 113 114 116 117 118 119 120 121 123 124 127 128 130 131 132 133 135 136 137 **P**5 6 **S** Memorial Hermann Healthcare System
Primary Contact: Juanita F. Romans, Chief Executive Officer
COO: Tom Flanagan, Chief Operating Officer
CFO: Barrie Strickland, Chief Financial Officer
CMO: William Peruzzi, M.D., Chief Medical Officer
CIO: David Bradshaw, Chief Information Officer
CHR: Vivian Kardow, Chief Human Resources Officer
Web address: www.mhhs.org
Control: Other not–for–profit (including NFP Corporation) **Service:** General Medical and Surgical

Staffed Beds: 766 **Admissions:** 32816 **Census:** 606 **Outpatient Visits:** 105614 **Births:** 4631 **Total Expense ($000):** 671127 **Payroll Expense ($000):** 209243 **Personnel:** 3928

☒ **MEMORIAL HERMANN MEMORIAL CITY HOSPITAL (450610)**, 921 Gessner Road, Zip 77024–9173; tel. 713/242–3000, (Total facility includes 24 beds in nursing home–type unit) **A**1 2 9 10 **F**3 12 13 15 18 20 22 24 25 26 27 30 31 32 33 35 38 42 43 44 46 49 51 54 55 56 57 59 63 68 70 72 73 74 75 76 77 78 79 80 82 84 86 96 98 99 100 102 105 106 107 108 109 116 117 118 119 120 121 124 133 135 136 137 **P**5 6 **S** Memorial Hermann Healthcare System
Primary Contact: David L. Jones, Interim Chief Executive Officer
COO: Keith N. Alexander, Assistant Vice President Operations
CFO: Lisa Kendler, Chief Financial Officer
CMO: Donald Gibson, Medical Director
CHR: Vicki Jones, Director Human Resources
Web address: www.memorialhermann.org
Control: Other not–for–profit (including NFP Corporation) **Service:** General Medical and Surgical

Staffed Beds: 343 **Admissions:** 18673 **Census:** 211 **Outpatient Visits:** 87741 **Births:** 3328 **Total Expense ($000):** 253770 **Payroll Expense ($000):** 70088 **Personnel:** 1299

MEMORIAL HERMANN NORTHWEST HOSPITAL See Memorial Hermann Southwest Hospital

☐ **MEMORIAL HERMANN SOUTHEAST (450184)**, 11800 Astoria, Zip 77089; tel. 281/929–6100, (Total facility includes 15 beds in nursing home–type unit) **A**1 9 10 **F**3 5 11 13 15 18 20 24 25 26 27 30 31 32 33 34 38 40 42 43 50 51 52 54 55 56 57 59 60 61 62 66 67 68 72 73 74 75 76 77 79 80 81 82 84 85 86 90 91 92 96 97 100 102 104 105 107 117 118 119 120 121 124 132 135 136 137 **P**5 6 **S** Memorial Hermann Healthcare System
COO: Jude Torchia, Chief Operating Officer
CFO: Douglas J. Arvin, Chief Financial Officer
Web address: www.memorialhermann.org
Control: Other not–for–profit (including NFP Corporation) **Service:** General Medical and Surgical

Staffed Beds: 265 **Admissions:** 12884 **Census:** 154 **Outpatient Visits:** 81822 **Births:** 1528 **Total Expense ($000):** 145320 **Payroll Expense ($000):** 53018 **Personnel:** 992

☒ **MEMORIAL HERMANN SOUTHWEST HOSPITAL (450184)**, 7600 Beechnut, Zip 77074–1850; tel. 713/456–5000, (Includes MEMORIAL HERMANN NORTHWEST HOSPITAL, 1635 North Loop West, Zip 77008; tel. 713/867–3380), (Total facility includes 16 beds in nursing home–type unit) **A**1 2 3 5 9 10 **F**3 8 13 15 17 18 20 22 25 26 27 30 31 32 33 34 36 38 40 41 43 44 46 47 49 50 51 55 56 57 59 60 62 63 68 70 72 73 74 75 76 77 79 81 82 85 86 96 97 98 99 100 101 102 103 104 105 106 107 108 109 112 114 116 117 118 119 120 121 124 135 136 137 **P**5 6 **S** Memorial Hermann Healthcare System
Primary Contact: Sonja Hagel, Chief Executive Officer
COO: Joe G. Baldwin, Chief Operating Officer
CFO: Roger Faculak, Chief Financial Officer
CMO: Maurice Leibman, M.D., Chief Medical Officer
CIO: David Bradshaw, Chief Information Officer
CHR: Terry Henske, Director Human Resources
Web address: www.memorialhermann.org
Control: Other not–for–profit (including NFP Corporation) **Service:** General Medical and Surgical

Staffed Beds: 485 **Admissions:** 24407 **Census:** 319 **Outpatient Visits:** 138407 **Births:** 4561 **Total Expense ($000):** 321920 **Payroll Expense ($000):** 110348 **Personnel:** 2060

☐ **MENNINGER CLINIC**, 2801 Gessner, Zip 77080, Mailing Address: P.O. Box 809045, Zip 77280; tel. 713/275–5000 **A**1 3 5 **F**26 88 89 119
Primary Contact: Ian Aitken, President and Chief Operating Officer
Web address: www.menningerclinic.com
Control: Other not–for–profit (including NFP Corporation) **Service:** Psychiatric

Staffed Beds: 130 **Admissions:** 901 **Census:** 106 **Outpatient Visits:** 0 **Births:** 0 **Total Expense ($000):** 38724 **Payroll Expense ($000):** 17407 **Personnel:** 331

☒ **METHODIST WILLOWBROOK HOSPITAL (450844)**, 18220 Tomball Parkway, Zip 77070; tel. 281/477–1000 **A**1 9 10 **F**3 13 15 18 20 25 26 30 31 32 33 34 35 38 41 43 49 55 56 57 60 62 63 68 71 72 73 74 75 77 78 79 80 81 82 86 96 97 100 103 107 119 121 124 135 136 137 **S** The Methodist Hospital System
Primary Contact: Andrew Cochrane, Chief Executive Officer
CFO: James Levermann, Chief Financial Officer
CHR: Sherene Thompson, Director Human Resources
Web address: www.methodisthealth.com
Control: Other not–for–profit (including NFP Corporation) **Service:** General Medical and Surgical

Staffed Beds: 119 **Admissions:** 9093 **Census:** 98 **Outpatient Visits:** 83565 **Births:** 2515 **Total Expense ($000):** 109650 **Payroll Expense ($000):** 46789 **Personnel:** 821

☒ △ **MICHAEL E. DEBAKEY VETERANS AFFAIRS MEDICAL CENTER**, 2002 Holcombe Boulevard, Zip 77030–4298; tel. 713/791–1414, (Total facility includes 120 beds in nursing home–type unit) (Nonreporting) **A**1 2 3 5 7 8 9 **S** Department of Veterans Affairs
Primary Contact: Edgar L. Tucker, Director
COO: Carlos Escobar, Associate Director
CFO: Jim Eddins, Financial Resources Manager
CIO: Kevin Lenamond, Information Management Service Line Executive
CHR: Charlotte Jones, Manager Human Resources
Web address: www.houston.va.gov
Control: Veterans Affairs, Government, federal **Service:** General Medical and Surgical

Staffed Beds: 859

NORTH CAMPUS See River Oaks Hospital

☒ **PARK PLAZA HOSPITAL (450659)**, 1313 Hermann Drive, Zip 77004–7092; tel. 713/527–5000 **A**1 2 9 10 **F**1 3 4 11 12 13 15 16 18 20 25 27 31 32 33 38 46 50 54 55 56 57 59 60 65 68 70 71 72 73 74 75 76 77 78 79 80 83 85 86 88 93 96 97 99 100 102 107 108 109 111 117 118 119 121 135 136 137 **S** TENET Healthcare Corporation
Primary Contact: Phillip E. Sowa, Chief Executive Officer
COO: John Tressa, Chief Operating Officer
CFO: Kirk Pogue, Chief Financial Officer
CIO: Terry Janis, Assistant Vice President
CHR: Lori Knowles, Director Human Resources
Web address: www.parkplazahospital.com
Control: Partnership, Investor–owned, for–profit **Service:** General Medical and Surgical

Staffed Beds: 218 **Admissions:** 7864 **Census:** 127 **Outpatient Visits:** 45104 **Births:** 1025 **Total Expense ($000):** 107054 **Payroll Expense ($000):** 41853 **Personnel:** 730

TX

 Many Facility Codes have changed. Please refer to the AHA Guide Code Chart.

★ **PLAZA SPECIALTY HOSPITAL (452046)**, 1300 Binz, Zip 77004; tel. 713/285–1000 **A**1 9 10 **F**1 3 25 27 31 32 43 44 54 68 73 75 76 77 80 82 119 124 137 **P**8 **S** TENET Healthcare Corporation
Primary Contact: Steven Barr, Chief Executive Officer
CFO: Charles R. Handley, Chief Financial Officer
CMO: Wasae S. Tabibi, M.D., President of Staff
CIO: Steve Peacock, Assistant Vice President
Web address: www.plazaspecialtyhospital.com
Control: Corporation, Investor–owned, for–profit **Service:** Long–Term Acute Care hospital

Staffed Beds: 57 **Admissions:** 349 **Census:** 23 **Outpatient Visits:** 0 **Births:** 0 **Total Expense ($000):** 17274 **Payroll Expense ($000):** 4920 **Personnel:** 81

QUENTIN MEASE HOSPITAL See Harris County Hospital District

RENAISSANCE HOSPITAL – HOUSTON (450795), 2807 Little York Road, Zip 77093–3495; tel. 713/697–7777 **A**9 10 **F**12 25 31 38 62 68 73 75 79 86 96 100 107 119 132 **P**8 **S** Renaissance Healthcare Systems
Primary Contact: Michael Smesny, President
COO: Nora Peralta, Chief Nursing Officer
CFO: John Lucia, Chief Financial Officer
CMO: Rafael Borges, Chief of Staff
CIO: Bill DuBrul, Director Information Technology
CHR: Cathy McCue, Director Human Resources
Control: Corporation, Investor–owned, for–profit **Service:** General Medical and Surgical

Staffed Beds: 39 **Admissions:** 849 **Census:** 10 **Outpatient Visits:** 12462 **Births:** 0 **Total Expense ($000):** 17430 **Payroll Expense ($000):** 6066 **Personnel:** 132

☐ **RIVER OAKS HOSPITAL (450378)**, (Formerly Twelve Oaks Medical Center), 4200 Twelve Oaks Drive, Zip 77027–6899; tel. 713/623–2500, (Includes NORTH CAMPUS; RIVER OAKS HOSPITAL – SHARPSTOWN CAMPUS, 6700 Bellaire, Zip 77074–4999; tel. 713/774–7611) **A**1 5 9 10 **F**3 11 12 13 18 20 22 25 27 32 38 40 43 46 54 57 59 60 62 66 68 70 72 73 74 76 77 79 80 88 93 96 97 100 103 107 118 119 121 135 136 137 **P**2 **S** Hospital Partners of America
Primary Contact: Chris M. Vasquez, Chief Executive Officer
CFO: Gregg Garrison, Chief Financial Officer
CMO: Timothy Castro, M.D., Chief of Staff
CIO: Stephen Farias, Director Information Services
CHR: Brenda Ray, Director Human Resources
Web address: www.twelveoaksmedicalcenter.com
Control: Partnership, Investor–owned, for–profit **Service:** General Medical and Surgical

Staffed Beds: 225 **Admissions:** 9742 **Census:** 110 **Outpatient Visits:** 38959 **Births:** 3234 **Total Expense ($000):** 108890 **Payroll Expense ($000):** 40780 **Personnel:** 688

RIVER OAKS HOSPITAL – SHARPSTOWN CAMPUS See River Oaks Hospital

☐ **RIVERSIDE GENERAL HOSPITAL (450446)**, 3204 Ennis Street, Zip 77004–3299; tel. 713/526–2441 **A**1 9 10 **F**4 5 25 26 31 32 33 38 54 55 57 60 82 88 89 90 91 93 95 119 121 132 135 **P**5
Primary Contact: Earnest Gibson, III, Administrator
CFO: Manny Ignacio, Controller
Web address: www.riversidegeneral.org
Control: Other not–for–profit (including NFP Corporation) **Service:** Psychiatric

Staffed Beds: 83 **Admissions:** 1172 **Census:** 31 **Outpatient Visits:** 3966 **Births:** 0 **Total Expense ($000):** 12600 **Payroll Expense ($000):** 6507 **Personnel:** 260

☐ **SELECT SPECIALTY HOSPITAL–HOUSTON HEIGHTS (452049)**, 1917 Ashland Street, Zip 77008–3994; tel. 713/861–6161 **A**1 9 10 **F**1 3 25 27 32 38 50 59 62 68 79 82 96 102 107 119 137 **P**8 **S** Select Medical Corporation
Primary Contact: Teresa L. Davis, Administrator
CFO: Traci Jameson, Manager Finance
CMO: Chi C. Mao, M.D., Ph.D., Medical Director
CHR: Pamela Reynolds, Director Human Resources
Web address: www.selectmedicalcorp.com
Control: Partnership, Investor–owned, for–profit **Service:** Long–Term Acute Care hospital

Staffed Beds: 242 **Admissions:** 2187 **Census:** 156 **Outpatient Visits:** 1016 **Births:** 0 **Total Expense ($000):** 71856 **Payroll Expense ($000):** 29943 **Personnel:** 613

SELECT SPECIALTY HOSPITAL–HOUSTON MEDICAL CENTER (452023), 6655 Travis Street, Suite 300, Zip 77030–1502, Mailing Address: 6500 Fannin Street, Suite 907, Zip 77030–1502; tel. 713/520–9595, (Nonreporting) **A**9 10 **S** Select Medical Corporation
Primary Contact: Vivian Bond, Administrator
Web address: www.selectmedicalcorp.com
Control: Corporation, Investor–owned, for–profit **Service:** Long–Term Acute Care hospital

Staffed Beds: 34

☐ **SELECT SPECIALTY HOSPITAL–HOUSTON WEST CAMPUS**, 9430 Old Katy Road, Zip 77055; tel. 713/984–2273, (Nonreporting) **A**1 9 **S** Select Medical Corporation
Primary Contact: Marinella Castroman, Administrator
Web address: www.selectmedicalcorp.com
Control: Corporation, Investor–owned, for–profit **Service:** Other specialty

Staffed Beds: 38

☐ **SHRINERS HOSPITALS FOR CHILDREN, HOUSTON**, 6977 Main Street, Zip 77030–3701; tel. 713/797–1616 **A**1 3 5 **F**3 25 28 33 43 55 56 57 58 62 64 66 72 73 77 79 80 81 82 84 85 86 114 119 120 121 123 132 135 137 **P**6 **S** Shriners Hospitals for Children
Primary Contact: Steven B. Reiter, Administrator
CFO: Lona Pope, Director Fiscal Services
CMO: Douglas A. Barnes, Chief of Staff
CHR: Lynn Clements, Director Human Resources
Web address: www.shrineshq.org
Control: Other not–for–profit (including NFP Corporation) **Service:** Children's orthopedic

Staffed Beds: 40 **Admissions:** 839 **Census:** 10 **Outpatient Visits:** 8263 **Births:** 0 **Total Expense ($000):** 15153 **Personnel:** 183

★ **SPRING BRANCH MEDICAL CENTER (450630)**, 8850 Long Point Road, Zip 77055–3082; tel. 713/467–6555 **A**1 9 10 **F**1 3 4 11 12 15 16 17 22 24 25 26 27 30 31 32 33 38 43 46 49 54 55 57 60 65 66 68 70 71 72 73 75 76 77 78 79 83 84 85 86 88 96 97 100 105 107 109 112 117 118 119 121 135 137 **P**7 **S** HCA
Primary Contact: Jay Woodall, Chief Executive Officer
CHR: Scott Doak, Human Resources Director
Web address: www.springbranchmedical.com
Control: Corporation, Investor–owned, for–profit **Service:** General Medical and Surgical

Staffed Beds: 224 **Admissions:** 6107 **Census:** 94 **Outpatient Visits:** 54515 **Births:** 0 **Total Expense ($000):** 121359 **Payroll Expense ($000):** 33897 **Personnel:** 528

☐ **ST. JOSEPH MEDICAL CENTER (450035)**, 1401 St. Joseph Parkway, Zip 77002–8321; tel. 713/757–1000, (Total facility includes 18 beds in nursing home–type unit) **A**1 3 5 9 10 **F**3 11 13 15 18 20 22 25 26 27 30 31 32 33 38 40 43 44 45 49 50 51 52 55 56 57 58 59 62 68 69 70 72 73 74 75 76 77 79 80 81 82 85 86 87 88 92 93 96 97 100 102 103 107 109 112 114 117 118 119 120 121 124 132 133 135 136 137 **P**2 **S** Hospital Partners of America
Primary Contact: Phillip D. Robinson, Chief Executive Officer
COO: Laura Fortin, Chief Operating Officer
CFO: Patrick J. Mathews, Chief Financial Officer
CIO: Robin Brown, Chief Information Officer and Compliance Officer
CHR: Kris Clatanoff, Director Human Resources
Web address: www.sjmetx.com
Control: Partnership, Investor–owned, for–profit **Service:** General Medical and Surgical

Staffed Beds: 362 **Admissions:** 14950 **Census:** 209 **Outpatient Visits:** 159994 **Births:** 4731 **Total Expense ($000):** 189524 **Payroll Expense ($000):** 67371 **Personnel:** 2141

TX

Hospital, Medicare Provider Number, Address, Telephone, Approval, Facility, and Physician Codes, Health Care System
★ American Hospital Association (AHA) membership
☐ The Joint Commission accreditation
○ American Osteopathic Association (AOA) accreditation
△ Commission on Accreditation of Rehabilitation Facilities (CARF) accreditation

★ △ **ST. LUKE'S EPISCOPAL HOSPITAL (450193)**, 6720 Bertner Avenue, Zip 77030–2697, Mailing Address: Box 20269, Zip 77225–0269; tel. 832/355–1000 **A**1 2 3 5 7 8 9 10 **F**3 8 11 12 13 14 15 17 18 20 22 24 25 26 27 30 31 32 33 35 37 38 39 41 43 44 46 47 48 49 50 51 53 54 55 56 57 58 59 60 62 63 66 68 72 73 74 75 76 77 79 80 81 82 84 85 86 90 96 97 98 99 100 102 103 104 105 106 107 108 109 111 114 116 118 119 120 121 124 126 127 128 129 131 134 135 136 137 **P**5 **S** St. Luke's Episcopal Health System
Primary Contact: David C. Pate, M.D., J.D., Chief Executive Officer
CFO: Steve Pickett, Chief Financial Officer
CMO: Angela Shippy, Medical Director
CIO: Jack Sandefur, Interim Chief Information Officer
CHR: Irene Helsinger, Senior Vice President and Chief Administrative Officer
Web address: www.stlukestexas.com
Control: Church–operated, Nongovernment, not–for profit **Service:** General Medical and Surgical

Staffed Beds: 718 **Admissions:** 32385 **Census:** 551 **Outpatient Visits:** 294211 **Births:** 2080 **Total Expense ($000):** 705902 **Payroll Expense ($000):** 268574 **Personnel:** 4825

★ **TEXAS CHILDREN'S HOSPITAL (453304)**, 6621 Fannin Street, Zip 77030–2399, Mailing Address: Box 300630, Zip 77230–0630; tel. 832/824–1000 **A**1 3 5 8 9 10 **F**3 7 9 11 12 17 19 21 23 25 26 27 28 31 32 33 36 37 38 48 49 50 55 56 57 58 59 60 61 62 63 66 69 70 71 72 73 75 76 77 78 79 80 81 82 83 84 86 87 89 90 91 94 96 100 102 103 106 107 114 118 119 120 121 123 125 126 127 128 129 130 132 133 135 137 **P**7
Primary Contact: Mark A. Wallace, President and Chief Executive Officer
COO: Randall P. Wright, Executive Vice President and Chief Operating Officer
CFO: Benjamin B. Melson, CPA, Executive Vice President and Chief Financial Officer
CMO: Ralph D. Feigin, M.D., Physician–in–Chief
CIO: David S. Finn, Vice President and Chief Information Officer
CHR: Linda Aldred, Senior Vice President
Web address: www.texaschildrenshospital.org
Control: Other not–for–profit (including NFP Corporation) **Service:** Children's general

Staffed Beds: 458 **Admissions:** 22128 **Census:** 396 **Outpatient Visits:** 1215424 **Births:** 0 **Total Expense ($000):** 746837 **Payroll Expense ($000):** 321664 **Personnel:** 10243

★ **TEXAS ORTHOPEDIC HOSPITAL (450804)**, 7401 South Main Street, Zip 77030–4509; tel. 713/799–8600 **A**1 3 5 9 10 **F**3 25 26 30 32 38 40 43 62 63 66 68 77 79 80 81 82 86 87 96 100 103 107 119 120 135 **S** HCA
Primary Contact: Alice G. Adams, RN, Chief Executive Officer
CFO: James Bills, Chief Financial Officer
CMO: James B. Bennett, M.D., Chief of Staff
Web address: www.texasorthopedic.com
Control: Partnership, Investor–owned, for–profit **Service:** Orthopedic

Staffed Beds: 49 **Admissions:** 2556 **Census:** 20 **Outpatient Visits:** 33033 **Births:** 0 **Total Expense ($000):** 56904 **Payroll Expense ($000):** 18047 **Personnel:** 353

TX

□ **TEXAS SPECIALTY HOSPITAL (452043)**, 6160 South Loop East, Zip 77087–1010; tel. 713/640–2400 **A**1 9 10 **F**1 3 25 26 27 30 31 32 54 62 68 73 75 80 119 137 **P**5 **S** Fundamental Long Term Care Holdings, LLC
Primary Contact: Patrick A. Auman, Ph.D., Executive Director
CFO: Betty Priestley, Business Officer Manager
CMO: Alfred Louis, M.D., Chief Medical Staff
CHR: Jacqueline Moten, Director Human Resources
Web address: www.thicare.com
Control: Corporation, Investor–owned, for–profit **Service:** General Medical and Surgical

Staffed Beds: 31 **Admissions:** 267 **Census:** 18 **Outpatient Visits:** 64 **Births:** 0 **Total Expense ($000):** 9072 **Payroll Expense ($000):** 3257 **Personnel:** 66

★ **THE METHODIST HOSPITAL (450358)**, 6565 Fannin Street, Zip 77030–2707; tel. 713/790–3311, (Total facility includes 25 beds in nursing home–type unit) **A**1 2 3 5 8 9 10 **F**3 5 9 11 12 13 14 15 17 18 20 22 24 25 26 27 29 30 31 32 33 34 35 36 37 38 41 42 43 44 45 46 47 48 49 50 51 52 53 54 55 56 57 58 59 60 61 62 63 66 68 69 71 72 73 74 75 76 77 78 79 80 81 82 85 86 87 88 90 92 93 96 97 98 99 100 102 103 104 105 106 107 108 109 111 112 114 116 117 118 119 120 121 124 125 126 127 128 129 130 131 132 134 135 136 137 **P**5 6 **S** The Methodist Hospital System
Primary Contact: Ronald G. Girotto, President and Chief Executive Officer
COO: Marc Boom, M.D., Senior Vice President and Chief Operating Officer
CFO: John E. Hagale, Executive Vice President, Chief Financial Officer and Chief Administrative Officer
CMO: Dirk Sostman, M.D., Executive Vice President
CIO: Matthew E. Fink, M.D., Interim Vice President
CHR: Lauren Rykert, Senior Vice President
Web address: www.methodisthealth.com
Control: Other not–for–profit (including NFP Corporation) **Service:** General Medical and Surgical

Staffed Beds: 966 **Admissions:** 38306 **Census:** 712 **Outpatient Visits:** 332704 **Births:** 1502 **Total Expense ($000):** 996780 **Payroll Expense ($000):** 309908 **Personnel:** 6265

★ **THE WOMAN'S HOSPITAL OF TEXAS (450674)**, 7600 Fannin Street, Zip 77054–1900; tel. 713/790–1234 **A**1 3 5 9 10 **F**3 13 15 25 38 46 52 56 58 68 70 71 73 74 75 76 79 80 81 82 86 96 97 106 107 116 119 121 135 136 **S** HCA
Primary Contact: Linda B. Russell, Chief Executive Officer
COO: Jennifer Garza, Chief Operating Officer
CFO: Teresa Finch, Chief Financial Officer
CMO: Eberhard Lotze, Chief Medical Officer
CHR: Arnita Crawford, Director Human Resources
Web address: www.womanshospital.com
Control: Partnership, Investor–owned, for–profit **Service:** Obstetrics and gynecology

Staffed Beds: 248 **Admissions:** 13937 **Census:** 193 **Outpatient Visits:** 55590 **Births:** 8870 **Total Expense ($000):** 129214 **Payroll Expense ($000):** 64624 **Personnel:** 954

□ **TOPS SURGICAL SPECIALTY HOSPITAL (450774)**, 17080 Red Oak Drive, Zip 77090; tel. 281/539–2900 **A**1 9 10 **F**3 15 25 30 31 32 37 38 46 62 66 76 77 79 80 84 96 97 99 102 107 131 **S** United Surgical Partners International
Primary Contact: Teresa R. Danna, RN, M.S.N., CHE, Chief Executive Officer
COO: Teresa R. Danna, R.N., MSN, CHE, Chief Executive Officer
CFO: Don Smith, Chief Financial Officer
CMO: Carl Battaglia, M.D., Medical Director
CIO: Miranda Primeaux, Manager Medical Records
CHR: Carolyn Colson, Manager Human Resources, Accounts Payable and Payroll
Web address: www.tops–hospital.com
Control: Partnership, Investor–owned, for–profit **Service:** General Medical and Surgical

Staffed Beds: 16 **Admissions:** 480 **Census:** 3 **Outpatient Visits:** 37585 **Births:** 0 **Total Expense ($000):** 22984 **Payroll Expense ($000):** 6842 **Personnel:** 119

□ **TRIUMPH HOSPITAL CENTRAL (452027)**, 105 Drew Avenue, Zip 77006; tel. 713/529–8922 **A**1 9 10 **F**1 3 25 26 32 33 54 59 75 80 81 82 96 119 137 **P**5 **S** Triumph HealthCare
Primary Contact: Claudia McCready, Chief Executive Officer
Web address: www.triumph–healthcare.com
Control: Corporation, Investor–owned, for–profit **Service:** Long–Term Acute Care hospital

Staffed Beds: 38 **Admissions:** 360 **Census:** 22 **Outpatient Visits:** 0 **Births:** 0 **Total Expense ($000):** 11217 **Payroll Expense ($000):** 3354 **Personnel:** 75

□ **TRIUMPH HOSPITAL NORTH HOUSTON (452074)**, 7407 North Freeway, Zip 77076; tel. 832/200–6000, (Includes TRIUMPH HOSPITAL WEST HOUSTON, 8850 Long Point Road, 5th Floor, Zip 77055, Mailing Address: 8850 Long Point Road, 6th Floor, Zip 77055; tel. 713/365–7800) **A**1 9 10 **F**1 3 7 25 26 31 33 46 48 49 59 72 73 75 76 77 82 86 96 107 119 133 137 **P**5 7 **S** Triumph HealthCare
Primary Contact: Michael R. Bullard, Chief Executive Officer
COO: Audrey Fisk, Chief Clinical Officer
CFO: Terry Hohmann, Chief Financial Officer
CIO: CeCe Mathews, Director Professional Relations
CHR: Adrienne Livingston, Director Human Resources
Web address: www.triumph–healthcare.com
Control: Partnership, Investor–owned, for–profit **Service:** General Medical and Surgical

Staffed Beds: 130 **Admissions:** 807 **Census:** 58 **Outpatient Visits:** 891 **Births:** 0 **Total Expense ($000):** 30854 **Payroll Expense ($000):** 9584 **Personnel:** 237

□ **TRIUMPH HOSPITAL NORTHWEST (452081)**, 205 Hollow Tree Lane, Zip 77090; tel. 832/249–2700, (Includes TRIUMPH HOSPITAL TOMBALL, 505 Graham Drive, Tomball, Zip 77375; tel. 281/255–5600; Eileen Branscome, Chief Executive Officer) **A**1 9 10 **F**1 3 25 27 31 33 46 47 48 49 55 57 62 68 72 73 75 76 77 82 86 96 107 137 **P**5 **S** Triumph HealthCare
Primary Contact: Bob Stein, Chief Executive Officer
Control: Partnership, Investor–owned, for–profit **Service:** General Medical and Surgical

Staffed Beds: 190 **Admissions:** 1124 **Census:** 74 **Outpatient Visits:** 276 **Births:** 0 **Total Expense ($000):** 33591 **Payroll Expense ($000):** 12177 **Personnel:** 408

★ **UNIVERSITY GENERAL HOSPITAL (670019)**, 7501 Fannin Street, Zip 77054; tel. 713/375–7000 **A**1 10 **F**3 12 18 20 25 33 38 43 46 49 55 56 57 68 73 77 79 80 81 96 97 98 100 102 103 107 118 119 124 137 **P**2
Primary Contact: Kelly Riedel, Chief Executive Officer
Web address: www.ughospital.com
Control: Individual, Investor–owned, for–profit **Service:** General Medical and Surgical

Staffed Beds: 72 **Admissions:** 1388 **Census:** 14 **Outpatient Visits:** 7508 **Births:** 0 **Total Expense ($000):** 61409 **Payroll Expense ($000):** 18145 **Personnel:** 245

★ **UNIVERSITY OF TEXAS HARRIS COUNTY PSYCHIATRIC CENTER (454076)**, 2800 South MacGregor Way, Zip 77021–1000, Mailing Address: P.O. Box 20249, Zip 77225–0249; tel. 713/741–5000 **A**1 3 5 9 10 **F**25 26 33 53 54 55 56 66 73 81 82 88 89 90 91 93 94 95 119 135 **P**6 **S** University of Texas System
Primary Contact: Pedro Ruiz, M.D., Interim Executive Director
COO: Lois Jean Moore, FACHE, Administrator
CFO: Judith Ghobrial, Chief Financial Officer
CMO: R. Andrew Harper, M.D., Medical Director
CIO: Geri Konigsberg, Director Public Information
CHR: Sherri Orioli, Director Personnel Systems
Web address: www.uth.tmc.edu
Control: State–Government, nonfederal **Service:** Psychiatric

Staffed Beds: 203 **Admissions:** 5500 **Census:** 163 **Outpatient Visits:** 11574 **Births:** 0 **Total Expense ($000):** 34586 **Payroll Expense ($000):** 18797

★ **UNIVERSITY OF TEXAS M. D. ANDERSON CANCER CENTER (450076)**, 1515 Holcombe Boulevard, Box 91, Zip 77030–4095; tel. 713/792–2121 **A**1 2 3 5 8 9 10 **F**3 8 11 14 15 22 24 25 26 27 28 30 31 32 33 34 35 36 37 38 41 42 43 44 45 46 47 48 49 50 53 55 56 57 58 59 62 64 66 68 69 72 73 75 76 77 78 79 80 81 82 83 84 86 87 89 90 91 92 93 94 96 97 99 100 101 102 103 104 105 106 107 108 109 110 111 112 114 116 118 119 121 123 124 125 130 134 135 136 137 **P**6 **S** University of Texas System
Primary Contact: John Mendelsohn, M.D., President
CFO: Dwain Morris, Vice President Finance and Accounting
CMO: Thomas Burke, M.D., Executive Vice President and Physician–in–Chief
CIO: Lynn H. Vogel, Vice President and Chief Information Officer
CHR: Jim Dorn, Vice President Human Resources
Web address: www.mdanderson.org
Control: State–Government, nonfederal **Service:** Cancer

Staffed Beds: 507 **Admissions:** 22257 **Census:** 447 **Outpatient Visits:** 930319 **Births:** 0 **Total Expense ($000):** 2393810 **Payroll Expense ($000):** 1116464 **Personnel:** 15975

★ **WEST HOUSTON MEDICAL CENTER (450644)**, 12141 Richmond Avenue, Zip 77082–2499; tel. 281/558–3444 **A**1 9 10 **F**3 11 13 15 18 20 22 24 25 26 30 32 37 38 43 46 50 51 53 54 55 57 62 68 71 72 73 74 75 76 77 78 79 80 81 85 86 88 92 93 96 100 104 105 107 109 112 118 119 121 133 134 135 136 137 **S** HCA
Primary Contact: Todd Caliva, Chief Executive Officer
CFO: Stanley K. Nord, Chief Financial Officer
CMO: Magdy Rizk, M.D., Chief of Staff
CIO: Sergio Almeida, Director Information Systems
CHR: Carol Melville, Director Human Resources
Web address: www.westhoustonmedical.com
Control: Partnership, Investor–owned, for–profit **Service:** General Medical and Surgical

Staffed Beds: 193 **Admissions:** 11100 **Census:** 153 **Outpatient Visits:** 108241 **Births:** 2270 **Total Expense ($000):** 107249 **Payroll Expense ($000):** 51792 **Personnel:** 742

□ **WEST OAKS HOSPITAL (454026)**, 6500 Hornwood Drive, Zip 77074–5095; tel. 713/995–0909 **A**1 9 10 **F**5 25 31 32 53 54 62 66 88 89 90 91 93 94 95 121 **S** Psychiatric Solutions
Primary Contact: Lucinda DeBruce, Chief Executive Officer
COO: Tim C. Simmons, Chief Operating Officer
CFO: Christy Amy, Chief Financial Officer
CMO: George Santos, M.D., Executive Medical Director
CHR: Janice Webster, Director Human Resources
Web address: www.psysolutions.com
Control: Corporation, Investor–owned, for–profit **Service:** Psychiatric

Staffed Beds: 144 **Admissions:** 4863 **Census:** 101 **Outpatient Visits:** 16018 **Births:** 0 **Total Expense ($000):** 22242 **Payroll Expense ($000):** 12245 **Personnel:** 299

HUMBLE—Harris County

★ **HEALTHSOUTH REHABILITATION HOSPITAL (453029)**, 19002 McKay Drive, Zip 77338–5701; tel. 281/446–6148 **A**1 9 10 **F**25 30 31 32 43 54 62 73 75 81 82 85 86 119 121 132 137 **S** HEALTHSOUTH Corporation
Primary Contact: Angela L. Simmons, Chief Executive Officer
CFO: Dave Renneker, Chief Financial Officer
CMO: Emile Mathurin, M.D., Medical Director
CHR: Valerie Wells, Manager Human Resources
Web address: www.healthsouth.com
Control: Corporation, Investor–owned, for–profit **Service:** Rehabilitation

Staffed Beds: 60 **Admissions:** 898 **Census:** 38 **Outpatient Visits:** 8728 **Births:** 0 **Total Expense ($000):** 10064 **Payroll Expense ($000):** 5866 **Personnel:** 95

KINGWOOD MEDICAL CENTER See Kingwood

★ **MEMORIAL HERMANN NORTHEAST (450684)**, 18951 Memorial North, Zip 77338–4297; tel. 281/540–7700 **A**1 2 9 10 **F**3 11 12 13 15 18 25 26 27 31 32 33 34 38 42 49 52 54 55 56 57 61 62 68 70 71 72 73 74 75 76 77 78 79 80 81 82 84 86 96 97 99 100 102 103 104 105 106 107 109 111 118 119 121 124 135 136 137 **S** Memorial Hermann Healthcare System
Primary Contact: Louis G. Smith, Jr., Chief Executive Officer
COO: Louis G. Smith, Chief Executive Officer
CFO: Brian Walton, Chief Financial Officer
CIO: David Bradshaw, Chief Information Officer
CHR: Stephanie Foster, Director Human Resources
Web address: www.memorialhermann.org
Control: Other not–for–profit (including NFP Corporation) **Service:** General Medical and Surgical

Staffed Beds: 243 **Admissions:** 12358 **Census:** 170 **Outpatient Visits:** 89471 **Births:** 2300 **Total Expense ($000):** 119813 **Payroll Expense ($000):** 54033 **Personnel:** 775

HUNT—Kerr County

LA HACIENDA TREATMENT CENTER, FM 1340, Zip 78024, Mailing Address: P.O. Box 1, Zip 78024–0001; tel. 830/238–4222 **F**4 5 25 26 33 52 53 57 73 81 82 90 121 **P**1
Primary Contact: Arthur Van Divier, Executive Director
COO: Richard Whitman, Chief Operating Officer
CFO: Lori Ditmar, Chief Financial Officer
CIO: David James, System Administrator
CHR: Julie Dunscomb, Human Resource Executive
Web address: www.lahacienda.com
Control: Partnership, Investor–owned, for–profit **Service:** Alcoholism and other chemical dependency

Staffed Beds: 9 **Admissions:** 428 **Census:** 2 **Outpatient Visits:** 0 **Births:** 0 **Total Expense ($000):** 2014 **Payroll Expense ($000):** 1022 **Personnel:** 148

HUNTSVILLE—Walker County

★ **HUNTSVILLE MEMORIAL HOSPITAL (450347)**, 110 Memorial Hospital Drive, Zip 77340–4362, Mailing Address: P.O. Box 4001, Zip 77342–4001; tel. 936/291–3411 **A**1 9 10 **F**3 11 13 15 24 25 28 30 33 38 50 51 54 55 56 57 61 62 64 66 68 73 74 75 77 79 80 81 82 84 85 86 92 93 94 96 97 100 102 107 119 120 121 130 131 134 135 136 137 **P**8 **S** Community Hospital Corporation
Primary Contact: Sally I. Nelson, Chief Executive Officer
CFO: Robert Gray, Assistant Administrator Financial Services
CIO: John Heeman, Director Information Systems
CHR: Diane L. Stevens, R.N., Director Human Resources
Web address: www.huntsvillememorial.com
Control: Other not–for–profit (including NFP Corporation) **Service:** General Medical and Surgical

Staffed Beds: 88 **Admissions:** 2869 **Census:** 34 **Outpatient Visits:** 69942 **Births:** 505 **Total Expense ($000):** 37360 **Payroll Expense ($000):** 16950 **Personnel:** 316

HURST—Tarrant County

□ **SOUTHWEST SURGICAL HOSPITAL (450886)**, 1612 Hurst Town Center Boulevard, Zip 76054; tel. 817/345–4100 **A**1 9 10 **F**3 12 25 34 38 41 43 49 51 55 56 57 63 66 72 73 75 77 79 80 81 82 84 85 118 119 120 121 132 135 137 **S** National Surgical Hospitals
Primary Contact: Trudy Wiig, Chief Executive Officer
CFO: Lisa Gildon, Chief Administrative Officer
CMO: Dale Brancel, M.D., Chief of Staff
CHR: Donna Irvin, Director Human Resources
Web address: www.swsurgery.com
Control: Partnership, Investor–owned, for–profit **Service:** Surgical

Staffed Beds: 23 **Admissions:** 332 **Census:** 2 **Outpatient Visits:** 4148 **Births:** 0 **Total Expense ($000):** 13273 **Payroll Expense ($000):** 3645 **Personnel:** 97

IRAAN—Pecos County

IRAAN GENERAL HOSPITAL (451307), 600 349 North, Zip 79744, Mailing Address: P.O. Box 665, Zip 79744–2057; tel. 432/639–2871 **A**9 10 18 **F**24 30 31 32 38 40 54 55 57 62 73 81 86 94 107 119 122
Primary Contact: Teresa Callahan, RN, M.S.N., Chief Executive Officer
CFO: Tami Burks, Chief Fiscal Services
CMO: Robert W. Garcia, M.D., Chief Medical Officer
CHR: Cathy Tucker, Director Human Resources
Web address: www.iraangeneralhospital.org
Control: Hospital district or authority, Government, nonfederal **Service:** General Medical and Surgical

Staffed Beds: 13 **Admissions:** 144 **Census:** 1 **Outpatient Visits:** 9761 **Total Expense ($000):** 3741 **Payroll Expense ($000):** 1480 **Personnel:** 35

TX

Hospital, Medicare Provider Number, Address, Telephone, Approval, Facility, and Physician Codes, Health Care System
★ American Hospital Association (AHA) membership
□ The Joint Commission accreditation
○ American Osteopathic Association (AOA) accreditation
△ Commission on Accreditation of Rehabilitation Facilities (CARF) accreditation

IRVING—Dallas County

★ **BAYLOR MEDICAL CENTER AT IRVING (450079)**, 1901 North MacArthur Boulevard, Zip 75061; tel. 972/579–8100 **A**1 9 10 **F**3 11 12 15 17 18 20 22 24 25 26 27 31 32 33 37 38 46 47 49 53 54 56 57 60 62 63 68 71 72 73 74 75 76 77 78 79 80 81 82 85 86 90 96 97 99 100 102 103 106 107 109 110 118 119 121 132 135 136 137 **S** Baylor Health Care System
Primary Contact: Cindy K. Schamp, President
CFO: Lucy Catala, Vice President Finance
CHR: Suzanne Sharp, Director Human Resources
Web address: www.baylorhealth.com
Control: Church–operated, Nongovernment, not–for profit **Service:** General Medical and Surgical

Staffed Beds: 209 **Admissions:** 11729 **Census:** 147 **Outpatient Visits:** 95621 **Births:** 2235 **Total Expense ($000):** 167767 **Payroll Expense ($000):** 61224 **Personnel:** 1272

☐ **IRVING COPPELL SURGICAL HOSPITAL (450874)**, 400 West Interstate 635, Zip 75063; tel. 972/868–4000 **A**1 9 10 **F**3 38 51 62 66 73 79 80 90 96 100 102 107 **S** United Surgical Partners International
Primary Contact: David Yoder, Chief Executive Officer
CFO: Gabrielle Holland, Director Finance
Web address: www.ic–sh.com
Control: Partnership, Investor–owned, for–profit **Service:** General Medical and Surgical

Staffed Beds: 12 **Admissions:** 251 **Census:** 2 **Outpatient Visits:** 8999 **Births:** 0 **Total Expense ($000):** 18134 **Payroll Expense ($000):** 4387 **Personnel:** 84

★ **LAS COLINAS MEDICAL CENTER (450822)**, 6800 North MacArthur Boulevard, Zip 75039–2422; tel. 972/969–2000 **A**1 9 10 **F**3 8 13 15 18 20 22 24 25 26 27 30 31 32 33 38 46 47 48 49 50 51 55 56 57 59 62 66 68 70 71 72 73 74 76 77 78 79 82 86 92 96 100 107 118 119 120 121 124 135 136 **S** HCA
Primary Contact: Daniela Decell, Chief Executive Officer
COO: Chip Zahn, Chief Operating Officer
CFO: Todd Gibson, Chief Financial Officer
Web address: www.lascolinasmedical.com
Control: Corporation, Investor–owned, for–profit **Service:** General Medical and Surgical

Staffed Beds: 80 **Admissions:** 3975 **Census:** 37 **Outpatient Visits:** 40455 **Births:** 1699 **Total Expense ($000):** 46775 **Payroll Expense ($000):** 17729 **Personnel:** 237

JACKSBORO—Jack County

FAITH COMMUNITY HOSPITAL (450241), 717 Magnolia Street, Zip 76458–1111; tel. 940/567–6633 **A**9 10 20 **F**7 11 24 30 31 32 38 40 55 61 75 86 96 107 119 122 **P**6
Primary Contact: Donald B. Hopkins, Administrator and Chief Executive Officer
COO: Jeff Miller, Chief Operating Officer
CFO: Margaret Wingo, Chief Financial Officer
CMO: S. Jamal, M.D., Medical Director
Web address: www.faithcommunityhospital.com
Control: Hospital district or authority, Government, nonfederal **Service:** General Medical and Surgical

Staffed Beds: 17 **Admissions:** 519 **Census:** 5 **Outpatient Visits:** 24935 **Births:** 0 **Total Expense ($000):** 5446 **Payroll Expense ($000):** 2514 **Personnel:** 76

JACKSONVILLE—Cherokee County

★ **EAST TEXAS MEDICAL CENTER JACKSONVILLE (450194)**, 501 South Ragsdale Street, Zip 75766–2413; tel. 903/541–5000 **A**1 9 10 20 **F**3 8 11 13 15 18 24 25 27 30 31 33 37 38 40 51 52 55 57 62 68 73 74 75 76 77 79 80 82 86 96 99 100 106 107 118 119 120 121 124 136 137 **P**7 8 **S** East Texas Medical Center Regional Healthcare System
Primary Contact: Jack R. Endres, Administrator
CFO: Greg Cummings, Chief Operating Officer and Chief Financial Officer
CHR: Elysia Epperson, Director Human Resources
Web address: www.etmc.org
Control: Other not–for–profit (including NFP Corporation) **Service:** General Medical and Surgical

Staffed Beds: 58 **Admissions:** 1968 **Census:** 20 **Outpatient Visits:** 31642 **Births:** 416 **Total Expense ($000):** 27751 **Payroll Expense ($000):** 10587 **Personnel:** 172

★ **MOTHER FRANCES HOSPITAL – JACKSONVILLE (451319)**, 2026 South Jackson, Zip 75766; tel. 903/541–4500 **A**1 9 10 18 **F**3 7 8 15 18 24 25 26 28 30 31 32 33 37 38 40 43 50 51 52 55 57 62 63 66 73 75 76 77 79 80 86 87 96 97 100 102 107 118 119 120 122 135 136 **P**5 6 7 8
Primary Contact: Thomas N. Cammack, Jr., Chief Administrative Officer
CMO: William Milawski, M.D., President Medical Staff
CHR: Davlin King, Team Leader Human Resources
Web address: www.tmfhs.org
Control: Other not–for–profit (including NFP Corporation) **Service:** General Medical and Surgical

Staffed Beds: 20 **Admissions:** 1142 **Census:** 11 **Outpatient Visits:** 71190 **Births:** 0 **Total Expense ($000):** 22392 **Payroll Expense ($000):** 6630 **Personnel:** 156

JASPER—Jasper County

★ **CHRISTUS JASPER MEMORIAL HOSPITAL (450573)**, 1275 Marvin Hancock Drive, Zip 75951–4995; tel. 409/384–5461 **A**1 9 10 **F**3 11 13 15 25 26 31 32 38 40 45 50 51 54 55 56 57 62 68 74 75 77 79 84 85 86 96 100 107 119 122 124 135 **P**8 **S** CHRISTUS Health
Primary Contact: Deborah Wiegand, RN, Chief Executive Officer
CFO: John Breidenthal, Chief Financial Officer
CHR: Kay Powell, Director Human Resources
Web address: www.christusjasper.org
Control: Church–operated, Nongovernment, not–for profit **Service:** General Medical and Surgical

Staffed Beds: 50 **Admissions:** 2283 **Census:** 24 **Outpatient Visits:** 84496 **Births:** 437 **Total Expense ($000):** 23389 **Payroll Expense ($000):** 10686 **Personnel:** 224

JOURDANTON—Atascosa County

★ **SOUTH TEXAS REGIONAL MEDICAL CENTER (450165)**, 1905 Highway 97 East, Zip 78026–1504; tel. 830/769–3515 **A**1 9 10 20 **F**3 11 13 15 18 24 25 26 30 31 32 33 37 38 40 55 56 57 61 62 66 68 73 74 75 77 79 80 86 96 97 100 102 107 118 119 121 122 135 136 137 **P**6 **S** Community Health Systems, Inc.
Primary Contact: Michael L. Pierce, CHE, Chief Executive Officer
COO: Gerardo Flores, Chief Nursing Officer and Chief Operating Officer
Web address: www.strmc.com
Control: Corporation, Investor–owned, for–profit **Service:** General Medical and Surgical

Staffed Beds: 67 **Admissions:** 3146 **Census:** 32 **Outpatient Visits:** 68230 **Births:** 268 **Total Expense ($000):** 36000 **Payroll Expense ($000):** 14586 **Personnel:** 285

JUNCTION—Kimble County

★ **KIMBLE HOSPITAL (451306)**, 2101 Main Street, Zip 76849–2101; tel. 325/446–3321 **A**9 10 18 **F**38 40 54 55 56 57 61 62 63 66 75 84 86 93 96 107 121 122 124 **P**5
Primary Contact: Marlene Jones, Chief Executive Officer
CFO: Rhett Fricke, Chief Financial Officer
CMO: Alberto Martinez, M.D., Chief of Staff
CIO: Anna Henry, Chief Information Officer
CHR: Gloria Blackard, Manager Human Resources
Control: Hospital district or authority, Government, nonfederal **Service:** General Medical and Surgical

Staffed Beds: 15 **Admissions:** 155 **Census:** 1 **Outpatient Visits:** 82056 **Births:** 0

KATY—Fort Bend County

★ **CHRISTUS ST. CATHERINE HOSPITAL (450832)**, 701 Fry Road, Zip 77450; tel. 281/599–5700 **A**1 9 10 **F**3 11 13 15 25 26 30 31 32 33 38 55 56 57 60 62 68 73 74 75 77 79 80 81 82 84 85 86 96 97 100 102 103 107 108 118 119 120 121 124 135 137 **P**8 **S** CHRISTUS Health
Primary Contact: Jack H. McCabe, FACHE, Chief Executive Officer
CFO: Buddy Whiddon, Chief Financial Officer
CHR: Dianne Mitchell, Manager Human Resources
Web address: www.christusstcatherine.org
Control: Church–operated, Nongovernment, not–for profit **Service:** General Medical and Surgical

Staffed Beds: 102 **Admissions:** 4927 **Census:** 45 **Outpatient Visits:** 64417 **Births:** 628 **Total Expense ($000):** 59950 **Payroll Expense ($000):** 25660 **Personnel:** 569

☐ **KATY REHABILITATION HOSPITAL (453097)**, 21720 Kingsland Boulevard, Zip 77450–2513; tel. 281/579–5555 **A**1 9 10 **F**3 25 62 82 85 86 96 100 102 119 137 **P**6
Primary Contact: Jenny Maxwell, Chief Executive Officer
CFO: Kayla Feazell, Controller
Control: Partnership, Investor–owned, for–profit **Service:** Rehabilitation

Staffed Beds: 30 **Admissions:** 548 **Census:** 19 **Outpatient Visits:** 18610 **Births:** 0 **Total Expense ($000):** 15663 **Payroll Expense ($000):** 7498 **Personnel:** 152

★ **MEMORIAL HERMANN KATY HOSPITAL (450847)**, 23900 Katy Freeway, Zip 77494; tel. 281/644–7000 **A**1 9 10 **F**3 8 11 13 15 25 26 30 31 32 33 37 38 40 46 49 55 57 60 62 63 64 66 67 68 71 73 74 75 77 79 84 86 92 96 97 100 102 106 107 119 121 135 136 **P**5 6 **S** Memorial Hermann Healthcare System
Primary Contact: Brian S. Barbe, Chief Executive Officer
CFO: Lisa Kendler, Chief Financial Officer
Web address: www.memorialhermann.org
Control: Other not–for–profit (including NFP Corporation) **Service:** General Medical and Surgical

Staffed Beds: 127 **Admissions:** 6858 **Census:** 62 **Outpatient Visits:** 52302 **Births:** 1888 **Total Expense ($000):** 57340 **Payroll Expense ($000):** 28875 **Personnel:** 590

TX

Many Facility Codes have changed. Please refer to the AHA Guide Code Chart.

KAUFMAN—Kaufman County

★ **TEXAS HEALTH PRESBYTERIAN HOSPITAL OF KAUFMAN (450292)**, (Formerly Presbyterian Hospital of Kaufman), 850 Highway 243 West, Zip 75142, Mailing Address: P.O. Box 1108, Zip 75142–1108; tel. 972/932–7200 **A**1 9 10 **F**3 8 11 13 15 24 25 26 31 32 33 38 40 43 50 55 56 57 63 66 68 73 74 77 79 80 81 82 84 86 92 96 97 100 102 106 107 119 121 124 135 137 **S** Texas Health Resources
Primary Contact: Patsy Youngs, President
COO: Krista Baty, Chief Nursing Officer
CFO: Jade Andrews, Director Finance
CMO: Mark Sij, D.O., President Medical Staff
CHR: Carolyn Whitehurst, Director Human Resources
Web address: www.texashealth.org
Control: Other not–for–profit (including NFP Corporation) **Service:** General Medical and Surgical

Staffed Beds: 68 **Admissions:** 2036 **Census:** 22 **Outpatient Visits:** 36372 **Births:** 245 **Total Expense ($000):** 26397 **Payroll Expense ($000):** 11659 **Personnel:** 226

KENEDY—Karnes County

OTTO KAISER MEMORIAL HOSPITAL (451364), 3349 South Highway 181, Zip 78119–5240; tel. 830/583–3401 **A**9 10 18 **F**11 15 25 32 38 46 55 57 61 62 79 84 86 96 100 107 121 122 124 **P**8
Primary Contact: Nancy Kinkler, Administrator and Chief Executive Officer
CFO: Beverly Montez, Business Office Manager
Web address: www.okmh.net
Control: Hospital district or authority, Government, nonfederal **Service:** General Medical and Surgical

Staffed Beds: 21 **Admissions:** 333 **Census:** 3 **Outpatient Visits:** 19416 **Births:** 0 **Total Expense ($000):** 2809 **Personnel:** 94

KERMIT—Winkler County

WINKLER COUNTY MEMORIAL HOSPITAL (451314), 821 Jeffee Drive, Zip 79745–4696, Mailing Address: Drawer H, Zip 79745–6008; tel. 432/586–5864 **A**9 10 18 **F**7 11 26 28 30 31 38 62 63 67 86 87 96 107 122
Primary Contact: Stan Wiley, Administrator
CFO: Jeanna Wilhelm, Controller
CMO: Niraj Choudhary, M.D., Chief of Staff
CIO: Keith Palmer, Assistant Administrator
Control: County–Government, nonfederal **Service:** General Medical and Surgical

Staffed Beds: 15 **Admissions:** 324 **Census:** 2 **Outpatient Visits:** 22978 **Births:** 0 **Total Expense ($000):** 4903 **Payroll Expense ($000):** 2444 **Personnel:** 75

KERRVILLE—Kerr County

KERRVILLE DIVISION See South Texas Veterans Health Care System, San Antonio

☐ **KERRVILLE STATE HOSPITAL (454014)**, 721 Thompson Drive, Zip 78028–5154; tel. 830/896–2211 **A**1 3 5 10 **F**11 26 31 32 37 41 43 50 54 55 56 66 73 81 82 87 88 91 93 119 121 124 135 **S** Texas Department of State Health Services
Primary Contact: Stephen R. Anfinson, Superintendent
CMO: Janet E. TRUE, M.D., Clinical Director
CIO: Mike Kellogg, Manager Information
Web address: www.dshs.state.tx.us/lmhhospitals/kerrvillesh
Control: State–Government, nonfederal **Service:** Psychiatric

Staffed Beds: 202 **Admissions:** 336 **Census:** 201 **Outpatient Visits:** 0 **Births:** 0 **Total Expense ($000):** 34723 **Payroll Expense ($000):** 18913 **Personnel:** 536

★ **PETERSON REGIONAL MEDICAL CENTER (450007)**, (Formerly Sid Peterson Memorial Hospital), 551 Hill Country Drive, Zip 78028–5398; tel. 830/896–4200 **A**1 9 10 19 20 **F**3 8 11 13 15 18 25 26 27 30 31 32 33 37 38 43 44 46 48 49 50 53 55 56 57 61 62 63 66 68 71 72 73 74 75 76 77 79 80 81 82 85 86 90 96 97 100 102 107 119 120 121 124 135 136 137 **P**8
Primary Contact: James Patrick Murray, Chief Executive Officer
CFO: Robert H. Walther, Chief Financial Officer
CMO: Eugene Clayton, Chief of Staff
CIO: Richard Cruthirds, Director Information Systems
CHR: Buddy Volpe, Director Human Resources
Web address: www.spmh.com
Control: Other not–for–profit (including NFP Corporation) **Service:** General Medical and Surgical

Staffed Beds: 112 **Admissions:** 5771 **Census:** 71 **Outpatient Visits:** 119408 **Births:** 483 **Total Expense ($000):** 64523 **Payroll Expense ($000):** 28712 **Personnel:** 688

KILGORE—Gregg County

★ **LAIRD MEMORIAL HOSPITAL (450488)**, 1612 South Henderson Boulevard, Zip 75662–3594; tel. 903/984–3505 **A**9 10 **F**3 11 13 15 25 26 31 32 33 38 40 43 54 55 57 62 63 66 73 74 77 78 79 82 88 90 91 93 94 95 96 99 100 107 118 135 136
Primary Contact: Bob S. Ellzey, FACHE, President and Chief Executive Officer
CFO: Tammy Welch, Chief Financial Officer
CHR: Brandy Richardson, Director Human Resources
Web address: www.lairdmemorialhospital.com
Control: Other not–for–profit (including NFP Corporation) **Service:** General Medical and Surgical

Staffed Beds: 60 **Admissions:** 1605 **Census:** 23 **Outpatient Visits:** 25962 **Births:** 467 **Total Expense ($000):** 16973 **Payroll Expense ($000):** 7844 **Personnel:** 225

KILLEEN—Bell County

★ **METROPLEX ADVENTIST HOSPITAL (450152)**, 2201 South Clear Creek Road, Zip 76549–4110; tel. 254/526–7523 **A**1 9 10 **F**3 4 11 15 18 20 24 25 26 30 31 32 33 38 43 53 55 56 57 61 66 68 73 74 75 76 77 79 80 81 82 86 88 89 90 91 92 93 94 95 96 97 100 102 103 106 107 118 119 120 121 124 135 137 **P**8 **S** Adventist Health System Sunbelt Health Care Corporation
Primary Contact: Kenneth A. Finch, President and Chief Executive Officer
CFO: Penny Johnson, Chief Financial Officer
CMO: Frederick Barnett, Chief of Staff
CIO: Dale Koebnick, Director Management Information Systems and Patient Access
CHR: Brenda Coley, Executive Director
Web address: www.mplex.org
Control: Church–operated, Nongovernment, not–for profit **Service:** General Medical and Surgical

Staffed Beds: 154 **Admissions:** 7954 **Census:** 79 **Outpatient Visits:** 103576 **Births:** 1391 **Total Expense ($000):** 80139 **Payroll Expense ($000):** 35645 **Personnel:** 806

KINGSVILLE—Kleberg County

★ **CHRISTUS SPOHN HOSPITAL KLEBERG (450163)**, 1311 General Cavazos Boulevard, Zip 78363–1197; tel. 361/595–1661 **A**1 9 10 20 **F**3 11 13 15 25 26 30 31 32 38 40 53 55 57 62 63 64 68 72 73 74 75 79 80 81 82 84 86 96 97 107 119 121 135 **P**7 8 **S** CHRISTUS Health
Primary Contact: Stephen Pautler, FACHE, Administrator
Web address: www.christusspohn.org
Control: Church–operated, Nongovernment, not–for profit **Service:** General Medical and Surgical

Staffed Beds: 100 **Admissions:** 4395 **Census:** 43 **Outpatient Visits:** 18370 **Births:** 282 **Total Expense ($000):** 34083 **Payroll Expense ($000):** 15987 **Personnel:** 281

TX

KINGWOOD—Harris County

★ **KINGWOOD MEDICAL CENTER (450775)**, 22999 U.S. Highway 59, Zip 77339; tel. 281/348–8000 **A**1 9 10 **F**3 7 11 13 15 17 18 20 22 24 25 27 30 31 32 33 38 43 49 51 55 56 57 59 66 68 70 71 72 73 74 75 76 77 79 81 82 84 85 86 87 96 97 100 102 105 106 107 112 117 118 119 120 121 135 136 **S** HCA
Primary Contact: Gay Nord, Chief Executive Officer
COO: Colin McRae, Chief Operating Officer
CFO: Bryan R. Lee, Chief Financial Officer
CMO: Chik–Fong Wei, M.D., Chief of Staff
Web address: www.kingwoodmedical.com
Control: Corporation, Investor–owned, for–profit **Service:** General Medical and Surgical

Staffed Beds: 169 **Admissions:** 7269 **Census:** 104 **Outpatient Visits:** 65774 **Births:** 985 **Total Expense ($000):** 82919 **Payroll Expense ($000):** 32558 **Personnel:** 565

☐ **KINGWOOD PINES HOSPITAL (454103)**, 2001 Ladbrook Drive, Zip 77339; tel. 281/358–1495 **A**1 9 10 **F**4 5 25 36 54 57 73 75 81 82 88 89 90 91 92 93 94 95 119 121 124 **S** Horizon Health Corporation
Primary Contact: Linda Hodgkins, Chief Executive Officer
CFO: Richard Kurzenberger, Chief Financial Officer
CMO: Gary E. Miller, M.D., Director Psychiatric Services
CHR: Marty Johnson, Director Human Resources
Control: Corporation, Investor–owned, for–profit **Service:** Psychiatric

Staffed Beds: 78 **Admissions:** 2759 **Census:** 65 **Outpatient Visits:** 1889 **Births:** 0 **Total Expense ($000):** 11843 **Payroll Expense ($000):** 6735 **Personnel:** 149

Hospital, Medicare Provider Number, Address, Telephone, Approval, Facility, and Physician Codes, Health Care System
★ American Hospital Association (AHA) membership
☐ The Joint Commission accreditation
○ American Osteopathic Association (AOA) accreditation
△ Commission on Accreditation of Rehabilitation Facilities (CARF) accreditation

KINGWOOD SPECIALTY HOSPITAL (670005), 300 Kingwood Medical Drive, Zip 77339; tel. 281/312–4000 **A**10 **F**3 38 51 62 66 77 79 80 81
Primary Contact: Steven L. Smith, Chief Executive Officer
Web address: www.kingwoodspecialtyhospital.com
Control: Corporation, Investor–owned, for–profit **Service:** General Medical and Surgical

Staffed Beds: 10 **Admissions:** 189 **Census:** 1 **Outpatient Visits:** 3783 **Births:** 0 **Total Expense ($000):** 6716 **Payroll Expense ($000):** 2294 **Personnel:** 44

KNOX CITY—Knox County

KNOX COUNTY HOSPITAL (450746), 701 South Fifth Street, Zip 79529, Mailing Address: P.O. Box 608, Zip 79529–0608; tel. 940/657–3535 **A**9 10 20 **F**7 11 24 28 32 38 40 52 53 55 57 61 73 86 87 122 **P**6
Primary Contact: Stephan A. Kuehler, Administrator
CFO: Dan Offutt, Financial Manager
CMO: Shirley Barretto, M.D., Chief of Staff
CIO: Sue Marion, Business Office Manager
Web address: www.knoxcountytx.net
Control: Hospital district or authority, Government, nonfederal **Service:** General Medical and Surgical

Staffed Beds: 14 **Admissions:** 327 **Census:** 3 **Outpatient Visits:** 30712 **Births:** 0 **Total Expense ($000):** 3843 **Payroll Expense ($000):** 1893 **Personnel:** 75

LA GRANGE—Fayette County

★ **ST. MARK'S MEDICAL CENTER (670004)**, One St. Mark's Place, Zip 78945; tel. 979/242–2200 **A**5 9 10 **F**11 13 15 25 26 27 31 32 33 38 40 50 55 57 63 64 68 73 74 76 77 79 82 86 96 100 103 107 119 121 122 134 135
Primary Contact: Carol Drozd, Interim President and Chief Executive Officer
CFO: Judy Woodward, Chief Financial Officer
CMO: Thomas Borgstedte, Chief of Staff
Web address: www.stmarksmedicalcenter.org
Control: Other not–for–profit (including NFP Corporation) **Service:** General Medical and Surgical

Staffed Beds: 48 **Admissions:** 2239 **Census:** 24 **Outpatient Visits:** 42544 **Births:** 365 **Total Expense ($000):** 24632 **Payroll Expense ($000):** 7410 **Personnel:** 180

TX

LAKE JACKSON—Brazoria County

⊠ **BRAZOSPORT REGIONAL HEALTH SYSTEM (450072)**, 100 Medical Drive, Zip 77566–9983; tel. 979/297–4411 **A**1 2 9 10 **F**3 11 13 15 18 20 24 25 26 27 32 35 38 40 50 57 59 61 67 68 73 74 75 76 77 79 80 85 86 96 97 100 106 107 108 109 118 119 121 133 135 136 137 **P**8 **S** QHR
Primary Contact: Daniel L. Buche, Chief Executive Officer
COO: Al Guevara, Vice President Operations
CFO: Daniel L. Smith, Vice President Fiscal Services
CMO: Howard La Roche, M.D., President Medical Staff
CIO: Lori Koepsel, Director Management Information Systems
CHR: Sheila Coggins, Director Human Resources
Web address: www.brhs.org
Control: Other not–for–profit (including NFP Corporation) **Service:** General Medical and Surgical

Staffed Beds: 156 **Admissions:** 6405 **Census:** 61 **Outpatient Visits:** 100688 **Births:** 860 **Total Expense ($000):** 72887 **Payroll Expense ($000):** 33406 **Personnel:** 687

LAMESA—Dawson County

MEDICAL ARTS HOSPITAL (450489), 1600 North Bryan Avenue, Zip 79331–3145; tel. 806/872–2183 **A**9 10 20 **F**11 13 14 15 24 25 30 31 32 33 38 40 55 57 61 62 74 79 82 86 96 107 119 122 134 135 137 **S** Covenant Health System
Primary Contact: Charles N. Butts, Chief Executive Officer
COO: Letha Hughes, Chief Operating Officer
CFO: Jay Vise, Chief Financial Officer
CMO: Griengsak Chow, M.D., Chief of Staff
CHR: Jo Beth Smith, Director Human Resources
Web address: www.medicalartshospital.org
Control: Hospital district or authority, Government, nonfederal **Service:** General Medical and Surgical

Staffed Beds: 29 **Admissions:** 517 **Census:** 6 **Outpatient Visits:** 162841 **Births:** 58 **Total Expense ($000):** 13330 **Payroll Expense ($000):** 6033 **Personnel:** 207

LAMPASAS—Lampasas County

⊠ **ROLLINS–BROOK COMMUNITY HOSPITAL (451323)**, 608 North Key Avenue, Zip 76550, Mailing Address: P.O. Box 589, Zip 76550; tel. 512/556–3682 **A**1 9 10 18 **F**3 15 25 26 30 33 38 55 57 60 73 75 79 82 86 96 102 107 119 121 122 135 **P**8 **S** Adventist Health System Sunbelt Health Care Corporation
Primary Contact: Jeffrey D. Villanueva, Vice President and Administrator
CFO: Janice Hagensicker, Chief Financial Officer
CHR: Brenda Coley, Executive Director
Web address: www.mplex.org
Control: Church–operated, Nongovernment, not–for profit **Service:** General Medical and Surgical

Staffed Beds: 25 **Admissions:** 886 **Census:** 11 **Outpatient Visits:** 14641 **Births:** 0 **Total Expense ($000):** 10629 **Payroll Expense ($000):** 3708 **Personnel:** 112

LAREDO—Webb County

☐ **DOCTORS HOSPITAL OF LAREDO (450643)**, 10700 McPherson Road, Zip 78045; tel. 956/523–2000, (Total facility includes 10 beds in nursing home–type unit) **A**1 2 9 10 **F**3 11 13 15 18 25 26 27 31 32 38 40 55 57 59 68 70 73 74 75 76 77 79 80 82 84 86 96 97 100 102 107 109 111 117 118 119 121 **P**5 **S** Universal Health Services, Inc.
Primary Contact: Elmo Lopez, Jr., Chief Executive Officer
COO: Eladio Montalvo, Chief Operating Officer
CFO: Dinah Gonzalez, Chief Financial Officer
CMO: J. Santiago–Guttierez, Chief of Staff
CIO: Maribel Mata, Director Information Services
CHR: Roseann Figueroa, Director Human Resources
Web address: www.doctorshosplaredo.com
Control: Partnership, Investor–owned, for–profit **Service:** General Medical and Surgical

Staffed Beds: 179 **Admissions:** 8168 **Census:** 95 **Outpatient Visits:** 64494 **Births:** 2776 **Total Expense ($000):** 71115 **Payroll Expense ($000):** 28421 **Personnel:** 617

⊠ **LAREDO MEDICAL CENTER (450029)**, 1700 East Saunders Avenue, Zip 78041–5401, Mailing Address: Drawer 2068, Zip 78044–2068; tel. 956/796–5000, (Total facility includes 18 beds in nursing home–type unit) **A**1 9 10 **F**3 8 11 13 15 18 20 22 24 25 26 27 30 31 32 33 38 40 42 46 49 50 51 53 54 55 56 57 59 61 62 66 68 70 72 73 74 75 76 77 79 80 81 82 84 85 86 96 97 100 102 107 108 109 111 117 118 119 124 135 136 137 **S** Community Health Systems, Inc.
Primary Contact: Abraham Martinez, Chief Executive Officer
CFO: Terry Fowler, Chief Financial Officer
CIO: Joe Rivera, Chief Information Officer
CHR: Linda Hickok, Director Human Resources
Web address: www.laredomedical.com
Control: Corporation, Investor–owned, for–profit **Service:** General Medical and Surgical

Staffed Beds: 326 **Admissions:** 16943 **Census:** 229 **Outpatient Visits:** 174597 **Births:** 3912 **Total Expense ($000):** 165051 **Payroll Expense ($000):** 52528 **Personnel:** 1267

☐ **LAREDO SPECIALTY HOSPITAL (670014)**, 2005 Bustamente Street, Zip 78041–5470; tel. 956/753–5353 **A**1 10 **F**1 3 25 26 30 52 73 75 80 81 82 117 119 137 **S** Ernest Health, Inc.
Primary Contact: Al Chapa, CHE, Chief Executive Officer
Web address: www.lsh.ernesthealth.com
Control: Partnership, Investor–owned, for–profit **Service:** Long–Term Acute Care hospital

Staffed Beds: 60 **Admissions:** 547 **Census:** 34 **Outpatient Visits:** 0 **Births:** 0 **Total Expense ($000):** 15516 **Payroll Expense ($000):** 6023 **Personnel:** 138

LEAGUE CITY—Galveston County

☐ **DEVEREUX TEXAS TREATMENT NETWORK (454085)**, 1150 Devereux Drive, Zip 77573–2043; tel. 281/335–1000 **A**1 9 10 **F**4 5 25 28 31 32 33 36 40 52 53 54 57 62 73 81 82 88 89 90 91 92 93 94 95 119 121 123 135 **S** Devereux
Primary Contact: Pamela E. Helm, Executive Director
CHR: Cynthia Carmichael, Director Human Resources
Web address: www.devereux.org
Control: Other not–for–profit (including NFP Corporation) **Service:** Children's hospital psychiatric

Staffed Beds: 70 **Admissions:** 393 **Census:** 67 **Outpatient Visits:** 8240 **Births:** 0 **Total Expense ($000):** 12164 **Payroll Expense ($000):** 3393 **Personnel:** 122

Many Facility Codes have changed. Please refer to the AHA Guide Code Chart.

LEVELLAND—Hockley County

★ **COVENANT HOSPITAL–LEVELLAND (450755)**, 1900 South College Avenue, Zip 79336–6508; tel. 806/894–4963 **A**9 10 **F**11 13 15 25 26 30 31 32 38 40 43 50 53 55 56 57 62 63 66 73 74 75 79 80 81 82 84 85 86 87 96 100 107 119 122 133 135 **P**4 **S** Covenant Health System
Primary Contact: Jerry Osburn, Administrator
CFO: John Dolan, Chief Financial Officer
CMO: Jeffrey Young, M.D., Chief of Staff
CIO: Joe Kenady, Chief Information Officer
CHR: Kathy McDonald, Director Personnel
Web address: www.covenanthealth.org
Control: Church–operated, Nongovernment, not–for profit **Service:** General Medical and Surgical

Staffed Beds: 22 **Admissions:** 1863 **Census:** 15 **Outpatient Visits:** 81180 **Births:** 330 **Total Expense ($000):** 16817 **Payroll Expense ($000):** 6064 **Personnel:** 178

LEWISVILLE—Denton County

☒ **MEDICAL CENTER OF LEWISVILLE (450669)**, 500 West Main, Zip 75057–3699; tel. 972/420–1000 **A**1 9 10 **F**3 13 15 18 23 24 25 27 30 31 32 33 38 46 49 55 57 66 68 70 72 73 74 75 76 77 79 80 82 84 85 86 96 97 100 102 107 118 119 120 121 135 **S** HCA
Primary Contact: Douglas Welch, President and Chief Executive Officer
CFO: Lisa Brodbeck, Chief Financial Officer
CIO: Shirley Archambeault, Chief Information Officer
CHR: Shelly Krueger, Director Human Resources
Web address: www.lewisvillemedical.com
Control: Corporation, Investor–owned, for–profit **Service:** General Medical and Surgical

Staffed Beds: 187 **Admissions:** 8704 **Census:** 106 **Outpatient Visits:** 59008 **Births:** 1944 **Total Expense ($000):** 122223 **Payroll Expense ($000):** 39929 **Personnel:** 694

LIBERTY—Liberty County

LIBERTY–DAYTON COMMUNITY HOSPITAL (451375), 1353 North Travis, Zip 77575–1353; tel. 936/336–7316 **A**9 10 18 **F**3 11 14 15 25 31 32 38 50 53 55 56 57 58 62 66 96 97 102 119 122 135
Primary Contact: Dan Yancy, Ph.D., Chief Executive Officer
CFO: Rachal Reel, Chief Financial Officer
CMO: Danny Kline, M.D., Chief Medical Staff
CIO: Dan Fox, Chief Information Officer
Web address: www.libertydaytonhospital.com
Control: Partnership, Investor–owned, for–profit **Service:** General Medical and Surgical

Staffed Beds: 25 **Admissions:** 721 **Census:** 7 **Outpatient Visits:** 14165 **Births:** 1 **Total Expense ($000):** 7686 **Payroll Expense ($000):** 3999 **Personnel:** 77

LINDEN—Cass County

★ **GOOD SHEPHERD MEDICAL CENTER–LINDEN (451302)**, 404 North Kaufman Street, Zip 75563–5235; tel. 903/756–5561 **A**9 10 18 **F**3 11 13 15 24 25 26 30 31 32 38 50 55 56 62 66 73 74 75 79 80 82 86 96 97 102 107 119 120 122 124 135 137
Primary Contact: Steven B. Webb, Interim Chief Executive Officer
CMO: R. Bruce LeGrow, M.D., Chief Medical Staff
Control: Other not–for–profit (including NFP Corporation) **Service:** General Medical and Surgical

Staffed Beds: 25 **Admissions:** 676 **Census:** 10 **Outpatient Visits:** 5074 **Births:** 66 **Total Expense ($000):** 8551 **Payroll Expense ($000):** 3610 **Personnel:** 94

LITTLEFIELD—Lamb County

★ **LAMB HEALTHCARE CENTER (450698)**, 1500 South Sunset, Zip 79339–4899; tel. 806/385–6411 **A**9 10 20 **F**13 25 31 32 33 38 40 55 57 61 62 73 74 79 81 82 84 96 107 121 122 123 136 **P**6 **S** Covenant Health System
Primary Contact: Jo Nell Wischkaemper, Administrator
CFO: Cindy Klein, Chief Financial Officer
CMO: Tony Hedges, M.D., Chief Medical Officer
CHR: Joan Williams, Administrative Assistant
Control: County–Government, nonfederal **Service:** General Medical and Surgical

Staffed Beds: 41 **Admissions:** 888 **Census:** 12 **Outpatient Visits:** 48740 **Births:** 130 **Total Expense ($000):** 10503 **Payroll Expense ($000):** 4285 **Personnel:** 140

LIVINGSTON—Polk County

□ **MEMORIAL MEDICAL CENTER – LIVINGSTON (450395)**, 1717 Highway 59 Bypass, Zip 77351–1257, Mailing Address: P.O. Box 1257, Zip 77351–1257; tel. 936/329–8700 **A**1 5 9 10 **F**3 11 13 15 25 31 32 33 38 40 50 55 56 57 61 62 66 68 73 74 77 79 80 84 96 97 99 100 102 107 119 121 135 **S** Memorial Health System of East Texas
Primary Contact: David LeMonte, Chief Executive Officer
CFO: Richard Ahrens, Chief Financial Officer
CMO: Charlene Smith, M.D., Chief of Staff
CIO: Shawn Gordon, Chief Information Officer
CHR: Tanya Tyler, Vice President Human Resources
Web address: www.memorialhealth.org
Control: Other not–for–profit (including NFP Corporation) **Service:** General Medical and Surgical

Staffed Beds: 66 **Admissions:** 3314 **Census:** 35 **Outpatient Visits:** 45378 **Births:** 336 **Total Expense ($000):** 32985 **Payroll Expense ($000):** 14177 **Personnel:** 266

LLANO—Llano County

★ **LLANO MEMORIAL HEALTHCARE SYSTEM (450219)**, 200 West Ollie Street, Zip 78643–2628; tel. 325/247–5040 **A**9 10 20 **F**3 7 11 13 15 28 30 31 32 33 38 40 55 56 57 61 73 74 75 79 80 82 86 96 107 118 119 135
Primary Contact: Kevin Leeper, Chief Executive Officer
COO: Linda Meredith, Chief Operating Officer
CFO: Charles Miffleton, Director Finance
CMO: Mike Cravey, M.D., Chief of Staff
CIO: Rodney Lott, Director Management Information Systems and Facility Operations
CHR: Pearl Oestreich, Director Human Resources
Web address: www.llanomemorial.org
Control: Hospital district or authority, Government, nonfederal **Service:** General Medical and Surgical

Staffed Beds: 30 **Admissions:** 1639 **Census:** 12 **Outpatient Visits:** 147475 **Births:** 334 **Total Expense ($000):** 26163 **Payroll Expense ($000):** 11409 **Personnel:** 310

LOCKNEY—Floyd County

★ **W. J. MANGOLD MEMORIAL HOSPITAL (451337)**, 320 North Main Street, Zip 79241–0037, Mailing Address: Box 37, Zip 79241–0037; tel. 806/652–3373 **A**9 10 18 **F**3 13 24 26 33 38 40 52 55 57 61 62 63 74 79 80 86 87 96 100 107 119 122 137 **P**4
Primary Contact: Sharon Hunt, Administrator
CFO: Jon Sorensen, Chief Financial Officer
CIO: Larry Mullins, Controller and Chief Information Officer
CHR: Marsha Allen, Director Human Resources
Web address: www.mangoldmemorial.org
Control: Hospital district or authority, Government, nonfederal **Service:** General Medical and Surgical

Staffed Beds: 25 **Admissions:** 513 **Census:** 4 **Outpatient Visits:** 26685 **Births:** 76 **Total Expense ($000):** 7126 **Payroll Expense ($000):** 3384 **Personnel:** 108

LONGVIEW—Gregg County

ACADIA PATHWAYS HOSPITAL (454105), 22 Bermuda Lane, Zip 75605; tel. 903/291–3456 **A**10 **F**25 88 89 90 91 92 93 94 95 119 **P**1
Primary Contact: Pamela M. Broughton, Administrator
Control: Individual, Investor–owned, for–profit **Service:** Psychiatric

Staffed Beds: 76 **Admissions:** 857 **Census:** 26 **Outpatient Visits:** 1099 **Births:** 0 **Total Expense ($000):** 7398 **Payroll Expense ($000):** 3614 **Personnel:** 103

☒ △ **GOOD SHEPHERD MEDICAL CENTER (450037)**, 700 East Marshall Avenue, Zip 75601–5571; tel. 903/315–2000 **A**1 7 9 10 **F**3 7 11 13 15 18 20 22 24 25 26 27 30 31 32 33 37 38 40 43 50 51 52 53 54 55 56 57 59 60 62 66 68 69 70 72 73 74 75 76 77 78 79 80 81 82 84 85 86 87 92 96 97 100 102 103 106 107 118 119 120 121 124 132 133 135 136 137 **P**8
Primary Contact: Joseph A. Reppert, Vice President and Chief Financial Officer
COO: Joseph A. Reppert, Vice President and Chief Financial Officer
CFO: Joseph A. Reppert, Vice President and Chief Financial Officer
CIO: Wiley Thomas, Director Information Systems
CHR: Mark Rainey, Director Human Resources
Web address: www.gsmc.org
Control: Other not–for–profit (including NFP Corporation) **Service:** General Medical and Surgical

Staffed Beds: 335 **Admissions:** 18506 **Census:** 241 **Outpatient Visits:** 156192 **Births:** 1994 **Total Expense ($000):** 207258 **Payroll Expense ($000):** 66006 **Personnel:** 1391

TX

Hospital, Medicare Provider Number, Address, Telephone, Approval, Facility, and Physician Codes, Health Care System

★ American Hospital Association (AHA) membership
□ The Joint Commission accreditation
○ American Osteopathic Association (AOA) accreditation
△ Commission on Accreditation of Rehabilitation Facilities (CARF) accreditation

★ **LONGVIEW REGIONAL MEDICAL CENTER (450702)**, 2901 North Fourth Street, Zip 75605–5191, Mailing Address: P.O. Box 14000, Zip 75607–4000; tel. 903/758–1818, (Total facility includes 15 beds in nursing home–type unit) **A**1 9 10 **F**3 8 11 12 13 15 17 18 20 22 24 25 26 27 30 31 32 38 40 49 50 55 56 57 60 62 63 65 68 72 73 74 76 77 79 80 81 82 84 96 97 100 102 103 106 107 112 116 117 118 119 135 137 **P**8 **S** Community Health Systems, Inc.
Primary Contact: Jim R. Kendrick, Chief Executive Officer
COO: Jill Bayless–Berney, Chief Operating Officer
CFO: Todd Johnson, Chief Financial Officer
CMO: James W. Sawyer, M.D., Chief of Staff
CIO: Keith Jarvis, Director Information Systems
CHR: Stella Barrow, Director Human Resources
Web address: www.longviewregional.com
Control: Corporation, Investor–owned, for–profit **Service:** General Medical and Surgical

Staffed Beds: 131 **Admissions:** 5559 **Census:** 65 **Outpatient Visits:** 45159 **Births:** 938 **Total Expense ($000):** 72877 **Payroll Expense ($000):** 28982 **Personnel:** 612

SELECT SPECIALTY HOSPITAL OF LONGVIEW (452087), 700 East Marshall Avenue, 1st Floor, Zip 75601; tel. 903/315–1111 **A**9 10 **F**1 3 24 25 38 73 75 80 119 137 **S** Select Medical Corporation
Primary Contact: Larry Donner, President and Chief Executive Officer
Web address: www.selectmedicalcorp.com
Control: Corporation, Investor–owned, for–profit **Service:** Long–Term Acute Care hospital

Staffed Beds: 32 **Admissions:** 363 **Census:** 26 **Outpatient Visits:** 0 **Births:** 0 **Total Expense ($000):** 11386 **Payroll Expense ($000):** 4848 **Personnel:** 90

LUBBOCK—Lubbock County

★ **COVENANT CHILDREN'S HOSPITAL (453306)**, 3610 21st Street, Zip 79410–1218; tel. 806/725–1011 **A**1 5 9 10 **F**3 26 27 28 30 31 32 38 40 50 57 70 71 79 83 84 **P**6 8 **S** Covenant Health System
Primary Contact: Melinda Clark, FACHE, President and Chief Executive Officer
COO: Brett Esrock, Executive Vice President and Chief Operating Officer
CFO: Craig Rucker, Senior Vice President and Chief Financial Officer
CMO: Robert J. Salem, M.D., Chief Medical Officer
CIO: Jim Reid, Vice President and Chief Information Officer
CHR: Jan Campbell, Senior Vice President Human Resources
Web address: www.covenanthealth.org
Control: Other not–for–profit (including NFP Corporation) **Service:** Children's general

Staffed Beds: 79 **Admissions:** 2454 **Census:** 44 **Outpatient Visits:** 26436 **Births:** 0 **Total Expense ($000):** 42566 **Payroll Expense ($000):** 10119 **Personnel:** 104

TX

★ **COVENANT MEDICAL CENTER (450040)**, 3615 19th Street, Zip 79410–1201, Mailing Address: P.O. Box 1201, Zip 79408–1201; tel. 806/725–1011, (Includes COVENANT MEDICAL CENTER–LAKESIDE, 4000 24th Street, Zip 79410–1894; tel. 806/725–6000) **A**1 2 5 6 9 10 **F**4 5 7 11 12 13 15 16 17 18 20 22 24 25 26 27 30 31 32 33 37 40 43 44 46 47 48 49 50 51 52 53 55 56 57 58 59 60 61 62 63 66 68 69 72 73 74 75 76 77 78 79 80 81 82 85 86 88 92 95 96 97 98 100 102 103 104 105 107 108 109 111 117 118 119 120 121 124 127 132 133 135 136 137 **P**6 8 **S** Covenant Health System
Primary Contact: Melinda Clark, FACHE, President and Chief Executive Officer
COO: Brett Esrock, Executive Vice President and Chief Operating Officer
CFO: Craig Rucker, Senior Vice President and Chief Financial Officer
CMO: Robert J. Salem, M.D., Chief Medical Officer
CIO: Jim Reid, Vice President and Chief Information Officer
CHR: Jan Campbell, Senior Vice President Human Resources
Web address: www.covenanthealth.org
Control: Other not–for–profit (including NFP Corporation) **Service:** General Medical and Surgical

Staffed Beds: 696 **Admissions:** 29100 **Census:** 456 **Outpatient Visits:** 270048 **Births:** 3204 **Total Expense ($000):** 519183 **Payroll Expense ($000):** 175565 **Personnel:** 3564

☐ **HIGHLAND COMMUNITY HOSPITAL (450162)**, (Formerly Highland Medical Center), 2412 50th Street, Zip 79412–2494; tel. 806/788–4100 **A**1 9 10 **F**3 11 12 25 31 32 33 38 40 46 49 50 55 57 62 66 68 73 75 77 79 82 86 96 100 107 119 135 137 **S** Shiloh Health Services, Inc.
Primary Contact: Charles Fulner, Administrator
CFO: Mark Havins, Chief Financial Officer
CMO: William T. Sisco, M.D., Chief of Staff
CIO: Paul Gilliery, Director Management Information Systems
CHR: Kelly Barnette, Director Human Resources
Web address: www.highlandcommunityhospital.com
Control: Partnership, Investor–owned, for–profit **Service:** General Medical and Surgical

Staffed Beds: 95 **Admissions:** 733 **Census:** 8 **Outpatient Visits:** 26364 **Births:** 0 **Total Expense ($000):** 17853 **Payroll Expense ($000):** 5904 **Personnel:** 119

LUBBOCK HEART HOSPITAL (450876), 4810 North Loop 289, Zip 79416; tel. 806/687–7777 **A**9 10 **F**3 17 18 20 22 25 30 32 38 55 57 59 79 97 103 107 124 135 137
Primary Contact: John McGreevy, Chief Executive Officer
Web address: www.lubbockhearthospital.com
Control: Partnership, Investor–owned, for–profit **Service:** Heart

Staffed Beds: 74 **Admissions:** 4953 **Census:** 44 **Outpatient Visits:** 11043 **Births:** 0 **Total Expense ($000):** 50881 **Payroll Expense ($000):** 16261 **Personnel:** 418

☐ **SOUTHWEST REGIONAL MEDICAL COMPLEX (452050)**, 1409 9th Street, Zip 79401–2601; tel. 806/767–9133 **A**1 9 10 **F**1 3 12 25 31 32 59 63 73 119 132 137 **S** Fundamental Long Term Care Holdings, LLC
Primary Contact: Deanna Graves, Chief Executive Officer
CMO: Vernon Farthing, M.D., Medical Director
CHR: Laua Dillon, Director Human Resources
Web address: www.ihsoflubbock.com
Control: Corporation, Investor–owned, for–profit **Service:** Long–Term Acute Care hospital

Staffed Beds: 30 **Admissions:** 329 **Census:** 23 **Outpatient Visits:** 7 **Births:** 0 **Total Expense ($000):** 8996 **Payroll Expense ($000):** 2957 **Personnel:** 107

SUNRISE CANYON HOSPITAL (454093), 1602 10th Street, Zip 79408–2828, Mailing Address: P.O. Box 2828, Zip 79408–2828; tel. 806/740–1407 **A**10 **F**30 31 32 81 88 91 93 119 132
Primary Contact: Mary Gerlach, Chief Operating Officer
Web address: www.lrl.mhmr.state.tx.us
Control: Other not–for–profit (including NFP Corporation) **Service:** Psychiatric

Staffed Beds: 30 **Admissions:** 593 **Census:** 23 **Outpatient Visits:** 0 **Births:** 0 **Total Expense ($000):** 4229 **Payroll Expense ($000):** 1633 **Personnel:** 37

★ **UNIVERSITY MEDICAL CENTER (450686)**, 602 Indiana Avenue, Zip 79415–3364, Mailing Address: P.O. Box 5980, Zip 79408–5980; tel. 806/775–8200 **A**1 2 3 5 8 9 10 **F**3 7 11 12 13 15 16 17 18 19 20 21 22 23 24 25 26 27 30 31 32 33 38 40 43 46 47 48 49 50 51 52 54 55 56 57 58 59 60 61 62 63 64 66 68 70 72 73 74 75 76 77 79 80 81 82 83 84 85 86 87 96 97 98 100 102 106 107 108 109 110 111 112 113 114 119 120 121 125 127 130 133 135 136 137
Primary Contact: David G. Allison, President and Chief Executive Officer
COO: Mark Funderburk, Executive Vice President and Chief Operating Officer
CFO: Jeff Dane, Executive Vice President and Chief Financial Officer
CIO: Bill Eubanks, Senior Vice President Information Systems
CHR: Adrienne Cozart, Vice President Human Resources
Web address: www.teamumc.org
Control: Hospital district or authority, Government, nonfederal **Service:** General Medical and Surgical

Staffed Beds: 413 **Admissions:** 23738 **Census:** 310 **Outpatient Visits:** 220864 **Births:** 2452 **Total Expense ($000):** 300726 **Payroll Expense ($000):** 114439 **Personnel:** 2360

LUFKIN—Angelina County

★ **MEMORIAL HEALTH SYSTEM OF EAST TEXAS (450211)**, 1201 West Frank Avenue, Zip 75904–3357, Mailing Address: P.O. Box 1447, Zip 75902–1447; tel. 936/634–8111 **A**1 2 9 10 19 **F**11 13 14 15 17 18 19 20 21 22 23 24 25 26 27 30 31 32 33 35 36 38 41 42 43 44 45 46 47 48 49 50 51 54 55 56 57 59 60 61 62 66 68 69 71 72 73 74 75 76 77 79 80 81 82 84 85 86 87 90 91 92 96 97 99 100 101 102 103 104 105 107 109 116 118 119 121 124 132 133 135 136 137 **P**5 7 **S** Memorial Health System of East Texas
Primary Contact: Bryant H. Krenek, Jr., President and Chief Executive Officer
COO: Richard Ahrens, Chief Operating Officer
CHR: Michael H. Taylor, Vice President Human Resources
Web address: www.memorialhealth.org
Control: Other not–for–profit (including NFP Corporation) **Service:** General Medical and Surgical

Staffed Beds: 180 **Admissions:** 8990 **Census:** 122 **Outpatient Visits:** 132901 **Births:** 697 **Total Expense ($000):** 137152 **Payroll Expense ($000):** 38976 **Personnel:** 917

MEMORIAL SPECIALTY HOSPITAL (452031), 1201 West Frank Avenue, Zip 75904; tel. 936/639–7975 **A**9 10 **F**1 3 25 27 30 31 50 60 66 72 73 80 81 119 134 **S** Memorial Health System of East Texas
Primary Contact: Brenda Broadway, Administrator
Web address: www.memorialhealth.org
Control: Other not–for–profit (including NFP Corporation) **Service:** Long–Term Acute Care hospital

Staffed Beds: 16 **Admissions:** 171 **Census:** 14 **Outpatient Visits:** 0 **Births:** 0 **Total Expense ($000):** 5890 **Payroll Expense ($000):** 3075 **Personnel:** 50

□★ **WOODLAND HEIGHTS MEDICAL CENTER (450484)**, 505 South John Redditt Drive, Zip 75904–3157, Mailing Address: P.O. Box 150610, Zip 75915–0610; tel. 936/634–8311 **A**1 9 10 19 **F**3 8 12 13 15 17 18 20 22 24 25 26 30 31 32 33 38 43 46 49 51 52 55 57 62 66 68 72 73 74 75 76 77 79 80 81 82 86 92 96 97 100 102 103 106 107 117 118 119 120 135 136 137 **P**5 7 **S** Community Health Systems, Inc.
Primary Contact: Lance Jones, Chief Executive Officer
COO: John Maxwell, Assistant Chief Executive Officer
CFO: Brian Russo, Chief Financial Officer
CMO: Jansen Todd, Chief of Staff
CIO: Sandy Williams, Director Information Systems
CHR: Sally McKinney, Director Human Resources
Web address: www.woodlandheights.net
Control: Partnership, Investor–owned, for–profit **Service:** General Medical and Surgical

Staffed Beds: 149 **Admissions:** 6087 **Census:** 91 **Outpatient Visits:** 49437 **Births:** 726 **Total Expense ($000):** 64253 **Payroll Expense ($000):** 26622 **Personnel:** 533

LULING—Caldwell County

□★ **SETON EDGAR B. DAVIS HOSPITAL (451371)**, (Formerly Edgar B. Davis Memorial Hospital), 130 Hays Street, Zip 78648–3207; tel. 830/875–7000 **A**1 9 10 18 **F**3 11 15 25 26 30 31 32 33 38 41 43 50 53 57 60 62 66 73 77 79 80 81 82 86 87 92 93 96 102 107 119 122 124 133 135 **P**8 **S** Ascension Health
Primary Contact: Neal Kelley, Administrator
COO: Michelle Berkhouse, Director Patient Care Services
CFO: Douglas D. Waite, Chief Financial Officer
CMO: Martin E. Weiner, M.D., Chief of Staff
CHR: Cheryl Williams, Human Resource Director
Web address: www.seton.net
Control: Church–operated, Nongovernment, not–for profit **Service:** General Medical and Surgical

Staffed Beds: 25 **Admissions:** 1493 **Census:** 15 **Outpatient Visits:** 60543 **Births:** 0 **Total Expense ($000):** 20378 **Payroll Expense ($000):** 8032 **Personnel:** 198

□ **WARM SPRINGS SPECIALTY HOSPITAL (452062)**, 200 Memorial Drive, Zip 78648; tel. 830/875–8400 **A**1 9 10 **F**1 3 25 52 62 86 119 122 **S** Vibra Healthcare
Primary Contact: Kurt Meyer, Chief Executive Officer
CFO: Jim Asberry, Chief Financial Officer
CIO: David Chionsini, Director Management Information Systems
Web address: www.warmsprings.org
Control: Partnership, Investor–owned, for–profit **Service:** Long–Term Acute Care hospital

Staffed Beds: 34 **Admissions:** 466 **Census:** 30 **Outpatient Visits:** 9127 **Births:** 0 **Total Expense ($000):** 12860 **Payroll Expense ($000):** 4890 **Personnel:** 125

MADISONVILLE—Madison County

□★ **MADISON ST. JOSEPH HEALTH CENTER (451316)**, 100 West Cross Street, Zip 77864–0698, Mailing Address: Box 698, Zip 77864–0698; tel. 936/348–2631 **A**1 9 10 18 **F**3 11 15 26 30 31 32 38 43 55 57 62 66 86 96 97 99 107 119 122 124 135 **P**6 **S** Franciscan Services Corporation
Primary Contact: Reed Edmundson, Administrator
Control: Church–operated, Nongovernment, not–for profit **Service:** General Medical and Surgical

Staffed Beds: 25 **Admissions:** 481 **Census:** 8 **Outpatient Visits:** 21356 **Births:** 0 **Total Expense ($000):** 7840 **Payroll Expense ($000):** 3965 **Personnel:** 98

MANSFIELD—Tarrant County

□ **KINDRED HOSPITAL–MANSFIELD (452019)**, 1802 Highway 157 North, Zip 76063–9555; tel. 817/473–6101 **A**1 9 10 **F**3 12 25 26 32 38 43 46 59 68 73 77 79 80 86 96 97 119 121 137 **S** Kindred Healthcare
Primary Contact: Dalton Stewart, Chief Executive Officer
CFO: Judy Baker, Chief Financial Officer
Web address: www.kindredmansfield.com
Control: Corporation, Investor–owned, for–profit **Service:** General Medical and Surgical

Staffed Beds: 55 **Admissions:** 376 **Census:** 29 **Outpatient Visits:** 447 **Births:** 0 **Total Expense ($000):** 14116 **Payroll Expense ($000):** 5391 **Personnel:** 95

★ **METHODIST MANSFIELD MEDICAL CENTER (670023)**, 2700 East Broad Street, Zip 76063–5899; tel. 682/622–2000 **A**9 10 **F**3 11 13 15 18 20 25 26 27 30 31 32 33 35 38 43 44 46 48 49 50 56 57 58 59 66 68 69 72 76 77 79 80 82 86 87 96 97 99 100 103 107 118 119 121 135 **P**1 7 **S** Methodist Health System
Primary Contact: Laura Irvine, President
Web address: www.mhd.com
Control: Other not–for–profit (including NFP Corporation) **Service:** General Medical and Surgical

Staffed Beds: 80 **Admissions:** 1939 **Census:** 20 **Outpatient Visits:** 25246 **Births:** 427 **Total Expense ($000):** 44971 **Payroll Expense ($000):** 22081 **Personnel:** 393

MARLIN—Falls County

★ **FALLS COMMUNITY HOSPITAL AND CLINIC (450348)**, 322 Coleman Street, Zip 76661–2358, Mailing Address: P.O. Box 60, Zip 76661–0060; tel. 254/803–3561 **A**9 10 20 **F**3 11 28 29 31 32 33 34 38 40 43 52 54 55 56 57 62 63 64 66 73 77 82 86 87 89 93 94 96 118 120 122 124 135 137
Primary Contact: Willis L. Reese, Administrator
COO: Julie Sharp, Chief Operations Officer
CFO: Willis L. Reese, Administrator
CMO: James Scott Crockett, M.D., Chief of Staff
CIO: Julie Sharp, Chief Operations Officer
CHR: Peggy Polster, Manager Personnel and Administrative Assistant
Web address: www.fallshospital.com
Control: Other not–for–profit (including NFP Corporation) **Service:** General Medical and Surgical

Staffed Beds: 32 **Admissions:** 1133 **Census:** 12 **Outpatient Visits:** 68756 **Births:** 4 **Total Expense ($000):** 11592 **Payroll Expense ($000):** 4688 **Personnel:** 148

MARSHALL—Harrison County

□★ **GOOD SHEPHERD MEDICAL CENTER–MARSHALL (450032)**, (Formerly Marshall Regional Medical Center), 811 South Washington Avenue, Zip 75670–5336, Mailing Address: P.O. Box 1599, Zip 75671–1599; tel. 903/927–6000 **A**1 9 10 **F**3 11 13 15 24 25 26 30 31 32 33 38 40 49 50 52 53 55 56 57 58 62 63 66 68 73 75 77 78 79 81 82 84 85 86 87 92 96 97 99 100 102 107 117 118 119 121 134 135 136 137 **P**7 8
Primary Contact: Russell J. Collier, President and Chief Executive Officer
CHR: Ginger Garrett, Administrative Director Human Resources
Web address: www.mrmc.net
Control: Other not–for–profit (including NFP Corporation) **Service:** General Medical and Surgical

Staffed Beds: 132 **Admissions:** 3799 **Census:** 41 **Outpatient Visits:** 93532 **Births:** 584 **Total Expense ($000):** 54415 **Payroll Expense ($000):** 17550 **Personnel:** 408

MCALLEN—Hidalgo County

□ **MCALLEN MEDICAL CENTER (450811)**, 301 West Expressway 83, Zip 78503–3045; tel. 956/632–4000, (Includes MCALLEN HEART HOSPITAL, 1900 South D. Street, Zip 78503; tel. 956/994–2000) **A**1 3 5 9 10 **F**3 4 11 12 13 15 17 18 20 22 25 26 27 31 32 38 40 41 43 44 46 49 50 55 56 57 58 59 62 68 70 71 72 73 74 75 76 77 79 80 81 82 83 84 86 88 89 90 91 92 93 96 97 100 102 103 106 107 119 121 127 135 136 **P**1 3 **S** Universal Health Services, Inc.
Primary Contact: Joe B. Riley, Chief Executive Officer
COO: Rebecca L. Ryder, R.N., Chief Operating Officer
CFO: Paul H. Ballard, Chief Financial Officer
Web address: www.mcallenmedicalcenter.com
Control: Partnership, Investor–owned, for–profit **Service:** General Medical and Surgical

Staffed Beds: 635 **Admissions:** 17968 **Census:** 246 **Outpatient Visits:** 33856 **Births:** 4049 **Total Expense ($000):** 185334 **Payroll Expense ($000):** 64359 **Personnel:** 1776

□★ **RIO GRANDE REGIONAL HOSPITAL (450711)**, 101 East Ridge Road, Zip 78503–1299; tel. 956/632–6000 **A**1 5 9 10 **F**3 8 11 12 13 15 17 18 20 22 25 26 27 31 32 33 37 38 47 49 50 51 53 54 55 56 57 59 62 66 68 69 70 71 72 73 74 76 77 79 80 82 83 84 86 96 97 99 100 102 107 119 121 135 136 137 **P**7 **S** HCA
Primary Contact: Stephen K. Jones, Jr., FACHE, Chief Executive Officer
COO: Robert A. Heifner, Chief Operation Officer
CFO: Bill Saller, Chief Financial Officer
CMO: Victor Bradley, M.D., Chief Medical Officer
CIO: Carlos DeLeon, Chief Information Officer
Web address: www.riohealth.com
Control: Partnership, Investor–owned, for–profit **Service:** General Medical and Surgical

Staffed Beds: 320 **Admissions:** 18386 **Census:** 210 **Outpatient Visits:** 72881 **Births:** 6219 **Total Expense ($000):** 113225 **Payroll Expense ($000):** 49324 **Personnel:** 819

TX

Hospital, Medicare Provider Number, Address, Telephone, Approval, Facility, and Physician Codes, Health Care System

★ American Hospital Association (AHA) membership
□ The Joint Commission accreditation
○ American Osteopathic Association (AOA) accreditation
△ Commission on Accreditation of Rehabilitation Facilities (CARF) accreditation

SOLARA HOSPITAL MCALLEN (452095), 301 West Expressway 83, Zip 78503–3045; tel. 956/632–4880 **A**10 **F**1 3 25 30 31 32 43 44 54 72 73 82 137 **P**5
Primary Contact: Richard Knowland, Chief Executive Officer
Control: Corporation, Investor–owned, for–profit **Service:** Long–Term Acute Care hospital

Staffed Beds: 78 **Admissions:** 772 **Census:** 59 **Outpatient Visits:** 0 **Births:** 0 **Total Expense ($000):** 22065 **Payroll Expense ($000):** 10070 **Personnel:** 181

MCCAMEY—Upton County

★ **MCCAMEY COUNTY HOSPITAL DISTRICT (451309)**, (Formerly McCamey Hospital), Highway 305 South, Zip 79752, Mailing Address: P.O. Box 1200, Zip 79752–1200; tel. 432/652–8626, (Total facility includes 30 beds in nursing home–type unit) **A**9 10 18 **F**3 31 38 55 57 62 63 64 86 117 122
Primary Contact: Jaime Ramirez, Chief Executive Officer
COO: Tana Robertson, Chief Operating Officer
CFO: Jodie Gulihur, Chief Financial Officer
CMO: Ramon Domingo, M.D., Chief of Staff
CIO: Billy Haun, Supervisor Information Technology
CHR: Judith Gulihur, Director Human Resources and Chief Financial Officer
Web address: www.mccameyhospital.org
Control: Hospital district or authority, Government, nonfederal **Service:** General Medical and Surgical

Staffed Beds: 44 **Admissions:** 85 **Census:** 27 **Outpatient Visits:** 12450 **Births:** 0 **Total Expense ($000):** 5272 **Payroll Expense ($000):** 2603 **Personnel:** 76

MCKINNEY—Collin County

★ **MEDICAL CENTER OF MCKINNEY (450403)**, 4500 Medical Center Drive, Zip 75069–3499; tel. 972/547–8000, (Includes WYSONG CAMPUS, 130 South Central Expressway, Zip 75070; tel. 972/548–5300) **A**1 9 10 **F**3 4 5 11 13 15 18 20 22 24 25 26 27 30 31 32 38 43 54 55 57 59 62 65 66 68 72 73 74 75 77 79 80 82 85 86 87 88 92 93 96 97 100 102 103 107 109 118 119 121 135 136 137 **S** HCA
Primary Contact: Ernest C. Lynch, III, Chief Executive Officer
COO: LaSharndra Barbarin, Chief Operating Officer
CFO: Dwayne Ray, Chief Financial Officer
CIO: Kevin Fletcher, Director Information Systems
CHR: Senta Miles, Director Human Resources
Web address: www.ncentralmedical.com
Control: Partnership, Investor–owned, for–profit **Service:** General Medical and Surgical

Staffed Beds: 222 **Admissions:** 13066 **Census:** 155 **Outpatient Visits:** 90827 **Births:** 1389 **Total Expense ($000):** 113641 **Payroll Expense ($000):** 48584 **Personnel:** 766

MESQUITE—Dallas County

☐ **DALLAS REGIONAL MEDICAL CENTER (450031)**, 1011 North Galloway Avenue, Zip 75149–2433; tel. 214/320–7000, (Includes MEDICAL CENTER OF MESQUITE, 1011 North Galloway Avenue, tel. 214/320–7000; MESQUITE COMMUNITY HOSPITAL, 3500 Interstate 30, Zip 75150–2696; tel. 972/698–3300) **A**1 9 10 **F**3 12 13 15 17 18 20 21 22 25 26 30 31 32 33 35 37 38 40 44 50 51 54 55 56 57 62 64 66 68 72 73 74 75 77 79 80 81 85 86 87 90 94 96 97 100 102 107 119 121 133 135 136 137 **P**5 **S** Health Management Associates
Primary Contact: Roy C. Vinson, Chief Executive Officer
COO: Kyllan Brown, Chief Operating Officer
CFO: Shane Wells, Chief Financial Officer
CMO: Alex Cowalha, M.D., Chief Medical Officer
CHR: Chris Layd, Director Human Resources
Control: Corporation, Investor–owned, for–profit **Service:** General Medical and Surgical

Staffed Beds: 292 **Admissions:** 11306 **Census:** 160 **Outpatient Visits:** 114961 **Births:** 2778 **Total Expense ($000):** 130258 **Payroll Expense ($000):** 56082 **Personnel:** 891

☐ **MESQUITE SPECIALTY HOSPITAL (670016)**, 1024 North Galloway Avenue, Zip 75149–2434; tel. 972/216–2300 **A**1 10 **F**1 3 25 32 62 73 75 82 86 119 137 **S** Ernest Health, Inc.
Primary Contact: Brenda M. Antwine, Chief Executive Officer
Web address: www.msh.ernesthealth.com
Control: Partnership, Investor–owned, for–profit **Service:** Long–Term Acute Care hospital

Staffed Beds: 40 **Admissions:** 313 **Census:** 28 **Outpatient Visits:** 51 **Births:** 0 **Total Expense ($000):** 8909 **Payroll Expense ($000):** 3599 **Personnel:** 139

MEXIA—Limestone County

★ **PARKVIEW REGIONAL HOSPITAL (450400)**, 600 South Bonham, Zip 76667–3608; tel. 254/562–0408 **A**1 9 10 20 **F**3 11 13 15 25 26 30 31 32 33 38 40 51 52 54 55 56 57 62 63 68 73 74 75 76 77 79 80 81 82 85 86 87 96 97 100 107 119 121 122 135 136 137 **S** LifePoint Hospitals, Inc.
Primary Contact: Jimmy D. Stuart, Chief Executive Officer
CFO: Michael Cheek, Chief Financial Officer
CMO: Kenneth Russell, Chief of Staff
Web address: www.parkviewregional.com
Control: Partnership, Investor–owned, for–profit **Service:** General Medical and Surgical

Staffed Beds: 50 **Admissions:** 2459 **Census:** 29 **Outpatient Visits:** 32348 **Births:** 73 **Total Expense ($000):** 23012 **Payroll Expense ($000):** 10126 **Personnel:** 226

MIDLAND—Midland County

☐ **DESERT SPRINGS MEDICAL CENTER (454049)**, 3300 South FM 1788, Zip 79706, Mailing Address: P.O. Box 60608, Zip 79711–0608; tel. 432/563–1200, (Nonreporting) **A**1 9 10 **S** Psychiatric Solutions
Primary Contact: James Baca, Chief Executive Officer
Web address: www.psysolutions.com/facilities/desertsprings/midland.html
Control: Corporation, Investor–owned, for–profit **Service:** Psychiatric

Staffed Beds: 64

★ **HEALTHSOUTH REHABILITATION HOSPITAL MIDLAND–ODESSA (453057)**, 1800 Heritage Boulevard, Zip 79707–9750; tel. 432/520–1600 **A**1 9 10 **F**3 25 32 55 57 61 62 85 86 119 120 132 137 **S** HEALTHSOUTH Corporation
Primary Contact: Ellen Shankles, Chief Executive Officer
Web address: www.healthsouth.com
Control: Corporation, Investor–owned, for–profit **Service:** Rehabilitation

Staffed Beds: 60 **Admissions:** 419 **Census:** 16 **Outpatient Visits:** 5491 **Births:** 0 **Total Expense ($000):** 6845 **Payroll Expense ($000):** 3781 **Personnel:** 119

★ **MIDLAND MEMORIAL HOSPITAL (450133)**, 2200 West Illinois Avenue, Zip 79701–6499; tel. 432/685–1111, (Includes MIDLAND MEMORIAL HOSPITAL–WEST CAMPUS, Zip 79703; tel. 432/522–3270) **A**1 2 3 5 9 10 **F**3 7 8 11 13 15 17 18 20 22 24 25 26 27 28 30 31 32 33 38 40 43 46 50 54 55 56 57 60 62 66 68 70 72 73 74 76 77 78 79 80 81 82 83 84 85 87 96 97 100 102 103 105 106 107 112 118 119 120 121 124 132 134 135 136 137 **P**8
Primary Contact: Russell Meyers, President and Chief Executive Officer
CFO: Lawrence A. Sanz, Senior Vice President Finance and Chief Financial Officer
CIO: David Whiles, Director Health Information Systems
CHR: Cori Moore, Director Human Resources
Web address: www.midland–memorial.com
Control: Hospital district or authority, Government, nonfederal **Service:** General Medical and Surgical

Staffed Beds: 217 **Admissions:** 10540 **Census:** 125 **Outpatient Visits:** 129183 **Births:** 1979 **Total Expense ($000):** 170599 **Payroll Expense ($000):** 60281 **Personnel:** 1290

MIDLAND MEMORIAL HOSPITAL (450133), 4214 Andrews Highway, Zip 79703–4861; tel. 432/685–1584, (Nonreporting) **A**9 10
Primary Contact: Russell Meyers, President and Chief Executive Officer
CFO: Lawrence A. Sanz, Senior Vice President Finance and Chief Financial Officer
CIO: David Whiles, Director Health Information Systems
CHR: Cori Moore, Director Human Resources
Web address: www.midland–memorial.com
Control: Corporation, Investor–owned, for–profit **Service:** General Medical and Surgical

Staffed Beds: 86

★ **REHABCARE REHABILITATION HOSPITAL - PERMIAN BASIN (453095)**, 207 Tradewinds Boulevard, Zip 79706; tel. 432/520–2333 **A**1 9 10 **F**3 30 62 66 72 73 75 82 85 86 91 119 **S** RehabCare Group, Inc.
Primary Contact: Dale R. Mulder, Chief Executive Officer
Web address: www.rehabcare.com
Control: Corporation, Investor–owned, for–profit **Service:** Rehabilitation

Staffed Beds: 38 **Admissions:** 638 **Census:** 19 **Outpatient Visits:** 3061 **Births:** 0 **Total Expense ($000):** 8680 **Payroll Expense ($000):** 4103 **Personnel:** 65

☐ **SELECT SPECIALTY HOSPITAL OF MIDLAND (452084)**, 4214 Andrews Highway, Suite 320, Zip 79703; tel. 432/522–3270 **A**1 9 10 **F**1 3 24 25 31 32 66 75 80 119 137 **S** Select Medical Corporation
Primary Contact: Paul E. Qualls, Jr., Chief Executive Officer
Web address: www.selectmedicalcorp.com
Control: Corporation, Investor–owned, for–profit **Service:** Long–Term Acute Care hospital

Staffed Beds: 29 **Admissions:** 331 **Census:** 24 **Outpatient Visits:** 0 **Births:** 0 **Total Expense ($000):** 9578 **Payroll Expense ($000):** 3765 **Personnel:** 65

Many Facility Codes have changed. Please refer to the AHA Guide Code Chart.

MINERAL WELLS—Palo Pinto County

⊠ **PALO PINTO GENERAL HOSPITAL (450565)**, 400 S.W. 25th Avenue, Zip 76067–9685; tel. 940/328–6403 **A**1 9 10 **F**11 13 15 17 24 25 28 30 31 32 38 40 42 44 46 51 52 53 55 56 57 61 62 63 64 66 67 69 72 73 74 75 76 77 79 81 82 86 96 97 100 102 107 118 119 120 122 124 135 136 **P**1
Primary Contact: Harris W. Brooks, Administrator and Chief Executive Officer
CFO: Dee Waldow, Chief Financial Officer
CMO: Mat Adams, Chief of Staff
CHR: Barbara Stagner, Director Human Resources
Web address: www.ppgh.com
Control: Hospital district or authority, Government, nonfederal **Service:** General Medical and Surgical

Staffed Beds: 42 **Admissions:** 2582 **Census:** 24 **Outpatient Visits:** 113387 **Births:** 537 **Total Expense ($000):** 32474 **Payroll Expense ($000):** 15239 **Personnel:** 337

MISSION—Hidalgo County

⊠ △ **MISSION REGIONAL MEDICAL CENTER (450176)**, 900 South Bryan Road, Zip 78572–6613; tel. 956/323–9000 **A**1 7 9 10 **F**3 11 13 15 18 20 25 26 27 30 31 32 33 38 40 46 49 50 55 56 57 59 62 63 65 66 68 70 72 73 74 75 77 79 80 82 84 85 86 96 97 99 100 103 106 107 119 121 135 136 137 **P**8
Primary Contact: Javier Iruegas, Chief Executive Officer
COO: Carlos Trevino, Chief Operating Officer
CIO: Major Raymond Bruels, Director Management Information Systems
CHR: Susan Willars, Vice President Human Resource
Web address: www.missionrmc.org
Control: Other not–for–profit (including NFP Corporation) **Service:** General Medical and Surgical

Staffed Beds: 237 **Admissions:** 11006 **Census:** 158 **Outpatient Visits:** 54457 **Births:** 3120 **Total Expense ($000):** 91079 **Payroll Expense ($000):** 39829 **Personnel:** 785

MONAHANS—Ward County

WARD MEMORIAL HOSPITAL (451373), 406 South Gary Street, Zip 79756–4798, Mailing Address: P.O. Box 40, Zip 79756–0040; tel. 432/943–2511 **A**9 10 18 **F**7 30 38 40 61 62 63 74 79 96 107 122 124 **P**5
Primary Contact: Viki Yates, Administrator
CFO: Leticia Rodriguez, Controller
CHR: Donna Lemon, Director Human Resources
Web address: www.wardmemorial.org
Control: County–Government, nonfederal **Service:** General Medical and Surgical

Staffed Beds: 25 **Admissions:** 365 **Census:** 3 **Outpatient Visits:** 17641 **Births:** 1 **Total Expense ($000):** 5279 **Payroll Expense ($000):** 3900 **Personnel:** 95

MORTON—Cochran County

★ **COCHRAN MEMORIAL HOSPITAL (451366)**, 201 East Grant Street, Zip 79346–3444; tel. 806/266–5565 **A**9 10 18 **F**31 38 40 55 56 57 63 **P**5 6
Primary Contact: Larry Turney, Administrator
CHR: Niona Tunney, Director Human Resources
Control: Hospital district or authority, Government, nonfederal **Service:** General Medical and Surgical

Staffed Beds: 18 **Admissions:** 85 **Census:** 1 **Outpatient Visits:** 6362 **Births:** 0 **Total Expense ($000):** 2873 **Payroll Expense ($000):** 1361 **Personnel:** 38

MOUNT PLEASANT—Titus County

⊠ **TITUS REGIONAL MEDICAL CENTER (450080)**, 2001 North Jefferson Avenue, Zip 75455–2398; tel. 903/577–6000, (Total facility includes 7 beds in nursing home–type unit) **A**1 9 10 19 **F**7 11 13 15 18 24 25 26 30 31 32 33 38 40 43 44 50 51 53 54 55 56 57 62 64 66 68 72 73 74 76 77 79 82 84 85 86 87 88 93 96 97 100 103 106 107 117 118 119 121 124 132 135 136 137 **P**8
Primary Contact: Ronald D. Davis, Chief Executive Officer
CFO: Duane Shafer, Chief Financial Officer
CMO: Colton Bradshaw, M.D., Chief of Staff
CIO: David Jones, Director Information Systems
CHR: Tony Piazza, Vice President Human Resources
Web address: www.titusregional.com
Control: Hospital district or authority, Government, nonfederal **Service:** General Medical and Surgical

Staffed Beds: 150 **Admissions:** 5408 **Census:** 67 **Outpatient Visits:** 64545 **Births:** 1130 **Total Expense ($000):** 45311 **Payroll Expense ($000):** 25450 **Personnel:** 496

MOUNT VERNON—Franklin County

★ **EAST TEXAS MEDICAL CENTER–MOUNT VERNON (450373)**, 500 Highway 37 South, Zip 75457–3602, Mailing Address: P.O. Box 477, Zip 75457–0477; tel. 903/537–8000 **A**9 10 **F**3 25 32 33 38 40 42 43 44 47 50 55 56 62 63 66 73 77 79 80 81 82 87 92 96 97 102 107 **P**7 **S** East Texas Medical Center Regional Healthcare System
Primary Contact: Stephen Pitts, Administrator
COO: Stephen Pitts, Administrator
CFO: Margaret Haak–Muse, Chief Financial Officer and Assistant Administrator
CMO: Michael Walker, D.O., Chief of Staff
CHR: Kathy Shelton, Director Human Resources
Web address: www.etmc.org
Control: Other not–for–profit (including NFP Corporation) **Service:** General Medical and Surgical

Staffed Beds: 30 **Admissions:** 569 **Census:** 5 **Outpatient Visits:** 12765 **Births:** 0 **Total Expense ($000):** 5521 **Payroll Expense ($000):** 2456 **Personnel:** 58

MUENSTER—Cooke County

MUENSTER MEMORIAL HOSPITAL (451335), 605 North Maple Street, Zip 76252–2424, Mailing Address: P.O. Box 370, Zip 76252–0370; tel. 940/759–2271 **A**9 10 18 **F**11 15 33 38 40 52 55 57 61 62 63 73 75 79 86 96 97 102 107 119 122 **P**8
Primary Contact: Lynn Heller, Administrator and Chief Executive Officer
CFO: Richard Teeter, Chief Financial Officer
CMO: Edd Advincula, M.D., Chief of Staff
CIO: Sheri Hutchins, Director Health Information Management
Control: Hospital district or authority, Government, nonfederal **Service:** General Medical and Surgical

Staffed Beds: 18 **Admissions:** 277 **Census:** 10 **Outpatient Visits:** 4714 **Births:** 0 **Total Expense ($000):** 5710 **Payroll Expense ($000):** 2033 **Personnel:** 80

MULESHOE—Bailey County

★ **MULESHOE AREA MEDICAL CENTER (451372)**, 708 South First Street, Zip 79347; tel. 806/272–4524 **A**9 10 18 **F**8 11 13 30 32 33 38 40 50 53 55 56 57 62 66 67 79 86 96 100 102 106 107 122 135 137 **S** Covenant Health System
Primary Contact: Ray Mason, Administrator and Chief Executive Officer
CMO: Bruce Purdy, M.D., Chief of Staff
Web address: www.mahdtx.org
Control: Hospital district or authority, Government, nonfederal **Service:** General Medical and Surgical

Staffed Beds: 25 **Admissions:** 937 **Census:** 7 **Outpatient Visits:** 69311 **Births:** 0 **Total Expense ($000):** 7054 **Payroll Expense ($000):** 2917 **Personnel:** 109

NACOGDOCHES—Nacogdoches County

⊠ **NACOGDOCHES MEDICAL CENTER (450656)**, 4920 N.E. Stallings, Zip 75965–1200, Mailing Address: P.O. Box 631604, Zip 75963–1604; tel. 936/569–9481 **A**1 9 10 19 **F**11 13 15 18 20 22 25 27 33 37 38 40 43 46 49 51 54 55 56 57 59 62 68 72 73 74 75 76 77 79 80 81 82 86 96 97 99 100 103 106 107 109 111 118 119 120 121 124 135 136 137 **S** TENET Healthcare Corporation
Primary Contact: Gary L. Stokes, Chief Executive Officer
COO: Jeb Jones, Chief Operating Officer
CFO: Rhonda Rogers, Chief Financial Officer
CMO: Gerard Ventura, M.D., Chief of Staff
CHR: Teresa Farrell, Director Human Resources
Web address: www.nacmedicalcenter.com
Control: Partnership, Investor–owned, for–profit **Service:** General Medical and Surgical

Staffed Beds: 109 **Admissions:** 5318 **Census:** 56 **Outpatient Visits:** 45322 **Births:** 709 **Total Expense ($000):** 51646 **Payroll Expense ($000):** 19615 **Personnel:** 410

□ **NACOGDOCHES MEMORIAL HOSPITAL (450508)**, 1204 North Mound Street, Zip 75961–4061; tel. 936/564–4611 **A**1 9 10 19 **F**3 7 11 13 15 18 20 22 24 25 26 27 31 32 38 40 42 49 50 55 56 57 59 60 61 62 66 68 72 74 75 76 77 78 79 80 81 84 85 86 96 97 100 102 106 107 118 119 121 135 136 137
Primary Contact: Tim Hayward, Administrator
CFO: Gina Oglesbee, Chief Financial Officer
CIO: Delia Mears, Assistant Administrator Marketing
Web address: www.nacmem.org
Control: Hospital district or authority, Government, nonfederal **Service:** General Medical and Surgical

Staffed Beds: 136 **Admissions:** 7114 **Census:** 97 **Outpatient Visits:** 70179 **Births:** 769 **Total Expense ($000):** 82117 **Payroll Expense ($000):** 32447 **Personnel:** 800

Hospital, Medicare Provider Number, Address, Telephone, Approval, Facility, and Physician Codes, Health Care System

★ American Hospital Association (AHA) membership
□ The Joint Commission accreditation
○ American Osteopathic Association (AOA) accreditation
△ Commission on Accreditation of Rehabilitation Facilities (CARF) accreditation

NASSAU BAY—Harris County

★ **CHRISTUS ST. JOHN HOSPITAL (450709)**, 18300 St. John Drive, Zip 77058–6302; tel. 281/333–5503 **A**1 5 9 10 **F**3 11 13 15 18 20 22 24 25 26 27 30 31 32 33 38 41 49 50 51 52 53 55 56 57 59 61 62 63 64 66 67 68 71 72 73 74 75 76 77 79 80 81 82 86 96 97 99 100 102 103 107 119 120 121 135 136 137 **P**8 **S** CHRISTUS Health
Primary Contact: Thomas Permetti, Chief Executive Officer
COO: Nancy Pittman, Chief Operating Officer
CFO: David Witt, Chief Financial Officer
CHR: Pamela Rhodes, Region Vice President Human Resources
Web address: www.christusstjohn.org
Control: Other not–for–profit (including NFP Corporation) **Service:** General Medical and Surgical

Staffed Beds: 134 **Admissions:** 5709 **Census:** 62 **Outpatient Visits:** 143308 **Births:** 399 **Total Expense ($000):** 81876 **Payroll Expense ($000):** 34577 **Personnel:** 657

NAVASOTA—Grimes County

★ **GRIMES ST. JOSEPH HEALTH CENTER (451322)**, 210 South Judson Street, Zip 77868–3704; tel. 936/825–6585 **A**1 9 10 18 **F**3 25 30 31 32 38 40 55 56 57 73 75 79 86 96 100 107 118 119 121 122 124 135 **S** Franciscan Services Corporation
Primary Contact: Dia Copeland, Administrator
COO: Anthony D. Pfitzer, FACHE, Chief Executive Officer
CFO: Lisa McNair, Senior Vice President and Chief Financial Officer
CMO: L. P. Scamardo, M.D., Chief of Staff
CHR: Michael Costo, Director Human Resources
Web address: www.st–joseph.org
Control: Church–operated, Nongovernment, not–for profit **Service:** General Medical and Surgical

Staffed Beds: 25 **Admissions:** 663 **Census:** 11 **Outpatient Visits:** 16841 **Births:** 0 **Total Expense ($000):** 7362 **Payroll Expense ($000):** 3805 **Personnel:** 93

NEDERLAND—Jefferson County

PROMISE SPECIALTY HOSPITAL OF SOUTHEAST TEXAS (452083), 2600 Highway 365, Zip 77627–6237; tel. 409/726–8700, (Nonreporting) **A**10 **S** Promise Healthcare
Primary Contact: James L. McEwen, Ph.D., Administrator
Web address: www.promise–southeasttexas.com
Control: Corporation, Investor–owned, for–profit **Service:** Long–Term Acute Care hospital

Staffed Beds: 25

NEW BRAUNFELS—Comal County

★ **CHRISTUS SANTA ROSA HOSPITAL – NEW BRAUNFELS (450059)**, (Formerly McKenna Memorial Hospital), 600 North Union Avenue, Zip 78130–4191; tel. 830/606–9111 **A**1 9 10 **F**3 8 11 13 15 18 24 25 26 27 30 31 32 38 43 44 49 50 53 55 56 57 61 62 68 72 73 74 75 76 77 79 80 81 82 86 92 96 100 102 103 104 105 107 118 119 121 124 133 135 136 137 **S** CHRISTUS Health
Primary Contact: Michael V. Williamson, FACHE, Interim Chief Executive Officer
CFO: Allen Strickland, Chief Financial Officer
CIO: Kim Deese, Vice President Information Systems
Web address: www.mckenna.org
Control: Other not–for–profit (including NFP Corporation) **Service:** General Medical and Surgical

Staffed Beds: 132 **Admissions:** 7291 **Census:** 69 **Outpatient Visits:** 97073 **Births:** 1053 **Total Expense ($000):** 79799 **Payroll Expense ($000):** 34211 **Personnel:** 713

NOCONA—Montague County

★ **NOCONA GENERAL HOSPITAL (450641)**, 100 Park Street, Zip 76255–3616; tel. 940/825–3235 **A**9 10 **F**7 11 15 24 25 26 30 31 32 33 38 40 43 50 52 55 56 57 61 62 73 79 81 82 86 87 96 97 102 107 119 122 135 137 **P**5
Primary Contact: Lance Meekins, Administrator
CFO: Lance Meekins, Administrator
CMO: Chance Dingler, M.D., Chief Medical Officer
CHR: Paula Monkres, Director Human Resources
Control: Hospital district or authority, Government, nonfederal **Service:** General Medical and Surgical

Staffed Beds: 30 **Admissions:** 910 **Census:** 11 **Outpatient Visits:** 17260 **Births:** 8 **Total Expense ($000):** 6230 **Payroll Expense ($000):** 3653 **Personnel:** 110

NORTH RICHLAND HILLS—Tarrant County

★ **NORTH HILLS HOSPITAL (450087)**, 4401 Booth Calloway Road, Zip 76180–7399; tel. 817/255–1000 **A**1 9 10 **F**3 8 11 12 13 15 17 18 20 22 24 25 26 27 31 32 38 52 54 55 56 57 62 68 73 74 75 76 77 78 79 80 81 82 85 86 96 97 99 100 102 107 112 119 121 135 136 137 **S** HCA
Primary Contact: Randolph Moresi, Chief Executive Officer
COO: Glenn Wallace, Chief Operating Officer
CFO: Kathleen Sweeney, Chief Financial Officer
CMO: Wesley Alderete, M.D., Chief of Staff
CIO: Ruben Castro, Director Information Systems
CHR: Cynthia Dang, Vice President Human Resources
Web address: www.northhillshospital.com
Control: Partnership, Investor–owned, for–profit **Service:** General Medical and Surgical

Staffed Beds: 176 **Admissions:** 8206 **Census:** 102 **Outpatient Visits:** 89215 **Births:** 1139 **Total Expense ($000):** 118985 **Payroll Expense ($000):** 36635 **Personnel:** 563

ODESSA—Ector County

★ **MEDICAL CENTER HOSPITAL (450132)**, 500 West Fourth Street, Zip 79761–5059, Mailing Address: P.O. Drawer 7239, Zip 79760–7239; tel. 432/640–4000 **A**1 2 3 5 8 9 10 **F**3 8 11 12 13 15 17 18 20 22 24 25 26 27 30 32 33 37 38 40 46 47 48 49 50 53 55 56 57 62 63 64 65 66 68 69 70 72 73 74 75 76 77 79 80 82 84 85 86 96 100 102 103 106 107 118 119 121 124 135 136 137 **P**6 8
Primary Contact: William W. Webster, Chief Executive Officer
COO: Tony Ruiz, Chief Operating Officer
CFO: Robert Abernethy, Chief Financial Officer
CMO: Bruce Becker, M.D., Chief Medical Officer
CIO: Gary Barnes, Chief Information Officer
CHR: Harvey Hudspeth, Executive Director Human Resources
Web address: www.mchodessa.com
Control: Hospital district or authority, Government, nonfederal **Service:** General Medical and Surgical

Staffed Beds: 311 **Admissions:** 13617 **Census:** 191 **Outpatient Visits:** 181418 **Births:** 1580 **Total Expense ($000):** 179185 **Payroll Expense ($000):** 67626 **Personnel:** 1465

□ **ODESSA REGIONAL MEDICAL CENTER (450661)**, (Formerly Odessa Regional Hospital), 520 East Sixth Street, Zip 79761–4565, Mailing Address: P.O. Box 4859, Zip 79760–4859; tel. 432/582–8000 **A**1 5 9 10 **F**3 13 15 17 18 19 20 21 22 23 25 31 32 33 38 40 46 49 50 55 57 62 68 70 73 74 77 79 81 82 84 96 97 100 103 107 112 113 114 119 135 136 **P**8 **S** IASIS Healthcare
Primary Contact: Matthew Roberts, Chief Executive Officer
COO: Stacey L. Gerig, Chief Operating Officer
CFO: Steve Bowerman, Chief Financial Officer
CHR: Jill Sparkman, Director Human Resources
Web address: www.odessaregionalmedicalcenter.com
Control: Partnership, Investor–owned, for–profit **Service:** General Medical and Surgical

Staffed Beds: 161 **Admissions:** 6074 **Census:** 64 **Outpatient Visits:** 53703 **Births:** 2290 **Total Expense ($000):** 89601 **Payroll Expense ($000):** 23815 **Personnel:** 622

★ **REGENCY HOSPITAL OF ODESSA (452085)**, 318 North Alleghaney, Suite 202, Zip 79761; tel. 432/552–4000 **A**1 9 10 **F**1 3 25 56 57 63 73 75 80 81 82 85 119 137 **P**5 **S** Regency Hospital Company
Primary Contact: Kay Peck, Chief Executive Officer
Web address: www.regencyhospital.com
Control: Corporation, Investor–owned, for–profit **Service:** General Medical and Surgical

Staffed Beds: 30 **Admissions:** 367 **Census:** 28 **Outpatient Visits:** 0 **Births:** 0 **Total Expense ($000):** 11881 **Payroll Expense ($000):** 5919 **Personnel:** 101

OLNEY—Young County

★ **HAMILTON HOSPITAL (451354)**, 903 West Hamilton Street, Zip 76374–1725, Mailing Address: P.O. Box 158, Zip 76374–0158; tel. 940/564–5521 **A**9 10 18 **F**7 11 13 24 25 38 40 52 55 74 75 79 81 84 86 96 119 122 135 137
Primary Contact: Michael K. Hare, Administrator
CMO: Mark L. Mankins, M.D., Chief of Staff
Web address: www.olneyhamiltonhospital.com
Control: Hospital district or authority, Government, nonfederal **Service:** General Medical and Surgical

Staffed Beds: 25 **Admissions:** 1028 **Census:** 11 **Outpatient Visits:** 5432 **Births:** 26 **Total Expense ($000):** 9058 **Payroll Expense ($000):** 4341 **Personnel:** 110

 Many Facility Codes have changed. Please refer to the AHA Guide Code Chart.

ORANGE—Orange County

CONTINUECARE HOSPITAL OF SOUTHEAST TEXAS (452093), 608 Strickland Drive, Zip 77630; tel. 409/883–9361 **A**10 **F**1 3 25 31 32 33 38 54 59 80 87 119 137
Primary Contact: Wade K. Lester, Chief Executive Officer
Control: Other not–for–profit (including NFP Corporation) **Service:** Long–Term Acute Care hospital

Staffed Beds: 30 **Admissions:** 162 **Census:** 16 **Outpatient Visits:** 0 **Births:** 0 **Total Expense ($000):** 4193 **Payroll Expense ($000):** 1575 **Personnel:** 43

★ **MEMORIAL HERMANN BAPTIST ORANGE HOSPITAL (450005)**, 608 Strickland Drive, Zip 77630–4717; tel. 409/883–9361 **A**1 9 10 **F**13 15 25 26 32 33 38 49 55 57 68 73 74 77 79 80 82 84 85 86 96 100 107 119 135 136 137 **S** Community Hospital Corporation
Primary Contact: Jarren Garrett, Interim Administrator
CFO: Gary Troutman, CPA, Chief Financial Officer
CMO: Victoria Gordon, M.D., Chief of Staff
CHR: April Seymour, Manager Human Resources
Web address: www.mhbh.org
Control: Other not–for–profit (including NFP Corporation) **Service:** General Medical and Surgical

Staffed Beds: 83 **Admissions:** 3173 **Census:** 38 **Outpatient Visits:** 31584 **Births:** 432 **Total Expense ($000):** 33689 **Payroll Expense ($000):** 11751 **Personnel:** 254

PALACIOS—Matagorda County

PALACIOS COMMUNITY MEDICAL CENTER (451332), 311 Green Street, Zip 77465–3214; tel. 361/972–2511 **A**9 10 18 **F**30 32 38 55 56 62 66 86 96 102 118 119 122 135 137 **P**3
Primary Contact: Kathy Nichols, Co–Administrator
Web address: www.palacioscommunitymedcenter.com
Control: Other not–for–profit (including NFP Corporation) **Service:** General Medical and Surgical

Staffed Beds: 10 **Admissions:** 127 **Census:** 1 **Outpatient Visits:** 5889 **Births:** 0 **Total Expense ($000):** 3799 **Payroll Expense ($000):** 1199 **Personnel:** 32

PALESTINE—Anderson County

★ **PALESTINE REGIONAL MEDICAL CENTER–EAST (450747)**, 2900 South Loop 256, Zip 75801–6958; tel. 903/731–1000 **A**1 9 10 19 20 **F**3 13 15 18 24 25 26 30 31 32 38 40 41 42 43 49 50 51 55 57 63 68 74 77 79 81 82 84 86 87 88 90 91 92 93 96 97 100 102 106 107 118 119 120 122 132 135 136 137 **S** LifePoint Hospitals, Inc.
Primary Contact: Tim Flusche, Chief Executive Officer
CIO: Rebecca Chou, Director Information Systems
Web address: www.palestineregional.com
Control: Partnership, Investor–owned, for–profit **Service:** General Medical and Surgical

Staffed Beds: 103 **Admissions:** 6146 **Census:** 54 **Outpatient Visits:** 74949 **Births:** 940 **Total Expense ($000):** 41367 **Payroll Expense ($000):** 20587 **Personnel:** 439

★ **PALESTINE REGIONAL REHABILITATION CENTER (453089)**, 4000 South Loop 256, Zip 75801–8467, Mailing Address: P.O. Box 4070, Zip 75802–4070; tel. 903/731–5100 **A**1 10 **F**3 7 30 31 32 41 81 82 85 86 **S** LifePoint Hospitals, Inc.
Primary Contact: Tim Flusche, Chief Executive Officer
CHR: Rhonda Beard, Director Human Resources
Web address: www.palestineregional.com
Control: Partnership, Investor–owned, for–profit **Service:** Rehabilitation

Staffed Beds: 17 **Admissions:** 186 **Census:** 6 **Outpatient Visits:** 5895 **Births:** 0 **Total Expense ($000):** 4201 **Payroll Expense ($000):** 2051 **Personnel:** 53

PAMPA—Gray County

□ **PAMPA REGIONAL MEDICAL CENTER (450099)**, One Medical Plaza, Zip 79065; tel. 806/665–3721, (Total facility includes 16 beds in nursing home–type unit) **A**1 9 10 20 **F**3 11 13 15 17 18 20 25 26 32 38 43 51 54 55 56 63 66 73 74 75 77 79 80 81 82 84 86 88 93 96 97 100 106 107 116 117 118 119 135 136 137 **P**8 **S** Signature Hospital Corporation
Primary Contact: Todd Lorenz, Chief Executive Officer
CMO: Kevin Sieck, M.D., Chief Medical Staff
CIO: Jeff Anderson, Director Information Services
CHR: Debbie Dixon, Director Human Resources
Web address: www.prmctx.com
Control: Partnership, Investor–owned, for–profit **Service:** General Medical and Surgical

Staffed Beds: 91 **Admissions:** 3112 **Census:** 38 **Outpatient Visits:** 20776 **Births:** 326 **Total Expense ($000):** 30251 **Payroll Expense ($000):** 11504 **Personnel:** 218

PARIS—Lamar County

★ **DUBUIS HOSPITAL OF PARIS (452082)**, 865 Deshong Drive, 5th Floor, Zip 75462; tel. 903/782–2960 **A**1 9 10 **F**1 3 25 31 32 **S** Dubuis Health System
Primary Contact: Holly Powell, Administrator
CMO: Robert Zimmerman, M.D., Medical Director
Web address: www.dubuis.org
Control: Church–operated, Nongovernment, not–for profit **Service:** Long–Term Acute Care hospital

Staffed Beds: 25 **Admissions:** 212 **Census:** 15 **Outpatient Visits:** 0 **Births:** 0 **Total Expense ($000):** 5117 **Payroll Expense ($000):** 1433 **Personnel:** 42

□ **PARIS REGIONAL MEDICAL CENTER (450196)**, 820 Clarksville Street, Zip 75460–9070; tel. 903/785–4521, (Includes PARIS REGIONAL MEDICAL CENTER, 865 Deshong Drive, Zip 75462–2097; tel. 903/737–1111; PARIS REGIONAL MEDICAL CENTER–SOUTH CAMPUS, Mailing Address: P.O. Box 9070, Zip 75461–9070; Andrew Knizley, Chief Executive Officer) **A**1 9 10 19 **F**3 8 11 13 15 18 20 22 24 25 26 27 30 31 32 33 34 37 38 43 49 51 52 53 55 56 57 59 62 64 66 68 71 72 73 74 75 76 77 79 80 81 82 84 85 86 87 92 94 96 97 100 107 119 121 124 133 134 135 136 137 **P**5 **S** Essent Healthcare
Primary Contact: Christopher W. Dux, Chief Executive Officer
COO: Barbara Butler, Chief Operating Officer
CFO: Ken Miller, Chief Financial Officer
CMO: Richard Bercher, M.D., Chief Medical Officer
Web address: www.parisrmc.com
Control: Partnership, Investor–owned, for–profit **Service:** General Medical and Surgical

Staffed Beds: 296 **Admissions:** 8734 **Census:** 117 **Outpatient Visits:** 88281 **Births:** 796 **Total Expense ($000):** 110253 **Payroll Expense ($000):** 32917 **Personnel:** 741

PASADENA—Harris County

★ **BAYSHORE MEDICAL CENTER (450097)**, 4000 Spencer Highway, Zip 77504–1294; tel. 713/359–2000 **A**1 2 9 10 **F**3 4 8 12 13 15 17 18 20 22 24 25 27 29 30 31 32 33 38 39 43 44 47 49 51 54 55 56 57 59 62 65 68 70 72 73 74 75 76 77 79 81 84 85 86 92 96 97 100 102 103 104 105 107 109 111 114 116 118 119 120 133 135 136 137 **S** HCA
Primary Contact: Jeffrey S. Holland, Chief Executive Officer
CFO: Patrick J. Mathews, Chief Financial Officer
CHR: Major Tommy Doss, Director Human Resources
Web address: www.bayshoremedical.com
Control: Partnership, Investor–owned, for–profit **Service:** General Medical and Surgical

Staffed Beds: 300 **Admissions:** 14747 **Census:** 206 **Outpatient Visits:** 125157 **Births:** 2644 **Total Expense ($000):** 140513 **Payroll Expense ($000):** 55586 **Personnel:** 946

□ **KINDRED HOSPITAL–BAY AREA (452039)**, 1004 Seymour Street, Zip 77506–2699; tel. 713/473–9700 **A**1 9 **F**1 3 25 31 32 68 80 96 102 119 137 **P**5 **S** Kindred Healthcare
Primary Contact: Melissa Miller, Administrator
CFO: Billy Wilcox, Chief Financial Officer
CHR: Nellie Moen, Human Resources Coordinator
Web address: www.kindredhealthcare.com
Control: Corporation, Investor–owned, for–profit **Service:** Long–Term Acute Care hospital

Staffed Beds: 78 **Admissions:** 626 **Census:** 42 **Outpatient Visits:** 0 **Total Expense ($000):** 17450 **Payroll Expense ($000):** 7030 **Personnel:** 132

TX

Hospital, Medicare Provider Number, Address, Telephone, Approval, Facility, and Physician Codes, Health Care System

★ American Hospital Association (AHA) membership
□ The Joint Commission accreditation
○ American Osteopathic Association (AOA) accreditation
△ Commission on Accreditation of Rehabilitation Facilities (CARF) accreditation

SURGERY SPECIALTY HOSPITALS OF AMERICA (450831), (Formerly Vista Medical Center Hospital), 4301B Vista, Zip 77504; tel. 713/378–3000 **A**10 **F**3 12 25 26 29 38 43 66 68 73 75 77 79 80 82 96 97 100 107 118 121 132 **P**8 **S** Dynacq Healthcare, Inc.
Primary Contact: Celia Barrera, Administrator
Control: Partnership, Investor–owned, for–profit **Service:** General Medical and Surgical

Staffed Beds: 37 **Admissions:** 197 **Census:** 1 **Outpatient Visits:** 3766 **Births:** 0 **Total Expense ($000):** 14977 **Payroll Expense ($000):** 4202 **Personnel:** 103

PEARSALL—Frio County

★ **FRIO REGIONAL HOSPITAL (450293)**, 200 South I. H. 35, Zip 78061–3998; tel. 830/334–3617 **A**9 10 **F**3 13 15 38 40 46 56 61 62 63 79 86 96 107
Primary Contact: Alan D. Holmes, Chief Executive Officer
CHR: Cayse Morse, Administrative Assistant
Web address: www.frioregionalhospital.com
Control: Other not–for–profit (including NFP Corporation) **Service:** General Medical and Surgical

Staffed Beds: 22 **Admissions:** 775 **Census:** 6 **Outpatient Visits:** 16180 **Births:** 179 **Total Expense ($000):** 7968 **Payroll Expense ($000):** 3228 **Personnel:** 97

PECOS—Reeves County

REEVES COUNTY HOSPITAL (450201), 2323 Texas Street, Zip 79772–7338; tel. 432/447–3551 **A**9 10 20 **F**3 7 11 13 31 33 38 40 55 59 62 66 68 74 79 80 82 86 96 102 107 119 120 122 135 136 **P**3
Primary Contact: Albert LaRochelle, Chief Executive Officer
CFO: Frank Seals, Chief Financial Officer
CMO: W. J. Bang, M.D., Chief of Staff
CHR: Nadine Smith, Director Human Resources
Web address: www.reevescountyhospital.com
Control: Hospital district or authority, Government, nonfederal **Service:** General Medical and Surgical

Staffed Beds: 25 **Admissions:** 684 **Census:** 7 **Outpatient Visits:** 23171 **Births:** 34 **Total Expense ($000):** 12979 **Payroll Expense ($000):** 5416 **Personnel:** 148

PERRYTON—Ochiltree County

★ **OCHILTREE GENERAL HOSPITAL (451359)**, 3101 Garrett Drive, Zip 79070–5393; tel. 806/435–3606 **A**9 10 18 **F**10 11 13 15 32 33 38 40 42 55 57 61 62 67 68 74 79 80 84 86 96 97 102 107 119 122 132 135 136 **P**1
Primary Contact: Wallace N. Boyd, Administrator
CIO: Dyan Harrison, Manager Health Information
Web address: www.ochiltreehospital.com
Control: Hospital district or authority, Government, nonfederal **Service:** General Medical and Surgical

Staffed Beds: 25 **Admissions:** 874 **Census:** 9 **Outpatient Visits:** 28817 **Births:** 198 **Total Expense ($000):** 9973 **Payroll Expense ($000):** 4184 **Personnel:** 120

PITTSBURG—Camp County

★ **EAST TEXAS MEDICAL CENTER PITTSBURG (451367)**, 414 Quitman Street, Zip 75686–1032; tel. 903/856–6663 **A**9 10 18 **F**3 11 12 24 25 33 38 40 50 55 57 62 66 68 79 80 84 86 87 96 97 103 107 117 118 119 122 **P**6 **S** East Texas Medical Center Regional Healthcare System
Primary Contact: W. Perry Henderson, Administrator
CFO: Thomas O'Gorman, Assistant Administrator and Chief Financial Officer
CMO: Rodney Burrow, M.D., Chief of Staff
CIO: Paula Anthony, Vice President Information Services
Web address: www.etmc.org
Control: Other not–for–profit (including NFP Corporation) **Service:** General Medical and Surgical

Staffed Beds: 25 **Admissions:** 1288 **Census:** 13 **Outpatient Visits:** 50432 **Births:** 0 **Total Expense ($000):** 13694 **Payroll Expense ($000):** 5407 **Personnel:** 133

PLAINVIEW—Hale County

ALLEGIANCE BEHAVIORAL HEALTH CENTER OF PLAINVIEW (454101), 2601 Dimmit Road, 4th Floor, Zip 79072; tel. 806/926–9191 **A**10 **F**25 33 54 62 88 91 93 94 **P**5
Primary Contact: Mel Beachy, Administrator
COO: Don Cameron, Chief Operating Officer
CFO: Jim Turgeon, Vice President Finance
CIO: Richard Merk, Executive Vice President
CHR: Rob Lindsey, Vice President Human Resources
Control: Corporation, Investor–owned, for–profit **Service:** Psychiatric

Staffed Beds: 20 **Admissions:** 237 **Census:** 12 **Outpatient Visits:** 5059 **Births:** 0 **Total Expense ($000):** 4665 **Payroll Expense ($000):** 1392 **Personnel:** 35

⊠ **COVENANT HOSPITAL PLAINVIEW (450539)**, 2601 Dimmitt Road, Zip 79072–1833; tel. 806/296–5531 **A**1 9 10 20 **F**3 11 13 15 18 24 25 26 27 30 31 32 33 37 38 40 41 43 50 51 53 54 55 56 57 60 62 63 66 68 73 74 75 76 77 79 80 81 82 84 86 87 96 97 100 107 118 119 120 121 122 123 135 137 **P**8 **S** Covenant Health System
Primary Contact: Jonathan O. Wade, Chief Executive Officer
COO: Todd Oberheu, Chief Operating Officer
CMO: Sergio Lara, Chief Medical Officer
CIO: Tim Branch, Manager Information Technology
CHR: Alice Sawayer, Director Human Resources
Web address: www.covenantplainview.org
Control: Church–operated, Nongovernment, not–for profit **Service:** General Medical and Surgical

Staffed Beds: 34 **Admissions:** 2055 **Census:** 19 **Outpatient Visits:** 52104 **Births:** 551 **Total Expense ($000):** 28032 **Payroll Expense ($000):** 8347 **Personnel:** 205

PLANO—Collin County

⊠ **BAYLOR REGIONAL MEDICAL CENTER AT PLANO (450890)**, 4700 Alliance Boulevard, Zip 75093; tel. 469/814–2000 **A**1 9 10 **F**3 12 15 17 18 20 22 25 26 30 31 32 33 38 43 44 46 49 55 57 62 68 72 73 76 77 78 79 80 81 82 86 96 97 99 100 102 106 107 118 119 121 135 136 **S** Baylor Health Care System
Primary Contact: Jerri Garison, RN, President
CMO: Lannie Hughes, M.D., Vice President Medical Affairs
Web address: www.baylorhealth.com
Control: Other not–for–profit (including NFP Corporation) **Service:** General Medical and Surgical

Staffed Beds: 94 **Admissions:** 5947 **Census:** 75 **Outpatient Visits:** 36041 **Births:** 0 **Total Expense ($000):** 139401 **Payroll Expense ($000):** 35586 **Personnel:** 670

⊠ **HEALTHSOUTH PLANO REHABILITATION HOSPITAL (453047)**, 2800 West 15th Street, Zip 75075–7526; tel. 972/612–9000, (Nonreporting) **A**1 9 10 **S** HEALTHSOUTH Corporation
Primary Contact: Duke Saldivar, CHE, Chief Executive Officer
CFO: Patricia Weigel, Controller
CMO: Richard Jones, M.D., Medical Director
CHR: April Maldonado, Manager Human Resources
Web address: www.healthsouth.com
Control: Partnership, Investor–owned, for–profit **Service:** Rehabilitation

Staffed Beds: 65

INTEGRA HOSPITAL PLANO (453099), 2301 Marsh Lane, Zip 75093; tel. 972/428–1600, (Nonreporting) **A**9 10
Primary Contact: Dorothy J. Elford, Chief Executive Officer
Web address: www.integrahospitalplano.com
Control: Corporation, Investor–owned, for–profit **Service:** Rehabilitation

Staffed Beds: 73

☐ **LIFECARE HOSPITALS OF PLANO**, 6800 Preston Road, Zip 75024; tel. 214/473–8822 **A**1 9 **F**1 3 25 38 43 44 54 59 62 73 75 80 81 86 96 102 103 107 119 137 **P**8 **S** LifeCare Management Services
Primary Contact: Kathleen Wallace, RN, M.S.N., Administrator and Chief Executive Officer
CMO: John Hughes, M.D., Medical Director
CHR: Alan Silva, Director Human Resources
Web address: www.lifecare–hospitals.com
Control: Partnership, Investor–owned, for–profit **Service:** Long–Term Acute Care hospital

Staffed Beds: 66 **Admissions:** 698 **Census:** 47 **Outpatient Visits:** 30 **Births:** 0 **Total Expense ($000):** 20755 **Payroll Expense ($000):** 11101 **Personnel:** 191

⊠ △ **MEDICAL CENTER OF PLANO (450651)**, 3901 West 15th Street, Zip 75075–7799; tel. 972/596–6800 **A**1 2 7 9 10 **F**3 11 13 15 17 18 20 22 24 25 26 27 30 31 32 33 38 40 43 46 48 49 51 52 53 55 56 57 59 60 62 68 70 72 73 74 75 76 77 79 80 81 82 84 85 96 97 99 100 101 102 103 105 106 107 112 114 118 119 121 124 135 136 137 **P**5 **S** HCA
Primary Contact: Harvey L. Fishero, President and Chief Executive Officer
COO: Winston Borland, Chief Operating Officer
CFO: Mark Atchley, Vice President and Chief Financial Officer
CIO: Michael Gfeller, Director Information Systems
CHR: Shanna Warren, Director
Web address: www.medicalcenterplano.com
Control: Partnership, Investor–owned, for–profit **Service:** General Medical and Surgical

Staffed Beds: 348 **Admissions:** 13656 **Census:** 196 **Outpatient Visits:** 130990 **Births:** 2945 **Total Expense ($000):** 177013 **Payroll Expense ($000):** 73298 **Personnel:** 1120

TX

☐ **PLANO SPECIALTY HOSPITAL (452054)**, 1621 Coit Road, Zip 75075; tel. 972/758–5200 **A**1 9 10 **F**1 3 25 30 31 37 43 44 73 80 81 82 119 124 137 **P**8 **S** Fundamental Long Term Care Holdings, LLC
Primary Contact: Neal Duncan, Administrator and Chief Executive Officer
Web address: www.planospecialtyhospital.com
Control: Corporation, Investor–owned, for–profit **Service:** Long–Term Acute Care hospital

Staffed Beds: 30 **Admissions:** 302 **Census:** 23 **Outpatient Visits:** 0 **Births:** 0 **Total Expense ($000):** 8717 **Payroll Expense ($000):** 4195 **Personnel:** 97

PRESBYTERIAN HOSPITAL OF PLANO See Texas Health Presbyterian Hospital of Plano

☐ **PRESBYTERIAN PLANO CENTER FOR DIAGNOSTIC & SURGERY (450891)**, 6020 West Parker Road, Zip 75093; tel. 972/403–2700 **A**1 9 10 **F**3 25 30 32 38 43 46 53 62 77 79 80 82 96 100 102 107 135 **P**1
Primary Contact: Larry Robertson, Chief Executive Officer
Web address: www.ppcds.com
Control: Partnership, Investor–owned, for–profit **Service:** General Medical and Surgical

Staffed Beds: 18 **Admissions:** 1370 **Census:** 6 **Outpatient Visits:** 16885 **Births:** 0 **Total Expense ($000):** 44116 **Payroll Expense ($000):** 8895 **Personnel:** 218

★☐ **TEXAS HEALTH PRESBYTERIAN HOSPITAL OF PLANO (450771)**, (Formerly Presbyterian Hospital of Plano), 6200 West Parker Road, Zip 75093–7914; tel. 972/981–8000, (Includes SEAY BEHAVIORAL HEALTH CENTER, 6200 West Parker Road, Zip 75093–7938; tel. 972/981–8000; Gayle Jensen–Savoie, Director Psychiatric Services) **A**1 9 10 **F**3 5 12 13 15 18 20 22 25 26 27 28 30 31 32 33 35 36 38 41 43 48 49 53 55 56 57 58 59 62 66 68 70 72 73 74 75 76 77 79 80 81 82 84 86 96 97 99 100 102 103 106 107 113 114 118 119 120 121 124 134 135 136 137 **P**8 **S** Texas Health Resources
Primary Contact: Philip M. Wentworth, FACHE, President
CFO: Ray Cassens, Vice President and Chief Financial Officer
CMO: Chet Wells, M.D., President Medical Staff
CHR: Deborah Diehl, Director Human Resources
Web address: www.texashealth.org
Control: Other not–for–profit (including NFP Corporation) **Service:** General Medical and Surgical

Staffed Beds: 342 **Admissions:** 15859 **Census:** 211 **Outpatient Visits:** 108333 **Births:** 4136 **Total Expense ($000):** 234972 **Payroll Expense ($000):** 89164 **Personnel:** 1446

☐ **THE HEART HOSPITAL BAYLOR PLANO (670025)**, 1100 Allied Drive, Zip 75093; tel. 469/814–3278 **A**1 9 **F**18 20 22 24 25 26 30 31 32 38 55 56 62 73 79 80 81 82 96 97 103 107 119 135
Primary Contact: Mark Valentine, Chief Executive Officer
Control: Partnership, Investor–owned, for–profit **Service:** Heart

Staffed Beds: 52 **Admissions:** 1076 **Census:** 16 **Outpatient Visits:** 1455 **Births:** 0 **Total Expense ($000):** 38920 **Payroll Expense ($000):** 7429 **Personnel:** 261

PORT ARTHUR—Jefferson County

★☐ **CHRISTUS HOSPITAL–ST. MARY**, 3600 Gates Boulevard, Zip 77642–3601, Mailing Address: P.O. Box 3696, Zip 77643–3696; tel. 409/985–7431, (Total facility includes 19 beds in nursing home–type unit) (Nonreporting) **A**1 9 **S** CHRISTUS Health
Primary Contact: Wayne Moore, Administrator
CFO: Bill Hecht, Chief Financial Officer
CIO: Robert Jacobs, Regional Director Information Management
CHR: Charles Foster, Regional Director Human Resources
Web address: www.christushospital.org
Control: Church–operated, Nongovernment, not–for profit **Service:** General Medical and Surgical

Staffed Beds: 202

★☐ **DUBUIS HOSPITAL OF PORT ARTHUR**, 3600 Gates Boulevard, Zip 77642; tel. 409/989–5300, (Nonreporting) **A**1 9 **S** Dubuis Health System
Primary Contact: Barbara Flournoy, Administrator
Web address: www.dubuis.org
Control: Church–operated, Nongovernment, not–for profit **Service:** Other specialty

Staffed Beds: 15

☐ **THE MEDICAL CENTER OF SOUTHEAST TEXAS (450518)**, 2555 Jimmy Johnson Boulevard, Zip 77640; tel. 409/724–7389 **A**1 9 10 **F**3 8 11 12 13 15 17 18 20 22 24 25 32 33 38 46 47 49 50 51 53 55 56 57 59 62 66 68 70 72 73 74 75 77 79 80 81 82 84 85 86 88 92 93 94 95 96 97 100 102 103 106 107 119 136 137 **P**2 **S** IASIS Healthcare
Primary Contact: Michael J. Landry, Chief Executive Officer
CFO: Max Owens, Chief Financial Officer
Web address: www.medicalcentersetexas.com
Control: Partnership, Investor–owned, for–profit **Service:** General Medical and Surgical

Staffed Beds: 224 **Admissions:** 7954 **Census:** 111 **Outpatient Visits:** 48185 **Births:** 1262 **Total Expense ($000):** 77650 **Payroll Expense ($000):** 31818 **Personnel:** 551

PORT LAVACA—Calhoun County

★ **MEMORIAL MEDICAL CENTER (451356)**, 815 North Virginia Street, Zip 77979–3025, Mailing Address: P.O. Box 25, Zip 77979–0025; tel. 361/552–6713 **A**9 10 18 **F**3 11 13 15 25 26 28 30 31 32 33 38 40 44 46 50 54 55 56 57 59 61 62 66 68 73 74 75 76 77 79 80 81 82 86 87 96 97 100 103 107 118 119 121 122 123 124 135 136 137 **P**5
Primary Contact: Elwood E. Currier, Jr., CHE, Administrator
CFO: Rhett Fricke, Chief Financial Officer
CMO: William Crowley, Chief of Staff
CIO: Bart Strauss, Chief Information Officer
CHR: Pat Trigg, Director Human Resources and Public Relations
Web address: www.mmcportlavaca.com
Control: County–Government, nonfederal **Service:** General Medical and Surgical

Staffed Beds: 25 **Admissions:** 1413 **Census:** 14 **Outpatient Visits:** 26781 **Births:** 126 **Total Expense ($000):** 22169 **Payroll Expense ($000):** 8637 **Personnel:** 199

QUANAH—Hardeman County

★ **HARDEMAN COUNTY MEMORIAL HOSPITAL (451352)**, 402 Mercer Street, Zip 79252–4026, Mailing Address: P.O. Box 90, Zip 79252–0090; tel. 940/663–2795 **A**9 10 18 **F**11 25 31 33 38 40 50 54 56 57 61 62 73 79 82 86 90 91 93 94 119 122 **P**5
Primary Contact: Scott Nail, Administrator
CFO: Butch Hall, Chief Financial Officer
CMO: Kevin Lane, D.O., Chief of Staff
Web address: www.quanahnet.com\hospital\navbarframe.htm
Control: Hospital district or authority, Government, nonfederal **Service:** General Medical and Surgical

Staffed Beds: 24 **Admissions:** 295 **Census:** 4 **Outpatient Visits:** 8598 **Births:** 0 **Total Expense ($000):** 7261 **Payroll Expense ($000):** 3381 **Personnel:** 95

QUITMAN—Wood County

★☐ **EAST TEXAS MEDICAL CENTER–QUITMAN (450547)**, 117 Winnsboro Street, Zip 75783–2144, Mailing Address: P.O. Box 1000, Zip 75783–1000; tel. 903/763–6300 **A**1 9 10 **F**3 11 13 15 24 25 30 31 32 33 38 40 50 55 57 62 63 64 66 74 77 79 80 82 87 96 97 99 100 102 107 119 122 **S** East Texas Medical Center Regional Healthcare System
Primary Contact: Christopher Stipe, FACHE, Administrator and Chief Executive Officer
CFO: Carol LaTurno, Chief Financial Officer
CMO: George Cathey, Chief Medical Staff
CHR: William Henry, Director Human Resources
Web address: www.etmc.org
Control: Other not–for–profit (including NFP Corporation) **Service:** General Medical and Surgical

Staffed Beds: 28 **Admissions:** 1314 **Census:** 13 **Outpatient Visits:** 50508 **Births:** 103 **Total Expense ($000):** 13965 **Payroll Expense ($000):** 6079 **Personnel:** 154

RANKIN—Upton County

RANKIN HOSPITAL DISTRICT (451329), 1105 Elizabeth Street, Zip 79778, Mailing Address: P.O. Box 327, Zip 79778–0327; tel. 432/693–2443 **A**9 10 18 **F**30 31 38 39 62 84
Primary Contact: Brent Wrinkle, Administrator
CMO: James Kirkpatrick, Chief of Staff
Control: Hospital district or authority, Government, nonfederal **Service:** General Medical and Surgical

Staffed Beds: 6 **Admissions:** 118 **Census:** 1 **Outpatient Visits:** 1585 **Births:** 0 **Total Expense ($000):** 2247 **Payroll Expense ($000):** 1007 **Personnel:** 25

Hospital, Medicare Provider Number, Address, Telephone, Approval, Facility, and Physician Codes, Health Care System
★ American Hospital Association (AHA) membership
☐ The Joint Commission accreditation
○ American Osteopathic Association (AOA) accreditation
△ Commission on Accreditation of Rehabilitation Facilities (CARF) accreditation

TX

REFUGIO—Refugio County

REFUGIO COUNTY MEMORIAL HOSPITAL (451317), 107 Swift Street, Zip 78377–2425; tel. 361/526–2321 **A**9 10 18 **F**3 7 25 30 31 32 38 40 55 60 62 73 79 81 82 86 87 96 107 122 135 **P**6
Primary Contact: Louis R. Willeke, Administrator
Control: Hospital district or authority, Government, nonfederal **Service:** General Medical and Surgical

Staffed Beds: 20 **Admissions:** 154 **Census:** 1 **Outpatient Visits:** 41147 **Births:** 0 **Total Expense ($000):** 9791 **Payroll Expense ($000):** 3292 **Personnel:** 102

RICHARDSON—Dallas County

★ **RELIANT REHABILITATION HOSPITAL NORTH TEXAS**, 3351 Waterview Parkway, Zip 75080; tel. 972/398–5700, (Nonreporting) **A**1
Primary Contact: Jim Ransom, Chief Executive Officer
Web address: www.relianthcp.com
Control: Partnership, Investor–owned, for–profit **Service:** Rehabilitation

Staffed Beds: 50

★ **RICHARDSON REGIONALMEDICAL CENTER (450537)**, 401 West Campbell Road, Zip 75080–3416; tel. 972/498–4000 **A**1 2 9 10 **F**3 4 5 11 13 15 17 18 20 22 25 26 27 30 31 32 33 36 37 38 43 46 49 54 55 56 57 62 63 64 66 68 72 73 74 75 76 77 79 80 81 82 85 86 87 88 90 91 92 93 94 95 96 97 98 100 101 103 107 108 109 111 112 114 118 119 120 121 124 135 136 137 **P**6
Primary Contact: Ronald L. Boring, President and Chief Executive Officer
CFO: Bob Simpson, Chief Financial Officer
CIO: Ron Franquiz, Director Information Systems
CHR: Connie Wright, Director Human Resources
Web address: www.richardsonregional.com
Control: Hospital district or authority, Government, nonfederal **Service:** General Medical and Surgical

Staffed Beds: 141 **Admissions:** 7641 **Census:** 92 **Outpatient Visits:** 65942 **Births:** 644 **Total Expense ($000):** 105845 **Payroll Expense ($000):** 38327 **Personnel:** 652

RICHMOND—Fort Bend County

□ △ **OAKBEND MEDICAL CENTER (450330)**, 1705 Jackson Street, Zip 77469–3289; tel. 281/341–3000, (Total facility includes 26 beds in nursing home–type unit) **A**1 2 7 9 10 **F**3 11 13 15 18 25 26 27 31 32 38 40 46 49 50 55 57 63 68 71 72 73 74 76 77 79 80 82 84 96 97 100 103 106 107 117 119 121 135 136 137 **P**6 8
Primary Contact: Joe Freudenberger, Chief Executive Officer
COO: Jody Jones Noirot, Chief Operating Officer
CFO: Susan Carruth, Chief Financial Officer
CMO: Douglas Thibodeaux, Chief Medical Officer
CHR: Nancy Retzlaff, Director Human Resources
Web address: www.oakbendmedcenter.org
Control: Hospital district or authority, Government, nonfederal **Service:** General Medical and Surgical

Staffed Beds: 153 **Admissions:** 5996 **Census:** 74 **Outpatient Visits:** 53554 **Births:** 1174 **Total Expense ($000):** 62907 **Payroll Expense ($000):** 23656 **Personnel:** 500

RIO GRANDE CITY—Starr County

★ **STARR COUNTY MEMORIAL HOSPITAL (450654)**, 2753 Hospital Court, Zip 78582–9801, Mailing Address: P.O. Box 78, Zip 78582–0078; tel. 956/487–5561 **A**5 9 10 20 **F**7 11 13 15 25 26 30 31 32 38 40 46 50 55 56 57 62 63 73 74 77 79 84 96 99 102 107 119 124 134 137
Primary Contact: Thalia H. Munoz, Administrator
CFO: Rafael Olivares, Controller
Web address: www.starrcountyhospital.com
Control: Hospital district or authority, Government, nonfederal **Service:** General Medical and Surgical

Staffed Beds: 48 **Admissions:** 2263 **Census:** 21 **Outpatient Visits:** 60390 **Births:** 507 **Total Expense ($000):** 19599 **Payroll Expense ($000):** 9034 **Personnel:** 225

ROCKDALE—Milam County

RICHARDS MEMORIAL HOSPITAL (451357), 1700 Brazos Street, Zip 76567–2517, Mailing Address: Drawer 1010, Zip 76567–1010; tel. 512/446–4500 **A**9 10 18 **F**8 10 11 31 34 38 40 47 49 50 51 55 57 62 66 73 76 77 79 80 82 86 87 96 97 100 103 107 118 119 120 122 136 137 **P**5 **S** Blackhawk Healthcare
Primary Contact: Jeffrey Madison, Administrator
CMO: John Weed, M.D., Medical Director
CIO: Jeremy Riney, Administrative Resident
CHR: Mary Hilton, Controller
Web address: www.richardsmemorial.org
Control: Corporation, Investor–owned, for–profit **Service:** General Medical and Surgical

Staffed Beds: 25 **Admissions:** 1239 **Census:** 13 **Outpatient Visits:** 20656 **Births:** 0 **Total Expense ($000):** 20503 **Payroll Expense ($000):** 6719 **Personnel:** 204

ROTAN—Fisher County

★ **FISHER COUNTY HOSPITAL DISTRICT (451313)**, 774 State Highway 70 North, Zip 79546–4019, Mailing Address: P.O. Drawer F, Zip 79546–4019; tel. 325/735–2256 **A**9 10 18 **F**7 24 28 31 32 33 34 36 38 40 52 55 56 57 62 64 73 86 87 96 107 122 **P**6
Primary Contact: Ella Raye Helms, Administrator
CFO: Debbie Hull, Assistant Administrator
CMO: C. M. Callan, M.D., Chief of Staff
Control: Hospital district or authority, Government, nonfederal **Service:** General Medical and Surgical

Staffed Beds: 10 **Admissions:** 244 **Census:** 3 **Outpatient Visits:** 19413 **Births:** 0 **Total Expense ($000):** 6002 **Payroll Expense ($000):** 2439 **Personnel:** 66

ROUND ROCK—Williamson County

★ **SCOTT AND WHITE AT UNIVERSITY MEDICAL CAMPUS (670034)**, (Formerly Scott and White University Medical Campus Hospital), 300 University Boulevard, Zip 78664; tel. 512/509–0200, (Nonreporting) **A**1 10 **S** Scott & White
Primary Contact: Ernest L. Bovio, Jr., Chief Executive Officer
Web address: www.scottandwhite.org
Control: Other not–for–profit (including NFP Corporation) **Service:** General Medical and Surgical

Staffed Beds: 72

★ **ST. DAVID'S ROUND ROCK MEDICAL CENTER (450718)**, 2400 Round Rock Avenue, Zip 78681–4097; tel. 512/341–1000 **A**1 5 9 10 **F**3 11 12 13 15 18 20 24 25 26 27 30 31 32 33 38 55 56 57 62 68 71 72 73 74 75 76 77 78 79 80 81 82 86 96 97 100 102 107 118 119 121 135 136 137 **S** HCA
Primary Contact: Deborah L. Ryle, Administrator and Chief Executive Officer
COO: Tad Hatton, Chief Operating Officer
CMO: David Martin, Vice President, Medical Staff Affairs
Web address: www.roundrockmc.com
Control: Other not–for–profit (including NFP Corporation) **Service:** General Medical and Surgical

Staffed Beds: 140 **Admissions:** 8413 **Census:** 92 **Outpatient Visits:** 82467 **Births:** 2346 **Total Expense ($000):** 101842 **Payroll Expense ($000):** 34593 **Personnel:** 545

ROWLETT—Rockwall County

★ **LAKE POINTE MEDICAL CENTER (450742)**, 6800 Scenic Drive, Zip 75088–4552, Mailing Address: P.O. Box 1550, Zip 75030–1550; tel. 972/412–2273 **A**1 9 10 **F**3 11 12 13 15 18 24 25 28 32 37 38 49 50 52 53 55 57 59 68 70 72 73 74 75 77 79 80 81 84 86 96 97 100 103 104 107 118 119 120 135 136 137 **S** TENET Healthcare Corporation
Primary Contact: Carolyn Jackson, Chief Executive Officer
CFO: Bryan Forry, Chief Financial Officer
CMO: Charles Mangum, Chief of Staff
CHR: Stephanie Talley, Associate Administrator and Director Human Resources
Web address: www.lakepointemedical.com
Control: Corporation, Investor–owned, for–profit **Service:** General Medical and Surgical

Staffed Beds: 112 **Admissions:** 6073 **Census:** 61 **Outpatient Visits:** 65474 **Births:** 993 **Total Expense ($000):** 65318 **Payroll Expense ($000):** 27264 **Personnel:** 558

RUSK—Cherokee County

□ **RUSK STATE HOSPITAL (454009)**, Jacksonville Highway North, Zip 75785, Mailing Address: P.O. Box 318, Zip 75785–0318; tel. 903/683–3421 **A**1 10 **F**3 26 30 31 32 37 41 50 66 73 81 82 88 93 119 124 135 137 **P**6 **S** Texas Department of State Health Services
Primary Contact: Ted Debbs, Administrator
COO: Lynda Roberson, Senior Program Director
CFO: Frances Long, Chief Financial Officer
CMO: Douglas Johnson, M.D., Clinical Director
CIO: Judy Garner, Director Community Relations
Web address: www.mhmr.state.tx.us/hospitals/rusksh/rusksh.html
Control: State–Government, nonfederal **Service:** Psychiatric

Staffed Beds: 335 **Admissions:** 1809 **Census:** 298 **Outpatient Visits:** 0 **Births:** 0 **Total Expense ($000):** 54953 **Payroll Expense ($000):** 30060 **Personnel:** 946

SAN ANGELO—Tom Green County

★ **RIVER CREST HOSPITAL (454064)**, 1636 Hunters Glen Road, Zip 76901–5016; tel. 325/949–5722 **A**1 9 10 **F**4 5 25 31 32 33 55 82 88 89 90 91 94 95 119 121 123 132 **S** Universal Health Services, Inc.
Primary Contact: Scott York, Chief Executive Officer
CFO: Frank Urban, Chief Financial Officer
CMO: John Crowley, M.D., Medical Director
CHR: Brenda Coats, Director Human Resources
Web address: www.rivercresthospital.com
Control: Corporation, Investor–owned, for–profit **Service:** Psychiatric

Staffed Beds: 80 **Admissions:** 2064 **Census:** 34 **Outpatient Visits:** 1112 **Births:** 0 **Total Expense ($000):** 6438 **Payroll Expense ($000):** 3283 **Personnel:** 93

TX

★ △ **SAN ANGELO COMMUNITY MEDICAL CENTER (450340)**, 3501 Knickerbocker Road, Zip 76904–7698; tel. 325/949–9511 **A**1 2 7 9 10 **F**3 8 11 13 15 17 18 20 22 24 25 26 27 28 30 31 32 33 37 38 40 41 43 44 45 46 49 50 51 52 53 54 55 56 57 59 60 62 63 66 68 70 71 72 73 74 75 76 77 78 79 80 81 82 83 84 85 86 87 96 97 100 102 106 107 118 119 120 121 122 133 135 136 137 **P**7 8 **S** Community Health Systems, Inc.
Primary Contact: Samuel G. Feazell, Chief Executive Officer
CFO: Jeff Casbeer, Chief Financial Officer
CMO: Cecil Jameson, R.N., Chief Clinical Officer
CHR: Lisa Bibb, Director Human Resources
Web address: www.sacmc.com
Control: Partnership, Investor–owned, for–profit **Service:** General Medical and Surgical

Staffed Beds: 171 **Admissions:** 7677 **Census:** 91 **Outpatient Visits:** 102530 **Births:** 1045 **Total Expense ($000):** 69523 **Payroll Expense ($000):** 25696 **Personnel:** 672

★ △ **SHANNON MEDICAL CENTER (450571)**, 120 East Harris Street, Zip 76903–5976; tel. 325/653–6741, (Includes SHANNON MEDICAL CENTER–ST. JOHN'S CAMPUS, 2018 Pulliam Street, Zip 76905–5197; tel. 915/659–7100), (Total facility includes 16 beds in nursing home–type unit) **A**1 2 7 9 10 **F**3 7 11 13 15 18 20 22 24 25 26 27 30 31 32 33 35 36 38 40 43 49 50 51 52 53 54 55 56 57 58 59 61 62 68 70 71 72 73 74 75 76 77 78 79 80 81 82 84 85 86 88 90 91 92 93 96 97 99 100 102 103 106 107 117 118 119 120 121 133 134 135 136 137
Primary Contact: Bryan Horner, President and Chief Executive Officer
CMO: Irvin Zeitler, D.O., Vice President Medical Affairs
CHR: Teresa Morgan, Assistant Vice President Human Resources
Web address: www.shannonhealth.com
Control: Other not–for–profit (including NFP Corporation) **Service:** General Medical and Surgical

Staffed Beds: 258 **Admissions:** 11758 **Census:** 161 **Outpatient Visits:** 110222 **Births:** 1122 **Total Expense ($000):** 144918 **Payroll Expense ($000):** 52239 **Personnel:** 1235

□ **TRIUMPH HOSPITAL SAN ANGELO (452064)**, 120 East Harris Avenue, 6th Floor, Zip 76903; tel. 325/659–3906 **A**1 9 10 **F**1 3 25 137 **S** Triumph HealthCare
Primary Contact: Steve Grappe, Chief Executive Officer
COO: Jerrie Smithwick, Chief Clinical Officer
CFO: Glen Powers, Chief Financial Officer
CMO: Dale Russwurm, Medical Staff President
CIO: Kevin Williams, Vice President Information Systems
CHR: Kurtis Neal, Director Human Resources
Web address: www.triumph–healthcare.com
Control: Corporation, Investor–owned, for–profit **Service:** Long–Term Acute Care hospital

Staffed Beds: 28 **Admissions:** 268 **Census:** 18 **Outpatient Visits:** 0 **Births:** 0 **Total Expense ($000):** 8175 **Payroll Expense ($000):** 2859 **Personnel:** 65

SAN ANTONIO—Bexar County

★ △ **BAPTIST HEALTH SYSTEM (450058)**, 111 Dallas Street, Zip 78205–1230; tel. 210/297–7000, (Includes NORTH CENTRAL BAPTIST HOSPITAL, 520 Madison Oak Drive, Zip 78258–3912; tel. 210/297–4000; John J. Cleary, Chief Executive Officer; NORTHEAST BAPTIST HOSPITAL, 8811 Village Drive, Zip 78217–5440; tel. 210/297–2000; Matthew Stone, Chief Executive Officer; SOUTHEAST BAPTIST HOSPITAL, 4214 East Southcross Boulevard, Zip 78222–3740; tel. 210/297–3000; Andrew M. Harris, Chief Executive Officer; ST. LUKE'S BAPTIST HOSPITAL, 7930 Floyd Curl Drive, Zip 78229–0100; tel. 210/297–5000; Graham D. Reeve, Chief Executive Officer) **A**1 2 3 5 6 7 9 10 **F**3 11 12 13 14 15 17 18 19 20 22 24 25 26 27 31 32 33 35 36 38 40 41 43 46 47 49 50 51 54 55 57 59 62 63 66 68 70 71 72 73 74 75 76 77 78 79 80 81 82 83 84 85 86 87 88 90 91 92 93 96 97 100 102 103 104 105 106 107 112 113 116 118 119 121 124 134 135 136 137 **P**8 **S** Vanguard Health System
Primary Contact: Keith L. Swinney, President
COO: Philip J. Noel, Assistant Administrator and Chief Operating Officer
CFO: Linda Kirks, Chief Financial Officer
CMO: Herman Williams, M.D., Chief Medical Officer
CIO: Gary Davis, Vice President Information Systems
CHR: Sarah Spinharney, Senior Vice President
Control: Partnership, Investor–owned, for–profit **Service:** General Medical and Surgical

Staffed Beds: 1189 **Admissions:** 63992 **Census:** 740 **Outpatient Visits:** 249995 **Births:** 9857 **Total Expense ($000):** 514815 **Payroll Expense ($000):** 238026 **Personnel:** 4345

★ **CHRISTUS SANTA ROSA CHILDREN'S HOSPITAL (453305)**, 333 North Santa Rosa Street, Zip 78207; tel. 210/704–2011 **A**9 10 **F**3 19 21 23 25 26 28 30 31 32 33 35 37 38 42 43 44 45 48 49 53 58 59 62 69 70 71 72 73 76 77 79 80 81 82 83 84 94 96 97 100 102 106 107 114 118 119 121 135 **S** CHRISTUS Health
Primary Contact: Richard Wayne, M.D., Vice President and Administrator
COO: Don A. Beeler, President and Chief Executive Officer
CFO: William Pack, Chief Financial Officer
CMO: Steve Martin, Chief Medical Information Officer
CIO: Steve Martin, Chief Information Officer
CHR: Fernando Fleites, Vice President Human Resources
Web address: www.christussantarosa.org
Control: Church–operated, Nongovernment, not–for profit **Service:** Children's general

Staffed Beds: 196 **Admissions:** 6140 **Census:** 120 **Outpatient Visits:** 113733 **Births:** 0 **Total Expense ($000):** 104342 **Payroll Expense ($000):** 41566 **Personnel:** 604

★ **CHRISTUS SANTA ROSA HEALTH CARE (450237)**, 333 North Santa Rosa Street, Zip 78207–3108; tel. 210/704–2011 **A**1 3 5 9 10 **F**3 11 13 15 17 18 20 22 24 25 26 30 31 32 33 35 38 40 48 49 59 62 68 69 72 73 74 75 76 77 79 80 81 82 85 86 97 100 102 106 107 114 118 119 121 126 127 129 135 136 **S** CHRISTUS Health
Primary Contact: Don A. Beeler, President and Chief Executive Officer
CFO: William Pack, Chief Financial Officer
CIO: Steve Martin, Chief Information Officer
CHR: Fernando Fleites, Vice President Human Resources
Web address: www.christussantarosa.org
Control: Church–operated, Nongovernment, not–for profit **Service:** General Medical and Surgical

Staffed Beds: 380 **Admissions:** 15750 **Census:** 227 **Outpatient Visits:** 90363 **Births:** 2191 **Total Expense ($000):** 178913 **Payroll Expense ($000):** 72471 **Personnel:** 1638

□ **COMPASS HOSPITAL (452045)**, 14743 Jones Maltsberger Avenue, Zip 78247–3713; tel. 210/402–0029 **A**1 9 10 **F**1 3 25 26 32 73 119 137 **P**5 **S** Psychiatric Solutions
Primary Contact: Alan J. Fisher, Chief Executive Officer
CFO: Laura Brown, Chief Financial Officer
CMO: Mark Nelson, M.D., Medical Director
CIO: Wendy Myers, Director Medical Records
CHR: Michael Langford, Director Human Resources
Web address: www.psysolutions.com
Control: Corporation, Investor–owned, for–profit **Service:** Long–Term Acute Care hospital

Staffed Beds: 35 **Admissions:** 402 **Census:** 25 **Outpatient Visits:** 0 **Births:** 0 **Total Expense ($000):** 9649 **Payroll Expense ($000):** 4345

★ **HEALTHSOUTH REHABILITATION INSTITUTE OF SAN ANTONIO (453031)**, 9119 Cinnamon Hill, Zip 78240–5401; tel. 210/691–0737 **A**1 9 10 **F**9 25 43 61 62 73 85 86 119 121 137 **P**5 **S** HEALTHSOUTH Corporation
Primary Contact: Lee A. Simpson, Jr., Chief Executive Officer
CFO: Larry Spriggs, Controller
CMO: Richard Senelick, M.D., Medical Director
CHR: Vanessa Tejada, Director Human Resources
Web address: www.healthsouth.com
Control: Corporation, Investor–owned, for–profit **Service:** Rehabilitation

Staffed Beds: 96 **Admissions:** 1357 **Census:** 59 **Outpatient Visits:** 11951 **Births:** 0 **Total Expense ($000):** 17150 **Payroll Expense ($000):** 8840 **Personnel:** 225

□ **INNOVA HOSPITAL – SAN ANTONIO (670021)**, 4243 East Southcross Boulevard, Zip 78222; tel. 210/368–7400, (Nonreporting) **A**1 10
Primary Contact: Chuck Cave, Chief Executive Officer
Web address: www.innovahealth.net
Control: Partnership, Investor–owned, for–profit **Service:** General Medical and Surgical

Staffed Beds: 6

□ **KINDRED HOSPITAL–SAN ANTONIO (452016)**, 3636 Medical Drive, Zip 78229–3184; tel. 210/616–0616 **A**1 9 10 **F**1 3 25 26 30 32 38 40 68 75 82 119 121 137 **S** Kindred Healthcare
Primary Contact: Edward L. Dyer, Chief Executive Officer
CFO: Ken Derrington, Chief Financial Officer
CMO: Michael Wooley, Medical Director
CHR: Brian Mosley, Human Resources and Payroll Coordinator
Web address: www.kindredhealthcare.com
Control: Partnership, Investor–owned, for–profit **Service:** Long–Term Acute Care hospital

Staffed Beds: 59 **Admissions:** 679 **Census:** 54 **Outpatient Visits:** 3 **Births:** 0 **Total Expense ($000):** 22452 **Payroll Expense ($000):** 9165 **Personnel:** 151

TX

Hospital, Medicare Provider Number, Address, Telephone, Approval, Facility, and Physician Codes, Health Care System
★ American Hospital Association (AHA) membership
□ The Joint Commission accreditation
○ American Osteopathic Association (AOA) accreditation
△ Commission on Accreditation of Rehabilitation Facilities (CARF) accreditation

☐ **LAUREL RIDGE TREATMENT CENTER (454060)**, 17720 Corporate Woods Drive, Zip 78259–3500; tel. 210/491–9400 **A**1 9 10 **F**5 25 31 36 88 89 90 91 93 95 119 **S** Psychiatric Solutions
Primary Contact: Dan Thomas, Chief Executive Officer
COO: Shawn Owens, Chief Operating Officer
CFO: Charles Braun, Chief Financial Officer
CMO: Benigno J. Fernandez, M.D., Executive Medical Director
CHR: Brenda Frederick, Director Human Resources
Web address: www.laurelridgetc.com
Control: Partnership, Investor–owned, for–profit **Service:** Psychiatric

Staffed Beds: 94 **Admissions:** 3077 **Census:** 64 **Outpatient Visits:** 11201 **Births:** 0 **Total Expense ($000):** 22731 **Payroll Expense ($000):** 12895 **Personnel:** 244

☐ **LIFECARE HOSPITALS OF SAN ANTONIO (452059)**, (Specialty Hospital), 8026 Floyd Curl Drive, Zip 78229; tel. 210/690–7000 **A**1 9 10 **F**1 3 25 73 75 80 81 82 87 96 102 119 137 **S** LifeCare Management Services
Primary Contact: Randall G. Stokes, Chief Executive Officer
CFO: Linda Garcia, Regional Chief Financial Officer
Web address: www.lifecare–hospitals.com
Control: Partnership, Investor–owned, for–profit **Service:** Other specialty

Staffed Beds: 62 **Admissions:** 378 **Census:** 34 **Outpatient Visits:** 0 **Births:** 0 **Total Expense ($000):** 18430 **Payroll Expense ($000):** 8261 **Personnel:** 194

★ **METHODIST AMBULATORY SURGERY HOSPITAL (450780)**, 9150 Huebner Road, Suite 100, Zip 78240–1545; tel. 210/575–5000 **A**1 9 10 **F**3 25 30 31 32 66 77 79 80 82 **P**8 **S** HCA
Primary Contact: Elaine F. Morris, Administrator
CFO: Tim Carr, Chief Financial Officer
Web address: www.mas.sahealth.com
Control: Partnership, Investor–owned, for–profit **Service:** Surgical

Staffed Beds: 23 **Admissions:** 485 **Census:** 3 **Outpatient Visits:** 9999 **Births:** 0 **Total Expense ($000):** 20011 **Payroll Expense ($000):** 6949 **Personnel:** 134

★ **METHODIST CHILDREN'S HOSPITAL OF SOUTH TEXAS**, 7700 Floyd Curl Drive, Zip 78229–3383; tel. 210/575–7000, (Nonreporting) **A**2 10 **S** HCA
Primary Contact: Mark McLoone, Chief Executive Officer
CFO: Nancy Meadows, Chief Financial Officer
CMO: Roby Joyce, M.D., Chairman Medical Board
CIO: Eddie Cuellar, Vice President Information Systems
CHR: Nancy Edgar, Vice President Human Resources
Web address: www.mch.sahealth.com/
Control: Partnership, Investor–owned, for–profit **Service:** General Medical and Surgical

Staffed Beds: 150

★ **METHODIST HOSPITAL (450388)**, 7700 Floyd Curl Drive, Zip 78229–3993; tel. 210/575–4000, (Includes METHODIST SPECIALTY AND TRANSPLANT HOSPITAL, 8026 Floyd Curl Drive, Zip 78229–3915; tel. 210/575–4000; NORTHEAST METHODIST HOSPITAL, 12412 Judson Road, Zip 78233–3255; tel. 210/650–4949) **A**1 2 3 5 9 10 **F**4 5 8 11 12 13 15 17 18 19 20 21 22 23 24 25 26 27 28 30 31 32 33 36 38 40 41 43 44 46 47 49 51 52 54 55 56 57 58 59 62 63 65 66 68 70 72 73 74 75 76 77 78 79 80 81 82 83 84 85 86 88 89 90 91 92 93 94 95 96 97 100 102 107 109 112 118 119 121 124 125 126 127 128 131 132 134 135 136 137 **S** HCA
Primary Contact: Michael E. Duffy, Chief Executive Officer
COO: Michael E. Beaver, Chief Operating Officer
CFO: Nancy Meadows, Chief Financial Officer
CMO: Russell Woodward, M.D., Chief Medical Officer
CIO: Eddie Cuellar, Vice President Information Systems
CHR: Nancy Edgar, Vice President Human Resources
Web address: www.sahealth.com
Control: Partnership, Investor–owned, for–profit **Service:** General Medical and Surgical

Staffed Beds: 1405 **Admissions:** 68173 **Census:** 988 **Outpatient Visits:** 398371 **Births:** 10695 **Total Expense ($000):** 879158 **Payroll Expense ($000):** 298669 **Personnel:** 6799

★ **METROPOLITAN METHODIST HOSPITAL**, 1310 McCullough Avenue, Zip 78212–2617; tel. 210/757–2200, (Total facility includes 16 beds in nursing home–type unit) (Nonreporting) **A**1 5 9 **S** HCA
Primary Contact: Dominic Dominguez, Chief Executive Officer
COO: Janice Simons, Chief Operating Officer
CFO: Charles Braun, Chief Financial Officer
CIO: Mike Angelico, Director Information Systems
Web address: www.metro.sahealth.com
Control: Partnership, Investor–owned, for–profit **Service:** General Medical and Surgical

Staffed Beds: 244

☐ **MISSION VISTA BEHAVIORAL HEALTH CENTER (454102)**, 14747 Jones Maltsberger, Zip 78247–3713; tel. 210/497–0004 **A**1 9 10 **F**4 5 25 32 73 94 119 **S** Psychiatric Solutions
Primary Contact: Dan Thomas, Chief Executive Officer
CFO: Laura Brown, Chief Financial Officer
CMO: Maria R. Sweeney, M.D., Medical Director
CIO: Wendy Myers, Director Medical Records
CHR: Michael Langford, Director Human Resources
Web address: www.missionvistabhc.com
Control: Corporation, Investor–owned, for–profit **Service:** Psychiatric

Staffed Beds: 34 **Admissions:** 682 **Census:** 22 **Outpatient Visits:** 1299 **Total Expense ($000):** 5140 **Payroll Expense ($000):** 2581

☐ **NIX HEALTH CARE SYSTEM (450130)**, 414 Navarro Street, Zip 78205–2522; tel. 210/271–1800 **A**1 3 5 9 10 **F**3 5 12 13 15 18 20 22 25 26 27 33 41 43 50 54 55 57 59 61 62 68 72 73 74 76 77 79 80 82 85 86 87 88 89 93 94 96 97 100 102 106 107 118 119 131 132 136 **S** Merit Health Systems
Primary Contact: John F. Strieby, Chief Executive Officer
CFO: Lester Surrock, Chief Financial Officer
CMO: Michael L. Jones, M.D., Chief of Staff
CIO: Steve Kinkaid, Vice President Technology
CHR: Richard Lance, Vice President Human Resources
Web address: www.nixhealth.com
Control: Partnership, Investor–owned, for–profit **Service:** General Medical and Surgical

Staffed Beds: 164 **Admissions:** 7678 **Census:** 110 **Outpatient Visits:** 81236 **Births:** 446 **Total Expense ($000):** 72285 **Payroll Expense ($000):** 29066 **Personnel:** 638

☐ **PROMISE HOSPITAL OF SAN ANTONIO (452090)**, 7400 Barlite Boulevard, 2nd Floor, Zip 78224; tel. 210/921–3550 **A**1 10 **F**1 3 25 26 30 119 137 **S** Promise Healthcare
Primary Contact: Karen Pitcher, Vice President and Chief Executive Officer
Web address: www.promise–sanantonio.com
Control: Corporation, Investor–owned, for–profit **Service:** Long–Term Acute Care hospital

Staffed Beds: 26 **Admissions:** 187 **Census:** 13 **Outpatient Visits:** 0 **Births:** 0 **Total Expense ($000):** 8124 **Payroll Expense ($000):** 3012 **Personnel:** 75

☐ **SAN ANTONIO STATE HOSPITAL (454011)**, 6711 South New Braunfels, Suite 100, Zip 78223–3006; tel. 210/531–7711 **A**1 5 10 **F**26 32 37 52 54 55 57 66 73 75 81 82 88 89 90 91 93 119 121 124 135 **P**1 **S** Texas Department of State Health Services
Primary Contact: Robert C. Arizpe, Superintendent
CFO: Helen S. Martinez, Assistant Superintendent Financial Operations
CMO: Terresa Stallworth, M.D., Clinical Director
CIO: Chris Stanush, Director Information and Quality Management
CHR: Margaret Barker, Human Resources Specialist
Web address: www.dshs.state.tx.us
Control: State–Government, nonfederal **Service:** Psychiatric

Staffed Beds: 302 **Admissions:** 2785 **Census:** 280 **Outpatient Visits:** 0 **Births:** 0 **Total Expense ($000):** 57942 **Payroll Expense ($000):** 30915 **Personnel:** 842

☐ **SELECT SPECIALTY HOSPITAL–SAN ANTONIO (452073)**, 111 Dallas Street, 4th Floor, Zip 78205; tel. 210/297–7185 **A**1 9 10 **F**1 25 31 32 1 107 119 126 137 24 30 31 **S** Select Medical Corporation
Primary Contact: Greg Floyd, Vice President
Web address: www.selectmedicalcorp.com
Control: Corporation, Investor–owned, for–profit **Service:** Long–Term Acute Care hospital

Staffed Beds: 44 **Admissions:** 618 **Census:** 41 **Outpatient Visits:** 0 **Births:** 0 **Total Expense ($000):** 18041288 **Payroll Expense ($000):** 5160515 **Personnel:** 108

☐ **SOUTH TEXAS SPINE AND SURGICAL HOSPITAL (450856)**, 18600 Hardy Oak Boulevard, Zip 78258; tel. 210/507–4090 **A**1 9 **F**3 25 32 35 38 43 62 66 73 75 77 79 80 81 82 **S** National Surgical Hospitals
Primary Contact: Debbie Kelly, Chief Executive Officer
CFO: Sylvia Garcia, Chief Accounting Officer
CHR: Sally Hall, Manager Human Resources
Web address: www.shst.net
Control: Partnership, Investor–owned, for–profit **Service:** General Medical and Surgical

Staffed Beds: 30 **Admissions:** 942 **Census:** 7 **Outpatient Visits:** 1940 **Births:** 0 **Total Expense ($000):** 20419 **Payroll Expense ($000):** 4130 **Personnel:** 92

★ △ **SOUTH TEXAS VETERANS HEALTH CARE SYSTEM**, 7400 Merton Minter Boulevard, Zip 78284–5799; tel. 210/617–5140, (Includes KERRVILLE DIVISION, 3600 Memorial Boulevard, Kerrville, Zip 78028; tel. 210/896–2020; SAN ANTONIO DIVISION), (Total facility includes 274 beds in nursing home–type unit) (Nonreporting) **A**1 2 3 5 7 8 **S** Department of Veterans Affairs
Primary Contact: Jose R. Coronado, FACHE, Director
CFO: I. M. Rachal, Chief Fiscal Service
CMO: Richard Bauer, M.D., Chief of Staff
CIO: Simon Willett, Director Administrative Operations
CHR: Leslie Cruthirds, Chief Human Resource Management Service
Web address: www.vasthcs.med.va.gov
Control: Veterans Affairs, Government, federal **Service:** General Medical and Surgical

Staffed Beds: 1112

□ △ **SOUTHWEST GENERAL HOSPITAL (450697)**, 7400 Barlite Boulevard, Zip 78224–1399; tel. 210/921–2000 **A**1 7 9 10 **F**3 12 13 15 18 25 26 30 31 32 33 35 38 40 46 50 51 54 55 57 62 63 68 70 73 74 75 76 77 79 80 82 85 86 88 90 92 93 95 96 97 100 107 118 119 121 132 135 136 137 **S** IASIS Healthcare
Primary Contact: Richard D. Gonzalez, Chief Executive Officer
COO: Trey Klawiter, Chief Operating Officer
CFO: Joe Sereno, Interim Chief Financial Officer
CMO: Damaso Oliva, M.D., Chief Medical Officer
CIO: Sam Sowder, Director Information Systems
CHR: Christina Rivera, Director Human Resources
Web address: www.swgeneralhospital.com
Control: Corporation, Investor–owned, for–profit **Service:** General Medical and Surgical

Staffed Beds: 215 **Admissions:** 8848 **Census:** 126 **Outpatient Visits:** 72173 **Births:** 2090 **Total Expense ($000):** 90855 **Payroll Expense ($000):** 38512 **Personnel:** 676

SOUTHWEST MENTAL HEALTH CENTER, 8535 Tom Slick, Zip 78229–3363; tel. 210/616–0300 **A**3 5 9 **F**25 31 32 88 89 91 92 94 95 119 **P**8
Primary Contact: Frederick W. Hines, President
CFO: Michael Bernick, Vice President Finance
CMO: Graham Rogeness, M.D., Medical Director
CHR: Gina Massey, Vice President Human Resources
Web address: www.smhc.org
Control: Other not–for–profit (including NFP Corporation) **Service:** Children's hospital psychiatric

Staffed Beds: 52 **Admissions:** 1432 **Census:** 35 **Outpatient Visits:** 3659 **Births:** 0 **Total Expense ($000):** 10366 **Payroll Expense ($000):** 6348 **Personnel:** 150

ST. LUKE'S BAPTIST HOSPITAL See Baptist Health System

□ **TEXAS CENTER FOR INFECTIOUS DISEASE (452033)**, 2303 S.E. Military Drive, Zip 78223–3597; tel. 210/534–8857 **A**1 10 **F**1 3 25 26 30 31 32 50 52 53 60 62 66 73 82 119 121 124 132 135 **P**4 6 **S** Texas Department of State Health Services
Primary Contact: James N. Elkins, FACHE, Director
COO: Peggy Perry, Assistant Director
CFO: Helen S. Martinez, Assistant Superintendent Financial Operations
CMO: David Griffith, M.D., Medical Director
CIO: Andre Avant, Director Information Services
CHR: Margaret Barker, Human Resources Specialist
Web address: www.dshs.state.tx.us/tcid/default/shtm
Control: State–Government, nonfederal **Service:** Tuberculosis and other respiratory diseases

Staffed Beds: 72 **Admissions:** 101 **Census:** 41 **Outpatient Visits:** 1112 **Births:** 0 **Total Expense ($000):** 11706 **Payroll Expense ($000):** 5026 **Personnel:** 144

□ **TEXAS SPECIALTY HOSPITAL AT SAN ANTONIO (452040)**, 7310 Oak Manor Drive, Zip 78229–4509; tel. 210/308–0261 **A**1 9 10 **F**1 3 24 25 30 31 32 43 59 73 119 137 **P**8 **S** Fundamental Long Term Care Holdings, LLC
Primary Contact: Yolanda Ochoa, Interim Administrator
CFO: Lydia Washington, Controller
CHR: Yolanda Ochoa, Director Human Resources
Web address: www.thicare.com
Control: Corporation, Investor–owned, for–profit **Service:** Long–Term Acute Care hospital

Staffed Beds: 30 **Admissions:** 236 **Census:** 17 **Outpatient Visits:** 0 **Births:** 0 **Total Expense ($000):** 6211 **Payroll Expense ($000):** 2957 **Personnel:** 72

★ **TEXSAN HEART HOSPITAL (450878)**, 6700 IH–10 West, Zip 78201; tel. 210/736–6700 **A**1 9 10 **F**3 17 18 20 22 25 30 38 46 55 57 79 96 107 124 136 **S** MedCath, Inc.
Primary Contact: P. Craig Desmond, President
CFO: Dinah Gonzalez, Chief Financial Officer
Web address: www.texsanhearthospital.com
Control: Partnership, Investor–owned, for–profit **Service:** Heart

Staffed Beds: 60 **Admissions:** 4000 **Census:** 37 **Outpatient Visits:** 5495 **Births:** 0 **Total Expense ($000):** 57320 **Payroll Expense ($000):** 18481 **Personnel:** 311

★ **UNIVERSITY HEALTH SYSTEM (450213)**, 4502 Medical Drive, Zip 78229–4493; tel. 210/358–4000, (Includes UNIVERSITY HEALTH CENTER – DOWNTOWN, tel. 210/358–3400; UNIVERSITY HOSPITAL, tel. 210/358–4000) **A**1 2 3 5 8 9 10 **F**3 4 7 11 13 14 15 16 17 18 20 22 24 25 26 27 28 30 31 32 33 36 37 38 40 41 43 46 47 48 49 50 51 52 53 54 55 56 57 58 59 60 62 63 64 66 68 70 71 72 73 74 75 76 77 78 79 80 81 82 83 84 85 86 87 88 90 91 92 94 96 97 98 100 102 103 106 107 113 114 118 119 121 124 127 128 129 130 131 132 133 134 135 136 137 **P**6
Primary Contact: George B. Hernandez, Jr., President and Chief Executive Officer
CFO: Peggy Deming, Executive Vice President and Chief Financial Officer
CMO: David Hnatow, M.D., President Medical and Dental Staff
CIO: John Blandford, Vice President Information Services
CHR: Theresa Scepanski, Vice President People and Organizational Development
Web address: www.universityhealthsystem.com
Control: Hospital district or authority, Government, nonfederal **Service:** General Medical and Surgical

Staffed Beds: 381 **Admissions:** 21869 **Census:** 357 **Outpatient Visits:** 452933 **Births:** 3231 **Total Expense ($000):** 745654 **Payroll Expense ($000):** 211286 **Personnel:** 4807

□ △ **WARM SPRINGS REHABILITATION HOSPITAL (453035)**, 5101 Medical Drive, Zip 78229–6098; tel. 210/616–0100, (Total facility includes 10 beds in nursing home–type unit) **A**1 3 5 7 9 10 **F**3 11 25 43 55 62 72 77 85 86 117 119 121 135 137 **S** Vibra Healthcare
Primary Contact: Dennis Falck, Chief Executive Officer
CFO: James Asberry, Chief Financial Officer
CMO: Alex Willingham, M.D., Medical Director
CIO: David Chionsini, Chief Information Officer
CHR: Helen Williams, System Director Human Resources
Web address: www.warmsprings.org
Control: Partnership, Investor–owned, for–profit **Service:** Rehabilitation

Staffed Beds: 65 **Admissions:** 1393 **Census:** 57 **Outpatient Visits:** 43722 **Births:** 0 **Total Expense ($000):** 22252 **Payroll Expense ($000):** 10064 **Personnel:** 223

★ **WILFORD HALL MEDICAL CENTER**, 2200 Bergquist Drive, Suite 1, Zip 78236–9908; tel. 210/292–7412, (Nonreporting) **A**1 2 3 5 9 **S** Department of the Air Force
Primary Contact: Brigadier General David G. Young, MC, USAF, Commander
COO: Colonel Randy B. Borg, MSC, USAF, Administrator
CMO: Colonel Sven T. Berg, M.D., Chief Medical Staff
CIO: Lieutenant Colonel Eric D. Huweart, Chief Information Systems
CHR: Lieutenant Colonel Laura L. Garner, Chief Human Resources
Control: Air Force, Government, federal **Service:** General Medical and Surgical

Staffed Beds: 284

SAN AUGUSTINE—San Augustine County

MEMORIAL MEDICAL CENTER – SAN AUGUSTINE (451360), 511 East Hospital Street, Zip 75972–2121, Mailing Address: P.O. Box 658, Zip 75972–0658; tel. 936/275–3446 **A**9 10 18 **F**3 24 25 31 32 33 38 55 57 62 84 92 96 107 121 122 **S** Memorial Health System of East Texas
Primary Contact: Darlene Williams, RN, Administrator
CFO: Richard Ahrens, Chief Financial Officer
Web address: www.memorialhealth.org
Control: Other not–for–profit (including NFP Corporation) **Service:** General Medical and Surgical

Staffed Beds: 18 **Admissions:** 672 **Census:** 5 **Outpatient Visits:** 17649 **Births:** 1 **Total Expense ($000):** 4390 **Payroll Expense ($000):** 1990 **Personnel:** 38

TX

Hospital, Medicare Provider Number, Address, Telephone, Approval, Facility, and Physician Codes, Health Care System
★ American Hospital Association (AHA) membership
□ The Joint Commission accreditation
○ American Osteopathic Association (AOA) accreditation
△ Commission on Accreditation of Rehabilitation Facilities (CARF) accreditation

SAN MARCOS—Hays County

★ **CENTRAL TEXAS MEDICAL CENTER (450272)**, 1301 Wonder World Drive, Zip 78666–7544; tel. 512/353–8979 **A**1 9 10 **F**11 13 15 18 20 22 25 26 28 30 31 32 33 37 38 41 42 43 49 50 52 53 54 55 56 57 59 61 62 63 66 68 73 74 75 77 78 79 81 82 86 87 93 96 97 100 102 104 105 106 107 118 119 120 121 135 137 **P**6 8 **S** Adventist Health System Sunbelt Health Care Corporation
Primary Contact: Gary L. Jepson, President and Chief Executive Officer
CFO: Richard Boggess, Chief Financial Officer
CHR: Debbie Cox, Director Human Resources
Web address: www.ctmc.org
Control: Church–operated, Nongovernment, not–for profit **Service:** General Medical and Surgical

Staffed Beds: 113 **Admissions:** 4953 **Census:** 47 **Outpatient Visits:** 70276 **Births:** 1180 **Total Expense ($000):** 59699 **Payroll Expense ($000):** 23092 **Personnel:** 511

SEGUIN—Guadalupe County

★ **GUADALUPE REGIONAL MEDICAL CENTER (450104)**, 1215 East Court Street, Zip 78155–5189; tel. 830/379–2411 **A**1 9 10 **F**3 5 11 12 13 15 24 25 26 27 32 38 40 42 43 44 45 46 49 50 51 52 54 56 61 62 65 66 68 72 73 74 75 76 77 79 80 81 82 85 86 93 94 96 97 100 102 107 118 119 121 132 135 137 **P**1
Primary Contact: Robert Haynes, Chief Executive Officer
COO: Lauren Carter, Associate Administrator
CFO: Penny Wallace, Chief Financial Officer
CMO: Steve White, M.D., Chief Medical Officer
CIO: Steve Ratliff, Director
CHR: Fay Bennett, Director
Web address: www.grmedcenter.com
Control: City–County, Government, nonfederal **Service:** General Medical and Surgical

Staffed Beds: 98 **Admissions:** 5238 **Census:** 56 **Outpatient Visits:** 108820 **Births:** 656 **Total Expense ($000):** 55164 **Payroll Expense ($000):** 25502 **Personnel:** 632

SEMINOLE—Gaines County

★ **MEMORIAL HOSPITAL (451358)**, 209 N.W. Eighth Street, Zip 79360–3447; tel. 432/758–5811 **A**9 10 18 **F**3 10 11 13 24 25 26 28 30 31 32 33 38 40 42 52 54 55 56 57 61 62 63 73 74 75 79 82 86 87 92 96 102 107 119 120 121 122 132 135 136 137 **P**7
Primary Contact: Betsy Briscoe, Interim Chief Executive Officer
CFO: Traci Anderson, Chief Financial Officer
CMO: Michael Watson, M.D., Chief of Staff
CHR: Jodie Wood, Director Human Resources
Web address: www.semmem.com
Control: Hospital district or authority, Government, nonfederal **Service:** General Medical and Surgical

Staffed Beds: 25 **Admissions:** 659 **Census:** 9 **Outpatient Visits:** 28238 **Births:** 205 **Total Expense ($000):** 15422 **Payroll Expense ($000):** 4392 **Personnel:** 155

SEYMOUR—Baylor County

★ **SEYMOUR HOSPITAL (450586)**, 200 Stadium Drive, Zip 76380–2344; tel. 940/889–5572 **A**9 10 20 **F**3 7 8 11 13 25 30 32 34 38 40 52 54 55 56 57 61 62 63 64 66 68 73 74 79 80 81 82 86 90 92 93 96 107 119 122 124 135 **P**1
Primary Contact: Leslie Hardin, Chief Executive Officer and Chief Financial Officer
CFO: Leslie Hardin, Chief Executive Officer and Chief Financial Officer
CMO: Richard Niles, Chief of Staff
CHR: Linda Hampton, Manager Human Resources
Control: Hospital district or authority, Government, nonfederal **Service:** General Medical and Surgical

Staffed Beds: 38 **Admissions:** 693 **Census:** 9 **Outpatient Visits:** 24903 **Births:** 46 **Total Expense ($000):** 5532 **Payroll Expense ($000):** 3302 **Personnel:** 103

SHAMROCK—Wheeler County

SHAMROCK GENERAL HOSPITAL (451340), 1000 South Main Street, Zip 79079–2896; tel. 806/256–2114 **A**9 10 18 **F**7 11 25 28 38 40 42 63 66 86 96 107 119 122 **P**4
Primary Contact: Wiley M. Fires, Administrator
CFO: Wiley M. Fires, Administrator
CHR: Cecille Williams, Assistant Administrator
Control: Hospital district or authority, Government, nonfederal **Service:** General Medical and Surgical

Staffed Beds: 13 **Admissions:** 361 **Census:** 3 **Outpatient Visits:** 18485 **Births:** 2 **Total Expense ($000):** 4142 **Payroll Expense ($000):** 1991 **Personnel:** 70

SHENANDOAH—Montgomery County

☐ **NEXUS SPECIALTY HOSPITAL (452057)**, 123 Vision Park Boulevard, Zip 77384; tel. 281/364–0317 **A**1 9 10 **F**1 3 25 32 68 73 80 82 119 135 137 **S** Nexus Health Systems
Primary Contact: Brian Holt, Chief Executive Officer
CFO: Rob Tyler, Chief Financial Officer
Web address: www.nexusspecialty.com
Control: Partnership, Investor–owned, for–profit **Service:** Long–Term Acute Care hospital

Staffed Beds: 75 **Admissions:** 559 **Census:** 44 **Outpatient Visits:** 14 **Births:** 0 **Total Expense ($000):** 19621 **Payroll Expense ($000):** 7832 **Personnel:** 234

SHERMAN—Grayson County

☐ **COMMUNITY SPECIALTY HOSPITAL (450393)**, 1111 Gallagher Drive, Zip 75090–1713; tel. 903/870–7000, (Total facility includes 22 beds in nursing home–type unit) **A**1 9 10 **F**25 26 31 32 33 41 50 52 54 55 56 57 62 72 75 77 81 82 85 88 89 91 93 94 95 117 119 121 132 135 **S** SeniorHealth Incorporated
Primary Contact: Travis W. Roderick, Administrator and Chief Executive Officer
CFO: Jan Bullock, Chief Financial Officer
Web address: www.cshsherman.com
Control: Other not–for–profit (including NFP Corporation) **Service:** Rehabilitation

Staffed Beds: 90 **Admissions:** 1723 **Census:** 50 **Outpatient Visits:** 1280 **Births:** 0 **Total Expense ($000):** 13756 **Payroll Expense ($000):** 6303 **Personnel:** 156

★ **WILSON N. JONES MEDICAL CENTER (450469)**, 500 North Highland Avenue, Zip 75092–7354; tel. 903/870–4611 **A**1 9 10 **F**3 11 13 15 17 18 20 22 24 25 26 27 30 31 33 38 44 49 52 53 54 55 57 58 60 62 68 72 74 75 76 77 78 79 81 82 84 86 96 97 100 106 107 119 121 135 136 137 **P**6
Primary Contact: Patrick D. Flynn, President and Chief Executive Officer
CFO: Mitch Mulvehill, Senior Vice President and Chief Financial Officer
CMO: Michael Isaac, M.D., President Medical Staff
CIO: Mel Ostlie, Chief Information Officer
CHR: Linda Creswell, Director Human Resources
Web address: www.wnj.org
Control: Other not–for–profit (including NFP Corporation) **Service:** General Medical and Surgical

Staffed Beds: 215 **Admissions:** 9807 **Census:** 125 **Outpatient Visits:** 71404 **Births:** 1098 **Total Expense ($000):** 108546 **Payroll Expense ($000):** 45583 **Personnel:** 890

SMITHVILLE—Bastrop County

★ **SMITHVILLE REGIONAL HOSPITAL (450143)**, 800 East Highway 71, Zip 78957; tel. 512/237–3214 **A**5 9 10 **F**3 11 15 25 30 31 32 38 40 52 55 57 61 62 66 68 75 77 79 82 84 86 96 97 99 100 102 107 119 132 135 137 **P**5
Primary Contact: Grady Hooper, Chief Executive Officer
CFO: Noralene Corder, Chief Financial Officer
CHR: Debbie Adkins, Director Human Resources
Web address: www.srhnet.org
Control: Hospital district or authority, Government, nonfederal **Service:** General Medical and Surgical

Staffed Beds: 33 **Admissions:** 1226 **Census:** 10 **Outpatient Visits:** 40004 **Births:** 0 **Total Expense ($000):** 16502 **Payroll Expense ($000):** 9293 **Personnel:** 246

SNYDER—Scurry County

★ **D. M. COGDELL MEMORIAL HOSPITAL (450073)**, 1700 Cogdell Boulevard, Zip 79549–6198; tel. 325/573–6374, (Total facility includes 24 beds in nursing home–type unit) **A**9 10 20 **F**8 10 11 13 15 24 25 26 27 30 31 38 40 46 52 54 55 56 57 61 62 63 66 68 73 74 75 79 80 81 82 86 96 97 102 107 108 119 122 135 136 137
Primary Contact: Evan Moore, FACHE, Chief Executive Officer
CFO: John Everett, Chief Financial Officer
CMO: Bid Cooper, M.D., Chief Medical Officer
CIO: Betty Woodard, Manager Health Information Management
CHR: Linda Warren, Director Human Resources
Web address: www.cogdellhospital.com
Control: County–Government, nonfederal **Service:** General Medical and Surgical

Staffed Beds: 73 **Admissions:** 1272 **Census:** 35 **Outpatient Visits:** 41642 **Births:** 158 **Total Expense ($000):** 15863 **Payroll Expense ($000):** 6694 **Personnel:** 207

Many Facility Codes have changed. Please refer to the AHA Guide Code Chart.

SONORA—Sutton County

★ **LILLIAN M. HUDSPETH MEMORIAL HOSPITAL (451324)**, 308 Hudspeth Avenue, Zip 76950–3399, Mailing Address: P.O. Box 455, Zip 76950–0455; tel. 325/387–2521 **A**9 10 18 **F**3 11 12 24 25 28 30 31 32 33 38 40 41 50 52 55 56 57 62 64 66 73 81 82 84 85 86 87 96 102 107 120 121 122 123 124 137
Primary Contact: Keith L. Butler, Chief Executive Officer
CFO: Michelle Schaefer, Chief Financial Officer
Web address: www.sonora–hospital.org
Control: Hospital district or authority, Government, nonfederal **Service:** General Medical and Surgical

Staffed Beds: 12 **Admissions:** 312 **Census:** 2 **Outpatient Visits:** 6536 **Births:** 0 **Total Expense ($000):** 4634 **Payroll Expense ($000):** 1883 **Personnel:** 55

SOUTHLAKE—Tarrant County

HARRIS METHODIST SOUTHLAKE CENTER FOR DIAGNOSTICS AND SURGERY (450888), 1545 East Southlake Boulevard, Zip 76092–6422; tel. 817/748–8700 **A**9 10 **F**3 25 26 38 62 72 77 79 80 96 100 102 107 135 **P**2
Primary Contact: Traci Bernard, President
Web address: www.hmsouthlake.com
Control: Partnership, Investor–owned, for–profit **Service:** Surgical

Staffed Beds: 6 **Admissions:** 472 **Census:** 3 **Outpatient Visits:** 10421 **Births:** 0 **Total Expense ($000):** 27215 **Payroll Expense ($000):** 5784 **Personnel:** 112

SPEARMAN—Hansford County

★ **HANSFORD HOSPITAL (451344)**, 707 South Roland Street, Zip 79081–3441; tel. 806/659–2535 **A**9 10 18 **F**11 27 28 30 38 40 42 54 55 56 57 61 62 63 66 67 76 86 96 119 122 **P**6
Primary Contact: Jerry Jasper, Chief Executive Officer
CFO: Scott Beedy, Chief Financial Officer
CMO: Mark Garnett, M.D., Chief of Staff
CHR: Jackie Nelson, Director Human Resources
Web address: www.hchd.net
Control: Hospital district or authority, Government, nonfederal **Service:** General Medical and Surgical

Staffed Beds: 20 **Admissions:** 197 **Census:** 2 **Outpatient Visits:** 18146 **Births:** 0 **Total Expense ($000):** 5177 **Payroll Expense ($000):** 2312 **Personnel:** 64

STAMFORD—Jones County

STAMFORD MEMORIAL HOSPITAL (450306), 1601 Columbia Street, Zip 79553, Mailing Address: P.O. Box 911, Zip 79553–0911; tel. 325/773–2725 **A**9 10 **F**11 37 38 40 42 43 52 55 61 62 73 79 81 84 86 87 93 120 122 135 137 **P**5
Primary Contact: Richard G. DeFoore, FACHE, Chief Executive Officer
CFO: Fran Tinnen, Chief Financial Officer
CMO: Michael Hart, M.D., Medical Director
CIO: Birgitta Neal, Data Entry and Information Technologist
CHR: Pam Bell, Director Human Resources
Control: Hospital district or authority, Government, nonfederal **Service:** General Medical and Surgical

Staffed Beds: 25 **Admissions:** 328 **Census:** 4 **Outpatient Visits:** 19725 **Births:** 0 **Total Expense ($000):** 5688 **Payroll Expense ($000):** 3340 **Personnel:** 140

STANTON—Martin County

MARTIN COUNTY HOSPITAL DISTRICT (451333), 610 North St. Peter Street, Zip 79782, Mailing Address: P.O. Box 640, Zip 79782–0640; tel. 432/756–3345 **A**9 10 18 **F**7 31 32 38 40 55 61 74 79 84 122
Primary Contact: Paul McKinney, Administrator
CFO: Alison Israel, Controller
Control: Hospital district or authority, Government, nonfederal **Service:** General Medical and Surgical

Staffed Beds: 20 **Admissions:** 336 **Census:** 3 **Outpatient Visits:** 16655 **Births:** 0 **Total Expense ($000):** 6729 **Payroll Expense ($000):** 2776 **Personnel:** 69

STEPHENVILLE—Erath County

★☐ **TEXAS HEALTH HARRIS METHODIST–ERATH COUNTY (450351)**, (Formerly Harris Methodist–Erath County), 411 North Belknap Street, Zip 76401–3415, Mailing Address: P.O. Box 1399, Zip 76401–1399; tel. 254/965–1500 **A**1 9 10 20 **F**3 11 13 15 25 26 30 31 32 33 38 40 50 51 55 56 57 63 68 73 74 75 76 77 79 81 84 86 96 97 100 102 106 107 118 119 122 124 135 137 **S** Texas Health Resources
Primary Contact: Christopher Leu, Chief Executive Officer
CFO: Carol Cross, Chief Financial Officer
CMO: Steve Erck, M.D., Chief of Staff
CHR: Linda Henderson, Director Human Resources
Web address: www.texashealth.org
Control: Other not–for–profit (including NFP Corporation) **Service:** General Medical and Surgical

Staffed Beds: 57 **Admissions:** 2781 **Census:** 25 **Outpatient Visits:** 26071 **Births:** 485 **Total Expense ($000):** 31442 **Payroll Expense ($000):** 13392 **Personnel:** 231

SUGAR LAND—Fort Bend County

★☐ **MEMORIAL HERMANN SUGAR LAND HOSPITAL (450848)**, 17500 West Grand Parkway South, Zip 77479; tel. 281/725–5000 **A**1 9 10 **F**3 8 11 13 14 15 25 26 27 30 31 32 33 34 35 37 38 40 41 42 43 46 47 48 49 50 51 52 53 54 55 56 57 59 62 66 68 70 72 73 74 75 76 77 79 80 81 82 86 87 96 99 100 102 107 118 119 120 124 135 136 **P**5 6 **S** Memorial Hermann Healthcare System
Primary Contact: Jim Brown, Chief Executive Officer
COO: Donita Fleming, Chief Operating Officer
CFO: Nancy Brock, Chief Financial Officer
CMO: William Riley, M.D., Chief of Staff
CHR: Patsy Jones, Director
Web address: www.memorialhermann.org
Control: Other not–for–profit (including NFP Corporation) **Service:** General Medical and Surgical

Staffed Beds: 77 **Admissions:** 3240 **Census:** 33 **Outpatient Visits:** 37869 **Births:** 692 **Total Expense ($000):** 51995 **Payroll Expense ($000):** 19554 **Personnel:** 395

★☐ **METHODIST SUGAR LAND HOSPITAL (450820)**, 16655 S.W. Freeway, Zip 77479–2343; tel. 281/274–7000 **A**1 9 10 **F**3 13 15 18 20 22 25 26 31 32 38 46 49 51 55 56 57 59 62 66 68 71 73 74 75 79 80 82 96 97 99 100 102 103 107 108 109 111 119 134 135 **S** The Methodist Hospital System
Primary Contact: Christopher Siebenaler, Acting Administrator and Chief Executive Officer
CFO: Lowell Stanton, Chief Financial Officer
CMO: Jeffrey Jackson, M.D., Medical Director
CHR: Luis Garcia, Director
Web address: www.methodisthealth.com
Control: Other not–for–profit (including NFP Corporation) **Service:** General Medical and Surgical

Staffed Beds: 54 **Admissions:** 5167 **Census:** 51 **Outpatient Visits:** 81095 **Births:** 1630 **Total Expense ($000):** 79462 **Payroll Expense ($000):** 34353 **Personnel:** 654

☐ **SUGAR LAND SURGICAL HOSPITAL (450860)**, 1211 Highway 6, Suite 70, Zip 77478; tel. 281/243–1000 **A**1 10 **F**1 3 4 16 17 25 38 43 55 57 62 65 68 70 71 73 77 78 79 80 81 82 83 84 85 87 88 100 107 117 119 **P**2 **S** United Surgical Partners International
Primary Contact: Madilyn Zbranek, RN, Chief Executive Officer
CFO: Raquel Hebert, Business Manager
CMO: Ken Thomson, M.D., Medical Director
CIO: Madilyn Zbranek, R.N., Chief Executive Officer
CHR: Jill Rajala, Director Nurses
Web address: www.sho–sugarland.com
Control: Partnership, Investor–owned, for–profit **Service:** General Medical and Surgical

Staffed Beds: 6 **Admissions:** 272 **Census:** 2 **Outpatient Visits:** 6565 **Births:** 0 **Total Expense ($000):** 15396 **Payroll Expense ($000):** 2553 **Personnel:** 55

TX

Hospital, Medicare Provider Number, Address, Telephone, Approval, Facility, and Physician Codes, Health Care System

★ American Hospital Association (AHA) membership
☐ The Joint Commission accreditation
○ American Osteopathic Association (AOA) accreditation
△ Commission on Accreditation of Rehabilitation Facilities (CARF) accreditation

☐ **TRIUMPH HOSPITAL SOUTHWEST (452080)**, 1550 First Colony Boulevard, Zip 77479; tel. 281/275–6000 **A**1 9 10 **F**1 3 25 27 31 32 33 38 55 62 63 68 73 75 82 86 96 119 137 **P**5 **S** Triumph HealthCare
Primary Contact: Michele Dionne, President and Chief Executive Officer
COO: Linda Fischer, Chief Clinical Officer
CFO: Paul Hanson, Chief Financial Officer
CMO: Subodh Bhuchar, M.D., Chief of Staff
CIO: David Stowers, Director Case Management
CHR: Nancy Carter, Director Human Resources
Web address: www.triumph–healthcare.com
Control: Partnership, Investor–owned, for–profit **Service:** Long–Term Acute Care hospital

Staffed Beds: 150 **Admissions:** 1565 **Census:** 111 **Outpatient Visits:** 1523 **Births:** 0 **Total Expense ($000):** 56118 **Payroll Expense ($000):** 19041 **Personnel:** 429

SULPHUR SPRINGS—Hopkins County

★ **HOPKINS COUNTY MEMORIAL HOSPITAL (450236)**, 115 Airport Road, Zip 75482–0115; tel. 903/885–7671 **A**9 10 **F**1 7 13 15 25 30 31 32 33 38 40 42 43 44 54 56 57 68 71 74 78 79 82 86 96 97 100 106 107 119 135 137
Primary Contact: Michael McAndrew, Chief Executive Officer
COO: Donna Geiken Wallace, Chief Operating Officer and Chief Financial Officer
CFO: Donna Geiken Wallace, Chief Operating Officer and Chief Financial Officer
CMO: James D. Doughtie, M.D., Chief Medical Staff
CIO: Brandon Gauntt, Director Information Systems
CHR: Donna Rudzik, Director Human Resources
Web address: www.hcmh.com
Control: Hospital district or authority, Government, nonfederal **Service:** General Medical and Surgical

Staffed Beds: 54 **Admissions:** 4288 **Census:** 42 **Outpatient Visits:** 50350 **Births:** 910 **Total Expense ($000):** 35177 **Payroll Expense ($000):** 15508 **Personnel:** 443

SWEENY—Brazoria County

SWEENY COMMUNITY HOSPITAL (451311), 305 North McKinney Street, Zip 77480–2895; tel. 979/548–3311 **A**9 10 18 **F**3 7 10 11 31 33 38 40 52 54 57 61 67 68 79 86 93 94 96 102 107 119 121 122 132
Primary Contact: William H. Barnes, Administrator
CFO: Delores Merchant, Director Financial Services
CMO: David Barr, M.D., Chief of Staff
CIO: Stuart Butler, Director Information Technology
CHR: Grace Baty, Director Human Resources
Web address: www.sweenyhospital.org
Control: Hospital district or authority, Government, nonfederal **Service:** General Medical and Surgical

Staffed Beds: 14 **Admissions:** 198 **Census:** 1 **Outpatient Visits:** 17544 **Births:** 0 **Total Expense ($000):** 7359 **Payroll Expense ($000):** 4433 **Personnel:** 113

SWEETWATER—Nolan County

⊡ **ROLLING PLAINS MEMORIAL HOSPITAL (450055)**, 200 East Arizona Street, Zip 79556–7199, Mailing Address: P.O. Box 690, Zip 79556–0690; tel. 325/235–1701 **A**1 9 10 20 **F**8 11 13 15 24 30 31 38 40 61 68 74 79 80 84 86 87 96 97 102 107 119 121 122 135
Primary Contact: Thomas F. Kennedy, Administrator
COO: Thomas F. Kennedy, Administrator
CFO: Rhonda Moses, Senior Director Finance
CMO: Judy Clayton, Chief of Staff
CHR: Gay Nell Cherry, Director Human Resources
Web address: www.rpmh.net
Control: Hospital district or authority, Government, nonfederal **Service:** General Medical and Surgical

Staffed Beds: 54 **Admissions:** 1909 **Census:** 22 **Outpatient Visits:** 95565 **Births:** 274 **Total Expense ($000):** 19807 **Payroll Expense ($000):** 9392 **Personnel:** 251

TAHOKA—Lynn County

★ **LYNN COUNTY HOSPITAL DISTRICT (451351)**, 2600 Lockwood, Zip 79373–1310, Mailing Address: Box 1310, Zip 79373–1310; tel. 806/998–4533 **A**9 10 18 **F**3 7 10 13 24 25 28 33 36 38 40 41 52 53 54 55 56 57 62 63 64 73 74 81 84 86 87 96 122 133 136 137 **P**5 8
Primary Contact: Jimmy L. Morris, Chief Executive Officer and Administrator
CFO: Donna Raindl, Manager Business Office
CMO: Donald Freitag, M.D., Chief Medical Officer
CIO: Tim Pledger, Director Information Technology
CHR: Amy Schuknecht, Manager Human Resources
Web address: www.lchdhealthcare.org
Control: Hospital district or authority, Government, nonfederal **Service:** General Medical and Surgical

Staffed Beds: 19 **Admissions:** 159 **Census:** 3 **Outpatient Visits:** 18849 **Births:** 9 **Total Expense ($000):** 4473 **Payroll Expense ($000):** 2333 **Personnel:** 97

TAYLOR—Williamson County

☐ **JOHNS COMMUNITY HOSPITAL (451374)**, 305 Mallard Lane, Zip 76574–1208; tel. 512/352–7611 **A**1 9 10 18 **F**3 11 15 25 31 38 40 56 57 61 62 68 79 80 81 86 87 96 97 102 107 119 122 **P**6
Primary Contact: Ernest Balla, RN, Administrator
CIO: Tim Tarbell, Assistant Administrator Support Services
Web address: www.johnscommunityhospital.org
Control: Other not–for–profit (including NFP Corporation) **Service:** General Medical and Surgical

Staffed Beds: 25 **Admissions:** 872 **Census:** 14 **Outpatient Visits:** 57552 **Births:** 0 **Total Expense ($000):** 14947 **Payroll Expense ($000):** 7764 **Personnel:** 181

TEMPLE—Bell County

⊡ △ **CENTRAL TEXAS VETERANS HEALTHCARE SYSTEM**, 1901 Veterans Memorial Drive, Zip 76504–7493; tel. 254/778–4811, (Includes OLIN E. TEAGUE VETERANS' CENTER; WACO VETERANS AFFAIRS HOSPITAL, 4800 Memorial Drive, Waco, Zip 76711–1397; tel. 254/752–6581), (Total facility includes 320 beds in nursing home–type unit) (Nonreporting) **A**1 2 3 5 7 8 9 **S** Department of Veterans Affairs
Primary Contact: Bruce A. Gordon, Director
COO: Thomas C. Smith, FACHE, Associate Director Resources
CFO: Val Martin, Chief Finance Services
CIO: Sandra Wright, Acting Chief Information Technology Services
CHR: James Basso, Chief Human Resources Officer
Web address: www.central–texas.med.va.gov
Control: Veterans Affairs, Government, federal **Service:** General Medical and Surgical

Staffed Beds: 1852

⊡ **KING'S DAUGHTERS HOSPITAL (450008)**, 1901 S.W. H. K. Dodgen Loop, Zip 76502–1896; tel. 254/771–8600 **A**1 9 10 **F**3 11 13 18 20 22 24 25 26 27 30 31 32 33 38 46 47 49 51 55 57 59 61 62 66 68 71 72 73 74 77 79 80 81 82 84 86 92 96 97 100 102 106 107 118 119 121 124 132 135 136 137 **P**5
Primary Contact: Tucker Bonner, President
CFO: Eric Lashbrook, Vice President Finance
CIO: Brian Stanford, Vice President
CHR: Ben Coldicutt, Vice President
Web address: www.kdhosp.org
Control: Other not–for–profit (including NFP Corporation) **Service:** General Medical and Surgical

Staffed Beds: 120 **Admissions:** 2500 **Census:** 21 **Outpatient Visits:** 32954 **Births:** 724 **Total Expense ($000):** 35466 **Payroll Expense ($000):** 14263 **Personnel:** 322

OLIN E. TEAGUE VETERANS' CENTER See Central Texas Veterans Healthcare System

⊡ △ **SCOTT AND WHITE MEMORIAL HOSPITAL (450054)**, 2401 South 31st Street, Zip 76508–0002; tel. 254/724–2111, (Total facility includes 49 beds in nursing home–type unit) **A**1 2 3 5 7 8 9 10 **F**3 4 5 7 11 12 13 14 15 17 18 20 22 25 26 27 30 31 32 33 35 36 37 38 39 40 41 42 43 46 48 49 50 51 55 56 57 58 59 60 61 62 63 66 68 70 71 72 74 75 76 77 79 80 81 82 83 84 85 86 88 90 92 96 97 98 99 100 102 103 105 106 107 109 111 112 113 114 116 117 118 119 120 121 125 127 130 131 132 134 135 136 137 **P**3 **S** Scott & White
Primary Contact: Patricia M. Currie, FACHE, Chief Hospital Services
COO: Donny Sequin, Chief Operating Officer
CFO: Dennis Laraway, Chief Financial Officer
CMO: Robert W. Pryor, M.D., Chief Medical Officer
CIO: William McCombs, Ph.D., Chief Information Officer
Web address: www.sw.org
Control: Other not–for–profit (including NFP Corporation) **Service:** General Medical and Surgical

Staffed Beds: 562 **Admissions:** 25448 **Census:** 357 **Outpatient Visits:** 994345 **Births:** 2435 **Total Expense ($000):** 504987 **Payroll Expense ($000):** 203974 **Personnel:** 6782

TERRELL—Kaufman County

☐ **RENAISSANCE HOSPITAL TERRELL (450683)**, 1551 Highway 34 South, Zip 75160–4833; tel. 972/563–7611 **A**1 9 10 **F**3 8 13 15 25 26 31 32 38 50 51 57 62 66 68 73 74 77 79 80 81 82 96 100 102 107 118 119 135 136 **S** Renaissance Healthcare Systems
Primary Contact: Sean Astolfo, Administrator
CMO: Reba Williams–White, Chief of Staff
CIO: Paul Ferguson, Director Information Systems
CHR: Patsy Branscum, Director Human Resources
Web address: www.renhealthcare.org
Control: Corporation, Investor–owned, for–profit **Service:** General Medical and Surgical

Staffed Beds: 106 **Admissions:** 2413 **Census:** 21 **Outpatient Visits:** 20935 **Births:** 296 **Total Expense ($000):** 17560 **Payroll Expense ($000):** 8171 **Personnel:** 195

TX

Many Facility Codes have changed. Please refer to the AHA Guide Code Chart.

□ **TERRELL STATE HOSPITAL (454006)**, 1200 East Brin Street, Zip 75160–2938; tel. 972/524–6452 **A**1 3 5 10 **F**26 30 31 32 37 55 56 66 73 81 82 88 89 90 91 92 93 119 121 124 135 **P**6 **S** Texas Department of State Health Services
Primary Contact: Fred Hale, Superintendent
COO: Joe Finch, Assistant Superintendent
CFO: Perry Harwell, Chief Financial Officer
CMO: Anthony Claxton, M.D., Clinical Director
CIO: Lidonna Bevins, Manager Facility Automation
Web address: www.dshs.state.tx.us
Control: State–Government, nonfederal **Service:** Psychiatric

Staffed Beds: 316 **Admissions:** 2710 **Census:** 313 **Outpatient Visits:** 0 **Births:** 0 **Total Expense ($000):** 55676 **Payroll Expense ($000):** 31207 **Personnel:** 880

TEXARKANA—Bowie County

★ **CHRISTUS ST. MICHAEL HEALTH SYSTEM (450801)**, 2600 St. Michael Drive, Zip 75503–2372; tel. 903/614–1000 **A**1 2 9 10 **F**3 11 13 15 17 18 20 22 25 26 27 30 31 32 33 38 43 44 49 52 53 54 55 56 57 59 62 63 65 66 68 69 72 73 74 75 76 77 79 80 81 82 84 96 97 98 99 100 102 103 106 107 108 109 111 112 118 119 120 121 124 132 133 135 136 137 **P**8 **S** CHRISTUS Health
Primary Contact: Chris Karam, President and Chief Executive Officer
COO: John Phillips, Vice President and Chief Operating Officer
CFO: Shawn Barnett, Vice President and Chief Financial Officer
CMO: Mike Finley, M.D., Vice President Medical Affairs
CHR: Pam Kennedy, Regional Director Human Resources
Web address: www.christusstmichael.org
Control: Church–operated, Nongovernment, not–for profit **Service:** General Medical and Surgical

Staffed Beds: 312 **Admissions:** 18734 **Census:** 212 **Outpatient Visits:** 112777 **Births:** 1351 **Total Expense ($000):** 185806 **Payroll Expense ($000):** 64581 **Personnel:** 1562

★ **CHRISTUS ST. MICHAEL REHABILITATION HOSPITAL (453065)**, 2400 St. Michael Drive, Zip 75503; tel. 903/614–4000 **A**1 9 10 **F**3 11 24 25 26 30 31 32 43 55 56 57 63 66 73 75 77 80 82 85 86 121 132 137 **S** CHRISTUS Health
Primary Contact: Aloma Gender, RN, M.S.N., Administrator and Director Nursing
CFO: Shawn Barnett, Vice President and Chief Financial Officer
CMO: Richard Sharp, M.D., Medical Director
CHR: Pamela J. White, Manager Customer Relations
Web address: www.christusstmichael.org
Control: Church–operated, Nongovernment, not–for profit **Service:** Rehabilitation

Staffed Beds: 50 **Admissions:** 1299 **Census:** 39 **Outpatient Visits:** 24968 **Births:** 0 **Total Expense ($000):** 19594 **Payroll Expense ($000):** 8402 **Personnel:** 149

★ **DUBUIS HOSPITAL OF TEXARKANA (452061)**, 2400 St. Michael Drive, 2nd Floor, Zip 75503–2372; tel. 903/614–7600 **A**1 9 10 **F**1 3 25 31 32 43 44 75 81 82 119 137 **S** Dubuis Health System
Primary Contact: David L. Adcock, FACHE, Administrator
Web address: www.dubuis.org
Control: Other not–for–profit (including NFP Corporation) **Service:** Long–Term Acute Care hospital

Staffed Beds: 30 **Admissions:** 324 **Census:** 26 **Outpatient Visits:** 0 **Births:** 0 **Total Expense ($000):** 10808 **Payroll Expense ($000):** 3360 **Personnel:** 85

★ **HEALTHSOUTH REHABILITATION HOSPITAL OF TEXARKANA (453053)**, 515 West 12th Street, Zip 75501–4416; tel. 903/793–0088 **A**1 9 10 **F**24 25 30 31 32 53 62 72 75 77 82 85 86 119 120 121 132 136 137 **S** HEALTHSOUTH Corporation
Primary Contact: Joanne Rose, Chief Executive Officer
CFO: Robbi Hudson, Controller
CHR: Ann Clapp, Manager Human Resources
Web address: www.healthsouth.com
Control: Corporation, Investor–owned, for–profit **Service:** Rehabilitation

Staffed Beds: 60 **Admissions:** 896 **Census:** 33 **Outpatient Visits:** 16203 **Births:** 0 **Total Expense ($000):** 10573 **Payroll Expense ($000):** 5863 **Personnel:** 151

★ **WADLEY REGIONAL MEDICAL CENTER (450200)**, 1000 Pine Street, Zip 75501–5170, Mailing Address: Box 1878, Zip 75504–1878; tel. 903/798–8000, (Total facility includes 13 beds in nursing home–type unit) **A**1 2 9 10 **F**3 11 12 13 15 18 20 22 24 25 26 27 31 32 33 37 38 41 43 49 50 51 54 55 56 57 59 60 62 63 64 66 68 70 71 72 73 74 76 77 79 80 81 82 84 87 88 93 94 96 97 99 100 102 107 111 117 118 119 121 124 135 136 137 **P**8 **S** Community Hospital Corporation
Primary Contact: Mike Lieb, Interim Chief Executive Officer
COO: Mike Lieb, Executive Vice President and Chief Operating Officer
CFO: Milton E. Aunan, CPA, Chief Financial Officer
CMO: Johnny Colley, Chief of Staff
CIO: Dan Schumann, Chief Information Officer
CHR: Debby Butler, Director Human Resources
Web address: www.wadleyhealth.com
Control: Other not–for–profit (including NFP Corporation) **Service:** General Medical and Surgical

Staffed Beds: 163 **Admissions:** 9279 **Census:** 112 **Outpatient Visits:** 104730 **Births:** 1523 **Total Expense ($000):** 89598 **Payroll Expense ($000):** 35863 **Personnel:** 747

TEXAS CITY—Galveston County

★ **MAINLAND MEDICAL CENTER (450530)**, 6801 E F Lowry Expressway, Zip 77591; tel. 409/938–5000 **A**1 3 5 9 10 **F**5 11 13 15 25 31 32 33 36 37 38 41 42 43 44 50 54 55 57 61 62 66 68 72 73 74 75 76 77 79 81 82 85 86 87 88 90 91 92 93 94 95 96 97 100 105 107 119 120 121 124 133 135 136 137 **S** HCA
Primary Contact: Melinda Stephenson, Chief Executive Officer
COO: Xoych Hurtado, Chief Operating Officer
CFO: Scott Bentley, Chief Financial Officer
CIO: Ley Samson, Director Management Information Systems
CHR: Jennifer Johnson, Director Human Resources
Web address: www.mainlandmedical.com
Control: Partnership, Investor–owned, for–profit **Service:** General Medical and Surgical

Staffed Beds: 218 **Admissions:** 9482 **Census:** 118 **Outpatient Visits:** 101389 **Births:** 743 **Total Expense ($000):** 82813 **Payroll Expense ($000):** 38364 **Personnel:** 659

THE WOODLANDS—Montgomery County

□ **ST LUKE'S COMMUNITY MEDICAL CENTER–THE WOODLANDS (450862)**, 17200 St. Luke's Way, Zip 77384; tel. 936/266–2000 **A**1 9 10 **F**3 11 13 15 18 20 22 25 26 30 33 36 38 49 50 55 56 57 58 62 66 68 70 72 73 74 77 79 80 82 84 96 97 98 99 100 102 106 107 112 116 118 119 124 134 135 136 **P**5 **S** St. Luke's Episcopal Health System
Primary Contact: Debra F. Sukin, Chief Executive Officer
COO: Debra F. Sukin, Chief Executive Officer
CFO: Mary Sue Lipham, Controller
CMO: Daniel Grimmer, Chief of Staff
CHR: Mona Tucker, Director Human Resources
Web address: www.stlukeswoodlands.com
Control: Church–operated, Nongovernment, not–for profit **Service:** General Medical and Surgical

Staffed Beds: 91 **Admissions:** 6913 **Census:** 71 **Outpatient Visits:** 51850 **Births:** 1771 **Total Expense ($000):** 86577 **Payroll Expense ($000):** 29895 **Personnel:** 575

THROCKMORTON—Throckmorton County

★ **THROCKMORTON COUNTY MEMORIAL HOSPITAL (451339)**, 802 North Minter Street, Zip 76483–5357, Mailing Address: P.O. Box 729, Zip 76483–0729; tel. 940/849–2151, (Nonreporting) **A**9 10 18
Primary Contact: Robert R. King, Administrator and Chief Executive Officer
COO: Robert R. King, Administrator and Chief Executive Officer
CFO: Silvia A. Tipton, Chief Financial Officer and Director Human Resources
CMO: Craig Beasley, M.D., Chief of Staff and Medical Officer
CIO: Amber Myer, Director Medical Records
CHR: Silvia A. Tipton, Chief Financial Officer and Director Human Resources
Control: County–Government, nonfederal **Service:** General Medical and Surgical

Staffed Beds: 14

TX

Hospital, Medicare Provider Number, Address, Telephone, Approval, Facility, and Physician Codes, Health Care System

★ American Hospital Association (AHA) membership
□ The Joint Commission accreditation
○ American Osteopathic Association (AOA) accreditation
△ Commission on Accreditation of Rehabilitation Facilities (CARF) accreditation

TOMBALL—Harris County

⊞ △ **TOMBALL REGIONAL HOSPITAL (450670)**, 605 Holderrieth Street, Zip 77375–0889, Mailing Address: P.O. Box 889, Zip 77375–6445; tel. 281/401–7500 **A**1 7 9 10 **F**2 3 8 10 13 14 15 17 18 20 22 24 25 26 31 32 38 39 43 49 50 51 52 56 57 59 61 62 68 70 73 74 76 77 78 79 80 81 82 84 85 88 90 91 92 93 95 96 97 99 100 102 103 107 109 111 113 115 117 118 119 120 121 135 137 **P**8
Primary Contact: L. Lynn LeBouef, President and Chief Executive Officer
COO: Keith Barber, CPA, Chief Operating Officer and Chief Financial Officer
CFO: Keith Barber, CPA, Chief Operating Officer and Chief Financial Officer
CIO: Marlene Pezzia, Director
CHR: Marcia Moore, Vice President
Web address: www.tomballhospital.org
Control: Hospital district or authority, Government, nonfederal **Service:** General Medical and Surgical

Staffed Beds: 289 **Admissions:** 13024 **Census:** 189 **Outpatient Visits:** 77243 **Births:** 864 **Total Expense ($000):** 153051 **Payroll Expense ($000):** 64924 **Personnel:** 1337

TRINITY—Trinity County

★ **EAST TEXAS MEDICAL CENTER TRINITY (450749)**, 317 Prospect Drive, Zip 75862, Mailing Address: P.O. Box 3169, Zip 75862; tel. 936/594–3541 **A**9 10 **F**11 25 31 32 38 40 62 66 96 100 107 135 **P**3 5 7 **S** East Texas Medical Center Regional Healthcare System
Primary Contact: Warren Robicheaux, Administrator
COO: Warren Robicheaux, Administrator
CFO: Jerry A. Dominguez, CPA, Chief Financial Officer
CMO: Amol Desh–Pande, Chief of Staff
CHR: Kathy Turner, Director Human Resources
Web address: www.etmc.org
Control: Other not–for–profit (including NFP Corporation) **Service:** General Medical and Surgical

Staffed Beds: 22 **Admissions:** 714 **Census:** 8 **Outpatient Visits:** 25208 **Births:** 0 **Total Expense ($000):** 6208 **Payroll Expense ($000):** 2999 **Personnel:** 73

TROPHY CLUB—Denton County

□ **BAYLOR MEDICAL CENTER AT TROPHY CLUB (450883)**, 2850 South Highway,114E, Zip 76262; tel. 817/837–4600 **A**1 9 **F**3 12 25 38 77 79 80 82 96 97 100 102 106 109 111 121 130 133 **S** Cirrus Health
Primary Contact: Lynn Warren, Chief Executive Officer
Web address: www.tc–mc.com
Control: Partnership, Investor–owned, for–profit **Service:** General Medical and Surgical

Staffed Beds: 14 **Admissions:** 422 **Census:** 2 **Outpatient Visits:** 5713 **Births:** 0 **Total Expense ($000):** 23475 **Payroll Expense ($000):** 5004 **Personnel:** 123

TX

TULIA—Swisher County

★ **SWISHER MEMORIAL HOSPITAL DISTRICT (451349)**, 539 Southeast Second, Zip 79088–2403, Mailing Address: P.O. Box 808, Zip 79088–0808; tel. 806/995–3581, (Nonreporting) **A**9 10 18
Primary Contact: James E. Koulovatos, Chief Executive Officer
COO: Debbie King, Assistant Administrator
CFO: Connie Wilhelm, Chief Financial Officer
CIO: Brad Roberts, Network Administrator
Web address: www.swisherhospital.com
Control: Hospital district or authority, Government, nonfederal **Service:** General Medical and Surgical

Staffed Beds: 20

TYLER—Smith County

⊞ △ **EAST TEXAS MEDICAL CENTER REHABILITATION CENTER (453072)**, 701 Olympic Plaza Circle, Zip 75701–1996; tel. 903/596–3000 **A**1 7 9 10 **F**3 24 25 26 32 52 55 56 73 81 85 86 119 120 121 137 **S** East Texas Medical Center Regional Healthcare System
Primary Contact: Eddie L. Howard, Vice President and Chief Operating Officer
CFO: James Blanton, Chief Financial Officer
CMO: Jerry Schwarzbach, M.D., Medical Director
CIO: Paula Anthony, Vice President Information Services
CHR: Mike Gray, Corporate Vice President Human Resources
Web address: www.etmc.org
Control: Other not–for–profit (including NFP Corporation) **Service:** Rehabilitation

Staffed Beds: 49 **Admissions:** 1072 **Census:** 38 **Outpatient Visits:** 59278 **Births:** 0 **Total Expense ($000):** 21793 **Payroll Expense ($000):** 10221 **Personnel:** 215

⊞ **EAST TEXAS MEDICAL CENTER SPECIALTY HOSPITAL (452051)**, 1000 South Beckham, 5th Floor, Zip 75701; tel. 903/596–3600 **A**1 9 10 **F**1 3 25 26 31 44 73 119 137 **S** East Texas Medical Center Regional Healthcare System
Primary Contact: Eddie L. Howard, Vice President, Chief Operating Officer and Administrator
CFO: James Blanton, Chief Financial Officer
CMO: J. David Johnson, Chief of Staff
CIO: Paula Anthony, Vice President Information Services
CHR: Mike Gray, Corporate Vice President Human Resources
Web address: www.etmc.org
Control: Other not–for–profit (including NFP Corporation) **Service:** Long–Term Acute Care hospital

Staffed Beds: 36 **Admissions:** 348 **Census:** 28 **Outpatient Visits:** 0 **Births:** 0 **Total Expense ($000):** 11005 **Payroll Expense ($000):** 3799 **Personnel:** 77

⊞ **EAST TEXAS MEDICAL CENTER TYLER (450083)**, 1000 South Beckham Street, Zip 75701–1996, Mailing Address: Box 6400, Zip 75711–6400; tel. 903/597–0351, (Includes EAST TEXAS MEDICAL CENTER BEHAVIORAL HEALTH CENTER, 4101 University Boulevard, Zip 75701–6600; tel. 903/566–8668) **A**1 2 5 9 10 **F**3 5 8 11 12 13 15 17 18 20 22 25 26 27 30 32 33 36 38 39 40 43 44 46 47 48 49 51 53 54 57 58 59 60 62 63 66 68 69 71 72 73 74 76 77 78 79 80 81 82 84 86 88 89 90 91 92 93 94 95 96 99 100 102 103 105 106 107 108 109 111 112 116 118 119 121 127 130 135 136 137 **S** East Texas Medical Center Regional Healthcare System
Primary Contact: Robert B. Evans, Administrator and Chief Executive Officer
CFO: Byron Hale, Chief Financial Officer
CMO: Duane Andrews, Chief of Staff
CIO: Paula Anthony, Vice President Information Services
CHR: Mike Gray, Corporate Vice President Human Resources
Web address: www.etmc.org
Control: Other not–for–profit (including NFP Corporation) **Service:** General Medical and Surgical

Staffed Beds: 422 **Admissions:** 20852 **Census:** 283 **Outpatient Visits:** 142499 **Births:** 685 **Total Expense ($000):** 296740 **Payroll Expense ($000):** 105201 **Personnel:** 3326

TEXAS SPINE & JOINT HOSPITAL (450864), 1814 Roseland Boulevard, Suite 100, Zip 75701; tel. 903/526–8754 **A**10 **F**3 8 25 30 37 38 43 75 77 79 80 81 96 100 135
Primary Contact: Tony Wahl, Chief Executive Officer
CFO: Greg Cummings, Chief Operating Officer and Chief Financial Officer
CMO: James Michaels, M.D., Chief of Staff
CHR: Sally Stuart, Manager Human Resources
Web address: www.tsjh.org
Control: Partnership, Investor–owned, for–profit **Service:** Orthopedic

Staffed Beds: 20 **Admissions:** 1388 **Census:** 10 **Outpatient Visits:** 13472 **Births:** 0 **Total Expense ($000):** 33917 **Payroll Expense ($000):** 8286 **Personnel:** 202

⊞ **TRINITY MOTHER FRANCES HEALTH SYSTEM (450102)**, 910 East Houston, Suite 500, Zip 75702–8369; tel. 903/593–8441 **A**1 2 9 10 **F**3 8 11 12 13 15 17 18 20 22 24 25 26 27 28 30 31 32 38 40 43 46 49 50 51 52 53 56 59 62 64 66 68 71 72 73 74 75 76 77 78 79 80 81 82 84 86 92 96 97 99 100 102 103 107 114 116 118 119 120 121 123 133 135 136 137 **P**5 6 7 8
Primary Contact: J. Lindsey Bradley, Jr., FACHE, President and Chief Administrative Officer
COO: Ray Thompson, Executive Vice President and Chief Operating Officer
CFO: William L. Bellenfant, Chief Financial Officer
CMO: David Teegarden, M.D., President and Chief Medical Officer
CIO: Lee Portwood, Vice President
CHR: Laura Owen, Senior Vice President
Web address: www.tmfhs.org
Control: Other not–for–profit (including NFP Corporation) **Service:** General Medical and Surgical

Staffed Beds: 370 **Admissions:** 20524 **Census:** 255 **Outpatient Visits:** 252395 **Births:** 2937 **Total Expense ($000):** 297544 **Payroll Expense ($000):** 103836 **Personnel:** 2553

⊞ **TRINITY MOTHER FRANCES REHABILITATION HOSPITAL (453056)**, (Formerly HEALTHSOUTH Rehabilitation Hospital–Tyler), 3131 Troup Highway, Zip 75701–8352; tel. 903/510–7000 **A**1 9 10 **F**9 24 25 30 31 32 43 54 61 62 72 75 77 82 85 86 119 120 121 132 136 137
S HEALTHSOUTH Corporation
Primary Contact: Sharla Anderson, Chief Executive Officer
CFO: Michael G. Treadway, Controller
CMO: Bradley Merritt, M.D., Medical Director
Web address: www.healthsouth.com
Control: Partnership, Investor–owned, for–profit **Service:** Rehabilitation

Staffed Beds: 62 **Admissions:** 1424 **Census:** 54 **Outpatient Visits:** 10122 **Births:** 0 **Total Expense ($000):** 13295 **Payroll Expense ($000):** 7606 **Personnel:** 163

TYLER CONTINUECARE HOSPITAL AT MOTHER FRANCES (452091), 800 East Dawson, 4th Floor, Zip 75701; tel. 903/531–4942 **A**10 **F**1 3 25 72 73 75 80 81 119 137
Primary Contact: Carl Lutz, Interim Chief Executive Officer
Web address: www.continuecare.org
Control: Other not–for–profit (including NFP Corporation) **Service:** Long–Term Acute Care hospital

Staffed Beds: 51 **Admissions:** 619 **Census:** 45 **Outpatient Visits:** 0 **Births:** 0 **Total Expense ($000):** 17938 **Payroll Expense ($000):** 7054 **Personnel:** 136

★□ **UNIVERSITY OF TEXAS HEALTH SCIENCE CENTER AT TYLER (450690)**, (Formerly University of Texas Health Center at Tyler), 11937 Highway 271, Zip 75708–3154; tel. 903/877–3451 **A**1 3 5 9 10 **F**3 8 11 15 18 20 22 25 26 27 28 31 32 33 38 49 50 52 54 55 56 57 58 62 63 66 68 72 73 75 76 79 80 81 82 86 87 94 96 100 103 105 107 118 119 121 123 124 135 136 137 **P**6 **S** University of Texas System
Primary Contact: Kirk A. Calhoun, M.D., President
COO: Robert Marshall, Vice President and Chief Operating Officer
CFO: Vernon Moore, Chief Business and Finance
CMO: David Coultas, M.D., Vice President Clinical Affairs
CIO: Vernon Moore, Chief Business and Finance
Web address: www.uthct.edu
Control: State–Government, nonfederal **Service:** General Medical and Surgical

Staffed Beds: 114 **Admissions:** 2521 **Census:** 35 **Outpatient Visits:** 154397 **Births:** 0 **Total Expense ($000):** 116328 **Payroll Expense ($000):** 52374 **Personnel:** 830

UVALDE—Uvalde County

★ **UVALDE COUNTY HOSPITAL AUTHORITY (450177)**, 1025 Garner Field Road, Zip 78801–1025; tel. 830/278–6251 **A**5 9 10 20 **F**3 11 13 15 17 25 26 27 31 32 37 38 40 42 50 53 54 55 57 62 65 68 71 74 79 80 81 82 83 84 85 86 94 96 97 100 102 106 107 119 121 122 135 136 137 **P**5
Primary Contact: James E. Buckner, Jr., CHE, Administrator
CFO: Valerie Lopez, CPA, Controller
CIO: Carolina Velasquez, Chief Information Officer
CHR: Charla Carter, Director Human Resources
Web address: www.umhtx.org
Control: Hospital district or authority, Government, nonfederal **Service:** General Medical and Surgical

Staffed Beds: 48 **Admissions:** 2198 **Census:** 24 **Outpatient Visits:** 57103 **Births:** 425 **Total Expense ($000):** 32944 **Payroll Expense ($000):** 15584 **Personnel:** 375

VAN HORN—Culberson County

★ **CULBERSON HOSPITAL (451338)**, Eisenhower–Farm Market Road 2185, Zip 79855, Mailing Address: P.O. Box 609, Zip 79855–0609; tel. 432/283–2760 **A**9 10 18 **F**7 11 31 38 55 86 96 107 122 137 **P**8 **S** Preferred Management Corporation
Primary Contact: Ladelle Bates, Chief Executive Officer
CMO: Paul E. Jackson, M.D., Chief Medical Staff
Control: Corporation, Investor–owned, for–profit **Service:** General Medical and Surgical

Staffed Beds: 14 **Admissions:** 250 **Census:** 2 **Outpatient Visits:** 4173 **Births:** 0 **Total Expense ($000):** 2952 **Payroll Expense ($000):** 1798 **Personnel:** 40

VERNON—Wilbarger County

□ **NORTH TEXAS STATE HOSPITAL (454008)**, Highway 70 Northwest, Zip 76384, Mailing Address: P.O. Box 2231, Zip 76384–2231; tel. 940/552–9901 **A**1 10 **F**11 26 30 31 32 37 41 54 55 66 73 81 82 88 89 93 119 121 124 135 **P**6 **S** Texas Department of State Health Services
Primary Contact: James E. Smith, Superintendent
Web address: www.mhmr.state.tx.us
Control: State–Government, nonfederal **Service:** Psychiatric

Staffed Beds: 616 **Admissions:** 2240 **Census:** 552 **Outpatient Visits:** 0 **Births:** 0 **Total Expense ($000):** 107246 **Payroll Expense ($000):** 61640 **Personnel:** 1972

WILBARGER GENERAL HOSPITAL (450584), 920 Hillcrest Drive, Zip 76384–3196; tel. 940/552–9351 **A**9 10 20 **F**3 11 15 25 30 31 32 33 38 43 54 55 56 59 61 68 79 80 81 82 84 86 93 96 100 102 107 119 121 122 124 137 **P**5
Primary Contact: Jonathon Voelkel, Administrator
CFO: Richard Thieman, Chief Financial Officer
Web address: www.wghospital.com
Control: Hospital district or authority, Government, nonfederal **Service:** General Medical and Surgical

Staffed Beds: 47 **Admissions:** 1260 **Census:** 12 **Outpatient Visits:** 29468 **Births:** 0 **Total Expense ($000):** 13759 **Payroll Expense ($000):** 5662 **Personnel:** 178

VICTORIA—Victoria County

★□ **CITIZENS MEDICAL CENTER (450023)**, 2701 Hospital Drive, Zip 77901–5749; tel. 361/573–9181, (Total facility includes 20 beds in nursing home–type unit) **A**1 2 9 10 **F**1 3 4 8 11 12 13 15 16 17 18 19 20 21 22 23 24 25 26 27 30 31 32 33 36 38 40 49 50 51 52 53 54 55 56 57 61 62 63 64 65 68 70 71 72 73 74 75 76 77 78 79 80 81 82 83 84 85 86 87 88 90 91 92 93 95 96 97 98 100 102 103 105 106 107 109 117 119 120 121 124 133 135 136 137 **P**6 8
Primary Contact: David P. Brown, Administrator
CFO: Phillip Hacker, Chief Financial Officer
CHR: Jim Heger, Director Human Resources
Web address: www.citizensmedicalcenter.org
Control: County–Government, nonfederal **Service:** General Medical and Surgical

Staffed Beds: 296 **Admissions:** 10518 **Census:** 143 **Outpatient Visits:** 98996 **Births:** 1011 **Total Expense ($000):** 112489 **Payroll Expense ($000):** 47582 **Personnel:** 1085

★□ **DETAR HEALTHCARE SYSTEM (450147)**, 506 East San Antonio Street, Zip 77901–6060, Mailing Address: P.O. Box 2089, Zip 77902–2089; tel. 361/575–7441, (Includes DETAR HOSPITAL NORTH, 101 Medical Drive, Zip 77904–3198; tel. 361/573–6100; William R. Blanchard, Chief Executive Officer), (Total facility includes 16 beds in nursing home–type unit) **A**1 9 10 **F**3 13 15 18 20 22 24 25 26 27 30 31 32 33 37 38 40 43 51 52 54 62 66 68 70 72 73 74 75 76 77 79 80 81 82 84 85 86 92 96 97 100 102 103 104 106 107 117 119 121 135 136 **P**3 5 7 8 **S** Community Health Systems, Inc.
Primary Contact: William R. Blanchard, Chief Executive Officer
COO: America Sherwood, Assistant Chief Executive Officer
CFO: Donald E. Hagan, Chief Financial Officer
CMO: William Hilbert, M.D., Chief of Staff
CIO: Kim Tompkins, Director Information Services
CHR: Kristina Toliusis, Director Human Resources
Web address: www.detar.com
Control: Corporation, Investor–owned, for–profit **Service:** General Medical and Surgical

Staffed Beds: 228 **Admissions:** 9426 **Census:** 113 **Outpatient Visits:** 79681 **Births:** 1371 **Total Expense ($000):** 101368 **Payroll Expense ($000):** 37583 **Personnel:** 807

□ **TRIUMPH HOSPITAL OF VICTORIA (452056)**, 506 East San Antonio Street, 3rd Floor, Zip 77901–6060, Mailing Address: 506 East San Antonio Street, 3rd Floor, Zip 77901–6060; tel. 361/575–1445 **A**1 9 10 **F**1 3 25 26 27 31 32 43 80 81 82 119 137 **S** Triumph HealthCare
Primary Contact: Tammy Barben, Chief Executive Officer
Web address: www.triumph–healthcare.com
Control: Corporation, Investor–owned, for–profit **Service:** Long–Term Acute Care hospital

Staffed Beds: 23 **Admissions:** 257 **Census:** 19 **Outpatient Visits:** 0 **Births:** 0 **Personnel:** 59

□ **VICTORIA WARM SPRINGS HOSPITAL (452094)**, 102 Medical Drive, Zip 77904; tel. 361/576–6200 **A**1 9 10 **F**1 3 25 73 75 80 86 121 124 137 **S** Vibra Healthcare
Primary Contact: Anne R. Leon, Administrator
CFO: Jim Asberry, Chief Financial Officer
CMO: John McNeill, Medical Director
CHR: Aimee Fehaver, Area Manager Human Resources
Web address: www.warmsprings.org
Control: Partnership, Investor–owned, for–profit **Service:** Long–Term Acute Care hospital

Staffed Beds: 26 **Admissions:** 367 **Census:** 22 **Outpatient Visits:** 3037 **Births:** 0 **Total Expense ($000):** 9032 **Payroll Expense ($000):** 3736 **Personnel:** 95

TX

Hospital, Medicare Provider Number, Address, Telephone, Approval, Facility, and Physician Codes, Health Care System

★ American Hospital Association (AHA) membership
□ The Joint Commission accreditation
○ American Osteopathic Association (AOA) accreditation
△ Commission on Accreditation of Rehabilitation Facilities (CARF) accreditation

WACO—McLennan County

☐ **DEPAUL CENTER (454032)**, 301 Londonderry Drive, Zip 76712; tel. 254/776–5970, (Nonreporting) **A**1 10 **S** Ascension Health
Web address: www.providence.ne/depaul
Control: Other not–for–profit (including NFP Corporation) **Service:** Psychiatric

Staffed Beds: 64

★ △ **HILLCREST BAPTIST MEDICAL CENTER (450101)**, 3000 Herring Avenue, Zip 76708–3299, Mailing Address: P.O. Box 5100, Zip 76708–0100; tel. 254/202–2000 **A**1 3 5 7 9 10 **F**3 8 9 11 12 13 15 17 18 20 22 24 25 26 27 30 31 32 38 40 42 43 48 49 50 51 52 53 54 55 56 57 58 59 60 61 62 63 66 68 70 72 73 74 75 76 77 78 79 80 81 82 84 85 86 92 96 97 100 102 103 104 105 106 107 113 118 119 120 121 133 134 135 136
Primary Contact: Glenn A. Robinson, Chief Executive Officer
COO: Jim Gebhart, FACHE, Chief Operating Officer
CFO: Richard Perkins, Chief Financial Officer
CIO: Richard Warren, Chief Information Officer
CHR: Bob Brace, Director Human Resources
Web address: www.hillcrest.net
Control: Church–operated, Nongovernment, not–for profit **Service:** General Medical and Surgical

Staffed Beds: 263 **Admissions:** 12043 **Census:** 149 **Outpatient Visits:** 177785 **Births:** 2524 **Total Expense ($000):** 160713 **Payroll Expense ($000):** 61763 **Personnel:** 1218

★ **PROVIDENCE HEALTH CENTER (450042)**, 6901 Medical Parkway, Zip 76712–7998, Mailing Address: P.O. Box 2589, Zip 76702–2589; tel. 254/751–4000, (Total facility includes 341 beds in nursing home–type unit) **A**1 2 3 5 9 10 **F**2 3 4 5 6 9 10 11 12 13 18 20 22 24 25 26 27 30 31 32 33 35 36 37 38 48 49 52 53 54 55 56 57 58 60 61 62 65 66 68 72 73 74 75 76 77 79 80 81 82 84 86 87 88 89 90 91 92 93 94 95 96 97 102 107 115 117 119 121 124 133 135 136 137 **P**5 6 **S** Ascension Health
Primary Contact: Kent A. Keahey, President and Chief Executive Officer
COO: Odis W. Nichols, Senior Vice President and Chief Operating Officer
CFO: Cheryl Sadro, Senior Vice President and Chief Financial Officer
CMO: T. Marc Barrett, Senior Vice President Medical Affairs
CIO: Jay Scherler, Director Information Systems and Vice President Business Services
CHR: Douglas J. Lennier, Vice President Human Resources
Web address: www.providence.net
Control: Church–operated, Nongovernment, not–for profit **Service:** General Medical and Surgical

Staffed Beds: 603 **Admissions:** 16682 **Census:** 493 **Outpatient Visits:** 247907 **Births:** 1487 **Total Expense ($000):** 186165 **Payroll Expense ($000):** 74412 **Personnel:** 1975

WACO VETERANS AFFAIRS HOSPITAL See Central Texas Veterans Healthcare System, Temple

TX

WAXAHACHIE—Ellis County

★ **BAYLOR MEDICAL CENTER AT WAXAHACHIE (450372)**, 1405 West Jefferson Street, Zip 75165–2275; tel. 972/923–7000 **A**1 9 10 **F**1 3 4 11 12 13 15 16 17 24 25 26 30 32 38 52 55 62 65 68 70 71 73 74 75 77 78 79 80 83 84 85 86 88 96 97 99 100 102 107 108 117 119 121 124 132 136 **S** Baylor Health Care System
Primary Contact: Jay Fox, President
CFO: Steve Roussel, Vice President Finance
CMO: Watson Roye, M.D., President Medical Staff
CIO: Gary Beazley, Coordinator Information Systems
Web address: www.bhcs.com
Control: Other not–for–profit (including NFP Corporation) **Service:** General Medical and Surgical

Staffed Beds: 56 **Admissions:** 3962 **Census:** 34 **Outpatient Visits:** 66670 **Births:** 858 **Total Expense ($000):** 53913 **Payroll Expense ($000):** 19520 **Personnel:** 322

WEATHERFORD—Parker County

★ **WEATHERFORD REGIONAL MEDICAL CENTER (450203)**, (Formerly Campbell Health System), 713 East Anderson Street, Zip 76086–9971; tel. 817/596–8751 **A**1 9 10 **F**3 13 17 24 25 27 30 31 32 33 38 40 49 52 55 57 61 68 73 74 75 76 77 79 80 86 96 97 100 102 107 119 121 122 124 135 137 **P**8 **S** Community Health Systems, Inc.
Primary Contact: Donnie L. Romine, Chief Executive Officer
CFO: Nancy Cooke, Chief Financial Officer
CMO: Jon–Paul Harmer, Chief Medical Staff
CIO: Merri Kober, Director Information Service
CHR: Richard Aguirre, Administrative Director Human Resources
Web address: www.weatherfordregional.com
Control: Corporation, Investor–owned, for–profit **Service:** General Medical and Surgical

Staffed Beds: 74 **Admissions:** 4962 **Census:** 46 **Outpatient Visits:** 64352 **Births:** 620 **Total Expense ($000):** 55385 **Payroll Expense ($000):** 20751 **Personnel:** 441

WEBSTER—Harris County

★ **CLEAR LAKE REGIONAL MEDICAL CENTER (450617)**, 500 Medical Center Boulevard, Zip 77598–4286; tel. 281/332–2511, (Includes ALVIN DIAGNOSTIC AND URGENT CARE CENTER, 301 Medic Lane, Alvin, Zip 77511–5597; tel. 281/331–6141) **A**1 5 9 10 **F**1 3 4 11 13 15 16 17 18 20 22 24 25 27 30 31 32 33 38 39 45 47 49 50 51 53 55 56 57 59 62 65 68 70 71 72 73 74 75 76 77 78 79 80 81 82 83 84 85 86 88 96 97 100 102 103 107 112 117 118 119 135 136 137 **S** HCA
Primary Contact: Donald A. Shaffett, Chief Executive Officer
COO: Randy Gross, Chief Operating Officer
CFO: Jeff Sliwinski, Chief Financial Officer
CMO: Richard Marietta, M.D., Medical Director
CIO: Ley Samson, Director Management Information Systems
CHR: Brad Horst, Director Human Resources
Web address: www.clearlakermc.com
Control: Partnership, Investor–owned, for–profit **Service:** General Medical and Surgical

Staffed Beds: 543 **Admissions:** 19237 **Census:** 259 **Outpatient Visits:** 137327 **Births:** 3900 **Total Expense ($000):** 190737 **Payroll Expense ($000):** 81204 **Personnel:** 1422

★ **CLEAR LAKE REHABILITATION HOSPITAL (453052)**, 655 East Medical Center Boulevard, Zip 77598–4328; tel. 281/286–1500 **A**1 9 10 **F**3 25 62 72 73 77 85 86 119 120 121 132 137 **S** RehabCare Group, Inc.
Primary Contact: Susan Schaetti, Interim Chief Executive Officer
CFO: Barbara Franco, Chief Financial Officer
CMO: Michael Rosenblatt, M.D., Medical Director
CIO: Barbara Franco, Chief Financial Officer
CHR: Dalia Nandin, Human Resources Manager
Web address: www.rehabcare.com
Control: Corporation, Investor–owned, for–profit **Service:** Rehabilitation

Staffed Beds: 59 **Admissions:** 1033 **Census:** 40 **Outpatient Visits:** 9557 **Births:** 0 **Total Expense ($000):** 13240 **Payroll Expense ($000):** 7094 **Personnel:** 155

WEIMAR—Colorado County

★ **COLORADO–FAYETTE MEDICAL CENTER (450438)**, 400 Youens Drive, Zip 78962–9561; tel. 979/725–9531 **A**3 5 9 10 **F**10 11 15 25 30 31 32 38 55 61 77 78 79 86 96 100 102 107 119 122 135
Primary Contact: Shannon McBride, Chief Executive Officer
COO: Betty Wick, Assistant Administrator
CFO: David Austin, Chief Financial Officer
CMO: Juan Carlos Ortega, M.D., Chief of Staff
Web address: www.cfmc–online.com
Control: Other not–for–profit (including NFP Corporation) **Service:** General Medical and Surgical

Staffed Beds: 24 **Admissions:** 909 **Census:** 11 **Outpatient Visits:** 36768 **Births:** 0 **Total Expense ($000):** 10217 **Payroll Expense ($000):** 3746 **Personnel:** 132

WELLINGTON—Collingsworth County

★ **COLLINGSWORTH GENERAL HOSPITAL (451355)**, 1014 15th Street, Zip 79095–3704, Mailing Address: P.O. Box 1112, Zip 79095–1112; tel. 806/447–2521 **A**9 10 18 **F**28 31 34 38 40 55 57 63 64 66 73 86 87 96 102 120 122 **S** Preferred Management Corporation
Primary Contact: Candy Powell, Administrator
CFO: Wanda Breedlove, Chief Financial Officer
CMO: John H. Thomas, M.D., Chief of Staff
Control: Corporation, Investor–owned, for–profit **Service:** General Medical and Surgical

Staffed Beds: 16 **Admissions:** 408 **Census:** 4 **Outpatient Visits:** 4886 **Births:** 1 **Total Expense ($000):** 2966 **Payroll Expense ($000):** 1340 **Personnel:** 52

WESLACO—Hidalgo County

★ **KNAPP MEDICAL CENTER (450128)**, 1401 East Eighth Street, Zip 78596–6640, Mailing Address: P.O. Box 1110, Zip 78599–1110; tel. 956/968–8567 **A**1 5 9 10 **F**3 8 11 12 13 15 25 26 27 32 33 37 38 40 41 42 43 44 47 49 50 51 54 55 56 57 59 62 68 71 72 73 74 75 76 77 79 80 81 82 84 86 96 97 99 100 102 106 107 119 120 121 123 124 132 135 136 137 **P**8
Primary Contact: James A. Summersett, III, FACHE, President and Chief Executive Officer
CFO: Curtis F. Haley, Chief Financial Officer
CIO: Gary Light, Chief Information Officer
Web address: www.knappmed.org
Control: Other not–for–profit (including NFP Corporation) **Service:** General Medical and Surgical

Staffed Beds: 202 **Admissions:** 12468 **Census:** 114 **Outpatient Visits:** 67458 **Births:** 1915 **Total Expense ($000):** 88983 **Payroll Expense ($000):** 36939 **Personnel:** 873

 Many Facility Codes have changed. Please refer to the AHA Guide Code Chart.

WESLACO REHABILITATION HOSPITAL (453091), 906 South James Street, Zip 78596; tel. 956/969–2222 **A**10 **F**3 85 **P**5
Primary Contact: Maggie E. Barreiro, Administrator
CMO: Pedro McDougal, M.D., Medical Director
CHR: Debbie Pendleton, Human Resources Specialist
Web address: www.weslacorehabhospital.com
Control: Partnership, Investor–owned, for–profit **Service:** Rehabilitation

Staffed Beds: 26 **Admissions:** 583 **Census:** 16 **Outpatient Visits:** 0 **Births:** 0 **Total Expense ($000):** 3046 **Payroll Expense ($000):** 1695 **Personnel:** 70

WHARTON—Wharton County

☐ **GULF COAST MEDICAL CENTER (450214)**, 10141 Highway 59, Zip 77488–3004; tel. 979/532–2500 **A**1 9 10 **F**11 18 20 25 30 31 32 38 40 43 49 62 68 74 75 76 77 79 86 96 97 102 106 107 109 118 119 135 **S** Signature Hospital Corporation
Primary Contact: Martin R. Slack, Chief Executive Officer
CFO: Gary Williams, Chief Financial Officer
CHR: Loretta Flynn, Director Human Resources
Web address: www.gulfcoastmedical.com
Control: Partnership, Investor–owned, for–profit **Service:** General Medical and Surgical

Staffed Beds: 96 **Admissions:** 2671 **Census:** 27 **Outpatient Visits:** 23502 **Births:** 565 **Total Expense ($000):** 28516 **Payroll Expense ($000):** 11706 **Personnel:** 225

WHEELER—Wheeler County

★ **PARKVIEW HOSPITAL (451334)**, 1000 Sweetwater Street, Zip 79096, Mailing Address: P.O. Box 1030, Zip 79096–1030; tel. 806/826–5581 **A**9 10 18 **F**3 7 10 30 31 37 38 40 55 61 63 66 86 96 102 107 119 122 137 **P**5
Primary Contact: Ann Fagan–Cook, Administrator and Chief Executive Officer
CIO: Sheryl Lane, Chief Information Officer
Web address: www.parkviewhosp.org
Control: Hospital district or authority, Government, nonfederal **Service:** General Medical and Surgical

Staffed Beds: 16 **Admissions:** 290 **Census:** 3 **Outpatient Visits:** 2866 **Births:** 0 **Total Expense ($000):** 4615 **Payroll Expense ($000):** 2094 **Personnel:** 65

WHITNEY—Hill County

LAKE WHITNEY MEDICAL CENTER (450270), 200 North San Jacinto Street, Zip 76692–2388, Mailing Address: P.O. Box 458, Zip 76692–0458; tel. 254/694–3165 **A**9 10 **F**3 5 7 11 33 38 55 61 62 63 66 82 84 85 89 90 91 92 93 94 96 102 119 122 135 137 **P**5 6
Primary Contact: Aman A. Shah, M.D., Administrator
COO: Tariq Mahmood, Chief Executive Officer
CFO: Joe White, Chief Financial Officer
CMO: Aman A. Shah, M.D., Administrator
CHR: Darleen Towers, Director Human Resources
Web address: www.lakewhitneychamber.com
Control: Corporation, Investor–owned, for–profit **Service:** General Medical and Surgical

Staffed Beds: 28 **Admissions:** 998 **Census:** 8 **Outpatient Visits:** 10685 **Births:** 0 **Total Expense ($000):** 6717 **Payroll Expense ($000):** 2667 **Personnel:** 124

WICHITA FALLS—Wichita County

★☐ **HEALTHSOUTH REHABILITATION HOSPITAL–WICHITA FALLS (453054)**, 3901 Armory Road, Zip 76302–2204; tel. 940/720–5700 **A**1 9 10 **F**3 25 26 31 32 34 41 43 50 55 56 57 66 72 73 75 77 81 82 85 86 121 132 135 137 **S** HEALTHSOUTH Corporation
Primary Contact: Michael L. Bullitt, Chief Executive Officer
COO: Michael L. Bullitt, Chief Executive Officer
CFO: John E. Bailey, Chief Financial Officer
CMO: Virgil Frardo, M.D., Medical Director
CHR: Kathleen Pirtle, Manager Human Resources
Web address: www.healthsouth.com
Control: Partnership, Investor–owned, for–profit **Service:** Rehabilitation

Staffed Beds: 63 **Admissions:** 1250 **Census:** 49 **Outpatient Visits:** 9956 **Births:** 0 **Total Expense ($000):** 12164 **Payroll Expense ($000):** 6533 **Personnel:** 170

☐ **KELL WEST REGIONAL HOSPITAL (450827)**, 5420 Kell West Boulevard, Zip 76310–1610; tel. 940/692–5888 **A**1 9 10 **F**3 30 31 32 38 43 49 50 51 72 73 76 77 79 80 82 96 102 107 108 119 134 **P**5
Primary Contact: Jerry Myers, M.D., Chief Executive Officer
COO: Diane Stewart, Chief Nursing Executive
CFO: Fran Lindemann, Director Finance
Web address: www.kellwest.com
Control: Partnership, Investor–owned, for–profit **Service:** General Medical and Surgical

Staffed Beds: 41 **Admissions:** 1461 **Census:** 16 **Outpatient Visits:** 25936 **Births:** 0 **Total Expense ($000):** 17442 **Payroll Expense ($000):** 6955 **Personnel:** 224

☐ **NORTH TEXAS STATE HOSPITAL, WICHITA FALLS CAMPUS (454008)**, 6515 Lake Road, Zip 76308–5419, Mailing Address: Box 300, Zip 76307–0300; tel. 940/692–1220, (Nonreporting) **A**1 10
Primary Contact: James E. Smith, Superintendent
CFO: Lisa Henry, Chief Financial Officer
Web address: www.mhmr.state.tx.us
Control: State–Government, nonfederal **Service:** Psychiatric

Staffed Beds: 381

☐ **RED RIVER HOSPITAL (454018)**, 1505 Eighth Street, Zip 76301–3106; tel. 940/322–3171 **A**1 9 10 **F**4 5 25 31 73 81 82 88 89 91 92 93 94 95 119 121 **S** SeniorHealth Incorporated
Primary Contact: Murray Browning, Chief Executive Officer
CFO: Doug Selser, Chief Financial Officer
CMO: Harvey C. Martin, M.D., Medical Director
CHR: Tracey Fehr, Executive Assistant and Director Human Resources
Web address: www.redriverhospital.com
Control: Partnership, Investor–owned, for–profit **Service:** Psychiatric

Staffed Beds: 66 **Admissions:** 1480 **Census:** 52 **Outpatient Visits:** 447 **Births:** 0 **Total Expense ($000):** 7402 **Payroll Expense ($000):** 4012 **Personnel:** 110

☐ **TEXAS SPECIALTY HOSPITAL AT WICHITA FALLS (452068)**, 1103 Grace Street, Zip 76301–4414; tel. 940/720–6633 **A**1 9 10 **F**1 3 25 26 27 43 54 73 75 80 81 82 90 119 132 137 **S** Fundamental Long Term Care Holdings, LLC
Primary Contact: Billy Blasingame, Administrator
Web address: www.thicare.com
Control: Corporation, Investor–owned, for–profit **Service:** Long–Term Acute Care hospital

Staffed Beds: 31 **Admissions:** 284 **Census:** 20 **Outpatient Visits:** 0 **Births:** 0 **Total Expense ($000):** 6941 **Payroll Expense ($000):** 2897 **Personnel:** 77

★☐ **UNITED REGIONAL HEALTH CARE SYSTEM (450010)**, 1600 Tenth Street, Zip 76301–4307; tel. 940/764–7000, (Includes UNITED REGIONAL HEALTH CARE SYSTEM–EIGHTH STREET CAMPUS, 1600 Eighth Street, Zip 76301–3164; UNITED REGIONAL HEALTH CARE SYSTEM–ELEVENTH STREET CAMPUS, 1600 11th Street, Zip 76301–9988; tel. 940/764–0055) **A**1 2 3 5 9 10 **F**3 11 12 13 15 17 18 19 20 22 24 25 26 27 28 30 31 32 33 37 38 40 41 43 46 47 48 49 50 51 52 55 56 57 59 60 62 63 66 68 71 72 73 74 75 76 77 78 79 80 81 82 84 86 92 96 97 99 100 102 103 104 105 106 107 108 109 110 111 112 118 119 120 121 123 133 135 136 137 **P**3
Primary Contact: Phyllis A. Cowling, President and Chief Executive Officer
COO: Nancy Townley, R.N., Senior Vice President Operations
CFO: Robert M. Pert, Vice President Finance and Chief Financial Officer
CIO: Jerry Marshall, Director Information Systems
CHR: Kristi Faulkner, Director Human Resources
Web address: www.urhcs.org
Control: Other not–for–profit (including NFP Corporation) **Service:** General Medical and Surgical

Staffed Beds: 346 **Admissions:** 16470 **Census:** 193 **Outpatient Visits:** 116930 **Births:** 2361 **Total Expense ($000):** 205236 **Payroll Expense ($000):** 83816 **Personnel:** 1584

WINNIE—Chambers County

WINNIE COMMUNITY HOSPITAL (451328), 538 Broadway, Zip 77665–1249, Mailing Address: P.O. Box 1249, Zip 77665–1249; tel. 409/296–6000 **A**9 10 18 **F**3 25 38 56 57 63 96 122 135 **P**6
Primary Contact: Shalia Hampton, Administrator
CFO: Rachal Reel, Chief Financial Officer
CMO: Mai El Mallah, M.D., Chief of Staff
CHR: Wanda Daigle, Director Human Resources
Web address: www.winniehospital.com
Control: Partnership, Investor–owned, for–profit **Service:** General Medical and Surgical

Staffed Beds: 25 **Admissions:** 554 **Census:** 4 **Outpatient Visits:** 5274 **Births:** 0 **Total Expense ($000):** 5590 **Payroll Expense ($000):** 2306 **Personnel:** 61

TX

Hospital, Medicare Provider Number, Address, Telephone, Approval, Facility, and Physician Codes, Health Care System
★ American Hospital Association (AHA) membership
☐ The Joint Commission accreditation
○ American Osteopathic Association (AOA) accreditation
△ Commission on Accreditation of Rehabilitation Facilities (CARF) accreditation

WINNSBORO—Wood County

⊠ **TEXAS HEALTH PRESBYTERIAN HOSPITAL OF WINNSBORO (450224)**, (Formerly Presbyterian Hospital of Winnsboro), 719 West Coke Road, Zip 75494–0628, Mailing Address: P.O. Box 628, Zip 75494–0628; tel. 903/342–5227 **A**1 9 10 **F**3 15 25 26 30 31 32 33 38 40 52 55 56 57 62 66 68 73 75 77 79 80 86 96 99 102 107 119 120 121 122 135 **S** Texas Health Resources
Primary Contact: Michael Sinclair, Administrator
CFO: Renae Thomas, Chief Financial Officer
CMO: Kim Burlingham, President Medical Staff
Web address: www.texashealth.org
Control: Church–operated, Nongovernment, not–for profit **Service:** General Medical and Surgical

Staffed Beds: 35 **Admissions:** 718 **Census:** 9 **Outpatient Visits:** 14993 **Births:** 0 **Total Expense ($000):** 14000 **Payroll Expense ($000):** 5691 **Personnel:** 94

WINTERS—Runnels County

NORTH RUNNELS HOSPITAL (451315), East Highway 53, Zip 79567, Mailing Address: P.O. Box 185, Zip 79567–0185; tel. 325/754–5551 **A**9 10 18 **F**7 11 34 38 55 57 61 63 64 66 87 107 122 **P**5
Primary Contact: Roland K. Rickard, Administrator
CFO: Harold Hudgens, Chief Financial Officer
CMO: Sarah Endicott, M.D., Chief of Staff
Control: Hospital district or authority, Government, nonfederal **Service:** General Medical and Surgical

Staffed Beds: 21 **Admissions:** 170 **Census:** 2 **Outpatient Visits:** 12605 **Births:** 0 **Total Expense ($000):** 3337 **Payroll Expense ($000):** 1581 **Personnel:** 57

WOODVILLE—Tyler County

★ **TYLER COUNTY HOSPITAL (450460)**, 1100 West Bluff Street, Zip 75979–4799, Mailing Address: P.O. Box 549, Zip 75979–0549; tel. 409/283–8141 **A**9 10 20 **F**1 4 10 11 16 17 26 30 31 32 38 40 55 61 62 65 68 70 71 78 79 83 84 85 88 96 102 107 117 135 **P**5
Primary Contact: Gayle D. Wright, Chief Executive Officer
CFO: Richard Wallace, Controller, Chief Financial Officer and Assistant Administrator
CIO: Rachel Haygood, Director Information Technology
CHR: Paul Gray, Director Human Resources
Web address: www.tchospital.us
Control: Hospital district or authority, Government, nonfederal **Service:** General Medical and Surgical

Staffed Beds: 25 **Admissions:** 954 **Census:** 10 **Outpatient Visits:** 21346 **Births:** 0 **Total Expense ($000):** 9216 **Payroll Expense ($000):** 4140 **Personnel:** 122

TX

YOAKUM—Lavaca County

★ **YOAKUM COMMUNITY HOSPITAL (451346)**, 1200 Carl Ramert Drive, Zip 77995–4198, Mailing Address: P.O. Box 753, Zip 77995–0753; tel. 361/293–2321 **A**9 10 18 **F**3 11 13 15 25 30 31 32 33 38 40 54 55 56 57 62 68 74 77 79 80 81 86 96 100 102 107 118 121 122 123 135 137 **S** Community Hospital Corporation
Primary Contact: Karen Barber, Chief Executive Officer
CFO: Robert Foret, Chief Financial Officer
CMO: Timothy Wagner, Chief Medical Staff
CHR: Karen Roznovsky, Administrative Assistant
Web address: www.yoakumhospital.org
Control: Other not–for–profit (including NFP Corporation) **Service:** General Medical and Surgical

Staffed Beds: 25 **Admissions:** 1126 **Census:** 13 **Outpatient Visits:** 17567 **Births:** 109 **Total Expense ($000):** 11630 **Payroll Expense ($000):** 4849 **Personnel:** 120

UTAH

AMERICAN FORK—Utah County

☒ **AMERICAN FORK HOSPITAL (460023)**, 170 North 1100 East, Zip 84003–2096; tel. 801/855–3300, (Total facility includes 12 beds in nursing home–type unit) **A**1 9 10 **F**3 11 13 15 25 27 28 30 31 32 36 37 38 40 41 43 48 49 53 55 56 57 61 62 68 70 73 74 75 76 79 80 81 82 84 86 87 96 99 100 102 104 105 107 111 117 119 120 121 123 133 135 136 137 **S** Intermountain Healthcare, Inc.
Primary Contact: Michael R. Olson, Administrator
CFO: Rodney Lisonbee, Chief Financial Officer
CIO: Diane Rindlisbacher, Manager Information Systems
Web address: www.intermountainhealthcare.org
Control: Other not–for–profit (including NFP Corporation) **Service:** General Medical and Surgical

Staffed Beds: 93 **Admissions:** 6641 **Census:** 49 **Outpatient Visits:** 152017 **Births:** 3299 **Total Expense ($000):** 70561 **Payroll Expense ($000):** 25842 **Personnel:** 557

BEAVER—Beaver County

BEAVER VALLEY HOSPITAL (460035), 1109 North 100 West, Zip 84713, Mailing Address: P.O. Box 1670, Zip 84713–1670; tel. 435/438–2531, (Total facility includes 36 beds in nursing home–type unit) (Nonreporting) **A**9 10 20
Primary Contact: Craig Val Davidson, CHE, Chief Executive Officer and Administrator
Web address: www.beaverutah.net
Control: City–Government, nonfederal **Service:** General Medical and Surgical

Staffed Beds: 57

BOUNTIFUL—Davis County

☒ **LAKEVIEW HOSPITAL (460042)**, 630 East Medical Drive, Zip 84010–4996; tel. 801/299–2200 **A**1 9 10 **F**3 5 11 13 15 17 18 25 27 30 31 32 36 38 46 47 48 49 52 55 56 57 62 63 68 71 72 73 75 77 79 80 81 82 86 88 92 93 96 97 100 102 106 107 119 120 121 135 136 137 **S** HCA
Primary Contact: Rand Kerr, Chief Executive Officer
CFO: Wayne Dalton, Chief Financial Officer
CHR: Julie Isom, Director Human Resources
Web address: www.lakeviewhospital.com
Control: Corporation, Investor–owned, for–profit **Service:** General Medical and Surgical

Staffed Beds: 116 **Admissions:** 4407 **Census:** 53 **Outpatient Visits:** 29166 **Births:** 479

SOUTH DAVIS COMMUNITY HOSPITAL (462003), 401 South 400 East, Zip 84010; tel. 801/295–2361, (Nonreporting) **A**10
Primary Contact: Richard G. Bennett, Administrator
CFO: Daniel J. Foster, Chief Financial Officer
CMO: Scott Southworth, M.D., Medical Director
CHR: Jamey Sulser, Director Human Resources
Web address: www.sdch.com
Control: Corporation, Investor–owned, for–profit **Service:** Long–Term Acute Care hospital

Staffed Beds: 39

BRIGHAM CITY—Box Elder County

☒ **BRIGHAM CITY COMMUNITY HOSPITAL (460017)**, 950 South Medical Drive, Zip 84302; tel. 435/734–9471 **A**1 9 10 **F**3 13 14 15 25 26 33 36 38 52 55 57 68 74 75 77 79 80 82 84 86 96 97 100 107 118 119 135 136 **S** HCA
Primary Contact: Mark B. Adams, Chief Executive Officer
COO: Richard Spuhler, Chief Financial Officer and Chief Operating Officer
CFO: Richard Spuhler, Chief Financial Officer and Chief Operating Officer
CMO: Ryan Stolworthy, Chief Medical Officer
CIO: Steve Reichard, Manager Information Systems
CHR: Kathy Worley, Director Human Resources
Web address: www.brighamcityhospital.com
Control: Corporation, Investor–owned, for–profit **Service:** General Medical and Surgical

Staffed Beds: 39 **Admissions:** 872 **Census:** 5 **Outpatient Visits:** 27583 **Births:** 346 **Total Expense ($000):** 14608 **Payroll Expense ($000):** 5789 **Personnel:** 103

CEDAR CITY—Iron County

☒ **VALLEY VIEW MEDICAL CENTER (460007)**, 1303 North Main Street, Zip 84720–3462; tel. 435/868–5000, (Nonreporting) **A**1 9 10 20 **S** Intermountain Healthcare, Inc.
Primary Contact: Jason Wilson, Administrator
CFO: Reed Sargent, Assistant Administrator Finance
Web address: www.ihc.com
Control: Other not–for–profit (including NFP Corporation) **Service:** General Medical and Surgical

Staffed Beds: 46

DELTA—Millard County

★ **DELTA COMMUNITY MEDICAL CENTER (461300)**, 126 South White Sage Avenue, Zip 84624–8928; tel. 435/864–5591 **A**9 10 18 **F**1 3 8 11 13 15 27 30 38 42 43 53 55 56 57 61 62 66 73 74 79 81 82 84 96 99 117 122 134 135 136 137 **P**5 **S** Intermountain Healthcare, Inc.
Primary Contact: James E. Beckstrand, Administrator
CFO: Chris Thompson, Chief Financial Officer
Web address: www.ihc.com
Control: Other not–for–profit (including NFP Corporation) **Service:** General Medical and Surgical

Staffed Beds: 20 **Admissions:** 475 **Census:** 3 **Outpatient Visits:** 13224 **Births:** 115 **Total Expense ($000):** 5139 **Payroll Expense ($000):** 2104 **Personnel:** 43

FILLMORE—Millard County

★ **FILLMORE COMMUNITY MEDICAL CENTER (461301)**, 674 South Highway 99, Zip 84631–9701; tel. 435/743–5591 **A**9 10 18 **F**3 8 11 13 15 25 27 30 31 32 36 38 42 43 50 54 55 56 57 61 62 65 66 73 74 79 81 82 84 86 96 99 117 122 134 135 136 137 **S** Intermountain Healthcare, Inc.
Primary Contact: James E. Beckstrand, Administrator
CFO: Chris Thompson, Chief Financial Officer
Web address: www.ihc.com
Control: Other not–for–profit (including NFP Corporation) **Service:** General Medical and Surgical

Staffed Beds: 20 **Admissions:** 283 **Census:** 13 **Outpatient Visits:** 9547 **Births:** 58 **Total Expense ($000):** 4866 **Payroll Expense ($000):** 2034 **Personnel:** 45

GUNNISON—Sanpete County

★ **GUNNISON VALLEY HOSPITAL (461306)**, 64 East 100 North, Zip 84634, Mailing Address: P.O. Box 759, Zip 84634–0759; tel. 435/528–7246 **A**9 10 18 **F**3 7 13 15 30 38 42 55 56 61 62 66 79 96 99 102 107 118 119 122 135 **P**6
Primary Contact: Greg Rosenvall, Administrator
CFO: Brian Murray, Chief Financial Officer
CHR: David Peterson, Manager Human Resources
Web address: www.gvhospital.org
Control: Hospital district or authority, Government, nonfederal **Service:** General Medical and Surgical

Staffed Beds: 25 **Admissions:** 906 **Census:** 9 **Outpatient Visits:** 32570 **Births:** 205 **Total Expense ($000):** 12420 **Payroll Expense ($000):** 5213 **Personnel:** 154

HEBER CITY—Wasatch County

★ **HEBER VALLEY MEDICAL CENTER (461307)**, 1485 South Highway 40, Zip 84032–3522; tel. 435/654–2500, (Nonreporting) **A**9 10 18 **S** Intermountain Healthcare, Inc.
Primary Contact: Ezra Segura, Administrator
Web address: www.ihc.com
Control: Other not–for–profit (including NFP Corporation) **Service:** General Medical and Surgical

Staffed Beds: 19

UT

Hospital, Medicare Provider Number, Address, Telephone, Approval, Facility, and Physician Codes, Health Care System

★ American Hospital Association (AHA) membership
□ The Joint Commission accreditation
○ American Osteopathic Association (AOA) accreditation
△ Commission on Accreditation of Rehabilitation Facilities (CARF) accreditation

KANAB—Kane County

KANE COUNTY HOSPITAL (460018), 355 North Main Street, Zip 84741–3238; tel. 435/644–5811 **A**9 10 20 **F**7 38 79 82 96 107 122
Primary Contact: Sherrie Pandya, Administrator
CFO: Steve Howells, Chief Financial Officer
CMO: Darin Ott, Chief of Staff
CHR: Laurali Noteman, Director Human Resources
Web address: www.kanecountyhospital.net
Control: Hospital district or authority, Government, nonfederal **Service:** General Medical and Surgical

Staffed Beds: 38 **Admissions:** 337 **Census:** 28 **Outpatient Visits:** 13568 **Births:** 81 **Total Expense ($000):** 8822 **Payroll Expense ($000):** 3670 **Personnel:** 101

LAYTON—Davis County

☐ **DAVIS HOSPITAL AND MEDICAL CENTER (460041)**, 1600 West Antelope Drive, Zip 84041–1142; tel. 801/807–1000 **A**1 9 10 **F**3 8 11 13 15 17 18 20 24 25 27 31 32 33 38 45 46 49 55 56 57 59 63 68 70 71 73 74 77 78 79 80 81 82 84 96 97 100 102 103 106 107 119 135 136 137 **P**6 **S** IASIS Healthcare
Primary Contact: Michael E. Jensen, President and Chief Executive Officer
COO: Dale Johns, Chief Operating Officer
CIO: Shane Williams, Director Information Systems
CHR: Kevin Mansfield, Director Human Resources
Web address: www.davishospital.com
Control: Corporation, Investor–owned, for–profit **Service:** General Medical and Surgical

Staffed Beds: 136 **Admissions:** 6639 **Census:** 58 **Outpatient Visits:** 143028 **Births:** 2536 **Personnel:** 612

LOGAN—Cache County

☒ **LOGAN REGIONAL HOSPITAL (460015)**, 1400 North 500 East, Zip 84341–2499; tel. 435/716–1000, (Total facility includes 14 beds in nursing home–type unit) **A**1 9 10 **F**3 8 11 13 15 17 18 24 25 27 30 31 32 33 34 35 38 40 43 46 49 50 51 55 56 57 59 62 64 66 68 71 73 74 75 76 77 79 80 81 84 86 88 89 90 92 93 94 95 96 97 99 100 102 103 107 108 109 111 117 118 119 120 121 124 135 136 137 **P**6 **S** Intermountain Healthcare, Inc.
Primary Contact: Robert C. Cash, CHE, Administrator
COO: Michael Clark, Operations Officer
CFO: Alan Robinson, Chief Financial Officer
CMO: Todd A. Brown, Medical Director
CIO: Dave Felts, Chief Information Systems
CHR: Jolene Clonts, Director Human Resources
Web address: www.ihc.com
Control: Other not–for–profit (including NFP Corporation) **Service:** General Medical and Surgical

Staffed Beds: 139 **Admissions:** 6644 **Census:** 58 **Outpatient Visits:** 236659 **Births:** 2561 **Total Expense ($000):** 87591 **Payroll Expense ($000):** 35694 **Personnel:** 836

MIDVALE—Salt Lake County

HIGHLAND RIDGE HOSPITAL, 7309 South 180 West, Zip 84047–3769; tel. 801/569–2153, (Nonreporting) **A**9 **S** Pioneer Behavioral Health
Primary Contact: Robert Beatty, Chief Operating Officer
COO: Robert Beatty, Chief Operating Officer
CFO: Sheri Sorenson, Business Office Manager
CMO: Sajid Faizi, Medical Director
CHR: Sharon Latar, Director Human Resources
Web address: www.highlandridgehospital.com
Control: Corporation, Investor–owned, for–profit **Service:** Psychiatric

Staffed Beds: 32

MILFORD—Beaver County

★ **MILFORD VALLEY MEMORIAL HOSPITAL (461305)**, 451 North Main Street, Zip 84751–0640, Mailing Address: P.O. Box 640, Zip 84751; tel. 435/387–2411, (Nonreporting) **A**9 10 18
Primary Contact: Craig Val Davidson, CHE, Chief Executive Officer
Control: Hospital district or authority, Government, nonfederal **Service:** General Medical and Surgical

Staffed Beds: 25

MOAB—Grand County

★ **ALLEN MEMORIAL HOSPITAL (461302)**, 719 West 400 North Street, Zip 84532–2297, Mailing Address: P.O. Box 998, Zip 84532–0998; tel. 435/259–7191, (Nonreporting) **A**9 10 18 **S** Rural Health Group
Primary Contact: Roy E. Barraclough, Administrator and Chief Executive Officer
COO: Vicki Gigliotti, Chief Clinical Officer
CFO: Ken Knight, Chief Financial Officer
CMO: Jonas Munger, Chief Medical Staff
CIO: Mike Foster, Manager Information Systems
CHR: Becky Striblen, Director Human Resources
Web address: www.amhmoab.org
Control: Other not–for–profit (including NFP Corporation) **Service:** General Medical and Surgical

Staffed Beds: 25

MONTICELLO—San Juan County

SAN JUAN HOSPITAL (461308), 380 West 100 North, Zip 84535, Mailing Address: P.O. Box 308, Zip 84535–0308; tel. 435/587–2116, (Nonreporting) **A**9 18
Primary Contact: Craig Preston, Chief Executive Officer
CFO: Lyman Duncan, Chief Financial Officer
CMO: James Redd, M.D., Chief Medical Officer
Control: County–Government, nonfederal **Service:** General Medical and Surgical

Staffed Beds: 25

MOUNT PLEASANT—Sanpete County

★ **SANPETE VALLEY HOSPITAL (461303)**, 1100 South Medical Drive, Zip 84647–2222; tel. 435/462–2441 **A**9 10 18 **F**3 13 15 25 30 31 32 33 37 38 40 50 55 56 57 62 63 64 65 66 73 74 75 79 80 82 87 96 107 118 119 122 124 135 **P**6 **S** Intermountain Healthcare, Inc.
Primary Contact: Bradley Howell, Administrator
CFO: Chris Thompson, Chief Financial Officer
CMO: Gary Cole, D.O., Medical Staff President
CIO: Michael Ence, Computer Specialist
CHR: Heather Hafen, Human Resource Manager
Web address: www.ihc.com
Control: Other not–for–profit (including NFP Corporation) **Service:** General Medical and Surgical

Staffed Beds: 18 **Admissions:** 830 **Census:** 6 **Outpatient Visits:** 27502 **Births:** 112 **Total Expense ($000):** 9729 **Payroll Expense ($000):** 4374 **Personnel:** 93

MURRAY—Salt Lake County

COTTONWOOD HOSPITAL MEDICAL CENTER See Intermountain Medical Center

☒ **INTERMOUNTAIN MEDICAL CENTER (460006)**, (Formerly Cottonwood Hospital Medical Center), 5121 South Cottonwood Street, Zip 84157; tel. 801/507–7000, (Nonreporting) **A**1 3 5 9 10 **S** Intermountain Healthcare, Inc.
Primary Contact: David Grauer, Administrator
Web address: www.ihc.com
Control: Other not–for–profit (including NFP Corporation) **Service:** General Medical and Surgical

Staffed Beds: 173

☐ **THE ORTHOPEDIC SPECIALTY HOSPITAL (460049)**, 5848 South 300 East, Zip 84107; tel. 801/314–4100, (Nonreporting) **A**1 9 10
Primary Contact: Bryan Johnson, Administrator
CFO: Ronald Jensen, Manager Hospital Finance
CMO: Jon Sundin, Medical Director
CIO: David Baird, Chief Information Officer
CHR: Tina Tasso, Manager Human Resources
Web address: www.intermountainhealthcare.org
Control: Partnership, Investor–owned, for–profit **Service:** Orthopedic

Staffed Beds: 14

NEPHI—Juab County

★ **CENTRAL VALLEY MEDICAL CENTER (461304)**, 48 West 1500 North, Zip 84648; tel. 435/623–3000 **A**9 10 18 **F**3 13 15 25 30 33 38 40 42 55 61 62 63 74 75 76 77 79 80 81 84 86 87 96 100 102 107 117 118 119 122 136 137 **P**6 **S** Rural Health Group
Primary Contact: Mark R. Stoddard, President
COO: John E. Gledhill, Chief Operating Officer
CFO: Brent Davis, Chief Financial Officer
CMO: Stanton Bailey, Chief of Staff
CIO: Ken Richens, Chief Information Officer
CHR: Brian Allsop, Director Human Resources
Web address: www.centralvalleymed.com
Control: Other not–for–profit (including NFP Corporation) **Service:** General Medical and Surgical

Staffed Beds: 25 **Admissions:** 911 **Census:** 9 **Outpatient Visits:** 73462 **Births:** 145 **Total Expense ($000):** 18990 **Payroll Expense ($000):** 6088 **Personnel:** 225

NORTH LOGAN—Cache County

☐ **CACHE VALLEY SPECIALTY HOSPITAL (460054)**, 2380 North 400 East, Zip 84341; tel. 435/713-9700, (Nonreporting) **A**1 9 10 **S** National Surgical Hospitals
Primary Contact: John C. Worley, Chief Executive Officer
CFO: David S. Geary, Chief Financial Officer
CMO: Brian Nelson, Chief Medical Officer
Web address: www.cvsh.com
Control: Corporation, Investor–owned, for–profit **Service:** General Medical and Surgical

Staffed Beds: 15

OGDEN—Weber County

★ **MCKAY–DEE HOSPITAL CENTER (460004)**, 4401 Harrison Boulevard, Zip 84403; tel. 801/387–2800 **A**1 2 9 10 **F**3 8 11 12 13 15 17 18 20 22 24 25 26 27 30 31 32 33 36 37 38 40 41 43 44 46 49 50 51 52 55 56 57 58 59 60 62 63 64 65 66 68 70 72 73 74 75 76 77 79 80 81 82 84 85 86 87 88 89 90 91 92 93 94 95 96 97 99 100 102 103 104 105 107 109 111 114 118 119 120 121 123 124 133 135 136 137 **P**6 **S** Intermountain Healthcare, Inc.
Primary Contact: Timothy T. Pehrson, Chief Executive Officer
CFO: Doug Smith, Chief Financial Officer
CMO: Richard Arbogast, M.D., Medical Director
CIO: Mary Gathers, Director Information Systems
CHR: Karen Burnett, Regional Director Human Resources
Web address: www.mckay–dee.org
Control: Other not–for–profit (including NFP Corporation) **Service:** General Medical and Surgical

Staffed Beds: 299 **Admissions:** 17328 **Census:** 194 **Outpatient Visits:** 219920 **Births:** 4049 **Total Expense ($000):** 259607 **Payroll Expense ($000):** 99523 **Personnel:** 2010

★ **OGDEN REGIONAL MEDICAL CENTER (460005)**, 5475 South 500 East, Zip 84405–6978; tel. 801/479–2111 **A**1 9 10 **F**3 4 5 11 13 14 15 17 18 20 22 24 25 26 27 30 31 32 33 36 38 40 41 43 50 52 54 55 56 57 61 65 66 70 72 73 74 75 76 77 79 80 81 82 84 86 96 97 100 103 106 107 109 111 117 118 119 121 124 135 136 **P**6 **S** HCA
Primary Contact: Mark B. Adams, Chief Executive Officer
COO: Dana Oaks, Chief Operating Officer
CFO: Judd Taylor, Chief Financial Officer
CMO: David Bierer, M.D., President
CIO: Sarah Dewitt, Director
CHR: Chris Bissenden, Director Human Resources
Web address: www.ogdenregional.com
Control: Corporation, Investor–owned, for–profit **Service:** General Medical and Surgical

Staffed Beds: 167 **Admissions:** 7484 **Census:** 86 **Total Expense ($000):** 88311 **Payroll Expense ($000):** 32488 **Personnel:** 744

OREM—Utah County

★ **OREM COMMUNITY HOSPITAL (460043)**, 331 North 400 West, Zip 84057–1999; tel. 801/224–4080 **A**1 9 10 **F**3 11 13 15 17 25 28 30 31 32 33 36 37 38 41 43 53 57 62 65 66 70 71 73 74 79 81 82 83 86 87 88 96 100 107 117 121 124 135 **S** Intermountain Healthcare, Inc.
Primary Contact: Ronald L. Liston, Administrator
COO: Ronald L. Liston, Administrator
CFO: Rodney Lisonbee, Chief Financial Officer
CMO: Neil Whitaker, M.D., Chief Medical Director
CIO: Diane Rindlisbacher, Manager Information Systems
CHR: Pam Niece, Director Human Resources
Web address: www.intermountainhealthcare.org
Control: Other not–for–profit (including NFP Corporation) **Service:** General Medical and Surgical

Staffed Beds: 18 **Admissions:** 1439 **Census:** 8 **Outpatient Visits:** 55600 **Births:** 1315 **Total Expense ($000):** 21524 **Payroll Expense ($000):** 7905 **Personnel:** 182

★ **TIMPANOGOS REGIONAL HOSPITAL (460052)**, 750 West 800 North, Zip 84059–3660; tel. 801/714–6000 **A**1 9 10 **F**3 11 13 15 17 18 20 22 24 25 27 30 35 38 47 49 55 56 57 68 70 71 74 77 79 80 82 84 96 97 99 100 103 107 119 135 **P**8 **S** HCA
Primary Contact: Keith D. Tintle, Chief Executive Officer
Web address: www.timpanogosregionalhospital.com
Control: Corporation, Investor–owned, for–profit **Service:** General Medical and Surgical

Staffed Beds: 69 **Admissions:** 4245 **Census:** 40 **Outpatient Visits:** 32355 **Births:** 1628 **Total Expense ($000):** 46728 **Payroll Expense ($000):** 17390 **Personnel:** 417

PANGUITCH—Garfield County

★ **GARFIELD MEMORIAL HOSPITAL AND CLINICS (460033)**, 200 North 400 East, Zip 84759, Mailing Address: P.O. Box 389, Zip 84759–0389; tel. 435/676–8811, (Total facility includes 30 beds in nursing home–type unit) (Nonreporting) **A**9 10 20 **S** Intermountain Healthcare, Inc.
Primary Contact: Alberto Vasquez, Administrator
CFO: Reed Sargent, Assistant Administrator Finance
Web address: www.ihc.com/xp/ihc/garfield
Control: Other not–for–profit (including NFP Corporation) **Service:** General Medical and Surgical

Staffed Beds: 41

PAYSON—Utah County

★ **MOUNTAIN VIEW HOSPITAL (460013)**, 1000 East 100 North, Zip 84651–1690; tel. 801/465–7000, (Nonreporting) **A**1 9 10 **S** HCA
Primary Contact: Kevin Johnson, Chief Executive Officer
COO: Kimball Anderson, FACHE, Chief Operating Officer
CFO: Steven R. Schramm, Chief Financial Officer
CMO: Joseph Dinkins, Chief Medical Staff
CHR: Wally Trotter, Director Human Resources
Web address: www.mvhpayson.com
Control: Corporation, Investor–owned, for–profit **Service:** General Medical and Surgical

Staffed Beds: 114

PRICE—Carbon County

★ **CASTLEVIEW HOSPITAL (460011)**, 300 North Hospital Drive, Zip 84501–4200; tel. 435/637–4800, (Total facility includes 8 beds in nursing home–type unit) (Nonreporting) **A**1 9 10 20 **S** LifePoint Hospitals, Inc.
Primary Contact: Jeffrey J. Manley, Chief Executive Officer
CFO: Craig M. Daniels, Chief Financial Officer
CMO: Glen Etzel, M.D., Chief of Staff
CIO: Harvey Peet, Director Information Systems
CHR: Dave Donaldson, Director Human Resources
Web address: www.castleviewhospital.net
Control: Corporation, Investor–owned, for–profit **Service:** General Medical and Surgical

Staffed Beds: 57

PROVO—Utah County

☐ **UTAH STATE HOSPITAL (464001)**, 1300 East Center Street, Zip 84606–3554, Mailing Address: P.O. Box 270, Zip 84603–0270; tel. 801/344–4400 **A**1 10 **F**26 30 54 56 73 75 81 82 88 89 90 91 93 119 124 132 135 **P**6
Primary Contact: Dallas Earnshaw, Chief Executive Officer
COO: Dallas Earnshaw, Chief Executive Officer
CFO: Mark Lomenick, Manager Finance
CMO: Richard Spencer, M.D., Clinical Director
CIO: Jill Hill, Director Information Technology
CHR: David Gardner, Manager Human Resources
Web address: www.ush.utah.gov
Control: State–Government, nonfederal **Service:** Psychiatric

Staffed Beds: 359 **Admissions:** 430 **Census:** 317 **Outpatient Visits:** 0 **Births:** 0 **Total Expense ($000):** 48663 **Payroll Expense ($000):** 25415 **Personnel:** 755

★ △ **UTAH VALLEY REGIONAL MEDICAL CENTER (460001)**, 1034 North 500 West, Zip 84604–3337; tel. 801/373–7850 **A**1 2 7 9 10 **F**3 11 13 15 17 18 19 20 21 22 23 24 25 26 27 28 30 31 32 33 36 37 38 40 41 42 43 44 48 49 50 51 52 53 54 55 56 57 58 59 60 61 62 66 67 68 70 72 73 74 75 76 79 80 81 82 83 84 85 86 87 88 89 90 91 92 93 94 95 96 97 99 100 102 103 104 105 106 107 109 111 118 119 120 121 122 123 133 135 136 137 **P**6 **S** Intermountain Healthcare, Inc.
Primary Contact: Steven Smoot, Administrator
COO: David Clark, Regional Vice President
CFO: Rodney Lisonbee, Chief Financial Officer
CMO: Neil Whitaker, M.D., Medical Director
CIO: Diane Rindlisbacher, Acting Manager Information Systems
CHR: Kenneth Walker, Director Human Resources
Web address: www.intermountainmail.org
Control: Other not–for–profit (including NFP Corporation) **Service:** General Medical and Surgical

Staffed Beds: 351 **Admissions:** 18750 **Census:** 240 **Outpatient Visits:** 327597 **Births:** 4756 **Total Expense ($000):** 310288 **Payroll Expense ($000):** 128316 **Personnel:** 2691

UT

Hospital, Medicare Provider Number, Address, Telephone, Approval, Facility, and Physician Codes, Health Care System

★ American Hospital Association (AHA) membership
☐ The Joint Commission accreditation
○ American Osteopathic Association (AOA) accreditation
△ Commission on Accreditation of Rehabilitation Facilities (CARF) accreditation

RICHFIELD—Sevier County

★ **SEVIER VALLEY MEDICAL CENTER (460026)**, 1000 North Main Street, Zip 84701–1843; tel. 435/896–8271 **A**1 9 10 20 **F**3 8 13 15 25 31 32 33 38 55 56 57 61 62 66 73 74 75 77 79 84 86 87 96 97 100 106 107 118 119 122 135 **P**6 8 **S** Intermountain Healthcare, Inc.
Primary Contact: Gary E. Beck, Administrator
CFO: Chris Thompson, Chief Financial Officer
CHR: Katey Nelson, Director Human Resources
Web address: www.intermountain.com
Control: Other not–for–profit (including NFP Corporation) **Service:** General Medical and Surgical

Staffed Beds: 27 **Admissions:** 926 **Census:** 6 **Outpatient Visits:** 50283 **Births:** 282 **Total Expense ($000):** 15578 **Payroll Expense ($000):** 5090 **Personnel:** 108

ROOSEVELT—Duchesne County

★ **UINTAH BASIN MEDICAL CENTER (460019)**, 250 West 300 North, 75–2, Zip 84066; tel. 435/722–6163, (Total facility includes 59 beds in nursing home–type unit) **A**9 10 20 **F**1 4 7 11 13 15 16 17 30 31 32 33 38 40 42 43 44 50 52 53 55 57 59 61 65 68 70 71 74 75 77 78 79 80 82 83 84 85 86 88 94 96 100 102 106 107 113 117 118 119 120 133 135 136 137 **P**7
Primary Contact: Bradley D. LeBaron, FACHE, President and Chief Executive Officer
CFO: Brent Hales, Chief Financial Officer
CMO: Jason Larsen, M.D., Chief Medical Staff
CHR: Randall Bennett, Assistant Administrator
Web address: www.ubmc.org
Control: Other not–for–profit (including NFP Corporation) **Service:** General Medical and Surgical

Staffed Beds: 97 **Admissions:** 1767 **Census:** 64 **Outpatient Visits:** 52473 **Births:** 556 **Total Expense ($000):** 45098 **Payroll Expense ($000):** 14598 **Personnel:** 468

SAINT GEORGE—Washington County

★ △ **DIXIE REGIONAL MEDICAL CENTER (460021)**, 1380 East Medical Center Drive, Zip 84790; tel. 435/251–1000 **A**1 2 7 9 10 19 20 **F**3 11 12 13 15 18 19 20 21 22 23 24 25 27 30 31 32 33 35 36 38 40 43 44 50 52 55 56 57 62 65 66 68 70 71 72 73 74 75 76 77 79 80 84 85 86 88 92 96 97 100 102 103 105 107 108 109 118 119 120 121 124 135 136 137 **P**5 **S** Intermountain Healthcare, Inc.
Primary Contact: Terri Kane, Administrator
CFO: Mary Hatch, Chief Financial Officer
CMO: Steven Van Norman, M.D., Medical Director
CIO: Lance Bedingford, Director Information Services
CHR: Vicki Wilson, Chief Human Resources Officer
Web address: www.intermountainhealthcare.org
Control: Other not–for–profit (including NFP Corporation) **Service:** General Medical and Surgical

Staffed Beds: 245 **Admissions:** 14637 **Census:** 147 **Outpatient Visits:** 375131 **Births:** 2853 **Total Expense ($000):** 207605 **Payroll Expense ($000):** 81057 **Personnel:** 2060

UT

SALT LAKE CITY—Salt Lake County

★ △ **LDS HOSPITAL (460010)**, Eighth Avenue and C Street, Zip 84143–0001; tel. 801/408–1100, (Nonreporting) **A**1 2 3 5 7 9 10 **S** Intermountain Healthcare, Inc.
Primary Contact: Mikelle D. Moore, CHE, Administrator
COO: Gary Pehrson, Chief Executive Officer
CFO: David M. Larsen, Chief Financial Officer
CMO: William L. Hamilton, Chief Medical Officer
CIO: David Baird, Chief Information Officer
CHR: Nancy Adams, Chief Human Resources Officer
Web address: www.ihc.com/xp/ihc/lds
Control: Other not–for–profit (including NFP Corporation) **Service:** General Medical and Surgical

Staffed Beds: 452

★ **PRIMARY CHILDREN'S MEDICAL CENTER (463301)**, 100 North Medical Drive, Zip 84113–1100; tel. 801/588–2000 **A**1 3 5 9 10 **F**3 5 9 11 19 21 23 25 26 27 28 30 31 32 33 36 37 38 40 41 43 44 48 49 50 56 57 58 62 63 66 70 72 73 75 76 77 79 80 81 82 83 84 86 88 89 90 91 92 94 95 96 97 100 102 104 105 106 107 112 114 118 119 121 123 125 126 128 130 131 135 137 **S** Intermountain Healthcare, Inc.
Primary Contact: Joseph Mott, Administrator and Chief Executive Officer
COO: Joe Mott, Chief Operating Officer
CFO: David Thompson, Chief Financial Officer
CMO: Ed Clark, M.D., Medical Director
CIO: Joe Hales, Director Information Systems
CHR: Albert Bennett Buckworth, Director Human Resources
Web address: www.ihc.com
Control: Other not–for–profit (including NFP Corporation) **Service:** Children's general

Staffed Beds: 252 **Admissions:** 13135 **Census:** 194 **Outpatient Visits:** 294806 **Births:** 0 **Total Expense ($000):** 296744 **Payroll Expense ($000):** 128192 **Personnel:** 2691

PROMISE SPECIALTY HOSPITAL OF SALT LAKE (462004), 3460 Pioneer Parkway, 5th Floor, Zip 84120; tel. 801/964–3551, (Nonreporting) **A**9 10
Primary Contact: Richard Luna, Chief Executive Officer
Web address: www.promise–saltlake.com
Control: Corporation, Investor–owned, for–profit **Service:** Long–Term Acute Care hospital

Staffed Beds: 54

☐ **SALT LAKE REGIONAL MEDICAL CENTER (460003)**, 1050 East South Temple, Zip 84102–1599; tel. 801/350–4111, (Nonreporting) **A**1 3 5 9 10 **S** IASIS Healthcare
Primary Contact: Jeff Frandsen, Chief Executive Officer
COO: Bart Adams, Chief Operating Officer
CFO: Ryan K. Smith, Chief Financial Officer
CMO: Steven W. Mintz, M.D., Chief of Staff
CIO: Mark Runyan, Director Information Services
CHR: Mary Moody, Director Human Resources
Web address: www.saltlakeregional.com
Control: Corporation, Investor–owned, for–profit **Service:** General Medical and Surgical

Staffed Beds: 138

☐ **SHRINERS HOSPITALS FOR CHILDREN–INTERMOUNTAIN**, Fairfax Road and Virginia Street, Zip 84103–4399; tel. 801/536–3500 **A**1 3 5 **F**3 31 33 43 57 58 62 66 73 75 77 79 80 81 82 84 86 119 121 123 135 **P**6 **S** Shriners Hospitals for Children
Primary Contact: J. Craig Patchin, Administrator
CFO: Randy Lindberg, Director Fiscal Services
CMO: James M. Roach, M.D., Chief of Staff
CHR: Russ Crockett, Director Human Resources
Web address: www.shriners.org
Control: Other not–for–profit (including NFP Corporation) **Service:** Children's orthopedic

Staffed Beds: 40 **Admissions:** 1347 **Census:** 14 **Outpatient Visits:** 6663 **Births:** 0 **Total Expense ($000):** 22767 **Payroll Expense ($000):** 11472 **Personnel:** 210

★ **ST. MARK'S HOSPITAL (460047)**, 1200 East 3900 South, Zip 84124–1390; tel. 801/268–7111 **A**1 2 9 10 **F**3 8 11 12 13 14 15 17 18 20 22 24 25 26 27 30 31 32 33 34 36 37 38 40 41 43 44 46 49 50 51 52 54 55 56 57 58 62 63 68 70 71 72 73 74 75 76 77 79 80 81 82 90 96 97 100 102 103 106 107 112 117 118 119 121 124 135 136 137 **S** HCA
Primary Contact: Steven B. Bateman, Chief Executive Officer
COO: Matt Dixon, Chief Operating Officer
CFO: Bryan McKinley, Chief Financial Officer
CMO: Brian Shiozawa, President Medical Staff
CIO: Jesse Trujillo, Director Information Systems
CHR: Robyn Opheikens, Assistant Administrator Human Resources
Web address: www.stmarkshospital.com
Control: Corporation, Investor–owned, for–profit **Service:** General Medical and Surgical

Staffed Beds: 297 **Admissions:** 15935 **Census:** 183 **Outpatient Visits:** 109520 **Births:** 3766 **Total Expense ($000):** 188839 **Payroll Expense ($000):** 70787 **Personnel:** 1256

★ △ **UNIVERSITY OF UTAH HEALTH CARE – HOSPITAL AND CLINICS (460009)**, 50 North Medical Drive, Zip 84132–0002; tel. 801/581–2121 **A**1 2 3 5 7 8 9 10 **F**3 5 6 8 14 15 16 17 18 20 22 24 25 26 27 30 33 34 36 37 38 40 41 43 44 46 47 48 49 50 51 53 54 55 56 57 58 59 60 61 62 63 66 68 69 70 72 73 74 75 76 77 79 80 81 82 85 86 87 88 89 90 92 93 94 95 96 97 98 99 100 102 103 104 105 107 108 109 113 114 116 118 119 120 121 124 125 126 127 128 129 130 131 133 134 135 136 137 **P**1
Primary Contact: David Entwistle, Chief Executive Officer
COO: Quinn McKenna, Chief Operating Officer
CFO: Gordon Crabtree, Chief Financial Officer
CMO: Thomas Miller, M.D., Medical Director
CIO: James Turnbull, Vice President and Chief Information Officer
CHR: Loretta Harper, Vice President Human Resources
Web address: www.uuhsc.utah.edu
Control: State–Government, nonfederal **Service:** General Medical and Surgical

Staffed Beds: 530 **Admissions:** 25448 **Census:** 417 **Outpatient Visits:** 806644 **Births:** 3277 **Total Expense ($000):** 641270 **Payroll Expense ($000):** 255377 **Personnel:** 6491

☐ △ **UNIVERSITY OF UTAH NEUROPSYCHIATRIC INSTITUTE (464009)**, 501 Chipeta Way, Zip 84108–1225; tel. 801/583–2500 **A**1 3 5 7 9 10 **F**4 5 25 30 31 32 33 54 55 88 89 90 91 92 93 94 95 119 121 **P**1 5 6
Primary Contact: Ross Van Vranken, Chief Executive Officer
CFO: Diana Goodell, Chief Financial Officer
Web address: www.med.utah.edu/uni
Control: State–Government, nonfederal **Service:** Psychiatric

Staffed Beds: 90 **Admissions:** 2923 **Census:** 70 **Outpatient Visits:** 8665 **Births:** 0 **Total Expense ($000):** 28833 **Payroll Expense ($000):** 12016 **Personnel:** 288

Many Facility Codes have changed. Please refer to the AHA Guide Code Chart.

▣ △ **VETERANS AFFAIRS SALT LAKE CITY HEALTH CARE SYSTEM**, 500 Foothill Drive, Zip 84148–0002; tel. 801/582–1565 **A**1 3 5 7 **F**3 5 8 18 20 22 24 25 26 33 34 36 37 38 41 42 43 44 45 46 47 48 49 50 52 53 54 55 56 57 58 59 60 61 62 68 72 73 75 76 77 79 80 81 82 85 86 87 88 90 91 92 93 94 95 96 97 100 107 108 119 121 122 124 126 132 133 135 136 137 **P**6 **S** Department of Veterans Affairs
Primary Contact: James R. Floyd, Director
COO: Robin Korogi, Associate Director
CFO: Patti Gire, Director Financial Management Services Center
CMO: Ronald J. Gebhart, M.D., Chief of Staff
CIO: Paul R. Smith, Chief Information Officer
CHR: Lisa Porter, Director Human Resources, Leadership and Education
Web address: www.va.gov/sta/guide/home.asp
Control: Veterans Affairs, Government, federal **Service:** General Medical and Surgical

Staffed Beds: 121 **Admissions:** 5381 **Census:** 91 **Outpatient Visits:** 401077 **Births:** 0 **Total Expense ($000):** 259167 **Payroll Expense ($000):** 98168 **Personnel:** 1525

SANDY—Salt Lake County

▣ **ALTA VIEW HOSPITAL (460044)**, 9660 South 1300 East, Zip 84094–3793; tel. 801/501–2600 **A**1 9 10 **F**3 12 13 15 25 30 31 32 33 36 37 38 41 46 47 48 49 50 55 56 57 62 66 68 73 74 75 77 79 80 82 86 87 92 96 97 99 100 102 103 107 118 119 121 124 132 135 136 137 **S** Intermountain Healthcare, Inc.
Primary Contact: Becky Kapp, Administrator
Web address: www.ihc.com
Control: Other not–for–profit (including NFP Corporation) **Service:** General Medical and Surgical

Staffed Beds: 72 **Admissions:** 5454 **Census:** 42 **Outpatient Visits:** 326569 **Births:** 2349 **Total Expense ($000):** 72574 **Payroll Expense ($000):** 29678

▣ **HEALTHSOUTH REHABILITATION HOSPITAL OF UTAH (463025)**, 8074 South 1300 East, Zip 84094–0743; tel. 801/561–3400 **A**1 10 **F**25 31 32 61 85 86 117 **S** HEALTHSOUTH Corporation
Primary Contact: Thomas Almerico, Chief Executive Officer
CFO: Daren Woolstenhulme, Chief Financial Officer
CMO: Joseph VickRoy, M.D., Medical Director
CHR: Kathy Whiting, Director Human Resources
Web address: www.healthsouth.com
Control: Corporation, Investor–owned, for–profit **Service:** Rehabilitation

Staffed Beds: 60 **Admissions:** 1291 **Census:** 47 **Outpatient Visits:** 13860 **Births:** 0 **Total Expense ($000):** 11771 **Payroll Expense ($000):** 7488 **Personnel:** 185

TOOELE—Tooele County

▣ **MOUNTAIN WEST MEDICAL CENTER (460014)**, 2055 North Main, Zip 84074–2794; tel. 435/843–3600, (Nonreporting) **A**1 9 10 20 **S** Community Health Systems, Inc.
Primary Contact: Kelly L. Duffin, Chief Executive Officer
CFO: Scott Banks, Chief Financial Officer
CMO: Greg Haroutunian, M.D., Chief of Staff
CHR: James Glade, Director Human Resources
Web address: www.mountainwestmc.com
Control: Corporation, Investor–owned, for–profit **Service:** General Medical and Surgical

Staffed Beds: 35

TREMONTON—Box Elder County

★ **BEAR RIVER VALLEY HOSPITAL (460039)**, 440 West 600 North, Zip 84337–2497; tel. 435/257–7441, (Total facility includes 38 beds in nursing home–type unit) (Nonreporting) **A**9 10 **S** Intermountain Healthcare, Inc.
Primary Contact: Eric Packer, Administrator
CHR: Joy Sadler, Director Human Resources
Web address: www.ihc.com
Control: Other not–for–profit (including NFP Corporation) **Service:** General Medical and Surgical

Staffed Beds: 58

VERNAL—Uintah County

▣ **ASHLEY REGIONAL MEDICAL CENTER (460030)**, (Formerly Ashley Valley Medical Center), 151 West 200 North, Zip 84078–1907; tel. 435/789–3342, (Nonreporting) **A**1 9 10 20 **S** LifePoint Hospitals, Inc.
Primary Contact: Si Hutt, Chief Executive Officer
COO: Mark Holyoak, Chief Clinical Officer
CFO: Chad Labrum, Chief Financial Officer
CMO: Michael Olsen, Chief of Staff
CIO: Mark Rich, Director Information Services
CHR: Deena Mansfield, Director Human Resources
Web address: www.ashleyregional.com
Control: Corporation, Investor–owned, for–profit **Service:** General Medical and Surgical

Staffed Beds: 31

WEST JORDAN—Salt Lake County

COPPER HILLS YOUTH CENTER, 5899 West Rivendell Drive, Zip 84088–5700; tel. 800/776–7116, (Nonreporting) **S** Horizon Health Corporation
Primary Contact: Michael Rowley, Chief Executive Officer
COO: Sig Evans, Chief Operating Officer
CFO: Bart Bennett, Chief Financial Officer
Web address: www.copperhillsyouthcenter.com
Control: Corporation, Investor–owned, for–profit **Service:** Children's hospital psychiatric

Staffed Beds: 98

☐ **JORDAN VALLEY MEDICAL CENTER (460051)**, (Formerly Jordan Valley Hospital), 3580 West 9000 South, Zip 84088–8811; tel. 801/561–8888, (Nonreporting) **A**1 9 10 **S** IASIS Healthcare
Primary Contact: Bryanie W. Swilley, Jr., Chief Executive Officer
COO: Jon Butterfield, Chief Operating Officer
CFO: Ben Cluff, Chief Financial Officer
CMO: B. Dee Allred, President Medical Staff
Web address: www.mc.com
Control: Partnership, Investor–owned, for–profit **Service:** General Medical and Surgical

Staffed Beds: 50

WEST VALLEY CITY—Salt Lake County

☐ **PIONEER VALLEY HOSPITAL (460008)**, 3460 South Pioneer Parkway, Zip 84120–2648; tel. 801/964–3100, (Nonreporting) **A**1 10 **S** IASIS Healthcare
Primary Contact: Bryanie W. Swilley, Jr., Chief Executive Officer
COO: Jon Butterfield, Chief Operating Officer
CFO: Jared Spackham, Chief Financial Officer
CMO: B. Dee Allred, President Medical Staff
CIO: Jodi DeJong, Director Marketing
CHR: Misty Birch, Director Human Resources
Web address: www.pioneervalleyhospital.com
Control: Corporation, Investor–owned, for–profit **Service:** General Medical and Surgical

Staffed Beds: 101

WOODS CROSS—Davis County

BENCHMARK BEHAVIORAL HEALTH SYSTEMS, 592 West 1350 South, Zip 84087–1665; tel. 801/299–5300, (Nonreporting) **A**9 **S** Psychiatric Solutions
Primary Contact: Barry W. Woodward, Chief Executive Officer
CFO: Darren Hedin, Chief Financial Officer
Web address: www.bbhsnet.com
Control: Corporation, Investor–owned, for–profit **Service:** Psychiatric

Staffed Beds: 77

Hospital, Medicare Provider Number, Address, Telephone, Approval, Facility, and Physician Codes, Health Care System
★ American Hospital Association (AHA) membership
☐ The Joint Commission accreditation
○ American Osteopathic Association (AOA) accreditation
△ Commission on Accreditation of Rehabilitation Facilities (CARF) accreditation

VERMONT

BARRE—Washington County

☒ **CENTRAL VERMONT MEDICAL CENTER (470001)**, Fisher Road, Zip 05641–9060, Mailing Address: P.O. Box 547, Zip 05641–0547; tel. 802/371–4100, (Total facility includes 153 beds in nursing home–type unit) **A**1 9 10 19 20 **F**3 8 11 13 15 24 25 26 27 30 31 32 33 38 41 43 44 46 50 51 52 55 56 57 62 66 68 73 74 75 79 80 81 82 84 86 87 88 89 90 91 92 93 94 96 97 100 102 103 104 105 106 107 113 117 118 119 120 121 124 132 135 136 137 **P**6 8
Primary Contact: Judith C. Tarr, President and Chief Executive Officer
CMO: Russell Davignon, M.D., Vice President Quality and Medical Affairs
CIO: Russell Davignon, M.D., Vice President Quality and Medical Affairs
CHR: Richard Theken, Vice President Human Resources
Web address: www.cvmc.hitchcock.org
Control: Other not–for–profit (including NFP Corporation) **Service:** General Medical and Surgical

Staffed Beds: 235 **Admissions:** 3228 **Census:** 40 **Outpatient Visits:** 306315 **Births:** 433 **Total Expense ($000):** 98217 **Payroll Expense ($000):** 49364 **Personnel:** 821

BENNINGTON—Bennington County

☒ **SOUTHWESTERN VERMONT MEDICAL CENTER (470012)**, 100 Hospital Drive East, Zip 5201; tel. 802/442–6361 **A**1 2 9 10 19 **F**3 8 13 15 17 24 25 27 28 30 31 32 33 34 38 40 42 43 44 55 56 57 60 61 62 68 71 73 74 75 76 77 79 80 81 82 84 86 87 89 90 91 92 93 94 95 96 97 98 100 102 104 105 107 109 111 112 118 119 120 121 124 132 133 135 136 **P**1 6
Primary Contact: Harvey M. Yorke, President and Chief Executive Officer
COO: Harvey M. Yorke, President and Chief Executive Officer
CFO: Tom Lenkowski, Vice President Finance and Chief Financial Officer
CMO: Mark Novotny, M.D., Chief Medical Officer
CIO: Richard Ogilvie, Chief Information Officer
CHR: Craig Ghidotti, Vice President Human Resources
Web address: www.svhealthcare.org
Control: Other not–for–profit (including NFP Corporation) **Service:** General Medical and Surgical

Staffed Beds: 99 **Admissions:** 4775 **Census:** 47 **Outpatient Visits:** 193371 **Births:** 500 **Total Expense ($000):** 92667 **Payroll Expense ($000):** 43018 **Personnel:** 730

BRATTLEBORO—Windham County

☒ **BRATTLEBORO MEMORIAL HOSPITAL (470011)**, 17 Belmont Avenue, Zip 05301–3498; tel. 802/257–0341 **A**1 9 10 **F**3 8 11 12 13 14 15 17 18 24 25 26 27 30 31 32 33 37 38 43 44 49 51 52 55 56 57 62 66 68 72 73 74 75 76 77 79 80 81 82 86 96 97 102 106 107 113 119 121 124 135 136 137
Primary Contact: Barry G. Beeman, President and Chief Executive Officer
CFO: Michael Rogers, Vice President Fiscal Services
CMO: Paul Righi, President Medical Staff
CIO: Jonathan Farina, Chief Information Officer
CHR: Michael Kelliher, Vice President Human Resources
Web address: www.bmhvt.org
Control: Other not–for–profit (including NFP Corporation) **Service:** General Medical and Surgical

Staffed Beds: 47 **Admissions:** 2030 **Census:** 21 **Outpatient Visits:** 81900 **Births:** 373 **Total Expense ($000):** 43510 **Payroll Expense ($000):** 15648 **Personnel:** 309

☒ **BRATTLEBORO RETREAT (474001)**, Anna Marsh Lane, Zip 5301, Mailing Address: P.O. Box 803, Zip 05302–0803; tel. 802/257–7785 **A**1 3 5 9 10 **F**3 5 25 30 31 32 33 50 52 53 54 55 57 62 66 73 88 89 90 91 93 94 95 119 121 132 **P**6
Primary Contact: Robert E. Simpson, Jr., M.P.H., President and Chief Executive Officer
COO: Robert G. Soucy, Chief Operating Officer
CFO: John E. Blaha, Vice President Finance and Chief Financial Officer
CMO: Gregory Miller, M.D., Vice President Medical Affairs
CHR: Kathleen Brooks, Director Human Resources
Web address: www.brattlebororetreat.org
Control: Other not–for–profit (including NFP Corporation) **Service:** Psychiatric

Staffed Beds: 71 **Admissions:** 2054 **Census:** 59 **Outpatient Visits:** 26773 **Births:** 0 **Total Expense ($000):** 34878 **Payroll Expense ($000):** 20516 **Personnel:** 333

BURLINGTON—Chittenden County

★ **FLETCHER ALLEN HEALTH CARE (470003)**, 111 Colchester Avenue, Zip 05401–1429; tel. 802/847–0000, (Includes FANNY ALLEN CAMPUS, 101 College Parkway, Colchester, Zip 05446–3035; tel. 802/655–1234; MEDICAL CENTER HOSPITAL CAMPUS, Colchester Avenue, Zip 05401; tel. 802/847–2345) **A**2 3 5 8 9 10 **F**3 4 5 6 7 9 11 12 13 15 16 17 18 19 20 21 22 23 24 25 26 27 28 30 31 32 33 34 37 38 40 41 43 44 46 47 48 49 50 51 53 54 55 56 57 58 59 60 62 63 64 66 68 70 71 72 73 74 75 76 77 79 80 81 82 83 84 85 86 87 88 89 90 91 92 93 94 95 96 97 99 100 102 103 104 105 106 107 108 109 111 112 113 114 118 119 120 121 124 125 127 130 131 132 133 134 135 136 137 **P**6
Primary Contact: Melinda Estes, M.D., President and Chief Executive Officer
COO: Angeline M. Marano, Senior Vice President and Chief Operating Officer
CFO: Roger Deshaies, Chief Financial Officer
CMO: John R. Brumsted, M.D., Chief Quality Officer
CIO: Charles Podesta, Vice President Information Services
CHR: Paul Macuga, Chief Human Resources Officer
Web address: www.fahc.org
Control: Other not–for–profit (including NFP Corporation) **Service:** General Medical and Surgical

Staffed Beds: 437 **Admissions:** 20031 **Census:** 320 **Outpatient Visits:** 1184433 **Births:** 2218 **Total Expense ($000):** 704025 **Payroll Expense ($000):** 351004 **Personnel:** 5177

COLCHESTER—Chittenden County

FANNY ALLEN CAMPUS See Fletcher Allen Health Care, Burlington

MIDDLEBURY—Addison County

☒ **PORTER MEDICAL CENTER (471307)**, 115 Porter Drive, Zip 05753–8606; tel. 802/388–4701 **A**1 9 10 18 **F**3 8 11 13 15 25 26 30 31 33 35 38 40 43 44 50 56 57 62 66 68 73 74 77 79 80 81 86 87 96 97 100 102 107 119 121 122 124 135 **P**6
Primary Contact: James L. Daily, President
COO: Patricia Jannene, Vice President Patient Care Services
CFO: Duncan Brines, Vice President Finance
CMO: Fred Kniffin, M.D., President Medical Staff
CIO: Ronald Hallman, Vice President Development and Public Relations
CHR: Dan Arseneau, Vice President Human Resources
Web address: www.portermedical.org
Control: Other not–for–profit (including NFP Corporation) **Service:** General Medical and Surgical

Staffed Beds: 25 **Admissions:** 1373 **Census:** 12 **Outpatient Visits:** 147181 **Births:** 301 **Total Expense ($000):** 45808 **Payroll Expense ($000):** 19989 **Personnel:** 482

MORRISVILLE—Lamoille County

★ **COPLEY HOSPITAL (471305)**, 528 Washington Highway, Zip 05661–9209; tel. 802/888–8888 **A**9 10 18 **F**13 15 24 25 26 27 30 31 32 33 37 38 55 56 57 62 63 68 72 73 74 75 76 77 79 80 81 86 96 99 107 119 120 122 135
Primary Contact: Melvyn Patashnick, President and Chief Executive Officer
CFO: Rassoul Rangaviz, Chief Financial Officer
CIO: Conrad Garven, Manager Information Services
CHR: April E. Tuck, Senior Director Human Resources
Web address: www.copleyvt.org
Control: Other not–for–profit (including NFP Corporation) **Service:** General Medical and Surgical

Staffed Beds: 25 **Admissions:** 1458 **Census:** 14 **Outpatient Visits:** 71849 **Births:** 313 **Total Expense ($000):** 39227 **Payroll Expense ($000):** 17034 **Personnel:** 299

NEWPORT—Orleans County

★ **NORTH COUNTRY HOSPITAL AND HEALTH CENTER (471304)**, 189 Prouty Drive, Zip 05855–9329; tel. 802/334–7331, (Total facility includes 23 beds in nursing home–type unit) **A**9 10 18 **F**11 15 24 26 27 34 38 43 44 52 56 59 68 72 73 74 75 76 77 79 84 86 94 96 97 99 100 107 117 118 119 120 122 124 135
Primary Contact: Kim Campbell, RN, Interim Chief Executive Officer
COO: Kim Campbell, R.N., Vice President Medical Group Operations
CFO: Robert L. Fotter, Vice President Finance
CMO: Chris Rickman, President Medical Staff
CIO: Ervin Goodwin, Manager Information Services
CHR: William Perket, Vice President Human Resources
Web address: www.nchsi.org
Control: Other not–for–profit (including NFP Corporation) **Service:** General Medical and Surgical

Staffed Beds: 48 **Admissions:** 1710 **Census:** 39 **Outpatient Visits:** 71807 **Births:** 225 **Total Expense ($000):** 54502 **Payroll Expense ($000):** 33080 **Personnel:** 455

VT

Many Facility Codes have changed. Please refer to the AHA Guide Code Chart.

RANDOLPH—Orange County

★ **GIFFORD MEDICAL CENTER (471301)**, 44 South Main Street, Zip 05060–1381, Mailing Address: P.O. Box 2000, Zip 05060–2000; tel. 802/728–7000, (Total facility includes 30 beds in nursing home–type unit) **A**2 9 10 18 **F**2 3 8 11 13 15 24 25 26 27 28 29 30 31 32 33 36 38 42 43 44 45 49 50 51 54 55 56 57 62 63 64 65 66 68 72 73 74 75 76 77 79 80 81 82 84 86 87 96 97 100 102 107 112 117 119 120 121 122 124 135 136 137 **P**6
Primary Contact: Joseph L. Woodin, President and Chief Executive Officer
COO: Margie Judd, Vice President Operations
CFO: David Sanville, Vice President Finance
CMO: Joshua Plavin, Director Medical Staff
CIO: John Brugger, Director Information Systems
CHR: Jeff Corrigan, Director Human Resources
Web address: www.giffordmed.org
Control: Other not–for–profit (including NFP Corporation) **Service:** General Medical and Surgical

Staffed Beds: 82 **Admissions:** 1469 **Census:** 45 **Outpatient Visits:** 55553 **Births:** 225 **Total Expense ($000):** 42138 **Payroll Expense ($000):** 19239 **Personnel:** 379

RUTLAND—Rutland County

★ **RUTLAND REGIONAL MEDICAL CENTER (470005)**, 160 Allen Street, Zip 05701–4595; tel. 802/775–7111 **A**1 2 9 10 19 20 **F**3 11 13 15 18 20 22 24 25 26 27 30 31 32 33 35 38 40 42 44 51 55 56 57 60 62 68 72 73 74 75 76 77 79 81 82 84 85 86 88 90 91 92 93 94 96 97 100 103 104 105 106 107 108 109 118 119 120 121 122 124 133 134 135 137
Primary Contact: Thomas W. Huebner, President and Chief Executive Officer
CFO: Ed Ogorzalek, Chief Financial Officer
CIO: Sherry Ravlin, Chief Information Officer
Web address: www.rrmc.org
Control: Other not–for–profit (including NFP Corporation) **Service:** General Medical and Surgical

Staffed Beds: 136 **Admissions:** 6553 **Census:** 87 **Outpatient Visits:** 172296 **Births:** 465 **Total Expense ($000):** 141685 **Payroll Expense ($000):** 62029 **Personnel:** 926

SAINT ALBANS—Franklin County

★ **NORTHWESTERN MEDICAL CENTER (470024)**, 133 Fairfield Street, Zip 05478–1734, Mailing Address: P.O. Box 1370, Zip 05478–1370; tel. 802/524–5911, (Nonreporting) **A**1 2 9 10 20 **S** QHR
Primary Contact: Peter A. Hofstetter, Chief Executive Officer
COO: Dan Petherbridge, Manager Support Services
CFO: Ted D. Sirotta, Chief Financial Officer
CIO: John Johnston, Chief Technology Officer
CHR: Mary Lou Beaulieu, Director Human Resources and Compliance Officer
Web address: www.nmcinc.org
Control: Other not–for–profit (including NFP Corporation) **Service:** General Medical and Surgical

Staffed Beds: 52

SAINT JOHNSBURY—Caledonia County

★ **NORTHEASTERN VERMONT REGIONAL HOSPITAL (471303)**, 1315 Hospital Drive, Zip 05819–9962, Mailing Address: P.O. Box 905, Zip 05819–9962; tel. 802/748–8141 **A**9 10 18 **F**3 11 13 15 17 24 25 26 30 31 32 33 38 41 42 44 50 51 56 57 62 63 66 68 72 73 74 75 77 79 81 82 84 86 96 97 99 100 102 107 119 120 121 122 124 135 136 **P**6
Primary Contact: Paul R. Bengtson, Chief Executive Officer
CFO: Robert Hersey, Chief Financial Officer
CIO: Andrea Lott, Vice President Information Services
CHR: Betty Ann Gwatkin, Vice President Human Resources
Web address: www.nvrh.org
Control: Other not–for–profit (including NFP Corporation) **Service:** General Medical and Surgical

Staffed Beds: 25 **Admissions:** 1546 **Census:** 14 **Outpatient Visits:** 119356 **Births:** 242 **Total Expense ($000):** 42782 **Payroll Expense ($000):** 18149 **Personnel:** 303

SPRINGFIELD—Windsor County

★ **SPRINGFIELD HOSPITAL (471306)**, 25 Ridgewood Road, Zip 05156–2003, Mailing Address: P.O. Box 2003, Zip 05156–2003; tel. 802/885–2151 **A**9 10 18 **F**2 3 5 13 15 24 25 28 30 31 32 33 34 35 36 38 43 44 45 50 52 53 54 55 56 57 60 62 63 68 73 74 75 77 79 80 81 82 84 86 87 88 90 91 92 93 94 95 96 97 102 107 119 121 122 124 133 134 135 136 137 **P**7
Primary Contact: Thomas Crawford, Chief Executive Officer
CFO: Laverne Lindamood, Director Finance
CMO: Mark C. Hamilton, M.D., President Medical Staff
Web address: www.springfieldhospital.org
Control: Other not–for–profit (including NFP Corporation) **Service:** General Medical and Surgical

Staffed Beds: 35 **Admissions:** 2289 **Census:** 26 **Outpatient Visits:** 190911 **Births:** 256 **Total Expense ($000):** 40148 **Payroll Expense ($000):** 17286 **Personnel:** 308

TOWNSHEND—Windham County

★ **GRACE COTTAGE HOSPITAL (471300)**, Route 35, Zip 05353–0216, Mailing Address: P.O. Box 216, Zip 05353–0216; tel. 802/365–7357, (Total facility includes 14 beds in nursing home–type unit) (Nonreporting) **A**10 18
Primary Contact: Mick Brant, Chief Executive Officer
CFO: Stephen A. Brown, Chief Financial Officer
CIO: David Booth, Director Information Systems
CHR: Tim McNulty, Vice President Human Resources
Web address: www.gracecottage.org
Control: Other not–for–profit (including NFP Corporation) **Service:** General Medical and Surgical

Staffed Beds: 33

WATERBURY—Washington County

VERMONT STATE HOSPITAL, 103 South Main Street, Zip 05671–2501; tel. 802/241–1000 **A**5 **F**26 57 63 73 75 81 82 88 92 93 119 121 132 135 **P**6
Primary Contact: Terry Rowe, Executive Director
Web address: www.healthvermont.gov
Control: State–Government, nonfederal **Service:** Psychiatric

Staffed Beds: 54 **Admissions:** 243 **Census:** 50 **Outpatient Visits:** 0 **Total Expense ($000):** 19106 **Payroll Expense ($000):** 10372 **Personnel:** 214

WHITE RIVER JUNCTION—Windsor County

★ **VETERANS AFFAIRS MEDICAL CENTER**, 215 North Main Street, Zip 05009–0001; tel. 802/295–9363 **A**1 3 5 8 9 **F**3 5 8 12 18 24 25 26 27 30 31 32 33 34 36 37 38 41 42 43 44 46 49 50 53 54 56 57 58 60 62 63 68 72 73 75 76 77 79 80 81 82 86 87 88 90 91 92 93 94 95 96 97 102 103 106 107 119 121 124 132 133 135 136 137 **P**1 6 **S** Department of Veterans Affairs
Primary Contact: Kathryn M. Harty, RN, M.S.N., Acting Director
COO: Sandra Davidson, Associate Director
CFO: Joan Wilmot, Chief Fiscal Officer
CMO: Eric Shirley, M.D., Chief of Staff
CIO: Matthew Rafus, Chief Information Officer
CHR: Kathy Masun, Chief Human Resources Officer
Web address: www.va.gov/sta/guide/home.asp
Control: Veterans Affairs, Government, federal **Service:** General Medical and Surgical

Staffed Beds: 60 **Admissions:** 2421 **Census:** 40 **Outpatient Visits:** 179323 **Births:** 0 **Total Expense ($000):** 105238 **Payroll Expense ($000):** 45635 **Personnel:** 646

WINDSOR—Windsor County

★ **MT. ASCUTNEY HOSPITAL AND HEALTH CENTER (471302)**, 289 County Road, Zip 05089–9702; tel. 802/674–6711, (Total facility includes 50 beds in nursing home–type unit) **A**9 10 18 **F**3 8 10 11 15 24 25 26 27 30 31 32 33 34 38 41 42 44 50 53 54 55 56 57 60 62 64 66 68 69 73 75 76 77 79 80 81 82 85 86 87 90 94 96 99 100 106 107 115 117 119 121 122 123 124 132 135 137 **P**6
Primary Contact: Richard Slusky, Chief Executive Officer
COO: Bennett J. Beres, Chief Operating Officer
CFO: Michael Long, Chief Financial Officer
CMO: Sikhar Banerjee, M.D., President Medical Staff
CIO: Tom Sims, Chief Information Officer
CHR: Jean Martaniuk, Director Personnel
Web address: www.mtascutneyhospital.org
Control: Other not–for–profit (including NFP Corporation) **Service:** General Medical and Surgical

Staffed Beds: 83 **Admissions:** 1092 **Census:** 70 **Outpatient Visits:** 92386 **Births:** 1 **Total Expense ($000):** 40750 **Payroll Expense ($000):** 19503 **Personnel:** 407

VT

Hospital, Medicare Provider Number, Address, Telephone, Approval, Facility, and Physician Codes, Health Care System

★ American Hospital Association (AHA) membership
□ The Joint Commission accreditation
○ American Osteopathic Association (AOA) accreditation
△ Commission on Accreditation of Rehabilitation Facilities (CARF) accreditation

VIRGINIA

ABINGDON—Washington County

★ **JOHNSTON MEMORIAL HOSPITAL (490053)**, 351 Court Street N.E., Zip 24210–2955; tel. 276/676–7000 **A**1 2 9 10 **F**3 11 13 14 15 24 25 26 27 30 33 35 38 43 44 49 50 51 53 55 56 57 60 61 62 66 68 70 72 73 74 75 76 77 79 80 81 82 86 93 96 97 99 100 102 103 106 107 108 109 111 119 120 121 124 133 134 135 136 137 **P**6 8
Primary Contact: Sean S. McMurray, FACHE, Chief Executive Officer
COO: Stephen K. Givens, Chief Operating Officer
CFO: Timothy Evans, Chief Financial Officer
CMO: Andrew Hawkins, M.D., President Medical Staff
CIO: Greg Copen, Director Management Information Services
CHR: Jackie G. Phipps, Executive Director Human Resources
Web address: www.jmh.org
Control: Other not–for–profit (including NFP Corporation) **Service:** General Medical and Surgical

Staffed Beds: 135 **Admissions:** 4968 **Census:** 48 **Outpatient Visits:** 114132 **Births:** 650 **Total Expense ($000):** 67382 **Payroll Expense ($000):** 25169 **Personnel:** 688

ALEXANDRIA—Independent City County

★ **INOVA ALEXANDRIA HOSPITAL (490040)**, 4320 Seminary Road, Zip 22304–1594; tel. 703/504–3000 **A**1 2 3 5 9 10 **F**3 4 11 13 14 15 17 18 20 22 24 25 26 27 30 31 32 33 36 38 39 41 43 44 48 49 50 51 55 56 57 58 59 60 62 63 64 65 66 67 68 70 72 73 74 75 76 77 78 79 80 81 82 84 85 86 90 92 96 97 100 102 104 105 106 107 108 109 111 117 118 119 120 121 124 135 136 137 **P**6 **S** Inova Health System
Primary Contact: Christine Candio, Chief Executive Officer
CFO: Thomas F. Knight, Chief Financial Officer
CMO: Stephen Rosenfeld, M.D., President Medical Staff
CIO: Nanci Little Gosnell, Vice President Information Services
CHR: Katy Reeves, Director Human Resources
Web address: www.inova.org
Control: Other not–for–profit (including NFP Corporation) **Service:** General Medical and Surgical

Staffed Beds: 334 **Admissions:** 16792 **Census:** 224 **Outpatient Visits:** 109427 **Births:** 3749 **Total Expense ($000):** 223428 **Payroll Expense ($000):** 106259 **Personnel:** 1517

★ △ **INOVA MOUNT VERNON HOSPITAL (490122)**, 2501 Parker's Lane, Zip 22306; tel. 703/664–7000 **A**1 2 5 7 9 10 **F**3 11 14 15 17 24 25 26 27 30 31 32 33 35 36 38 41 43 44 46 47 48 50 52 55 56 57 58 59 60 62 66 67 68 72 73 75 76 77 78 79 80 81 82 85 86 88 90 91 92 93 94 96 97 99 100 102 103 106 107 119 120 121 124 135 137 **S** Inova Health System
Primary Contact: Barbara J. Doyle, Senior Vice President and Chief Executive Officer
CFO: Edward Healey, Associate Administrator Finance and Chief Financial Officer
CMO: Ali Ganjei, M.D., President Medical Staff
CHR: Bev Sugar, Associate Administrator and Director Human Resources
Web address: www.inova.org
Control: Other not–for–profit (including NFP Corporation) **Service:** General Medical and Surgical

Staffed Beds: 237 **Admissions:** 7876 **Census:** 148 **Outpatient Visits:** 76709 **Births:** 0 **Total Expense ($000):** 132128 **Payroll Expense ($000):** 57168 **Personnel:** 933

ARLINGTON—Arlington County

★ **VIRGINIA HOSPITAL CENTER – ARLINGTON (490050)**, 1701 North George Mason Drive, Zip 22205–3698; tel. 703/558–5000, (Nonreporting) **A**1 2 3 5 9 10
Primary Contact: James B. Cole, Chief Executive Officer
COO: Carl Bahnlein, Executive Vice President and Chief Operating Officer
CFO: Robin Norman, Senior Vice President and Chief Financial Officer
CMO: Archie McPherson, M.D., Vice President and Chief Medical Officer
CIO: David Crutchfield, Vice President and Chief Information Officer
CHR: Michael Malone, Vice President Administrative Services
Web address: www.virginiahospitalcenter.com
Control: Other not–for–profit (including NFP Corporation) **Service:** General Medical and Surgical

Staffed Beds: 264

BEDFORD—Independent City County

★ **BEDFORD MEMORIAL HOSPITAL (490088)**, 1613 Oakwood Street, Zip 24523–0688, Mailing Address: P.O. Box 688, Zip 24523–0688; tel. 540/586–2441, (Total facility includes 111 beds in nursing home–type unit) (Nonreporting) **A**1 9 10 **S** Carilion Clinic
Primary Contact: Georgia Watts, Interim Chief Executive Officer
CFO: Donald E. Lorton, Executive Vice President
CMO: E. Allen Joslyn, M.D., Chief Medical Officer
Web address: www.bmhva.com
Control: Other not–for–profit (including NFP Corporation) **Service:** General Medical and Surgical

Staffed Beds: 161

BIG STONE GAP—Wise County

★ **WELLMONT LONESOME PINE HOSPITAL (490114)**, 1990 Holton Avenue East, Zip 24219–0230; tel. 276/523–3111 **A**1 9 10 **F**11 13 15 25 28 30 31 32 33 38 42 44 46 49 50 54 55 57 62 68 73 74 75 76 77 79 80 81 82 84 86 96 97 100 102 107 108 109 119 120 121 124 135 136 **P**5 **S** Wellmont Health System
Primary Contact: Robert G. Polahar, President
CFO: Scarlett Dixon, Chief Financial Officer
Web address: www.wellmont.org
Control: Other not–for–profit (including NFP Corporation) **Service:** General Medical and Surgical

Staffed Beds: 60 **Admissions:** 3406 **Census:** 34 **Outpatient Visits:** 39925 **Births:** 261 **Total Expense ($000):** 31710 **Payroll Expense ($000):** 13620 **Personnel:** 279

BLACKSBURG—Montgomery County

★ **MONTGOMERY REGIONAL HOSPITAL (490110)**, 3700 South Main Street, Zip 24060–7081, Mailing Address: P.O. Box 90004, Zip 24062–9004; tel. 540/951–1111 **A**1 9 10 **F**3 13 15 17 18 24 25 26 27 33 34 35 38 40 43 48 49 53 55 56 57 62 68 72 73 74 75 76 77 79 80 81 84 86 96 97 100 102 103 106 107 119 120 121 135 136 137 **S** HCA
Primary Contact: Scott Hill, Chief Executive Officer
COO: David Cashwell, Chief Operating Officer
CFO: Tim Haasken, Chief Financial Officer
CMO: C Y Davis, Chief Medical Officer
CHR: Pat Guy, Director Human Resources
Web address: www.mrhospital.com
Control: Corporation, Investor–owned, for–profit **Service:** General Medical and Surgical

Staffed Beds: 89 **Admissions:** 4824 **Census:** 56

BURKEVILLE—Nottoway County

☐ **PIEDMONT GERIATRIC HOSPITAL (490134)**, 5001 East Patrick Henry Highway, Zip 23922–0427, Mailing Address: P.O. Box 427, Zip 23922–0427; tel. 434/767–4401, (Nonreporting) **A**1 9 10 **S** Virginia Department of Mental Health
Primary Contact: Stephen M. Herrick, Ph.D., Director
CFO: James G. Ayers, Chief Financial Officer
CMO: Hugo Falcon, M.D., Director Medical Services
CHR: Michael Wimsatt, Director Human Resources
Web address: www.pgh.dmhmrsas.virginia.gov
Control: State–Government, nonfederal **Service:** Other specialty

Staffed Beds: 150

CATAWBA—Roanoke County

☐ **CATAWBA HOSPITAL (490135)**, 5525 Catawba Hospital Drive, Zip 24070–2115, Mailing Address: P.O. Box 200, Zip 24070–0200; tel. 540/375–4200 **A**1 9 10 **F**25 26 30 31 32 33 36 37 41 50 66 73 75 88 93 119 135 **P**6 **S** Virginia Department of Mental Health
Primary Contact: Jack L. Wood, Director
COO: Charles Law, Director Information Technology Services
CFO: Charles Law, Director Information Technology Services
CMO: Yad Jabbarpour, M.D., Chief of Staff
CIO: Charles Law, Director Information Technology Services
CHR: Patricia Ebbett, Chief Human Resources Officer
Web address: www.catawba.dmhmrsas.virginia.gov
Control: State–Government, nonfederal **Service:** Psychiatric

Staffed Beds: 110 **Admissions:** 284 **Census:** 107 **Outpatient Visits:** 0 **Births:** 0 **Total Expense ($000):** 21891 **Payroll Expense ($000):** 11774 **Personnel:** 281

Many Facility Codes have changed. Please refer to the AHA Guide Code Chart.

CHARLOTTESVILLE—Independent City County

☒ **MARTHA JEFFERSON HOSPITAL (490077)**, 459 Locust Avenue, Zip 22902–9940; tel. 434/982–7000 **A**1 2 5 9 10 **F**3 8 13 15 18 20 24 25 26 27 30 31 32 33 34 38 43 44 46 48 49 50 52 53 55 56 57 61 62 66 68 72 73 74 76 77 79 80 81 82 84 86 87 96 97 99 100 102 103 106 107 109 111 113 118 119 121 124 133 134 135 136 137 **P**1
Primary Contact: James E. Haden, President and Chief Executive Officer
COO: Elliot H. Kuida, Vice President and Chief Operating Officer
CFO: J. Michael Burris, Vice President Corporate Services and Chief Financial Officer
CMO: F. Michael Ashby, M.D., Vice President and Medical Director
CIO: Marijo Lecker, Vice President
CHR: Susan M. Cabell–Mains, Vice President Administration
Web address: www.marthajefferson.org
Control: Other not–for–profit (including NFP Corporation) **Service:** General Medical and Surgical

Staffed Beds: 149 **Admissions:** 9932 **Census:** 91 **Outpatient Visits:** 304765 **Births:** 1819 **Total Expense ($000):** 165291 **Payroll Expense ($000):** 73492 **Personnel:** 1232

☒ **UNIVERSITY OF VIRGINIA MEDICAL CENTER (490009)**, 1215 Lee Street, Zip 22908–0001, Mailing Address: P.O. Box 800809, Zip 22908–0809; tel. 434/924–0211 **A**1 2 3 5 8 10 **F**3 5 6 7 8 9 11 12 13 15 16 17 18 19 20 21 22 23 24 25 26 27 28 30 31 32 33 34 35 36 37 38 40 41 42 43 44 45 46 47 48 49 50 51 53 54 55 56 57 58 59 60 61 62 63 64 66 68 69 70 71 72 73 74 75 76 77 78 79 80 81 82 83 84 85 86 87 88 89 90 91 92 93 94 96 97 99 100 102 103 104 105 106 107 108 109 111 112 113 114 116 118 119 120 121 123 124 125 126 127 128 129 130 131 132 134 135 136 137 **P**3 4
Primary Contact: R. Edward Howell, Vice President and Chief Executive Officer
COO: Margaret M. Van Bree, Dr.PH, Chief Operations Officer
CFO: Larry Fitzgerald, Chief Financial Officer
CMO: Susan E. Kirk, M.D., Associate Dean
CIO: Barbara Baldwin, Chief Information Officer
Web address: www.healthsystem.virginia.edu
Control: State–Government, nonfederal **Service:** General Medical and Surgical

Staffed Beds: 579 **Admissions:** 30133 **Census:** 474 **Outpatient Visits:** 1578433 **Births:** 1813 **Total Expense ($000):** 828474 **Payroll Expense ($000):** 301799 **Personnel:** 6186

☒ **UVA–HEALTHSOUTH REHABILITATION HOSPITAL (493029)**, 515 Ray C. Hunt Drive, Zip 22903; tel. 434/244–2000, (Nonreporting) **A**1 3 5 10 **S** HEALTHSOUTH Corporation
Primary Contact: Thomas J. Cook, Chief Executive Officer
Web address: www.healthsystem.virginia.edu/internet/pmr/pmrneo.cfm
Control: Corporation, Investor–owned, for–profit **Service:** Rehabilitation

Staffed Beds: 50

CHESAPEAKE—Independent City County

☒ **CHESAPEAKE GENERAL HOSPITAL (490120)**, 736 Battlefield Boulevard North, Zip 23320–4941, Mailing Address: P.O. Box 2028, Zip 23327–2028; tel. 757/312–8121 **A**1 2 9 10 **F**2 3 6 8 10 11 12 13 15 18 20 24 25 26 27 32 33 34 38 41 42 43 50 52 53 54 55 56 57 60 61 62 66 67 68 69 72 73 74 75 76 77 79 80 81 82 84 86 88 92 93 95 96 97 100 102 106 107 108 109 111 118 119 121 124 130 131 132 135 136 137
Primary Contact: Christopher R. Mosley, President and Chief Executive Officer
COO: Elaine Griffiths, Vice President Patient Services and Chief Nursing Officer
CFO: Michael Corcoran, Chief Financial Officer
CIO: Ken Deans, Chief Information Officer
CHR: Wynn Dixon, Vice President Operations
Web address: www.chesapeakeregional.com
Control: Hospital district or authority, Government, nonfederal **Service:** General Medical and Surgical

Staffed Beds: 310 **Admissions:** 16382 **Census:** 230 **Outpatient Visits:** 185862 **Births:** 3267 **Total Expense ($000):** 200826 **Payroll Expense ($000):** 79380 **Personnel:** 1793

CHRISTIANSBURG—Montgomery County

☒ **CARILION NEW RIVER VALLEY MEDICAL CENTER (490042)**, 2900 Lamb Circle, Zip 24073–5041, Mailing Address: P.O. Box 5, Radford, Zip 24143; tel. 540/731–2000 **A**1 9 10 19 **F**5 12 13 15 18 24 25 26 27 31 32 33 38 40 42 43 44 47 48 49 50 51 54 55 56 57 61 62 63 68 72 73 74 75 77 79 80 84 86 88 92 93 94 95 96 97 100 102 103 105 107 112 118 119 121 124 135 136 137 **S** Carilion Clinic
Primary Contact: Don Halliwill, President and Administrator
CFO: Rob Vaughan, Chief Financial Officer
CMO: Dennis Means, Vice President Medical Affairs
CIO: Daniel Borchi, Chief Information Officer
CHR: Patti Jurkus, Director Human Resources
Web address: www.carilion.com
Control: Other not–for–profit (including NFP Corporation) **Service:** General Medical and Surgical

Staffed Beds: 146 **Admissions:** 7492 **Census:** 86 **Outpatient Visits:** 102575 **Births:** 1152 **Total Expense ($000):** 110802 **Payroll Expense ($000):** 44455 **Personnel:** 889

CLINTWOOD—Dickenson County

★ **DICKENSON COMMUNITY HOSPITAL (491303)**, 312 Hospital Drive, Zip 24228, Mailing Address: P.O. Box 1440, Zip 24228–1440; tel. 276/926–0300 **A**9 10 18 **F**3 11 25 26 38 50 55 62 66 68 73 80 81 87 96 107 119 122 135 **P**6
Primary Contact: Lee Turner, Executive Director
CFO: Christy Fleming, Controller
CMO: Erin Mullins, Chief Medical Staff
CHR: Valerie Colyer, Director Human Resources
Web address: www.dchosp.com
Control: Other not–for–profit (including NFP Corporation) **Service:** General Medical and Surgical

Staffed Beds: 15 **Admissions:** 762 **Census:** 7 **Outpatient Visits:** 31207 **Births:** 0 **Total Expense ($000):** 9346 **Payroll Expense ($000):** 3803 **Personnel:** 93

CULPEPER—Culpeper County

☒ **CULPEPER REGIONAL HOSPITAL (490019)**, 501 Sunset Lane, Zip 22701–3917, Mailing Address: Box 592, Zip 22701–0592; tel. 540/829–4100 **A**1 9 10 **F**3 7 8 11 13 15 24 25 26 30 31 32 33 34 35 36 38 42 43 44 45 50 55 56 57 61 62 66 68 72 73 74 75 76 77 79 80 82 84 86 92 96 97 100 102 107 112 119 121 122 124 132 134 135 137 **P**6 8
Primary Contact: H. Lee Kirk, Jr., President and Chief Executive Officer
COO: Patricia Mullins, Senior Vice President Operations
CFO: Samuel Morgan, Senior Vice President Financial Operations
CMO: Eric Mowatt–Larssen, President Medical Staff
CIO: Brian Rock, Director Information Systems
CHR: Susan Edwards, Director Human Resources
Web address: www.culpeperhospital.com
Control: Other not–for–profit (including NFP Corporation) **Service:** General Medical and Surgical

Staffed Beds: 60 **Admissions:** 3804 **Census:** 38 **Outpatient Visits:** 36658 **Births:** 532 **Total Expense ($000):** 52028 **Payroll Expense ($000):** 23701 **Personnel:** 533

DANVILLE—Independent City County

☒ **DANVILLE REGIONAL MEDICAL CENTER (490075)**, 142 South Main Street, Zip 24541–2922; tel. 434/799–2100, (Total facility includes 35 beds in nursing home–type unit) **A**1 2 6 9 10 **F**3 4 5 11 13 14 15 17 18 20 22 24 25 26 27 30 31 32 33 38 42 43 49 50 52 53 55 56 57 58 59 60 61 62 66 68 73 74 75 76 77 79 80 81 82 84 85 86 87 88 90 91 92 94 95 96 97 100 102 103 104 106 107 109 111 112 117 119 121 124 133 135 136 **P**6 8 **S** LifePoint Hospitals, Inc.
Primary Contact: Jerel T. Humphrey, Chief Executive Officer
CFO: Mark T. Anderson, Chief Financial Officer
CIO: David Cartwright, Director Management Information Systems
CHR: MaDena DuChemin, Assistant Administrator Human Resources
Web address: www.danvilleregional.org
Control: Corporation, Investor–owned, for–profit **Service:** General Medical and Surgical

Staffed Beds: 173 **Admissions:** 10001 **Census:** 166 **Outpatient Visits:** 137743 **Births:** 966 **Total Expense ($000):** 147080 **Payroll Expense ($000):** 50387 **Personnel:** 1044

VA

Hospital, Medicare Provider Number, Address, Telephone, Approval, Facility, and Physician Codes, Health Care System
★ American Hospital Association (AHA) membership
□ The Joint Commission accreditation
○ American Osteopathic Association (AOA) accreditation
△ Commission on Accreditation of Rehabilitation Facilities (CARF) accreditation

☐ **SOUTHERN VIRGINIA MENTAL HEALTH INSTITUTE (494017)**, 382 Taylor Drive, Zip 24541–4023; tel. 434/799–6220 **A**1 9 10 **F**88 124 135 **S** Virginia Department of Mental Health
Primary Contact: David M. Lyon, Director
CFO: Wade Hopkins, Administrator
CMO: B. R. Ashby, M.D., President and Chief Executive Officer
CIO: Bracken Jones, Director Information Technology
CHR: Pauline Wasiuk, Director Human Resources
Web address: www.svmhi.dmhmrsas.virginia.gov
Control: State–Government, nonfederal **Service:** Psychiatric

Staffed Beds: 72 **Admissions:** 497 **Census:** 69 **Outpatient Visits:** 0 **Births:** 0 **Total Expense ($000):** 12330 **Payroll Expense ($000):** 6717 **Personnel:** 172

EMPORIA—Independent City County

★ **SOUTHERN VIRGINIA REGIONAL MEDICAL CENTER (490097)**, 727 North Main Street, Zip 23847–1482; tel. 434/348–4400 **A**1 9 10 **F**3 11 15 24 25 26 27 32 37 38 43 49 55 57 61 62 68 75 76 79 80 84 86 88 93 94 96 102 107 112 118 119 122 135 137 **P**5 **S** Community Health Systems, Inc.
Primary Contact: Douglas T. Arbour, Chief Executive Officer
COO: Douglas T. Arbour, Chief Executive Officer
CFO: Michael Cotton, Chief Financial Officer
CMO: Adolph Flowers, Chief of Staff
CIO: Tracy Bullock, Director Management Information Systems
CHR: Becky Parrish, Director Human Resources
Web address: www.svrmc.com
Control: Corporation, Investor–owned, for–profit **Service:** General Medical and Surgical

Staffed Beds: 80 **Admissions:** 2887 **Census:** 35 **Outpatient Visits:** 26593 **Births:** 0 **Total Expense ($000):** 33112 **Payroll Expense ($000):** 11146 **Personnel:** 321

FAIRFAX—Independent City County

★ △ **INOVA FAIR OAKS HOSPITAL (490101)**, 3600 Joseph Siewick Drive, Zip 22033–1798; tel. 703/391–3600 **A**1 2 3 5 7 9 10 **F**3 11 12 13 15 25 26 27 28 30 31 32 33 35 37 38 40 41 43 44 46 47 48 49 50 51 55 56 57 59 60 61 62 66 67 68 70 72 73 74 75 76 77 78 79 80 81 82 84 86 87 90 92 96 97 100 102 106 107 118 119 120 121 135 136 137 **S** Inova Health System
Primary Contact: John L. Fitzgerald, Chief Executive Officer
COO: Pam Capobianco, Chief Operating Officer
CFO: Bill Bane, Assistant Vice President and Chief Financial Officer
CIO: Geoffrey Brown, Chief Information Officer
Web address: www.inova.org
Control: Other not–for–profit (including NFP Corporation) **Service:** General Medical and Surgical

Staffed Beds: 196 **Admissions:** 13371 **Census:** 131 **Outpatient Visits:** 104553 **Births:** 3896 **Total Expense ($000):** 182074 **Payroll Expense ($000):** 75129 **Personnel:** 1188

FALLS CHURCH—Independent City County

CAPITAL HOSPICE (490129), 6565 Arlington Boulevard, Suite 500, Zip 22042; tel. 703/538–2065, (Nonreporting) **A**5 10
Primary Contact: Malene S. Davis, RN, President and Chief Executive Officer
CFO: David Schwind, Chief Financial Officer
CIO: Diane Rigsby, Chief Information Officer
Web address: www.capitalhospice.org
Control: Other not–for–profit (including NFP Corporation) **Service:** Other specialty

Staffed Beds: 15

★ **DOMINION HOSPITAL (494023)**, 2960 Sleepy Hollow Road, Zip 22044–2001; tel. 703/536–2000 **A**1 9 10 **F**25 30 33 56 88 89 90 91 92 95 119 **S** HCA
Primary Contact: Suzanne B. Jackson, Chief Executive Officer
CFO: Edward R. Stojakovich, Chief Financial Officer
CMO: Gary Litovitz, Medical Director
CIO: Cyndi Hite, Director Information Services
CHR: Lesley Channell, Assistant Vice President Human Resources
Web address: www.dominionhospital.com
Control: Corporation, Investor–owned, for–profit **Service:** Psychiatric

Staffed Beds: 91 **Admissions:** 1891 **Census:** 44 **Outpatient Visits:** 6107 **Births:** 0 **Total Expense ($000):** 14572 **Payroll Expense ($000):** 8463 **Personnel:** 106

★ **INOVA FAIRFAX HOSPITAL (490063)**, 3300 Gallows Road, Zip 22042–3300; tel. 703/776–4001 **A**1 2 3 5 8 9 10 **F**3 4 5 7 8 11 12 13 14 15 17 18 19 20 21 22 23 24 25 26 27 28 30 31 32 33 34 35 36 37 38 39 40 41 42 43 44 45 46 47 48 49 50 51 53 54 55 56 57 58 59 60 62 63 64 66 67 68 70 71 72 73 74 75 76 77 78 79 80 81 82 83 84 85 86 87 88 89 90 91 92 93 94 95 96 97 98 99 100 102 103 104 105 106 107 108 109 111 112 114 116 119 120 121 123 124 125 126 127 129 130 131 133 134 135 136 137 **P**6 **S** Inova Health System
Primary Contact: Reuven Pasternak, M.D., Chief Executive Officer
COO: Toni R. Ardabell, R.N., Chief Operating Officer
CFO: Ronald Ewald, Chief Financial Officer
CMO: Joseph Hallal, M.D., President, Medical Staff
CIO: Geoffrey Brown, Vice President Information Systems
CHR: Hugo Aguas, Vice President Human Resources
Web address: www.inova.org
Control: Other not–for–profit (including NFP Corporation) **Service:** General Medical and Surgical

Staffed Beds: 927 **Admissions:** 54527 **Census:** 748 **Outpatient Visits:** 367122 **Births:** 11746 **Total Expense ($000):** 918315 **Payroll Expense ($000):** 374778 **Personnel:** 5831

☐ **NORTHERN VIRGINIA MENTAL HEALTH INSTITUTE (494010)**, 3302 Gallows Road, Zip 22042–3398; tel. 703/207–7110, (Nonreporting) **A**1 5 9 10 **S** Virginia Department of Mental Health
Primary Contact: Lynn Delacy, RN, Ph.D., Facility Director
CFO: Anne Baxter, Fiscal Services Director
CMO: R. Maximilien del Rio, Medical Director
CHR: Betsy Thompson, Director Human Resources
Web address: www.nvmhi.dmhmrsas.virginia.gov
Control: State–Government, nonfederal **Service:** Psychiatric

Staffed Beds: 137

FARMVILLE—Prince Edward County

★ **SOUTHSIDE COMMUNITY HOSPITAL (490090)**, 800 Oak Street, Zip 23901–1199; tel. 434/392–8811 **A**1 3 5 9 10 20 **F**3 11 13 15 25 26 30 31 32 33 38 40 41 50 51 55 56 57 59 61 62 66 68 69 72 73 74 75 77 79 80 81 82 84 86 96 97 100 102 106 107 118 119 120 121 122 135 137 **P**6
Primary Contact: Gwen S. Eddleman, FACHE, Ed.D., President and Chief Executive Officer
COO: Claudia Meinhard, Chief Nursing Officer
CFO: William L. Bass, Vice President Finance and Chief Financial Officer
Web address: www.sch–farmville.org
Control: Other not–for–profit (including NFP Corporation) **Service:** General Medical and Surgical

Staffed Beds: 88 **Admissions:** 4376 **Census:** 39 **Outpatient Visits:** 51678 **Births:** 437 **Total Expense ($000):** 40749 **Payroll Expense ($000):** 17994 **Personnel:** 382

FISHERSVILLE—Augusta County

☐ **AUGUSTA HEALTH CARE (490018)**, 78 Medical Center Drive, Zip 22939–2332, Mailing Address: P.O. Box 1000, Zip 22939–1000; tel. 540/932–4000 **A**1 2 3 5 9 10 19 20 **F**1 2 3 4 5 7 11 13 15 16 17 24 25 26 27 30 31 32 33 34 37 38 42 43 46 48 49 51 52 54 55 56 57 58 60 61 62 65 66 68 70 71 72 73 74 75 76 77 78 79 80 81 82 83 84 85 86 87 88 89 90 91 92 93 94 95 96 97 100 102 103 104 105 106 107 108 109 111 117 118 119 120 121 124 132 133 135 136 137 **P**6
Primary Contact: Mary N. Mannix, President and Chief Executive Officer
COO: David E. Deering, Senior Vice President and Chief Operating Officer
CFO: John R. Heider, Vice President Finance
CMO: Fred Castello, M.D., Chief Medical Officer
CIO: Martin Morehouse, Director
CHR: Sue Krzastek, Vice President Human Resources
Web address: www.augustamed.com
Control: Other not–for–profit (including NFP Corporation) **Service:** General Medical and Surgical

Staffed Beds: 178 **Admissions:** 10954 **Census:** 134 **Outpatient Visits:** 434070 **Births:** 1243 **Total Expense ($000):** 193115 **Payroll Expense ($000):** 78044 **Personnel:** 1858

WOODROW WILSON REHABILITATION CENTER, Mailing Address: P.O. Box 1500, Zip 22939–1500; tel. 540/332–7000, (Nonreporting)
Primary Contact: Richard Luck, Ed.D., Facility Director
COO: Richard Luck, Ed.D., Facility Director
CFO: Ernie Steidle, Chief Operating Officer
CMO: Mammen Mathew, Chief Rehabilitation Medicine
CIO: Keith Burt, Marketing Director
CHR: Debbie Mitchell, Human Resource Director
Web address: www.wwrc.net
Control: State–Government, nonfederal **Service:** Rehabilitation

Staffed Beds: 30

VA

FORT BELVOIR—Fairfax County

★ **DEWITT ARMY COMMUNITY HOSPITAL**, 9501 Farrell Road, Zip 22060–5901; tel. 703/805–0510, (Nonreporting) **A**1 3 5 **S** Department of the Army, Office of the Surgeon General
Primary Contact: Colonel Kenneth Canestrini, Commander
CMO: Lieutenant Colonel Mark D. Harris, Deputy Commander Clinical Services
CIO: Terrance Branch, Chief Information Management
Web address: www.dewitt.wramc.amedd.army.mil
Control: Army, Government, federal **Service:** General Medical and Surgical

Staffed Beds: 46

FRANKLIN—Independent City County

★ **SOUTHAMPTON MEMORIAL HOSPITAL (490092)**, 100 Fairview Drive, Zip 23851–1206, Mailing Address: P.O. Box 817, Zip 23851–0817; tel. 757/569–6100, (Total facility includes 131 beds in nursing home–type unit) (Nonreporting) **A**1 9 10 20 **S** Community Health Systems, Inc.
Primary Contact: David W. Fuller, Chief Executive Officer
CFO: Steve Ramey, Chief Financial Officer
CMO: Daniel Peak, M.D., Chief Medical Staff
CHR: Elizabeth Parrish, Director Human Resources
Web address: www.smhfranklin.com
Control: Corporation, Investor–owned, for–profit **Service:** General Medical and Surgical

Staffed Beds: 203

FREDERICKSBURG—Independent City County

★ **MARY WASHINGTON HOSPITAL (490022)**, 1001 Sam Perry Boulevard, Zip 22401–3354; tel. 540/741–1100 **A**1 2 9 10 19 20 **F**3 11 12 13 15 17 18 20 22 24 25 26 27 30 31 32 33 34 38 41 42 43 44 45 46 47 48 49 50 51 54 55 56 57 58 59 60 61 62 66 68 69 70 72 73 74 75 76 77 79 80 81 82 84 86 88 89 90 92 96 97 100 102 103 104 106 107 116 118 119 120 124 135 136 137 **P**6 8
Primary Contact: Fred M. Rankin, III, President and Chief Executive Officer
COO: Walter J. Kiwall, Executive Vice President and Chief Operating Officer
CFO: Sean Barden, Executive Vice President and Chief Financial Officer
CMO: J. Thomas Ryan, M.D., Executive Vice President Medical Affairs
CIO: Steve Cooley, Vice President Information Services
CHR: Kathryn Wall, Executive Vice President Human Resources and Organizational Development
Web address: www.medicorp.org
Control: Other not–for–profit (including NFP Corporation) **Service:** General Medical and Surgical

Staffed Beds: 412 **Admissions:** 29139 **Census:** 306 **Outpatient Visits:** 355761 **Births:** 4077 **Total Expense ($000):** 364908 **Payroll Expense ($000):** 124925 **Personnel:** 2876

☐ **SNOWDEN AT FREDERICKSBURG (494028)**, 1200 Sam Perry Boulevard, Zip 22401; tel. 540/741–3900, (Nonreporting) **A**1 9 10
Primary Contact: Jim King, Chief Executive Officer
Control: Other not–for–profit (including NFP Corporation) **Service:** Psychiatric

Staffed Beds: 30

FRONT ROYAL—Warren County

★ **WARREN MEMORIAL HOSPITAL (490033)**, 1000 Shenandoah Avenue, Zip 22630–3598; tel. 540/636–0300, (Total facility includes 120 beds in nursing home–type unit) **A**1 9 10 **F**3 11 13 15 24 25 26 30 31 33 34 38 43 50 54 55 56 57 62 63 65 68 73 74 75 77 79 80 81 82 84 86 96 97 100 102 106 107 117 119 121 124 135 136 137 **S** Valley Health System
Primary Contact: Patrick B. Nolan, President and Chief Executive Officer
CFO: Mark Bower, Vice President
CMO: Robert Meltredt, M.D., Vice President Medical Affairs
CHR: Adrienne McKenna, Vice President and Human Resources Officer
Web address: www.valleyhealthlink.com
Control: Other not–for–profit (including NFP Corporation) **Service:** General Medical and Surgical

Staffed Beds: 166 **Admissions:** 2770 **Census:** 137 **Outpatient Visits:** 68000 **Births:** 236 **Total Expense ($000):** 50064 **Payroll Expense ($000):** 23045 **Personnel:** 411

GALAX—Independent City County

★ **TWIN COUNTY REGIONAL HOSPITAL (490115)**, 200 Hospital Drive, Zip 24333–2283; tel. 276/236–8181 **A**1 9 10 20 **F**3 13 14 15 24 25 26 27 30 32 33 38 42 50 51 52 55 56 61 62 66 68 73 74 76 77 79 80 82 84 86 88 90 91 92 93 94 96 97 100 102 107 118 119 121 122 124 135 136 137 **P**5 8
Primary Contact: Jon D. Applebaum, President and Chief Executive Officer
COO: Sandy Moretz, R.N., Vice President Patient Care Services and Chief Operating Officer
CFO: Nelson L. Montgomery, Chief Financial Officer
CMO: Jack G. Brock, M.D., Chief of Staff
CIO: Jack Roberts, Director Information Systems
CHR: Ruth Ann Lewis, Vice President Human Resources
Web address: www.tcrh.org
Control: Other not–for–profit (including NFP Corporation) **Service:** General Medical and Surgical

Staffed Beds: 86 **Admissions:** 4218 **Census:** 46 **Outpatient Visits:** 61407 **Births:** 430 **Total Expense ($000):** 44074 **Payroll Expense ($000):** 21711 **Personnel:** 574

GLOUCESTER—Gloucester County

☐ **RIVERSIDE WALTER REED HOSPITAL (490130)**, 7519 Hospital Drive, Zip 23061–4178, Mailing Address: P.O. Box 1130, Zip 23061–1130; tel. 804/693–8800 **A**1 9 10 **F**3 11 15 24 25 30 31 32 33 38 40 41 42 49 50 51 55 57 62 68 73 75 77 79 80 81 82 86 96 97 99 100 102 106 107 108 109 111 119 121 135 **P**6 **S** Riverside Health System
Primary Contact: Robert E. Bryant, Vice President and Administrator
CHR: Kent Taylor, Director Human Resources
Web address: www.riversideonline.com
Control: Other not–for–profit (including NFP Corporation) **Service:** General Medical and Surgical

Staffed Beds: 24 **Admissions:** 2448 **Census:** 24 **Outpatient Visits:** 82484 **Births:** 0 **Total Expense ($000):** 31142 **Payroll Expense ($000):** 12241 **Personnel:** 212

GRUNDY—Buchanan County

★ **BUCHANAN GENERAL HOSPITAL (490127)**, Mailing Address: Route 5, Box 20, Zip 24614–9611; tel. 276/935–1000 **A**1 9 10 20 **F**3 15 25 27 38 46 55 57 61 68 76 77 79 86 96 97 102 106 107 119 121 124 135
Primary Contact: Joan Jamison, Chief Executive Officer
CFO: Kim Boyd, Chief Financial Officer
CMO: Dinkar Patel, Chief of Staff
CIO: Rita Ramey, Director Information Systems
CHR: Wanda Stiltner, Director Human Resources
Web address: www.bgh.org
Control: Other not–for–profit (including NFP Corporation) **Service:** General Medical and Surgical

Staffed Beds: 134 **Admissions:** 2565 **Census:** 32 **Outpatient Visits:** 47461 **Births:** 0 **Total Expense ($000):** 24484 **Payroll Expense ($000):** 10383 **Personnel:** 281

HAMPTON—Independent City County

★ **RIVERSIDE BEHAVIORAL HEALTH CENTER (494001)**, 2244 Executive Drive, Zip 23666–2430; tel. 757/827–1001 **A**1 9 10 **F**4 5 25 88 89 90 91 92 93 94 **P**5 **S** Riverside Health System
Primary Contact: Debora S. Tanner, Vice President and Administrator
CFO: Vonnie James, Director Finance and Support Services
CMO: Anthony Caterine, M.D., Executive Medical Director
Web address: www.riversideonline.com
Control: Corporation, Investor–owned, for–profit **Service:** Psychiatric

Staffed Beds: 79 **Admissions:** 2328 **Census:** 79 **Outpatient Visits:** 5617 **Births:** 0 **Total Expense ($000):** 17057 **Payroll Expense ($000):** 10420 **Personnel:** 262

★ **SENTARA CAREPLEX HOSPITAL (490093)**, 3000 Coliseum Drive, Zip 23666–5963; tel. 757/736–2656 **A**1 2 5 9 10 **F**3 8 11 12 13 15 18 20 24 25 26 27 30 31 32 33 34 35 37 38 39 40 41 43 44 45 49 50 51 52 53 55 56 57 58 59 60 62 63 66 68 69 72 73 74 75 76 77 78 79 80 81 82 86 90 96 97 99 100 102 104 105 106 107 108 109 111 118 119 120 121 133 135 136 137 **S** Sentara Healthcare
Primary Contact: Debra A. Flores, Vice President and Administrator
CFO: Cheryl Larner, Chief Financial Officer
CMO: Gary R. Yates, M.D., Chief Medical Officer
Web address: www.sentara.com
Control: Other not–for–profit (including NFP Corporation) **Service:** General Medical and Surgical

Staffed Beds: 200 **Admissions:** 11265 **Census:** 162 **Outpatient Visits:** 479522 **Births:** 933 **Total Expense ($000):** 197160 **Payroll Expense ($000):** 76295 **Personnel:** 1408

VA

Hospital, Medicare Provider Number, Address, Telephone, Approval, Facility, and Physician Codes, Health Care System

★ American Hospital Association (AHA) membership
☐ The Joint Commission accreditation
○ American Osteopathic Association (AOA) accreditation
△ Commission on Accreditation of Rehabilitation Facilities (CARF) accreditation

★ **U. S. AIR FORCE HOSPITAL**, 45 Pine Street, Zip 23665–2080; tel. 757/764–6969, (Nonreporting) **S** Department of the Air Force
Primary Contact: Colonel David C. Houglum, MC, Administrator
COO: Colonel Paul Ziaya, Commander
CMO: Colonel June Carraher, Chief Hospital Services
CIO: Major Charles Chapdelaine, Chief of Information Management and Technology
Control: Air Force, Government, federal **Service:** General Medical and Surgical

Staffed Beds: 59

★ △ **VETERANS AFFAIRS MEDICAL CENTER**, 100 Emancipation Drive, Zip 23667–0001; tel. 757/722–9961, (Total facility includes 120 beds in nursing home–type unit) (Nonreporting) **A**1 2 3 5 7 **S** Department of Veterans Affairs
Primary Contact: Wanda Mims, Director
COO: Lorraine B. Price, Associate Director
CFO: Terry Grew, Chief Business Office
CMO: Val Gibberman, Acting Chief of Staff
CIO: Cary Parks, Chief Information Resource Management
Web address: www.va.gov/sta/guide/home.asp
Control: Veterans Affairs, Government, federal **Service:** General Medical and Surgical

Staffed Beds: 485

HARRISONBURG—Independent City County

★ **ROCKINGHAM MEMORIAL HOSPITAL (490004)**, 235 Cantrell Avenue, Zip 22801–3293; tel. 540/433–4100 **A**1 2 5 6 9 10 19 **F**5 8 11 13 15 17 18 20 22 24 25 26 27 30 31 32 33 34 36 38 42 43 49 50 52 53 55 56 57 61 62 66 68 69 72 73 74 75 76 77 79 81 82 84 86 87 88 92 94 95 97 99 107 108 109 111 112 118 119 120 121 123 124 135 136 137 **P**4
Primary Contact: James D. Krauss, President and Chief Executive Officer
COO: Richard L. Haushalter, Chief Operating Officer
CFO: Richard L. Haushalter, Chief Operating Officer
CMO: Dale Carroll, M.D., Senior Vice President Medical Affairs and Performance Improvement
CIO: Mike Rozmus, Director Information Systems
CHR: Mark Zimmerman, Vice President Human Resources Development
Web address: www.rmhonline.com
Control: Other not–for–profit (including NFP Corporation) **Service:** General Medical and Surgical

Staffed Beds: 244 **Admissions:** 13946 **Census:** 150 **Outpatient Visits:** 478222 **Births:** 1725 **Total Expense ($000):** 223614 **Payroll Expense ($000):** 99751 **Personnel:** 1871

HOPEWELL—Independent City County

★ **JOHN RANDOLPH MEDICAL CENTER (490020)**, 411 West Randolph Road, Zip 23860–2938; tel. 804/541–1600 **A**1 2 9 10 **F**3 5 11 15 17 18 24 25 26 27 30 31 32 36 37 38 41 49 50 53 55 56 57 62 67 68 72 73 75 76 77 79 80 81 82 86 88 90 91 92 93 94 95 96 97 99 100 102 103 106 107 119 120 121 124 133 135 137 **S** HCA
Primary Contact: Elwood Bernard Boone, III, Chief Executive Officer
COO: Dia Nichols, Chief Operating Officer
CFO: Chigger Bynum, Chief Financial Officer
CHR: MaDena DuChemin, Assistant Administrator Human Resources
Web address: www.johnrandolphmed.com
Control: Corporation, Investor–owned, for–profit **Service:** General Medical and Surgical

Staffed Beds: 132 **Admissions:** 5240 **Census:** 89 **Outpatient Visits:** 72824 **Births:** 0 **Personnel:** 537

HOT SPRINGS—Bath County

★ **BATH COMMUNITY HOSPITAL (491300)**, (Formerly Bath County Community Hospital), 83 Park Drive, Zip 24445, Mailing Address: P.O. Drawer Z, Zip 24445; tel. 540/839–7000 **A**1 9 10 18 **F**3 7 15 24 33 38 42 50 52 55 57 61 62 73 75 77 79 86 92 96 100 107 117 119 120 122 124 132
Primary Contact: Deborah Lipes, RN, Chief Executive Officer
CFO: James A. Greer, Chief Financial Officer
CMO: James Redington, M.D., Chief of Staff
CIO: Tracy Bartley, Manager Information Technology
CHR: Patricia Foutz, Director Human Resources
Web address: www.bcchospital.org
Control: Other not–for–profit (including NFP Corporation) **Service:** General Medical and Surgical

Staffed Beds: 25 **Admissions:** 541 **Census:** 8 **Outpatient Visits:** 10614 **Births:** 0 **Total Expense ($000):** 11869 **Payroll Expense ($000):** 5394 **Personnel:** 122

KILMARNOCK—Lancaster County

★ **RAPPAHANNOCK GENERAL HOSPITAL (490123)**, 101 Harris Drive, Zip 22482, Mailing Address: P.O. Box 1449, Zip 22482–1449; tel. 804/435–8000 **A**1 9 10 20 **F**3 8 11 15 25 26 27 28 30 31 32 37 38 44 54 55 57 60 61 62 66 68 73 75 76 77 79 81 82 86 88 90 91 92 93 94 95 96 97 100 102 107 119 120 121 122 135 137 **P**3 4
Primary Contact: James M. Holmes, Jr., President and Chief Executive Officer
Web address: www.rgh–hospital.com
Control: Other not–for–profit (including NFP Corporation) **Service:** General Medical and Surgical

Staffed Beds: 76 **Admissions:** 2267 **Census:** 33 **Outpatient Visits:** 58425 **Births:** 0 **Total Expense ($000):** 32111 **Payroll Expense ($000):** 14370 **Personnel:** 336

LEBANON—Russell County

★ **RUSSELL COUNTY MEDICAL CENTER (490002)**, 58 Carroll Street, Zip 24266–4510, Mailing Address: P.O. Box 3600, Zip 24266–3600; tel. 276/883–8000, (Nonreporting) **A**1 9 10
Primary Contact: Jeffrey H. Whitton, Chief Executive Officer
CFO: Mother Superior John Doyle, Chief Financial Officer
CMO: Matthew Cheng, M.D., Chief of Staff
CIO: Tammy Bratcher, Director Information Systems
CHR: Phyllis Kiser, Director Human Resources
Web address: www.rcmc.net
Control: Corporation, Investor–owned, for–profit **Service:** General Medical and Surgical

Staffed Beds: 78

LEESBURG—Loudoun County

★ **INOVA LOUDOUN HOSPITAL (490043)**, 44045 Riverside Parkway, Zip 20176–2799, Mailing Address: P.O. Box 6000, Zip 20176–6000; tel. 703/858–6000 **A**1 2 9 10 **F**3 8 11 13 15 18 19 24 25 26 27 28 30 31 32 33 38 39 41 48 49 53 54 55 56 57 59 62 66 68 69 71 72 73 74 75 76 77 79 80 81 82 84 86 88 90 91 92 93 94 95 96 97 100 102 103 106 107 108 109 111 119 120 121 124 135 136 137 **P**6 **S** Inova Health System
Primary Contact: Randall L. Kelley, Chief Executive Officer
COO: Susan Carroll, Chief Operating Officer
CFO: Glenn Zirbser, Chief Financial Officer
CMO: Christopher Chiantella, Chief of Staff
CIO: Nancy Mengel, Director Information Technology
CHR: Roxanne Cole, Director Human Resources and Guest Services
Web address: www.loudounhospital.org
Control: Other not–for–profit (including NFP Corporation) **Service:** General Medical and Surgical

Staffed Beds: 155 **Admissions:** 11020 **Census:** 122 **Outpatient Visits:** 122559 **Births:** 2509 **Total Expense ($000):** 162146 **Payroll Expense ($000):** 70854 **Personnel:** 1201

NORTH SPRINGS BEHAVIORAL HEALTHCARE, (Formerly Whisper Ridge at Leesburg), 42009 Victory Lane, Zip 20176–6269; tel. 703/777–0800 **F**88 89 **P**6 **S** Psychiatric Solutions
Primary Contact: Scott Zeiter, Chief Executive Officer
CFO: Bill Gitzen, Chief Financial Officer
CMO: Edgardo Francisco, M.D., Medical Director
Web address: www.northspringleesburg.com
Control: Corporation, Investor–owned, for–profit **Service:** Children's hospital psychiatric

Staffed Beds: 77 **Admissions:** 73 **Census:** 52 **Outpatient Visits:** 0 **Births:** 0

LEXINGTON—Independent City County

★ **CARILION STONEWALL JACKSON HOSPITAL (491304)**, (Formerly Stonewall Jackson Hospital), 1 Health Circle, Zip 24450–2492; tel. 540/458–3300 **A**1 9 10 18 **F**11 13 15 24 25 26 30 31 32 33 38 43 55 56 57 61 67 68 73 74 75 77 79 86 96 100 102 107 119 122 135 **S** Carilion Clinic
Primary Contact: Thomas W. McNamara, D.O., President and Chief Executive Officer
CFO: David L. Jones, Chief Financial Officer
CMO: Lyle McClung, Chief of Staff
Web address: www.sjhospital.com
Control: Other not–for–profit (including NFP Corporation) **Service:** General Medical and Surgical

Staffed Beds: 25 **Admissions:** 1568 **Census:** 16 **Outpatient Visits:** 32672 **Births:** 315 **Total Expense ($000):** 27524 **Payroll Expense ($000):** 10841 **Personnel:** 249

VA

Many Facility Codes have changed. Please refer to the AHA Guide Code Chart.

LOW MOOR—Alleghany County

▣ **ALLEGHANY REGIONAL HOSPITAL (490126)**, One ARH Lane, Zip 24457, Mailing Address: P.O. Box 7, Zip 24457–0007; tel. 540/862–6011, (Nonreporting) **A**1 9 10 20 **S** HCA
Primary Contact: Timothy C. Tobin, President and Chief Executive Officer
CFO: Joe Jeans, Chief Financial Officer
CMO: Hassan Honainy, M.D., President Medical Staff
CIO: Jeffrey Steelman, Director Information Systems
Web address: www.alleghanyregional.com
Control: Corporation, Investor–owned, for–profit **Service:** General Medical and Surgical

Staffed Beds: 146

LURAY—Page County

▣ **PAGE MEMORIAL HOSPITAL (491307)**, 200 Memorial Drive, Zip 22835–1005; tel. 540/743–4561, (Nonreporting) **A**1 9 10 18
Primary Contact: Travis Clark, Chief Executive Officer
CFO: Phillip Graybeal, Chief Financial Officer
Web address: www.pagememorialhospital.org
Control: Other not–for–profit (including NFP Corporation) **Service:** General Medical and Surgical

Staffed Beds: 25

LYNCHBURG—Independent City County

★ △ **CENTRA HEALTH (490021)**, 1920 Atherholt Road, Zip 24501–1104; tel. 434/200–4700, (Includes LYNCHBURG GENERAL HOSPITAL, 1901 Tate Springs Road, Zip 24501–1167; tel. 434/200–3000; VIRGINIA BAPTIST HOSPITAL, 3300 Rivermont Avenue, Zip 24503–2053; tel. 434/200–4000), (Total facility includes 36 beds in nursing home–type unit) **A**2 3 5 6 7 9 10 **F**1 3 5 7 10 11 13 15 17 18 20 22 24 25 26 27 31 32 33 38 40 42 43 50 54 55 56 57 59 61 62 66 68 69 70 72 73 74 75 76 77 79 80 82 84 85 86 88 89 90 92 94 96 97 99 100 102 103 107 109 110 112 117 118 119 121 124 132 135 137 **P**6 7
Primary Contact: George W. Dawson, President and Chief Executive Officer
CFO: Lewis C. Addison, Senior Vice President and Chief Financial Officer
CMO: Chalmers Nunn, M.D., Chief Medical Officer and Senior Vice President
CIO: Ben Clark, Vice President and Chief Information Officer
CHR: Jan Walker, Director Human Resources
Web address: www.centrahealth.com
Control: Other not–for–profit (including NFP Corporation) **Service:** General Medical and Surgical

Staffed Beds: 577 **Admissions:** 27241 **Census:** 714 **Outpatient Visits:** 116339 **Births:** 2544 **Total Expense ($000):** 364598 **Payroll Expense ($000):** 159146 **Personnel:** 3071

MADISON HEIGHTS—Amherst County

CENTRAL VIRGINIA TRAINING CENTER (490108), 210 East Colony Road, Zip 24572–2005, Mailing Address: P.O. Box 1098, Lynchburg, Zip 24505–1098; tel. 434/947–6326, (Total facility includes 104 beds in nursing home–type unit) (Nonreporting) **A**10 **S** Virginia Department of Mental Health
Primary Contact: Denise D. Micheletti, RN, Acting Director
COO: Denise D. Micheletti, Acting Director
CFO: Charles Felmlee, Assistant Director Fiscal Services
CMO: Balraj Bawa, Assistant Director Medical Services
CHR: Burchkhard Blob, Manager Human Resources
Web address: www.cvtc.dmhmrsas.virginia.gov/
Control: State–Government, nonfederal **Service:** Institution for mental retardation

Staffed Beds: 1112

MANASSAS—Independent City County

★ **PRINCE WILLIAM HOSPITAL (490045)**, 8700 Sudley Road, Zip 20110–4418, Mailing Address: P.O. Box 2610, Zip 20108–0867; tel. 703/369–8000 **A**2 9 10 **F**3 5 8 10 11 13 15 22 24 25 26 27 28 30 31 32 33 34 36 37 38 41 50 52 53 55 56 57 61 62 66 68 70 72 73 74 75 76 77 79 80 81 82 84 86 88 89 90 91 92 93 94 95 96 100 102 103 106 107 118 119 121 123 124 135 137
Primary Contact: Michael J. Schwartz, President and Chief Executive Officer
COO: Cynda Tipple, Chief Operating Officer
CFO: Robert Riley, Chief Financial Officer
CMO: Richard D. Travers, M.D., Vice President Medical Affairs
CIO: Mark Fehling, Chief Information Officer
CHR: Terry Lovell, Vice President Human Resources
Web address: www.pwhs.org
Control: Other not–for–profit (including NFP Corporation) **Service:** General Medical and Surgical

Staffed Beds: 168 **Admissions:** 10788 **Census:** 119 **Outpatient Visits:** 202575 **Births:** 2393 **Total Expense ($000):** 149154 **Payroll Expense ($000):** 73754 **Personnel:** 1040

MARION—Smyth County

▣ **SMYTH COUNTY COMMUNITY HOSPITAL (490038)**, 565 Radio Hill Road, Zip 24354–3526, Mailing Address: P.O. Box 880, Zip 24354–0880; tel. 276/782–1234, (Total facility includes 109 beds in nursing home–type unit) **A**1 9 10 20 **F**3 10 11 15 17 24 25 26 30 31 32 38 43 44 46 47 48 54 55 56 57 61 62 63 65 66 68 73 74 75 77 79 80 82 84 86 87 96 100 107 117 119 121 122 124 135 137 **S** Mountain States Health Alliance
Primary Contact: Lindy P. White, President and Chief Executive Officer
CFO: Allen Harris, Chief Financial Officer
Web address: www.scchosp.org
Control: Other not–for–profit (including NFP Corporation) **Service:** General Medical and Surgical

Staffed Beds: 168 **Admissions:** 1874 **Census:** 86 **Outpatient Visits:** 84009 **Births:** 225 **Total Expense ($000):** 33818 **Payroll Expense ($000):** 13226 **Personnel:** 493

□ **SOUTHWESTERN VIRGINIA MENTAL HEALTH INSTITUTE (490105)**, 340 Bagley Circle, Zip 24354–3390; tel. 276/783–1200, (Nonreporting) **A**1 9 10 **S** Virginia Department of Mental Health
Primary Contact: Cynthia McKaskey, Ph.D., Director
Control: State–Government, nonfederal **Service:** Psychiatric

Staffed Beds: 266

MARTINSVILLE—Independent City County

▣ **MEMORIAL HOSPITAL (490079)**, 320 Hospital Drive, Zip 24112–1981, Mailing Address: P.O. Box 4788, Zip 24115–4788; tel. 276/666–7200, (Nonreporting) **A**1 2 9 10 19 **S** LifePoint Hospitals, Inc.
Primary Contact: Joseph Roach, Chief Executive Officer
COO: William Haugh, Administrator
CFO: Brandy Hanners, Chief Financial Officer
CIO: Jeff Butker, Chief Information Officer
CHR: Sherry Schofield, Director Human Resources
Web address: www.martinsvillehospital.com
Control: Corporation, Investor–owned, for–profit **Service:** General Medical and Surgical

Staffed Beds: 212

MECHANICSVILLE—Hanover County

▣ **MEMORIAL REGIONAL MEDICAL CENTER (490069)**, 8260 Atlee Road, Zip 23116–1844; tel. 804/764–6000 **A**1 2 5 9 10 **F**3 10 11 13 15 17 18 20 22 24 25 26 27 28 29 30 31 32 33 34 36 38 40 42 43 44 45 46 49 50 53 54 55 56 57 58 59 60 61 62 63 66 68 72 73 74 75 76 77 79 80 81 82 84 86 87 90 92 96 97 100 102 104 105 106 107 119 120 121 124 135 136 137 **P**7 **S** Bon Secours Health System, Inc.
Primary Contact: Michael Robinson, Executive Vice President and Administrator
COO: Charles Malloy, Vice President Operations
CFO: Peter Gallagher, Vice President and Chief Financial Officer
CMO: Roger Cappello, Vice President Medical Affairs
CHR: Bonnie Shelor, Vice President Human Resources
Web address: www.bonsecours.com
Control: Other not–for–profit (including NFP Corporation) **Service:** General Medical and Surgical

Staffed Beds: 225 **Admissions:** 12682 **Census:** 160 **Outpatient Visits:** 117723 **Births:** 1850 **Total Expense ($000):** 186920 **Payroll Expense ($000):** 62685 **Personnel:** 1138

▣ **SHELTERING ARMS REHABILITATION HOSPITAL (493025)**, 8254 Atlee Road, Zip 23116–1844; tel. 804/764–7055, (Nonreporting) **A**1 5 10
Primary Contact: James E. Sok, FACHE, President and Chief Executive Officer
COO: Michael J. McDonnell, Vice President and Chief Operating Officer
CFO: Michael Boemmel, Vice President and Chief Financial Officer
CMO: Albert Jones, M.D., Medical Director Hanover Hospital
CHR: Kelly Lewis, Associate Vice President Human Resources
Web address: www.shelteringarms.com
Control: Other not–for–profit (including NFP Corporation) **Service:** Rehabilitation

Staffed Beds: 40

VA

Hospital, Medicare Provider Number, Address, Telephone, Approval, Facility, and Physician Codes, Health Care System

★ American Hospital Association (AHA) membership
□ The Joint Commission accreditation
○ American Osteopathic Association (AOA) accreditation
△ Commission on Accreditation of Rehabilitation Facilities (CARF) accreditation

MIDLOTHIAN—Chesterfield County

★ **BON SECOURS ST. FRANCIS MEDICAL CENTER (490136)**, 13710 St. Francis Boulevard, Zip 23114; tel. 804/594–7300, (Nonreporting) **A**1 9 10 **S** Bon Secours Health System, Inc.
Primary Contact: Teresa Edwards, Executive Vice President and Administrator
COO: Peter J. Bernard, Chief Executive Officer
CFO: Peter Gallagher, Chief Financial Officer
CIO: Mike Lokie, Project Director
CHR: Linda Martin, R.N., Administrative Director Human Resources
Web address: www.bonsecours.com/sfmc/default.asp
Control: Other not–for–profit (including NFP Corporation) **Service:** General Medical and Surgical

Staffed Beds: 130

NASSAWADOX—Northampton County

☐ **SHORE MEMORIAL HOSPITAL (490037)**, 9507 Hospital Avenue, Zip 23413–1821, Mailing Address: P.O. Box 17, Zip 23413–0017; tel. 757/414–8000, (Total facility includes 149 beds in nursing home–type unit) (Nonreporting) **A**1 2 9 10 20
Primary Contact: Joseph P. Zager, President and Chief Executive Officer
COO: Gene Erb, Senior Vice President and Chief Operating Officer
CFO: Patrick Yearty, Vice President Fiscal Services
CMO: John Bulette, M.D., President Medical Staff
CIO: Rob Gayman, Director Information Systems
CHR: Charles Waters, Director Human Resources
Web address: www.shorehealthservices.org
Control: Other not–for–profit (including NFP Corporation) **Service:** General Medical and Surgical

Staffed Beds: 256

NEW KENT—New Kent County

☐ **CUMBERLAND HOSPITAL (493300)**, 9407 Cumberland Road, Zip 23124–0150; tel. 804/966–2242, (Nonreporting) **A**1 10 **S** Psychiatric Solutions
Primary Contact: Patrice Gay Brooks, Chief Executive Officer
COO: Jay Maguire, Director Nursing
CFO: Joanne Rial, Chief Financial Officer
CMO: Daniel N. Davidow, M.D., Medical Director
CIO: Elizabeth Peak, Director Standards and Regulatory Compliance
CHR: Sophie Webb, Director Human Resources
Web address: www.cumberlandhospital.com
Control: Corporation, Investor–owned, for–profit **Service:** Children's rehabilitation

Staffed Beds: 132

NEWPORT NEWS—Independent City County

KEYSTONE NEWPORT NEWS, 17579 Warwick Boulevard, Zip 23603–1343; tel. 757/888–0400, (Nonreporting)
Primary Contact: Robert J. Lehmann, Chief Executive Officer
Web address: www.keystonenewportnews.com
Control: Corporation, Investor–owned, for–profit **Service:** Psychiatric

Staffed Beds: 68

VA

★ **MARY IMMACULATE HOSPITAL (490041)**, 2 Bernardine Drive, Zip 23602–4499; tel. 757/886–6000, (Includes ST. FRANCIS NURSING CENTER), (Total facility includes 115 beds in nursing home–type unit) **A**1 9 10 **F**3 11 13 15 18 20 24 25 26 30 31 32 33 38 41 42 43 44 46 50 51 53 55 56 57 60 62 65 66 68 70 71 72 73 74 75 76 77 79 80 81 82 86 92 96 97 100 102 106 107 119 120 121 132 134 135 136 137 **S** Bon Secours Health System, Inc.
Primary Contact: Patricia L. Robertson, Executive Vice President and Administrator
CMO: Rob Ryan, M.D., Medical Director
CIO: Laishy Williams Carlson, Chief Information Officer
Web address: www.bonsecourshamptonroads.com
Control: Other not–for–profit (including NFP Corporation) **Service:** General Medical and Surgical

Staffed Beds: 225 **Admissions:** 6487 **Census:** 167 **Outpatient Visits:** 83388 **Births:** 919 **Total Expense ($000):** 95047 **Payroll Expense ($000):** 34387

★ **RIVERSIDE REGIONAL MEDICAL CENTER (490052)**, 500 J. Clyde Morris Boulevard, Zip 23601–1976; tel. 757/594–2000, (Includes RIVERSIDE PSYCHIATRIC INSTITUTE) **A**1 2 3 5 6 9 10 12 13 **F**3 11 12 13 15 17 18 20 22 24 25 26 27 28 30 31 32 33 36 37 38 40 41 42 43 49 50 51 53 54 55 57 58 59 60 61 62 68 70 72 73 74 75 76 77 79 80 81 82 84 86 87 96 97 99 100 102 103 104 105 106 107 108 109 111 112 116 118 119 121 130 131 133 135 136 137 **P**6 **S** Riverside Health System
Primary Contact: Golden H. Bethune, RN, Executive Vice President and Administrator
CFO: Wade Broughman, Executive Vice President and Chief Financial Officer
CMO: Barry L. Gross, M.D., Executive Vice President and Chief Medical Officer
CIO: John T. Stanley, Vice President Planning and Information Systems
CHR: Larry Boyles, Senior Vice President
Web address: www.riverside–online.com
Control: Other not–for–profit (including NFP Corporation) **Service:** General Medical and Surgical

Staffed Beds: 205 **Admissions:** 18664 **Census:** 203 **Outpatient Visits:** 254237 **Births:** 2921 **Total Expense ($000):** 309657 **Payroll Expense ($000):** 124905 **Personnel:** 1474

★ △ **RIVERSIDE REHABILITATION INSTITUTE (493027)**, 245 Chesapeake Avenue, Zip 23607–6038; tel. 757/928–8000 **A**1 5 7 10 **F**11 25 26 30 31 33 41 55 57 62 72 73 75 77 80 81 82 85 86 107 119 121 135 **P**6 **S** Riverside Health System
Primary Contact: Anne T. Moffat, Administrator
COO: Richard J. Pearce, President and Chief Executive Officer
CFO: Wade Broughman, Executive Vice President and Chief Financial Officer
CMO: Mark Ross, Chief Medical Officer
CIO: John T. Stanley, Vice President Planning and Information Systems
CHR: Ashleigh Pigford, Director Human Resources
Web address: www.riverside–online.com
Control: Other not–for–profit (including NFP Corporation) **Service:** Rehabilitation

Staffed Beds: 26 **Admissions:** 667 **Census:** 26 **Outpatient Visits:** 6732 **Births:** 0 **Total Expense ($000):** 11726 **Payroll Expense ($000):** 6297 **Personnel:** 117

NORFOLK—Independent City County

★ △ **BON SECOURS–DEPAUL MEDICAL CENTER (490011)**, 150 Kingsley Lane, Zip 23505–4650; tel. 757/889–5000, (Total facility includes 24 beds in nursing home–type unit) **A**1 2 3 5 7 9 10 **F**3 11 13 15 18 20 25 26 27 30 31 32 33 37 38 41 43 44 46 50 51 53 54 55 56 57 59 60 62 64 66 68 72 73 74 76 77 79 80 81 82 85 86 87 92 96 97 99 100 102 106 107 109 117 118 119 120 121 132 134 135 136 137 **P**6 **S** Bon Secours Health System, Inc.
Primary Contact: Daniel Duggan, Executive Vice President and Administrator
COO: David P. Setchel, Vice President Operations
CFO: Joe Buchheit, Interim Chief Financial Officer
CIO: Lynne Zultansky, Director Corporate Communications and Media Relations
CHR: John Mashinski, Senior Vice President Human Resources
Web address: www.bonsecourshamptonroads.com
Control: Other not–for–profit (including NFP Corporation) **Service:** General Medical and Surgical

Staffed Beds: 238 **Admissions:** 7471 **Census:** 114 **Outpatient Visits:** 130130 **Births:** 959 **Total Expense ($000):** 119048 **Payroll Expense ($000):** 44724 **Personnel:** 611

★ **CHILDREN'S HOSPITAL OF THE KING'S DAUGHTERS (493301)**, 601 Children's Lane, Zip 23507–1969; tel. 757/668–7000 **A**1 3 5 9 10 **F**3 7 11 12 19 21 23 25 26 27 28 32 33 36 37 38 41 43 44 46 47 48 49 50 51 53 55 56 57 58 59 60 62 66 70 71 72 73 75 76 77 78 79 80 81 82 83 84 85 86 87 89 90 91 92 94 96 97 100 102 106 107 114 118 119 120 121 123 125 127 130 131 132 135 137 **P**1 6
Primary Contact: James D. Dahling, President and Chief Executive Officer
CFO: Dennis Ryan, Senior Vice President and Chief Financial Officer
CMO: Al Finch, M.D., Executive Medical Director
CIO: Debbie Barnes, Vice President and Chief Information Officer
CHR: David Bowers, Vice President Support Services
Web address: www.chkd.org
Control: Other not–for–profit (including NFP Corporation) **Service:** Children's general

Staffed Beds: 170 **Admissions:** 6254 **Census:** 145 **Outpatient Visits:** 219920 **Births:** 0 **Total Expense ($000):** 202426 **Payroll Expense ($000):** 96158 **Personnel:** 1882

HOSPITAL FOR EXTENDED RECOVERY (492007), 600 Gresham Drive, Suite 700, Zip 23507; tel. 757/388–1700, (Nonreporting) **A**10
Primary Contact: Linda Stones, Chief Executive Officer
Control: Corporation, Investor–owned, for–profit **Service:** Long–Term Acute Care hospital

Staffed Beds: 35

Many Facility Codes have changed. Please refer to the AHA Guide Code Chart.

★ **LAKE TAYLOR TRANSITIONAL CARE HOSPITAL (492001)**, 1309 Kempsville Road, Zip 23502–2286; tel. 757/461–5001, (Total facility includes 192 beds in nursing home–type unit) **A**3 5 10 **F**1 3 11 25 26 37 42 43 44 59 60 65 73 77 80 107 117 119 135 137
Primary Contact: Thomas J. Orsini, President and Chief Executive Officer
CFO: Robert W. Fogg, Director Finance
CMO: Antoine A. Arrage, M.D., Director Medical Services
CIO: Mark Davis, Director Information Systems
CHR: LeeAnn Lowman, Director Human Resources
Web address: www.laketaylor.org
Control: Hospital district or authority, Government, nonfederal **Service:** Long–Term Acute Care hospital

Staffed Beds: 293 **Admissions:** 1181 **Census:** 247 **Outpatient Visits:** 0 **Births:** 0 **Total Expense ($000):** 29032 **Payroll Expense ($000):** 12859 **Personnel:** 434

NORFOLK PSYCHIATRIC CENTER, 860 Kempsville Road, Zip 23502–3980; tel. 757/461–4565, (Nonreporting)
Primary Contact: Arlene Manzella, Administrator
Control: Corporation, Investor–owned, for–profit **Service:** Psychiatric

Staffed Beds: 77

★□ **SENTARA LEIGH HOSPITAL (490046)**, 830 Kempsville Road, Zip 23502–3920; tel. 757/466–6000 **A**1 3 5 9 10 **F**3 8 9 11 12 13 15 18 20 24 25 26 27 30 31 32 33 34 35 36 37 38 39 40 41 43 44 45 49 50 51 53 55 56 57 58 59 60 62 63 66 68 69 72 73 74 75 76 77 79 80 81 82 86 90 92 96 97 98 100 102 104 105 106 107 111 119 120 121 130 134 135 136 137 **S** Sentara Healthcare
Primary Contact: Mark A. Szalwinski, Vice President and Administrator
COO: Howard P. Kern, President and Chief Operating Officer
CFO: Robert Broermann, Senior Vice President and Chief Financial Officer
CMO: Gary R. Yates, M.D., Chief Medical Officer
CIO: Bert Reese, Chief Information Officer
CHR: Michael V. Taylor, Senior Vice President Human Resources
Web address: www.sentara.com
Control: Other not–for–profit (including NFP Corporation) **Service:** General Medical and Surgical

Staffed Beds: 233 **Admissions:** 14617 **Census:** 180 **Outpatient Visits:** 312830 **Births:** 2995 **Total Expense ($000):** 182085 **Payroll Expense ($000):** 68588 **Personnel:** 1236

★□ **SENTARA NORFOLK GENERAL HOSPITAL (490007)**, 600 Gresham Drive, Zip 23507; tel. 757/388–3000 **A**1 2 3 5 6 8 9 10 **F**2 3 7 8 9 11 12 13 15 16 17 18 20 22 24 25 26 27 30 31 32 33 34 36 37 38 39 40 41 43 44 45 46 49 50 51 53 54 55 56 57 58 59 60 62 63 64 66 68 69 72 73 74 75 76 77 79 80 81 82 85 86 87 88 90 92 93 94 95 96 97 98 100 102 103 104 105 106 107 108 109 111 112 116 118 119 120 121 124 125 126 127 130 131 133 134 135 136 137 **S** Sentara Healthcare
Primary Contact: Mary L. Blunt, Vice President and Administrator
COO: Pamela Robertson, Vice President Operations
CFO: Robert Broermann, Senior Vice President and Chief Financial Officer
CMO: Gene Burke, M.D., Vice President Medical Affairs
CIO: Bert Reese, Chief Information Officer
Web address: www.sentara.com
Control: Other not–for–profit (including NFP Corporation) **Service:** General Medical and Surgical

Staffed Beds: 464 **Admissions:** 24742 **Census:** 411 **Outpatient Visits:** 472249 **Births:** 2829 **Total Expense ($000):** 521734 **Payroll Expense ($000):** 206155 **Personnel:** 3391

NORTON—Independent City County

□ **MOUNTAIN VIEW REGIONAL MEDICAL CENTER (490027)**, Third Street N.E., Zip 24273–1131, Mailing Address: P.O. Box 620, Zip 24273–0620; tel. 276/679–9100, (Total facility includes 43 beds in nursing home–type unit) (Nonreporting) **A**1 9 10 **S** Wellmont Health System
Primary Contact: David L. Brash, Chief Executive Officer
CFO: James Rooy, Chief Financial Officer
CMO: Ted Thompson, M.D., Chief of Staff
CIO: Teresa Stough, Chief Information Officer
CHR: Barbara Stanley, Director Human Resources
Web address: www.mountainviewregional.org
Control: Other not–for–profit (including NFP Corporation) **Service:** General Medical and Surgical

Staffed Beds: 133

★ ○ △ **NORTON COMMUNITY HOSPITAL (490001)**, 100 15th Street N.W., Zip 24273–1699; tel. 276/679–9600 **A**7 9 10 11 12 13 **F**3 11 12 13 15 24 25 26 28 30 31 32 33 34 36 38 43 50 51 52 53 54 55 56 57 61 62 63 66 68 73 74 75 77 79 80 81 82 85 86 87 96 100 102 106 107 118 119 120 121 122 123 124 135 136 137
Primary Contact: Craig B. James, Chief Executive Officer
CFO: Barbara B. Hale, Chief Financial Officer
CMO: Erin Mullins, Chief Medical Staff
CIO: Judy Lawson, Director Information Services
CHR: Valeri Colyer, Director Human Resources
Web address: www.nchosp.org
Control: Other not–for–profit (including NFP Corporation) **Service:** General Medical and Surgical

Staffed Beds: 48 **Admissions:** 5621 **Census:** 47 **Outpatient Visits:** 91515 **Births:** 502 **Total Expense ($000):** 47431 **Payroll Expense ($000):** 19150 **Personnel:** 527

PEARISBURG—Giles County

★□ **CARILION GILES MEMORIAL HOSPITAL (491302)**, 1 Taylor Avenue, Zip 24134–1932; tel. 540/921–6000 **A**1 9 10 18 **F**3 11 15 24 25 26 30 32 33 34 37 38 50 55 56 57 62 63 66 68 73 75 77 79 81 82 86 96 100 102 107 117 119 122 124 132 135 **S** Carilion Clinic
Primary Contact: James E. Tyler, Vice President and Administrator
CMO: John Tamminen, M.D., President Medical Staff
CHR: Carrie Boggess, Human Resource Generalist
Web address: www.carilion.com
Control: Other not–for–profit (including NFP Corporation) **Service:** General Medical and Surgical

Staffed Beds: 25 **Admissions:** 1193 **Census:** 13 **Outpatient Visits:** 24193 **Births:** 0 **Total Expense ($000):** 20524 **Payroll Expense ($000):** 8461 **Personnel:** 183

PENNINGTON GAP—Lee County

□ **LEE REGIONAL MEDICAL CENTER (490012)**, West Morgan Avenue, Zip 24277–0070, Mailing Address: P.O. Box 70, Zip 24277–0070; tel. 276/546–1440, (Nonreporting) **A**1 9 10 20 **S** Wellmont Health System
Primary Contact: Joseph J. Peluso, Chief Executive Officer
CFO: Marc Nakagawa, Chief Financial Officer
Web address: www.leeregional.com
Control: Other not–for–profit (including NFP Corporation) **Service:** General Medical and Surgical

Staffed Beds: 50

PETERSBURG—Independent City County

□ **CENTRAL STATE HOSPITAL (490104)**, 26317 West Washington Street, Zip 23803, Mailing Address: P.O. Box 4030, Zip 23803–4030; tel. 804/524–7000 **A**1 5 9 10 **F**26 88 92 119 **P**6 **S** Virginia Department of Mental Health
Primary Contact: Charles M. Davis, M.D., Director
CMO: Ronald O. Forbes, M.D., Medical Director
CHR: Tracy Salisbury, Director Human Resources
Web address: www.csh.dmhmrsas.virginia.gov
Control: State–Government, nonfederal **Service:** Psychiatric

Staffed Beds: 277 **Admissions:** 670 **Census:** 246 **Outpatient Visits:** 0 **Births:** 0 **Total Expense ($000):** 49427 **Payroll Expense ($000):** 30249 **Personnel:** 798

★ **POPLAR SPRINGS HOSPITAL (494022)**, 350 Poplar Drive, Zip 23805–4657, Mailing Address: P.O. Box 3060, Zip 23805–3060; tel. 804/733–6874, (Nonreporting) **A**9 10 **S** Horizon Health Corporation
Primary Contact: Richard Clark, Chief Executive Officer
CFO: Bettie Hill, Chief Financial Officer
CHR: Morris Mitchell, Director Human Resources
Web address: www.poplarsprings.com
Control: Corporation, Investor–owned, for–profit **Service:** Psychiatric

Staffed Beds: 120

Hospital, Medicare Provider Number, Address, Telephone, Approval, Facility, and Physician Codes, Health Care System
★ American Hospital Association (AHA) membership
□ The Joint Commission accreditation
○ American Osteopathic Association (AOA) accreditation
△ Commission on Accreditation of Rehabilitation Facilities (CARF) accreditation

★ **SOUTHSIDE REGIONAL MEDICAL CENTER (490067)**, 200 Medical Park Boulevard, Zip 23805; tel. 804/862–5000, (Total facility includes 20 beds in nursing home–type unit) (Nonreporting) **A**1 6 9 10 **S** Community Health Systems, Inc.
Primary Contact: David J. Fikse, Chief Executive Officer
COO: Douglas J. Moyer, Associate Chief Executive Officer
CFO: Stephen Embree, Chief Financial Officer
CMO: Loknath Shandilya, Chief of Staff
CIO: Jake Dorst, Director Management Information Systems
CHR: Irene Buskey, Director Human Resources
Web address: www.srmconline.com
Control: Corporation, Investor–owned, for–profit **Service:** General Medical and Surgical

Staffed Beds: 283

PORTSMOUTH—Independent City County

★ △ **MARYVIEW MEDICAL CENTER (490017)**, 3636 High Street, Zip 23707–3270; tel. 757/398–2200, (Total facility includes 120 beds in nursing home–type unit) **A**2 3 5 7 9 10 **F**3 4 5 8 11 12 13 15 17 18 20 22 24 25 26 27 30 31 32 33 34 36 37 38 39 41 42 43 44 46 50 51 53 55 56 57 59 60 61 62 64 65 66 68 72 73 74 75 76 77 79 80 81 82 85 86 87 88 89 90 91 92 93 94 95 96 97 99 100 102 103 106 107 109 112 116 117 118 119 120 121 123 124 132 133 134 135 136 **P**6 **S** Bon Secours Health System, Inc.
Primary Contact: Susan MacLeod, Executive Vice President
CFO: Greg Simia, Chief Financial Officer
CIO: Terri Spence, Chief Information Officer
CHR: Vickie Humphries, Director Human Resources
Web address: www.bonsecourshamptonroads.com
Control: Other not–for–profit (including NFP Corporation) **Service:** General Medical and Surgical

Staffed Beds: 466 **Admissions:** 15281 **Census:** 325 **Outpatient Visits:** 177943 **Births:** 1118 **Total Expense ($000):** 214417 **Payroll Expense ($000):** 78896

★ **NAVAL MEDICAL CENTER**, 620 John Paul Jones Circle, Zip 23708–2197; tel. 757/953–7424, (Nonreporting) **A**1 2 3 5 **S** Bureau of Medicine and Surgery, Department of the Navy
Primary Contact: Rear Admiral Thomas Cullison, Commander
COO: Captain Peter E. Kopacz, Director Administration
CFO: Commander Manuel Naguit, Director Resources
CMO: Captain Kevin Knoop, Director Medical Education
CIO: Lieutenant Commander Richard Makarski, Chief Information Officer
CHR: Jane Ackiss, Site Manager Human Resources
Web address: www.www–nmcp.med.navy.mil
Control: Navy, Government, federal **Service:** General Medical and Surgical

Staffed Beds: 274

PULASKI—Independent City County

★ **PULASKI COMMUNITY HOSPITAL (490116)**, 2400 Lee Highway, Zip 24301–0759, Mailing Address: P.O. Box 759, Zip 24301–0759; tel. 540/994–8100, (Total facility includes 12 beds in nursing home–type unit) **A**1 2 9 10 **F**3 8 13 15 24 25 26 27 30 31 32 33 38 47 50 55 56 57 68 71 72 73 74 75 76 77 79 80 81 82 86 96 97 100 102 107 109 111 117 119 120 121 124 132 135 136 137 **P**6 **S** HCA
Primary Contact: W. Mark Rader, Chief Executive Officer
COO: Kathleen Kirk, Chief Operating Officer
CFO: Tom Lawhorne, Chief Financial Officer
CMO: Stuart Goldstein, Chief of Staff
CIO: Dan Cheverton, Director Information Systems
CHR: Jana Beckner, Director Human Resource
Web address: www.pulaskicommunityhospital.com
Control: Corporation, Investor–owned, for–profit **Service:** General Medical and Surgical

Staffed Beds: 55 **Admissions:** 2522 **Census:** 25 **Outpatient Visits:** 55626 **Births:** 57 **Total Expense ($000):** 34153 **Payroll Expense ($000):** 13349 **Personnel:** 350

RESTON—Fairfax County

★ **RESTON HOSPITAL CENTER (490107)**, 1850 Town Center Parkway, Zip 20190–3210; tel. 703/689–9000 **A**1 2 9 10 **F**3 12 13 15 18 25 26 27 30 31 32 33 34 38 41 43 46 47 49 51 52 55 56 57 58 62 67 68 70 72 73 74 75 76 77 79 80 81 82 84 86 96 97 99 100 103 106 107 108 109 110 111 119 120 121 124 134 135 136 **S** HCA
Primary Contact: William A. Adams, President and Chief Executive Officer
COO: Jane Raymond, Vice President and Chief Operating Officer
CFO: Edward R. Stojakovich, Chief Financial Officer
CMO: Walter R. Zolkiwsky, M.D., Vice President Medical Affairs
CIO: Paresh Shah, Director Information Systems
CHR: Lesley Channell, Assistant Vice President Human Resources
Web address: www.restonhospital.com
Control: Corporation, Investor–owned, for–profit **Service:** General Medical and Surgical

Staffed Beds: 187 **Admissions:** 11091 **Census:** 120 **Outpatient Visits:** 98640 **Births:** 2974 **Total Expense ($000):** 174855 **Payroll Expense ($000):** 57329 **Personnel:** 736

RICHLANDS—Tazewell County

★ **CLINCH VALLEY MEDICAL CENTER (490060)**, 2949 West Front Street, Zip 24641–2099; tel. 276/596–6000, (Total facility includes 14 beds in nursing home–type unit) **A**1 9 10 **F**3 13 14 15 17 18 24 25 26 27 30 32 33 37 38 46 49 54 55 56 57 59 60 62 68 72 73 74 75 76 77 79 80 81 82 84 85 86 87 96 97 100 103 106 107 108 109 117 118 119 121 124 132 135 136 137 **S** LifePoint Hospitals, Inc.
Primary Contact: David B. Darden, Chief Executive Officer
CFO: Bob Haralson, Chief Financial Officer
CMO: Tushar Patel, Chief of Staff
CIO: Chris Perkins, Director Information Services
CHR: John Knowles, Director Human Resources
Web address: www.clinchvalleymedicalcenter.com
Control: Corporation, Investor–owned, for–profit **Service:** General Medical and Surgical

Staffed Beds: 140 **Admissions:** 5571 **Census:** 64 **Outpatient Visits:** 58646 **Births:** 492 **Personnel:** 488

RICHMOND—Independent City County

★ **BON SECOURS ST. MARY'S HOSPITAL (490059)**, 5801 Bremo Road, Zip 23226–1907; tel. 804/285–2011 **A**1 2 3 5 9 10 **F**3 8 11 12 13 15 17 18 20 22 24 25 26 27 30 31 32 34 35 38 41 42 43 44 46 47 49 50 51 54 55 56 57 59 62 66 68 70 71 72 73 74 76 77 79 80 81 82 83 84 88 92 93 96 97 99 100 102 104 105 106 107 112 116 120 121 134 135 136 **P**7 8 **S** Bon Secours Health System, Inc.
Primary Contact: Michael K. Kerner, Executive Vice President and Administrator
COO: Thomas L. Koenig, Vice President and Chief Operating Officer
CFO: Peter Gallagher, Chief Financial Officer
CMO: Mark Bladergroen, M.D., Vice President Medical Affairs
CIO: Jeff Burke, Chief Information Officer
CHR: Paul Catucci, Director Human Resources
Web address: www.bonsecours.com
Control: Church–operated, Nongovernment, not–for profit **Service:** General Medical and Surgical

Staffed Beds: 391 **Admissions:** 21547 **Census:** 276 **Outpatient Visits:** 91853 **Births:** 2867 **Total Expense ($000):** 298125 **Payroll Expense ($000):** 97909 **Personnel:** 1613

★ **BON SECOURS–RICHMOND COMMUNITY HOSPITAL (490094)**, 1500 North 28th Street, Zip 23223–5396, Mailing Address: P.O. Box 27184, Zip 23261–7184; tel. 804/225–1700 **A**1 6 9 10 **F**15 25 26 27 31 33 36 38 41 43 49 50 55 56 57 60 62 66 68 75 76 77 79 80 81 82 86 88 90 91 92 93 94 95 96 97 99 100 103 105 106 107 119 121 132 135 **P**6 **S** Bon Secours Health System, Inc.
Primary Contact: Michael Robinson, Executive Vice President and Administrator
COO: Charles Malloy, Vice President Operations
CFO: Peter Gallagher, Senior Vice President and Chief Financial Officer
CIO: Jeff Burke, Chief Information Officer
CHR: Shelia White, Director Human Resources
Web address: www.bonsecours.com
Control: Church–operated, Nongovernment, not–for profit **Service:** General Medical and Surgical

Staffed Beds: 101 **Admissions:** 2981 **Census:** 53 **Outpatient Visits:** 36925 **Births:** 0 **Total Expense ($000):** 41583 **Payroll Expense ($000):** 13643 **Personnel:** 199

★ **CHILDREN'S HOSPITAL (493302)**, 2924 Brook Road, Zip 23220–1298; tel. 804/321–7474, (Nonreporting) **A**3 5 9 10
Primary Contact: Leslie G. Wyatt, President and Chief Executive Officer
COO: Leslie G. Wyatt, President and Chief Executive Officer
CFO: Samuel G. Weidman, Executive Vice President and Chief Financial Officer
CMO: Eugenio A. Monasterio, Medical Director
CIO: Greg Friedman, Director Information Technology
CHR: Karen Bennett, Vice President, Human Resources and Compliance
Web address: www.childrenshosp–richmond.org
Control: Other not–for–profit (including NFP Corporation) **Service:** Children's rehabilitation

Staffed Beds: 36

★ **CJW MEDICAL CENTER (490112)**, 7101 Jahnke Road, Zip 23225–4044; tel. 804/320–3911, (Includes CHIPPENHAM MEDICAL CENTER; JOHNSTON–WILLIS HOSPITAL, 1401 Johnston–Willis Drive, Zip 23235; tel. 804/330–2000) **A**1 2 3 5 9 10 **F**3 5 11 13 15 17 18 20 22 24 25 26 27 30 31 33 34 35 36 38 40 41 43 44 46 48 49 50 52 53 54 55 56 57 58 59 62 66 68 69 70 71 72 73 74 75 76 77 78 79 80 81 82 83 84 85 86 87 88 89 90 91 92 93 94 95 96 97 99 100 102 103 106 107 108 109 111 112 114 118 119 120 121 124 133 135 136 137 **P**7 **S** HCA
Primary Contact: Peter A. Marmerstein, Chief Executive Officer
COO: Dia Nichols, Chief Operating Officer
CFO: David McClung, Chief Financial Officer
CMO: David Geckle, M.D., Chairman Medical Staff
CIO: Steven Smith, Healthcare Director Information Services
CHR: Kris Lukish, Human Resources Officer
Web address: www.cjwmedical.com
Control: Corporation, Investor–owned, for–profit **Service:** General Medical and Surgical

Staffed Beds: 758 **Admissions:** 29929 **Census:** 484 **Outpatient Visits:** 172110 **Births:** 3321 **Total Expense ($000):** 396498 **Payroll Expense ($000):** 146396 **Personnel:** 2795

HALLMARK YOUTHCARE – RICHMOND, 12800 West Creek Parkway, Zip 23238–1116; tel. 804/784–2200, (Nonreporting)
Primary Contact: A. Scott Cork, Chief Executive Officer
Web address: www.hallmarkyouthcare.org
Control: Corporation, Investor–owned, for–profit **Service:** Psychiatric

Staffed Beds: 84

★ **HEALTHSOUTH REHABILITATION HOSPITAL OF VIRGINIA (493028)**, 5700 Fitzhugh Avenue, Zip 23226–1877; tel. 804/288–5700 **A**1 10 **F**43 54 55 56 59 62 72 73 75 77 85 86 121 135 **P**4 5 **S** HEALTHSOUTH Corporation
Primary Contact: Jeff Ruskan, II, Chief Executive Officer
CFO: Chuck Fraley, Controller
CIO: Marjorie Morris, Director Information Management
Web address: www.healthsouth.com
Control: Corporation, Investor–owned, for–profit **Service:** Rehabilitation

Staffed Beds: 40 **Admissions:** 749 **Census:** 35 **Outpatient Visits:** 9345 **Births:** 0

★ **HENRICO DOCTORS' HOSPITAL (490118)**, 1602 Skipwith Road, Zip 23229–5205; tel. 804/289–4500, (Includes HENRICO DOCTORS' HOSPITAL – FOREST; HENRICO DOCTORS' HOSPITAL – PARHAM, 7700 East Parham Road, Zip 23294–4301; tel. 804/747–5600) **A**1 2 9 10 **F**3 12 13 15 17 18 20 22 24 25 26 27 30 31 32 33 38 41 43 46 50 51 53 55 56 57 62 63 66 68 69 70 71 72 73 74 75 76 77 79 80 81 82 84 85 86 96 97 99 100 102 103 105 106 107 109 111 113 116 118 119 120 121 124 127 133 134 135 136 137 **S** HCA
Primary Contact: David Williams, Chief Executive Officer
COO: Lisa R. Valentine, Chief Operating Officer
CFO: Christopher Denton, Chief Financial Officer
CIO: Daniel Patton, Director Information Systems
CHR: Steven Burgess, Administrator Human Resources
Web address: www.henricodoctorshospital.com
Control: Corporation, Investor–owned, for–profit **Service:** General Medical and Surgical

Staffed Beds: 533 **Admissions:** 17320 **Census:** 265 **Outpatient Visits:** 151953 **Births:** 3188 **Personnel:** 1644

★ △ **HUNTER HOLMES MCGUIRE VETERANS AFFAIRS MEDICAL CENTER**, 1201 Broad Rock Boulevard, Zip 23249–0002; tel. 804/675–5000, (Total facility includes 98 beds in nursing home–type unit) **A**1 2 3 5 7 8 **F**3 4 5 11 15 17 18 20 22 24 25 26 27 31 32 36 37 38 41 42 43 44 46 49 50 51 53 54 55 56 57 58 59 60 61 62 63 64 66 68 72 73 75 76 77 78 79 81 82 85 86 87 88 90 91 92 93 94 96 97 100 102 106 107 109 111 117 118 119 121 124 126 129 132 134 135 136 137 **P**6 **S** Department of Veterans Affairs
Primary Contact: Michael B. Phaup, Director
COO: Deanne Seekins, Associate Director
CFO: Roger T. Vergne, Chief Fiscal Service
CMO: Judy Brannen, M.D., Interim Chief of Staff
CIO: Katherine Gianola, M.D., Associate Chief of Staff Information Technology
CHR: Ted Knicely, Chief Human Resource Management
Web address: www.va.gov/sta/guide/home.asp
Control: Veterans Affairs, Government, federal **Service:** General Medical and Surgical

Staffed Beds: 415 **Admissions:** 6698 **Census:** 158 **Outpatient Visits:** 406625 **Births:** 0 **Total Expense ($000):** 268437 **Payroll Expense ($000):** 125895 **Personnel:** 2279

JOHNSTON–WILLIS HOSPITAL See CJW Medical Center

★ **RETREAT HOSPITAL (490071)**, 2621 Grove Avenue, Zip 23220–4308; tel. 804/254–5100 **A**1 2 9 10 **F**8 15 18 25 26 27 33 38 42 43 44 46 55 56 68 72 73 75 76 77 79 80 82 86 96 99 100 102 106 107 119 121 134 135 137 **S** HCA
Primary Contact: William E. Caldwell, Jr., Chief Executive Officer
CFO: Sean Thomson, Chief Financial Officer
Web address: www.retreathospital.com
Control: Corporation, Investor–owned, for–profit **Service:** General Medical and Surgical

Staffed Beds: 113 **Admissions:** 3726 **Census:** 73 **Outpatient Visits:** 28517

★ **VCU HEALTH SYSTEM (490032)**, 1250 East Marshall Street, Zip 23219, Mailing Address: P.O. Box 980510, Zip 23298–0510; tel. 804/828–9000 **A**1 2 3 5 8 9 10 **F**3 6 7 8 9 11 12 13 15 16 17 18 19 20 21 22 23 24 25 26 27 28 30 31 32 33 34 35 36 37 38 40 41 43 44 45 46 47 49 50 51 52 53 54 55 56 57 58 59 60 61 62 64 66 68 69 70 71 72 73 74 75 76 77 78 79 80 81 82 83 84 85 86 87 88 89 90 91 92 93 94 95 96 97 98 99 100 102 103 104 105 106 107 108 109 111 112 113 114 116 118 119 120 121 123 124 125 126 127 128 129 130 131 132 133 134 135 136 137 **P**6
Primary Contact: John Duval, Chief Executive Officer
CFO: Dominic J. Puleo, Executive Vice President Finance and Chief Financial Officer
CMO: Ron Clark, M.D., Vice President Clinical Activities and Chief Medical Officer
CHR: Maria Curran, Vice President Human Resources
Web address: www.vcuhealth.org
Control: Hospital district or authority, Government, nonfederal **Service:** General Medical and Surgical

Staffed Beds: 708 **Admissions:** 29721 **Census:** 494 **Outpatient Visits:** 537772 **Births:** 2112 **Total Expense ($000):** 697732 **Payroll Expense ($000):** 273350 **Personnel:** 6182

ROANOKE—Independent City County

★ △ **CARILION MEDICAL CENTER (490024)**, (Formerly Carilion Roanoke Memorial Hospital), Belleview at Jefferson Street, Zip 24014, Mailing Address: P.O. Box 13367, Zip 24033–3367; tel. 540/981–7000, (Includes CARILION ROANOKE COMMUNITY HOSPITAL, 101 Elm Avenue S.E., Zip 24013–2230, Mailing Address: P.O. Box 12946, Zip 24029–2946; tel. 540/985–8000; ROANOKE MEMORIAL REHABILITATION CENTER, South Jefferson and McClanahan Streets, Mailing Address: P.O. Box 13367, Zip 24033) **A**1 2 3 5 7 8 9 10 12 13 **F**3 5 8 9 11 12 13 15 17 18 20 22 24 25 26 27 28 30 31 32 33 34 35 36 37 38 40 41 42 43 44 46 47 48 49 50 51 52 53 54 55 56 57 58 59 60 61 62 63 64 66 68 69 70 71 72 73 74 75 76 77 79 80 81 82 83 84 85 86 87 88 89 90 91 92 93 94 95 96 97 100 102 103 105 106 107 108 109 111 112 113 114 116 118 119 120 121 123 124 132 133 135 136 137 **P**6 **S** Carilion Clinic
Primary Contact: Edward G. Murphy, M.D., President and Chief Executive Officer
COO: Nancy Howell Agee, Chief Operating Officer
CFO: Donald E. Lorton, Executive Vice President and Chief Financial Officer
CMO: Mark D. Werner, M.D., Executive Vice President and Chief Medical Officer
CIO: Daniel Barchi, Senior Vice President and Chief Information Officer
CHR: Bruce Boggs, Senior Vice President and Director Human Resources
Web address: www.carilion.com
Control: Other not–for–profit (including NFP Corporation) **Service:** General Medical and Surgical

Staffed Beds: 589 **Admissions:** 33118 **Census:** 479 **Outpatient Visits:** 194379 **Births:** 3528 **Total Expense ($000):** 624425 **Payroll Expense ($000):** 241768 **Personnel:** 4646

ROCKY MOUNT—Franklin County

★ **CARILION FRANKLIN MEMORIAL HOSPITAL (490089)**, 180 Floyd Avenue, Zip 24151–1389; tel. 540/483–5277 **A**1 9 10 **F**11 13 15 24 25 26 31 32 33 38 42 43 44 50 57 59 61 66 68 73 74 75 79 82 86 96 102 107 119 121 124 135 **S** Carilion Clinic
Primary Contact: William D. Jacobsen, Chief Executive Officer
Web address: www.carilion.com
Control: Other not–for–profit (including NFP Corporation) **Service:** General Medical and Surgical

Staffed Beds: 37 **Admissions:** 2049 **Census:** 19 **Outpatient Visits:** 45257 **Births:** 279 **Total Expense ($000):** 31918 **Payroll Expense ($000):** 12361 **Personnel:** 259

VA

Hospital, Medicare Provider Number, Address, Telephone, Approval, Facility, and Physician Codes, Health Care System

★ American Hospital Association (AHA) membership
□ The Joint Commission accreditation
○ American Osteopathic Association (AOA) accreditation
△ Commission on Accreditation of Rehabilitation Facilities (CARF) accreditation

SALEM—Independent City County

★ **LEWIS–GALE MEDICAL CENTER (490048)**, 1900 Electric Road, Zip 24153–7494; tel. 540/776–4000, (Includes LEWIS–GALE PAVILION, 1902 Braeburn Drive, Zip 24153–7391; tel. 703/772–2800), (Nonreporting) **A**1 2 9 10 **S** HCA
Primary Contact: Victor Giovanetti, Chief Executive Officer
COO: Charlotte Tyson, Chief Operating Officer
CFO: Angela D. Hoke–Reynolds, Chief Financial Officer
CMO: Nelson Greene, M.D., President Medical Staff
CIO: Beth Cole, Director Information Services
Web address: www.lewis–gale.com
Control: Corporation, Investor–owned, for–profit **Service:** General Medical and Surgical

Staffed Beds: 521

MOUNT REGIS CENTER, 405 Kimball Avenue, Zip 24153–6299; tel. 540/389–4761, (Nonreporting) **A**9 **S** Pioneer Behavioral Health
Primary Contact: Gail S. Basham, Chief Executive Officer
CFO: Jenna Ratcliff, Manager Business Office
CMO: Mukesh Patel, M.D., Chief of Staff
CHR: Angie Miller, Coordinator Human Resources
Web address: www.mtregis.com
Control: Corporation, Investor–owned, for–profit **Service:** Alcoholism and other chemical dependency

Staffed Beds: 25

★ **VETERANS AFFAIRS MEDICAL CENTER**, 1970 Roanoke Boulevard, Zip 24153–6478; tel. 540/982–2463, (Total facility includes 90 beds in nursing home–type unit) (Nonreporting) **A**1 2 3 5 8 **S** Department of Veterans Affairs
Primary Contact: Stephen L. Lemons, Ed.D., Director
CFO: Richard J. Schroeder, Chief Financial Officer
Web address: www.va.gov/sta/guide/home.asp
Control: Veterans Affairs, Government, federal **Service:** General Medical and Surgical

Staffed Beds: 282

SOUTH BOSTON—Independent City County

★ **HALIFAX REGIONAL HEALTH SYSTEM (490013)**, 2204 Wilborn Avenue, Zip 24592–1638; tel. 434/517–3100, (Total facility includes 19 beds in nursing home–type unit) **A**1 9 10 19 20 **F**3 4 11 13 14 15 24 25 27 30 31 32 42 49 54 55 56 57 61 62 68 73 74 75 76 77 79 80 82 84 86 87 89 90 91 92 93 94 96 97 100 103 106 107 112 117 118 119 120 121 124 135 137 **P**6 7 8
Primary Contact: Chris A. Lumsden, Chief Executive Officer
COO: Thomas S. Kluge, Chief Operating Officer
CFO: Stewart R. Nelson, Chief Financial Officer
CMO: James F. Witko, M.D., Chief Medical Officer
CIO: William Zirkle, Information Systems Manager
CHR: Catherine Howard, Director Human Resources
Web address: www.hrhs.org
Control: Other not–for–profit (including NFP Corporation) **Service:** General Medical and Surgical

Staffed Beds: 128 **Admissions:** 4669 **Census:** 80 **Outpatient Visits:** 90970 **Births:** 473 **Total Expense ($000):** 73113 **Payroll Expense ($000):** 29351 **Personnel:** 632

SOUTH HILL—Mecklenburg County

★ **COMMUNITY MEMORIAL HEALTHCENTER (490098)**, 125 Buena Vista Circle, Zip 23970–0090, Mailing Address: P.O. Box 90, Zip 23970–0090; tel. 434/447–3151, (Total facility includes 161 beds in nursing home–type unit) **A**1 9 10 20 **F**3 4 11 13 15 24 25 26 27 28 30 31 32 33 36 37 38 42 43 44 46 49 50 52 54 55 56 57 59 60 61 62 63 66 68 72 73 74 75 76 77 79 80 81 82 86 87 88 90 91 92 93 96 97 100 102 106 107 119 120 121 122 124 132 135 136 137 **P**8
Primary Contact: W. Scott Burnette, President and Chief Executive Officer
COO: Edward Brandenburg, Vice President Operations and Human Resources
CFO: Ronald E. Tatum, Chief Financial Officer
CMO: Wallace J. Horne, M.D., Vice President Medical Affairs
CIO: Mark Clemmons, Director Information Systems
CHR: Edward Brandenburg, Vice President Operations and Human Resources
Web address: www.cmh–sh.org
Control: Other not–for–profit (including NFP Corporation) **Service:** General Medical and Surgical

Staffed Beds: 284 **Admissions:** 6069 **Census:** 223 **Outpatient Visits:** 100327 **Births:** 317 **Total Expense ($000):** 68049 **Payroll Expense ($000):** 28360 **Personnel:** 672

STAUNTON—Independent City County

COMMONWEALTH CENTER FOR CHILDREN AND ADOLESCENTS, 1355 Richmond Road, Zip 24401–1091, Mailing Address: Box 4000, Zip 24402–4000; tel. 540/332–2100, (Nonreporting) **A**3 5 9 **S** Virginia Department of Mental Health
Primary Contact: William J. Tuell, M.S.N., Facility Director
Web address: www.ccca.dmhmrsas.virginia.gov
Control: State–Government, nonfederal **Service:** Children's other specialty

Staffed Beds: 60

☐ **WESTERN STATE HOSPITAL (490106)**, 1301 Richmond Avenue, Zip 24401–9146, Mailing Address: P.O. Box 2500, Zip 24402–2500; tel. 540/332–8000 **A**1 3 5 9 10 **F**3 26 31 32 37 82 88 91 119 121 132 135 **S** Virginia Department of Mental Health
Primary Contact: Jack W. Barber, M.D., Director
CFO: David Mawyer, Chief Financial Officer
CMO: Mary Clare Smith, M.D., Medical Director
CIO: Sharon Johnson, Director Health Information Management
CHR: Anita Jackson, Director Human Resources
Web address: www.wsh.dmhmrsas.virginia.gov/
Control: State–Government, nonfederal **Service:** Psychiatric

Staffed Beds: 260 **Admissions:** 620 **Census:** 241 **Outpatient Visits:** 0 **Births:** 0 **Total Expense ($000):** 51323 **Payroll Expense ($000):** 30347 **Personnel:** 720

STUART—Patrick County

☐ **R. J. REYNOLDS–PATRICK COUNTY MEMORIAL HOSPITAL (491306)**, 18688 Jeb Stuart Highway, Zip 24171–1559; tel. 276/694–3151, (Total facility includes 25 beds in nursing home–type unit) (Nonreporting) **A**1 9 10 18
Primary Contact: Janice F. Wilkins, Administrator
COO: Janice F. Wilkins, Administrator
CFO: Christine Olszewski, Chief Financial Officer
CMO: Ralph Kramer, M.D., Chief Medical Staff
CIO: Nova Coleman, Director Information Systems
CHR: Carolyn Belcher, Executive Assistant and Coordinator Human Resources
Web address: www.rjrhospital.com
Control: Other not–for–profit (including NFP Corporation) **Service:** General Medical and Surgical

Staffed Beds: 50

SUFFOLK—Independent City County

★ **SENTARA OBICI HOSPITAL (490044)**, 2800 Godwin Boulevard, Zip 23434–4323, Mailing Address: P.O. Box 1100, Zip 23439–1100; tel. 757/934–4000 **A**1 5 9 10 **F**3 11 13 15 18 20 24 25 26 27 30 31 32 33 38 40 45 48 49 50 51 55 56 57 58 62 67 68 72 73 74 75 76 77 79 80 86 88 89 92 96 97 99 100 102 106 107 108 109 111 118 119 121 135 136 137 **P**6 **S** Sentara Healthcare
Primary Contact: Rosemary C. Check, Vice President and Administrator
COO: Chet M. Hart, Senior Vice President and Chief Operating Officer
CFO: William A. Carpenter, Senior Vice President and Chief Financial Officer
CMO: Brian Gruber, M.D., President of the Medical Staff
CIO: Chip Mills, Director, Information Technology
CHR: Sandra Lane, Vice President Human Resources
Web address: www.sentara.com/Sentara/HospitalsFacilities/Hospitals/Obici
Control: Other not–for–profit (including NFP Corporation) **Service:** General Medical and Surgical

Staffed Beds: 138 **Admissions:** 8484 **Census:** 104 **Outpatient Visits:** 150895 **Births:** 1312 **Total Expense ($000):** 111558 **Payroll Expense ($000):** 48225 **Personnel:** 969

TAPPAHANNOCK—Essex County

☐ **RIVERSIDE TAPPAHANNOCK HOSPITAL (490084)**, 618 Hospital Road, Zip 22560–5000; tel. 804/443–3311, (Total facility includes 25 beds in nursing home–type unit) **A**1 9 10 20 **F**3 11 15 25 27 31 32 33 36 38 40 41 42 43 49 50 51 54 55 56 57 61 62 68 73 75 76 77 79 80 81 82 86 87 96 97 100 102 104 105 106 107 117 119 120 121 122 124 135 137 **P**6 **S** Riverside Health System
Primary Contact: Elizabeth J. Martin, Vice President and Administrator
COO: Elizabeth J. Martin, Vice President and Administrator
CFO: Jeri Sibley, Revenue Cycle Director
CMO: Randy Ferrance, M.D., Medical Staff President
CHR: Jaime Cook, Human Resources Director
Web address: www.riverside–online.com
Control: Other not–for–profit (including NFP Corporation) **Service:** General Medical and Surgical

Staffed Beds: 42 **Admissions:** 2016 **Census:** 20 **Outpatient Visits:** 55447 **Births:** 0 **Total Expense ($000):** 29778 **Payroll Expense ($000):** 10882 **Personnel:** 220

TAZEWELL—Tazewell County

★ **TAZEWELL COMMUNITY HOSPITAL (490117)**, 141 Ben Bolt Avenue, Zip 24651–9700; tel. 276/988–8700 **A**1 9 10 **F**3 11 15 24 25 26 31 33 37 38 44 51 55 57 61 62 63 66 68 73 79 80 82 96 100 102 107 122 124 135 **S** Carilion Clinic
Primary Contact: Christopher L. Wearmouth, FACHE, President and Chief Executive Officer
CFO: Melinda Fanning, Director Financial Services
CMO: Mary Anne Smith, M.D., Chief of Staff
CHR: Shelley Keene Hicks, Director Human Resources
Web address: www.tazecommhospital.org
Control: Other not–for–profit (including NFP Corporation) **Service:** General Medical and Surgical

Staffed Beds: 34 **Admissions:** 1185 **Census:** 10 **Outpatient Visits:** 36370 **Births:** 0 **Total Expense ($000):** 13688 **Payroll Expense ($000):** 6167 **Personnel:** 185

VIRGINIA BEACH—Independent City County

★ **SENTARA BAYSIDE HOSPITAL (490119)**, 800 Independence Boulevard, Zip 23455–6076; tel. 757/363–6100 **A**1 3 5 9 10 **F**3 11 15 18 20 24 25 26 27 30 31 32 33 34 36 37 38 39 40 41 44 48 49 50 51 55 56 57 58 59 60 62 63 66 68 69 72 73 75 76 77 79 80 82 86 90 92 96 97 100 102 106 107 111 118 119 121 134 135 136 137 **S** Sentara Healthcare
Primary Contact: Stephen D. Porter, Vice President and Administrator
COO: Howard P. Kern, Chief Operating Officer
CFO: Robert Broermann, Senior Vice President and Chief Financial Officer
CMO: Thomas H. Scott, M.D., Vice President Medical Affairs
CIO: Bert Reese, Chief Information Officer
CHR: Michael V. Taylor, Vice President Human Resources
Web address: www.sentara.com
Control: Other not–for–profit (including NFP Corporation) **Service:** General Medical and Surgical

Staffed Beds: 97 **Admissions:** 5443 **Census:** 62 **Outpatient Visits:** 256447 **Births:** 0 **Total Expense ($000):** 89231 **Payroll Expense ($000):** 35674 **Personnel:** 653

★ **SENTARA VIRGINIA BEACH GENERAL HOSPITAL (490057)**, (Formerly Virginia Beach General Hospital), 1060 First Colonial Road, Zip 23454–3002; tel. 757/395–8000 **A**1 2 3 5 9 10 **F**3 11 13 15 17 18 20 22 24 25 26 27 30 31 32 33 34 35 36 37 38 40 41 43 44 45 46 47 49 50 51 52 55 56 57 58 59 60 62 63 66 68 69 72 73 74 75 76 77 79 80 81 82 84 86 90 92 96 97 98 100 102 106 107 109 111 112 118 119 120 121 130 131 133 134 135 136 137 **S** Sentara Healthcare
Primary Contact: Raymond G. Troiano, M.D., Vice President and Administrator
COO: R. William Hoefer, Vice President Operations
CFO: Mary Robinson, Director Finance
CHR: Michelle Meekins, Manager Human Resources
Web address: www.sentara.com
Control: Other not–for–profit (including NFP Corporation) **Service:** General Medical and Surgical

Staffed Beds: 251 **Admissions:** 13932 **Census:** 209 **Outpatient Visits:** 322141 **Births:** 1799 **Total Expense ($000):** 214408 **Payroll Expense ($000):** 81255 **Personnel:** 1508

□ **VIRGINIA BEACH PSYCHIATRIC CENTER (494025)**, 1100 First Colonial Road, Zip 23454; tel. 757/496–6000, (Nonreporting) **A**1 9 10 **S** Psychiatric Solutions
Primary Contact: Denise Webb, Administrator
Web address: www.absfirst.com
Control: Corporation, Investor–owned, for–profit **Service:** Psychiatric

Staffed Beds: 100

WARRENTON—Fauquier County

★ **FAUQUIER HOSPITAL (490023)**, 500 Hospital Drive, Zip 20186–3099; tel. 540/316–5000, (Nonreporting) **A**1 9 10
Primary Contact: Rodger H. Baker, President and Chief Executive Officer
CFO: Lionel J. Phillips, Vice President Financial Services
CMO: Adam Winick, M.D., President Medical Staff
CIO: Donna Staton, Chief Information Officer
CHR: Susan B. Smith, Interim Director Human Resources
Web address: www.fauquierhospital.org
Control: Other not–for–profit (including NFP Corporation) **Service:** General Medical and Surgical

Staffed Beds: 86

WILLIAMSBURG—Independent City County

□ **EASTERN STATE HOSPITAL (490109)**, 4601 Ironbound Road, Zip 23188–2652; tel. 757/253–5161, (Total facility includes 210 beds in nursing home–type unit) (Nonreporting) **A**1 3 5 9 10 **S** Virginia Department of Mental Health
Primary Contact: John M. Favret, Director
CFO: E. Clifford Love, Director Fiscal Services
CMO: Guillermo Schrader, M.D., Acting Medical Director
CIO: Barbara Lambert, Director Healthcare Compliance
CHR: Rosemary Travers, Manager Human Resources
Web address: www.esh.dmhmrsas.virginia. gov
Control: State–Government, nonfederal **Service:** Psychiatric

Staffed Beds: 471

★ **SENTARA WILLIAMSBURG COMMUNITY HOSPITAL (490066)**, 100 Sentara Circle, Zip 23188; tel. 757/984–6000 **A**1 2 9 10 **F**3 8 11 13 15 18 20 24 25 26 27 30 31 32 33 34 36 37 38 39 40 41 43 44 45 49 50 51 53 54 55 56 57 58 59 60 62 63 66 67 68 72 73 74 75 76 77 79 80 81 82 84 85 86 90 92 96 97 100 102 106 107 111 112 118 119 120 121 124 133 135 136 137 **S** Sentara Healthcare, Norfolk, VA
Primary Contact: Robert L. Graves, Vice President and Administrator
CFO: Andreas Roehrle, Chief Financial Officer
CMO: James Sammons, M.D., Vice President Medical Affairs
CIO: Thomas Ewing, Director Information Technology
CHR: Nicole Miller, Manager Human Resources
Web address: www.sentara.com
Control: Other not–for–profit (including NFP Corporation) **Service:** General Medical and Surgical

Staffed Beds: 120 **Admissions:** 7042 **Census:** 76 **Outpatient Visits:** 220049 **Births:** 964 **Total Expense ($000):** 101878 **Payroll Expense ($000):** 36812 **Personnel:** 671

WINCHESTER—Independent City County

★ △ **WINCHESTER MEDICAL CENTER (490005)**, 1840 Amherst Street, Zip 22601–2540, Mailing Address: P.O. Box 3340, Zip 22604–3340; tel. 540/536–8000, (Nonreporting) **A**1 2 7 9 10 19 **S** Valley Health System
Primary Contact: Reese Jackson, President and Chief Executive Officer
CFO: J. Craig Lewis, Senior Vice President and Chief Financial Officer
CMO: Terry Sinclair, M.D., Senior Vice President Medical Staff Affairs
CIO: Joan Roscoe, Chief Information Officer
CHR: Adrienne McKenna, Vice President and Human Resources Officer
Web address: www.valleyhealthlink.com
Control: Other not–for–profit (including NFP Corporation) **Service:** General Medical and Surgical

Staffed Beds: 411

WOODBRIDGE—Prince William County

★ **POTOMAC HOSPITAL (490113)**, 2300 Opitz Boulevard, Zip 22191–3399; tel. 703/670–1313 **A**1 2 9 10 **F**3 8 11 12 13 15 18 20 24 25 26 27 30 31 32 33 38 42 43 44 45 49 55 57 59 66 68 69 70 72 73 74 76 77 79 80 82 84 92 96 97 99 100 102 103 106 107 119 121 124 135 136
Primary Contact: William Mason Moss, President
CFO: Paula Brown, Senior Vice President Corporate Finance
CMO: Ali Mortazavi, M.D., President Medical Staff
CIO: Khali Bouharoun, Vice President and Director Management Information Systems
CHR: Charles W. Ramey, Vice President
Web address: www.potomachospital.com
Control: Other not–for–profit (including NFP Corporation) **Service:** General Medical and Surgical

Staffed Beds: 183 **Admissions:** 10849 **Census:** 123 **Outpatient Visits:** 140825 **Births:** 2326 **Total Expense ($000):** 144573 **Payroll Expense ($000):** 55730 **Personnel:** 1119

WOODSTOCK—Shenandoah County

★ **SHENANDOAH MEMORIAL HOSPITAL (491305)**, 759 South Main Street, Zip 22664–1127; tel. 540/459–1100 **A**1 9 10 18 **F**3 11 13 15 25 26 30 31 32 33 38 43 50 52 55 57 62 63 66 68 73 74 75 77 79 81 82 86 87 89 90 94 96 97 100 102 106 107 119 121 122 124 135 136 137 **P**6 **S** Valley Health System
Primary Contact: Floyd Heater, Chief Executive Officer
CFO: Virginia Kilmer, Chief Financial Officer
CMO: Donald Jansen, M.D., Vice President Medical Affairs
CIO: Donna Brill, Director Information Systems
CHR: Charles Walton, Corporate Director Human Resources
Web address: www.valleyhealthlink.com
Control: Other not–for–profit (including NFP Corporation) **Service:** General Medical and Surgical

Staffed Beds: 23 **Admissions:** 1772 **Census:** 17 **Outpatient Visits:** 106484 **Births:** 333 **Total Expense ($000):** 39674 **Payroll Expense ($000):** 17668 **Personnel:** 460

Hospital, Medicare Provider Number, Address, Telephone, Approval, Facility, and Physician Codes, Health Care System
★ American Hospital Association (AHA) membership
□ The Joint Commission accreditation
○ American Osteopathic Association (AOA) accreditation
△ Commission on Accreditation of Rehabilitation Facilities (CARF) accreditation

WYTHEVILLE—Wythe County

★ **WYTHE COUNTY COMMUNITY HOSPITAL (490111)**, 600 West Ridge Road, Zip 24382–1099; tel. 276/228–0200, (Total facility includes 8 beds in nursing home–type unit) **A**1 9 10 20 **F**3 11 13 15 17 24 25 26 28 30 31 32 33 38 42 44 47 49 50 53 54 55 56 57 60 61 62 63 66 68 73 74 75 76 77 79 81 82 84 85 86 87 90 92 96 97 100 102 106 107 117 118 119 120 121 122 135 136 137 **S** LifePoint Hospitals, Inc.
Primary Contact: Eric Deaton, Chief Executive Officer
CFO: John D. White, Chief Financial Officer
CMO: W T Kilgore, Chief of Staff
CIO: Andrea Harless, Director Information Services
CHR: John Knowles, Director Human Resources
Web address: www.wcch.org
Control: Corporation, Investor–owned, for–profit **Service:** General Medical and Surgical

Staffed Beds: 90 **Admissions:** 2857 **Census:** 32 **Outpatient Visits:** 32013 **Births:** 243 **Total Expense ($000):** 33987 **Payroll Expense ($000):** 13142 **Personnel:** 318

VA

WASHINGTON

ABERDEEN—Grays Harbor County

□ **GRAYS HARBOR COMMUNITY HOSPITAL (500031)**, 915 Anderson Drive, Zip 98520–1097; tel. 360/532–8330, (Total facility includes 60 beds in nursing home–type unit) (Nonreporting) **A**1 9 10
Primary Contact: John Mitchell, President and Chief Executive Officer
COO: Thomas Hightower, Chief Operating Officer
CFO: Tim Howden, Interim Chief Financial Officer
CMO: Bill Hofmann, M.D., Chief Medical Staff
CIO: Scott Quigley, Director Information Services
CHR: Julie Feller, Director Human Resources
Web address: www.ghchwa.org
Control: Other not–for–profit (including NFP Corporation) **Service:** General Medical and Surgical

Staffed Beds: 172

ANACORTES—Skagit County

★□ **ISLAND HOSPITAL (500007)**, 1211 24th Street, Zip 98221–2590; tel. 360/299–1300, (Nonreporting) **A**1 2 5 9 10
Primary Contact: Vincent Oliver, Administrator
CFO: Peter Swanson, Assistant Administrator Fiscal Services
CMO: Shawna Laursen, M.D., Chief of Staff
CIO: Tom Bluhm, Director Information Systems
CHR: Mike Bruggeman, Director Human Resources
Web address: www.islandhospital.org
Control: Hospital district or authority, Government, nonfederal **Service:** General Medical and Surgical

Staffed Beds: 43

ARLINGTON—Snohomish County

□ **CASCADE VALLEY HOSPITAL AND CLINICS (500060)**, 330 South Stillaguamish Avenue, Zip 98223–1642; tel. 360/435–2133, (Nonreporting) **A**1 9 10
Primary Contact: W. Clark Jones, Administrator
CFO: Ardis Schmiege, Chief Financial Officer
CMO: David Janeway, President Medical Staff
CIO: Heather Logan, Assistant Administrator Diagnostic and Support Services
CHR: Connie DiGregorio, Assistant Administrator
Web address: www.cascadevalley.org
Control: Hospital district or authority, Government, nonfederal **Service:** General Medical and Surgical

Staffed Beds: 48

AUBURN—King County

□ **AUBURN REGIONAL MEDICAL CENTER (500015)**, 202 North Division, Plaza One, Zip 98001–4908; tel. 253/833–7711, (Nonreporting) **A**1 2 9 10 **S** Universal Health Services, Inc.
Primary Contact: Leonard Freehof, Chief Executive Officer
CIO: Denis Uhler, Information Systems Manager
Web address: www.auburnregional.com
Control: Corporation, Investor–owned, for–profit **Service:** General Medical and Surgical

Staffed Beds: 120

BELLEVUE—King County

★□ **OVERLAKE HOSPITAL MEDICAL CENTER (500051)**, 1035 116th Avenue N.E., Zip 98004–4686; tel. 425/688–5000 **A**1 2 5 9 10 **F**3 8 11 12 13 15 17 18 19 20 22 25 26 27 30 32 33 34 35 36 38 40 43 44 46 47 48 49 50 54 55 56 57 58 60 62 66 68 70 71 72 73 74 75 76 77 79 81 82 86 87 88 89 90 91 92 93 94 95 96 97 99 102 103 106 107 109 111 119 121 123 133 134 135 136 137 **P**6
Primary Contact: Craig L. Hendrickson, President and Chief Executive Officer
COO: David E. Schultz, Chief Operating Officer and Administrator
CFO: Gary McLaughlin, Vice President Finance and Chief Financial Officer
CHR: Lisa Brock, Vice President Human Resources
Web address: www.overlakehospital.org
Control: Other not–for–profit (including NFP Corporation) **Service:** General Medical and Surgical

Staffed Beds: 232 **Admissions:** 17290 **Census:** 166 **Outpatient Visits:** 295859 **Births:** 4137 **Total Expense ($000):** 260365 **Payroll Expense ($000):** 114204 **Personnel:** 1688

BELLINGHAM—Whatcom County

★□ △ **ST. JOSEPH HOSPITAL (500030)**, 2901 Squalicum Parkway, Zip 98225–1898; tel. 360/734–5400 **A**1 2 7 9 10 **F**2 3 4 5 8 11 13 15 17 18 20 22 24 25 26 27 30 31 32 33 36 38 40 42 43 44 45 46 47 48 49 50 51 54 55 56 57 59 60 62 63 66 68 72 73 74 75 76 77 79 80 81 82 84 85 86 87 88 90 91 92 93 94 95 96 97 98 100 101 102 103 104 105 106 107 108 109 110 111 112 119 121 124 132 135 137 **P**6 **S** PeaceHealth
Primary Contact: Nancy Steiger, Chief Executive Officer and Chief Mission Officer
COO: Stephen R. Omta, Chief Operating Officer
CFO: Dale Zender, Regional Vice President Finance and Chief Financial Officer
CMO: James Hopper, Chief of Staff
CIO: Kelly Lundy, Director Information Services
CHR: Shawna Unger, Interim Vice President Human Resources
Web address: www.peacehealth.org
Control: Other not–for–profit (including NFP Corporation) **Service:** General Medical and Surgical

Staffed Beds: 243 **Admissions:** 14979 **Census:** 158 **Outpatient Visits:** 97030 **Births:** 2022 **Total Expense ($000):** 243615 **Payroll Expense ($000):** 106222 **Personnel:** 2112

BREMERTON—Kitsap County

★□ **HARRISON MEDICAL CENTER (500039)**, 2520 Cherry Avenue, Zip 98310–4270; tel. 360/377–3911 **A**1 2 9 10 **F**3 11 13 18 20 22 25 26 27 30 31 32 33 35 36 37 38 40 41 43 44 48 49 50 52 53 54 55 56 57 60 61 62 63 66 68 72 73 74 75 76 77 79 80 81 82 84 86 87 88 89 90 91 92 93 96 97 102 106 107 108 109 118 119 121 124 133 135 136 137 **P**6
Primary Contact: Scott W. Bosch, President and Chief Executive Officer
COO: Patty Cochrell, Vice President and Chief Operating Officer
CFO: James S. Rowson, Vice President Operations and Chief Financial Officer
CMO: Ronald Morris, M.D., Chief Medical Officer
CIO: Adar Palis, Chief Information Officer
CHR: Rebecca Kelly, Vice President Human Resources
Web address: www.harrisonhospital.org
Control: Other not–for–profit (including NFP Corporation) **Service:** General Medical and Surgical

Staffed Beds: 254 **Admissions:** 17048 **Census:** 171 **Outpatient Visits:** 178811 **Births:** 2081 **Total Expense ($000):** 227732 **Payroll Expense ($000):** 98783 **Personnel:** 1404

★□ **NAVAL HOSPITAL**, One Boone Road, Zip 98312–1898; tel. 360/475–4239, (Nonreporting) **A**1 3 5 9 **S** Bureau of Medicine and Surgery, Department of the Navy
Primary Contact: Captain Catherine A. Wilson, Commanding Officer
COO: Lieutenant Kirk Houser, Director Administration
CFO: Judith Hogan, Comptroller and Director Resources and Logistics
CIO: Patrick Flaherty, Director Management Information
Web address: www.nh_bremerton.med.navy.mil
Control: Navy, Government, federal **Service:** General Medical and Surgical

Staffed Beds: 51

BREWSTER—Okanogan County

OKANOGAN DOUGLAS DISTRICT HOSPITAL (501324), 507 Hospital Way, Zip 98812–0577, Mailing Address: P.O. Box 577, Zip 98812–0577; tel. 509/689–2517, (Nonreporting) **A**9 10 18
Primary Contact: Dale E. Polla, Administrator
COO: Sandy Walter, Chief Operating Officer
CFO: Jennifer Munson, Chief Financial Officer
CMO: Eric Haeger, President Medical Staff
CIO: Christopher Freel, Chief Information Technologist
CHR: Janeen Reding, Director Human Resources
Web address: www.oddh.org
Control: Hospital district or authority, Government, nonfederal **Service:** General Medical and Surgical

Staffed Beds: 20

WA

Hospital, Medicare Provider Number, Address, Telephone, Approval, Facility, and Physician Codes, Health Care System

★ American Hospital Association (AHA) membership
□ The Joint Commission accreditation
○ American Osteopathic Association (AOA) accreditation
△ Commission on Accreditation of Rehabilitation Facilities (CARF) accreditation

BURIEN—King County

▣ **HIGHLINE MEDICAL CENTER (500011)**, 16251 Sylvester Road S.W., Zip 98166–3052; tel. 206/244–9970, (Includes HIGHLINE SPECIALTY CENTER, 12844 MILITARY ROAD FORK, TUKWILA, ZIP 98168; MARK BENEDUM, ADMINISTRATOR), (Total facility includes 31 beds in nursing home–type unit) (Nonreporting) **A**1 2 9 10
Primary Contact: Mark Benedum, Chief Executive Officer
CFO: Don Halterman, Administrator Finance and Chief Financial Officer
Web address: www.hchnet.org
Control: Other not–for–profit (including NFP Corporation) **Service:** General Medical and Surgical

Staffed Beds: 192

CENTRALIA—Lewis County

▣ **PROVIDENCE CENTRALIA HOSPITAL (500019)**, 914 South Scheuber Road, Zip 98531–9027; tel. 360/736–2803, (Total facility includes 29 beds in nursing home–type unit) (Nonreporting) **A**1 9 10 20 **S** Providence Health & Services
Primary Contact: Cindy Mayo, Chief Executive
CFO: Thomas Risse, Chief Financial Officer
CIO: Stacy Steck, Chief Information Officer
CHR: Susan Meenk, Assistant Administrator Service Area
Web address: www.providence.org
Control: Church–operated, Nongovernment, not–for profit **Service:** General Medical and Surgical

Staffed Beds: 133

CHELAN—Chelan County

★ **LAKE CHELAN COMMUNITY HOSPITAL (501334)**, 503 East Highland Avenue, Zip 98816–0908, Mailing Address: P.O. Box 908, Zip 98816–0908; tel. 509/682–3300 **A**9 10 18 **F**4 7 8 10 13 30 31 32 33 38 40 41 42 61 64 74 79 82 96 97 100 102 107 119 122 132 135 137
Primary Contact: David M. Bernier, Ph.D., FACHE, Chief Executive Officer
CFO: Karen Spurgeon, Chief Financial Officer
CMO: Louise Simons, Chief Medical Staff
CIO: Ross Hurd, Chief Information Officer
CHR: Nancy Young, Director Human Resources
Web address: www.lakechelancommunityhospital.com
Control: Hospital district or authority, Government, nonfederal **Service:** General Medical and Surgical

Staffed Beds: 24 **Admissions:** 698 **Census:** 15 **Outpatient Visits:** 4662
Births: 93 **Total Expense ($000):** 13441 **Payroll Expense ($000):** 7313
Personnel: 162

CHEWELAH—Stevens County

★ **ST. JOSEPH'S HOSPITAL (501309)**, 500 East Webster Street, Zip 99109–0197, Mailing Address: P.O. Box 197, Zip 99109–0197; tel. 509/935–8211, (Nonreporting) **A**9 10 18 **S** Providence Health & Services
Primary Contact: Gary V. Peck, Administrator
CFO: Chris Hargis, Chief Financial Officer
Web address: www.sjhospital.org
Control: Church–operated, Nongovernment, not–for profit **Service:** General Medical and Surgical

Staffed Beds: 25

CLARKSTON—Asotin County

▣ **TRI–STATE MEMORIAL HOSPITAL (501332)**, 1221 Highland Avenue, Zip 99403–0189, Mailing Address: P.O. Box 189, Zip 99403–0189; tel. 509/758–5511 **A**1 9 10 18 **F**3 8 11 15 25 30 31 32 33 35 38 40 42 49 51 55 57 59 61 62 68 73 77 79 82 96 99 100 103 107 118 119 121 122 133 135 136 137
Primary Contact: Christopher Noland, FACHE, Chief Executive Officer and Administrator
COO: Sister Mary Croghan, FACHE, Assistant Administrator and Chief Operating Officer
CFO: Alex Town, Chief Financial Officer
Web address: www.tristatehospital.org
Control: Other not–for–profit (including NFP Corporation) **Service:** General Medical and Surgical

Staffed Beds: 25 **Admissions:** 1676 **Census:** 19 **Outpatient Visits:** 73455
Births: 0 **Total Expense ($000):** 39685 **Payroll Expense ($000):** 13021
Personnel: 305

COLFAX—Whitman County

★ **WHITMAN HOSPITAL AND MEDICAL CENTER (501327)**, 1200 West Fairview, Zip 99111–9579; tel. 509/397–3435 **A**9 10 18 **F**8 11 13 15 25 26 27 30 33 38 46 51 54 56 57 62 67 73 74 75 76 77 79 80 82 96 100 102 117 119 122 124 137 **S** Providence Health & Services
Primary Contact: Jon R. Davis, FACHE, Chief Executive Officer
CFO: Jim Heilsberg, Chief Financial Officer and Chief Information Officer
CMO: H. Graeme French, M.D., Chief Medical Officer
CIO: Jim Heilsberg, Chief Financial Officer and Chief Information Officer
CHR: Linda Ledgerwood, Director Human Resources
Web address: www.whitmanhospital.com
Control: Hospital district or authority, Government, nonfederal **Service:** General Medical and Surgical

Staffed Beds: 25 **Admissions:** 869 **Census:** 8 **Outpatient Visits:** 18423
Births: 53 **Total Expense ($000):** 17223 **Payroll Expense ($000):** 7289
Personnel: 171

COLVILLE—Stevens County

★ **MOUNT CARMEL HOSPITAL (501326)**, 982 East Columbia Street, Zip 99114–3352; tel. 509/684–2561 **A**9 10 18 **F**11 13 15 25 26 30 31 32 38 40 41 43 44 55 56 57 62 68 73 74 75 77 79 80 81 82 86 96 97 103 106 107 111 120 121 122 124 135 137 **P**6 **S** Providence Health & Services
Primary Contact: Robert D. Campbell, Jr., President
CFO: Chris Hargis, Chief Financial Officer
CMO: Ramon Canto, M.D., Chief of Staff
CIO: Theron DePaulo, Manager Information Systems
CHR: Linda Grittner, Manager Human Resources
Web address: www.mtcarmelhospital.org
Control: Church–operated, Nongovernment, not–for profit **Service:** General Medical and Surgical

Staffed Beds: 25 **Admissions:** 1216 **Census:** 11 **Outpatient Visits:** 35527
Births: 211 **Total Expense ($000):** 26187 **Payroll Expense ($000):** 11431
Personnel: 166

COUPEVILLE—Island County

★ **WHIDBEY GENERAL HOSPITAL (501339)**, 101 North Main Street, Zip 98239; tel. 360/678–5151, (Nonreporting) **A**2 9 10 18
Primary Contact: Scott Rhine, Administrator and Chief Executive Officer
COO: Tom Tomasino, Chief Operating Officer
CFO: Joe Vessey, Chief Financial Officer
CMO: Chris Bibby, Chief of Staff
CIO: Tom Tomasino, Assistant Administrator and Chief Information Officer
CHR: Carolyn Pape, Director Human Resources
Web address: www.whidbeygen.org
Control: Hospital district or authority, Government, nonfederal **Service:** General Medical and Surgical

Staffed Beds: 25

DAVENPORT—Lincoln County

★ **LINCOLN HOSPITAL (501305)**, 10 Nicholls Street, Zip 99122–9729; tel. 509/725–7101, (Total facility includes 68 beds in nursing home–type unit) (Nonreporting) **A**9 10 18
Primary Contact: Thomas J. Martin, Chief Executive Officer
CMO: Ralph Monteagudo, M.D., Chief of Staff
CIO: Elliott Donson, Chief Information Specialist
CHR: Janelle Hiccox, Director Human Resources
Web address: www.lincolnhospital.org
Control: Hospital district or authority, Government, nonfederal **Service:** General Medical and Surgical

Staffed Beds: 89

DAYTON—Columbia County

DAYTON GENERAL HOSPITAL (501302), 1012 South Third Street, Zip 99328–1696; tel. 509/382–2531, (Nonreporting) **A**9 10 18
Primary Contact: Charles A. Button, Chief Executive Officer
CFO: Gary Schroeder, Chief Financial Officer
Web address: www.cchd–wa.org
Control: Hospital district or authority, Government, nonfederal **Service:** General Medical and Surgical

Staffed Beds: 25

EDMONDS—Snohomish County

🞕 **STEVENS HEALTHCARE (500026)**, 21601 76th Avenue West, Zip 98026–7506; tel. 425/640–4000 **A**1 2 9 10 **F**3 7 8 11 12 13 15 18 20 24 25 26 27 33 38 40 49 55 56 57 63 66 73 74 75 76 77 78 79 80 82 83 85 86 88 92 94 95 96 100 103 106 107 118 119 121 124 135 137 **P**6 7
Primary Contact: Michael C. Carter, President and Chief Executive Officer
CFO: Gary L. Wangsmo, Vice President and Chief Financial Officer
CMO: Tim Roddy, M.D., Vice President Medical Affairs
CIO: Fred Grannan, Director Information Services
CHR: John Omel, Vice President Human Resources
Web address: www.stevenshealthcare.org
Control: Hospital district or authority, Government, nonfederal **Service:** General Medical and Surgical

Staffed Beds: 129 **Admissions:** 7844 **Census:** 91 **Outpatient Visits:** 102044 **Births:** 1149 **Total Expense ($000):** 144163 **Payroll Expense ($000):** 59921 **Personnel:** 1038

ELLENSBURG—Kittitas County

★ **KITTITAS VALLEY COMMUNITY HOSPITAL (501333)**, 603 South Chestnut Street, Zip 98926–3875; tel. 509/962–7302, (Nonreporting) **A**9 10 18
Primary Contact: Eric Jensen, Chief Executive Officer
COO: Eric Jensen, Chief Executive Officer
CFO: Harold Brockman, Chief Financial Officer
CMO: Craig Wilson, Chief Nursing and Patient Care Services Officer
CHR: Lisa McDaniel, Assistant Administrator Human Resources
Web address: www.kvch.com
Control: Hospital district or authority, Government, nonfederal **Service:** General Medical and Surgical

Staffed Beds: 25

ENUMCLAW—King County

★ **ENUMCLAW REGIONAL HOSPITAL (501335)**, 1450 Battersby Avenue, Zip 98022–0218, Mailing Address: P.O. Box 218, Zip 98022–0218; tel. 360/825–2505 **A**9 10 18 **F**3 13 15 33 38 40 62 66 68 74 77 79 80 96 97 100 102 107 135 **S** Catholic Health Initiatives
Primary Contact: Dennis Popp, Chief Operating Officer and Administrator
COO: Dennis Popp, Administrator and Chief Executive Officer
CFO: Philip Hjembo, Assistant Administrator Fiscal Services and Chief Financial Officer
CHR: Jerilyn Ray, Manager Human Resources
Web address: www.fhshealth.org
Control: Other not–for–profit (including NFP Corporation) **Service:** General Medical and Surgical

Staffed Beds: 25 **Admissions:** 1174 **Census:** 9 **Outpatient Visits:** 32487 **Births:** 230 **Total Expense ($000):** 21546 **Payroll Expense ($000):** 9672 **Personnel:** 157

EPHRATA—Grant County

★ **COLUMBIA BASIN HOSPITAL (501317)**, 200 Nat Washington Way, Zip 98823–1973; tel. 509/754–4631, (Total facility includes 29 beds in nursing home–type unit) **A**9 10 18 **F**10 11 15 25 28 30 31 32 33 38 40 54 55 56 57 62 63 73 75 86 87 96 107 117 119 122 124 135 **P**6
Primary Contact: Donald W. James, Ph.D., Administrator
CFO: Rhonda Handley, Chief Financial Officer
CMO: Lowell C. Allred, Chief of Staff
CHR: Suzanne Little, Human Resources Specialist
Web address: www.columbiabasinhospital.org
Control: Hospital district or authority, Government, nonfederal **Service:** General Medical and Surgical

Staffed Beds: 54 **Admissions:** 225 **Census:** 40 **Outpatient Visits:** 15204 **Births:** 0 **Total Expense ($000):** 4209 **Payroll Expense ($000):** 5325

EVERETT—Snohomish County

🞕 △ **PROVIDENCE EVERETT MEDICAL CENTER (500014)**, 1321 Colby Avenue, Zip 98206–1147, Mailing Address: P.O. Box 1147, Zip 98206–1147; tel. 425/261–2000, (Includes PROVIDENCE EVERETT MEDICAL CENTER – COLBY CAMPUS, 1321 Colby Avenue, Zip 98206; tel. 425/261–2000; PROVIDENCE EVERETT MEDICAL CENTER – PACIFIC CAMPUS, Pacific and Nassau Streets, Zip 98201) **A**1 2 7 9 10 **F**3 4 5 8 11 13 15 17 18 20 22 25 26 27 28 30 31 32 33 34 36 38 40 41 43 44 45 50 52 53 55 56 57 59 62 64 66 68 70 72 73 74 75 76 77 78 79 80 81 82 84 85 86 87 96 97 98 100 102 104 105 106 107 109 111 118 119 121 124 135 136 137 **P**6 8 **S** Providence Health & Services
Primary Contact: David Brooks, Chief Operating Officer
CFO: Dave Mast, Chief Financial Officer
CMO: Lawrence Schecter, M.D., Chief Medical Officer
Web address: www.providence.org
Control: Church–operated, Nongovernment, not–for profit **Service:** General Medical and Surgical

Staffed Beds: 362 **Admissions:** 24674 **Census:** 275 **Outpatient Visits:** 264022 **Births:** 4080 **Total Expense ($000):** 423074 **Payroll Expense ($000):** 177262 **Personnel:** 2437

FEDERAL WAY—King County

🞕 **ST. FRANCIS HOSPITAL (500141)**, 34515 Ninth Avenue South, Zip 98003–6799; tel. 253/944–8100 **A**1 2 9 10 **F**3 8 11 12 13 15 20 25 26 27 31 32 33 34 36 38 39 40 41 44 46 47 49 50 51 53 55 57 62 68 72 73 75 76 77 79 80 81 82 86 88 92 96 97 99 100 102 106 107 109 111 118 119 121 124 134 135 136 **P**6 **S** Catholic Health Initiatives
Primary Contact: Sister Anne McNamara, Chief Operating Officer
COO: Sister Anne McNamara, Chief Operating Officer
CFO: Mike Fitzgerald, Chief Financial Officer
CMO: Mike Newcomb, D.O., Senior Vice President Medical Affairs
CIO: Bruce Elkington, Vice President Information Technology
CHR: David Lawson, Vice President Human Resources
Web address: www.fhshealth.org
Control: Church–operated, Nongovernment, not–for profit **Service:** General Medical and Surgical

Staffed Beds: 110 **Admissions:** 7846 **Census:** 73 **Outpatient Visits:** 89954 **Births:** 1424 **Total Expense ($000):** 119741 **Payroll Expense ($000):** 53784 **Personnel:** 677

FORKS—Clallam County

FORKS COMMUNITY HOSPITAL (501325), 530 Bogachiel Way, Zip 98331–9120; tel. 360/374–6271, (Nonreporting) **A**9 10 18
Primary Contact: Camille Scott, Administrator
COO: John Sherrett, Chief Financial Officer and Chief Operating Officer
CFO: John Sherrett, Chief Financial Officer and Chief Operating Officer
CIO: Roger Harrison, Manager Information Services
CHR: Geoff Roach, Director Human Resources
Web address: www.forkshospital.org
Control: Hospital district or authority, Government, nonfederal **Service:** General Medical and Surgical

Staffed Beds: 45

GOLDENDALE—Klickitat County

★ **KLICKITAT VALLEY HEALTH SERVICES (501316)**, 310 South Roosevelt Avenue, Zip 98620–9201; tel. 509/773–4022, (Nonreporting) **A**9 10 18 **S** Brim Healthcare, Inc.
Primary Contact: John E. Rohrer, Interim Chief Executive Officer
CFO: Wade Sturgeon, Chief Financial Officer
CMO: Michael Garnett, M.D., Chief of Staff
CHR: Gwyn Miller, Director Human Resources
Web address: www.kvhealth.net
Control: Hospital district or authority, Government, nonfederal **Service:** General Medical and Surgical

Staffed Beds: 25

GRAND COULEE—Grant County

COULEE COMMUNITY HOSPITAL (501308), 411 Fortuyn Road, Zip 99133–8718; tel. 509/633–1753 **A**9 10 18 **F**33 38 46 57 63 74 77 79 80 82 87 96 99 107 119 122 136 137 **P**6
Primary Contact: Tom Jensen, Chief Executive Officer
CFO: Debbie Bigelow, Chief Financial Officer
CMO: Jacob Chaffee, M.D., Chief of Staff
CIO: Chrys Hakola, Chief Human Resources and Information Officer
CHR: Chrys Hakola, Chief Human Resources and Information Officer
Web address: www.couleecommhosp.org
Control: Hospital district or authority, Government, nonfederal **Service:** General Medical and Surgical

Staffed Beds: 25 **Admissions:** 403 **Census:** 17 **Births:** 90

WA

Hospital, Medicare Provider Number, Address, Telephone, Approval, Facility, and Physician Codes, Health Care System

★ American Hospital Association (AHA) membership
□ The Joint Commission accreditation
○ American Osteopathic Association (AOA) accreditation
△ Commission on Accreditation of Rehabilitation Facilities (CARF) accreditation

ILWACO—Pacific County

★ **OCEAN BEACH HOSPITAL (501314)**, 174 First Avenue North, Zip 98624–0258, Mailing Address: P.O. Drawer H, Zip 98624–0258; tel. 360/642–3181, (Nonreporting) **A**9 10 18
Primary Contact: Linda Kaino, Interim Chief Executive Officer
COO: Julie Oakes, R.N., Chief Operating Officer
CFO: Edward A. Norris, Chief Financial Officer
CMO: Albert Fabiano, M.D., Chief Medical Officer
CIO: Julie Oakes, R.N., Manager Risk and Quality
CHR: Mary Ward–Riggs, Director Human Resources
Web address: www.oceanbeachhospital.net
Control: Hospital district or authority, Government, nonfederal **Service:** General Medical and Surgical

Staffed Beds: 15

KENNEWICK—Benton County

⊡ **KENNEWICK GENERAL HOSPITAL (500053)**, 900 South Auburn Street, Zip 99336–6128, Mailing Address: P.O. Box 6128, Zip 99336–6128; tel. 509/586–6111, (Nonreporting) **A**1 2 9 10
Primary Contact: Glen Marshall, Chief Executive Officer
CFO: Terry Litke, Chief Financial Officer
CHR: Russ Keefer, Chief Human Resources Officer
Web address: www.kennewickgeneral.com
Control: Hospital district or authority, Government, nonfederal **Service:** General Medical and Surgical

Staffed Beds: 101

KIRKLAND—King County

⊡ **EVERGREEN HEALTHCARE (500124)**, 12040 N.E. 128th Street, Zip 98034–9917; tel. 425/899–1000, (Nonreporting) **A**1 2 3 5 9 10
Primary Contact: Steven E. Brown, FACHE, Chief Executive Officer
COO: David S. Danielson, Senior Vice President Operations
CFO: Chrissy Yamada, CPA, Senior Vice President Finance
CMO: Mitch Weinberg, M.D., Chief of Staff
CIO: Tom Martin, Vice President Chief Information Officer
Web address: www.evergreenhealthcare.org
Control: Hospital district or authority, Government, nonfederal **Service:** General Medical and Surgical

Staffed Beds: 230

☐ **FAIRFAX HOSPITAL (504002)**, 10200 N.E. 132nd Street, Zip 98034–2899; tel. 425/821–2000 **A**1 9 10 **F**4 5 25 33 36 88 89 90 91 92 94 95 119 **P**6 **S** Psychiatric Solutions
Primary Contact: Ron Escarda, Chief Executive Officer
COO: Mike Zauner, Chief Operating Officer
CFO: Pam Rhoads, Chief Financial Officer
CMO: William Adams, M.D., Medical Director
CHR: Anne Schreiber, Manager Human Resources
Web address: www.fairfaxhospital.com
Control: Corporation, Investor–owned, for–profit **Service:** Psychiatric

Staffed Beds: 95 **Admissions:** 2302 **Census:** 65 **Outpatient Visits:** 1880 **Births:** 0

LEAVENWORTH—Chelan County

CASCADE MEDICAL CENTER (501313), 817 Commercial Street, Zip 98826, Mailing Address: P.O. Box 330, Zip 98826; tel. 509/548–5815 **A**9 10 18 **F**7 15 38 62 63 66 86 87 96 122 137 **P**6
Primary Contact: Douglas Williams, Administrator
COO: Eugene Suksi, Chief Operating Officer
CFO: Alan MacPhee, Chief Financial Officer
CHR: Lance Heise, Director Human Resources
Web address: www.cascademedicalcenter.org
Control: Hospital district or authority, Government, nonfederal **Service:** General Medical and Surgical

Staffed Beds: 7 **Admissions:** 136 **Census:** 2 **Total Expense ($000):** 7975 **Payroll Expense ($000):** 4408 **Personnel:** 79

LONGVIEW—Cowlitz County

⊡ **ST. JOHN MEDICAL CENTER (500041)**, 1615 Delaware Street, Zip 98632–2310, Mailing Address: P.O. Box 3002, Zip 98632–3002; tel. 360/414–2000, (Nonreporting) **A**1 2 9 10 **S** PeaceHealth
Primary Contact: Medrice Coluccio, Chief Executive Officer
COO: James Meskew, Chief Operating Officer
CFO: Sy Johnson, Chief Financial Officer
Web address: www.peacehealth.org
Control: Church–operated, Nongovernment, not–for profit **Service:** General Medical and Surgical

Staffed Beds: 202

MCCLEARY—Grays Harbor County

★ **MARK REED HOSPITAL (501304)**, 322 South Birch Street, Zip 98557–9522; tel. 360/495–3244, (Nonreporting) **A**9 10 18
Primary Contact: Renee K. Dunham, Chief Executive Officer
CFO: Georgette Hiles, Accountant
CMO: R. Samantha Ritchie, M.D., President Medical Staff
CIO: David Gibson, Chief Information Officer
CHR: Mindy Portchy, Manager Human Resources
Web address: www.markreedhospital.com
Control: Corporation, Investor–owned, for–profit **Service:** General Medical and Surgical

Staffed Beds: 6

MEDICAL LAKE—Spokane County

☐ **EASTERN STATE HOSPITAL (504004)**, Maple Street, Zip 99022–0045, Mailing Address: P.O. Box 800, Zip 99022–0800; tel. 509/299–3121, (Nonreporting) **A**1 9 10
Primary Contact: Harold E. Wilson, Chief Executive Officer
Web address: www.www1.dsgs.wa.gov/mentalhealth/eshfaqs.shtml
Control: State–Government, nonfederal **Service:** Psychiatric

Staffed Beds: 319

MONROE—Snohomish County

⊡ **VALLEY GENERAL HOSPITAL (500084)**, 14701 179th S.E., Zip 98272–1108, Mailing Address: P.O. Box 646, Zip 98272–0646; tel. 360/794–7497, (Nonreporting) **A**1 9 10
Primary Contact: Mark D. Judy, Chief Executive Officer
CFO: John Beltz, Chief Financial Officer
CMO: William Thot, M.D., President Medical Staff
CIO: Kathy Nelson, Director Marketing and Strategic Planning
CHR: Joan Catlett, Director Human Resources
Web address: www.valleygeneral.com
Control: Hospital district or authority, Government, nonfederal **Service:** General Medical and Surgical

Staffed Beds: 68

MORTON—Lewis County

★ **MORTON GENERAL HOSPITAL (501319)**, 521 Adams Street, Zip 98356, Mailing Address: Drawer C, Zip 98356–0019; tel. 360/496–5112, (Total facility includes 30 beds in nursing home–type unit) (Nonreporting) **A**9 10 18
Primary Contact: Ron DeArth, Superintendent
CFO: Tim Cournyer, Chief Financial Officer
CHR: Shannon Kelly, Director Human Resources
Control: Hospital district or authority, Government, nonfederal **Service:** General Medical and Surgical

Staffed Beds: 55

MOSES LAKE—Grant County

★ **SAMARITAN HEALTHCARE (500033)**, 801 East Wheeler Road, Zip 98837–1899; tel. 509/765–5606 **A**9 10 20 **F**8 13 15 26 32 33 38 40 53 55 56 57 62 66 68 73 74 75 77 79 81 82 84 87 97 100 102 107 119 121 133 135 **P**6
Primary Contact: John R. White, President and Chief Executive Officer
CFO: Robert Reeder, Interim Chief Financial Officer
CIO: Michael Cloutier, Director Information Systems
CHR: Kim Garza, Director Human Resources
Web address: www.samaritanhealthcare.com
Control: Hospital district or authority, Government, nonfederal **Service:** General Medical and Surgical

Staffed Beds: 50 **Admissions:** 3563 **Census:** 27 **Outpatient Visits:** 86523 **Births:** 1108 **Total Expense ($000):** 53444 **Payroll Expense ($000):** 24910 **Personnel:** 458

MOUNT VERNON—Skagit County

⊡ **SKAGIT VALLEY HOSPITAL (500003)**, 1415 East Kincaid Street, Zip 98273, Mailing Address: P.O. Box 1376, Zip 98273–1376; tel. 360/424–4111 **A**1 2 9 10 19 **F**3 6 9 11 13 18 20 24 25 26 27 30 31 32 33 34 35 37 38 40 41 43 44 45 46 49 50 53 55 56 57 59 62 66 68 72 73 74 75 76 77 79 80 81 82 86 88 95 108 109 111 118 119 121 124 135 136 137 **P**6
Primary Contact: Gregg A. Davidson, Chief Executive Officer
COO: Lori Harlow, Chief Operating Officer
CFO: Thomas Litaker, Chief Financial Officer
CMO: Richard Abbott, M.D., Medical Advisor Quality Improvement
CIO: Doug Riley, Director Information Services
CHR: Elizabeth Feingold, Director Human Resources
Web address: www.skagitvalleyhospital.org
Control: Hospital district or authority, Government, nonfederal **Service:** General Medical and Surgical

Staffed Beds: 115 **Admissions:** 8847 **Census:** 78 **Outpatient Visits:** 106518 **Births:** 1322 **Total Expense ($000):** 120160 **Payroll Expense ($000):** 45739 **Personnel:** 817

NEWPORT—Pend Oreille County

NEWPORT HOSPITAL AND HEALTH SERVICES (501310), 714 West Pine Street, Zip 99156–9046; tel. 509/447–2441, (Total facility includes 50 beds in nursing home–type unit) **A**9 10 18 **F**3 8 10 11 13 15 30 31 38 55 56 57 62 63 73 74 79 80 82 84 86 87 96 102 107 117 119 122 135 **P**6
Primary Contact: Thomas W. Wilbur, Chief Executive Officer and Superintendent
COO: Ginny Monroe, Chief Operating Officer
CFO: Kim Manus, Assistant Administrator and Chief Financial Officer
CMO: Jeremy Lewis, D.O., Chief Medical Staff
CIO: Roger Rasmussen, Chief Administrative Officer
CHR: Roger Rasmussen, Chief Administrative Officer
Web address: www.phd1.org
Control: Hospital district or authority, Government, nonfederal **Service:** General Medical and Surgical

Staffed Beds: 75 **Admissions:** 758 **Census:** 47 **Outpatient Visits:** 59328 **Births:** 112

OAK HARBOR—Island County

★□ **NAVAL HOSPITAL**, 3475 North Saratoga Street, Zip 98278–8800; tel. 360/257–9500, (Nonreporting) **A**1 9 **S** Bureau of Medicine and Surgery, Department of the Navy
Primary Contact: Captain Colin Chinn, Commanding Officer
CFO: Lieutenant Gerald Hall, Director Resource Management
CMO: Commander Stephen Cooley, M.D., Chairman, Executive Committee of the Medical Staff
CIO: Gregory Carruth, Head Information Management
CHR: Kathy Vass, Head Human Resources
Web address: www.nhoh.med.navy.mil
Control: Navy, Government, federal **Service:** General Medical and Surgical

Staffed Beds: 29

ODESSA—Lincoln County

ODESSA MEMORIAL HEALTHCARE CENTER (501307), 502 East Amende Drive, Zip 99159–0368, Mailing Address: P.O. Box 368, Zip 99159–0368; tel. 509/982–2611, (Total facility includes 23 beds in nursing home–type unit) (Nonreporting) **A**9 10 18
Primary Contact: Mark Barglof, Administrator
CFO: Carol Schott, Chief Financial Officer and Assistant Administrator
CMO: Linda J. Powel, M.D., Medical Director
Web address: www.odessahealth.org
Control: Hospital district or authority, Government, nonfederal **Service:** General Medical and Surgical

Staffed Beds: 48

OLYMPIA—Thurston County

□ **CAPITAL MEDICAL CENTER (500139)**, 3900 Capital Mall Drive S.W., Zip 98502–5026, Mailing Address: P.O. Box 19002, Zip 98507–9002; tel. 360/754–5858, (Total facility includes 9 beds in nursing home–type unit) (Nonreporting) **A**1 9 10 **S** Capella Healthcare
Primary Contact: Michael Motte, Chief Executive Officer
COO: Lynn Peoples, Interim Chief Nursing Officer
CFO: Brian Anderson, Chief Financial Officer
CMO: Rojesh Sharangpani, M.D., Chief of Staff
CIO: Renee Crotty, Coordinator Marketing and Public Relations
CHR: Dana Vandewege, Director Human Resources
Web address: www.capitalmedical.com
Control: Partnership, Investor–owned, for–profit **Service:** General Medical and Surgical

Staffed Beds: 99

★□ △ **PROVIDENCE ST. PETER HOSPITAL (500024)**, 413 Lilly Road N.E., Zip 98506–5166; tel. 360/491–9480 **A**1 3 5 7 9 10 **F**1 3 4 5 11 12 13 15 16 17 18 20 22 24 25 26 30 31 32 33 34 36 38 40 41 45 49 51 52 53 55 56 57 58 59 60 62 64 65 68 70 71 72 73 74 75 76 77 78 79 80 81 82 83 84 85 86 87 88 89 90 91 92 94 95 96 97 98 100 102 104 106 107 117 118 119 120 121 122 123 124 133 135 136 **P**6 **S** Providence Health & Services
Primary Contact: James Leonard, Administrator
CFO: Thomas Risse, Chief Financial Officer
CMO: Mike Matlock, M.D., Chief Medical Officer
CIO: Stacy Steck, Chief Information Officer
CHR: Susan Meenk, Service Area Assistant Administrator
Web address: www.providence.org/swsa/facilities/st_peter_hospital
Control: Church–operated, Nongovernment, not–for profit **Service:** General Medical and Surgical

Staffed Beds: 338 **Admissions:** 18648 **Census:** 228 **Outpatient Visits:** 286313 **Births:** 2227 **Total Expense ($000):** 278960 **Payroll Expense ($000):** 114790 **Personnel:** 1774

OMAK—Okanogan County

★ **MID-VALLEY HOSPITAL (501328)**, 810 Jasmine, Zip 98841–0793, Mailing Address: P.O. Box 793, Zip 98841–0793; tel. 509/826–1760 **A**3 5 9 10 18 **F**11 13 15 25 30 31 32 38 40 43 62 66 68 74 79 82 84 86 96 97 107 122 **P**6
Primary Contact: Michael Billings, Administrator
CFO: Scott Attridge, Controller
CMO: Daman Chugh, M.D., Chief Medical Officer
CIO: Kelly Cariker, Manager
CHR: Norene Van Brunt, Manager Human Resources
Web address: www.mvhealth.org
Control: Hospital district or authority, Government, nonfederal **Service:** General Medical and Surgical

Staffed Beds: 30 **Admissions:** 1383 **Census:** 12 **Outpatient Visits:** 49034 **Births:** 253 **Total Expense ($000):** 25605 **Payroll Expense ($000):** 12408

OTHELLO—Adams County

★ **OTHELLO COMMUNITY HOSPITAL (501318)**, 315 North 14th Street, Zip 99344–1297; tel. 509/488–2636 **A**9 10 18 **F**3 7 11 13 15 26 38 40 66 67 74 79 86 96 99 102 107 122 134 137
Primary Contact: Harold S. Geller, Administrator
CFO: Leon Walsh, Director Finance
CHR: Kurt Richter, Chief Human Resources Officer
Web address: www.othellocommunityhospital.org
Control: Hospital district or authority, Government, nonfederal **Service:** General Medical and Surgical

Staffed Beds: 25 **Admissions:** 1306 **Census:** 7 **Outpatient Visits:** 26544 **Births:** 594 **Total Expense ($000):** 14459 **Payroll Expense ($000):** 6730 **Personnel:** 146

PASCO—Franklin County

★□ △ **LOURDES MEDICAL CENTER (501337)**, 520 North Fourth Avenue, Zip 99301–2568, Mailing Address: P.O. Box 2568, Zip 99302–2568; tel. 509/547–7704 **A**1 2 7 9 10 18 **F**3 11 13 15 17 26 33 35 38 40 43 51 56 57 59 62 72 73 74 75 76 77 79 80 81 84 85 86 96 97 100 107 118 119 120 121 122 135 136 **S** Ascension Health
Primary Contact: John Serle, President and Chief Executive Officer
CFO: Frank Becker, Chief Financial Officer
CHR: Craig Pearsall, Director Human Resources
Web address: www.lourdesonline.org
Control: Church–operated, Nongovernment, not–for profit **Service:** General Medical and Surgical

Staffed Beds: 35 **Admissions:** 2132 **Census:** 21 **Outpatient Visits:** 57485 **Births:** 415 **Total Expense ($000):** 52961 **Payroll Expense ($000):** 24453

POMEROY—Garfield County

★ **GARFIELD COUNTY PUBLIC HOSPITAL DISTRICT (501301)**, 66 North Sixth Street, Zip 99347–0880; tel. 509/843–1591, (Total facility includes 20 beds in nursing home–type unit) (Nonreporting) **A**9 10 18
Primary Contact: Andrew Craigie, Chief Executive Officer
CFO: Mel Ahrens, Chief Financial Officer
CMO: Syed Zafar, M.D., Chief Medical Officer
CIO: Jorie Gaines, Manager Information
CHR: Linda Duckett, Assistant Controller
Web address: www.garfieldcountyphd.org
Control: Hospital district or authority, Government, nonfederal **Service:** General Medical and Surgical

Staffed Beds: 45

PORT ANGELES—Clallam County

★□ **OLYMPIC MEDICAL CENTER (500072)**, 939 Caroline Street, Zip 98362–3997; tel. 360/417–7000 **A**1 2 9 10 19 20 **F**11 13 15 17 24 27 30 31 32 38 40 43 49 50 55 57 61 62 63 68 72 73 74 75 76 77 79 80 81 82 84 85 86 87 96 97 100 102 107 108 109 118 119 124 135 136 137 **P**6
Primary Contact: Eric Lewis, Chief Executive Officer
CMO: R. Scott Kennedy, M.D., Chief Medical Officer
CIO: Evan Boyd, Director Information Technology
CHR: Richard Neuman, Assistant Administrator
Web address: www.olympicmedical.org
Control: Hospital district or authority, Government, nonfederal **Service:** General Medical and Surgical

Staffed Beds: 78 **Admissions:** 4569 **Census:** 45 **Outpatient Visits:** 209650 **Births:** 473 **Total Expense ($000):** 111642 **Payroll Expense ($000):** 49743 **Personnel:** 853

WA

Hospital, Medicare Provider Number, Address, Telephone, Approval, Facility, and Physician Codes, Health Care System

★ American Hospital Association (AHA) membership
□ The Joint Commission accreditation
○ American Osteopathic Association (AOA) accreditation
△ Commission on Accreditation of Rehabilitation Facilities (CARF) accreditation

PORT TOWNSEND—Jefferson County

★ **JEFFERSON HEALTHCARE (501323)**, 834 Sheridan Avenue, Zip 98368–2443; tel. 360/385–2200, (Nonreporting) **A**9 10 18
Primary Contact: Victor J. Dirksen, Administrator
COO: Paula Dowdle, Chief Operating Officer
CFO: James Chaney, Chief Financial Officer
CMO: Todd Carlson, M.D., Chief Medical Officer
CHR: Beki Lischalk, Director Human Resources
Web address: www.jeffersonhealthcare.org
Control: Hospital district or authority, Government, nonfederal **Service:** General Medical and Surgical

Staffed Beds: 25

PROSSER—Benton County

★ **PROSSER MEMORIAL HOSPITAL (501312)**, 723 Memorial Street, Zip 99350–1593; tel. 509/786–2222, (Total facility includes 36 beds in nursing home–type unit) (Nonreporting) **A**9 10 18
Primary Contact: James Tavary, Administrator
CFO: Julie Petersen, Director Financial Services
CIO: Dan Harter, Manager Information Systems
CHR: Sharon Cloos, Manager Human Resources
Web address: www.prossermemorial.com
Control: Hospital district or authority, Government, nonfederal **Service:** General Medical and Surgical

Staffed Beds: 62

PULLMAN—Whitman County

☐ **PULLMAN REGIONAL HOSPITAL (501331)**, 835 S.E. Bishop Boulevard, Zip 99163–5512; tel. 509/332–2541 **A**1 9 10 18 **F**3 13 15 25 26 30 31 32 33 34 36 38 40 41 47 51 52 55 56 57 62 66 68 72 73 74 75 76 77 79 81 82 84 86 88 91 92 94 95 96 97 99 100 102 106 107 118 119 120 121 122 133 135 **P**4
Primary Contact: Scott K. Adams, Chief Executive Officer
CFO: Steven Febus, Chief Financial Officer
CMO: Kim Guida, M.D., President Medical Staff
CHR: Bernadette Berney, Director Human Resources
Web address: www.pullmanhospital.org
Control: Hospital district or authority, Government, nonfederal **Service:** General Medical and Surgical

Staffed Beds: 25 **Admissions:** 1470 **Census:** 12 **Outpatient Visits:** 49966 **Births:** 381 **Total Expense ($000):** 36087 **Payroll Expense ($000):** 15704 **Personnel:** 288

PUYALLUP—Pierce County

⊡ △ **GOOD SAMARITAN COMMUNITY HEALTHCARE (500079)**, 407 14th Avenue S.E., Zip 98372–0118, Mailing Address: P.O. Box 1247, Zip 98371–1247; tel. 253/697–4000 **A**1 2 7 9 10 **F**13 18 20 24 25 26 27 30 31 32 38 40 42 44 46 50 53 56 57 61 62 63 68 69 71 72 73 74 75 76 77 78 79 80 81 82 85 86 90 96 97 100 102 103 104 105 107 118 119 135 137 **P**6
Primary Contact: John R. Long, Jr., President
COO: John R. Long, President and Chief Executive Officer
CFO: Kim Lintott, Vice President
CMO: Donald Mott, M.D., Chief Medical Officer
CIO: Florence Chang, Vice President Information Technology
CHR: Sarah Horsman, Vice President Human Resources
Web address: www.goodsamhealth.org
Control: Other not–for–profit (including NFP Corporation) **Service:** General Medical and Surgical

Staffed Beds: 221 **Admissions:** 14624 **Census:** 152 **Outpatient Visits:** 203692 **Births:** 2112 **Total Expense ($000):** 235291 **Payroll Expense ($000):** 109024 **Personnel:** 1484

QUINCY—Grant County

★ **QUINCY VALLEY MEDICAL CENTER (501320)**, 908 10th Avenue S.W., Zip 98848–1376; tel. 509/787–3531, (Total facility includes 22 beds in nursing home–type unit) (Nonreporting) **A**9 10 18
Primary Contact: Mehdi Merred, Administrator
CFO: Ken Kiehn, Controller
CMO: Peter Himmel, M.D., Chief Medical Officer
CIO: Ruth Vance, Director Information Systems
CHR: Alene Adams, Director Human Resources
Web address: www.quincyhospital.org
Control: County–Government, nonfederal **Service:** General Medical and Surgical

Staffed Beds: 47

REDMOND—King County

☐ **GROUP HEALTH EASTSIDE HOSPITAL (500052)**, 2700 152nd Avenue N.E., Zip 98052–5560; tel. 425/883–5151, (Nonreporting) **A**1 9 10
Primary Contact: Scott Armstrong, President and Chief Executive Officer
CFO: Ric Magnuson, Executive Vice President and Chief Financial Officer
CMO: Michael Soman, M.D., Executive Medical Director
CIO: Ernie Hood, Vice President and Chief Information Officer
Web address: www.ghc.org
Control: Other not–for–profit (including NFP Corporation) **Service:** General Medical and Surgical

Staffed Beds: 125

RENTON—King County

⊡ **VALLEY MEDICAL CENTER (500088)**, 400 South 43rd Street, Zip 98055–5784; tel. 425/228–3450 **A**1 2 3 5 9 10 **F**3 8 11 12 13 15 18 20 24 25 26 27 28 30 31 32 33 34 35 36 38 40 43 46 47 49 50 51 52 53 55 56 57 58 62 66 68 70 71 72 73 74 75 76 77 79 80 81 82 84 86 87 90 91 94 96 97 100 102 103 105 106 107 108 109 111 112 116 118 119 120 121 124 133 135 136 137 **P**8
Primary Contact: Richard D. Roodman, Chief Executive Officer
COO: Paul Hayes, R.N., Chief Operating Officer
CFO: Michael Bernstein, Chief Financial Officer
CIO: Phil Perry, Chief Information Officer
CHR: Barbara Mitchell, Administrator Organizational Development
Web address: www.valleymed.org
Control: Hospital district or authority, Government, nonfederal **Service:** General Medical and Surgical

Staffed Beds: 170 **Admissions:** 16281 **Census:** 147 **Outpatient Visits:** 562110 **Births:** 3844 **Total Expense ($000):** 306262 **Payroll Expense ($000):** 131883 **Personnel:** 1994

REPUBLIC—Ferry County

★ **FERRY COUNTY MEMORIAL HOSPITAL (501322)**, 36 Klondike Road, Zip 99166–9701; tel. 509/775–3333, (Total facility includes 14 beds in nursing home–type unit) (Nonreporting) **A**9 10 18
Primary Contact: Ronald O'Halloran, Administrator
CFO: Marvel Brenner, Chief Financial Officer
CHR: Kelly Leslie, Human Resources Officer
Web address: www.fcphd.org
Control: Hospital district or authority, Government, nonfederal **Service:** General Medical and Surgical

Staffed Beds: 39

RICHLAND—Benton County

⊡ △ **KADLEC MEDICAL CENTER (500058)**, 888 Swift Boulevard, Zip 99352–3542; tel. 509/946–4611 **A**1 2 7 9 10 **F**3 11 13 15 18 20 22 24 25 26 27 31 32 34 38 40 43 46 47 48 49 50 51 55 62 66 68 70 73 74 75 76 77 79 80 81 82 84 85 86 87 96 97 99 100 102 104 105 106 107 114 119 135 137 **S** QHR
Primary Contact: Rand J. Wortman, President and Chief Executive Officer
COO: Lane A. Savitch, President
CFO: Julie Meek, Vice President Finance
CMO: Fred Bower, M.D., Chief of Staff
CIO: David Roach, Vice President Information Systems
CHR: Jeff Clark, Vice President Human Resources
Web address: www.kadlecmed.org
Control: Other not–for–profit (including NFP Corporation) **Service:** General Medical and Surgical

Staffed Beds: 181 **Admissions:** 9886 **Census:** 111 **Outpatient Visits:** 156258 **Births:** 2052 **Total Expense ($000):** 182937 **Payroll Expense ($000):** 69093 **Personnel:** 1246

★ **LOURDES COUNSELING CENTER (504008)**, 1175 Carondelet Drive, Zip 99352–3396; tel. 509/943–9104 **A**9 10 **F**5 25 30 31 32 36 53 58 62 88 89 90 91 93 94 95 119 121 123 124 **P**6 **S** Ascension Health
Primary Contact: Barbara Mead, Executive Director
CFO: Frank Becker, Chief Financial Officer
Web address: www.lourdesonline.org
Control: Church–operated, Nongovernment, not–for profit **Service:** Psychiatric

Staffed Beds: 32 **Admissions:** 672 **Census:** 23 **Outpatient Visits:** 49349 **Births:** 0 **Total Expense ($000):** 14148 **Payroll Expense ($000):** 7169 **Personnel:** 153

RITZVILLE—Adams County

EAST ADAMS RURAL HOSPITAL (501311), 903 South Adams Street, Zip 99169–2298; tel. 509/659–1200, (Nonreporting) **A**9 10 18
Primary Contact: Paul Lewis, Administrator
CFO: Sandi Lehman, Chief Financial Officer
CIO: Kellie Ottman, Manager Information Services
Web address: www.earh.com
Control: Hospital district or authority, Government, nonfederal **Service:** General Medical and Surgical

Staffed Beds: 10

Many Facility Codes have changed. Please refer to the AHA Guide Code Chart.

SEATTLE—King County

★ △ **CHILDREN'S HOSPITAL AND REGIONAL MEDICAL CENTER (503300)**, 4800 Sand Point Way N.E., Zip 98105–0371, Mailing Address: Box 5371, Zip 98105–0371; tel. 206/987–2000 **A**1 2 3 5 7 8 9 10 **F**3 7 8 9 19 21 23 25 26 27 28 30 31 32 33 34 36 37 38 40 43 44 46 52 53 55 56 58 59 60 61 62 63 64 66 69 70 72 73 75 76 77 79 80 81 82 83 84 85 86 87 88 89 90 91 92 94 95 96 97 100 103 105 107 114 116 118 119 120 121 123 125 126 127 128 130 131 132 133 135 137
Primary Contact: Thomas N. Hansen, M.D., Chief Executive Officer
COO: Patrick J. Hagan, President and Chief Operating Officer
CFO: Kelly Wallace, Senior Vice President and Chief Financial Officer
CMO: David Fisher, M.D., Vice President and Medical Director
CIO: John Dwight, Chief Information Officer
CHR: Charles Sims, Director Human Resources
Web address: www.seattlechildrens.org
Control: Other not–for–profit (including NFP Corporation) **Service:** Children's general

Staffed Beds: 250 **Admissions:** 12785 **Census:** 186 **Outpatient Visits:** 219784 **Total Expense ($000):** 421122 **Payroll Expense ($000):** 172448 **Personnel:** 2573

★ △ **HARBORVIEW MEDICAL CENTER (500064)**, 325 Ninth Avenue, Box 359717, Zip 98104–2499; tel. 206/731–3000 **A**1 3 5 7 8 9 10 **F**3 5 8 16 17 18 20 25 26 27 30 31 32 33 36 37 38 40 43 44 46 49 50 54 55 56 57 58 60 62 63 64 66 68 72 73 75 76 77 78 79 80 81 82 83 84 85 86 87 88 90 91 92 93 94 95 96 97 100 102 106 107 112 116 118 119 120 121 124 133 135 136 137 **P**6
Primary Contact: Johnese Spisso, Interim Chief Executive Officer
COO: Johnese Spisso, Chief Operating Officer
CFO: Lori J. Mitchell, Chief Financial Officer
CMO: Scott Barnhart, M.D., Medical Director
CIO: James Fine, M.D., Executive Director Clinical Computing
CHR: Janelle Browne, Executive Director Health Sciences and Human Resources
Web address: www.uwmedicine.org
Control: County–Government, nonfederal **Service:** General Medical and Surgical

Staffed Beds: 368 **Admissions:** 18538 **Census:** 365 **Outpatient Visits:** 310395 **Births:** 0 **Total Expense ($000):** 511268 **Payroll Expense ($000):** 278179 **Personnel:** 4518

★ **KINDRED HOSPITAL SEATTLE (502002)**, 10631 8th Avenue N.E., Zip 98125–0716; tel. 206/364–2050 **A**1 9 10 **F**1 30 31 32
S Kindred Healthcare
Primary Contact: Greg Davis, Chief Executive Officer
CFO: Scott Eyler, Chief Financial Officer
Web address: www.kindredhealthcare.com
Control: Corporation, Investor–owned, for–profit **Service:** Long–Term Acute Care hospital

Staffed Beds: 42 **Admissions:** 316 **Census:** 25 **Outpatient Visits:** 0 **Births:** 0 **Total Expense ($000):** 13846 **Payroll Expense ($000):** 5324

★ △ **NORTHWEST HOSPITAL AND MEDICAL CENTER (500001)**, 1550 North 115th Street, Zip 98133–9733; tel. 206/364–0500 **A**1 2 3 5 7 9 10 **F**3 11 12 13 15 17 18 20 22 24 25 26 27 30 31 32 33 34 36 38 40 46 47 48 49 52 53 54 55 56 57 58 62 63 66 68 70 71 72 73 74 75 76 77 78 79 81 85 86 87 88 93 94 95 96 97 100 102 103 104 106 107 112 116 119 120 121 135 136 137 **P**6 7
Primary Contact: C. W. Schneider, President and Chief Executive Officer
CFO: Robert Steigmeyer, Vice President and Chief Financial Officer
CMO: Greg Schroedl, M.D., Vice President Medical and Chief Quality Officer
Web address: www.nwhospital.org
Control: Other not–for–profit (including NFP Corporation) **Service:** General Medical and Surgical

Staffed Beds: 187 **Admissions:** 9661 **Census:** 116 **Outpatient Visits:** 424429 **Births:** 1067 **Total Expense ($000):** 194555 **Payroll Expense ($000):** 76977 **Personnel:** 1348

★ **REGIONAL HOSPITAL FOR RESPIRATORY AND COMPLEX CARE (502001)**, 12844 Military Road South, Zip 98168–9981; tel. 206/248–4548 **A**1 9 10 **F**1
Primary Contact: Barbara Hostetler, Interim Chief Executive Officer
CFO: Gregg Terreson, Controller
CMO: Robert L. Clark, M.D., Medical Director
CHR: Valerie Albano, Manager Human Resources
Web address: www.regionalhospital.org
Control: Other not–for–profit (including NFP Corporation) **Service:** Children's Long–Term Acute Care

Staffed Beds: 31 **Admissions:** 154 **Census:** 27 **Outpatient Visits:** 0 **Births:** 0 **Total Expense ($000):** 20572 **Payroll Expense ($000):** 8063 **Personnel:** 98

SCHICK SHADEL HOSPITAL (500134), 12101 Ambaum Boulevard S.W., Zip 98146–2699, Mailing Address: Box 48149, Zip 98148–0149; tel. 206/244–8100, (Nonreporting) **A**9 10
Primary Contact: Elaine Oksendahl, Administrator
CFO: Jack Brinkerhoff, Chief Financial Officer
CMO: James W. Smith, M.D., Medical Director
CIO: Henry Brown, Director Plant Operations and Information Technology
Web address: www.schickshadel.com
Control: Corporation, Investor–owned, for–profit **Service:** Alcoholism and other chemical dependency

Staffed Beds: 48

□ **SEATTLE CANCER CARE ALLIANCE (500138)**, 825 Eastlake Avenue East, Zip 98109, Mailing Address: P.O. Box 19023, Zip 98109–1023; tel. 206/288–1400, (Nonreporting) **A**1 2 9 10
Primary Contact: Fred R. Appelbaum, M.D., Executive Director
COO: Norm Hubbard, Executive Vice President
CFO: Jonathan Tingstad, Vice President and Chief Financial Officer
CMO: Marc Stewart, M.D., Vice President and Medical Director
CIO: Kelly Martin, Director Information Technology
CHR: Han Nachtrieb, Vice President Human Resources
Web address: www.seattlecca.org
Control: Other not–for–profit (including NFP Corporation) **Service:** Cancer

Staffed Beds: 20

★ **SWEDISH HEALTH SERVICES (500027)**, 747 Broadway Avenue, Zip 98122–4307; tel. 206/386–6000, (Includes SWEDISH MEDICAL CENTER–BALLARD, 5300 Tallman Avenue N.W., Zip 98107–3932; tel. 206/782–2700; SWEDISH MEDICAL CENTER–FIRST HILL) **A**1 2 3 5 9 10 **F**3 4 5 8 11 12 13 15 18 19 20 21 22 23 24 25 26 27 28 30 31 32 33 34 36 38 39 41 42 43 44 46 47 49 50 51 54 55 56 57 58 59 60 61 62 64 66 68 69 70 71 72 73 74 75 76 77 79 80 81 82 83 84 86 87 90 92 96 97 98 99 100 102 104 106 107 108 109 110 111 112 114 116 118 119 120 121 123 124 125 127 130 131 132 135 136 137 **P**6
Primary Contact: Rodney F. Hochman, M.D., Chief Executive Officer
COO: Calvin K. Knight, Chief Operating Officer
CFO: Ronald K. Sperling, Chief Financial Officer
CMO: Nancy Auer, M.D., Chief Medical Officer
CIO: Janice Newell, Interim Chief Information Officer
CHR: Joanne Suffis, Interim Vice President Human Resources
Web address: www.swedish.org
Control: Other not–for–profit (including NFP Corporation) **Service:** General Medical and Surgical

Staffed Beds: 615 **Admissions:** 34208 **Census:** 393 **Outpatient Visits:** 448687 **Births:** 7909 **Total Expense ($000):** 706537 **Payroll Expense ($000):** 295807 **Personnel:** 4212

★ △ **SWEDISH MEDICAL CENTER–CHERRY HILL CAMPUS (500025)**, (Formerly Swedish Medical Center Providence Campus), 500 17th Avenue, Zip 98122–5711; tel. 206/320–2000 **A**1 2 3 5 7 9 10 **F**3 8 11 15 18 20 22 24 25 26 27 30 31 32 33 38 41 43 44 46 50 52 55 56 57 58 59 60 62 63 64 66 68 69 72 73 75 76 77 79 80 81 82 85 86 87 88 90 91 92 93 94 95 96 97 98 99 100 101 107 108 109 111 112 118 121 132 135 137
Primary Contact: Marcel C. Loh, Chief Operating Officer
COO: Marcel C. Loh, Chief Operating Officer
CFO: Ronald K. Sperling, Chief Financial Officer
CMO: Nancy Auer, M.D., Chief Medical Officer
CIO: Janice Newell, Chief Information Officer
Web address: www.swedish.org
Control: Other not–for–profit (including NFP Corporation) **Service:** General Medical and Surgical

Staffed Beds: 224 **Admissions:** 8920 **Census:** 113 **Outpatient Visits:** 123973 **Births:** 0 **Total Expense ($000):** 262034 **Payroll Expense ($000):** 102585 **Personnel:** 1288

★ △ **UNIVERSITY OF WASHINGTON MEDICAL CENTER (500008)**, 1959 Northeast Pacific Street, Box 356151, Zip 98195–6151; tel. 206/598–3300 **A**1 2 3 5 7 8 9 10 **F**3 8 9 11 12 13 15 17 18 20 22 23 24 25 26 27 30 31 32 33 34 37 38 41 43 44 46 47 48 49 50 51 53 54 55 56 57 58 59 60 62 63 66 68 70 72 73 74 75 76 77 78 79 80 81 82 85 86 87 88 90 91 92 93 94 96 97 99 100 102 103 104 105 106 107 108 109 111 112 114 116 119 120 121 125 126 127 128 129 130 131 133 134 135 136 137 **P**6
Primary Contact: Stephen P. Zieniewicz, Executive Director
CFO: Paul Ishizuka, Associate Executive Director and Chief Financial Officer
CMO: Ed Walker, M.D., Medical Director
CHR: Mason Hudson, Assistant Director Human Resources
Web address: www.uwmedicine.org/Facilities/UWMedicalCenter/
Control: State–Government, nonfederal **Service:** General Medical and Surgical

Staffed Beds: 390 **Admissions:** 18866 **Census:** 317 **Outpatient Visits:** 359311 **Births:** 1833 **Total Expense ($000):** 593801 **Payroll Expense ($000):** 241189 **Personnel:** 3896

WA

Hospital, Medicare Provider Number, Address, Telephone, Approval, Facility, and Physician Codes, Health Care System

★ American Hospital Association (AHA) membership
□ The Joint Commission accreditation
○ American Osteopathic Association (AOA) accreditation
△ Commission on Accreditation of Rehabilitation Facilities (CARF) accreditation

★ △ **VETERANS AFFAIRS PUGET SOUND HEALTH CARE SYSTEM**, 1660 South Columbian Way, Zip 98108–1597; tel. 206/762–1010, (Includes VETERANS AFFAIRS PUGET SOUND HEALTH CARE SYSTEM–AMERICAN LAKE DIVISION, Tacoma, Zip 98493; tel. 253/582–8440), (Total facility includes 131 beds in nursing home–type unit) **A**1 2 3 5 7 8 9 **F**1 3 5 6 7 17 18 20 22 24 25 26 27 29 32 33 36 37 38 41 42 43 44 50 51 52 53 54 55 56 57 60 61 62 63 66 68 72 73 75 76 77 78 79 80 81 85 88 90 92 93 94 95 96 97 100 102 106 107 108 118 119 121 124 125 130 133 135 136 137 **P**6
S Department of Veterans Affairs
Primary Contact: Stan Johnson, Director
CFO: Kenneth J. Hudson, Chief Financial Officer
CMO: Gordon Starkebaum, M.D., Chief of Staff
CIO: Glenn Zwinger, Manager Information Systems Services
Web address: www.va.gov/sta/guide/home.asp
Control: Veterans Affairs, Government, federal **Service:** General Medical and Surgical

Staffed Beds: 504 **Admissions:** 9155 **Census:** 202 **Outpatient Visits:** 645623 **Births:** 0 **Total Expense ($000):** 425049 **Payroll Expense ($000):** 250161 **Personnel:** 3330

★ △ **VIRGINIA MASON MEDICAL CENTER (500005)**, 1100 Ninth Avenue, Zip 98101–2756, Mailing Address: P.O. Box 900, Zip 98111–0900; tel. 206/223–6600, (Total facility includes 35 beds in nursing home–type unit) **A**1 2 3 5 7 9 10 **F**2 3 8 9 12 15 18 20 22 23 24 25 26 27 28 30 31 32 33 34 35 38 43 44 46 47 48 49 51 53 54 56 57 59 60 61 62 63 65 66 68 69 72 73 75 76 77 79 80 81 82 85 86 87 90 93 94 96 97 98 99 100 101 102 103 104 105 106 107 108 109 111 112 113 114 116 117 118 119 120 121 124 125 127 130 131 133 134 135 136 137 **P**6
Primary Contact: Gary Kaplan, President
COO: Sarah Patterson, Executive Vice President and Administrator
CFO: Craig Goodrich, Chief Financial Officer
CIO: Bill Poppy, Senior Vice President
Web address: www.vmmc.org
Control: Other not–for–profit (including NFP Corporation) **Service:** General Medical and Surgical

Staffed Beds: 324 **Admissions:** 17752 **Census:** 243 **Outpatient Visits:** 840176 **Births:** 0 **Total Expense ($000):** 625101 **Payroll Expense ($000):** 327285 **Personnel:** 4309

☐ **WEST SEATTLE PSYCHIATRIC HOSPITAL (504009)**, 2600 S.W. Holden Street, Zip 98126–3505; tel. 206/933–7199, (Nonreporting) **A**1 9 10
Primary Contact: David Johnson, Chief Executive Officer
CFO: Lisa Yamilkoski, Chief Financial Officer
CMO: Jeff Skolnick, M.D., Chief Medical Officer
CIO: Linda Johnson, Director Information Systems
CHR: Judi Mitchell, Vice President Human Resources
Web address: www.highlinementalhealth.org
Control: Other not–for–profit (including NFP Corporation) **Service:** Psychiatric

Staffed Beds: 40

SEDRO WOOLLEY—Skagit County

★ **UNITED GENERAL HOSPITAL (501329)**, 2000 Hospital Drive, Zip 98284–4327; tel. 360/856–6021 **A**1 9 10 18 **F**3 15 25 27 30 31 32 33 38 52 55 56 57 62 66 68 73 76 79 81 86 93 96 97 102 107 108 109 111 118 119 122 132 135
Primary Contact: Greg Reed, Chief Executive Officer
CFO: Michael W. Bonthuis, Chief Financial Officer
CMO: Daryl Vogel, M.D., Chief Medical Officer
CHR: Tracie Skrinde, Director Human Resources
Web address: www.unitedgeneral.org
Control: Hospital district or authority, Government, nonfederal **Service:** General Medical and Surgical

Staffed Beds: 35 **Admissions:** 1687 **Census:** 20 **Outpatient Visits:** 100849 **Births:** 2 **Total Expense ($000):** 39523 **Payroll Expense ($000):** 15847 **Personnel:** 291

WA

SHELTON—Mason County

★ **MASON GENERAL HOSPITAL (501336)**, 901 Mountain View Drive, Building 1, Zip 98584–1668, Mailing Address: P.O. Box 1668, Zip 98584–1668; tel. 360/426–1611 **A**1 9 10 18 **F**11 13 15 25 26 31 32 38 55 66 73 77 79 80 81 96 100 119 121 135
Primary Contact: G. Robert Appel, Chief Executive Officer
COO: Diane Stillman, Chief Operating Officer
CFO: Eric Moll, Chief Financial Officer
CIO: Brian Conklin, Director Information Systems
CHR: Claudia Hawley, Director Human Resources
Web address: www.masongeneral.com
Control: Hospital district or authority, Government, nonfederal **Service:** General Medical and Surgical

Staffed Beds: 25 **Admissions:** 1770 **Census:** 15 **Outpatient Visits:** 52545 **Total Expense ($000):** 48827 **Payroll Expense ($000):** 21913 **Personnel:** 375

SNOQUALMIE—King County

SNOQUALMIE VALLEY HOSPITAL (501338), 9575 Ethan Wade Way S.E., Zip 98065–9577, Mailing Address: P.O. Box 2021, Zip 98065–2021; tel. 425/831–2300, (Nonreporting) **A**9 10 18
Primary Contact: Rodger McCollum, Chief Executive Officer
Control: Hospital district or authority, Government, nonfederal **Service:** General Medical and Surgical

Staffed Beds: 18

SOUTH BEND—Pacific County

WILLAPA HARBOR HOSPITAL (501303), 800 Alder Street, Zip 98586–0438, Mailing Address: P.O. Box 438, Zip 98586–0438; tel. 360/875–4502, (Nonreporting) **A**9 10 18
Primary Contact: Carole Halsan, Chief Executive Officer
CFO: Terry Stone, Chief Financial Officer and Chief Information Officer
CIO: Terry Stone, Chief Financial Officer and Chief Information Officer
Web address: www.willapaharborhospital.com
Control: Hospital district or authority, Government, nonfederal **Service:** General Medical and Surgical

Staffed Beds: 26

SPOKANE—Spokane County

★ **DEACONESS MEDICAL CENTER–SPOKANE (500044)**, 800 West Fifth Avenue, Zip 99204–2803, Mailing Address: P.O. Box 248, Zip 99210–0248; tel. 509/458–5800 **A**1 2 3 5 9 10 **F**3 11 13 15 17 18 20 22 24 25 26 27 33 38 39 40 43 44 50 51 52 53 54 57 59 62 64 65 66 68 70 71 72 74 76 77 79 80 81 82 87 96 97 100 101 107 111 112 118 119 120 121 132 133 135 137 **S** Empire Health Services
Primary Contact: Robert Quist, Chief Executive Officer
COO: Michael T. Liepman, Chief Operating Officer
CFO: Garman E. Lutz, Chief Financial Officer
CIO: Paul Fitzpatrick, Manager Information Technology
Web address: www.deaconess–spokane.org
Control: Other not–for–profit (including NFP Corporation) **Service:** General Medical and Surgical

Staffed Beds: 265 **Admissions:** 12048 **Census:** 179 **Outpatient Visits:** 179726 **Births:** 2187

★ **HOLY FAMILY HOSPITAL (500077)**, North 5633 Lidgerwood Street, Zip 99208–2533; tel. 509/482–0111 **A**1 2 9 10 **F**3 8 11 12 13 15 17 18 20 25 26 27 30 31 32 33 36 37 38 40 42 43 44 46 47 48 49 50 52 54 55 56 57 58 59 60 62 66 68 71 72 73 74 75 76 77 79 80 81 82 84 86 87 90 96 97 107 109 111 118 119 120 121 124 132 135 136 137 **P**7 **S** Providence Health & Services
Primary Contact: Thomas Corley, President
COO: Cathy J. Simchuk, Vice President Clinical and Facility Operations
CFO: Janis H. Simpson, Chief Financial Officer
CMO: Chris Tullis, M.D., President
CIO: Mark Vogelsang, Director Information Services
CHR: Kellie Sheldon, Vice President Human Resources
Web address: www.holy–family.org
Control: Church–operated, Nongovernment, not–for profit **Service:** General Medical and Surgical

Staffed Beds: 199 **Admissions:** 9704 **Census:** 106 **Outpatient Visits:** 125595 **Births:** 1272 **Total Expense ($000):** 136488 **Payroll Expense ($000):** 53303 **Personnel:** 890

★ **SACRED HEART MEDICAL CENTER (500054)**, 101 West Eighth Avenue, Zip 99204–2364, Mailing Address: P.O. Box 2555, Zip 99220–2555; tel. 509/474–3040 **A**1 2 3 5 9 10 **F**3 11 12 13 15 17 18 19 20 21 22 23 25 26 27 30 31 32 38 40 43 44 46 47 48 49 51 52 54 55 59 62 66 68 70 72 73 74 76 77 79 80 81 83 84 88 89 90 92 93 94 95 96 97 98 99 100 102 103 104 106 107 108 111 112 116 119 126 127 128 129 130 135 136 137 **P**6 **S** Providence Health & Services
Primary Contact: Michael D. Wilson, President
COO: Elaine Couture, Chief Operating Officer
CFO: Kevin Walstrom, Chief Financial Officer
CMO: Jeff Collins, M.D., Chief Medical Officer
CHR: Patrick Clary, Vice President Human Resources
Web address: www.shmc.org
Control: Church–operated, Nongovernment, not–for profit **Service:** General Medical and Surgical

Staffed Beds: 623 **Admissions:** 29486 **Census:** 410 **Outpatient Visits:** 145063 **Births:** 1331 **Total Expense ($000):** 494628 **Payroll Expense ($000):** 199794 **Personnel:** 3273

☐ **SHRINERS HOSPITALS FOR CHILDREN–SPOKANE**, 911 West Fifth Avenue, Zip 99204, Mailing Address: P.O. Box 2472, Zip 99210–2472; tel. 509/455–7844, (Nonreporting) **A**1 **S** Shriners Hospitals for Children
Primary Contact: Gene Raynaud, Administrator
CFO: Margreta Kilgore, Director Fiscal Services
CMO: Paul Caskey, M.D., Chief of Staff
CIO: Jeremy Long, Manager Information Systems
CHR: Odetta Curtis, Director Human Resources
Web address: www.shrinershospital.org
Control: Other not–for–profit (including NFP Corporation) **Service:** Children's orthopedic

Staffed Beds: 30

★ △ **ST. LUKE'S REHABILITATION INSTITUTE (503025)**, 711 South Cowley Street, Zip 99202–1388; tel. 509/473–6000 **A**1 7 10 **F**11 24 25 26 30 31 32 40 58 62 66 72 73 75 77 81 82 85 86 119 120 121 132 135
Primary Contact: Thomas M. Fritz, Administrator and Chief Executive Officer
COO: Gary J. Smith, Ph.D., Chief Operating Officer
CFO: John D. Craig, Chief Financial Officer
CMO: Stefan Humphries, M.D., Medical Director
CIO: Fred Galusha, Chief Information Officer
CHR: Alan Wagner, Director Human Resources
Web address: www.st–lukes.org
Control: Other not–for–profit (including NFP Corporation) **Service:** Rehabilitation

Staffed Beds: 80 **Admissions:** 1516 **Census:** 60 **Outpatient Visits:** 66320 **Births:** 0 **Total Expense ($000):** 32029 **Payroll Expense ($000):** 18275 **Personnel:** 440

★ **VALLEY HOSPITAL AND MEDICAL CENTER (500119)**, 12606 East Mission Avenue, Zip 99216–1090; tel. 509/924–6650, (Nonreporting) **A**1 2 9 10 **S** Empire Health Services
Primary Contact: Robert Quist, Chief Executive Officer
Web address: www.valleyhospital.org
Control: Other not–for–profit (including NFP Corporation) **Service:** General Medical and Surgical

Staffed Beds: 93

★ **VETERANS AFFAIRS MEDICAL CENTER**, North 4815 Assembly Street, Zip 99205–6197; tel. 509/434–7000, (Total facility includes 34 beds in nursing home–type unit) **A**1 **F**1 3 5 8 10 12 15 17 18 25 26 27 33 36 37 38 42 43 44 46 47 48 49 53 54 55 56 57 63 68 69 73 75 76 77 79 81 82 86 87 88 92 93 94 95 96 97 103 107 118 119 121 124 132 133 134 135 136 137 **S** Department of Veterans Affairs
Primary Contact: Sharon M. Helman, Director
COO: Ken Eigen, Chief Engineering and Technology
CFO: Michael Gatham, Chief Financial Officer
CMO: Jacy Ryan, M.D., Chief Medical Service
CHR: Jacqueline Ross, Acting Chief Human Resources Officer
Web address: www.va.gov/sta/guide/home.asp
Control: Veterans Affairs, Government, federal **Service:** General Medical and Surgical

Staffed Beds: 66 **Admissions:** 945 **Census:** 13 **Outpatient Visits:** 215971 **Births:** 0

SUNNYSIDE—Yakima County

★ **SUNNYSIDE COMMUNITY HOSPITAL (501330)**, 1016 Tacoma Avenue, Zip 98944–0719, Mailing Address: P.O. Box 719, Zip 98944–0719; tel. 509/837–1500, (Nonreporting) **A**9 10 18 **S** Brim Healthcare, Inc.
Primary Contact: Jon D. Smiley, Chief Executive Officer
CFO: Jim Schlenker, Chief Financial Officer
CMO: Coke R. Smith, M.D., Chief of Staff
CIO: Salvador Betancourt, Manager Information Systems
CHR: Lisa Gray, Director Human Resources
Web address: www.sunnysidehospital.com
Control: Corporation, Investor–owned, for–profit **Service:** General Medical and Surgical

Staffed Beds: 25

TACOMA—Pierce County

ALLENMORE HOSPITAL See Tacoma General Hospital

★ **MADIGAN ARMY MEDICAL CENTER**, Fitzsimmons Drive, Building 9040, Zip 98431–1100; tel. 253/968–1110 **A**1 2 3 5 **F**3 5 7 11 12 13 14 15 17 18 19 20 22 24 25 26 27 28 29 30 31 32 33 34 36 37 38 40 41 43 46 48 49 50 51 52 53 54 55 56 57 58 59 60 62 63 65 66 68 70 71 72 73 74 75 76 77 79 80 81 82 84 86 87 88 90 91 92 93 94 95 96 97 100 102 104 105 106 107 108 113 114 118 119 120 121 124 131 133 135 136 137 **P**6 **S** Department of the Army, Office of the Surgeon General
Primary Contact: Brigadier General Sheila R. Baxter, Commanding General
CFO: Lieutenant Colonel Bryan Longmuir, Chief Resource Management
CMO: Colonel George McClure, M.D., Deputy Commander for Clinical Operations
CIO: Lieutenant Colonel Craig Anderson, Chief Information Management
CHR: David Aiken, Chief Human Resources Officer
Web address: www.mamc.amedd.army.mil
Control: Army, Government, federal **Service:** General Medical and Surgical

Staffed Beds: 205 **Admissions:** 11095 **Census:** 115 **Outpatient Visits:** 907155 **Births:** 1974 **Total Expense ($000):** 351689 **Payroll Expense ($000):** 172128

☐ **MARY BRIDGE CHILDREN'S HOSPITAL AND HEALTH CENTER (503301)**, 317 Martin Luther King Jr. Way, Zip 98405–0299, Mailing Address: Box 5299, Zip 98415–0299; tel. 253/403–1400 **A**1 3 5 9 10 **F**19 23 24 25 26 27 28 30 31 32 33 36 38 40 48 53 55 56 57 62 63 64 66 69 72 73 76 77 79 83 84 90 92 96 100 104 105 107 114 118 119 120 121 133 135 **P**6 **S** MultiCare Health System
Primary Contact: Mady Murrey, Vice President and Administrator
COO: George J. Brown, M.D., Chief Operating Officer
CFO: Vince Schmitz, Senior Vice President and Chief Financial Officer
CMO: Lester Reed, M.D., Vice President Medical Affairs
CIO: Florence Chang, Senior Vice President and Chief Information Officer
CHR: Sarah Horsman, Senior Vice President Human Potential
Web address: www.multicare.org/marybridge
Control: Other not–for–profit (including NFP Corporation) **Service:** Children's general

Staffed Beds: 67 **Admissions:** 3990 **Census:** 38 **Outpatient Visits:** 75468 **Births:** 0 **Total Expense ($000):** 92279 **Payroll Expense ($000):** 44989 **Personnel:** 325

★ **ST. CLARE HOSPITAL (500021)**, 11315 Bridgeport Way S.W., Zip 98499–3004; tel. 253/588–1711 **A**1 2 9 10 **F**3 12 15 25 26 27 31 32 33 36 38 41 44 49 50 53 55 56 57 62 68 72 73 75 76 77 78 79 80 81 82 86 92 96 97 102 106 107 118 119 121 123 124 135 136 **P**6 **S** Catholic Health Initiatives
Primary Contact: Kathy Bressler, Chief Operating Officer
COO: Kathy Bressler, Chief Operating Officer
CFO: Mike Fitzgerald, Chief Financial Officer
CMO: Mike Newcomb, D.O., Senior Vice President Medical Affairs
CIO: Bruce Elkington, Vice President Information Technology
CHR: David Lawson, Vice President Human Resources
Web address: www.fhshealth.org
Control: Church–operated, Nongovernment, not–for profit **Service:** General Medical and Surgical

Staffed Beds: 98 **Admissions:** 6878 **Census:** 75 **Outpatient Visits:** 66230 **Births:** 0 **Total Expense ($000):** 90859 **Payroll Expense ($000):** 41548 **Personnel:** 565

★ △ **ST. JOSEPH MEDICAL CENTER (500108)**, 1717 South J Street, Zip 98405–3004, Mailing Address: P.O. Box 2197, Zip 98401–2197; tel. 253/426–4101 **A**1 2 5 7 9 10 **F**12 13 15 17 18 20 22 24 25 26 27 31 32 33 34 36 38 40 41 43 44 45 46 47 49 53 55 56 57 59 62 66 68 70 72 73 74 75 76 77 78 79 80 81 82 85 86 88 89 92 94 96 97 100 102 103 106 107 112 116 118 119 121 123 124 125 134 135 136 **P**6 **S** Catholic Health Initiatives
Primary Contact: Syd Bersante, Chief Operating Officer
COO: Syd Bersante, Chief Operating Officer
CFO: Mike Fitzgerald, Chief Financial Officer
CMO: Mike Newcomb, D.O., Senior Vice President Medical Affairs
CIO: Bruce Elkington, Vice President Information Technology
CHR: David Lawson, Vice President Human Resources
Web address: www.fhshealth.org
Control: Church–operated, Nongovernment, not–for profit **Service:** General Medical and Surgical

Staffed Beds: 305 **Admissions:** 21629 **Census:** 252 **Outpatient Visits:** 459309 **Births:** 3772 **Total Expense ($000):** 394527 **Payroll Expense ($000):** 170959 **Personnel:** 2939

WA

Hospital, Medicare Provider Number, Address, Telephone, Approval, Facility, and Physician Codes, Health Care System
★ American Hospital Association (AHA) membership
☐ The Joint Commission accreditation
○ American Osteopathic Association (AOA) accreditation
△ Commission on Accreditation of Rehabilitation Facilities (CARF) accreditation

★ **TACOMA GENERAL HOSPITAL (500129)**, 315 Martin Luther King Jr. Way, Zip 98405–0299, Mailing Address: P.O. Box 5299, Zip 98415–0299; tel. 253/403–1000, (Includes ALLENMORE HOSPITAL, South 19th and Union Avenue, Zip 98405, Mailing Address: P.O. Box 11414, Zip 98411–0414; tel. 253/403–2323) **A**1 3 5 9 10 **F**7 8 13 15 17 18 19 20 21 22 23 24 25 26 27 28 30 31 32 33 36 38 40 42 43 44 46 47 48 49 55 56 57 61 62 68 69 70 71 72 73 74 75 76 77 78 79 80 81 82 86 87 96 97 100 102 103 104 105 107 109 111 116 118 119 120 121 124 133 135 **P**6 **S** MultiCare Health System
Primary Contact: Diane Cecchettini, RN, President and Chief Executive Officer
COO: George J. Brown, M.D., Vice President Acute Care Service and Facilities
CFO: Vince Schmitz, Vice President and Chief Financial Officer
CMO: Lester Reed, M.D., Chief Medical Officer
CIO: Florence Chang, Vice President Information Technologies
CHR: Sarah Horsman, Vice President Human Resources
Web address: www.multicare.org
Control: Other not–for–profit (including NFP Corporation) **Service:** General Medical and Surgical

Staffed Beds: 404 **Admissions:** 17975 **Census:** 227 **Outpatient Visits:** 176805 **Births:** 3149 **Total Expense ($000):** 338203 **Payroll Expense ($000):** 171025 **Personnel:** 1420

VETERANS AFFAIRS PUGET SOUND HEALTH CARE SYSTEM–AMERICAN LAKE DIVISION See Veterans Affairs Puget Sound Health Care System, Seattle

□ **WESTERN STATE HOSPITAL (504003)**, 9601 Steilacoom Boulevard S.W., Zip 98498–7213; tel. 253/582–8900 **A**1 9 10 **F**37 81 88 91 92 93
Primary Contact: Andrew J. Phillips, Ed.D., Chief Executive Officer
COO: Dale Thompson, Chief Operating Officer
CFO: Nancy Skaar, Chief Financial Officer
CMO: Margaret Dean, M.D., Acting Medical Director
CHR: John Black, Administrator Human Resources
Web address: www.dshs.wa.gov/mentalhealth/wsh.shtml
Control: State–Government, nonfederal **Service:** Psychiatric

Staffed Beds: 897 **Admissions:** 1609 **Census:** 828 **Outpatient Visits:** 0 **Births:** 0 **Total Expense ($000):** 164960 **Payroll Expense ($000):** 104177 **Personnel:** 2045

TONASKET—Okanogan County

★ **NORTH VALLEY HOSPITAL (501321)**, 203 South Western Avenue, Zip 98855; tel. 509/486–2151, (Total facility includes 58 beds in nursing home–type unit) **A**9 10 18 **F**10 13 15 25 30 38 52 54 62 73 74 77 79 80 85 86 96 107 117 122 124
Primary Contact: Warner H. Bartleson, Administrator
CFO: Bomi Bharucha, Chief Financial Officer
CMO: Justina Bolz, M.D., Chief Medical Staff
CIO: Carlos Antuna, Manager Information Systems
CHR: Jan Gonzales, Director Human Resources
Web address: www.nvhospital.org
Control: Hospital district or authority, Government, nonfederal **Service:** General Medical and Surgical

Staffed Beds: 85 **Admissions:** 796 **Census:** 52 **Outpatient Visits:** 8514 **Births:** 83 **Total Expense ($000):** 13832 **Payroll Expense ($000):** 6517 **Personnel:** 152

TOPPENISH—Yakima County

★ **TOPPENISH COMMUNITY HOSPITAL (500037)**, 502 West Fourth Avenue, Zip 98948–0672, Mailing Address: P.O. Box 672, Zip 98948–0672; tel. 509/865–3105 **A**1 9 10 **F**13 15 25 30 31 38 68 74 77 79 84 96 99 107 123 135 **S** Health Management Associates
Primary Contact: Michael P. Curran, Chief Executive Officer
CFO: Caroline Wong, Chief Financial Officer
CHR: Stefanie Durand, Director Human Resources
Web address: www.hma–corp.com
Control: Corporation, Investor–owned, for–profit **Service:** General Medical and Surgical

Staffed Beds: 40 **Admissions:** 2191 **Census:** 15 **Outpatient Visits:** 60000 **Births:** 605 **Personnel:** 184

VANCOUVER—Clark County

★ **LEGACY SALMON CREEK HOSPITAL (500150)**, 2211 N.E. 139th Street, Zip 98686–2742; tel. 360/487–1000 **A**1 9 10 **F**3 11 13 15 18 20 25 26 27 28 30 31 32 36 38 41 46 49 50 62 66 68 70 72 73 74 76 77 78 79 80 81 82 84 86 96 97 99 100 102 104 105 106 107 108 109 119 135 136 **P**8 **S** Legacy Health System
Primary Contact: Jonathan Avery, Chief Administrative Officer
COO: Ted Schreck, Senior Vice President and Chief Operating Officer
CFO: Pamela S. Vukovich, Senior Vice President and Chief Financial Officer
CMO: Jack Cioffi, M.D., Interim Chief Medical Officer
CIO: Richard Gibson, M.D., Chief Information Officer
CHR: Sonja Steves, Vice President Human Resources and Marketing
Web address: www.legacyhealth.org
Control: Other not–for–profit (including NFP Corporation) **Service:** General Medical and Surgical

Staffed Beds: 139 **Admissions:** 8156 **Census:** 81 **Outpatient Visits:** 73230 **Births:** 1666 **Total Expense ($000):** 109439 **Payroll Expense ($000):** 43046 **Personnel:** 671

★ △ **SOUTHWEST WASHINGTON MEDICAL CENTER (500050)**, 400 N.E. Mother Joseph Place, Zip 98664–3200, Mailing Address: P.O. Box 1600, Zip 98668–1600; tel. 360/256–2000, (Includes VANCOUVER MEMORIAL CAMPUS, 3400 Main Street, Zip 98663; tel. 206/696–5000) **A**1 2 3 5 7 9 10 **F**3 11 12 13 15 17 18 20 22 24 25 26 27 30 31 32 33 38 39 40 41 42 43 44 49 50 51 53 55 56 57 58 59 60 61 62 63 66 68 71 72 73 74 75 76 77 79 80 81 82 84 85 86 87 88 89 90 91 92 93 94 95 96 97 98 99 100 102 103 104 105 107 109 110 112 119 120 121 124 133 134 135 136 137 **P**5 6
Primary Contact: Joseph M. Kortum, President and Chief Executive Officer
COO: Rainy Atkins, Chief Operating Officer
CFO: David Willie, Chief Financial Officer
CMO: Gilbert Rodriguez, M.D., Chief Medical Officer
CIO: Petra Knowles, Chief Information Officer
CHR: Cheri Meyerhofer, Vice President Human Resources
Web address: www.swmedicalcenter.org
Control: Other not–for–profit (including NFP Corporation) **Service:** General Medical and Surgical

Staffed Beds: 360 **Admissions:** 20969 **Census:** 235 **Outpatient Visits:** 331491 **Births:** 3946 **Total Expense ($000):** 382763 **Payroll Expense ($000):** 168110 **Personnel:** 2621

WALLA WALLA—Walla Walla County

★ **JONATHAN M. WAINWRIGHT MEMORIAL VA MEDICAL CENTER**, 77 Wainwright Drive, Zip 99362–3994; tel. 509/525–5200, (Total facility includes 30 beds in nursing home–type unit) (Nonreporting) **A**1 9 **S** Department of Veterans Affairs
Primary Contact: Sharon M. Helman, Director
COO: Sharon M. Helman, Director
CFO: Ron Preszler, Manager Business Office
CMO: Donald L. Rowberg, M.D., Chief of Staff
CIO: Gary Ramer, Manager Information Management
Web address: www.va.gov/sta/guide/home.asp
Control: Veterans Affairs, Government, federal **Service:** General Medical and Surgical

Staffed Beds: 44

★ △ **ST. MARY MEDICAL CENTER (500002)**, 401 West Poplar Street, Zip 99362, Mailing Address: Box 1477, Zip 99362; tel. 509/525–3320 **A**1 2 7 9 10 19 **F**3 8 11 13 15 17 18 24 25 26 27 38 40 44 49 59 61 62 68 71 73 74 75 76 77 79 80 84 85 86 96 99 100 102 105 106 107 109 111 117 118 119 121 133 135 136 137 **P**6 **S** Providence Health & Services
Primary Contact: Steven A. Burdick, Chief Executive Officer
CFO: Michael Parenteau, Vice President Finance
CMO: John Reike, M.D., Vice President Physician Group
CIO: Kathleen Obenland, Director Public Affairs
CHR: Susan Blackburn, Vice President Human Resources and Support Services
Web address: www.smmc.com
Control: Church–operated, Nongovernment, not–for profit **Service:** General Medical and Surgical

Staffed Beds: 99 **Admissions:** 4797 **Census:** 58 **Outpatient Visits:** 129249 **Births:** 576 **Total Expense ($000):** 106008 **Payroll Expense ($000):** 47241 **Personnel:** 825

STATE PENITENTIARY HOSPITAL, Mailing Address: Box 520, Zip 99362; tel. 509/525–3610, (Nonreporting)
Primary Contact: Pat Rima, Health Care Manager
Control: State–Government, nonfederal **Service:** Hospital unit of an institution (prison hospital, college infirmary, etc.)

Staffed Beds: 36

★ **WALLA WALLA GENERAL HOSPITAL (500049)**, 1025 South Second Avenue, Zip 99362–1398, Mailing Address: P.O. Box 1398, Zip 99362–1398; tel. 509/525–0480, (Nonreporting) **A**1 2 9 10 **S** Adventist Health
Primary Contact: Monty E. Knittel, President and Chief Executive Officer
CFO: Duane Meidinger, Vice President Finance
CIO: Gary Dietz, Director Information Systems
Web address: www.wwgh.com
Control: Church–operated, Nongovernment, not–for profit **Service:** General Medical and Surgical

Staffed Beds: 40

Many Facility Codes have changed. Please refer to the AHA Guide Code Chart.

WENATCHEE—Chelan County

★ **CENTRAL WASHINGTON HOSPITAL (500016)**, 1201 South Miller Street, Zip 98801–1948, Mailing Address: P.O. Box 1887, Zip 98807–1887; tel. 509/662–1511, (Total facility includes 30 beds in nursing home–type unit) **A**1 9 10 12 13 19 **F**3 13 15 17 18 20 22 24 25 26 31 32 33 37 38 40 42 43 46 51 55 56 57 59 61 62 66 67 68 72 73 74 75 76 77 79 80 81 82 84 86 87 96 100 102 107 114 117 119 135 136 137 **P**6
Primary Contact: John T. Evans, Jr., President and Chief Executive Officer
COO: John B. Hamilton, Executive Vice President and Chief Operating Officer
CFO: Steven R. Jacobs, Chief Financial Officer
CIO: Darryl Higa, Chief Information Officer
CHR: Jack Powers, Director Human Resources
Web address: www.cwhs.com
Control: Other not–for–profit (including NFP Corporation) **Service:** General Medical and Surgical

Staffed Beds: 159 **Admissions:** 9792 **Census:** 95 **Births:** 2100 **Total Expense ($000):** 154498 **Payroll Expense ($000):** 69983

△ **WENATCHEE VALLEY HOSPITAL (500148)**, 820 North Chelan Avenue, Zip 98807–9881; tel. 509/663–8711, (Nonreporting) **A**5 7 9 10
Primary Contact: Shaun Koos, Administrator
COO: Kevin Gilbert, R.N., Director Surgical and Operations
CFO: John Doyle, Chief Financial Officer
CMO: Stuart Freed, M.D., Medical Director
CIO: Mall Boyd, Director Marketing
CHR: Alan Patterson, Director Human Resources
Web address: www.wvclinic.com
Control: Corporation, Investor–owned, for–profit **Service:** General Medical and Surgical

Staffed Beds: 20

WHITE SALMON—Klickitat County

SKYLINE HOSPITAL (501315), 211 Skyline Drive, Zip 98672–0099, Mailing Address: P.O. Box 99, Zip 98672–0099; tel. 509/493–1101 **A**9 10 18 **F**13 15 17 38 40 55 62 65 74 79 84 87 96 107 117 120 122 **P**5
Primary Contact: Michael J. Madden, Superintendent and Chief Executive Officer
CFO: Brenda Schneider, Chief Financial Officer
CMO: Ray J. FitzSimmons, M.D., Chief Medical Officer
CHR: Robin Loomis, Manager Human Resources
Web address: www.skylinehospital.com
Control: City–County, Government, nonfederal **Service:** General Medical and Surgical

Staffed Beds: 25 **Admissions:** 683 **Census:** 5 **Births:** 66 **Total Expense ($000):** 12150 **Payroll Expense ($000):** 6993 **Personnel:** 170

YAKIMA—Yakima County

□ △ **YAKIMA REGIONAL MEDICAL AND CARDIAC CENTER (500012)**, 110 South Ninth Avenue, Zip 98902–3397; tel. 509/575–5000, (Nonreporting) **A**1 2 3 5 7 9 10 **S** Health Management Associates
Primary Contact: Monte J. Bostwick, Chief Executive Officer
COO: Sean Richardson, Chief Operating Officer
CFO: Vicky Swank, Chief Financial Officer
CMO: Robert Rockwell, M.D., Chief of Staff
Web address: www.yakimaregional.org
Control: Corporation, Investor–owned, for–profit **Service:** General Medical and Surgical

Staffed Beds: 169

★ **YAKIMA VALLEY MEMORIAL HOSPITAL (500036)**, 2811 Tieton Drive, Zip 98902–3761; tel. 509/575–8000, (Nonreporting) **A**1 2 3 5 9 10
Primary Contact: Richard W. Linneweh, Jr., President and Chief Executive Officer
COO: Russ Myers, Vice President and Chief Operating Officer
CFO: John G. Vornbrock, Senior Vice President and Chief Financial Officer
CMO: Jan Lange, M.D., Medical Director
CIO: James Aberle, Vice President Support Services and Chief Information Officer
CHR: Kathy Franz, Director Human Resources
Web address: www.yakimamemorial.org
Control: Other not–for–profit (including NFP Corporation) **Service:** General Medical and Surgical

Staffed Beds: 218

WA

Hospital, Medicare Provider Number, Address, Telephone, Approval, Facility, and Physician Codes, Health Care System

★ American Hospital Association (AHA) membership
□ The Joint Commission accreditation
○ American Osteopathic Association (AOA) accreditation
△ Commission on Accreditation of Rehabilitation Facilities (CARF) accreditation

WEST VIRGINIA

BECKLEY—Raleigh County

☐ **BECKLEY APPALACHIAN REGIONAL HOSPITAL (510062)**, 306 Stanaford Road, Zip 25801–3142; tel. 304/255–3000 **A**1 9 10 **F**3 11 15 17 18 25 26 27 30 31 32 33 36 37 38 40 41 43 50 55 56 57 60 61 62 63 68 72 73 75 76 77 79 80 81 82 85 86 87 88 89 90 91 92 93 96 97 100 102 106 107 118 119 135 **P**6 **S** Appalachian Regional Healthcare
Primary Contact: Rocco K. Massey, Community Chief Executive Officer
CMO: Richard Wisman, M.D., Chief of Staff
CHR: Sue Thomas, Manager Human Resources
Web address: www.arh.org
Control: Other not–for–profit (including NFP Corporation) **Service:** General Medical and Surgical

Staffed Beds: 163 **Admissions:** 6854 **Census:** 116 **Outpatient Visits:** 82632 **Births:** 0 **Total Expense ($000):** 63135 **Payroll Expense ($000):** 24963 **Personnel:** 621

★ **RALEIGH GENERAL HOSPITAL (510070)**, 1710 Harper Road, Zip 25801–3397; tel. 304/256–4100 **A**1 9 10 19 **F**3 13 15 17 18 25 26 31 32 33 38 40 49 55 56 57 59 62 68 73 74 76 77 79 80 82 84 86 96 97 100 102 103 106 107 119 120 121 135 136 **S** LifePoint Hospitals, Inc.
Primary Contact: Karen L. Bowling, Chief Executive Officer
COO: Joseph G. Koch, Vice President and Chief Operating Officer
CFO: Tom Steslicki, Vice President and Chief Financial Officer
CMO: Juddson Lindley, M.D., President Medical Staff
CIO: Lou Worrell, Director Information Systems
CHR: Debbie Christian, Director Human Resources
Web address: www.raleighgeneral.com
Control: Corporation, Investor–owned, for–profit **Service:** General Medical and Surgical

Staffed Beds: 229 **Admissions:** 12930 **Census:** 151 **Outpatient Visits:** 108675 **Births:** 1698 **Total Expense ($000):** 101934 **Payroll Expense ($000):** 41177 **Personnel:** 841

★ **VETERANS AFFAIRS MEDICAL CENTER**, 200 Veterans Avenue, Zip 25801–6499; tel. 304/255–2121, (Total facility includes 50 beds in nursing home–type unit) **A**1 9 **F**2 3 5 8 12 25 26 27 32 33 36 37 38 42 43 44 45 50 52 54 55 56 57 60 61 62 63 65 66 68 69 73 76 77 79 80 81 82 86 87 90 91 92 93 94 96 97 102 106 107 119 121 124 132 133 134 135 136 137 **P**6 **S** Department of Veterans Affairs
CFO: G. Darrell Harvey, Chief Fiscal Services
Web address: www.va.gov/sta/guide/home.asp
Control: Veterans Affairs, Government, federal **Service:** General Medical and Surgical

Staffed Beds: 90 **Admissions:** 1911 **Census:** 73 **Outpatient Visits:** 149730 **Births:** 0 **Total Expense ($000):** 78342 **Payroll Expense ($000):** 25008 **Personnel:** 643

BERKELEY SPRINGS—Morgan County

★ **MORGAN COUNTY WAR MEMORIAL HOSPITAL (511309)**, 109 War Memorial Drive, Zip 25411–1718; tel. 304/258–1234, (Total facility includes 16 beds in nursing home–type unit) **A**9 10 18 **F**3 15 24 25 30 31 32 33 38 43 52 55 56 57 61 62 73 75 79 80 81 86 87 96 100 102 107 117 119 121 122 124 135 137 **P**6 **S** Valley Health System
Primary Contact: John H. Borg, Administrator
CFO: David Applewood, Chief Financial Officer and Compliance Officer
CIO: Janet Fagan, Data Processing Director
CHR: Helen Miller, Human Resources Director
Web address: www.warmemorialhospital.com
Control: County–Government, nonfederal **Service:** General Medical and Surgical

Staffed Beds: 41 **Admissions:** 634 **Census:** 24 **Outpatient Visits:** 36426 **Births:** 0 **Total Expense ($000):** 14792 **Payroll Expense ($000):** 5695 **Personnel:** 139

BLUEFIELD—Mercer County

★ **BLUEFIELD REGIONAL MEDICAL CENTER (510071)**, 500 Cherry Street, Zip 24701–3390; tel. 304/327–1100 **A**1 9 10 19 **F**3 8 13 15 17 18 24 25 26 27 30 31 32 38 40 49 50 54 55 56 57 59 62 66 68 72 73 74 75 76 77 79 80 81 84 96 97 99 103 106 107 118 119 121 124 133 135 136 137 **P**1
Primary Contact: Lynn W. Whitteker, Chief Executive Officer
COO: Rex Hardy, Vice President Ancillary Services
CFO: Patti Gusler, Vice President Finance
CMO: Joel Shor, M.D., Chief of Staff
CIO: Rose Lasker, Director Information Services
CHR: Sandee Cheynet, Vice President Administrative Services
Web address: www.bluefield.org
Control: Other not–for–profit (including NFP Corporation) **Service:** General Medical and Surgical

Staffed Beds: 240 **Admissions:** 6398 **Census:** 75 **Outpatient Visits:** 117733 **Births:** 753 **Total Expense ($000):** 71240 **Payroll Expense ($000):** 30401 **Personnel:** 743

BUCKEYE—Pocahontas County

★ **POCAHONTAS MEMORIAL HOSPITAL (511314)**, Mailing Address: Rural Route 2, Box 52 W, Zip 24924; tel. 304/799–7400 **A**9 10 18 **F**3 11 26 30 31 32 38 54 55 56 57 61 62 79 81 82 86 96 107 117 119 121 122 133
Primary Contact: Donald Muhlenthaler, FACHE, President and Chief Executive Officer
COO: Donald Muhlenthaler, FACHE, President and Chief Executive Officer
CFO: Greg Curry, Director Finance
CMO: William Browning, D.O., Chief of Staff
CIO: Sara Casto, Executive Secretary
CHR: Sara Casto, Executive Secretary
Web address: www.wvha.com/web/pmh/index.htm
Control: County–Government, nonfederal **Service:** General Medical and Surgical

Staffed Beds: 25 **Admissions:** 454 **Census:** 5 **Outpatient Visits:** 14709 **Births:** 0 **Total Expense ($000):** 7207 **Payroll Expense ($000):** 3684 **Personnel:** 101

BUCKHANNON—Upshur County

★ **ST. JOSEPH'S HOSPITAL OF BUCKHANNON (510053)**, 1 Amalia Drive, Zip 26201–2222; tel. 304/473–2000, (Total facility includes 16 beds in nursing home–type unit) **A**1 9 10 **F**3 11 13 15 25 26 27 30 31 32 33 38 40 41 42 43 44 50 55 56 57 61 62 63 68 73 74 76 79 80 82 84 96 102 107 117 118 119 121 124 135 **P**6
Primary Contact: Sue E. Johnson–Phillippe, Interim Chief Executive Officer
CFO: Renee Hofer, Vice President Fiscal Services
CMO: Patrick Galey, M.D., Chief of Staff
CIO: Brian Williams, Director Information Systems
CHR: Allen Wilson, Director Human Resources
Web address: www.stj.net
Control: Other not–for–profit (including NFP Corporation) **Service:** General Medical and Surgical

Staffed Beds: 69 **Admissions:** 1798 **Census:** 30 **Outpatient Visits:** 115036 **Births:** 375 **Total Expense ($000):** 31288 **Payroll Expense ($000):** 13697 **Personnel:** 339

CHARLESTON—Kanawha County

★ △ **CHARLESTON AREA MEDICAL CENTER (510022)**, 501 Morris Street, Zip 25301–1300, Mailing Address: P.O. Box 1547, Zip 25326–1547; tel. 304/388–5432, (Includes GENERAL HOSPITAL, 501 Morris Street, Zip 25301, Mailing Address: Box 1393, Zip 25325; tel. 304/388–6203; Michael D. Williams, Vice President and Administrator; MEMORIAL HOSPITAL, 3200 MacCorkle Avenue S.E., Zip 25304; tel. 304/388–5432; William D. Adams, Vice President and Administrator; WOMEN AND CHILDREN'S HOSPITAL, 800 Pennsylvania Avenue, Zip 25302; tel. 304/388–2286; Sarah Llewellyn, Vice President and Administrator) **A**1 2 3 5 7 8 9 10 12 13 **F**3 8 9 11 12 13 15 17 18 20 22 24 25 26 27 28 31 32 33 36 37 38 40 41 43 44 46 47 48 49 50 51 53 54 55 56 57 59 60 62 63 66 68 70 72 73 74 75 76 77 79 80 81 82 83 84 85 86 87 88 89 90 91 92 93 94 96 97 100 102 103 104 105 106 107 112 113 114 116 118 119 120 121 123 124 127 130 132 133 135 136 137 **P**7 **S** Charleston Area Medical Center Health System, Inc.
Primary Contact: David L. Ramsey, President and Chief Executive Officer
COO: Glenn Crotty, M.D., Executive Vice President and Chief Operating Officer
CFO: Larry C. Hudson, Executive Vice President and Chief Financial Officer
CMO: Elizabeth Spangler, M.D., Vice President Medical Affairs
CIO: Lynn Brookshire, Vice President Information Services and Chief Information Officer
CHR: Beth A. Samples, Vice President Human Resources
Web address: www.camc.org
Control: Other not–for–profit (including NFP Corporation) **Service:** General Medical and Surgical

Staffed Beds: 776 **Admissions:** 35372 **Census:** 526 **Outpatient Visits:** 557867 **Births:** 2712 **Total Expense ($000):** 604575 **Payroll Expense ($000):** 231476 **Personnel:** 5032

☐ **EYE AND EAR CLINIC OF CHARLESTON (510059)**, 1306 Kanawha Boulevard East, Zip 25301–3001, Mailing Address: P.O. Box 2271, Zip 25328–2271; tel. 304/343–4371 **A**1 10 **F**31 32 37 79 131
Primary Contact: Christina Arvon, Administrator and Chief Executive Officer
CMO: James W. Candill, M.D., President Medical Staff
Control: Corporation, Investor–owned, for–profit **Service:** General Medical and Surgical

Staffed Beds: 21 **Admissions:** 4 **Census:** 1 **Outpatient Visits:** 6477 **Births:** 0 **Total Expense ($000):** 6448 **Payroll Expense ($000):** 2423 **Personnel:** 63

GENERAL HOSPITAL See Charleston Area Medical Center

WV

☒ **HIGHLAND HOSPITAL (514001)**, 300 56th Street S.E., Zip 25304–2361, Mailing Address: P.O. Box 4107, Zip 25364–4107; tel. 304/926–1600 **A**1 9 10 **F**25 30 31 32 33 55 73 88 89 91 95 119 **P**6
Primary Contact: David M. McWatters, Administrator
CFO: Lisa Layden, Director of Finance
CMO: Charles Weise, M.D., Medical Director
CIO: Pearl McWatters, Director Information Services
Web address: www.highlandhosp.com
Control: Other not–for–profit (including NFP Corporation) **Service:** Psychiatric

Staffed Beds: 58 **Admissions:** 1127 **Census:** 32 **Outpatient Visits:** 4249 **Births:** 0 **Total Expense ($000):** 8915 **Payroll Expense ($000):** 5027 **Personnel:** 155

MEMORIAL HOSPITAL See Charleston Area Medical Center

☒ **SAINT FRANCIS HOSPITAL (510031)**, 333 Laidley Street, Zip 25301–1628, Mailing Address: P.O. Box 471, Zip 25322–0471; tel. 304/347–6500, (Total facility includes 10 beds in nursing home–type unit) **A**1 9 10 **F**3 15 18 20 25 26 30 31 32 38 43 44 46 49 51 55 56 57 59 62 66 67 68 72 73 77 79 81 82 86 87 96 97 99 100 103 104 107 117 118 119 120 124 132 134 135 136 137
Primary Contact: Dan Lauffer, FACHE, Chief Executive Officer
COO: Tim Bess, Chief Operating Officer
CFO: Renee Cross, Chief Financial Officer
CMO: David Santrock, M.D., President Medical Staff
CIO: Jane Harless, Director Information Services
CHR: Cathy McCarthy, Director Human Resources
Web address: www.stfrancishospital.com
Control: Other not–for–profit (including NFP Corporation) **Service:** General Medical and Surgical

Staffed Beds: 123 **Admissions:** 3485 **Census:** 62 **Outpatient Visits:** 61331 **Births:** 0 **Total Expense ($000):** 54916 **Payroll Expense ($000):** 19189 **Personnel:** 643

☒ **SELECT SPECIALTY HOSPITAL–CHARLESTON (512002)**, 333 Laidley Street, Zip 25301–1628; tel. 304/720–7234 **A**1 9 10 **F**1 25 31 32 72 73 77 80 119 137 **S** Select Medical Corporation
Primary Contact: Frank Weber, Chief Executive Officer
Web address: www.selectmedicalcorp.com
Control: Corporation, Investor–owned, for–profit **Service:** Long–Term Acute Care hospital

Staffed Beds: 32 **Admissions:** 396 **Census:** 27 **Outpatient Visits:** 0 **Births:** 0 **Total Expense ($000):** 13566 **Payroll Expense ($000):** 4760 **Personnel:** 110

WOMEN AND CHILDREN'S HOSPITAL See Charleston Area Medical Center

CLARKSBURG—Harrison County

☒ **LOUIS A. JOHNSON VETERANS AFFAIRS MEDICAL CENTER**, 1 Medical Center Drive, Zip 26301–4199; tel. 304/623–3461, (Total facility includes 27 beds in nursing home–type unit) (Nonreporting) **A**1 3 5 9 **S** Department of Veterans Affairs
Primary Contact: William E. Cox, Director
COO: Frank Miles, Associate Director
CFO: William Salser, Chief Financial Officer
CMO: Glenn R. Snider, M.D., Chief of Staff
CIO: Paul Williams, Chief Information Management
Web address: www.va.gov/sta/guide/home.asp
Control: Veterans Affairs, Government, federal **Service:** General Medical and Surgical

Staffed Beds: 98

☒ **UNITED HOSPITAL CENTER (510006)**, 3 Hospital Plaza, Zip 26301, Mailing Address: P.O. Box 1680, Zip 26302–1680; tel. 304/624–2121 **A**1 2 3 5 9 10 12 13 19 20 **F**3 5 11 13 15 17 18 20 24 25 26 27 30 32 34 36 37 38 42 43 44 46 48 49 51 53 55 56 57 58 59 61 62 63 66 68 72 73 74 75 76 77 79 80 81 82 84 86 87 88 89 90 91 92 93 94 96 97 98 100 102 103 104 105 106 107 108 109 111 117 118 119 121 135 137 **P**6 8 **S** West Virginia United Health System
Primary Contact: Bruce C. Carter, President
COO: Michael Tillman, Vice President Patient Services and Chief Operating Officer
CFO: Douglas Coffman, Vice President and Chief Financial Officer
CMO: Eric Radcliffe, M.D., Medical Director
CIO: Ed Collins, Chief Information Officer
CHR: Tim Allen, Vice President Human Resources
Web address: www.uhcwv.org
Control: Other not–for–profit (including NFP Corporation) **Service:** General Medical and Surgical

Staffed Beds: 311 **Admissions:** 13736 **Census:** 202 **Outpatient Visits:** 398258 **Births:** 914 **Total Expense ($000):** 162044 **Payroll Expense ($000):** 69384 **Personnel:** 1501

ELKINS—Randolph County

☒ **DAVIS MEMORIAL HOSPITAL (510030)**, Gorman Avenue and Reed Street, Zip 26241, Mailing Address: P.O. Box 1484, Zip 26241–1484; tel. 304/636–3300 **A**1 9 10 20 **F**11 13 15 18 25 26 27 30 31 32 33 38 43 49 51 53 54 55 56 57 61 62 66 67 68 69 72 73 74 75 76 77 79 80 81 82 84 86 96 97 98 100 102 104 105 106 107 109 111 118 119 124 135 136 137 **P**8
Primary Contact: Mark Doak, President and Chief Executive Officer
COO: D. Parker Haddix, Chief Operating Officer
CFO: Rebecca Hammer, Chief Financial Officer
CMO: John Henderson, M.D., Chief Medical Officer
CIO: Steve Crowl, Acting Chief Information Officer
CHR: Judith L. Williams, Director Human Resources
Web address: www.davishealthcare.com
Control: Other not–for–profit (including NFP Corporation) **Service:** General Medical and Surgical

Staffed Beds: 90 **Admissions:** 5421 **Census:** 55 **Outpatient Visits:** 147802 **Births:** 449 **Total Expense ($000):** 74636 **Payroll Expense ($000):** 30400 **Personnel:** 678

FAIRMONT—Marion County

☒ **FAIRMONT GENERAL HOSPITAL (510047)**, 1325 Locust Avenue, Zip 26554–1435; tel. 304/367–7100 **A**1 2 9 10 19 20 **F**3 4 5 11 13 15 17 18 24 25 26 27 30 31 32 33 36 38 40 41 43 44 48 49 50 51 55 56 57 61 62 63 66 67 72 73 74 75 76 77 79 80 81 82 84 86 88 89 90 91 92 93 94 96 97 100 102 103 105 106 107 119 120 121 123 124 132 135 136 137 **P**7
Primary Contact: Albert Pilkington, III, Chief Executive Officer
CFO: Mike Sengewalt, Senior Vice President and Chief Financial Officer
CMO: Joedy Daristotle, M.D., Chief of Staff
CHR: George Perich, Vice President Human Resources and Legal Services
Web address: www.fghi.com
Control: Other not–for–profit (including NFP Corporation) **Service:** General Medical and Surgical

Staffed Beds: 161 **Admissions:** 6147 **Census:** 89 **Outpatient Visits:** 188701 **Births:** 347 **Total Expense ($000):** 73157 **Payroll Expense ($000):** 24581 **Personnel:** 626

GASSAWAY—Braxton County

★ **BRAXTON COUNTY MEMORIAL HOSPITAL (511308)**, 100 Hoylman Drive, Zip 26624–9320; tel. 304/364–5156 **A**9 10 18 **F**3 8 11 15 26 28 30 31 32 33 38 40 55 56 57 61 62 73 79 87 96 97 102 119 122 135 136 **P**6
Primary Contact: Ben Vincent, FACHE, Administrator
CFO: Kimber Knight, Chief Financial Officer
CMO: Russell L. Stewart, M.D., D.O., Chief Medical Officer
Web address: www.braxtonmemorial.org
Control: Other not–for–profit (including NFP Corporation) **Service:** General Medical and Surgical

Staffed Beds: 25 **Admissions:** 526 **Census:** 6 **Outpatient Visits:** 31655 **Births:** 0 **Total Expense ($000):** 13719 **Payroll Expense ($000):** 5764 **Personnel:** 141

GLEN DALE—Marshall County

☒ **REYNOLDS MEMORIAL HOSPITAL (510013)**, 800 Wheeling Avenue, Zip 26038–1697; tel. 304/845–3211, (Total facility includes 20 beds in nursing home–type unit) **A**1 9 10 **F**3 11 13 15 18 24 26 30 31 32 37 38 40 44 52 54 55 56 57 61 62 63 68 72 73 74 75 76 77 78 79 80 81 84 86 96 97 100 102 106 107 117 119 121 124 135 137 **P**8
Primary Contact: John Sicurella, Chief Executive Officer
COO: Jay E. Prager, Chief Operating Officer
CFO: William Robert Hunt, Chief Financial Officer
CMO: Robert B. Wade, M.D., President Medical Staff
CIO: Warren Kelley, Chief Information Officer
Web address: www.reynoldsmemorial.com
Control: Other not–for–profit (including NFP Corporation) **Service:** General Medical and Surgical

Staffed Beds: 127 **Admissions:** 2916 **Census:** 50 **Outpatient Visits:** 72792 **Births:** 188 **Total Expense ($000):** 33470 **Payroll Expense ($000):** 15646 **Personnel:** 374

WV

Hospital, Medicare Provider Number, Address, Telephone, Approval, Facility, and Physician Codes, Health Care System
★ American Hospital Association (AHA) membership
□ The Joint Commission accreditation
○ American Osteopathic Association (AOA) accreditation
△ Commission on Accreditation of Rehabilitation Facilities (CARF) accreditation

GRAFTON—Taylor County

GRAFTON CITY HOSPITAL (511307), 500 Market Street, Zip 26354–1187; tel. 304/265–0400, (Total facility includes 76 beds in nursing home–type unit) **A**9 10 18 **F**11 15 25 26 27 28 30 31 32 33 37 38 40 44 45 52 53 54 55 56 57 60 62 63 65 73 75 76 77 79 81 82 86 87 90 91 92 93 94 95 96 97 100 107 117 119 120 121 122 123 124 132 133 135 136 137 **P**6
Primary Contact: Jeffrey Lilley, Administrator
COO: Patrick Shaw, Chief Operating Officer
CFO: Brian Kelbaugh, Chief Financial Officer
CMO: Christopher Villaraza, M.D., Chief Medical Staff
CIO: Anna Lee White, Health Information Management Officer
CHR: Missey Kimbrew, Director Human Resources
Web address: www.graftonhospital.com
Control: City–Government, nonfederal **Service:** General Medical and Surgical

Staffed Beds: 101 **Admissions:** 1008 **Census:** 83 **Outpatient Visits:** 39678 **Births:** 0 **Total Expense ($000):** 15061 **Payroll Expense ($000):** 8402 **Personnel:** 291

GRANTSVILLE—Calhoun County

★ **MINNIE HAMILTON HEALTHCARE CENTER (511303)**, 186 Hospital Drive, Zip 26147; tel. 304/354–9244, (Total facility includes 24 beds in nursing home–type unit) **A**9 10 18 **F**3 7 11 15 25 26 28 30 31 32 33 34 37 38 41 43 50 52 54 55 56 57 60 62 63 64 66 73 81 82 86 87 89 91 96 97 107 118 119 121 122 123 124 132 135 136 137 **P**6
Primary Contact: Barbara Lay, Chief Executive Officer
CFO: Edward Lawaty, Compliance Officer
CMO: Vishwanath Hande, M.D., Chief Medical Officer
CIO: Steve Whited, Chief Operating Officer
CHR: Sheila Gherke, Director Human Resources
Web address: www.mhhcc.com
Control: Other not–for–profit (including NFP Corporation) **Service:** General Medical and Surgical

Staffed Beds: 42 **Admissions:** 338 **Census:** 29 **Outpatient Visits:** 61358 **Births:** 0 **Total Expense ($000):** 12866 **Payroll Expense ($000):** 7918 **Personnel:** 220

HINTON—Summers County

□ **SUMMERS COUNTY APPALACHIAN REGIONAL HOSPITAL (511310)**, Terrace Street, Zip 25951–2407, Mailing Address: Drawer 940, Zip 25951–0940; tel. 304/466–1000, (Total facility includes 36 beds in nursing home–type unit) **A**1 9 10 18 **F**11 15 25 26 28 30 31 32 33 34 38 40 41 43 50 53 54 55 56 57 61 62 63 65 69 79 81 82 85 86 87 96 107 117 119 122 135 136 137 **P**6 **S** Appalachian Regional Healthcare
Primary Contact: Wesley Dangerfield, Community Chief Executive Officer
CFO: Janett Green, Assistant Administrator
CMO: Stanley Day, M.D., President Medical Staff
CIO: Jeff Brady, Chief Information Officer
CHR: Nancy Whitlock, Manager Human Resources
Web address: www.arh.org
Control: Other not–for–profit (including NFP Corporation) **Service:** General Medical and Surgical

Staffed Beds: 61 **Admissions:** 665 **Census:** 41 **Outpatient Visits:** 24535 **Births:** 0 **Total Expense ($000):** 12901 **Payroll Expense ($000):** 5151 **Personnel:** 141

HUNTINGTON—Cabell County

★ **CABELL HUNTINGTON HOSPITAL (510055)**, 1340 Hal Greer Boulevard, Zip 25701–0195; tel. 304/526–2000, (Total facility includes 15 beds in nursing home–type unit) **A**1 2 3 5 9 10 12 13 **F**3 7 11 12 13 15 16 17 18 24 25 26 27 30 31 32 33 34 35 36 37 38 40 41 42 43 44 46 47 48 49 50 51 53 54 55 56 57 59 60 61 62 64 66 68 69 70 71 72 73 74 75 76 77 79 80 81 82 83 84 86 87 96 97 98 99 100 102 103 104 105 106 107 108 109 111 113 114 116 117 118 119 120 121 124 133 134 135 136 137 **P**8
Primary Contact: Brent A. Marsteller, President and Chief Executive Officer
COO: T. Douglas Lawson, Senior Vice President and Chief Operating Officer
CFO: David M. Ward, Senior Vice President and Chief Financial Officer
CMO: Hoyt J. Burdick, M.D., Vice President Medical Affairs
CIO: Sanjay Shah, Vice President and Chief Information Officer
CHR: Barry Tourigny, Director Human Resources
Web address: www.cabellhuntington.org
Control: Other not–for–profit (including NFP Corporation) **Service:** General Medical and Surgical

Staffed Beds: 276 **Admissions:** 22067 **Census:** 200 **Outpatient Visits:** 380348 **Births:** 2627 **Total Expense ($000):** 259734 **Payroll Expense ($000):** 99786 **Personnel:** 1945

□ **CORNERSTONE HOSPITAL OF HUNTINGTON (512003)**, 2900 First Avenue, Two East, Zip 25702; tel. 304/399–2600 **A**1 9 10 **F**1 3 25 137 **P**8 **S** Cornerstone Healthcare Group
Primary Contact: Tony Aluise, Chief Executive Officer
CFO: Brandi Lusher, Chief Financial Officer
CMO: William Beam, M.D., Chief of Staff
Web address: www.cornerstonehealthcaregroup.com
Control: Corporation, Investor–owned, for–profit **Service:** General Medical and Surgical

Staffed Beds: 28 **Admissions:** 291 **Census:** 21 **Outpatient Visits:** 0 **Births:** 0 **Total Expense ($000):** 9406 **Payroll Expense ($000):** 3009 **Personnel:** 54

★ **HEALTHSOUTH HUNTINGTON REHABILITATION HOSPITAL (513028)**, 6900 West Country Club Drive, Zip 25705–2000; tel. 304/733–1060 **A**1 10 **F**25 33 57 85 86 135 **S** HEALTHSOUTH Corporation
Primary Contact: Michael E. Zuliani, Chief Executive Officer
Web address: www.healthsouthhuntington.com
Control: Corporation, Investor–owned, for–profit **Service:** Rehabilitation

Staffed Beds: 52 **Admissions:** 990 **Census:** 40 **Outpatient Visits:** 6591 **Births:** 0 **Total Expense ($000):** 9620 **Payroll Expense ($000):** 4933 **Personnel:** 139

□ **MILDRED MITCHELL–BATEMAN HOSPITAL (514009)**, 1530 Norway Avenue, Zip 25705–1358, Mailing Address: P.O. Box 448, Zip 25709–0448; tel. 304/525–7801 **A**1 9 10 **F**11 26 75 88 89 95 119 135
Primary Contact: Mary Beth Carlisle, Chief Executive Officer
CFO: James Spencer, Chief Financial Officer
CMO: Shahid Masood, M.D., Clinical Director
CIO: Elias Majdalani, Director Management Information Systems
CHR: Kieth Anne Worden, Director Human Resources
Web address: www.batemanhospital.org
Control: State–Government, nonfederal **Service:** Psychiatric

Staffed Beds: 90 **Admissions:** 650 **Census:** 90 **Outpatient Visits:** 0 **Births:** 0 **Total Expense ($000):** 26109 **Payroll Expense ($000):** 12768 **Personnel:** 325

□ **RIVER PARK HOSPITAL (514008)**, 1230 Sixth Avenue, Zip 25701–2312, Mailing Address: P.O. Box 1875, Zip 25719–1875; tel. 304/526–9111 **A**1 9 10 **F**25 31 33 36 38 40 56 88 89 90 91 92 93 119 132 **S** Horizon Health Corporation
Primary Contact: Patrick D. Burrows, CPA, Chief Executive Officer
CFO: Drew Hefner, Chief Financial Officer
CMO: David J. Humphreys, M.D., Medical Director
CIO: Ian Wiley, Network Administrator
CHR: Mary Stratton, Director Human Resources
Web address: www.riverparkhospital.net/home.htm
Control: Corporation, Investor–owned, for–profit **Service:** Psychiatric

Staffed Beds: 147 **Admissions:** 1477 **Census:** 106 **Outpatient Visits:** 0 **Births:** 0 **Total Expense ($000):** 16960 **Payroll Expense ($000):** 9075 **Personnel:** 272

★ **ST. MARY'S MEDICAL CENTER (510007)**, 2900 First Avenue, Zip 25702–1272; tel. 304/526–1234, (Total facility includes 19 beds in nursing home–type unit) **A**1 2 3 5 9 10 **F**3 11 12 13 15 17 18 20 22 24 25 26 27 28 30 31 32 33 34 38 40 43 44 46 47 49 50 52 55 56 57 59 61 62 64 66 68 71 72 73 74 75 76 77 79 80 81 82 84 86 88 90 91 92 93 96 97 99 100 102 103 106 107 108 109 111 112 116 117 118 119 121 122 124 134 135 136 137 **P**8
Primary Contact: Michael G. Sellards, President and Chief Executive Officer
CFO: Todd Campbell, Vice President Financial Affairs and Chief Financial Officer
CMO: Tyson Smith, M.D., Vice President Medical Affairs
CIO: James Jordan, Director Information Systems
CHR: Susan Beth McKenzie, Vice President Human Resources
Web address: www.st-marys.org
Control: Church–operated, Nongovernment, not–for profit **Service:** General Medical and Surgical

Staffed Beds: 355 **Admissions:** 16623 **Census:** 257 **Outpatient Visits:** 221968 **Births:** 462 **Total Expense ($000):** 257660 **Payroll Expense ($000):** 92106 **Personnel:** 1968

★ **VETERANS AFFAIRS MEDICAL CENTER**, 1540 Spring Valley Drive, Zip 25704–9300; tel. 304/429–6741, (Nonreporting) **A**1 3 5 9 **S** Department of Veterans Affairs
Primary Contact: Edward H. Seiler, Director
CMO: Joseph Pellecchia, M.D., Chief of Staff
CIO: Gary Henderson, Chief Information Resources Management Services
Web address: www.va.gov/sta/guide/home.asp
Control: Veterans Affairs, Government, federal **Service:** General Medical and Surgical

Staffed Beds: 80

Many Facility Codes have changed. Please refer to the AHA Guide Code Chart.

HURRICANE—Putnam County

★ **TEAYS VALLEY HOSPITAL (510085)**, 1400 Hospital Drive, Zip 25526–9210; tel. 304/757–1700 **A**1 9 10 **F**3 11 12 15 24 25 30 31 32 33 37 38 43 44 46 47 50 54 55 56 57 62 63 68 72 73 75 77 79 80 82 86 87 90 92 96 97 100 103 106 107 112 119 120 121 124 134 135 137 **S** Charleston Area Medical Center Health System, Inc.
Primary Contact: Albert H. Michaels, Chief Executive Officer
COO: Randall H. Hodges, Vice President
CFO: Larry C. Hudson, Executive Vice President and Chief Financial Officer
CMO: Tom Horsman, M.D., Administrator Medical Staff
CIO: Lynn Brookshire, Vice President Information Services and Chief Information Officer
CHR: Scott Lannan, Chief Human Resources Officer
Web address: www.camc.org
Control: Other not–for–profit (including NFP Corporation) **Service:** General Medical and Surgical

Staffed Beds: 53 **Admissions:** 2703 **Census:** 37 **Outpatient Visits:** 65038 **Births:** 0 **Total Expense ($000):** 40728 **Payroll Expense ($000):** 13384 **Personnel:** 300

KEYSER—Mineral County

☐ **POTOMAC VALLEY HOSPITAL (511315)**, 167 South Mineral Street, Zip 26726–2699; tel. 304/788–3141 **A**1 9 10 18 **F**3 15 24 25 26 38 42 53 55 56 57 62 68 79 80 82 86 96 97 102 107 119 122 124 135 **S** Mid Atlantic Health Management, Inc.
Primary Contact: Michael Makosky, Administrator
CFO: Marian Cardwell, Chief Financial Officer
Web address: www.potomacvalleyhospital.com
Control: Corporation, Investor–owned, for–profit **Service:** General Medical and Surgical

Staffed Beds: 25 **Admissions:** 1032 **Census:** 9 **Outpatient Visits:** 41451 **Births:** 0 **Total Expense ($000):** 14321 **Payroll Expense ($000):** 5887 **Personnel:** 205

KINGWOOD—Preston County

★ **PRESTON MEMORIAL HOSPITAL (511312)**, 300 South Price Street, Zip 26537–1495; tel. 304/329–1400 **A**9 10 18 **F**3 11 13 15 25 26 33 38 40 44 52 55 57 61 62 72 73 74 75 79 86 96 97 100 102 106 107 118 119 121 122 124 135 **P**5
Primary Contact: Michael S. Thompson, Chief Executive Officer
CFO: Melissa Lockwood, Chief Financial Officer
CIO: Beth Horne, System Administrator Information Technology
CHR: Michele Weimer, Director Human Resources
Web address: www.prestonmemorial.org
Control: Other not–for–profit (including NFP Corporation) **Service:** General Medical and Surgical

Staffed Beds: 25 **Admissions:** 857 **Census:** 8 **Outpatient Visits:** 55590 **Births:** 133 **Total Expense ($000):** 13559 **Payroll Expense ($000):** 7202 **Personnel:** 213

LOGAN—Logan County

★ **LOGAN REGIONAL MEDICAL CENTER (510048)**, 20 Hospital Drive, Zip 25601–3473; tel. 304/831–1101 **A**1 9 10 20 **F**3 11 13 15 24 25 27 30 31 32 33 38 40 49 53 55 56 57 62 68 72 73 74 75 76 77 79 81 82 84 85 86 87 96 97 100 102 103 107 118 119 122 124 135 136 **P**6 **S** LifePoint Hospitals, Inc.
Primary Contact: Kevin N. Fowler, Chief Executive Officer
CFO: Donald E. McDaniel, Chief Financial Officer
Web address: www.loganregionalmedicalcenter.com
Control: Corporation, Investor–owned, for–profit **Service:** General Medical and Surgical

Staffed Beds: 129 **Admissions:** 6676 **Census:** 86 **Outpatient Visits:** 100246 **Births:** 391 **Total Expense ($000):** 69876 **Payroll Expense ($000):** 21723 **Personnel:** 615

MADISON—Boone County

★ **BOONE MEMORIAL HOSPITAL (511313)**, 701 Madison Avenue, Zip 25130–1699; tel. 304/369–1230 **A**1 9 10 18 **F**11 15 24 30 31 32 38 40 55 56 79 96 97 107 119 120 122 136
Primary Contact: Tommy H. Mullins, Administrator
CFO: Randy Foxx, Chief Financial Officer
CMO: John Cook, Chief of Staff
CIO: Susan Shreve, Executive Director Information Technology
Web address: www.bmh.org
Control: County–Government, nonfederal **Service:** General Medical and Surgical

Staffed Beds: 25 **Admissions:** 1014 **Census:** 10 **Outpatient Visits:** 50070 **Births:** 0 **Total Expense ($000):** 10263 **Payroll Expense ($000):** 5246 **Personnel:** 172

MARTINSBURG—Berkeley County

★ **CITY HOSPITAL (510008)**, Dry Run Road, Zip 25401, Mailing Address: P.O. Box 1418, Zip 25402–1418; tel. 304/264–1000, (Total facility includes 19 beds in nursing home–type unit) **A**1 2 3 5 9 10 **F**3 11 13 15 18 24 25 26 27 30 31 32 33 36 38 40 46 49 51 52 55 57 58 62 68 72 73 74 75 76 77 79 80 81 82 84 86 88 90 92 94 96 99 100 102 103 106 107 117 118 119 120 121 124 134 135 136 137 **P**8 **S** West Virginia United Health System
Primary Contact: Anthony Zelenka, Administrator
CFO: Gary W. Broadwater, Chief Financial Officer
Web address: www.cityhospital.org
Control: Other not–for–profit (including NFP Corporation) **Service:** General Medical and Surgical

Staffed Beds: 159 **Admissions:** 7178 **Census:** 97 **Outpatient Visits:** 176015 **Births:** 1011 **Total Expense ($000):** 97688 **Payroll Expense ($000):** 41174 **Personnel:** 931

★ △ **VETERANS AFFAIRS MEDICAL CENTER**, 510 Butler Avenue, Zip 25401–0205; tel. 304/263–0811, (Nonreporting) **A**1 3 5 7 9 **S** Department of Veterans Affairs
Primary Contact: Pedro Garcia, Director
CFO: Jody Slonaker, Chief Fiscal Section
CIO: Debe Gantt, Chief Information Resource Management
CHR: Steve Childs, Chief Business Programs and Operations
Web address: www.va.gov/sta/guide/home.asp
Control: Veterans Affairs, Government, federal **Service:** General Medical and Surgical

Staffed Beds: 559

MONTGOMERY—Fayette County

★ **MONTGOMERY GENERAL HOSPITAL (511318)**, 401 Sixth Avenue, Zip 25136–0270, Mailing Address: P.O. Box 270, Zip 25136–0270; tel. 304/442–5151, (Total facility includes 44 beds in nursing home–type unit) **A**1 9 10 18 **F**11 15 25 26 31 32 33 38 49 52 55 62 65 68 75 79 82 86 87 96 100 107 117 118 119 120 124 135 137 **P**6 8
Primary Contact: Vickie Gay, Chief Executive Officer
CFO: Sherri Murray, Chief Financial Officer
CMO: Traci Acklin, M.D., Chief of Staff
CIO: Kevin Sexton, Information Systems Director
CHR: LeeAnn Snyder, Vice President Human Resources
Web address: www.mghwv.net
Control: Other not–for–profit (including NFP Corporation) **Service:** General Medical and Surgical

Staffed Beds: 69 **Admissions:** 1259 **Census:** 40 **Outpatient Visits:** 64507 **Births:** 0 **Total Expense ($000):** 19684 **Payroll Expense ($000):** 8821 **Personnel:** 202

MORGANTOWN—Monongalia County

CHESTNUT RIDGE HOSPITAL See West Virginia University Hospitals

★ **HEALTHSOUTH MOUNTAINVIEW REGIONAL REHABILITATION HOSPITAL (513030)**, 1160 Van Voorhis Road, Zip 26505–3437; tel. 304/598–1100 **A**1 5 10 **F**3 9 12 24 25 26 30 31 32 43 53 54 55 57 62 72 73 75 76 77 81 82 85 86 90 119 120 121 135 137 **S** HEALTHSOUTH Corporation
Primary Contact: John C. Forester, Chief Executive Officer
CFO: Jason Gizzi, Controller
CMO: Russell Biundo, M.D., Medical Director
CIO: Rita D' Aurora, R.N., Risk Manager and Quality Assurance – Health Information Management Director
CHR: Trish Plevich, Human Resource Director
Web address: www.healthsouth.com
Control: Corporation, Investor–owned, for–profit **Service:** Rehabilitation

Staffed Beds: 96 **Admissions:** 1496 **Census:** 75 **Outpatient Visits:** 14718 **Births:** 0 **Total Expense ($000):** 22711 **Payroll Expense ($000):** 10962 **Personnel:** 261

★ **MONONGALIA GENERAL HOSPITAL (510024)**, 1200 J. D. Anderson Drive, Zip 26505–3486; tel. 304/598–1200 **A**1 9 10 19 **F**3 13 15 17 18 20 22 24 25 26 27 28 30 31 32 33 34 38 42 43 44 50 51 52 53 55 56 57 62 63 68 72 73 74 75 76 77 79 80 81 82 84 96 97 100 102 103 106 107 118 119 121 124 133 134 135 136 137 **P**6 8
Primary Contact: David J. Robertson, Chief Executive Officer
CFO: Nicholas Grubbs, Chief Financial Officer
Web address: www.monhealthsys.org
Control: Other not–for–profit (including NFP Corporation) **Service:** General Medical and Surgical

Staffed Beds: 175 **Admissions:** 9230 **Census:** 106 **Outpatient Visits:** 136099 **Births:** 695 **Total Expense ($000):** 148865 **Payroll Expense ($000):** 53002 **Personnel:** 1092

WV

Hospital, Medicare Provider Number, Address, Telephone, Approval, Facility, and Physician Codes, Health Care System

★ American Hospital Association (AHA) membership
☐ The Joint Commission accreditation
○ American Osteopathic Association (AOA) accreditation
△ Commission on Accreditation of Rehabilitation Facilities (CARF) accreditation

★ **WEST VIRGINIA UNIVERSITY HOSPITALS (510001)**, Medical Center Drive, Zip 26506–4749; tel. 304/598–4000, (Includes CHESTNUT RIDGE HOSPITAL, 930 Chestnut Ridge Road, Zip 26505–2854; tel. 304/293–4000), (Total facility includes 20 beds in nursing home–type unit) **A**1 2 3 5 8 9 10 12 13 19 **F**3 4 5 11 12 13 15 17 18 19 20 21 22 23 24 25 26 27 30 31 32 33 34 36 37 38 40 43 44 49 50 51 55 57 59 60 62 66 68 70 72 73 74 75 76 77 78 79 80 81 82 83 84 88 89 90 91 92 93 95 96 97 102 103 106 107 109 111 112 116 117 118 119 121 125 134 135 136 **P**6 **S** West Virginia United Health System
Primary Contact: Bruce McClymonds, President and Chief Executive Officer
CFO: David Salsberry, Vice President and Chief Financial Officer
CMO: Niti Armistead, M.D., Vice President Medical Staff Affairs
CIO: Michael Balassone, Vice President Information Technology
CHR: Charlotte Bennett, Vice President Human Resources
Web address: www.health.wvu.edu
Control: Other not–for–profit (including NFP Corporation) **Service:** General Medical and Surgical

Staffed Beds: 486 **Admissions:** 22797 **Census:** 385 **Outpatient Visits:** 520570 **Births:** 1382 **Total Expense ($000):** 466002 **Payroll Expense ($000):** 165332 **Personnel:** 3931

NEW MARTINSVILLE—Wetzel County

★ **WETZEL COUNTY HOSPITAL (510072)**, 3 East Benjamin Drive, Zip 26155–2758; tel. 304/455–8000, (Total facility includes 10 beds in nursing home–type unit) **A**1 9 10 **F**3 15 24 27 30 31 32 38 40 50 55 56 57 62 63 68 73 75 77 79 80 86 96 97 102 107 117 119 121 122 135 137 **P**6
Primary Contact: George G. Couch, Chief Executive Officer
CFO: David K. McCartney, CPA, Chief Financial Officer
CIO: Amy Fraizer, Supervisor Management Information Systems
CHR: Sarah Boley, Director Human Resources
Web address: www.wetzelcountyhospital.com
Control: County–Government, nonfederal **Service:** General Medical and Surgical

Staffed Beds: 51 **Admissions:** 1467 **Census:** 18 **Outpatient Visits:** 100056 **Births:** 8 **Total Expense ($000):** 21233 **Payroll Expense ($000):** 9809 **Personnel:** 242

OAK HILL—Fayette County

★ **PLATEAU MEDICAL CENTER (511317)**, 430 Main Street, Zip 25901–3455; tel. 304/469–8600 **A**1 9 10 18 **F**3 15 25 26 31 38 46 62 66 68 73 75 79 80 82 84 86 87 96 102 107 135 **S** Community Health Systems, Inc.
Primary Contact: David V. Bunch, Chief Executive Officer
CFO: Heather Carr, Chief Financial Officer
CMO: Scott Keffer, M.D., Chief of Staff
CIO: Steve Bowen, Director Information Systems
CHR: Tammie Miller, Director Marketing and Public Relations
Web address: www.plateaumedicalcenter.com
Control: Corporation, Investor–owned, for–profit **Service:** General Medical and Surgical

Staffed Beds: 25 **Admissions:** 1584 **Census:** 16 **Outpatient Visits:** 26787 **Births:** 0 **Total Expense ($000):** 19429 **Payroll Expense ($000):** 7496 **Personnel:** 171

PARKERSBURG—Wood County

★ **CAMDEN–CLARK MEMORIAL HOSPITAL (510058)**, 800 Garfield Avenue, Zip 26101–5378, Mailing Address: P.O. Box 718, Zip 26102–0718; tel. 304/424–2111, (Total facility includes 25 beds in nursing home–type unit) **A**1 2 9 10 **F**3 7 11 13 15 17 18 24 25 26 27 28 30 31 32 33 35 38 40 42 43 44 46 48 49 51 52 55 56 57 59 61 62 63 66 68 72 73 74 75 76 77 79 80 81 82 84 86 88 91 92 93 96 97 100 104 105 106 107 108 109 112 114 117 119 120 121 124 135 136 137 **P**6
Primary Contact: Michael A. King, President and Chief Executive Officer
COO: Michael A. King, President and Chief Executive Officer
CFO: Allen R. Butcher, Vice President Finance
CMO: Jennifer Leavitt, D.O., President Medical Staff
CIO: Josh Woods, Director Information Systems
CHR: Tom Heller, Vice President Human Resources
Web address: www.ccmh.org
Control: Other not–for–profit (including NFP Corporation) **Service:** General Medical and Surgical

Staffed Beds: 330 **Admissions:** 10489 **Census:** 134 **Outpatient Visits:** 298129 **Births:** 1404 **Total Expense ($000):** 137300 **Payroll Expense ($000):** 53369 **Personnel:** 1242

★ **HEALTHSOUTH WESTERN HILLS REHABILITATION CENTER (513027)**, 3 Western Hills Drive, Zip 26101–8122; tel. 304/420–1300 **A**1 10 **F**25 30 31 32 53 62 73 77 85 86 119 120 121 135 136 137 **S** HEALTHSOUTH Corporation
Primary Contact: Dean Hatcher, Chief Executive Officer
CFO: Sam Minehart, Assistant Controller
CMO: Kalapala Rao, M.D., Medical Director
CHR: Candace Ross, Human Resource Coordinator
Web address: www.healthsouth.com
Control: Corporation, Investor–owned, for–profit **Service:** Rehabilitation

Staffed Beds: 40 **Admissions:** 1022 **Census:** 37 **Outpatient Visits:** 18924 **Births:** 0 **Total Expense ($000):** 9417 **Payroll Expense ($000):** 5457 **Personnel:** 139

★ **ST. JOSEPH'S HOSPITAL (510033)**, 1824 Murdoch Avenue, Zip 26101–3246, Mailing Address: P.O. Box 327, Zip 26102–0327; tel. 304/424–4111 **A**1 9 10 **F**3 13 15 17 18 20 22 24 25 26 27 28 30 31 32 33 38 40 43 44 50 51 55 56 57 62 66 68 72 73 74 76 77 79 80 81 82 84 92 96 97 100 102 106 107 114 118 119 121 123 135 136 **P**6 **S** Signature Hospital Corporation
Primary Contact: Alan N. King, FACHE, Chief Executive Officer
CFO: Donna Sands, Chief Financial Officer
CIO: Brandon Holbert, Director Information Systems
CHR: Joseph Johnston, Director Human Resources
Web address: www.stjosephs–hospital.com
Control: Partnership, Investor–owned, for–profit **Service:** General Medical and Surgical

Staffed Beds: 194 **Admissions:** 6440 **Census:** 82 **Outpatient Visits:** 70049 **Births:** 327 **Total Expense ($000):** 96001 **Payroll Expense ($000):** 30140 **Personnel:** 714

PETERSBURG—Grant County

★ **GRANT MEMORIAL HOSPITAL (510026)**, Route 55 West, Zip 26847, Mailing Address: P.O. Box 1019, Zip 26847–1019; tel. 304/257–1026, (Total facility includes 10 beds in nursing home–type unit) **A**9 10 20 **F**3 7 11 13 15 24 25 26 28 31 32 33 34 38 40 41 42 43 44 50 52 55 56 57 61 62 63 66 68 73 74 75 77 79 80 81 82 84 86 96 97 102 106 107 117 119 121 122 136 **P**6
Primary Contact: Robert L. Harman, Chief Executive Officer
COO: Mary Beth Barr, R.N., Chief Operating Officer
CFO: Sandy Michaels, Chief Financial Officer
CMO: Bruce Leslie, M.D., Chief of Staff
CIO: Jenny McKinney, Director Information Systems
CHR: Roanie Arbaugh, Director Human Resources
Web address: www.grantmemorial.com
Control: County–Government, nonfederal **Service:** General Medical and Surgical

Staffed Beds: 57 **Admissions:** 1989 **Census:** 25 **Outpatient Visits:** 91804 **Births:** 304 **Total Expense ($000):** 23889 **Payroll Expense ($000):** 10949 **Personnel:** 325

PHILIPPI—Barbour County

★ **BROADDUS HOSPITAL (511300)**, 1 Healthcare Drive, Zip 26416–1051, Mailing Address: P.O. Box 930, Zip 26416–1051; tel. 304/457–1760, (Total facility includes 60 beds in nursing home–type unit) **A**9 10 18 **F**15 25 26 28 30 31 32 33 38 55 56 57 62 63 73 75 80 86 87 96 107 117 119 122 124 135 137
Primary Contact: Jeffrey A. Powelson, Chief Executive Officer
CFO: Cathy Kalar, Chief Financial Officer
CHR: Penny Brown, Human Resources Representative
Web address: www.davishealthsystem.org/
Control: Other not–for–profit (including NFP Corporation) **Service:** General Medical and Surgical

Staffed Beds: 72 **Admissions:** 387 **Census:** 60 **Outpatient Visits:** 24092 **Births:** 0 **Total Expense ($000):** 11309 **Payroll Expense ($000):** 4170 **Personnel:** 145

POINT PLEASANT—Mason County

★ **PLEASANT VALLEY HOSPITAL (510012)**, 2520 Valley Drive, Zip 25550–2083; tel. 304/675–4340, (Total facility includes 100 beds in nursing home–type unit) **A**1 9 10 **F**2 3 11 13 15 17 24 25 26 27 30 31 32 33 34 37 38 40 41 42 44 50 52 54 55 56 57 61 62 65 66 68 72 73 74 75 76 77 79 80 81 82 84 85 86 87 96 97 100 102 103 106 107 113 117 118 119 120 121 132 134 135 136 137 **P**7 8
Primary Contact: Alvin R. Lawson, J.D., FACHE, President and Chief Executive Officer
COO: Sandy Wood, Vice President Patient Services
CFO: Thomas Schauer, Chief Financial Officer
CMO: Shrikart Vaidya, M.D., President Medical Staff
CIO: Paula Brooker, Director Information Services
CHR: Matthew Keefer, Director Human Resources
Web address: www.pvalley.org
Control: Other not–for–profit (including NFP Corporation) **Service:** General Medical and Surgical

Staffed Beds: 201 **Admissions:** 5098 **Census:** 139 **Outpatient Visits:** 196269 **Births:** 207 **Total Expense ($000):** 63601 **Payroll Expense ($000):** 30021 **Personnel:** 720

PRINCETON—Mercer County

★ **HEALTHSOUTH SOUTHERN HILLS REHABILITATION HOSPITAL (513026)**, 120 Twelfth Street, Zip 24740–2312; tel. 304/487–8000 **A**1 10 **F**24 25 30 31 53 54 55 57 59 62 72 73 77 81 82 85 86 119 120 121 132 136 137 **S** HEALTHSOUTH Corporation
Primary Contact: Sharon Boggess, Chief Executive Officer
CFO: Derondah Bradley, Controller
CMO: Carl Shelton, M.D., Medical Director
Web address: www.healthsouth.com
Control: Corporation, Investor–owned, for–profit **Service:** Rehabilitation

Staffed Beds: 60 **Admissions:** 1001 **Census:** 35 **Outpatient Visits:** 8306 **Births:** 0 **Total Expense ($000):** 7901 **Payroll Expense ($000):** 394 **Personnel:** 129

 Many Facility Codes have changed. Please refer to the AHA Guide Code Chart.

★ **PRINCETON COMMUNITY HOSPITAL (510046)**, 122 12th Street, Zip 24740–2352, Mailing Address: P.O. Box 1369, Zip 24740–1369; tel. 304/487–7000 **A**1 2 9 10 12 19 **F**3 11 12 13 15 17 25 26 27 28 30 31 32 33 37 38 40 41 49 50 51 52 55 56 57 58 61 62 68 72 73 74 75 76 77 79 80 81 82 84 86 88 90 91 92 93 96 97 99 100 102 103 105 106 107 118 119 120 121 123 124 130 131 133 135 136 **P**1
Primary Contact: Wayne B. Griffith, FACHE, Chief Executive Officer
CFO: Frank J. Sinicrope, Vice President Financial Services
CIO: Danny Farley, Director Information Services
CHR: D. Darlene Huffman, Director Human Resources
Web address: www.pchonline.org
Control: City–Government, nonfederal **Service:** General Medical and Surgical

Staffed Beds: 188 **Admissions:** 7972 **Census:** 102 **Outpatient Visits:** 168604 **Births:** 556 **Total Expense ($000):** 88325 **Payroll Expense ($000):** 33983 **Personnel:** 937

RANSON—Jefferson County

★ **JEFFERSON MEMORIAL HOSPITAL (511319)**, 300 South Preston Street, Zip 25438–1699; tel. 304/728–1600, (Total facility includes 20 beds in nursing home–type unit) **A**3 5 9 10 18 **F**3 11 13 15 25 26 30 31 32 33 38 40 46 49 51 55 56 57 61 62 68 72 73 74 75 79 80 81 82 86 96 100 102 107 117 118 119 121 124 135 137 **P**8 **S** West Virginia United Health System
Primary Contact: Roger M. Eitelman, Chief Executive Officer
CMO: Jan Kletter, M.D., Medical Staff President
CIO: Todd Smoot, Chief Information Officer
CHR: Becky Nucilli, Director Human Resources
Web address: www.jeffmem.com
Control: Other not–for–profit (including NFP Corporation) **Service:** General Medical and Surgical

Staffed Beds: 45 **Admissions:** 1957 **Census:** 26 **Outpatient Visits:** 61595 **Births:** 317 **Total Expense ($000):** 37450 **Payroll Expense ($000):** 15714 **Personnel:** 319

RIPLEY—Jackson County

☐ **JACKSON GENERAL HOSPITAL (510018)**, Pinnell Street, Zip 25271–1009, Mailing Address: P.O. Box 720, Zip 25271–0720; tel. 304/372–2731 **A**1 9 10 **F**3 11 15 17 24 25 26 30 31 32 33 38 50 55 56 57 62 66 73 79 80 86 96 102 107 121 122 **P**6
Primary Contact: Sandra Elza, Chief Executive Officer
COO: Stephanie McCoy, Chief Operating Officer
CFO: Angela Frame, Chief Financial Officer
CIO: Warren Johnson, System Administrator
CHR: Kimberli Lanham, Director Human Resources
Web address: www.jacksongeneral.com
Control: Other not–for–profit (including NFP Corporation) **Service:** General Medical and Surgical

Staffed Beds: 36 **Admissions:** 1727 **Census:** 19 **Outpatient Visits:** 44975 **Births:** 0 **Total Expense ($000):** 22594 **Payroll Expense ($000):** 10876 **Personnel:** 250

ROMNEY—Hampshire County

☐ **HAMPSHIRE MEMORIAL HOSPITAL (511311)**, 549 Center Avenue, Zip 26757–1199; tel. 304/822–4561, (Total facility includes 30 beds in nursing home–type unit) **A**1 9 10 18 **F**15 30 31 32 38 54 55 57 60 79 86 96 107 117 119 121 122 **P**4 **S** Valley Health System
Primary Contact: Roberta D. McCauley, Chief Executive Officer
CFO: Marian Cardwell, Chief Financial Officer
Control: Corporation, Investor–owned, for–profit **Service:** General Medical and Surgical

Staffed Beds: 44 **Admissions:** 408 **Census:** 32 **Outpatient Visits:** 26866 **Births:** 0 **Total Expense ($000):** 9307 **Payroll Expense ($000):** 3227 **Personnel:** 107

RONCEVERTE—Greenbrier County

★ ○ **GREENBRIER VALLEY MEDICAL CENTER (510002)**, 202 Maplewood Avenue, Zip 24970–0497, Mailing Address: P.O. Box 497, Zip 24970–0497; tel. 304/647–4411 **A**1 9 10 11 12 13 19 20 **F**13 15 18 24 25 31 32 38 49 51 55 66 68 74 79 81 82 84 96 97 100 102 104 107 118 121 122 135 137 **P**2 6 **S** Community Health Systems, Inc.
Primary Contact: Brenda Hamilton, Interim Chief Executive Officer
CFO: Angela Swearingen, Chief Financial Officer
CMO: Craig Bookout, M.D., Chief of Staff
CIO: Joe Sams, Director Information Systems
CHR: Melissa Williams, Director Human Resources
Web address: www.gvmc.com
Control: Corporation, Investor–owned, for–profit **Service:** General Medical and Surgical

Staffed Beds: 112 **Admissions:** 4498 **Census:** 50 **Outpatient Visits:** 56989 **Births:** 561 **Total Expense ($000):** 41117 **Payroll Expense ($000):** 16806 **Personnel:** 406

SISTERSVILLE—Tyler County

★ **SISTERSVILLE GENERAL HOSPITAL (511304)**, 314 South Wells Street, Zip 26175–1098; tel. 304/652–2611 **A**9 10 18 **F**3 7 11 15 24 25 26 28 30 31 32 33 37 38 40 42 43 44 45 50 52 55 57 62 63 77 82 86 87 96 107 118 119 121 122 124 135 **P**6
Primary Contact: Lynn McCormick, Administrator
COO: Mike Hall, Chief Operating Officer
CFO: Stephen Smith, Chief Financial Officer
CMO: Tom Gilligan, M.D., Chief of Staff
CHR: Mary Beth Neff, Director Human Resources
Web address: www.wvha.com/web/sgh
Control: City–Government, nonfederal **Service:** General Medical and Surgical

Staffed Beds: 12 **Admissions:** 207 **Census:** 2 **Outpatient Visits:** 20075 **Births:** 0 **Total Expense ($000):** 7685 **Payroll Expense ($000):** 4350 **Personnel:** 124

SOUTH CHARLESTON—Kanawha County

★ **THOMAS MEMORIAL HOSPITAL (510029)**, 4605 MacCorkle Avenue S.W., Zip 25309–1398; tel. 304/766–3600, (Total facility includes 19 beds in nursing home–type unit) **A**1 3 5 9 10 **F**3 5 8 11 13 15 17 18 25 26 27 28 30 31 32 33 36 38 43 44 45 46 47 48 49 52 53 55 56 57 59 61 62 66 67 68 70 72 73 74 75 76 77 79 80 81 82 84 86 88 89 90 91 92 93 94 95 96 97 99 100 103 106 107 108 109 111 112 117 118 119 120 133 135 137
Primary Contact: Stephen P. Dexter, President and Chief Executive Officer
CFO: Charles O. Covert, Vice President Finance
Web address: www.thomaswv.org
Control: Other not–for–profit (including NFP Corporation) **Service:** General Medical and Surgical

Staffed Beds: 216 **Admissions:** 10889 **Census:** 159 **Outpatient Visits:** 210999 **Births:** 906 **Total Expense ($000):** 136456 **Payroll Expense ($000):** 50904 **Personnel:** 1158

SPENCER—Roane County

★ **ROANE GENERAL HOSPITAL (511306)**, 200 Hospital Drive, Zip 25276–1060; tel. 304/927–4444, (Total facility includes 35 beds in nursing home–type unit) **A**1 9 10 18 **F**3 11 13 15 24 31 32 33 38 40 52 55 56 57 62 74 79 87 96 107 117 119 122 **P**6
Primary Contact: Douglas E. Bentz, Chief Executive Officer
COO: Ann Kendall, R.N., Vice President Clinical Services
CFO: Louise Ward, Vice President Financial and Support Services
CMO: Kenneth Seen, M.D., Chief Medical Staff
CIO: Tonja Prine, Executive Director Information Systems
CHR: Denise Higgs, Director Human Resources
Web address: www.roanegeneralhospital.com
Control: Other not–for–profit (including NFP Corporation) **Service:** General Medical and Surgical

Staffed Beds: 60 **Admissions:** 728 **Census:** 39 **Outpatient Visits:** 56849 **Births:** 123 **Total Expense ($000):** 19163 **Payroll Expense ($000):** 9854 **Personnel:** 227

SUMMERSVILLE—Nicholas County

★ **SUMMERSVILLE MEMORIAL HOSPITAL (510082)**, 400 Fairview Heights Road, Zip 26651–0400; tel. 304/872–2891, (Total facility includes 52 beds in nursing home–type unit) **A**9 10 20 **F**3 11 13 15 24 27 30 32 33 38 40 43 44 45 46 54 55 56 57 62 63 66 68 74 77 79 80 81 82 84 86 87 96 100 102 107 117 118 119 120 121 122 124 135 136 **P**6
Primary Contact: Deborah A. Hill, RN, Chief Executive Officer
CFO: Dora Douglas, Chief Financial Officer
CMO: Robert Fleer, M.D., Chief of Staff
CIO: Mike Ellison, Information Systems Lead
CHR: David Henderson, Director Human Resources
Web address: www.summersvillememorial.org
Control: City–Government, nonfederal **Service:** General Medical and Surgical

Staffed Beds: 105 **Admissions:** 2067 **Census:** 78 **Outpatient Visits:** 118333 **Births:** 300 **Total Expense ($000):** 36995 **Payroll Expense ($000):** 17981 **Personnel:** 545

WV

Hospital, Medicare Provider Number, Address, Telephone, Approval, Facility, and Physician Codes, Health Care System

★ American Hospital Association (AHA) membership
☐ The Joint Commission accreditation
○ American Osteopathic Association (AOA) accreditation
△ Commission on Accreditation of Rehabilitation Facilities (CARF) accreditation

WEBSTER SPRINGS—Webster County

★ **WEBSTER COUNTY MEMORIAL HOSPITAL (511301)**, 324 Miller Mountain Drive, Zip 26288–1087, Mailing Address: P.O. Box 312, Zip 26288–0312; tel. 304/847–5682 **A**9 10 18 **F**7 15 26 31 33 38 55 56 57 64 82 84 86 87 96 102 107 117 119 122 **P**6
Primary Contact: Annette M. Keenan, Chief Executive Officer
CMO: Robert Mace, M.D., Chief of Staff
CIO: Margaret W. Short, Chief Information Officer
Web address: www.wcmhwv.com
Control: County–Government, nonfederal **Service:** General Medical and Surgical

Staffed Beds: 15 **Admissions:** 263 **Census:** 2 **Outpatient Visits:** 37867 **Births:** 1 **Total Expense ($000):** 6009 **Payroll Expense ($000):** 4110 **Personnel:** 96

WEIRTON—Brooke County

▣ **WEIRTON MEDICAL CENTER (510023)**, 601 Colliers Way, Zip 26062–5091; tel. 304/797–6000, (Total facility includes 33 beds in nursing home–type unit) **A**1 9 10 **F**3 5 9 11 13 15 17 18 20 24 25 26 28 30 31 32 33 37 38 40 43 46 47 48 49 50 51 52 53 54 55 56 57 59 60 61 62 66 68 72 73 74 75 77 79 80 81 84 86 87 88 89 90 91 92 93 94 95 96 97 100 102 106 107 117 119 120 121 124 132 134 135 136 137 **P**6
Primary Contact: Joseph Endrich, M.D., President and Chief Executive Officer
CFO: Michael S. Miller, Vice President Finance
CIO: Richard Lucas, Director Information Services
CHR: Jennifer Anderson, Director Human Resources
Web address: www.weirtonmedical.com
Control: Other not–for–profit (including NFP Corporation) **Service:** General Medical and Surgical

Staffed Beds: 238 **Admissions:** 7961 **Census:** 111 **Outpatient Visits:** 209589 **Births:** 365 **Total Expense ($000):** 88010 **Payroll Expense ($000):** 38256 **Personnel:** 891

WELCH—McDowell County

WELCH COMMUNITY HOSPITAL (510086), 454 McDowell Street, Zip 24801–2097; tel. 304/436–8461, (Total facility includes 59 beds in nursing home–type unit) **A**9 10 20 **F**3 13 15 25 31 32 33 38 50 55 57 62 63 64 65 66 68 73 74 79 81 82 87 96 107 119 135 136 **P**6
Primary Contact: Walter J. Garrett, Administrator
CFO: Carla Parent, Chief Financial Officer
Control: State–Government, nonfederal **Service:** General Medical and Surgical

Staffed Beds: 108 **Admissions:** 894 **Census:** 60 **Outpatient Visits:** 35965 **Births:** 85 **Total Expense ($000):** 41702 **Payroll Expense ($000):** 8702 **Personnel:** 318

WESTON—Lewis County

▣ **STONEWALL JACKSON MEMORIAL HOSPITAL (510038)**, 230 Hospital Plaza, Zip 26452–8558; tel. 304/269–8000 **A**1 9 10 20 **F**11 13 15 24 25 26 27 30 31 32 38 40 50 54 55 57 61 62 66 68 73 76 77 79 80 81 86 96 97 100 102 106 107 118 119 120 121 122 124 134 135 136 137 **P**8
Primary Contact: David D. Shaffer, Chief Executive Officer
CFO: Dodie Arbogest, Controller
CIO: Harriett Williams, Director Management Information
CHR: Aimee Green, Director Human Resources
Web address: www.stonewallhospital.com
Control: Other not–for–profit (including NFP Corporation) **Service:** General Medical and Surgical

Staffed Beds: 70 **Admissions:** 3491 **Census:** 39 **Outpatient Visits:** 72826 **Births:** 290 **Total Expense ($000):** 31579 **Payroll Expense ($000):** 14968 **Personnel:** 342

☐ **WILLIAM R. SHARPE, JR. HOSPITAL (514010)**, 936 Sharpe Hospital Road, Zip 26452–8550; tel. 304/269–1210 **A**1 5 9 10 **F**11 26 31 32 54 58 81 82 88 90 91 93 119 121 132 135 **P**6
Primary Contact: Kevin P. Stalnaker, Chief Executive Officer
CFO: Steve Benson, Chief Financial Officer
CMO: Robert Keefover, M.D., Chief Medical Officer
CIO: Terry Small, Chief Compliance Officer
CHR: Debbie Cook, Director Human Resources
Web address: www.wvdhhr.org/sharpe
Control: State–Government, nonfederal **Service:** Psychiatric

Staffed Beds: 150 **Admissions:** 802 **Census:** 150 **Outpatient Visits:** 0 **Births:** 0 **Total Expense ($000):** 32024 **Payroll Expense ($000):** 12702 **Personnel:** 465

WHEELING—Ohio County

☐ **OHIO VALLEY MEDICAL CENTER (510039)**, 2000 Eoff Street, Zip 26003–3870; tel. 304/234–0123 **A**1 2 3 5 9 10 12 13 **F**3 5 9 11 13 15 17 18 24 25 26 27 30 31 32 33 34 36 37 38 40 41 43 44 45 46 47 48 49 50 51 52 54 55 56 57 58 59 60 62 63 66 68 72 73 75 76 77 79 80 81 82 83 84 86 87 88 89 90 91 92 93 94 95 96 100 102 103 104 105 106 107 109 111 114 118 119 120 121 123 124 132 135 136 **P**6 **S** Ohio Valley Health Services and Education Corporation
Primary Contact: Brian K. Felici, President and Chief Executive Officer
CFO: David T. Baranik, Senior Vice President and Chief Financial Officer
CIO: Robert Panichi, Chief Information Officer
Web address: www.ohiovalleymedicalcenter.com
Control: Other not–for–profit (including NFP Corporation) **Service:** General Medical and Surgical

Staffed Beds: 179 **Admissions:** 7257 **Census:** 103 **Outpatient Visits:** 171016 **Births:** 559 **Total Expense ($000):** 85546 **Payroll Expense ($000):** 35262 **Personnel:** 848

★ **PETERSON REHABILITATION HOSPITAL (513025)**, Homestead Avenue, Zip 26003; tel. 304/234–0500, (Total facility includes 150 beds in nursing home–type unit) **A**10 **F**55 56 85 86 117 119 121 132 137
Primary Contact: Patricia B. Speak, Administrator
Control: Corporation, Investor–owned, for–profit **Service:** Rehabilitation

Staffed Beds: 172 **Admissions:** 541 **Census:** 147 **Outpatient Visits:** 1861 **Births:** 0 **Total Expense ($000):** 15219 **Payroll Expense ($000):** 5193 **Personnel:** 154

▣ **WHEELING HOSPITAL (510050)**, 1 Medical Park, Zip 26003–0708; tel. 304/243–3000, (Total facility includes 24 beds in nursing home–type unit) **A**1 2 9 10 12 13 **F**3 11 13 15 17 18 20 22 24 25 26 27 28 31 32 33 34 38 40 41 44 49 50 52 53 55 56 57 58 60 61 62 63 64 68 72 73 74 75 76 77 79 80 81 82 84 86 87 96 97 100 102 106 107 108 109 111 117 118 119 120 121 124 132 135 136 137 **P**5
Primary Contact: Ronald L. Violi, Chief Executive Officer
COO: Scott McKeets, Chief Operating Officer
CFO: Jim Murdy, Chief Financial Officer
CMO: Angelo Georges, M.D., President Medical and Dental Staff
CIO: David Rapp, Chief Information Officer
CHR: Susan Falbo, Vice President Human Resources
Web address: www.wheelinghospital.com
Control: Other not–for–profit (including NFP Corporation) **Service:** General Medical and Surgical

Staffed Beds: 276 **Admissions:** 11648 **Census:** 148 **Outpatient Visits:** 425428 **Births:** 812 **Total Expense ($000):** 178422 **Payroll Expense ($000):** 71993 **Personnel:** 1839

WILLIAMSON—Mingo County

☐ **WILLIAMSON MEMORIAL HOSPITAL (510077)**, 859 Alderson Street, Zip 25661–3215, Mailing Address: P.O. Box 1980, Zip 25661–1980; tel. 304/235–2500 **A**1 9 10 **F**3 13 15 18 24 25 26 31 32 38 50 51 55 56 57 59 60 66 68 73 75 79 82 86 96 97 100 102 107 118 119 120 135 **P**6 7 **S** Health Management Associates
Primary Contact: Todd Hubler, Interim Chief Executive Officer
CFO: Todd Hubler, Controller
CMO: Manuel Angco, M.D., Chief of Staff
CHR: Tina Jackson, Manager Human Resources
Web address: www.hmawmh.com
Control: Corporation, Investor–owned, for–profit **Service:** General Medical and Surgical

Staffed Beds: 76 **Admissions:** 2797 **Census:** 30 **Outpatient Visits:** 37918 **Births:** 119 **Total Expense ($000):** 27128 **Payroll Expense ($000):** 10754 **Personnel:** 316

WISCONSIN

AMERY—Polk County

★ **AMERY REGIONAL MEDICAL CENTER (521308)**, 225 Scholl Court, Zip 54001–1292; tel. 715/268–8000 **A**9 10 18 **F**11 13 15 17 24 30 31 32 34 38 40 43 52 53 56 62 68 73 74 75 76 79 81 82 84 85 86 96 97 107 119 120 133 **P**6 **S** QHR
Primary Contact: Michael Karuschak, Jr., Chief Executive Officer
CFO: Scott D. Edin, Chief Financial Officer
CMO: Craig Johnson, M.D., Chief Medical Officer
CIO: Bill Lehner, Director Management Information Systems
CHR: Joanne Jackson, Administrator Human Resources and Community Relations
Web address: www.amerymedicalcenter.org
Control: Other not–for–profit (including NFP Corporation) **Service:** General Medical and Surgical

Staffed Beds: 25 **Admissions:** 1385 **Census:** 11 **Outpatient Visits:** 83777 **Births:** 177 **Total Expense ($000):** 31529 **Payroll Expense ($000):** 10627 **Personnel:** 279

ANTIGO—Langlade County

□ **LANGLADE MEMORIAL HOSPITAL (521350)**, 112 East Fifth Avenue, Zip 54409–2796; tel. 715/623–2331 **A**1 3 5 9 10 18 **F**2 10 11 13 15 17 24 25 31 38 42 43 52 53 54 56 59 62 67 68 73 74 75 76 78 79 81 82 84 86 96 97 100 104 106 107 119 120 133 136
Primary Contact: David R. Schneider, Executive Director
CFO: Pat Tincher, Director Finance
CMO: Noel Deep, M.D., Chief Medical Staff
CHR: Janelle Markgraf, Vice President Human Resources
Web address: www.langladememorial.org
Control: Church–operated, Nongovernment, not–for profit **Service:** General Medical and Surgical

Staffed Beds: 25 **Admissions:** 1381 **Census:** 13 **Outpatient Visits:** 49004 **Births:** 248 **Total Expense ($000):** 41130 **Payroll Expense ($000):** 17136 **Personnel:** 339

APPLETON—Outagamie County

□ **APPLETON MEDICAL CENTER (520160)**, 1818 North Meade Street, Zip 54911–3496; tel. 920/731–4101 **A**1 3 5 9 10 **F**3 8 9 11 13 15 17 25 26 27 30 31 32 35 39 40 41 43 44 46 47 48 49 52 54 59 62 67 68 72 73 74 75 76 77 78 79 80 81 82 84 86 87 96 98 100 104 105 107 108 109 110 111 112 114 119 120 132 133 135 136 137 **S** ThedaCare, Inc.
Primary Contact: Kathryn Correia, Senior Vice President
COO: Matthew Furlan, Chief Operating Officer
CFO: Tim Olson, Senior Vice President Finance
CIO: Keith Livingston, Senior Vice President and Chief Information Officer
CHR: J. Michael Gautney, Manager Human Resources
Web address: www.thedacare.org
Control: Other not–for–profit (including NFP Corporation) **Service:** General Medical and Surgical

Staffed Beds: 142 **Admissions:** 8222 **Census:** 91 **Outpatient Visits:** 125378 **Births:** 1024 **Total Expense ($000):** 149819 **Payroll Expense ($000):** 55238 **Personnel:** 1060

★□ △ **ST. ELIZABETH HOSPITAL (520009)**, 1506 South Oneida Street, Zip 54915–1397; tel. 920/738–2000 **A**1 2 3 5 7 10 **F**4 5 6 9 11 13 15 17 24 25 30 31 32 34 38 40 43 54 56 62 65 67 68 70 73 74 75 76 78 79 81 82 83 84 86 88 89 90 92 93 94 95 96 97 100 106 107 119 120 133 136 **S** Wheaton Franciscan Healthcare
Primary Contact: Travis Andersen, President
CFO: Jeff Badger, Chief Financial Officer
CMO: Ronald Molony, M.D., Vice President Medical Affairs
CIO: Will Weider, Chief Information Officer
CHR: Vince Gallucci, Senior Vice President Human Resources
Web address: www.affinityhealth.org
Control: Church–operated, Nongovernment, not–for profit **Service:** General Medical and Surgical

Staffed Beds: 197 **Admissions:** 8046 **Census:** 99 **Outpatient Visits:** 74557 **Births:** 1141 **Total Expense ($000):** 112662 **Payroll Expense ($000):** 46246 **Personnel:** 764

ARCADIA—Trempealeau County

FRANCISCAN SKEMP HEALTHCARE–ARCADIA CAMPUS (521306), 464 South St. Joseph Avenue, Zip 54612–1401; tel. 608/323–3341 **A**9 10 18 **F**4 11 13 24 30 31 32 38 43 54 56 62 65 74 75 76 78 79 81 82 84 86 96 119 120 **S** Mayo Foundation
Primary Contact: Darlene Feltes, Administrator
CHR: Del Long, Human Resources Administrator
Web address: www.mayohealthsystem.com
Control: Church–operated, Nongovernment, not–for profit **Service:** General Medical and Surgical

Staffed Beds: 25 **Admissions:** 391 **Census:** 76 **Outpatient Visits:** 23505 **Births:** 52 **Total Expense ($000):** 5054 **Payroll Expense ($000):** 2536 **Personnel:** 45

ASHLAND—Ashland County

★□ **MEMORIAL MEDICAL CENTER – ASHLAND (520173)**, 1615 Maple Lane, Zip 54806–3689; tel. 715/685–5500 **A**1 9 10 **F**3 4 5 11 13 15 17 26 30 31 37 38 40 49 54 55 57 62 66 68 74 75 76 78 79 80 81 84 85 86 88 89 90 91 92 93 94 95 96 100 102 106 107 119 120 121 124 133 137 **P**6
Primary Contact: Daniel J. Hymans, President
COO: Daniel H. Adams, Vice President and Chief Operating Officer
CFO: Les Whiteaker, Vice President and Chief Financial Officer
CMO: Peter Areson, M.D., President Medical Staff
CIO: Todd Reynolds, Chief Information Officer
CHR: Kathy Carlson, Director Human Resources
Web address: www.ashlandmmc.com
Control: Other not–for–profit (including NFP Corporation) **Service:** General Medical and Surgical

Staffed Beds: 100 **Admissions:** 3090 **Census:** 34 **Outpatient Visits:** 27022 **Births:** 294 **Total Expense ($000):** 41410 **Payroll Expense ($000):** 19506 **Personnel:** 388

BALDWIN—St. Croix County

★ **BALDWIN AREA MEDICAL CENTER (521347)**, 730 10th Avenue, Zip 54002, Mailing Address: P.O. Box 300, Zip 54002; tel. 715/684–3311 **A**9 10 18 **F**11 13 15 17 24 25 30 31 32 34 38 40 43 52 56 62 68 73 74 75 76 78 79 81 82 84 85 86 96 97 107 119 120
Primary Contact: Gregory T. Burns, Chief Executive Officer
CFO: Karen Traynor, Chief Financial Officer
CMO: Joel Stoeckeler, M.D., Chief of Staff
CIO: Scott Swedien, Director Information Services
CHR: Trudy Acterhof, Director Human Resources
Web address: www.baldwinhospital.com
Control: Other not–for–profit (including NFP Corporation) **Service:** General Medical and Surgical

Staffed Beds: 25 **Admissions:** 1239 **Census:** 10 **Outpatient Visits:** 40549 **Births:** 83 **Total Expense ($000):** 22745 **Payroll Expense ($000):** 9406 **Personnel:** 185

BARABOO—Sauk County

★□ **ST. CLARE HOSPITAL AND HEALTH SERVICES (520057)**, 707 14th Street, Zip 53913–1597; tel. 608/356–1400 **A**1 3 5 9 10 **F**4 5 11 13 15 24 25 30 31 32 34 36 38 43 52 54 56 59 62 67 68 73 74 75 76 78 79 81 86 88 92 93 94 96 97 106 107 119 120 133 **S** SSM Health Care
Primary Contact: Sandra L. Anderson, President
CFO: Troy Walker, Director Finance
CIO: Alan Steevens, Director Information Management
CHR: Jason Stelzer, Director Human Resources
Web address: www.stclare.com
Control: Church–operated, Nongovernment, not–for profit **Service:** General Medical and Surgical

Staffed Beds: 77 **Admissions:** 2576 **Census:** 28 **Outpatient Visits:** 72750 **Births:** 301 **Total Expense ($000):** 45362 **Payroll Expense ($000):** 20304 **Personnel:** 365

WI

Hospital, Medicare Provider Number, Address, Telephone, Approval, Facility, and Physician Codes, Health Care System

★ American Hospital Association (AHA) membership
□ The Joint Commission accreditation
○ American Osteopathic Association (AOA) accreditation
△ Commission on Accreditation of Rehabilitation Facilities (CARF) accreditation

BARRON—Barron County

☐ **LUTHER MIDELFORT NORTHLAND (521315)**, (Formerly Barron Medical Center), 1222 Woodland Avenue, Zip 54812–1798; tel. 715/537–3186, (Total facility includes 32 beds in nursing home–type unit) (Nonreporting) **A**1 9 10 18 **S** Mayo Foundation
Primary Contact: Maurita Sullivan, Administrator
CFO: Kristy Hanson, Assistant Administrator and Controller
Web address: www.luthermidelfortnorthland.org
Control: Other not–for–profit (including NFP Corporation) **Service:** General Medical and Surgical

Staffed Beds: 57

BEAVER DAM—Dodge County

★ **BEAVER DAM COMMUNITY HOSPITALS (520076)**, 707 South University Avenue, Zip 53916–3089; tel. 920/887–7181, (Total facility includes 123 beds in nursing home–type unit) **A**1 9 10 19 **F**4 6 8 13 15 16 17 27 28 30 31 32 41 42 43 44 50 54 55 56 57 61 62 63 64 65 67 68 70 72 73 75 76 77 78 79 80 81 82 85 86 88 96 102 106 107 117 118 119 120 121 122 124 132 135 136 137
Primary Contact: Kimberly J. Miller, FACHE, President and Chief Executive Officer
CFO: Scott Abrams, Vice President Finance
CIO: Carol Ciancio, Director Health Information Systems
CHR: Tam Cohen, Director Employee Services
Web address: www.bdch.org
Control: Other not–for–profit (including NFP Corporation) **Service:** General Medical and Surgical

Staffed Beds: 210 **Admissions:** 2643 **Census:** 140 **Outpatient Visits:** 70751 **Births:** 439 **Total Expense ($000):** 57090 **Payroll Expense ($000):** 22218 **Personnel:** 585

BELOIT—Rock County

☐ **BELOIT MEMORIAL HOSPITAL (520100)**, 1969 West Hart Road, Zip 53511–2299; tel. 608/364–5011 **A**1 9 10 **F**3 5 6 8 9 11 13 14 15 17 25 27 30 31 32 33 34 40 43 44 47 49 51 52 53 54 55 56 57 59 61 62 63 66 68 72 73 74 75 76 77 78 79 80 81 82 84 85 86 87 89 90 91 92 93 94 96 99 100 102 103 104 105 106 107 109 111 118 119 120 121 124 133 135 136 137 **P**1
Primary Contact: Gregory K. Britton, President and Chief Executive Officer
CFO: David A. Bolen, Vice President Finance
Web address: www.beloitmemorialhospital.org
Control: Other not–for–profit (including NFP Corporation) **Service:** General Medical and Surgical

Staffed Beds: 124 **Admissions:** 5104 **Census:** 61 **Outpatient Visits:** 151128 **Births:** 771 **Total Expense ($000):** 88628 **Payroll Expense ($000):** 38124 **Personnel:** 817

BERLIN—Green Lake County

☐ **BERLIN MEMORIAL HOSPITAL (521355)**, 225 Memorial Drive, Zip 54923–1295; tel. 920/361–1313, (Includes JULIETTE MANOR NURSING HOME, COMMUNITY CLINICS), (Total facility includes 81 beds in nursing home–type unit) **A**1 9 10 18 **F**10 11 13 15 17 24 25 30 31 32 38 40 43 53 54 56 61 62 65 67 68 73 74 75 76 78 79 81 83 84 86 96 97 100 106 107 115 117 119 120 133 136
Primary Contact: Douglas I. Guy, President and Chief Executive Officer
COO: Mary P. Hansen, Vice President Acute Care
CFO: Thomas P. Krystowiak, Vice President Finance
CIO: Greg Beltran, Director Information Technology
Web address: www.communityhealthnetwork.org
Control: Other not–for–profit (including NFP Corporation) **Service:** General Medical and Surgical

Staffed Beds: 106 **Admissions:** 2051 **Census:** 87 **Outpatient Visits:** 65141 **Births:** 245 **Total Expense ($000):** 45825 **Payroll Expense ($000):** 22007 **Personnel:** 283

BLACK RIVER FALLS—Jackson County

☐ **BLACK RIVER MEMORIAL HOSPITAL (521333)**, 711 West Adams Street, Zip 54615–9113; tel. 715/284–5361 **A**1 9 10 18 **F**3 4 8 13 26 30 31 32 33 39 42 44 50 54 55 56 57 61 62 63 66 67 69 73 74 75 77 78 79 80 81 84 85 86 87 96 100 103 104 105 107 118 119 120 121 122 124 132 133 135 137
Primary Contact: Stanley J. Gaynor, Chief Executive Officer
CFO: Robert Daley, Chief Financial Officer
CMO: Howard Spegman, M.D., Chief of Staff
CIO: Robert Daley, Chief Financial Officer
CHR: Holly Fredrickson, Human Resources Director
Web address: www.blackriverhospital.com
Control: Other not–for–profit (including NFP Corporation) **Service:** General Medical and Surgical

Staffed Beds: 25 **Admissions:** 930 **Census:** 8 **Outpatient Visits:** 30075 **Births:** 167 **Total Expense ($000):** 20378 **Payroll Expense ($000):** 9100 **Personnel:** 198

BLOOMER—Chippewa County

☐ **LUTHER MIDELFORT CHIPPEWA VALLEY (521314)**, (Formerly Bloomer Memorial Medical Center), 1501 Thompson Street, Zip 54724–1299; tel. 715/568–2000, (Total facility includes 42 beds in nursing home–type unit) **A**1 9 10 18 **F**1 3 8 15 25 26 31 32 33 40 54 55 56 57 62 63 65 66 72 73 75 77 78 79 80 81 82 84 85 86 87 96 102 103 107 117 118 119 121 122 124 133 135 137 **S** Mayo Foundation
Primary Contact: Colleen Skold, Administrator
COO: Jennifer Abernathy, Assistant Administrator
CFO: Michele Eberle, Assistant Administrator
CHR: Christine Krizan, Director Human Resource
Web address: www.bloomermedicalcenter.org
Control: Other not–for–profit (including NFP Corporation) **Service:** General Medical and Surgical

Staffed Beds: 54 **Admissions:** 535 **Census:** 50 **Outpatient Visits:** 24973 **Births:** 0 **Total Expense ($000):** 13030 **Payroll Expense ($000):** 5696 **Personnel:** 132

BOSCOBEL—Grant County

BOSCOBEL AREA HEALTH CARE (521344), 205 Parker Street, Zip 53805–1698; tel. 608/375–4112, (Total facility includes 66 beds in nursing home–type unit) **A**9 10 18 **F**3 4 5 11 13 15 27 33 36 40 43 50 53 54 55 56 57 62 65 66 68 73 74 75 76 78 79 80 81 82 84 85 86 87 88 89 90 91 93 94 96 99 100 102 103 107 117 118 119 121 122 124 133 135 **P**6
Primary Contact: John Russel, Administrator
CFO: Rita Moore, Manager Accounting
CMO: Thomas Pelz, M.D., Chief of Staff
CIO: Mathew Young, Information Systems Technician
CHR: Dennis Carpenter, Director Human Resources
Web address: www.boscobelhealth.com
Control: Other not–for–profit (including NFP Corporation) **Service:** General Medical and Surgical

Staffed Beds: 101 **Admissions:** 1237 **Census:** 71 **Outpatient Visits:** 4625 **Births:** 65 **Total Expense ($000):** 15468 **Payroll Expense ($000):** 7688 **Personnel:** 140

BROOKFIELD—Waukesha County

★ △ **WHEATON FRANCISCAN HEALTHCARE – ELMBROOK MEMORIAL (520170)**, 19333 West North Avenue, Zip 53045–4198; tel. 262/785–2000 **A**1 7 9 10 **F**3 4 15 16 17 26 27 30 31 32 33 38 41 43 44 45 46 49 50 54 55 56 57 62 63 65 68 72 73 75 76 77 78 79 80 81 82 86 87 90 94 96 98 99 100 102 103 105 106 107 108 109 119 120 121 124 132 134 135 136 **S** Wheaton Franciscan Healthcare
Primary Contact: Kimry A. Johnsrud, President
CFO: Annette Schiebel, Controller
CHR: Nathan Albertson, Director Human Resources
Web address: www.wfhealthcare.org
Control: Church–operated, Nongovernment, not–for profit **Service:** General Medical and Surgical

Staffed Beds: 88 **Admissions:** 5434 **Census:** 60 **Outpatient Visits:** 87482 **Births:** 600 **Total Expense ($000):** 121816 **Payroll Expense ($000):** 33682 **Personnel:** 610

BURLINGTON—Racine County

★ **AURORA MEMORIAL HOSPITAL OF BURLINGTON (520059)**, 252 McHenry Street, Zip 53105–1828; tel. 262/767–6000 **A**1 9 10 **F**3 11 13 15 17 25 26 30 31 32 33 34 35 38 41 43 44 46 49 50 51 52 54 55 56 57 58 62 63 66 68 72 73 74 77 78 79 80 81 82 84 86 90 96 100 102 105 106 107 112 119 120 121 123 124 134 135 137 **S** Aurora Health Care
Primary Contact: Kathleen Skowlund, RN, M.S., Administrator and Chief Nurse Executive
COO: Loren J. Anderson, Executive Vice President
CFO: E. Stuart Arnett, Vice President Finance and Chief Financial Officer
CMO: James Moran, M.D., President Medical Staff
CIO: Jean Chase, Regional Manager Information Services
CHR: Gene Krauklis, Regional Vice President Human Resources
Web address: www.aurorahealthcare.org
Control: Other not–for–profit (including NFP Corporation) **Service:** General Medical and Surgical

Staffed Beds: 65 **Admissions:** 3247 **Census:** 29 **Outpatient Visits:** 67762 **Births:** 313 **Total Expense ($000):** 59618 **Payroll Expense ($000):** 22131 **Personnel:** 539

CHILTON—Calumet County

☐ **CALUMET MEDICAL CENTER (521317)**, 614 Memorial Drive, Zip 53014–1597; tel. 920/849–2386 **A**1 10 18 **F**7 11 15 24 25 30 32 34 38 40 43 54 56 62 67 73 75 76 78 79 81 82 84 86 92 96 107 119 120 133 136
Primary Contact: Jennifer Weber, Interim President and Chief Executive Officer
CHR: Susan Jorgensen, Director Support Services
Web address: www.affinityhealth.org
Control: Other not–for–profit (including NFP Corporation) **Service:** General Medical and Surgical

Staffed Beds: 15 **Admissions:** 567 **Census:** 6 **Outpatient Visits:** 102192 **Births:** 0 **Total Expense ($000):** 13213 **Payroll Expense ($000):** 6326 **Personnel:** 134

 Many Facility Codes have changed. Please refer to the AHA Guide Code Chart.

CHIPPEWA FALLS—Chippewa County

★ **ST. JOSEPH'S HOSPITAL (520017)**, 2661 County Highway I, Zip 54729–1498; tel. 715/723–1811 **A**1 9 10 **F**3 4 13 15 16 17 26 30 31 32 38 42 43 50 54 55 61 62 65 68 69 70 73 75 76 77 78 79 81 82 83 88 92 96 100 102 107 118 119 121 124 135 136 137 **S** Hospital Sisters Health System
Primary Contact: David B. Fish, Executive Vice President and Administrator
COO: Raymond B. Myers, Assistant Administrator
CFO: Robert Koehler, Manager Financial Services
CMO: Michael Walton, M.D., Chief of Staff
CIO: Kevin Groskreutz, Coordinator Information Systems
CHR: Carolyn Craft, Division Manager Human and Support Services
Web address: www.stjoeschipfalls.com
Control: Church–operated, Nongovernment, not–for profit **Service:** General Medical and Surgical

Staffed Beds: 102 **Admissions:** 3700 **Census:** 39 **Outpatient Visits:** 70379 **Births:** 521 **Total Expense ($000):** 50682 **Payroll Expense ($000):** 23866 **Personnel:** 505

COLUMBUS—Columbia County

★ **COLUMBUS COMMUNITY HOSPITAL (521338)**, 1515 Park Avenue, Zip 53925–2402; tel. 920/623–2200 **A**1 9 10 18 **F**13 15 16 17 24 25 30 31 32 38 54 56 62 68 73 74 75 76 78 79 81 83 84 86 96 107 119 133 136
Primary Contact: Edward A. Harding, FACHE, President and Chief Executive Officer
CMO: Bruce A. Kraus, M.D., Chief of Staff
CIO: Lori Cherrier, Director Health Information
CHR: Ann Roundy, Director Employee Services
Web address: www.cch–inc.com
Control: Other not–for–profit (including NFP Corporation) **Service:** General Medical and Surgical

Staffed Beds: 25 **Admissions:** 1215 **Census:** 13 **Outpatient Visits:** 25195 **Births:** 68 **Total Expense ($000):** 21289 **Payroll Expense ($000):** 10277 **Personnel:** 177

CUBA CITY—Grant County

SOUTHWEST HEALTH CENTER NURSING HOME See Southwest Health Center, Platteville

CUDAHY—Milwaukee County

AURORA ST. LUKE'S SOUTH SHORE See Aurora St. Luke's Medical Center, Milwaukee

CUMBERLAND—Barron County

□ **CUMBERLAND MEMORIAL HOSPITAL (521353)**, 1110 Seventh Avenue, Zip 54829–9133; tel. 715/822–2741, (Total facility includes 50 beds in nursing home–type unit) **A**1 9 10 18 **F**3 4 16 17 30 31 32 38 43 44 45 54 55 56 63 65 68 70 72 73 74 75 77 78 79 80 81 82 83 85 86 94 97 102 115 117 118 119 120 121 122 124 137 **P**6
Primary Contact: Debora A. Kunferman, Administrator and Chief Executive Officer
COO: Robert J. Hansen, Administrator and Chief Executive Officer
CFO: Angela Martens, Controller
CMO: Barbara Ankarlo, M.D., Chief of Staff
CHR: Hilary Butzler, Director Human Resources
Web address: www.cumberlandhealthcare.com
Control: Other not–for–profit (including NFP Corporation) **Service:** General Medical and Surgical

Staffed Beds: 85 **Admissions:** 1464 **Census:** 66 **Outpatient Visits:** 9689 **Births:** 72 **Total Expense ($000):** 13023 **Payroll Expense ($000):** 6584 **Personnel:** 94

DARLINGTON—Lafayette County

MEMORIAL HOSPITAL OF LAFAYETTE COUNTY (521312), 800 Clay Street, Zip 53530–1228, Mailing Address: P.O. Box 70, Zip 53530–0070; tel. 608/776–4466 **A**9 10 18 **F**1 3 11 13 15 25 27 28 30 31 32 33 40 43 54 55 59 62 66 72 73 74 77 78 79 80 81 82 84 85 86 92 96 100 104 105 107 119 120 122 133
Primary Contact: Sherry Kudronowicz, Administrator
CFO: David Meister, Assistant Administrator Finance
Web address: www.mhlc–mhf.org
Control: County–Government, nonfederal **Service:** General Medical and Surgical

Staffed Beds: 25 **Admissions:** 718 **Census:** 5 **Outpatient Visits:** 2997 **Births:** 42 **Total Expense ($000):** 9594 **Payroll Expense ($000):** 2539 **Personnel:** 83

DODGEVILLE—Iowa County

★ **UPLAND HILLS HEALTH (521352)**, 800 Compassion Way, Zip 53533–0800, Mailing Address: P.O. Box 800, Zip 53533–0800; tel. 608/930–8000, (Total facility includes 44 beds in nursing home–type unit) **A**1 9 10 18 **F**2 3 11 13 15 17 25 30 31 32 38 42 43 52 54 56 57 61 62 63 65 68 73 74 75 76 77 78 79 80 81 82 83 84 85 86 87 96 97 102 104 107 117 118 119 120 122 133 135 136
Primary Contact: Phyllis Fritsch, Administrator
COO: Steve McCarthy, Assistant Administrator Business Operations
CFO: Karl Pustina, Assistant Administrator Finance
CIO: Karen Thuli, Coordinator Information Systems
CHR: Troy Marx, Director Human Resources
Web address: www.uplandhillshealth.org
Control: Other not–for–profit (including NFP Corporation) **Service:** General Medical and Surgical

Staffed Beds: 69 **Admissions:** 1350 **Census:** 52 **Outpatient Visits:** 47803 **Births:** 298 **Total Expense ($000):** 22067 **Payroll Expense ($000):** 9573 **Personnel:** 203

DURAND—Pepin County

★ **CHIPPEWA VALLEY HOSPITAL AND OAKVIEW CARE CENTER (521307)**, 1220 Third Avenue West, Zip 54736–1600, Mailing Address: P.O. Box 224, Zip 54736–0224; tel. 715/672–4211, (Total facility includes 58 beds in nursing home–type unit) **A**9 10 18 **F**15 25 38 54 56 67 73 79 81 82 96 100 117 119 **S** Adventist Health System Sunbelt Health Care Corporation
Primary Contact: Douglas R. Peterson, President and Chief Executive Officer
Web address: www.keepingyouwell.com
Control: Church–operated, Nongovernment, not–for profit **Service:** General Medical and Surgical

Staffed Beds: 83 **Admissions:** 631 **Census:** 62 **Outpatient Visits:** 9732 **Births:** 0 **Total Expense ($000):** 9748 **Payroll Expense ($000):** 3419 **Personnel:** 77

EAGLE RIVER—Vilas County

★ **EAGLE RIVER MEMORIAL HOSPITAL (521300)**, 201 Hospital Road, Zip 54521–8835; tel. 715/479–7411 **A**9 10 18 **F**7 8 11 15 26 28 30 31 32 33 40 44 52 54 55 56 57 62 67 69 73 77 79 81 84 87 96 99 103 107 121 122 133 135 **S** Marian Health System
Primary Contact: Sheila Clough, President
CFO: Jack P. Sutliff, Vice President and Chief Financial Officer
CMO: Michael Byrnes, M.D., Chief of Staff
CHR: Michelle Cornelius, Vice President Human Resources
Web address: www.ministryhealth.org
Control: Other not–for–profit (including NFP Corporation) **Service:** General Medical and Surgical

Staffed Beds: 10 **Admissions:** 745 **Census:** 6 **Outpatient Visits:** 29975 **Births:** 0 **Total Expense ($000):** 12762 **Payroll Expense ($000):** 4649 **Personnel:** 93

EAU CLAIRE—Eau Claire County

□ **LUTHER HOSPITAL (520070)**, 1221 Whipple Street, Zip 54702–4105, Mailing Address: P.O. Box 5, Zip 54702–0005; tel. 715/838–3311 **A**1 2 3 5 9 10 **F**4 5 11 13 15 17 24 30 31 32 38 40 43 51 52 56 59 62 68 70 73 74 75 76 78 79 81 82 84 86 88 89 90 91 92 93 94 95 96 97 100 106 107 119 136 **S** Mayo Foundation
Primary Contact: Randall L. Linton, M.D., President and Chief Executive Officer
COO: John M. Dickey, Chief Administrative Officer
CFO: Paul Bammel, Vice President
CMO: Terrance Borman, M.D., Medical Director
CIO: Brian Foster, Chief Information Officer
CHR: Blythe Loyd, Vice President
Web address: www.mhs.mayo.edu
Control: Other not–for–profit (including NFP Corporation) **Service:** General Medical and Surgical

Staffed Beds: 172 **Admissions:** 9299 **Census:** 106 **Outpatient Visits:** 144426 **Births:** 753 **Total Expense ($000):** 162183 **Payroll Expense ($000):** 65857 **Personnel:** 1447

□ **OAKLEAF SURGICAL HOSPITAL (520196)**, 3802 West Oakwood Mall Drive, Zip 54701; tel. 715/831–8130 **A**1 9 10 **F**43 51 62 73 78 79 107 119 **S** National Surgical Hospitals
Primary Contact: Michael McClain, Chief Executive Officer
Web address: www.oakleafmedical.com
Control: Partnership, Investor–owned, for–profit **Service:** General Medical and Surgical

Staffed Beds: 13 **Admissions:** 530 **Census:** 4 **Outpatient Visits:** 6798 **Births:** 0 **Total Expense ($000):** 18676 **Payroll Expense ($000):** 5920 **Personnel:** 86

WI

Hospital, Medicare Provider Number, Address, Telephone, Approval, Facility, and Physician Codes, Health Care System

★ American Hospital Association (AHA) membership
□ The Joint Commission accreditation
○ American Osteopathic Association (AOA) accreditation
△ Commission on Accreditation of Rehabilitation Facilities (CARF) accreditation

▣ △ **SACRED HEART HOSPITAL (520013)**, 900 West Clairemont Avenue, Zip 54701–6122; tel. 715/829–4121 **A**1 2 3 5 7 9 10 19 **F**3 4 6 15 16 17 26 27 28 30 31 32 33 37 38 43 44 45 46 48 49 50 54 55 56 57 62 63 65 66 67 68 70 72 73 75 76 77 78 79 80 81 82 83 85 86 88 89 90 91 93 96 97 98 100 102 104 105 106 107 108 109 111 112 116 118 119 121 123 124 134 135 136 137 **S** Hospital Sisters Health System
Primary Contact: Stephen F. Ronstrom, Executive Vice President and Administrator
CFO: Patricia Huettl, Assistant Administrator Financial Services
CMO: Greg Heiler, M.D., President Medical Staff
CHR: Robert Hassemer, Division Director Human Resources
Web address: www.sacredhearthospital-ec.org
Control: Church–operated, Nongovernment, not–for profit **Service:** General Medical and Surgical

Staffed Beds: 220 **Admissions:** 10019 **Census:** 133 **Outpatient Visits:** 133019 **Births:** 1138 **Total Expense ($000):** 144091 **Payroll Expense ($000):** 57476 **Personnel:** 1038

EDGERTON—Rock County

★ **EDGERTON HOSPITAL AND HEALTH SERVICES (521319)**, 313 Stoughton Road, Zip 53534–1198; tel. 608/884–3441, (Total facility includes 61 beds in nursing home–type unit) **A**9 10 18 **F**15 30 31 32 54 56 61 62 67 68 75 78 79 81 85 86 96 97 107 117 133 **P**5 **S** Brim Healthcare, Inc.
Primary Contact: James O. Pernau, Chief Executive Officer
CFO: Charles Roader, Vice President Finance
CMO: Thomas Berentsen, M.D., Chief of Staff
CIO: Sheryl Rucker, Chief Information Officer
CHR: Brad Young, Director Human Resources
Web address: www.edgertonhospital.com
Control: Other not–for–profit (including NFP Corporation) **Service:** General Medical and Surgical

Staffed Beds: 86 **Admissions:** 605 **Census:** 23 **Outpatient Visits:** 7035 **Births:** 0 **Total Expense ($000):** 15698 **Payroll Expense ($000):** 7690 **Personnel:** 123

ELKHORN—Walworth County

▣ △ **AURORA LAKELAND MEDICAL CENTER (520102)**, W3985 County Road NN, Zip 53121–4389; tel. 262/741–2000 **A**1 7 9 10 **F**3 11 13 15 17 25 26 27 30 31 32 33 34 35 38 41 43 44 50 51 54 55 56 57 58 62 63 66 68 72 73 74 76 77 78 79 80 81 82 84 85 86 90 96 100 102 104 105 106 107 118 119 120 121 124 135 137 **S** Aurora Health Care
Primary Contact: Kathleen Skowlund, RN, M.S., Administrator and Chief Nurse Executive
COO: Loren J. Anderson, Executive Vice President
CFO: E. Stuart Arnett, Regional Vice President Finance
CMO: Chad Kort, M.D., President Medical Staff
CIO: Jean Chase, Regional Manager Information Services
CHR: Gene Krauklis, Regional Vice President Human Resources
Web address: www.aurorahealthcare.org
Control: Other not–for–profit (including NFP Corporation) **Service:** General Medical and Surgical

Staffed Beds: 75 **Admissions:** 4667 **Census:** 45 **Outpatient Visits:** 62802 **Births:** 812 **Total Expense ($000):** 59000 **Payroll Expense ($000):** 21800 **Personnel:** 446

FOND DU LAC—Fond Du Lac County

▣ △ **AGNESIAN HEALTHCARE (520088)**, 430 East Division Street, Zip 54935–0385, Mailing Address: P.O. Box 385, Zip 54936–0385; tel. 920/929–2300 **A**1 2 7 9 10 20 **F**2 4 6 15 16 17 30 31 32 42 43 54 56 61 62 65 67 68 70 73 75 76 78 79 81 82 85 86 89 90 91 92 93 94 95 96 97 100 106 107 114 119 120 136 **P**3 6
Primary Contact: Robert A. Fale, President and Chief Executive Officer
CFO: Steven N. Little, Chief Financial Officer
CHR: Norma Tirado, Vice President Employee and Information Services
Web address: www.agnesian.com
Control: Church–operated, Nongovernment, not–for profit **Service:** General Medical and Surgical

Staffed Beds: 175 **Admissions:** 8275 **Census:** 93 **Outpatient Visits:** 177207 **Births:** 951 **Total Expense ($000):** 224957 **Payroll Expense ($000):** 77467 **Personnel:** 1073

FOND DU LAC COUNTY MENTAL HEALTH CENTER (524025), 459 East First Street, Zip 54935–4599; tel. 920/929–3571 **A**9 10 **F**4 30 31 32 36 88 89 92 93 119 **P**6
Primary Contact: Don Stout, Administrator
Control: County–Government, nonfederal **Service:** Psychiatric

Staffed Beds: 25 **Admissions:** 1088 **Census:** 14 **Outpatient Visits:** 369 **Births:** 0 **Total Expense ($000):** 3261 **Payroll Expense ($000):** 1805 **Personnel:** 42

FORT ATKINSON—Jefferson County

▣ **FORT HEALTHCARE (520071)**, 611 East Sherman Avenue, Zip 53538–1998; tel. 920/568–5000, (Total facility includes 28 beds in nursing home–type unit) **A**1 9 10 **F**3 5 11 13 15 17 25 27 30 31 32 33 40 43 44 52 53 54 55 56 57 61 62 66 68 73 74 75 76 77 78 79 80 81 82 83 84 85 86 96 100 103 106 107 108 117 118 119 120 121 124 133 134 135 136 **P**1 5
Primary Contact: Michael S. Wallace, President and Chief Executive Officer
CFO: James J. Nelson, Senior Vice President Finance and Strategic Planning
CIO: James E. Dahl, Manager Information Systems
Web address: www.forthealthcare.com
Control: Other not–for–profit (including NFP Corporation) **Service:** General Medical and Surgical

Staffed Beds: 100 **Admissions:** 3450 **Census:** 46 **Outpatient Visits:** 165369 **Births:** 466 **Total Expense ($000):** 81408 **Payroll Expense ($000):** 31687 **Personnel:** 607

FRIENDSHIP—Adams County

MOUNDVIEW MEMORIAL HOSPITAL & CLINICS (521309), 402 West Lake Street, Zip 53934–0040, Mailing Address: P.O. Box 40, Zip 53934–0040; tel. 608/339–3331, (Total facility includes 18 beds in nursing home–type unit) **A**9 10 18 **F**2 3 4 6 15 16 17 26 28 30 31 32 33 38 39 41 43 44 46 50 54 55 56 57 58 61 62 63 64 65 68 69 70 73 75 76 77 78 79 81 82 86 87 96 97 100 102 106 107 117 119 120 121 122 123 124 132 134 135 137 **P**5 6
Primary Contact: Janet M. Brown, Chief Executive Officer
CFO: Rodney Munger, Director Finance
CIO: Jim Frankowiak, Chief Information Officer
Web address: www.moundview.org
Control: Other not–for–profit (including NFP Corporation) **Service:** General Medical and Surgical

Staffed Beds: 43 **Admissions:** 537 **Census:** 23 **Outpatient Visits:** 25160 **Births:** 0 **Total Expense ($000):** 13586 **Payroll Expense ($000):** 5275 **Personnel:** 146

GLENDALE—Milwaukee County

ORTHOPAEDIC HOSPITAL OF WISCONSIN – GLENDALE (520194), 575 West River Woods Parkway, Zip 53212; tel. 414/961–6800 **A**9 10 **F**8 26 30 36 41 43 52 62 66 77 78 79 80 81 86 97 100 120 **P**2
Primary Contact: Brian J. Cramer, Chief Executive Officer
Web address: www.ohow.org
Control: Partnership, Investor–owned, for–profit **Service:** General Medical and Surgical

Staffed Beds: 7 **Admissions:** 371 **Census:** 1 **Outpatient Visits:** 31380 **Births:** 0 **Total Expense ($000):** 13883 **Payroll Expense ($000):** 5273 **Personnel:** 91

GRANTSBURG—Burnett County

★ **BURNETT MEDICAL CENTER (521331)**, 257 West St. George Avenue, Zip 54840–7827; tel. 715/463–5353, (Total facility includes 53 beds in nursing home–type unit) **A**9 10 18 **F**2 3 13 15 25 27 30 31 32 33 54 55 57 62 65 66 73 74 75 76 78 79 80 81 82 84 85 86 87 96 117 119 120 122 133 **P**6 **S** Brim Healthcare, Inc.
Primary Contact: Timothy J. Wick, Chief Executive Officer
CFO: Charles J. Faught, Chief Financial Officer
CHR: Amy Fossum, Director Human Resources
Web address: www.burnettmedicalcenter.com
Control: Other not–for–profit (including NFP Corporation) **Service:** General Medical and Surgical

Staffed Beds: 70 **Admissions:** 572 **Census:** 56 **Outpatient Visits:** 34400 **Births:** 49 **Total Expense ($000):** 10683 **Payroll Expense ($000):** 4708 **Personnel:** 86

GREEN BAY—Brown County

▣ △ **AURORA BAYCARE MEDICAL CENTER (520193)**, 2845 Greenbrier Road, Zip 54311, Mailing Address: P.O. Box 8900, Zip 54308; tel. 920/288–8000 **A**1 2 7 9 10 **F**3 8 13 15 17 25 26 27 30 31 32 33 34 38 40 41 43 46 47 49 50 52 53 55 56 57 58 62 63 68 70 72 73 74 76 77 78 79 80 81 82 84 85 86 96 98 99 100 102 103 105 106 107 109 111 112 118 119 120 121 124 133 135 136 137 **S** Aurora Health Care
Primary Contact: Daniel T. Meyer, Chief Administrative Officer
CFO: Sandra Ewald, Vice President Finance
CMO: Robert Griesser, M.D., Chief of Staff
CIO: Chuck Geurts, Manager Management Information Services
CHR: Gwen Baumel, Vice President Human Resources
Web address: www.aurorabaycare.com
Control: Partnership, Investor–owned, for–profit **Service:** General Medical and Surgical

Staffed Beds: 160 **Admissions:** 8685 **Census:** 89 **Outpatient Visits:** 141123 **Births:** 1643 **Total Expense ($000):** 166567 **Payroll Expense ($000):** 54490 **Personnel:** 1206

★ **BELLIN MEMORIAL HOSPITAL (520049)**, 744 South Webster Avenue, Zip 54301–3581, Mailing Address: P.O. Box 23400, Zip 54305–3400; tel. 920/433–3500 **A**1 9 10 **F**11 13 15 17 24 25 30 31 32 34 38 40 43 51 52 53 54 56 61 62 73 74 75 76 78 79 81 82 84 85 97 100 106 107 119 120 133 **P**6 8
Primary Contact: George Kerwin, President
CFO: Jim Dietsche, Executive Vice President and Chief Financial Officer
CMO: Christopher Watson, M.D., Chief Medical Officer
CIO: Randy Ronsman, Team Leader Information Services
CHR: Ken Peters, Team Leader Human Resources Management
Web address: www.bellin.org
Control: Church–operated, Nongovernment, not–for profit **Service:** General Medical and Surgical

Staffed Beds: 191 **Admissions:** 7846 **Census:** 87 **Outpatient Visits:** 139966 **Births:** 1234 **Total Expense ($000):** 218832 **Payroll Expense ($000):** 96826 **Personnel:** 1686

□ **BELLIN PSYCHIATRIC CENTER (524038)**, 301 East St. Joseph Street, Zip 54301–2241, Mailing Address: P.O. Box 23725, Zip 54305–3725; tel. 920/433–3630 **A**1 9 10 **F**4 5 25 30 31 32 36 53 54 56 81 82 88 89 90 91 92 93 94 95 119 **P**6
Primary Contact: Linda Roethle, President
CFO: Kevin McGurk, Controller
CMO: Anthony Marchlewski, M.D., President Medical and Psychological Staff
CIO: Randy Ronsman, Team Leader Information Services
Web address: www.bellin.org
Control: Church–operated, Nongovernment, not–for profit **Service:** Psychiatric

Staffed Beds: 53 **Admissions:** 1699 **Census:** 24 **Outpatient Visits:** 50879 **Births:** 0 **Total Expense ($000):** 13016 **Payroll Expense ($000):** 8242 **Personnel:** 130

BROWN COUNTY HUMAN SERVICES MENTAL HEALTH CENTER (524014), 2900 St. Anthony Drive, Zip 54311–5899; tel. 920/468–1136 **A**10 **F**4 5 73 88 91 92 93 94 119
Primary Contact: Earlene Ronk, Administrator
Web address: www.co.brown.wi.us/
Control: County–Government, nonfederal **Service:** Psychiatric

Staffed Beds: 25 **Admissions:** 1365 **Census:** 18 **Outpatient Visits:** 2109 **Births:** 0 **Total Expense ($000):** 5658 **Payroll Expense ($000):** 2785 **Personnel:** 70

★ **ST. MARY'S HOSPITAL MEDICAL CENTER (520097)**, 1726 Shawano Avenue, Zip 54303–3282; tel. 920/498–4200 **A**1 9 10 **F**3 4 15 20 21 26 27 30 31 32 33 38 41 43 44 46 47 48 49 50 55 56 57 62 65 66 67 68 69 70 72 73 74 76 77 78 79 80 81 82 84 86 87 88 92 96 97 102 103 104 105 106 107 111 114 119 121 123 124 132 134 135 136 137 **P**2 **S** Hospital Sisters Health System
Primary Contact: James G. Coller, FACHE, President and Chief Executive Officer
CFO: John Miller, Chief Financial Officer
CIO: Tanya Townsend, Chief Information Officer
Web address: www.stmgb.org
Control: Church–operated, Nongovernment, not–for profit **Service:** General Medical and Surgical

Staffed Beds: 94 **Admissions:** 5905 **Census:** 53 **Outpatient Visits:** 83217 **Births:** 659 **Total Expense ($000):** 95661 **Payroll Expense ($000):** 38566 **Personnel:** 638

★ △ **ST. VINCENT HOSPITAL (520075)**, 835 South Van Buren Street, Zip 54307–3508, Mailing Address: P.O. Box 13508, Zip 54307–3508; tel. 920/433–0111 **A**1 2 7 9 10 **F**3 4 15 16 17 26 27 28 30 31 32 33 35 37 41 43 44 46 49 50 54 56 57 58 61 62 63 64 65 66 68 70 72 73 74 75 76 77 78 79 80 81 83 84 86 87 88 96 97 99 100 101 102 103 104 105 106 107 108 109 110 112 116 118 119 121 123 124 135 136 137 **P**2 **S** Hospital Sisters Health System
Primary Contact: Thomas R. Bayer, Chief Operating Officer
COO: James G. Coller, FACHE, Executive Vice President and Administrator
CFO: Karl Appleton, Assistant Administrator and Chief Financial Officer
CMO: Kenneth Johnson, M.D., President Medical Staff
CIO: Tanya Townsend, Chief Information Officer
CHR: Jean Marsch, Director Human Resources
Web address: www.stvgh.org
Control: Church–operated, Nongovernment, not–for profit **Service:** General Medical and Surgical

Staffed Beds: 255 **Admissions:** 10785 **Census:** 152 **Outpatient Visits:** 198112 **Births:** 1009 **Total Expense ($000):** 227575 **Payroll Expense ($000):** 94293 **Personnel:** 1689

HARTFORD—Washington County

★ **AURORA MEDICAL CENTER OF WASHINGTON COUNTY (520038)**, 1032 East Sumner Street, Zip 53027–1698; tel. 262/673–2300 **A**1 2 9 10 **F**2 3 8 11 13 17 25 26 28 30 31 32 33 35 37 38 40 41 43 44 46 47 48 49 50 52 54 55 56 57 58 62 63 66 68 72 73 74 75 77 78 79 80 81 82 84 86 87 96 97 102 106 107 118 119 120 121 122 123 124 132 135 137 **S** Aurora Health Care
Primary Contact: Jeff Euclide, Interim Administrator
CMO: Majdi Abu–Salih, M.D., Chief of Staff
CHR: Tom TerHorst, Director Human Resources
Web address: www.aurorahealthcare.org
Control: Other not–for–profit (including NFP Corporation) **Service:** General Medical and Surgical

Staffed Beds: 55 **Admissions:** 2529 **Census:** 23 **Outpatient Visits:** 57884 **Births:** 347 **Total Expense ($000):** 48963 **Payroll Expense ($000):** 16832 **Personnel:** 344

HAYWARD—Sawyer County

★ **HAYWARD AREA MEMORIAL HOSPITAL AND NURSING HOME (521336)**, 11040 North State Road 77, Zip 54843–6391; tel. 715/934–4321, (Total facility includes 76 beds in nursing home–type unit) **A**9 10 18 **F**3 4 8 15 16 27 30 31 32 33 43 54 62 65 68 70 73 74 76 78 79 80 81 86 87 88 92 96 103 106 107 117 119 121 122 123 124 135 137
Primary Contact: Barbara A. Peickert, RN, Chief Executive Officer
Web address: www.hamhnh.com
Control: Other not–for–profit (including NFP Corporation) **Service:** General Medical and Surgical

Staffed Beds: 101 **Admissions:** 1620 **Census:** 83 **Outpatient Visits:** 23563 **Births:** 189 **Total Expense ($000):** 21818 **Payroll Expense ($000):** 10135 **Personnel:** 150

HILLSBORO—Vernon County

★ **ST. JOSEPH'S COMMUNITY HEALTH SERVICES (521304)**, 400 Water Avenue, Zip 54634–0527, Mailing Address: P.O. Box 527, Zip 54634–0527; tel. 608/489–8000, (Total facility includes 28 beds in nursing home–type unit) **A**9 10 18 **F**2 4 15 16 17 31 32 54 56 62 65 68 70 73 74 75 78 79 81 83 85 86 88 96 117 119 120 **P**6
Primary Contact: Billy J. Bruce, Jr., Chief Executive Officer and President
CFO: Tom Jones, Interim Chief Financial Officer
CMO: Sheila A. Patel, M.D., Chief of Staff
CHR: Kristie McCoic, Director Human Resources
Web address: www.stjhealthcare.org
Control: Church–operated, Nongovernment, not–for profit **Service:** General Medical and Surgical

Staffed Beds: 34 **Admissions:** 508 **Census:** 40 **Outpatient Visits:** 17654 **Births:** 34 **Total Expense ($000):** 10568 **Payroll Expense ($000):** 4241 **Personnel:** 111

HUDSON—St. Croix County

□ **HUDSON HOSPITAL (521335)**, 405 Stageline Road, Zip 54016–1600; tel. 715/531–6000 **A**1 9 10 18 **F**3 5 13 15 27 34 35 40 43 46 52 54 56 57 72 73 74 76 77 78 79 80 81 82 84 86 96 100 102 107 118 119 121 122 124 132 135 137
Primary Contact: Marian M. Furlong, RN, Chief Executive Officer
CFO: Sheila Proehl, Chief Financial Officer
CMO: Gregory Young, M.D., Chief of Staff
CHR: Carolyn Milbrath, Director Human Resources
Web address: www.hudsonhospital.org
Control: Other not–for–profit (including NFP Corporation) **Service:** General Medical and Surgical

Staffed Beds: 12 **Admissions:** 1385 **Census:** 11 **Outpatient Visits:** 27630 **Births:** 412 **Total Expense ($000):** 34261 **Payroll Expense ($000):** 12218 **Personnel:** 223

JANESVILLE—Rock County

★ **MERCY HEALTH SYSTEM (520066)**, 1000 Mineral Point Avenue, Zip 53547–2982, Mailing Address: P.O. Box 5003, Zip 53547–5003; tel. 608/756–6000, (Total facility includes 28 beds in nursing home–type unit) (Nonreporting) **A**1 2 9 10
Primary Contact: Javon R. Bea, President and Chief Executive Officer
CFO: Joseph D. Nemeth, Vice President and Chief Financial Officer
Web address: www.mercyhealthsystem.org
Control: Other not–for–profit (including NFP Corporation) **Service:** General Medical and Surgical

Staffed Beds: 195

Hospital, Medicare Provider Number, Address, Telephone, Approval, Facility, and Physician Codes, Health Care System
★ American Hospital Association (AHA) membership
□ The Joint Commission accreditation
○ American Osteopathic Association (AOA) accreditation
△ Commission on Accreditation of Rehabilitation Facilities (CARF) accreditation

KENOSHA—Kenosha County

★ **AURORA MEDICAL CENTER (520189)**, 10400 South 75th Street, Zip 53142; tel. 262/948–5600 **A**1 2 9 10 **F**3 6 8 11 13 15 17 25 26 30 31 32 33 34 35 38 41 43 44 46 47 48 49 50 51 53 54 55 56 57 58 62 63 66 68 72 73 74 77 78 79 80 81 82 84 86 90 96 99 100 102 103 104 105 106 107 109 111 112 118 119 120 121 124 134 135 137 **S** Aurora Health Care
Primary Contact: Christine Olson, Administrator
CFO: Stuart Arnett, Vice President Finance
CMO: Alfred J. Capelli, M.D., President Medical Staff
CIO: Jean Chase, Regional Manager Information Services
CHR: Gene Krauklis, Regional Vice President Human Resources
Web address: www.aurorahealthcare.org
Control: Other not–for–profit (including NFP Corporation) **Service:** General Medical and Surgical

Staffed Beds: 73 **Admissions:** 5594 **Census:** 48 **Outpatient Visits:** 96245 **Births:** 1256 **Total Expense ($000):** 80726 **Payroll Expense ($000):** 27765 **Personnel:** 596

☐ **CHILDREN'S HOSPITAL OF WISCONSIN (523301)**, 6308 Eighth Avenue, 6th Floor, Zip 53143–5082; tel. 262/656–2261 **A**1 9 10 **F**3 25 30 31 32 33 66 80 81 82 84 87 119 **P**4
Primary Contact: Jon E. Vice, President and Chief Executive Officer
Web address: www.chw.org
Control: Other not–for–profit (including NFP Corporation) **Service:** Children's general

Staffed Beds: 21 **Admissions:** 1238 **Census:** 4 **Outpatient Visits:** 1837 **Births:** 0 **Total Expense ($000):** 4900 **Payroll Expense ($000):** 1313 **Personnel:** 24

☐ **UNITED HEALTH SYSTEM–KENOSHA CAMPUS (520021)**, 6308 Eighth Avenue, Zip 53143–5082; tel. 262/656–2011, (Nonreporting) **A**1 9 10
Primary Contact: Richard O. Schmidt, Jr., President and Chief Executive Officer
Control: Other not–for–profit (including NFP Corporation) **Service:** General Medical and Surgical

Staffed Beds: 151

LA CROSSE—La Crosse County

☐ **FRANCISCAN SKEMP HEALTHCARE–LA CROSSE CAMPUS (520004)**, 700 West Avenue South, Zip 54601–4783; tel. 608/785–0940, (Total facility includes 23 beds in nursing home–type unit) **A**1 2 9 10 **F**4 5 6 11 13 15 17 24 25 30 31 32 34 36 38 40 42 43 51 52 53 54 56 61 62 67 68 70 73 74 75 76 78 79 81 82 83 84 85 86 88 89 90 91 92 93 94 96 97 100 106 107 114 117 119 120 133 136 **P**6 **S** Mayo Foundation
Primary Contact: Robert Nesse, M.D., President and Chief Executive Officer
COO: Ronald R. Paczkowski, Executive Vice President
CFO: Tom Tiggelaar, Vice President Finance
CMO: P. Stephen Shultz, M.D., Vice President Medical Affairs
CIO: Daniel Schaefer, Vice President Systems, Process and Support Services
CHR: Del Long, Administrator Human Resources
Web address: www.franciscanskemp.org
Control: Church–operated, Nongovernment, not–for profit **Service:** General Medical and Surgical

Staffed Beds: 198 **Admissions:** 7741 **Census:** 93 **Outpatient Visits:** 70841 **Births:** 727 **Total Expense ($000):** 129649 **Payroll Expense ($000):** 58594 **Personnel:** 1272

★ △ **GUNDERSEN LUTHERAN MEDICAL CENTER (520087)**, 1900 South Avenue, Zip 54601–9980; tel. 608/782–7300 **A**1 2 3 5 7 8 9 10 **F**4 5 9 11 13 16 17 24 25 30 31 32 34 36 38 40 42 43 51 54 56 59 60 61 67 68 70 74 75 76 78 79 81 82 83 84 85 86 88 89 90 91 92 93 94 119 136
Primary Contact: Jeffrey E. Thompson, M.D., Chief Executive Officer
CFO: Jerry Arndt, Senior Vice President Business Services
CMO: Julio J. Bird, M.D., Chief Medical Officer
CIO: Deb Rislow, Director Information Systems
CHR: Kathy Klock, Senior Vice President Operations and Human Resources
Web address: www.gundluth.org
Control: Other not–for–profit (including NFP Corporation) **Service:** General Medical and Surgical

Staffed Beds: 258 **Admissions:** 14378 **Census:** 154 **Outpatient Visits:** 191010 **Births:** 1628 **Total Expense ($000):** 259011 **Payroll Expense ($000):** 82485 **Personnel:** 1552

LADYSMITH—Rusk County

★ **RUSK COUNTY MEMORIAL HOSPITAL AND NURSING HOME (521328)**, 900 College Avenue West, Zip 54848–2116; tel. 715/532–5561, (Total facility includes 50 beds in nursing home–type unit) **A**9 10 18 **F**3 11 13 15 17 25 40 43 52 54 62 65 68 74 75 78 79 80 84 85 86 87 96 99 100 102 117 119 122 133 137
Primary Contact: J. Michael Shaw, Chief Executive Officer
CFO: Judith Strop, Director Finance
CMO: John Ziemer, M.D., Chief of Staff
CHR: Rita Telitz, Director Human Resources
Web address: www.ruskhospital.org
Control: County–Government, nonfederal **Service:** General Medical and Surgical

Staffed Beds: 75 **Admissions:** 865 **Census:** 69 **Outpatient Visits:** 33352 **Births:** 79 **Total Expense ($000):** 14497 **Payroll Expense ($000):** 6132 **Personnel:** 112

LAKE GENEVA—Walworth County

☐ **MERCY WALWORTH HOSPITAL AND MEDICAL CENTER (521357)**, N2950 State Road 67, Zip 53147; tel. 262/245–0535 **A**1 9 10 18 **F**4 13 15 16 30 31 32 43 53 56 62 65 68 73 74 75 76 78 79 81 85 86 88 89 90 91 93 94 96 100 107 114 119 120 **P**5 6
Primary Contact: Jennifer Hallatt, Director
Web address: www.mercyhealthsystem.org
Control: Other not–for–profit (including NFP Corporation) **Service:** General Medical and Surgical

Staffed Beds: 6 **Admissions:** 298 **Census:** 2 **Outpatient Visits:** 111676 **Births:** 0 **Total Expense ($000):** 32328 **Payroll Expense ($000):** 7107 **Personnel:** 177

LANCASTER—Grant County

★ **GRANT REGIONAL HEALTH CENTER (521322)**, 507 South Monroe Street, Zip 53813–2054; tel. 608/723–2143 **A**1 9 10 18 **F**3 11 13 15 25 30 31 32 33 34 39 40 43 52 54 55 57 62 67 68 73 74 75 76 79 80 81 82 84 85 86 96 107 118 119 120 121 122 124 135 **P**6 **S** Brim Healthcare, Inc.
Primary Contact: Nicole Clapp, RN, M.S.N., FACHE, President and Chief Executive Officer
CFO: Van Osborn, Chief Financial Officer
CMO: Eric Stader, M.D., Chief of Staff
CIO: David Chitwood, Coordinator Information Systems
CHR: Sheri Fischer, Manager Human Resources
Web address: www.grantregional.com
Control: Other not–for–profit (including NFP Corporation) **Service:** General Medical and Surgical

Staffed Beds: 25 **Admissions:** 734 **Census:** 5 **Outpatient Visits:** 25315 **Births:** 145 **Total Expense ($000):** 13477 **Payroll Expense ($000):** 5924 **Personnel:** 122

MADISON—Dane County

☐ **MENDOTA MENTAL HEALTH INSTITUTE (524008)**, 301 Troy Drive, Zip 53704–1599; tel. 608/301–1000 **A**1 3 5 10 **F**6 13 17 30 43 54 56 65 70 73 78 81 82 83 85 88 89 90 91 93 94 95 119 **P**6
Primary Contact: Greg Van Rybroek, Chief Executive Officer
CFO: Stacie Schiereck, Manager Business Office
CMO: Kenneth Casimir, M.D., Medical Director
Web address: www.dhfs.state.wi.us
Control: State–Government, nonfederal **Service:** Psychiatric

Staffed Beds: 264 **Admissions:** 1449 **Census:** 255 **Outpatient Visits:** 27284 **Births:** 0 **Total Expense ($000):** 63950 **Payroll Expense ($000):** 37653 **Personnel:** 718

★ △ **MERITER HOSPITAL (520089)**, 202 South Park Street, Zip 53715–1599; tel. 608/417–6000 **A**1 3 5 7 9 10 **F**1 3 4 5 9 11 13 15 17 25 26 27 30 31 32 33 34 35 37 40 43 44 45 47 48 49 52 53 54 55 56 57 58 62 63 68 70 73 74 76 78 79 81 82 83 84 85 86 88 89 90 91 92 93 94 95 96 100 102 103 106 107 114 119 121 133 135 136 137 **P**6
Primary Contact: James L. Woodward, President and Chief Administrative Officer
CFO: Linda Hoff, Chief Financial Officer
CMO: Geoff Priest, M.D., Senior Vice President Medical Affairs
CHR: Mary Nick, Vice President Human Resources
Web address: www.meriter.com
Control: Other not–for–profit (including NFP Corporation) **Service:** General Medical and Surgical

Staffed Beds: 357 **Admissions:** 17560 **Census:** 205 **Outpatient Visits:** 183164 **Births:** 3796 **Total Expense ($000):** 268454 **Payroll Expense ($000):** 116433 **Personnel:** 1874

WI

★ **ST. MARY'S HOSPITAL (520083)**, 700 South Park Street, Zip 53715–0450; tel. 608/251–6100 **A**1 3 5 9 10 **F**7 11 13 17 24 25 30 31 32 36 38 40 43 56 59 68 70 73 74 76 78 79 81 82 83 84 86 88 90 93 96 97 106 107 119 133 **S** SSM Health Care
Primary Contact: Frank D. Byrne, M.D., President
COO: Jon Rozenfeld, Executive Vice President and Chief Operating Officer
CFO: Charlie Johnson, Vice President Finance and Chief Financial Officer
CIO: Major Dave Lundal, Vice President and Regional Chief Information Officer
CHR: Linda Taplin Statz, Director Human Resources
Web address: www.stmarysmadison.com
Control: Other not–for–profit (including NFP Corporation) **Service:** General Medical and Surgical

Staffed Beds: 338 **Admissions:** 22041 **Census:** 259 **Outpatient Visits:** 95563 **Births:** 3486 **Total Expense ($000):** 278036 **Payroll Expense ($000):** 106837 **Personnel:** 1828

★ △ **UNIVERSITY OF WISCONSIN HOSPITAL AND CLINICS (520098)**, 600 Highland Avenue, Zip 53792–0002; tel. 608/263–6400, (Includes UNIVERSITY OF WISCONSIN CHILDREN'S HOSPITAL) **A**1 3 5 7 8 9 10 12 13 **F**1 3 4 6 8 15 16 17 20 21 26 27 28 30 31 32 33 37 38 41 43 44 45 46 47 48 49 50 54 55 56 57 61 62 65 66 68 69 70 72 73 75 76 77 78 79 80 81 82 83 86 87 88 90 92 93 94 96 97 99 100 101 102 103 104 105 106 107 108 109 111 112 113 114 116 118 119 120 121 123 124 125 126 127 128 129 131 132 134 135 136 137 **P**3
Primary Contact: Donna Katen–Bahensky, President and Chief Executive Officer
CFO: Gary Eiler, Senior Vice President and Chief Financial Officer
CMO: Carl J. Getto, M.D., Senior Vice President Medical Affairs and Associate Dean Hospital Affairs
CIO: Michael Sauk, Chief Information Officer
CHR: Jan Bultema, Vice President Human Resources
Web address: www.uwhospital.org
Control: Other not–for–profit (including NFP Corporation) **Service:** General Medical and Surgical

Staffed Beds: 467 **Admissions:** 23259 **Census:** 356 **Outpatient Visits:** 755823 **Births:** 0 **Total Expense ($000):** 766936 **Payroll Expense ($000):** 304776 **Personnel:** 5902

★ **WILLIAM S. MIDDLETON MEMORIAL VETERANS HOSPITAL**, 2500 Overlook Terrace, Zip 53705–2286; tel. 608/256–1901 **A**1 3 5 **F**3 6 8 13 16 17 20 26 27 37 38 43 44 46 47 48 50 54 55 57 58 61 62 63 65 68 70 72 73 75 76 77 78 79 80 81 82 85 86 87 88 90 91 92 93 94 96 97 100 102 103 107 118 119 121 124 132 135 136 137 **P**6 **S** Department of Veterans Affairs
Primary Contact: Deborah A. Thompson, Director
COO: Allen R. Ackers, Associate Director
CFO: Abraham Rabinowitz, Assistant Finance Officer
CMO: Alan J. Bridges, M.D., Chief of Staff
CIO: Randall Margenau, Chief Information Officer
CHR: Kathleen Hendricks, Coordinator Human Resources
Web address: www.madison.med.va.gov
Control: Veterans Affairs, Government, federal **Service:** General Medical and Surgical

Staffed Beds: 86 **Admissions:** 3772 **Census:** 62 **Outpatient Visits:** 263299 **Births:** 0 **Total Expense ($000):** 195533 **Payroll Expense ($000):** 96539 **Personnel:** 1262

MANITOWOC—Manitowoc County

★ **HOLY FAMILY MEMORIAL MEDICAL CENTER (520107)**, 2300 Western Avenue, Zip 54220, Mailing Address: P.O. Box 1450, Zip 54221–1450; tel. 920/320–2011 **A**1 2 9 10 **F**2 3 4 5 11 13 15 17 25 26 27 28 30 31 32 33 34 40 41 42 43 44 46 48 49 50 51 52 53 54 55 57 59 61 62 66 68 73 74 75 76 77 78 79 80 81 84 85 86 88 89 90 91 92 93 94 96 100 102 103 104 107 109 111 118 119 120 121 124 132 133 135 136 137 **S** Franciscan Sisters of Christian Charity HealthCare Ministry, Inc
Primary Contact: Mark P. Herzog, President and Chief Executive Officer
CFO: Patrick J. Brandel, Chief Financial Officer
CMO: Steve Driggers, M.D., Chief Medical Officer
CIO: Ed Bauknecht, Director Management Information Systems
Web address: www.hfmhealth.org
Control: Church–operated, Nongovernment, not–for profit **Service:** General Medical and Surgical

Staffed Beds: 67 **Admissions:** 4331 **Census:** 41 **Outpatient Visits:** 148228 **Births:** 331 **Total Expense ($000):** 112208 **Payroll Expense ($000):** 56122 **Personnel:** 864

MARINETTE—Marinette County

★ **BAY AREA MEDICAL CENTER (520113)**, 3100 Shore Drive, Zip 54143–4297; tel. 715/735–6621 **A**1 9 10 20 **F**3 7 8 11 13 15 17 25 26 27 30 31 39 40 53 54 55 57 59 62 68 73 74 75 76 78 79 80 81 82 84 86 87 96 100 102 104 107 118 119 120 133 135 136
Primary Contact: David Olson, President and Chief Executive Officer
COO: Bernie VanCourt, Chief Operating Officer
CFO: Dan Carlson, Chief Financial Officer
CIO: Pete Eisenzoph, Director Information Technology
CHR: Curt Oberholtzer, Assistant Administrator Human Resources and Organizational Development
Web address: www.bamc.org
Control: Other not–for–profit (including NFP Corporation) **Service:** General Medical and Surgical

Staffed Beds: 99 **Admissions:** 4174 **Census:** 44 **Outpatient Visits:** 77548 **Births:** 365 **Total Expense ($000):** 88471 **Payroll Expense ($000):** 38100 **Personnel:** 518

MARSHFIELD—Wood County

NORWOOD HEALTH CENTER (524019), 1600 North Chestnut Avenue, Zip 54449–1499; tel. 715/384–2188, (Total facility includes 45 beds in nursing home–type unit) **A**10 **F**3 4 88 89 90 91 92 93 95 117 **P**6
Primary Contact: Rhonda Kozik, Administrator
CFO: Lynn Dehmlow, Manager Accounting
CHR: Barb Shoemaker, Administrative Assistant
Web address: www.co.wood.wi.us/norwood/index.htm
Control: County–Government, nonfederal **Service:** Psychiatric

Staffed Beds: 67 **Admissions:** 690 **Census:** 39 **Outpatient Visits:** 0 **Births:** 0 **Total Expense ($000):** 2994 **Payroll Expense ($000):** 1646 **Personnel:** 60

★ △ **SAINT JOSEPH'S HOSPITAL (520037)**, 611 St. Joseph Avenue, Zip 54449–1898; tel. 715/387–1713 **A**1 2 3 5 7 9 10 20 **F**3 4 5 6 7 9 11 13 16 17 21 25 26 27 30 31 32 33 34 36 40 41 43 44 45 49 50 52 54 55 56 57 59 60 62 63 66 67 68 70 72 73 74 75 76 77 78 79 80 81 82 83 84 85 86 88 90 91 92 93 97 100 101 104 105 106 107 108 109 111 112 116 118 119 121 124 125 132 133 135 136 137 **S** Marian Health System
Primary Contact: Michael A. Schmidt, President
CFO: John Skaden, Chief Financial Officer
CIO: Steve Pelton, Chief Information Officer
CHR: Layton Anderson, Regional Director Human Resources
Web address: www.stjosephs–marshfield.org
Control: Church–operated, Nongovernment, not–for profit **Service:** General Medical and Surgical

Staffed Beds: 319 **Admissions:** 17812 **Census:** 247 **Outpatient Visits:** 84406 **Births:** 1204 **Total Expense ($000):** 257496 **Payroll Expense ($000):** 90445 **Personnel:** 1956

MAUSTON—Juneau County

□ **MILE BLUFF MEDICAL CENTER (520109)**, 1050 Division Street, Zip 53948–1997; tel. 608/847–6161, (Total facility includes 132 beds in nursing home–type unit) **A**1 9 10 20 **F**10 11 13 15 24 31 32 38 43 53 54 56 59 61 62 73 74 75 76 78 79 81 82 84 86 90 96 97 100 104 106 107 115 117 119 120 133 **P**5 6
Primary Contact: James M. O'Keefe, President and Chief Executive Officer
Web address: www.milebluff.com
Control: Other not–for–profit (including NFP Corporation) **Service:** General Medical and Surgical

Staffed Beds: 169 **Admissions:** 2527 **Census:** 148 **Outpatient Visits:** 93243 **Births:** 200 **Total Expense ($000):** 40403 **Payroll Expense ($000):** 20865 **Personnel:** 400

MEDFORD—Taylor County

★ **MEMORIAL HEALTH CENTER (521324)**, 135 South Gibson Street, Zip 54451–1696; tel. 715/748–8100, (Includes MEMORIAL NURSING HOME), (Total facility includes 97 beds in nursing home–type unit) **A**1 9 10 18 **F**2 3 4 15 16 17 27 30 31 32 33 43 50 54 55 56 57 62 65 66 73 74 75 76 78 79 81 82 84 85 86 87 88 96 102 115 117 118 119 120 121 122 124 135 136
Primary Contact: Gregory A. Olson, President and Chief Executive Officer
CMO: Cathy Reuter, M.D., Medical Director
CIO: Dave Zoromski, Director Information Systems
CHR: Angela Hupf, Vice President Human Resources and Marketing
Web address: www.memhc.com
Control: Other not–for–profit (including NFP Corporation) **Service:** General Medical and Surgical

Staffed Beds: 122 **Admissions:** 972 **Census:** 104 **Outpatient Visits:** 38611 **Births:** 249 **Total Expense ($000):** 23967 **Payroll Expense ($000):** 10643 **Personnel:** 193

Hospital, Medicare Provider Number, Address, Telephone, Approval, Facility, and Physician Codes, Health Care System

★ American Hospital Association (AHA) membership
□ The Joint Commission accreditation
○ American Osteopathic Association (AOA) accreditation
△ Commission on Accreditation of Rehabilitation Facilities (CARF) accreditation

MENOMONEE FALLS—Waukesha County

★ △ **COMMUNITY MEMORIAL HOSPITAL (520103)**, W180 N8085 Town Hall Road, Zip 53051–3518, Mailing Address: P.O. Box 408, Zip 53052–0408; tel. 262/251–1000 **A**1 2 3 5 7 9 10 **F**3 4 5 8 11 13 15 17 25 26 27 30 31 32 33 34 36 37 40 41 43 44 46 47 48 49 50 51 52 54 55 56 57 58 59 62 64 66 67 68 70 72 73 74 75 76 77 78 79 80 81 83 84 85 86 87 88 90 91 92 93 94 95 96 100 103 105 107 108 109 111 114 118 119 120 121 124 134 135 136 137
Primary Contact: William E. Bestor, President and Chief Executive Officer
CFO: Lisa A. Heider, Vice President Finance and Chief Information Officer
CMO: Michael Unger, M.D., Vice President Medical Affairs
CIO: Lisa A. Heider, Vice President and Chief Information Officer
CHR: John Zorbini, Vice President Human Resources
Web address: www.communitymemorial.com
Control: Other not–for–profit (including NFP Corporation) **Service:** General Medical and Surgical

Staffed Beds: 200 **Admissions:** 9509 **Census:** 113 **Outpatient Visits:** 92317 **Births:** 844 **Total Expense ($000):** 146700 **Payroll Expense ($000):** 55055 **Personnel:** 1035

MENOMONIE—Dunn County

☐ **RED CEDAR MEDICAL CENTER–MAYO HEALTH SYSTEM (521340)**, 2321 Stout Road, Zip 54751–2397; tel. 715/235–5531 **A**1 3 5 9 10 18 **F**3 11 13 15 17 32 34 38 40 43 54 55 56 57 62 64 66 68 73 74 75 77 78 79 80 81 82 84 85 86 96 118 119 120 121 122 124 135 136 **S** Mayo Foundation
Primary Contact: Hank Simpson, M.D., Chief Executive Officer
COO: Steve Lindberg, Chief Administrative Officer
CFO: Jeanie Lubinsky, Chief Financial Officer
CMO: Mark Deyo Svendsen, M.D., Medical Director
CIO: Frank Wrogg, Director Information Technology
CHR: LeAnn Wurtzel, Director Human Resources
Web address: www.rcmc–mhs.org
Control: Other not–for–profit (including NFP Corporation) **Service:** General Medical and Surgical

Staffed Beds: 25 **Admissions:** 1343 **Census:** 12 **Outpatient Visits:** 42351 **Births:** 298 **Total Expense ($000):** 50157 **Payroll Expense ($000):** 25454 **Personnel:** 505

MEQUON—Ozaukee County

★ **COLUMBIA CENTER (520195)**, 13125 North Port Washington Road, Zip 53097; tel. 262/243–7408 **A**9 10 **F**3 4 8 30 31 32 43 56 62 65 74 78 80 81 82 107 114 121
Primary Contact: Karen J. Casey, RN, M.S., President and Chief Executive Officer
CMO: Anna Windsor, M.D., Medical Staff President
Web address: www.columbiacenter.org
Control: Other not–for–profit (including NFP Corporation) **Service:** General Medical and Surgical

Staffed Beds: 23 **Admissions:** 562 **Census:** 4 **Outpatient Visits:** 384 **Births:** 562 **Total Expense ($000):** 5420 **Payroll Expense ($000):** 1874 **Personnel:** 52

★ **COLUMBIA ST. MARY'S OZAUKEE HOSPITAL (520027)**, 13111 North Port Washington Road, Zip 53097–2416; tel. 262/243–7300, (Nonreporting) **A**1 9 10 **S** Ascension Health
Primary Contact: Leo P. Brideau, President and Chief Executive Officer
COO: Therese B. Pandl, Executive Vice President Operations and Chief Operating Officer
CMO: David Shapiro, M.D., Vice President Medical Affairs and Chief Medical Officer
CIO: Mary Paul, Chief Information Officer
CHR: Cheryl Hill, Vice President Human Resources
Web address: www.columbia–stmarys.com
Control: Church–operated, Nongovernment, not–for profit **Service:** General Medical and Surgical

Staffed Beds: 116

MERRILL—Lincoln County

★ **GOOD SAMARITAN HEALTH CENTER OF MERRILL (521339)**, 601 Center Avenue South, Zip 54452–3404; tel. 715/536–5511 **A**1 9 10 18 **F**3 4 8 15 16 17 26 27 31 43 50 54 55 56 57 62 65 67 68 73 74 75 76 77 78 79 80 81 82 86 88 96 100 102 106 107 119 121 122 135 136 **S** Marian Health System
Primary Contact: Michael Hammer, President and Chief Operating Officer
CFO: Michele Ruesch, Chief Financial Officer
Web address: www.ministryhealth.org
Control: Church–operated, Nongovernment, not–for profit **Service:** General Medical and Surgical

Staffed Beds: 11 **Admissions:** 1013 **Census:** 10 **Outpatient Visits:** 34428 **Births:** 0 **Total Expense ($000):** 22154 **Payroll Expense ($000):** 10377 **Personnel:** 208

MILWAUKEE—Milwaukee County

★ △ **AURORA SINAI MEDICAL CENTER (520064)**, 945 North 12th Street, Zip 53233–1337, Mailing Address: P.O. Box 342, Zip 53201–0342; tel. 414/219–2000 **A**1 2 3 5 7 8 9 10 **F**1 3 5 6 8 11 13 15 17 25 26 27 30 31 32 33 34 35 36 37 38 39 40 41 43 49 50 53 54 55 56 57 62 63 66 67 68 70 72 73 74 76 77 78 79 80 81 82 84 85 86 87 90 92 93 94 96 97 99 100 102 105 106 107 114 118 119 120 121 124 132 133 135 136 137 **S** Aurora Health Care
Primary Contact: Leonard E. Wilk, Administrator
CFO: Kevin Jones, Director Finance
Web address: www.aurorahealthcare.org
Control: Other not–for–profit (including NFP Corporation) **Service:** General Medical and Surgical

Staffed Beds: 195 **Admissions:** 10045 **Census:** 114 **Outpatient Visits:** 288269 **Births:** 2813 **Total Expense ($000):** 191879 **Payroll Expense ($000):** 64219 **Personnel:** 1270

★ △ **AURORA ST. LUKE'S MEDICAL CENTER (520138)**, 2900 West Oklahoma Avenue, Zip 53215–4330, Mailing Address: P.O. Box 2901, Zip 53201–2901; tel. 414/649–6000, (Includes AURORA ST. LUKE'S SOUTH SHORE, 5900 South Lake Drive, Cudahy, Zip 53110–8903; tel. 414/769–9000) **A**1 2 3 5 7 8 9 10 **F**1 3 4 5 6 11 15 17 25 26 27 30 31 32 33 34 35 36 38 39 40 41 43 46 47 49 50 51 53 54 55 56 57 62 63 64 66 67 68 72 73 76 77 78 79 80 81 82 84 85 86 87 88 90 91 92 93 94 95 96 97 98 99 100 102 103 104 105 106 107 108 109 111 112 116 118 119 121 124 125 126 127 128 129 130 131 132 133 134 135 137 **S** Aurora Health Care
Primary Contact: Mary O'Brien, Administrator
Web address: www.aurorahealthcare.org
Control: Other not–for–profit (including NFP Corporation) **Service:** General Medical and Surgical

Staffed Beds: 733 **Admissions:** 39418 **Census:** 524 **Outpatient Visits:** 494196 **Births:** 0 **Total Expense ($000):** 780744 **Payroll Expense ($000):** 245309 **Personnel:** 4836

★ **CHILDREN'S HOSPITAL OF WISCONSIN (523300)**, 9000 West Wisconsin Avenue, Zip 53226–4810, Mailing Address: P.O. Box 1997, Zip 53201–1997; tel. 414/266–2000 **A**1 3 5 8 9 10 **F**3 9 20 21 24 25 26 27 28 30 31 32 33 34 36 37 39 40 41 43 44 46 47 48 49 50 51 53 55 56 57 58 59 60 62 63 66 69 70 72 73 75 76 77 79 80 81 82 83 84 86 87 89 90 94 96 97 98 99 100 101 102 103 104 105 106 107 108 109 110 111 112 118 119 120 121 123 125 126 127 128 129 130 131 132 133 135 137 **P**4
Primary Contact: Jon E. Vice, President and Chief Executive Officer
COO: Cinthia S. Christensen, Executive Vice President and Chief Operating Officer
CFO: Timothy L. Birkenstock, Treasurer and Chief Financial Officer
CMO: Michael Gutzeit, M.D., Chief Medical Officer
CIO: Michael Jones, Vice President and Chief Information Officer
CHR: Peggy Niemer, Vice President Human Resources
Web address: www.chw.org
Control: Other not–for–profit (including NFP Corporation) **Service:** Children's general

Staffed Beds: 236 **Admissions:** 22190 **Census:** 216 **Outpatient Visits:** 311352 **Births:** 0 **Total Expense ($000):** 343183 **Payroll Expense ($000):** 115945 **Personnel:** 2141

★ △ **CLEMENT J. ZABLOCKI VETERANS AFFAIRS MEDICAL CENTER**, 5000 West National Avenue, Zip 53295; tel. 414/384–2000, (Total facility includes 196 beds in nursing home–type unit) (Nonreporting) **A**1 2 3 5 7 **S** Department of Veterans Affairs
Primary Contact: Glen W. Grippen, Director
COO: Larry L. Berkeley, Associate Director
CMO: Michael Erdmann, M.D., Chief of Staff
CIO: Chris Houterman, Chief Information Officer
CHR: Wayne Davis, Chief Human Resources
Web address: www.va.gov/sta/guide/home.asp
Control: Veterans Affairs, Government, federal **Service:** General Medical and Surgical

Staffed Beds: 566

★ **COLUMBIA ST. MARY'S COLUMBIA HOSPITAL (520051)**, 2025 East Newport Avenue, Zip 53211–2990; tel. 414/961–3300 **A**1 2 3 5 9 10 **F**3 4 6 8 15 16 17 26 27 28 29 30 31 32 33 35 38 39 41 43 44 45 46 48 49 50 53 54 55 56 57 62 65 66 68 70 72 73 74 76 77 78 79 81 84 85 86 87 88 89 90 91 92 93 94 95 96 97 99 100 101 102 103 104 106 107 116 118 119 121 123 124 131 132 135 136 137 **P**6 **S** Ascension Health
Primary Contact: Leo P. Brideau, President and Chief Executive Officer
COO: Therese B. Pandl, Executive Vice President Operations and Chief Operating Officer
CFO: Charles J. Dreher, Vice President Finance and Chief Financial Officer
CMO: David Shapiro, M.D., Vice President Medical Affairs and Chief Medical Officer
CIO: Mary Paul, Chief Information Officer
CHR: Cheryl Hill, Vice President Human Resources
Web address: www.columbia–stmarys.com
Control: Other not–for–profit (including NFP Corporation) **Service:** General Medical and Surgical

Staffed Beds: 248 **Admissions:** 8280 **Census:** 111 **Outpatient Visits:** 239850 **Births:** 0 **Total Expense ($000):** 183855 **Payroll Expense ($000):** 75446 **Personnel:** 1038

 Many Facility Codes have changed. Please refer to the AHA Guide Code Chart.

★□ **COLUMBIA ST. MARY'S MILWAUKEE HOSPITAL (520051)**, 2323 North Lake Drive, Zip 53211–9682, Mailing Address: P.O. Box 503, Zip 53201–0503; tel. 414/291–1000 **A**1 2 9 10 **F**3 4 8 15 16 17 26 27 28 29 30 31 32 33 37 38 39 41 44 45 48 49 50 53 54 55 56 57 62 64 65 66 68 70 72 73 75 76 77 78 79 80 81 82 85 87 88 94 96 97 99 100 101 102 103 106 107 108 109 111 112 119 121 124 130 132 135 136 137 **P**6 **S** Ascension Health
Primary Contact: Leo P. Brideau, President and Chief Executive Officer
COO: Therese B. Pandl, Executive Vice President Operations and Chief Operating Officer
CFO: Charles J. Dreher, Vice President Finance and Chief Financial Officer
CMO: David Shapiro, M.D., Vice President Medical Affairs and Chief Medical Officer
CIO: Mary Paul, Chief Information Officer
CHR: Cheryl Hill, Vice President Human Resources
Web address: www.columbia–stmarys.com
Control: Church–operated, Nongovernment, not–for profit **Service:** General Medical and Surgical

Staffed Beds: 226 **Admissions:** 9857 **Census:** 130 **Outpatient Visits:** 427959 **Births:** 2953 **Total Expense ($000):** 251608 **Payroll Expense ($000):** 117981 **Personnel:** 1904

★□ △ **FROEDTERT MEMORIAL LUTHERAN HOSPITAL (520177)**, 9200 West Wisconsin Avenue, Zip 53226–3596, Mailing Address: P.O. Box 26099, Zip 53226–3596; tel. 414/805–3000 **A**1 2 3 5 7 8 9 10 **F**6 11 13 15 17 24 25 30 31 32 36 38 40 43 51 53 54 56 59 62 68 73 74 75 76 78 79 81 82 85 86 90 91 92 93 94 96 97 100 104 106 107 113 114 119 120 125 126 127 129 130 133 136
Primary Contact: William D. Petasnick, President and Chief Executive Officer
COO: Catherine Buck, Executive Vice President Operations
CFO: Blaine J. O'Connell, Senior Vice President Finance
CMO: Andrew J. Norton, M.D., Senior Vice President Medical Affairs
CIO: Lisa A. Heider, Interim Chief Information Officer
CHR: Elizabeth J. Forman, Vice President Human Resources
Web address: www.froedtert.com
Control: Other not–for–profit (including NFP Corporation) **Service:** General Medical and Surgical

Staffed Beds: 451 **Admissions:** 25188 **Census:** 354 **Outpatient Visits:** 484007 **Births:** 1600 **Total Expense ($000):** 604186 **Payroll Expense ($000):** 192349 **Personnel:** 3723

□ **KINDRED HOSPITAL–MILWAUKEE (522004)**, 5017 South 110th Street, Zip 53228–3131; tel. 414/427–8282 **A**1 9 10 **F**1 25 32 38 54 56 68 73 81 82 85 90 119 **S** Kindred Healthcare
Primary Contact: Linda Newberry–Ferguson, Chief Executive Officer
COO: Christine Ninu, Chief Operating Officer
CFO: Sharon Rand, Chief Financial Officer
CMO: Scott Fenske, M.D., Medical Director
Web address: www.khmilwaukee.com
Control: Corporation, Investor–owned, for–profit **Service:** Children's Long–Term Acute Care

Staffed Beds: 56 **Admissions:** 398 **Census:** 31 **Outpatient Visits:** 0 **Births:** 0 **Total Expense ($000):** 13882 **Payroll Expense ($000):** 5873 **Personnel:** 116

□ **LIFECARE HOSPITALS OF MILWAUKEE (522007)**, 5000 West Chambers Street, 8th Floor, Zip 53210; tel. 414/447–3600 **A**1 9 10 **F**1 3 25 80 81 103 137 **S** LifeCare Management Services
Primary Contact: Steven J. Schultz, Chief Executive Officer
COO: Jennifer Culotta, Ph.D., Chief Clinical Officer and Director of Nursing
CMO: Russell Harland, M.D., Medical Director
CHR: Marland Henderson, Director
Web address: www.lifecare–hospitals.com
Control: Corporation, Investor–owned, for–profit **Service:** Children's Long–Term Acute Care

Staffed Beds: 34 **Admissions:** 296 **Census:** 22 **Outpatient Visits:** 0 **Births:** 0 **Total Expense ($000):** 10662 **Payroll Expense ($000):** 4644 **Personnel:** 79

★ **MILWAUKEE COUNTY BEHAVIORAL HEALTH DIVISION (524001)**, 9455 Watertown Plank Road, Zip 53226–3559; tel. 414/257–6995, (Total facility includes 72 beds in nursing home–type unit) **A**3 5 10 **F**31 32 65 67 88 89 90 91 92 93 94 95 117
Primary Contact: John Chianelle, Administrator
CFO: Michael Kreuser, Director Fiscal Services
CMO: Thomas Harding, M.D., Medical Director
CIO: William Borja, Chief Information Officer
Web address: www.milwaukeecounty.org
Control: County–Government, nonfederal **Service:** Psychiatric

Staffed Beds: 216 **Admissions:** 2727 **Census:** 231 **Outpatient Visits:** 14957 **Births:** 0 **Total Expense ($000):** 145391 **Payroll Expense ($000):** 33082 **Personnel:** 880

★□ △ **SACRED HEART REHABILITATION INSTITUTE (523025)**, 2025 East Newport Avenue, Zip 53211–2906; tel. 414/298–6700 **A**1 7 9 10 **F**16 17 30 31 32 53 54 56 62 65 73 78 81 83 85 86 119 120 **P**6 **S** Ascension Health
Primary Contact: Jack Burke, Administrator
COO: Therese B. Pandl, Executive Vice President Operations and Chief Operating Officer
CFO: Charles J. Dreher, Vice President Finance and Chief Financial Officer
CMO: David Shapiro, M.D., Vice President Medical Affairs and Chief Medical Officer
CIO: Mary Paul, Chief Information Officer
CHR: Cheryl Hill, Vice President Human Resources
Web address: www.columbia–stmarys.com
Control: Church–operated, Nongovernment, not–for profit **Service:** Rehabilitation

Staffed Beds: 49 **Admissions:** 536 **Census:** 20 **Outpatient Visits:** 8020 **Births:** 0 **Total Expense ($000):** 11664 **Payroll Expense ($000):** 5237 **Personnel:** 83

SELECT SPECIALTY HOSPITAL (522006), 8901 West Lincoln Avenue, 6th Floor, Zip 53227; tel. 414/328–7700 **A**9 10 **F**1 3 17 25 26 34 43 54 68 73 75 76 78 80 81 82 85 90 93 119 137 **S** Select Medical Corporation
Primary Contact: Dennis Mattes, Chief Executive Officer
COO: Mary Puetzer, Chief Operating Officer
CMO: Jeffrey Aldred, M.D., Medical Director
CHR: Chris Froh, Senior Coordinator Human Resources
Web address: www.selectmedicalcorp.com
Control: Corporation, Investor–owned, for–profit **Service:** Children's Long–Term Acute Care

Staffed Beds: 34 **Admissions:** 394 **Census:** 28 **Outpatient Visits:** 0 **Births:** 0 **Total Expense ($000):** 14201 **Payroll Expense ($000):** 4193 **Personnel:** 92

★□ △ **WHEATON FRANCISCAN HEALTHCARE – ST. FRANCIS (520078)**, 3237 South 16th Street, Zip 53215–4592; tel. 414/647–5000 **A**1 2 7 9 10 **F**4 13 15 17 30 31 32 43 53 54 56 62 65 68 70 73 75 76 78 79 81 82 86 89 90 91 92 93 94 95 96 97 100 106 107 119 120 136 **S** Wheaton Franciscan Healthcare
Primary Contact: Debra Standridge, President
COO: Debra Standridge, President
CFO: Michael Petitt, Director Finance
CIO: Gregory Smith, Senior Vice President and Chief Information Officer
CHR: Christopher Morris, Director Human Resources
Web address: www.stfrancishospital.net
Control: Church–operated, Nongovernment, not–for profit **Service:** General Medical and Surgical

Staffed Beds: 192 **Admissions:** 9426 **Census:** 110 **Outpatient Visits:** 155926 **Births:** 1227 **Total Expense ($000):** 141575 **Payroll Expense ($000):** 51955 **Personnel:** 1006

★□ △ **WHEATON FRANCISCAN HEALTHCARE – ST. JOSEPH (520136)**, 5000 West Chambers Street, Zip 53210–9988; tel. 414/447–2000, (Nonreporting) **A**1 2 3 5 7 9 10 **S** Wheaton Franciscan Healthcare
Primary Contact: Ronald Groepper, President
CFO: Patty Allen, Vice President Business and Ambulatory Services
CMO: Rita Hanson, M.D., Vice President Medical Affairs
CIO: Patrick Henkhaus, Regional Director Information Services
CHR: Shakila Shimp, Director Human Resources
Web address: www.whfc.org
Control: Church–operated, Nongovernment, not–for profit **Service:** General Medical and Surgical

Staffed Beds: 396

MONROE—Green County

□ **THE MONROE CLINIC (520028)**, 515 22nd Avenue, Zip 53566–1598; tel. 608/324–1000 **A**1 9 10 **F**3 5 6 8 9 11 13 15 17 26 27 28 30 31 32 33 34 36 38 40 41 42 43 46 49 50 53 54 55 56 57 61 62 66 68 73 74 75 76 77 78 79 80 81 82 83 84 85 86 87 89 90 91 92 93 94 96 103 107 114 118 119 120 121 124 133 134 135 136 137 **P**6
Primary Contact: Michael B. Sanders, President and Chief Executive Officer
CFO: Julie Wilke, Chief Financial Officer
CIO: Carrie Blum, Director Information Systems
CHR: Julie Allemagne, Human Resources Officer
Web address: www.monroeclinic.org
Control: Other not–for–profit (including NFP Corporation) **Service:** General Medical and Surgical

Staffed Beds: 61 **Admissions:** 3321 **Census:** 29 **Outpatient Visits:** 206736 **Births:** 390 **Total Expense ($000):** 103078 **Payroll Expense ($000):** 49874 **Personnel:** 800

Hospital, Medicare Provider Number, Address, Telephone, Approval, Facility, and Physician Codes, Health Care System

★ American Hospital Association (AHA) membership
□ The Joint Commission accreditation
○ American Osteopathic Association (AOA) accreditation
△ Commission on Accreditation of Rehabilitation Facilities (CARF) accreditation

NEENAH—Winnebago County

★ **CHILDREN'S HOSPITAL OF WISCONSIN–FOX VALLEY (523302)**, 130 Second Avenue, 3rd Floor South, Zip 54956; tel. 920/969–7900 **A**1 9 10 **F**3 25 30 31 32 33 55 56 57 58 63 70 78 80 81 82 84 87 119 121 135 **P**6
Primary Contact: Jon E. Vice, President and Chief Executive Officer
Web address: www.chw.org
Control: Other not–for–profit (including NFP Corporation) **Service:** Children's general

Staffed Beds: 41 **Admissions:** 1448 **Census:** 20 **Outpatient Visits:** 3619 **Births:** 0 **Total Expense ($000):** 14584 **Payroll Expense ($000):** 5391 **Personnel:** 71

□ △ **THEDA CLARK MEDICAL CENTER (520045)**, 130 Second Street, Zip 54956–2883, Mailing Address: P.O. Box 2021, Zip 54957–2021; tel. 920/729–3100 **A**1 2 7 9 10 **F**3 4 5 7 8 9 11 13 15 17 25 26 27 30 31 32 35 39 40 41 43 44 46 47 48 49 52 54 59 62 67 68 72 73 74 75 76 77 78 79 80 81 82 85 86 87 88 89 91 92 93 94 95 96 98 100 105 107 108 109 110 111 112 114 119 120 132 133 135 136 137 **S** ThedaCare, Inc.
Primary Contact: Kathryn Correia, Senior Vice President
COO: Matthew Furlan, Chief Operating Officer
CFO: Tim Olson, Senior Vice President Finance
CIO: Keith Livingston, Senior Vice President and Chief Information Officer
CHR: Maureen Pistone, Senior Vice President Human Resources
Web address: www.thedacare.org
Control: Other not–for–profit (including NFP Corporation) **Service:** General Medical and Surgical

Staffed Beds: 168 **Admissions:** 8122 **Census:** 86 **Outpatient Visits:** 87736 **Births:** 1348 **Total Expense ($000):** 133078 **Payroll Expense ($000):** 51736 **Personnel:** 962

NEILLSVILLE—Clark County

MEMORIAL MEDICAL CENTER – NEILLSVILLE (521323), 216 Sunset Place, Zip 54456–1799; tel. 715/743–3101, (Includes NEILLSVILLE MEMORIAL HOME), (Total facility includes 99 beds in nursing home–type unit) **A**9 10 18 **F**3 6 11 13 15 31 32 35 38 40 43 54 55 56 57 61 62 63 65 66 73 74 75 77 79 80 81 82 86 87 96 97 107 117 119 120 121 122 133 137 **P**6
Primary Contact: Scott Polenz, Chief Executive Officer
COO: Scott Polenz, Chief Executive Officer
CFO: Kelly Moen, Chief Financial Officer
CMO: Timothy Meyer, M.D., Chief of Staff
CIO: Jim Griepentrog, Director Information Systems
CHR: Tamie Zarak, Director Human Resources
Web address: www.mmcneillsville.com
Control: Other not–for–profit (including NFP Corporation) **Service:** General Medical and Surgical

Staffed Beds: 124 **Admissions:** 956 **Census:** 92 **Outpatient Visits:** 6319 **Births:** 47 **Total Expense ($000):** 11325 **Payroll Expense ($000):** 5167 **Personnel:** 131

NEW LONDON—Outagamie County

□ **NEW LONDON FAMILY MEDICAL CENTER (521326)**, 1405 Mill Street, Zip 54961–2155, Mailing Address: P.O. Box 307, Zip 54961–0307; tel. 920/531–2000 **A**1 9 10 18 **F**3 7 8 11 13 15 25 26 30 31 32 33 39 43 44 55 57 62 64 66 73 74 77 78 79 80 81 82 84 85 86 87 96 107 120 121 122 130 132 135 137 **S** ThedaCare, Inc.
Primary Contact: William Schmidt, President and Chief Executive Officer
CFO: Cindy Mischler, Vice President Finance
CMO: Paul Hoell, M.D., President Medical Staff
Web address: www.newlondon.thedacare.org
Control: Other not–for–profit (including NFP Corporation) **Service:** General Medical and Surgical

Staffed Beds: 25 **Admissions:** 1142 **Census:** 10 **Outpatient Visits:** 39894 **Births:** 139 **Total Expense ($000):** 19520 **Payroll Expense ($000):** 8910 **Personnel:** 164

NEW RICHMOND—St. Croix County

★ **WESTFIELDS HOSPITAL (521345)**, 535 Hospital Road, Zip 54017–1495; tel. 715/246–2101 **A**9 10 18 **F**1 13 15 24 25 31 32 36 38 40 43 54 56 62 67 68 73 74 76 78 79 81 82 84 85 86 96 100 107 119 120 **P**5 **S** HealthPartners
Primary Contact: Jean M. Needham, President
CFO: David Kuehn, Chief Financial Officer
CIO: Kim Rosario, Chief Information Officer
CHR: Chris Riba, Human Resource Manager
Web address: www.holyfamilyhospital.org
Control: Other not–for–profit (including NFP Corporation) **Service:** General Medical and Surgical

Staffed Beds: 25 **Admissions:** 1266 **Census:** 12 **Outpatient Visits:** 24830 **Births:** 161 **Total Expense ($000):** 23126 **Payroll Expense ($000):** 8971 **Personnel:** 169

OCONOMOWOC—Waukesha County

★ △ **OCONOMOWOC MEMORIAL HOSPITAL (520062)**, 791 Summit Avenue, Zip 53066–3896; tel. 262/569–9400 **A**1 2 7 9 10 **F**2 3 8 11 13 15 17 25 26 27 28 30 31 32 33 35 40 43 44 46 49 54 55 56 57 58 62 66 68 72 73 74 75 76 77 78 79 80 81 82 84 85 86 87 92 96 98 99 100 101 102 103 106 107 108 109 111 118 119 121 124 132 133 134 135 136 137 **S** ProHealth Care
Primary Contact: John R. Robertstad, FACHE, President and Chief Executive Officer
COO: Mary Jo O'Malley, R.N., MS, Vice President Operations
CFO: Nan Nelson, Vice President Finance
CMO: Brian Lipman, M.D., Chief of Staff
CIO: William Miller, Vice President Information Services
CHR: Nadine Guirl, Senior Vice President Human Resources
Web address: www.oconomowocmemorial.org
Control: Other not–for–profit (including NFP Corporation) **Service:** General Medical and Surgical

Staffed Beds: 74 **Admissions:** 4751 **Census:** 41 **Outpatient Visits:** 95191 **Births:** 782 **Total Expense ($000):** 80139 **Payroll Expense ($000):** 26679 **Personnel:** 450

□ **ROGERS MEMORIAL HOSPITAL (524018)**, 34700 Valley Road, Zip 53066–4599; tel. 262/646–4411 **A**1 3 5 9 10 **F**13 31 32 56 65 70 73 78 81 82 84 89 90 91 93 94 95 119
Primary Contact: David L. Moulthrop, Ph.D., President and Chief Executive Officer
COO: Paul A. Mueller, Chief Operating Officer
CFO: Gerald A. Noll, Chief Financial Officer
CMO: Kambiz Pahlavan, M.D., Chief Medical Officer
CIO: Wayne Mattson, Management Information Systems Specialist
CHR: Renee Patterson, Vice President of Employment and Training Services
Web address: www.rogershospital.org
Control: Other not–for–profit (including NFP Corporation) **Service:** Psychiatric

Staffed Beds: 90 **Admissions:** 1362 **Census:** 28 **Outpatient Visits:** 32346 **Births:** 0 **Total Expense ($000):** 25251 **Payroll Expense ($000):** 14906 **Personnel:** 150

OCONTO—Oconto County

BOND HEALTH CENTER (521356), 820 Arbutus Avenue, Zip 54153, Mailing Address: P.O. Box 357, Zip 54153–0357; tel. 920/835–1100 **A**9 10 18 **F**3 30 31 32 33 40 50 55 56 57 63 87 102 118 122 133 **P**8
Primary Contact: Laura Cormier, Director
Web address: www.bondhealth.org
Control: Other not–for–profit (including NFP Corporation) **Service:** General Medical and Surgical

Staffed Beds: 4 **Admissions:** 61 **Census:** 1 **Outpatient Visits:** 2931 **Births:** 0 **Total Expense ($000):** 2849 **Payroll Expense ($000):** 1374 **Personnel:** 21

OCONTO FALLS—Oconto County

★ **COMMUNITY MEMORIAL HOSPITAL (521310)**, 855 South Main Street, Zip 54154–1296; tel. 920/846–3444 **A**9 10 18 **F**11 13 15 24 25 31 32 38 40 43 54 56 73 74 75 78 79 81 82 83 84 85 86 96 97 100 107 119 136 **P**6 **S** Brim Healthcare, Inc.
Primary Contact: James Van Dornick, Chief Executive Officer
COO: Kay Kuchta, Chief Nursing Officer
CFO: Bill Beaston, Chief Financial Officer
CMO: R. Scott Liebl, M.D., Chief of Staff
CIO: Andy Miller, Chief Information Officer
CHR: Trisha Brown, Manager Human Resources
Web address: www.cmhospital.org
Control: Other not–for–profit (including NFP Corporation) **Service:** General Medical and Surgical

Staffed Beds: 25 **Admissions:** 1360 **Census:** 13 **Outpatient Visits:** 67551 **Births:** 97 **Total Expense ($000):** 26687 **Payroll Expense ($000):** 10927 **Personnel:** 212

OSCEOLA—Polk County

OSCEOLA MEDICAL CENTER (521318), 301 River Street, Zip 54020, Mailing Address: P.O. Box 218, Zip 54020–0218; tel. 715/294–2111 **A**9 10 18 **F**11 13 15 24 25 38 40 54 56 62 68 73 74 75 76 79 81 84 86 96 107 **P**6
Primary Contact: Jeffrey K. Meyer, Chief Executive Officer
CFO: Cathy Bukowski, Chief Financial Officer
CMO: Rob Dybvig, M.D., Chief Medical Officer
CIO: Shawn Kammerud, Manager Information Services
CHR: Margie Evenson, Manager Human Resources
Web address: www.osceolamedicalcenter.com
Control: Other not–for–profit (including NFP Corporation) **Service:** General Medical and Surgical

Staffed Beds: 16 **Admissions:** 741 **Census:** 6 **Outpatient Visits:** 29467 **Births:** 86 **Total Expense ($000):** 17668 **Payroll Expense ($000):** 6962 **Personnel:** 178

OSHKOSH—Winnebago County

★□ **AURORA MEDICAL CENTER OF OSHKOSH (520198)**, 855 North Westhaven Drive, Zip 54904; tel. 920/456–6000 **A**1 9 10 **F**3 8 11 13 15 17 25 26 30 31 32 35 38 40 43 47 49 52 54 56 66 68 69 70 72 73 74 77 78 79 80 81 82 84 86 96 98 99 100 101 102 103 105 106 107 109 110 111 118 119 134 135 136 137 **S** Aurora Health Care
Primary Contact: Frances R. Finley, Vice President and Chief Administrative Officer
CFO: Robin Pedersen, Vice President Finance
CHR: Linda Mingus, Director Human Resources
Web address: www.aurorahealthcare.com
Control: Other not–for–profit (including NFP Corporation) **Service:** General Medical and Surgical

Staffed Beds: 71 **Admissions:** 3498 **Census:** 31 **Outpatient Visits:** 85089 **Births:** 771 **Total Expense ($000):** 65479 **Payroll Expense ($000):** 23654 **Personnel:** 510

□ △ **MERCY MEDICAL CENTER (520048)**, 500 South Oakwood Road, Zip 54903–3370, Mailing Address: P.O. Box 3370, Zip 54903–3370; tel. 920/223–2000 **A**1 2 7 10 **F**3 4 5 11 13 15 16 17 25 26 27 30 31 32 33 36 37 40 41 43 44 46 47 48 49 50 51 52 54 55 56 57 62 63 65 66 68 73 74 76 78 79 81 82 83 85 86 88 93 94 96 99 100 101 102 105 106 107 108 109 110 111 118 119 120 121 123 133 135 136 137
Primary Contact: Daniel Neufelder, Chief Executive Officer
CFO: Jeff Badger, Chief Financial Officer
CMO: Mark W. Kehrberg, M.D., Senior Vice President and Chief Medical Officer
CIO: Will Weider, Chief Information Officer
CHR: Vince Gallucci, Senior Vice President Human Resources
Web address: www.affinityhealth.org
Control: Church–operated, Nongovernment, not–for profit **Service:** General Medical and Surgical

Staffed Beds: 172 **Admissions:** 6272 **Census:** 71 **Outpatient Visits:** 62948 **Births:** 631 **Total Expense ($000):** 95957 **Payroll Expense ($000):** 37586 **Personnel:** 578

OSSEO—Trempealeau County

□ **LUTHER MIDELFORT OAKRIDGE (521302)**, 13025 Eighth Street, Zip 54758–7673, Mailing Address: P.O. Box 70, Zip 54758–0070; tel. 715/597–3121, (Total facility includes 50 beds in nursing home–type unit) **A**1 9 10 18 **F**2 6 7 10 11 24 25 30 31 32 38 40 54 56 67 73 78 81 82 84 85 86 96 115 117 119 **S** Mayo Foundation
Primary Contact: Michael Ryan, Administrator
COO: Michael Ryan, Administrator
Web address: www.luthermidelfortoakridge.com
Control: Other not–for–profit (including NFP Corporation) **Service:** General Medical and Surgical

Staffed Beds: 104 **Admissions:** 264 **Census:** 54 **Outpatient Visits:** 10735 **Births:** 1 **Total Expense ($000):** 8011 **Payroll Expense ($000):** 3977 **Personnel:** 98

PARK FALLS—Price County

★ **FLAMBEAU HOSPITAL (521325)**, 98 Sherry Avenue, Zip 54552–1467, Mailing Address: P.O. Box 310, Zip 54552–0310; tel. 715/762–2484 **A**9 10 18 **F**3 8 11 13 14 15 17 25 26 27 30 31 32 42 43 44 50 52 54 55 56 57 61 62 66 67 68 69 72 73 74 75 78 79 81 82 84 85 86 96 99 102 107 119 120 121 122 132 133 135 137 **S** Marian Health System
Primary Contact: David A. Grundstrom, Chief Administrative Officer
CFO: James R. Braun, Chief Financial Officer
CHR: Barb Michalski, Manager Human Resources
Web address: www.flambeauhospital.org
Control: Other not–for–profit (including NFP Corporation) **Service:** General Medical and Surgical

Staffed Beds: 25 **Admissions:** 1020 **Census:** 11 **Outpatient Visits:** 32369 **Births:** 36 **Total Expense ($000):** 17629 **Payroll Expense ($000):** 7030 **Personnel:** 176

PLATTEVILLE—Grant County

★□ **SOUTHWEST HEALTH CENTER (521354)**, 1400 Eastside Road, Zip 53818–9800; tel. 608/348–2331, (Includes SOUTHWEST HEALTH CENTER NURSING HOME, 808 South Washington Street, Cuba City, Zip 53807; tel. 608/744–2161), (Total facility includes 84 beds in nursing home–type unit) (Nonreporting) **A**1 9 10 18 **S** Brim Healthcare, Inc.
Primary Contact: Anne K. Klawiter, President and Chief Executive Officer
CFO: James Ehasz, Chief Financial Officer
CMO: Michael Connelly, M.D., Chief of Staff
CHR: Tammy Gore, Manager Human Resources
Web address: www.southwesthealth.org
Control: Other not–for–profit (including NFP Corporation) **Service:** General Medical and Surgical

Staffed Beds: 119

PLEASANT PRAIRIE—Kenosha County

★□ **UNITED HOSPITAL SYSTEM, ST. CATHERINE'S MEDICAL CENTER CAMPUS**, 9555 76th Street, Zip 53158; tel. 262/656–2011 **A**1 2 9 10 **F**4 6 15 16 17 30 31 32 43 54 56 62 65 68 73 76 78 79 81 82 84 86 88 96 97 100 106 107 119 136 **P**5 6 **S** Wheaton Franciscan Healthcare
Primary Contact: Richard O. Schmidt, Jr., President and Chief Executive Officer
Web address: www.uhsi.org
Control: Other not–for–profit (including NFP Corporation) **Service:** General Medical and Surgical

Staffed Beds: 189 **Admissions:** 9391 **Census:** 108 **Outpatient Visits:** 334951 **Births:** 733 **Total Expense ($000):** 178353 **Payroll Expense ($000):** 79826 **Personnel:** 1429

PORTAGE—Columbia County

□ **DIVINE SAVIOR HEALTHCARE (520041)**, 2817 New Pinery Road, Zip 53901–0387, Mailing Address: P.O. Box 387, Zip 53901–0387; tel. 608/742–4131, (Total facility includes 110 beds in nursing home–type unit) **A**1 9 10 **F**3 13 15 16 17 26 27 30 31 32 33 41 46 48 50 53 54 55 56 57 61 62 65 66 67 68 72 73 75 76 78 79 80 81 82 86 87 88 92 96 100 103 105 106 107 117 118 119 120 121 122 124 132 134 135 136 137 **P**6
Primary Contact: Michael Decker, President and Chief Executive Officer
Web address: www.dshealthcare.com
Control: Church–operated, Nongovernment, not–for profit **Service:** General Medical and Surgical

Staffed Beds: 162 **Admissions:** 2481 **Census:** 110 **Outpatient Visits:** 129509 **Births:** 313 **Total Expense ($000):** 48531 **Payroll Expense ($000):** 22820 **Personnel:** 478

PRAIRIE DU CHIEN—Crawford County

★□ **PRAIRIE DU CHIEN MEMORIAL HOSPITAL (521330)**, 705 East Taylor Street, Zip 53821–2196; tel. 608/357–2000 **A**1 9 10 18 **F**2 4 15 16 17 30 31 32 42 54 61 62 65 67 68 70 73 74 75 78 79 81 82 86 88 96 100 119 120
Primary Contact: Harold W. Brown, Chief Executive Officer
COO: M. Connie Achenbach, Assistant Administrator and Chief Operating Officer
CFO: Dave Breitbach, Chief Financial Officer
CHR: Laurie Hampton, Director Human Resources
Web address: www.pdcmemorialhospital.org
Control: Other not–for–profit (including NFP Corporation) **Service:** General Medical and Surgical

Staffed Beds: 10 **Admissions:** 1335 **Census:** 20 **Outpatient Visits:** 31019 **Births:** 168 **Total Expense ($000):** 22274 **Payroll Expense ($000):** 11191 **Personnel:** 239

PRAIRIE DU SAC—Sauk County

★□ **SAUK PRAIRIE MEMORIAL HOSPITAL (520095)**, 80 First Street, Zip 53578–1599; tel. 608/643–3311 **A**1 9 10 **F**3 4 8 11 13 15 17 25 26 28 30 31 32 34 38 40 50 52 53 54 55 56 57 62 66 67 68 73 74 76 77 78 79 80 81 84 85 86 87 96 102 106 107 118 119 120 121 122 133 135 **P**6
Primary Contact: Larry Schroeder, Chief Executive Officer
CMO: John McAuliffe, M.D., Medical Director
CHR: Robbi Murphy, Director Human Resources
Web address: www.spmh.org
Control: Other not–for–profit (including NFP Corporation) **Service:** General Medical and Surgical

Staffed Beds: 17 **Admissions:** 2357 **Census:** 20 **Outpatient Visits:** 50761 **Births:** 275 **Total Expense ($000):** 33935 **Payroll Expense ($000):** 15100 **Personnel:** 344

RACINE—Racine County

★□ △ **WHEATON FRANCISCAN HEALTHCARE – ALL SAINTS (520096)**, (Formerly All Saints Healthcare), 3801 Spring Street, Zip 53405–1690; tel. 262/687–4011, (Total facility includes 50 beds in nursing home–type unit) **A**1 2 3 5 7 9 10 **F**4 6 15 16 17 30 32 43 53 54 56 62 65 68 70 73 75 76 78 79 81 82 83 86 88 89 90 91 92 94 95 96 97 100 104 106 107 117 119 120 136 **P**6 **S** Wheaton Franciscan Healthcare
Primary Contact: Kenneth R. Buser, President and Chief Executive Officer
COO: Susan Boland, Senior Vice President and Chief Operating Officer
CFO: John Skeans, Vice President Finance and Chief Financial Officer
CIO: Joanne Bisterfeldt, Chief Information Officer
Web address: www.allsaintshealth.com
Control: Church–operated, Nongovernment, not–for profit **Service:** General Medical and Surgical

Staffed Beds: 389 **Admissions:** 16871 **Census:** 262 **Outpatient Visits:** 446577 **Births:** 1983 **Total Expense ($000):** 355090 **Payroll Expense ($000):** 168842 **Personnel:** 2614

Hospital, Medicare Provider Number, Address, Telephone, Approval, Facility, and Physician Codes, Health Care System

★ American Hospital Association (AHA) membership
□ The Joint Commission accreditation
○ American Osteopathic Association (AOA) accreditation
△ Commission on Accreditation of Rehabilitation Facilities (CARF) accreditation

REEDSBURG—Sauk County

★ **REEDSBURG AREA MEDICAL CENTER (521351)**, 2000 North Dewey Street, Zip 53959–1097; tel. 608/524–6487 **A**1 9 10 18 **F**3 8 11 13 15 17 25 26 27 30 31 32 33 34 36 38 40 43 46 48 50 52 56 62 64 68 74 75 76 77 78 79 80 81 83 84 86 87 96 97 102 106 118 119 121 122 133 135 **P**6
Primary Contact: Robert Van Meeteren, President and Chief Executive Officer
Web address: www.ramchealth.com
Control: Other not–for–profit (including NFP Corporation) **Service:** General Medical and Surgical

Staffed Beds: 25 **Admissions:** 2144 **Census:** 18 **Outpatient Visits:** 58913 **Births:** 275 **Total Expense ($000):** 31386 **Payroll Expense ($000):** 12926 **Personnel:** 284

RHINELANDER—Oneida County

★ **SACRED HEART–ST. MARY'S HOSPITALS (520019)**, 2251 North Shore Drive, Zip 54501–3998; tel. 715/361–2000, (Includes ST. MARY'S HOSPITAL) **A**1 9 10 20 **F**5 13 15 17 24 25 30 31 32 38 43 56 62 67 68 73 74 75 76 78 79 81 82 84 88 89 90 91 92 93 94 95 96 97 100 104 106 107 119 120 133 136 **S** Marian Health System
Primary Contact: Monica Hilt, President and Chief Operating Officer
COO: William A. Erickson, Vice President and Chief Operating Officer
CFO: Jack P. Sutliff, Vice President and Chief Financial Officer
Web address: www.ministryhealth.org
Control: Church–operated, Nongovernment, not–for profit **Service:** General Medical and Surgical

Staffed Beds: 45 **Admissions:** 4242 **Census:** 40 **Outpatient Visits:** 73914 **Births:** 363 **Total Expense ($000):** 96235 **Payroll Expense ($000):** 39776 **Personnel:** 570

RICE LAKE—Barron County

★ **LAKEVIEW MEDICAL CENTER (520011)**, 1100 North Main Street, Zip 54868–1238; tel. 715/234–1515 **A**1 9 10 20 **F**3 16 17 30 31 42 43 55 56 61 63 65 66 67 68 73 77 78 79 80 81 83 86 88 96 102 106 107 118 119 120 121 122 135 137
Primary Contact: Edward H. Wolf, President and Chief Executive Officer
COO: Howard P. Johnson, MS, Vice President and Chief Operating Officer
CFO: Jacqueline Klein, Vice President Finance
CIO: Brad Gerrits, Director Information Systems
CHR: Howard P. Johnson, MS, Vice President and Chief Operating Officer
Web address: www.lakeviewmedical.com
Control: Other not–for–profit (including NFP Corporation) **Service:** General Medical and Surgical

Staffed Beds: 69 **Admissions:** 2774 **Census:** 24 **Outpatient Visits:** 49607 **Births:** 457 **Total Expense ($000):** 37583 **Payroll Expense ($000):** 17887 **Personnel:** 332

RICHLAND CENTER—Richland County

☐ **RICHLAND HOSPITAL (521341)**, 333 East Second Street, Zip 53581–1899; tel. 608/647–6321 **A**1 9 10 18 **F**6 13 15 17 24 31 32 38 40 54 56 62 68 73 74 75 76 78 79 81 84 96 100 107 119 120
Primary Contact: Steven R. Nockerts, Chief Executive Officer
CFO: Charles Aber, Chief Financial Officer
CMO: Kay Balink, M.D., Chief of Staff
CIO: Jerry Cooper, Manager Data Processing
CHR: Rhonda Sutton, Director Human Resources
Web address: www.richlandhospital.com
Control: Other not–for–profit (including NFP Corporation) **Service:** General Medical and Surgical

Staffed Beds: 25 **Admissions:** 1509 **Census:** 14 **Outpatient Visits:** 22843 **Births:** 202 **Total Expense ($000):** 25379 **Payroll Expense ($000):** 10869 **Personnel:** 238

RIPON—Fond Du Lac County

★ **RIPON MEDICAL CENTER (521321)**, 933 Newbury Street, Zip 54971–1798, Mailing Address: P.O. Box 390, Zip 54971–0390; tel. 920/748–3101 **A**1 9 10 18 **F**3 8 11 15 17 25 31 32 33 38 40 43 51 52 53 54 55 56 57 62 66 67 68 73 75 76 77 78 79 80 81 82 83 84 86 87 90 94 96 102 107 119 120 121 122 123 124 133 135 **S** Brim Healthcare, Inc.
Primary Contact: Jean Surguy, Interim Chief Executive Officer
CFO: Bobbie Pollesch, Chief Financial Officer
CIO: Wayne Johnston, Director Information Systems
CHR: George Truell, Director Human Resources
Web address: www.riponmedicalcenter.com
Control: Other not–for–profit (including NFP Corporation) **Service:** General Medical and Surgical

Staffed Beds: 23 **Admissions:** 755 **Census:** 9 **Outpatient Visits:** 37735 **Births:** 0 **Total Expense ($000):** 15970 **Payroll Expense ($000):** 6618 **Personnel:** 137

RIVER FALLS—St. Croix County

★ **RIVER FALLS AREA HOSPITAL (521349)**, 1629 East Division Street, Zip 54022–1571; tel. 715/425–6155 **A**1 9 10 18 **F**13 15 24 25 31 32 38 43 52 56 62 74 75 76 78 79 81 82 84 85 86 96 107 119 120 136 **S** Allina Hospitals & Clinics
Primary Contact: Randy Farrow, President
CFO: Tom Halada, Director Finance
CHR: Kristen Stoehr, Manager Human Resources
Web address: www.allina.com
Control: Other not–for–profit (including NFP Corporation) **Service:** General Medical and Surgical

Staffed Beds: 25 **Admissions:** 1658 **Census:** 11 **Outpatient Visits:** 17416 **Births:** 267 **Total Expense ($000):** 23821 **Payroll Expense ($000):** 9258 **Personnel:** 141

SHAWANO—Shawano County

★ **SHAWANO MEDICAL CENTER (521346)**, 309 North Bartlette Street, Zip 54166; tel. 715/526–2111 **A**1 9 10 18 **F**3 4 15 16 17 26 30 31 32 33 37 42 43 44 54 55 56 57 62 65 68 73 74 75 78 79 80 81 82 86 87 88 92 96 100 102 107 118 120 121 122 124 135 **P**5 **S** Brim Healthcare, Inc.
Primary Contact: James E. Baer, FACHE, Chief Executive Officer
CFO: Vince Studer, Chief Financial Officer
CMO: Tod Lewis, M.D., President Medical Staff
CIO: Ken Zade, Manager Information Technology
CHR: Mark Gabavics, Director Human Resources
Web address: www.shawanomed.org
Control: Other not–for–profit (including NFP Corporation) **Service:** General Medical and Surgical

Staffed Beds: 25 **Admissions:** 2065 **Census:** 16 **Outpatient Visits:** 46979 **Births:** 405 **Total Expense ($000):** 31173 **Payroll Expense ($000):** 13323 **Personnel:** 252

SHEBOYGAN—Sheboygan County

★ **AURORA SHEBOYGAN MEMORIAL MEDICAL CENTER (520035)**, 2629 North Seventh Street, Zip 53083–4998; tel. 920/451–5000 **A**1 2 9 10 **F**3 4 5 8 11 13 15 17 25 26 27 30 31 32 33 38 40 41 43 48 49 50 52 53 54 56 57 62 68 72 73 74 76 77 78 79 80 81 82 84 86 88 89 90 91 92 93 94 96 100 103 104 105 106 107 118 119 121 124 133 135 136 **S** Aurora Health Care
Primary Contact: Bobbe Teigen, Vice President and Chief Administrative Officer
CFO: Robin Pedersen, Vice President Finance
CMO: John T. Livermore, M.D., President Medical Staff
CIO: Steve Serketich, Manager Information Services
CHR: Carla LaFever, Director Human Resources
Web address: www.aurorahealthcare.org
Control: Other not–for–profit (including NFP Corporation) **Service:** General Medical and Surgical

Staffed Beds: 135 **Admissions:** 6327 **Census:** 59 **Outpatient Visits:** 78180 **Births:** 1170 **Total Expense ($000):** 81176 **Payroll Expense ($000):** 29482 **Personnel:** 668

★ △ **ST. NICHOLAS HOSPITAL (520044)**, 3100 Superior Avenue, Zip 53081; tel. 920/459–8300 **A**1 2 7 9 10 **F**3 4 15 16 17 26 27 30 31 32 37 38 41 42 43 44 49 53 54 55 56 57 61 62 63 65 66 68 70 72 73 74 75 76 77 78 79 80 81 82 85 86 88 96 100 102 106 107 109 118 119 121 124 135 136 137 **P**5 **S** Hospital Sisters Health System
Primary Contact: Mary T. Brasseaux, Chief Executive Officer
CFO: Donald R. Pieters, Assistant Administrator Financial and Support Services
CMO: Vytas K. Kerpe, M.D., President Medical Staff
CHR: Christine F. Jensema, Administrative Director Human Resources
Web address: www.stnicholashospital.org
Control: Church–operated, Nongovernment, not–for profit **Service:** General Medical and Surgical

Staffed Beds: 78 **Admissions:** 3281 **Census:** 37 **Outpatient Visits:** 108323 **Births:** 282 **Total Expense ($000):** 59688 **Payroll Expense ($000):** 23008 **Personnel:** 387

SHELL LAKE—Washburn County

☐ **INDIANHEAD MEDICAL CENTER (521342)**, 113 Fourth Avenue, Zip 54871, Mailing Address: P.O. Box 300, Zip 54871–0300; tel. 715/468–7833 **A**1 9 10 18 **F**11 13 15 17 24 30 31 32 38 54 56 61 62 68 74 75 76 78 79 81 82 84 96 107 119 120 **P**5 **S** Mid Atlantic Health Management, Inc.
Primary Contact: Paul Naglosky, Administrator
CFO: Michael Elliott, Controller
CMO: Allan Haesemeyer, M.D., Chief of Staff
CHR: Gwen Nielsen, Manager Human Resources
Control: Corporation, Investor–owned, for–profit **Service:** General Medical and Surgical

Staffed Beds: 25 **Admissions:** 571 **Census:** 4 **Outpatient Visits:** 11345 **Births:** 20 **Total Expense ($000):** 5495 **Payroll Expense ($000):** 2276 **Personnel:** 67

Many Facility Codes have changed. Please refer to the AHA Guide Code Chart.

SPARTA—Monroe County

□ **FRANCISCAN SKEMP HEALTHCARE–SPARTA CAMPUS (521305)**, 310 West Main Street, Zip 54656–2171; tel. 608/269–2132 **A**1 9 10 18 **F**3 11 13 15 26 27 30 31 32 40 55 56 57 62 63 65 66 73 74 75 76 77 78 79 80 81 82 84 86 87 96 107 119 122 124 136 **P**8 **S** Mayo Foundation
Primary Contact: Robert M. Tracey, Administrator
Web address: www.mayohealthsystem.com
Control: Church–operated, Nongovernment, not–for profit **Service:** General Medical and Surgical

Staffed Beds: 25 **Admissions:** 476 **Census:** 6 **Outpatient Visits:** 31812
Births: 90 **Total Expense ($000):** 9927 **Payroll Expense ($000):** 5406
Personnel: 99

SPOONER—Washburn County

★ **SPOONER HEALTH SYSTEM (521332)**, 819 Ash Street, Zip 54801–1299; tel. 715/635–2111, (Total facility includes 90 beds in nursing home–type unit) **A**9 10 18 **F**3 4 15 16 27 30 31 32 33 38 44 50 54 55 56 57 61 62 65 66 67 68 69 70 73 76 78 79 80 81 82 85 86 96 97 100 102 107 117 119 121 122 124 135 137 **S** Brim Healthcare, Inc.
Primary Contact: Michael Schafer, Chief Executive Officer and Administrator
CFO: Rebecca Busch, Chief Financial Officer
CHR: Cindy Rouzer, Human Resources Director
Web address: www.spoonerhealthsystem.com
Control: Other not–for–profit (including NFP Corporation) **Service:** General Medical and Surgical

Staffed Beds: 115 **Admissions:** 922 **Census:** 95 **Outpatient Visits:** 16005
Births: 83 **Total Expense ($000):** 11228 **Payroll Expense ($000):** 5705
Personnel: 127

ST. CROIX FALLS—Polk County

ST. CROIX REGIONAL MEDICAL CENTER (521337), 235 State Street, Zip 54024–9400; tel. 715/483–3261 **A**9 10 18 **F**4 6 13 15 16 17 30 31 32 43 54 56 62 65 68 70 73 75 76 78 79 81 82 85 86 88 89 90 91 93 94 96 97 100 104 106 107 114 120 136 **P**5
Primary Contact: Leonard B. Libis, Chief Executive Officer
CFO: John Tremble, Chief Financial Officer
CMO: William Beyer, M.D., Chief Medical Officer
CIO: Duane Laabs, Director Management Information
CHR: Cathy Gray, Executive Director Human Resources
Web address: www.scrmc.org
Control: Other not–for–profit (including NFP Corporation) **Service:** General Medical and Surgical

Staffed Beds: 15 **Admissions:** 1741 **Census:** 13 **Outpatient Visits:** 127131
Births: 312 **Total Expense ($000):** 41309 **Payroll Expense ($000):** 13876
Personnel: 324

STANLEY—Chippewa County

★ **OUR LADY OF VICTORY HOSPITAL (521311)**, 1120 Pine Street, Zip 54768–0220, Mailing Address: P.O. Box 220, Zip 54768–0220; tel. 715/644–5571 **A**9 10 18 **F**3 15 17 26 31 32 40 44 50 55 56 57 63 68 73 75 78 79 80 81 82 84 85 86 87 96 102 119 120 121 122 133 135 **P**6 **S** Marian Health System
Primary Contact: Cynthia Eichman, President and Chief Executive Officer
CFO: Linda Klapperich, Director Financial Services
CIO: Eric Haglund, Director Information Systems
Web address: www.ministryhealth.org
Control: Other not–for–profit (including NFP Corporation) **Service:** General Medical and Surgical

Staffed Beds: 24 **Admissions:** 629 **Census:** 10 **Outpatient Visits:** 24740
Births: 0 **Total Expense ($000):** 18300 **Payroll Expense ($000):** 6805
Personnel: 117

STEVENS POINT—Portage County

★□ **SAINT MICHAEL'S HOSPITAL (520002)**, 900 Illinois Avenue, Zip 54481–3196; tel. 715/346–5000 **A**1 9 10 19 **F**4 5 13 15 17 24 25 30 31 32 38 40 43 51 54 56 59 62 68 70 73 74 75 76 78 79 81 82 83 84 86 88 89 90 91 92 93 94 95 96 97 100 104 106 107 114 119 120 133 **S** Marian Health System
Primary Contact: Bradley Neet, President
COO: Bradley Neet, President and Chief Operating Officer
CFO: William J. Hinner, Vice President Fiscal Services and Chief Financial Officer
CIO: Will Weider, Chief Information Officer
Web address: www.saintmichaelshospital.org
Control: Church–operated, Nongovernment, not–for profit **Service:** General Medical and Surgical

Staffed Beds: 48 **Admissions:** 4151 **Census:** 36 **Outpatient Visits:** 458249
Births: 685 **Total Expense ($000):** 151172 **Payroll Expense ($000):** 42362
Personnel: 932

STOUGHTON—Dane County

□ **STOUGHTON HOSPITAL ASSOCIATION (521343)**, 900 Ridge Street, Zip 53589–1896; tel. 608/873–6611 **A**1 9 10 18 **F**3 4 6 8 11 15 17 25 26 30 31 33 34 38 39 43 53 54 55 56 57 62 66 68 75 77 78 79 80 81 82 84 85 86 88 93 96 100 102 107 118 119 120 121 122 133 135 136 137
Primary Contact: Terrence Brenny, President and Chief Executive Officer
COO: Kristi Hund, Vice President Patient Services
CFO: Karen Myers, Vice President Financial Services
CMO: Richard Hill, M.D., Chief of Staff
CIO: Karen Myers, Vice President Financial Services
CHR: Chris Schmitz, Manager Human Resources
Web address: www.stoughtonhospital.com
Control: Other not–for–profit (including NFP Corporation) **Service:** General Medical and Surgical

Staffed Beds: 32 **Admissions:** 1425 **Census:** 19 **Outpatient Visits:** 41043
Births: 0 **Total Expense ($000):** 27168 **Payroll Expense ($000):** 11902
Personnel: 259

STURGEON BAY—Door County

★□ **DOOR COUNTY MEMORIAL HOSPITAL (521358)**, 323 South 18th Avenue, Zip 54235–1495; tel. 920/743–5566, (Total facility includes 30 beds in nursing home–type unit) **A**1 9 10 18 **F**2 3 11 13 15 17 25 26 27 28 30 31 32 33 37 40 43 44 54 55 56 57 60 62 63 64 66 68 73 74 75 76 77 78 79 80 81 82 84 85 86 87 96 99 100 102 105 107 114 117 118 119 121 122 124 133 134 137 **P**1 **S** Marian Health System
Primary Contact: Gerald M. Worrick, President and Chief Executive Officer
CFO: Robert C. Scieszinski, Vice President Finance
CIO: Mary Lopas, Chief Information Officer
CHR: Sandy McKuen, Vice President Human Resources
Web address: www.dcmh.org
Control: Church–operated, Nongovernment, not–for profit **Service:** General Medical and Surgical

Staffed Beds: 55 **Admissions:** 2110 **Census:** 46 **Outpatient Visits:** 71762
Births: 184 **Total Expense ($000):** 46116 **Payroll Expense ($000):** 23103
Personnel: 486

SUPERIOR—Douglas County

★□ **ST. MARY'S HOSPITAL OF SUPERIOR (521329)**, 3500 Tower Avenue, Zip 54880–5395; tel. 715/395–5400 **A**1 9 10 18 **F**4 15 16 17 30 31 32 54 56 62 65 68 70 73 74 75 76 78 79 81 82 86 88 96 107 119 120 **S** Essentia Health
Primary Contact: Mary Shaw, Chief Operating Officer
Web address: www.smdc.org
Control: Other not–for–profit (including NFP Corporation) **Service:** General Medical and Surgical

Staffed Beds: 25 **Admissions:** 611 **Census:** 14 **Outpatient Visits:** 48664
Births: 0 **Total Expense ($000):** 27963 **Payroll Expense ($000):** 14198
Personnel: 194

TOMAH—Monroe County

★□ **TOMAH MEMORIAL HOSPITAL (521320)**, 321 Butts Avenue, Zip 54660–1412; tel. 608/372–2181 **A**1 9 10 18 **F**3 11 13 26 27 31 32 33 40 41 42 43 44 54 55 56 57 62 67 73 74 75 77 78 79 80 81 82 84 86 96 100 103 107 119 122 124 133 137 **S** Brim Healthcare, Inc.
Primary Contact: Philip Stuart, Administrator and Chief Executive Officer
CFO: Joseph Zeps, Vice President Finance
Web address: www.tomahhospital.org
Control: Other not–for–profit (including NFP Corporation) **Service:** General Medical and Surgical

Staffed Beds: 25 **Admissions:** 1242 **Census:** 11 **Outpatient Visits:** 19403
Births: 269 **Total Expense ($000):** 20714 **Payroll Expense ($000):** 8020
Personnel: 223

WI

Hospital, Medicare Provider Number, Address, Telephone, Approval, Facility, and Physician Codes, Health Care System
★ American Hospital Association (AHA) membership
□ The Joint Commission accreditation
○ American Osteopathic Association (AOA) accreditation
△ Commission on Accreditation of Rehabilitation Facilities (CARF) accreditation

★ △ **VETERANS AFFAIRS MEDICAL CENTER**, 500 East Veterans Street, Zip 54660; tel. 608/372–3971, (Total facility includes 200 beds in nursing home–type unit) **A**1 7 **F**3 6 16 17 26 30 31 32 33 37 41 42 43 44 45 50 53 54 55 56 57 61 62 63 64 65 66 68 72 73 74 75 76 78 80 81 82 83 84 85 86 87 88 90 91 92 93 94 107 117 119 120 121 124 132 135 136 137 **S** Department of Veterans Affairs
Primary Contact: Jerald D. Molnar, Acting Medical Center Director
COO: Jerald D. Molnar, Associate Director
CFO: Donna Welch, Line Manager Resources Service
CMO: David Houlihan, M.D., Chief of Staff
CIO: John Hina, Information Technologist
CHR: Susan Peters, Personnel Specialist
Web address: www.va.gov/tomahvamc
Control: Veterans Affairs, Government, federal **Service:** General Medical and Surgical

Staffed Beds: 271 **Admissions:** 1135 **Census:** 196 **Outpatient Visits:** 149413 **Births:** 0 **Total Expense ($000):** 83308 **Payroll Expense ($000):** 39363 **Personnel:** 784

TOMAHAWK—Lincoln County

☐ **SACRED HEART HOSPITAL (521313)**, 401 West Mohawk Drive, Zip 54487; tel. 715/453–7700 **A**1 9 10 18 **F**15 17 24 25 30 31 32 38 43 52 54 56 62 68 73 75 78 79 81 82 84 86 89 90 91 92 93 94 95 96 107 119 120 136
Control: Church–operated, Nongovernment, not–for profit **Service:** General Medical and Surgical

Staffed Beds: 9 **Admissions:** 658 **Census:** 6 **Outpatient Visits:** 15607 **Births:** 0 **Total Expense ($000):** 11021 **Payroll Expense ($000):** 5228 **Personnel:** 84

TWO RIVERS—Manitowoc County

★ **AURORA MEDICAL CENTER – MANITOWOC COUNTY (520034)**, 5000 Memorial Drive, Zip 54241–2399; tel. 920/794–5000 **A**1 9 10 **F**3 11 13 25 26 27 30 31 32 33 34 38 40 41 43 44 48 49 50 54 55 56 57 62 73 74 76 77 78 79 80 81 82 84 86 96 102 107 109 111 118 119 120 121 122 124 132 133 135 136 137 **S** Aurora Health Care
Primary Contact: Steve Long, Vice President and Chief Administrative Officer
CFO: Sandra Ewald, Vice President Finance
Web address: www.aurorahealthcare.org
Control: Other not–for–profit (including NFP Corporation) **Service:** General Medical and Surgical

Staffed Beds: 63 **Admissions:** 2678 **Census:** 28 **Outpatient Visits:** 51745 **Births:** 310 **Total Expense ($000):** 41452 **Payroll Expense ($000):** 15373 **Personnel:** 342

VIROQUA—Vernon County

VERNON MEMORIAL HEALTHCARE (521348), 507 South Main Street, Zip 54665–2096; tel. 608/637–2101 **A**9 10 18 **F**3 5 13 15 25 30 31 32 33 34 35 40 42 43 52 54 55 56 57 61 73 74 75 77 78 79 81 82 84 86 87 96 102 107 119 120 121 122 124 133 135 **P**6
Primary Contact: Garith W. Steiner, Chief Executive Officer and Administrator
COO: Kyle Bakkum, Chief Operating Officer
CFO: Mary Koenig, Chief Financial Officer
CIO: Julie Steiner, Manager Marketing and Public Relations
CHR: Kay Starr, Manager Human Resources
Web address: www.vmh.org
Control: Other not–for–profit (including NFP Corporation) **Service:** General Medical and Surgical

Staffed Beds: 17 **Admissions:** 1561 **Census:** 13 **Outpatient Visits:** 74642 **Births:** 177 **Total Expense ($000):** 36942 **Payroll Expense ($000):** 16473 **Personnel:** 239

WATERFORD—Racine County

☐ **LAKEVIEW SPECIALTY HOSPITAL AND REHABILITATION CENTER (522005)**, 1701 Sharp Road, Zip 53185; tel. 262/534–7297, (Nonreporting) **A**1 10
Primary Contact: Tony Merka, President and Chief Executive Officer
Web address: www.lakeviewsystem.com
Control: Corporation, Investor–owned, for–profit **Service:** Long–Term Acute Care hospital

Staffed Beds: 39

WATERTOWN—Dodge County

★ **WATERTOWN MEMORIAL HOSPITAL (520116)**, 125 Hospital Drive, Zip 53098–3384; tel. 920/261–4210 **A**1 9 10 **F**2 3 5 10 11 13 15 17 25 31 32 33 34 35 40 43 53 54 55 56 57 61 62 63 66 67 68 69 73 74 75 76 77 78 79 81 82 83 84 86 94 96 100 101 102 106 107 115 118 119 120 121 122 124 132 133 135 136 137 **P**7 8
Primary Contact: John P. Kosanovich, President
CFO: John Graf, Senior Vice President
CMO: Mohamed Yafai, M.D., Chief of Staff
CIO: Jennifer Laughlin, Vice President and Chief Information Officer
CHR: Duane Floyd, Vice President Human Resources and Support Services
Web address: www.wahs.com
Control: Other not–for–profit (including NFP Corporation) **Service:** General Medical and Surgical

Staffed Beds: 51 **Admissions:** 2693 **Census:** 29 **Outpatient Visits:** 138858 **Births:** 343 **Total Expense ($000):** 52822 **Payroll Expense ($000):** 24844 **Personnel:** 487

WAUKESHA—Waukesha County

WAUKESHA COUNTY MENTAL HEALTH CENTER (524026), 25042 West Northview Road, Zip 53186; tel. 262/548–7950 **A**10 **F**4 30 31 32 88 119
Primary Contact: William T. Pratt, Administrator
Control: County–Government, nonfederal **Service:** Psychiatric

Staffed Beds: 28 **Admissions:** 1112 **Census:** 126 **Outpatient Visits:** 0 **Births:** 0 **Total Expense ($000):** 5196 **Payroll Expense ($000):** 2465 **Personnel:** 58

★ △ **WAUKESHA MEMORIAL HOSPITAL (520008)**, 725 American Avenue, Zip 53188–5099; tel. 262/928–1000 **A**1 2 3 5 7 9 10 **F**4 6 11 13 15 17 24 25 30 31 32 38 40 43 53 54 56 62 67 68 70 73 74 75 76 78 79 81 84 85 86 88 89 90 91 92 93 95 96 97 100 104 106 107 119 120 133 136 **S** ProHealth Care
Primary Contact: Edward A. Olson, President and Chief Executive Officer
CFO: Robert W. Mlynarek, Vice President Finance
CMO: James D. Gardner, M.D., Vice President Medical Staff
CIO: William Miller, Vice President Information Services
Web address: www.waukeshamemorial.org
Control: Other not–for–profit (including NFP Corporation) **Service:** General Medical and Surgical

Staffed Beds: 330 **Admissions:** 16955 **Census:** 207 **Outpatient Visits:** 299415 **Births:** 2242 **Total Expense ($000):** 309598 **Payroll Expense ($000):** 103370 **Personnel:** 1894

WAUPACA—Waupaca County

★ **RIVERSIDE MEDICAL CENTER (521334)**, 800 Riverside Drive, Zip 54981–1999; tel. 715/258–1000 **A**1 9 10 18 **F**11 13 15 17 24 25 38 43 54 56 62 68 74 75 76 78 79 81 82 83 84 85 96 107 119 133 136
Primary Contact: Craig A. Kantos, Chief Executive Officer
CFO: Kerry Lee Blanke, Director Financial Services
CMO: Joseph McCausland, D.O., Chief of Staff
CIO: Cathy Reynertson, Manager Management Information Systems
CHR: Kevin Gossens, Director Human Resources
Web address: www.riversidemedical.org
Control: Other not–for–profit (including NFP Corporation) **Service:** General Medical and Surgical

Staffed Beds: 25 **Admissions:** 1717 **Census:** 14 **Outpatient Visits:** 50684 **Births:** 204 **Total Expense ($000):** 27335 **Payroll Expense ($000):** 12142 **Personnel:** 244

WAUPUN—Fond Du Lac County

★ **WAUPUN MEMORIAL HOSPITAL (521327)**, 620 West Brown Street, Zip 53963–1799; tel. 920/324–5581 **A**1 9 10 18 **F**4 15 16 30 31 32 43 53 56 62 65 67 68 70 73 74 78 79 81 96 97 100 104 107 119
Primary Contact: DeAnn Thurmer, Chief Operating Officer
CFO: Steven N. Little, Chief Financial Officer
Web address: www.agnesian.com
Control: Church–operated, Nongovernment, not–for profit **Service:** General Medical and Surgical

Staffed Beds: 25 **Admissions:** 1195 **Census:** 11 **Outpatient Visits:** 42190 **Births:** 138 **Total Expense ($000):** 22248 **Payroll Expense ($000):** 8391 **Personnel:** 173

WI

WAUSAU—Marathon County

★ △ **ASPIRUS WAUSAU HOSPITAL (520030)**, 333 Pine Ridge Boulevard, Zip 54401–4187, Mailing Address: P.O. Box 1847, Zip 54402–1847; tel. 715/847–2121 **A**1 2 3 5 7 9 10 **F**3 4 8 15 16 17 26 30 31 32 33 42 43 44 45 46 49 50 54 55 56 57 62 65 66 68 69 70 72 73 75 76 77 78 79 80 81 82 83 84 85 86 88 89 90 92 93 94 95 96 99 100 101 102 103 104 106 107 108 109 111 116 118 119 121 134 135 136 137
Primary Contact: Duane L. Erwin, President and Chief Executive Officer
COO: Diane Postler–Slattery, Ph.D., Chief Operating Officer
CFO: Sidney C. Sczygelski, Senior Vice President Finance and Chief Financial Officer
CMO: Jamie Roche, M.D., Interim Senior Vice President Medical Affairs
CIO: Alan Wyman, Vice President Information Technology
CHR: Roger Lucas, Vice President Human Resources
Web address: www.aspirus.org
Control: Other not–for–profit (including NFP Corporation) **Service:** General Medical and Surgical

Staffed Beds: 252 **Admissions:** 14659 **Census:** 165 **Outpatient Visits:** 97512 **Births:** 1240 **Total Expense ($000):** 237545 **Payroll Expense ($000):** 85226 **Personnel:** 1966

NORTH CENTRAL HEALTH CARE FACILITIES (524017), 1100 Lakeview Drive, Zip 54403–6799; tel. 715/848–4600, (Total facility includes 320 beds in nursing home–type unit) **A**9 10 **F**4 5 6 25 31 32 33 36 53 54 62 73 81 86 88 89 90 91 92 93 94 95 117 119 121 132 135
Primary Contact: Gary Bezucha, FACHE, Chief Executive Officer
CFO: Brenda Glodowski, Chief Financial Officer
Web address: www.norcen.org
Control: County–Government, nonfederal **Service:** Psychiatric

Staffed Beds: 358 **Admissions:** 1360 **Census:** 318 **Outpatient Visits:** 208995 **Births:** 0 **Total Expense ($000):** 39980 **Payroll Expense ($000):** 16894 **Personnel:** 268

WAUWATOSA—Milwaukee County

★ **AURORA PSYCHIATRIC HOSPITAL (524000)**, 1220 Dewey Avenue, Zip 53213–2598; tel. 414/454–6600 **A**1 9 10 **F**4 5 25 26 30 31 32 33 41 50 53 57 62 66 73 81 82 88 89 90 91 92 94 95 119 121 124 **S** Aurora Health Care
Primary Contact: Peter Carlson, Administrator
CFO: David Eager, Vice President Finance
CMO: Anthony Meyer, M.D., Medical Director
CIO: Philip Loftus, Ph.D., Vice President and Chief Information Officer
CHR: Barbara Molthen, Director Human Resources
Web address: www.aurorahealthcare.org
Control: Other not–for–profit (including NFP Corporation) **Service:** Psychiatric

Staffed Beds: 68 **Admissions:** 3610 **Census:** 42 **Outpatient Visits:** 93557 **Births:** 0 **Total Expense ($000):** 27551 **Payroll Expense ($000):** 13518 **Personnel:** 284

★ **THE WISCONSIN HEART HOSPITAL (520199)**, 10000 West Bluemound Road, Zip 53226; tel. 414/778–7800 **A**1 9 10 **F**17 25 30 31 32 34 36 38 56 62 79 81 86 96 119 **P**8 **S** Wheaton Franciscan Healthcare
Primary Contact: Norma J. McCutcheon, President
CFO: Greg Kopp, Vice President Business and Support Services
CHR: Robert Bauer, Manager Human Resources
Web address: www.twhh.org
Control: Partnership, Investor–owned, for–profit **Service:** General Medical and Surgical

Staffed Beds: 30 **Admissions:** 2082 **Census:** 17 **Outpatient Visits:** 8254 **Births:** 0 **Total Expense ($000):** 53517 **Payroll Expense ($000):** 12342 **Personnel:** 219

WEST ALLIS—Milwaukee County

★ △ **AURORA WEST ALLIS MEDICAL CENTER (520139)**, (Formerly West Allis Memorial Hospital), 8901 West Lincoln Avenue, Zip 53227–0901, Mailing Address: P.O. Box 27901, Zip 53227–0901; tel. 414/328–6000 **A**1 2 7 9 10 **F**1 2 3 11 13 15 25 26 27 30 31 32 33 34 35 38 40 41 43 49 50 51 53 54 55 56 57 62 63 68 70 72 73 74 76 77 78 79 80 81 82 84 85 86 87 90 92 96 97 99 100 102 106 107 109 111 113 114 116 118 119 121 123 124 135 136 137 **S** Aurora Health Care
Primary Contact: Richard A. Kellar, Administrator
CFO: David Eager, Vice President Finance
Web address: www.aurorahealthcare.org
Control: Other not–for–profit (including NFP Corporation) **Service:** General Medical and Surgical

Staffed Beds: 227 **Admissions:** 12588 **Census:** 149 **Outpatient Visits:** 157626 **Births:** 3121 **Total Expense ($000):** 176804 **Payroll Expense ($000):** 51583 **Personnel:** 1016

WEST BEND—Washington County

★ **ST. JOSEPH'S COMMUNITY HOSPITAL OF WEST BEND (520063)**, 3200 Pleasant Valley Road, Zip 53095; tel. 262/334–5533 **A**1 9 10 **F**3 4 15 26 27 30 31 32 33 41 44 46 47 48 49 50 53 55 56 57 65 66 67 68 72 73 74 75 76 77 78 79 80 81 85 88 90 92 93 96 100 102 103 105 107 108 109 118 119 121 124 132 135 137
Primary Contact: Michael J. Laird, FACHE, President
CFO: Mike Malzewski, Chief Financial Officer
CHR: Deb Lauenstein, Vice President Human Resources and Marketing
Web address: www.synergyhealth.org
Control: Other not–for–profit (including NFP Corporation) **Service:** General Medical and Surgical

Staffed Beds: 80 **Admissions:** 4847 **Census:** 57 **Outpatient Visits:** 70676 **Births:** 707 **Total Expense ($000):** 72154 **Payroll Expense ($000):** 28705 **Personnel:** 516

WESTON—Marathon County

★ **SAINT CLARE'S HOSPITAL (520202)**, 3400 Ministry Parkway, Zip 54476; tel. 715/393–3000 **A**1 9 **F**3 7 13 16 17 25 26 27 30 31 32 33 35 37 38 40 41 43 44 50 51 55 56 57 62 66 68 70 72 73 74 77 78 79 80 81 82 83 84 119 121 124 132 135 137 **P**6 8 **S** Marian Health System
Primary Contact: Mary T. Krueger, President
CMO: Larry T. Hegland, M.D., Chief Medical Officer
Web address: www.ministryhealth.org
Control: Church–operated, Nongovernment, not–for profit **Service:** General Medical and Surgical

Staffed Beds: 37 **Admissions:** 2146 **Census:** 19 **Outpatient Visits:** 8639 **Births:** 410 **Total Expense ($000):** 83296 **Payroll Expense ($000):** 30075 **Personnel:** 426

WHITEHALL—Trempealeau County

TRI–COUNTY MEMORIAL HOSPITAL (521316), 18601 Lincoln Street, Zip 54773–0065; tel. 715/538–4361, (Total facility includes 75 beds in nursing home–type unit) **A**9 10 18 **F**3 8 15 16 17 26 27 30 31 32 39 44 46 54 55 56 57 62 63 65 66 67 70 73 75 76 78 80 81 83 86 87 96 99 100 103 107 115 117 119 122 124 135 137
Primary Contact: Brian Theiler, President and Chief Executive Officer
CFO: Curtis A. Johnson, CPA, FACHE, Director Finance
Web address: www.gundluth.org
Control: Other not–for–profit (including NFP Corporation) **Service:** General Medical and Surgical

Staffed Beds: 100 **Admissions:** 575 **Census:** 70 **Outpatient Visits:** 4286 **Births:** 0 **Total Expense ($000):** 11931 **Payroll Expense ($000):** 5806 **Personnel:** 88

WILD ROSE—Waushara County

WILD ROSE COMMUNITY MEMORIAL HOSPITAL (521303), 601 Grove Avenue, Zip 54984, Mailing Address: P.O. Box 243, Zip 54984–0243; tel. 920/622–3257 **A**9 10 18 **F**10 11 15 25 30 31 38 40 43 54 56 62 73 75 78 79 81 84 85 86 89 90 91 92 93 94 96 107 133
Primary Contact: Donald Caves, President
CFO: Thomas P. Krystowiak, Vice President Finance
CMO: Dan Fifield, M.D., Chief of Staff
CHR: Karen M. West, Administrator Support Services
Web address: www.wildrosehospital.org
Control: Other not–for–profit (including NFP Corporation) **Service:** General Medical and Surgical

Staffed Beds: 25 **Admissions:** 317 **Census:** 3 **Outpatient Visits:** 16736 **Births:** 0 **Total Expense ($000):** 9264 **Payroll Expense ($000):** 3303 **Personnel:** 100

WINNEBAGO—Winnebago County

☐ **WINNEBAGO MENTAL HEALTH INSTITUTE (524002)**, Mailing Address: Box 9, Zip 54985–0009; tel. 920/235–4910 **A**1 10 **F**17 43 56 65 68 70 78 81 82 83 85 89 90 91 93 119 **P**6
Primary Contact: Joann B. O'Connor, Director and Chief Executive Officer
CMO: Randy Kerswill, M.D., Medical Director
CIO: Greg Schneider, Director Information Technology
CHR: Frances Dujon–Reynolds, Director Human Resources
Web address: www.dhfs.state.wi.us/mh_winnebago
Control: State–Government, nonfederal **Service:** Psychiatric

Staffed Beds: 242 **Admissions:** 1561 **Census:** 239 **Outpatient Visits:** 0 **Births:** 0 **Total Expense ($000):** 55183 **Payroll Expense ($000):** 31926 **Personnel:** 673

Hospital, Medicare Provider Number, Address, Telephone, Approval, Facility, and Physician Codes, Health Care System

★ American Hospital Association (AHA) membership
☐ The Joint Commission accreditation
○ American Osteopathic Association (AOA) accreditation
△ Commission on Accreditation of Rehabilitation Facilities (CARF) accreditation

WISCONSIN RAPIDS—Wood County

★ **RIVERVIEW HOSPITAL ASSOCIATION (520033)**, 410 Dewey Street, Zip 54494–4715, Mailing Address: P.O. Box 8080, Zip 54494–8080; tel. 715/423–6060, (Total facility includes 114 beds in nursing home–type unit) (Nonreporting) **A**1 9 10
Primary Contact: Celse A. Berard, President
CFO: Michael Bovee, Vice President Finance
CIO: Marge Tell, Director Information Services
CHR: Tom Hunsberger, Vice President Human Resources
Web address: www.rhahealthcare.org
Control: Other not–for–profit (including NFP Corporation) **Service:** General Medical and Surgical

Staffed Beds: 183

WOODRUFF—Oneida County

★ **HOWARD YOUNG MEDICAL CENTER (520091)**, 240 Maple Street, Zip 54568, Mailing Address: P.O. Box 470, Zip 54568–0470; tel. 715/356–8000 **A**1 9 10 **F**3 5 7 8 11 13 15 16 17 26 30 31 32 33 34 43 49 50 52 54 55 56 59 62 68 72 73 74 75 76 77 78 79 80 81 82 83 84 85 86 92 94 96 100 103 106 107 118 119 120 121 122 132 135 136 137 **S** Marian Health System
Primary Contact: Sheila Clough, President
CFO: Jack P. Sutliff, Vice President and Chief Financial Officer
CIO: Tom Wise, Director Information Technology Services
CHR: Michele Cornelius, Director Human Resources
Web address: www.ministryhealth.org
Control: Other not–for–profit (including NFP Corporation) **Service:** General Medical and Surgical

Staffed Beds: 65 **Admissions:** 3749 **Census:** 38 **Outpatient Visits:** 76447 **Births:** 343 **Total Expense ($000):** 58481 **Payroll Expense ($000):** 22733 **Personnel:** 452

WYOMING

AFTON—Lincoln County

★ **STAR VALLEY MEDICAL CENTER (531313)**, 901 Adams Street, Zip 83110–0579, Mailing Address: P.O. Box 579, Zip 83110–0579; tel. 307/885–5800, (Total facility includes 24 beds in nursing home–type unit) **A**9 10 18 **F**3 8 11 13 15 25 27 30 31 38 40 51 54 55 62 63 65 66 72 73 74 75 76 77 79 82 87 96 100 107 118 119 122 135 **P**6
Primary Contact: J. Steve Perry, Chief Executive Officer
CFO: Ken Brough, Chief Financial Officer
CMO: Scott Bennett, D.O., Chief of Staff
CIO: Marty Ashton, Chief Information Officer
CHR: Joel Johnson, Director Human Resources
Web address: www.svmcwy.org
Control: Hospital district or authority, Government, nonfederal **Service:** General Medical and Surgical

Staffed Beds: 40 **Admissions:** 657 **Census:** 28 **Outpatient Visits:** 13952 **Births:** 121 **Total Expense ($000):** 14855 **Payroll Expense ($000):** 6505 **Personnel:** 140

BASIN—Big Horn County

SOUTH BIG HORN COUNTY HOSPITAL (531301), 388 South U.S. Highway 20, Zip 82410; tel. 307/568–3311, (Total facility includes 37 beds in nursing home–type unit) **A**9 10 18 **F**31 32 38 62 87 96 117 119 **P**4
Primary Contact: Jackie Claudson, Administrator
Web address: www.midwayclinic.com
Control: Hospital district or authority, Government, nonfederal **Service:** General Medical and Surgical

Staffed Beds: 43 **Admissions:** 121 **Census:** 33 **Outpatient Visits:** 1265 **Births:** 0 **Total Expense ($000):** 2899 **Payroll Expense ($000):** 2194 **Personnel:** 56

BUFFALO—Johnson County

★ **JOHNSON COUNTY HEALTHCARE CENTER (531308)**, 497 West Lott Street, Zip 82834–1691; tel. 307/684–6188, (Total facility includes 50 beds in nursing home–type unit) **A**9 10 18 **F**6 11 13 15 24 27 30 32 38 42 55 61 65 68 74 76 77 79 84 96 107 119 122
Primary Contact: Sandy Ward, Administrator
CFO: Sandy Ward, Administrator
CMO: Doziier Tabb, M.D., Chief of Staff
CIO: Laurie Hansen, Director Administrative Services
CHR: Karen Ferguson, Director Human Resources
Web address: www.buffalowyoming.com/hospital/
Control: Hospital district or authority, Government, nonfederal **Service:** General Medical and Surgical

Staffed Beds: 75 **Admissions:** 553 **Census:** 55 **Outpatient Visits:** 11924 **Births:** 60 **Total Expense ($000):** 13576 **Payroll Expense ($000):** 7027 **Personnel:** 176

CASPER—Natrona County

☐ **WYOMING BEHAVIORAL INSTITUTE (534004)**, 2521 East 15th Street, Zip 82609–4126; tel. 800/457–9312 **A**1 9 10 **F**4 31 32 55 56 57 88 89 90 91 92 93 94 95 119 **S** Universal Health Services, Inc.
Primary Contact: Bill Sexton, Chief Executive Officer
CFO: Carmel Bickford, Chief Financial Officer
CMO: Steven Brown, M.D., Medical Director
Web address: www.wbihelp.com
Control: Corporation, Investor–owned, for–profit **Service:** Psychiatric

Staffed Beds: 70 **Admissions:** 1171 **Census:** 50 **Outpatient Visits:** 0 **Births:** 0 **Total Expense ($000):** 9942 **Payroll Expense ($000):** 5236 **Personnel:** 32

☒ **WYOMING MEDICAL CENTER (530012)**, 1233 East Second Street, Zip 82601–2988; tel. 307/577–7201, (Total facility includes 15 beds in nursing home–type unit) **A**1 9 10 20 **F**3 7 11 13 18 20 22 24 25 26 27 30 31 32 33 38 40 46 49 50 51 55 57 59 60 66 68 72 74 77 79 80 81 82 84 85 87 92 96 97 100 102 106 107 108 109 111 112 117 118 119 121 124 133 135 136 137 **P**6
Primary Contact: Vickie Diamond, President and Chief Executive Officer
CFO: Nancy Brandt, Chief Financial Officer
CIO: Don Claunch, Chief Information Officer
Web address: www.wmcnet.org
Control: Other not–for–profit (including NFP Corporation) **Service:** General Medical and Surgical

Staffed Beds: 205 **Admissions:** 9245 **Census:** 114 **Outpatient Visits:** 76075 **Births:** 1162 **Total Expense ($000):** 146039 **Payroll Expense ($000):** 57806 **Personnel:** 1181

CHEYENNE—Laramie County

☒ △ **CHEYENNE REGIONAL MEDICAL CENTER (530014)**, 214 East 23rd Street, Zip 82001–3790; tel. 307/634–2273, (Total facility includes 12 beds in nursing home–type unit) **A**1 3 5 7 9 10 19 20 **F**5 11 12 13 15 18 20 22 24 25 26 27 28 30 31 32 33 38 40 42 43 44 45 46 47 48 49 51 52 55 56 57 59 61 66 68 72 73 74 75 76 77 79 80 82 84 85 86 88 89 90 91 92 93 94 95 96 97 100 102 103 107 108 109 111 117 118 119 124 135 136 137 **P**6
Primary Contact: Charles F. Harms, Chief Executive Officer
CFO: Kimberly Webb, Vice President Fiscal Services
CIO: David Squires, Chief Information Officer
CHR: Phyllis Bell, Vice President Human Resources
Web address: www.crmcwy.org
Control: County–Government, nonfederal **Service:** General Medical and Surgical

Staffed Beds: 217 **Admissions:** 11641 **Census:** 133 **Outpatient Visits:** 105226 **Births:** 1273 **Total Expense ($000):** 167410 **Payroll Expense ($000):** 70730 **Personnel:** 1345

☒ **VETERANS AFFAIRS MEDICAL CENTER**, 2360 East Pershing Boulevard, Zip 82001–5392; tel. 307/778–7550, (Total facility includes 50 beds in nursing home–type unit) **A**1 9 **F**3 5 8 11 25 26 27 30 32 33 36 37 42 43 44 46 50 54 55 60 62 64 65 66 68 73 75 76 77 79 80 81 82 85 86 87 90 91 93 94 96 97 100 107 117 118 119 121 124 132 135 136 137 **P**6 **S** Department of Veterans Affairs
Primary Contact: David M. Kilpatrick, M.D., Director
COO: Robert Anselmi, Director Environmental Care
CFO: Melvin Cranford, Acting Chief Fiscal Services
CMO: Roger Johnson, M.D., Chief of Staff
CIO: Chad Cartwright, Chief Information Resource Management Systems
CHR: Sandra Willoughby, Chief Human Resources
Web address: www.va.gov/sta/guide/home.asp
Control: Veterans Affairs, Government, federal **Service:** General Medical and Surgical

Staffed Beds: 71 **Admissions:** 1085 **Census:** 92 **Outpatient Visits:** 148794 **Births:** 0 **Personnel:** 436

CODY—Park County

★ **WEST PARK HOSPITAL (531312)**, 707 Sheridan Avenue, Zip 82414–3409; tel. 307/527–7501, (Total facility includes 97 beds in nursing home–type unit) **A**9 10 18 **F**3 4 5 7 11 13 15 25 26 27 31 32 33 34 37 38 40 42 43 44 46 54 57 59 61 62 63 66 68 73 74 75 76 77 79 80 81 82 86 87 89 90 91 92 93 94 95 96 97 100 103 106 107 117 119 120 121 122 123 124 132 133 134 135 136 137 **S** QHR
Primary Contact: Douglas A. McMillan, Administrator and Chief Executive Officer
CFO: Patrick G. McConnell, Chief Financial Officer
CHR: Dick Smith, Director Human Resources
Web address: www.westparkhospital.org
Control: Hospital district or authority, Government, nonfederal **Service:** General Medical and Surgical

Staffed Beds: 140 **Admissions:** 1976 **Census:** 89 **Outpatient Visits:** 64208 **Births:** 217 **Total Expense ($000):** 37347 **Payroll Expense ($000):** 16524 **Personnel:** 317

Hospital, Medicare Provider Number, Address, Telephone, Approval, Facility, and Physician Codes, Health Care System

★ American Hospital Association (AHA) membership
☐ The Joint Commission accreditation
○ American Osteopathic Association (AOA) accreditation
△ Commission on Accreditation of Rehabilitation Facilities (CARF) accreditation

DOUGLAS—Converse County

★ **MEMORIAL HOSPITAL OF CONVERSE COUNTY (531302)**, 111 South Fifth Street, Zip 82633–1450, Mailing Address: P.O. Box 1450, Zip 82633–1450; tel. 307/358–2122 **A**9 10 18 **F**3 7 8 13 15 25 28 30 31 32 33 38 40 50 57 62 68 73 74 77 79 80 81 82 96 99 103 107 122 124 135 136 137 **P**6
Primary Contact: Thomas Nordwick, President and Chief Executive Officer
CFO: Curtis R. Dugger, Chief Financial Officer
CMO: Dennis Yutani, M.D., Chief of Staff
CIO: Dave Patterson, Director
CHR: Linda York, Manager Human Resources
Web address: www.conversehospital.com
Control: County–Government, nonfederal **Service:** General Medical and Surgical

Staffed Beds: 25 **Admissions:** 877 **Census:** 10 **Outpatient Visits:** 26879 **Births:** 101 **Total Expense ($000):** 26167 **Payroll Expense ($000):** 11199 **Personnel:** 288

EVANSTON—Uinta County

★ **EVANSTON REGIONAL HOSPITAL (530032)**, 190 Arrowhead Drive, Zip 82930–9266; tel. 307/789–3636 **A**1 9 10 20 **F**11 15 25 30 31 32 33 38 40 56 59 63 64 68 72 73 74 75 77 79 80 81 82 84 96 97 103 107 118 122 123 135 **P**6 **S** Community Health Systems, Inc.
Primary Contact: Ben Quinton, Chief Executive Officer
CFO: Darin Malchus, Chief Financial Officer
CMO: Tom Laucomer, M.D., Chief of Staff
CHR: Mark Hiatt, Director Marketing and Human Resources
Web address: www.evanstonregionalhospital.com
Control: Corporation, Investor–owned, for–profit **Service:** General Medical and Surgical

Staffed Beds: 36 **Admissions:** 1521 **Census:** 8 **Outpatient Visits:** 27073 **Births:** 297 **Total Expense ($000):** 16225 **Payroll Expense ($000):** 6508 **Personnel:** 198

△ **WYOMING STATE HOSPITAL (532002)**, 830 Highway 150 South, Zip 82931–5341, Mailing Address: P.O. Box 177, Zip 82931–0177; tel. 307/789–3464 **A**7 9 10 **F**5 25 26 30 31 32 33 36 50 54 62 73 75 81 82 88 90 91 92 93 94 119 121 124 132 **P**6
Primary Contact: Pablo Hernandez, M.D., Administrator
CFO: Paul Mullenax, Business Manager
CIO: Steve Baldwin, Manager Information Technology
CHR: Bob Stahl, Manager Human Resources
Web address: www.mentalhealth.state.wy.us/hospital/index.html
Control: State–Government, nonfederal **Service:** Psychiatric

Staffed Beds: 166 **Admissions:** 307 **Census:** 72 **Outpatient Visits:** 0 **Births:** 0 **Total Expense ($000):** 28072 **Payroll Expense ($000):** 14139 **Personnel:** 436

GILLETTE—Campbell County

★ **CAMPBELL COUNTY MEMORIAL HOSPITAL (530002)**, 501 South Burma Avenue, Zip 82716–3426, Mailing Address: P.O. Box 3011, Zip 82717–3011; tel. 307/682–8811, (Total facility includes 137 beds in nursing home–type unit) **A**1 9 10 20 **F**5 6 7 11 13 15 24 25 26 27 30 32 33 36 38 40 42 43 51 52 53 54 55 56 57 59 61 62 63 66 67 68 69 71 73 74 75 76 77 79 80 81 82 83 86 87 88 89 90 91 92 93 94 95 96 97 98 99 100 102 103 104 107 109 111 115 118 119 120 121 122 124 132 135 136 137 **P**6
Primary Contact: Robert A. Morasko, Chief Executive Officer
COO: Andy Fitzgerald, Executive Vice President
CFO: Andy Fitzgerald, Executive Vice President
CIO: Stevan Bailey, Manager Information Systems
CHR: John A. Fitch, Vice President Human Resources
Web address: www.ccmh.net
Control: Hospital district or authority, Government, nonfederal **Service:** General Medical and Surgical

Staffed Beds: 227 **Admissions:** 3812 **Census:** 156 **Outpatient Visits:** 148522 **Births:** 739 **Total Expense ($000):** 81303 **Payroll Expense ($000):** 39729 **Personnel:** 812

JACKSON—Teton County

★ **ST. JOHN'S MEDICAL CENTER AND LIVING CENTER (530015)**, 625 East Broadway Street, Zip 83001, Mailing Address: P.O. Box 428, Zip 83001–0428; tel. 307/733–3636, (Total facility includes 60 beds in nursing home–type unit) **A**1 9 10 20 **F**3 11 12 13 15 25 26 27 30 31 32 33 38 39 40 42 43 46 51 52 55 56 57 61 65 66 68 73 74 75 76 79 82 86 87 96 97 100 102 107 119 134 135
Primary Contact: James P. Schuessler, Chief Executive Officer
CFO: Robert Flake, Chief Financial Officer
CIO: David Witton, Manager
CHR: Michelle Byers, Manager Human Resources
Web address: www.tetonhospital.org
Control: Hospital district or authority, Government, nonfederal **Service:** General Medical and Surgical

Staffed Beds: 112 **Admissions:** 3230 **Census:** 74 **Outpatient Visits:** 45640 **Births:** 490 **Total Expense ($000):** 57143 **Payroll Expense ($000):** 22510 **Personnel:** 396

KEMMERER—Lincoln County

★ **SOUTH LINCOLN MEDICAL CENTER (530017)**, 711 Onyx Street, Zip 83101–3214, Mailing Address: P.O. Box 390, Zip 83101–0390; tel. 307/877–4401, (Total facility includes 24 beds in nursing home–type unit) **A**9 10 20 **F**3 7 13 15 28 37 38 40 55 56 57 63 66 73 75 77 79 84 86 87 96 100 102 107 117 118 122 135 137 **P**6
Primary Contact: Eric Boley, Administrator and Chief Executive Officer
CFO: Curtis Nielson, Chief Financial Officer
CMO: G. Christopher Krell, M.D., Chief of Staff
CIO: Kristin Housley, Chief Management Information Systems
CHR: Kristine Richardson, Administrative Assistant and Coordinator Personnel
Web address: www.southlincolnmedical.com
Control: Hospital district or authority, Government, nonfederal **Service:** General Medical and Surgical

Staffed Beds: 40 **Admissions:** 248 **Census:** 27 **Outpatient Visits:** 32521 **Births:** 53 **Total Expense ($000):** 12401 **Payroll Expense ($000):** 6825 **Personnel:** 151

LANDER—Fremont County

★ **LANDER REGIONAL HOSPITAL (530010)**, (Formerly Lander Valley Medical Center), 1320 Bishop Randall Drive, Zip 82520–3996; tel. 307/332–4420 **A**1 9 10 20 **F**3 11 13 15 24 25 26 27 31 33 37 38 40 55 68 74 75 77 78 79 80 82 85 86 88 89 96 97 100 107 117 119 122 136 **P**5 **S** LifePoint Hospitals, Inc.
Primary Contact: Phil Eaton, Chief Executive Officer
CFO: Ann Huhnke, Chief Financial Officer
CMO: Greg Clifford, M.D., Emergency Services Director
CIO: Keith Blair, M.D., Information Systems Manager
CHR: Carolyn Livingston, Manager
Web address: www.landerhospital.com
Control: Corporation, Investor–owned, for–profit **Service:** General Medical and Surgical

Staffed Beds: 98 **Admissions:** 2651 **Census:** 29 **Outpatient Visits:** 31883 **Births:** 319 **Total Expense ($000):** 22057 **Payroll Expense ($000):** 10183 **Personnel:** 197

LARAMIE—Albany County

★ **IVINSON MEMORIAL HOSPITAL (530025)**, 255 North 30th Street, Zip 82072; tel. 307/742–2141, (Total facility includes 8 beds in nursing home–type unit) **A**1 9 10 20 **F**11 13 15 24 25 26 27 30 31 32 36 38 50 54 55 56 57 59 68 71 73 74 75 76 77 79 80 84 86 88 96 97 98 100 102 106 107 108 109 111 117 118 119 121 122 124 135 136 **P**8 **S** QHR
Primary Contact: Carol Dozier, Chief Executive Officer
CFO: Nick Braccino, Interim Chief Financial Officer
CMO: Brian Horst, M.D., Chief of Staff
CHR: Holly Zajic, Director Human Resources
Web address: www.ivinsonhospital.org
Control: Hospital district or authority, Government, nonfederal **Service:** General Medical and Surgical

Staffed Beds: 99 **Admissions:** 2559 **Census:** 23 **Outpatient Visits:** 43683 **Births:** 441 **Total Expense ($000):** 42077 **Payroll Expense ($000):** 17808 **Personnel:** 340

LOVELL—Big Horn County

★ **NORTH BIG HORN HOSPITAL DISTRICT (531309)**, 1115 Lane 12, Zip 82431–9537; tel. 307/548–5200, (Total facility includes 85 beds in nursing home–type unit) **A**9 10 18 **F**3 6 7 10 15 24 25 30 38 54 55 57 62 63 64 66 73 75 79 80 81 82 86 87 96 102 107 119 120 121 122 132 134 135 136 **P**6
Primary Contact: Peter Birkholz, Chief Executive Officer
CFO: Daphne Hartman, Chief Financial Officer
CMO: David E. Hoffman, M.D., Chief of Staff
CIO: Eileen Fink, Health Information Officer
CHR: Barbara Shumway, Human Resources Officer
Web address: www.nbhh.com
Control: Hospital district or authority, Government, nonfederal **Service:** General Medical and Surgical

Staffed Beds: 100 **Admissions:** 495 **Census:** 78 **Outpatient Visits:** 6193 **Births:** 0 **Total Expense ($000):** 10777 **Payroll Expense ($000):** 6032 **Personnel:** 170

LUSK—Niobrara County

NIOBRARA HEALTH AND LIFE CENTER (531314), 921 Ballencee Avenue, Zip 82225, Mailing Address: P.O. Box 780, Zip 82225–0780; tel. 307/334–2711 **A**9 10 18 **F**3 38 96 107 117 119 121 124
Primary Contact: Bob Brummond, Administrator
Web address: www.niobrarahospital.com
Control: Hospital district or authority, Government, nonfederal **Service:** General Medical and Surgical

Staffed Beds: 24 **Admissions:** 188 **Census:** 11 **Outpatient Visits:** 1041 **Births:** 0 **Total Expense ($000):** 3737 **Payroll Expense ($000):** 1750

NEWCASTLE—Weston County

★ **WESTON COUNTY HEALTH SERVICES (531303)**, 1124 Washington Boulevard, Zip 82701–2996; tel. 307/746–4491, (Total facility includes 51 beds in nursing home–type unit) **A**9 10 18 **F**1 4 16 17 30 32 38 42 54 55 57 61 65 68 70 71 74 77 78 79 83 84 85 87 88 96 100 107 117 122 **P**5
S Regional Health
Primary Contact: Kevin Stiffarm, Chief Executive Officer
CIO: Clara Varner, Manager Business Office
CHR: Shirley Parks, Coordinator Human Resources
Web address: www.wchs-wy.org
Control: Hospital district or authority, Government, nonfederal **Service:** General Medical and Surgical

Staffed Beds: 86 **Admissions:** 266 **Census:** 51 **Outpatient Visits:** 1923
Births: 1 **Personnel:** 114

POWELL—Park County

★ **POWELL VALLEY HEALTHCARE (531310)**, 777 Avenue H, Zip 82435–2296; tel. 307/754–2267, (Total facility includes 100 beds in nursing home–type unit) **A**9 10 18 **F**7 10 11 13 15 24 25 30 32 33 38 40 42 43 54 55 56 61 62 68 74 77 79 80 96 97 100 107 117 119 120 121 122 124 133 135 136 137 **P**1
S Brim Healthcare, Inc.
Primary Contact: Rod Barton, Chief Executive Officer
CFO: Steve Ramsey, Chief Financial Officer
CMO: Michael Tracy, M.D., Chief of Staff
CIO: Denise Roberson, Director Information Systems
CHR: Tami Lineback, Director Human Resources
Web address: www.pvhc.org
Control: Other not–for–profit (including NFP Corporation) **Service:** General Medical and Surgical

Staffed Beds: 125 **Admissions:** 1243 **Census:** 104 **Outpatient Visits:** 23669
Births: 237 **Total Expense ($000):** 30810 **Payroll Expense ($000):** 17027
Personnel: 330

RAWLINS—Carbon County

★ **MEMORIAL HOSPITAL OF CARBON COUNTY (530009)**, 2221 West Elm Street, Zip 82301–0460, Mailing Address: P.O. Box 460, Zip 82301–0460; tel. 307/324–8213, (Total facility includes 10 beds in nursing home–type unit) **A**9 10 20 **F**3 7 11 13 15 25 26 27 30 32 33 38 40 54 55 56 57 61 65 66 68 74 75 76 77 79 80 82 86 96 100 107 119 121 122 135
Primary Contact: Patricia L. Carter, Chief Executive Officer
CFO: Florence Kostic, Chief Financial Officer
CMO: Kenneth Schulze, M.D., Chief of Staff
CHR: Beverly Young, Director Human Resources
Web address: www.imhcc.com
Control: County–Government, nonfederal **Service:** General Medical and Surgical

Staffed Beds: 45 **Admissions:** 1721 **Census:** 22 **Outpatient Visits:** 26407
Births: 126 **Total Expense ($000):** 16562 **Payroll Expense ($000):** 8915
Personnel: 191

RIVERTON—Fremont County

★☐ **RIVERTON MEMORIAL HOSPITAL (530008)**, 2100 West Sunset Drive, Zip 82501–2274; tel. 307/856–4161 **A**1 9 10 20 **F**3 11 12 13 15 25 27 31 32 38 51 55 57 66 68 73 74 75 77 79 80 86 96 97 102 107 118 119 121 122 124 134 135 137 **P**7 **S** LifePoint Hospitals, Inc.
Primary Contact: James Christian Smolik, Chief Executive Officer
CFO: Susan Goetzinger, Chief Financial Officer
CIO: Tim Foley, Director Information Systems
CHR: Norma Atwood, Director Human Resources
Web address: www.riverton–hospital.com
Control: Corporation, Investor–owned, for–profit **Service:** General Medical and Surgical

Staffed Beds: 49 **Admissions:** 1866 **Census:** 15 **Outpatient Visits:** 33084
Births: 301 **Total Expense ($000):** 18726 **Payroll Expense ($000):** 7294
Personnel: 150

ROCK SPRINGS—Sweetwater County

★☐ **MEMORIAL HOSPITAL OF SWEETWATER COUNTY (530011)**, 1200 College Drive, Zip 82901–5868, Mailing Address: P.O. Box 1359, Zip 82902–1359; tel. 307/362–3711 **A**1 9 10 20 **F**3 11 13 15 25 26 27 32 38 40 43 48 55 56 57 59 68 73 74 76 77 79 82 83 84 85 86 87 96 100 102 107 118 119 124 135 **S** Brim Healthcare, Inc.
Primary Contact: Kevin Hawk, Chief Executive Officer
COO: Linda Simmons, Chief Nursing Officer and Vice President Operations
CMO: Daryl Kaan, M.D., President Medical Staff
CHR: Lisa Clark, Director Human Resources
Web address: www.sweetwatermedicalcenter.com
Control: County–Government, nonfederal **Service:** General Medical and Surgical

Staffed Beds: 99 **Admissions:** 2381 **Census:** 17 **Outpatient Visits:** 90109
Births: 607 **Total Expense ($000):** 31714 **Payroll Expense ($000):** 13430
Personnel: 299

SHERIDAN—Sheridan County

☐ **SHERIDAN MEMORIAL HOSPITAL (530006)**, 1401 West Fifth Street, Zip 82801–2799; tel. 307/672–1000 **A**1 9 10 20 **F**3 11 13 15 24 25 30 31 33 38 40 42 46 52 55 57 61 68 72 73 74 76 77 79 80 82 84 86 92 94 96 97 100 102 107 109 111 117 118 119 120 121 122 124 134 135 137
Primary Contact: Michael McCafferty, Chief Executive Officer
CFO: Ed Johlman, Chief Financial Officer
CMO: Barry Wohl, M.D., Chief of Staff
CIO: Deb Anderson, Manager Information Systems
CHR: Len Gross, Manager Human Resources
Web address: www.sheridanhospital.org
Control: County–Government, nonfederal **Service:** General Medical and Surgical

Staffed Beds: 62 **Admissions:** 2704 **Census:** 30 **Outpatient Visits:** 37230
Births: 412 **Total Expense ($000):** 41271 **Payroll Expense ($000):** 17919
Personnel: 500

★☐ **VETERANS AFFAIRS MEDICAL CENTER**, 1898 Fort Road, Zip 82801–8320; tel. 307/672–3473, (Total facility includes 50 beds in nursing home–type unit) **A**1 5 9 **F**4 5 25 26 27 29 31 32 33 36 37 42 43 44 45 50 54 60 62 64 65 66 73 75 76 78 81 82 86 87 88 90 91 92 93 94 95 96 100 102 107 118 119 121 124 132 133 135 136 137 **S** Department of Veterans Affairs
Primary Contact: Debra L. Hirschman, Director
CFO: William Brayton, Manager Finance
CMO: Wendell Robison, M.D., Chief of Staff
CIO: Kaylene Zimmer, Chief Information Officer
CHR: Randy Wilson, Manager Human Resources
Web address: www.va.gov/sta/guide/home.asp
Control: Veterans Affairs, Government, federal **Service:** Psychiatric

Staffed Beds: 203 **Admissions:** 1639 **Census:** 58 **Outpatient Visits:** 98666
Births: 0 **Personnel:** 167

SUNDANCE—Crook County

★ **CROOK COUNTY MEDICAL SERVICES DISTRICT (531311)**, 713 Oak Street, Zip 82729, Mailing Address: P.O. Box 517, Zip 82729–0517; tel. 307/283–3501, (Total facility includes 32 beds in nursing home–type unit) **A**9 10 18 **F**2 7 31 38 42 54 55 56 57 61 65 81 86 107 119 122 **P**6
Primary Contact: Doris Brown, Chief Executive Officer
CMO: Keith Noback, M.D., Chief of Staff
CHR: Patricia Feist, Manager Human Resources
Web address: www.crookcountymedical.com
Control: Hospital district or authority, Government, nonfederal **Service:** General Medical and Surgical

Staffed Beds: 48 **Admissions:** 146 **Census:** 31 **Outpatient Visits:** 10802
Births: 0 **Total Expense ($000):** 5662 **Payroll Expense ($000):** 3362
Personnel: 102

THERMOPOLIS—Hot Springs County

★ **HOT SPRINGS COUNTY MEMORIAL HOSPITAL (531304)**, 150 East Arapahoe Street, Zip 82443–2498; tel. 307/864–3121 **A**9 10 18 **F**3 11 13 15 24 25 27 30 31 38 40 46 56 57 61 62 66 68 73 74 76 77 79 80 81 84 96 97 100 102 107 112 117 118 119 122 132 135 **S** Brim Healthcare, Inc.
Primary Contact: Trudy Chittick, Chief Executive Officer
COO: Belenda Willson, Chief Operating Officer
CFO: Alan W. Streeter, Chief Financial Officer
CIO: Tim Knight, Director Information Technology
CHR: Patti Jeunehomme, Director Human Resources
Web address: www.hscmh.org
Control: County–Government, nonfederal **Service:** General Medical and Surgical

Staffed Beds: 25 **Admissions:** 564 **Census:** 6 **Outpatient Visits:** 25190
Births: 53 **Total Expense ($000):** 10494 **Payroll Expense ($000):** 4410
Personnel: 104

Hospital, Medicare Provider Number, Address, Telephone, Approval, Facility, and Physician Codes, Health Care System
★ American Hospital Association (AHA) membership
☐ The Joint Commission accreditation
○ American Osteopathic Association (AOA) accreditation
△ Commission on Accreditation of Rehabilitation Facilities (CARF) accreditation

WY

TORRINGTON—Goshen County

★ **COMMUNITY HOSPITAL (531307)**, 2000 Campbell Drive, Zip 82240–1597; tel. 307/532–4181 **A**9 10 18 **F**3 8 11 13 15 25 26 30 31 32 33 34 38 40 44 46 55 57 62 66 68 73 75 77 79 82 96 107 117 118 119 120 121 122 124 134 135 **P**5 6 **S** Banner Health
Primary Contact: Marilyn Schock, Interim Chief Executive Officer
CFO: Steve Smith, Chief Financial Officer
CMO: Richard Campbell, D.O., Chief of Staff
CIO: Rod Miller, Chief Information Technology
CHR: Sandy Dugger, Director Human Resources
Web address: www.bannerhealth.com
Control: Other not–for–profit (including NFP Corporation) **Service:** General Medical and Surgical

Staffed Beds: 25 **Admissions:** 1164 **Census:** 13 **Outpatient Visits:** 27740 **Births:** 101 **Total Expense ($000):** 14061 **Payroll Expense ($000):** 5889 **Personnel:** 127

WHEATLAND—Platte County

★ **PLATTE COUNTY MEMORIAL HOSPITAL (531305)**, 201 14th Street, Zip 82201–3201, Mailing Address: P.O. Box 848, Zip 82201–0848; tel. 307/322–3636, (Total facility includes 43 beds in nursing home–type unit) **A**1 9 10 18 **F**3 13 15 25 26 30 31 32 38 40 46 47 48 49 55 62 65 73 74 79 84 96 102 107 117 118 119 121 122 **S** Banner Health
Primary Contact: Gavin H. Carmichael, FACHE, Chief Executive Officer
CIO: Robin Wood, Director Information Systems
CHR: Mark Winger, Manager People Resources
Web address: www.bannerhealth.com
Control: Other not–for–profit (including NFP Corporation) **Service:** General Medical and Surgical

Staffed Beds: 68 **Admissions:** 572 **Census:** 36 **Outpatient Visits:** 20258 **Births:** 57 **Total Expense ($000):** 12447 **Payroll Expense ($000):** 6211 **Personnel:** 93

WORLAND—Washakie County

★ **WASHAKIE MEDICAL CENTER (531306)**, 400 South 15th Street, Zip 82401–3531, Mailing Address: P.O. Box 700, Zip 82401–0700; tel. 307/347–3221 **A**9 10 18 **F**3 11 13 15 24 25 33 38 40 43 55 57 62 66 68 73 74 75 77 79 80 82 86 87 96 99 100 102 107 118 119 122 124 134 135 137 **P**6 **S** Banner Health
Primary Contact: Margie Molitor, RN, Chief Executive Officer
CFO: Joe Devin, Chief Financial Officer
CMO: Vernon Miller, M.D., Chief of Staff
CHR: Sandra Colman, Manager Human Resources
Web address: www.washakiemedicalcenter.com
Control: Other not–for–profit (including NFP Corporation) **Service:** General Medical and Surgical

Staffed Beds: 25 **Admissions:** 985 **Census:** 10 **Outpatient Visits:** 26522 **Births:** 79 **Total Expense ($000):** 15321 **Payroll Expense ($000):** 6293 **Personnel:** 115

 Many Facility Codes have changed. Please refer to the AHA Guide Code Chart.

Hospitals in Areas Associated with the United States, by Area

AMERICAN SAMOA

PAGO PAGO—American Samoa County

LYNDON B. JOHNSON TROPICAL MEDICAL CENTER (640001), Zip 96799; tel. 684/633–1222, (Nonreporting) **A**10
Primary Contact: Iotamo T. Saleapaga, M.D., Director Health
Control: State–Government, nonfederal **Service:** General Medical and Surgical

Staffed Beds: 125

GUAM

AGANA—Guam County

★ **U. S. NAVAL HOSPITAL**, Mailing Address: PSC 490, Box 7607, FPO, AP, Zip 96538–1600; tel. 671/344–9340, (Nonreporting) **S** Bureau of Medicine and Surgery, Department of the Navy
Primary Contact: Captain Kathleen A. Rief, Commanding Officer
Web address: www.usnhguam.med.navy.mil
Control: Navy, Government, federal **Service:** General Medical and Surgical

Staffed Beds: 55

TAMUNING—Guam County

★ **GUAM MEMORIAL HOSPITAL AUTHORITY (650001)**, 850 Governor Carlos G. Camacho Road, Zip 96913; tel. 671/647–2108, (Total facility includes 30 beds in nursing home–type unit) **A**10 **F**3 13 14 15 18 20 22 24 25 26 27 31 32 38 43 55 56 59 62 63 66 68 70 71 73 74 75 78 79 81 82 83 84 86 96 97 103 107 117 119 132 135 137
Primary Contact: Peter John Diaz Camacho, M.P.H., Administrator and Chief Executive Officer
COO: Wilfred Aflague, Chief Financial Officer
CMO: James J. Stadler, M.D., Associate Administrator of Medical Services
CIO: Vince Quichocho, Manager Information Systems
CHR: Elizabeth Claros, Personnel Services Administrator
Web address: www.gmha.org
Control: Hospital district or authority, Government, nonfederal **Service:** General Medical and Surgical

Staffed Beds: 208 **Admissions:** 11186 **Census:** 180 **Outpatient Visits:** 332454 **Births:** 2487 **Total Expense ($000):** 62441 **Payroll Expense ($000):** 45972 **Personnel:** 878

MARSHALL ISLANDS

KWAJALEIN ISLAND—Marshall Islands County

KWAJALEIN HOSPITAL, U.S. Army Kwajalein Atoll, Zip 96960, Mailing Address: Box 1702, APO, AP, Zip 96555–5000; tel. 805/355–2225, (Nonreporting) **S** Department of the Army, Office of the Surgeon General
Primary Contact: Elaine McMahon, Administrator
Control: Army, Government, federal **Service:** General Medical and Surgical

Staffed Beds: 14

NORTHERN MARIANA ISLANDS

SAIPAN—Northern Mariana Island County

COMMONWEALTH HEALTH CENTER (660001), Navy Hill Road, Zip 96950, Mailing Address: P.O. Box 409, Zip 96950; tel. 670/234–8950, (Nonreporting) **A**10
Primary Contact: Joseph C. Santos, M.P.H., Deputy Secretary for Hospital Administration
Web address: www.dphsaipan.com
Control: Corporation, Investor–owned, for–profit **Service:** Other specialty

Staffed Beds: 86

PUERTO RICO

AGUADILLA—Aguadilla County

★□ **HOSPITAL BUEN SAMARITANO (400079)**, Carr Aguadilla San Juan, Zip 605; tel. 787/819–0844 **A**1 5 9 10 **F**3 13 14 15 26 38 46 48 49 57 60 68 73 74 77 79 80 82 84 96 99 107 118 135
Primary Contact: Marco Reyes, Executive Director
Control: Other not–for–profit (including NFP Corporation) **Service:** General Medical and Surgical

Staffed Beds: 142 **Admissions:** 8161 **Census:** 107 **Births:** 629 **Total Expense ($000):** 33965 **Payroll Expense ($000):** 9348 **Personnel:** 488

AIBONITO—Aibonito County

★□ **MENNONITE GENERAL HOSPITAL (400018)**, Calle Jose C. Vasquez, Zip 705, Mailing Address: P.O. Box 373130, Cayey, Zip 00737–3130; tel. 787/535–1001, (Nonreporting) **A**1 9 10
Primary Contact: Pedro Melendez, Administrator
COO: Marta R Mercado Suro, Chief Operating Officer
CFO: Jose E. Solivan, Chief Financial Officer
CMO: Victor Hernandez Miranda, M.D., Chief of Staff
CIO: Daniza Morales, Manager Information System
CHR: Evelyn Padilla Ortiz, Director Human Resources
Web address: www.hospitalmenonita.com
Control: Other not–for–profit (including NFP Corporation) **Service:** General Medical and Surgical

Staffed Beds: 131

ARECIBO—Arecibo County

★□ **HOSPITAL DR. CAYETANO COLL Y TOSTE (400087)**, 129 San Luis Avenue, Zip 612, Mailing Address: P.O. Box 659, Zip 613; tel. 787/650–7272, (Nonreporting) **A**1 9 10
Primary Contact: Homar Perez, Chief Executive Officer and Vice President Administration
COO: Maritza Rodriguez, Chief Financial Officer
CFO: Luis Curbelo, Director Finance
CMO: Ada S. Miranda, M.D., Medical Director
CIO: Vicent Ortiz, Chief Information Officer
CHR: Carmen Sanchez, Director Human Resources
Web address: www.cayetano@xsn.net
Control: Corporation, Investor–owned, for–profit **Service:** General Medical and Surgical

Staffed Beds: 188

HOSPITAL DR. SUSONI (400117), 55 Nicomedes Rivera Street, Zip 612, Mailing Address: P.O. Box 145200, Zip 614; tel. 787/878–1010, (Nonreporting) **A**9 10
Primary Contact: Vivian Solivan, Administrator
CFO: Vivian Aceuedo, CPA, Chief Financial Director
CMO: Ada S. Miranda, M.D., Medical Director
CIO: Mayra Montano, Director Information Systems
CHR: Patria Nieves, Director
Control: State–Government, nonfederal **Service:** General Medical and Surgical

Staffed Beds: 131

Hospital, Medicare Provider Number, Address, Telephone, Approval, Facility, and Physician Codes, Health Care System

★ American Hospital Association (AHA) membership
□ The Joint Commission accreditation
○ American Osteopathic Association (AOA) accreditation
△ Commission on Accreditation of Rehabilitation Facilities (CARF) accreditation

HOSPITAL EL BUEN PASTOR, 52 De Diego, Zip 00612–4503, Mailing Address: P.O. Box 413, Zip 00612–0413; tel. 787/878–2730, (Nonreporting) **A**9
Primary Contact: Hector Mercado, Executive Director
Control: Corporation, Investor–owned, for–profit **Service:** General Medical and Surgical

Staffed Beds: 48

ARROYO—Arroyo County

★ **LAFAYETTE HOSPITAL (400026)**, Central Lafayette, Zip 714, Mailing Address: P.O. Box 207, Zip 714; tel. 787/839–3232 **A**9 10 **F**3 38 62 68 79 96 107 **P**5
Primary Contact: Francisco Santiago–Vega, Consultor
CFO: Francisco Vazquez, General Manager and Executive Director
CIO: Francisco Vazquez, General Manager and Executive Director
Control: Corporation, Investor–owned, for–profit **Service:** General Medical and Surgical

Staffed Beds: 39 **Admissions:** 2109 **Census:** 26 **Outpatient Visits:** 18676 **Births:** 42 **Total Expense ($000):** 9554 **Payroll Expense ($000):** 2986 **Personnel:** 157

BAYAMON—Bayamon County

☒ **HOSPITAL HERMANOS MELENDEZ (400032)**, Route 2, KM 11–7, Zip 960, Mailing Address: P.O. Box 306, Zip 960; tel. 787/620–8181, (Nonreporting) **A**1 9 10
Primary Contact: Waleska Crespo, Administrator
CFO: Luz D. Medina, Controller
CMO: Norma Ortiz, M.D., Medical Director
CIO: Leticia Santana, Administrator Medical Records
Web address: www.hospitalhermanosmelendez.net
Control: Corporation, Investor–owned, for–profit **Service:** General Medical and Surgical

Staffed Beds: 211

HOSPITAL MATILDE BRENES (400102), Extension Hermanas Davila, Zip 960, Mailing Address: P.O. Box 2957, Zip 960; tel. 787/622–5420, (Nonreporting) **A**9 10
Primary Contact: Pedro Rivera, Administrator
Control: Corporation, Investor–owned, for–profit **Service:** General Medical and Surgical

Staffed Beds: 91

☒ **HOSPITAL SAN PABLO (400109)**, Calle Santa Cruz 70, Zip 00961–7020, Mailing Address: P.O. Box 236, Zip 00960–0236; tel. 787/740–4747 **A**1 3 5 9 10 **F**17 18 20 22 25 27 38 46 49 51 56 68 70 71 72 74 76 77 79 81 82 83 84 96 99 100 108 116 119 135
Primary Contact: Rogelio Diaz, Chief Executive Officer and Managing Director
Web address: www.sanpablo.com
Control: Corporation, Investor–owned, for–profit **Service:** General Medical and Surgical

Staffed Beds: 410 **Admissions:** 17069 **Census:** 317 **Outpatient Visits:** 86790 **Births:** 1617

☒ **HOSPITAL UNIVERSITARIO DR. RAMON RUIZ ARNAU (400105)**, Avenue Laurel, Santa Juanita, Zip 956; tel. 787/787–5151, (Nonreporting) **A**1 3 5 10 **S** Puerto Rico Department of Health
Primary Contact: Rafael Garcia, Chief Executive Officer
CFO: Elsie Morales, Chief Financial Officer
CMO: Hector Cintron Principe, M.D., Director
CIO: Irma Duprey, Administrator Medical Records
CHR: Aurea De Leon, Chief Human Resources Officer
Control: State–Government, nonfederal **Service:** General Medical and Surgical

Staffed Beds: 70

★ **MEPSI CENTER (404002)**, Carretera Numero 2 K 8–2, Zip 00959–6089, Mailing Address: P.O. Box 600089, Zip 00960–0089; tel. 787/793–3030, (Nonreporting) **A**10
Primary Contact: Jorge A. Torres, Administrator
CFO: Noel Ortiz, Finance Director and Controller
Web address: www.mepsicenter.com
Control: Corporation, Investor–owned, for–profit **Service:** Psychiatric

Staffed Beds: 450

CAGUAS—Caguas County

☐ **HOSPITAL INTERAMERICANO DE MEDICINA AVANZADA (400120)**, Avenida Luis Munoz Marin, Zip 726, Mailing Address: P.O. Box 4980, Zip 726; tel. 787/653–3434, (Nonreporting) **A**1 5 9 10
Primary Contact: Carlos M. Pineiro, President
CFO: Luis A. Arroyo, Finance Senior Director
CIO: Fernando Mora, Management Information Systems Vice President
Control: Partnership, Investor–owned, for–profit **Service:** General Medical and Surgical

Staffed Beds: 300

CAROLINA—Carolina County

☒ **HOSPITAL DE LA UNIVERSIDAD DE PUERTO RICO/DR. FEDERICO TRILLA (400112)**, 65th Infanteria, KM 8 3, Zip 984, Mailing Address: P.O. Box 6021, Zip 984; tel. 787/757–1800, (Nonreporting) **A**1 3 5 9 10
Primary Contact: Jorge Torres Otero, Chief Executive Officer
COO: Diraida Maldonado, Administrator
CFO: Hector Ortiz, Chief Financial Officer
CMO: Marina Roman, M.D., Medical Director
CIO: Francisco Perez, Manager Management Information Systems
CHR: Betzaida Jimenez, Director Human Resources
Web address: www.hospitalupr.org
Control: Corporation, Investor–owned, for–profit **Service:** General Medical and Surgical

Staffed Beds: 197

CASTANER—Lares County

★ **CASTANER GENERAL HOSPITAL (400010)**, KM 64–2, Route 135, Zip 631, Mailing Address: P.O. Box 1003, Zip 631; tel. 787/829–5010, (Nonreporting) **A**5 10
Primary Contact: Domingo Monroig, Administrator
COO: Agustin Ponce, Supervisor Maintenance
CFO: Ernesto Montes, Director Finance
CMO: Jose O. Rodriguez, M.D., Medical Director
CIO: Domingo Monroig, Administrator
CHR: Nydimar Salcedo, Chief Human Resources Officer
Control: Other not–for–profit (including NFP Corporation) **Service:** General Medical and Surgical

Staffed Beds: 24

CAYEY—Cayey County

☐ **HOSPITAL MENONITA DE CAYEY (400013)**, 4 H. Mendoza Street, Zip 00736–3801, Mailing Address: P.O. Box 373130, Zip 00737–3130; tel. 787/263–1001 **A**1 9 10 **F**12 18 38 39 46 59 68 72 74 77 79 84 100
Primary Contact: Pedro Melendez, Administrator
COO: Leda Marta R Mercado, Chief Operating Officer
CFO: Jose E. Solivan, Chief Financial Officer
CMO: Luis J Rodriquez Saenz, M.D., Medical Director
CIO: Daniza Morales, Chief Information Officer
CHR: Evelyn Padilla Ortiz, Director Human Resources
Web address: www.hospitalmenonita.com
Control: Other not–for–profit (including NFP Corporation) **Service:** General Medical and Surgical

Staffed Beds: 145 **Admissions:** 10004 **Census:** 133 **Outpatient Visits:** 100521 **Births:** 1188 **Total Expense ($000):** 48607 **Payroll Expense ($000):** 16786

CIDRA—Cidra County

☐ **FIRST HOSPITAL PANAMERICANO (404004)**, State Road 787 KM 1 5, Zip 739, Mailing Address: P.O. Box 1400, Zip 739; tel. 787/739–5555, (Nonreporting) **A**1 3 5 10 **S** Psychiatric Solutions
Primary Contact: Marta Rivera, Executive Director
COO: Tim McCarthy, Executive Vice President
CFO: Gabriel Rivera, Controller
CMO: Ramon Parrilla, M.D., Chief Medical Officer
CIO: Carlos Nunez, Director Management Information Systems
CHR: Shirley Ayala, Director Human Resources
Web address: www.firsthospitalpr.org
Control: Corporation, Investor–owned, for–profit **Service:** Psychiatric

Staffed Beds: 153

COTO LAUREL—Ponce County

HOSPITAL SAN CRISTOBAL (400113), 506 Carr Road, Zip 780; tel. 787/848–2100, (Nonreporting) **A**5 9 10
Primary Contact: Pedro L. Benetti–Loyola, Administrator
COO: Pedro L. Benetti–Loyola, Administrator
CFO: Marian Collazo, Director Finance
CMO: Ramon Rodriguez Rivas, M.D., Medical Director
CIO: Emilio Diaz, Director Information Systems
CHR: Candie Rodriguez, Director Human Resources
Web address: www.hospitalsancristobal.com
Control: Corporation, Investor–owned, for–profit **Service:** Other specialty

Staffed Beds: 103

FAJARDO—Fajardo County

☒ **HOSPITAL SAN PABLO DEL ESTE (400125)**, Avenida General Valero, 404, Zip 738, Mailing Address: P.O. Box 1028, Zip 00738–1028; tel. 787/863–0505, (Nonreporting) **A**1 9 10
Primary Contact: Jose Carballo, Executive Administrator
COO: Maria Elena Rodriguez, Patient Relations Director
CFO: Luis A. Arroyo, Chief Financial Officer
CMO: Manuel Navas, M.D., Medical Director
CHR: Vilma Rodriguez, Human Resources Director
Web address: www.sanpablo.com
Control: Corporation, Investor–owned, for–profit **Service:** General Medical and Surgical

Staffed Beds: 136

GUAYAMA—Guayama County

☒ **HOSPITAL EPISCOPAL CRISTO REDENTOR (400048)**, Avenue Pedro Albesus, Zip 784, Mailing Address: PO Box 10011, Zip 00785–1006; tel. 787/864–4300 **A**1 5 9 10 **F**3 7 8 13 14 17 18 22 38 68 70 73 74 79 81 84 86 96 100 107 118 119 135
Primary Contact: Guillermo J. Martin, President and Chief Executive Officer
COO: Wilfredo Rabelo, Chief Operating Officer
CFO: Carlos Porrata, CPA, Chief Financial Officer
CMO: Gerson Jimenez, M.D., Medical Director
CHR: Ivette Lacot, Director Human Resources
Control: Church–operated, Nongovernment, not–for profit **Service:** General Medical and Surgical

Staffed Beds: 365 **Admissions:** 10686 **Census:** 49 **Outpatient Visits:** 97589 **Births:** 0 **Total Expense ($000):** 107250 **Payroll Expense ($000):** 31082 **Personnel:** 1335

★ **HOSPITAL SANTA ROSA (400009)**, Veterans Avenue, Zip 784, Mailing Address: P.O. Box 10008, Zip 785; tel. 787/864–0101 **A**9 10 **F**38 68 74 86 96 98 99 100 107 119
Primary Contact: Herson E. Morales, Executive Director
CFO: Edwin De Jesus, Comptroller
CMO: Joaquin Pales, President
CIO: Waleska Rolon, Manager
Control: Other not–for–profit (including NFP Corporation) **Service:** General Medical and Surgical

Staffed Beds: 89 **Admissions:** 3758 **Census:** 41 **Outpatient Visits:** 39859 **Births:** 151 **Total Expense ($000):** 13126 **Payroll Expense ($000):** 4339

HUMACAO—Humacao County

☐ **FONT MARTELO HOSPITAL (400005)**, 3 Font Martelo Street, Zip 00791–3342, Mailing Address: P.O. Box 639, Zip 00792–0639; tel. 787/656–2424, (Nonreporting) **A**1 9 10
Primary Contact: Aixa Irizarry, Executive Director
COO: Carlos M. Pineiro, President
CFO: Luis A. Arroyo, Chief Financial Officer
CMO: Julio Ortiz–McWilliams, M.D., Medical Director
CIO: Giovanni Piereschi, Vice President Management Information Systems
CHR: Iris Abreu, Supervisor Human Resources
Control: Corporation, Investor–owned, for–profit **Service:** General Medical and Surgical

Staffed Beds: 64

HOSPITAL DR. DOMINGUEZ (400011), 300 Font Martelo Street, Zip 00791–3230, Mailing Address: P.O. Box 699, Zip 00792–0699; tel. 787/852–0505, (Nonreporting) **A**9 10
Primary Contact: Miguel A. Solivan, Administrator
CFO: Ivonne Rivera, Director Finance
CMO: Carmelo Herrero, M.D., Medical Director
CHR: Ivonne Lopez, Director Human Resources
Control: Corporation, Investor–owned, for–profit **Service:** General Medical and Surgical

Staffed Beds: 60

★ **RYDER MEMORIAL HOSPITAL (400007)**, 355 Font Martelo Street, Zip 00791–3249, Mailing Address: P.O. Box 859, Zip 00792–0859; tel. 787/852–0768, (Total facility includes 56 beds in nursing home–type unit) **A**10 **F**6 8 10 13 15 18 20 26 27 30 32 37 38 39 42 53 57 60 61 62 63 68 70 71 72 73 74 75 76 77 79 82 84 86 87 89 90 96 97 100 102 103 107 115 117 119 132 135
Primary Contact: Jose R. Feliciano, Chief Executive Officer
CFO: Jose O. Ortiz, Chief Financial Officer
CMO: Juan F. Gonzalez–Diaz, M.D., Medical Director
CIO: Joseph V. Cruz, Chief Information Officer
CHR: Maria Figueroa, Director Human Resources
Web address: www.hryder@prtc.net
Control: Other not–for–profit (including NFP Corporation) **Service:** General Medical and Surgical

Staffed Beds: 221 **Admissions:** 8920 **Census:** 129 **Outpatient Visits:** 107198 **Births:** 1670 **Total Expense ($000):** 54868

MANATI—Manati County

DOCTORS CENTER (400118), KM 47–7, Zip 674, Mailing Address: P.O. Box 30532, Zip 674; tel. 787/854–3322, (Nonreporting) **A**9 10
Primary Contact: Pedro Rivera, Administrator
Control: Corporation, Investor–owned, for–profit **Service:** General Medical and Surgical

Staffed Beds: 150

☐ **HOSPITAL MANATI MEDICAL CENTER (400114)**, Calle Hernandez, Carrion 668, Zip 674, Mailing Address: P.O. Box 1142, Zip 00674–1142; tel. 787/621–3700, (Nonreporting) **A**1 3 5 9 10
Primary Contact: Jorge Galva, Executive Director
CFO: Noriselle Rivera–Pol, Vice President Finance
CMO: Luis R. Rosa–Toledo, M.D., Medical Director
CIO: Alberto Medina, Information Technology Senior Consultant
CHR: Nilda Paravisini, Director Human Resources
Control: Corporation, Investor–owned, for–profit **Service:** Other specialty

Staffed Beds: 178

MAYAGUEZ—Mayaguez County

☒ **BELLA VISTA HOSPITAL (400014)**, State Road 349, Zip 680, Mailing Address: P.O. Box 1750, Zip 681; tel. 787/834–6000 **A**1 9 10 **F**3 8 13 14 15 18 25 26 27 38 55 68 72 74 76 77 79 80 81 82 84 96 97 100 102 107 118 134 135 137
Primary Contact: Jesus Nieves, Chief Executive Officer
CFO: Enrique Rivera, Chief Financial Officer
CMO: Miguel Cruz, M.D., Medical Director
CHR: Benjamin Astacio, Director Human Resources
Web address: www.bvhpr.com
Control: Church–operated, Nongovernment, not–for profit **Service:** General Medical and Surgical

Staffed Beds: 157 **Admissions:** 7645 **Census:** 116 **Outpatient Visits:** 41069 **Births:** 625 **Personnel:** 710

CLINICA ESPANOLA (400024), Barrio La Quinta, Zip 680, Mailing Address: P.O. Box 490, Zip 00681–0490; tel. 787/832–0442, (Nonreporting) **A**10
Primary Contact: Emigdio Inigo–Agostini, M.D., Board President
Control: Corporation, Investor–owned, for–profit **Service:** General Medical and Surgical

Staffed Beds: 89

☐ **DR. RAMON E. BETANCES HOSPITAL–MAYAGUEZ MEDICAL CENTER BRANCH (400103)**, 410 Hostos Avenue, Zip 00680–1501; tel. 787/834–8656, (Nonreporting) **A**1 3 5 10
Primary Contact: Julio Andino Rodriguez, Chief Executive Officer
CFO: Carlos Muniz, Director Finance
Control: State–Government, nonfederal **Service:** General Medical and Surgical

Staffed Beds: 144

★ **HOSPITAL PEREA (400123)**, 15 Basora Street, Zip 681, Mailing Address: P.O. Box 170, Zip 681; tel. 787/834–0101, (Nonreporting) **A**9 10 **S** United Medical Corporation
Primary Contact: Rafael Alvarado, Chief Executive Officer
CFO: Joannie Garcia, CPA, Finance Director
CMO: Humberto Olivencia, M.D., Medical Director
Web address: www.paviahealth.com/perea_hospital.htm
Control: Corporation, Investor–owned, for–profit **Service:** General Medical and Surgical

Staffed Beds: 103

Hospital, Medicare Provider Number, Address, Telephone, Approval, Facility, and Physician Codes, Health Care System

★ American Hospital Association (AHA) membership
☐ The Joint Commission accreditation
○ American Osteopathic Association (AOA) accreditation
△ Commission on Accreditation of Rehabilitation Facilities (CARF) accreditation

MOCA—Moca County

HOSPITAL SAN CARLOS BORROMEO (400111), 550 Concepcion Bera Ayala, Zip 676; tel. 787/877–8000 **A**9 10 **F**8 15 25 26 38 43 46 55 57 62 68 73 74 75 77 79 80 81 84 96 100 102 107 119 135
Primary Contact: Javier Malave, Administrator
Web address: www.hospitalsancarlos.org
Control: Other not–for–profit (including NFP Corporation) **Service:** General Medical and Surgical

Staffed Beds: 106 **Admissions:** 5857 **Census:** 74 **Outpatient Visits:** 34242 **Births:** 1121 **Total Expense ($000):** 23314 **Payroll Expense ($000):** 8270 **Personnel:** 402

PONCE—Ponce County

★ **DR. PILA'S HOSPITAL (400003)**, Avenida Las Americas, Zip 731, Mailing Address: P.O. Box 1910, Zip 00733–1910; tel. 787/848–5600, (Nonreporting) **A**1 3 5 9 10
Primary Contact: Melvin Lamboy, Chief Executive Officer
Web address: www.drpila.com
Control: Other not–for–profit (including NFP Corporation) **Service:** General Medical and Surgical

Staffed Beds: 169

★ **HOSPITAL DE DAMAS (400022)**, Ponce by Pass, Zip 731; tel. 787/840–8686, (Total facility includes 19 beds in nursing home–type unit) **A**1 3 5 9 10 **F**17 18 20 22 38 59 61 68 70 74 79 83 84 96 107 117 118 119 135
Primary Contact: Enrique A. Vicens Rivera, Jr., Executive Director
CFO: Julio Colon, Director Finance
CMO: Pedro Benitez, M.D., Medical Director
CIO: Bienvenido Ortiz, Coordinator Information Systems
CHR: Gilberto Cuevas, Director Human Resources
Web address: www.hospitaldamas.com
Control: Other not–for–profit (including NFP Corporation) **Service:** General Medical and Surgical

Staffed Beds: 269 **Admissions:** 14074 **Census:** 198 **Outpatient Visits:** 43704 **Births:** 1731 **Total Expense ($000):** 66061 **Payroll Expense ($000):** 31187 **Personnel:** 1029

★ **HOSPITAL ONCOLOGICO ANDRES GRILLASCA (400028)**, Centro Medico De Ponce, Zip 733, Mailing Address: P.O. Box 331324, Zip 00733–1324; tel. 787/848–0800, (Nonreporting) **A**1 3 5 9 10
Primary Contact: Manuel J. Vazquez, Executive Administrator
COO: Elyonel Ponton Cruz, Finance Director
CFO: Elyonel Ponton Cruz, Finance Director
CMO: Roberto Velasquez, M.D., Medical Director
CIO: Maria T. Teissonniere, Public Relations Director
CHR: Carlos T. Santiago, Director Human Resources
Control: Other not–for–profit (including NFP Corporation) **Service:** Cancer

Staffed Beds: 49

★ **ST. LUKE'S EPISCOPAL HOSPITAL (400002)**, 917 Tito Castro Avenue, Zip 00731–4717, Mailing Address: P.O. Box 336810, Zip 00733–6810; tel. 787/844–2080 **A**1 9 10 **F**3 7 8 13 14 17 18 22 32 38 68 70 73 74 79 81 84 86 96 100 107 118 119 135
Primary Contact: Guillermo J. Martin, President and Chief Executive Officer
COO: Jorge De Jesus, Associate Chief Operating Officer
CFO: Aristides Castro, Chief Financial Officer
CMO: Gilberto Rodriguez, M.D., Medical Director
CHR: Juan Salazar, Director Human Resources
Control: Church–operated, Nongovernment, not–for profit **Service:** General Medical and Surgical

Staffed Beds: 205 **Admissions:** 17805 **Census:** 194 **Outpatient Visits:** 97589 **Births:** 0 **Total Expense ($000):** 107250 **Payroll Expense ($000):** 31082 **Personnel:** 1332

SAN GERMAN—San German County

★ **HOSPITAL DE LA CONCEPCION (400021)**, Carr 2, Km 173, Bo Cain Alto, Zip 00683–3920, Mailing Address: P.O. Box 285, Zip 00683–0285; tel. 787/892–1860 **A**1 3 5 9 10 **F**3 15 25 49 68 70 74 79 84 96 100 103 107 119 134
Primary Contact: Felicita Bonilla, Administrator
CFO: Lizmari Calderon, Director Finance
CMO: Ivan Acosta, M.D., Medical Director
CIO: Aaron Mendez, Director Management Information Systems
CHR: Jorge Rodriguez Diaz, Director Human Resources
Web address: www.hospitalconcepcion.org
Control: Church–operated, Nongovernment, not–for profit **Service:** General Medical and Surgical

Staffed Beds: 167 **Admissions:** 9315 **Census:** 137 **Outpatient Visits:** 43960 **Births:** 855 **Total Expense ($000):** 51825 **Payroll Expense ($000):** 18920 **Personnel:** 791

HOSPITAL METROPOLITANO SAN GERMAN (400126), Calle Javilla Al Costado Parque de Bombas, Zip 683; tel. 787/892–5300, (Nonreporting) **A**9 10
Primary Contact: Ramon Lopez–Maldonado, Chief Executive Officer
Control: Corporation, Investor–owned, for–profit **Service:** Other specialty

Staffed Beds: 40

SAN JUAN—San Juan County

★ **ASHFORD PRESBYTERIAN COMMUNITY HOSPITAL (400001)**, 1451 Ashford Avenue Condado, Zip 907, Mailing Address: P.O. Box 9020032, Zip 00902–0032; tel. 787/721–2160 **A**1 9 10 **F**3 11 13 15 25 26 28 33 38 48 49 51 52 56 66 68 70 73 74 79 80 82 83 84 86 87 96 100 107 112 119 135 **P**4
Primary Contact: Pedro J. Gonzalez, Executive Director
COO: Marilyn Morales, Assistant Administrator and Chief Operating Officer
CFO: Milagros Ortiz, CPA, Chief Financial Officer
CMO: Francisco de Torres, M.D., Medical Director
CIO: Arnaldo Quinones, Chief Information Officer
CHR: Irma Carrillo, Director Human Resources
Web address: www.presbypr.com
Control: Other not–for–profit (including NFP Corporation) **Service:** General Medical and Surgical

Staffed Beds: 201 **Admissions:** 12050 **Census:** 163 **Outpatient Visits:** 108885 **Births:** 3629 **Total Expense ($000):** 59685 **Payroll Expense ($000):** 19763 **Personnel:** 753

★ **AUXILIO MUTUO HOSPITAL (400016)**, Ponce De Leon Avenue, Zip 00918–1000, Mailing Address: P.O. Box 191227, Zip 00919–1227; tel. 787/758–2000 **A**1 5 9 10 **F**3 15 17 18 20 22 25 26 27 38 46 52 59 68 70 72 73 74 75 76 77 79 81 82 83 84 86 96 97 98 99 100 105 107 118 119 120 121 126 127 128 130 135 137
Primary Contact: Jorge L. Matta Serrano, Administrator
COO: Carmen Martin, Associate Administrator
CFO: Maria L. Marti, Director Fiscal Services
CMO: Jose Isado, M.D., Medical Director
CIO: Edgardo Rodriguez, Director Management Information Systems
CHR: Maria Vega, Director Human Resources
Web address: www.auxiliopr.com
Control: Other not–for–profit (including NFP Corporation) **Service:** General Medical and Surgical

Staffed Beds: 515 **Admissions:** 24098 **Census:** 403 **Outpatient Visits:** 1900887 **Births:** 2130 **Personnel:** 1936

★ **CARDIOVASCULAR CENTER OF PUERTO RICO AND THE CARIBBEAN (400124)**, Americo Miranda Centro Medico, Zip 936, Mailing Address: P.O. Box 366528, Zip 00936–6528; tel. 787/754–8500, (Nonreporting) **A**1 9 10 **S** Puerto Rico Department of Health
Primary Contact: Humberto M. Monserrate, Executive Director
COO: Ivette Nunez Lopez, Executive Subdirector
CFO: Maria de Lourdes Alegria, Comptroller
CMO: Jose E. Novoa, M.D., Medical Director
CIO: Eugenio Torres Ayala, Director Information Systems
CHR: Hector Troche Garcia, Director Human Resources
Web address: www.cardiovascular.gobierno.pr
Control: State–Government, nonfederal **Service:** General Medical and Surgical

Staffed Beds: 121

DOCTORS' CENTER HOSPITAL SAN JUAN (400006), (Formerly Doctors Hospital), 1395 San Rafael Street, Zip 00909–2518, Mailing Address: Box 11338, Santurce Station, Zip 00910–1338; tel. 787/723–2950 **A**9 10 **F**38 68 74 84 96 97 107 119
Primary Contact: Alfredo E. Volckers, Executive Director
COO: Juan Carlos Latorre, Administrator
CFO: Alejandro Santiago, Director Finance
CMO: Lourdes Feliciano, M.D., Chairman
CIO: Antonio Sisco, Chief Information Officer
CHR: Carmen Perez, Director Human Resources
Control: Corporation, Investor–owned, for–profit **Service:** General Medical and Surgical

Staffed Beds: 89 **Admissions:** 1728 **Census:** 24 **Outpatient Visits:** 4823 **Births:** 134 **Total Expense ($000):** 12627 **Payroll Expense ($000):** 3501 **Personnel:** 237

★ **HEALTHSOUTH REHABILITATION HOSPITAL (403025)**, University Hospital, 3rd Floor, Zip 923, Mailing Address: P.O. Box 70344, Zip 923; tel. 787/274–5100, (Nonreporting) **A**3 5 10 **S** HEALTHSOUTH Corporation
Primary Contact: Daniel Del Castillo, Chief Executive Officer
CMO: Edwardo Ramos, M.D., Medical Director
CHR: Frances Fuentes, Coordinator Human Resources
Control: Corporation, Investor–owned, for–profit **Service:** Rehabilitation

Staffed Beds: 32

★ **HOSPITAL DEL MAESTRO (400004)**, 550 Sergio Cuevas, Zip 00918–3741, Mailing Address: P.O. Box 364708, Zip 00936–4708; tel. 787/758–8383, (Nonreporting) **A**1 9 10
Primary Contact: Milton Maldonado, Administrator
COO: Milton Maldonado, Administrator
CFO: Marisol Vargas, Director Finance
CMO: Jose Montalvo, M.D., Medical Director
CIO: Laura Rodriguez, Director Medical Records
CHR: Orlando Santiago, Human Resources Officer
Control: Corporation, Investor–owned, for–profit **Service:** General Medical and Surgical

Staffed Beds: 250

☒ **HOSPITAL METROPOLITAN (400106)**, (Formerly Fundacion Hospital Metropolitan), 1785 Route 21, Zip 922, Mailing Address: P.O. Box 11981, Zip 922; tel. 787/782–9999, (Nonreporting) **A**1 9 10
Primary Contact: Gilberto Gonzalez, Chief Executive Officer
CFO: Maritza Rodriguez, Chief Financial Officer
CMO: Maria de los Angeles Correa, M.D., Medical Director
CIO: Abel Velez, Chief Information Officer
Control: Corporation, Investor–owned, for–profit **Service:** General Medical and Surgical

Staffed Beds: 130

☒ **HOSPITAL PAVIA–HATO REY (400128)**, (Formerly Hato Rey Community Hospital), Mailing Address: 435 Ponce De Leon, Hato Rey, Zip 00917–3428; tel. 787/754–0909, (Nonreporting) **A**1 3 5 9 **S** United Medical Corporation
Primary Contact: Astro Munoz, Chief Executive Officer
Web address: www.paviahealth.com
Control: Corporation, Investor–owned, for–profit **Service:** General Medical and Surgical

Staffed Beds: 180

☒ **HOSPITAL PAVIA–SANTURCE (400019)**, 1462 Asia Street, Zip 00909–2143, Mailing Address: Box 11137, Santurce Station, Zip 00910–1137; tel. 787/727–6060, (Nonreporting) **A**1 9 10 **S** United Medical Corporation
Primary Contact: Henry Ruberte, Executive Director
CFO: Francisco Espina, Finance Director
Web address: www.paviahealth.com
Control: Corporation, Investor–owned, for–profit **Service:** General Medical and Surgical

Staffed Beds: 309

★ **HOSPITAL SAN FRANCISCO (400098)**, 371 Avenida De Diego, Zip 00923–1711, Mailing Address: P.O. Box 29025, Zip 00929–0025; tel. 787/767–2528 **A**9 10 **F**3 25 26 38 68 79 83 84 96 106
Primary Contact: Karen Z. Artau, Vice President of Administration
CFO: Carmen S. Oliveras, Director Finance
CMO: Hector L. Cotto, M.D., Medical Director
CIO: Deborah Nieves, Management Information Systems Director
CHR: Sugehi Santiago, Director
Web address: www.sanpablo.com
Control: Corporation, Investor–owned, for–profit **Service:** General Medical and Surgical

Staffed Beds: 139 **Admissions:** 6725 **Census:** 104 **Outpatient Visits:** 42207 **Births:** 0 **Total Expense ($000):** 25064 **Payroll Expense ($000):** 10847 **Personnel:** 398

HOSPITAL SAN GERARDO (400121), El Senorial Mail Station 250, Winston Churchill Avenue 138, Rio Piedras, Zip 926; tel. 787/761–8383, (Nonreporting) **A**9 10
Primary Contact: Lorenzo Bosques, Administrator
Control: Other not–for–profit (including NFP Corporation) **Service:** Chronic disease

Staffed Beds: 60

☒ **I. GONZALEZ MARTINEZ ONCOLOGIC HOSPITAL (400012)**, Puerto Rico Medical Center, Hato Rey, Zip 935, Mailing Address: P.O. Box 191811, Zip 00919–1811; tel. 787/765–2382, (Nonreporting) **A**1 2 3 5 9 10
Primary Contact: Milagros Vargas, Executive Director
COO: Felix Ortiz, Administrator
CFO: Yolanda Quinones, Director Finance
CMO: Carlos Chevere, M.D., Medical Director
CHR: Luz Maria Hernandez, Director Human Resources
Control: Other not–for–profit (including NFP Corporation) **Service:** General Medical and Surgical

Staffed Beds: 47

★ **INDUSTRIAL HOSPITAL**, Puerto Rico Medical Center, Zip 936, Mailing Address: P.O. Box 365028, Zip 936; tel. 787/764–3660 **A**9 **F**3 8 16 18 34 38 62 72 73 75 77 79 85 86 94 119 132 137 **P**5 6
Primary Contact: Jane Vega De Diaz, Executive Director
CFO: Robert Bernier Casanova, Chief Financial Officer
CMO: Carmen Carrasquillo, M.D., Medical Director
CHR: Sonia M. Lebron, Human Resources Specialist
Control: State–Government, nonfederal **Service:** General Medical and Surgical

Staffed Beds: 121 **Admissions:** 3013 **Census:** 74 **Outpatient Visits:** 157342 **Personnel:** 629

SAN CARLOS GENERAL HOSPITAL (400017), 1822 Ponce De Leon Avenue, Zip 00909–1906, Mailing Address: Call Box 8410, Zip 00910–8410; tel. 787/727–5858, (Nonreporting) **A**9 10
Primary Contact: Pedro J. Gonzalez, Executive Director
Control: Corporation, Investor–owned, for–profit **Service:** General Medical and Surgical

Staffed Beds: 66

☒ **SAN JORGE CHILDREN'S HOSPITAL**, 252 San Jorge Street, Santurce, Zip 00912–3310; tel. 787/727–1000, (Nonreporting) **A**1 5 9 **S** United Medical Corporation
Primary Contact: Domingo Cruz Vivaldi, Senior Vice President Operations
CFO: Jose Marrero, Director Finance
CMO: Luis Clavell, M.D., Medical Director
CIO: Jorge Calderon, Chief Information Systems
CHR: Ana Acevedo, Supervisor Human Resources
Web address: www.sanjorgechildrenhospital.com
Control: Corporation, Investor–owned, for–profit **Service:** Children's general

Staffed Beds: 125

☒ **SAN JUAN CAPESTRANO HOSPITAL (404005)**, Mailing Address: Rural Route 2, Box 11, Zip 926; tel. 787/760–0222 **A**1 10 **F**2 4 5 25 36 88 89 90 91 92 93 94 95 119 121 **S** Universal Health Services, Inc.
Primary Contact: Laura Vargas, Chief Executive Officer and Managing Director
CFO: Julia Cruz, Chief Financial Officer
CMO: Luis Dorta, M.D., Medical Director
CIO: Ana Morandeira, Director Marketing
CHR: Luis Rivera, Administrator
Web address: www.sjcapestrano.com
Control: Corporation, Investor–owned, for–profit **Service:** Psychiatric

Staffed Beds: 108 **Admissions:** 4861 **Census:** 98 **Outpatient Visits:** 33668 **Births:** 0 **Total Expense ($000):** 15609 **Payroll Expense ($000):** 6290 **Personnel:** 234

☒ **SAN JUAN CITY HOSPITAL (400015)**, Puerto Rico Medical Center, Zip 928, Mailing Address: PMB 79, P.O. Box 70344, Zip 00936–8344; tel. 787/766–2222, (Nonreporting) **A**1 3 5 10
Primary Contact: Myrna Boysen, Executive Director
COO: Fernando Sosa, Chief Operating Officer
CFO: Juan Gonzalez, Chief Financial Officer
CMO: Ana Barletta, M.D., Medical Director
CIO: Julio Motta, Chief Information Officer
CHR: Mildred Oritz, Chief Human Resources Officer
Web address: www.massalud.com
Control: City–Government, nonfederal **Service:** General Medical and Surgical

Staffed Beds: 267

★ **STATE PSYCHIATRIC HOSPITAL (404006)**, Monacillos Avenue, Zip 936, Mailing Address: Call Box 2100, Caparra Heights Station, Zip 00922–2100; tel. 787/766–4646, (Nonreporting) **A**3 5 10
Primary Contact: Lisette Diaz, Executive Director
CMO: Diana Diaz, M.D., Medical Director
CHR: Idalia Garcia, Chief Human Resources Officer
Control: State–Government, nonfederal **Service:** Psychiatric

Staffed Beds: 153

★ **UNIVERSITY HOSPITAL (400061)**, Mailing Address: P.O. Box 2116, Zip 922; tel. 787/754–0101, (Nonreporting) **A**3 5 10 **S** Puerto Rico Department of Health
Primary Contact: Roberto Burgos, Executive Director
COO: Roberto Burgos, Executive Director
CFO: Janet Baez, Director
CMO: Ricardo Moscoso, M.D., Medical Director
CIO: Josue Martinez, Coordinator Information Systems
CHR: Wanda Maldonado, Director Human Resources
Control: State–Government, nonfederal **Service:** General Medical and Surgical

Staffed Beds: 262

☒ **UNIVERSITY PEDIATRIC HOSPITAL (403301)**, Barrio Monacenno, Carretera 22, Rio Piedras, Zip 935, Mailing Address: P.O. Box 2129, San Juan, Zip 00922–2129; tel. 787/777–3535, (Nonreporting) **A**1 5 9 10 **S** Puerto Rico Department of Health
Primary Contact: Sylvette Llovet, Executive Director
COO: Sylvette Llovet, Executive Director
CFO: Blanca Olmo, Director Finance
CMO: Concepcion Q. De Longo, M.D., Medical Director
Control: State–Government, nonfederal **Service:** Children's general

Staffed Beds: 145

Hospital, Medicare Provider Number, Address, Telephone, Approval, Facility, and Physician Codes, Health Care System

★ American Hospital Association (AHA) membership
☐ The Joint Commission accreditation
○ American Osteopathic Association (AOA) accreditation
△ Commission on Accreditation of Rehabilitation Facilities (CARF) accreditation

★ △ **VETERANS AFFAIRS MEDICAL CENTER**, 10 Casia Street, Zip 00921–3201; tel. 787/641–7582, (Total facility includes 149 beds in nursing home–type unit) (Nonreporting) **A**1 2 3 5 7 8 9 **S** Department of Veterans Affairs
Primary Contact: Nancy Reissener, Acting Director
CFO: Ricardo Ochoa, Chief Fiscal Officer
CMO: Sandra C. Gracia, M.D., Chief of Staff
CIO: Manuel Negron, Chief Information Technology Service
CHR: Damaris Tosado, Manager Human Resources
Web address: www.va.gov/visn8/sanjuan
Control: Veterans Affairs, Government, federal **Service:** General Medical and Surgical

Staffed Beds: 479

VEGA BAJA—Vega Baja County

★ **WILMA N. VAZQUEZ MEDICAL CENTER (400115)**, KM 39 1/2 Road 2, Call Box 7001, Zip 694; tel. 787/858–1580, (Total facility includes 20 beds in nursing home–type unit) **A**9 10 **F**3 38 59 62 63 68 75 79 82 84 86 96 97 100 107 117 119 135 137 **P**8
Primary Contact: Ramon J. Vilar, Administrator
COO: Jose O. Pabon, Director Operations
CFO: Youdie Reynolds–Gossette, Controller
CMO: Jaime Rodriguez Solis, M.D., President Medical Staff
CIO: Miguel Aponte, Supervisor Management Information Systems
CHR: Aymette Garcia, Manager Human Resources
Control: Corporation, Investor–owned, for–profit **Service:** General Medical and Surgical

Staffed Beds: 110 **Admissions:** 4581 **Census:** 66 **Outpatient Visits:** 35038 **Births:** 3 **Total Expense ($000):** 17584 **Payroll Expense ($000):** 5712 **Personnel:** 295

YAUCO—Yauco County

★ **HOSPITAL METROPOLITANO DR. TITO MATTEI (400110)**, Carretera 128 KM 1, Zip 698, Mailing Address: P.O. Box 68, Zip 698; tel. 787/856–1000 **A**1 5 9 10 **F**3 7 8 13 15 33 37 38 43 49 59 60 68 73 74 75 77 79 80 81 82 84 86 88 89 90 91 92 93 96 105 107 118 119 **P**5 7
Primary Contact: Pedro Barez, Chief Executive Officer
CFO: Elizabeth Gonzalez, Chief Financial Officer
CMO: Manuel Ramirez Soto, M.D., Medical Director
CIO: Edson Ortiz, Chief Information Officer
CHR: Nannete Acosta, Director Human Resources
Web address: www.hmyauco.com
Control: Individual, Investor–owned, for–profit **Service:** General Medical and Surgical

Staffed Beds: 130 **Admissions:** 6091 **Census:** 73 **Outpatient Visits:** 61234 **Births:** 680

VIRGIN ISLANDS

CHRISTIANSTED—St. Croix County

★ **GOVERNOR JUAN F. LOUIS HOSPITAL (480002)**, 4007 Estate Diamond Ruby, Zip 00820–4421; tel. 340/778–6311, (Nonreporting) **A**1 10
Primary Contact: Gregory Calliste, FACHE, Ph.D., President and Chief Executive Officer
COO: Darice Plaskett, R.N., Chief Operating Officer and Vice President Patient Care Services
CFO: Anthony Saul, CPA, Chief Financial Officer
CMO: Kendall Griffith, M.D., Medical Director
CIO: Reuben D. Molloy, Chief Information Officer
CHR: Joan Jean–Baptiste, Vice President Human Resources
Web address: www.jflusvi.org
Control: State–Government, nonfederal **Service:** General Medical and Surgical

Staffed Beds: 165

SAINT THOMAS—St. Thomas County

★ **SCHNEIDER REGIONAL MEDICAL CENTER (480001)**, (Formerly Roy Lester Schneider Hospital), 9048 Sugar Estate, Charlotte Amalie, Zip 802; tel. 340/776–8311, (Nonreporting) **A**1 10
Primary Contact: Amos W. Carty, Jr., Chief Executive Officer
CFO: Peter R. Najawicz, Chief Financial Officer
CMO: Thelma Ruth Watson, M.D., Medical Director
CIO: J. C. Creque, Director Management Information Systems
CHR: Marlene J. Adams, Director Human Resources
Web address: www.rlshospital.org
Control: State–Government, nonfederal **Service:** General Medical and Surgical

Staffed Beds: 123

Many Facility Codes have changed. Please refer to the AHA Guide Code Chart.

U.S. Government Hospitals Outside the United States, by Area

GERMANY

Heidelberg: ★ Heidelberg Army Community Hospital, APO, CMR 242, AE 09042

Landstuhl: ★ Landstuhl Army Regional Medical Center, APO, CMR 402, AE 09180

Wuerzburg: ★ Wuerzburg Army Community Hospital, APO, USAMEDDAC Wuerzburg, Ut 26610, AE 09244

ICELAND

Keflavilk: ★ U. S. Naval Hospital–Keflavilk, FPO, PSC 1003, Box 8, AE 09728–0308

ITALY

Naples: ★ U. S. Naval Hospital, FPO, AE 09619

JAPAN

Yokosuka: ★ U. S. Naval Hospital, FPO, Box 1487, AP 96350

KOREA

Seoul: ★ U. S. Army Community Hospital Seoul, APO, 121st General Hospital, AP 96205

Yongsan: Medcom 18th Commander, Facilities Division Eamc L EM, APO, AP 96205

SPAIN

Rota: ★ U. S. Naval Hospital, Rota, FPO, PSC 819, Box 18, AE 09645–2500

TAIWAN

Taipei: U. S. Naval Hospital Taipei, Taipei, No 300 Shin–Pai Road, Sec 2

Index of Hospitals

This section is an index of all hospitals in alphabetical order by hospital name, followed by the city, state, and page reference to the hospital's listing in Section A.

A

B

C

D

E

F

G

H

I

J

K

L

M

N

O

P

Q

R

S

T

U

V

W

Y

Z

Index of Health Care Professionals

This section is an index of the key health care professionals for the hospitals and/or health care systems listed in this publication. The index is in alphabetical order, by individual, followed by the title, institutional affiliation, city, state and page reference to the hospital and/or health care system listing in section A and/or B.

A

B

C

D

E

F

G

H

HEATHERLY, John
  Assistant Administrator Support Services, Hunt Memorial Hospital District, Greenville, TX, p. A572
  Assistant Administrator Human and Support Services Director, Presbyterian Hospital of Commerce, Commerce, TX, p. A560
HEATHERLY, Neil A., CHE, Chief Executive Officer, StoneCrest Medical Center, Smyrna, TN, p. A548
HEATHERLY, Steve, Executive Vice President Finance and Operations, Swain County Hospital, Bryson City, NC, p. A424
HEATHERLY–LLOYD, Sara, Chief Operating Officer, St. Mary's Medical Center of Campbell County, La Follette, TN, p. A541
HEATON, Lisa, Administrator and Chief Nursing Officer, Johnson County Community Hospital, Mountain City, TN, p. A544
HEAUKULANI, Ed, Manager Information Technology, Kona Community Hospital, Kealakekua, HI, p. A155
HEBBELER, Gregory P.
  Chief Financial Officer, Methodist Hospital, Henderson, KY, p. A236
  Chief Financial Officer, Methodist Hospital Union County, Morganfield, KY, p. A241
HEBEL, Barbara, Director Human Resources, Doylestown Hospital, Doylestown, PA, p. A495
HEBERT, FACHE, Erie J., Senior Vice President, West Jefferson Medical Center, Marrero, LA, p. A255
HEBERT, Gerard, Chief Financial Officer, Natchitoches Regional Medical Center, Natchitoches, LA, p. A256
HEBERT, Katherine, Administrator and Chief Executive Officer, Lafayette General Surgical Hospital, Lafayette, LA, p. A252
HEBERT, Kim, Chief Financial Officer, Our Lady of Lourdes Regional Medical Center, Lafayette, LA, p. A253
HEBERT, Michael, Director Technology, MetroWest Medical Center, Framingham, MA, p. A282
HEBERT, Raquel, Business Manager, Sugar Land Surgical Hospital, Sugar Land, TX, p. A597
HEBERT, Timothy, Director Human Resources, Teche Regional Medical Center, Morgan City, LA, p. A256
HEBURN, William R., Interim Chief Executive Officer, Trinity Medical Center, Birmingham, AL, p. A17
HECHT, Bill
  Chief Financial Officer, CHRISTUS Hospital–St. Elizabeth, Beaumont, TX, p. A555
  Chief Financial Officer, CHRISTUS Hospital–St. Mary, Port Arthur, TX, p. A591
  Chief Financial Officer, CHRISTUS St. Patrick Hospital of Lake Charles, Lake Charles, LA, p. A253
HECHT, M.D., Melvyn L., Medical Director and Chief Medical Officer, Youville Hospital and Rehabilitation Center, Cambridge, MA, p. A281
HECHT, M.D., Michael, Medical Director, Tucson Heart Hospital, Tucson, AZ, p. A38
HECK, George L., President and Chief Executive Officer, Coffee Regional Medical Center, Douglas, GA, p. A142
HECK, M.D., Michael, Chief Medical Officer, Fairview Range Regional Health Services, Hibbing, MN, p. A315
HECK, Terry
  Vice President Finance and Chief Financial Officer, Saint Joseph Regional Medical Center, South Bend, IN, p. A199
  Chief Financial Officer, Saint Joseph Regional Medical Center–Mishawaka Campus, Mishawaka, IN, p. A196
  Vice President Finance and Chief Financial Officer, Saint Joseph Regional Medical Center–Plymouth Campus, Plymouth, IN, p. A198
HECKATHORNE, Daniel R., Associate Administrator and Chief Financial Officer, Pioneers Memorial Healthcare District, Brawley, CA, p. A53
HECKENLIVELY, Gretchin, Director Financial Services, Tri–County Area Hospital, Lexington, NE, p. A364
HECKER, Lisa, Director Human Resources, Hedrick Medical Center, Chillicothe, MO, p. A338
HECKERMAN, Ray, Chief Executive Officer and Managing Director, Coastal Harbor Treatment Center, Savannah, GA, p. A149
HECKERT, Brian, Medical Center Director, Wm. Jennings Bryan Dorn Veterans Affairs Medical Center, Columbia, SC, p. A521
HECKERT Jr., Robert J., Chief Executive Officer, Gerald Champion Regional Medical Center, Alamogordo, NM, p. A391
HECKEY, M.D., Robert, Chief of Staff, Sutter Medical Center of Santa Rosa, Chanate Campus, Santa Rosa, CA, p. A86
HECKMAN, Katie, Director Community Relations, Saint Joseph Berea, Berea, KY, p. A232
HEDBERG, M.D., Peter, Chief of Staff, Medical Center of Southeastern Oklahoma, Durant, OK, p. A469
HEDDE, M.D., Charles C., Vice President Medical Affairs, Good Samaritan Hospital, Vincennes, IN, p. A200
HEDDEN, Elizabeth A., Chief Financial Officer, Johnson Memorial Hospital, Franklin, IN, p. A190
HEDDERMAN, Michael, Senior Vice President Finance and Chief Financial Officer, Marianjoy Rehabilitation Hospital, Wheaton, IL, p. A185
HEDGES, David, Chief Financial Officer, Southwestern Regional Medical Center, Tulsa, OK, p. A480
HEDGES, M.D., Tony, Chief Medical Officer, Lamb Healthcare Center, Littlefield, TX, p. A583
HEDGES, M.D., Wesley, President Medical Staff, Mercy Hospital of Tiffin, Tiffin, OH, p. A462
HEDIN, Darren, Chief Financial Officer, Benchmark Behavioral Health Systems, Woods Cross, UT, p. A609
HEDRICK, M.D., William, Chief Medical Officer, Rehabilitation Hospital of Fort Wayne, Fort Wayne, IN, p. A190
HEDSTROM, Marjorie, Associate Director Operations, Veterans Affairs Central Iowa Health Care System, Des Moines, IA, p. A206
HEEMAN, John, Director Information Systems, Huntsville Memorial Hospital, Huntsville, TX, p. A579
HEER, John R., President and Chief Executive Officer, North Mississippi Health Services, Inc., Tupelo, MS, p. B85
HEFFERNAN, Rebecca, Director Human Resources, MetroWest Medical Center, Framingham, MA, p. A282
HEFFERS, Margaret, Assistant Vice President Human Resources, Geisinger Wyoming Valley Medical Center, Wilkes–Barre, PA, p. A514
HEFFLINGER, Larry, Director Information Systems, Fulton County Health Center, Wauseon, OH, p. A464
HEFFNER, John, Chief Executive Officer, Select Specialty Hospital of Savannah, Savannah, GA, p. A149
HEFNER, Drew, Chief Financial Officer, River Park Hospital, Huntington, WV, p. A638
HEGER, Jim, Director Human Resources, Citizens Medical Center, Victoria, TX, p. A601
HEGGEM, M.D., Mark, Medical Director, Riverwood HealthCare Center, Aitkin, MN, p. A310
HEGLAND, M.D., Larry T., Chief Medical Officer, Saint Clare's Hospital, Weston, WI, p. A657
HEGLAND, Sandra, Chief Executive Officer, HEALTHSOUTH Bakersfield Rehabilitation Hospital, Bakersfield, CA, p. A51
HEIDER, M.D., Allison, Chief of Staff, Cox Monett Hospital, Monett, MO, p. A345
HEIDER, John R., Vice President Finance, Augusta Health Care, Fishersville, VA, p. A614
HEIDER, Lisa A.
  Vice President Finance and Chief Information Officer, Community Memorial Hospital, Menomonee Falls, WI, p. A650
  Interim Chief Information Officer, Froedtert Memorial Lutheran Hospital, Milwaukee, WI, p. A651
HEIDT, Robert, Director Information Systems, Pembina County Memorial Hospital and Wedgewood Manor, Cavalier, ND, p. A440
HEIFNER, Robert A., Chief Operation Officer, Rio Grande Regional Hospital, McAllen, TX, p. A585
HEILER, M.D., Greg, President Medical Staff, Sacred Heart Hospital, Eau Claire, WI, p. A646
HEILSBERG, Jim, Chief Financial Officer and Chief Information Officer, Whitman Hospital and Medical Center, Colfax, WA, p. A626
HEIMAN, Thomas, Assistant Vice President Information Services, John T. Mather Memorial Hospital, Port Jefferson, NY, p. A416
HEINDEL, Michael, Chief Operating Officer, North Vista Hospital, North Las Vegas, NV, p. A373
HEINEMANN, Don, Associate Administrator and Chief Operating Officer, Blount Memorial Hospital, Maryville, TN, p. A542
HEINRICH, D.O., Mark T., President Medical Staff, Oroville Hospital, Oroville, CA, p. A74
HEINRICH, Michael G., Senior Vice President Finance and Chief Financial Officer, Mercy Iowa City, Iowa City, IA, p. A208
HEINRICHS, CPA, Alice, Chief Financial Officer, Hamilton Hospital, Webster City, IA, p. A215
HEINSOHN, M.D., Carmel, Medical Director, Bournewood Health System, Brookline, MA, p. A280
HEINTZELMAN, Gayle M., President and Chief Executive Officer, Mercy Hospital Clermont, Batavia, OH, p. A445
HEINZE, Kyle, Coordinator Information Technology, Riveredge Hospital, Forest Park, IL, p. A171
HEINZMAN, Jerry, Senior Vice President and Chief Financial Officer, Sampson Regional Medical Center, Clinton, NC, p. A426
HEISE, Lance, Director Human Resources, Cascade Medical Center, Leavenworth, WA, p. A628
HEISE, Teresa, Coordinator Management Information Systems, Pender Community Hospital, Pender, NE, p. A368
HEISER, Eric, Chief Information Resource Management, Royal C. Johnson Veterans Memorial Medical Center, Sioux Falls, SD, p. A531
HEISLER, M.D., Michael, Chief Medical Officer, Emory Eastside Medical Center, Snellville, GA, p. A150
HEISMEYER, Joyce, Chief Executive Officer, Allen County Hospital, Iola, KS, p. A221
HEITZENRATER, James F., President, Saint Joseph Mount Sterling, Mount Sterling, KY, p. A241
HELDRETH, Karen, Director Data Processing, Parkview Hospital, El Reno, OK, p. A470
HELGERSON, Bryce R., Chief Administrative Officer, Legacy Mount Hood Medical Center, Gresham, OR, p. A484
HELLA, Timothy, Director Information Management, Otsego Memorial Hospital, Gaylord, MI, p. A296
HELLER, Lisa, Manager Human Resources and Payroll, Mercy Medical Center–New Hampton, New Hampton, IA, p. A211
HELLER, Lynn, Administrator and Chief Executive Officer, Muenster Memorial Hospital, Muenster, TX, p. A587
HELLER, Michael, Chief Financial Officer, Corry Memorial Hospital, Corry, PA, p. A494
HELLER, Tom, Vice President Human Resources, Camden–Clark Memorial Hospital, Parkersburg, WV, p. A640
HELLER, M.D., Virginia, Medical Director, Parkside Hospital, Tulsa, OK, p. A479
HELLERSTEDT, Wayne P., Chief Executive Officer, Helen Newberry Joy Hospital, Newberry, MI, p. A302
HELLSTERN, Anne, Associate Administrator and Chief Operating Officer, East Ohio Regional Hospital, Martins Ferry, OH, p. A458
HELLYER, Nancy R., Chief Executive Officer, Saint Joseph Regional Medical Center–Plymouth Campus, Plymouth, IN, p. A198
HELM, Ben, Interim Chief Financial Officer, Haskell County Healthcare System, Stigler, OK, p. A478
HELM, Pamela E., Executive Director, Devereux Texas Treatment Network, League City, TX, p. A582
HELM, Richard, Chief Information Officer, Jellico Community Hospital, Jellico, TN, p. A539
HELMAN, Sharon M.
  Director, Jonathan M. Wainwright Memorial VA Medical Center, Walla Walla, WA, p. A634
  Director, Jonathan M. Wainwright Memorial VA Medical Center, Walla Walla, WA, p. A634
  Director, Veterans Affairs Medical Center, Spokane, WA, p. A633
HELMANDOLLAR, Billy, Director Information Services, Wallace Thomson Hospital, Union, SC, p. A526
HELMINIAK, Clare, Clinical Director, U. S. Public Health Service Indian Hospital, Parker, AZ, p. A33
HELMS, Candace, Director Information Services, Good Samaritan Medical Center, West Palm Beach, FL, p. A133
HELMS, Ella Raye, Administrator, Fisher County Hospital District, Rotan, TX, p. A592
HELMS, Sheryl, Vice President Human Resources, Good Samaritan Regional Medical Center, Corvallis, OR, p. A483
HELSEL, David S., M.D., Chief Executive Officer, Spring Grove Hospital Center, Baltimore, MD, p. A269
HELSINGER, Irene, Senior Vice President and Chief Administrative Officer, St. Luke's Episcopal Hospital, Houston, TX, p. A578
HELTON, Deirdre, Director Human Resources, Lakeway Regional Hospital, Morristown, TN, p. A544
HELTON, Michelle, Director Human Resources, Wallace Thomson Hospital, Union, SC, p. A526
HELTON, Stephanie, Chief Financial Officer, Weatherford Regional Hospital, Weatherford, OK, p. A480
HELWIG, Ann M., Chief Executive Officer, Knoxville Hospital & Clinics, Knoxville, IA, p. A209
HEMBREE, Greg, Chief Financial Officer, South Georgia Medical Center, Valdosta, GA, p. A151
HEMETER, Donald, Administrator, Wayne General Hospital, Waynesboro, MS, p. A335
HEMKER, Robert
  Chief Financial Officer, Palomar Medical Center, Escondido, CA, p. A57
  Chief Financial Officer, Pomerado Hospital, Poway, CA, p. A77
HEMMING, Stuart, Chief Operating Officer, Portsmouth Regional Hospital, Portsmouth, NH, p. A378
HEMPLER, Shannan, Director Human Resources, Norton County Hospital, Norton, KS, p. A224
HEMPLING, Randall, Chief Executive Officer, MountainView Regional Medical Center, Las Cruces, NM, p. A393
HEMSCHOOT, Ed, Director Information Systems, Montgomery Hospital Medical Center, Norristown, PA, p. A504
HENDERSON, Andre, Director Information Systems, Mission Community Hospital–San Fernando Campus, Los Angeles, CA, p. A67
HENDERSON, Anita, Director Human Resources, Pennock Hospital, Hastings, MI, p. A298

I

J

K

L

M

N

O

P

Q

R

S

T

U

V

W

X

Y

Z

AHA Membership Categories

The American Hospital Association is primarily an organization of hospitals and related institutions. Its object, according to its bylaws, is "to promote high–quality health care and health services for all the people through leadership in the development of public policy, leadership in the representation and advocacy of hospital and health care organization interests, and leadership in the provision of services to assist hospitals and health care organizations in meeting the health care needs of their communities."

The major source of income for the AHA is its membership dues, which are established by the membership through the Board of Trustees. The types of membership are described in the following paragraphs.

Institutional Members

Type I–Hospitals or health services organizations or systems which provide a continuum of integrated, community health resources and which include at least one licensed hospital that is owned, leased, managed or religiously sponsored.

Type I members include hospitals, health care systems, integrated delivery systems, and physician hospital organizations (PHOs) and health maintenance organizations (HMOs) wholly or partially owned by or owning a member hospital or system. A Type I member hospital, health care system or integrated delivery system may, at its discretion and upon approval of a membership application by the Association chief executive officer, extend membership to the health care provider organizations, other than a hospital that it owns, leases, or fully controls.

Type II–Freestanding Health Care Provider Organizations

These are health provider organizations, other than registered hospitals, that provide patient care services, including, but not limited to, ambulatory, preventive, rehabilitative, specialty, post–acute and continuing care, as well as physician groups, health insurance services, and staff and group model health maintenance organizations without a hospital component. Type II members are not owned or controlled by a Type I hospital, health care system or integrated delivery system member. They may, however, be part of an organization eligible for, but not holding, Type I membership.

Type III–Other Organizations

Type III membership includes organizations interested in the objectives of the Association, but not eligible for Type I or Type II membership. Organizations eligible for Type III membership shall include, but not be limited to, associations, societies, foundations, corporations, educational and academic institutions, companies, government agencies, international health providers, and organizations having an interest in and a desire to support the objectives of the Association.

Provisional Members

Hospitals that are in the planning or construction stage and that, on completion, will be eligible for institutional membership type I or type II. Provisional membership may also be granted to applicant institutions that cannot, at present, meet the requirements of type I or type II membership.

Government Institution Group Members

Groups of government hospitals operated by the same unit of government may obtain institutional membership under a group plan. Membership dues are based on a special schedule set forth in the bylaws of the AHA.

Contracting Hospitals

The AHA also provides membership services to certain hospitals that are prevented from holding membership because of legal or other restrictions.

Other Institutional Members

Types IA

Hospitals

U.S. hospitals and hospitals in areas associated with the U.S. that are type IA members of the American Hospital Association are included in the list of hospitals in section A. Canadian types I members of the American Hospital Association are listed below.

Canada

ALBERTA

Lamont: LAMONT HEALTH CARE CENTRE, P.O. Bag 10, Zip T0B 2R0; tel. 780/895–2211; Harold James, Executive Director

MANITOBA

Winnipeg: RIVERVIEW HEALTH CENTRE, 1 Morley Avenue East, Zip R3L 2P4; tel. 204/452–3411; Norman R. Kasian, President and Chief Executive Officer

ONTARIO

Alliston: STEVENSON MEMORIAL HOSPITAL, 200 Fletcher Crescent, Zip L9R 1W7; tel. 705/435–6281; Gary Ryan, Executive Director

London: ST. JOSEPH'S HEALTH CENTRE, P.O. Box 5777, Zip N6A 4V2; tel. 519/646–6000; Clifford A. Nordal, President and Chief Executive Officer

North York: BAYCREST CENTRE–GERIATRIC CARE, 3560 Bathurst Street, Zip M6A 2E1; tel. 416/785–2500; William E. Reichman, President and Chief Executive Officer

Renfrew: RENFREW VICTORIA HOSPITAL, 499 Raglan Street North, Zip K7V 1P6; tel. 613/432–4851; Randy V. Penney, Executive Director

Thornhill: SHOULDICE HOSPITAL, 7750 Bayview Avenue, Zip L3T 4A3; tel. 905/889–1125; Alan O'Dell, Administrator

Toronto: MOUNT SINAI HOSPITAL, 600 University Avenue, Zip M5G 1X5; tel. 416/596–4200; Joseph Mapa, FACHE, Executive Vice President and Chief Operating Officer

TORONTO REHABILITATION INSTITUTE, 550 University Avenue, Zip M5G 2A2; tel. 416/597–5111; Mark Rochon, President and Chief Executive Officer

QUEBEC

Montreal: MOUNT SINAI HOSPITAL CENTER, 5690 Cavendish Cote St–Luc', Zip H4W 1S7; tel. 514/369–2222; Joseph Rothbart, Executive Director

Associated University Programs in Health Administration

CALIFORNIA

San Diego: CALIFORNIA COLLEGE SAN DIEGO, 2820 Camino Del Rio South, Suite 300, Zip 92108–3821; tel. 619/295–5784; Jeff Welsh, President

San Francisco: GOLDEN GATE UNIVERSITY, 536 Mission Street, University Library, Zip 94105–2968; tel. 415/442–7242; Steven Dunlap, Head Techinical Services

CONNECTICUT

Hartford: RENSSELAER POLYTECHNIC INSTITUTE, 275 Windsor Street, Zip 06410; tel. 203/548–5346; Gregory M. Sparzo, Senior Program Manager

IOWA

Iowa City: DEPARTMENT OF HEALTH MANAGEMENT AND POLICY, UNIVERSITY OF IOWA, 200 Hawkins Drive, E211 GH, Zip 52242; tel. 319/384–5120; Barry Greene, Interim Head

KANSAS

Shawnee Mission: ROCKHURST UNIVERSITY CONTINUING EDUCATION CENTER, 6901 West 63rd Street, Zip 66202; tel. 913/432–7755; William M. Sutton, Training Consultant

MAINE

Standish: SAINT JOSEPH'S COLLEGE OF MAINE, 278 Whites Bridge Road, Zip 04084–5263; tel. 207/893–7983; John R. Pratt, Director Health Administration

MARYLAND

Bethesda: NAVAL SCHOOL OF HEALTH SCIENCES, Naval Medical Command, National Region, Zip 20889–5611; tel. 301/295–1251

MISSOURI

Saint Louis: WASHINGTON UNIVERSITY, SCHOOL OF MEDICINE, 4547 Clayton Avenue, Zip 63110; tel. 314/362–2477; Stuart Boxerman, Interim Director

PENNSYLVANIA

University Park: PENNSYLVANIA STATE UNIVERSITY, 116 Henderson Building, Zip 16802; tel. 814/863–2859; Diane Brannon, Ph.D., Interim Department Head, Health Policy and Administration

TEXAS

Brooks AFB: U. S. AIR FORCE SCHOOL OF AEROSPACE MEDICINE, USAFSAM–CCE, Zip 78235–5301; tel. 210/536–4251; Colonel Richard E. Bachmann, Jr., Commander

San Antonio: ARMY–BAYLOR UNIVERSITY PROGRAM IN HEALTH CARE ADMINISTRATION, tel. 210/221–6443; Lieutenant Colonel M. Nicholas Coppola, Program Director

TRINITY UNIVERSITY, One Trinity Place, #58, Zip 78212–7200; tel. 210/736–8107; Mary E. Stefl, Ph.D., Chairman

Sheppard AFB: U. S. AIR FORCE SCHOOL OF HEALTH CARE SCIENCES, Building 1900, MSTL/114, Academic Library, Zip 76311; tel. 817/851–2511

PUERTO RICO

San Juan: SCHOOL OF PUBLIC HEALTH, P.O. Box 5067, Zip 00936; tel. 809/767–9626; Orlando Nieves, Dean

Hospital Schools of Nursing

ILLINOIS

Canton: GRAHAM HOSPITAL School of Nursing

NEW JERSEY

Plainfield: MUHLENBERG REGIONAL MEDICAL CENTER School of Nursing

NEW YORK

Elmira: ARNOT–OGDEN MEMORIAL HOSPITAL School of Nursing

PENNSYLVANIA

New Castle: JAMESON HOSPITAL School of Nursing

Pittsburgh: WESTERN PENNSYLVANIA HOSPITAL School of Nursing

Nonhospital Preacute and Postacute Care Facilities

ALABAMA

Fort Rucker: LYSTER U. S. ARMY HEALTH CLINIC, Andrews Lane, Building 301, Zip 36362–5000; tel. 334/255–7361; Colonel Suzan Denny, Commanding Officer

Montgomery: MAXWELL CLINIC, 330 Kirkpatrick Avenue East, Zip 36112–6219; tel. 334/953–7801; Colonel Bart O. Iddins, Commander

ALASKA

Anchorage: DEPARTMENT OF VETERANS AFFAIRS ALASKA MEDICAL AND REGIONAL OFFICE CENTER, 2925 Debarr Road, Zip 99508–2989; tel. 907/257–6930; Alonzo M. Poteet, III., Director

ARIZONA

Davis–Monthan AFB: U. S. AIR FORCE CLINIC, 4175 South Alamo Avenue, Zip 85707–4405; tel. 520/228–2930

Fort Huachuca: RAYMOND W. BLISS ARMY HEALTH CENTER, 45001 Winrow Avenue, Zip 85613–7040; tel. 520/533–2350; Colonel Thomas W. Smith, M.D., MSC, Commander

Glendale: U. S. AIR FORCE HOSPITAL LUKE, Luke AFB, 7219 North Litchfield Road, Zip 85309–1525; tel. 623/856–7502; Colonel Schuyler K. Geller, Commander

ARKANSAS

Jacksonville: U. S. AIR FORCE CLINIC LITTLE ROCK, Little Rock AFB, Zip 72099–5057; tel. 501/987–7411; Colonel Rebecca A. Russell, USAF, Commander

Little Rock: CENTRAL ARKANSAS RADIATION THERAPY INSTITUTE, P.O. Box 55050, Zip 72215; tel. 501/664–8573; Janice E. Burford, President and Chief Executive Officer

CALIFORNIA

Beale AFB: U. S. AIR FORCE HOSPITAL, 15301 Warren Shingle Road, Zip 95903–1907; tel. 530/634–4838; Lieutenant Colonel Robert G. Quinn, MSC, USAF, FACHE, Administrator

Edwards AFB: U. S. AIR FORCE CLINIC, 30 Hospital Road, Building 5500, Zip 93524–1730; tel. 661/277–2010; Colonel Sally Petty, Commander

Los Angeles: DEPARTMENT OF VETERANS AFFAIRS, OUTPATIENT CLINIC, 351 East Temple Street, Room A–102, Zip 90012; tel. 213/253–5000; Jules Morevac, Ph.D., Director

Martinez: VETERANS AFFAIRS NORTHERN CALIFORNIA HEALTH SYSTEM, 150 Muir Road, Zip 94553; tel. 925/372–2000; Lawrence S. Sandler, Director

Port Hueneme: NAVAL AMBULATORY CARE CENTER, Zip 93043; tel. 805/982–6301; Major Frederick White, Officer–in–Charge

San Francisco: VETERANS AFFAIRS OUTPATIENT CLINIC, 4150 Clement Street, Zip 94121; tel. 415/221–4810; Lawrence C. Stewart, Director

Sepulveda: VETERANS AFFAIRS MEDICAL CENTER, 16111 Plummer Street, Zip 91343; tel. 818/891–7711; Charles M. Doorman, Acting Director

Vandenberg AFB: U. S. AIR FORCE HOSPITAL, 338 South Dakota Street, Zip 93437–6307; tel. 805/606–1110; Colonel Alan D. Newton, Commander

Winterhaven: U. S. PUBLIC HEALTH SERVICE INDIAN HOSPITAL, P.O. Box 1368, Zip 85366–1368; tel. 760/572–0217; Kent Smalley, M.D., Acting Chief Executive Officer and Clinical Director

CONNECTICUT

Groton: NAVAL HOSPITAL, 1 Wahoo Drive, Box 600, Zip 06349–5600; tel. 860/694–3261

Newington: VETERANS AFFAIRS MEDICAL CENTER–NEWINGTON CAMPUS, 555 Willard Avenue, Zip 06111–2600; tel. 860/666–6951; Roger L. Johnson, Director

DELAWARE

Dover: U. S. AIR FORCE HOSPITAL DOVER, 300 Tuskegee Boulevard, Zip 19902–7307; tel. 302/677–2525; Colonel Genanne Hansen–Bayless, Administrator

New Castle: CHRISTIANA CARE VISITING NURSE ASSOCIATION, One Reads Way, Zip 19720; tel. 302/327–8200; Lynn C. Jones, President

PHYSICAL THERAPY PLUS, 1 Reads Way, Suite 300, Zip 19720; tel. 302/326–8755; Stephen Rombach, Director

Newark: CHRISTIANA CARE IMAGING CENTER, 4751 Ogletown–Stanton Road, Zip 19713; tel. 302/731–9800; Charles Baxter, Director

CHRISTIANA INFUSION SERVICES, 200 Hygeia Drive, Zip 19713; Barbara Knightly, Director

CHRISTIANA SURGICENTER, 4755 Ogletown–Stanton Road, Zip 19718; tel. 302/733–6900; Margaret Wojcik, Coordinator

HEALTH CARE CENTER AT CHRISTIANA, 200 Hygeia Drive, Zip 19714

Wilmington: EUGENE DUPONT PREVENTIVE MEDICINE AND REHABILITATION INSTITUTE, 3506 Kennett Pike, Zip 19807; tel. 302/655–4041

FLORIDA

Jacksonville: BAPTIST HOME HEALTH CARE, 3563 Philips Highway, Suite 202, Zip 32207; tel. 904/202–4300; Diane Jones, Director

BAPTIST OCCUPATIONAL HEALTH, 1325 San Marco Boulevard, Suite 301, Zip 32207; tel. 904/202–2395; Donna Snider, Director

BAPTIST PRIMARY CARE, 3563 Philips Highway, Suite 101, Zip 32207; tel. 904/376–3744; Mother Superior Berl O'Malley, Administrator

PAVILION INFUSION THERAPY, 3563 Philips Highway, Suite 202, Zip 32207; tel. 904/202–5730; Diane Jones, Director

PSYCHIATRIC AND PSYCHOLOGICAL CARE, 4160 University Boulevard South, Zip 32216; tel. 904/376–3800; Mark A. Masters, Ph.D., Director

Key West: NAVAL REGIONAL MEDICAL CLINIC, 1500 Douglas Circle, Zip 33040; tel. 305/293–4613; Commander Stephen Lanier, Officer–in–Charge

MacDill AFB: U. S. AIR FORCE HOSPITAL, 8415 Bayshore Boulevard, Zip 33621–1607; tel. 813/827–9521

Tyndall AFB: U. S. AIR FORCE CLINIC, 340 Magnolia Avenue, Zip 32403–5612; tel. 850/283–7515; Colonel Michael J. Murphy, Commander

GEORGIA

Calhoun: ALLIANT HEALTH PLANS, INC., 401 South Wall Street, Suite 201, Zip 30701; tel. 706/629–8848; Jeff Myers, Chief Executive Officer

GEORGIA HEALTH PLUS, 401 South Wall Street, Suite 201, Zip 30701; tel. 706/629–1833; Jeff Myers, Chief Executive Officer

Moody AFB: U. S. AIR FORCE HOSPITAL MOODY, 3278 Mitchell Boulevard, Zip 31699–1500; tel. 229/257–3772

Robins AFB: U. S. AIR FORCE CLINIC, 655 Seventh Street, Zip 31098–2227; tel. 912/327–7996; Colonel John A. Lee, USAF, MSC, Commander

Rome: CENTREX, 420 East Second Avenue, Zip 30161; tel. 706/235–1006; Dee B. Russell, M.D., Chief Executive Officer

COMMUNITY HOSPICECARE, P.O. Box 233, Zip 30162–0233; tel. 706/232–0807; Kurt Stuenkel, FACHE, President and Chief Executive Officer

FLOYD HOME HEALTH AGENCY, P.O. Box 6248, Zip 30162–6248; tel. 706/802–4600; Kurt Stuenkel, FACHE, President and Chief Executive Officer

FLOYD MEDICAL OUTPATIENT SURGERY, P.O. Box 233, Zip 30162–0233; tel. 706/802–2070; Kurt Stuenkel, FACHE, President and Chief Executive Officer

FLOYD REHABILITATION CENTER, P.O. Box 233, Zip 30162–0233; tel. 706/802–2091; Kurt Stuenkel, FACHE, President and Chief Executive Officer

HAWAII

Honolulu: KAISER MOANALUA, 3288 Moanalua Road, Zip 96819–1469; tel. 808/432–0000; Melodee J. Deutsch, M.S., M.P.H., Director of Quality

VETERANS AFFAIRS MEDICAL REGIONAL OFFICE, 459 Patterson Road, Zip 96819; tel. 808/541–1582

Pearl Harbor: NAVAL REGIONAL MEDICAL CLINIC, Box 121, Building 1750, Zip 96860–5080; tel. 808/471–3025; Captain Joseph Moore, Commanding Officer

IDAHO

Mountain Home AFB: U. S. AIR FORCE CLINIC, 90 Hope Drive, Building 600, Zip 83648–5300; tel. 208/828–7610; Lieutenant Colonel Gregory W. Carson, Administrator

ILLINOIS

Great Lakes: NAVAL HOSPITAL, 3001A Sixth Street, Zip 60088–5230; tel. 847/688–4560; Captain Thomas E. McGue, Commanding Officer

KANSAS

Fort Leavenworth: MUNSON ARMY HEALTH CENTER, 550 Pope Avenue, Zip 66027–2332; tel. 913/684–6420; Colonel William Davis, Commander

Wichita: U. S. AIR FORCE HOSPITAL, 59570 Leavenworth Street, Suite 6E4, Zip 67221–5300; tel. 316/759–5421

LOUISIANA

Barksdale AFB: U. S. AIR FORCE CLINIC, 243 Curtiss Road, Suite 100, Zip 71110–5300; tel. 318/456–6004; Colonel James M. Benge, Commander

New Orleans: NAVAL MEDICAL CLINIC, 1 Sanctuary Drive, Zip 70142–5300; tel. 504/678–2400

MAINE

Damariscotta: MILES MEDICAL GROUP, INC., 35 Miles Street, Zip 04543; tel. 207/563–1234; Stacey Miller–Friant, Director

Kennebunk: SOUTHERN MAINE HEALTH AND HOME SERVICES, P.O. Box 739, Zip 04043; tel. 207/985–4767; Elaine Brady, RN, Executive Director

MARYLAND

Annapolis: NAVAL MEDICAL CLINIC, 50 Rodgers Road, Zip 21402; tel. 410/293–1330; Captain Francis R. MacMahon, MC, USN, Commanding Officer

Baltimore: ST. AGNES HEALTH SERVICES, 900 Caton Avenue, Zip 21229; tel. 410/368–2945; Peter Clay, Senior Vice President Managed Care

ST. AGNES HOME CARE AND HOSPICE, 3421 Benson Avenue, Suite G100, Zip 21227; tel. 410/368–2825; Robin Dowell, Director

Fort George G Meade: KIMBROUGH ARMY HEALTH CENTER, 2480 Llewellyn Avenue, Zip 20755; tel. 301/677–4171; Colonel Billie J. Mielcarek, Commanding Officer

Fort Howard: VETERANS AFFAIRS MARYLAND HEALTH CARE SYSTEM–FORT HOWARD DIVISION, 9600 North Point Road, Zip 21052–9989; tel. 410/477–1800; Patricia Vicari, Director

Patuxent River: NAVAL MEDICAL CLINIC, 47149 Buse Road, Zip 20670–5370; tel. 301/342–1418; Captain Ralph A. Puckett, MC, USN, Commanding Officer

MASSACHUSETTS

Boston: JOSLIN CLINIC, INC., One Joslin Place, Zip 02215; tel. 617/732–2400; C. Ronald Kahn, M.D., President and Chief Executive Officer

Springfield: BAY STATE VISITING NURSE ASSOCIATION AND HOSPICE, 50 Maple Street, Zip 01105; tel. 413/781–5070; Ruth Odgren, President

MICHIGAN

Big Rapids: MECOSTA HEALTH SERVICES, 650 Linden Street, Zip 49307; tel. 231/796–3200; Gail Bullard, Director

Detroit: ST. JOHN DETROIT RIVERVIEW CENTER, 7733 East Jefferson Avenue, Zip 48214–2598; tel. 313/499–4000; Joseph M. Tasse, FACHE, President and Chief Executive Officer

ST. JOHN NORTHEAST COMMUNITY HOSPITAL, 4777 East Outer Drive, Zip 48234–0401; tel. 313/369–9100

Port Huron: TRI–HOSPITAL E.M.S., 309 Grand River Street, Zip 48060; tel. 313/985–7115; Ken Cummings, Chief Executive Officer

WILLOW ENTERPRISES, INC., 1221 Pine Grove Avenue, Zip 48060; tel. 313/989–3737

Sault Sainte Marie: SAULT SAINTE MARIE TRIBAL HEALTH AND HUMAN SERVICES CENTER, 2864 Ashmun Street, Zip 49783; tel. 906/495–5651; Russell Vizina, Division Director Health

Vicksburg: BRONSON VICKSBURG HOSPITAL, 13326 North Boulevard, Zip 49097–1099; tel. 269/649–2321; Frank J. Sardone, President and Chief Executive Officer

MINNESOTA

Bemidji: BEMIDJI SAME DAY SURGERY, 1233 34th Street N.W., Zip 56601; tel. 218/333–5000; Randy D. Beck, Executive Partner

MERITCARE DIALYSIS CTR BEMIDJI, 1300 Anne Street N.W., Zip 56601; tel. 218/333–5000; Maria Regnier

MERITCARE PHYSICAL THERAPY BEMIDJI, 3604 Bemidji Avenue North, Zip 56601; tel. 218/333–5000; Don Martin

MERITCARE RADIATION ONCOLOGY PHYSICS, 1233 34th Street N.W., Zip 56601; tel. 218/333–4600; Randy D. Beck, Executive Partner

Detroit Lakes: MERITCARE DIALYSIS CENTER DETROIT LAKES, 1027 Washington Avenue, Zip 56501; tel. 218/847–0825; Roger L. Gilbertson, M.D., President and Chief Executive Officer

MERITCARE PHYSICAL THERAPY DETROIT LAKES, 1245 Washington Avenue, Zip 56501; tel. 218/846–2000; Brenda Muckenhirn

Morris: MERITCARE DIALYSIS CENTER MORRIS, P.O. Box 660, Zip 56267–0660; tel. 320/586–2832; Maria Regnier

Pelican Rapids: MERITCARE HOME HEALTH CARE PELICAN RAPIDS, P.O. Box 737, Zip 56572–0737; tel. 218/863–2273; Marsha Sjulstad

Saint Paul: HEALTHEAST CARE, INC., 1690 University Avenue W, Suite 370, Zip 55104–3729; tel. 651/232–5070

HEALTHEAST HOME CARE, INC., 1700 University Avenue, Zip 55104; tel. 651/232–2800; Ann M. Schrader, Vice President and Administrator

HEALTHEAST MEDICAL RESEARCH INSTITUTE, 559 Capitol Boulevard, Zip 55103; tel. 651/232–2300; Timothy H. Hanson, President and Chief Executive Officer

MISSISSIPPI

Columbus: U. S. AIR FORCE CLINIC, 201 Independence, Suite 235, Zip 39701–5300; tel. 662/434–2297; Colonel Dave Armstrong, Commander

MISSOURI

Independence: SURGI–CARE CENTER OF INDEPENDENCE, 2311 Redwood Avenue, Zip 64057; tel. 816/373–7995

Whiteman AFB: U. S. AIR FORCE CLINIC WHITEMAN, 331 Sijan Avenue, Zip 65305–5001; tel. 660/687–1194; Lieutenant Colonel David Wilmot, USAF, MSC, Administrator

MONTANA

Malmstrom AFB: U. S. AIR FORCE CLINIC, Zip 59402–5300; tel. 406/731–3863; Colonel David L. Doty, Administrator

Miles City: VETERANS AFFAIRS MEDICAL CENTER, 210 South Winchester Avenue, Zip 59301–4742; tel. 406/232–3060

NEBRASKA

Grand Island: GRAND ISLAND DIVISION, 2211 North Broadwell Avenue, Zip 68803–2196; tel. 308/382–3660; Gary N. Nugent, Chief Executive Officer

North Platte: GREAT PLAINS PHO, INC., P.O. Box 1167, Zip 69103; tel. 308/535–7496; Todd Hlavaty, M.D., Chairman

Offutt AFB: EHRLING BERGQUIST HOSPITAL, 2501 Capehart Road, Zip 68113–2160; tel. 402/294–7312; Colonel Howard Googins, Deputy Commander

NEW HAMPSHIRE

Portsmouth: NAVAL MEDICAL CLINIC, Building H–1, Zip 03801; tel. 207/439–1000; Captain F. M. Richardson, Commanding Officer

NEW JERSEY

Atlantic City: ATLANTICARE SURGERY CENTER, 1925 Pacific Avenue, Zip 08401; tel. 609/407–2200; William Aarons, M.D., President

Egg Harbor City: ATLANTICARE BEHAVIORAL HEALTH, 2511 Fire Road, Suite B10, Zip 08234; tel. 609/272–6392; Theodore Stryker, President and Chief Executive Officer

ATLANTICARE HEALTH SERVICES, 2500 English Creek Avenue, Building C., Zip 08234; tel. 609/272–6392; Donald Parker, President and Chief Executive Officer

Fort Monmouth: PATTERSON ARMY HEALTH CLINIC, Stephenson Avenue, Building 1075, Zip 07703–5504; tel. 908/532–1266; Colonel Don Speers, Commander

Millburn: ATLANTIC HOME CARE AND HOSPICE, 33 Bleeker Street, Zip 07041; tel. 973/379–8400; Susan Quinn, Administrator

Morristown: ALLIANCE IMAGING CENTER, 65 Maple Street, Zip 07960; tel. 973/267–5700; Barbara Picorale, Administrator

Succasunna: DIALYSIS CENTER OF NORTHWEST NEW JERSEY, 170 Righter Road, Zip 07876; tel. 973/584–1117; Carol Cahill, Administrator

NEW MEXICO

Albuquerque: ALBUQUERQUE IHS HEALTH CENTER, 801 Vassar Drive N.E., Zip 87106–2799; tel. 505/248–4000; Maria Rickert, Chief Executive Officer

Cannon AFB: U. S. AIR FORCE CLINIC, 208 West Casablanca Avenue, Zip 88103–5300; tel. 505/784–6318; Lieutenant Colonel Michelle Pufall, Administrator

Holloman AFB: U. S. AIR FORCE CLINIC, 280 First Street, Zip 88330–8273; tel. 505/572–5587

Kirtland AFB: U. S. AIR FORCE CLINIC–KIRTLAND, 2050 A. Second Street S.E., Zip 87117–5559; tel. 505/846–3547; Colonel Regina Aune, Commander

NEW YORK

Bronx: MORRISANIA DIAGNOSTIC AND TREATMENT CENTER, 1225 Gerard Avenue, Zip 10452; tel. 718/960–2777; Victor Hernandez, Administrator

SEGUNDO RUIZ BELVIS DIAGNOSTIC AND TREATMENT CENTER, 545 East 142nd Street, Zip 10454; tel. 718/579–4000; Victor Hernandez, Administrator

Brooklyn: CUMBERLAND DIAGNOSTIC AND TREATMENT CENTER, 100 North Portland Avenue, Zip 11205; tel. 718/260–7500; K. Candis Best, Administrator

DR. SUSAN SMITH NURSING REHABILITATION CENTER, 594 Albany Avenue, Zip 11203; tel. 718/245–7000; Ruth Ogieste, Administrator

EAST NEW YORK DIAGNOSTIC AND TREATMENT CENTER, 2094 Pitkin Avenue, Zip 11207; tel. 718/240–0400; Yvette Isaac, Administrator

Cheektowaga: MCAULEY SETON HOME CARE, 2875 Union Road, Suite 14, Zip 14227; tel. 716/685–4870; Mark A. Sullivan, President and Senior Administrative Officer

MERCY HOME CARE, 2875 Union Road, Suite 14, Zip 14227; tel. 716/685–4870; Mark A. Sullivan, President and Senior Administrative Officer

Fort Drum: 11050 MOUNT BELVEDERE BOULEVARD, 11050 Mount Belvedere Boulevard, Zip 13602–5004; tel. 315/772–4024; Colonel John M. Wempe, Commander

New York: RENAISSANCE DIAGNOSTIC AND TREATMENT CENTER, 215 West 125 Street, Zip 10027; tel. 212/932–6500; Rose Garcia, Administrator

Tuckahoe: HOME NURSING ASSOCIATION OF WESTCHESTER, 69 Main Street, Zip 10707; tel. 919/961–2818; Mary Wehrberger, Director

NORTH CAROLINA

Cherry Point: NAVAL HOSPITAL, PSC Box 8023, Zip 28533–0023; tel. 252/466–0266; Captain Eleanor V. Valentin, MSC, USN, Commanding Officer

Seymour Johnson AFB: U. S. AIR FORCE HOSPITAL SEYMOUR JOHNSON, 1050 Curtis Avenue, Zip 27531–5300; tel. 919/722–1812; Colonel Donna M. Lake, Commanding Officer

NORTH DAKOTA

Grand Forks AFB: U. S. AIR FORCE HOSPITAL, 220 G. Street, Zip 58205–6332; tel. 701/747–5391

Jamestown: MERITCARE PHYSICAL THERAPY, 904 Fifth Avenue N.E., Zip 58401; tel. 702/253–4000; Jim Schaefer, Regional Clinic Manager

Minot: U. S. AIR FORCE REGIONAL HOSPITAL, 10 Missile Avenue, Zip 58705–5024; tel. 701/723–5103; Colonel Lawrence Riddles, Commander

OHIO

Cleveland: KAISER PERMANENTE, 1001 Lakeside, Zip 44114; tel. 216/362–2000; Patricia Kennedy–Scott, President

Columbus: OHIOHEALTH GROUP, 445 Hutchinson Avenue, Suite 300, Zip 43235–5677; tel. 614/566–0123; John Burns, Chief Executive Officer

VETERANS AFFAIRS OUTPATIENT CLINIC, 543 Taylor Avenue, Zip 43203–1278; tel. 614/257–5200; Lillian Thone, Chief Executive Officer

Worthington: HOMEREACH, 404 East Wilson Bridge Road, Suite H., Zip 43085; tel. 614/566–0888; Fran Baby, Vice President Home and Hospice Services

OKLAHOMA

Altus: U. S. AIR FORCE CLINIC ALTUS, 301 North First Street, Zip 73523–5005; tel. 580/481–5204; Colonel Charles W. Cotta, USAF, Commander

Clinton: U. S. PUBLIC HEALTH SERVICE INDIAN HOSPITAL, Route 1, Box 3060, Zip 73601–9303; tel. 580/323–2884; Terri Schmidt, Director

Enid: U. S. AIR FORCE CLINIC, Vance AFB, Building 810, Zip 73705–5000; tel. 405/249–7494; Lieutenant Colonel Andrew F. Love, MSC, USAF, Commander Medical Group

Eufaula: EUFALA INDIAN HEALTH CENTER, 800 Forest Avenue, Zip 74432; tel. 918/689–2547; Shelly Crow, Health System Administrator

Okmulgee: OKMULGEE INDIAN HEALTH SYSTEM, 1313 East 20th, Zip 74447; tel. 918/758–1926; Steve Landsberry, Administrator

Sapulpa: SAPULPA INDIAN HEALTH CENTER, 1125 East Clevelend, Zip 74066; tel. 918/224–9310; Judy Aaron, Health System Administrator
Tinker AFB: U. S. AIR FORCE HOSPITAL TINKER, 5700 Arnold Street, Zip 73145; tel. 405/736–2084; Colonel Lloyd A. Reinke, Commander
Tulsa: WARREN CLINIC, 6600 South Yale Avenue, Zip 74136; tel. 918/502–7300; James Kaltenbachner, Senior Vice President

PENNSYLVANIA

Chester: COMMUNITY HOSPITAL, DIVISION OF THE CROZER–CHESTER MEDICAL CENTER, Ninth and Wilson Streets, Zip 19013–2098; tel. 610/494–0700; Kevin Caputo, M.D., Vice President Operations
Dallastown: WELLSPAN MEDICAL GROUP, Zip 17313; tel. 717/851–6515
Warminster: ABINGTON MEMORIAL HEALTH CENTER – WARMINSTER CAMPUS, 225 Newtown Road, Zip 18974–5221; tel. 215/441–6600; Katie Farrell, Chief Executive Officer
York: SOUTH CENTRAL PREFERRED, 45 Monument Road, Suite 200, Zip 17403; tel. 717/741–9511; Charles H. Chodroff, M.D., Executive Director
WELLSPAN HEALTH CARE SERVICES, 1001 South George Street, Zip 17405; tel. 717/851–2121; Bruce M. Bartels, President

RHODE ISLAND

Newport: NAVAL HOSPITAL, 1 Riggs Road, Zip 02841–1002; tel. 401/841–3771; Captain Andre Greedan, Deputy Commander

SOUTH CAROLINA

Shaw AFB: U. S. AIR FORCE HOSPITAL SHAW, 431 Meadowlark Street, Zip 29152–5019; tel. 803/895–6324; Colonel Troy Molnar, Commander

SOUTH DAKOTA

Ellsworth AFB: U. S. AIR FORCE CLINIC, 2900 Doolittle Drive, Zip 57706–4821; tel. 605/385–3201; Colonel Chris Gray, Commanding Officer

TEXAS

Abilene: U. S. AIR FORCE CLINIC, 7th Medical Group, Dyess AFB, Zip 79607–1367; tel. 915/696–5429; Major John G. Wiseman, Administrator
Corpus Christi: NAVAL HOSPITAL, 10651 East Street, Zip 78419–5131; tel. 361/961–2688; Captain James P. Rice, Commanding Officicer
NORTHWEST REGIONAL HOSPITAL, 13725 Northwest Boulevard, Zip 78410–5199; tel. 361/241–4243
Dallas: SURGICARE OF TRAVIS CENTER, INC., 13355 Noel Road, Suite 650, Zip 75240–6694; tel. 713/520–1782
El Paso: VETERANS AFFAIRS HEALTHCARE CENTER, 5001 North Piedras Street, Zip 79930–4211; tel. 915/564–6100; Edward Valenzuela, Director
Houston: GRAMERCY OUTPATIENT SURGERY CENTER. LTD., 2727 Gramercy, Zip 77025; Carol Simons, Administrator
WEST HOUSTON SURGICARE, 970 Campbell Road, Zip 77024; tel. 713/461–3547
Laughlin AFB: U. S. AIR FORCE HOSPITAL, 590 Mitchell Boulevard, Zip 78843–5200; tel. 210/298–6311
San Antonio: U. S. AIR FORCE CLINIC BROOKS, Building 615, Zip 78235–5300; tel. 210/536–2087; Lieutenant Colonel Donald Sampson, Commanding Officer
Sheppard AFB: U. S. AIR FORCE REGIONAL HOSPITAL–SHEPPARD, 149 Hart Street, Suite 1, Zip 76311–3478; tel. 940/676–5874; Lieutenant Colonel Lance Rogers, Administrator
Universal City: U. S. AIR FORCE CLINIC RANDOLPH, 221 3rd Street West, Zip 78150–4801; tel. 210/652–5701; Lieutenant Colonel Dennis E. Franks, Administrator
Webster: BAY AREA SURGICARE CENTER, 502 Medical Center Boulevard, Zip 77598; tel. 281/332–2433

VIRGINIA

Fort Lee: KENNER ARMY HEALTH CENTER, 700 24th Street, Zip 23801–1716; tel. 804/734–9256; Colonel Nancy Gilmore–Lee, Commander
Quantico: NAVAL REGIONAL MEDICAL CLINIC, 3259 Catlin Avenue, Zip 22134; tel. 703/784–1699; Captain Joan Queen, Commanding Officer

WASHINGTON

Fairchild AFB: U. S. AIR FORCE CLINIC, 701 Hospital Loop, Suite 102, Zip 99011–8701; tel. 509/247–5217; Colonel Barbara Jefts, Commanding Officer

WISCONSIN

Green Bay: UNITY HOSPICE, P.O. Box 28345, Zip 54324–8345; tel. 920/494–0225; Donald Seibel, Executive Director

WYOMING

Cheyenne: U. S. AIR FORCE HOSPITAL, 6900 Alden Drive, Zip 82005–3913; tel. 307/773–2045; Major Brenda Bullard, Administrator

Provisional Hospitals

This listing includes organizations that, as of June 1, 2008, were in the planning or construction stage and that, on completion, will be eligible for Type I institutional membership. Some hospitals are granted provisional membership for reasons related to other Association requirements. Hospitals classified as provisional members for reasons other than being under construction are indicated by a bullet (●).

KANSAS

Greensburg: KIOWA COUNTY MEMORIAL HOSPITAL, P.O. Box 616, Zip 67054–0616; tel. 620/723–3341; Mary Sweet, Administrator

KENTUCKY

Louisville: NORTON SOUTHWEST HOSPITAL, 9700 Stonestreet Road, Zip 40272; tel. 502/933–8100; Thomas D. Kmetz, President

MICHIGAN

Novi: ST. JOHN PROVIDENCE PARK HOSPITAL, 47601 Grand River Avenue, Zip 48374; tel. 248/465–4100; Robert F. Casalou, President

OHIO

Cincinnati: THE LINDER CENTER OF HOPE, 3200 Burnett Avenue, 6 Ridgeway, Zip 45229; tel. 513/585–8668; Paul Keck, M.D., President and Chief Executive Officer

TEXAS

El Paso: SIERRA PROVIDENCE EASTSIDE HOSPITAL, 2400 Trawood Drive, Zip 79936; tel. 915/577–8000; Sally Hurt–Steffen, Chief Executive Officer

Rockwall: PRESBYTERIAN HOSPITAL OF ROCKWALL, 3150 Horizon Road, Zip 75032; tel. 972/772–6212; Kenneth R. Teel, President

Associate Members

Ambulatory Centers and Home Care Agencies

United States

FLORIDA

NEMOURS CHILDREN'S CLINIC, 807 Children's Way, Jacksonville, Zip 32207; tel. 904/390–3600; Traci Pezall, Associate Administrator

NEW HAMPSHIRE

DARTMOUTH COLLEGE HEALTH SERVICE, 7 Rope Ferry Road, Hanover, Zip 03755–1421; tel. 603/650–1400; John H. Turco, M.D., Director

WASHINGTON

PACIFIC MEDICAL CENTERS, 1200 12th Avenue South, Seattle, Zip 98144; tel. 206/621–4489; Harvey W. Smith, President and Chief Executive Officer

Philippines

DEPARTMENT OF VETERANS AFFAIRS, OUTPATIENT CLINIC, Manila, Zip 96440; tel. 632/521–7116

Blue Cross Plans

United States

ARIZONA

BLUE CROSS AND BLUE SHIELD OF ARIZONA, Box 13466, Phoenix, Zip 85002–3466; tel. 602/864–4100; Richard Boals, President and Chief Financial Officer

NEW YORK

EXCELLUS HEALTH PLAN, INC., 165 Court Street, Rochester, Zip 14647; tel. 585/327–6540; David Mack, Senior Vice President Corporate Relations

PENNSYLVANIA

CAPITAL BLUE CROSS, 2500 Elmerton Avenue, Harrisburg, Zip 17110; tel. 717/541–7000; Anita Smith, President and Chief Executive Officer

HIGHMARK BLUE CROSS BLUE SHIELD, 120 Fifth Avenue Place, Suite 3014, Pittsburgh, Zip 15222; tel. 412/544–7646; Sandra R. Tomlinson, Senior Vice President, Provider Services

INDEPENDENCE BLUE CROSS, 1901 Market Street, Philadelphia, Zip 19103; tel. 215/241–3300; Denise Dodd–Healy, Manager

Other Members

UNITED STATES

Alliance:

PREMIER, INC., 3 Westbrook Corporate Center, 9th Floor, San Diego, California Zip 92130; tel. 858/481–2727; Richard A. Norling, Chief Executive Officer; www.premierinc.com

THE NEW JERSEY COUNCIL OF TEACHING HOSPITALS, 154 West State Street, Trenton, New Jersey Zip 08608; tel. 609/656–9600; J. Richard Goldstein, M.D., President; www.njcth.org

UNIVERSITY HEALTHSYSTEM CONSORTIUM, INC., 2001 Spring Road, Suite 700, Oak Brook, Illinois Zip 60523; tel. 630/954–1700; Irene M. Thompson, President and Chief Executive Officer; www.uhc.edu

VHA, INC., P.O. Box 140909, Irving, Texas Zip 75014–0909; tel. 972/830–0000; Curtis W. Nonomaque, President and Chief Executive Officer; www.vha.com

Architecture:

BURT HILL, 400 Morgan Center, 101 East Diamond Street, Butler, Pennsylvania Zip 16001–5977; tel. 724/285–4761; John E. Brock, Vice President; www.burthill.com

EARL SWENSSON ASSOCIATES, INC., 2100 West End Avenue, Suite 1200, Nashville, Tennessee Zip 37203; tel. 615/329–9445; Richard L. Miller, President; www.esarch.com

HDR ARCHITECTURE, 8404 Indian Hills Drive, Omaha, Nebraska Zip 68114; tel. 402/399–1000; Jim Pine, Executive Vice President; www.hdrinc.com

KARLSBERGER COMPANIES, 99 East Main Street, Columbus, Ohio Zip 43215–5189; tel. 614/461–9500; Mitchel R. Levitt, Executive Vice President; www.karlsberger.com

MATTHEI AND COLIN ASSOCIATES, 332 South Michigan Avenue, Suite 614, Chicago, Illinois Zip 60604; tel. 312/939–4002; Ronald G. Kobold, Managing Partner

MESSER CONSTRUCTION COMPANY, 5158 Fishwick Drive, Cincinnati, Ohio Zip 45216; tel. 513/242–1541; Tiffany Witham, Director Marketing; www.messer.com

PERKINS & WILL, INC., 330 North Wabash, Suite 3600, Chicago, Illinois Zip 60611; tel. 312/755–0770; Jean Mah, Principal and National Market Sector Manager; www.perkinswill.com

REES ASSOCIATES, INC., 9211 Lake Hefner Parkway, Suite 300, Oklahoma City, Oklahoma Zip 73120; tel. 405/942–7337; Melanie Compton, Senior Associate

SMITHGROUP, INC., 301 Battery Street, San Francisco, California Zip 94104–4250; tel. 415/227–0100; James T. Hannon, Senior Vice President; www.sf.smithgroup.com

VITETTA ARCHITECTS & ENGINEERS, 4747 South Broad Street, Philadelphia, Pennsylvania Zip 19112; tel. 215/218–4747; Vincent Della Donna, Director Healthcare; www.vitetta.com

Bank:

BANK OF AMERICA, 101 South Tryon Street, Charlotte, North Carolina Zip 28255–0001; tel. 704/388–2255; Gayle Higaki, Senior Vice President; www.bankofamerica.com

Communication Systems Org:

AT & T, 1010 Wilshire Boulevard, Room 1240, Los Angeles, California Zip 90017; tel. 805/648–2463; Pat Pothier, Associate Director Medical

Construction Firm:

BE & K BUILDING GROUP, INC., 10 Cadillac Drive, Suite 460, Brentwood, Tennessee Zip 37027–5096; tel. 615/742–6610; Burk Waugh, Principal In Charge and Executive Vice President

HBE CORPORATION, P.O. Box 419039, Saint Louis, Missouri Zip 63141; tel. 314/567–9000; Stephen G. Dailey, Senior Vice President

Consulting Firm:

ARAMARK HEALTHCARE, 1101 Market Street, Philadelphia, Pennsylvania Zip 19107–2988; tel. 215/238–4054; Anthony C. Stanowski, Vice President Industrial Relations; www.aramark.com

BEACON PARTNERS, 97 Libbey Parkway, Suite 310, Weymouth, Massachusetts Zip 02189; tel. 781/982–8400; Jay M. Tolchinsky, Director Marketing and Communications; www.beaconpartners.com

BLIS, INC., 333 South State Street, Suite V, 459, Lake Oswego, Oregon Zip 97034; tel. 503/342–2444; Regi Schindler, President and Chief Executive Officer; www.bliscompany.com

BOLDT CONSULTING SERVICES, 1110 North Old World 3rd Street, Suite 610, Milwaukee, Wisconsin Zip 53203; tel. 414/276–4666; Kenneth R. Greve, Principal; www.boldtconsulting.com

BURWOOD GROUP, INC., 20 North Clark Street, Suite 1950, Chicago, Illinois Zip 60602; tel. 312/327–4600; Mark Theoharous, President; www.burwood.com

DARWIN, 10015 Old Columbia Road, Suite B–215, Columbia, Maryland Zip 21046; tel. 443/283–1153; Walter H. Killian, Owner

DST TECHNOLOGIES, INC., 330 West 9th Street, 7th Floor, Kansas City, Missouri Zip 64105; tel. 816/843–8024; Michelle Crowl, Corporate Marketing Coordinator; www.dstawd.com

ERNST & YOUNG, 5 Times Square, 14th Floor, New York, New York Zip 10036–6530; tel. 212/773–3000; Frank Bresz, Senior Manager; www.ey.com/global/content.nsf/us/home

EXECUTIVE HEALTH RESOURCES, INC., 15 Campus Boulevard, Suite 200, Newtown Square, Pennsylvania Zip 19073; tel. 610/446–6100; Robert Corrato, M.D., President and Chief Executive Officer; www.ehrdocs.com

GETWELLNETWORK, INC., 7920 Norfolk Avenue, 11th Floor, Bethesda, Maryland Zip 20814–2500; tel. 240/482–3200; Michael B. O'Neil, Jr., President and Chief Executive Officer; www.getwellnetwork.com

HEALTHLINK, AN IBM COMPANY, P.O. Box 10760, Burke, Texas Zip 22009; tel. 703/866–3570; Doug O'Boyle, Healthcare Market Intelligence Analyst

HEIDRICK AND STRUGGLES, 233 South Wacker, Suite 7000, Chicago, Illinois Zip 60606; tel. 312/372–8811; Richard P. Gustafson, Partner

ICF INTERNATIONAL, 9300 Lee Highway, Fairfax, Virginia Zip 22031; tel. 703/218–2658; Jean Hand, Senior Associate; www.icfi.com

KAUFMAN HALL, 5202 Old Orchard Road, Suite 700, Skokie, Illinois Zip 60077; tel. 847/441–8780; Jason Sussman, Partner; www.kaufmanhall.com

KURT SALMON ASSOCIATES, 1355 Peachtree Street N.E., Suite 900, Atlanta, Georgia Zip 30309–0900; tel. 404/892–0321; C. B. Souther, Communication Director; www.kurtsalmon.com

LATHAM AND WATKINS, LLP, 633 West 5th Street, Suite 4000, Los Angeles, California Zip 90071; tel. 213/485–1234; Daniel K. Settelmayer, Partner; www.lw.com

LEXECON, 332 South Michigan Avenue, Suite 1300, Chicago, Illinois Zip 60604; tel. 312/322–0200; Ben Brighoff, Senior Analyst; www.lexecon.com

MARSHALL ERDMAN & ASSOCIATES, INC., P.O. Box 44975, Madison, Wisconsin Zip 53744–4975; tel. 608/238–0211; Scott Ransom, President and Chief Executive Officer; www.erdman.com

MCKESSON HBO, 5995 Windward Parkway, Alpharetta, Georgia Zip 30005; tel. 404/338–3519; Louise Smith, RN, Manager, Regulatory Assessment and Operations

NAVIGANT CONSULTING, 200 South Wacker Drive, Suite 2620, Chicago, Illinois Zip 60606–7481; tel. 312/583–5700; Sheila Story, Research Coordinator

PHOENIX HEALTH SYSTEMS, INC., 910 Clopper Road, Suite 165, Gaithersburg, Maryland Zip 20878; tel. 301/869–7300; Darin LeGrange, Chief Executive Officer; www.phoenixhealth.com

PREMISE, 76 Batterson Park Road, Farmington, Connecticut Zip 06032; tel. 860/246–3000; Andrew Canepari, Director Marketing; www.premiseusa.com

PRESS GANEY ASSOCIATES, INC., 404 Columbia Place, South Bend, Indiana Zip 46601; tel. 800/232–8032; Dan Farrell, Director Marketing; www.pressganey.com

RWD, 5440 Corporate Drive, Suite 400, Troy, Michigan Zip 48098; tel. 248/267–1001; Mike Brown, Manager Lean Solutions; www.rwd.com

STOCKAMP AND ASSOCIATES, INC., 6000 S.W. Meadows Road, Suite 300, Lake Oswego, Oregon Zip 97035; tel. 503/303–1200; Karen Andrews, Senior Marketing Manager; www.stockamp.com

THE CENTER FOR MULTICULTURAL COMPETENCE IN HEALTHCARE ORGANIZATIONS, 4555 Lake Forest Drive, Suite 650, Cincinnati, Ohio Zip 45242; tel. 513/563–3004; Lawrence W. James, President and Chief Executive Officer; www.cmcho.com

THE FOSTER GROUP, INC., 180 North Stetson Avenue, Suite 3470, Chicago, Illinois Zip 60601–6702; tel. 312/609–1009; David Hillenmeyer, Healthcare Services Partner; www.thefostergroup.com

THE HSM GROUP, LTD, 8777 East Via de Ventura #188, Scottsdale, Arizona Zip 85258; tel. 480/947–8078; Sheryl Bronkesh, President; www.hsmgroup.com

THE QUAMMEN GROUP, 1400 South Orlando Avenue, Suite 204, Winter Park, Florida Zip 32789; tel. 407/539–2015; Lynne S. Moore, Manager; www.quammengroup.com

WIPFLI LLP, P.O. Box 690, Eau Claire, Wisconsin Zip 54702–0690; tel. 715/858–3407; Sylvia Weise; www.wipfli.com

Information Systems:

3M HEALTH INFORMATION SYSTEMS, 575 West Murray Boulevard, Murray, Utah Zip 84157; tel. 801/265–4330; Katherina Holzhauser, Vice President Marketing; www.3mhis.com

CERNER CORPORATION, 2800 Rockcreek Parkway, Kansas City, Missouri Zip 64117; tel. 816/221–1024; Judy Sorio Jeffers, Marketing Manager; www.cerner.com

KPMG LLP, 303 East Wacker Drive, 19th Floor, Chicago, Illinois Zip 60601; tel. 312/665–2073; Edward J. Giniat, Partner

THOMSON HEALTHCARE, 6200 South Syracuse Way, Suite 300, Greenwood Village, Colorado Zip 80111–4740; tel. 303/486–6400; Tara Sweitzer, Manager, Events and Tradeshows; www.thomsonhealthcare.com

Insurance Broker:

AMERICAN FIDELITY ASSURANCE COMPANY, 2000 North Classen Boulevard, Oklahoma City, Oklahoma Zip 73106; tel. 877/967–5748; Barry Koonce, National Sales Director; www.af-group.com

AON'S AFFINITY INSURANCE SERVICES, INC., 300 South Wacker Drive, Suite 700, Chicago, Illinois Zip 60606; tel. 312/381–2806; Mark A. Brostowitz, Senior Vice President; www.aon.com

BOSTON MUTUAL LIFE INSURANCE COMPANY, 120 Royall Street, Canton, Massachusetts Zip 02021; tel. 781/828–7000; Peter Tillson, Vice President; www.bostonmutual.com

DYE & ESKIN, 1324 Vincent Place, Mc Lean, Virginia Zip 22101; tel. 703/556–0744; Major Rick Eskin, President

G. E. FINANCIAL, GE Appliance Park Building, Suite 100, Louisville, Kentucky Zip 40225; tel. 502/254–1756; Greg Miller, Director Business Development; www.ge.com

ING EMPLOYEE BENEFITS, 20 Washington Avenue South, Minneapolis, Minnesota Zip 55401; tel. 612/372–1122; Steve Pitzer, Vice President

LOCKTON COMPANIES, 444 West 47th Street, Suite 900, Kansas City, Missouri Zip 64112–1906; tel. 816/960–9000; Becky Sullivan, Senior Vice President and Unit Manager; www.lockton.com

LOYAL INSURANCE, 423 Westport Road, Suite 201, Kansas City, Missouri Zip 64111; tel. 816/841–3597; Michael Reidy, Vice President

NEBCO, 1264 Knollwood Drive West, West Chester, Rhode Island Zip 19380; tel. 877/739–3330; James M. Mattison, Vice President; www.nebenefit.com

PRINCIPAL FINANCIAL GROUP, 711 High Street, Des Moines, Iowa Zip 50392–5440; tel. 515/248–4455; Pat Burch, Senior Technical Consultant; www.goldfarb@shands.ufl.edu

THE ALLEN J. FLOOD COMPANIES, INC., 2 Madison Avenue, Larchmont, New York Zip 10538; tel. 914/834–9326; Allen J. Flood, President; www.ajfusa.com

UNITED CONCORDIA COMPANY, INC., 4401 Deer Path Road, Harrisburg, Pennsylvania Zip 17110; tel. 717/260–6800; Brett Altland, Product Development Analyst; www.ucci.com

WESTROPE, 801 West 47th Street, Suite 500, Kansas City, Missouri Zip 64112; tel. 816/842–8222; Phil Holderness, Senior Vice President; www.westrope.com

Manufacturer/Supplier:

ABBOTT LABORATORIES, 100 Abbott Park Road, Abbott Park, Illinois Zip 60064; tel. 847/937–4537; William D. Motley, Jr., Divisional Vice President; www.abbott.com

AMGEN, INC., 1840 Dehavilland Drive, Department 631, Thousand Oaks, California Zip 91320; tel. 805/447–2106; Rob Jacobson, President and Chief Executive Officer; www.amgen.com

APCO GRAPHICS, INC., 388 Grant Street S.E., Atlanta, Georgia Zip 30312; tel. 404/688–9000; Christopher McArthur, Manager Marketing; www.apcosigns.com

BAXTER HEALTHCARE CORPORATION, Route 120 and Wilson Road, Round Lake, Illinois Zip 60073; tel. 847/270–5440; Ali Corbett, Vice President Strategic and Professional Relations; www.baxter.com

BONDTECH CORPORATION, 2400 North Highway 27, Somerset, Kentucky Zip 42502; tel. 606/677–2616; Lisa Clark, Sales Manager; www.bondtech.net

ELI LILLY AND COMPANY, Lilly Corporate Center, Suite 18, Indianapolis, Indiana Zip 46285–4113; tel. 317/277–8173; Keith Mason, Associate Advocacy and Professional Relations; www.lilly.com

GE HEALTHCARE, 3000 North Grandview Boulevard, Waukesha, Wisconsin Zip 53188; tel. 262/312–7915; Patrick Connolly, Information Management and Strategy Manager; www.gehealthcare.com

HERMAN MILLER, INC., 2690 Misty Morning Lane, Roswell, Georgia Zip 30076; tel. 404/680–8136; Tom Livengood, Vice President Sales

HILL–ROM, 1069 State Route 46 East, Batesville, Indiana Zip 47006–9167; tel. 812/934–7958; Thomas J. Jeffers, Director Government Relations; www.hill–rom.com

JOHNSON & JOHNSON, 425 Hoes Lane, Piscataway, New Jersey Zip 08855; tel. 732/562–3058; Cathi Brozena, Manager Professional Affairs

KEY SURGICAL, INC., 11000 West 78th Street, Suite 100, Eden Prairie, Minnesota Zip 55344–2114; tel. 952/914–9789; Brian O'Connell, President; www.keysurgical.com

MERCK & COMPANY INC., MARKETING INFORMATION CENTER, P.O. Box 4, West Point, Pennsylvania Zip 19486; tel. 215/652–3244; Harry Rieck, Executive Director

OTSUKA AMERICA PHARMACEUTICAL, INC., 2440 Research Boulevard, Rockville, Maryland Zip 20850; tel. 301/990–0030; Debra Kaufmann, Director Corporate Communications; www.otsuka.com

PFIZER U.S. PHARMACEUTICALS GROUP, 235 East 42nd Street, New York, New York Zip 10017; tel. 212/573–3192; John A. Tara, Vice President Institutional Accounts

SANOFI AVENTIS, 300 Somerset Corporate Boulevard, Bridgewater, New Jersey Zip 08807; tel. 908/243–6000; Annette Schmidt, Coordinator Professional and Association Markets; www.sanofi–aventis.com

SENTINEL DOOR CONTROLS, 3020–D Hutchison McDonald Road, Charlotte, North Carolina Zip 28269; tel. 800/327–7848; David J. Scopel, Brand Development Manager; www.sentineldoor.com

SPECIALTY MEDICAL ELECTRONICS, INC., 69 Tupelo Trace, Mandeville, Louisiana Zip 70471; tel. 504/464–1134; Ralph A. Marshall, III, President

Metro Health Care Assn:

HOSPITAL ASSOCIATION OF SOUTHERN CALIFORNIA, 201 North Figueroa Street, 4th Floor, Los Angeles, California Zip 90071–3322; tel. 213/538–0700; James D. Barber, President

Other:

3N, 505 North Brand Boulevard, Suite 700, Glendale, California Zip 91203; tel. 818/230–9728; Steve Kirchmeier, Vice President Healthcare; www.3nonline.com

901 EAST ST. LOUIS STREET, SUITE 1800, P.O. Box 1900, Springfield, Missouri Zip 65801–1900; tel. 417/831–7283; Melanie K. Miller Short, Niche Marketing Specialist; www.bkd.com

ACS HEALTHCARE SOLUTIONS, 5225 Auto Club Drive, Dearborn, Michigan Zip 48126; tel. 248/386–8300; Julie Heintz, Marketing Manager; www.acs–hcs.com

AEROSCOUT, 1300 Island Drive, Suite 202, Redwood City, California Zip 94065; tel. 650/596–2994; Gabi Daniely, Vice President Marketing and Product Strategy; www.aeroscout.com

AMERICA DEVELOPMENT, 14881 Quorum Drive, Suite 200, Dallas, Texas Zip 75254; tel. 972/490–9190; Paula Marie Jones, President; www.america–development.com

AMERICA'S BLOOD CENTERS, 725 15th Street N.W., Suite 700, Washington, District of Columbia Zip 20005; tel. 202/393–5725; Jim MacPherson, Executive Director

AMERICAN ACADEMY OF PHYSICIAN ASSISTANTS, 950 North Washington Street, Alexandria, Virginia Zip 22314; tel. 703/836–2272; Bill Leinweber, Chief Executive Officer; www.aapa.org

AMERICAN ASSOCIATION OF NURSE ANESTHETISTS, 222 South Prospect Avenue, Park Ridge, Illinois Zip 60068–4001; tel. 847/692–7050; Jeff Beutler, M.S., Executive Director; www.aana.com

AMERICAN BOARD OF INTERNAL MEDICINE, 510 Walnut Street, Suite 1700, Philadelphia, Pennsylvania Zip 19106; tel. 215/446–3500; Kevin P. Caviston, Strategic Relations Liaison; www.abim.org

AMERICAN BOARD OF MEDICAL SPECIALTIES, 1007 Church Street, Suite 404, Evanston, Illinois Zip 60201–5913; tel. 847/491–9091; Stephen H. Miller, M.D., M.P.H., President; www.abms.org

AMERICAN COLLEGE OF HEALTHCARE EXECUTIVES, One North Franklin, Suite 1700, Chicago, Illinois Zip 60606–3491; tel. 312/424–2800; Thomas C. Dolan, Ph.D., FACHE, President and Chief Executive Officer; www.ache.org

AMERICAN DENTAL EDUCATION ASSOCIATION, 1400 K. Street N.W., Suite 1100, Washington, District of Columbia Zip 20005; tel. 202/289–7201; Richard Valachovic, Executive Director; www.adea.org

AMERICAN HEALTH INFORMATION MANAGEMENT ASSOCIATION, 233 North Michigan Avenue, Suite 2150, Chicago, Illinois Zip 60601–5519; tel. 312/233–1100; David A. Sweet, Director Library Services

AMERICAN RED CROSS BIOMEDICAL SERVICES, 2025 East Street, N.W., Washington, District of Columbia Zip 20006; tel. 703/206–6000; Avele Conlogue, Office Manager

AMERICAN SOCIETY OF HEALTH SYSTEM PHARMACISTS, 7272 Wisconsin Avenue, Bethesda, Maryland Zip 20814; tel. 301/657–3000; Henri R. Manasse, Ph.D., Sc.D., Executive Vice President and Chief Executive Officer

AMERICAN TECHNOLOGIES, INC., 21410 North 15th Lane, Suite 112, Phoenix, Arizona Zip 85027; tel. 623/434–9445; Jeff Moore, General Manager; www.amer–tech.com

AMERINET, INC., 2060 Craigshire Road, Saint Louis, Missouri Zip 63146; tel. 800/388–2638; Todd Ebert, President; www.amerinet–gpo.com

AMN HEALTHCARE, INC., 12400 High Bluff Drive, Suite 100, San Diego, California Zip 92130–3581; tel. 866/871–8519; Steve Wehn, Senior Vice President of Corporate Development

ANOTO, INC., 200 Friberg Parkway Suite 3003, Westborough, Massachusetts Zip 01581–3954; tel. 781/890–1555; Virginia Carpenter, Marketing Manager Healthcare; www.anoto.com

APIC, 1275 K. Street N.W., Suite 1000, Washington, District of Columbia Zip 20005–4006; tel. 202/789–1890; Kathy L. Warye, Chief Executive Officer; www.apic.org

APTIUM ONCOLOGY, INC., 8201 Beverly Boulevard, Los Angeles, California Zip 90048; tel. 323/966–3400; Michele Bollinger, Vice President Business Development and Consulting; www.aptiumoncology.com

ARC GROUP ASSOCIATES, 500 Old York Road, Suite 10, Jenkintown, Pennsylvania Zip 19046; tel. 215/881–9500; Eric Malakoff, Vice President Sales and Marketing; www.arcgroup.net

ARMED FORCES INSTITUTE OF PATHOLOGY, 6825 16th Street N.W., Building 54, Washington, District of Columbia Zip 20306–6000; tel. 202/782–2100; Colonel Renata Greenspan, Director; www.afip.osd.mil

ASSOCIATION OF PERIOPERATIVE REGISTERED NURSES, 2170 South Parker Road, Suite 300, Denver, Colorado Zip 80231; tel. 303/755–6304; Linda Groah, RN, M.S.N., Executive Director and Chief Executive Officer; www.aorn.org

ASSOCIATION OF UNIVERSITY PROGRAMS IN HEALTH ADMINISTRATION, 1911 North Fort Myer Drive, Suite 503, Arlington, Virginia Zip 22201–2543; tel. 703/894–0940; Lydia Reed, President and Chief Executive Officer; www.aupha.org

AVAILITY, LLC, 7406 Fullerton Street, Suite 300, Jacksonville, Florida Zip 32256–0857; tel. 904/470–4984; Tony Shepse, Manager Marketing; www.availity.com

AVP, INC., 7734 Hedge Lane Terrace, Shawnee Mission, Kansas Zip 66227–3017; tel. 913/441–0769; Jeff Perry, Executive Vice President Sales and Marketing; www.avpco.com

BLUE BELL BIO–MEDICAL, 1260 Industrial Drive, Van Wert, Ohio Zip 45891; tel. 800/258–3235; Konnie Rutschilling, Chief Executive Officer; www.bluebellcarts.com

BLUE CROSS AND BLUE SHIELD ASSOCIATION, 225 North Michigan Avenue, Chicago, Illinois Zip 60601–7680; tel. 312/297–6000; Scott P. Serota, President and Chief Executive Officer; www.bcbs.com

BRIGHT HORIZONS FAMILY SOLUTIONS, 200 Talcott Avenue South, Watertown, Massachusetts Zip 02472; tel. 617/673–8000; Jamie Garofano, Marketing Coordinator; www.brighthorizons.com

BROADCAST MUSIC, INC., 10 Music Square East, Nashville, Tennessee Zip 37203–4399; tel. 615/401–2874; Sebastian Pittman, Director General Licensing; www.bmi.com

BUXTON, 2651 South Polaris Drive, Fort Worth, Texas Zip 76137; tel. 817/332–3681; Charles Wetzel, Chief Operating Officer; www.buxtonco.com

C. R. BARD, 730 Central Avenue, Murray Hill, New Jersey Zip 07974; tel. 908/277–8018; James L. Natale, Senior Vice President; www.crbard.com

C2P GROUP, LLC, 511 East John Carpenter Freeway, Suite 500, Irving, Texas Zip 75062; tel. 214/260–3200; Kelli Mulloy, Marketing Assistant; www.c2pgroup.com

CAMBIO HEALTH SOLUTIONS, LLC, 100 Westwood Place, Suite 350, Brentwood, Tennessee Zip 37027; tel. 615/324–8500; Thomas W. Singleton, President; www.cambiohealth.com

CARDON HEALTHCARE NETWORK, INC., P.O. Box 4950, The Woodlands, Texas Zip 77387; tel. 281/296–8911; Scott Wiley, Executive Vice President; www.cardonhealthcare.com

CAREFX CORPORATION, 8767 East Via de Ventura, Suite 390, Scottsdale, Arizona Zip 85258; tel. 480/833–5010; David Ward, Vice President Business Development; www.carefx.com

CCM ADVISORS, LLC, 190 South LaSalle Street, Suite 2800, Chicago, Illinois Zip 60603; tel. 312/444–6200; Michael Randall, Director Sales and Marketing; www.ahafunds.org

CERTIPHI SCREENING, INC., 1105 Industrial Highway, Southampton, Pennsylvania Zip 18966; tel. 888/260–1370; Tony D'Orazio, President6; www.certiphi.com

CHAN HEALTHCARE AUDITORS, 231 South Bemiston Avenue, Suite 300, Saint Louis, Missouri Zip 63105; tel. 314/802–2008; Michael G. Brown, Senior Manager, Knowledge Management; www.chanllc.com

The members listed in **bold** *are Associate Advantage members.*

CISCO SYSTEMS, 165 Needletree Lane, Glastonbury, California Zip 06033; tel. 860/657–8127; Michael Haymaker, Director Healthcare Industry Marketing; www.cisco.com

CLAREDI CORPORATION, 2525 Lake Park Boulevard, Salt Lake City, Utah Zip 84120; tel. 801/982–3001; www.claredi.com

COMMERCE INSURANCE SERVICES, INC., 13 Emery Avenue, Randolph, New Jersey Zip 07869; tel. 877/396–3800; Mary Donohue, Senior Vice President Healthcare; www.commercescienceandtechnology.com

COMMUNITY OF DOCTORS.COM, 12073 30th Avenue S.W., Seattle, Washington Zip 98146; tel. 206/243–3611; Michael Steiner, M.D., President

COMPREHENSIVE PHARMACY SERVICES, 6409 North Quail Hollow Road, Memphis, Tennessee Zip 38120–1414; tel. 901/748–0470; Donald Nickleson, President

COMPUTER ASSOCIATES, 4601 Touchton Road East, Suite 3210, Islandia, New York Zip 11749; tel. 631/342–6000; Michael McDermand, Vice President Healthcare; www.ca.com

CONCENTRIC RECEIVABLES MANAGEMENT, LTD., 1220 Blalock Road, Suite 310, Houston, Texas Zip 77055; tel. 713/973–0591; Robert Gitomer, President; www.concentricreceivables.com

CONCUITY, INCORPORATED, 150 North Fairway Drive, Suite 146, Vernon Hills, Illinois Zip 60061–1860; tel. 847/465–6003; James Farrar, Vice President Sales; www.concuity.com

COOPER SIGNAGE & GRAPHICS, INC., 3680 Hewatt Court S.W., Snellville, Georgia Zip 30039; tel. 800/297–2324; Randy R. Cooper, President; www.sinsystems.org

COVENANT HOSPICE, 5041 North 12th Avenue, Pensacola, Florida Zip 32504; tel. 850/433–2155; Dale O. Knee, President and Chief Executive Officer; www.covenanthospice.org

CRANEWARE, INC., 5770 Hoffner Avenue, Suite 102, Orlando, Florida Zip 32822; tel. 407/384–1711; Derek Morkel, Chief Executive Officer US Operations; www.craneware.com

DAVITA, INC., 1423 Pacific Avenue, Tacoma, Washington Zip 98402; tel. 800/477–1916; Daniel Evans, Director Acute Support Services and Marketing; www.davita.com

DEPARTMENT OF AIR FORCE MEDICAL SERVICE, HQ USAF/SG, Bolling AFB, District of Columbia Zip 20332–6188; tel. 202/545–6700

DEPARTMENT OF THE ARMY, OFFICE OF THE SURGEON GENERAL, 5109 Leesburg Pike, Falls Church, Virginia Zip 22041–3258; tel. 202/690–6467; Lieutenant General Kevin C. Kiley, M.D., Surgeon General

DEPARTMENT OF THE NAVY, BUREAU OF MEDICINE AND SURGERY, 2300 East Street N.W., Washington, District of Columbia Zip 20372–5300; tel. 202/762–3701; Rear Admiral Adam M. Robinson, Jr., Surgeon General

DEPARTMENT OF VETERANS AFFAIRS, 201 Walnut Avenue, Suite 201, Vallejo, California Zip 94592–1107; Linda Pierce, Director, Sierra Pacific Network

DEPARTMENT OF VETERANS AFFAIRS, 810 Vermont Avenue N.W., Washington, District of Columbia Zip 20420; tel. 202/273–5400; Michael J. Kussman, M.D., Acting Undersecretary of Health

DEVELOPMENT DIMENSIONS INTERNATIONAL, 1225 Washington Pike, Bridgeville, Pennsylvania Zip 15017–2838; tel. 412/257–3623; Colby Fazio, Marketing Consultant; www.ddiworld.com

DHHS, PUBLIC HEALTH SERVICE, INDIAN HEALTH SERVICE, DIVISION OF BUSINESS OFFICE ENHANCEMENT, 12300 Twinbrook Parkway, Suite 360–57, Rockville, Maryland Zip 20852; tel. 301/443–0227; Frank Martin, Management Analyst; www.ihs.gov

DILIGENT, A DIVISION OF ARJO, 50 North Gary Avenue, Roselle, Illinois Zip 60172; tel. 800/323–1245; Andrew Hepburn, Vice President; www.arjousa.com

DIVERSIFIED INVESTMENT ADVISORS, 4 Manhattanville Road, Purchase, New York Zip 10577; tel. 914/697–8952; Eric Henon, Vice President; www.divinvest.com

DLA PIPER RUDNICK GRAY CARY US, LLP, 1200 Nineteenth Street N.W., Washington, District of Columbia Zip 20036–2412; tel. 202/861–3900; Deborah Gersh, Partner

DMJM H&N, INC., 515 South Flower Street, 9th Floor, Los Angeles, California Zip 90071; tel. 213/593–8429; Fred Gans, Vice President; www.dmjmhn.aecom.com

DNV HEALTHCARE, INC., 16340 Park Ten Place, Suite 100, Houston, Texas Zip 77084; tel. 281/721–6869; Yehuda Dror, Chief Executive Officer; www.dnvhealthcareinc.com

DUOS TECHNOLOGIES, 6622 Southpoint Drive South, Suite 310, Jacksonville, Florida Zip 32216; tel. 904/861–2711; Alison Myers, Senior Healthcare Account Executive; www.duostech.com

EDOCUMENT RESOURCES, 6101 Baker Road, Suite 207, Minnetonka, Minnesota Zip 55345; tel. 952/607–3500; Mark Rubin, Director Healthcare Sales; www.edocumentresources.com

EMERGENCY CONSULTANTS, INC., 4075 Copper Ridge Drive, Traverse City, Michigan Zip 49684–4796; tel. 800/253–1795; James Johnson, M.D., President; www.eci–med.com

ERNST & YOUNG, 1811 Von Karman Avenue, Suite 1000, Irvine, California Zip 92612; tel. 949/437–0220; Dee Balle, Jr., Partner

FASTAFF NURSING, 6501 South Fiddlers Green Circle, Suite 200, Greenwood Village, Colorado Zip 80111; tel. 800/736–8773; Sheryl Hinton, Director Marketing; www.fastaff.com

GHN – ONLINE, 12655 North Central Expressway, Suite 550, Dallas, Texas Zip 75243; tel. 214/696–5717; Jennifer Millikin, Director Marketing; www.ghnonline.com

GLAXOSMITHKLINE, Five Moore Drive, Research Traingle Park, North Carolina Zip 27709–3398; tel. 919/483–2031; Ronald Sorrentino, Segment Vice President; www.gsk.com

GREENHOUSE, 303 West Erie Street, Suite 400, Chicago, Illinois Zip 60610; tel. 312/278–6010; Patti Bridge, Accounts Director

GULDMANN INC., 5525 Johns Road, Suite 905, Tampa, Florida Zip 33634–4307; tel. 813/880–0619; Anders Drechsler, President; www.guldmann.com

H. R. S. INTERNATIONAL, 25 East Washington, 6th Floor, Chicago, Illinois Zip 60602; tel. 312/236–7770; Carrie Parks, Marketing Specialist; www.hrsolutions.com

HAWAII MEDICAL SERVICE ASSOCIATION, P.O. Box 860, Honolulu, Hawaii Zip 96808–0860; tel. 808/948–5482; Gina Marting, Manager Facility Reimbursement

HEALTHCARE APPRAISERS, INC., 75 N.W. 1st Avenue, Suite 201, Delray Beach, Florida Zip 33444–2609; tel. 561/330–3488; Curtis H. Bernstein, Senior Associate; www.ncfmv.com

HEALTHCARE MANAGEMENT SYSTEMS, INC., 3102 West End Avenue, Suite 400, Nashville, Tennessee Zip 37203; tel. 615/383–7300; Christy Wright, Marketing Manager; www.hmstn.com

HEALTHCARE.COM, INC., 1749 N.E. Miami Court, Suite 604, Miami, Florida Zip 33132; tel. 305/371–9724; Jose Vargas, Chief Operating Officer; www.healthcare.com

HIPAA ACADEMY, 14225 University Avenue, Suite 240, Waukee, Iowa Zip 50263; tel. 515/453–8247; Lorna L. Waggoner, Director Business Development

HOOPER, LUNDY & BOOKMAN, INC., 1875 Century Park East, Suite 1600, Los Angeles, California Zip 90067; tel. 310/551–8111; Lloyd Bookman, Partner; www.health–law.com

HOSPITAL INVENTORIES SPECIALISTS, INC., 3615 West Waters Avenue, Tampa, Florida Zip 33614; tel. 800/284–7690; Julie Stoddard, Sales and Marketing Representative; www.hisi.com

HQ ACC/SGMS, 162 Dodd, Suite 100, Langley AFB, Virginia Zip 23665–1995

HQ AETC/SGAL, 63 Main Circle, Suite 3, Randolph AFB, Texas Zip 78150–4549

HQ AFMC/SGAR, 4225 Logistics Avenue, N–209, Dayton, Ohio Zip 45433–5761; tel. 937/656–3655; Alice Rohrbach

HQ AFSPC/SGAL, 150 Vandenberg Street, Suite 1105, Petterson AFB, Colorado Zip 80914–4550

HQ AMC/SGSL, 203 West Losey Street, Room 1180, Scott A F B, Illinois Zip 62225–5219

HQ PACAF/SGAL, 25 East Street, Suite D1, Hickam AFB, Hawaii Zip 96853–5418

HQ USAFA/SGAL, Pinion Drive, Building 4102, Suite 3, U South A F Academy, Colorado Zip 80840–2325

HR SOLUTIONS, INC., 25 East Washington Street, Suite 600, Chicago, Illinois Zip 60602; tel. 312/236–7170; Chris Dustin, Executive Vice President; www.hrsolutionsinc.com

HYLAND SOFTWARE, INC., 28500 Clemens Road, Westlake, Ohio Zip 44145; tel. 440/788–5814; Michael Kortan, Director Health Care Solutions; www.onbase.com

IKON OFFICE SOLUTIONS, INC., 70 Valley Stream Parkway, Malvern, Pennsylvania Zip 19355; tel. 610/296–8000; Will Nicolls, Manager Process Improvement; www.ikon.com

INTERNATIONAL ASSOCIATION FOR HEALTHCARE SECURITY AND SAFETY, P.O. Box 5038, Glendale Heights, Illinois Zip 60139; tel. 630/529–3913; Nancy Felesena, Executive Assistant; www.iahss.org

IRONPORT, 950 Elm Avenue, San Bruno, California Zip 94066; tel. 650/989–6500; Michael Weir; www.ironport.com

J. STEPHENS MAYHUGH AND ASSOCIATES, INC., P.O. Box 77458, Baton Rouge, Louisiana Zip 70879; tel. 225/295–7000; Melanie Johnson, Chief Executive Officer

JANI–KING, 16885 Dallas Parkway, Addison, Texas Zip 75001; tel. 972/991–0900; Mark Regna, Director Healthcare Services; www.janiking.com

JONES LANG LASALLE, 200 East Randolph Drive, Chicago, Illinois Zip 60601; tel. 312/228–2598; Donald D. Hamilton, Managing Director; www.joneslanglasalle.com

KEPPLER SPEAKERS, 4350 North Fairfax Drive, Suite 700, Arlington, Virginia Zip 22203; tel. 703/516–4000; Donna Berger, Associate, Healthcare Division

KROLL ONTRACK, INC., 18350 Mount Langley Street, Suite 110, Fountain Valley, California Zip 92708; tel. 800/872–2599; William Miller, Manager Business Development; www.krollontrack.com

LIKO, INC., 122 Grove Street, Franklin, Massachusetts Zip 02038; tel. 508/553–3993; Melissa Nowitz, Senior Marketing Communications Specialist; www.liko.com

LIVEPROCESS, 271 Grove Avenue, Building D., Verona, New Jersey Zip 07044; tel. 973/571–2500; Nathaniel Weiss, Chief Executive Officer; www.liveprocess.com

LODGENET ENTERTAINMENT CORPORATION, 3900 West Innovation Street, Sioux Falls, South Dakota Zip 57107; tel. 605/988–1418; Major Gary Kolbeck, Vice President Healthcare Business Development; www.lodgenet.com

LOGICARE CORPORATION, 2125 Heights Drive, Eau Claire, Wisconsin Zip 54701; tel. 800/848–0099; Debbie Foss, Director Marketing; www.logicare.com

LYON SOFTWARE, 5800 Monroe Street, Building E., Sylvania, Ohio Zip 43560–2209; tel. 419/882–7184; Douglas W. Lyon, CPA, President; www.lyonsoftware.com

MAGELLAN HEALTH SERVICES, 6950 Columbia Gateway Drive, Columbia, Missouri Zip 21046; tel. 314/387–4000; Rick Lee, President Employer Solutions; www.magellanhealth.com

MARSH AFFINITY GROUP SERVICES, 1440 Renaissance Drive, Park Ridge, Illinois Zip 60068; tel. 847/803–3100; Gordon P. Hall, Vice President

MEDEFINANCE, INC., 15950 North Dallas Parkway, Suite 1375, Dallas, California Zip 75248; tel. 310/647–1300; Marcia Shields, Director Marketing Communications; www.medefinance.com

MEDEM, INC., 100 Pine Street, 3rd Floor, San Francisco, California Zip 94111; tel. 415/644–3915; Jason W. Best, Vice President Marketing; www.medem.com

MEDFONE, INC., 3305 Jerusalem Avenue, Wantagh, New York Zip 11793; tel. 516/679–7641; Stacey Horowitz, Manager Marketing; www.medfone.com

MEDICAL PROPERTIES TRUST, 1000 Urban Center Drive, Suite 501, Birmingham, Alabama Zip 35242; tel. 205/969–3755; R. Steven Hamner, Executive Vice President and Chief Financial Officer; www.medicalpropertiestrust.com

MEDICAL PROTECTIVE, 5814 Reed Road, Fort Wayne, Indiana Zip 46835; tel. 260/486–0814; Timothy Krautheim, Hospital Sales Leader; www.medpro.com

MEDIMPACT HEALTHCARE SYSTEMS, INC, 10680 Treena Street, San Diego, California Zip 92128; tel. 858/566–2727; Dale Brown, Senior Vice President Business Development; www.medimpact.com

MEDITRACT, Two Union Square, Suite 304, Chattanooga, Tennessee Zip 37402; tel. 423/267–9300; Scott R. Jeffery, Chief Operating Officer; www.meditract.com

MEMORIAL BLOOD CENTERS, 737 Pelham Boulevard, Saint Paul, Minnesota Zip 55114–1739; tel. 612/871–3300; Donald C. Berglund, Chief Executive Officer; www.memorialbloodcenters.org

MID–CONTINENT GENERAL AGENCY, INC., 3131 Eastside, Suite 600, Houston, Texas Zip 77098; tel. 713/639–6200; Lawrence M. Keefe, Senior Vice President; www.mid–continentga.com

MIDPARK HEALTHCARE PARKING LOGISTICS, 55 Quincy Place, N.W., Washington, District of Columbia Zip 20001; tel. 202/462–1204; Brian Macklin, Director; www.hospitalparking.net

MODERN HEALTHCARE, 360 North Michigan Avenue, Chicago, Illinois Zip 60601–3806; tel. 312/649–5491; Fawn Lopez, Publisher; www.modernhealthcare.com

MRI INTERNATIONAL, INC./CLAIMS SERVICING OF AMERICA, 5330 South Durango Drive, Las Vegas, Nevada Zip 89113–1835; tel. 702/396–8822; Linda Martinez

MYRON STEVES INSURANCE SOLUTIONS, 3131 Eastside, Suite 600, Houston, Texas Zip 77098; tel. 713/351–8201; Buddy Steves, Vice Chairman; www.myronsteves.com

NATIONAL CENTER FOR HEALTHCARE LEADERSHIP, 515 North State Street, Suite 2000, Chicago, Illinois Zip 60610; tel. 312/755–5017; Marie E. Sinioris, President and Chief Executive Officer; www.nchl.org

NATIONAL CERTIFICATION CORPORATION, 142 East Ontario, Suite 1700, Chicago, Illinois Zip 60611; tel. 312/951–0207; Betty Burns, Executive Director; www.nccnet.org

NATIONAL CITY BANK, 1 North Franklin, Suite 2500, Chicago, Illinois Zip 60606; tel. 312/384–4619; John B. Weber, Senior Vice President Healthcare; www.nationalcity.com

NATIONAL RESEARCH CORPORATION, 1245 Q. Street, Lincoln, Nebraska Zip 68508; tel. 402/475–2525; Jessica Meyer, Area Manager; www.nationalresearch.com

NAVAL REGIONAL MEDICAL CENTER, PSC 1005, Box 36, FPO, APO/FPO Europe Zip 09593–0136

NEW HEIGHTS GROUP, LLC, 41 Sundance Drive, Santa Fe, New Mexico Zip 87506; tel. 505/690–8433; Howard J. Gershon, Principal; www.reach–newheights.com

NOBLIS, 3150 Fairview Park South, Falls Church, Virginia Zip 22042; tel. 703/610–2255; Alan Dowling, M.D., Executive Director; www.mitretek.org

NORTH CENTRAL HEALTH SERVICES, INC., P.O. Box 528, Lafayette, Indiana Zip 47902; tel. 765/423–1604; John R. Walling, President and Chief Executive Officer; www.nchsi.com

NOTIFYMD, INC., 318 Seaboard Lane, Suite 310, Franklin, Tennessee Zip 37067; tel. 866/438–1799; Michael T. Sandwith, Vice President Sales; www.notifymd.com

NOVAMED, LLC, 4 Westchester Plaza, Elmsford, New York Zip 10523; tel. 914/789–2100; Peter M. Derrico, President; www.novamed–usa.com

NUMEROF & ASSOCIATES, INC., Four City Place Drive, Suite 430, Saint Louis, Missouri Zip 63141; tel. 314/997–1587; Rita E. Numerof, M.D., President; www.nai–consulting.com

OLYMPUS AMERICA, INC., 3500 Corporate Parkway, Center Valley, Pennsylvania Zip 18034–0610; tel. 484/896–5000; Steven K. Wendt, Senior Manager National Accounts

PERKINELMER GENETICS, INC., P.O. Box 219, Bridgeville, Pennsylvania Zip 15017; tel. 412/220–2300; Joseph M. Quashnock, Ph.D., Laboratory Director; www.perkinelmergenetics.com

PEROT SYSTEMS HEALTHCARE, 26 Century Boulevard, Suite 400, Nashville, Tennessee Zip 37214–3683; tel. 800/659–8883; Ann Clark, Director Membership; www.perotsystems.com/revenuecycle

PILAT, 496 Route 22 West, Lebanon, New Jersey Zip 08833; tel. 908/823–9417; Travis Lupo, Director Business Development; www.pilat–nai.com

POLICY TECHNOLOGIES INTERNATIONAL, INC., 2687 South 2000 West, Rexburg, Idaho Zip 83440; tel. 208/359–8123; Anthony Tietjen, Director Marketing; www.policytech.com

PORTFOLIO RECOVERY ASSOCIATES, INC., 130 Corporate Boulevard, Norfolk, Virginia Zip 23502; tel. 757/351–3065; David Foster, Vice President Healthcare Acquisitions; www.portfoliorecovery.com

PRACTICE MANAGEMENT INFORMATION CORPORATION, 4727 Wilshire Boulevard – 300, Los Angeles, California Zip 90010; tel. 323/954–0224; James B. Davis, President; www.pmiconline.com

PREMIERE GLOBAL SERVICES, 3280 Peachtree Road N.W., Suite 1000, Atlanta, Georgia Zip 30305–2422; tel. 404/543–9449; Mark H. Horne, Vice President Marketing, Notifications and Reminders; www.premiereglobal.com

PROCTER AND GAMBLE COMPANY, 8700 Mason–Montgomery Road, Box 2071, Mason, Ohio Zip 45040–9462; tel. 513/622–4672; John E. Roney, Associate Director

PURCHASE COMMANDER, LLC, 8845 Red Oak Boulevard, Charlotte, North Carolina Zip 28217; tel. 866/787–9992; Ted Matson, FACHE, Managing Partner; www.purchasecommander.com

QUADRAMED CORPORATION, 12110 Sunset Hills Road, Suite 600, Reston, Virginia Zip 20190; tel. 800/393–0278; Brooke Kane, Marketing Manager; www.quadramed.com

R. S. I., 1001 Cromwell Bridge Road, Suite 200, Baltimore, Maryland Zip 21286; tel. 800/787–9669; Peter Callan, Chief Operating Officer; www.rsirecruit.com

RF TECHNOLOGIES, 3125 North 126th Street, Brookfield, Wisconsin Zip 53005; tel. 800/669–9946; Kathie Vick, Manager Marketing; www.rft.com

ROSARIO INCORPORATED, 3500 Vest Mill Road, Winston Salem, North Carolina Zip 27103; tel. 866/279–8485; Sandra R. Rosario, President and Chief Executive Officer; www.rosarioinc.com

RSI ENTERPRISES, INC., 3838 North Central Avenue, Suite 1700, Phoenix, Arizona Zip 85012; tel. 602/263–4000; Roxanne Giannerini, President; www.rsico.com

RURAL HEALTH RESOURCE CENTER, 600 East Superior Street, Suite 404, Duluth, Minnesota Zip 55802; tel. 218/727–9390; Terry J. Hill, Executive Director; www.ruralcenter.org

RYCAN, P.O. Box 306, Marshall, Minnesota Zip 56258–0306; tel. 800/201–3324; Jody Heard, Sales Executive; www.rycan.com

SECUREACH SYSTEMS, INC., 60 Public Square, Suite 250, Medina, Ohio Zip 44256; tel. 330/721–8255; Steven Pap, M.D., President; www.secureachsystems.com

SEI, 1 Freedom Valley Drive, Oaks, Pennsylvania Zip 19456; tel. 610/676–3593; David Alexander, Director Lead Generation; www.seic.com

SIMPLEX GRINNELL, 50 Technology Drive, Westminster, Massachusetts Zip 01441; tel. 978/731–8486; Suzanne Rahall, Marketing Manager, Healthcare Communications; www.simplexgrinnell.com

SMITHS MEDICAL CRITICAL CARE, 160 Weymouth Street, Rockland, Massachusetts Zip 02370–1136; tel. 781/878–8011; John Mueckler, Market Research Manager; www.smiths–medical.com

STERLING SERVICES GROUP, 259 North Radnor–Chester Road, Suite 130, Radnor, Pennsylvania Zip 19087; tel. 484/588–4000; Graeme A. Crothall, President and Chief Executive Officer

SUBWAY, 325 Bic Drive, Milford, Connecticut Zip 06461; tel. 800/888–4848; Joanne Kilgore, Global Account Manager; www.subway.com

SURGICAL INFORMATION SYSTEMS, 11605 Haynes Bridge Road, Alpharetta, Georgia Zip 30004; tel. 678/507–1706; Kelly R. Pinkerton, Manager Marketing; www.sisfirst.com

TANDBERG, 29 Norfolk Avenue, Peabody, New York Zip 01960; tel. 978/531–1516; Joe D'Iorio, Healthcare Manager; www.tandberg.com

TEAMHEALTH, 1900 Winston Road, Suite 300, Knoxville, Tennessee Zip 37919; tel. 865/293–5486; Tracy Young, Vice President Marketing; www.teamhealth.com

TESTSOURCE, 4344 Plainfield Avenue N.E., Grand Rapids, Michigan Zip 49525; tel. 800/691–3737; Mark Wiersma, President; www.testsource.com

THE ADVISORY BOARD COMPANY, 2445 M. Street N.W., Washington, District of Columbia Zip 20037–2403; tel. 202/266–5600; Scott Fassbach, Chief Research Officer; www.advisory.com

THE AMERICAN COLLEGE OF OBSTETRICIANS AND GYNECOLOGISTS, 409 12th Street, S.W., Washington, District of Columbia Zip 20024–2188; tel. 202/863–2525; Ralph W. Hale, M.D., Executive Vice President; www.acog.org

THE EXIGENCE GROUP, 6653 Main Street, Williamsville, New York Zip 14221; tel. 716/204–4500; Susan S. Luff, Director Recruitment and Marketing; www.exigencellc.com

THE GOVERNANCE INSTITUTE, 6333 Greenwich Drive, Suite 200, San Diego, California Zip 92122; tel. 858/909–0811; Jona Raasch, President and Chief Executive Officer; www.governanceinstitute.com

THE JEWISH GUILD FOR THE BLIND, 15 West 65th Street, New York, New York Zip 10023; tel. 212/769–6200; Alan R. Morse, J.D., Ph.D., President and Chief Executive Officer; www.jgb.org

THE RISK MANAGEMENT AND PATIENT SAFETY INSTITUTE, 6215 West St. Joseph Highway, Lansing, Michigan Zip 48917; tel. 517/886–8352; Patricia A. Dextrom, Merchandising Manager

THE WALKER COMPANY, 4848 Hastings Drive, Lake Oswego, Oregon Zip 97035; tel. 503/534–9461; Larry W. Walker, Principal; www.walkercompany.com

THE WHITING TURNER CONTRACTING COMPANY, 300 East Joppa Road, Baltimore, Maryland Zip 21286; tel. 410/337–7422; Kim Bates, Market Coordinator; www.whiting–turner.com

THERADOC, 257 East 200 South, Suite 600, Salt Lake City, Utah Zip 84111; tel. 801/415–4400; Jerry Engelson; www.theradoc.com

THEREX, INC., 341 Cool Springs Boulevard, Franklin, Tennessee Zip 37067; tel. 615/236–2550; Michael G. Skiera, President and Chief Executive Officer; www.therex.us

THERMO USCS, 120 Bishop's Way, Brookfield, Wisconsin Zip 53008; tel. 262/784–5600; Christine Miller, Executive Vice President Healthcare Group; www.thermo.com

TRANSUNION, LLC, 445 Hutchinson Avenue, Suite 800, Columbus, Ohio Zip 43235; tel. 614/785–6411; Martin Callahan, Vice President Business Development; www.transunion.com

U. S. ARMY MEDICAL COMMAND, 2050 Worth Road, Suite 10, San Antonio, Texas Zip 78234–6010; tel. 210/221–2212; Ann Russell Potter

UNIFORM DATA SYSTEM FOR MEDICAL REHABILITATION, 270 Northpointe Parkway, Suite 300, Amherst, New York Zip 14228; tel. 716/817–7800; Beth Christiansen, Associate Product Manager; www.udsmr.org

UNITED HEALTH GROUP, 5901 Lincoln Drive, Edina, Minnesota Zip 55436; tel. 952/992–4605; Nick Hilger, Senior Vice President Strategic Development; www.uhc.com

UNITED HOSPITAL FUND OF NEW YORK, 350 Fifth Avenue, 23rd Floor, New York, New York Zip 10118; tel. 212/494–0700; James R. Tallon, Jr., President

VANGUARD MODULAR BUILDING SYSTEMS, LLC, 100 Lindenwood Drive, Suite 200, Malvern, Pennsylvania Zip 19355; tel. 610/232–2920; Cathy L. Conti, Director Marketing and Training; www.vanguardmodular.com

VERSUS TECHNOLOGY, INC., 2600 Miller Creek Road, Traverse City, Michigan Zip 49684; tel. 231/946–5868; Stephanie Bertschy, Director Marketing; www.versustech.com

VERTICAL CLAIMS MANAGEMENT, L.L.C., Three Gateway Center, 15 North, Pittsburgh, Pennsylvania Zip 15222; tel. 800/501–6248; Clare Bello, President; www.vcm–llc.com

VETERANS AFFAIRS EASTERN REGION OFFICE, 9600 North Point Road, Fort Howard, Maryland Zip 21052

VIRTUAL HEALTHCARE STAFFING, 350 Sansome Street, Suite 240, San Francisco, California Zip 94104–1306; tel. 866/761–6091; Leslie King, Operations Manager

VISION INTEGRATED GRAPHICS GROUP, 8301 West 183rd Street, Tinley Park, Illinois Zip 60487–9606; tel. 708/429–2000; Bruce Brankle, Senior Account Executive; www.visionps.com

VISN 1 OFFICE, 200 Spring Road, Building 61, Bedford, Massachusetts Zip 01730

VISN 10 OFFICE, 11500 Northlake Drive, Suite 200, Cincinnati, Ohio Zip 45259–1655

VISN 11 OFFICE, P.O. Box 134002, Ann Arbor, Michigan Zip 48113–4002; Linda Belton, Network Director

VISN 12 OFFICE, P.O. Box 5000, Building 18, Hines, Illinois Zip 60141–5000; tel. 708/202–8400; Renee Oshinski, Acting Network Director

VISN 15 OFFICE, 4801 Linwood Boulevard, Kansas City, Missouri Zip 64128

VISN 16 OFFICE, 1600 East Woodrow Wilson Drive, Suite A, 3rd Floor, Jackson, Mississippi Zip 39216; tel. 601/364–7901; Rica Lewis Payton, Deputy Network Director

VISN 17 OFFICE, 2301 East Lamar Boulevard, Suite 650, Arlington, Texas Zip 76006–7435

VISN 18 OFFICE, 6950 East Williams Field Road, Mesa, Arizona Zip 85212–6033; tel. 602/222–2681; Patricia A. McKlem, Director; www.va.gov/VISN18

VISN 19 OFFICE, 4100 East Mississippi Avenue, Suite 510, Glendale, Colorado Zip 80222

VISN 2 OFFICE, P.O. Box 8980, Albany, New York Zip 12208–0980; tel. 518/626–5000

VISN 20 OFFICE, P.O. Box 1035, Portland, Oregon Zip 97207

VISN 21 OFFICE, 201 Walnut Avenue, Mare Island, California Zip 94592

VISN 22 OFFICE, 5901 East Seventh Street, Long Beach, California Zip 90822; tel. 562/826–8000; Kenneth J. Clark, FACHE, Director

VISN 23 OFFICE, 5445 Minnehaha Avenue South, 2nd Floor, Minneapolis, Minnesota Zip 55417; tel. 612/727–5967; Robert A. Petzel, M.D., Network Director; www.visn23.med.va.gov

VISN 3 OFFICE, 130 West Kingsbridge Road, Building 16, Bronx, New York Zip 10468; tel. 718/584–9000; James J. Farsetta, FACHE, Director
VISN 4 OFFICE, Delafield Road, Pittsburgh, Pennsylvania Zip 15240
VISN 5 OFFICE, 849 International Drive, Suite 275, Linthicum Heights, Maryland Zip 21090
VISN 6 OFFICE, 300 West Morgan Street, Suite 1402, Durham, North Carolina Zip 27701
VISN 7 OFFICE, 3700 Crestwood Parkway N.E., Suite 260, Duluth, Georgia Zip 30096–5585
VISN 8 OFFICE, P.O. Box 406, Bay Pines, Florida Zip 33744
VISN 9 OFFICE, 1310 24th Avenue South, Nashville, Tennessee Zip 37212–2637
VOCERA COMMUNICATIONS, 525 Race Street, Suite 150, San Jose, California Zip 95126–3495; tel. 408/882–5100; Diana Harman, Sales Administrator; www.vocera.com
VOLTAGE SECURITY, 1070 Arastradero Road, Palo Alto, California Zip 94304; tel. 650/543–1280; Lisa Snyders, Marketing Program Manager; www.voltage.com
WALGREENS HEALTH SERVICES, 1411 Lake Cook Road, MS L414, Deerfield, Illinois Zip 60015; tel. 847/374–2640; Kathy Tavitian, Director Health Care Real Estate; www.walgreens.com
WATERGUARD, 8485 – 15th Way North, Saint Petersburg, Florida Zip 33702; tel. 727/577–0441; Thomas H. Carson, President; www.waterguardsb.com
WITT/KIEFFER, 2015 Spring Road, Suite 510, Oak Brook, Illinois Zip 60523; tel. 630/990–1370; Susan G. Nalepa, Vice President
ZURICH, 12222 Merit Drive, Dallas, Texas Zip 75251; tel. 214/866–1373; Paula Holman, Vice President Healthcare; www.zurichna.com

Recruitment Services:

CEJKA SEARCH, 4 City Place Drive, Suite 300, Saint Louis, Missouri Zip 63141; tel. 800/678–7858; Gretchen A. Harman, Manager Creative and Media Resources; www.cejkasearch.com
DIVERSIFIED SEARCH RAY AND BERNDTSON, One Commerce Square, 2005 Market Street, Suite 3300, Philadelphia, Pennsylvania Zip 19103; tel. 800/423–3932; Sandra L. Goldman, Vice President; www.diversifiedsearch.com

School of Nursing:

CONEMAUGH VALLEY MEDICAL CENTER SCHOOL OF NURSING, 1086 Franklin Street, Johnstown, Pennsylvania Zip 15905; tel. 814/534–9844; Louise Pugliese, Director School of Nursing

CANADA

Other:

700, 10216–124 STREET, 700, 10216–124 Street, Edmonton, Alberta Zip T5N 4A3; tel. 780/482–7200; Neill Orr, Director Marketing; www.ormed.com
CDI COMPUTER DEALERS, INC., 130 Town Center Boulevard, Markhan, Ontario Zip L6G 1B8; tel. 905/946–3851; Mark Glazer, Account Manager Medical Sales; www.cdicomputers.com
DARCOR CASTERS, 7 Staffordshire Place, Toronto, Ontario Zip M8W 1T1; tel. 416/255–8563; Cheryl Campbell, Regional Sales Manager
HALOGEN SOFTWARE CORPORATION, 495 March Road, Suite 500, Ottawa, Ontario Zip K2K 3G1; tel. 613/270–1011; Lorna Daly, Channel Manager Healthcare; www.halogensoftware.com
ST. JOSEPH'S HEALTH CARE SYSTEM, P.O. Box 155, LCD 1, Hamilton, Ontario Zip L8L 7V7; tel. 905/528–0138; Brian Guest, Executive Director

Provincial Hospital Assn:

ONTARIO HOSPITAL ASSOCIATION, 200 Front Street W, Suite 2800, Toronto, Ontario Zip M5V 3L1; tel. 416/205–1300; Warren Di Clemente, Vice President Educational Services and Operations; www.oha.com

FOREIGN

BAHAMAS

Other:

PRINCESS MARGARET HOSPITAL, P.O. Box N–8200, Nassau, tel. 242/322–2861; Coralie Adderley, Chief Hospital Administrator; www.phabahamas.org

BAHRAIN

Other:

INTERNATIONAL HOSPITAL OF BAHRAIN, P.O. Box 1084, Manama, F. S. Zeerah, M.D., President

BERMUDA

Other:

KING EDWARD VII MEMORIAL HOSPITAL, P.O. Box HM1023, Hamilton, L. Keitha Bassett, Health Sciences Librarian

BRAZIL

Construction Firm:

W. TORRE ENGENHARIA E CONSTRUCAO, S. A., Rua George Eastman, Suite 280, Sao Paulo, Zip 05690; Marcos Gurgel, Manager Business Development; www.wtorre.com.br

Other:

HOSPITAL ISRAELITA ALBERT EINSTEIN, Avenue Albert Einstein, 627, Sao Paulo 05651–901, Jairo Tabacow Hidal, M.D., Vice President; www.einstein.br
HOSPITAL SAMARITANO, Rua Conselheiro Brotero, 1486, Sao Paulo, Zip 01232–010; Jose Antonio de Lima, M.D., General Superintendent; www.samaritano.com.br

CAYMAN ISLANDS

Insurance Broker:

ATLAS INSURANCE MANAGEMENT, P.O. Box 699, Sagicor House, George Town, Zip KY1–1107; tel. 345/945–5556; Martin Eveleigh, Chairman; www.atlascaptives.com

CHINA

Other:

CHINA INTERNATIONAL CAPITAL CORPORATION, 1 Jian Guo Men Wai Avenue, China World Tower 2, 28th Floor, Beijing, Gu Yue, Associate; www.cicc.com.cn
ELECTRICAL AND MECHANICAL SERVICES DEPARTMENT, HONGKONG SPECIAL ADMINISTRATIVE REGION GOVERNMENT, 3 Lok Man Road, Chai Wan, Hongkong, Alfred Sit Wing–hang, Health Sector Manager
TAI AN TRADITIONAL CHINESE MEDICINE HOSPITAL, Wanda Plaza Jian Guo Men Wai 93, Room 2103, Building 5, Chaonyang District Beijing, Zip 100021; Wen He, Healthcare Tour Director

COLUMBIA

Other:

ASOCIACION COLOMBIANA DE HOSPITALES Y CLINICAS, Carrera 4, No 73–15, Bogota, Juan Carlos Giraldo Valencia, Director General; www.achc.org.co

ECUADOR

Other:

HOSPITAL VOZANDES – QUITO, Villengua 022–37, Casilla17–17–691, Quito, tel. 719/590–9800; Gustavo Struve; www.hcjb.org
JUNTA DE BENEFICENCIA DE GUAYAQUIL, P.O. Box 09–01–789, Guayaquil, Lautaro Aspiazu Wright, Director; www.jbg.org.ec

GERMANY

Other:

HQ USAFE/SGPXL, Unit 3050, Box 130, Ramstein AB, Zip 09094–5001
INTERNATIONAL SPINE CLINIC BERLIN, Tauentzienstr 17, Berlin 10789, Munther Sabarini, M.D., Ph.D., Medical Director; www.spine–clinic.de

GREAT BRITAIN

Other:

BYOTROL PLC, 100 Corporate Drive, Suite J., Spartanburg, Zip 29303; Jerry Bennett, M.D., President; www.byotrol.com

GREECE

Other:

DIAGNOSTIC AND THERAPEUTIC CENTRE OF ATHENS HYGEIA, S A, 4 Erythrou Stavrou & Kifissiap, Athens, C. Kitsionas, Executive Director
ERASINIO HOSPITAL S.A., 110 Vasilisis Sofias, Athens 115 27, Constantin Mavros, Ph.D., Chief Executive Officer and Managing Director
IASO OBSTETRICS–GYNECOLOGY–SURGERY–DIAGNOSTICS–TREATMENT & RESEARCH CENTER GENERAL CLINIC S.A., 37–39 Kifissias Avenue, Maroussi Athens, Zip 15123; Takis Gianniris, Chief Executive Officer

ISRAEL

Other:

HADASSAH MEDICAL ORGANIZATION, Box 12000, Jerusalem, Zip 91120; Shlomo Mor–Yosef, Director General; www.hadassah.org.il
S.A.R.E.L. SUPPLIES AND SERVICES FOR MEDICINE LTD., P.O. Box 8466, Netanya 42504, Johsua Trounovsky, Assistant General Manager; www.sarel.co.il

JAPAN

Other:

KAMEDA MEDICAL CENTER AND CLINICS, 929 Higashi–Cho, Kamogawa City, Zip 296–8602; John C. Wocher, Executive Vice President; www.kameda.com
NAVAL REGIONAL MEDICAL CENTER, U.S. Naval Base, FPO, Zip 96362
ST. LUKE'S INTERNATIONAL HOSPITAL, 10–1 Akashi–Cho, Chuo–Ku, Tokyo 104, Shigeaki Hinohara, M.D., Honorary President

JORDAN

Other:

SPECIALTY HOSPITAL, P.O. Box 930186, Amman, Zip 11193; Fawzi Al–Hammouri, M.D., General Manager; www.specialty–hospital.com

LEBANON

Other:

AMERICAN UNIVERSITY OF BEIRUT MEDICAL CENTER, 3 Dag Hammarskjold Plaza, 8th Floor, New York, Zip 10017–2303; Munthir Kuzayli, Medical Center Director
SAINT GEORGE HOSPITAL, P.O. Box 166378, Beirut, Zip 1100–2807; Ziad Kamel, Administrative Director; www.stgeorgehospital.org

MEXICO

Consulting Firm:

ASOCIACION NACIONAL DE HOSPITALES PRIVADOS, Av Ejercito Nacional Mexicano No 613 Col Granada, Mexico City, Roberto Simon Sauma, President

Other:

INTERNATIONAL HEALTH SERVICES, Paseo Cristina 129–A, Monterrey, tel. 210/922–1141; Ivan Lourido, Chief Executive Officer; www.ihsamerica.org
SHRINERS HOSPITAL FOR CHILDREN, Av Del Iman 257, Col Pedregal de Santa Ursula, Delegacion Coyoacan, Mexico City, Zip 04600; Araceli Nagore, RN, Administrator
UNIVERSIDAD AUTONOMA DE GUADALAJARA, 110 Gallery Circle, San Antonio, Zip 78258–3310; tel. 210/366–1611; Susana Leano, Dean

NETHERLANDS ANTILLES

Other:

SINT MAARTEN MEDICAL CENTER FOUNDATION, Welgelegen Road 30 Ut 1 Cay Hill, Sint Maarten, tel. 599/543–1111; George Scot, M.D., General Director

PANAMA

Other:

CLINICA SAN FERNANDO, S. A., Dept PTY 1663, P.O. Box 25207, Miami, Zip 33102–5207; tel. 507/229–1699; Edgardo Fernandez, M.D., Medical Director; www.hospitalsanfernando.com

PERU

Other:

BRITISH AMERICAN HOSPITAL, Avenue Alfredo Salazar 3 Era, Lima 27, tel. 511/712–3000; Gonzalo Garrido–Lecca, Director; www.clinangloamericana.com.pe

PHILIPPINES

Other:

ST. LUKE'S MEDICAL CENTER, 279 East Rodriguez Sr Boulevard, Quezon City, Jose F. G. Ledesma, Chief Executive Officer

SAUDI ARABIA

Other:

ABDUL RAHMAN AL MISHARI GENERAL HOSPITAL, Olaya, Riyadh 11564, Abdul Rahman Al Mishari, M.D., President
DR. KHALID IDRISS HOSPITAL, P.O. Box 75, Jeddah, Zip 21411; Bassem Abdulaziz, Administration Director; www.kih–sa.com

TURKEY

Other:

ANADOLU MEDICAL CENTER, Anadolu Caddesi No 1 Bayramoglu Cikisi, Cayirova Mevkii, Gebze, Kocaeli, Zip 41400; Murat Dayanikli, M.D., Chief Executive Officer; www.anadolusaglik.org

UNITED ARAB EMIRATES

Other:

AMERICAN HOSPITAL–DUBAI, P.O. Box 59, Dubai, Saeed M. Almulla, Chairman

VENEZUELA

Other:

POLICLINICA METROPOLITANA, C.A., Calle A–1, URB, Caurimare, Caracas 1060, Pedro Del Medico, M.D., Medical Director

Notes

Notes

Notes

Notes

Notes

Notes

B

Health Care Systems, Networks and Alliances

Introduction

This section includes listings for networks, health care systems and alliances.

Health Care Systems

To reflect the diversity that exists among health care organizations, this publication uses the term health care system to identify both multihospital and diversified single hospital systems.

Multihospital Systems

A multihospital health care system is two or more hospitals owned, leased, sponsored, or contract managed by a central organization.

Single Hospital Systems

Single, freestanding member hospitals may be categorized as health care systems by bringing into membership three or more, and at least 25 percent, of their owned or leased non–hospital preacute and postacute health care organizations. (For purposes of definition, health care delivery is the availability of professional healthcare staff during all hours of the organization's operations). Organizations provide, or provide and finance, diagnostic, therapeutic, and/or consultative patient or client services that normally precede or follow acute, inpatient, hospitalization; or that serve to prevent or substitute for such hospitalization. These services are provided in either a freestanding facility not eligible for licensure as a hospital under state statue or through one that is a subsidiary of a hospital.

The first part of this section is an alphabetical list of multihospital health care systems. Each system listed contains two or more hospitals, which are listed under the system by state. Data for this section were compiled from the 2007 *Annual Survey* and the membership information base as published in section A of the *AHA Guide.*

One of the following codes appears after the name of each system listed to indicate the type of organizational control reported by that system:

- **CC** Catholic (Roman) church–related system, not–for–profit
- **CO** Other church–related system, not–for–profit
- **NP** Other not–for–profit system, including nonfederal, governmental systems
- **IO** Investor–owned, for profit system
- **FG** Federal Government

One of the following codes appears after the name of each hospital to indicate how that hospital is related to the system:

- **O** Owned
- **L** Leased
- **S** Sponsored
- **CM** Contract–managed

Health System Classification System

An identification system for Health Systems was developed jointly by the American Hospital Association's Health Research and Education Trust and Health Forum, and the University of California-Berkeley.[1] A health system is assigned to one of five categories based on how much they differentiate and centeralize their hospital services, physician arrangements, and provider-based insurance products. Differentiation refers to the number of different products or services that the organization offers. Centralization refers to whether decision-making and service delivery emanate from the system level more so than individual hospitals.

Categories:

Centralized Health System: A delivery system in which the system centrally organizes individual hospital service delivery, physician arrangements, and insurance product development. The number of different products/services that are offered across the system is moderate.

Centralized Physician/Insurance Health System: A delivery system with highly centralized physician arrangements and insurance product development. Within this group, hospital services are relatively decentralized with individual hospitals having discretion over the array of services they offer. The number of different products/services that are offered across the system is moderate.

Moderately Centralized Health System: A delivery system that is distinguished by the presence of both centralized and decentralized activity for hospital services, physician arrangements, and insurance product development. For example, a system within this group may have centralized care of expensive, high technology services, such as open heart surgery, but allows individual hospitals to provide an array of other health services based on local needs. The number of different products/services that are offered across the system is moderate.

Decentralized Health System: A delivery system with a high degree of decentralized of hospital services, physician arrangements, and insurance product development. Within this group, systems may lack an overarching structure for coordination. Service and product differentiation is high, which may explain why centralization is hard to achieve. In this group, the system may simply service a role in sharing information and providing administrative support to highly developed local delivery systems centered around hospitals.

Independent Hospital System: A delivery system with limited differentiation in hospital services, physician arrangements, and insurance product development. These systems are largely horizontal affiliations of autonomous hospitals.

No Assignment: For some systems sufficient data from the Annual Survey were not available to determine a cluster assignment.

The second part of this section lists health care systems indexed geographically by state and city. Every effort has been made to be as inclusive and accurate as possible. However, as in all efforts of this type, there may be omissions. For further information, write to the section for Health Care Systems, American Hospital Association, One North Franklin, Chicago, IL 60606–3401.

Networks

The *AHA Guide* shows listings of networks. A network is defined as a group of hospitals, physicians, other providers, insurers and/or community agencies that work together to coordinate and deliver a broad spectrum of services to their community. Organizations listed represent the lead or hub of the network activity. Networks are listed by state, then alphabetically by name including participating partners.

The network identification process has purposely been designed to capture networks of varying organization type. Sources include but are not limited to the following: *AHA Annual Survey,* national, state and metropolitan associations, national news and periodical searches, and the networks and their health care providers themselves. Therefore, networks are included regardless of whether a hospital or healthcare system is the network lead. When an individual hospital does appear in the listing, it is indicative of the role the hospital plays as the network lead. In addition, the network listing is **not** mutually exclusive of the hospital, health care system or alliance listings within this publication.

Networks are very fluid in their composition as goals evolve and partners change. Therefore, some of the networks included in this listing may have dissolved, reformed, or simply been renamed as this section was being produced for publication.

The network identification process is an ongoing and responsive initiative. As more information is collected and validated, it will be made available in other venues, in addition to the *AHA Guide.* For more information concerning the network identification process, please contact The American Hospital Association Resource Center at 312/422–2050.

Alliances

An alliance is a formal organization, usually owned by shareholders/members, that works on behalf of its individual members in the provision of services and products and in the promotion of activities and ventures. The organization functions under a set of bylaws or other written rules to which each member agrees to abide.

Alliances are listed alphabetically by name. Its members are listed alphabetically by state, city, and then by member name.

[1] Bazzoli, CJ; Shortell, SM; Dubbs, N; Chan, C; and Kralovec, P; "A Taxonomy of Health networks and Systems: Bringing Order Out of Chaos" *Health Services Research,* February; 1999

Section B

Statistics for Multihospital Health Care Systems and their Hospitals

The following tables describing multihospital health care systems refer to information in section B of the 2009 *AHA Guide*.

Table 1 shows the number of multihospital health care systems by type of control. Table 2 provides a breakdown of the number of systems that own, lease, sponsor or contract manage hospitals within each control category. Table 3 gives the number of hospitals and beds in each control category as well as total hospitals and beds. Finally, Table 4 shows the percentage of hospitals and beds in each control category.

For more information on multihospital health care systems, please write to the Section for Health Care Systems, One North Franklin, Chicago, Illinois 60606–3401 or call 312/422–3000.

Table 1. Multihospital Health Care Systems, by Type of Organizaton Control

Type of Control	Code	Number of Systems
Catholic (Roman) church–related	CC	40
Other church–related	CO	12
Subtotal, church–related		52
Other not–for–profit	NP	259
Subtotal, not–for–profit		311
Investor Owned	IO	74
Federal Government	FG	5
Total		390

Table 2. Multihospital Health Care Systems, by Type of Ownership and Control

Type of Ownership	Catholic Church–Related (CC)	Other Church–Related (CO)	Total Church–Related (CC + CO)	Other Not–for–Profit (NP)	Total Not–for–Profit (CC, CO, + NP)	Investor–Owned (IO)	Federal Govern–ment	All Systems
Systems that only own, lease or sponsor	35	11	46	228	274	64	5	343
Systems that only contract–manage	0	0	0	1	1	1	0	2
Systems that manage, own, lease, or sponsor	5	1	6	30	36	9	0	45
Total	40	12	52	259	311	74	5	390

Table 3. Hospitals and Beds in Multihospital Health Care Systems, by Type of Ownership and Control

	Catholic Church–Related (CC)		Other Church–Related (CO)		Total Church–Related (CC + CO)		Other Not–for–Profit (NP)		Total Not–for–Profit (CC, CO, + NP)		Investor–Owned (IO)		Federal Govern–ment		All Systems	
Type of Ownership	H	B	H	B	H	B	H	B	H	B	H	B	H	B	H	B
Owned, leased or sponsored	521	102,328	100	21,572	621	123,900	1,195	273,126	1,816	397,026	1,146	137,487	214	46,764	3,176	581,277
Contract–managed	36	1,720	1	268	37	1,988	92	7,815	129	9,803	176	12,608	0	0	305	22,411
Total	557	104,048	101	21,840	658	125,888	1,287	280,941	1,945	406,829	1,322	150,095	214	46,764	3,481	603,688

H = *hospitals;* **B** = *beds.*

Table 4. Hospitals and Beds in Multihospital Health Care Systems, by Type of Ownership and Control as a Percentage of All Systems

	Catholic Church–Related (CC)		Other Church–Related (CO)		Total Church–Related (CC + CO)		Other Not–for–Profit (NP)		Total Not–for–Profit (CC, CO, + NP)		Investor–Owned (IO)		Federal Govern–ment		All Systems	
Type of Ownership	H	B	H	B	H	B	H	B	H	B	H	B	H	B	H	B
Owned, leased or sponsored	16.4	17.6	3.1	3.7	19.6	21.3	37.6	47.0	57.2	68.3	36.1	23.7	6.7	8.0	100.0	100.0
Contract–managed	11.8	7.7	0.3	1.2	12.1	8.9	30.2	34.9	42.3	43.7	57.7	56.3	0.0	0.0	100.0	100.0
Total	16.0	17.2	2.9	3.6	18.9	20.9	37.0	46.5	55.9	67.4	38.0	24.9	6.1	7.7	100.0	100.0

H = *hospitals;* **B** = *beds.*
*Please note that figures may not always equal the provided subtotal or total percentages due to rounding.

Health Care Systems and Their Hospitals

0071: ACCORD HEALTH CARE CORPORATION (IO)
14010 Roosevelt Road, Clearwater, FL Zip 33762; tel. 727/573–1755; Stephen H. Noble, President

GEORGIA: STEWART–WEBSTER HOSPITAL (O, 25 beds) 300 Alston Street, Richland, GA Zip 31825–1406, Mailing Address: P.O. Box 190, Zip 31825–0190; tel. 229/887–3366; Stephen H. Noble, President

WHEELER COUNTY HOSPITAL (O, 25 beds) 111 Third Street, Glenwood, GA Zip 30428–2301, Mailing Address: P.O. Box 398, Zip 30428–0398; tel. 912/523–5113; William Posey, Administrator

Owned, leased, sponsored:	2 hospitals	50 beds
Contract–managed:	0 hospitals	0 beds
Totals:	2 hospitals	50 beds

★0235: ADVENTIST HEALTH (CO)
2100 Douglas Boulevard, Roseville, CA Zip 95661–3898, Mailing Address: P.O. Box 619002, Zip 95661–9002; tel. 916/781–2000; Robert G. Carmen, President
(Moderately Centralized Health System)

CALIFORNIA: CENTRAL VALLEY GENERAL HOSPITAL (O, 49 beds) 1025 North Douty Street, Hanford, CA Zip 93230–3722, Mailing Address: P.O. Box 480, Zip 93232–0480; tel. 559/583–2100; Douglas L. Lafferty, Administrator
Web address: www.hanfordhealth.com

FEATHER RIVER HOSPITAL (O, 101 beds) 5974 Pentz Road, Paradise, CA Zip 95969–5509; tel. 530/877–9361; A. Wayne Ferch, President and Chief Executive Officer
Web address: www.frhosp.org

FRANK R. HOWARD MEMORIAL HOSPITAL (L, 25 beds) One Madrone Street, Willits, CA Zip 95490–4225; tel. 707/459–6801; Kevin R. Erich, President and Chief Executive Officer
Web address: www.howardhospital.com

GLENDALE ADVENTIST MEDICAL CENTER (O, 396 beds) 1509 Wilson Terrace, Glendale, CA Zip 91206–4098; tel. 818/409–8000; Morre Dean, President and Chief Executive Officer
Web address: www.glendaleadventist.com

HANFORD COMMUNITY MEDICAL CENTER (O, 121 beds) 450 North Greenfield Avenue, Hanford, CA Zip 93230–3513, Mailing Address: P.O. Box 240, Zip 93232–0240; tel. 559/582–9000; Richard L. Rawson, President and Chief Executive Officer
Web address: www.hanfordhealth.com

REDBUD COMMUNITY HOSPITAL (O, 25 beds) 15630 18th Avenue, Clearlake, CA Zip 95422–9339, Mailing Address: P.O. Box 6720, Zip 95422–6720; tel. 707/994–6486; JoAline Olson, RN, President and Chief Executive Officer
Web address: www.adventisthealth.org

SAN JOAQUIN COMMUNITY HOSPITAL (O, 166 beds) 2615 Chester Avenue, Bakersfield, CA Zip 93301–2006, Mailing Address: P.O. Box 2615, Zip 93303–2615; tel. 661/395–3000; Robert J. Beehler, President and Chief Executive Officer
Web address: www.sanjoaquinhospital.org

SELMA COMMUNITY HOSPITAL (O, 57 beds) 1141 Rose Avenue, Selma, CA Zip 93662–3241; tel. 559/891–1000; Richard L. Rawson, President and Chief Executive Officer
Web address: www.selmahospital.org

SIMI VALLEY HOSPITAL AND HEALTH CARE SERVICES (O, 181 beds) 2975 North Sycamore Drive, Simi Valley, CA Zip 93065–1201; tel. 805/955–6000; Gary G. Irish, President and Chief Executive Officer
Web address: www.simivalleyhospital.com

SONORA REGIONAL MEDICAL CENTER (O, 147 beds) 1000 Greenley Road, Sonora, CA Zip 95370–4819; tel. 209/536–5000; Lary Davis, President and Chief Executive Officer
Web address: www.sonorahospital.org

SOUTH COAST MEDICAL CENTER (O, 83 beds) 31872 Coast Highway, Laguna Beach, CA Zip 92651–6775; tel. 949/499–1311; Bruce C. Christian, President and Chief Executive Officer
Web address: www.southcoastmedcenter.com

ST. HELENA HOSPITAL (O, 140 beds) 10 Woodland Road, Saint Helena, CA Zip 94574; tel. 707/963–3611; JoAline Olson, RN, President and Chief Executive Officer
Web address: www.sthelenahospital.org

ST. HELENA HOSPITAL–CENTER FOR BEHAVIORAL HEALTH (O, 61 beds) 525 Oregon Street, Vallejo, CA Zip 94590–3201; tel. 707/648–2200; JoAline Olson, RN, President and Chief Executive Officer
Web address: www.sthelenahospital.org/Behavioral/

UKIAH VALLEY MEDICAL CENTER (O, 65 beds) 275 Hospital Drive, Ukiah, CA Zip 95482–4531; tel. 707/462–3111; Terry M. Burns, President and Chief Executive Officer
Web address: www.adventisthealth.org

WHITE MEMORIAL MEDICAL CENTER (O, 277 beds) 1720 Cesar E Chavez Avenue, Los Angeles, CA Zip 90033–2481; tel. 323/268–5000; Beth D. Zachary, President and Chief Executive Officer
Web address: www.whitememorial.com

HAWAII: CASTLE MEDICAL CENTER (O, 160 beds) 640 Ulukahiki Street, Kailua, HI Zip 96734–4498; tel. 808/263–5500; Kevin Roberts, President and Chief Executive Officer
Web address: www.castlemed.com

OREGON: ADVENTIST MEDICAL CENTER (O, 252 beds) 10123 S.E. Market Street, Portland, OR Zip 97216–2599; tel. 503/257–2500; Deryl L. Jones, President
Web address: www.adventisthealthnw.com

TILLAMOOK COUNTY GENERAL HOSPITAL (L, 25 beds) 1000 Third Street, Tillamook, OR Zip 97141–3430; tel. 503/842–4444; Larry Davy, President and Chief Executive Officer
Web address: www.tcgh.com

WASHINGTON: WALLA WALLA GENERAL HOSPITAL (O, 40 beds) 1025 South Second Avenue, Walla Walla, WA Zip 99362–1398, Mailing Address: P.O. Box 1398, Zip 99362–1398; tel. 509/525–0480; Monty E. Knittel, President and Chief Executive Officer
Web address: www.wwgh.com

Owned, leased, sponsored:	19 hospitals	2371 beds
Contract–managed:	0 hospitals	0 beds
Totals:	19 hospitals	2371 beds

★4165: ADVENTIST HEALTH SYSTEM SUNBELT HEALTH CARE CORPORATION (CO)
111 North Orlando Avenue, Winter Park, FL Zip 32789–3675; tel. 407/975–1401; Donald L. Jernigan, Ph.D., President and Chief Executive Officer
(Decentralized Health System)

COLORADO: AVISTA ADVENTIST HOSPITAL (O, 85 beds) 100 Health Park Drive, Louisville, CO Zip 80027–9583; tel. 303/673–1000; John Sackett, Chief Executive Officer
Web address: www.avistahosp.org

LITTLETON ADVENTIST HOSPITAL (O, 134 beds) 7700 South Broadway Street, Littleton, CO Zip 80122–2628; tel. 303/730–8900; Kenneth J. Bacon, Chief Executive Officer
Web address: www.centura.org

PARKER ADVENTIST HOSPITAL (O, 10 beds) 9395 Crown Crest Boulevard, Parker, CO Zip 80138; tel. 303/269–4000; Terry Forde, Chief Executive Officer
Web address: www.parkerhospital.org

PORTER ADVENTIST HOSPITAL (O, 220 beds) 2525 South Downing Street, Denver, CO Zip 80210–5876; tel. 303/778–1955; James W. Boyle, Chief Executive Officer
Web address: www.centura.org

FLORIDA: FLORIDA HOSPITAL (O, 1906 beds) 601 East Rollins Street, Orlando, FL Zip 32803–1489; tel. 407/303–6611; Lars D. Houmann, President
Web address: www.flhosp.org

For explanation of codes following names, see page B2.
★ Indicates Type III membership in the American Hospital Association.

FLORIDA HOSPITAL – DE LAND (O, 156 beds) 701 West Plymouth Avenue, De Land, FL Zip 32720; tel. 386/943–4522; Daryl Tol, President and Chief Executive Officer
Web address: www.fhdeland.org

FLORIDA HOSPITAL FISH MEMORIAL (O, 139 beds) 1055 Saxon Boulevard, Orange City, FL Zip 32763–8468; tel. 386/917–5000; Joe Johnson, President and Chief Executive Officer
Web address: www.fhfishmemorial.org

FLORIDA HOSPITAL HEARTLAND MEDICAL CENTER (O, 234 beds) 4200 Sun'n Lake Boulevard, Sebring, FL Zip 33872–1986, Mailing Address: P.O. Box 9400, Zip 33871–9400; tel. 863/314–4466; Timothy W. Cook, President and Chief Executive Officer
Web address: www.flhosp–heartland.org

FLORIDA HOSPITAL WATERMAN (O, 182 beds) 1000 Waterman Way, Tavares, FL Zip 32778–5266; tel. 352/253–3333; Kenneth R. Mattison, President and Chief Executive Officer
Web address: www.fhwat.org

FLORIDA HOSPITAL WAUCHULA (O, 25 beds) 533 West Carlton Street, Wauchula, FL Zip 33873; tel. 863/773–3101; Linda Adler, Administrator
Web address: www.flhosp–heartland.org/Facilities/Wauchula.htm

FLORIDA HOSPITAL ZEPHYRHILLS (O, 154 beds) 7050 Gall Boulevard, Zephyrhills, FL Zip 33541–1399; tel. 813/788–0411; John R. Harding, President and Chief Executive Officer
Web address: www.fhzep.org

FLORIDA HOSPITAL–FLAGLER (O, 99 beds) 60 Memorial Medical Parkway, Palm Coast, FL Zip 32164; tel. 386/586–2000; David Ottati, President and Chief Executive Officer
Web address: www.fhms.com

FLORIDA HOSPITAL–ORMOND MEMORIAL (O, 324 beds) 875 Sterthaus Avenue, Ormond Beach, FL Zip 32174–5197; tel. 386/676–6000; Darlinda Copeland, Chief Operating Officer
Web address: www.memorial–health.com

GEORGIA: EMORY–ADVENTIST HOSPITAL (O, 57 beds) 3949 South Cobb Drive S.E., Smyrna, GA Zip 30080–6300; tel. 770/434–0710; Dennis Kiley, President
Web address: www.emoryadventist.org

GORDON HOSPITAL (O, 69 beds) 1035 Red Bud Road, Calhoun, GA Zip 30701–2082, Mailing Address: P.O. Box 12938, Zip 30703–7013; tel. 706/629–2895; Carlene Jamerson, President and Chief Executive Officer
Web address: www.gordonhospital.com

ILLINOIS: ADVENTIST GLENOAKS HOSPITAL (O, 141 beds) 701 Winthrop Avenue, Glendale Heights, IL Zip 60139–1403; tel. 630/545–8000; Brinsley B. Lewis, Chief Executive Officer
Web address: www.keepingyouwell.com

ADVENTIST HINSDALE HOSPITAL (O, 353 beds) 120 North Oak Street, Hinsdale, IL Zip 60521–3890; tel. 630/856–9000; David Crane, President and Chief Executive Officer
Web address: www.keepingyouwell.com

ADVENTIST LA GRANGE MEMORIAL HOSPITAL (O, 180 beds) 5101 South Willow Spring Road, La Grange, IL Zip 60525–2680; tel. 708/245–9000; Rick Wright, FACHE, CPA, Chief Executive Officer
Web address: www.keepingyouwell.com

KANSAS: SHAWNEE MISSION MEDICAL CENTER (O, 317 beds) 9100 West 74th Street, Shawnee Mission, KS Zip 66204–4004, Mailing Address: Box 2923, Zip 66201–1323; tel. 913/676–2000; Samuel H. Turner, Sr., Chief Executive Officer
Web address: www.shawneemission.org

KENTUCKY: MANCHESTER MEMORIAL HOSPITAL (O, 63 beds) 210 Marie Langdon Drive, Manchester, KY Zip 40962–9156; tel. 606/598–5104; Dennis Meyers, President and Chief Executive Officer
Web address: www.manchestermemorial.com

NORTH CAROLINA: PARK RIDGE HOSPITAL (O, 98 beds) Naples Road, Fletcher, NC Zip 28732, Mailing Address: P.O. Box 1569, Zip 28732–1569; tel. 828/684–8501; Jimm Bunch, President and Chief Executive Officer
Web address: www.parkridgehospital.org

TENNESSEE: JELLICO COMMUNITY HOSPITAL (L, 39 beds) 188 Hospital Lane, Jellico, TN Zip 37762–4400; tel. 423/784–7252; David A. Butler, President and Chief Executive Officer
Web address: www.jellicohospital.com

TAKOMA REGIONAL HOSPITAL (O, 100 beds) 401 Takoma Avenue, Greeneville, TN Zip 37743–4647; tel. 423/639–3151; Carlyle L. E. Walton, President
Web address: www.takoma.org

TEXAS: CENTRAL TEXAS MEDICAL CENTER (O, 113 beds) 1301 Wonder World Drive, San Marcos, TX Zip 78666–7544; tel. 512/353–8979; Gary L. Jepson, President and Chief Executive Officer
Web address: www.ctmc.org

HUGULEY MEMORIAL MEDICAL CENTER (O, 207 beds) 11801 South Freeway, Fort Worth, TX Zip 76134, Mailing Address: P.O. Box 6337, Zip 76115–6337; tel. 817/293–9110; Peter M. Weber, President and Chief Executive Officer
Web address: www.huguley.org

METROPLEX ADVENTIST HOSPITAL (O, 154 beds) 2201 South Clear Creek Road, Killeen, TX Zip 76549–4110; tel. 254/526–7523; Kenneth A. Finch, President and Chief Executive Officer
Web address: www.mplex.org

ROLLINS–BROOK COMMUNITY HOSPITAL (O, 25 beds) 608 North Key Avenue, Lampasas, TX Zip 76550, Mailing Address: P.O. Box 589, Zip 76550; tel. 512/556–3682; Jeffrey D. Villanueva, Vice President and Administrator
Web address: www.mplex.org

WISCONSIN: CHIPPEWA VALLEY HOSPITAL AND OAKVIEW CARE CENTER (O, 83 beds) 1220 Third Avenue West, Durand, WI Zip 54736–1600, Mailing Address: P.O. Box 224, Zip 54736–0224; tel. 715/672–4211; Douglas R. Peterson, President and Chief Executive Officer
Web address: www.keepingyouwell.com

Owned, leased, sponsored:	28 hospitals	5667 beds
Contract–managed:	0 hospitals	0 beds
Totals:	28 hospitals	5667 beds

Section B

★0214: ADVENTIST HEALTHCARE (NP)

1801 Research Boulevard, Suite 400, Rockville, MD Zip 20850; tel. 301/315–3030; William G. Robertson, President and Chief Executive Officer
(Moderately Centralized Health System)

MARYLAND: ADVENTIST REHABILITATION HOSPITAL OF MARYLAND (O, 73 beds) 9909 Medical Center Drive, Rockville, MD Zip 20850; tel. 240/864–6000; Doris B. Reinhart, Vice President and Administrator
Web address: www.adventisthealthcare.com

POTOMAC RIDGE BEHAVIORAL HEALTH SYSTEM (O, 181 beds) 14901 Broschart Road, Rockville, MD Zip 20850–3395; tel. 301/251–4500; Sako Maki, President
Web address: www.potomacridge.com

SHADY GROVE ADVENTIST HOSPITAL (O, 243 beds) 9901 Medical Center Drive, Rockville, MD Zip 20850–3395; tel. 301/279–6000; Dennis Hansen, Interim President
Web address: www.adventisthealthcare.com

WASHINGTON ADVENTIST HOSPITAL (O, 210 beds) 7600 Carroll Avenue, Takoma Park, MD Zip 20912–6392; tel. 301/891–7600; Jere D. Stocks, President
Web address: www.adventisthealthcare.com

NEW JERSEY: HACKETTSTOWN REGIONAL MEDICAL CENTER (O, 99 beds) 651 Willow Grove Street, Hackettstown, NJ Zip 07840–1792; tel. 908/852–5100; Gene C. Milton, President and Chief Executive Officer
Web address: www.hrmcnj.org

Owned, leased, sponsored:	5 hospitals	806 beds
Contract–managed:	0 hospitals	0 beds
Totals:	5 hospitals	806 beds

★0064: ADVOCATE HEALTH CARE (NP)

2025 Windsor Drive, Oak Brook, IL Zip 60523; tel. 630/990–5018; James H. Skogsbergh, President and Chief Executive Officer
(Moderately Centralized Health System)

ILLINOIS: ADVOCATE BETHANY HOSPITAL (O, 54 beds) 3435 West Van Buren Street, Chicago, IL Zip 60624–3399; tel. 773/265–7700; Lena Dobbs–Johnson, President
Web address: www.advocatehealth.com

For explanation of codes following names, see page B2.
★ Indicates Type III membership in the American Hospital Association.

ADVOCATE CHRIST MEDICAL CENTER (O, 678 beds) 4440 West 95th Street, Oak Lawn, IL Zip 60453–2699; tel. 708/684–8000; Kenneth W. Lukhard, President
Web address: www.advocatehealth.com/christ

ADVOCATE GOOD SAMARITAN HOSPITAL (O, 325 beds) 3815 Highland Avenue, Downers Grove, IL Zip 60515–1590; tel. 630/275–5900; David S. Fox, President
Web address: www.advocatehealth.com

ADVOCATE GOOD SHEPHERD HOSPITAL (O, 142 beds) 450 West Highway 22, Barrington, IL Zip 60010–1901; tel. 847/381–0123; Karen A. Lambert, President
Web address: www.advocatehealth.com

ADVOCATE ILLINOIS MASONIC MEDICAL CENTER (O, 348 beds) 836 West Wellington Avenue, Chicago, IL Zip 60657–5193; tel. 773/975–1600; Susan Nordstrom Lopez, President
Web address: www.advocatehealth.com

ADVOCATE LUTHERAN GENERAL HOSPITAL (O, 584 beds) 1775 Dempster Street, Park Ridge, IL Zip 60068–1174; tel. 847/723–2210; Bruce C. Campbell, President
Web address: www.advocatehealth.com

ADVOCATE SOUTH SUBURBAN HOSPITAL (O, 240 beds) 17800 South Kedzie Avenue, Hazel Crest, IL Zip 60429–0989; tel. 708/799–8000; Ann Errichetti, M.D., President
Web address: www.advocatehealth.com/ssub/

ADVOCATE TRINITY HOSPITAL (O, 195 beds) 2320 East 93rd Street, Chicago, IL Zip 60617–9984; tel. 773/967–2000; Jonathan R. Bruss, Interim Administrator
Web address: www.advocatehealth.com/trinity

Owned, leased, sponsored:	8 hospitals	2566 beds
Contract-managed:	0 hospitals	0 beds
Totals:	8 hospitals	2566 beds

0312: AHMC, INC (IO)
100 South Raymond Avenue, Alhambra, CA Zip 91801–3199; tel. 626/458–4789; Jonathan Wu, M.D., President and Chairman
(Independent Hospital System)

CALIFORNIA: ALHAMBRA HOSPITAL MEDICAL CENTER (O, 144 beds) 100 South Raymond Avenue, Alhambra, CA Zip 91801–3199, Mailing Address: P.O. Box 510, Zip 91802–0510; tel. 626/570–1606; Iris Lai, Chief Executive Officer
Web address: www.alhambrahospital.com

GARFIELD MEDICAL CENTER (O, 210 beds) 525 North Garfield Avenue, Monterey Park, CA Zip 91754–1205; tel. 626/573–2222; Philip A. Cohen, Chief Executive Officer
Web address: www.garfieldmedicalcenter.com

GREATER EL MONTE COMMUNITY HOSPITAL (O, 117 beds) 1701 Santa Anita Avenue, El Monte, CA Zip 91733–3411; tel. 626/579–7777; Philip A. Cohen, Chief Executive Officer
Web address: www.greaterelmonte.com

MONTEREY PARK HOSPITAL (O, 101 beds) 900 South Atlantic Boulevard, Monterey Park, CA Zip 91754–4780; tel. 626/570–9000; Philip A. Cohen, Chief Executive Officer
Web address: www.montereyparkhosp.com

SAN GABRIEL VALLEY MEDICAL CENTER (O, 231 beds) 438 West Las Tunas Drive, San Gabriel, CA Zip 91776–1216, Mailing Address: P.O. Box 1507, Zip 91778–1507; tel. 626/289–5454; Makoto Nakayama, Chief Executive Officer
Web address: www.sgvmc.org

WHITTIER HOSPITAL MEDICAL CENTER (O, 104 beds) 9080 Colima Road, Whittier, CA Zip 90605–1600; tel. 562/945–3561; Howard Ternes, Chief Executive Officer
Web address: www.whittierhospital.com

Owned, leased, sponsored:	6 hospitals	907 beds
Contract-managed:	0 hospitals	0 beds
Totals:	6 hospitals	907 beds

0247: AKRON GENERAL HEALTH SYSTEM (NP)
400 Wabash Avenue, Akron, OH Zip 44307–2433; tel. 330/344–6000; Alan J. Bleyer, President and Chief Executive Officer
(Moderately Centralized Health System)

OHIO: AKRON GENERAL MEDICAL CENTER (O, 473 beds) 400 Wabash Avenue, Akron, OH Zip 44307–2433; tel. 330/344–6000; Alan J. Bleyer, President and Chief Executive Officer
Web address: www.akrongeneral.org

EDWIN SHAW REHAB (O, 161 beds) 1621 Flickinger Road, Akron, OH Zip 44312–4495; tel. 330/784–1271; Cathy M. Ceccio, M.S.N., President
Web address: www.edwinshaw.com

LODI COMMUNITY HOSPITAL (O, 25 beds) 225 Elyria Street, Lodi, OH Zip 44254–1096; tel. 330/948–1222; Thomas Whelan, President
Web address: www.lodihospital.com

Owned, leased, sponsored:	3 hospitals	659 beds
Contract-managed:	0 hospitals	0 beds
Totals:	3 hospitals	659 beds

0225: ALAMEDA MEDICAL CENTER (NP)
15400 Foothill Boulevard, San Leandro, CA Zip 94578; tel. 510/677–7920; Wright L. Lassiter, III, Chief Executive Officer
(Independent Hospital System)

CALIFORNIA: ALAMEDA COUNTY MEDICAL CENTER–FAIRMONT CAMPUS (O, 399 beds) 15400 Foothill Boulevard, San Leandro, CA Zip 94578–1009; tel. 510/895–4200; Wright L. Lassiter, III, Chief Executive Officer
Web address: www.acmedctr.org

ALAMEDA COUNTY MEDICAL CENTER–HIGHLAND CAMPUS (O, 399 beds) 1411 East 31st Street, Oakland, CA Zip 94602–1018; tel. 510/437–4800; Wright L. Lassiter, III, Chief Executive Officer
Web address: www.acmedctr.org

Owned, leased, sponsored:	2 hospitals	798 beds
Contract-managed:	0 hospitals	0 beds
Totals:	2 hospitals	798 beds

1685: ALBERT EINSTEIN HEALTHCARE NETWORK (NP)
5501 Old York Road, Philadelphia, PA Zip 19141–3098; tel. 215/456–7890; Barry R. Freedman, President and Chief Executive Officer

PENNSYLVANIA: ALBERT EINSTEIN MEDICAL CENTER (O, 701 beds) 5501 Old York Road, Philadelphia, PA Zip 19141–3098; tel. 215/456–7890; A. Susan Bernini, Chief Operating Officer
Web address: www.einstein.edu

BELMONT CENTER FOR COMPREHENSIVE TREATMENT (O, 146 beds) 4200 Monument Road, Philadelphia, PA Zip 19131–1625; tel. 215/877–2000; Sharon A. Bergen, Chief Operating Officer
Web address: www.einstein.edu

MOSS REHAB, EINSTEIN AT ELKINS PARK (O, 158 beds) 60 East Township Line Road, Elkins Park, PA Zip 19027–2220; tel. 215/663–6000; Ruth Lefton, Chief Operating Officer
Web address: www.einstein.edu

Owned, leased, sponsored:	3 hospitals	1005 beds
Contract-managed:	0 hospitals	0 beds
Totals:	3 hospitals	1005 beds

0278: ALEGENT HEALTH (CO)
1010 North 96th Street, Suite 200, Omaha, NE Zip 68154; tel. 402/343–4300; Wayne A. Sensor, President and Chief Executive Officer
(Centralized Physician/Insurance Health System)

IOWA: ALEGENT HEALTH COMMUNITY MEMORIAL HOSPITAL (O, 25 beds) 631 North Eighth Street, Missouri Valley, IA Zip 51555–1199; tel. 712/642–2784; Robert R. Sellers, Regional Administrator
Web address: www.alegent.org

For explanation of codes following names, see page B2.
★ Indicates Type III membership in the American Hospital Association.

ALEGENT HEALTH MERCY HOSPITAL (S, 22 beds) 603 Rosary Drive, Corning, IA Zip 50841–1685, Mailing Address: P.O. Box 368, Zip 50841–0368; tel. 641/322–3121; James C. Ruppert, Regional Administrator
Web address: www.alegent.com

ALEGENT HEALTH MERCY HOSPITAL (S, 147 beds) 800 Mercy Drive, Council Bluffs, IA Zip 51503–3128, Mailing Address: P.O. Box 1C, Zip 51502–3001; tel. 712/328–5000; Marie E. Knedler, RN, Vice President and Chief Operating Officer
Web address: www.alegent.com/mercy

NEBRASKA: ALEGENT HEALTH BERGAN MERCY MEDICAL CENTER (S, 304 beds) 7500 Mercy Road, Omaha, NE Zip 68124–2319; tel. 402/398–6060; David Tew, Chief Operating Officer
Web address: www.alegent.com/bergan

ALEGENT HEALTH IMMANUEL MEDICAL CENTER (O, 471 beds) 6901 North 72nd Street, Omaha, NE Zip 68122–1799; tel. 402/572–2121; Ann Schumacher, Vice President and Chief Operating Officer
Web address: www.alegent.com/immanuel

ALEGENT HEALTH LAKESIDE HOSPITAL (O, 83 beds) 16901 Lakeside Hills Court, Omaha, NE Zip 68130–2318; tel. 402/717–8000; Cindy Alloway, RN, Vice President and Chief Operating Officer
Web address: www.alegent.org

ALEGENT HEALTH–MEMORIAL HOSPITAL (O, 25 beds) 104 West 17th Street, Schuyler, NE Zip 68661–1396; tel. 402/352–2441; Connie Peters, RN, Regional Health Administrator
Web address: www.alegent.org

ALEGENT–HEALTH MIDLANDS HOSPITAL (O, 121 beds) 11111 South 84th Street, Papillion, NE Zip 68046–4157; tel. 402/593–3000; Kevin Nokels, Vice President and Chief Operating Officer
Web address: www.alegent.org/midlands

MEMORIAL COMMUNITY HOSPITAL AND HEALTH SYSTEM (O, 25 beds) 810 North 22nd Street, Blair, NE Zip 68008–1199, Mailing Address: P.O. Box 250, Zip 68008–0250; tel. 402/426–2182; Sally Harvey, RN, Regional Administrator
Web address: www.mchhs.org

Owned, leased, sponsored:	9 hospitals	1223 beds
Contract–managed:	0 hospitals	0 beds
Totals:	9 hospitals	1223 beds

0065: ALEXIAN BROTHERS HEALTH SYSTEM (CC)

3040 Salt Creek Lane, Arlington Heights, IL Zip 60005; tel. 847/463–8910; Brother Thomas Keusenkothen, President and Chief Executive Officer
(Independent Hospital System)

ILLINOIS: ALEXIAN BROTHERS BEHAVIORAL HEALTH HOSPITAL (O, 94 beds) 1650 Moon Lake Boulevard, Hoffman Estates, IL Zip 60194–5000; tel. 847/882–1600; Bruce Anderson, President and Chief Executive Officer
Web address: www.abbhh.org

ALEXIAN BROTHERS MEDICAL CENTER (O, 348 beds) 800 Biesterfield Road, Elk Grove Village, IL Zip 60007–3397; tel. 847/437–5500; John P. Werrbach, Acting President and Chief Executive Officer
Web address: www.alexian.org

ST. ALEXIUS MEDICAL CENTER (O, 211 beds) 1555 Barrington Road, Hoffman Estates, IL Zip 60194–1018; tel. 847/843–2000; Edward M. Goldberg, President and Chief Executive Officer
Web address: www.stalexius.org

Owned, leased, sponsored:	3 hospitals	653 beds
Contract–managed:	0 hospitals	0 beds
Totals:	3 hospitals	653 beds

0317: ALLIANT MANAGEMENT SERVICES (IO)

2501 Nelson Miller Parkway, Suite 104, Louisville, KY Zip 40223; tel. 502/992–3525; Chris West, President and Chief Executive Officer
(Moderately Centralized Health System)

FAIRFIELD MEMORIAL HOSPITAL (C, 163 beds) 303 N.W. 11th Street, Fairfield, IL Zip 62837–1203; tel. 618/842–2611; Katherine Bunting, Chief Executive Officer
Web address: www.fairfieldmemorial.org

FAYETTE COUNTY HOSPITAL (O, 110 beds) 650 West Taylor Street, Vandalia, IL Zip 62471–1296; tel. 618/283–1231; Gregory D. Starnes, Chief Executive Officer
Web address: www.fayettecountyhospital.org

FERRELL HOSPITAL COMMUNITY FOUNDATION (C, 25 beds) 1201 Pine Street, Eldorado, IL Zip 62930–1634; tel. 618/273–3361; William Hartley, FACHE, President and Chief Executive Officer
Web address: www.ferrellhosp.org

FRANKLIN HOSPITAL (C, 25 beds) 201 Bailey Lane, Benton, IL Zip 62812–1999; tel. 618/439–3161; Hervey E. Davis, Chief Executive Officer
Web address: www.franklinhospital.net

PARIS COMMUNITY HOSPITAL (C, 25 beds) 721 East Court Street, Paris, IL Zip 61944–2420; tel. 217/465–4141; Randy Simmons, President and Chief Executive Officer
Web address: www.pariscommunityhospital.com

WABASH GENERAL HOSPITAL DISTRICT (C, 25 beds) 1418 College Drive, Mount Carmel, IL Zip 62863–2638; tel. 618/262–8621; Jay Purvis, Administrator
Web address: www.wabashgeneral.com

INDIANA: GIBSON GENERAL HOSPITAL (C, 70 beds) 1808 Sherman Drive, Princeton, IN Zip 47670–1043; tel. 812/385–3401; Emmett C. Schuster, President and Chief Executive Officer
Web address: www.gibsongeneral.com

PERRY COUNTY MEMORIAL HOSPITAL (C, 25 beds) 1 Hospital Road, Tell City, IN Zip 47586–0362; tel. 812/547–7011; Joseph A. Stuber, President and Chief Executive Officer
Web address: www.pchospital.org

WABASH COUNTY HOSPITAL (C, 50 beds) 710 North East Street, Wabash, IN Zip 46992–1924, Mailing Address: P.O. Box 548, Zip 46992–0548; tel. 260/563–3131; Marilyn J. Custer–Mitchell, President and Chief Executive Officer
Web address: www.wchospital.com

KENTUCKY: BRECKINRIDGE MEMORIAL HOSPITAL (C, 43 beds) 1011 Old Highway 60, Hardinsburg, KY Zip 40143–2597; tel. 270/756–7000; John E. Monnahan, President and Chief Executive Officer
Web address: www.breckhealth.org

CAVERNA MEMORIAL HOSPITAL (C, 25 beds) 1501 South Dixie Street, Horse Cave, KY Zip 42749–1477; tel. 270/786–2191; Alan B. Alexander, Chief Executive Officer
Web address: www.cavernahospital.com

MUHLENBERG COMMUNITY HOSPITAL (C, 135 beds) 440 Hopkinsville Street, Greenville, KY Zip 42345–1172, Mailing Address: P.O. Box 387, Zip 42345–0387; tel. 270/338–8000; George E. Walz, CHE, Interim Chief Executive Officer
Web address: www.mchky.org

THE JAMES B. HAGGIN MEMORIAL HOSPITAL (C, 59 beds) 464 Linden Avenue, Harrodsburg, KY Zip 40330–1862; tel. 859/734–5441; Earl J. Motzer, Ph.D., FACHE, Chief Executive Officer
Web address: www.hagginhosp.org

TWIN LAKES REGIONAL MEDICAL CENTER (C, 75 beds) 910 Wallace Avenue, Leitchfield, KY Zip 42754–1499; tel. 270/259–9400; Stephen L. Meredith, Chief Executive Officer
Web address: www.tlrmc.com

Owned, leased, sponsored:	1 hospital	110 beds
Contract–managed:	13 hospitals	745 beds
Totals:	14 hospitals	855 beds

★0041: ALLINA HOSPITALS & CLINICS (NP)

2925 Chicago Avenue, Minneapolis, MN Zip 55407, Mailing Address: P.O. Box 43, Zip 55440; tel. 612/262–5000; Richard R. Pettingill, President and Chief Executive Officer
(Moderately Centralized Health System)

MINNESOTA: ABBOTT NORTHWESTERN HOSPITAL (O, 637 beds) 800 East 28th Street, Minneapolis, MN Zip 55407–3799; tel. 612/863–4000; Jeffrey D. Peterson, President and Chief Executive Officer
Web address: www.abbottnorthwestern.com

BUFFALO HOSPITAL (O, 40 beds) 303 Catlin Street, Buffalo, MN Zip 55313–1947; tel. 763/682–1212; Steve Hatkin, President
Web address: www.buffalohospital.org

For explanation of codes following names, see page B2.
★ Indicates Type III membership in the American Hospital Association.

Section B

CAMBRIDGE MEDICAL CENTER (O, 78 beds) 701 South Dellwood Street, Cambridge, MN Zip 55008–1920; tel. 763/689–7700; Dennis J. Doran, President
Web address: www.allina.com/ahs/cambridge.nsf

HUTCHINSON AREA HEALTH CARE (C, 179 beds) 1095 Highway 15 South, Hutchinson, MN Zip 55350–3182; tel. 320/234–5000; Mary Ellen Wells, President
Web address: www.hahc–hmc.com

MERCY HOSPITAL (O, 264 beds) 4050 Coon Rapids Boulevard, Coon Rapids, MN Zip 55433–2586; tel. 763/236–6000; Thomas O'Connor, President
Web address: www.allinamercy.org

NEW ULM MEDICAL CENTER (O, 35 beds) 1324 Fifth Street North, New Ulm, MN Zip 56073–1553, Mailing Address: P.O. Box 577, Zip 56073–0577; tel. 507/233–1000; Lori L. Wightman, President
Web address: www.newulmmedicalcenter.com

OWATONNA HOSPITAL (O, 43 beds) 903 South Oak Street, Owatonna, MN Zip 55060–3234; tel. 507/451–3850; Dorothy Erdmann, President
Web address: www.owatonnahospital.com

PHILLIPS EYE INSTITUTE (O, 10 beds) 2215 Park Avenue, Minneapolis, MN Zip 55404–3756; tel. 612/775–8800; David B. Orbuch, President
Web address: www.allina.com

ST. FRANCIS REGIONAL MEDICAL CENTER (O, 86 beds) 1455 St. Francis Avenue, Shakopee, MN Zip 55379–3380; tel. 952/403–3000; Michael A. Baumgartner, President
Web address: www.stfrancis–shakopee.com

UNITED HOSPITAL (O, 449 beds) 333 North Smith Avenue, Saint Paul, MN Zip 55102–2389; tel. 651/241–8000; Mark G. Mishek, President
Web address: www.allina.com

UNITY HOSPITAL (O, 237 beds) 550 Osborne Road N.E., Fridley, MN Zip 55432–2799; tel. 763/236–5000; Rickie L. Ressler, RN, President
Web address: www.allina.com

WISCONSIN: RIVER FALLS AREA HOSPITAL (O, 25 beds) 1629 East Division Street, River Falls, WI Zip 54022–1571; tel. 715/425–6155; Randy Farrow, President
Web address: www.allina.com

Owned, leased, sponsored:	11 hospitals	1904 beds
Contract-managed:	1 hospital	179 beds
Totals:	12 hospitals	2083 beds

0187: ALTA HEALTHCARE SYSTEM (IO)
11500 West Olympic Boulevard, Suite 502, Los Angeles, CA Zip 90064; tel. 562/925–0201; David Topper, Chief Executive Officer
(Independent Hospital System)

CALIFORNIA: HOLLYWOOD COMMUNITY HOSPITAL (O, 45 beds) 6245 De Longpre Avenue, Los Angeles, CA Zip 90028–9001; tel. 323/462–2271; Michael Sarian, Chief Executive Officer
Web address: www.hollywoodcommunityhospital.com

LOS ANGELES COMMUNITY HOSPITAL (O, 180 beds) 4081 East Olympic Boulevard, Los Angeles, CA Zip 90023–3330; tel. 323/267–0477; David Topper, Chief Executive Officer

Owned, leased, sponsored:	2 hospitals	225 beds
Contract-managed:	0 hospitals	0 beds
Totals:	2 hospitals	225 beds

2295: AMERICAN PROVINCE OF LITTLE COMPANY OF MARY SISTERS (CC)
9350 South California Avenue, Evergreen Park, IL Zip 60805–2595; tel. 708/229–5491; Sister Kathleen McIntyre, Province Leader
(Moderately Centralized Health System)

ILLINOIS: LITTLE COMPANY OF MARY HOSPITAL AND HEALTH CARE CENTERS (O, 294 beds) 2800 West 95th Street, Evergreen Park, IL Zip 60805–2795; tel. 708/422–6200; Dennis A. Reilly, President and Chief Executive Officer
Web address: www.lcmh.org

INDIANA: MEMORIAL HOSPITAL AND HEALTH CARE CENTER (O, 129 beds) 800 West Ninth Street, Jasper, IN Zip 47546–2516; tel. 812/482–2345; Raymond W. Snowden, President and Chief Executive Officer
Web address: www.mhhcc.org

Owned, leased, sponsored:	2 hospitals	423 beds
Contract-managed:	0 hospitals	0 beds
Totals:	2 hospitals	423 beds

0316: AMERIS HEALTH SYSTEMS (IO)
1114 17th Avenue South, Suite 205, Nashville, TN Zip 37212–2215; tel. 615/327–4440; Sam Lewis, Chairman and Chief Executive Officer
(Moderately Centralized Health System)

ALABAMA: SUMMIT HOSPITAL (O, 70 beds) 4401 Riverchase Drive, Phenix City, AL Zip 36867; tel. 334/732–3000; Greg Griffith, Chief Executive Officer
Web address: www.summithospital.net

ARKANSAS: GREAT RIVER MEDICAL CENTER (O, 111 beds) 1520 North Division Street, Blytheville, AR Zip 72315–1448, Mailing Address: P.O. Box 108, Zip 72316–0108; tel. 870/838–7300; Michael G. Layfield, Chief Executive Officer
Web address: www.greatrivermc.com

SOUTH MISSISSIPPI COUNTY REGIONAL MEDICAL CENTER (O, 25 beds) 611 West Lee Avenue, Osceola, AR Zip 72370–3001, Mailing Address: P.O. Box 607, Zip 72370–0607; tel. 870/563–7000; Franklin G. Schupp, Chief Executive Officer

GEORGIA: SMITH NORTHVIEW HOSPITAL (C, 31 beds) 4280 North Valdosta Road, Valdosta, GA Zip 31602, Mailing Address: P.O. Box 10010, Zip 31604; tel. 229/671–2000; Larry R. Jeter, Chief Executive Officer
Web address: www.smithhospital.com

Owned, leased, sponsored:	3 hospitals	206 beds
Contract-managed:	1 hospital	31 beds
Totals:	4 hospitals	237 beds

• 0389: ANMED HEALTH (NP)
800 North Fant Street, Anderson, SC Zip 29621–5793; tel. 864/512–1000; John A. Miller, Jr., FACHE, President

SOUTH CAROLINA: ANMED HEALTH MEDICAL CENTER (O, 369 beds) 800 North Fant Street, Anderson, SC Zip 29621–5793; tel. 864/512–1000; John A. Miller, Jr., FACHE, President
Web address: www.anmedhealth.org

Owned, leased, sponsored:	1 hospital	369 beds
Contract-managed:	0 hospitals	0 beds
Totals:	1 hospital	369 beds

0145: APPALACHIAN REGIONAL HEALTHCARE (NP)
2285 Executive Drive, Suite 400, Lexington, KY Zip 40505, Mailing Address: P.O. Box 8086, Zip 40533–8086; tel. 859/226–2440; Jerry Haynes, President and Chief Executive Officer
(Decentralized Health System)

KENTUCKY: HARLAN ARH HOSPITAL (O, 130 beds) 81 Ball Park Road, Harlan, KY Zip 40831–1792; tel. 606/573–8100; Dan Stone, Chief Executive Officer
Web address: www.arh.org

HAZARD ARH REGIONAL MEDICAL CENTER (O, 308 beds) 100 Medical Center Drive, Hazard, KY Zip 41701–1000; tel. 606/439–6600; Donald R. Fields, Senior Community Chief Executive Officer
Web address: www.arh.org

MCDOWELL ARH HOSPITAL (O, 35 beds) Route 122, McDowell, KY Zip 41647, Mailing Address: P.O. Box 247, Zip 41647–0247; tel. 606/377–3400; Russel Barker, Community Chief Executive Officer
Web address: www.arh.org

MIDDLESBORO APPALACHIAN REGIONAL HOSPITAL (O, 96 beds) 3600 West Cumberland Avenue, Middlesboro, KY Zip 40965–2614, Mailing Address: P.O. Box 340, Zip 40965–0340; tel. 606/242–1100; Susan Roman, Community Chief Executive Officer
Web address: www.arh.org/middlesboro

For explanation of codes following names, see page B2.
★ Indicates Type III membership in the American Hospital Association.
● Single hospital health care system

MORGAN COUNTY APPALACHIAN REGIONAL HOSPITAL (L, 25 beds) 476 Liberty Road, West Liberty, KY Zip 41472–2049, Mailing Address: P.O. Box 579, Zip 41472–0579; tel. 606/743–3186; Stephen M. Gavalchik, Community Chief Executive Officer
Web address: www.arh.org

WHITESBURG APPALACHIAN REGIONAL HOSPITAL (O, 82 beds) 240 Hospital Road, Whitesburg, KY Zip 41858–1254; tel. 606/633–3600; Ellen Wright, Community Chief Executive Officer
Web address: www.arh.org/whitesburg

WILLIAMSON ARH HOSPITAL (O, 138 beds) 260 Hospital Drive, South Williamson, KY Zip 41503–4072; tel. 606/237–1710; Timothy A. Hatfield, Community Chief Executive Officer
Web address: www.arh.org

WEST VIRGINIA: BECKLEY APPALACHIAN REGIONAL HOSPITAL (O, 163 beds) 306 Stanaford Road, Beckley, WV Zip 25801–3142; tel. 304/255–3000; Rocco K. Massey, Community Chief Executive Officer
Web address: www.arh.org

SUMMERS COUNTY APPALACHIAN REGIONAL HOSPITAL (L, 61 beds) Terrace Street, Hinton, WV Zip 25951–2407, Mailing Address: Drawer 940, Zip 25951–0940; tel. 304/466–1000; Wesley Dangerfield, Community Chief Executive Officer
Web address: www.arh.org

Owned, leased, sponsored:	9 hospitals	1038 beds
Contract-managed:	0 hospitals	0 beds
Totals:	9 hospitals	1038 beds

★0104: ARCHBOLD MEDICAL CENTER (NP)

910 South Broad Street, Thomasville, GA Zip 31792–6113; tel. 229/228–2739; J. Perry Mustian, Interim President
(Centralized Physician/Insurance Health System)

GEORGIA: BROOKS COUNTY HOSPITAL (L, 25 beds) 903 North Court Street, Quitman, GA Zip 31643–1315, Mailing Address: P.O. Box 5000, Zip 31643–5000; tel. 229/263–4171; LaDon Toole, Administrator
Web address: www.archbold.org

EARLY MEMORIAL HOSPITAL (L, 152 beds) 11740 Columbia Street, Blakely, GA Zip 39823–9604; tel. 229/723–4241; Robin Rau, Administrator
Web address: www.archbold.org

GRADY GENERAL HOSPITAL (L, 48 beds) 1155 Fifth Street S.E., Cairo, GA Zip 39828–0360, Mailing Address: P.O. Box 360, Zip 39828–0360; tel. 229/377–1150; LaDon Toole, Administrator
Web address: www.archbold.org

JOHN D. ARCHBOLD MEMORIAL HOSPITAL (O, 328 beds) Gordon Avenue at Mimosa Drive, Thomasville, GA Zip 31792–6113, Mailing Address: P.O. Box 1018, Zip 31799–1018; tel. 229/228–2000; J. Perry Mustian, President and Chief Executive Officer
Web address: www.archbold.org

MITCHELL COUNTY HOSPITAL (L, 181 beds) 90 Stephens Street, Camilla, GA Zip 31730, Mailing Address: P.O. Box 639, Zip 31730–0639; tel. 229/336–5284; Mark E. Kimball, Administrator
Web address: www.archbold.org

Owned, leased, sponsored:	5 hospitals	734 beds
Contract-managed:	0 hospitals	0 beds
Totals:	5 hospitals	734 beds

★0069: ARDENT HEALTH SERVICES (IO)

1 Burton Hills Boulevard, Suite 250, Nashville, TN Zip 37215; tel. 615/296–3000; David T. Vandewater, President and Chief Executive Officer
(Moderately Centralized Health System)

NEW MEXICO: LOVELACE MEDICAL CENTER–DOWNTOWN (O, 128 beds) 601 Martin Luther King Jr. Avenue N.E., Albuquerque, NM Zip 87102–3670, Mailing Address: P.O. Box 25555, Zip 87125–0555; tel. 505/727–8000; Clay Holderman, Chief Executive Officer
Web address: www.albuquerquehospital.com

LOVELACE REHABILITATION HOSPITAL (O, 62 beds) 505 Elm Street N.E., Albuquerque, NM Zip 87102–2500; tel. 505/727–4700; Ulrike Berzau, Chief Executive Officer
Web address: www.lovelace.com

LOVELACE WESTSIDE HOSPITAL (O, 48 beds) 10501 Golf Course Road N.W., Albuquerque, NM Zip 87114–5000, Mailing Address: P.O. Box 25555, Zip 87125–0555; tel. 505/727–2000; Troy Greer, Chief Executive Officer
Web address: www.lovelacesandia.com

LOVELACE WOMEN'S HOSPITAL (O, 84 beds) 4701 Montgomery Boulevard N.E., Albuquerque, NM Zip 87109–1251, Mailing Address: P.O. Box 25555, Zip 87125–0555; tel. 505/727–7800; Sheri Milone, Chief Executive Officer and Administrator
Web address: www.lovelacesandia.com

OKLAHOMA: BAILEY MEDICAL CENTER (C, 67 beds) 10502 North 110th East Avenue, Owasso, OK Zip 74055; tel. 918/376–8000; Dee Renshaw, Chief Executive Officer
Web address: www.baileymedicalcenter.com

CUSHING REGIONAL HOSPITAL (O, 88 beds) 1027 East Cherry Street, Cushing, OK Zip 74023–4101, Mailing Address: P.O. Box 1409, Zip 74023–1409; tel. 918/225–2915; Ron Cackler, President and Chief Executive Officer
Web address: www.hillcrest.com

HENRYETTA MEDICAL CENTER (O, 41 beds) Dewey Bartlett and Main Streets, Henryetta, OK Zip 74437–6820, Mailing Address: P.O. Box 1269, Zip 74437–1269; tel. 918/652–4463; Eric N. Looper, Chief Executive Officer
Web address: www.hillcrest.com/henryetta

HILLCREST MEDICAL CENTER (O, 418 beds) 1120 South Utica, Tulsa, OK Zip 74104–4090; tel. 918/579–1000; Steve Dobbs, Chief Executive Officer
Web address: www.hillcrest.com

HILLCREST SPECIALTY HOSPITAL (O, 84 beds) 1145 South Utica Avenue, Suite 1200, Tulsa, OK Zip 74104; tel. 918/579–7260; Tracy Ferlet, Chief Executive Officer
Web address: www.hillcrestspecialty.com

OKLAHOMA STATE UNIVERSITY MEDICAL CENTER (O, 331 beds) 744 West Ninth Street, Tulsa, OK Zip 74127–9990; tel. 918/587–2561; Earl Denning, Chief Executive Officer
Web address: www.osu–medcenter.com

Owned, leased, sponsored:	9 hospitals	1284 beds
Contract-managed:	1 hospital	67 beds
Totals:	10 hospitals	1351 beds

★0094: ASANTE HEALTH SYSTEM (NP)

2650 Siskiyou Boulevard, Suite 200, Medford, OR Zip 97504–8170; tel. 541/789–4100; Roy G. Vinyard, FACHE, President and Chief Executive Officer
(Moderately Centralized Health System)

OREGON: ROGUE VALLEY MEDICAL CENTER (O, 312 beds) 2825 East Barnett Road, Medford, OR Zip 97504–8332; tel. 541/789–7000; Kent L. Brown, FACHE, Chief Executive Officer
Web address: www.asante.org

THREE RIVERS COMMUNITY HOSPITAL AND HEALTH CENTER (O, 115 beds) 500 S.W. Ramsey Avenue, Grants Pass, OR Zip 97527; tel. 541/472–7000; Paul Janke, FACHE, Chief Executive Officer
Web address: www.asante.org

Owned, leased, sponsored:	2 hospitals	427 beds
Contract-managed:	0 hospitals	0 beds
Totals:	2 hospitals	427 beds

★0198: ASCENSION HEALTH (CC)

4600 Edmundson Road, Saint Louis, MO Zip 63134–3806; tel. 314/733–8000; Anthony R. Tersigni, Ed.D., FACHE, President and Chief Executive Officer
(Decentralized Health System)

ALABAMA: PROVIDENCE HOSPITAL (S, 349 beds) 6801 Airport Boulevard, Mobile, AL Zip 36608–3785, Mailing Address: P.O. Box 850429, Zip 36685–0429; tel. 251/633–1000; Clark P. Christianson, President and Chief Executive Officer
Web address: www.providencehospital.org

For explanation of codes following names, see page B2.
★ Indicates Type III membership in the American Hospital Association.

Section B

ST. VINCENT'S BIRMINGHAM (S, 372 beds) 810 St. Vincent's Drive, Birmingham, AL Zip 35205–1695, Mailing Address: P.O. Box 12407, Zip 35202–2407; tel. 205/939–7000; Neeysa Biddle, President and Chief Operating Officer
Web address: www.stv.org

ST. VINCENT'S BLOUNT (S, 40 beds) 150 Gilbreath, Oneonta, AL Zip 35121–2534, Mailing Address: P.O. Box 1000, Zip 35121–1000; tel. 205/274–3000; Sean Tinney, President and Chief Operating Officer
Web address: www.stvhs.com

ST. VINCENT'S EAST (S, 282 beds) 50 Medical Park East Drive, Birmingham, AL Zip 35235–9987; tel. 205/838–3000; Todd S. Kennedy, President and Chief Operating Officer
Web address: www.medicalcentereast.com

ST. VINCENT'S ST. CLAIR (S, 72 beds) 2805 Doctor John Haynes Drive, Pell City, AL Zip 35125–1499; tel. 205/338–3301; Terrell Vick, President and Chief Operating Officer
Web address: www.stclairregional.com

ARIZONA: CARONDELET HOLY CROSS HOSPITAL (S, 72 beds) 1171 West Target Range Road, Nogales, AZ Zip 85621–2496; tel. 520/285–3000; Richard Polheber, Chief Executive Officer
Web address: www.carondelet.org

CARONDELET ST. JOSEPH'S HOSPITAL (S, 251 beds) 350 North Wilmot Road, Tucson, AZ Zip 85711–2678; tel. 520/296–3211; Gregory R. Angle, Chief Executive Officer
Web address: www.carondelet.org

CARONDELET ST. MARY'S HOSPITAL (S, 429 beds) 1601 West St. Mary's Road, Tucson, AZ Zip 85745–2682; tel. 520/872–3000; Odette Bolano, Chief Executive Officer
Web address: www.carondelet.org

TUCSON HEART HOSPITAL (S, 58 beds) 4888 North Stone Avenue, Tucson, AZ Zip 85704; tel. 520/696–2328; Edward W. Myers, Chief Executive Officer
Web address: www.tucsonhearthospital.com

CONNECTICUT: ST. VINCENT'S MEDICAL CENTER (S, 312 beds) 2800 Main Street, Bridgeport, CT Zip 06606–4292; tel. 203/576–5454; Susan L. Davis, RN, Ed.D., President and Chief Executive Officer
Web address: www.stvincents.org

DISTRICT OF COLUMBIA: PROVIDENCE HOSPITAL (S, 533 beds) 1150 Varnum Street N.E., Washington, DC Zip 20017–2180; tel. 202/269–7000; Julius D. Spears, Jr., President and Chief Executive Officer
Web address: www.provhosp.org

FLORIDA: SACRED HEART HOSPITAL OF PENSACOLA (S, 458 beds) 5151 North Ninth Avenue, Pensacola, FL Zip 32504–8795, Mailing Address: P.O. Box 2700, Zip 32513–2700; tel. 850/416–7000; Debbie Bostic, President
Web address: www.sacred–heart.org

SACRED HEART HOSPITAL ON THE EMERALD COAST (S, 50 beds) 7800 Highway 98 West, Destin, FL Zip 32550; tel. 850/278–3000; Roger L. Hall, Chief Executive Officer
Web address: www.sacredheartemerald.org

ST. LUKE'S HOSPITAL (O, 214 beds) 4201 Belfort Road, Jacksonville, FL Zip 32216; tel. 904/296–3700; Michael D. Holmes, Chief Operating Officer
Web address: www.stlukesjax.com

ST. VINCENT'S MEDICAL CENTER (S, 455 beds) 1 Shircliff Way, Jacksonville, FL Zip 32204–2982, Mailing Address: P.O. Box 2982, Zip 32203–2982; tel. 904/308–7300; Scott Whalen, Ph.D., Chief Executive Officer
Web address: www.jaxhealth.com

IDAHO: ST. JOSEPH REGIONAL MEDICAL CENTER (S, 149 beds) 415 Sixth Street, Lewiston, ID Zip 83501–0816; tel. 208/743–2511; Howard A. Hayes, President and Chief Executive Officer
Web address: www.sjrmc.org

ILLINOIS: SAINT ANTHONY HOSPITAL (S, 151 beds) 2875 West 19th Street, Chicago, IL Zip 60623–3596; tel. 773/484–1000; Guy Medaglia, President and Chief Executive Officer
Web address: www.saintanthonyhospital.org

INDIANA: SAINT JOHN'S HEALTH SYSTEM (S, 209 beds) 2015 Jackson Street, Anderson, IN Zip 46016–4339; tel. 765/649–2511; Thomas J. VanOsdol, Interim President
Web address: www.stjohnshealthsystem.org

ST VINCENT SETON SPECIALTY HOSPITAL (O, 74 beds) 8050 Township Line Road, Indianapolis, IN Zip 46260; tel. 317/415–8353; Peter H. Alexander, Administrator

ST. ELIZABETH ANN SETON SPECIALTY CARE HOSPITAL (S, 31 beds) 3700 Washington Avenue, Evansville, IN Zip 47750; tel. 812/485–4000; Timothy A. Flesch, President and Chief Executive Officer

ST. JOSEPH HOSPITAL (S, 136 beds) 1907 West Sycamore Street, Kokomo, IN Zip 46901–4197, Mailing Address: P.O. Box 9010, Zip 46904–9010; tel. 765/452–5611; Kathlene A. Young, M.S., FACHE, Interim President
Web address: www.stjosephhospital.net

ST. MARY'S WARRICK HOSPITAL (S, 35 beds) 1116 Millis Avenue, Boonville, IN Zip 47601–0629, Mailing Address: P.O. Box 629, Zip 47601–0629; tel. 812/897–4800; Carol Godsey, Administrator
Web address: www.stmarys.org

ST. MARY'S MEDICAL CENTER OF EVANSVILLE (S, 455 beds) 3700 Washington Avenue, Evansville, IN Zip 47750–0002; tel. 812/485–4000; Timothy A. Flesch, President and Chief Executive Officer
Web address: www.stmarys.org

ST. VINCENT CARMEL HOSPITAL (S, 104 beds) 13500 North Meridian Street, Carmel, IN Zip 46032; tel. 317/582–7000; Michael D. Chittenden, President
Web address: www.stvincent.org

ST. VINCENT CLAY HOSPITAL (S, 25 beds) 1206 East National Avenue, Brazil, IN Zip 47834–2797, Mailing Address: P.O. Box 489, Zip 47834–0489; tel. 812/442–2500; Jerry Laue, Administrator
Web address: www.stvincent.org

ST. VINCENT FRANKFORT HOSPITAL (S, 25 beds) 1300 South Jackson Street, Frankfort, IN Zip 46041–3394, Mailing Address: P.O. Box 669, Zip 46041–0669; tel. 765/656–3000; Thomas Crawford, Chief Executive Officer
Web address: www.stvincent.org

ST. VINCENT HEART CENTER OF INDIANA (S, 80 beds) 10580 North Meridian Street, Indianapolis, IN Zip 46290; tel. 317/583–5000; John Stewart, Chief Executive Officer
Web address: www.theheartcenter.com

ST. VINCENT INDIANAPOLIS HOSPITAL (S, 744 beds) 2001 West 86th Street, Indianapolis, IN Zip 46260–1991, Mailing Address: P.O. Box 40970, Zip 46240–0970; tel. 317/338–2345; Kyle De Fur, FACHE, President
Web address: www.stvincent.org

ST. VINCENT JENNINGS HOSPITAL (S, 25 beds) 301 Henry Street, North Vernon, IN Zip 47265–1097; tel. 812/352–4200; Joseph E. Roche, Administrator
Web address: www.stvincent.org

ST. VINCENT MERCY HOSPITAL (S, 25 beds) 1331 South A Street, Elwood, IN Zip 46036–1942; tel. 765/552–4600; Deborah Y. Rasper, FACHE, Administrator
Web address: www.stvincent.org

ST. VINCENT PEDIATRIC REHABILITATION CENTER (S, 20 beds) 1707 West 86th Street, Indianapolis, IN Zip 46240, Mailing Address: P.O. Box 40407, Zip 46240; tel. 317/415–5500; Anne Coleman, Administrator

ST. VINCENT RANDOLPH HOSPITAL (S, 20 beds) 473 Greenville Avenue, Winchester, IN Zip 47394–2235, Mailing Address: P.O. Box 407, Zip 47394–0407; tel. 765/584–0004; Francis G. Albarano, Administrator
Web address: www.stvincent.org

ST. VINCENT WILLIAMSPORT HOSPITAL (S, 16 beds) 412 North Monroe Street, Williamsport, IN Zip 47993–0215; tel. 765/762–4000; Jane Craigin, Chief Executive Officer
Web address: www.stvincent.org

ST. VINCENT WOMEN'S HOSPITAL (S, 60 beds) 8111 Township Line Road, Indianapolis, IN Zip 46260–8043; tel. 317/415–8111; Anne Coleman, Administrator
Web address: www.stvincent.org

MARYLAND: ST. AGNES HEALTHCARE (S, 351 beds) 900 Caton Avenue, Baltimore, MD Zip 21229–5299; tel. 410/368–6000; Bonnie Phipps, President and Chief Executive Officer
Web address: www.stagnes.org

MICHIGAN: BORGESS MEDICAL CENTER (S, 392 beds) 1521 Gull Road, Kalamazoo, MI Zip 49048–1640; tel. 269/226–7000; Paul A. Spaude, FACHE, President and Chief Executive Officer
Web address: www.borgess.com

BORGESS–LEE MEMORIAL HOSPITAL (S, 25 beds) 420 West High Street, Dowagiac, MI Zip 49047–1907; tel. 269/782–8681; Joy Strand, Chief Executive Officer
Web address: www.borgess.com

BORGESS–PIPP HOSPITAL (O, 43 beds) 411 Naomi Street, Plainwell, MI Zip 49080–9911; tel. 269/685–6811; ,
Web address: www.borgess.com

For explanation of codes following names, see page B2.
★ Indicates Type III membership in the American Hospital Association.

BRIGHTON HOSPITAL (S, 92 beds) 12851 East Grand River Avenue, Brighton, MI Zip 48116–8596; tel. 810/227–1211; Denise Bertin-Epp, Chief Executive Officer
Web address: www.stjohn.org/brighton/

CARELINK OF JACKSON (S, 30 beds) 110 North Elm Avenue, Jackson, MI Zip 49202–3595; tel. 517/787–1440; Victoria Webster, Vice President and Chief Operating Officer
Web address: www.carelinkofjackson.org

GENESYS REGIONAL MEDICAL CENTER (S, 410 beds) One Genesys Parkway, Grand Blanc, MI Zip 48439–8066; tel. 810/606–5000; Elizabeth Aderholdt, President
Web address: www.genesys.org

PROVIDENCE HOSPITAL AND MEDICAL CENTER (S, 453 beds) 16001 West Nine Mile Road, Southfield, MI Zip 48075–4854, Mailing Address: Box 2043, Zip 48037–2043; tel. 248/424–3000; Michael Wiemann, M.D., Senior Vice President and Chief Medical Officer
Web address: www.providence–stjohnhealth.org

ST. JOHN HOSPITAL AND MEDICAL CENTER (S, 612 beds) 22101 Moross Road, Detroit, MI Zip 48236–2172; tel. 313/343–4000; David B. Stephens, President and Chief Executive Officer
Web address: www.stjohn.org

ST. JOHN MACOMB HOSPITAL (S, 353 beds) 11800 East Twelve Mile Road, Warren, MI Zip 48093–3494; tel. 586/573–5000; Patricia A. Maryland, Dr.P.h., President and Chief Executive Officer
Web address: www.stjohn.org

ST. JOHN NORTH SHORES HOSPITAL (S, 60 beds) 26755 Ballard Road, Harrison Township, MI Zip 48045–2458; tel. 586/465–5501; David Sessions, Administrator
Web address: www.stjohn.org

ST. JOHN OAKLAND HOSPITAL (S, 159 beds) 27351 Dequindre, Madison Heights, MI Zip 48071–3499; tel. 248/967–7000; Joseph M. Tasse, FACHE, President
Web address: www.stjohn.org

ST. JOHN RIVER DISTRICT HOSPITAL (S, 68 beds) 4100 River Road, East China, MI Zip 48054–2909; tel. 810/329–7111; Frank W. Poma, President
Web address: www.stjohn.org

ST. JOSEPH HEALTH SYSTEM (S, 20 beds) 200 Hemlock Street, Tawas City, MI Zip 48763–9360, Mailing Address: P.O. Box 659, Zip 48764–0659; tel. 989/362–3411; Patrick Murtha, President and Chief Executive Officer
Web address: www.sjhsys.org

ST. MARY'S OF MICHIGAN (S, 268 beds) 800 South Washington Avenue, Saginaw, MI Zip 48601–2594; tel. 989/776–8000; Andrew W. Allen, Interim President and Chief Executive Officer
Web address: www.saintmarys–saginaw.org

ST. MARY'S OF MICHIGAN STANDISH HOSPITAL (S, 68 beds) 805 West Cedar Street, Standish, MI Zip 48658–9526; tel. 989/846–4521; Sheri Leaman–Case, Administrator and Chief Executive Officer
Web address: www.stmarysofmichigan.org/standish

MISSOURI: ST. JOSEPH MEDICAL CENTER (S, 242 beds) 1000 Carondelet Drive, Kansas City, MO Zip 64114–4673; tel. 816/942–4400; Scott Kashman, Chief Executive Officer
Web address: www.carondelethealth.org

ST. MARY'S MEDICAL CENTER (S, 139 beds) 201 West R. D. Mize Road, Blue Springs, MO Zip 64014–2518; tel. 816/228–5900; Robin M. Schluter, Chief Executive Officer
Web address: www.carondelethealth.org

NEW YORK: MOUNT ST. MARY'S HOSPITAL AND HEALTH CENTER (S, 373 beds) 5300 Military Road, Lewiston, NY Zip 14092–1997; tel. 716/297–4800; Judith A. Maness, FACHE, President and Chief Executive Officer
Web address: www.msmh.org

OUR LADY OF LOURDES MEMORIAL HOSPITAL (S, 169 beds) 169 Riverside Drive, Binghamton, NY Zip 13905–4198; tel. 607/798–5111; John D. O'Neil, President and Chief Executive Officer
Web address: www.lourdes.com

ST. MARY'S HOSPITAL (S, 177 beds) 1300 Massachusetts Avenue, Troy, NY Zip 12180–1695; tel. 518/268–5000; Gino J. Pazzaglini, FACHE, President and Chief Executive Officer
Web address: www.setonhealth.org

ST. MARY'S HOSPITAL (S, 143 beds) 427 Guy Park Avenue, Amsterdam, NY Zip 12010–1095; tel. 518/842–1900; Victor Giulianelli, FACHE, President and Chief Executive Officer
Web address: www.smha.org

PENNSYLVANIA: GOOD SAMARITAN REGIONAL MEDICAL CENTER (S, 136 beds) 700 East Norwegian Street, Pottsville, PA Zip 17901–2798; tel. 570/621–4000; Bernard G. Koval, President and Chief Executive Officer
Web address: www.gsrmc.com

TENNESSEE: BAPTIST HOSPITAL (S, 425 beds) 2000 Church Street, Nashville, TN Zip 37236–0002; tel. 615/284–5555; Bernard Sherry, President and Chief Executive Officer
Web address: www.baptisthospital.com

HICKMAN COMMUNITY HOSPITAL (S, 65 beds) 135 East Swan Street, Centerville, TN Zip 37033–1446; tel. 931/729–4271; Jack M. Keller, Administrator
Web address: www.hickmanhospital.com

MIDDLE TENNESSEE MEDICAL CENTER (S, 199 beds) 400 North Highland Avenue, Murfreesboro, TN Zip 37130–3854, Mailing Address: P.O. Box 1178, Zip 37133–1178; tel. 615/396–4100; Gordon B. Ferguson, CHE, President and Chief Executive Officer
Web address: www.mtmc.org

SAINT THOMAS HOSPITAL (S, 420 beds) 4220 Harding Road, Nashville, TN Zip 37205–2095, Mailing Address: P.O. Box 380, Zip 37202–0380; tel. 615/222–2111; Les A. Donahue, Chief Executive Officer
Web address: www.stthomas.org

TEXAS: DELL CHILDREN'S MEDICAL CENTER OF CENTRAL TEXAS (S, 168 beds) 4900 Mueller Boulevard, Austin, TX Zip 78723; tel. 512/324–0000; Robert I. Bonar, Jr., President and Chief Executive Officer
Web address: www.dellchildrens.net

DEPAUL CENTER (O, 64 beds) 301 Londonderry Drive, Waco, TX Zip 76712; tel. 254/776–5970; ,
Web address: www.providence.ne/depaul

PROVIDENCE HEALTH CENTER (S, 603 beds) 6901 Medical Parkway, Waco, TX Zip 76712–7998, Mailing Address: P.O. Box 2589, Zip 76702–2589; tel. 254/751–4000; Kent A. Keahey, President and Chief Executive Officer
Web address: www.providence.net

SETON EDGAR B. DAVIS HOSPITAL (S, 25 beds) 130 Hays Street, Luling, TX Zip 78648–3207; tel. 830/875–7000; Neal Kelley, Administrator
Web address: www.seton.net

SETON HIGHLAND LAKES (S, 25 beds) 3201 South Water Street, Burnet, TX Zip 78611–7219, Mailing Address: P.O. Box 1219, Zip 78611–7219; tel. 512/715–3000; Scott O. Fuller, Vice President and Administrator
Web address: www.seton.net

SETON MEDICAL CENTER (S, 455 beds) 1201 West 38th Street, Austin, TX Zip 78705–1056; tel. 512/324–1000; John C. Brindley, President and Chief Executive Officer
Web address: www.seton.net

SETON NORTHWEST HOSPITAL (S, 124 beds) 11113 Research Boulevard, Austin, TX Zip 78759–7513; tel. 512/324–6000; Charles E. Durant, Jr., FACHE, Administrator
Web address: www.seton.net

SETON SHOAL CREEK HOSPITAL (S, 89 beds) 3501 Mills Avenue, Austin, TX Zip 78731–6391; tel. 512/324–2000; Alan Isaacson, Vice President and Chief Operating Officer
Web address: www.seton.net

SETON SOUTHWEST HEALTHCARE CENTER (S, 17 beds) 7900 F. M. 1826, Austin, TX Zip 78737; tel. 512/324–9000; Maria Faria, FACHE, Administrator
Web address: www.seton.net

UNIVERSITY MEDICAL CENTER AT BRACKENRIDGE (S, 372 beds) 601 East 15th Street, Austin, TX Zip 78701–1996; tel. 512/324–7000; Jesus Garza, President and Chief Executive Officer
Web address: www.seton.net

WASHINGTON: LOURDES COUNSELING CENTER (S, 32 beds) 1175 Carondelet Drive, Richland, WA Zip 99352–3396; tel. 509/943–9104; Barbara Mead, Executive Director
Web address: www.lourdesonline.org

LOURDES MEDICAL CENTER (S, 35 beds) 520 North Fourth Avenue, Pasco, WA Zip 99301–2568, Mailing Address: P.O. Box 2568, Zip 99302–2568; tel. 509/547–7704; John Serle, President and Chief Executive Officer
Web address: www.lourdesonline.org

WISCONSIN: COLUMBIA ST. MARY'S COLUMBIA HOSPITAL (S, 248 beds) 2025 East Newport Avenue, Milwaukee, WI Zip 53211–2990; tel. 414/961–3300; Leo P. Brideau, President and Chief Executive Officer
Web address: www.columbia–stmarys.com

For explanation of codes following names, see page B2.
★ Indicates Type III membership in the American Hospital Association.

COLUMBIA ST. MARY'S MILWAUKEE HOSPITAL (S, 226 beds) 2323 North Lake Drive, Milwaukee, WI Zip 53211–9682, Mailing Address: P.O. Box 503, Zip 53201–0503; tel. 414/291–1000; Leo P. Brideau, President and Chief Executive Officer
Web address: www.columbia-stmarys.com

COLUMBIA ST. MARY'S OZAUKEE HOSPITAL (S, 116 beds) 13111 North Port Washington Road, Mequon, WI Zip 53097–2416; tel. 262/243–7300; Leo P. Brideau, President and Chief Executive Officer
Web address: www.columbia-stmarys.com

SACRED HEART REHABILITATION INSTITUTE (S, 49 beds) 2025 East Newport Avenue, Milwaukee, WI Zip 53211–2906; tel. 414/298–6700; Jack Burke, Administrator
Web address: www.columbia-stmarys.com

Owned, leased, sponsored:	77 hospitals	14871 beds
Contract-managed:	0 hospitals	0 beds
Totals:	77 hospitals	14871 beds

0229: ASSOCIATED HEALTHCARE SYSTEMS, INC. (IO)
214 Overlook Court, Suite 260, Gainesville, GA Zip 30501; tel. 770/297–1252; A. Ronald Turner, President and Chief Executive Officer
(Independent Hospital System)

GEORGIA: BERRIEN COUNTY HOSPITAL (O, 171 beds) 1221 East McPherson Avenue, Nashville, GA Zip 31639–2326, Mailing Address: P.O. Box 665, Zip 31639–0665; tel. 229/543–7100; James D. Janek, Chief Executive Officer
Web address: www.berrienhospital.com

LOUISIANA: SABINE MEDICAL CENTER (O, 44 beds) 240 Highland Drive, Many, LA Zip 71449–3718; tel. 318/256–7383; Patrick W. Gandy, Chief Executive Officer
Web address: www.sabinemedicalcenter.net

TENNESSEE: THREE RIVERS HOSPITAL (O, 25 beds) 451 Highway 13 South, Waverly, TN Zip 37185–2149, Mailing Address: P.O. Box 437, Zip 37185–2149; tel. 931/296–4203; R. Kent Koster, Chief Executive Officer
Web address: www.threerivershospital.org

TRINITY HOSPITAL (O, 25 beds) 5001 East Main Street, Erin, TN Zip 37061–0489, Mailing Address: P.O. Box 489, Zip 37061–0489; tel. 931/289–4211; Yvette Gillespie, Chief Executive Officer
Web address: www.trinityhospitaltn.com

Owned, leased, sponsored:	4 hospitals	265 beds
Contract-managed:	0 hospitals	0 beds
Totals:	4 hospitals	265 beds

★0865: ATLANTIC HEALTH (NP)
475 South Street, Morristown, NJ Zip 07962, Mailing Address: P.O. Box 1905, Zip 07962–1905; tel. 973/660–3270; Joseph A. Trunfio, Ph.D., President and Chief Executive Officer
(Moderately Centralized Health System)

NEW JERSEY: MORRISTOWN MEMORIAL HOSPITAL (O, 626 beds) 100 Madison Avenue, Morristown, NJ Zip 07962–1956; tel. 973/971–5000; Joseph A. Trunfio, Ph.D., President and Chief Executive Officer
Web address: www.atlantichealth.org/cons/hospitals/at_MMH

OVERLOOK HOSPITAL (O, 373 beds) 99 Beauvoir Avenue, Summit, NJ Zip 07902–0220; tel. 908/522–2000; Alan R. Lieber, Chief Operating Officer
Web address: www.atlantichealth.org/cons/hospitals/at_OH

Owned, leased, sponsored:	2 hospitals	999 beds
Contract-managed:	0 hospitals	0 beds
Totals:	2 hospitals	999 beds

• ★0293: ATLANTICARE (NP)
2500 English Creek Avenue, Building 500, Suite 501, Egg Harbor Township, NJ Zip 08234; tel. 609/407–2300; David P. Tilton, President and Chief Executive Officer
(Centralized Physician/Insurance Health System)

ATLANTICARE REGIONAL MEDICAL CENTER (O, 494 beds) 1925 Pacific Avenue, Atlantic City, NJ Zip 08401–6713; tel. 609/345–4000; David P. Tilton, President and Chief Executive Officer
Web address: www.atlanticare.org

Owned, leased, sponsored:	1 hospital	494 beds
Contract-managed:	0 hospitals	0 beds
Totals:	1 hospital	494 beds

0360: AURORA BEHAVIORAL HEALTH CARE (IO)
4238 Green River Road, Corona, CA Zip 92882; tel. 951/549–8032; Soon K. Kim, M.D., President and Chief Executive Officer

ARIZONA: AURORA BEHAVIORAL HEALTH SYSTEM–GLENDALE (O, 90 beds) 6015 West Peoria Avenue, Glendale, AZ Zip 85302–1201; tel. 623/344–4400; Jane Blum, Interim Chief Executive Officer
Web address: www.aurorabehavioral.com

CALIFORNIA: AURORA CHARTER OAK HOSPITAL (O, 82 beds) 1161 East Covina Boulevard, Covina, CA Zip 91724–1599; tel. 626/966–1632; Todd A. Smith, Chief Executive Officer
Web address: www.aurorabehavioral.com

AURORA LAS ENCINAS HOSPITAL (O, 138 beds) 2900 East Del Mar Boulevard, Pasadena, CA Zip 91107–4399; tel. 626/795–9901; Linda Parks, Chief Executive Officer
Web address: www.lasencinashospital.com

AURORA SAN DIEGO HOSPITAL (O, 80 beds) 11878 Avenue of Industry, San Diego, CA Zip 92128–3423; tel. 858/487–3200; James S. Plummer, Chief Executive Officer
Web address: www.aurorasandiego.com

AURORA VISTA DEL MAR HOSPITAL (O, 87 beds) 801 Seneca Street, Ventura, CA Zip 93001–1411; tel. 805/653–6434; Mayla Krebsbach, Chief Executive Officer
Web address: www.vistadelmarhospital.com

ILLINOIS: AURORA CHICAGO LAKESHORE HOSPITAL (O, 108 beds) 4840 North Marine Drive, Chicago, IL Zip 60640–4296; tel. 773/878–9700; C. Alan Eaks, Chief Executive Officer
Web address: www.chicagolakeshorehospital.com

Owned, leased, sponsored:	6 hospitals	585 beds
Contract-managed:	0 hospitals	0 beds
Totals:	6 hospitals	585 beds

★2215: AURORA HEALTH CARE (NP)
3000 West Montana, Milwaukee, WI Zip 53215–3268, Mailing Address: P.O. Box 343910, Zip 53234–3910; tel. 414/647–3000; Nick Turkal, M.D., President and Chief Executive Officer
(Centralized Health System)

WISCONSIN: AURORA BAYCARE MEDICAL CENTER (O, 160 beds) 2845 Greenbrier Road, Green Bay, WI Zip 54311, Mailing Address: P.O. Box 8900, Zip 54308; tel. 920/288–8000; Daniel T. Meyer, Chief Administrative Officer
Web address: www.aurorabaycare.com

AURORA LAKELAND MEDICAL CENTER (O, 75 beds) W3985 County Road NN, Elkhorn, WI Zip 53121–4389; tel. 262/741–2000; Kathleen Skowlund, RN, M.S., Administrator and Chief Nurse Executive
Web address: www.aurorahealthcare.org

AURORA MEDICAL CENTER (O, 73 beds) 10400 South 75th Street, Kenosha, WI Zip 53142; tel. 262/948–5600; Christine Olson, Administrator
Web address: www.aurorahealthcare.org

AURORA MEDICAL CENTER – MANITOWOC COUNTY (O, 63 beds) 5000 Memorial Drive, Two Rivers, WI Zip 54241–2399; tel. 920/794–5000; Steve Long, Vice President and Chief Administrative Officer
Web address: www.aurorahealthcare.org

AURORA MEDICAL CENTER OF OSHKOSH (O, 71 beds) 855 North Westhaven Drive, Oshkosh, WI Zip 54904; tel. 920/456–6000; Frances R. Finley, Vice President and Chief Administrative Officer
Web address: www.aurorahealthcare.com

AURORA MEDICAL CENTER OF WASHINGTON COUNTY (O, 55 beds) 1032 East Sumner Street, Hartford, WI Zip 53027–1698; tel. 262/673–2300; Jeff Euclide, Interim Administrator
Web address: www.aurorahealthcare.org

For explanation of codes following names, see page B2.
★ Indicates Type III membership in the American Hospital Association.
• Single hospital health care system

AURORA MEMORIAL HOSPITAL OF BURLINGTON (O, 65 beds) 252 McHenry Street, Burlington, WI Zip 53105–1828; tel. 262/767–6000; Kathleen Skowlund, RN, M.S., Administrator and Chief Nurse Executive
Web address: www.aurorahealthcare.org

AURORA PSYCHIATRIC HOSPITAL (O, 68 beds) 1220 Dewey Avenue, Wauwatosa, WI Zip 53213–2598; tel. 414/454–6600; Peter Carlson, Administrator
Web address: www.aurorahealthcare.org

AURORA SHEBOYGAN MEMORIAL MEDICAL CENTER (O, 135 beds) 2629 North Seventh Street, Sheboygan, WI Zip 53083–4998; tel. 920/451–5000; Bobbe Teigen, Vice President and Chief Administrative Officer
Web address: www.aurorahealthcare.org

AURORA SINAI MEDICAL CENTER (O, 195 beds) 945 North 12th Street, Milwaukee, WI Zip 53233–1337, Mailing Address: P.O. Box 342, Zip 53201–0342; tel. 414/219–2000; Leonard E. Wilk, Administrator
Web address: www.aurorahealthcare.org

AURORA ST. LUKE'S MEDICAL CENTER (O, 733 beds) 2900 West Oklahoma Avenue, Milwaukee, WI Zip 53215–4330, Mailing Address: P.O. Box 2901, Zip 53201–2901; tel. 414/649–6000; Mary O'Brien, Administrator
Web address: www.aurorahealthcare.org

AURORA WEST ALLIS MEDICAL CENTER (O, 227 beds) 8901 West Lincoln Avenue, West Allis, WI Zip 53227–0901, Mailing Address: P.O. Box 27901, Zip 53227–0901; tel. 414/328–6000; Richard A. Kellar, Administrator
Web address: www.aurorahealthcare.org

Owned, leased, sponsored:	12 hospitals	1920 beds
Contract-managed:	0 hospitals	0 beds
Totals:	12 hospitals	1920 beds

★5255: AVERA HEALTH (CC)
3900 West Avera Drive, Suite 301, Sioux Falls, SD Zip 57108; tel. 605/322–4700; John T. Porter, President and Chief Executive Officer
(Decentralized Health System)

IOWA: AVERA HOLY FAMILY HEALTH (O, 25 beds) 826 North Eighth Street, Estherville, IA Zip 51334–1598; tel. 712/362–2631; William Bumgarner, Chief Executive Officer
Web address: www.avera-holyfamily.org

FLOYD VALLEY HOSPITAL/AVERA HEALTH (C, 25 beds) 714 Lincoln Street N.E., Le Mars, IA Zip 51031–0010, Mailing Address: P.O. Box 10, Zip 51031–0010; tel. 712/546–7871; Michael T. Donlin, Administrator
Web address: www.floydvalleyhospital.org

HEGG MEMORIAL HEALTH CENTER/AVERA HEALTH (C, 85 beds) 1202 21st Avenue, Rock Valley, IA Zip 51247–1497; tel. 712/476–8000; Glenn Zevenbergen, Chief Executive Officer
Web address: www.heggmemorialhealthcenter.org

OSCEOLA COMMUNITY HOSPITAL (C, 25 beds) Ninth Avenue North, Sibley, IA Zip 51249–0258, Mailing Address: P.O. Box 258, Zip 51249–0258; tel. 712/754–2574; Janet Dykstra, Administrator
Web address: www.osceolacommunityhospital.org

SIOUX CENTER COMMUNITY HOSPITAL/HEALTH CENTER (C, 90 beds) 605 South Main Avenue, Sioux Center, IA Zip 51250–1398; tel. 712/722–1271; Wayne Muth, Interim Chief Executive Officer
Web address: www.schospital.org

MINNESOTA: AVERA MARSHALL REGIONAL MEDICAL CENTER (C, 111 beds) 300 South Bruce Street, Marshall, MN Zip 56258–3900; tel. 507/532–9661; Mary Maertens, Chief Executive Officer
Web address: www.wmmc.org

PIPESTONE COUNTY MEDICAL CENTER/AVERA HEALTH (C, 68 beds) 916 4th Avenue S.W., Pipestone, MN Zip 56164–0370; tel. 507/825–6125; Bradley D. Burris, Chief Executive Officer
Web address: www.pcmchealth.org

TYLER HEALTHCARE CENTER/AVERA HEALTH (C, 52 beds) 240 Willow Street, Tyler, MN Zip 56178–0280, Mailing Address: P.O. Box 280, Zip 56178–0280; tel. 507/247–5521; Dale K. Kruger, Chief Executive Officer and Chief Financial Officer
Web address: www.averamckennan.org/amck/regionalfacilities/tyler/

NEBRASKA: AVERA ST. ANTHONY'S HOSPITAL (O, 27 beds) 300 North 2nd Street, O'Neill, NE Zip 68763–1569; tel. 402/336–2611; Ronald J. Cork, President and Chief Executive Officer
Web address: www.avera–sta.org

SOUTH DAKOTA: AVERA DELLS AREA HEALTH CENTER (L, 20 beds) 909 North Iowa Avenue, Dell Rapids, SD Zip 57022–1231; tel. 605/428–5431; James A. Faulwell, Chief Executive Officer and Administrator
Web address: www.avera.org

AVERA GREGORY HEALTHCARE CENTER (O, 80 beds) 400 Park Avenue, Gregory, SD Zip 57533–0400, Mailing Address: P.O. Box 408, Zip 57533–0408; tel. 605/835–8394; Jack Williams, Jr., Chief Executive Officer
Web address: www.gregoryhealthcare.org

AVERA HAND COUNTY MEMORIAL HOSPITAL & CLINIC (C, 42 beds) 300 West Fifth Street, Miller, SD Zip 57362–1238; tel. 605/853–2421; Bryan Breitling, Administrator
Web address: www.avera.org

AVERA MCKENNAN HOSPITAL AND UNIVERSITY HEALTH CENTER (O, 531 beds) 800 East 21st Street, Sioux Falls, SD Zip 57105–1096, Mailing Address: P.O. Box 5045, Zip 57117–5045; tel. 605/322–8000; Fredrick Slunecka, Regional President
Web address: www.averamckennan.org

AVERA QUEEN OF PEACE (O, 199 beds) 525 North Foster, Mitchell, SD Zip 57301–2999; tel. 605/995–2000; Thomas P. Rasmusson, Regional President
Web address: www.averaqueenofpeace.org

AVERA SACRED HEART HOSPITAL (O, 293 beds) 501 Summit Avenue, Yankton, SD Zip 57078–3899; tel. 605/668–8000; Pamela J. Rezac, Regional President
Web address: www.averasacredheart.com

AVERA ST. BENEDICT HEALTH CENTER (O, 100 beds) 401 Glynn Drive, Parkston, SD Zip 57366–2031; tel. 605/928–3311; Gale Walker, President and Chief Executive Officer
Web address: www.averastbenedict.org

AVERA ST. LUKE'S (O, 265 beds) 305 South State Street, Aberdeen, SD Zip 57402–4450; tel. 605/622–5000; Ronald L. Jacobson, Regional President
Web address: www.averastlukes.org

AVERA WESKOTA MEMORIAL MEDICAL CENTER (L, 14 beds) 604 First Street N.E., Wessington Springs, SD Zip 57382; tel. 605/539–1201; Kayleen R. Lee, Chief Executive Officer
Web address: www.averaweskota.org

EUREKA COMMUNITY HEALTH SERVICES/AVERA (C, 6 beds) 410 Ninth Street, Eureka, SD Zip 57437–0517, Mailing Address: P.O. Box 517, Zip 57437–0517; tel. 605/284–2661; Robert A. Dockter, Administrator

FLANDREAU MEDICAL CENTER/AVERA HEALTH (L, 18 beds) 214 North Prairie Avenue, Flandreau, SD Zip 57028–1243; tel. 605/997–2433; Paul Lewis, Administrator and Chief Executive Officer
Web address: www.flandreaumedical.org

LANDMANN–JUNGMAN MEMORIAL HOSPITAL (C, 19 beds) 600 Billars Street, Scotland, SD Zip 57059–2026; tel. 605/583–2226; Jay Plucker, Administrator
Web address: www.ljmh.org

MARSHALL COUNTY HEALTHCARE CENTER/AVERA HEALTH (C, 18 beds) 413 Ninth Street, Britton, SD Zip 57430; tel. 605/448–2253; Stephanie Reasy, Administrator
Web address: www.avera.org

MILBANK AREA HOSPITAL/AVERA HEALTH (L, 25 beds) 901 East Virgil Avenue, Milbank, SD Zip 57252; tel. 605/432–4538; Marc Lemon, Administrator

PLATTE HEALTH CENTER/AVERA HEALTH (C, 63 beds) 601 East Seventh, Platte, SD Zip 57369–2123, Mailing Address: P.O. Box 200, Zip 57369–0200; tel. 605/337–3364; Mark Burket, Chief Executive Officer
Web address: www.phcavera.org

ST. MICHAEL'S HOSPITAL (C, 25 beds) 410 West 16th Avenue, Tyndall, SD Zip 57066, Mailing Address: P.O. Box 27, Zip 57066–0027; tel. 605/589–3341; Carol Deurmier, Chief Executive Officer

WAGNER COMMUNITY MEMORIAL HOSPITAL – AVERA (C, 20 beds) 513 Third Street S.W., Wagner, SD Zip 57380, Mailing Address: P.O. Box 280, Zip 57380–0280; tel. 605/384–3611; Bryan Slaba, Chief Executive Officer
Web address: www.avera.org

Owned, leased, sponsored:	12 hospitals	1597 beds
Contract-managed:	14 hospitals	649 beds
Totals:	26 hospitals	2246 beds

Section B

For explanation of codes following names, see page B2.
★ Indicates Type III membership in the American Hospital Association.

★0194: BANNER HEALTH (NP)
1441 North 12th Street, Phoenix, AZ Zip 85006, Mailing Address: P.O. Box 25489, Zip 85002–5489; tel. 602/747–4000; Peter S. Fine, FACHE, President and Chief Executive Officer
(Decentralized Health System)

ALASKA: FAIRBANKS MEMORIAL HOSPITAL (L, 207 beds) 1650 Cowles Street, Fairbanks, AK Zip 99701–5998; tel. 907/452–8181; Michael K. Powers, FACHE, Chief Executive Officer
Web address: www.bannerhealth.com

ARIZONA: BANNER BAYWOOD MEDICAL CENTER (O, 340 beds) 6644 East Baywood Avenue, Mesa, AZ Zip 85206–1797; tel. 480/321–2000; Don A. Evans, FACHE, Chief Executive Officer
Web address: www.bannerhealth.com

BANNER BEHAVIORAL HEALTH HOSPITAL – SCOTTSDALE (O, 92 beds) 7575 East Earll Drive, Scottsdale, AZ Zip 85251–6915; tel. 480/941–7500; Patricia A. Little–Upah, Chief Executive Officer
Web address: www.bannerhealth.com

BANNER DESERT MEDICAL CENTER (O, 518 beds) 1400 South Dobson Road, Mesa, AZ Zip 85202–9879; tel. 480/512–3000; Todd S. Werner, Chief Executive Officer
Web address: www.bannerhealth.com

BANNER ESTRELLA MEDICAL CENTER (O, 172 beds) 9201 West Thomas Road, Phoenix, AZ Zip 85037–3332; tel. 623/327–4000; Kathy Bollinger, Chief Executive Officer
Web address: www.bannerhealth.com

BANNER GATEWAY MEDICAL CENTER (O, 176 beds) 1900 North Higley Road, Gilbert, AZ Zip 85234; tel. 480/543–2000; Rebecca C. Kuhn, Chief Executive Officer
Web address: www.bannerhealth.com

BANNER GOOD SAMARITAN MEDICAL CENTER (O, 601 beds) 1111 East McDowell Road, Phoenix, AZ Zip 85006–2666, Mailing Address: P.O. Box 2989, Zip 85062–2989; tel. 602/239–2000; Larry E. Volkmar, Chief Executive Officer
Web address: www.bannerhealth.com

BANNER HEART HOSPITAL (O, 111 beds) 6750 East Baywood Avenue, Mesa, AZ Zip 85206; tel. 480/854–5000; John L. Harrington, Jr., FACHE, Chief Executive Officer
Web address: www.bannerhealth.com

BANNER THUNDERBIRD MEDICAL CENTER (O, 376 beds) 5555 West Thunderbird Road, Glendale, AZ Zip 85306–4696; tel. 602/865–5555; Thomas C. Dickson, Chief Executive Officer
Web address: www.bannerhealth.com

PAGE HOSPITAL (C, 25 beds) 501 North Navajo Drive, Page, AZ Zip 86040, Mailing Address: P.O. Box 1447, Zip 86040–1447; tel. 928/645–2424; Sandy Haryasz, RN, Chief Executive Officer
Web address: www.bannerhealth.com

CALIFORNIA: BANNER LASSEN MEDICAL CENTER (O, 25 beds) 1800 Spring Ridge Drive, Susanville, CA Zip 96130–4809; tel. 530/252–2000; Richard L. Smith, Chief Executive Officer
Web address: www.bannerhealth.com

COLORADO: EAST MORGAN COUNTY HOSPITAL (L, 15 beds) 2400 West Edison Street, Brush, CO Zip 80723–1640; tel. 970/842–6200; Christopher J. Rogers, Chief Executive Officer
Web address: www.emchbrush.com

MCKEE MEDICAL CENTER (O, 132 beds) 2000 Boise Avenue, Loveland, CO Zip 80538–4281, Mailing Address: P.O. Box 830, Zip 80539–0830; tel. 970/669–4640; Richard O. Sutton, Chief Executive Officer
Web address: www.mckeeloveland.com

NORTH COLORADO MEDICAL CENTER (L, 282 beds) 1801 16th Street, Greeley, CO Zip 80631–5199; tel. 970/352–4121; Richard O. Sutton, Chief Executive Officer
Web address: www.ncmcgreeley.com

STERLING REGIONAL MEDCENTER (O, 36 beds) 615 Fairhurst Street, Sterling, CO Zip 80751–0500; tel. 970/522–0122; Michelle L. Joy, Chief Executive Officer
Web address: www.bannerhealth.com

NEBRASKA: OGALLALA COMMUNITY HOSPITAL (L, 18 beds) 2601 North Spruce Street, Ogallala, NE Zip 69153–2465; tel. 308/284–4011; Bob S. Edwards, Jr., Chief Executive Officer
Web address: www.bannerhealth.com

NEVADA: BANNER CHURCHILL COMMUNITY HOSPITAL (O, 40 beds) 801 East Williams Avenue, Fallon, NV Zip 89406–3052; tel. 775/423–3151; Charles Myers, Chief Executive Officer
Web address: www.bannerhealth.com

WYOMING: COMMUNITY HOSPITAL (O, 25 beds) 2000 Campbell Drive, Torrington, WY Zip 82240–1597; tel. 307/532–4181; Marilyn Schock, Interim Chief Executive Officer
Web address: www.bannerhealth.com

PLATTE COUNTY MEMORIAL HOSPITAL (L, 68 beds) 201 14th Street, Wheatland, WY Zip 82201–3201, Mailing Address: P.O. Box 848, Zip 82201–0848; tel. 307/322–3636; Gavin H. Carmichael, FACHE, Chief Executive Officer
Web address: www.bannerhealth.com

WASHAKIE MEDICAL CENTER (L, 25 beds) 400 South 15th Street, Worland, WY Zip 82401–3531, Mailing Address: P.O. Box 700, Zip 82401–0700; tel. 307/347–3221; Margie Molitor, RN, Chief Executive Officer
Web address: www.washakiemedicalcenter.com

Owned, leased, sponsored:	19 hospitals	3259 beds
Contract-managed:	1 hospital	25 beds
Totals:	20 hospitals	3284 beds

★0005: BAPTIST HEALTH (CO)
800 Prudential Drive, Jacksonville, FL Zip 32207; tel. 904/202–4011; Hugh Greene, President and Chief Executive Officer
(Moderately Centralized Health System)

FLORIDA: BAPTIST MEDICAL CENTER (O, 579 beds) 800 Prudential Drive, Jacksonville, FL Zip 32207–8203; tel. 904/202–2000; Joseph M. Mitrick, FACHE, Administrator
Web address: www.e–baptisthealth.com

BAPTIST MEDICAL CENTER BEACHES (O, 146 beds) 1350 13th Avenue South, Jacksonville Beach, FL Zip 32250–3205; tel. 904/627–2900; Mark F. Slyter, FACHE, Administrator
Web address: www.e–baptisthealth.com

BAPTIST MEDICAL CENTER NASSAU (O, 32 beds) 1250 South 18th Street, Fernandina Beach, FL Zip 32034–3098; tel. 904/321–3500; Jim L. Mayo, FACHE, Administrator
Web address: www.e–baptisthealth.com

Owned, leased, sponsored:	3 hospitals	757 beds
Contract-managed:	0 hospitals	0 beds
Totals:	3 hospitals	757 beds

★0150: BAPTIST HEALTH (NP)
301 Brown Springs Road, Montgomery, AL Zip 36117; tel. 334/273–4400; W. Russell Tyner, President and Chief Executive Officer

ALABAMA: BAPTIST MEDICAL CENTER EAST (O, 150 beds) 400 Taylor Road, Montgomery, AL Zip 36117–3512, Mailing Address: P.O. Box 241267, Zip 36124–1267; tel. 334/277–8330; Mindy Burdick, Administrator
Web address: www.baptistfirst.org

BAPTIST MEDICAL CENTER SOUTH (O, 400 beds) 2105 East South Boulevard, Montgomery, AL Zip 36116–2498, Mailing Address: Box 11010, Zip 36111–0010; tel. 334/288–2100; Lynne Parker, Administrator
Web address: www.baptistfirst.org

PRATTVILLE BAPTIST HOSPITAL (O, 50 beds) 124 South Memorial Drive, Prattville, AL Zip 36067–3619, Mailing Address: P.O. Box 681630, Zip 36067–1638; tel. 334/365–0651; Ginger Henry, Administrator
Web address: www.baptistfirst.org

Owned, leased, sponsored:	3 hospitals	600 beds
Contract-managed:	0 hospitals	0 beds
Totals:	3 hospitals	600 beds

★0355: BAPTIST HEALTH (NP)
9601 Interstate 630, Exit 7, Little Rock, AR Zip 72205–7299; tel. 501/202–2000; Russell D. Harrington, Jr., President and Chief Executive Officer
(Centralized Health System)

For explanation of codes following names, see page B2.
★ Indicates Type III membership in the American Hospital Association.

ARKANSAS: BAPTIST HEALTH MEDICAL CENTER – NORTH LITTLE ROCK (O, 220 beds) 3333 Springhill Drive, North Little Rock, AR Zip 72117–2922; tel. 501/202–3000; Harrison M. Dean, FACHE, Senior Vice President and Administrator
Web address: www.baptist–health.org

BAPTIST HEALTH MEDICAL CENTER–ARKADELPHIA (L, 25 beds) 3050 Twin Rivers Drive, Arkadelphia, AR Zip 71923–4299; tel. 870/245–2622; Greg Stubblefield, Interim Administrator
Web address: www.baptist–health.org

BAPTIST HEALTH MEDICAL CENTER–HEBER SPRINGS (O, 25 beds) 1800 Bypass Road, Heber Springs, AR Zip 72543–9135; tel. 501/887–3000; Edward L. Lacy, FACHE, Vice President and Administrator

BAPTIST HEALTH MEDICAL CENTER–LITTLE ROCK (O, 721 beds) 9601 Interstate 630, Exit 7, Little Rock, AR Zip 72205–7299; tel. 501/202–2000; Steven Douglas Weeks, FACHE, Senior Vice President and Administrator
Web address: www.baptist–health.org

BAPTIST HEALTH REHABILITATION INSTITUTE (O, 100 beds) 9601 Interstate 630, Exit 7, Little Rock, AR Zip 72205–7249; tel. 501/202–7000; Greg Crain, Vice President
Web address: www.baptist–health.com

Owned, leased, sponsored:	5 hospitals	1091 beds
Contract–managed:	0 hospitals	0 beds
Totals:	5 hospitals	1091 beds

★0185: BAPTIST HEALTH CARE CORPORATION (NP)

1717 North E Street, Suite 320, Pensacola, FL Zip 32501–6335; tel. 850/469–7643; Alfred G. Stubblefield, President
(Centralized Health System)

ALABAMA: ATMORE COMMUNITY HOSPITAL (L, 51 beds) 401 Medical Park Drive, Atmore, AL Zip 36502–3091; tel. 251/368–2500; Robert E. Gowing, Administrator
Web address: www.ebaptisthealthcare.org

FLORIDA: BAPTIST HOSPITAL (O, 435 beds) 1000 West Moreno, Pensacola, FL Zip 32501–2393, Mailing Address: P.O. Box 17500, Zip 32522–7500; tel. 850/434–4011; Mark Faulkner, Administrator
Web address: www.ebaptisthealthcare.org

GULF BREEZE HOSPITAL (O, 60 beds) 1110 Gulf Breeze Parkway, Gulf Breeze, FL Zip 32561; tel. 850/934–2000; Robert Harriman, Administrator
Web address: www.e–baptisthealthcare.org

JAY HOSPITAL (L, 55 beds) 14114 South Alabama Street, Jay, FL Zip 32565–1070; tel. 850/675–8000; Michael T. Hutchins, Administrator
Web address: www.bhcpns.org/jayhospital/

Owned, leased, sponsored:	4 hospitals	601 beds
Contract–managed:	0 hospitals	0 beds
Totals:	4 hospitals	601 beds

★0122: BAPTIST HEALTH SOUTH FLORIDA (NP)

6855 Red Road, Suite 600, Coral Gables, FL Zip 33143–3632; tel. 786/662–7111; Brian E. Keeley, President and Chief Executive Officer
(Moderately Centralized Health System)

BAPTIST HOSPITAL OF MIAMI (O, 584 beds) 8900 North Kendall Drive, Miami, FL Zip 33176–2197; tel. 786/596–1960; Bo Boulenger, Chief Executive Officer
Web address: www.baptisthealth.net

DOCTORS HOSPITAL (O, 148 beds) 5000 University Drive, Coral Gables, FL Zip 33146–2094; tel. 305/308–3000; Lincoln S. Mendez, Chief Executive Officer
Web address: www.baptisthealth.net

HOMESTEAD HOSPITAL (O, 120 beds) 975 Baptist Way, Homestead, FL Zip 33033–7600; tel. 786/243–8000; Bill Duquette, Chief Executive Officer
Web address: www.baptisthealth.net

MARINERS HOSPITAL (O, 42 beds) 91500 Overseas Highway, Tavernier, FL Zip 33070–2547; tel. 305/434–1582; Nelson Lazo, Chief Executive Officer
Web address: www.baptisthealth.net

SOUTH MIAMI HOSPITAL (O, 324 beds) 6200 S.W. 73rd Street, Miami, FL Zip 33143–9990; tel. 786/662–4000; Javier Hernandez–Lichtl, Chief Executive Officer
Web address: www.baptisthealth.net

Owned, leased, sponsored:	5 hospitals	1218 beds
Contract–managed:	0 hospitals	0 beds
Totals:	5 hospitals	1218 beds

0345: BAPTIST HEALTH SYSTEM (CO)

3201 4th Avenue South, Birmingham, AL Zip 35222, Mailing Address: P.O. Box 830605, Zip 35283–0605; tel. 205/715–5319; M. Shane Spees, President and Chief Executive Officer
(Moderately Centralized Health System)

ALABAMA: CITIZENS BAPTIST MEDICAL CENTER (O, 106 beds) 604 Stone Avenue, Talladega, AL Zip 35160–2217, Mailing Address: P.O. Box 978, Zip 35161–0978; tel. 256/362–8111; Steven Gautney, President
Web address: www.bhsala.com

PRINCETON BAPTIST MEDICAL CENTER (O, 368 beds) 701 Princeton Avenue S.W., Birmingham, AL Zip 35211–1305; tel. 205/783–3000; Betsy Postlethwait, Interim President
Web address: www.bhsala.com

SHELBY BAPTIST MEDICAL CENTER (O, 176 beds) 1000 First Street North, Alabaster, AL Zip 35007–0488; tel. 205/620–8100; David C. Wilson, President
Web address: www.bhsala.com

WALKER BAPTIST MEDICAL CENTER (O, 212 beds) 3400 Highway 78 East, Jasper, AL Zip 35501–8956, Mailing Address: P.O. Box 3547, Zip 35502–3547; tel. 205/387–4000; Joel W. Tate, FACHE, President
Web address: www.bhsala.com

Owned, leased, sponsored:	4 hospitals	862 beds
Contract–managed:	0 hospitals	0 beds
Totals:	4 hospitals	862 beds

★0315: BAPTIST HEALTHCARE SYSTEM (CO)

4007 Kresge Way, Louisville, KY Zip 40207–4677; tel. 502/896–5000; Tommy J. Smith, President and Chief Executive Officer
(Centralized Physician/Insurance Health System)

KENTUCKY: BAPTIST HOSPITAL EAST (O, 407 beds) 4000 Kresge Way, Louisville, KY Zip 40207–4676; tel. 502/897–8100; Susan Stout Tamme, FACHE, President
Web address: www.baptisteast.com

BAPTIST HOSPITAL NORTHEAST (O, 82 beds) 1025 New Moody Lane, La Grange, KY Zip 40031–0559; tel. 502/222–5388; Dennis B. Johnson, Administrator
Web address: www.baptistnortheast.com

BAPTIST REGIONAL MEDICAL CENTER (O, 263 beds) 1 Trillium Way, Corbin, KY Zip 40701–8420; tel. 606/528–1212; John S. Henson, President
Web address: www.baptistregional.com

CENTRAL BAPTIST HOSPITAL (O, 347 beds) 1740 Nicholasville Road, Lexington, KY Zip 40503–1499; tel. 859/260–6100; William G. Sisson, President
Web address: www.centralbap.com

HARDIN MEMORIAL HOSPITAL (C, 268 beds) 913 North Dixie Avenue, Elizabethtown, KY Zip 42701; tel. 270/737–1212; David L. Gray, President
Web address: www.hmh.net

WESTERN BAPTIST HOSPITAL (O, 288 beds) 2501 Kentucky Avenue, Paducah, KY Zip 42003–3200; tel. 270/575–2100; Larry O. Barton, FACHE, President
Web address: www.westernbaptist.com

Owned, leased, sponsored:	5 hospitals	1387 beds
Contract–managed:	1 hospital	268 beds
Totals:	6 hospitals	1655 beds

★1625: BAPTIST MEMORIAL HEALTH CARE CORPORATION (NP)

350 North Humphreys Boulevard, Memphis, TN Zip 38120–2177; tel. 901/227–5117; Stephen Curtis Reynolds, President and Chief Executive Officer
(Moderately Centralized Health System)

Section B

For explanation of codes following names, see page B2.
★ Indicates Type III membership in the American Hospital Association.

ARKANSAS: NEA BAPTIST MEMORIAL HOSPITAL (O, 104 beds) 3024 Stadium Boulevard, Jonesboro, AR Zip 72401–7493; tel. 870/972–7000; Paul Betz, Chief Executive Officer
Web address: www.neamedicalcenter.com

MISSISSIPPI: BAPTIST MEMORIAL HOSPITAL–BOONEVILLE (L, 66 beds) 100 Hospital Street, Booneville, MS Zip 38829–3359; tel. 662/720–5000; Larkin Kennedy, Administrator and Chief Executive Officer
Web address: www.bmhcc.org

BAPTIST MEMORIAL HOSPITAL–DESOTO (O, 305 beds) 7601 Southcrest Parkway, Southaven, MS Zip 38671–4742; tel. 662/772–4000; Randy King, Administrator and Chief Executive Officer
Web address: www.bmhcc.org

BAPTIST MEMORIAL HOSPITAL–GOLDEN TRIANGLE (O, 328 beds) 2520 Fifth Street North, Columbus, MS Zip 39705–2095, Mailing Address: P.O. Box 1307, Zip 39703–1307; tel. 662/244–1000; Paul Cade, Interim Administrator and Chief Executive Officer
Web address: www.bmhcc.org

BAPTIST MEMORIAL HOSPITAL–NORTH MISSISSIPPI (L, 203 beds) 2301 South Lamar Boulevard, Oxford, MS Zip 38655–5373, Mailing Address: P.O. Box 946, Zip 38655–0946; tel. 662/232–8100; Jim Ainsworth, Interim Administrator and Chief Executive Officer
Web address: www.bmhcc.org

BAPTIST MEMORIAL HOSPITAL–UNION COUNTY (L, 153 beds) 200 Highway 30 West, New Albany, MS Zip 38652–3197; tel. 662/538–7631; James Huffman, Administrator and Chief Executive Officer
Web address: www.bmhcc.org

TENNESSEE: BAPTIST MEMORIAL HOSPITAL – MEMPHIS (O, 633 beds) 6019 Walnut Grove Road, Memphis, TN Zip 38120–2173; tel. 901/226–5000; Jason Little, Administrator and Chief Executive Officer
Web address: www.baptistonline.org

BAPTIST MEMORIAL HOSPITAL FOR WOMEN (O, 140 beds) 6225 Humphreys Boulevard, Memphis, TN Zip 38120–2373; tel. 901/227–9000; Anita Vaughn, Administrator and Chief Executive Officer
Web address: www.bmhcc.org

BAPTIST MEMORIAL HOSPITAL–COLLIERVILLE (O, 61 beds) 1500 West Poplar Avenue, Collierville, TN Zip 38017–0601; tel. 901/861–9400; Glenn Baker, Administrator and Chief Executive Officer
Web address: www.bmhcc.org

BAPTIST MEMORIAL HOSPITAL–HUNTINGDON (O, 45 beds) 631 R. B. Wilson Drive, Huntingdon, TN Zip 38344–1675; tel. 731/986–4461; Susan M. Breeden, Administrator and Chief Executive Officer
Web address: www.bmhcc.org

BAPTIST MEMORIAL HOSPITAL–LAUDERDALE (O, 35 beds) 326 Asbury Avenue, Ripley, TN Zip 38063–9701; tel. 731/221–2200; Daryl Blalack, Administrator and Chief Executive Officer
Web address: www.lauderdale.baptistonline.org

BAPTIST MEMORIAL HOSPITAL–TIPTON (O, 50 beds) 1995 Highway 51 South, Covington, TN Zip 38019–3635; tel. 901/476–2621; Barry Bondurant, Administrator and Chief Executive Officer
Web address: www.bmhcc.org

BAPTIST MEMORIAL HOSPITAL–UNION CITY (O, 85 beds) 1201 Bishop Street, Union City, TN Zip 38261–5403, Mailing Address: P.O. Box 310, Zip 38281–0310; tel. 731/884–8601; Donald Hutson, Administrator and Chief Executive Officer
Web address: www.bmhcc.org

BAPTIST MEMORIAL RESTORATIVE CARE HOSPITAL (O, 30 beds) 6019 Walnut Grove Road, Memphis, TN Zip 38120; tel. 901/226–1400; Janice Hill, Administrator
Web address: www.baptistonline.org/facilities/restorativecare

BAPTIST REHABILITATION–GERMANTOWN (O, 51 beds) 2100 Exeter Road, Germantown, TN Zip 38138–3978; tel. 901/757–1350; Susan Stralka, Administrator and Chief Executive Officer
Web address: www.bmhcc.org

Owned, leased, sponsored:	15 hospitals	2289 beds
Contract–managed:	0 hospitals	0 beds
Totals:	15 hospitals	2289 beds

★0095: BAYLOR HEALTH CARE SYSTEM (CO)

3500 Gaston Avenue, Dallas, TX Zip 75246; tel. 214/820–0111; Joel T. Allison, President and Chief Executive Officer
(Centralized Health System)

TEXAS: BAYLOR ALL SAINTS MEDICAL CENTER AT FORT WORTH (O, 393 beds) 1400 Eighth Avenue, Fort Worth, TX Zip 76104–4192; tel. 817/926–2544; Steven R. Newton, President and Chief Executive Officer
Web address: www.baylorhealth.com

BAYLOR INSTITUTE FOR REHABILITATION (O, 100 beds) 909 North Washington Avenue, Dallas, TX Zip 75246–2018; tel. 214/820–9300; Jon C. Skinner, President
Web address: www.bhcs.com

BAYLOR MEDICAL CENTER AT GARLAND (O, 214 beds) 2300 Marie Curie Boulevard, Garland, TX Zip 75042–5706; tel. 972/487–5000; James D. Thaxton, President
Web address: www.baylorhealth.com

BAYLOR MEDICAL CENTER AT IRVING (L, 209 beds) 1901 North MacArthur Boulevard, Irving, TX Zip 75061; tel. 972/579–8100; Cindy K. Schamp, President
Web address: www.baylorhealth.com

BAYLOR MEDICAL CENTER AT WAXAHACHIE (O, 56 beds) 1405 West Jefferson Street, Waxahachie, TX Zip 75165–2275; tel. 972/923–7000; Jay Fox, President
Web address: www.bhcs.com

BAYLOR REGIONAL MEDICAL CENTER AT GRAPEVINE (O, 233 beds) 1650 West College Street, Grapevine, TX Zip 76051–1650; tel. 817/481–1588; Doug Lawson, President
Web address: www.bhcs.com

BAYLOR REGIONAL MEDICAL CENTER AT PLANO (O, 94 beds) 4700 Alliance Boulevard, Plano, TX Zip 75093; tel. 469/814–2000; Jerri Garison, RN, President
Web address: www.baylorhealth.com

BAYLOR SPECIALTY HOSPITAL (O, 98 beds) 3504 Swiss Avenue, Dallas, TX Zip 75204–6224; tel. 214/820–9700; Scott Peek, President
Web address: www.bhcs.com

BAYLOR UNIVERSITY MEDICAL CENTER (O, 923 beds) 3500 Gaston Avenue, Dallas, TX Zip 75246–2088; tel. 214/820–0111; John B. McWhorter, III, President
Web address: www.baylorhealth.com

OUR CHILDREN'S HOUSE AT BAYLOR (O, 54 beds) 3504 Swiss Avenue, Dallas, TX Zip 75204–6219; tel. 214/820–9838; Scott Peek, President
Web address: www.bhcs.com

Owned, leased, sponsored:	10 hospitals	2374 beds
Contract–managed:	0 hospitals	0 beds
Totals:	10 hospitals	2374 beds

★1095: BAYSTATE HEALTH, INC. (NP)

759 Chestnut Street, Springfield, MA Zip 01199–0001; tel. 413/794–0000; Mark R. Tolosky, FACHE, J.D., President and Chief Executive Officer
(Centralized Physician/Insurance Health System)

MASSACHUSETTS: BAYSTATE FRANKLIN MEDICAL CENTER (O, 90 beds) 164 High Street, Greenfield, MA Zip 01301–2613; tel. 413/773–0211; Charles Gijanto, President
Web address: www.baystatehealth.com

BAYSTATE MARY LANE HOSPITAL (O, 31 beds) 85 South Street, Ware, MA Zip 01082–1697; tel. 413/967–6211; Christine Shirtcliff, FACHE, President
Web address: www.baystatehealth.com

BAYSTATE MEDICAL CENTER (O, 653 beds) 759 Chestnut Street, Springfield, MA Zip 01199–0001; tel. 413/794–0000; Mark R. Tolosky, FACHE, J.D., President and Chief Executive Officer
Web address: www.baystatehealth.com

Owned, leased, sponsored:	3 hospitals	774 beds
Contract–managed:	0 hospitals	0 beds
Totals:	3 hospitals	774 beds

★9575: BEAUMONT HOSPITALS (NP)

3601 West Thirteen Mile Road, Royal Oak, MI Zip 48073–6769; tel. 248/551–5000; Kenneth J. Matzick, President and Chief Executive Officer
(Moderately Centralized Health System)

For explanation of codes following names, see page B2.
★ Indicates Type III membership in the American Hospital Association.

MICHIGAN: BEAUMONT HOSPITAL – ROYAL OAK (O, 1061 beds) 3601 West Thirteen Mile Road, Royal Oak, MI Zip 48073–6769; tel. 248/898–5000; John D. Labriola, Senior Vice President and Director
Web address: www.beaumonthospitals.com

BEAUMONT HOSPITAL – TROY (O, 346 beds) 44201 Dequindre Road, Troy, MI Zip 48085; tel. 248/964–5000; Thomas Brisse, Senior Vice President and Hospital Director
Web address: www.beaumonthospitals.com

BEAUMONT HOSPITAL GROSSE POINTE (O, 234 beds) 468 Cadieux Road, Grosse Pointe, MI Zip 48230–1592; tel. 313/343–1000; Richard P. Swaine, Chief Executive Officer
Web address: www.bschealth.com

Owned, leased, sponsored:	3 hospitals	1641 beds
Contract–managed:	0 hospitals	0 beds
Totals:	3 hospitals	1641 beds

0545: BENEDICTINE SISTERS OF THE ANNUNCIATION (CC)

7520 University Drive, Bismarck, ND Zip 58504–9653; tel. 701/255–1520; Sister Susan Berger, Prioress
(Moderately Centralized Health System)

NORTH DAKOTA: GARRISON MEMORIAL HOSPITAL (S, 50 beds) 407 Third Avenue S.E., Garrison, ND Zip 58540–0039; tel. 701/463–2275; Dean Mattern, President and Chief Executive Officer
Web address: www.garrisonmh.com

ST. ALEXIUS MEDICAL CENTER (S, 280 beds) 900 East Broadway, Bismarck, ND Zip 58501–4586, Mailing Address: P.O. Box 5510, Zip 58506–5510; tel. 701/530–7000; Andrew L. Wilson, President and Chief Executive Officer
Web address: www.st.alexius.org

Owned, leased, sponsored:	2 hospitals	330 beds
Contract–managed:	0 hospitals	0 beds
Totals:	2 hospitals	330 beds

★2435: BERKSHIRE HEALTH SYSTEMS, INC. (NP)

725 North Street, Pittsfield, MA Zip 01201–4124; tel. 413/447–2743; David E. Phelps, President and Chief Executive Officer
(Centralized Health System)

MASSACHUSETTS: BERKSHIRE MEDICAL CENTER (O, 283 beds) 725 North Street, Pittsfield, MA Zip 01201–4124; tel. 413/447–2000; Helen Downey, RN, Chief Operating Officer and Chief Nursing Officer
Web address: www.berkshirehealthsystems.com

FAIRVIEW HOSPITAL (O, 25 beds) 29 Lewis Avenue, Great Barrington, MA Zip 01230–1713; tel. 413/528–0790; Eugene A. Dellea, President
Web address: www.berkshirehealthsystems.com

Owned, leased, sponsored:	2 hospitals	308 beds
Contract–managed:	0 hospitals	0 beds
Totals:	2 hospitals	308 beds

★0051: BJC HEALTHCARE (NP)

4444 Forest Park Avenue, Suite 500, Saint Louis, MO Zip 63108–2259; tel. 314/286–2000; Steven H. Lipstein, President and Chief Executive Officer
(Moderately Centralized Health System)

ILLINOIS: ALTON MEMORIAL HOSPITAL (O, 240 beds) One Memorial Drive, Alton, IL Zip 62002–6722; tel. 618/463–7311; David A. Braasch, President
Web address: www.altonmemorialhospital.org

CLAY COUNTY HOSPITAL (C, 22 beds) 911 Stacy Burk Drive, Flora, IL Zip 62839–1823, Mailing Address: P.O. Box 280, Zip 62839–0280; tel. 618/662–2131; Susan G. Batchelor, President
Web address: www.claycountyhospital.org

MISSOURI: BARNES–JEWISH HOSPITAL (O, 1207 beds) One Barnes–Jewish Hospital Plaza, Saint Louis, MO Zip 63110–1003; tel. 314/747–3000; Andrew A. Ziskind, M.D., President
Web address: www.barnesjewish.org

BARNES–JEWISH ST. PETERS HOSPITAL (O, 101 beds) 10 Hospital Drive, Saint Peters, MO Zip 63376–1659; tel. 636/916–9000; David Ross, President
Web address: www.bjsph.org/

BARNES–JEWISH WEST COUNTY HOSPITAL (O, 79 beds) 12634 Olive Boulevard, Saint Louis, MO Zip 63141–6337; tel. 314/996–8000; Larry Tracy, Vice President and Chief Operating Officer
Web address: www.barnesjewishwestcounty.org

BOONE HOSPITAL CENTER (L, 349 beds) 1600 East Broadway, Columbia, MO Zip 65201–5844; tel. 573/815–8000; Daniel J. Rothery, President
Web address: www.boone.org

CHRISTIAN HOSPITAL (O, 244 beds) 11133 Dunn Road, Saint Louis, MO Zip 63136–6119; tel. 314/653–5000; Ronald B. McMullen, President
Web address: www.bjc.org

MISSOURI BAPTIST HOSPITAL–SULLIVAN (O, 55 beds) 751 Sappington Bridge Road, Sullivan, MO Zip 63080–2354; tel. 573/468–4186; Tony Schwarm, President
Web address: www.missouribaptistsullivan.org

MISSOURI BAPTIST MEDICAL CENTER (O, 418 beds) 3015 North Ballas Road, Saint Louis, MO Zip 63131–2329; tel. 314/996–5000; Joan Magruder, President
Web address: www.missouribaptistmedicalcenter.org

PARKLAND HEALTH CENTER (O, 94 beds) 1101 West Liberty Street, Farmington, MO Zip 63640–1921; tel. 573/756–6451; Richard L. Conklin, President
Web address: www.parklandhealthcenter.org

PARKLAND HEALTH CENTER–BONNE TERRE (O, 3 beds) 7245 Raider Road, Bonne Terre, MO Zip 63628–3767; tel. 573/358–1400; Richard L. Conklin, President
Web address: www.parklandhealthcenter.org

PROGRESS WEST HEALTHCARE CENTER (O, 34 beds) Two Progress Point, Saint Charles, MO Zip 63368–2208; tel. 636/344–2273; John Antes, President
Web address: www.progresswesthealthcare.org

ST. LOUIS CHILDREN'S HOSPITAL (O, 250 beds) One Children's Place, Saint Louis, MO Zip 63110–1002; tel. 314/454–6000; Lee F. Fetter, President and Senior Executive Officer
Web address: www.stlouischildrens.org

Owned, leased, sponsored:	12 hospitals	3074 beds
Contract–managed:	1 hospital	22 beds
Totals:	13 hospitals	3096 beds

0377: BLACKHAWK HEALTHCARE (IO)

6836 Bee Caves Road, Suite 202, Austin, TX Zip 78746; tel. 512/617–6363; Matthew Q. Hainline, Chief Executive Officer

OKLAHOMA: MANGUM COMMUNITY HOSPITAL (O, 21 beds) One Wickersham Drive, Mangum, OK Zip 73554–9116, Mailing Address: P.O. Box 280, Zip 73554–0280; tel. 580/782–3353; Brian Roland, Chief Executive Officer
Web address: www.mangumhealth.com

TEXAS: RICHARDS MEMORIAL HOSPITAL (O, 25 beds) 1700 Brazos Street, Rockdale, TX Zip 76567–2517, Mailing Address: Drawer 1010, Zip 76567–1010; tel. 512/446–4500; Jeffrey Madison, Administrator
Web address: www.richardsmemorial.org

Owned, leased, sponsored:	2 hospitals	46 beds
Contract–managed:	0 hospitals	0 beds
Totals:	2 hospitals	46 beds

0300: BLUE MOUNTAIN HEALTH SYSTEM (NP)

211 North 12th Street, Lehighton, PA Zip 18235–1138; tel. 610/377–1300; Andrew E. Harris, Chief Executive Officer

For explanation of codes following names, see page B2.
★ Indicates Type III membership in the American Hospital Association.

Section B

PENNSYLVANIA: GNADEN HUETTEN MEMORIAL HOSPITAL (O, 182 beds) 211 North 12th Street, Lehighton, PA Zip 18235–1138; tel. 610/377–1300; Andrew E. Harris, Chief Executive Officer
Web address: www.bluemountainhealthsystem.org

PALMERTON HOSPITAL (O, 59 beds) 135 Lafayette Avenue, Palmerton, PA Zip 18071–1596; tel. 610/826–3141; Andrew E. Harris, Chief Executive Officer
Web address: www.palmertonhospital.com

Owned, leased, sponsored:	2 hospitals	241 beds
Contract-managed:	0 hospitals	0 beds
Totals:	2 hospitals	241 beds

• ★0053: BLUE WATER HEALTH SERVICES CORPORATION (NP)
1221 Pine Grove Avenue, Port Huron, MI Zip 48061–5011; tel. 810/989–3717; Thomas D. DeFauw, FACHE, President and Chief Executive Officer
(Independent Hospital System)

MICHIGAN: PORT HURON HOSPITAL (O, 186 beds) 1221 Pine Grove Avenue, Port Huron, MI Zip 48061–5011; tel. 810/987–5000; Thomas D. DeFauw, FACHE, President and Chief Executive Officer
Web address: www.porthuronhospital.org

Owned, leased, sponsored:	1 hospital	186 beds
Contract-managed:	0 hospitals	0 beds
Totals:	1 hospital	186 beds

★5085: BON SECOURS HEALTH SYSTEM, INC. (CC)
1505 Marriottsville Road, Marriottsville, MD Zip 21104–1399; tel. 410/442–5511; Richard Statuto, President and Chief Executive Officer
(Decentralized Health System)

KENTUCKY: OUR LADY OF BELLEFONTE HOSPITAL (O, 214 beds) St. Christopher Drive, Ashland, KY Zip 41101–7071, Mailing Address: P.O. Box 789, Zip 41105–0789; tel. 606/833–3333; Mark M. Gordon, Chief Executive Officer
Web address: www.olbh.com

MARYLAND: BON SECOURS BALTIMORE HEALTH SYSTEM (O, 141 beds) 2000 West Baltimore Street, Baltimore, MD Zip 21223–1597; tel. 410/362–3000; Samuel Lee Ross, M.D., Chief Executive Officer
Web address: www.bonsecours.org

NEW YORK: BON SECOURS COMMUNITY HOSPITAL (O, 187 beds) 160 East Main Street, Port Jervis, NY Zip 12771–2245, Mailing Address: P.O. Box 1014, Zip 12771–1014; tel. 845/858–7000; Leah Cerkvenik, Executive Vice President, Administrator and Chief Executive Officer
Web address: www.bonsecourscommunityhosp.org

GOOD SAMARITAN HOSPITAL (O, 308 beds) 255 Lafayette Avenue, Suffern, NY Zip 10901–4869; tel. 845/368–5000; Dominick M. Stanzione, Chief Executive Officer
Web address: www.goodsamhosp.org

ST. ANTHONY COMMUNITY HOSPITAL (O, 73 beds) 15 Maple Avenue, Warwick, NY Zip 10990–5180; tel. 845/987–5173; Thomas R. Brunelle, Executive Vice President and Administrator
Web address: www.stanthonycommunityhosp.org

SOUTH CAROLINA: BON SECOURS ST. FRANCIS HEALTH SYSTEM (O, 245 beds) One St. Francis Drive, Greenville, SC Zip 29601–3207; tel. 864/255–1000; Valinda Rutledge, Chief Executive Officer
Web address: www.stfrancishealth.org

VIRGINIA: BON SECOURS ST. FRANCIS MEDICAL CENTER (O, 130 beds) 13710 St. Francis Boulevard, Midlothian, VA Zip 23114; tel. 804/594–7300; Teresa Edwards, Executive Vice President and Administrator
Web address: www.bonsecours.com/sfmc/default.asp

BON SECOURS ST. MARY'S HOSPITAL (O, 391 beds) 5801 Bremo Road, Richmond, VA Zip 23226–1907; tel. 804/285–2011; Michael K. Kerner, Executive Vice President and Administrator
Web address: www.bonsecours.com

Bon SECOURS–DEPAUL MEDICAL CENTER (O, 238 beds) 150 Kingsley Lane, Norfolk, VA Zip 23505–4650; tel. 757/889–5000; Daniel Duggan, Executive Vice President and Administrator
Web address: www.bonsecourshamptonroads.com

BON SECOURS–RICHMOND COMMUNITY HOSPITAL (O, 101 beds) 1500 North 28th Street, Richmond, VA Zip 23223–5396, Mailing Address: P.O. Box 27184, Zip 23261–7184; tel. 804/225–1700; Michael Robinson, Executive Vice President and Administrator
Web address: www.bonsecours.com

MARY IMMACULATE HOSPITAL (O, 225 beds) 2 Bernardine Drive, Newport News, VA Zip 23602–4499; tel. 757/886–6000; Patricia L. Robertson, Executive Vice President and Administrator
Web address: www.bonsecourshamptonroads.com

MARYVIEW MEDICAL CENTER (O, 466 beds) 3636 High Street, Portsmouth, VA Zip 23707–3270; tel. 757/398–2200; Susan MacLeod, Executive Vice President
Web address: www.bonsecourshamptonroads.com

MEMORIAL REGIONAL MEDICAL CENTER (O, 225 beds) 8260 Atlee Road, Mechanicsville, VA Zip 23116–1844; tel. 804/764–6000; Michael Robinson, Executive Vice President and Administrator
Web address: www.bonsecours.com

Owned, leased, sponsored:	13 hospitals	2944 beds
Contract-managed:	0 hospitals	0 beds
Totals:	13 hospitals	2944 beds

• 2455: BRADFORD HEALTH SERVICES (IO)
2101 Magnolia Avenue South, Suite 518, Birmingham, AL Zip 35205; tel. 205/251–7753; Jerry W. Crowder, President and Chief Executive Officer

ALABAMA: BRADFORD HEALTH SERVICES AT HUNTSVILLE (O, 84 beds) 1600 Browns Ferry Road, Madison, AL Zip 35758–9769, Mailing Address: P.O. Box 176, Zip 35758–0176; tel. 256/461–7272; Bob Hinds, Executive Director
Web address: www.bradfordhealth.com

Owned, leased, sponsored:	1 hospital	84 beds
Contract-managed:	0 hospitals	0 beds
Totals:	1 hospital	84 beds

0371: BRIDGE REGIONAL HEALTH SYSTEM (IO)
29 East 29th Street, Bayonne, NJ Zip 07002; tel. 201/858–5000; Daniel A. Kane, Dr.P.h., Acting Chief Executive Officer

NEW JERSEY: BAYONNE MEDICAL CENTER (O, 206 beds) 29 East 29th Street, Bayonne, NJ Zip 07002–4699; tel. 201/858–5000; Daniel A. Kane, Dr.P.h., President and Chief Executive Officer
Web address: www.bayonnemedicalcenter.org

NEW YORK: RICHMOND UNIVERSITY MEDICAL CENTER (O, 449 beds) 355 Bard Avenue, Staten Island, NY Zip 10310–1699; tel. 718/818–1234; Richard J. Murphy, President and Chief Executive Officer
Web address: www.svcmc.org/statenisland/

Owned, leased, sponsored:	2 hospitals	655 beds
Contract-managed:	0 hospitals	0 beds
Totals:	2 hospitals	655 beds

★0585: BRIM HEALTHCARE, INC. (IO)
105 Westwood Place, Suite 300, Brentwood, TN Zip 37027; tel. 615/309–6053; Dave Woodland, President
(Decentralized Health System)

ALABAMA: LAWRENCE MEDICAL CENTER (C, 37 beds) 202 Hospital Street, Moulton, AL Zip 35650, Mailing Address: P.O. Box 39, Zip 35650–0039; tel. 256/974–2200; Thomas Dunning, Chief Executive Officer
Web address: www.attentushealthcare.com/lawrencemedicalcenter.htm

ARIZONA: COBRE VALLEY COMMUNITY HOSPITAL (C, 25 beds) 5880 South Hospital Drive, Globe, AZ Zip 85501–9454; tel. 928/425–3261; Neal Jensen, Chief Executive Officer
Web address: www.cvchospital.com

For explanation of codes following names, see page B2.
★ Indicates Type III membership in the American Hospital Association.
• Single hospital health care system

SUMMIT HEALTHCARE REGIONAL MEDICAL CENTER (C, 66 beds) 2200 East Show Low Lake Road, Show Low, AZ Zip 85901–7800; tel. 928/537–4375; Thomas D. Plantz, Chief Executive Officer
Web address: www.nrmc.org

CALIFORNIA: HAZEL HAWKINS MEMORIAL HOSPITAL (C, 113 beds) 911 Sunset Drive, Hollister, CA Zip 95023–5695; tel. 831/637–5711; Ken Underwood, Chief Executive Officer
Web address: www.hazelhawkins.com

HI–DESERT MEDICAL CENTER (C, 144 beds) 6601 White Feather Road, Joshua Tree, CA Zip 92252–6601; tel. 760/366–3711; Larry L. Meyer, Interim Chief Executive Officer
Web address: www.hdmc.org

PIONEERS MEMORIAL HEALTHCARE DISTRICT (C, 107 beds) 207 West Legion Road, Brawley, CA Zip 92227–7780; tel. 760/351–3333; Richard L. Mendoza, Chief Executive Officer
Web address: www.pmhd.org

SAN GORGONIO MEMORIAL HOSPITAL (C, 77 beds) 600 North Highland Springs Avenue, Banning, CA Zip 92220–3046; tel. 951/845–1121; Jonathan Brenn, Chief Executive Officer
Web address: www.sgmh.org

GEORGIA: EMANUEL MEDICAL HOSPITAL (C, 108 beds) 117 Kite Road, Swainsboro, GA Zip 30401–3231, Mailing Address: P.O. Box 879, Zip 30401–0879; tel. 478/237–9911; Leonard W. Daugherty, Chief Executive Officer
Web address: www.emanuelmedical.org

ROCKDALE MEDICAL CENTER (C, 154 beds) 1412 Milstead Avenue N.E., Conyers, GA Zip 30012; tel. 770/918–3000; Michael S. Potter, FACHE, Chief Executive Officer
Web address: www.rockdalemedicalcenter.org

UPSON REGIONAL MEDICAL CENTER (C, 115 beds) 801 West Gordon Street, Thomaston, GA Zip 30286–2831, Mailing Address: P.O. Box 1059, Zip 30286–1059; tel. 706/647–8111; Gene B. Wright, Chief Executive Officer
Web address: www.urmc.org

ILLINOIS: CARLINVILLE AREA HOSPITAL (C, 25 beds) 1001 East Morgan Street, Carlinville, IL Zip 62626–1499; tel. 217/854–3141; Kenneth G. Reid, President and Chief Executive Officer
Web address: www.cahcare.com

HAMMOND–HENRY HOSPITAL (C, 80 beds) 600 North College Avenue, Geneseo, IL Zip 61254–1099; tel. 309/944–4625; Bradley Solberg, FACHE, Chief Executive Officer
Web address: www.hammondhenry.com

HILLSBORO AREA HOSPITAL (C, 65 beds) 1200 East Tremont Street, Hillsboro, IL Zip 62049–1900; tel. 217/532–6111; Rex H. Brown, Chief Executive Officer
Web address: www.hillsboroareahospital.org

LOUISIANA: DE SOTO REGIONAL HEALTH SYSTEM (C, 49 beds) 207 Jefferson Street, Mansfield, LA Zip 71052–2603, Mailing Address: P.O. Box 1636, Zip 71052–2603; tel. 318/871–3100; John Domansky, Interim Chief Executive Officer
Web address: www.desotoregional.com

IBERIA MEDICAL CENTER (C, 83 beds) 2315 East Main Street, New Iberia, LA Zip 70560–4031, Mailing Address: P.O. Box 13338, Zip 70562–3338; tel. 337/364–0441; John A. Tucker, Chief Executive Officer
Web address: www.iberiamedicalcenter.com

LADY OF THE SEA GENERAL HOSPITAL (C, 25 beds) 200 West 134th Place, Cut Off, LA Zip 70345–4145; tel. 985/632–6401; Don Werner, Chief Executive Officer
Web address: www.losgh.org

MONTANA: BARRETT HOSPITAL & HEALTHCARE (C, 20 beds) 90 Highway 91 South, Dillon, MT Zip 59725–3597; tel. 406/683–3000; Steve Hannah, Chief Executive Officer
Web address: www.barretthospital.org

MINERAL COMMUNITY HOSPITAL (C, 25 beds) 1208 6th Avenue East, Superior, MT Zip 59872–9603, Mailing Address: P.O. Box 66, Zip 59872–0066; tel. 406/822–4841; Barry Kenfield, Interim Chief Executive Officer

ROUNDUP MEMORIAL HEALTHCARE (C, 48 beds) 1202 Third Street West, Roundup, MT Zip 59072–1816, Mailing Address: P.O. Box 40, Zip 59072–0040; tel. 406/323–2302; Lee Rhodes, Chief Executive Officer

NEBRASKA: TRI–VALLEY HEALTH SYSTEM (C, 51 beds) 1305 West Highway 6 and 34, Cambridge, NE Zip 69022–0488, Mailing Address: P.O. Box 488, Zip 69022–0488; tel. 308/697–3329; Carol H. Hanes, Chief Executive Officer
Web address: www.trivalleyhealth.com

NEW MEXICO: UNION COUNTY GENERAL HOSPITAL (C, 21 beds) 301 Harding Street, Clayton, NM Zip 88415–3321, Mailing Address: P.O. Box 489, Zip 88415–0489; tel. 575/374–2585; Stephen J. Campbell, Administrator
Web address: www.unioncountygeneral.com

NEW YORK: ADIRONDACK MEDICAL CENTER (C, 263 beds) 2233 State Route 86, Saranac Lake, NY Zip 12983, Mailing Address: P.O. Box 471, Zip 12983–0471; tel. 518/891–4141; Chandler M. Ralph, President and Chief Executive Officer
Web address: www.amccares.org

SCHUYLER HOSPITAL (C, 145 beds) 220 Steuben Street, Montour Falls, NY Zip 14865–9709; tel. 607/535–7121; V. Richard Stelzer, Jr., FACHE, President and Chief Executive Officer
Web address: www.schuylerhospital.org

OKLAHOMA: HOLDENVILLE GENERAL HOSPITAL (C, 25 beds) 100 McDougal Drive, Holdenville, OK Zip 74848–9700; tel. 405/379–4200; Alden M. Vandeveer, Jr., CHE, Chief Executive Officer
Web address: www.holdenvillegeneral.org

OREGON: BLUE MOUNTAIN HOSPITAL (C, 68 beds) 170 Ford Road, John Day, OR Zip 97845–2009; tel. 541/575–1311; Robert Houser, FACHE, Chief Executive Officer
Web address: www.bluemountainhospital.org

WASHINGTON: KLICKITAT VALLEY HEALTH SERVICES (C, 25 beds) 310 South Roosevelt Avenue, Goldendale, WA Zip 98620–9201; tel. 509/773–4022; John E. Rohrer, Interim Chief Executive Officer
Web address: www.kvhealth.net

SUNNYSIDE COMMUNITY HOSPITAL (C, 25 beds) 1016 Tacoma Avenue, Sunnyside, WA Zip 98944–0719, Mailing Address: P.O. Box 719, Zip 98944–0719; tel. 509/837–1500; Jon D. Smiley, Chief Executive Officer
Web address: www.sunnysidehospital.com

WISCONSIN: BURNETT MEDICAL CENTER (C, 70 beds) 257 West St. George Avenue, Grantsburg, WI Zip 54840–7827; tel. 715/463–5353; Timothy J. Wick, Chief Executive Officer
Web address: www.burnettmedicalcenter.com

COMMUNITY MEMORIAL HOSPITAL (C, 25 beds) 855 South Main Street, Oconto Falls, WI Zip 54154–1296; tel. 920/846–3444; James Van Dornick, Chief Executive Officer
Web address: www.cmhospital.org

EDGERTON HOSPITAL AND HEALTH SERVICES (C, 86 beds) 313 Stoughton Road, Edgerton, WI Zip 53534–1198; tel. 608/884–3441; James O. Pernau, Chief Executive Officer
Web address: www.edgertonhospital.com

GRANT REGIONAL HEALTH CENTER (C, 25 beds) 507 South Monroe Street, Lancaster, WI Zip 53813–2054; tel. 608/723–2143; Nicole Clapp, RN, M.S.N., FACHE, President and Chief Executive Officer
Web address: www.grantregional.com

RIPON MEDICAL CENTER (C, 23 beds) 933 Newbury Street, Ripon, WI Zip 54971–1798, Mailing Address: P.O. Box 390, Zip 54971–0390; tel. 920/748–3101; Jean Surguy, Interim Chief Executive Officer
Web address: www.riponmedicalcenter.com

SHAWANO MEDICAL CENTER (C, 25 beds) 309 North Bartlette Street, Shawano, WI Zip 54166; tel. 715/526–2111; James E. Baer, FACHE, Chief Executive Officer
Web address: www.shawanomed.org

SOUTHWEST HEALTH CENTER (C, 119 beds) 1400 Eastside Road, Platteville, WI Zip 53818–9800; tel. 608/348–2331; Anne K. Klawiter, President and Chief Executive Officer
Web address: www.southwesthealth.org

SPOONER HEALTH SYSTEM (C, 115 beds) 819 Ash Street, Spooner, WI Zip 54801–1299; tel. 715/635–2111; Michael Schafer, Chief Executive Officer and Administrator
Web address: www.spoonerhealthsystem.com

TOMAH MEMORIAL HOSPITAL (C, 25 beds) 321 Butts Avenue, Tomah, WI Zip 54660–1412; tel. 608/372–2181; Philip Stuart, Administrator and Chief Executive Officer
Web address: www.tomahhospital.org

For explanation of codes following names, see page B2.
★ Indicates Type III membership in the American Hospital Association.

Section B

WYOMING: HOT SPRINGS COUNTY MEMORIAL HOSPITAL (C, 25 beds) 150 East Arapahoe Street, Thermopolis, WY Zip 82443–2498; tel. 307/864–3121; Trudy Chittick, Chief Executive Officer
Web address: www.hscmh.org

MEMORIAL HOSPITAL OF SWEETWATER COUNTY (C, 99 beds) 1200 College Drive, Rock Springs, WY Zip 82901–5868, Mailing Address: P.O. Box 1359, Zip 82902–1359; tel. 307/362–3711; Kevin Hawk, Chief Executive Officer
Web address: www.sweetwatermedicalcenter.com

POWELL VALLEY HEALTHCARE (C, 125 beds) 777 Avenue H, Powell, WY Zip 82435–2296; tel. 307/754–2267; Rod Barton, Chief Executive Officer
Web address: www.pvhc.org

Owned, leased, sponsored:	0 hospitals	0 beds
Contract–managed:	39 hospitals	2751 beds
Totals:	39 hospitals	2751 beds

★0595: BRONSON HEALTHCARE GROUP, INC. (NP)

One Healthcare Plaza, Kalamazoo, MI Zip 49007–5345; tel. 269/341–6000; Frank J. Sardone, President and Chief Executive Officer
(Centralized Physician/Insurance Health System)

MICHIGAN: BRONSON LAKEVIEW HOSPITAL (O, 155 beds) 408 Hazen Street, Paw Paw, MI Zip 49079–0209, Mailing Address: P.O. Box 209, Zip 49079–0209; tel. 269/657–3141; Frank J. Sardone, President and Chief Executive Officer
Web address: www.bronsonhealth.com/lakeview

BRONSON METHODIST HOSPITAL (O, 356 beds) 601 John Street, Kalamazoo, MI Zip 49007–5345; tel. 269/341–6000; Frank J. Sardone, President and Chief Executive Officer
Web address: www.bronsonhealth.com

Owned, leased, sponsored:	2 hospitals	511 beds
Contract–managed:	0 hospitals	0 beds
Totals:	2 hospitals	511 beds

★3115: BROWARD HEALTH (NP)

303 S.E. 17th Street, Fort Lauderdale, FL Zip 33316–2510; tel. 954/355–5100; Frank P. Nask, President and Chief Executive Officer
(Centralized Health System)

FLORIDA: BROWARD GENERAL MEDICAL CENTER (O, 640 beds) 1600 South Andrews Avenue, Fort Lauderdale, FL Zip 33316–2510; tel. 954/355–4400; ,
Web address: www.nbhd.org

CORAL SPRINGS MEDICAL CENTER (O, 182 beds) 3000 Coral Hills Drive, Coral Springs, FL Zip 33065; tel. 954/344–3000; Patrick Maloney, Chief Executive Officer
Web address: www.browardhealth.org

IMPERIAL POINT MEDICAL CENTER (O, 180 beds) 6401 North Federal Highway, Fort Lauderdale, FL Zip 33308–1495; tel. 954/776–8500; Calvin E. Glidewell, Jr., Chief Executive Officer
Web address: www.browardhealth.org

NORTH BROWARD MEDICAL CENTER (O, 360 beds) 201 Sample Road, Deerfield Beach, FL Zip 33064–3502; tel. 954/941–8300; Pauline Grant, Chief Executive Officer
Web address: www.nbhd.org

Owned, leased, sponsored:	4 hospitals	1362 beds
Contract–managed:	0 hospitals	0 beds
Totals:	4 hospitals	1362 beds

★0400: BRYANLGH HEALTH SYSTEM (NP)

1600 South 48th Street, Lincoln, NE Zip 68506; tel. 402/489–0200; Kimberly A. Russel, President and Chief Executive Officer

NEBRASKA: BRYANLGH MEDICAL CENTER (O, 349 beds) 1600 South 48th Street, Lincoln, NE Zip 68506–1299; tel. 402/489–0200; Craig M. Ames, President and Chief Operating Officer
Web address: www.bryanlgh.org

CRETE AREA MEDICAL CENTER (O, 25 beds) 2910 Betten Drive, Crete, NE Zip 68333–0220, Mailing Address: P.O. Box 220, Zip 68333–0220; tel. 402/826–2102; Carol Friesen, Chief Executive Officer
Web address: www.creteareamedicalcenter.com

Owned, leased, sponsored:	2 hospitals	374 beds
Contract–managed:	0 hospitals	0 beds
Totals:	2 hospitals	374 beds

9655: BUREAU OF MEDICINE AND SURGERY, DEPARTMENT OF THE NAVY (FG)

2300 East Street N.W., Washington, DC Zip 20372–5300; tel. 202/762–3701; Rear Admiral Adam M. Robinson, Jr., Commanding Officer
(Independent Hospital System)

CALIFORNIA: NAVAL HOSPITAL (O, 16 beds) 937 Franklin Avenue, Lemoore, CA Zip 93246–5004; tel. 559/998–4201; Captain Stephen Mandia, Commanding Officer
Web address: www.lemoore.med.navy.mil

NAVAL HOSPITAL (O, 66 beds) Camp Pendleton, CA Mailing Address: Box 555191, Zip 92055–5191; tel. 760/725–1304; Captain Steven M. Nichols, Commanding Officer
Web address: www.cpen.med.navy.mil

NAVAL HOSPITAL (O, 29 beds) Twentynine Palms, CA Mailing Address: Box 788250, MCAGCC, Zip 92278–8250; tel. 760/830–2190; Captain Don Albia, Commanding Officer
Web address: www.nhtp.med.navy.mil/nhtp

NAVAL MEDICAL CENTER (O, 285 beds) 34800 Bob Wilson Drive, San Diego, CA Zip 92134–5000; tel. 619/532–6400; Captain Christine S. Hunter, Commander
Web address: www.nmcsd.med.navy.mil

FLORIDA: NAVAL HOSPITAL (O, 76 beds) 2080 Child Street, Jacksonville, FL Zip 32214–5000; tel. 904/542–7300; Captain Raquel Bono, Commanding Officer
Web address: www.navalhospitaljax.com

NAVAL HOSPITAL (O, 30 beds) 6000 West Highway 98, Pensacola, FL Zip 32512–0003; tel. 850/505–6413; Captain Maryalice Morro, Commanding Officer
Web address: www.psaweb.pcola.med.navy.mil

GUAM: U. S. NAVAL HOSPITAL (O, 55 beds) Agana, GU Mailing Address: PSC 490, Box 7607, FPO, APZip 96538–1600; tel. 671/344–9340; Captain Kathleen A. Rief, Commanding Officer
Web address: www.usnhguam.med.navy.mil

MARYLAND: NATIONAL NAVAL MEDICAL CENTER (O, 240 beds) 8901 Wisconsin Avenue, Bethesda, MD Zip 20889–5600; tel. 301/295–5800; Rear Admiral Richard Jeffries, Commanding Officer
Web address: www.bethesda.med.navy.mil

NORTH CAROLINA: NAVAL HOSPITAL (O, 117 beds) Camp Lejeune, NC Mailing Address: P.O. Box 10100, Zip 28547–0100; tel. 910/450–4300; Captain Mark C. Olesen, Commanding Officer
Web address: www.lej–www.med.navy.mil

SOUTH CAROLINA: NAVAL HOSPITAL (O, 20 beds) 1 Pinckney Boulevard, Beaufort, SC Zip 29902–6148; tel. 843/228–5301; Captain James Hoffower, Commanding Officer

VIRGINIA: NAVAL MEDICAL CENTER (O, 274 beds) 620 John Paul Jones Circle, Portsmouth, VA Zip 23708–2197; tel. 757/953–7424; Rear Admiral Thomas Cullison, Commander
Web address: www.www–nmcp.med.navy.mil

WASHINGTON: NAVAL HOSPITAL (O, 51 beds) One Boone Road, Bremerton, WA Zip 98312–1898; tel. 360/475–4239; Captain Catherine A. Wilson, Commanding Officer
Web address: www.nh_bremerton.med.navy.mil

NAVAL HOSPITAL (O, 29 beds) 3475 North Saratoga Street, Oak Harbor, WA Zip 98278–8800; tel. 360/257–9500; Captain Colin Chinn, Commanding Officer
Web address: www.nhoh.med.navy.mil

Owned, leased, sponsored:	13 hospitals	1288 beds
Contract–managed:	0 hospitals	0 beds
Totals:	13 hospitals	1288 beds

For explanation of codes following names, see page B2.
★ Indicates Type III membership in the American Hospital Association.

0077: CAMBRIDGE HEALTH FOUNDATION (IO)
1120 Cypress Station Drive, Houston, TX Zip 77090; tel. 281/893–7200; Deo Shanker, CPA, President
(Independent Hospital System)

TEXAS: INTRACARE MEDICAL CENTER HOSPITAL (O, 120 beds) 7601 Fannin Street, Houston, TX Zip 77054–1905; tel. 713/790–0949; Terry Scovill, Chief Executive Officer
Web address: www.intracarehospital.com

INTRACARE NORTH HOSPITAL (O, 68 beds) 1120 Cypress Station Drive, Houston, TX Zip 77090–3031; tel. 281/893–7200; Teisha York, Chief Executive Officer
Web address: www.intracare.org

Owned, leased, sponsored:	2 hospitals	188 beds
Contract-managed:	0 hospitals	0 beds
Totals:	2 hospitals	188 beds

0113: CANCER TREATMENT CENTERS OF AMERICA (IO)
1336 Basswood Road, Schaumburg, IL Zip 60173; tel. 847/342–7400; Stephen B. Bonner, President and Chief Executive Officer
(Independent Hospital System)

ILLINOIS: MIDWESTERN REGIONAL MEDICAL CENTER (O, 73 beds) 2520 Elisha Avenue, Zion, IL Zip 60099–2587; tel. 847/872–4561; Roger C. Cary, President and Chief Executive Officer
Web address: www.cancercenter.com

OKLAHOMA: SOUTHWESTERN REGIONAL MEDICAL CENTER (O, 42 beds) 10109 East 79th Street, Tulsa, OK Zip 74133; tel. 918/286–5000; Steve Mackin, President and Chief Executive Officer
Web address: www.cancercenter.com

Owned, leased, sponsored:	2 hospitals	115 beds
Contract-managed:	0 hospitals	0 beds
Totals:	2 hospitals	115 beds

★0124: CAPE COD HEALTHCARE, INC. (NP)
88 Lewis Bay Road, Hyannis, MA Zip 02601–5210; tel. 508/862–5010; Richard Salluzzo, M.D., President and Chief Executive Officer
(Centralized Health System)

MASSACHUSETTS: CAPE COD HOSPITAL (O, 268 beds) 27 Park Street, Hyannis, MA Zip 02601–5203; tel. 508/771–1800; Margaret Hanson, RN, Chief Administrative Officer
Web address: www.capecodhealth.org

FALMOUTH HOSPITAL (O, 95 beds) 100 Ter Heun Drive, Falmouth, MA Zip 02540–2599; tel. 508/548–5300; Susan M. Wing, Chief Operating Officer
Web address: www.capecodhealth.org

Owned, leased, sponsored:	2 hospitals	363 beds
Contract-managed:	0 hospitals	0 beds
Totals:	2 hospitals	363 beds

0337: CAPELLA HEALTHCARE (IO)
501 Corporate Center Drive, Suite 200, Franklin, TN Zip 37067; tel. 615/764–3000; Daniel S. Slipkovich, Chief Executive Officer
(Moderately Centralized Health System)

ALABAMA: HARTSELLE MEDICAL CENTER (O, 120 beds) 201 Pine Street N.W., Hartselle, AL Zip 35640–2309, Mailing Address: P.O. Box 969, Zip 35640–0969; tel. 256/773–6511; Jeff G. Rains, Chief Executive Officer
Web address: www.hartsellemedicalcenter.com

JACKSONVILLE MEDICAL CENTER (O, 56 beds) 1701 Pelham Road South, Jacksonville, AL Zip 36265–3399, Mailing Address: P.O. Box 999, Zip 36265–0999; tel. 256/435–4970; Roger Collins, Chief Executive Officer
Web address: www.jmchealth.com

PARKWAY MEDICAL CENTER (O, 120 beds) 1874 Beltline Road S.W., Decatur, AL Zip 35601–5509, Mailing Address: P.O. Box 2211, Zip 35609–2211; tel. 256/350–2211; Sherry J. Jones, Interim Chief Executive Officer
Web address: www.pmcrecruitment.com

WOODLAND MEDICAL CENTER (O, 70 beds) 1910 Cherokee Avenue S.W., Cullman, AL Zip 35055–5502; tel. 256/739–3500; George F. Naylor, III, FACHE, Chief Executive Officer
Web address: www.woodlandmedicalcenter.com

ARKANSAS: NATIONAL PARK MEDICAL CENTER (O, 181 beds) 1910 Malvern Avenue, Hot Springs, AR Zip 71901–7799; tel. 501/321–1000; Jerry D. Mabry, Chief Executive Officer
Web address: www.nationalparkmedical.com

SAINT MARY'S REGIONAL MEDICAL CENTER (O, 153 beds) 1808 West Main Street, Russellville, AR Zip 72801–2724; tel. 479/968–2841; Mike McCoy, Chief Executive Officer
Web address: www.saintmarysregional.com

MISSOURI: MINERAL AREA REGIONAL MEDICAL CENTER (O, 98 beds) 1212 Weber Road, Farmington, MO Zip 63640–3325; tel. 573/756–4581; Philip H. Walkley, Jr., FACHE, Chief Executive Officer
Web address: www.marmc.org

OKLAHOMA: MUSKOGEE REGIONAL MEDICAL CENTER (L, 245 beds) 300 Rockefeller Drive, Muskogee, OK Zip 74401–5081; tel. 918/682–5501; Stephen W. Mahan, Chief Executive Officer
Web address: www.muskogeehealth.com

SOUTHWESTERN MEDICAL CENTER (O, 166 beds) 5602 S.W. Lee Boulevard, Lawton, OK Zip 73505–9635, Mailing Address: P.O. Box 7290, Zip 73506–7290; tel. 580/531–4700; Jon C. O'Shaughnessy, Chief Executive Officer
Web address: www.swmconline.com

OREGON: WILLAMETTE VALLEY MEDICAL CENTER (O, 88 beds) 2700 S.E. Stratus Avenue, McMinnville, OR Zip 97128–6498; tel. 503/472–6131; Rosemari Davis, Chief Executive Officer
Web address: www.wvmcweb.com

TENNESSEE: GRANDVIEW MEDICAL CENTER (O, 68 beds) 1000 Highway 28, Jasper, TN Zip 37347–3638; tel. 423/837–9500; Daniel Aranda, Chief Executive Officer
Web address: www.grandviewhospital.com

RIVER PARK HOSPITAL (O, 125 beds) 1559 Sparta Road, McMinnville, TN Zip 37110–1399; tel. 931/815–4000; John R. McLain, Chief Executive Officer
Web address: www.riverparkhospital.com

WHITE COUNTY COMMUNITY HOSPITAL (O, 24 beds) 401 Sewell Road, Sparta, TN Zip 38583–1299; tel. 931/738–9211; Joel Taylor, Chief Executive Officer
Web address: www.whitecountyhospital.com

WASHINGTON: CAPITAL MEDICAL CENTER (O, 99 beds) 3900 Capital Mall Drive S.W., Olympia, WA Zip 98502–5026, Mailing Address: P.O. Box 19002, Zip 98507–9002; tel. 360/754–5858; Michael Motte, Chief Executive Officer
Web address: www.capitalmedical.com

Owned, leased, sponsored:	14 hospitals	1613 beds
Contract-managed:	0 hospitals	0 beds
Totals:	14 hospitals	1613 beds

0297: CAPITAL HEALTH SYSTEM (NP)
750 Brunswick Avenue, Trenton, NJ Zip 08638–4174; tel. 609/394–6000; Al Maghazehe, Chief Executive Officer
(Moderately Centralized Health System)

NEW JERSEY: CAPITAL HEALTH SYSTEM AT FULD (O, 195 beds) 750 Brunswick Avenue, Trenton, NJ Zip 08638–4174; tel. 609/394–6000; Al Maghazehe, Chief Executive Officer
Web address: www.capitalhealth.org

Section B

For explanation of codes following names, see page B2.
★ Indicates Type III membership in the American Hospital Association.

CAPITAL HEALTH SYSTEM AT MERCER (O, 235 beds) 446 Bellevue Avenue, Trenton, NJ Zip 08618–4597, Mailing Address: P.O. Box 1658, Zip 08607–1658; tel. 609/394–4000; Al Maghazehe, Chief Executive Officer
Web address: www.capitalhealth.org

Owned, leased, sponsored:	2 hospitals	430 beds
Contract–managed:	0 hospitals	0 beds
Totals:	2 hospitals	430 beds

★**0262: CARDINAL HEALTH SYSTEM** (NP)
2401 University Avenue, Muncie, IN Zip 47303; tel. 765/747–3139; Kelly N. Stanley, President and Chief Executive Officer
(Centralized Physician/Insurance Health System)

INDIANA: BALL MEMORIAL HOSPITAL (O, 356 beds) 2401 University Avenue, Muncie, IN Zip 47303–3499; tel. 765/747–3111; Brent L. Batman, President
Web address: www.accesschs.org

BLACKFORD COMMUNITY HOSPITAL (O, 15 beds) 410 Pilgrim Boulevard, Hartford City, IN Zip 47348–1897; tel. 765/348–0300; Steven J. West, Chief Executive Officer
Web address: www.blackfordcommunityhospital.org

JAY COUNTY HOSPITAL (C, 35 beds) 500 West Votaw Street, Portland, IN Zip 47371–1322; tel. 260/726–7131; Joe Johnston, Chief Executive Officer
Web address: www.jaycountyhospital.com

Owned, leased, sponsored:	2 hospitals	371 beds
Contract–managed:	1 hospital	35 beds
Totals:	3 hospitals	406 beds

0301: CARDINAL HILL HEALTHCARE SYSTEM (NP)
2050 Versailes Road, Lexington, KY Zip 40504; tel. 859/254–5701; Kerry G. Gillihan, FACHE, President and Chief Executive Officer
(Independent Hospital System)

KENTUCKY: CARDINAL HILL REHABILITATION HOSPITAL (O, 108 beds) 2050 Versailles Road, Lexington, KY Zip 40504–1499; tel. 859/254–5701; Kerry G. Gillihan, FACHE, President and Chief Executive Officer
Web address: www.cardinalhill.org

CARDINAL HILL SPECIALTY HOSPITAL (O, 32 beds) 85 North Grand Avenue, Fort Thomas, KY Zip 41075; tel. 859/572–3880; Janice Bauer, Administrator
Web address: www.iglou.com/cardinalhill/ltach.html

Owned, leased, sponsored:	2 hospitals	140 beds
Contract–managed:	0 hospitals	0 beds
Totals:	2 hospitals	140 beds

★**0099: CARE NEW ENGLAND HEALTH SYSTEM** (NP)
45 Willard Avenue, Providence, RI Zip 02905–3218; tel. 401/453–7900; John J. Hynes, President and Chief Executive Officer
(Centralized Health System)

RHODE ISLAND: BUTLER HOSPITAL (O, 117 beds) 345 Blackstone Boulevard, Providence, RI Zip 02906–4829; tel. 401/455–6200; Patricia R. Recupero, J.D., M.D., President and Chief Executive Officer
Web address: www.butler.org

KENT COUNTY MEMORIAL HOSPITAL (O, 320 beds) 455 Tollgate Road, Warwick, RI Zip 02886–2770; tel. 401/737–7000; Mark E. Crevier, President and Chief Executive Officer
Web address: www.kentri.org

WOMEN & INFANTS HOSPITAL OF RHODE ISLAND (O, 197 beds) 101 Dudley Street, Providence, RI Zip 02905–2499; tel. 401/274–1100; Constance A. Howes, President and Chief Executive Officer
Web address: www.womenandinfants.org

Owned, leased, sponsored:	3 hospitals	634 beds
Contract–managed:	0 hospitals	0 beds
Totals:	3 hospitals	634 beds

★**0070: CARILION CLINIC** (NP)
Belleview at Jefferson Street, Roanoke, VA Zip 24014, Mailing Address: P.O. Box 13727, Zip 24036–3727; tel. 540/981–7893; Edward G. Murphy, M.D., President and Chief Executive Officer
(Independent Hospital System)

VIRGINIA: BEDFORD MEMORIAL HOSPITAL (O, 161 beds) 1613 Oakwood Street, Bedford, VA Zip 24523–0688, Mailing Address: P.O. Box 688, Zip 24523–0688; tel. 540/586–2441; Georgia Watts, Interim Chief Executive Officer
Web address: www.bmhva.com

CARILION FRANKLIN MEMORIAL HOSPITAL (O, 37 beds) 180 Floyd Avenue, Rocky Mount, VA Zip 24151–1389; tel. 540/483–5277; William D. Jacobsen, Chief Executive Officer
Web address: www.carilion.com

CARILION GILES MEMORIAL HOSPITAL (O, 25 beds) 1 Taylor Avenue, Pearisburg, VA Zip 24134–1932; tel. 540/921–6000; James E. Tyler, Vice President and Administrator
Web address: www.carilion.com

CARILION MEDICAL CENTER (O, 589 beds) Belleview at Jefferson Street, Roanoke, VA Zip 24014, Mailing Address: P.O. Box 13367, Zip 24033–3367; tel. 540/981–7000; Edward G. Murphy, M.D., President and Chief Executive Officer
Web address: www.carilion.com

CARILION NEW RIVER VALLEY MEDICAL CENTER (O, 146 beds) 2900 Lamb Circle, Christiansburg, VA Zip 24073–5041, Mailing Address: P.O. Box 5, Radford, Zip 24143; tel. 540/731–2000; Don Halliwill, President and Administrator
Web address: www.carilion.com

CARILION STONEWALL JACKSON HOSPITAL (O, 25 beds) 1 Health Circle, Lexington, VA Zip 24450–2492; tel. 540/458–3300; Thomas W. McNamara, D.O., President and Chief Executive Officer
Web address: www.sjhospital.com

TAZEWELL COMMUNITY HOSPITAL (C, 34 beds) 141 Ben Bolt Avenue, Tazewell, VA Zip 24651–9700; tel. 276/988–8700; Christopher L. Wearmouth, FACHE, President and Chief Executive Officer
Web address: www.tazecommhospital.org

Owned, leased, sponsored:	6 hospitals	983 beds
Contract–managed:	1 hospital	34 beds
Totals:	7 hospitals	1017 beds

★**0141: CARITAS CHRISTI HEALTH CARE** (NP)
736 Cambridge Street, Boston, MA Zip 02135–2997; tel. 617/789–2500; Ralph de la Torre, M.D., President and Chief Executive Officer
(Moderately Centralized Health System)

MASSACHUSETTS: CARITAS CARNEY HOSPITAL (S, 133 beds) 2100 Dorchester Avenue, Dorchester, MA Zip 02124–5666; tel. 617/296–4000; Daniel H. O'Leary, M.D., President
Web address: www.carneyhospital.org

CARITAS GOOD SAMARITAN MEDICAL CENTER (S, 258 beds) 235 North Pearl Street, Brockton, MA Zip 02301–1794; tel. 508/427–3000; John J. Holiver, President
Web address: www.caritasgoodsam.org

CARITAS HOLY FAMILY HOSPITAL AND MEDICAL CENTER (S, 255 beds) 70 East Street, Methuen, MA Zip 01844–4597; tel. 978/687–0151; Thomas K. Sager, President and Chief Executive Officer
Web address: www.holyfamilyhosp.org

CARITAS NORWOOD HOSPITAL (S, 264 beds) 800 Washington Street, Norwood, MA Zip 02062–3487; tel. 781/769–4000; John B. Chessare, M.D., M.P.H., President
Web address: www.caritasnorwood.org

CARITAS ST. ELIZABETH'S MEDICAL CENTER (S, 338 beds) 736 Cambridge Street, Brighton, MA Zip 02135–2997; tel. 617/789–3000; Christopher M. O'Connor, President
Web address: www.semc.org

SAINT ANNE'S HOSPITAL (S, 108 beds) 795 Middle Street, Fall River, MA Zip 02721–1798; tel. 508/674–5741; Richard L. Cunningham, Interim Chief Executive Officer
Web address: www.saintanneshospital.org

For explanation of codes following names, see page B2.
★ Indicates Type III membership in the American Hospital Association.

Owned, leased, sponsored:	6 hospitals	1356 beds
Contract-managed:	0 hospitals	0 beds
Totals:	6 hospitals	1356 beds

★0705: CAROLINAS HEALTHCARE SYSTEM (NP)
1000 Blythe Boulevard, Charlotte, NC Zip 28203–5871, Mailing Address: P.O. Box 32861, Zip 28232–2861; tel. 704/355–2000; Michael C. Tarwater, President and Chief Executive Officer
(Moderately Centralized Health System)

NORTH CAROLINA: ANSON COMMUNITY HOSPITAL (O, 125 beds) 500 Morven Road, Wadesboro, NC Zip 28170–2745; tel. 704/694–5131; Frederick G. Thompson, Ph.D., Administrator and Chief Executive Officer
Web address: www.carolinashealthcare.org

CAROLINAS MEDICAL CENTER (O, 874 beds) 1000 Blythe Boulevard, Charlotte, NC Zip 28203–5871, Mailing Address: P.O. Box 32861, Zip 28232–2861; tel. 704/355–2000; Suzanne H. Freeman, RN, President
Web address: www.carolinasmedicalcenter.org

CAROLINAS MEDICAL CENTER–LINCOLN (O, 92 beds) 200 Gamble Drive, Lincolnton, NC Zip 28092–4421, Mailing Address: P.O. Box 677, Zip 28093–0677; tel. 704/735–3071; Peter W. Acker, President and Chief Executive Officer
Web address: www.cmc–lincoln.org

CAROLINAS MEDICAL CENTER–MERCY (O, 157 beds) 2001 Vail Avenue, Charlotte, NC Zip 28207–1289; tel. 704/304–5000; Phyllis Wingate–Jones, Administrator
Web address: www.carolinashealthcare.org

CAROLINAS MEDICAL CENTER–NORTHEAST (O, 418 beds) 920 Church Street North, Concord, NC Zip 28025–2983; tel. 704/403–3000; Mark Nantz, President and Chief Executive Officer
Web address: www.northeastmedical.org

CAROLINAS MEDICAL CENTER–PINEVILLE (O, 109 beds) 10628 Park Road, Charlotte, NC Zip 28210; tel. 704/543–2000; Christopher R. Hummer, Administrator
Web address: www.carolinashealthcare.org

CAROLINAS MEDICAL CENTER–UNION (L, 241 beds) 600 Hospital Drive, Monroe, NC Zip 28112–6000, Mailing Address: P.O. Box 5003, Zip 28111–5003; tel. 704/283–3100; Michael Lutes, President
Web address: www.cmc–union.org

CAROLINAS MEDICAL CENTER–UNIVERSITY (O, 130 beds) 8800 North Tryon Street, Charlotte, NC Zip 28262–8415, Mailing Address: P.O. Box 560727, Zip 28256–0727; tel. 704/863–6000; W. Spencer Lilly, Vice President and Administrator
Web address: www.carolinashealthcare.org

CAROLINAS REHABILITATION (O, 159 beds) 1100 Blythe Boulevard, Charlotte, NC Zip 28203–5864; tel. 704/355–4300; C. Curtis Copenhaver, Vice President and Administrator
Web address: www.carolinashealthcare.org

CLEVELAND REGIONAL MEDICAL CENTER (L, 309 beds) 201 East Grover Street, Shelby, NC Zip 28150; tel. 704/487–3000; John E. Young, President and Chief Executive Officer
Web address: www.clevelandregional.org

COLUMBUS REGIONAL HEALTHCARE SYSTEM (C, 151 beds) 500 Jefferson Street, Whiteville, NC Zip 28472–9987; tel. 910/642–8011; Henry Hawthorne, III, President and Chief Executive Officer
Web address: www.crhealthcare.org

CRAWLEY MEMORIAL HOSPITAL (C, 60 beds) 315 West College Avenue, Boiling Springs, NC Zip 28017, Mailing Address: P.O. Box 996, Zip 28017–0996; tel. 704/434–9466; Angela M. Orsky, President
Web address: www.carolinas.org

GRACE HOSPITAL (C, 269 beds) 2201 South Sterling Street, Morganton, NC Zip 28655–4058; tel. 828/580–5000; Kenneth W. Wood, President and Chief Executive Officer
Web address: www.gracehcs.org

KINGS MOUNTAIN HOSPITAL (L, 72 beds) 706 West King Street, Kings Mountain, NC Zip 28086–2708; tel. 704/739–3601; John E. Young, President and Chief Executive Officer
Web address: www.carolinas.org

VALDESE GENERAL HOSPITAL (O, 163 beds) 720 Malcolm Boulevard, Valdese, NC Zip 28690, Mailing Address: P.O. Box 700, Zip 28690–0700; tel. 828/874–2251; Kenneth W. Wood, President and Chief Executive Officer
Web address: www.blueridgehealth.org

SOUTH CAROLINA: BON SECOURS–ST. FRANCIS XAVIER HOSPITAL (C, 145 beds) 2095 Henry Tecklenburg Drive, Charleston, SC Zip 29414–0001; tel. 843/402–1000; Allen P. Carroll, Administrator
Web address: www.ropersaintfrancis.com

ROPER HOSPITAL (C, 342 beds) 316 Calhoun Street, Charleston, SC Zip 29401–1125; tel. 843/724–2000; Matthew J. Severance, Chief Executive Officer
Web address: www.ropersaintfrancis.com

WALLACE THOMSON HOSPITAL (C, 220 beds) 322 West South Street, Union, SC Zip 29379–2857, Mailing Address: P.O. Box 789, Zip 29379–0789; tel. 864/427–0351; William H. Leonard, Chief Executive Officer
Web address: www.wallacethomson.com

Owned, leased, sponsored:	12 hospitals	2849 beds
Contract-managed:	6 hospitals	1187 beds
Totals:	18 hospitals	4036 beds

★0250: CASCADE HEALTHCARE COMMUNITY (NP)
2500 N.E. Neff Road, Bend, OR Zip 97701–6015; tel. 541/382–4321; James A. Diegel, FACHE, President and Chief Executive Officer
(Centralized Physician/Insurance Health System)

OREGON: CASCADE HEALTHCARE COMMUNITY ST. CHARLES MEDICAL CENTER – BEND (O, 261 beds) 2500 N.E. Neff Road, Bend, OR Zip 97701–6015; tel. 541/382–4321; James A. Diegel, FACHE, President and Chief Executive Officer
Web address: www.scmc.org

CASCADE HEALTHCARE COMMUNITY ST. CHARLES MEDICAL CENTER – REDMOND (O, 48 beds) 1253 North Canal Boulevard, Redmond, OR Zip 97756–1395; tel. 541/548–8131; James A. Diegel, FACHE, President and Chief Executive Officer
Web address: www.cascadehealthcare.org

PIONEER MEMORIAL HOSPITAL (O, 25 beds) 1201 N.E. Elm Street, Prineville, OR Zip 97754–1206; tel. 541/447–6254; Donald J. Wee, Executive Director
Web address: www.cascadehealthcare.org

Owned, leased, sponsored:	3 hospitals	334 beds
Contract-managed:	0 hospitals	0 beds
Totals:	3 hospitals	334 beds

6545: CATHEDRAL HEALTHCARE SYSTEM, INC. (CC)
1160 Raymond Boulevard, Newark, NJ Zip 07102; tel. 973/690–3600; Father Ronald Rozniak, Interim President and Chief Executive Officer
(Independent Hospital System)

NEW JERSEY: COLUMBUS HOSPITAL (O, 206 beds) 495 North 13th Street, Newark, NJ Zip 07107–1397; tel. 973/268–1400; Patricia Fehring White, Administrator
Web address: www.cathedralhealth.org

SAINT MICHAEL'S MEDICAL CENTER (O, 223 beds) 268 Dr. Martin Luther King Jr. Boulevard, Newark, NJ Zip 07102–2094; tel. 973/877–5000; Felicia Karsos, Administrator
Web address: www.cathedralhealthcare.org

Owned, leased, sponsored:	2 hospitals	429 beds
Contract-managed:	0 hospitals	0 beds
Totals:	2 hospitals	429 beds

★0136: CATHOLIC HEALTH EAST (CC)
3805 West Chester Pike, Suite 100, Newtown Square, PA Zip 19073; tel. 610/355–2000; Robert V. Stanek, President and Chief Executive Officer
(Moderately Centralized Health System)

ALABAMA: MERCY MEDICAL (O, 156 beds) 101 Villa Drive, Daphne, AL Zip 36526–1090, Mailing Address: P.O. Box 1090, Zip 36526–1090; tel. 251/621–4200; Mary Kay Polys, President and Chief Executive Officer

Section B

For explanation of codes following names, see page B2.
★ Indicates Type III membership in the American Hospital Association.

DELAWARE: ST. FRANCIS HOSPITAL (O, 298 beds) Seventh and Clayton Streets, Wilmington, DE Zip 19805–0500, Mailing Address: P.O. Box 2500, Zip 19805–0500; tel. 302/421–4100; Clarence R. LaLiberty, Jr., President and Chief Executive Officer
Web address: www.stfrancishealthcare.org

FLORIDA: HOLY CROSS HOSPITAL (O, 436 beds) 4725 North Federal Highway, Fort Lauderdale, FL Zip 33308–4668, Mailing Address: P.O. Box 23460, Zip 33307–3460; tel. 954/771–8000; John C. Johnson, Chief Executive Officer
Web address: www.holy-cross.com

MERCY HOSPITAL (O, 357 beds) 3663 South Miami Avenue, Miami, FL Zip 33133–4237; tel. 305/854–4400; John E. Matuska, President and Chief Executive Officer
Web address: www.mercymiami.com

SOUTH FLORIDA BAPTIST HOSPITAL (S, 147 beds) 301 North Alexander Street, Plant City, FL Zip 33563–9058, Mailing Address: Drawer H, Zip 33564–9058; tel. 813/757–1200; Isaac Mallah, President and Chief Executive Officer
Web address: www.sjbhealth.org

ST. ANTHONY'S HOSPITAL (S, 370 beds) 1200 Seventh Avenue North, Saint Petersburg, FL Zip 33705–1388, Mailing Address: P.O. Box 12588, Zip 33733–2588; tel. 727/825–1100; William G. Ulbricht, President
Web address: www.stanthonys.org

ST. JOSEPH'S HOSPITAL (S, 883 beds) 3001 West Dr. Martin Luther King Jr. Boulevard, Tampa, FL Zip 33607–6387, Mailing Address: P.O. Box 4227, Zip 33677–4227; tel. 813/870–4000; Isaac Mallah, President and Chief Executive Officer
Web address: www.sjbhealth.org

GEORGIA: SAINT JOSEPH'S HOSPITAL OF ATLANTA (O, 410 beds) 5665 Peachtree Dunwoody Road N.E., Atlanta, GA Zip 30342–1764; tel. 404/851–7001; Kirk G. Wilson, President and Chief Executive Officer
Web address: www.stjosephsatlanta.org

ST. MARY'S HEALTH CARE SYSTEM (O, 188 beds) 1230 Baxter Street, Athens, GA Zip 30606–3791; tel. 706/389–3000; Thomas E. Fitz, Jr., FACHE, President and Chief Executive Officer
Web address: www.stmarysathens.com

MAINE: MERCY HOSPITAL OF PORTLAND (O, 168 beds) 144 State Street, Portland, ME Zip 04101–3795; tel. 207/879–3000; Eileen F. Skinner, FACHE, President and Chief Executive Officer
Web address: www.mercyhospital.com

MASSACHUSETTS: MERCY MEDICAL CENTER (O, 325 beds) 271 Carew Street, Springfield, MA Zip 01104–2398, Mailing Address: P.O. Box 9012, Zip 01102–9012; tel. 413/748–9000; Vincent J. McCorkle, CHE, President and Chief Executive Officer
Web address: www.mercycares.com

NEW JERSEY: LOURDES MEDICAL CENTER OF BURLINGTON COUNTY (O, 188 beds) 218–A Sunset Road, Willingboro, NJ Zip 08046–1162; tel. 609/835–2900; Eugene Johnson, Chief Administrative Officer
Web address: www.lourdesnet.org

OUR LADY OF LOURDES MEDICAL CENTER (O, 391 beds) 1600 Haddon Avenue, Camden, NJ Zip 08103–3117; tel. 856/757–3500; Mark T. Bateman, Chief Administrative Officer
Web address: www.lourdesnet.org

ST. FRANCIS MEDICAL CENTER (O, 165 beds) 601 Hamilton Avenue, Trenton, NJ Zip 08629–1986; tel. 609/599–5000; Gerard J. Jablonowski, President and Chief Executive Officer
Web address: www.stfrancismedical.org

NEW YORK: ST. JAMES MERCY HOSPITAL (O, 212 beds) 411 Canisteo Street, Hornell, NY Zip 14843–2197; tel. 607/324–8000; Mary E. LaRowe, FACHE, President and Chief Executive Officer
Web address: www.stjamesmercy.org

ST. PETER'S HOSPITAL (O, 762 beds) 315 South Manning Boulevard, Albany, NY Zip 12208–1789; tel. 518/525–1550; Steven P. Boyle, President and Chief Executive Officer
Web address: www.stpetershealthcare.org

PENNSYLVANIA: MARIAN COMMUNITY HOSPITAL (O, 80 beds) 100 Lincoln Avenue, Carbondale, PA Zip 18407–2198; tel. 570/281–1000; Mary Theresa Vautrinot, President and Chief Executive Officer
Web address: www.marianhospital.org

MERCY FITZGERALD HOSPITAL (O, 413 beds) 1500 South Lansdowe Avenue, Darby, PA Zip 19023; tel. 610/237–4000; Brian Finestein, Executive Director
Web address: www.mercyhealth.org

MERCY SUBURBAN HOSPITAL (O, 141 beds) 2701 DeKalb Pike, Norristown, PA Zip 19401–1820; tel. 610/278–2000; Lisa Mallon, Chief Executive Officer
Web address: www.mercyhealth.org

NAZARETH HOSPITAL (O, 233 beds) 2601 Holme Avenue, Philadelphia, PA Zip 19152–2096; tel. 215/335–6672; Christina Fitz–Patrick, RN, President and Chief Executive Officer
Web address: www.nazarethhospital.org

ST. AGNES CONTINUING CARE CENTER (O, 96 beds) 1900 South Broad Street, Philadelphia, PA Zip 19145–2304; tel. 215/339–4100; Mary Ann Papa, Vice President and General Manager Long Term Care Hospital
Web address: www.stagnesccc.org

ST. MARY MEDICAL CENTER (O, 294 beds) Langhorne–Newtown Road, Langhorne, PA Zip 19047–1295; tel. 215/710–2000; Gregory T. Wozniak, President and Chief Executive Officer
Web address: www.stmaryhealthcare.org

Owned, leased, sponsored:	22 hospitals	6713 beds
Contract-managed:	0 hospitals	0 beds
Totals:	22 hospitals	6713 beds

★**0092: CATHOLIC HEALTH INITIATIVES** (CC)
1999 Broadway, Suite 4000, Denver, CO Zip 80202–4004; tel. 303/298–9100; Kevin E. Lofton, President and Chief Executive Officer
(Decentralized Health System)

ARKANSAS: ST. ANTHONY'S MEDICAL CENTER (S, 35 beds) 4 Hospital Drive, Morrilton, AR Zip 72110–4510; tel. 501/977–2300; Christina Hockaday, FACHE, Chief Executive Officer
Web address: www.stanthonysmorrilton.com/

ST. VINCENT INFIRMARY MEDICAL CENTER (S, 542 beds) Two St. Vincent Circle, Little Rock, AR Zip 72205–5499; tel. 501/552–3000; Peter D. Banko, FACHE, President and Chief Executive Officer
Web address: www.stvincenthealth.com

ST. VINCENT MEDICAL CENTER–NORTH (S, 50 beds) 2215 Wildwood Avenue, Sherwood, AR Zip 72120; tel. 501/552–7100; Randall R. Cason, FACHE, Administrator and Chief Executive Officer
Web address: www.stvincenthealth.com

COLORADO: MERCY REGIONAL MEDICAL CENTER (S, 82 beds) 1010 Three Springs Boulevard, Durango, CO Zip 81301–5089; tel. 970/247–4311; Kirk Dignum, Ph.D., President and Chief Executive Officer
Web address: www.mercydurango.org

PENROSE–ST. FRANCIS HEALTH SERVICES (S, 443 beds) 2215 North Cascade Avenue, Colorado Springs, CO Zip 80907–6799, Mailing Address: P.O. Box 7021, Zip 80933–7021; tel. 719/776–5000; Philip Shaw, Interim Chief Executive Officer
Web address: www.penrosestfrancis.org

ST. ANTHONY CENTRAL HOSPITAL (S, 265 beds) 4231 West 16th Avenue, Denver, CO Zip 80204–4098; tel. 303/629–3511; Peter E. Makowski, Chief Executive Officer
Web address: www.stanthonyhosp.org

ST. ANTHONY NORTH HOSPITAL (S, 123 beds) 2551 West 84th Avenue, Westminster, CO Zip 80031; tel. 303/426–2151; James F. Dover, FACHE, Chief Executive Officer
Web address: www.stanthonynorth.org

ST. ANTHONY SUMMIT MEDICAL CENTER (S, 22 beds) 340 Peak One Drive, Frisco, CO Zip 80443, Mailing Address: P.O. Box 738, Zip 80443–0738; tel. 970/668–3300; Paul J. Chodkowski, Chief Executive Officer
Web address: www.summitmedicalcenter.org

ST. MARY–CORWIN MEDICAL CENTER (S, 254 beds) 1008 Minnequa Avenue, Pueblo, CO Zip 81004–3798; tel. 719/560–4000; Michael J. Stenger, Chief Executive Officer
Web address: www.centura.org

ST. THOMAS MORE HOSPITAL (S, 49 beds) 1338 Phay Avenue, Canon City, CO Zip 81212–2221; tel. 719/285–2000; Diane Swagger, RN, President and Chief Executive Officer
Web address: www.stmhospital.org

IDAHO: MERCY MEDICAL CENTER (S, 118 beds) 1512 12th Avenue Road, Nampa, ID Zip 83686–6008; tel. 208/463–5000; Joseph Messmer, President and Chief Executive Officer
Web address: www.mercynampa.org

For explanation of codes following names, see page B2.
★ Indicates Type III membership in the American Hospital Association.

IOWA: MERCY CAPITOL (S, 62 beds) 603 East 12th Street, Des Moines, IA Zip 50309–5515; tel. 515/643–1000; David H. Vellinga, FACHE, President and Chief Executive Officer

MERCY MEDICAL CENTER–CENTERVILLE (S, 54 beds) 1 St. Joseph's Drive, Centerville, IA Zip 52544–8055; tel. 641/437–4111; Clinton J. Christianson, President and Chief Executive Officer
Web address: www.mercycenterville.org

MERCY MEDICAL CENTER–DES MOINES (S, 584 beds) 1111 6th Avenue, Des Moines, IA Zip 50314–2611; tel. 515/247–3121; David H. Vellinga, FACHE, President and Chief Executive Officer
Web address: www.mercydesmoines.org

KANSAS: CENTRAL KANSAS MEDICAL CENTER (S, 61 beds) 3515 Broadway Street, Great Bend, KS Zip 67530–3633; tel. 620/792–2511; Sharon Lind, President and Chief Executive Officer
Web address: www.ckmc.org

ST. CATHERINE HOSPITAL (S, 101 beds) 401 East Spuce Street, Garden City, KS Zip 67846–5679; tel. 620/272–2561; Scott J. Taylor, President and Chief Executive Officer
Web address: www.stcath–hosp.org

ST. JOHN'S MAUDE NORTON MEMORIAL HOSPITAL (S, 18 beds) 220 North Pennsylvania Street, Columbus, KS Zip 66725–1110; tel. 620/429–2545; Cindy Neely, Administrator

ST. JOSEPH MEMORIAL HOSPITAL (S, 55 beds) 923 Carroll Avenue, Larned, KS Zip 67550; tel. 620/285–3161; Teri Thomas, Administrator
Web address: www.ckmc.org

KENTUCKY: CONTINUING CARE HOSPITAL (S, 30 beds) 150 North Eagle Creek Drive, 5th Floor, Lexington, KY Zip 40509; tel. 859/967–5744; Tonja Williams, President and Chief Executive Officer

FLAGET MEMORIAL HOSPITAL (S, 52 beds) 4305 New Shepherdsville Road, Bardstown, KY Zip 40004; tel. 502/350–5000; Bruce A. Klockars, CHE, President
Web address: www.flaget.com

OUR LADY OF THE WAY HOSPITAL (S, 25 beds) 11203 Main Street, Martin, KY Zip 41649–0910; tel. 606/285–6400; Kathy Stumbo, Chief Executive Officer
Web address: www.olwh.org

SAINT JOSEPH – LONDON (S, 89 beds) 310 East Ninth Street, London, KY Zip 40741–1299; tel. 606/878–6520; Virginia B. Dempsey, Chief Executive Officer
Web address: www.marymount.com

SAINT JOSEPH BEREA (S, 25 beds) 305 Estill Street, Berea, KY Zip 40403–1909; tel. 859/986–3151; Eugene A. Woods, President and Chief Executive Officer
Web address: www.bereahospital.com

SAINT JOSEPH HOSPITAL (S, 366 beds) One St. Joseph Drive, Lexington, KY Zip 40504–3754; tel. 859/278–3436; Eugene A. Woods, President and Chief Executive Officer
Web address: www.sjhlex.org

SAINT JOSEPH HOSPITAL EAST (S, 144 beds) 150 North Eagle Creek Drive, Lexington, KY Zip 40509–1807; tel. 859/268–4800; Eric Gilliam, Administrator
Web address: www.sjhlex.org

SAINT JOSEPH MOUNT STERLING (O, 56 beds) 50 Sterling Avenue, Mount Sterling, KY Zip 40353–1158, Mailing Address: P.O. Box 7, Zip 40353–0007; tel. 859/497–6000; James F. Heitzenrater, President
Web address: www.sjhlex.org

MARYLAND: ST. JOSEPH MEDICAL CENTER (S, 364 beds) 7601 Osler Drive, Towson, MD Zip 21204–7582; tel. 410/337–1000; John Kerr Tolmie, President and Chief Executive Officer
Web address: www.sjmcmd.org

MINNESOTA: ALBANY AREA HOSPITAL AND MEDICAL CENTER (S, 17 beds) 300 Third Avenue, Albany, MN Zip 56307–9363; tel. 320/845–2121; Nicholas R. Brandner, Administrator
Web address: www.albanyareahospital.com

LAKEWOOD HEALTH CENTER (S, 61 beds) 600 Main Avenue South, Baudette, MN Zip 56623–2855; tel. 218/634–2120; SharRay Feickert, President and Chief Executive Officer
Web address: www.lakewoodhealthcenter.org

ST. FRANCIS HEALTHCARE CAMPUS (S, 145 beds) 2400 St. Francis Drive, Breckenridge, MN Zip 56520–1298; tel. 218/643–3000; David A. Nelson, President and Chief Executive Officer
Web address: www.sfcare.org

ST. GABRIEL'S HOSPITAL (S, 167 beds) 815 Second Street S.E., Little Falls, MN Zip 56345–3596; tel. 320/632–5441; Carl P. Vaagenes, President and Chief Executive Officer
Web address: www.stgabriels.com

ST. JOSEPH'S AREA HEALTH SERVICES (S, 25 beds) 600 Pleasant Avenue, Park Rapids, MN Zip 56470–1432; tel. 218/732–3311; Benjamin Koppelman, President and Chief Executive Officer
Web address: www.sjahs.org

MISSOURI: ST. JOHN'S REGIONAL MEDICAL CENTER (S, 367 beds) 2727 McClelland Boulevard, Joplin, MO Zip 64804–1626; tel. 417/781–2727; George P. Caralis, President and Chief Executive Officer
Web address: www.stj.com

NEBRASKA: GOOD SAMARITAN HEALTH SYSTEMS (S, 238 beds) 10 East 31st Street, Kearney, NE Zip 68847–2926, Mailing Address: P.O. Box 1990, Zip 68848–1990; tel. 308/865–7100; John Allen, President and Chief Executive Officer
Web address: www.gshs.org

RICHARD H. YOUNG HOSPITAL (S, 67 beds) 1755 Prairie View Place, Kearney, NE Zip 68848; tel. 308/865–2000; ,
Web address: www.gshs.org

SAINT ELIZABETH REGIONAL MEDICAL CENTER (S, 257 beds) 555 South 70th Street, Lincoln, NE Zip 68510–2494; tel. 402/219–8000; Robert J. Lanik, President and Chief Executive Officer
Web address: www.saintelizabethonline.com

SAINT FRANCIS MEDICAL CENTER (S, 179 beds) 2620 West Faidley Avenue, Grand Island, NE Zip 68803–4297, Mailing Address: P.O. Box 9804, Zip 68802–9804; tel. 308/384–4600; Daniel P. McElligott, FACHE, President and Chief Executive Officer
Web address: www.saintfrancisgi.org

ST. MARY'S COMMUNITY HOSPITAL (S, 18 beds) 1314 Third Avenue, Nebraska City, NE Zip 68410–1999; tel. 402/873–3321; Daniel J. Kelly, President and Chief Executive Officer
Web address: www.stmaryshospitalnecity.org

NEW JERSEY: SAINT CLARE'S HOSPITAL (O, 607 beds) 400 West Blackwell Street, Dover, NJ Zip 7801; tel. 973/625–6000; Leslie D. Hirsch, FACHE, President and Chief Executive Officer
Web address: www.saintclares.org

NORTH DAKOTA: CARRINGTON HEALTH CENTER (S, 49 beds) 800 North Fourth Street, Carrington, ND Zip 58421–1217, Mailing Address: P.O. Box 461, Zip 58421–0461; tel. 701/652–3141; Mariann Doeling, RN, Executive Vice President
Web address: www.carringtonhealthcenter.net

LISBON AREA HEALTH SERVICES (S, 25 beds) 905 Main Street, Lisbon, ND Zip 58054–0353, Mailing Address: P.O. Box 353, Zip 58054–0353; tel. 701/683–5241; Jeffrey S. Drop, Senior Vice President and Division Executive Officer

MERCY HOSPITAL (S, 35 beds) 1031 Seventh Street N.E., Devils Lake, ND Zip 58301–2798; tel. 701/662–2131; Marlene J. Krein, President and Chief Executive Officer
Web address: www.mercyhospitaldl.com

MERCY HOSPITAL (S, 25 beds) 570 Chautauqua Boulevard, Valley City, ND Zip 58072–3199; tel. 701/845–6400; ,
Web address: www.mercyhospital.biz

MERCY MEDICAL CENTER (S, 86 beds) 1301 15th Avenue West, Williston, ND Zip 58801–3896; tel. 701/774–7400; Dennis Goebel, President and Chief Executive Officer
Web address: www.mercy–williston.org

OAKES COMMUNITY HOSPITAL (S, 20 beds) 1200 North Seventh Street, Oakes, ND Zip 58474–2502; tel. 701/742–3291; Major James Gabriel, Administrator
Web address: www.oakeshospital.com

ST. JOSEPH'S HOSPITAL AND HEALTH CENTER (S, 49 beds) 30 Seventh Street West, Dickinson, ND Zip 58601–4399; tel. 701/456–4000; Claudia Ann Eisenmann, President and Chief Executive Officer
Web address: www.stjoeshospital.org

OHIO: GOOD SAMARITAN HOSPITAL (S, 499 beds) 375 Dixmyth Avenue, Cincinnati, OH Zip 45220–2489; tel. 513/872–1400; John S. Prout, President and Chief Executive Officer
Web address: www.trihealth.com

For explanation of codes following names, see page B2.
★ Indicates Type III membership in the American Hospital Association.

Section B

GOOD SAMARITAN HOSPITAL (S, 353 beds) 2222 Philadelphia Drive, Dayton, OH Zip 45406–1813; tel. 937/278–2612; James R. Pancoast, President and Chief Executive Officer
Web address: www.goodsamdayton.com

OREGON: HOLY ROSARY MEDICAL CENTER (S, 49 beds) 351 S.W. Ninth Street, Ontario, OR Zip 97914–2693; tel. 541/881–7000; Mark F. Dalley, Administrator and Chief Executive Officer
Web address: www.holyrosary–ontario.org

MERCY MEDICAL CENTER (S, 163 beds) 2700 Stewart Parkway, Roseburg, OR Zip 97470–1297; tel. 541/673–0611; Kelly C. Morgan, President and Chief Executive Officer
Web address: www.mercyrose.org

ST. ANTHONY HOSPITAL (S, 25 beds) 1601 S.E. Court Avenue, Pendleton, OR Zip 97801–3297; tel. 541/276–5121; Theodore P. Fox, President and Chief Executive Officer
Web address: www.sahpendleton.org

ST. ELIZABETH HEALTH SERVICES (S, 75 beds) 3325 Pocahontas Road, Baker City, OR Zip 97814–1464; tel. 541/523–6461; George Winn, President and Chief Executive Officer
Web address: www.stelizabethhealth.com

PENNSYLVANIA: ST. JOSEPH MEDICAL CENTER (S, 232 beds) 2500 Bernville Road, Reading, PA Zip 19605, Mailing Address: P.O. Box 316, Zip 19603–0316; tel. 610/378–2000; John R. Morahan, President and Chief Executive Officer
Web address: www.thefutureofhealthcare.org

SOUTH DAKOTA: GETTYSBURG MEMORIAL HOSPITAL (S, 60 beds) 606 East Garfield Avenue, Gettysburg, SD Zip 57442–1398; tel. 605/765–2480; Mark Schmidt, Executive Director
Web address: www.st–marys.com

ST. MARY'S HEALTHCARE CENTER (S, 165 beds) 800 East Dakota Avenue, Pierre, SD Zip 57501–3313; tel. 605/224–3100; Chad Cooper, Chief Executive Officer
Web address: www.st–marys.com

TENNESSEE: MEMORIAL HEALTH CARE SYSTEM (S, 405 beds) 2525 De Sales Avenue, Chattanooga, TN Zip 37404–3322; tel. 423/495–8656; Debra L. Moore, Interim Chief Executive Officer
Web address: www.memorial.org

WASHINGTON: ENUMCLAW REGIONAL HOSPITAL (O, 25 beds) 1450 Battersby Avenue, Enumclaw, WA Zip 98022–0218, Mailing Address: P.O. Box 218, Zip 98022–0218; tel. 360/825–2505; Dennis Popp, Chief Operating Officer and Administrator
Web address: www.fhshealth.org

ST. CLARE HOSPITAL (S, 98 beds) 11315 Bridgeport Way S.W., Tacoma, WA Zip 98499–3004; tel. 253/588–1711; Kathy Bressler, Chief Operating Officer
Web address: www.fhshealth.org

ST. FRANCIS HOSPITAL (S, 110 beds) 34515 Ninth Avenue South, Federal Way, WA Zip 98003–6799; tel. 253/944–8100; Sister Anne McNamara, Chief Operating Officer
Web address: www.fhshealth.org

ST. JOSEPH MEDICAL CENTER (S, 305 beds) 1717 South J Street, Tacoma, WA Zip 98405–3004, Mailing Address: P.O. Box 2197, Zip 98401–2197; tel. 253/426–4101; Syd Bersante, Chief Operating Officer
Web address: www.fhshealth.org

Owned, leased, sponsored:	60 hospitals	9070 beds
Contract–managed:	0 hospitals	0 beds
Totals:	60 hospitals	9070 beds

0233: CATHOLIC HEALTH SERVICES OF LONG ISLAND (CC)

1 Huntington Quadrangle, Suite 4C04, Rockville Centre, NY Zip 11570; tel. 516/705–3700; James Harden, President and Chief Executive Officer
(Centralized Physician/Insurance Health System)

NEW YORK: GOOD SAMARITAN HOSPITAL MEDICAL CENTER (O, 531 beds) 1000 Montauk Highway, West Islip, NY Zip 11795–4958; tel. 631/376–3000; William Allison, President and Chief Executive Officer
Web address: www.good–samaritan–hospital.org

MERCY MEDICAL CENTER (O, 387 beds) 1000 North Village Avenue, Rockville Centre, NY Zip 11570–1098; tel. 516/705–2525; Alan D. Guerci, M.D., Chief Executive Officer
Web address: www.mercymedicalcenter.chsli.org

ST. CATHERINE OF SIENA MEDICAL CENTER (O, 503 beds) 50 Route 25–A, Smithtown, NY Zip 11787–1398; tel. 631/862–3000; Sharon A. Kennish, Executive Director and Administrative Officer
Web address: www.stcatherinemedicalcenter.org

ST. CHARLES HOSPITAL (O, 289 beds) 200 Belle Terre Road, Port Jefferson, NY Zip 11777–1928; tel. 631/474–6000; James O'Connor, President and Chief Executive Officer
Web address: www.stcharleshospital.chsli.org

ST. FRANCIS HOSPITAL (O, 311 beds) 100 Port Washington Boulevard, Roslyn, NY Zip 11576–1348; tel. 516/562–6000; Alan D. Guerci, M.D., Chief Executive Officer
Web address: www.stfrancisheartcenter.chsli.org

Owned, leased, sponsored:	5 hospitals	2021 beds
Contract–managed:	0 hospitals	0 beds
Totals:	5 hospitals	2021 beds

★0234: CATHOLIC HEALTH SYSTEM (CC)

2121 Main Street, Suite 300, Buffalo, NY Zip 14214; tel. 716/862–2410; Joseph D. McDonald, President and Chief Executive Officer
(Centralized Physician/Insurance Health System)

KENMORE MERCY HOSPITAL (O, 313 beds) 2950 Elmwood Avenue, Kenmore, NY Zip 14217–1390; tel. 716/447–6100; Mary Hoffman, President and Chief Executive Officer
Web address: www.chsbuffalo.org

MERCY HOSPITAL (O, 420 beds) 565 Abbott Road, Buffalo, NY Zip 14220–2095; tel. 716/826–7000; Charles J. Urlaub, President and Chief Executive Officer
Web address: www.chsbuffalo.org

SISTERS OF CHARITY HOSPITAL OF BUFFALO (O, 325 beds) 2157 Main Street, Buffalo, NY Zip 14214–2692; tel. 716/862–1000; Peter U. Bergmann, President and Chief Executive Officer
Web address: www.chsbuffalo.org

ST. JOSEPH HOSPITAL (O, 127 beds) 2605 Harlem Road, Cheektowaga, NY Zip 14225–4097; tel. 716/891–2400; James M. Millard, President and Senior Administrative Officer
Web address: www.chsbuffalo.org

Owned, leased, sponsored:	4 hospitals	1185 beds
Contract–managed:	0 hospitals	0 beds
Totals:	4 hospitals	1185 beds

★5155: CATHOLIC HEALTHCARE PARTNERS (CC)

615 Elsinore Place, Cincinnati, OH Zip 45202; tel. 513/639–2800; Michael D. Connelly, President and Chief Executive Officer
(Moderately Centralized Health System)

KENTUCKY: LOURDES HOSPITAL (O, 256 beds) 1530 Lone Oak Road, Paducah, KY Zip 42003–7900, Mailing Address: P.O. Box 7100, Zip 42002–7100; tel. 270/444–2444; Steven Grinnell, President and Chief Executive Officer
Web address: www.lourdes–pad.org

MARCUM AND WALLACE MEMORIAL HOSPITAL (O, 25 beds) 60 Mercy Court, Irvine, KY Zip 40336–1331; tel. 606/723–2115; Susan Starling, President and Chief Executive Officer
Web address: www.marcumandwallace.org

OHIO: ALLEN COMMUNITY HOSPITAL (O, 25 beds) 200 West Lorain Street, Oberlin, OH Zip 44074–1077; tel. 440/775–1211; Susan Bowers, RN, President
Web address: www.ehealthconnection.com/lorain

COMMUNITY HEALTH PARTNERS REGIONAL MEDICAL CENTER (O, 291 beds) 3700 Kolbe Road, Lorain, OH Zip 44053–1697; tel. 440/960–4000; Edwin M. Oley, President and Chief Executive Officer
Web address: www.community–health–partners.com

For explanation of codes following names, see page B2.
★ Indicates Type III membership in the American Hospital Association.

INSTITUTE FOR ORTHOPAEDIC SURGERY (O, 3 beds) 801 Medical Drive, Suite B., Lima, OH Zip 45804; tel. 419/224–7586; Mark McDonald, M.D., President
Web address: www.ioshospital.com

MERCY HOSPITAL ANDERSON (O, 160 beds) 7500 State Road, Cincinnati, OH Zip 45255–2492; tel. 513/624–4500; Patricia A. Schroer, President and Chief Executive Officer
Web address: www.e–mercy.com

MERCY HOSPITAL CLERMONT (O, 114 beds) 3000 Hospital Drive, Batavia, OH Zip 45103–1921; tel. 513/732–8200; Gayle M. Heintzelman, President and Chief Executive Officer
Web address: www.e–mercy.com

MERCY HOSPITAL FAIRFIELD (O, 207 beds) 3000 Mack Road, Fairfield, OH Zip 45014; tel. 513/870–7000; Thomas S. Urban, President and Chief Executive Officer
Web address: www.e–mercy.com

MERCY HOSPITAL MOUNT AIRY (O, 160 beds) 2446 Kipling Avenue, Cincinnati, OH Zip 45239–6650; tel. 513/853–5000; Paul C. Hiltz, President and Chief Executive Officer
Web address: www.e–mercy.com

MERCY HOSPITAL OF DEFIANCE (O, 23 beds) 1404 East Second Street, Defiance, OH Zip 43512; tel. 419/782–8444; William A. Sutton, Administrator
Web address: www.ehealthconnection.com/regions/toledo/

MERCY HOSPITAL OF TIFFIN (O, 70 beds) 45 St. Lawrence Drive, Tiffin, OH Zip 44883–0727; tel. 419/447–3130; Dale E. Thornton, M.P.H., CHE, President and Chief Executive Officer
Web address: www.mercyweb.org

MERCY HOSPITAL OF WILLARD (O, 25 beds) 110 East Howard Street, Willard, OH Zip 44890–1611; tel. 419/964–5000; Robert E. Gospodarek, President and Chief Executive Officer
Web address: www.mercyweb.org

MERCY HOSPITAL WESTERN HILLS (O, 181 beds) 3131 Queen City Avenue, Cincinnati, OH Zip 45238–2396; tel. 513/389–5000; Patrick A. Kowalski, President and Chief Executive Officer
Web address: www.e–mercy.com

MERCY MEMORIAL HOSPITAL (O, 25 beds) 904 Scioto Street, Urbana, OH Zip 43078–2200; tel. 937/653–5231; Jeanne Bowman, Administrator and Chief Nursing Officer
Web address: www.mercy–health.org

SPECIALTY HOSPITAL OF LORAIN (O, 30 beds) 205 West 20th Street, Suite 200, Amherst, OH Zip 44001; tel. 440/988–6260; Julia M. Meeks, President and Chief Executive Officer
Web address: www.specialtyhospitaloflorain.com

SPRINGFIELD REGIONAL MEDICAL CENTER – FOUNTAIN CAMPUS (O, 154 beds) 1343 North Fountain Boulevard, Springfield, OH Zip 45501–1380; tel. 937/390–5000; George N. Miller, Jr., President and Chief Executive Officer
Web address: www.mercy–health.org

SPRINGFIELD REGIONAL MEDICAL CENTER – HIGH STREET CAMPUS (O, 215 beds) 2615 East High Street, Springfield, OH Zip 45505–1422, Mailing Address: P.O. Box 1228, Zip 45501–1228; tel. 937/325–0531; George N. Miller, Jr., Regional President and Chief Executive Officer
Web address: www.communityhospital.com

ST. ANNE MERCY HOSPITAL (O, 128 beds) 3404 West Sylvania Avenue, Toledo, OH Zip 43623; tel. 419/407–2663; Richard R. Evens, President and Chief Executive Officer
Web address: www.mercyweb.org

ST. CHARLES MERCY HOSPITAL (O, 294 beds) 2600 Navarre Avenue, Oregon, OH Zip 43616–3297; tel. 419/696–7200; Carol A. Whittaker, President and Chief Executive Officer
Web address: www.mercyweb.org

ST. ELIZABETH BOARDMAN HEALTH CENTER (O, 108 beds) 8401 Market Street, Boardman, OH Zip 44512–6777; tel. 330/729–2929; Eugenia Aubel, President
Web address:
www.ehealthconnection.com/regions/youngstown/content/show_facility.asp?facility_id=190

ST. ELIZABETH HEALTH CENTER (O, 418 beds) 1044 Belmont Avenue, Youngstown, OH Zip 44504–1096, Mailing Address: P.O. Box 1790, Zip 44501–1790; tel. 330/746–7211; Robert W. Shroder, President and Chief Executive Officer
Web address: www.hmpartners.org

ST. JOSEPH HEALTH CENTER (O, 162 beds) 667 Eastland Avenue S.E., Warren, OH Zip 44484–4531; tel. 330/841–4000; Robert W. Shroder, President and Chief Executive Officer
Web address: www.hmpartners.org

ST. RITA'S MEDICAL CENTER (O, 413 beds) 730 West Market Street, Lima, OH Zip 45801–4670; tel. 419/227–3361; James P. Reber, President and Chief Executive Officer
Web address: www.stritas.org

ST. VINCENT MERCY MEDICAL CENTER (O, 462 beds) 2213 Cherry Street, Toledo, OH Zip 43608–2691; tel. 419/251–3232; Michael L. McEachern, President and Chief Executive Officer
Web address: www.mercyweb.org

PENNSYLVANIA: MERCY HOSPITAL OF SCRANTON (O, 230 beds) 746 Jefferson Avenue, Scranton, PA Zip 18501–1697; tel. 570/348–7100; John M. Starcher, Interim President and Chief Executive Officer
Web address: www.mhs–nepa.com

MERCY SPECIAL CARE HOSPITAL (O, 68 beds) 128 West Washington Street, Nanticoke, PA Zip 18634–3113; tel. 570/735–5000; Robert D. Williams, Administrator
Web address: www.mercyhealthpartners.com

TENNESSEE: BAPTIST HOSPITAL FOR WOMEN (O, 16 beds) 10820 Parkside Drive, Knoxville, TN Zip 37922–1956; tel. 865/218–7090; David E. Loving, Chief Administrative Officer
Web address: www.baptistoneword.org/women

BAPTIST HOSPITAL OF COCKE COUNTY (O, 103 beds) 435 Second Street, Newport, TN Zip 37821–3799; tel. 423/625–2200; Patricia Ketterman, RN, Interim Administrator
Web address: www.baptistoneword.org/

BAPTIST HOSPITAL OF EAST TENNESSEE (O, 212 beds) 137 Blount Avenue S.E., Knoxville, TN Zip 37920–1643, Mailing Address: P.O. Box 1788, Zip 37901–1788; tel. 865/632–5011; Jeffrey A. Ashin, Chief Executive Officer
Web address: www.baptistoneword.org

BAPTIST HOSPITAL WEST (O, 75 beds) 10820 Parkside Drive, Knoxville, TN Zip 37922–1956; tel. 865/218–7011; David E. Loving, Chief Administrative Officer
Web address: www.baptistoneword.org/west

ST. MARY'S JEFFERSON MEMORIAL HOSPITAL (L, 30 beds) 110 Hospital Drive, Jefferson City, TN Zip 37760–5281; tel. 865/471–2500; Michael C. Hicks, Administrator
Web address: www.jeffersonhealthinc.com

ST. MARY'S MEDICAL CENTER (O, 407 beds) 900 East Oak Hill Avenue, Knoxville, TN Zip 37917–4556; tel. 865/545–8000; Debra K. London, President and Chief Executive Officer
Web address: www.mercy.com

ST. MARY'S MEDICAL CENTER OF CAMPBELL COUNTY (O, 164 beds) 923 East Central Avenue, La Follette, TN Zip 37766–3106, Mailing Address: P.O. Box 1301, Zip 37766–1301; tel. 423/907–1200; H. Alan Watson, FACHE, Chief Executive Officer
Web address: www.stmaryshealth.com

ST. MARY'S MEDICAL CENTER OF SCOTT COUNTY (L, 54 beds) 18797 Alberta Avenue, Oneida, TN Zip 37841–2127, Mailing Address: P.O. Box 4939, Zip 37841–4939; tel. 423/569–8521; H. Alan Watson, FACHE, Interim Chief Executive Officer
Web address: www.stmaryshealth.com

Owned, leased, sponsored:	34 hospitals	5308 beds
Contract–managed:	0 hospitals	0 beds
Totals:	34 hospitals	5308 beds

★5205: CATHOLIC HEALTHCARE WEST (CC)
185 Berry Street, Suite 300, San Francisco, CA Zip 94107–1773; tel. 415/438–5500; Lloyd H. Dean, President and Chief Executive Officer
(Decentralized Health System)

ARIZONA: CHANDLER REGIONAL MEDICAL CENTER (O, 208 beds) 475 South Dobson Road, Chandler, AZ Zip 85224–4230; tel. 480/728–3000; David G. Covert, President
Web address: www.chandlerregional.com

For explanation of codes following names, see page B2.
★ Indicates Type III membership in the American Hospital Association.

MERCY GILBERT MEDICAL CENTER (S, 92 beds) 3555 South Val Vista Road, Gilbert, AZ Zip 85296; tel. 480/728–8000; Laurie Eberst, RN, President and Chief Executive Officer
Web address: www.mercygilbert.org

ST. JOSEPH'S HOSPITAL AND MEDICAL CENTER (S, 690 beds) 350 West Thomas Road, Phoenix, AZ Zip 85013–4496, Mailing Address: P.O. Box 2071, Zip 85001–2071; tel. 602/406–3000; Linda A. Hunt, President
Web address: www.ichosestjoes.com

CALIFORNIA: ARROYO GRANDE COMMUNITY HOSPITAL (O, 65 beds) 345 South Halcyon Road, Arroyo Grande, CA Zip 93420–3899; tel. 805/489–4261; Richard Castro, President
Web address: www.arroyograndehospital.org

BAKERSFIELD MEMORIAL HOSPITAL (O, 339 beds) 420 34th Street, Bakersfield, CA Zip 93301–2237, Mailing Address: P.O. Box 1888, Zip 93303–1888; tel. 661/327–1792; Jon Van Boening, President
Web address: www.chw.edu

CALIFORNIA HOSPITAL MEDICAL CENTER (O, 316 beds) 1401 South Grand Avenue, Los Angeles, CA Zip 90015–3010; tel. 213/748–2411; Mark A. Meyers, President
Web address: www.chmcla.org

COMMMUNITY HOSPITAL OF SAN BERNARDINO (O, 292 beds) 1805 Medical Center Drive, San Bernardino, CA Zip 92411–1214; tel. 909/887–6333; Diane Nitta, Administrator
Web address: www.chsb.org

DOMINICAN HOSPITAL (S, 281 beds) 1555 Soquel Drive, Santa Cruz, CA Zip 95065–1794; tel. 831/462–7700; Nanette Mickiewicz, M.D., President and Chief Medical Officer
Web address: www.dominicanhospital.org

FRENCH HOSPITAL MEDICAL CENTER (O, 112 beds) 1911 Johnson Avenue, San Luis Obispo, CA Zip 93401–4131; tel. 805/543–5353; Alan Iftiniuk, President
Web address: www.frenchmedicalcenter.org

GLENDALE MEMORIAL HOSPITAL AND HEALTH CENTER (O, 334 beds) 1420 South Central Avenue, Glendale, CA Zip 91204–2594; tel. 818/502–1900; Catherine M. Pelley, President
Web address: www.glendalememorial.com

MARIAN MEDICAL CENTER (S, 262 beds) 1400 East Church Street, Santa Maria, CA Zip 93454–5906; tel. 805/739–3000; Charles J. Cova, President
Web address: www.marianmedicalcenter.org

MARK TWAIN ST. JOSEPH'S HOSPITAL (O, 26 beds) 768 Mountain Ranch Road, San Andreas, CA Zip 95249–9707; tel. 209/754–3521; Feliciano Jiron, President
Web address: www.marktwainhospital.com

MERCY GENERAL HOSPITAL (S, 342 beds) 4001 J Street, Sacramento, CA Zip 95819–3600; tel. 916/453–4545; Denny W. Powell, President
Web address: www.mercygeneral.org

MERCY HOSPITAL (S, 269 beds) 2215 Truxtun Avenue, Bakersfield, CA Zip 93301–3698, Mailing Address: P.O. Box 119, Zip 93302–0119; tel. 661/632–5000; Russell V. Judd, President
Web address: www.mercybakersfield.org

MERCY HOSPITAL OF FOLSOM (S, 85 beds) 1650 Creekside Drive, Folsom, CA Zip 95630–3405; tel. 916/983–7400; Donald C. Hudson, President
Web address: www.mercyfolsom.org

MERCY MEDICAL CENTER MERCED (S, 160 beds) 301 East 13th Street, Merced, CA Zip 95340–6211; tel. 209/385–7000; David S. Dunham, President
Web address: www.mercymercedcares.org

MERCY MEDICAL CENTER MOUNT SHASTA (S, 80 beds) 914 Pine Street, Mount Shasta, CA Zip 96067–2143; tel. 530/926–6111; Chuck Gersdorf, President
Web address: www.mercy.org

MERCY MEDICAL CENTER REDDING (S, 250 beds) 2175 Rosaline Avenue, Redding, CA Zip 96001–2509, Mailing Address: P.O. Box 496009, Zip 96049–6009; tel. 530/225–6000; Richard J. Barnett, President
Web address: www.mercy.org

MERCY SAN JUAN MEDICAL CENTER (S, 260 beds) 6501 Coyle Avenue, Carmichael, CA Zip 95608–0306, Mailing Address: P.O. Box 479, Zip 95608–0479; tel. 916/537–5000; Brian K. Ivie, President
Web address: www.mercysanjuan.org

METHODIST HOSPITAL OF SACRAMENTO (O, 326 beds) 7500 Hospital Drive, Sacramento, CA Zip 95823–5477; tel. 916/423–3000; Timothy M. Moran, President
Web address: www.methodistsacramento.org

NORTHRIDGE HOSPITAL MEDICAL CENTER–ROSCOE BOULEVARD CAMPUS (O, 371 beds) 18300 Roscoe Boulevard, Northridge, CA Zip 91328–4167; tel. 818/885–8500; Michael L. Wall, President
Web address: www.northridgehospital.org

OAK VALLEY HOSPITAL DISTRICT (O, 150 beds) 350 South Oak Street, Oakdale, CA Zip 95361–3519; tel. 209/847–3011; John P. Friel, President and Chief Executive Officer
Web address: www.oakvalleycares.org

SAINT FRANCIS MEMORIAL HOSPITAL (O, 210 beds) 900 Hyde Street, San Francisco, CA Zip 94109–4899, Mailing Address: P.O. Box 7726, Zip 94120–7726; tel. 415/353–6000; Thomas G. Hennessy, President
Web address: www.saintfrancismemorial.org

SEQUOIA HOSPITAL (O, 205 beds) 170 Alameda De Las Pulgas, Redwood City, CA Zip 94062–2799; tel. 650/369–5811; Glenna L. Vaskelis, President and Administrator
Web address: www.sequoiahospital.org

SIERRA NEVADA MEMORIAL HOSPITAL (O, 121 beds) 155 Glasson Way, Grass Valley, CA Zip 95945–5723, Mailing Address: P.O. Box 1029, Zip 95945–1029; tel. 530/274–6000; Katherine Medeiros, President and Chief Executive Officer
Web address: www.snmh.org

ST. BERNARDINE MEDICAL CENTER (S, 250 beds) 2101 North Waterman Avenue, San Bernardino, CA Zip 92404–4836; tel. 909/883–8711; Steven R. Barron, President
Web address: www.stbernardinemedicalcenter.com

ST. ELIZABETH COMMUNITY HOSPITAL (S, 65 beds) 2550 Sister Mary Columba Drive, Red Bluff, CA Zip 96080–4397; tel. 530/529–8000; Jon W. Halfhide, President
Web address: www.mercy.org

ST. JOHN'S PLEASANT VALLEY HOSPITAL (S, 171 beds) 2309 Antonio Avenue, Camarillo, CA Zip 93010–1414; tel. 805/389–5800; Gerard Conway, President
Web address: www.catholichealthcarewest.org

ST. JOHN'S REGIONAL MEDICAL CENTER (S, 230 beds) 1600 North Rose Avenue, Oxnard, CA Zip 93030–3723; tel. 805/988–2500; T. Michael Murray, President
Web address: www.chw.edu

ST. JOSEPH'S BEHAVIORAL HEALTH CENTER (S, 35 beds) 2510 North California Street, Stockton, CA Zip 95204–5502; tel. 209/461–2000; Paul Rains, President
Web address: www.stjosephscanhelp.org

ST. JOSEPH'S MEDICAL CENTER (S, 294 beds) 1800 North California Street, Stockton, CA Zip 95204–6019, Mailing Address: P.O. Box 213008, Zip 95213–3008; tel. 209/943–2000; Donald J. Wiley, President
Web address: www.stjosephsCARES.org

ST. MARY MEDICAL CENTER (S, 287 beds) 1050 Linden Avenue, Long Beach, CA Zip 90813, Mailing Address: P.O. Box 887, Zip 90813–0887; tel. 562/491–9000; Christopher DiCicco, President
Web address: www.stmarymedicalcenter.org

ST. MARY'S MEDICAL CENTER (S, 232 beds) 450 Stanyan Street, San Francisco, CA Zip 94117–1079; tel. 415/668–1000; Anna Cheung, Interim President
Web address: www.stmarysmedicalcenter.com

WOODLAND HEALTHCARE (O, 111 beds) 1325 Cottonwood Street, Woodland, CA Zip 95695–5199; tel. 530/662–3961; H. Kevin Vaziri, President
Web address: www.woodlandhealthcare.org

NEVADA: SAINT MARY'S REGIONAL MEDICAL CENTER (O, 269 beds) 235 West Sixth Street, Reno, NV Zip 89503; tel. 775/770–3000; Michael J. Uboldi, President
Web address: www.saintmarysreno.com

ST. ROSE DOMINCIAN HOSPITALS – SAN MARTIN CAMPUS (O, 147 beds) 8280 West Warm Springs Road, Las Vegas, NV Zip 89113; tel. 702/492–8000; Victoria J. VanMeetren, President
Web address: www.strosehospitals.org

ST. ROSE DOMINICAN HOSPITALS – ROSE DE LIMA CAMPUS (S, 145 beds) 102 East Lake Mead Parkway, Henderson, NV Zip 89015–5524; tel. 702/616–5000; Renato V. Baciarelli, President
Web address: www.strosecares.com

ST. ROSE DOMINICAN HOSPITALS – SIENA CAMPUS (S, 245 beds) 3001 St. Rose Parkway, Henderson, NV Zip 89052; tel. 702/616–5000; Rod A. Davis, President and Chief Executive Officer
Web address: www.strosehospitals.com

For explanation of codes following names, see page B2.
★ Indicates Type III membership in the American Hospital Association.

Owned, leased, sponsored:	38 hospitals	8327 beds
Contract-managed:	0 hospitals	0 beds
Totals:	38 hospitals	8327 beds

★0298: CENTEGRA HEALTH SYSTEM (NP)
385 Millennium Drive, Crystal Lake, IL Zip 60012; tel. 815/788-5825; Michael S. Eesley, President and Chief Executive Officer
(Centralized Health System)

ILLINOIS: CENTEGRA MEMORIAL MEDICAL CENTER (O, 145 beds) 3701 Doty Road, Woodstock, IL Zip 60098-3797, Mailing Address: P.O. Box 1990, Zip 60098-1990; tel. 815/338-2500; Michael S. Eesley, President and Chief Executive Officer
Web address: www.centegra.org

CENTEGRA NORTHERN ILLINOIS MEDICAL CENTER (O, 156 beds) 4201 Medical Center Drive, McHenry, IL Zip 60050-9506; tel. 815/344-5000; Michael S. Eesley, President and Chief Executive Officer
Web address: www.centegra.org

Owned, leased, sponsored:	2 hospitals	301 beds
Contract-managed:	0 hospitals	0 beds
Totals:	2 hospitals	301 beds

★0184: CENTRACARE HEALTH SYSTEM (NP)
1406 Sixth Avenue North, Saint Cloud, MN Zip 56303; tel. 320/251-2700; Terence Pladson, M.D., President and Chief Executive Officer
(Moderately Centralized Health System)

MINNESOTA: LONG PRAIRIE MEMORIAL HOSPITAL AND HOME (O, 122 beds) 20 Ninth Street S.E., Long Prairie, MN Zip 56347-1404; tel. 320/732-2141; Roger B. Oberg, Administrator
Web address: www.centracare.com

MELROSE AREA HOSPITAL – CENTRACARE (L, 93 beds) 11 North Fifth Avenue West, Melrose, MN Zip 56352-1098; tel. 320/256-4231; Joan D. Jackson, Chief Executive Officer
Web address: www.centracare.com

ST. CLOUD HOSPITAL (O, 447 beds) 1406 Sixth Avenue North, Saint Cloud, MN Zip 56303-1901; tel. 320/251-2700; Craig J. Broman, President
Web address: www.centracare.com

Owned, leased, sponsored:	3 hospitals	662 beds
Contract-managed:	0 hospitals	0 beds
Totals:	3 hospitals	662 beds

★0955: CHARLESTON AREA MEDICAL CENTER HEALTH SYSTEM, INC. (NP)
501 Morris Street, Charleston, WV Zip 25301-1300, Mailing Address: P.O. Box 1547, Zip 25326-1547; tel. 304/388-5432; David L. Ramsey, President and Chief Executive Officer
(Independent Hospital System)

WEST VIRGINIA: CHARLESTON AREA MEDICAL CENTER (O, 776 beds) 501 Morris Street, Charleston, WV Zip 25301-1300, Mailing Address: P.O. Box 1547, Zip 25326-1547; tel. 304/388-5432; David L. Ramsey, President and Chief Executive Officer
Web address: www.camc.org

TEAYS VALLEY HOSPITAL (O, 53 beds) 1400 Hospital Drive, Hurricane, WV Zip 25526-9210; tel. 304/757-1700; Albert H. Michaels, Chief Executive Officer
Web address: www.camc.org

Owned, leased, sponsored:	2 hospitals	829 beds
Contract-managed:	0 hospitals	0 beds
Totals:	2 hospitals	829 beds

0331: CHILDREN'S HOSPITALS AND CLINICS OF MINNESOTA (NP)
2525 Chicago Avenue South, Minneapolis, MN Zip 55404; tel. 612/813-6100; Alan L. Goldbloom, M.D., President and Chief Executive Officer
(Independent Hospital System)

MINNESOTA: CHILDREN'S HOSPITALS AND CLINICS OF MINNESOTA (O, 193 beds) 2525 Chicago Avenue South, Minneapolis, MN Zip 55404-9976; tel. 612/813-6100; Alan L. Goldbloom, M.D., President and Chief Executive Officer
Web address: www.childrenshc.org

CHILDREN'S HOSPITALS AND CLINICS OF MINNESOTA (O, 133 beds) 345 North Smith Avenue, Saint Paul, MN Zip 55102-2392; tel. 651/220-6000; Alan L. Goldbloom, M.D., President and Chief Executive Officer
Web address: www.childrensmn.org

Owned, leased, sponsored:	2 hospitals	326 beds
Contract-managed:	0 hospitals	0 beds
Totals:	2 hospitals	326 beds

● ★0131: CHRISTIANA CARE HEALTH SYSTEM (NP)
501 West 14th Street, Wilmington, DE Zip 19801, Mailing Address: P.O. Box 1668, Zip 19899; tel. 302/733-1000; Robert J. Laskowski, M.D., President and Chief Executive Officer
(Independent Hospital System)

DELAWARE: CHRISTIANA CARE HEALTH SYSTEM (O, 1011 beds) 501 West 14th Street, Wilmington, DE Zip 19801; tel. 302/428-2570; Robert J. Laskowski, M.D., President and Chief Executive Officer
Web address: www.christianacare.org

Owned, leased, sponsored:	1 hospital	1011 beds
Contract-managed:	0 hospitals	0 beds
Totals:	1 hospital	1011 beds

★0192: CHRISTUS HEALTH (CC)
6363 North Highway 161, Suite 450, Irving, TX Zip 75038; tel. 877/980-0100; Thomas C. Royer, M.D., President and Chief Executive Officer
(Decentralized Health System)

ARKANSAS: MAGNOLIA HOSPITAL (C, 70 beds) 101 Hospital Drive, Magnolia, AR Zip 71753-2416, Mailing Address: P.O. Box 629, Zip 71753-0629; tel. 870/235-3000; Terry L. Amstutz, FACHE, Chief Executive Officer
Web address: www.magnoliahospital.org

LOUISIANA: CHRISTUS COUSHATTA HEALTH CARE CENTER (O, 25 beds) 1635 Marvel Street, Coushatta, LA Zip 71019-9022, Mailing Address: P.O. Box 589, Zip 71019-0589; tel. 318/932-2000; Karen Mixon, RN, Administrator
Web address: www.christuscoushatta.org

CHRISTUS SCHUMPERT HEALTH SYSTEM (O, 488 beds) One St. Mary Place, Shreveport, LA Zip 71101-4399; tel. 318/681-4500; Charles J. Paine, M.D., President and Chief Executive Officer
Web address: www.christusschumpert.org

CHRISTUS ST. FRANCES CABRINI HOSPITAL (O, 246 beds) 3330 Masonic Drive, Alexandria, LA Zip 71301-3899; tel. 318/487-1122; Stephen F. Wright, President and Chief Executive Officer
Web address: www.christushealth.org/sfcabrini

CHRISTUS ST. PATRICK HOSPITAL OF LAKE CHARLES (O, 288 beds) 524 South Ryan Street, Lake Charles, LA Zip 70601-5799, Mailing Address: P.O. Box 3401, Zip 70602-3401; tel. 337/436-2511; Ellen M. Jones, President and Chief Executive Officer
Web address: www.stpatrickhospital.org

NATCHITOCHES REGIONAL MEDICAL CENTER (C, 211 beds) 501 Keyser Avenue, Natchitoches, LA Zip 71457-6036, Mailing Address: P.O. Box 2009, Zip 71457-2009; tel. 318/214-4200; Mark E. Marley, CHE, Chief Executive Officer
Web address: www.natchitocheshospital.org

TEXAS: CHRISTUS HOSPITAL–ST. ELIZABETH (O, 610 beds) 2830 Calder Avenue, Beaumont, TX Zip 77702-1809, Mailing Address: P.O. Box 5405, Zip 77726-5405; tel. 409/892-7171; Ellen M. Jones, President and Chief Executive Officer
Web address: www.christushospital.org

Section B

For explanation of codes following names, see page B2.
★ Indicates Type III membership in the American Hospital Association.
● Single hospital health care system

CHRISTUS HOSPITAL–ST. MARY (O, 202 beds) 3600 Gates Boulevard, Port Arthur, TX Zip 77642–3601, Mailing Address: P.O. Box 3696, Zip 77643–3696; tel. 409/985–7431; Wayne Moore, Administrator
Web address: www.christushospital.org

CHRISTUS JASPER MEMORIAL HOSPITAL (L, 50 beds) 1275 Marvin Hancock Drive, Jasper, TX Zip 75951–4995; tel. 409/384–5461; Deborah Wiegand, RN, Chief Executive Officer
Web address: www.christusjasper.org

CHRISTUS SANTA ROSA CHILDREN'S HOSPITAL (O, 196 beds) 333 North Santa Rosa Street, San Antonio, TX Zip 78207; tel. 210/704–2011; Richard Wayne, M.D., Vice President and Administrator
Web address: www.christussantarosa.org

CHRISTUS SANTA ROSA HEALTH CARE (O, 380 beds) 333 North Santa Rosa Street, San Antonio, TX Zip 78207–3108; tel. 210/704–2011; Don A. Beeler, President and Chief Executive Officer
Web address: www.christussantarosa.org

CHRISTUS SANTA ROSA HOSPITAL – NEW BRAUNFELS (O, 132 beds) 600 North Union Avenue, New Braunfels, TX Zip 78130–4191; tel. 830/606–9111; Michael V. Williamson, FACHE, Interim Chief Executive Officer
Web address: www.mckenna.org

CHRISTUS SPOHN HOSPITAL ALICE (O, 152 beds) 2500 East Main Street, Alice, TX Zip 78332–4794; tel. 361/661–8000; Mark Casanova, Chief Operating Officer
Web address: www.christusspohn.org/locations_alice.htm

CHRISTUS SPOHN HOSPITAL BEEVILLE (L, 63 beds) 1500 East Houston Street, Beeville, TX Zip 78102–5312; tel. 361/354–2000; Jerry Rodriguez, Vice President and Chief Operating Officer
Web address: www.christusspohn.org

CHRISTUS SPOHN HOSPITAL CORPUS CHRISTI MEMORIAL (O, 809 beds) 2606 Hospital Boulevard, Corpus Christi, TX Zip 78405–1818, Mailing Address: P.O. Box 5280, Zip 78465–5280; tel. 361/902–4000; Estela Chapa, FACHE, Vice President and Chief Operating Officer
Web address: www.christusspohn.org

CHRISTUS SPOHN HOSPITAL KLEBERG (O, 100 beds) 1311 General Cavazos Boulevard, Kingsville, TX Zip 78363–1197; tel. 361/595–1661; Stephen Pautler, FACHE, Administrator
Web address: www.christuspohn.org

CHRISTUS ST. CATHERINE HOSPITAL (O, 102 beds) 701 Fry Road, Katy, TX Zip 77450; tel. 281/599–5700; Jack H. McCabe, FACHE, Chief Executive Officer
Web address: www.christusstcatherine.org

CHRISTUS ST. JOHN HOSPITAL (O, 134 beds) 18300 St. John Drive, Nassau Bay, TX Zip 77058–6302; tel. 281/333–5503; Thomas Permetti, Chief Executive Officer
Web address: www.christusstjohn.org

CHRISTUS ST. MICHAEL HEALTH SYSTEM (O, 312 beds) 2600 St. Michael Drive, Texarkana, TX Zip 75503–2372; tel. 903/614–1000; Chris Karam, President and Chief Executive Officer
Web address: www.christusstmichael.org

CHRISTUS ST. MICHAEL REHABILITATION HOSPITAL (O, 50 beds) 2400 St. Michael Drive, Texarkana, TX Zip 75503; tel. 903/614–4000; Aloma Gender, RN, M.S.N., Administrator and Director Nursing
Web address: www.christusstmichael.org

RICE MEDICAL CENTER (C, 25 beds) 600 South Austin Road, Eagle Lake, TX Zip 77434–3298, Mailing Address: P.O. Box 277, Zip 77434–0277; tel. 979/234–5571; Susan Hernandez, RN, Interim Administrator
Web address: www.ricemedicalcenter.org

Owned, leased, sponsored:	18 hospitals	4339 beds
Contract-managed:	3 hospitals	306 beds
Totals:	21 hospitals	4645 beds

0350: CIRRUS HEALTH (IO)

9301 North Central Expressway, Suite 360, Dallas, TX Zip 75231, Mailing Address: 9301 North Central Expressway, Suite360, Zip 75231; tel. 214/217–0100; Timothy Parris, President and Chief Executive Officer
(Independent Hospital System)

BAYLOR MEDICAL CENTER AT TROPHY CLUB (O, 14 beds) 2850 South Highway,114E, Trophy Club, TX Zip 76262; tel. 817/837–4600; Lynn Warren, Chief Executive Officer
Web address: www.tc–mc.com

NORTH TEXAS HOSPITAL (O, 16 beds) 2801 South Mayhill Road, Denton, TX Zip 76208; tel. 940/220–0600; Randy B. Bacus, FACHE, Chief Executive Officer and Administrator
Web address: www.northtexashospital.com

Owned, leased, sponsored:	2 hospitals	30 beds
Contract-managed:	0 hospitals	0 beds
Totals:	2 hospitals	30 beds

0101: CITRUS VALLEY HEALTH PARTNERS (NP)

210 West San Bernardino Road, Covina, CA Zip 91723; tel. 626/331–7331; James T. Yoshioka, President and Chief Executive Officer
(Independent Hospital System)

CALIFORNIA: CITRUS VALLEY MEDICAL CENTER–INTER–COMMUNITY CAMPUS (O, 252 beds) 210 West San Bernardino Road, Covina, CA Zip 91723–1901, Mailing Address: P.O. Box 6108, Zip 91722–5108; tel. 626/331–7331; James T. Yoshioka, President and Chief Executive Officer
Web address: www.cvhp.org

CITRUS VALLEY MEDICAL CENTER–QUEEN OF THE VALLEY CAMPUS (O, 263 beds) 1115 South Sunset Avenue, West Covina, CA Zip 91790–3940, Mailing Address: P.O. Box 1980, Zip 91793–1980; tel. 626/962–4011; James T. Yoshioka, President and Chief Executive Officer
Web address: www.cvhp.org

FOOTHILL PRESBYTERIAN HOSPITAL–MORRIS L. JOHNSTON MEMORIAL (O, 106 beds) 250 South Grand Avenue, Glendora, CA Zip 91741–4218; tel. 626/963–8411; Larry S. Fetters, Administrator
Web address: www.cvhp.org

Owned, leased, sponsored:	3 hospitals	621 beds
Contract-managed:	0 hospitals	0 beds
Totals:	3 hospitals	621 beds

★0231: CLARIAN HEALTH (NP)

I–65 at 21st Street, Indianapolis, IN Zip 46202–5250, Mailing Address: P.O. Box 1367, Zip 46206–1367; tel. 317/962–5900; Daniel F. Evans, Jr., President and Chief Executive Officer
(Centralized Physician/Insurance Health System)

INDIANA: BEDFORD REGIONAL MEDICAL CENTER (O, 25 beds) 2900 West 16th Street, Bedford, IN Zip 47421–3583; tel. 812/275–1200; Bradford W. Dykes, President and Chief Executive Officer
Web address: www.brmchealthcare.com

CLARIAN HEALTH PARTNERS (O, 1380 beds) I–65 at 21st Street, Indianapolis, IN Zip 46202–5250, Mailing Address: P.O. Box 1367, Zip 46206–1367; tel. 317/962–2000; Daniel F. Evans, Jr., President and Chief Executive Officer
Web address: www.clarian.org

CLARIAN NORTH MEDICAL CENTER (O, 154 beds) 11700 North Meridian Avenue, Carmel, IN Zip 46032; tel. 317/688–2000; Jonathan R. Goble, President and Chief Executive Officer
Web address: www.clariannorth.com

CLARIAN WEST MEDICAL CENTER (O, 86 beds) 1111 North Ronald Reagan Parkway, Avon, IN Zip 46123; tel. 317/217–3000; Alfonso W. Gatmaitan, Chief Executive Officer
Web address: www.clarian.org

GOSHEN GENERAL HOSPITAL (O, 123 beds) 200 High Park Avenue, Goshen, IN Zip 46526–4899, Mailing Address: P.O. Box 139, Zip 46527–0139; tel. 574/533–2141; James O. Dague, President and Chief Executive Officer
Web address: www.goshenhealth.org

LA PORTE REGIONAL HEALTH SYSTEM (O, 227 beds) 1007 Lincolnway, La Porte, IN Zip 46350–3201, Mailing Address: P.O. Box 250, Zip 46352–0250; tel. 219/326–1234; Michael E. Haley, President and Chief Executive Officer
Web address: www.laportehealth.org

For explanation of codes following names, see page B2.
★ Indicates Type III membership in the American Hospital Association.

Section B

TIPTON HOSPITAL (C, 25 beds) 1000 South Main Street, Tipton, IN Zip 46072–9799; tel. 765/675–8500; Michael Harlowe, President and Chief Executive Officer
Web address: www.tiptonhospital.org

Owned, leased, sponsored:	6 hospitals	1995 beds
Contract-managed:	1 hospital	25 beds
Totals:	7 hospitals	2020 beds

0212: CLEVELAND CLINIC HEALTH SYSTEM (NP)
9500 Euclid, Cleveland, OH Zip 44195–5108; tel. 216/444–2200; Delos Cosgrove, M.D., President and Chief Executive Officer
(Centralized Health System)

FLORIDA: CLEVELAND CLINIC FLORIDA (O, 150 beds) 3100 Weston Road, Weston, FL Zip 33331–3602; tel. 954/689–5000; Bernardo Fernandez, M.D., Chief Executive Officer
Web address: www.clevelandclinic.org/florida

OHIO: CLEVELAND CLINIC CHILDREN'S HOSPITAL FOR REHABILITATION (O, 25 beds) Cleveland, OH Mailing Address: 2801 Martin Luther King Jr. Drive, Zip 44104–3865; tel. 216/721–5400; David Kenagny, M.D., Medical Director
Web address: www.clevelandclinic.org/childrenshospital

CLEVELAND CLINIC FOUNDATION (O, 1080 beds) 9500 Euclid Avenue, Cleveland, OH Zip 44195–5108; tel. 216/444–2200; Delos Cosgrove, M.D., President and Chief Executive Officer
Web address: www.clevelandclinic.org

EUCLID HOSPITAL (O, 190 beds) 18901 Lake Shore Boulevard, Euclid, OH Zip 44119–1090; tel. 216/531–9000; Robert Stall, President
Web address: www.euclidhospital.org

FAIRVIEW HOSPITAL (O, 410 beds) 18101 Lorain Avenue, Cleveland, OH Zip 44111–5656; tel. 216/476–7000; Fred M. DeGrandis, Chief Executive Officer
Web address: www.fairviewhospital.org

HILLCREST HOSPITAL (O, 361 beds) 6780 Mayfield Road, Cleveland, OH Zip 44124–2202; tel. 440/449–4500; Jeffrey A. Leimgruber, President
Web address: www.hillcresthospital.org

HURON HOSPITAL (O, 197 beds) 13951 Terrace Road, Cleveland, OH Zip 44112–4399; tel. 216/761–3300; A. Gus Kious, M.D., Chief Administrative Officer
Web address: www.meridia.org

LAKEWOOD HOSPITAL (O, 271 beds) 14519 Detroit Avenue, Lakewood, OH Zip 44107–4383; tel. 216/521–4200; Jack D. Gustin, President
Web address: www.lakewoodhospital.org

LUTHERAN HOSPITAL (O, 191 beds) 1730 West 25th Street, Cleveland, OH Zip 44113–3170; tel. 216/696–4300; David Perse, M.D., President
Web address: www.lutheranhospital.org

MARYMOUNT HOSPITAL (O, 282 beds) 12300 McCracken Road, Garfield Heights, OH Zip 44125–2975; tel. 216/581–0500; David J. Kilarski, President and Chief Executive Officer
Web address: www.marymount.org

SOUTH POINTE HOSPITAL (O, 259 beds) 20000 Harvard Road, Warrensville Heights, OH Zip 44122–7099; tel. 216/491–6000; David J. Kilarski, President and Chief Executive Officer
Web address: www.southpointehospital.org

Owned, leased, sponsored:	11 hospitals	3416 beds
Contract-managed:	0 hospitals	0 beds
Totals:	11 hospitals	3416 beds

★0152: COFFEE HEALTH GROUP (NP)
205 Marengo Street, Florence, AL Zip 35630–6033; tel. 256/768–9413; Carl W. Bailey, President and Chief Executive Officer
(Independent Hospital System)

ALABAMA: ELIZA COFFEE MEMORIAL HOSPITAL (O, 289 beds) 205 Marengo Street, Florence, AL Zip 35630–6033, Mailing Address: P.O. Box 818, Zip 35631–0818; tel. 256/768–9191; Carl W. Bailey, Administrator
Web address: www.chgroup.org

SHOALS HOSPITAL (O, 95 beds) 201 Avalon Avenue, Muscle Shoals, AL Zip 35661–2805, Mailing Address: P.O. Box 3359, Zip 35662–3359; tel. 256/386–1600; Jody Pigg, Interim Administrator

Owned, leased, sponsored:	2 hospitals	384 beds
Contract-managed:	0 hospitals	0 beds
Totals:	2 hospitals	384 beds

0076: COLLEGE HEALTH ENTERPRISES (IO)
11627 Telegraph Road, Suite 200, Santa Fe Springs, CA Zip 90670; tel. 562/923–9449; Barry J. Weiss, Chairman of the Board

CALIFORNIA: COLLEGE HOSPITAL (O, 157 beds) 10802 College Place, Cerritos, CA Zip 90703–1579; tel. 562/924–9581; Stephen Witt, Chief Executive Officer
Web address: www.collegehospitals.com

COLLEGE HOSPITAL COSTA MESA (O, 122 beds) 301 Victoria Street, Costa Mesa, CA Zip 92627–7131; tel. 949/642–2734; Wayne M. Lingenfelter, Ed.D., Chief Executive Officer
Web address: www.collegehospitalcm.com

Owned, leased, sponsored:	2 hospitals	279 beds
Contract-managed:	0 hospitals	0 beds
Totals:	2 hospitals	279 beds

★0161: COLUMBUS REGIONAL HEALTHCARE SYSTEM (NP)
707 Center Street, Suite 400, Columbus, GA Zip 31901; tel. 706/660–6100; Larry Sanders, FACHE, Chairman and Chief Executive Officer
(Centralized Physician/Insurance Health System)

GEORGIA: DOCTORS HOSPITAL OF COLUMBUS (O, 171 beds) 616 19th Street, Columbus, GA Zip 31901–1528, Mailing Address: P.O. Box 2188, Zip 31902–2188; tel. 706/494–4262; Lance B. Duke, FACHE, Interim Chief Executive Officer
Web address: www.doctorshospital.net

THE MEDICAL CENTER (O, 497 beds) 710 Center Street, Columbus, GA Zip 31901–1527, Mailing Address: P.O. Box 951, Zip 31902–0951; tel. 706/571–1000; Lance B. Duke, FACHE, President and Chief Executive Officer
Web address: www.columbusregional.com

Owned, leased, sponsored:	2 hospitals	668 beds
Contract-managed:	0 hospitals	0 beds
Totals:	2 hospitals	668 beds

0401: COMMUNITY HEALTH NETWORK (NP)
1500 North Ritter Street, Indianapolis, IN Zip 46219; tel. 317/355–1411; William E. Corley, President

INDIANA: COMMUNITY HOSPITAL EAST (O, 233 beds) 1500 North Ritter Avenue, Indianapolis, IN Zip 46219–3095; tel. 317/355–1411; Anita J. Harden, Administrator
Web address: www.ecommunity.org

COMMUNITY HOSPITAL NORTH (O, 389 beds) 7150 Clearvista Drive, Indianapolis, IN Zip 46256; tel. 317/621–6262; Barbara Summers, Chief Executive Officer
Web address: www.ecommunity.org

COMMUNITY HOSPITAL OF ANDERSON AND MADISON COUNTY (O, 173 beds) 1515 North Madison Avenue, Anderson, IN Zip 46011–3453; tel. 765/642–8011; William C. Vanness, II, M.D., President
Web address: www.ecommunity.org

COMMUNITY HOSPITAL SOUTH (O, 108 beds) 1402 East County Line Road South, Indianapolis, IN Zip 46227; tel. 317/887–7000; Michael Blanchet, President
Web address: www.ecommunity.com

INDIANA HEART HOSPITAL (O, 56 beds) 8075 North Shadeland Avenue, Indianapolis, IN Zip 46256; tel. 317/621–8000; Thomas A. Malasto, Chief Executive Officer
Web address: www.hearthospital.com

Owned, leased, sponsored:	5 hospitals	959 beds
Contract-managed:	0 hospitals	0 beds
Totals:	5 hospitals	959 beds

For explanation of codes following names, see page B2.
★ Indicates Type III membership in the American Hospital Association.

Section B

★0080: COMMUNITY HEALTH SYSTEMS, INC. (IO)
4000 Meridian Boulevard, Franklin, TN Zip 37067, Mailing Address: P.O. Box 689020, Zip 37068–9020; tel. 615/465–7000; Wayne T. Smith, Chairman, President and Chief Executive Officer
(Decentralized Health System)

ALABAMA: CHEROKEE MEDICAL CENTER (O, 60 beds) 400 Northwood Drive, Centre, AL Zip 35960–1023; tel. 256/927–5531; Jeff Noblin, FACHE, Chief Executive Officer
Web address: www.cherokeemedicalcenter.com

CRESTWOOD MEDICAL CENTER (O, 120 beds) One Hospital Drive, Huntsville, AL Zip 35801–3403; tel. 256/882–3100; Pamela Hudson, M.D., Chief Executive Officer
Web address: www.crestwoodmedcenter.com

DEKALB REGIONAL MEDICAL CENTER (O, 115 beds) 200 Medical Center Drive, Fort Payne, AL Zip 35968–3415, Mailing Address: P.O. Box 680778, Zip 35968–1608; tel. 256/845–3150; J. Peter Selman, Chief Executive Officer
Web address: www.dekalbregional.com

FLOWERS HOSPITAL (O, 235 beds) 4370 West Main Street, Dothan, AL Zip 36305–4000, Mailing Address: P.O. Box 6907, Zip 36302–6907; tel. 334/793–5000; Keith Granger, President and Chief Executive Officer
Web address: www.flowershospital.com

GADSDEN REGIONAL MEDICAL CENTER (O, 264 beds) 1007 Goodyear Avenue, Gadsden, AL Zip 35903–1195; tel. 256/494–4000; Douglas P. DeGraaf, Chief Executive Officer
Web address: www.gadsdenregional.com

L. V. STABLER MEMORIAL HOSPITAL (O, 72 beds) 29 L. V. Stabler Drive, Greenville, AL Zip 36037–3800; tel. 334/382–2671; Bobby Ginn, Chief Executive Officer
Web address: www.lvstabler.com

MEDICAL CENTER ENTERPRISE (O, 117 beds) 400 North Edwards Street, Enterprise, AL Zip 36330; tel. 334/347–0584; Jeffrey M. Brannon, Chief Executive Officer
Web address: www.mcehospital.com

SOUTH BALDWIN REGIONAL MEDICAL CENTER (L, 110 beds) 1613 North McKenzie Street, Foley, AL Zip 36535–2299; tel. 251/949–3400; Rich McAuliffe, Chief Executive Officer
Web address: www.southbaldwinrmc.com

TRINITY MEDICAL CENTER (O, 375 beds) 800 Montclair Road, Birmingham, AL Zip 35213–1984; tel. 205/592–1000; William R. Heburn, Interim Chief Executive Officer
Web address: www.bhsala.com

ALASKA: MAT–SU REGIONAL MEDICAL CENTER (O, 74 beds) 2500 South Woodworth Loop, Palmer, AK Zip 99645, Mailing Address: P.O. Box 1687, Zip 99645–1687; tel. 907/746–8600; Norman F. Stephens, Chief Executive Officer
Web address: www.matsuregional.com

ARIZONA: NORTHWEST MEDICAL CENTER (O, 244 beds) 6200 North La Cholla Boulevard, Tucson, AZ Zip 85741–3599; tel. 520/742–9000; Paul Kappelman, Chief Executive Officer
Web address: www.northwestmedicalcenter.com

NORTHWEST MEDICAL CENTER, ORO VALLEY (O, 70 beds) 1551 East Tangerine Road, Oro Valley, AZ Zip 85737; tel. 520/901–3500; Shawn G. Strash, Chief Executive Officer
Web address: www.nmcorovalley.com

PAYSON REGIONAL MEDICAL CENTER (L, 44 beds) 807 South Ponderosa Street, Payson, AZ Zip 85541–5599; tel. 928/474–3222; R. Chris Wolf, Chief Executive Officer
Web address: www.paysonhospital.com

WESTERN ARIZONA REGIONAL MEDICAL CENTER (O, 139 beds) 2735 Silver Creek Road, Bullhead City, AZ Zip 86442–8303; tel. 928/763–2273; Barry S. Schneider, Chief Executive Officer
Web address: www.warmc.com

ARKANSAS: FORREST CITY MEDICAL CENTER (O, 70 beds) 1601 Newcastle Road, Forrest City, AR Zip 72335, Mailing Address: P.O. Box 667, Zip 72336–0667; tel. 870/261–0000; Brett Kinman, Chief Executive Officer
Web address: www.chs.net

HARRIS HOSPITAL (O, 83 beds) 1205 McLain Street, Newport, AR Zip 72112–3533; tel. 870/523–8911; Claude E. Camp, III, Chief Executive Officer
Web address: www.harrishospital.com

HELENA REGIONAL MEDICAL CENTER (L, 100 beds) 1801 Martin Luther King Drive, Helena, AR Zip 72342, Mailing Address: P.O. Box 788, Zip 72342–0788; tel. 870/338–5800; Thomas E. Fewell, Chief Executive Officer
Web address: www.helenarmc.com

MEDICAL CENTER OF SOUTH ARKANSAS (O, 140 beds) 700 West Grove Street, El Dorado, AR Zip 71730–4416, Mailing Address: P.O. Box 1998, Zip 71731–1998; tel. 870/863–2000; Luther J. Lewis, FACHE, Chief Executive Officer
Web address: www.themedcenter.net

NORTHWEST MEDICAL CENTER (O, 179 beds) 609 West Maple Avenue, Springdale, AR Zip 72764; tel. 479/751–5711; Daniel E. McKay, Chief Executive Officer
Web address: www.northwesthealth.com

NORTHWEST MEDICAL CENTER – BENTONVILLE (O, 91 beds) 3000 Medical Center Parkway, Bentonville, AR Zip 72712; tel. 479/553–1000; ,
Web address: www.northwesthealth.com

WILLOW CREEK WOMEN'S HOSPITAL (O, 30 beds) 4301 Greathouse Springs Road, Johnson, AR Zip 72741–0544, Mailing Address: P.O. Box 544, Zip 72741–0544; tel. 479/684–3000; Gary N. Looper, Chief Executive Officer
Web address: www.northwesthealth.com

CALIFORNIA: BARSTOW COMMUNITY HOSPITAL (L, 56 beds) 555 South Seventh Street, Barstow, CA Zip 92311–3043; tel. 760/256–1761; Michael K. Stewart, Chief Executive Officer
Web address: www.barstowhospital.com

FALLBROOK HOSPITAL (L, 179 beds) 624 East Elder Street, Fallbrook, CA Zip 92028–3099; tel. 760/728–1191; Fred Capozello, Jr., Interim Chief Executive Officer
Web address: www.fallbrookhospital.com

WATSONVILLE COMMUNITY HOSPITAL (O, 74 beds) 75 Nielson Street, Watsonville, CA Zip 95076–2468; tel. 831/724–4741; Jae Dale, Interim Chief Executive Officer
Web address: www.watsonvillehospital.com

FLORIDA: LAKE WALES MEDICAL CENTERS (O, 126 beds) 410 South 11th Street, Lake Wales, FL Zip 33853–4256; tel. 863/676–1433; Michael Yungmann, Chief Executive Officer
Web address: www.lakewalesmedicalcenter.com

NORTH OKALOOSA MEDICAL CENTER (O, 110 beds) 151 Redstone Avenue S.E., Crestview, FL Zip 32539–6026; tel. 850/689–8100; David S. Sanders, Chief Executive Officer
Web address: www.northokaloosa.com

GEORGIA: FANNIN REGIONAL HOSPITAL (O, 50 beds) 2855 Old Highway 5, Blue Ridge, GA Zip 30513–6248; tel. 706/632–3711; Scott M. Smith, Chief Executive Officer
Web address: www.fanninregionalhospital.com

TRINITY HOSPITAL OF AUGUSTA (O, 105 beds) 2260 Wrightsboro Road, Augusta, GA Zip 30904–4726; tel. 706/481–7000; James A. Cruickshank, Chief Executive Officer
Web address: www.trinityofaugusta.com

ILLINOIS: CROSSROADS COMMUNITY HOSPITAL (O, 41 beds) 8 Doctors Park Road, Mount Vernon, IL Zip 62864–6224; tel. 618/244–5500; M. Edward Cunningham, Chief Executive Officer
Web address: www.crossroadscommunityhospital.com

GALESBURG COTTAGE HOSPITAL (O, 150 beds) 695 North Kellogg Street, Galesburg, IL Zip 61401–2885; tel. 309/343–8131; Kenneth Hutchenrider, Chief Executive Officer
Web address: www.cottagehospital.com

GATEWAY REGIONAL MEDICAL CENTER (O, 327 beds) 2100 Madison Avenue, Granite City, IL Zip 62040–4799; tel. 618/798–3000; John W. Sanders, Chief Executive Officer
Web address: www.gatewayregional.net

HEARTLAND REGIONAL MEDICAL CENTER (O, 92 beds) 3333 West DeYoung, Marion, IL Zip 62959; tel. 618/998–7000; Timothy E. Schmidt, Chief Executive Officer
Web address: www.heartlandregional.com

RED BUD REGIONAL HOSPITAL (O, 140 beds) 325 Spring Street, Red Bud, IL Zip 62278–1194; tel. 618/282–3831; Robert Honeycutt, Chief Executive Officer
Web address: www.redbudhospital.com

For explanation of codes following names, see page B2.
★ Indicates Type III membership in the American Hospital Association.

UNION COUNTY HOSPITAL (O, 47 beds) 517 North Main Street, Anna, IL Zip 62906–1696; tel. 618/833–4511; James R. Farris, CHE, Chief Executive Officer
Web address: www.unioncountyhospital.com

VISTA MEDICAL CENTER EAST (O, 209 beds) 1324 North Sheridan Road, Waukegan, IL Zip 60085–2181; tel. 847/360–4000; Barbara J. Martin, RN, President and Chief Executive Officer
Web address: www.vistahealth.com

VISTA MEDICAL CENTER WEST (O, 67 beds) 2615 Washington Street, Waukegan, IL Zip 60085–4988; tel. 847/249–3900; Barbara J. Martin, RN, President and Chief Executive Officer
Web address: www.vistahealth.com

INDIANA: BLUFFTON REGIONAL MEDICAL CENTER (O, 79 beds) 303 South Main Street, Bluffton, IN Zip 46714–2529; tel. 260/824–3210; Thomas A. Clark, Chief Executive Officer
Web address: www.blufftonregional.com

DUKES MEMORIAL HOSPITAL (O, 25 beds) 275 West 12th Street, Peru, IN Zip 46970–1698; tel. 765/472–8000; Debra Close, Chief Executive Officer
Web address: www.dukesmemorialhosp.com

DUPONT HOSPITAL (O, 122 beds) 2520 East Dupont Road, Fort Wayne, IN Zip 46825; tel. 260/416–3000; Michael H. Schatzlein, M.D., Chief Executive Officer
Web address: www.theduponthospital.com

KOSCIUSKO COMMUNITY HOSPITAL (O, 72 beds) 2101 East Dubois Drive, Warsaw, IN Zip 46580–3288; tel. 574/267–3200; Stephen R. Miller, Chief Executive Officer
Web address: www.kch.com

LUTHERAN HOSPITAL OF INDIANA (O, 435 beds) 7950 West Jefferson Boulevard, Fort Wayne, IN Zip 46804–1677; tel. 260/435–7001; Joseph M. Dorko, Chief Executive Officer
Web address: www.lutheran–hosp.com

PORTER–VALPARAISO HOSPITAL CAMPUS (O, 276 beds) 814 La Porte Avenue, Valparaiso, IN Zip 46383–5898; tel. 219/263–4600; Jonathan Nalli, Chief Executive Officer
Web address: www.porterhealth.org

REHABILITATION HOSPITAL OF FORT WAYNE (O, 36 beds) 7970 West Jefferson Boulevard, Fort Wayne, IN Zip 46804–4140; tel. 260/435–6100; Ted Scholten, Interim Chief Operating Officer
Web address: www.rehabhospital.com

ST. JOSEPH HOSPITAL (O, 201 beds) 700 Broadway, Fort Wayne, IN Zip 46802–1493; tel. 260/425–3000; Kirk M. Ray, Chief Executive Officer
Web address: www.stjoehospital.com

KENTUCKY: KENTUCKY RIVER MEDICAL CENTER (L, 54 beds) 540 Jett Drive, Jackson, KY Zip 41339–9620; tel. 606/666–6000; Donald Rentfro, Chief Executive Officer
Web address: www.kentuckyrivermc.com

PARKWAY REGIONAL HOSPITAL (O, 70 beds) 2000 Holiday Lane, Fulton, KY Zip 42041–8468; tel. 270/472–2522; Stephen Lunn, Chief Executive Officer
Web address: www.parkwayregionalhospital.com

THREE RIVERS MEDICAL CENTER (O, 80 beds) Highway 644, Louisa, KY Zip 41230–9632, Mailing Address: P.O. Box 769, Zip 41230–0769; tel. 606/638–9451; Greg Kiser, Chief Executive Officer
Web address: www.threeriversmedicalcenter.com

LOUISIANA: BYRD REGIONAL HOSPITAL (O, 60 beds) 1020 Fertitta Boulevard, Leesville, LA Zip 71446–4697; tel. 337/239–9041; Roger C. LeDoux, Chief Executive Officer
Web address: www.byrdregional.com

NORTHERN LOUISIANA MEDICAL CENTER (O, 99 beds) 401 East Vaughn Avenue, Ruston, LA Zip 71270–5950, Mailing Address: P.O. Drawer 1368, Zip 71273–1368; tel. 318/254–2100; Doug Sills, Chief Executive Officer
Web address: www.northernlouisianamedicalcenter.com

WOMEN AND CHILDREN'S HOSPITAL (O, 118 beds) 4200 Nelson Road, Lake Charles, LA Zip 70605–4118; tel. 337/474–6370; William L. Willis, Chief Executive Officer
Web address: www.women–childrens.com

MISSISSIPPI: RIVER REGION MEDICAL CENTER (O, 324 beds) 2100 Highway 61 North, Vicksburg, MS Zip 39183, Mailing Address: P.O. Box 590, Zip 39181–0590; tel. 601/883–5000; Phillip A. Clendenin, Chief Executive Officer
Web address: www.riverregion.com

WESLEY MEDICAL CENTER (O, 211 beds) 5001 Hardy Street, Hattiesburg, MS Zip 39402–1366, Mailing Address: P.O. Box 16509, Zip 39404–6509; tel. 601/268–8000; Ronald T. Seal, Chief Executive Officer
Web address: www.wesley.com

MISSOURI: MOBERLY REGIONAL MEDICAL CENTER (O, 100 beds) 1515 Union Avenue, Moberly, MO Zip 65270–9449; tel. 660/263–8400; Kevin Clement, Chief Executive Officer
Web address: www.moberlyhospital.com

NORTHEAST REGIONAL MEDICAL CENTER (L, 115 beds) 315 South Osteopathy, Kirksville, MO Zip 63501–8599, Mailing Address: P.O. Box C8502, Zip 63501–8599; tel. 660/785–1000; Bob Moore, FACHE, Chief Executive Officer
Web address: www.nermc.com

NEVADA: MESA VIEW REGIONAL HOSPITAL (O, 25 beds) 1299 Bertha Howe Avenue, Mesquite, NV Zip 89027; tel. 702/346–8040; Sue Conley, Chief Executive Officer
Web address: www.mesaviewhospital.com

NEW JERSEY: MEMORIAL HOSPITAL OF SALEM COUNTY (O, 110 beds) 310 Woodstown Road, Salem, NJ Zip 08079–2080; tel. 856/935–1000; James L. Angle, Chief Executive Officer
Web address: www.salemhospitalnj.org

NEW MEXICO: ALTA VISTA REGIONAL HOSPITAL (O, 42 beds) 104 Legion Drive, Las Vegas, NM Zip 87701; tel. 505/426–3500; Richard Grogan, Chief Executive Officer
Web address: www.altavistaregionalhospital.com

CARLSBAD MEDICAL CENTER (O, 127 beds) 2430 West Pierce Street, Carlsbad, NM Zip 88220–3597; tel. 505/887–4100; Janet Carbary, Interim Chief Executive Officer
Web address: www.carlsbadmedicalcenter.com

EASTERN NEW MEXICO MEDICAL CENTER (L, 162 beds) 405 West Country Club Road, Roswell, NM Zip 88201–9981; tel. 505/622–8170; Bradley McGrath, Chief Executive Officer
Web address: www.enmmc.com

LEA REGIONAL MEDICAL CENTER (O, 214 beds) 5419 North Lovington Highway, Hobbs, NM Zip 88240–9125, Mailing Address: P.O. Box 3000, Zip 88240–3000; tel. 505/492–5000; Larry W. Payton, Chief Executive Officer
Web address: www.learegional.com

MIMBRES MEMORIAL HOSPITAL (O, 119 beds) 900 West Ash Street, Deming, NM Zip 88030–4098, Mailing Address: P.O. Box 710, Zip 88031–0710; tel. 505/546–2761; John M. Gallagher, Chief Executive Officer
Web address: www.mimbresmemorial.com

MOUNTAINVIEW REGIONAL MEDICAL CENTER (O, 131 beds) 4311 East Lohman Avenue, Las Cruces, NM Zip 88011; tel. 505/556–7600; Randall Hempling, Chief Executive Officer
Web address: www.mountainviewregional.com

NORTH CAROLINA: MARTIN GENERAL HOSPITAL (L, 49 beds) 310 South McCaskey Road, Williamston, NC Zip 27892–2150, Mailing Address: P.O. Box 1128, Zip 27892–1128; tel. 252/809–6179; Glenn Carney, Chief Executive Officer
Web address: www.martingeneral.com

OHIO: AFFINITY MEDICAL CENTER, DOCTORS CAMPUS (O, 166 beds) 400 Austin Avenue N.W., Massillon, OH Zip 44646–3554; tel. 330/837–7200; Ronald L. Bierman, Chief Executive Officer
Web address: www.drshospital.com

AFFINITY MEDICAL CENTER, MASSILLON CAMPUS (O, 128 beds) 875 Eighth Street N.E., Massillon, OH Zip 44646–8503, Mailing Address: P.O. Box 805, Zip 44648–8503; tel. 330/832–8761; Ronald L. Bierman, Chief Executive Officer
Web address: www.mchosp.org

OKLAHOMA: CLAREMORE REGIONAL HOSPITAL (O, 71 beds) 1202 North Muskogee Place, Claremore, OK Zip 74017–3036; tel. 918/341–2556; David Chaussard, Chief Executive Officer
Web address: www.claremorereghospital.com

DEACONESS HOSPITAL (O, 273 beds) 5501 North Portland Avenue, Oklahoma City, OK Zip 73112–2099; tel. 405/604–6000; Cathryn A. Hibbs, Chief Executive Officer
Web address: www.deaconessokc.com

PONCA CITY MEDICAL CENTER (O, 85 beds) 1900 North 14th Street, Ponca City, OK Zip 74601–2035; tel. 580/765–3321; Dennis Barts, Chief Executive Officer
Web address: www.poncamedcenter.com

For explanation of codes following names, see page B2.
★ Indicates Type III membership in the American Hospital Association.

SOUTHCREST HOSPITAL (O, 148 beds) 8801 South 101st East Avenue, Tulsa, OK Zip 74133; tel. 918/294–4000; Anthony R. Young, Chief Executive Officer
Web address: www.southcresthospital.com

WOODWARD REGIONAL HOSPITAL (L, 68 beds) 900 17th Street, Woodward, OK Zip 73801–2423; tel. 580/256–5511; Lavah Lowe, Interim Chief Executive Officer
Web address: www.woodwardhospital.com

OREGON: MCKENZIE–WILLAMETTE MEDICAL CENTER (O, 112 beds) 1460 G Street, Springfield, OR Zip 97477–4197; tel. 541/726–4400; Maurine Cate, Chief Executive Officer
Web address: www.mckweb.com

PENNSYLVANIA: BERWICK HOSPITAL CENTER (O, 341 beds) 701 East 16th Street, Berwick, PA Zip 18603–2397; tel. 570/759–5000; John Kristel, Chief Executive Officer
Web address: www.berwick–hospital.com

BRANDYWINE HOSPITAL (O, 164 beds) 201 Reeceville Road, Coatesville, PA Zip 19320–1536; tel. 610/383–8000; Mark A. Benz, Chief Executive Officer
Web address: www.brandywinehospital.com

CHESTNUT HILL HEALTH SYSTEM (O, 212 beds) 8835 Germantown Avenue, Philadelphia, PA Zip 19118–2765; tel. 215/248–8200; M. Brooks Turkel, Chief Executive Officer
Web address: www.chh.org

EASTON HOSPITAL (O, 221 beds) 250 South 21st Street, Easton, PA Zip 18042–3892; tel. 610/250–4000; Angela M. Marchi, FACHE, President and Chief Executive Officer
Web address: www.easton–hospital.com

JENNERSVILLE REGIONAL HOSPITAL (O, 59 beds) 1015 West Baltimore Pike, West Grove, PA Zip 19390–9499; tel. 610/869–1000; Charles A. Davis, Chief Executive Officer
Web address: www.jennersville.com

LOCK HAVEN HOSPITAL (O, 171 beds) 24 Cree Drive, Lock Haven, PA Zip 17745–2699; tel. 570/893–5000; Cindy Segar–Gorr, RN, M.S., Chief Executive Officer
Web address: www.lockhavenhospital.com

PHOENIXVILLE HOSPITAL (O, 136 beds) 140 Nutt Road, Phoenixville, PA Zip 19460–3900, Mailing Address: P.O. Box 3001, Zip 19460–3001; tel. 610/983–1000; Stephen M. Tullman, Chief Executive Officer
Web address: www.phoenixvillehospital.com

POTTSTOWN MEMORIAL MEDICAL CENTER (O, 226 beds) 1600 East High Street, Pottstown, PA Zip 19464–5093; tel. 610/327–7000; Steven MacLauchlan, Chief Executive Officer
Web address: www.pottstownmemorial.com

SUNBURY COMMUNITY HOSPITAL (O, 121 beds) 350 North Eleventh Street, Sunbury, PA Zip 17801–0737; tel. 570/286–3333; Cornelio R. Catena, Interim Chief Executive Officer
Web address: www.schopc.org

SOUTH CAROLINA: CAROLINAS HOSPITAL SYSTEM (O, 334 beds) 805 Pamplico Highway, Florence, SC Zip 29505–6050, Mailing Address: P.O. Box 100550, Zip 29501–0550; tel. 843/674–5000; James O'Laughlin, Chief Executive Officer
Web address: www.carolinashospital.com

CHESTERFIELD GENERAL HOSPITAL (L, 59 beds) 711 Chesterfield Highway, Cheraw, SC Zip 29520; tel. 843/537–7881; Vance Reynolds, Chief Executive Officer
Web address: www.chesterfieldgeneral.com

MARLBORO PARK HOSPITAL (L, 102 beds) 1138 Cheraw Highway, Bennettsville, SC Zip 29512–0738, Mailing Address: P.O. Box 738, Zip 29512–0738; tel. 843/479–2881; Todd Blanchard, Chief Executive Officer
Web address: www.marlboroparkhospital.com

MARY BLACK MEMORIAL HOSPITAL (O, 182 beds) 1700 Skylyn Drive, Spartanburg, SC Zip 29307–1061, Mailing Address: P.O. Box 3217, Zip 29304–3217; tel. 864/573–3000; Phillip L. Wright, FACHE, Chief Executive Officer
Web address: www.maryblack.org

SPRINGS MEMORIAL HOSPITAL (O, 204 beds) 800 West Meeting Street, Lancaster, SC Zip 29720–2298; tel. 803/286–1481; Tom R. McDougal, Chief Executive Officer
Web address: www.springsmemorial.com

TENNESSEE: BEDFORD COUNTY MEDICAL CENTER (O, 177 beds) 845 Union Street, Shelbyville, TN Zip 37160–2609; tel. 931/685–5433; Daniel Buckner, Interim Chief Executive Officer
Web address: www.bcmctn.com

DYERSBURG REGIONAL MEDICAL CENTER (O, 105 beds) 400 Tickle Street, Dyersburg, TN Zip 38024–3182; tel. 731/285–2410; Greg Lowe, Chief Executive Officer
Web address: www.dyersburgregionalmc.com

GATEWAY MEDICAL CENTER (O, 198 beds) 651 Dunlop Lane, Clarksville, TN Zip 37040–5015, Mailing Address: P.O. Box 31629, Zip 37043–0028; tel. 931/502–1000; Michael L. Mullins, Chief Executive Officer
Web address: www.ghsystem.com

HAYWOOD PARK COMMUNITY HOSPITAL (O, 44 beds) 2545 North Washington Avenue, Brownsville, TN Zip 38012–1697; tel. 731/772–4110; Kim Anthony, Chief Executive Officer
Web address: www.haywoodparkcommunity.com

HENDERSON COUNTY COMMUNITY HOSPITAL (O, 45 beds) 200 West Church Street, Lexington, TN Zip 38351–2014; tel. 731/968–3646; Holly Clark, Chief Executive Officer
Web address: www.hendersoncchospital.com

LAKEWAY REGIONAL HOSPITAL (O, 100 beds) 726 McFarland Street, Morristown, TN Zip 37814–3990; tel. 423/586–2302; Priscilla Millis, Chief Executive Officer
Web address: www.lakewayregionalhospital.com

MCKENZIE REGIONAL HOSPITAL (O, 31 beds) 161 Hospital Drive, McKenzie, TN Zip 38201–1636; tel. 731/352–5344; David D. Rasmussen, Chief Executive Officer
Web address: www.mckenzieregionalhospital.com

MCNAIRY REGIONAL HOSPITAL (O, 41 beds) 705 East Poplar Avenue, Selmer, TN Zip 38375–1828; tel. 731/645–3221; Pamela W. Roberts, Chief Executive Officer
Web address: www.mcnairyregionalhospital.com

REGIONAL HOSPITAL OF JACKSON (O, 127 beds) 367 Hospital Boulevard, Jackson, TN Zip 38305–2081; tel. 731/661–2000; Stephen Grubbs, Chief Executive Officer
Web address: www.regionalhospital.com

SKYRIDGE MEDICAL CENTER (O, 209 beds) 2305 Chambliss Avenue N.W., Cleveland, TN Zip 37311–3847, Mailing Address: P.O. Box 3060, Zip 37320–3060; tel. 423/559–6000; R. Coleman Foss, Chief Executive Officer
Web address: www.skyridgemedicalcenter.net

VOLUNTEER COMMUNITY HOSPITAL (O, 65 beds) 161 Mount Pelia Road, Martin, TN Zip 38237–0967; tel. 731/587–4261; Steve Westenhofer, Chief Executive Officer
Web address: www.volunteercommunityhospital.com

TEXAS: ABILENE REGIONAL MEDICAL CENTER (O, 205 beds) 6250 Highway 83–84 at Antilley Road, Abilene, TX Zip 79606–5299; tel. 325/695–9900; Michael D. Murphy, Chief Executive Officer
Web address: www.abileneregional.com

BIG BEND REGIONAL MEDICAL CENTER (O, 25 beds) 2600 Highway 118 North, Alpine, TX Zip 79830–2002; tel. 432/837–3447; Michael J. Ellis, Chief Executive Officer
Web address: www.bigbendhealthcare.com

BROWNWOOD REGIONAL MEDICAL CENTER (O, 168 beds) 1501 Burnet Drive, Brownwood, TX Zip 76801–5933, Mailing Address: P.O. Box 760, Zip 76804–0760; tel. 325/646–8541; Matt T. Maxfield, FACHE, Chief Executive Officer
Web address: www.brmc–cares.com

CEDAR PARK REGIONAL MEDICAL CENTER (O, 75 beds) 1490 East Whitestone Boulevard, Cedar Park, TX Zip 78613–2274; tel. 512/528–7000; David G. Klein, M.D., Chief Executive Officer
Web address: www.cedarparkregional.com

CLEVELAND REGIONAL MEDICAL CENTER (L, 98 beds) 300 East Crockett Street, Cleveland, TX Zip 77327–4062, Mailing Address: P.O. Box 1688, Zip 77328–1688; tel. 281/593–1811; Jude Torchia, Chief Executive Officer
Web address: www.clevelandregionalmedicalcenter.com

COLLEGE STATION MEDICAL CENTER (O, 150 beds) 1604 Rock Prairie Road, College Station, TX Zip 77845–8345, Mailing Address: P.O. Box 10000, Zip 77842–3500; tel. 979/764–5100; Thomas W. Jackson, Chief Executive Officer
Web address: www.csmedcenter.com

For explanation of codes following names, see page B2.
★ Indicates Type III membership in the American Hospital Association.

Section B

DETAR HEALTHCARE SYSTEM (O, 228 beds) 506 East San Antonio Street, Victoria, TX Zip 77901–6060, Mailing Address: P.O. Box 2089, Zip 77902–2089; tel. 361/575–7441; William R. Blanchard, Chief Executive Officer
Web address: www.detar.com

HILL REGIONAL HOSPITAL (O, 84 beds) 101 Circle Drive, Hillsboro, TX Zip 76645–2670; tel. 254/580–8950; Jan McClure, Chief Executive Officer
Web address: www.chs.net

LAKE GRANBURY MEDICAL CENTER (L, 59 beds) 1310 Paluxy Road, Granbury, TX Zip 76048–5699; tel. 817/573–2273; David Orcutt, Chief Executive Officer
Web address: www.lakegranburymedicalcenter.com

LAREDO MEDICAL CENTER (O, 326 beds) 1700 East Saunders Avenue, Laredo, TX Zip 78041–5401, Mailing Address: Drawer 2068, Zip 78044–2068; tel. 956/796–5000; Abraham Martinez, Chief Executive Officer
Web address: www.laredomedical.com

LONGVIEW REGIONAL MEDICAL CENTER (O, 131 beds) 2901 North Fourth Street, Longview, TX Zip 75605–5191, Mailing Address: P.O. Box 14000, Zip 75607–4000; tel. 903/758–1818; Jim R. Kendrick, Chief Executive Officer
Web address: www.longviewregional.com

NAVARRO REGIONAL HOSPITAL (O, 148 beds) 3201 West State Highway 22, Corsicana, TX Zip 75110–2469; tel. 903/654–6800; Xavier Villarreal, Chief Executive Officer
Web address: www.navarrohospital.com

PRESBYTERIAN HOSPITAL OF DENTON (O, 208 beds) 3000 I. 35 North, Denton, TX Zip 76201–3798; tel. 940/898–7000; Stan C. Morton, Chief Executive Officer
Web address: www.dentonhospital.com

SAN ANGELO COMMUNITY MEDICAL CENTER (O, 171 beds) 3501 Knickerbocker Road, San Angelo, TX Zip 76904–7698; tel. 325/949–9511; Samuel G. Feazell, Chief Executive Officer
Web address: www.sacmc.com

SCENIC MOUNTAIN MEDICAL CENTER (O, 122 beds) 1601 West 11th Place, Big Spring, TX Zip 79720–4198; tel. 432/263–1211; George N. Parsley, Chief Executive Officer
Web address: www.smmccares.com

SOUTH TEXAS REGIONAL MEDICAL CENTER (O, 67 beds) 1905 Highway 97 East, Jourdanton, TX Zip 78026–1504; tel. 830/769–3515; Michael L. Pierce, CHE, Chief Executive Officer
Web address: www.strmc.com

WEATHERFORD REGIONAL MEDICAL CENTER (O, 74 beds) 713 East Anderson Street, Weatherford, TX Zip 76086–9971; tel. 817/596–8751; Donnie L. Romine, Chief Executive Officer
Web address: www.weatherfordregional.com

WOODLAND HEIGHTS MEDICAL CENTER (O, 149 beds) 505 South John Redditt Drive, Lufkin, TX Zip 75904–3157, Mailing Address: P.O. Box 150610, Zip 75915–0610; tel. 936/634–8311; Lance Jones, Chief Executive Officer
Web address: www.woodlandheights.net

UTAH: MOUNTAIN WEST MEDICAL CENTER (O, 35 beds) 2055 North Main, Tooele, UT Zip 84074–2794; tel. 435/843–3600; Kelly L. Duffin, Chief Executive Officer
Web address: www.mountainwestmc.com

VIRGINIA: SOUTHAMPTON MEMORIAL HOSPITAL (O, 203 beds) 100 Fairview Drive, Franklin, VA Zip 23851–1206, Mailing Address: P.O. Box 817, Zip 23851–0817; tel. 757/569–6100; David W. Fuller, Chief Executive Officer
Web address: www.smhfranklin.com

SOUTHERN VIRGINIA REGIONAL MEDICAL CENTER (O, 80 beds) 727 North Main Street, Emporia, VA Zip 23847–1482; tel. 434/348–4400; Douglas T. Arbour, Chief Executive Officer
Web address: www.svrmc.com

SOUTHSIDE REGIONAL MEDICAL CENTER (L, 283 beds) 200 Medical Park Boulevard, Petersburg, VA Zip 23805; tel. 804/862–5000; David J. Fiske, Chief Executive Officer
Web address: www.srmconline.com

WEST VIRGINIA: GREENBRIER VALLEY MEDICAL CENTER (O, 112 beds) 202 Maplewood Avenue, Ronceverte, WV Zip 24970–0497, Mailing Address: P.O. Box 497, Zip 24970–0497; tel. 304/647–4411; Brenda Hamilton, Interim Chief Executive Officer
Web address: www.gvmc.com

PLATEAU MEDICAL CENTER (O, 25 beds) 430 Main Street, Oak Hill, WV Zip 25901–3455; tel. 304/469–8600; David V. Bunch, Chief Executive Officer
Web address: www.plateaumedicalcenter.com

WYOMING: EVANSTON REGIONAL HOSPITAL (O, 36 beds) 190 Arrowhead Drive, Evanston, WY Zip 82930–9266; tel. 307/789–3636; Ben Quinton, Chief Executive Officer
Web address: www.evanstonregionalhospital.com

Owned, leased, sponsored:	121 hospitals	15948 beds
Contract–managed:	0 hospitals	0 beds
Totals:	121 hospitals	15948 beds

0249: COMMUNITY HEALTHCARE SYSTEM (NP)

901 MacArthur Boulevard, Hammond, IN Zip 46321–2959; tel. 219/836–1600; Donald Powers, Chairman, President and Chief Executive Officer
(Independent Hospital System)

INDIANA: COMMUNITY HOSPITAL (O, 367 beds) 901 MacArthur Boulevard, Munster, IN Zip 46321–2959; tel. 219/836–1600; Donald P. Fesko, Administrator
Web address: www.comhs.org

ST. CATHERINE HOSPITAL (O, 200 beds) 4321 Fir Street, East Chicago, IN Zip 46312–3097; tel. 219/392–7000; JoAnn Birdzell, President and Chief Executive Officer
Web address: www.stcatherinehospital.org

ST. MARY MEDICAL CENTER (O, 186 beds) 1500 South Lake Park Avenue, Hobart, IN Zip 46342–6699; tel. 219/942–0551; Janice Ryba, Administrator
Web address: www.comhs.org

Owned, leased, sponsored:	3 hospitals	753 beds
Contract–managed:	0 hospitals	0 beds
Totals:	3 hospitals	753 beds

0384: COMMUNITY HOSPITAL CORPORATION (NP)

5180 Tennyson Parkway, Suite 500, Plano, TX Zip 75024; tel. 972/943–6400; Michael D. Williams, President and Chief Executive Officer

TEXAS: HUNTSVILLE MEMORIAL HOSPITAL (C, 88 beds) 110 Memorial Hospital Drive, Huntsville, TX Zip 77340–4362, Mailing Address: P.O. Box 4001, Zip 77342–4001; tel. 936/291–3411; Sally I. Nelson, Chief Executive Officer
Web address: www.huntsvillememorial.com

MEMORIAL HERMANN BAPTIST BEAUMONT HOSPITAL (C, 408 beds) 3080 College Street, Beaumont, TX Zip 77701–4689, Mailing Address: P.O. Box 1591, Zip 77704–1591; tel. 409/212–5000; David N. Parmer, President and Chief Executive Officer
Web address: www.mhbh.org

MEMORIAL HERMANN BAPTIST ORANGE HOSPITAL (C, 83 beds) 608 Strickland Drive, Orange, TX Zip 77630–4717; tel. 409/883–9361; Jarren Garrett, Interim Administrator
Web address: www.mhbh.org

VAL VERDE REGIONAL MEDICAL CENTER (C, 86 beds) 801 Bedell Avenue, Del Rio, TX Zip 78840–4185, Mailing Address: P.O. Box 1527, Zip 78840–1527; tel. 830/775–8566; Jack F. Houghton, Chief Executive Officer
Web address: www.vvrmc.org

WADLEY REGIONAL MEDICAL CENTER (C, 163 beds) 1000 Pine Street, Texarkana, TX Zip 75501–5170, Mailing Address: Box 1878, Zip 75504–1878; tel. 903/798–8000; Mike Lieb, Interim Chief Executive Officer
Web address: www.wadleyhealth.com

YOAKUM COMMUNITY HOSPITAL (C, 25 beds) 1200 Carl Ramert Drive, Yoakum, TX Zip 77995–4198, Mailing Address: P.O. Box 753, Zip 77995–0753; tel. 361/293–2321; Karen Barber, Chief Executive Officer
Web address: www.yoakumhospital.org

Owned, leased, sponsored:	0 hospitals	0 beds
Contract–managed:	6 hospitals	853 beds
Totals:	6 hospitals	853 beds

For explanation of codes following names, see page B2.
★ Indicates Type III membership in the American Hospital Association.

Section B

1085: COMMUNITY MEDICAL CENTERS (NP)
Fresno and Maddy Drive, Fresno, CA Zip 93721, Mailing Address: P.O. Box 1232, Zip 93715–1232; tel. 559/459–6000; Tim A. Joslin, President and Chief Executive Officer

CALIFORNIA: CLOVIS COMMUNITY MEDICAL CENTER (O, 76 beds) 2755 Herndon Avenue, Clovis, CA Zip 93611–6800; tel. 559/324–4000; Craig Castro, Administrator
Web address: www.communitymedical.org

COMMUNITY BEHAVIORAL HEALTH CENTER (O, 60 beds) 7171 North Cedar Avenue, Fresno, CA Zip 93720–3311; tel. 559/449–8000; Dawan Haubursin, Chief Executive Officer
Web address: www.communitymedical.org

COMMUNITY REGIONAL MEDICAL CENTER (O, 460 beds) 2823 Fresno Street, Fresno, CA Zip 93721–1324, Mailing Address: P.O. Box 1232, Zip 93715–1232; tel. 559/459–6000; John M. Chubb, Chief Executive Officer
Web address: www.communitymedical.org

Owned, leased, sponsored:	3 hospitals	596 beds
Contract-managed:	0 hospitals	0 beds
Totals:	3 hospitals	596 beds

0339: CONEMAUGH HEALTH SYSTEM (NP)
1086 Franklin Street, Johnstown, PA Zip 15905–4398; tel. 814/534–9000; Scott A. Becker, President and Chief Executive Officer
(Centralized Physician/Insurance Health System)

PENNSYLVANIA: MEMORIAL MEDICAL CENTER (O, 538 beds) 1086 Franklin Street, Johnstown, PA Zip 15905–4398; tel. 814/534–9000; Steven E. Tucker, President
Web address: www.conemaugh.org

MEMORIAL MEDICAL CENTER – LEE CAMPUS (O, 212 beds) 320 Main Street, Johnstown, PA Zip 15901–1694; tel. 814/533–0123; Steven E. Tucker, President
Web address: www.conemaugh.org

MEYERSDALE MEDICAL CENTER (O, 20 beds) 200 Hospital Drive, Meyersdale, PA Zip 15552–1249; tel. 814/634–5911; Mary L. Libengood, President
Web address: www.conemaugh.org

MINERS MEDICAL CENTER (O, 30 beds) 290 Haida Avenue, Hastings, PA Zip 16646, Mailing Address: P.O. Box 689, Zip 16646–0689; tel. 814/247–3100; William R. Crowe, President
Web address: www.minersmedicalcenter.org

Owned, leased, sponsored:	4 hospitals	800 beds
Contract-managed:	0 hospitals	0 beds
Totals:	4 hospitals	800 beds

0014: CONNECTICUT DEPARTMENT OF MENTAL HEALTH AND ADDICTION SERVICES (NP)
410 Capitol Avenue, Hartford, CT Zip 06106, Mailing Address: P.O. Box 341431, Zip 06134–1431; tel. 860/418–7000; Thomas A. Kirk, Jr., Ph.D., Commissioner
(Independent Hospital System)

CONNECTICUT: CEDARCREST HOSPITAL (O, 145 beds) 525 Russell Road, Newington, CT Zip 06111–1595; tel. 860/666–4613; Brenda Thorington, Chief Executive Officer

CONNECTICUT MENTAL HEALTH CENTER (O, 33 beds) 34 Park Street, New Haven, CT Zip 06508–1842, Mailing Address: P.O. Box 1842, Zip 06508–1842; tel. 203/974–7144; Selby Jacobs, M.D., Director
Web address: www.dmhas.state.ct.us/lmha.htm

CONNECTICUT VALLEY HOSPITAL (O, 537 beds) Eastern Drive, Middletown, CT Zip 06457–3947, Mailing Address: P.O. Box 351, Zip 06457–0351; tel. 860/262–5000; Luis B. Perez, Chief Executive Officer

SOUTHWEST CONNECTICUT MENTAL HEALTH SYSTEM (O, 62 beds) 97 Middle Street, Bridgeport, CT Zip 6604; tel. 203/551–7400; James M. Pisciotta, Chief Executive Officer

Owned, leased, sponsored:	4 hospitals	777 beds
Contract-managed:	0 hospitals	0 beds
Totals:	4 hospitals	777 beds

★0127: CONTINUUM HEALTH PARTNERS (NP)
555 West 57th Street, New York, NY Zip 10019; tel. 212/523–8130; Stanley Brezenoff, President and Chief Executive Officer
(Decentralized Health System)

NEW YORK: BETH ISRAEL MEDICAL CENTER (O, 1077 beds) First Avenue and 16th Street, New York, NY Zip 10003–3803; tel. 212/420–2000; David J. Shulkin, M.D., President and Chief Executive Officer
Web address: www.bethisraelny.org

LONG ISLAND COLLEGE HOSPITAL (O, 352 beds) 339 Hicks Street, Brooklyn, NY Zip 11201–5509; tel. 718/780–1000; Rita Battles, President and Chief Executive Officer
Web address: www.wehealny.org

NEW YORK EYE AND EAR INFIRMARY (O, 32 beds) 310 East 14th Street, New York, NY Zip 10003–4201; tel. 212/979–4000; D. McWilliams Kessler, President and Chief Executive Officer
Web address: www.nyee.edu

ST. LUKE'S–ROOSEVELT HOSPITAL CENTER (O, 702 beds) 1111 Amsterdam Avenue, New York, NY Zip 10025; tel. 212/523–4000; Frank J. Cracolici, President and Chief Executive Officer
Web address: www.slrhc.org

Owned, leased, sponsored:	4 hospitals	2163 beds
Contract-managed:	0 hospitals	0 beds
Totals:	4 hospitals	2163 beds

0016: COOK COUNTY BUREAU OF HEALTH SERVICES (NP)
1900 West Polk Street, Suite 200, Chicago, IL Zip 60612; tel. 312/864–6820; Robert Simon, M.D., Chief
(Moderately Centralized Health System)

ILLINOIS: JOHN H. STROGER JR. HOSPITAL OF COOK COUNTY (O, 460 beds) 1901 West Harrison Street, Chicago, IL Zip 60612–3785; tel. 312/864–6000; Johnny C. Brown, Chief Operating Officer
Web address: www.ccbhs.org

OAK FOREST HOSPITAL OF COOK COUNTY (O, 456 beds) 15900 South Cicero Avenue, Oak Forest, IL Zip 60452–4006; tel. 708/687–7200; Sylvia Edwards, Chief Operating Officer
Web address: www.cookcountygov.com

PROVIDENT HOSPITAL OF COOK COUNTY (O, 119 beds) 500 East 51st Street, Chicago, IL Zip 60615–2494; tel. 312/572–2000; Sidney Thomas, Chief Operating Officer
Web address: www.ccbhs.org/pages/ProvidentHospitalofCookCounty.htm

Owned, leased, sponsored:	3 hospitals	1035 beds
Contract-managed:	0 hospitals	0 beds
Totals:	3 hospitals	1035 beds

0905: CORNERSTONE HEALTHCARE GROUP (IO)
816 Congress Avenue, Suite 400, Austin, TX Zip 78701; tel. 512/533–2400; Timothy P. Hall, President and Chief Executive Officer
(Independent Hospital System)

ARIZONA: CORNERSTONE HOSPITAL OF SOUTHEAST ARIZONA (O, 54 beds) 7220 East Rosewood Drive, Tucson, AZ Zip 85710; tel. 520/546–4595; James Mikes, Interim Chief Executive Officer
Web address: www.cornerstonehealthcaregroup.com

LOUISIANA: CORNERSTONE HOSPITAL OF BOSSIER CITY (O, 54 beds) 4900 Medical Drive, Bossier City, LA Zip 71112–4596; tel. 318/747–9500; Sheri Burnette, RN, Chief Executive Officer and Administrator
Web address: www.cornerstonehealthcaregroup.com

CORNERSTONE HOSPITAL OF SOUTHWEST LOUISIANA (O, 30 beds) 703 Cypress Street, Sulphur, LA Zip 70663; tel. 337/527–1102; W. Darrell Jean, Chief Executive Officer
Web address: www.cornerstonehealthcaregroup.com

For explanation of codes following names, see page B2.
★ Indicates Type III membership in the American Hospital Association.

CORNERSTONE HOSPITAL–WEST MONROE (O, 40 beds) 6198 Cypress Street, West Monroe, LA Zip 71291–9010; tel. 318/396–5600; Chris Simpson, Chief Executive Officer
Web address: www.cornerstonehealthcaregroup.com

TEXAS: CORNERSTONE HOSPITAL OF AUSTIN (O, 95 beds) 4207 Burnet Road, Austin, TX Zip 78756–3396; tel. 512/706–1900; Mary Ann Lee, Chief Executive Officer
Web address: www.cornerstonehealthcaregroup.com

WEST VIRGINIA: CORNERSTONE HOSPITAL OF HUNTINGTON (O, 28 beds) 2900 First Avenue, Two East, Huntington, WV Zip 25702; tel. 304/399–2600; Tony Aluise, Chief Executive Officer
Web address: www.cornerstonehealthcaregroup.com

Owned, leased, sponsored:	6 hospitals	301 beds
Contract-managed:	0 hospitals	0 beds
Totals:	6 hospitals	301 beds

★0103: COTTAGE HEALTH SYSTEM (NP)

Pueblo at Bath Streets, Santa Barbara, CA Zip 93105, Mailing Address: P.O. Box 689, Zip 93102–0689; tel. 805/569–7290; Ronald C. Werft, President and Chief Executive Officer
(Independent Hospital System)

CALIFORNIA: GOLETA VALLEY COTTAGE HOSPITAL (O, 177 beds) 351 South Patterson Avenue, Santa Barbara, CA Zip 93111–2496, Mailing Address: Box 6306, Zip 93160–6306; tel. 805/967–3411; Ronald C. Werft, President and Chief Executive Officer
Web address: www.sbch.org

SANTA BARBARA COTTAGE HOSPITAL (O, 353 beds) Pueblo at Bath Streets, Santa Barbara, CA Zip 93105–4390, Mailing Address: P.O. Box 689, Zip 93102–0689; tel. 805/682–7111; Ronald C. Werft, President and Chief Executive Officer
Web address: www.cottagehealthsystem.org

SANTA YNEZ VALLEY COTTAGE HOSPITAL (O, 20 beds) 2050 Viborg Road, Solvang, CA Zip 93463–2295; tel. 805/688–6431; Wende Cappetta, Administrator
Web address: www.cottagehealthsystem.org

Owned, leased, sponsored:	3 hospitals	550 beds
Contract-managed:	0 hospitals	0 beds
Totals:	3 hospitals	550 beds

★0123: COVENANT HEALTH (NP)

100 Fort Sanders West Boulevard, Knoxville, TN Zip 37922; tel. 865/531–5555; Anthony L. Spezia, President and Chief Executive Officer
(Centralized Physician/Insurance Health System)

TENNESSEE: FORT LOUDOUN MEDICAL CENTER (L, 32 beds) 550 Fort Loudoun Medical Center Drive, Lenoir City, TN Zip 37772–5673; tel. 865/271–6000; Jeffrey Feike, President and Chief Administrative Officer
Web address: www.covenanthealth.com

FORT SANDERS REGIONAL MEDICAL CENTER (O, 351 beds) 1901 Clinch Avenue S.W., Knoxville, TN Zip 37916–2394; tel. 865/541–1111; Keith Altshuler, President and Chief Administrative Officer
Web address: www.covenanthealth.com

FORT SANDERS–SEVIER MEDICAL CENTER (L, 108 beds) 709 Middle Creek Road, Sevierville, TN Zip 37862–5016, Mailing Address: P.O. Box 8005, Zip 37864–8005; tel. 865/429–6100; Ellen Wilhoit, President and Chief Administrative Officer
Web address: www.covenanthealth.com

METHODIST MEDICAL CENTER OF OAK RIDGE (O, 225 beds) 990 Oak Ridge Turnpike, Oak Ridge, TN Zip 37830–6976, Mailing Address: P.O. Box 2529, Zip 37831–2529; tel. 865/835–1000; Michael Belbeck, President and Chief Administrative Officer
Web address: www.mmcoakridge.com

PARKWEST MEDICAL CENTER (O, 274 beds) 9352 Park West Boulevard, Knoxville, TN Zip 37923–4325, Mailing Address: P.O. Box 22993, Zip 37933–0993; tel. 865/373–1000; Rick Lassiter, President and Chief Administrative Officer
Web address: www.yesparkwest.com

Owned, leased, sponsored:	5 hospitals	990 beds
Contract-managed:	0 hospitals	0 beds
Totals:	5 hospitals	990 beds

★0036: COVENANT HEALTH SYSTEM (NP)

3615 19th Street, Lubbock, TX Zip 79410–1201; tel. 806/725–0447; Melinda Clark, FACHE, President and Chief Executive Officer
(Decentralized Health System)

NEW MEXICO: NOR–LEA GENERAL HOSPITAL (C, 12 beds) 1600 North Main Avenue, Lovington, NM Zip 88260–2871; tel. 505/396–6611; David B. Shaw, Chief Executive Officer and Administrator
Web address: www.nlgh.org

ROOSEVELT GENERAL HOSPITAL (C, 22 beds) 14121 U.S. Highway 70, Portales, NM Zip 88130, Mailing Address: P.O. Box 868, Zip 88130–0868; tel. 575/359–1800; James P. D'Agostino, Chief Executive Officer

TEXAS: COVENANT CHILDREN'S HOSPITAL (O, 79 beds) 3610 21st Street, Lubbock, TX Zip 79410–1218; tel. 806/725–1011; Melinda Clark, FACHE, President and Chief Executive Officer
Web address: www.covenanthealth.org

COVENANT HOSPITAL PLAINVIEW (L, 34 beds) 2601 Dimmitt Road, Plainview, TX Zip 79072–1833; tel. 806/296–5531; Jonathan O. Wade, Chief Executive Officer
Web address: www.covenantplainview.org

COVENANT HOSPITAL–LEVELLAND (L, 22 beds) 1900 South College Avenue, Levelland, TX Zip 79336–6508; tel. 806/894–4963; Jerry Osburn, Administrator
Web address: www.covenanthealth.org

COVENANT MEDICAL CENTER (O, 696 beds) 3615 19th Street, Lubbock, TX Zip 79410–1201, Mailing Address: P.O. Box 1201, Zip 79408–1201; tel. 806/725–1011; Melinda Clark, FACHE, President and Chief Executive Officer
Web address: www.covenanthealth.org

CROSBYTON CLINIC HOSPITAL (C, 25 beds) 710 West Main Street, Crosbyton, TX Zip 79322–2143; tel. 806/675–2382; Steve Beck, Chief Executive Officer

LAMB HEALTHCARE CENTER (C, 41 beds) 1500 South Sunset, Littlefield, TX Zip 79339–4899; tel. 806/385–6411; Jo Nell Wischkaemper, Administrator

MEDICAL ARTS HOSPITAL (C, 29 beds) 1600 North Bryan Avenue, Lamesa, TX Zip 79331–3145; tel. 806/872–2183; Charles N. Butts, Chief Executive Officer
Web address: www.medicalartshospital.org

MULESHOE AREA MEDICAL CENTER (C, 25 beds) 708 South First Street, Muleshoe, TX Zip 79347; tel. 806/272–4524; Ray Mason, Administrator and Chief Executive Officer
Web address: www.mahdtx.org

YOAKUM COUNTY HOSPITAL (C, 22 beds) 412 Mustang Avenue, Denver City, TX Zip 79323–2750, Mailing Address: P.O. Drawer 1130, Zip 79323–1130; tel. 806/592–2121; Clay Taylor, Chief Executive Officer
Web address: www.ych.us

Owned, leased, sponsored:	4 hospitals	831 beds
Contract-managed:	7 hospitals	176 beds
Totals:	11 hospitals	1007 beds

★5885: COVENANT HEALTH SYSTEMS, INC. (CC)

420 Bedford Street, Lexington, MA Zip 02420–1502; tel. 781/862–1634; David R. Lincoln, President and Chief Executive Officer
(Moderately Centralized Health System)

MAINE: ST. MARY'S REGIONAL MEDICAL CENTER (O, 171 beds) 330 Sabattus Street, Lewiston, ME Zip 4240, Mailing Address: P.O. Box 291, Zip 04243–0291; tel. 207/777–8100; Lee T. Myles, Chief Executive Officer
Web address: www.stmarysmaine.com

MASSACHUSETTS: YOUVILLE HOSPITAL AND REHABILITATION CENTER (O, 150 beds) 1575 Cambridge Street, Cambridge, MA Zip 02138–4398; tel. 617/876–4344; Daniel P. Leahey, President and Chief Executive Officer
Web address: www.youville.org

For explanation of codes following names, see page B2.
★ Indicates Type III membership in the American Hospital Association.

Section B

NEW HAMPSHIRE: ST. JOSEPH HOSPITAL (O, 144 beds) 172 Kinsley Street, Nashua, NH Zip 03060–3688; tel. 603/882–3000; Peter B. Davis, President and Chief Executive Officer
Web address: www.stjosephhealthcare.com

Owned, leased, sponsored:	3 hospitals	465 beds
Contract–managed:	0 hospitals	0 beds
Totals:	3 hospitals	465 beds

0179: COXHEALTH (NP)
1423 North Jefferson Avenue, Springfield, MO Zip 65802–1988; tel. 417/269–3108; Robert H. Bezanson, President and Chief Executive Officer
(Centralized Health System)

MISSOURI: COX MONETT HOSPITAL (O, 25 beds) 801 Lincoln Avenue, Monett, MO Zip 65708–1641; tel. 417/235–3144; Gregory D. Johnson, Administrator and Chief Executive Officer
Web address: www.coxhealth.com

LESTER E. COX MEDICAL CENTERS (O, 623 beds) 1423 North Jefferson Street, Springfield, MO Zip 65802–1988; tel. 417/269–3000; Robert H. Bezanson, President and Chief Executive Officer
Web address: www.coxhealth.com

Owned, leased, sponsored:	2 hospitals	648 beds
Contract–managed:	0 hospitals	0 beds
Totals:	2 hospitals	648 beds

★0008: CROZER–KEYSTONE HEALTH SYSTEM (NP)
100 West Sproul Road, Springfield, PA Zip 19064; tel. 610/338–8205; Joan K. Richards, President and Chief Executive Officer
(Moderately Centralized Health System)

PENNSYLVANIA: CROZER–CHESTER MEDICAL CENTER (O, 554 beds) One Medical Center Boulevard, Upland, PA Zip 19013–3995; tel. 610/447–2000; Joseph Saunders, President
Web address: www.crozer.org

DELAWARE COUNTY MEMORIAL HOSPITAL (O, 214 beds) 501 North Lansdowne Avenue, Drexel Hill, PA Zip 19026–1114; tel. 610/284–8100; William McCune, President
Web address: www.crozer.org

Owned, leased, sponsored:	2 hospitals	768 beds
Contract–managed:	0 hospitals	0 beds
Totals:	2 hospitals	768 beds

0334: CYPRESS HEALTH SYSTEMS (IO)
106 Preston Day Circle, Benton, LA Zip 71006; tel. 318/965–9914; Kim B. Bird, President and Chief Executive Officer
(Independent Hospital System)

FLORIDA: NATURE COAST REGIONAL HOSPITAL (O, 40 beds) 125 S.W. Seventh Street, Williston, FL Zip 32696–2403; tel. 352/528–2801; Kim B. Bird, Administrator
Web address: www.cypress–of–fl.com

MONTANA: POWELL COUNTY MEDICAL CENTER (O, 35 beds) 1101 Texas Avenue, Deer Lodge, MT Zip 59722–1828; tel. 406/846–2212; Mike Walsh, Chief Executive Officer
Web address: www.pcmh.org

NORTH DAKOTA: SAKAKAWEA MEDICAL CENTER (O, 25 beds) 510 Eighth Avenue N.E., Hazen, ND Zip 58545–4637; tel. 701/748–2225; James L. Marshall, Chief Executive Officer
Web address: www.sakmedcenter.com

OKLAHOMA: FAIRVIEW REGIONAL MEDICAL CENTER (O, 25 beds) 523 East State Road, Fairview, OK Zip 73737–1498, Mailing Address: P.O. Box 548, Zip 73737–0548; tel. 580/227–3721; Roger Knak, Administrator
Web address: www.fairviewhospital.net

Owned, leased, sponsored:	4 hospitals	125 beds
Contract–managed:	0 hospitals	0 beds
Totals:	4 hospitals	125 beds

★1075: DAUGHTERS OF CHARITY HEALTH SYSTEM (CC)
26000 Altamont Road, Los Altos Hills, CA Zip 94022; tel. 650/917–4500; Robert Issai, President and Chief Executive Officer
(Moderately Centralized Health System)

CALIFORNIA: O'CONNOR HOSPITAL (O, 248 beds) 2105 Forest Avenue, San Jose, CA Zip 95128–1471; tel. 408/947–2500; Robert H. Curry, President and Chief Executive Officer
Web address: www.oconnorhospital.org

SETON MEDICAL CENTER (O, 263 beds) 1900 Sullivan Avenue, Daly City, CA Zip 94015–2229; tel. 650/992–4000; Bernadette M. Smith, President and Chief Executive Officer
Web address: www.setonmedicalcenter.org

SETON MEDICAL CENTER COASTSIDE (O, 121 beds) 600 Marine Boulevard, Moss Beach, CA Zip 94038–9641; tel. 650/563–7100; Bernadette M. Smith, President and Chief Executive Officer
Web address: www.setonmedicalcenter.com/coastside

ST. FRANCIS MEDICAL CENTER (O, 384 beds) 3630 East Imperial Highway, Lynwood, CA Zip 90262–2636; tel. 310/900–8900; Gerald T. Kozai, President
Web address: www.dochs.org

ST. LOUISE REGIONAL HOSPITAL (O, 83 beds) 9400 No Name Uno, Gilroy, CA Zip 95020–3528; tel. 408/848–2000; Joanne E. Allen, President and Chief Executive Officer
Web address: www.dochs.org

ST. VINCENT MEDICAL CENTER (O, 318 beds) 2131 West Third Street, Los Angeles, CA Zip 90057–7992, Mailing Address: P.O. Box 57992, Zip 90057–7992; tel. 213/484–7111; Catherine Fickes, RN, President and Chief Executive Officer
Web address: www.stvincentmedicalcenter.com

Owned, leased, sponsored:	6 hospitals	1417 beds
Contract–managed:	0 hospitals	0 beds
Totals:	6 hospitals	1417 beds

1825: DCH HEALTH SYSTEM (NP)
809 University Boulevard East, Tuscaloosa, AL Zip 35401; tel. 205/759–7111; Bryan N. Kindred, President and Chief Executive Officer
(Moderately Centralized Health System)

ALABAMA: DCH REGIONAL MEDICAL CENTER (O, 455 beds) 809 University Boulevard East, Tuscaloosa, AL Zip 35401–9961; tel. 205/759–7111; William H. Cassels, Administrator
Web address: www.dchsystem.com

FAYETTE MEDICAL CENTER (L, 169 beds) 1653 Temple Avenue North, Fayette, AL Zip 35555–1314, Mailing Address: P.O. Drawer 710, Zip 35555–0710; tel. 205/932–5966; Barry S. Cochran, FACHE, Administrator
Web address: www.dchsystem.com

NORTHPORT MEDICAL CENTER (O, 196 beds) 2700 Hospital Drive, Northport, AL Zip 35476; tel. 205/333–4500; Luke Standeffer, Administrator
Web address: www.dchsystem.com

Owned, leased, sponsored:	3 hospitals	820 beds
Contract–managed:	0 hospitals	0 beds
Totals:	3 hospitals	820 beds

★0313: DEACONESS HEALTH SYSTEM (NP)
600 Mary Street, Evansville, IN Zip 47747; tel. 812/450–5000; Linda E. White, President and Chief Executive Officer
(Centralized Health System)

INDIANA: DEACONESS HOSPITAL (O, 541 beds) 600 Mary Street, Evansville, IN Zip 47747–0001; tel. 812/450–5000; Harry L. Smith, Jr., President and Chief Executive Officer
Web address: www.deaconess.com

THE WOMEN'S HOSPITAL (O, 74 beds) 4199 Gateway Boulevard, Newburgh, IN Zip 47630; tel. 812/842–4200; Christina M. Ryan, Chief Executive Officer
Web address: www.deaconess.com

For explanation of codes following names, see page B2.
★ Indicates Type III membership in the American Hospital Association.

Owned, leased, sponsored:	2 hospitals	615 beds
Contract-managed:	0 hospitals	0 beds
Totals:	2 hospitals	615 beds

0330: DEKALB REGIONAL HEALTH SYSTEM (NP)

2701 North Decatur Road, Decatur, GA Zip 30033; tel. 404/501–1000; Eric P. Norwood, President and Chief Executive Officer
(Independent Hospital System)

GEORGIA: DEKALB MEDICAL CENTER (O, 417 beds) 2701 North Decatur Road, Decatur, GA Zip 30033–5995; tel. 404/501–1000; Eric P. Norwood, President and Chief Executive Officer
Web address: www.dekalbmedicalcenter.org

DEKALB MEDICAL CENTER AT DECATUR (O, 76 beds) 450 North Candler Street, Decatur, GA Zip 30030–2671; tel. 404/501–6700; Brent Robinson, Vice President
Web address: www.dekalbmedicalcenter.org

DEKALB MEDICAL CENTER AT HILLANDALE (O, 100 beds) 2801 DeKalb Medical Parkway, Lithonia, GA Zip 30058; tel. 404/501–8700; Clay Fowler, Vice President and Administrator
Web address: www.dekalbmedicalcenter.org

Owned, leased, sponsored:	3 hospitals	593 beds
Contract-managed:	0 hospitals	0 beds
Totals:	3 hospitals	593 beds

9495: DEPARTMENT OF THE AIR FORCE (FG)

1420 Pentagon, Room 4E1084, Washington, DC Zip 20330–1420; tel. 202/767–4765; Lieutenant General James G. Roudebush, M.D., Surgeon General
(Independent Hospital System)

ALASKA: U. S. AIR FORCE REGIONAL HOSPITAL (O, 64 beds) 5955 Zeamer Avenue, Elmendorf AFB, AK Zip 99506–3700; tel. 907/560–6260; Colonel Elisha Powell, Commander
Web address: www.elmendorf.af.mil/

CALIFORNIA: DAVID GRANT MEDICAL CENTER (O, 84 beds) 101 Bodin Circle, Travis AFB, CA Zip 94535–1800; tel. 707/423–7300; Colonel Michael R. Skidmore, Administrator

COLORADO: U. S. AIR FORCE ACADEMY HOSPITAL (O, 27 beds) 4102 Pinion Drive, USAF Academy, CO Zip 80840–4000; tel. 719/333–5102; Colonel Alan B. Berg, Commander
Web address: www.usafa.af.mil

FLORIDA: U. S. AIR FORCE REGIONAL HOSPITAL (O, 61 beds) 307 Boatner Road, Suite 114, Eglin AFB, FL Zip 32542–1282; tel. 850/883–8221; Tama Van Decar, M.D., Commander
Web address: www.eglin.af.mil

ILLINOIS: SCOTT MEDICAL CENTER (O, 18 beds) 310 West Losey Street, Scott AFB, IL Zip 62225–5252; tel. 618/256–7000; Colonel Diane C. Ritter, Commanding Officer
Web address: www.public.scott.amc.af.mil

MARYLAND: MALCOLM GROW MEDICAL CENTER (O, 60 beds) 1050 West Perimeter, Andrews AFB, MD Zip 20762–6600, Mailing Address: 1050 West Perimeter, Suite A1–19, Zip 20762–6600; tel. 240/857–3001; Colonel Robert I. Miller, Commanding Officer
Web address: www.mgmc.af.mil

MISSISSIPPI: U. S. AIR FORCE MEDICAL CENTER KEESLER (O, 185 beds) 301 Fisher Street, Suite 1A132, Keesler AFB, MS Zip 39534–2519; tel. 228/377–1110; Colonel Anthony S. Lonigro, MSC, USAF, Administrator
Web address: www.keesler.af.mil

NEVADA: MIKE O'CALLAGHAN FEDERAL HOSPITAL (O, 102 beds) 4700 Las Vegas Boulevard North, Suite 2419, Nellis AFB, NV Zip 89191–6601; tel. 702/653–2000; Colonel Christian Benjamin, USAF, MC, Commander

OHIO: WRIGHT PATTERSON MEDICAL CENTER (O, 70 beds) 4881 Sugar Maple Drive, Wright-Patterson AFB, OH Zip 45433–5529; tel. 937/257–9133; Colonel Mark S. White, Administrator
Web address: www.wpmc1.wpafb.af.mil

TEXAS: WILFORD HALL MEDICAL CENTER (O, 284 beds) 2200 Bergquist Drive, Suite 1, San Antonio, TX Zip 78236–9908; tel. 210/292–7412; Brigadier General David G. Young, MC, USAF, Commander

VIRGINIA: U. S. AIR FORCE HOSPITAL (O, 59 beds) 45 Pine Street, Hampton, VA Zip 23665–2080; tel. 757/764–6969; Colonel David C. Houglum, MC, Administrator

Owned, leased, sponsored:	11 hospitals	1014 beds
Contract-managed:	0 hospitals	0 beds
Totals:	11 hospitals	1014 beds

9395: DEPARTMENT OF THE ARMY, OFFICE OF THE SURGEON GENERAL (FG)

5109 Leesburg Pike, Falls Church, VA Zip 22041; tel. 703/681–3000; Lieutenant General Eric B. Schoomaker, Surgeon General
(Moderately Centralized Health System)

ALASKA: BASSETT ARMY COMMUNITY HOSPITAL (O, 24 beds) 1060 Gaffney Road, Box 7400, Fort Wainwright, AK Zip 99703–7400, Mailing Address: 1060 Gaffney Road, Building 7440, Zip 99703–7440; tel. 907/361–5172; Lieutenant Colonel Jeffrey Hillard, Deputy Commander for Administration
Web address: www.alaska.amedd.army.mil

CALIFORNIA: WEED ARMY COMMUNITY HOSPITAL (O, 27 beds) Inner Loop Road and 4th Street, Bl 166, Fort Irwin, CA Zip 92310–5065, Mailing Address: P.O. Box 105109, Zip 92310–5109; tel. 760/380–3108; Colonel Margaret Bates, Commanding Officer
Web address: www.irwin.amedd.army.mil

COLORADO: EVANS U. S. ARMY COMMUNITY HOSPITAL (O, 78 beds) 1650 Cochrane Circle, Building 7500, Fort Carson, CO Zip 80913–5101; tel. 719/526–7200; Colonel John Cho, Commander
Web address: www.evans.amedd.army.mil

DISTRICT OF COLUMBIA: WALTER REED ARMY MEDICAL CENTER (O, 256 beds) 6900 Georgia Avenue N.W., Washington, DC Zip 20307–5001; tel. 202/782–6395; Colonel Patricia Horoho, Commander
Web address: www.wramc.amedd.army.mil

GEORGIA: DWIGHT DAVID EISENHOWER ARMY MEDICAL CENTER (O, 95 beds) Hospital Drive, Fort Gordon, GA Zip 30905–5650; tel. 706/787–5811; Brigadier General Donald M. Bradshaw, Commander
Web address: www.ddeamc.amedd.army.mil

MARTIN ARMY COMMUNITY HOSPITAL (O, 57 beds) 7950 Martin Loop, Fort Benning, GA Zip 31905–6100; tel. 706/544–2516; Colonel Margaret Rivera, Commander
Web address: www.martin.amedd.army.mil

WINN ARMY COMMUNITY HOSPITAL (O, 79 beds) 1061 Harmon Avenue, Hinesville, GA Zip 31314–5611; tel. 912/435–6965; Colonel John P. Collins, Commander
Web address: www.winn.amedd.army.mil/

HAWAII: TRIPLER ARMY MEDICAL CENTER (O, 180 beds) 1 Jarret White Road, Honolulu, HI Zip 96859–5000; tel. 808/433–6661; ,
Web address: www.tamc.amedd.army.mil

KANSAS: IRWIN ARMY COMMUNITY HOSPITAL (O, 44 beds) 600 Caisson Hill Road, Junction City, KS Zip 66442–5037; tel. 785/239–7000; Colonel Dawn Smith, Chief Executive Officer
Web address: www.iach.amedd.army.mil/

KENTUCKY: COLONEL FLORENCE A. BLANCHFIELD ARMY COMMUNITY HOSPITAL (O, 66 beds) 650 Joel Drive, Fort Campbell, KY Zip 42223; tel. 270/798–8040; Colonel Richard Thomas, Commander
Web address: www.campbell.amedd.army.mil/

IRELAND ARMY COMMUNITY HOSPITAL (O, 76 beds) 289 Ireland Avenue, Fort Knox, KY Zip 40121–5111; tel. 502/624–0467; Colonel Rhonda Earls, Commander
Web address: www.iach.knox.amedd.army.mil/

LOUISIANA: BAYNE–JONES ARMY COMMUNITY HOSPITAL (O, 44 beds) 1585 Third Street, Fort Polk, LA Zip 71459–5110; tel. 337/531–3928; Colonel William K. Statz, Commander
Web address: www.polk.amedd.army.mil

For explanation of codes following names, see page B2.
★ Indicates Type III membership in the American Hospital Association.

Section B

MARSHALL ISLANDS: KWAJALEIN HOSPITAL (O, 14 beds) U.S. Army Kwajalein Atoll, Kwajalein Island, MH Zip 96960, Mailing Address: Box 1702, APO, APZip 96555–5000; tel. 805/355–2225; Elaine McMahon, Administrator

MISSOURI: GENERAL LEONARD WOOD ARMY COMMUNITY HOSPITAL (O, 42 beds) 126 Missouri Avenue, Fort Leonard Wood, MO Zip 65473–8952; tel. 573/596–0414; Lieutenant Colonel Margaret Toillion, Interim Deputy Commander
Web address: www.amedd.army.mil

NEW YORK: KELLER ARMY COMMUNITY HOSPITAL (O, 31 beds) 900 Washington Road, West Point, NY Zip 10996–1197; tel. 845/938–5169; Colonel Van Coots, Commanding Officer
Web address: www.usma.edu/meddac/

NORTH CAROLINA: WOMACK ARMY MEDICAL CENTER (O, 156 beds) Normandy Drive, Fort Bragg, NC Zip 28307–5000; tel. 910/907–6000; Colonel Terry Walters, Commander
Web address: www.wamc.amedd.army.mil/

OKLAHOMA: REYNOLDS ARMY COMMUNITY HOSPITAL (O, 46 beds) 4301 Mow Way Road, Fort Sill, OK Zip 73503–6300; tel. 580/458–3000; Colonel Ellen E. Forster, Commander
Web address: www.rach.sill.amedd.army.mil

SOUTH CAROLINA: MONCRIEF ARMY COMMUNITY HOSPITAL (O, 60 beds) 4500 Stuart Street, Fort Jackson, SC Zip 29207–5720; tel. 803/751–2284; Colonel James A. Mundy, Commander
Web address: www.moncrief.amedd.army.mil

TEXAS: BROOKE ARMY MEDICAL CENTER (O, 226 beds) 3851 Roger Brookes Drive, Fort Sam Houston, TX Zip 78234–6200; tel. 210/916–4141; Brigadier General James K. Gilman, Commander
Web address: www.bamc.amedd.army.mil

CARL R. DARNALL ARMY MEDICAL CENTER (O, 109 beds) 36000 Darnall Loop, Fort Hood, TX Zip 76544–4752; tel. 254/288–8000; Colonel Casper P. Jones, III, Commander
Web address: www.hood–meddac.army.mil

WILLIAM BEAUMONT ARMY MEDICAL CENTER (O, 209 beds) 5005 North Piedras Street, El Paso, TX Zip 79920–5001; tel. 915/569–2121; Colonel John A. Powell, Commanding Officer
Web address: www.wbamc.amedd.army.mil

VIRGINIA: DEWITT ARMY COMMUNITY HOSPITAL (O, 46 beds) 9501 Farrell Road, Fort Belvoir, VA Zip 22060–5901; tel. 703/805–0510; Colonel Kenneth Canestrini, Commander
Web address: www.dewitt.wramc.amedd.army.mil

WASHINGTON: MADIGAN ARMY MEDICAL CENTER (O, 205 beds) Fitzsimmons Drive, Building 9040, Tacoma, WA Zip 98431–1100; tel. 253/968–1110; Brigadier General Sheila R. Baxter, Commanding General
Web address: www.mamc.amedd.army.mil

Owned, leased, sponsored:	23 hospitals	2170 beds
Contract–managed:	0 hospitals	0 beds
Totals:	23 hospitals	2170 beds

9295: DEPARTMENT OF VETERANS AFFAIRS (FG)

810 Vermont Avenue N.W., Washington, DC Zip 20420; tel. 202/273–5781; Michael J. Kussman, M.D., Acting Undersecretary for Health
(Decentralized Health System)

ALABAMA: CENTRAL ALABAMA VETERANS HEALTH CARE SYSTEM (O, 330 beds) 215 Perry Hill Road, Montgomery, AL Zip 36109–3798; tel. 334/272–4670; N. Rao Chava, M.D., Director
Web address: www.va.gov/sta/guide/home.asp

VETERANS AFFAIRS MEDICAL CENTER (O, 144 beds) 700 South 19th Street, Birmingham, AL Zip 35233–1927; tel. 205/933–8101; Robert W. Ratliff, Ph.D., FACHE, Interim Director
Web address: www.va.gov/sta/guide/home.asp

VETERANS AFFAIRS MEDICAL CENTER (O, 381 beds) 3701 Loop Road, Tuscaloosa, AL Zip 35404–5015; tel. 205/554–2000; Alan J. Tyler, M.S., FACHE, Director
Web address: www.tuscaloosa.va.gov

ARIZONA: NORTHERN ARIZONA VA HEALTH CARE SYSTEM (O, 236 beds) 500 Highway 89 North, Prescott, AZ Zip 86313–5000; tel. 928/445–4860; Susan Angell, Ph.D., Director
Web address: www.va.gov/sta/guide/home.asp

PHOENIX VETERANS AFFAIRS HEALTH CARE SYSTEM (O, 177 beds) 650 East Indian School Road, Phoenix, AZ Zip 85012–1892; tel. 602/277–5551; Donald F. Moore, Medical Center Director
Web address: www.phoenix.med.va.gov

SOUTHERN ARIZONA VETERANS AFFAIRS HEALTH CARE SYSTEM (O, 283 beds) 3601 South 6th Avenue, Tucson, AZ Zip 85723–0002; tel. 520/792–1450; Jonathan H. Gardner, Chief Executive Officer
Web address: www.tucson.va.gov

ARKANSAS: CENTRAL ARKANSAS VETERANS HEALTHCARE SYSTEM (O, 583 beds) 4300 West Seventh Street, Little Rock, AR Zip 72205–5484; tel. 501/257–1000; Michael R. Winn, Director
Web address: www.va.gov/sta/guide/home.asp

VETERANS AFFAIRS MEDICAL CENTER (O, 70 beds) 1100 North College Avenue, Fayetteville, AR Zip 72703–6995; tel. 479/443–4301; Kathleen R. Fogarty, M.S., Director
Web address: www.va.gov/sta/guide/home.asp

CALIFORNIA: JERRY L. PETTIS MEMORIAL VETERANS MEDICAL CENTER (O, 205 beds) 11201 Benton Street, Loma Linda, CA Zip 92357; tel. 909/825–7084; Dwight Evans, M.D., Acting Director
Web address: www.lomalinda.va.gov

VETERANS AFFAIRS GREATER LOS ANGELES HEALTHCARE SYSTEM (O, 1327 beds) 11301 Wilshire Boulevard, Los Angeles, CA Zip 90073–1003; tel. 310/478–3711; Donna M. Beiter, RN, M.S.N., Acting Director
Web address: www.va.gov/sta/guide/home.asp

VETERANS AFFAIRS LONG BEACH HEALTHCARE SYSTEM (O, 333 beds) 5901 East Seventh Street, Long Beach, CA Zip 90822–5201; tel. 562/826–8000; Isabel Duff, M.S., Acting Director
Web address: www.va.gov/sta/guide/home.asp

VETERANS AFFAIRS MEDICAL CENTER (O, 125 beds) 2615 East Clinton Avenue, Fresno, CA Zip 93703–2223; tel. 559/225–6100; Alan S. Perry, Director
Web address: www.va.gov/sta/guide/home.asp

VETERANS AFFAIRS MEDICAL CENTER (O, 244 beds) 4150 Clement Street, San Francisco, CA Zip 94121–1598; tel. 415/221–4810; Sheila M. Cullen, Director
Web address: www.va.gov/sta/guide/home.asp

VETERANS AFFAIRS PALO ALTO HEALTH CARE SYSTEM (O, 967 beds) 3801 Miranda Avenue, Palo Alto, CA Zip 94304–1207; tel. 650/493–5000; Elizabeth Joyce Freeman, Director
Web address: www.va.gov/sta/guide/home.asp

VETERANS AFFAIRS SAN DIEGO HEALTHCARE SYSTEM (O, 238 beds) 3350 LaJolla Village Drive, San Diego, CA Zip 92161–0002; tel. 858/552–8585; Gary J. Rossio, Director
Web address: www.sandiego.va.gov

COLORADO: VETERANS AFFAIRS EASTERN COLORADO HEALTH CARE SYSTEM (O, 222 beds) 1055 Clermont Street, Denver, CO Zip 80220–3877; tel. 303/399–8020; Lynette A. Roff, Director
Web address: www.va.gov/sta/guide/home.asp

VETERANS AFFAIRS MEDICAL CENTER (O, 53 beds) 2121 North Avenue, Grand Junction, CO Zip 81501–6499; tel. 970/242–0731; William R. Berryman, M.D., Acting Director
Web address: www.va.gov/sta/guide/home.asp

CONNECTICUT: VETERANS AFFAIRS CONNECTICUT HEALTHCARE SYSTEM–NEW HAVEN DIVISION (O, 200 beds) 950 Campbell Avenue, West Haven, CT Zip 06516–2770; tel. 203/932–5711; Roger L. Johnson, Director
Web address: www.va.gov/sta/guide/home.asp

DELAWARE: VETERANS AFFAIRS MEDICAL CENTER (O, 120 beds) 1601 Kirkwood Highway, Wilmington, DE Zip 19805–4989; tel. 302/994–2511; Charles M. Dorman, FACHE, Director
Web address: www.va.gov/wilmington

DISTRICT OF COLUMBIA: VETERANS AFFAIRS MEDICAL CENTER (O, 291 beds) 50 Irving Street N.W., Washington, DC Zip 20422–0002; tel. 202/745–8100; Fernando O. Rivera, Director
Web address: www.va.gov/sta/guide/home.asp

For explanation of codes following names, see page B2.
★ Indicates Type III membership in the American Hospital Association.

FLORIDA: JAMES A. HALEY VETERANS HOSPITAL (O, 321 beds) 13000 Bruce B. Downs Boulevard, Tampa, FL Zip 33612–4798; tel. 813/972–2000; Stephen M. Lucas, FACHE, Director
Web address: www.va.gov/visn8/tampa

MALCOM RANDALL VETERANS AFFAIRS MEDICAL CENTER (O, 535 beds) 1601 S.W. Archer Road, Gainesville, FL Zip 32608–1197; tel. 352/376–1611; Frederick L. Malphurs, Director
Web address: www.va.gov/visn8/nfsg

VETERANS AFFAIRS MEDICAL CENTER (O, 461 beds) 10000 Bay Pines Boulevard, Bay Pines, FL Zip 33744, Mailing Address: P.O. Box 5005, Zip 33744–5005; tel. 727/398–6661; Wallace M. Hopkins, FACHE, Director
Web address: www.baypines.va.gov/

VETERANS AFFAIRS MEDICAL CENTER (O, 231 beds) 7305 North Military Trail, West Palm Beach, FL Zip 33410–6400; tel. 561/422–8262; Charleen R. Szabo, FACHE, Director
Web address: www.va.gov/sta/guide/home.asp

VETERANS AFFAIRS MEDICAL CENTER (O, 339 beds) 1201 N.W. 16th Street, Miami, FL Zip 33125–1624; tel. 305/575–7000; Mary D. Berrocal, Director
Web address: www.va.gov/miami

VETERANS AFFAIRS MEDICAL CENTER (O, 360 beds) 619 South Marion Avenue, Lake City, FL Zip 32025–5898; tel. 386/755–3016; Thomas A. Cappello, M.P.H., FACHE, Director
Web address: www.va.gov/sta/guide/home.asp

GEORGIA: CARL VINSON VETERANS AFFAIRS MEDICAL CENTER (O, 339 beds) 1826 Veterans Boulevard, Dublin, GA Zip 31021–3620; tel. 478/272–1210; Kelly O. Duke, Acting Director
Web address: www.va.gov/sta/guide/home.asp

VETERANS AFFAIRS MEDICAL CENTER (O, 239 beds) 1670 Clairmont Road, Decatur, GA Zip 30033–4004; tel. 404/321–6111; Thomas A. Cappello, M.P.H., FACHE, Director
Web address: www.va.gov/sta/guide/home.asp

VETERANS AFFAIRS MEDICAL CENTER (O, 470 beds) 1 Freedom Way, Augusta, GA Zip 30904–6285; tel. 706/733–0188; John S. Goldman, Associate Director
Web address: www.va.gov/sta/guide/home.asp

IDAHO: VETERANS AFFAIRS MEDICAL CENTER (O, 176 beds) 500 West Fort Street, Boise, ID Zip 83702–4598; tel. 208/422–1000; Dewayne Hamlin, Director
Web address: www.va.gov/directory/guide/home.asp

ILLINOIS: JESSE BROWN VETERANS AFFAIRS CHICAGO HEALTH CARE SYSTEM (O, 241 beds) 820 South Damen, Chicago, IL Zip 60612–3776; tel. 312/569–8387; James S. Jones, Medical Center Director
Web address: www.va.gov/sta/guide/home.asp

VETERANS AFFAIRS EDWARD HINES, JR. HOSPITAL (O, 484 beds) Fifth Avenue and Roosevelt Road, Hines, IL Zip 60141–5000, Mailing Address: P.O. Box 5000, Zip 60141–5000; tel. 708/202–8387; Nathan L. Geraths, Director
Web address: www.va.gov/sta/guide/home.asp

VETERANS AFFAIRS ILLIANA HEALTH CARE SYSTEM (O, 346 beds) 1900 East Main Street, Danville, IL Zip 61832–5198; tel. 217/554–3000; Michael E. Hamilton, Director
Web address: www.va.gov/sta/guide/home.asp

VETERANS AFFAIRS MEDICAL CENTER (O, 103 beds) 3001 Green Bay Road, North Chicago, IL Zip 60064–3049; tel. 847/688–1900; Patrick L. Sullivan, Director
Web address: www.va.gov/sta/guide/home.asp

VETERANS AFFAIRS MEDICAL CENTER (O, 115 beds) 2401 West Main Street, Marion, IL Zip 62959–1194; tel. 618/997–5311; Robert D. Morrel, Director
Web address: www.va.gov/sta/guide/home.asp

INDIANA: RICHARD L. ROUDEBUSH VETERANS AFFAIRS MEDICAL CENTER (O, 144 beds) 1481 West Tenth Street, Indianapolis, IN Zip 46202–2884; tel. 317/554–0000; Thomas Mattice, Director
Web address: www.va.gov/sta/guide/home.asp

VETERANS AFFAIRS NORTHERN INDIANA HEALTH CARE SYSTEM (O, 255 beds) 2121 Lake Avenue, Fort Wayne, IN Zip 46805–5347; tel. 260/460–1310; Cathi Spivey–Paul, Director
Web address: www.va.gov/sta/guide/home.asp

IOWA: VETERANS AFFAIRS CENTRAL IOWA HEALTH CARE SYSTEM (O, 227 beds) 3600 30th Street, Des Moines, IA Zip 50310–5774; tel. 515/699–5999; Donald C. Cooper, Director
Web address: www.va.centra/iowa.va.gov

VETERANS AFFAIRS MEDICAL CENTER (O, 93 beds) 601 Highway 6 West, Iowa City, IA Zip 52246–2208; tel. 319/338–0581; Barry Sharp, Director
Web address: www.va.gov/sta/guide/home.asp

KANSAS: ROBERT J. DOLE VETERANS AFFAIRS MEDICAL CENTER (O, 81 beds) 5500 East Kellogg, Wichita, KS Zip 67218; tel. 316/685–2221; Thomas J. Sanders, CHE, Director
Web address: www.va.gov/sta/guide/home.asp

VETERANS AFFAIRS EASTERN KANSAS HEALTH CARE SYSTEM (O, 351 beds) 2200 Gage Boulevard, Topeka, KS Zip 66622–0002; tel. 785/350–3111; Marie L. Weldon, FACHE, Director
Web address: www.va.gov/sta/guide/home.asp

KENTUCKY: VETERANS AFFAIRS MEDICAL CENTER–LEXINGTON (O, 199 beds) 1101 Veterans Drive, Lexington, KY Zip 40502; tel. 859/233–4511; Sandy Nielsen, Director
Web address: www.va.gov/sta/guide/home.asp

VETERANS AFFAIRS MEDICAL CENTER–LOUISVILLE (O, 110 beds) 800 Zorn Avenue, Louisville, KY Zip 40206–1499; tel. 502/287–4000; Wayne L. Pfeffer, FACHE, Director
Web address: www.louisville.va.gov

LOUISIANA: OVERTON BROOKS VETERANS AFFAIRS MEDICAL CENTER (O, 124 beds) 510 East Stoner Avenue, Shreveport, LA Zip 71101–4295; tel. 318/221–8411; George M. Moore, Jr., Director
Web address: www.va.gov/sta/guide/home.asp

VETERANS AFFAIRS MEDICAL CENTER (O, 292 beds) 2495 Shreveport Highway, 71 North, Pineville, LA Zip 71360, Mailing Address: P.O. Box 69004, Alexandria, Zip 71306–9004; tel. 318/473–0010; Barbara C. Watkins, Director
Web address: www.va.gov/sta/guide/home.asp

MAINE: VETERANS AFFAIRS MEDICAL CENTER (O, 167 beds) 1 VA Center, Togus, ME Zip 4330; tel. 207/623–8411; Brian Stiller, Director
Web address: www.visn1.med.va.gov/togus/

MARYLAND: VETERANS AFFAIRS MARYLAND HEALTH CARE SYSTEM–BALTIMORE DIVISION (O, 727 beds) 10 North Greene Street, Baltimore, MD Zip 21201–1524; tel. 410/605–7001; Dennis H. Smith, Director
Web address: www.va.gov/sta/guide/home.asp

MASSACHUSETTS: BROCKTON VETERANS AFFAIRS MEDICAL CENTER (O, 502 beds) 940 Belmont Street, Brockton, MA Zip 02401–5596; tel. 508/583–4500; Michael E. Lawson, Director
Web address: www.va.gov/sta/guide/home.asp

EDITH NOURSE ROGERS MEMORIAL VETERANS HOSPITAL (O, 453 beds) 200 Springs Road, Bedford, MA Zip 01730–1198; tel. 781/687–2000; Karen Y. Waghorn, Director
Web address: www.va.gov/sta/guide/home.asp

VETERANS AFFAIRS BOSTON HEALTHCARE SYSTEM (O, 502 beds) 1400 VFW Parkway, Boston, MA Zip 2132; tel. 617/232–9500; Michael M. Lawson, Director
Web address: www.va.gov/sta/guide/home.asp

VETERANS AFFAIRS MEDICAL CENTER (O, 167 beds) 421 North Main Street, Leeds, MA Zip 01053–9764; tel. 413/584–4040; Gary M. De Gasta, Acting Director
Web address: www.va.gov/sta/guide/home.asp

MICHIGAN: ALEDA E. LUTZ VETERANS AFFAIRS MEDICAL CENTER (O, 114 beds) 1500 Weiss Street, Saginaw, MI Zip 48602–5298; tel. 989/497–2500; Gabriel Perez, Medical Director
Web address: www.va.gov/sta/guide/home.asp

JOHN D. DINGELL VETERANS AFFAIRS MEDICAL CENTER (O, 217 beds) 4646 John R Street, Detroit, MI Zip 48201–1932; tel. 313/576–1000; Pamela Reeves, M.D., Director
Web address: www.va.gov/sta/guide/home.asp

VETERANS AFFAIRS ANN ARBOR HEALTHCARE SYSTEM (O, 136 beds) 2215 Fuller Road, Ann Arbor, MI Zip 48105–2399; tel. 734/769–7100; Lou Ann Atkins, Director
Web address: www.va.gov/sta/guide/home.asp

VETERANS AFFAIRS MEDICAL CENTER (O, 368 beds) 5500 Armstrong Road, Battle Creek, MI Zip 49015; tel. 269/966–5600; Alice L. Wood, Director
Web address: www.va.gov/sta/guide/home.asp

VETERANS AFFAIRS MEDICAL CENTER (O, 57 beds) 325 East H Street, Iron Mountain, MI Zip 49801–4792; tel. 906/774–3300; Michael Murphy, Director
Web address: www.va.gov/sta/guide/home.asp

For explanation of codes following names, see page B2.
★ Indicates Type III membership in the American Hospital Association.

MINNESOTA: VETERANS AFFAIRS MEDICAL CENTER (O, 365 beds) One Veterans Drive, Minneapolis, MN Zip 55417–2399; tel. 612/725–2000; Steven P. Kleinglass, Director
Web address: www.va.gov/sta/guide/home.asp

VETERANS AFFAIRS MEDICAL CENTER (O, 388 beds) 4801 Veterans Drive, Saint Cloud, MN Zip 56303–2099; tel. 320/252–1670; Barry I. Bahl, Director
Web address: www.visn13.med.va.gov

MISSISSIPPI: G.V. MONTGOMERY VETERANS AFFAIRS MEDICAL CENTER (O, 443 beds) 1500 East Woodrow Wilson Drive, Jackson, MS Zip 39216–5199; tel. 601/364–1201; Richard J. Baltz, FACHE, Center Director
Web address: www.va.gov

VETERANS AFFAIRS GULF COAST VETERANS HEALTH CARE SYSTEM (O, 552 beds) 400 Veterans Avenue, Biloxi, MS Zip 39531–2410; tel. 228/523–5000; Charles E. Sepich, FACHE, Director
Web address: www.va.gov/biloxi

MISSOURI: HARRY S. TRUMAN MEMORIAL VETERANS HOSPITAL (O, 118 beds) 800 Hospital Drive, Columbia, MO Zip 65201–5275; tel. 573/814–6000; Sallie Houser–Hanfelder, FACHE, Director
Web address: www.va.gov/cmo

JOHN J. PERSHING VETERANS AFFAIRS MEDICAL CENTER (O, 58 beds) 1500 North Westwood Boulevard, Poplar Bluff, MO Zip 63901–3318; tel. 573/686–4151; Nancy Arnold, RN, Director
Web address: www.va.gov/sta/guide/home.asp

VETERANS AFFAIRS MEDICAL CENTER (O, 339 beds) 915 North Grand, Saint Louis, MO Zip 63106–1621; tel. 314/652–4100; Glen E. Struchtemeyer, Director
Web address: www.va.gov/sta/guide/home.asp

VETERANS AFFAIRS MEDICAL CENTER (O, 157 beds) 4801 East Linwood Boulevard, Kansas City, MO Zip 64128–2226; tel. 816/861–4700; Kent D. Hill, Director
Web address: www.va.gov/sta/guide/home.asp

MONTANA: VETERANS AFFAIRS MONTANA HEALTH CARE SYSTEM (O, 80 beds) 1892 Williams Street, Fort Harrison, MT Zip 59636; tel. 406/442–6410; Joseph Underkofler, Director
Web address: www.va.gov/sta/guide/home.asp

NEBRASKA: VETERANS AFFAIRS MEDICAL CENTER (O, 202 beds) 4101 Woolworth Avenue, Omaha, NE Zip 68105–1873; tel. 402/346–8800; Albert B. Washko, Director
Web address: www.va.gov/sta/guide/home.asp

VETERANS AFFAIRS NEBRASKA–WESTERN IOWA HEALTH CARE SYSTEM (O, 186 beds) 600 South 70th Street, Lincoln, NE Zip 68510–2493; tel. 402/489–3802; Denise Harrison, Site Manager
Web address: www.va.gov/sta/guide/home.asp

NEVADA: VETERANS AFFAIRS SIERRA NEVADA HEALTH CARE SYSTEM (O, 116 beds) 1000 Locust Street, Reno, NV Zip 89502–2597; tel. 775/786–7200; Kurt W. Schlegelmilch, M.D., FACHE, Director
Web address: www.va.gov/sta/guide/home.asp

VETERANS AFFAIRS SOUTHERN NEVADA HEALTHCARE SYSTEM (O, 52 beds) North Las Vegas, NV Mailing Address: P.O. Box 360001, Zip 89036; tel. 702/636–3000; John Bright, Director
Web address: www.va.gov/sta/guide/home.asp

NEW HAMPSHIRE: VETERANS AFFAIRS MEDICAL CENTER (O, 90 beds) 718 Smyth Road, Manchester, NH Zip 03104–4098; tel. 603/624–4366; Marc Levenson, Administrator
Web address: www.va.gov/sta/guide/home.asp

NEW JERSEY: VETERANS AFFAIRS NEW JERSEY HEALTH CARE SYSTEM (O, 684 beds) 385 Tremont Avenue, East Orange, NJ Zip 07018–1095; tel. 973/676–1000; Kenneth H. Mizrach, Director
Web address: www.va.gov/sta/guide/home.asp

NEW MEXICO: VETERANS AFFAIRS MEDICAL CENTER (O, 307 beds) 1501 San Pedro S.E., Albuquerque, NM Zip 87108–5138; tel. 505/265–1711; George Marnell, Director
Web address: www.southwest.va.gov/albuquerque/

NEW YORK: VETERANS ADMINISTRATION NEW YORK HARBOR HEALTHCARE SYSTEM (O, 547 beds) 800 Poly Place, Brooklyn, NY Zip 11209–7104; tel. 718/630–3500; John J. Donnellan, Jr., Director
Web address: www.va.gov/sta/guide/home.asp

VETERANS AFFAIRS HUDSON VALLEY HEALTH CARE SYSTEM–F.D. ROOSEVELT HOSPITAL (O, 383 beds) Montrose, NY Mailing Address: P.O. Box 100, Zip 10548–0110; tel. 914/737–4400; Robert Walton, Acting Director
Web address: www.va.gov/sta/guide/home.asp

VETERANS AFFAIRS MEDICAL CENTER (O, 177 beds) 113 Holland Avenue, Albany, NY Zip 12208–3473; tel. 518/626–5000; Mary–Ellen Piche, Director
Web address: www.va.gov/sta/guide/home.asp

VETERANS AFFAIRS MEDICAL CENTER (O, 344 beds) 76 Veterans Avenue, Bath, NY Zip 14810–0842; tel. 607/664–4000; David J. West, Director
Web address: www.va.gov/sta/guide/home.asp

VETERANS AFFAIRS MEDICAL CENTER (O, 218 beds) 400 Fort Hill Avenue, Canandaigua, NY Zip 14424–1197; tel. 585/394–2000; Craig Howard, Acting Director
Web address: www.va.gov/sta/guide/home.asp

VETERANS AFFAIRS MEDICAL CENTER (O, 330 beds) 130 West Kingsbridge Road, Bronx, NY Zip 10468–3992; tel. 718/584–9000; Maryann Musumeci, Director
Web address: www.va.gov/sta/guide/home.asp

VETERANS AFFAIRS MEDICAL CENTER (O, 331 beds) 79 Middleville Road, Northport, NY Zip 11768–2293; tel. 631/261–4400; Robert Schuster, Director
Web address: www.va.gov/sta/guide/home.asp

VETERANS AFFAIRS MEDICAL CENTER (O, 167 beds) 800 Irving Avenue, Syracuse, NY Zip 13210–2796; tel. 315/425–4400; James Cody, Director
Web address: www.va.gov/sta/guide/home.asp

VETERANS AFFAIRS WESTERN NEW YORK HEALTHCARE SYSTEM–BATAVIA DIVISION (O, 158 beds) 222 Richmond Avenue, Batavia, NY Zip 14020–1288; tel. 585/297–1000; Michael S. Finegan, Director
Web address: www.va.gov/visns/visn02

VETERANS AFFAIRS WESTERN NEW YORK HEALTHCARE SYSTEM–BUFFALO DIVISION (O, 233 beds) 3495 Bailey Avenue, Buffalo, NY Zip 14215–1129; tel. 716/834–9200; Michael S. Finegan, Director
Web address: www.va.gov/visns/visn02

NORTH CAROLINA: DURHAM VETERANS AFFAIRS MEDICAL CENTER (O, 232 beds) 508 Fulton Street, Durham, NC Zip 27705–3897; tel. 919/286–0411; Ralph T. Gigliotti, Director
Web address: www.va.gov/sta/guide/facility.asp?id=43

VETERANS AFFAIRS MEDICAL CENTER (O, 159 beds) 2300 Ramsey Street, Fayetteville, NC Zip 28301–3899; tel. 910/822–7059; Janet S. Stout, Director
Web address: www.va.gov/sta/guide/home.asp

VETERANS AFFAIRS MEDICAL CENTER (O, 196 beds) 1100 Tunnel Road, Asheville, NC Zip 28805–2087; tel. 828/298–7911; Susan Pendergrass, Director
Web address: www.va.gov/sta/guide/home.asp

VETERANS AFFAIRS MEDICAL CENTER (O, 533 beds) 1601 Brenner Avenue, Salisbury, NC Zip 28144–2559; tel. 704/638–9000; Carolyn L. Adams, Director
Web address: www.va.gov/sta/guide/home.asp

NORTH DAKOTA: VETERANS AFFAIRS MEDICAL CENTER (O, 77 beds) 2101 Elm Street, Fargo, ND Zip 58102–2498; tel. 701/232–3241; Robert P. McDivitt, FACHE, Director
Web address: www.va.gov/sta/guide/home.asp

OHIO: VETERANS AFFAIRS MEDICAL CENTER (O, 671 beds) 10701 East Boulevard, Cleveland, OH Zip 44106–1702; tel. 216/791–3800; William D. Montague, Director
Web address: www.va.gov/sta/guide/home.asp

VETERANS AFFAIRS MEDICAL CENTER (O, 297 beds) 17273 State Route 104, Chillicothe, OH Zip 45601–8608; tel. 740/773–1141; Jeffrey T. Gering, Medical Center Director
Web address: www.va.gov/sta/guide/home.asp

VETERANS AFFAIRS MEDICAL CENTER (O, 277 beds) 3200 Vine Street, Cincinnati, OH Zip 45220–2288; tel. 513/861–3100; Linda Smith, Director
Web address: www.va.gov/sta/guide/home.asp

VETERANS AFFAIRS MEDICAL CENTER (O, 500 beds) 4100 West Third Street, Dayton, OH Zip 45428–1002; tel. 937/268–6511; Guy B. Richardson, Director
Web address: www.va.gov/sta/guide/home.asp

For explanation of codes following names, see page B2.
★ Indicates Type III membership in the American Hospital Association.

OKLAHOMA: JACK C. MONTGOMERY VETERANS AFFAIRS MEDICAL CENTER (O, 88 beds) 1011 Honor Heights Drive, Muskogee, OK Zip 74401–1399; tel. 918/683–3261; Adam C. Walmus, Director
Web address: www.visn16.med.va.gov/muskogee.asp

VETERANS AFFAIRS MEDICAL CENTER (O, 205 beds) 921 N.E. 13th Street, Oklahoma City, OK Zip 73104–5028; tel. 405/270–0501; David P. Wood, Medical Center Director
Web address: www.va.gov/sta/guide/home.asp

OREGON: VETERANS AFFAIRS MEDICAL CENTER (O, 221 beds) 3710 S.W. U.S. Veterans Hospital Road, Portland, OR Zip 97239; tel. 503/220–8262; James Tuchschmidt, M.D., Director
Web address: www.va.gov/sta/guide/home.asp

VETERANS AFFAIRS ROSEBURG HEALTHCARE SYSTEM (O, 157 beds) 913 N.W. Garden Valley Boulevard, Roseburg, OR Zip 97470–6513; tel. 541/440–1000; Susan Yeager, Director
Web address: www.va.gov/sta/guide/home.asp

PENNSYLVANIA: JAMES E. VAN ZANDT VETERANS AFFAIRS MEDICAL CENTER (O, 68 beds) 2907 Pleasant Valley Boulevard, Altoona, PA Zip 16602–4377; tel. 814/943–8164; Anthony Bennett, Director
Web address: www.va.gov/sta/guide/home.asp

VETERANS AFFAIRS MEDICAL CENTER (O, 126 beds) 325 New Castle Road, Butler, PA Zip 16001–2480; tel. 724/287–4781; Patricia Nealon, Director
Web address: www.va.gov/sta/guide/home.asp

VETERANS AFFAIRS MEDICAL CENTER (O, 472 beds) 1400 Black Horse Hill Road, Coatesville, PA Zip 19320–2040; tel. 610/384–7711; Gary W. Devansky, Director
Web address: www.va.gov/sta/guide/home.asp

VETERANS AFFAIRS MEDICAL CENTER (O, 78 beds) 135 East 38th Street, Erie, PA Zip 16504–1596; tel. 814/860–2576; Michael Adelman, M.D., Director
Web address: www.va.gov/sta/guide/home.asp

VETERANS AFFAIRS MEDICAL CENTER (O, 213 beds) 1700 South Lincoln Avenue, Lebanon, PA Zip 17042–7529; tel. 717/272–6621; Robert W. Callahan, Jr., Director
Web address: www.va.gov/sta/guide/home.asp

VETERANS AFFAIRS MEDICAL CENTER (O, 389 beds) University and Woodland Avenues, Philadelphia, PA Zip 19104–4594; tel. 215/823–5800; Michael J. Sullivan, Director

VETERANS AFFAIRS MEDICAL CENTER (O, 174 beds) 1111 East End Boulevard, Wilkes–Barre, PA Zip 18711–0026; tel. 570/824–3521; C. Gene Molino, Acting Director
Web address: www.va.gov/vamcwb

VETERANS AFFAIRS PITTSBURGH HEALTHCARE SYSTEM (O, 692 beds) Delafield Road, Pittsburgh, PA Zip 15240–1001; tel. 412/688–6000; Terry Gerigk Wolf, Director
Web address: www.va.gov/pittsburgh

PUERTO RICO: VETERANS AFFAIRS MEDICAL CENTER (O, 479 beds) 10 Casia Street, San Juan, PR Zip 00921–3201; tel. 787/641–7582; Nancy Reissener, Acting Director
Web address: www.va.gov/visn8/sanjuan

RHODE ISLAND: VETERANS AFFAIRS MEDICAL CENTER (O, 73 beds) 830 Chalkstone Avenue, Providence, RI Zip 02908–4799; tel. 401/457–3042; Vincent Ng, Director
Web address: www.va.gov/sta/guide/home.asp

SOUTH CAROLINA: RALPH H. JOHNSON VETERANS AFFAIRS MEDICAL CENTER (O, 98 beds) 109 Bee Street, Charleston, SC Zip 29401–5799; tel. 843/577–5011; John E. Barilich, Director
Web address: www.va.gov/sta/guide/home.asp

WM. JENNINGS BRYAN DORN VETERANS AFFAIRS MEDICAL CENTER (O, 109 beds) 6439 Garners Ferry Road, Columbia, SC Zip 29209–1639; tel. 803/776–4000; Brian Heckert, Medical Center Director
Web address: www.va.gov/sta/guide/home.asp

SOUTH DAKOTA: ROYAL C. JOHNSON VETERANS MEMORIAL MEDICAL CENTER (O, 103 beds) 2501 West 22nd Street, Sioux Falls, SD Zip 57105–9920, Mailing Address: P.O. Box 5046, Zip 57117–5046; tel. 605/336–3230; Paul Bockelman, Director
Web address: www.visn23.med.va.gov

VETERANS AFFAIRS BLACK HILLS HEALTH CARE SYSTEM (O, 322 beds) 113 Comanche Road, Fort Meade, SD Zip 57741–1099; tel. 605/347–2511; Peter P. Henry, FACHE, Director
Web address: www.va.gov/sta/guide/home.asp

TENNESSEE: JAMES H. QUILLEN VETERANS AFFAIRS MEDICAL CENTER (O, 603 beds) Mountain Home, TN Mailing Address: P.O. Box 4000, Zip 37684–4000; tel. 423/926–1171; John W. McFadden, Interim Director
Web address: www.va.gov

VETERANS AFFAIRS MEDICAL CENTER (O, 280 beds) 1030 Jefferson Avenue, Memphis, TN Zip 38104–2193; tel. 901/523–8990; Patricia O. Pittman, Director
Web address: www.va.gov/sta/guide/home.asp

VETERANS AFFAIRS TENNESSEE VALLEY HEALTHCARE SYSTEM (O, 498 beds) 1310 24th Avenue South, Nashville, TN Zip 37212–2637; tel. 615/327–4751; Juan A. Morales, Interim Director
Web address: www.tennesseevalley.va.gov

TEXAS: AMARILLO VETERANS AFFAIRS HEALTH CARE SYSTEM (O, 189 beds) 6010 Amarillo Boulevard West, Amarillo, TX Zip 79106–1992; tel. 806/355–9703; Gracie Specks, Acting Director
Web address: www.va.gov/sta/guide/home.asp

CENTRAL TEXAS VETERANS HEALTHCARE SYSTEM (O, 1852 beds) 1901 Veterans Memorial Drive, Temple, TX Zip 76504–7493; tel. 254/778–4811; Bruce A. Gordon, Director
Web address: www.central–texas.med.va.gov

MICHAEL E. DEBAKEY VETERANS AFFAIRS MEDICAL CENTER (O, 859 beds) 2002 Holcombe Boulevard, Houston, TX Zip 77030–4298; tel. 713/791–1414; Edgar L. Tucker, Director
Web address: www.houston.va.gov

SOUTH TEXAS VETERANS HEALTH CARE SYSTEM (O, 1112 beds) 7400 Merton Minter Boulevard, San Antonio, TX Zip 78284–5799; tel. 210/617–5140; Jose R. Coronado, FACHE, Director
Web address: www.vasthcs.med.va.gov

VETERANS AFFAIRS NORTH TEXAS HEALTH CARE SYSTEM (O, 875 beds) 4500 South Lancaster Road, Dallas, TX Zip 75216–7167; tel. 214/742–8387; Betty Bolin Brown, Ed.D., Director
Web address: www.va.gov/sta/guide/home.asp

WEST TEXAS VA HEALTH CARE SYSTEM (O, 189 beds) 300 Veterans Boulevard, Big Spring, TX Zip 79720–5500; tel. 432/263–7361; Michael L. Bell, Director
Web address: www.va.gov/sta/guide/home.asp

UTAH: VETERANS AFFAIRS SALT LAKE CITY HEALTH CARE SYSTEM (O, 121 beds) 500 Foothill Drive, Salt Lake City, UT Zip 84148–0002; tel. 801/582–1565; James R. Floyd, Director
Web address: www.va.gov/sta/guide/home.asp

VERMONT: VETERANS AFFAIRS MEDICAL CENTER (O, 60 beds) 215 North Main Street, White River Junction, VT Zip 05009–0001; tel. 802/295–9363; Kathryn M. Harty, RN, M.S.N., Acting Director
Web address: www.va.gov/sta/guide/home.asp

VIRGINIA: HUNTER HOLMES MCGUIRE VETERANS AFFAIRS MEDICAL CENTER (O, 415 beds) 1201 Broad Rock Boulevard, Richmond, VA Zip 23249–0002; tel. 804/675–5000; Michael B. Phaup, Director
Web address: www.va.gov/sta/guide/home.asp

VETERANS AFFAIRS MEDICAL CENTER (O, 485 beds) 100 Emancipation Drive, Hampton, VA Zip 23667–0001; tel. 757/722–9961; Wanda Mims, Director
Web address: www.va.gov/sta/guide/home.asp

VETERANS AFFAIRS MEDICAL CENTER (O, 282 beds) 1970 Roanoke Boulevard, Salem, VA Zip 24153–6478; tel. 540/982–2463; Stephen L. Lemons, Ed.D., Director
Web address: www.va.gov/sta/guide/home.asp

WASHINGTON: JONATHAN M. WAINWRIGHT MEMORIAL VA MEDICAL CENTER (O, 44 beds) 77 Wainwright Drive, Walla Walla, WA Zip 99362–3994; tel. 509/525–5200; Sharon M. Helman, Director
Web address: www.va.gov/sta/guide/home.asp

VETERANS AFFAIRS MEDICAL CENTER (O, 66 beds) North 4815 Assembly Street, Spokane, WA Zip 99205–6197; tel. 509/434–7000; Sharon M. Helman, Director
Web address: www.va.gov/sta/guide/home.asp

VETERANS AFFAIRS PUGET SOUND HEALTH CARE SYSTEM (O, 504 beds) 1660 South Columbian Way, Seattle, WA Zip 98108–1597; tel. 206/762–1010; Stan Johnson, Director
Web address: www.va.gov/sta/guide/home.asp

Section B

For explanation of codes following names, see page B2.
★ Indicates Type III membership in the American Hospital Association.

WEST VIRGINIA: LOUIS A. JOHNSON VETERANS AFFAIRS MEDICAL CENTER (O, 98 beds) 1 Medical Center Drive, Clarksburg, WV Zip 26301–4199; tel. 304/623–3461; William E. Cox, Director
Web address: www.va.gov/sta/guide/home.asp

VETERANS AFFAIRS MEDICAL CENTER (O, 90 beds) 200 Veterans Avenue, Beckley, WV Zip 25801–6499; tel. 304/255–2121; ,
Web address: www.va.gov/sta/guide/home.asp

VETERANS AFFAIRS MEDICAL CENTER (O, 80 beds) 1540 Spring Valley Drive, Huntington, WV Zip 25704–9300; tel. 304/429–6741; Edward H. Seiler, Director
Web address: www.va.gov/sta/guide/home.asp

VETERANS AFFAIRS MEDICAL CENTER (O, 559 beds) 510 Butler Avenue, Martinsburg, WV Zip 25401–0205; tel. 304/263–0811; Pedro Garcia, Director
Web address: www.va.gov/sta/guide/home.asp

WISCONSIN: CLEMENT J. ZABLOCKI VETERANS AFFAIRS MEDICAL CENTER (O, 566 beds) 5000 West National Avenue, Milwaukee, WI Zip 53295; tel. 414/384–2000; Glen W. Grippen, Director
Web address: www.va.gov/sta/guide/home.asp

VETERANS AFFAIRS MEDICAL CENTER (O, 271 beds) 500 East Veterans Street, Tomah, WI Zip 54660; tel. 608/372–3971; Jerald D. Molnar, Acting Medical Center Director
Web address: www.va.gov/tomahvamc

WILLIAM S. MIDDLETON MEMORIAL VETERANS HOSPITAL (O, 86 beds) 2500 Overlook Terrace, Madison, WI Zip 53705–2286; tel. 608/256–1901; Deborah A. Thompson, Director
Web address: www.madison.med.va.gov

WYOMING: VETERANS AFFAIRS MEDICAL CENTER (O, 71 beds) 2360 East Pershing Boulevard, Cheyenne, WY Zip 82001–5392; tel. 307/778–7550; David M. Kilpatrick, M.D., Director
Web address: www.va.gov/sta/guide/home.asp

VETERANS AFFAIRS MEDICAL CENTER (O, 203 beds) 1898 Fort Road, Sheridan, WY Zip 82801–8320; tel. 307/672–3473; Debra L. Hirschman, Director
Web address: www.va.gov/sta/guide/home.asp

Owned, leased, sponsored:	135 hospitals	41067 beds
Contract-managed:	0 hospitals	0 beds
Totals:	135 hospitals	41067 beds

★2145: DETROIT MEDICAL CENTER (NP)

3990 John R., Detroit, MI Zip 48201; tel. 313/745–1250; Michael Duggan, President and Chief Executive Officer
(Centralized Health System)

MICHIGAN: CHILDREN'S HOSPITAL OF MICHIGAN (O, 225 beds) 3901 Beaubien Boulevard, Detroit, MI Zip 48201–9985; tel. 313/745–5437; Herman B. Gray, M.D., President
Web address: www.chmkids.org

DETROIT RECEIVING HOSPITAL AND UNIVERSITY HEALTH CENTER (O, 217 beds) 4201 St. Antoine Boulevard, Detroit, MI Zip 48201–2194; tel. 313/745–3603; Iris Taylor, Ph.D., President
Web address: www.dmc.org

HARPER UNIVERSITY HOSPITAL (O, 471 beds) 3990 John R. Street, Detroit, MI Zip 48201–9027; tel. 313/745–8040; Brooks Bock, M.D., President
Web address: www.harperhospital.org

HURON VALLEY–SINAI HOSPITAL (O, 153 beds) 1 William Carls Drive, Commerce Township, MI Zip 48382–2201; tel. 248/937–3300; Lynn M. Torossian, President
Web address: www.hvsh.org

REHABILITATION INSTITUTE OF MICHIGAN (O, 62 beds) 261 Mack Boulevard, Detroit, MI Zip 48201–2495; tel. 313/745–1203; Terry Reiley, President
Web address: www.rimrehab.org

SINAI–GRACE HOSPITAL (O, 380 beds) 6071 West Outer Drive, Detroit, MI Zip 48235–2679; tel. 313/966–3300; Conrad L. Mallett, Jr., President
Web address: www.sinaigrace.org

Owned, leased, sponsored:	6 hospitals	1508 beds
Contract-managed:	0 hospitals	0 beds
Totals:	6 hospitals	1508 beds

0845: DEVEREUX (NP)

444 Devereux Drive, Villanova, PA Zip 19085, Mailing Address: P.O. Box 638, Zip 19085–0638; tel. 610/520–3000; Robert Q. Kreider, President and Chief Executive Officer
(Independent Hospital System)

FLORIDA: DEVEREUX HOSPITAL AND CHILDREN'S CENTER OF FLORIDA (O, 100 beds) 8000 Devereux Drive, Melbourne, FL Zip 32940–7907; tel. 321/242–9100; Mark Halal, Administrator
Web address: www.devereux.org

GEORGIA: DEVEREUX GEORGIA TREATMENT NETWORK (O, 187 beds) 1291 Stanley Road N.W., Kennesaw, GA Zip 30152–4359, Mailing Address: P.O. Box 1688, Zip 30156–8688; tel. 770/427–0147; Mario Bolivar, Executive Director
Web address: www.devereuxga.org

PENNSYLVANIA: DEVEREUX CHILDREN'S BEHAVIORAL HEALTH CENTER (O, 13 beds) 655 Sugartown Road, Malvern, PA Zip 19355–0275, Mailing Address: P.O. Box 275, Zip 19355–0275; tel. 484/595–6777; Walter J. Grono, Executive Director
Web address: www.devereux.org

TEXAS: DEVEREUX TEXAS TREATMENT NETWORK (O, 70 beds) 1150 Devereux Drive, League City, TX Zip 77573–2043; tel. 281/335–1000; Pamela E. Helm, Executive Director
Web address: www.devereux.org

Owned, leased, sponsored:	4 hospitals	370 beds
Contract-managed:	0 hospitals	0 beds
Totals:	4 hospitals	370 beds

0029: DIMENSIONS HEALTHCARE SYSTEM (NP)

3001 Hospital Drive, 3rd Floor, Cheverly, MD Zip 20785; tel. 301/583–4000; G. T. Dunlop Ecker, President and Chief Executive Officer
(Independent Hospital System)

MARYLAND: LAUREL REGIONAL HOSPITAL (O, 124 beds) 7300 Van Dusen Road, Laurel, MD Zip 20707–9266; tel. 301/725–4300; Douglas Shepherd, FACHE, President
Web address: www.laurelregionalhospital.org

PRINCE GEORGE'S HOSPITAL CENTER (O, 395 beds) 3001 Hospital Drive, Cheverly, MD Zip 20785–1189; tel. 301/618–2000; John A. O'Brien, FACHE, President
Web address: www.princegeorgeshospital.org

Owned, leased, sponsored:	2 hospitals	519 beds
Contract-managed:	0 hospitals	0 beds
Totals:	2 hospitals	519 beds

0010: DIVISION OF MENTAL HEALTH SERVICES, DEPARTMENT OF HUMAN SERVICES, STATE OF NEW JERSEY (NP)

Capital Center, P.O. Box 727, Trenton, NJ Zip 08625–0727; tel. 609/777–0702; Kevin Martone, Assistant Commissioner
(Independent Hospital System)

NEW JERSEY: ANCORA PSYCHIATRIC HOSPITAL (O, 709 beds) 301 Spring Garden Road, Ancora, NJ Zip 08037–9699; tel. 609/561–1700; LaTanya Wood El, Chief Executive Officer
Web address: www.peoplefirstnurses.nj.gov/ancora.htm

GREYSTONE PARK PSYCHIATRIC HOSPITAL (O, 557 beds) 99 Central Avenue, Morris Plains, NJ Zip 07950–1005, Mailing Address: P.O. Box A, Zip 07950–1005; tel. 973/538–1800; Janet Monroe, Chief Executive Officer
Web address: www.state.nj.us/humanservices/pfnurse/greystone.htm

SENATOR GARRETT W. HAGEDORN PSYCHIATRIC HOSPITAL (O, 288 beds) 200 Sanatorium Road, Glen Gardner, NJ Zip 08826–3291; tel. 908/537–2141; Debra A. Smith, Chief Executive Officer

TRENTON PSYCHIATRIC HOSPITAL (O, 436 beds) Route 29 and Sullivan Way, Trenton, NJ Zip 08628–3425, Mailing Address: P.O. Box 7500, West Trenton, Zip 08628–7500; tel. 609/633–1500; Teresa A. McQuaide, Chief Executive Officer

For explanation of codes following names, see page B2.
★ Indicates Type III membership in the American Hospital Association.

Owned, leased, sponsored:	4 hospitals	1990 beds
Contract-managed:	0 hospitals	0 beds
Totals:	4 hospitals	1990 beds

★0226: DUBUIS HEALTH SYSTEM (CC)
10333 Richmond Avenue, Suite 300, Houston, TX Zip 77042; tel. 713/339-7000; Ellen Smith, President and Chief Executive Officer
(Independent Hospital System)

ARKANSAS: ADVANCE CARE HOSPITAL (O, 27 beds) 300 Werner Street, 3rd Floor East, Hot Springs National Park, AR Zip 71913; tel. 501/609-4300; Keith Rogers, Administrator
Web address: www.dubuis.org

ADVANCE CARE HOSPITAL OF FORT SMITH (C, 25 beds) 7301 Rogers Avenue, 4th Floor, Fort Smith, AR Zip 72917; tel. 479/314-4900; Susan Legg, Administrator
Web address: www.dubuis.org

GEORGIA: SOUTHERN CRESCENT HOSPITAL FOR SPECIALTY CARE (C, 30 beds) 11 Upper Riverdale Road S.W., 6th Floor, Riverdale, GA Zip 30274; tel. 770/897-7603; Janice Hamilton-Crawford, Administrator

LOUISIANA: DUBUIS HOSPITAL OF ALEXANDRIA (O, 33 beds) 3330 Masonic Drive, 4th Floor, Alexandria, LA Zip 71301; tel. 318/448-6505; Michelle Hamilton, Administrator
Web address: www.dubuis.org

DUBUIS HOSPITAL OF LAKE CHARLES (O, 24 beds) 524 South Ryan, 5th Floor, Lake Charles, LA Zip 70601-5725; tel. 337/491-7752; Ronald E. Hand, Administrator

DUBUIS HOSPITAL OF SHREVEPORT (O, 36 beds) One St. Mary Place, 6th Floor, Shreveport, LA Zip 71101; tel. 318/221-3802; Berry Gilbert, Administrator
Web address: www.dubuis.org

MISSOURI: DUBUIS HOSPITAL OF ST. LOUIS (C, 54 beds) 13190 South Outer Forty Road, Chesterfield, MO Zip 63017-5917; tel. 314/392-6380; John F. Brothers, Interim Administrator
Web address: www.dubuis.org

TEXAS: DUBUIS HOSPITAL OF BEAUMONT (O, 51 beds) 2830 Calder Avenue, 4th Floor, Beaumont, TX Zip 77702; tel. 409/899-8154; Barbara Flournoy, Administrator
Web address: www.dubuis.org

DUBUIS HOSPITAL OF CORPUS CHRISTI (O, 22 beds) 600 Elizabeth Street, 5rd Floor, Corpus Christi, TX Zip 78404, Mailing Address: 600 Elizabeth Street, 3rd Floor, Zip 78404; tel. 361/881-3223; Diane Kaiser, Administrator
Web address: www.dubuis.org

DUBUIS HOSPITAL OF HOUSTON (O, 30 beds) 1919 Labranch 7GWS Street, Houston, TX Zip 77002; tel. 713/756-8660; Marissa Henry, Administrator
Web address: www.dubuis.org

DUBUIS HOSPITAL OF PARIS (O, 25 beds) 865 Deshong Drive, 5th Floor, Paris, TX Zip 75462; tel. 903/782-2960; Holly Powell, Administrator
Web address: www.dubuis.org

DUBUIS HOSPITAL OF PORT ARTHUR (O, 15 beds) 3600 Gates Boulevard, Port Arthur, TX Zip 77642; tel. 409/989-5300; Barbara Flournoy, Administrator
Web address: www.dubuis.org

DUBUIS HOSPITAL OF TEXARKANA (O, 30 beds) 2400 St. Michael Drive, 2nd Floor, Texarkana, TX Zip 75503-2372; tel. 903/614-7600; David L. Adcock, FACHE, Administrator
Web address: www.dubuis.org

Owned, leased, sponsored:	10 hospitals	293 beds
Contract-managed:	3 hospitals	109 beds
Totals:	13 hospitals	402 beds

★0190: DUKE UNIVERSITY HEALTH SYSTEM (NP)
Erwin Road, Durham, NC Zip 27710, Mailing Address: P.O. Box 3701, Zip 27710-3701; tel. 919/684-2255; Victor J. Dzau, M.D., President and Chief Executive Officer
(Centralized Health System)

NORTH CAROLINA: DUKE RALEIGH HOSPITAL (O, 146 beds) 3400 Wake Forest Road, Raleigh, NC Zip 27609-7373, Mailing Address: P.O. Box 28280, Zip 27611-8280; tel. 919/954-3000; Douglas B. Vinsel, Chief Executive Officer
Web address: www.dukehealthraleigh.org

DUKE UNIVERSITY HOSPITAL (O, 784 beds) 2301 Erwin Road, Durham, NC Zip 27710-0001, Mailing Address: P.O. Box 3708, Zip 27710-3708; tel. 919/684-8111; William J. Fulkerson, M.D., Chief Executive Officer
Web address: www.dukehealth.org

DURHAM REGIONAL HOSPITAL (L, 201 beds) 3643 North Roxboro Road, Durham, NC Zip 27704-2763; tel. 919/470-4000; Kerry Watson, Chief Executive Officer
Web address: www.durhamregional.org

PERSON MEMORIAL HOSPITAL (C, 110 beds) 615 Ridge Road, Roxboro, NC Zip 27573-4630; tel. 336/599-2121; Jamie W. Guin, Jr., Chief Executive Officer
Web address: www.personhospital.com

Owned, leased, sponsored:	3 hospitals	1131 beds
Contract-managed:	1 hospital	110 beds
Totals:	4 hospitals	1241 beds

0286: DYNACQ HEALTHCARE, INC. (IO)
10304 Interstate 10 East, Suite 369, Houston, TX Zip 77029; tel. 713/673-6432; Chiu Moon Chan, Chairman, President and Chief Executive Officer
(Independent Hospital System)

LOUISIANA: VISTA SURGICAL HOSPITAL OF BATON ROUGE (O, 39 beds) 9032 Perkins Road, Baton Rouge, LA Zip 70810; tel. 225/819-4100; Alan A. Beauchamp, Chief Executive Officer
Web address: www.dynacq.com

TEXAS: SURGERY SPECIALTY HOSPITALS OF AMERICA (O, 37 beds) 4301B Vista, Pasadena, TX Zip 77504; tel. 713/378-3000; Celia Barrera, Administrator

VISTA HOSPITAL OF DALLAS (O, 29 beds) 2696 West Walnut Street, Garland, TX Zip 75042-6499; tel. 972/665-3000; Alan A. Beauchamp, Chief Executive Officer
Web address: www.vista-hospital-dallas.com

Owned, leased, sponsored:	3 hospitals	105 beds
Contract-managed:	0 hospitals	0 beds
Totals:	3 hospitals	105 beds

★1895: EAST TEXAS MEDICAL CENTER REGIONAL HEALTHCARE SYSTEM (NP)
1000 South Beckham Street, Tyler, TX Zip 75701-1996, Mailing Address: P.O. Box 6400, Zip 75711-6400; tel. 903/535-6211; Elmer G. Ellis, FACHE, President and Chief Executive Officer
(Centralized Physician/Insurance Health System)

EAST TEXAS MEDICAL CENTER ATHENS (L, 117 beds) 2000 South Palestine Street, Athens, TX Zip 75751-5610; tel. 903/676-1000; Patrick L. Wallace, Administrator
Web address: www.etmc.org

EAST TEXAS MEDICAL CENTER CARTHAGE (L, 37 beds) 409 Cottage Road, Carthage, TX Zip 75633-1466, Mailing Address: P.O. Box 549, Zip 75633-0549; tel. 903/693-3841; Gary Mikeal Hudson, Administrator
Web address: www.etmc.org

EAST TEXAS MEDICAL CENTER CLARKSVILLE (L, 36 beds) 3000 West Main Street, Clarksville, TX Zip 75426, Mailing Address: P.O. Box 1270, Zip 75426-1270; tel. 903/427-6400; John S. Hart, Administrator
Web address: www.etmc.org

EAST TEXAS MEDICAL CENTER CROCKETT (L, 49 beds) 1100 Loop 304 East, Crockett, TX Zip 75835-1810; tel. 936/546-3862; Terry Cutler, Administrator and Chief Operating Officer
Web address: www.etmc.org

EAST TEXAS MEDICAL CENTER FAIRFIELD (L, 20 beds) 125 Newman Street, Fairfield, TX Zip 75840-1499; tel. 903/389-2121; Ruth Cook, Administrator
Web address: www.etmc.org

For explanation of codes following names, see page B2.
★ Indicates Type III membership in the American Hospital Association.

Section B

EAST TEXAS MEDICAL CENTER JACKSONVILLE (O, 58 beds) 501 South Ragsdale Street, Jacksonville, TX Zip 75766–2413; tel. 903/541–5000; Jack R. Endres, Administrator
Web address: www.etmc.org

EAST TEXAS MEDICAL CENTER PITTSBURG (L, 25 beds) 414 Quitman Street, Pittsburg, TX Zip 75686–1032; tel. 903/856–6663; W. Perry Henderson, Administrator
Web address: www.etmc.org

EAST TEXAS MEDICAL CENTER REHABILITATION CENTER (O, 49 beds) 701 Olympic Plaza Circle, Tyler, TX Zip 75701–1996; tel. 903/596–3000; Eddie L. Howard, Vice President and Chief Operating Officer
Web address: www.etmc.org

EAST TEXAS MEDICAL CENTER SPECIALTY HOSPITAL (O, 36 beds) 1000 South Beckham, 5th Floor, Tyler, TX Zip 75701; tel. 903/596–3600; Eddie L. Howard, Vice President, Chief Operating Officer and Administrator
Web address: www.etmc.org

EAST TEXAS MEDICAL CENTER TRINITY (L, 22 beds) 317 Prospect Drive, Trinity, TX Zip 75862, Mailing Address: P.O. Box 3169, Zip 75862; tel. 936/594–3541; Warren Robicheaux, Administrator
Web address: www.etmc.org

EAST TEXAS MEDICAL CENTER TYLER (O, 422 beds) 1000 South Beckham Street, Tyler, TX Zip 75701–1996, Mailing Address: Box 6400, Zip 75711–6400; tel. 903/597–0351; Robert B. Evans, Administrator and Chief Executive Officer
Web address: www.etmc.org

EAST TEXAS MEDICAL CENTER–GILMER (O, 37 beds) 712 North Wood Street, Gilmer, TX Zip 75644; tel. 903/841–7100; Michael W. Pruitt, Chief Executive Officer
Web address: www.etmc.org

EAST TEXAS MEDICAL CENTER–MOUNT VERNON (L, 30 beds) 500 Highway 37 South, Mount Vernon, TX Zip 75457–3602, Mailing Address: P.O. Box 477, Zip 75457–0477; tel. 903/537–8000; Stephen Pitts, Administrator
Web address: www.etmc.org

EAST TEXAS MEDICAL CENTER–QUITMAN (L, 28 beds) 117 Winnsboro Street, Quitman, TX Zip 75783–2144, Mailing Address: P.O. Box 1000, Zip 75783–1000; tel. 903/763–6300; Christopher Stipe, FACHE, Administrator and Chief Executive Officer
Web address: www.etmc.org

Owned, leased, sponsored:	14 hospitals	966 beds
Contract–managed:	0 hospitals	0 beds
Totals:	14 hospitals	966 beds

★0270: EASTERN CONNECTICUT HEALTH NETWORK (NP)
71 Haynes Street, Manchester, CT Zip 06040; tel. 860/533–3400; Peter J. Karl, President and Chief Executive Officer
(Independent Hospital System)

CONNECTICUT: MANCHESTER MEMORIAL HOSPITAL (O, 148 beds) 71 Haynes Street, Manchester, CT Zip 06040–4188; tel. 860/646–1222; Peter J. Karl, President and Chief Executive Officer
Web address: www.echn.org

ROCKVILLE GENERAL HOSPITAL (O, 59 beds) 31 Union Street, Vernon Rockville, CT Zip 06066–3160; tel. 860/872–0501; Peter J. Karl, President and Chief Executive Officer
Web address: www.echn.org

Owned, leased, sponsored:	2 hospitals	207 beds
Contract–managed:	0 hospitals	0 beds
Totals:	2 hospitals	207 beds

★0555: EASTERN MAINE HEALTHCARE SYSTEMS (NP)
43 Whiting Hill Road, Brewer, ME Zip 04412; tel. 207/973–7045; M. Michelle Hood, President and Chief Executive Officer
(Centralized Health System)

MAINE: ACADIA HOSPITAL (O, 93 beds) 268 Stillwater Avenue, Bangor, ME Zip 04401–3945, Mailing Address: P.O. Box 422, Zip 04402–0422; tel. 207/973–6100; Dorothy E. Hill, Chief Executive Officer
Web address: www.acadiahospital.org

AROOSTOOK MEDICAL CENTER (O, 132 beds) 140 Academy Street, Presque Isle, ME Zip 04769–3171, Mailing Address: P.O. Box 151, Zip 04769–0151; tel. 207/768–4000; David A. Peterson, President and Chief Executive Officer
Web address: www.tamc.org

BLUE HILL MEMORIAL HOSPITAL (O, 25 beds) 57 Water Street, Blue Hill, ME Zip 04614–0823, Mailing Address: P.O. Box 823, Zip 04614–0823; tel. 207/374–3400; Timothy Garrity, FACHE, President and Chief Executive Officer
Web address: www.bhmh.org

CHARLES A. DEAN MEMORIAL HOSPITAL AND NURSING HOME (O, 36 beds) 364 Pritham Avenue, Greenville, ME Zip 04441–1395, Mailing Address: P.O. Box 1129, Zip 04441–1129; tel. 207/695–5200; Geno Murray, President and Chief Executive Officer
Web address: www.cadean.org

EASTERN MAINE MEDICAL CENTER (O, 349 beds) 489 State Street, Bangor, ME Zip 04401–6674, Mailing Address: P.O. Box 404, Zip 04402–0404; tel. 207/973–7000; Deborah Carey Johnson, RN, President and Chief Executive Officer
Web address: www.emh.org

INLAND HOSPITAL (O, 46 beds) 200 Kennedy Memorial Drive, Waterville, ME Zip 04901–4595; tel. 207/861–3000; John Dalton, President and Chief Executive Officer
Web address: www.inlandhospital.org

SEBASTICOOK VALLEY HOSPITAL (O, 25 beds) 447 North Main Street, Pittsfield, ME Zip 04967–1199; tel. 207/487–5141; John C. May, Chief Executive Officer
Web address: www.sebasticookhospital.org

Owned, leased, sponsored:	7 hospitals	706 beds
Contract–managed:	0 hospitals	0 beds
Totals:	7 hospitals	706 beds

★0256: EMORY HEALTHCARE (NP)
1440 Clifton Road, N.E., Suite 420, Atlanta, GA Zip 30322–1102, Mailing Address: 1440 Clifton Road N.E., Suite 420, Zip 30322–1102; tel. 404/778–5000; John T. Fox, Chief Executive Officer
(Centralized Health System)

GEORGIA: EMORY CRAWFORD LONG HOSPITAL (O, 439 beds) 550 Peachtree Street N.E., Atlanta, GA Zip 30308; tel. 404/686–4411; John T. Fox, Chief Executive Officer
Web address: www.emoryhealthcare.org

EMORY UNIVERSITY HOSPITAL (O, 548 beds) 1364 Clifton Road N.E., Atlanta, GA Zip 30322–1102; tel. 404/712–2000; John T. Fox, Chief Executive Officer
Web address: www.emoryhealthcare.org

WESLEY WOODS CENTER OF EMORY UNIVERSITY (O, 344 beds) 1821 Clifton Road N.E., Atlanta, GA Zip 30329–5102; tel. 404/728–6200; Albert K. Blackwelder, FACHE, Chief Operating Officer
Web address: www.emory.org

Owned, leased, sponsored:	3 hospitals	1331 beds
Contract–managed:	0 hospitals	0 beds
Totals:	3 hospitals	1331 beds

★0945: EMPIRE HEALTH SERVICES (NP)
West 800 Fifth Avenue, Spokane, WA Zip 99204, Mailing Address: P.O. Box 248, Zip 99210–0248; tel. 509/473–7965; C. E. Bilbrey, Interim Chief Executive Officer
(Independent Hospital System)

WASHINGTON: DEACONESS MEDICAL CENTER–SPOKANE (O, 265 beds) 800 West Fifth Avenue, Spokane, WA Zip 99204–2803, Mailing Address: P.O. Box 248, Zip 99210–0248; tel. 509/458–5800; Robert Quist, Chief Executive Officer
Web address: www.deaconess–spokane.org

VALLEY HOSPITAL AND MEDICAL CENTER (O, 93 beds) 12606 East Mission Avenue, Spokane, WA Zip 99216–1090; tel. 509/924–6650; Robert Quist, Chief Executive Officer
Web address: www.valleyhospital.org

For explanation of codes following names, see page B2.
★ Indicates Type III membership in the American Hospital Association.

Owned, leased, sponsored:	2 hospitals	358 beds
Contract-managed:	0 hospitals	0 beds
Totals:	2 hospitals	358 beds

0164: ENVISION HOSPITAL CORPORATION (IO)
6730 North Scottsdale Road, Suite 290, Scottsdale, AZ Zip 85253; tel. 480/348–9800; Paul R. Tuft, Chairman and Chief Executive Officer
(Independent Hospital System)

CALIFORNIA: PACIFICA HOSPITAL OF THE VALLEY (O, 221 beds) 9449 San Fernando Road, Sun Valley, CA Zip 91352–1421; tel. 818/767–3310; Casey Fatch, Chief Executive Officer
Web address: www.pacificahospital.com

ILLINOIS: MICHAEL REESE HOSPITAL AND MEDICAL CENTER (O, 364 beds) 2929 South Ellis Avenue, Chicago, IL Zip 60616–3376; tel. 312/791–2000; Enrique Beckmann, M.D., Ph.D., Chief Executive Officer
Web address: www.michaelreesehospital.com

MISSOURI: FOREST PARK COMMUNITY HOSPITAL (O, 178 beds) 6150 Oakland Avenue, Saint Louis, MO Zip 63139–3215; tel. 314/768–3000; Jordan Tenenbaum, Chief Executive Officer
Web address: www.forestparkhospital.com

ST. ALEXIUS HOSPITAL (O, 169 beds) 3933 South Broadway, Saint Louis, MO Zip 63118–4601; tel. 314/865–3333; Robert S. Adcock, Chief Executive Officer
Web address: www.stalexiushospital.com

Owned, leased, sponsored:	4 hospitals	932 beds
Contract-managed:	0 hospitals	0 beds
Totals:	4 hospitals	932 beds

0525: ERLANGER HEALTH SYSTEM (NP)
975 East Third Street, Chattanooga, TN Zip 37403; tel. 423/778–7000; James L. Brexler, President and Chief Executive Officer
(Centralized Physician/Insurance Health System)

TENNESSEE: ERLANGER BLEDSOE HOSPITAL (C, 29 beds) 71 Wheeler Avenue, Pikeville, TN Zip 37367, Mailing Address: P.O. Box 699, Zip 37367–0699; tel. 423/447–2112; Stephanie Boynton, Administrator
Web address: www.erlanger.org

ERLANGER MEDICAL CENTER (O, 551 beds) 975 East Third Street, Chattanooga, TN Zip 37403–2112; tel. 423/778–7000; James L. Brexler, President and Chief Executive Officer
Web address: www.erlanger.org

Owned, leased, sponsored:	1 hospital	551 beds
Contract-managed:	1 hospital	29 beds
Totals:	2 hospitals	580 beds

0382: ERNEST HEALTH, INC. (IO)
7770 Jefferson Street N.E., Suite 320, Albuquerque, NM Zip 87109; tel. 505/856–5300; Darby Brockette, Chief Executive Officer

ARIZONA: MOUNTAIN VALLEY REGIONAL REHABILITATION HOSPITAL (O, 40 beds) 3700 North Windsong Drive, Prescott Valley, AZ Zip 86314; tel. 928/759–8800; Kelly Silberschlag, Chief Executive Officer
Web address: www.mvrrh.ernesthealth.com

COLORADO: NORTHERN COLORADO REHABILITATION HOSPITAL (O, 40 beds) 4401 Union Street, Johnstown, CO Zip 80534; tel. 970/619–3400; Dennis R. Shelby, Chief Executive Officer
Web address: www.ncrh.ernesthealth.com

NEW MEXICO: REHABILITATION HOSPITAL OF SOUTHERN NEW MEXICO (O, 40 beds) 4441 East Lohman Avenue, Las Cruces, NM Zip 88011; tel. 575/521–6400; Tony Hernandez, Chief Executive Officer
Web address: www.rhsnm.ernesthealth.com

TEXAS: LAREDO SPECIALTY HOSPITAL (O, 60 beds) 2005 Bustamente Street, Laredo, TX Zip 78041–5470; tel. 956/753–5353; Al Chapa, CHE, Chief Executive Officer
Web address: www.lsh.ernesthealth.com

MESQUITE SPECIALTY HOSPITAL (O, 40 beds) 1024 North Galloway Avenue, Mesquite, TX Zip 75149–2434; tel. 972/216–2300; Brenda M. Antwine, Chief Executive Officer
Web address: www.msh.ernesthealth.com

SOUTH TEXAS REHABILITATION HOSPITAL (O, 40 beds) 425 East Alton Gloor Boulevard, Brownsville, TX Zip 78526; tel. 956/554–6000; Jessie Eason Gonzales, Chief Executive Officer
Web address: www.strh.ernesthealth.com

Owned, leased, sponsored:	6 hospitals	260 beds
Contract-managed:	0 hospitals	0 beds
Totals:	6 hospitals	260 beds

0241: ESSENT HEALTHCARE (IO)
3100 West End Avenue, Suite 900, Nashville, TN Zip 37203; tel. 615/312–5100; Michael W. Browder, President and Chief Executive Officer
(Independent Hospital System)

CONNECTICUT: SHARON HOSPITAL (O, 78 beds) 50 Hospital Hill Road, Sharon, CT Zip 06069–0789, Mailing Address: P.O. Box 789, Zip 06069–0789; tel. 860/364–4141; Charles Therrien, Chief Executive Officer
Web address: www.sharonhospital.com

MASSACHUSETTS: MERRIMACK VALLEY HOSPITAL (O, 90 beds) 140 Lincoln Avenue, Haverhill, MA Zip 01830–6798; tel. 978/374–2000; Michael F. Collins, M.D., Chief Executive Officer
Web address: www.merrimackvalleyhospital.com

NASHOBA VALLEY MEDICAL CENTER (O, 57 beds) 200 Groton Road, Ayer, MA Zip 01432–3300; tel. 978/784–9000; Steven P. Roach, Chief Executive Officer
Web address: www.nashobamed.com

PENNSYLVANIA: SOUTHWEST REGIONAL MEDICAL CENTER (O, 45 beds) Seventh Street and Bonar Avenue, Waynesburg, PA Zip 15370–1697; tel. 724/627–3101; Cynthia Cowie, Chief Executive Officer
Web address: www.sw-rmc.com

TEXAS: PARIS REGIONAL MEDICAL CENTER (O, 296 beds) 820 Clarksville Street, Paris, TX Zip 75460–9070; tel. 903/785–4521; Christopher W. Dux, Chief Executive Officer
Web address: www.parisrmc.com

Owned, leased, sponsored:	5 hospitals	566 beds
Contract-managed:	0 hospitals	0 beds
Totals:	5 hospitals	566 beds

0396: ESSENTIA HEALTH (NP)
502 East Second Street, Duluth, MN Zip 55805; tel. 218/786–8376; Peter E. Person, M.D., Chief Executive Officer

IDAHO: CLEARWATER VALLEY HOSPITAL AND CLINICS (O, 23 beds) 301 Cedar, Orofino, ID Zip 83544–9029; tel. 208/476–4555; Casey Meza, Chief Executive Officer
Web address: www.smh-cvhc.org

ST. BENEDICTS FAMILY MEDICAL CENTER (O, 65 beds) 709 North Lincoln Street, Jerome, ID Zip 83338–1851, Mailing Address: P.O. Box 586, Zip 83338–0586; tel. 208/324–4301; Alan Stevenson, Administrator
Web address: www.stbenshospital.org

ST. MARY'S HOSPITAL (O, 28 beds) Lewiston and North Streets, Cottonwood, ID Zip 83522–9750, Mailing Address: P.O. Box 137, Zip 83522–0137; tel. 208/962–3251; Casey Meza, Chief Executive Officer
Web address: www.stmaryshospital.net

MINNESOTA: BRIDGES MEDICAL CENTER (O, 14 beds) 201 9th Street West, Ada, MN Zip 56510–1243; tel. 218/784–5000; Dan Rohrbach, Chief Executive Officer
Web address: www.bridgesmed.com

GRACEVILLE HEALTH CENTER (O, 65 beds) 115 West Second Street, Graceville, MN Zip 56240–0157, Mailing Address: P.O. Box 157, Zip 56240–0157; tel. 320/748–7223; A. Todd Howell, Administrator and Chief Executive Officer
Web address: www.gracevillehealth.com

For explanation of codes following names, see page B2.
★ Indicates Type III membership in the American Hospital Association.

Section B

MILLER–DWAN MEDICAL CENTER (O, 154 beds) 502 East Second Street, Duluth, MN Zip 55805–1982; tel. 218/727–8762; Rocklon B. Chapin, Executive Vice President and Chief Operating Officer
Web address: www.miller–dwan.com

PINE MEDICAL CENTER (O, 94 beds) 109 Court Avenue South, Sandstone, MN Zip 55072–5120; tel. 320/245–2212; Timothy E. Zwickey, Administrator and Chief Executive Officer
Web address: www.pinemedical.org

ST. JOSEPH'S MEDICAL CENTER (O, 162 beds) 523 North Third Street, Brainerd, MN Zip 56401–3098; tel. 218/829–2861; Jani Wiebolt, President and Chief Executive Officer
Web address: www.sjmcmn.org

ST. MARY'S MEDICAL CENTER (O, 337 beds) 407 East Third Street, Duluth, MN Zip 55805–1984; tel. 218/786–4000; Peter E. Person, M.D., President and Chief Executive Officer
Web address: www.smdc.org

ST. MARY'S REGIONAL HEALTH CENTER (O, 154 beds) 1027 Washington Avenue, Detroit Lakes, MN Zip 56501–3598; tel. 218/847–5611; Thomas R. Thompson, Chief Executive Officer
Web address: www.smrhc.com

MONTANA: CENTRAL MONTANA HOSPITAL (O, 20 beds) 1411 9th Street South, Great Falls, MT Zip 59405; tel. 406/216–8000; Jane Drolet, Administrator

NORTH DAKOTA: INNOVIS HEALTH (O, 96 beds) 3000 32nd Avenue South, Fargo, ND Zip 58103; tel. 701/364–8000; Greg Glasner, M.D., Chief Executive Officer
Web address: www.innovishealth.com

WISCONSIN: ST. MARY'S HOSPITAL OF SUPERIOR (O, 25 beds) 3500 Tower Avenue, Superior, WI Zip 54880–5395; tel. 715/395–5400; Mary Shaw, Chief Operating Officer
Web address: www.smdc.org

Owned, leased, sponsored:	13 hospitals	1237 beds
Contract–managed:	0 hospitals	0 beds
Totals:	13 hospitals	1237 beds

2395: EXCELA HEALTH (NP)
532 West Pittsburgh Street, Greensburg, PA Zip 15601; tel. 724/832–5050; David S. Gallatin, Chief Executive Officer
(Centralized Health System)

PENNSYLVANIA: EXCELA FRICK HOSPITAL (O, 83 beds) 508 South Church Street, Mount Pleasant, PA Zip 15666–1790; tel. 724/547–1500; David S. Gallatin, Chief Executive Officer
Web address: www.frickhospital.org

EXCELA HEALTH WESTMORELAND HOSPITAL AT JEANNETTE (O, 149 beds) 600 Jefferson Avenue, Jeannette, PA Zip 15644–2599; tel. 724/527–3551; Julie A. Hester, Administrator

EXCELA LATROBE AREA HOSPITAL (O, 164 beds) 121 West Second Avenue, Latrobe, PA Zip 15650–1096; tel. 724/537–1000; Kim N. Hollon, FACHE, Chief Executive Officer
Web address: www.excelahealth.org

EXCELA WESTMORELAND REGIONAL HOSPITAL (O, 299 beds) 532 West Pittsburgh Street, Greensburg, PA Zip 15601–2282; tel. 724/832–4000; David S. Gallatin, Chief Executive Officer
Web address: www.excelahealth.org

Owned, leased, sponsored:	4 hospitals	695 beds
Contract–managed:	0 hospitals	0 beds
Totals:	4 hospitals	695 beds

★0134: EXEMPLA HEALTHCARE, INC. (NP)
2420 West 26th Avenue, Suite 100–D, Denver, CO Zip 80211; tel. 303/813–5000; Jeffrey D. Selberg, President and Chief Executive Officer
(Moderately Centralized Health System)

COLORADO: EXEMPLA GOOD SAMARITAN MEDICAL CENTER (O, 150 beds) 200 Exempla Circle, Lafayette, CO Zip 80026; tel. 303/689–4000; David Hamm, President and Chief Executive Officer
Web address: www.exempla.org

EXEMPLA LUTHERAN MEDICAL CENTER (O, 543 beds) 8300 West 38th Avenue, Wheat Ridge, CO Zip 80033–6005; tel. 303/425–4500; Robert H. Malte, President and Chief Executive Officer
Web address: www.exempla.org

EXEMPLA SAINT JOSEPH HOSPITAL (C, 436 beds) 1835 Franklin Street, Denver, CO Zip 80218–1191; tel. 303/837–7111; Robert A. Minkin, CHE, President and Chief Executive Officer
Web address: www.exempla.org

Owned, leased, sponsored:	2 hospitals	693 beds
Contract–managed:	1 hospital	436 beds
Totals:	3 hospitals	1129 beds

★1325: FAIRVIEW HEALTH SERVICES (NP)
2450 Riverside Avenue, Minneapolis, MN Zip 55454–1400; tel. 612/672–6300; Mark A. Eustis, President and Chief Executive Officer
(Centralized Physician/Insurance Health System)

MINNESOTA: FAIRVIEW LAKES REGIONAL HEALTH CARE (O, 55 beds) 5200 Fairview Boulevard, Wyoming, MN Zip 55092–8013; tel. 651/982–7000; Daniel K. Anderson, President
Web address: www.fairview.org/lakes/flrmc.htm

FAIRVIEW NORTHLAND MEDICAL CENTER (O, 54 beds) 911 Northland Drive, Princeton, MN Zip 55371–2173; tel. 763/389–1313; Michael Youso, President
Web address: www.fairview.org/northland/

FAIRVIEW RANGE REGIONAL HEALTH SERVICES (O, 107 beds) 750 East 34th Street, Hibbing, MN Zip 55746–4600; tel. 218/262–4881; Lawrence W. Pfaff, President and Chief Executive Officer
Web address: www.range.fairview.org

FAIRVIEW RED WING MEDICAL CENTER (O, 135 beds) 701 Fairview Boulevard, Red Wing, MN Zip 55066–2848, Mailing Address: P.O. Box 95, Zip 55066–0095; tel. 651/267–5000; Scott Wordelman, President and Chief Executive Officer
Web address: www.fairview.org

FAIRVIEW RIDGES HOSPITAL (O, 149 beds) 201 East Nicollet Boulevard, Burnsville, MN Zip 55337–5799; tel. 952/892–2000; Beth Krehbiel, President and Chief Executive Officer
Web address: www.fairview.org

FAIRVIEW SOUTHDALE HOSPITAL (O, 357 beds) 6401 France Avenue South, Edina, MN Zip 55435–2199; tel. 952/924–5000; Bradley Beard, President
Web address: www.fairview.org

UNIVERSITY OF MINNESOTA MEDICAL CENTER, FAIRVIEW (O, 819 beds) 2450 Riverside Avenue, Minneapolis, MN Zip 55454–1400; tel. 612/672–6000; Gordon L. Alexander, President
Web address: www.fairview.org

Owned, leased, sponsored:	7 hospitals	1676 beds
Contract–managed:	0 hospitals	0 beds
Totals:	7 hospitals	1676 beds

0397: FINGER LAKES HEALTH (NP)
196 North Street, Geneva, NY Zip 14456; tel. 315/787–4053; James J. Dooley, President and Chief Executive Officer

NEW YORK: GENEVA GENERAL HOSPITAL (O, 119 beds) 196 North Street, Geneva, NY Zip 14456–1694; tel. 315/787–4000; James J. Dooley, President and Chief Executive Officer
Web address: www.flhealth.org

SOLDIERS AND SAILORS MEMORIAL HOSPITAL OF YATES COUNTY (O, 186 beds) 418 North Main Street, Penn Yan, NY Zip 14527–1085; tel. 315/531–2000; James J. Dooley, President and Chief Executive Officer
Web address: www.flhealth.org

Owned, leased, sponsored:	2 hospitals	305 beds
Contract–managed:	0 hospitals	0 beds
Totals:	2 hospitals	305 beds

For explanation of codes following names, see page B2.
★ Indicates Type III membership in the American Hospital Association.

★0243: FIRSTHEALTH OF THE CAROLINAS (NP)
155 Memorial Drive, Pinehurst, NC Zip 28374–8710, Mailing Address: P.O. Box 3000, Zip 28374–3000; tel. 910/715–1000; Charles T. Frock, Chief Executive Officer
(Centralized Physician/Insurance Health System)

NORTH CAROLINA: FIRSTHEALTH MONTGOMERY MEMORIAL HOSPITAL (O, 25 beds) 520 Allen Street, Troy, NC Zip 27371–2802, Mailing Address: P.O. Box 486, Zip 27371–0486; tel. 910/572–1301; Kerry A. Hensley, RN, President
Web address: www.firsthealth.org

FIRSTHEALTH MOORE REGIONAL HOSPITAL (O, 356 beds) 155 Memorial Drive, Pinehurst, NC Zip 28374–8710, Mailing Address: P.O. Box 3000, Zip 28374–3000; tel. 910/715–1000; Stuart Voelpel, President and Chief Operating Officer
Web address: www.firsthealth.org

FIRSTHEALTH RICHMOND MEMORIAL HOSPITAL (O, 141 beds) 925 Long Drive, Rockingham, NC Zip 28379–4815; tel. 910/417–3000; John J. Jackson, President
Web address: www.firsthealth.org

Owned, leased, sponsored:	3 hospitals	522 beds
Contract-managed:	0 hospitals	0 beds
Totals:	3 hospitals	522 beds

0378: FIVE STAR QUALITY CARE (IO)
400 Centre Street, Newton, MA Zip 02458–2076; tel. 617/796–8387

MASSACHUSETTS: BRAINTREE REHABILITATION HOSPITAL (O, 187 beds) 250 Pond Street, Braintree, MA Zip 2184; tel. 781/848–5353; Randy Doherty, Administrator
Web address: www.braintreerehabhospital.com

NEW ENGLAND REHABILITATION HOSPITAL (O, 210 beds) Two Rehabilitation Way, Woburn, MA Zip 01801–6098; tel. 781/935–5050; Joel Rudin, Chief Executive Officer
Web address: www.newenglandrehab.com

Owned, leased, sponsored:	2 hospitals	397 beds
Contract-managed:	0 hospitals	0 beds
Totals:	2 hospitals	397 beds

0174: FORUM HEALTH (NP)
3530 Belmont Avenue, Suite 7, Youngstown, OH Zip 44505; tel. 330/884–1044; Lowell W. Johnson, President and Chief Executive Officer
(Independent Hospital System)

OHIO: FORUM HEALTH TRUMBULL MEMORIAL HOSPITAL (O, 292 beds) 1350 East Market Street, Warren, OH Zip 44482–6628; tel. 330/841–9011; Todd Hickey, CHE, Interim Chief Executive Officer
Web address: www.forumhealth.org

FORUM HILLSIDE REHABILITATION HOSPITAL (O, 47 beds) 8747 Squires Lane N.E., Warren, OH Zip 44484–1649; tel. 330/841–3700; Marilyn Titus, Vice President and Chief Operating Officer
Web address: www.forumhealth.org

WESTERN RESERVE CARE SYSTEM (O, 373 beds) 500 Gypsy Lane, Youngstown, OH Zip 44501–0240, Mailing Address: P.O. Box 990, Zip 44501–0990; tel. 330/747–1444; Keith T. Ghezzi, M.D., President and Chief Executive Officer
Web address: www.forumhealth.org

Owned, leased, sponsored:	3 hospitals	712 beds
Contract-managed:	0 hospitals	0 beds
Totals:	3 hospitals	712 beds

★1475: FRANCISCAN MISSIONARIES OF OUR LADY HEALTH SYSTEM, INC. (CC)
4200 Essen Lane, Baton Rouge, LA Zip 70809; tel. 225/923–2701; John J. Finan, Jr., President and Chief Executive Officer
(Moderately Centralized Health System)

LOUISIANA: ASSUMPTION COMMUNITY HOSPITAL (O, 6 beds) 135 Highway 402, Napoleonville, LA Zip 70390; tel. 985/369–3600; Wayne M. Arboneaux, Chief Executive Officer
Web address: www.ololrmc.com

OUR LADY OF LOURDES REGIONAL MEDICAL CENTER (O, 217 beds) 611 St. Landry Street, Lafayette, LA Zip 70506–4627, Mailing Address: P.O. Box 4027, Zip 70502–4027; tel. 337/289–2000; William F. Barrow, II, President and Chief Executive Officer
Web address: www.lourdes.net

OUR LADY OF THE LAKE REGIONAL MEDICAL CENTER (O, 1006 beds) 5000 Hennessy Boulevard, Baton Rouge, LA Zip 70808–4350; tel. 225/765–6565; K. Scott Wester, FACHE, President and Chief Executive Officer
Web address: www.ololrmc.com

ST. ELIZABETH HOSPITAL (O, 66 beds) 1125 West Highway 30, Gonzales, LA Zip 70737; tel. 225/647–5000; Dolores LeJeune, Chief Executive Officer
Web address: www.steh.com

ST. FRANCIS MEDICAL CENTER (O, 415 beds) 309 Jackson Street, Monroe, LA Zip 71201–7407, Mailing Address: P.O. Box 1901, Zip 71210–1901; tel. 318/327–4000; Sister Kathleen Cain, Interim President and Chief Executive Officer
Web address: www.stfran.com

ST. PATRICK'S PSYCHIATRIC HOSPITAL (O, 24 beds) 3421 Medical Park Drive, Monroe, LA Zip 71203–2355; tel. 318/327–4686; Cindy J. Rogers, FACHE, Chief Executive Officer
Web address: www.stpatrickshospital.net

Owned, leased, sponsored:	6 hospitals	1734 beds
Contract-managed:	0 hospitals	0 beds
Totals:	6 hospitals	1734 beds

★5375: FRANCISCAN SERVICES CORPORATION (CC)
6832 Convent Boulevard, Sylvania, OH Zip 43560–2897; tel. 419/882–8373; John W. O'Connell, President
(Centralized Physician/Insurance Health System)

OHIO: TRINITY HEALTH SYSTEM (S, 308 beds) 380 Summit Avenue, Steubenville, OH Zip 43952–2699; tel. 740/283–7000; Fred B. Brower, President and Chief Executive Officer
Web address: www.trinityhealth.com

TEXAS: BURLESON ST. JOSEPH HEALTH CENTER (S, 25 beds) 1101 Woodson Drive, Caldwell, TX Zip 77836–1052, Mailing Address: P.O. Drawer 360, Zip 77836–0360; tel. 979/567–3245; Reed Edmundson, Administrator
Web address: www.st-joseph.org/

GRIMES ST. JOSEPH HEALTH CENTER (S, 25 beds) 210 South Judson Street, Navasota, TX Zip 77868–3704; tel. 936/825–6585; Dia Copeland, Administrator
Web address: www.st-joseph.org

MADISON ST. JOSEPH HEALTH CENTER (S, 25 beds) 100 West Cross Street, Madisonville, TX Zip 77864–0698, Mailing Address: Box 698, Zip 77864–0698; tel. 936/348–2631; Reed Edmundson, Administrator

ST. JOSEPH REGIONAL HEALTH CENTER (S, 253 beds) 2801 Franciscan Drive, Bryan, TX Zip 77802–2599; tel. 979/776–3777; Anthony D. Pfitzer, FACHE, Chief Executive Officer
Web address: www.st-joseph.org

TRINITY COMMUNITY MEDICAL CENTER OF BRENHAM (S, 60 beds) 700 Medical Parkway, Brenham, TX Zip 77833–5498; tel. 979/836–6173; John L. Simms, President and Chief Executive Officer
Web address: www.trinitymed.org

Owned, leased, sponsored:	6 hospitals	696 beds
Contract-managed:	0 hospitals	0 beds
Totals:	6 hospitals	696 beds

★1455: FRANCISCAN SISTERS OF CHRISTIAN CHARITY HEALTHCARE MINISTRY, INC (CC)
1415 South Rapids Road, Manitowoc, WI Zip 54220–9302; tel. 920/684–7071; Sister Laura J. Wolf, President
(Moderately Centralized Health System)

For explanation of codes following names, see page B2.
★ Indicates Type III membership in the American Hospital Association.

NEBRASKA: ST. FRANCIS MEMORIAL HOSPITAL (O, 92 beds) 430 North Monitor Street, West Point, NE Zip 68788–1595; tel. 402/372–2404; Ronald O. Briggs, FACHE, President and Chief Executive Officer
Web address: www.fcswp.org

OHIO: GENESIS HEALTHCARE SYSTEM (O, 395 beds) 2951 Maple Avenue, Zanesville, OH Zip 43701–2881; tel. 740/454–5000; Matthew J. Perry, President and Chief Executive Officer
Web address: www.genesishcs.org

WISCONSIN: HOLY FAMILY MEMORIAL MEDICAL CENTER (O, 67 beds) 2300 Western Avenue, Manitowoc, WI Zip 54220, Mailing Address: P.O. Box 1450, Zip 54221–1450; tel. 920/320–2011; Mark P. Herzog, President and Chief Executive Officer
Web address: www.hfmhealth.org

Owned, leased, sponsored:	3 hospitals	554 beds
Contract-managed:	0 hospitals	0 beds
Totals:	3 hospitals	554 beds

★0271: FREEMAN HEALTH SYSTEM (NP)

1102 West 32nd Street, Joplin, MO Zip 64804; tel. 417/347–1111; Gary D. Duncan, President and Chief Executive Officer
(Centralized Health System)

MISSOURI: FREEMAN HEALTH SYSTEM (O, 326 beds) 1102 West 32nd Street, Joplin, MO Zip 64804–3503; tel. 417/347–1111; Gary D. Duncan, President and Chief Executive Officer
Web address: www.freemanhealth.com

FREEMAN NEOSHO HOSPITAL (O, 25 beds) 113 West Hickory Street, Neosho, MO Zip 64850–1705; tel. 417/455–4352; Daxton Holcomb, Chief Executive Officer
Web address: www.freemanhealth.com

Owned, leased, sponsored:	2 hospitals	351 beds
Contract-managed:	0 hospitals	0 beds
Totals:	2 hospitals	351 beds

2115: FREMONT–RIDEOUT HEALTH GROUP (NP)

989 Plumas Street, Yuba City, CA Zip 95991; tel. 530/751–4010; Thomas P. Hayes, President and Chief Executive Officer
(Independent Hospital System)

CALIFORNIA: FREMONT MEDICAL CENTER (O, 90 beds) 989 Plumas Street, Yuba City, CA Zip 95991–4087; tel. 530/751–4000; Theresa Hamilton, Chief Executive Officer
Web address: www.frhg.org

RIDEOUT MEMORIAL HOSPITAL (O, 222 beds) 726 Fourth Street, Marysville, CA Zip 95901–5600, Mailing Address: P.O. Box 2128, Zip 95901–2128; tel. 530/749–4300; Theresa Hamilton, Chief Executive Officer
Web address: www.frhg.org

Owned, leased, sponsored:	2 hospitals	312 beds
Contract-managed:	0 hospitals	0 beds
Totals:	2 hospitals	312 beds

0182: FUNDAMENTAL LONG TERM CARE HOLDINGS, LLC (IO)

930 Ridgebrook Road, Sparks Glencoe, MD Zip 21152; tel. 410/773–1000; W. Bradley Bennett, President and Chief Executive Officer
(Independent Hospital System)

KANSAS: SPECIALTY HOSPITAL OF MID–AMERICA (O, 52 beds) 6509 West 103rd Street, Overland Park, KS Zip 66212–1728; tel. 913/649–3701; Karen Leverich, Chief Executive Officer
Web address: www.thicare.com/SpecHospOfMidAmerica/

WICHITA SPECIALTY HOSPITAL (O, 26 beds) 8080 East Pawnee Street, Wichita, KS Zip 67207–5475; tel. 316/682–0004; Phyllis Williams, Chief Executive Officer
Web address: www.fundltc.com

NEVADA: HARMON MEDICAL AND REHABILITATION HOSPITAL (O, 118 beds) 2170 East Harmon Avenue, Las Vegas, NV Zip 89119; tel. 702/794–0100; Darrin Cook, Administrator

HORIZON SPECIALTY HOSPITAL (O, 25 beds) 640 Desert Lane, Las Vegas, NV Zip 89106; tel. 702/382–3155; Frank Bellinger, Chief Executive Officer and Administrator

NEW MEXICO: SPECIALTY HOSPITAL OF ALBUQUERQUE (O, 25 beds) 235 Elm Street N.E., Albuquerque, NM Zip 87102; tel. 505/842–5550; Kathi Gleim, Chief Executive Officer

OKLAHOMA: EDMOND SPECIALTY HOSPITAL (O, 37 beds) 1100 East Ninth Street, Edmond, OK Zip 73034–5755; tel. 405/341–8150; Phyllis Williams, Chief Executive Officer
Web address: www.thicare.com/EdmondSpecialty/

TEXAS: PLANO SPECIALTY HOSPITAL (O, 30 beds) 1621 Coit Road, Plano, TX Zip 75075; tel. 972/758–5200; Neal Duncan, Administrator and Chief Executive Officer
Web address: www.planospecialtyhospital.com

SOUTHWEST REGIONAL MEDICAL COMPLEX (O, 30 beds) 1409 9th Street, Lubbock, TX Zip 79401–2601; tel. 806/767–9133; Deanna Graves, Chief Executive Officer
Web address: www.ihsoflubbock.com

SPECIALTY HOSPITAL AT PLUM CREEK (O, 47 beds) 5601 Plum Creek Drive, Amarillo, TX Zip 79124–1801; tel. 806/351–1000; Thomas P. Harlan, Chief Executive Officer

TEXAS SPECIALTY HOSPITAL (O, 31 beds) 6160 South Loop East, Houston, TX Zip 77087–1010; tel. 713/640–2400; Patrick A. Auman, Ph.D., Executive Director
Web address: www.thicare.com

TEXAS SPECIALTY HOSPITAL AT DALLAS (O, 66 beds) 7955 Harry Hines Boulevard, Dallas, TX Zip 75235–3395; tel. 214/637–0000; Cathy Campbell, Chief Executive Officer
Web address: www.thicare.com

TEXAS SPECIALTY HOSPITAL AT SAN ANTONIO (O, 30 beds) 7310 Oak Manor Drive, San Antonio, TX Zip 78229–4509; tel. 210/308–0261; Yolanda Ochoa, Interim Administrator
Web address: www.thicare.com

TEXAS SPECIALTY HOSPITAL AT WICHITA FALLS (O, 31 beds) 1103 Grace Street, Wichita Falls, TX Zip 76301–4414; tel. 940/720–6633; Billy Blasingame, Administrator
Web address: www.thicare.com

Owned, leased, sponsored:	13 hospitals	548 beds
Contract-managed:	0 hospitals	0 beds
Totals:	13 hospitals	548 beds

★5570: GEISINGER HEALTH SYSTEM (NP)

100 North Academy Avenue, Danville, PA Zip 17822; tel. 570/271–6211; Glenn Steele, Jr., M.D., Ph.D., President and Chief Executive Officer
(Centralized Physician/Insurance Health System)

PENNSYLVANIA: GEISINGER MEDICAL CENTER (O, 392 beds) 100 North Academy Avenue, Danville, PA Zip 17822–2201; tel. 570/271–6211; E. Lynn Miller, Chief Administrative Officer
Web address: www.geisinger.org

GEISINGER SOUTH WILKES–BARRE (O, 112 beds) 25 Church Street, Wilkes–Barre, PA Zip 18765–0999; tel. 570/826–3100; Cynthia Brylinsky, Vice President, Administration
Web address: www.geisinger.org

GEISINGER WYOMING VALLEY MEDICAL CENTER (O, 148 beds) 1000 East Mountain Drive, Wilkes–Barre, PA Zip 18711–0027; tel. 570/826–7300; Lissa Bryan–Smith, Chief Administrative Officer
Web address: www.geisinger.org

Owned, leased, sponsored:	3 hospitals	652 beds
Contract-managed:	0 hospitals	0 beds
Totals:	3 hospitals	652 beds

★0311: GENESIS HEALTH SYSTEM (NP)

1227 East Rusholme Street, Davenport, IA Zip 52803–2498; tel. 563/421–1000; Douglas P. Cropper, Chief Executive Officer
(Centralized Health System)

For explanation of codes following names, see page B2.
★ Indicates Type III membership in the American Hospital Association.

ILLINOIS: GENESIS MEDICAL CENTER, ILLINI CAMPUS (O, 110 beds) 801 Illini Drive, Silvis, IL Zip 61282–1893; tel. 309/792–9363; Charles E. Bruhn, Administrator
Web address: www.genesishealth.com

IOWA: GENESIS MEDICAL CENTER, DEWITT (O, 86 beds) 1118 11th Street, De Witt, IA Zip 52742–1296; tel. 563/659–4200; Jeffrey M. Cooper, Vice President, DeWitt Operations
Web address: www.genesishealth.com

GENESIS MEDICAL CENTER–DAVENPORT (O, 414 beds) 1227 East Rusholme Street, Davenport, IA Zip 52803–2498; tel. 563/421–1000; Douglas P. Cropper, Chief Executive Officer
Web address: www.genesishealth.com

Owned, leased, sponsored:	3 hospitals	610 beds
Contract–managed:	0 hospitals	0 beds
Totals:	3 hospitals	610 beds

0283: GILLIARD HEALTH SERVICES (IO)

3091 Carter Hill Road, Montgomery, AL Zip 36111; tel. 334/265–5009; William G. McKenzie, President, Chief Executive Officer and Chairman
(Independent Hospital System)

ALABAMA: EVERGREEN MEDICAL CENTER (O, 44 beds) 101 Crestview Avenue, Evergreen, AL Zip 36401–0706, Mailing Address: P.O. Box 706, Zip 36401–0706; tel. 251/578–2480; Robert J. Humphrey, Administrator
Web address: www.evergreenmedical.org

JACKSON MEDICAL CENTER (O, 26 beds) 220 Hospital Drive, Jackson, AL Zip 36545–2459, Mailing Address: P.O. Box 428, Zip 36545–0428; tel. 251/246–9021; Teresa F. Grimes, Administrator
Web address: www.jacksonmedicalcenter.com

TROY REGIONAL MEDICAL CENTER (O, 78 beds) 1330 Highway 231 South, Troy, AL Zip 36081–1224; tel. 334/670–5000; Russell Eldridge, Chief Executive Officer

Owned, leased, sponsored:	3 hospitals	148 beds
Contract–managed:	0 hospitals	0 beds
Totals:	3 hospitals	148 beds

★1535: GREAT PLAINS HEALTH ALLIANCE, INC. (NP)

625 Third Street, Phillipsburg, KS Zip 67661–2138, Mailing Address: P.O. Box 366, Zip 67661–0366; tel. 785/543–2111; Roger S. John, President and Chief Executive Officer
(Decentralized Health System)

KANSAS: ASHLAND HEALTH CENTER (C, 47 beds) 709 Oak Street, Ashland, KS Zip 67831–0188, Mailing Address: P.O. Box 188, Zip 67831–0188; tel. 620/635–2241; Daryl Marshall, Administrator
Web address: www.ashlandks.com/healthserv.htm

CHEYENNE COUNTY HOSPITAL (L, 16 beds) 210 West First Street, Saint Francis, KS Zip 67756–0547, Mailing Address: P.O. Box 547, Zip 67756–0547; tel. 785/332–2104; Leslie Lacy, Administrator
Web address: www.cheyennecountyhospital.com

COMANCHE COUNTY HOSPITAL (C, 14 beds) 202 South Frisco Street, Coldwater, KS Zip 67029, Mailing Address: HC 65, Box 8A, Zip 67029; tel. 620/582–2144; Nancy Zimmerman, RN, Administrator
Web address: www.gpha.com

ELLINWOOD DISTRICT HOSPITAL (L, 25 beds) 605 North Main Street, Ellinwood, KS Zip 67526–1440; tel. 620/564–2548; Joyce Schulte, Chief Executive Officer
Web address: www.ellinwood.org

FREDONIA REGIONAL HOSPITAL (C, 34 beds) 1527 Madison Street, Fredonia, KS Zip 66736–1751, Mailing Address: P.O. Box 579, Zip 66736–0579; tel. 620/378–2121; Terry Deschaine, Chief Executive Officer
Web address: www.gpha.com

GRISELL MEMORIAL HOSPITAL DISTRICT ONE (C, 46 beds) 210 South Vermont Avenue, Ransom, KS Zip 67572; tel. 785/731–2231; Kristine Ochs, RN, Administrator
Web address: www.gpha.com

LANE COUNTY HOSPITAL (C, 31 beds) 235 West Vine, Dighton, KS Zip 67839–0969, Mailing Address: P.O. Box 969, Zip 67839–0969; tel. 620/397–5321; Donna McGowan, Administrator
Web address: www.gpha.com

MEDICINE LODGE MEMORIAL HOSPITAL (C, 25 beds) 710 North Walnut Street, Medicine Lodge, KS Zip 67104–1019; tel. 620/886–3771; Kevin A. White, Administrator

MINNEOLA DISTRICT HOSPITAL (C, 54 beds) 212 Main Street, Minneola, KS Zip 67865–0127, Mailing Address: P.O. Box 127, Zip 67865–0127; tel. 620/885–4264; Cynthia K. Schneider, Interim Administrator and Chief Executive Officer
Web address: www.minneolakansas.com

OSBORNE COUNTY MEMORIAL HOSPITAL (C, 25 beds) 424 West New Hampshire Street, Osborne, KS Zip 67473–0070, Mailing Address: P.O. Box 70, Zip 67473–0070; tel. 785/346–2121; Kiley Floyd, Administrator
Web address: www.ocmh.org

OTTAWA COUNTY HEALTH CENTER (L, 52 beds) 215 East Eighth, Minneapolis, KS Zip 67467–1999, Mailing Address: P.O. Box 290, Zip 67467–0290; tel. 785/392–2122; Joy Johnson, RN, Administrator
Web address: www.ottawacountyhealthcenter.com

PHILLIPS COUNTY HOSPITAL (L, 58 beds) 1150 State Street, Phillipsburg, KS Zip 67661–1799, Mailing Address: P.O. Box 607, Zip 67661–0607; tel. 785/543–5226; Heather L. Harper, Administrator
Web address: www.phillipshospital.org

RAWLINS COUNTY HEALTH CENTER (C, 24 beds) 707 Grant Street, Atwood, KS Zip 67730–4700, Mailing Address: P.O. Box 47, Zip 67730–4700; tel. 785/626–3211; Deanna Freeman, Administrator and Chief Executive Officer
Web address: www.rchc.us

REPUBLIC COUNTY HOSPITAL (L, 63 beds) 2420 G Street, Belleville, KS Zip 66935–2400; tel. 785/527–2254; Blaine K. Miller, Administrator
Web address: www.rphospital.org

SABETHA COMMUNITY HOSPITAL (L, 25 beds) 14th and Oregon Streets, Sabetha, KS Zip 66534–0229, Mailing Address: P.O. Box 229, Zip 66534–0229; tel. 785/284–2121; Lora Key, Chief Executive Officer
Web address: www.sabethahospital.com

SATANTA DISTRICT HOSPITAL (C, 57 beds) 401 South Cheyenne Street, Satanta, KS Zip 67870–0159, Mailing Address: P.O. Box 159, Zip 67870–0159; tel. 620/649–2761; Curt Colson, Administrator
Web address: www.satantahospital.org

SMITH COUNTY MEMORIAL HOSPITAL (L, 53 beds) 614 South Main Street, Smith Center, KS Zip 66967–0349, Mailing Address: P.O. Box 349, Zip 66967–0349; tel. 785/282–6845; Carolyn K. Hess, RN, Administrator
Web address: www.gpha.com

TREGO COUNTY–LEMKE MEMORIAL HOSPITAL (C, 62 beds) 320 North 13th Street, Wakeeney, KS Zip 67672–2099; tel. 785/743–2182; Jean Dean, Administrator
Web address: www.tclmh.com

NEBRASKA: HARLAN COUNTY HEALTH SYSTEM (C, 25 beds) 717 North Brown Street, Alma, NE Zip 68920–0836, Mailing Address: P.O. Box 836, Zip 68920–0836; tel. 308/928–2151; Allen Van Driel, CHE, Administrator
Web address: www.gpha.com

Owned, leased, sponsored:	7 hospitals	292 beds
Contract–managed:	12 hospitals	444 beds
Totals:	19 hospitals	736 beds

★1555: GREENVILLE HOSPITAL SYSTEM (NP)

701 Grove Road, Greenville, SC Zip 29605–4211; tel. 864/455–7000; Michael C. Riordan, President and Chief Executive Officer
(Moderately Centralized Health System)

SOUTH CAROLINA: ALLEN BENNETT MEMORIAL HOSPITAL (O, 146 beds) 313 Memorial Drive, Greer, SC Zip 29650–1521; tel. 864/848–8200; Phil Feisal, Administrator
Web address: www.ghs.org

GREENVILLE MEMORIAL HOSPITAL (O, 777 beds) 701 Grove Road, Greenville, SC Zip 29605–4295; tel. 864/455–7000; Greg Rusnak, Chief Operating Officer
Web address: www.ghs.org

HILLCREST HOSPITAL (O, 43 beds) 729 S.E. Main Street, Simpsonville, SC Zip 29681–3280; tel. 864/967–6100; Dennis R. Burns, FACHE, Administrator
Web address: www.ghs.org

For explanation of codes following names, see page B2.
★ Indicates Type III membership in the American Hospital Association.

Section B

PATEWOOD MEMORIAL HOSPITAL (O, 72 beds) 175 Patewood Drive, Greenville, SC Zip 29605; tel. 864/797–0112; Scott R. Jones, Administrator

Owned, leased, sponsored:	4 hospitals	1038 beds
Contract–managed:	0 hospitals	0 beds
Totals:	4 hospitals	1038 beds

★0675: GUTHRIE HEALTHCARE SYSTEM (NP)
Guthrie Square, Sayre, PA Zip 18840; tel. 570/882–4312; Mark Stensager, President and Chief Executive Officer
(Centralized Health System)

NEW YORK: CORNING HOSPITAL (O, 82 beds) 176 Denison Parkway East, Corning, NY Zip 14830–2899; tel. 607/937–7200; Shirley P. Magana, President and Chief Operating Officer
Web address: www.corninghospital.com

PENNSYLVANIA: ROBERT PACKER HOSPITAL (O, 224 beds) 1 Guthrie Square, Sayre, PA Zip 18840–1698; tel. 570/888–6666; Marie T. Droege, President and Chief Operating Officer
Web address: www.guthrie.org

TROY COMMUNITY HOSPITAL (O, 25 beds) 100 John Street, Troy, PA Zip 16947–0036; tel. 570/297–2121; Staci Covey, Administrator
Web address: www.guthrie.org

Owned, leased, sponsored:	3 hospitals	331 beds
Contract–managed:	0 hospitals	0 beds
Totals:	3 hospitals	331 beds

0303: HACKLEY HEALTH SYSTEM (NP)
2700 Clinton Street, Muskegon, MI Zip 49442; tel. 231/726–3511; Gordon A. Mudler, President and Chief Executive Officer
(Centralized Physician/Insurance Health System)

MICHIGAN: HACKLEY HOSPITAL (O, 181 beds) 1700 Clinton Street, Muskegon, MI Zip 49443–3302, Mailing Address: P.O. Box 3302, Zip 49443–3302; tel. 231/726–3511; Gordon A. Mudler, President and Chief Executive Officer
Web address: www.hackley.org

HACKLEY LAKESHORE HOSPITAL (O, 24 beds) 72 South State Street, Shelby, MI Zip 49455–1299; tel. 231/861–2156; Jay Bryan, Chief Executive Officer
Web address: www.hackley.org

Owned, leased, sponsored:	2 hospitals	205 beds
Contract–managed:	0 hospitals	0 beds
Totals:	2 hospitals	205 beds

★3555: HAWAII HEALTH SYSTEMS CORPORATION (NP)
3675 Kilauea Avenue, Honolulu, HI Zip 96816; tel. 808/733–4151; Thomas M. Driskill, Jr., President and Chief Executive Officer
(Moderately Centralized Health System)

HAWAII: HALE HO'OLA HAMAKUA (O, 52 beds) 45–547 Plumeria Street, Honokaa, HI Zip 96727–6902; tel. 808/775–7211; Jeanne Abe, Administrator
Web address: www.hhsc.org

HILO MEDICAL CENTER (O, 271 beds) 1190 Waianuenue Avenue, Hilo, HI Zip 96720–2095; tel. 808/974–4700; Ronald J. Schurra, Regional Chief Executive Officer
Web address: www.hmc.hhsc.org

KAU HOSPITAL (O, 21 beds) 1 Kamani Street, Pahala, HI Zip 96777, Mailing Address: P.O. Box 40, Zip 96777–0040; tel. 808/928–8331; Merilyn Harris, Administrator
Web address: www.hhsc.org

KAUAI VETERANS MEMORIAL HOSPITAL (O, 45 beds) Waimea Canyon Road, Waimea, HI Zip 96796, Mailing Address: P.O. Box 337, Zip 96796–0337; tel. 808/338–9431; Orianna A. Skomoroch, Regional Chief Executive Officer
Web address: www.kvmh.hhsc.org

KOHALA HOSPITAL (O, 26 beds) 54–383 Hospital Road, Kohala, HI Zip 96755, Mailing Address: P.O. Box 10, Kapaau, Zip 96755–0010; tel. 808/889–6211; Donald Lewis, Administrator
Web address: www.koh.hhsc.org

KONA COMMUNITY HOSPITAL (O, 88 beds) 79–1019 Haukapila Street, Kealakekua, HI Zip 96750–7920; tel. 808/322–9311; Earl Greenia, Regional Chief Executive Officer
Web address: www.kch.hhsc.org

KULA HOSPITAL (O, 5 beds) 100 Keokea Place, Kula, HI Zip 96790–7450; tel. 808/878–1221; Lee Johnson, Administrator
Web address: www.hhsc.org

LANAI COMMUNITY HOSPITAL (O, 14 beds) 628 Seventh Street, Lanai City, HI Zip 96763–0650, Mailing Address: P.O. Box 630650, Zip 96763–0650; tel. 808/565–6411; John Schaumburg, Administrator
Web address: www.lch.hhsc.org

LEAHI HOSPITAL (O, 190 beds) 3675 Kilauea Avenue, Honolulu, HI Zip 96816–2398; tel. 808/733–8000; Vincent H. S. Lee, FACHE, Regional Chief Executive Officer
Web address: www.hhsc.org

MAUI MEMORIAL MEDICAL CENTER (O, 203 beds) 221 Mahalani Street, Wailuku, HI Zip 96793–2581; tel. 808/244–9056; Wesley Lo, Regional Chief Executive Officer
Web address: www.mmmc.hhsc.org

SAMUEL MAHELONA MEMORIAL HOSPITAL (O, 14 beds) 4800 Kawaihau Road, Kapaa, HI Zip 96746–1998; tel. 808/822–4961; Orianna A. Skomoroch, Regional Chief Executive Officer
Web address: www.smmh.hhsc.org

Owned, leased, sponsored:	11 hospitals	929 beds
Contract–managed:	0 hospitals	0 beds
Totals:	11 hospitals	929 beds

0266: HAWAII PACIFIC HEALTH (NP)
55 Merchant Street, Honolulu, HI Zip 96813; tel. 808/535–7414; Charles A. Sted, President and Chief Executive Officer
(Independent Hospital System)

KAPIOLANI MEDICAL CENTER AT PALI MOMI (O, 116 beds) 98–1079 Moanalua Road, Aiea, HI Zip 96701–4713; tel. 808/486–6000; Raymond Vara, Chief Executive Officer
Web address: www.kapiolani.org

KAPIOLANI MEDICAL CENTER FOR WOMEN & CHILDREN (O, 225 beds) 1319 Punahou Street, Honolulu, HI Zip 96826–1032; tel. 808/983–6000; Raymond Vara, Chief Executive Officer
Web address: www.kapiolani.org

STRAUB CLINIC & HOSPITAL (O, 143 beds) 888 South King Street, Honolulu, HI Zip 96813–3083; tel. 808/522–4000; Raymond Vara, Chief Executive Officer
Web address: www.straubhealth.org

WILCOX MEMORIAL HOSPITAL (O, 71 beds) 3–3420 Kuhio Highway, Lihue, HI Zip 96766–1099; tel. 808/245–1100; Kathleen Clark, President and Chief Executive Officer
Web address: www.wilcoxhealth.org

Owned, leased, sponsored:	4 hospitals	555 beds
Contract–managed:	0 hospitals	0 beds
Totals:	4 hospitals	555 beds

★0048: HCA (IO)
One Park Plaza, Nashville, TN Zip 37203–1548; tel. 615/344–9551; Jack O. Bovender, Jr., Chairman and Chief Executive Officer
(Decentralized Health System)

ALASKA: ALASKA REGIONAL HOSPITAL (O, 129 beds) 2801 Debarr Road, Anchorage, AK Zip 99508–2997, Mailing Address: P.O. Box 143889, Zip 99514–3889; tel. 907/264–1754; Edward H. Lamb, FACHE, President and Chief Executive Officer
Web address: www.alaskaregional.com

CALIFORNIA: GOOD SAMARITAN HOSPITAL (O, 328 beds) 2425 Samaritan Drive, San Jose, CA Zip 95124–3997, Mailing Address: P.O. Box 240002, Zip 95154–2402; tel. 408/559–2011; William K. Piche, Chief Executive Officer
Web address: www.goodsamsanjose.com

LOS ROBLES HOSPITAL AND MEDICAL CENTER (O, 273 beds) 215 West Janss Road, Thousand Oaks, CA Zip 91360–1847; tel. 805/497–2727; Jim Sherman, President and Chief Executive Officer
Web address: www.losrobleshospital.com

For explanation of codes following names, see page B2.
★ Indicates Type III membership in the American Hospital Association.

Section B

REGIONAL MEDICAL CENTER OF SAN JOSE (O, 184 beds) 225 North Jackson Avenue, San Jose, CA Zip 95116–1691; tel. 408/259–5000; William L. Gilbert, Chief Executive Officer
Web address: www.regionalmedicalsanjose.com

RIVERSIDE COMMUNITY HOSPITAL (O, 373 beds) 4445 Magnolia Avenue, Riverside, CA Zip 92501–4199, Mailing Address: P.O. Box 1669, Zip 92502–1669; tel. 951/788–3000; Michael A. Rembis, FACHE, President and Chief Executive Officer
Web address: www.riversidecommunityhospital.com

WEST HILLS HOSPITAL AND MEDICAL CENTER (O, 114 beds) 7300 Medical Center Drive, Canoga Park, CA Zip 91307–1910; tel. 818/676–4000; Beverly Gilmore, President and Chief Executive Officer
Web address: www.westhillshospital.com

COLORADO: MEDICAL CENTER OF AURORA (O, 314 beds) 1501 South Potomac Street, Aurora, CO Zip 80012–5499; tel. 303/695–2600; John Hill, President and Chief Executive Officer
Web address: www.auroramed.com

NORTH SUBURBAN MEDICAL CENTER (O, 118 beds) 9191 Grant Street, Thornton, CO Zip 80229–4341; tel. 303/451–7800; Todd Steward, President and Chief Executive Officer
Web address: www.northsuburban.com

PRESBYTERIAN–ST. LUKE'S MEDICAL CENTER (O, 400 beds) 1719 East 19th Avenue, Denver, CO Zip 80218–1281; tel. 303/839–6000; Madeleine Roberson, President and Chief Executive Officer
Web address: www.pslmc.com

ROSE MEDICAL CENTER (O, 294 beds) 4567 East Ninth Avenue, Denver, CO Zip 80220–3941; tel. 303/320–2121; Kenneth H. Feiler, President and Chief Executive Officer
Web address: www.rosebabies.com

SKY RIDGE MEDICAL CENTER (O, 150 beds) 10101 Ridge Gate Parkway, Lone Tree, CO Zip 80124; tel. 720/225–1000; Maureen Tarrant, Chief Executive Officer
Web address: www.skyridgemedcenter.com

SPALDING REHABILITATION HOSPITAL (O, 50 beds) 900 Potomac Street, Aurora, CO Zip 80011–6716; tel. 303/367–1166; Cynthia Kreutz, President and Chief Executive Officer
Web address: www.spaldingrehab.com

SWEDISH MEDICAL CENTER (O, 350 beds) 501 East Hampden Avenue, Englewood, CO Zip 80113; tel. 303/788–5000; Mary M. White, President and Chief Executive Officer
Web address: www.swedishhospital.com

FLORIDA: AVENTURA HOSPITAL AND MEDICAL CENTER (O, 359 beds) 20900 Biscayne Boulevard, Aventura, FL Zip 33180–1407; tel. 305/682–7000; Heather J. Rohan, Chief Executive Officer
Web address: www.aventurahospital.com

BLAKE MEDICAL CENTER (O, 263 beds) 2020 59th Street West, Bradenton, FL Zip 34209–4669; tel. 941/792–6611; Daniel J. Friedrich, III, Chief Executive Officer
Web address: www.blakemedicalcenter.com

BRANDON REGIONAL HOSPITAL (O, 367 beds) 119 Oakfield Drive, Brandon, FL Zip 33511–5799; tel. 813/681–5551; Michael M. Fencel, Chief Executive Officer
Web address: www.brandonhospital.com

CAPITAL REGIONAL MEDICAL CENTER (O, 177 beds) 2626 Capital Medical Boulevard, Tallahassee, FL Zip 32308–4499; tel. 850/325–5000; Sharon L. Roush, Chief Executive Officer
Web address: www.capitalregionalmedicalcenter.com

CENTRAL FLORIDA REGIONAL HOSPITAL (O, 226 beds) 1401 West Seminole Boulevard, Sanford, FL Zip 32771–6764; tel. 407/321–4500; Rodney R. Smith, Chief Executive Officer
Web address: www.centralfloridaregional.com

COLUMBIA HOSPITAL (O, 250 beds) 2201 45th Street, West Palm Beach, FL Zip 33407–2069; tel. 561/842–6141; Valerie A. Jackson, Chief Executive Officer
Web address: www.columbiahospital.com

COMMUNITY HOSPITAL (O, 267 beds) 5637 Marine Parkway, New Port Richey, FL Zip 34652–4331, Mailing Address: P.O. Box 996, Zip 34656–0996; tel. 727/848–1733; Kathryn Gillette, Chief Executive Officer
Web address: www.communityhospitalnpr.com

DOCTORS HOSPITAL OF SARASOTA (O, 168 beds) 5731 Bee Ridge Road, Sarasota, FL Zip 34233–5056; tel. 941/342–1100; Robert C. Meade, Chief Executive Officer
Web address: www.doctorsofsarasota.com

EDWARD WHITE HOSPITAL (O, 113 beds) 2323 Ninth Avenue North, Saint Petersburg, FL Zip 33713–6898, Mailing Address: P.O. Box 12018, Zip 33733–2018; tel. 727/323–1111; Roland Metivier, Chief Executive Officer
Web address: www.edwardwhitehospital.com

ENGLEWOOD COMMUNITY HOSPITAL (O, 100 beds) 700 Medical Boulevard, Englewood, FL Zip 34223–3978; tel. 941/475–6571; Wendy H. Brandon, Chief Executive Officer
Web address: www.englewoodcommunityhospital.com

FAWCETT MEMORIAL HOSPITAL (O, 238 beds) 21298 Olean Boulevard, Port Charlotte, FL Zip 33952–6765, Mailing Address: P.O. Box 494960, Punta Gorda, Zip 33949–4960; tel. 941/629–1181; Thomas J. Rice, President and Chief Executive Officer
Web address: www.fawcetthospital.com

FORT WALTON BEACH MEDICAL CENTER (O, 257 beds) 1000 Mar–Walt Drive, Fort Walton Beach, FL Zip 32547–6795; tel. 850/862–1111; Wayne F. Campbell, Chief Executive Officer
Web address: www.fwbmedicalcenter.com

GULF COAST MEDICAL CENTER (O, 176 beds) 449 West 23rd Street, Panama City, FL Zip 32405–4593, Mailing Address: P.O. Box 15309, Zip 32406–5309; tel. 850/769–8341; Todd Gallati, Chief Executive Officer
Web address: www.egulfcoastmedical.com

J. F. K. MEDICAL CENTER (O, 424 beds) 5301 South Congress Avenue, Atlantis, FL Zip 33462–1197; tel. 561/965–7300; Gina Melby, Chief Executive Officer
Web address: www.jfkmc.com

KENDALL REGIONAL MEDICAL CENTER (O, 300 beds) 11750 Bird Road, Miami, FL Zip 33175–3530; tel. 305/223–3000; Mauricio E. Sirvent, Chief Executive Officer
Web address: www.kendallmed.com

LAKE CITY MEDICAL CENTER (O, 67 beds) 340 N.W. Commerce Drive, Lake City, FL Zip 32055–3718; tel. 386/719–9000; John Deardorff, Chief Executive Officer
Web address: www.lakecitymedical.com

LARGO MEDICAL CENTER (O, 243 beds) 201 14th Street S.W., Largo, FL Zip 33770–3133, Mailing Address: P.O. Box 2905, Zip 33779–2905; tel. 727/588–5200; Richard H. Satcher, President and Chief Executive Officer
Web address: www.largomedical.com

LAWNWOOD REGIONAL MEDICAL CENTER (O, 331 beds) 1700 South 23rd Street, Fort Pierce, FL Zip 34950–0188; tel. 772/461–4000; Thomas R. Pentz, President and Chief Executive Officer
Web address: www.lawnwoodmed.com

MEMORIAL HOSPITAL JACKSONVILLE (O, 353 beds) 3625 University Boulevard South, Jacksonville, FL Zip 32216–4240, Mailing Address: P.O. Box 16325, Zip 32216–6325; tel. 904/399–6111; James B. Wood, President and Chief Executive Officer
Web address: www.memorialhospitaljax.com

NORTH FLORIDA REGIONAL MEDICAL CENTER (O, 278 beds) 6500 Newberry Road, Gainesville, FL Zip 32605–4392, Mailing Address: P.O. Box 147006, Zip 32614–7006; tel. 352/333–4000; James R. Thomas, Chief Executive Officer
Web address: www.nfrmc.com

NORTHSIDE HOSPITAL AND HEART INSTITUTE (O, 288 beds) 6000 49th Street North, Saint Petersburg, FL Zip 33709–2145; tel. 727/521–4411; Ward Boston, III, Chief Executive Officer
Web address: www.northsidehospital.com

NORTHWEST MEDICAL CENTER (O, 215 beds) 2801 North State Road 7, Margate, FL Zip 33063; tel. 954/978–4000; Dianne Aleman, Chief Executive Officer
Web address: www.northwestmed.com

OAK HILL HOSPITAL (O, 204 beds) 11375 Cortez Boulevard, Brooksville, FL Zip 34613, Mailing Address: P.O. Box 5300, Spring Hill, Zip 34611–5300; tel. 352/596–6632; Mickey Smith, Chief Executive Officer
Web address: www.oakhillhospital.com

For explanation of codes following names, see page B2.
★ Indicates Type III membership in the American Hospital Association.

OCALA REGIONAL MEDICAL CENTER (O, 270 beds) 1431 S.W. First Avenue, Ocala, FL Zip 34474–4058, Mailing Address: P.O. Box 2200, Zip 34478–2200; tel. 352/401–1000; H. Rex Etheredge, President and Chief Executive Officer
Web address: www.ocalaregional.com

ORANGE PARK MEDICAL CENTER (O, 230 beds) 2001 Kingsley Avenue, Orange Park, FL Zip 32073–5156; tel. 904/276–8500; Thomas R. Pentz, President and Chief Executive Officer
Web address: www.opmedical.com

OSCEOLA REGIONAL MEDICAL CENTER (O, 156 beds) 700 West Oak Street, Kissimmee, FL Zip 34741–4996; tel. 407/846–2266; E. Tim Cook, Chief Executive Officer
Web address: www.osceolaregional.com

PALMS WEST HOSPITAL (O, 175 beds) 13001 Southern Boulevard, Loxahatchee, FL Zip 33470–1150; tel. 561/798–3300; Bland Eng, Chief Executive Officer
Web address: www.palmswesthospital.com

PLANTATION GENERAL HOSPITAL (O, 264 beds) 401 N.W. 42nd Avenue, Plantation, FL Zip 33317–2882; tel. 954/587–5010; Barbara Simmons, RN, Chief Executive Officer
Web address: www.plantationgeneral.com

RAULERSON HOSPITAL (O, 100 beds) 1796 Highway 441 North, Okeechobee, FL Zip 34972–1918, Mailing Address: P.O. Box 1307, Zip 34973–1307; tel. 863/763–2151; Robert H. Lee, President
Web address: www.raulersonhospital.com

REGIONAL MEDICAL CENTER–BAYONET POINT (O, 280 beds) 14000 Fivay Road, Hudson, FL Zip 34667–7199; tel. 727/863–2411; Stephen A. Rector, Chief Executive Officer
Web address: www.rmchealth.com

SOUTH BAY HOSPITAL (O, 112 beds) 4016 State Road 674, Sun City Center, FL Zip 33573–5298; tel. 813/634–3301; Stephen J. Daugherty, Chief Executive Officer
Web address: www.southbayhospital.com

SPECIALTY HOSPITAL JACKSONVILLE (O, 62 beds) 4901 Richard Street, Jacksonville, FL Zip 32207–7328; tel. 904/737–3120; Barbara Walsh, Chief Executive Officer
Web address: www.specialtyhospitaljax.com

ST. LUCIE MEDICAL CENTER (O, 194 beds) 1800 S.E. Tiffany Avenue, Port St. Lucie, FL Zip 34952–7580; tel. 772/335–4000; Gary Cantrell, President and Chief Executive Officer
Web address: www.stluciemed.com

ST. PETERSBURG GENERAL HOSPITAL (O, 219 beds) 6500 38th Avenue North, Saint Petersburg, FL Zip 33710–1629; tel. 727/384–1414; Robert B. Conroy, Jr., Chief Executive Officer
Web address: www.stpetegeneral.com

TWIN CITIES HOSPITAL (O, 65 beds) 2190 Highway 85 North, Niceville, FL Zip 32578–1045; tel. 850/678–4131; David Whalen, Chief Executive Officer
Web address: www.tchealthcare.com

UNIVERSITY HOSPITAL AND MEDICAL CENTER (O, 271 beds) 7201 North University Drive, Tamarac, FL Zip 33321–2996; tel. 954/721–2200; Lee B. Chaykin, Chief Executive Officer
Web address: www.uhmchealth.com

WEST FLORIDA HOSPITAL (O, 339 beds) 8383 North Davis Highway, Pensacola, FL Zip 32514–6088; tel. 850/494–4000; Dennis A. Taylor, Chief Executive Officer
Web address: www.westfloridahospital.com

WESTSIDE REGIONAL MEDICAL CENTER (O, 204 beds) 8201 West Broward Boulevard, Plantation, FL Zip 33324–9937; tel. 954/473–6600; MaryLynn Swartz, Chief Executive Officer
Web address: www.westsideregional.com

GEORGIA: CARTERSVILLE MEDICAL CENTER (O, 80 beds) 960 Joe Frank Harris Parkway, Cartersville, GA Zip 30120–2129, Mailing Address: P.O. Box 200008, Zip 30120–9001; tel. 770/382–1530; Keith Sandlin, Chief Executive Officer
Web address: www.cartersvillemedical.com

COLISEUM MEDICAL CENTERS (O, 227 beds) 350 Hospital Drive, Macon, GA Zip 31217–3871; tel. 478/765–7000; Allen Golson, Chief Executive Officer
Web address: www.coliseumhealthsystem.com

COLISEUM NORTHSIDE HOSPITAL (O, 103 beds) 400 Charter Boulevard, Macon, GA Zip 31210–4853, Mailing Address: P.O. Box 4627, Zip 31208–4627; tel. 478/757–8200; Mark Nichols, FACHE, Chief Executive Officer
Web address: www.coliseumhealthsystem.com

COLISEUM PSYCHIATRIC CENTER (O, 34 beds) 340 Hospital Drive, Macon, GA Zip 31217–8002; tel. 478/741–1355; James W. Eyler, FACHE, Chief Executive Officer
Web address: www.coliseumhealthsystem.com

DOCTORS HOSPITAL (O, 242 beds) 3651 Wheeler Road, Augusta, GA Zip 30909–6426; tel. 706/651–3232; C. Shayne George, President and Chief Executive Officer
Web address: www.doctors–hospital.net

EMORY EASTSIDE MEDICAL CENTER (O, 218 beds) 1700 Medical Way, Snellville, GA Zip 30078–2195, Mailing Address: P.O. Box 587, Zip 30078–0587; tel. 770/979–0200; Kimberly Ryan, Chief Executive Officer
Web address: www.emoryeastside.com

EMORY JOHNS CREEK HOSPITAL (O, 76 beds) 6325 Hospital Parkway, Johns Creek, GA Zip 30097; tel. 678/474–7000; John Quinlivan, Chief Executive Officer
Web address: www.emoryjohnscreek.com

FAIRVIEW PARK HOSPITAL (O, 168 beds) 200 Industrial Boulevard, Dublin, GA Zip 31021–2997, Mailing Address: P.O. Box 1408, Zip 31040–1408; tel. 478/275–2000; Donald R. Avery, FACHE, President and Chief Executive Officer
Web address: www.fairviewparkhospital.com

HUGHSTON ORTHOPEDIC HOSPITAL (O, 100 beds) 100 Frist Court, Columbus, GA Zip 31908–7188, Mailing Address: P.O. Box 7188, Zip 31908–7188; tel. 706/576–2101; Donald R. Avery, FACHE, President and Chief Executive Officer
Web address: www.hughstonsports.com

PALMYRA MEDICAL CENTERS (O, 170 beds) 2000 Palmyra Road, Albany, GA Zip 31702–1908, Mailing Address: P.O. Box 1908, Zip 31702–1908; tel. 229/434–2000; Bud Wethington, Chief Executive Officer
Web address: www.palmyramedicalcenters.com

POLK MEDICAL CENTER (O, 18 beds) 424 North Main Street, Cedartown, GA Zip 30125–2698; tel. 770/748–2500; Steven C. Hoelscher, Chief Executive Officer
Web address: www.polkmedicalcenter.com

REDMOND REGIONAL MEDICAL CENTER (O, 230 beds) 501 Redmond Road, Rome, GA Zip 30165–7001, Mailing Address: Box 107001, Zip 30164–7001; tel. 706/291–0291; Brenda M. Waltz, FACHE, Chief Executive Officer
Web address: www.redmondregional.com

IDAHO: EASTERN IDAHO REGIONAL MEDICAL CENTER (O, 294 beds) 3100 Channing Way, Idaho Falls, ID Zip 83404–7533, Mailing Address: P.O. Box 2077, Zip 83403–2077; tel. 208/529–6111; Douglas Crabtree, Chief Executive Officer
Web address: www.eirmc.com

WEST VALLEY MEDICAL CENTER (O, 122 beds) 1717 Arlington, Caldwell, ID Zip 83605–4864; tel. 208/459–4641; Kathy D. Moore, Chief Executive Officer
Web address: www.westvalleymedctr.com

INDIANA: TERRE HAUTE REGIONAL HOSPITAL (O, 231 beds) 3901 South Seventh Street, Terre Haute, IN Zip 47802–4299; tel. 812/232–0021; Christopher J. Hill, Chief Executive Officer
Web address: www.regionalhospital.com

KANSAS: ALLEN COUNTY HOSPITAL (O, 25 beds) 101 South First Street, Iola, KS Zip 66749–3505, Mailing Address: P.O. Box 540, Zip 66749–0540; tel. 620/365–1000; Joyce Heismeyer, Chief Executive Officer
Web address: www.allencountyhospital.com

MENORAH MEDICAL CENTER (O, 158 beds) 5721 West 119th Street, Overland Park, KS Zip 66209–3722; tel. 913/498–6000; Steven D. Wilkinson, President and Chief Executive Officer
Web address: www.menorahmedicalcenter.com

OVERLAND PARK REGIONAL MEDICAL CENTER (O, 244 beds) 10500 Quivira Road, Overland Park, KS Zip 66215–2306, Mailing Address: P.O. Box 15959, Zip 66215–5959; tel. 913/541–5000; Steven M. Anderson, CHE, Chief Executive Officer
Web address: www.oprmc.com

WESLEY MEDICAL CENTER (O, 529 beds) 550 North Hillside, Wichita, KS Zip 67214–4976; tel. 316/962–2000; Hugh C. Tappan, President and Chief Executive Officer
Web address: www.wesleymc.com

For explanation of codes following names, see page B2.
★ Indicates Type III membership in the American Hospital Association.

KENTUCKY: FRANKFORT REGIONAL MEDICAL CENTER (O, 148 beds) 299 King's Daughters Drive, Frankfort, KY Zip 40601–4186; tel. 502/875–5240; Chip Peal, Chief Executive Officer
Web address: www.frankfortregional.com

GREENVIEW REGIONAL HOSPITAL (O, 211 beds) 1801 Ashley Circle, Bowling Green, KY Zip 42104–3384; tel. 270/793–1000; Mark A. Marsh, Chief Executive Officer
Web address: www.greenviewhospital.com

LOUISIANA: AVOYELLES HOSPITAL (O, 47 beds) 4231 Highway 1192, Marksville, LA Zip 71351, Mailing Address: P.O. Box 249, Zip 71351–0249; tel. 318/253–8611; David M. Mitchel, Chief Executive Officer
Web address: www.avoyelleshospital.com

DAUTERIVE HOSPITAL (O, 103 beds) 600 North Lewis Street, New Iberia, LA Zip 70563; tel. 337/365–7311; Alan J. Fabian, Chief Executive Officer
Web address: www.dauterivehospital.com

LAKEVIEW REGIONAL MEDICAL CENTER (O, 159 beds) 95 East Fairway Drive, Covington, LA Zip 70433–7507; tel. 985/867–3800; Jason E. Cobb, FACHE, Chief Executive Officer
Web address: www.lakeviewregional.com

OAKDALE COMMUNITY HOSPITAL (O, 59 beds) 130 North Hospital Drive, Oakdale, LA Zip 71463, Mailing Address: P.O. Box 629, Zip 71463–0629; tel. 318/335–3700; John W. Stigall, Chief Executive Officer
Web address: www.oakdalecommunityhospital.com

RAPIDES REGIONAL MEDICAL CENTER (O, 343 beds) 211 Fourth Street, Alexandria, LA Zip 71301; tel. 318/473–3000; A. C. Buchanan, President and Chief Executive Officer
Web address: www.rapidesregional.com

SAVOY MEDICAL CENTER (O, 180 beds) 801 Poinciana Avenue, Mamou, LA Zip 70554–2298; tel. 337/468–5261; Cristina Rivera, Chief Executive Officer
Web address: www.savoymedicalcenter.com

SOUTHWEST MEDICAL CENTER (O, 142 beds) 2810 Ambassador Caffery Parkway, Lafayette, LA Zip 70506; tel. 337/981–2949; Kyle J. Viator, Chief Executive Officer
Web address: www.southwestmc.com

TULANE UNIVERSITY HOSPITAL AND CLINIC (O, 331 beds) 1415 Tulane Avenue, New Orleans, LA Zip 70112–2605; tel. 504/988–5263; Robert Lynch, M.D., Chief Executive Officer
Web address: www.tuhc.com

TULANE–LAKESIDE HOSPITAL (O, 116 beds) 4700 I–10 Service Road, Metairie, LA Zip 70001–1269; tel. 504/780–8282; Stephen Robinson, Administrator
Web address: www.hcahealthcare.com

WINN PARISH MEDICAL CENTER (O, 60 beds) 301 West Boundary Street, Winnfield, LA Zip 71483–3427, Mailing Address: P.O. Box 152, Zip 71483–0152; tel. 318/648–3000; H. J. Gaspard, Chief Executive Officer
Web address: www.winnparishmedical.com

WOMEN'S AND CHILDREN'S HOSPITAL (O, 161 beds) 4600 Ambassador Caffery Parkway, Lafayette, LA Zip 70508–6923, Mailing Address: P.O. Box 88030, Zip 70598–8030; tel. 337/521–9100; Kathy J. Bobbs, Chief Executive Officer
Web address: www.womens–childrens.com

MISSISSIPPI: GARDEN PARK MEDICAL CENTER (O, 130 beds) 15200 Community Road, Gulfport, MS Zip 39503–3085, Mailing Address: P.O. Box 1240, Zip 39502–1240; tel. 228/575–7000; William E. Peaks, Chief Executive Officer
Web address: www.gpmedical.com

MISSOURI: CENTERPOINT MEDICAL CENTER (O, 221 beds) 19600 East 39th Street, Independence, MO Zip 64057; tel. 816/698–7000; Carolyn W. Caldwell, President and Chief Executive Officer

LAFAYETTE REGIONAL HEALTH CENTER (O, 25 beds) 1500 State Street, Lexington, MO Zip 64067–1107; tel. 660/259–2203; Bret Kolman, CPA, Chief Executive Officer
Web address: www.lafayetteregionalhealthcenter.com

LEE'S SUMMIT MEDICAL CENTER (O, 64 beds) 2100 S.E. Blue Parkway, Lee's Summit, MO Zip 64063; tel. 816/282–5000; Damond Boatright, Chief Executive Officer
Web address: www.leessummitmedicalcenter.com

RESEARCH BELTON HOSPITAL (O, 38 beds) 17065 South 71 Highway, Belton, MO Zip 64012–4631; tel. 816/348–1200; Todd Krass, Chief Executive Officer
Web address: www.researchbeltonhospital.com

RESEARCH MEDICAL CENTER (O, 383 beds) 2316 East Meyer Boulevard, Kansas City, MO Zip 64132–1136; tel. 816/276–4000; Kevin J. Hicks, President and Chief Executive Officer
Web address: www.researchmedicalcenter.com

RESEARCH MEDICAL CENTER – BROOKSIDE CAMPUS (O, 265 beds) 6601 Rockhill Road, Kansas City, MO Zip 64131–1197; tel. 816/276–7000; Kevin J. Hicks, President and Chief Executive Officer
Web address: www.b–lmc.com

RESEARCH PSYCHIATRIC CENTER (O, 100 beds) 2323 East 63rd Street, Kansas City, MO Zip 64130–3462; tel. 816/444–8161; Todd Krass, President and Chief Executive Officer
Web address: www.researchpsychiatriccenter.com

NEVADA: MOUNTAINVIEW HOSPITAL (O, 235 beds) 3100 North Tenaya Way, Las Vegas, NV Zip 89128–0436; tel. 702/255–5000; William Wagnon, Chief Executive Officer
Web address: www.mountainview–hospital.com

SOUTHERN HILLS HOSPITAL AND MEDICAL CENTER (O, 139 beds) 9300 West Sunset Road, Las Vegas, NV Zip 89148; tel. 702/880–2100; Stephen E. Dixon, Chief Executive Officer
Web address: www.southernhillshospital.com

SUNRISE HOSPITAL AND MEDICAL CENTER (O, 645 beds) 3186 Maryland Parkway, Las Vegas, NV Zip 89109–2306, Mailing Address: P.O. Box 98530, Zip 89193–8530; tel. 702/731–8000; Sylvia Young, Chief Executive Officer
Web address: www.sunrisehospital.com

NEW HAMPSHIRE: PARKLAND MEDICAL CENTER (O, 82 beds) One Parkland Drive, Derry, NH Zip 03038–2750; tel. 603/432–1500; Anne Jamieson, Chief Executive Officer
Web address: www.parklandmedicalcenter.com

PORTSMOUTH REGIONAL HOSPITAL (O, 165 beds) 333 Borthwick Avenue, Portsmouth, NH Zip 03801–7004; tel. 603/436–5110; William J. Schuler, Chief Executive Officer
Web address: www.portsmouthhospital.com

OKLAHOMA: EDMOND MEDICAL CENTER (O, 92 beds) 1 South Bryant Street, Edmond, OK Zip 73034–4798; tel. 405/341–6100; Tayo Fichtl, Chief Executive Officer
Web address: www.edmondhospital.com

OU MEDICAL CENTER (O, 587 beds) 1200 Everett Drive, Oklahoma City, OK Zip 73104–5047, Mailing Address: P.O. Box 26307, Zip 73126; tel. 405/271–5911; Cole C. Eslyn, FACHE, President and Chief Executive Officer
Web address: www.oumedcenter.com

SOUTH CAROLINA: COLLETON MEDICAL CENTER (O, 131 beds) 501 Robertson Boulevard, Walterboro, SC Zip 29488–5714; tel. 843/782–2000; Mitchell P. Mongell, Chief Executive Officer
Web address: www.colletonmedical.com

GRAND STRAND REGIONAL MEDICAL CENTER (O, 221 beds) 809 82nd Parkway, Myrtle Beach, SC Zip 29572–1413; tel. 843/692–1000; Doug White, Chief Executive Officer
Web address: www.grandstrandmed.com

TRIDENT MEDICAL CENTER (O, 281 beds) 9330 Medical Plaza Drive, Charleston, SC Zip 29406–9195; tel. 843/797–7000; Terry J. Gunn, President and Chief Executive Officer
Web address: www.tridenthealthsystem.com

TENNESSEE: CENTENNIAL MEDICAL CENTER AND PARTHENON PAVILION (O, 572 beds) 2300 Patterson Street, Nashville, TN Zip 37203–1528; tel. 615/342–1000; Thomas L. Herron, FACHE, Chief Executive Officer
Web address: www.centennialmedicalcenter.com

CENTENNIAL MEDICAL CENTER AT ASHLAND CITY (O, 8 beds) 313 North Main Street, Ashland City, TN Zip 37015–1358; tel. 615/792–3030; Renaye Smith, Administrator
Web address: www.centennialmedicalcenter.com

HENDERSONVILLE MEDICAL CENTER (O, 70 beds) 355 New Shackle Island Road, Hendersonville, TN Zip 37075–2393; tel. 615/338–1000; Regina Bartlett, Chief Executive Officer
Web address: www.hendersonvillemedicalcenter.com

HORIZON MEDICAL CENTER (O, 116 beds) 111 Highway 70 East, Dickson, TN Zip 37055–2033; tel. 615/446–0446; John A. Marshall, Chief Executive Officer
Web address: www.horizonmedicalcenter.com

For explanation of codes following names, see page B2.
★ Indicates Type III membership in the American Hospital Association.

Section B

PARKRIDGE MEDICAL CENTER (O, 185 beds) 2333 McCallie Avenue, Chattanooga, TN Zip 37404–3285; tel. 423/698–6061; Darrell W. Moore, CHE, Chief Executive Officer
Web address: www.parkridgemedicalcenter.com

SKYLINE MADISON CAMPUS (O, 284 beds) 500 Hospital Drive, Madison, TN Zip 37115–5032; tel. 615/865–2373; Michael W. Garfield, Chief Executive Officer
Web address: www.skylinemadison.com

SKYLINE MEDICAL CENTER (O, 288 beds) 3441 Dickerson Pike, Nashville, TN Zip 37207–2539; tel. 615/769–2000; Michael W. Garfield, Chief Executive Officer
Web address: www.skylinemedicalcenter.com

SOUTHERN HILLS MEDICAL CENTER (O, 120 beds) 391 Wallace Road, Nashville, TN Zip 37211–4859; tel. 615/781–4000; Thomas H. Ozburn, Chief Executive Officer
Web address: www.southernhills.com

STONECREST MEDICAL CENTER (O, 75 beds) 200 StoneCrest Boulevard, Smyrna, TN Zip 37167–6810; tel. 615/768–2000; Neil A. Heatherly, CHE, Chief Executive Officer
Web address: www.stonecrestmedical.com

SUMMIT MEDICAL CENTER (O, 188 beds) 5655 Frist Boulevard, Hermitage, TN Zip 37076–2053; tel. 615/316–3000; Jeffrey T. Whitehorn, Chief Executive Officer
Web address: www.summitmedctr.com

TEXAS: BAYSHORE MEDICAL CENTER (O, 300 beds) 4000 Spencer Highway, Pasadena, TX Zip 77504–1294; tel. 713/359–2000; Jeffrey S. Holland, Chief Executive Officer
Web address: www.bayshoremedical.com

CLEAR LAKE REGIONAL MEDICAL CENTER (O, 543 beds) 500 Medical Center Boulevard, Webster, TX Zip 77598–4286; tel. 281/332–2511; Donald A. Shaffett, Chief Executive Officer
Web address: www.clearlakermc.com

CONROE REGIONAL MEDICAL CENTER (O, 267 beds) 504 Medical Boulevard, Conroe, TX Zip 77304, Mailing Address: P.O. Box 1538, Zip 77305–1538; tel. 936/539–1111; Jerry A. Nash, Chief Executive Officer
Web address: www.conroeregional.com

CORPUS CHRISTI MEDICAL CENTER (O, 362 beds) 3315 South Alameda Street, Corpus Christi, TX Zip 78411–1883, Mailing Address: P.O. Box 8991, Zip 78468–8991; tel. 361/761–1400; James T. Montgomery, CHE, Chief Executive Officer
Web address: www.ccmedicalcenter.com

DEL SOL MEDICAL CENTER (O, 289 beds) 10301 Gateway West, El Paso, TX Zip 79925–7798; tel. 915/595–9000; Jacob Cintron, Chief Executive Officer
Web address: www.delsolmedicalcenter.com

DENTON REGIONAL MEDICAL CENTER (O, 208 beds) 3535 South 1–35 East, Denton, TX Zip 76210; tel. 940/384–3535; Caleb F. O'Rear, Chief Executive Officer
Web address: www.dentonregional.com

EAST HOUSTON REGIONAL MEDICAL CENTER (O, 131 beds) 13111 East Freeway, Houston, TX Zip 77015–5820; tel. 713/393–2000; Clay Franklin, Chief Executive Officer
Web address: www.easthoustonrmc.com

GREEN OAKS HOSPITAL (O, 105 beds) 7808 Clodus Fields Drive, Dallas, TX Zip 75251–2206; tel. 972/991–9504; Thomas M. Collins, Chief Executive Officer
Web address: www.greenoakspsych.com

KINGWOOD MEDICAL CENTER (O, 169 beds) 22999 U.S. Highway 59, Kingwood, TX Zip 77339; tel. 281/348–8000; Gay Nord, Chief Executive Officer
Web address: www.kingwoodmedical.com

LAS COLINAS MEDICAL CENTER (O, 80 beds) 6800 North MacArthur Boulevard, Irving, TX Zip 75039–2422; tel. 972/969–2000; Daniela Decell, Chief Executive Officer
Web address: www.lascolinasmedical.com

LAS PALMAS MEDICAL CENTER (O, 261 beds) 1801 North Oregon Street, El Paso, TX Zip 79902–3591; tel. 915/521–1200; Hank Hernandez, Chief Executive Officer
Web address: www.laspalmashealth.com

MAINLAND MEDICAL CENTER (O, 218 beds) 6801 E F Lowry Expressway, Texas City, TX Zip 77591; tel. 409/938–5000; Melinda Stephenson, Chief Executive Officer
Web address: www.mainlandmedical.com

MEDICAL CENTER OF ARLINGTON (O, 266 beds) 3301 Matlock Road, Arlington, TX Zip 76015–2998; tel. 817/465–3241; Patrick D. Brilliant, Chief Executive Officer
Web address: www.medicalcenterarlington.com

MEDICAL CENTER OF LEWISVILLE (O, 187 beds) 500 West Main, Lewisville, TX Zip 75057–3699; tel. 972/420–1000; Douglas Welch, President and Chief Executive Officer
Web address: www.lewisvillemedical.com

MEDICAL CENTER OF MCKINNEY (O, 222 beds) 4500 Medical Center Drive, McKinney, TX Zip 75069–3499; tel. 972/547–8000; Ernest C. Lynch, III, Chief Executive Officer
Web address: www.ncentralmedical.com

MEDICAL CENTER OF PLANO (O, 348 beds) 3901 West 15th Street, Plano, TX Zip 75075–7799; tel. 972/596–6800; Harvey L. Fishero, President and Chief Executive Officer
Web address: www.medicalcenterplano.com

MEDICAL CITY DALLAS HOSPITAL (O, 542 beds) 7777 Forest Lane, Dallas, TX Zip 75230–2598; tel. 972/566–7000; Britt Berrett, President and Chief Executive Officer
Web address: www.medicalcityhospital.com

METHODIST AMBULATORY SURGERY HOSPITAL (O, 23 beds) 9150 Huebner Road, Suite 100, San Antonio, TX Zip 78240–1545; tel. 210/575–5000; Elaine F. Morris, Administrator
Web address: www.mas.sahealth.com

METHODIST CHILDREN'S HOSPITAL OF SOUTH TEXAS (O, 150 beds) 7700 Floyd Curl Drive, San Antonio, TX Zip 78229–3383; tel. 210/575–7000; Mark McLoone, Chief Executive Officer
Web address: www.mch.sahealth.com/

METHODIST HOSPITAL (O, 1405 beds) 7700 Floyd Curl Drive, San Antonio, TX Zip 78229–3993; tel. 210/575–4000; Michael E. Duffy, Chief Executive Officer
Web address: www.sahealth.com

METROPOLITAN METHODIST HOSPITAL (O, 244 beds) 1310 McCullough Avenue, San Antonio, TX Zip 78212–2617; tel. 210/757–2200; Dominic Dominguez, Chief Executive Officer
Web address: www.metro.sahealth.com

NORTH HILLS HOSPITAL (O, 176 beds) 4401 Booth Calloway Road, North Richland Hills, TX Zip 76180–7399; tel. 817/255–1000; Randolph Moresi, Chief Executive Officer
Web address: www.northhillshospital.com

PLAZA MEDICAL CENTER OF FORT WORTH (O, 211 beds) 900 Eighth Avenue, Fort Worth, TX Zip 76104–3986; tel. 817/336–2100; Troy Villarreal, Chief Executive Officer
Web address: www.plazamedicalcenter.com

RIO GRANDE REGIONAL HOSPITAL (O, 320 beds) 101 East Ridge Road, McAllen, TX Zip 78503–1299; tel. 956/632–6000; Stephen K. Jones, Jr., FACHE, Chief Executive Officer
Web address: www.riohealth.com

SPRING BRANCH MEDICAL CENTER (O, 224 beds) 8850 Long Point Road, Houston, TX Zip 77055–3082; tel. 713/467–6555; Jay Woodall, Chief Executive Officer
Web address: www.springbranchmedical.com

ST. DAVID'S GEORGETOWN HOSPITAL (O, 96 beds) 2000 Scenic Drive, Georgetown, TX Zip 78626–7793; tel. 512/943–3000; Hugh Brown, Chief Executive Officer
Web address: www.stdavidsgeorgetown.com

ST. DAVID'S MEDICAL CENTER (O, 326 beds) 919 East 32nd Street, Austin, TX Zip 78705–2709, Mailing Address: P.O. Box 4039, Zip 78765–4039; tel. 512/476–7111; C. David Huffstutler, President
Web address: www.stdavids.com

ST. DAVID'S NORTH AUSTIN MEDICAL CENTER (O, 228 beds) 12221 MoPac Expressway North, Austin, TX Zip 78758–2496; tel. 512/901–1000; Donald H. Wilkerson, Chief Executive Officer
Web address: www.northaustin.com

ST. DAVID'S REHABILITATION CENTER (O, 62 beds) 1005 East 32nd Street, Austin, TX Zip 78705–2705, Mailing Address: P.O. Box 4270, Zip 78765–4270; tel. 512/867–5100; Diane Owens, Administrator
Web address: www.stdavids.com

ST. DAVID'S ROUND ROCK MEDICAL CENTER (O, 140 beds) 2400 Round Rock Avenue, Round Rock, TX Zip 78681–4097; tel. 512/341–1000; Deborah L. Ryle, Administrator and Chief Executive Officer
Web address: www.roundrockmc.com

For explanation of codes following names, see page B2.
★ Indicates Type III membership in the American Hospital Association.

ST. DAVID'S SOUTH AUSTIN HOSPITAL (O, 222 beds) 901 West Ben White Boulevard, Austin, TX Zip 78704–6903; tel. 512/447–2211; Erol R. Akdamar, Chief Executive Officer
Web address: www.southaustinhospital.com

TEXAS ORTHOPEDIC HOSPITAL (O, 49 beds) 7401 South Main Street, Houston, TX Zip 77030–4509; tel. 713/799–8600; Alice G. Adams, RN, Chief Executive Officer
Web address: www.texasorthopedic.com

THE WOMAN'S HOSPITAL OF TEXAS (O, 248 beds) 7600 Fannin Street, Houston, TX Zip 77054–1900; tel. 713/790–1234; Linda B. Russell, Chief Executive Officer
Web address: www.womanshospital.com

VALLEY REGIONAL MEDICAL CENTER (O, 214 beds) 100A Alton Gloor Boulevard, Brownsville, TX Zip 78526–3346, Mailing Address: P.O. Box 3710, Zip 78521–3710; tel. 956/350–7101; David Handley, Chief Executive Officer
Web address: www.valleyregionalmedicalcenter.com

WEST HOUSTON MEDICAL CENTER (O, 193 beds) 12141 Richmond Avenue, Houston, TX Zip 77082–2499; tel. 281/558–3444; Todd Caliva, Chief Executive Officer
Web address: www.westhoustonmedical.com

UTAH: BRIGHAM CITY COMMUNITY HOSPITAL (O, 39 beds) 950 South Medical Drive, Brigham City, UT Zip 84302; tel. 435/734–9471; Mark B. Adams, Chief Executive Officer
Web address: www.brighamcityhospital.com

LAKEVIEW HOSPITAL (O, 116 beds) 630 East Medical Drive, Bountiful, UT Zip 84010–4996; tel. 801/299–2200; Rand Kerr, Chief Executive Officer
Web address: www.lakeviewhospital.com

MOUNTAIN VIEW HOSPITAL (O, 114 beds) 1000 East 100 North, Payson, UT Zip 84651–1690; tel. 801/465–7000; Kevin Johnson, Chief Executive Officer
Web address: www.mvhpayson.com

OGDEN REGIONAL MEDICAL CENTER (O, 167 beds) 5475 South 500 East, Ogden, UT Zip 84405–6978; tel. 801/479–2111; Mark B. Adams, Chief Executive Officer
Web address: www.ogdenregional.com

ST. MARK'S HOSPITAL (O, 297 beds) 1200 East 3900 South, Salt Lake City, UT Zip 84124–1390; tel. 801/268–7111; Steven B. Bateman, Chief Executive Officer
Web address: www.stmarkshospital.com

TIMPANOGOS REGIONAL HOSPITAL (O, 69 beds) 750 West 800 North, Orem, UT Zip 84059–3660; tel. 801/714–6000; Keith D. Tintle, Chief Executive Officer
Web address: www.timpanogosregionalhospital.com

VIRGINIA: ALLEGHANY REGIONAL HOSPITAL (O, 146 beds) One ARH Lane, Low Moor, VA Zip 24457, Mailing Address: P.O. Box 7, Zip 24457–0007; tel. 540/862–6011; Timothy C. Tobin, President and Chief Executive Officer
Web address: www.alleghanyregional.com

CJW MEDICAL CENTER (O, 758 beds) 7101 Jahnke Road, Richmond, VA Zip 23225–4044; tel. 804/320–3911; Peter A. Marmerstein, Chief Executive Officer
Web address: www.cjwmedical.com

DOMINION HOSPITAL (O, 91 beds) 2960 Sleepy Hollow Road, Falls Church, VA Zip 22044–2001; tel. 703/536–2000; Suzanne B. Jackson, Chief Executive Officer
Web address: www.dominionhospital.com

HENRICO DOCTORS' HOSPITAL (O, 533 beds) 1602 Skipwith Road, Richmond, VA Zip 23229–5205; tel. 804/289–4500; David Williams, Chief Executive Officer
Web address: www.henricodoctorshospital.com

JOHN RANDOLPH MEDICAL CENTER (O, 132 beds) 411 West Randolph Road, Hopewell, VA Zip 23860–2938; tel. 804/541–1600; Elwood Bernard Boone, III, Chief Executive Officer
Web address: www.johnrandolphmed.com

LEWIS–GALE MEDICAL CENTER (O, 521 beds) 1900 Electric Road, Salem, VA Zip 24153–7494; tel. 540/776–4000; Victor Giovanetti, Chief Executive Officer
Web address: www.lewis–gale.com

MONTGOMERY REGIONAL HOSPITAL (O, 89 beds) 3700 South Main Street, Blacksburg, VA Zip 24060–7081, Mailing Address: P.O. Box 90004, Zip 24062–9004; tel. 540/951–1111; Scott Hill, Chief Executive Officer
Web address: www.mrhospital.com

PULASKI COMMUNITY HOSPITAL (O, 55 beds) 2400 Lee Highway, Pulaski, VA Zip 24301–0759, Mailing Address: P.O. Box 759, Zip 24301–0759; tel. 540/994–8100; W. Mark Rader, Chief Executive Officer
Web address: www.pulaskicommunityhospital.com

RESTON HOSPITAL CENTER (O, 187 beds) 1850 Town Center Parkway, Reston, VA Zip 20190–3210; tel. 703/689–9000; William A. Adams, President and Chief Executive Officer
Web address: www.restonhospital.com

RETREAT HOSPITAL (O, 113 beds) 2621 Grove Avenue, Richmond, VA Zip 23220–4308; tel. 804/254–5100; William E. Caldwell, Jr., Chief Executive Officer
Web address: www.retreathospital.com

Owned, leased, sponsored:	162 hospitals	35177 beds
Contract–managed:	0 hospitals	0 beds
Totals:	162 hospitals	35177 beds

★0082: HEALTH ALLIANCE OF GREATER CINCINNATI (NP)
3200 Burnet Avenue, Cincinnati, OH Zip 45229; tel. 513/585–6000; Kenneth Hanover, President and Chief Executive Officer
(Centralized Physician/Insurance Health System)

OHIO: DRAKE CENTER (O, 278 beds) 151 West Galbraith Road, Cincinnati, OH Zip 45216–1015; tel. 513/418–2500; Karen Bankston, Ph.D., Senior Vice President
Web address: www.drakecenter.com

FORT HAMILTON HOSPITAL (O, 185 beds) 630 Eaton Avenue, Hamilton, OH Zip 45013–2770; tel. 513/867–2000; Lynn M. Oswald, FACHE, Senior Vice President
Web address: www.forthamiltonhospital.com

JEWISH HOSPITAL (O, 209 beds) 4777 East Galbraith Road, Cincinnati, OH Zip 45236–2725; tel. 513/686–3000; M. Aurora Lambert, Senior Vice President
Web address: www.health–alliance.com/jewish.html

UNIVERSITY HOSPITAL (O, 438 beds) 234 Goodman Street, Cincinnati, OH Zip 45219–2316; tel. 513/584–1000; Lee Ann Liska, Executive Director and Senior Vice President
Web address: www.health–alliance.com/Univ_control.html

Owned, leased, sponsored:	4 hospitals	1110 beds
Contract–managed:	0 hospitals	0 beds
Totals:	4 hospitals	1110 beds

0328: HEALTH FIRST, INC. (NP)
6450 U.S. Highway 1, Rockledge, FL Zip 32955; tel. 321/434–7000; Michael D. Means, President and Chief Executive Officer
(Centralized Physician/Insurance Health System)

FLORIDA: CAPE CANAVERAL HOSPITAL (O, 145 beds) 701 West Cocoa Beach Causeway, Cocoa Beach, FL Zip 32931–5595, Mailing Address: P.O. Box 320069, Zip 32932–0069; tel. 321/799–7111; Roy Wright, FACHE, President and Chief Executive Officer
Web address: www.health–first.org

HOLMES REGIONAL MEDICAL CENTER (O, 514 beds) 1350 South Hickory Street, Melbourne, FL Zip 32901–3276; tel. 321/434–7000; Jerry Senne, FACHE, President
Web address: www.health–first.org

Owned, leased, sponsored:	2 hospitals	659 beds
Contract–managed:	0 hospitals	0 beds
Totals:	2 hospitals	659 beds

1775: HEALTH MANAGEMENT ASSOCIATES (IO)
5811 Pelican Bay Boulevard, Suite 500, Naples, FL Zip 34108; tel. 239/598–3131; Burke W. Whitman, President and Chief Executive Officer
(Decentralized Health System)

For explanation of codes following names, see page B2.
★ Indicates Type III membership in the American Hospital Association.

Section B

ALABAMA: RIVERVIEW REGIONAL MEDICAL CENTER (O, 190 beds) 600 South Third Street, Gadsden, AL Zip 35901–5399, Mailing Address: P.O. Box 268, Zip 35999–0268; tel. 256/543–5200; J. Matthew Hayes, Executive Director
Web address: www.riverviewregional.com

STRINGFELLOW MEMORIAL HOSPITAL (L, 125 beds) 301 East 18th Street, Anniston, AL Zip 36207–0038, Mailing Address: P.O. Box 38, Zip 36207–0038; tel. 256/235–8900; Linda P. Burdette, Chief Executive Officer
Web address: www.stringfellowhealth.com

ARKANSAS: SOUTHWEST REGIONAL MEDICAL CENTER (O, 79 beds) 11401 Interstate 30, Little Rock, AR Zip 72209–7056; tel. 501/455–7100; Nancy C. Fodi, FACHE, Chief Executive Officer
Web address: www.hma–corp.com

SUMMIT MEDICAL CENTER (L, 103 beds) East Main and South 20th Streets, Van Buren, AR Zip 72956–5715, Mailing Address: P.O. Box 409, Zip 72957–0409; tel. 479/474–3401; Pamela Tahan, Chief Executive Officer
Web address: www.summitmedicalcenter.net

FLORIDA: BARTOW REGIONAL MEDICAL CENTER (O, 72 beds) 2200 Osprey Boulevard, Bartow, FL Zip 33830–3308, Mailing Address: P.O. Box 1050, Zip 33830–1050; tel. 863/533–8111; Justin Davis, Chief Executive Officer
Web address: www.bartowregional.com

BROOKSVILLE REGIONAL HOSPITAL (L, 91 beds) 17240 Cortez Boulevard, Brooksville, FL Zip 34601, Mailing Address: P.O. Box 37, Zip 34605–0037; tel. 352/796–5111; Kathy A. Burke, Chief Executive Officer
Web address: www.brooksvilleregionalhospital.org

CHARLOTTE REGIONAL MEDICAL CENTER (O, 208 beds) 809 East Marion Avenue, Punta Gorda, FL Zip 33950–3898, Mailing Address: P.O. Box 51–1328, Zip 33951–1328; tel. 941/639–3131; Brad K. Nurkin, Chief Executive Officer
Web address: www.charlotteregional.com

FISHERMEN'S HOSPITAL (L, 46 beds) 3301 Overseas Highway, Marathon, FL Zip 33050–0068; tel. 305/743–5533; Kim Bassett, Chief Executive Officer
Web address: www.fishermenshospital.com

HEART OF FLORIDA REGIONAL MEDICAL CENTER (O, 142 beds) 40100 Highway 27, Davenport, FL Zip 33837–5902, Mailing Address: P.O. Box 67, Haines City, Zip 33845–0067; tel. 863/422–4971; James R. Beatty, Chief Executive Officer
Web address: www.heartofflorida.com

HIGHLANDS REGIONAL MEDICAL CENTER (L, 126 beds) 3600 South Highlands Avenue, Sebring, FL Zip 33870–5495, Mailing Address: Drawer 2066, Zip 33871–2066; tel. 863/471–5800; Robert Mahaffey, Chief Executive Officer
Web address: www.highlandsregional.com

LEHIGH REGIONAL MEDICAL CENTER (O, 71 beds) 1500 Lee Boulevard, Lehigh Acres, FL Zip 33936–4897; tel. 239/369–2101; Jose Morillo, Chief Executive Officer
Web address: www.lehighregional.com

LOWER KEYS MEDICAL CENTER (L, 100 beds) 5900 College Road, Key West, FL Zip 33040–4396, Mailing Address: P.O. Box 9107, Zip 33041–9107; tel. 305/294–5531; Nicki Will, Ph.D., President and Chief Executive Officer
Web address: www.lkmc.com

PASCO REGIONAL MEDICAL CENTER (O, 90 beds) 13100 Fort King Road, Dade City, FL Zip 33525–5294; tel. 352/521–1100; Stan Holm, Chief Executive Officer
Web address: www.pascoregionalmc.com

PEACE RIVER REGIONAL MEDICAL CENTER (O, 296 beds) 2500 Harbor Boulevard, Port Charlotte, FL Zip 33952–5396; tel. 941/766–4122; David McCormack, Chief Executive Officer
Web address: www.peaceriverregional.com

PHYSICIANS REGIONAL MEDICAL CENTER – PINE RIDGE (O, 70 beds) 6101 Pine Ridge Road, Naples, FL Zip 34119; tel. 239/348–4000; Geoffrey D. Moebius, Chief Executive Officer
Web address: www.physiciansregional.com

SANTA ROSA MEDICAL CENTER (O, 129 beds) 1450 Berryhill Road, Milton, FL Zip 32570–4028, Mailing Address: P.O. Box 648, Zip 32572–0648; tel. 850/626–7762; M. P. Gandy, Jr., Chief Executive Officer
Web address: www.santarosamedicalcenter.org

SEBASTIAN RIVER MEDICAL CENTER (O, 119 beds) 13695 North U.S. Highway 1, Sebastian, FL Zip 32958–3230, Mailing Address: Box 780838, Zip 32978–0838; tel. 772/589–3186; Emily Holliman, Chief Executive Officer
Web address: www.sebastianrivermedical.com

SEVEN RIVERS REGIONAL MEDICAL CENTER (O, 128 beds) 6201 North Suncoast Boulevard, Crystal River, FL Zip 34428–6712; tel. 352/795–6560; Joyce Brancato, Chief Executive Officer
Web address: www.srrmc.com

SPRING HILL REGIONAL HOSPITAL (L, 75 beds) 10461 Quality Drive, Brooksville, FL Zip 34609–9634; tel. 352/688–8200; Jason N. Roeback, Chief Executive Officer
Web address: www.springhillregionalhospital.org

ST. CLOUD REGIONAL MEDICAL CENTER (O, 84 beds) 2906 17th Street, Saint Cloud, FL Zip 34769–6099; tel. 407/892–2135; Thomas D. Barb, Chief Executive Officer
Web address: www.stcloudregional.com

VENICE REGIONAL MEDICAL CENTER (O, 394 beds) 540 The Rialto, Venice, FL Zip 34285–2900; tel. 941/485–7711; Melody Trimble, Chief Executive Officer
Web address: www.veniceregional.com

GEORGIA: BARROW REGIONAL MEDICAL CENTER (O, 56 beds) 316 North Broad Street, Winder, GA Zip 30680–2150, Mailing Address: P.O. Box 688, Zip 30680–0688; tel. 770/867–3400; Joe Clancy, Chief Executive Officer
Web address: www.barrowregional.com

EAST GEORGIA REGIONAL MEDICAL CENTER (O, 150 beds) 1499 Fair Road, Statesboro, GA Zip 30458, Mailing Address: P.O. Box 1048, Zip 30459–1048; tel. 912/486–1000; Robert F. Bigley, Chief Executive Officer
Web address: www.egrmc.com

WALTON REGIONAL MEDICAL CENTER (O, 115 beds) 330 Alcovy Street, Monroe, GA Zip 30655–2140, Mailing Address: P.O. Box 1346, Zip 30655–1346; tel. 770/267–8461; Gary Lang, Chief Executive Officer
Web address: www.walton.org

KENTUCKY: PAUL B. HALL REGIONAL MEDICAL CENTER (O, 72 beds) 625 James S Trimble Boulevard, Paintsville, KY Zip 41240–0000; tel. 606/789–3511; Deborah L. Trimble, Chief Executive Officer
Web address: www.pbhrmc.com

MISSISSIPPI: BILOXI REGIONAL MEDICAL CENTER (L, 153 beds) 150 Reynoir Street, Biloxi, MS Zip 39530–4199, Mailing Address: P.O. Box 128, Zip 39533–0128; tel. 228/432–1571; Timothy W. Mitchell, Chief Executive Officer
Web address: www.hmamississippi.com

CENTRAL MISSISSIPPI MEDICAL CENTER (L, 429 beds) 1850 Chadwick Drive, Jackson, MS Zip 39204–3479, Mailing Address: P.O. Box 59001, Zip 39204–9001; tel. 601/376–1000; Joe D. Pinion, Chief Executive Officer
Web address: www.centralmississippimedicalcenter.com

CROSSGATES RIVER OAKS HOSPITAL (L, 134 beds) 350 Crossgates Boulevard, Brandon, MS Zip 39042–2698; tel. 601/825–2811; J. Allen Tyra, Chief Executive Officer
Web address: www.rankinmedcenter.com

GILMORE MEMORIAL REGIONAL MEDICAL CENTER (O, 95 beds) 1105 Earl Frye Boulevard, Amory, MS Zip 38821–0459, Mailing Address: P.O. Box 459, Zip 38821–0459; tel. 662/256–7111; Dwayne Blaylock, Chief Executive Officer
Web address: www.gilmorehealth.com

MADISON COUNTY MEDICAL CENTER (O, 67 beds) Highway 16 East, Canton, MS Zip 39046–8823, Mailing Address: P.O. Box 1607, Zip 39046–1607; tel. 601/859–1331; Joseph Weaver, Chief Executive Officer
Web address: www.madisonregionalmedicalcenter.com

NATCHEZ COMMUNITY HOSPITAL (O, 101 beds) 129 Jefferson Davis Boulevard, Natchez, MS Zip 39120–5100, Mailing Address: P.O. Box 1203, Zip 39121–1203; tel. 601/445–6200; Timothy Trottier, Chief Executive Officer
Web address: www.hmamississippi.com

NORTHWEST MISSISSIPPI REGIONAL MEDICAL CENTER (L, 195 beds) 1970 Hospital Drive, Clarksdale, MS Zip 38614–7204, Mailing Address: P.O. Box 1218, Zip 38614–1218; tel. 662/627–3211; Mark W. Caton, Chief Executive Officer
Web address: www.nwmsregionalmedcenter.com

RILEY HOSPITAL (O, 140 beds) 1102 21st Avenue, Meridian, MS Zip 39301–4096, Mailing Address: P.O. Box 1810, Zip 39301–1810; tel. 601/693–2511; Kerry Tirman, Chief Executive Officer
Web address: www.hmamississippi.com

For explanation of codes following names, see page B2.
★ Indicates Type III membership in the American Hospital Association.

RIVER OAKS HOSPITAL (O, 109 beds) 1030 River Oaks Drive, Jackson, MS Zip 39232, Mailing Address: P.O. Box 5100, Zip 39296–5100; tel. 601/932–1030; Davis A. Richards, III, President and Chief Executive Officer
Web address: www.riveroakshospital.org

WOMAN'S HOSPITAL AT RIVER OAKS (O, 60 beds) 1026 North Flowood Drive, Jackson, MS Zip 39232, Mailing Address: P.O. Box 4546, Zip 39296–4546; tel. 601/932–1000; Sherry J. Pitts, Chief Executive Officer
Web address: www.womanshospitalms.com

MISSOURI: POPLAR BLUFF REGIONAL MEDICAL CENTER (O, 255 beds) 2620 North Westwood Boulevard, Poplar Bluff, MO Zip 63901–3396, Mailing Address: P.O. Box 88, Zip 63901–0088; tel. 573/686–5311; Bruce Eady, Chief Executive Officer
Web address: www.poplarbluffregional.com

TWIN RIVERS REGIONAL MEDICAL CENTER (O, 116 beds) 1301 First Street, Kennett, MO Zip 63857–2508, Mailing Address: P.O. Box 728, Zip 63857–0728; tel. 573/888–4522; John W. McClellan, Chief Executive Officer
Web address: www.twinriversmedctr.com

NORTH CAROLINA: DAVIS REGIONAL MEDICAL CENTER (O, 149 beds) 218 Old Mocksville Road, Statesville, NC Zip 28625–1930, Mailing Address: P.O. Box 1823, Zip 28687–1823; tel. 704/873–0281; Karen Metz, Chief Executive Officer
Web address: www.davisregional.com

FRANKLIN REGIONAL MEDICAL CENTER (O, 59 beds) 100 Hospital Drive, Louisburg, NC Zip 27549–2256, Mailing Address: P.O. Box 609, Zip 27549–0609; tel. 919/497–8401; Michael H. McNair, Chief Executive Officer
Web address: www.franklinregionalmedicalctr.com

LAKE NORMAN REGIONAL MEDICAL CENTER (O, 129 beds) 171 Fairview Road, Mooresville, NC Zip 28117–9500, Mailing Address: P.O. Box 3250, Zip 28117–3250; tel. 704/660–4000; J. Michael Cowling, Chief Executive Officer
Web address: www.lnrmc.com

SANDHILLS REGIONAL MEDICAL CENTER (O, 64 beds) 1000 West Hamlet Avenue, Hamlet, NC Zip 28345–4522, Mailing Address: P.O. Box 1109, Zip 28345–1109; tel. 910/205–8000; Andrew L. Davis, Chief Executive Officer
Web address: www.hma–corp.com

OKLAHOMA: MEDICAL CENTER OF SOUTHEASTERN OKLAHOMA (O, 120 beds) 1800 University Boulevard, Durant, OK Zip 74701–3006, Mailing Address: P.O. Box 1207, Zip 74702–1207; tel. 580/924–3080; Jacquelyn Harms, RN, Chief Executive Officer
Web address: www.mcso.com

MIDWEST REGIONAL MEDICAL CENTER (L, 255 beds) 2825 Parklawn Drive, Midwest City, OK Zip 73110–4258; tel. 405/610–4411; Douglas Arnold, Chief Executive Officer
Web address: www.midwestregional.com

PENNSYLVANIA: CARLISLE REGIONAL MEDICAL CENTER (O, 103 beds) 361 Alexander Spring Road, Carlisle, PA Zip 17013–3661; tel. 717/249–1212; Nathan Staggs, Chief Executive Officer
Web address: www.chhs.org/home/default.asp

HEART OF LANCASTER REGIONAL MEDICAL CENTER (O, 139 beds) 1500 Highlands Avenue, Lititz, PA Zip 17543; tel. 717/625–5000; Rebecca T. Brewer, FACHE, Interim Chief Executive Officer
Web address: www.chol.org

LANCASTER REGIONAL MEDICAL CENTER (O, 226 beds) 250 College Avenue, Lancaster, PA Zip 17603, Mailing Address: P.O. Box 3434, Zip 17604–3434; tel. 717/291–8211; Rebecca T. Brewer, FACHE, Interim Chief Executive Officer
Web address: www.lancasterregional.com

SOUTH CAROLINA: CAROLINA PINES REGIONAL MEDICAL CENTER (O, 120 beds) 1304 West BoBo Newsom Highway, Hartsville, SC Zip 29550–4710; tel. 843/339–2100; David L. Castleberry, Chief Executive Officer
Web address: www.cprmc.com

CHESTER REGIONAL MEDICAL CENTER (O, 156 beds) 1 Medical Park Drive, Chester, SC Zip 29706–9799; tel. 803/581–3151; Patrice L. Tavernier, Chief Executive Officer
Web address: www.chospital.org

UPSTATE CAROLINA MEDICAL CENTER (O, 125 beds) 1530 North Limestone Street, Gaffney, SC Zip 29340–4738; tel. 864/487–4271; Joe D. Howell, Executive Director
Web address: www.upstatecarolina.org

TENNESSEE: HARTON REGIONAL MEDICAL CENTER (O, 104 beds) 1801 North Jackson Street, Tullahoma, TN Zip 37388–2201; tel. 931/393–3000; Kenneth Ward, Interim Chief Executive Officer
Web address: www.hartonmedicalcenter.com

JAMESTOWN REGIONAL MEDICAL CENTER (O, 85 beds) 436 Central Avenue West, Jamestown, TN Zip 38556–3031, Mailing Address: P.O. Box 1500, Zip 38556–1500; tel. 931/879–8171; John Lee, Chief Executive Officer
Web address: www.jamestownregional.org

UNIVERSITY MEDICAL CENTER (O, 245 beds) 1411 Baddour Parkway, Lebanon, TN Zip 37087–2595; tel. 615/444–8262; Vincent T. Cherry, Jr., Chief Executive Director
Web address: www.universitymedicalcenter.com

TEXAS: DALLAS REGIONAL MEDICAL CENTER (O, 292 beds) 1011 North Galloway Avenue, Mesquite, TX Zip 75149–2433; tel. 214/320–7000; Roy C. Vinson, Chief Executive Officer

WASHINGTON: TOPPENISH COMMUNITY HOSPITAL (O, 40 beds) 502 West Fourth Avenue, Toppenish, WA Zip 98948–0672, Mailing Address: P.O. Box 672, Zip 98948–0672; tel. 509/865–3105; Michael P. Curran, Chief Executive Officer
Web address: www.hma–corp.com

YAKIMA REGIONAL MEDICAL AND CARDIAC CENTER (O, 169 beds) 110 South Ninth Avenue, Yakima, WA Zip 98902–3397; tel. 509/575–5000; Monte J. Bostwick, Chief Executive Officer
Web address: www.yakimaregional.org

WEST VIRGINIA: WILLIAMSON MEMORIAL HOSPITAL (O, 76 beds) 859 Alderson Street, Williamson, WV Zip 25661–3215, Mailing Address: P.O. Box 1980, Zip 25661–1980; tel. 304/235–2500; Todd Hubler, Interim Chief Executive Officer
Web address: www.hmawmh.com

Owned, leased, sponsored:	56 hospitals	7641 beds
Contract–managed:	0 hospitals	0 beds
Totals:	56 hospitals	7641 beds

★0307: HEALTH QUEST SYSTEMS, INC. (NP)

45 Reade Place, Poughkeepsie, NY Zip 12601; tel. 845/431–5601; Michael T. Weber, President and Chief Executive Officer
(Moderately Centralized Health System)

NEW YORK: NORTHERN DUTCHESS HOSPITAL (O, 68 beds) 6511 Springbrook Avenue, Rhinebeck, NY Zip 12572–5002, Mailing Address: P.O. Box 5002, Zip 12572–5002; tel. 845/876–3001; Denise George, RN, President and Chief Executive Officer
Web address: www.ndhosp.com

PUTNAM HOSPITAL CENTER (O, 144 beds) 670 Stoneleigh Avenue, Carmel, NY Zip 10512–9948; tel. 845/279–5711; Donna McGregor, President and Chief Executive Officer
Web address: www.putnamhospital.org

VASSAR BROTHERS MEDICAL CENTER (O, 355 beds) 45 Reade Place, Poughkeepsie, NY Zip 12601–3990; tel. 845/454–8500; Daniel Z. Aronzon, M.D., President and Chief Executive Officer
Web address: www.vassarbrothers.org

Owned, leased, sponsored:	3 hospitals	567 beds
Contract–managed:	0 hospitals	0 beds
Totals:	3 hospitals	567 beds

★2185: HEALTHEAST CARE SYSTEM (NP)

559 Capitol Boulevard, 6–South, Saint Paul, MN Zip 55103–0000; tel. 651/232–2300; Timothy H. Hanson, President and Chief Executive Officer
(Centralized Health System)

MINNESOTA: BETHESDA HOSPITAL (O, 140 beds) 559 Capitol Boulevard, Saint Paul, MN Zip 55103–2101; tel. 651/232–2000; Catherine Barr, Chief Executive Officer
Web address: www.healtheast.org

For explanation of codes following names, see page B2.
★ Indicates Type III membership in the American Hospital Association.

Section B

ST. JOHN'S HOSPITAL (O, 193 beds) 1575 Beam Avenue, Saint Paul, MN Zip 55109–1126; tel. 651/232–7000; Scott North, Chief Executive Officer
Web address: www.stjohnshospital-mn.org

ST. JOSEPH'S HOSPITAL (O, 258 beds) 69 West Exchange Street, Saint Paul, MN Zip 55102–1053; tel. 651/232–3000; Sara J. Criger, Chief Executive Officer
Web address: www.healtheast.org

WOODWINDS HEALTH CAMPUS (O, 78 beds) 1925 Woodwinds Drive, Woodbury, MN Zip 55125; tel. 651/232–0100; Julie A. Schmidt, Chief Executive Officer
Web address: www.woodwinds.org

Owned, leased, sponsored:	4 hospitals	669 beds
Contract-managed:	0 hospitals	0 beds
Totals:	4 hospitals	669 beds

0342: HEALTHPARTNERS (NP)

8100 34th Avenue South, Bloomington, MN Zip 55440; tel. 952/883–7463; Mary K. Brainerd, President and Chief Executive Officer
(Independent Hospital System)

REGIONS HOSPITAL (O, 416 beds) 640 Jackson Street, Saint Paul, MN Zip 55101–2595; tel. 651/254–3456; Brock D. Nelson, President and Chief Executive Officer
Web address: www.regionshospital.com

WISCONSIN: WESTFIELDS HOSPITAL (O, 25 beds) 535 Hospital Road, New Richmond, WI Zip 54017–1495; tel. 715/246–2101; Jean M. Needham, President
Web address: www.holyfamilyhospital.org

Owned, leased, sponsored:	2 hospitals	441 beds
Contract-managed:	0 hospitals	0 beds
Totals:	2 hospitals	441 beds

0296: HEALTHPLUS (IO)

509 West Tidwell Road, Houston, TX Zip 77091; tel. 713/490–0700; Wilton M. Burt, President and Chief Executive Officer
(Independent Hospital System)

CALIFORNIA: EAST LOS ANGELES DOCTORS HOSPITAL (O, 127 beds) 4060 East Whittier Boulevard, Los Angeles, CA Zip 90023–2526; tel. 323/268–5514; Araceli Lonergan, Chief Executive Officer
Web address: www.elalax.com

MEMORIAL HOSPITAL OF GARDENA (O, 107 beds) 1145 West Redondo Beach Boulevard, Gardena, CA Zip 90247–3528; tel. 310/532–4200; Steve Popkin, Chief Executive Officer

Owned, leased, sponsored:	2 hospitals	234 beds
Contract-managed:	0 hospitals	0 beds
Totals:	2 hospitals	234 beds

★0023: HEALTHSOUTH CORPORATION (IO)

One Healthsouth Parkway, Birmingham, AL Zip 35243; tel. 205/967–7116; Jay Grinney, President
(Decentralized Health System)

ALABAMA: HEALTHSOUTH LAKESHORE REHABILITATION HOSPITAL (O, 100 beds) 3800 Ridgeway Drive, Birmingham, AL Zip 35209–5599; tel. 205/868–2000; Terrence E. Brown, Chief Executive Officer
Web address: www.healthsouth.com

HEALTHSOUTH REHABILITATION HOSPITAL (O, 34 beds) 1736 East Main Street, Dothan, AL Zip 36301, Mailing Address: P.O. Box 6708, Zip 36302–6708; tel. 334/712–6333; Margaret A. Futch, Chief Executive Officer
Web address: www.healthsouth.com

HEALTHSOUTH REHABILITATION HOSPITAL OF MONTGOMERY (O, 80 beds) 4465 Narrow Lane Road, Montgomery, AL Zip 36116–2900; tel. 334/284–7700; Linda Wade, Chief Executive Officer
Web address: www.healthsouth.com

HEALTHSOUTH REHABILITATION HOSPITAL OF NORTH ALABAMA (O, 50 beds) 107 Governors Drive S.W., Huntsville, AL Zip 35801–4329; tel. 256/535–2300; Douglas H. Beverly, CHE, Chief Executive Officer
Web address: www.healthsouth.com

HEALTHSOUTH REHABILITATION OF GADSDEN (O, 40 beds) 801 Goodyear Avenue, Gadsden, AL Zip 35903; tel. 256/439–5000; Michael W. Thompson, Chief Executive Officer
Web address: www.healthsouth.com

REGIONAL REHABILITATION HOSPITAL (O, 38 beds) 3715 Highway 280/431 North, Phenix City, AL Zip 36867; tel. 334/732–2200; Jill Jordan, Chief Executive Officer
Web address: www.regionalrehabhospital.com

ARIZONA: HEALTHSOUTH REHABILITATION HOSPITAL OF SOUTHERN ARIZONA (O, 60 beds) 1921 West Hospital Drive, Tucson, AZ Zip 85704–7806; tel. 520/742–2800; Martha Gerganoff, Chief Executive Officer
Web address: www.healthsouth.com

HEALTHSOUTH REHABILITATION INSTITUTE OF TUCSON (O, 80 beds) 2650 North Wyatt Drive, Tucson, AZ Zip 85712–6108; tel. 520/325–1300; Jeffrey Christensen, Chief Executive Officer
Web address: www.healthsouth.com

HEALTHSOUTH SCOTTSDALE REHABILITATION HOSPITAL (O, 46 beds) 9630 East Shea Boulevard, Scottsdale, AZ Zip 85260; tel. 480/551–5400; Richard Schulz, Chief Executive Officer
Web address: www.healthsouth.com

HEALTHSOUTH VALLEY OF THE SUN REHABILITATION HOSPITAL (O, 60 beds) 13460 North 67th Avenue, Glendale, AZ Zip 85304–1042; tel. 623/878–8800; Beth Bacher, Chief Executive Officer
Web address: www.healthsouth.com

YUMA REHABILITATION HOSPITAL (O, 41 beds) 901 West 24th Street, Yuma, AZ Zip 85364; tel. 928/726–5000; Steve Smith, Chief Executive Officer
Web address: www.yumarehabhospital.com

ARKANSAS: HEALTHSOUTH REHABILITATION HOSPITAL (O, 60 beds) 153 East Monte Painter Drive, Fayetteville, AR Zip 72703–4002; tel. 479/444–2200; Jerry Alexander, Chief Executive Officer
Web address: www.healthsouth.com

HEALTHSOUTH REHABILITATION HOSPITAL OF FORT SMITH (O, 80 beds) 1401 South J Street, Fort Smith, AR Zip 72901–5155; tel. 479/785–3300; Julianne Stec, Chief Executive Officer
Web address: www.healthsouth.com

HEALTHSOUTH REHABILITATION HOSPITAL OF JONESBORO (O, 67 beds) 1201 Fleming Avenue, Jonesboro, AR Zip 72401–4311, Mailing Address: P.O. Box 1680, Zip 72403–1680; tel. 870/932–0440; Donna Harris, Chief Executive Officer
Web address: www.healthsouth.com

ST. VINCENT REHABILITATION HOSPITAL (S, 60 beds) 2201 Wildwood Avenue, Sherwood, AR Zip 72120–5074, Mailing Address: P.O. Box 6930, Zip 72124–6930; tel. 501/834–1800; Lee Frazier, Chief Executive Officer
Web address: www.healthsouth.com

CALIFORNIA: HEALTHSOUTH BAKERSFIELD REHABILITATION HOSPITAL (O, 40 beds) 5001 Commerce Drive, Bakersfield, CA Zip 93309–0689; tel. 661/323–5500; Sandra Hegland, Chief Executive Officer
Web address: www.healthsouth.com

HEALTHSOUTH TUSTIN REHABILITATION HOSPITAL (O, 48 beds) 14851 Yorba Street, Tustin, CA Zip 92780–2925; tel. 714/832–9200; David Mulhern, Chief Executive Officer
Web address: www.healthsouth.com

COLORADO: HEALTHSOUTH REHABILITATION HOSPITAL OF COLORADO SPRINGS (O, 64 beds) 325 Parkside Drive, Colorado Springs, CO Zip 80910; tel. 719/630–8000; William B. Mohon, Chief Executive Officer
Web address: www.healthsouth.com

FLORIDA: HEALTHSOUTH EMERALD COAST REHABILITATION HOSPITAL (O, 75 beds) 1847 Florida Avenue, Panama City, FL Zip 32405–4640; tel. 850/914–8600; Tony N. Bennett, Chief Executive Officer
Web address: www.healthsouthpanamacity.com

HEALTHSOUTH REHABILITATION HOSPITAL (O, 60 beds) 901 North Clearwater-Largo Road, Largo, FL Zip 33770–4126; tel. 727/586–2999; Elaine D. Ebaugh, Chief Executive Officer
Web address: www.healthsouth.com

For explanation of codes following names, see page B2.
★ Indicates Type III membership in the American Hospital Association.

HEALTHSOUTH REHABILITATION HOSPITAL (O, 60 beds) 20601 Old Cutler Road, Miami, FL Zip 33189–2400; tel. 305/251–3800; Elizabeth L. Izquierdo, CPA, Chief Executive Officer
Web address: www.healthsouthmiami.com

HEALTHSOUTH REHABILITATION HOSPITAL OF SARASOTA (O, 76 beds) 6400 Edgelake Drive, Sarasota, FL Zip 34240–8813; tel. 941/921–8600; Daniel A. Eppley, FACHE, Chief Executive Officer
Web address: www.healthsouthsarasota.com

HEALTHSOUTH REHABILITATION HOSPITAL OF SPRING HILL (O, 60 beds) 12440 Cortez Boulevard, Brooksville, FL Zip 34613–2628; tel. 352/592–4250; Lori Bedard, Chief Executive Officer
Web address: www.healthsouth.com

HEALTHSOUTH REHABILITATION HOSPITAL OF TALLAHASSEE (O, 70 beds) 1675 Riggins Road, Tallahassee, FL Zip 32308–5315; tel. 850/656–4800; Robert F. Jernigan, Jr., Chief Executive Officer
Web address: www.healthsouth.com

HEALTHSOUTH SEA PINES REHABILITATION HOSPITAL (O, 90 beds) 101 East Florida Avenue, Melbourne, FL Zip 32901–9966; tel. 321/984–4600; Denise B. McGrath, Chief Executive Officer
Web address: www.healthsouthseapines.com

HEALTHSOUTH SUNRISE REHABILITATION HOSPITAL (O, 116 beds) 4399 Nob Hill Road, Fort Lauderdale, FL Zip 33351–5899; tel. 954/749–0300; Kevin R. Conn, Chief Executive Officer
Web address: www.healthsouth.com

HEALTHSOUTH TREASURE COAST REHABILITATION HOSPITAL (O, 90 beds) 1600 37th Street, Vero Beach, FL Zip 32960–6549; tel. 772/778–2100; Patricia Parden, Chief Executive Officer
Web address: www.healthsouthtreasurecoast.com

ILLINOIS: VAN MATRE HEALTHSOUTH REHABILITATION HOSPITAL (O, 40 beds) 950 South Mulford Road, Rockford, IL Zip 61108; tel. 815/381–8500; Daniel B. Woloszyn, Chief Executive Officer
Web address: www.healthsouth.com

INDIANA: HEALTHSOUTH DEACONESS REHABILITATION HOSPITAL (O, 80 beds) 4100 Covert Avenue, Evansville, IN Zip 47714–5567, Mailing Address: P.O. Box 5349, Zip 47716–5349; tel. 812/476–9983; Barbara Butler, Chief Executive Officer
Web address: www.healthsouth.com

KANSAS: KANSAS REHABILITATION HOSPITAL (O, 79 beds) 1504 S.W. Eighth Avenue, Topeka, KS Zip 66606–1632; tel. 785/235–6600; Paul Livingston, Chief Executive Officer
Web address: www.kansasrehab.com

MID–AMERICA REHABILITATION HOSPITAL (O, 80 beds) 5701 West 110th Street, Shawnee Mission, KS Zip 66211–2503; tel. 913/491–2400; Kristen De Hart, Chief Executive Officer
Web address: www.healthsouth.com

WESLEY REHABILITATION HOSPITAL (O, 65 beds) 8338 West 13th Street North, Wichita, KS Zip 67212–2984; tel. 316/729–9999; Pamela Stanberry, Chief Executive Officer
Web address: www.wesleyrehabhospital.com

KENTUCKY: HEALTHSOUTH NORTHERN KENTUCKY REHABILITATION HOSPITAL (O, 40 beds) 201 Medical Village Drive, Edgewood, KY Zip 41017–3407; tel. 859/341–2044; Brenda Gosney, Chief Executive Officer
Web address: www.healthsouth.com

HEALTHSOUTH REHABILITATION HOSPITAL OF CENTRAL KENTUCKY (O, 40 beds) 134 Heartland Drive, Elizabethtown, KY Zip 42701–2778; tel. 270/769–3100; Eileen Nelson, Chief Executive Officer
Web address: www.healthsouth.com

LOUISIANA: HEALTHSOUTH REHABILITATION HOSPITAL OF ALEXANDRIA (O, 47 beds) 104 North Third Street, Alexandria, LA Zip 71301–8581; tel. 318/449–1370; William Bush, Interim Chief Executive Officer
Web address: www.healthsouth.com

HEALTHSOUTH REHABILITATION HOSPITAL OF BATON ROUGE (O, 80 beds) 8595 United Plaza Boulevard, Baton Rouge, LA Zip 70809–2251; tel. 225/927–0567; David M. Snyder, Chief Executive Officer
Web address: www.healthsouth.com

HEALTHSOUTH SPECIALTY HOSPITAL OF NORTH LOUISIANA (O, 90 beds) 1401 Ezell Street, Ruston, LA Zip 71270–7221; tel. 318/251–3126; Mark J. Rice, Chief Executive Officer
Web address: www.healthsouth.com

MAINE: NEW ENGLAND REHABILITATION HOSPITAL OF PORTLAND (O, 90 beds) 335 Brighton Avenue, Portland, ME Zip 04102–9735; tel. 207/775–4000; Amy Morse, Chief Executive Officer
Web address: www.healthsouth.com

MARYLAND: HEALTHSOUTH CHESAPEAKE REHABILITATION HOSPITAL (O, 42 beds) 220 Tilghman Road, Salisbury, MD Zip 21804–1921; tel. 410/546–4600; Gary Crowley, Chief Executive Officer
Web address: www.healthsouth.com

MASSACHUSETTS: FAIRLAWN REHABILITATION HOSPITAL (O, 110 beds) 189 May Street, Worcester, MA Zip 01602–4399; tel. 508/791–6351; Peter M. Mantegazza, Chief Executive Officer
Web address: www.fairlawnrehab.org

HEALTHSOUTH REHABILITATION HOSPITAL OF WESTERN MASSACHUSETTS (O, 53 beds) 14 Chestnut Place, Ludlow, MA Zip 01056–3460; tel. 413/589–7581; R. David Richer, Chief Executive Officer
Web address: www.healthsouth.com

MISSOURI: HOWARD A. RUSK REHABILITATION CENTER (O, 60 beds) 315 Business Loop 70 West, Columbia, MO Zip 65203–3248; tel. 573/817–2703; Gary Payne, Chief Executive Officer
Web address: www.healthsouth.com

THE REHABILITATION INSTITUTE OF ST. LOUIS (O, 80 beds) 4455 Duncan Avenue, Saint Louis, MO Zip 63110–1111; tel. 314/658–3800; Barbara Jacobsmeyer, Chief Executive Officer
Web address: www.healthsouth.com

NEVADA: HEALTHSOUTH HOSPITAL OF TENAYA (O, 70 beds) 2500 North Tenaya, Las Vegas, NV Zip 89128; tel. 702/562–2021; Kenneth D'Amico, Chief Executive Officer
Web address: www.healthsouth.com

HEALTHSOUTH REHABILITATION HOSPITAL – HENDERSON (O, 60 beds) 10301 Jeffreys Street, Henderson, NV Zip 89052; tel. 702/939–9400; William Schoonmaker, Chief Executive Officer
Web address: www.healthsouth.com

HEALTHSOUTH REHABILITATION HOSPITAL–LAS VEGAS (O, 79 beds) 1250 South Valley View Boulevard, Las Vegas, NV Zip 89102–1861; tel. 702/877–8898; Cheryl Williams, Chief Executive Officer
Web address: www.healthsouth.com

NEW HAMPSHIRE: HEALTHSOUTH REHABILITATION HOSPITAL (O, 50 beds) 254 Pleasant Street, Concord, NH Zip 03301–2508; tel. 603/226–9800; Catherine Devaney, Chief Executive Officer
Web address: www.healthsouth.com

NEW JERSEY: HEALTHSOUTH REHABILITATION HOSPITAL OF NEW JERSEY (O, 131 beds) 14 Hospital Drive, Toms River, NJ Zip 08755–6470; tel. 732/244–3100; Patricia Ostaszewski, Chief Executive Officer
Web address: www.healthsouth.com

REHABILITATION HOSPITAL OF TINTON FALLS (O, 60 beds) 2 Centre Plaza, Tinton Falls, NJ Zip 7724; tel. 732/460–5320; Linda A. Savino, Chief Executive Officer
Web address: www.rehabnj.com

NEW MEXICO: HEALTHSOUTH REHABILITATION HOSPITAL (O, 60 beds) 7000 Jefferson N.E., Albuquerque, NM Zip 87109–4357; tel. 505/344–9478; Sylvia K. Kelly, Chief Executive Officer
Web address: www.healthsouth.com

PENNSYLVANIA: GEISINGER HEALTHSOUTH REHABILITATION HOSPITAL (O, 40 beds) 2 Rehab Lane, Danville, PA Zip 17821; tel. 570/271–6733; Lorie Dillon, Chief Executive Officer
Web address: www.healthsouth.com

HEALTHSOUTH HARMARVILLE REHABILITATION HOSPITAL (O, 202 beds) Guys Run Road, Pittsburgh, PA Zip 15238–0460, Mailing Address: P.O. Box 11460, Zip 15238–0460; tel. 412/828–1300; Kenneth J. Anthony, Chief Executive Officer
Web address: www.healthsouth.com

HEALTHSOUTH HOSPITAL OF PITTSBURGH (O, 89 beds) 2380 McGinley Road, Monroeville, PA Zip 15146–4400; tel. 412/856–2400; Cynthia Eiseman, Chief Executive Officer
Web address: www.healthsouth.com

HEALTHSOUTH NITTANY VALLEY REHABILITATION HOSPITAL (O, 85 beds) 550 West College Avenue, Pleasant Gap, PA Zip 16823–7416; tel. 814/359–3421; Susan Hartman, Chief Executive Officer
Web address: www.nittanyvalleyrehab.com

Section B

For explanation of codes following names, see page B2.
★ Indicates Type III membership in the American Hospital Association.

HEALTHSOUTH READING REHABILITATION HOSPITAL (O, 95 beds) 1623 Morgantown Road, Reading, PA Zip 19607–9455; tel. 610/796–6000; Richard Kruczek, Chief Executive Officer
Web address: www.healthsouthreading.com

HEALTHSOUTH REGIONAL SPECIALTY HOSPITAL (O, 46 beds) 4950 Wilson Lane, Mechanicsburg, PA Zip 17055; tel. 717/697–7706; Brent Burger, Chief Executive Officer
Web address: www.healthsouth.com

HEALTHSOUTH REHABILITATION HOSPITAL (O, 31 beds) 303 Camp Meeting Road, Sewickley, PA Zip 15143–8322; tel. 412/741–9500; Marlene Hughes, Chief Executive Officer
Web address: www.healthsouth.com

HEALTHSOUTH REHABILITATION HOSPITAL OF ALTOONA (O, 70 beds) 2005 Valley View Boulevard, Altoona, PA Zip 16602–4598; tel. 814/944–3535; Scott Filler, Chief Executive Officer
Web address: www.healthsouthaltoona.com

HEALTHSOUTH REHABILITATION HOSPITAL OF ERIE (O, 108 beds) 143 East Second Street, Erie, PA Zip 16507–1501; tel. 814/878–1200; John Ferritto, Chief Executive Officer
Web address: www.healthsouth.com

HEALTHSOUTH REHABILITATION HOSPITAL OF MECHANICSBURG (O, 103 beds) 175 Lancaster Boulevard, Mechanicsburg, PA Zip 17055–0736, Mailing Address: P.O. Box 2016, Zip 17055–2016; tel. 717/691–3700; Gregory P. Toot, Chief Executive Officer
Web address: www.healthsouth.com

HEALTHSOUTH REHABILITATION HOSPITAL OF YORK (O, 88 beds) 1850 Normandie Drive, York, PA Zip 17408; tel. 717/767–6941; Mark Freeburn, Chief Executive Officer
Web address: www.healthsouth.com

PUERTO RICO: HEALTHSOUTH REHABILITATION HOSPITAL (O, 32 beds) University Hospital, 3rd Floor, San Juan, PR Zip 923, Mailing Address: P.O. Box 70344, Zip 923; tel. 787/274–5100; Daniel Del Castillo, Chief Executive Officer

SOUTH CAROLINA: ANMED HEALTH REHABILITATION HOSPITAL (O, 37 beds) 1 Spring Back Way, Anderson, SC Zip 29621; tel. 864/716–2600; Michele M. Skripps, Chief Executive Officer
Web address: www.anmedhealth.org

HEALTHSOUTH REHABILITATION HOSPITAL (O, 96 beds) 2935 Colonial Drive, Columbia, SC Zip 29203–6811; tel. 803/254–7777; James H. Rogers, FACHE, Chief Executive Officer
Web address: www.healthsouth.com

HEALTHSOUTH REHABILITATION HOSPITAL (O, 88 beds) 900 East Cheves Street, Florence, SC Zip 29506–2704; tel. 843/679–9000; Jeanette Filpi, Chief Executive Officer
Web address: www.healthsouth.com

HEALTHSOUTH REHABILITATION HOSPITAL (O, 40 beds) 1795 Frank Gaston Boulevard, Rock Hill, SC Zip 29732; tel. 803/362–3500; Anthony W. Jackson, Chief Executive Officer
Web address: www.healthsouth.com

HEALTHSOUTH REHABILITATION HOSPITAL OF CHARLESTON (O, 46 beds) 9181 Medcom Street, Charleston, SC Zip 29406–9168; tel. 843/820–7777; Troy Powell, Chief Executive Officer
Web address: www.healthsouthcharleston.com

TENNESSEE: HEALTHSOUTH CANE CREEK REHABILITATION HOSPITAL (O, 40 beds) 180 Mt Pelia Road, Martin, TN Zip 38237–3812; tel. 731/587–4231; William P. Macri, Chief Executive Officer
Web address: www.healthsouth.com

HEALTHSOUTH CHATTANOOGA REHABILITATION HOSPITAL (O, 46 beds) 2412 McCallie Avenue, Chattanooga, TN Zip 37404–3398; tel. 423/698–0221; Scott Rowe, Chief Executive Officer
Web address: www.healthsouth.com

HEALTHSOUTH REHABILITATION HOSPITAL (O, 50 beds) 113 Cassel Drive, Kingsport, TN Zip 37660–3775; tel. 423/246–7240; Terri Alsbrook, Chief Executive Officer
Web address: www.healthsouth.com

HEALTHSOUTH REHABILITATION HOSPITAL (O, 80 beds) 1282 Union Avenue, Memphis, TN Zip 38104–3414; tel. 901/722–2000; Traci Willis, Chief Executive Officer
Web address: www.healthsouth.com

HEALTHSOUTH REHABILITATION HOSPITAL (O, 40 beds) 4100 Austin Peay Highway, Memphis, TN Zip 38128–2503; tel. 901/213–5400; John R. Borden, Chief Executive Officer
Web address: www.healthsouth.com

VANDERBILT STALLWORTH REHABILITATION HOSPITAL (O, 80 beds) 2201 Childrens Way, Nashville, TN Zip 37212–3165; tel. 615/320–7600; Susan Heath, Chief Executive Officer
Web address: www.healthsouth.com

TEXAS: HEALTHSOUTH HOSPITAL FOR SPECIALIZED SURGERY (O, 7 beds) 5400 La Branch Street, Houston, TX Zip 77004–6836; tel. 713/528–6800; Trent Gastineau, Chief Executive Officer
Web address: www.healthsouth.com

HEALTHSOUTH HOSPITAL OF HOUSTON (O, 74 beds) 17506 Red Oak Drive, Houston, TX Zip 77090–7721; tel. 281/580–1212; Aleen D. Arabit, Chief Executive Officer
Web address: www.healthsouth.com

HEALTHSOUTH MEDICAL CENTER (O, 73 beds) 2124 Research Row, Dallas, TX Zip 75235–2504; tel. 214/904–6100; Daniel L. Gideon, CHE, Chief Executive Officer
Web address: www.healthsouth.com

HEALTHSOUTH PLANO REHABILITATION HOSPITAL (O, 65 beds) 2800 West 15th Street, Plano, TX Zip 75075–7526; tel. 972/612–9000; Duke Saldivar, CHE, Chief Executive Officer
Web address: www.healthsouth.com

HEALTHSOUTH REHABILITATION HOSPITAL (O, 60 beds) 1212 West Lancaster Avenue, Fort Worth, TX Zip 76102–4510; tel. 817/870–2336; Jon McPike, Chief Executive Officer
Web address: www.healthsouth.com

HEALTHSOUTH REHABILITATION HOSPITAL (O, 60 beds) 19002 McKay Drive, Humble, TX Zip 77338–5701; tel. 281/446–6148; Angela L. Simmons, Chief Executive Officer
Web address: www.healthsouth.com

HEALTHSOUTH REHABILITATION HOSPITAL MIDLAND–ODESSA (O, 60 beds) 1800 Heritage Boulevard, Midland, TX Zip 79707–9750; tel. 432/520–1600; Ellen Shankles, Chief Executive Officer
Web address: www.healthsouth.com

HEALTHSOUTH REHABILITATION HOSPITAL OF ARLINGTON (O, 65 beds) 3200 Matlock Road, Arlington, TX Zip 76015–2911; tel. 817/468–4000; Jessica Knox, Chief Executive Officer
Web address: www.healthsouth.com

HEALTHSOUTH REHABILITATION HOSPITAL OF AUSTIN (O, 50 beds) 1215 Red River Street, Austin, TX Zip 78701–1921; tel. 512/474–5700; Robert A. Prehn, Ph.D., Chief Executive Officer
Web address: www.healthsouthaustin.com

HEALTHSOUTH REHABILITATION HOSPITAL OF BEAUMONT (O, 61 beds) 3340 Plaza 10 Boulevard, Beaumont, TX Zip 77707–2551; tel. 409/835–0835; Bill Klamforth, Chief Executive Officer
Web address: www.healthsouth.com

HEALTHSOUTH REHABILITATION HOSPITAL OF NORTH HOUSTON (O, 84 beds) 18550 I 45 South, Conroe, TX Zip 77384; tel. 281/364–2000; Russell Bailey, Chief Executive Officer
Web address: www.healthsouth.com

HEALTHSOUTH REHABILITATION HOSPITAL OF TEXARKANA (O, 60 beds) 515 West 12th Street, Texarkana, TX Zip 75501–4416; tel. 903/793–0088; Joanne Rose, Chief Executive Officer
Web address: www.healthsouth.com

HEALTHSOUTH REHABILITATION HOSPITAL–CITYVIEW (O, 62 beds) 6701 Oakmont Boulevard, Fort Worth, TX Zip 76132–2957; tel. 817/370–4700; Barbara Mobley, Chief Executive Officer
Web address: www.healthsouth.com

HEALTHSOUTH REHABILITATION HOSPITAL–WICHITA FALLS (O, 63 beds) 3901 Armory Road, Wichita Falls, TX Zip 76302–2204; tel. 940/720–5700; Michael L. Bullitt, Chief Executive Officer
Web address: www.healthsouth.com

HEALTHSOUTH REHABILITATION INSTITUTE OF SAN ANTONIO (O, 96 beds) 9119 Cinnamon Hill, San Antonio, TX Zip 78240–5401; tel. 210/691–0737; Lee A. Simpson, Jr., Chief Executive Officer
Web address: www.healthsouth.com

TRINITY MOTHER FRANCES REHABILITATION HOSPITAL (O, 62 beds) 3131 Troup Highway, Tyler, TX Zip 75701–8352; tel. 903/510–7000; Sharla Anderson, Chief Executive Officer
Web address: www.healthsouth.com

For explanation of codes following names, see page B2.
★ Indicates Type III membership in the American Hospital Association.

UTAH: HEALTHSOUTH REHABILITATION HOSPITAL OF UTAH (O, 60 beds) 8074 South 1300 East, Sandy, UT Zip 84094–0743; tel. 801/561–3400; Thomas Almerico, Chief Executive Officer
Web address: www.healthsouth.com

VIRGINIA: HEALTHSOUTH REHABILITATION HOSPITAL OF VIRGINIA (O, 40 beds) 5700 Fitzhugh Avenue, Richmond, VA Zip 23226–1877; tel. 804/288–5700; Jeff Ruskan, II, Chief Executive Officer
Web address: www.healthsouth.com

UVA–HEALTHSOUTH REHABILITATION HOSPITAL (O, 50 beds) 515 Ray C. Hunt Drive, Charlottesville, VA Zip 22903; tel. 434/244–2000; Thomas J. Cook, Chief Executive Officer
Web address: www.healthsystem.virginia.edu/internet/pmr/pmrneo.cfm

WEST VIRGINIA: HEALTHSOUTH HUNTINGTON REHABILITATION HOSPITAL (O, 52 beds) 6900 West Country Club Drive, Huntington, WV Zip 25705–2000; tel. 304/733–1060; Michael E. Zuliani, Chief Executive Officer
Web address: www.healthsouthhuntington.com

HEALTHSOUTH MOUNTAINVIEW REGIONAL REHABILITATION HOSPITAL (O, 96 beds) 1160 Van Voorhis Road, Morgantown, WV Zip 26505–3437; tel. 304/598–1100; John C. Forester, Chief Executive Officer
Web address: www.healthsouth.com

HEALTHSOUTH SOUTHERN HILLS REHABILITATION HOSPITAL (O, 60 beds) 120 Twelfth Street, Princeton, WV Zip 24740–2312; tel. 304/487–8000; Sharon Boggess, Chief Executive Officer
Web address: www.healthsouth.com

HEALTHSOUTH WESTERN HILLS REHABILITATION CENTER (O, 40 beds) 3 Western Hills Drive, Parkersburg, WV Zip 26101–8122; tel. 304/420–1300; Dean Hatcher, Chief Executive Officer
Web address: www.healthsouth.com

Owned, leased, sponsored:	96 hospitals	6363 beds
Contract–managed:	0 hospitals	0 beds
Totals:	96 hospitals	6363 beds

★9505: HENRY FORD HEALTH SYSTEM (NP)

One Ford Place, Detroit, MI Zip 48202–3450; tel. 313/876–8708; Nancy M. Schlichting, President and Chief Executive Officer
(Centralized Physician/Insurance Health System)

MICHIGAN: HENRY FORD COTTAGE HOSPITAL (O, 63 beds) 159 Kercheval Avenue, Grosse Pointe Farms, MI Zip 48236–3692; tel. 313/640–1000; Denise Allar, Interim Administrator
Web address: www.bonsecourscottage.org

HENRY FORD HOSPITAL (O, 768 beds) 2799 West Grand Boulevard, Detroit, MI Zip 48202–2689; tel. 313/916–2600; Anthony A. Armada, President and Chief Executive Officer
Web address: www.henryfordhealth.org

HENRY FORD KINGSWOOD HOSPITAL (O, 80 beds) 10300 West Eight Mile Road, Ferndale, MI Zip 48220–2198; tel. 248/398–3200; Richard T. Young, FACHE, Chief Operating Officer
Web address: www.henryford.com

HENRY FORD MACOMB HOSPITAL (O, 419 beds) Clinton Township, MI Barbara Rossmann, President and Chief Executive Officer
Web address: www.stjoe-macomb.com

HENRY FORD MACOMB HOSPITAL–WARREN CAMPUS (O, 137 beds) 13355 East Ten Mile Road, Warren, MI Zip 48089–2065; tel. 586/759–7300; Barbara Rossmann, President and Chief Executive Officer
Web address: www.bicountyhospital.org

HENRY FORD WEST BLOOMFIELD HOSPITAL (O, 300 beds) 6777 West Maple Road, West Bloomfield, MI Zip 48322; tel. 248/661–4100; Gerard van Grinsven, President and Chief Executive Officer
Web address: www.henryford.com

HENRY FORD WYANDOTTE HOSPITAL (O, 344 beds) 2333 Biddle Avenue, Wyandotte, MI Zip 48192–4693; tel. 734/246–6000; James J. Sexton, FACHE, President and Chief Executive Officer
Web address: www.henryfordhealth.org

Owned, leased, sponsored:	7 hospitals	2111 beds
Contract–managed:	0 hospitals	0 beds
Totals:	7 hospitals	2111 beds

0309: HERITAGE VALLEY HEALTH SYSTEM (NP)

1000 Dutch Ridge Road, Beaver, PA Zip 15009–9727; tel. 724/773–2024; Norman F. Mitry, President and Chief Executive Officer

PENNSYLVANIA: HERITAGE VALLEY BEAVER (O, 300 beds) 1000 Dutch Ridge Road, Beaver, PA Zip 15009–9727; tel. 724/728–7000; Norman F. Mitry, President and Chief Executive Officer
Web address: www.heritagevalley.org

SEWICKLEY VALLEY HOSPITAL, (A DIVISION OF VALLEY MEDICAL FACILITIES) (O, 175 beds) 720 Blackburn Road, Sewickley, PA Zip 15143–1459; tel. 412/741–6600; Norman F. Mitry, President and Chief Executive Officer
Web address: www.heritagevalley.org

Owned, leased, sponsored:	2 hospitals	475 beds
Contract–managed:	0 hospitals	0 beds
Totals:	2 hospitals	475 beds

0306: HORIZON HEALTH CORPORATION (IO)

1500 Waters Ridge Drive, Lewisville, TX Zip 75057; tel. 972/420–8222; Ken Newman, President and Chief Executive Officer
(Independent Hospital System)

DELAWARE: MEADOW WOOD BEHAVIORAL HEALTH SYSTEM (O, 53 beds) 575 South Dupont Highway, New Castle, DE Zip 19720–4600; tel. 302/328–3330; Kim Whitelock, Chief Executive Officer
Web address: www.horizonhealth.com

GEORGIA: FOCUS BY–THE–SEA (O, 101 beds) 2927 Demere Road, Saint Simons Island, GA Zip 31522–1620; tel. 912/638–1999; Ronald Mays, Chief Executive Officer
Web address: www.focushealthcare.com

INDIANA: MICHIANA BEHAVIORAL HEALTH CENTER (O, 76 beds) 1800 North Oak Road, Plymouth, IN Zip 46563–3492; tel. 574/936–3784; Bryan W. Lett, Chief Executive Officer
Web address: www.michianabhc.com

OHIO: FOCUS HEALTHCARE OF OHIO (O, 42 beds) 1725 Timber Line Road, Maumee, OH Zip 43537–4015; tel. 419/891–9333; Gene Riegle, Chief Executive Officer
Web address: www.focushealthcare.com

WINDSOR–LAURELWOOD CENTER FOR BEHAVIORAL MEDICINE (O, 160 beds) 35900 Euclid Avenue, Willoughby, OH Zip 44094–4648; tel. 440/953–3000; David Fletcher–Janzen, Chief Executive Officer
Web address: www.laurelwoodhospital.com

PENNSYLVANIA: FRIENDS BEHAVIORAL HEALTH SYSTEM (O, 219 beds) 4641 Roosevelt Boulevard, Philadelphia, PA Zip 19124–2399; tel. 215/831–4600; Arris S. Veronie, Chief Executive Officer
Web address: www.fbhs.org

SOUTH CAROLINA: LIGHTHOUSE CARE CENTER OF CONWAY (O, 44 beds) 152 Waccamaw Medical Park Drive, Conway, SC Zip 29520; tel. 843/347–8871; Fran Sauvageau, Chief Executive Officer

TEXAS: KINGWOOD PINES HOSPITAL (O, 78 beds) 2001 Ladbrook Drive, Kingwood, TX Zip 77339; tel. 281/358–1495; Linda Hodgkins, Chief Executive Officer

UTAH: COPPER HILLS YOUTH CENTER (O, 98 beds) 5899 West Rivendell Drive, West Jordan, UT Zip 84088–5700; tel. 800/776–7116; Michael Rowley, Chief Executive Officer
Web address: www.copperhillsyouthcenter.com

VIRGINIA: POPLAR SPRINGS HOSPITAL (O, 120 beds) 350 Poplar Drive, Petersburg, VA Zip 23805–4657, Mailing Address: P.O. Box 3060, Zip 23805–3060; tel. 804/733–6874; Richard Clark, Chief Executive Officer

WEST VIRGINIA: RIVER PARK HOSPITAL (O, 147 beds) 1230 Sixth Avenue, Huntington, WV Zip 25701–2312, Mailing Address: P.O. Box 1875, Zip 25719–1875; tel. 304/526–9111; Patrick D. Burrows, CPA, Chief Executive Officer
Web address: www.riverparkhospital.net/home.htm

Owned, leased, sponsored:	11 hospitals	1138 beds
Contract–managed:	0 hospitals	0 beds
Totals:	11 hospitals	1138 beds

Section B

For explanation of codes following names, see page B2.
★ Indicates Type III membership in the American Hospital Association.

0348: HOSPITAL MANAGEMENT CONSULTING, LLC (IO)
4254 North Trafficway, Kansas City, MO Zip 64116–4541; tel. 816/474–7800; Lawrence J. Arthur, President
(Independent Hospital System)

KANSAS: OSWEGO MEDICAL CENTER (O, 12 beds) 800 Barker Drive, Oswego, KS Zip 67356–9033; tel. 620/795–2921; Daniel Hiben, Chief Executive Officer
Web address: www.oswegomedical.com

MISSOURI: ELLETT MEMORIAL HOSPITAL (C, 25 beds) 610 North Ohio Avenue, Appleton City, MO Zip 64724–1609, Mailing Address: P.O. Box 6, Zip 64724–0006; tel. 660/476–2111; Stephanie Lyon, RN, Administrator
Web address: www.ellettmemorial.com

I–70 MEDICAL CENTER (C, 15 beds) 105 Hospital Drive, Sweet Springs, MO Zip 65351–2229; tel. 660/335–4700; Ronald D. Baker, Chief Executive Officer
Web address: www.i70medcenter.com

OKLAHOMA: DRUMRIGHT REGIONAL HOSPITAL (C, 15 beds) 610 West Bypass Street, Drumright, OK Zip 74030; tel. 918/382–2300; Darrel Morris, Chief Executive Officer

Owned, leased, sponsored:	1 hospital	12 beds
Contract-managed:	3 hospitals	55 beds
Totals:	4 hospitals	67 beds

0289: HOSPITAL PARTNERS OF AMERICA (IO)
2815 Coliseum Centre Drive, Suite 150, Charlotte, NC Zip 28217–1378; tel. 704/424–6800; Todd Johnson, President and Chief Executive Officer
(Moderately Centralized Health System)

CALIFORNIA: SHASTA REGIONAL MEDICAL CENTER (O, 125 beds) 1100 Butte Street, Redding, CA Zip 96001–0853, Mailing Address: P.O. Box 496072, Zip 96049–6072; tel. 530/244–5400; Philip G. Dionne, Chief Executive Officer

LOUISIANA: MONROE SURGICAL HOSPITAL (O, 10 beds) 2408 Broadmoor Boulevard, Monroe, LA Zip 71201, Mailing Address: P.O. Box 4887, Zip 71211–4887; tel. 318/410–0002; Alan Daugherty, Administrator
Web address: www.monroesurgical.com

TEXAS: AUSTIN SURGICAL HOSPITAL (O, 23 beds) 3003 Bee Caves Road, Austin, TX Zip 78746; tel. 512/314–3800; Todd Mann, Chief Executive Officer
Web address: www.austinsurgicalhospital.com

RHD MEMORIAL MEDICAL CENTER (L, 118 beds) Seven Medical Parkway, Dallas, TX Zip 75234, Mailing Address: P.O. Box 819094, Zip 75381–9094; tel. 972/247–1000; Kenneth Howell, Chief Executive Officer
Web address: www.rhdmemorial.com

RIVER OAKS HOSPITAL (O, 225 beds) 4200 Twelve Oaks Drive, Houston, TX Zip 77027–6899; tel. 713/623–2500; Chris M. Vasquez, Chief Executive Officer
Web address: www.twelveoaksmedicalcenter.com

ST. JOSEPH MEDICAL CENTER (O, 362 beds) 1401 St. Joseph Parkway, Houston, TX Zip 77002–8321; tel. 713/757–1000; Phillip D. Robinson, Chief Executive Officer
Web address: www.sjmetx.com

TRINITY MEDICAL CENTER (L, 149 beds) 4343 North Josey Lane, Carrollton, TX Zip 75010–4691; tel. 972/492–1010; Spencer Turner, Chief Executive Officer
Web address: www.trinitymedicalcenter.com

Owned, leased, sponsored:	7 hospitals	1012 beds
Contract-managed:	0 hospitals	0 beds
Totals:	7 hospitals	1012 beds

★5355: HOSPITAL SISTERS HEALTH SYSTEM (CC)
Springfield, IL Mailing Address: P.O. Box 19456, Zip 62794–9456; tel. 217/523–4747; Stephanie S. McCutcheon, President and Chief Executive Officer
(Moderately Centralized Health System)

ILLINOIS: SAINT ANTHONY'S HEALTH CENTER (S, 229 beds) 1 Saint Anthony's Way, Alton, IL Zip 62002–4579, Mailing Address: P.O. Box 340, Zip 62002–0340; tel. 618/465–2571; Mark F. Weber, FACHE, President
Web address: www.sahc.org

ST. ANTHONY'S MEMORIAL HOSPITAL (O, 146 beds) 503 North Maple Street, Effingham, IL Zip 62401–2099; tel. 217/342–2121; Daniel J. Woods, President and Chief Executive Officer
Web address: www.stanthonyshospital.org

ST. ELIZABETH'S HOSPITAL (O, 260 beds) 211 South Third Street, Belleville, IL Zip 62220–1998; tel. 618/234–2120; Kevin Shrake, Interim President and Chief Executive Officer
Web address: www.steliz.org

ST. FRANCIS HOSPITAL (O, 36 beds) 1215 Franciscan Drive, Litchfield, IL Zip 62056–1799, Mailing Address: P.O. Box 1215, Zip 62056–1215; tel. 217/324–2191; Daniel L. Perryman, President and Chief Executive Officer
Web address: www.stfrancis–litchfield.org

ST. JOHN'S HOSPITAL (O, 465 beds) 800 East Carpenter Street, Springfield, IL Zip 62769–0002; tel. 217/544–6464; Robert P. Ritz, Chief Executive Officer
Web address: www.st–johns.org

ST. JOSEPH'S HOSPITAL (O, 60 beds) 9515 Holy Cross Lane, Breese, IL Zip 62230–0099; tel. 618/526–4511; Lowell Jones, Interim Administrator
Web address: www.stjoebreese.com

ST. JOSEPH'S HOSPITAL (O, 55 beds) 1515 Main Street, Highland, IL Zip 62249–1656; tel. 618/654–7421; Claudio Fort, Executive Vice President and Administrator
Web address: www.stjosephshighland.com

ST. MARY'S HOSPITAL (O, 226 beds) 1800 East Lake Shore Drive, Decatur, IL Zip 62521–3883; tel. 217/464–2966; Kevin F. Kast, President and Chief Executive Officer
Web address: www.stmarys–hospital.com

ST. MARY'S HOSPITAL (O, 116 beds) 111 Spring Street, Streator, IL Zip 61364–3399; tel. 815/673–2311; Richard J. Carlson, Interim President and Chief Executive Officer
Web address: www.stmaryshospital.org

WISCONSIN: SACRED HEART HOSPITAL (O, 220 beds) 900 West Clairemont Avenue, Eau Claire, WI Zip 54701–6122; tel. 715/829–4121; Stephen F. Ronstrom, Executive Vice President and Administrator
Web address: www.sacredhearthospital–ec.org

ST. JOSEPH'S HOSPITAL (O, 102 beds) 2661 County Highway I, Chippewa Falls, WI Zip 54729–1498; tel. 715/723–1811; David B. Fish, Executive Vice President and Administrator
Web address: www.stjoeschipfalls.com

ST. MARY'S HOSPITAL MEDICAL CENTER (O, 94 beds) 1726 Shawano Avenue, Green Bay, WI Zip 54303–3282; tel. 920/498–4200; James G. Coller, FACHE, President and Chief Executive Officer
Web address: www.stmgb.org

ST. NICHOLAS HOSPITAL (O, 78 beds) 3100 Superior Avenue, Sheboygan, WI Zip 53081; tel. 920/459–8300; Mary T. Brasseaux, Chief Executive Officer
Web address: www.stnicholashospital.org

ST. VINCENT HOSPITAL (O, 255 beds) 835 South Van Buren Street, Green Bay, WI Zip 54307–3508, Mailing Address: P.O. Box 13508, Zip 54307–3508; tel. 920/433–0111; Thomas R. Bayer, Chief Operating Officer
Web address: www.stvgh.org

Owned, leased, sponsored:	14 hospitals	2342 beds
Contract-managed:	0 hospitals	0 beds
Totals:	14 hospitals	2342 beds

0347: HOWARD REGIONAL HEALTH SYSTEM (NP)
3500 South Lafountain Street, Kokomo, IN Zip 46902, Mailing Address: P.O. Box 9011, Zip 46904–9011; tel. 765/453–0702; James P. Alender, President and Chief Executive Officer
(Independent Hospital System)

INDIANA: HOWARD REGIONAL HEALTH SYSTEM (O, 150 beds) 3500 South Lafountain Street, Kokomo, IN Zip 46904–9011, Mailing Address: P.O. Box 9011, Zip 46904–9011; tel. 765/453–0702; James P. Alender, President and Chief Executive Officer
Web address: www.howardregional.org

For explanation of codes following names, see page B2.
★ Indicates Type III membership in the American Hospital Association.

HOWARD REGIONAL HEALTH SYSTEM WEST CAMPUS SPECIALTY HOSPITAL (O, 30 beds) 829 North Dixon Road, Kokomo, IN Zip 46901–7709; tel. 765/452–6700; Michelle L. Russell, Vice President and Administrator
Web address: www.howardregional.org

Owned, leased, sponsored:	2 hospitals	180 beds
Contract-managed:	0 hospitals	0 beds
Totals:	2 hospitals	180 beds

0201: IASIS HEALTHCARE (IO)
117 Seaboard Lane, Building E., Franklin, TN Zip 37067; tel. 615/844–2747; David R. White, Chairman and Chief Executive Officer
(Moderately Centralized Health System)

ARIZONA: ST. LUKE'S BEHAVIORAL HEALTH CENTER (O, 85 beds) 1800 East Van Buren, Phoenix, AZ Zip 85006–3742; tel. 602/251–8546; Gregory L. Jahn, RN, Chief Executive Officer
Web address: www.iasishealthcare.com

ST. LUKE'S MEDICAL CENTER (O, 225 beds) 1800 East Van Buren Street, Phoenix, AZ Zip 85006–3742; tel. 602/251–8100; Brent A. Cope, Chief Executive Officer
Web address: www.stlukesmedcenter.com

TEMPE ST. LUKE'S HOSPITAL (O, 110 beds) 1500 South Mill Avenue, Tempe, AZ Zip 85281–6699; tel. 480/784–5510; Bill R. Porter, Chief Executive Officer
Web address: www.tempestlukehospital.com

FLORIDA: MEMORIAL HOSPITAL OF TAMPA (O, 180 beds) 2901 Swann Avenue, Tampa, FL Zip 33609–4057; tel. 813/873–6400; John J. Mainieri, Chief Executive Officer
Web address: www.memorialhospitaltampa.com

PALMS OF PASADENA HOSPITAL (O, 307 beds) 1501 Pasadena Avenue South, Saint Petersburg, FL Zip 33707–3798; tel. 727/381–1000; James E. Purcell, III, Chief Executive Officer
Web address: www.palmspasadena.com

TOWN AND COUNTRY HOSPITAL (O, 200 beds) 6001 Webb Road, Tampa, FL Zip 33615–3291; tel. 813/888–7060; Michael J. Landry, Chief Executive Officer
Web address: www.townandcountryhospital.com

LOUISIANA: GLENWOOD REGIONAL MEDICAL CENTER (O, 231 beds) 503 McMillan Road, West Monroe, LA Zip 71291–5327, Mailing Address: P.O. Box 35805, Zip 71294–5805; tel. 318/329–4200; Ronald J. Elder, Chief Executive Officer
Web address: www.grmc.com

NEVADA: NORTH VISTA HOSPITAL (O, 198 beds) 1409 East Lake Mead Boulevard, North Las Vegas, NV Zip 89030–7197; tel. 702/649–7711; Anthony Marinello, Chief Executive Officer
Web address: www.northvistahospital.com

TEXAS: ODESSA REGIONAL MEDICAL CENTER (O, 161 beds) 520 East Sixth Street, Odessa, TX Zip 79761–4565, Mailing Address: P.O. Box 4859, Zip 79760–4859; tel. 432/582–8000; Matthew Roberts, Chief Executive Officer
Web address: www.odessaregionalmedicalcenter.com

SOUTHWEST GENERAL HOSPITAL (O, 215 beds) 7400 Barlite Boulevard, San Antonio, TX Zip 78224–1399; tel. 210/921–2000; Richard D. Gonzalez, Chief Executive Officer
Web address: www.swgeneralhospital.com

THE MEDICAL CENTER OF SOUTHEAST TEXAS (O, 224 beds) 2555 Jimmy Johnson Boulevard, Port Arthur, TX Zip 77640; tel. 409/724–7389; Michael J. Landry, Chief Executive Officer
Web address: www.medicalcentersetexas.com

UTAH: DAVIS HOSPITAL AND MEDICAL CENTER (O, 136 beds) 1600 West Antelope Drive, Layton, UT Zip 84041–1142; tel. 801/807–1000; Michael E. Jensen, President and Chief Executive Officer
Web address: www.davishospital.com

JORDAN VALLEY MEDICAL CENTER (O, 50 beds) 3580 West 9000 South, West Jordan, UT Zip 84088–8811; tel. 801/561–8888; Bryanie W. Swilley, Jr., Chief Executive Officer
Web address: www.mc.com

PIONEER VALLEY HOSPITAL (O, 101 beds) 3460 South Pioneer Parkway, West Valley City, UT Zip 84120–2648; tel. 801/964–3100; Bryanie W. Swilley, Jr., Chief Executive Officer
Web address: www.pioneervalleyhospital.com

SALT LAKE REGIONAL MEDICAL CENTER (O, 138 beds) 1050 East South Temple, Salt Lake City, UT Zip 84102–1599; tel. 801/350–4111; Jeff Frandsen, Chief Executive Officer
Web address: www.saltlakeregional.com

Owned, leased, sponsored:	15 hospitals	2561 beds
Contract-managed:	0 hospitals	0 beds
Totals:	15 hospitals	2561 beds

2025: INFIRMARY HEALTH SYSTEM (NP)
5 Mobile Infirmary Circle, Mobile, AL Zip 36607–3520; tel. 251/435–5500; E. Chandler Bramlett, Jr., Chief Executive Officer
(Independent Hospital System)

ALABAMA: INFIRMARY WEST AT KNOLLWOOD (O, 182 beds) 5600 Girby Road, Mobile, AL Zip 36693–3398; tel. 251/660–5120; Ormond Thompson, Administrator
Web address: www.southalabama.edu/usakph/index.html

MOBILE INFIRMARY MEDICAL CENTER (O, 704 beds) 5 Mobile Infirmary Drive North, Mobile, AL Zip 36607–3513, Mailing Address: P.O. Box 2144, Zip 36652–2144; tel. 251/435–2400; E. Chandler Bramlett, Jr., Chief Executive Officer
Web address: www.mobileinfirmary.org

NORTH BALDWIN INFIRMARY (L, 130 beds) 1815 Hand Avenue, Bay Minette, AL Zip 36507–4110, Mailing Address: P.O. Box 1409, Zip 36507–1409; tel. 251/937–5521; William J. McLaughlin, Administrator
Web address: www.mobileinfirmary.org

THOMAS HOSPITAL (L, 129 beds) 750 Morphy Avenue, Fairhope, AL Zip 36532–1812, Mailing Address: P.O. Drawer 929, Zip 36533–0929; tel. 251/928–2375; Philip L. Cusa, Administrator
Web address: www.thomashospital.com

Owned, leased, sponsored:	4 hospitals	1145 beds
Contract-managed:	0 hospitals	0 beds
Totals:	4 hospitals	1145 beds

★1305: INOVA HEALTH SYSTEM (NP)
8110 Gatehouse Road, Falls Church, VA Zip 22042; tel. 703/289–2069; J. Knox Singleton, President and Chief Executive Officer
(Centralized Health System)

VIRGINIA: INOVA ALEXANDRIA HOSPITAL (O, 334 beds) 4320 Seminary Road, Alexandria, VA Zip 22304–1594; tel. 703/504–3000; Christine Candio, Chief Executive Officer
Web address: www.inova.org

INOVA FAIR OAKS HOSPITAL (O, 196 beds) 3600 Joseph Siewick Drive, Fairfax, VA Zip 22033–1798; tel. 703/391–3600; John L. Fitzgerald, Chief Executive Officer
Web address: www.inova.org

INOVA FAIRFAX HOSPITAL (O, 927 beds) 3300 Gallows Road, Falls Church, VA Zip 22042–3300; tel. 703/776–4001; Reuven Pasternak, M.D., Chief Executive Officer
Web address: www.inova.org

INOVA LOUDOUN HOSPITAL (O, 155 beds) 44045 Riverside Parkway, Leesburg, VA Zip 20176–2799, Mailing Address: P.O. Box 6000, Zip 20176–6000; tel. 703/858–6000; Randall L. Kelley, Chief Executive Officer
Web address: www.loudounhospital.org

INOVA MOUNT VERNON HOSPITAL (O, 237 beds) 2501 Parker's Lane, Alexandria, VA Zip 22306; tel. 703/664–7000; Barbara J. Doyle, Senior Vice President and Chief Executive Officer
Web address: www.inova.org

Owned, leased, sponsored:	5 hospitals	1849 beds
Contract-managed:	0 hospitals	0 beds
Totals:	5 hospitals	1849 beds

For explanation of codes following names, see page B2.
★ Indicates Type III membership in the American Hospital Association.

Section B

0333: INTEGRATED HEALTHCARE (IO)
1301 North Tustin Avenue, Santa Ana, CA Zip 92705; tel. 714/953–3652; Larry B. Anderson, President
(Independent Hospital System)

CALIFORNIA: CHAPMAN MEDICAL CENTER (O, 114 beds) 2601 East Chapman Avenue, Orange, CA Zip 92869–3206; tel. 714/633–0011; Doug Norris, Chief Executive Officer
Web address: www.chapmanmedicalcenter.com

COASTAL COMMUNITIES HOSPITAL (O, 178 beds) 2701 South Bristol Street, Santa Ana, CA Zip 92704–6201; tel. 714/754–5454; Craig G. Myers, Chief Executive Officer
Web address: www.coastalcommhospital.com

WESTERN MEDICAL CENTER ANAHEIM (O, 181 beds) 1025 South Anaheim Boulevard, Anaheim, CA Zip 92805–5806; tel. 714/533–6220; Josh D. Luke, Ph.D., CHE, Chief Executive Officer
Web address: www.westernmedanaheim.com

WESTERN MEDICAL CENTER–SANTA ANA (O, 287 beds) 1001 North Tustin Avenue, Santa Ana, CA Zip 92705–3577; tel. 714/835–3555; Daniel Brothman, Chief Executive Officer
Web address: www.westernmedicalcenter.com

Owned, leased, sponsored:	4 hospitals	760 beds
Contract-managed:	0 hospitals	0 beds
Totals:	4 hospitals	760 beds

★0305: INTEGRIS HEALTH (NP)
3366 N.W. Expressway, Suite 800, Oklahoma City, OK Zip 73112–9756; tel. 405/949–6068; Stanley F. Hupfeld, President and Chief Executive Officer
(Moderately Centralized Health System)

OKLAHOMA: INTEGRIS BAPTIST MEDICAL CENTER (O, 570 beds) 3300 N.W. Expressway, Oklahoma City, OK Zip 73112–4481; tel. 405/949–3011; Chris Hammes, President
Web address: www.integris–health.com

INTEGRIS BAPTIST REGIONAL HEALTH CENTER (O, 99 beds) 200 Second Street S.W., Miami, OK Zip 74354–6830, Mailing Address: P.O. Box 1207, Zip 74355–1207; tel. 918/542–6611; Joel A. Hart, FACHE, President
Web address: www.integris–health.com

INTEGRIS BASS BAPTIST HEALTH CENTER (O, 151 beds) 600 South Monroe Street, Enid, OK Zip 73701–7211, Mailing Address: P.O. Box 3168, Zip 73702–3168; tel. 580/233–2300; Jeffrey S. Tarrant, FACHE, President
Web address: www.integris–health.com

INTEGRIS BASS PAVILION (O, 24 beds) 401 South Third, Enid, OK Zip 73701; tel. 580/249–4260; Jeffrey S. Tarrant, FACHE, President
Web address: www.integris–health.com/integris/en–us/locations/bass–enid

INTEGRIS BLACKWELL REGIONAL HOSPITAL (L, 34 beds) 710 South 13th Street, Blackwell, OK Zip 74631–3700; tel. 580/363–2311; Rex Van Meter, President
Web address: www.integris–health.com

INTEGRIS CANADIAN VALLEY REGIONAL HOSPITAL (O, 44 beds) 1201 Health Center Parkway, Yukon, OK Zip 73099; tel. 405/717–6800; James D. Moore, FACHE, President
Web address: www.integris–health.com

INTEGRIS CLINTON REGIONAL HOSPITAL (L, 49 beds) 100 North 30th Street, Clinton, OK Zip 73601–3117, Mailing Address: P.O. Box 1569, Zip 73601–1569; tel. 580/323–2363; Jerry Jones, President
Web address: www.integris–health.com

INTEGRIS GROVE GENERAL HOSPITAL (O, 50 beds) 1310 South Main Street, Grove, OK Zip 74344–1310; tel. 918/786–2243; Greg Martin, President
Web address: www.integris–health.com

INTEGRIS MARSHALL COUNTY MEDICAL CENTER (L, 21 beds) 1 Hospital Drive, Madill, OK Zip 73446, Mailing Address: P.O. Box 827, Zip 73446–0827; tel. 580/795–3384; Karen Reynolds, Administrator
Web address: www.integris–health.com

INTEGRIS MAYES COUNTY MEDICAL CENTER (L, 39 beds) 111 North Bailey Street, Pryor, OK Zip 74361–4211, Mailing Address: P.O. Box 278, Zip 74362–0278; tel. 918/825–1600; W. Charles Jordan, President
Web address: www.integris–health.com

INTEGRIS SEMINOLE MEDICAL CENTER (O, 32 beds) 2401 Wrangler Boulevard, Seminole, OK Zip 74868–1917; tel. 405/303–4000; C. David Hill, President
Web address: www.seminolemedicalcenter.com

INTEGRIS SOUTHWEST MEDICAL CENTER (O, 358 beds) 4401 South Western, Oklahoma City, OK Zip 73109–3441; tel. 405/636–7000; Patricia Dorris, President
Web address: www.integris–health.com

Owned, leased, sponsored:	12 hospitals	1471 beds
Contract-managed:	0 hospitals	0 beds
Totals:	12 hospitals	1471 beds

★1815: INTERMOUNTAIN HEALTHCARE, INC. (NP)
36 South State Street, 22nd Floor, Salt Lake City, UT Zip 84111–1453; tel. 801/442–2000; William H. Nelson, President and Chief Executive Officer
(Decentralized Health System)

IDAHO: CASSIA REGIONAL MEDICAL CENTER (O, 25 beds) 1501 Hiland Avenue, Burley, ID Zip 83318–2648; tel. 208/678–4444; Kenneth Harman, Administrator
Web address: www.ihc.com

UTAH: ALTA VIEW HOSPITAL (O, 72 beds) 9660 South 1300 East, Sandy, UT Zip 84094–3793; tel. 801/501–2600; Becky Kapp, Administrator
Web address: www.ihc.com

AMERICAN FORK HOSPITAL (O, 93 beds) 170 North 1100 East, American Fork, UT Zip 84003–2096; tel. 801/855–3300; Michael R. Olson, Administrator
Web address: www.intermountainhealthcare.org

BEAR RIVER VALLEY HOSPITAL (O, 58 beds) 440 West 600 North, Tremonton, UT Zip 84337–2497; tel. 435/257–7441; Eric Packer, Administrator
Web address: www.ihc.com

DELTA COMMUNITY MEDICAL CENTER (O, 20 beds) 126 South White Sage Avenue, Delta, UT Zip 84624–8928; tel. 435/864–5591; James E. Beckstrand, Administrator
Web address: www.ihc.com

DIXIE REGIONAL MEDICAL CENTER (O, 245 beds) 544 South 400 East, Saint George, UT Zip 84790; tel. 435/251–1000; Terri Kane, Administrator
Web address: www.intermountainhealthcare.org

FILLMORE COMMUNITY MEDICAL CENTER (O, 20 beds) 674 South Highway 99, Fillmore, UT Zip 84631–9701; tel. 435/743–5591; James E. Beckstrand, Administrator
Web address: www.ihc.com

GARFIELD MEMORIAL HOSPITAL AND CLINICS (C, 41 beds) 200 North 400 East, Panguitch, UT Zip 84759, Mailing Address: P.O. Box 389, Zip 84759–0389; tel. 435/676–8811; Alberto Vasquez, Administrator
Web address: www.ihc.com/xp/ihc/garfield

HEBER VALLEY MEDICAL CENTER (O, 19 beds) 1485 South Highway 40, Heber City, UT Zip 84032–3522; tel. 435/654–2500; Ezra Segura, Administrator
Web address: www.ihc.com

INTERMOUNTAIN MEDICAL CENTER (O, 173 beds) 5121 South Cottonwood Street, Murray, UT Zip 84157; tel. 801/507–7000; David Grauer, Administrator
Web address: www.ihc.com

LDS HOSPITAL (O, 452 beds) Eighth Avenue and C Street, Salt Lake City, UT Zip 84143–0001; tel. 801/408–1100; Mikelle D. Moore, CHE, Administrator
Web address: www.ihc.com/xp/ihc/lds

LOGAN REGIONAL HOSPITAL (O, 139 beds) 1400 North 500 East, Logan, UT Zip 84341–2499; tel. 435/716–1000; Robert C. Cash, CHE, Administrator
Web address: www.ihc.com

MCKAY–DEE HOSPITAL CENTER (O, 299 beds) 4401 Harrison Boulevard, Ogden, UT Zip 84403; tel. 801/387–2800; Timothy T. Pehrson, Chief Executive Officer
Web address: www.mckay–dee.org

OREM COMMUNITY HOSPITAL (O, 18 beds) 331 North 400 West, Orem, UT Zip 84057–1999; tel. 801/224–4080; Ronald L. Liston, Administrator
Web address: www.intermountainhealthcare.org

PRIMARY CHILDREN'S MEDICAL CENTER (O, 252 beds) 100 North Medical Drive, Salt Lake City, UT Zip 84113–1100; tel. 801/588–2000; Joseph Mott, Administrator and Chief Executive Officer
Web address: www.ihc.com

For explanation of codes following names, see page B2.
★ Indicates Type III membership in the American Hospital Association.

SANPETE VALLEY HOSPITAL (O, 18 beds) 1100 South Medical Drive, Mount Pleasant, UT Zip 84647–2222; tel. 435/462–2441; Bradley Howell, Administrator
Web address: www.ihc.com

SEVIER VALLEY MEDICAL CENTER (O, 27 beds) 1000 North Main Street, Richfield, UT Zip 84701–1843; tel. 435/896–8271; Gary E. Beck, Administrator
Web address: www.intermountain.com

UTAH VALLEY REGIONAL MEDICAL CENTER (O, 351 beds) 1034 North 500 West, Provo, UT Zip 84604–3337; tel. 801/373–7850; Steven Smoot, Administrator
Web address: www.intermountainmail.org

VALLEY VIEW MEDICAL CENTER (O, 46 beds) 1303 North Main Street, Cedar City, UT Zip 84720–3462; tel. 435/868–5000; Jason Wilson, Administrator
Web address: www.ihc.com

Owned, leased, sponsored:	18 hospitals	2327 beds
Contract-managed:	1 hospital	41 beds
Totals:	19 hospitals	2368 beds

★0061: IOWA HEALTH SYSTEM (NP)
1200 Pleasant Street, Des Moines, IA Zip 50309–1453; tel. 515/241–6161; William B. Leaver, President and Chief Executive Officer
(Decentralized Health System)

ILLINOIS: TRINITY MEDICAL CENTER–WEST (O, 314 beds) 2701 17th Street, Rock Island, IL Zip 61201–5393; tel. 309/779–5000; Andrea Y. Coleman, President and Chief Executive Officer
Web address: www.trinityqc.com

IOWA: ALLEN MEMORIAL HOSPITAL (O, 225 beds) 1825 Logan Avenue, Waterloo, IA Zip 50703–1916; tel. 319/235–3941; Richard A. Seidler, FACHE, Chief Executive Officer
Web address: www.allenhospital.org

BUENA VISTA REGIONAL MEDICAL CENTER (C, 35 beds) 1525 West Fifth Street, Storm Lake, IA Zip 50588–0309, Mailing Address: P.O. Box 309, Zip 50588–0309; tel. 712/732–4030; Todd Hudspeth, Chief Executive Officer
Web address: www.bvrmc.org

CLARKE COUNTY HOSPITAL (C, 25 beds) 800 South Fillmore Street, Osceola, IA Zip 50213–1619; tel. 641/342–2184; Brian Evans, Chief Executive Officer
Web address: www.clarkehosp.org

COMMUNITY MEMORIAL HOSPITAL (C, 25 beds) 909 West First Street, Sumner, IA Zip 50674–1203, Mailing Address: P.O. Box 148, Zip 50674–0148; tel. 563/578–3275; Mary Wells, Administrator

DALLAS COUNTY HOSPITAL (C, 25 beds) 610 10th Street, Perry, IA Zip 50220–2221; tel. 515/465–3547; Laurie A. Conner, Chief Executive Officer
Web address: www.dallascohospital.org

FINLEY HOSPITAL (O, 137 beds) 350 North Grandview Avenue, Dubuque, IA Zip 52001–6392; tel. 563/582–1881; John E. Knox, FACHE, President and Chief Executive Officer
Web address: www.finleyhospital.org

GREATER REGIONAL MEDICAL CENTER (C, 34 beds) 1700 West Townline, Creston, IA Zip 50801–1099; tel. 641/782–7091; Monte Neitzel, Administrator and Chief Executive Officer
Web address: www.greaterregional.org

GREENE COUNTY MEDICAL CENTER (C, 97 beds) 1000 West Lincolnway, Jefferson, IA Zip 50129–1697; tel. 515/386–2114; Karen L. Bossard, FACHE, Administrator and Chief Executive Officer
Web address: www.gcmchealth.com

GRUNDY COUNTY MEMORIAL HOSPITAL (C, 80 beds) 201 East J Avenue, Grundy Center, IA Zip 50638–2096; tel. 319/824–5421; Pamela K. Delagardelle, Chief Executive Officer
Web address: www.grundyhospital.com

GUTHRIE COUNTY HOSPITAL (C, 25 beds) 710 North 12th Street, Guthrie Center, IA Zip 50115–1544; tel. 641/332–2201; Gerald D. Neal, Chief Executive Officer and Administrator
Web address: www.gcho.org

GUTTENBERG MUNICIPAL HOSPITAL (C, 23 beds) 200 Main Street, Guttenberg, IA Zip 52052–0550, Mailing Address: P.O. Box 550, Zip 52052–0550; tel. 563/252–1121; Kimberley A. Gau, Chief Executive Officer
Web address: www.guttenberghospital.org

HUMBOLDT COUNTY MEMORIAL HOSPITAL (C, 49 beds) 1000 North 15th Street, Humboldt, IA Zip 50548–1008; tel. 515/332–4200; Steven Colerick, Chief Executive Officer
Web address: www.humboldthospital.org

IOWA LUTHERAN HOSPITAL (O, 219 beds) 700 East University Avenue, Des Moines, IA Zip 50316–2392; tel. 515/263–5612; Eric T. Crowell, President and Chief Executive Officer
Web address: www.iowahealth.org

IOWA METHODIST MEDICAL CENTER (O, 444 beds) 1200 Pleasant Street, Des Moines, IA Zip 50309–9976; tel. 515/241–6212; Eric T. Crowell, President and Chief Executive Officer
Web address: www.iowahealth.org

JACKSON COUNTY REGIONAL HEALTH CENTER (C, 43 beds) 700 West Grove Street, Maquoketa, IA Zip 52060–0910; tel. 563/652–2474; Curt Coleman, CHE, FACHE, Chief Executive Officer
Web address: www.jcrhc.org

JONES REGIONAL MEDICAL CENTER (O, 25 beds) 104 Broadway Place, Anamosa, IA Zip 52205–1100; tel. 319/462–6131; Sean J. Williams, Chief Executive Officer
Web address: www.jonesregional.org

LORING HOSPITAL (C, 50 beds) 211 Highland Avenue, Sac City, IA Zip 50583–0217; tel. 712/662–7105; Michael S. Ketcham, President and Chief Executive Officer
Web address: www.loringhospital.org

POCAHONTAS COMMUNITY HOSPITAL (C, 20 beds) 606 N.W. Seventh, Pocahontas, IA Zip 50574–1099; tel. 712/335–3501; James D. Roetman, President and Chief Executive Officer
Web address: www.pocahontashospital.org

ST. LUKE'S HOSPITAL (O, 390 beds) 1026 A Avenue N.E., Cedar Rapids, IA Zip 52402–3026, Mailing Address: P.O. Box 3026, Zip 52406–3026; tel. 319/369–7211; Theodore E. Townsend, President and Chief Executive Officer
Web address: www.crstlukes.org

ST. LUKE'S REGIONAL MEDICAL CENTER (O, 146 beds) 2720 Stone Park Boulevard, Sioux City, IA Zip 51104–2000; tel. 712/279–3500; Peter W. Thoreen, President and Chief Executive Officer
Web address: www.stlukes.org

TRINITY AT TERRACE PARK (O, 69 beds) 4500 Utica Ridge Road, Bettendorf, IA Zip 52722–1626; tel. 563/742–5000; Andrea Y. Coleman, President and Chief Executive Officer
Web address: www.trinityqc.com

TRINITY REGIONAL MEDICAL CENTER (O, 133 beds) 802 Kenyon Road, Fort Dodge, IA Zip 50501–5795; tel. 515/573–3101; Tom Tibbitts, President
Web address: www.trmc.org

Owned, leased, sponsored:	10 hospitals	2102 beds
Contract-managed:	13 hospitals	531 beds
Totals:	23 hospitals	2633 beds

7775: JEFFERSON HEALTH SYSTEM (NP)
259 Radnor–Chester Road, Suite 290, Radnor, PA Zip 19087–5288; tel. 610/225–6200; Joseph T. Sebastianelli, President and Chief Executive Officer
(Centralized Health System)

For explanation of codes following names, see page B2.
★ Indicates Type III membership in the American Hospital Association.

Section B

PENNSYLVANIA: BRYN MAWR HOSPITAL (O, 311 beds) 130 South Bryn Mawr Avenue, Bryn Mawr, PA Zip 19010–3160; tel. 610/526–3000; Andrea F. Gilbert, CHE, President
Web address: www.brynmawrhospital.org

BRYN MAWR REHABILITATION HOSPITAL (O, 148 beds) 414 Paoli Pike, Malvern, PA Zip 19355–3300, Mailing Address: P.O. Box 3007, Zip 19355–3300; tel. 610/251–5400; Donna Phillips, President
Web address: www.mainlinehealth.org

FRANKFORD HOSPITAL OF THE CITY OF PHILADELPHIA (O, 486 beds) Knights and Red Lion Roads, Philadelphia, PA Zip 19114–4208; tel. 215/612–4000; Roy A. Powell, President
Web address: www.frankfordhospitals.org

LANKENAU HOSPITAL (O, 331 beds) 100 Lancaster Avenue West, Wynnewood, PA Zip 19096–3411; tel. 610/645–2000; Elaine Thompson, Ph.D., President
Web address: www.mainlinehealth.org

MAGEE REHABILITATION HOSPITAL (O, 96 beds) 1513 Race Street, Philadelphia, PA Zip 19102–1177; tel. 215/587–3000; Jack A. Carroll, Ph.D., President and Chief Executive Officer
Web address: www.mageerehab.org

PAOLI HOSPITAL (O, 157 beds) 255 West Lancaster Avenue, Paoli, PA Zip 19301–1792; tel. 610/648–1000; Barbara J. Tachovsky, President
Web address: www.mainlinehealth.org

THOMAS JEFFERSON UNIVERSITY HOSPITAL (O, 933 beds) 111 South 11th Street, Philadelphia, PA Zip 19107–5096; tel. 215/955–6000; Thomas J. Lewis, CHE, President and Chief Executive Officer
Web address: www.jeffersonhospital.org

Owned, leased, sponsored:	7 hospitals	2462 beds
Contract-managed:	0 hospitals	0 beds
Totals:	7 hospitals	2462 beds

★0052: JEWISH HOSPITAL & ST. MARY'S HEALTHCARE (NP)

200 Abraham Flexner Way, Louisville, KY Zip 40202–1886; tel. 502/587–4011; Robert L. Shircliff, President and Chief Executive Officer
(Moderately Centralized Health System)

INDIANA: CLARK MEMORIAL HOSPITAL (C, 241 beds) 1220 Missouri Avenue, Jeffersonville, IN Zip 47130–3743, Mailing Address: P.O. Box 69, Zip 47131–0069; tel. 812/282–6631; Martin Padgett, President and Chief Executive Officer
Web address: www.clarkmemorial.org

SCOTT MEMORIAL HOSPITAL (C, 25 beds) 1415 North Gardner Street, Scottsburg, IN Zip 47170–0430, Mailing Address: Box 430, Zip 47170–0430; tel. 812/752–3456; Clifford D. Nay, Executive Director
Web address: www.scottmemorial.com

SOUTHERN INDIANA REHABILITATION HOSPITAL (O, 60 beds) 3104 Blackiston Boulevard, New Albany, IN Zip 47150–9579; tel. 812/941–8300; Randy L. Napier, President and Chief Executive Officer
Web address: www.sirh.org

KENTUCKY: FRAZIER REHAB INSTITUTE (O, 135 beds) 220 Abraham Flexner Way, Louisville, KY Zip 40202–1887; tel. 502/582–7400; Joanne Berryman, Senior Vice President
Web address: www.frazierrehab.org

JEWISH HOSPITAL (O, 442 beds) 200 Abraham Flexner Way, Louisville, KY Zip 40202–1886; tel. 502/587–4011; Martin J. Bonick, President and Chief Executive Officer
Web address: www.jewishhospital.org

JEWISH HOSPITAL–SHELBYVILLE (O, 76 beds) 727 Hospital Drive, Shelbyville, KY Zip 40065–1699; tel. 502/647–4000; Michael L. Collins, President and Chief Executive Officer
Web address: www.jhsmh.org

OUR LADY OF PEACE (O, 206 beds) 2020 Newburg Road, Louisville, KY Zip 40205–1879; tel. 502/451–3330; JoAnne D. Maamry, Chief Executive Officer
Web address: www.jhsmh.org

STS. MARY & ELIZABETH HOSPITAL (O, 236 beds) 1850 Bluegrass Avenue, Louisville, KY Zip 40215–1199; tel. 502/361–6000; Thomas Gessel, Chief Executive Officer
Web address: www.jhsmh.org

TAYLOR REGIONAL HOSPITAL (C, 90 beds) 1700 Old Lebanon Road, Campbellsville, KY Zip 42718–9600; tel. 270/465–3561; Jane Wheatley, Chief Executive Officer
Web address: www.trhosp.org

Owned, leased, sponsored:	6 hospitals	1155 beds
Contract-managed:	3 hospitals	356 beds
Totals:	9 hospitals	1511 beds

★0218: JOHN C. LINCOLN HEALTH NETWORK (NP)

250 East Dunlap Avenue, Phoenix, AZ Zip 85020–2446; tel. 602/943–2381; Dan C. Coleman, President and Chief Executive Officer
(Centralized Health System)

ARIZONA: JOHN C. LINCOLN DEER VALLEY HOSPITAL (O, 174 beds) 19829 North 27th Avenue, Phoenix, AZ Zip 85027–4002; tel. 623/879–6100; Tim Tracy, Chief Executive Officer
Web address: www.jcl.com

JOHN C. LINCOLN NORTH MOUNTAIN HOSPITAL (O, 266 beds) 250 East Dunlap Avenue, Phoenix, AZ Zip 85020–2446; tel. 602/943–2381; Bruce E. Pearson, Chief Executive Officer
Web address: www.jcl.com

Owned, leased, sponsored:	2 hospitals	440 beds
Contract-managed:	0 hospitals	0 beds
Totals:	2 hospitals	440 beds

★0324: JOHN MUIR HEALTH (NP)

1400 Treat Boulevard, Walnut Creek, CA Zip 94597–2142; tel. 925/941–2100; J. Kendall Anderson, President and Chief Executive Officer
(Centralized Health System)

CALIFORNIA: JOHN MUIR BEHAVIORAL HEALTH (O, 70 beds) 2740 Grant Street, Concord, CA Zip 94520; tel. 925/674–4100; Elizabeth Stallings, Chief Operating Officer
Web address: www.johnmuirhealth.com

JOHN MUIR MEDICAL CENTER, CONCORD (O, 202 beds) 2540 East Street, Concord, CA Zip 94520; tel. 925/682–8200; Thomas M. Harlan, President and Chief Administrative Officer
Web address: www.johnmuirhealth.com

JOHN MUIR MEDICAL CENTER, WALNUT CREEK (O, 324 beds) 1601 Ygnacio Valley Road, Walnut Creek, CA Zip 94598–3194; tel. 925/939–3000; Jane Willemsen, Chief Administrative Officer
Web address: www.jmmdhs.com/index.php/jmmdhs_jmmc.html

Owned, leased, sponsored:	3 hospitals	596 beds
Contract-managed:	0 hospitals	0 beds
Totals:	3 hospitals	596 beds

★1015: JOHNS HOPKINS HEALTH SYSTEM (NP)

733 North Broadway, BRB 104, Baltimore, MD Zip 21205; tel. 410/955–5000; Ronald R. Peterson, President
(Centralized Physician/Insurance Health System)

MARYLAND: HOWARD COUNTY GENERAL HOSPITAL (O, 203 beds) 5755 Cedar Lane, Columbia, MD Zip 21044–2999; tel. 410/740–7890; Victor A. Broccolino, President and Chief Executive Officer
Web address: www.hcgh.org

JOHNS HOPKINS BAYVIEW MEDICAL CENTER (O, 560 beds) 4940 Eastern Avenue, Baltimore, MD Zip 21224–2780; tel. 410/550–0100; Gregory F. Schaffer, President
Web address: www.hopkinsbayview.org

JOHNS HOPKINS HOSPITAL (O, 920 beds) 600 North Wolfe Street, Baltimore, MD Zip 21287–2182; tel. 410/955–5000; Ronald R. Peterson, President
Web address: www.hopkinsmedicine.org

Owned, leased, sponsored:	3 hospitals	1683 beds
Contract-managed:	0 hospitals	0 beds
Totals:	3 hospitals	1683 beds

For explanation of codes following names, see page B2.
★ Indicates Type III membership in the American Hospital Association.

★2105: KAISER FOUNDATION HOSPITALS (NP)
One Kaiser Plaza, Oakland, CA Zip 94612–3600; tel. 510/271–5910; George C. Halvorson, M.D., Chairman and Chief Executive Officer
(Decentralized Health System)

CALIFORNIA: KAISER FOUNDATION HOSPITAL (O, 264 beds) 2200 O'Farrell Street, San Francisco, CA Zip 94115–3358; tel. 415/833–2000; Christine Robisch, Senior Vice President and Service Area Manager
Web address: www.kaiserpermanente.org

KAISER FOUNDATION HOSPITAL (O, 117 beds) 401 Bicentennial Way, Santa Rosa, CA Zip 95403–2192; tel. 707/571–4000; Judy Coffey, Senior Vice President and Service Area Manager
Web address: www.kaiserpermanente.org

KAISER FOUNDATION HOSPITAL (O, 455 beds) 4867 Sunset Boulevard, Los Angeles, CA Zip 90027–5969; tel. 323/783–4011; Mark E. Costa, Executive Director
Web address: www.kaiserpermanente.org

KAISER FOUNDATION HOSPITAL (O, 341 beds) 280 West MacArthur Boulevard, Oakland, CA Zip 94611–5693; tel. 510/752–1000; Bettie L. Coles, RN, Senior Vice President and Area Manager
Web address: www.kaiserpermanente.org

KAISER FOUNDATION HOSPITAL (O, 257 beds) 1425 South Main Street, Walnut Creek, CA Zip 94596–5300; tel. 925/295–4000; Sandra H. Small, RN, Senior Vice President and Service Area Manager
Web address: www.kaiserpermanente.org

KAISER FOUNDATION HOSPITAL (O, 199 beds) 25825 South Vermont Avenue, Harbor City, CA Zip 90710–3599; tel. 310/325–5111; Jan F. Boyd, Executive Director
Web address: www.kaiserpermanente.org

KAISER FOUNDATION HOSPITAL (O, 168 beds) 1150 Veterans Boulevard, Redwood City, CA Zip 94063–2037; tel. 650/299–2000; Linda Jensen, Senior Vice President and Area Manager
Web address: www.kaiserpermanente.org

KAISER FOUNDATION HOSPITAL (O, 410 beds) 2025 Morse Avenue, Sacramento, CA Zip 95825–2115; tel. 916/973–5000; Deborah Aspling, Senior Vice President and Service Area Manager
Web address: www.kp.org

KAISER FOUNDATION HOSPITAL (O, 161 beds) 6600 Bruceville Road, Sacramento, CA Zip 95823–4671; tel. 916/688–2430; Max Villalobos, Area Manager and Chief Operating Officer
Web address: www.kp.org

KAISER FOUNDATION HOSPITAL (O, 107 beds) 99 Montecillo Road, San Rafael, CA Zip 94903–3308; tel. 415/444–2000; Judy Coffey, Senior Vice President and Service Area Manager
Web address: www.kaiserpermanente.org

KAISER FOUNDATION HOSPITAL (O, 286 beds) 700 Lawrence Expressway, Santa Clara, CA Zip 75051–5173; tel. 408/236–6400; Mary Ann Barnes, Vice President and Service Area Manager
Web address: www.kaiserpermanente.org

KAISER FOUNDATION HOSPITAL (O, 105 beds) 1200 El Camino Real, South San Francisco, CA Zip 94080–3299; tel. 650/742–2000; Linda Jensen, Senior Vice President and Service Area Manager
Web address: www.kaiserpermanente.org

KAISER FOUNDATION HOSPITAL (O, 205 beds) 13652 Cantara Street, Panorama City, CA Zip 91402–5497; tel. 818/375–2000; Dennis C. Benton, Executive Director
Web address: www.kaiserpermanente.org

KAISER FOUNDATION HOSPITAL (O, 218 beds) 5601 DeSoto Avenue, Woodland Hills, CA Zip 91365–6701; tel. 818/719–3800; Cathy A. Casas, Executive Director
Web address: www.kaiserpermanente.org

KAISER FOUNDATION HOSPITAL – FONTANA (O, 379 beds) 9961 Sierra Avenue, Fontana, CA Zip 92335–6720; tel. 909/427–5000; Greg Christian, Executive Director
Web address: www.kaiserpermanente.org

KAISER FOUNDATION HOSPITAL – FRESNO (O, 169 beds) 7300 North Fresno Street, Fresno, CA Zip 93720–2941; tel. 559/448–4500; Susan A. Ryan, Senior Vice President and Service Area Manager
Web address: www.kaiserpermanente.org

KAISER FOUNDATION HOSPITAL – HAYWARD (O, 208 beds) 27400 Hesperian Boulevard, Hayward, CA Zip 94545–4235; tel. 510/784–4000; Colleen McKeown, Senior Vice President and Service Area Manager
Web address: www.kaiserpermanente.org

KAISER FOUNDATION HOSPITAL – MANTECA (O, 99 beds) 1777 West Yosemite Avenue, Manteca, CA Zip 95337–5187; tel. 209/825–3500; Corwin Harper, Senior Vice President and Service Area Manager
Web address: www.kaiserpermanente.org

KAISER FOUNDATION HOSPITAL – ORANGE COUNTY (O, 176 beds) 441 North Lakeview Avenue, Anaheim, CA Zip 92807–3089; tel. 714/279–4000; Julie K. Miller–Phipps, Senior Vice President and Executive Director
Web address: www.kp.org

KAISER FOUNDATION HOSPITAL – SAN DIEGO (O, 392 beds) 4647 Zion Avenue, San Diego, CA Zip 92120–2507; tel. 619/528–5000; Nathaniel L. Oubre, Jr., Senior Vice President and Executive Director
Web address: www.kaiserpermanente.org

KAISER FOUNDATION HOSPITAL – SAN JOSE MEDICAL CENTER (O, 228 beds) 250 Hospital Parkway, San Jose, CA Zip 95119–1199; tel. 408/972–7000; Terry L. Austen, Senior Vice President and Area Manager
Web address: www.kaiserpermanente.org

KAISER FOUNDATION HOSPITAL AND REHABILITATION CENTER (O, 270 beds) 975 Sereno Drive, Vallejo, CA Zip 94589–2441; tel. 707/651–1000; Steven Stricker, M.D., Administrator and Chief Executive Officer
Web address: www.kaiserpermanente.org

KAISER FOUNDATION HOSPITAL–BALDWIN PARK (O, 222 beds) 1011 Baldwin Park Boulevard, Baldwin Park, CA Zip 91706–5806; tel. 626/851–1011; Margaret H. Pierce, Executive Director
Web address: www.kp.org

KAISER FOUNDATION HOSPITAL–BELLFLOWER (O, 218 beds) 9400 East Rosecrans Avenue, Bellflower, CA Zip 90706–2246; tel. 562/461–3000; Jane Finley, Senior Vice President and Executive Director
Web address: www.kaiserpermanente.org

KAISER FOUNDATION HOSPITAL–RIVERSIDE (O, 215 beds) 10800 Magnolia Avenue, Riverside, CA Zip 92505–3000; tel. 951/353–2000; Vita M. Willett, Executive Director
Web address: www.kaiserpermanente.org

KAISER FOUNDATION HOSPITAL–WEST LOS ANGELES (O, 172 beds) 6041 Cadillac Avenue, Los Angeles, CA Zip 90034–1702; tel. 323/857–2201; Gloria Blackburn, Executive Director
Web address: www.kaiserpermanente.org

HAWAII: KAISER PERMANENTE MEDICAL CENTER (O, 217 beds) 3288 Moanalua Road, Honolulu, HI Zip 96819–1469; tel. 808/432–0000; Susan R. Murray, Regional Administrator
Web address: www.kaiserpermanente.org

OREGON: KAISER SUNNYSIDE MEDICAL CENTER (O, 233 beds) 10180 S.E. Sunnyside Road, Clackamas, OR Zip 97015–9303; tel. 503/652–2880; William Butcher, Administrator and Chief Executive Officer
Web address: www.kaiserpermanente.org

Owned, leased, sponsored:	28 hospitals	6491 beds
Contract–managed:	0 hospitals	0 beds
Totals:	28 hospitals	6491 beds

★0258: KETTERING HEALTH NETWORK (NP)
3965 Southern Boulevard, Dayton, OH Zip 45429–1221; tel. 937/395–8150; Francisco J. Perez, FACHE, Network Chief Executive Officer
(Centralized Health System)

OHIO: CHARLES F. KETTERING MEMORIAL HOSPITAL (O, 507 beds) 3535 Southern Boulevard, Kettering, OH Zip 45429; tel. 937/298–4331; Fred M. Manchur, President
Web address: www.kmcnetwork.org

GRANDVIEW HOSPITAL AND MEDICAL CENTER (O, 318 beds) 405 Grand Avenue, Dayton, OH Zip 45405–4796; tel. 937/226–3200; Roy G. Chew, Ph.D., President
Web address: www.kmcnetwork.org

GREENE MEMORIAL HOSPITAL (O, 204 beds) 1141 North Monroe Drive, Xenia, OH Zip 45385–1600; tel. 937/352–2000; Michael R. Stephens, President
Web address: www.greenehealth.org

Section B

For explanation of codes following names, see page B2.
★ Indicates Type III membership in the American Hospital Association.

KETTERING MEDICAL CENTER–SYCAMORE (O, 136 beds) 2150 Leiter Road, Miamisburg, OH Zip 45342; tel. 937/866–0551; Richard Haas, Senior Executive Officer
Web address: www.kmcnetwork.org

Owned, leased, sponsored:	4 hospitals	1165 beds
Contract-managed:	0 hospitals	0 beds
Totals:	4 hospitals	1165 beds

0026: KINDRED HEALTHCARE (IO)
680 South Fourth Street, Louisville, KY Zip 40202–2412; tel. 502/596–7300; Paul J. Diaz, President and Chief Executive Officer
(Independent Hospital System)

ARIZONA: KINDRED HOSPITAL – TUCSON (O, 51 beds) 355 North Wilmot Road, Tucson, AZ Zip 85711–2635; tel. 520/584–4500; Heidi Miller, Chief Executive Officer
Web address: www.kindredhealthcare.com

KINDRED HOSPITAL ARIZONA – PHOENIX (O, 58 beds) 40 East Indianola Avenue, Phoenix, AZ Zip 85012–2059; tel. 602/280–7000; Scott Floden, Chief Executive Officer
Web address: www.kindredhealthcare.com

KINDRED HOSPITAL ARIZONA–SCOTTSDALE (O, 50 beds) 11250 North 92nd Street, Scottsdale, AZ Zip 85260; tel. 480/391–4040; Scott Floden, Chief Executive Officer
Web address: www.kindredhealthcare.com

CALIFORNIA: KINDRED HOSPITAL SAN GABRIEL VALLEY (O, 76 beds) 845 North Lark Ellen Avenue, West Covina, CA Zip 91791–1069; tel. 626/339–5451; Norman J. Andrews, Administrator
Web address: www.kindredhealthcare.com

KINDRED HOSPITAL SANTA ANA (O, 54 beds) 1901 North College Avenue, Santa Ana, CA Zip 92706–2334; tel. 714/564–7800; Diana C. Hanyak, Administrator
Web address: www.kindredhealthcare.com

KINDRED HOSPITAL–BREA (O, 48 beds) 875 North Brea Boulevard, Brea, CA Zip 92821–2699; tel. 714/529–6842; Kathleen Smith, Administrator
Web address: www.kindredhealthcare.com

KINDRED HOSPITAL–LOS ANGELES (O, 81 beds) 5525 West Slauson Avenue, Los Angeles, CA Zip 90056–1067; tel. 310/642–0325; Trude Williams, RN, Administrator
Web address: www.kindredhealthcare.com

KINDRED HOSPITAL–ONTARIO (O, 91 beds) 550 North Monterey Avenue, Ontario, CA Zip 91764–3399; tel. 909/391–0333; Peter J. Adamo, Chief Executive Officer
Web address: www.kindredhealthcare.com

KINDRED HOSPITAL–SACRAMENTO (O, 31 beds) 223 Fargo Way, Folsom, CA Zip 95630–2961; tel. 916/351–9151; Virginia Matthews, Chief Executive Officer
Web address: www.kindredhealthcare.com

KINDRED HOSPITAL–SAN DIEGO (O, 70 beds) 1940 El Cajon Boulevard, San Diego, CA Zip 92104–1096; tel. 619/543–4500; Natalie Germuska, Chief Executive Officer
Web address: www.kindredsandiego.com

KINDRED HOSPITAL–SAN FRANCISCO BAY AREA (O, 80 beds) 2800 Benedict Drive, San Leandro, CA Zip 94577–6840; tel. 510/357–8300; Michael P. Lawson, FACHE, Chief Executive Officer
Web address: www.kindredhospitalsfba.com

KINDRED HOSPITAL–WESTMINSTER (O, 99 beds) 200 Hospital Circle, Westminster, CA Zip 92683–3910; tel. 714/893–4541; Adam Darvish, M.P.H., Executive Director
Web address: www.kindredhealthcare.com

COLORADO: KINDRED HOSPITAL–DENVER (O, 55 beds) 1920 High Street, Denver, CO Zip 80218–1213; tel. 303/320–5871; April Myers, Chief Executive Officer
Web address: www.kh–denver.com

FLORIDA: KINDRED HOSPITAL – CENTRAL TAMPA (O, 73 beds) 4801 North Howard Avenue, Tampa, FL Zip 33603–1484; tel. 813/874–7575; Brian L. Pugh, Interim Chief Executive Officer
Web address: www.kindredhealthcare.com

KINDRED HOSPITAL BAY AREA –TAMPA (O, 73 beds) 4555 South Manhattan Avenue, Tampa, FL Zip 33611–2397; tel. 813/839–6341; Sally Hoffmann, Chief Executive Officer
Web address: www.kindredhealthcare.com

KINDRED HOSPITAL NORTH FLORIDA (O, 60 beds) 801 Oak Street, Green Cove Springs, FL Zip 32043–4317; tel. 904/284–9230; Tim Simpson, Executive Director
Web address: www.khnorthflorida.com

KINDRED HOSPITAL OCALA (O, 31 beds) 1500 S.W. 1st Avenue, Ocala, FL Zip 34474; tel. 352/369–0513; Angelica Cotshott, Administrator
Web address: www.kindredhealthcare.com

KINDRED HOSPITAL SOUTH FLORIDA–CORAL GABLES (O, 53 beds) 5190 S.W. Eighth Street, Coral Gables, FL Zip 33134–2495; tel. 305/445–1364; Charles Doten, Chief Executive Officer
Web address: www.kindredhealthcare.com

KINDRED HOSPITAL SOUTH FLORIDA–FORT LAUDERDALE (O, 64 beds) 1516 East Las Olas Boulevard, Fort Lauderdale, FL Zip 33301–2399; tel. 954/764–8900; Theodore L. Welding, Chief Executive Officer
Web address: www.kindredhealthcare.com

KINDRED HOSPITAL SOUTH FLORIDA–HOLLYWOOD (O, 124 beds) 1859 Van Buren Street, Hollywood, FL Zip 33020–5127; tel. 954/920–9000; Chris Clements, Chief Executive Officer
Web address: www.kindredhealthcare.com

KINDRED HOSPITAL–BAY AREA ST. PETERSBURG (O, 112 beds) 3030 Sixth Street South, Saint Petersburg, FL Zip 33705–3720; tel. 727/894–8719; Pamela M. Riter, RN, Chief Executive Officer
Web address: www.kindredstpete.com

GEORGIA: KINDRED HOSPITAL–ATLANTA (O, 70 beds) 705 Juniper Street N.E., Atlanta, GA Zip 30365–2500; tel. 404/873–2871; Tim E. Merritt, Chief Executive Officer
Web address: www.kindredhealthcare.com

ILLINOIS: KINDRED CHICAGO CENTRAL HOSPITAL (O, 76 beds) 4058 West Melrose Street, Chicago, IL Zip 60641–4797; tel. 773/736–7000; Sandra Yule, Administrator
Web address: www.kindredhealthcare.com

KINDRED HOSPITAL CHICAGO NORTH (O, 164 beds) 2544 West Montrose Avenue, Chicago, IL Zip 60618–1589; tel. 773/267–2622; Larry Foster, Chief Executive Officer
Web address: www.kindredhealthcare.com

KINDRED HOSPITAL CHICAGO NORTHLAKE (O, 86 beds) 365 East North Avenue, Northlake, IL Zip 60164–2628; tel. 708/345–8100; Timothy Page, Chief Executive Officer
Web address: www.kindredhealthcare.com

KINDRED HOSPITAL–SYCAMORE (O, 69 beds) 225 Edward Street, Sycamore, IL Zip 60178–2197; tel. 815/895–2144; Cindy Smith, Chief Executive Officer
Web address: www.kindredhealthcare.com

INDIANA: KINDRED HOSPITAL INDIANAPOLIS SOUTH (O, 36 beds) 607 Greenwood Spring Drive, Greenwood, IN Zip 46143–1400; tel. 317/888–8155; Mona Euler, Chief Executive Officer
Web address: www.kindredhealthcare.com

KINDRED HOSPITAL–INDIANAPOLIS (O, 59 beds) 1700 West 10th Street, Indianapolis, IN Zip 46222–3802; tel. 317/636–4400; Dennis Nicely, Administrator
Web address: www.kindredhealthcare.com

KENTUCKY: KINDRED HOSPITAL LOUISVILLE AT JEWISH HOSPITAL (O, 30 beds) 200 Abraham Flexner Way, 2nd Floor, Louisville, KY Zip 40202; tel. 502/587–3999; Jack Nicholson, Chief Executive Officer
Web address: www.kindredhealthcare.com

KINDRED HOSPITAL–LOUISVILLE (O, 156 beds) 1313 St. Anthony Place, Louisville, KY Zip 40204–1765; tel. 502/587–7001; Lourene Money, Interim Chief Executive Officer
Web address: www.kindredhealthcare.com

LOUISIANA: KINDRED HOSPITAL – NEW ORLEANS (O, 55 beds) 3601 Coliseum Street, New Orleans, LA Zip 70115–3606; tel. 504/899–1555; Jan Turk, Chief Executive Officer
Web address: www.kindredhealthcare.com

MASSACHUSETTS: KINDRED HOSPITAL BOSTON NORTH SHORE (O, 50 beds) 15 King Street, Peabody, MA Zip 01960–4268; tel. 978/531–2900; Thomas Dowley, Interim Chief Executive Officer
Web address: www.kindredbns.com

For explanation of codes following names, see page B2.
★ Indicates Type III membership in the American Hospital Association.

KINDRED HOSPITAL NORTHEAST–NATICK (O, 23 beds) 67 Union Street, 6th Floor, Natick, MA Zip 1760; tel. 508/650–7630; Robert A. Gundersen, Chief Executive Officer
Web address: www.kindredhealthcare.com

KINDRED HOSPITAL NORTHEAST–STOUGHTON (O, 10 beds) 909 Sumner Street, 1st Floor, Stoughton, MA Zip 2072; tel. 781/297–8200; James MacKenzie, Administrator
Web address: www.kindredhealthcare.com

KINDRED HOSPITAL PARK VIEW (O, 284 beds) 1400 State Street, Springfield, MA Zip 01109–2589; tel. 413/726–6700; Karen O. Moore, RN, M.S., Chief Executive Officer
Web address: www.kindredhealthcare.com

KINDRED HOSPITAL PARK VIEW–CENTRAL MASSACHUSETTS (O, 10 beds) 111 Huntoon Memorial Highway, Rochdale, MA Zip 1542; tel. 508/892–6000; Scott MacLean, Administrator
Web address: www.kindredhealthcare.com

KINDRED HOSPITAL–BOSTON (O, 36 beds) 1515 Commonwealth Avenue, Boston, MA Zip 02135–3696; tel. 617/254–1100; Jacqueline Arocho, Chief Executive Officer
Web address: www.kindredhealthcare.com

MISSOURI: KINDRED HOSPITAL KANSAS CITY (O, 130 beds) 8701 Troost Avenue, Kansas City, MO Zip 64131–2767; tel. 816/995–2000; Cindy Mostaffa, Chief Executive Officer
Web address: www.kindredhospitalkc.com

KINDRED HOSPITAL–ST. LOUIS (O, 98 beds) 4930 Lindell Boulevard, Saint Louis, MO Zip 63108–1510; tel. 314/361–8700; Peter Miller, FACHE, Chief Executive Officer
Web address: www.kindredhealthcare.com

NEVADA: KINDRED HOSPITAL LAS VEGAS–SAHARA (O, 144 beds) 5110 West Sahara Avenue, Las Vegas, NV Zip 89146–3406; tel. 702/871–1418; Jennifer Schomburg, Administrator
Web address: www.kindredhealthcare.com

NEW JERSEY: KINDRED HOSPITAL NEW JERSEY – RAHWAY (O, 28 beds) 865 Stone Street, Rahway, NJ Zip 7065; tel. 732/453–2950; Janet Biedron, Chief Executive Officer

KINDRED HOSPITAL NEW JERSEY – WAYNE (O, 38 beds) 224 Hamburg Turnpike, Wayne, NJ Zip 7470; tel. 973/636–7200; Robert Meyers, Chief Executive Officer
Web address: www.kindredhealthcare.com

NEW MEXICO: KINDRED HOSPITAL – ALBUQUERQUE (O, 61 beds) 700 High Street N.E., Albuquerque, NM Zip 87102–2565; tel. 505/242–4444; Charles Tozer, Interim Chief Executive Officer
Web address: www.kindredhealthcare.com

NORTH CAROLINA: KINDRED HOSPITAL–GREENSBORO (O, 124 beds) 2401 Southside Boulevard, Greensboro, NC Zip 27406–3311; tel. 336/271–2800; David M. Polunas, Chief Executive Officer
Web address: www.kindredhealthcare.com

OKLAHOMA: KINDRED HOSPITAL– OKLAHOMA CITY (O, 93 beds) 1407 North Robinson Avenue, Oklahoma City, OK Zip 73103; tel. 405/232–8000; Gayla Campbell, Chief Executive Officer
Web address: www.kindredoklahoma.com

PENNSYLVANIA: KINDRED HOSPITAL – DELAWARE COUNTY (O, 43 beds) 1500 Landsdowne Avenue, 6th Floor, Darby, PA Zip 19023, Mailing Address: 1500 Lansdowne Avenue, 6th Floor, Zip 19023; tel. 610/237–5780; Garrett Arneson, Chief Executive Officer
Web address: www.kindredhealthcare.com

KINDRED HOSPITAL–HERITAGE VALLEY (O, 35 beds) 1000 Dutch Ridge Road, Beaver, PA Zip 15009; tel. 724/773–8210; Timothy Bugin, Administrator
Web address: www.kindredhealthcare.com

KINDRED HOSPITAL–PHILADELPHIA (O, 52 beds) 6129 Palmetto Street, Philadelphia, PA Zip 19111–5729; tel. 215/722–8555; Margaret M. Murphy, Chief Executive Officer
Web address: www.kindredhealthcare.com

KINDRED HOSPITAL–PITTSBURGH (O, 63 beds) 7777 Steubenville Pike, Oakdale, PA Zip 15071–3409; tel. 412/494–5500; Susan Colpo, Chief Executive Officer
Web address: www.kindredhealthcare.com

KINDRED HOSPITAL–WOMING VALLEY (O, 36 beds) 575 North River Street, 7th Floor, Wilkes–Barre, PA Zip 18764; tel. 570/552–7620; Erin Pica, Chief Executive Officer
Web address: www.kindredhealthcare.com

TENNESSEE: KINDRED HOSPITAL – NASHVILLE (O, 60 beds) 1412 County Hospital Road, Nashville, TN Zip 37218; tel. 615/687–2600; Michael L. Moody, Chief Executive Officer
Web address: www.kindredhealthcare.com

KINDRED HOSPITAL–CHATTANOOGA (O, 44 beds) 709 Walnut Street, Chattanooga, TN Zip 37402–1961; tel. 423/266–7721; William J. Bryant, Chief Executive Officer
Web address: www.kindredhealthcare.com

TEXAS: KINDRED HOSPITAL – DALLAS (O, 130 beds) 9525 Greenville Avenue, Dallas, TX Zip 75243–4116; tel. 214/355–2600; Robert M. Smart, Chief Executive Officer
Web address: www.kindredhealthcare.com

KINDRED HOSPITAL TARRANT COUNTY–ARLINGTON (O, 79 beds) 1000 North Cooper Street, Arlington, TX Zip 76011–5540; tel. 817/548–3400; Christina Richard, Administrator
Web address: www.kindredhealthcare.com

KINDRED HOSPITAL TARRANT COUNTY–FORT WORTH SOUTHWEST (O, 57 beds) 7800 Oakmont Boulevard, Fort Worth, TX Zip 76132–4299; tel. 817/346–0094; Audra Early, Chief Executive Officer
Web address: www.kindredhealthcare.com

KINDRED HOSPITAL–BAY AREA (O, 78 beds) 1004 Seymour Street, Pasadena, TX Zip 77506–2699; tel. 713/473–9700; Melissa Miller, Administrator
Web address: www.kindredhealthcare.com

KINDRED HOSPITAL–HOUSTON (O, 92 beds) 6441 Main Street, Houston, TX Zip 77030–1596; tel. 713/790–0500; Randy E. Johnson, Chief Executive Officer
Web address: www.kindredhealthcare.com

KINDRED HOSPITAL–HOUSTON NORTHWEST (O, 84 beds) 11297 Fallbrook Drive, Houston, TX Zip 77065–4292; tel. 281/897–8114; Mary Anne Craig, Chief Executive Officer
Web address: www.kindredhealthcare.com

KINDRED HOSPITAL–MANSFIELD (O, 55 beds) 1802 Highway 157 North, Mansfield, TX Zip 76063–9555; tel. 817/473–6101; Dalton Stewart, Chief Executive Officer
Web address: www.kindredmansfield.com

KINDRED HOSPITAL–SAN ANTONIO (O, 59 beds) 3636 Medical Drive, San Antonio, TX Zip 78229–3184; tel. 210/616–0616; Edward L. Dyer, Chief Executive Officer
Web address: www.kindredhealthcare.com

WASHINGTON: KINDRED HOSPITAL SEATTLE (O, 42 beds) 10631 8th Avenue N.E., Seattle, WA Zip 98125–0716; tel. 206/364–2050; Greg Davis, Chief Executive Officer
Web address: www.kindredhealthcare.com

WISCONSIN: KINDRED HOSPITAL–MILWAUKEE (O, 56 beds) 5017 South 110th Street, Milwaukee, WI Zip 53228–3131; tel. 414/427–8282; Linda Newberry–Ferguson, Chief Executive Officer
Web address: www.khmilwaukee.com

Owned, leased, sponsored:	62 hospitals	4429 beds
Contract–managed:	0 hospitals	0 beds
Totals:	62 hospitals	4429 beds

★0149: KISH HEALTH SYSTEM (NP)

1 Kish Hospital Drive, De Kalb, IL Zip 60115–4939, Mailing Address: P.O. Box 707, Zip 60115–4939; tel. 815/756–1521; Kevin P. Poorten, President and Chief Executive Officer
(Independent Hospital System)

ILLINOIS: KISHWAUKEE COMMUNITY HOSPITAL (O, 100 beds) One Kish Hospital Drive, De Kalb, IL Zip 60115–4939, Mailing Address: P.O. Box 707, Zip 60115–0707; tel. 815/756–1521; Brad Copple, Administrator
Web address: www.kishhospital.org

VALLEY WEST COMMUNITY HOSPITAL (O, 25 beds) 11 East Pleasant Avenue, Sandwich, IL Zip 60548–0901; tel. 815/786–8484; Brad Copple, Administrator
Web address: www.vwch.org

Owned, leased, sponsored:	2 hospitals	125 beds
Contract–managed:	0 hospitals	0 beds
Totals:	2 hospitals	125 beds

For explanation of codes following names, see page B2.
★ Indicates Type III membership in the American Hospital Association.

Section B

0056: LAKELAND HEALTHCARE (NP)
1234 Napier Avenue, Saint Joseph, MI Zip 49085–2158; tel. 269/983–8300; Joseph A. Wasserman, President and Chief Executive Officer

MICHIGAN: LAKELAND REGIONAL MEDICAL CENTER–ST. JOSEPH (O, 671 beds) 1234 Napier Avenue, Saint Joseph, MI Zip 49085–2112; tel. 269/983–8300; Joseph A. Wasserman, President and Chief Executive Officer
Web address: www.lakelandhealth.org

LAKELAND SPECIALTY HOSPITAL, BERRIEN CENTER (O, 221 beds) 6418 Dean's Hill Road, Berrien Center, MI Zip 49102–9704; tel. 269/473–3003; Joseph A. Wasserman, President and Chief Executive Officer
Web address: www.lakelandhealth.org

Owned, leased, sponsored:	2 hospitals	892 beds
Contract-managed:	0 hospitals	0 beds
Totals:	2 hospitals	892 beds

• 0393: LANDMARK HOSPITALS (NP)
3255 Independence Street, Cape Girardeau, MO Zip 63701–4904; tel. 573/335–1091; William Kapp, M.D., President

MISSOURI: LANDMARK HOSPITAL (O, 25 beds) 3255 Independence Street, Cape Girardeau, MO Zip 63701–4904; tel. 573/335–1091; Deborah Sabella, Chief Executive Officer
Web address: www.landmarkhospitals.com

Owned, leased, sponsored:	1 hospital	25 beds
Contract-managed:	0 hospitals	0 beds
Totals:	1 hospital	25 beds

0369: LEE MEMORIAL HEALTH SYSTEM (NP)
2776 Cleveland Avenue, Fort Myers, FL Zip 33901; tel. 239/332–1111; James R. Nathan, President and Chief Executive Officer

FLORIDA: CAPE CORAL HOSPITAL (O, 209 beds) 636 Del Prado Boulevard, Cape Coral, FL Zip 33990–2695; tel. 239/574–2323; James R. Nathan, President
Web address: www.leememorial.org

GULF COAST HOSPITAL (O, 107 beds) 13681 Doctors Way, Fort Myers, FL Zip 33912–4309; tel. 239/768–5000; James R. Nathan, President and Chief Executive Officer
Web address: www.gulfcoasthospital.com

LEE MEMORIAL HOSPITAL (O, 1574 beds) 2776 Cleveland Avenue, Fort Myers, FL Zip 33901–5855, Mailing Address: P.O. Box 2218, Zip 33902–2218; tel. 239/332–1111; James R. Nathan, President and Chief Executive Officer
Web address: www.leememorial.org

SOUTHWEST FLORIDA REGIONAL MEDICAL CENTER (O, 279 beds) 2727 Winkler Avenue, Fort Myers, FL Zip 33901–9396; tel. 239/939–1147; Douglas R. Luckett, Chief Executive Officer
Web address: www.swfrmc.com

Owned, leased, sponsored:	4 hospitals	2169 beds
Contract-managed:	0 hospitals	0 beds
Totals:	4 hospitals	2169 beds

★2755: LEGACY HEALTH SYSTEM (NP)
1919 N.W. Lovejoy Street, Portland, OR Zip 97209–1503; tel. 503/415–5600; Pamela S. Vukovich, Interim President and Chief Executive Officer
(Centralized Health System)

OREGON: LEGACY EMANUEL HOSPITAL AND HEALTH CENTER (O, 401 beds) 2801 North Gantenbein Avenue, Portland, OR Zip 97227–1674; tel. 503/413–2200; April Whitworth, Chief Administrative Officer
Web address: www.legacyhealth.org

LEGACY GOOD SAMARITAN HOSPITAL AND MEDICAL CENTER (O, 263 beds) 1015 N.W. 22nd Avenue, Portland, OR Zip 97210–3099; tel. 503/413–7711; Tony Melaragno, M.D., Chief Administrative Officer
Web address: www.legacyhealth.org

LEGACY MERIDIAN PARK HOSPITAL (O, 133 beds) 19300 S.W. 65th Avenue, Tualatin, OR Zip 97062–9741; tel. 503/692–1212; Allyson Anderson, Chief Administrative Officer
Web address: www.legacyhealth.org

LEGACY MOUNT HOOD MEDICAL CENTER (O, 81 beds) 24800 S.E. Stark, Gresham, OR Zip 97030–0154; tel. 503/667–1122; Bryce R. Helgerson, Chief Administrative Officer
Web address: www.legacyhealth.org

WASHINGTON: LEGACY SALMON CREEK HOSPITAL (O, 139 beds) 2211 N.E. 139th Street, Vancouver, WA Zip 98686–2742; tel. 360/487–1000; Jonathan Avery, Chief Administrative Officer
Web address: www.legacyhealth.org

Owned, leased, sponsored:	5 hospitals	1017 beds
Contract-managed:	0 hospitals	0 beds
Totals:	5 hospitals	1017 beds

★0370: LEHIGH VALLEY HOSPITAL AND HEALTH NETWORK (NP)
1200 South Cedar Crest Boulevard, Allentown, PA Zip 18103, Mailing Address: P.O. Box 689, Zip 18105–0689; tel. 610/402–8000; Elliot J. Sussman, M.D., President and Chief Executive Officer

PENNSYLVANIA: LEHIGH VALLEY HOSPITAL (O, 701 beds) 1200 South Cedar Crest Boulevard, Allentown, PA Zip 18105–6248, Mailing Address: P.O. Box 689, Zip 18105–0689; tel. 610/402–8000; Elliot J. Sussman, M.D., President and Chief Executive Officer
Web address: www.lvhhn.org

LEHIGH VALLEY HOSPITAL–MUHLENBERG (O, 156 beds) 2545 Schoenersville Road, Bethlehem, PA Zip 18017–7384; tel. 484/884–2201; Elliot J. Sussman, M.D., President and Chief Executive Officer
Web address: www.lvhhn.org

Owned, leased, sponsored:	2 hospitals	857 beds
Contract-managed:	0 hospitals	0 beds
Totals:	2 hospitals	857 beds

0206: LIBERTY MANAGEMENT GROUP, INC. (IO)
19 Spear Road, Suite 305, Ramsey, NJ Zip 07446; tel. 201/236–8880; William J. Hartigan, President and Chief Executive Officer
(Independent Hospital System)

NEW YORK: HOLLISWOOD HOSPITAL (C, 110 beds) 87–37 Palermo Street, Jamaica, NY Zip 11423–1209; tel. 718/776–8181; Jeffrey Borenstein, M.D., Chief Executive Officer and Medical Director
Web address: www.holliswoodhospital.com

OKLAHOMA: ROLLING HILLS HOSPITAL (O, 40 beds) 1000 Rolling Hills Lane, Ada, OK Zip 74820–9415; tel. 580/436–3600; Brian Beutin, M.S., Chief Executive Officer
Web address: www.rollinghillshospital.com

Owned, leased, sponsored:	1 hospital	40 beds
Contract-managed:	1 hospital	110 beds
Totals:	2 hospitals	150 beds

0173: LIBERTYHEALTH (NP)
355 Grand Street, Jersey City, NJ Zip 07302; tel. 201/915–2000; Jonathan M. Metsch, Dr.P.h., President and Chief Executive Officer
(Centralized Health System)

NEW JERSEY: LIBERTYHEALTH–JERSEY CITY MEDICAL CENTER (O, 324 beds) 355 Grand Street, Jersey City, NJ Zip 7302; tel. 201/915–2000; E. Stephen Kirby, Interim Chief Executive Officer
Web address: www.libertyhcs.org

LIBERTYHEALTH–MEADOWLANDS HOSPITAL MEDICAL CENTER (O, 163 beds) 55 Meadowland Parkway, Secaucus, NJ Zip 07094–1580; tel. 201/392–3100; Joseph F. Scott, Chief Executive Officer
Web address: www.libertyhcs.com

For explanation of codes following names, see page B2.
★ Indicates Type III membership in the American Hospital Association.
• Single hospital health care system

Owned, leased, sponsored:	2 hospitals	487 beds
Contract-managed:	0 hospitals	0 beds
Totals:	2 hospitals	487 beds

★0158: LIFEBRIDGE HEALTH (NP)
2401 West Belvedere Avenue, Baltimore, MD Zip 21215; tel. 410/601–5134; Warren A. Green, President and Chief Executive Officer
(Centralized Health System)

MARYLAND: LEVINDALE HEBREW GERIATRIC CENTER AND HOSPITAL (O, 443 beds) 2434 West Belvedere Avenue, Baltimore, MD Zip 21215–5299; tel. 410/466–8700; Ronald Rothstein, President and Chief Operating Officer
Web address: www.sinai–balt.com

NORTHWEST HOSPITAL CENTER (O, 230 beds) 5401 Old Court Road, Randallstown, MD Zip 21133–5185; tel. 410/521–2200; Erik G. Wexler, President and Chief Operating Officer
Web address: www.lifebridgehealth.org

SINAI HOSPITAL OF BALTIMORE (O, 439 beds) 2401 West Belvedere Avenue, Baltimore, MD Zip 21215–5271; tel. 410/601–9000; Neil M. Meltzer, President and Chief Operating Officer
Web address: www.lifebridgehealth.org

Owned, leased, sponsored:	3 hospitals	1112 beds
Contract-managed:	0 hospitals	0 beds
Totals:	3 hospitals	1112 beds

0191: LIFECARE MANAGEMENT SERVICES (IO)
5560 Tennyson Parkway, Plano, TX Zip 75024; tel. 469/241–2100; Wayne McAlister, Chairman of the Board and Chief Executive Officer
(Independent Hospital System)

COLORADO: COLORADO ACUTE LONG TERM HOSPITAL (O, 24 beds) 1601 North Lowell Boulevard, Denver, CO Zip 80204–1545; tel. 303/899–5166; Kent Ashley, Chief Executive Officer
Web address: www.lifecare–hospitals.com

LOUISIANA: LIFECARE HOSPITALS OF SHREVEPORT (O, 130 beds) 9320 Linwood Avenue, Shreveport, LA Zip 71106–7003; tel. 318/688–8504; Keith Cox, CHE, Chief Executive Officer
Web address: www.lifecare–hospitals.com

MICHIGAN: LIFECARE HOSPITALS OF WEST MICHIGAN (O, 20 beds) 1700 Oak Avenue, 3rd Floor, Muskegon, MI Zip 49442; tel. 231/777–6202; Jevne Conover, Administrator
Web address: www.lifecare–hospitals.com

NEVADA: TAHOE PACIFIC HOSPITALS (O, 50 beds) 10405 Double R Boulevard, Reno, NV Zip 89512; tel. 775/355–5970; Phil Greenhill, Chief Executive Officer
Web address: www.lifecare–hospitals.com

NORTH CAROLINA: LIFECARE HOSPITALS OF NORTH CAROLINA (O, 50 beds) 1051 Noell Lane, Rocky Mount, NC Zip 27804–1761; tel. 252/451–2300; Kevin S. Cooper, RN, Chief Executive Officer and Administrator
Web address: www.lifecare–hospitals.com

OHIO: LIFECARE HOSPITAL OF DAYTON (O, 42 beds) 4000 Miamisburg–Centerville Road, Miamisburg, OH Zip 45342; tel. 937/384–8300; Brent Martin, Chief Executive Officer
Web address: www.lifecare–hospitals.com

PENNSYLVANIA: LIFECARE HOSPITALS OF CHESTER COUNTY (O, 39 beds) 400 East Marshall Street, West Chester, PA Zip 19380; tel. 484/826–0400; Rosalie Cox, Chief Executive Officer
Web address: www.lifecare–hospitals.com

LIFECARE HOSPITALS OF PITTSBURGH (O, 159 beds) 225 Penn Avenue, Pittsburgh, PA Zip 15221–2173; tel. 412/247–2424; Richard Pletz, Chief Executive Officer
Web address: www.lifecare–hospitals.com

TEXAS: LIFECARE HOSPITALS OF FORT WORTH (O, 80 beds) 6201 Overton Ridge Boulevard, Fort Worth, TX Zip 76132; tel. 817/370–6078; Barbara Schmidt, Chief Executive Officer
Web address: www.lifecare–hospitals.com

LIFECARE HOSPITALS OF NORTH TEXAS–DALLAS (O, 64 beds) 6161 Harry Hines Boulevard, Suite 100, Dallas, TX Zip 75235–5306; tel. 214/525–6300; Edward Downs, Chief Executive Officer
Web address: www.lifecare–hospitals.com

LIFECARE HOSPITALS OF PLANO (O, 66 beds) 6800 Preston Road, Plano, TX Zip 75024; tel. 214/473–8822; Kathleen Wallace, RN, M.S.N., Administrator and Chief Executive Officer
Web address: www.lifecare–hospitals.com

LIFECARE HOSPITALS OF SAN ANTONIO (O, 62 beds) 8026 Floyd Curl Drive, San Antonio, TX Zip 78229; tel. 210/690–7000; Randall G. Stokes, Chief Executive Officer
Web address: www.lifecare–hospitals.com

LIFECARE HOSPITALS OF SOUTH TEXAS (O, 94 beds) 333 West Freddy Gonzalez Drive, Edinburg, TX Zip 78539–6132; tel. 956/388–1800; David L. Tupper, Chief Executive Officer
Web address: www.lifecare–hospitals.com

WISCONSIN: LIFECARE HOSPITALS OF MILWAUKEE (O, 34 beds) 5000 West Chambers Street, 8th Floor, Milwaukee, WI Zip 53210; tel. 414/447–3600; Steven J. Schultz, Chief Executive Officer
Web address: www.lifecare–hospitals.com

Owned, leased, sponsored:	14 hospitals	914 beds
Contract-managed:	0 hospitals	0 beds
Totals:	14 hospitals	914 beds

★0180: LIFEPOINT HOSPITALS, INC. (IO)
103 Powell Court, Suite 200, Brentwood, TN Zip 37027; tel. 615/372–8500; William F. Carpenter, III, President and Chief Executive Officer
(Moderately Centralized Health System)

ALABAMA: ANDALUSIA REGIONAL HOSPITAL (O, 87 beds) 849 South Three Notch Street, Andalusia, AL Zip 36420–5325, Mailing Address: P.O. Box 760, Zip 36420–0760; tel. 334/222–8466; Mark J. Dooley, Chief Executive Officer
Web address: www.andalusiaregionalhospital.com

LAKELAND COMMUNITY HOSPITAL (O, 47 beds) Highway 195 East, Haleyville, AL Zip 35565–9536, Mailing Address: P.O. Box 780, Zip 35565–0780; tel. 205/486–5213; Christine R. Stewart, Chief Executive Officer
Web address: www.lifepointhospitals.com

NORTHWEST MEDICAL CENTER (O, 66 beds) 1530 U.S. Highway 43, Winfield, AL Zip 35594–5056; tel. 205/487–7000; Chuck Spann, Chief Executive Officer
Web address: www.northwestmedcenter.com

RUSSELLVILLE HOSPITAL (O, 100 beds) 15155 Highway 43, Russellville, AL Zip 35653–1975, Mailing Address: P.O. Box 1089, Zip 35653–1089; tel. 256/332–1611; Christine R. Stewart, Chief Executive Officer
Web address: www.russellvillehospital.com

VAUGHAN REGIONAL MEDICAL CENTER (O, 149 beds) 1015 Medical Center Parkway, Selma, AL Zip 36701–6352; tel. 334/418–4100; Barry L. Keel, Chief Executive Officer
Web address: www.uabsfm.org/vaughan.html

ARIZONA: HAVASU REGIONAL MEDICAL CENTER (O, 138 beds) 101 Civic Center Lane, Lake Havasu City, AZ Zip 86403–5683; tel. 928/855–8185; Ruth A. McDaniel, Interim Chief Executive Officer
Web address: www.havasuregional.com

VALLEY VIEW MEDICAL CENTER (O, 60 beds) 5330 South Highway 95, Fort Mohave, AZ Zip 86426; tel. 928/788–2273; Jim Matney, Chief Executive Officer
Web address: www.valleyviewmedicalcenter.net

COLORADO: COLORADO PLAINS MEDICAL CENTER (L, 50 beds) 1000 Lincoln Street, Fort Morgan, CO Zip 80701–3298; tel. 970/867–3391; Michael A. Anaya, Sr., FACHE, Chief Executive Officer
Web address: www.coloradoplainsmedicalcenter.com

FLORIDA: PUTNAM COMMUNITY MEDICAL CENTER (O, 141 beds) Highway 20 West, Palatka, FL Zip 32177–8118, Mailing Address: P.O. Box 778, Zip 32178–0778; tel. 386/328–5711; Bruce A. Baldwin, Chief Executive Officer
Web address: www.pcmcfl.com

For explanation of codes following names, see page B2.
★ Indicates Type III membership in the American Hospital Association.

Section B

INDIANA: STARKE MEMORIAL HOSPITAL (L, 49 beds) 102 East Culver Road, Knox, IN Zip 46534–2299, Mailing Address: P.O. Box 339, Zip 46534–0339; tel. 574/772–6231; Michael J. Meadows, Chief Executive Officer
Web address: www.starkememorial.com

KANSAS: WESTERN PLAINS MEDICAL COMPLEX (O, 99 beds) 3001 Avenue A, Dodge City, KS Zip 67801–6508, Mailing Address: P.O. Box 1478, Zip 67801–1478; tel. 620/225–8400; John E. Walker, President and Chief Executive Officer
Web address: www.westernplainsmc.com

KENTUCKY: BLUEGRASS COMMUNITY HOSPITAL (O, 25 beds) 360 Amsden Avenue, Versailles, KY Zip 40383–1286; tel. 859/873–3111; Kathy Love, Chief Executive Officer
Web address: www.lifepointhospitals.com

BOURBON COMMUNITY HOSPITAL (O, 58 beds) 9 Linville Drive, Paris, KY Zip 40361–2196; tel. 859/987–3600; Ronald Tyrer, Interim Chief Executive Officer
Web address: www.bourbonhospital.com

GEORGETOWN COMMUNITY HOSPITAL (O, 75 beds) 1140 Lexington Road, Georgetown, KY Zip 40324–9362; tel. 502/868–1100; Barry A. Papania, Chief Executive Officer
Web address: www.georgetowncommunityhospital.com

JACKSON PURCHASE MEDICAL CENTER (O, 107 beds) 1099 Medical Center Circle, Mayfield, KY Zip 42066–1179; tel. 270/251–4100; Mary Jo Lewis, Chief Executive Officer
Web address: www.jacksonpurchase.com

LAKE CUMBERLAND REGIONAL HOSPITAL (O, 259 beds) 305 Langdon Street, Somerset, KY Zip 42501–2750, Mailing Address: P.O. Box 620, Zip 42502–2750; tel. 606/679–7441; Jeffrey G. Seraphine, CHE, Chief Executive Officer
Web address: www.lakecrmc.com

LOGAN MEMORIAL HOSPITAL (O, 92 beds) 1625 South Nashville Road, Russellville, KY Zip 42276–8834, Mailing Address: P.O. Box 10, Zip 42276–0010; tel. 270/726–4011; Greg Moore, Chief Executive Officer
Web address: www.loganmemorial.com

MEADOWVIEW REGIONAL MEDICAL CENTER (O, 101 beds) 989 Medical Park Drive, Maysville, KY Zip 41056–8750; tel. 606/759–5311; Chad Patrick, Chief Executive Officer
Web address: www.meadowviewregional.com

SPRING VIEW HOSPITAL (O, 60 beds) 320 Loretto Road, Lebanon, KY Zip 40033–0320; tel. 270/692–3161; Michael T. Sherrod, Chief Executive Officer
Web address: www.springviewhospital.com

LOUISIANA: ACADIAN MEDICAL CENTER (O, 42 beds) 3501 Highway 190 East, Eunice, LA Zip 70535–3628; tel. 337/580–7500; James P. Frazier, III, M.D., Chief Executive Officer
Web address: www.acadianmedicalcenter.com

DOCTOR'S HOSPITAL OF OPELOUSAS (O, 171 beds) 3983 I–49 South Service Road, Opelousas, LA Zip 70570–8975; tel. 337/948–2100; Phillip Young, FACHE, Chief Executive Officer
Web address: www.doctorshospital.com

MINDEN MEDICAL CENTER (O, 159 beds) 1 Medical Plaza, Minden, LA Zip 71055–3330, Mailing Address: P.O. Box 5003, Zip 71058–5003; tel. 318/377–2321; George E. French, III, CHE, Chief Executive Officer
Web address: www.mindenmedicalcenter.com

RIVER PARISHES HOSPITAL (O, 72 beds) 500 Rue de Sante, La Place, LA Zip 70068–5420; tel. 985/652–7000; Charlotte W. Dupre', Chief Executive Officer
Web address: www.riverparisheshospital.com

TECHE REGIONAL MEDICAL CENTER (L, 127 beds) 1125 Marguerite Street, Morgan City, LA Zip 70380–1855, Mailing Address: P.O. Box 2308, Zip 70381–2308; tel. 985/384–2200; Scott M. Smith, Chief Executive Officer
Web address: www.techeregional.com

VILLE PLATTE MEDICAL CENTER (O, 60 beds) 800 East Main Street, Ville Platte, LA Zip 70586–4618, Mailing Address: P.O. Box 349, Zip 70586–0349; tel. 337/363–5684; Brian L. Riddle, Sr., Chief Executive Officer
Web address: www.vpmc.com

MISSISSIPPI: BOLIVAR MEDICAL CENTER (L, 156 beds) 901 East Sunflower Road, Cleveland, MS Zip 38732–9722, Mailing Address: P.O. Box 1380, Zip 38732–1380; tel. 662/846–0061; Stephen Nichols, Chief Executive Officer
Web address: www.bolivarmedical.com

NEVADA: NORTHEASTERN NEVADA REGIONAL HOSPITAL (O, 50 beds) 2001 Errecart Boulevard, Elko, NV Zip 89801–3499; tel. 775/738–5151; David L. Henson, Chief Executive Officer
Web address: www.nnrhospital.com

NEW MEXICO: LOS ALAMOS MEDICAL CENTER (O, 47 beds) 3917 West Road, Los Alamos, NM Zip 87544–2293; tel. 505/662–4201; Sandra C. Podley, Chief Executive Officer
Web address: www.losalamosmedicalcenter.com

MEMORIAL MEDICAL CENTER (L, 198 beds) 2450 South Telshor Boulevard, Las Cruces, NM Zip 88011–5076; tel. 575/522–8641; Paul F. Herzog, Chief Executive Officer
Web address: www.mmclc.org

TENNESSEE: ATHENS REGIONAL MEDICAL CENTER (O, 97 beds) 1114 West Madison Avenue, Athens, TN Zip 37303–4150, Mailing Address: P.O. Box 250, Zip 37371–0250; tel. 423/745–1411; John R. Workman, Chief Executive Officer
Web address: www.athensrmc.com

CROCKETT HOSPITAL (O, 98 beds) U.S. Highway 43 South, Lawrenceburg, TN Zip 38464–0847, Mailing Address: P.O. Box 847, Zip 38464–0847; tel. 931/762–6571; Jack S. Buck, Chief Executive Officer
Web address: www.crocketthospital.com

HILLSIDE HOSPITAL (O, 50 beds) 1265 East College Street, Pulaski, TN Zip 38478–4500; tel. 931/363–7531; James H. Edmondson, Chief Executive Officer
Web address: www.hillsidehospital.com

LIVINGSTON REGIONAL HOSPITAL (O, 72 beds) 315 Oak Street, Livingston, TN Zip 38570, Mailing Address: P.O. Box 550, Zip 38570–0550; tel. 931/823–5611; Timothy W. McGill, Chief Executive Officer
Web address: www.livingston–hospital.com

SOUTHERN TENNESSEE MEDICAL CENTER (O, 153 beds) 185 Hospital Road, Winchester, TN Zip 37398–9504; tel. 931/967–8200; William Russell Spray, Chief Executive Officer
Web address: www.southerntennessee.com

TEXAS: ENNIS REGIONAL MEDICAL CENTER (L, 56 beds) 2201 West Lampasas Street, Ennis, TX Zip 75119; tel. 972/875–0900; David Anderson, Chief Executive Officer
Web address: www.ennisregional.com

PALESTINE REGIONAL MEDICAL CENTER–EAST (O, 103 beds) 2900 South Loop 256, Palestine, TX Zip 75801–6958; tel. 903/731–1000; Tim Flusche, Chief Executive Officer
Web address: www.palestineregional.com

PALESTINE REGIONAL REHABILITATION CENTER (O, 17 beds) 4000 South Loop 256, Palestine, TX Zip 75801–8467, Mailing Address: P.O. Box 4070, Zip 75802–4070; tel. 903/731–5100; Tim Flusche, Chief Executive Officer
Web address: www.palestineregional.com

PARKVIEW REGIONAL HOSPITAL (L, 50 beds) 600 South Bonham, Mexia, TX Zip 76667–3608; tel. 254/562–0408; Jimmy D. Stuart, Chief Executive Officer
Web address: www.parkviewregional.com

UTAH: ASHLEY REGIONAL MEDICAL CENTER (O, 31 beds) 151 West 200 North, Vernal, UT Zip 84078–1907; tel. 435/789–3342; Si Hutt, Chief Executive Officer
Web address: www.ashleyregional.com

CASTLEVIEW HOSPITAL (O, 57 beds) 300 North Hospital Drive, Price, UT Zip 84501–4200; tel. 435/637–4800; Jeffrey J. Manley, Chief Executive Officer
Web address: www.castleviewhospital.net

VIRGINIA: CLINCH VALLEY MEDICAL CENTER (O, 140 beds) 2949 West Front Street, Richlands, VA Zip 24641–2099; tel. 276/596–6000; David B. Darden, Chief Executive Officer
Web address: www.clinchvalleymedicalcenter.com

DANVILLE REGIONAL MEDICAL CENTER (O, 173 beds) 142 South Main Street, Danville, VA Zip 24541–2922; tel. 434/799–2100; Jerel T. Humphrey, Chief Executive Officer
Web address: www.danvilleregional.org

For explanation of codes following names, see page B2.
★ Indicates Type III membership in the American Hospital Association.

MEMORIAL HOSPITAL (O, 212 beds) 320 Hospital Drive, Martinsville, VA Zip 24112–1981, Mailing Address: P.O. Box 4788, Zip 24115–4788; tel. 276/666–7200; Joseph Roach, Chief Executive Officer
Web address: www.martinsvillehospital.com

WYTHE COUNTY COMMUNITY HOSPITAL (L, 90 beds) 600 West Ridge Road, Wytheville, VA Zip 24382–1099; tel. 276/228–0200; Eric Deaton, Chief Executive Officer
Web address: www.wcch.org

WEST VIRGINIA: LOGAN REGIONAL MEDICAL CENTER (O, 129 beds) 20 Hospital Drive, Logan, WV Zip 25601–3473; tel. 304/831–1101; Kevin N. Fowler, Chief Executive Officer
Web address: www.loganregionalmedicalcenter.com

RALEIGH GENERAL HOSPITAL (O, 229 beds) 1710 Harper Road, Beckley, WV Zip 25801–3397; tel. 304/256–4100; Karen L. Bowling, Chief Executive Officer
Web address: www.raleighgeneral.com

WYOMING: LANDER REGIONAL HOSPITAL (O, 98 beds) 1320 Bishop Randall Drive, Lander, WY Zip 82520–3996; tel. 307/332–4420; Phil Eaton, Chief Executive Officer
Web address: www.landerhospital.com

RIVERTON MEMORIAL HOSPITAL (O, 49 beds) 2100 West Sunset Drive, Riverton, WY Zip 82501–2274; tel. 307/856–4161; James Christian Smolik, Chief Executive Officer
Web address: www.riverton–hospital.com

Owned, leased, sponsored:	48 hospitals	4749 beds
Contract–managed:	0 hospitals	0 beds
Totals:	48 hospitals	4749 beds

0060: LIFESPAN CORPORATION (NP)

167 Point Street, Providence, RI Zip 02903–4771; tel. 401/444–3500; George A. Vecchione, President
(Moderately Centralized Health System)

RHODE ISLAND: EMMA PENDLETON BRADLEY HOSPITAL (O, 51 beds) 1011 Veterans Memorial Parkway, East Providence, RI Zip 02915–5099; tel. 401/432–1000; Daniel J. Wall, President and Chief Executive Officer
Web address: www.lifespan.org

MIRIAM HOSPITAL (O, 247 beds) 164 Summit Avenue, Providence, RI Zip 02906–2895; tel. 401/793–2500; Kathleen C. Hittner, M.D., President and Chief Executive Officer
Web address: www.lifespan.org

NEWPORT HOSPITAL (O, 119 beds) 11 Friendship Street, Newport, RI Zip 02840–2299; tel. 401/846–6400; Arthur J. Sampson, President and Chief Executive Officer
Web address: www.newporthospital.org

RHODE ISLAND HOSPITAL (O, 632 beds) 593 Eddy Street, Providence, RI Zip 02903–4900; tel. 401/444–4000; George A. Vecchione, Interim Chief Executive Officer
Web address: www.lifespan.org

Owned, leased, sponsored:	4 hospitals	1049 beds
Contract–managed:	0 hospitals	0 beds
Totals:	4 hospitals	1049 beds

2175: LOMA LINDA UNIVERSITY ADVENTIST HEALTH SCIENCES CENTER (NP)

11175 Campus Street, Loma Linda, CA Zip 92354; tel. 909/558–7572; Richard H. Hart, President and Chief Executive Officer
(Moderately Centralized Health System)

CALIFORNIA: LOMA LINDA UNIVERSITY BEHAVIORAL MEDICINE CENTER (O, 89 beds) 1710 Barton Road, Redlands, CA Zip 92373–5304; tel. 909/558–9200; Ruthita J. Fike, Chief Executive Officer
Web address: www.llu.edu

LOMA LINDA UNIVERSITY MEDICAL CENTER (O, 739 beds) 11234 Anderson Street, Loma Linda, CA Zip 92354–2870, Mailing Address: P.O. Box 2000, Zip 92354–0200; tel. 909/558–4000; Ruthita J. Fike, Chief Executive Officer
Web address: www.llumc.edu

Owned, leased, sponsored:	2 hospitals	828 beds
Contract–managed:	0 hospitals	0 beds
Totals:	2 hospitals	828 beds

5755: LOS ANGELES COUNTY–DEPARTMENT OF HEALTH SERVICES (NP)

313 North Figueroa Street, Room 912, Los Angeles, CA Zip 90012–2691; tel. 213/240–8101; Bruce A. Chernof, M.D., Director and Chief Medical Officer
(Independent Hospital System)

LAC/UNIVERSITY OF SOUTHERN CALIFORNIA MEDICAL CENTER (O, 676 beds) 1200 North State Street, Los Angeles, CA Zip 90033–1029; tel. 323/226–2622; Pete Delgado, Chief Executive Officer
Web address: www.lacusc.org

LAC–HARBOR–UNIVERSITY OF CALIFORNIA AT LOS ANGELES MEDICAL CENTER (O, 343 beds) 1000 West Carson Street, Torrance, CA Zip 90502–2004; tel. 310/222–2345; Miguel Ortiz–Marroquin, Interim Chief Executive Officer
Web address: www.humc.edu

LAC–OLIVE VIEW–UCLA MEDICAL CENTER (O, 226 beds) 14445 Olive View Drive, Sylmar, CA Zip 91342–1495; tel. 818/364–1555; Gretchen McGinley, Interim Chief Executive Officer
Web address: www.ladhs.org

RANCHO LOS AMIGOS NATIONAL REHABILITATION CENTER (O, 207 beds) 7601 East Imperial Highway, Downey, CA Zip 90242–3496; tel. 562/401–7022; Jorge Orozco, Chief Executive Officer
Web address: www.rancho.org

Owned, leased, sponsored:	4 hospitals	1452 beds
Contract–managed:	0 hospitals	0 beds
Totals:	4 hospitals	1452 beds

0047: LOUISIANA STATE HOSPITALS (NP)

210 State Street, New Orleans, LA Zip 70118–5797; tel. 504/897–4616; Shelby Price, Chief Executive Officer
(Independent Hospital System)

LOUISIANA: CENTRAL LOUISIANA STATE HOSPITAL (O, 132 beds) 242 West Shamrock Avenue, Pineville, LA Zip 71361–5031, Mailing Address: P.O. Box 5031, Zip 71360–5031; tel. 318/484–6200; Patrick Kelly, Chief Executive Officer
Web address: www.dhh.la.gov/omh/inpatient–serv/clsh.htm

EASTERN LOUISIANA MENTAL HEALTH SYSTEM (O, 515 beds) 4502 Highway 951, Jackson, LA Zip 70748–5842, Mailing Address: P.O. Box 498, Zip 70748–0498; tel. 225/634–0100; Mark Anders, Chief Executive Officer
Web address: www.dhh.louisiana.gov/offices/locations.asp?ID=62&Detail=126

NEW ORLEANS ADOLESCENT HOSPITAL (O, 30 beds) 210 State Street, New Orleans, LA Zip 70118–5797; tel. 504/897–3400; Shelby Price, Chief Executive Officer

SOUTHEAST LOUISIANA HOSPITAL (O, 151 beds) 23515 Highway 190, Mandeville, LA Zip 70448–5612, Mailing Address: P.O. Box 3850, Zip 70470–3850; tel. 985/626–6300; Patricia Gonzales, Chief Executive Officer
Web address: www.dhh.state.la.us/offices/?ID=335

Owned, leased, sponsored:	4 hospitals	828 beds
Contract–managed:	0 hospitals	0 beds
Totals:	4 hospitals	828 beds

★0320: LRG HEALTHCARE (NP)

80 Highland Street, Laconia, NH Zip 03246–3298; tel. 603/524–3211; Thomas Clairmont, President
(Independent Hospital System)

NEW HAMPSHIRE: FRANKLIN REGIONAL HOSPITAL (O, 31 beds) 15 Aiken Avenue, Franklin, NH Zip 03235–1299; tel. 603/934–2060; Thomas Clairmont, President
Web address: www.lrgh.org

Section B

For explanation of codes following names, see page B2.
★ Indicates Type III membership in the American Hospital Association.

LAKES REGION GENERAL HOSPITAL (O, 113 beds) 80 Highland Street, Laconia, NH Zip 03246–3298; tel. 603/524–3211; Thomas Clairmont, President
Web address: www.lrgh.org

Owned, leased, sponsored:	2 hospitals	144 beds
Contract-managed:	0 hospitals	0 beds
Totals:	2 hospitals	144 beds

★0715: LSU HEALTH SCIENCES CENTER (NP)
8550 United Plaza Boulevard, 4th Floor, Baton Rouge, LA Zip 70809; tel. 225/922–0490; Michael K. Butler, M.D., Acting Chief Executive Officer
(Independent Hospital System)

LOUISIANA: EARL K. LONG MEDICAL CENTER (O, 146 beds) 5825 Airline Highway, Baton Rouge, LA Zip 70805–2498; tel. 225/358–1000; Kathy A. Viator, Interim Administrator
Web address: www.lsuhsc.edu

HUEY P. LONG MEDICAL CENTER (O, 60 beds) 352 Hospital Boulevard, Pineville, LA Zip 71360, Mailing Address: P.O. Box 5352, Zip 71361–5352; tel. 318/448–0811; Gary L. Crockett, Administrator
Web address: www.lsuhsc.edu/hcsd/hpl

LALLIE KEMP MEDICAL CENTER (O, 25 beds) 52579 Highway 51 South, Independence, LA Zip 70443–2231; tel. 985/878–9421; Sherre Pack-Hookfin, Administrator
Web address: www.lsuhospitals.org

LEONARD J. CHABERT MEDICAL CENTER (O, 85 beds) 1978 Industrial Boulevard, Houma, LA Zip 70363–7094; tel. 985/873–2200; Rhonda G. Green, Administrator
Web address: www.lsuhsc.edu/hcsd/ljc

LSU BOGALUSA MEDICAL CENTER (O, 66 beds) 433 Plaza Street, Bogalusa, LA Zip 70427–3793; tel. 985/730–6700; Kurt M. Scott, FACHE, Administrator

MEDICAL CENTER OF LOUISIANA AT NEW ORLEANS (O, 145 beds) 2021 Perdido Street, New Orleans, LA Zip 70112–1396; tel. 504/903–3000; Dwayne Thomas, M.D., Administrator
Web address: www.mclno.org

UNIVERSITY MEDICAL CENTER (O, 124 beds) 2390 West Congress Street, Lafayette, LA Zip 70506–4298, Mailing Address: P.O. Box 69300, Zip 70596–9300; tel. 337/261–6001; Lawrence T. Dorsey, Administrator
Web address: www.lsuhospitals.org

WALTER OLIN MOSS REGIONAL MEDICAL CENTER (O, 36 beds) 1000 Walters Street, Lake Charles, LA Zip 70605–4647; tel. 337/475–8100; Patrick C. Robinson, M.D., Administrator

Owned, leased, sponsored:	8 hospitals	687 beds
Contract-managed:	0 hospitals	0 beds
Totals:	8 hospitals	687 beds

★5305: MARIAN HEALTH SYSTEM (CC)
1923 South Utica Avenue, Tulsa, OK Zip 74104, Mailing Address: P.O. Box 4753, Zip 74159–0753; tel. 918/742–9988; Sister M. Therese Gottschalk, President
(Moderately Centralized Health System)

MINNESOTA: SAINT ELIZABETH'S MEDICAL CENTER (O, 168 beds) 1200 Grant Boulevard West, Wabasha, MN Zip 55981–1098; tel. 651/565–4531; Thomas Crowley, President and Chief Executive Officer
Web address: www.stelizabethswabasha.org

OKLAHOMA: JANE PHILLIPS MEDICAL CENTER (O, 137 beds) 3500 East Frank Phillips Boulevard, Bartlesville, OK Zip 74006–2409; tel. 918/333–7200; David R. Stire, President and Chief Executive Officer
Web address: www.jpmc.org

ST. JOHN MEDICAL CENTER (O, 560 beds) 1923 South Utica Avenue, Tulsa, OK Zip 74104–6502; tel. 918/744–2345; S. Charles Anderson, President and Chief Executive Officer
Web address: www.sjmc.org

ST. JOHN OWASSO (O, 24 beds) 12451 East 100th Street North, Owasso, OK Zip 74055; tel. 918/274–5000; David Phillips, President and Chief Executive Officer
Web address: www.stjohnowasso.com

ST. JOHN SAPULPA (O, 25 beds) 519 South Division Street, Sapulpa, OK Zip 74066–4501, Mailing Address: P.O. Box 1368, Zip 74067–1368; tel. 918/224–4280; Raymond L. Replogle, President and Chief Executive Officer
Web address: www.sjmc.org

WISCONSIN: DOOR COUNTY MEMORIAL HOSPITAL (O, 55 beds) 323 South 18th Avenue, Sturgeon Bay, WI Zip 54235–1495; tel. 920/743–5566; Gerald M. Worrick, President and Chief Executive Officer
Web address: www.dcmh.org

EAGLE RIVER MEMORIAL HOSPITAL (O, 10 beds) 201 Hospital Road, Eagle River, WI Zip 54521–8835; tel. 715/479–7411; Sheila Clough, President
Web address: www.ministryhealth.org

FLAMBEAU HOSPITAL (O, 25 beds) 98 Sherry Avenue, Park Falls, WI Zip 54552–1467, Mailing Address: P.O. Box 310, Zip 54552–0310; tel. 715/762–2484; David A. Grundstrom, Chief Administrative Officer
Web address: www.flambeauhospital.org

GOOD SAMARITAN HEALTH CENTER OF MERRILL (O, 11 beds) 601 Center Avenue South, Merrill, WI Zip 54452–3404; tel. 715/536–5511; Michael Hammer, President and Chief Operating Officer
Web address: www.ministryhealth.org

HOWARD YOUNG MEDICAL CENTER (O, 65 beds) 240 Maple Street, Woodruff, WI Zip 54568, Mailing Address: P.O. Box 470, Zip 54568–0470; tel. 715/356–8000; Sheila Clough, President
Web address: www.ministryhealth.org

OUR LADY OF VICTORY HOSPITAL (O, 24 beds) 1120 Pine Street, Stanley, WI Zip 54768–0220, Mailing Address: P.O. Box 220, Zip 54768–0220; tel. 715/644–5571; Cynthia Eichman, President and Chief Executive Officer
Web address: www.ministryhealth.org

SACRED HEART–ST. MARY'S HOSPITALS (O, 45 beds) 2251 North Shore Drive, Rhinelander, WI Zip 54501–3998; tel. 715/361–2000; Monica Hilt, President and Chief Operating Officer
Web address: www.ministryhealth.org

SAINT CLARE'S HOSPITAL (O, 37 beds) 3400 Ministry Parkway, Weston, WI Zip 54476; tel. 715/393–3000; Mary T. Krueger, President
Web address: www.ministryhealth.org

SAINT JOSEPH'S HOSPITAL (O, 319 beds) 611 St. Joseph Avenue, Marshfield, WI Zip 54449–1898; tel. 715/387–1713; Michael A. Schmidt, President
Web address: www.stjosephs-marshfield.org

SAINT MICHAEL'S HOSPITAL (O, 48 beds) 900 Illinois Avenue, Stevens Point, WI Zip 54481–3196; tel. 715/346–5000; Bradley Neet, President
Web address: www.saintmichaelshospital.org

Owned, leased, sponsored:	15 hospitals	1553 beds
Contract-managed:	0 hospitals	0 beds
Totals:	15 hospitals	1553 beds

★1975: MARSHALL COUNTY HEALTH CARE AUTHORITY (NP)
227 Britany Road, Guntersville, AL Zip 35976; tel. 256/894–6615; Gary R. Gore, Chief Executive Officer

ALABAMA: MARSHALL MEDICAL CENTER NORTH (O, 90 beds) 8000 Alabama Highway 69, Guntersville, AL Zip 35976; tel. 256/753–8000; Cheryl M. Hays, FACHE, Administrator
Web address: www.mmcenters.com

MARSHALL MEDICAL CENTER SOUTH (O, 102 beds) U.S. Highway 431 North, Boaz, AL Zip 35957–0999, Mailing Address: P.O. Box 758, Zip 35957–0758; tel. 256/593–8310; John D. Anderson, Administrator
Web address: www.mmcs.org

Owned, leased, sponsored:	2 hospitals	192 beds
Contract-managed:	0 hospitals	0 beds
Totals:	2 hospitals	192 beds

0013: MASSACHUSETTS DEPARTMENT OF MENTAL HEALTH (NP)
25 Staniford Street, Boston, MA Zip 02114–2575; tel. 617/626–8123; Elizabeth Childs, M.D., Commissioner

MASSACHUSETTS: DR. J. CORRIGAN MENTAL HEALTH CENTER (O, 16 beds) 49 Hillside Street, Fall River, MA Zip 02720–5266; tel. 508/235–7200; Steve Figueiredo, Interim Director

For explanation of codes following names, see page B2.
★ Indicates Type III membership in the American Hospital Association.

TAUNTON STATE HOSPITAL (O, 185 beds) 60 Hodges Avenue Extension, Taunton, MA Zip 02780–3034, Mailing Address: P.O. Box 4007, Zip 02780–4007; tel. 508/977–3000; Roberta H. Guez, Administrator and Chief Operating Officer

WESTBOROUGH STATE HOSPITAL (O, 220 beds) Lyman Street, Westborough, MA Zip 01581–0288, Mailing Address: P.O. Box 288, Zip 01581–0288; tel. 508/616–2100; Joel Skolnick, Chief Operating Officer

WORCESTER STATE HOSPITAL (O, 126 beds) 305 Belmont Street, Worcester, MA Zip 01604–1695; tel. 508/368–3300; Anthony Riccitelli, Chief Operating Officer

Owned, leased, sponsored:	4 hospitals	547 beds
Contract-managed:	0 hospitals	0 beds
Totals:	4 hospitals	547 beds

0280: MASSACHUSETTS DEPARTMENT OF PUBLIC HEALTH (NP)
250 Washington Street, Boston, MA Zip 02108–4619; tel. 617/624–6000; John Auerbach, Commissioner
(Independent Hospital System)

LEMUEL SHATTUCK HOSPITAL (O, 260 beds) 170 Morton Street, Jamaica Plain, MA Zip 02130–3787; tel. 617/522–8110; Paul Romary, Chief Executive Officer
Web address: www.shattuckhospital.org

MASSACHUSETTS HOSPITAL SCHOOL (O, 86 beds) 3 Randolph Street, Canton, MA Zip 02021–2397; tel. 781/828–2440; Katherine Ann Chmiel, RN, M.S., Chief Executive Officer
Web address: www.state.ma.us/dph/hosp/mhs.htm

TEWKSBURY HOSPITAL (O, 720 beds) 365 East Street, Tewksbury, MA Zip 01876–1998; tel. 978/851–7321; Sandra Akers, Chief Executive Officer
Web address: www.state.ma.us/dph/hosp/th.htm

WESTERN MASSACHUSETTS HOSPITAL (O, 80 beds) 91 East Mountain Road, Westfield, MA Zip 1085; tel. 413/562–4131; Blake M. Molleur, Chief Executive Officer
Web address: www.mass.gov/dph/hosp/wmh.htm

Owned, leased, sponsored:	4 hospitals	1146 beds
Contract-managed:	0 hospitals	0 beds
Totals:	4 hospitals	1146 beds

★1875: MAYO FOUNDATION (NP)
200 S.W. First Street, Rochester, MN Zip 55905–0002; tel. 507/284–2511; Denis A. Cortese, M.D., President and Chief Executive Officer
(Moderately Centralized Health System)

ARIZONA: MAYO CLINIC HOSPITAL (O, 217 beds) 5777 East Mayo Boulevard, Phoenix, AZ Zip 85054–4502; tel. 480/515–6296; Thomas C. Bour, Administrator
Web address: www.mayoclinic.org

FLORIDA: MAYO CLINIC JACKSONVILLE (L, 313 beds) 4500 San Pablo Road, Jacksonville, FL Zip 32224; tel. 904/953–2000; Hilary G. Mathews, Administrator
Web address: www.mayoclinic.org

IOWA: FLOYD COUNTY MEDICAL CENTER (C, 25 beds) 800 Eleventh Street, Charles City, IA Zip 50616–3499; tel. 641/228–6830; Bill D. Faust, Administrator

MINNESOTA: ALBERT LEA MEDICAL CENTER (O, 129 beds) 404 West Fountain Street, Albert Lea, MN Zip 56007–2473; tel. 507/373–2384; Mark Ciota, M.D., Chief Executive Officer
Web address: www.almedcenter.org

AUSTIN MEDICAL CENTER (O, 82 beds) 1000 First Drive N.W., Austin, MN Zip 55912–2904; tel. 507/437–4551; Timothy Johnson, M.D., President and Chief Executive Officer
Web address: www.austinmedicalcenter.org

CANNON FALLS MEDICAL CENTER (C, 21 beds) 1116 West Mill Street, Cannon Falls, MN Zip 55009–1898; tel. 507/263–4221; Glenn Christian, Administrator
Web address: www.cannonhealth.org/

FAIRMONT MEDICAL CENTER–MAYO HEALTH SYSTEM (O, 97 beds) 800 Medical Center Drive, Fairmont, MN Zip 56031–0800; tel. 507/238–8100; Barbara Allen, M.D., President and Chief Executive Officer
Web address: www.fairmontmedicalcenter.org

IMMANUEL ST. JOSEPH'S–MAYO HEALTH SYSTEM (O, 174 beds) 1025 Marsh Street, Mankato, MN Zip 56002–8673, Mailing Address: P.O. Box 8673, Zip 56002–8673; tel. 507/625–4031; Greg Kutcher, M.D., President and Chief Executive Officer
Web address: www.isj–mhs.org

LAKE CITY MEDICAL CENTER–MAYO (O, 111 beds) 500 West Grant Street, Lake City, MN Zip 55041–1143; tel. 651/345–3321; Thomas J. Witt, M.D., President and Chief Executive Officer
Web address: www.lakecitymedicalcenter.org

ROCHESTER METHODIST HOSPITAL (O, 335 beds) 201 West Center Street, Rochester, MN Zip 55902–3084; tel. 507/266–7890; Lynn Frederick, Administrator
Web address: www.mayoclinic.org

SAINT MARYS HOSPITAL (O, 797 beds) 1216 Second Street S.W., Rochester, MN Zip 55902–1970; tel. 507/255–5123; Lynn Frederick, Administrator
Web address: www.mayoclinic.org

SPRINGFIELD MEDICAL CENTER–MAYO HEALTH SYSTEM (O, 24 beds) 625 North Jackson Avenue, Springfield, MN Zip 56087–1714, Mailing Address: P.O. Box 146, Zip 56087–0146; tel. 507/723–6201; Scott D. Thoreson, Administrator
Web address: www.smc–mhs.org

ST. JAMES MEDICAL CENTER (C, 13 beds) 1101 Moulton and Parsons Drive, Saint James, MN Zip 56081; tel. 507/375–3261; Matthew Grimshaw, Administrator
Web address: www.stjmc–mhs.org

WASECA MEDICAL CENTER (O, 25 beds) 501 North State Street, Waseca, MN Zip 56093–2811; tel. 507/835–1210; Michael Milbrath, Executive Vice President
Web address: www.wmc–mhs.org

WISCONSIN: FRANCISCAN SKEMP HEALTHCARE–ARCADIA CAMPUS (O, 25 beds) 464 South St. Joseph Avenue, Arcadia, WI Zip 54612–1401; tel. 608/323–3341; Darlene Feltes, Administrator
Web address: www.mayohealthsystem.com

FRANCISCAN SKEMP HEALTHCARE–LA CROSSE CAMPUS (O, 198 beds) 700 West Avenue South, La Crosse, WI Zip 54601–4783; tel. 608/785–0940; Robert Nesse, M.D., President and Chief Executive Officer
Web address: www.franciscanskemp.org

FRANCISCAN SKEMP HEALTHCARE–SPARTA CAMPUS (O, 25 beds) 310 West Main Street, Sparta, WI Zip 54656–2171; tel. 608/269–2132; Robert M. Tracey, Administrator
Web address: www.mayohealthsystem.com

LUTHER HOSPITAL (O, 172 beds) 1221 Whipple Street, Eau Claire, WI Zip 54702–4105, Mailing Address: P.O. Box 5, Zip 54702–0005; tel. 715/838–3311; Randall L. Linton, M.D., President and Chief Executive Officer
Web address: www.mhs.mayo.edu

LUTHER MIDELFORT CHIPPEWA VALLEY (O, 54 beds) 1501 Thompson Street, Bloomer, WI Zip 54724–1299; tel. 715/568–2000; Colleen Skold, Administrator
Web address: www.bloomermedicalcenter.org

LUTHER MIDELFORT NORTHLAND (O, 57 beds) 1222 Woodland Avenue, Barron, WI Zip 54812–1798; tel. 715/537–3186; Maurita Sullivan, Administrator
Web address: www.luthermidelfortnorthland.org

LUTHER MIDELFORT OAKRIDGE (C, 104 beds) 13025 Eighth Street, Osseo, WI Zip 54758–7673, Mailing Address: P.O. Box 70, Zip 54758–0070; tel. 715/597–3121; Michael Ryan, Administrator
Web address: www.luthermidelfortoakridge.com

RED CEDAR MEDICAL CENTER–MAYO HEALTH SYSTEM (O, 25 beds) 2321 Stout Road, Menomonie, WI Zip 54751–2397; tel. 715/235–5531; Hank Simpson, M.D., Chief Executive Officer
Web address: www.rcmc–mhs.org

Owned, leased, sponsored:	18 hospitals	2860 beds
Contract-managed:	4 hospitals	163 beds
Totals:	22 hospitals	3023 beds

For explanation of codes following names, see page B2.
★ Indicates Type III membership in the American Hospital Association.

0252: MCLAREN HEALTH CARE CORPORATION (NP)
G3235 Beecher Road, Suite B., Flint, MI Zip 48532; tel. 810/342–1100; Philip A. Incarnati, President and Chief Executive Officer
(Centralized Physician/Insurance Health System)

MICHIGAN: BAY REGIONAL MEDICAL CENTER (O, 320 beds) 1900 Columbus Avenue, Bay City, MI Zip 48708–6880; tel. 989/894–3000; Alice Gerard, President and Chief Executive Officer
Web address: www.bayregional.org

INGHAM REGIONAL MEDICAL CENTER (O, 352 beds) 401 West Greenlawn Avenue, Lansing, MI Zip 48910–2819; tel. 517/334–2121; Robert N. Wright, President and Chief Executive Officer
Web address: www.irmc.org

LAPEER REGIONAL MEDICAL CENTER (O, 222 beds) 1375 North Main Street, Lapeer, MI Zip 48446–1376; tel. 810/667–5500; Barton Buxton, President and Chief Executive Officer
Web address: www.lapeerhospital.org

MCLAREN REGIONAL MEDICAL CENTER (O, 324 beds) 401 South Ballenger Highway, Flint, MI Zip 48532–3685; tel. 810/342–2000; Donald C. Kooy, President and Chief Executive Officer
Web address: www.mclarenregional.org

MOUNT CLEMENS REGIONAL MEDICAL CENTER (O, 288 beds) 1000 Harrington Boulevard, Mount Clemens, MI Zip 48043–2992; tel. 586/493–8000; Mark S. O'Halla, President and Chief Executive Officer
Web address: www.mcrmc.org

POH REGIONAL MEDICAL CENTER (O, 268 beds) 50 North Perry Street, Pontiac, MI Zip 48342–2253; tel. 248/338–5000; Patrick Lamberti, Chief Executive Officer
Web address: www.pohmedical.org

Owned, leased, sponsored:	6 hospitals	1774 beds
Contract-managed:	0 hospitals	0 beds
Totals:	6 hospitals	1774 beds

0200: MEDCATH, INC. (IO)
10720 Sikes Place, Suite 300, Charlotte, NC Zip 28277–8143; tel. 704/708–6600; O. Edwin French, President and Chief Executive Officer
(Independent Hospital System)

ARIZONA: ARIZONA HEART HOSPITAL (O, 59 beds) 1930 East Thomas Road, Phoenix, AZ Zip 85016; tel. 602/532–1000; James R. Resendez, Chief Executive Officer
Web address: www.azheart.com

ARKANSAS: ARKANSAS HEART HOSPITAL (O, 84 beds) 1701 South Shackleford Road, Little Rock, AR Zip 72211–4335; tel. 501/219–7000; Charlie Smith, President
Web address: www.arheart.com

CALIFORNIA: BAKERSFIELD HEART HOSPITAL (O, 46 beds) 3001 Sillect Avenue, Bakersfield, CA Zip 93308–6337; tel. 661/316–6000; Richard Priore, Interim Chief Executive Officer
Web address: www.bakersfieldhearthospital.com

LOUISIANA: HEART HOSPITAL OF LAFAYETTE (O, 32 beds) 1105 Kaliste Saloom, Lafayette, LA Zip 70508; tel. 337/521–1000; Karen O. Wyble, Interim President
Web address: www.hearthospitaloflafayette.com

LOUISIANA MEDICAL CENTER AND HEART HOSPITAL (O, 58 beds) 64030 Highway 434, Lacombe, LA Zip 70445; tel. 985/690–7500; William W. Fox, III, President
Web address: www.louisianahearthospital.com

NEW MEXICO: HEART HOSPITAL OF NEW MEXICO (O, 55 beds) 504 Elm Street, Albuquerque, NM Zip 87102; tel. 505/724–2000; Ronald C. Winger, President
Web address: www.hearthospitalnm.com

OHIO: DAYTON HEART HOSPITAL (O, 47 beds) 707 South Edwin C. Moses Boulevard, Dayton, OH Zip 45408; tel. 937/221–8000; ,
Web address: www.daytonhearthospital.com

SOUTH DAKOTA: AVERA HEART HOSPITAL OF SOUTH DAKOTA (O, 55 beds) 4500 West 69th Street, Sioux Falls, SD Zip 57108–8148; tel. 605/977–7000; Jon Soderholm, President
Web address: www.southdakotaheart.com

TEXAS: HARLINGEN MEDICAL CENTER (O, 88 beds) 5501 South Expressway 77, Harlingen, TX Zip 78550; tel. 956/365–1000; Daniel P. McLean, President and Chief Executive Officer
Web address: www.harlingenmedicalcenter.com

HEART HOSPITAL OF AUSTIN (O, 58 beds) 3801 North Lamar Boulevard, Austin, TX Zip 78756; tel. 512/407–7000; David Laird, President
Web address: www.hearthospitalofaustin.com

TEXSAN HEART HOSPITAL (O, 60 beds) 6700 IH–10 West, San Antonio, TX Zip 78201; tel. 210/736–6700; P. Craig Desmond, President
Web address: www.texsanhearthospital.com

Owned, leased, sponsored:	11 hospitals	642 beds
Contract-managed:	0 hospitals	0 beds
Totals:	11 hospitals	642 beds

0391: MEDCENTRAL HEALTH SYSTEM (NP)
335 Glessner Avenue, Mansfield, OH Zip 44903; tel. 419/526–8000; James E. Meyer, President and Chief Executive Officer

OHIO: MEDCENTRAL – MANSFIELD HOSPITAL (O, 308 beds) 335 Glessner Avenue, Mansfield, OH Zip 44903–2265; tel. 419/526–8000; James E. Meyer, President and Chief Executive Officer
Web address: www.medcentral.org

MEDCENTRAL – SHELBY HOSPITAL (O, 25 beds) 20 Morris Road, Shelby, OH Zip 44875; tel. 419/342–5015; Ron Distl, Chief Executive Officer
Web address: www.medcentral.org/body.cfm?id=153

Owned, leased, sponsored:	2 hospitals	333 beds
Contract-managed:	0 hospitals	0 beds
Totals:	2 hospitals	333 beds

★0154: MEDSTAR HEALTH (NP)
5565 Sterrett Place, 5th Floor, Columbia, MD Zip 21044; tel. 410/772–6500; Kenneth A. Samet, President and Chief Executive Officer
(Centralized Health System)

DISTRICT OF COLUMBIA: MEDSTAR-GEORGETOWN MEDICAL CENTER (O, 390 beds) 3800 Reservoir Road N.W., Washington, DC Zip 20007–2197; tel. 202/444–3000; M. Joy Drass, M.D., President
Web address: www.georgetownuniversityhospital.org

NATIONAL REHABILITATION HOSPITAL (O, 137 beds) 102 Irving Street N.W., Washington, DC Zip 20010–2949; tel. 202/877–1000; Edward A. Eckenhoff, President and Chief Executive Officer
Web address: www.nrhrehab.org

WASHINGTON HOSPITAL CENTER (O, 841 beds) 110 Irving Street N.W., Washington, DC Zip 20010–2975; tel. 202/877–7000; James F. Caldas, President
Web address: www.whcenter.org

MARYLAND: FRANKLIN SQUARE HOSPITAL CENTER (O, 347 beds) 9000 Franklin Square Drive, Baltimore, MD Zip 21237–2998; tel. 443/777–7000; Carl J. Schindelar, President
Web address: www.franklinsquare.org

GOOD SAMARITAN HOSPITAL OF MARYLAND (O, 315 beds) 5601 Loch Raven Boulevard, Baltimore, MD Zip 21239–2995; tel. 410/532–8000; Lawrence M. Beck, President
Web address: www.goodsam–md.org

HARBOR HOSPITAL (O, 240 beds) 3001 South Hanover Street, Baltimore, MD Zip 21225–1290; tel. 410/350–3200; Joseph M. Oddis, President
Web address: www.harborhospital.org

MONTGOMERY GENERAL HOSPITAL (O, 149 beds) 18101 Prince Philip Drive, Olney, MD Zip 20832–1512; tel. 301/774–8882; Peter W. Monge, President
Web address: www.montgomerygeneral.com

UNION MEMORIAL HOSPITAL (O, 273 beds) 201 East University Parkway, Baltimore, MD Zip 21218–2895; tel. 410/554–2000; Harrison J. Rider, III, President
Web address: www.unionmemorial.org

Owned, leased, sponsored:	8 hospitals	2692 beds
Contract-managed:	0 hospitals	0 beds
Totals:	8 hospitals	2692 beds

For explanation of codes following names, see page B2.
★ Indicates Type III membership in the American Hospital Association.

0084: MEMORIAL HEALTH SERVICES (NP)
2801 Atlantic Avenue, Long Beach, CA Zip 90806, Mailing Address: P.O. Box 1428, Zip 90801–1428; tel. 562/933–2000; Barry S. Arbuckle, Ph.D., President and Chief Executive Officer
(Centralized Health System)

CALIFORNIA: ANAHEIM MEMORIAL MEDICAL CENTER (O, 223 beds) 1111 West La Palma Avenue, Anaheim, CA Zip 92801–2881; tel. 714/774–1450; Byron F. Schweigert, Interim Chief Executive Officer
Web address: www.memorialcare.org

LONG BEACH MEMORIAL MEDICAL CENTER (O, 462 beds) 2801 Atlantic Avenue, Long Beach, CA Zip 90806–1737, Mailing Address: P.O. Box 1428, Zip 90801–1428; tel. 562/933–2000; Terry A. Belmont, Chief Executive Officer
Web address: www.memorialcare.org

MILLER CHILDREN'S HOSPITAL (O, 308 beds) 2801 Atlantic Avenue, Long Beach, CA Zip 90806; tel. 562/933–5437; Terry A. Belmont, Chief Executive Officer
Web address: www.memorialcare.org

ORANGE COAST MEMORIAL MEDICAL CENTER (O, 224 beds) 9920 Talbert Avenue, Fountain Valley, CA Zip 92708–5153; tel. 714/378–7000; Marcia Manker, Chief Executive Officer
Web address: www.memorialcare.org

SADDLEBACK MEMORIAL MEDICAL CENTER (O, 252 beds) 24451 Health Center Drive, Laguna Hills, CA Zip 92653–3689; tel. 949/837–4500; Steve Geidt, Chief Executive Officer
Web address: www.memorialcare.org

SADDLEBACK MEMORIAL MEDICAL CENTER – SAN CLEMENTE CAMPUS (O, 73 beds) 654 Camino De Los Mares, San Clemente, CA Zip 92673–2827; tel. 949/496–1122; Liz Bear, Administrator
Web address: www.sanclementehospital.com

Owned, leased, sponsored:	6 hospitals	1542 beds
Contract–managed:	0 hospitals	0 beds
Totals:	6 hospitals	1542 beds

★0086: MEMORIAL HEALTH SYSTEM (NP)
701 North First Street, Springfield, IL Zip 62781–0001; tel. 217/788–3000; Edgar J. Curtis, RN, President and Chief Executive Officer
(Centralized Physician/Insurance Health System)

ILLINOIS: ABRAHAM LINCOLN MEMORIAL HOSPITAL (O, 25 beds) 315 8th Street, Lincoln, IL Zip 62656–2698; tel. 217/732–2161; Dolan Dalpoas, President and Chief Executive Officer
Web address: www.almh.org

MEMORIAL MEDICAL CENTER (O, 446 beds) 701 North First Street, Springfield, IL Zip 62781–0001; tel. 217/788–3000; Edgar J. Curtis, RN, Executive Vice President and Chief Operating Officer
Web address: www.memorialmedical.com

TAYLORVILLE MEMORIAL HOSPITAL (O, 45 beds) 201 East Pleasant Street, Taylorville, IL Zip 62568–1597; tel. 217/824–3331; Daniel J. Raab, President and Chief Executive Officer
Web address: www.taylorvillememorial.org

Owned, leased, sponsored:	3 hospitals	516 beds
Contract–managed:	0 hospitals	0 beds
Totals:	3 hospitals	516 beds

0176: MEMORIAL HEALTH SYSTEM OF EAST TEXAS (NP)
1201 West Frank Avenue, Lufkin, TX Zip 75904–3357; tel. 936/634–8111; Bryant H. Krenek, Jr., President and Chief Executive Officer
(Moderately Centralized Health System)

TEXAS: MEMORIAL HEALTH SYSTEM OF EAST TEXAS (O, 180 beds) 1201 West Frank Avenue, Lufkin, TX Zip 75904–3357, Mailing Address: P.O. Box 1447, Zip 75902–1447; tel. 936/634–8111; Bryant H. Krenek, Jr., President and Chief Executive Officer
Web address: www.memorialhealth.org

MEMORIAL MEDICAL CENTER – LIVINGSTON (O, 66 beds) 1717 Highway 59 Bypass, Livingston, TX Zip 77351–1257, Mailing Address: P.O. Box 1257, Zip 77351–1257; tel. 936/329–8700; David LeMonte, Chief Executive Officer
Web address: www.memorialhealth.org

MEMORIAL MEDICAL CENTER – SAN AUGUSTINE (O, 18 beds) 511 East Hospital Street, San Augustine, TX Zip 75972–2121, Mailing Address: P.O. Box 658, Zip 75972–0658; tel. 936/275–3446; Darlene Williams, RN, Administrator
Web address: www.memorialhealth.org

MEMORIAL SPECIALTY HOSPITAL (O, 16 beds) 1201 West Frank Avenue, Lufkin, TX Zip 75904; tel. 936/639–7975; Brenda Broadway, Administrator
Web address: www.memorialhealth.org

Owned, leased, sponsored:	4 hospitals	280 beds
Contract–managed:	0 hospitals	0 beds
Totals:	4 hospitals	280 beds

★0083: MEMORIAL HEALTHCARE SYSTEM (NP)
3501 Johnson Street, Hollywood, FL Zip 33021–5421; tel. 954/985–5805; Frank V. Sacco, FACHE, President and Chief Executive Officer
(Centralized Health System)

FLORIDA: MEMORIAL HOSPITAL MIRAMAR (O, 128 beds) 1901 S.W. 172nd Avenue, Miramar, FL Zip 33029; tel. 954/538–5000; Aurelio Fernandez, Administrator
Web address: www.mhs.net

MEMORIAL HOSPITAL PEMBROKE (L, 149 beds) 7800 Sheridan Street, Pembroke Pines, FL Zip 33024–2536; tel. 954/962–9650; Zeff Ross, Interim Administrator
Web address: www.mhs–net.com

MEMORIAL HOSPITAL WEST (O, 299 beds) 703 North Flamingo Road, Pembroke Pines, FL Zip 33028–1014; tel. 954/436–5000; Kennon Hetlage, Chief Executive Officer Administrator
Web address: www.mhs.net

MEMORIAL REGIONAL HOSPITAL (O, 690 beds) 3501 Johnson Street, Hollywood, FL Zip 33021–5421; tel. 954/987–2000; Rodney E. Miller, Sr., Administrator
Web address: www.mhs.net

MEMORIAL REGIONAL HOSPITAL SOUTH (O, 120 beds) 3600 Washington Street, Hollywood, FL Zip 33021–8216; tel. 954/966–4500; Douglas Zaren, FACHE, Administrator
Web address: www.memorialregionalsouth.com

Owned, leased, sponsored:	5 hospitals	1386 beds
Contract–managed:	0 hospitals	0 beds
Totals:	5 hospitals	1386 beds

★2645: MEMORIAL HERMANN HEALTHCARE SYSTEM (NP)
7737 S.W. Freeway, Suite 200, Houston, TX Zip 77074–1800; tel. 713/456–5550; Daniel J. Wolterman, President and Chief Executive Officer
(Centralized Health System)

TEXAS: MEMORIAL HERMANN – THE INSTITUTE FOR REHABILITATION AND RESEARCH (O, 98 beds) 1333 Moursund, Houston, TX Zip 77030–3405; tel. 713/797–5278; Carl E. Josehart, Chief Executive Officer
Web address: www.memorialhermann.org/locations/tirr.html

MEMORIAL HERMANN HOSPITAL (O, 766 beds) 6411 Fannin, Houston, TX Zip 77030–1501; tel. 713/704–4000; Juanita F. Romans, Chief Executive Officer
Web address: www.mhhs.org

MEMORIAL HERMANN KATY HOSPITAL (O, 127 beds) 23900 Katy Freeway, Katy, TX Zip 77494; tel. 281/644–7000; Brian S. Barbe, Chief Executive Officer
Web address: www.memorialhermann.org

MEMORIAL HERMANN MEMORIAL CITY HOSPITAL (L, 343 beds) 921 Gessner Road, Houston, TX Zip 77024–9173; tel. 713/242–3000; David L. Jones, Interim Chief Executive Officer
Web address: www.memorialhermann.org

For explanation of codes following names, see page B2.
★ Indicates Type III membership in the American Hospital Association.

Section B

MEMORIAL HERMANN NORTHEAST (L, 243 beds) 18951 Memorial North, Humble, TX Zip 77338–4297; tel. 281/540–7700; Louis G. Smith, Jr., Chief Executive Officer
Web address: www.memorialhermann.org

MEMORIAL HERMANN SOUTHEAST (O, 265 beds) 11800 Astoria, Houston, TX Zip 77089; tel. 281/929–6100; ,
Web address: www.memorialhermann.org

MEMORIAL HERMANN SOUTHWEST HOSPITAL (O, 485 beds) 7600 Beechnut, Houston, TX Zip 77074–1850; tel. 713/456–5000; Sonja Hagel, Chief Executive Officer
Web address: www.memorialhermann.org

MEMORIAL HERMANN SUGAR LAND HOSPITAL (O, 77 beds) 17500 West Grand Parkway South, Sugar Land, TX Zip 77479; tel. 281/725–5000; Jim Brown, Chief Executive Officer
Web address: www.memorialhermann.org

Owned, leased, sponsored:	8 hospitals	2404 beds
Contract-managed:	0 hospitals	0 beds
Totals:	8 hospitals	2404 beds

★0257: MERIDIAN HEALTH (NP)
1350 Campus Parkway, Neptune, NJ Zip 07753; tel. 732/751–7510; John K. Lloyd, President and Chief Executive Officer
(Centralized Health System)

NEW JERSEY: JERSEY SHORE UNIVERSITY MEDICAL CENTER (O, 453 beds) 1945 Route 33, Neptune, NJ Zip 07754–0397; tel. 732/775–5500; Steven G. Littleson, President
Web address: www.meridianhealth.com

OCEAN MEDICAL CENTER (O, 229 beds) 425 Jack Martin Boulevard, Brick Township, NJ Zip 8724; tel. 732/840–2200; W. Peter Daniels, President
Web address: www.meridianhealth.com

RIVERVIEW MEDICAL CENTER (O, 278 beds) 1 Riverview Plaza, Red Bank, NJ Zip 07701–9982; tel. 732/741–2700; Timothy J. Hogan, President
Web address: www.meridianhealth.com

Owned, leased, sponsored:	3 hospitals	960 beds
Contract-managed:	0 hospitals	0 beds
Totals:	3 hospitals	960 beds

0291: MERIT HEALTH SYSTEMS (IO)
333 East Main Street, Suite 300, Louisville, KY Zip 40202; tel. 502/753–0890; Tyree Wilburn, Chaiman, President and Chief Executive Officer
(Independent Hospital System)

ILLINOIS: LINCOLN PARK HOSPITAL (O, 158 beds) 550 Webster Avenue, Chicago, IL Zip 60614–9980; tel. 773/883–2000; Frank G. DeLisi, III, CHE, Chief Executive Officer
Web address: www.lincolnparkhospital.com

NEW JERSEY: MOUNTAINSIDE HOSPITAL (O, 233 beds) 1 Bay Avenue, Montclair, NJ Zip 07042–4898; tel. 973/429–6000; C. Barry Dykes, President and Chief Executive Officer
Web address: www.mountainsidenow.com

TEXAS: NIX HEALTH CARE SYSTEM (O, 164 beds) 414 Navarro Street, San Antonio, TX Zip 78205–2522; tel. 210/271–1800; John F. Strieby, Chief Executive Officer
Web address: www.nixhealth.com

Owned, leased, sponsored:	3 hospitals	555 beds
Contract-managed:	0 hospitals	0 beds
Totals:	3 hospitals	555 beds

★0287: MERITCARE HEALTH SYSTEM (NP)
801 Broadway North, Fargo, ND Zip 58122; tel. 701/234–2000; Roger L. Gilbertson, M.D., President and Chief Executive Officer
(Moderately Centralized Health System)

MINNESOTA: CLEARWATER HEALTH SERVICES (C, 95 beds) 203 Fourth Street N.W., Bagley, MN Zip 56621–8307; tel. 218/694–6501; Bonnie Anderson, Interim Chief Executive Officer
Web address: www.clearwaterhs.com

MAHNOMEN HEALTH CENTER (C, 66 beds) 414 West Jefferson Avenue, Mahnomen, MN Zip 56557–4912, Mailing Address: P.O. Box 396, Zip 56557–0396; tel. 218/935–2511; Susan Klabo, Administrator
Web address: www.mahnomenhealthcenter.com

PERHAM MEMORIAL HOSPITAL AND HOME (C, 115 beds) 665 Third Street S.W., Perham, MN Zip 56573–1199; tel. 218/346–4500; Chuck Hofius, Chief Executive Officer and Administrator
Web address: www.pmhh.com

NORTH DAKOTA: HILLSBORO MEDICAL CENTER (C, 62 beds) 12 Third Street S.E., Hillsboro, ND Zip 58045, Mailing Address: P.O. Box 609, Zip 58045–0609; tel. 701/636–4501; Patricia Dirk, Administrator
Web address: www.hillsboromedicalcenter.com

MERITCARE MEDICAL CENTER (O, 447 beds) 720 Fourth Street North, Fargo, ND Zip 58122; tel. 701/234–6000; Roger L. Gilbertson, M.D., President and Chief Executive Officer
Web address: www.meritcare.com

Owned, leased, sponsored:	1 hospital	447 beds
Contract-managed:	4 hospitals	338 beds
Totals:	5 hospitals	785 beds

★2735: METHODIST HEALTH SYSTEM (NP)
1441 North Beckley Avenue, Dallas, TX Zip 75203–1201, Mailing Address: P.O. Box 655999, Zip 75265–5999; tel. 214/947–8181; Stephen L. Mansfield, Ph.D., FACHE, President and Chief Executive Officer
(Independent Hospital System)

TEXAS: METHODIST CHARLTON MEDICAL CENTER (O, 240 beds) 3500 West Wheatland Road, Dallas, TX Zip 75237–3460, Mailing Address: Box 225357, Zip 75222–5357; tel. 214/947–7777; Zachary Chandler, President
Web address: www.mhs.com

METHODIST DALLAS MEDICAL CENTER (O, 488 beds) 1441 North Beckley Avenue, Dallas, TX Zip 75203–1201, Mailing Address: Box 655999, Zip 75265–5999; tel. 214/947–8181; Michael A. Mayo, FACHE, President
Web address: www.mhd.com

METHODIST MANSFIELD MEDICAL CENTER (O, 80 beds) 2700 East Broad Street, Mansfield, TX Zip 76063–5899; tel. 682/622–2000; Laura Irvine, President
Web address: www.mhd.com

Owned, leased, sponsored:	3 hospitals	808 beds
Contract-managed:	0 hospitals	0 beds
Totals:	3 hospitals	808 beds

9345: METHODIST LE BONHEUR HEALTHCARE (CO)
1211 Union Avenue, Suite 700, Memphis, TN Zip 38104–6600; tel. 901/516–0543; Gary S. Shorb, President and Chief Executive Officer
(Moderately Centralized Health System)

TENNESSEE: METHODIST EXTENDED CARE HOSPITAL (O, 36 beds) 225 South Claybrook Street, Memphis, TN Zip 38104–3537; tel. 901/516–2152; Sandra Bailey, Administrator
Web address: www.methodisthealth.org

METHODIST HEALTHCARE–FAYETTE HOSPITAL (O, 1336 beds) 214 Lakeview Drive, Somerville, TN Zip 38068–9737; tel. 901/516–4000; David Crislip, Administrator
Web address: www.methodisthealth.org

METHODIST UNIVERSITY HOSPITAL (O, 1359 beds) 1265 Union Avenue, Memphis, TN Zip 38104; tel. 901/516–7000; Kevin M. Spiegel, FACHE, Chief Executive Officer
Web address: www.methodisthealth.org

Owned, leased, sponsored:	3 hospitals	2731 beds
Contract-managed:	0 hospitals	0 beds
Totals:	3 hospitals	2731 beds

For explanation of codes following names, see page B2.
★ Indicates Type III membership in the American Hospital Association.

0208: MID ATLANTIC HEALTH MANAGEMENT, INC. (IO)
1220 Butterworth Court, Stevensville, MD Zip 21666–2504; tel. 410/643–3393; Harold A. McBee, Jr., President
(Independent Hospital System)

WEST VIRGINIA: POTOMAC VALLEY HOSPITAL (O, 25 beds) 167 South Mineral Street, Keyser, WV Zip 26726–2699; tel. 304/788–3141; Michael Makosky, Administrator
Web address: www.potomacvalleyhospital.com

WISCONSIN: INDIANHEAD MEDICAL CENTER (O, 25 beds) 113 Fourth Avenue, Shell Lake, WI Zip 54871, Mailing Address: P.O. Box 300, Zip 54871–0300; tel. 715/468–7833; Paul Naglosky, Administrator

Owned, leased, sponsored:	2 hospitals	50 beds
Contract–managed:	0 hospitals	0 beds
Totals:	2 hospitals	50 beds

★0001: MIDMICHIGAN HEALTH (NP)
4005 Orchard Drive, Midland, MI Zip 48670–0001; tel. 989/839–3000; Terence F. Moore, President
(Independent Hospital System)

MICHIGAN: GRATIOT MEDICAL CENTER (O, 127 beds) 300 East Warwick Drive, Alma, MI Zip 48801–1096; tel. 989/463–1101; Mark E. Bush, President and Chief Executive Officer
Web address: www.gratiothealth.com

MIDMICHIGAN MEDICAL CENTER–CLARE (O, 55 beds) 703 North McEwan Street, Clare, MI Zip 48617–1409; tel. 989/802–5000; Lawrence F. Barco, President
Web address: www.midmichigan.org

MIDMICHIGAN MEDICAL CENTER–GLADWIN (O, 25 beds) 515 South Quarter Street, Gladwin, MI Zip 48624–1918; tel. 989/426–9286; Ray Stover, Executive Vice President
Web address: www.midmichigan.org

MIDMICHIGAN MEDICAL CENTER–MIDLAND (O, 222 beds) 4005 Orchard Drive, Midland, MI Zip 48670–0001; tel. 989/839–3000; Gregory H. Rogers, Senior Vice President and Treasurer
Web address: www.midmichigan.org

Owned, leased, sponsored:	4 hospitals	429 beds
Contract–managed:	0 hospitals	0 beds
Totals:	4 hospitals	429 beds

0368: MINNESOTA DEPARMENT OF HUMAN SERVICES (NP)
540 Cedar Street, Saint Paul, MN Zip 55164–0980, Mailing Address: P.O. Box 64980, Zip 55164–0980; tel. 651/431–2369; Michael Tessneer, Chief Executive Officer

MINNESOTA: ANOKA–METROPOLITAN REGIONAL TREATMENT CENTER (O, 227 beds) 3301 Seventh Avenue, Anoka, MN Zip 55303–1119; tel. 763/712–4000; David Hartford, Administrator
Web address: www.health.state.mn.us

COMMUNITY BEHAVIORAL HEALTH HOSPITAL – ALEXANDRIA (O, 16 beds) 1610 8th Avenue East, Alexandria, MN Zip 55308; tel. 320/335–6201; John A. Cosco, Ph.D., FACHE, Administrator
Web address: www.health.state.mn.us

COMMUNITY BEHAVIORAL HEALTH HOSPITAL – FERGUS FALLS (O, 138 beds) 1801 West Alcott Avenue, Fergus Falls, MN Zip 56538–0478, Mailing Address: P.O. Box 478, Zip 56538–0478; tel. 218/332–5001; Derrick A. Jones, Administrator

COMMUNITY BEHAVIORAL HEALTH HOSPITAL – ROCHESTER (O, 16 beds) 251 Wood Lake Drive S.E., Rochester, MN Zip 55904; tel. 507/206–2561; Rod Kornrumpf, Regional Administrator
Web address: www.health.state.mn.us

COMMUNITY BEHAVIORAL HEALTH HOSPITAL – ST. PETER (O, 560 beds) 2000 Klein Street, Saint Peter, MN Zip 56082–5800; tel. 507/933–5001; Carol Olson, Administrator
Web address: www.health.state.mn.us

WILLMAR ADULT MENTAL HEALTH PROGRAM (O, 164 beds) 1550 Highway 71 N.E., Willmar, MN Zip 56201; tel. 320/231–5100; Sandra J. Butturff, Site Director

Owned, leased, sponsored:	6 hospitals	1121 beds
Contract–managed:	0 hospitals	0 beds
Totals:	6 hospitals	1121 beds

2855: MISSIONARY BENEDICTINE SISTERS AMERICAN PROVINCE (CC)
300 North 18th Street, Norfolk, NE Zip 68701–3687; tel. 402/371–3438; Sister Kevin Hermsen, Prioress
(Moderately Centralized Health System)

NEBRASKA: FAITH REGIONAL HEALTH SERVICES (O, 245 beds) 2700 West Norfolk Avenue, Norfolk, NE Zip 68701, Mailing Address: P.O. Box 869, Zip 68702–0869; tel. 402/644–7201; Michael Hammond, Interim Chief Executive Officer
Web address: www.frhs.org

PROVIDENCE MEDICAL CENTER (O, 25 beds) 1200 Providence Road, Wayne, NE Zip 68787–1299; tel. 402/375–3800; Marcile Thomas, Administrator
Web address: www.providencemedical.com

Owned, leased, sponsored:	2 hospitals	270 beds
Contract–managed:	0 hospitals	0 beds
Totals:	2 hospitals	270 beds

0336: MISSISSIPPI BAPTIST HEALTH SYSTEM (NP)
1225 North State Street, Jackson, MS Zip 39202–2002; tel. 601/968–1000; Kurt W. Metzner, President and Chief Executive Officer
(Moderately Centralized Health System)

MISSISSIPPI: MISSISSIPPI BAPTIST MEDICAL CENTER (O, 638 beds) 1225 North State Street, Jackson, MS Zip 39202–2002; tel. 601/968–1000; C. Gerald Cotton, President
Web address: www.mbhs.org

MISSISSIPPI HOSPITAL FOR RESTORATIVE CARE (O, 25 beds) 1225 North State Street, Jackson, MS Zip 39202–2097, Mailing Address: P.O. Box 23695, Zip 39225–3695; tel. 601/968–1000; David Jackson, Chief Executive Officer
Web address: www.mbhs.org

Owned, leased, sponsored:	2 hospitals	663 beds
Contract–managed:	0 hospitals	0 beds
Totals:	2 hospitals	663 beds

0017: MISSISSIPPI STATE DEPARTMENT OF MENTAL HEALTH (NP)
1101 Robert East Lee Building, 239 North Lamar Street, Jackson, MS Zip 39201–1101; tel. 601/359–1288; Edwin C. LeGrand, III, Executive Director
(Independent Hospital System)

EAST MISSISSIPPI STATE HOSPITAL (O, 334 beds) 4555 Highland Park Drive, Meridian, MS Zip 39307–5498, Mailing Address: Box 4128, West Station, Zip 39304–4128; tel. 601/482–6186; Charles Carlisle, Director
Web address: www.emsh.state.ms.us

MISSISSIPPI STATE HOSPITAL (O, 1119 beds) 3550 Highway 468 West, Whitfield, MS Zip 39193, Mailing Address: P.O. Box 157–A, Zip 39193–0157; tel. 601/351–8000; James G. Chastain, CHE, Director
Web address: www.msh.state.ms.us

NORTH MISSISSIPPI STATE HOSPITAL (O, 50 beds) 1937 Briar Ridge Road, Tupelo, MS Zip 38804; tel. 662/690–4200; Paul A. Callens, Ph.D., Director
Web address: www.nmsh.state.ms.us

SOUTH MISSISSIPPI STATE HOSPITAL (O, 50 beds) 823 Highway 589, Purvis, MS Zip 39475–4194; tel. 601/794–0100; Wynona C. Winfield, Director
Web address: www.smsh.state.ms.us

Owned, leased, sponsored:	4 hospitals	1553 beds
Contract–managed:	0 hospitals	0 beds
Totals:	4 hospitals	1553 beds

Section B

For explanation of codes following names, see page B2.
★ Indicates Type III membership in the American Hospital Association.

Section B

0343: MONTEFIORE HEALTH SYSTEM (NP)
111 East 210th Street, New York, NY Zip 10467–2490; tel. 718/920–4321; Spencer Foreman, M.D., President
(Centralized Physician/Insurance Health System)

NEW YORK: MONTEFIORE MEDICAL CENTER (O, 1094 beds) 111 East 210th Street, Bronx, NY Zip 10467–2490; tel. 718/920–4321; Steven M. Safyer, M.D., President and Chief Executive Officer
Web address: www.montefiore.org

OUR LADY OF MERCY MEDICAL CENTER (O, 341 beds) 600 East 233rd Street, Bronx, NY Zip 10466–2697; tel. 718/920–9000; Richard Celiberti, President and Chief Executive Officer
Web address: www.ourladyofmercy.com

Owned, leased, sponsored:	2 hospitals	1435 beds
Contract-managed:	0 hospitals	0 beds
Totals:	2 hospitals	1435 beds

1335: MORTON PLANT MEASE HEALTH CARE (NP)
300 Pinellas Street, Clearwater, FL Zip 33756, Mailing Address: P.O. Box 210, Zip 33756–0210; tel. 727/462–7000; Philip K. Beauchamp, FACHE, President and Chief Executive Officer

FLORIDA: MEASE COUNTRYSIDE HOSPITAL (O, 100 beds) 3231 McMullen–Booth Road, Safety Harbor, FL Zip 34695–1098, Mailing Address: P.O. 1098, Zip 34695–1098; tel. 727/725–6111; Philip K. Beauchamp, FACHE, President and Chief Executive Officer
Web address: www.mpmhealth.com

MEASE HOSPITAL DUNEDIN (O, 258 beds) 601 Main Street, Dunedin, FL Zip 34698–5891, Mailing Address: P.O. Box 760, Zip 34697–0760; tel. 727/733–1111; Philip K. Beauchamp, FACHE, President and Chief Executive Officer
Web address: www.mpmhealth.com

MORTON PLANT HOSPITAL (S, 742 beds) 300 Pinellas Street, Clearwater, FL Zip 33756–3825, Mailing Address: P.O. Box 210, Zip 34657–0210; tel. 727/462–7000; Philip K. Beauchamp, FACHE, President and Chief Executive Officer
Web address: www.mortonplant.com

MORTON PLANT NORTH BAY HOSPITAL (S, 122 beds) 6600 Madison Street, New Port Richey, FL Zip 34652–1900; tel. 727/842–8468; Philip K. Beauchamp, FACHE, President and Chief Executive Officer
Web address: www.mpmhealth.com

Owned, leased, sponsored:	4 hospitals	1222 beds
Contract-managed:	0 hospitals	0 beds
Totals:	4 hospitals	1222 beds

0167: MOUNTAIN STATES HEALTH ALLIANCE (NP)
701 North State of Franklin, Suite 1, Johnson City, TN Zip 37604; tel. 423/431–1040; Dennis Vonderfecht, President and Chief Executive Officer
(Centralized Health System)

TENNESSEE: INDIAN PATH MEDICAL CENTER (O, 216 beds) 2000 Brookside Drive, Kingsport, TN Zip 37660–4682; tel. 423/857–7000; Monty E. McLaurin, President and Chief Executive Officer
Web address: www.msha.com

JOHNSON CITY MEDICAL CENTER (O, 443 beds) 400 North State of Franklin Road, Johnson City, TN Zip 37604–6094; tel. 423/431–6111; John W. Melton, Senior Vice President Operations and Chief Executive Officer
Web address: www.msha.com

JOHNSON CITY SPECIALTY HOSPITAL (O, 36 beds) 203 East Watauga Avenue, Johnson City, TN Zip 37601–4651; tel. 423/434–1400; Rhonda Mann, Director Nursing and Operations
Web address: www.jcmc.com

JOHNSON COUNTY COMMUNITY HOSPITAL (O, 2 beds) 1901 South Shady Street, Mountain City, TN Zip 37683–2271; tel. 423/727–1100; Lisa Heaton, Administrator and Chief Nursing Officer
Web address: www.msha.com

NORTH SIDE HOSPITAL (O, 88 beds) 401 Princeton Road, Johnson City, TN Zip 37601–2097; tel. 423/854–5600; Rhonda Mann, Administrator, Director and Chief Nursing Officer
Web address: www.msha.com

QUILLEN REHABILITATION HOSPITAL (O, 60 beds) 2511 Wesley Street, Johnson City, TN Zip 37601–1723; tel. 423/283–0700; John W. Melton, Senior Vice President Operations and Chief Executive Officer
Web address: www.msha.com

SYCAMORE SHOALS HOSPITAL (O, 121 beds) 1501 West Elk Avenue, Elizabethton, TN Zip 37643–2874; tel. 423/542–1300; Dwayne Taylor, Chief Executive Officer
Web address: www.msha.com

WOODRIDGE HOSPITAL (O, 75 beds) 403 State of Franklin Road, Johnson City, TN Zip 37604–6034; tel. 423/431–7060; Jeffrey N. Dice, Assistant Vice President
Web address: www.msha.com

VIRGINIA: SMYTH COUNTY COMMUNITY HOSPITAL (O, 168 beds) 565 Radio Hill Road, Marion, VA Zip 24354–3526, Mailing Address: P.O. Box 880, Zip 24354–0880; tel. 276/782–1234; Lindy P. White, President and Chief Executive Officer
Web address: www.scchosp.org

Owned, leased, sponsored:	9 hospitals	1209 beds
Contract-managed:	0 hospitals	0 beds
Totals:	9 hospitals	1209 beds

6555: MULTICARE HEALTH SYSTEM (NP)
315 Martin Luther King Jr. Way, Tacoma, WA Zip 98415, Mailing Address: P.O. Box 5299, Zip 98415–0299; tel. 253/403–1000; Diane Cecchettini, RN, President and Chief Executive Officer
(Centralized Physician/Insurance Health System)

WASHINGTON: MARY BRIDGE CHILDREN'S HOSPITAL AND HEALTH CENTER (O, 67 beds) 317 Martin Luther King Jr. Way, Tacoma, WA Zip 98405–0299, Mailing Address: Box 5299, Zip 98415–0299; tel. 253/403–1400; Mady Murrey, Vice President and Administrator
Web address: www.multicare.org/marybridge

TACOMA GENERAL HOSPITAL (O, 404 beds) 315 Martin Luther King Jr. Way, Tacoma, WA Zip 98405–0299, Mailing Address: P.O. Box 5299, Zip 98415–0299; tel. 253/403–1000; Diane Cecchettini, RN, President and Chief Executive Officer
Web address: www.multicare.org

Owned, leased, sponsored:	2 hospitals	471 beds
Contract-managed:	0 hospitals	0 beds
Totals:	2 hospitals	471 beds

★1465: MUNSON HEALTHCARE (NP)
1105 Sixth Street, Traverse City, MI Zip 49684–2386; tel. 231/935–6502; K. Douglas Deck, President and Chief Executive Officer
(Centralized Physician/Insurance Health System)

MICHIGAN: KALKASKA MEMORIAL HEALTH CENTER (O, 96 beds) 419 South Coral Street, Kalkaska, MI Zip 49646–2500; tel. 231/258–7500; James D. Austin, FACHE, Administrator
Web address: www.munsonhealthcare.org

MUNSON MEDICAL CENTER (O, 391 beds) 1105 Sixth Street, Traverse City, MI Zip 49684–2386; tel. 231/935–5000; Edwin Ness, President and Chief Executive Officer
Web address: www.munsonhealthcare.org

PAUL OLIVER MEMORIAL HOSPITAL (O, 48 beds) 224 Park Avenue, Frankfort, MI Zip 49635–9658; tel. 231/352–2200; James D. Austin, FACHE, Administrator
Web address: www.munsonhealthcare.org

Owned, leased, sponsored:	3 hospitals	535 beds
Contract-managed:	0 hospitals	0 beds
Totals:	3 hospitals	535 beds

0248: MUSC MEDICAL CENTER OF MEDICAL UNIVERSITY OF SOUTH CAROLINA (NP)
169 Ashley Avenue, Charleston, SC Zip 29425–5836; tel. 843/792–2300; Stuart Smith, Vice President Clinical Operations and Executive Director
(Moderately Centralized Health System)

For explanation of codes following names, see page B2.
★ Indicates Type III membership in the American Hospital Association.

SOUTH CAROLINA: CHARLESTON MEMORIAL HOSPITAL (O, 20 beds) 326 Calhoun Street, Charleston, SC Zip 29401–1189; tel. 843/792–2300; John Franklin, Director
Web address: www.musc.edu

MUSC MEDICAL CENTER OF MEDICAL UNIVERSITY OF SOUTH CAROLINA (O, 596 beds) 169 Ashley Avenue, Charleston, SC Zip 29425; tel. 843/792–2300; Stuart Smith, Vice President Clinical Operations and Executive Director
Web address: www.muschealth.com

Owned, leased, sponsored:	2 hospitals	616 beds
Contract–managed:	0 hospitals	0 beds
Totals:	2 hospitals	616 beds

0261: NATIONAL SURGICAL HOSPITALS (IO)

30 South Wacker Drive, Suite 2302, Chicago, IL Zip 60606; tel. 312/627–8400; John G. Rex–Waller, President and Chief Executive Officer
(Independent Hospital System)

ARIZONA: ARIZONA SPINE AND JOINT HOSPITAL (O, 23 beds) 4620 East Baseline Road, Mesa, AZ Zip 85206; tel. 480/832–4770; Peggy Wellman, Acting Chief Executive Officer
Web address: www.azspineandjoint.com

IDAHO: NORTHWEST SPECIALTY HOSPITAL (O, 12 beds) 1593 East Polston Avenue, Post Falls, ID Zip 83854; tel. 208/262–2300; ,
Web address: www.northwestspecialtyhospital.com

MICHIGAN: SOUTHEAST MICHIGAN SURGICAL HOSPITAL (O, 13 beds) 21230 Dequindre, Warren, MI Zip 48091–2287; tel. 586/427–1000; John Kolozsvary, Chief Executive Officer
Web address: www.nshinc.com

NORTH CAROLINA: NORTH CAROLINA SPECIALTY HOSPITAL (O, 14 beds) 3916 Ben Franklin Boulevard, Durham, NC Zip 27704; tel. 919/956–9300; Randi L. Pisko, Chief Executive Officer
Web address: www.ncspecialty.com

TEXAS: EL PASO SPECIALTY HOSPITAL (O, 31 beds) 1755 Curie Drive, El Paso, TX Zip 79902; tel. 915/533–7465; Paul Gallagher, Chief Executive Officer
Web address: www.elpasospecialtyhospital.com

SOUTH TEXAS SPINE AND SURGICAL HOSPITAL (O, 30 beds) 18600 Hardy Oak Boulevard, San Antonio, TX Zip 78258; tel. 210/507–4090; Debbie Kelly, Chief Executive Officer
Web address: www.shst.net

SOUTHWEST SURGICAL HOSPITAL (O, 23 beds) 1612 Hurst Town Center Boulevard, Hurst, TX Zip 76054; tel. 817/345–4100; Trudy Wiig, Chief Executive Officer
Web address: www.swsurgery.com

UTAH: CACHE VALLEY SPECIALTY HOSPITAL (O, 15 beds) 2380 North 400 East, North Logan, UT Zip 84341; tel. 435/713–9700; John C. Worley, Chief Executive Officer
Web address: www.cvsh.com

WISCONSIN: OAKLEAF SURGICAL HOSPITAL (O, 13 beds) 3802 West Oakwood Mall Drive, Eau Claire, WI Zip 54701; tel. 715/831–8130; Michael McClain, Chief Executive Officer
Web address: www.oakleafmedical.com

Owned, leased, sponsored:	9 hospitals	174 beds
Contract–managed:	0 hospitals	0 beds
Totals:	9 hospitals	174 beds

★9265: NEBRASKA METHODIST HEALTH SYSTEM, INC. (CO)

8511 West Dodge Road, Omaha, NE Zip 68114; tel. 402/354–5411; John M. Fraser, President and Chief Executive Officer
(Moderately Centralized Health System)

IOWA: JENNIE EDMUNDSON HOSPITAL (O, 118 beds) 933 East Pierce Street, Council Bluffs, IA Zip 51503–4652, Mailing Address: P.O. Box 2C, Zip 51502–3002; tel. 712/396–6000; Steven P. Baumert, President and Chief Executive Officer
Web address: www.bestcare.org

NEBRASKA: NEBRASKA METHODIST HOSPITAL (O, 334 beds) 8303 Dodge Street, Omaha, NE Zip 68114–4199; tel. 402/354–4000; Stephen L. Goeser, President and Chief Executive Officer
Web address: www.bestcare.org

Owned, leased, sponsored:	2 hospitals	452 beds
Contract–managed:	0 hospitals	0 beds
Totals:	2 hospitals	452 beds

★0213: NEW HANOVER HEALTH NETWORK (NP)

2131 South 17th Street, Wilmington, NC Zip 28401–9000; tel. 910/343–7040; John K. Barto, Jr., President and Chief Executive Officer
(Moderately Centralized Health System)

NORTH CAROLINA: NEW HANOVER REGIONAL MEDICAL CENTER (O, 646 beds) 2131 South 17th Street, Wilmington, NC Zip 28401–7483, Mailing Address: P.O. Box 9000, Zip 28402–9000; tel. 910/343–7000; John K. Barto, Jr., President and Chief Executive Officer
Web address: www.nhhn.org

PENDER MEMORIAL HOSPITAL (C, 68 beds) 507 Freemont Street, Burgaw, NC Zip 28425–5131; tel. 910/259–5451; David Long, Administrator
Web address: www.pendermemorial.org

Owned, leased, sponsored:	1 hospital	646 beds
Contract–managed:	1 hospital	68 beds
Totals:	2 hospitals	714 beds

★3075: NEW YORK CITY HEALTH AND HOSPITALS CORPORATION (NP)

125 Worth Street, Room 514, New York, NY Zip 10013–4006; tel. 212/788–3321; Alan D. Aviles, President
(Moderately Centralized Health System)

NEW YORK: BELLEVUE HOSPITAL CENTER (O, 788 beds) 462 First Avenue, New York, NY Zip 10016–9198; tel. 212/562–4141; Lynda D. Curtis, Senior Vice President and Executive Director
Web address: www.nyc.gov/bellevue

COLER–GOLDWATER SPECIALTY HOSPITAL AND NURSING FACILITY (O, 2013 beds) One Main Street, New York, NY Zip 10044; tel. 212/318–8000; Claude Ritman, Executive Director
Web address: www.coler–goldwater.org

CONEY ISLAND HOSPITAL (O, 351 beds) 2601 Ocean Parkway, Brooklyn, NY Zip 11235–7795; tel. 718/616–3000; Peter Wolf, Senior Vice President and Executive Director
Web address: www.ci.nyc.ny.us/html/hhc/html/coneyisland.html

ELMHURST HOSPITAL CENTER (O, 527 beds) 79–01 Broadway, Flushing, NY Zip 11373–1368; tel. 718/334–4000; Chris D. Constantino, Executive Director
Web address: www.elmhursthospitalcenter.org

HARLEM HOSPITAL CENTER (O, 286 beds) 506 Lenox Avenue, New York, NY Zip 10037–1894; tel. 212/939–1000; John M. Palmer, Ph.D., Executive Director
Web address: www.nyclink.org/hhc

JACOBI MEDICAL CENTER (O, 457 beds) Pelham Parkway South and Eastchester Road, Bronx, NY Zip 10461–1197; tel. 718/918–5000; William P. Walsh, Senior Vice President and Executive Director
Web address: www.nyc.gov/html/hhc/jacobi/home.html

KINGS COUNTY HOSPITAL CENTER (O, 616 beds) 451 Clarkson Avenue, Brooklyn, NY Zip 11203–2097; tel. 718/245–3131; Jean G. Leon, RN, Senior Vice President and Executive Director
Web address: www.ci.nyc.ny.us/html/hhc/html/kings.html

LINCOLN MEDICAL AND MENTAL HEALTH CENTER (O, 332 beds) 234 East 149th Street, Bronx, NY Zip 10451–9998; tel. 718/579–5700; Jose R. Sanchez, Senior Vice President and Executive Director

METROPOLITAN HOSPITAL CENTER (O, 333 beds) 1901 First Avenue, New York, NY Zip 10029–7496; tel. 212/423–6262; Meryl Weinberg, Executive Director
Web address: www.nyc.gov/html/hhc/metropolitan.html

NORTH CENTRAL BRONX HOSPITAL (O, 213 beds) 3424 Kossuth Avenue, Bronx, NY Zip 10467–2489; tel. 718/519–3500; Arthur Wagner, Executive Director
Web address: www.ci.nyc.ny.us/html/hhc/html/northcentralbronx.html

For explanation of codes following names, see page B2.
★ Indicates Type III membership in the American Hospital Association.

QUEENS HOSPITAL CENTER (O, 261 beds) 82–68 164th Street, Jamaica, NY Zip 11432–1104; tel. 718/883–3000; Antonio D. Martin, Executive Director
Web address: www.ci.nyc.ny.us/html/hhc/html/facilities/queens.shtml

WOODHULL MEDICAL AND MENTAL HEALTH CENTER (O, 406 beds) 760 Broadway Street, Brooklyn, NY Zip 11206–5383; tel. 718/963–8000; Iris Jimenez–Hernandez, Senior Vice President and Executive Director
Web address: www.nyc.gov/html/hhc

Owned, leased, sponsored:	12 hospitals	6583 beds
Contract–managed:	0 hospitals	0 beds
Totals:	12 hospitals	6583 beds

0142: NEW YORK PRESBYTERIAN HEALTHCARE SYSTEM (NP)

525 East 68th Street, New York, NY Zip 10021–4885; tel. 212/746–3745; Herbert Pardes, M.D., President and Chief Executive Officer
(Moderately Centralized Health System)

BROOKLYN HOSPITAL CENTER (S, 653 beds) 121 DeKalb Avenue, Brooklyn, NY Zip 11201–5493; tel. 718/250–8000; Richard B. Becker, M.D., President and Chief Executive Officer
Web address: www.tbh.org

GRACIE SQUARE HOSPITAL (S, 157 beds) 420 East 76th Street, New York, NY Zip 10021–3104; tel. 212/988–4400; Frank Bruno, Chief Executive Officer
Web address: www.nygsh.org

HOSPITAL FOR SPECIAL SURGERY (S, 162 beds) 535 East 70th Street, New York, NY Zip 10021–4898; tel. 212/606–1000; Louis A. Shapiro, President and Chief Executive Officer
Web address: www.hss.edu

NEW YORK COMMUNITY HOSPITAL (S, 125 beds) 2525 Kings Highway, Brooklyn, NY Zip 11229–1798, Mailing Address: 2513 Avenue O, Zip 11210; tel. 718/692–5300; Lin H. Mo, President and Chief Executive Officer
Web address: www.nych.com

NEW YORK HOSPITAL QUEENS (S, 439 beds) 56–45 Main Street, Flushing, NY Zip 11355–5000; tel. 718/670–1231; Stephen S. Mills, President and Chief Executive Officer
Web address: www.nyhq.org

NEW YORK METHODIST HOSPITAL (S, 576 beds) 506 Sixth Street, Brooklyn, NY Zip 11215–3645; tel. 718/780–3000; Mark J. Mundy, President and Chief Executive Officer
Web address: www.nym.org

NEW YORK WESTCHESTER SQUARE MEDICAL CENTER (S, 169 beds) 2475 St. Raymond Avenue, Bronx, NY Zip 10461–3198; tel. 718/430–7300; Alan Kopman, President and Chief Executive Officer
Web address: www.nywsmc.org

NEW YORK–PRESBYTERIAN HOSPITAL (O, 2207 beds) 525 East 68th Street, New York, NY Zip 10021–4885; tel. 212/746–5454; Herbert Pardes, M.D., President and Chief Executive Officer
Web address: www.nyp.org

NYACK HOSPITAL (S, 267 beds) 160 North Midland Avenue, Nyack, NY Zip 10960–1998; tel. 845/348–2000; David H. Freed, President and Chief Executive Officer
Web address: www.nyackhospital.org

Owned, leased, sponsored:	9 hospitals	4755 beds
Contract–managed:	0 hospitals	0 beds
Totals:	9 hospitals	4755 beds

0009: NEW YORK STATE OFFICE OF MENTAL HEALTH (NP)

44 Holland Avenue, Albany, NY Zip 12229–3411; tel. 518/474–4403; Michael F. Hogan, Ph.D., Commissioner
(Independent Hospital System)

BRONX CHILDREN'S PSYCHIATRIC CENTER (O, 75 beds) 1000 Waters Place, Bronx, NY Zip 10461–2799; tel. 718/239–3600; Mark D. Bienstock, Executive Director
Web address: www.omh.state.ny.us

BRONX PSYCHIATRIC CENTER (O, 450 beds) 1500 Waters Place, Bronx, NY Zip 10461–2796; tel. 718/931–0600; Pamela Turner, Interim Executive Director
Web address: www.omh.state.ny.us

BROOKLYN CHILDREN'S PSYCHRIC CENTER (O, 36 beds) 1819 Bergen Street, Brooklyn, NY Zip 11233–4513; tel. 718/221–4500; Diane Aman, Acting Executive Director

BUFFALO PSYCHIATRIC CENTER (O, 240 beds) 400 Forest Avenue, Buffalo, NY Zip 14213–1298; tel. 716/885–2261; Thomas Dodson, Executive Director
Web address: www.omh.state.ny.us

CAPITAL DISTRICT PSYCHIATRIC CENTER (O, 200 beds) 75 New Scotland Avenue, Albany, NY Zip 12208–3474; tel. 518/447–9611; Lewis Campbell, Executive Director
Web address: www.omh.state.ny.us/omhweb/facilities/cdpc/facility.htm

CENTRAL NEW YORK PSYCHIATRIC CENTER (O, 206 beds) Marcy, NY Mailing Address: P.O. Box 300, Zip 13403–0300; tel. 315/736–3620; Donald Sawyer, Ph.D., Executive Director
Web address: www.omh.state.ny.us/

CREEDMOOR PSYCHIATRIC CENTER (O, 420 beds) Jamaica, NY Mailing Address: 80–45 Winchester Boulevard, Queens Village, Zip 11427–2199; tel. 718/264–3600; Kathleen Iverson, Executive Director
Web address: www.omh.state.ny.us

ELMIRA PSYCHIATRIC CENTER (O, 93 beds) 100 Washington Street, Elmira, NY Zip 14901–2898; tel. 607/737–4739; William Benedict, Executive Director
Web address: www.omh.state.ny.us/omhweb/facilities/elpc/facility.htm

GREATER BINGHAMTON HEALTH CENTER (O, 168 beds) 425 Robinson Street, Binghamton, NY Zip 13901–4198; tel. 607/724–1391; Margaret R. Dugan, Executive Director
Web address: www.omh.state.ny.us

HUDSON RIVER PSYCHIATRIC CENTER (O, 460 beds) 10 Ross Circle, Poughkeepsie, NY Zip 12601–1078; tel. 845/452–8000; Jean L. Wolfersteig, Acting Executive Director
Web address: www.omh.state.ny.us

KINGSBORO PSYCHIATRIC CENTER (O, 290 beds) 681 Clarkson Avenue, Brooklyn, NY Zip 11203–2199; tel. 718/221–7395; Martin Darcy, Executive Director
Web address: www.omh.state.ny.us/omhweb/facilities/kbpc/facility/htm

MANHATTAN PSYCHIATRIC CENTER–WARD'S ISLAND (O, 745 beds) 600 East 125th Street, New York, NY Zip 10035–9998; tel. 646/672–6767; Stephen Rabinowitz, Acting Executive Director

MID–HUDSON FORENSIC PSYCHIATRIC CENTER (O, 268 beds) Route 17M, New Hampton, NY Zip 10958, Mailing Address: P.O. Box 158, Zip 10958–0158; tel. 845/374–8700; Howard Holanchock, Executive Director
Web address: www.omh.state.ny.us

MOHAWK VALLEY PSYCHIATRIC CENTER (O, 614 beds) 1400 Noyes Street, Utica, NY Zip 13502–3803; tel. 315/738–3800; Collen A. Sawyer, RN, M.S.N., Executive Director
Web address: www.omh.state.ny.us/omhweb/facilities/mvpc/facility.htm

NEW YORK STATE PSYCHIATRIC INSTITUTE (O, 58 beds) 1051 Riverside Drive, New York, NY Zip 10032–2695; tel. 212/543–5000; Jeffrey A. Lieberman, M.D., Executive Director
Web address: www.nyspi.org

PILGRIM PSYCHIATRIC CENTER (O, 569 beds) 998 Crooked Hill Road, Brentwood, NY Zip 11717–1087; tel. 631/761–3500; Dean R. Weinstock, RN, Executive Director
Web address: www.omh.state.ny.us/omhweb/facilities/pgpc/facility.htm

QUEENS CHILDREN'S PSYCHIATRIC CENTER (O, 84 beds) 74–03 Commonwealth Boulevard, Jamaica, NY Zip 11426–1890; tel. 718/264–4506; Keith Little, Acting Executive Director
Web address: www.omh.state.ny.us

RICHARD H. HUTCHINGS PSYCHIATRIC CENTER (O, 131 beds) 620 Madison Street, Syracuse, NY Zip 13210–2319; tel. 315/426–3632; Colleen Sawyer, Executive Director
Web address: www.omh.state.ny.us

ROCHESTER PSYCHIATRIC CENTER (O, 180 beds) 1111 Elmwood Avenue, Rochester, NY Zip 14620–3005; tel. 585/241–1200; Michael P. Zuber, Ph.D., Executive Director
Web address: www.omh.state.ny.us/omhweb/facilities/ropc/facility.htm

ROCKLAND CHILDREN'S PSYCHIATRIC CENTER (O, 54 beds) 599 Convent Road, Orangeburg, NY Zip 10962; tel. 845/359–7400; Raul Silva, M.D., Executive Director

ROCKLAND PSYCHIATRIC CENTER (O, 525 beds) 140 Old Orangeburg Road, Orangeburg, NY Zip 10962–0071; tel. 845/359–1000; James H. Bopp, Executive Director

For explanation of codes following names, see page B2.
★ Indicates Type III membership in the American Hospital Association.

SAGAMORE CHILDREN'S PSYCHIATRIC CENTER (O, 69 beds) 197 Half Hollow Road, Dix Hills, NY Zip 11746–5861; tel. 631/370–1700; Dennis Dubey, Ph.D., Executive Director
Web address: www.omh.state.ny.us/ombweb/facilities/scpc/facility.htm

SOUTH BEACH PSYCHIATRIC CENTER (O, 316 beds) 777 Seaview Avenue, Staten Island, NY Zip 10305–3499; tel. 718/667–2300; William Henri, Executive Director
Web address: www.omh.state.ny.us

ST. LAWRENCE PSYCHIATRIC CENTER (O, 114 beds) 1 Chimney Point Drive, Ogdensburg, NY Zip 13669–2291; tel. 315/541–2001; Samua A. Bastien, IV, Ph.D., Executive Director
Web address: www.omh.state.ny.us/omhweb/facilities/slpc/facility.htm

WESTERN NEW YORK CHILDREN'S PSYCHIATRIC CENTER (O, 46 beds) 1010 East and West Road, West Seneca, NY Zip 14224–3698; tel. 716/677–7000; Kathe Hayes, Executive Director
Web address: www.omh.state.ny.us

Owned, leased, sponsored:	25 hospitals	6411 beds
Contract-managed:	0 hospitals	0 beds
Totals:	25 hospitals	6411 beds

0353: NEXUS HEALTH SYSTEMS (IO)

One Riverway, Suite 600, Houston, TX Zip 77056; tel. 713/355–6111; John W. Cassidy, M.D., President, Chief Executive Officer and Chief Medical Officer
(Independent Hospital System)

CALIFORNIA: HEALTHBRIDGE CHILDRENS REHABILITATION HOSPITAL (O, 6 beds) 393 South Tustin Street, Orange, CA Zip 92868; tel. 714/289–2400; Ronelo Mysburgh, Administrator
Web address: www.nhsltd.com/HealthBridge–Orange/Default.htm

TEXAS: HEALTHBRIDGE CHILDREN'S HOSPITAL OF HOUSTON (O, 24 beds) 2929 Woodland Park Drive, Houston, TX Zip 77082; tel. 281/293–7774; Geoffrey Swaby, Administrator
Web address: www.nhsltd.com/HealthBridge–Houston/Default.htm

NEXUS SPECIALTY HOSPITAL (O, 75 beds) 123 Vision Park Boulevard, Shenandoah, TX Zip 77384; tel. 281/364–0317; Brian Holt, Chief Executive Officer
Web address: www.nexusspecialty.com

Owned, leased, sponsored:	3 hospitals	105 beds
Contract-managed:	0 hospitals	0 beds
Totals:	3 hospitals	105 beds

0349: NOLAND HEALTH SERVICES, INC. (NP)

600 Corporate Parkway, Suite 1000, Birmingham, AL Zip 35242; tel. 205/783–8484; Gary M. Glasscock, President and Chief Executive Officer

ALABAMA: LONG TERM HOSPITAL OF ANNISTON (O, 34 beds) 400 East 10th Street, 4th Floor, Anniston, AL Zip 36207; tel. 256/741–6141; Bob Notarianni, Administrator
Web address: www.nolandhealth.com

LONG TERM HOSPITAL OF BIRMINGHAM (O, 23 beds) 50 Medical Park East Drive, 8th Floor, Birmingham, AL Zip 35235; tel. 205/808–5100; Xavier Ritchie, Administrator
Web address: www.nolandhealth.com

LONG TERM HOSPITAL OF DOTHAN (O, 30 beds) 1108 Ross Clark Circle, 4th Floor, Dothan, AL Zip 36302; tel. 334/699–4300; Kaye Burke, Administrator
Web address: www.nolandhealth.com

LONG TERM HOSPITAL OF MONTGOMERY (O, 36 beds) 1725 Pine Street, 5 North, Montgomery, AL Zip 36106–1109, Mailing Address: P.O. Box 11649, Zip 36111–1649; tel. 334/240–0532; Ray Owens, Administrator
Web address: www.nolandhealth.com

LONG TERM HOSPITAL OF TUSCALOOSA (O, 27 beds) 809 Unviersity Boulevard East, 4th Floor, Tuscaloosa, AL Zip 35401, Mailing Address: 809 University Boulevard East, 4th Floor, Zip 35401; tel. 205/759–7241; Bob Notarianni, Administrator
Web address: www.nolandhealth.com

Owned, leased, sponsored:	5 hospitals	150 beds
Contract-managed:	0 hospitals	0 beds
Totals:	5 hospitals	150 beds

★0221: NORTH CAROLINA BAPTIST HOSPITAL (NP)

Medical Center Boulevard, Winston–Salem, NC Zip 27157; tel. 336/716–2011; Donny C. Lambeth, Interim President
(Moderately Centralized Health System)

NORTH CAROLINA: HOOTS MEMORIAL HOSPITAL (L, 22 beds) 624 West Main Street, Yadkinville, NC Zip 27055–7804, Mailing Address: P.O. Box 68, Zip 27055–0068; tel. 336/679–2041; Lance C. Labine, President
Web address: www.bgsm.edu/hoots/

NORTH CAROLINA BAPTIST HOSPITAL (WAKE FOREST UNIVERSITY BAPTIST MEDICAL CENTER) (O, 965 beds) Medical Center Boulevard, Winston–Salem, NC Zip 27157–0001; tel. 336/716–2011; Donny C. Lambeth, Interim President
Web address: www.wfubmc.edu

STOKES–REYNOLDS MEMORIAL HOSPITAL (L, 65 beds) 1570 Highway 8 and 89 North, Danbury, NC Zip 27016, Mailing Address: P.O. Box 10, Zip 27016–0010; tel. 336/593–2831; Lance C. Labine, President
Web address: www.wfubmc.edu/stokes

Owned, leased, sponsored:	3 hospitals	1052 beds
Contract-managed:	0 hospitals	0 beds
Totals:	3 hospitals	1052 beds

★0032: NORTH MISSISSIPPI HEALTH SERVICES, INC. (NP)

830 South Gloster Street, Tupelo, MS Zip 38801–4996; tel. 662/377–3136; John R. Heer, President and Chief Executive Officer
(Centralized Physician/Insurance Health System)

ALABAMA: NORTH MISSISSIPPI MEDICAL CENTER–HAMILTON (O, 57 beds) 1256 Military Street South, Hamilton, AL Zip 35570–5001; tel. 205/921–6200; Donald J. Jones, Administrator
Web address: www.nmhs.net

MISSISSIPPI: CALHOUN HEALTH SERVICES (C, 150 beds) 140 Burke–Calhoun City Road, Calhoun City, MS Zip 38916–9690; tel. 662/628–6611; James P. Franklin, Administrator
Web address: www.nmhs.net/calhoun_city

NORTH MISSISSIPPI MEDICAL CENTER – TUPELO (O, 726 beds) 830 South Gloster Street, Tupelo, MS Zip 38801–4934; tel. 662/377–3000; Charles D. Stokes, FACHE, President
Web address: www.nmhs.net

NORTH MISSISSIPPI MEDICAL CENTER–EUPORA (O, 73 beds) 70 Medical Plaza, Eupora, MS Zip 39744–2215; tel. 662/258–6221; John R. Jones, Administrator
Web address: www.nmhs.net/eupora

NORTH MISSISSIPPI MEDICAL CENTER–IUKA (O, 48 beds) 1777 Curtis Drive, Iuka, MS Zip 38852–1001, Mailing Address: P.O. Box 860, Zip 38852–0860; tel. 662/423–6051; Fred A. Truesdale, Jr., Administrator
Web address: www.nmhs.net

NORTH MISSISSIPPI MEDICAL CENTER–PONTOTOC HOSPITAL AND NURSING HOME (L, 69 beds) 176 South Main Street, Pontotoc, MS Zip 38863–3311, Mailing Address: P.O. Box 790, Zip 38863–0790; tel. 662/488–7640; Fred B. Hood, FACHE, Administrator
Web address: www.nmhs.net

NORTH MISSISSIPPI MEDICAL CENTER–WEST POINT (O, 60 beds) 835 Medical Center Drive, West Point, MS Zip 39773–9320; tel. 662/495–2300; W. Kent Rogers, Administrator
Web address: www.nmhs.net

Owned, leased, sponsored:	6 hospitals	1033 beds
Contract-managed:	1 hospital	150 beds
Totals:	7 hospitals	1183 beds

Section B

For explanation of codes following names, see page B2.
★ Indicates Type III membership in the American Hospital Association.

★0062: NORTH SHORE–LIJ HEALTH SYSTEM (NP)
145 Community Drive, Great Neck, NY Zip 11021; tel. 516/465–8100; Michael J. Dowling, President and Chief Executive Officer
(Centralized Health System)

NEW YORK: FOREST HILLS HOSPITAL (O, 199 beds) Forest Hills, NY Mailing Address: 102–01 66th Road, Zip 11375–2029; tel. 718/830–4000; Robert T. Hettenbach, Executive Director
Web address: www.northshorelij.com

FRANKLIN HOSPITAL (O, 356 beds) 900 Franklin Avenue, Valley Stream, NY Zip 11580–2190; tel. 516/256–6000; Deborah Tascone, RN, M.S., Executive Director
Web address: www.fhmc.org

GLEN COVE HOSPITAL (O, 265 beds) 101 St. Andrews Lane, Glen Cove, NY Zip 11542–2254; tel. 516/674–7300; Dennis Connors, Executive Director
Web address: www.northshorelij.com

HUNTINGTON HOSPITAL (S, 303 beds) 270 Park Avenue, Huntington, NY Zip 11743–2799; tel. 631/351–2200; Kevin F. Lawlor, President and Chief Executive Officer
Web address: www.hunthosp.org

LONG ISLAND JEWISH MEDICAL CENTER (O, 840 beds) 270–05 76th Avenue, New Hyde Park, NY Zip 11040–1496; tel. 718/470–7000; John Steel, Executive Director
Web address: www.lij.edu

NORTH SHORE UNIVERSITY HOSPITAL (O, 798 beds) 300 Community Drive, Manhasset, NY Zip 11030–3876; tel. 516/562–0100; Susan Somerville, RN, Executive Director
Web address: www.northshorelij.com

NORTH SHORE UNIVERSITY HOSPITAL AT PLAINVIEW (O, 211 beds) 888 Old Country Road, Plainview, NY Zip 11803–4978; tel. 516/719–3000; Deborah Tascone, RN, M.S., Executive Director
Web address: www.northshorelij.com

NORTH SHORE UNIVERSITY HOSPITAL AT SYOSSET (O, 79 beds) 221 Jericho Turnpike, Syosset, NY Zip 11791–4567; tel. 516/496–6400; Deborah Tascone, RN, M.S., Executive Director
Web address: www.northshorelij.com

SOUTHSIDE HOSPITAL (O, 296 beds) 301 East Main Street, Bay Shore, NY Zip 11706–8458; tel. 631/968–3000; Winifred Mack, Executive Director
Web address: www.southsidehospital.org

STATEN ISLAND UNIVERSITY HOSPITAL (S, 672 beds) 475 Seaview Avenue, Staten Island, NY Zip 10305–9998; tel. 718/226–9000; Anthony C. Ferreri, President and Chief Executive Officer
Web address: www.siuh.edu

Owned, leased, sponsored:	10 hospitals	4019 beds
Contract–managed:	0 hospitals	0 beds
Totals:	10 hospitals	4019 beds

★2075: NORTHBAY HEALTHCARE SYSTEM (NP)
1200 B. Gale Wilson Boulevard, Fairfield, CA Zip 94533–3587; tel. 707/429–7809; Gary J. Passama, President and Chief Executive Officer
(Independent Hospital System)

CALIFORNIA: NORTHBAY MEDICAL CENTER (O, 107 beds) 1200 B. Gale Wilson Boulevard, Fairfield, CA Zip 94533–3587; tel. 707/429–3600; Deborah Sugiyama, President
Web address: www.northbay.org

NORTHBAY VACAVALLEY HOSPITAL (O, 48 beds) 1000 Nut Tree Road, Vacaville, CA Zip 95687–4100; tel. 707/446–4000; Deborah Sugiyama, President
Web address: www.northbay.org

Owned, leased, sponsored:	2 hospitals	155 beds
Contract–managed:	0 hospitals	0 beds
Totals:	2 hospitals	155 beds

★0281: NORTHERN ARIZONA HEALTHCARE (NP)
1200 North Beaver Street, Flagstaff, AZ Zip 86001; tel. 928/773–2001; James Puffenberger, President and Chief Executive Officer
(Moderately Centralized Health System)

ARIZONA: FLAGSTAFF MEDICAL CENTER (O, 271 beds) 1200 North Beaver Street, Flagstaff, AZ Zip 86001–3198; tel. 928/779–3366; William T. Bradel, President
Web address: www.flagstaffmedicalcenter.com

VERDE VALLEY MEDICAL CENTER (O, 110 beds) 269 South Candy Lane, Cottonwood, AZ Zip 86326–4170; tel. 928/639–6000; James J. Sinek, President
Web address: www.nahealth.com

Owned, leased, sponsored:	2 hospitals	381 beds
Contract–managed:	0 hospitals	0 beds
Totals:	2 hospitals	381 beds

★2285: NORTON HEALTHCARE (NP)
234 East Gray Street, Suite 225, Louisville, KY Zip 40202, Mailing Address: P.O. Box 35070, Zip 40232–5070; tel. 502/629–8000; Stephen A. Williams, President
(Centralized Physician/Insurance Health System)

KENTUCKY: NORTON AUDUBON HOSPITAL (O, 268 beds) One Audubon Plaza Drive, Louisville, KY Zip 40217–1397, Mailing Address: P.O. Box 17550, Zip 40217–0550; tel. 502/636–7111; Thomas D. Kmetz, President
Web address: www.nortonhealthcare.org

NORTON HOSPITAL (O, 649 beds) 200 East Chestnut Street, Louisville, KY Zip 40202–1800, Mailing Address: P.O. Box 35070, Zip 40232–5070; tel. 502/629–8000; Kevin S. Wardell, President
Web address: www.nortonhealthcare.org

NORTON SUBURBAN HOSPITAL (O, 348 beds) 4001 Dutchmans Lane, Louisville, KY Zip 40207–4799; tel. 502/893–1000; John D. Harryman, President
Web address: www.nortonhealthcare.com

Owned, leased, sponsored:	3 hospitals	1265 beds
Contract–managed:	0 hospitals	0 beds
Totals:	3 hospitals	1265 beds

★0139: NOVANT HEALTH (NP)
2085 Frontis Plaza Boulevard, Winston–Salem, NC Zip 27103–3090; tel. 336/718–2023; Paul M. Wiles, President and Chief Executive Officer
(Centralized Health System)

NORTH CAROLINA: BRUNSWICK COMMUNITY HOSPITAL (L, 60 beds) 1 Medical Center Drive, Supply, NC Zip 28462–3350, Mailing Address: P.O. Box 139, Zip 28462–0139; tel. 910/755–8121; Denise B. Mihal, RN, President
Web address: www.brunswickcommunityhospital.com

FORSYTH MEDICAL CENTER (O, 852 beds) 3333 Silas Creek Parkway, Winston–Salem, NC Zip 27103–3090; tel. 336/718–5000; Gregory J. Beier, President and Chief Executive Officer
Web address: www.novanthealth.org

MEDICAL PARK HOSPITAL (O, 22 beds) 1950 South Hawthorne Road, Winston–Salem, NC Zip 27103–3993, Mailing Address: P.O. Box 24728, Zip 27114–4728; tel. 336/718–0600; Timothy S. Shelton, Administrator
Web address: www.novanthealth.org

PRESBYTERIAN HOSPITAL (O, 529 beds) 200 Hawthorne Lane, Charlotte, NC Zip 28204–2528, Mailing Address: P.O. Box 33549, Zip 28233–3549; tel. 704/384–4000; Carl S. Armato, President and Chief Executive Officer
Web address: www.presbyterian.org

PRESBYTERIAN HOSPITAL HUNTERSVILLE (O, 50 beds) 10030 Gilead Road, Huntersville, NC Zip 28078, Mailing Address: P.O. Box 3508, Zip 28070–3508; tel. 704/316–4000; Jeffrey T. Lindsay, Vice President and Administrator
Web address: www.novanthealth.org

For explanation of codes following names, see page B2.
★ Indicates Type III membership in the American Hospital Association.

PRESBYTERIAN HOSPITAL–MATTHEWS (O, 102 beds) 1500 Matthews Township Parkway, Matthews, NC Zip 28105–4656, Mailing Address: P.O. Box 3310, Zip 28106–3310; tel. 704/384–6500; Derrick Mark Billings, President
Web address: www.presbyterian.org

PRESBYTERIAN–ORTHOPAEDIC HOSPITAL (O, 80 beds) 1901 Randolph Road, Charlotte, NC Zip 28207–1195; tel. 704/316–2000; Tanya S. Blackmon, Vice President and Administrator

ROWAN REGIONAL MEDICAL CENTER (O, 180 beds) 612 Mocksville Avenue, Salisbury, NC Zip 28144–2799; tel. 704/210–5000; Charles W. Elliott, Jr., Chief Executive Officer
Web address: www.rowan.org

THOMASVILLE MEDICAL CENTER (O, 94 beds) 207 Old Lexington Road, Thomasville, NC Zip 27360–3428, Mailing Address: P.O. Box 789, Zip 27361–0789; tel. 336/472–2000; Gabrielle K. Causby, President
Web address: www.thomasvillemedicalcenter.org

Owned, leased, sponsored:	9 hospitals	1969 beds
Contract–managed:	0 hospitals	0 beds
Totals:	9 hospitals	1969 beds

★1165: OAKWOOD HEALTHCARE, INC. (NP)
One Parklane Boulevard, Suite 1000E, Dearborn, MI Zip 48126; tel. 313/253–6050; Brian M. Connolly, President and Chief Executive Officer
(Decentralized Health System)

MICHIGAN: OAKWOOD ANNAPOLIS HOSPITAL (O, 193 beds) 33155 Annapolis Avenue, Wayne, MI Zip 48184–2493; tel. 734/467–4000; Kathleen Cronin, RN, Interim President
Web address: www.oakwood.org

OAKWOOD HERITAGE HOSPITAL (O, 153 beds) 10000 Telegraph Road, Taylor, MI Zip 48180–3349; tel. 313/295–5000; Michael Geheb, M.D., Division President
Web address: www.oakwood.org

OAKWOOD HOSPITAL AND MEDICAL CENTER–DEARBORN (O, 594 beds) 18101 Oakwood Boulevard, Dearborn, MI Zip 48124–4093, Mailing Address: P.O. Box 2500, Zip 48123–2500; tel. 313/593–7000; Michael Geheb, M.D., Division President
Web address: www.oakwood.org

OAKWOOD SOUTHSHORE MEDICAL CENTER (O, 129 beds) 5450 Fort Street, Trenton, MI Zip 48183–4625; tel. 734/671–3800; Edith M. Hughes, Division President
Web address: www.oakwood.org

Owned, leased, sponsored:	4 hospitals	1069 beds
Contract–managed:	0 hospitals	0 beds
Totals:	4 hospitals	1069 beds

★0359: OCHSNER HEALTH SYSTEM (NP)
1514 Jefferson Highway, New Orleans, LA Zip 70121; tel. 800/874–8984; Patrick J. Quinlan, M.D., Chief Executive Officer

LOUISIANA: OCHSNER BAPTIST MEDICAL CENTER (O, 10 beds) New Orleans, LA Robert Wolterman, Chief Executive Officer
Web address: www.ochsner.org

OCHSNER MEDICAL CENTER (O, 390 beds) 1514 Jefferson Highway, New Orleans, LA Zip 70121–2484; tel. 504/842–3000; Patrick J. Quinlan, M.D., Chief Executive Officer
Web address: www.ochsner.org

OCHSNER MEDICAL CENTER – KENNER (O, 106 beds) 180 West Esplanade Avenue, Kenner, LA Zip 70065–6001; tel. 504/468–8600; Paolo Zambito, Chief Executive Officer
Web address: www.ochsner.org/body.cfm?id=1397

OCHSNER MEDICAL CENTER – WEST BANK (O, 132 beds) 2500 Belle Chase Highway, Gretna, LA Zip 70056–7196; tel. 504/392–3131; Michael O'Bryan, M.D., Chief Executive Officer
Web address: www.ochsner.org/westbank

OCHSNER MEDICAL CENTER–BATON ROUGE (O, 164 beds) 17000 Medical Center Drive, Baton Rouge, LA Zip 70816–3224; tel. 225/752–2470; Mitch Wasden, Chief Executive Officer
Web address: www.ochsner.org/page.cfm?id=103

OCHSNER ST. ANNE GENERAL HOSPITAL (O, 35 beds) 4608 Highway 1, Raceland, LA Zip 70394–2623; tel. 985/537–6841; Milton D. Bourgeois, Jr., Chief Executive Officer
Web address: www.stannegeneral.com

Owned, leased, sponsored:	6 hospitals	837 beds
Contract–managed:	0 hospitals	0 beds
Totals:	6 hospitals	837 beds

0388: OCONEE REGIONAL HEALTH SYSTEM (NP)
821 North Cobb Street, Milledgeville, GA Zip 31061; tel. 478/454–3505; Jean Aycock, President and Chief Executive Officer

GEORGIA: JASPER MEMORIAL HOSPITAL (O, 67 beds) 898 College Street, Monticello, GA Zip 31064–1298; tel. 706/468–6411; David J. Owens, Chief Executive Officer
Web address: www.jaspermemorialhospital.org

OCONEE REGIONAL MEDICAL CENTER (O, 106 beds) 821 North Cobb Street, Milledgeville, GA Zip 31061–2351, Mailing Address: P.O. Box 690, Zip 31061–0690; tel. 478/454–3500; Jean Aycock, President and Chief Executive Officer
Web address: www.oconeeregional.com

Owned, leased, sponsored:	2 hospitals	173 beds
Contract–managed:	0 hospitals	0 beds
Totals:	2 hospitals	173 beds

★0251: OHIO STATE UNIVERSITY HEALTH SYSTEM (NP)
370 West Ninth Avenue, Columbus, OH Zip 43210–1240; tel. 614/247–5555; Peter E. Geier, Chief Executive Officer
(Moderately Centralized Health System)

OHIO: JAMES CANCER HOSPITAL AND SOLOVE RESEARCH INSTITUTE (O, 163 beds) 300 West Tenth Avenue, Columbus, OH Zip 43210–1240; tel. 614/293–3300; Dennis J. Smith, Chief Operating Officer
Web address: www.jamesline.com

OHIO STATE UNIVERSITY HOSPITALS EAST (O, 172 beds) 1492 East Broad Street, Columbus, OH Zip 43205–1546; tel. 614/257–3000; Elizabeth Seely, Executive Director
Web address: www.medicalcenter.osu.edu

OHIO STATE UNIVERSITY MEDICAL CENTER (O, 732 beds) 370 West 9th Avenue, Columbus, OH Zip 43210–1240; tel. 614/293–8000; Peter E. Geier, Chief Operating Officer
Web address: www.osumedcenter.edu

Owned, leased, sponsored:	3 hospitals	1067 beds
Contract–managed:	0 hospitals	0 beds
Totals:	3 hospitals	1067 beds

3315: OHIO VALLEY HEALTH SERVICES AND EDUCATION CORPORATION (NP)
2000 Eoff Street, Wheeling, WV Zip 26003; tel. 304/234–8383; Brian K. Felici, President and Chief Executive Officer
(Moderately Centralized Health System)

EAST OHIO REGIONAL HOSPITAL (O, 172 beds) 90 North Fourth Street, Martins Ferry, OH Zip 43935–1648; tel. 740/633–1100; Brian K. Felici, President and Chief Executive Officer
Web address: www.eorh–online.com

WEST VIRGINIA: OHIO VALLEY MEDICAL CENTER (O, 179 beds) 2000 Eoff Street, Wheeling, WV Zip 26003–3870; tel. 304/234–0123; Brian K. Felici, President and Chief Executive Officer
Web address: www.ohiovalleymedicalcenter.com

Owned, leased, sponsored:	2 hospitals	351 beds
Contract–managed:	0 hospitals	0 beds
Totals:	2 hospitals	351 beds

For explanation of codes following names, see page B2.
★ Indicates Type III membership in the American Hospital Association.

Section B

★0162: OHIOHEALTH (NP)
1087 Dennison Avenue, Columbus, OH Zip 43201; tel. 614/544–5430; David P. Blom, President and Chief Executive Officer
(Moderately Centralized Health System)

OHIO: DOCTORS HOSPITAL (O, 193 beds) 5100 West Broad Street, Columbus, OH Zip 43228–1607; tel. 614/544–1000; Michael L. Reichfield, President
Web address: www.ohiohealth.com

DOCTORS HOSPITAL NELSONVILLE (O, 70 beds) 1950 Mount Saint Mary Drive, Nelsonville, OH Zip 45764–1193; tel. 740/753–1931; Steve Swart, Administrator
Web address: www.ohiohealth.com

GRADY MEMORIAL HOSPITAL (O, 61 beds) 561 West Central Avenue, Delaware, OH Zip 43015–1485; tel. 740/369–8711; Steven J. Garlock, President
Web address: www.ohiohealth.com

GRANT MEDICAL CENTER (O, 404 beds) 111 South Grant Avenue, Columbus, OH Zip 43215–1898; tel. 614/566–9000; Karen H. Connors, President
Web address: www.ohiohealth.com

HARDIN MEMORIAL HOSPITAL (O, 25 beds) 921 East Franklin Street, Kenton, OH Zip 43326–2099, Mailing Address: P.O. Box 710, Zip 43326–0710; tel. 419/673–0761; Mark R. Seckinger, Administrator and Chief Executive Officer
Web address: www.hardinmemorial.org

MARION GENERAL HOSPITAL (O, 204 beds) 1000 McKinley Park Drive, Marion, OH Zip 43302–6397; tel. 740/383–8400; Ronald J. Bachman, President and Chief Executive Officer
Web address: www.mariongeneral.com

MORROW COUNTY HOSPITAL (C, 53 beds) 651 West Marion Road, Mount Gilead, OH Zip 43338–1027; tel. 419/946–5015; Diana D. Fisher, President and Chief Executive Officer
Web address: www.morrowcountyhospital.com

RIVERSIDE METHODIST HOSPITAL (O, 826 beds) 3535 Olentangy River Road, Columbus, OH Zip 43214–3998; tel. 614/566–5000; Bruce P. Hagen, President
Web address: www.ohiohealth.com

Owned, leased, sponsored:	7 hospitals	1783 beds
Contract-managed:	1 hospital	53 beds
Totals:	8 hospitals	1836 beds

0018: OKLAHOMA STATE DEPARTMENT OF MENTAL HEALTH AND SUBSTANCE ABUSE SERVICES (NP)
1200 N.E. 13th Street, Oklahoma City, OK Zip 73117, Mailing Address: P.O. Box 53277, Zip 73152–3277; tel. 405/522–3908; Terri White, Commissioner

OKLAHOMA: GRIFFIN MEMORIAL HOSPITAL (O, 132 beds) 900 East Main Street, Norman, OK Zip 73071–5305, Mailing Address: P.O. Box 151, Zip 73070–0151; tel. 405/321–4880; Don Bowen, Executive Director
Web address: www.odmhsas.org

NORTHWESTERN CENTER FOR BEHAVIORAL HEALTH (O, 28 beds) 1222 10th Street, Suite 211, Woodward, OK Zip 73801; tel. 580/571–3233; Trudy Hoffman, Executive Director

OKLAHOMA FORENSIC CENTER (O, 221 beds) Vinita, OK Mailing Address: P.O. Box 69, Zip 74301–0069; tel. 918/256–7841; William T. Burkett, Chief Executive Officer

Owned, leased, sponsored:	3 hospitals	381 beds
Contract-managed:	0 hospitals	0 beds
Totals:	3 hospitals	381 beds

3355: ORLANDO HEALTH (NP)
1414 Kuhl Avenue, Orlando, FL Zip 32806–2093; tel. 407/841–5111; John Hillenmeyer, President and Chief Executive Officer
(Moderately Centralized Health System)

FLORIDA: ORLANDO REGIONAL MEDICAL CENTER (O, 1387 beds) 1414 Kuhl Avenue, Orlando, FL Zip 32806–2093; tel. 407/841–5111; Sherrie Sitarik, President
Web address: www.orhs.org

ORLANDO REGIONAL SOUTH SEMINOLE HOSPITAL (O, 206 beds) 555 West State Road 434, Longwood, FL Zip 32750–4999; tel. 407/767–1200; Stephen M. Glazier, President
Web address: www.orhs.org

SOUTH LAKE HOSPITAL (O, 104 beds) 1099 Citrus Tower Boulevard, Clermont, FL Zip 34711–2787; tel. 352/394–4071; Leslie Longacre, Chief Executive Officer
Web address: www.southlakehospital.com

Owned, leased, sponsored:	3 hospitals	1697 beds
Contract-managed:	0 hospitals	0 beds
Totals:	3 hospitals	1697 beds

★5335: OSF HEALTHCARE SYSTEM (CC)
800 N.E. Glen Oak Avenue, Peoria, IL Zip 61603–3200; tel. 309/655–2850; James M. Moore, Chief Executive Officer
(Centralized Physician/Insurance Health System)

ILLINOIS: OSF SAINT ANTHONY MEDICAL CENTER (O, 238 beds) 5666 East State Street, Rockford, IL Zip 61108–2472; tel. 815/226–2000; David A. Schertz, Administrator
Web address: www.osfhealth.com

OSF SAINT FRANCIS MEDICAL CENTER (O, 566 beds) 530 N.E. Glen Oak Avenue, Peoria, IL Zip 61637–0001; tel. 309/655–2000; Keith E. Steffen, President and Chief Executive Officer
Web address: www.osfsaintfrancis.org

OSF SAINT JAMES – JOHN W. ALBRECHT MEDICAL CENTER (O, 42 beds) 2500 West Reynolds, Pontiac, IL Zip 61764–2194; tel. 815/842–2828; David T. Ochs, President and Chief Executive Officer
Web address: www.osfsaintjames.org

OSF ST. JOSEPH MEDICAL CENTER (O, 157 beds) 2200 East Washington Street, Bloomington, IL Zip 61701–4323; tel. 309/662–3311; Kenneth J. Natzke, President and Chief Executive Officer
Web address: www.osfstjoseph.org

OSF ST. MARY MEDICAL CENTER (O, 99 beds) 3333 North Seminary Street, Galesburg, IL Zip 61401–1299; tel. 309/344–3161; Richard S. Kowalski, Administrator and Chief Executive Officer
Web address: www.osfstmary.org

MICHIGAN: OSF ST. FRANCIS HOSPITAL (O, 48 beds) 3401 Ludington Street, Escanaba, MI Zip 49829–1377; tel. 906/786–3311; Peter G. Jennings, Chief Executive Officer
Web address: www.osfstfrancis.org

Owned, leased, sponsored:	6 hospitals	1150 beds
Contract-managed:	0 hospitals	0 beds
Totals:	6 hospitals	1150 beds

● 0367: PACER HEALTH CORPORATION (IO)
7759 N.W. 146th Street, Miami Lakes, FL Zip 33016; tel. 305/828–7660; Rainier Gonzalez, Chairman and Chief Executive Officer

KENTUCKY: KNOX COUNTY HOSPITAL (O, 41 beds) 80 Hospital Drive, Barbourville, KY Zip 40906–1317, Mailing Address: P.O. Box 10, Zip 40906–0160; tel. 606/546–4175; Rebecca Lewis, Chief Executive Officer
Web address: www.knoxcohospital.com

Owned, leased, sponsored:	1 hospital	41 beds
Contract-managed:	0 hospitals	0 beds
Totals:	1 hospital	41 beds

0435: PACIFIC HEALTH CORPORATION (IO)
14642 Newport Avenue, Suite 388, Tustin, CA Zip 92780; tel. 714/669–2085; James W. Young, President and Chief Executive Officer
(Independent Hospital System)

CALIFORNIA: ANAHEIM GENERAL HOSPITAL (O, 126 beds) 3350 West Ball Road, Anaheim, CA Zip 92804–3799; tel. 714/827–6700; Michael Hartman, Chief Executive Officer

For explanation of codes following names, see page B2.
★ Indicates Type III membership in the American Hospital Association.
● Single hospital health care system

BELLFLOWER MEDICAL CENTER (O, 110 beds) 9542 East Artesia Boulevard, Bellflower, CA Zip 90706–6511; tel. 562/925–8355; James Linhares, Chief Executive Officer

LOS ANGELES METROPOLITAN MEDICAL CENTER (O, 213 beds) 2231 South Western Avenue, Los Angeles, CA Zip 90018–1302; tel. 323/730–7300; John V. Fenton, Chief Executive Officer
Web address: www.lammc.com

TUSTIN HOSPITAL AND MEDICAL CENTER (O, 64 beds) 14662 Newport Avenue, Tustin, CA Zip 92680–6064; tel. 714/838–9600; R. Michael Hartman, Chief Executive Officer
Web address: www.tustinhospital.com

Owned, leased, sponsored:	4 hospitals	513 beds
Contract-managed:	0 hospitals	0 beds
Totals:	4 hospitals	513 beds

★4155: PALMETTO HEALTH (NP)
1301 Taylor Street, Suite 9–A, Columbia, SC Zip 29201, Mailing Address: P.O. Box 2266, Zip 29202–2266; tel. 803/296–2100; Charles D. Beaman, Jr., President and Chief Executive Officer
(Centralized Physician/Insurance Health System)

SOUTH CAROLINA: PALMETTO HEALTH BAPTIST EASLEY (O, 88 beds) 200 Fleetwood Drive, Easley, SC Zip 29640–2076, Mailing Address: P.O. Box 2129, Zip 29641–2129; tel. 864/442–7200; Roddey E. Gettys, III, Executive Vice President and Chief Operating Officer
Web address: www.palmettohealth.org

PALMETTO HEALTH BAPTIST/COLUMBIA (O, 441 beds) Taylor at Marion Street, Columbia, SC Zip 29220–0001; tel. 803/296–5010; James M. Bridges, Executive Vice President and Chief Operating Officer
Web address: www.palmettohealth.org

PALMETTO HEALTH RICHLAND (O, 643 beds) Five Richland Medical Park Drive, Columbia, SC Zip 29203–6897, Mailing Address: P.O. Box 2266, Zip 29203–2266; tel. 803/434–7000; John Singerling, Executive Vice President and Chief Operating Officer
Web address: www.palmettohealth.org

Owned, leased, sponsored:	3 hospitals	1172 beds
Contract-managed:	0 hospitals	0 beds
Totals:	3 hospitals	1172 beds

★7555: PALOMAR POMERADO HEALTH (NP)
15255 Innovation Drive, Suite 204, San Diego, CA Zip 92128–3410; tel. 858/675–5100; Michael H. Covert, FACHE, Chief Executive Officer
(Moderately Centralized Health System)

CALIFORNIA: PALOMAR MEDICAL CENTER (O, 315 beds) 555 East Valley Parkway, Escondido, CA Zip 92025–3084; tel. 760/739–3000; Gerald E. Bracht, Chief Administrative Officer
Web address: www.pph.org

POMERADO HOSPITAL (O, 204 beds) 15615 Pomerado Road, Poway, CA Zip 92064–2460; tel. 858/613–4000; David A. Tam, M.D., FACHE, Chief Administrative Officer
Web address: www.pph.org

Owned, leased, sponsored:	2 hospitals	519 beds
Contract-managed:	0 hospitals	0 beds
Totals:	2 hospitals	519 beds

★1985: PARK NICOLLET HEALTH SERVICES (NP)
6500 Excelsior Boulevard, Saint Louis Park, MN Zip 55426–4702; tel. 952/993–5000; David K. Wessner, President and Chief Executive Officer
(Independent Hospital System)

MINNESOTA: GLENCOE REGIONAL HEALTH SERVICES (C, 135 beds) 1805 Hennepin Avenue North, Glencoe, MN Zip 55336–1416; tel. 320/864–3121; Jon D. Braband, President and Chief Executive Officer
Web address: www.grhsonline.com

METHODIST HOSPITAL (O, 426 beds) 6500 Excelsior Boulevard, Saint Louis Park, MN Zip 55426–4702; tel. 952/993–5000; David K. Wessner, President and Chief Executive Officer
Web address: www.parknicollet.com

Owned, leased, sponsored:	1 hospital	426 beds
Contract-managed:	1 hospital	135 beds
Totals:	2 hospitals	561 beds

★0159: PARKVIEW HEALTH (NP)
10501 Corporate Drive, Fort Wayne, IN Zip 46845, Mailing Address: P.O. Box 5600, Zip 46895–5600; tel. 260/373–7001; Michael J. Packnett, President and Chief Executive Officer
(Centralized Physician/Insurance Health System)

INDIANA: PARKVIEW HOSPITAL (O, 673 beds) 2200 Randallia Drive, Fort Wayne, IN Zip 46805–4699; tel. 260/373–4000; Sue Ehinger, Chief Operating Officer
Web address: www.parkview.com

PARKVIEW HUNTINGTON HOSPITAL (O, 36 beds) 2001 Stults Road, Huntington, IN Zip 46750–3696; tel. 260/355–3000; Darlene Garrett, Chief Operating Officer
Web address: www.parkview.com

PARKVIEW LAGRANGE HOSPITAL (O, 25 beds) 207 North Townline Road, LaGrange, IN Zip 46761–1325; tel. 260/463–2143; Robert T. Myers, Chief Operating Officer
Web address: www.parkview.com

PARKVIEW NOBLE HOSPITAL (O, 31 beds) 401 Sawyer Road, Kendallville, IN Zip 46755–2293, Mailing Address: P.O. Box 728, Zip 46755–0728; tel. 260/347–8700; David C. Hunter, Chief Operating Officer
Web address: www.parkview.com

PARKVIEW WHITLEY HOSPITAL (O, 118 beds) 353 North Oak Street, Columbia City, IN Zip 46725–1623; tel. 260/248–9000; John K. Meister, Chief Operating Officer
Web address: www.parkview.com

Owned, leased, sponsored:	5 hospitals	883 beds
Contract-managed:	0 hospitals	0 beds
Totals:	5 hospitals	883 beds

★1785: PARTNERS HEALTHCARE SYSTEM, INC. (NP)
800 Boylston Street, Suite 1150, Boston, MA Zip 02199–8001; tel. 617/278–1004; James J. Mongan, M.D., President and Chief Executive Officer
(Moderately Centralized Health System)

MASSACHUSETTS: BRIGHAM AND WOMEN'S HOSPITAL (O, 746 beds) 75 Francis Street, Boston, MA Zip 02115–6195; tel. 617/732–5500; Gary L. Gottlieb, M.D., President
Web address: www.brighamandwomens.org

FAULKNER HOSPITAL (O, 104 beds) Boston, MA Mailing Address: 1153 Centre Sreet, Zip 02130–3400; tel. 617/983–7000; David J. Trull, President and Chief Executive Officer
Web address: www.faulknerhospital.org

MARTHA'S VINEYARD HOSPITAL (O, 25 beds) One Hospital Road, Oak Bluffs, MA Zip 2557, Mailing Address: P.O. Box 1477, Zip 02557–1477; tel. 508/693–0410; Timothy J. Walsh, Chief Executive Officer
Web address: www.marthasvineyardhospital.org

MASSACHUSETTS GENERAL HOSPITAL (O, 907 beds) 55 Fruit Street, Boston, MA Zip 02114–2696; tel. 617/726–2000; Peter L. Slavin, M.D., President
Web address: www.massgeneral.org

MCLEAN HOSPITAL (O, 172 beds) 115 Mill Street, Belmont, MA Zip 02478-9106; tel. 617/855–2000; Scott L. Rauch, M.D., President
Web address: www.mclean.harvard.edu

NANTUCKET COTTAGE HOSPITAL (O, 19 beds) 57 Prospect Street, Nantucket, MA Zip 02554–2799; tel. 508/825–8100; Sylvia Getman, President and Chief Executive Officer
Web address: www.nantuckethospital.org

NEWTON–WELLESLEY HOSPITAL (O, 226 beds) 2014 Washington Street, Newton Lower Falls, MA Zip 02462–1699; tel. 617/243–6000; Michael Jellinek, M.D., President
Web address: www.nwh.org

Section B

For explanation of codes following names, see page B2.
★ Indicates Type III membership in the American Hospital Association.

NORTH SHORE MEDICAL CENTER (O, 415 beds) 81 Highland Avenue, Salem, MA Zip 01970–2768; tel. 978/741–1200; Robert G. Norton, CHE, President and Chief Executive Officer
Web address: www.nsmc.partners.org

SHAUGHNESSY–KAPLAN REHABILITATION HOSPITAL (O, 160 beds) Dove Avenue, Salem, MA Zip 01970–2999; tel. 978/745–9000; Maureen Banks, President
Web address: www.shaughnessy–kaplan.org

SPAULDING REHABILITATION HOSPITAL (O, 196 beds) 125 Nashua Street, Boston, MA Zip 02114–1198; tel. 617/573–7000; Judith C. Waterston, M.S., President
Web address: www.spauldingrehab.org

Owned, leased, sponsored:	10 hospitals	2970 beds
Contract–managed:	0 hospitals	0 beds
Totals:	10 hospitals	2970 beds

★5415: PEACEHEALTH (CC)
14432 S.E. Eastgate Way, Suite 300, Bellevue, WA Zip 98007–6412; tel. 425/747–1711; Alan R. Yordy, President and Chief Mission Officer
(Moderately Centralized Health System)

ALASKA: KETCHIKAN GENERAL HOSPITAL (L, 54 beds) 3100 Tongass Avenue, Ketchikan, AK Zip 99901–5746; tel. 907/225–5171; Patrick J. Branco, Chief Executive Officer
Web address: www.peacehealth.org

OREGON: COTTAGE GROVE COMMUNITY HOSPITAL (O, 14 beds) 1515 Village Drive, Cottage Grove, OR Zip 97424; tel. 541/942–0511; Randall L. Mee, RN, Chief Executive Officer
Web address: www.peacehealth.org

PEACE HARBOR HOSPITAL (O, 21 beds) 400 Ninth Street, Florence, OR Zip 97439–7398; tel. 541/997–8412; James R. Barnhart, Chief Executive Officer
Web address: www.peacehealth.org

SACRED HEART MEDICAL CENTER (O, 476 beds) 1255 Hilyard Street, Eugene, OR Zip 97401–3700, Mailing Address: P.O. Box 10905, Zip 97440–0905; tel. 541/686–7300; Jill Hoggard Green, RN, Ph.D., Administrator and Chief Executive Officer
Web address: www.peacehealth.org

WASHINGTON: ST. JOHN MEDICAL CENTER (O, 202 beds) 1615 Delaware Street, Longview, WA Zip 98632–2310, Mailing Address: P.O. Box 3002, Zip 98632–3002; tel. 360/414–2000; Medrice Coluccio, Chief Executive Officer
Web address: www.peacehealth.org

ST. JOSEPH HOSPITAL (O, 243 beds) 2901 Squalicum Parkway, Bellingham, WA Zip 98225–1898; tel. 360/734–5400; Nancy Steiger, Chief Executive Officer and Chief Mission Officer
Web address: www.peacehealth.org

Owned, leased, sponsored:	6 hospitals	1010 beds
Contract–managed:	0 hospitals	0 beds
Totals:	6 hospitals	1010 beds

★0314: PHOEBE PUTNEY HEALTH SYSTEM (NP)
417 Third Avenue, Albany, GA Zip 31702; tel. 229/312–1000; Joel Wernick, President and Chief Executive Officer
(Centralized Health System)

GEORGIA: PHOEBE PUTNEY MEMORIAL HOSPITAL (O, 439 beds) 417 Third Avenue, Albany, GA Zip 31701–1828, Mailing Address: P.O. Box 1828, Zip 31703–1828; tel. 229/883–1800; Joel Wernick, President and Chief Executive Officer
Web address: www.phoebeputney.com

PHOEBE WORTH MEDICAL CENTER (O, 25 beds) 807 South Isabella Street, Sylvester, GA Zip 31791–0545, Mailing Address: P.O. Box 545, Zip 31791–0545; tel. 229/776–6961; Keith J. Petersen, Chief Executive Officer
Web address: www.phobeputney.com

Owned, leased, sponsored:	2 hospitals	464 beds
Contract–managed:	0 hospitals	0 beds
Totals:	2 hospitals	464 beds

★0310: PIEDMONT HEALTHCARE (NP)
2001 Peachtree Road N.E., Suite 400, Atlanta, GA Zip 30309; tel. 404/605–3215; R. Timothy Stack, FACHE, President and Chief Executive Officer
(Moderately Centralized Health System)

PIEDMONT FAYETTE HOSPITAL (O, 106 beds) 1255 Highway 54 West, Fayetteville, GA Zip 30214; tel. 770/719–7000; W. Darrell Cutts, President and Chief Executive Officer
Web address: www.fayettehospital.org

PIEDMONT HOSPITAL (O, 441 beds) 1968 Peachtree Road N.W., Atlanta, GA Zip 30309–1231; tel. 404/605–5000; Robert W. Maynard, President and Chief Executive Officer
Web address: www.piedmonthospital.org

PIEDMONT MOUNTAINSIDE HOSPITAL (O, 48 beds) 1266 Highway 515 South, Jasper, GA Zip 30143; tel. 706/692–2441; Ed Lovern, President and Chief Executive Officer
Web address: www.piedmontmountainsidehospital.org

PIEDMONT NEWNAN HOSPITAL (O, 271 beds) 60 Hospital Road, Newnan, GA Zip 30263–1210, Mailing Address: P.O. Box 997, Zip 30264–0997; tel. 770/253–1912; G. Michael Bass, President and Chief Executive Officer
Web address: www.newnanhospital.org

Owned, leased, sponsored:	4 hospitals	866 beds
Contract–managed:	0 hospitals	0 beds
Totals:	4 hospitals	866 beds

0091: PIONEER BEHAVIORAL HEALTH (IO)
200 Lake Street, Suite 102, Peabody, MA Zip 01960–4780; tel. 978/536–2777; Bruce A. Shear, President and Chief Executive Officer
(Independent Hospital System)

MICHIGAN: HARBOR OAKS HOSPITAL (O, 64 beds) 35031 23 Mile Road, New Baltimore, MI Zip 48047–2097; tel. 586/725–5777; Tina Lesnik, Chief Operating Officer
Web address: www.harboroaks.com

UTAH: HIGHLAND RIDGE HOSPITAL (O, 32 beds) 7309 South 180 West, Midvale, UT Zip 84047–3769; tel. 801/569–2153; Robert Beatty, Chief Operating Officer
Web address: www.highlandridgehospital.com

VIRGINIA: MOUNT REGIS CENTER (O, 25 beds) 405 Kimball Avenue, Salem, VA Zip 24153–6299; tel. 540/389–4761; Gail S. Basham, Chief Executive Officer
Web address: www.mtregis.com

Owned, leased, sponsored:	3 hospitals	121 beds
Contract–managed:	0 hospitals	0 beds
Totals:	3 hospitals	121 beds

0326: PIONEER HEALTH SERVICES (IO)
301 Eighth Avenue S.W., Magee, MS Zip 39111, Mailing Address: P.O. Box 1100, Zip 39111; tel. 601/849–6440; Joseph S. McNulty, President and Chief Executive Officer
(Independent Hospital System)

MISSISSIPPI: PIONEER COMMUNITY HOSPITAL OF ABERDEEN (O, 35 beds) 400 South Chestnut Street, Aberdeen, MS Zip 39730–3335, Mailing Address: P.O. Box 548, Zip 39730–0747; tel. 662/369–2455; Steven M. Fontaine, Administrator
Web address: www.pchaberdeen.com

S. E. LACKEY MEMORIAL HOSPITAL (O, 55 beds) 330 Broad Street, Forest, MS Zip 39074–0428, Mailing Address: P.O. Box 428, Zip 39074–0428; tel. 601/469–4151; Donna Riser, Administrator
Web address: www.selackey.com

For explanation of codes following names, see page B2.
★ Indicates Type III membership in the American Hospital Association.

Owned, leased, sponsored:	2 hospitals	90 beds
Contract-managed:	0 hospitals	0 beds
Totals:	2 hospitals	90 beds

0381: POUDRE VALLEY HEALTH SYSTEM (NP)
1809 East Harmony Road, Fort Collins, CO Zip 80528; tel. 970/297-6701; Rulon F. Stacey, President and Chief Executive Officer

COLORADO: MEDICAL CENTER OF THE ROCKIES (O, 136 beds) 2500 Rocky Mountain Avenue, Loveland, CO Zip 80538; tel. 970/624-2500; George E. Hayes, Chief Executive Officer
Web address: www.medctrrockies.org

POUDRE VALLEY HOSPITAL (O, 233 beds) 1024 South Lemay Avenue, Fort Collins, CO Zip 80524-3998; tel. 970/495-7000; Kevin L. Unger, FACHE, President and Chief Executive Officer
Web address: www.pvhs.org

Owned, leased, sponsored:	2 hospitals	369 beds
Contract-managed:	0 hospitals	0 beds
Totals:	2 hospitals	369 beds

0240: PREFERRED MANAGEMENT CORPORATION (IO)
120 West MacArthur, Suite 121, Shawnee, OK Zip 74804-2028; tel. 405/878-0202; Donald Freeman, Vice President and Chief Executive Officer
(Independent Hospital System)

OKLAHOMA: ARBUCKLE MEMORIAL HOSPITAL (C, 25 beds) 2011 West Broadway Street, Sulphur, OK Zip 73086-4221; tel. 580/622-2161; Darin Farrell, Chief Executive Officer
Web address: www.arbucklehospital.com/

TEXAS: COLLINGSWORTH GENERAL HOSPITAL (L, 16 beds) 1014 15th Street, Wellington, TX Zip 79095-3704, Mailing Address: P.O. Box 1112, Zip 79095-1112; tel. 806/447-2521; Candy Powell, Administrator

CULBERSON HOSPITAL (L, 14 beds) Eisenhower-Farm Market Road 2185, Van Horn, TX Zip 79855, Mailing Address: P.O. Box 609, Zip 79855-0609; tel. 432/283-2760; Ladelle Bates, Chief Executive Officer

PARMER COUNTY COMMUNITY HOSPITAL (C, 15 beds) 1307 Cleveland Street, Friona, TX Zip 79035-1121; tel. 806/250-2754; Brandon L. Gatlin, Administrator

SABINE COUNTY HOSPITAL (L, 25 beds) Highway 83 West, Hemphill, TX Zip 75948, Mailing Address: P.O. Box 750, Zip 75948-0750; tel. 409/787-3300; Deanna Lathrop, Interim Chief Executive Officer

SCHLEICHER COUNTY MEDICAL CENTER (L, 14 beds) 400 West Murchison, Eldorado, TX Zip 76936, Mailing Address: Box V, Zip 76936; tel. 325/853-2507; Sharon Dietz, Administrator

Owned, leased, sponsored:	4 hospitals	69 beds
Contract-managed:	2 hospitals	40 beds
Totals:	6 hospitals	109 beds

★3505: PRESBYTERIAN HEALTHCARE SERVICES (CO)
2501 Buena Vista, S.E., Albuquerque, NM Zip 87106, Mailing Address: P.O. Box 26666, Zip 87125-6666; tel. 505/841-1234; James H. Hinton, President and Chief Executive Officer
(Centralized Physician/Insurance Health System)

NEW MEXICO: DR. DAN C. TRIGG MEMORIAL HOSPITAL (L, 25 beds) 301 East Miel De Luna Avenue, Tucumcari, NM Zip 88401-3810, Mailing Address: P.O. Box 608, Zip 88401-0608; tel. 505/461-7003; Hoyt Skabelund, Administrator
Web address: www.phs.org

ESPANOLA HOSPITAL (O, 80 beds) 1010 Spruce Street, Espanola, NM Zip 87532-2746; tel. 505/753-7111; Derrick Yu, Administrator
Web address: www.phs.org

LINCOLN COUNTY MEDICAL CENTER (L, 25 beds) 211 Sudderth Drive, Ruidoso, NM Zip 88345-6043, Mailing Address: P.O. Box 8000, Zip 88345-8000; tel. 505/257-7381; James P. Gibson, Administrator
Web address: www.phs.org

PLAINS REGIONAL MEDICAL CENTER (O, 106 beds) 2100 Martin Luther King, Jr. Boulevard, Clovis, NM Zip 88101-9412, Mailing Address: P.O. Box 1688, Zip 88101-1688; tel. 505/769-2141; Hoyt Skabelund, Administrator
Web address: www.phs.org

PRESBYTERIAN HOSPITAL (O, 552 beds) 1100 Central Avenue S.E., Albuquerque, NM Zip 87106-4934, Mailing Address: P.O. Box 26666, Zip 87125-6666; tel. 505/841-1234; Lauren Cates, Vice President Central New Mexico Operations
Web address: www.phs.org

PRESBYTERIAN KASEMAN HOSPITAL (O, 124 beds) 8300 Constitution Avenue N.E., Albuquerque, NM Zip 87110-7624, Mailing Address: P.O. Box 26666, Zip 87125-6666; tel. 505/291-2000; Matt Pehrson, Administrative Director
Web address: www.phs.org

SOCORRO GENERAL HOSPITAL (O, 24 beds) 1202 Highway 60 West, Socorro, NM Zip 87801, Mailing Address: P.O. Box 1009, Zip 87801-1009; tel. 505/835-1140; Bo Beames, Administrator
Web address: www.phs.org/facilities/facsocorro.htm

Owned, leased, sponsored:	7 hospitals	936 beds
Contract-managed:	0 hospitals	0 beds
Totals:	7 hospitals	936 beds

0357: PRIME HEALTHCARE SERVICES (IO)
16850 Bear Valley Road, Wildomar, CA Zip 92395; tel. 760/241-8000; Lex Reddy, President and Chief Executive Officer
(Independent Hospital System)

CALIFORNIA: CENTINELA HOSPITAL MEDICAL CENTER (O, 369 beds) 555 East Hardy Street, Inglewood, CA Zip 90301-4011, Mailing Address: P.O. Box 720, Zip 90307-0720; tel. 310/673-4660; Von L. Crockett, President and Chief Executive Officer
Web address: www.centinelamed.com

CHINO VALLEY MEDICAL CENTER (O, 126 beds) 5451 Walnut Avenue, Chino, CA Zip 91710-2672; tel. 909/464-8600; Lex Reddy, Chief Executive Officer
Web address: www.cvmc.com

DESERT VALLEY HOSPITAL (O, 83 beds) 16850 Bear Valley Road, Victorville, CA Zip 92395; tel. 760/241-8000; Lex Reddy, President and Chief Executive Officer
Web address: www.dvmc.com

ENCINO-TARZANA REGIONAL MEDICAL CENTER-ENCINO CAMPUS (O, 151 beds) 16237 Ventura Boulevard, Encino, CA Zip 91436-2201; tel. 818/995-5000; Dale Surowitz, Chief Executive Officer
Web address: www.encino-tarzana.com

GARDEN GROVE HOSPITAL AND MEDICAL CENTER (O, 74 beds) 12601 Garden Grove Boulevard, Garden Grove, CA Zip 92843-1908; tel. 714/537-5160; Maxine T. Cooper, Chief Executive Officer
Web address: www.gardengrovehospital.com

HUNTINGTON BEACH HOSPITAL (O, 145 beds) 17772 Beach Boulevard, Huntington Beach, CA Zip 92647-6819; tel. 714/842-1473; Sofia Abrina, Administrator and Chief Nursing Officer
Web address: www.hbhospital.com

LA PALMA INTERCOMMUNITY HOSPITAL (O, 141 beds) 7901 Walker Street, La Palma, CA Zip 90623-1722, Mailing Address: P.O. Box 5850, Buena Park, Zip 90622-5850; tel. 714/670-7400; Virgis Narbutas, Chief Executive Officer
Web address: www.lapalmaintercommunityhospital.com

MONTCLAIR HOSPITAL MEDICAL CENTER (O, 102 beds) 5000 San Bernardino Street, Montclair, CA Zip 91763-2326; tel. 909/625-5411; Gregory Brentano, Chief Executive Officer
Web address: www.dhmcm.com

PARADISE VALLEY HOSPITAL (O, 301 beds) 2400 East Fourth Street, National City, CA Zip 91950-2099; tel. 619/470-4321; Luis Leon, Chief Executive Officer
Web address: www.paradisevalleyhospital.org

SAN DIMAS COMMUNITY HOSPITAL (O, 64 beds) 1350 West Covina Boulevard, San Dimas, CA Zip 91773-3219; tel. 909/599-6811; Dan Bowers, Chief Executive Officer
Web address: www.sandimashospital.com

SHERMAN OAKS HOSPITAL (O, 112 beds) 4929 Van Nuys Boulevard, Sherman Oaks, CA Zip 91403-1702; tel. 818/981-7111; Lex Reddy, President and Chief Executive Officer
Web address: www.shermanoakshospital.com

For explanation of codes following names, see page B2.
★ Indicates Type III membership in the American Hospital Association.

WEST ANAHEIM MEDICAL CENTER (O, 219 beds) 3033 West Orange Avenue, Anaheim, CA Zip 92804–3184; tel. 714/827–3000; Virgis Narbutas, Chief Executive Officer
Web address: www.westanaheimmedctr.com

Owned, leased, sponsored:	12 hospitals	1887 beds
Contract–managed:	0 hospitals	0 beds
Totals:	12 hospitals	1887 beds

★0153: PROHEALTH CARE (NP)

N17 W24100 Riverwood Drive, Suite 130, Waukesha, WI Zip 53188; tel. 262/928–2244; Rexford W. Titus, III, President and Chief Executive Officer
(Moderately Centralized Health System)

WISCONSIN: OCONOMOWOC MEMORIAL HOSPITAL (O, 74 beds) 791 Summit Avenue, Oconomowoc, WI Zip 53066–3896; tel. 262/569–9400; John R. Robertstad, FACHE, President and Chief Executive Officer
Web address: www.oconomowocmemorial.org

WAUKESHA MEMORIAL HOSPITAL (O, 330 beds) 725 American Avenue, Waukesha, WI Zip 53188–5099; tel. 262/928–1000; Edward A. Olson, President and Chief Executive Officer
Web address: www.waukeshamemorial.org

Owned, leased, sponsored:	2 hospitals	404 beds
Contract–managed:	0 hospitals	0 beds
Totals:	2 hospitals	404 beds

★0197: PROMEDICA HEALTH SYSTEM (NP)

1801 Richards Road, Toledo, OH Zip 43607; tel. 419/469–3800; Alan W. Brass, FACHE, Chief Executive Officer and President
(Centralized Physician/Insurance Health System)

MICHIGAN: BIXBY MEDICAL CENTER (O, 66 beds) 818 Riverside Avenue, Adrian, MI Zip 49221–1496; tel. 517/265–0900; Gregory Corbett, President
Web address: www.promedica.org

HERRICK MEDICAL CENTER (O, 60 beds) 500 East Pottawatamie Street, Tecumseh, MI Zip 49286–2097; tel. 517/424–3000; Gregory Corbett, President
Web address: www.promedica.org

OHIO: BAY PARK COMMUNITY HOSPITAL (O, 70 beds) 2801 Bay Park Drive, Oregon, OH Zip 43616; tel. 419/690–7900; Bill Mueller, President
Web address: www.promedica.org

DEFIANCE REGIONAL MEDICAL CENTER (O, 35 beds) 1200 Ralston Avenue, Defiance, OH Zip 43512–1396; tel. 419/783–6955; Timothy Jakacki, President and Chief Executive Officer
Web address: www.promedica.org

FLOWER HOSPITAL (O, 225 beds) 5200 Harroun Road, Sylvania, OH Zip 43560–2196; tel. 419/824–1444; Kevin C. Webb, FACHE, President
Web address: www.promedica.org

FOSTORIA COMMUNITY HOSPITAL (O, 25 beds) 501 Van Buren Street, Fostoria, OH Zip 44830–0907, Mailing Address: P.O. Box 907, Zip 44830–0907; tel. 419/435–7734; Timothy Jakacki, President and Chief Executive Officer
Web address: www.promedica.org

THE TOLEDO HOSPITAL (O, 587 beds) 2142 North Cove Boulevard, Toledo, OH Zip 43606–3896; tel. 419/291–4000; Barbara Steele, Chief Executive Officer
Web address: www.promedica.org

Owned, leased, sponsored:	7 hospitals	1068 beds
Contract–managed:	0 hospitals	0 beds
Totals:	7 hospitals	1068 beds

0230: PROMISE HEALTHCARE (IO)

999 Yamato Road, 3rd Floor, Boca Raton, FL Zip 33431; tel. 561/869–3100; Howard B. Koslow, President and Chief Executive Officer
(Independent Hospital System)

ARIZONA: PROMISE HOSPITAL OF PHOENIX (O, 40 beds) 1800 East Van Buren Street, 2nd Floor, Phoenix, AZ Zip 85007; tel. 602/716–5000; Kevin Nicholson, Chief Executive Officer
Web address: www.promise–phoenix.com

ARKANSAS: DE QUEEN MEDICAL CENTER (O, 35 beds) 1306 Collin Raye Drive, De Queen, AR Zip 71832–2198; tel. 870/584–4111; Layne Webb, Chief Executive Officer
Web address: www.dequeenmedicalcenter.com

CALIFORNIA: PROMISE HOSPITAL OF EAST LOS ANGELES, SUBURBAN MEDICAL CENTER CAMPUS (O, 182 beds) 16453 South Colorado Avenue, Paramount, CA Zip 90723–5000; tel. 562/531–3110; Richard McCarthy, Chief Executive Officer
Web address: www.promiseeastla.com

LOUISIANA: DEQUINCY MEMORIAL HOSPITAL (O, 19 beds) 110 West Fourth Street, DeQuincy, LA Zip 70633–3508, Mailing Address: P.O. Box 1166, Zip 70633–1166; tel. 337/786–1200; Michael Ashford, Administrator
Web address: www.dequincyhospital.com

PROMISE HOSPITAL OF BATON ROUGE (O, 29 beds) 17000 Medical Center Drive, 3rd Floor, Baton Rouge, LA Zip 70816; tel. 225/236–5440; Craig Boudreaux, Jr., Chief Executive Officer
Web address: www.promise–batonrouge.com

PROMISE HOSPITAL OF MISS LOU (O, 40 beds) 6818–A Highway 84, Ferriday, LA Zip 71334–5101; tel. 318/757–7575; Lee Huckaby, Chief Executive Officer
Web address: www.camelothealthcare.net

PROMISE SPECIALTY HOSPITAL OF SHREVEPORT (O, 146 beds) 1800 Irving Place, Shreveport, LA Zip 71101–4608; tel. 318/425–4096; Martin C. Milner, Chief Executive Officer
Web address: www.promise–shreveport.com

MISSISSIPPI: PROMISE HOSPITAL OF VICKSBURG (O, 35 beds) 1111 North Frontage Road, 2nd Floor, Vicksburg, MS Zip 39180; tel. 601/619–3526; Lee Huckaby, Chief Executive Officer
Web address: www.promise–vicksburg.com

TEXAS: PROMISE HOSPITAL OF SAN ANTONIO (O, 26 beds) 7400 Barlite Boulevard, 2nd Floor, San Antonio, TX Zip 78224; tel. 210/921–3550; Karen Pitcher, Vice President and Chief Executive Officer
Web address: www.promise–sanantonio.com

PROMISE SPECIALTY HOSPITAL OF SOUTHEAST TEXAS (O, 25 beds) 2600 Highway 365, Nederland, TX Zip 77627–6237; tel. 409/726–8700; James L. McEwen, Ph.D., Administrator
Web address: www.promise–southeasttexas.com

Owned, leased, sponsored:	10 hospitals	577 beds
Contract–managed:	0 hospitals	0 beds
Totals:	10 hospitals	577 beds

★0132: PROVENA HEALTH (CO)

19065 Hickory Creek Drive, Suite 300, Mokena, IL Zip 60448; tel. 708/478–6300; Steven L. Hunter, President and Chief Executive Officer
(Moderately Centralized Health System)

ILLINOIS: PROVENA COVENANT MEDICAL CENTER (O, 202 beds) 1400 West Park Street, Urbana, IL Zip 61801–2396; tel. 217/337–2000; David Bertauski, President and Chief Executive Officer
Web address: www.provenacovenant.org

PROVENA MERCY MEDICAL CENTER (O, 261 beds) 1325 North Highland Avenue, Aurora, IL Zip 60506–1449; tel. 630/859–2222; William A. Brown, FACHE, President and Chief Executive Officer
Web address: www.provenamercy.com

PROVENA SAINT JOSEPH HOSPITAL (O, 179 beds) 77 North Airlite Street, Elgin, IL Zip 60123–4912; tel. 847/695–3200; William A. Brown, FACHE, President and Chief Executive Officer
Web address: www.provenahealth.com

PROVENA SAINT JOSEPH MEDICAL CENTER (O, 462 beds) 333 North Madison Street, Joliet, IL Zip 60435–6595; tel. 815/725–7133; Jeffrey Brickman, President and Chief Executive Officer
Web address: www.provenasaintjoe.org

PROVENA ST. MARY'S HOSPITAL (O, 143 beds) 500 West Court Street, Kankakee, IL Zip 60901–3661; tel. 815/937–2400; Jeffrey Brickman, President and Chief Executive Officer
Web address: www.provena–stmarys.com

For explanation of codes following names, see page B2.
★ Indicates Type III membership in the American Hospital Association.

PROVENA UNITED SAMARITANS MEDICAL CENTER (O, 158 beds) 812 North Logan, Danville, IL Zip 61832–3788; tel. 217/443–5000; David Bertauski, President and Chief Executive Officer
Web address: www.provenausmc.org

Owned, leased, sponsored:	6 hospitals	1405 beds
Contract–managed:	0 hospitals	0 beds
Totals:	6 hospitals	1405 beds

★0344: PROVIDENCE HEALTH & SERVICES (CC)
506 Second Avenue, Suite 1200, Seattle, WA Zip 98104–2329; tel. 206/464–3355; John F. Koster, M.D., President and Chief Executive Officer
(Decentralized Health System)

ALASKA: PROVIDENCE ALASKA MEDICAL CENTER (O, 364 beds) 3200 Providence Drive, Anchorage, AK Zip 99508–4615, Mailing Address: P.O. Box 196604, Zip 99519–6604; tel. 907/562–2211; E. Al Parrish, Vice President and Chief Executive Officer
Web address: www.providence.org/alaska/pamc/default.htm

PROVIDENCE KODIAK ISLAND MEDICAL CENTER (L, 25 beds) 1915 East Rezanof Drive, Kodiak, AK Zip 99615–6602; tel. 907/486–3281; Donald J. Rush, Chief Executive Officer
Web address: www.providence.org

PROVIDENCE SEWARD MEDICAL CENTER (L, 6 beds) 417 First Avenue, Seward, AK Zip 99664, Mailing Address: P.O. Box 365, Zip 99664–0365; tel. 907/224–5205; Kathy Kloster, Administrator
Web address: www.providence.org

CALIFORNIA: LITTLE COMPANY OF MARY HOSPITAL (O, 272 beds) 4101 Torrance Boulevard, Torrance, CA Zip 90503–4698; tel. 310/540–7676; Michael Hunn, Administrator
Web address: www.lcmweb.org

LITTTLE COMPANY OF MARY – SAN PEDRO HOSPITAL (O, 335 beds) 1300 West Seventh Street, San Pedro, CA Zip 90732–3505; tel. 310/832–3311; Nancy Carlson, Administrator
Web address: www.lcmhs.org

PROVIDENCE HOLY CROSS MEDICAL CENTER (O, 254 beds) 15031 Rinaldi Street, San Fernando, CA Zip 91346–9600; tel. 818/365–8051; Kerry Carmody, Chief Executive
Web address: www.providence.org/losangeles/facilities/providence_holy_cross/

PROVIDENCE SAINT JOSEPH MEDICAL CENTER (O, 448 beds) 501 South Buena Vista Street, Burbank, CA Zip 91505–4866; tel. 818/843–5111; Barry A. Wolfman, Chief Executive
Web address: www.providence.org

MONTANA: COMMUNITY HOSPITAL OF ANACONDA (C, 87 beds) 401 West Pennsylvania Street, Anaconda, MT Zip 59711–1931; tel. 406/563–8500; Steve McNeece, Chief Executive Officer

ST. JOSEPH HOSPITAL (S, 22 beds) 6 Thirteenth Avenue East, Polson, MT Zip 59860–5316, Mailing Address: P.O. Box 1010, Zip 59860–1010; tel. 406/883–5377; John W. Glueckert, President
Web address: www.saintjoes.org

ST. PATRICK HOSPITAL (S, 185 beds) 500 West Broadway, Missoula, MT Zip 59802–4096, Mailing Address: P.O. Box 4587, Zip 59806–4587; tel. 406/543–7271; Jeff Fee, Chief Executive Officer
Web address: www.saintpatrick.org

OREGON: PROVIDENCE HOOD RIVER MEMORIAL HOSPITAL (O, 25 beds) 811 13th Street, Hood River, OR Zip 97031–1204, Mailing Address: P.O. Box 149, Zip 97031–0149; tel. 541/386–3911; Ty W. Erickson, Chief Executive Officer
Web address: www.providence.org/hoodriver

PROVIDENCE MEDFORD MEDICAL CENTER (O, 135 beds) 1111 Crater Lake Avenue, Medford, OR Zip 97504–6241; tel. 541/732–5000; Thomas S. Hanenburg, Chief Executive
Web address: www.providence.org

PROVIDENCE MILWAUKIE HOSPITAL (O, 66 beds) 10150 S.E. 32nd Avenue, Milwaukie, OR Zip 97222–6593; tel. 503/513–8300; Theron Park, Administrator
Web address: www.providence.org

PROVIDENCE NEWBERG MEDICAL CENTER (O, 40 beds) 1001 Providence Drive, Newberg, OR Zip 97132–7485; tel. 503/537–1555; Larry Bowe, Chief Executive, Yamhill Service Area
Web address: www.phsor.org

PROVIDENCE PORTLAND MEDICAL CENTER (O, 409 beds) 4805 N.E. Glisan Street, Portland, OR Zip 97213–2967; tel. 503/215–1111; Lisa Vance, Administrator
Web address: www.providence.org

PROVIDENCE SEASIDE HOSPITAL (L, 47 beds) 725 South Wahanna Road, Seaside, OR Zip 97138–7735; tel. 503/717–7000; William P. Sexton, Chief Executive
Web address: www.providence.org

PROVIDENCE ST. VINCENT MEDICAL CENTER (O, 523 beds) 9205 S.W. Barnes Road, Portland, OR Zip 97225–6661; tel. 503/216–1234; Janice Burger, Administrator
Web address: www.providence.org/portland/hospitals

WASHINGTON: HOLY FAMILY HOSPITAL (S, 199 beds) North 5633 Lidgerwood Street, Spokane, WA Zip 99208–2533; tel. 509/482–0111; Thomas Corley, President
Web address: www.holy–family.org

MOUNT CARMEL HOSPITAL (S, 25 beds) 982 East Columbia Street, Colville, WA Zip 99114–3352; tel. 509/684–2561; Robert D. Campbell, Jr., President
Web address: www.mtcarmelhospital.org

PROVIDENCE CENTRALIA HOSPITAL (O, 133 beds) 914 South Scheuber Road, Centralia, WA Zip 98531–9027; tel. 360/736–2803; Cindy Mayo, Chief Executive
Web address: www.providence.org

PROVIDENCE EVERETT MEDICAL CENTER (O, 362 beds) 1321 Colby Avenue, Everett, WA Zip 98206–1147, Mailing Address: P.O. Box 1147, Zip 98206–1147; tel. 425/261–2000; David Brooks, Chief Operating Officer
Web address: www.providence.org

PROVIDENCE ST. PETER HOSPITAL (O, 338 beds) 413 Lilly Road N.E., Olympia, WA Zip 98506–5166; tel. 360/491–9480; James Leonard, Administrator
Web address: www.providence.org/swsa/facilities/st_peter_hospital

SACRED HEART MEDICAL CENTER (S, 623 beds) 101 West Eighth Avenue, Spokane, WA Zip 99204–2364, Mailing Address: P.O. Box 2555, Zip 99220–2555; tel. 509/474–3040; Michael D. Wilson, President
Web address: www.shmc.org

ST. JOSEPH'S HOSPITAL (S, 25 beds) 500 East Webster Street, Chewelah, WA Zip 99109–0197, Mailing Address: P.O. Box 197, Zip 99109–0197; tel. 509/935–8211; Gary V. Peck, Administrator
Web address: www.sjhospital.org

ST. MARY MEDICAL CENTER (S, 99 beds) 401 West Poplar Street, Walla Walla, WA Zip 99362, Mailing Address: Box 1477, Zip 99362; tel. 509/525–3320; Steven A. Burdick, Chief Executive Officer
Web address: www.smmc.com

WHITMAN HOSPITAL AND MEDICAL CENTER (C, 25 beds) 1200 West Fairview, Colfax, WA Zip 99111–9579; tel. 509/397–3435; Jon R. Davis, FACHE, Chief Executive Officer
Web address: www.whitmanhospital.com

Owned, leased, sponsored:	24 hospitals	4960 beds
Contract–managed:	2 hospitals	112 beds
Totals:	26 hospitals	5072 beds

0263: PSYCHIATRIC SOLUTIONS (IO)
6640 Carothers Parkway, Suite 500, Franklin, TN Zip 37067; tel. 615/312–5700; Joey Jacobs, President and Chief Executive Officer
(Independent Hospital System)

ALABAMA: HILL CREST BEHAVIORAL HEALTH SERVICES (O, 55 beds) 6869 Fifth Avenue South, Birmingham, AL Zip 35212–1866; tel. 205/833–9000; Steve McCabe, Chief Executive Officer
Web address: www.psysolutions.com

LAUREL OAKS BEHAVIORAL HEALTH CENTER (O, 24 beds) 700 East Cottonwood Road, Dothan, AL Zip 36301; tel. 334/794–7373; Russell C. Dean, Jr., Chief Executive Officer
Web address: www.psysolutions.com

For explanation of codes following names, see page B2.
★ Indicates Type III membership in the American Hospital Association.

Section B

ARKANSAS: PINNACLE POINTE HOSPITAL (O, 102 beds) 11501 Financial Center Parkway, Little Rock, AR Zip 72211–3715; tel. 501/223–3322; Lisa Evans, Chief Executive Officer
Web address: www.psysolutions.com

CALIFORNIA: ALHAMBRA HOSPITAL (O, 85 beds) 4619 North Rosemead Boulevard, Rosemead, CA Zip 91770–1478, Mailing Address: P.O. Box 369, Zip 91770–0369; tel. 626/286–1191; Peggy Minnick, RN, Chief Executive Officer
Web address: www.ardenthealth.com

CANYON RIDGE HOSPITAL (O, 59 beds) 5353 G Street, Chino, CA Zip 91710–5250; tel. 909/590–3700; Peggy Minnick, RN, Chief Executive Officer
Web address: www.psysolutions.com

FREMONT HOSPITAL (O, 78 beds) 39001 Sundale Drive, Fremont, CA Zip 94538–2005; tel. 510/796–1100; Jay R. Kellison, Chief Executive Officer
Web address: www.fremonthospital.com

HERITAGE OAKS HOSPITAL (O, 76 beds) 4250 Auburn Boulevard, Sacramento, CA Zip 95841–4164; tel. 916/489–3336; Kenneth A. Meibert, Chief Executive Officer
Web address: www.psysolutions.com/facilities/heritageoaks/index.html

SIERRA VISTA HOSPITAL (O, 72 beds) 8001 Bruceville Road, Sacramento, CA Zip 95823–2329; tel. 916/288–0300; Nancy Purtell, Chief Executive Officer

COLORADO: CEDAR SPRINGS BEHAVIORAL HEALTH SYSTEM (O, 110 beds) 2135 Southgate Road, Colorado Springs, CO Zip 80906–2693; tel. 719/633–4114; Elaine Crnkovic, Chief Executive Officer
Web address: www.psysolutions.com

FLORIDA: ATLANTIC SHORES HOSPITAL (O, 86 beds) 4545 North Federal Highway, Fort Lauderdale, FL Zip 33308–5274; tel. 954/771–2711; Steve Shell, Administrator
Web address: www.atlanticshoreshospital.com

FORT LAUDERDALE HOSPITAL (O, 100 beds) 1601 East Las Olas Boulevard, Fort Lauderdale, FL Zip 33301–2393; tel. 954/463–4321; Ali A. Elhaj, Ph.D., Chief Executive Officer
Web address: www.psysolutions.com

SANDYPINES (O, 80 beds) 11301 S.E. Tequesta Terrace, Tequesta, FL Zip 33469–8146; tel. 561/744–0211; John W. Thompson, Ph.D., Chief Executive Officer
Web address: www.psysolutions.com

WINDMOOR HEALTHCARE OF CLEARWATER (O, 100 beds) 11300 U.S. 19 North, Clearwater, FL Zip 33764; tel. 727/541–2646; Wendy Merson, Chief Executive Officer
Web address: www.windmoor–healthcare.com

IDAHO: INTERMOUNTAIN HOSPITAL (O, 140 beds) 303 North Allumbaugh Street, Boise, ID Zip 83704–9266; tel. 208/377–8400; Richard A. Bangert, Chief Executive Officer
Web address: www.psysolutions.com

ILLINOIS: RIVEREDGE HOSPITAL (O, 210 beds) 8311 West Roosevelt Road, Forest Park, IL Zip 60130–2500; tel. 708/771–7000; Carey Carlock, Chief Executive Officer
Web address: www.psysolutions.com

STREAMWOOD HOSPITAL (O, 134 beds) 1400 East Irving Park Road, Streamwood, IL Zip 60107–3203; tel. 630/837–9000; Cynthia A. Meyer, Chief Executive Officer
Web address: www.streamwoodhospital.com

INDIANA: MEADOWS HOSPITAL (O, 66 beds) 3600 North Prow Road, Bloomington, IN Zip 47404; tel. 812/331–8000; Kurt A. Isaacson, Chief Executive Officer
Web address: www.psysolutions.com

VALLE VISTA HOSPITAL (O, 98 beds) 898 East Main Street, Greenwood, IN Zip 46143–1400; tel. 317/887–1348; David Bell, Chief Executive Officer
Web address: www.vallevistahospital.com

WELLSTONE REGIONAL HOSPITAL (O, 100 beds) 2700 Vissing Park Road, Jeffersonville, IN Zip 47130; tel. 812/284–8000; Dean T. Saling, President and Chief Executive Officer
Web address: www.psysolutions.com/facilities/wellstone/

KENTUCKY: CUMBERLAND HALL HOSPITAL (O, 48 beds) 210 West 17th Street, Hopkinsville, KY Zip 42240–1999; tel. 270/886–1919; Catherine Willner, Chief Executive Officer
Web address: www.psysolutions.com

LOUISIANA: BRENTWOOD HOSPITAL (O, 160 beds) 1006 Highland Avenue, Shreveport, LA Zip 71101–4103; tel. 318/618–7500; J. Paul Smith, Chief Executive Officer
Web address: www.psysolutions.com

MICHIGAN: HAVENWYCK HOSPITAL (O, 181 beds) 1525 University Drive, Auburn Hills, MI Zip 48326–2675; tel. 248/373–9200; Robert A. Kercorian, Chief Executive Officer
Web address: www.havenwyckhospital.com

MISSISSIPPI: ALLIANCE HEALTH CENTER (O, 122 beds) 5000 Highway 39 North, Meridian, MS Zip 39301; tel. 601/483–6211; William M. Patterson, Chief Executive Officer
Web address: www.psysolutions.com

BRENTWOOD BEHAVIORAL HEALTHCARE OF MISSISSIPPI (O, 107 beds) 3531 East Lakeland Drive, Jackson, MS Zip 39296–9794; tel. 601/936–2024; Michael J. Carney, Chief Executive Officer
Web address: www.psysolutions.com

MISSOURI: HEARTLAND BEHAVIORAL HEALTH SERVICES (O, 159 beds) 1500 West Ashland Street, Nevada, MO Zip 64772–1710; tel. 417/667–2666; Michael D. Ham, Chief Executive Officer
Web address: www.psysolutions.com/heartland/site/index.html

NEVADA: MONTEVISTA HOSPITAL (O, 80 beds) 5900 West Rochelle Avenue, Las Vegas, NV Zip 89103–3327; tel. 702/364–1111; Ingrid L. Whipple, Chief Executive Officer
Web address: www.montevistahospital.com

WEST HILLS HOSPITAL (O, 95 beds) 1240 East Ninth Street, Reno, NV Zip 89512–2997, Mailing Address: P.O. Box 30012, Zip 89520–3012; tel. 775/323–0478; Jeffrey Rice, Chief Executive Officer
Web address: www.psysolutions.com/facilities/westhills/

WILLOW SPRINGS CENTER (O, 76 beds) 690 Edison Way, Reno, NV Zip 89502–4135; tel. 775/858–3303; Jim Serratt, Chief Executive Officer
Web address: www.psysolutions.com/facilities/willowsprings/index.html

NEW JERSEY: SUMMIT OAKS HOSPITAL (O, 90 beds) 19 Prospect Street, Summit, NJ Zip 07902–0100; tel. 908/522–7000; James P. Gallagher, Chief Executive Officer

NEW MEXICO: MESILLA VALLEY HOSPITAL (O, 121 beds) 3751 Del Rey Boulevard, Las Cruces, NM Zip 88012–8526; tel. 505/382–3500; Margaret McCowen, Chief Executive Officer
Web address: www.mesillavalleyhospital.com

PEAK BEHAVIORAL HEALTH SERVICES (O, 36 beds) 5065 McNut Road, Santa Teresa, NM Zip 88008; tel. 505/589–3000; Bruce Waldo, Chief Executive Officer
Web address: www.psysolutions.com/facilities/peak/index.html

NORTH CAROLINA: BRYNN MARR HOSPITAL (O, 87 beds) 192 Village Drive, Jacksonville, NC Zip 28546–7299; tel. 910/577–1400; Sarah Wiltgen, Chief Executive Officer
Web address: www.brynnmarr.org

HOLLY HILL HOSPITAL (O, 108 beds) 3019 Falstaff Road, Raleigh, NC Zip 27610–1812; tel. 919/250–7000; Robert L. Turner, Ph.D., Chief Executive Officer
Web address: www.hollyhillhospital.com

OHIO: BELMONT PINES HOSPITAL (O, 46 beds) 615 Churchill–Hubbard Road, Youngstown, OH Zip 44505–1379; tel. 330/759–2700; George H. Perry, Ph.D., Chief Executive Officer
Web address: www.belmontpines.com

OKLAHOMA: SHADOW MOUNTAIN BEHAVIORAL HEALTH SYSTEM (O, 100 beds) 6262 South Sheridan Road, Tulsa, OK Zip 74133–4099; tel. 918/492–8200; Kevin A. Burgess, Chief Executive Officer
Web address: www.psysolutions.com

PENNSYLVANIA: BROOKE GLEN BEHAVIORAL HOSPITAL (O, 146 beds) 7170 Lafayette Avenue, Fort Washington, PA Zip 19034–0209; tel. 215/641–5300; Mark Schor, Chief Executive Officer
Web address: www.brookeglenbehavioral.com

PUERTO RICO: FIRST HOSPITAL PANAMERICANO (O, 153 beds) State Road 787 KM 1 5, Cidra, PR Zip 739, Mailing Address: P.O. Box 1400, Zip 739; tel. 787/739–5555; Marta Rivera, Executive Director
Web address: www.firsthospitalpr.org

SOUTH CAROLINA: PALMETTO LOWCOUNTRY BEHAVIORAL HEALTH (O, 70 beds) 2777 Speissegger Drive, Charleston, SC Zip 29405–8299; tel. 843/747–5830; Cherie Tolley, Chief Executive Officer
Web address: www.plbhs.com

For explanation of codes following names, see page B2.
★ Indicates Type III membership in the American Hospital Association.

THREE RIVERS BEHAVIORAL HEALTH (O, 86 beds) 2900 Sunset Boulevard, West Columbia, SC Zip 29169–3422; tel. 803/796–9911; R. Andy Hanner, Chief Executive Officer
Web address: www.psysolutions.com/facilities/threerivers/site/

TENNESSEE: CUMBERLAND HALL PSYCHIATRIC HOSPITAL (O, 64 beds) 7351 Standifer Gap Road, Chattanooga, TN Zip 37421; tel. 423/499–9007; Stephanie Austin, Chief Executive Officer
Web address: www.psysolutions.com

NASHVILLE REHABILITATION HOSPITAL (O, 37 beds) 1034 West Eastland Avenue, Nashville, TN Zip 37206–3238; tel. 615/226–4330; B. Touby Witzky, Chief Executive Officer
Web address: www.nrhcares.com

TEXAS: COMPASS HOSPITAL (O, 35 beds) 14743 Jones Maltsberger Avenue, San Antonio, TX Zip 78247–3713; tel. 210/402–0029; Alan J. Fisher, Chief Executive Officer
Web address: www.psysolutions.com

CYPRESS CREEK HOSPITAL (O, 64 beds) 17750 Cali Drive, Houston, TX Zip 77090–2700; tel. 281/586–7600; Diane P. Reidy, Chief Executive Officer
Web address: www.psysolutions.com

DESERT SPRINGS MEDICAL CENTER (O, 64 beds) 3300 South FM 1788, Midland, TX Zip 79706, Mailing Address: P.O. Box 60608, Zip 79711–0608; tel. 432/563–1200; James Baca, Chief Executive Officer
Web address: www.psysolutions.com/facilities/desertsprings/midland.html

HICKORY TRAIL HOSPITAL (O, 86 beds) 2000 North Old Hickory Trail, De Soto, TX Zip 75115–2242; tel. 972/298–7323; Shanti Carter, Chief Executive Officer
Web address: www.cedarshospital.com

LAUREL RIDGE TREATMENT CENTER (O, 94 beds) 17720 Corporate Woods Drive, San Antonio, TX Zip 78259–3500; tel. 210/491–9400; Dan Thomas, Chief Executive Officer
Web address: www.laurelridgetc.com

MILLWOOD HOSPITAL (O, 120 beds) 1011 North Cooper Street, Arlington, TX Zip 76011–5517; tel. 817/261–3121; John Baker, Chief Executive Officer
Web address: www.millwoodhospital.com

MISSION VISTA BEHAVIORAL HEALTH CENTER (O, 34 beds) 14747 Jones Maltsberger, San Antonio, TX Zip 78247–3713; tel. 210/497–0004; Dan Thomas, Chief Executive Officer
Web address: www.missionvistabhc.com

TEXAS NEUROREHAB CENTER (O, 47 beds) 1106 West Dittmar, Austin, TX Zip 78745–6388, Mailing Address: P.O. Box 150459, Zip 78715–0459; tel. 512/444–4835; Edgar E. Prettyman, XPsyD, Chief Executive Officer
Web address: www.psysolutions.com

WEST OAKS HOSPITAL (O, 144 beds) 6500 Hornwood Drive, Houston, TX Zip 77074–5095; tel. 713/995–0909; Lucinda DeBruce, Chief Executive Officer
Web address: www.psysolutions.com

UTAH: BENCHMARK BEHAVIORAL HEALTH SYSTEMS (O, 77 beds) 592 West 1350 South, Woods Cross, UT Zip 84087–1665; tel. 801/299–5300; Barry W. Woodward, Chief Executive Officer
Web address: www.bbhsnet.com

VIRGINIA: CUMBERLAND HOSPITAL (O, 132 beds) 9407 Cumberland Road, New Kent, VA Zip 23124–0150; tel. 804/966–2242; Patrice Gay Brooks, Chief Executive Officer
Web address: www.cumberlandhospital.com

NORTH SPRINGS BEHAVIORAL HEALTHCARE (O, 77 beds) 42009 Victory Lane, Leesburg, VA Zip 20176–6269; tel. 703/777–0800; Scott Zeiter, Chief Executive Officer
Web address: www.northspringleesburg.com

VIRGINIA BEACH PSYCHIATRIC CENTER (O, 100 beds) 1100 First Colonial Road, Virginia Beach, VA Zip 23454; tel. 757/496–6000; Denise Webb, Administrator
Web address: www.absfirst.com

WASHINGTON: FAIRFAX HOSPITAL (O, 95 beds) 10200 N.E. 132nd Street, Kirkland, WA Zip 98034–2899; tel. 425/821–2000; Ron Escarda, Chief Executive Officer
Web address: www.fairfaxhospital.com

Owned, leased, sponsored:	55 hospitals	5116 beds
Contract-managed:	0 hospitals	0 beds
Totals:	55 hospitals	5116 beds

★0011: PUERTO RICO DEPARTMENT OF HEALTH (NP)
Building A – Medical Center, San Juan, PR Zip 00936, Mailing Address: Call Box 70184, Zip 00936; tel. 787/274–7676; Rosa Perez Perdomo, M.D., M.P.H., Ph.D., Secretary of Health
(Independent Hospital System)

PUERTO RICO: CARDIOVASCULAR CENTER OF PUERTO RICO AND THE CARIBBEAN (O, 121 beds) Americo Miranda Centro Medico, San Juan, PR Zip 936, Mailing Address: P.O. Box 366528, Zip 00936–6528; tel. 787/754–8500; Humberto M. Monserrate, Executive Director
Web address: www.cardiovascular.gobierno.pr

HOSPITAL UNIVERSITARIO DR. RAMON RUIZ ARNAU (O, 70 beds) Avenue Laurel, Santa Juanita, Bayamon, PR Zip 956; tel. 787/787–5151; Rafael Garcia, Chief Executive Officer

UNIVERSITY HOSPITAL (O, 262 beds) San Juan, PR Mailing Address: P.O. Box 2116, Zip 922; tel. 787/754–0101; Roberto Burgos, Executive Director

UNIVERSITY PEDIATRIC HOSPITAL (O, 145 beds) Barrio Monacenno, Carretera 22, Rio Piedras, PR Zip 935, Mailing Address: P.O. Box 2129, San Juan, Zip 00922–2129; tel. 787/777–3535; Sylvette Llovet, Executive Director

Owned, leased, sponsored:	4 hospitals	598 beds
Contract-managed:	0 hospitals	0 beds
Totals:	4 hospitals	598 beds

★0002: QHR (IO)
5800 Tennyson Parkway, Plano, TX Zip 75024; tel. 214/473–3700; John C. Stinson, President and Chief Executive Officer
(Decentralized Health System)

ALABAMA: MONROE COUNTY HOSPITAL (C, 62 beds) 1901 South Alabama Avenue, Monroeville, AL Zip 36460, Mailing Address: P.O. Box 886, Zip 36461–0886; tel. 251/575–3111; Vincent B. DiFranco, Chief Executive Officer
Web address: www.mchcare.com

ALASKA: BARTLETT REGIONAL HOSPITAL (C, 65 beds) 3260 Hospital Drive, Juneau, AK Zip 99801–7808; tel. 907/586–2611; Shawn Morrow, Chief Executive Officer
Web address: www.bartletthospital.org

ARKANSAS: CHICOT MEMORIAL HOSPITAL (C, 25 beds) 2729 Highway 65 and 82 South, Lake Village, AR Zip 71653; tel. 870/265–5351; Bruce A. Bennett, Interim Chief Executive Officer
Web address: www.chicotmemorial.com

HOWARD MEMORIAL HOSPITAL (C, 25 beds) 800 West Leslie Street, Nashville, AR Zip 71852–0381, Mailing Address: P.O. Box 381, Zip 71852–0381; tel. 870/845–4400; Brian E. Bickel, President and Chief Executive Officer

MENA REGIONAL HEALTH SYSTEM (C, 65 beds) 311 North Morrow Street, Mena, AR Zip 71953–2516; tel. 479/394–6100; Leland E. Farnell, Interim Chief Executive Officer
Web address: www.menaregional.com

NORTH METRO MEDICAL CENTER (C, 111 beds) 1400 West Braden Street, Jacksonville, AR Zip 72076–3788; tel. 501/985–7000; Scott M. Landrum, Chief Executive Officer
Web address: www.rebsamenmedicalcenter.com

SPARKS REGIONAL MEDICAL CENTER (C, 303 beds) 1311 South I Street, Fort Smith, AR Zip 72901–4995, Mailing Address: P.O. Box 17006, Zip 72917–7006; tel. 479/441–4000; Frederick D. Woodrell, FACHE, Chief Executive Officer
Web address: www.sparks.org

COLORADO: ARKANSAS VALLEY REGIONAL MEDICAL CENTER (C, 155 beds) 1100 Carson Avenue, La Junta, CO Zip 81050–2799; tel. 719/383–6000; Lynn Crowell, Chief Executive Officer
Web address: www.avrmc.org

COMMUNITY HOSPITAL (C, 40 beds) 2021 North 12th Street, Grand Junction, CO Zip 81501–2999; tel. 970/242–0920; Wesley White, President
Web address: www.gjhosp.org

MEMORIAL HOSPITAL (C, 25 beds) 785 Russell Street, Craig, CO Zip 81625–9906; tel. 970/824–9411; George A. Rohrich, Chief Executive Officer
Web address: www.thememorialhospital.com

For explanation of codes following names, see page B2.
★ Indicates Type III membership in the American Hospital Association.

MONTROSE MEMORIAL HOSPITAL (C, 63 beds) 800 South Third Street, Montrose, CO Zip 81401–4291; tel. 970/249–2211; Kenneth E. S. Platou, Chief Executive Officer
Web address: www.montrosehospital.com

MT. SAN RAFAEL HOSPITAL (C, 25 beds) 410 Benedicta Avenue, Trinidad, CO Zip 81082–2093; tel. 719/846–9213; James Robertson, Chief Executive Officer
Web address: www.msrhc.org

PARKVIEW MEDICAL CENTER (C, 293 beds) 400 West 16th Street, Pueblo, CO Zip 81003–2781; tel. 719/584–4000; C. W. Smith, President and Chief Executive Officer
Web address: www.parkviewmc.org

PIONEERS MEDICAL CENTER (C, 47 beds) 345 Cleveland Street, Meeker, CO Zip 81641–3238; tel. 970/878–5047; Robert W. Omer, FACHE, Chief Executive Officer
Web address: www.pioneershospital.com

PROWERS MEDICAL CENTER (C, 25 beds) 401 Kendall Drive, Lamar, CO Zip 81052–3993; tel. 719/336–4343; Theodore Kubicki, Chief Executive Officer
Web address: www.prowersmedical.com

SOUTHWEST MEMORIAL HOSPITAL (C, 49 beds) 1311 North Mildred Road, Cortez, CO Zip 81321–2299; tel. 970/565–6666; Nelson Toebbe, Interim Chief Executive Officer
Web address: www.swhealth.org

Section B

FLORIDA: HENDRY REGIONAL MEDICAL CENTER (C, 25 beds) 524 West Sagamore Avenue, Clewiston, FL Zip 33440–3094; tel. 863/983–9121; Craig R. Cudworth, Chief Executive Officer
Web address: www.hendryregional.org

JACKSON HOSPITAL (C, 62 beds) 4250 Hospital Drive, Marianna, FL Zip 32446–1939, Mailing Address: P.O. Box 1608, Zip 32447–1608; tel. 850/526–2200; David L. Hample, Chief Executive Officer
Web address: www.jacksonhosp.com

GEORGIA: ELBERT MEMORIAL HOSPITAL (C, 52 beds) 4 Medical Drive, Elberton, GA Zip 30635–1897; tel. 706/283–3151; Mark LeNeave, Chief Executive Officer
Web address: www.emhcare.net

HABERSHAM COUNTY MEDICAL CENTER (C, 159 beds) 541 Historic Highway 441, Demorest, GA Zip 30535–3118, Mailing Address: P.O. Box 37, Zip 30535–0037; tel. 706/754–2161; C. Richard Dwozan, Chief Executive Officer
Web address: www.hcmcmed.org

MCDUFFIE REGIONAL MEDICAL CENTER (C, 35 beds) 521 Hill Street S.W., Thomson, GA Zip 30824–2199; tel. 706/595–1411; Douglas C. Keir, Chief Executive Officer
Web address: www.mrmc.org

IDAHO: BENEWAH COMMUNITY HOSPITAL (C, 19 beds) 229 South Seventh Street, Saint Maries, ID Zip 83861–1803; tel. 208/245–5551; Brian Nall, Chief Executive Officer
Web address: www.bchmed.org

GRITMAN MEDICAL CENTER (C, 25 beds) 700 South Main Street, Moscow, ID Zip 83843–3047; tel. 208/882–4511; Jeffrey W. Martin, Chief Executive Officer
Web address: www.gritman.org

SHOSHONE MEDICAL CENTER (C, 25 beds) 25 Jacobs Gulch, Kellogg, ID Zip 83837–2096; tel. 208/784–1221; David B. Selman, FACHE, Chief Executive Officer
Web address: www.shomed.org

STEELE MEMORIAL MEDICAL CENTER (C, 18 beds) 203 South Daisy, Salmon, ID Zip 83467–4109, Mailing Address: P.O. Box 700, Zip 83467–0700; tel. 208/756–5600; Victoria A. Alexander, Chief Executive Officer
Web address: www.steelemh.org

ILLINOIS: COMMUNITY MEMORIAL HOSPITAL (C, 25 beds) 400 Caldwell Street, Staunton, IL Zip 62088–1499; tel. 618/635–2200; Susie Campbell, Chief Executive Officer
Web address: www.stauntonhospital.org

CRAWFORD MEMORIAL HOSPITAL (C, 65 beds) 1000 North Allen Street, Robinson, IL Zip 62454–1167; tel. 618/544–3131; Donald E. Annis, Chief Executive Officer
Web address: www.crawfordmh.com

GIBSON AREA HOSPITAL AND HEALTH SERVICES (C, 67 beds) 1120 North Melvin Street, Gibson City, IL Zip 60936, Mailing Address: P.O. Box 429, Zip 60936–0429; tel. 217/784–4251; Robert C. Schmitt, II, Chief Executive Officer
Web address: www.gibsonhospital.org

LAWRENCE COUNTY MEMORIAL HOSPITAL (C, 35 beds) 2200 West State Street, Lawrenceville, IL Zip 62439–1853; tel. 618/943–1000; Doug Florkowski, Chief Executive Officer

PEKIN HOSPITAL (C, 110 beds) 600 South 13th Street, Pekin, IL Zip 61554–5098; tel. 309/347–1151; Kevin R. Andrews, Chief Executive Officer
Web address: www.pekinhospital.org

INDIANA: DAVIESS COMMUNITY HOSPITAL (C, 80 beds) 1314 East Walnut Street, Washington, IN Zip 47501–2198, Mailing Address: P.O. Box 760, Zip 47501–0760; tel. 812/254–2760; Louis H. Bremer, Jr., Interim Chief Executive Officer
Web address: www.dchosp.org

SULLIVAN COUNTY COMMUNITY HOSPITAL (C, 25 beds) 2200 North Section Street, Sullivan, IN Zip 47882, Mailing Address: P.O. Box 10, Zip 47882–0010; tel. 812/268–4311; Michelle Sly–Smith, Chief Executive Officer
Web address: www.schosp.com

IOWA: BOONE COUNTY HOSPITAL (C, 39 beds) 1015 Union Street, Boone, IA Zip 50036–4821; tel. 515/432–3140; Joseph S. Smith, Chief Executive Officer
Web address: www.boonehospital.com

FORT MADISON COMMUNITY HOSPITAL (C, 50 beds) 5445 Avenue O, Fort Madison, IA Zip 52627–0174, Mailing Address: P.O. Box 174, Zip 52627–0174; tel. 319/372–6530; C. James Platt, Chief Executive Officer
Web address: www.fmchosp.com

KNOXVILLE HOSPITAL & CLINICS (C, 25 beds) 1002 South Lincoln Street, Knoxville, IA Zip 50138–3155; tel. 641/842–2151; Ann M. Helwig, Chief Executive Officer
Web address: www.kach.org

KANSAS: COFFEYVILLE REGIONAL MEDICAL CENTER (C, 105 beds) 1400 West Fourth, Coffeyville, KS Zip 67337–0856; tel. 620/251–1200; Gerald J. Marquette, Jr., Chief Executive Officer
Web address: www.crmcinc.com

NEOSHO MEMORIAL REGIONAL MEDICAL CENTER (C, 25 beds) 629 South Plummer, Chanute, KS Zip 66720–0426, Mailing Address: P.O. Box 426, Zip 66720–0426; tel. 620/431–4000; Dennis Franks, FACHE, Chief Executive Officer
Web address: www.nmrmc.com

NEWMAN REGIONAL HEALTH (C, 122 beds) 1201 West 12th Avenue, Emporia, KS Zip 66801–2597; tel. 620/343–6800; Joyce Grove–Hein, Interim Chief Executive Officer
Web address: www.newmanrh.org

ST. LUKE HOSPITAL AND LIVING CENTER (C, 42 beds) 535 South Freeborn, Marion, KS Zip 66861–1299; tel. 620/382–2177; Jeremy Armstrong, CHE, Chief Executive Officer
Web address: www.slhmarion.org

KENTUCKY: CALDWELL COUNTY HOSPITAL (C, 25 beds) 101 Hospital Drive, Princeton, KY Zip 42445–0410; tel. 270/365–0300; Charles D. Lovell, Jr., President and Chief Executive Officer
Web address: www.caldwellhosp.org

CRITTENDEN COUNTY HOSPITAL (C, 48 beds) 520 West Gum Street, Marion, KY Zip 42064–6201, Mailing Address: P.O. Box 386, Zip 42064–0386; tel. 270/965–5281; Jim Christensen, Chief Executive Officer
Web address: www.crittenden–health.org

FLEMING COUNTY HOSPITAL (C, 52 beds) 920 Elizaville Avenue, Flemingsburg, KY Zip 41041, Mailing Address: P.O. Box 388, Zip 41041–0388; tel. 606/849–5000; David R. Sirk, Chief Executive Officer
Web address: www.flemingcountyhospital.org

JENNIE STUART MEDICAL CENTER (C, 139 beds) 320 West 18th Street, Hopkinsville, KY Zip 42241–2400, Mailing Address: P.O. Box 2400, Zip 42241–2400; tel. 270/887–0100; Terry Peeples, Chief Executive Officer
Web address: www.jsmc.org

MARSHALL COUNTY HOSPITAL (C, 59 beds) 503 George McClain Drive, Benton, KY Zip 42025–1399, Mailing Address: P.O. Box 630, Zip 42025–0630; tel. 270/527–4800; Kathy Long, Chief Executive Officer
Web address: www.marshallcountyhospital.org

For explanation of codes following names, see page B2.
★ Indicates Type III membership in the American Hospital Association.

MONROE COUNTY MEDICAL CENTER (C, 49 beds) 529 Capp Harlan Road, Tompkinsville, KY Zip 42167–1840; tel. 270/487–9231; Vicky McFall, Chief Executive Officer
Web address: www.mcmccares.com

OHIO COUNTY HOSPITAL (C, 25 beds) 1211 Main Street, Hartford, KY Zip 42347–1619; tel. 270/298–7411; Blaine Pieper, Chief Executive Officer
Web address: www.ohiocountyhospital.com

LOUISIANA: FRANKLIN FOUNDATION HOSPITAL (C, 25 beds) 1097 Northwest Boulevard, Franklin, LA Zip 70538–3724, Mailing Address: P.O. Box 577, Zip 70538–0577; tel. 337/828–0760; Cindy Bradley, Interim Chief Executive Officer
Web address: www.franklinfoundation.org

OPELOUSAS GENERAL HEALTH SYSTEM (C, 163 beds) 539 East Prudhomme Street, Opelousas, LA Zip 70570, Mailing Address: P.O. Box 1389, Zip 70571–1389; tel. 337/948–3011; Gerald A. Fornoff, Chief Executive Officer
Web address: www.opelousasgeneral.com

THIBODAUX REGIONAL MEDICAL CENTER (C, 144 beds) 602 North Acadia Road, Thibodaux, LA Zip 70301–4847, Mailing Address: P.O. Box 1118, Zip 70302–1118; tel. 985/447–5500; Greg K. Stock, Chief Executive Officer
Web address: www.thibodaux.com

MAINE: CALAIS REGIONAL HOSPITAL (O, 25 beds) 22 Hospital Lane, Calais, ME Zip 04619–1398; tel. 207/454–7521; Ray H. Davis, Jr., Chief Executive Officer
Web address: www.calaishospital.com

CARY MEDICAL CENTER (C, 49 beds) 163 Van Buren Road, Suite 1, Caribou, ME Zip 04736–2599; tel. 207/498–3111; Kris A. Doody, RN, Chief Executive Officer
Web address: www.carymedicalcenter.org

DOWN EAST COMMUNITY HOSPITAL (C, 25 beds) Upper Court Street, Machias, ME Zip 4654, Mailing Address: Rural Route 1, Box 11, Zip 04654–9702; tel. 207/255–3356; Wayne Dodwell, Chief Executive Officer
Web address: www.dech.org

MILLINOCKET REGIONAL HOSPITAL (C, 25 beds) 200 Somerset Street, Millinocket, ME Zip 04462–1298; tel. 207/723–5161; Marie E. Vienneau, RN, Chief Executive Officer
Web address: www.mrhme.org

PARKVIEW ADVENTIST MEDICAL CENTER (C, 55 beds) 329 Maine Street, Brunswick, ME Zip 04011–3398; tel. 207/373–2000; Theodore M. Lewis, President and Chief Executive Officer
Web address: www.parkviewamc.org

PENOBSCOT VALLEY HOSPITAL (C, 25 beds) 7 Transalpine Road, Lincoln, ME Zip 04457–0368, Mailing Address: P.O. Box 368, Zip 04457–0368; tel. 207/794–3321; David A. Shannon, Chief Executive Officer
Web address: www.pvhhealthcare.org

MICHIGAN: ALLEGAN GENERAL HOSPITAL (C, 34 beds) 555 Linn Street, Allegan, MI Zip 49010–1594; tel. 269/673–8424; Gerald J. Barbini, President and Chief Executive Officer
Web address: www.aghosp.org

COMMUNITY HOSPITAL (C, 46 beds) 400 Medical Park Drive, Watervliet, MI Zip 49098–9225; tel. 269/463–3111; Ray Cruse, Interim Chief Executive Officer
Web address: www.communityhospitalwatervliet.com

HAYES GREEN BEACH MEMORIAL HOSPITAL (C, 25 beds) 321 East Harris Street, Charlotte, MI Zip 48813–1697; tel. 517/543–1050; Matthew Rush, President and Chief Executive Officer
Web address: www.hgbhealth.com

MARLETTE REGIONAL HOSPITAL (C, 84 beds) 2770 Main Street, Marlette, MI Zip 48453–0307, Mailing Address: P.O. Box 307, Zip 48453–0307; tel. 989/635–4000; Michael A. Kozar, Chief Executive Officer
Web address: www.marlettecommunityhospital.com

MECOSTA COUNTY MEDICAL CENTER (C, 64 beds) 605 Oak Street, Big Rapids, MI Zip 49307–2099; tel. 231/796–8691; Thomas E. Daugherty, Administrator
Web address: www.mcmcbr.com

STURGIS HOSPITAL (C, 49 beds) 916 Myrtle, Sturgis, MI Zip 49091–2001; tel. 269/651–7824; Robert J. LaBarge, Chief Executive Officer
Web address: www.sturgishospital.com

THREE RIVERS HEALTH (C, 60 beds) 701 South Health Parkway, Three Rivers, MI Zip 49093–9362; tel. 269/278–1145; Matthew Chambers, President and Chief Executive Officer
Web address: www.threerivershealth.org

MINNESOTA: FALLS MEMORIAL HOSPITAL (C, 25 beds) 1400 Highway 71, International Falls, MN Zip 56649–2189; tel. 218/283–4481; Bonnie Erickson, Interim Chief Executive Officer
Web address: www.fmh–mn.com

MISSISSIPPI: HANCOCK MEDICAL CENTER (C, 41 beds) 149 Drinkwater Boulevard, Bay Saint Louis, MS Zip 39521–2790, Mailing Address: P.O. Box 2790, Zip 39521–2790; tel. 228/467–8600; Hal W. Leftwich, FACHE, Administrator
Web address: www.hmc.org

KING'S DAUGHTERS MEDICAL CENTER (C, 99 beds) 427 Highway 51 North, Brookhaven, MS Zip 39601–2600, Mailing Address: P.O. Box 948, Zip 39602–0948; tel. 601/833–6011; Alvin Hoover, FACHE, Chief Executive Officer
Web address: www.kdmc.org

NATCHEZ REGIONAL MEDICAL CENTER (C, 132 beds) 54 Seargent S Prentiss Drive, Natchez, MS Zip 39120–4726; tel. 601/443–2100; Scott Phillips, Chief Executive Officer
Web address: www.natchezregional.com

NESHOBA COUNTY GENERAL HOSPITAL (C, 200 beds) 1001 Holland Avenue, Philadelphia, MS Zip 39350–2161, Mailing Address: P.O. Box 648, Zip 39350–0648; tel. 601/663–1200; Karen A. Fiducia, Interim Chief Executive Officer
Web address: www.neshobageneral.com

MISSOURI: NEVADA REGIONAL MEDICAL CENTER (C, 63 beds) 800 South Ash Street, Nevada, MO Zip 64772–3223; tel. 417/667–3355; Judith K. Feuquay, Chief Executive Officer
Web address: www.nrmchealth.com

MONTANA: CENTRAL MONTANA MEDICAL CENTER (C, 124 beds) 408 Wendell Avenue, Lewistown, MT Zip 59457–2261; tel. 406/538–7711; David M. Faulkner, Chief Executive Officer
Web address: www.cmmccares.com

NORTH VALLEY HOSPITAL (C, 25 beds) 1600 Hospital Way, Whitefish, MT Zip 59937–2958; tel. 406/863–3500; Craig E. Aasved, Chief Executive Officer
Web address: www.nvhosp.org

NEBRASKA: GREAT PLAINS REGIONAL MEDICAL CENTER (C, 96 beds) 601 West Leota Street, North Platte, NE Zip 69101–6598, Mailing Address: P.O. Box 1167, Zip 69103–1167; tel. 308/696–8000; Lucinda A. Bradley, Chief Executive Officer
Web address: www.gprmc.com

MEMORIAL HEALTH CENTER (C, 88 beds) 645 Osage Street, Sidney, NE Zip 69162–1799; tel. 308/254–5825; Danielle Gearhart, Chief Executive Officer
Web address: www.memorialhealthcenter.org

PHELPS MEMORIAL HEALTH CENTER (C, 25 beds) 1215 Tibbals Street, Holdrege, NE Zip 68949–1280; tel. 308/995–2211; Mark Harrel, Chief Executive Officer
Web address: www.phelpsmemorial.com

NEW MEXICO: CIBOLA GENERAL HOSPITAL (C, 25 beds) 1016 Roosevelt Avenue, Grants, NM Zip 87020–2104; tel. 505/287–4446; Kenneth Cochran, RN, FACHE, Chief Executive Officer
Web address: www.cibolahospital.com

GERALD CHAMPION REGIONAL MEDICAL CENTER (C, 99 beds) 2669 North Scenic Drive, Alamogordo, NM Zip 88310–8799; tel. 575/439–6100; Robert J. Heckert, Jr., Chief Executive Officer
Web address: www.gcrmc.org

HOLY CROSS HOSPITAL (C, 47 beds) 1397 Weimer Road, Taos, NM Zip 87571–6284, Mailing Address: P.O. Box DD, Zip 87571–6284; tel. 575/758–8883; Warren K. Spellman, Chief Executive Officer
Web address: www.taoshospital.org

NORTH CAROLINA: ALLEGHANY MEMORIAL HOSPITAL (C, 25 beds) 233 Doctors Street, Sparta, NC Zip 28675–0009, Mailing Address: P.O. Box 9, Zip 28675–0009; tel. 336/372–5511; Ralph Castillo, Chief Executive Officer
Web address: www.amhsparta.org

For explanation of codes following names, see page B2.
★ Indicates Type III membership in the American Hospital Association.

ASHE MEMORIAL HOSPITAL (C, 85 beds) 200 Hospital Avenue, Jefferson, NC Zip 28640–9244; tel. 336/846–7101; R. D. Williams, Administrator and Chief Executive Officer
Web address: www.ashememorial.org

JOHNSTON MEMORIAL HOSPITAL (C, 167 beds) 509 North Bright Leaf Boulevard, Smithfield, NC Zip 27577–1376, Mailing Address: P.O. Box 1376, Zip 27577–1376; tel. 919/934–8171; Kevin L. Rogols, CHE, President and Chief Executive Officer
Web address: www.johnstonmemorial.org

MOREHEAD MEMORIAL HOSPITAL (C, 224 beds) 117 East King's Highway, Eden, NC Zip 27288–5299; tel. 336/623–9711; Robert Enders, President
Web address: www.morehead.org

NORTHERN HOSPITAL OF SURRY COUNTY (C, 120 beds) 830 Rockford Street, Mount Airy, NC Zip 27030–5365, Mailing Address: P.O. Box 1101, Zip 27030–1101; tel. 336/719–7000; William B. James, Chief Executive Officer
Web address: www.northernhospital.com

RUTHERFORD HOSPITAL (C, 116 beds) 288 South Ridgecrest Avenue, Rutherfordton, NC Zip 28139–3097; tel. 828/286–5000; David Bixler, President
Web address: www.rutherfordhosp.org

OHIO: KNOX COMMUNITY HOSPITAL (C, 96 beds) 1330 Coshocton Road, Mount Vernon, OH Zip 43050–1495; tel. 740/393–9000; Bruce D. White, Chief Executive Officer
Web address: www.knoxcommhosp.org

MEMORIAL HOSPITAL (C, 102 beds) 715 South Taft Avenue, Fremont, OH Zip 43420–3200; tel. 419/332–7321; John A. Gorman, Chief Executive Officer
Web address: www.fremontmemorial.org

SELBY GENERAL HOSPITAL (C, 35 beds) 1106 Colegate Drive, Marietta, OH Zip 45750–1323; tel. 740/568–2000; Robert M. Peterson, Chief Executive Officer
Web address: www.selbygeneralhospital.com

WOOSTER COMMUNITY HOSPITAL (C, 150 beds) 1761 Beall Avenue, Wooster, OH Zip 44691–2342; tel. 330/263–8100; William E. Sheron, Chief Executive Officer
Web address: www.woosterhospital.org

OKLAHOMA: CHOCTAW MEMORIAL HOSPITAL (C, 34 beds) 1405 East Kirk Road, Hugo, OK Zip 74743–3603; tel. 580/317–9500; Davie Lloyd, Chief Executive Officer

KINGFISHER REGIONAL HOSPITAL (C, 25 beds) 500 South Ninth Street, Kingfisher, OK Zip 73750–3528, Mailing Address: P.O. Box 59, Zip 73750–0059; tel. 405/375–3141; Damon Benson, Chief Executive Officer and Administrator
Web address: www.kingfisherhospital.com

LOGAN MEDICAL CENTER (C, 25 beds) Highway 33 West at Academy Road, Guthrie, OK Zip 73044–3700, Mailing Address: P.O. Box 1017, Zip 73044–1017; tel. 405/282–6700; K. Steven Rowley, CHE, Chief Executive Officer
Web address: www.loganhosp.com

OKMULGEE MEMORIAL HOSPITAL (C, 66 beds) 1401 Morris Drive, Okmulgee, OK Zip 74447–6419, Mailing Address: P.O. Box 1038, Zip 74447–1038; tel. 918/756–4233; Rex Jones, Chief Executive Officer
Web address: www.okmulgeehospital.com

PERRY MEMORIAL HOSPITAL (C, 26 beds) 501 14th Street, Perry, OK Zip 73077–5099; tel. 580/336–3541; Joe Duerr, Chief Executive Officer
Web address: www.pmh–ok.org

PURCELL MUNICIPAL HOSPITAL (C, 30 beds) 1500 North Green Avenue, Purcell, OK Zip 73080–1699, Mailing Address: P.O. Box 511, Zip 73080–0511; tel. 405/527–6524; ,
Web address: www.purcellhospital.com

SAYRE MEMORIAL HOSPITAL (C, 35 beds) 501 East Washington Street, Sayre, OK Zip 73662–1337; tel. 580/928–5541; Jason Anglin, Chief Executive Officer
Web address: www.sayrehospital.org

SHARE MEDICAL CENTER (C, 102 beds) 800 Share Drive, Alva, OK Zip 73717–3699, Mailing Address: P.O. Box 727, Zip 73717–0727; tel. 580/327–2800; Barbara Oestmann, Chief Executive Officer
Web address: www.smcok.com

PENNSYLVANIA: CLARION HOSPITAL (C, 83 beds) One Hospital Drive, Clarion, PA Zip 16214–8599; tel. 814/226–9500; Byron Quinton, Chief Executive Officer
Web address: www.clarionhospital.org

J. C. BLAIR MEMORIAL HOSPITAL (C, 73 beds) 1225 Warm Springs Avenue, Huntingdon, PA Zip 16652–2398; tel. 814/643–2290; Kevin P. Calhoun, Chief Executive Officer
Web address: www.jcblair.org

JERSEY SHORE HOSPITAL (C, 25 beds) 1020 Thompson Street, Jersey Shore, PA Zip 17740–1794; tel. 570/398–0100; Carey W. Plummer, President and Chief Executive Officer
Web address: www.jsh.org

MEMORIAL HOSPITAL (C, 161 beds) One Hospital Drive, Towanda, PA Zip 18848–9702; tel. 570/265–2191; Gary A. Baker, President
Web address: www.memorialhospital.org

SOUTH CAROLINA: ABBEVILLE AREA MEDICAL CENTER (C, 25 beds) 901 West Greenwood Street, Abbeville, SC Zip 29620–0887, Mailing Address: P.O. Box 887, Zip 29620–0887; tel. 864/366–5011; Richard D. Osmus, Chief Executive Officer
Web address: www.abbevilleareamc.com

GEORGETOWN MEMORIAL HOSPITAL (C, 136 beds) 606 Black River Road, Georgetown, SC Zip 29440–3368, Mailing Address: Drawer 421718, Zip 29442–1718; tel. 843/527–7000; Bruce P. Bailey, Chief Executive Officer
Web address: www.gmhsc.com

NEWBERRY COUNTY MEMORIAL HOSPITAL (C, 48 beds) 2669 Kinard Street, Newberry, SC Zip 29108–0497, Mailing Address: P.O. Box 497, Zip 29108–0497; tel. 803/276–7570; Lynn W. Beasley, President and Chief Executive Officer
Web address: www.newberryhospital.org

REGIONAL MEDICAL CENTER OF ORANGEBURG AND CALHOUN COUNTIES (C, 266 beds) 3000 St. Matthews Road, Orangeburg, SC Zip 29118–1470; tel. 803/395–2200; Thomas C. Dandridge, President and Chief Executive Officer
Web address: www.trmchealth.org

WACCAMAW COMMUNITY HOSPITAL (C, 111 beds) 4070 Highway 17 Bypass, Murrells Inlet, SC Zip 29576, Mailing Address: P.O. Drawer 3350, Zip 29576; tel. 843/652–1000; Gayle L. Resetar, Chief Operating Officer
Web address: www.gmhsc.com

SOUTH DAKOTA: HURON REGIONAL MEDICAL CENTER (C, 25 beds) 172 Fourth Street S.E., Huron, SD Zip 57350–2590; tel. 605/353–6200; John L. Single, Chief Executive Officer
Web address: www.huronregional.org

TENNESSEE: LINCOLN COUNTY HEALTH SYSTEM (C, 327 beds) 106 Medical Center Boulevard, Fayetteville, TN Zip 37334–2684; tel. 931/438–1100; Gary G. Kendrick, Chief Executive Officer
Web address: www.lchealthsystem.com

MACON COUNTY GENERAL HOSPITAL (C, 25 beds) 204 Medical Drive, Lafayette, TN Zip 37083–1799, Mailing Address: P.O. Box 378, Zip 37083–0378; tel. 615/666–2147; Dennis A. Wolford, FACHE, Chief Executive Officer
Web address: www.mcgh.net

RHEA MEDICAL CENTER (C, 114 beds) 9400 Rhea County Highway, Dayton, TN Zip 37321–7922; tel. 423/775–1121; Kennedy L. Croom, Jr., Administrator and Chief Executive Officer
Web address: www.rheamedical.org

TEXAS: BRAZOSPORT REGIONAL HEALTH SYSTEM (C, 156 beds) 100 Medical Drive, Lake Jackson, TX Zip 77566–9983; tel. 979/297–4411; Daniel L. Buche, Chief Executive Officer
Web address: www.brhs.org

MATAGORDA COUNTY HOSPITAL DISTRICT (C, 60 beds) 1115 Avenue G, Bay City, TX Zip 77414–3544; tel. 979/245–6383; Daryle Voss, Chief Executive Officer
Web address: www.matagordageneral.org

MEMORIAL HOSPITAL (C, 34 beds) 1110 Sarah Dewitt Drive, Gonzales, TX Zip 78629–2021, Mailing Address: P.O. Box 587, Zip 78629–0587; tel. 830/672–7581; Charles Norris, Chief Executive Officer
Web address: www.gonzaleshealthcare.com

For explanation of codes following names, see page B2.
★ Indicates Type III membership in the American Hospital Association.

VERMONT: NORTHWESTERN MEDICAL CENTER (C, 52 beds) 133 Fairfield Street, Saint Albans, VT Zip 05478–1734, Mailing Address: P.O. Box 1370, Zip 05478–1370; tel. 802/524–5911; Peter A. Hofstetter, Chief Executive Officer
Web address: www.nmcinc.org

WASHINGTON: KADLEC MEDICAL CENTER (C, 181 beds) 888 Swift Boulevard, Richland, WA Zip 99352–3542; tel. 509/946–4611; Rand J. Wortman, President and Chief Executive Officer
Web address: www.kadlecmed.org

WISCONSIN: AMERY REGIONAL MEDICAL CENTER (C, 25 beds) 225 Scholl Court, Amery, WI Zip 54001–1292; tel. 715/268–8000; Michael Karuschak, Jr., Chief Executive Officer
Web address: www.amerymedicalcenter.org

WYOMING: IVINSON MEMORIAL HOSPITAL (C, 99 beds) 255 North 30th Street, Laramie, WY Zip 82072; tel. 307/742–2141; Carol Dozier, Chief Executive Officer
Web address: www.ivinsonhospital.org

WEST PARK HOSPITAL (C, 140 beds) 707 Sheridan Avenue, Cody, WY Zip 82414–3409; tel. 307/527–7501; Douglas A. McMillan, Administrator and Chief Executive Officer
Web address: www.westparkhospital.org

Owned, leased, sponsored:	1 hospital	25 beds
Contract–managed:	114 hospitals	8601 beds
Totals:	115 hospitals	8626 beds

★0040: QUEEN'S HEALTH SYSTEMS (NP)
1099 Alakea Street, Suite 1100, Honolulu, HI Zip 96813; tel. 808/535–5448; Arthur A. Ushijima, President and Chief Executive Officer
(Moderately Centralized Health System)

HAWAII: MOLOKAI GENERAL HOSPITAL (O, 15 beds) Kaunakakai, HI Mailing Address: P.O. Box 408, Zip 96748–0408; tel. 808/553–5331; Janice Kalanihuia, President
Web address: www.queens.org

QUEEN'S MEDICAL CENTER (O, 470 beds) 1301 Punchbowl Street, Honolulu, HI Zip 96813–2499; tel. 808/538–9011; Arthur A. Ushijima, President
Web address: www.queens.org

Owned, leased, sponsored:	2 hospitals	485 beds
Contract–managed:	0 hospitals	0 beds
Totals:	2 hospitals	485 beds

★0260: REGENCY HOSPITAL COMPANY (IO)
30000 Mill Creek Avenue, Suite 250, Alpharetta, GA Zip 30022; tel. 770/772–4345; William L. Anderson, President and Chief Executive Officer
(Independent Hospital System)

ARKANSAS: REGENCY HOSPITAL OF NORTHWEST ARKANSAS (O, 25 beds) 1125 North College, Fayetteville, AR Zip 72703; tel. 479/713–7000; Michael A. McLean, Chief Executive Officer
Web address: www.regencyhospital.com

REGENCY HOSPITAL OF SPRINGDALE (O, 25 beds) 609 West Maple Avenue, 6th Floor, Springdale, AR Zip 72764; tel. 479/757–2600; Michael A. McLean, Chief Executive Officer
Web address: www.regencyhospital.com

GEORGIA: REGENCY HOSPITAL OF CENTRAL GEORGIA (O, 34 beds) 700 Spring Street, Macon, GA Zip 31201; tel. 478/633–8260; Susan Smith, RN,
Web address: www.regencyhospital.com

REGENCY HOSPITAL OF SOUTH ATLANTA (O, 37 beds) 1170 Cleveland Avenue, 4th Floor, East Point, GA Zip 30344; tel. 404/466–6250; Paul C. Miller, Chief Executive Officer
Web address: www.regencyhospital.com

INDIANA: REGENCY HOSPITAL OF NORTHWEST INDIANA (O, 25 beds) 4321 Fir Street, 4th Floor, East Chicago, IN Zip 46312; tel. 219/392–7790; Beverly Foster, Chief Executive Officer
Web address: www.regencyhospital.com

REGENCY HOSPITAL OF PORTER COUNTY (O, 23 beds) 3630 Willow Road, Portage, IN Zip 46368; tel. 219/364–3800; Beverly Foster, Chief Executive Officer
Web address: www.regencyhospital.com

LOUISIANA: REGENCY HOSPITAL OF COVINGTON (O, 38 beds) 195 Highland Park Entrance, Covington, LA Zip 70433; tel. 985/867–3977; Timothy Burke, Chief Executive Officer
Web address: www.regencyhospital.com

MINNESOTA: REGENCY HOSPITAL OF MINNEAPOLIS (O, 54 beds) 1300 Hidden Lakes Parkway, Golden Valley, MN Zip 55422–4299; tel. 763/588–2750; Deborah Graves, RN, Chief Executive Officer
Web address: www.regencyhospital.com

MISSISSIPPI: REGENCY HOSPITAL OF HATTIESBURG (O, 33 beds) 125 South 25th Avenue, Hattiesburg, MS Zip 39401; tel. 601/288–8510; Douglas L. Johnson, FACHE, Chief Executive Officer
Web address: www.regencyhospital.com/hattiesburg

REGENCY HOSPITAL OF JACKSON (O, 36 beds) 971 Lakeland Drive, Jackson, MS Zip 39216; tel. 601/364–6200; Tommy Jackson, Chief Executive Officer
Web address: www.regencyhospital.com

REGENCY HOSPITAL OF MERIDIAN (O, 40 beds) 1102 Constitution Avenue, 2nd Floor, Meridian, MS Zip 39301; tel. 601/484–7900; Benny Costello, Chief Executive Officer
Web address: www.regencyhospital.com

OHIO: REGENCY HOSPITAL OF AKRON (O, 36 beds) 155 Fifth Street N.E., Barberton, OH Zip 44203; tel. 330/861–2065; Andrew Escamilla, Chief Executive Officer
Web address: www.regencyhospital.com

REGENCY HOSPITAL OF CINCINNATI (O, 15 beds) 311 Straight Street, 8th Floor, Cincinnati, OH Zip 45219; tel. 513/559–5900; Russell Dean, Chief Executive Officer
Web address: www.regencyhospital.com

REGENCY HOSPITAL OF RAVENNA (O, 19 beds) 6847 North Chestnut Street, Ravenna, OH Zip 44266; tel. 330/296–2350; Andrew Escamilla, Chief Executive Officer
Web address: www.regencyhospital.com

SOUTH CAROLINA: REGENCY HOSPITAL OF FLORENCE (O, 40 beds) 121 East Cedar Street, Florence, SC Zip 29506; tel. 843/661–3499; Timothy T. Poore, Interim Chief Executive Officer
Web address: www.regencyhospital.com

REGENCY HOSPITAL OF GREENVILLE (O, 32 beds) One St. Francis Drive, 4th Floor, Greenville, SC Zip 29601; tel. 864/255–1438; Stephanie James, Chief Executive Officer
Web address: www.regencyhospital.com

TEXAS: REGENCY HOSPITAL OF FORT WORTH (O, 41 beds) 6801 Oakmont Boulevard, Fort Worth, TX Zip 76132; tel. 817/840–2500; Denise Scurlock, Chief Executive Officer
Web address: www.regencyhospital.com

REGENCY HOSPITAL OF NORTH DALLAS (O, 41 beds) 2225 Parker Road, Carrollton, TX Zip 75010; tel. 972/236–6800; Judith Schiros, Chief Executive Officer
Web address: www.regencyhospital.com

REGENCY HOSPITAL OF ODESSA (O, 30 beds) 318 North Alleghaney, Suite 202, Odessa, TX Zip 79761; tel. 432/552–4000; Kay Peck, Chief Executive Officer
Web address: www.regencyhospital.com

Owned, leased, sponsored:	19 hospitals	624 beds
Contract–managed:	0 hospitals	0 beds
Totals:	19 hospitals	624 beds

8495: REGIONAL HEALTH (NP)
353 Fairmont Boulevard, Rapid City, SD Zip 57701, Mailing Address: P.O. Box 6000, Zip 57709–6000; tel. 605/719–1000; Charles Hart, M.D., President and Chief Executive Officer
(Moderately Centralized Health System)

SOUTH DAKOTA: CUSTER REGIONAL HOSPITAL (L, 87 beds) 1039 Montgomery Street, Custer, SD Zip 57730–1397; tel. 605/673–2229; Jason Petik, Chief Executive Officer
Web address: www.custerhospital.org

Section B

For explanation of codes following names, see page B2.
★ Indicates Type III membership in the American Hospital Association.

HANS P. PETERSON MEMORIAL HOSPITAL (C, 48 beds) 503 West Pine Street, Philip, SD Zip 57567, Mailing Address: P.O. Box 790, Zip 57567–0790; tel. 605/859–2511; Kent Olson, Administrator and Chief Executive Officer
Web address: www.rcrh.org/Facilities/Hospitals/HPPMemorial.asp

LEAD–DEADWOOD REGIONAL HOSPITAL (O, 18 beds) 61 Charles Street, Deadwood, SD Zip 57732–1303; tel. 605/722–6101; Sherry Bea Smith, RN, Chief Executive Officer
Web address: www.rcrh.org

RAPID CITY REGIONAL HOSPITAL (O, 372 beds) 353 Fairmont Boulevard, Rapid City, SD Zip 57701–7393, Mailing Address: P.O. Box 6000, Zip 57709–6000; tel. 605/719–1000; Timothy H. Sughrue, Chief Executive Officer
Web address: www.rcrh.org

SPEARFISH REGIONAL HOSPITAL (O, 32 beds) 1440 North Main Street, Spearfish, SD Zip 57783–1504; tel. 605/644–4000; Larry W. Veitz, Chief Executive Officer
Web address: www.rcrh.org

STURGIS REGIONAL HOSPITAL (O, 108 beds) 949 Harmon Street, Sturgis, SD Zip 57785–2452; tel. 605/720–2400; Van Hyde, Chief Executive Officer

WYOMING: WESTON COUNTY HEALTH SERVICES (C, 86 beds) 1124 Washington Boulevard, Newcastle, WY Zip 82701–2996; tel. 307/746–4491; Kevin Stiffarm, Chief Executive Officer
Web address: www.wchs-wy.org

Owned, leased, sponsored:	5 hospitals	617 beds
Contract–managed:	2 hospitals	134 beds
Totals:	7 hospitals	751 beds

★0363: REHABCARE GROUP, INC. (IO)

7733 Forsyth Boulevard, Saint Louis, MO Zip 63105; tel. 800/677–1238; John H. Short, Ph.D., President and Chief Executive Officer

FLORIDA: WEST GABLES REHABILITATION HOSPITAL (O, 60 beds) 2525 S.W. 75th Avenue, Miami, FL Zip 33155; tel. 305/262–6800; Ismael Roque–Velasco, M.D., Chief Executive Officer
Web address: www.rehabcare.com/portfolio/long_term_acute_care/westgables.htm

LOUISIANA: LOUISIANA SPECIALTY HOSPITAL (O, 56 beds) 1111 Medical Center Boulevard, 7th Floor, Marrero, LA Zip 70072, Mailing Address: 1111 Medical Center Boulecvard, 7th Floor, Zip 70072; tel. 504/349–2584; Stephanie T. Wells, CPA, Chief Executive Officer
Web address: www.rehabcare.com

MEADOWBROOK SPECIALTY HOSPITAL OF LAFAYETTE (O, 70 beds) 204 Energy Parkway, Lafayette, LA Zip 70508; tel. 337/232–1905; R. Christopher Fox, Chief Executive Officer and Administrator
Web address: www.rehabcare.com

OKLAHOMA: TULSA SPECIALTY HOSPITAL (O, 60 beds) 3219 South 79th East Avenue, Tulsa, OK Zip 74145–1312; tel. 918/663–8183; Ginger Creech, Chief Executive Officer
Web address: www.mbhealth.com

TEXAS: CLEAR LAKE REHABILITATION HOSPITAL (O, 59 beds) 655 East Medical Center Boulevard, Webster, TX Zip 77598–4328; tel. 281/286–1500; Susan Schaetti, Interim Chief Executive Officer
Web address: www.rehabcare.com

NORTHWEST TEXAS REHABILITATION HOSPITAL (O, 42 beds) 7200 West 9th Avenue, Amarillo, TX Zip 79106; tel. 806/468–2900; Mark A. Kelly, Chief Executive Officer and Administrator
Web address: www.rehabcare.com

REHABCARE OF ARLINGTON (O, 24 beds) 2601 West Randol Mill Road, Arlington, TX Zip 76012; tel. 817/804–4400; Susan Schaetti, Chief Executive Officer
Web address: www.rehabcare.com/portfolio/long_term_acute_care/Arlington.htm

REHABCARE REHABILITATION HOSPITAL – PERMIAN BASIN (O, 38 beds) 207 Tradewinds Boulevard, Midland, TX Zip 79706; tel. 432/520–2333; Dale R. Mulder, Chief Executive Officer
Web address: www.rehabcare.com

Owned, leased, sponsored:	8 hospitals	409 beds
Contract–managed:	0 hospitals	0 beds
Totals:	8 hospitals	409 beds

0373: RENAISSANCE HEALTHCARE SYSTEMS (IO)

14440 John F. Kennedy Boulevard, Houston, TX Zip 77032; tel. 832/886–1900; Michael Smesny, Chief Executive Officer

RENAISSANCE HOSPITAL (O, 72 beds) 5500 39th Street, Groves, TX Zip 77619–9805; tel. 409/962–5733; Chris McMahon, Administrator
Web address: www.renhealthcare.org

RENAISSANCE HOSPITAL – HOUSTON (O, 39 beds) 2807 Little York Road, Houston, TX Zip 77093–3495; tel. 713/697–7777; Michael Smesny, President

RENAISSANCE HOSPITAL OF DALLAS (O, 108 beds) 2929 South Hampton Road, Dallas, TX Zip 75224; tel. 214/623–4400; Sammy E. Davis, Chief Executive Officer
Web address: www.dallas.renhealthcare.org

RENAISSANCE HOSPITAL TERRELL (L, 106 beds) 1551 Highway 34 South, Terrell, TX Zip 75160–4833; tel. 972/563–7611; Sean Astolfo, Administrator
Web address: www.renhealthcare.org

Owned, leased, sponsored:	4 hospitals	325 beds
Contract–managed:	0 hospitals	0 beds
Totals:	4 hospitals	325 beds

2625: RENOWN HEALTH (NP)

77 Pringle Way, Reno, NV Zip 89502–1474; tel. 775/982–4100; James I. Miller, President and Chief Executive Officer
(Centralized Health System)

NEVADA: RENOWN REGIONAL MEDICAL CENTER (O, 517 beds) 1155 Mill Street, Reno, NV Zip 89502; tel. 775/982–4100; James I. Miller, President and Chief Executive Officer
Web address: www.renown.org

RENOWN REHABILITATION HOSPITAL (O, 62 beds) 1495 Mill Street, Reno, NV Zip 89502–1449; tel. 775/982–3500; Troy Smith, Interim Administrator
Web address: www.renown.org

RENOWN SOUTH MEADOWS MEDICAL CENTER (O, 76 beds) 10101 Double R Boulevard, Reno, NV Zip 89521; tel. 775/982–7000; Alan C. Olive, Chief Executive Officer
Web address: www.renown.org

Owned, leased, sponsored:	3 hospitals	655 beds
Contract–managed:	0 hospitals	0 beds
Totals:	3 hospitals	655 beds

0290: RESURGENCE HEALTH GROUP (IO)

1400 Buford Highway, Building R–3, Sugar Hill, GA Zip 30518; tel. 770/904–6731; Philip H. Eastman, III, President
(Independent Hospital System)

ALABAMA: SOUTHWEST ALABAMA MEDICAL CENTER (O, 27 beds) 33700 Highway 43, Thomasville, AL Zip 36784–3351; tel. 334/636–4311; Anne S. Thompson, Chief Executive Officer
Web address: www.resurgencehealthgroup.com

GEORGIA: FLINT RIVER COMMUNITY HOSPITAL (O, 49 beds) 509 Sumter Street, Montezuma, GA Zip 31063–0770, Mailing Address: P.O. Box 770, Zip 31063–0770; tel. 478/472–3100; Laurie Hair, Chief Executive Officer and Chief Financial Officer
Web address: www.resurgencehealthgroup.com

Owned, leased, sponsored:	2 hospitals	76 beds
Contract–managed:	0 hospitals	0 beds
Totals:	2 hospitals	76 beds

0171: RESURRECTION HEALTH CARE (CC)

7435 West Talcott Avenue, Chicago, IL Zip 60631; tel. 773/792–5150; Joseph F. Toomey, President and Chief Executive Officer
(Moderately Centralized Health System)

For explanation of codes following names, see page B2.
★ Indicates Type III membership in the American Hospital Association.

ILLINOIS: HOLY FAMILY MEDICAL CENTER (O, 165 beds) 100 North River Road, Des Plaines, IL Zip 60016–1255; tel. 847/297–1800; John D. Baird, Chief Executive Officer
Web address: www.reshealth.org

OUR LADY OF THE RESURRECTION MEDICAL CENTER (O, 237 beds) 5645 West Addison Street, Chicago, IL Zip 60634–4455; tel. 773/282–7000; Ivette Estrada, Executive Vice President and Chief Executive Officer
Web address: www.reshealthcare.org

RESURRECTION MEDICAL CENTER (O, 406 beds) 7435 West Talcott Avenue, Chicago, IL Zip 60631–3746; tel. 773/774–8000; Sister Donna Marie Wolowicki, Executive Vice President and Chief Executive Officer
Web address: www.reshealthcare.org

SAINT FRANCIS HOSPITAL (O, 232 beds) 355 Ridge Avenue, Evanston, IL Zip 60202–3399; tel. 847/316–4000; Jeffrey J. Murphy, Executive Vice President and Chief Executive Officer
Web address: www.reshealth.org

SAINT JOSEPH HOSPITAL (O, 347 beds) 2900 North Lake Shore Drive, Chicago, IL Zip 60657–6274; tel. 773/665–3000; Ronald E. Struxness, Chief Executive Officer
Web address: www.reshealth.org

SAINTS MARY & ELIZABETH MEDICAL CENTER, CLAREMONT AVENUE (O, 246 beds) 1431 North Claremont Avenue, Chicago, IL Zip 60622–1791; tel. 773/278–2000; Margaret McDermott, Chief Executive Officer
Web address: www.reshealthcare.org

SAINTS MARY & ELIZABETH MEDICAL CENTER, DIVISION STREET (O, 313 beds) 2233 West Division Street, Chicago, IL Zip 60622–3086; tel. 312/770–2000; Margaret McDermott, Chief Executive Officer
Web address: www.stmaryofnazareth.org

WEST SUBURBAN MEDICAL CENTER (O, 152 beds) 3 Erie Court, Oak Park, IL Zip 60302–2599; tel. 708/383–6200; Jay E. Kreuzer, FACHE, President and Chief Executive Officer
Web address: www.wsmc.reshealth.org

WESTLAKE HOSPITAL (O, 181 beds) 1225 Lake Street, Melrose Park, IL Zip 60160–4000; tel. 708/681–3000; Patricia Shehorn, Chief Executive Officer
Web address: www.reshealth.org

Owned, leased, sponsored:	9 hospitals	2279 beds
Contract-managed:	0 hospitals	0 beds
Totals:	9 hospitals	2279 beds

4810: RIVERSIDE HEALTH SYSTEM (NP)
701 Town Center Drive, Suite 1000, Newport News, VA Zip 23606; tel. 757/534–7000; Richard J. Pearce, President and Chief Executive Officer
(Centralized Health System)

VIRGINIA: RIVERSIDE BEHAVIORAL HEALTH CENTER (O, 79 beds) 2244 Executive Drive, Hampton, VA Zip 23666–2430; tel. 757/827–1001; Debora S. Tanner, Vice President and Administrator
Web address: www.riversideonline.com

RIVERSIDE REGIONAL MEDICAL CENTER (O, 205 beds) 500 J. Clyde Morris Boulevard, Newport News, VA Zip 23601–1976; tel. 757/594–2000; Golden H. Bethune, RN, Executive Vice President and Administrator
Web address: www.riverside–online.com

RIVERSIDE REHABILITATION INSTITUTE (O, 26 beds) 245 Chesapeake Avenue, Newport News, VA Zip 23607–6038; tel. 757/928–8000; Anne T. Moffat, Administrator
Web address: www.riverside–online.com

RIVERSIDE TAPPAHANNOCK HOSPITAL (O, 42 beds) 618 Hospital Road, Tappahannock, VA Zip 22560–5000; tel. 804/443–3311; Elizabeth J. Martin, Vice President and Administrator
Web address: www.riverside–online.com

RIVERSIDE WALTER REED HOSPITAL (O, 24 beds) 7519 Hospital Drive, Gloucester, VA Zip 23061–4178, Mailing Address: P.O. Box 1130, Zip 23061–1130; tel. 804/693–8800; Robert E. Bryant, Vice President and Administrator
Web address: www.riversideonline.com

Owned, leased, sponsored:	5 hospitals	376 beds
Contract-managed:	0 hospitals	0 beds
Totals:	5 hospitals	376 beds

0268: ROBERT WOOD JOHNSON HEALTH SYSTEM & NETWORK (NP)
1 Robert Wood Johnson Place, New Brunswick, NJ Zip 08903–2601; tel. 732/828–3000; Stephen K. Jones, President and Chief Executive Officer
(Moderately Centralized Health System)

NEW JERSEY: CHILDREN'S SPECIALIZED HOSPITAL (O, 126 beds) 150 New Providence Road, Mountainside, NJ Zip 07092–2590; tel. 908/233–3720; Amy B. Mansue, President and Chief Executive Officer
Web address: www.childrens–specialized.org

ROBERT WOOD JOHNSON UNIVERSITY HOSPITAL (O, 610 beds) 1 Robert Wood Johnson Place, New Brunswick, NJ Zip 08903–2601; tel. 732/828–3000; Stephen K. Jones, President and Chief Executive Officer
Web address: www.rwjuh.edu

ROBERT WOOD JOHNSON UNIVERSITY HOSPITAL AT HAMILTON (O, 270 beds) One Hamilton Health Place, Hamilton, NJ Zip 08690–3599; tel. 609/586–7900; Ellen Guarnieri, President and Chief Executive Officer
Web address: www.rwjhamilton.org

ROBERT WOOD JOHNSON UNIVERSITY HOSPITAL AT RAHWAY (O, 165 beds) 865 Stone Street, Rahway, NJ Zip 07065–2797; tel. 732/381–4200; Kirk C. Tice, President and Chief Executive Officer
Web address: www.rahwayhospital.com

Owned, leased, sponsored:	4 hospitals	1171 beds
Contract-managed:	0 hospitals	0 beds
Totals:	4 hospitals	1171 beds

★0109: RURAL HEALTH GROUP (IO)
48 West 1500 North, Nephi, UT Zip 84648–1226; tel. 435/623–4924; Mark R. Stoddard, President and Chairman
(Independent Hospital System)

NEVADA: DESERT VIEW REGIONAL MEDICAL CENTER (O, 24 beds) 360 South Lola Lane, Pahrump, NV Zip 89048; tel. 775/751–7500; Susan Davila, Administrator and Chief Executive Officer
Web address: www.dvrmc.org

UTAH: ALLEN MEMORIAL HOSPITAL (L, 25 beds) 719 West 400 North Street, Moab, UT Zip 84532–2297, Mailing Address: P.O. Box 998, Zip 84532–0998; tel. 435/259–7191; Roy E. Barraclough, Administrator and Chief Executive Officer
Web address: www.amhmoab.org

CENTRAL VALLEY MEDICAL CENTER (L, 25 beds) 48 West 1500 North, Nephi, UT Zip 84648; tel. 435/623–3000; Mark R. Stoddard, President
Web address: www.centralvalleymed.com

Owned, leased, sponsored:	3 hospitals	74 beds
Contract-managed:	0 hospitals	0 beds
Totals:	3 hospitals	74 beds

0220: RUSH HEALTH SYSTEMS (NP)
1314 19th Avenue, Meridian, MS Zip 39301; tel. 601/483–0011; Wallace Strickland, President and Chief Executive Officer
(Independent Hospital System)

MISSISSIPPI: RUSH FOUNDATION HOSPITAL (O, 182 beds) 1314 19th Avenue, Meridian, MS Zip 39301–4195; tel. 601/483–0011; Wallace Strickland, President and Chief Executive Officer
Web address: www.rushhealthsystems.org

SCOTT REGIONAL HOSPITAL (O, 30 beds) 317 Highway 13 South, Morton, MS Zip 39117–3353, Mailing Address: P.O. Box 259, Zip 39117–0259; tel. 601/732–6301; Michael R. Edwards, Chief Executive Officer

SPECIALTY HOSPITAL OF MERIDIAN (O, 49 beds) 1314 19th Avenue, Meridian, MS Zip 39301–4116; tel. 601/703–4211; Wallace Strickland, President and Chief Executive Officer
Web address: www.rushhealthsystems.org

Owned, leased, sponsored:	3 hospitals	261 beds
Contract-managed:	0 hospitals	0 beds
Totals:	3 hospitals	261 beds

Section B

For explanation of codes following names, see page B2.
★ Indicates Type III membership in the American Hospital Association.

Section B

★3855: RUSH UNIVERSITY MEDICAL CENTER (NP)
1653 West Congress Parkway, Chicago, IL Zip 60612–3864; tel. 312/942–5000; Larry J. Goodman, M.D., President and Chief Executive Officer
(Moderately Centralized Health System)

ILLINOIS: RUSH NORTH SHORE MEDICAL CENTER (O, 234 beds) 9600 Gross Point Road, Skokie, IL Zip 60076–1257; tel. 847/677–9600; James T. Frankenbach, President and Chief Executive Officer
Web address: www.rnsmc.org

RUSH UNIVERSITY MEDICAL CENTER (O, 676 beds) 1653 West Congress Parkway, Chicago, IL Zip 60612–3833; tel. 312/942–5000; Larry J. Goodman, M.D., President and Chief Executive Officer
Web address: www.rush.edu

RUSH–COPLEY MEDICAL CENTER (O, 157 beds) 2000 Ogden Avenue, Aurora, IL Zip 60504–4206; tel. 630/978–6200; Barry C. Finn, President and Chief Executive Officer
Web address: www.rushcopley.com

Owned, leased, sponsored:	3 hospitals	1067 beds
Contract–managed:	0 hospitals	0 beds
Totals:	3 hospitals	1067 beds

★0118: SAINT BARNABAS HEALTH CARE SYSTEM (NP)
95 Old Short Hills Road, West Orange, NJ Zip 07052; tel. 973/322–4001; Ronald J. Del Mauro, President and Chief Executive Officer
(Centralized Health System)

NEW JERSEY: CLARA MAASS MEDICAL CENTER (O, 426 beds) One Clara Maass Drive, Belleville, NJ Zip 07109–3557; tel. 973/450–2000; Thomas A. Biga, Executive Director
Web address: www.sbhcs.com

COMMUNITY MEDICAL CENTER (O, 495 beds) 99 Route 37 West, Toms River, NJ Zip 08755–6423; tel. 732/557–8000; Mark D. Pilla, Executive Director
Web address: www.sbhcs.com

KIMBALL MEDICAL CENTER (O, 302 beds) 600 River Avenue, Lakewood, NJ Zip 08701–4281; tel. 732/363–1900; Joe Hicks, Executive Director
Web address: www.sbhcs.com

MONMOUTH MEDICAL CENTER (O, 324 beds) 300 Second Avenue, Long Branch, NJ Zip 07740–6303; tel. 732/222–5200; Frank J. Vozos, M.D., FACS, Executive Director
Web address: www.sbhcs.com

NEWARK BETH ISRAEL MEDICAL CENTER (O, 407 beds) 201 Lyons Avenue, Newark, NJ Zip 07112–2027; tel. 973/926–7000; John A. Brennan, M.D., Executive Director
Web address: www.sbhcs.com

SAINT BARNABAS MEDICAL CENTER (O, 601 beds) 94 Old Short Hills Road, Livingston, NJ Zip 07039–5668; tel. 973/322–5000; John F. Bonamo, M.D., Executive Director
Web address: www.sbhcs.com

Owned, leased, sponsored:	6 hospitals	2555 beds
Contract–managed:	0 hospitals	0 beds
Totals:	6 hospitals	2555 beds

0351: SAINT CATHERINE HEALTHCARE, LLC (IO)
101 Broad Street, Ashland, PA Zip 17921; tel. 570/875–2000; Robert C. Marquardt, FACHE, Chief Operating Officer
(Independent Hospital System)

INDIANA: SAINT CATHERINE REGIONAL HOSPITAL (O, 77 beds) 2200 Market Street, Charlestown, IN Zip 47111–0009, Mailing Address: P.O. Box 9, Zip 47111–0009; tel. 812/256–3301; Michael J. Funk, President and Chief Executive Officer
Web address: www.stchc.com/scrh/

PENNSYLVANIA: SAINT CATHERINE MEDICAL CENTER FOUNTAIN SPRINGS (O, 79 beds) 101 Broad Street, Ashland, PA Zip 17921–0000; tel. 570/875–2000; Robert C. Marquardt, FACHE, President and Chief Executive Officer

Owned, leased, sponsored:	2 hospitals	156 beds
Contract–managed:	0 hospitals	0 beds
Totals:	2 hospitals	156 beds

0318: SAINT FRANCIS CARE, INC. (NP)
114 Woodland Street, Hartford, CT Zip 06105; tel. 860/714–5541; Christopher M. Dadlez, President and Chief Executive Officer
(Moderately Centralized Health System)

CONNECTICUT: MOUNT SINAI REHABILITATION HOSPITAL (O, 46 beds) 490 Blue Hills Avenue, Hartford, CT Zip 6112; tel. 860/714–3500; Christopher M. Dadlez, President and Chief Executive Officer
Web address: www.stfranciscare.org

SAINT FRANCIS HOSPITAL AND MEDICAL CENTER (O, 542 beds) 114 Woodland Street, Hartford, CT Zip 06105–1208; tel. 860/714–4000; Christopher M. Dadlez, President and Chief Executive Officer
Web address: www.saintfranciscare.com

Owned, leased, sponsored:	2 hospitals	588 beds
Contract–managed:	0 hospitals	0 beds
Totals:	2 hospitals	588 beds

★0254: SAINT FRANCIS HEALTH SYSTEM (NP)
6161 South Yale Avenue, Tulsa, OK Zip 74136–1902; tel. 918/494–8454; Jake Henry, Jr., President and Chief Executive Officer
(Centralized Physician/Insurance Health System)

OKLAHOMA: LAUREATE PSYCHIATRIC CLINIC AND HOSPITAL (O, 75 beds) 6655 South Yale Avenue, Tulsa, OK Zip 74136–3329; tel. 918/481–4000; John M. Robson, Executive Director
Web address: www.laureate.com

SAINT FRANCIS HEART HOSPITAL (O, 40 beds) 10501 East 91st Street South, Tulsa, OK Zip 74133; tel. 918/307–6000; Joseph H. Neely, Senior Vice President and Administrator
Web address: www.saintfrancisheart.com

SAINT FRANCIS HOSPITAL (O, 682 beds) 6161 South Yale Avenue, Tulsa, OK Zip 74136–1902; tel. 918/494–2200; Lynn Sund, Administrator
Web address: www.saintfrancis.com

Owned, leased, sponsored:	3 hospitals	797 beds
Contract–managed:	0 hospitals	0 beds
Totals:	3 hospitals	797 beds

0120: SAINT LUKE'S HEALTH SYSTEM (NP)
10920 Elm Avenue, Kansas City, MO Zip 64134–4108; tel. 816/932–2000; G. Richard Hastings, President and Chief Executive Officer
(Centralized Health System)

KANSAS: ANDERSON COUNTY HOSPITAL (O, 47 beds) 421 South Maple, Garnett, KS Zip 66032–1334, Mailing Address: P.O. Box 309, Zip 66032–0309; tel. 785/448–3131; Dennis A. Hachenberg, FACHE, Chief Executive Officer
Web address: www.saint–lukes.org

CUSHING MEMORIAL HOSPITAL (O, 49 beds) 711 Marshall Street, Leavenworth, KS Zip 66048–3235; tel. 913/684–1100; Ronald L. Baker, Chief Executive Officer
Web address: www.cushinghospital.org

SAINT LUKE'S SOUTH HOSPITAL (O, 95 beds) 12300 Metcalf Avenue, Overland Park, KS Zip 66213; tel. 913/317–7000; Julie Quirin, Chief Executive Officer
Web address: www.saint–lukes.org

MISSOURI: CRITTENTON CHILDREN'S CENTER (O, 46 beds) 10918 Elm Avenue, Kansas City, MO Zip 64134–4108; tel. 816/765–6600; Stephen W. Churchill, M.D., Chief Executive Officer and Medical Director
Web address: www.saintlukeshealthsystem.org/app/hpcrittenton.asp

HEDRICK MEDICAL CENTER (O, 25 beds) 100 Central Avenue, Chillicothe, MO Zip 64601–1554; tel. 660/646–1480; Brian J. Johnston, FACHE, Chief Executive Officer
Web address: www.saintlukeshealthsystem.org

For explanation of codes following names, see page B2.
★ Indicates Type III membership in the American Hospital Association.

SAINT LUKE'S CANCER INSTITUTE (O, 30 beds) 4323 Wornall Road, Kansas City, MO Zip 64111–3214; tel. 816/932–2823; Jeffrey Wieman, M.D., Chief Executive Officer
Web address: www.saint–lukes.org

SAINT LUKE'S EAST–LEE'S SUMMIT (O, 57 beds) 100 N.E. Saint Luke's Boulevard, Lee's Summit, MO Zip 64086–6000; tel. 816/347–5000; George A. Pagels, M.D., President and Chief Executive Officer
Web address: www.saint–lukes.org

SAINT LUKE'S HOSPITAL OF KANSAS CITY (O, 404 beds) 4401 Wornall Road, Kansas City, MO Zip 64111–3238; tel. 816/932–2000; G. Richard Hastings, Chief Executive Officer
Web address: www.saint–lukes.org

SAINT LUKE'S NORTHLAND HOSPITAL (O, 134 beds) 5830 N.W. Barry Road, Kansas City, MO Zip 64154–2778; tel. 816/891–6000; N. Gary Wages, FACHE, President and Chief Executive Officer
Web address: www.saint–lukes.org

SAINT LUKE'S NORTHLAND HOSPITAL–SMITHVILLE CAMPUS (O, 51 beds) 601 South 169 Highway, Smithville, MO Zip 64089–9317; tel. 816/532–3700; Don Sipes, Chief Executive Officer
Web address: www.saintlukeshealthsystem.org

WRIGHT MEMORIAL HOSPITAL (O, 25 beds) 701 East First Street, Trenton, MO Zip 64683–2402, Mailing Address: P.O. Box 628, Zip 64683–0628; tel. 660/359–5621; Karen S. Cole, FACHE, Chief Executive Officer
Web address: www.saintlukeshealthsystem.org

Owned, leased, sponsored:	11 hospitals	963 beds
Contract–managed:	0 hospitals	0 beds
Totals:	11 hospitals	963 beds

0403: SALEM HEALTH (NP)
665 Winter S.E., Salem, OR Zip 97301–3959; tel. 503/561–5200

OREGON: SALEM HOSPITAL (O, 417 beds) 665 Winter Street S.E., Salem, OR Zip 97301–3959, Mailing Address: P.O. Box 14001, Zip 97309–5014; tel. 503/561–5200; Norman F. Gruber, President and Chief Executive Officer
Web address: www.salemhospital.org

WEST VALLEY HOSPITAL (O, 6 beds) 525 S.E. Washington Street, Dallas, OR Zip 97338–2899, Mailing Address: P.O. Box 378, Zip 97338–0378; tel. 503/623–8301; Eric Buckland, CHE, Site Administrator
Web address: www.westvalleyhospital.org

Owned, leased, sponsored:	2 hospitals	423 beds
Contract–managed:	0 hospitals	0 beds
Totals:	2 hospitals	423 beds

★0186: SAMARITAN HEALTH SERVICES (NP)
3600 N.W. Samaritan Drive, Corvallis, OR Zip 97330, Mailing Address: P.O. Box 1068, Zip 97339; tel. 541/768–5001; Larry A. Mullins, FACHE, President and Chief Executive Officer
(Centralized Physician/Insurance Health System)

GOOD SAMARITAN REGIONAL MEDICAL CENTER (O, 185 beds) 3600 N.W. Samaritan Drive, Corvallis, OR Zip 97330–3737, Mailing Address: P.O. Box 1068, Zip 97339–1068; tel. 541/768–5111; Steven W. Jasperson, Chief Executive Officer
Web address: www.samhealth.org

SAMARITAN ALBANY GENERAL HOSPITAL (O, 67 beds) 1046 West Sixth Avenue, Albany, OR Zip 97321–1999; tel. 541/812–4000; David G. Triebes, Chief Executive Officer
Web address: www.samhealth.org

SAMARITAN LEBANON COMMUNITY HOSPITAL (O, 25 beds) 525 North Santiam Highway, Lebanon, OR Zip 97355–4363, Mailing Address: P.O. Box 739, Zip 97355–0739; tel. 541/258–2101; Becky A. Pape, RN, Chief Executive Officer
Web address: www.samhealth.org

SAMARITAN NORTH LINCOLN HOSPITAL (C, 25 beds) 3043 N.E. 28th Street, Lincoln City, OR Zip 97367–4523, Mailing Address: P.O. Box 767, Zip 97367–0767; tel. 541/994–3661; Sue Massart, Chief Executive Officer
Web address: www.samhealth.org

SAMARITAN PACIFIC COMMUNITIES HOSPITAL (C, 42 beds) 930 S.W. Abbey Street, Newport, OR Zip 97365–4820, Mailing Address: P.O. Box 945, Zip 97365–4820; tel. 541/265–2244; David C. Bigelow, Chief Executive Officer
Web address: www.samhealth.org

Owned, leased, sponsored:	3 hospitals	277 beds
Contract–managed:	2 hospitals	67 beds
Totals:	5 hospitals	344 beds

★0078: SANFORD HEALTH (NP)
1305 West 18th Street, Sioux Falls, SD Zip 57105–0496, Mailing Address: P.O. Box 5039, Zip 57117–5039; tel. 605/333–1000; Kelby K. Krabbenhoft, President and Chief Executive Officer
(Decentralized Health System)

IOWA: ORANGE CITY AREA HEALTH SYSTEM (C, 104 beds) 1000 Lincoln Circle S.E., Orange City, IA Zip 51041–1398; tel. 712/737–4984; Martin W. Guthmiller, Chief Executive Officer
Web address: www.ochealthsystem.org

SANFORD MERRILL MEDICAL CENTER (L, 16 beds) 801 South Greene Street, Rock Rapids, IA Zip 51246–1998; tel. 712/472–2591; Gordon U. Smith, Chief Executive Officer
Web address: www.merrillpioneer.org

SANFORD SHELDON MEDICAL CENTER (O, 95 beds) 118 North Seventh Avenue, Sheldon, IA Zip 51201–1235, Mailing Address: P.O. Box 250, Zip 51201–0250; tel. 712/324–5041; Charles R. Miller, Chief Executive Officer
Web address: www.nwiowahealthcenter.org

MINNESOTA: MURRAY COUNTY MEDICAL CENTER (C, 25 beds) 2042 Juniper Avenue, Slayton, MN Zip 56172–1016; tel. 507/836–6111; Meldon L. Snow, Chief Executive Officer
Web address: www.murraycountymed.org

ORTONVILLE AREA HEALTH SERVICES (C, 81 beds) 450 Eastvold Avenue, Ortonville, MN Zip 56278–1133; tel. 320/839–2502; Richard M. Ash, Chief Executive Officer
Web address: www.ortonvilleareahealth.org

SANFORD CANBY MEDICAL CENTER (L, 100 beds) 112 St. Olaf Avenue South, Canby, MN Zip 56220–1433; tel. 507/223–7277; Robert J. Salmon, Chief Executive Officer
Web address: www.sanfordcanby.org

SANFORD JACKSON MEDICAL CENTER (L, 20 beds) 1430 North Highway, Jackson, MN Zip 56143–1098; tel. 507/847–2420; Mary J. Ruyter, Chief Executive Officer
Web address: www.sanfordjackson.org

SANFORD TRACY MEDICAL CENTER (L, 25 beds) 251 Fifth Street East, Tracy, MN Zip 56175–1536; tel. 507/629–3200; Richard E. Nordahl, Administrator and Chief Executive Officer
Web address: www.tracyareamedical.org

SANFORD WESTBROOK MEDICAL CENTER (L, 6 beds) 920 Bell Avenue, Westbrook, MN Zip 56183–0188, Mailing Address: P.O. Box 188, Zip 56183–0188; tel. 507/274–6121; Richard E. Nordahl, Administrator and Chief Executive Officer
Web address: www.westbrookhealthcenter.org

SIOUX VALLEY LUVERNE MEDICAL CENTER (O, 25 beds) 1600 North Kniss, Luverne, MN Zip 56156–2519; tel. 507/283–2321; Mark Henke, Chief Executive Officer
Web address: www.sanfordluverne.org

WINDOM AREA HOSPITAL (C, 25 beds) 2150 Hospital Drive, Windom, MN Zip 56101–0339, Mailing Address: P.O. Box 339, Zip 56101–0339; tel. 507/831–2400; Geraldine S. Burmeister, Chief Executive Officer
Web address: www.windomareahospital.com

WORTHINGTON REGIONAL HOSPITAL (C, 64 beds) 1018 Sixth Avenue, Worthington, MN Zip 56187–2202, Mailing Address: P.O. Box 997, Zip 56187–0997; tel. 507/372–2941; Melvin J. Platt, Chief Executive Officer
Web address: www.worthingtonhospital.com

NEBRASKA: NIOBRARA VALLEY HOSPITAL (C, 20 beds) 401 South Fifth Street, Lynch, NE Zip 68746–0118, Mailing Address: P.O. Box 118, Zip 68746–0118; tel. 402/569–2451; Kelly Kalkowski, Chief Executive Officer
Web address: www.ci.lynch.ne.us/health.htm

For explanation of codes following names, see page B2.
★ Indicates Type III membership in the American Hospital Association.

WEST HOLT MEMORIAL HOSPITAL (C, 18 beds) 406 West Neely Street, Atkinson, NE Zip 68713–0200; tel. 402/925–2811; John N. Olson, Chief Executive Officer
Web address: www.westholtmed.org

SOUTH DAKOTA: CANTON–INWOOD MEMORIAL HOSPITAL (L, 18 beds) 440 North Hiawatha Drive, Canton, SD Zip 57013–9404; tel. 605/987–2621; Eric C. Hilmoe, Chief Executive Officer
Web address: www.cantoninwoodhospital.org

COMMUNITY MEMORIAL HOSPITAL (C, 16 beds) 809 Jackson Street, Burke, SD Zip 57523, Mailing Address: P.O. Box 319, Zip 57523–0319; tel. 605/775–2621; Jim Frank, Chief Executive Officer

PIONEER MEMORIAL HOSPITAL AND HEALTH SERVICES (C, 64 beds) 315 North Washington Street, Viborg, SD Zip 57070–2002, Mailing Address: P.O. Box 368, Zip 57070–0368; tel. 605/326–5161; Georgia C. Pokorney, Chief Executive Officer
Web address: www.pioneermemorial.org

SANFORD DEUEL COUNTY MEDICAL CENTER (L, 20 beds) 701 Third Avenue South, Clear Lake, SD Zip 57226–2016; tel. 605/874–2141; Robert J. Salmon, Chief Executive Officer
Web address: www.deuelcountymemorial.org

SANFORD MID DAKOTA MEDICAL CENTER (O, 72 beds) 300 South Byron Boulevard, Chamberlain, SD Zip 57325–9741; tel. 605/234–5511; Maureen K. Cadwell, Chief Executive Officer
Web address: www.sanfordmiddakota.org

SANFORD UNIVERSITY OF SOUTH DAKOTA MEDICAL CENTER (O, 451 beds) 1305 West 18th Street, Sioux Falls, SD Zip 57105–0496, Mailing Address: P.O. Box 5039, Zip 57117–5039; tel. 605/333–1000; Charles O'Brien, M.D., President
Web address: www.sanfordhealth.org

SANFORD VERMILLION MEDICAL CENTER (L, 114 beds) 20 South Plum Street, Vermillion, SD Zip 57069–3346; tel. 605/624–2611; Timothy J. Tracy, Chief Executive Officer

SANFORD WEBSTER MEDICAL CENTER (L, 25 beds) 1401 West 1st Street, Webster, SD Zip 57274–1816, Mailing Address: P.O. Box 489, Zip 57274–0489; tel. 605/345–3336; Kyle Richards, Chief Executive Officer
Web address: www.sanfordhealth.org

WINNER REGIONAL HEALTHCARE CENTER (C, 106 beds) 745 East Eighth Street, Winner, SD Zip 57580–2677; tel. 605/842–7100; Michael L. Hall, Chief Executive Officer
Web address: www.winnerregional.org

Owned, leased, sponsored:	13 hospitals	987 beds
Contract-managed:	10 hospitals	523 beds
Totals:	23 hospitals	1510 beds

0398: SCOTT & WHITE (NP)

2401 South 31st Street, Temple, TX Zip 76508; tel. 254/724–2111; Alfred B. Knight, M.D., Chief Executive Officer

TEXAS: SCOTT AND WHITE AT UNIVERSITY MEDICAL CAMPUS (O, 72 beds) 300 University Boulevard, Round Rock, TX Zip 78664; tel. 512/509–0200; Ernest L. Bovio, Jr., Chief Executive Officer
Web address: www.scottandwhite.org

SCOTT AND WHITE MEMORIAL HOSPITAL (O, 562 beds) 2401 South 31st Street, Temple, TX Zip 76508–0002; tel. 254/724–2111; Patricia M. Currie, FACHE, Chief Hospital Services
Web address: www.sw.org

Owned, leased, sponsored:	2 hospitals	634 beds
Contract-managed:	0 hospitals	0 beds
Totals:	2 hospitals	634 beds

★0037: SCOTTSDALE HEALTHCARE (NP)

3621 Wells Fargo Avenue, Scottsdale, AZ Zip 85251–5607; tel. 480/882–4000; Thomas J. Sadvary, FACHE, President and Chief Executive Officer
(Centralized Physician/Insurance Health System)

ARIZONA: SCOTTSDALE HEALTHCARE SHEA (O, 405 beds) 9003 East Shea Boulevard, Scottsdale, AZ Zip 85260–6771; tel. 480/323–3000; Peggy Reiley, Senior Vice President and Chief Clinical Officer
Web address: www.shc.org

SCOTTSDALE HEALTHCARE THOMPSON PEAK (O, 64 beds) 7400 East Thompson Peak Parkway, Scottsdale, AZ Zip 85255; tel. 480/324–7000; Jean Knoedler, Vice President and Administrator
Web address: www.scottsdalehealthcare.org

SCOTTSDALE HEALTHCARE–OSBORN (O, 337 beds) 7400 East Osborn Road, Scottsdale, AZ Zip 85251–6403; tel. 480/882–4000; Gary E. Baker, Senior Vice President and Administrator
Web address: www.shc.org

Owned, leased, sponsored:	3 hospitals	806 beds
Contract-managed:	0 hospitals	0 beds
Totals:	3 hospitals	806 beds

★1505: SCRIPPS HEALTH (NP)

4275 Campus Point Court, San Diego, CA Zip 92121; tel. 858/678–7200; Chris D. Van Gorder, FACHE, President and Chief Executive Officer
(Centralized Health System)

CALIFORNIA: SCRIPPS GREEN HOSPITAL (O, 173 beds) 10666 North Torrey Pines Road, La Jolla, CA Zip 92037–1093; tel. 858/455–9100; Robin Brown, Senior Vice President and Chief Executive
Web address: www.scrippshealth.org

SCRIPPS MEMORIAL HOSPITAL–ENCINITAS (O, 134 beds) 354 Santa Fe Drive, Encinitas, CA Zip 92024–5182, Mailing Address: P.O. Box 230817, Zip 92023–0817; tel. 760/633–6501; Carl J. Etter, Senior Vice President and Chief Executive
Web address: www.scrippshealth.org

SCRIPPS MEMORIAL HOSPITAL–LA JOLLA (O, 301 beds) 9888 Genesee Avenue, La Jolla, CA Zip 92037–1200, Mailing Address: P.O. Box 28, Zip 92038–0028; tel. 858/626–4123; Gary G. Fybel, Senior Vice President and Chief Executive
Web address: www.scrippshealth.org

SCRIPPS MERCY HOSPITAL (O, 420 beds) 4077 Fifth Avenue, San Diego, CA Zip 92103–2105; tel. 619/294–8111; Thomas A. Gammiere, Senior Vice President and Chief Executive
Web address: www.scrippshealth.org

Owned, leased, sponsored:	4 hospitals	1028 beds
Contract-managed:	0 hospitals	0 beds
Totals:	4 hospitals	1028 beds

0181: SELECT MEDICAL CORPORATION (IO)

4714 Old Gettysburg Road, Mechanicsburg, PA Zip 17055; tel. 717/972–1100; Robert Ortenzio, Chief Executive Officer
(Moderately Centralized Health System)

ALABAMA: SELECT SPECIALTY HOSPITAL–BIRMINGHAM (O, 38 beds) 800 Montclair Road, Birmingham, AL Zip 35213; tel. 205/599–4600; Craig L. Johnson, CHE, Chief Executive Officer
Web address: www.selectmedicalcorp.com

ARIZONA: SELECT SPECIALTY HOSPITAL – PHOENIX (O, 48 beds) 350 West Thomas Road, Phoenix, AZ Zip 85013; tel. 602/406–6800; Beth Liguori, Chief Executive Officer
Web address: www.selectmedicalcorp.com

SELECT SPECIALTY HOSPITAL–PHOENIX DOWNTOWN (O, 33 beds) 1012 East Wiletta Street, 4th Floor, Phoenix, AZ Zip 85006; tel. 602/239–6134; Sharon Anthony, Chief Executive Officer
Web address: www.selectmedicalcorp.com

SELECT SPECIALTY HOSPITAL–SCOTTSDALE (O, 29 beds) 7400 Osborn Road, 3 West, Scottsdale, AZ Zip 85021–6403; tel. 480/675–6040; Sharon Anthony, Chief Executive Officer
Web address: www.selectmedicalcorp.com

ARKANSAS: SELECT SPECIALTY HOSPITAL – FORT SMITH (O, 34 beds) 1131 South I Street, Fort Smith, AR Zip 72917; tel. 479/441–3960; Cindy McLain, Chief Executive Officer
Web address: www.selectmedicalcorp.com

SELECT SPECIALTY HOSPITAL–LITTLE ROCK (O, 43 beds) 2 St. Vincent Circle, 6th Floor, Little Rock, AR Zip 72204; tel. 501/661–4198; Maureen Henneken, Chief Executive Officer
Web address: www.selectmedicalcorp.com

For explanation of codes following names, see page B2.
★ Indicates Type III membership in the American Hospital Association.

COLORADO: SELECT SPECIALTY HOSPITAL – DENVER (O, 65 beds) 1719 East 19th Avenue, 5th Floor, Denver, CO Zip 80218; tel. 303/563–3700; Lynn Dawson, Chief Executive Officer
Web address: www.selectmedicalcorp.com

DELAWARE: SELECT SPECIALTY HOSPITAL WILMINGTON (O, 35 beds) 7 Clayton Street, 5th Floor, Wilmington, DE Zip 19801; tel. 302/421–4545; Carol Chrisman, Chief Executive Officer
Web address: www.selectmedicalcorp.com

FLORIDA: SELECT SPECIALTY HOSPITAL OF MIAMI (O, 40 beds) 955 N.W. 3rd Street, Miami, FL Zip 33128; tel. 305/416–5700; Dionisio Bencomo, Chief Executive Officer
Web address: www.selectmedicalcorp.com

SELECT SPECIALTY HOSPITAL OF ORLANDO (O, 35 beds) 2250 Bedford Road, Orlando, FL Zip 32803; tel. 407/303–7869; Rose O'Neil, Chief Executive Officer
Web address: www.selectmedicalcorp.com

SELECT SPECIALTY HOSPITAL OF PANAMA CITY (O, 30 beds) 615 North Bonita Avenue, 3rd Floor, Panama City, FL Zip 32401; tel. 850/767–3180; Debra R. Gibson, Chief Executive Officer
Web address: www.selectmedicalcorp.com

GEORGIA: SELECT SPECIALTY HOSPITAL (O, 30 beds) 1537 Walton Way, Augusta, GA Zip 30901; tel. 706/774–7101; Brian Davis, Chief Executive Officer
Web address: www.selectmedicalcorp.com

SELECT SPECIALTY HOSPITAL OF SAVANNAH (O, 40 beds) 5353 Reynolds Street, 4 South, Savannah, GA Zip 31405; tel. 912/819–7972; John Heffner, Chief Executive Officer
Web address: www.selectmedicalcorp.com

SELECT SPECIALTY HOSPITAL–ATLANTA (O, 30 beds) 550 Peachtree Street N.E., Atlanta, GA Zip 30327; tel. 404/350–4623; Phil Greenhill, Chief Executive Officer
Web address: www.selectmedicalcorp.com

INDIANA: SELECT SPECIALTY HOSPITAL (O, 32 beds) 700 Broadway, 7th Floor, Fort Wayne, IN Zip 46802; tel. 260/425–3810; Darlene Degener, Chief Executive Officer
Web address: www.selectmedicalcorp.com

SELECT SPECIALTY HOSPITAL OF BEECH GROVE (O, 40 beds) 1600 Albany Street, Suite 200, Beech Grove, IN Zip 46107; tel. 317/783–8913; Cheryl G. Gentry, Chief Executive Officer
Web address: www.selectmedicalcorp.com

SELECT SPECIALTY HOSPITAL OF EVANSVILLE (O, 60 beds) 600 Mary Street, Suite 3325, Evansville, IN Zip 47747; tel. 812/450–5270; Tracy Conroy, Chief Executive Officer
Web address: www.selectmedicalcorp.com

SELECT SPECIALTY HOSPITAL OF INDIANAPOLIS (O, 54 beds) 1701 North Senate Boulevard, Building C, 7th Floor, Greenwood, IN Zip 46143; tel. 317/884–2599; Mary L. Jackson–Boustani, Chief Executive Officer
Web address: www.selectmedicalcorp.com

SELECT SPECIALTY HOSPITAL OF NORTHWEST INDIANA (O, 70 beds) 5454 Hohman Avenue, 5th Floor, Hammond, IN Zip 46320; tel. 219/937–9900; Scott Deig, Interim Chief Executive Officer
Web address: www.selectmedicalcorp.com

IOWA: SELECT SPECIALTY HOSPITAL–QUAD CITIES (O, 50 beds) 1111 West Kimberly Road, Davenport, IA Zip 52806–5711; tel. 563/468–2000; Kerry McLane, Interim Chief Executive Officer
Web address: www.selectmedicalcorp.com

KANSAS: 929 NORTH ST FRANCIS STREET, 5 SW (O, 60 beds) 929 North St. Francis Street, 5 S.W., Wichita, KS Zip 67208, Mailing Address: 929 North St. Francis Street, 5 S.W., Zip 67208; tel. 316/268–5593; David Cross, Chief Executive Officer
Web address: www.selectmedicalcorp.com

SELECT SPECIALTY HOSPITAL – KANSAS CITY (O, 40 beds) 10550 Quivira Road, Overland Park, KS Zip 66215; tel. 913/541–5886; Sheryl Laing, Interim Administrator
Web address: www.selectmedicalcorp.com

SELECT SPECIALTY HOSPITAL – TOPEKA (O, 34 beds) 1700 S.W. Seventh Street, Suite 840, Topeka, KS Zip 66606–1660; tel. 785/295–5551; Mark Davis, Chief Executive Officer
Web address: www.selectmedicalcorp.com

SELECT SPECIALTY HOSPITAL OF WICHITA (O, 35 beds) 3243 East Murdock, Suite 103, Wichita, KS Zip 67208; tel. 316/688–3900; David Cross, Chief Executive Officer
Web address: www.selectmedicalcorp.com

KENTUCKY: SELECT SPECIALTY HOSPITAL OF LEXINGTON (O, 41 beds) 310 South Limeston Street, 3rd Floor, Lexington, KY Zip 40509; tel. 859/226–7178; Seth A. Sauve, Chief Executive Officer
Web address: www.selectmedicalcorp.com

MICHIGAN: SELECT SPECIALTY HOSPITAL – GROSSE POINTE (O, 30 beds) 159 Kercheval Avenue, Grosse Pointe, MI Zip 48236; tel. 313/640–2220; Linda Steiger, Chief Executive Officer

SELECT SPECIALTY HOSPITAL OF KALAMAZOO (O, 25 beds) 601 John Street, Kalamazoo, MI Zip 49007; tel. 269/836–1300; Robert C. Desotelle, Chief Executive Officer
Web address: www.selectmedicalcorp.com

SELECT SPECIALTY HOSPITAL OF WESTERN MICHIGAN (O, 32 beds) 1700 Clinton Street, Suite S2, Muskegon, MI Zip 49442; tel. 231/728–5811; Jonathan Cohee, Interim Chief Executive Officer
Web address: www.selectmedicalcorp.com

SELECT SPECIALTY HOSPITAL–ANN ARBOR (O, 36 beds) 5301 East Huron River Drive, 5th Floor, Ypsilanti, MI Zip 48197; tel. 734/712–0103; Carol Littleton, Chief Executive Officer

SELECT SPECIALTY HOSPITAL–BATTLE CREEK (O, 32 beds) 300 North Avenue, 6th Floor, Battle Creek, MI Zip 49016; tel. 269/565–8900; Dave Gehringer, Chief Executive Officer
Web address: www.selectmedicalcorp.com

SELECT SPECIALTY HOSPITAL–DOWNRIVER (O, 32 beds) 10000 Telegraph Road, Taylor, MI Zip 48180; tel. 313/375–7075; Robert Padalino, Chief Executive Officer
Web address: www.selectmedicalcorp.com

SELECT SPECIALTY HOSPITAL–FLINT (O, 32 beds) One Hurley Plaza, 11th Floor, Flint, MI Zip 48503; tel. 810/237–6793; Lorie Powell, Chief Executive Officer
Web address: www.selectmedicalcorp.com

SELECT SPECIALTY HOSPITAL–MACOMB (O, 32 beds) 215 North Avenue, Mount Clemens, MI Zip 48043; tel. 586/307–9000; Linda Steiger, Chief Executive Officer

SELECT SPECIALTY HOSPITAL–NORTHWEST DETROIT (O, 36 beds) 6071 West Outer Drive, Detroit, MI Zip 48235; tel. 313/966–4747; Sandra Baumchen, Chief Executive Officer
Web address: www.selectmedicalcorp.com

SELECT SPECIALTY HOSPITAL–PONTIAC (O, 32 beds) 44405 Woodward Avenue, 8th Floor, Pontiac, MI Zip 48341, Mailing Address: 4405 Woodward Avenue, 8th Floor, Zip 48341; tel. 248/452–5206; Peggy Kingston, Chief Executive Officer and Administrator

SELECT SPECIALTY HOSPITAL–SAGINAW (O, 32 beds) 1447 North Harrison Street, Saginaw, MI Zip 48602; tel. 989/583–4850; Jonathan Cohee, Chief Executive Officer
Web address: www.selectmedicalcorp.com

MISSISSIPPI: SELECT SPECIALTY HOSPITAL – GULFPORT (O, 61 beds) 1520 Broad Avenue, Suite 300, Gulfport, MS Zip 39501, Mailing Address: 1521 Broad Avenue, Suite 300, Zip 39501; tel. 228/575–7500; Ray Owens, Chief Executive Officer
Web address: www.selectmedicalcorp.com

SELECT SPECIALTY HOSPITAL OF JACKSON (O, 53 beds) 5903 Ridgewood Road, Jackson, MS Zip 39211; tel. 601/899–3800; Aaron Anothayanontha, Chief Executive Officer
Web address: www.selectmedicalcorp.com

MISSOURI: SELECT SPECIALTY HOSPITAL (O, 33 beds) 6150 Oakland Avenue, 5th Floor, Saint Louis, MO Zip 63139–3297; tel. 314/768–3513; Megan Schmidt, Chief Executive Officer
Web address: www.selectmedicalcorp.com

SELECT SPECIALTY HOSPITAL – WESTERN MISSOURI (O, 34 beds) 2316 East Meyer Boulevard, 3 West, Kansas City, MO Zip 64132; tel. 816/276–9444; Larry Brown, Chief Executive Officer
Web address: www.selectmedicalcorp.com

NEBRASKA: SELECT SPECIALTY HOSPITAL – OMAHA NORTH (O, 36 beds) 6901 North 72nd Street, 7th Floor West, Omaha, NE Zip 68122; tel. 402/572–2714; Thomas N. Theroult, Administrator
Web address: www.selectmedicalcorp.com

For explanation of codes following names, see page B2.
★ Indicates Type III membership in the American Hospital Association.

SELECT SPECIALTY HOSPITAL–OMAHA (O, 30 beds) 11111 South 84th Street, 6th Floor, Papillion, NE Zip 68046; tel. 402/898–2700; Thomas N. Theroult, Chief Executive Officer
Web address: www.selectmedicalcorp.com

NEW JERSEY: KESSLER INSTITUTE FOR REHABILITATION (O, 322 beds) 1199 Pleasant Valley Way, West Orange, NJ Zip 07052–1419; tel. 973/731–3600; Robert Brehm, President
Web address: www.kessler–rehab.com

SELECT SPECIALTY HOSPITAL OF NORTHEAST (O, 25 beds) 96 Parkway, Rochelle Park, NJ Zip 7662; tel. 201/221–2351; Barbara E. Hannan, Chief Executive Officer
Web address: www.selectmedicalcorp.com

NORTH CAROLINA: SELECT SPECIALTY HOSPITAL OF DURHAM (O, 30 beds) 3643 North Roxboro Road, 6th Floor, Durham, NC Zip 27704; tel. 919/470–9000; Matthew Womble, Chief Executive Officer
Web address: www.selectmedicalcorp.com

SELECT SPECIALTY HOSPITAL OF WINSTON–SALEM (O, 25 beds) 3333 Silas Creek Parkway, 6th Floor, Winston–Salem, NC Zip 27103; tel. 336/718–6300; Marion Reef, Chief Executive Officer
Web address: www.selectmedicalcorp.com

OHIO: SELECT SPECIALTY HOSPITAL (O, 36 beds) 375 Dixmyth Avenue, Cincinnati, OH Zip 45220; tel. 513/487–4105; Damian Jones, Administrator and Chief Executive
Web address: www.selectmedicalcorp.com

SELECT SPECIALTY HOSPITAL–AKRON (O, 34 beds) 525 East Market Street, Akron, OH Zip 44309–3617; tel. 330/375–4390; Gregory T. Storer, Chief Executive Officer
Web address: www.selectmedicalcorp.com

SELECT SPECIALTY HOSPITAL–COLUMBUS (O, 50 beds) 410 West 10th Avenue, 11th Floor, Columbus, OH Zip 43210; tel. 614/293–6931; Dan West, Chief Executive Officer
Web address: www.selectmedicalcorp.com

SELECT SPECIALTY HOSPITAL–COLUMBUS (O, 37 beds) 111 South Grant Avenue, 5th Floor, Columbus, OH Zip 43215; tel. 614/566–8211; Mary Burkett, Interim Chief Executive Officer
Web address: www.selectmedicalcorp.com

SELECT SPECIALTY HOSPITAL–COLUMBUS (O, 44 beds) 1492 East Broad Street, 8th Floor, Columbus, OH Zip 43205; tel. 614/252–4440; Craig A. Hoover, Chief Executive Officer
Web address: www.selectmedicalcorp.com

SELECT SPECIALTY HOSPITAL–NORTHEAST OHIO (O, 31 beds) 400 Wabash Avenue, 9th Floor, Akron, OH Zip 44307; tel. 330/344–6910; Pat Mahovich, Chief Executive Officer
Web address: www.selectmedicalcorp.com

SELECT SPECIALTY HOSPITAL–YOUNGSTOWN (O, 31 beds) 1044 Belmont Avenue, Youngstown, OH Zip 44501; tel. 330/480–2349; MaryJo Shuntich, Chief Executive Officer
Web address: www.selectmedicalcorp.com

SELECT SPECIALTY HOSPITAL–ZANESVILLE (O, 35 beds) 800 Forest Avenue, 6th Floor, Zanesville, OH Zip 43701; tel. 740/588–7888; Linda Supplee, Chief Executive Officer
Web address: www.selectmedicalcorp.com

OKLAHOMA: SELECT SPECIALTY HOSPITAL – TULSA (O, 30 beds) 744 West Ninth Street, Tulsa, OK Zip 74127–9096; tel. 918/502–1400; David Bennett, Chief Executive Officer

SELECT SPECIALTY HOSPITAL–OKLAHOMA CITY (O, 72 beds) 3524 N.W. 56th Stret, Oklahoma City, OK Zip 73112–4510; tel. 405/606–6700; Connie Strickland, Administrator
Web address: www.selectmedicalcorp.com

PENNSYLVANIA: SELECT SPECIALTY HOSPITAL (O, 32 beds) 200 Lothrop Street, E824, Pittsburgh, PA Zip 15213; tel. 412/586–9819; Keith J. Weinhold, Chief Executive Officer
Web address: www.selectmedicalcorp.com

SELECT SPECIALTY HOSPITAL – JOHNSTOWN (O, 38 beds) 320 Main Street, Johnstown, PA Zip 15901; tel. 814/534–7300; Marylee Dadey, Chief Executive Officer
Web address: www.selectmedicalcorp.com

SELECT SPECIALTY HOSPITAL – YORK (O, 23 beds) 1001 South George Street, York, PA Zip 17403–3676; tel. 717/851–2661; Marcia Medlin, Chief Executive Officer
Web address: www.selectmedicalcorp.com

SELECT SPECIALTY HOSPITAL OF GREENSBURG (O, 31 beds) 532 West Pittsburgh Street, Greensburg, PA Zip 15601; tel. 724/832–4210; Anthony Martino, Chief Executive Officer
Web address: www.selectmedicalcorp.com

SELECT SPECIALTY HOSPITAL OF MCKEESPORT (O, 30 beds) 1500 Fifth Avenue, McKeesport, PA Zip 15132; tel. 412/664–2900; Tina Ruskewicz, Chief Executive Officer
Web address: www.selectmedicalcorp.com

SELECT SPECIALTY HOSPITAL–CAMP HILL (O, 31 beds) 503 North 21st Street, 5th Floor, Camp Hill, PA Zip 17011; tel. 717/972–4560; Marcia Medlin, Chief Executive Officer
Web address: www.selectmedicalcorp.com

SELECT SPECIALTY HOSPITAL–DANVILLE (O, 30 beds) 100 North Academy Avenue, 3rd Floor, Danville, PA Zip 17822–3050; tel. 570/214–9657; Brian Mann, Chief Executive Officer
Web address: www.selectmedicalcorp.com

SELECT SPECIALTY HOSPITAL–ERIE (O, 35 beds) 201 State Street, Erie, PA Zip 16550; tel. 814/877–2774; Anne Frew, Chief Executive Officer
Web address: www.selectmedicalcorp.com

SOUTH DAKOTA: SELECT SPECIALTY HOSPITAL–SIOUX FALLS (O, 24 beds) 800 East 21st Street, Suite 3300, Sioux Falls, SD Zip 57105; tel. 605/322–3500; Carol Ulmer, Chief Executive Officer
Web address: www.selectmedicalcorp.com

TENNESSEE: SELECT SPECIALTY HOSPITAL OF NASHVILLE (O, 37 beds) 2021 Church Street, Nashville, TN Zip 37203–2016; tel. 615/284–4599; Edward T. Stinson, Chief Executive Officer
Web address: www.selectmedicalcorp.com

SELECT SPECIALTY HOSPITAL–KNOXVILLE (O, 35 beds) 1901 Clinch Avenue, Suite 404, Knoxville, TN Zip 37916; tel. 865/541–2615; Vanda Scott, Chief Executive Officer
Web address: www.selectmedicalcorp.com

SELECT SPECIALTY HOSPITAL–MEMPHIS (O, 30 beds) 5959 Park Avenue, 12th Floor, Memphis, TN Zip 38119–5200; tel. 901/684–4110; David Key, Chief Executive Officer
Web address: www.selectmedicalcorp.com

SELECT SPECIALTY HOSPITAL–NORTH KNOXVILLE (O, 33 beds) 900 East Oak Hill Avenue, Knoxville, TN Zip 37917; tel. 865/541–2615; Vanda Scott, Chief Executive Officer
Web address: www.selectmedicalcorp.com

SELECT SPECIALTY HOSPITAL–TRICITIES (O, 33 beds) One Medical Park Boulevard, 5th Floor, Bristol, TN Zip 37620–8964; tel. 423/844–5900; Christopher E. Anderson, Chief Executive Officer
Web address: www.selectmedicalcorp.com

TEXAS: SELECT SPECIALTY HOSPITAL – DALLAS (O, 60 beds) 10 Medical Parkway, Suite 205, Dallas, TX Zip 75234–7845; tel. 972/488–9167; Joy Dier, RN, M.S., Administrator and Chief Executive Officer
Web address: www.selectmedicalcorp.com

SELECT SPECIALTY HOSPITAL OF LONGVIEW (O, 32 beds) 700 East Marshall Avenue, 1st Floor, Longview, TX Zip 75601; tel. 903/315–1111; Larry Donner, President and Chief Executive Officer
Web address: www.selectmedicalcorp.com

SELECT SPECIALTY HOSPITAL OF MIDLAND (O, 29 beds) 4214 Andrews Highway, Suite 320, Midland, TX Zip 79703; tel. 432/522–3270; Paul E. Qualls, Jr., Chief Executive Officer
Web address: www.selectmedicalcorp.com

SELECT SPECIALTY HOSPITAL–CONROE (O, 46 beds) 506 Medical Center Boulevard, Conroe, TX Zip 77304; tel. 936/538–3154; Sandra Stephens, RN, Administrator and Chief Executive Officer
Web address: www.selectmedicalcorp.com

SELECT SPECIALTY HOSPITAL–HOUSTON HEIGHTS (O, 242 beds) 1917 Ashland Street, Houston, TX Zip 77008–3994; tel. 713/861–6161; Teresa L. Davis, Administrator
Web address: www.selectmedicalcorp.com

SELECT SPECIALTY HOSPITAL–HOUSTON MEDICAL CENTER (O, 34 beds) 6655 Travis Street, Suite 300, Houston, TX Zip 77030–1502, Mailing Address: 6500 Fannin Street, Suite 907, Zip 77030–1502; tel. 713/520–9595; Vivian Bond, Administrator
Web address: www.selectmedicalcorp.com

SELECT SPECIALTY HOSPITAL–HOUSTON WEST CAMPUS (O, 38 beds) 9430 Old Katy Road, Houston, TX Zip 77055; tel. 713/984–2273; Marinella Castroman, Administrator
Web address: www.selectmedicalcorp.com

For explanation of codes following names, see page B2.
★ Indicates Type III membership in the American Hospital Association.

SELECT SPECIALTY HOSPITAL–SAN ANTONIO (O, 44 beds) 111 Dallas Street, 4th Floor, San Antonio, TX Zip 78205; tel. 210/297–7185; Greg Floyd, Vice President
Web address: www.selectmedicalcorp.com

SELECT SPECIALTY HOSPITAL–SOUTH DALLAS (O, 100 beds) 800 Kirkwood Drive, De Soto, TX Zip 75115; tel. 972/780–6500; James Camp, Chief Executive Officer
Web address: www.selectmedicalcorp.com

WEST VIRGINIA: SELECT SPECIALTY HOSPITAL–CHARLESTON (O, 32 beds) 333 Laidley Street, Charleston, WV Zip 25301–1628; tel. 304/720–7234; Frank Weber, Chief Executive Officer
Web address: www.selectmedicalcorp.com

WISCONSIN: SELECT SPECIALTY HOSPITAL (O, 34 beds) 8901 West Lincoln Avenue, 6th Floor, Milwaukee, WI Zip 53227; tel. 414/328–7700; Dennis Mattes, Chief Executive Officer
Web address: www.selectmedicalcorp.com

Owned, leased, sponsored:	81 hospitals	3579 beds
Contract–managed:	0 hospitals	0 beds
Totals:	81 hospitals	3579 beds

0374: SENIORHEALTH INCORPORATED (IO)
49 Music Square West, Suite 502, Nashville, TN Zip 37203; tel. 615/321–5577; Kevin D. Lee, President and Chief Executive Officer

TEXAS: COMMUNITY SPECIALTY HOSPITAL (O, 90 beds) 1111 Gallagher Drive, Sherman, TX Zip 75090–1713; tel. 903/870–7000; Travis W. Roderick, Administrator and Chief Executive Officer
Web address: www.cshsherman.com

MAYHILL HOSPITAL (O, 57 beds) 2809 South Mayhill Road, Denton, TX Zip 76208–5910; tel. 940/239–3000; William W. Brattvet, Administrator
Web address: www.mayhillhospital.com

RED RIVER HOSPITAL (O, 66 beds) 1505 Eighth Street, Wichita Falls, TX Zip 76301–3106; tel. 940/322–3171; Murray Browning, Chief Executive Officer
Web address: www.redriverhospital.com

REHABILITATION HOSPITAL OF GREENVILLE (O, 16 beds) 4215 Joe Ramsey Boulevard, 7th Floor, Greenville, TX Zip 75401; tel. 903/408–1770; Lorraine Cook, Administrator
Web address: www.seniorhealthrehab.com

Owned, leased, sponsored:	4 hospitals	229 beds
Contract–managed:	0 hospitals	0 beds
Totals:	4 hospitals	229 beds

★2565: SENTARA HEALTHCARE (NP)
6015 Poplar Hall Drive, Norfolk, VA Zip 23502–3819; tel. 757/455–7000; David L. Bernd, Chief Executive Officer
(Centralized Health System)

VIRGINIA: SENTARA BAYSIDE HOSPITAL (O, 97 beds) 800 Independence Boulevard, Virginia Beach, VA Zip 23455–6076; tel. 757/363–6100; Stephen D. Porter, Vice President and Administrator
Web address: www.sentara.com

SENTARA CAREPLEX HOSPITAL (O, 200 beds) 3000 Coliseum Drive, Hampton, VA Zip 23666–5963; tel. 757/736–2656; Debra A. Flores, Vice President and Administrator
Web address: www.sentara.com

SENTARA LEIGH HOSPITAL (O, 233 beds) 830 Kempsville Road, Norfolk, VA Zip 23502–3920; tel. 757/466–6000; Mark A. Szalwinski, Vice President and Administrator
Web address: www.sentara.com

SENTARA NORFOLK GENERAL HOSPITAL (O, 464 beds) 600 Gresham Drive, Norfolk, VA Zip 23507; tel. 757/388–3000; Mary L. Blunt, Vice President and Administrator
Web address: www.sentara.com

SENTARA OBICI HOSPITAL (O, 138 beds) 2800 Godwin Boulevard, Suffolk, VA Zip 23434–4323, Mailing Address: P.O. Box 1100, Zip 23439–1100; tel. 757/934–4000; Rosemary C. Check, Vice President and Administrator
Web address: www.sentara.com/Sentara/HospitalsFacilities/Hospitals/Obici

SENTARA VIRGINIA BEACH GENERAL HOSPITAL (O, 251 beds) 1060 First Colonial Road, Virginia Beach, VA Zip 23454–3002; tel. 757/395–8000; Raymond G. Troiano, M.D., Vice President and Administrator
Web address: www.sentara.com

SENTARA WILLIAMSBURG COMMUNITY HOSPITAL (O, 120 beds) 100 Sentara Circle, Williamsburg, VA Zip 23188; tel. 757/984–6000; Robert L. Graves, Vice President and Administrator
Web address: www.sentara.com

Owned, leased, sponsored:	7 hospitals	1503 beds
Contract–managed:	0 hospitals	0 beds
Totals:	7 hospitals	1503 beds

★0111: SHANDS HEALTHCARE (NP)
1600 S.W. Archer Road, Gainesville, FL Zip 32610–0326; tel. 352/265–8929; Timothy M. Goldfarb, Chief Executive Officer
(Moderately Centralized Health System)

FLORIDA: SHANDS AGH (O, 269 beds) 801 S.W. Second Avenue, Gainesville, FL Zip 32601–6289; tel. 352/733–0111; Francis A. Pommett, Jr., Administrator
Web address: www.shands.org/hospitals/agh

SHANDS AT THE UNIVERSITY OF FLORIDA (O, 734 beds) 1600 S.W. Archer Road, Gainesville, FL Zip 32610–0326, Mailing Address: P.O. Box 100326, Zip 32610–0326; tel. 352/265–0111; Timothy J. Goldfarb, Chief Executive Officer
Web address: www.shands.org

SHANDS JACKSONVILLE MEDICAL CENTER (O, 599 beds) 655 West Eighth Street, Jacksonville, FL Zip 32209–6595; tel. 904/244–0411; James R. Burkhart, FACHE, President and Chief Executive Officer
Web address: www.shandsjacksonville.org

SHANDS LAKE SHORE (L, 94 beds) 368 N.E. Franklin Street, Lake City, FL Zip 32055–3047; tel. 386/754–8000; Rhonda Kay Sherrod, RN, M.S.N., Administrator
Web address: www.shands.org

SHANDS LIVE OAK (O, 15 beds) 1100 S.W. 11th Street, Live Oak, FL Zip 32060–3608; tel. 386/362–0800; Russell A. Test, Administrator
Web address: www.shands.org

SHANDS REHAB HOSPITAL (O, 121 beds) 4101 N.W. 89th Boulevard, Gainesville, FL Zip 32606–3813; tel. 352/265–5491; Marina T. Cecchini, Administrator
Web address: www.shands.org

SHANDS STARKE (O, 25 beds) 922 East Call Street, Starke, FL Zip 32091–3699; tel. 904/368–2300; Jeannie Baker, Administrator
Web address: www.shands.org

Owned, leased, sponsored:	7 hospitals	1857 beds
Contract–managed:	0 hospitals	0 beds
Totals:	7 hospitals	1857 beds

★2065: SHARP HEALTHCARE (NP)
8695 Spectrum Center Boulevard, San Diego, CA Zip 92123–1489; tel. 858/499–4000; Michael Murphy, President and Chief Executive Officer
(Moderately Centralized Health System)

CALIFORNIA: SHARP CHULA VISTA MEDICAL CENTER (O, 330 beds) 751 Medical Center Court, Chula Vista, CA Zip 91911–6699, Mailing Address: P.O. Box 1297, Zip 91912–1297; tel. 619/482–5800; Christopher L. Boyd, Chief Executive Officer
Web address: www.sharp.com

SHARP CORONADO HOSPITAL AND HEALTH CENTER (C, 175 beds) 250 Prospect Place, Coronado, CA Zip 92118–1999; tel. 619/522–3600; Marcia K. Hall, Chief Executive Officer
Web address: www.sharp.com

SHARP GROSSMONT HOSPITAL (C, 445 beds) 5555 Grossmont Center Drive, La Mesa, CA Zip 91942–3019, Mailing Address: P.O. Box 158, Zip 91944–0158; tel. 619/740–6000; Michele T. Tarbet, RN, Chief Executive Officer
Web address: www.sharp.com

Section B

For explanation of codes following names, see page B2.
★ Indicates Type III membership in the American Hospital Association.

SHARP MARY BIRCH HOSPITAL FOR WOMEN (O, 169 beds) 3003 Health Center Drive, San Diego, CA Zip 92123; tel. 858/939–3400; Mary Henrikson, Senior Vice President and Chief Executive Officer
Web address: www.sharp.com

SHARP MEMORIAL HOSPITAL (O, 488 beds) 7901 Frost Street, San Diego, CA Zip 92123–2701; tel. 858/939–3400; Tim Smith, Chief Executive Officer
Web address: www.sharp.com

Owned, leased, sponsored:	3 hospitals	987 beds
Contract–managed:	2 hospitals	620 beds
Totals:	5 hospitals	1607 beds

0383: SHILOH HEALTH SERVICES, INC. (NP)
2412 50th Street, Lubbock, TX Zip 79412–2494; tel. 806/788–4060; James R. Cheek, President

LOUISIANA: RIVER WEST MEDICAL CENTER (O, 75 beds) 59355 River West Drive, Plaquemine, LA Zip 70764–0737, Mailing Address: P.O. Box 737, Zip 70764–0737; tel. 225/687–9222; James P. Jeansonne, Chief Executive Officer
Web address: www.riverwestmc.com

TEXAS: HIGHLAND COMMUNITY HOSPITAL (O, 95 beds) 2412 50th Street, Lubbock, TX Zip 79412–2494; tel. 806/788–4100; Charles Fulner, Administrator
Web address: www.highlandcommunityhospital.com

Owned, leased, sponsored:	2 hospitals	170 beds
Contract–managed:	0 hospitals	0 beds
Totals:	2 hospitals	170 beds

0304: SHORE HEALTH SYSTEM (NP)
219 South Washington Street, Easton, MD Zip 21601; tel. 410/822–1000; Joseph P. Ross, President and Chief Executive Officer
(Independent Hospital System)

MARYLAND: DORCHESTER GENERAL HOSPITAL (O, 46 beds) 300 Byrn Street, Cambridge, MD Zip 21613–1908; tel. 410/228–5511; Joseph P. Ross, President and Chief Executive Officer
Web address: www.shorehealth.org

MEMORIAL HOSPITAL AT EASTON MARYLAND (O, 123 beds) 219 South Washington Street, Easton, MD Zip 21601–2996; tel. 410/822–1000; Joseph P. Ross, President and Chief Executive Officer
Web address: www.shorehealth.org

Owned, leased, sponsored:	2 hospitals	169 beds
Contract–managed:	0 hospitals	0 beds
Totals:	2 hospitals	169 beds

4125: SHRINERS HOSPITALS FOR CHILDREN (NP)
2900 Rocky Point Drive, Tampa, FL Zip 33607–1435, Mailing Address: P.O. Box 31356, Zip 33631–3356; tel. 813/281–0300; James M. Full, FACHE, Executive Vice President and Chief Operating Officer
(Independent Hospital System)

CALIFORNIA: SHRINERS HOSPITALS FOR CHILDREN, LOS ANGELES (O, 60 beds) 3160 Geneva Street, Los Angeles, CA Zip 90020–1199; tel. 213/388–3151; Terence T. Cunningham, FACHE, Administrator
Web address: www.shrinehg.org

SHRINERS HOSPITALS FOR CHILDREN, NORTHERN CALIFORNIA (O, 40 beds) 2425 Stockton Boulevard, Sacramento, CA Zip 95817–2215; tel. 916/453–2000; Margaret Bryan, Administrator
Web address: www.shrinershq.org

FLORIDA: SHRINERS HOSPITALS FOR CHILDREN, TAMPA (O, 60 beds) 12502 USF Pine Drive, Tampa, FL Zip 33612–9499; tel. 813/972–2250; Alice Reed Lanford, RN, M.S.N., FACHE, Administrator
Web address: www.shrinershq.org

HAWAII: SHRINERS HOSPITALS FOR CHILDREN, HONOLULU (O, 40 beds) 1310 Punahou Street, Honolulu, HI Zip 96826–1099; tel. 808/941–4466; Stanley B. Berry, FACHE, Administrator
Web address: www.shrinershq.org

ILLINOIS: SHRINERS HOSPITALS FOR CHILDREN–CHICAGO (O, 36 beds) 2211 North Oak Park Avenue, Chicago, IL Zip 60707–3392; tel. 773/622–5400; James Cohick, Administrator
Web address: www.shrinershospitals.org

KENTUCKY: SHRINERS HOSPITALS FOR CHILDREN–LEXINGTON (O, 50 beds) 1900 Richmond Road, Lexington, KY Zip 40502–1298; tel. 859/266–2101; Tony Lewgood, Administrator
Web address: www.shrinershq.com

LOUISIANA: SHRINERS HOSPITALS FOR CHILDREN, SHREVEPORT (O, 45 beds) 3100 Samford Avenue, Shreveport, LA Zip 71103–4289; tel. 318/222–5704; Garry K. Green, Administrator
Web address: www.shriners.com

MASSACHUSETTS: SHRINERS HOSPITALS FOR CHILDREN, SPRINGFIELD (O, 20 beds) 516 Carew Street, Springfield, MA Zip 01104–2396; tel. 413/787–2000; Mark L. Niederpruem, FACHE, Administrator
Web address: www.shrinershq.org

SHRINERS HOSPITALS FOR CHILDREN–BOSTON (O, 30 beds) 51 Blossom Street, Boston, MA Zip 2114; tel. 617/722–3000; C. Thomas D'Esmond, Administrator
Web address: www.shrinershospitals.org

MINNESOTA: SHRINERS HOSPITALS FOR CHILDREN, TWIN CITIES (O, 40 beds) 2025 East River Parkway, Minneapolis, MN Zip 55414–3696; tel. 612/596–6100; Charles C. Lobeck, Administrator
Web address: www.shrinershq.org

MISSOURI: SHRINERS HOSPITALS FOR CHILDREN, ST. LOUIS (O, 42 beds) 2001 South Lindbergh Boulevard, Saint Louis, MO Zip 63131–3597; tel. 314/432–3600; John W. O'Shaughnessy, FACHE, Administrator
Web address: www.shrinershq.org

OHIO: SHRINERS HOSPITALS FOR CHILDREN, SHRINERS BURNS HOSPITAL, CINCINNATI (O, 30 beds) 3229 Burnet Avenue, Cincinnati, OH Zip 45229–3095; tel. 513/872–6000; Ronald R. Hitzler, Administrator
Web address: www.shrinershq.org

OREGON: SHRINERS HOSPITALS FOR CHILDREN, PORTLAND (O, 22 beds) 3101 S.W. Sam Jackson Park Road, Portland, OR Zip 97239; tel. 503/241–5090; Gayle Littlejohn, Interim Administrator
Web address: www.shcc.org

PENNSYLVANIA: SHRINERS HOSPITALS FOR CHILDREN, ERIE (O, 30 beds) 1645 West 8th Street, Erie, PA Zip 16505–5007; tel. 814/875–8700; Richard W. Brzuz, FACHE, Administrator
Web address: www.shrinershq.org

SHRINERS HOSPITALS FOR CHILDREN, PHILADELPHIA (O, 80 beds) 3551 North Broad Street, Philadelphia, PA Zip 19140–4131; tel. 215/430–4000; Ernest N. Perilli, Administrator
Web address: www.shrinershq.org

SOUTH CAROLINA: SHRINERS HOSPITALS FOR CHILDREN, GREENVILLE (O, 50 beds) 950 West Faris Road, Greenville, SC Zip 29605–4277; tel. 864/271–3444; Gary F. Fraley, Administrator
Web address: www.shrinershq.org

TEXAS: SHRINERS HOSPITALS FOR CHILDREN, GALVESTON BURNS HOSPITAL (O, 30 beds) 815 Market Street, Galveston, TX Zip 77550–2725; tel. 409/770–6600; John A. Swartwout, Administrator
Web address: www.shrinershq.org

SHRINERS HOSPITALS FOR CHILDREN, HOUSTON (O, 40 beds) 6977 Main Street, Houston, TX Zip 77030–3701; tel. 713/797–1616; Steven B. Reiter, Administrator
Web address: www.shrineshq.org

UTAH: SHRINERS HOSPITALS FOR CHILDREN–INTERMOUNTAIN (O, 40 beds) Fairfax Road and Virginia Street, Salt Lake City, UT Zip 84103–4399; tel. 801/536–3500; J. Craig Patchin, Administrator
Web address: www.shriners.org

WASHINGTON: SHRINERS HOSPITALS FOR CHILDREN–SPOKANE (O, 30 beds) 911 West Fifth Avenue, Spokane, WA Zip 99204, Mailing Address: P.O. Box 2472, Zip 99210–2472; tel. 509/455–7844; Gene Raynaud, Administrator
Web address: www.shrinershospital.org

Owned, leased, sponsored:	20 hospitals	815 beds
Contract–managed:	0 hospitals	0 beds
Totals:	20 hospitals	815 beds

For explanation of codes following names, see page B2.
★ Indicates Type III membership in the American Hospital Association.

0376: SIGNATURE HOSPITAL CORPORATION (IO)
12160 North Abrams Road, Dallas, TX Zip 75243;
tel. 214/580–8800; Charles R. Miller, Chief Executive Officer

ARKANSAS: MEDICAL PARK HOSPITAL (O, 79 beds) 2001 South Main Street, Hope, AR Zip 71801–8194; tel. 870/777–2323; Faye Hughes, Interim Chief Executive Officer
Web address: www.mphhope.com

TEXAS: GULF COAST MEDICAL CENTER (O, 96 beds) 10141 Highway 59, Wharton, TX Zip 77488–3004; tel. 979/532–2500; Martin R. Slack, Chief Executive Officer
Web address: www.gulfcoastmedical.com

PAMPA REGIONAL MEDICAL CENTER (O, 91 beds) One Medical Plaza, Pampa, TX Zip 79065; tel. 806/665–3721; Todd Lorenz, Chief Executive Officer
Web address: www.prmctx.com

WEST VIRGINIA: ST. JOSEPH'S HOSPITAL (O, 194 beds) 1824 Murdoch Avenue, Parkersburg, WV Zip 26101–3246, Mailing Address: P.O. Box 327, Zip 26102–0327; tel. 304/424–4111; Alan N. King, FACHE, Chief Executive Officer
Web address: www.stjosephs–hospital.com

Owned, leased, sponsored:	4 hospitals	460 beds
Contract–managed:	0 hospitals	0 beds
Totals:	4 hospitals	460 beds

★0284: SINAI HEALTH SYSTEM (NP)
California Avenue at 15th Street, Chicago, IL Zip 60608;
tel. 773/542–2000; Alan H. Channing, President and Chief Executive Officer

ILLINOIS: MOUNT SINAI HOSPITAL (O, 291 beds) California Avenue and 15th Street, Chicago, IL Zip 60608–1610; tel. 773/542–2000; Alan H. Channing, President and Chief Executive Officer
Web address: www.sinai.org

SCHWAB REHABILITATION HOSPITAL (O, 75 beds) 1401 South California Boulevard, Chicago, IL Zip 60608–1612; tel. 773/522–2010; Alan H. Channing, President and Chief Executive Officer
Web address: www.schwabrehab.org

Owned, leased, sponsored:	2 hospitals	366 beds
Contract–managed:	0 hospitals	0 beds
Totals:	2 hospitals	366 beds

5125: SISTERS OF CHARITY HEALTH SYSTEM (CC)
2351 East 22nd Street, Cleveland, OH Zip 44115–3197;
tel. 216/696–5560; Sister Judith Ann Karam, President and Chief Executive Officer
(Moderately Centralized Health System)

OHIO: MERCY MEDICAL CENTER (O, 345 beds) 1320 Mercy Drive N.W., Canton, OH Zip 44708–2641; tel. 330/489–1000; Thomas E. Cecconi, President and Chief Executive
Web address: www.cantonmercy.com

ST. JOHN WEST SHORE HOSPITAL (O, 183 beds) 29000 Center Ridge Road, Cleveland, OH Zip 44145–5219; tel. 440/835–8000; Cliff J. Coker, President
Web address: www.sjws.net

ST. VINCENT CHARITY HOSPITAL (O, 182 beds) 2351 East 22nd Street, Cleveland, OH Zip 44115–3111; tel. 216/861–6200; Jeffrey S. Jeney, President and Chief Executive Officer
Web address: www.svch.net

SOUTH CAROLINA: SISTERS OF CHARITY PROVIDENCE HOSPITALS (O, 258 beds) 2435 Forest Drive, Columbia, SC Zip 29204–2098; tel. 803/865–4500; George A. Zara, President and Chief Executive Officer
Web address: www.provhosp.com

Owned, leased, sponsored:	4 hospitals	968 beds
Contract–managed:	0 hospitals	0 beds
Totals:	4 hospitals	968 beds

★5095: SISTERS OF CHARITY OF LEAVENWORTH HEALTH SYSTEM (CC)
9801 Renner Boulevard, Suite 100, Lenexa, KS Zip 66219;
tel. 913/895–2800; William M. Murray, President
(Moderately Centralized Health System)

CALIFORNIA: SAINT JOHN'S HEALTH CENTER (O, 228 beds) 1328 Twenty Second Street, Santa Monica, CA Zip 90404–2091; tel. 310/829–5511; Lourdes Lazatin, President and Chief Executive Officer
Web address: www.stjohns.org

COLORADO: ST. MARY'S HOSPITAL AND MEDICAL CENTER (O, 280 beds) 2635 North 7th Street, Grand Junction, CO Zip 81501–8204, Mailing Address: P.O. Box 1628, Zip 81502–1628; tel. 970/244–2273; Robert W. Ladenburger, President and Chief Executive Officer
Web address: www.stmarygj.com

KANSAS: PROVIDENCE MEDICAL CENTER (O, 257 beds) 8929 Parallel Parkway, Kansas City, KS Zip 66112–1636; tel. 913/596–4000; Michael A. Dorsey, President and Chief Executive Officer
Web address: www.providence–health.org

SAINT JOHN HOSPITAL (O, 43 beds) 3500 South Fourth Street, Leavenworth, KS Zip 66048–5043; tel. 913/680–6000; Greg Madsen, Administrator
Web address: www.providence–health.org/sjh

ST. FRANCIS HEALTH CENTER (O, 283 beds) 1700 West Seventh Street, Topeka, KS Zip 66606–1690; tel. 785/295–8000; Michael E. Schrader, President and Chief Executive Officer
Web address: www.stfrancistopeka.org

MONTANA: HOLY ROSARY HEALTHCARE (O, 99 beds) 2600 Wilson Street, Miles City, MT Zip 59301–5094; tel. 406/233–2600; Greg A. Nielsen, Chief Executive Officer
Web address: www.holyrosaryhealthcare.org

ST. JAMES HEALTHCARE (O, 65 beds) 400 South Clark Street, Butte, MT Zip 59702–3300, Mailing Address: P.O. Box 3300, Zip 59702–3300; tel. 406/723–2500; James Kiser, II, President and Chief Executive Officer
Web address: www.stjameshealthcare.org

ST. VINCENT HEALTHCARE (O, 234 beds) 1233 North 30th Street, Billings, MT Zip 59101–0165, Mailing Address: P.O. Box 35200, Zip 59107–5200; tel. 406/237–7000; James T. Paquette, President and Chief Executive Officer
Web address: www.svh–mt.org

Owned, leased, sponsored:	8 hospitals	1489 beds
Contract–managed:	0 hospitals	0 beds
Totals:	8 hospitals	1489 beds

5805: SISTERS OF MARY OF THE PRESENTATION HEALTH SYSTEM (CC)
1102 Page Drive S.W., Fargo, ND Zip 58106–0007, Mailing Address: P.O. Box 10007, Zip 58106–0007; tel. 701/237–9290; Aaron Alton, President and Chief Executive Officer
(Independent Hospital System)

ILLINOIS: ST. MARGARET'S HOSPITAL (O, 86 beds) 600 East First Street, Spring Valley, IL Zip 61362–2034; tel. 815/664–5311; Tim Muntz, President and Chief Executive Officer
Web address: www.st–margarets.com

NORTH DAKOTA: PRESENTATION MEDICAL CENTER (O, 25 beds) 213 Second Avenue N.E., Rolla, ND Zip 58367–7153, Mailing Address: P.O. Box 759, Zip 58367–0759; tel. 701/477–3161; Kimber Wraalstad, President and Chief Executive Officer
Web address: www.pmc–rolla.com

ST. ALOISIUS MEDICAL CENTER (O, 131 beds) 325 East Brewster Street, Harvey, ND Zip 58341–1605; tel. 701/324–4651; Rockford Zastoupil, President and Chief Executive Officer
Web address: www.staloisius.com

ST. ANDREW'S HEALTH CENTER (O, 25 beds) 316 Ohmer Street, Bottineau, ND Zip 58318–1018; tel. 701/228–9300; Jodi Atkinson, President and Chief Executive Officer
Web address: www.standrewshealth.com

Owned, leased, sponsored:	4 hospitals	267 beds
Contract–managed:	0 hospitals	0 beds
Totals:	4 hospitals	267 beds

For explanation of codes following names, see page B2.
★ Indicates Type III membership in the American Hospital Association.

Section B

★5185: SISTERS OF MERCY HEALTH SYSTEM (CC)
14528 South Outer 40, Suite 100, Chesterfield, MO Zip 63017–5743; tel. 314/579–6100; John Sullivan, Chief Executive Officer
(Decentralized Health System)

ARKANSAS: MERCY HOSPITAL OF SCOTT COUNTY (O, 24 beds) 1341 West 6th Street, Waldron, AR Zip 72958–7001; tel. 479/637–4135; Jim L. Maddox, Administrator
Web address: www.stedwardmercy.com

MERCY HOSPITAL–TURNER MEMORIAL (L, 25 beds) 801 West River Street, Ozark, AR Zip 72949–3000; tel. 479/667–4138; Jim L. Maddox, Administrator
Web address: www.gravettehospital.org

MERCY MEDICAL CENTER (O, 133 beds) 2710 Rife Medical Lane, Rogers, AR Zip 72758; tel. 479/338–8000; George Flynn, Chief Executive Officer
Web address: www.mercyhealthnwa.smhs.com

NORTH LOGAN MERCY HOSPITAL (L, 16 beds) 500 East Academy, Paris, AR Zip 72855–4099; tel. 479/963–6101; Jim L. Maddox, Administrator
Web address: www.stedwardmercy.com

ST. EDWARD MERCY MEDICAL CENTER (O, 389 beds) 7301 Rogers Avenue, Fort Smith, AR Zip 72903–4189, Mailing Address: P.O. Box 17000, Zip 72917–7000; tel. 479/314–6000; Jerry L. Stevenson, FACHE, Chief Executive Officer
Web address: www.stedwardmercy.com

ST. JOHN'S HOSPITAL–BERRYVILLE (L, 25 beds) 214 Carter Street, Berryville, AR Zip 72616–4303; tel. 870/423–3355; Kristy K. Noble, FACHE, President
Web address: www.stjohnsberryville.com

ST. JOSEPH'S MERCY HEALTH CENTER (O, 264 beds) 300 Werner Street, Hot Springs National Park, AR Zip 71913–9937, Mailing Address: P.O. Box 29001, Zip 71913–9001; tel. 501/622–1000; Timothy J. Johnsen, President and Chief Executive Officer
Web address: www.saintjosephs.com

KANSAS: MERCY HEALTH CENTER–FORT SCOTT (O, 72 beds) 401 Woodland Hills Boulevard, Fort Scott, KS Zip 66701–8797; tel. 620/223–2200; John T. Woodrich, Chief Executive Officer
Web address: www.mercykansas.com

MISSOURI: ST. JOHN'S HOSPITAL (O, 623 beds) 1235 East Cherokee Street, Springfield, MO Zip 65804–2263; tel. 417/820–2000; Jon Swope, President
Web address: www.stjohns.com

ST. JOHN'S HOSPITAL – AURORA (L, 25 beds) 500 Porter Street, Aurora, MO Zip 65605–2365; tel. 417/678–2122; Gary W. Jordan, President
Web address: www.stjohns.com/aboutus/aurora.aspx

ST. JOHN'S HOSPITAL – CASSVILLE (L, 18 beds) 94 Main Street, Cassville, MO Zip 65625–1610; tel. 417/847–6000; Gary W. Jordan, President
Web address: www.southbarrycountyhospital.com

ST. JOHN'S HOSPITAL – LEBANON (O, 48 beds) 100 Hospital Drive, Lebanon, MO Zip 65536–9210; tel. 417/533–6100; Michael J. Gillen, President
Web address: www.stjohnslebanon.com

ST. JOHN'S MERCY HOSPITAL (O, 169 beds) 901 East Fifth Street, Washington, MO Zip 63090–3127; tel. 636/239–8000; Terri L. McLain, FACHE, President
Web address: www.stjohnsmercy.org

ST. JOHN'S MERCY MEDICAL CENTER (O, 822 beds) 615 South New Ballas Road, Saint Louis, MO Zip 63141–8277; tel. 314/569–6000; Margaret DeNarvaez, President and Chief Executive Officer
Web address: www.stjohnsmercy.org

ST. JOHN'S ST. FRANCIS HOSPITAL (O, 20 beds) 100 West Highway 60, Mountain View, MO Zip 65548–7125; tel. 417/934–7000; Douglas R. Trembath, President
Web address: www.stjohns.com/aboutus/stfrancis.aspx

OKLAHOMA: MERCY HEALTH CENTER (O, 338 beds) 4300 West Memorial Road, Oklahoma City, OK Zip 73120–8362; tel. 405/755–1515; Diana Smalley, President
Web address: www.mercyok.net

MERCY MEMORIAL HEALTH CENTER (O, 159 beds) 1011 14th Avenue N.W., Ardmore, OK Zip 73401–1889; tel. 580/223–5400; Bobby G. Thompson, President and Chief Executive Officer
Web address: www.mercyok.net

Owned, leased, sponsored:	17 hospitals	3170 beds
Contract-managed:	0 hospitals	0 beds
Totals:	17 hospitals	3170 beds

5955: SISTERS OF SAINT FRANCIS (CC)
2500 Grant Boulevard, Syracuse, NY Zip 13208–1713; tel. 315/634–7000; Sister Grace Anne Dillenschneider, Assistant General Minister
(Independent Hospital System)

HAWAII: HAWAII MEDICAL CENTER EAST (S, 240 beds) 2230 Liliha Street, Honolulu, HI Zip 96817–9979, Mailing Address: P.O. Box 30100, Zip 96820–0100; tel. 808/547–6011; Danelo R. Canete, M.D., Chief Executive Officer
Web address: www.stfrancishawaii.org

HAWAII MEDICAL CENTER–WEST (S, 102 beds) 91–2141 Fort Weaver Road, Ewa Beach, HI Zip 96706–1993; tel. 808/678–7000; Danelo R. Canete, M.D., Chief Executive Officer
Web address: www.sfhs–hi.org

NEW YORK: ST. ELIZABETH MEDICAL CENTER (S, 190 beds) 2209 Genesee Street, Utica, NY Zip 13501–5999; tel. 315/798–8100; Sister M. Johanna DeLelys, President and Chief Executive Officer
Web address: www.stemc.org

ST. JOSEPH'S HOSPITAL HEALTH CENTER (S, 431 beds) 301 Prospect Avenue, Syracuse, NY Zip 13203–1895; tel. 315/448–5111; Theodore M. Pasinski, President
Web address: www.sjhsyr.org

Owned, leased, sponsored:	4 hospitals	963 beds
Contract-managed:	0 hospitals	0 beds
Totals:	4 hospitals	963 beds

5345: SISTERS OF ST. FRANCIS HEALTH SERVICES, INC. (CC)
1515 Dragoon Trail, Mishawaka, IN Zip 46546–1290, Mailing Address: P.O. Box 1290, Zip 46546–1290; tel. 574/256–3935; Kevin D. Leahy, President and Chief Executive Officer
(Independent Hospital System)

ILLINOIS: ST. JAMES HOSPITAL AND HEALTH CENTERS (O, 494 beds) Olympia Fields, IL Seth C. R. Warren, President
Web address: www.stjameshhc.org

INDIANA: FRANCISCAN PHYSICIANS HOSPITAL (O, 32 beds) 701 Superior Avenue, Munster, IN Zip 46321–4029; tel. 219/924–1300; Barbara M. Greene, President
Web address: www.heartlandmemorial.org

SAINT ANTHONY MEMORIAL (O, 168 beds) 301 West Homer Street, Michigan City, IN Zip 46360–4358; tel. 219/879–8511; James Callaghan, III, M.D., President
Web address: www.saintanthonymemorial.org

SAINT MARGARET MERCY HEALTHCARE CENTERS (O, 624 beds) 5454 Hohman Avenue, Hammond, IN Zip 46320–1999; tel. 219/933–2074; Thomas J. Gryzbek, President
Web address: www.smmhc.com

ST. ANTHONY MEDICAL CENTER (O, 234 beds) 1201 South Main Street, Crown Point, IN Zip 46307–8483; tel. 219/738–2100; David Ruskowski, President
Web address: www.stanthonymedicalcenter.com

ST. CLARE MEDICAL CENTER (O, 83 beds) 1710 Lafayette Road, Crawfordsville, IN Zip 47933–1099; tel. 765/362–2800; Jim Siemers, Chief Executive Officer
Web address: www.stclaremedical.org

ST. ELIZABETH REGIONAL HEALTH (O, 451 beds) 2400 South Street, Lafayette, IN Zip 47904–3027; tel. 765/447–6811; Terrance E. Wilson, President and Chief Executive Officer
Web address: www.ste.org

ST. FRANCIS HOSPITAL AND HEALTH CENTERS – NORTH CAMPUS (O, 434 beds) 1600 Albany Street, Beech Grove, IN Zip 46107–1593; tel. 317/787–3311; Robert J. Brody, President and Chief Executive Officer
Web address: www.stfrancishospitals.org

For explanation of codes following names, see page B2.
★ Indicates Type III membership in the American Hospital Association.

ST. FRANCIS HOSPITAL–MOORESVILLE (O, 54 beds) 1201 Hadley Road N.W., Mooresville, IN Zip 46158–1789; tel. 317/831–1160; D. Keith Jewell, Interim Executive Director

Owned, leased, sponsored:	9 hospitals	2574 beds
Contract-managed:	0 hospitals	0 beds
Totals:	9 hospitals	2574 beds

★8855: SOLARIS HEALTH SYSTEM (NP)
80 James Street, 2nd Floor, Edison, NJ Zip 08820–3998; tel. 732/632–1501; John P. McGee, President and Chief Executive Officer
(Independent Hospital System)

NEW JERSEY: JFK JOHNSON REHABILITATION INSTITUTE (O, 92 beds) 65 James Street, Edison, NJ Zip 08818–3059; tel. 732/321–7050; Anthony Cuzzola, Vice President Rehabilitation Services
Web address: www.solarishs.org

JFK MEDICAL CENTER (O, 325 beds) 65 James Street, Edison, NJ Zip 08818–3059; tel. 732/321–7000; Scott Gebhard, Executive Vice President and Chief Operating Officer
Web address: www.solarishs.org

MUHLENBERG REGIONAL MEDICAL CENTER (O, 184 beds) Park Avenue and Randolph Road, North Plainfield, NJ Zip 7060; tel. 908/668–2000; Nancy A. Fiamingo, Senior Vice President and Chief Operating Officer
Web address: www.solarishs.org

Owned, leased, sponsored:	3 hospitals	601 beds
Contract-managed:	0 hospitals	0 beds
Totals:	3 hospitals	601 beds

0358: SOUND SHORE HEALTH SYSTEM (NP)
16 Guion Place, New Rochelle, NY Zip 10801–5500; tel. 914/632–5000; John R. Spicer, President and Chief Executive Officer

NEW YORK: MOUNT VERNON HOSPITAL (O, 132 beds) 12 North Seventh Avenue, Mount Vernon, NY Zip 10550–2098; tel. 914/664–8000; John R. Spicer, President and Chief Executive Officer
Web address: www.sshsw.org

SOUND SHORE MEDICAL CENTER OF WESTCHESTER (O, 356 beds) 16 Guion Place, New Rochelle, NY Zip 10801–5500; tel. 914/632–5000; John R. Spicer, President and Chief Executive Officer
Web address: www.sshsw.org

Owned, leased, sponsored:	2 hospitals	488 beds
Contract-managed:	0 hospitals	0 beds
Totals:	2 hospitals	488 beds

0151: SOUTH JERSEY HEALTHCARE (NP)
2950 College Drive, Suite 1E, Vineland, NJ Zip 08360; tel. 856/641–8000; Chester B. Kaletkowski, President and Chief Executive Officer
(Moderately Centralized Health System)

NEW JERSEY: SOUTH JERSEY HEALTHCARE – ELMER HOSPITAL (O, 91 beds) 501 West Front Street, Elmer, NJ Zip 08318–1090; tel. 856/363–1000; Chester B. Kaletkowski, President and Chief Executive Officer
Web address: www.sjhealthcare.net

SOUTH JERSEY HEALTHCARE – REGIONAL MEDICAL CENTER (O, 421 beds) 1505 West Sherman Avenue, Vineland, NJ Zip 8360; tel. 856/641–8000; Chester B. Kaletkowski, President and Chief Executive Officer
Web address: www.sjhealthcare.net

Owned, leased, sponsored:	2 hospitals	512 beds
Contract-managed:	0 hospitals	0 beds
Totals:	2 hospitals	512 beds

0253: SOUTHEAST GEORGIA HEALTH SYSTEM (NP)
2415 Parkwood Drive, Brunswick, GA Zip 31520–4252, Mailing Address: P.O. Box 1518, Zip 31521–1518; tel. 912/466–7000; Gary R. Colberg, FACHE, President and Chief Executive Officer
(Independent Hospital System)

GEORGIA: SOUTHEAST GEORGIA HEALTH SYSTEM BRUNSWICK CAMPUS (O, 273 beds) 2415 Parkwood Drive, Brunswick, GA Zip 31520–4252, Mailing Address: P.O. Box 1518, Zip 31521–1518; tel. 912/466–7000; Gary R. Colberg, FACHE, President and Chief Executive Officer
Web address: www.sghs.org

SOUTHEAST GEORGIA HEALTH SYSTEM CAMDEN CAMPUS (O, 40 beds) 2000 Dan Proctor Drive, Saint Marys, GA Zip 31558–3810; tel. 912/576–6200; Howard W. Sepp, Jr., FACHE, Vice President and Administrator
Web address: www.sghs.org

Owned, leased, sponsored:	2 hospitals	313 beds
Contract-managed:	0 hospitals	0 beds
Totals:	2 hospitals	313 beds

4175: SOUTHERN ILLINOIS HOSPITAL SERVICES (NP)
1239 East Main Street, Carbondale, IL Zip 62901, Mailing Address: P.O. Box 3988, Zip 62902–3988; tel. 618/457–5200; Thomas J. Firestone, M.D., President and Chief Executive Officer
(Independent Hospital System)

ILLINOIS: HERRIN HOSPITAL (O, 94 beds) 201 South 14th Street, Herrin, IL Zip 62948–3631; tel. 618/942–2171; Becky Ashton, Administrator
Web address: www.sih.net

MEMORIAL HOSPITAL OF CARBONDALE (O, 142 beds) 405 West Jackson Street, Carbondale, IL Zip 62901–1467, Mailing Address: P.O. Box 10000, Zip 62902–9000; tel. 618/549–0721; George Maroney, Senior Vice President and Administrator
Web address: www.sih.net

ST. JOSEPH MEMORIAL HOSPITAL (O, 25 beds) 2 South Hospital Drive, Murphysboro, IL Zip 62966–3333; tel. 618/684–3156; Scott Seaborn, Administrator
Web address: www.sih.net

Owned, leased, sponsored:	3 hospitals	261 beds
Contract-managed:	0 hospitals	0 beds
Totals:	3 hospitals	261 beds

1245: SPARROW HEALTH SYSTEM (NP)
1215 East Michigan Avenue, Lansing, MI Zip 48912; tel. 517/364–1000; Dennis A. Swan, President and Chief Executive Officer

MICHIGAN: CLINTON MEMORIAL HOSPITAL (O, 25 beds) 805 South Oakland Street, Saint Johns, MI Zip 48879–0260; tel. 989/224–6881; Edward Bruun, President and Chief Executive Officer
Web address: www.clintonmemorial.org

SPARROW HOSPITAL (O, 560 beds) 1215 East Michigan Avenue, Lansing, MI Zip 48912–1811, Mailing Address: P.O. Box 30480, Zip 48909–7980; tel. 517/364–1000; Dennis A. Swan, President and Chief Executive Officer
Web address: www.sparrow.org

SPARROW SPECIALTY HOSPITAL (O, 36 beds) 1210 West Saginaw Street, Lansing, MI Zip 48915, Mailing Address: P.O. Box 85201, Zip 48915; tel. 517/364–6800; Kira Carter, President and Chief Executive Officer
Web address: www.sparrowspecialty.org

Owned, leased, sponsored:	3 hospitals	621 beds
Contract-managed:	0 hospitals	0 beds
Totals:	3 hospitals	621 beds

★4195: SPARTANBURG REGIONAL HEALTHCARE SYSTEM (NP)
101 East Wood Street, Spartanburg, SC Zip 29303–3016; tel. 864/560–6000; Ingo Angermeier, FACHE, President and Chief Executive Officer
(Moderately Centralized Health System)

Section B

For explanation of codes following names, see page B2.
★ Indicates Type III membership in the American Hospital Association.

SOUTH CAROLINA: SPARTANBURG HOSPITAL FOR RESTORATIVE CARE (O, 82 beds) 389 Serpentine Drive, Spartanburg, SC Zip 29303–3026; tel. 864/560–3280; Anita M. Butler, Chief Executive Officer
Web address: www.srhs.com

SPARTANBURG REGIONAL MEDICAL CENTER (O, 518 beds) 101 East Wood Street, Spartanburg, SC Zip 29303–3016; tel. 864/560–6000; Ingo Angermeier, FACHE, President and Chief Executive Officer
Web address: www.srhs.com

Owned, leased, sponsored:	2 hospitals	600 beds
Contract-managed:	0 hospitals	0 beds
Totals:	2 hospitals	600 beds

0352: SPECIALTY HOSPITALS OF AMERICA, LLC (IO)
155 Fleet Street, Portsmouth, NH Zip 03801; tel. 603/570–4888; Eric F. Rieseberg, President
(Independent Hospital System)

DISTRICT OF COLUMBIA: SPECIALTY HOSPITAL OF WASHINGTON (O, 177 beds) 700 Constitution Avenue N.E., Washington, DC Zip 20002–6058; tel. 202/546–5700; Susan P. Bailey, RN, Chief Executive Officer
Web address: www.specialtyhospitalofwashington.com

SPECIALTY HOSPITALS OF WASHINGTON–HADLEY (O, 82 beds) 4601 Martin Luther King Jr. Avenue, S.W., Washington, DC Zip 20032–1199; tel. 202/574–5700; Irving B. Sawyers, Jr., Chief Executive Officer

UNITED MEDICAL CENTER (O, 303 beds) 1310 Southern Avenue S.E., Washington, DC Zip 20032–4699; tel. 202/574–6000; Gary L. Rowe, Chief Executive Officer
Web address: www.greatersoutheast.org

Owned, leased, sponsored:	3 hospitals	562 beds
Contract-managed:	0 hospitals	0 beds
Totals:	3 hospitals	562 beds

★0177: SPECTRUM HEALTH (NP)
100 Michigan Street N.E., Grand Rapids, MI Zip 49503–2551; tel. 616/391–1774; Richard C. Breon, President and Chief Executive Officer
(Centralized Physician/Insurance Health System)

MICHIGAN: SPECTRUM HEALTH (O, 987 beds) 100 Michigan Street N.E., Grand Rapids, MI Zip 49503; tel. 616/774–7444; Matthew Van Vranken, President
Web address: www.spectrum-health.org

SPECTRUM HEALTH REED CITY HOSPITAL (O, 79 beds) 300 North Patterson Road, Reed City, MI Zip 49677–0075, Mailing Address: P.O. Box 75, Zip 49677–0075; tel. 231/832–3271; Thomas D. Kaufman, President and Chief Executive Officer
Web address: www.reedcity.spectrum-health.org

SPECTRUM HEALTH–SPECIAL CARE HOSPITAL (O, 36 beds) 750 Fuller Avenue N.E., Grand Rapids, MI Zip 49503–1995; tel. 616/486–3000; Don Romain, Chief Executive Officer
Web address: www.kentcommunity.spectrum-health.org

SPECTRUM HEALTH–UNITED MEMORIAL (O, 141 beds) 615 South Bower Street, Greenville, MI Zip 48838–2628; tel. 616/754–4691; Paul Bonis, Chief Executive Officer
Web address: www.umha.org

Owned, leased, sponsored:	4 hospitals	1243 beds
Contract-managed:	0 hospitals	0 beds
Totals:	4 hospitals	1243 beds

★5455: SSM HEALTH CARE (CC)
477 North Lindbergh Boulevard, Saint Louis, MO Zip 63141–7813; tel. 314/994–7800; Sister Mary Jean Ryan, President and Chief Executive Officer
(Decentralized Health System)

ILLINOIS: GOOD SAMARITAN REGIONAL HEALTH CENTER (O, 139 beds) 605 North 12th Street, Mount Vernon, IL Zip 62864–2899; tel. 618/242–4600; Leo F. Childers, Jr., FACHE, President
Web address: www.smgsi.com

ST. FRANCIS HOSPITAL & HEALTH CENTER (O, 282 beds) 12935 South Gregory Street, Blue Island, IL Zip 60406–2470; tel. 708/597–2000; Colleen Kannaday, FACHE, President
Web address: www.stfrancisblueisland.com

ST. MARY'S HOSPITAL (O, 114 beds) 400 North Pleasant Avenue, Centralia, IL Zip 62801–3091; tel. 618/436–8000; Bruce Merrell, FACHE, President
Web address: www.smgsi.com

MISSOURI: SSM CARDINAL GLENNON CHILDREN'S MEDICAL CENTER (O, 176 beds) 1465 South Grand Boulevard, Saint Louis, MO Zip 63104–1095; tel. 314/577–5600; Douglas A. Ries, FACHE, President
Web address: www.cardinalglennon.com

SSM DEPAUL HEALTH CENTER (O, 457 beds) 12303 DePaul Drive, Bridgeton, MO Zip 63044–2588; tel. 314/344–6000; Patrice L. Komoroski, M.S.N., RN, President
Web address: www.ssmdepaul.com

SSM ST. JOSEPH HEALTH CENTER (O, 297 beds) 300 First Capitol Drive, Saint Charles, MO Zip 63301–2844; tel. 636/947–5000; Gaspare Calvaruso, President
Web address: www.ssmstjoseph.com

SSM ST. JOSEPH HOSPITAL OF KIRKWOOD (O, 187 beds) 525 Couch Avenue, Saint Louis, MO Zip 63122–5536; tel. 314/966–1500; Sherry Hausmann, President
Web address: www.st josephkirkwood.com

SSM ST. JOSEPH HOSPITAL WEST (O, 129 beds) 100 Medical Plaza, Lake Saint Louis, MO Zip 63367–1366; tel. 636/625–5200; Verna Meacham, Interim President
Web address: www.ssmstjoseph.com

SSM ST. MARY'S HEALTH CENTER (O, 293 beds) 6420 Clayton Road, Saint Louis, MO Zip 63117–1811; tel. 314/768–8000; William M. Jennings, President
Web address: www.stmarys-stlouis.com

ST. FRANCIS HOSPITAL AND HEALTH SERVICES (O, 57 beds) 2016 South Main Street, Maryville, MO Zip 64468–2655; tel. 660/562–2600; Gray Cox, President
Web address: www.stfrancismaryville.com

ST. MARYS HEALTH CENTER (O, 167 beds) 100 St. Marys Medical Plaza, Jefferson City, MO Zip 65101–1602; tel. 573/761–7000; R. Brent VanConia, President
Web address: www.stmarys-jeffcity.com

OKLAHOMA: BONE AND JOINT HOSPITAL (O, 11 beds) 1111 North Dewey Avenue, Oklahoma City, OK Zip 73103–2615; tel. 405/552–9100; Chad Aduddell, President
Web address: www.boneandjoint.com

ST. ANTHONY HOSPITAL (O, 499 beds) 1000 North Lee Street, Oklahoma City, OK Zip 73102–1080, Mailing Address: P.O. Box 205, Zip 73101–0205; tel. 405/272–7000; Joe Hodges, President
Web address: www.saintsok.com

WISCONSIN: ST. CLARE HOSPITAL AND HEALTH SERVICES (O, 77 beds) 707 14th Street, Baraboo, WI Zip 53913–1597; tel. 608/356–1400; Sandra L. Anderson, President
Web address: www.stclare.com

ST. MARY'S HOSPITAL (O, 338 beds) 700 South Park Street, Madison, WI Zip 53715–0450; tel. 608/251–6100; Frank D. Byrne, M.D., President
Web address: www.stmarysmadison.com

Owned, leased, sponsored:	15 hospitals	3223 beds
Contract-managed:	0 hospitals	0 beds
Totals:	15 hospitals	3223 beds

For explanation of codes following names, see page B2.
★ Indicates Type III membership in the American Hospital Association.

★5425: ST. JOSEPH HEALTH SYSTEM (CC)
500 South Main Street, Suite 1000, Orange, CA Zip 92868, Mailing Address: P.O. Box 14132, Zip 92863–1532; tel. 714/347–7500; Deborah A. Proctor, President and Chief Executive Officer
(Moderately Centralized Health System)

CALIFORNIA: MISSION HOSPITAL (O, 284 beds) 27700 Medical Center Road, Mission Viejo, CA Zip 92691–6426; tel. 949/364–1400; Peter F. Bastone, President and Chief Executive Officer
Web address: www.mission4health.com

PETALUMA VALLEY HOSPITAL (L, 59 beds) 400 North McDowell Boulevard, Petaluma, CA Zip 94954–2369; tel. 707/778–1111; George Perez, President and Chief Executive Officer
Web address: www.stjosephhealth.org/petalumavalley

QUEEN OF THE VALLEY MEDICAL CENTER (O, 179 beds) 1000 Trancas Street, Napa, CA Zip 94558–2906, Mailing Address: P.O. Box 2340, Zip 94558–2340; tel. 707/252–4411; Dennis Sisto, President and Chief Executive Officer
Web address: www.thequeen.org

REDWOOD MEMORIAL HOSPITAL (O, 25 beds) 3300 Renner Drive, Fortuna, CA Zip 95540–3198; tel. 707/725–3361; Joseph M. Mark, President and Chief Executive Officer
Web address: www.stjosepheureka.org

SANTA ROSA MEMORIAL HOSPITAL (O, 337 beds) 1165 Montgomery Drive, Santa Rosa, CA Zip 95405–4897, Mailing Address: P.O. Box 522, Zip 95402–0522; tel. 707/546–3210; George Perez, President and Chief Executive Officer
Web address: www.stjosephhealth.org

ST. JOSEPH HOSPITAL (O, 125 beds) 2700 Dolbeer Street, Eureka, CA Zip 95501–4799; tel. 707/445–8121; Joseph M. Mark, President and Chief Executive Officer
Web address: www.stjosepheureka.org

ST. JOSEPH HOSPITAL (O, 366 beds) 1100 West Stewart Drive, Orange, CA Zip 92668–3891, Mailing Address: P.O. Box 5600, Zip 92613–5600; tel. 714/633–9111; Larry K. Ainsworth, President and Chief Executive Officer
Web address: www.sjo.org

ST. JUDE MEDICAL CENTER (O, 359 beds) 101 East Valencia Mesa Drive, Fullerton, CA Zip 92835–3809; tel. 714/992–3000; Lee Penrose, President and Chief Executive Officer
Web address: www.stjudemedicalcenter.org

ST. MARY MEDICAL CENTER (O, 177 beds) 18300 Highway 18, Apple Valley, CA Zip 92307–2206, Mailing Address: P.O. Box 7025, Zip 92307–0725; tel. 760/242–2311; Jason Barker, President and Chief Executive Officer

Owned, leased, sponsored:	9 hospitals	1911 beds
Contract-managed:	0 hospitals	0 beds
Totals:	9 hospitals	1911 beds

0269: ST. JOSEPH'S HEALTHCARE SYSTEM (CC)
703 Main Street, Paterson, NJ Zip 07503–2691; tel. 973/754–2000; William A. McDonald, President and Chief Executive Officer
(Moderately Centralized Health System)

NEW JERSEY: ST. JOSEPH'S REGIONAL MEDICAL CENTER (O, 651 beds) 703 Main Street, Paterson, NJ Zip 07503–2691; tel. 973/754–2000; William A. McDonald, President and Chief Executive Officer
Web address: www.stjosephshealth.org

ST. JOSEPH'S WAYNE HOSPITAL (O, 136 beds) 224 Hamburg Turnpike, Wayne, NJ Zip 07470–2100; tel. 973/942–6900; William A. McDonald, President and Chief Executive Officer
Web address: www.sjwh.net

Owned, leased, sponsored:	2 hospitals	787 beds
Contract-managed:	0 hospitals	0 beds
Totals:	2 hospitals	787 beds

0302: ST. LUKE'S EPISCOPAL HEALTH SYSTEM (NP)
6624 Fannin Street, Suite 1100, Houston, TX Zip 77030; tel. 832/355–7661; Beryl Vallejo, RN, Dr.P.h., Senior Vice President and Chief Quality Officer
(Centralized Physician/Insurance Health System)

TEXAS: ST LUKE'S COMMUNITY MEDICAL CENTER–THE WOODLANDS (O, 91 beds) 17200 St. Luke's Way, The Woodlands, TX Zip 77384; tel. 936/266–2000; Debra F. Sukin, Chief Executive Officer
Web address: www.stlukeswoodlands.com

ST. LUKE'S EPISCOPAL HOSPITAL (O, 718 beds) 6720 Bertner Avenue, Houston, TX Zip 77030–2697, Mailing Address: Box 20269, Zip 77225–0269; tel. 832/355–1000; David C. Pate, M.D., J.D., Chief Executive Officer
Web address: www.stlukestexas.com

Owned, leased, sponsored:	2 hospitals	809 beds
Contract-managed:	0 hospitals	0 beds
Totals:	2 hospitals	809 beds

★0356: ST. LUKE'S HEALTH SYSTEM (NP)
420 West Idaho Street, Boise, ID Zip 83702; tel. 208/381–1832; Edwin E. Dahlberg, President and Chief Executive Officer
(Moderately Centralized Health System)

IDAHO: ELMORE MEDICAL CENTER (C, 63 beds) 895 North Sixth East Street, Mountain Home, ID Zip 83647–2207, Mailing Address: P.O. Box 1270, Zip 83647–1270; tel. 208/587–8401; Gregory L. Maurer, Administrator
Web address: www.elmoremedicalcenter.org

GOODING COUNTY MEMORIAL HOSPITAL (C, 14 beds) 1120 Montana Street, Gooding, ID Zip 83330–1858; tel. 208/934–4433; Earl Fitzpatrick, Chief Executive Officer
Web address: www.goodinghospital.org

MCCALL MEMORIAL HOSPITAL (C, 15 beds) 1000 State Street, McCall, ID Zip 83638–3704; tel. 208/634–2221; Karen J. Kellie, RN, President and Administrator
Web address: www.mccallhosp.org

ST. LUKE'S MAGIC VALLEY REGIONAL MEDICAL CENTER (O, 191 beds) 650 Addison Avenue West, Twin Falls, ID Zip 83301–5444, Mailing Address: P.O. Box 409, Zip 83303–0409; tel. 208/737–2000; Mark Schwartz, Chief Executive Officer
Web address: www.mvrmc.org

ST. LUKE'S REGIONAL MEDICAL CENTER (O, 475 beds) 190 East Bannock Street, Boise, ID Zip 83712–6298; tel. 208/381–2222; Gary Fletcher, Chief Executive Officer
Web address: www.slrmc.org

ST. LUKE'S WOOD RIVER MEDICAL CENTER (O, 25 beds) 100 Hospital Drive, Ketchum, ID Zip 83340, Mailing Address: P.O. Box 100, Zip 83340; tel. 208/727–8800; Bruce C. Jensen, Chief Executive Officer
Web address: www.slrmc.org

Owned, leased, sponsored:	3 hospitals	691 beds
Contract-managed:	3 hospitals	92 beds
Totals:	6 hospitals	783 beds

0264: ST. VINCENT HEALTH SYSTEM (CC)
232 West 25th Street, Erie, PA Zip 16544–0002; tel. 814/452–5000; C. Angela Bontempo, President and Chief Executive Officer
(Moderately Centralized Health System)

NEW YORK: WESTFIELD MEMORIAL HOSPITAL (O, 19 beds) 189 East Main Street, Westfield, NY Zip 14787–1195; tel. 716/326–4921; C. Angela Bontempo, President and Chief Executive Officer
Web address: www.wmhinc.org

PENNSYLVANIA: SAINT VINCENT HEALTH CENTER (O, 456 beds) 232 West 25th Street, Erie, PA Zip 16544–0002; tel. 814/452–5000; C. Angela Bontempo, President and Chief Executive Officer
Web address: www.svhs.org

Owned, leased, sponsored:	2 hospitals	475 beds
Contract-managed:	0 hospitals	0 beds
Totals:	2 hospitals	475 beds

For explanation of codes following names, see page B2.
★ Indicates Type III membership in the American Hospital Association.

Section B

0156: STANFORD HEALTH CARE (NP)
300 Pasteur Drive, Palo Alto, CA Zip 94304–2299;
tel. 650/723–4000; Martha H. Marsh, President and Chief Executive Officer
(Moderately Centralized Health System)

CALIFORNIA: LUCILE SALTER PACKARD CHILDREN'S HOSPITAL AT STANFORD (O, 264 beds) 725 Welch Road, Palo Alto, CA Zip 94304–1601; tel. 650/497–8000; Christopher G. Dawes, President and Chief Executive Officer
Web address: www.lpch.org

STANFORD HOSPITAL AND CLINICS (O, 467 beds) 300 Pasteur Drive, Palo Alto, CA Zip 94304–2299; tel. 650/723–4000; Martha H. Marsh, President and Chief Executive Officer
Web address: www.stanfordhospital.com/

Owned, leased, sponsored:	2 hospitals	731 beds
Contract-managed:	0 hospitals	0 beds
Totals:	2 hospitals	731 beds

0223: STRONG MEMORIAL HOSPITAL (NP)
601 Elmwood Avenue, Rochester, NY Zip 14642–0002;
tel. 585/275–2100; Steven I. Goldstein, General Director and Chief Executive Officer
(Centralized Physician/Insurance Health System)

NEW YORK: HIGHLAND HOSPITAL OF ROCHESTER (O, 261 beds) 1000 South Avenue, Rochester, NY Zip 14620–2782; tel. 585/473–2200; Steven I. Goldstein, President and Chief Executive Officer
Web address: www.stronghealth.com

STRONG MEMORIAL HOSPITAL OF THE UNIVERSITY OF ROCHESTER (O, 1006 beds) 601 Elmwood Avenue, Rochester, NY Zip 14642–0002; tel. 585/275–2100; Steven I. Goldstein, President and Chief Executive Officer
Web address: www.urmc.rochester.edu

Owned, leased, sponsored:	2 hospitals	1267 beds
Contract-managed:	0 hospitals	0 beds
Totals:	2 hospitals	1267 beds

0399: SUMMA HEALTH SYSTEM (NP)
525 East Market Street, Akron, OH Zip 44309–2090;
tel. 330/375–3000; Thomas J. Strauss, President and Chief Executive Officer

OHIO: CUYAHOGA FALLS GENERAL HOSPITAL (O, 105 beds) 1900 23rd Street, Cuyahoga Falls, OH Zip 44223–1499; tel. 330/971–7000; Kathleen A. Rice, President and Chief Operating Officer
Web address: www.summahealth.org

ROBINSON MEMORIAL HOSPITAL (O, 115 beds) 6847 North Chestnut Street, Ravenna, OH Zip 44266–1204, Mailing Address: P.O. Box 1204, Zip 44266–1204; tel. 330/297–0811; Stephen Colecchi, President and Chief Executive Officer
Web address: www.robinsonmemorial.org

SUMMA BARBERTON CITIZENS HOSPITAL (O, 245 beds) 155 Fifth Street N.E., Barberton, OH Zip 44203–3332; tel. 330/615–3000; Willard P. Roderick, Chief Executive Officer
Web address: www.barbhosp.com

SUMMA HEALTH SYSTEM (O, 481 beds) Akron, OH Thomas J. Strauss, President and Chief Executive Officer
Web address: www.summahealth.org

WADSWORTH–RITTMAN HOSPITAL (O, 67 beds) 195 Wadsworth Road, Wadsworth, OH Zip 44281–9505; tel. 330/334–1504; James W. Pope, FACHE, President and Chief Executive Officer
Web address: www.wrhhs.org

Owned, leased, sponsored:	5 hospitals	1013 beds
Contract-managed:	0 hospitals	0 beds
Totals:	5 hospitals	1013 beds

★0189: SUMMIT HEALTH (NP)
112 North Seventh Street, Chambersburg, PA Zip 17201;
tel. 717/267–7138; Norman B. Epstein, FACHE, President
(Independent Hospital System)

PENNSYLVANIA: CHAMBERSBURG HOSPITAL (O, 240 beds) 112 North Seventh Street, Chambersburg, PA Zip 17201–0187; tel. 717/267–3000; Norman B. Epstein, FACHE, President
Web address: www.summithealth.org

WAYNESBORO HOSPITAL (O, 64 beds) 501 East Main Street, Waynesboro, PA Zip 17268–2394; tel. 717/765–4000; Kenneth L. Shur, FACHE, Vice President and Chief Operating Officer
Web address: www.summithealth.org

Owned, leased, sponsored:	2 hospitals	304 beds
Contract-managed:	0 hospitals	0 beds
Totals:	2 hospitals	304 beds

0292: SUMNER REGIONAL HEALTH SYSTEMS (NP)
255 Airport Road, Gallatin, TN Zip 37066; tel. 615/328–6695;
William T. Sugg, President and Chief Executive Officer
(Independent Hospital System)

TENNESSEE: RIVERVIEW REGIONAL MEDICAL CENTER NORTH (O, 63 beds) 158 Hospital Drive, Carthage, TN Zip 37030–1096; tel. 615/735–1560; Edward J. Sanford, Chief Executive Officer

RIVERVIEW REGIONAL MEDICAL CENTER SOUTH (O, 25 beds) 130 Lebanon Highway, Carthage, TN Zip 37030–2955, Mailing Address: P.O. Box 319, Zip 37030–0319; tel. 615/735–9815; Edward J. Sanford, Chief Executive Officer
Web address: www.sumner.org

SUMNER REGIONAL MEDICAL CENTER (O, 155 beds) 555 Hartsville Pike, Gallatin, TN Zip 37066–2449, Mailing Address: P.O. Box 1558, Zip 37066–1558; tel. 615/452–4210; Bruce James, Administrator
Web address: www.sumner.org

TROUSDALE MEDICAL CENTER (O, 25 beds) 500 Church Street, Hartsville, TN Zip 37074–2936, Mailing Address: P.O. Box 319, Carthage, Zip 37030–0319; tel. 615/374–2221; William D. Mize, Administrator
Web address: www.trousdale.org

Owned, leased, sponsored:	4 hospitals	268 beds
Contract-managed:	0 hospitals	0 beds
Totals:	4 hospitals	268 beds

★0030: SUN HEALTH CORPORATION (NP)
13180 North 103rd Drive, Sun City, AZ Zip 85351–3038, Mailing Address: P.O. Box 1278, Zip 85372–1278; tel. 623/876–5301;
Leland W. Peterson, President and Chief Executive Officer
(Centralized Physician/Insurance Health System)

ARIZONA: 10401 WEST THUNDERBIRD BOULEVARD (O, 436 beds) 10401 West Thunderbird Boulevard, Sun City, AZ Zip 85351–3092, Mailing Address: P.O. Box 1690, Zip 85372–1690; tel. 623/977–7211; Nancy L. Burton, Chief Executive Officer
Web address: www.sunhealth.org

SUN HEALTH DEL E. WEBB HOSPITAL (O, 332 beds) 14502 West Meeker Boulevard, Sun City West, AZ Zip 85375–5299, Mailing Address: P.O. Box 5169, Sun City, Zip 85375–5169; tel. 623/214–4000; Jo Adkins, Chief Executive Officer
Web address: www.sunhealth.org

Owned, leased, sponsored:	2 hospitals	768 beds
Contract-managed:	0 hospitals	0 beds
Totals:	2 hospitals	768 beds

0210: SUN HEALTHCARE GROUP (IO)
18831 Von Karman, Suite 400, Irvine, CA Zip 92612;
tel. 949/255–7100; Richard K. Matros, Chairman of the Board and Chief Executive Officer

CALIFORNIA: CONTINENTAL REHABILITATION HOSPITAL (O, 110 beds) 555 Washington Street, San Diego, CA Zip 92103; tel. 619/260–8300; Nancy Wiewiora, Interim Chief Executive Officer
Web address: www.continentalrehab.com

For explanation of codes following names, see page B2.
★ Indicates Type III membership in the American Hospital Association.

ROBERT H. BALLARD REHABILITATION HOSPITAL (O, 60 beds) 1760 West 16th Street, San Bernardino, CA Zip 92411; tel. 909/473–1200; Robert Herrick, Chief Executive Officer
Web address: www.ballardhospital.com

IDAHO: SUNHEALTH BEHAVIORAL HEALTH SYSTEM FOR BOISE (O, 22 beds) 8050 Northview Street, Boise, ID Zip 83704; tel. 208/327–0504; Phil Herink, Chief Executive Officer

Owned, leased, sponsored:	3 hospitals	192 beds
Contract-managed:	0 hospitals	0 beds
Totals:	3 hospitals	192 beds

0237: SUNLINK HEALTH SYSTEMS (IO)
900 Circle 75 Parkway, Suite 1300, Atlanta, GA Zip 30339; tel. 770/933–7000; Robert M. Thornton, Jr., Chief Executive Officer
(Independent Hospital System)

ALABAMA: CHILTON MEDICAL CENTER (O, 30 beds) 1010 Lay Dam Road, Clanton, AL Zip 35045–2306; tel. 205/755–2500; Rob Followell, Chief Executive Officer
Web address: www.sunlinkhealth.com

GEORGIA: CHESTATEE REGIONAL HOSPITAL (O, 49 beds) 227 Mountain Drive, Dahlonega, GA Zip 30533–1606; tel. 706/864–6136; Alan E. George, Chief Executive Officer
Web address: www.chestateeregionalhospital.com

MEMORIAL HOSPITAL OF ADEL (O, 155 beds) 706 North Parrish Avenue, Adel, GA Zip 31620–0677; tel. 229/896–8000; William Hawley, Chief Executive Officer
Web address: www.sunlinkhealth.com

NORTH GEORGIA MEDICAL CENTER (O, 150 beds) 1362 South Main Street, Ellijay, GA Zip 30540–0346, Mailing Address: P.O. Box 2239, Zip 30540–0346; tel. 706/276–4741; Jeffrey Dunn, Chief Executive Officer
Web address: www.northgeorgiamedicalcenter.com

MISSISSIPPI: TRACE REGIONAL HOSPITAL (O, 84 beds) Highway 8 East, Houston, MS Zip 38851–9396, Mailing Address: P.O. Box 626, Zip 38851–0626; tel. 662/456–3700; Gary L. Staten, Chief Executive Officer
Web address: www.traceregional.com

MISSOURI: CALLAWAY COMMUNITY HOSPITAL (O, 35 beds) 10 South Hospital Drive, Fulton, MO Zip 65251–2510; tel. 573/642–3376; John T. Graves, CHE, Chief Executive Officer
Web address: www.sunlinkhealth.com/callaway.html

MISSOURI SOUTHERN HEALTHCARE (L, 45 beds) 1200 North One Mile Road, Dexter, MO Zip 63841–1000; tel. 573/624–5566; James P. Crawford, Jr., Chief Executive Officer

Owned, leased, sponsored:	7 hospitals	548 beds
Contract-managed:	0 hospitals	0 beds
Totals:	7 hospitals	548 beds

★8795: SUTTER HEALTH (NP)
2200 River Plaza Drive, Sacramento, CA Zip 95833; tel. 916/733–8800; Patrick E. Fry, Chief Executive Officer
(Moderately Centralized Health System)

CALIFORNIA: ALTA BATES SUMMIT MEDICAL CENTER (O, 527 beds) 2450 Ashby Avenue, Berkeley, CA Zip 94705–2067; tel. 510/204–4444; Warren J. Kirk, President and Chief Executive Officer
Web address: www.altabates.com

ALTA BATES SUMMIT MEDICAL CENTER – SUMMIT CAMPUS (O, 408 beds) 350 Hawthorne Avenue, Oakland, CA Zip 94609–3100; tel. 510/655–4000; Warren J. Kirk, President and Chief Executive Officer
Web address: www.altabatessummit.com

CALIFORNIA PACIFIC MEDICAL CENTER (C, 798 beds) 2333 Buchanan Street, San Francisco, CA Zip 94115–1925, Mailing Address: P.O. Box 7999, Zip 94120–7999; tel. 415/563–4321; Martin Brotman, M.D., President and Chief Executive Officer
Web address: www.cpmc.org

MARIN GENERAL HOSPITAL (O, 235 beds) 250 Bon Air Road, Greenbrae, CA Zip 94904–1784, Mailing Address: P.O. Box 8010, San Rafael, Zip 94912–8010; tel. 415/925–7000; David Bradley, Chief Executive Officer
Web address: www.maringeneral.sutterhealth.org

MEMORIAL MEDICAL CENTER (O, 417 beds) Modesto, CA Mailing Address: P.O. Box 942, Zip 95353–0942; tel. 209/526–4500; David P. Benn, Chief Executive Officer
Web address: www.memorialmedicalcenter.org

MENLO PARK SURGICAL HOSPITAL (O, 12 beds) 570 Willow Road, Menlo Park, CA Zip 94025–2617; tel. 650/324–8500; Kathleen Palange, Administrator and Chief Executive Officer
Web address: www.pamf.org/mpsh

MILLS–PENINSULA HEALTH SERVICES (O, 389 beds) 1783 El Camino Real, Burlingame, CA Zip 94010–3282; tel. 650/696–5400; Robert W. Merwin, Chief Executive Officer
Web address: www.mills–peninsula.org

NOVATO COMMUNITY HOSPITAL (O, 47 beds) 180 Rowland Way, Novato, CA Zip 94945–5009, Mailing Address: P.O. Box 1108, Zip 94948–1108; tel. 415/209–1300; Anne L. Hosfeld, Chief Administrative Officer
Web address: www.novatocommunity.sutterhealth.org

ST. LUKE'S HOSPITAL (O, 229 beds) 3555 Cesar Chavez Street, San Francisco, CA Zip 94110–4490; tel. 415/647–8600; Martin Brotman, M.D., President and Chief Executive Officer
Web address: www.stlukes–sf.org

SUTTER AMADOR HOSPITAL (O, 52 beds) 200 Mission Boulevard, Jackson, CA Zip 95642–2132; tel. 209/223–7500; Anne Platt, Chief Executive Officer
Web address: www.sutteramador.com

SUTTER AUBURN FAITH HOSPITAL (O, 86 beds) 11815 Education Street, Auburn, CA Zip 95602–2410; tel. 530/888–4500; Mitchell J. Hanna, Chief Administrative Officer
Web address: www.sutterhealth.org

SUTTER CENTER FOR PSYCHIATRY (O, 69 beds) 7700 Folsom Boulevard, Sacramento, CA Zip 95826–2608; tel. 916/386–3000; Diane Gail Stewart, Chief Administrative Officer
Web address: www.sutterpsychiatry.org

SUTTER COAST HOSPITAL (O, 59 beds) 800 East Washington Boulevard, Crescent City, CA Zip 95531–8359; tel. 707/464–8511; John E. Menaugh, Chief Executive Officer
Web address: www.sutterhealth.org

SUTTER DAVIS HOSPITAL (O, 48 beds) 2000 Sutter Place, Davis, CA Zip 95616–6201, Mailing Address: P.O. Box 1617, Zip 95617–1617; tel. 530/756–6440; Janet Wagner, RN, Chief Administrative Officer
Web address: www.sutterhealth.org

SUTTER DELTA MEDICAL CENTER (O, 107 beds) 3901 Lone Tree Way, Antioch, CA Zip 94509–6253; tel. 925/779–7200; Gary D. Rapaport, Chief Executive Officer
Web address: www.sutterdelta.org

SUTTER LAKESIDE HOSPITAL (O, 53 beds) 5176 Hill Road East, Lakeport, CA Zip 95453–6300; tel. 707/262–5001; Kelly Mather, Chief Executive Officer
Web address: www.sutterlake.org

SUTTER MATERNITY AND SURGERY CENTER OF SANTA CRUZ (O, 28 beds) 2900 Chanticleer Avenue, Santa Cruz, CA Zip 95065–1816; tel. 831/477–2200; Richard Nichols, Administrator
Web address: www.suttermatsurg.org

SUTTER MEDICAL CENTER OF SANTA ROSA, CHANATE CAMPUS (O, 143 beds) 3325 Chanate Road, Santa Rosa, CA Zip 95404–1707; tel. 707/576–4000; Michael J. Cohill, Chief Executive Officer
Web address: www.sutterhealth.org

SUTTER MEDICAL CENTER, SACRAMENTO (O, 659 beds) 5151 F Street, Sacramento, CA Zip 95819–3295; tel. 916/454–3333; Thomas C. Gagen, Chief Executive Officer
Web address: www.sutterhealth.org

SUTTER ROSEVILLE MEDICAL CENTER (O, 172 beds) One Medical Plaza, Roseville, CA Zip 95661–3037; tel. 916/781–1000; Patrick R. Brady, Chief Executive Officer
Web address: www.sutterroseville.org

SUTTER SOLANO MEDICAL CENTER (O, 111 beds) 300 Hospital Drive, Vallejo, CA Zip 94589–2517, Mailing Address: P.O. Box 3189, Zip 94589–3189; tel. 707/554–4444; Theresa Glubka, Chief Executive Officer
Web address: www.suttersolano.org

SUTTER TRACY COMMUNITY HOSPITAL (O, 82 beds) 1420 North Tracy Boulevard, Tracy, CA Zip 95376–3497; tel. 209/835–1500; David M. Thompson, Chief Executive Officer
Web address: www.suttertracy.org

For explanation of codes following names, see page B2.
★ Indicates Type III membership in the American Hospital Association.

HAWAII: KAHI MOHALA BEHAVIORAL HEALTH (O, 88 beds) 91–2301 Old Fort Weaver Road, Ewa Beach, HI Zip 96706–3602; tel. 808/671–8511; Leonard Licina, Chief Executive Officer
Web address: www.kahi.org

Owned, leased, sponsored:	22 hospitals	4021 beds
Contract–managed:	1 hospital	798 beds
Totals:	23 hospitals	4819 beds

0379: TAHOE FOREST HEALTH SYSTEM (NP)

10121 Pine Avenue, Truckee, CA Zip 96161; tel. 530/587–6011; Robert A. Schapper, Chief Executive Officer

CALIFORNIA: TAHOE FOREST HOSPITAL DISTRICT (O, 61 beds) 10121 Pine Avenue, Truckee, CA Zip 96161–4856, Mailing Address: P.O. Box 759, Zip 96160–0759; tel. 530/587–6011; Robert A. Schapper, Chief Executive Officer
Web address: www.tfhd.com

NEVADA: INCLINE VILLAGE COMMUNITY HOSPITAL (O, 4 beds) 880 Alder Avenue, Incline Village, NV Zip 89450; tel. 775/833–4100; Peter A. Basler, Chief Executive Officer
Web address: www.tfhd.com

Owned, leased, sponsored:	2 hospitals	65 beds
Contract–managed:	0 hospitals	0 beds
Totals:	2 hospitals	65 beds

★0341: TANNER HEALTH SYSTEM (NP)

705 Dixie Street, Carrollton, GA Zip 30117–3818; tel. 770/836–9580; Loy M. Howard, President and Chief Executive Officer

GEORGIA: HIGGINS GENERAL HOSPITAL (L, 25 beds) 200 Allen Memorial Drive, Bremen, GA Zip 30110–2012, Mailing Address: P.O. Box 655, Zip 30110–0655; tel. 770/537–5851; Michael Alexander, Administrator
Web address: www.tanner.org

TANNER MEDICAL CENTER (O, 176 beds) 705 Dixie Street, Carrollton, GA Zip 30117–3818; tel. 770/836–9666; Loy M. Howard, President and Chief Executive Officer
Web address: www.tanner.org

TANNER MEDICAL CENTER–VILLA RICA (O, 39 beds) 601 Dallas Road, Villa Rica, GA Zip 30180–1202, Mailing Address: P.O. Box 638, Zip 30180–0638; tel. 770/456–3100; Larry N. Steed, FACHE, Administrator
Web address: www.tanner.org

Owned, leased, sponsored:	3 hospitals	240 beds
Contract–managed:	0 hospitals	0 beds
Totals:	3 hospitals	240 beds

★0169: TEMPLE UNIVERSITY HEALTH SYSTEM (NP)

2450 West Hunting Park Avenue, 4th Floor, Philadelphia, PA Zip 19129; tel. 215/707–0900; Joseph W. Marshall, III, President and Chief Executive Officer
(Centralized Health System)

PENNSYLVANIA: JEANES HOSPITAL (O, 198 beds) 7600 Central Avenue, Philadelphia, PA Zip 19111–2499; tel. 215/728–2000; Linda J. Grass, Executive Director and Chief Executive Officer
Web address: www.jeanes.com

TEMPLE EAST, NORTHEASTERN HOSPITAL (O, 187 beds) 2301 East Allegheny Avenue, Philadelphia, PA Zip 19134–4497; tel. 215/291–3000; John J. Buckley, Executive Director and Chief Executive Officer
Web address: www.health.temple.edu/northeastern.html

TEMPLE UNIVERSITY HOSPITAL (O, 678 beds) 3401 North Broad Street, Philadelphia, PA Zip 19140–5192; tel. 215/707–2000; Robert E. Pezzoli, Interim Chief Executive Officer
Web address: www.health.temple.edu/tuh/

Owned, leased, sponsored:	3 hospitals	1063 beds
Contract–managed:	0 hospitals	0 beds
Totals:	3 hospitals	1063 beds

★0063: TENET HEALTHCARE CORPORATION (IO)

13737 Noel Road, Suite 100, Dallas, TX Zip 75240–2200; tel. 469/893–2200; Trevor Fetter, President and Chief Executive Officer
(Decentralized Health System)

ALABAMA: BROOKWOOD MEDICAL CENTER (O, 586 beds) 2010 Brookwood Medical Center Drive, Birmingham, AL Zip 35209–6875; tel. 205/877–1000; Garry L. Gause, Chief Executive Officer
Web address: www.brookwood–medical.com

CALIFORNIA: COMMUNITY HOSPITAL OF LOS GATOS (L, 77 beds) 815 Pollard Road, Los Gatos, CA Zip 95032–1438; tel. 408/378–6131; Gary Honts, Chief Executive Officer
Web address: www.communityhospitallg.com

DESERT REGIONAL MEDICAL CENTER (L, 331 beds) 1150 North Indian Canyon Drive, Palm Springs, CA Zip 92262–4872, Mailing Address: P.O. Box 2739, Zip 92263–2739; tel. 760/323–6511; Karolee M. Sowle, RN, Chief Executive Officer
Web address: www.desertmedctr.com

DOCTORS HOSPITAL OF MANTECA (O, 73 beds) 1205 East North Street, Manteca, CA Zip 95336–4900; tel. 209/823–3111; Mark P. Lisa, FACHE, Chief Executive Officer
Web address: www.doctorsmanteca.com

DOCTORS MEDICAL CENTER (O, 456 beds) 1441 Florida Avenue, Modesto, CA Zip 95350–4418, Mailing Address: P.O. Box 4138, Zip 95352–4138; tel. 209/578–1211; Dennis M. Litos, Chief Executive Officer
Web address: www.dmc–modesto.com

FOUNTAIN VALLEY REGIONAL HOSPITAL AND MEDICAL CENTER (O, 400 beds) 17100 Euclid Street, Fountain Valley, CA Zip 92708–4043; tel. 714/966–7200; Deborah C. Keel, Chief Executive Officer
Web address: www.fountainvalleyhospital.com

IRVINE REGIONAL HOSPITAL AND MEDICAL CENTER (L, 176 beds) 16200 Sand Canyon Avenue, Irvine, CA Zip 92618–3714; tel. 949/753–2000; Donald A. Lorack, Jr., Chief Executive Officer
Web address: www.irvineregionalhospital.com

JOHN F. KENNEDY MEMORIAL HOSPITAL (O, 145 beds) 47111 Monroe Street, Indio, CA Zip 92201; tel. 760/347–6191; John J. Ferrelli, Chief Executive Officer
Web address: www.jfkmemorialhosp.com

LAKEWOOD REGIONAL MEDICAL CENTER (O, 157 beds) 3700 East South Street, Lakewood, CA Zip 90712–1498, Mailing Address: P.O. Box 6070, Zip 90714–6070; tel. 562/531–2550; Mark Korth, Chief Executive Officer
Web address: www.lakewoodregional.com

LOS ALAMITOS MEDICAL CENTER (O, 167 beds) 3751 Katella Avenue, Los Alamitos, CA Zip 90720–3164; tel. 562/598–1311; Michele Finney, Chief Executive Officer

PLACENTIA–LINDA HOSPITAL (O, 114 beds) 1301 North Rose Drive, Placentia, CA Zip 92870–3899; tel. 714/993–2000; Kent G. Clayton, President and Chief Executive Officer
Web address: www.placentialinda.com

SAN RAMON REGIONAL MEDICAL CENTER (O, 123 beds) 6001 Norris Canyon Road, San Ramon, CA Zip 94583–5400; tel. 925/275–9200; Gary Sloan, Chief Executive Officer
Web address: www.sanramonmedctr.com

SIERRA VISTA REGIONAL MEDICAL CENTER (O, 165 beds) 1010 Murray Street, San Luis Obispo, CA Zip 93405–8800, Mailing Address: P.O. Box 1367, Zip 93406–1367; tel. 805/546–7600; Candace L. Markwith, Chief Executive Officer
Web address: www.sierravistaregional.com

TWIN CITIES COMMUNITY HOSPITAL (O, 114 beds) 1100 Las Tablas Road, Templeton, CA Zip 93465–9704; tel. 805/434–3500; Richard D. Lyons, Chief Executive Officer
Web address: www.twincitieshospital.com

UNIVERSITY OF SOUTHERN CALIFORNIA–NORRIS COMPREHENSIVE CANCER CENTER AND HOSPITAL (L, 60 beds) 1441 Eastlake Avenue, Los Angeles, CA Zip 90033–3804; tel. 323/865–3000; Debbie Walsh, Chief Operating Officer
Web address: www.uscnorris.com

USC UNIVERSITY HOSPITAL (L, 162 beds) 1500 San Pablo Street, Los Angeles, CA Zip 90033–4587; tel. 323/442–8500; Debbie Walsh, Chief Executive Officer
Web address: www.uscuh.com

For explanation of codes following names, see page B2.
★ Indicates Type III membership in the American Hospital Association.

FLORIDA: CORAL GABLES HOSPITAL (O, 256 beds) 3100 Douglas Road, Coral Gables, FL Zip 33134–6990; tel. 305/445–8461; Jay S. Miranda, Chief Executive Officer
Web address: www.coralgableshospital.com

DELRAY MEDICAL CENTER (O, 403 beds) 5352 Linton Boulevard, Delray Beach, FL Zip 33484–6580; tel. 561/498–4440; Robert M. Krieger, Chief Executive Officer
Web address: www.delraymedicalctr.com

FLORIDA MEDICAL CENTER (O, 459 beds) 5000 West Oakland Park Boulevard, Fort Lauderdale, FL Zip 33313–1585; tel. 954/735–6000; Robert Haley, Chief Executive Officer
Web address: www.floridamedicalctr.com

GOOD SAMARITAN MEDICAL CENTER (O, 174 beds) Flagler Drive at Palm Beach Lakes Boulevard, West Palm Beach, FL Zip 33401–3499; tel. 561/655–5511; Mark Nosacka, Chief Executive Officer
Web address: www.goodsamaritanmc.com

HIALEAH HOSPITAL (O, 378 beds) 651 East 25th Street, Hialeah, FL Zip 33013–3878; tel. 305/693–6100; Ralph A. Aleman, Chief Executive Officer
Web address: www.hialeahhosp.com

NORTH SHORE MEDICAL CENTER (O, 357 beds) 1100 N.W. 95th Street, Miami, FL Zip 33150–2098; tel. 305/835–6000; Manuel Linares, Chief Executive Officer
Web address: www.northshoremedical.com

PALM BEACH GARDENS MEDICAL CENTER (L, 199 beds) 3360 Burns Road, Palm Beach Gardens, FL Zip 33410–4304; tel. 561/622–1411; David A. Pettit, Chief Executive Officer

PALMETTO GENERAL HOSPITAL (O, 360 beds) 2001 West 68th Street, Hialeah, FL Zip 33016–1898; tel. 305/823–5000; Ana J. Mederos, Chief Executive Officer
Web address: www.palmettogeneral.com

PINECREST REHABILITATION HOSPITAL (O, 90 beds) 5360 Linton Boulevard, Delray Beach, FL Zip 33484–6538; tel. 561/495–0400; Robert M. Krieger, Chief Executive Officer
Web address: www.pinecrestrehab.com

ST. MARY'S MEDICAL CENTER (O, 463 beds) 901 45th Street, West Palm Beach, FL Zip 33407–2495, Mailing Address: P.O. Box 24620, Zip 33416–4620; tel. 561/844–6300; Davide M. Carbone, Chief Executive Officer
Web address: www.stmarysmc.com

WEST BOCA MEDICAL CENTER (O, 185 beds) 21644 State Road 7, Boca Raton, FL Zip 33428–1899; tel. 561/488–8000; Walt Mickens, Chief Executive Officer
Web address: www.westbocamedctr.com

GEORGIA: ATLANTA MEDICAL CENTER (O, 403 beds) 303 Parkway Drive N.E., Atlanta, GA Zip 30312–1212; tel. 404/265–4000; William T. Moore, Chief Executive Officer
Web address: www.atlantamedcenter.com

NORTH FULTON REGIONAL HOSPITAL (L, 195 beds) 3000 Hospital Boulevard, Roswell, GA Zip 30076–3899; tel. 770/751–2500; Joe Austin, Chief Executive Officer
Web address: www.northfultonregional.com

SOUTH FULTON MEDICAL CENTER (O, 260 beds) 1170 Cleveland Avenue, Atlanta, GA Zip 30344–3665; tel. 404/466–1170; James Clements, Chief Executive Officer
Web address: www.southfultonmedicalcenter.com

SPALDING REGIONAL MEDICAL CENTER (O, 160 beds) 601 South Eighth Street, Griffin, GA Zip 30224–4294, Mailing Address: P.O. Drawer V, Zip 30224–1168; tel. 770/228–2721; John A. Quinn, Chief Executive Officer
Web address: www.spaldingregional.com

SYLVAN GROVE HOSPITAL (L, 21 beds) 1050 McDonough Road, Jackson, GA Zip 30233–1599; tel. 770/775–7861; John A. Quinn, Chief Executive Officer
Web address: www.sylvangrovehospital.com

LOUISIANA: NORTHSHORE REGIONAL MEDICAL CENTER (L, 165 beds) 100 Medical Center Drive, Slidell, LA Zip 70461–8572; tel. 985/646–5025; Alan Cason, Chief Executive Officer
Web address: www.northshoremedctr.com

MISSOURI: DES PERES HOSPITAL (O, 143 beds) 2345 Dougherty Ferry Road, Saint Louis, MO Zip 63122–3313; tel. 314/966–9100; Michele C. Meyer, Chief Executive Officer
Web address: www.despereshospital.com

SAINT LOUIS UNIVERSITY HOSPITAL (O, 332 beds) 3635 Vista at Grand Boulevard, Saint Louis, MO Zip 63110–0250, Mailing Address: P.O. Box 15250, Zip 63110–0250; tel. 314/577–8000; Crystal L. Haynes, Chief Executive Officer
Web address: www.sluhospital.com

NEBRASKA: CREIGHTON UNIVERSITY MEDICAL CENTER (O, 334 beds) 601 North 30th Street, Omaha, NE Zip 68131–2197; tel. 402/449–5021; Linda Neu Ollis, FACHE, Administrator and Chief Operating Officer
Web address: www.saintjosephhospital.com

NORTH CAROLINA: CENTRAL CAROLINA HOSPITAL (O, 129 beds) 1135 Carthage Street, Sanford, NC Zip 27330–4111; tel. 919/774–2100; Doug Doris, Chief Executive Officer
Web address: www.centralcarolinahosp.com

FRYE REGIONAL MEDICAL CENTER (L, 322 beds) 420 North Center Street, Hickory, NC Zip 28601–5049; tel. 828/322–6070; Michael R. Blackburn, Chief Executive Officer
Web address: www.fryemedctr.com

PENNSYLVANIA: HAHNEMANN UNIVERSITY HOSPITAL (O, 483 beds) Broad and Vine Streets, Philadelphia, PA Zip 19102–1192; tel. 215/762–7000; Michael P. Halter, Chief Executive Officer
Web address: www.hahnemannhospital.com

ST. CHRISTOPHER'S HOSPITAL FOR CHILDREN (O, 124 beds) Erie Avenue at Front Street, Philadelphia, PA Zip 19134–1095; tel. 215/427–5000; Bernadette M. Mangan, Chief Executive Officer
Web address: www.stchristophershospital.com

SOUTH CAROLINA: COASTAL CAROLINA HOSPITAL (O, 41 beds) 1000 Medical Center Drive, Hardeeville, SC Zip 29927; tel. 843/784–8000; Teresa C. Urquhart, Chief Executive Officer
Web address: www.coastalcarolinamedicalcenter.com

EAST COOPER REGIONAL MEDICAL CENTER (O, 106 beds) 1200 Johnnie Dodds Boulevard, Mount Pleasant, SC Zip 29464–3294; tel. 843/881–0100; Andrea L. Wozniak, RN, FACHE, Chief Executive Officer
Web address: www.eastcoopermedctr.com

HILTON HEAD HOSPITAL (O, 93 beds) 25 Hospital Center Boulevard, Hilton Head Island, SC Zip 29926–2738, Mailing Address: P.O. Box 21117, Zip 29925–1117; tel. 843/681–6122; Elizabeth Lamkin, President and Chief Executive Officer
Web address: www.hiltonheadregional.com

PIEDMONT MEDICAL CENTER (O, 266 beds) 222 Herlong Avenue, Rock Hill, SC Zip 29732–1952; tel. 803/329–1234; Charles F. Miller, President and Chief Executive Officer
Web address: www.piedmonthealth.com

TENNESSEE: SAINT FRANCIS HOSPITAL (O, 533 beds) 5959 Park Avenue, Memphis, TN Zip 38119–5198, Mailing Address: P.O. Box 171808, Zip 38187–1808; tel. 901/765–1000; David L. Archer, Chief Executive Officer
Web address: www.saintfrancishosp.com

SAINT FRANCIS HOSPITAL–BARTLETT (O, 100 beds) 2986 Kate Bond Road, Bartlett, TN Zip 38133–4003; tel. 901/820–7000; Kem Mullins, Chief Executive Officer
Web address: www.saintfrancisbartlett.com

TEXAS: CENTENNIAL MEDICAL CENTER (O, 108 beds) 12505 Lebanon Road, Frisco, TX Zip 75035–8298; tel. 972/963–3333; William C. Henning, Chief Executive Officer
Web address: www.centennialmedcenter.com

CYPRESS FAIRBANKS MEDICAL CENTER (O, 170 beds) 10655 Steepletop Drive, Houston, TX Zip 77065–4297; tel. 281/890–4285; Terry J. Wheeler, Chief Executive Officer
Web address: www.cyfairhospital.com

DOCTORS HOSPITAL AT WHITE ROCK LAKE (O, 156 beds) 9440 Poppy Drive, Dallas, TX Zip 75218–3694; tel. 214/324–6100; Mitch Edgeworth, Chief Executive Officer
Web address: www.doctorshospitaldallas.com

HOUSTON NORTHWEST MEDICAL CENTER (O, 369 beds) 710 FM 1960 West, Houston, TX Zip 77090–3496; tel. 281/440–1000; Drew Kahn, Chief Executive Officer
Web address: www.hnmc.com

LAKE POINTE MEDICAL CENTER (O, 112 beds) 6800 Scenic Drive, Rowlett, TX Zip 75088–4552, Mailing Address: P.O. Box 1550, Zip 75030–1550; tel. 972/412–2273; Carolyn Jackson, Chief Executive Officer
Web address: www.lakepointemedical.com

Section B

For explanation of codes following names, see page B2.
★ Indicates Type III membership in the American Hospital Association.

NACOGDOCHES MEDICAL CENTER (O, 109 beds) 4920 N.E. Stallings, Nacogdoches, TX Zip 75965–1200, Mailing Address: P.O. Box 631604, Zip 75963–1604; tel. 936/569–9481; Gary L. Stokes, Chief Executive Officer
Web address: www.nacmedicalcenter.com

PARK PLAZA HOSPITAL (O, 218 beds) 1313 Hermann Drive, Houston, TX Zip 77004–7092; tel. 713/527–5000; Phillip E. Sowa, Chief Executive Officer
Web address: www.parkplazahospital.com

PLAZA SPECIALTY HOSPITAL (O, 57 beds) 1300 Binz, Houston, TX Zip 77004; tel. 713/285–1000; Steven Barr, Chief Executive Officer
Web address: www.plazaspecialtyhospital.com

PROVIDENCE MEMORIAL HOSPITAL (O, 359 beds) 2001 North Oregon Street, El Paso, TX Zip 79902–3368; tel. 915/577–6011; Irene Chavez, Chief Executive Officer
Web address: www.sphn.com

SIERRA MEDICAL CENTER (O, 334 beds) 1625 Medical Center Drive, El Paso, TX Zip 79902–5044; tel. 915/747–4000; Edmundo Castaneda, Chief Executive Officer
Web address: www.sphn.com

SIERRA PROVIDENCE PHYSICAL REHABILITATION HOSPITAL (O, 42 beds) 1740 Curie Drive, El Paso, TX Zip 79902–2900; tel. 915/544–3399; John Harris, President
Web address: www.sphn.com

Owned, leased, sponsored:	57 hospitals	12874 beds
Contract-managed:	0 hospitals	0 beds
Totals:	57 hospitals	12874 beds

0020: TEXAS DEPARTMENT OF STATE HEALTH SERVICES (NP)
1100 West 49th Street, Austin, TX Zip 78756–3199; tel. 512/458–7111; David L. Lakey, M.D., Commissioner
(Independent Hospital System)

AUSTIN STATE HOSPITAL (O, 299 beds) 4110 Guadalupe Street, Austin, TX Zip 78751–4296; tel. 512/452–0381; Carl Schock, Superintendent
Web address: www.mhmr.state.tx.us

BIG SPRING STATE HOSPITAL (O, 200 beds) 1901 North Highway 87, Big Spring, TX Zip 79720; tel. 432/267–8216; Edward Moughon, Superintendent
Web address: www.dshs.state.tx.us/mhhospitals/bigspringSH/bigspringsh.html

EL PASO PSYCHIATRIC CENTER (O, 74 beds) 4615 Alameda Avenue, El Paso, TX Zip 79905–2702; tel. 915/532–2202; Zulema Carrillo, Chief Executive Officer

KERRVILLE STATE HOSPITAL (O, 202 beds) 721 Thompson Drive, Kerrville, TX Zip 78028–5154; tel. 830/896–2211; Stephen R. Anfinson, Superintendent
Web address: www.dshs.state.tx.us/lmhhospitals/kerrvillesh

NORTH TEXAS STATE HOSPITAL (O, 616 beds) Highway 70 Northwest, Vernon, TX Zip 76384, Mailing Address: P.O. Box 2231, Zip 76384–2231; tel. 940/552–9901; James E. Smith, Superintendent
Web address: www.mhmr.state.tx.us

RIO GRANDE STATE CENTER/SOUTH TEXAS HEALTH CARE SYSTEM (O, 132 beds) 1401 South Rangerville Road, Harlingen, TX Zip 78552–7638; tel. 956/364–8000; Sonia Hernandez-Keeble, Superintendent
Web address: www.dshs.state.tx.us/mhospital/riograndesc/default.shtm

RUSK STATE HOSPITAL (O, 335 beds) Jacksonville Highway North, Rusk, TX Zip 75785, Mailing Address: P.O. Box 318, Zip 75785–0318; tel. 903/683–3421; Ted Debbs, Administrator
Web address: www.mhmr.state.tx.us/hospitals/rusksh/rusksh.html

SAN ANTONIO STATE HOSPITAL (O, 302 beds) 6711 South New Braunfels, Suite 100, San Antonio, TX Zip 78223–3006; tel. 210/531–7711; Robert C. Arizpe, Superintendent
Web address: www.dshs.state.tx.us

TERRELL STATE HOSPITAL (O, 316 beds) 1200 East Brin Street, Terrell, TX Zip 75160–2938; tel. 972/524–6452; Fred Hale, Superintendent
Web address: www.dshs.state.tx.us

TEXAS CENTER FOR INFECTIOUS DISEASE (O, 72 beds) 2303 S.E. Military Drive, San Antonio, TX Zip 78223–3597; tel. 210/534–8857; James N. Elkins, FACHE, Director
Web address: www.dshs.state.tx.us/tcid/default/shtm

Owned, leased, sponsored:	10 hospitals	2548 beds
Contract-managed:	0 hospitals	0 beds
Totals:	10 hospitals	2548 beds

★0129: TEXAS HEALTH RESOURCES (NP)
612 East Lamar Boulevard, Suite 900, Arlington, TX Zip 76011; tel. 817/462–7900; Douglas D. Hawthorne, FACHE, Chief Executive Officer
(Decentralized Health System)

HARRIS CONTINUED CARE HOSPITAL (O, 10 beds) 1301 Pennsylvania Avenue, 4th Floor, Fort Worth, TX Zip 76104–2190; tel. 817/250–5500; Susan Louise Baldwin, RN, FACHE, President and Chief Nursing Officer
Web address: www.texashealth.org

TEXAS HEALTH ARLINGTON MEMORIAL HOSPITAL (O, 344 beds) 800 West Randol Mill Road, Arlington, TX Zip 76012–2503; tel. 817/548–6100; Kirk King, CHE, President
Web address: www.arlingtonmemorial.org

TEXAS HEALTH HARRIS METHODIST FORT WORTH (O, 603 beds) 1301 Pennsylvania Avenue, Fort Worth, TX Zip 76104–2895; tel. 817/250–2000; Oscar Amparan, President
Web address: www.texashealth.org

TEXAS HEALTH HARRIS METHODIST NORTHWEST (O, 31 beds) 108 Denver Trail, Azle, TX Zip 76020–3697; tel. 817/444–8600; Winjie Tang Miao, President
Web address: www.harrismethodisthospitals.org

TEXAS HEALTH HARRIS METHODIST SOUTHWEST (O, 156 beds) 6100 Harris Parkway, Fort Worth, TX Zip 76132–4199; tel. 817/433–6550; Brett McClung, President
Web address: www.texashealth.org

TEXAS HEALTH HARRIS METHODIST–ERATH COUNTY (O, 57 beds) 411 North Belknap Street, Stephenville, TX Zip 76401–3415, Mailing Address: P.O. Box 1399, Zip 76401–1399; tel. 254/965–1500; Christopher Leu, Chief Executive Officer
Web address: www.texashealth.org

TEXAS HEALTH HARRIS METHODIST–HEB (O, 228 beds) 1600 Hospital Parkway, Bedford, TX Zip 76022–6913, Mailing Address: P.O. Box 669, Zip 76095–0669; tel. 817/685–4000; Deborah Paganelli, CHE, President
Web address: www.texashealth.org

TEXAS HEALTH PRESBYTERIAN HOSPITAL OF ALLEN (O, 62 beds) 1105 Central Expressway North, Allen, TX Zip 75013; tel. 972/747–1000; Sheila A. McKinney, President
Web address: www.texashealth.org

TEXAS HEALTH PRESBYTERIAN HOSPITAL OF DALLAS (O, 655 beds) 8200 Walnut Hill Lane, Dallas, TX Zip 75231–4402; tel. 214/345–6789; Mark H. Merrill, President
Web address: www.texashealth.org

TEXAS HEALTH PRESBYTERIAN HOSPITAL OF KAUFMAN (O, 68 beds) 850 Highway 243 West, Kaufman, TX Zip 75142, Mailing Address: P.O. Box 1108, Zip 75142–1108; tel. 972/932–7200; Patsy Youngs, President
Web address: www.texashealth.org

TEXAS HEALTH PRESBYTERIAN HOSPITAL OF PLANO (O, 342 beds) 6200 West Parker Road, Plano, TX Zip 75093–7914; tel. 972/981–8000; Philip M. Wentworth, FACHE, President
Web address: www.texashealth.org

TEXAS HEALTH PRESBYTERIAN HOSPITAL OF WINNSBORO (O, 35 beds) 719 West Coke Road, Winnsboro, TX Zip 75494–0628, Mailing Address: P.O. Box 628, Zip 75494–0628; tel. 903/342–5227; Michael Sinclair, Administrator
Web address: www.texashealth.org

WALLS REGIONAL HOSPITAL (O, 48 beds) 201 Walls Drive, Cleburne, TX Zip 76033–4008; tel. 817/641–2551; Blake Kretz, President
Web address: www.texashealth.org

Owned, leased, sponsored:	13 hospitals	2639 beds
Contract-managed:	0 hospitals	0 beds
Totals:	13 hospitals	2639 beds

For explanation of codes following names, see page B2.
★ Indicates Type III membership in the American Hospital Association.

★7235: THE METHODIST HOSPITAL SYSTEM (CO)
6565 Fannin Street, D–200, Houston, TX Zip 77030–2707; tel. 713/441–2221; Ronald G. Girotto, President and Chief Executive Officer
(Independent Hospital System)

METHODIST SUGAR LAND HOSPITAL (O, 54 beds) 16655 S.W. Freeway, Sugar Land, TX Zip 77479–2343; tel. 281/274–7000; Christopher Siebenaler, Acting Administrator and Chief Executive Officer
Web address: www.methodisthealth.com

METHODIST WILLOWBROOK HOSPITAL (O, 119 beds) 18220 Tomball Parkway, Houston, TX Zip 77070; tel. 281/477–1000; Andrew Cochrane, Chief Executive Officer
Web address: www.methodisthealth.com

SAN JACINTO METHODIST HOSPITAL (O, 268 beds) 4401 Garth Road, Baytown, TX Zip 77521–3160; tel. 281/420–8600; Donna Gares, RN, Interim President and Chief Executive Officer
Web address: www.methodisthealth.com

THE METHODIST HOSPITAL (O, 966 beds) 6565 Fannin Street, Houston, TX Zip 77030–2707; tel. 713/790–3311; Ronald G. Girotto, President and Chief Executive Officer
Web address: www.methodisthealth.com

Owned, leased, sponsored:	4 hospitals	1407 beds
Contract–managed:	0 hospitals	0 beds
Totals:	4 hospitals	1407 beds

0346: THE SCHUSTER GROUP (IO)
3555 N.W. 58th Street, Suite 1000, Oklahoma City, OK Zip 73112; tel. 405/917–0300; Mike Schuster, President and Chief Executive Officer
(Independent Hospital System)

OKLAHOMA: JOHNSTON MEMORIAL HOSPITAL (O, 21 beds) 1000 South Byrd Street, Tishomingo, OK Zip 73460–3299; tel. 580/371–2327; Mary Owen, RN, Administrator

PHYSICIANS' HOSPITAL IN ANADARKO (O, 25 beds) 1002 Central Boulevard East, Anadarko, OK Zip 73005–4496; tel. 405/247–2551; Joe Swart, Administrator

PRAGUE MUNICIPAL HOSPITAL (O, 19 beds) 1322 Klabzuba Avenue, Prague, OK Zip 74864–9005, Mailing Address: P.O. Drawer S, Zip 74864–9005; tel. 405/567–4922; Joan Walters, RN, M.S.N., Administrator
Web address: www.praguehospital.com

STROUD REGIONAL MEDICAL CENTER (C, 22 beds) Highway 66 West, Stroud, OK Zip 74079, Mailing Address: P.O. Box 530, Zip 74079–0530; tel. 918/968–3571; Beverly Ash, Chief Executive Officer

Owned, leased, sponsored:	3 hospitals	65 beds
Contract–managed:	1 hospital	22 beds
Totals:	4 hospitals	87 beds

2445: THEDACARE, INC. (NP)
122 East College Avenue, Appleton, WI Zip 54911, Mailing Address: P.O. Box 8025, Zip 54912; tel. 920/830–5880; John S. Toussaint, M.D., President and Chief Executive Officer
(Centralized Physician/Insurance Health System)

WISCONSIN: APPLETON MEDICAL CENTER (O, 142 beds) 1818 North Meade Street, Appleton, WI Zip 54911–3496; tel. 920/731–4101; Kathryn Correia, Senior Vice President
Web address: www.thedacare.org

NEW LONDON FAMILY MEDICAL CENTER (O, 25 beds) 1405 Mill Street, New London, WI Zip 54961–2155, Mailing Address: P.O. Box 307, Zip 54961–0307; tel. 920/531–2000; William Schmidt, President and Chief Executive Officer
Web address: www.newlondon.thedacare.org

THEDA CLARK MEDICAL CENTER (O, 168 beds) 130 Second Street, Neenah, WI Zip 54956–2883, Mailing Address: P.O. Box 2021, Zip 54957–2021; tel. 920/729–3100; Kathryn Correia, Senior Vice President
Web address: www.thedacare.org

Owned, leased, sponsored:	3 hospitals	335 beds
Contract–managed:	0 hospitals	0 beds
Totals:	3 hospitals	335 beds

0354: TLC HEALTH NETWORK (NP)
100 Memorial Drive, Gowanda, NY Zip 14070; tel. 716/532–3377; Louis J. Frascella, President and Chief Executive Officer
(Independent Hospital System)

NEW YORK: LAKE SHORE HEALTH CARE CENTER (O, 576 beds) 845 Route 5 and 20, Irving, NY Zip 14081–9716; tel. 716/951–7000; Louis J. Frascella, President and Chief Executive Officer
Web address: www.tlchealth.org

TRI–COUNTY MEMORIAL HOSPITAL (O, 576 beds) 100 Memorial Drive, Gowanda, NY Zip 14070–1194; tel. 716/532–3377; Louis J. Frascella, President and Chief Executive Officer
Web address: www.tlchealth.org

Owned, leased, sponsored:	2 hospitals	1152 beds
Contract–managed:	0 hospitals	0 beds
Totals:	2 hospitals	1152 beds

★0219: TRINITY HEALTH (CC)
27870 Cabot Drive, Novi, MI Zip 48377; tel. 248/489–5004; Joseph R. Swedish, President and Chief Executive Officer
(Decentralized Health System)

CALIFORNIA: SAINT AGNES MEDICAL CENTER (O, 434 beds) 1303 East Herndon Avenue, Fresno, CA Zip 93720–3309; tel. 559/450–3000; Thomas E. Anderson, President and Chief Executive Officer
Web address: www.samc.com

IDAHO: CASCADE MEDICAL CENTER (C, 10 beds) 402 Old State Highway, Cascade, ID Zip 83611, Mailing Address: P.O. Box 1330, Zip 83611–1330; tel. 208/382–4242; William C. Behnke, Jr., Administrator

SAINT ALPHONSUS REGIONAL MEDICAL CENTER (O, 351 beds) 1055 North Curtis Road, Boise, ID Zip 83706–1370; tel. 208/367–2121; Sandra B. Bruce, President and Chief Executive Officer
Web address: www.saintalphonsus.org

ILLINOIS: MORRISON COMMUNITY HOSPITAL (C, 60 beds) 303 North Jackson Street, Morrison, IL Zip 61270–3042; tel. 815/772–4003; John R. Perushek, Chief Executive Officer

INDIANA: SAINT JOSEPH REGIONAL MEDICAL CENTER (O, 267 beds) 801 East LaSalle, South Bend, IN Zip 46617–2800; tel. 574/237–7111; Lori Price, Chief Operating Officer
Web address: www.sjmed.com

SAINT JOSEPH REGIONAL MEDICAL CENTER–MISHAWAKA CAMPUS (O, 78 beds) 215 West Fourth Street, Mishawaka, IN Zip 46544–1999; tel. 574/259–2431; Steven A. Rose, RN, Executive Vice President
Web address: www.sjmed.com

SAINT JOSEPH REGIONAL MEDICAL CENTER–PLYMOUTH CAMPUS (O, 45 beds) 1915 Lake Avenue, Plymouth, IN Zip 46563–9905, Mailing Address: P.O. Box 670, Zip 46563–9905; tel. 574/936–3181; Nancy R. Hellyer, Chief Executive Officer
Web address: www.sjmed.com

IOWA: BAUM HARMON MERCY HOSPITAL (O, 13 beds) 255 North Welch Avenue, Primghar, IA Zip 51245–1034, Mailing Address: P.O. Box 528, Zip 51245–0528; tel. 712/957–2300; Robert Monical, Chief Executive Officer and Administrator
Web address: www.baumharmon.org

BELMOND MEDICAL CENTER (C, 22 beds) 403 First Street S.E., Belmond, IA Zip 50421–1201; tel. 641/444–3223; Nancy Gabrielson, Administrator
Web address: www.belmondmedicalcenter.com

CENTRAL COMMUNITY HOSPITAL (C, 16 beds) 901 Davidson Street N.W., Elkader, IA Zip 52043–9015; tel. 563/245–7000; Frances J. Zichal, Chief Executive Officer
Web address: www.centralcommunityhospital.com

ELLSWORTH MUNICIPAL HOSPITAL (C, 35 beds) 110 Rocksylvania Avenue, Iowa Falls, IA Zip 50126–2400; tel. 641/648–4631; John O'Brien, Administrator
Web address: www.emhia.com

For explanation of codes following names, see page B2.
★ Indicates Type III membership in the American Hospital Association.

FRANKLIN GENERAL HOSPITAL (C, 77 beds) 1720 Central Avenue East, Hampton, IA Zip 50441–1859; tel. 641/456–5000; Mark Klosterman, Chief Executive Officer
Web address: www.franklingeneral.com

HANCOCK COUNTY MEMORIAL HOSPITAL (C, 25 beds) 532 First Street N.W., Britt, IA Zip 50423; tel. 641/843–5000; Vance Jackson, FACHE, Administrator and Chief Executive Officer
Web address: www.hancockmemhospital.com

HAWARDEN COMMUNITY HOSPITAL (C, 18 beds) 1111 11th Street, Hawarden, IA Zip 51023–1999; tel. 712/551–3100; Chad Markham, Chief Executive Officer
Web address: www.hawardencommunityhospital.org

KOSSUTH REGIONAL HEALTH CENTER (C, 22 beds) 1515 South Phillips Street, Algona, IA Zip 50511–3649; tel. 515/295–2451; Scott A. Curtis, Administrator and Chief Executive Officer
Web address: www.krhc.com

MERCY MEDICAL CENTER–CLINTON (O, 341 beds) 1410 North Fourth Street, Clinton, IA Zip 52732–2940; tel. 563/244–5555; Donna M. Oliver, President and Chief Executive Officer
Web address: www.mercyclinton.com

MERCY MEDICAL CENTER–DUBUQUE (O, 303 beds) 250 Mercy Drive, Dubuque, IA Zip 52001–7360; tel. 563/589–8000; Russell M. Knight, President and Chief Executive Officer
Web address: www.mercydubuque.com

MERCY MEDICAL CENTER–DYERSVILLE (S, 25 beds) 1111 Third Street S.W., Dyersville, IA Zip 52040; tel. 319/875–7101; Russell M. Knight, President and Chief Executive Officer
Web address: www.mercydubuque.com/dyersville

MERCY MEDICAL CENTER–NEW HAMPTON (O, 18 beds) 308 North Maple Avenue, New Hampton, IA Zip 50659–1142; tel. 641/394–4121; Bruce Roesler, Chief Executive Officer
Web address: www.mercynewhampton.com

MERCY MEDICAL CENTER–NORTH IOWA (O, 241 beds) 1000 Fourth Street S.W., Mason City, IA Zip 50401–2800; tel. 641/422–7000; James G. FitzPatrick, President and Chief Executive Officer
Web address: www.mercynorthiowa.com

MERCY MEDICAL CENTER–SIOUX CITY (O, 258 beds) 801 Fifth Street, Sioux City, IA Zip 51101–1326, Mailing Address: P.O. Box 3168, Zip 51102–3168; tel. 712/279–2010; Paul Dougherty, President and Chief Executive Officer
Web address: www.mercysiouxcity.com

MITCHELL COUNTY REGIONAL HEALTH CENTER (C, 25 beds) 616 North Eighth Street, Osage, IA Zip 50461–1498; tel. 641/732–6000; Sandy Leggett, Chief Executive Officer
Web address: www.mitchellcohospital–clinics.com

PALO ALTO COUNTY HEALTH SYSTEM (C, 47 beds) 3201 First Street, Emmetsburg, IA Zip 50536; tel. 712/852–5500; Thomas J. Lee, Chief Executive Officer
Web address: www.pachs.com

REGIONAL HEALTH SERVICES OF HOWARD COUNTY (C, 25 beds) 235 Eighth Avenue West, Cresco, IA Zip 52136–1098; tel. 563/547–2101; David Hartberg, Chief Executive Officer
Web address: www.rhshc.com

MARYLAND: HOLY CROSS HOSPITAL (O, 425 beds) 1500 Forest Glen Road, Silver Spring, MD Zip 20910–1487; tel. 301/754–7000; Kevin J. Sexton, President and Chief Executive Officer
Web address: www.holycrosshealth.org

MICHIGAN: BATTLE CREEK HEALTH SYSTEM (O, 211 beds) Battle Creek, MI tel. 269/966–8000; Patrick R. Garrett, President and Chief Executive Officer
Web address: www.bchealth.com

MERCY HEALTH PARTNERS (O, 230 beds) 1500 East Sherman Boulevard, Muskegon, MI Zip 49443; tel. 231/672–2000; Roger Spoelman, President and Chief Executive Officer
Web address: www.mghp.com

MERCY HOSPITAL (O, 119 beds) 2601 Electric Avenue, Port Huron, MI Zip 48060–6518; tel. 810/985–1500; Peter Karadjoff, President and Chief Executive Officer
Web address: www.mercyporthuron.com

MERCY HOSPITAL CADILLAC (O, 65 beds) 400 Hobart Street, Cadillac, MI Zip 49601–9596; tel. 231/876–7200; John L. MacLeod, President and Chief Executive Officer
Web address: www.munsonhealthcare.org

MERCY HOSPITAL GRAYLING (O, 95 beds) 1100 East Michigan Avenue, Grayling, MI Zip 49738–1398; tel. 989/348–5461; Stephanie J. Riemer–Matuzak, Chief Executive Officer
Web address: www.mercygrayling.munsonhealthcare.org

SAINT JOSEPH MERCY LIVINGSTON HOSPITAL (O, 83 beds) 620 Byron Road, Howell, MI Zip 48843–1093; tel. 517/545–6000; Garry C. Faja, President and Chief Executive Officer
Web address: www.sjmh.com/who/mcphersn.shtml

SAINT JOSEPH MERCY SALINE HOSPITAL (O, 40 beds) 400 West Russell Street, Saline, MI Zip 48176–1101; tel. 734/429–1500; Kathleen Rhine, Executive Director
Web address: www.sjmercyhealth.org

SAINT MARY'S HEALTH CARE (O, 336 beds) 200 Jefferson Avenue S.E., Grand Rapids, MI Zip 49503–4598; tel. 616/685–6090; Philip H. McCorkle, Jr., President and Chief Executive Officer
Web address: www.smhealthcare.org

ST. JOSEPH MERCY HOSPITAL (O, 529 beds) 5301 McAuley Drive, Ypsilanti, MI Zip 48197, Mailing Address: P.O. Box 995, Ann Arbor, Zip 48106–0995; tel. 734/712–3456; Garry C. Faja, President and Chief Executive Officer
Web address: www.sjmercyhealth.org

ST. JOSEPH MERCY OAKLAND (O, 403 beds) 44405 Woodward Avenue, Pontiac, MI Zip 48341–2985; tel. 248/858–3000; Jack Weiner, President and Chief Executive Officer
Web address: www.stjoesoakland.com

ST. MARY MERCY HOSPITAL (O, 293 beds) 36475 West Five Mile Road, Livonia, MI Zip 48154–1988; tel. 734/655–4800; David A. Spivey, President and Chief Executive Officer
Web address: www.stmarymercy.org

NEBRASKA: OAKLAND MERCY HOSPITAL (O, 18 beds) 601 East Second Street, Oakland, NE Zip 68045–1499; tel. 402/685–5601; Timothy Fischer, Administrator and Chief Executive Officer
Web address: www.oaklandhospital.org

PENDER COMMUNITY HOSPITAL (C, 137 beds) 603 Earl Street, Pender, NE Zip 68047–0100, Mailing Address: P.O. Box 100, Zip 68047–0100; tel. 402/385–3083; Michael Hansen, FACHE, Administrator and Chief Executive Officer
Web address: www.pendercommunityhospital.com

OHIO: FAYETTE COUNTY MEMORIAL HOSPITAL (C, 25 beds) 1430 Columbus Avenue, Washington Court House, OH Zip 43160–1791; tel. 740/335–1210; Lyndon J. Christman, Administrator
Web address: www.fcmh.org

MOUNT CARMEL (O, 760 beds) Columbus, OH Mailing Address: 793 West State Street, Zip 43222–1551; tel. 614/234–5000; Claus von Zychlin, President and Chief Executive Officer
Web address: www.mountcarmelhealth.com

MOUNT CARMEL NEW ALBANY SURGICAL HOSPITAL (O, 42 beds) 7333 Smith's Mill Road, New Albany, OH Zip 43054; tel. 614/775–6600; Richard D'Enbeau, Chief Operating Officer
Web address: www.newalbanysurgicalhospital.com

MOUNT CARMEL ST. ANN'S (O, 273 beds) 500 South Cleveland Avenue, Westerville, OH Zip 43081–8998; tel. 614/898–4000; Claus von Zychlin, Executive Vice President and Chief Operating Officer
Web address: www.mountcarmelhealth.com

Owned, leased, sponsored:	28 hospitals	6296 beds
Contract–managed:	14 hospitals	544 beds
Totals:	42 hospitals	6840 beds

0319: TRIUMPH HEALTHCARE (IO)

7333 North Freeway, Suite 500, Houston, TX Zip 77076; tel. 713/807–8686; Charles Allen, President and Chief Executive
(Independent Hospital System)

COLORADO: TRIUMPH HOSPITAL AURORA (O, 29 beds) 700 Potomac Street, Aurora, CO Zip 80012; tel. 720/857–8333; Jay Quebedeaux, Chief Executive Officer
Web address: www.triumph–healthcare.com

MICHIGAN: TRIUMPH HOSPITAL DETROIT (O, 65 beds) 4777 East Outer Drive, Detroit, MI Zip 48234; tel. 313/369–5800; Kim Knight, Chief Executive Officer
Web address: www.triumph–healthcare.com

For explanation of codes following names, see page B2.
★ Indicates Type III membership in the American Hospital Association.

NORTH DAKOTA: TRIUMPH HOSPITAL – CENTRAL DAKOTAS (O, 41 beds) 1000 18th Street N.W., Mandan, ND Zip 58554; tel. 701/667–2000; Cora Pifer, Chief Executive Officer
Web address: www.triumph–healthcare.com

TRIUMPH HOSPITAL – FARGO (O, 31 beds) 1720 University Drive South, Fargo, ND Zip 58103; tel. 701/241–9099; Custer Huseby, Chief Executive Officer
Web address: www.triumph–healthcare.com

OHIO: TRIUMPH HOSPITAL LIMA (O, 26 beds) 730 West Market Street, 6th Floor, Lima, OH Zip 45801; tel. 419/224–1888; Kimberly Thomas, Chief Executive Officer
Web address: www.triumph–healthcare.com

TRIUMPH HOSPITAL MANSFIELD (O, 17 beds) 335 Glessner Avenue, 5th Floor, Mansfield, OH Zip 44903; tel. 419/526–0777; Kimberly Thomas, Chief Executive Officer
Web address: www.triumph–healthcare.com

PENNSYLVANIA: TRIUMPH HOSPITAL EASTON (O, 31 beds) 250 South 21st Street, 3rd Floor, Easton, PA Zip 18042; tel. 610/250–4724; Linda Luther, Chief Executive Officer
Web address: www.triumph–healthcare.com

TEXAS: MEMORIAL HERMANN CONTINUING CARE HOSPITAL (L, 191 beds) 3043 Gessner Drive, Houston, TX Zip 77080–2597; tel. 713/462–2515; Joe G. Baldwin, Chief Executive Officer
Web address: www.memorialhermann.org

TRIUMPH HOSPITAL AMARILLO (O, 97 beds) 2828 West 27th Avenue, Amarillo, TX Zip 79109; tel. 806/351–1600; Ronda L. Crow, RN, Chief Executive Officer
Web address: www.triumph–healthcare.com

TRIUMPH HOSPITAL CENTRAL (O, 38 beds) 105 Drew Avenue, Houston, TX Zip 77006; tel. 713/529–8922; Claudia McCready, Chief Executive Officer
Web address: www.triumph–healthcare.com

TRIUMPH HOSPITAL EAST HOUSTON (O, 230 beds) 15101 East Freeway, Channelview, TX Zip 77530; tel. 832/200–5500; Mike Files, Chief Executive Officer
Web address: www.triumph–healthcare.com

TRIUMPH HOSPITAL EL PASO (O, 29 beds) 1740 Curie Drive, El Paso, TX Zip 79902; tel. 915/351–9044; Jay Quintana, Chief Executive Officer
Web address: www.triumph–healthcare.com

TRIUMPH HOSPITAL NORTH HOUSTON (O, 130 beds) 7407 North Freeway, Houston, TX Zip 77076; tel. 832/200–6000; Michael R. Bullard, Chief Executive Officer
Web address: www.triumph–healthcare.com

TRIUMPH HOSPITAL NORTHWEST (O, 190 beds) 205 Hollow Tree Lane, Houston, TX Zip 77090; tel. 832/249–2700; Bob Stein, Chief Executive Officer

TRIUMPH HOSPITAL OF VICTORIA (O, 23 beds) 506 East San Antonio Street, 3rd Floor, Victoria, TX Zip 77901–6060, Mailing Address: 506 East San Antonio Street, 3rd Floor, Zip 77901–6060; tel. 361/575–1445; Tammy Barben, Chief Executive Officer
Web address: www.triumph–healthcare.com

TRIUMPH HOSPITAL SAN ANGELO (O, 28 beds) 120 East Harris Avenue, 6th Floor, San Angelo, TX Zip 76903; tel. 325/659–3906; Steve Grappe, Chief Executive Officer
Web address: www.triumph–healthcare.com

TRIUMPH HOSPITAL SOUTHWEST (O, 150 beds) 1550 First Colony Boulevard, Sugar Land, TX Zip 77479; tel. 281/275–6000; Michele Dionne, President and Chief Executive Officer
Web address: www.triumph–healthcare.com

Owned, leased, sponsored:	17 hospitals	1346 beds
Contract–managed:	0 hospitals	0 beds
Totals:	17 hospitals	1346 beds

★9255: TRUMAN MEDICAL CENTERS (NP)

2301 Holmes Street, Kansas City, MO Zip 64108–2677; tel. 816/404–1000; John W. Bluford, President and Chief Executive Officer
(Moderately Centralized Health System)

MISSOURI: TRUMAN MEDICAL CENTER–HOSPITAL HILL (O, 229 beds) 2301 Holmes Street, Kansas City, MO Zip 64108–2640; tel. 816/404–1000; John W. Bluford, President and Chief Executive Officer
Web address: www.trumed.org

TRUMAN MEDICAL CENTER–LAKEWOOD (O, 301 beds) 7900 Lee's Summit Road, Kansas City, MO Zip 64139–1236; tel. 816/404–7000; John W. Bluford, President and Chief Executive Officer
Web address: www.trumanmed.org

Owned, leased, sponsored:	2 hospitals	530 beds
Contract–managed:	0 hospitals	0 beds
Totals:	2 hospitals	530 beds

0238: TY COBB HEALTHCARE SYSTEM, INC. (NP)

461 Cook Street, Suite A., Royston, GA Zip 30662, Mailing Address: P.O. Box 589, Zip 30662; tel. 706/245–1825; Charles T. Adams, Chief Executive Officer
(Independent Hospital System)

GEORGIA: COBB MEMORIAL HOSPITAL (O, 331 beds) 521 Franklin Springs Street, Royston, GA Zip 30662–3909, Mailing Address: P.O. Box 589, Zip 30662–0589; tel. 706/245–5071; John M. Herron, Administrator
Web address: www.tycobbhealthcare.org

HART COUNTY HOSPITAL (L, 174 beds) Gibson and Cade Streets, Hartwell, GA Zip 30643–0280, Mailing Address: P.O. Box 280, Zip 30643–0280; tel. 706/856–6100; Jerry R. Wise, Administrator and Vice President
Web address: www.tycobbhealthcare.org

Owned, leased, sponsored:	2 hospitals	505 beds
Contract–managed:	0 hospitals	0 beds
Totals:	2 hospitals	505 beds

9195: U. S. INDIAN HEALTH SERVICE (FG)

801 Thompson Avenue, Rockville, MD Zip 20852; tel. 301/443–1083; Major Robert McSwain, Acting Director
(Independent Hospital System)

ARIZONA: CHINLE COMPREHENSIVE HEALTH CARE FACILITY (O, 60 beds) Highway 191, Chinle, AZ Zip 86503, Mailing Address: P.O. Drawer PH, Zip 86503; tel. 928/674–7011; Ronald Tso, Chief Executive Officer
Web address: www.ihs.gov

FORT DEFIANCE INDIAN HEALTH SERVICE HOSPITAL (O, 39 beds) Fort Defiance, AZ Mailing Address: P.O. Box 649, Zip 86504–0649; tel. 928/729–8014; Franklin R. Freeland, Ed.D., Chief Executive Officer

HOPI HEALTH CARE CENTER (O, 15 beds) Keams Canyon, AZ Mailing Address: P.O. Box 4000, Polacca, Zip 86042; tel. 928/737–6000; Daryl Melvin, Chief Executive Officer
Web address: www.ihs.gov/index.asp

U. S. PUBLIC HEALTH SERVICE INDIAN HOSPITAL (O, 20 beds) Parker, AZ Mailing Address: Route 1, Box 12, Zip 85344; tel. 928/669–2137; Timothy Taylor, Chief Executive Officer
Web address: www.ihs.gov

U. S. PUBLIC HEALTH SERVICE INDIAN HOSPITAL (O, 34 beds) Sells, AZ Mailing Address: P.O. Box 548, Zip 85634–0548; tel. 520/383–7251; Priscilla Whitethorne, Service Unit Director
Web address: www.ihs.gov

U. S. PUBLIC HEALTH SERVICE INDIAN HOSPITAL (O, 8 beds) San Carlos, AZ Mailing Address: P.O. Box 208, Zip 85550–0208; tel. 928/475–2371; Nella J. Ben, Chief Executive Officer
Web address: www.ihs.gov

U. S. PUBLIC HEALTH SERVICE INDIAN HOSPITAL–WHITERIVER (O, 40 beds) 200 West Hospital Drive, Whiteriver, AZ Zip 85941–0860, Mailing Address: State Route 73, Box 860, Zip 85941–0860; tel. 928/338–4911; Michelle Martinez, Interim Chief Executive Officer
Web address: www.ihs.gov

U. S. PUBLIC HEALTH SERVICE PHOENIX INDIAN MEDICAL CENTER (O, 127 beds) 4212 North 16th Street, Phoenix, AZ Zip 85016–5389; tel. 602/263–1200; Vincent A. Berkley, M.D., Chief Executive Officer
Web address: www.ihs.gov

Section B

For explanation of codes following names, see page B2.
★ Indicates Type III membership in the American Hospital Association.

MARYLAND: NATIONAL INSTITUTES OF HEALTH CLINICAL CENTER (O, 234 beds) 9000 Rockville Pike, Building 10, Room 6–2551, Bethesda, MD Zip 20892–1504; tel. 301/496–4000; John I. Gallin, M.D., Director, NIH Clinical Center
Web address: www.clinicalcenter.nih.gov

MINNESOTA: U. S. PUBLIC HEALTH SERVICE INDIAN HOSPITAL (O, 11 beds) 7th Street and Grant Utley Avenue N.W., Cass Lake, MN Zip 56633, Mailing Address: Rural Route 3, Box 211, Zip 56633; tel. 218/335–3200; Earl Cournoyer, Interim Chief Executive Officer
Web address: www.ihs.gov

U.S. PUBLIC HEALTH SERVICE INDIAN HOSPITAL (O, 19 beds) Highway 1, Redlake, MN Zip 56671, Mailing Address: P.O. Box 497, Zip 56671–0497; tel. 218/679–3912; Constance James, Chief Executive Officer
Web address: www.ihs.gov

MONTANA: CROW/NORTHERN CHEYENNE HOSPITAL (O, 24 beds) Crow Agency, MT Mailing Address: P.O. Box 9, Zip 59022–0009; tel. 406/638–2626; Charlene Johnson, Service Unit Director

FORT BELKNAP U. S. PUBLIC HEALTH SERVICE INDIAN HOSPITAL (O, 6 beds) Rural Route 1, Box 67, Harlem, MT Zip 59526; tel. 406/353–3100; Daryl A. Brockie, Director
Web address: www.ihs.gov

U. S. PUBLIC HEALTH SERVICE BLACKFEET COMMUNITY HOSPITAL (O, 25 beds) Saint Mary, MT Mailing Address: P.O. Box 760, Browning, Zip 59417–0760; tel. 406/338–6100; James Kennedy, Chief Executive Officer
Web address: www.phs.ihs.gov

NEBRASKA: U. S. PUBLIC HEALTH SERVICE INDIAN HOSPITAL (O, 30 beds) Highway 7577, Winnebago, NE Zip 68071; tel. 402/878–2231; Sheriann Moore, Service Unit Director
Web address: www.ihs.gov

NEW MEXICO: ACOMA–CANONCITO–LAGUNA HOSPITAL (O, 7 beds) San Fidel, NM Mailing Address: P.O. Box 130, Zip 87049–0130; tel. 505/552–5300; William Thorne, Jr., Chief Executive Officer

GALLUP INDIAN MEDICAL CENTER (O, 65 beds) 516 East Nizhoni Boulevard, Gallup, NM Zip 87301–5748, Mailing Address: P.O. Box 1337, Zip 87305–1337; tel. 505/722–1000; Bennie C. Yazzie, Interim Chief Executive Officer
Web address: www.ihs.gov/facilitiesservices/areaoffices/navajo/naihs–hcc–gallup.asp

MESCALERO PUBLIC HEALTH SERVICE INDIAN HOSPITAL (O, 13 beds) Mescalero, NM Mailing Address: Box 210, Zip 88340–0210; tel. 505/671–4441; Dorlynn Simmons, Chief Executive Officer
Web address: www.ihs.gov

NORTHERN NAVAJO MEDICAL CENTER (O, 64 beds) Shiprock, NM Mailing Address: P.O. Box 160, Zip 87420–0160; tel. 505/368–6001; George C. Baacke, II, M.D., Acting Chief Executive Officer
Web address: www.home.nnmc.ihs.gov/

PHS SANTA FE INDIAN HOSPITAL (O, 39 beds) 1700 Cerrillos Road, Santa Fe, NM Zip 87505–3554; tel. 505/988–9821; Robert J. Lyon, Chief Executive Officer

U. S. PUBLIC HEALTH SERVICE INDIAN HOSPITAL (O, 12 beds) Crownpoint, NM Mailing Address: P.O. Box 358, Zip 87313–0358; tel. 505/786–5291; Fannessa Comer, Acting Chief Executive Officer
Web address: www.ihs.gov

U. S. PUBLIC HEALTH SERVICE INDIAN HOSPITAL (O, 32 beds) Route 301 North B. Street, Zuni, NM Zip 87327, Mailing Address: P.O. Box 467, Zip 87327–0467; tel. 505/782–4431; Jean Othole, Chief Executive Officer
Web address: www.ihs.gov

NORTH DAKOTA: PUBLIC HEALTH SERVICE INDIAN HOSPITAL – QUENTIN N. BURDICK MEMORIAL HEALTH FACILITY (O, 27 beds) 2 Blocks North of Highway 5, Belcourt, ND Zip 58316, Mailing Address: P.O. Box 160, Zip 58316–0160; tel. 701/477–6111; David L. Quincy, Chief Executive Officer
Web address: www.ihs.gov

U. S. PUBLIC HEALTH SERVICE INDIAN HOSPITAL (O, 14 beds) N 10 North River Road, Fort Yates, ND Zip 58538, Mailing Address: P.O. Box J, Zip 58538; tel. 701/854–3831; Tim Yellow, Director
Web address: www.ihs.gov

OKLAHOMA: CLAREMORE INDIAN HOSPITAL (O, 46 beds) 101 South Moore Avenue, Claremore, OK Zip 74017–5091; tel. 918/342–6200; Marty Smith, Interim Chief Executive Officer
Web address: www.ihs.gov

LAWTON INDIAN HOSPITAL (O, 26 beds) 1515 Lawrie Tatum Road, Lawton, OK Zip 73507–3099; tel. 580/353–0350; Greg Ketcher, Acting Chief Executive Officer
Web address: www.ihs.gov

WILLIAM W. HASTINGS INDIAN HOSPITAL (O, 60 beds) 100 South Bliss Avenue, Tahlequah, OK Zip 74464–3399; tel. 918/458–3100; Edwin McLemore, Chief Executive Officer

SOUTH DAKOTA: INDIAN HEALTH SERVICE HOSPITAL (O, 19 beds) 3200 Canyon Lake Drive, Rapid City, SD Zip 57702–8197; tel. 605/355–2280; Lorraine Jewett, Administrator
Web address: www.ihs.gov

U. S. PUBLIC HEALTH SERVICE INDIAN HOSPITAL (O, 11 beds) 317 Main Street, Eagle Butte, SD Zip 57625–1012, Mailing Address: P.O. Box 1012, Zip 57625–1012; tel. 605/964–7724; Charlene Red Thunder, Chief Executive Officer
Web address: www.ihs.gov

U. S. PUBLIC HEALTH SERVICE INDIAN HOSPITAL (O, 45 beds) Pine Ridge, SD Mailing Address: P.O. Box 1201, Zip 57770–1201; tel. 605/867–5131; William Pourier, Service Unit Director
Web address: www.ihs.gov

U. S. PUBLIC HEALTH SERVICE INDIAN HOSPITAL (O, 35 beds) Highway 18, Soldier Creek Road, Rosebud, SD Zip 57570; tel. 605/747–2231; Shelly Harris, Chief Executive Officer
Web address: www.ihs.gov

U. S. PUBLIC HEALTH SERVICE INDIAN HOSPITAL (O, 18 beds) Chestnut Street, Sisseton, SD Zip 57262, Mailing Address: P.O. Box 189, Zip 57262–0189; tel. 605/698–7606; Richard Huff, Administrator
Web address: www.ihs.gov

Owned, leased, sponsored:	32 hospitals	1225 beds
Contract-managed:	0 hospitals	0 beds
Totals:	32 hospitals	1225 beds

9105: UAB HEALTH SYSTEM (NP)

500 22nd Street South, Suite 408, Birmingham, AL Zip 35233; tel. 205/975–5362; Ray Watts, M.D., Interim Chief Executive Officer
(Moderately Centralized Health System)

ALABAMA: CALLAHAN EYE FOUNDATION HOSPITAL (O, 20 beds) 1720 University Boulevard, Birmingham, AL Zip 35233–1816; tel. 205/325–8100; Raymond Butler, President
Web address: www.health.uab.edu/eyes

MEDICAL WEST (O, 214 beds) 995 Ninth Avenue S.W., Bessemer, AL Zip 35022–4527; tel. 205/481–7000; Timothy J. Thornton, Chief Executive Officer
Web address: www.uabmedicalwest.org

UAB HIGHLANDS (O, 73 beds) 1201 11th Avenue South, Birmingham, AL Zip 35205–5299; tel. 205/930–7000; Robert Cofield, Chief Operating Officer
Web address: www.health.uab.edu

UNIVERSITY OF ALABAMA HOSPITAL (O, 908 beds) 1802 Sixth Avenue South, Birmingham, AL Zip 35210; tel. 205/934–4011; Michael Waldrum, M.D., Chief Executive Officer
Web address: www.health.uab.edu

Owned, leased, sponsored:	4 hospitals	1215 beds
Contract-managed:	0 hospitals	0 beds
Totals:	4 hospitals	1215 beds

0390: UK HEALTHCARE (NP)

800 Rose Street, Lexington, KY Zip 40536–0293; tel. 859/323–5000; Michael Karpf, M.D., Executive Vice President Health Affairs

KENTUCKY: UK HEALTHCARE GOOD SAMARITAN HOSPITAL (O, 271 beds) 310 South Limestone Street, Lexington, KY Zip 40508–3008; tel. 859/226–7000; Frank Beirne, Chief Executive Officer
Web address: www.samaritanhospital.com

UNIVERSITY OF KENTUCKY HOSPITAL (O, 473 beds) 800 Rose Street, N100, Lexington, KY Zip 40536–0293; tel. 859/323–5000; Murray B. Clark, Jr., Associate Vice President Operations and Hospital Administration
Web address: www.ukhealthcare.uky.edu

For explanation of codes following names, see page B2.
★ Indicates Type III membership in the American Hospital Association.

Owned, leased, sponsored:	2 hospitals	744 beds
Contract-managed:	0 hospitals	0 beds
Totals:	2 hospitals	744 beds

★0224: UMASS MEMORIAL HEALTH CARE, INC. (NP)
1 Biotech Park, Worcester, MA Zip 01605–2982; tel. 508/334–0100; John G. O'Brien, President and Chief Executive Officer
(Moderately Centralized Health System)

MASSACHUSETTS: CLINTON HOSPITAL (O, 41 beds) 201 Highland Street, Clinton, MA Zip 01510–1096; tel. 978/368–3000; Sheila Daly, President and Chief Executive Officer
Web address: www.clintonhospital.org

HEALTH ALLIANCE HOSPITALS (O, 97 beds) 60 Hospital Road, Leominster, MA Zip 01453–8004; tel. 978/466–2000; Patrick L. Muldoon, FACHE, President and Chief Executive Officer
Web address: www.healthalliance.com

UMASS MEMORIAL MEDICAL CENTER (O, 723 beds) 119 Belmont Street, Worcester, MA Zip 01605–2982; tel. 508/334–1000; Walter Ettinger, M.D., President and Chief Executive Officer
Web address: www.umassmemorial.org

UMASS MEMORIAL–MARLBOROUGH HOSPITAL (O, 67 beds) 157 Union Street, Marlborough, MA Zip 01752–1297; tel. 508/481–5000; John Polanowicz, President and Chief Executive Officer
Web address: www.marlboroughhospital.org

WING MEMORIAL HOSPITAL AND MEDICAL CENTERS (O, 52 beds) 40 Wright Street, Palmer, MA Zip 01069–1138; tel. 413/283–7651; Charles E. Cavagnaro, III, M.D., President and Chief Executive Officer
Web address: www.winghealth.org

Owned, leased, sponsored:	5 hospitals	980 beds
Contract-managed:	0 hospitals	0 beds
Totals:	5 hospitals	980 beds

★0288: UNITED HEALTH SERVICES (NP)
10–42 Mitchell Avenue, Binghamton, NY Zip 13903; tel. 607/762–2200; Matthew J. Salanger, President and Chief Executive Officer
(Moderately Centralized Health System)

NEW YORK: CHENANGO MEMORIAL HOSPITAL (O, 138 beds) 179 North Broad Street, Norwich, NY Zip 13815–1097; tel. 607/337–4111; Drake M. Lamen, M.D., President and Chief Executive Officer
Web address: www.chenangomemorial.com

DELAWARE VALLEY HOSPITAL (O, 25 beds) 1 Titus Place, Walton, NY Zip 13856–1498; tel. 607/865–2100; David J. Polge, President and Chief Executive Officer
Web address: www.uhs.net

UNITED HEALTH SERVICES HOSPITALS–BINGHAMTON (O, 465 beds) 10–42 Mitchell Avenue, Binghamton, NY Zip 13903–1678; tel. 607/763–6000; Matthew J. Salanger, President and Chief Executive Officer
Web address: www.uhs.net

Owned, leased, sponsored:	3 hospitals	628 beds
Contract-managed:	0 hospitals	0 beds
Totals:	3 hospitals	628 beds

9605: UNITED MEDICAL CORPORATION (IO)
603 Main Street, Windermere, FL Zip 34786–3548, Mailing Address: P.O. Box 1100, Zip 34786–1100; tel. 407/876–2200; Donald R. Dizney, Chairman and Chief Executive Officer
(Independent Hospital System)

FLORIDA: TEN BROECK HOSPITAL JACKSONVILLE (O, 99 beds) 6300 Beach Boulevard, Jacksonville, FL Zip 32216–2782; tel. 904/724–9202; Paul Andrews, Chief Executive Officer
Web address: www.tenbroeck.com

KENTUCKY: TEN BROECK DUPONT (O, 66 beds) 1405 Browns Lane, Louisville, KY Zip 40207; tel. 502/896–0495; John Hollinsworth, Executive Director

TEN BROECK HOSPITAL (O, 94 beds) 8521 Old LaGrange Road, Louisville, KY Zip 40242–3800; tel. 502/426–6380; John Hollinsworth, Executive Director
Web address: www.tenbroeck.com

PUERTO RICO: HOSPITAL PAVIA–HATO REY (O, 180 beds) San Juan, PR Mailing Address: 435 Ponce De Leon, Hato Rey, Zip 00917–3428; tel. 787/754–0909; Astro Munoz, Chief Executive Officer
Web address: www.paviahealth.com

HOSPITAL PAVIA–SANTURCE (O, 309 beds) 1462 Asia Street, San Juan, PR Zip 00909–2143, Mailing Address: Box 11137, Santurce Station, Zip 00910–1137; tel. 787/727–6060; Henry Ruberte, Executive Director
Web address: www.paviahealth.com

HOSPITAL PEREA (O, 103 beds) 15 Basora Street, Mayaguez, PR Zip 681, Mailing Address: P.O. Box 170, Zip 681; tel. 787/834–0101; Rafael Alvarado, Chief Executive Officer
Web address: www.paviahealth.com/perea_hospital.htm

SAN JORGE CHILDREN'S HOSPITAL (O, 125 beds) 252 San Jorge Street, Santurce, San Juan, PR Zip 00912–3310; tel. 787/727–1000; Domingo Cruz Vivaldi, Senior Vice President Operations
Web address: www.sanjorgechildrenhospital.com

Owned, leased, sponsored:	7 hospitals	976 beds
Contract-managed:	0 hospitals	0 beds
Totals:	7 hospitals	976 beds

0338: UNITED REHAB CORPORATION (IO)
9707 Shelbyville Road, Louisville, KY Zip 40223; tel. 502/426–2242; Kyle White, President and Chief Executive Officer
(Independent Hospital System)

KENTUCKY: GATEWAY REHABILITATION HOSPITAL (O, 40 beds) 5940 Merchant Street, Florence, KY Zip 41042; tel. 859/426–2400; Jim Burcham, Chief Executive Officer
Web address: www.gatewaylouisville.com

TEXAS: HIGHLANDS REGIONAL REHABILITATION HOSPITAL (O, 41 beds) 1395 George Dieter Drive, El Paso, TX Zip 79936; tel. 915/298–7222; William G. Collins, Chief Executive Officer

Owned, leased, sponsored:	2 hospitals	81 beds
Contract-managed:	0 hospitals	0 beds
Totals:	2 hospitals	81 beds

0322: UNITED SURGICAL PARTNERS INTERNATIONAL (IO)
15305 Dallas Parkway, Suite 1600, Addison, TX Zip 75001–6491; tel. 972/713–3500; William H. Wilcox, President and Chief Executive Officer
(Independent Hospital System)

ARIZONA: ARIZONA ORTHOPEDIC SURGICAL HOSPITAL (O, 16 beds) 2905 West Warner Road, Chandler, AZ Zip 85224; tel. 480/603–9000; Chris Hartshorn, Chief Executive Officer
Web address: www.azosh.com

OKLAHOMA: OKLAHOMA CENTER FOR ORTHOPEDIC AND MULTI–SPECIALTY SURGERY (O, 10 beds) 8100 South Walker, Suite C., Oklahoma City, OK Zip 73139, Mailing Address: P.O. Box 890609, Zip 73189; tel. 405/602–6500; Teri Philbrick, Chief Executive Officer

TEXAS: BAYLOR MEDICAL CENTER AT FRISCO (O, 68 beds) 5601 Warren Parkway, Frisco, TX Zip 75034; tel. 214/618–2000; William A. Keaton, Chief Executive Officer
Web address: www.bmcf.com

IRVING COPPELL SURGICAL HOSPITAL (O, 12 beds) 400 West Interstate 635, Irving, TX Zip 75063; tel. 972/868–4000; David Yoder, Chief Executive Officer
Web address: www.ic–sh.com

MARY SHIELS HOSPITAL (O, 14 beds) 3515 Howell Street, Dallas, TX Zip 75204–2895; tel. 214/443–3000; Suzanne Greever, Chief Executive Officer
Web address: www.maryshiels.com

For explanation of codes following names, see page B2.
★ Indicates Type III membership in the American Hospital Association.

Section B

SUGAR LAND SURGICAL HOSPITAL (O, 6 beds) 1211 Highway 6, Suite 70, Sugar Land, TX Zip 77478; tel. 281/243–1000; Madilyn Zbranek, RN, Chief Executive Officer
Web address: www.sho–sugarland.com

TOPS SURGICAL SPECIALTY HOSPITAL (O, 16 beds) 17080 Red Oak Drive, Houston, TX Zip 77090; tel. 281/539–2900; Teresa R. Danna, RN, M.S.N., CHE, Chief Executive Officer
Web address: www.tops–hospital.com

Owned, leased, sponsored:	7 hospitals	142 beds
Contract–managed:	0 hospitals	0 beds
Totals:	7 hospitals	142 beds

9555: UNIVERSAL HEALTH SERVICES, INC. (IO)
367 South Gulph Road, King of Prussia, PA Zip 19406–0958, Mailing Address: P.O. Box 61558, Zip 19406–0958; tel. 610/768–3300; Alan B. Miller, President and Chief Executive Officer
(Decentralized Health System)

ALASKA: NORTH STAR BEHAVIORAL HEALTH SYSTEM (O, 74 beds) 2530 DeBarr Road, Anchorage, AK Zip 99508–2948; tel. 907/258–7575; James Shill, Chief Executive Officer and Managing Director
Web address: www.northstarbehavioral.com

ARKANSAS: RIVENDELL BEHAVIORAL HEALTH SERVICES OF ARKANSAS (O, 77 beds) 100 Rivendell Drive, Benton, AR Zip 72019–9100; tel. 501/316–1255; Scott Williams, Administrator and Chief Executive Officer
Web address: www.rivendellofarkansas.com

THE BRIDGEWAY (L, 98 beds) 21 Bridgeway Road, North Little Rock, AR Zip 72113–9516; tel. 501/771–1500; Jennifer Nolan, Chief Executive Officer
Web address: www.thebridgeway.com

CALIFORNIA: CORONA REGIONAL MEDICAL CENTER (O, 228 beds) 800 South Main Street, Corona, CA Zip 92882–3420; tel. 951/737–4343; Kenneth I. Rivers, Chief Executive Officer
Web address: www.coronaregional.com

DEL AMO HOSPITAL (O, 70 beds) 23700 Camino Del Sol, Torrance, CA Zip 90505–5000; tel. 310/530–1151; Lisa K. Montes, Chief Executive Officer and Managing Director
Web address: www.delamohospital.com

INLAND VALLEY MEDICAL CENTER (L, 80 beds) 36485 Inland Valley Drive, Wildomar, CA Zip 92595–9700; tel. 951/677–1111; Dennis M. Knox, Chief Executive Officer
Web address: www.ivrmc–rsmc.com

LANCASTER COMMUNITY HOSPITAL (O, 78 beds) 43830 10th Street West, Lancaster, CA Zip 93534–4895; tel. 661/948–4781; Robert J. Trautman, Chief Executive Officer
Web address: www.lancastercommunityhospital.net

RANCHO SPRINGS MEDICAL CENTER (O, 51 beds) 25500 Medical Center Drive, Murrieta, CA Zip 92562–5965; tel. 951/696–6000; Linda Bradley, Chief Executive Officer and Managing Director
Web address: www.swhcs.com

COLORADO: HIGHLANDS BEHAVIORAL HEALTH SYSTEM (O, 86 beds) 8565 South Poplar Way, Highlands Ranch, CO Zip 80130; tel. 720/348–2800; ,
Web address: www.highlandsbhs.com

DELAWARE: DOVER BEHAVIORAL HEALTH SYSTEM (O, 56 beds) 725 Horsepond Road, Dover, DE Zip 19901; tel. 302/741–0140; ,
Web address: www.doverbehavioral.com

ROCKFORD CENTER (O, 92 beds) 100 Rockford Drive, Newark, DE Zip 19713–2121; tel. 302/996–5480; John F. McKenna, Chief Executive Officer and Managing Director
Web address: www.rockfordcenter.com

DISTRICT OF COLUMBIA: GEORGE WASHINGTON UNIVERSITY HOSPITAL (O, 326 beds) 900 23rd Street N.W., Washington, DC Zip 20037–2377; tel. 202/715–4000; Trent Crable, Interim Chief Executive Officer
Web address: www.gwhospital.com

FLORIDA: LAKEWOOD RANCH MEDICAL CENTER (O, 120 beds) 8330 Lakewood Ranch Boulevard, Bradenton, FL Zip 34202; tel. 941/782–2100; Linda S. Widra, FACHE, Ph.D., RN, Interim Chief Executive Officer
Web address: www.lakewoodranchmedicalcenter.com

MANATEE MEMORIAL HOSPITAL (O, 512 beds) 206 Second Street East, Bradenton, FL Zip 34208–1000; tel. 941/746–5111; Moody L. Chisholm, Chief Executive Officer
Web address: www.manateememorial.com

WELLINGTON REGIONAL MEDICAL CENTER (L, 108 beds) 10101 Forest Hill Boulevard, West Palm Beach, FL Zip 33414–6199; tel. 561/798–8500; Kevin DiLallo, Chief Executive Officer and Managing Director
Web address: www.wellingtonregional.com

GEORGIA: ANCHOR HOSPITAL (O, 74 beds) 5454 Yorktowne Drive, Atlanta, GA Zip 30349–5305; tel. 770/991–6044; Jennifer Morgan, Chief Executive Officer and Managing Director
Web address: www.anchorhospital.com

COASTAL HARBOR TREATMENT CENTER (O, 132 beds) 1150 Cornell Avenue, Savannah, GA Zip 31406–2797; tel. 912/354–3911; Ray Heckerman, Chief Executive Officer and Managing Director
Web address: www.coastalharbor.com

PEACHFORD BEHAVIORAL HEALTH SYSTEM (O, 224 beds) 2151 Peachford Road, Atlanta, GA Zip 30338–6599; tel. 770/455–3200; Matthew Crouch, Chief Executive Officer and Managing Director
Web address: www.peachfordhospital.com

TURNING POINT HOSPITAL (O, 59 beds) 3015 Veterans Parkway S.E., Moultrie, GA Zip 31768–6705, Mailing Address: P.O. Box 1177, Zip 31776–1177; tel. 229/985–4815; Ben Marion, Chief Executive Officer and Managing Director
Web address: www.turningpointcare.com

ILLINOIS: HARTGROVE HOSPITAL (O, 128 beds) 520 North Ridgeway Avenue, Chicago, IL Zip 60624–1299; tel. 773/722–3113; Steven Airhart, Chief Executive Officer and Managing Director
Web address: www.uhsinc.com

THE PAVILION (O, 46 beds) 809 West Church Street, Champaign, IL Zip 61820–3399; tel. 217/373–1700; Joseph Sheehy, Chief Executive Officer and Managing Director
Web address: www.info@pavilionhospital.com

KENTUCKY: LINCOLN TRAIL BEHAVIORAL HEALTH SYSTEM (O, 67 beds) 3909 South Wilson Road, Radcliff, KY Zip 40160–9714, Mailing Address: P.O. Box 369, Zip 40159–0369; tel. 270/351–9444; Charles L. Webb, Jr., Administrator
Web address: www.lincolnbehavioral.com

RIDGE BEHAVIORAL HEALTH SYSTEM (O, 110 beds) 3050 Rio Dosa Drive, Lexington, KY Zip 40509–9990; tel. 859/269–2325; Nina W. Eisner, Chief Executive Officer and Managing Director
Web address: www.ridgebhs.com

RIVENDELL BEHAVIORAL HEALTH (O, 84 beds) 1035 Porter Pike, Bowling Green, KY Zip 42103; tel. 270/843–1199; Janice Richardson, Chief Executive Officer and Managing Director
Web address: www.rivendellbehavioral.com

LOUISIANA: RIVER OAKS HOSPITAL (O, 121 beds) 1525 River Oaks Road West, New Orleans, LA Zip 70123–2199; tel. 504/734–1740; Evelyn Nolting, Chief Executive Officer and Managing Director
Web address: www.riveroakshospital.com

MASSACHUSETTS: ARBOUR H. R. I. HOSPITAL (O, 68 beds) 227 Babcock Street, Brookline, MA Zip 02146–6799; tel. 617/731–3200; Patrick Moallemian, Chief Executive Officer and Managing Director
Web address: www.arbourhealth.com

ARBOUR HOSPITAL (O, 118 beds) 49 Robinwood Avenue, Boston, MA Zip 02130–2156, Mailing Address: P.O. Box 9, Zip 2130; tel. 617/522–4400; Joseph Murphy, Chief Executive Officer
Web address: www.arbourhealth.com

ARBOUR–FULLER HOSPITAL (O, 46 beds) 200 May Street, Attleboro, MA Zip 02703–5515; tel. 508/761–8500; Robert Mansfield, Chief Executive Officer
Web address: www.arbourhealth.com

PEMBROKE HOSPITAL (O, 80 beds) 199 Oak Street, Pembroke, MA Zip 02359–1953; tel. 781/826–8161; Paul Zani, Chief Executive Officer and Managing Director

WESTWOOD LODGE HOSPITAL (O, 65 beds) 45 Clapboardtree Street, Westwood, MA Zip 02090–2930; tel. 781/762–7764; Robert W. Spiegel, Chief Executive Officer and Managing Director
Web address: www.arbourhealth.com

For explanation of codes following names, see page B2.
★ Indicates Type III membership in the American Hospital Association.

MICHIGAN: FOREST VIEW PSYCHIATRIC HOSPITAL (O, 62 beds) 1055 Medical Park Drive S.E., Grand Rapids, MI Zip 49546–8323; tel. 616/942–9610; Wayne T. Miller, Chief Executive Officer and Managing Director
Web address: www.forestviewhospital.com

MISSISSIPPI: PARKWOOD BEHAVIORAL HEALTH SYSTEM (O, 128 beds) 8135 Goodman Road, Olive Branch, MS Zip 38654–2199; tel. 662/895–4900; M. Andrew Mayo, Ph.D., Chief Executive Officer and Managing Director
Web address: www.parkwoodbhs.com

MISSOURI: TWO RIVERS PSYCHIATRIC HOSPITAL (O, 105 beds) 5121 Raytown Road, Kansas City, MO Zip 64133–2141; tel. 816/382–6300; Norma Ferris, Chief Executive Officer and Managing Director
Web address: www.tworivershospital.com

NEVADA: DESERT SPRINGS HOSPITAL MEDICAL CENTER (O, 346 beds) 2075 East Flamingo Road, Las Vegas, NV Zip 89119–5121; tel. 702/733–8800; Samuel Kaufman, Chief Executive Officer and Managing Director
Web address: www.desertspringshospital.net

NORTHERN NEVADA MEDICAL CENTER (O, 80 beds) 2375 East Prater Way, Sparks, NV Zip 89434–9900; tel. 775/331–7000; Mark W. Crawford, Interim Chief Executive Officer
Web address: www.nnmc.com

SPRING MOUNTAIN SAHARA (O, 30 beds) 5460 West Sahara, Las Vegas, NV Zip 89146; tel. 702/216–8900; ,
Web address: www.springmountainsahara.com

SPRING VALLEY HOSPITAL MEDICAL CENTER (O, 210 beds) 5400 South Rainbow Boulevard, Las Vegas, NV Zip 89118; tel. 702/853–3000; Leonard Freehof, Chief Executive Officer and Managing Director
Web address: www.springvalleyhospital.com

SUMMERLIN HOSPITAL MEDICAL CENTER (O, 148 beds) 657 Town Center Drive, Las Vegas, NV Zip 89144; tel. 702/233–7000; Tim Hingtgen, Chief Executive Officer and Managing Director
Web address: www.summerlinhospital.org

VALLEY HOSPITAL MEDICAL CENTER (O, 365 beds) 620 Shadow Lane, Las Vegas, NV Zip 89106–4119; tel. 702/388–4000; Gregory E. Boyer, Chief Executive Officer and Managing Director
Web address: www.valleyhospital.net

NEW JERSEY: HAMPTON BEHAVIORAL HEALTH CENTER (O, 100 beds) 650 Rancocas Road, Westampton Township, NJ Zip 08060–5613; tel. 609/267–7000; Craig Hilton, Chief Executive Officer
Web address: www.hamptonhospital.com

NORTH CAROLINA: OLD VINEYARD BEHAVIORAL HEALTH SERVICES (O, 108 beds) 3637 Old Vineyard Road, Winston–Salem, NC Zip 27104–4835; tel. 336/794–3550; Wesley E. Mason, III, Chief Executive Officer
Web address: www.oldvineyard.net

OKLAHOMA: CEDAR RIDGE HOSPITAL (O, 36 beds) 6501 N.E. 50th Street, Oklahoma City, OK Zip 73141; tel. 405/605–6111; John A. Holter, Chief Executive Officer

ST. MARY'S REGIONAL MEDICAL CENTER (O, 176 beds) 305 South Fifth Street, Enid, OK Zip 73701–5899, Mailing Address: Box 232, Zip 73702–0232; tel. 580/233–6100; Rick Wallace, FACHE, Chief Executive Officer and Managing Director
Web address: www.stmarysregional.com

PENNSYLVANIA: CENTRAL MONTGOMERY MEDICAL CENTER (O, 125 beds) 100 Medical Campus Drive, Lansdale, PA Zip 19446–1200; tel. 215/368–2100; James D. Wilson, Chief Executive Officer
Web address: www.cmmc–uhs.com

CLARION PSYCHIATRIC CENTER (O, 74 beds) 2 Hospital Drive, Clarion, PA Zip 16214; tel. 814/226–9545; Curtis J. Dyer, Chief Executive Officer
Web address: www.clarioncenter.com

FAIRMOUNT BEHAVIORAL HEALTH SYSTEM (O, 182 beds) 561 Fairthorne Avenue, Philadelphia, PA Zip 19128–2499; tel. 215/487–4000; Geoff Botak, Chief Executive Officer and Managing Director
Web address: www.fairmountbhs.com

FOUNDATIONS BEHAVIORAL HEALTH (O, 94 beds) 833 East Butler Avenue, Doylestown, PA Zip 18901–2280; tel. 215/345–0444; Robert Weinhold, Chief Executive Officer
Web address: www.fbh.com

HORSHAM CLINIC (O, 138 beds) 722 East Butler Pike, Ambler, PA Zip 19002–2310; tel. 215/643–7800; Phyllis Weisfield, Chief Executive Officer and Managing Director
Web address: www.horshamclinic.com

KEYSTONE CENTER (O, 119 beds) 2001 Providence Avenue, Chester, PA Zip 19013–5504; tel. 610/876–9000; Michael Salazar, XPsyD, Chief Executive Officer and Managing Director
Web address: www.keystonecenter.net

MEADOWS PSYCHIATRIC CENTER (O, 101 beds) 132 The Meadows Drive, Centre Hall, PA Zip 16828–9798; tel. 814/364–2161; Larry Grimes, Chief Executive Officer
Web address: www.themeadows.net

PUERTO RICO: SAN JUAN CAPESTRANO HOSPITAL (O, 108 beds) San Juan, PR Mailing Address: Rural Route 2, Box 11, Zip 926; tel. 787/760–0222; Laura Vargas, Chief Executive Officer and Managing Director
Web address: www.sjcapestrano.com

SOUTH CAROLINA: AIKEN REGIONAL MEDICAL CENTERS (O, 230 beds) 302 University Parkway, Aiken, SC Zip 29801–2757; tel. 803/641–5000; Kathryn D. Justyn, Chief Executive Officer and Managing Director
Web address: www.aikenregional.com

CAROLINA CENTER FOR BEHAVIORAL HEALTH (O, 89 beds) 2700 East Phillips Road, Greer, SC Zip 29650–4816; tel. 864/235–2335; John Willingham, Chief Executive Officer and Managing Director
Web address: www.thecarolinacenter.com

TENNESSEE: LAKESIDE BEHAVIORAL HEALTH SYSTEM (O, 295 beds) 2911 Brunswick Road, Memphis, TN Zip 38133–4199; tel. 901/377–4700; Shelley A. Nowak, Chief Executive Officer
Web address: www.lakesidebhs.com

TEXAS: CORNERSTONE REGIONAL HOSPITAL (L, 14 beds) 2302 Cornerstone Boulevard, Edinburg, TX Zip 78539–8471; tel. 956/618–4444; Alma Medina, RN, Interim Chief Executive Officer

DOCTORS HOSPITAL OF LAREDO (O, 179 beds) 10700 McPherson Road, Laredo, TX Zip 78045; tel. 956/523–2000; Elmo Lopez, Jr., Chief Executive Officer
Web address: www.doctorshosplaredo.com

EDINBURG REGIONAL MEDICAL CENTER (O, 848 beds) 1102 West Trenton Road, Edinburg, TX Zip 78539–6199; tel. 956/388–6000; Linda Resendez, RN, Chief Executive Officer
Web address: www.edinburgregional.com

FORT DUNCAN REGIONAL MEDICAL CENTER (O, 101 beds) 3333 North Foster Maldonado Boulevard, Eagle Pass, TX Zip 78852; tel. 830/773–5321; Rene Lopez, Chief Executive Officer
Web address: www.fortduncanmedicalcenter.com

GLEN OAKS HOSPITAL (O, 54 beds) 301 East Division, Greenville, TX Zip 75402–4199; tel. 903/454–6000; Joel Klein, Chief Executive Officer and Managing Director
Web address: www.glenoakshospital.com

MCALLEN MEDICAL CENTER (L, 635 beds) 301 West Expressway 83, McAllen, TX Zip 78503–3045; tel. 956/632–4000; Joe B. Riley, Chief Executive Officer
Web address: www.mcallenmedicalcenter.com

NORTHWEST TEXAS HEALTHCARE SYSTEM (O, 419 beds) 1501 South Coulter Avenue, Amarillo, TX Zip 79106–1790, Mailing Address: P.O. Box 1110, Zip 79175–1110; tel. 806/354–1000; Frank Lopez, FACHE, Chief Executive Officer and Managing Director
Web address: www.nwtexashealthcare.com

RIVER CREST HOSPITAL (O, 80 beds) 1636 Hunters Glen Road, San Angelo, TX Zip 76901–5016; tel. 325/949–5722; Scott York, Chief Executive Officer
Web address: www.rivercresthospital.com

TEXOMA MEDICAL CENTER (O, 205 beds) 1000 Memorial Drive, Denison, TX Zip 75020–2035, Mailing Address: P.O. Box 890, Zip 75021–9988; tel. 903/416–4000; W. Mackey Watkins, M.D., President and Chief Executive Officer
Web address: www.texomamedicalcenter.net

TIMBERLAWN MENTAL HEALTH SYSTEM (O, 144 beds) 4600 Samuell Boulevard, Dallas, TX Zip 75228–6800; tel. 214/381–7181; Craig Nuckles, Chief Executive Officer, Managing and Regional Vice President
Web address: www.timberlawn.com

WASHINGTON: AUBURN REGIONAL MEDICAL CENTER (O, 120 beds) 202 North Division, Plaza One, Auburn, WA Zip 98001–4908; tel. 253/833–7711; Leonard Freehof, Chief Executive Officer
Web address: www.auburnregional.com

For explanation of codes following names, see page B2.
★ Indicates Type III membership in the American Hospital Association.

Section B

WYOMING: WYOMING BEHAVIORAL INSTITUTE (O, 70 beds) 2521 East 15th Street, Casper, WY Zip 82609–4126; tel. 800/457–9312; Bill Sexton, Chief Executive Officer
Web address: www.wbihelp.com

Owned, leased, sponsored:	66 hospitals	9796 beds
Contract–managed:	0 hospitals	0 beds
Totals:	66 hospitals	9796 beds

0246: UNIVERSITY COMMUNITY HEALTH (NP)
3100 East Fletcher Avenue, Tampa, FL Zip 33613; tel. 813/971–6000; Norman V. Stein, President and Chief Executive Officer
(Independent Hospital System)

FLORIDA: HELEN ELLIS MEMORIAL HOSPITAL (O, 168 beds) 1395 South Pinellas Avenue, Tarpon Springs, FL Zip 34689–3721; tel. 727/942–5000; Donald D. Evans, Chief Executive Officer
Web address: www.hemh.com

UNIVERSITY COMMUNITY HOSPITAL (O, 306 beds) 3100 East Fletcher Avenue, Tampa, FL Zip 33613–4688; tel. 813/971–6000; Larry J. Archbell, Chief Executive Officer
Web address: www.uch.org

UNIVERSITY COMMUNITY HOSPITAL–CARROLLWOOD (O, 57 beds) 7171 North Dale Mabry Highway, Tampa, FL Zip 33614–2699; tel. 813/932–2222; Norman V. Stein, Interim Chief Executive Officer
Web address: www.uch.org

Owned, leased, sponsored:	3 hospitals	531 beds
Contract–managed:	0 hospitals	0 beds
Totals:	3 hospitals	531 beds

★0217: UNIVERSITY HEALTH SYSTEMS OF EASTERN CAROLINA (NP)
2100 Stantonsburg Road, Greenville, NC Zip 27834, Mailing Address: P.O. Box 6028, Zip 27835–6028; tel. 252/847–4100; Dave C. McRae, Chief Executive Officer
(Moderately Centralized Health System)

NORTH CAROLINA: BERTIE MEMORIAL HOSPITAL (L, 6 beds) 1403 South King Street, Windsor, NC Zip 27983–1726, Mailing Address: P.O. Box 40, Zip 27983–1726; tel. 252/794–6600; Jeffrey N. Sackrison, FACHE, President
Web address: www.bertie.uhseast.com

CHOWAN HOSPITAL (L, 67 beds) 211 Virginia Road, Edenton, NC Zip 27932–0629, Mailing Address: P.O. Box 629, Zip 27932–0629; tel. 252/482–8451; Jeffrey N. Sackrison, FACHE, President
Web address: www.uhseast.com

HERITAGE HOSPITAL (O, 117 beds) 111 Hospital Drive, Tarboro, NC Zip 27886–2011; tel. 252/641–7700; Wendell H. Baker, Jr., President
Web address: www.heritage.uhseast.com

PITT COUNTY MEMORIAL HOSPITAL (O, 737 beds) 2100 Stantonsburg Road, Greenville, NC Zip 27834, Mailing Address: P.O. Box 6028, Zip 27835–6028; tel. 252/847–4100; Stephen J. Lawler, President
Web address: www.uhseast.com

ROANOKE–CHOWAN HOSPITAL (L, 102 beds) 500 South Academy Street, Ahoskie, NC Zip 27910–3261, Mailing Address: P.O. Box 1385, Zip 27910–1385; tel. 252/209–3000; Susan S. Lassiter, President
Web address: www.uhseast.com

THE OUTER BANKS HOSPITAL (O, 19 beds) 4800 South Croatan Highway, Nags Head, NC Zip 27959–9704; tel. 252/449–4500; D. Van Smith, Jr., President
Web address: www.theouterbankshospital.com

Owned, leased, sponsored:	6 hospitals	1048 beds
Contract–managed:	0 hospitals	0 beds
Totals:	6 hospitals	1048 beds

0112: UNIVERSITY HOSPITALS (NP)
11100 Euclid Avenue, Cleveland, OH Zip 44106–5000; tel. 216/844–1000; Thomas F. Zenty, III, Chief Executive Officer
(Centralized Physician/Insurance Health System)

OHIO: SOUTHWEST GENERAL HEALTH CENTER (O, 300 beds) 18697 Bagley Road, Middleburg Heights, OH Zip 44130–3497; tel. 440/816–8000; Thomas A. Selden, President and Chief Executive Officer
Web address: www.swgeneral.com

UNIVERSITY HOSPITALS BEDFORD MEDICAL CENTER (O, 77 beds) 44 Blaine Avenue, Cleveland, OH Zip 44146–2709; tel. 440/735–3900; Sean McKibben, President
Web address: www.uhhsbmc.com

UNIVERSITY HOSPITALS CASE MEDICAL CENTER (O, 649 beds) 11100 Euclid Avenue, Cleveland, OH Zip 44106–2602; tel. 216/844–1000; Fred C. Rothstein, M.D., President
Web address: www.UHhospitals.org

UNIVERSITY HOSPITALS CONNEAUT MEDICAL CENTER (O, 25 beds) 158 West Main Road, Conneaut, OH Zip 44030–2039; tel. 440/593–1131; Laurie Delgado, President and Chief Executive Officer
Web address: www.uhhs.com

UNIVERSITY HOSPITALS EXTENDED CARE CAMPUS (O, 214 beds) 12340 Bass Lake Road, Chardon, OH Zip 44024–8327; tel. 440/285–4040; Susan V. Juris, President and Chief Executive Officer
Web address: www.heatherhill.com

UNIVERSITY HOSPITALS GEAUGA REGIONAL HOSPITAL (O, 137 beds) 13207 Ravenna Road, Chardon, OH Zip 44024–7032; tel. 440/269–6000; Richard J. Frenchie, President and Chief Executive Officer
Web address: www.uhhsgrh.com

UNIVERSITY HOSPITALS GENEVA MEDICAL CENTER (O, 25 beds) 870 West Main Street, Geneva, OH Zip 44041–1295; tel. 440/466–1141; Laurie Delgado, President and Chief Executive Officer
Web address: www.uhhs.com

UNIVERSITY HOSPITALS RICHMOND MEDICAL CENTER (O, 80 beds) 27100 Chardon Road, Cleveland, OH Zip 44143–1116; tel. 440/585–6500; Michael Szubski, Interim President
Web address: www.uhhsrh.org

Owned, leased, sponsored:	8 hospitals	1507 beds
Contract–managed:	0 hospitals	0 beds
Totals:	8 hospitals	1507 beds

★6405: UNIVERSITY OF CALIFORNIA–SYSTEMWIDE ADMINISTRATION (NP)
1111 Franklin Street, 11th Floor, Oakland, CA Zip 94607–5200; tel. 510/987–9071; William Gurtner, Vice President Clinical Services
(Moderately Centralized Health System)

CALIFORNIA: SANTA MONICA–UCLA MEDICAL CENTER AND ORTHOPAEDIC HOSPITAL (O, 236 beds) 1250 16th Street, Santa Monica, CA Zip 90404; tel. 310/319–4000; Posie Carpenter, RN, M.S.N., Chief Administrative Officer
Web address: www.healthcare.ucla.edu

UCSF MEDICAL CENTER (O, 642 beds) 500 Parnassus Avenue, San Francisco, CA Zip 94143–0296, Mailing Address: 500 Parnassus Avenue, Box 0296, Zip 94143–0296; tel. 415/476–1000; Mark R. Laret, Chief Executive Officer
Web address: www.ucsfhealth.org

UNIVERSITY OF CALIFORNIA LOS ANGELES MEDICAL CENTER (L, 595 beds) 10833 Le Conte Avenue, Los Angeles, CA Zip 90095–3075; tel. 310/825–9111; David Feinberg, M.D., Chief Executive Officer
Web address: www.uclahealth.org

UNIVERSITY OF CALIFORNIA LOS ANGELES NEUROPSYCHIATRIC HOSPITAL (O, 69 beds) 760 Westwood Plaza, Los Angeles, CA Zip 90095–8353; tel. 310/825–0511; Fawzy I. Fawzy, M.D., Chief Executive Officer
Web address: www.npi.ucla.edu

UNIVERSITY OF CALIFORNIA SAN DIEGO MEDICAL CENTER (O, 519 beds) 200 West Arbor Drive, San Diego, CA Zip 92103–8970; tel. 619/543–6222; Richard Liekweg, Chief Executive Officer
Web address: www.health.ucsd.edu

UNIVERSITY OF CALIFORNIA, DAVIS MEDICAL CENTER (O, 565 beds) 2315 Stockton Boulevard, Sacramento, CA Zip 95817–2282; tel. 916/734–2011; Ann Madden Rice, Chief Executive Officer
Web address: www.ucdmc.ucdavis.edu

UNIVERSITY OF CALIFORNIA, IRVINE MEDICAL CENTER (O, 348 beds) 101 The City Drive, Orange, CA Zip 92868–3298; tel. 714/456–6011; Maureen Zehntner, RN, Interim Chief Executive Officer
Web address: www.ucihealth.com

For explanation of codes following names, see page B2.
★ Indicates Type III membership in the American Hospital Association.

Owned, leased, sponsored:	7 hospitals	2974 beds
Contract-managed:	0 hospitals	0 beds
Totals:	7 hospitals	2974 beds

★0216: UNIVERSITY OF MARYLAND MEDICAL SYSTEM (NP)

250 West Pratt Street, 24th Floor, Baltimore, MD Zip 21201–1595; tel. 410/328–8667; Edmond F. Notebaert, President and Chief Executive Officer
(Centralized Health System)

MARYLAND: BALTIMORE WASHINGTON MEDICAL CENTER (O, 277 beds) 301 Hospital Drive, Glen Burnie, MD Zip 21061–5899; tel. 410/787–4000; James R. Walker, FACHE, President and Chief Executive Officer
Web address: www.bwmc.umms.org

KERNAN ORTHOPAEDICS AND REHABILITATION (O, 133 beds) 2200 Kernan Drive, Baltimore, MD Zip 21207–6697; tel. 410/448–2500; James E. Ross, FACHE, Chief Executive Officer
Web address: www.kernan.org

MARYLAND GENERAL HOSPITAL (O, 238 beds) 827 Linden Avenue, Baltimore, MD Zip 21201–4681; tel. 410/225–8000; Sylvia Smith Johnson, President and Chief Executive Officer
Web address: www.marylandgeneral.org

MT. WASHINGTON PEDIATRIC HOSPITAL (O, 70 beds) 1708 West Rogers Avenue, Baltimore, MD Zip 21209–4537; tel. 410/578–8600; Sheldon J. Stein, President and Chief Executive Officer
Web address: www.mwph.org

UNIVERSITY OF MARYLAND MEDICAL CENTER (O, 666 beds) 22 South Greene Street, Baltimore, MD Zip 21201–1595; tel. 410/328–8667; Jeffrey A. Rivest, President and Chief Executive Officer
Web address: www.umm.edu

UNIVERSITY SPECIALTY HOSPITAL (O, 180 beds) 601 South Charles Street, Baltimore, MD Zip 21230–3898; tel. 410/547–8500; James L. Warner, Vice President
Web address: www.umm.edu/ush/

Owned, leased, sponsored:	6 hospitals	1564 beds
Contract-managed:	0 hospitals	0 beds
Totals:	6 hospitals	1564 beds

★0227: UNIVERSITY OF MISSOURI HEALTH CARE (NP)

One Hospital Drive, DC 031, Columbia, MO Zip 65212–0001; tel. 573/884–8738; James H. Ross, Chief Executive Officer
(Centralized Health System)

MISSOURI: CAPITAL REGION MEDICAL CENTER (O, 114 beds) 1125 Madison Street, Jefferson City, MO Zip 65101–5227, Mailing Address: P.O. Box 1128, Zip 65102–1128; tel. 573/632–5000; Edward F. Farnsworth, FACHE, President
Web address: www.crmc.org

COLUMBIA REGIONAL HOSPITAL (O, 176 beds) 404 Keene Street, Columbia, MO Zip 65201–6626; tel. 573/875–9000; Keri Simon, Executive Director
Web address: www.columbiaregional.org

COOPER COUNTY MEMORIAL HOSPITAL (C, 49 beds) 17651 B Highway, Boonville, MO Zip 65233–2839, Mailing Address: P.O. Box 88, Zip 65233–0088; tel. 660/882–7461; Jeffrey L. Durham, Interim Chief Executive Officer

MISSOURI REHABILITATION CENTER (O, 115 beds) 600 North Main Street, Mount Vernon, MO Zip 65712–1004; tel. 417/466–3711; Steve Patterson, Executive Director
Web address: www.muhealth.org/~MOrehab

UNIVERSITY OF MISSOURI HOSPITALS AND CLINICS (O, 282 beds) One Hospital Drive, Columbia, MO Zip 65212–0001; tel. 573/882–4141; James H. Ross, Chief Executive Officer
Web address: www.muhealth.org

Owned, leased, sponsored:	4 hospitals	687 beds
Contract-managed:	1 hospital	49 beds
Totals:	5 hospitals	736 beds

★0168: UNIVERSITY OF PENNSYLVANIA HEALTH SYSTEM (NP)

399 South 34th Street, 21st Floor, Philadelphia, PA Zip 19104–4385; tel. 215/662–2203; Ralph W. Muller, President and Chief Executive Officer
(Centralized Health System)

PENNSYLVANIA: HOSPITAL OF THE UNIVERSITY OF PENNSYLVANIA (O, 694 beds) 3400 Spruce Street, Philadelphia, PA Zip 19104–4283; tel. 215/662–4000; Garry L. Scheib, Executive Director
Web address: www.pennhealth.com

PENNSYLVANIA HOSPITAL (O, 434 beds) 800 Spruce Street, Philadelphia, PA Zip 19107–6192; tel. 215/829–3000; Kathleen Kinslow, Ed.D., Executive Director
Web address: www.pahosp.com

PRESBYTERIAN MEDICAL CENTER OF THE UNIVERSITY OF PENNSYLVANIA HEALTH SYSTEM (O, 279 beds) 39th and Market Street, Philadelphia, PA Zip 19104–2699; tel. 215/662–8000; Michele M. Volpe, Executive Director and Chief Executive Officer
Web address: www.health.upenn.edu/pmc

Owned, leased, sponsored:	3 hospitals	1407 beds
Contract-managed:	0 hospitals	0 beds
Totals:	3 hospitals	1407 beds

★0057: UNIVERSITY OF SOUTH ALABAMA HOSPITALS (NP)

2451 Filligim Street, Mobile, AL Zip 36617; tel. 251/471–7000; Stanley K. Hammack, Associate Vice President Hospital Affairs and Chief Executive Officer
(Independent Hospital System)

ALABAMA: UNIVERSITY OF SOUTH ALABAMA CHILDREN'S AND WOMEN'S HOSPITAL (O, 198 beds) 1700 Center Street, Mobile, AL Zip 36604–3301; tel. 251/415–1000; Becky DeVillier, Administrator
Web address: www.southalabama.edu/usacwh

UNIVERSITY OF SOUTH ALABAMA MEDICAL CENTER (O, 137 beds) 2451 Fillingim Street, Mobile, AL Zip 36617–2293; tel. 251/471–7000; Beth Anderson, Administrator
Web address: www.usahospitals.org

Owned, leased, sponsored:	2 hospitals	335 beds
Contract-managed:	0 hospitals	0 beds
Totals:	2 hospitals	335 beds

★0033: UNIVERSITY OF TEXAS SYSTEM (NP)

601 Colorado Street, Suite 205, Austin, TX Zip 78701–2982; tel. 512/499–4224; Kenneth Shine, M.D., Executive Vice Chancellor
(Moderately Centralized Health System)

TEXAS: UNIVERSITY OF TEXAS HARRIS COUNTY PSYCHIATRIC CENTER (O, 203 beds) 2800 South MacGregor Way, Houston, TX Zip 77021–1000, Mailing Address: P.O. Box 20249, Zip 77225–0249; tel. 713/741–5000; Pedro Ruiz, M.D., Interim Executive Director
Web address: www.uth.tmc.edu

UNIVERSITY OF TEXAS HEALTH SCIENCE CENTER AT TYLER (O, 114 beds) 11937 Highway 271, Tyler, TX Zip 75708–3154; tel. 903/877–3451; Kirk A. Calhoun, M.D., President
Web address: www.uthct.edu

UNIVERSITY OF TEXAS M. D. ANDERSON CANCER CENTER (O, 507 beds) 1515 Holcombe Boulevard, Box 91, Houston, TX Zip 77030–4095; tel. 713/792–2121; John Mendelsohn, M.D., President
Web address: www.mdanderson.org

UNIVERSITY OF TEXAS MEDICAL BRANCH HOSPITALS (O, 679 beds) 301 University Boulevard, Galveston, TX Zip 77555–0518; tel. 409/772–1011; Karen H. Sexton, RN, Ph.D., Vice President and Chief Executive Officer
Web address: www.utmb.edu

Owned, leased, sponsored:	4 hospitals	1503 beds
Contract-managed:	0 hospitals	0 beds
Totals:	4 hospitals	1503 beds

Section B

For explanation of codes following names, see page B2.
★ Indicates Type III membership in the American Hospital Association.

0137: UPMC (NP)
600 Grent Street, U.S. Steel Tower, Suite 6262, Pittsburgh, PA Zip 15219, Mailing Address: 600 Grant Stret, U.S. Steel Tower, Suite 6262, Zip 15219; tel. 412/647–4800; Jeffrey A. Romoff, President and Chief Executive Officer
(Centralized Physician/Insurance Health System)

PENNSYLVANIA: CHILDREN'S HOSPITAL OF PITTSBURGH OF UPMC (O, 260 beds) 3705 Fifth Avenue at De Soto Street, Pittsburgh, PA Zip 15213–2583; tel. 412/692–5325; Roger A. Oxendale, President
Web address: www.chp.edu

MAGEE–WOMENS HOSPITAL OF UPMC (O, 278 beds) 300 Halket Street, Pittsburgh, PA Zip 15213–3180; tel. 412/641–1000; Leslie C. Davis, President
Web address: www.magee.edu

UPMC BEDFORD MEMORIAL (O, 27 beds) 10455 Lincoln Highway, Everett, PA Zip 15537–7046; tel. 814/623–6161; Roger P. Winn, President
Web address: www.bedford.org

UPMC BRADDOCK (O, 176 beds) 400 Holland Avenue, Braddock, PA Zip 15104–1598; tel. 412/636–5000; Cynthia M. Dorundo, President
Web address: www.upmc.edu

UPMC HORIZON (O, 187 beds) Greenville, PA Neil Yuhas, President
Web address: www.horizon.upmc.com

UPMC MCKEESPORT (O, 209 beds) 1500 Fifth Avenue, McKeesport, PA Zip 15132–2482; tel. 412/664–2000; Ronald H. Ott, President
Web address: www.mckeesport.upmc.com

UPMC MERCY (O, 413 beds) 1400 Locust Street, Pittsburgh, PA Zip 15219–5166; tel. 412/232–8111; Kenneth A. Eshak, President and Chief Executive Officer
Web address: www.upmc.com/HospitalsFacilities/HFHome/Hospitals/Mercy/

UPMC NORTHWEST (O, 159 beds) 100 Fairfield Drive, Seneca, PA Zip 16346; tel. 814/676–7600; Neil E. Todhunter, President
Web address: www.northwest.upmc.com

UPMC PASSAVANT (O, 346 beds) 9100 Babcock Boulevard, Pittsburgh, PA Zip 15237–5815; tel. 412/367–6700; Teresa A. Petrick, President
Web address: www.upmc.edu/passavant

UPMC PRESBYTERIAN (O, 1501 beds) 200 Lothrop Street, Pittsburgh, PA Zip 15213–2585; tel. 412/647–2345; John Innocenti, President and Chief Executive Officer
Web address: www.upmc.edu

UPMC SOUTH SIDE (O, 150 beds) 2000 Mary Street, Pittsburgh, PA Zip 15203–2095; tel. 412/488–5550; Nancy Magee, President
Web address: www.upmc.com

UPMC ST. MARGARET (O, 240 beds) 815 Freeport Road, Pittsburgh, PA Zip 15215–3399; tel. 412/784–4000; David T. Martin, President
Web address: www.horizon.upmc.com

Owned, leased, sponsored:	12 hospitals	3946 beds
Contract–managed:	0 hospitals	0 beds
Totals:	12 hospitals	3946 beds

★0038: UPPER CHESAPEAKE HEALTH SYSTEM (NP)
520 Upper Chesapeake Drive, Suite 405, Bel Air, MD Zip 21014–4324; tel. 443/643–3303; Lyle Ernest Sheldon, FACHE, President and Chief Executive Officer
(Independent Hospital System)

MARYLAND: HARFORD MEMORIAL HOSPITAL (O, 108 beds) 501 South Union Avenue, Havre De Grace, MD Zip 21078–3493; tel. 443/843–5000; Lyle Ernest Sheldon, FACHE, President and Chief Executive Officer
Web address: www.uchs.org

UPPER CHESAPEAKE MEDICAL CENTER (O, 168 beds) 500 Upper Chesapeake Drive, Bel Air, MD Zip 21014–4324; tel. 443/643–1000; Lyle Ernest Sheldon, FACHE, President and Chief Executive Officer
Web address: www.uchs.org

Owned, leased, sponsored:	2 hospitals	276 beds
Contract–managed:	0 hospitals	0 beds
Totals:	2 hospitals	276 beds

0386: VALLEY BAPTIST HEALTH SYSTEM (NP)
2101 Pease Street, Harlingen, TX Zip 78550; tel. 956/389–1100; James G. Springfield, FACHE, President and Chief Executive Officer

TEXAS: VALLEY BAPTIST MEDICAL CENTER–BROWNSVILLE (O, 243 beds) 1040 West Jefferson Street, Brownsville, TX Zip 78520–5829, Mailing Address: P.O. Box 3590, Zip 78523–3590; tel. 956/698–5400; Leslie Bingham, Senior Vice President and Chief Executive Officer
Web address: www.valleybaptist.net/brownsville/

VALLEY BAPTIST MEDICAL CENTER–HARLINGEN (O, 481 beds) 2101 Pease Street, Harlingen, TX Zip 78550–8307, Mailing Address: P.O. Drawer 2588, Zip 78551–2588; tel. 956/389–1100; Jim D. Wesson, Senior Vice President and Chief Executive Officer
Web address: www.valleybaptist.net

Owned, leased, sponsored:	2 hospitals	724 beds
Contract–managed:	0 hospitals	0 beds
Totals:	2 hospitals	724 beds

★0043: VALLEY HEALTH SYSTEM (NP)
1117 East Devonshire Avenue, Hemet, CA Zip 92543; tel. 951/652–2811; Fred M. Harder, Chief Executive Officer
(Independent Hospital System)

CALIFORNIA: HEMET VALLEY MEDICAL CENTER (O, 395 beds) 1117 East Devonshire Avenue, Hemet, CA Zip 92543–3083; tel. 951/652–2811; Fred M. Harder, Chief Executive Officer
Web address: www.valleyhealthsystem.com

MENIFEE VALLEY MEDICAL CENTER (O, 82 beds) 28400 McCall Boulevard, Sun City, CA Zip 92585–9537; tel. 951/679–8888; Thomas E. Dougherty, Administrator
Web address: www.valleyhealthsystem.com

MORENO VALLEY COMMUNITY HOSPITAL (O, 101 beds) 27300 Iris Avenue, Moreno Valley, CA Zip 92555–4800; tel. 951/243–0811; Corey A. Seale, Administrator
Web address: www.valleyhealthsystem.com

Owned, leased, sponsored:	3 hospitals	578 beds
Contract–managed:	0 hospitals	0 beds
Totals:	3 hospitals	578 beds

★0128: VALLEY HEALTH SYSTEM (NP)
190 Campus Boulevard, Suite 220, Winchester, VA Zip 22601, Mailing Address: P.O. Box 3340, Zip 22604–1334; tel. 540/536–8024; Michael J. Halseth, President and Chief Executive Officer
(Independent Hospital System)

VIRGINIA: SHENANDOAH MEMORIAL HOSPITAL (O, 23 beds) 759 South Main Street, Woodstock, VA Zip 22664–1127; tel. 540/459–1100; Floyd Heater, Chief Executive Officer
Web address: www.valleyhealthlink.com

WARREN MEMORIAL HOSPITAL (O, 166 beds) 1000 Shenandoah Avenue, Front Royal, VA Zip 22630–3598; tel. 540/636–0300; Patrick B. Nolan, President and Chief Executive Officer
Web address: www.valleyhealthlink.com

WINCHESTER MEDICAL CENTER (O, 411 beds) 1840 Amherst Street, Winchester, VA Zip 22601–2540, Mailing Address: P.O. Box 3340, Zip 22604–3340; tel. 540/536–8000; Reese Jackson, President and Chief Executive Officer
Web address: www.valleyhealthlink.com

WEST VIRGINIA: HAMPSHIRE MEMORIAL HOSPITAL (O, 44 beds) 549 Center Avenue, Romney, WV Zip 26757–1199; tel. 304/822–4561; Roberta D. McCauley, Chief Executive Officer

MORGAN COUNTY WAR MEMORIAL HOSPITAL (C, 41 beds) 109 War Memorial Drive, Berkeley Springs, WV Zip 25411–1718; tel. 304/258–1234; John H. Borg, Administrator
Web address: www.warmemorialhospital.com

Owned, leased, sponsored:	4 hospitals	644 beds
Contract–managed:	1 hospital	41 beds
Totals:	5 hospitals	685 beds

For explanation of codes following names, see page B2.
★ Indicates Type III membership in the American Hospital Association.

• 0387: VANDERBILT HEALTHCARE (NP)
1211 22nd Avenue South, Nashville, TN Zip 37232; tel. 615/322–5000; Larry Goldberg, Executive Director and Chief Executive Officer

TENNESSEE: VANDERBILT UNIVERSITY MEDICAL CENTER (O, 833 beds) 1211 22nd Avenue South, Nashville, TN Zip 37232–2102; tel. 615/322–5000; Larry Goldberg, Executive Director and Chief Executive Officer
Web address: www.vanderbilt.edu

Owned, leased, sponsored:	1 hospital	833 beds
Contract-managed:	0 hospitals	0 beds
Totals:	1 hospital	833 beds

0193: VANGUARD HEALTH SYSTEM (IO)
20 Burton Hills Boulevard, Suite 10, Nashville, TN Zip 37215; tel. 615/665–6000; Charles N. Martin, Jr., Chairman and Chief Executive Officer
(Moderately Centralized Health System)

ARIZONA: ARROWHEAD HOSPITAL (O, 155 beds) 18701 North 67th Avenue, Glendale, AZ Zip 85308–5722; tel. 623/561–1000; Jonathan W. Bartlett, Chief Executive Officer
Web address: www.arrowheadhospital.com

MARYVALE HOSPITAL MEDICAL CENTER (O, 226 beds) 5102 West Campbell Avenue, Phoenix, AZ Zip 85031–1799; tel. 623/848–5000; Jeff R. Egbert, Chief Executive Officer
Web address: www.maryvalehospital.com

PARADISE VALLEY HOSPITAL (O, 142 beds) 3929 East Bell Road, Phoenix, AZ Zip 85032–2196; tel. 602/923–5000; Steve Sisto, Chief Executive Officer
Web address: www.paradisevalleyhospital.com

PHOENIX BAPTIST HOSPITAL (O, 215 beds) 2000 West Bethany Home Road, Phoenix, AZ Zip 85015–2110; tel. 602/249–0212; Bruce F. Buchanan, FACHE, Chief Executive Officer
Web address: www.phoenixbaptisthospital.com

WEST VALLEY HOSPITAL (O, 106 beds) 13677 West McDowell Road, Goodyear, AZ Zip 85338; tel. 623/882–1500; Thomas W. Keller, Chief Executive Officer
Web address: www.wvhospital.com

ILLINOIS: LOUIS A. WEISS MEMORIAL HOSPITAL (O, 172 beds) 4646 North Marine Drive, Chicago, IL Zip 60640–1501; tel. 773/878–8700; Frank L. Molinaro, Chief Executive Officer
Web address: www.weisshospital.com

MACNEAL HOSPITAL (O, 240 beds) 3249 South Oak Park Avenue, Berwyn, IL Zip 60402–0715; tel. 708/783–9100; Brian J. Lemon, Chief Executive Officer
Web address: www.macneal.com

MASSACHUSETTS: METROWEST MEDICAL CENTER (O, 407 beds) 115 Lincoln Street, Framingham, MA Zip 01702–6342; tel. 508/383–1000; Andrei Soran, Chief Executive Officer
Web address: www.mwmc.com

SAINT VINCENT HOSPITAL AT WORCESTER MEDICAL CENTER (O, 351 beds) 123 Summer Street, Worcester, MA Zip 1608; tel. 508/363–5000; John E. Smithhisler, CHE, President and Chief Executive Officer
Web address: www.stvincenthospital.com

TEXAS: BAPTIST HEALTH SYSTEM (O, 1189 beds) 111 Dallas Street, San Antonio, TX Zip 78205–1230; tel. 210/297–7000; Keith L. Swinney, President

Owned, leased, sponsored:	10 hospitals	3203 beds
Contract-managed:	0 hospitals	0 beds
Totals:	10 hospitals	3203 beds

5435: VIA CHRISTI HEALTH SYSTEM (CC)
3720 East Bayley, Wichita, KS Zip 67218–3002; tel. 316/858–4900; Kevin P. Conlin, President and Chief Executive Officer
(Centralized Health System)

KANSAS: KANSAS SURGERY AND RECOVERY CENTER (O, 32 beds) 2770 North Webb Road, Wichita, KS Zip 67226–8112; tel. 316/634–0090; Ely Bartal, M.D., Chief Executive Officer
Web address: www.ksrc.org

MERCY REGIONAL HEALTH CENTER (O, 121 beds) 1823 College Avenue, Manhattan, KS Zip 66502, Mailing Address: P.O. Box 1289, Zip 66505–1289; tel. 785/776–3322; Richard L. Allen, President and Chief Executive Officer
Web address: www.mercyregional.org

MT. CARMEL REGIONAL MEDICAL CENTER (O, 129 beds) 1102 East Centennial Drive, Pittsburg, KS Zip 66762–6643; tel. 620/232–0109; Jonathan S. Davis, FACHE, President and Chief Executive Officer
Web address: www.mtcarmel.org

VIA CHRISTI REGIONAL MEDICAL CENTER (O, 749 beds) 929 North St. Francis Street, Wichita, KS Zip 67214–3882; tel. 316/268–5000; Laurie Labarca, Interim President and Chief Executive Officer
Web address: www.via–christi.org

VIA CHRISTI REHABILITATION CENTER (O, 60 beds) 1151 North Rock Road, Wichita, KS Zip 67206–1262; tel. 316/634–3400; Laurie Labarca, Chief Operating Officer
Web address: www.via–christi.org

Owned, leased, sponsored:	5 hospitals	1091 beds
Contract-managed:	0 hospitals	0 beds
Totals:	5 hospitals	1091 beds

0046: VIAHEALTH (NP)
1425 Portland Avenue, 5th Floor, Rochester, NY Zip 14621; tel. 585/922–4437; Mark C. Clement, President and Chief Executive Officer
(Moderately Centralized Health System)

NEW YORK: NEWARK–WAYNE COMMUNITY HOSPITAL (O, 263 beds) Driving Park Avenue, Newark, NY Zip 14513, Mailing Address: P.O. Box 111, Zip 14513–0111; tel. 315/332–2022; Annette B. Leahy, President and Chief Executive Officer
Web address: www.viahealth.org

ROCHESTER GENERAL HOSPITAL (O, 494 beds) 1425 Portland Avenue, Rochester, NY Zip 14621–3099; tel. 585/922–4000; Mark C. Clement, President and Chief Executive Officer
Web address: www.viahealth.org/

Owned, leased, sponsored:	2 hospitals	757 beds
Contract-managed:	0 hospitals	0 beds
Totals:	2 hospitals	757 beds

0299: VIBRA HEALTHCARE (IO)
4550 Lena Drive, Suite 225, Mechanicsburg, PA Zip 17055; tel. 717/591–5700; Brad Hollinger, Chairman and Chief Executive Officer
(Independent Hospital System)

CALIFORNIA: KENTFIELD REHABILITATION AND SPECIALTY HOSPITAL (O, 60 beds) 1125 Sir Francis Drake Boulevard, San Rafael, CA Zip 94904–1455; tel. 415/456–9680; Ann Gors, Chief Executive Officer
Web address: www.kentfieldrehab.com

NORTHERN CALIFORNIA REHABILITATION HOSPITAL (O, 76 beds) 2801 Eureka Way, Redding, CA Zip 96001; tel. 530/246–9000; Chris Jones, Chief Executive Officer
Web address: www.norcalrehab.com

SAN JOAQUIN VALLEY REHABILITATION HOSPITAL (O, 60 beds) 7173 North Sharon Avenue, Fresno, CA Zip 93720–3329; tel. 559/436–3600; Edward C. Palacios, Chief Executive Officer
Web address: www.sjvrehab.com

COLORADO: NORTH VALLEY HOSPITALS (O, 117 beds) 8451 Pearl Street, Thornton, CO Zip 80229–4804; tel. 303/288–3000; Kathleen Cahill, Chief Executive Officer
Web address: www.northvalleyrehab.com

KENTUCKY: SOUTHERN KENTUCKY REHABILITATION HOSPITAL (O, 60 beds) 1300 Campbell Lane, Bowling Green, KY Zip 42104–4162; tel. 270/782–6900; Joanna Thomas, Chief Executive Officer
Web address: www.skyrehab.com

For explanation of codes following names, see page B2.
★ Indicates Type III membership in the American Hospital Association.
• Single hospital health care system

MASSACHUSETTS: NEW BEDFORD REHABILITATION HOSPITAL (O, 90 beds) 4499 Acushnet Avenue, New Bedford, MA Zip 2745; tel. 508/995–6900; Edward B. Leary, Chief Executive Officer
Web address: www.newbedfordrehab.com

NEW JERSEY: MARLTON REHABILITATION HOSPITAL (O, 46 beds) 92 Brick Road, Marlton, NJ Zip 08053–2177; tel. 856/988–8778; David T. Shannon, Chief Executive Officer
Web address: www.marltonrehab.com

OHIO: ST. FRANCIS HEALTH CARE CENTRE (C, 186 beds) 401 North Broadway, Green Springs, OH Zip 44836–9653; tel. 419/639–2626; Kim D. Eicher, Chief Executive Officer
Web address: www.sfhcc.org

TEXAS: VIBRA SPECIALTY HOSPITAL OF DALLAS (O, 60 beds) 1950 Record Crossing Road, Dallas, TX Zip 75235–6223; tel. 214/638–1500; Paul P. Hall, Jr., Chief Executive Officer
Web address: www.vshdallas.com

VICTORIA WARM SPRINGS HOSPITAL (O, 26 beds) 102 Medical Drive, Victoria, TX Zip 77904; tel. 361/576–6200; Anne R. Leon, Administrator
Web address: www.warmsprings.org

WARM SPRINGS REHABILITATION HOSPITAL (O, 65 beds) 5101 Medical Drive, San Antonio, TX Zip 78229–6098; tel. 210/616–0100; Dennis Falck, Chief Executive Officer
Web address: www.warmsprings.org

WARM SPRINGS SPECIALTY HOSPITAL (O, 34 beds) 200 Memorial Drive, Luling, TX Zip 78648; tel. 830/875–8400; Kurt Meyer, Chief Executive Officer
Web address: www.warmsprings.org

Owned, leased, sponsored:	11 hospitals	694 beds
Contract–managed:	1 hospital	186 beds
Totals:	12 hospitals	880 beds

0012: VIRGINIA DEPARTMENT OF MENTAL HEALTH (NP)
1220 Bank Street, Richmond, VA Zip 23219, Mailing Address: P.O. Box 1797, Zip 23218–1797; tel. 804/786–3921; James S. Reinhard, M.D., Commissioner
(Independent Hospital System)

VIRGINIA: CATAWBA HOSPITAL (O, 110 beds) 5525 Catawba Hospital Drive, Catawba, VA Zip 24070–2115, Mailing Address: P.O. Box 200, Zip 24070–0200; tel. 540/375–4200; Jack L. Wood, Director
Web address: www.catawba.dmhmrsas.virginia.gov

CENTRAL STATE HOSPITAL (O, 277 beds) 26317 West Washington Street, Petersburg, VA Zip 23803, Mailing Address: P.O. Box 4030, Zip 23803–4030; tel. 804/524–7000; Charles M. Davis, M.D., Director
Web address: www.csh.dmhmrsas.virginia.gov

CENTRAL VIRGINIA TRAINING CENTER (O, 1112 beds) 210 East Colony Road, Madison Heights, VA Zip 24572–2005, Mailing Address: P.O. Box 1098, Lynchburg, Zip 24505–1098; tel. 434/947–6326; Denise D. Micheletti, RN, Acting Director
Web address: www.cvtc.dmhmrsas.virginia.gov/

COMMONWEALTH CENTER FOR CHILDREN AND ADOLESCENTS (O, 60 beds) 1355 Richmond Road, Staunton, VA Zip 24401–1091, Mailing Address: Box 4000, Zip 24402–4000; tel. 540/332–2100; William J. Tuell, M.S.N., Facility Director
Web address: www.ccca.dmhmrsas.virginia.gov

EASTERN STATE HOSPITAL (O, 471 beds) 4601 Ironbound Road, Williamsburg, VA Zip 23188–2652; tel. 757/253–5161; John M. Favret, Director
Web address: www.esh.dmhmrsas.virginia. gov

NORTHERN VIRGINIA MENTAL HEALTH INSTITUTE (O, 137 beds) 3302 Gallows Road, Falls Church, VA Zip 22042–3398; tel. 703/207–7110; Lynn Delacy, RN, Ph.D., Facility Director
Web address: www.nvmhi.dmhmrsas.virginia.gov

PIEDMONT GERIATRIC HOSPITAL (O, 150 beds) 5001 East Patrick Henry Highway, Burkeville, VA Zip 23922–0427, Mailing Address: P.O. Box 427, Zip 23922–0427; tel. 434/767–4401; Stephen M. Herrick, Ph.D., Director
Web address: www.pgh.dmhmrsas.virginia.gov

SOUTHERN VIRGINIA MENTAL HEALTH INSTITUTE (O, 72 beds) 382 Taylor Drive, Danville, VA Zip 24541–4023; tel. 434/799–6220; David M. Lyon, Director
Web address: www.svmhi.dmhmrsas.virginia.gov

SOUTHWESTERN VIRGINIA MENTAL HEALTH INSTITUTE (O, 266 beds) 340 Bagley Circle, Marion, VA Zip 24354–3390; tel. 276/783–1200; Cynthia McKaskey, Ph.D., Director

WESTERN STATE HOSPITAL (O, 260 beds) 1301 Richmond Avenue, Staunton, VA Zip 24401–9146, Mailing Address: P.O. Box 2500, Zip 24402–2500; tel. 540/332–8000; Jack W. Barber, M.D., Director
Web address: www.wsh.dmhmrsas.virginia.gov/

Owned, leased, sponsored:	10 hospitals	2915 beds
Contract–managed:	0 hospitals	0 beds
Totals:	10 hospitals	2915 beds

★6725: VIRTUA HEALTH (NP)
50 Lake Center Executive Park, Suite 401, Marlton, NJ Zip 08053; tel. 856/355–0010; Richard P. Miller, President and Chief Executive Officer
(Independent Hospital System)

NEW JERSEY: VIRTUA MEMORIAL HOSPITAL BURLINGTON COUNTY (O, 326 beds) 175 Madison Avenue, Mount Holly, NJ Zip 08060–2099; tel. 609/267–0700; Stephen Kolesk, M.D., Vice President and Chief Operating Officer
Web address: www.virtua.org

VIRTUA WEST JERSEY HOSPITAL–BERLIN (O, 84 beds) 100 Townsend Avenue, Berlin, NJ Zip 08009–9035; tel. 856/322–3000; Christopher A. Chekouras, Vice President and Chief Operating Officer
Web address: www.virtua.org

VIRTUA WEST JERSEY HOSPITAL–MARLTON (O, 165 beds) 90 Brick Road, Marlton, NJ Zip 08053–9697; tel. 856/355–6000; Gary L. Long, Vice President and Chief Operating Officer
Web address: www.virtua.org

VIRTUA WEST JERSEY HOSPITAL–VOORHEES (O, 258 beds) 101 Carnie Boulevard, Voorhees, NJ Zip 08043–1597; tel. 856/325–3000; Michael S. Kotzen, Vice President and Chief Operating Officer
Web address: www.virtua.org

Owned, leased, sponsored:	4 hospitals	833 beds
Contract–managed:	0 hospitals	0 beds
Totals:	4 hospitals	833 beds

★6705: WAKEMED (NP)
3000 New Bern Avenue, Raleigh, NC Zip 27610; tel. 919/350–8000; William K. Atkinson, II, President and Chief Executive Officer
(Moderately Centralized Health System)

NORTH CAROLINA: BETSY JOHNSON REGIONAL HOSPITAL (C, 101 beds) 800 Tilghman Drive, Dunn, NC Zip 28334–5599, Mailing Address: Drawer 1706, Zip 28335–1706; tel. 910/892–7161; Kenneth E. Bryan, President and Chief Executive Officer
Web address: www.bjrh.org

WAKEMED CARY HOSPITAL (O, 150 beds) 1900 Kildaire Farm Road, Cary, NC Zip 27511; tel. 919/350–2300;

WAKEMED RALEIGH CAMPUS (O, 612 beds) 3000 New Bern Avenue, Raleigh, NC Zip 27610–1295; tel. 919/350–8000; William K. Atkinson, II, President and Chief Executive Officer
Web address: www.wakemed.org

Owned, leased, sponsored:	2 hospitals	762 beds
Contract–managed:	1 hospital	101 beds
Totals:	3 hospitals	863 beds

0188: WELLMONT HEALTH SYSTEM (NP)
1905 American Way, Kingsport, TN Zip 37662–0224; tel. 423/230–8200
(Moderately Centralized Health System)

KENTUCKY: JENKINS COMMUNITY HOSPITAL (O, 25 beds) Main Street, Jenkins, KY Zip 41537–9614, Mailing Address: P.O. Box 472, Zip 41537–0472; tel. 606/832–2171; Sherrie L. Newcomb, Administrator

For explanation of codes following names, see page B2.
★ Indicates Type III membership in the American Hospital Association.

TENNESSEE: WELLMONT BRISTOL REGIONAL MEDICAL CENTER (O, 348 beds) 1 Medical Park Boulevard, Bristol, TN Zip 37620–7434; tel. 423/844–1121; Barton A. Hove, President
Web address: www.wellmont.org

WELLMONT HANCOCK COUNTY HOSPITAL (O, 10 beds) 1517 Main Street, Highway 33, Sneedville, TN Zip 37869; tel. 423/921–7023; Troy Clark, Chief Executive Officer
Web address: www.wellmont.org

WELLMONT HAWKINS COUNTY MEMORIAL HOSPITAL (L, 50 beds) 851 Locust Street, Rogersville, TN Zip 37857–2407, Mailing Address: P.O. Box 130, Zip 37857–0130; tel. 423/921–7000; Fred L. Pelle, FACHE, President
Web address: www.wellmont.org

WELLMONT HOLSTON VALLEY MEDICAL CENTER (O, 317 beds) 130 West Ravine Street, Kingsport, TN Zip 37660, Mailing Address: P.O. Box 238, Zip 37662–0238; tel. 423/224–4000; Blaine L. Douglas, Chief Executive Officer
Web address: www.wellmont.org

VIRGINIA: LEE REGIONAL MEDICAL CENTER (O, 50 beds) West Morgan Avenue, Pennington Gap, VA Zip 24277–0070, Mailing Address: P.O. Box 70, Zip 24277–0070; tel. 276/546–1440; Joseph J. Peluso, Chief Executive Officer
Web address: www.leeregional.com

MOUNTAIN VIEW REGIONAL MEDICAL CENTER (O, 133 beds) Third Street N.E., Norton, VA Zip 24273–1131, Mailing Address: P.O. Box 620, Zip 24273–0620; tel. 276/679–9100; David L. Brash, Chief Executive Officer
Web address: www.mountainviewregional.org

WELLMONT LONESOME PINE HOSPITAL (O, 60 beds) 1990 Holton Avenue East, Big Stone Gap, VA Zip 24219–0230; tel. 276/523–3111; Robert G. Polahar, President
Web address: www.wellmont.org

Owned, leased, sponsored:	8 hospitals	993 beds
Contract-managed:	0 hospitals	0 beds
Totals:	8 hospitals	993 beds

★0068: WELLSPAN HEALTH (NP)

45 Monument Road, Suite 200, York, PA Zip 17403; tel. 717/851–2121; Bruce M. Bartels, President
(Centralized Physician/Insurance Health System)

PENNSYLVANIA: GETTYSBURG HOSPITAL (O, 95 beds) 147 Gettys Street, Gettysburg, PA Zip 17325–2534; tel. 717/334–2121; Kevin H. Mosser, M.D., Chief Executive Officer
Web address: www.wellspan.org

YORK HOSPITAL (O, 517 beds) 1001 South George Street, York, PA Zip 17405–3645; tel. 717/851–2345; Richard L. Seim, President and Chief Executive Officer
Web address: www.wellspan.org

Owned, leased, sponsored:	2 hospitals	612 beds
Contract-managed:	0 hospitals	0 beds
Totals:	2 hospitals	612 beds

★0995: WELLSTAR HEALTH SYSTEM (NP)

805 Sandy Plains Road, Marietta, GA Zip 30066; tel. 770/792–5012; Gregory L. Simone, M.D., President and Chief Executive Officer
(Centralized Health System)

GEORGIA: WELLSTAR COBB HOSPITAL (O, 378 beds) 3950 Austell Road, Austell, GA Zip 30106–1121; tel. 770/732–4000; Randy Cook, Senior Vice President and Administrator
Web address: www.wellstar.org

WELLSTAR DOUGLAS HOSPITAL (O, 98 beds) 8954 Hospital Drive, Douglasville, GA Zip 30134–2282; tel. 770/949–1500; J. Michael Poore, Vice President and Administrator
Web address: www.wellstar.org

WELLSTAR KENNESTONE HOSPITAL (O, 604 beds) 677 Church Street, Marietta, GA Zip 30060–1148; tel. 770/793–5000; Candice Saunders, Senior Vice President and Administrator
Web address: www.wellstar.org

WELLSTAR PAULDING HOSPITAL (O, 216 beds) 600 West Memorial Drive, Dallas, GA Zip 30132–1335; tel. 770/445–4411; John Law, Administrator
Web address: www.wellstar.org

WELLSTAR WINDY HILL HOSPITAL (O, 42 beds) 2540 Windy Hill Road, Marietta, GA Zip 30067–8632; tel. 770/644–1000; Lou Little, Vice President and Administrator
Web address: www.wellstar.org

Owned, leased, sponsored:	5 hospitals	1338 beds
Contract-managed:	0 hospitals	0 beds
Totals:	5 hospitals	1338 beds

★0199: WEST PENN ALLEGHENY HEALTH SYSTEM (NP)

3200 East North Avenue, Pittsburgh, PA Zip 15212; tel. 412/359–8588; Christopher Olivia, M.D., President and Chief Executive Officer
(Moderately Centralized Health System)

PENNSYLVANIA: ALLEGHENY GENERAL HOSPITAL (O, 473 beds) 320 East North Avenue, Pittsburgh, PA Zip 15212–4756; tel. 412/359–3131; Connie M. Cibrone, President and Chief Executive Officer
Web address: www.wpahs.org

ALLE–KISKI MEDICAL CENTER (O, 250 beds) 1301 Carlisle Street, Natrona Heights, PA Zip 15065–1192; tel. 724/224–5100; Michael Harlovic, RN, Interim President and Chief Executive Officer
Web address: www.wpahs.org

CANONSBURG GENERAL HOSPITAL (O, 104 beds) 100 Medical Boulevard, Canonsburg, PA Zip 15317–9762; tel. 724/745–6100; Kim Malinky, President and Chief Executive Officer
Web address: www.wpahs.org

WESTERN PENNSYLVANIA HOSPITAL (O, 448 beds) 4800 Friendship Avenue, Pittsburgh, PA Zip 15224–1722; tel. 412/578–5000; Dawn M. Gideon, President and Chief Executive Officer
Web address: www.wpahs.org

WESTERN PENNSYLVANIA HOSPITAL – FORBES REGIONAL CAMPUS (O, 264 beds) 2570 Haymaker Road, Monroeville, PA Zip 15146–3592; tel. 412/858–2000; Dawn M. Gideon, President and Chief Executive Officer
Web address: www.wpahs.org

Owned, leased, sponsored:	5 hospitals	1539 beds
Contract-managed:	0 hospitals	0 beds
Totals:	5 hospitals	1539 beds

★0004: WEST TENNESSEE HEALTHCARE (NP)

620 Skyline Drive, Jackson, TN Zip 38301–3901; tel. 731/541–5000; Richard H. Parks, FACHE, President and Chief Executive Officer
(Centralized Health System)

TENNESSEE: BOLIVAR GENERAL HOSPITAL (O, 23 beds) 650 Nuckolls Road, Bolivar, TN Zip 38008–1532, Mailing Address: P.O. Box 509, Zip 38008–0509; tel. 731/658–3100; Ruby Kirby, Administrator
Web address: www.wth.net

CAMDEN GENERAL HOSPITAL (O, 25 beds) 175 Hospital Drive, Camden, TN Zip 38320–1617; tel. 731/584–6135; Denny R. Smith, Administrator
Web address: www.wth.net

GIBSON GENERAL HOSPITAL (O, 34 beds) 200 Hospital Drive, Trenton, TN Zip 38382–3313; tel. 731/855–7900; Sherry Scruggs, Administrator
Web address: www.wth.net

HUMBOLDT GENERAL HOSPITAL (O, 35 beds) 3525 Chere Carol Road, Humboldt, TN Zip 38343–3699; tel. 731/784–2321; Bill Kail, Administrator
Web address: www.wth.net

JACKSON–MADISON COUNTY GENERAL HOSPITAL (O, 644 beds) 708 West Forest Avenue, Jackson, TN Zip 38301–3956; tel. 731/541–5000; Richard H. Parks, FACHE, President and Chief Executive Officer
Web address: www.wth.org

MILAN GENERAL HOSPITAL (O, 28 beds) 4039 South Highland, Milan, TN Zip 38358–3167; tel. 731/686–1591; John M. Carruth, Administrator
Web address: www.wth.net

For explanation of codes following names, see page B2.
★ Indicates Type III membership in the American Hospital Association.

PATHWAYS OF TENNESSEE (O, 25 beds) 238 Summar Drive, Jackson, TN Zip 38301–3982; tel. 731/541–8200; Pam Henson, Executive Director
Web address: www.wth.net

Owned, leased, sponsored:	7 hospitals	814 beds
Contract-managed:	0 hospitals	0 beds
Totals:	7 hospitals	814 beds

★0119: WEST VIRGINIA UNITED HEALTH SYSTEM (NP)
1000 Technology Drive, Suite 2320, Fairmont, WV Zip 26554; tel. 304/368–2700; J. Thomas Jones, President and Chief Executive Officer
(Moderately Centralized Health System)

WEST VIRGINIA: CITY HOSPITAL (O, 159 beds) Dry Run Road, Martinsburg, WV Zip 25401, Mailing Address: P.O. Box 1418, Zip 25402–1418; tel. 304/264–1000; Anthony Zelenka, Administrator
Web address: www.cityhospital.org

JEFFERSON MEMORIAL HOSPITAL (O, 45 beds) 300 South Preston Street, Ranson, WV Zip 25438–1699; tel. 304/728–1600; Roger M. Eitelman, Chief Executive Officer
Web address: www.jeffmem.com

UNITED HOSPITAL CENTER (O, 311 beds) 3 Hospital Plaza, Clarksburg, WV Zip 26301, Mailing Address: P.O. Box 1680, Zip 26302–1680; tel. 304/624–2121; Bruce C. Carter, President
Web address: www.uhcwv.org

WEST VIRGINIA UNIVERSITY HOSPITALS (O, 486 beds) Medical Center Drive, Morgantown, WV Zip 26506–4749; tel. 304/598–4000; Bruce McClymonds, President and Chief Executive Officer
Web address: www.health.wvu.edu

Owned, leased, sponsored:	4 hospitals	1001 beds
Contract-managed:	0 hospitals	0 beds
Totals:	4 hospitals	1001 beds

★0323: WESTCARE HEALTH SYSTEM (NP)
68 Hospital Road, Sylva, NC Zip 28779; tel. 828/586–7000; Mark T. Leonard, Chief Executive Officer
(Independent Hospital System)

NORTH CAROLINA: HARRIS REGIONAL HOSPITAL (O, 200 beds) 68 Hospital Road, Sylva, NC Zip 28779–2795; tel. 828/586–7000; Mark T. Leonard, Chief Executive Officer
Web address: www.westcare.org

SWAIN COUNTY HOSPITAL (O, 25 beds) 45 Plateau Street, Bryson City, NC Zip 28713–6784; tel. 828/488–4013; Ronald A. Sloan, Administrator
Web address: www.westcare.org

Owned, leased, sponsored:	2 hospitals	225 beds
Contract-managed:	0 hospitals	0 beds
Totals:	2 hospitals	225 beds

★0372: WESTERN MARYLAND HEALTH SYSTEM (NP)
Cumberland, MD Mailing Address: P.O. Box 539, Zip 21502; tel. 301/723–4200; Barry P. Ronan, President

MARYLAND: MEMORIAL HOSPITAL AND MEDICAL CENTER OF CUMBERLAND (O, 151 beds) 600 Memorial Avenue, Cumberland, MD Zip 21502–3797; tel. 301/723–4000; Thomas C. Dowdell, FACHE, Senior Vice President and Chief Operating Officer
Web address: www.wmhs.com

WMHS BRADDOCK HOSPITAL (O, 256 beds) 900 Seton Drive, Cumberland, MD Zip 21502–1874; tel. 301/723–4200; Thomas C. Dowdell, FACHE, Senior Vice President and Chief Operating Officer
Web address: www.wmhs.com

Owned, leased, sponsored:	2 hospitals	407 beds
Contract-managed:	0 hospitals	0 beds
Totals:	2 hospitals	407 beds

★6745: WHEATON FRANCISCAN HEALTHCARE (CC)
26W171 Roosevelt Road, Wheaton, IL Zip 60189–0667, Mailing Address: P.O. Box 667, Zip 60189–0667; tel. 630/462–9271; John D. Oliverio, President and Chief Executive Officer
(Decentralized Health System)

ILLINOIS: MARIANJOY REHABILITATION HOSPITAL (O, 120 beds) 26 West 171 Roosevelt Road, Wheaton, IL Zip 60187–0795, Mailing Address: P.O. Box 795, Zip 60189–0795; tel. 630/909–8000; Kathleen C. Yosko, President and Chief Executive Officer
Web address: www.marianjoy.org

RUSH OAK PARK HOSPITAL (O, 177 beds) 520 South Maple Avenue, Oak Park, IL Zip 60304–1097; tel. 708/383–9300; Bruce M. Elegant, President and Chief Executive Officer
Web address: www.roph.org

IOWA: COVENANT MEDICAL CENTER (O, 275 beds) 3421 West Ninth Street, Waterloo, IA Zip 50702–5499; tel. 319/272–8000; Jack Dusenbery, President and Chief Executive Officer
Web address: www.covhealth.com

MERCY HOSPITAL OF FRANCISCAN SISTERS (O, 62 beds) 201 Eighth Avenue S.E., Oelwein, IA Zip 50662–2447; tel. 319/283–6000; Katherine Hintz, Administrator
Web address: www.covhealth.com

SARTORI MEMORIAL HOSPITAL (O, 66 beds) 515 College Street, Cedar Falls, IA Zip 50613–2500; tel. 319/268–3000; Sherri Greenwood, Administrator
Web address: www.covhealth.com

WISCONSIN: ST. ELIZABETH HOSPITAL (O, 197 beds) 1506 South Oneida Street, Appleton, WI Zip 54915–1397; tel. 920/738–2000; Travis Andersen, President
Web address: www.affinityhealth.org

THE WISCONSIN HEART HOSPITAL (O, 30 beds) 10000 West Bluemound Road, Wauwatosa, WI Zip 53226; tel. 414/778–7800; Norma J. McCutcheon, President
Web address: www.twhh.org

UNITED HOSPITAL SYSTEM, ST. CATHERINE'S MEDICAL CENTER CAMPUS (O, 189 beds) 9555 76th Street, Pleasant Prairie, WI Zip 53158; tel. 262/656–2011; Richard O. Schmidt, Jr., President and Chief Executive Officer
Web address: www.uhsi.org

WHEATON FRANCISCAN HEALTHCARE – ALL SAINTS (O, 389 beds) 3801 Spring Street, Racine, WI Zip 53405–1690; tel. 262/687–4011; Kenneth R. Buser, President and Chief Executive Officer
Web address: www.allsaintshealth.com

WHEATON FRANCISCAN HEALTHCARE – ELMBROOK MEMORIAL (O, 88 beds) 19333 West North Avenue, Brookfield, WI Zip 53045–4198; tel. 262/785–2000; Kimry A. Johnsrud, President
Web address: www.wfhealthcare.org

WHEATON FRANCISCAN HEALTHCARE – ST. FRANCIS (S, 192 beds) 3237 South 16th Street, Milwaukee, WI Zip 53215–4592; tel. 414/647–5000; Debra Standridge, President
Web address: www.stfrancishospital.net

WHEATON FRANCISCAN HEALTHCARE – ST. JOSEPH (O, 396 beds) 5000 West Chambers Street, Milwaukee, WI Zip 53210–9988; tel. 414/447–2000; Ronald Groepper, President
Web address: www.whfc.org

Owned, leased, sponsored:	12 hospitals	2181 beds
Contract-managed:	0 hospitals	0 beds
Totals:	12 hospitals	2181 beds

1945: WILLIS–KNIGHTON HEALTH SYSTEM (NP)
2600 Greenwood Road, Shreveport, LA Zip 71130–2600; tel. 318/212–4000; James K. Elrod, President and Chief Executive Officer
(Independent Hospital System)

LOUISIANA: WILLIS–KNIGHTON BOSSIER HEALTH CENTER (O, 115 beds) 2400 Hospital Drive, Bossier City, LA Zip 71111; tel. 318/212–7000; Cliff LeBlanc, Administrator
Web address: www.wkhs.com/wkb/

For explanation of codes following names, see page B2.
★ Indicates Type III membership in the American Hospital Association.

WILLIS–KNIGHTON MEDICAL CENTER (O, 651 beds) 2600 Greenwood Road, Shreveport, LA Zip 71103–2600, Mailing Address: P.O. Box 32600, Zip 71130–2600; tel. 318/212–4600; Jaf Fielder, Vice President and Administrator
Web address: www.wkhs.com

Owned, leased, sponsored:	2 hospitals	766 beds
Contract-managed:	0 hospitals	0 beds
Totals:	2 hospitals	766 beds

0282: WUESTHOFF HEALTH SYSTEM (NP)
110 Longwood Avenue, Rockledge, FL Zip 32955; tel. 321/636–2211; Emil P. Miller, President and Chief Executive Officer
(Centralized Health System)

FLORIDA: WUESTHOFF MEDICAL CENTER – MELBOURNE (O, 115 beds) 250 North Wickham Road, Melbourne, FL Zip 32935; tel. 321/752–1200; Donald McKenna, Administrator
Web address: www.wuesthoff.org

WUESTHOFF MEDICAL CENTER – ROCKLEDGE (O, 291 beds) 110 Longwood Avenue, Rockledge, FL Zip 32955–2887, Mailing Address: P.O. Box 565002, Mail Stop 1, Zip 32956–5002; tel. 321/636–2211; Chantal Leconte, Administrator
Web address: www.wuesthoff.org

Owned, leased, sponsored:	2 hospitals	406 beds
Contract-managed:	0 hospitals	0 beds
Totals:	2 hospitals	406 beds

★0157: YALE NEW HAVEN HEALTH SYSTEM (NP)
789 Howard Avenue, New Haven, CT Zip 06519; tel. 203/688–4608; Marna P. Borgstrom, President and Chief Executive Officer
(Moderately Centralized Health System)

CONNECTICUT: BRIDGEPORT HOSPITAL (O, 354 beds) 267 Grant Street, Bridgeport, CT Zip 06610–0120, Mailing Address: P.O. Box 5000, Zip 06610–5000; tel. 203/384–3000; Robert J. Trefry, President and Chief Executive Officer
Web address: www.bridgeporthospital.org

GREENWICH HOSPITAL (O, 174 beds) 5 Perryridge Road, Greenwich, CT Zip 06830–4697; tel. 203/863–3000; Frank A. Corvino, President and Chief Executive Officer
Web address: www.greenhosp.org

YALE–NEW HAVEN HOSPITAL (O, 881 beds) 20 York Street, New Haven, CT Zip 06510–3202; tel. 203/688–4242; Marna P. Borgstrom, President and Chief Executive Officer
Web address: www.ynhh.org

Owned, leased, sponsored:	3 hospitals	1409 beds
Contract-managed:	0 hospitals	0 beds
Totals:	3 hospitals	1409 beds

0211: YOUTH AND FAMILY CENTERED SERVICES (IO)
1705 Capital of Texas Highway South, Austin, TX Zip 78746; tel. 512/327–1119; Kevin P. Sheehan, Chairman, President and Chief Executive Officer
(Independent Hospital System)

MISSOURI: LAKELAND REGIONAL HOSPITAL (O, 60 beds) 440 South Market Street, Springfield, MO Zip 65806–2026; tel. 417/865–5581; Rick Crump, Chief Executive Officer
Web address: www.yfcs.com/facilities/lakeland/index.html

PENNSYLVANIA: SOUTHWOOD PSYCHIATRIC HOSPITAL (O, 174 beds) 2575 Boyce Plaza Road, Pittsburgh, PA Zip 15241–3925; tel. 412/257–2290; Barbara L. Callaghan, Chief Executive Officer
Web address: www.southwoodhospital.com

Owned, leased, sponsored:	2 hospitals	234 beds
Contract-managed:	0 hospitals	0 beds
Totals:	2 hospitals	234 beds

Section B

For explanation of codes following names, see page B2.
★ Indicates Type III membership in the American Hospital Association.

Headquarters of Health Care Systems

Geographically

United States

ALABAMA

Birmingham: BAPTIST HEALTH SYSTEM 3201 4th Avenue South, Zip 35222, Mailing Address: P.O. Box 830605, Zip 35283–0605; tel. 205/715–5319; M. Shane Spees, President and Chief Executive Officer, p. B15

BRADFORD HEALTH SERVICES 2101 Magnolia Avenue South, Suite 518, Zip 35205; tel. 205/251–7753; Jerry W. Crowder, President and Chief Executive Officer, p. B18

★ HEALTHSOUTH CORPORATION One Healthsouth Parkway, Zip 35243; tel. 205/967–7116; Jay Grinney, President, p. B60

NOLAND HEALTH SERVICES, INC. 600 Corporate Parkway, Suite 1000, Zip 35242; tel. 205/783–8484; Gary M. Glasscock, President and Chief Executive Officer, p. B85

UAB HEALTH SYSTEM 500 22nd Street South, Suite 408, Zip 35233; tel. 205/975–5362; Ray Watts, M.D., Interim Chief Executive Officer, p. B122

Florence: ★ COFFEE HEALTH GROUP 205 Marengo Street, Zip 35630–6033; tel. 256/768–9413; Carl W. Bailey, President and Chief Executive Officer, p. B31

Guntersville: ★ MARSHALL COUNTY HEALTH CARE AUTHORITY 227 Britany Road, Zip 35976; tel. 256/894–6615; Gary R. Gore, Chief Executive Officer, p. B76

Mobile: INFIRMARY HEALTH SYSTEM 5 Mobile Infirmary Circle, Zip 36607–3520; tel. 251/435–5500; E. Chandler Bramlett, Jr., Chief Executive Officer, p. B65

★ UNIVERSITY OF SOUTH ALABAMA HOSPITALS 2451 Filligim Street, Zip 36617; tel. 251/471–7000; Stanley K. Hammack, Associate Vice President Hospital Affairs and Chief Executive Officer, p. B127

Montgomery: ★ BAPTIST HEALTH 301 Brown Springs Road, Zip 36117; tel. 334/273–4400; W. Russell Tyner, President and Chief Executive Officer, p. B14

GILLIARD HEALTH SERVICES 3091 Carter Hill Road, Zip 36111; tel. 334/265–5009; William G. McKenzie, President, Chief Executive Officer and Chairman, p. B51

Tuscaloosa: DCH HEALTH SYSTEM 809 University Boulevard East, Zip 35401; tel. 205/759–7111; Bryan N. Kindred, President and Chief Executive Officer, p. B38

ARIZONA

Flagstaff: ★ NORTHERN ARIZONA HEALTHCARE 1200 North Beaver Street, Zip 86001; tel. 928/773–2001; James Puffenberger, President and Chief Executive Officer, p. B86

Phoenix: ★ BANNER HEALTH 1441 North 12th Street, Zip 85006, Mailing Address: P.O. Box 25489, Zip 85002–5489; tel. 602/747–4000; Peter S. Fine, FACHE, President and Chief Executive Officer, p. B14

★ JOHN C. LINCOLN HEALTH NETWORK 250 East Dunlap Avenue, Zip 85020–2446; tel. 602/943–2381; Dan C. Coleman, President and Chief Executive Officer, p. B68

Scottsdale: ENVISION HOSPITAL CORPORATION 6730 North Scottsdale Road, Suite 290, Zip 85253; tel. 480/348–9800; Paul R. Tuft, Chairman and Chief Executive Officer, p. B47

★ SCOTTSDALE HEALTHCARE 3621 Wells Fargo Avenue, Zip 85251–5607; tel. 480/882–4000; Thomas J. Sadvary, FACHE, President and Chief Executive Officer, p. B104

Sun City: ★ SUN HEALTH CORPORATION 13180 North 103rd Drive, Zip 85351–3038, Mailing Address: P.O. Box 1278, Zip 85372–1278; tel. 623/876–5301; Leland W. Peterson, President and Chief Executive Officer, p. B114

ARKANSAS

Little Rock: ★ BAPTIST HEALTH 9601 Interstate 630, Exit 7, Zip 72205–7299; tel. 501/202–2000; Russell D. Harrington, Jr., President and Chief Executive Officer, p. B14

CALIFORNIA

Alhambra: AHMC, INC 100 South Raymond Avenue, Zip 91801–3199; tel. 626/458–4789; Jonathan Wu, M.D., President and Chairman, p. B6

Corona: AURORA BEHAVIORAL HEALTH CARE 4238 Green River Road, Zip 92882; tel. 951/549–8032; Soon K. Kim, M.D., President and Chief Executive Officer, p. B12

Covina: CITRUS VALLEY HEALTH PARTNERS 210 West San Bernardino Road, Zip 91723; tel. 626/331–7331; James T. Yoshioka, President and Chief Executive Officer, p. B30

Fairfield: ★ NORTHBAY HEALTHCARE SYSTEM 1200 B. Gale Wilson Boulevard, Zip 94533–3587; tel. 707/429–7809; Gary J. Passama, President and Chief Executive Officer, p. B86

Fresno: COMMUNITY MEDICAL CENTERS Fresno and Maddy Drive, Zip 93721, Mailing Address: P.O. Box 1232, Zip 93715–1232; tel. 559/459–6000; Tim A. Joslin, President and Chief Executive Officer, p. B36

Hemet: ★ VALLEY HEALTH SYSTEM 1117 East Devonshire Avenue, Zip 92543; tel. 951/652–2811; Fred M. Harder, Chief Executive Officer, p. B128

Irvine: SUN HEALTHCARE GROUP 18831 Von Karman, Suite 400, Zip 92612; tel. 949/255–7100; Richard K. Matros, Chairman of the Board and Chief Executive Officer, p. B114

Loma Linda: LOMA LINDA UNIVERSITY ADVENTIST HEALTH SCIENCES CENTER 11175 Campus Street, Zip 92354; tel. 909/558–7572; Richard H. Hart, President and Chief Executive Officer, p. B75

Long Beach: MEMORIAL HEALTH SERVICES 2801 Atlantic Avenue, Zip 90806, Mailing Address: P.O. Box 1428, Zip 90801–1428; tel. 562/933–2000; Barry S. Arbuckle, Ph.D., President and Chief Executive Officer, p. B79

Los Altos Hills: ★ DAUGHTERS OF CHARITY HEALTH SYSTEM 26000 Altamont Road, Zip 94022; tel. 650/917–4500; Robert Issai, President and Chief Executive Officer, p. B38

Los Angeles: ALTA HEALTHCARE SYSTEM 11500 West Olympic Boulevard, Suite 502, Zip 90064; tel. 562/925–0201; David Topper, Chief Executive Officer, p. B8

LOS ANGELES COUNTY–DEPARTMENT OF HEALTH SERVICES 313 North Figueroa Street, Room 912, Zip 90012–2691; tel. 213/240–8101; Bruce A. Chernof, M.D., Director and Chief Medical Officer, p. B75

Oakland: ★ KAISER FOUNDATION HOSPITALS One Kaiser Plaza, Zip 94612–3600; tel. 510/271–5910; George C. Halvorson, M.D., Chairman and Chief Executive Officer, p. B69

★ UNIVERSITY OF CALIFORNIA–SYSTEMWIDE ADMINISTRATION 1111 Franklin Street, 11th Floor, Zip 94607–5200; tel. 510/987–9071; William Gurtner, Vice President Clinical Services, p. B126

Orange: ★ ST. JOSEPH HEALTH SYSTEM 500 South Main Street, Suite 1000, Zip 92868, Mailing Address: P.O. Box 14132, Zip 92863–1532; tel. 714/347–7500; Deborah A. Proctor, President and Chief Executive Officer, p. B113

Palo Alto: STANFORD HEALTH CARE 300 Pasteur Drive, Zip 94304–2299; tel. 650/723–4000; Martha H. Marsh, President and Chief Executive Officer, p. B114

Roseville: ★ ADVENTIST HEALTH 2100 Douglas Boulevard, Zip 95661–3898, Mailing Address: P.O. Box 619002, Zip 95661–9002; tel. 916/781–2000; Robert G. Carmen, President, p. B4

Sacramento: ★ SUTTER HEALTH 2200 River Plaza Drive, Zip 95833; tel. 916/733–8800; Patrick E. Fry, Chief Executive Officer, p. B115

San Diego: ★ PALOMAR POMERADO HEALTH 15255 Innovation Drive, Suite 204, Zip 92128–3410; tel. 858/675–5100; Michael H. Covert, FACHE, Chief Executive Officer, p. B89

★ SCRIPPS HEALTH 4275 Campus Point Court, Zip 92121; tel. 858/678–7200; Chris D. Van Gorder, FACHE, President and Chief Executive Officer, p. B104

★ SHARP HEALTHCARE 8695 Spectrum Center Boulevard, Zip 92123–1489; tel. 858/499–4000; Michael Murphy, President and Chief Executive Officer, p. B107

San Francisco: ★ CATHOLIC HEALTHCARE WEST 185 Berry Street, Suite 300, Zip 94107–1773; tel. 415/438–5500; Lloyd H. Dean, President and Chief Executive Officer, p. B27

San Leandro: ALAMEDA MEDICAL CENTER 15400 Foothill Boulevard, Zip 94578; tel. 510/677–7920; Wright L. Lassiter, III, Chief Executive Officer, p. B6

Santa Ana: INTEGRATED HEALTHCARE 1301 North Tustin Avenue, Zip 92705; tel. 714/953–3652; Larry B. Anderson, President, p. B66

Santa Barbara: ★ COTTAGE HEALTH SYSTEM Pueblo at Bath Streets, Zip 93105, Mailing Address: P.O. Box 689, Zip 93102–0689; tel. 805/569–7290; Ronald C. Werft, President and Chief Executive Officer, p. B37

Santa Fe Springs: COLLEGE HEALTH ENTERPRISES 11627 Telegraph Road, Suite 200, Zip 90670; tel. 562/923–9449; Barry J. Weiss, Chairman of the Board, p. B31

Truckee: TAHOE FOREST HEALTH SYSTEM 10121 Pine Avenue, Zip 96161; tel. 530/587–6011; Robert A. Schapper, Chief Executive Officer, p. B116

Tustin: PACIFIC HEALTH CORPORATION 14642 Newport Avenue, Suite 388, Zip 92780; tel. 714/669–2085; James W. Young, President and Chief Executive Officer, p. B88

Walnut Creek: ★ JOHN MUIR HEALTH 1400 Treat Boulevard, Zip 94597–2142; tel. 925/941–2100; J. Kendall Anderson, President and Chief Executive Officer, p. B68

Wildomar: PRIME HEALTHCARE SERVICES 16850 Bear Valley Road, Zip 92395; tel. 760/241–8000; Lex Reddy, President and Chief Executive Officer, p. B91

Yuba City: FREMONT–RIDEOUT HEALTH GROUP 989 Plumas Street, Zip 95991; tel. 530/751–4010; Thomas P. Hayes, President and Chief Executive Officer, p. B50

COLORADO

Denver: ★ CATHOLIC HEALTH INITIATIVES 1999 Broadway, Suite 4000, Zip 80202–4004; tel. 303/298–9100; Kevin E. Lofton, President and Chief Executive Officer, p. B24

★ EXEMPLA HEALTHCARE, INC. 2420 West 26th Avenue, Suite 100–D, Zip 80211; tel. 303/813–5000; Jeffrey D. Selberg, President and Chief Executive Officer, p. B48

Fort Collins: POUDRE VALLEY HEALTH SYSTEM 1809 East Harmony Road, Zip 80528; tel. 970/297–6701; Rulon F. Stacey, President and Chief Executive Officer, p. B91

CONNECTICUT

Hartford: CONNECTICUT DEPARTMENT OF MENTAL HEALTH AND ADDICTION SERVICES 410 Capitol Avenue, Zip 06106, Mailing Address: P.O. Box 341431, Zip 06134–1431; tel. 860/418–7000; Thomas A. Kirk, Jr., Ph.D., Commissioner, p. B36

SAINT FRANCIS CARE, INC. 114 Woodland Street, Zip 06105; tel. 860/714–5541; Christopher M. Dadlez, President and Chief Executive Officer, p. B102

Manchester: ★ EASTERN CONNECTICUT HEALTH NETWORK 71 Haynes Street, Zip 06040; tel. 860/533–3400; Peter J. Karl, President and Chief Executive Officer, p. B46

New Haven: ★ YALE NEW HAVEN HEALTH SYSTEM 789 Howard Avenue, Zip 06519; tel. 203/688–4608; Marna P. Borgstrom, President and Chief Executive Officer, p. B133

DELAWARE

Wilmington: ★ CHRISTIANA CARE HEALTH SYSTEM 501 West 14th Street, Zip 19801, Mailing Address: P.O. Box 1668, Zip 19899; tel. 302/733–1000; Robert J. Laskowski, M.D., President and Chief Executive Officer, p. B29

DISTRICT OF COLUMBIA

Washington: BUREAU OF MEDICINE AND SURGERY, DEPARTMENT OF THE NAVY 2300 East Street N.W., Zip 20372–5300; tel. 202/762–3701; Rear Admiral Adam M. Robinson, Jr., Commanding Officer, p. B20

DEPARTMENT OF THE AIR FORCE 1420 Pentagon, Room 4E1084, Zip 20330–1420; tel. 202/767–4765; Lieutenant General James G. Roudebush, M.D., Surgeon General, p. B39

DEPARTMENT OF VETERANS AFFAIRS 810 Vermont Avenue N.W., Zip 20420; tel. 202/273–5781; Michael J. Kussman, M.D., Acting Undersecretary for Health, p. B40

FLORIDA

Boca Raton: PROMISE HEALTHCARE 999 Yamato Road, 3rd Floor, Zip 33431; tel. 561/869–3100; Howard B. Koslow, President and Chief Executive Officer, p. B92

Clearwater: ACCORD HEALTH CARE CORPORATION 14010 Roosevelt Road, Zip 33762; tel. 727/573–1755; Stephen H. Noble, President, p. B4

MORTON PLANT MEASE HEALTH CARE 300 Pinellas Street, Zip 33756, Mailing Address: P.O. Box 210, Zip 33756–0210; tel. 727/462–7000; Philip K. Beauchamp, FACHE, President and Chief Executive Officer, p. B82

Coral Gables: ★ BAPTIST HEALTH SOUTH FLORIDA 6855 Red Road, Suite 600, Zip 33143–3632; tel. 786/662–7111; Brian E. Keeley, President and Chief Executive Officer, p. B15

Fort Lauderdale: ★ BROWARD HEALTH 303 S.E. 17th Street, Zip 33316–2510; tel. 954/355–5100; Frank P. Nask, President and Chief Executive Officer, p. B20

Fort Myers: LEE MEMORIAL HEALTH SYSTEM 2776 Cleveland Avenue, Zip 33901; tel. 239/332–1111; James R. Nathan, President and Chief Executive Officer, p. B72

Gainesville: ★ SHANDS HEALTHCARE 1600 S.W. Archer Road, Zip 32610–0326; tel. 352/265–8929; Timothy M. Goldfarb, Chief Executive Officer, p. B107

Hollywood: ★ MEMORIAL HEALTHCARE SYSTEM 3501 Johnson Street, Zip 33021–5421; tel. 954/985–5805; Frank V. Sacco, FACHE, President and Chief Executive Officer, p. B79

Jacksonville: ★ BAPTIST HEALTH 800 Prudential Drive, Zip 32207; tel. 904/202–4011; Hugh Greene, President and Chief Executive Officer, p. B14

Miami: JACKSON HEALTH SYSTEM 1611 N.W. 12th Avenue, Zip 33136–1094; tel. 305/585–1111; Marvin O'Quinn, President and Chief Executive Officer, p. B67

Miami Lakes: PACER HEALTH CORPORATION 7759 N.W. 146th Street, Zip 33016; tel. 305/828–7660; Rainier Gonzalez, Chairman and Chief Executive Officer, p. B88

Naples: HEALTH MANAGEMENT ASSOCIATES 5811 Pelican Bay Boulevard, Suite 500, Zip 34108; tel. 239/598–3131; Burke W. Whitman, President and Chief Executive Officer, p. B57

Orlando: ORLANDO HEALTH 1414 Kuhl Avenue, Zip 32806–2093; tel. 407/841–5111; John Hillenmeyer, President and Chief Executive Officer, p. B88

Pensacola: ★ BAPTIST HEALTH CARE CORPORATION 1717 North E Street, Suite 320, Zip 32501–6335; tel. 850/469–7643; Alfred G. Stubblefield, President, p. B15

Rockledge: HEALTH FIRST, INC. 6450 U.S. Highway 1, Zip 32955; tel. 321/434–7000; Michael D. Means, President and Chief Executive Officer, p. B57

WUESTHOFF HEALTH SYSTEM 110 Longwood Avenue, Zip 32955; tel. 321/636–2211; Emil P. Miller, President and Chief Executive Officer, p. B133

Tampa: SHRINERS HOSPITALS FOR CHILDREN 2900 Rocky Point Drive, Zip 33607–1435, Mailing Address: P.O. Box 31356, Zip 33631–3356; tel. 813/281–0300; James M. Full, FACHE, Executive Vice President and Chief Operating Officer, p. B108

UNIVERSITY COMMUNITY HEALTH 3100 East Fletcher Avenue, Zip 33613; tel. 813/971–6000; Norman V. Stein, President and Chief Executive Officer, p. B126

Windermere: UNITED MEDICAL CORPORATION 603 Main Street, Zip 34786–3548, Mailing Address: P.O. Box 1100, Zip 34786–1100; tel. 407/876–2200; Donald R. Dizney, Chairman and Chief Executive Officer, p. B123

Winter Park: ★ ADVENTIST HEALTH SYSTEM SUNBELT HEALTH CARE CORPORATION 111 North Orlando Avenue, Zip 32789–3675; tel. 407/975–1401; Donald L. Jernigan, Ph.D., President and Chief Executive Officer, p. B4

GEORGIA

Albany: ★ PHOEBE PUTNEY HEALTH SYSTEM 417 Third Avenue, Zip 31702; tel. 229/312–1000; Joel Wernick, President and Chief Executive Officer, p. B90

Alpharetta: ★ REGENCY HOSPITAL COMPANY 30000 Mill Creek Avenue, Suite 250, Zip 30022; tel. 770/772–4345; William L. Anderson, President and Chief Executive Officer, p. B99

Atlanta: ★ EMORY HEALTHCARE 1440 Clifton Road, N.E., Suite 420, Zip 30322–1102, Mailing Address: 1440 Clifton Road N.E., Suite 420, Zip 30322–1102; tel. 404/778–5000; John T. Fox, Chief Executive Officer, p. B46

★ PIEDMONT HEALTHCARE 2001 Peachtree Road N.E., Suite 400, Zip 30309; tel. 404/605–3215; R. Timothy Stack, FACHE, President and Chief Executive Officer, p. B90

SUNLINK HEALTH SYSTEMS 900 Circle 75 Parkway, Suite 1300, Zip 30339; tel. 770/933–7000; Robert M. Thornton, Jr., Chief Executive Officer, p. B115

Brunswick: SOUTHEAST GEORGIA HEALTH SYSTEM 2415 Parkwood Drive, Zip 31520–4252, Mailing Address: P.O. Box 1518, Zip 31521–1518; tel. 912/466–7000; Gary R. Colberg, FACHE, President and Chief Executive Officer, p. B111

Carrollton: ★ TANNER HEALTH SYSTEM 705 Dixie Street, Zip 30117–3818; tel. 770/836–9580; Loy M. Howard, President and Chief Executive Officer, p. B116

Columbus: ★ COLUMBUS REGIONAL HEALTHCARE SYSTEM 707 Center Street, Suite 400, Zip 31901; tel. 706/660–6100; Larry Sanders, FACHE, Chairman and Chief Executive Officer, p. B31

Decatur: DEKALB REGIONAL HEALTH SYSTEM 2701 North Decatur Road, Zip 30033; tel. 404/501–1000; Eric P. Norwood, President and Chief Executive Officer, p. B39

Gainesville: ASSOCIATED HEALTHCARE SYSTEMS, INC. 214 Overlook Court, Suite 260, Zip 30501; tel. 770/297–1252; A. Ronald Turner, President and Chief Executive Officer, p. B12

Marietta: ★ WELLSTAR HEALTH SYSTEM 805 Sandy Plains Road, Zip 30066; tel. 770/792–5012; Gregory L. Simone, M.D., President and Chief Executive Officer, p. B131

Milledgeville: OCONEE REGIONAL HEALTH SYSTEM 821 North Cobb Street, Zip 31061; tel. 478/454–3505; Jean Aycock, President and Chief Executive Officer, p. B87

Royston: TY COBB HEALTHCARE SYSTEM, INC. 461 Cook Street, Suite A., Zip 30662, Mailing Address: P.O. Box 589, Zip 30662; tel. 706/245–1825; Charles T. Adams, Chief Executive Officer, p. B121

Sugar Hill: RESURGENCE HEALTH GROUP 1400 Buford Highway, Building R–3, Zip 30518; tel. 770/904–6731; Philip H. Eastman, III, President, p. B100

Thomasville: ★ ARCHBOLD MEDICAL CENTER 910 South Broad Street, Zip 31792–6113; tel. 229/228–2739; J. Perry Mustian, Interim President, p. B9

HAWAII

Honolulu: ★ HAWAII HEALTH SYSTEMS CORPORATION 3675 Kilauea Avenue, Zip 96816; tel. 808/733–4151; Thomas M. Driskill, Jr., President and Chief Executive Officer, p. B52

HAWAII PACIFIC HEALTH 55 Merchant Street, Zip 96813; tel. 808/535–7414; Charles A. Sted, President and Chief Executive Officer, p. B52

★ QUEEN'S HEALTH SYSTEMS 1099 Alakea Street, Suite 1100, Zip 96813; tel. 808/535–5448; Arthur A. Ushijima, President and Chief Executive Officer, p. B99

IDAHO

Boise: ★ ST. LUKE'S HEALTH SYSTEM 420 West Idaho Street, Zip 83702; tel. 208/381–1832; Edwin E. Dahlberg, President and Chief Executive Officer, p. B113

ILLINOIS

Arlington Heights: ALEXIAN BROTHERS HEALTH SYSTEM 3040 Salt Creek Lane, Zip 60005; tel. 847/463–8910; Brother Thomas Keusenkothen, President and Chief Executive Officer, p. B7

Carbondale: SOUTHERN ILLINOIS HOSPITAL SERVICES 1239 East Main Street, Zip 62901, Mailing Address: P.O. Box 3988, Zip 62902–3988; tel. 618/457–5200; Thomas J. Firestone, M.D., President and Chief Executive Officer, p. B111

Chicago: COOK COUNTY BUREAU OF HEALTH SERVICES 1900 West Polk Street, Suite 200, Zip 60612; tel. 312/864–6820; Robert Simon, M.D., Chief, p. B36

NATIONAL SURGICAL HOSPITALS 30 South Wacker Drive, Suite 2302, Zip 60606; tel. 312/627–8400; John G. Rex–Waller, President and Chief Executive Officer, p. B83

RESURRECTION HEALTH CARE 7435 West Talcott Avenue, Zip 60631; tel. 773/792–5150; Joseph F. Toomey, President and Chief Executive Officer, p. B100

★ RUSH UNIVERSITY MEDICAL CENTER 1653 West Congress Parkway, Zip 60612–3864; tel. 312/942–5000; Larry J. Goodman, M.D., President and Chief Executive Officer, p. B102

★ SINAI HEALTH SYSTEM California Avenue at 15th Street, Zip 60608; tel. 773/542–2000; Alan H. Channing, President and Chief Executive Officer, p. B109

Crystal Lake: ★ CENTEGRA HEALTH SYSTEM 385 Millennium Drive, Zip 60012; tel. 815/788–5825; Michael S. Eesley, President and Chief Executive Officer, p. B29

De Kalb: ★ KISH HEALTH SYSTEM 1 Kish Hospital Drive, Zip 60115–4939, Mailing Address: P.O. Box 707, Zip 60115–4939; tel. 815/756–1521; Kevin P. Poorten, President and Chief Executive Officer, p. B71

Evergreen Park: AMERICAN PROVINCE OF LITTLE COMPANY OF MARY SISTERS 9350 South California Avenue, Zip 60805–2595; tel. 708/229–5491; Sister Kathleen McIntyre, Province Leader, p. B8

Mokena: ★ PROVENA HEALTH 19065 Hickory Creek Drive, Suite 300, Zip 60448; tel. 708/478–6300; Steven L. Hunter, President and Chief Executive Officer, p. B92

Oak Brook: ★ ADVOCATE HEALTH CARE 2025 Windsor Drive, Zip 60523; tel. 630/990–5018; James H. Skogsbergh, President and Chief Executive Officer, p. B5

Peoria: ★ OSF HEALTHCARE SYSTEM 800 N.E. Glen Oak Avenue, Zip 61603–3200; tel. 309/655–2850; James M. Moore, Chief Executive Officer, p. B88

Schaumburg: CANCER TREATMENT CENTERS OF AMERICA 1336 Basswood Road, Zip 60173; tel. 847/342–7400; Stephen B. Bonner, President and Chief Executive Officer, p. B21

Springfield: ★ HOSPITAL SISTERS HEALTH SYSTEM Mailing Address: P.O. Box 19456, Zip 62794–9456; tel. 217/523–4747; Stephanie S. McCutcheon, President and Chief Executive Officer, p. B64

★ MEMORIAL HEALTH SYSTEM 701 North First Street, Zip 62781–0001; tel. 217/788–3000; Edgar J. Curtis, RN, President and Chief Executive Officer, p. B79

Wheaton: ★ WHEATON FRANCISCAN HEALTHCARE 26W171 Roosevelt Road, Zip 60189–0667, Mailing Address: P.O. Box 667, Zip 60189–0667; tel. 630/462–9271; John D. Oliverio, President and Chief Executive Officer, p. B132

INDIANA

Evansville: ★ DEACONESS HEALTH SYSTEM 600 Mary Street, Zip 47747; tel. 812/450–5000; Linda E. White, President and Chief Executive Officer, p. B38

Fort Wayne: ★ PARKVIEW HEALTH 10501 Corporate Drive, Zip 46845, Mailing Address: P.O. Box 5600, Zip 46895–5600; tel. 260/373–7001; Michael J. Packnett, President and Chief Executive Officer, p. B89

Hammond: COMMUNITY HEALTHCARE SYSTEM 901 MacArthur Boulevard, Zip 46321–2959; tel. 219/836–1600; Donald Powers, Chairman, President and Chief Executive Officer, p. B35

Indianapolis: ★ CLARIAN HEALTH I–65 at 21st Street, Zip 46202–5250, Mailing Address: P.O. Box 1367, Zip 46206–1367; tel. 317/962–5900; Daniel F. Evans, Jr., President and Chief Executive Officer, p. B30

COMMUNITY HEALTH NETWORK 1500 North Ritter Street, Zip 46219; tel. 317/355–1411; William E. Corley, President, p. B31

Kokomo: HOWARD REGIONAL HEALTH SYSTEM 3500 South Lafountain Street, Zip 46902, Mailing Address: P.O. Box 9011, Zip 46904–9011; tel. 765/453–0702; James P. Alender, President and Chief Executive Officer, p. B64

Mishawaka: SISTERS OF ST. FRANCIS HEALTH SERVICES, INC. 1515 Dragoon Trail, Zip 46546–1290, Mailing Address: P.O. Box 1290, Zip 46546–1290; tel. 574/256–3935; Kevin D. Leahy, President and Chief Executive Officer, p. B110

Muncie: ★ CARDINAL HEALTH SYSTEM 2401 University Avenue, Zip 47303; tel. 765/747–3139; Kelly N. Stanley, President and Chief Executive Officer, p. B22

IOWA

Davenport: ★ GENESIS HEALTH SYSTEM 1227 East Rusholme Street, Zip 52803–2498; tel. 563/421–1000; Douglas P. Cropper, Chief Executive Officer, p. B50

Des Moines: ★ IOWA HEALTH SYSTEM 1200 Pleasant Street, Zip 50309–1453; tel. 515/241–6161; William B. Leaver, President and Chief Executive Officer, p. B67

KANSAS

Lenexa: ★ SISTERS OF CHARITY OF LEAVENWORTH HEALTH SYSTEM 9801 Renner Boulevard, Suite 100, Zip 66219; tel. 913/895–2800; William M. Murray, President, p. B109

Phillipsburg: ★ GREAT PLAINS HEALTH ALLIANCE, INC. 625 Third Street, Zip 67661–2138, Mailing Address: P.O. Box 366, Zip 67661–0366; tel. 785/543–2111; Roger S. John, President and Chief Executive Officer, p. B51

Wichita: VIA CHRISTI HEALTH SYSTEM 3720 East Bayley, Zip 67218–3002; tel. 316/858–4900; Kevin P. Conlin, President and Chief Executive Officer, p. B129

KENTUCKY

Lexington: APPALACHIAN REGIONAL HEALTHCARE 2285 Executive Drive, Suite 400, Zip 40505, Mailing Address: P.O. Box 8086, Zip 40533–8086; tel. 859/226–2440; Jerry Haynes, President and Chief Executive Officer, p. B8

CARDINAL HILL HEALTHCARE SYSTEM 2050 Versailes Road, Zip 40504; tel. 859/254–5701; Kerry G. Gillihan, FACHE, President and Chief Executive Officer, p. B22

UK HEALTHCARE 800 Rose Street, Zip 40536–0293; tel. 859/323–5000; Michael Karpf, M.D., Executive Vice President Health Affairs, p. B122

Louisville: ALLIANT MANAGEMENT SERVICES 2501 Nelson Miller Parkway, Suite 104, Zip 40223; tel. 502/992–3525; Chris West, President and Chief Executive Officer, p. B7

★ BAPTIST HEALTHCARE SYSTEM 4007 Kresge Way, Zip 40207–4677; tel. 502/896–5000; Tommy J. Smith, President and Chief Executive Officer, p. B15

★ JEWISH HOSPITAL & ST. MARY'S HEALTHCARE 200 Abraham Flexner Way, Zip 40202–1886; tel. 502/587–4011; Robert L. Shircliff, President and Chief Executive Officer, p. B68

KINDRED HEALTHCARE 680 South Fourth Street, Zip 40202–2412; tel. 502/596–7300; Paul J. Diaz, President and Chief Executive Officer, p. B70

MERIT HEALTH SYSTEMS 333 East Main Street, Suite 300, Zip 40202; tel. 502/753–0890; Tyree Wilburn, Chaiman, President and Chief Executive Officer, p. B80

★ NORTON HEALTHCARE 234 East Gray Street, Suite 225, Zip 40202, Mailing Address: P.O. Box 35070, Zip 40232–5070; tel. 502/629–8000; Stephen A. Williams, President, p. B86

UNITED REHAB CORPORATION 9707 Shelbyville Road, Zip 40223; tel. 502/426–2242; Kyle White, President and Chief Executive Officer, p. B123

LOUISIANA

Baton Rouge: ★ FRANCISCAN MISSIONARIES OF OUR LADY HEALTH SYSTEM, INC. 4200 Essen Lane, Zip 70809; tel. 225/923–2701; John J. Finan, Jr., President and Chief Executive Officer, p. B49

★ LSU HEALTH SCIENCES CENTER 8550 United Plaza Boulevard, 4th Floor, Zip 70809; tel. 225/922–0490; Michael K. Butler, M.D., Acting Chief Executive Officer, p. B76

Benton: CYPRESS HEALTH SYSTEMS 106 Preston Day Circle, Zip 71006; tel. 318/965–9914; Kim B. Bird, President and Chief Executive Officer, p. B38

New Orleans: LOUISIANA STATE HOSPITALS 210 State Street, Zip 70118–5797; tel. 504/897–4616; Shelby Price, Chief Executive Officer, p. B75

★ OCHSNER HEALTH SYSTEM 1514 Jefferson Highway, Zip 70121; tel. 800/874–8984; Patrick J. Quinlan, M.D., Chief Executive Officer, p. B87

Shreveport: WILLIS–KNIGHTON HEALTH SYSTEM 2600 Greenwood Road, Zip 71130–2600; tel. 318/212–4000; James K. Elrod, President and Chief Executive Officer, p. B132

MAINE

Brewer: ★ EASTERN MAINE HEALTHCARE SYSTEMS 43 Whiting Hill Road, Zip 04412; tel. 207/973–7045; M. Michelle Hood, President and Chief Executive Officer, p. B46

MARYLAND

Baltimore: ★ JOHNS HOPKINS HEALTH SYSTEM 733 North Broadway, BRB 104, Zip 21205; tel. 410/955–5000; Ronald R. Peterson, President, p. B68

★ LIFEBRIDGE HEALTH 2401 West Belvedere Avenue, Zip 21215; tel. 410/601–5134; Warren A. Green, President and Chief Executive Officer, p. B73

★ UNIVERSITY OF MARYLAND MEDICAL SYSTEM 250 West Pratt Street, 24th Floor, Zip 21201–1595; tel. 410/328–8667; Edmond F. Notebaert, President and Chief Executive Officer, p. B127

Bel Air: ★ UPPER CHESAPEAKE HEALTH SYSTEM 520 Upper Chesapeake Drive, Suite 405, Zip 21014–4324; tel. 443/643–3303; Lyle Ernest Sheldon, FACHE, President and Chief Executive Officer, p. B128

Cheverly: DIMENSIONS HEALTHCARE SYSTEM 3001 Hospital Drive, 3rd Floor, Zip 20785; tel. 301/583–4000; G. T. Dunlop Ecker, President and Chief Executive Officer, p. B44

Columbia: ★ MEDSTAR HEALTH 5565 Sterrett Place, 5th Floor, Zip 21044; tel. 410/772–6500; Kenneth A. Samet, President and Chief Executive Officer, p. B78

Cumberland: ★ WESTERN MARYLAND HEALTH SYSTEM Mailing Address: P.O. Box 539, Zip 21502; tel. 301/723–4200; Barry P. Ronan, President, p. B132

Easton: SHORE HEALTH SYSTEM 219 South Washington Street, Zip 21601; tel. 410/822–1000; Joseph P. Ross, President and Chief Executive Officer, p. B108

Marriottsville: ★ BON SECOURS HEALTH SYSTEM, INC. 1505 Marriottsville Road, Zip 21104–1399; tel. 410/442–5511; Richard Statuto, President and Chief Executive Officer, p. B18

Rockville: ★ ADVENTIST HEALTHCARE 1801 Research Boulevard, Suite 400, Zip 20850; tel. 301/315–3030; William G. Robertson, President and Chief Executive Officer, p. B5

U. S. INDIAN HEALTH SERVICE 801 Thompson Avenue, Zip 20852; tel. 301/443–1083; Major Robert McSwain, Acting Director, p. B121

Sparks Glencoe: FUNDAMENTAL LONG TERM CARE HOLDINGS, LLC 930 Ridgebrook Road, Zip 21152; tel. 410/773–1000; W. Bradley Bennett, President and Chief Executive Officer, p. B50

Stevensville: MID ATLANTIC HEALTH MANAGEMENT, INC. 1220 Butterworth Court, Zip 21666–2504; tel. 410/643–3393; Harold A. McBee, Jr., President, p. B81

MASSACHUSETTS

Boston: ★ CARITAS CHRISTI HEALTH CARE 736 Cambridge Street, Zip 02135–2997; tel. 617/789–2500; Ralph de la Torre, M.D., President and Chief Executive Officer, p. B22

MASSACHUSETTS DEPARTMENT OF MENTAL HEALTH 25 Staniford Street, Zip 02114–2575; tel. 617/626–8123; Elizabeth Childs, M.D., Commissioner, p. B76

MASSACHUSETTS DEPARTMENT OF PUBLIC HEALTH 250 Washington Street, Zip 02108–4619; tel. 617/624–6000; John Auerbach, Commissioner, p. B77

★ PARTNERS HEALTHCARE SYSTEM, INC. 800 Boylston Street, Suite 1150, Zip 02199–8001; tel. 617/278–1004; James J. Mongan, M.D., President and Chief Executive Officer, p. B89

Hyannis: ★ CAPE COD HEALTHCARE, INC. 88 Lewis Bay Road, Zip 02601–5210; tel. 508/862–5010; Richard Salluzzo, M.D., President and Chief Executive Officer, p. B21

Lexington: ★ COVENANT HEALTH SYSTEMS, INC. 420 Bedford Street, Zip 02420–1502; tel. 781/862–1634; David R. Lincoln, President and Chief Executive Officer, p. B37

Newton: FIVE STAR QUALITY CARE 400 Centre Street, Zip 02458–2076; tel. 617/796–8387; , p. B49

Peabody: PIONEER BEHAVIORAL HEALTH 200 Lake Street, Suite 102, Zip 01960–4780; tel. 978/536–2777; Bruce A. Shear, President and Chief Executive Officer, p. B90

Pittsfield: ★ BERKSHIRE HEALTH SYSTEMS, INC. 725 North Street, Zip 01201–4124; tel. 413/447–2743; David E. Phelps, President and Chief Executive Officer, p. B17

Springfield: ★ BAYSTATE HEALTH, INC. 759 Chestnut Street, Zip 01199–0001; tel. 413/794–0000; Mark R. Tolosky, FACHE, J.D., President and Chief Executive Officer, p. B16

Worcester: ★ UMASS MEMORIAL HEALTH CARE, INC. 1 Biotech Park, Zip 01605–2982; tel. 508/334–0100; John G. O'Brien, President and Chief Executive Officer, p. B123

MICHIGAN

Dearborn: ★ OAKWOOD HEALTHCARE, INC. One Parklane Boulevard, Suite 1000E, Zip 48126; tel. 313/253–6050; Brian M. Connolly, President and Chief Executive Officer, p. B87

Detroit: ★ DETROIT MEDICAL CENTER 3990 John R., Zip 48201; tel. 313/745–1250; Michael Duggan, President and Chief Executive Officer, p. B44

★ HENRY FORD HEALTH SYSTEM One Ford Place, Zip 48202–3450; tel. 313/876–8708; Nancy M. Schlichting, President and Chief Executive Officer, p. B63

Flint: MCLAREN HEALTH CARE CORPORATION G3235 Beecher Road, Suite B., Zip 48532; tel. 810/342–1100; Philip A. Incarnati, President and Chief Executive Officer, p. B78

Grand Rapids: ★ SPECTRUM HEALTH 100 Michigan Street N.E., Zip 49503–2551; tel. 616/391–1774; Richard C. Breon, President and Chief Executive Officer, p. B112

Kalamazoo: ★ BRONSON HEALTHCARE GROUP, INC. One Healthcare Plaza, Zip 49007–5345; tel. 269/341–6000; Frank J. Sardone, President and Chief Executive Officer, p. B20

Lansing: SPARROW HEALTH SYSTEM 1215 East Michigan Avenue, Zip 48912; tel. 517/364–1000; Dennis A. Swan, President and Chief Executive Officer, p. B111

Midland: ★ MIDMICHIGAN HEALTH 4005 Orchard Drive, Zip 48670–0001; tel. 989/839–3000; Terence F. Moore, President, p. B81

Muskegon: HACKLEY HEALTH SYSTEM 2700 Clinton Street, Zip 49442; tel. 231/726–3511; Gordon A. Mudler, President and Chief Executive Officer, p. B52

Novi: ★ TRINITY HEALTH 27870 Cabot Drive, Zip 48377; tel. 248/489–5004; Joseph R. Swedish, President and Chief Executive Officer, p. B119

Port Huron: ★ BLUE WATER HEALTH SERVICES CORPORATION 1221 Pine Grove Avenue, Zip 48061–5011; tel. 810/989–3717; Thomas D. DeFauw, FACHE, President and Chief Executive Officer, p. B18

Royal Oak: ★ BEAUMONT HOSPITALS 3601 West Thirteen Mile Road, Zip 48073–6769; tel. 248/551–5000; Kenneth J. Matzick, President and Chief Executive Officer, p. B16

Saint Joseph: LAKELAND HEALTHCARE 1234 Napier Avenue, Zip 49085–2158; tel. 269/983–8300; Joseph A. Wasserman, President and Chief Executive Officer, p. B72

Traverse City: ★ MUNSON HEALTHCARE 1105 Sixth Street, Zip 49684–2386; tel. 231/935–6502; K. Douglas Deck, President and Chief Executive Officer, p. B82

MINNESOTA

Bloomington: HEALTHPARTNERS 8100 34th Avenue South, Zip 55440; tel. 952/883–7463; Mary K. Brainerd, President and Chief Executive Officer, p. B60

Duluth: ESSENTIA HEALTH 502 East Second Street, Zip 55805; tel. 218/786–8376; Peter E. Person, M.D., Chief Executive Officer, p. B47

Minneapolis: ★ ALLINA HOSPITALS & CLINICS 2925 Chicago Avenue, Zip 55407, Mailing Address: P.O. Box 43, Zip 55440; tel. 612/262–5000; Richard R. Pettingill, President and Chief Executive Officer, p. B7

CHILDREN'S HOSPITALS AND CLINICS OF MINNESOTA 2525 Chicago Avenue South, Zip 55404; tel. 612/813–6100; Alan L. Goldbloom, M.D., President and Chief Executive Officer, p. B29

★ FAIRVIEW HEALTH SERVICES 2450 Riverside Avenue, Zip 55454–1400; tel. 612/672–6300; Mark A. Eustis, President and Chief Executive Officer, p. B48

Rochester: ★ MAYO FOUNDATION 200 S.W. First Street, Zip 55905–0002; tel. 507/284–2511; Denis A. Cortese, M.D., President and Chief Executive Officer, p. B77

Saint Cloud: ★ CENTRACARE HEALTH SYSTEM 1406 Sixth Avenue North, Zip 56303; tel. 320/251–2700; Terence Pladson, M.D., President and Chief Executive Officer, p. B29

Saint Louis Park: ★ PARK NICOLLET HEALTH SERVICES 6500 Excelsior Boulevard, Zip 55426–4702; tel. 952/993–5000; David K. Wessner, President and Chief Executive Officer, p. B89

Saint Paul: ★ HEALTHEAST CARE SYSTEM 559 Capitol Boulevard, 6–South, Zip 55103–0000; tel. 651/232–2300; Timothy H. Hanson, President and Chief Executive Officer, p. B59

MINNESOTA DEPARMENT OF HUMAN SERVICES 540 Cedar Street, Zip 55164–0980, Mailing Address: P.O. Box 64980, Zip 55164–0980; tel. 651/431–2369; Michael Tessneer, Chief Executive Officer, p. B81

MISSISSIPPI

Jackson: MISSISSIPPI BAPTIST HEALTH SYSTEM 1225 North State Street, Zip 39202–2002; tel. 601/968–1000; Kurt W. Metzner, President and Chief Executive Officer, p. B81

MISSISSIPPI STATE DEPARTMENT OF MENTAL HEALTH 1101 Robert East Lee Building, 239 North Lamar Street, Zip 39201–1101; tel. 601/359–1288; Edwin C. LeGrand, III, Executive Director, p. B81

Magee: PIONEER HEALTH SERVICES 301 Eighth Avenue S.W., Zip 39111, Mailing Address: P.O. Box 1100, Zip 39111; tel. 601/849–6440; Joseph S. McNulty, President and Chief Executive Officer, p. B90

Meridian: RUSH HEALTH SYSTEMS 1314 19th Avenue, Zip 39301; tel. 601/483–0011; Wallace Strickland, President and Chief Executive Officer, p. B101

Tupelo: ★ NORTH MISSISSIPPI HEALTH SERVICES, INC. 830 South Gloster Street, Zip 38801–4996; tel. 662/377–3136; John R. Heer, President and Chief Executive Officer, p. B85

MISSOURI

Cape Girardeau: LANDMARK HOSPITALS 3255 Independence Street, Zip 63701–4904; tel. 573/335–1091; William Kapp, M.D., President, p. B72

Chesterfield: ★ SISTERS OF MERCY HEALTH SYSTEM 14528 South Outer 40, Suite 100, Zip 63017–5743; tel. 314/579–6100; John Sullivan, Chief Executive Officer, p. B110

Columbia: ★ UNIVERSITY OF MISSOURI HEALTH CARE One Hospital Drive, DC 031, Zip 65212–0001; tel. 573/884–8738; James H. Ross, Chief Executive Officer, p. B127

Joplin: ★ FREEMAN HEALTH SYSTEM 1102 West 32nd Street, Zip 64804; tel. 417/347–1111; Gary D. Duncan, President and Chief Executive Officer, p. B50

Kansas City: HOSPITAL MANAGEMENT CONSULTING, LLC 4254 North Trafficway, Zip 64116–4541; tel. 816/474–7800; Lawrence J. Arthur, President, p. B64

SAINT LUKE'S HEALTH SYSTEM 10920 Elm Avenue, Zip 64134–4108; tel. 816/932–2000; G. Richard Hastings, President and Chief Executive Officer, p. B102

★ TRUMAN MEDICAL CENTERS 2301 Holmes Street, Zip 64108–2677; tel. 816/404–1000; John W. Bluford, President and Chief Executive Officer, p. B121

Saint Louis: ★ ASCENSION HEALTH 4600 Edmundson Road, Zip 63134–3806; tel. 314/733–8000; Anthony R. Tersigni, Ed.D., FACHE, President and Chief Executive Officer, p. B9

★ BJC HEALTHCARE 4444 Forest Park Avenue, Suite 500, Zip 63108–2259; tel. 314/286–2000; Steven H. Lipstein, President and Chief Executive Officer, p. B17

★ REHABCARE GROUP, INC. 7733 Forsyth Boulevard, Zip 63105; tel. 800/677–1238; John H. Short, Ph.D., President and Chief Executive Officer, p. B100

★ SSM HEALTH CARE 477 North Lindbergh Boulevard, Zip 63141–7813; tel. 314/994–7800; Sister Mary Jean Ryan, President and Chief Executive Officer, p. B112

Springfield: COXHEALTH 1423 North Jefferson Avenue, Zip 65802–1988; tel. 417/269–3108; Robert H. Bezanson, President and Chief Executive Officer, p. B38

NEBRASKA

Lincoln: ★ BRYANLGH HEALTH SYSTEM 1600 South 48th Street, Zip 68506; tel. 402/489–0200; Kimberly A. Russel, President and Chief Executive Officer, p. B20

Norfolk: MISSIONARY BENEDICTINE SISTERS AMERICAN PROVINCE 300 North 18th Street, Zip 68701–3687; tel. 402/371–3438; Sister Kevin Hermsen, Prioress, p. B81

Omaha: ALEGENT HEALTH 1010 North 96th Street, Suite 200, Zip 68154; tel. 402/343–4300; Wayne A. Sensor, President and Chief Executive Officer, p. B6

★ NEBRASKA METHODIST HEALTH SYSTEM, INC. 8511 West Dodge Road, Zip 68114; tel. 402/354–5411; John M. Fraser, President and Chief Executive Officer, p. B83

NEVADA

Reno: RENOWN HEALTH 77 Pringle Way, Zip 89502–1474; tel. 775/982–4100; James I. Miller, President and Chief Executive Officer, p. B100

NEW HAMPSHIRE

Laconia: ★ LRGHEALTHCARE 80 Highland Street, Zip 03246–3298; tel. 603/524–3211; Thomas Clairmont, President, p. B75

Portsmouth: SPECIALTY HOSPITALS OF AMERICA, LLC 155 Fleet Street, Zip 03801; tel. 603/570–4888; Eric F. Rieseberg, President, p. B112

NEW JERSEY

Bayonne: BRIDGE REGIONAL HEALTH SYSTEM 29 East 29th Street, Zip 07002; tel. 201/858–5000; Daniel A. Kane, Dr.P.h., Acting Chief Executive Officer, p. B18

Edison: ★ SOLARIS HEALTH SYSTEM 80 James Street, 2nd Floor, Zip 08820–3998; tel. 732/632–1501; John P. McGee, President and Chief Executive Officer, p. B111

Egg Harbor Township: ★ ATLANTICARE 2500 English Creek Avenue, Building 500, Suite 501, Zip 08234; tel. 609/407–2300; David P. Tilton, President and Chief Executive Officer, p. B12

Jersey City: LIBERTYHEALTH 355 Grand Street, Zip 07302; tel. 201/915–2000; Jonathan M. Metsch, Dr.P.h., President and Chief Executive Officer, p. B72

Marlton: ★ VIRTUA HEALTH 50 Lake Center Executive Park, Suite 401, Zip 08053; tel. 856/355–0010; Richard P. Miller, President and Chief Executive Officer, p. B130

Morristown: ★ ATLANTIC HEALTH 475 South Street, Zip 07962, Mailing Address: P.O. Box 1905, Zip 07962–1905; tel. 973/660–3270; Joseph A. Trunfio, Ph.D., President and Chief Executive Officer, p. B12

Neptune: ★ MERIDIAN HEALTH 1350 Campus Parkway, Zip 07753; tel. 732/751–7510; John K. Lloyd, President and Chief Executive Officer, p. B80

New Brunswick: ROBERT WOOD JOHNSON HEALTH SYSTEM & NETWORK 1 Robert Wood Johnson Place, Zip 08903–2601; tel. 732/828–3000; Stephen K. Jones, President and Chief Executive Officer, p. B101

Newark: CATHEDRAL HEALTHCARE SYSTEM, INC. 1160 Raymond Boulevard, Zip 07102; tel. 973/690–3600; Father Ronald Rozniak, Interim President and Chief Executive Officer, p. B23

Paterson: ST. JOSEPH'S HEALTHCARE SYSTEM 703 Main Street, Zip 07503–2691; tel. 973/754–2000; William A. McDonald, President and Chief Executive Officer, p. B113

Ramsey: LIBERTY MANAGEMENT GROUP, INC. 19 Spear Road, Suite 305, Zip 07446; tel. 201/236–8880; William J. Hartigan, President and Chief Executive Officer, p. B72

Trenton: CAPITAL HEALTH SYSTEM 750 Brunswick Avenue, Zip 08638–4174; tel. 609/394–6000; Al Maghazehe, Chief Executive Officer, p. B21

DIVISION OF MENTAL HEALTH SERVICES, DEPARTMENT OF HUMAN SERVICES, STATE OF NEW JERSEY Capital Center, P.O. Box 727, Zip 08625–0727; tel. 609/777–0702; Kevin Martone, Assistant Commissioner, p. B44

Vineland: SOUTH JERSEY HEALTHCARE 2950 College Drive, Suite 1E, Zip 08360; tel. 856/641–8000; Chester B. Kaletkowski, President and Chief Executive Officer, p. B111

West Orange: ★ SAINT BARNABAS HEALTH CARE SYSTEM 95 Old Short Hills Road, Zip 07052; tel. 973/322–4001; Ronald J. Del Mauro, President and Chief Executive Officer, p. B102

NEW MEXICO

Albuquerque: ERNEST HEALTH, INC. 7770 Jefferson Street N.E., Suite 320, Zip 87109; tel. 505/856–5300; Darby Brockette, Chief Executive Officer, p. B47

★ PRESBYTERIAN HEALTHCARE SERVICES 2501 Buena Vista, S.E., Zip 87106, Mailing Address: P.O. Box 26666, Zip 87125–6666; tel. 505/841–1234; James H. Hinton, President and Chief Executive Officer, p. B91

NEW YORK

Albany: NEW YORK STATE OFFICE OF MENTAL HEALTH 44 Holland Avenue, Zip 12229–3411; tel. 518/474–4403; Michael F. Hogan, Ph.D., Commissioner, p. B84

Binghamton: ★ UNITED HEALTH SERVICES 10–42 Mitchell Avenue, Zip 13903; tel. 607/762–2200; Matthew J. Salanger, President and Chief Executive Officer, p. B123

Buffalo: ★ CATHOLIC HEALTH SYSTEM 2121 Main Street, Suite 300, Zip 14214; tel. 716/862–2410; Joseph D. McDonald, President and Chief Executive Officer, p. B26

Geneva: FINGER LAKES HEALTH 196 North Street, Zip 14456; tel. 315/787–4053; James J. Dooley, President and Chief Executive Officer, p. B48

Gowanda: TLC HEALTH NETWORK 100 Memorial Drive, Zip 14070; tel. 716/532–3377; Louis J. Frascella, President and Chief Executive Officer, p. B119

Great Neck: ★ NORTH SHORE–LIJ HEALTH SYSTEM 145 Community Drive, Zip 11021; tel. 516/465–8100; Michael J. Dowling, President and Chief Executive Officer, p. B86

New Rochelle: SOUND SHORE HEALTH SYSTEM 16 Guion Place, Zip 10801–5500; tel. 914/632–5000; John R. Spicer, President and Chief Executive Officer, p. B111

New York: ★ CONTINUUM HEALTH PARTNERS 555 West 57th Street, Zip 10019; tel. 212/523–8130; Stanley Brezenoff, President and Chief Executive Officer, p. B36

MONTEFIORE HEALTH SYSTEM 111 East 210th Street, Zip 10467–2490; tel. 718/920–4321; Spencer Foreman, M.D., President, p. B82

★ NEW YORK CITY HEALTH AND HOSPITALS CORPORATION 125 Worth Street, Room 514, Zip 10013–4006; tel. 212/788–3321; Alan D. Aviles, President, p. B83

NEW YORK PRESBYTERIAN HEALTHCARE SYSTEM 525 East 68th Street, Zip 10021–4885; tel. 212/746–3745; Herbert Pardes, M.D., President and Chief Executive Officer, p. B84

Poughkeepsie: ★ HEALTH QUEST SYSTEMS, INC. 45 Reade Place, Zip 12601; tel. 845/431–5601; Michael T. Weber, President and Chief Executive Officer, p. B59

Rochester: STRONG MEMORIAL HOSPITAL 601 Elmwood Avenue, Zip 14642–0002; tel. 585/275–2100; Steven I. Goldstein, General Director and Chief Executive Officer, p. B114

VIAHEALTH 1425 Portland Avenue, 5th Floor, Zip 14621; tel. 585/922–4437; Mark C. Clement, President and Chief Executive Officer, p. B129

Rockville Centre: CATHOLIC HEALTH SERVICES OF LONG ISLAND 1 Huntington Quadrangle, Suite 4C04, Zip 11570; tel. 516/705–3700; James Harden, President and Chief Executive Officer, p. B26

Syracuse: SISTERS OF SAINT FRANCIS 2500 Grant Boulevard, Zip 13208–1713; tel. 315/634–7000; Sister Grace Anne Dillenschneider, Assistant General Minister, p. B110

NORTH CAROLINA

Charlotte: ★ CAROLINAS HEALTHCARE SYSTEM 1000 Blythe Boulevard, Zip 28203–5871, Mailing Address: P.O. Box 32861, Zip 28232–2861; tel. 704/355–2000; Michael C. Tarwater, President and Chief Executive Officer, p. B23

HOSPITAL PARTNERS OF AMERICA 2815 Coliseum Centre Drive, Suite 150, Zip 28217–1378; tel. 704/424–6800; Todd Johnson, President and Chief Executive Officer, p. B64

MEDCATH, INC. 10720 Sikes Place, Suite 300, Zip 28277–8143; tel. 704/708–6600; O. Edwin French, President and Chief Executive Officer, p. B78

Durham: ★ DUKE UNIVERSITY HEALTH SYSTEM Erwin Road, Zip 27710, Mailing Address: P.O. Box 3701, Zip 27710–3701; tel. 919/684–2255; Victor J. Dzau, M.D., President and Chief Executive Officer, p. B45

Greenville: ★ UNIVERSITY HEALTH SYSTEMS OF EASTERN CAROLINA 2100 Stantonsburg Road, Zip 27834, Mailing Address: P.O. Box 6028, Zip 27835–6028; tel. 252/847–4100; Dave C. McRae, Chief Executive Officer, p. B126

Pinehurst: ★ FIRSTHEALTH OF THE CAROLINAS 155 Memorial Drive, Zip 28374–8710, Mailing Address: P.O. Box 3000, Zip 28374–3000; tel. 910/715–1000; Charles T. Frock, Chief Executive Officer, p. B49

Raleigh: ★ WAKEMED 3000 New Bern Avenue, Zip 27610; tel. 919/350–8000; William K. Atkinson, II, President and Chief Executive Officer, p. B130

Sylva: ★ WESTCARE HEALTH SYSTEM 68 Hospital Road, Zip 28779; tel. 828/586–7000; Mark T. Leonard, Chief Executive Officer, p. B132

Wilmington: ★ NEW HANOVER HEALTH NETWORK 2131 South 17th Street, Zip 28401–9000; tel. 910/343–7040; John K. Barto, Jr., President and Chief Executive Officer, p. B83

Winston–Salem: ★ NORTH CAROLINA BAPTIST HOSPITAL Medical Center Boulevard, Zip 27157; tel. 336/716–2011; Donny C. Lambeth, Interim President, p. B85

★ NOVANT HEALTH 2085 Frontis Plaza Boulevard, Zip 27103–3090; tel. 336/718–2023; Paul M. Wiles, President and Chief Executive Officer, p. B86

NORTH DAKOTA

Bismarck: BENEDICTINE SISTERS OF THE ANNUNCIATION 7520 University Drive, Zip 58504–9653; tel. 701/255–1520; Sister Susan Berger, Prioress, p. B17

Fargo: ★ MERITCARE HEALTH SYSTEM 801 Broadway North, Zip 58122; tel. 701/234–2000; Roger L. Gilbertson, M.D., President and Chief Executive Officer, p. B80

SISTERS OF MARY OF THE PRESENTATION HEALTH SYSTEM 1102 Page Drive S.W., Zip 58106–0007, Mailing Address: P.O. Box 10007, Zip 58106–0007; tel. 701/237–9290; Aaron Alton, President and Chief Executive Officer, p. B109

OHIO

Akron: AKRON GENERAL HEALTH SYSTEM 400 Wabash Avenue, Zip 44307–2433; tel. 330/344–6000; Alan J. Bleyer, President and Chief Executive Officer, p. B6

SUMMA HEALTH SYSTEM 525 East Market Street, Zip 44309–2090; tel. 330/375–3000; Thomas J. Strauss, President and Chief Executive Officer, p. B114

Cincinnati: ★ CATHOLIC HEALTHCARE PARTNERS 615 Elsinore Place, Zip 45202; tel. 513/639–2800; Michael D. Connelly, President and Chief Executive Officer, p. B26

★ HEALTH ALLIANCE OF GREATER CINCINNATI 3200 Burnet Avenue, Zip 45229; tel. 513/585–6000; Kenneth Hanover, President and Chief Executive Officer, p. B57

Cleveland: CLEVELAND CLINIC HEALTH SYSTEM 9500 Euclid, Zip 44195–5108; tel. 216/444–2200; Delos Cosgrove, M.D., President and Chief Executive Officer, p. B31

SISTERS OF CHARITY HEALTH SYSTEM 2351 East 22nd Street, Zip 44115–3197; tel. 216/696–5560; Sister Judith Ann Karam, President and Chief Executive Officer, p. B109

UNIVERSITY HOSPITALS 11100 Euclid Avenue, Zip 44106–5000; tel. 216/844–1000; Thomas F. Zenty, III, Chief Executive Officer, p. B126

Columbus: ★ OHIO STATE UNIVERSITY HEALTH SYSTEM 370 West Ninth Avenue, Zip 43210–1240; tel. 614/247–5555; Peter E. Geier, Chief Executive Officer, p. B87

★ OHIOHEALTH 1087 Dennison Avenue, Zip 43201; tel. 614/544–5430; David P. Blom, President and Chief Executive Officer, p. B88

Dayton: ★ KETTERING HEALTH NETWORK 3965 Southern Boulevard, Zip 45429–1221; tel. 937/395–8150; Francisco J. Perez, FACHE, Network Chief Executive Officer, p. B69

Mansfield: MEDCENTRAL HEALTH SYSTEM 335 Glessner Avenue, Zip 44903; tel. 419/526–8000; James E. Meyer, President and Chief Executive Officer, p. B78

Sylvania: ★ FRANCISCAN SERVICES CORPORATION 6832 Convent Boulevard, Zip 43560–2897; tel. 419/882–8373; John W. O'Connell, President, p. B49

Toledo: ★ PROMEDICA HEALTH SYSTEM 1801 Richards Road, Zip 43607; tel. 419/469–3800; Alan W. Brass, FACHE, Chief Executive Officer and President, p. B92

Youngstown: FORUM HEALTH 3530 Belmont Avenue, Suite 7, Zip 44505; tel. 330/884–1044; Lowell W. Johnson, President and Chief Executive Officer, p. B49

OKLAHOMA

Oklahoma City: ★ INTEGRIS HEALTH 3366 N.W. Expressway, Suite 800, Zip 73112–9756; tel. 405/949–6068; Stanley F. Hupfeld, President and Chief Executive Officer, p. B66

OKLAHOMA STATE DEPARTMENT OF MENTAL HEALTH AND SUBSTANCE ABUSE SERVICES 1200 N.E. 13th Street, Zip 73117, Mailing Address: P.O. Box 53277, Zip 73152–3277; tel. 405/522–3908; Terri White, Commissioner, p. B88

THE SCHUSTER GROUP 3555 N.W. 58th Street, Suite 1000, Zip 73112; tel. 405/917–0300; Mike Schuster, President and Chief Executive Officer, p. B119

Shawnee: PREFERRED MANAGEMENT CORPORATION 120 West MacArthur, Suite 121, Zip 74804–2028; tel. 405/878–0202; Donald Freeman, Vice President and Chief Executive Officer, p. B91

Tulsa: ★ MARIAN HEALTH SYSTEM 1923 South Utica Avenue, Zip 74104, Mailing Address: P.O. Box 4753, Zip 74159–0753; tel. 918/742–9988; Sister M. Therese Gottschalk, President, p. B76

★ SAINT FRANCIS HEALTH SYSTEM 6161 South Yale Avenue, Zip 74136–1902; tel. 918/494–8454; Jake Henry, Jr., President and Chief Executive Officer, p. B102

OREGON

Bend: ★ CASCADE HEALTHCARE COMMUNITY 2500 N.E. Neff Road, Zip 97701–6015; tel. 541/382–4321; James A. Diegel, FACHE, President and Chief Executive Officer, p. B23

Corvallis: ★ SAMARITAN HEALTH SERVICES 3600 N.W. Samaritan Drive, Zip 97330, Mailing Address: P.O. Box 1068, Zip 97339; tel. 541/768–5001; Larry A. Mullins, FACHE, President and Chief Executive Officer, p. B103

Medford: ★ ASANTE HEALTH SYSTEM 2650 Siskiyou Boulevard, Suite 200, Zip 97504–8170; tel. 541/789–4100; Roy G. Vinyard, FACHE, President and Chief Executive Officer, p. B9

Portland: ★ LEGACY HEALTH SYSTEM 1919 N.W. Lovejoy Street, Zip 97209–1503; tel. 503/415–5600; Pamela S. Vukovich, Interim President and Chief Executive Officer, p. B72

Salem: SALEM HEALTH 665 Winter S.E., Zip 97301–3959; tel. 503/561–5200; , p. B103

PENNSYLVANIA

Allentown: ★ LEHIGH VALLEY HOSPITAL AND HEALTH NETWORK 1200 South Cedar Crest Boulevard, Zip 18103, Mailing Address: P.O. Box 689, Zip 18105–0689; tel. 610/402–8000; Elliot J. Sussman, M.D., President and Chief Executive Officer, p. B72

Ashland: SAINT CATHERINE HEALTHCARE, LLC 101 Broad Street, Zip 17921; tel. 570/875–2000; Robert C. Marquardt, FACHE, Chief Operating Officer, p. B102

Beaver: HERITAGE VALLEY HEALTH SYSTEM 1000 Dutch Ridge Road, Zip 15009–9727; tel. 724/773–2024; Norman F. Mitry, President and Chief Executive Officer, p. B63

Chambersburg: ★ SUMMIT HEALTH 112 North Seventh Street, Zip 17201; tel. 717/267–7138; Norman B. Epstein, FACHE, President, p. B114

Danville: ★ GEISINGER HEALTH SYSTEM 100 North Academy Avenue, Zip 17822; tel. 570/271–6211; Glenn Steele, Jr., M.D., Ph.D., President and Chief Executive Officer, p. B50

Erie: ST. VINCENT HEALTH SYSTEM 232 West 25th Street, Zip 16544–0002; tel. 814/452–5000; C. Angela Bontempo, President and Chief Executive Officer, p. B113

Greensburg: EXCELA HEALTH 532 West Pittsburgh Street, Zip 15601; tel. 724/832–5050; David S. Gallatin, Chief Executive Officer, p. B48

Johnstown: CONEMAUGH HEALTH SYSTEM 1086 Franklin Street, Zip 15905–4398; tel. 814/534–9000; Scott A. Becker, President and Chief Executive Officer, p. B36

King of Prussia: UNIVERSAL HEALTH SERVICES, INC. 367 South Gulph Road, Zip 19406–0958, Mailing Address: P.O. Box 61558, Zip 19406–0958; tel. 610/768–3300; Alan B. Miller, President and Chief Executive Officer, p. B124

Lehighton: BLUE MOUNTAIN HEALTH SYSTEM 211 North 12th Street, Zip 18235–1138; tel. 610/377–1300; Andrew E. Harris, Chief Executive Officer, p. B17

Mechanicsburg: SELECT MEDICAL CORPORATION 4714 Old Gettysburg Road, Zip 17055; tel. 717/972–1100; Robert Ortenzio, Chief Executive Officer, p. B104

VIBRA HEALTHCARE 4550 Lena Drive, Suite 225, Zip 17055; tel. 717/591–5700; Brad Hollinger, Chairman and Chief Executive Officer, p. B129

Newtown Square: ★ CATHOLIC HEALTH EAST 3805 West Chester Pike, Suite 100, Zip 19073; tel. 610/355–2000; Robert V. Stanek, President and Chief Executive Officer, p. B23

Philadelphia: ALBERT EINSTEIN HEALTHCARE NETWORK 5501 Old York Road, Zip 19141–3098; tel. 215/456–7890; Barry R. Freedman, President and Chief Executive Officer, p. B6

★ TEMPLE UNIVERSITY HEALTH SYSTEM 2450 West Hunting Park Avenue, 4th Floor, Zip 19129; tel. 215/707–0900; Joseph W. Marshall, III, President and Chief Executive Officer, p. B116

★ UNIVERSITY OF PENNSYLVANIA HEALTH SYSTEM 399 South 34th Street, 21st Floor, Zip 19104–4385; tel. 215/662–2203; Ralph W. Muller, President and Chief Executive Officer, p. B127

Pittsburgh: UPMC 600 Grent Street, U.S. Steel Tower, Suite 6262, Zip 15219, Mailing Address: 600 Grant Stret, U.S. Steel Tower, Suite 6262, Zip 15219; tel. 412/647–4800; Jeffrey A. Romoff, President and Chief Executive Officer, p. B128

★ WEST PENN ALLEGHENY HEALTH SYSTEM 3200 East North Avenue, Zip 15212; tel. 412/359–8588; Christopher Olivia, M.D., President and Chief Executive Officer, p. B131

Radnor: JEFFERSON HEALTH SYSTEM 259 Radnor–Chester Road, Suite 290, Zip 19087–5288; tel. 610/225–6200; Joseph T. Sebastianelli, President and Chief Executive Officer, p. B67

Sayre: ★ GUTHRIE HEALTHCARE SYSTEM Guthrie Square, Zip 18840; tel. 570/882–4312; Mark Stensager, President and Chief Executive Officer, p. B52

Springfield: ★ CROZER–KEYSTONE HEALTH SYSTEM 100 West Sproul Road, Zip 19064; tel. 610/338–8205; Joan K. Richards, President and Chief Executive Officer, p. B38

Villanova: DEVEREUX 444 Devereux Drive, Zip 19085, Mailing Address: P.O. Box 638, Zip 19085–0638; tel. 610/520–3000; Robert Q. Kreider, President and Chief Executive Officer, p. B44

York: ★ WELLSPAN HEALTH 45 Monument Road, Suite 200, Zip 17403; tel. 717/851–2121; Bruce M. Bartels, President, p. B131

PUERTO RICO

San Juan: ★ PUERTO RICO DEPARTMENT OF HEALTH Building A – Medical Center, Zip 00936, Mailing Address: Call Box 70184, Zip 00936; tel. 787/274–7676; Rosa Perez Perdomo, M.D., M.P.H., Ph.D., Secretary of Health, p. B95

RHODE ISLAND

Providence: ★ CARE NEW ENGLAND HEALTH SYSTEM 45 Willard Avenue, Zip 02905–3218; tel. 401/453–7900; John J. Hynes, President and Chief Executive Officer, p. B22

LIFESPAN CORPORATION 167 Point Street, Zip 02903–4771; tel. 401/444–3500; George A. Vecchione, President, p. B75

SOUTH CAROLINA

Anderson: ANMED HEALTH 800 North Fant Street, Zip 29621–5793; tel. 864/512–1000; John A. Miller, Jr., FACHE, President, p. B8

Charleston: MUSC MEDICAL CENTER OF MEDICAL UNIVERSITY OF SOUTH CAROLINA 169 Ashley Avenue, Zip 29425–5836; tel. 843/792–2300; Stuart Smith, Vice President Clinical Operations and Executive Director, p. B82

Columbia: ★ PALMETTO HEALTH 1301 Taylor Street, Suite 9–A, Zip 29201, Mailing Address: P.O. Box 2266, Zip 29202–2266; tel. 803/296–2100; Charles D. Beaman, Jr., President and Chief Executive Officer, p. B89

Greenville: ★ GREENVILLE HOSPITAL SYSTEM 701 Grove Road, Zip 29605–4211; tel. 864/455–7000; Michael C. Riordan, President and Chief Executive Officer, p. B51

Spartanburg: ★ SPARTANBURG REGIONAL HEALTHCARE SYSTEM 101 East Wood Street, Zip 29303–3016; tel. 864/560–6000; Ingo Angermeier, FACHE, President and Chief Executive Officer, p. B111

SOUTH DAKOTA

Rapid City: REGIONAL HEALTH 353 Fairmont Boulevard, Zip 57701, Mailing Address: P.O. Box 6000, Zip 57709–6000; tel. 605/719–1000; Charles Hart, M.D., President and Chief Executive Officer, p. B99

Sioux Falls: ★ AVERA HEALTH 3900 West Avera Drive, Suite 301, Zip 57108; tel. 605/322–4700; John T. Porter, President and Chief Executive Officer, p. B13

★ SANFORD HEALTH 1305 West 18th Street, Zip 57105–0496, Mailing Address: P.O. Box 5039, Zip 57117–5039; tel. 605/333–1000; Kelby K. Krabbenhoft, President and Chief Executive Officer, p. B103

TENNESSEE

Brentwood: ★ BRIM HEALTHCARE, INC. 105 Westwood Place, Suite 300, Zip 37027; tel. 615/309–6053; Dave Woodland, President, p. B18

★ LIFEPOINT HOSPITALS, INC. 103 Powell Court, Suite 200, Zip 37027; tel. 615/372–8500; William F. Carpenter, III, President and Chief Executive Officer, p. B73

Chattanooga: ERLANGER HEALTH SYSTEM 975 East Third Street, Zip 37403; tel. 423/778–7000; James L. Brexler, President and Chief Executive Officer, p. B47

Franklin: CAPELLA HEALTHCARE 501 Corporate Center Drive, Suite 200, Zip 37067; tel. 615/764–3000; Daniel S. Slipkovich, Chief Executive Officer, p. B21

★ COMMUNITY HEALTH SYSTEMS, INC. 4000 Meridian Boulevard, Zip 37067, Mailing Address: P.O. Box 689020, Zip 37068–9020; tel. 615/465–7000; Wayne T. Smith, Chairman, President and Chief Executive Officer, p. B32

IASIS HEALTHCARE 117 Seaboard Lane, Building E., Zip 37067; tel. 615/844–2747; David R. White, Chairman and Chief Executive Officer, p. B65

PSYCHIATRIC SOLUTIONS 6640 Carothers Parkway, Suite 500, Zip 37067; tel. 615/312–5700; Joey Jacobs, President and Chief Executive Officer, p. B93

Gallatin: SUMNER REGIONAL HEALTH SYSTEMS 255 Airport Road, Zip 37066; tel. 615/328–6695; William T. Sugg, President and Chief Executive Officer, p. B114

Jackson: ★ WEST TENNESSEE HEALTHCARE 620 Skyline Drive, Zip 38301–3901; tel. 731/541–5000; Richard H. Parks, FACHE, President and Chief Executive Officer, p. B131

Johnson City: MOUNTAIN STATES HEALTH ALLIANCE 701 North State of Franklin, Suite 1, Zip 37604; tel. 423/431–1040; Dennis Vonderfecht, President and Chief Executive Officer, p. B82

Kingsport: WELLMONT HEALTH SYSTEM 1905 American Way, Zip 37662–0224; tel. 423/230–8200; , p. B130

Knoxville: ★ COVENANT HEALTH 100 Fort Sanders West Boulevard, Zip 37922; tel. 865/531–5555; Anthony L. Spezia, President and Chief Executive Officer, p. B37

Memphis: ★ BAPTIST MEMORIAL HEALTH CARE CORPORATION 350 North Humphreys Boulevard, Zip 38120–2177; tel. 901/227–5117; Stephen Curtis Reynolds, President and Chief Executive Officer, p. B15

METHODIST LE BONHEUR HEALTHCARE 1211 Union Avenue, Suite 700, Zip 38104–6600; tel. 901/516–0543; Gary S. Shorb, President and Chief Executive Officer, p. B80

Nashville: AMERIS HEALTH SYSTEMS 1114 17th Avenue South, Suite 205, Zip 37212–2215; tel. 615/327–4440; Sam Lewis, Chairman and Chief Executive Officer, p. B8

★ ARDENT HEALTH SERVICES 1 Burton Hills Boulevard, Suite 250, Zip 37215; tel. 615/296–3000; David T. Vandewater, President and Chief Executive Officer, p. B9

BEHAVIORAL CENTERS OF AMERICA 3100 West End Street, Suite 1000, Zip 37203; tel. 615/463–3200; Edward A. Stack, President and Chief Executive Officer, p. B17

ESSENT HEALTHCARE 3100 West End Avenue, Suite 900, Zip 37203; tel. 615/312–5100; Michael W. Browder, President and Chief Executive Officer, p. B47

★ HCA One Park Plaza, Zip 37203–1548; tel. 615/344–9551; Jack O. Bovender, Jr., Chairman and Chief Executive Officer, p. B52

SENIORHEALTH INCORPORATED 49 Music Square West, Suite 502, Zip 37203; tel. 615/321–5577; Kevin D. Lee, President and Chief Executive Officer, p. B107

VANDERBILT HEALTHCARE 1211 22nd Avenue South, Zip 37232; tel. 615/322–5000; Larry Goldberg, Executive Director and Chief Executive Officer, p. B129

VANGUARD HEALTH SYSTEM 20 Burton Hills Boulevard, Suite 10, Zip 37215; tel. 615/665–6000; Charles N. Martin, Jr., Chairman and Chief Executive Officer, p. B129

TEXAS

Addison: UNITED SURGICAL PARTNERS INTERNATIONAL 15305 Dallas Parkway, Suite 1600, Zip 75001–6491; tel. 972/713–3500; William H. Wilcox, President and Chief Executive Officer, p. B123

Arlington: ★ TEXAS HEALTH RESOURCES 612 East Lamar Boulevard, Suite 900, Zip 76011; tel. 817/462–7900; Douglas D. Hawthorne, FACHE, Chief Executive Officer, p. B118

Austin: BLACKHAWK HEALTHCARE 6836 Bee Caves Road, Suite 202, Zip 78746; tel. 512/617–6363; Matthew Q. Hainline, Chief Executive Officer, p. B17

CORNERSTONE HEALTHCARE GROUP 816 Congress Avenue, Suite 400, Zip 78701; tel. 512/533–2400; Timothy P. Hall, President and Chief Executive Officer, p. B36

ST. DAVID'S HEALTHCARE SYSTEM 98 San Jacinto Boulevard, Suite 1800, Zip 78701; tel. 512/708–9700; Jon M. Foster, President and Chief Executive Officer, p. B112

TEXAS DEPARTMENT OF STATE HEALTH SERVICES 1100 West 49th Street, Zip 78756–3199; tel. 512/458–7111; David L. Lakey, M.D., Commissioner, p. B118

★ UNIVERSITY OF TEXAS SYSTEM 601 Colorado Street, Suite 205, Zip 78701–2982; tel. 512/499–4224; Kenneth Shine, M.D., Executive Vice Chancellor, p. B127

YOUTH AND FAMILY CENTERED SERVICES 1705 Capital of Texas Highway South, Zip 78746; tel. 512/327–1119; Kevin P. Sheehan, Chairman, President and Chief Executive Officer, p. B133

Dallas: ★ BAYLOR HEALTH CARE SYSTEM 3500 Gaston Avenue, Zip 75246; tel. 214/820–0111; Joel T. Allison, President and Chief Executive Officer, p. B16

CIRRUS HEALTH 9301 North Central Expressway, Suite 360, Zip 75231, Mailing Address: 9301 North Central Expressway, Suite360, Zip 75231; tel. 214/217–0100; Timothy Parris, President and Chief Executive Officer, p. B30

★ METHODIST HEALTH SYSTEM 1441 North Beckley Avenue, Zip 75203–1201, Mailing Address: P.O. Box 655999, Zip 75265–5999; tel. 214/947–8181; Stephen L. Mansfield, Ph.D., FACHE, President and Chief Executive Officer, p. B80

SIGNATURE HOSPITAL CORPORATION 12160 North Abrams Road, Zip 75243; tel. 214/580–8800; Charles R. Miller, Chief Executive Officer, p. B109

★ TENET HEALTHCARE CORPORATION 13737 Noel Road, Suite 100, Zip 75240–2200; tel. 469/893–2200; Trevor Fetter, President and Chief Executive Officer, p. B116

Harlingen: VALLEY BAPTIST HEALTH SYSTEM 2101 Pease Street, Zip 78550; tel. 956/389–1100; James G. Springfield, FACHE, President and Chief Executive Officer, p. B128

Houston: CAMBRIDGE HEALTH FOUNDATION 1120 Cypress Station Drive, Zip 77090; tel. 281/893–7200; Deo Shanker, CPA, President, p. B21

★ DUBUIS HEALTH SYSTEM 10333 Richmond Avenue, Suite 300, Zip 77042; tel. 713/339–7000; Ellen Smith, President and Chief Executive Officer, p. B45

DYNACQ HEALTHCARE, INC. 10304 Interstate 10 East, Suite 369, Zip 77029; tel. 713/673–6432; Chiu Moon Chan, Chairman, President and Chief Executive Officer, p. B45

HEALTHPLUS 509 West Tidwell Road, Zip 77091; tel. 713/490–0700; Wilton M. Burt, President and Chief Executive Officer, p. B60

★ MEMORIAL HERMANN HEALTHCARE SYSTEM 7737 S.W. Freeway, Suite 200, Zip 77074–1800; tel. 713/456–5550; Daniel J. Wolterman, President and Chief Executive Officer, p. B79

NEXUS HEALTH SYSTEMS One Riverway, Suite 600, Zip 77056; tel. 713/355–6111; John W. Cassidy, M.D., President, Chief Executive Officer and Chief Medical Officer, p. B85

RENAISSANCE HEALTHCARE SYSTEMS 14440 John F. Kennedy Boulevard, Zip 77032; tel. 832/886–1900; Michael Smesny, Chief Executive Officer, p. B100

ST. LUKE'S EPISCOPAL HEALTH SYSTEM 6624 Fannin Street, Suite 1100, Zip 77030; tel. 832/355–7661; Beryl Vallejo, RN, Dr.P.h., Senior Vice President and Chief Quality Officer, p. B113

★ THE METHODIST HOSPITAL SYSTEM 6565 Fannin Street, D–200, Zip 77030–2707; tel. 713/441–2221; Ronald G. Girotto, President and Chief Executive Officer, p. B119

TRIUMPH HEALTHCARE 7333 North Freeway, Suite 500, Zip 77076; tel. 713/807–8686; Charles Allen, President and Chief Executive, p. B120

Irving: ★ CHRISTUS HEALTH 6363 North Highway 161, Suite 450, Zip 75038; tel. 877/980–0100; Thomas C. Royer, M.D., President and Chief Executive Officer, p. B29

Lewisville: HORIZON HEALTH CORPORATION 1500 Waters Ridge Drive, Zip 75057; tel. 972/420–8222; Ken Newman, President and Chief Executive Officer, p. B63

Lubbock: ★ COVENANT HEALTH SYSTEM 3615 19th Street, Zip 79410–1201; tel. 806/725–0447; Melinda Clark, FACHE, President and Chief Executive Officer, p. B37

SHILOH HEALTH SERVICES, INC. 2412 50th Street, Zip 79412–2494; tel. 806/788–4060; James R. Cheek, President, p. B108

Lufkin: MEMORIAL HEALTH SYSTEM OF EAST TEXAS 1201 West Frank Avenue, Zip 75904–3357; tel. 936/634–8111; Bryant H. Krenek, Jr., President and Chief Executive Officer, p. B79

Plano: COMMUNITY HOSPITAL CORPORATION 5180 Tennyson Parkway, Suite 500, Zip 75024; tel. 972/943–6400; Michael D. Williams, President and Chief Executive Officer, p. B35

LIFECARE MANAGEMENT SERVICES 5560 Tennyson Parkway, Zip 75024; tel. 469/241–2100; Wayne McAlister, Chairman of the Board and Chief Executive Officer, p. B73

★ QHR 5800 Tennyson Parkway, Zip 75024; tel. 214/473–3700; John C. Stinson, President and Chief Executive Officer, p. B95

Temple: SCOTT & WHITE 2401 South 31st Street, Zip 76508; tel. 254/724–2111; Alfred B. Knight, M.D., Chief Executive Officer, p. B104

Tyler: ★ EAST TEXAS MEDICAL CENTER REGIONAL HEALTHCARE SYSTEM 1000 South Beckham Street, Zip 75701–1996, Mailing Address: P.O. Box 6400, Zip 75711–6400; tel. 903/535–6211; Elmer G. Ellis, FACHE, President and Chief Executive Officer, p. B45

UTAH

Nephi: ★ RURAL HEALTH GROUP 48 West 1500 North, Zip 84648–1226; tel. 435/623–4924; Mark R. Stoddard, President and Chairman, p. B101

Salt Lake City: ★ INTERMOUNTAIN HEALTHCARE, INC. 36 South State Street, 22nd Floor, Zip 84111–1453; tel. 801/442–2000; William H. Nelson, President and Chief Executive Officer, p. B66

VIRGINIA

Falls Church: DEPARTMENT OF THE ARMY, OFFICE OF THE SURGEON GENERAL 5109 Leesburg Pike, Zip 22041; tel. 703/681–3000; Lieutenant General Eric B. Schoomaker, Surgeon General, p. B39

★ INOVA HEALTH SYSTEM 8110 Gatehouse Road, Zip 22042; tel. 703/289–2069; J. Knox Singleton, President and Chief Executive Officer, p. B65

Newport News: RIVERSIDE HEALTH SYSTEM 701 Town Center Drive, Suite 1000, Zip 23606; tel. 757/534–7000; Richard J. Pearce, President and Chief Executive Officer, p. B101

Norfolk: ★ SENTARA HEALTHCARE 6015 Poplar Hall Drive, Zip 23502–3819; tel. 757/455–7000; David L. Bernd, Chief Executive Officer, p. B107

Richmond: VIRGINIA DEPARTMENT OF MENTAL HEALTH 1220 Bank Street, Zip 23219, Mailing Address: P.O. Box 1797, Zip 23218–1797; tel. 804/786–3921; James S. Reinhard, M.D., Commissioner, p. B130

Roanoke: ★ CARILION CLINIC Belleview at Jefferson Street, Zip 24014, Mailing Address: P.O. Box 13727, Zip 24036–3727; tel. 540/981–7893; Edward G. Murphy, M.D., President and Chief Executive Officer, p. B22

Winchester: ★ VALLEY HEALTH SYSTEM 190 Campus Boulevard, Suite 220, Zip 22601, Mailing Address: P.O. Box 3340, Zip 22604–1334; tel. 540/536–8024; Michael J. Halseth, President and Chief Executive Officer, p. B128

WASHINGTON

Bellevue: ★ PEACEHEALTH 14432 S.E. Eastgate Way, Suite 300, Zip 98007–6412; tel. 425/747–1711; Alan R. Yordy, President and Chief Mission Officer, p. B90

Seattle: ★ PROVIDENCE HEALTH & SERVICES 506 Second Avenue, Suite 1200, Zip 98104–2329; tel. 206/464–3355; John F. Koster, M.D., President and Chief Executive Officer, p. B93

Spokane: ★ EMPIRE HEALTH SERVICES West 800 Fifth Avenue, Zip 99204, Mailing Address: P.O. Box 248, Zip 99210–0248; tel. 509/473–7965; C. E. Bilbrey, Interim Chief Executive Officer, p. B46

Tacoma: MULTICARE HEALTH SYSTEM 315 Martin Luther King Jr. Way, Zip 98415, Mailing Address: P.O. Box 5299, Zip 98415–0299; tel. 253/403–1000; Diane Cecchettini, RN, President and Chief Executive Officer, p. B82

WEST VIRGINIA

Charleston: ★ CHARLESTON AREA MEDICAL CENTER HEALTH SYSTEM, INC. 501 Morris Street, Zip 25301–1300, Mailing Address: P.O. Box 1547, Zip 25326–1547; tel. 304/388–5432; David L. Ramsey, President and Chief Executive Officer, p. B29

Fairmont: ★ WEST VIRGINIA UNITED HEALTH SYSTEM 1000 Technology Drive, Suite 2320, Zip 26554; tel. 304/368–2700; J. Thomas Jones, President and Chief Executive Officer, p. B132

Wheeling: OHIO VALLEY HEALTH SERVICES AND EDUCATION CORPORATION 2000 Eoff Street, Zip 26003; tel. 304/234–8383; Brian K. Felici, President and Chief Executive Officer, p. B87

WISCONSIN

Appleton: THEDACARE, INC. 122 East College Avenue, Zip 54911, Mailing Address: P.O. Box 8025, Zip 54912; tel. 920/830–5880; John S. Toussaint, M.D., President and Chief Executive Officer, p. B119

Manitowoc: ★ FRANCISCAN SISTERS OF CHRISTIAN CHARITY HEALTHCARE MINISTRY, INC 1415 South Rapids Road, Zip 54220–9302; tel. 920/684–7071; Sister Laura J. Wolf, President, p. B49

Milwaukee: ★ AURORA HEALTH CARE 3000 West Montana, Zip 53215–3268, Mailing Address: P.O. Box 343910, Zip 53234–3910; tel. 414/647–3000; Nick Turkal, M.D., President and Chief Executive Officer, p. B12

Waukesha: ★ PROHEALTH CARE N17 W24100 Riverwood Drive, Suite 130, Zip 53188; tel. 262/928–2244; Rexford W. Titus, III, President and Chief Executive Officer, p. B92

Networks and their Hospitals

ALASKA

KETCHIKAN GENERAL HOSPITAL
3100 Tongass Avenue, Ketchikan, AK 99901; tel. 907/225–5171; Pat Branco, Chief Executive Officer

KETCHIKAN GENERAL HOSPITAL, 3100 Tongass Avenue, Ketchikan, AK, Zip 99901–5746; tel. 907/225–5171; Patrick J. Branco, Chief Executive Officer

ARIZONA

NORTHERN ARIZONA HEALTHCARE
1200 North Beaver Street, Flagstaff, AZ 86001; tel. 928/779–3366; James Puffenberger, President

FLAGSTAFF MEDICAL CENTER, 1200 North Beaver Street, Flagstaff, AZ, Zip 86001–3198; tel. 928/779–3366; William T. Bradel, President

VERDE VALLEY MEDICAL CENTER, 269 South Candy Lane, Cottonwood, AZ, Zip 86326–4170; tel. 928/639–6000; James J. Sinek, President

CALIFORNIA

LITTLE COMPANY OF MARY HEALTH SERVICES
4101 Torrance Boulevard, Torrance, CA 90503; tel. 310/543–5868; Michael Hunn, Chief Executive Officer

LITTLE COMPANY OF MARY – SAN PEDRO HOSPITAL, 1300 West Seventh Street, San Pedro, CA, Zip 90732–3505; tel. 310/832–3311; Nancy Carlson, Administrator

LITTLE COMPANY OF MARY HOSPITAL, 4101 Torrance Boulevard, Torrance, CA, Zip 90503–4698; tel. 310/540–7676; Michael Hunn, Administrator

COLORADO

COMMUNITY HEALTH PROVIDERS ORGANIZATION
2021 North 12th Street, Grand Junction, CO 81501; tel. 970/256–6200; Heather Gray, Administrator

COMMUNITY HOSPITAL, 2021 North 12th Street, Grand Junction, CO, Zip 81501–2999; tel. 970/242–0920; Wesley White, President

HCA HEALTHONE, LLC
4900 South Monaco Street, Suite 380, Denver, CO 80237; tel. 303/788–2500; Jeffrey A. Dorsey, President and Chief Executive Officer

MEDICAL CENTER OF AURORA, 1501 South Potomac Street, Aurora, CO, Zip 80012–5499; tel. 303/695–2600; John Hill, President and Chief Executive Officer

NORTH SUBURBAN MEDICAL CENTER, 9191 Grant Street, Thornton, CO, Zip 80229–4341; tel. 303/451–7800; Todd Steward, President and Chief Executive Officer

PRESBYTERIAN–ST. LUKE'S MEDICAL CENTER, 1719 East 19th Avenue, Denver, CO, Zip 80218–1281; tel. 303/839–6000; Madeleine Roberson, President and Chief Executive Officer

ROSE MEDICAL CENTER, 4567 East Ninth Avenue, Denver, CO, Zip 80220–3941; tel. 303/320–2121; Kenneth H. Feiler, President and Chief Executive Officer

SKY RIDGE MEDICAL CENTER, 10101 Ridge Gate Parkway, Lone Tree, CO, Zip 80124; tel. 720/225–1000; Maureen Tarrant, Chief Executive Officer

SPALDING REHABILITATION HOSPITAL, 900 Potomac Street, Aurora, CO, Zip 80011–6716; tel. 303/367–1166; Cynthia Kreutz, President and Chief Executive Officer

SWEDISH MEDICAL CENTER, 501 East Hampden Avenue, Englewood, CO, Zip 80113; tel. 303/788–5000; Mary M. White, President and Chief Executive Officer

CONNECTICUT

DANBURY HEALTH SYSTEMS, INC.
24 Hospital Avenue, Danbury, CT 06810; tel. 203/797–7066; Frank J. Kelly, President and Chief Executive Officer

DANBURY HOSPITAL, 24 Hospital Avenue, Danbury, CT, Zip 06810–6099; tel. 203/739–7000; Frank J. Kelly, President and Chief Executive Officer

EASTERN CONNECTICUT HEALTH NETWORK, INC.
71 Haynes Street, Manchester, CT 06040; tel. 860/533–3400; Peter J. Karl, President and Chief Executive Officer

MANCHESTER MEMORIAL HOSPITAL, 71 Haynes Street, Manchester, CT, Zip 06040–4188; tel. 860/646–1222; Peter J. Karl, President and Chief Executive Officer

ROCKVILLE GENERAL HOSPITAL, 31 Union Street, Vernon Rockville, CT, Zip 06066–3160; tel. 860/872–0501; Peter J. Karl, President and Chief Executive Officer

HARTFORD HEALTH CARE CORPORATION
80 Seymour Street, P.O. Box 5037, Hartford, CT 06102; tel. 860/545–2100; Elliot Joseph, President and Chief Executive Officer

HARTFORD HOSPITAL, 80 Seymour Street, Hartford, CT, Zip 06102–5037, Mailing Address: P.O. Box 5037, Zip 06102–5037; tel. 860/545–5000; Elliot T. Joseph, President and Chief Executive Officer

HOSPITAL FOR SPECIAL CARE, 2150 Corbin Avenue, New Britain, CT, Zip 06053–2298; tel. 860/223–2761; David Crandall, FACHE, President and Chief Executive Officer

HOSPITAL OF SAINT RAPHAEL, 1450 Chapel Street, New Haven, CT, Zip 06511–1450; tel. 203/789–3000; David W. Benfer, FACHE, President and Chief Executive Officer

JOHNSON MEMORIAL HOSPITAL, 201 Chestnut Hill Road, Stafford Springs, CT, Zip 06076–4005; tel. 860/684–4251; Peter Betts, Interim President and Chief Executive Officer

MIDDLESEX HOSPITAL, 28 Crescent Street, Middletown, CT, Zip 06457–3650; tel. 860/358–6000; Robert Gerard Kiely, President and Chief Executive Officer

MIDSTATE MEDICAL CENTER, 435 Lewis Avenue, Meriden, CT, Zip 06451–2101; tel. 203/694–8200; Lucille A. Janatka, President and Chief Executive Officer

ST. VINCENT'S MEDICAL CENTER, 2800 Main Street, Bridgeport, CT, Zip 06606–4292; tel. 203/576–5454; Susan L. Davis, RN, Ed.D., President and Chief Executive Officer

STAMFORD HOSPITAL, 30 Shelburne Road, Stamford, CT, Zip 6902, Mailing Address: P.O. Box 9317, Zip 06904–9317; tel. 203/276–1000; Brian G. Grissler, President and Chief Executive Officer

THE CHARLOTTE HUNGERFORD HOSPITAL, 540 Litchfield Street, Torrington, CT, Zip 06790–0988, Mailing Address: P.O. Box 988, Zip 06790–0988; tel. 860/496–6666; Daniel J. McIntyre, President and Chief Executive Officer

THE HOSPITAL OF CENTRAL CONNECTICUT, 100 Grand Street, New Britain, CT, Zip 06052–2017, Mailing Address: P.O. Box 100, Zip 06050–0100; tel. 860/224–5011; Laurence A. Tanner, President and Chief Executive Officer

WINDHAM COMMUNITY MEMORIAL HOSPITAL, 112 Mansfield Avenue, Willimantic, CT, Zip 06226–2040; tel. 860/456–9116; Richard A. Brvenik, FACHE, President and Chief Executive Officer

ST. MARY'S HOSPITAL INTEGRATED DELIVERY NETWORK
56 Franklin Street, Waterbury, CT 06702; tel. 203/709–6000; Chad Wable, Executive Vice President and Strategy Development and System Operations

SAINT MARY'S HOSPITAL, 56 Franklin Street, Waterbury, CT, Zip 06706–1281; tel. 203/709–6000

FLORIDA

MID–FLORIDA MEDICAL SERVICES
200 Avenue F. Northeast, Winter Haven, FL 33881; tel. 863/297–1899; Lance Anastasio, President

WINTER HAVEN HOSPITAL, 200 Avenue F. N.E., Winter Haven, FL, Zip 33881–4193; tel. 863/293–1121; Lance W. Anastasio, President

GEORGIA

EMORY HEALTHCARE
1365 Clifton Road Northeast, Atlanta, GA 30322; tel. 404/778–7777; Michael Johns, M.D., Chief Executive Officer

EMORY CRAWFORD LONG HOSPITAL, 550 Peachtree Street N.E., Atlanta, GA, Zip 30308; tel. 404/686–4411; John T. Fox, Chief Executive Officer

EMORY UNIVERSITY HOSPITAL, 1364 Clifton Road N.E., Atlanta, GA, Zip 30322–1102; tel. 404/712–2000; John T. Fox, Chief Executive Officer

WESLEY WOODS CENTER OF EMORY UNIVERSITY, 1821 Clifton Road N.E., Atlanta, GA, Zip 30329–5102; tel. 404/728–6200; Albert K. Blackwelder, FACHE, Chief Operating Officer

GEORGIA FIRST NETWORK
1899 Powers Ferry, Atlanta, GA 30339; tel. 678/742–9100; Gary Hutchins, Chief Executive Officer

APPLING HEALTHCARE SYSTEM, 163 East Tollison Street, Baxley, GA, Zip 31513–2898; tel. 912/367–9841; Dale Spell, Chief Executive Officer

ATHENS REGIONAL MEDICAL CENTER, 1199 Prince Avenue, Athens, GA, Zip 30606–2793; tel. 706/475–7000; John A. Drew, President and Chief Executive Officer

BROOKS COUNTY HOSPITAL, 903 North Court Street, Quitman, GA, Zip 31643–1315, Mailing Address: P.O. Box 5000, Zip 31643–5000; tel. 229/263–4171; LaDon Toole, Administrator

CRISP REGIONAL HOSPITAL, 902 North Seventh Street, Cordele, GA, Zip 31015–5007; tel. 229/276–3100; D. Wayne Martin, President and Chief Executive Officer

EARLY MEMORIAL HOSPITAL, 11740 Columbia Street, Blakely, GA, Zip 39823–9604; tel. 229/723–4241; Robin Rau, Administrator

EFFINGHAM HOSPITAL, 459 Highway 119 South, Springfield, GA, Zip 31329–3021, Mailing Address: P.O. Box 386, Zip 31329–0386; tel. 912/754–6451; Norma J. Morgan, Chief Executive Officer

ELBERT MEMORIAL HOSPITAL, 4 Medical Drive, Elberton, GA, Zip 30635–1897; tel. 706/283–3151; Mark LeNeave, Chief Executive Officer

EMORY CRAWFORD LONG HOSPITAL, 550 Peachtree Street N.E., Atlanta, GA, Zip 30308; tel. 404/686–4411; John T. Fox, Chief Executive Officer

EMORY EASTSIDE MEDICAL CENTER, 1700 Medical Way, Snellville, GA, Zip 30078–2195, Mailing Address: P.O. Box 587, Zip 30078–0587; tel. 770/979–0200; Kimberly Ryan, Chief Executive Officer

EMORY UNIVERSITY HOSPITAL, 1364 Clifton Road N.E., Atlanta, GA, Zip 30322–1102; tel. 404/712–2000; John T. Fox, Chief Executive Officer

EMORY–ADVENTIST HOSPITAL, 3949 South Cobb Drive S.E., Smyrna, GA, Zip 30080–6300; tel. 770/434–0710; Dennis Kiley, President

FAIRVIEW PARK HOSPITAL, 200 Industrial Boulevard, Dublin, GA, Zip 31021–2997, Mailing Address: P.O. Box 1408, Zip 31040–1408; tel. 478/275–2000; Donald R. Avery, FACHE, President and Chief Executive Officer

FLOYD MEDICAL CENTER, 304 Turner McCall Boulevard, Rome, GA, Zip 30165–2734, Mailing Address: P.O. Box 233, Zip 30162–0233; tel. 706/509–5000; Kurt Stuenkel, FACHE, President and Chief Executive Officer

GRADY GENERAL HOSPITAL, 1155 Fifth Street S.E., Cairo, GA, Zip 39828–0360, Mailing Address: P.O. Box 360, Zip 39828–0360; tel. 229/377–1150; LaDon Toole, Administrator

HABERSHAM COUNTY MEDICAL CENTER, 541 Historic Highway 441, Demorest, GA, Zip 30535–3118, Mailing Address: P.O. Box 37, Zip 30535–0037; tel. 706/754–2161; C. Richard Dwozan, Chief Executive Officer

HIGGINS GENERAL HOSPITAL, 200 Allen Memorial Drive, Bremen, GA, Zip 30110–2012, Mailing Address: P.O. Box 655, Zip 30110–0655; tel. 770/537–5851; Michael Alexander, Administrator

HOUSTON MEDICAL CENTER, 1601 Watson Boulevard, Warner Robins, GA, Zip 31093–3431, Mailing Address: P.O. Box 2886, Zip 31099–2886; tel. 478/922–4281; Anthony Alford, D.O., FACHE, Chief Executive Officer

JOHN D. ARCHBOLD MEMORIAL HOSPITAL, Gordon Avenue at Mimosa Drive, Thomasville, GA, Zip 31792–6113, Mailing Address: P.O. Box 1018, Zip 31799–1018; tel. 229/228–2000; J. Perry Mustian, President and Chief Executive Officer

LIBERTY REGIONAL MEDICAL CENTER, 462 East G. Miles Parkway, Hinesville, GA, Zip 31313, Mailing Address: P.O. Box 919, Zip 31313; tel. 912/369–9438; H. Scott Kroell, Jr., Chief Executive Officer

LOUIS SMITH MEMORIAL HOSPITAL, 852 West Thigpen Avenue, Lakeland, GA, Zip 31635–1099; tel. 229/482–3110; Neil W. Ginty, Administrator

MEDICAL CENTER OF CENTRAL GEORGIA, 777 Hemlock Street, Macon, GA, Zip 31201–2155, Mailing Address: P.O. Box 6000, Zip 31208–6000; tel. 478/633–1000; A. Donald Faulk, Jr., FACHE, President

MEDICAL COLLEGE OF GEORGIA HEALTH, 1120 15th Street, Augusta, GA, Zip 30912–5000; tel. 706/721–0211; Donald F. Snell, President and Chief Executive Officer

MITCHELL COUNTY HOSPITAL, 90 Stephens Street, Camilla, GA, Zip 31730, Mailing Address: P.O. Box 639, Zip 31730–0639; tel. 229/336–5284; Mark E. Kimball, Administrator

NEWTON MEDICAL CENTER, 5126 Hospital Drive, Covington, GA, Zip 30014–2567; tel. 770/786–7053; James F. Weadick, Administrator and Chief Executive Officer

NORTHSIDE HOSPITAL, 1000 Johnson Ferry Road N.E., Atlanta, GA, Zip 30342–1611; tel. 404/851–8000; Robert Quattrocchi, President and Chief Executive Officer

OCONEE REGIONAL MEDICAL CENTER, 821 North Cobb Street, Milledgeville, GA, Zip 31061–2351, Mailing Address: P.O. Box 690, Zip 31061–0690; tel. 478/454–3500; Jean Aycock, President and Chief Executive Officer

PALMYRA MEDICAL CENTERS, 2000 Palmyra Road, Albany, GA, Zip 31702–1908, Mailing Address: P.O. Box 1908, Zip 31702–1908; tel. 229/434–2000; Bud Wethington, Chief Executive Officer

SOUTH GEORGIA MEDICAL CENTER, 2501 North Patterson Street, Valdosta, GA, Zip 31602–1735, Mailing Address: P.O. Box 1727, Zip 31603–1727; tel. 229/333–1000; James McGahee, Administrator and Chief Executive Officer

SOUTHEAST GEORGIA HEALTH SYSTEM BRUNSWICK CAMPUS, 2415 Parkwood Drive, Brunswick, GA, Zip 31520–4252, Mailing Address: P.O. Box 1518, Zip 31521–1518; tel. 912/466–7000; Gary R. Colberg, FACHE, President and Chief Executive Officer

SOUTHEAST GEORGIA HEALTH SYSTEM CAMDEN CAMPUS, 2000 Dan Proctor Drive, Saint Marys, GA, Zip 31558–3810; tel. 912/576–6200; Howard W. Sepp, Jr., FACHE, Vice President and Administrator

SOUTHERN REGIONAL MEDICAL CENTER, 11 Upper Riverdale Road S.W., Riverdale, GA, Zip 30274–2615; tel. 770/991–8000; Edward J. Bonn, President and Chief Executive Officer

SPALDING REGIONAL MEDICAL CENTER, 601 South Eighth Street, Griffin, GA, Zip 30224–4294, Mailing Address: P.O. Drawer V, Zip 30224–1168; tel. 770/228–2721; John A. Quinn, Chief Executive Officer

ST. JOSEPH'S/CANDLER, CANDLER HOSPITAL, 5353 Reynolds Street, Savannah, GA, Zip 31405–6013; tel. 912/819–6000; Paul P. Hinchey, President and Chief Executive Officer

TANNER MEDICAL CENTER, 705 Dixie Street, Carrollton, GA, Zip 30117–3818; tel. 770/836–9666; Loy M. Howard, President and Chief Executive Officer

TANNER MEDICAL CENTER–VILLA RICA, 601 Dallas Road, Villa Rica, GA, Zip 30180–1202, Mailing Address: P.O. Box 638, Zip 30180–0638; tel. 770/456–3100; Larry N. Steed, FACHE, Administrator

TATTNALL COMMUNITY HOSPITAL, 247 South Main Street, Reidsville, GA, Zip 30453; tel. 912/557–1000; Karen O'Neal, Chief Executive Officer

THE MEDICAL CENTER, 710 Center Street, Columbus, GA, Zip 31901–1527, Mailing Address: P.O. Box 951, Zip 31902–0951; tel. 706/571–1000; Lance B. Duke, FACHE, President and Chief Executive Officer

TIFT REGIONAL MEDICAL CENTER, 901 East 18th Street, Tifton, GA, Zip 31794–3648, Mailing Address: Drawer 747, Zip 31793–0747; tel. 229/382–7120; William T. Richardson, President and Chief Executive Officer

UPSON REGIONAL MEDICAL CENTER, 801 West Gordon Street, Thomaston, GA, Zip 30286–2831, Mailing Address: P.O. Box 1059, Zip 30286–1059; tel. 706/647–8111; Gene B. Wright, Chief Executive Officer

WALTON REGIONAL MEDICAL CENTER, 330 Alcovy Street, Monroe, GA, Zip 30655–2140, Mailing Address: P.O. Box 1346, Zip 30655–1346; tel. 770/267–8461; Gary Lang, Chief Executive Officer

WEST GEORGIA HEALTH SYSTEM, 1514 Vernon Road, La Grange, GA, Zip 30240–4199; tel. 706/882–1411; Gerald N. Fulks, President and Chief Executive Officer

ST. JOSEPH'S/CANDLER HEALTH SYSTEM, INC.
5353 Reynolds Street, Savannah, GA 31412; tel. 912/819–6000; Paul Hinchey, President

APPLING HEALTHCARE SYSTEM, 163 East Tollison Street, Baxley, GA, Zip 31513–2898; tel. 912/367–9841; Dale Spell, Chief Executive Officer

EFFINGHAM HOSPITAL, 459 Highway 119 South, Springfield, GA, Zip 31329–3021, Mailing Address: P.O. Box 386, Zip 31329–0386; tel. 912/754–6451; Norma J. Morgan, Chief Executive Officer

EMORY UNIVERSITY HOSPITAL, 1364 Clifton Road N.E., Atlanta, GA, Zip 30322–1102; tel. 404/712–2000; John T. Fox, Chief Executive Officer

LIBERTY REGIONAL MEDICAL CENTER, 462 East G. Miles Parkway, Hinesville, GA, Zip 31313, Mailing Address: P.O. Box 919, Zip 31313; tel. 912/369–9438; H. Scott Kroell, Jr., Chief Executive Officer

MEADOWS REGIONAL MEDICAL CENTER, 1703 Meadows Lane, Vidalia, GA, Zip 30474–8915, Mailing Address: P.O. Box 1048, Zip 30475–1048; tel. 912/537–8921; Alan Kent, Chief Executive Officer

ST. JOSEPH'S/CANDLER, CANDLER HOSPITAL, 5353 Reynolds Street, Savannah, GA, Zip 31405–6013; tel. 912/819–6000; Paul P. Hinchey, President and Chief Executive Officer

WILLINGWAY HOSPITAL, 311 Jones Mill Road, Statesboro, GA, Zip 30458–4765; tel. 912/764–6236; Jimmy Mooney, Chief Executive Officer

IDAHO

NORTH IDAHO HEALTH NETWORK
700 Ironwood Drive, Suite 210, Coeur D'Alene, ID 83814; tel. 208/666–3212; Richard McMaster, Executive Director

BENEWAH COMMUNITY HOSPITAL, 229 South Seventh Street, Saint Maries, ID, Zip 83861–1803; tel. 208/245–5551; Brian Nall, Chief Executive Officer

BONNER GENERAL HOSPITAL, 520 North Third Avenue, Sandpoint, ID, Zip 83864–0877, Mailing Address: Box 1448, Zip 83864–0877; tel. 208/263–1441; Sheryl Rickard, Chief Executive Officer

BOUNDARY COMMUNITY HOSPITAL, 6640 Kaniksu Street, Bonners Ferry, ID, Zip 83805–7532; tel. 208/267–3141; Craig A. Johnson, Chief Executive Officer and Chief Financial Officer

KOOTENAI MEDICAL CENTER, 2003 Lincoln Way, Coeur D'Alene, ID, Zip 83814–2677; tel. 208/666–2000; Joseph E. Morris, Chief Executive Officer

SHOSHONE MEDICAL CENTER, 25 Jacobs Gulch, Kellogg, ID, Zip 83837–2096; tel. 208/784–1221; David B. Selman, FACHE, Chief Executive Officer

ILLINOIS

FELICIAN SERVICES, INC.
3800 W. Peterson, Chicago, IL 53215; tel. 773/463–3020; Sr. Mary Clarette Stryzewski, President

WHEATON FRANCISCAN HEALTHCARE – ST. FRANCIS, 3237 South 16th Street, Milwaukee, WI, Zip 53215–4592; tel. 414/647–5000; Debra Standridge, President

SWEDISH AMERICAN HEALTH SYSTEM
1313 East State Street, Rockford, IL 61104; tel. 815/968–4400; Dr. Bill Gorski, President and Chief Executive Officer

SWEDISHAMERICAN HOSPITAL, 1401 East State Street, Rockford, IL, Zip 61104–2315; tel. 815/968–4400; William R. Gorski, M.D., President and Chief Executive Officer

INDIANA

MEMORIAL HEALTH SYSTEM
100 Navarre, Suite 1100, South Bend, IN 46601; tel. 574/647–1000; Phillip Newbold, President and Chief Executive Officer

MEMORIAL HOSPITAL OF SOUTH BEND, 615 North Michigan Street, South Bend, IN, Zip 46601–9986; tel. 574/647–1000; Philip A. Newbold, President and Chief Executive Officer

ST. VINCENT HEALTH
8425 Harcourt Road, Indianapolis, IN 46260; tel. 317/338–7080; Vincent Caponi, Chief Executive Officer

SAINT JOHN'S HEALTH SYSTEM, 2015 Jackson Street, Anderson, IN, Zip 46016–4339; tel. 765/649–2511; Thomas J. VanOsdol, Interim President

ST VINCENT SETON SPECIALTY HOSPITAL, 1907 West Sycamore Street, 4th Floor, Lafayette, IN, Zip 47904; tel. 765/236–8900; Peter H. Alexander, Administrator

ST. JOSEPH HOSPITAL, 1907 West Sycamore Street, Kokomo, IN, Zip 46901–4197, Mailing Address: P.O. Box 9010, Zip 46904–9010; tel. 765/452–5611; Kathlene A. Young, M.S., FACHE, Interim President

ST. VINCENT CARMEL HOSPITAL, 13500 North Meridian Street, Carmel, IN, Zip 46032; tel. 317/582–7000; Michael D. Chittenden, President

ST. VINCENT CLAY HOSPITAL, 1206 East National Avenue, Brazil, IN, Zip 47834–2797, Mailing Address: P.O. Box 489, Zip 47834–0489; tel. 812/442–2500; Jerry Laue, Administrator

ST. VINCENT FRANKFORT HOSPITAL, 1300 South Jackson Street, Frankfort, IN, Zip 46041–3394, Mailing Address: P.O. Box 669, Zip 46041–0669; tel. 765/656–3000; Thomas Crawford, Chief Executive Officer

ST. VINCENT INDIANAPOLIS HOSPITAL, 2001 West 86th Street, Indianapolis, IN, Zip 46260–1991, Mailing Address: P.O. Box 40970, Zip 46240–0970; tel. 317/338–2345; Kyle De Fur, FACHE, President

ST. VINCENT JENNINGS HOSPITAL, 301 Henry Street, North Vernon, IN, Zip 47265–1097; tel. 812/352–4200; Joseph E. Roche, Administrator

ST. VINCENT MERCY HOSPITAL, 1331 South A Street, Elwood, IN, Zip 46036–1942; tel. 765/552–4600; Deborah Y. Rasper, FACHE, Administrator

ST. VINCENT RANDOLPH HOSPITAL, 473 Greenville Avenue, Winchester, IN, Zip 47394–2235, Mailing Address: P.O. Box 407, Zip 47394–0407; tel. 765/584–0004; Francis G. Albarano, Administrator

ST. VINCENT WILLIAMSPORT HOSPITAL, 412 North Monroe Street, Williamsport, IN, Zip 47993–0215; tel. 765/762–4000; Jane Craigin, Chief Executive Officer

SUBURBAN HEALTH ORGANIZATION
2780 Waterfront Parkway, East Drive, Suite 300, Indianapolis, IN 46214; tel. 317/692–5222; Julie M. Carmichael, President

HANCOCK REGIONAL HOSPITAL, 801 North State Street, Greenfield, IN, Zip 46140–1270, Mailing Address: P.O. Box 827, Zip 46140–0827; tel. 317/462–5544; Robert C. Keen, Ph.D., FACHE, President and Chief Executive Officer

HENDRICKS REGIONAL HEALTH, 1000 East Main Street, Danville, IN, Zip 46122–0409, Mailing Address: P.O. Box 409, Zip 46122–0409; tel. 317/745–4451; Dennis W. Dawes, FACHE, President

HENRY COUNTY HOSPITAL, 1000 North 16th Street, New Castle, IN, Zip 47362–4319, Mailing Address: P.O. Box 490, Zip 47362–0490; tel. 765/521–0890; Blake A. Dye, President and Chief Executive Officer

MORGAN HOSPITAL AND MEDICAL CENTER, 2209 John R. Wooden Drive, Martinsville, IN, Zip 46151–1840, Mailing Address: P.O. Box 1717, Zip 46151–1717; tel. 765/342–8441; Thomas W. Laux, President and Chief Executive Officer

RIVERVIEW HOSPITAL, 395 Westfield Road, Noblesville, IN, Zip 46060–1425, Mailing Address: P.O. Box 220, Zip 46061–0220; tel. 317/773–0760; Patricia K. Fox, President and Chief Executive Officer

WESTVIEW HOSPITAL, 3630 Guion Road, Indianapolis, IN, Zip 46222–1699; tel. 317/924–6661; Jerry L. Porter, Chief Executive Officer

WITHAM MEMORIAL HOSPITAL, 2605 North Lebanon Street, Lebanon, IN, Zip 46052, Mailing Address: P.O. Box 1200, Zip 46052–3005; tel. 765/485–8000; Raymond V. Ingham, Ph.D., President and Chief Executive Officer

IOWA

GENESIS HEALTH SYSTEM
1227 East Rusholme Street, Davenport, IA 52803; tel. 563/421–1000; Douglas P. Cropper, Chief Executive Officer

GENESIS MEDICAL CENTER, DEWITT, 1118 11th Street, De Witt, IA, Zip 52742–1296; tel. 563/659–4200; Jeffrey M. Cooper, Vice President, DeWitt Operations

GENESIS MEDICAL CENTER, ILLINI CAMPUS, 801 Illini Drive, Silvis, IL, Zip 61282–1893; tel. 309/792–9363; Charles E. Bruhn, Administrator

GENESIS MEDICAL CENTER–DAVENPORT, 1227 East Rusholme Street, Davenport, IA, Zip 52803–2498; tel. 563/421–1000; Douglas P. Cropper, Chief Executive Officer

MERCY HEALTH NETWORK – NORTH IOWA
1000 4th Street, Southwest, Mason City, IA 50401; tel. 641/422–7000; James FitzPatrick, President and Chief Executive Officer

BELMOND MEDICAL CENTER, 403 First Street S.E., Belmond, IA, Zip 50421–1201; tel. 641/444–3223; Nancy Gabrielson, Administrator

ELLSWORTH MUNICIPAL HOSPITAL, 110 Rocksylvania Avenue, Iowa Falls, IA, Zip 50126–2400; tel. 641/648–4631; John O'Brien, Administrator

FRANKLIN GENERAL HOSPITAL, 1720 Central Avenue East, Hampton, IA, Zip 50441–1859; tel. 641/456–5000; Mark Klosterman, Chief Executive Officer

HANCOCK COUNTY MEMORIAL HOSPITAL, 532 First Street N.W., Britt, IA, Zip 50423; tel. 641/843–5000; Vance Jackson, FACHE, Administrator and Chief Executive Officer

KOSSUTH REGIONAL HEALTH CENTER, 1515 South Phillips Street, Algona, IA, Zip 50511–3649; tel. 515/295–2451; Scott A. Curtis, Administrator and Chief Executive Officer

MERCY MEDICAL CENTER–NEW HAMPTON, 308 North Maple Avenue, New Hampton, IA, Zip 50659–1142; tel. 641/394–4121; Bruce Roesler, Chief Executive Officer

MERCY MEDICAL CENTER–NORTH IOWA, 1000 Fourth Street S.W., Mason City, IA, Zip 50401–2800; tel. 641/422–7000; James G. FitzPatrick, President and Chief Executive Officer

MITCHELL COUNTY REGIONAL HEALTH CENTER, 616 North Eighth Street, Osage, IA, Zip 50461–1498; tel. 641/732–6000; Sandy Leggett, Chief Executive Officer

PALO ALTO COUNTY HEALTH SYSTEM, 3201 First Street, Emmetsburg, IA, Zip 50536; tel. 712/852–5500; Thomas J. Lee, Chief Executive Officer

REGIONAL HEALTH SERVICES OF HOWARD COUNTY, 235 Eighth Avenue West, Cresco, IA, Zip 52136–1098; tel. 563/547–2101; David Hartberg, Chief Executive Officer

MERCY NETWORK
400 University, Des Moines, IA 50309; tel. 515/247–3121; Sara Drobnick, Vice President

ADAIR COUNTY MEMORIAL HOSPITAL, 609 S.E. Kent Street, Greenfield, IA, Zip 50849–9454; tel. 641/743–2123; Myrna Erb-Gundel, Administrator

AUDUBON COUNTY MEMORIAL HOSPITAL, 515 Pacific Street, Audubon, IA, Zip 50025–1052; tel. 712/563–2611; Thomas G. Smith, Administrator and Chief Executive Officer

DAVIS COUNTY HOSPITAL, 507 North Madison Street, Bloomfield, IA, Zip 52537–1271; tel. 641/664–2145; Deborah Herzberg, RN, M.S., CHE, Chief Executive Officer

HAMILTON HOSPITAL, 800 Ohio Street, Webster City, IA, Zip 50595–2824, Mailing Address: P.O. Box 430, Zip 50595–0430; tel. 515/832–9400; Palmer Schneider, Administrator

MADISON COUNTY HEALTHCARE SYSTEM, 300 Hutchings Street, Winterset, IA, Zip 50273–2199; tel. 515/462–2373; Marcia Harris, Chief Executive Officer

MANNING REGIONAL HEALTHCARE CENTER, 410 Main Street, Manning, IA, Zip 51455–1093; tel. 712/655–2072; Darrell E. Vondrak, Interim Chief Executive Officer

MERCY MEDICAL CENTER–CENTERVILLE, 1 St. Joseph's Drive, Centerville, IA, Zip 52544–8055; tel. 641/437–4111; Clinton J. Christianson, President and Chief Executive Officer

MERCY MEDICAL CENTER–DES MOINES, 1111 6th Avenue, Des Moines, IA, Zip 50314–2611; tel. 515/247–3121; David H. Vellinga, FACHE, President and Chief Executive Officer

MONROE COUNTY HOSPITAL, 1901 South Alabama Avenue, Monroeville, AL, Zip 36460, Mailing Address: P.O. Box 886, Zip 36461–0886; tel. 251/575–3111; Vincent B. DiFranco, Chief Executive Officer

RINGGOLD COUNTY HOSPITAL, 211 Shellway Drive, Mount Ayr, IA, Zip 50854–1299; tel. 641/464–3226; Gordon W. Winkler, Administrator

ST. ANTHONY REGIONAL HOSPITAL, 311 South Clark Street, Carroll, IA, Zip 51401–3038, Mailing Address: P.O. Box 628, Zip 51401–0628; tel. 712/792–3581; Gary P. Riedmann, FACHE, President and Chief Executive Officer

STORY COUNTY MEDICAL CENTER, 630 Sixth Street, Nevada, IA, Zip 50201–2266; tel. 515/382–2111; Todd Willert, Administrator

WAYNE COUNTY HOSPITAL, 417 South East Street, Corydon, IA, Zip 50060–1860, Mailing Address: P.O. Box 305, Zip 50060–0305; tel. 641/872–2260; Brian D. Burnside, Chief Executive Officer

KANSAS

GREAT PLAINS HEALTH ALLIANCE
P.O. Box 366, Phillipsberg, KS 67661; tel. 800/432–2779; Roger John, President

SATANTA DISTRICT HOSPITAL, 401 South Cheyenne Street, Satanta, KS, Zip 67870–0159, Mailing Address: P.O. Box 159, Zip 67870–0159; tel. 620/649–2761; Curt Colson, Administrator

HEALTH INNOVATIONS NETWORK OF KANSAS
1500 S. W. 10th Avenue, Topeka, KS 66604; tel. 785/354–6137; Kristi Grosser, Network Operations Director

CLAY COUNTY MEDICAL CENTER, 617 Liberty Street, Clay Center, KS, Zip 67432–0512, Mailing Address: P.O. Box 512, Zip 67432–0512; tel. 785/632–2144; Ron Bender, Chief Executive Officer

COFFEY COUNTY HOSPITAL, 801 North Fourth Street, Burlington, KS, Zip 66839–0189, Mailing Address: P.O. Box 189, Zip 66839–0189; tel. 620/364–2121; Dennis L. George, Chief Executive Officer

COMMUNITY HEALTH CARE SYSTEM, 120 West Eighth Street, Onaga, KS, Zip 66521–0120; tel. 785/889–4272; Greg Unruh, Chief Executive Officer

COMMUNITY MEMORIAL HEALTHCARE, 708 North 18th Street, Marysville, KS, Zip 66508–1338; tel. 785/562–2311; Curtis R. Hawkinson, Chief Executive Officer

GEARY COMMUNITY HOSPITAL, 1102 St. Mary's Road, Junction City, KS, Zip 66441–4196, Mailing Address: P.O. Box 490, Zip 66441–0490; tel. 785/238–1204; David K. Bradley, FACHE, Chief Executive Officer

HERINGTON MUNICIPAL HOSPITAL, 100 East Helen Street, Herington, KS, Zip 67449–1606; tel. 785/258–2207; Richard Q. Bergling, Chief Executive Officer

HIAWATHA COMMUNITY HOSPITAL, 300 Utah Street, Hiawatha, KS, Zip 66434–2314; tel. 785/742–2131; John Moore, Administrator

HOLTON COMMUNITY HOSPITAL, 1110 Columbine Drive, Holton, KS, Zip 66436–1545; tel. 785/364–2116; Ron Marshall, Interim Chief Executive Officer

HORTON COMMUNITY HOSPITAL, 240 West 18th Street, Horton, KS, Zip 66439–1245; tel. 785/486–2642; Dale A. White, Chief Executive Officer

JEFFERSON COUNTY MEMORIAL HOSPITAL, 408 Delaware Street, Winchester, KS, Zip 66097–4003; tel. 913/774–4340; LaMont Cook, Administrator

KANSAS REHABILITATION HOSPITAL, 1504 S.W. Eighth Avenue, Topeka, KS, Zip 66606–1632; tel. 785/235–6600; Paul Livingston, Chief Executive Officer

MORRIS COUNTY HOSPITAL, 600 North Washington Street, Council Grove, KS, Zip 66846–0275, Mailing Address: P.O. Box 275, Zip 66846–0275; tel. 620/767–6811; James H. Reagan, Jr., Ph.D., Chief Executive Officer

NEMAHA VALLEY COMMUNITY HOSPITAL, 1600 Community Drive, Seneca, KS, Zip 66538–9739; tel. 785/336–6181; Stan Regehr, President and Chief Executive Officer

SABETHA COMMUNITY HOSPITAL, 14th and Oregon Streets, Sabetha, KS, Zip 66534–0229, Mailing Address: P.O. Box 229, Zip 66534–0229; tel. 785/284–2121; Lora Key, Chief Executive Officer

STORMONT–VAIL HEALTHCARE, 1500 S.W. Tenth Avenue, Topeka, KS, Zip 66604–1353; tel. 785/354–6000; Maynard F. Oliverius, President and Chief Executive Officer

WASHINGTON COUNTY HOSPITAL, 304 East Third Street, Washington, KS, Zip 66968–2033; tel. 785/325–2211; Everett Lutjemeier, Administrator

HUGHES MEDICAL CENTER
2220 Canterbury Drive, Hays, KS 67601; tel. 785/623–2300; Jodi A. Schmidt, Vice President and Chief Development Officer

CHEYENNE COUNTY HOSPITAL, 210 West First Street, Saint Francis, KS, Zip 67756–0547, Mailing Address: P.O. Box 547, Zip 67756–0547; tel. 785/332–2104; Leslie Lacy, Administrator

CITIZENS MEDICAL CENTER, 100 East College Drive, Colby, KS, Zip 67701–3799; tel. 785/462–7511; Janice McCart, Chief Executive Officer

CLARA BARTON HOSPITAL, 250 West Ninth Street, Hoisington, KS, Zip 67544–1706; tel. 620/653–2114; W. Charles Waters, President and Chief Executive Officer

EDWARDS COUNTY HOSPITAL AND HEALTHCARE CENTER, 620 West Eighth Street, Kinsley, KS, Zip 67547–2329, Mailing Address: P.O. Box 99, Zip 67547–0099; tel. 620/659–3621; Ann Zielinski, Chief Executive Officer

GOVE COUNTY MEDICAL CENTER, 520 West Fifth Street, Quinter, KS, Zip 67752–0129, Mailing Address: P.O. Box 129, Zip 67752–0129; tel. 785/754–3341; Paul Davis, Administrator

GRAHAM COUNTY HOSPITAL, 304 West Prout Street, Hill City, KS, Zip 67642–1435, Mailing Address: P.O. Box 339, Zip 67642–0339; tel. 785/421–2121; Shaun Keef, Administrator and Chief Executive Officer

GRISELL MEMORIAL HOSPITAL DISTRICT ONE, 210 South Vermont Avenue, Ransom, KS, Zip 67572; tel. 785/731–2231; Kristine Ochs, RN, Administrator

HARLAN COUNTY HEALTH SYSTEM, 717 North Brown Street, Alma, NE, Zip 68920–0836, Mailing Address: P.O. Box 836, Zip 68920–0836; tel. 308/928–2151; Allen Van Driel, CHE, Administrator

LANE COUNTY HOSPITAL, 235 West Vine, Dighton, KS, Zip 67839–0969, Mailing Address: P.O. Box 969, Zip 67839–0969; tel. 620/397–5321; Donna McGowan, Administrator

LOGAN COUNTY HOSPITAL, 211 Cherry Street, Oakley, KS, Zip 67748–1201; tel. 785/672–3211; Scott Buck, Administrator

MINNEOLA DISTRICT HOSPITAL, 212 Main Street, Minneola, KS, Zip 67865–0127, Mailing Address: P.O. Box 127, Zip 67865–0127; tel. 620/885–4264; Cynthia K. Schneider, Interim Administrator and Chief Executive Officer

NESS COUNTY HOSPITAL, 312 Custer Street, Ness City, KS, Zip 67560–1654; tel. 785/798–2291; Kyle Hahn, Administrator

NORTON COUNTY HOSPITAL, 102 East Holme, Norton, KS, Zip 67654–0250, Mailing Address: P.O. Box 250, Zip 67654–0250; tel. 785/877–3351; Richard Miller, Administrator and Chief Executive Officer

PHILLIPS COUNTY HOSPITAL, 1150 State Street, Phillipsburg, KS, Zip 67661–1799, Mailing Address: P.O. Box 607, Zip 67661–0607; tel. 785/543–5226; Heather L. Harper, Administrator

RAWLINS COUNTY HEALTH CENTER, 707 Grant Street, Atwood, KS, Zip 67730–4700, Mailing Address: P.O. Box 47, Zip 67730–4700; tel. 785/626–3211; Deanna Freeman, Administrator and Chief Executive Officer

ROOKS COUNTY HEALTH CENTER, 304 South Colorado Avenue, Plainville, KS, Zip 67663–0389; tel. 785/434–4553; Julie Price, Chief Executive Officer and Chief Financial Officer

RUSH COUNTY MEMORIAL HOSPITAL, 801 Locust Street, La Crosse, KS, Zip 67548–9673, Mailing Address: P.O. Box 520, Zip 67548–0520; tel. 785/222–2545; George Stover, Administrator and Chief Executive Officer

RUSSELL REGIONAL HOSPITAL, 200 South Main Street, Russell, KS, Zip 67665–2997; tel. 785/483–3131; Shelley Boden, Administrator and Chief Executive Officer

SCOTT COUNTY HOSPITAL, 310 East Third Street, Scott City, KS, Zip 67871–1203; tel. 620/872–5811; Mark Burnett, President and Chief Executive Officer

SHERIDAN COUNTY HEALTH COMPLEX, 826 18th Street, Hoxie, KS, Zip 67740–0167, Mailing Address: P.O. Box 167, Zip 67740–0167; tel. 785/675–3281; Joe Stratton, Chief Executive Officer

SMITH COUNTY MEMORIAL HOSPITAL, 614 South Main Street, Smith Center, KS, Zip 66967–0349, Mailing Address: P.O. Box 349, Zip 66967–0349; tel. 785/282–6845; Carolyn K. Hess, RN, Administrator

TREGO COUNTY–LEMKE MEMORIAL HOSPITAL, 320 North 13th Street, Wakeeney, KS, Zip 67672–2099; tel. 785/743–2182; Jean Dean, Administrator

WAMEGO CITY HOSPITAL, 711 Genn Drive, Wamego, KS, Zip 66547–1179; tel. 785/456–2295; John R. Broberg, Interim Chief Executive Officer

MED–OP, INC.
205 E. 7th Street, Hays, KS 67601; tel. 785/621–4510; David Britain, Executive Director

CITIZENS MEDICAL CENTER, 100 East College Drive, Colby, KS, Zip 67701–3799; tel. 785/462–7511; Janice McCart, Chief Executive Officer

CLARA BARTON HOSPITAL, 250 West Ninth Street, Hoisington, KS, Zip 67544–1706; tel. 620/653–2114; W. Charles Waters, President and Chief Executive Officer

DECATUR COUNTY HOSPITAL AND CEDAR LIVING CENTER, 810 West Columbia Street, Oberlin, KS, Zip 67749–2450, Mailing Address: P.O. Box 268, Zip 67749–0268; tel. 785/475–2208; Lynn Doeden, Chief Executive Officer

EDWARDS COUNTY HOSPITAL AND HEALTHCARE CENTER, 620 West Eighth Street, Kinsley, KS, Zip 67547–2329, Mailing Address: P.O. Box 99, Zip 67547–0099; tel. 620/659–3621; Ann Zielinski, Chief Executive Officer

GOODLAND REGIONAL MEDICAL CENTER, 220 West Second Street, Goodland, KS, Zip 67735–1602; tel. 785/890–3625; Jay P. Jolly, Chief Executive Officer

GOVE COUNTY MEDICAL CENTER, 520 West Fifth Street, Quinter, KS, Zip 67752–0129, Mailing Address: P.O. Box 129, Zip 67752–0129; tel. 785/754–3341; Paul Davis, Administrator

GRAHAM COUNTY HOSPITAL, 304 West Prout Street, Hill City, KS, Zip 67642–1435, Mailing Address: P.O. Box 339, Zip 67642–0339; tel. 785/421–2121; Shaun Keef, Administrator and Chief Executive Officer

HAYS MEDICAL CENTER, 2220 Canterbury Drive, Hays, KS, Zip 67601–2342, Mailing Address: P.O. Box 8100, Zip 67601–8100; tel. 785/623–5000; John H. Jeter, M.D., President and Chief Executive Officer

HOSPITAL DISTRICT NUMBER ONE OF RICE COUNTY, 619 South Clark Street, Lyons, KS, Zip 67554–0828, Mailing Address: P.O. Box 828, Zip 67554–0828; tel. 620/257–5173; Robert L. Mullen, Chief Executive Officer

LOGAN COUNTY HOSPITAL, 211 Cherry Street, Oakley, KS, Zip 67748–1201; tel. 785/672–3211; Scott Buck, Administrator

NESS COUNTY HOSPITAL, 312 Custer Street, Ness City, KS, Zip 67560–1654; tel. 785/798–2291; Kyle Hahn, Administrator

NORTON COUNTY HOSPITAL, 102 East Holme, Norton, KS, Zip 67654–0250, Mailing Address: P.O. Box 250, Zip 67654–0250; tel. 785/877–3351; Richard Miller, Administrator and Chief Executive Officer

ROOKS COUNTY HEALTH CENTER, 304 South Colorado Avenue, Plainville, KS, Zip 67663–0389; tel. 785/434–4553; Julie Price, Chief Executive Officer and Chief Financial Officer

RUSH COUNTY MEMORIAL HOSPITAL, 801 Locust Street, La Crosse, KS, Zip 67548–9673, Mailing Address: P.O. Box 520, Zip 67548–0520; tel. 785/222–2545; George Stover, Administrator and Chief Executive Officer

RUSSELL REGIONAL HOSPITAL, 200 South Main Street, Russell, KS, Zip 67665–2997; tel. 785/483–3131; Shelley Boden, Administrator and Chief Executive Officer

SCOTT COUNTY HOSPITAL, 310 East Third Street, Scott City, KS, Zip 67871–1203; tel. 620/872–5811; Mark Burnett, President and Chief Executive Officer

SHERIDAN COUNTY HEALTH COMPLEX, 826 18th Street, Hoxie, KS, Zip 67740–0167, Mailing Address: P.O. Box 167, Zip 67740–0167; tel. 785/675–3281; Joe Stratton, Chief Executive Officer

STAFFORD DISTRICT HOSPITAL, 502 South Buckeye Street, Stafford, KS, Zip 67578–2035, Mailing Address: P.O. Box 190, Zip 67578–0190; tel. 620/234–5221; Vernon Minnis, Administrator and Chief Executive Officer

MID-KANSAS HEALTH NETWORK
3515 Broadway, Great Bend, KS 67530; tel. 620/792–2511; Charlene Koochel, Executive Assistant

CENTRAL KANSAS MEDICAL CENTER, 3515 Broadway Street, Great Bend, KS, Zip 67530–3633; tel. 620/792–2511; Sharon Lind, President and Chief Executive Officer

ELLINWOOD DISTRICT HOSPITAL, 605 North Main Street, Ellinwood, KS, Zip 67526–1440; tel. 620/564–2548; Joyce Schulte, Chief Executive Officer

NESS COUNTY HOSPITAL, 312 Custer Street, Ness City, KS, Zip 67560–1654; tel. 785/798–2291; Kyle Hahn, Administrator

ST. JOSEPH MEMORIAL HOSPITAL, 923 Carroll Avenue, Larned, KS, Zip 67550; tel. 620/285–3161; Teri Thomas, Administrator

NEK CENTER FOR HEALTH & WELLNESS
240 West 18th Street, Horton, KS 66439; tel. 785/486–2642; Dale White, Chief Executive Officer

COMMUNITY HEALTH CARE SYSTEM, 120 West Eighth Street, Onaga, KS, Zip 66521–0120; tel. 785/889–4272; Greg Unruh, Chief Executive Officer

COMMUNITY MEMORIAL HEALTHCARE, 708 North 18th Street, Marysville, KS, Zip 66508–1338; tel. 785/562–2311; Curtis R. Hawkinson, Chief Executive Officer

GEARY COMMUNITY HOSPITAL, 1102 St. Mary's Road, Junction City, KS, Zip 66441–4196, Mailing Address: P.O. Box 490, Zip 66441–0490; tel. 785/238–1204; David K. Bradley, FACHE, Chief Executive Officer

HOLTON COMMUNITY HOSPITAL, 1110 Columbine Drive, Holton, KS, Zip 66436–1545; tel. 785/364–2116; Ron Marshall, Interim Chief Executive Officer

HORTON COMMUNITY HOSPITAL, 240 West 18th Street, Horton, KS, Zip 66439–1245; tel. 785/486–2642; Dale A. White, Chief Executive Officer

MERCY REGIONAL HEALTH CENTER, 1823 College Avenue, Manhattan, KS, Zip 66502, Mailing Address: P.O. Box 1289, Zip 66505–1289; tel. 785/776–3322; Richard L. Allen, President and Chief Executive Officer

MORRIS COUNTY HOSPITAL, 600 North Washington Street, Council Grove, KS, Zip 66846–0275, Mailing Address: P.O. Box 275, Zip 66846–0275; tel. 620/767–6811; James H. Reagan, Jr., Ph.D., Chief Executive Officer

NEMAHA VALLEY COMMUNITY HOSPITAL, 1600 Community Drive, Seneca, KS, Zip 66538–9739; tel. 785/336–6181; Stan Regehr, President and Chief Executive Officer

ST. FRANCIS HEALTH CENTER, 1700 West Seventh Street, Topeka, KS, Zip 66606–1690; tel. 785/295–8000; Michael E. Schrader, President and Chief Executive Officer

WAMEGO CITY HOSPITAL, 711 Genn Drive, Wamego, KS, Zip 66547–1179; tel. 785/456–2295; John R. Broberg, Interim Chief Executive Officer

PIONEER HEALTH NETWORK, INC.
P.O. Box 1787, Garden City, KS 67846; tel. 620/276–7700; Jason Friesen, Executive Director

ASHLAND HEALTH CENTER, 709 Oak Street, Ashland, KS, Zip 67831–0188, Mailing Address: P.O. Box 188, Zip 67831–0188; tel. 620/635–2241; Daryl Marshall, Administrator

BOB WILSON MEMORIAL GRANT COUNTY HOSPITAL, 415 North Main Street, Ulysses, KS, Zip 67880–2133; tel. 620/356–1266; Robert B. Ohlen, Chief Executive Officer

GREELEY COUNTY HEALTH SERVICES, 506 Third Street, Tribune, KS, Zip 67879–0338, Mailing Address: P.O. Box 338, Zip 67879–0338; tel. 620/376–4221; Todd Burch, Administrator and Chief Executive Officer

HAMILTON COUNTY HOSPITAL, East Avenue G and Huser Street, Syracuse, KS, Zip 67878–0948, Mailing Address: P.O. Box 948, Zip 67878–0948; tel. 620/384–7461; Todd Burch, Administrator and Chief Executive Officer

HODGEMAN COUNTY HEALTH CENTER, 809 Bramley Street, Jetmore, KS, Zip 67854–9320, Mailing Address: P.O. Box 310, Zip 67854–0310; tel. 620/357–8361; Phillip W. Lowe, Chief Executive Officer

KEARNY COUNTY HOSPITAL, 500 Thorpe Street, Lakin, KS, Zip 67860; tel. 620/355–7111; John Loebl, Chief Executive Officer

LANE COUNTY HOSPITAL, 235 West Vine, Dighton, KS, Zip 67839–0969, Mailing Address: P.O. Box 969, Zip 67839–0969; tel. 620/397–5321; Donna McGowan, Administrator

MEADE DISTRICT HOSPITAL, 510 East Carthage Street, Meade, KS, Zip 67864–0820, Mailing Address: P.O. Box 820, Zip 67864–0820; tel. 620/873–2141; Michael P. Thomas, Administrator

MORTON COUNTY HEALTH SYSTEM, 445 Hilltop Street, Elkhart, KS, Zip 67950–0937, Mailing Address: P.O. Box 937, Zip 67950–0937; tel. 620/697–2141; Leonard Hernandez, Chief Executive Officer

SATANTA DISTRICT HOSPITAL, 401 South Cheyenne Street, Satanta, KS, Zip 67870–0159, Mailing Address: P.O. Box 159, Zip 67870–0159; tel. 620/649–2761; Curt Colson, Administrator

SCOTT COUNTY HOSPITAL, 310 East Third Street, Scott City, KS, Zip 67871–1203; tel. 620/872–5811; Mark Burnett, President and Chief Executive Officer

SOUTHWEST MEDICAL CENTER, 315 West 15th Street, Liberal, KS, Zip 67901–1340, Mailing Address: Box 1340, Zip 67905–1340; tel. 620/624–1651; Norman Lambert, Chief Executive Officer

ST. CATHERINE HOSPITAL, 401 East Spuce Street, Garden City, KS, Zip 67846–5679; tel. 620/272–2561; Scott J. Taylor, President and Chief Executive Officer

STANTON COUNTY HEALTH CARE FACILITY, 404 North Chestnut Street, Johnson, KS, Zip 67855–0779, Mailing Address: P.O. Box 779, Zip 67855–0779; tel. 620/492–6250; Shae Veach, Administrator

STEVENS COUNTY HOSPITAL, 1006 South Jackson Street, Hugoton, KS, Zip 67951–2842, Mailing Address: P.O. Box 10, Zip 67951–0010; tel. 620/544–8511; Linda Stalcup, Chief Executive Officer

WICHITA COUNTY HEALTH CENTER, 211 East Earl Street, Leoti, KS, Zip 67861–9620; tel. 620/375–2233; Victoria J. Hahn, Administrator and Chief Executive Officer

SUNFLOWER HEALTH NETWORK
139 North Penn, Salina, KS 67401; tel. 785/452–6102; Heather Fuller, Executive Director

CLAY COUNTY MEDICAL CENTER, 617 Liberty Street, Clay Center, KS, Zip 67432–0512, Mailing Address: P.O. Box 512, Zip 67432–0512; tel. 785/632–2144; Ron Bender, Chief Executive Officer

CLOUD COUNTY HEALTH CENTER, 1100 Highland Drive, Concordia, KS, Zip 66901–3923; tel. 785/243–1234; James E. Wahlmeier, President and Chief Executive Officer

ELLSWORTH COUNTY MEDICAL CENTER, 1604 Aylward Street, Ellsworth, KS, Zip 67439–0087, Mailing Address: P.O. Box 87, Zip 67439–0087; tel. 785/472–3111; Roger W. Pearson, Administrator

HERINGTON MUNICIPAL HOSPITAL, 100 East Helen Street, Herington, KS, Zip 67449–1606; tel. 785/258–2207; Richard Q. Bergling, Chief Executive Officer

HILLSBORO COMMUNITY MEDICAL CENTER, 701 South Main Street, Hillsboro, KS, Zip 67063–1595; tel. 620/947–3114; Michael J. Ryan, Chief Executive Officer

JEWELL COUNTY HOSPITAL, 100 Crestvue Avenue, Mankato, KS, Zip 66956–2407, Mailing Address: P.O. Box 327, Zip 66956–0327; tel. 785/378–3137; Doyle McKimmy, Administrator

LINCOLN COUNTY HOSPITAL, 624 North Second Street, Lincoln, KS, Zip 67455–1738, Mailing Address: P.O. Box 406, Zip 67455–0406; tel. 785/524–4403; Greg R. McNeil, Chief Executive Officer

LINDSBORG COMMUNITY HOSPITAL, 605 West Lincoln Street, Lindsborg, KS, Zip 67456–2328; tel. 785/227–3308; Larry VanDer Wege, Administrator and Chief Executive Officer

MEMORIAL HEALTH SYSTEM, 511 N.E. Tenth Street, Abilene, KS, Zip 67410; tel. 785/263–2100; Mark A. Miller, Chief Executive Officer

MEMORIAL HOSPITAL, 1000 Hospital Drive, McPherson, KS, Zip 67460–2321; tel. 620/241–2250; James R. Chromik, Interim Administrator

MITCHELL COUNTY HOSPITAL HEALTH SYSTEMS, 400 West Eighth, Beloit, KS, Zip 67420–1605, Mailing Address: P.O. Box 399, Zip 67420–0399; tel. 785/738–2266; David Dick, Chief Executive Officer

OSBORNE COUNTY MEMORIAL HOSPITAL, 424 West New Hampshire Street, Osborne, KS, Zip 67473–0070, Mailing Address: P.O. Box 70, Zip 67473–0070; tel. 785/346–2121; Kiley Floyd, Administrator

OTTAWA COUNTY HEALTH CENTER, 215 East Eighth, Minneapolis, KS, Zip 67467–1999, Mailing Address: P.O. Box 290, Zip 67467–0290; tel. 785/392–2122; Joy Johnson, RN, Administrator

REPUBLIC COUNTY HOSPITAL, 2420 G Street, Belleville, KS, Zip 66935–2400; tel. 785/527–2254; Blaine K. Miller, Administrator

SALINA REGIONAL HEALTH CENTER, 400 South Santa Fe Avenue, Salina, KS, Zip 67401–4198, Mailing Address: P.O. Box 5080, Zip 67401–5080; tel. 785/452–7000; Micheal Terry, President and Chief Executive Officer

SMITH COUNTY MEMORIAL HOSPITAL, 614 South Main Street, Smith Center, KS, Zip 66967–0349, Mailing Address: P.O. Box 349, Zip 66967–0349; tel. 785/282–6845; Carolyn K. Hess, RN, Administrator

KENTUCKY

COMMONWEALTH HEALTH CORPORATION
800 Park Street, Bowling Green, KY 42101; tel. 270/745–1500; John Desmarais, President and Chief Executive Officer

MEDICAL CENTER AT SCOTTSVILLE, 456 Burnley Road, Scottsville, KY, Zip 42164–6355; tel. 270/622–2800; Eric Hagan, RN, Vice President and Administrator

THE MEDICAL CENTER AT BOWLING GREEN, 250 Park Street, Bowling Green, KY, Zip 42101–1795, Mailing Address: P.O. Box 90010, Zip 42102–9010; tel. 270/745–1000; Connie Smith, Chief Executive Officer

THE MEDICAL CENTER AT FRANKLIN, 1100 Brookhaven Road, Franklin, KY, Zip 42134–2746; tel. 270/598–4800; Clara M. Sumner, Chief Executive Officer

COMMUNITY CARE NETWORK
110 A. Second Street, Henderson, KY 42420; tel. 502/827–7380; Elizabeth Johnson, Director of Marketing

Section B

CALDWELL COUNTY HOSPITAL, 101 Hospital Drive, Princeton, KY, Zip 42445–0410; tel. 270/365–0300; Charles D. Lovell, Jr., President and Chief Executive Officer

CRITTENDEN COUNTY HOSPITAL, 520 West Gum Street, Marion, KY, Zip 42064–6201, Mailing Address: P.O. Box 386, Zip 42064–0386; tel. 270/965–5281; Jim Christensen, Chief Executive Officer

JENNIE STUART MEDICAL CENTER, 320 West 18th Street, Hopkinsville, KY, Zip 42241–2400, Mailing Address: P.O. Box 2400, Zip 42241–2400; tel. 270/887–0100; Terry Peeples, Chief Executive Officer

LIVINGSTON HOSPITAL AND HEALTHCARE SERVICES, 131 Hospital Drive, Salem, KY, Zip 42078–8043; tel. 270/988–2299; Michael J. Budnick, FACHE, Chief Executive Officer

METHODIST HOSPITAL, 1305 North Elm Street, Henderson, KY, Zip 42420–2775, Mailing Address: P.O. Box 48, Zip 42420–0048; tel. 270/827–7700; Bruce D. Begley, Executive Director

METHODIST HOSPITAL UNION COUNTY, 4604 Highway 60 West, Morganfield, KY, Zip 42437–9570; tel. 270/389–5000; Patrick Donahue, Administrator

MURRAY–CALLOWAY COUNTY HOSPITAL, 803 Poplar Street, Murray, KY, Zip 42071–2432; tel. 270/762–1100; Keith E. Bailey, Chief Executive Officer

REGIONAL MEDICAL CENTER OF HOPKINS COUNTY, 900 Hospital Drive, Madisonville, KY, Zip 42431–1694; tel. 270/825–5100; E. Berton Whitaker, Chief Executive Officer

STS. MARY & ELIZABETH HOSPITAL, 1850 Bluegrass Avenue, Louisville, KY, Zip 40215–1199; tel. 502/361–6000; Thomas Gessel, Chief Executive Officer

THE MEDICAL CENTER AT FRANKLIN, 1100 Brookhaven Road, Franklin, KY, Zip 42134–2746; tel. 270/598–4800; Clara M. Sumner, Chief Executive Officer

ST. ELIZABETH MEDICAL CENTER
1 Medical Village Drive, Edgewood, KY 41017; tel. 859/301–2000; Joseph W. Gross, President

ST. ELIZABETH MEDICAL CENTER–GRANT COUNTY, 238 Barnes Road, Williamstown, KY, Zip 41097–9460; tel. 859/824–8240; Chris Carle, Administrator

ST. ELIZABETH MEDICAL CENTER–SOUTH, 1 Medical Village Drive, Covington, KY, Zip 41017–3403; tel. 859/301–2000; Joseph W. Gross, FACHE, President and Chief Executive Officer

MAINE

BLUE HILL MEMORIAL HOSPITAL
P.O. Box 823, Blue Hill, ME 04614; tel. 207/374–3400; Timothy Gamity, FACHE, President and Chief Executive Officer

BLUE HILL MEMORIAL HOSPITAL, 57 Water Street, Blue Hill, ME, Zip 04614–0823, Mailing Address: P.O. Box 823, Zip 04614–0823; tel. 207/374–3400; Timothy Garrity, FACHE, President and Chief Executive Officer

MAINE NETWORK FOR HEALTH
Key Plaza, 23 Water Street, Bangor, ME 04401; tel. 207/942–2844; Stephen P. Ryan, President and Chief Executive Officer

ACADIA HOSPITAL, 268 Stillwater Avenue, Bangor, ME, Zip 04401–3945, Mailing Address: P.O. Box 422, Zip 04402–0422; tel. 207/973–6100; Dorothy E. Hill, Chief Executive Officer

AROOSTOOK MEDICAL CENTER, 140 Academy Street, Presque Isle, ME, Zip 04769–3171, Mailing Address: P.O. Box 151, Zip 04769–0151; tel. 207/768–4000; David A. Peterson, President and Chief Executive Officer

BLUE HILL MEMORIAL HOSPITAL, 57 Water Street, Blue Hill, ME, Zip 04614–0823, Mailing Address: P.O. Box 823, Zip 04614–0823; tel. 207/374–3400; Timothy Garrity, FACHE, President and Chief Executive Officer

CHARLES A. DEAN MEMORIAL HOSPITAL AND NURSING HOME, 364 Pritham Avenue, Greenville, ME, Zip 04441–1395, Mailing Address: P.O. Box 1129, Zip 04441–1129; tel. 207/695–5200; Geno Murray, President and Chief Executive Officer

EASTERN MAINE MEDICAL CENTER, 489 State Street, Bangor, ME, Zip 04401–6674, Mailing Address: P.O. Box 404, Zip 04402–0404; tel. 207/973–7000; Deborah Carey Johnson, RN, President and Chief Executive Officer

HOULTON REGIONAL HOSPITAL, 20 Hartford Street, Houlton, ME, Zip 04730–9998; tel. 207/532–9471; Thomas J. Moakler, Chief Executive Officer

INLAND HOSPITAL, 200 Kennedy Memorial Drive, Waterville, ME, Zip 04901–4595; tel. 207/861–3000; John Dalton, President and Chief Executive Officer

MILLINOCKET REGIONAL HOSPITAL, 200 Somerset Street, Millinocket, ME, Zip 04462–1298; tel. 207/723–5161; Marie E. Vienneau, RN, Chief Executive Officer

MOUNT DESERT ISLAND HOSPITAL, 10 Wayman Lane, Bar Harbor, ME, Zip 04609–0008, Mailing Address: P.O. Box 8, Zip 04609–0008; tel. 207/288–5081; Arthur J. Blank, President and Chief Executive Officer

NORTHERN MAINE MEDICAL CENTER, 194 East Main Street, Fort Kent, ME, Zip 04743–1497; tel. 207/834–3155; Martin B. Bernstein, Chief Executive Officer

SEBASTICOOK VALLEY HOSPITAL, 447 North Main Street, Pittsfield, ME, Zip 04967–1199; tel. 207/487–5141; John C. May, Chief Executive Officer

SYNERNET, INC.
222 St. John Street, Suite 329, Portland, ME 04102; tel. 207/771–3456; Gerald Vicenzi, President and Chief Executive Officer

FRANKLIN MEMORIAL HOSPITAL, 111 Franklin Health Commons, Farmington, ME, Zip 04938–9990; tel. 207/778–6031; Richard A. Batt, President and Chief Executive Officer

HENRIETTA D. GOODALL HOSPITAL, 25 June Street, Sanford, ME, Zip 04073–2645; tel. 207/324–4310; Darlene Stromstad, FACHE, Chief Executive Officer

MOUNT DESERT ISLAND HOSPITAL, 10 Wayman Lane, Bar Harbor, ME, Zip 04609–0008, Mailing Address: P.O. Box 8, Zip 04609–0008; tel. 207/288–5081; Arthur J. Blank, President and Chief Executive Officer

NORTHERN MAINE MEDICAL CENTER, 194 East Main Street, Fort Kent, ME, Zip 04743–1497; tel. 207/834–3155; Martin B. Bernstein, Chief Executive Officer

PENOBSCOT BAY MEDICAL CENTER, 6 Glen Cove Drive, Rockport, ME, Zip 04856–4240; tel. 207/596–8000; Roy A. Hitchings, Jr., FACHE, President and Chief Executive Officer

REDINGTON–FAIRVIEW GENERAL HOSPITAL, Fairview Avenue, Skowhegan, ME, Zip 4976, Mailing Address: P.O. Box 468, Zip 04976–0468; tel. 207/474–5121; Richard Willett, Chief Executive Officer

ST. JOSEPH HOSPITAL, 360 Broadway, Bangor, ME, Zip 04401–3897, Mailing Address: P.O. Box 403, Zip 04402–0403; tel. 207/262–1000; Sister Mary Norberta Malinowski, President

MASSACHUSETTS

LAHEY CLINIC MEDICAL CENTER
41 Mall Road, Burlington, MA 01805; tel. 781/744–5796; David M. Barrett, M.D., President and Chief Executive Officer

LAHEY CLINIC HOSPITAL, 41 Mall Road, Burlington, MA, Zip 01805–0001; tel. 781/744–5100; David M. Barrett, M.D., Chief Executive Officer

NORTHEAST HEALTH SYSTEM
85 Herrick Street, Beverly, MA 01915; tel. 978/922–3000; Steven R. Laverty, President

ADDISON GILBERT HOSPITAL, 298 Washington Street, Gloucester, MA, Zip 01930–4887; tel. 978/283–4000

BEVERLY HOSPITAL, 85 Herrick Street, Beverly, MA, Zip 01915–1777; tel. 978/922–3000; Stephen R. Laverty, President and Chief Executive Officer

SISTERS OF PROVIDENCE HEALTH SYSTEM
271 Carew Street, Springfield, MA 01104; tel. 413/748–9000; Vincent McCorkle, President and Chief Executive Officer

MERCY MEDICAL CENTER, 271 Carew Street, Springfield, MA, Zip 01104–2398, Mailing Address: P.O. Box 9012, Zip 01102–9012; tel. 413/748–9000; Vincent J. McCorkle, CHE, President and Chief Executive Officer

MICHIGAN

GENESYS HEALTH SYSTEM
One Genesys Parkway, Grand Blanc, MI 48439; tel. 810/606–5000; Mark Taylor, President and Chief Executive Officer

GENESYS REGIONAL MEDICAL CENTER, One Genesys Parkway, Grand Blanc, MI, Zip 48439–8066; tel. 810/606–5000; Elizabeth Aderholdt, President

HOSPITAL NETWORK, INC.
6212 American Avenue, Portage, MI 49002; tel. 269/329–3200; Gregory Hedegore, President and Chief Executive Officer

ALLEGAN GENERAL HOSPITAL, 555 Linn Street, Allegan, MI, Zip 49010–1594; tel. 269/673–8424; Gerald J. Barbini, President and Chief Executive Officer

BRONSON METHODIST HOSPITAL, 601 John Street, Kalamazoo, MI, Zip 49007–5345; tel. 269/341–6000; Frank J. Sardone, President and Chief Executive Officer

OAKLAWN HOSPITAL, 200 North Madison Street, Marshall, MI, Zip 49068–1199; tel. 269/781–4271; Rob Covert, President and Chief Executive Officer

PENNOCK HOSPITAL, 1009 West Green Street, Hastings, MI, Zip 49058–1790; tel. 269/945–3451; Sheryl Lewis Blake, FACHE, Chief Executive Officer

STURGIS HOSPITAL, 916 Myrtle, Sturgis, MI, Zip 49091–2001; tel. 269/651–7824; Robert J. LaBarge, Chief Executive Officer

LAKELAND REGIONAL HEALTH SYSTEM
1234 Napier Avenue, St. Joseph, MI 49085; tel. 269/983–0999; Joseph Wasserman, President and Chief Executive Officer

LAKELAND REGIONAL MEDICAL CENTER–ST. JOSEPH, 1234 Napier Avenue, Saint Joseph, MI, Zip 49085–2112; tel. 269/983–8300; Joseph A. Wasserman, President and Chief Executive Officer

ST. JOHN HEALTH
28000 Dequindre, Warren, MI 48092; tel. 586/753–0500; Patricia Maryland, President and Chief Executive Officer

PROVIDENCE HOSPITAL AND MEDICAL CENTER, 16001 West Nine Mile Road, Southfield, MI, Zip 48075–4854, Mailing Address: Box 2043, Zip 48037–2043; tel. 248/424–3000; Michael Wiemann, M.D., Senior Vice President and Chief Medical Officer

ST. JOHN NORTH SHORES HOSPITAL, 26755 Ballard Road, Harrison Township, MI, Zip 48045–2458; tel. 586/465–5501; David Sessions, Administrator

ST. JOHN OAKLAND HOSPITAL, 27351 Dequindre, Madison Heights, MI, Zip 48071–3499; tel. 248/967–7000; Joseph M. Tasse, FACHE, President

ST. JOHN RIVER DISTRICT HOSPITAL, 4100 River Road, East China, MI, Zip 48054–2909; tel. 810/329–7111; Frank W. Poma, President

MISSOURI

FREEMAN HEALTH SYSTEM
1102 West 32nd, Joplin, MO 64804; tel. 417/347–1111; Gary Duncan, President and Chief Executive Officer

FREEMAN HEALTH SYSTEM, 1102 West 32nd Street, Joplin, MO, Zip 64804–3503; tel. 417/347–1111; Gary D. Duncan, President and Chief Executive Officer

FREEMAN NEOSHO HOSPITAL, 113 West Hickory Street, Neosho, MO, Zip 64850–1705; tel. 417/455–4352; Daxton Holcomb, Chief Executive Officer

HEARTLAND HEALTH
5325 Faraon Street, St. Joseph, MO 64506; tel. 816/271–6000; Lowell C. Kruse, President and Chief Executive Officer

HEARTLAND REGIONAL MEDICAL CENTER, 5325 Faraon Street, Saint Joseph, MO, Zip 64506–3488; tel. 816/271–6000; Lowell C. Kruse, President and Chief Executive Officer

ST. JOHN'S MERCY HEALTH CARE
615 S. New Ballas Road, St. Louis, MO 63141; tel. 314/251–6000; Ms. Denny DeNarvaez, President and Chief Executive Officer

ST. JOHN'S MERCY HOSPITAL, 901 East Fifth Street, Washington, MO, Zip 63090–3127; tel. 636/239–8000; Terri L. McLain, FACHE, President

ST. JOHN'S MERCY MEDICAL CENTER, 615 South New Ballas Road, Saint Louis, MO, Zip 63141–8277; tel. 314/569–6000; Margaret DeNarvaez, President and Chief Executive Officer

MONTANA

MONTANA HEALTH NETWORK INC.
11 South 7th Street, Suite 160, Miles City, MT 59301; tel. 406/232–1420; Janet Bastian, Chief Executive Officer

BEARTOOTH HOSPITAL AND HEALTH CENTER, 600 West 20th Street, Red Lodge, MT, Zip 59068, Mailing Address: P.O. Box 590, Zip 59068–0590; tel. 406/446–2345; Kelley Evans, Administrator

BILLINGS CLINIC, 2800 10th Avenue North, Billings, MT, Zip 59101, Mailing Address: P.O. Box 37000, Zip 59107–7000; tel. 406/657–4000; Nicholas Wolter, M.D., Chief Executive Officer

CENTRAL MONTANA MEDICAL CENTER, 408 Wendell Avenue, Lewistown, MT, Zip 59457–2261; tel. 406/538–7711; David M. Faulkner, Chief Executive Officer

DANIELS MEMORIAL HEALTHCARE CENTER, 105 Fifth Avenue East, Scobey, MT, Zip 59263, Mailing Address: P.O. Box 400, Zip 59263–0400; tel. 406/487–2296; Steve Hubbard, Interim Chief Executive Officer

FALLON MEDICAL COMPLEX, 202 South 4th Street West, Baker, MT, Zip 59313–0820, Mailing Address: P.O. Box 820, Zip 59313–0820; tel. 406/778–3331; David Espeland, Chief Executive Officer

FRANCES MAHON DEACONESS HOSPITAL, 621 Third Street South, Glasgow, MT, Zip 59230–2699; tel. 406/228–3500; Randall G. Holom, Chief Executive Officer

GLENDIVE MEDICAL CENTER, 202 Prospect Drive, Glendive, MT, Zip 59330–1999; tel. 406/345–3306; Scott Duke, Chief Executive Officer

HOLY ROSARY HEALTHCARE, 2600 Wilson Street, Miles City, MT, Zip 59301–5094; tel. 406/233–2600; Greg A. Nielsen, Chief Executive Officer

MCCONE COUNTY HEALTH CENTER, Circle, MT, Mailing Address: P.O. Box 48, Zip 59215–0048; tel. 406/485–3381; Nancy Hansen, Administrator

PHILLIPS COUNTY HOSPITAL, 417 South Fourth East, Malta, MT, Zip 59538, Mailing Address: P.O. Box 640, Zip 59538–0640; tel. 406/654–1100; Ward C. VanWichen, Chief Executive Officer

ROOSEVELT MEDICAL CENTER, 818 Second Avenue East, Culbertson, MT, Zip 59218, Mailing Address: P.O. Box 419, Zip 59218–0419; tel. 406/787–6401; Audrey Stromberg, Administrator

ROUNDUP MEMORIAL HEALTHCARE, 1202 Third Street West, Roundup, MT, Zip 59072–1816, Mailing Address: P.O. Box 40, Zip 59072–0040; tel. 406/323–2302; Lee Rhodes, Chief Executive Officer

SHERIDAN MEMORIAL HOSPITAL, 440 West Laurel Avenue, Plentywood, MT, Zip 59254–1596; tel. 406/765–1420; Wayne Nelson, Chief Executive Officer

SIDNEY HEALTH CENTER, 216 14th Avenue S.W., Sidney, MT, Zip 59270–3586; tel. 406/488–2100; Richard Haraldson, Chief Executive Officer

STILLWATER COMMUNITY HOSPITAL, 44 West Fourth Avenue North, Columbus, MT, Zip 59019–7126, Mailing Address: P.O. Box 959, Zip 59019–0959; tel. 406/322–5316; Tim Russell, Administrator

NEBRASKA

ALEGENT HEALTH
1010 North 96th Street Suite 200, Omaha, NE 68114; tel. 402/343–4410; Wayne A. Sensor, Chief Executive Officer

ALEGENT HEALTH BERGAN MERCY MEDICAL CENTER, 7500 Mercy Road, Omaha, NE, Zip 68124–2319; tel. 402/398–6060; David Tew, Chief Operating Officer

ALEGENT HEALTH COMMUNITY MEMORIAL HOSPITAL, 631 North Eighth Street, Missouri Valley, IA, Zip 51555–1199; tel. 712/642–2784; Robert R. Sellers, Regional Administrator

ALEGENT HEALTH IMMANUEL MEDICAL CENTER, 6901 North 72nd Street, Omaha, NE, Zip 68122–1799; tel. 402/572–2121; Ann Schumacher, Vice President and Chief Operating Officer

ALEGENT HEALTH MERCY HOSPITAL, 603 Rosary Drive, Corning, IA, Zip 50841–1685, Mailing Address: P.O. Box 368, Zip 50841–0368; tel. 641/322–3121; James C. Ruppert, Regional Administrator

ALEGENT HEALTH MERCY HOSPITAL, 800 Mercy Drive, Council Bluffs, IA, Zip 51503–3128, Mailing Address: P.O. Box 1C, Zip 51502–3001; tel. 712/328–5000; Marie E. Knedler, RN, Vice President and Chief Operating Officer

ALEGENT HEALTH–MEMORIAL HOSPITAL, 104 West 17th Street, Schuyler, NE, Zip 68661–1396; tel. 402/352–2441; Connie Peters, RN, Regional Health Administrator

ALEGENT–HEALTH MIDLANDS HOSPITAL, 11111 South 84th Street, Papillion, NE, Zip 68046–4157; tel. 402/593–3000; Kevin Nokels, Vice President and Chief Operating Officer

BLUE RIVER VALLEY HEALTH NETWORK
2222 Lincoln Avenue, York, NE 68467; tel. 402/362–0445; Charles Schulz, President

ANNIE JEFFREY MEMORIAL COUNTY HEALTH CENTER, 531 Beebe Street, Osceola, NE, Zip 68651, Mailing Address: P.O. Box 428, Zip 68651–0428; tel. 402/747–2031; Joseph W. Lohrman, Chief Executive Officer

BOONE COUNTY HEALTH CENTER, 723 West Fairview Street, Albion, NE, Zip 68620–1725, Mailing Address: P.O. Box 151, Zip 68620–0151; tel. 402/395–2191; Victor N. Lee, FACHE, President and Chief Executive Officer

BRODSTONE MEMORIAL HOSPITAL, 520 East Tenth Street, Superior, NE, Zip 68978–1225, Mailing Address: P.O. Box 187, Zip 68978–0187; tel. 402/879–3281; John E. Keelan, Administrator and Chief Executive Officer

BUTLER COUNTY HEALTH CARE CENTER, 372 South Ninth Street, David City, NE, Zip 68632–2199; tel. 402/367–1200; Donald T. Naiberk, Administrator

COMMUNITY MEMORIAL HOSPITAL, 1579 Midland Street, Syracuse, NE, Zip 68446–9732, Mailing Address: P.O. Box N, Zip 68446; tel. 402/269–2011; Michael Harvey, Chief Executive Officer

CRETE AREA MEDICAL CENTER, 2910 Betten Drive, Crete, NE, Zip 68333–0220, Mailing Address: P.O. Box 220, Zip 68333–0220; tel. 402/826–2102; Carol Friesen, Chief Executive Officer

FILLMORE COUNTY HOSPITAL, 1325 H Street, Geneva, NE, Zip 68361–1325, Mailing Address: P.O. Box 193, Zip 68361–0193; tel. 402/759–3167; Paul Utemark, Chief Executive Officer

HENDERSON HEALTH CARE SERVICES, 1621 Front Street, Henderson, NE, Zip 68371; tel. 402/723–4512; Marianna Harris, Administrator

HOWARD COUNTY COMMUNITY HOSPITAL, 1113 Sherman Street, Saint Paul, NE, Zip 68873–1536, Mailing Address: P.O. Box 406, Zip 68873–0406; tel. 308/754–4421; Arthur H. Frable, Chief Executive Officer

JEFFERSON COMMUNITY HEALTH CENTER, 2200 H Street, Fairbury, NE, Zip 68352–1119, Mailing Address: P.O. Box 277, Zip 68352–0277; tel. 402/729–3351; William L. Welch, FACHE, Chief Executive Officer

JOHNSON COUNTY HOSPITAL, 202 High Street, Tecumseh, NE, Zip 68450–0599, Mailing Address: P.O. Box 599, Zip 68450–0599; tel. 402/335–3361; Diane Newman, Administrator

LITZENBERG MEMORIAL COUNTY HOSPITAL, 1715 26th Street, Central City, NE, Zip 68826–9620, Mailing Address: Route 2, Box 1, Zip 68826–0001; tel. 308/946–3015; Michael R. Bowman, Administrator

MEMORIAL HEALTH CARE SYSTEMS, 300 North Columbia Avenue, Seward, NE, Zip 68434–9907; tel. 402/643–2971; Roger J. Reamer, Chief Executive Officer

MEMORIAL HOSPITAL, 1423 Seventh Street, Aurora, NE, Zip 68818–1197; tel. 402/694–3171; Diane R. Keller, Chief Executive Officer

THAYER COUNTY HEALTH SERVICES, 120 Park Avenue, Hebron, NE, Zip 68370–2019, Mailing Address: P.O. Box 49, Zip 68370–0049; tel. 402/768–6041; Joyce Beck, Administrator

VALLEY COUNTY HEALTH SYSTEM, 217 Westridge Drive, Ord, NE, Zip 68862–1675; tel. 308/728–3211; Larry Schrage, Chief Executive Officer

WARREN MEMORIAL HOSPITAL, 905 Second Street, Friend, NE, Zip 68359–1198; tel. 402/947–2541; John W. Wilson, Chief Executive Officer

YORK GENERAL HOSPITAL, 2222 North Lincoln Avenue, York, NE, Zip 68467–1095; tel. 402/362–6671; Charles K. Schulz, Chief Executive Officer

CENTRAL NEBRASKA PRIMARY
1518 J. Street, Ord, NE 68862; tel. 308/728–3011; Victoria Bauer, Executive Director

BOX BUTTE GENERAL HOSPITAL, 2101 Box Butte Avenue, Alliance, NE, Zip 69301–0810, Mailing Address: P.O. Box 810, Zip 69301–0810; tel. 308/762–6660; Dan Griess, Chief Executive Officer

VALLEY COUNTY HEALTH SYSTEM, 217 Westridge Drive, Ord, NE, Zip 68862–1675; tel. 308/728–3211; Larry Schrage, Chief Executive Officer

NORTHEAST HEALTH SERVICES
P.O. Box 186, Creighton, NE 68729; tel. 402/358–5700; Paul Hurd, President

CREIGHTON AREA HEALTH SERVICES, 1503 Main Street, Creighton, NE, Zip 68729–0186, Mailing Address: P.O. Box 186, Zip 68729–0186; tel. 402/358–5700; Jeff Lingerfelt, Chief Executive Officer

OSMOND GENERAL HOSPITAL, 402 North Maple Street, Osmond, NE, Zip 68765–0429, Mailing Address: P.O. Box 429, Zip 68765–0429; tel. 402/748–3393; Celine M. Mlady, Chief Executive Officer

PLAINVIEW AREA HEALTH SYSTEM, 704 North Third Street, Plainview, NE, Zip 68769, Mailing Address: P.O. Box 489, Zip 68769–0489; tel. 402/582–4245; Becky Lambrecht, Administrator

REGIONAL CARE, INC.
905 W. 27th Street, Scottsbluff, NE 69361; tel. 308/635–2260; Steve Hetzel, President

BOX BUTTE GENERAL HOSPITAL, 2101 Box Butte Avenue, Alliance, NE, Zip 69301–0810, Mailing Address: P.O. Box 810, Zip 69301–0810; tel. 308/762–6660; Dan Griess, Chief Executive Officer

CHADRON COMMUNITY HOSPITAL AND HEALTH SERVICES, 821 Morehead Street, Chadron, NE, Zip 69337–2599; tel. 308/432–5586; Harold L. Krueger, Jr., Chief Executive Officer

GARDEN COUNTY HEALTH SERVICES, 1100 West Second Street, Oshkosh, NE, Zip 69154, Mailing Address: P.O. Box 320, Zip 69154–0320; tel. 308/772–3283; Carol A. Kraus, Chief Executive Officer

GORDON MEMORIAL HOSPITAL, 300 East Eighth Street, Gordon, NE, Zip 69343–9990; tel. 308/282–0401; Kay Garcia, Chief Executive Officer

KIMBALL HEALTH SERVICES, 505 South Burg Street, Kimball, NE, Zip 69145–1398; tel. 308/235–1952; Julie Schnell, Chief Executive Officer

MORRILL COUNTY COMMUNITY HOSPITAL, 1313 S Street, Bridgeport, NE, Zip 69336–0579, Mailing Address: P.O. Box 579, Zip 69336–0579; tel. 308/262–1616; Julia Morrow, Administrator

REGIONAL WEST MEDICAL CENTER, 4021 Avenue B, Scottsbluff, NE, Zip 69361–4695; tel. 308/635–3711; Todd Sorensen, M.D., Chief Executive Officer

RURAL NEBRASKA HEALTHCARE NETWORK
821 Morehead Street, Chadron, NE 69337; tel. 308/432–5586; Harold L. Krueger, Chief Executive Officer

BOX BUTTE GENERAL HOSPITAL, 2101 Box Butte Avenue, Alliance, NE, Zip 69301–0810, Mailing Address: P.O. Box 810, Zip 69301–0810; tel. 308/762–6660; Dan Griess, Chief Executive Officer

CHADRON COMMUNITY HOSPITAL AND HEALTH SERVICES, 821 Morehead Street, Chadron, NE, Zip 69337–2599; tel. 308/432–5586; Harold L. Krueger, Jr., Chief Executive Officer

GARDEN COUNTY HEALTH SERVICES, 1100 West Second Street, Oshkosh, NE, Zip 69154, Mailing Address: P.O. Box 320, Zip 69154–0320; tel. 308/772–3283; Carol A. Kraus, Chief Executive Officer

GORDON MEMORIAL HOSPITAL, 300 East Eighth Street, Gordon, NE, Zip 69343–9990; tel. 308/282–0401; Kay Garcia, Chief Executive Officer

KIMBALL HEALTH SERVICES, 505 South Burg Street, Kimball, NE, Zip 69145–1398; tel. 308/235–1952; Julie Schnell, Chief Executive Officer

MEMORIAL HEALTH CENTER, 645 Osage Street, Sidney, NE, Zip 69162–1799; tel. 308/254–5825; Danielle Gearhart, Chief Executive Officer

MORRILL COUNTY COMMUNITY HOSPITAL, 1313 S Street, Bridgeport, NE, Zip 69336–0579, Mailing Address: P.O. Box 579, Zip 69336–0579; tel. 308/262–1616; Julia Morrow, Administrator

PERKINS COUNTY HEALTH SERVICES, 900 Lincoln Avenue, Grant, NE, Zip 69140–9799; tel. 308/352–7200; Pam Holm, RN, Administrator

REGIONAL WEST MEDICAL CENTER, 4021 Avenue B, Scottsbluff, NE, Zip 69361–4695; tel. 308/635–3711; Todd Sorensen, M.D., Chief Executive Officer

NEVADA

SAINT MARY'S HEALTH NETWORK
235 West Sixth Street, Reno, NV 89520; tel. 775/770–3000; Michael J. Uboldi, President

SAINT MARY'S REGIONAL MEDICAL CENTER, 235 West Sixth Street, Reno, NV, Zip 89503; tel. 775/770–3000; Michael J. Uboldi, President

NEW HAMPSHIRE

CARING COMMUNITY NETWORK OF THE TWIN RIVERS
c/o Health First 841 Central Street, Franklin, NH 03235; tel. 603/934–0177; Rick Silverberg, Managing Director

FRANKLIN REGIONAL HOSPITAL, 15 Aiken Avenue, Franklin, NH, Zip 03235–1299; tel. 603/934–2060; Thomas Clairmont, President

HEALTHLINK
80 Highland Street, Laconia, NH 03246; tel. 603/527–2801; Thomas Clairmont, President

CATHOLIC MEDICAL CENTER, 100 McGregor Street, Manchester, NH, Zip 03102–3770; tel. 603/668–3545; Alyson Pitman Giles, President and Chief Executive Officer

CONCORD HOSPITAL, 250 Pleasant Street, Concord, NH, Zip 03301–2598; tel. 603/225–2711; Michael B. Green, President and Chief Executive Officer

DARTMOUTH–HITCHCOCK MEDICAL CENTER, One Medical Center Drive, Lebanon, NH, Zip 03756–0001; tel. 603/650–5000; Nancy A. Formella, President

ELLIOT HOSPITAL, One Elliot Way, Manchester, NH, Zip 03103–3599; tel. 603/669–5300; Douglas F. Dean, Jr., President and Chief Executive Officer

LAKES REGION GENERAL HOSPITAL, 80 Highland Street, Laconia, NH, Zip 03246–3298; tel. 603/524–3211; Thomas Clairmont, President

NEW JERSEY

ATLANTICARE
2500 English Creek Avenue, Building 500, Suite 501, Egg Harbor Township, NJ 08234; tel. 609/272–6316; George F. Lynn, President Emeritus

ATLANTICARE REGIONAL MEDICAL CENTER, 1925 Pacific Avenue, Atlantic City, NJ, Zip 08401–6713; tel. 609/345–4000; David P. Tilton, President and Chief Executive Officer

CAPE REGIONAL HEALTH SYSTEM
Two Stone Habor Boulevard, Cape May, NJ 08210; tel. 609/463–2266; Joanne Carrocino, President and Chief Executive Officer

CAPE REGIONAL MEDICAL CENTER, Two Stone Harbor Boulevard, Cape May Court House, NJ, Zip 08210–9990; tel. 609/463–2000; Joanne Carrocino, FACHE, President and Chief Executive Officer

QUALCARE, INC.
242 Old Brunswick Road, Piscataway, NJ 08854; tel. 908/562–2800; Jerry Eisenberg, Network Contact

CAPITAL HEALTH SYSTEM AT MERCER, 446 Bellevue Avenue, Trenton, NJ, Zip 08618–4597, Mailing Address: P.O. Box 1658, Zip 08607–1658; tel. 609/394–4000; Al Maghazehe, Chief Executive Officer

CHILTON MEMORIAL HOSPITAL, 97 West Parkway, Pompton Plains, NJ, Zip 07444–1696; tel. 973/831–5000; Deborah K. Zastocki, FACHE, President and Chief Executive Officer

CHRIST HOSPITAL, 176 Palisade Avenue, Jersey City, NJ, Zip 07306–1196, Mailing Address: P.O. Box J–1, Zip 07306–1196; tel. 201/795–8200; Peter A. Kelly, President and Chief Executive Officer

CLARA MAASS MEDICAL CENTER, One Clara Maass Drive, Belleville, NJ, Zip 07109–3557; tel. 973/450–2000; Thomas A. Biga, Executive Director

DEBORAH HEART AND LUNG CENTER, 200 Trenton Road, Browns Mills, NJ, Zip 08015–1799; tel. 609/893–6611; John R. Ernst, President and Chief Executive Officer

ENGLEWOOD HOSPITAL AND MEDICAL CENTER, 350 Engle Street, Englewood, NJ, Zip 07631–1898; tel. 201/894–3000; Douglas A. Duchak, President and Chief Executive Officer

HACKETTSTOWN REGIONAL MEDICAL CENTER, 651 Willow Grove Street, Hackettstown, NJ, Zip 07840–1792; tel. 908/852–5100; Gene C. Milton, President and Chief Executive Officer

JFK MEDICAL CENTER, 65 James Street, Edison, NJ, Zip 08818–3059; tel. 732/321–7000; Scott Gebhard, Executive Vice President and Chief Operating Officer

MEMORIAL HOSPITAL OF SALEM COUNTY, 310 Woodstown Road, Salem, NJ, Zip 08079–2080; tel. 856/935–1000; James L. Angle, Chief Executive Officer

MUHLENBERG REGIONAL MEDICAL CENTER, Park Avenue and Randolph Road, North Plainfield, NJ, Zip 7060; tel. 908/668–2000; Nancy A. Fiamingo, Senior Vice President and Chief Operating Officer

OCEAN MEDICAL CENTER, 425 Jack Martin Boulevard, Brick Township, NJ, Zip 8724; tel. 732/840–2200; W. Peter Daniels, President

PIEDMONT MOUNTAINSIDE HOSPITAL, 1266 Highway 515 South, Jasper, GA, Zip 30143; tel. 706/692–2441; Ed Lovern, President and Chief Executive Officer

RARITAN BAY MEDICAL CENTER, 530 New Brunswick Avenue, Perth Amboy, NJ, Zip 8861; tel. 732/442–3700; Michael R. D'Agnes, President and Chief Executive Officer

RIVERVIEW MEDICAL CENTER, 1 Riverview Plaza, Red Bank, NJ, Zip 07701–9982; tel. 732/741–2700; Timothy J. Hogan, President

ROBERT WOOD JOHNSON UNIVERSITY HOSPITAL, 1 Robert Wood Johnson Place, New Brunswick, NJ, Zip 08903–2601; tel. 732/828–3000; Stephen K. Jones, President and Chief Executive Officer

SAINT MICHAEL'S MEDICAL CENTER, 268 Dr. Martin Luther King Jr. Boulevard, Newark, NJ, Zip 07102–2094; tel. 973/877–5000; Felicia Karsos, Administrator

SOUTH JERSEY HEALTHCARE – REGIONAL MEDICAL CENTER, 1505 West Sherman Avenue, Vineland, NJ, Zip 8360; tel. 856/641–8000; Chester B. Kaletkowski, President and Chief Executive Officer

ST. MARY'S HOSPITAL, 350 Boulevard, Passaic, NJ, Zip 7055; tel. 973/365–4300; Colene Y. Daniel, M.S., M.P.H., FACHE, President and Chief Executive Officer

UNIVERSITY MEDICAL CENTER AT PRINCETON, 253 Witherspoon Street, Princeton, NJ, Zip 08540–3213; tel. 609/497–4000; Vincent D. Joseph, President

UNIVERSITY OF MEDICINE AND DENTISTRY OF NEW JERSEY–UNIVERSITY HOSPITAL, 150 Bergen Street, Newark, NJ, Zip 07103–2496; tel. 973/972–4300; Darlene L. Cox, President and Chief Executive Officer

VIRTUA WEST JERSEY HOSPITAL–BERLIN, 100 Townsend Avenue, Berlin, NJ, Zip 08009–9035; tel. 856/322–3000; Christopher A. Chekouras, Vice President and Chief Operating Officer

VIRTUA WEST JERSEY HOSPITAL–MARLTON, 90 Brick Road, Marlton, NJ, Zip 08053–9697; tel. 856/355–6000; Gary L. Long, Vice President and Chief Operating Officer

NEW YORK

ALLEGANY WESTERN STEUBEN RURAL HEALTH NETWORK, INC.
85 North Main, Suite 4, Wellsville, NY 14895; tel. 585/593–5223; Carrie Whitwood, Executive Director

JONES MEMORIAL HOSPITAL, 191 North Main Street, Wellsville, NY, Zip 14895–1197, Mailing Address: P.O. Box 72, Zip 14895–0072; tel. 585/593–1100; Eva Benedict, President and Chief Executive Officer

ST. JAMES MERCY HOSPITAL, 411 Canisteo Street, Hornell, NY, Zip 14843–2197; tel. 607/324–8000; Mary E. LaRowe, FACHE, President and Chief Executive Officer

ARNOT HEALTH
600 Roe Avenue, Elmira, NY 14905; tel. 607/737–4100; Anthony J. Cooper, FACHE, President

ARNOT OGDEN MEDICAL CENTER, 600 Roe Avenue, Elmira, NY, Zip 14905–1629; tel. 607/737–4100; Anthony J. Cooper, FACHE, President and Chief Executive Officer

BASSETT HEALTHCARE
1 Atwell Road, Cooperstown, NY 13326; tel. 607/547–3100; William F. Streck, M.D., President and Chief Executive Officer

COBLESKILL REGIONAL HOSPITAL, 178 Grandview Drive, Cobleskill, NY, Zip 12043; tel. 518/254–3456; Eric H. Stein, FACHE, President and Chief Executive Officer

LITTLE FALLS HOSPITAL, 140 Burwell Street, Little Falls, NY, Zip 13365–1725; tel. 315/823–1000; Jonathan I. Lawrence, President and Chief Executive Officer

MARY IMOGENE BASSETT HOSPITAL, One Atwell Road, Cooperstown, NY, Zip 13326–1394; tel. 607/547–3100; William F. Streck, M.D., President and Chief Executive Officer

O'CONNOR HOSPITAL, 460 Andes Road, State Route 28, Delhi, NY, Zip 13753; tel. 607/746–0300

MOHAWK VALLEY NETWORK, INC.
P.O. Box 4308, Utica, NY 13504; tel. 315/624–5116; Keith A. Fenstemacher, President and Chief Executive Officer

FAXTON–ST. LUKE'S HEALTHCARE, 1676 Sunset Avenue, Utica, NY, Zip 13502–5475, Mailing Address: P.O. Box 479, Zip 13503–0479; tel. 315/624–6000; Keith A. Fenstemacher, President and Chief Executive Officer

MOUNT SINAI NYU HEALTH NETWORK
One Gustave L. Levy Place, Box #1220, New York, NY 10029; tel. 212/659–8888; Kenneth Davis, President and Chief Executive Officer

COMMUNITY HOSPITAL AT DOBBS FERRY, 128 Ashford Avenue, Dobbs Ferry, NY, Zip 10522–1896; tel. 914/693–0700; Ronald Corti, President and Chief Executive Officer

ELMHURST HOSPITAL CENTER, 79–01 Broadway, Flushing, NY, Zip 11373–1368; tel. 718/334–4000; Chris D. Constantino, Executive Director

ENGLEWOOD HOSPITAL AND MEDICAL CENTER, 350 Engle Street, Englewood, NJ, Zip 07631–1898; tel. 201/894–3000; Douglas A. Duchak, President and Chief Executive Officer

LIBERTYHEALTH–JERSEY CITY MEDICAL CENTER, 355 Grand Street, Jersey City, NJ, Zip 7302; tel. 201/915–2000; E. Stephen Kirby, Interim Chief Executive Officer

LIBERTYHEALTH–MEADOWLANDS HOSPITAL MEDICAL CENTER, 55 Meadowland Parkway, Secaucus, NJ, Zip 07094–1580; tel. 201/392–3100; Joseph F. Scott, Chief Executive Officer

LUTHERAN MEDICAL CENTER, 150 55th Street, Brooklyn, NY, Zip 11220–2570; tel. 718/630–7000; Wendy Z. Goldstein, President and Chief Executive Officer

MORRISTOWN MEMORIAL HOSPITAL, 100 Madison Avenue, Morristown, NJ, Zip 07962–1956; tel. 973/971–5000; Joseph A. Trunfio, Ph.D., President and Chief Executive Officer

MOUNT SINAI HOSPITAL, One Gustave L. Levy Place, New York, NY, Zip 10029–6574; tel. 212/241–6500; Burton P. Drayer, M.D., President

NORTH GENERAL HOSPITAL, 1879 Madison Avenue, New York, NY, Zip 10035–2745; tel. 212/423–4000; Samuel J. Daniel, M.D., President and Chief Executive Officer

NYU HOSPITAL FOR JOINT DISEASES, 301 East 17th Street, New York, NY, Zip 10003–3890; tel. 212/598–6000; David A. Dibner, FACHE, Senior Vice President Operations

OVERLOOK HOSPITAL, 99 Beauvoir Avenue, Summit, NJ, Zip 07902–0220; tel. 908/522–2000; Alan R. Lieber, Chief Operating Officer

PHELPS MEMORIAL HOSPITAL CENTER, 701 North Broadway, Sleepy Hollow, NY, Zip 10591–1096; tel. 914/366–3000; Keith F. Safian, President and Chief Executive Officer

QUEENS HOSPITAL CENTER, 82–68 164th Street, Jamaica, NY, Zip 11432–1104; tel. 718/883–3000; Antonio D. Martin, Executive Director

ST. JOHN'S RIVERSIDE HOSPITAL, 967 North Broadway, Yonkers, NY, Zip 10701–1399; tel. 914/964–4444; James Foy, President and Chief Executive Officer

ST. JOSEPH'S REGIONAL MEDICAL CENTER, 703 Main Street, Paterson, NJ, Zip 07503–2691; tel. 973/754–2000; William A. McDonald, President and Chief Executive Officer

ST. LUKE'S CORNWALL HOSPITAL – NEWBURGH CAMPUS, 70 Dubois Street, Newburgh, NY, Zip 12550–4898; tel. 845/561–4400; Allan E. Atzrott, President and Chief Executive Officer

THE MOUNT SINAI HOSPITAL OF QUEENS, 25–10 30th Avenue, Long Island City, NY, Zip 11102–2495; tel. 718/932–1000; Caryn A. Schwab, Executive Director

VASSAR BROTHERS MEDICAL CENTER, 45 Reade Place, Poughkeepsie, NY, Zip 12601–3990; tel. 845/454–8500; Daniel Z. Aronzon, M.D., President and Chief Executive Officer

VETERANS AFFAIRS MEDICAL CENTER, 130 West Kingsbridge Road, Bronx, NY, Zip 10468–3992; tel. 718/584–9000; Maryann Musumeci, Director

NORTHERN NY RURAL HEALTH CARE ALLIANCE
200 Washington Street, Suite 300, Watertown, NY 13601; tel. 315/786–0565; James C. Bellinger, Chairman

CARTHAGE AREA HOSPITAL, 1001 West Street, Carthage, NY, Zip 13619–9703; tel. 315/493–1000; Walter S. Becker, Chief Executive Officer

RIVER HOSPITAL, 4 Fuller Street, Alexandria Bay, NY, Zip 13607; tel. 315/482–2511; Ben Moore, III, President and Chief Executive Officer

SAMARITAN MEDICAL CENTER, 830 Washington Street, Watertown, NY, Zip 13601–4066; tel. 315/785–4000; Thomas H. Carman, President and Chief Executive Officer

STELLARIS HEALTH
1 North Greenwich Road, Armonk, NY 10504; tel. 914/273–2850; Arthur Nizza, President and Chief Executive Officer

LAWRENCE HOSPITAL CENTER, 55 Palmer Avenue, Bronxville, NY, Zip 10708–3491; tel. 914/787–1000; Edward M. Dinan, President and Chief Executive Officer

NORTHERN WESTCHESTER HOSPITAL, 400 East Main Street, Mount Kisco, NY, Zip 10549–3477; tel. 914/666–1200; Joel Seligman, President and Chief Executive Officer

PHELPS MEMORIAL HOSPITAL CENTER, 701 North Broadway, Sleepy Hollow, NY, Zip 10591–1096; tel. 914/366–3000; Keith F. Safian, President and Chief Executive Officer

WHITE PLAINS HOSPITAL CENTER, Davis Avenue and Post Road, White Plains, NY, Zip 10601–4699; tel. 914/681–0600; Jon B. Schandler, President and Chief Executive Officer

THE RURAL HEALTH NETWORK OF OSWEGO COUNTY
239 Oneida Street, Fulton, NY 13069; tel. 315/598–4710; Ellen Holst, Health Director

ALBERT LINDLEY LEE MEMORIAL HOSPITAL, 510 South Fourth Street, Fulton, NY, Zip 13069–2994; tel. 315/591–9400; Dennis A. Casey, Executive Director

OSWEGO HOSPITAL, 110 West Sixth Street, Oswego, NY, Zip 13126–9985; tel. 315/349–5511; Ann C. Gilpin, President and Chief Executive Officer

NORTH CAROLINA

BLADEN COUNTY HOSPITAL
P.O. Box 398, Elizabethtown, NC 28337; tel. 910/862–5179; David Masterson, Chief Executive Officer

BLADEN COUNTY HOSPITAL, 501 South Poplar Street, Elizabethtown, NC, Zip 28337–0398, Mailing Address: P.O. Box 398, Zip 28337–0398; tel. 910/862–5100; David J. Masterson, Chief Executive Officer

MISSION HEALTH SYSTEM AND HOSPITAL
509 Biltmore Avenue, Asheville, NC 28801; tel. 828/213–1144; Joe Damore, President and Chief Executive Officer

BLUE RIDGE REGIONAL HOSPITAL, 125 Hospital Drive, Spruce Pine, NC, Zip 28777, Mailing Address: P.O. Drawer 9, Zip 28777; tel. 828/765–4201; Keith S. Holtsclaw, Chief Executive Officer

MCDOWELL HOSPITAL, 430 Rankin Drive, Marion, NC, Zip 28752–4989, Mailing Address: P.O. Box 730, Zip 28752–0730; tel. 828/659–5000; Edward J. Hannon, Chief Executive Officer

MISSION HOSPITAL, 509 Biltmore Avenue, Asheville, NC, Zip 28801–4690; tel. 828/213–1111; Joseph F. Damore, President and Chief Executive Officer

WNC HEALTH NETWORK, INC.
501 Biltmore Avenue, Asheville, NC 28801; tel. 828/257–2983; Gary Bowers, Executive Director

ALAMANCE REGIONAL MEDICAL CENTER, 1240 Huffman Mill Road, Burlington, NC, Zip 27216–0202, Mailing Address: P.O. Box 202, Zip 27216–0202; tel. 336/538–7000; John G. Currin, Jr., President

ANGEL MEDICAL CENTER, 120 Riverview Street, Franklin, NC, Zip 28734, Mailing Address: P.O. Box 1209, Zip 28744; tel. 828/524–8411; Donald D. Sandoval, FACHE, Chief Executive Officer

ANMED HEALTH MEDICAL CENTER, 800 North Fant Street, Anderson, SC, Zip 29621–5793; tel. 864/512–1000; John A. Miller, Jr., FACHE, President

ANMED HEALTH REHABILITATION HOSPITAL, 1 Spring Back Way, Anderson, SC, Zip 29621; tel. 864/716–2600; Michele M. Skripps, Chief Executive Officer

BLADEN COUNTY HOSPITAL, 501 South Poplar Street, Elizabethtown, NC, Zip 28337–0398, Mailing Address: P.O. Box 398, Zip 28337–0398; tel. 910/862–5100; David J. Masterson, Chief Executive Officer

BLOWING ROCK HOSPITAL, Chestnut Street, Blowing Rock, NC, Zip 28605–0148, Mailing Address: Box 148, Zip 28605–0148; tel. 828/295–3136; Timothy R. Ford, Chief Executive Officer

BLUE RIDGE REGIONAL HOSPITAL, 125 Hospital Drive, Spruce Pine, NC, Zip 28777, Mailing Address: P.O. Drawer 9, Zip 28777; tel. 828/765–4201; Keith S. Holtsclaw, Chief Executive Officer

BUCHANAN GENERAL HOSPITAL, Grundy, VA, Mailing Address: Route 5, Box 20, Zip 24614–9611; tel. 276/935–1000; Joan Jamison, Chief Executive Officer

CALDWELL MEMORIAL HOSPITAL, 321 Mulberry Street S.W., Lenoir, NC, Zip 28645–5720, Mailing Address: P.O. Box 1890, Zip 28645–1890; tel. 828/757–5100; Laura J. Easton, President and Chief Executive Officer

CAPE FEAR VALLEY HEALTH SYSTEM, 1638 Owen Drive, Fayetteville, NC, Zip 28304–3431, Mailing Address: P.O. Box 2000, Zip 28302–2000; tel. 910/609–4000; Joyce P. Korzen, RN, Interim Chief Executive Officer

CAREPARTNERS REHABILITATION HOSPITAL, 68 Sweeten Creek Road, Asheville, NC, Zip 28803–1599, Mailing Address: P.O. Box 5779, Zip 28813–5779; tel. 828/277–4800; Charles D. Norvell, President and Chief Executive Officer

CARTERET GENERAL HOSPITAL, 3500 Arendell Street, Morehead City, NC, Zip 28557–1619, Mailing Address: P.O. Box 1619, Zip 28557–1619; tel. 252/808–6000; Frederick A. Odell, III, FACHE, President

CATAWBA VALLEY MEDICAL CENTER, 810 Fairgrove Church Road S.E., Hickory, NC, Zip 28602–9643; tel. 828/326–3000; J. Anthony Rose, President and Chief Executive Officer

CHARLES A. CANNON JR. MEMORIAL HOSPITAL, 434 Hospital Drive, Linville, NC, Zip 28646, Mailing Address: P.O. Box 767, Zip 28646; tel. 828/737–7000; Chuck Mantooth, Chief Executive Officer

CHEROKEE INDIAN HOSPITAL AUTHORITY, Hospital Road, Cherokee, NC, Zip 28719, Mailing Address: Caller Box C–268, Zip 28719; tel. 828/497–9163; Casey Cooper, Chief Executive Officer

COMMUNITY MEMORIAL HEALTHCENTER, 125 Buena Vista Circle, South Hill, VA, Zip 23970–0090, Mailing Address: P.O. Box 90, Zip 23970–0090; tel. 434/447–3151; W. Scott Burnette, President and Chief Executive Officer

FIRSTHEALTH MONTGOMERY MEMORIAL HOSPITAL, 520 Allen Street, Troy, NC, Zip 27371–2802, Mailing Address: P.O. Box 486, Zip 27371–0486; tel. 910/572–1301; Kerry A. Hensley, RN, President

FIRSTHEALTH MOORE REGIONAL HOSPITAL, 155 Memorial Drive, Pinehurst, NC, Zip 28374–8710, Mailing Address: P.O. Box 3000, Zip 28374–3000; tel. 910/715–1000; Stuart Voelpel, President and Chief Operating Officer

FIRSTHEALTH RICHMOND MEMORIAL HOSPITAL, 925 Long Drive, Rockingham, NC, Zip 28379–4815; tel. 910/417–3000; John J. Jackson, President

GRANVILLE MEDICAL CENTER, 1010 College Street, Oxford, NC, Zip 27565–2507, Mailing Address: P.O. Box 947, Zip 27565–0947; tel. 919/690–3000; L. Lee Isley, Chief Executive Officer

HALIFAX REGIONAL MEDICAL CENTER, 250 Smith Church Road, Roanoke Rapids, NC, Zip 27870, Mailing Address: P.O. Box 1089, Zip 27870; tel. 252/535–8011; William Mahone, V, President and Chief Executive Officer

HARRIS REGIONAL HOSPITAL, 68 Hospital Road, Sylva, NC, Zip 28779–2795; tel. 828/586–7000; Mark T. Leonard, Chief Executive Officer

HAYWOOD REGIONAL MEDICAL CENTER, 262 Leroy George Drive, Clyde, NC, Zip 28721–9434; tel. 828/456–7311; Alton T. Byers, Chief Executive Officer

HIGHLANDS–CASHIERS HOSPITAL, 190 Hospital Drive, Highlands, NC, Zip 28741–7600, Mailing Address: P.O. Drawer 190, Zip 28741–0190; tel. 828/526–1200; Kenneth A. Shull, FACHE, President and Chief Executive Officer

IREDELL MEMORIAL HOSPITAL, 557 Brookdale Drive, Statesville, NC, Zip 28677–1828, Mailing Address: P.O. Box 1828, Zip 28687–1828; tel. 704/873–5661; Ed Rush, President and Chief Executive Officer

JOHNSTON MEMORIAL HOSPITAL, 351 Court Street N.E., Abingdon, VA, Zip 24210–2955; tel. 276/676–7000; Sean S. McMurray, FACHE, Chief Executive Officer

LENOIR MEMORIAL HOSPITAL, 100 Airport Road, Kinston, NC, Zip 28501–1634, Mailing Address: P.O. Box 1678, Zip 28503–1678; tel. 252/522–7000; Gary E. Black, President and Chief Executive Officer

LEXINGTON MEDICAL CENTER, 2720 Sunset Boulevard, West Columbia, SC, Zip 29169–4816; tel. 803/791–2000; Michael J. Biediger, President and Chief Executive Officer

LORIS COMMUNITY HOSPITAL, 3655 Mitchell Street, Box 690001, Loris, SC, Zip 29569–9601; tel. 843/716–7000; J. Timothy Browne, President and Chief Executive Officer

MARGARET R. PARDEE MEMORIAL HOSPITAL, 800 North Justice Street, Hendersonville, NC, Zip 28791–2563; tel. 828/696–1000; Kris Hoce, Chief Executive Officer

MARIA PARHAM MEDICAL CENTER, 566 Ruin Creek Road, Henderson, NC, Zip 27536–2957; tel. 252/438–4143; Robert G. Singletary, President and Chief Executive Officer

MCDOWELL HOSPITAL, 430 Rankin Drive, Marion, NC, Zip 28752–4989, Mailing Address: P.O. Box 730, Zip 28752–0730; tel. 828/659–5000; Edward J. Hannon, Chief Executive Officer

MISSION HOSPITAL, 509 Biltmore Avenue, Asheville, NC, Zip 28801–4690; tel. 828/213–1111; Joseph F. Damore, President and Chief Executive Officer

MURPHY MEDICAL CENTER, 4130 U.S. Highway 64 East, Murphy, NC, Zip 28906–7917; tel. 828/837–8161; Mike Stevenson, Administrator

PARK RIDGE HOSPITAL, Naples Road, Fletcher, NC, Zip 28732, Mailing Address: P.O. Box 1569, Zip 28732–1569; tel. 828/684–8501; Jimm Bunch, President and Chief Executive Officer

RANDOLPH HOSPITAL, 364 White Oak Street, Asheboro, NC, Zip 27203–5400, Mailing Address: P.O. Box 1048, Zip 27204–1048; tel. 336/625–5151; Robert E. Morrison, President

RUTHERFORD HOSPITAL, 288 South Ridgecrest Avenue, Rutherfordton, NC, Zip 28139–3097; tel. 828/286–5000; David Bixler, President

SELF REGIONAL HEALTHCARE, 1325 Spring Street, Greenwood, SC, Zip 29646–3860; tel. 864/725–4111; M. John Heydel, President and Chief Executive Officer

SOUTHEASTERN REGIONAL MEDICAL CENTER, 300 West 27th Street, Lumberton, NC, Zip 28358–3017, Mailing Address: P.O. Box 1408, Zip 28359–1408; tel. 910/671–5000; Joann Anderson, President and Chief Executive Officer

SPARTANBURG REGIONAL MEDICAL CENTER, 101 East Wood Street, Spartanburg, SC, Zip 29303–3016; tel. 864/560–6000; Ingo Angermeier, FACHE, President and Chief Executive Officer

ST. LUKE'S HOSPITAL, 101 Hospital Drive, Columbus, NC, Zip 28722–9473; tel. 828/894–3311; C. Cameron Highsmith, President and Chief Executive Officer

STANLY REGIONAL MEDICAL CENTER, 301 Yadkin Street, Albemarle, NC, Zip 28001–3448, Mailing Address: P.O. Box 1489, Zip 28002–1489; tel. 704/984–4000; Alfred P. Taylor, Chief Executive Officer

TRANSYLVANIA COMMUNITY HOSPITAL, Hospital Drive, Brevard, NC, Zip 28712–1116, Mailing Address: Box 1116, Zip 28712–1116; tel. 828/884–9111; Robert J. Bednarek, President and Chief Executive Officer

TWIN COUNTY REGIONAL HOSPITAL, 200 Hospital Drive, Galax, VA, Zip 24333–2283; tel. 276/236–8181; Jon D. Applebaum, President and Chief Executive Officer

WATAUGA MEDICAL CENTER, Deerfield Road, Boone, NC, Zip 28607–2600, Mailing Address: P.O. Box 2600, Zip 28607–2600; tel. 828/262–4100; Richard G. Sparks, President

WAYNE MEMORIAL HOSPITAL, 2700 Wayne Memorial Drive, Goldsboro, NC, Zip 27534, Mailing Address: P.O. Box 8001, Zip 27533; tel. 919/736–1110; J. William Paugh, President and Chief Executive Officer

WILSON MEDICAL CENTER, 1705 Tarboro Street, S.W., Wilson, NC, Zip 27893–3428; tel. 252/399–8040; Richard E. Hudson, FACHE, President and Chief Executive Officer

NORTH DAKOTA

MEDCENTER ONE
300 North 7th Street, Bismarck, ND 58506; tel. 701/323–6000; James Cooper, President and Chief Executive Officer

MEDCENTER ONE, 300 North Seventh Street, Bismarck, ND, Zip 58501–4439, Mailing Address: P.O. Box 5525, Zip 58506–5525; tel. 701/323–6000; James C. Cooper, President and Chief Executive Officer

MERIT CARE HEALTH SYSTEM
720 Fourth Street North, Fargo, ND 58122; tel. 701/234–2600; Dr. Roger Gilbertson, M.D., Chief Executive Officer

MERITCARE MEDICAL CENTER, 720 Fourth Street North, Fargo, ND, Zip 58122; tel. 701/234–6000; Roger L. Gilbertson, M.D., President and Chief Executive Officer

OHIO

BLANCHARD VALLEY HEALTH ASSOCIATION
145 West Wallace, Findlay, OH 45840; tel. 419/423–5201; Scott Malaney, President and Chief Executive Officer

BLANCHARD VALLEY HEALTH SYSTEM, 1900 South Main Street, Findlay, OH, Zip 45840; tel. 419/423–4500; Scott C. Malaney, President and Chief Executive Officer

BLUFFTON REGIONAL MEDICAL CENTER, 303 South Main Street, Bluffton, IN, Zip 46714–2529; tel. 260/824–3210; Thomas A. Clark, Chief Executive Officer

CLEVELAND HEALTH NETWORK
6000 W. Creek Road, Suite 20, Independence, OH 44131; tel. 216/986–1100; Dennis Pijor, Executive Vice President and Chief Operating Officer

AFFINITY MEDICAL CENTER, DOCTORS CAMPUS, 400 Austin Avenue N.W., Massillon, OH, Zip 44646–3554; tel. 330/837–7200; Ronald L. Bierman, Chief Executive Officer

AKRON CHILDREN'S HOSPITAL, One Perkins Square, Akron, OH, Zip 44308–1062; tel. 330/543–1000; William H. Considine, President

AMHERST HOSPITAL, 254 Cleveland Avenue, Amherst, OH, Zip 44001–1620; tel. 440/988–6000; Kevin C. Martin, President and Chief Executive Officer

ASHTABULA COUNTY MEDICAL CENTER, 2420 Lake Avenue, Ashtabula, OH, Zip 44004–4954; tel. 440/997–2262; Kevin J. Miller, FACHE, President and Chief Executive Officer

CLEVELAND CLINIC CHILDREN'S HOSPITAL FOR REHABILITATION, Cleveland, OH, Mailing Address: 2801 Martin Luther King Jr. Drive, Zip 44104–3865; tel. 216/721–5400; David Kenagny, M.D., Medical Director

CLEVELAND CLINIC FOUNDATION, 9500 Euclid Avenue, Cleveland, OH, Zip 44195–5108; tel. 216/444–2200; Delos Cosgrove, M.D., President and Chief Executive Officer

CUYAHOGA FALLS GENERAL HOSPITAL, 1900 23rd Street, Cuyahoga Falls, OH, Zip 44223–1499; tel. 330/971–7000; Kathleen A. Rice, President and Chief Operating Officer

EMH REGIONAL MEDICAL CENTER, 630 East River Street, Elyria, OH, Zip 44035–5902; tel. 440/329–7500; Kevin C. Martin, President and Chief Executive Officer

EUCLID HOSPITAL, 18901 Lake Shore Boulevard, Euclid, OH, Zip 44119–1090; tel. 216/531–9000; Robert Stall, President

FAIRVIEW HOSPITAL, 18101 Lorain Avenue, Cleveland, OH, Zip 44111–5656; tel. 216/476–7000; Fred M. DeGrandis, Chief Executive Officer

FIRELANDS REGIONAL HEALTH SYSTEM, 1111 Hayes Avenue, Sandusky, OH, Zip 44870; tel. 419/557–7400; Charles A. Stark, FACHE, President and Chief Executive Officer

FISHER–TITUS MEDICAL CENTER, 272 Benedict Avenue, Norwalk, OH, Zip 44857–2374; tel. 419/668–8101; Patrick J. Martin, President and Chief Executive Officer

HAMOT MEDICAL CENTER, 201 State Street, Erie, PA, Zip 16550–0002; tel. 814/877–6000; John T. Malone, President and Chief Executive Officer

HILLCREST HOSPITAL, 6780 Mayfield Road, Cleveland, OH, Zip 44124–2202; tel. 440/449–4500; Jeffrey A. Leimgruber, President

HURON HOSPITAL, 13951 Terrace Road, Cleveland, OH, Zip 44112–4399; tel. 216/761–3300; A. Gus Kious, M.D., Chief Administrative Officer

LAKEWOOD HOSPITAL, 14519 Detroit Avenue, Lakewood, OH, Zip 44107–4383; tel. 216/521–4200; Jack D. Gustin, President

LUTHERAN HOSPITAL, 1730 West 25th Street, Cleveland, OH, Zip 44113–3170; tel. 216/696–4300; David Perse, M.D., President

MARYMOUNT HOSPITAL, 12300 McCracken Road, Garfield Heights, OH, Zip 44125–2975; tel. 216/581–0500; David J. Kilarski, President and Chief Executive Officer

METROHEALTH MEDICAL CENTER, 2500 MetroHealth Drive, Cleveland, OH, Zip 44109–1998; tel. 216/778–7800; Mark J. Moran, Interim President and Chief Executive Officer

PARMA COMMUNITY GENERAL HOSPITAL, 7007 Powers Boulevard, Parma, OH, Zip 44129–5495; tel. 440/743–3000; Patricia A. Ruflin, President and Chief Executive Officer

SOUTH POINTE HOSPITAL, 20000 Harvard Road, Warrensville Heights, OH, Zip 44122–7099; tel. 216/491–6000; David J. Kilarski, President and Chief Executive Officer

ST. ELIZABETH HEALTH CENTER, 1044 Belmont Avenue, Youngstown, OH, Zip 44504–1096, Mailing Address: P.O. Box 1790, Zip 44501–1790; tel. 330/746–7211; Robert W. Shroder, President and Chief Executive Officer

ST. JOSEPH HEALTH CENTER, 667 Eastland Avenue S.E., Warren, OH, Zip 44484–4531; tel. 330/841–4000; Robert W. Shroder, President and Chief Executive Officer

SUMMA BARBERTON CITIZENS HOSPITAL, 155 Fifth Street N.E., Barberton, OH, Zip 44203–3332; tel. 330/615–3000; Willard P. Roderick, Chief Executive Officer

SUMMA HEALTH SYSTEM, Akron, OH, Thomas J. Strauss, President and Chief Executive Officer

WADSWORTH–RITTMAN HOSPITAL, 195 Wadsworth Road, Wadsworth, OH, Zip 44281–9505; tel. 330/334–1504; James W. Pope, FACHE, President and Chief Executive Officer

COMPREHENSIVE HEALTHCARE OF OHIO, INC.
630 East River Street, Elyria, OH 44035; tel. 440/329–7700; Kevin Martin, President and Chief Executive Officer

AMHERST HOSPITAL, 254 Cleveland Avenue, Amherst, OH, Zip 44001–1620; tel. 440/988–6000; Kevin C. Martin, President and Chief Executive Officer

EMH REGIONAL MEDICAL CENTER, 630 East River Street, Elyria, OH, Zip 44035–5902; tel. 440/329–7500; Kevin C. Martin, President and Chief Executive Officer

LAKE HOSPITAL SYSTEM
10 East Washington, Painesville, OH 44077; tel. 440/354–2400; Cynthia Moore–Hardy, President and Chief Executive Officer

LAKE HOSPITAL SYSTEM, 10 East Washington, Painesville, OH, Zip 44077–3472; tel. 440/354–2400; Cynthia Ann Moore–Hardy, President and Chief Executive Officer

MERCY HEALTH PARTNERS – SOUTHWEST OHIO
4600 McAuley Place, Cincinnati, OH 45242; tel. 513/981–6000; James May, President and Chief Executive Officer

MERCY HOSPITAL ANDERSON, 7500 State Road, Cincinnati, OH, Zip 45255–2492; tel. 513/624–4500; Patricia A. Schroer, President and Chief Executive Officer

MERCY HOSPITAL CLERMONT, 3000 Hospital Drive, Batavia, OH, Zip 45103–1921; tel. 513/732–8200; Gayle M. Heintzelman, President and Chief Executive Officer

MERCY HOSPITAL FAIRFIELD, 3000 Mack Road, Fairfield, OH, Zip 45014; tel. 513/870–7000; Thomas S. Urban, President and Chief Executive Officer

MERCY HOSPITAL MOUNT AIRY, 2446 Kipling Avenue, Cincinnati, OH, Zip 45239–6650; tel. 513/853–5000; Paul C. Hiltz, President and Chief Executive Officer

MERCY HOSPITAL WESTERN HILLS, 3131 Queen City Avenue, Cincinnati, OH, Zip 45238–2396; tel. 513/389–5000; Patrick A. Kowalski, President and Chief Executive Officer

NORTHWEST OHIO SHARED SERVICES
2200 Jefferson Avenue, Toledo, OH 43624; tel. 419/251–2138; Scott Fry, President and Chief Executive Officer

BELLEVUE HOSPITAL, 1400 West Main Street, Bellevue, OH, Zip 44811–1028, Mailing Address: P.O. Box 8004, Zip 44811–8004; tel. 419/483–4040; Michael K. Winthrop, President

FIRELANDS REGIONAL HEALTH SYSTEM, 1111 Hayes Avenue, Sandusky, OH, Zip 44870; tel. 419/557–7400; Charles A. Stark, FACHE, President and Chief Executive Officer

FISHER–TITUS MEDICAL CENTER, 272 Benedict Avenue, Norwalk, OH, Zip 44857–2374; tel. 419/668–8101; Patrick J. Martin, President and Chief Executive Officer

FULTON COUNTY HEALTH CENTER, 725 South Shoop Avenue, Wauseon, OH, Zip 43567–1701; tel. 419/335–2015; E. Dean Beck, Administrator

HENRY COUNTY HOSPITAL, 11600 State Route 424, Napoleon, OH, Zip 43545–9399; tel. 419/592–4015; Kimberly Bordenkircher, Chief Executive Officer

MEMORIAL HOSPITAL, 715 South Taft Avenue, Fremont, OH, Zip 43420–3200; tel. 419/332–7321; John A. Gorman, Chief Executive Officer

MERCY HOSPITAL OF TIFFIN, 45 St. Lawrence Drive, Tiffin, OH, Zip 44883–0727; tel. 419/447–3130; Dale E. Thornton, M.P.H., CHE, President and Chief Executive Officer

MERCY HOSPITAL OF WILLARD, 110 East Howard Street, Willard, OH, Zip 44890–1611; tel. 419/964–5000; Robert E. Gospodarek, President and Chief Executive Officer

ST. ANNE MERCY HOSPITAL, 3404 West Sylvania Avenue, Toledo, OH, Zip 43623; tel. 419/407–2663; Richard R. Evens, President and Chief Executive Officer

ST. CHARLES MERCY HOSPITAL, 2600 Navarre Avenue, Oregon, OH, Zip 43616–3297; tel. 419/696–7200; Carol A. Whittaker, President and Chief Executive Officer

ST. LUKE'S HOSPITAL, 5901 Monclova Road, Maumee, OH, Zip 43537–1899; tel. 419/893–5911; Daniel L. Wakeman, President and Chief Executive Officer

ST. VINCENT MERCY MEDICAL CENTER, 2213 Cherry Street, Toledo, OH, Zip 43608–2691; tel. 419/251–3232; Michael L. McEachern, President and Chief Executive Officer

THE UNIVERSITY OF TOLEDO MEDICAL CENTER, 3000 Arlington Avenue, Toledo, OH, Zip 43614–5805; tel. 419/383–4000; Mark J. Chastang, Executive Director

WOOD COUNTY HOSPITAL, 950 West Wooster Street, Bowling Green, OH, Zip 43402–2603; tel. 419/354–8900; Stanley R. Korducki, President

OHIO STATE HEALTH NETWORK
660 Ackerman Rd. Suite 601F, Columbus, OH 43218; tel. 614/293–3756; Joann Ort, Executive Director

BARNESVILLE HOSPITAL ASSOCIATION, 639 West Main Street, Barnesville, OH, Zip 43713–0309, Mailing Address: P.O. Box 309, Zip 43713–0309; tel. 740/425–3941; Richard L. Doan, CHE, Chief Executive Officer

BUCYRUS COMMUNITY HOSPITAL, 629 North Sandusky Avenue, Bucyrus, OH, Zip 44820–1821; tel. 419/562–4677; Gerard D. Klein, President and Chief Executive Officer

MADISON COUNTY HOSPITAL, 210 North Main Street, London, OH, Zip 43140–1115; tel. 740/845–7000; Fred L. Kolb, Chief Executive Officer

MARY RUTAN HOSPITAL, 205 Palmer Avenue, Bellefontaine, OH, Zip 43311–2281; tel. 937/592–4015; Mandy C. Goble, President and Chief Executive Officer

MERCER COUNTY JOINT TOWNSHIP COMMUNITY HOSPITAL, 800 West Main Street, Coldwater, OH, Zip 45828–1698; tel. 419/678–2341; James A. Wermert, Chief Executive Officer

OHIO STATE UNIVERSITY MEDICAL CENTER, 370 West 9th Avenue, Columbus, OH, Zip 43210–1240; tel. 614/293–8000; Peter E. Geier, Chief Operating Officer

TWIN CITY HOSPITAL, 819 North First Street, Dennison, OH, Zip 44621–1098; tel. 740/922–2800; Marge Jentes, Chief Executive Officer

WYANDOT MEMORIAL HOSPITAL, 885 North Sandusky Avenue, Upper Sandusky, OH, Zip 43351–1098; tel. 419/294–4991; Joseph A. D'Ettorre, Chief Executive Officer

TRIHEALTH INC.
619 Oak Street Corporate Administration, Cincinnati, OH 45206; tel. 513/569–6507; John Prout, President and Chief Executive Officer

BETHESDA NORTH HOSPITAL, 10500 Montgomery Road, Cincinnati, OH, Zip 45242–4402; tel. 513/745–1111; John S. Prout, President and Chief Executive Officer

GOOD SAMARITAN HOSPITAL, 375 Dixmyth Avenue, Cincinnati, OH, Zip 45220–2489; tel. 513/872–1400; John S. Prout, President and Chief Executive Officer

WEST CENTRAL OHIO REGIONAL HEALTHCARE ALLIANCE, LLC
2615 Ft. Amanda Road, Lima, OH 45804; tel. 419/226–9085; Robin Johnson, Executive Director

JOINT TOWNSHIP DISTRICT MEMORIAL HOSPITAL, 200 St. Clair Street, Saint Marys, OH, Zip 45885–2400; tel. 419/394–3335; Kevin W. Harlan, President

MARY RUTAN HOSPITAL, 205 Palmer Avenue, Bellefontaine, OH, Zip 43311–2281; tel. 937/592–4015; Mandy C. Goble, President and Chief Executive Officer

MERCER COUNTY JOINT TOWNSHIP COMMUNITY HOSPITAL, 800 West Main Street, Coldwater, OH, Zip 45828–1698; tel. 419/678–2341; James A. Wermert, Chief Executive Officer

ST. RITA'S MEDICAL CENTER, 730 West Market Street, Lima, OH, Zip 45801–4670; tel. 419/227–3361; James P. Reber, President and Chief Executive Officer

VAN WERT COUNTY HOSPITAL, 1250 South Washington Street, Van Wert, OH, Zip 45891–2599; tel. 419/238–2390; Mark J. Minick, President and Chief Executive Officer

OKLAHOMA

MERCY HEALTH SYSTEM OF OKLAHOMA
4300 West Memorial Road, Oklahoma City, OK 73120; tel. 405/752–3756; Diana Smalleg, President and Chief Executive Officer

MERCY HEALTH CENTER, 4300 West Memorial Road, Oklahoma City, OK, Zip 73120–8362; tel. 405/755–1515; Diana Smalley, President

MERCY MEMORIAL HEALTH CENTER, 1011 14th Avenue N.W., Ardmore, OK, Zip 73401–1889; tel. 580/223–5400; Bobby G. Thompson, President and Chief Executive Officer

OKLAHOMA HEART HOSPITAL, 4050 West Memorial Road, Oklahoma City, OK, Zip 73120; tel. 405/608–3200; John Harvey, M.D., Chief Executive Officer

OREGON

HEALTH FUTURE, LLC
777 Murphy Road, Medford, OR 97504; tel. 541/772–3062; Mary Kay Chess, Executive Director

BAY AREA HOSPITAL, 1775 Thompson Road, Coos Bay, OR, Zip 97420–2198; tel. 541/269–8111; Daniel L. Smith, President and Chief Executive Officer

CASCADE HEALTHCARE COMMUNITY ST. CHARLES MEDICAL CENTER – BEND, 2500 N.E. Neff Road, Bend, OR, Zip 97701–6015; tel. 541/382–4321; James A. Diegel, FACHE, President and Chief Executive Officer

CASCADE HEALTHCARE COMMUNITY ST. CHARLES MEDICAL CENTER – REDMOND, 1253 North Canal Boulevard, Redmond, OR, Zip 97756–1395; tel. 541/548–8131; James A. Diegel, FACHE, President and Chief Executive Officer

COQUILLE VALLEY HOSPITAL, 940 East Fifth Street, Coquille, OR, Zip 97423–1699; tel. 541/396–3101; Dennis G. Zielinski, Chief Executive Officer and Administrator

GOOD SHEPHERD HEALTHCARE SYSTEM, 610 N.W. 11th Street, Hermiston, OR, Zip 97838–9696; tel. 541/667–3400; Dennis E. Burke, President

GRANDE RONDE HOSPITAL, 900 Sunset Drive, La Grande, OR, Zip 97850–1362, Mailing Address: P.O. Box 3290, Zip 97850–3290; tel. 541/963–8421; James A. Mattes, President and Chief Executive Officer

IDAHO FALLS RECOVERY CENTER, 1957 East 17th Street, Idaho Falls, ID, Zip 83404–6429; tel. 208/529–5285; Lindee Hokanson, Administrator

LAKE DISTRICT HOSPITAL, 700 South J Street, Lakeview, OR, Zip 97630–1679; tel. 541/947–2114; Gordon Ensley, Chief Executive Officer

LODI MEMORIAL HOSPITAL, 975 South Fairmont Avenue, Lodi, CA, Zip 95240–5179, Mailing Address: P.O. Box 3004, Zip 95241–1908; tel. 209/334–3411; Joseph P. Harrington, Chief Executive Officer

MID–COLUMBIA MEDICAL CENTER, 1700 East 19th Street, The Dalles, OR, Zip 97058–3316; tel. 541/296–1111; Duane Francis, President

OHSU HOSPITAL, 3181 S.W. Sam Jackson Park Road, Portland, OR, Zip 97201–3098; tel. 503/494–8311; Peter F. Rapp, Vice President and Executive Director

ROGUE VALLEY MEDICAL CENTER, 2825 East Barnett Road, Medford, OR, Zip 97504–8332; tel. 541/789–7000; Kent L. Brown, FACHE, Chief Executive Officer

SILVERTON HOSPITAL, 342 Fairview Street, Silverton, OR, Zip 97381–1993; tel. 503/873–1500; Gary W. Pulsipher, Vice President and Chief Executive Officer

SKY LAKES MEDICAL CENTER, 2865 Daggett Avenue, Klamath Falls, OR, Zip 97601–1180; tel. 541/882–6311; Paul R. Stewart, Chief Executive Officer

ST. ANTHONY HOSPITAL, 1601 S.E. Court Avenue, Pendleton, OR, Zip 97801–3297; tel. 541/276–5121; Theodore P. Fox, President and Chief Executive Officer

THREE RIVERS COMMUNITY HOSPITAL AND HEALTH CENTER, 500 S.W. Ramsey Avenue, Grants Pass, OR, Zip 97527; tel. 541/472–7000; Paul Janke, FACHE, Chief Executive Officer

TUALITY HEALTHCARE, 335 S.E. Eighth Avenue, Hillsboro, OR, Zip 97123–4246; tel. 503/681–1111; Richard Stenson, President and Chief Executive Officer

INTERCOMMUNITY HEALTH NETWORK
3600 N.W. Samaritan Drive, Corvallis, OR 97330; tel. 541/768–5377; Larry Mullins, President and Chief Executive Officer

GOOD SAMARITAN REGIONAL MEDICAL CENTER, 3600 N.W. Samaritan Drive, Corvallis, OR, Zip 97330–3737, Mailing Address: P.O. Box 1068, Zip 97339–1068; tel. 541/768–5111; Steven W. Jasperson, Chief Executive Officer

SAMARITAN ALBANY GENERAL HOSPITAL, 1046 West Sixth Avenue, Albany, OR, Zip 97321–1999; tel. 541/812–4000; David G. Triebes, Chief Executive Officer

SAMARITAN LEBANON COMMUNITY HOSPITAL, 525 North Santiam Highway, Lebanon, OR, Zip 97355–4363, Mailing Address: P.O. Box 739, Zip 97355–0739; tel. 541/258–2101; Becky A. Pape, RN, Chief Executive Officer

SAMARITAN NORTH LINCOLN HOSPITAL, 3043 N.E. 28th Street, Lincoln City, OR, Zip 97367–4523, Mailing Address: P.O. Box 767, Zip 97367–0767; tel. 541/994–3661; Sue Massart, Chief Executive Officer

SAMARITAN PACIFIC COMMUNITIES HOSPITAL, 930 S.W. Abbey Street, Newport, OR, Zip 97365–4820, Mailing Address: P.O. Box 945, Zip 97365–4820; tel. 541/265–2244; David C. Bigelow, Chief Executive Officer

PENNSYLVANIA

DUBOIS REGIONAL MEDICAL
P.O. Box 447, DuBois, PA 15801; tel. 814/371–2200; Raymond A. Graeca, President

DUBOIS REGIONAL MEDICAL CENTER, 100 Hospital Avenue, Du Bois, PA, Zip 15801–1440, Mailing Address: P.O. Box 447, Zip 15801–0447; tel. 814/371–2200; Raymond A. Graeca, President and Chief Executive Officer

LAUREL HEALTH SYSTEM
22 Walnut Street, Wellsboro, PA 16901; tel. 570/723–0500; Ronald Butler, President and Chief Executive Officer

SOLDIERS AND SAILORS MEMORIAL HOSPITAL, 32–36 Central Avenue, Wellsboro, PA, Zip 16901–1899; tel. 570/724–1631; Jan E. Fisher, President and Chief Executive Officer

SAINT VINCENT HEALTH SYSTEM
232 West 25th Street, Erie, PA 16544; tel. 814/452–5000; C. Angela Bontempo, Chief Executive Officer

SAINT VINCENT HEALTH CENTER, 232 West 25th Street, Erie, PA, Zip 16544–0002; tel. 814/452–5000; C. Angela Bontempo, President and Chief Executive Officer

WESTFIELD MEMORIAL HOSPITAL, 189 East Main Street, Westfield, NY, Zip 14787–1195; tel. 716/326–4921; C. Angela Bontempo, President and Chief Executive Officer

VANTAGE HEALTHCARE NETWORK, INC.
18282 Technology Dr., Suite 202, Meadville, PA 16335; tel. 814/337–0000; Gerald P. Alonge, Chief Executive Officer and Administrator

BRADFORD REGIONAL MEDICAL CENTER, 116 Interstate Parkway, Bradford, PA, Zip 16701–0218; tel. 814/368–4143; George E. Leonhardt, CHE, President and Chief Executive Officer

BROOKVILLE HOSPITAL, 100 Hospital Road, Brookville, PA, Zip 15825–1367; tel. 814/849–2312; John Sutika, President and Chief Executive Officer

CLARION HOSPITAL, One Hospital Drive, Clarion, PA, Zip 16214–8599; tel. 814/226–9500; Byron Quinton, Chief Executive Officer

CORRY MEMORIAL HOSPITAL, 612 West Smith Street, Corry, PA, Zip 16407–1196; tel. 814/664–4641; Barbara Nichols, RN, President and Chief Executive Officer

DUBOIS REGIONAL MEDICAL CENTER, 100 Hospital Avenue, Du Bois, PA, Zip 15801–1440, Mailing Address: P.O. Box 447, Zip 15801–0447; tel. 814/371–2200; Raymond A. Graeca, President and Chief Executive Officer

ELK REGIONAL HEALTH CENTER, 763 Johnsonburg Road, Saint Marys, PA, Zip 15857–3498; tel. 814/788–8000; Gregory Bauer, President and Chief Executive Officer

ELLWOOD CITY HOSPITAL, 724 Pershing Street, Ellwood City, PA, Zip 16117–1474; tel. 724/752–0081; Raymond J. Beck, President and Chief Executive Officer

HAMOT MEDICAL CENTER, 201 State Street, Erie, PA, Zip 16550–0002; tel. 814/877–6000; John T. Malone, President and Chief Executive Officer

JAMESON HOSPITAL, 1211 Wilmington Avenue, New Castle, PA, Zip 16105–2595; tel. 724/658–9001; Thomas White, President and Chief Executive Officer

KANE COMMUNITY HOSPITAL, 4372 Route 6, Kane, PA, Zip 16735–9654; tel. 814/837–8585; J. Gary Rhodes, FACHE, Chief Executive Officer

MEADVILLE MEDICAL CENTER, 751 Liberty Street, Meadville, PA, Zip 16335–2555; tel. 814/333–5000; Anthony J. DeFail, FACHE, President and Chief Executive Officer

MILLCREEK COMMUNITY HOSPITAL, 5515 Peach Street, Erie, PA, Zip 16509–2695; tel. 814/864–4031; Mary L. Eckert, President and Chief Executive Officer

PUNXSUTAWNEY AREA HOSPITAL, 81 Hillcrest Drive, Punxsutawney, PA, Zip 15767–2616; tel. 814/938–1800; Daniel D. Blough, Jr., Chief Executive Officer

SAINT VINCENT HEALTH CENTER, 232 West 25th Street, Erie, PA, Zip 16544–0002; tel. 814/452–5000; C. Angela Bontempo, President and Chief Executive Officer

TITUSVILLE AREA HOSPITAL, 406 West Oak Street, Titusville, PA, Zip 16354–1404; tel. 814/827–1851; Anthony J. Nasralla, FACHE, President and Chief Executive Officer

UPMC BEDFORD MEMORIAL, 10455 Lincoln Highway, Everett, PA, Zip 15537–7046; tel. 814/623–6161; Roger P. Winn, President

UPMC BRADDOCK, 400 Holland Avenue, Braddock, PA, Zip 15104–1598; tel. 412/636–5000; Cynthia M. Dorundo, President

UPMC HORIZON, Greenville, PA, Neil Yuhas, President

UPMC MCKEESPORT, 1500 Fifth Avenue, McKeesport, PA, Zip 15132–2482; tel. 412/664–2000; Ronald H. Ott, President

UPMC NORTHWEST, 100 Fairfield Drive, Seneca, PA, Zip 16346; tel. 814/676–7600; Neil E. Todhunter, President

UPMC PASSAVANT, 9100 Babcock Boulevard, Pittsburgh, PA, Zip 15237–5815; tel. 412/367–6700; Teresa A. Petrick, President

UPMC PASSAVANT CRANBERRY, One St. Francis Way, Cranberry, PA, Zip 16066; tel. 724/772–5300; Teresa A. Petrick, President

UPMC SOUTH SIDE, 2000 Mary Street, Pittsburgh, PA, Zip 15203–2095; tel. 412/488–5550; Nancy Magee, President

UPMC ST. MARGARET, 815 Freeport Road, Pittsburgh, PA, Zip 15215–3399; tel. 412/784–4000; David T. Martin, President

WARREN GENERAL HOSPITAL, Two Crescent Park West, Warren, PA, Zip 16365–0068, Mailing Address: P.O. Box 68, Zip 16365–0068; tel. 814/723–4973; John P. Papalia, CHE, Chief Executive Officer

SOUTH DAKOTA

REGIONAL HEALTH NETWORK
353 Fairmont Boulevard, P.O. Box 6000, Rapid City, SD 57701; tel. 605/719–1000; Rick Giesel, Chief Executive Officer

BENNETT COUNTY HOSPITAL AND NURSING HOME, 102 Major Allen Street, Martin, SD, Zip 57551, Mailing Address: P.O. Box 70, Zip 57551; tel. 605/685–6622; Joseph Caldwell, Administrator

CAMPBELL COUNTY MEMORIAL HOSPITAL, 501 South Burma Avenue, Gillette, WY, Zip 82716–3426, Mailing Address: P.O. Box 3011, Zip 82717–3011; tel. 307/682–8811; Robert A. Morasko, Chief Executive Officer

CHADRON COMMUNITY HOSPITAL AND HEALTH SERVICES, 821 Morehead Street, Chadron, NE, Zip 69337–2599; tel. 308/432–5586; Harold L. Krueger, Jr., Chief Executive Officer

CROOK COUNTY MEDICAL SERVICES DISTRICT, 713 Oak Street, Sundance, WY, Zip 82729, Mailing Address: P.O. Box 517, Zip 82729–0517; tel. 307/283–3501; Doris Brown, Chief Executive Officer

CUSTER REGIONAL HOSPITAL, 1039 Montgomery Street, Custer, SD, Zip 57730–1397; tel. 605/673–2229; Jason Petik, Chief Executive Officer

FIVE COUNTIES HOSPITAL, 405 Sixth Avenue West, Lemmon, SD, Zip 57638–1318, Mailing Address: P.O. Box 479, Zip 57638–0479; tel. 605/374–3871; Jannette Van Beek, Administrator and Chief Executive Officer

GORDON MEMORIAL HOSPITAL, 300 East Eighth Street, Gordon, NE, Zip 69343–9990; tel. 308/282–0401; Kay Garcia, Chief Executive Officer

LEAD–DEADWOOD REGIONAL HOSPITAL, 61 Charles Street, Deadwood, SD, Zip 57732–1303; tel. 605/722–6101; Sherry Bea Smith, RN, Chief Executive Officer

SPEARFISH REGIONAL HOSPITAL, 1440 North Main Street, Spearfish, SD, Zip 57783–1504; tel. 605/644–4000; Larry W. Veitz, Chief Executive Officer

STURGIS REGIONAL HOSPITAL, 949 Harmon Street, Sturgis, SD, Zip 57785–2452; tel. 605/720–2400; Van Hyde, Chief Executive Officer

U. S. PUBLIC HEALTH SERVICE INDIAN HOSPITAL, Pine Ridge, SD, Mailing Address: P.O. Box 1201, Zip 57770–1201; tel. 605/867–5131; William Pourier, Service Unit Director

WESTON COUNTY HEALTH SERVICES, 1124 Washington Boulevard, Newcastle, WY, Zip 82701–2996; tel. 307/746–4491; Kevin Stiffarm, Chief Executive Officer

TEXAS

HEALTHCARE PARTNERS OF EAST TEXAS, INC
426 N. Center Street, Longview, TX 75601; tel. 903/238–8845; Mark Hobgood, Executive Director

ATLANTA MEMORIAL HOSPITAL, Highway 77 at South William, Atlanta, TX, Zip 75551, Mailing Address: P.O. Box 1049, Zip 75551–1049; tel. 903/799–3000; Tom Crow, Administrator

CHRISTUS ST. MICHAEL HEALTH SYSTEM, 2600 St. Michael Drive, Texarkana, TX, Zip 75503–2372; tel. 903/614–1000; Chris Karam, President and Chief Executive Officer

COZBY–GERMANY HOSPITAL, 707 North Waldrip Street, Grand Saline, TX, Zip 75140–1555; tel. 903/962–4242; Ronald J. Ensor, Chief Executive Officer

DUBUIS HOSPITAL OF TEXARKANA, 2400 St. Michael Drive, 2nd Floor, Texarkana, TX, Zip 75503–2372; tel. 903/614–7600; David L. Adcock, FACHE, Administrator

EAST TEXAS MEDICAL CENTER ATHENS, 2000 South Palestine Street, Athens, TX, Zip 75751–5610; tel. 903/676–1000; Patrick L. Wallace, Administrator

EAST TEXAS MEDICAL CENTER CARTHAGE, 409 Cottage Road, Carthage, TX, Zip 75633–1466, Mailing Address: P.O. Box 549, Zip 75633–0549; tel. 903/693–3841; Gary Mikeal Hudson, Administrator

EAST TEXAS MEDICAL CENTER CLARKSVILLE, 3000 West Main Street, Clarksville, TX, Zip 75426, Mailing Address: P.O. Box 1270, Zip 75426–1270; tel. 903/427–6400; John S. Hart, Administrator

EAST TEXAS MEDICAL CENTER CROCKETT, 1100 Loop 304 East, Crockett, TX, Zip 75835–1810; tel. 936/546–3862; Terry Cutler, Administrator and Chief Operating Officer

EAST TEXAS MEDICAL CENTER FAIRFIELD, 125 Newman Street, Fairfield, TX, Zip 75840–1499; tel. 903/389–2121; Ruth Cook, Administrator

EAST TEXAS MEDICAL CENTER JACKSONVILLE, 501 South Ragsdale Street, Jacksonville, TX, Zip 75766–2413; tel. 903/541–5000; Jack R. Endres, Administrator

EAST TEXAS MEDICAL CENTER PITTSBURG, 414 Quitman Street, Pittsburg, TX, Zip 75686–1032; tel. 903/856–6663; W. Perry Henderson, Administrator

EAST TEXAS MEDICAL CENTER REHABILITATION CENTER, 701 Olympic Plaza Circle, Tyler, TX, Zip 75701–1996; tel. 903/596–3000; Eddie L. Howard, Vice President and Chief Operating Officer

EAST TEXAS MEDICAL CENTER TRINITY, 317 Prospect Drive, Trinity, TX, Zip 75862, Mailing Address: P.O. Box 3169, Zip 75862; tel. 936/594–3541; Warren Robicheaux, Administrator

EAST TEXAS MEDICAL CENTER TYLER, 1000 South Beckham Street, Tyler, TX, Zip 75701–1996, Mailing Address: Box 6400, Zip 75711–6400; tel. 903/597–0351; Robert B. Evans, Administrator and Chief Executive Officer

EAST TEXAS MEDICAL CENTER–MOUNT VERNON, 500 Highway 37 South, Mount Vernon, TX, Zip 75457–3602, Mailing Address: P.O. Box 477, Zip 75457–0477; tel. 903/537–8000; Stephen Pitts, Administrator

EAST TEXAS MEDICAL CENTER–QUITMAN, 117 Winnsboro Street, Quitman, TX, Zip 75783–2144, Mailing Address: P.O. Box 1000, Zip 75783–1000; tel. 903/763–6300; Christopher Stipe, FACHE, Administrator and Chief Executive Officer

GOOD SHEPHERD MEDICAL CENTER, 700 East Marshall Avenue, Longview, TX, Zip 75601–5571; tel. 903/315–2000; Joseph A. Reppert, Vice President and Chief Financial Officer

GOOD SHEPHERD MEDICAL CENTER–LINDEN, 404 North Kaufman Street, Linden, TX, Zip 75563–5235; tel. 903/756–5561; Steven B. Webb, Interim Chief Executive Officer

GOOD SHEPHERD MEDICAL CENTER–MARSHALL, 811 South Washington Avenue, Marshall, TX, Zip 75670–5336, Mailing Address: P.O. Box 1599, Zip 75671–1599; tel. 903/927–6000; Russell J. Collier, President and Chief Executive Officer

HENDERSON MEMORIAL HOSPITAL, 300 Wilson Street, Henderson, TX, Zip 75652–5956; tel. 903/657–7541; Mark Leitner, Chief Executive Officer

HOPKINS COUNTY MEMORIAL HOSPITAL, 115 Airport Road, Sulphur Springs, TX, Zip 75482–0115; tel. 903/885–7671; Michael McAndrew, Chief Executive Officer

HOWARD MEMORIAL HOSPITAL, 800 West Leslie Street, Nashville, AR, Zip 71852–0381, Mailing Address: P.O. Box 381, Zip 71852–0381; tel. 870/845–4400; Brian E. Bickel, President and Chief Executive Officer

HUNTSVILLE MEMORIAL HOSPITAL, 110 Memorial Hospital Drive, Huntsville, TX, Zip 77340–4362, Mailing Address: P.O. Box 4001, Zip 77342–4001; tel. 936/291–3411; Sally I. Nelson, Chief Executive Officer

LAIRD MEMORIAL HOSPITAL, 1612 South Henderson Boulevard, Kilgore, TX, Zip 75662–3594; tel. 903/984–3505; Bob S. Ellzey, FACHE, President and Chief Executive Officer

LITTLE RIVER MEMORIAL HOSPITAL, 451 West Locke Street, Ashdown, AR, Zip 71822–3398; tel. 870/898–5011; David Deaton, Administrator and Chief Executive Officer

MAGNOLIA HOSPITAL, 101 Hospital Drive, Magnolia, AR, Zip 71753–2416, Mailing Address: P.O. Box 629, Zip 71753–0629; tel. 870/235–3000; Terry L. Amstutz, FACHE, Chief Executive Officer

MCCURTAIN MEMORIAL HOSPITAL, 1301 Lincoln Road, Idabel, OK, Zip 74745–7341; tel. 580/286–7623; Bristol Messer, Chief Executive Officer

MEMORIAL HEALTH SYSTEM OF EAST TEXAS, 1201 West Frank Avenue, Lufkin, TX, Zip 75904–3357, Mailing Address: P.O. Box 1447, Zip 75902–1447; tel. 936/634–8111; Bryant H. Krenek, Jr., President and Chief Executive Officer

MEMORIAL MEDICAL CENTER – LIVINGSTON, 1717 Highway 59 Bypass, Livingston, TX, Zip 77351–1257, Mailing Address: P.O. Box 1257, Zip 77351–1257; tel. 936/329–8700; David LeMonte, Chief Executive Officer

MEMORIAL MEDICAL CENTER – SAN AUGUSTINE, 511 East Hospital Street, San Augustine, TX, Zip 75972–2121, Mailing Address: P.O. Box 658, Zip 75972–0658; tel. 936/275–3446; Darlene Williams, RN, Administrator

NACOGDOCHES MEMORIAL HOSPITAL, 1204 North Mound Street, Nacogdoches, TX, Zip 75961–4061; tel. 936/564–4611; Tim Hayward, Administrator

PALESTINE REGIONAL MEDICAL CENTER–EAST, 2900 South Loop 256, Palestine, TX, Zip 75801–6958; tel. 903/731–1000; Tim Flusche, Chief Executive Officer

PARIS REGIONAL MEDICAL CENTER, 820 Clarksville Street, Paris, TX, Zip 75460–9070; tel. 903/785–4521; Christopher W. Dux, Chief Executive Officer

SABINE COUNTY HOSPITAL, Highway 83 West, Hemphill, TX, Zip 75948, Mailing Address: P.O. Box 750, Zip 75948–0750; tel. 409/787–3300; Deanna Lathrop, Interim Chief Executive Officer

SHELBY REGIONAL MEDICAL CENTER, 602 Hurst Street, Center, TX, Zip 75935–3414, Mailing Address: P.O. Box 1749, Zip 75935–1749; tel. 936/598–2781; Gary L. Stokes, Chief Executive Officer

TITUS REGIONAL MEDICAL CENTER, 2001 North Jefferson Avenue, Mount Pleasant, TX, Zip 75455–2398; tel. 903/577–6000; Ronald D. Davis, Chief Executive Officer

TYLER COUNTY HOSPITAL, 1100 West Bluff Street, Woodville, TX, Zip 75979–4799, Mailing Address: P.O. Box 549, Zip 75979–0549; tel. 409/283–8141; Gayle D. Wright, Chief Executive Officer

REGIONAL HEALTHCARE ALLIANCE
530 S. Beckham, Tyler, TX 75701; tel. 903/531–4449; John Webb, President

ATLANTA MEMORIAL HOSPITAL, Highway 77 at South William, Atlanta, TX, Zip 75551, Mailing Address: P.O. Box 1049, Zip 75551–1049; tel. 903/799–3000; Tom Crow, Administrator

BAYLOR UNIVERSITY MEDICAL CENTER, 3500 Gaston Avenue, Dallas, TX, Zip 75246–2088; tel. 214/820–0111; John B. McWhorter, III, President

CHILDREN'S MEDICAL CENTER OF DALLAS, 1935 Medical District Drive, Dallas, TX, Zip 75235–7794; tel. 214/456–7000; Christopher J. Durovich, President and Chief Executive Officer

COZBY–GERMANY HOSPITAL, 707 North Waldrip Street, Grand Saline, TX, Zip 75140–1555; tel. 903/962–4242; Ronald J. Ensor, Chief Executive Officer

GOOD SHEPHERD MEDICAL CENTER, 700 East Marshall Avenue, Longview, TX, Zip 75601–5571; tel. 903/315–2000; Joseph A. Reppert, Vice President and Chief Financial Officer

GOOD SHEPHERD MEDICAL CENTER–LINDEN, 404 North Kaufman Street, Linden, TX, Zip 75563–5235; tel. 903/756–5561; Steven B. Webb, Interim Chief Executive Officer

HENDERSON MEMORIAL HOSPITAL, 300 Wilson Street, Henderson, TX, Zip 75652–5956; tel. 903/657–7541; Mark Leitner, Chief Executive Officer

HOPKINS COUNTY MEMORIAL HOSPITAL, 115 Airport Road, Sulphur Springs, TX, Zip 75482–0115; tel. 903/885–7671; Michael McAndrew, Chief Executive Officer

LAIRD MEMORIAL HOSPITAL, 1612 South Henderson Boulevard, Kilgore, TX, Zip 75662–3594; tel. 903/984–3505; Bob S. Ellzey, FACHE, President and Chief Executive Officer

MOTHER FRANCES HOSPITAL – JACKSONVILLE, 2026 South Jackson, Jacksonville, TX, Zip 75766; tel. 903/541–4500; Thomas N. Cammack, Jr., Chief Administrative Officer

NACOGDOCHES MEDICAL CENTER, 4920 N.E. Stallings, Nacogdoches, TX, Zip 75965–1200, Mailing Address: P.O. Box 631604, Zip 75963–1604; tel. 936/569–9481; Gary L. Stokes, Chief Executive Officer

PALESTINE REGIONAL MEDICAL CENTER–EAST, 2900 South Loop 256, Palestine, TX, Zip 75801–6958; tel. 903/731–1000; Tim Flusche, Chief Executive Officer

PARIS REGIONAL MEDICAL CENTER, 820 Clarksville Street, Paris, TX, Zip 75460–9070; tel. 903/785–4521; Christopher W. Dux, Chief Executive Officer

TITUS REGIONAL MEDICAL CENTER, 2001 North Jefferson Avenue, Mount Pleasant, TX, Zip 75455–2398; tel. 903/577–6000; Ronald D. Davis, Chief Executive Officer

TRINITY MOTHER FRANCES HEALTH SYSTEM, 910 East Houston, Suite 500, Tyler, TX, Zip 75702–8369; tel. 903/593–8441; J. Lindsey Bradley, Jr., FACHE, President and Chief Administrative Officer

TRINITY MOTHER FRANCES REHABILITATION HOSPITAL, 3131 Troup Highway, Tyler, TX, Zip 75701–8352; tel. 903/510–7000; Sharla Anderson, Chief Executive Officer

TYLER CONTINUECARE HOSPITAL AT MOTHER FRANCES, 800 East Dawson, 4th Floor, Tyler, TX, Zip 75701; tel. 903/531–4942; Carl Lutz, Interim Chief Executive Officer

UNIVERSITY OF TEXAS HEALTH SCIENCE CENTER AT TYLER, 11937 Highway 271, Tyler, TX, Zip 75708–3154; tel. 903/877–3451; Kirk A. Calhoun, M.D., President

ST. DAVID'S HEALTH NETWORK
98 San Jacinto Blvd., Austin, TX 78701; tel. 512/708–9700; Jon M. Foster, Chief Executive Officer

ST. DAVID'S GEORGETOWN HOSPITAL, 2000 Scenic Drive, Georgetown, TX, Zip 78626–7793; tel. 512/943–3000; Hugh Brown, Chief Executive Officer

ST. DAVID'S MEDICAL CENTER, 919 East 32nd Street, Austin, TX, Zip 78705–2709, Mailing Address: P.O. Box 4039, Zip 78765–4039; tel. 512/476–7111; C. David Huffstutler, President

ST. DAVID'S NORTH AUSTIN MEDICAL CENTER, 12221 MoPac Expressway North, Austin, TX, Zip 78758–2496; tel. 512/901–1000; Donald H. Wilkerson, Chief Executive Officer

ST. DAVID'S REHABILITATION CENTER, 1005 East 32nd Street, Austin, TX, Zip 78705–2705, Mailing Address: P.O. Box 4270, Zip 78765–4270; tel. 512/867–5100; Diane Owens, Administrator

ST. DAVID'S ROUND ROCK MEDICAL CENTER, 2400 Round Rock Avenue, Round Rock, TX, Zip 78681–4097; tel. 512/341–1000; Deborah L. Ryle, Administrator and Chief Executive Officer

ST. DAVID'S SOUTH AUSTIN HOSPITAL, 901 West Ben White Boulevard, Austin, TX, Zip 78704–6903; tel. 512/447–2211; Erol R. Akdamar, Chief Executive Officer

VIRGINIA

CENTRAL VIRGINIA HEALTH NETWORK
2201 West Broad Street Suite 202, Richmond, VA 23220; tel. 804/359–4500; Michael Matthews, Chief Executive Officer

BON SECOURS ST. MARY'S HOSPITAL, 5801 Bremo Road, Richmond, VA, Zip 23226–1907; tel. 804/285–2011; Michael K. Kerner, Executive Vice President and Administrator

BON SECOURS–RICHMOND COMMUNITY HOSPITAL, 1500 North 28th Street, Richmond, VA, Zip 23223–5396, Mailing Address: P.O. Box 27184, Zip 23261–7184; tel. 804/225–1700; Michael Robinson, Executive Vice President and Administrator

COMMUNITY MEMORIAL HEALTHCENTER, 125 Buena Vista Circle, South Hill, VA, Zip 23970–0090, Mailing Address: P.O. Box 90, Zip 23970–0090; tel. 434/447–3151; W. Scott Burnette, President and Chief Executive Officer

MEMORIAL REGIONAL MEDICAL CENTER, 8260 Atlee Road, Mechanicsville, VA, Zip 23116–1844; tel. 804/764–6000; Michael Robinson, Executive Vice President and Administrator

RAPPAHANNOCK GENERAL HOSPITAL, 101 Harris Drive, Kilmarnock, VA, Zip 22482, Mailing Address: P.O. Box 1449, Zip 22482–1449; tel. 804/435–8000; James M. Holmes, Jr., President and Chief Executive Officer

SHELTERING ARMS REHABILITATION HOSPITAL, 8254 Atlee Road, Mechanicsville, VA, Zip 23116–1844; tel. 804/764–7055; James E. Sok, FACHE, President and Chief Executive Officer

SOUTHSIDE COMMUNITY HOSPITAL, 800 Oak Street, Farmville, VA, Zip 23901–1199; tel. 434/392–8811; Gwen S. Eddleman, FACHE, Ed.D., President and Chief Executive Officer

UNIVERSITY OF VIRGINIA MEDICAL CENTER, 1215 Lee Street, Charlottesville, VA, Zip 22908–0001, Mailing Address: P.O. Box 800809, Zip 22908–0809; tel. 434/924–0211; R. Edward Howell, Vice President and Chief Executive Officer

VIRGINIA HEALTH NETWORK
7400 Beaufont Springs Drive, Suite 505, Richmond, VA 23225; tel. 804/320–3837; James Brittain, President

ALLEGHANY REGIONAL HOSPITAL, One ARH Lane, Low Moor, VA, Zip 24457, Mailing Address: P.O. Box 7, Zip 24457–0007; tel. 540/862–6011; Timothy C. Tobin, President and Chief Executive Officer

AUGUSTA HEALTH CARE, 78 Medical Center Drive, Fishersville, VA, Zip 22939–2332, Mailing Address: P.O. Box 1000, Zip 22939–1000; tel. 540/932–4000; Mary N. Mannix, President and Chief Executive Officer

BATH COMMUNITY HOSPITAL, 83 Park Drive, Hot Springs, VA, Zip 24445, Mailing Address: P.O. Drawer Z, Zip 24445; tel. 540/839–7000; Deborah Lipes, RN, Chief Executive Officer

BEDFORD MEMORIAL HOSPITAL, 1613 Oakwood Street, Bedford, VA, Zip 24523–0688, Mailing Address: P.O. Box 688, Zip 24523–0688; tel. 540/586–2441; Georgia Watts, Interim Chief Executive Officer

BON SECOURS ST. FRANCIS MEDICAL CENTER, 13710 St. Francis Boulevard, Midlothian, VA, Zip 23114; tel. 804/594–7300; Teresa Edwards, Executive Vice President and Administrator

BON SECOURS ST. MARY'S HOSPITAL, 5801 Bremo Road, Richmond, VA, Zip 23226–1907; tel. 804/285–2011; Michael K. Kerner, Executive Vice President and Administrator

BON SECOURS–DEPAUL MEDICAL CENTER, 150 Kingsley Lane, Norfolk, VA, Zip 23505–4650; tel. 757/889–5000; Daniel Duggan, Executive Vice President and Administrator

BON SECOURS–RICHMOND COMMUNITY HOSPITAL, 1500 North 28th Street, Richmond, VA, Zip 23223–5396, Mailing Address: P.O. Box 27184, Zip 23261–7184; tel. 804/225–1700; Michael Robinson, Executive Vice President and Administrator

BUCHANAN GENERAL HOSPITAL, Grundy, VA, Mailing Address: Route 5, Box 20, Zip 24614–9611; tel. 276/935–1000; Joan Jamison, Chief Executive Officer

CARILION FRANKLIN MEMORIAL HOSPITAL, 180 Floyd Avenue, Rocky Mount, VA, Zip 24151–1389; tel. 540/483–5277; William D. Jacobsen, Chief Executive Officer

CARILION GILES MEMORIAL HOSPITAL, 1 Taylor Avenue, Pearisburg, VA, Zip 24134–1932; tel. 540/921–6000; James E. Tyler, Vice President and Administrator

CARILION MEDICAL CENTER, Belleview at Jefferson Street, Roanoke, VA, Zip 24014, Mailing Address: P.O. Box 13367, Zip 24033–3367; tel. 540/981–7000; Edward G. Murphy, M.D., President and Chief Executive Officer

CARILION NEW RIVER VALLEY MEDICAL CENTER, 2900 Lamb Circle, Christiansburg, VA, Zip 24073–5041, Mailing Address: P.O. Box 5, Radford, Zip 24143; tel. 540/731–2000; Don Halliwill, President and Administrator

CARILION STONEWALL JACKSON HOSPITAL, 1 Health Circle, Lexington, VA, Zip 24450–2492; tel. 540/458–3300; Thomas W. McNamara, D.O., President and Chief Executive Officer

CHESAPEAKE GENERAL HOSPITAL, 736 Battlefield Boulevard North, Chesapeake, VA, Zip 23320–4941, Mailing Address: P.O. Box 2028, Zip 23327–2028; tel. 757/312–8121; Christopher R. Mosley, President and Chief Executive Officer

CHILDREN'S HOSPITAL, 2924 Brook Road, Richmond, VA, Zip 23220–1298; tel. 804/321–7474; Leslie G. Wyatt, President and Chief Executive Officer

CHILDREN'S HOSPITAL OF THE KING'S DAUGHTERS, 601 Children's Lane, Norfolk, VA, Zip 23507–1969; tel. 757/668–7000; James D. Dahling, President and Chief Executive Officer

CJW MEDICAL CENTER, 7101 Jahnke Road, Richmond, VA, Zip 23225–4044; tel. 804/320–3911; Peter A. Marmerstein, Chief Executive Officer

CLINCH VALLEY MEDICAL CENTER, 2949 West Front Street, Richlands, VA, Zip 24641–2099; tel. 276/596–6000; David B. Darden, Chief Executive Officer

COMMUNITY MEMORIAL HEALTHCENTER, 125 Buena Vista Circle, South Hill, VA, Zip 23970–0090, Mailing Address: P.O. Box 90, Zip 23970–0090; tel. 434/447–3151; W. Scott Burnette, President and Chief Executive Officer

CULPEPER REGIONAL HOSPITAL, 501 Sunset Lane, Culpeper, VA, Zip 22701–3917, Mailing Address: Box 592, Zip 22701–0592; tel. 540/829–4100; H. Lee Kirk, Jr., President and Chief Executive Officer

DOMINION HOSPITAL, 2960 Sleepy Hollow Road, Falls Church, VA, Zip 22044–2001; tel. 703/536–2000; Suzanne B. Jackson, Chief Executive Officer

FAUQUIER HOSPITAL, 500 Hospital Drive, Warrenton, VA, Zip 20186–3099; tel. 540/316–5000; Rodger H. Baker, President and Chief Executive Officer

HEALTHSOUTH REHABILITATION HOSPITAL OF VIRGINIA, 5700 Fitzhugh Avenue, Richmond, VA, Zip 23226–1877; tel. 804/288–5700; Jeff Ruskan, II, Chief Executive Officer

HENRICO DOCTORS' HOSPITAL, 1602 Skipwith Road, Richmond, VA, Zip 23229–5205; tel. 804/289–4500; David Williams, Chief Executive Officer

INOVA ALEXANDRIA HOSPITAL, 4320 Seminary Road, Alexandria, VA, Zip 22304–1594; tel. 703/504–3000; Christine Candio, Chief Executive Officer

INOVA FAIR OAKS HOSPITAL, 3600 Joseph Siewick Drive, Fairfax, VA, Zip 22033–1798; tel. 703/391–3600; John L. Fitzgerald, Chief Executive Officer

INOVA FAIRFAX HOSPITAL, 3300 Gallows Road, Falls Church, VA, Zip 22042–3300; tel. 703/776–4001; Reuven Pasternak, M.D., Chief Executive Officer

INOVA LOUDOUN HOSPITAL, 44045 Riverside Parkway, Leesburg, VA, Zip 20176–2799, Mailing Address: P.O. Box 6000, Zip 20176–6000; tel. 703/858–6000; Randall L. Kelley, Chief Executive Officer

INOVA MOUNT VERNON HOSPITAL, 2501 Parker's Lane, Alexandria, VA, Zip 22306; tel. 703/664–7000; Barbara J. Doyle, Senior Vice President and Chief Executive Officer

JOHN RANDOLPH MEDICAL CENTER, 411 West Randolph Road, Hopewell, VA, Zip 23860–2938; tel. 804/541–1600; Elwood Bernard Boone, III, Chief Executive Officer

JOHNSTON MEMORIAL HOSPITAL, 351 Court Street N.E., Abingdon, VA, Zip 24210–2955; tel. 276/676–7000; Sean S. McMurray, FACHE, Chief Executive Officer

MARTHA JEFFERSON HOSPITAL, 459 Locust Avenue, Charlottesville, VA, Zip 22902–9940; tel. 434/982–7000; James E. Haden, President and Chief Executive Officer

MARY IMMACULATE HOSPITAL, 2 Bernardine Drive, Newport News, VA, Zip 23602–4499; tel. 757/886–6000; Patricia L. Robertson, Executive Vice President and Administrator

MARY WASHINGTON HOSPITAL, 1001 Sam Perry Boulevard, Fredericksburg, VA, Zip 22401–3354; tel. 540/741–1100; Fred M. Rankin, III, President and Chief Executive Officer

MARYVIEW MEDICAL CENTER, 3636 High Street, Portsmouth, VA, Zip 23707–3270; tel. 757/398–2200; Susan MacLeod, Executive Vice President

MEMORIAL HOSPITAL, 320 Hospital Drive, Martinsville, VA, Zip 24112–1981, Mailing Address: P.O. Box 4788, Zip 24115–4788; tel. 276/666–7200; Joseph Roach, Chief Executive Officer

MEMORIAL REGIONAL MEDICAL CENTER, 8260 Atlee Road, Mechanicsville, VA, Zip 23116–1844; tel. 804/764–6000; Michael Robinson, Executive Vice President and Administrator

MOUNT REGIS CENTER, 405 Kimball Avenue, Salem, VA, Zip 24153–6299; tel. 540/389–4761; Gail S. Basham, Chief Executive Officer

MOUNTAIN VIEW REGIONAL MEDICAL CENTER, Third Street N.E., Norton, VA, Zip 24273–1131, Mailing Address: P.O. Box 620, Zip 24273–0620; tel. 276/679–9100; David L. Brash, Chief Executive Officer

NORTHERN HOSPITAL OF SURRY COUNTY, 830 Rockford Street, Mount Airy, NC, Zip 27030–5365, Mailing Address: P.O. Box 1101, Zip 27030–1101; tel. 336/719–7000; William B. James, Chief Executive Officer

POTOMAC HOSPITAL, 2300 Opitz Boulevard, Woodbridge, VA, Zip 22191–3399; tel. 703/670–1313; William Mason Moss, President

PRINCE WILLIAM HOSPITAL, 8700 Sudley Road, Manassas, VA, Zip 20110–4418, Mailing Address: P.O. Box 2610, Zip 20108–0867; tel. 703/369–8000; Michael J. Schwartz, President and Chief Executive Officer

PULASKI COMMUNITY HOSPITAL, 2400 Lee Highway, Pulaski, VA, Zip 24301–0759, Mailing Address: P.O. Box 759, Zip 24301–0759; tel. 540/994–8100; W. Mark Rader, Chief Executive Officer

R. J. REYNOLDS–PATRICK COUNTY MEMORIAL HOSPITAL, 18688 Jeb Stuart Highway, Stuart, VA, Zip 24171–1559; tel. 276/694–3151; Janice F. Wilkins, Administrator

RAPPAHANNOCK GENERAL HOSPITAL, 101 Harris Drive, Kilmarnock, VA, Zip 22482, Mailing Address: P.O. Box 1449, Zip 22482–1449; tel. 804/435–8000; James M. Holmes, Jr., President and Chief Executive Officer

RESTON HOSPITAL CENTER, 1850 Town Center Parkway, Reston, VA, Zip 20190–3210; tel. 703/689–9000; William A. Adams, President and Chief Executive Officer

RETREAT HOSPITAL, 2621 Grove Avenue, Richmond, VA, Zip 23220–4308; tel. 804/254–5100; William E. Caldwell, Jr., Chief Executive Officer

RIVERSIDE BEHAVIORAL HEALTH CENTER, 2244 Executive Drive, Hampton, VA, Zip 23666–2430; tel. 757/827–1001; Debora S. Tanner, Vice President and Administrator

RIVERSIDE REGIONAL MEDICAL CENTER, 500 J. Clyde Morris Boulevard, Newport News, VA, Zip 23601–1976; tel. 757/594–2000; Golden H. Bethune, RN, Executive Vice President and Administrator

RIVERSIDE REHABILITATION INSTITUTE, 245 Chesapeake Avenue, Newport News, VA, Zip 23607–6038; tel. 757/928–8000; Anne T. Moffat, Administrator

RIVERSIDE TAPPAHANNOCK HOSPITAL, 618 Hospital Road, Tappahannock, VA, Zip 22560–5000; tel. 804/443–3311; Elizabeth J. Martin, Vice President and Administrator

RIVERSIDE WALTER REED HOSPITAL, 7519 Hospital Drive, Gloucester, VA, Zip 23061–4178, Mailing Address: P.O. Box 1130, Zip 23061–1130; tel. 804/693–8800; Robert E. Bryant, Vice President and Administrator

RUSSELL COUNTY MEDICAL CENTER, 58 Carroll Street, Lebanon, VA, Zip 24266–4510, Mailing Address: P.O. Box 3600, Zip 24266–3600; tel. 276/883–8000; Jeffrey H. Whitton, Chief Executive Officer

SENTARA BAYSIDE HOSPITAL, 800 Independence Boulevard, Virginia Beach, VA, Zip 23455–6076; tel. 757/363–6100; Stephen D. Porter, Vice President and Administrator

SENTARA CAREPLEX HOSPITAL, 3000 Coliseum Drive, Hampton, VA, Zip 23666–5963; tel. 757/736–2656; Debra A. Flores, Vice President and Administrator

SENTARA LEIGH HOSPITAL, 830 Kempsville Road, Norfolk, VA, Zip 23502–3920; tel. 757/466–6000; Mark A. Szalwinski, Vice President and Administrator

SENTARA NORFOLK GENERAL HOSPITAL, 600 Gresham Drive, Norfolk, VA, Zip 23507; tel. 757/388–3000; Mary L. Blunt, Vice President and Administrator

SENTARA OBICI HOSPITAL, 2800 Godwin Boulevard, Suffolk, VA, Zip 23434–4323, Mailing Address: P.O. Box 1100, Zip 23439–1100; tel. 757/934–4000; Rosemary C. Check, Vice President and Administrator

SENTARA VIRGINIA BEACH GENERAL HOSPITAL, 1060 First Colonial Road, Virginia Beach, VA, Zip 23454–3002; tel. 757/395–8000; Raymond G. Troiano, M.D., Vice President and Administrator

SENTARA WILLIAMSBURG COMMUNITY HOSPITAL, 100 Sentara Circle, Williamsburg, VA, Zip 23188; tel. 757/984–6000; Robert L. Graves, Vice President and Administrator

SHELTERING ARMS REHABILITATION HOSPITAL, 8254 Atlee Road, Mechanicsville, VA, Zip 23116–1844; tel. 804/764–7055; James E. Sok, FACHE, President and Chief Executive Officer

SHORE MEMORIAL HOSPITAL, 9507 Hospital Avenue, Nassawadox, VA, Zip 23413–1821, Mailing Address: P.O. Box 17, Zip 23413–0017; tel. 757/414–8000; Joseph P. Zager, President and Chief Executive Officer

SMYTH COUNTY COMMUNITY HOSPITAL, 565 Radio Hill Road, Marion, VA, Zip 24354–3526, Mailing Address: P.O. Box 880, Zip 24354–0880; tel. 276/782–1234; Lindy P. White, President and Chief Executive Officer

SOUTHAMPTON MEMORIAL HOSPITAL, 100 Fairview Drive, Franklin, VA, Zip 23851–1206, Mailing Address: P.O. Box 817, Zip 23851–0817; tel. 757/569–6100; David W. Fuller, Chief Executive Officer

SOUTHERN VIRGINIA REGIONAL MEDICAL CENTER, 727 North Main Street, Emporia, VA, Zip 23847–1482; tel. 434/348–4400; Douglas T. Arbour, Chief Executive Officer

SOUTHSIDE COMMUNITY HOSPITAL, 800 Oak Street, Farmville, VA, Zip 23901–1199; tel. 434/392–8811; Gwen S. Eddleman, FACHE, Ed.D., President and Chief Executive Officer

SOUTHSIDE REGIONAL MEDICAL CENTER, 200 Medical Park Boulevard, Petersburg, VA, Zip 23805; tel. 804/862–5000; David J. Fikse, Chief Executive Officer

TAZEWELL COMMUNITY HOSPITAL, 141 Ben Bolt Avenue, Tazewell, VA, Zip 24651–9700; tel. 276/988–8700; Christopher L. Wearmouth, FACHE, President and Chief Executive Officer

TWIN COUNTY REGIONAL HOSPITAL, 200 Hospital Drive, Galax, VA, Zip 24333–2283; tel. 276/236–8181; Jon D. Applebaum, President and Chief Executive Officer

UNIVERSITY OF VIRGINIA MEDICAL CENTER, 1215 Lee Street, Charlottesville, VA, Zip 22908–0001, Mailing Address: P.O. Box 800809, Zip 22908–0809; tel. 434/924–0211; R. Edward Howell, Vice President and Chief Executive Officer

UVA–HEALTHSOUTH REHABILITATION HOSPITAL, 515 Ray C. Hunt Drive, Charlottesville, VA, Zip 22903; tel. 434/244–2000; Thomas J. Cook, Chief Executive Officer

VCU HEALTH SYSTEM, 1250 East Marshall Street, Richmond, VA, Zip 23219, Mailing Address: P.O. Box 980510, Zip 23298–0510; tel. 804/828–9000; John Duval, Chief Executive Officer

VIRGINIA HOSPITAL CENTER – ARLINGTON, 1701 North George Mason Drive, Arlington, VA, Zip 22205–3698; tel. 703/558–5000; James B. Cole, Chief Executive Officer

WYTHE COUNTY COMMUNITY HOSPITAL, 600 West Ridge Road, Wytheville, VA, Zip 24382–1099; tel. 276/228–0200; Eric Deaton, Chief Executive Officer

WASHINGTON

GROUP HEALTH COOPERATIVE
320 Westlake Ave. N., Suite 100, Seattle, WA 98109; tel. 206/326–3000; Scott Armstrong, Chief Executive Officer

CASCADE VALLEY HOSPITAL AND CLINICS, 330 South Stillaguamish Avenue, Arlington, WA, Zip 98223–1642; tel. 360/435–2133; W. Clark Jones, Administrator

CHILDREN'S HOSPITAL AND REGIONAL MEDICAL CENTER, 4800 Sand Point Way N.E., Seattle, WA, Zip 98105–0371, Mailing Address: Box 5371, Zip 98105–0371; tel. 206/987–2000; Thomas N. Hansen, M.D., Chief Executive Officer

DAYTON GENERAL HOSPITAL, 1012 South Third Street, Dayton, WA, Zip 99328–1696; tel. 509/382–2531; Charles A. Button, Chief Executive Officer

DEACONESS MEDICAL CENTER–SPOKANE, 800 West Fifth Avenue, Spokane, WA, Zip 99204–2803, Mailing Address: P.O. Box 248, Zip 99210–0248; tel. 509/458–5800; Robert Quist, Chief Executive Officer

GROUP HEALTH EASTSIDE HOSPITAL, 2700 152nd Avenue N.E., Redmond, WA, Zip 98052–5560; tel. 425/883–5151; Scott Armstrong, President and Chief Executive Officer

HARRISON MEDICAL CENTER, 2520 Cherry Avenue, Bremerton, WA, Zip 98310–4270; tel. 360/377–3911; Scott W. Bosch, President and Chief Executive Officer

HOLY FAMILY HOSPITAL, North 5633 Lidgerwood Street, Spokane, WA, Zip 99208–2533; tel. 509/482–0111; Thomas Corley, President

ISLAND HOSPITAL, 1211 24th Street, Anacortes, WA, Zip 98221–2590; tel. 360/299–1300; Vincent Oliver, Administrator

KADLEC MEDICAL CENTER, 888 Swift Boulevard, Richland, WA, Zip 99352–3542; tel. 509/946–4611; Rand J. Wortman, President and Chief Executive Officer

KENNEWICK GENERAL HOSPITAL, 900 South Auburn Street, Kennewick, WA, Zip 99336–6128, Mailing Address: P.O. Box 6128, Zip 99336–6128; tel. 509/586–6111; Glen Marshall, Chief Executive Officer

KITTITAS VALLEY COMMUNITY HOSPITAL, 603 South Chestnut Street, Ellensburg, WA, Zip 98926–3875; tel. 509/962–7302; Eric Jensen, Chief Executive Officer

KOOTENAI MEDICAL CENTER, 2003 Lincoln Way, Coeur D'Alene, ID, Zip 83814–2677; tel. 208/666–2000; Joseph E. Morris, Chief Executive Officer

LOURDES MEDICAL CENTER, 520 North Fourth Avenue, Pasco, WA, Zip 99301–2568, Mailing Address: P.O. Box 2568, Zip 99302–2568; tel. 509/547–7704; John Serle, President and Chief Executive Officer

MARY BRIDGE CHILDREN'S HOSPITAL AND HEALTH CENTER, 317 Martin Luther King Jr. Way, Tacoma, WA, Zip 98405–0299, Mailing Address: Box 5299, Zip 98415–0299; tel. 253/403–1400; Mady Murrey, Vice President and Administrator

NORTHWEST SPECIALTY HOSPITAL, 1593 East Polston Avenue, Post Falls, ID, Zip 83854; tel. 208/262–2300

OVERLAKE HOSPITAL MEDICAL CENTER, 1035 116th Avenue N.E., Bellevue, WA, Zip 98004–4686; tel. 425/688–5000; Craig L. Hendrickson, President and Chief Executive Officer

PROSSER MEMORIAL HOSPITAL, 723 Memorial Street, Prosser, WA, Zip 99350–1593; tel. 509/786–2222; James Tavary, Administrator

PROVIDENCE CENTRALIA HOSPITAL, 914 South Scheuber Road, Centralia, WA, Zip 98531–9027; tel. 360/736–2803; Cindy Mayo, Chief Executive

PROVIDENCE EVERETT MEDICAL CENTER, 1321 Colby Avenue, Everett, WA, Zip 98206–1147, Mailing Address: P.O. Box 1147, Zip 98206–1147; tel. 425/261–2000; David Brooks, Chief Operating Officer

PROVIDENCE ST. PETER HOSPITAL, 413 Lilly Road N.E., Olympia, WA, Zip 98506–5166; tel. 360/491–9480; James Leonard, Administrator

PULLMAN REGIONAL HOSPITAL, 835 S.E. Bishop Boulevard, Pullman, WA, Zip 99163–5512; tel. 509/332–2541; Scott K. Adams, Chief Executive Officer

SACRED HEART MEDICAL CENTER, 101 West Eighth Avenue, Spokane, WA, Zip 99204–2364, Mailing Address: P.O. Box 2555, Zip 99220–2555; tel. 509/474–3040; Michael D. Wilson, President

SKAGIT VALLEY HOSPITAL, 1415 East Kincaid Street, Mount Vernon, WA, Zip 98273, Mailing Address: P.O. Box 1376, Zip 98273–1376; tel. 360/424–4111; Gregg A. Davidson, Chief Executive Officer

ST. FRANCIS HOSPITAL, 34515 Ninth Avenue South, Federal Way, WA, Zip 98003–6799; tel. 253/944–8100; Sister Anne McNamara, Chief Operating Officer

ST. JOSEPH HOSPITAL, 2901 Squalicum Parkway, Bellingham, WA, Zip 98225–1898; tel. 360/734–5400; Nancy Steiger, Chief Executive Officer and Chief Mission Officer

ST. JOSEPH MEDICAL CENTER, 1717 South J Street, Tacoma, WA, Zip 98405–3004, Mailing Address: P.O. Box 2197, Zip 98401–2197; tel. 253/426–4101; Syd Bersante, Chief Operating Officer

ST. MARY MEDICAL CENTER, 401 West Poplar Street, Walla Walla, WA, Zip 99362, Mailing Address: Box 1477, Zip 99362; tel. 509/525–3320; Steven A. Burdick, Chief Executive Officer

SUNNYSIDE COMMUNITY HOSPITAL, 1016 Tacoma Avenue, Sunnyside, WA, Zip 98944–0719, Mailing Address: P.O. Box 719, Zip 98944–0719; tel. 509/837–1500; Jon D. Smiley, Chief Executive Officer

TOPPENISH COMMUNITY HOSPITAL, 502 West Fourth Avenue, Toppenish, WA, Zip 98948–0672, Mailing Address: P.O. Box 672, Zip 98948–0672; tel. 509/865–3105; Michael P. Curran, Chief Executive Officer

UNITED GENERAL HOSPITAL, 2000 Hospital Drive, Sedro Woolley, WA, Zip 98284–4327; tel. 360/856–6021; Greg Reed, Chief Executive Officer

VALLEY HOSPITAL AND MEDICAL CENTER, 12606 East Mission Avenue, Spokane, WA, Zip 99216–1090; tel. 509/924–6650; Robert Quist, Chief Executive Officer

VIRGINIA MASON MEDICAL CENTER, 1100 Ninth Avenue, Seattle, WA, Zip 98101–2756, Mailing Address: P.O. Box 900, Zip 98111–0900; tel. 206/223–6600; Gary Kaplan, President

WALLA WALLA GENERAL HOSPITAL, 1025 South Second Avenue, Walla Walla, WA, Zip 99362–1398, Mailing Address: P.O. Box 1398, Zip 99362–1398; tel. 509/525–0480; Monty E. Knittel, President and Chief Executive Officer

WHIDBEY GENERAL HOSPITAL, 101 North Main Street, Coupeville, WA, Zip 98239; tel. 360/678–5151; Scott Rhine, Administrator and Chief Executive Officer

WHITMAN HOSPITAL AND MEDICAL CENTER, 1200 West Fairview, Colfax, WA, Zip 99111–9579; tel. 509/397–3435; Jon R. Davis, FACHE, Chief Executive Officer

YAKIMA REGIONAL MEDICAL AND CARDIAC CENTER, 110 South Ninth Avenue, Yakima, WA, Zip 98902–3397; tel. 509/575–5000; Monte J. Bostwick, Chief Executive Officer

YAKIMA VALLEY MEMORIAL HOSPITAL, 2811 Tieton Drive, Yakima, WA, Zip 98902–3761; tel. 509/575–8000; Richard W. Linneweh, Jr., President and Chief Executive Officer

LINCOLN HEALTH DEPARTMENT
90 Nicholls Street, Davenport, WA 99122; tel. 509/725–1001; Ed Dzedzy, Public Health Administration

LINCOLN HOSPITAL, 10 Nicholls Street, Davenport, WA, Zip 99122–9729; tel. 509/725–7101; Thomas J. Martin, Chief Executive Officer

ODESSA MEMORIAL HEALTHCARE CENTER, 502 East Amende Drive, Odessa, WA, Zip 99159–0368, Mailing Address: P.O. Box 368, Zip 99159–0368; tel. 509/982–2611; Mark Barglof, Administrator

WEST VIRGINIA

EASTERN PANHANDLE INTEGRATED DELIVERY SYSTEM
109 Tavern Rd. P.O. Box 758, Martinsburg, WV 25401; tel. 304/262–0201; Jeffrey Debord, Chairman

HEALTH PARTNERS NETWORK, INC.
1000 Technology Drive, Suite 2320, Fairmont, WV 26554; tel. 304/368–2740; William G. Maclean, Chief Operating Officer

BROADDUS HOSPITAL, 1 Healthcare Drive, Philippi, WV, Zip 26416–1051, Mailing Address: P.O. Box 930, Zip 26416–1051; tel. 304/457–1760; Jeffrey A. Powelson, Chief Executive Officer

CAMDEN–CLARK MEMORIAL HOSPITAL, 800 Garfield Avenue, Parkersburg, WV, Zip 26101–5378, Mailing Address: P.O. Box 718, Zip 26102–0718; tel. 304/424–2111; Michael A. King, President and Chief Executive Officer

CITY HOSPITAL, Dry Run Road, Martinsburg, WV, Zip 25401, Mailing Address: P.O. Box 1418, Zip 25402–1418; tel. 304/264–1000; Anthony Zelenka, Administrator

DAVIS MEMORIAL HOSPITAL, Gorman Avenue and Reed Street, Elkins, WV, Zip 26241, Mailing Address: P.O. Box 1484, Zip 26241–1484; tel. 304/636–3300; Mark Doak, President and Chief Executive Officer

FAIRMONT GENERAL HOSPITAL, 1325 Locust Avenue, Fairmont, WV, Zip 26554–1435; tel. 304/367–7100; Albert Pilkington, III, Chief Executive Officer

GRAFTON CITY HOSPITAL, 500 Market Street, Grafton, WV, Zip 26354–1187; tel. 304/265–0400; Jeffrey Lilley, Administrator

HEALTHSOUTH HUNTINGTON REHABILITATION HOSPITAL, 6900 West Country Club Drive, Huntington, WV, Zip 25705–2000; tel. 304/733–1060; Michael E. Zuliani, Chief Executive Officer

HEALTHSOUTH MOUNTAINVIEW REGIONAL REHABILITATION HOSPITAL, 1160 Van Voorhis Road, Morgantown, WV, Zip 26505–3437; tel. 304/598–1100; John C. Forester, Chief Executive Officer

HEALTHSOUTH WESTERN HILLS REHABILITATION CENTER, 3 Western Hills Drive, Parkersburg, WV, Zip 26101–8122; tel. 304/420–1300; Dean Hatcher, Chief Executive Officer

JEFFERSON MEMORIAL HOSPITAL, 300 South Preston Street, Ranson, WV, Zip 25438–1699; tel. 304/728–1600; Roger M. Eitelman, Chief Executive Officer

MINNIE HAMILTON HEALTHCARE CENTER, 186 Hospital Drive, Grantsville, WV, Zip 26147; tel. 304/354–9244; Barbara Lay, Chief Executive Officer

ST. JOSEPH'S HOSPITAL OF BUCKHANNON, 1 Amalia Drive, Buckhannon, WV, Zip 26201–2222; tel. 304/473–2000; Sue E. Johnson–Phillippe, Interim Chief Executive Officer

STONEWALL JACKSON MEMORIAL HOSPITAL, 230 Hospital Plaza, Weston, WV, Zip 26452–8558; tel. 304/269–8000; David D. Shaffer, Chief Executive Officer

UNITED HOSPITAL CENTER, 3 Hospital Plaza, Clarksburg, WV, Zip 26301, Mailing Address: P.O. Box 1680, Zip 26302–1680; tel. 304/624–2121; Bruce C. Carter, President

WEST VIRGINIA UNIVERSITY HOSPITALS, Medical Center Drive, Morgantown, WV, Zip 26506–4749; tel. 304/598–4000; Bruce McClymonds, President and Chief Executive Officer

PARTNERS IN HEALTH NETWORK, INC.
501 Morris Street, Charleston, WV 25301; tel. 304/388–7385; Bob Whitler, Executive Director

BOONE MEMORIAL HOSPITAL, 701 Madison Avenue, Madison, WV, Zip 25130–1699; tel. 304/369–1230; Tommy H. Mullins, Administrator

BRAXTON COUNTY MEMORIAL HOSPITAL, 100 Hoylman Drive, Gassaway, WV, Zip 26624–9320; tel. 304/364–5156; Ben Vincent, FACHE, Administrator

CHARLESTON AREA MEDICAL CENTER, 501 Morris Street, Charleston, WV, Zip 25301–1300, Mailing Address: P.O. Box 1547, Zip 25326–1547; tel. 304/388–5432; David L. Ramsey, President and Chief Executive Officer

HIGHLAND HOSPITAL, 300 56th Street S.E., Charleston, WV, Zip 25304–2361, Mailing Address: P.O. Box 4107, Zip 25364–4107; tel. 304/926–1600; David M. McWatters, Administrator

JACKSON GENERAL HOSPITAL, Pinnell Street, Ripley, WV, Zip 25271–1009, Mailing Address: P.O. Box 720, Zip 25271–0720; tel. 304/372–2731; Sandra Elza, Chief Executive Officer

MONTGOMERY GENERAL HOSPITAL, 401 Sixth Avenue, Montgomery, WV, Zip 25136–0270, Mailing Address: P.O. Box 270, Zip 25136–0270; tel. 304/442–5151; Vickie Gay, Chief Executive Officer

ROANE GENERAL HOSPITAL, 200 Hospital Drive, Spencer, WV, Zip 25276–1060; tel. 304/927–4444; Douglas E. Bentz, Chief Executive Officer

STONEWALL JACKSON MEMORIAL HOSPITAL, 230 Hospital Plaza, Weston, WV, Zip 26452–8558; tel. 304/269–8000; David D. Shaffer, Chief Executive Officer

SUMMERSVILLE MEMORIAL HOSPITAL, 400 Fairview Heights Road, Summersville, WV, Zip 26651–0400; tel. 304/872–2891; Deborah A. Hill, RN, Chief Executive Officer

TEAYS VALLEY HOSPITAL, 1400 Hospital Drive, Hurricane, WV, Zip 25526–9210; tel. 304/757–1700; Albert H. Michaels, Chief Executive Officer

WEBSTER COUNTY MEMORIAL HOSPITAL, 324 Miller Mountain Drive, Webster Springs, WV, Zip 26288–1087, Mailing Address: P.O. Box 312, Zip 26288–0312; tel. 304/847–5682; Annette M. Keenan, Chief Executive Officer

WISCONSIN

AFFINITY HEALTH SYSTEM
1570 Midway Place, Menasha, WI 54954; tel. 920/720–1713; Daniel E. Neufelder, Chief Executive Officer

CALUMET MEDICAL CENTER, 614 Memorial Drive, Chilton, WI, Zip 53014–1597; tel. 920/849–2386; Jennifer Weber, Interim President and Chief Executive Officer

MERCY MEDICAL CENTER, 500 South Oakwood Road, Oshkosh, WI, Zip 54903–3370, Mailing Address: P.O. Box 3370, Zip 54903–3370; tel. 920/223–2000; Daniel Neufelder, Chief Executive Officer

ST. ELIZABETH HOSPITAL, 1506 South Oneida Street, Appleton, WI, Zip 54915–1397; tel. 920/738–2000; Travis Andersen, President

ASPIRUS, INC.
425 Pine Ridge Boulevard, Wausau, WI 54401; tel. 715/847–2121; Duane L. Erwin, President and Chief Executive Officer

ASPIRUS ONTONAGON HOSPITAL, 601 Seventh Street, Ontonagon, MI, Zip 49953–1496; tel. 906/884–8000; Mike Gutsch, Chief Executive Officer

ASPIRUS WAUSAU HOSPITAL, 333 Pine Ridge Boulevard, Wausau, WI, Zip 54401–4187, Mailing Address: P.O. Box 1847, Zip 54402–1847; tel. 715/847–2121; Duane L. Erwin, President and Chief Executive Officer

COLUMBIA ST. MARY'S
2025 E. Newport Ave., Milwaukee, WI 53211; tel. 414/961–3300; Leo Brideau, President and Chief Executive Officer

COLUMBIA ST. MARY'S COLUMBIA HOSPITAL, 2025 East Newport Avenue, Milwaukee, WI, Zip 53211–2990; tel. 414/961–3300; Leo P. Brideau, President and Chief Executive Officer

COLUMBIA ST. MARY'S MILWAUKEE HOSPITAL, 2323 North Lake Drive, Milwaukee, WI, Zip 53211–9682, Mailing Address: P.O. Box 503, Zip 53201–0503; tel. 414/291–1000; Leo P. Brideau, President and Chief Executive Officer

COLUMBIA ST. MARY'S OZAUKEE HOSPITAL, 13111 North Port Washington Road, Mequon, WI, Zip 53097–2416; tel. 262/243–7300; Leo P. Brideau, President and Chief Executive Officer

SACRED HEART REHABILITATION INSTITUTE, 2025 East Newport Avenue, Milwaukee, WI, Zip 53211–2906; tel. 414/298–6700; Jack Burke, Administrator

COMMUNITY HEALTH NETWORK, INC.
225 Memorial Drive, Berlin, WI 54923; tel. 920/361–5580; Douglas I. Guy, Chief Executive Officer

BERLIN MEMORIAL HOSPITAL, 225 Memorial Drive, Berlin, WI, Zip 54923–1295; tel. 920/361–1313; Douglas I. Guy, President and Chief Executive Officer

WILD ROSE COMMUNITY MEMORIAL HOSPITAL, 601 Grove Avenue, Wild Rose, WI, Zip 54984, Mailing Address: P.O. Box 243, Zip 54984–0243; tel. 920/622–3257; Donald Caves, President

GUNDERSON LUTHERAN HEALTH SYSTEM
1900 South Avenue, LaCrosse, WI 54601; tel. 608/782–7300; Jeffrey Thompson, M.D., Chief Executive Officer

GUNDERSEN LUTHERAN MEDICAL CENTER, 1900 South Avenue, La Crosse, WI, Zip 54601–9980; tel. 608/782–7300; Jeffrey E. Thompson, M.D., Chief Executive Officer

PALMER LUTHERAN HEALTH CENTER, 112 Jefferson Street, West Union, IA, Zip 52175–1022; tel. 563/422–3811; Debrah Chensvold, President and Chief Executive Officer

TRI–COUNTY MEMORIAL HOSPITAL, 18601 Lincoln Street, Whitehall, WI, Zip 54773–0065; tel. 715/538–4361; Brian Theiler, President and Chief Executive Officer

MERCY ALLIANCE, INC.
1000 Mineral Point Avenue, Janesville, WI 53548; tel. 608/756–6080; Javon R. Bea, President and Chief Executive Officer

MERCY HARVARD HOSPITAL, 901 Grant Street, Harvard, IL, Zip 60033–1898, Mailing Address: P.O. Box 850, Zip 60033–0850; tel. 815/943–5431; Sue Ripsch, Chief Operating Officer

MERCY HEALTH SYSTEM, 1000 Mineral Point Avenue, Janesville, WI, Zip 53547–2982, Mailing Address: P.O. Box 5003, Zip 53547–5003; tel. 608/756–6000; Javon R. Bea, President and Chief Executive Officer

MERCY WALWORTH HOSPITAL AND MEDICAL CENTER, N2950 State Road 67, Lake Geneva, WI, Zip 53147; tel. 262/245–0535; Jennifer Hallatt, Director

MINISTRY HEALTH CARE
11925 West Lake Park Drive, Suite 100, Milwaukee, WI 53224; tel. 414/359–1060; Nicholas Desien, President and Chief Executive Officer

CALUMET MEDICAL CENTER, 614 Memorial Drive, Chilton, WI, Zip 53014–1597; tel. 920/849–2386; Jennifer Weber, Interim President and Chief Executive Officer

DOOR COUNTY MEMORIAL HOSPITAL, 323 South 18th Avenue, Sturgeon Bay, WI, Zip 54235–1495; tel. 920/743–5566; Gerald M. Worrick, President and Chief Executive Officer

EAGLE RIVER MEMORIAL HOSPITAL, 201 Hospital Road, Eagle River, WI, Zip 54521–8835; tel. 715/479–7411; Sheila Clough, President

FLAMBEAU HOSPITAL, 98 Sherry Avenue, Park Falls, WI, Zip 54552–1467, Mailing Address: P.O. Box 310, Zip 54552–0310; tel. 715/762–2484; David A. Grundstrom, Chief Administrative Officer

GOOD SAMARITAN HEALTH CENTER OF MERRILL, 601 Center Avenue South, Merrill, WI, Zip 54452–3404; tel. 715/536–5511; Michael Hammer, President and Chief Operating Officer

HOWARD YOUNG MEDICAL CENTER, 240 Maple Street, Woodruff, WI, Zip 54568, Mailing Address: P.O. Box 470, Zip 54568–0470; tel. 715/356–8000; Sheila Clough, President

MERCY MEDICAL CENTER, 500 South Oakwood Road, Oshkosh, WI, Zip 54903–3370, Mailing Address: P.O. Box 3370, Zip 54903–3370; tel. 920/223–2000; Daniel Neufelder, Chief Executive Officer

OUR LADY OF VICTORY HOSPITAL, 1120 Pine Street, Stanley, WI, Zip 54768–0220, Mailing Address: P.O. Box 220, Zip 54768–0220; tel. 715/644–5571; Cynthia Eichman, President and Chief Executive Officer

SACRED HEART HOSPITAL, 401 West Mohawk Drive, Tomahawk, WI, Zip 54487; tel. 715/453–7700

SACRED HEART–ST. MARY'S HOSPITALS, 2251 North Shore Drive, Rhinelander, WI, Zip 54501–3998; tel. 715/361–2000; Monica Hilt, President and Chief Operating Officer

SAINT CLARE'S HOSPITAL, 3400 Ministry Parkway, Weston, WI, Zip 54476; tel. 715/393–3000; Mary T. Krueger, President

SAINT ELIZABETH'S MEDICAL CENTER, 1200 Grant Boulevard West, Wabasha, MN, Zip 55981–1098; tel. 651/565–4531; Thomas Crowley, President and Chief Executive Officer

SAINT JOSEPH'S HOSPITAL, 611 St. Joseph Avenue, Marshfield, WI, Zip 54449–1898; tel. 715/387–1713; Michael A. Schmidt, President

SAINT MICHAEL'S HOSPITAL, 900 Illinois Avenue, Stevens Point, WI, Zip 54481–3196; tel. 715/346–5000; Bradley Neet, President

ST. ELIZABETH HOSPITAL, 1506 South Oneida Street, Appleton, WI, Zip 54915–1397; tel. 920/738–2000; Travis Andersen, President

WHEATON FRANCISCAN HEALTHCARE
400 W. River Woods Parkway, Glendale, WI 53212; tel. 414/465–3000; John Olivero, President and Chief Executive Officer

THE WISCONSIN HEART HOSPITAL, 10000 West Bluemound Road, Wauwatosa, WI, Zip 53226; tel. 414/778–7800; Norma J. McCutcheon, President

WHEATON FRANCISCAN HEALTHCARE – ALL SAINTS, 3801 Spring Street, Racine, WI, Zip 53405–1690; tel. 262/687–4011; Kenneth R. Buser, President and Chief Executive Officer

WHEATON FRANCISCAN HEALTHCARE – ELMBROOK MEMORIAL, 19333 West North Avenue, Brookfield, WI, Zip 53045–4198; tel. 262/785–2000; Kimry A. Johnsrud, President

WHEATON FRANCISCAN HEALTHCARE – ST. FRANCIS, 3237 South 16th Street, Milwaukee, WI, Zip 53215–4592; tel. 414/647–5000; Debra Standridge, President

WHEATON FRANCISCAN HEALTHCARE – ST. JOSEPH, 5000 West Chambers Street, Milwaukee, WI, Zip 53210–9988; tel. 414/447–2000; Ronald Groepper, President

WHEATON FRANCISCAN HEALTHCARE–ALL SAINTS
3801 Spring Street, Racine, WI 53405; tel. 262/636–4011; Ken Buser, President and Chief Executive Officer

WHEATON FRANCISCAN HEALTHCARE – ALL SAINTS, 3801 Spring Street, Racine, WI, Zip 53405–1690; tel. 262/687–4011; Kenneth R. Buser, President and Chief Executive Officer

Alliances

ALLIANCE OF INDEPENDENT ACADEMIC MEDICAL CENTERS

233 East Erie Street, Ste 306, Chicago, IL Zip 60611; tel. 312/988–7572; Ms. Nancie Noie Thompson, Executive Director

ARIZONA

Phoenix
Member
Maricopa Integrated Health System
St. Joseph's Hospital and Medical Center

CALIFORNIA

Los Angeles
Member
Cedars–Sinai Medical Center

CONNECTICUT

Hartford
Member
Saint Francis Hospital and Medical Center

DELAWARE

Wilmington
Member
Christiana Care Health System

DISTRICT OF COLUMBIA

Washington
Member
National Rehabilitation Hospital
Washington Hospital Center

FLORIDA

Miami
Member
Miami Children's Hospital

Miami Beach
Member
Mount Sinai Medical Center

ILLINOIS

Oak Brook
Member
Advocate Health Care

Peoria
Member
OSF Saint Francis Medical Center

LOUISIANA

New Orleans
Member
Ochsner Medical Center

MARYLAND

Baltimore
Sinai Hospital of Baltimore
Member
Franklin Square Hospital Center
Good Samaritan Hospital of Maryland
Harbor Hospital
Union Memorial Hospital

Columbia
Member
MedStar Health

MASSACHUSETTS

Springfield
Member
Baystate Medical Center

MICHIGAN

Dearborn
Member
Oakwood Healthcare, Inc.

Grand Rapids
Member
Spectrum Health

Royal Oak
Member
Beaumont Hospital – Royal Oak

MISSOURI

Kansas City
Member
Saint Luke's Hospital of Kansas City

Saint Louis
Member
St. John's Mercy Medical Center

NEW JERSEY

Morristown
Member
Atlantic Health

Neptune
Member
Jersey Shore University Medical Center
Meridian Health

NEW YORK

Brooklyn
Member
Maimonides Medical Center

Mineola
Member
Winthrop–University Hospital

Rochester
Member
Rochester General Hospital

NORTH CAROLINA

Charlotte
Member
Carolinas Medical Center

OHIO

Akron
Member
Akron General Medical Center

Columbus
Member
Riverside Methodist Hospital

PENNSYLVANIA

Bethlehem
Member
St. Luke's Hospital – Bethlehem Campus

Pittsburgh
Member
Western Pennsylvania Hospital

York
Member
York Hospital

TEXAS

Dallas
Member
Baylor Health Care System

VIRGINIA

Falls Church
Member
Inova Fairfax Hospital

CATHOLIC CEO HEALTHCARE CONNECTION

3333 Warrenville Rd, Ste 200, Lisle, IL Zip 60532; tel. 630/799–8315; Mr. Roger N. Butler, Executive Director

CALIFORNIA

Orange
Member
St. Joseph Health System

San Francisco
Member
Catholic Healthcare West

COLORADO

Denver
Member
Catholic Health Initiatives

ILLINOIS

Mokena
Member
Provena Health

Wheaton
Member
Wheaton Franciscan Healthcare

INDIANA

Mishawaka
Member
Sisters of St. Francis Health Services, Inc.

KANSAS

Lenexa
Shareholder
Sisters of Charity of Leavenworth Health System

Wichita
Member
Via Christi Health System

LOUISIANA

Baton Rouge
Member
Franciscan Missionaries of Our Lady Health System, Inc.

MARYLAND

Marriottsville
Member
Bon Secours Health System, Inc.

MASSACHUSETTS

Lexington
Member
Covenant Health Systems, Inc.

MICHIGAN

Novi
Member
Trinity Health

MISSOURI

Chesterfield
Member
Sisters of Mercy Health System

Saint Louis
Member
Ascension Health

OHIO

Cincinnati
Member
Catholic Healthcare Partners

Sylvania
Member
Franciscan Services Corporation

PENNSYLVANIA

Newtown Square
Member
Catholic Health East

SOUTH DAKOTA

Sioux Falls
Member
Avera Health

TEXAS

Irving
Member
CHRISTUS Health

WASHINGTON

Bellevue
Member
PeaceHealth

WISCONSIN

Manitowoc
Member
Franciscan Sisters of Christian Charity HealthCare Ministry, Inc

CHILD HEALTH CORPORATION OF AMERICA

6803 West 64th Street, Ste 208, Shawnee Mission, KS Zip 66202; tel. 913/262–1436; Mr. Don C. Black, President and Chief Executive Officer

ALABAMA

Birmingham
Member
The Children's Hospital of Alabama

ARIZONA

Phoenix
Member
Phoenix Children's Hospital

ARKANSAS

Little Rock
Member
Arkansas Children's Hospital

CALIFORNIA

Los Angeles
Member
Childrens Hospital Los Angeles

Madera
Member
Children's Hospital Central California

Oakland
Member
Children's Hospital and Research Center at Oakland

Orange
Member
Children's Hospital of Orange County

Palo Alto
Member
Lucile Salter Packard Children's Hospital at Stanford

San Diego
Member
Rady Children's Hospital and Health Center

COLORADO

Aurora
Member
The Children's Hospital

CONNECTICUT

Hartford
Member
Connecticut Children's Medical Center

DISTRICT OF COLUMBIA

Washington
Member
Children's National Medical Center

FLORIDA

Miami
Member
Miami Children's Hospital

Saint Petersburg
Member
All Children's Hospital

GEORGIA

Atlanta
Member
Children's Healthcare of Atlanta

ILLINOIS

Chicago
Member
Children's Memorial Hospital

LOUISIANA

New Orleans
Member
Children's Hospital

MASSACHUSETTS

Boston
Member
Children's Hospital Boston

MICHIGAN

Detroit
Member
Children's Hospital of Michigan

MINNESOTA

Minneapolis
Member
Children's Hospitals and Clinics of Minnesota

MISSOURI

Kansas City
Member
Children's Mercy Hospitals and Clinics

Saint Louis
Member
St. Louis Children's Hospital

NEBRASKA

Omaha
Member
Children's Hospital

OHIO

Akron
Member
Akron Children's Hospital

Cincinnati
Member
Cincinnati Children's Hospital Medical Center

Columbus
Member
Nationwide Children's Hospital

Dayton
Member
Children's Medical Center

PENNSYLVANIA

Philadelphia
Member
Children's Hospital of Philadelphia

Pittsburgh
Member
Children's Hospital of Pittsburgh of UPMC

TENNESSEE

Memphis
Member
Le Bonheur Children's Medical Center
St. Jude Children's Research Hospital

TEXAS

Corpus Christi
Member
Driscoll Children's Hospital

Dallas
Member
Children's Medical Center of Dallas

Fort Worth
Member
Cook Children's Medical Center

Houston
Member
Texas Children's Hospital

VIRGINIA

Norfolk
Member
Children's Hospital of The King's Daughters

WASHINGTON

Seattle
Member
Children's Hospital and Regional Medical Center

WISCONSIN

Milwaukee
Member
Children's Hospital of Wisconsin

HOSPITAL NETWORK, INC.

4510 Commercial Avenue, Portage, MI Zip 49002; tel. 269/341–8888; Mr. George Angelidis, President and Chief Executive Officer

MICHIGAN

Allegan
Member
Allegan General Hospital

Hastings
Member
Pennock Hospital

Kalamazoo
Member
Bronson Healthcare Group, Inc.
Bronson Methodist Hospital

Marshall
Member
Oaklawn Hospital

Sturgis
Member
Sturgis Hospital

Vicksburg
Member
Bronson Vicksburg Hospital

MEDI–SOTA, INC.

669 Sixth Street, Suite 3, Dawson, MN Zip 56232; tel. 320/769–2269

MINNESOTA

Arlington
Member
Sibley Medical Center

Benson
Member
Swift County–Benson Hospital

Canby
Member
Sanford Canby Medical Center

Dawson
Member
Johnson Memorial Health Services

Glencoe
Member
Glencoe Regional Health Services

Graceville
Member
Graceville Health Center

Granite Falls
Member
Granite Falls Municipal Hospital and Manor

Hendricks
Member
Hendricks Community Hospital

Litchfield
Member
Meeker County Memorial Hospital

Madelia
Member
Madelia Community Hospital

Marshall
Member
Avera Marshall Regional Medical Center

Montevideo
Member
Chippewa County–Montevideo Hospital

Olivia
Member
RC Hospital and Clinics

Ortonville
Member
Ortonville Area Health Services

Paynesville
Member
Paynesville Area Health Care System

Perham
Member
Perham Memorial Hospital and Home

Pipestone
Member
Pipestone County Medical Center/Avera Health

Redwood Falls
Member
Redwood Area Hospital

Slayton
Member
Murray County Medical Center

Sleepy Eye
Member
Sleepy Eye Medical Center

Tracy
Member
Sanford Tracy Medical Center

Tyler
Member
Tyler Healthcare Center/Avera Health

Willmar
Member
Rice Memorial Hospital

Windom
Member
Windom Area Hospital

SOUTH DAKOTA

Watertown
Member
Prairie Lakes Healthcare System

NORTH REGION HEALTH ALLIANCE

120 East Bridge Avenue, Warren, MN Zip 56762; tel. 218/745–5343; Mr. Jon E. Linnell, Chief Executive Officer

MINNESOTA

Ada
Member
Bridges Medical Center

Bagley
Member
Clearwater Health Services

Baudette
Member
LakeWood Health Center

Crookston
Member
Riverview Healthcare Association

Fosston
Member
First Care Medical Services

Hallock
Member
Kittson Memorial Healthcare Center

Roseau
Member
LifeCare Medical Center

Thief River Falls
Member
MeritCare Thief River Falls Northwest Medical Center

Warren
Member
North Valley Health Center

NORTH DAKOTA

Cavalier
Member
Pembina County Memorial Hospital and Wedgewood Manor

Cooperstown
Member
Cooperstown Medical Center

Devils Lake
Member
Mercy Hospital

Grafton
Member
Unity Medical Center

Grand Forks
Member
Altru Health System

Hillsboro
Member
Hillsboro Medical Center

Langdon
Member
Cavalier County Memorial Hospital

Mayville
Member
Union Hospital

McVille
Member
Nelson County Health System

Northwood
Member
Northwood Deaconess Health Center

Park River
Member
First Care Health Center

PREMIER, INC.

3 Westbrook Corporate Center, 9th Floor, San Diego, CA Zip 92130; tel. 858/481–2727; Mr. Richard A. Norling, Chief Executive Officer

ALABAMA

Dothan
Owner
Southeast Alabama Medical Center

Opelika
Owner
East Alabama Medical Center

ALASKA

Fairbanks
Member
Fairbanks Memorial Hospital

Ketchikan
Member
Ketchikan General Hospital

ARIZONA

Chandler
Chandler Regional Mecical Center

Gilbert
Mercy Gilbert Medical Center

Glendale
Banner Thunderbird Medical Center

Mesa
Banner Desert Medical Center
Banner Heart Hospital
Member
Banner Baywood Medical Center

Page
Page Hospital

Phoenix
Banner Estrella Medical Center
Banner Good Samaritan Medical Center
St. Joseph's Hospital and Medical Center
Owner
Banner Health

Scottsdale
Banner Behavioral Health Hospital – Scottsdale

Sun City
10401 West Thunderbird Boulevard
Sun Health Corporation

Sun City West
Sun Health Del E. Webb Hospital

ARKANSAS

Pine Bluff
Owner
Jefferson Regional Medical Center

CALIFORNIA

Arroyo Grande
Member
Arroyo Grande Community Hospital

Bakersfield
Bakersfield Memorial Hospital
Mercy Hospital
Member
San Joaquin Community Hospital

Camarillo
St. John's Pleasant Valley Hospital

Carmichael
Mercy San Juan Medical Center

Chula Vista
Member
Sharp Chula Vista Medical Center

Clearlake
Member
Redbud Community Hospital

Coronado
Member
Sharp Coronado Hospital and Health Center

Daly City
Seton Medical Center

Folsom
Mercy Hospital of Folsom

Gilroy
St. Louise Regional Hospital

Glendale
Member
Glendale Adventist Medical Center
Glendale Memorial Hospital and Health Center

Grass Valley
Sierra Nevada Memorial Hospital

Hanford
Central Valley General Hospital
Member
Hanford Community Medical Center

La Mesa
Member
Sharp Grossmont Hospital

Laguna Beach
Member
South Coast Medical Center

Long Beach
St. Mary Medical Center

Los Altos Hills
Daughters of Charity Health System

Los Angeles
St. Vincent Medical Center
Member
California Hospital Medical Center
White Memorial Medical Center

Lynwood
St. Francis Medical Center

Merced
Mercy Medical Center Merced

Moss Beach
Seton Medical Center Coastside

Mount Shasta
Mercy Medical Center Mount Shasta

Northridge
Member
Northridge Hospital Medical Center–Roscoe Boulevard Campus

Oakdale
Oak Valley Hospital District

Oceanside
Tri–City Medical Center

Orange
Owner
St. Joseph Health System

Oxnard
St. John's Regional Medical Center

Paradise
Member
Feather River Hospital

Rancho Mirage
Owner
Eisenhower Medical Center

Red Bluff
St. Elizabeth Community Hospital

Redding
Mercy Medical Center Redding

Redwood City
Sequoia Hospital

Roseville
Owner
Adventist Health

Sacramento
Mercy General Hospital
Methodist Hospital of Sacramento

Saint Helena
Member
St. Helena Hospital

San Andreas
Mark Twain St. Joseph's Hospital

San Bernardino
Commmunity Hospital of San Bernardino
St. Bernardine Medical Center

Section B

San Diego
Member
Sharp Memorial Hospital
Owner
Palomar Pomerado Health
Sharp Healthcare

San Francisco
Saint Francis Memorial Hospital
St. Mary's Medical Center
Owner
Catholic Healthcare West

San Gabriel
Member
San Gabriel Valley Medical Center

San Jose
O'Connor Hospital

San Luis Obispo
Member
French Hospital Medical Center

Santa Cruz
Dominican Hospital

Santa Maria
Marian Medical Center

Selma
Member
Selma Community Hospital

Simi Valley
Member
Simi Valley Hospital and Health Care Services

Sonora
Member
Sonora Regional Medical Center

Stockton
St. Joseph's Behavioral Health Center
St. Joseph's Medical Center

Susanville
Member
Banner Lassen Medical Center

Ukiah
Member
Ukiah Valley Medical Center

Vallejo
Member
St. Helena Hospital–Center for Behavioral Health

Willits
Member
Frank R. Howard Memorial Hospital

Woodland
Woodland Healthcare

COLORADO

Brush
Member
East Morgan County Hospital

Denver
Porter Adventist Hospital

Greeley
Member
North Colorado Medical Center

Littleton
Littleton Adventist Hospital

Louisville
Avista Adventist Hospital

Loveland
Member
McKee Medical Center

Parker
Parker Adventist Hospital

Sterling
Member
Sterling Regional MedCenter

CONNECTICUT

Hartford
Owner
Saint Francis Hospital and Medical Center

New Haven
Member
Hospital of Saint Raphael

Waterbury
Saint Mary's Hospital

DELAWARE

Dover
Owner
Bayhealth Medical Center

Lewes
Owner
Beebe Medical Center

Wilmington
Member
Alfred I. duPont Hospital for Children

DISTRICT OF COLUMBIA

Washington
Owner
Sibley Memorial Hospital

FLORIDA

Clearwater
Morton Plant Hospital

Coral Gables
Doctors Hospital
Owner
Baptist Health South Florida

Coral Springs
Member
Coral Springs Medical Center

De Land
Member
Florida Hospital – De Land

Deerfield Beach
Member
North Broward Medical Center

Dunedin
Member
Mease Hospital Dunedin

Fernandina Beach
Member
Baptist Medical Center Nassau

Fort Lauderdale
Member
Broward General Medical Center
Imperial Point Medical Center
Owner
Broward Health

Gainesville
Member
AvMed–Santa Fe

Hollywood
Member
Memorial Regional Hospital

Homestead
Member
Homestead Hospital

Jacksonville
Baptist Health
Baptist Medical Center

Jacksonville Beach
Member
Baptist Medical Center Beaches

Miami
Member
Baptist Hospital of Miami
South Miami Hospital

Miami Beach
Owner
Mount Sinai Medical Center

Miramar
Memorial Hospital Miramar

Naples
Owner
Naples Community Hospital

New Port Richey
Member
Morton Plant North Bay Hospital

Orange City
Member
Florida Hospital Fish Memorial

Orlando
Member
Florida Hospital

Ormond Beach
Member
Florida Hospital–Ormond Memorial

Palm Coast
Member
Florida Hospital–Flagler

Pembroke Pines
Member
Memorial Hospital Pembroke
Memorial Hospital West

Plant City
Member
South Florida Baptist Hospital

Safety Harbor
Member
Mease Countryside Hospital

Saint Petersburg
Member
Bayfront Medical Center
St. Anthony's Hospital

Sebring
Member
Florida Hospital Heartland Medical Center

Tampa
Member
H. Lee Moffitt Cancer Center and Research Institute
St. Joseph's Hospital

Tavares
Member
Florida Hospital Waterman

Tavernier
Member
Mariners Hospital

Vero Beach
Owner
Indian River Medical Center

Wauchula
Florida Hospital Wauchula

Weston
Member
Cleveland Clinic Florida

Winter Haven
Owner
Winter Haven Hospital

Winter Park
Owner
Adventist Health System Sunbelt Health Care Corporation

Zephyrhills
Member
Florida Hospital Zephyrhills

GEORGIA

Brunswick
Southeast Georgia Health System
Member
Southeast Georgia Health System Brunswick Campus

Calhoun
Member
Gordon Hospital

Columbus
Owner
St. Francis Hospital

Fort Oglethorpe
Owner
Hutcheson Medical Center

La Grange
Owner
West Georgia Health System

Saint Marys
Member
Southeast Georgia Health System Camden Campus

Savannah
Owner
Memorial Health
St. Joseph's/Candler, Candler Hospital

Smyrna
Member
Emory–Adventist Hospital

HAWAII

Honolulu
Owner
Kuakini Medical Center

Kailua
Castle Medical Center

Kamuela
North Hawaii Community Hospital

IDAHO

Coeur D'Alene
Kootenai Medical Center

Moscow
Member
Gritman Medical Center

Post Falls
Northwest Specialty Hospital

ILLINOIS

Arlington Heights
Alexian Brothers Health System

Blue Island
Member
St. Francis Hospital & Health Center

Centralia
Member
St. Mary's Hospital

Chicago
Resurrection Health Care
Saint Joseph Hospital
Saints Mary & Elizabeth Medical Center, Claremont Avenue
Saints Mary & Elizabeth Medical Center, Division Street
Schwab Rehabilitation Hospital
Sinai Health System
Member
Our Lady of the Resurrection Medical Center
Resurrection Medical Center
Owner
Mercy Hospital and Medical Center
Mount Sinai Hospital

Des Plaines
Holy Family Medical Center

Elk Grove Village
Member
Alexian Brothers Medical Center

Evanston
Saint Francis Hospital

Glendale Heights
Adventist GlenOaks Hospital

Hinsdale
Member
Adventist Hinsdale Hospital

Hoffman Estates
Alexian Brothers Behavioral Health Hospital
St. Alexius Medical Center

La Grange
Adventist La Grange Memorial Hospital

Melrose Park
Westlake Hospital
Member
Gottlieb Memorial Hospital

Mount Vernon
Member
Good Samaritan Regional Health Center

Oak Park
West Suburban Medical Center

Peoria
Owner
Methodist Health Services Corporation

Urbana
Owner
Carle Foundation Hospital

Winfield
Owner
Central DuPage Hospital

INDIANA

Gary
Owner
Methodist Hospitals

Princeton
Member
Gibson General Hospital

IOWA

Ames
Member
Mary Greeley Medical Center

Charles City
Member
Floyd County Medical Center

Corning
Member
Alegent Health Mercy Hospital

Council Bluffs
Member
Alegent Health Mercy Hospital

Davenport
Member
Genesis Medical Center–Davenport

De Witt
Member
Genesis Medical Center, DeWitt

Estherville
Member
Avera Holy Family Health

Fairfield
Member
Jefferson County Hospital

Iowa City
Member
Mercy Iowa City

Le Mars
Floyd Valley Hospital/Avera Health

Manchester
Member
Regional Medical Center

Maquoketa
Member
Jackson County Regional Health Center

Marshalltown
Member
Marshalltown Medical & Surgical Center

Missouri Valley
Owner
Alegent Health Community Memorial Hospital

Mount Pleasant
Henry County Health Center

Newton
Member
Skiff Medical Center

Oskaloosa
Member
Mahaska Health Partnership

Ottumwa
Member
Ottumwa Regional Health Center

Pella
Member
Pella Regional Health Center

Rock Valley
Member
Hegg Memorial Health Center/Avera Health

Sibley
Member
Osceola Community Hospital

Sioux Center
Sioux Center Community Hospital/Health Center

West Burlington
Member
Great River Medical Center

KENTUCKY

Ashland
King's Daughters Medical Center
Our Lady of Bellefonte Hospital

Bowling Green
Commonwealth Regional Specialty Hospital

Corbin
Member
Baptist Regional Medical Center

Covington
St. Elizabeth Medical Center–South

Danville
Ephraim McDowell Regional Medical Center

Elizabethtown
Member
Hardin Memorial Hospital

Glasgow
Owner
T. J. Samson Community Hospital

Henderson
Owner
Methodist Hospital

Irvine
Member
Marcum and Wallace Memorial Hospital

La Grange
Member
Baptist Hospital Northeast

Lexington
Member
Central Baptist Hospital

Louisville
Norton Audubon Hospital
Norton Southwest Hospital
Norton Suburban Hospital
Member
Baptist Hospital East
Norton Hospital
University of Louisville Hospital
Owner
Baptist Healthcare System
Norton Healthcare

Madisonville
Regional Medical Center of Hopkins County

Manchester
Member
Manchester Memorial Hospital

Murray
Owner
Murray–Calloway County Hospital

Paducah
Member
Lourdes Hospital
Western Baptist Hospital

Salem
Member
Livingston Hospital and Healthcare Services

LOUISIANA

Baton Rouge
Baton Rouge General Medical Center
Member
Woman's Hospital

Columbia
Caldwell Memorial Hospital

Hammond
Member
North Oaks Medical Center

Houma
Owner
Terrebonne General Medical Center

Lafayette
Owner
Lafayette General Medical Center

Marrero
Owner
West Jefferson Medical Center

New Orleans
Owner
Touro Infirmary

West Monroe
Owner
Glenwood Regional Medical Center

Zachary
Lane Regional Medical Center

MAINE

Bangor
St. Joseph Hospital

MARYLAND

Annapolis
Owner
Anne Arundel Medical Center

Baltimore
Greater Baltimore Medical Center
Member
Bon Secours Baltimore Health System
Mercy Medical Center
Sinai Hospital of Baltimore

Bethesda
Owner
Suburban Hospital Healthcare System

Columbia
Owner
Howard County General Hospital

Cumberland
Western Maryland Health System
Owner
Memorial Hospital and Medical Center of Cumberland
WMHS Braddock Hospital

Elkton
Owner
Union Hospital

Frederick
Owner
Frederick Memorial Hospital

Hagerstown
Owner
Washington County Health System

La Plata
Civista Health

Lanham
Owner
Doctors Community Hospital

Marriottsville
Owner
Bon Secours Health System, Inc.

Olney
Owner
Montgomery General Hospital

Randallstown
Member
Northwest Hospital Center

Rockville
Adventist Rehabilitation Hospital of Maryland
Potomac Ridge Behavioral Health System
Member
Shady Grove Adventist Hospital
Owner
Adventist HealthCare

Salisbury
Owner
Peninsula Regional Health System

Takoma Park
Member
Washington Adventist Hospital

Westminster
Owner
Carroll Hospital Center

MASSACHUSETTS

Andover
Yankee Alliance

Attleboro
Member
Sturdy Memorial Hospital

Boston
Member
Beth Israel Deaconess Medical Center
Boston Medical Center

Brockton
Member
Signature Healthcare Brockton Hospital

Cambridge
Member
Youville Hospital and Rehabilitation Center

Fall River
Owner
Southcoast Hospitals Group

Great Barrington
Member
Fairview Hospital

Greenfield
Member
Baystate Franklin Medical Center

Lowell
Member
Saints Medical Center

North Adams
North Adams Regional Hospital

Pittsfield
Member
Berkshire Medical Center

Springfield
Member
Baystate Medical Center
Owner
Baystate Health, Inc.

Ware
Member
Baystate Mary Lane Hospital

Winchester
Member
Winchester Hospital

MICHIGAN

Bay City
Bay Regional Medical Center

Detroit
Member
Henry Ford Hospital
Owner
Henry Ford Health System

Ferndale
Henry Ford Kingswood Hospital

Flint
McLaren Health Care Corporation
Owner
McLaren Regional Medical Center

Grosse Pointe
Member
Beaumont Hospital Grosse Pointe

Grosse Pointe Farms
Member
Henry Ford Cottage Hospital

Lansing
Member
Ingham Regional Medical Center
Owner
Sparrow Hospital

Lapeer
Member
Lapeer Regional Medical Center

Rochester
Member
Crittenton Hospital Medical Center

Warren
Member
Henry Ford Macomb Hospital–Warren Campus

Wyandotte
Member
Henry Ford Wyandotte Hospital

MINNESOTA

Burnsville
Member
Fairview Ridges Hospital

Edina
Member
Fairview Southdale Hospital

Fairmont
Member
Fairmont Medical Center–Mayo Health System

Glencoe
Member
Glencoe Regional Health Services

Hibbing
Member
Fairview Range Regional Health Services

Marshall
Avera Marshall Regional Medical Center

Minneapolis
Member
University of Minnesota Medical Center, Fairview
Owner
Fairview Health Services

Pipestone
Member
Pipestone County Medical Center/Avera Health

Princeton
Member
Fairview Northland Medical Center

Red Wing
Member
Fairview Red Wing Medical Center

Saint Louis Park
Methodist Hospital
Member
Park Nicollet Health Services

Tyler
Member
Tyler Healthcare Center/Avera Health

Wyoming
Member
Fairview Lakes Regional Health Care

MISSISSIPPI

Grenada
Owner
Grenada Lake Medical Center

Jackson
Mississippi Baptist Health System
Mississippi Hospital for Restorative Care
Owner
Mississippi Baptist Medical Center
University Hospitals and Clinics, University of Mississippi Medical Center

Laurel
Owner
South Central Regional Medical Center

Meridian
Specialty Hospital of Meridian
Member
Rush Foundation Hospital
Owner
Rush Health Systems

Picayune
Member
Highland Community Hospital

MISSOURI

Bridgeton
SSM DePaul Health Center

Jefferson City
Member
St. Marys Health Center

Lake Saint Louis
Member
SSM St. Joseph Hospital West

Maryville
Member
St. Francis Hospital and Health Services

Saint Charles
Member
SSM St. Joseph Health Center

Saint Louis
Member
SSM Cardinal Glennon Children's Medical Center
SSM St. Joseph Hospital of Kirkwood
SSM St. Mary's Health Center
Owner
SSM Health Care

NEBRASKA

Blair
Memorial Community Hospital and Health System

Ogallala
Member
Ogallala Community Hospital

Omaha
Alegent Health
Alegent Health Lakeside Hospital
Owner
Alegent Health Bergan Mercy Medical Center
Alegent Health Immanuel Medical Center

O'Neill
Member
Avera St. Anthony's Hospital

Papillion
Owner
Alegent–Health Midlands Hospital

Schuyler
Owner
Alegent Health–Memorial Hospital

NEVADA

Fallon
Member
Banner Churchill Community Hospital

Henderson
St. Rose Dominican Hospitals – Rose de Lima Campus
St. Rose Dominican Hospitals – Siena Campus

NEW HAMPSHIRE

Manchester
Member
Catholic Medical Center
Elliot Hospital

Nashua
Member
St. Joseph Hospital

NEW JERSEY

Hackettstown
Member
Hackettstown Regional Medical Center

Secaucus
Member
LibertyHealth–Meadowlands Hospital Medical Center

NEW MEXICO

Albuquerque
Member
Presbyterian Hospital
Presbyterian Kaseman Hospital
Owner
Presbyterian Healthcare Services

Clovis
Member
Plains Regional Medical Center

Espanola
Member
Espanola Hospital

Ruidoso
Member
Lincoln County Medical Center

Socorro
Member
Socorro General Hospital

Tucumcari
Member
Dr. Dan C. Trigg Memorial Hospital

NEW YORK

Albany
Member
Albany Medical Center

Batavia
Member
United Memorial Medical Center

Bath
Member
Ira Davenport Memorial Hospital

Brockport
Member
Lakeside Memorial Hospital

Bronx
St. Barnabas Hospital

Buffalo
Member
Brylin Hospitals

Canandaigua
Member
Thompson Health

Carthage
Carthage Area Hospital

Clifton Springs
Member
Clifton Springs Hospital and Clinic

Corning
Member
Corning Hospital

Dansville
Member
Nicholas H. Noyes Memorial Hospital

Elizabethtown
Member
Elizabethtown Community Hospital

Elmira
Member
Arnot Ogden Medical Center
St. Joseph's Hospital

Geneva
Geneva General Hospital

Glens Falls
Member
Glens Falls Hospital

Hornell
Member
St. James Mercy Hospital

Lockport
Lockport Memorial Hospital

Medina
Member
Medina Memorial Hospital

Montour Falls
Member
Schuyler Hospital

Newark
Newark–Wayne Community Hospital

Olean
Olean General Hospital

Penn Yan
Member
Soldiers and Sailors Memorial Hospital of Yates County

Plattsburgh
Member
Champlain Valley Physicians Hospital Medical Center

Port Jervis
Bon Secours Community Hospital

Rochester
Highland Hospital of Rochester
Rochester Psychiatric Center
Strong Memorial Hospital of the University of Rochester
Unity Hospital
Member
Rochester General Hospital
Owner
ViaHealth

Suffern
Good Samaritan Hospital

Syracuse
Member
Upstate Medical University

Troy
Member
Samaritan Hospital

Warwick
St. Anthony Community Hospital

Wellsville
Jones Memorial Hospital

NORTH CAROLINA

Albemarle
Owner
Stanly Regional Medical Center

Asheboro
Owner
Randolph Hospital

Asheville
Owner
Mission Hospital

Boone
Owner
Watauga Medical Center

Bryson City
Member
Swain County Hospital

Burlington
Owner
Alamance Regional Medical Center

Clyde
Owner
Haywood Regional Medical Center

Fayetteville
Cape Fear Valley Health System

Fletcher
Member
Park Ridge Hospital

Gastonia
Owner
Gaston Memorial Hospital

Goldsboro
Owner
Wayne Memorial Hospital

Hendersonville
Owner
Margaret R. Pardee Memorial Hospital

Hickory
Owner
Catawba Valley Medical Center

Kinston
Owner
Lenoir Memorial Hospital

Lumberton
Owner
Southeastern Regional Medical Center

Pinehurst
FirstHealth of the Carolinas
Owner
FirstHealth Moore Regional Hospital

Roanoke Rapids
Owner
Halifax Regional Medical Center

Rockingham
FirstHealth Richmond Memorial Hospital

Statesville
Owner
Iredell Memorial Hospital

Sylva
WestCare Health System
Owner
Harris Regional Hospital

Troy
Owner
FirstHealth Montgomery Memorial Hospital

Wilmington
Owner
New Hanover Regional Medical Center

Wilson
Owner
Wilson Medical Center

OHIO

Akron
Owner
Summa Health System

Amherst
Specialty Hospital of Lorain

Batavia
Member
Mercy Hospital Clermont

Cincinnati
Mercy Hospital Mount Airy
Mercy Hospital Western Hills
Member
Mercy Hospital Anderson
Owner
Bethesda North Hospital
Catholic Healthcare Partners
Good Samaritan Hospital

Cleveland
Cleveland Clinic Health System
Member
Cleveland Clinic Children's Hospital for Rehabilitation
Fairview Hospital
Lutheran Hospital
MetroHealth Medical Center
Owner
Cleveland Clinic Foundation
Hillcrest Hospital
Huron Hospital

Dayton
Grandview Hospital and Medical Center
Kettering Health Network

Defiance
Mercy Hospital of Defiance

Elyria
Member
EMH Regional Medical Center

Euclid
Member
Euclid Hospital

Fairfield
Mercy Hospital Fairfield

Garfield Heights
Member
Marymount Hospital

Kettering
Charles F. Kettering Memorial Hospital

Lakewood
Member
Lakewood Hospital

Lima
Institute for Orthopaedic Surgery
Member
St. Rita's Medical Center

Lorain
Member
Community Health Partners Regional Medical Center

Miamisburg
Kettering Medical Center–Sycamore

Oberlin
Member
Allen Community Hospital

Oregon
Member
St. Charles Mercy Hospital

Parma
Member
Parma Community General Hospital

Springfield
Springfield Regional Medical Center – High Street Campus
Member
Springfield Regional Medical Center – Fountain Campus

Tiffin
Member
Mercy Hospital of Tiffin

Toledo
St. Anne Mercy Hospital
Member
St. Vincent Mercy Medical Center

Urbana
Member
Mercy Memorial Hospital

Warren
Member
St. Joseph Health Center

Warrensville Heights
Owner
South Pointe Hospital

Willard
Member
Mercy Hospital of Willard

Youngstown
Member
St. Elizabeth Health Center

OKLAHOMA

Oklahoma City
Member
Bone and Joint Hospital
St. Anthony Hospital

Tulsa
Saint Francis Heart Hospital
Member
Laureate Psychiatric Clinic and Hospital
Owner
Saint Francis Hospital

OREGON

Cottage Grove
Cottage Grove Community Hospital

Eugene
Member
Sacred Heart Medical Center

Florence
Member
Peace Harbor Hospital

Medford
Providence Medford Medical Center

Portland
Member
Adventist Medical Center

Salem
Member
Salem Hospital

Tillamook
Member
Tillamook County General Hospital

PENNSYLVANIA

Bethlehem
Owner
St. Luke's Hospital – Bethlehem Campus

Bryn Mawr
Member
Bryn Mawr Hospital
Bryn Mawr Hospital

Canonsburg
Canonsburg General Hospital

Corry
Member
Corry Memorial Hospital

Danville
Member
Geisinger Health System
Geisinger Medical Center

Du Bois
DuBois Regional Medical Center

Ellwood City
Ellwood City Hospital

Erie
Member
Millcreek Community Hospital
Saint Vincent Health Center

Greensburg
Excela Health
Excela Westmoreland Regional Hospital

Greenville
UPMC Horizon

Kane
Member
Kane Community Hospital

Kittanning
ACMH

Latrobe
Excela Latrobe Area Hospital

Malvern
Member
Bryn Mawr Rehabilitation Hospital

Meadville
Member
Meadville Medical Center

Monroeville
Member
Western Pennsylvania Hospital – Forbes Regional Campus

Mount Pleasant
Excela Frick Hospital

Nanticoke
Member
Mercy Special Care Hospital

Natrona Heights
Alle–Kiski Medical Center

Paoli
Member
Paoli Hospital

Philadelphia
Frankford Hospital of the City of Philadelphia
Magee Rehabilitation Hospital
Member
Albert Einstein Medical Center
Thomas Jefferson University Hospital

Pittsburgh
Allegheny General Hospital
West Penn Allegheny Health System
Owner
Western Pennsylvania Hospital

Radnor
Owner
Jefferson Health System

Scranton
Member
Mercy Hospital of Scranton

Seneca
UPMC Northwest

Titusville
Member
Titusville Area Hospital

Warren
Owner
Warren General Hospital

Wilkes–Barre
Member
Geisinger South Wilkes–Barre
Geisinger Wyoming Valley Medical Center

Wynnewood
Member
Lankenau Hospital

SOUTH CAROLINA

Anderson
Owner
AnMed Health Medical Center

Columbia
Palmetto Health Baptist/Columbia
Member
Palmetto Health Richland
Owner
Palmetto Health

Conway
Owner
Conway Medical Center

Easley
Palmetto Health Baptist Easley

Florence
Owner
McLeod Health

Greenville
Bon Secours St. Francis Health System
Member
Greenville Memorial Hospital
Owner
Greenville Hospital System

Greenwood
Owner
Self Regional Healthcare

Greer
Member
Allen Bennett Memorial Hospital

Spartanburg
Owner
Spartanburg Regional Medical Center

West Columbia
Owner
Lexington Medical Center

SOUTH DAKOTA

Aberdeen
Member
Avera St. Luke's

Britton
Member
Marshall County Healthcare Center/Avera Health

Dell Rapids
Member
Avera Dells Area Health Center

Eureka
Member
Eureka Community Health Services/Avera

Flandreau
Member
Flandreau Medical Center/Avera Health

Gregory
Member
Avera Gregory Healthcare Center

Milbank
Member
Milbank Area Hospital/Avera Health

Miller
Member
Avera Hand County Memorial Hospital & Clinic

Mitchell
Member
Avera Queen of Peace

Parkston
Member
Avera St. Benedict Health Center

Platte
Member
Platte Health Center/Avera Health

Rapid City
Owner
Rapid City Regional Hospital

Scotland
Member
Landmann–Jungman Memorial Hospital

Sioux Falls
Member
Avera McKennan Hospital and University Health Center
Owner
Avera Health

Tyndall
Member
St. Michael's Hospital

Wagner
Member
Wagner Community Memorial Hospital – Avera

Wessington Springs
Member
Avera Weskota Memorial Medical Center

Yankton
Member
Avera Sacred Heart Hospital

TENNESSEE

Carthage
Riverview Regional Medical Center North
Riverview Regional Medical Center South

Elizabethton
Sycamore Shoals Hospital

Etowah
Member
Woods Memorial Hospital

Gallatin
Sumner Regional Health Systems
Owner
Sumner Regional Medical Center

Greeneville
Member
Takoma Regional Hospital

Hartsville
Trousdale Medical Center

Jefferson City
Member
St. Mary's Jefferson Memorial Hospital

Jellico
Member
Jellico Community Hospital

Johnson City
Johnson City Specialty Hospital
North Side Hospital
Quillen Rehabilitation Hospital
Woodridge Hospital
Member
Johnson City Medical Center
Owner
Mountain States Health Alliance

Kingsport
Indian Path Medical Center

Knoxville
Baptist Hospital for Women
Baptist Hospital West
Member
St. Mary's Medical Center

La Follette
Member
St. Mary's Medical Center of Campbell County

Madison
Skyline Madison Campus

Maryville
Owner
Blount Memorial Hospital

Memphis
Methodist Extended Care Hospital
Member
Methodist Le Bonheur Healthcare
Methodist University Hospital

Mountain City
Johnson County Community Hospital

Nashville
Owner
Vanderbilt University Medical Center

Newport
Member
Baptist Hospital of Cocke County

Somerville
Owner
Methodist Healthcare–Fayette Hospital

Tazewell
Member
Claiborne County Hospital

TEXAS

Abilene
Owner
Hendrick Health System

Allen
Texas Health Presbyterian Hospital of Allen

Arlington
Texas Health Arlington Memorial Hospital
Texas Health Resources

Azle
Member
Texas Health Harris Methodist Northwest

Bedford
Member
Texas Health Harris Methodist–HEB

Cleburne
Member
Walls Regional Hospital

Dallas
University of Texas Southwestern Medical Center
Member
Methodist Charlton Medical Center
Methodist Dallas Medical Center
Texas Health Presbyterian Hospital of Dallas
Owner
Methodist Health System

Denison
Owner
Texoma Medical Center

El Paso
Owner
R. E. Thomason General Hospital

Fort Worth
Harris Continued Care Hospital
Member
Huguley Memorial Medical Center
Texas Health Harris Methodist Fort Worth
Texas Health Harris Methodist Southwest

Henderson
Member
Henderson Memorial Hospital

Houston
Harris County Hospital District
St. Luke's Episcopal Health System
Member
The Methodist Hospital
Owner
St. Luke's Episcopal Hospital
The Methodist Hospital System
University of Texas M. D. Anderson Cancer Center

Kaufman
Member
Texas Health Presbyterian Hospital of Kaufman

Killeen
Member
Metroplex Adventist Hospital

Lampasas
Rollins–Brook Community Hospital

Livingston
Member
Memorial Medical Center – Livingston

Lubbock
Owner
University Medical Center

Lufkin
Memorial Specialty Hospital
Owner
Memorial Health System of East Texas

Nacogdoches
Owner
Nacogdoches Memorial Hospital

Plano
Member
Texas Health Presbyterian Hospital of Plano

San Augustine
Member
Memorial Medical Center – San Augustine

San Marcos
Member
Central Texas Medical Center

Stephenville
Member
Texas Health Harris Methodist–Erath County

The Woodlands
St Luke's Community Medical Center–The Woodlands

Weslaco
Owner
Knapp Medical Center

Winnsboro
Member
Texas Health Presbyterian Hospital of Winnsboro

VIRGINIA

Abingdon
Owner
Johnston Memorial Hospital

Bedford
Member
Bedford Memorial Hospital

Chesapeake
Owner
Chesapeake General Hospital

Christiansburg
Member
Carilion New River Valley Medical Center

Front Royal
Member
Warren Memorial Hospital

Galax
Owner
Twin County Regional Hospital

Lexington
Member
Carilion Stonewall Jackson Hospital

Marion
Owner
Smyth County Community Hospital

Mechanicsville
Member
Memorial Regional Medical Center

Midlothian
Bon Secours St. Francis Medical Center

Newport News
Member
Mary Immaculate Hospital

Norfolk
Member
Bon Secours–DePaul Medical Center

Pearisburg
Member
Carilion Giles Memorial Hospital

Portsmouth
Member
Maryview Medical Center

Richmond
Member
Bon Secours St. Mary's Hospital
Bon Secours–Richmond Community Hospital

Roanoke
Member
Carilion Medical Center
Owner
Carilion Clinic

Rocky Mount
Member
Carilion Franklin Memorial Hospital

South Hill
Owner
Community Memorial Healthcenter

Suffolk
Owner
Sentara Obici Hospital

Tazewell
Member
Tazewell Community Hospital

Winchester
Member
Winchester Medical Center
Owner
Valley Health System

Woodstock
Member
Shenandoah Memorial Hospital

WASHINGTON

Anacortes
Island Hospital

Arlington
Cascade Valley Hospital and Clinics

Bellevue
Member
Overlake Hospital Medical Center
Owner
PeaceHealth

Bellingham
Member
St. Joseph Hospital

Bremerton
Harrison Medical Center

Burien
Member
Highline Medical Center

Centralia
Member
Providence Centralia Hospital

Chelan
Member
Lake Chelan Community Hospital

Clarkston
Member
Tri–State Memorial Hospital

Colfax
Member
Whitman Hospital and Medical Center

Coupeville
Member
Whidbey General Hospital

Davenport
Member
Lincoln Hospital

Dayton
Dayton General Hospital

Edmonds
Member
Stevens Healthcare

Ellensburg
Kittitas Valley Community Hospital

Ephrata
Member
Columbia Basin Hospital

Everett
Member
Providence Everett Medical Center

Federal Way
St. Francis Hospital

Grand Coulee
Member
Coulee Community Hospital

Kennewick
Kennewick General Hospital

Longview
Member
St. John Medical Center

Medical Lake
Eastern State Hospital

Moses Lake
Member
Samaritan Healthcare

Mount Vernon
Skagit Valley Hospital

Newport
Member
Newport Hospital and Health Services

Odessa
Member
Odessa Memorial Healthcare Center

Olympia
Member
Providence St. Peter Hospital

Othello
Member
Othello Community Hospital

Pasco
Lourdes Medical Center

Prosser
Member
Prosser Memorial Hospital

Pullman
Member
Pullman Regional Hospital

Quincy
Member
Quincy Valley Medical Center

Redmond
Member
Group Health Eastside Hospital

Renton
Member
Valley Medical Center

Republic
Member
Ferry County Memorial Hospital

Richland
Member
Kadlec Medical Center

Ritzville
Member
East Adams Rural Hospital

Seattle
Virginia Mason Medical Center

Sedro Woolley
United General Hospital

Spokane
Member
Holy Family Hospital
Sacred Heart Medical Center
Valley Hospital and Medical Center

Sunnyside
Sunnyside Community Hospital

Tacoma
Mary Bridge Children's Hospital and Health Center
St. Clare Hospital
St. Joseph Medical Center

Tonasket
Member
North Valley Hospital

Toppenish
Member
Toppenish Community Hospital

Vancouver
Member
Southwest Washington Medical Center

Walla Walla
Member
St. Mary Medical Center
Walla Walla General Hospital

Yakima
Yakima Valley Memorial Hospital

WEST VIRGINIA

Berkeley Springs
Member
Morgan County War Memorial Hospital

Bluefield
Owner
Bluefield Regional Medical Center

Buckhannon
Member
St. Joseph's Hospital of Buckhannon

Clarksburg
Member
United Hospital Center

Elkins
Owner
Davis Memorial Hospital

Fairmont
Owner
West Virginia United Health System

Huntington
Cabell Huntington Hospital
Owner
St. Mary's Medical Center

Martinsburg
Member
City Hospital

Morgantown
West Virginia University Hospitals
Owner
Monongalia General Hospital

Parkersburg
Owner
Camden–Clark Memorial Hospital

Point Pleasant
Owner
Pleasant Valley Hospital

Ranson
Member
Jefferson Memorial Hospital

South Charleston
Owner
Thomas Memorial Hospital

Weirton
Owner
Weirton Medical Center

WISCONSIN

Baraboo
Member
St. Clare Hospital and Health Services

Boscobel
Boscobel Area Health Care

Burlington
Member
Aurora Memorial Hospital of Burlington

Durand
Member
Chippewa Valley Hospital and Oakview Care Center

Elkhorn
Member
Aurora Lakeland Medical Center

Green Bay
Aurora BayCare Medical Center

Hartford
Member
Aurora Medical Center of Washington County

Kenosha
Aurora Medical Center

Madison
Member
St. Mary's Hospital

Milwaukee
Member
Aurora Sinai Medical Center
Aurora St. Luke's Medical Center
Owner
Aurora Health Care

Oshkosh
Aurora Medical Center of Oshkosh

Sheboygan
Member
Aurora Sheboygan Memorial Medical Center

Two Rivers
Member
Aurora Medical Center – Manitowoc County

Wauwatosa
Aurora Psychiatric Hospital

West Allis
Member
Aurora West Allis Medical Center

WYOMING

Torrington
Member
Community Hospital

Wheatland
Platte County Memorial Hospital

Worland
Member
Washakie Medical Center

SYNERNET, INC.

222 St John Street, Portland, ME Zip 04102; tel. 207/775–6081; Mr. Paul I. Davis, III, President

MAINE

Bangor
Affiliate
St. Joseph Hospital

Bar Harbor
Affiliate
Mount Desert Island Hospital

Biddeford
Affiliate
Southern Maine Medical Center

Boothbay Harbor
Owner
St. Andrews Hospital and Healthcare Center

Brunswick
Affiliate
Mid Coast Hospital

Damariscotta
Owner
Miles Memorial Hospital

Farmington
Owner
Franklin Memorial Hospital

Fort Kent
Affiliate
Northern Maine Medical Center

Norway
Owner
Stephens Memorial Hospital

Portland
Owner
Maine Medical Center
New England Rehabilitation Hospital of Portland

Rockport
Affiliate
Penobscot Bay Medical Center

Sanford
Owner
Henrietta D. Goodall Hospital

Skowhegan
Affiliate
Redington–Fairview General Hospital

Waterville
Affiliate
MaineGeneral Medical Center–Waterville Campus

Westbrook
Owner
Spring Harbor Hospital

THE NEW JERSEY COUNCIL OF TEACHING HOSPITALS

154 West State Street, Trenton, NJ Zip 08608; tel. 609/656–9600; Dr. J. Richard Goldstein , M.D., President

NEW JERSEY

Camden
Member
Cooper Health System

Hamilton
Member
Robert Wood Johnson University Hospital at Hamilton

Morristown
Member
Atlantic Health

Neptune
Member
Meridian Health

New Brunswick
Member
Robert Wood Johnson University Hospital

Newark
Member
University of Medicine and Dentistry of New Jersey–University Hospital

Paterson
Member
St. Joseph's Regional Medical Center

Phillipsburg
Member
Warren Hospital

Somerville
Member
Somerset Medical Center

UNIVERSITY HEALTHSYSTEM CONSORTIUM, INC.

2001 Spring Road, Suite 700, Oak Brook, IL Zip 60523; tel. 630/954–1700; Ms. Irene M. Thompson, President and Chief Executive Officer

ALABAMA

Birmingham
Member
University of Alabama Hospital

Mobile
Affiliate
Infirmary West at Knollwood
Member
University of South Alabama Medical Center

ARIZONA

Tucson
Member
University Medical Center

ARKANSAS

Little Rock
Member
UAMS Medical Center

CALIFORNIA

Downey
Affiliate
Rancho Los Amigos National Rehabilitation Center

Los Angeles
Member
King–Harbor's Health Center
LAC/University of Southern California Medical Center
University of California Los Angeles Medical Center

Martinez
Affiliate
Contra Costa Regional Medical Center

Orange
Member
University of California, Irvine Medical Center

Palo Alto
Lucile Salter Packard Children's Hospital at Stanford
Member
Stanford Hospital and Clinics

Sacramento
Member
University of California, Davis Medical Center

San Diego
Member
University of California San Diego Medical Center

San Francisco
Affiliate
University of California–San Francisco Mount Zion Medical Center
Member
San Francisco General Hospital Medical Center

San Jose
Affiliate
Santa Clara Valley Medical Center

San Leandro
Affiliate
Alameda County Medical Center–Fairmont Campus

Santa Monica
Affiliate
Santa Monica–UCLA Medical Center and Orthopaedic Hospital

Sylmar
Affiliate
LAC–Olive View–UCLA Medical Center

Torrance
Member
LAC–Harbor–University of California at Los Angeles Medical Center

Valencia
Affiliate
Henry Mayo Newhall Memorial Hospital

COLORADO

Aurora
Member
University of Colorado Hospital

Denver
Affiliate
National Jewish Medical and Research Center
Member
Denver Health Medical Center

CONNECTICUT

Farmington
Member
University of Connecticut Health Center, John Dempsey Hospital

New Haven
Member
Yale–New Haven Hospital

DISTRICT OF COLUMBIA

Washington
Member
Howard University Hospital
MedStar–Georgetown Medical Center

FLORIDA

Gainesville
Affiliate
Shands AGH
Member
Shands at the University of Florida

Lake City
Affiliate
Shands Lake Shore

Live Oak
Affiliate
Shands Live Oak

Starke
Affiliate
Shands Starke

Tampa
Member
Tampa General Hospital

GEORGIA

Atlanta
Wesley Woods Center of Emory University
Member
Emory Crawford Long Hospital
Emory University Hospital

Section B

Augusta
Member
Medical College of Georgia Health

ILLINOIS

Chicago
Affiliate
Louis A. Weiss Memorial Hospital
Member
University of Chicago Medical Center
University of Illinois Medical Center at Chicago

Maywood
Member
Loyola University Medical Center

INDIANA

Indianapolis
Member
Clarian Health Partners
Wishard Health Services

IOWA

Iowa City
Member
University of Iowa Hospitals and Clinics

KANSAS

Kansas City
Member
University of Kansas Hospital

KENTUCKY

Lexington
Member
University of Kentucky Hospital

LOUISIANA

Shreveport
Member
LSU Medical Center–University Hospital

MARYLAND

Baltimore
Maryland General Hospital
Mt. Washington Pediatric Hospital
Affiliate
Kernan Orthopaedics and Rehabilitation
Member
University of Maryland Medical Center

Glen Burnie
Baltimore Washington Medical Center

MASSACHUSETTS

Boston
Faulkner Hospital
Member
Brigham and Women's Hospital
Massachusetts General Hospital

Clinton
Affiliate
Clinton Hospital

Marlborough
Affiliate
UMass Memorial–Marlborough Hospital

Newton Lower Falls
Newton–Wellesley Hospital

Salem
North Shore Medical Center

MICHIGAN

Ann Arbor
Member
University of Michigan Hospitals and Health Centers

MINNESOTA

Burnsville
Fairview Ridges Hospital

Edina
Fairview Southdale Hospital

Hibbing
Fairview Range Regional Health Services

Minneapolis
Affiliate
Hennepin County Medical Center

MISSOURI

Boonville
Cooper County Memorial Hospital

Columbia
Columbia Regional Hospital
Member
University of Missouri Hospitals and Clinics

Jefferson City
Capital Region Medical Center

Kansas City
Truman Medical Center–Hospital Hill
Truman Medical Center–Lakewood

NEBRASKA

Omaha
Member
Nebraska Medical Center

NEVADA

Las Vegas
Affiliate
University Medical Center

NEW JERSEY

New Brunswick
Member
Robert Wood Johnson University Hospital

Newark
Member
University of Medicine and Dentistry of New Jersey–University Hospital

NEW MEXICO

Albuquerque
University of New Mexico Hospitals

NEW YORK

Albany
Member
Albany Medical Center

Brooklyn
Kings County Hospital Center
Member
SUNY Downstate Medical Center University Hospital of Brooklyn

Flushing
Elmhurst Hospital Center

New York
Bellevue Hospital Center
New York–Presbyterian Hospital

Stony Brook
Member
Stony Brook University Hospital

Syracuse
Member
Upstate Medical University

NORTH CAROLINA

Ahoskie
Affiliate
Roanoke–Chowan Hospital

Chapel Hill
Member
University of North Carolina Hospitals

Edenton
Chowan Hospital

Greenville
Member
Pitt County Memorial Hospital

Tarboro
Heritage Hospital

Windsor
Affiliate
Bertie Memorial Hospital

Winston–Salem
Old Vineyard Behavioral Health Services
Member
North Carolina Baptist Hospital (Wake Forest University Baptist Medical Center)

OHIO

Canton
Mercy Medical Center

Chardon
Affiliate
University Hospitals Geauga Regional Hospital

Cincinnati
Member
University Hospital

Cleveland
St. John West Shore Hospital
St. Vincent Charity Hospital
University Hospitals Richmond Medical Center
Affiliate
University Hospitals Bedford Medical Center
Member
University Hospitals Case Medical Center

Columbus
Member
Ohio State University Medical Center

Conneaut
Affiliate
University Hospitals Conneaut Medical Center

Geneva
Affiliate
University Hospitals Geneva Medical Center

Middleburg Heights
Southwest General Health Center

Toledo
Member
The University of Toledo Medical Center

Waverly
Affiliate
Pike Community Hospital

Willoughby
Affiliate
Windsor–Laurelwood Center for Behavioral Medicine

OREGON

Portland
Member
OHSU Hospital

PENNSYLVANIA

Philadelphia
Affiliate
Friends Behavioral Health System
Presbyterian Medical Center of the University of Pennsylvania Health System
Thomas Jefferson University Hospital
Member
Hospital of the University of Pennsylvania

Phoenixville
Affiliate
Phoenixville Hospital

Pittsburgh
Member
UPMC Presbyterian

SOUTH CAROLINA

Charleston
Affiliate
Charleston Memorial Hospital
Member
MUSC Medical Center of Medical University of South Carolina

TENNESSEE

Knoxville
Member
University of Tennessee Medical Center

TEXAS

Baytown
San Jacinto Methodist Hospital

Galveston
Member
University of Texas Medical Branch Hospitals

Houston
Methodist Willowbrook Hospital
The Methodist Hospital

Sugar Land
Methodist Sugar Land Hospital

Tyler
Affiliate
University of Texas Health Science Center at Tyler

UTAH

Salt Lake City
Member
University of Utah Health Care – Hospital and Clinics

VIRGINIA

Charlottesville
Member
University of Virginia Medical Center

Richmond
Member
VCU Health System

WASHINGTON

Seattle
Member
Harborview Medical Center
University of Washington Medical Center

WISCONSIN

Antigo
Affiliate
Langlade Memorial Hospital

Madison
Member
University of Wisconsin Hospital and Clinics

Medford
Affiliate
Memorial Health Center

Merrill
Affiliate
Good Samaritan Health Center of Merrill

Milwaukee
Member
Froedtert Memorial Lutheran Hospital

Wausau
Affiliate
Aspirus Wausau Hospital

VANTAGE HEALTH GROUP

265 Conneaut Lake Road, Meadville, PA Zip 16335; tel. 814/337–0000; Mr. David C. Petno, Vice President Business Development

PENNSYLVANIA

Corry
Member
Corry Memorial Hospital

Du Bois
Member
DuBois Regional Medical Center

Ellwood City
Member
Ellwood City Hospital

Erie
Member
Millcreek Community Hospital
Saint Vincent Health Center

Greenville
Member
UPMC Horizon

Kane
Member
Kane Community Hospital

Kittanning
Member
ACMH

Meadville
Member
Meadville Medical Center

Seneca
Member
UPMC Northwest

Titusville
Member
Titusville Area Hospital

Warren
Member
Warren General Hospital

VHA, INC.

220 East Las Colinas Boulevard, Irving, TX Zip 75039–5500; tel. 972/830–0000; Mr. Curtis W. Nonomaque, President and Chief Executive Officer

ALABAMA

Alabaster
Shelby Baptist Medical Center

Anniston
Partner
Northeast Alabama Regional Medical Center

Athens
Partner
Athens–Limestone Hospital

Atmore
Atmore Community Hospital

Bay Minette
North Baldwin Infirmary

Birmingham
Princeton Baptist Medical Center
Trinity Medical Center
Shareholder
Baptist Health System

Boaz
Marshall Medical Center South

Brewton
D. W. McMillan Memorial Hospital

Carrollton
Pickens County Medical Center

Centre
Cherokee Medical Center

Chatom
Washington County Hospital and Nursing Home

Cullman
Partner
Cullman Regional Medical Center

Decatur
Decatur General Hospital

Fairhope
Thomas Hospital

Fayette
Fayette Medical Center

Florence
Coffee Health Group

Fort Payne
DeKalb Regional Medical Center

Grove Hill
Grove Hill Memorial Hospital

Guntersville
Marshall Medical Center North
Partner
Marshall County Health Care Authority

Hamilton
North Mississippi Medical Center–Hamilton

Huntsville
Huntsville Hospital

Jasper
Walker Baptist Medical Center

Luverne
Crenshaw Community Hospital

Mobile
Mobile Infirmary Medical Center

Montgomery
Baptist Medical Center East
Shareholder
Baptist Medical Center South

Moulton
Lawrence Medical Center

Muscle Shoals
Shoals Hospital

Northport
Northport Medical Center

Opp
Mizell Memorial Hospital

Ozark
Dale Medical Center

Prattville
Prattville Baptist Hospital

Scottsboro
Partner
Highlands Medical Center

Sylacauga
Coosa Valley Medical Center

Talladega
Citizens Baptist Medical Center

Tuscaloosa
DCH Regional Medical Center
Partner
DCH Health System

Union Springs
Bullock County Hospital

ALASKA

Anchorage
Providence Alaska Medical Center

Cordova
Cordova Community Medical Center

Kodiak
Providence Kodiak Island Medical Center

Seward
Providence Seward Medical Center

Valdez
Providence Valdez Medical Center

Wrangell
Wrangell Medical Center

ARIZONA

Bisbee
Copper Queen Community Hospital

Phoenix
Mayo Clinic Hospital

Safford
Mt. Graham Regional Medical Center

Tucson
Tucson Medical Center

ARKANSAS

Arkadelphia
Baptist Health Medical Center–Arkadelphia

Booneville
Booneville Community Hospital

Clinton
Ozark Health Medical Center

Conway
Partner
Conway Regional Medical Center

Eureka Springs
Eureka Springs Hospital

Fayetteville
Partner
Washington Regional Medical Center

Forrest City
Forrest City Medical Center

Fort Smith
Shareholder
Sparks Regional Medical Center

Heber Springs
Baptist Health Medical Center–Heber Springs

Jonesboro
Partner
St. Bernards Medical Center

Little Rock
Baptist Health Medical Center–Little Rock
Shareholder
Baptist Health

North Little Rock
Baptist Health Medical Center – North Little Rock

Paragould
Partner
Arkansas Methodist Medical Center

Piggott
Piggott Community Hospital

Walnut Ridge
Lawrence Memorial Hospital

Wynne
CrossRidge Community Hospital

CALIFORNIA

Alameda
Alameda Hospital

Anaheim
Partner
Anaheim Memorial Medical Center

Antioch
Sutter Delta Medical Center

Arcadia
Methodist Hospital of Southern California

Auburn
Sutter Auburn Faith Hospital

Berkeley
Alta Bates Medical Center–Herrick Campus
Alta Bates Summit Medical Center

Section B

Burbank
Providence Saint Joseph Medical Center

Burlingame
Mills–Peninsula Health Services

Clovis
Clovis Community Medical Center

Concord
John Muir Medical Center, Concord

Covina
Citrus Valley Health Partners
Citrus Valley Medical Center–Inter–Community Campus

Crescent City
Sutter Coast Hospital

Davis
Sutter Davis Hospital

El Centro
El Centro Regional Medical Center

Encinitas
Scripps Memorial Hospital–Encinitas

Fountain Valley
Orange Coast Memorial Medical Center

Fresno
Community Regional Medical Center
Shareholder
Community Medical Centers

Glendora
Foothill Presbyterian Hospital–Morris L. Johnston Memorial

Greenbrae
Marin General Hospital

Jackson
Sutter Amador Hospital

La Jolla
Scripps Green Hospital
Shareholder
Scripps Memorial Hospital–La Jolla

Laguna Hills
Saddleback Memorial Medical Center

Lakeport
Sutter Lakeside Hospital

Lancaster
Partner
Antelope Valley Hospital

Long Beach
Long Beach Memorial Medical Center
Shareholder
Memorial Health Services

Los Angeles
Shareholder
Cedars–Sinai Medical Center

Modesto
Partner
Memorial Medical Center

Monterey
Community Hospital of the Monterey Peninsula

Napa
Queen of the Valley Medical Center

Newport Beach
Shareholder
Hoag Memorial Hospital Presbyterian

Novato
Novato Community Hospital

Oakland
Alta Bates Summit Medical Center – Summit Campus

Pasadena
Huntington Memorial Hospital

Pleasanton
ValleyCare Medical Center

Pomona
Partner
Pomona Valley Hospital Medical Center

Roseville
Sutter Roseville Medical Center

Sacramento
Sutter Medical Center, Sacramento
Shareholder
Sutter Health

San Diego
Scripps Health
Scripps Mercy Hospital

San Fernando
Providence Holy Cross Medical Center

San Francisco
California Pacific Medical Center–Davies Campus
Chinese Hospital
St. Luke's Hospital
Shareholder
California Pacific Medical Center

San Pedro
Litttle Company of Mary – San Pedro Hospital

Santa Barbara
Cottage Health System
Goleta Valley Cottage Hospital
Partner
Santa Barbara Cottage Hospital

Santa Cruz
Sutter Maternity and Surgery Center of Santa Cruz

Santa Rosa
Sutter Medical Center of Santa Rosa, Chanate Campus

Sonoma
Sonoma Valley Hospital

Torrance
Little Company of Mary Hospital
Partner
Torrance Memorial Medical Center

Tracy
Sutter Tracy Community Hospital

Turlock
Partner
Emanuel Medical Center

Vallejo
Sutter Solano Medical Center

Van Nuys
Partner
Valley Presbyterian Hospital

Walnut Creek
John Muir Health
John Muir Medical Center, Walnut Creek

Whittier
Partner
Presbyterian Intercommunity Hospital

COLORADO

Alamosa
Partner
San Luis Valley Regional Medical Center

Aspen
Partner
Aspen Valley Hospital District

Boulder
Partner
Boulder Community Hospital

Colorado Springs
Partner
Memorial Health System

Denver
Exempla Healthcare, Inc.
Exempla Saint Joseph Hospital

Englewood
Craig Hospital

Estes Park
Estes Park Medical Center

Fort Collins
Poudre Valley Hospital

Grand Junction
Partner
Community Hospital

Gunnison
Partner
Gunnison Valley Hospital

Haxtun
Haxtun Hospital District

La Jara
Conejos County Hospital

Lafayette
Exempla Good Samaritan Medical Center

Longmont
Partner
Longmont United Hospital

Rangely
Rangely District Hospital

Steamboat Springs
Partner
Yampa Valley Medical Center

Vail
Shareholder
Vail Valley Medical Center

Wheat Ridge
Shareholder
Exempla Lutheran Medical Center

Yuma
Yuma District Hospital

CONNECTICUT

Bridgeport
Bridgeport Hospital

Danbury
Partner
Danbury Hospital

Greenwich
Partner
Greenwich Hospital

Hartford
Connecticut Children's Medical Center
Shareholder
Hartford Hospital

Manchester
Eastern Connecticut Health Network
Manchester Memorial Hospital

Meriden
Partner
MidState Medical Center

Middletown
Partner
Middlesex Hospital

New Britain
Hospital for Special Care

New Haven
Yale New Haven Health System
Yale–New Haven Hospital

New Milford
New Milford Hospital

Putnam
Day Kimball Hospital

Stamford
Partner
Stamford Hospital

Torrington
Partner
The Charlotte Hungerford Hospital

Vernon Rockville
Rockville General Hospital

Waterbury
Partner
Waterbury Hospital

DISTRICT OF COLUMBIA

Washington
MedStar–Georgetown Medical Center
Washington Hospital Center

FLORIDA

Boca Raton
Partner
Boca Raton Community Hospital

Boynton Beach
Partner
Bethesda Memorial Hospital

Cape Coral
Cape Coral Hospital

Clermont
South Lake Hospital

Cocoa Beach
Cape Canaveral Hospital

Daytona Beach
Atlantic Medical Center
Halifax–Fish Community Health
Shareholder
Halifax Health Medical Center

Fort Myers
Partner
Lee Memorial Hospital

Gainesville
Shands AGH
Shands at the University of Florida
Shands HealthCare
Shands Rehab Hospital

Gulf Breeze
Gulf Breeze Hospital

Inverness
Partner
Citrus Memorial Health System

Jacksonville
Mayo Clinic Jacksonville
Shands Jacksonville Medical Center

Jay
Jay Hospital

Lake City
Shands Lake Shore

Lakeland
Shareholder
Lakeland Regional Medical Center

Largo
Sun Coast Hospital

Leesburg
Leesburg Regional Medical Center

Live Oak
Shands Live Oak

Longwood
Orlando Regional South Seminole Hospital

Melbourne
Palm Bay Community Hospital
Shareholder
Holmes Regional Medical Center

New Smyrna Beach
Bert Fish Medical Center

Ocala
Partner
Munroe Regional Medical Center

Ocoee
Health Central

Orlando
Orlando Regional Medical Center
Shareholder
Orlando Health

Panama City
Bay Medical Center

Pensacola
Baptist Hospital
Shareholder
Baptist Health Care Corporation

Rockledge
Health First, Inc.

Sarasota
Partner
Sarasota Memorial Hospital

Starke
Shands Starke

Tallahassee
Shareholder
Tallahassee Memorial HealthCare

Tampa
Partner
University Community Hospital

Tarpon Springs
Helen Ellis Memorial Hospital

The Villages
The Villages Regional Hospital

Titusville
Partner
Parrish Medical Center

GEORGIA

Albany
Phoebe Putney Health System
Partner
Phoebe Putney Memorial Hospital

Americus
Sumter Regional Hospital

Athens
Partner
Athens Regional Medical Center

Atlanta
Partner
Northside Hospital
Shareholder
Piedmont Hospital

Augusta
University Health Care System

Austell
WellStar Cobb Hospital

Blakely
Early Memorial Hospital

Cairo
Grady General Hospital

Camilla
Mitchell County Hospital

Chatsworth
Murray Medical Center

Cochran
Bleckley Memorial Hospital

Columbus
Columbus Regional Healthcare System
Columbus Specialty Hospital
Partner
The Medical Center

Cordele
Crisp Regional Hospital

Cuthbert
Southwest Georgia Regional Medical Center

Dallas
WellStar Paulding Hospital

Dalton
Partner
Hamilton Medical Center

Decatur
Partner
DeKalb Medical Center

Douglas
Coffee Regional Medical Center

Douglasville
WellStar Douglas Hospital

Fitzgerald
Dorminy Medical Center

Gainesville
Northeast Georgia Medical Center

Hawkinsville
Taylor Regional Hospital

Homerville
Clinch Memorial Hospital

Jasper
Piedmont Mountainside Hospital

Lakeland
Louis Smith Memorial Hospital

Lawrenceville
Partner
Gwinnett Hospital System

Macon
Partner
Medical Center of Central Georgia

Marietta
WellStar Health System
WellStar Windy Hill Hospital
Partner
WellStar Kennestone Hospital

Moultrie
Colquitt Regional Medical Center

Newnan
Piedmont Newnan Hospital

Perry
Perry Hospital

Quitman
Brooks County Hospital

Riverdale
Partner
Southern Regional Medical Center

Rome
Specialty Hospital
Partner
Floyd Medical Center

Sylvester
Phoebe Worth Medical Center

Thomasville
Partner
Archbold Medical Center
John D. Archbold Memorial Hospital

Tifton
Tift Regional Medical Center

Valdosta
Partner
South Georgia Medical Center

Warner Robins
Houston Medical Center

HAWAII

Honolulu
Queen's Medical Center

Kaunakakai
Molokai General Hospital

IDAHO

American Falls
Harms Memorial Hospital District

Arco
Lost Rivers District Hospital

Blackfoot
Bingham Memorial Hospital

Boise
Idaho Elks Rehabilitation Hospital
Shareholder
St. Luke's Regional Medical Center

Bonners Ferry
Boundary Community Hospital

Coeur D'Alene
Partner
Kootenai Medical Center

Emmett
Walter Knox Memorial Hospital

Gooding
Gooding County Memorial Hospital

Grangeville
Syringa General Hospital

Ketchum
St. Luke's Wood River Medical Center

Malad City
Oneida County Hospital

Montpelier
Bear Lake Memorial Hospital

Mountain Home
Elmore Medical Center

Pocatello
Portneuf Medical Center

Preston
Franklin County Medical Center

Rupert
Minidoka Memorial Hospital and Extended Care Facility

Sandpoint
Partner
Bonner General Hospital

Twin Falls
Partner
St. Luke's Magic Valley Regional Medical Center

Weiser
Weiser Memorial Hospital

ILLINOIS

Arlington Heights
Partner
Northwest Community Hospital

Belleville
Partner
Memorial Hospital

Carbondale
Memorial Hospital of Carbondale
Partner
Southern Illinois Hospital Services

Chester
Memorial Hospital

Chicago
Partner
Swedish Covenant Hospital
Shareholder
Northwestern Memorial Hospital

De Kalb
Kish Health System
Partner
Kishwaukee Community Hospital

Decatur
Decatur Memorial Hospital

Dixon
Partner
Katherine Shaw Bethea Hospital

Elgin
Partner
Sherman Hospital

Elmhurst
Partner
Elmhurst Memorial Hospital

Eureka
Eureka Community Hospital

Evanston
Evanston Northwestern Healthcare

Evergreen Park
Partner
Little Company of Mary Hospital and Health Care Centers

Flora
Clay County Hospital

Freeport
Partner
FHN Memorial Hospital

Geneseo
Hammond–Henry Hospital

Geneva
Delnor–Community Hospital

Greenville
Greenville Regional Hospital

Harvey
Shareholder
Ingalls Memorial Hospital

Herrin
Herrin Hospital

Jacksonville
Partner
Passavant Area Hospital

Jerseyville
Jersey Community Hospital

Joliet
Partner
Silver Cross Hospital

Kankakee
Partner
Riverside Medical Center

Lake Forest
Partner
Lake Forest Hospital

Lincoln
Abraham Lincoln Memorial Hospital

Macomb
Partner
McDonough District Hospital

Maryville
Partner
Anderson Hospital

Mendota
Mendota Community Hospital

Monticello
John and Mary Kirby Hospital

Murphysboro
St. Joseph Memorial Hospital

Naperville
Edward Hospital

Normal
Partner
BroMenn Healthcare System

Peoria
Partner
Proctor Hospital

Pittsfield
Illini Community Hospital

Quincy
Partner
Blessing Hospital

Salem
Salem Township Hospital

Sandwich
Valley West Community Hospital

Shelbyville
Shelby Memorial Hospital

Springfield
Shareholder
Memorial Medical Center

Taylorville
Taylorville Memorial Hospital

Vandalia
Fayette County Hospital

INDIANA

Anderson
Community Hospital of Anderson and Madison County

Batesville
Margaret Mary Community Hospital

Bedford
Bedford Regional Medical Center

Bloomington
Partner
Bloomington Hospital

Clinton
West Central Community Hospital

Columbia City
Parkview Whitley Hospital

Columbus
Partner
Columbus Regional Hospital

Danville
Partner
Hendricks Regional Health

Elkhart
Partner
Elkhart General Hospital

Evansville
Shareholder
Deaconess Hospital

Fort Wayne
Parkview Health
Partner
Parkview Hospital

Goshen
Goshen General Hospital

Greenfield
Hancock Regional Hospital

Greensburg
Decatur County Memorial Hospital

Hartford City
Blackford Community Hospital

Huntington
Parkview Huntington Hospital

Indianapolis
Community Hospital East
Community Hospital North
Indiana Heart Hospital
Methodist Hospital
Westview Hospital
Shareholder
Clarian Health Partners

Kendallville
Parkview Noble Hospital

Kokomo
Partner
Howard Regional Health System

La Porte
Partner
La Porte Regional Health System

Lafayette
St. Elizabeth Regional Health
Partner
Lafayette Home Hospital

LaGrange
Parkview LaGrange Hospital

Madison
Partner
King's Daughters' Hospital and Health Services

Marion
Partner
Marion General Hospital

Martinsville
Morgan Hospital and Medical Center

Muncie
Cardinal Health System
Shareholder
Ball Memorial Hospital

New Albany
Partner
Floyd Memorial Hospital and Health Services

New Castle
Henry County Hospital

Newburgh
The Women's Hospital

Noblesville
Partner
Riverview Hospital

Paoli
Bloomington Hospital of Orange County

Portland
Jay County Hospital

Richmond
Partner
Reid Hospital and Health Care Services

Shelbyville
Major Hospital

South Bend
Madison Center and Hospital
Memorial Hospital of South Bend

Terre Haute
Partner
Union Hospital

Tipton
Tipton Hospital

Valparaiso
Partner
Porter–Valparaiso Hospital Campus

Vincennes
Partner
Good Samaritan Hospital

IOWA

Atlantic
Shareholder
Cass County Memorial Hospital

Council Bluffs
Shareholder
Jennie Edmundson Hospital

Decorah
Winneshiek Medical Center

Hamburg
Grape Community Hospital

Harlan
Partner
Myrtue Medical Center

Keokuk
Shareholder
Keokuk Area Hospital

Le Mars
Partner
Floyd Valley Hospital/Avera Health

Muscatine
Unity HealthCare

Onawa
Partner
Burgess Health Center

Orange City
Orange City Area Health System

Red Oak
Shareholder
Montgomery County Memorial Hospital

Rock Rapids
Sanford Merrill Medical Center

Sheldon
Sanford Sheldon Medical Center

Sioux City
Shareholder
St. Luke's Regional Medical Center

West Union
Palmer Lutheran Health Center

KANSAS

Abilene
Memorial Health System

Atchison
Shareholder
Atchison Hospital

Atwood
Rawlins County Health Center

Belleville
Republic County Hospital

Beloit
Mitchell County Hospital Health Systems

Clay Center
Clay County Medical Center

Colby
Shareholder
Citizens Medical Center

Coldwater
Comanche County Hospital

Concordia
Cloud County Health Center

Dighton
Lane County Hospital

Ellinwood
Ellinwood District Hospital

Ellsworth
Ellsworth County Medical Center

Fredonia
Fredonia Regional Hospital

Garnett
Anderson County Hospital

Goodland
Goodland Regional Medical Center

Greensburg
Kiowa County Memorial Hospital

Hays
Shareholder
Hays Medical Center

Herington
Herington Municipal Hospital

Hiawatha
Partner
Hiawatha Community Hospital

Hill City
Graham County Hospital

Hillsboro
Hillsboro Community Medical Center

Hoisington
Clara Barton Hospital

Hoxie
Sheridan County Health Complex

Hutchinson
Shareholder
Hutchinson Hospital Corporation

Junction City
Geary Community Hospital

Kinsley
Edwards County Hospital and Healthcare Center

La Crosse
Rush County Memorial Hospital

Lawrence
Lawrence Memorial Hospital

Leavenworth
Cushing Memorial Hospital

Leoti
Wichita County Health Center

Liberal
Shareholder
Southwest Medical Center

Lincoln
Lincoln County Hospital

Lindsborg
Lindsborg Community Hospital

Lyons
Hospital District Number One of Rice County

Mankato
Jewell County Hospital

McPherson
Memorial Hospital

Medicine Lodge
Medicine Lodge Memorial Hospital

Minneapolis
Ottawa County Health Center

Minneola
Minneola District Hospital

Ness City
Ness County Hospital

Norton
Norton County Hospital

Oakley
Logan County Hospital

Osborne
Osborne County Memorial Hospital

Overland Park
Saint Luke's South Hospital

Parsons
Partner
Labette Health

Phillipsburg
Phillips County Hospital
Shareholder
Great Plains Health Alliance, Inc.

Pittsburg
Mt. Carmel Regional Medical Center

Plainville
Rooks County Health Center

Pratt
Shareholder
Pratt Regional Medical Center

Quinter
Gove County Medical Center

Ransom
Grisell Memorial Hospital District One

Russell
Russell Regional Hospital

Sabetha
Sabetha Community Hospital

Saint Francis
Cheyenne County Hospital

Salina
Partner
Salina Regional Health Center

Smith Center
Smith County Memorial Hospital

Stafford
Stafford District Hospital

Topeka
Shareholder
Stormont–Vail HealthCare

Tribune
Greeley County Health Services

Wakeeney
Trego County–Lemke Memorial Hospital

Wichita
Partner
Via Christi Health System

KENTUCKY

Florence
St. Luke Hospital West

Fort Thomas
Partner
St. Luke Hospital East

Harlan
Harlan ARH Hospital

Hazard
Hazard ARH Regional Medical Center

Lexington
Appalachian Regional Healthcare

McDowell
McDowell ARH Hospital

Middlesboro
Middlesboro Appalachian Regional Hospital

Pikeville
Pikeville Medical Center

South Williamson
Williamson ARH Hospital

West Liberty
Morgan County Appalachian Regional Hospital

Whitesburg
Whitesburg Appalachian Regional Hospital

LOUISIANA

Amite
Hood Memorial Hospital

Baton Rouge
Franciscan Missionaries of Our Lady Health System, Inc.
Member
Our Lady of the Lake Regional Medical Center
Partner
Woman's Hospital

Bossier City
Willis–Knighton Bossier Health Center

Bunkie
Bunkie General Hospital

Church Point
Acadia–St. Landry Hospital

Columbia
Citizens Medical Center

Covington
Partner
St. Tammany Parish Hospital

Crowley
Partner
American Legion Hospital

De Ridder
Partner
Beauregard Memorial Hospital

Ferriday
Riverland Medical Center

Franklinton
Riverside Medical Center

Gonzales
St. Elizabeth Hospital

Greensburg
St. Helena Parish Hospital

Jennings
Jennings American Legion Hospital

Jonesboro
Jackson Parish Hospital

Lafayette
Partner
Our Lady of Lourdes Regional Medical Center

Lake Charles
Partner
Lake Charles Memorial Hospital

Mansfield
De Soto Regional Health System

Monroe
Partner
St. Francis Medical Center

Napoleonville
Assumption Community Hospital

Natchitoches
Natchitoches Regional Medical Center

New Iberia
Iberia Medical Center

New Orleans
Shareholder
Ochsner Medical Center

New Roads
Pointe Coupee General Hospital

Oak Grove
West Carroll Memorial Hospital

Olla
Hardtner Medical Center

Shreveport
Willis–Knighton Health System
Shareholder
Willis–Knighton Medical Center

Slidell
Partner
Slidell Memorial Hospital

Sulphur
Partner
West Calcasieu Cameron Hospital

Vivian
North Caddo Medical Center

MAINE

Augusta
MaineGeneral Medical Center–Augusta Campus

Bangor
Acadia Hospital
Eastern Maine Medical Center

Bar Harbor
Mount Desert Island Hospital

Biddeford
Shareholder
Southern Maine Medical Center

Blue Hill
Blue Hill Memorial Hospital

Brewer
Partner
Eastern Maine Healthcare Systems

Bridgton
Bridgton Hospital

Brunswick
Mid Coast Hospital

Damariscotta
Miles Memorial Hospital

Dover–Foxcroft
Mayo Regional Hospital

Ellsworth
Maine Coast Memorial Hospital

Greenville
Charles A. Dean Memorial Hospital and Nursing Home

Houlton
Houlton Regional Hospital

Lewiston
Shareholder
Central Maine Medical Center

Norway
Stephens Memorial Hospital

Pittsfield
Sebasticook Valley Hospital

Portland
Shareholder
Maine Medical Center

Presque Isle
Aroostook Medical Center

Rockport
Penobscot Bay Medical Center

Rumford
Rumford Hospital

Waterville
Inland Hospital
Shareholder
MaineGeneral Medical Center–Waterville Campus

Westbrook
Spring Harbor Hospital

York
York Hospital

MARYLAND

Baltimore
Franklin Square Hospital Center
Good Samaritan Hospital of Maryland
Harbor Hospital
Union Memorial Hospital

Bel Air
Upper Chesapeake Medical Center
Partner
Upper Chesapeake Health System

Cambridge
Dorchester General Hospital

Columbia
MedStar Health

Easton
Shore Health System
Partner
Memorial Hospital at Easton Maryland

Havre De Grace
Harford Memorial Hospital

Prince Frederick
Calvert Memorial Hospital

MASSACHUSETTS

Belmont
McLean Hospital

Beverly
Partner
Beverly Hospital

Boston
Brigham and Women's Hospital
Faulkner Hospital
Massachusetts General Hospital
Spaulding Rehabilitation Hospital
Partner
Massachusetts Eye and Ear Infirmary
Shareholder
Partners HealthCare System, Inc.
Tufts Medical Center

Burlington
Partner
Lahey Clinic Hospital

Cambridge
Partner
Mount Auburn Hospital

Clinton
Clinton Hospital

Concord
Partner
Emerson Hospital

East Sandwich
Rehabilitation Hospital of the Cape and Islands

Falmouth
Falmouth Hospital

Gardner
Partner
Heywood Hospital

Hyannis
Cape Cod Healthcare, Inc.
Partner
Cape Cod Hospital

Lawrence
Owner
Lawrence General Hospital

Leominster
Partner
Health Alliance Hospitals

Lowell
Partner
Lowell General Hospital

Marlborough
UMass Memorial–Marlborough Hospital

Melrose
Hallmark Health System
Partner
Melrose–Wakefield Hospital

Nantucket
Nantucket Cottage Hospital

Newton Lower Falls
Newton–Wellesley Hospital

Northampton
Cooley Dickinson Hospital

Palmer
Wing Memorial Hospital and Medical Centers

Plymouth
Jordan Hospital

Salem
North Shore Medical Center
Shaughnessy–Kaplan Rehabilitation Hospital

South Weymouth
Partner
South Shore Hospital

Southbridge
Partner
Harrington Memorial Hospital

Worcester
UMass Memorial Health Care, Inc.

MICHIGAN

Adrian
Bixby Medical Center

Allegan
Allegan General Hospital

Bad Axe
Huron Medical Center

Caro
Caro Community Hospital

Cass City
Hills and Dales General Hospital

Cheboygan
Cheboygan Memorial Hospital

Dearborn
Member
Oakwood Healthcare, Inc.
Partner
Oakwood Hospital and Medical Center–Dearborn

Detroit
St. John Detroit Riverview Center
Partner
St. John Hospital and Medical Center

East China
St. John River District Hospital

Fremont
Gerber Memorial Health Services

Gaylord
Otsego Memorial Hospital

Grand Haven
North Ottawa Community Hospital

Grand Rapids
Mary Free Bed Rehabilitation Hospital
Spectrum Health

Greenville
Spectrum Health–United Memorial

Harrison Township
St. John North Shores Hospital

Hastings
Pennock Hospital

Holland
Partner
Holland Hospital

Ionia
Ionia County Memorial Hospital

Jackson
Allegiance Health

Kalamazoo
Partner
Bronson Healthcare Group, Inc.
Bronson Methodist Hospital

Ludington
Memorial Medical Center of West Michigan

Madison Heights
St. John Oakland Hospital

Marshall
Oaklawn Hospital

Monroe
Partner
Mercy Memorial Hospital System

Muskegon
Partner
Hackley Hospital

Owosso
Partner
Memorial Healthcare

Petoskey
Northern Michigan Regional Hospital

Port Huron
Port Huron Hospital
Partner
Blue Water Health Services Corporation

Reed City
Spectrum Health Reed City Hospital

Royal Oak
Shareholder
Beaumont Hospital – Royal Oak

Saginaw
Covenant Medical Center

Saint Joseph
Lakeland Regional Medical Center–St. Joseph

Sandusky
McKenzie Memorial Hospital

Shelby
Hackley Lakeshore Hospital

South Haven
South Haven Community Hospital

Southfield
Providence Hospital and Medical Center

Taylor
Oakwood Heritage Hospital

Tecumseh
Herrick Medical Center

Trenton
Oakwood Southshore Medical Center

Troy
Beaumont Hospital – Troy

Vicksburg
Bronson Vicksburg Hospital

Warren
St. John Macomb Hospital

Wayne
Oakwood Annapolis Hospital

West Branch
Partner
West Branch Regional Medical Center

Wyoming
Metro Health Hospital

Zeeland
Zeeland Community Hospital

MINNESOTA

Albert Lea
Albert Lea Medical Center

Arlington
Sibley Medical Center

Austin
Austin Medical Center

Bemidji
Partner
North Country Regional Hospital

Benson
Swift County–Benson Hospital

Blue Earth
United Hospital District

Buffalo
Buffalo Hospital

Cambridge
Cambridge Medical Center

Canby
Sanford Canby Medical Center

Coon Rapids
Mercy Hospital

Duluth
Partner
St. Luke's Hospital

Fairmont
Fairmont Medical Center–Mayo Health System

Fergus Falls
Partner
Lake Region Healthcare Corporation

Fosston
First Care Medical Services

Fridley
Unity Hospital

Hallock
Kittson Memorial Healthcare Center

Hutchinson
Hutchinson Area Health Care

Jackson
Sanford Jackson Medical Center

Lake City
Lake City Medical Center–Mayo

Long Prairie
Long Prairie Memorial Hospital and Home

Luverne
Sioux Valley Luverne Medical Center

Madelia
Madelia Community Hospital

Mahnomen
Mahnomen Health Center

Mankato
Partner
Immanuel St. Joseph's–Mayo Health System

Melrose
Melrose Area Hospital – CentraCare

Minneapolis
Abbott Northwestern Hospital
Shareholder
Allina Hospitals & Clinics

Morris
Stevens Community Medical Center

New Ulm
New Ulm Medical Center

Ortonville
Ortonville Area Health Services

Owatonna
Owatonna Hospital

Paynesville
Paynesville Area Health Care System

Perham
Perham Memorial Hospital and Home

Redwood Falls
Redwood Area Hospital

Robbinsdale
North Memorial Health Care

Rochester
Mayo Foundation
Rochester Methodist Hospital
Saint Marys Hospital

Roseau
LifeCare Medical Center

Saint Cloud
CentraCare Health System
Partner
St. Cloud Hospital

Saint James
St. James Medical Center

Saint Paul
Bethesda Hospital
St. Joseph's Hospital
United Hospital
Shareholder
HealthEast Care System

Saint Peter
St. Peter Community Hospital

Shakopee
St. Francis Regional Medical Center

Slayton
Murray County Medical Center

Springfield
Springfield Medical Center–Mayo Health System

Tracy
Sanford Tracy Medical Center

Waconia
Partner
Ridgeview Medical Center

Warren
North Valley Health Center

Waseca
Waseca Medical Center

Westbrook
Sanford Westbrook Medical Center

Willmar
Partner
Rice Memorial Hospital

Windom
Windom Area Hospital

Worthington
Worthington Regional Hospital

MISSISSIPPI

Batesville
Tri–Lakes Medical Center

Booneville
Baptist Memorial Hospital–Booneville

Calhoun City
Calhoun Health Services

Columbus
Baptist Memorial Hospital–Golden Triangle

Corinth
Magnolia Regional Health Center

Eupora
North Mississippi Medical Center–Eupora

Greenwood
Partner
Greenwood Leflore Hospital

Gulfport
Partner
Memorial Hospital at Gulfport

Hattiesburg
Partner
Forrest General Hospital

Jackson
Partner
St. Dominic–Jackson Memorial Hospital

McComb
Partner
Southwest Mississippi Regional Medical Center

Meridian
Partner
Jeff Anderson Regional Medical Center

Monticello
Lawrence County Hospital

New Albany
Baptist Memorial Hospital–Union County

Oxford
Baptist Memorial Hospital–North Mississippi

Pascagoula
Singing River Hospital System

Pontotoc
North Mississippi Medical Center–Pontotoc Hospital and Nursing Home

Ripley
Tippah County Hospital

Southaven
Baptist Memorial Hospital–Desoto

Starkville
Oktibbeha County Hospital

Tylertown
Walthall County General Hospital

West Point
North Mississippi Medical Center–West Point

MISSOURI

Bolivar
Partner
Citizens Memorial Hospital

Branson
Partner
Skaggs Community Health Center

Brookfield
General John J. Pershing Memorial Hospital

Cameron
Partner
Cameron Regional Medical Center

Cape Girardeau
Partner
Saint Francis Medical Center

Carthage
Partner
McCune–Brooks Regional Hospital

Chillicothe
Hedrick Medical Center

Columbia
Boone Hospital Center

Crystal City
Jefferson Memorial Hospital

Florissant
Northwest HealthCare

Joplin
Freeman Health System
Freeman Hospital East
Partner
Freeman Hospital West

Kansas City
Crittenton Children's Center
Saint Luke's Northland Hospital
Shareholder
Saint Luke's Health System
Saint Luke's Hospital of Kansas City

Lamar
Barton County Memorial Hospital

Liberty
Partner
Liberty Hospital

Marshall
Fitzgibbon Hospital

Monett
Cox Monett Hospital

Neosho
Freeman Neosho Hospital

Potosi
Washington County Memorial Hospital

Saint Louis
Barnes–Jewish Hospital
Barnes–Jewish West County Hospital
Christian Hospital
Missouri Baptist Medical Center
St. Louis Children's Hospital
Shareholder
BJC HealthCare

Section B

Saint Peters
Barnes–Jewish St. Peters Hospital

Salem
Salem Memorial District Hospital

Sikeston
Missouri Delta Medical Center

Smithville
Saint Luke's Northland Hospital–Smithville Campus

Springfield
CoxHealth
Lester E. Cox Medical Center North
Shareholder
Lester E. Cox Medical Centers

Ste Genevieve
Ste. Genevieve County Memorial Hospital

Sullivan
Missouri Baptist Hospital–Sullivan

Trenton
Wright Memorial Hospital

MONTANA

Big Timber
Pioneer Medical Center

Billings
Partner
Billings Clinic

Bozeman
Partner
Bozeman Deaconess Hospital

Forsyth
Rosebud Health Care Center

Glasgow
Frances Mahon Deaconess Hospital

Glendive
Partner
Glendive Medical Center

Great Falls
Benefis Healthcare System

Hamilton
Partner
Marcus Daly Memorial Hospital

Helena
Partner
St. Peter's Hospital

Livingston
Livingston Memorial Hospital

Missoula
Partner
Community Medical Center

Plentywood
Sheridan Memorial Hospital

Red Lodge
Beartooth Hospital and Health Center

Ronan
Partner
St. Luke Community Hospital

Scobey
Daniels Memorial Healthcare Center

Sidney
Partner
Sidney Health Center

NEBRASKA

Alliance
Box Butte General Hospital

Alma
Harlan County Health System

Atkinson
West Holt Memorial Hospital

Beatrice
Partner
Beatrice Community Hospital and Health Center

Bridgeport
Morrill County Community Hospital

Broken Bow
Jennie M. Melham Memorial Medical Center

Columbus
Partner
Columbus Community Hospital

Crete
Crete Area Medical Center

David City
Butler County Health Care Center

Falls City
Community Medical Center

Franklin
Franklin County Memorial Hospital

Hastings
Partner
Mary Lanning Memorial Hospital

Lexington
Partner
Tri–County Area Hospital

Lincoln
BryanLGH Medical Center
Partner
Madonna Rehabilitation Hospital

Lynch
Niobrara Valley Hospital

McCook
Partner
Community Hospital

Minden
Kearney County Health Services

Neligh
Antelope Memorial Hospital

Norfolk
Partner
Faith Regional Health Services

Omaha
Shareholder
Nebraska Methodist Hospital

Oshkosh
Garden County Health Services

Osmond
Osmond General Hospital

Plainview
Plainview Area Health System

Scottsbluff
Partner
Regional West Medical Center

Sidney
Partner
Memorial Health Center

Tilden
Tilden Community Hospital

York
Partner
York General Hospital

NEW HAMPSHIRE

Claremont
Valley Regional Hospital

Colebrook
Upper Connecticut Valley Hospital

Concord
Concord Hospital

Dover
Partner
Wentworth–Douglass Hospital

Keene
Partner
Cheshire Medical Center

Lancaster
Weeks Medical Center

Lebanon
Alice Peck Day Memorial Hospital
Dartmouth–Hitchcock Medical Center

Nashua
Partner
Southern New Hampshire Medical Center

New London
New London Hospital

Peterborough
Monadnock Community Hospital

Rochester
Partner
Frisbie Memorial Hospital

NEW JERSEY

Bayonne
Bayonne Medical Center

Brick Township
Ocean Medical Center

Camden
Partner
Our Lady of Lourdes Medical Center

East Orange
East Orange Division

Edison
Solaris Health System

Flemington
Partner
Hunterdon Medical Center

Hackettstown
Partner
Hackettstown Regional Medical Center

Neptune
Jersey Shore University Medical Center
Meridian Health

Newton
Partner
Newton Memorial Hospital

North Plainfield
Partner
Muhlenberg Regional Medical Center

Phillipsburg
Partner
Warren Hospital

Pompton Plains
Partner
Chilton Memorial Hospital

Red Bank
Riverview Medical Center

Ridgewood
Valley Hospital

Somers Point
Partner
Shore Memorial Hospital

Trenton
Capital Health System
Capital Health System at Fuld
Capital Health System at Mercer

Vineland
South Jersey Healthcare
South Jersey Healthcare – Regional Medical Center

Willingboro
Lourdes Medical Center of Burlington County

Woodbury
Partner
Underwood–Memorial Hospital

NEW MEXICO

Artesia
Artesia General Hospital

Farmington
Partner
San Juan Regional Medical Center

Gallup
Partner
Rehoboth McKinley Christian Health Care Services

Santa Fe
St. Vincent Regional Medical Center

NEW YORK

Binghamton
Shareholder
United Health Services Hospitals–Binghamton

Bronxville
Lawrence Hospital Center

Brooklyn
New York Community Hospital
Wyckoff Heights Medical Center
Partner
Brooklyn Hospital Center

Buffalo
Roswell Park Cancer Institute

Cobleskill
Partner
Cobleskill Regional Hospital

Cooperstown
Partner
Mary Imogene Bassett Hospital

Corning
Corning Hospital
Elmira
St. Joseph's Hospital
Flushing
New York Hospital Queens
Geneva
Partner
Geneva General Hospital
Hamilton
Community Memorial Hospital
Ithaca
Partner
Cayuga Medical Center at Ithaca
Jamestown
Woman's Christian Association Hospital
Little Falls
Little Falls Hospital
Malone
Alice Hyde Medical Center
Middletown
Orange Regional Medical Center
Mount Kisco
Partner
Northern Westchester Hospital
New York
New York Downtown Hospital
New York–Presbyterian Hospital
Rockefeller University Hospital
Shareholder
New York–Presbyterian/Columbia University Medical Center
Norwich
Chenango Memorial Hospital
Ogdensburg
Claxton–Hepburn Medical Center
Penn Yan
Soldiers and Sailors Memorial Hospital of Yates County
Potsdam
Canton–Potsdam Hospital
Rochester
Strong Memorial Hospital
Strong Memorial Hospital of the University of Rochester
Unity Hospital
Partner
Highland Hospital of Rochester
Sleepy Hollow
Phelps Memorial Hospital Center
Syracuse
Community–General Hospital of Greater Syracuse
Partner
Crouse Hospital
Utica
Faxton–St. Luke's Healthcare
Walton
Delaware Valley Hospital
Watertown
Partner
Samaritan Medical Center
White Plains
Partner
White Plains Hospital Center

NORTH CAROLINA

Ahoskie
Roanoke–Chowan Hospital
Cary
WakeMed Cary Hospital
Charlotte
Carolinas Medical Center
Carolinas Medical Center–Mercy
Carolinas Medical Center–Pineville
Carolinas Medical Center–University
Presbyterian Hospital
Presbyterian–Orthopaedic Hospital
Shareholder
Carolinas HealthCare System
Concord
Shareholder
Carolinas Medical Center–Northeast
Edenton
Chowan Hospital
Greenville
Shareholder
Pitt County Memorial Hospital
High Point
Shareholder
High Point Regional Health System
Huntersville
Presbyterian Hospital Huntersville
Kings Mountain
Kings Mountain Hospital
Lincolnton
Carolinas Medical Center–Lincoln
Matthews
Presbyterian Hospital–Matthews
Monroe
Carolinas Medical Center–Union
Morganton
Blue Ridge HealthCare
Grace Hospital
Nags Head
The Outer Banks Hospital
New Bern
Shareholder
Craven Regional Medical Center
North Wilkesboro
Wilkes Regional Medical Center
Raleigh
WakeMed
Partner
WakeMed Raleigh Campus
Rocky Mount
Partner
Nash Health Care Systems
Salisbury
Partner
Rowan Regional Medical Center
Shelby
Cleveland Regional Medical Center
Tarboro
Heritage Hospital
Thomasville
Partner
Thomasville Medical Center
Valdese
Valdese General Hospital
Wadesboro
Anson Community Hospital
Windsor
Bertie Memorial Hospital
Winston–Salem
Forsyth Medical Center
Medical Park Hospital
Novant Health

NORTH DAKOTA

Bismarck
Partner
MedCenter One
Fargo
MeritCare Health System
MeritCare Medical Center
Grafton
Unity Medical Center
Grand Forks
Partner
Altru Health System
Hillsboro
Hillsboro Medical Center
Jamestown
Partner
Jamestown Hospital
Minot
Trinity Health

OHIO

Akron
Akron General Health System
Shareholder
Akron General Medical Center
Athens
O'Bleness Memorial Hospital
Bellaire
Belmont Community Hospital
Bowling Green
Bowling Green University Medical Center
Cambridge
Partner
Southeastern Ohio Regional Medical Center
Cincinnati
Health Alliance of Greater Cincinnati
Jewish Hospital
Shareholder
Christ Hospital
Cleveland
University Hospitals Case Medical Center
Columbus
Doctors Hospital
Grant Medical Center
Riverside Methodist Hospital
Member
OhioHealth
Dayton
Miami Valley Hospital
Partner
Good Samaritan Hospital
Defiance
Defiance Regional Medical Center
Delaware
Grady Memorial Hospital
Dover
Partner
Union Hospital
Findlay
Blanchard Valley Health System
Fostoria
Fostoria Community Hospital
Franklin
Partner
Atrium Medical Center
Fremont
Partner
Memorial Hospital
Galion
Galion Community Hospital
Hamilton
Partner
Fort Hamilton Hospital
Kenton
Hardin Memorial Hospital
Lima
Partner
Lima Memorial Health System
Lodi
Lodi Community Hospital
Mansfield
MedCentral – Mansfield Hospital
Marion
Marion General Hospital
Massillon
Affinity Medical Center, Massillon Campus
Maumee
Partner
St. Luke's Hospital
Mount Gilead
Morrow County Hospital
Nelsonville
Doctors Hospital Nelsonville
Newark
Partner
Licking Memorial Hospital
Norwalk
Fisher–Titus Medical Center
Oregon
Bay Park Community Hospital
Painesville
Partner
Lake Hospital System
Portsmouth
Southern Ohio Medical Center
Ravenna
Robinson Memorial Hospital

Section B

Steubenville
Partner
Trinity Health System

Sylvania
Flower Hospital

Toledo
ProMedica Health System
Shareholder
The Toledo Hospital

Troy
Partner
Upper Valley Medical Center

Warren
Forum Hillside Rehabilitation Hospital

Wauseon
Fulton County Health Center

Xenia
Partner
Greene Memorial Hospital

Youngstown
Forum Health
Western Reserve Care System

Zanesville
Partner
Genesis HealthCare System

OKLAHOMA

Ada
Partner
Valley View Regional Hospital

Altus
Partner
Jackson County Memorial Hospital

Blackwell
Integris Blackwell Regional Hospital

Carnegie
Carnegie Tri–County Municipal Hospital

Chickasha
Partner
Grady Memorial Hospital

Clinton
Integris Clinton Regional Hospital

Duncan
Partner
Duncan Regional Hospital

El Reno
Parkview Hospital

Elk City
Great Plains Regional Medical Center

Enid
Integris Bass Baptist Health Center
Integris Bass Pavilion

Frederick
Memorial Hospital and Physician Group

Guymon
Partner
Memorial Hospital of Texas County

Hobart
Elkview General Hospital

Lawton
Partner
Comanche County Memorial Hospital

Madill
Integris Marshall County Medical Center

McAlester
Partner
McAlester Regional Health Center

Miami
Integris Baptist Regional Health Center

Muskogee
Partner
Muskogee Regional Medical Center

Oklahoma City
Integris Baptist Medical Center
INTEGRIS Health
Integris Southwest Medical Center
Oklahoma Spine Hospital

Pryor
Integris Mayes County Medical Center

Shawnee
Unity Health Center

Stillwater
Partner
Stillwater Medical Center

Yukon
INTEGRIS Canadian Valley Regional Hospital

OREGON

Hillsboro
Partner
Tuality Healthcare

Hood River
Providence Hood River Memorial Hospital

Medford
Providence Medford Medical Center

Milwaukie
Providence Milwaukie Hospital

Newberg
Providence Newberg Medical Center

Portland
Providence Portland Medical Center
Providence St. Vincent Medical Center

Seaside
Providence Seaside Hospital

Silverton
Silverton Hospital

PENNSYLVANIA

Abington
Partner
Abington Memorial Hospital

Allentown
Shareholder
Lehigh Valley Hospital

Beaver
Heritage Valley Beaver
Heritage Valley Health System

Bethlehem
Lehigh Valley Hospital–Muhlenberg

Bradford
Bradford Regional Medical Center

Butler
Partner
Butler Health System

Chambersburg
Chambersburg Hospital
Summit Health

Clairton
Jefferson Regional Medical Center

Drexel Hill
Delaware County Memorial Hospital

Du Bois
DuBois Regional Medical Center

East Stroudsburg
Pocono Medical Center

Ephrata
Partner
Ephrata Community Hospital

Erie
Shareholder
Hamot Medical Center

Gettysburg
Gettysburg Hospital

Hanover
Hanover Hospital

Harrisburg
Community Hospital
PinnacleHealth System

Indiana
Indiana Regional Medical Center

Jenkintown
Holy Redeemer Hospital and Medical Center

Johnstown
Memorial Medical Center

Lancaster
Partner
Lancaster General Hospital

Lebanon
The Good Samaritan Hospital

Lehighton
Gnaden Huetten Memorial Hospital

Lewisburg
Evangelical Community Hospital

Media
Riddle Memorial Hospital

Meyersdale
Meyersdale Medical Center

New Castle
Jameson Hospital

Norristown
Partner
Montgomery Hospital Medical Center

Philadelphia
Albert Einstein Medical Center
Friends Behavioral Health System
Hospital of the University of Pennsylvania
Jeanes Hospital
Presbyterian Medical Center of the University of Pennsylvania Health System
Temple East, Northeastern Hospital
Temple University Health System
Temple University Hospital
University of Pennsylvania Health System
Shareholder
Pennsylvania Hospital

Pittsburgh
Partner
St. Clair Memorial Hospital

Renovo
Bucktail Medical Center

Ridgway
Ridgway Health Center

Saint Marys
Elk Regional Health Center

Sayre
Robert Packer Hospital
Shareholder
Guthrie Healthcare System

Scranton
Partner
Community Medical Center

Sellersville
Partner
Grand View Hospital

Sewickley
Sewickley Valley Hospital, (A Division of Valley Medical Facilities)

Sharon
Partner
Sharon Regional Health System

State College
Mount Nittany Medical Center

Troy
Troy Community Hospital

Uniontown
Partner
Uniontown Hospital

Upland
Crozer–Chester Medical Center

Waynesboro
Waynesboro Hospital

West Chester
Partner
Chester County Hospital

West Reading
Reading Hospital and Medical Center

Williamsport
Divine Providence Hospital
Partner
Susquehanna Health System

Windber
Windber Medical Center

York
Partner
WellSpan Health
Shareholder
York Hospital

RHODE ISLAND

East Providence
Emma Pendleton Bradley Hospital

Newport
Newport Hospital

Pawtucket
Memorial Hospital of Rhode Island

Providence
Butler Hospital
Miriam Hospital
Women & Infants Hospital of Rhode Island
Shareholder
Lifespan Corporation
Rhode Island Hospital

Warwick
Kent County Memorial Hospital

SOUTH CAROLINA

Charleston
Bon Secours–St. Francis Xavier Hospital
Roper Hospital

Varnville
Hampton Regional Medical Center

SOUTH DAKOTA

Burke
Community Memorial Hospital

Canton
Canton–Inwood Memorial Hospital

Chamberlain
Sanford Mid Dakota Medical Center

Clear Lake
Sanford Deuel County Medical Center

Sioux Falls
Sanford Health
Shareholder
Sanford University of South Dakota Medical Center

Vermillion
Sanford Vermillion Medical Center

Viborg
Pioneer Memorial Hospital and Health Services

Watertown
Prairie Lakes Healthcare System

Webster
Sanford Webster Medical Center

Winner
Winner Regional Healthcare Center

TENNESSEE

Bolivar
Bolivar General Hospital

Camden
Camden General Hospital

Chattanooga
Erlanger Health System
Erlanger North Hospital

Collierville
Baptist Memorial Hospital–Collierville

Columbia
Partner
Maury Regional Hospital

Covington
Baptist Memorial Hospital–Tipton

Franklin
Williamson Medical Center

Harriman
Roane Medical Center

Humboldt
Humboldt General Hospital

Huntingdon
Baptist Memorial Hospital–Huntingdon

Jackson
Shareholder
Jackson–Madison County General Hospital

Knoxville
Covenant Health
East Tennessee Children's Hospital
Fort Sanders Regional Medical Center
Parkwest Medical Center

Lenoir City
Fort Loudoun Medical Center

Lewisburg
Marshall Medical Center

Louisville
Peninsula Hospital

Memphis
Baptist Memorial Health Care Corporation
Baptist Memorial Hospital – Memphis
Baptist Memorial Hospital for Women

Milan
Milan General Hospital

Oak Ridge
Partner
Methodist Medical Center of Oak Ridge

Oneida
St. Mary's Medical Center of Scott County

Paris
Henry County Medical Center

Parsons
Decatur County General Hospital

Pikeville
Erlanger Bledsoe Hospital

Ripley
Baptist Memorial Hospital–Lauderdale

Savannah
Hardin Medical Center

Sevierville
Fort Sanders–Sevier Medical Center

Trenton
Gibson General Hospital

Union City
Baptist Memorial Hospital–Union City

Waynesboro
Wayne Medical Center

TEXAS

Amarillo
Partner
Baptist St. Anthony Health System

Andrews
Permian Regional Medical Center

Angleton
Angleton Danbury Medical Center

Atlanta
Atlanta Memorial Hospital

Beaumont
Memorial Hermann Baptist Beaumont Hospital

Bellville
Bellville General Hospital

Dallas
Baylor Jack and Jane Hamilton Heart and Vascular Hospital
Baylor Specialty Hospital
Baylor University Medical Center
Children's Medical Center of Dallas
Shareholder
Baylor Health Care System

Del Rio
Val Verde Regional Medical Center

Electra
Electra Memorial Hospital

Floresville
Connally Medical Center

Fort Worth
Shareholder
Baylor All Saints Medical Center at Fort Worth

Gainesville
North Texas Medical Center

Garland
Baylor Medical Center at Garland

Gatesville
Coryell Memorial Hospital

Grapevine
Partner
Baylor Regional Medical Center at Grapevine

Harlingen
Partner
Valley Baptist Medical Center–Harlingen

Henrietta
Clay County Memorial Hospital

Houston
Memorial Hermann Healthcare System
Memorial Hermann Hospital
Memorial Hermann Northwest Hospital
Shareholder
Memorial Hermann Southwest Hospital

Humble
Memorial Hermann Northeast

Huntsville
Huntsville Memorial Hospital

Irving
Partner
Baylor Medical Center at Irving

Jacksonville
Mother Frances Hospital – Jacksonville

Katy
Memorial Hermann Katy Hospital

Kilgore
Laird Memorial Hospital

La Grange
St. Mark's Medical Center

Levelland
Covenant Hospital–Levelland

Longview
Partner
Good Shepherd Medical Center

Lubbock
Covenant Children's Hospital
Covenant Medical Center
Covenant Medical Center–Lakeside
Shareholder
Covenant Health System

Marshall
Partner
Good Shepherd Medical Center–Marshall

Midland
Midland Memorial Hospital
Partner
Midland Memorial Hospital

Odessa
Medical Center Hospital

Orange
Continuecare Hospital of Southeast Texas
Memorial Hermann Baptist Orange Hospital

Pearsall
Frio Regional Hospital

Plainview
Covenant Hospital Plainview

Plano
Baylor Regional Medical Center at Plano

Richardson
Partner
Richardson RegionalMedical Center

Richmond
OakBend Medical Center

Rockdale
Richards Memorial Hospital

San Antonio
Baptist Health System

Sherman
Partner
Wilson N. Jones Medical Center

Sugar Land
Memorial Hermann Sugar Land Hospital

Sulphur Springs
Hopkins County Memorial Hospital

Sweeny
Sweeny Community Hospital

Temple
Partner
King's Daughters Hospital

Texarkana
Partner
Wadley Regional Medical Center

Tyler
Tyler Continuecare Hospital at Mother Frances
Partner
Trinity Mother Frances Health System

Vernon
Wilbarger General Hospital

Waco
Partner
Hillcrest Baptist Medical Center

Waxahachie
Baylor Medical Center at Waxahachie

Wichita Falls
Partner
United Regional Health Care System
United Regional Health Care System–Eighth Street Campus

Yoakum
Yoakum Community Hospital

Section B

VERMONT

Barre
Partner
Central Vermont Medical Center

Bennington
Southwestern Vermont Medical Center

Burlington
Shareholder
Fletcher Allen Health Care

Morrisville
Copley Hospital

Newport
North Country Hospital and Health Center

Randolph
Gifford Medical Center

Rutland
Partner
Rutland Regional Medical Center

Saint Johnsbury
Northeastern Vermont Regional Hospital

Windsor
Mt. Ascutney Hospital and Health Center

VIRGINIA

Charlottesville
Partner
Martha Jefferson Hospital

Fredericksburg
Mary Washington Hospital

Hampton
Sentara CarePlex Hospital

Harrisonburg
Partner
Rockingham Memorial Hospital

Lynchburg
Centra Health

Norfolk
Sentara Leigh Hospital
Sentara Norfolk General Hospital
Shareholder
Sentara Healthcare

Virginia Beach
Sentara Bayside Hospital
Sentara Virginia Beach General Hospital

Williamsburg
Sentara Williamsburg Regional Center

WASHINGTON

Aberdeen
Grays Harbor Community Hospital

Centralia
Providence Centralia Hospital

Everett
Providence Everett Medical Center

Morton
Morton General Hospital

Olympia
Providence St. Peter Hospital

Seattle
Providence Health & Services

Tacoma
Tacoma General Hospital
Shareholder
MultiCare Health System

Wenatchee
Central Washington Hospital

Yakima
Partner
Yakima Valley Memorial Hospital

WEST VIRGINIA

Beckley
Beckley Appalachian Regional Hospital

Charleston
Charleston Area Medical Center
Women and Children's Hospital
Shareholder
Charleston Area Medical Center Health System, Inc.

Gassaway
Braxton County Memorial Hospital

Glen Dale
Partner
Reynolds Memorial Hospital

Hinton
Summers County Appalachian Regional Hospital

Madison
Boone Memorial Hospital

Montgomery
Montgomery General Hospital

Princeton
Partner
Princeton Community Hospital

Ripley
Jackson General Hospital

Spencer
Roane General Hospital

Wheeling
Partner
Wheeling Hospital

WISCONSIN

Appleton
Appleton Medical Center
Shareholder
ThedaCare, Inc.

Arcadia
Franciscan Skemp Healthcare–Arcadia Campus

Barron
Luther Midelfort Northland

Beaver Dam
Partner
Beaver Dam Community Hospitals

Beloit
Partner
Beloit Memorial Hospital

Bloomer
Luther Midelfort Chippewa Valley

Eau Claire
Partner
Luther Hospital

Green Bay
Partner
Bellin Memorial Hospital

La Crosse
Franciscan Skemp Healthcare
Franciscan Skemp Healthcare–La Crosse Campus
Shareholder
Gundersen Lutheran Medical Center

Madison
St. Mary's Hospital
Shareholder
Meriter Hospital

Menomonee Falls
Partner
Community Memorial Hospital

Menomonie
Red Cedar Medical Center–Mayo Health System

Milwaukee
Partner
Froedtert Memorial Lutheran Hospital

New London
New London Family Medical Center

Oconomowoc
Oconomowoc Memorial Hospital

Osseo
Luther Midelfort Oakridge

Rice Lake
Partner
Lakeview Medical Center

River Falls
River Falls Area Hospital

Sparta
Franciscan Skemp Healthcare–Sparta Campus

St Croix Falls
St. Croix Regional Medical Center

Watertown
Partner
Watertown Memorial Hospital

Waukesha
ProHealth Care
Waukesha Memorial Hospital

West Bend
Owner
St. Joseph's Community Hospital of West Bend

Whitehall
Tri–County Memorial Hospital

WYOMING

Afton
Star Valley Medical Center

Buffalo
Johnson County Healthcare Center

Casper
Partner
Wyoming Medical Center

Cheyenne
Partner
Cheyenne Regional Medical Center

Douglas
Memorial Hospital of Converse County

Gillette
Campbell County Memorial Hospital

Jackson
St. John's Medical Center and Living Center

Kemmerer
South Lincoln Medical Center

Laramie
Partner
Ivinson Memorial Hospital

Lovell
North Big Horn Hospital District

Rawlins
Memorial Hospital of Carbon County

YANKEE ALLIANCE

300 Brickstone Square, 5th Floor, Andover, MA Zip 01810–1429; tel. 978/475–2000; Mr. R. Paul O'Neill, President

CONNECTICUT

New Haven
Member
Hospital of Saint Raphael

MAINE

Bangor
Member
St. Joseph Hospital

MASSACHUSETTS

Attleboro
Affiliate
Sturdy Memorial Hospital

Boston
Member
Boston Medical Center

Brockton
Member
Signature Healthcare Brockton Hospital

Cambridge
Member
Youville Hospital and Rehabilitation Center

Fall River
Member
Charlton Memorial Hospital
Southcoast Hospitals Group

Great Barrington
Member
Fairview Hospital

Lowell
Member
Saints Medical Center

New Bedford
Member
St. Luke's Hospital

North Adams
Affiliate
North Adams Regional Hospital

Pittsfield
Member
Berkshire Medical Center

Wareham
Member
Tobey Hospital

Winchester
Member
Winchester Hospital

NEW HAMPSHIRE

Manchester
Affiliate
Catholic Medical Center
Elliot Hospital

Nashua
Member
St. Joseph Hospital

NEW YORK

Albany
Member
Albany Medical Center

Elizabethtown
Affiliate
Elizabethtown Community Hospital

Glens Falls
Member
Glens Falls Hospital

Plattsburgh
Affiliate
Champlain Valley Physicians Hospital Medical Center

Troy
Member
Samaritan Hospital

Section B

C

Health Organizations, Agencies, and Providers

Section C

†List supplied by The Joint Commission

Description of Lists

This section of AHA Guide was compiled to provide a directory of information useful to the health care field.

National and International Organizations

The national and international lists include many types of voluntary organizations concerned with matters of interest to the health care field. The organizational information includes address, telephone number, FAX number, and the primary contact. The information was obtained directly from the organizations.

Organizations are searchable by state, then city within state, and ''kind of organization.''

We present these organization listings simply as a convenient directory. Inclusion or omission of any organization's name indicates neither approval nor disapproval by Health Forum LLC, an American Hospital Association company.

United States Government Agencies

National agencies concerned with health–related matters are listed by the major department of government under which the different functions fall.

State and Local Organizations and Agencies

The lists of organizations in states, associated areas, and provinces include Blue Cross and Blue Shield plans, group purchasing organizations, hospital associations and councils, hospital licensure agencies, medical and nursing licensure agencies, quality improvement organizations, state health planning and development agencies, and statewide health coordinating councils.

There are many active local organizations that do not fall within these categories. Contact the hospital association of the state or province for information about such additional groups. The hospital association and councils listed have offices with full-time executives.

The selected state and provincial government agencies include those within state departments of health and welfare, and other agencies, such as comprehensive health planning, mental health, and vocational rehabilitation.

Other Providers

Lists of State Government Agencies for Managed Care Organizations, Freestanding Hospices, and Freestanding Ambulatory Surgery Centers (FASC's) are provided as a resource for obtaining the most current list of agencies in various states. A list of Freestanding Ambulatory Surgery Centers is provided.

Lists of The Joint Commission Accredited Long Term Care Organizations and Joint Commission Accredited Behavioral Health Organizations are provided for your information.

These lists are provided simply as a convenient reference. Inclusion or omission of any organization's name indicates neither approval or disapproval by Health Forum L.L.C.

National Organizations

A

AARP, 601 E. Street, N.W., Washington, DC 20049; tel. 202/434–2277; FAX. 888/836–3985; William D. Novelli, Chief Executive Officer

Academic Pediatric Association, 6728 Old McLean Village Drive, McLean, VA 22101; tel. 703/556–9222; FAX. 703/556–8729; Marge Degnon, Executive Director

AcademyHealth, 1150 17th Street N.W., Suite 600, Washington, DC 20036; tel. 202/292–6756; FAX. 202/282–6856; Bonnie J. Austin, Director

Accreditation Association for Ambulatory Health Care, 5250 Old Orchard Rd., Suite 200, Skokie, IL 60077; tel. 847/853–6060; FAX. 847/853–9028; John E. Burke, Ph. D., Executive Director

Accreditation Council for Pharmacy Education, 20 North Clark Street, Suite 2500, Chicago, IL 60602-5109; tel. 312/664–3575; FAX. 312/664–4652; Peter H. Vlasses, Pharm. D., BCPS, FCCP, Executive Director

Acute Long Term Hospital Association, 625 Slaters Lane, Suite 302, Alexandria, VA 22314; tel. 703/518–9900; FAX. 703/518–9980; William Walters, Chief Executive Officer

Advanced Medical Technology Association, 701 Pennsylvania Avenue, N.W., Suite 800, Washington, DC 20004; tel. 202/783–8700; FAX. 202/783–8750; Stephen J. Ubl, President

Aerospace Medical Association, 320 South Henry Street, Alexandria, VA 22314-3579; tel. 703/739–2240; FAX. 703/739–9652; Russell B. Rayman, M.D., Executive Director

Alcoholics Anonymous World Services, Inc., P.O. Box 459, New York, NY 10163; tel. 212/870–3400; FAX. 202/870–3003; Greg Muth, General Manager

Alexander Graham Bell Association for the Deaf & Hard Of Hearing, 3417 Volta Place, NW, Washington, DC 20007; tel. 202/337–5220; FAX. 202/337–8314; Corrine Abbott, Chief Advancement Officer

Allergy Associates, 2004 Grand Avenue, Baldwin, NY 11510; tel. 516/223–7656; FAX. 516/223–0583; Joe D' Amore, MD, President

Alliance for Children & Families, 11700 West Lake Park Drive, Milwaukee, WI 53224; tel. 414/359–1040; FAX. 414/359–1074; Peter B. Goldberg, President and CEO

Alzheimer's Association, (Alzheimer's Disease and Related Disorders Association, Inc.), 225 North Michigan Avenue, Suite 1700, Chicago, IL 60601; tel. 312/335–8700; FAX. 312/335–1110; Elizabeth Gould, Clinical Care

America's Blood Centers, 725 15th Street, N.W., Suite 700, Washington, DC 20005-2109; tel. 202/393–5725; FAX. 202/393–1282; Jim MacPherson, CEO

America's Health Insurance Plans, 601 Pennsylvania Ave. NW, South Bldg, Suite 500, Washington, DC 20004; tel. 202/778–3200; FAX. 202/778–8486; Charles W. Stellar, Executive Vice President

American Academy for Cerebral Palsy and Developmental Medicine, 555 E. Wells Street, Suite 1100, Milwaukee, WI 53202; tel. 414/918–3014; FAX. 414/276–2146; Tracy Burr, Executive Director

American Academy of Allergy, Asthma and Immunology, 555 East Wells Street, Suite 1100, Milwaukee, WI 53202; tel. 414/272–6071; FAX. 414/272–6070; Kay Whalen, Executive Director

American Academy of Child and Adolescent Psychiatry, 3615 Wisconsin Avenue, N.W., Washington, DC 20016; tel. 202/966–7300; FAX. 202/966–2891; Virginia Q. Anthony, Executive Director

American Academy of Dental Practice Administration, 1063 Whippoorwill Lane, Palatine, IL 60067; tel. 847/934–4404; Kathleen Uebel, Executive Director

American Academy of Dermatology, 930 East Woodfield Road, Schaumburg, IL 60173; tel. 847/330–0230; FAX. 847/330–0050; Robert S. Bolan, Ph D, Interim Executive Director

American Academy of Family Physicians, 11400 Tomahawk Creek Parkway, Leawood, KS 66211; tel. 913/906–6000; FAX. 913/906–6083

American Academy of Medical Administrators, 701 Lee Street, Suite 600, Des Plaines, IL 60016; tel. 847/759–8601; FAX. 847/759–8602; Renee Schleicher, CAE, President and CEO

American Academy of Neurology, 1080 Montreal Avenue, St. Paul, MN 55116-2325; tel. 651/695–1940; FAX. 612/695–2791; Catherine Rydell, Executive Director

American Academy of Ophthalmology, 655 Beach Street, P.O. Box 7424, San Francisco, CA 94120; tel. 415/561–8500; FAX. 415/561–8533; H. Dunbar Hoskins, Jr., M.D., Executive Vice President

American Academy of Optometry, 6110 Executive Boulevard, Suite 506, Rockville, MD 20852; tel. 301/984–1441; FAX. 301/984–4737; Lois Schoenbrun, CAE, FAAO Executive Director

American Academy of Oral Medicine, P.O. Box 2016, Edmonds, WA 98020-9516; tel. 425/778–6162; FAX. 425/771–9588; Jane Kantor, CMP, Executive Director

American Academy of Orthopedic Surgeons, 6300 North River Road, Rosemont, IL 60018-4262; tel. 847/823–7186; FAX. 847/823–8125; Karen L. Hackett, FACHE, CAE, Chief Executive Officer

American Academy of Otolaryngic Allergy, 1990 M. Street, NW, Suite 680, Washington, DC 20036; tel. 202/955–5010; FAX. 202/955–5016; Jami Lucas, Executive Director

American Academy of Otolaryngology-Head and Neck Surgery, Inc., One Prince Street, Alexandria, VA 22314; tel. 703/836–4444; FAX. 703/519–1553; David R. Nielsen, MD, FACS, CEO and Executive Vice President

American Academy of Pain Management, 13947 Mono Way, Suite A, Sonora, CA 95370-2807; tel. 209/533–9744; FAX. 209/533–9750; Kathryn A. Padgett, Ph.D., Executive Director

American Academy of Pediatrics, 141 Northwest Point Boulevard, Elk Grove Village, IL 60007-1098; tel. 847/434–4000; FAX. 847/434–8000; Errol R. Alden MD., Executive Director & CEO

American Academy of Physical Medicine and Rehabilitation, 330 N. Wabash Ave, Suite 2500, Chicago, IL 60611-7617; tel. 312/464–9700; FAX. 312/464–0227; Thomas E. Stautzenbach, CAE, Executive Director

American Academy of Physician Assistants, 950 North Washington Street, Alexandria, VA 22314-1552; tel. 703/836–2272; FAX. 703/684–1924; William F. Leinweber, Executive Vice President/CEO

American Academy of Psychoanalysis And Dynamic Psychiatry, One Regency Drive, P.O. Box 30, Bloomfield, CT 06002; tel. 888/691–8281; FAX. 860/286–0787; Jacquelyn T. Coleman, CAE, Executive Director

American Aging Association, The Sally Balin Medical Center, 110 Chesley Drive, Media, PA 19063; tel. 610/627–2626; FAX. 610/565–9747; Arthur K. Balin, M.D., Ph D., FACP

American Alliance for Health, Physical Education, Recreation & Dance, 1900 Association Drive, Reston, VA 20191; tel. 703/476–3400; FAX. 703/476–9527; Michael G. Davis, CEO

American Ambulance Association, 8201 Greensboro Drive, Suite 300, McLean, VA 22102; tel. 703/610–9000; FAX. 703/610–9005; Maria Bianchi, Executive Vice President

American Art Therapy Association, Inc., 11160 - C1 South Lakes Drive, Suite 813, Reston, VA 20191; tel. 703/212–2238; Peg Dunn-Snow, PhD, ATR-BC, President

American Association for Clinical Chemistry, Inc. (AACC), 1850 K Street, NW, Washington, DC 20006; tel. 202/857–0717; FAX. 202/877–5093; Richard Flaherty, Executive Vice President

American Association for Dental Research, 1619 Duke Street, Alexandria, VA 22314-3406; tel. 703/548–0066; FAX. 703/548–1883; Christopher Fox, Executive Director

American Association For Homecare, 2011 Crystal Drive, Suite 725, Arlington, VA 22202-3709; tel. 703/836–6263; FAX. 703/836–6730; Michael Reinemer, Vice President

American Association for Laboratory Animal Science, AALAS, 9190 Crestwyn Hills Drive, Memphis, TN 38125; tel. 901/754–8620; FAX. 901/753–0046; Ann T. Turner, PHD, CAE, Executive Director

American Association for Respiratory Care, 9425 N. MacArthur, Suite 100, Irving, TX 75063; tel. 972/243–2272; FAX. 972/484–2720; Sam P. Giordano, Executive Director

American Association for the Advancement of Science, 1200 New York Avenue, N.W., Washington, DC 20005; tel. 202/326–6640; FAX. 202/371–9526; Alan Leshner, Chief Executive Officer

American Association for the Surgery of Trauma, 633 N. Saint Clair Street, Suite 2600, Chicago, IL 60611; tel. 800/789–4006; FAX. 312/202–5013; Sharon Gautschy, AAST Executive Director

American Association of Ambulatory Surgery Centers, P.O. Box 5271, Johnson City, TN 37602-5271; tel. 423/915–1001; FAX. 423/282–9712; Craig Jeffries, Esq Executive Director

American Association of Anatomists, Department of Anatomy, University of Mississippi Medical Center, Jackson, MS 39216-4505; tel. 601/984–1640; FAX. 601/984–1655; Duaine E. Haines, Secretary-Treasury

American Association of Bioanalysts, 906 Olive, Suite 1200, St. Louis, MO 63101-1434; tel. 314/241–1445; FAX. 314/241–1449; Mark S. Birenbaum, Ph.D., Administrator

American Association of Certified Orthoptists, Tennessee Lions Eye Center, 1211 21st Ave. South, Nashville, TN 37212; tel. 615/936–1034; FAX. 615/936–2118; Ronald Biernacki, C.O., President

American Association of Colleges of Nursing, One DuPont Circle, N.W., Suite 530, Washington, DC 20036; tel. 202/463–6930; FAX. 202/785–8320; Geraldine Bednash, Ph.D., RN, FAAN, Executive Director

American Association of Colleges of Osteopathic Medicine, 5550 Friendship Boulevard, Suite 310, Chevy Chase, MD 20815-7231; tel. 301/968–4100; FAX. 301/968–4101; Stephen C. Shannon, DO, MPH, President and Chief Executive Officer

American Association of Colleges of Pharmacy, 1727 King Street, Alexandria, VA 22314-2700; tel. 703/739–2330; FAX. 703/836–8982; Lucinda Maine, Ph.D., Executive Vice President

American Association of Colleges of Podiatric Medicine, 15850 Crabbs Branch Way, Suite 320, Rockville, MD 20855-2622; tel. 301/948–9760; FAX. 301/948–1928

American Association of Critical-Care Nurses, 101 Columbia, Aliso Viejo, CA 92656-1491; tel. 949/362–2000; FAX. 949/362–2020; Wanda L. Johansson, RN, MN, CEO

American Association of Dental Consultants, Inc., 10032 Wind Hill Drive, Greenville, IN 47124; tel. 812/923–2600; FAX. 812/923–2900; Judy Salisbury, Executive Director

American Association of Endodontists, 211 East Chicago Avenue, Suite 1100, Chicago, IL 60611-2691; tel. 312/266–7255; FAX. 312/266–9867; Trina Anderson, Executive Assistant to the Executive Director

American Association of Healthcare Administrative Management, 11240 Waples Mill Road, Suite 200, Fairfax, VA 22030; tel. 703/281–4043; FAX. 703/359–7562; Sharon Galler, Executive Director

American Association of Healthcare Consultants, 5938 N. Drake Ave., Chicago, IL 60659; tel. 888/350–2242; FAX. 773/463–3552; Linda Campbell, CAE, Executive Director

American Association of Homes and Services for the Aging, 2519 Connecticut Avenue, NW, Washington, DC 20008-1520; tel. 202/783–2242; FAX. 202/783–2255; William L. (Larry) Minnix Jr., D. Min, President and CEO

American Association of Kidney Patients, 3505 E. Frontage Road, Suite 315, Tampa, FL 33607; tel. 800/749–2257; FAX. 813/636–8122; Kris Robinson, Executive Director

American Association of Medical Assistants, 20 North Wacker Drive, Suite 1575, Chicago, IL 60606; tel. 312/899–1500; FAX. 312/899–1259; Donald A. Balasa, JD, MBA, Executive Director, Legal Counsel

American Association of Nurse Anesthetists, 222 South Prospect Avenue, Park Ridge, IL 60068-4001; tel. 847/692–7050; FAX. 847/692–6968; Jeffery M. Beutler, CRNA, MS, Executive Director

American Association of Occupational Health Nurses, Inc., 2920 Brandywine Road, Suite 100, Atlanta, GA 30341; tel. 770/455–7757; FAX. 770/455–7271; Ann R. Cox, CAE, Executive Director

American Association of Oral and Maxillofacial Surgeons, 9700 West Bryn Mawr Avenue, Rosemont, IL 60018-5701; tel. 847/678–6200; FAX. 847/678–6286; Robert C. Rinaldi, Ph.D., Executive Director

American Association of Orthodontists, 401 North Lindbergh Boulevard, St. Louis, MO 63141-7816; tel. 314/993–1700; FAX. 314/997–1745; Chris P. Vranas, Executive Director

American Association of Pastoral Counselors, 9504A Lee Highway, Fairfax, VA 22031-2303; tel. 703/385–6967; FAX. 703/352–7725; Douglas M. Ronsheim, D.Min, Executive Director

American Association of Physicists in Medicine, One Physics Ellipse, College Park, MD 20740-3846; tel. 301/209–3350; FAX. 301/209–0862; Angela R. Keyser, Executive Director

American Association of Plastic Surgeons, 900 Cummings Center, Suite 221U, Beverly, MA 01915; tel. 978/927–8330; FAX. 978/524–0461; Aurelie Alger, JD, Executive Director

American Association of Poison Control Centers, 515 King Street, Suite 510, Alexandria, MD 22314; tel. 703/894–1858; FAX. 703/683–2812; Jim Hirt, Executive Director

American Association of Psychiatric Technicians, Inc., A.A.P.T., 1220 S St., Suite 100, Sacramento, CA 95814-7138; tel. 800/391–7589; FAX. 916/329–9145; Debi Loger, Executive Director

American Association of Public Health Dentistry, A.A.P.H.D. National Office, 3085 Stevenson Drive, Springfield, IL 62703; tel. 217/529–6941; FAX. 217/529–9120; Pamela J. Tolson, CAE, Executive Director

American Association on Intellectual and Developmental Disabilities (AAIDD), 444 North Capitol Street, N.W., Suite 846, Washington, DC 20001-1512; tel. 202/387–1968; FAX. 202/387–2193; M. Doreen Croser, Executive Director

American Baptist Homes and Caring Ministries, P.O. Box 851 (National Ministries), Valley Forge, PA 19482-0851; tel. 610/768–2430; FAX. 610/768–2453; Rev. Aundreia Alexander, Director

American Board of Allergy and Immunology, 111 S. Independence Mall East, Suite 701, Philadelphia, PA 19106-3699; tel. 866/264–5568; FAX. 215/592–9411; John W. Yunginger, M.D., President

American Board of Anesthesiology, 4101 Lake Boone Trail, Suite 510, Raleigh, NC 27607-7506; tel. 919/881–2570; FAX. 919/881–2575; Francis P. Hughes, Ph.D., Executive Director

American Board of Cardiovascular Perfusion, 207 North 25th Avenue, Hattiesburg, MS 39401; tel. 601/582–2227; FAX. 601/582–2271; Beth A. Richmond, Ph.D., Mark G. Richmond, Ed.D., Executive Co-Directors

American Board of Colon and Rectal Surgery, 20600 Eureka Road, Suite 600, Taylor, MI 48180; tel. 734/282–9400; FAX. 734/282–9402; David J. Schoetz, M.D., Executive Director

American Board of Dermatology, Inc., Henry Ford Health System, One Ford Place, Detroit, MI 48202-3450; tel. 313/874–1088; FAX. 313/872–3221; Antoinette F. Hood, M.D., Executive Director

American Board of Emergency Medicine, 3000 Coolidge Road, East Lansing, MI 48823; tel. 517/332–4800; FAX. 517/332–2234; Mary Ann Reinhart, Ph.D., Executive Director

American Board of Family Medicine, Inc., 2228 Young Drive, Lexington, KY 40505; tel. 859/269–5626; FAX. 859/335–7501; James Puffer, M.D., President & CEO

American Board of Internal Medicine, 510 Walnut Street, Suite 1700, Philadelphia, PA 19106-3699; tel. 215/446–3500; FAX. 215/446–3473; Christine K. Cassel, M.D., President

American Board of Medical Specialties, 1007 Church Street, Suite 404, Evanston, IL 60201-5913; tel. 847/491–9091; FAX. 847/328–3596; Stephen H. Miller, M.D., MPH, President

American Board of Neurological Surgery, 6550 Fannin Street, Suite 2139, Houston, TX 77030; tel. 713/441–6015; FAX. 713/794–0207; Mary Louise Sanderson, Administrator

American Board of Nuclear Medicine, 4555 Forest Park Blvd, Suite 119, St. Louis, MO 63108; tel. 314/367–2225; Henry D. Royal, M.D., Executive Director

American Board of Ophthalmology, 111 Presidential Boulevard, Suite 241, Bala Cynwyd, PA 19004; tel. 610/664–1175; FAX. 610/664–6503; John G. Clarkson, M.D., Executive Director

American Board of Oral and Maxillofacial Surgery, 625 North Michigan Avenue, Suite 1820, Chicago, IL 60611; tel. 312/642–0070; FAX. 312/642–8584; Cheryl E. Mounts, Executive Secretary

American Board of Orthopedic Surgery, Inc., 400 Silver Cedar Court, Chapel Hill, NC 27514; tel. 919/929–7103; FAX. 919/942–8988; Shepard R. Hurwitz, M.D., Executive Director

American Board of Pathology, One Urban Centre, 4830 West Kennedy Boulevard, Suite 690, Tampa, FL 33622-5915; tel. 813/286–2444; FAX. 813/289–5279; Betsy D. Bennett M.D Ph D., Executive Vice President

American Board of Pediatrics, Inc., 111 Silver Cedar Court, Chapel Hill, NC 27514; tel. 919/929–0461; FAX. 919/929–9255; James A. Stockman III, M.D., President

American Board of Physical Medicine and Rehabilitation, 3015 Allegro Park, Lake SW, Rochester, MN 55902; tel. 507/282–1776; FAX. 507/282–9242; Anthony M. Tarvestad, JD, Executive Director

American Board of Podiatric Surgery, 445 Fillmore Street, San Francisco, CA 94117-3404; tel. 415/553–7800; FAX. 415/553–7801; James A. Lamb, Executive Director

American Board of Preventive Medicine, Inc., 111 West Jackson Blvd., Suite 1110, Chicago, IL 60604; tel. 312/939–2276; FAX. 312/939–2218; James M. Vanderploeg, M.D., M.P.H.

American Board of Prosthodontics, P.O. Box 271894, West Hartford, CT 06127-1894; tel. 860/679–2649; FAX. 860/206–1169; Thomas D. Taylor, D.D.S., M.S.D., Executive Director

American Board of Psychiatry and Neurology, Inc., 500 Lake Cook Road, Suite 335, Deerfield, IL 60015; tel. 847/945–7900; FAX. 847/945–1146; Stephen C. Scheiber, M.D., Executive Vice President

American Board of Quality Assurance and Utilization Review, 2120 Range Road, Clearwater, FL 33765; tel. 727/298–8777; FAX. 727/449–0555; H.E. Hartsell, Chief Operating Officer

American Board of Radiology, 5441 E. Williams Blvd, Suite 200, Tucson, AZ 85711; tel. 520/790–2900; FAX. 520/790–3200; Gary J. Becker, M.D., Executive Director

American Board of Surgery, Inc., 1617 John F. Kennedy Boulevard, Suite 860, Philadelphia, PA 19103; tel. 215/568–4000; FAX. 215/563–5718; Frank R. Lewis, M.D., Executive Director

American Board of Thoracic Surgery, 633 N. St. Clair Street, Suite 2320, Chicago, IL 60611; tel. 312/202–5900; FAX. 312/202–5960; William A. Gay, Jr., M.D., Executive Director

American Broncho-Esophagological Association, Office of the Secretary, Stanford University School of Medicine, Division of Pediatric Otolaryngology, Stanford, CA 94305-5739; tel. 650/725–6500; FAX. 650/725–8502; Peter Koltai, M.D., Secretary

American Burn Association, 625 North Michigan Avenue, Suite 2550, Chicago, IL 60611; tel. 312/642–9260; FAX. 312/642–9130; John Krichbaum, JD, Executive Director

American Cancer Society, 1599 Clifton Road, N.E., Atlanta, GA 30329; tel. 404/320–3333; Gerald P. Murphy, M.D., Senior Vice President

American Center for the Alexander Technique, Inc., 39 W. 14th Street, #507, New York, NY 10011; tel. 212/633–2229; FAX. 212/633–2239; Jane Tomkiewicz, Executive Director

American Chiropractic Association, 1701 Clarendon Boulevard, Arlington, VA 22209; tel. 703/276–8800; FAX. 703/243–2593; Kevin P. Corcoran, CAE, Executive Vice President

American Cleft Palate-Craniofacial Association, 1504 E. Franklin St., Suite 102, Chapel Hill, NC 27514; tel. 919/933–9044; FAX. 919/933–9604; Nancy C. Smythe, Executive Director

American College Health Association, P.O. Box 28937, Baltimore, MD 21240-8937; tel. 410/859–1500; FAX. 410/859–1510; Doyle E. Randol, MS, Executive Director

American College of Allergy, Asthma and Immunology, 85 West Algonquin Road, Suite 550, Arlington Heights, IL 60005; tel. 847/427–1200; FAX. 847/427–1294; James R. Slawny, Executive Director

American College of Apothecaries, P.O. Box 341266, Bartlett, TN 38184; tel. 901/383–8119; FAX. 901/383–8882; D. C. Huffman, Jr., Ph.D., Executive Vice President

American College of Cardiology, 2400 N Street, NW, Washington, DC 20037; tel. 202/375–6180; FAX. 202/375–6819; Jack Lewin, MD, CEO

American College of Cardiovascular Nursing, 11219 Rice Creek Road, Riverview, FL 33569; tel. 813/677–1116; FAX. 813/671–8912; Jonni Cooper, BSN, MBA, PhD, FACCN-III, Chief Executive Officer

American College of Chest Physicians, 3300 Dundee Road, Northbrook, IL 60062-2348; tel. 847/498–1400; FAX. 847/498–5460; Alvin Lever, Executive Vice President and CEO

American College of Dentists, 839J Quince Orchard Boulevard, Gaithersburg, MD 20878-1614; tel. 301/977–3223; FAX. 301/977–3330; Stephen A. Ralls, D.D.S.

American College of Emergency Physicians, P.O. Box 619911, Dallas, TX 75261-9911; tel. 972/550–0911; FAX. 972/580–2816; Michael E. Gallery, Ph.D, CAE, Interim Executive Director

American College of Foot and Ankle Surgeons, 8725 W. Higgins Rd, Suite 555, Chicago, IL 60631; tel. 773/693–9300; FAX. 773/693–9304; J.C. Mahaffey, CAE, Executive Director

American College of Gastroenterology, P.O. Box 342260, Bethesda, MD 208272260; tel. 301/263–9000; FAX. 703/931–4520; Thomas F. Fise, Executive Director

American College of Healthcare Executives, One North Franklin, Suite 1700, Chicago, IL 60606-3491; tel. 312/424–2800; FAX. 312/424–0023; Thomas C. Dolan, Ph.D., FACHE, CAE, President and CEO

American College of Mohs Surgery, 555 E. Wells, Suite 1100, Milwaukee, WI 53202-3823; tel. 414/347–1103; FAX. 414/272–6070; Georganne Dixon, Executive Director

American College of Nurse-Midwives, Silver Spring Metro Plaza, 8403 Colesville Rd, Ste.1550, Silver Spring, MD 20910-6374; tel. 240/485–1800; FAX. 240/485–1818; Lorrie Kline Kaplan, Executive Director

American College of Obstetricians and Gynecologists, 409 12th Street, S.W., Washington, DC 20090-6920; tel. 202/638–5577; FAX. 202/484–5107; Ralph W. Hale, M.D., Executive Vice President

American College of Occupational and Environmental Medicine, (Includes Occupational & Environmental Health Fnd. & The Occupational Physicians Scholarship Fund), 25 Northwest Point Blvd, Suite 700, Elk Grove Village, IL 60007; tel. 847/818–1800; FAX. 847/818–9266; Barry S. Eisenberg, CAE., Executive Director

American College of Physician Executives, 400 N. Ashley Drive, Suite 400, Tampa, FL 33602; tel. 813/287–2000; FAX. 813/287–8993; Roger S. Schenke, Executive Vice President

American College of Physician Executives, 4890 West Kennedy Boulevard, Suite 200, Tampa, FL 33619-2575; tel. 813/287–2000; FAX. 813/287–8993; Roger S. Schenke, Executive Vice President

American College of Physicians, 190 North Independence Mall West, Philadelphia, PA 19106-1572; tel. 215/351–2800; FAX. 215/351–2829; John Tooker, M.D., MBA, F.A.C.P., Executive VP, CEO

American College of Preventive Medicine, 1307 New York Avenue, N.W., Suite 200, Washington, DC 20005; tel. 202/466–2044; FAX. 202/466–2662; Jordan H. Richland, MPH, Executive Director

American College of Radiology, 1891 Preston White Drive, Reston, VA 20191-4397; tel. 703/648–8900; FAX. 703/648–9176; Harvey L. Neiman, M.D., Executive Director

American College of Rheumatology, 1800 Century Place, Suite 250, Atlanta, GA 30345; tel. 404/633–3777; FAX. 404/633–1870; Lynn Bonfiglio, Director of Membership

American College of Sports Medicine, P.O. Box 1440, Indianapolis, IN 46206-1440; tel. 317/637–9200; FAX. 317/634–7817; James R. Whitehead, Executive Vice President

American College of Surgeons, 633 N. Saint Clair Street, Chicago, IL 60611; tel. 312/202–5000; FAX. 312/202–5001; Thomas R. Russell, M.D., Executive Director

American Congress of Rehabilitation Medicine, 6801 Lake Plaza Drive, Suite B205, Indianapolis, IN 46220; tel. 317/915–2250; FAX. 317/915–2245; Richard D. Morgan, MBA

American Dental Assistants Association, 35 E. Wacker Driver, Suite 1730, Chicago, IL 60601; tel. 312/541–1550; FAX. 312/541–1496; Lawrence H. Sepin, Executive Director

American Dental Association, 211 East Chicago Avenue, Chicago, IL 60611; tel. 312/440–2500; FAX. 312/440–7494; James B. Bramson, DDS, Executive Director

American Dental Education Association, 1400 K. Street NW, Suite 1100, Washington, DC 20005; tel. 202/289–7201; FAX. 202/289–7204; Jack Bresch, Director, Center for Public Policy and Advocacy

American Dental Society of Anesthesiology, Inc., 211 East Chicago Avenue, Suite 780, Chicago, IL 60611; tel. 312/664–8270; FAX. 312/224–8624; R. Knight Charlton, Executive Director

American Diabetes Association, Inc., 1701 N. Beauregard Street, Alexandria, VA 22311; tel. 703/549–1500; FAX. 703/836–7439; Michael D. Farley, CFRE, Interim Chief Executive Officer

American Dietetic Association, 120 South Riverside Plaza, Suite 2000, Chicago, IL 60606-6995; tel. 312/899–0040; FAX. 312/899–4765; Ronald S. Moen, Chief Executive Officer

American Foundation for Aging Research, North Carolina State University, Biochemistry Department, Raleigh, NC 27695-7622; tel. 919/515–5679; FAX. 919/515–2047; Paul F. Agris, President & Jaime Vodvarka, Program Assistant

American Foundation for the Blind, Inc., 11 Penn Plaza, Suite 300, New York, NY 10001; tel. 212/502–7600; FAX. 212/502–7770; Liz Greco - Rocks, Vice President, Communications

American Group Psychotherapy Association, Inc., 25 East 21st Street, Sixth Floor, New York, NY 10010; tel. 212/477–2677; FAX. 212/979–6627; Marsha S. Block, CAE, Chief Executive Officer

American Head and Neck Society, 11300 W. Olympic Blvd #600, Los Angles, CA 90064; tel. 310/437–0559; FAX. 310/437–0585; Erin Schwarz, Executive Director

American Headache Society, 19 Mantua Road, Mt. Royal, NJ 08061; tel. 856/423–0043; FAX. 856/423–0082; Linda McGillicuddy, Executive Director

American Health Care Association, 1201 L Street, N.W., Washington, DC 20005; tel. 202/842–4444; FAX. 202/842–3860; Charles H. Roadman II, M.D., President and CEO

American Health Information Management Association (AHIMA), 233 North Michigan Avenue, 21st Floor, Chicago, IL 60601-5800; tel. 312/233–1100; FAX. 312/233–1090; Linda Kloss, R.H.I.A., C.A.E.

American Health Lawyers Association, 1025 Connecticut Avenue, N.W., Suite 600, Washington, DC 20036; tel. 202/833–1100; FAX. 202/833–1105; Peter M. Leibold, Esq, Executive Vice President and CEO

American Health Planning Association, 7245 Arlington Boulevard, Suite 300, Falls Church, VA 22042; tel. 703/573–3103; FAX. 703/573–3103; Dean Montgomery, Director

American Healthcare Radiology Administrators, 490 - B Boston, Post Road, Suite 101, Sudbury, MA 01776; tel. 978/443–7591; FAX. 978/443–8046; Mary S. Reitter, Executive Director

American Heart Association, Inc., 7272 Greenville Avenue, Dallas, TX 75231; tel. 214/706–1574; FAX. 214/373–9818; Rose Marie Robertson, MD, FAHA, Chief Science Officer

American Hospital Association, 325 Seventh Street, NW, Suite 700, Washington, DC 20004; tel. 202/626–2363; FAX. 202/626–2303; Richard Umbdenstock, President and CEO

American Hospital Association, One North Franklin Street, Chicago, IL 60606-3491; tel. 312/422–3000; FAX. 312/422–4796; Richard Umbdenstock, President and CEO

American Hospital Association, Washington Office, 325 Seventh Street, N.W., Suite 700, Washington, DC 20004; tel. 202/638–1100; FAX. 202/626–2355; Rick Pollack, Executive Vice President

American International Health Alliance, 1250 Eye Street, NW, Suite 350, Washington, DC 20005; tel. 202/789–1136; FAX. 202/789–1277; James P. Smith, Executive Director

American Laryngological Association, Department of Otolaryngology/MonteFiore Medical Center, 3400 Bainbridge Ave, 3rd fl, Bronx, NY 10467-2404; tel. 718/920–8453; FAX. 718/405–9014; Marvin D. Fried MD, Secretary

American Library Association, 50 East Huron Street, Chicago, IL 60611; tel. 312/280–5044; FAX. 312/944–8520; Debra Davis, Director

American Lung Association, 61 Broadway, New York, NY 10006; tel. 212/315–8700; FAX. 212/315–8800; John L. Kirkwood, Pres. & CEO

American Lung Association of Ohio Southwest Region, 4050 Executive Park Drive, Suite 402, Cincinnati, OH 45241; tel. 513/985–3990; FAX. 513/985–3995; Gale Steitz, Regional Program Director

American Medical Association, 515 North State Street, Chicago, IL 60610; tel. 312/464–5000; FAX. 312/464–4184

American Medical Association Alliance, 515 North State Street, 9th Floor, Chicago, IL 60610; tel. 312/464–4470; FAX. 312/464–5020; Hazel J. Lewis, Executive Director

American Medical Group Association, 1422 Duke Street, Alexandria, VA 22314-3403; tel. 703/838–0033; FAX. 703/548–1890; Donald W. Fisher, Ph.D., President and CEO

American Medical Student Association/Foundation, 1902 Association Drive, Reston, VA 20191; tel. 703/620–6600; FAX. 703/620–5873; Paul R. Wright, Executive Director

American Medical Technologists, 10700 W. Higgins Rd., Rosemont, IL 60018; tel. 847/823–5169; FAX. 847/823–0458; Christopher Damon, Executive Director

American Medical Women's Association, 100 North 20th Street, 4th Floor, Philadelphia, PA 19103; tel. 215/320–3716; FAX. 215/564–2175; Rebecca Mathis, Associate Director

American Medical Writers Association, 40 West Gude Drive #101, Rockville, MD 20850-1192; tel. 301/294–5303; FAX. 301/294–9006

American Music Therapy Association, 8455 Colesville Road, Suite 1000, Silver Spring, MD 20910; tel. 301/589–3300; FAX. 301/589–5175; Andrea Farbman, Ed.D., Executive Director

American National Standards Institute, 25 West 43rd Street, Fourth Floor, New York, NY 10036; tel. 212/642–4900; FAX. 212/398–0023; S. Joe Bhatia, President and CEO

American Nephrology Nurses' Association, East Holly Avenue, P.O. Box 56, Pitman, NJ 08071; tel. 856/256–2320; FAX. 856/589–7463

American Neurological Association, 5841 Cedar Lake Road, Suite 204, Minneapolis, MN 55416; tel. 952/545–6284; FAX. 952/545–6073; Lori Peterson, Executive Director

American Occupational Therapy Association, Inc., 4720 Montgomery Lane, P.O. Box 31220, Bethesda, MD 20824-1220; tel. 301/652–2682; FAX. 301/652–7711; Frederick P. Somers, Executive Director

American Ophthalmological Society, P.O. Box 193940, San Francisco, CA 94119-3940; tel. 415/561–8578; FAX. 415/561–8531; Thomas J. Liesegang, M.D., Secretary-Treasurer

American Optometric Association, 243 North Lindbergh Boulevard, St. Louis, MO 63141; tel. 314/991–4100; FAX. 314/991–4101; Michael D. Jones, O.D., Executive Director

American Organization of Nurse Executives (AONE), 325 7th Street, NW, Washington, DC 20004; tel. 202/626–2240; FAX. 202/638–5499; Pamela Thompson, MS, RN, FAAN, Chief Executive Officer

American Orthopsychiatric Association, Department of Psychology, Box 871104, Tempe, AZ 85287-1104; tel. 480/965–0380; FAX. 480/965–8544; Nicole Bruno, Director

American Orthoptic Council, 3914 Nakoma Road, Madison, WI 53711; tel. 608/233–5383; FAX. 608/263–4247; Leslie France, Administrator

American Osteopathic Association, 142 East Ontario Street, Chicago, IL 60611; tel. 312/202–8003; FAX. 312/202–8303; John B. Crosby, J.D., Executive Director

American Otological Society, Inc., Administrative Office, 3096 Riverdale Rd., The Villages, FL 32162; tel. 352/751–0932; FAX. 352/751–0696; Shirley Gossard, Administrator

American Parkinson Disease Association, Inc., 135 Parkinson Ave, Parkinson Plaza, Staten Island, NY 10305; tel. 800/223–2732; FAX. 718/981–4399; G. Maestrone, D.V.M., Scientific and Medical Affairs Director

American Pediatric Society, Inc., 3400 Research Forest Drive, Suite B7, The Woodlands, TX 77381; tel. 281/419–0052; FAX. 281/419–0082; Kathy Cannon, Associate Executive Director

American Pharmacists Association, 1100 15th Street NW, Suite 400, Washington, DC 20005; tel. 202/628–4410; FAX. 202/429–6300; John A. Gans, Pharm.D., Executive Vice President

American Physical Therapy Association, 1111 North Fairfax Street, Alexandria, VA 22314; tel. 703/684–2782; FAX. 703/684–7343; Francis J. Mallon, Esq., Chief Executive Officer

American Physiological Society, 9650 Rockville Pike, Bethesda, MD 20814-3991; tel. 301/634–7118; FAX. 301/634–7241; Martin Frank, Ph.D., Executive Director

American Podiatric Medical Association, 9312 Old Georgetown Road, Bethesda, MD 20814-1698; tel. 301/571–9200; FAX. 301/530–2752; Glenn B. Gastwirth, DPM, Executive Director

American Psychiatric Association, 1000 Wilson Boulevard, Suite 1825, Arlington, VA 22209; tel. 703/907–7300; FAX. 703/907–1085; James H. Scully Jr., M.D., Medical Director

American Psychoanalytic Association, 309 East 49th Street, New York, NY 10017; tel. 212/752–0450; FAX. 212/593–0571; Dean K. Stein, Executive Director

American Psychological Association, 750 First Street, N.E., Washington, DC 20002-4242; tel. 202/336–5800; FAX. 202/336–5797; Russ Newman, Ph.D., JD, Executive Director For Professional Practice

American Psychosomatic Society, 6728 Old McLean Village Drive, McLean, VA 22101-3906; tel. 703/556–9222; FAX. 703/556–8729; George K. Degnon, Executive Director

American Public Health Association, 800 I. Street, NW, Washington, DC 20001-3710; tel. 202/777–2430; FAX. 202/777–2532; Georges C. Benjamin, MD, FACP, FACEP(E), Executive Director

American Public Human Services Association, 810 First Street, N.E., Suite 500, Washington, DC 20002; tel. 202/682–0100; FAX. 202/289–6555; Jerry W. Friedman, Executive Director

American Red Cross, National Headquarters, 2025 E. Street, NW, Washington, DC 20006; tel. 202/303–4498; FAX. 703/206–7765

American Registry of Medical Assistants, 69 Southwick Road, Westfield, MA 01085-4729; tel. 800/527–2762; FAX. 413/562–9021; Annette H. Heyman, R.M.A., Director

American Registry of Radiologic Technologists, 1255 Northland Drive, St. Paul, MN 55120; tel. 651/687–0048; Jerry B. Reid, Ph.D., Executive Director

American Rhinologic Society, University of North Carolina, CB 7070 Room G0142, Chapel Hill, NC 25799-7070; tel. 919/966–3342; FAX. 919/966–7941; Brent Senior, M.D., Secretary

American Roentgen Ray Society, 44211 Slate Stone Court, Leesburg, VA 20176; tel. 703/729–3353; FAX. 703/729–4839; Susan Brown Cappitelli, Executive Director

American School Health Association, 7263 S.R. 43, P.O. Box 708, Kent, OH 44240-0708; tel. 330/678–1601; FAX. 330/678–4526; Susan Wooley, Ph.D., CHES, Executive Director

American Society for Adolescent Psychiatry, P.O. Box 570218, Dallas, TX 75357-0218; tel. 972/613–0985; FAX. 972/613–5532; Frances M. Roton, Executive Director

American Society for Anesthesiologists, 520 N. Northwest Highway, Park Ridge, IL 60068; tel. 847/825–5586; FAX. 847/825–2085; John Thorner, J.D., CAE, Executive Vice President

American Society for Biochemistry and Molecular Biology, Inc., 9650 Rockville Pike, Bethesda, MD 20814-3996; tel. 301/634–7145; FAX. 301/634–7126; Charles C. Hancock, Executive Officer

American Society for Clinical Laboratory Science, 6701 Democracy Boulevard, Suite 300, Bethesda, MD 20817; tel. 301/657–2768; FAX. 301/657–2909; Elissa Passiment, Vice President

American Society for Clinical Pathology, (Includes Board of Registry), 33 W. Monroe Street, Suite 1600, Chicago, IL 60603; tel. 312/541–4999; FAX. 312/541–4767; John R. Ball, MD, JD Executive Vice President

American Society for Clinical Pharmacology and Therapeutics, 528 North Washington Street, Alexandria, VA 22314; tel. 703/836–6981; FAX. 703/836–5223; Sharon J. Swan, CAE, Executive Director

American Society for Cytotechnology, 1500 Sunday Drive, Suite 102, Raleigh, NC 27607; tel. 800/948–3947; FAX. 919/787–4916; Beth Denny, Executive Director

American Society for Healthcare Engineering (ASHE), One North Franklin St., 28th Floor, Chicago, IL 60606; tel. 312/422–3812; FAX. 312/422–4571; Dale Woodin, CHFM, SASHE, Executive Director

American Society for Healthcare Environmental Services (ASHES), 1 N. Franklin Street, Suite 2800, Chicago, IL 60606; tel. 312/422–3862; FAX. 312/422–4578; Patti Costello, Executive Director

American Society for Healthcare Food Service Administrators (ASHFSA), 455 S. Fourth Street, Suite 650, Louisville, KY 40202; tel. 800/620–6422; FAX. 502/589–3602; Keith Howard, Executive VP

American Society for Healthcare Human Resources Administration (ASHHRA), One North Franklin, 31st Floor, Chicago, IL 60606; tel. 312/422–3728; FAX. 312/422–4577; Shirley Armistead, Project Specialist

American Society for Healthcare Risk Management (ASHRM), One North Franklin, 31st Floor, Chicago, IL 60606; tel. 312/422–3989; FAX. 312/422–4580; Elizabeth Summy, M.Sc., CAE, Executive Director

American Society for Investigative Pathology, 9650 Rockville Pike, Bethesda, MD 20814-3993; tel. 301/634–7130; FAX. 301/634–7990; Mark E. Sobel, M.D., Ph.D, Executive Director

American Society for Laser Medicine and Surgery, Inc., 2100 Stewart Avenue, Suite 240, Wausau, WI 54401; tel. 715/845–9283; FAX. 715/848–2493; J. Stuart Nelson, M.D., Ph.D., Secretary

American Society for Microbiology, 1752 North Street, NW, Washington, DC 20036; tel. 202/924–9265; FAX. 202/942–9333; Michael I. Goldberg, Ph.D., Executive Director

American Society for Pharmacology and Experimental Therapeutic, 9650 Rockville Pike, Bethesda, MD 20814-3995; tel. 301/634–7060; FAX. 301/634–7061; Christine K. Carrico, Ph. D., Executive Officer

American Society for Public Administration, 1301 Pennsylvania Ave., NW, Suite 840, Washington, DC 20004; tel. 202/393–7878; FAX. 202/638–4952; Antoinette Samuel, CAE

American Society for Reproductive Medicine, 1209 Montgomery Highway, Birmingham, AL 35216-2809; tel. 205/978–5000; FAX. 205/978–5005; Robert W. Rebar, M.D., Executive Director

American Society for the Advancement of Anesthesia and Sedation in Dentistry, Six East Union Avenue, P.O. Box 551, Bound Brook, NJ 08805; tel. 732/469–9050; FAX. 732/271–1985; David Crystal, D.D.S., Executive Secretary

American Society for Therapeutic Radiology and Oncology, 8280 Willow Oaks Corporate Drive, Suite 500, Fairfax, VA 22031; tel. 703/502–1550; FAX. 703/502–7852; Laura Thevenot, Chief Executive Officer

American Society of Anesthesiologists, 520 North Northwest Highway, Park Ridge, IL 60068; tel. 847/825–5586; FAX. 847/825–2085; John A. Thorner, J.D., CAE, Executive Vice President

American Society of Colon and Rectal Surgeons, 85 West Algonquin Road, Suite 550, Arlington Heights, IL 60005; tel. 847/290–9184; FAX. 847/290–9203; James Slawny, Executive Director

American Society of Consultant Pharmacists, 1321 Duke Street, Alexandria, VA 22314-3563; tel. 703/739–1300; FAX. 703/739–1321; John Feather, Executive Director

American Society of Cytopathology, 400 West Ninth Street, Suite 201, Wilmington, DE 19801; tel. 302/429–8802; FAX. 302/429–8807; Elizabeth A. Jenkins, Co-Executive Director

American Society of Directors of Volunteer Services (ASDVS), One North Franklin, 31st Floor, Chicago, IL 60606; tel. 312/422–3938; FAX. 312/422–4577; Audrey L. Harris, Executive Director

American Society of Electroneurodiagnostic Technologists, Inc., 6501 E. Commerce Ave, Suite 120, Kansas City, MO 64120; tel. 816/931–1120; FAX. 816/931–1145; Sheila R. Navis, CAE, Executive Director

American Society of Health-System Pharmacists, 7272 Wisconsin Avenue, Bethesda, MD 20814; tel. 301/664–8794; FAX. 301/664–8877; Henri R. Manasse, Jr., Executive VP and CEO

American Society of Internal Medicine, 2011 Pennsylvania Avenue, N.W., Suite 800, Washington, DC 20006-1808; tel. 202/835–2746; FAX. 202/835–0443

American Society of Law, Medicine & Ethics, 765 Commonwealth Avenue, Suite 1634, Boston, MA 02215; tel. 617/262–4990; FAX. 617/437–7596; Benjamin W. Moulton, JD, MPH, Executive Director

American Society of Neuroimaging, 5841 Cedar Lake Road, Suite 204, Minneapolis, MN 55416; tel. 952/545–6291; FAX. 952/545–6073; Kris McDowell, Associate Executive Director

American Society of Plastic Surgeons, 444 East Algonquin Road, Arlington Heights, IL 60005; tel. 847/228–9900; FAX. 847/228–9131; Executive Director

American Society of Radiologic Technologists, 15000 Central Avenue, S.E., Albuquerque, NM 87123-3909; tel. 505/298–4500; FAX. 505/298–5063; DuVonne Campbell, Executive Vice President

American Speech-Language-Hearing Association, 2200 Research Blvd., Rockville, MD 20850-3289; tel. 301/296–5700; FAX. 301/296–8587

American Surgical Association, 900 Cummings Center, Suite 221-U, Beverly, MA 01915; tel. 978/927–8330; FAX. 978/524–0461; Robert P. Jones, Ed.D., Executive Director

American Thoracic Society, 61 Broadway, New York, NY 10006-2755; tel. 212/315–6444; FAX. 212/315–8630; Stephen C. Crane, Ph.D., MPH, Executive Director

American Trauma Society, 7611 S. Osborne Road, Suite 202, Upper Marlboro, MD 20772-2656; tel. 800/556–7890; FAX. 301/574–4301; Harry Teter, Executive Director PR Dept.

American Urological Association, Inc., 1000 Corporate Boulevard, Linthicum, MD 21090; tel. 410/689–3700; Michael Sheppard, Executive Director

amfAR, The Foundation for AIDS Research, 120 Wall Street, 13th Floor, New York, NY 10005-3902; tel. 212/806–1600; FAX. 212/806–1601; Donald Kaplan, Director, Program Communications

AORN, Association of Peri Operative Registered Nurses, 2170 South Parker Road, Suite 300, Denver, CO 80231-5711; tel. 303/755–6300; FAX. 303/750–2927; Linda Groah, RN, Executive Director

Arthritis Foundation, 1330 West Peachtree Street, Suite 100, Atlanta, GA 30309; tel. 404/872–7100; FAX. 404/965–7712; John H. Klippel, M.D., President and CEO

Association for Applied Psychophysiology and Biofeedback, 10200 West 44th Avenue, Suite 304, Wheat Ridge, CO 80033; tel. 303/422–8436; FAX. 303/422–8894; David Stumph, Executive Director

Association for Clinical Pastoral Education, Inc., 1549 Clairmont Road, Suite 103, Decatur, GA 30033; tel. 404/320–1472; FAX. 404/320–0849; Teresa E. Snorton, Executive Director

Association for Community Health Improvement (ACHI), 180 Montgomery Street, Suite 1520, San Francisco, CA 94104; tel. 415/248–8411; FAX. 415/296–0519; Michael Bilton, Director

Association for Healthcare Philanthropy, 313 Park Avenue, Suite 400, Falls Church, VA 22046; tel. 703/532–6243; FAX. 703/532–7170

Association for Healthcare Resource & Materials Management (AHRMM), One North Franklin St., Suite 2800, Chicago, IL 60606-3491; tel. 312/422–3840; FAX. 312/422–4573; Deborah L. Sprindzunas, Executive Director

Association for Hospital Medical Education, 109 Brush Creek Road, Irwin, PA 15642; tel. 724/864–7321; FAX. 724/864–6153; Margie Kleppick, Executive Director

Association for Professionals in Infection Control and Epidemiology, 1275 K Street, NW, Suite 1000, Washington, DC 20005; tel. 202/789–1890; FAX. 202/789–1899; Kathy L. Warye, CEO

Association for the Advancement of Automotive Medicine (AAAM), P.O. Box 4176, Barrington, IL 60146; tel. 847/844–3880; FAX. 847/844–3884; Irene Herzau, Executive Director

Association of American Medical Colleges, 2450 N Street, N.W., Washington, DC 20037-1127; tel. 202/828–0400; FAX. 202/828–1125; Darrell G. Kirch, M.D., President and CEO

Association of American Physicians and Surgeons, Inc., 1601 North Tucson Boulevard, Suite Nine, Tucson, AZ 85716; tel. 520/327–4885; FAX. 520/325–4230; Jane M. Orient, M.D., Executive Director

Association of American Veterinary Medical Colleges, 1101 Vermont Ave, NW, Suite 301, Washington, DC 20005; tel. 202/371–9195; FAX. 202/842–0773; Dr. Michael Chaddock, Deputy Executive Director

Association of Community Cancer Centers, 11600 Nebel Street, Suite 201, Rockville, MD 20852-2557; tel. 301/984–9496; FAX. 301/770–1949; Christian Downs, JD, MHA, Executive Director

Association of Environmental Health Academic Programs, 2632 SE 25th Avenue, Suite F, Portland, OR 97202; tel. 503/235–6047; FAX. 503/235–7300; Yalonda Sinde, Executive Director

Association of Healthcare Administrative Professionals, One North Franklin Street, Chicago, IL 60606; tel. 312/422–3701; FAX. 312/422–4577; Elizabeth Summy, Associate Vice President

Association of Occupational & Environmental Clinics, 1010 Vermont Avenue, N.W. # 513, Washington, DC 20005; tel. 202/347–4976; Katherine Kirkland, MPH, Executive Director

Section C

Association of Professional Chaplains, 1701 East Woodfield Road, Suite 400, Schaumburg, IL 60173-5109; tel. 847/240–1014; FAX. 847/240–1015; Josephine N. Schrader, CAE, IOM, Executive Director

Association of Public Health Laboratories, 8515 Georgia Avenue, Suite 700, Silver Spring, MD 20910; tel. 240/485–2747; FAX. 240/485–2700; Scott J. Becker, MS, Executive Director

Association of Schools of Allied Health Professions, 4400 Jennifer Street, N.W., Suite 333, Washington, DC 20015; tel. 202/237–6481; FAX. 202/237–6485; Thomas W. Elwood, Dr. P.H., Executive Director

Association of Schools of Public Health, 1101 15th Street, N.W., Suite 910, Washington, DC 20005; tel. 202/296–1099; FAX. 202/296–1252; Harrison C. Spencer, MD, MPH, President and CEO

Association of Schools of Public Health, 1101 15th Street NW, Suite 910, Washington; tel. 202/296–1099; FAX. 202/296–1252; Allison J. Foster, MBA, CAE, Deputy Executive Director

Association of Specialized and Cooperative Library Agencies, 50 East Huron Street, Chicago, IL 60611; tel. 312/280–4399; FAX. 312/944–8085; Cathleen Bourdon, ASCLA, Executive Director

Association of State & Territorial Health Officials, 2231 Crystal Drive, Suite 450, Arlington, VA 22202; tel. 202/371–9090; FAX. 571/527–3189; Paul E. Jarris, MD, MBA, Executive Director

Association of State and Territorial Health Officials, 2231 Crystal Drive, Suite 450, Washington, DC 20005-4006; tel. 202/371–9090; FAX. 571/527–3189; Paul E. Jarris, MD, MBA, Executive Director

Association of Surgical Technologists, Inc., 6 West Dry Creek Circle, Suite 200, Littleton, CO 80120; tel. 303/694–9130; FAX. 303/694–9169; William J. Teutsch, CAE, CEO

Association of University Programs in Health Administration, 2000 14th St., N., Suite 780, Arlington, VA 22201; tel. 703/894–0940; FAX. 703/894–0941; Lydia Reed, MBA, CAE, President and CEO

Asthma and Allergy Foundation of America, 1233 20th Street, NW, Suite 402, Washington, DC 20036; tel. 800–7–ASTHMA; FAX. 202/466–8940; William McLin, Executive Director

B

Bereavement and Advance Care Planning Services, Gundersen Lutheran Medical Foundation, 1900 South Avenue-Alex, La Crosse, WI 54601; tel. 608/775–4747; FAX. 608/775–5137; Rana Limbo, Director

Biological Stain Commission, Inc., University of Rochester Medical Center, Department Pathology, Rochester, NY 14642-0001; tel. 585/275–6335; FAX. 585/442–8993; David P. Penney, Ph.D., Treasurer

Birth Defect Research for Children, 800 Celebration Avenue, Suite 225, Celebration, FL 34747; tel. 407/566–8304; FAX. 407/566–8341; Betty Mekdeci, Executive Director

Blinded Veterans Association, 477 H Street, N.W., Washington, DC 20001; tel. 202/371–8880; FAX. 202/371–8258; Thomas H. Miller, Executive Director

Blue Cross and Blue Shield Association, 225 N. Michigan Avenue, Chicago, IL 60601; tel. 312/297–6000; FAX. 312/297–6120; Scott Serota, President and CEO

Brady Center to Prevent Gun Violence, 1225 Eye Street, N.W., Suite 1100, Washington, DC 20005; tel. 202/289–7319; FAX. 202/408–1851; Paul Helmke, President

C

California Distance Learning Health Network, 9245 Sky Park Court, Suite 100, San Diego, CA 92123; tel. 619/594–3364; FAX. 619/594–2111; Violet Macias-Reynolds, M.S. M.Ed, Executive Director

CARE Program(Community Action for a Renewed Environment Program), Mail Code 8001A, EPA, Washington, DC 20460; tel. 877/227–3909

Catholic Health Association of the United States, 1875 Eye Street NW, Suite 1000, Washington, DC 20006-5409; tel. 202/296–3993; FAX. 202/296–3997; Sr. Carol Keehan, DC, President and CEO

Catholic Medical Association, 2020 Pennsylvania Avenue, NW, Suite 864, Washington, DC 20006; tel. 703/988–0588; FAX. 702/830–1308; Executive Director

Center for American Nurses, 8515 Georgia Ave., Suite 400, Silver Spring, MD 20910; tel. 301/628–5243; FAX. 301/628–5297; Wylecia Wiggs Harris, MBA, CAE, Executive Director

Center for Health Administration Studies, University of Chicago, 969 East 60th Street, Chicago, IL 60637; tel. 773/702–7104; FAX. 773/702–7222; Kristiana Raube, Ph.D., Director

Center for Healthcare Governance, 1 N. Franklin Street, 29th Floor, Chicago, IL 60606; tel. 888/540–6111; FAX. 312/422–4650; John R. Combes, M.D., President and Chief Operating Officer

Center for Healthy Aging, c/o National Council on Aging, 1901 L Street, NW, 4th Floor, Washington, DC 20036; tel. 202/479–1200; FAX. 202/479–0735; Nancy Whitelaw, PhD, Director, Center for Healthy Aging

Central Surgical Association, University of Chicago, 5841 S. Maryland m/c 5094, Chicago, IL 60637; tel. 773/702–6237; FAX. 773/702–6120; Fabrizio Michelassi, Secretary-CSA

Children's Eye Foundation, 1527 West State Highway, Suite 500, #216, Grapevine, TX 76051; tel. 817/891–1144; FAX. 817/329–5532; Robert D. Gross, MBA, M.D., President

Christian Record Services, Inc., 4444 South 52nd Street, Lincoln, NE 68516; tel. 402/488–0981; FAX. 402/488–1902; Dwayne Bullock, Treasurer

College of American Pathologists, 325 Waukegan Road, Northfield, IL 60093-2750; tel. 847/832–7000; FAX. 847/832–8151; Stephen R. Myers, Interim Executive Vice President

Commission on Accreditation of Rehabilitation Facilities, 4891 East Grant Road, Tucson, AZ 85712; tel. 202/587–5001; FAX. 202/587–5009; Christine MacDonell, Managing Director

Community Anti-Drug Coalitions of America, 625 Slaters Lane, Suite 300, Alexandria, VA 22314; tel. 800/542–2322; FAX. 703/706–0565; Arthur T. Dean, Chairman and CEO

Community Health Accreditation Program, 1300 19th Street, Suite 150, Washington, DC 20036; tel. 202/862–3413; FAX. 202/862–3419

Consortium of African American Public Health Programs (CAAPHP), Morehouse School of Medicine, 720 Westview Drive, S.W., National Center for Primary Care, Atlanta, GA 30310-1495; tel. 404/752–1835; FAX. 404/756–8829; C. Abeo Jones, PhD, MPH, MBA, Program Coordinator

Cooley's Anemia Foundation, Inc., 330 Seventh Avenue, Suite 900, New York, NY 10001; tel. 800/522–7222; FAX. 212/279–5999; Gina Cioffi, National Executive Director

Corporate Angel Network, Inc., CAN (Arranges Free Air Transportation for Cancer Patients Traveling To or From Treatment), Westchester County Airport, One Loop Road, White Plains, NY 10604; tel. 914/328–1313; FAX. 914/328–4226; Vicki Blucher, Director of Volunteers

Council of Medical Specialty Societies, 51 Sherwood Terrace, Suite M, Lake Bluff, IL 60044; tel. 847/295–3456; FAX. 847/295–3759; Norman B. Kahn, Jr., M.D., EVP, and CEO

Council on Education for Public Health, 800 Eye Street, NW, Suite 202, Washington, DC 20001-3710; tel. 202/789–1050; FAX. 202/789–1895; Laura Rasar King, Executive Director

Crohn's & Colitis Foundation of America, Inc., 386 Park Avenue, S., 17th Floor, New York, NY 10016-8804; tel. 800/932–2423; FAX. 212/779–4098; Richard J. Geswell, President and CEO

Cystic Fibrosis Foundation, 6931 Arlington Road, Bethesda, MD 20814; tel. 301/951–4422; FAX. 301/951–6378; Robert J. Beall, Ph.D., President and CEO

D

Damien Dutton Society for Leprosy Aid, Inc., 616 Bedford Avenue, Bellmore, NY 11710; tel. 516/221–5829; FAX. 516/221–5909; Howard Crouch, President

Depression and Bipolar Support Alliance, 730 North Franklin Street, Suite 501, Chicago, IL 60610; tel. 312/642–0049; FAX. 312/642–7243; Susan Bergeson, President

Dietary Managers Association, 406 Surrey Woods Drive, St. Charles, IL 60174; tel. 630/587–6336; FAX. 630/587–6308; William St. John, President

Dysautonomia Foundation, Inc., 315 W. 39th Street, Suite 701, New York, NY 10018; tel. 212/279–1066; FAX. 212/279–2066; David Brenner, Executive Director

E

Easter Seals, Inc., 230 West Monroe Street, Suite 1800, Chicago, IL 60606-4802; tel. 312/726–6200; FAX. 312/726–1494; James E. Williams, Jr., President and CEO

ECRI Institute, 5200 Butler Pike, Plymouth Meeting, PA 19462; tel. 610/825–6000; FAX. 610/834–1275; Jeffery C. Lerner, Ph.D., CEO & President

Educational Commission for Foreign Medical Graduates, 3624 Market Street, Philadelphia, PA 19104-2685; tel. 215/386–5900; FAX. 215/387–9963; James A. Hallock, M.D., President and CEO

Ehlers-Danlos National Foundation, P.O. Box 13157, Richmond, VA 23225; tel. 804/276–9940; FAX. 804/276–9940; Susan L. Stephenson, Patient Advocate

Emergency Nurses Association, 915 Lee Street, Des Plaines, IL 60016; tel. 847/460–4000; FAX. 847/460–4006; David Westman, CPA, MBA, Executive Director

Epilepsy Foundation, 8301 Professional Place-East, Landover, MD 20785; tel. 301/459–3700; FAX. 301/577–2684; Eric Hargis, Chief Executive Officer

Epilepsy Foundation of Connecticut, 386 Main Street, Middletown, CT 06457; tel. 860/346–1924; FAX. 860/346–1928; Linda Wallace

F

Federated Ambulatory Surgery Association, 1012 Cameron Street, Alexandria, VA 22314; tel. 703/836–8808; FAX. 703/549–0976; Kathy Bryant, Executive Director

Federation of American Hospitals, 801 Pennsylvania Ave N.W., Suite 245, Washington, DC 20004; tel. 202/624–1500; FAX. 202/737–6832; Chip Kahn, President

Federation of State Medical Boards of the United States, Inc., P.O. Box 619850, Dallas, TX 75261-9850; tel. 817/868–4000; FAX. 817/868–4097; James N. Thompson, MD, President and CEO

Financial Accounting Standards Board, 401 Merritt 7, P.O. Box 5116, Norwalk, CT 06856-5116; tel. 203/847–0700; FAX. 203/849–9714

Foundation for Chiropractic Education and Research, 1330 Beacon Street, Suite 315, Brookline, MA 02446-3202; tel. 617/734–3397; FAX. 617/734–0989; Anthony L. Rosner, Ph.D., L.L. D,. Hon. Director of Research and Education

G

Gerontological Society of America, 1200 L St., NW, Suite 901, Washington, DC 20005-4018; tel. 202/842–1275; FAX. 202/842–1150; Linda Krogh Harootyan, Interim Executive Director

Great Plains Health Alliance, Inc., 625 Third Street, Box 366, Phillipsburg, KS 67661; tel. 785/543–2111; FAX. 785/543–5098; Roger S. John, President and CEO

Guide Dog Users, Inc., 14311 Astrodome Dr., Silver Spring, MD 20906-2245; tel. 888/858–1008; FAX. 301/871–7591; Jane Sheehan, Office Manager

H

Health Industry Distributors Association, 310 Montgomery Street, Alexandria, VA 22314-1516; tel. 703/549–4432; FAX. 703/549–6495; Matthew J. Rowan, President & Chief Executive Officer

Health Research and Educational Trust, One North Franklin, Chicago, IL 60606; tel. 312/422–2622; FAX. 312/422–4568; John Combs, Interim President

Healthcare Financial Management Association, Two Westbrook Corporate Center, Suite 700, Westchester, IL 60154; tel. 708/531–9600; FAX. 708/531–0032; Richard L. Clarke, DHA, FHFMA, President and CEO

Healthcare Information and Management Systems Society (HIMSS), 230 East Ohio Street, Suite 500, Chicago, IL 60611-3201; tel. 312/664–4467; FAX. 312/664–6143; H. Stephen Lieber, President, CEO

HealthCare Partnership, Inc., Quality Healthcare Partnership Inc., # 3 Bradley Park Court, Suite C, Columbus, GA 31904; tel. 706/323–1777; FAX. 706/324–5025; James N. Railey, President

HEAR Center, 301 East Del Mar Boulevard, Pasadena, CA 91101; tel. 626/796–2016; FAX. 626/796–2320; Ellen Simon, Executive Director

Histochemical Society, Inc., P.O. Box 85630, University Station, Seattle, WA 98195-1630; tel. 206/616–5894; FAX. 206/616–5842; W.L. Stahl, Ph.D., Executive Director

Huntington's Disease Society of America, Inc., 505 Eighth Avenue, Suite 902, New York, NY 10018; tel. 800/345–HDSA; FAX. 212/239–3430; Barbara T. Boyle, National Executive Director/CEO

I

iKeepSafe Internet Safety Coalition, 4607 N. 40th Street, Arlington, VA 22207; tel. 703/536–1637; FAX. 703/852–7100; Marsali S. Hancock, President

Infusion Nurses Society, 315 Norwood Park South, Norwood, MA 02062; tel. 781/440–9408; FAX. 781/440–9409; Mary Alexander, Chief Executive Officer

Institute for Diversity in Health Management, One North Franklin Street, 30th Floor, Chicago, IL 60606; tel. 312/422–2690; FAX. 312/895–2561; Frederick D. Hobby, President and CEO

Institute of Medicine, 500 Fifth Street, N.W., Washington, DC 20001; tel. 202/334–2352; FAX. 202/334–1412; Harvey V. Fineberg, M.D., Ph.D., President

Institutes for the Achievement of Human Potential, 8801 Stenton Avenue, Wyndmoor, PA 19038; tel. 215/233–2050; FAX. 215/233–3940; Coralee Thompson, M.D.

International Childbirth Education Association, Inc., P.O. Box 20048, Minneapolis, MN 55420-0048; tel. 612/854–8660; FAX. 612/854–8772

International College of Surgeons/United States Section, 1516 North Lake Shore Drive, Chicago, IL 60610-1694; tel. 312/787–6274; FAX. 312/787–9289; Maggie Kearney, Meeting and Publications Manager

International Council for Health, Physical Education, Recreation, Sport and Dance, 1900 Association Drive, Reston, VA 20191; tel. 703/476–3486; FAX. 703/476–9527; Dr. Dong Ja Yang, President

L

Lupus Foundation of America, Inc., 2000 L Street, NW, Suite 710, Washington, DC 20036; tel. 202/349–1155; FAX. 202/349–1156; Karen Johnson, Health Educator

M

March of Dimes, 1275 Mamaroneck Avenue, White Plains, NY 10605; tel. 914/428–7100; Vincent Sampugnaro, Senior Vice President of Human Resources

March of Dimes Foundation, 1275 Mamaroneck Avenue, White Plains, NY 10605; tel. 914/428–7100; FAX. 914/428–8203; Jennifer L. Howse, Ph.D., President

Medic Alert Foundation International, 2323 Colorado Avenue, Turlock, CA 95382; tel. 800/432–5378; FAX. 209/669–2495; Ramesh Srinvasar, Vice President Business Development & Marketing

Medical Fitness Association, P.O. Box 73103, Richmond, VA 23235; tel. 804/897–5701; FAX. 804/897–5704; Cary Wing, Ed.D., Executive Director

Medical Group Management Association, 104 Inverness Terrace, E., Englewood, CO 80112-5306; tel. 877/275–6462; FAX. 303/643–4427; William F. Jessee, MD, FACMPE, President and CEO

Medical Library Association, 65 East Wacker Place, Suite 1900, Chicago, IL 60601-7298; tel. 312/419–9094; FAX. 312/419–8950; Carla J. Funk, Executive Director

Men's Health Network, P.O. Box 75972, Washington, DC 20013; tel. 202/543–6461; Theresa Morrow, Director- Marketing and External Affairs

Mental Health America, (formerly known as the National Mental Health Association), 2000 N. Beauregard Street, 6th Floor, Alexandria, VA 22311; tel. 703/684–7722; FAX. 703/684–5968; David L. Shern, Ph.D., President and CEO

Midwives Alliance of North America, 611 Pennsylvania Avenue, SE # 1700, Washington, DC 200034303; tel. 888/923–6262; President, Geradine Simkins

Muscular Dystrophy Association, 3300 East Sunrise Drive, Tucson, AZ 85718; tel. 520/529–2000; FAX. 520/529–5300; Gerald C. Weinberg, President & CEO

N

National Academy of Sciences, Division on Earth and Life Studies, 500 Fifth St., NW-Keck 654, Washington, DC 20001; tel. 202/334–2500; FAX. 202/334–3362; Warren R. Muir, PH.D, Executive Director

National Accreditation Council for Agencies Serving the Blind, 21475 Lorain Road, Suite300, Fairview, OH 44126; tel. 440/409–0340; Steven K. Hegedeos Executive Director

National Accrediting Agency for Clinical Laboratory Sciences, 8410 West Bryn Mawr, Suite 670, Chicago, IL 60631-3415; tel. 773/714–8880; FAX. 773/714–8886; Dianne M. Cearlock, CEO

National Alliance for Hispanic Health, 1501 16th Street N.W., Washington, DC 20036; tel. 202/387–5000; FAX. 202/797–4353; Mr. Adolph Falcón, Vice President for Science and Policy

National Alliance for the Mentally Ill (NAMI), 2107 Wilson Blvd, Suite 300, Arlington, VA 22201-3042; tel. 703/524–7600; FAX. 703/524–9094; Michael J. Fitzpatrick, M.S.W., Executive Director

National Assembly on School Based Health Care, 666 11th Street, NW, Suite 735, Washington, DC 20001; tel. 202/638–5872; FAX. 202/638–5879; John Schlitt, Executive Director

National Association for Home Care & Hospice, 228 Seventh Street, S.E., Washington, DC 20003; tel. 202/547–7424; FAX. 202/547–3540; Val J. Halamandaris, President

National Association for Practical Nurse Education and Service, Mail Processing, 1940 Duke Street, Alexandria, VA 22314; tel. 703/933–1003; FAX. 703/933–1004; Patrick Mahan, Executive Director

National Association Medical Staff Services, 2025 M Street, NW, Suite 800, Washington, DC 20036; tel. 202/367–1196; FAX. 202/367–2196; Megan Cohen, Executive Director

National Association of Boards of Pharmacy, 1600 Feehanville Dr., Mt. Prospect, IL 60056; tel. 847/391–4406; FAX. 847/391–4502; Carmen A. Catizone, R.Ph., M.S., Executive Director/ Secretary

National Association of Children's Hospitals and Related Institutes, 401 Wythe Street, Alexandria, VA 22314; tel. 703/684–1355; FAX. 703/684–1589; Lawrence A. McAndrews, President and CEO

National Association of County and City Health Officials, 1100 17th Street, NW, 2nd Floor, Washington, DC 20036; tel. 202/783–5550; FAX. 202/783–1583; Angela Ablorh-Odjidja, MHS, Program Manager, Community Health Team

National Association of Dental Assistants, 900 South Washington Street, Suite G13, Falls Church, VA 22046; tel. 703/237–8616; FAX. 703/533–1153; S. Young, Director

National Association of Dental Laboratories, (Includes National Board for Certification in Dental Laboratory Technology), 325 John Knox Rd, #L 103, Tallahassee, FL 32303; tel. 800/950–1150; FAX. 850/222–0053; Bennett Napier, CAE, Co-Executive Director

National Association of Health Services Executives, 8630 Fenton Street, Suite 126, Silver Spring, MD 20910; tel. 202/628–3953; FAX. 301/588–0011; Ozzie Jenkins, CMP, Association Manager

National Association of Psychiatric Health Systems, 701 13th Street, N.W., Suite 950, Washington, DC 20005-3903; tel. 202/393–6700; FAX. 202/783–6041; Mark J. Covall, Executive Director

National Association of Social Workers, 750 First Street, N.E., Suite 700, Washington, DC 20002; tel. 202/336–8200; FAX. 202/336–8313; Elizabeth Clark, Ph.D., ACSW, MPH, Executive Director

National Association of State Mental Health Program Directors, 66 Canal Center Plaza, Suite 302, Alexandria, VA 22314; tel. 703/739–9333; FAX. 703/548–9517; Robert W. Glover, Ph.D., Executive Director

National Biosafety and Biocontainment Training Program, Three Dunwoody Park, Suite 103, Atlanta, GA 30338; tel. 678/781–5241; FAX. 678/781–5242; Murray L. Cohen, PhD, MPH, CIH, NBBTP Executive Director

National Board for Respiratory Care, NBRC Executive Office, 18000 W. 105th Street, Olathe, KS 66061-7543; tel. 913/895–4900; FAX. 913/895–4650; Gary A. Smith, Executive Director

National Board of Anesthesiology, Inc, 11817 Summit, Kansas, MO 64114; tel. 785/842–7067; FAX. 816/836–8953; R. Scott Richart, JD, Executive Director

National Board of Medical Examiners, 3750 Market Street, Philadelphia, PA 19104; tel. 215/590–9500; FAX. 215/590–9430; Donald E. Melnick, M.D., President

National Board of Public Health Examiners, 1101 15th Street, N.W., Suite 910, Washington, DC 20005; tel. 866/514–7569; FAX. 202/296–1252; Cynthia Godes, Interim Board Administrator

National Council of State Boards of Nursing, 111 E. Wacker Dr., Suite 2900, Chicago, IL 60601; tel. 312/525–3600; FAX. 312/279–1032; Kathy Apple, Executive Director

National Council on Aging, Inc., NCOA Headquarters, 1901 L Street, N.W., 4th Floor, Washington, DC 20024; tel. 202/479–1200; FAX. 202/479–0735; James P. Firman, Ed. D., President & CEO

National Council on Alcoholism and Drug Dependence, Inc., 22 Cortland Street, 8th floor, New York, NY 1000; tel. 212/269–7797; FAX. 212/269–7510; Robert J. Lindsey, M.Ed., CEAP President

National Council on Radiation Protection and Measurements, 7910 Woodmont Avenue, Suite 400, Bethesda, MD 20814; tel. 301/657–2652; FAX. 301/907–8768; David A. Schauer, Executive Director

National Dental Association, 3517 16th Street, NW, Washington, DC 20010; tel. 202/588–1697; FAX. 202/588–1244; Robert S. Johns, Executive Director

National Environmental Health Association, 720 South Colorado Boulevard, North Tower, Suite 1000-N, Denver, CO 80246-1926; tel. 303/756–9090; FAX. 303/691–9490; Nelson Fabian, Executive Director

National Federation of Licensed Practical Nurses, 605 Poole Dr., Garner, NC 27529; tel. 919/779–0046; FAX. 919/779–5642; Charlene Barbour, Executive Director

National Fire Protection Association, P.O. Box 9101, One Batterymarck Park, Quincy, MA 02269-9101; tel. 617/770–3000; FAX. 617/770–7110; Richard P. Bielen, P.E. Chief Systems and Applications Engineer

National Gaucher Foundation, 2227 Idlewood Road, Suite 12, Tucker, GA 30084; tel. 800/504–3189; FAX. 770/934–2911; Rhonda Buyers, Executive Director & CEO

National Headache Foundation, 820 N. Orleans, Suite 217, Chicago, IL 60610-3132; tel. 888/NHF–5552; FAX. 312/640–9049; Suzanne Simons, Executive Director

National Health Council, Inc., 1730 M Street, N.W., Suite 500, Washington, DC 20036; tel. 202/785–3910; FAX. 202/785–5923; Myrl Weinberg, CAE, President

National Hemophilia Foundation, 116 West 32nd Street, 11th Floor, New York, NY 10001; tel. 212/328–3700; FAX. 212/328–3795; Alan J. Kinniburgh, PH.D, CEO

National Institute for Jewish Hospice, Central Telephone Network, P.O. Box 48025, Los Angeles, CA 90048; tel. 800/446–4448; FAX. 516/791–6999; Shirley Lamm, Executive Director

National Institute for Occupational Safety and Health, 395 E Street, S.W., Suite 9200, Washington, DC 20201; tel. 202/245–0625; John Howard, MD, Director

National Kidney Foundation, 30 East 33rd Street, New York, NY 10016; tel. 800/622–9010; FAX. 212/779–0068; John Davis, Chief Executive Officer

National Multiple Sclerosis Society, 733 Third Avenue, New York, NY 10017; tel. 212/986–3240; FAX. 212/986–7981; Dwayne Howell, Executive Vice President

National Organization for Rare Disorders, 55 Kenosia Avenue, PO Box 1968, Danbury, CT 06813-1968; tel. 203/744–0100; FAX. 203/798–2291; Names Peter L. Saltonstal, President and CEO

National Parkinson Foundation, Inc., 1501 Northwest Ninth Avenue, Miami, FL 33136-1494; tel. 800/327–4545; FAX. 305/243–5540; Pamela Olmo, Director of Finance & Administration

National Perinatal Association, 2090 Linglestown Rd, Suite 107, Harrisburg, PA 17110; tel. 888/971–3295; FAX. 717/920–1390; Sharon Chesna, President

National Reference Center for Bioethics Literature, Kennedy Institute of Ethics, Georgetown University, Box 571212, Washington, DC 20057-1212; tel. 202/687–3885; FAX. 202/687–6770; Doris Goldstein, M.L.S., M.A., Director of Library and Information Services

National Registry of Emergency Medical Technicians, 6610 Busch Boulevard, P.O. Box 29233, Columbus, OH 43229; tel. 614/888–4484; FAX. 614/888–8920; William E. Brown, Jr., Executive Director

National Rehabilitation Association, (Includes Nine National Divisions and 58 Affiliate Chapters), 633 South Washington Street, Alexandria, VA 22314; tel. 703/836–0850; FAX. 703/836–0848; Linda R. Winslow, Executive Director

National Resident Matching Program, 2450 N Street, N.W., Washington, DC 1127; tel. 202/828–0676; FAX. 202/828–4797; Mona M. Signer, Executive Director

National Rural Health Association, 1108 K. Street NW, 2nd Floor, Washington, DC 20005; tel. 202/639–0550; FAX. 202/639–0559; Alan Morgan, Chief Executive Officer

National Safety Council, 1121 Spring Lake Drive, Itasca, IL 60143-3201; tel. 800/621–7619; FAX. 630/285–0797; Customer Service Department

National Stroke Association, 9707 E Easter Lane, Building B, Centennial, CO 80112; tel. 303/754–0902; FAX. 303/649–1328; Suzanne Sparks, Executive Assistant to the CEO

National Student Nurses' Association, Inc., 45 Main Street, Suite 606, Brooklyn, NY 11201; tel. 718/210–0705; FAX. 718/210–0710; Diane J. Mancino, Ed.D., RN, CAE, Executive Director

National Tay-Sachs and Allied Diseases Association, 2001 Beacon Street, Suite 204, Brighton, MA 02135; tel. 800/90–NTSAD; FAX. 617/277–0134; Susan R. Kahn, Executive Director

National Women's Health Network, 514 10th Street NW, Suite 400, Washington, DC 20004; tel. 202/347–1140; FAX. 202/347–1168; Cynthia Pearson, Executive Director

New England Gerontological Association, One Cutts Road, Durham, NH 03824-3102; tel. 603/868–5757; Eugene E. Tillock, Ed.D., Executive Director

New York State Nurses Association, NYSNA, 11 Cornel Road, Latham, NY 12110-1499; tel. 518/782–9400; FAX. 518/782–9530; Gene Tranbarger Ed. D., RN

NSF International, 789 Dixboro Road, P.O. Box 130140, Ann Arbor, MI 48113-0140; tel. 313/769–8010; FAX. 313/769–0109; Dennis R. Mangino, Ph. D., President and CEO

O

Osteogenesis Imperfecta Foundation, Inc., 804 West Diamond Avenue, Suite 210, Gaithersburg, MD 20878; tel. 301/947–0083; FAX. 301/947–0456; Tracy Smith Hart, CEO

P

Pan American Health Organization, Pan American Sanitary Bureau, Regional Office of the World Health Organization, 525 23rd Street, N.W., Washington, DC 20037; tel. 202/974–3000; FAX. 202/974–3663; Dr. Mirta Roses Periago, Director

Parkinson's Disease Foundation, Inc, (Formerly United Parkinson Foundation), 833 West Washington Boulevard, Chicago, IL 60607; tel. 800/457–6676; FAX. 312/733–1896; Jeanne Rosner, Director

Partnership for Food Safety Education, 50 F Street N.W., 6th Floor, Washington, DC 20001; tel. 202/220–0651; Shelly Feist, Executive Director

Partnership for Prevention, 1015 18th Street N.W., Suite 300, Washington, DC 20036; tel. 202/833–0009; FAX. 202/833–0113; John M. Clymer, President

Physician Executive Management Center, 3403 West Fletcher Avenue, Tampa, FL 33618-2813; tel. 813/963–1800; FAX. 813/264–2207; David R. Kirschman, President

Pilot Dogs, Inc., 625 West Town Street, Columbus, OH 43215; tel. 614/221–6367; FAX. 614/221–1577; J. Jay Gray, Executive Director

Practice Greenhealth, 1901 N. Moore Street, Suite 509, Arlington, VA 22209; FAX. 866/379–8705; Robert Jarboe, Executive Director

Prevent Blindness America, 211 W. Wacker Drive, Suite 1700, Chicago, IL 60606; tel. 800/331–2020; FAX. 312/363–6052; Hugh Parry, President & Chief Executive Officer

Public Health Foundation, 1300 L STREET N.W., SUITE 800, Washington, DC 20005; tel. 202/218–4400; FAX. 202/218–4409; Sue Madden, Deputy Executive Director

Public Relations Society of America, 33 Maiden Lane 11th Floor, New York, NY 10038-5150; tel. 212/460–1400; FAX. 212/995–0757; Catherine A. Bolton, Executive Director and COO

R

Radiological Society of North America, Inc., 820 Jorie Boulevard, Oak Brook, IL 60523-2251; tel. 630/571–2670; FAX. 630/571–7837; Natalie Boden, Director of Marketing & Communications

Recording for the Blind and Dyslexic, 20 Roszel Road, Princeton, NJ 08540; tel. 866/732–3585; FAX. 609/520–7990; Richard O. Scribner, President

Renal Physicians Association, 1700 Rockville Pike, Suite 220, Rockville, MD 20852; tel. 301/468–3515; FAX. 301/468–3511; Dale Singer, MHA, Executive Director

Robert Wood Johnson Foundation, P.O. Box 2316, Route One and College Road East, Princeton, NJ 08543-2316; tel. 877/843–7953; FAX. 888/727–1966; Richard J. Toth, Director, Office of Proposal Management

S

Safe Kids Worldwide, 1301 Pennsylvania Avenue, N.W., Suite 1000, Washington, DC 20004; tel. 202/662–0600; FAX. 202/393–2072; Mitchell R. Stoller, President and Chief Executive Officer

Shriners Hospitals for Children, P.O. Box 31356, Tampa, FL 33631-3356; tel. 813/281–8110; FAX. 813/281–8113; James M. Full, FACHE, Executive Vice President & CEO

Society for Academic Emergency Medicine, 901 North Washington Avenue, Lansing, MI 48906; tel. 517/485–5484; FAX. 517/485–0801; Barbara A. Mulder, Associate Executive Director

Society for Adolescent Medicine, Inc., 1916 NW Copper Oaks Circle, Blue Springs, MO 64015; tel. 816/224–8010; FAX. 816/224–8009; Edie Moore, Executive Director

Society for Healthcare Consumer Advocacy (SHCA), One North Franklin, 28th Floor, Chicago, IL 60606; tel. 312/422–3700; FAX. 312/422–4577; Elizabeth Summy, Associate Vice President

Society for Healthcare Strategy and Market Development, of the American Hospital Association, One North Franklin, 28th Floor, Chicago, IL 60606; tel. 312/422–3740; FAX. 312/422–4579; Lauren A. Barnett, Executive Director

Society for Occupational and Environmental Health, 6728 Old McLean Village Drive, McLean, VA 22101; tel. 703/556–9222; FAX. 703/556–8729; Connie MacKay, Account Manager

Society for Pediatric Pathology, 3643 Walton Way Extension, Augusta, GA 30909; tel. 706/364–3375; FAX. 706/733–8033; Kerry Crockett, Director of Convention and Meeting Services

Society for Social Work Leadership in Health Care (SSWLHC), 100 North 20th Street, Suite 400, Philadelphia, PA 19103; FAX. 215/545–8107; Vaughn Wurst, Account Executive

Society of Critical Care Medicine, 500 Midway Drive, Mount Prospect, IL 60056; tel. 847/827–6869; FAX. 847/827–6886; David J. Martin, CAE, Chief Executive Officer/EVP

Society of Neurological Surgeons, 3303 SW Bond Ave., Portland, OR 97239; tel. 503/494–7978; Kim J. Burchiel, M.D., F.A.C.S., Secretary

Society of Nuclear Medicine, 1850 Samuel Morse Drive, Reston, VA 20190-5316; tel. 703/708–9000; FAX. 703/708–9777; Mike Nelson, COO

Society of University Otolaryngologists-Head and Neck Surgeons, USC School of Medicine, Department of Otolaryngology, Los Angeles, CA 90033; tel. 323/226–7315; FAX. 323/226–2780; Donna Hoffman, M.A., Executive Director

Southeastern Healthcare Association, 4150 Carmichael Court, P.O. Box 11126, Montgomery, AL 36111-0126; tel. 334/260–8600; FAX. 205/260–0023; Tommy R. McDougal, FACHE, President

Special Care Dentistry Association, 401 N. Michigan Avenue, Suite 2200, Chicago, IL 60611; tel. 312/527–6764; FAX. 312/673–6663; Kristen Smith, Executive Director

Special Care Dentistry Association, 401 N. Michigan Ave, 22nd Floor, Chicago, IL 60611; tel. 312/527–6764; FAX. 312/673–6663; Kaye Englebrecht

Spina Bifida Association, 4590 MacArthur Boulevard, N.W., Washington, DC 20007; tel. 800/621–3141; FAX. 202/944–3295; Sherry Arvin, Information and Referral Coordinator

Susan G. Komen Breast Cancer Foundation, 5005 LBJ Freeway, Suite 250, Dallas, TX 75244; tel. 800/465–6636; Kimberly Simpson, Chief Operating Officer

T

Technologist Section, Society of Nuclear Medicine, 1850 Samuel Morse Drive, Reston, VA 20190; tel. 703/708–9000; FAX. 703/708–9013; Virginia M. Pappas, Executive Director

The American Association of Immunologists, Inc., 9650 Rockville Pike, Bethesda, MD 20814; tel. 301/634–7178; FAX. 301/634–7887; M. Michele Hogan, Ph.D., Executive Director

The American Board of Obstetrics and Gynecology, Inc., 2915 Vine Street, Dallas, TX 75204; tel. 214/871–1619; FAX. 214/871–1943; Dr. Norman F. Gant, Executive Director

The American Board of Pediatric Dentistry, 325 E. Washington Street, Suite 208, Iowa City, IA 52240-3960; tel. 319/341–8488; FAX. 319/341–9499; Arthur J. Nowak, Executive Director

The American Board of Plastic Surgery, Inc., Seven Penn Center, Suite 400, 1635 Market Street, Philadelphia, PA 19103-2204; tel. 215/587–9322; FAX. 215/587–9622; Terry M. Cullison, RN, MSN, Administrator

The American Board of Professional Disability Consultants, 1350 Beverly Road, Suite 115-327, McLean, VA 22101; tel. 703/790–8644; Taras J. Cerkevitch, Ph.D., Director, Operations

The American Board of Urology, Inc., 2216 Ivy Road, Suite 210, Charlottesville, VA 22903; tel. 434/979–0059; FAX. 434/979–0266; Stuart S. Howards, M.D., Executive Secretary

The American Orthopaedic Association, 6300 North River Road, Suite 505, Rosemont, IL 60018-4263; tel. 847/318–7330; FAX. 847/318–7339; Camille Murray, Education and Membership Manager

The Arc of the United States, 1010 Wayne Ave, Suite 650, Silver Spring, MD 60910; tel. 301/565–3842; FAX. 301/565–3843; John Foley, Acting Executive Director

The Association for Research in Vision and Ophthalmology, 12300 Twinbrook Parkway, Suite 250, Rockville, MD 20852-1606; tel. 240/221–2900; FAX. 240/221–0370; Joanne G. Angle, Executive Director

The Association of Medical Illustrators, 810 E. 10th Street, P.O. Box 1897, Lawrence, KS 66044; tel. 866/393–4264; FAX. 785/843–1274; Vanessa Reilly, Executive Director

The Association of Women's Health, Obstetric and Neonatal Nurses, 2000 L. Street, NW, Suite 740, Washington, DC 20036; tel. 202/261–2400; FAX. 202/728–0575; Gail G. Kincaide, Executive Director

The Christopher and Dana Reeve Foundation Paralysis Resource Center, Short Hills Plaza, 636 Morris Turnpike, Suite #3A, Short Hills, NJ 07078-7503; tel. 800/539–7309; Angela Cantillon, Associate Director-Operations

The Duke Endowment, 100 North Tryon Street, Suite 3500, Charlotte, NC 28202; tel. 704/376–0291; FAX. 704/376–9336; Eugene W. Cochrane, Jr., President

The Endocrine Society, 8401 Connecticut Ave, Suite 900, Chevy Chase, MD 20815; tel. 301/941–0200; FAX. 301/941–0259; Susan Koppi, Director, Public Affairs

The Foundation Fighting Blindness, Inc., 11435 Cronhill Drive, Owings Mill,, MD 21117-2220; tel. 410/568–0150; FAX. 410/363–3159; William T. Schmidt, CEO

The Foundation for Ichthyosis and Related Skin Types, Inc., (F.I.R.S.T.), 1364 Welsh Road, G2, North Wales, PA 19454; tel. 215/619–0670; FAX. 215/619–0780; Jean Pickford, Executive Director

The International Dyslexia Association, (Formerly The Orton Dyslexia Society), 40 York Road, 4th Floor, Baltimore, MD 21204; tel. 410/296–0232; FAX. 410/321–5069; Judith Dudek, Director, Marketing and Membership

The Joint Commission, One Renaissance Boulevard, Oakbrook Terrace, IL 60181; tel. 630/792–5000; FAX. 630/792–5005; Mark R. Chassin, M.D., MPP, MPH, President

The Leukemia & Lymphoma Society, 1311 Mamaroneck Avenue, White Plains, NY 10650; tel. 914/949–5213; FAX. 914/949–6691; John E. Walter, President and CEO

The Mended Hearts, Inc., 7272 Greenville Avenue, Dallas, TX 75231; tel. 214/706–1442; FAX. 214/706–5245; Tim Elsner, Executive Director

The National Academies, 500 Fifth St. N.W., Washington, DC' 20001; tel. 202/334–2000; Harvey V. Fineberg, President, Institute of Medicine

The National Commission for Health Education Credentialing, Inc., 1541 Alta Drive, Suite 303, Whitehall, PA 18052-5642; tel. 484/223–0770; FAX. 800/813–0727; Linda Lysoby, MS, CHES, Executive Director

The Salvation Army National Corporation, 615 Slaters Lane, P.O. Box 269, Alexandria, VA 22313; tel. 703/684–5500; FAX. 703/519–5889; Major Ronald R. Foreman, National Social Services Secretary

The Seeing Eye, Inc., P.O. Box 375, Morristown, NJ 07963-0375; tel. 973/539–4425; FAX. 973/539–0922; Kenneth Rosenthal, President

The Southwestern Surgical Congress, P.O. Box 24425, Overland Park, KS 66223; tel. 913/402–7102; FAX. 913/402–7103; Nonie Lowry, Administrative Manager

The Vision Council of America, 1700 Diagonal Road, Suite 500, Alexandria, VA 22314; tel. 703/548–4560; FAX. 703/548–4580; Ed Greene, Chief Executive Officer

U

UCLA Medical Center, Neurosurgery, Box 956901, Room 74-134 CHS, Los Angeles, CA 90095-6901; tel. 301/794–1222; FAX. 310/825–7245; Donald P. Becker, M.D.

United Cerebral Palsy Associations, Inc., 1660 L Street, N.W., Suite 700, Washington, DC 20036; tel. 800/872–5827; FAX. 202/776–0414; Stephen Bennett, President and CEO

United Methodist Association of Health and Welfare Ministries, 407 Corporate Center Dr., Suite B, Vandalia, OH 45377; tel. 937/227–9494; FAX. 937/222–7364; Mearle L. Griffith, President and CEO

United Way of America, 701 North Fairfax Street, Alexandria, VA 22314-2045; tel. 703/836–7100; FAX. 703/683–7846; Brian A. Gallagher, President and CEO

USP, 12601 Twinbrook Parkway, Rockville, MD 20852; tel. 301/816–8368; FAX. 301/816–8511; Arline M. Bilbo, Director, Member and Professional Relations

W

Western Orthopedic Association, 154-A W. Foothill Boulevard, # 107, Upland, CA 91786; tel. 866/962–1388; FAX. 410/494–0515; Chuck Freitag, Executive Director

International Organizations

ARGENTINA

Argentinean Association of Dermatology (AAD), Asociacion Argentina De Dermatologia, Mexico 1720, 1100 Buenos Aires, Argentina; tel. 1143812737; FAX. 1143831153; Dra. Lidia Ester Valle, Chairman

Camara Argentina De Empresas De Salud, (Argentina Hospital Association), Tucuman 1668, 2 Piso, C.P. 1050, Buenos Aires; tel. 541143725915; FAX. 541143723229; Norberto Larroca-President

AUSTRALIA

Australian Healthcare Association, 99 Northbourne Ave, Suite 4, Level 1, Turner, 26120; tel. 1261620780; FAX. 1261620779; Prue Power, Executive Director

BELGIUM

Verbond der Verzorgingsinstellingen V.Z.W., 1, Guimardstraat, Brussels 1040, Belgium; FAX. 2 5135269; G. Van Oevelen, President

BRAZIL

Fraternidade Crista De Doentes E Deficientes, Cap. Correa Pacheco 134, Americana, SP, Brazil; tel. 0 194 619754; Salete Inês Milan, National Coordinator

CANADA

Association of Physicians of English Canada, Association des Medecins de langue francaise du Canada, 8355 St. Laurent Boulevard, Montreal, PQ H2P 2Z6; tel. 514/388–2228; FAX. 514/388–5335; Gilles Lapiene, Financial Director

Canadian Anesthesiologists' Society (CAS), 1 Eglinton Avenue East,, Suite 208, Toronto, ON M4P 3A1; tel. 416/480–0602; FAX. 416/480–0320; S. Stanley Mandarich, Executive Director

Canadian Association of Pathologists (CAP), 774 Echo Drive, Ottawa, ON K1S 5N8; tel. 613/730–6230; FAX. 613/730–1116; Dr. Bruce Burns, Secretary-Treasurer

Canadian Association of Social Workers, 383 Parkdale Avenue, Suite 402, Ottawa, ON K1Y 4R4; tel. 613/729–6668; FAX. 613/729–9608; Eugenia Repetur Moreno, Executive Director

Canadian Blood Services, Head Office, 1800 Alta Vista Drive, Ottawa, ON K1G 4J5; tel. 613/739–2300; FAX. 613/731–1411; Dr. Graham D. Sher, CEO

Canadian Cancer Society (CCS), 10 Alcorn Ave, Suite 200, Toronto, ON; tel. 416/961–7223; FAX. 416/961–4189; Barbara Whylie, Chief Executive Officer

Canadian Cardiovascular Society, 222 Queen Street, Suite 1403, Ottawa, ON K1P 5V9; tel. 613/569–3407; FAX. 613/569–6574; Anne Fegruson, CEO

Canadian Council of the Blind (CCB), (Conseil Canadien des Aveugles---CCA), 396 Cooper Street, Office 401, Ottawa, ON K2P 2H7; tel. 613/567–0311; FAX. 613/567–2728; Harold Schnellert, National President

Canadian Council on Social Development, (Conseil Canadien de Developpement Social), 190 O'Connor St, Suite 100, Ottawa, ON; tel. 613/236–8977; FAX. 613/236–2750; Nancy Perkins, Communications Coordinator

Canadian Dental Association, 1815 Alta Vista Drive, Ottawa, ON K1G 3Y6; tel. 613/523–1770; FAX. 613/521–5572; Dr. Deborah Stymiest, President

Canadian Health Information Management Association, 148 Fullarton Street, Suite 1404, London, ON; tel. 519/438–6700; FAX. 519/438–7001; Gail Crook, CEO & Registrar

Canadian Healthcare Association, 17 York Street, Ottawa, ON K1N 9J6; tel. 613/241–8005; FAX. 613/241–5055; Pamela C. Fralick, MA, President and CEO

Canadian Medical Engineering Consultants, 594 Bush Street, Belfountain, ON; tel. 519/927–3286; FAX. 519/927–9440; A. M. Dolan, President

Canadian Mental Health Association, (Association Canadien pour la Sante Mentale), Phenix Professional Building, 595 Montreal Road, Suite 303, Ottawa, ON; tel. 6137457550; FAX. 613/745–5522; Dr. Taylor Alexander, CEO

Canadian National Institute for the Blind, CNIB National Office, 1929 Bayview Avenue, Toronto, ON; tel. 800/563–2642; FAX. 416/480–7700; Jim Sanders, President & CEO

Canadian Nurses Association, 50 Driveway, Ottawa, ON K2P 1E2; tel. 613/237–2133; FAX. 613/237–3520; Lucille Auffrey, RN, MN, CEO

Canadian Orthopaedic Association, 4150 St. Catherine St. West, Suite 360, Westmount, PQ; tel. 514/874–9003; FAX. 514/874–0464; Douglas C. Thomson, CEO

Canadian Pharmacists Association, 1785 Alta Vista Drive, Ottawa, ON K1G 3Y6; tel. 613/523–7877; FAX. 613/523–0445; Jeff Poston, Executive Director

Canadian Physiotherapy Association, National Office, 2345 Yonge Street, Suite 410, Toronto, ON M4P 2E5; tel. 416/932–1888; FAX. 416/932–9708; Michel Landry, President

Canadian Psychiatric Association, 701-141 Laurier Ave W., Suite 701, Ottawa, ON KIP5J3; tel. 613/234–2815; FAX. 613/234–9857; Dr. Patrick J. White, President

Canadian Public Health Association, 1565 Carling Avenue, Suite 400, Ottawa, ON K1Z 8R1; tel. 613/725–3769; FAX. 613/725–9826; Debra Lynkowski, Chief Executive Officer

Canadian Society for Medical Laboratory Science, P.O. Box 2830, LCD 1, Hamilton, ON L8N 3N8; tel. 905/528–8642; FAX. 905/528–4968; Susan Atkinson, PresidentSusan Atkinson, President

Canadian Society of Hospital Pharmacists, 30 Concourse Gate, Unit 3, Ottawa, ON K2E7V7; tel. 613/736–9733; FAX. 613/736–5660; Janet Lett, Executive Assistant

Catholic Health Association of Canada, 1247 Kilborn Place, Ottawa, ON K1H 6K9; tel. 613/731–7148; FAX. 613/731–7797; Gerald Lewis, President & CEO

College des medecins du Quebec, 2170, boulevard Rene-Levesque Ouest, Montreal, PQ H3H 2T8; tel. 514/933–4441; FAX. 514/993–3112; Andre Garon, M.D., Secretary General

Dietitians of Canada/Les dietetistes du Canada, 480 University Avenue, Suite 604, Toronto, ON M5G 1V2; tel. 416/596–0857; FAX. 416/596–0603; Marsha Sharp, Chief Executive Officer

National Cancer Institute of Canada, 10 Alcorn Avenue, Suite 200, Toronto, ON M4V 3B1; tel. 416/961–7223; FAX. 416/961–4189; Barbara Whylie, CEO

The Canadian Hearing Society(La Societe Canadienne de l'Ouie, 271 Spadina Road, Toronto, ON M5R 2V3; tel. 416/928–2500; FAX. 416/928–2523; Kelly Duffin, President & CEO

The Canadian Medical Association, 1867 Alta Vista Drive, Ottawa, ON K1G 3Y60G8; tel. 613/731–9331; FAX. 613/731–7314; Colin J. McMillian, M.D., President

The College of Family Physicians of Canada, 2630 Skymark Avenue, Mississauga, ON L4W 5A4; tel. 905/629–0900; FAX. 905/629–0893; Dr. Calvin Gutkin, Executive Director and Chief Executive Officer

The College of Physicians and Surgeons of New Brunswick, One Hampton Road, Suite 300, Rothesay, NB E2E 5K8; tel. 506/849–5050; FAX. 506/849–5069; Ed Schollenberg, M.D., Registrar

The Royal College of Physicians and Surgeons of Canada, 774 Echo Drive, Ottawa, ON K1S 5N8; tel. 613/730–8177; FAX. 613/730–8300; Dr. M. Andrew Padmos, FRCPC, CEO

World Federation of Hemophilia, 1425 Rene Levesque Blvd. West, Suite 1010, Montreal, QC H3G 1T7; tel. 514/8757944; FAX. 514/8758916; Claudia Black, CEO & Executive Director

COSTA RICA

Asociacion Coctarricense De Hospitales, (Costa Rica Hospital Association), Aparatado 267-1005, Barrio Mexico San Jose Costa Rica, Costa Rica; tel. 5062214919; FAX. 506/255–0363; Dr. Kenneth Gonzalez Arias, Presidente

DENMARK

Amtsradsforeningen, Dampfaergevej 22, Postboks 2593, Copenhagen; tel. +453529 8196; FAX. +453529 8337; Peder Ring, Assistant Director

Danish Dental Association, Amaliegade 17, Postboks 143, Copenhagen K; Per Graverson, Chief Executive

Danish Regions, DAMPFAEORGEVEJ 22, P.O. Box 2593, Copenhagen; tel. +4535298100; FAX. +4535298300; Peter Ring, Assistant Director

National Committee for Danish Hospitals, Dampfaergevej 22, Postboks 2593, Denmark; tel. 45 35298196; FAX. 45 35298337; Peder Ring, Assistant Director

ENGLAND

British Medical Association (BMA), BMA House, Tavistock Square, London, WCIH 9JP; tel. 02073874499; FAX. 02073836400; Mr. Tony Bourne, Chief Executive/Secretary

European Association of Poisons/Centres and Clinical Toxicology, Hopitaux Universitaires de Strasbourg, Hospital de Hautepierre, Cedex; tel. 33/388127906; FAX. 33/388127908; Prof. Philippe Hantson, President

Institute of Healthcare Management, IHM 18-21 Morley Street, London, SE 17Q2; Ms. Susan Hodgetts, Chief Executive

King's Fund, 11-13 Cavendish Square, London, England, W1G 0AN; tel. 020 73072400; FAX. 020 73072801; Niall Dickson, Chief Executive Officer

Nuffield Trust, 59 New Cavendish Street, London W1G 7LP; tel. 02076318450; FAX. 02076318451; Dr Jennifer Dixon, Director

FINLAND

National Research and Development Centre for Welfare and Health (STAKES), P.O. Box 220, FI-00531 Helsinki, Lintulahdenkuja 4, Helsinki; tel. 3589396710; FAX. 3589761307; Matti Heikkilä, Director General

FRANCE

Federation Hospitaliere De France, (France Hospital Association), 1 bis, Rue Cabanis, Paris, 75014; Pascal Garel- Deputy Director

International Hospital Federation, Immeuble JB SAY, 13 Chemin du Levant, F-01210 Ferney-Voltaire; tel. 3345042600; FAX. 3345042601; Professor Per-Gunnar Svensson, Director General

World Medical Association, 13, ch. du Levant, CIB - Bâtiment A, Voltaire; tel. 33450407575; FAX. 33450405937; Dr. Otmar Kloiber, Secretary General

GERMANY

Deutsche Krankenhausgesellschaft, (German Hospital Federation), Wegelystrabe 3, D - 10623, Berlin; tel. +4930398040; FAX. 493039087307; Jorg Robbers, Managing Director

International Academy of CytologyUniversity of Freiburg, Burgenderster. 1, Freiburg, 79104; tel. 497612923801; FAX. 497612923802; Volker Schneider, M.D., FIAC, Secretary General

HUNGARY

Magyar Korhazszovetseg, (Hungarian Hospital Association), 1113 Budapest, Ibrahim u. 19., Hungary; Dr. Zoltan Ajkay, President

INDIA

Indian Hospital Association, B-401 Sarita Vihar, New Delhi, 110044; FAX. 91–11–694126; Dr. P.Ghez, Secretary General

INDONESIA

Indonesian Hospital Association (PERSI), Jl. Blvd. Artha Gading A-7A No. 28, Kelapa Gading, Jakarta, Utara, 14240; Dr. A.W. Boediarso, SKM, MBA, President

ITALY

Federazione Italiana delle Aziende Sanitarie e Ospedaliere (FIASO), (Italy Hospital Association), Corso Vi Horis Emmanuele II n. 24, Roma, 00186; Dott. Francesco Ripa di Meana, Presidente

KOREA

Korean Hospital Association, (Mapo Hyun Dai Building), 35-1 Mapo-dong, Korea; tel. 2 7187521; FAX. 2 7187522; (Internation Cooperation Officer)

MEXICO

Asociacion Mexicana De Hospitales AC, (Mexico Hospital Association), Queretaro 210, Mexico City, 06700; tel. 55740135; FAX. 55841882; LIC. Francisco Spindola Salazar, Manager

MONGOLIA

Mongolian Hospital Association, P.O. Box 48/146, MHSW Olympic Street, Mongolia; Dr. Sodor Sonin, Minister of Health, Vice President

NORWAY

Norsk Sykehus Helsetjenesten, (Norway Hospital Association), Nedre Slottsgt 7, 0157 Oslo, Norske Kommuners sentralforbund, Vika Oslo 1

PANAMA

Asociacion Panamena De Hospitales Privados, (Panama Hospital Association), Apartado 07503, Panama, Panama; Rodrigo A. Moreno, President

PERU

Peruvian Hospital Association, Av. Dos De Mayo 8502 Of. 203, San Isidro, Lima; tel. 14 419546; Arturo Vasi Paez, President

PHILIPPINES

Philippine Hospital Association, 14 Kamias Road, Quezon City-1, Philippines; tel. 2 9227674/75; Thelma Navarrete-Clemente, M.D., M.H.A., President

SOUTH AFRICA

Provincial Administration, Health Services Branch, P.O. Box 517, South Africa; tel. 051/4055818; FAX. 051/304958; Dr. J. H. Kotze

South African Hospital Federation, Department of Health, Facilities Planning, Private Bag X828, Pretoria 0001, South Africa; tel. 0123120678; FAX. 0123123157; R.E. Lawrenee

SWEDEN

Federation of Swedish County Councils, S-118 82 Stockholm, Sweden; tel. +4684527200; FAX. +4684527210; Kicki Nilsson, Assistant

SWITZERLAND

H+ Die Spitaler der Schweiz, (Swiss Hospital Association), Lorrainestrasse 4 A, Bern; Geschaeftsstelle

THE NETHERLANDS

International Federation of Oto-Rhino-Laryngological Societies, P.O. Box 115, 2300 AC Leiden, Leiden; Emelie, Administrator

UNITED STATES

Association for Assessment and Accreditation of Laboratory Animal Care International, 5283 Corporate Drive, Suite 203, Frederick, MD 217032879; tel. 301/696–9626; FAX. 301/696–9627; Lynn C. Anderson D.V.M., Executive Director Executive Director

ASTM International, 100 Barr Harbor Drive, West Conshohocken, PA 19428-2959; tel. 610/832–9672; FAX. 610/832–9666; Kenneth C. Pearson, Vice President

Honor Society of Nursing, Sigma Theta Tau International, 550 West North Street, Indianapolis, IN 46202; tel. 317/634–8171; FAX. 317/634–8188; Patricia Thompson, Chief Executive Officer

International Aid, 17011 West Hickory, Spring Lake, MI 49456-9712; tel. 616/846–7490; FAX. 616/846–3842; Rev Miles D. Fish, President

International Association for Dental Research, 1619 Duke Street, Alexandria, VA 22314-3406; tel. 703/548–0066; FAX. 703/548–1883; Christopher H. Fox, Executive Director

International Association of Healthcare Central Service Materiel Management, 2113 W. Institute Place, Suite 307, Chicago, IL 60610; tel. 312/440–0078; FAX. 3124409474; Betty Hnna, Executive Director

International Association of Society for Quality of Life Research, 6728 Old McLean Village Drive, McLean, VA 22101; tel. 703/556–9222; FAX. 703/556–8729; Laura Degnon, Executive Director

International Council on Social Welfare, 750 First Street, N.E., Washington, DC 20002; tel. 202/336–8274; FAX. 202/336–8311; Helen Whetzel, Secretary; Margery Carpenter, Volunteer Coordinator

International Essential Tremor Foundation, P. O. Box 14005, Lenexa, KS 66285-4005; tel. 913/341–3880; FAX. 913/341–1296; Catherine S. Rice, Executive Director

International Executive Housekeepers Association, Inc., 1001 Eastwind Drive, Suite 301, Westerville, OH 43081-3361; tel. 800/200–6342; FAX. 614/895–1248; Beth Risinger, CEO/ Executive Director

Rehabilitation International, 25 East 21st Street, New York, NY 10010; tel. 212/420–1500; FAX. 212/505–0871; Tomas Lagerwall, Secretary General

World Federation of Public Health Associations, c/o APHA, 800 I Street NW, Washington, DC 20001-3710; tel. 202/777–2486; FAX. 202/777–2533; Georges C. Benjamin, MD, FACP, FACEP (Emeritus), Executive Director

VENEZUELA

Latin American Association for the Study of the Liver (LAASL), P.O. Box 51890, Sabana Grande, Venezuela; tel. 58–2–9799380; FAX. 58–2–9799380; Dr. Miguel A. Garassini, President

U. S. GOVERNMENT AGENCIES

The following information is based on data available as of June, 2008.
For more information about U.S. government agencies, consult the U.S. Government Manual, *available from the Office of the* Federal Register, *National Archives and Records Service, Washington, DC 20408. A telephone directory of the U.S. Department of Health and Human Services is available from the Superintendent of Documents, Government Printing Office, Washington, DC 20402. Additional assistance may be obtained by contacting the American Hospital Association's Washington office, 325 Seventh Street, N.W., Washington, DC 20004.*

Executive Office of the President, The White House
1600 Pennsylvania Avenue NW
Washington, DC 20500
202/456-1414
George W. Bush, President of the United States
http://www.whitehouse.gov

Office of the Vice President of the United States
Old Executive Office Building
Washington, DC 20501
202/452-2326
Richard B. Cheney, Vice President of the United States
http://www.whitehouse.gov/vicepresident/

Centers for Disease Control and Prevention
1600 Clifton Road
Atlanta, GA 30333
404/498-1515
Dr. Julie L. Gerberding, Director
http://www.cdc.gov

Centers for Medicare & Medicaid Services
200 Independence
Washington, DC 20201
877/267-2323
Kerry N. Weems, Acting Administrator
http://www.cms.gov

Council of Economic Advisors
Old Executive Office Building
Washington, DC 20502
202/395-5084
Dr. Edward P. Lazear, Chairman
http://www.whitehouse.gov/cea/

Council on Environmental Quality
722 Jackson Place, NW
Washington, DC 20503
202/395-5750
James Connaughton, Chairman
http://www.whitehouse.gov/ceq

Department of Agriculture
1400 Independence Avenue, S.W.
Washington, DC 20250
202/720-3631
Ed Schafer, Secretary of Agriculture
http://www.usda.gov

Department of Commerce
1401 Constitution Avenue NW
Washington, DC 20230
202/482-2000
Carlos Gutierrez, Secretary of Commerce
http://www.doc.gov

Department of Defense
Office of the Secretary
The Pentagon
Washington, DC 20301-1155
703/545-6700
Dr. Robert M. Gates, Secretary of Defense
http://www.defenselink.mil

Department of Education
400 Maryland Avenue SW
Washington, DC 20202
800/USA-LEAR
Margaret Spellings, Secretary of Education
http://www.ed.gov

Department of Energy
1000 Independence Avenue SW
Washington, DC 20585
800/342-5363
Samuel Bodman, Secretary of Energy
http://www.doe.gov

Department of Health and Human Services
200 Independence Avenue SW
Washington, DC 20201
202/619-0257
Mike Leavitt, Secretary of Health and Human Services
http://www.dhhs.gov

Department of Justice
950 Pennsylvinia Ave NW
Washington, DC 20530-0001
202/514-2000
Michael B. Mukasey, The Attorney General
http://www.usdoj.gov

Department of Labor
Frances Perkins Building
200 Constitution Avenue NW
Washington, DC 20210
202/693-6000
Elaine L. Chao, Labor Secretary
http://www.dol.gov

Department of State
2201 C. Street NW
Washington, DC 20520
202/647-4000
Condoleezza Rice, Secretary of State
http://www.state.gov

Department of the Air Force
1670 Air Force Pentagon
Washington, DC 20330-1670
202/720-3631
Michael W. Wynne, Secretary of the Air Force
http://www.af.mil/main/welcome.asp

Department of the ARMY
The Pentagon
Washington, DC 20310
703/545-6700
Pete Geren, Acting Secretary of the ARMY
http://www.army.mil

Department of the NAVY
1000 Navy Pentagon
Washington, DC 20350-1000
703/545-6700
Donald C. Winter, Secretary of the NAVY
http://www.navy.mil

Department of the Treasury
1500 Pennsylvania NW,
Washington, DC 20220
202/622-2000
Henry M. Paulson Jr., Secretary of the Treasury
http://www.treas.gov

Drug Enforcement Administration
2401 Jefferson Davis Highway
Alexander, VA 22301
202/307-1000
Michele Leonhart, Acting Administrator

Environmental Protection Agency
Ariel Rios Building
1200 Pennsylvania Ave., NW
Washington, DC 20460
202/564-4700
Stephen L. Johnson, Administrator
http://www.epa.gov

Equal Employment Opportunity Commission
1801 L. Street NW
Washington, DC 20507
202/663-4900
Naomi C. Earp, Chairwoman
http://www.eeoc.gov

Food and Drug Administration
5600 Fishers Lane
Rockville, MD 20857-0001
301/443-1544
Andrew C. von Eschenbach, Commissioner
http://www.fda.gov

Health Resources and Services Administration
5600 Fishers Lane
Rockville, MD 20857
301/443-2194
Elizabeth M. Duke, Administrator
http://www.hrsa.gov

Office of Management and Budget
725 17th St, NW
Washington, DC 20503
202/395-3080
Jim Nussle, Director
http://www.whitehouse.gov/omb/

Office of National Drug Control Policy
Executive Office of the President
Washington, DC 20503
202/395-6700
John P. Walters, Director
http://www.whitehousedrugpolicy.gov

Substance Abuse and Mental Health Services Administration
1 Choke Cherry RD
Room 8-1036
Rockville, MD 20857
240/276-2000
Terry Cline, Administrator
http://www.samhsa.gov

Blue Cross–Blue Shield Plans

The following listing is based on information provided by the agencies themselves and the Blue Cross and Blue Shield Association. Inclusion or omission of any organization's name indicates neither approval nor disapproval by Health Forum LLC, an American Hospital Association Company.

United States

ALABAMA: Blue Cross and Blue Shield of Alabama, 450 Riverchase Parkway, East, Birmingham, AL 35244; tel. 205/220–2100; G. Phillip Pope, President and CEO

ALASKA: Premera Blue Cross Blue Shield of Alaska, 2550 Denali Street, Suite 1404, Anchorage, AK 99503; tel. 907/258–5065 (See Washington- Premera Blue Cross for additional information)

ARIZONA: Blue Cross and Blue Shield of Arizona, 2444 West Las Palmaritas Drive, Phoenix, AZ 85021-4872; tel. 602/864–4100; Richard L. Boals, President and CEO

ARKANSAS: Arkansas Blue Cross and Blue Shield, 601 Gaines Street, Little Rock, AR 72201; tel. 501/378–2000; Robert Shoptaw, CEO

CALIFORNIA: Blue Cross of California, 21555 Oxnard Street, Woodland Hills, CA 91367; tel. 818/234–3612 (See Indiana- WellPoint, Inc. for additional information)
Blue Shield of California, 50 Beale Street, San Francisco, CA 94105; tel. 415/229–5000; Bruce G. Bodaken, Chairman, President and CEO

COLORADO: Anthem Blue Cross and Blue Shield, 700 Broadway, Denver, CO 80273; tel. 303/831–2131 (See Indiana- WellPoint, Inc. for additional information)

CONNECTICUT: Anthem Blue Cross and Blue Shield, 370 Bassett Road, North Haven, CT 06473; tel. 203/239–4911 (See Indiana- WellPoint, Inc. for additional information)

DELAWARE: Blue Cross Blue Shield of Delaware, 800 Delaware Avenue, Suite 900, Wilmington, DE 19801; tel. 302/421–3000; Timothy J. Constantine, President and CEO

DISTRICT OF COLUMBIA: CareFirst BlueCross BlueShield, Washington, DC (See Maryland- CareFirst BlueCross BlueShield for additional information)

FLORIDA: Blue Cross and Blue Shield of Florida, 4800 Deerwood Campus Parkway, Jacksonville, FL 32246-8273; tel. 904/791–6111; Robert I. Lufrano, M.D., Chairman, CEO and President

GEORGIA: Blue Cross and Blue Shield of Georgia, Capital City Plaza, 3350 Peachtree Rd NE, Atlanta, GA 30326; tel. 404/842–8000 (See Indiana- WellPoint, Inc. for additional information)

HAWAII: Blue Cross and Blue Shield of Hawaii, (Hawaii Medical Service Association), 818 Keeaumoku Street, Honolulu, HI 96814; tel. 808/948–5110; Robert P. Hiam, President and CEO

IDAHO: Blue Cross of Idaho Health Service, 3000 East Pine Avenue, Meridian, ID 83642-5995; tel. 208/345–4550; Ray Flachbart, President and CEO
Regence BlueShield of Idaho, 1602 21st Avenue, Lewiston, ID 83501; tel. 208/746–2671; John M. Stellmon, President

ILLINOIS: Health Care Service Corporation, (Blue Cross and Blue Shield Plans in Illinois, New Mexico, Oklahoma and Texas), 300 East Randolph Street, Chicago, IL 60601-5099; tel. 312/653–6000; Raymond F. McCaskey, Chief Executive Officer

INDIANA: WellPoint, Inc., 120 Monument Circle, Indianapolis, IN 46204; tel. 317/488–6000; Angela F. Braly, President and CEO

IOWA: Wellmark Blue Cross and Blue Shield of Iowa, 636 Grand Avenue, Des Moines, IA 50309; tel. 515/245–4500; John D. Forsyth, Chairman and CEO

KANSAS: Blue Cross and Blue Shield of Kansas, 1133 Topeka Boulevard, Topeka, KS 66629-0001; tel. 785/291–7000; Andrew C. Corbin, President and CEO

KENTUCKY: Anthem Blue Cross and Blue Shield, 13550 Triton Park Blvd., Louisville, KY 40223-2011; tel. 502/889–2000 (See Indiana- WellPoint, Inc. for additional Information)

LOUISIANA: Blue Cross and Blue Shield of Louisiana, 5525 Reitz Avenue, Baton Rouge, LA 70809-3802; tel. 225/295–3307; Gery J. Barry, President and CEO

MAINE: Anthem Blue Cross and Blue Shield, 2 Gannett Drive, South Portland, ME 04106-6911; tel. 207/822–7000 (See Indiana- WellPoint, Inc. for additional information)

MARYLAND: CareFirst BlueCross BlueShield, 10455 Mill Run Circle, Owings Mills, MD 21117; tel. 410/581–3000; Chester E. Burrell, President and CEO

MASSACHUSETTS: Blue Cross and Blue Shield of Massachusetts, Inc., Landmark Center, 401 Park Drive, Boston, MA 02215; tel. 617/246–5000; Cleve L. Killingsworth, Chairman, President and CEO

MICHIGAN: Blue Cross Blue Shield of Michigan, 600 East Lafayette Blvd., Detroit, MI 48226-2998; tel. 313/225–9000; Daniel J. Loepp, President and CEO

MINNESOTA: Blue Cross and Blue Shield of Minnesota, 3535 Blue Cross Road, St. Paul, MN 55122; tel. 651/662–8000; Mark W. Banks, M.D., CEO

MISSISSIPPI: BlueCross BlueShield of Mississippi, 3545 Lakeland Drive, Flowood, MS 39232-9799; tel. 601/932–3704; Richard J. Hale, President and CEO

MISSOURI: Anthem Blue Cross and Blue Shield, 1831 Chestnut Street, St. Louis, MO 63103; tel. 314/923–4444 (See Indiana- WellPoint, Inc. for additional information)
Blue Cross and Blue Shield of Kansas City, 2301 Main Street, Kansas City, MO 64108; tel. 816/395–2222; Tom Bowser, President and CEO

MONTANA: Blue Cross and Blue Shield of Montana, 560 North Park Avenue, Helena, MT 59601; tel. 406/444–8200; Sherry L. Cladouhos, President and CEO

NEBRASKA: Blue Cross and Blue Shield of Nebraska, 7261 Mercy Road, Omaha, NE 68124; tel. 402/390–1800; Steven S. Martin, President and CEO

NEVADA: Anthem Blue Cross and Blue Shield, 6900 West Cliff Drive, Las Vegas, NV 89145; tel. 702/228–2583 (See Indiana- WellPoint, Inc. for additional information)

NEW HAMPSHIRE: Anthem Blue Cross and Blue Shield, 3000 Goffs Falls Rd, Manchester, NH 03111; tel. 603/695–7000 (See Indiana- WellPoint, Inc. for additional information)

NEW JERSEY: Horizon Blue Cross and Blue Shield of New Jersey, Inc., 3 Penn Plaza East, Newark, NJ 07105; tel. 973/466–4000; William J. Marino, President and CEO

NEW MEXICO: Blue Cross and Blue Shield of New Mexico, 5701 Balloon Fiesta Parkway N.E., Albuquerque, NM 87113; tel. 505/291–3500 (See Illinois- Health Care Service Corporation for additional information)

NEW YORK: Empire Blue Cross and Blue Shield, 165 Broadway, New York, NY 10006; tel. 212/476–1000 (See Indiana- WellPoint, Inc. for additional information)
Excellus BlueCross BlueShield, 165 Court Street, Rochester, NY 14647; tel. 585/454–1700; David H. Klein, President and CEO
HealthNow New York Inc., d/b/a BlueCross BlueShield of Western New York and BlueShield of Northeastern New York, 257 W. Genesee Street, Buffalo, NY 14202; tel. 716/887–6900; Alphonso O'Neil-White, President and CEO

NORTH CAROLINA: BlueCross BlueShield of North Carolina, 5901 Chapel Hill Road, Durham, NC 27707; tel. 800/446–8053; Robert J. Greczyn, Jr., President and CEO

NORTH DAKOTA: Blue Cross Blue Shield of North Dakota, 4510 13th Avenue South, Fargo, ND 58121-0001; tel. 701/282–1100; Michael B. Unhjem, President and CEO

OHIO: Anthem Blue Cross and Blue Shield, 4361 Irwin Simpson Rd., Mason, OH 45040; tel. 513/872–8100 (See Indiana- WellPoint, Inc. for additional information)

OKLAHOMA: BlueCross BlueShield of Oklahoma, 1215 South Boulder Avenue, Tulsa, OK 74119-2800; tel. 918/560–3500 (See Illinois- Health Care Service Corporation for additional information)

OREGON: Regence, BlueCross BlueShield of Oregon, 100 SW Market Street, Portland, OR 97201; tel. 503/225–5221; Mark B. Ganz, President and CEO

PENNSYLVANIA: Blue Cross of Northeastern Pennsylvania, 19 North Main Street, Wilkes-Barre, PA 18711; tel. 570/200–4300; Denise S. Cesare, President and CEO
Capital BlueCross, 2500 Elmerton Avenue, Harrisburg, PA 17177-9799; tel. 717/541–7000; Anita M. Smith, President and CEO
Highmark, Inc., 120 Fifth Avenue, Pittsburgh, PA 15222-3099; tel. 412/544–7000; Kenneth R. Melani, M.D., President and CEO
Independence Blue Cross, 1901 Market Street, Philadelphia, PA 19103; tel. 215/241–2400; Joseph A. Frick, President and CEO

RHODE ISLAND: Blue Cross & Blue Shield of Rhode Island, 444 Westminster Street, Providence, RI 02903-3279; tel. 401/459–1000; James E. Purcell, President and Chief Executive Officer

SOUTH CAROLINA: Blue Cross and Blue Shield of South Carolina, I-20 East at Alpine Road, Columbia, SC 29219; tel. 803/788–3860; M. Edward Sellers, Chairman and CEO

SOUTH DAKOTA: Wellmark Blue Cross and Blue Shield of South Dakota, 1601 West Madison Street, Sioux Falls, SD 57104; tel. 605/373–7200 (See Iowa- Wellmark Blue Cross and Blue Shield for additional information)

TENNESSEE: BlueCross BlueShield of Tennessee, Inc., 801 Pine Street, Chattanooga, TN 37402; tel. 423/535–5600; Vicky B. Gregg, President and CEO

TEXAS: Blue Cross and Blue Shield of Texas, 901 S. Central Expressway, Richardson, TX 75080; tel. 972/766–6900 (See Illinois- Health Care Service Corporation for additional information)

UTAH: Regence BlueCross BlueShield of Utah, 2890 E. Cottonwood Parkway, Salt Lake City, UT 84121; tel. 801/333–2000 (See Oregon- Regence BlueCross BlueShield of Oregon for additional information)

VERMONT: BlueCross BlueShield of Vermont, Mailing Address: P.O. Box 186, Montpelier, VT 05601-0186; tel. 802/223–6131; William R. Milnes, Jr., President and CEO

VIRGINIA: Anthem Blue Cross and Blue Shield, 2015 Staples Mill Road, Richmond, VA 23230; tel. 804/354–7000 (See Indiana- WellPoint, Inc. for additional information)

WASHINGTON: Premera Blue Cross, 7001 220th St. S.W. Bldg. 3, Mountlake Terrace, WA 98043-2124; tel. 425/918–4000; H. R. Brereton Barlow, President and CEO
Regence Blue Shield, 1800 Ninth Avenue, Seattle, WA 98101; tel. 206/464–3600 (See Oregon- The Regence Group for additional information)

WEST VIRGINIA: Mountain State Blue Cross & Blue Shield, Inc., 700 Market Square, Parkersburg, WV 26101; tel. 304/424–7700 (See Pennsylvania- Highmark, Inc. for additional information)

WISCONSIN: Anthem Blue Cross and Blue Shield, 401 West Michigan Street, Milwaukee, WI 53203; tel. 414/226–5000 (See Indiana- WellPoint, Inc. for additional information)

WYOMING: Blue Cross and Blue Shield of Wyoming, 4000 House Avenue, Cheyenne, WY 82001-2266; tel. 307/634–1393; Tim J. Crilly, President and CEO

U.S. Associated Areas

PUERTO RICO: Triple-S Management Corporation, 1441 F.D. Roosevelt Avenue, San Juan, PR 00920; tel. 787/749–4949; Ramon M. Ruiz-Comas, CPA, President and CEO

Section C

Group Purchasing Organizations

The following list of Group Purchasing Organizations is derived from the AHA Annual Survey of Hospitals. It reflects Group Purchasing Organizations serving hospitals. Inclusion or omission of any organization's name indicates neither approval nor disapproval by Health Forum LLC, an American Hospital Association company.

A

Advantage Healthcare Net, 2100 South Columbia Road, Suite 104, Grand Forks, ND 58201; tel. 800/548–2744; F. Wade Johnson, Vice President & Chief Operating Officer; www.advantage-healthcare.net

Affiliated Materiel Services, P.O. Box 1300, Bangor, ME 04402-1300; tel. 207/973–6730; FAX. 207/973–6763; Daryl Briggs, Director of Logistics; www.bigbluea.com/ams.htm

AHC
see Aurora Health Care

Alaska Federal Health Care Partnership, 1919 Bragaw St., Anchorage, AK 99508; tel. 907/729–4480; Philip W. Ginder, Deputy Director; www.afhcp.org

All Health, 4750 Lindle Road, P.O. Box 8800, Harrisburg, PA 17105-8800; tel. 800/377–8200; D. Patrick Mazzolla, President & CEO; www.all-health.com

Allegiance Health Care Corporation
see CardinalHealth

Allen Health System, 1825 Logan Avenue, Waterloo, IA 50703-1916; tel. 319/235–3941; Rick Seidler, President & CEO; www.allenhospital.org

Alliant Purchasing, LLC, 2650 Eastpoint Parkway, Suite 320, Louisville, KY 40223; tel. 502/992–3525; FAX. 502/992–3526; Joe Broyles, Executive Director; www.alliantpurchasing.com

Amerinet, Inc., 2060 Craigshire Road, St. Louis, MO 63146; tel. 800/388–2638; Todd Ebert, President & CEO; www.amerinet-gpo.com

AmerisourceBergen, 1300 Morris Drive, Suite 100, Chesterbrook, PA 19087; tel. 800/829–3132; R. David Yost, CEO; www.amerisourcebergen.com

APG
see Alliance Purchasing Group

Associated Purchasing Services, 7015 College Blvd Suite 150, Overland Park, MO 66211; tel. 913/327–8730; FAX. 913/327–7210; Tom Bell, President & CEO; www.apskc.org

Aurora Health Care, 3031 West Montana Street, P.O. Box 343910, Milwaukee, WI 53234-3910; tel. 414/647–3313; Ron Buettner, C.P.M., Purchasing Agent; www.aurorahealthcare.org

Avera PACE, 3900 West Avera Drive, Suite 100, Sioux Falls, SD 57108-5721; tel. 800/657–8095; Mary Kuper, Executive Director; www.averapace.com

B

Bergen Brunswig Drug Company
see AmerisourceBergen

Boone Hospital Center, 1600 East Broadway, Columbia, MO 65201; tel. 573/815–3210; FAX. 573/815–2638; Daniel J. Rothery, President; www.boone.org

Brim Healthcare Inc., 105 Westwood Place, Suite 300, Brentwood, TN 37027; tel. 800/228–0647; Dave Woodland, President; www.brimhealthcare.com

Broadlane, 13727 Noel Road, Suite 1400, Dallas, TX 75240; tel. 972/813–8200; FAX. 972/813–8199; Charles E. Saunders, M.D., CEO & Chairman; www.broadlane.com

BuyPower
see Broadlane

C

Capital Region Health Care, 250 Pleasant Street, Concord, NH 03301-2598; tel. 603/225–2711; Kevin McCarthy, Vice President, Materials Management; www.concordhospital.org

CardinalHealth, 7000 Cardinal Place, Dublin, OH 43017; tel. 800/234–8701; www.cardinal.com

Catholic Materials Management Alliance
see Consorta, Inc.

Central Kansas Medical Center, 3515 Broadway, Great Bend, KS 67530; tel. 620/792–2511; Chris Thomas, FACHE President/CEO; www.ckmc.org

CHAMPS Management Services, 1226 Huron Road East, Cleveland, OH 44115; tel. 216/255–3680; Laura Gronowski, Senior Vice President; www.chanet.org

CHCA
see Child Health Corporation of America

Child Health Corporation of America, 6803 West 64th Street, Shawnee Mission, KS 66202; tel. 913/262–1436; FAX. 913/262–1575; Don C. Black, President & CEO; www.chca.com

Coastal Cooperative of New Jersey, L.L.C., Monmouth Shores Corporate Park, 1350 Campus Parkway, Wall, NJ 07753; tel. 732/751–3404; Frederick J. Tavani, Jr. CMRP Director

COHR
see MasterPlan

Connecticut Hospital Association Shared Services Program, 110 Barnes Road, P.O. Box 90, Wallingford, CT 06492-0090; tel. 203/294–7380; FAX. 203/265–9130; Diane Mase, Assistant Vice President; www.chassp.com

Consorta, Inc., 1475 East Woodfield Road, Suite 400, Schaumburg, IL 60173; tel. 800/342–5333; John W. Strong, President & CEO; www.consorta.com

Cooperative Health Services of Florida
see LeeSar & Cooperative Services of Florida

D

Dartmouth-Hitchcock Alliance, One Medical Center Drive, Lebanon, NH 03756-1000; tel. 630/650–5000; Nancy A. Formella, President; www.dartmouth-hitchcock.org

Department of Defense
see United States Department of Defense

Department of Veteran Affairs (VISN 9)Mid South Healthcare Network, 1801 West End Ave Suite 1100, Nashville, TN 37203; tel. 615/695–2200; FAX. 615/695–2210; John Dandridge, Jr., Director; vaww.va.gov/visn9

Department of Veterans Affairs
see United States Department of Veterans Affairs

Direct Sourcing Solutions, Inc., 26261 Evergreen Road, Suite 250, Southfield, MI 48076; tel. 248/208–8375; B.P. Thacker, CEO; www.directsourcing.com

DSSI
see Direct Sourcing Solutions, Inc.

E

East Texas Medical Center Regional Healthcare System, 1000 South Beckham Avenue, Tyler, TX 75701; tel. 903/597–0351; Elmer G. Ellis, President & CEO; www.etmc.org

F

FirstChoice Cooperative, 4815 Troup Highway, Tyler, TX 75703; tel. 800/250–3457; Freddie Sanchez, Chairman; www.fccoop.org

Frontier Health, Center of Tri-Cities Business Park, P.O. Box 9054, Gray, TN 37615-6205; tel. 423/467–3600; E. Douglas Varney, President & CEO; www.frontierhealth.org

G

General Services Commission
see Texas Building & Procurement Commission

Georgia Shared Services
see Shared Services Healthcare, Inc.

Greater New York Hospital Association, 555 West 57th Street, 15th floor, New York, NY 10019; tel. 212/258–5330; Alfred J. LoBiondo, Senior Vice President, Supply Chain Management; www.gnyha.org

GSA & Consolidated
see United States General Services Administration

H

HCSC
see Hospital Central Services Cooperative

Health Enterprises, 4250 Glass Road, N.E., Cedar Rapids, IA 52402; tel. 319/368–3619; Eric L. Lothe, President & CEO; www.healthenterprises.org

Health Purchasing Group
see HealthTrust Purchasing Group

Health Services Corporation of America
see MedAssets HSCA

Healthcare Purchasing Partners International, 125 East John Carpenter Freeway, Irving, TX 75062-2324; tel. 888/538–4662; Eldon Petersen, President; www.hppigpo.com.

Healthcare Services of New England, Inc., 859 Willard Street, Suite 510, Quincy, MA 02169-7428; tel. 888/848–4763; Martha A. Dula, President & CEO; www.hsne.com

HealthTrust Purchasing Group, 155 Franklin Road, Suite 400, Brentwood, TN 37027; tel. 615/344–3000; Jim Fitzgerald, President & CEO; www.healthtrustpg.com

Hospital Central Services Cooperative, 2171 28th Street, S.W., Allentown, PA 18103; tel. 800/444–4272; FAX. 610/971–2919; J. Michael Lee, President & CEO; www.hcsc.org/index.shtml

Hospital Council of Western Pennsylvania, 500 Commonwealth Drive, Warrendale, PA 15086; tel. 800/704–8434; FAX. 724/772–8339; A.J. Harper, President; www.hcwp.org

Hospital Shared Services (HSS), 900 South Broadway, Suite 100, Denver, CO 80209; tel. 303/603–3000; FAX. 303/282–4200; George Schiel, President; www.hss-us.com

Hospital Shared Services Association, 300 Elliott Avenue West, Suite 300, Seattle, WA 98119; tel. 206/285–3937; John White, President; www.hssagroup.org

HPG
see HealthTrust Purchasing Group

HPPI
see Healthcare Purchasing Partners International

HPS, 3275 North M-37 Highway, P.O. Box 247, Middleville, MI 49333-0040; tel. 800/632–4572; Jerry Welsh, President & CEO; www.hpsnet.com

HSCA
see MedAssets HSCA

HSNE
see Healthcare Services of New England, Inc.

HSS
see Hospital Shared Services

HSSA
see Hospital Shared Services Association

I

Idaho Department of Health and Welfare, 450 West State Street, P.O. Box 83720, Boise, ID 83720-0036; tel. 208/334–5500; FAX. 208/334–6558; Richard M. Armstrong, Director; www.healthandwelfare.idaho.gov

InSource
see MedAssets HSCA

Iroquois Healthcare Alliance
see United Iroquois Shared Services

J

Jane Phillips Medical Center, 3500 S.E. Frank Phillips Boulevard, Bartlesville, OK 74006; tel. 918/333–7200; David Stire, President & CEO; www.jpmc.org

Jewish Hospital Healthcare Services, Regional Service Center, 5000 Commerce Crossing Drive, Louisville, KY 40299; tel. 502/962–6349; Alan Broude, President; www.jhhs.org

L

Lake Erie Regional Cooperative, 2142 North Cove Boulevard, Toledo, OH 43606; tel. 419/291–3450; FAX. 491/291–4313; Robert J. Kolodgy, President; www.lercnet.org

Lake Erie Regional Cooperative
see Lake Erie Health Alliance

LeeSar & Cooperative Services of Florida, 401 Leonard Boulevard North, Lehigh Acres, FL 33971; tel. 239/303–3402; Robert Simpson, President; leesar@aol.com

Louisiana Office of State Purchasing & Travel, 1201 North 3rd Street, Suite 2-160, P.O. Box 94095, Baton Rouge, LA 70804-9095; tel. 225/342–8010; Denise M. Lea, State Purchasing Director; www.state.la.us/osp/osp.htm

M

Maine, Division of Purchases, Burton Cross Building, 4th Floor, 9 State House Station, Augusta, ME 04333; tel. 207/624–7340; Betty M. Lamoreau, Director; www.state.me.us/purchase

Managed Health Care Associates, Inc., 25-A Vreeland Road, Suite 203, P.O. Box 789, Florham Park, NJ 07932-0789; tel. 800/642–3020; Douglas Present, CEO; www.mhainc.com

Massachusetts Alliance for State Pharmaceutical Buying, 1 Ashburton Place, Room 1017, Boston, MA 02108-1552; tel. 617/720–3328; Brian Putnam, Procurement Manager; www.maspb.com

MasterPlan, 21540 Plummer Street, Chatsworth, CA 91311-4103; tel. 800/950–2647; Bruce Cree, Chairman & CEO; www.masterplan-inc.com

MCHC
see Metropolitan Chicago Healthcare Council, Group

McKesson Corporation, One Post Street, San Francisco, CA 94104; tel. 415/983–8300; John H. Hammergren, Chairman, President & CEO; www.mckesson.com

Med Assets HSCA, 100 North Point Center East, Suite 200, Alpharetta, GA 30022; tel. 678/323–2500; John Bardis, Chairman, President & CEO; www.medassets.com

MedEcon
see Managed Health Care Associates, Inc.

Medical Logistics Command
see United States Naval Medical Logistics Command

Mercy Memorial Health Center, 1011 Fourteenth Avenue, N.W., Ardmore, OK 73401; tel. 580/223–5400; Bobby G. Thompson, President & CEO; www.mercyok.com/mmhc

Mercy Resource Management, Inc., 280 Shuman Boulevard, Suite 110, Naperville, IL 60563-8401; tel. 630/778–2150; Michael D. Gray, President & CEO; www.mrmi.org

Metropolitan Chicago Healthcare Council, Group Purchasing Services, 222 South Riverside Plaza, Suite 1900, Chicago, IL 60606; tel. 312/906–6122; FAX. 312/993–0779; Ron Michalak, Manager Supply Chain; www.mchc.org

MHA
see Managed Health Care Associates, Inc.

MHA Ventures, Inc., P.O. Box 5119, Helena, MT 59604; tel. 406/442–1911; FAX. 406/443–3894; Dick Brown, Executive Dir. or Jeff Springer, Dir. of Business Development; www.mtha.org/ventures1.htm

Midsouth Healthcare Network
see United States Department of Veterans Affairs

Minnesota Multi-State Contracting Alliance for Pharmacy, 50 Sherburne Avenue, Room 112, St. Paul, MN 55155; tel. 651/296–2600; Paul Stembler, Manager; www.mmd.admin.state.mn.us/mmcap

Missouri Procurement Office, 301 West High, Room 630, P.O. Box 809, Jefferson City, MO 65102-0809; tel. 573/751–2387; James Miluski, Director; www.oa.mo.gov/purch/purch.htm

MMCAP
see Minnesota Multi-State Contracting for Pharmacy

N

National Acquisition Center
see United States Department of Veterans Affairs NAC

Navajo Area Indian Health Service, P.O. Box 9020, Window Rock, AZ 86515; tel. 928/871–5811; John Hubbard, Jr., Director; www.ihs.gov/FacilitiesServices/AreaOffices/Navajo

NCHA Strategic Partners, P.O. Box 4449, Cary, NC 27519-4449; tel. 919/677–4131; FAX. 919/677–4111; Veda Williams, Director; www.nchastrategicpartners.org

New Jersey Hospital Association, 760 Alexander Road, P.O. Box 1, Princeton, NJ 08543; tel. 888/221–2182; Marilyn Zacks, Director of Materials Services; www.njha.com/corporate.services/bs.materials.aspx

New Mexico General Services Department, State Purchasing Division , P.O. Box 26110, Santa Fe, NM 87502-0110; tel. 505/827–0472; Michael C. Vinyard, State Purchasing Agent; www.state.nm.us/clients/spd/spd.html

New York City Health & Hospitals Corporation, 125 Worth Street, New York, NY 10013; tel. 212/788–3321; FAX. 212/788–0040; Alan D. Aviles, President; www.nyc.gov/html/hhc/home.html

New York University Purchasing Services & Contract Administration, 726 Broadway 2nd Floor, New York, NY 10003; tel. 212/998–1030; John Sexton, President; www.nyu.edu/purchasing.services

North Carolina Department of Correction, Division of Departmental Purchasing & Services, 2020 Yonkers Road, 4227 Mail Service Center, Raleigh, NC 27699-4227; tel. 919/716–3250; Barbara Baker, Chief Procurement Officer & Budget Officer; www.doc.state.nc.us/purchasing/index.htm

North Dakota Healthcare Association, P.O. Box 7340, Bismarck, ND 58507; tel. 701/224–9732; FAX. 701/224–9529; Arnold Thomas, President; www.ndha.org

Northern Michigan Supply Alliance, LLC, 2651 Aero Park Drive, Traverse City, MI 49686-9101; tel. 231/935–8233; FAX. 231/947–2436; Mark Deponio, President; www.nmsa-mi.org

NOVATION, 125 East John Carpenter Freeway, Irving, TX 75062-2324; tel. 888/766–8283; Joellyn Willis, President; www.novationco.com

O

Oklahoma Department of Central Services, 2401 Lincoln Boulevard, Suite 206, Oklahoma City, OK 73105; tel. 405/521–2121; John S. Richard, Director; www.dcs.ok.gov

Owens & Minor, 9120 Lockwood Blvd., Mechanicsville, VA 23116; tel. 804/723–7000; Craig R. Smith President & CEO; www.owens-minor.com

P

PACE
see Avera PACE

Peconic Bay Medical Center, 1300 Roanoke Ave, Riverhead, NY 11901; tel. 631/548–6889; FAX. 631/369–7119; Peter E. Joss, Director

Phoenix Area Indian Health Services, Two Renaissance Square, 40 North Central Ave, Phoenix, AZ 85004-4424; tel. 602/364–5039; Don J. Davis, Area Director; www.ihs.gov/FacilitiesServices/AreaOffices/Phoenix/index.cfm

PPG
see Professionals' Purchasing Group, Inc.

Premier, 700 Commerce Drive, Suite 100, Oak Brook, IL 60523; tel. 630/891–4100; Robert A. Norling, President and CEO; www.premierinc.com/groupbuy

Professionals' Purchasing Group, Inc., 2904 Eastpoint Parkway, Louisville, KY 40223; tel. 800/333–1774; John Deweese, President; www.ppginc.net/index.htm

Purchase Connection
see MedAssets HSCA

S

Seagate Alliance, LLC, 3445 Winton Place, Suite 222, Rochester, NY 14623; tel. 585/273–8180; FAX. 585/475–0266; Diane H. Ashley, President & CEO; www.seagatealliance.com

Shared Health Services Corporation, 2635 Hemstock Street, LaCrosse, WI 54603; tel. 680/781–4410; FAX. 608/781–4412; Wade Turner, Executive Director; www.shsc-gpo.com

Shared Services Healthcare, Inc., 2300 Windy Ridge Parkway, Suite 5605, Atlanta, GA 30339; tel. 800/827–0340; Bill Bedsole, CEO; www.sharedservices.org

Sun Healthcare Group, 18831 Von Karman, Suite 400, Irvine, CA 92612; tel. 800/729–6600; Richard K. Matos, Chairman & CEO; www.sunh.com/Production/shg/index.asp

T

Texas Building & Procurement Commission, 1711 San Jacinto, Austin, TX 78701; tel. 512/463–6363; Tom Beard, Chairman; www.tbpc.state.tx.us

The CHI Group of Superior Consultant Company, 130 South First Street, Ann Arbor, MI 48104; tel. 734/761–3912; www.superiorconsultant.com/solutions/Chi/TheChiGroup.asp

U

UHC
see University Healthsystem Consortium

United Iroquois Shared Service, 17 Halfmoon Executive Park Drive, Clifton Park, NY 12065; tel. 518/383–5060; J. Edward "Jed" Potocar, Executive Vice President, UISS; www.iroquois.org/uiss.htm

United States Department of Defense, Defense Supply Center Philadelphia, 700 Robbins Avenue, Philadelphia, PA 19111-5092; tel. 888/352–2255; Col. Raymond V. Mason, U.S.A., Commander; www.dscp.dla.mil

United States Department of Veterans Affairs National Acquisition Center, P. O. Box 76, Building 37, Hines, IL 60141; tel. 708/786–5157; FAX. 708/786–5148; Craig Robinson, Executive Director & COO; www1.va.gov/oamm/nac/index.htm

United States Department of Veterans Affairs Veterans Integrated Services Network (VISN)

United States General Services Administration (Consolidated), 400 15th S.W., Auburn, WA 98001-6599; tel. 800/241–7246; Warren Jayashi, Business Management Specialist; www.gsa.gov

United States Naval Medical Logistics Command, Fort Detrick, MD 21702-5015; tel. 301/619–2157; nmlc.med.navy.mil

Universal Hospital Services, Inc., 7700 France Ave. S., Suite 275, Edina, MN 55435; tel. 800/847–7368; Gary D. Blackford, Chairman & CEO; www.uhs.com

University Healthsystem Consortium, 2001 Spring Road, Suite 700, Oak Brook, IL 60523; tel. 630/954–1700; Irene M. Thompson, President & CEO; www.uhc.edu

Upper Peninsula Health Care Network, 228 West Washington Street Suite 2, Marquette, MI 49855; tel. 906/225–3146; Gerald A. Messana, Executive Director; www.uphcn.org

VA Great Lakes Acquisition Center, 5000 West National Avenue, Building No. 5, Milwaukee, WI 53295-0005; tel. 414/902–5400

V

VA System
see United States Department of Veterans Affairs

VA: Desert Pacific Healthcare Network, 5901 East 7th Street, Long Beach, CA 90822; tel. 562/826–5963; John Bright, Acting Network Director; www.visn22.med.va.gov/home.htm

Vector Amerinet
see Amerinet, Inc.

VHA, Inc., 220 East Las Colinas Boulevard, Irving, TX 75039-5500; tel. 972/830–0000; Curt Nonomaque, President & CEO; www.vha.com.

Virginia Department of Mental Health, Mental Retardation, and Substance Abuse Services, Office of Administrative Services, P.O. Box 1797, Richmond, VA 23218-1797; tel. 804/786–3915; Joy Lazarus, Director, OAS; www.dmhmrsas.virginia.gov

VISN 1: VA New England Healthcare System, 200 Springs Road, Building No. 61, Bedford, MA 01730; tel. 781/687–3400; Jeanette Chirico-Post, M.D., Network Director; www.visn1.med.va.gov/default.htm

VISN 2: VA Healthcare Network Upstate New York, P.O. Box 8980, Albany, NY 12202-8980; tel. 518/626–7300; William F. Feeley, Network Director; www1.va.gov/visns/visn02

VISN 4: VA Stars & Stripes Healthcare Network, VAMC, Delafield Road, Pittsburgh, PA 15240; tel. 412/784–3939; Charleen R. Szabo, Acting Network Director; www.starsandstripes.med.va.gov/visn4

VISN 12: Great Lakes Health Care System, P.O. Box 5000, Building No. 18, Hines, IL 60141-5000; tel. 708/202–8400; FAX. 708/202–8424; James W. Roseborough; www.visn12.va.gov

VISN 15: VA Heartland Network, 1201 Walnut Street, Suite 800, Kansas City, MO 64106; tel. 816/701–3000; FAX. 816/221–0930; Peter L. Almenoff, M.D., Director; www1.va.gov/directory/guide/region.asp?ID=1015

V

Voluntary Hospital Association
see VHA

W

West Virginia Health Services , 100 Association Drive, Charleston, WV 25311; tel. 304/295–7450; Richard L. Miller, President; www.wvha.org

Wisconsin Valley Health Network, LLC, 3000 Westhill Drive, Suite 300, Wausau, WI 54401; tel. 715/847–2999

Hospital Associations

The following list of state and metropolitan hospital associations is derived from the American Hospital Association. For additional information visit the American Hospital Association website: www.aha.org.

United States

ALABAMA: Alabama Hospital Association, 500 North East Boulevard, Montgomery, AL 36117; tel. 334/272–8781; FAX. 334/270–9527; J. Michael Horsley, President and CEO

ALASKA: Alaska State Hospital and Nursing Home Association, 426 Main Street, Juneau, AK 99801; tel. 907/586–1790; FAX. 907/463–3573; Rod Betit, President and CEO

ARIZONA: Arizona Hospital and Healthcare Association, 2901 North Central Avenue, Suite 900, Phoenix, AZ 85012-2729; tel. 602/445–4300; FAX. 602/445–4299; John R. Rivers, President and CEO

ARKANSAS: Arkansas Hospital Association, 419 Natural Resources Drive, Little Rock, AR 72205-1539; tel. 501/224–7878; FAX. 501/224–0519; Phil E. Matthews, President and CEO

CALIFORNIA: California Hospital Association, 1215 K. Street, Suite 800, Sacramento, CA 95814; tel. 916/552–7547; FAX. 916/552–7618; C. Duane Dauner, President and CEO

Hospital Association of San Diego and Imperial Counties, 5575 Ruffin Road, Suite 225, San Diego, CA 92123; tel. 858/614–0200; FAX. 858/614–0201; Steven A. Escoboza, President and CEO

Hospital Association of Southern California, 515 South Figueroa Street, Suite 1300, Los Angeles, CA 90071-3322; tel. 213/538–0700; FAX. 213/629–4272; James D. Barber, President and CEO

Hospital Council of Northern and Central California, 1215 K Street, Suite 730, Sacramento, CA 95814; tel. 916/552–7608; FAX. 916/552–2618; Arthur A. Sponseller, President and CEO

COLORADO: Colorado Health and Hospital Association, 7335 East Orchard Road, Suite 100, Greenwood Village, CO 80111; tel. 720/489–1630; FAX. 720/489–9400; Steven Summer, President & CEO

CONNECTICUT: Connecticut Hospital Association, 110 Barnes Road, P.O. Box 90, Wallingford, CT 06492-0090; tel. 203/265–7611; FAX. 203/269–7713; Jennifer Jackson, President and CEO

DELAWARE: Delaware Healthcare Association, 1280 South Governors Avenue, Dover, DE 19904-4802; tel. 302/674–2853; FAX. 302/734–2731; Wayne A. Smith, President and CEO

DISTRICT OF COLUMBIA: District of Columbia Hospital Association, 1250 Eye Street, N.W., Suite 700, Washington, DC 20005-3930; tel. 202/682–1581; FAX. 202/371–8151; Robert A. Malson, President

FLORIDA: Florida Hospital Association, 306 East College Avenue, Tallahassee, FL 32301; tel. 850/222–9800; FAX. 850/561–6230; Wayne NeSmith, President

South Florida Hospital and Healthcare Association, Inc, 6030 Hollywood Blvd., Suite 140, Hollywood, FL 33024; tel. 954/964–1660; FAX. 954/962–1260; Linda S. Quick, President

GEORGIA: Georgia Hospital Association (GHA), 1675 Terrell Mill Road, Marietta, GA 30067; tel. 770/249–4500; FAX. 770/955–5801; Joseph A. Parker, President

HAWAII: Healthcare Association of Hawaii, 932 Ward Avenue, Suite 430, Honolulu, HI 96814-2126; tel. 808/521–8961; FAX. 808/599–2879; Richard E. Meiers, President and CEO

IDAHO: Idaho Hospital Association, 615 N. Seventh Street, Boise, ID 83701-1278; tel. 208/338–5100; FAX. 208/338–7800; Steven A. Millard, President

ILLINOIS: Illinois Hospital Association, 1151 East Warrenville Road, P.O. Box 3015, Naperville, IL 60566-7015; tel. 630/276–5400; FAX. 630/276–5431; Kenneth C. Robbins, President

Metropolitan Chicago Healthcare Council, 222 South Riverside Plaza, 19th Floor, Chicago, IL 60606; tel. 312/906–6100; FAX. 312/993–1501; Kevin Scanlan, President/CEO

INDIANA: Indiana Hospital Association, 1 American Square, Suite 1900, Indianapolis, IN 46282; tel. 317/633–4870; FAX. 317/633–4875; Douglas J. Leonard, FACHE, President

IOWA: Iowa Hospital Association, 100 East Grand Avenue, Suite 100, Des Moines, IA 50309-1835; tel. 515/288–1955; FAX. 515/283–9366; Kirk Norris, President

KANSAS: Kansas Hospital Association, 215 SE 8th Street, Topeka, KS 66603; tel. 785/233–7436; FAX. 785/233–6955; Thomas L. Bell, President

KENTUCKY: Kentucky Hospital Association, 2501 Nelson Miller Parkway, P.O. Box 436629, Louisville, KY 40253-6629; tel. 502/426–6220; FAX. 502/426–6226; Michael T. Rust, President

LOUISIANA: Louisiana Hospital Association, 9521 Brookline Avenue, Baton Rouge, LA 70809-1431; tel. 225/928–0026; FAX. 225/923–1004; John Matessino, President & CEO

Metropolitan Hospital Council of New Orleans, 2450 Severn Avenue, Suite 210, Metairie, LA 70001; tel. 504/837–1171; FAX. 504/837–1174; Paul Salles, President

MAINE: Maine Hospital Association, 33 Fuller Road, Augusta, ME 04330; tel. 207/622–4794; FAX. 207/622–3073; Steven R. Michaud, President

MARYLAND: Maryland Hospital Association, 6820 Deerpath Road, Elkridge, MD 21075-6234; tel. 410/379–6200; FAX. 410/379–8239; Carmela Coyle, President and CEO

Healthcare Council of the National Capital Area, 8201 Corporate Drive, Suite 250, Landover, MD 20785-2229; tel. 301/731–4700; FAX. 301/731–8286; Joseph P. Burns, President and CEO

MASSACHUSETTS: Massachusetts Hospital Association, Five New England Executive Park, Burlington, MA 01803; tel. 781/272–6000; FAX. 781/272–8000; Lynn Nicholas, FACHE, President and CEO

MICHIGAN: Michigan Health & Hospital Association, 6215 West St. Joseph Highway, Lansing, MI 48917; tel. 517/323–3443; FAX. 517/323–0946; Spencer C. Johnson, President

Hospital Council of East Central Michigan, 315 Mullholland Street, Bay City, MI 48703; tel. 989/891–8810; FAX. 989/891–8161; Elizabeth S. Schnettler, President

North Central Council of MHA, 616 Petoskey St., Suite 208, Petoskey, MI 49770; tel. 231/439–9812; FAX. 231/439–9813; Elizabeth Gertz, Executive Director

Upper Peninsula Hospital Council, 6215 West St. Joseph Highway, Lansing, MI 48917; tel. 517/323–3443; FAX. 517/323–0946; Clark R. Ballard, President

MINNESOTA: Minnesota Hospital Association, 2550 University Avenue, W., Suite 350S, St. Paul, MN 55114-1900; tel. 651/641–1121; FAX. 651/659–1477; Bruce J. Rueben, President

MISSISSIPPI: Mississippi Hospital Association, 116 Woodgreen Crossing, P.O. Box 1909, Madison, MS 39130; tel. 800/289–8884; FAX. 601/368–3200; Sam W. Cameron, President and CEO

MISSOURI: Missouri Hospital Association, P.O. Box 60, Jefferson City, MO 65102-0060; tel. 573/893–3700; FAX. 573/893–2809; Marc D. Smith, President

MONTANA: MHA...An Association of Montana Health Care Providers, 1720 Ninth Avenue, P.O. Box 5119, Helena, MT 59601; tel. 406/442–1911; FAX. 406/443–3894; Dick Brown, President

NEBRASKA: Nebraska Hospital Association, 3255 Salt Creek Circle, Suite 100, Lincoln, NE 68504; tel. 402/742–8140; FAX. 402/742–8191; Laura J. Redoutey, FACHE, President

NEVADA: Nevada Hospital Association, 5250 Neil Road, Suite 302, Reno, NV 89502; tel. 775/827–0184; FAX. 775/827–0190; Bill M. Welch, President and CEO

NEW HAMPSHIRE: New Hampshire Hospital Association, Foundation for Healthy Communities, 125 Airport Road, Concord, NH 03301-7300; tel. 603/225–0900; FAX. 603/225–4346; Michael J. Hill, President

NEW JERSEY: New Jersey Hospital Association, P.O. Box One, 760 Alexander Road, Princeton, NJ 08543-0001; tel. 609/275–4000; FAX. 609/452–8097; Elizabeth A. Ryah, Esq., President and CEO

NEW MEXICO: New Mexico Hospital Association, 2121 Osuna Road, N.E., Albuquerque, NM 87113; tel. 505/343–0010; FAX. 505/343–0012; Jeff Dye, President and CEO

NEW YORK: Healthcare Association of New York State, One Empire Drive, Rensselaer, NY 12144; tel. 518/431–7600; FAX. 518/431–7915; Daniel Sisto, President

Greater New York Hospital Association, 555 West 57 Street, 15th Floor, New York, NY 10019; tel. 212/246–7100; FAX. 212/262–6350; Kenneth E. Raske, President

Iroquois Healthcare Alliance, 17 Halfmoon Executive Park Drive, Clifton Park, NY 12065; tel. 518/383–5060; FAX. 518/383–2616; Gary J. Fitzgerald, President

Nassau-Suffolk Hospital Council, Inc, 1383 Veterans Memorial Highway, Suite 26, Hauppauge, NY 11788; tel. 631/435–3000; FAX. 631/435–2343; Wendy Darwell, VP/COO

Northern Metropolitan Hospital Association, 400 Stony Brook Court, Newburgh, NY 12550; tel. 845/562–7520; FAX. 845/562–0187; Neil Abitabilo, President

Rochester Regional Healthcare Association, 3445 Winton Place, Suite 222, Rochester, NY 14623; tel. 585/273–8180; FAX. 585/475–0266; Diane H. Ashley, President and CEO

Western New York Healthcare Association, 1876 Niagara Falls Boulevard, Tonawanda, NY 14150-6439; tel. 716/512–7105; FAX. 716/695–0073; John E. Bartimole, President

NORTH CAROLINA: North Carolina Hospital Association, P.O. Box 4449, Cary, NC 27519-4449; tel. 919/677–2400; FAX. 919/677–4200; William A. Pully, President

NORTH DAKOTA: North Dakota Healthcare Association, P.O. Box 7340, Bismarck, ND 58507; tel. 701/224–9732; FAX. 701/224–9529; Arnold R. Thomas, President

OHIO: Ohio Hospital Association, 155 East Broad Street, Floor 15, Columbus, OH 43215; tel. 614/221–7614; FAX. 614/221–4771; James R. Castle, President and CEO

Greater Cincinnati Health Council, 2100 Sherman Avenue, Suite 100, Cincinnati, OH 45212-2775; tel. 513/531–0200; FAX. 513/531–0278; Colleen K. O'Toole, President

Greater Dayton Area Hospital Association, 2 River Place, Suite 400, Dayton, OH 45405; tel. 937/228–1000; FAX. 937/228–1035; Bryan J. Bucklew, President & CEO

Hospital Council of Northwest Ohio, 3231 Central Park West Drive, Suite 200, Toledo, OH 43617; tel. 419/842–0800; FAX. 419/843–8889; W. Scott Fry, President and CEO

The Center for Health Affairs, 1226 Huron Road East, Cleveland, OH 44115; tel. 216/696–6900; FAX. 216/696–1875; William T. (Bill) Ryan, President and CEO

OKLAHOMA: Oklahoma Hospital Association, 4000 Lincoln Boulevard, Oklahoma City, OK 73105; tel. 405/427–9537; FAX. 405/424–4507; Craig W. Jones, President

OREGON: Oregon Association of Hospitals and Health Systems, 4000 Kruse Way Place, Building 2, Suite 100, Lake Oswego, OR 97035-2543; tel. 503/636–2204; FAX. 503/636–8310; Andy Davidson, President & CEO

PENNSYLVANIA: The Hospital & Healthsystem Association of Pennsylvania, 4750 Lindle Road, P.O. Box 8600, Harrisburg, PA 17105-8600; tel. 717/564–9200; FAX. 717/561–5334; Caroyln F. Scanlan, President and CEO

The Delaware Valley Healthcare Council of HAP, 1835 Market Street, 10th Floor, Philadelphia, PA 19103; tel. 215/563–2229; FAX. 215/563–2442; Kenneth J. Braithwaite, Senior Vice President, Regional Executive

RHODE ISLAND: Hospital Association of Rhode Island, 100 Midway Road, Suite 21, Cranston, RI 02920; tel. 401/946–7887; FAX. 401/946–8188; Edward Quinlan, President

SOUTH CAROLINA: South Carolina Hospital Association, 1000 Center Point Road, Columbia, SC 29210-5802; tel. 803/796–3080; FAX. 803/796–2938; Thorton Kirby, President

SOUTH DAKOTA: South Dakota Association of Healthcare Organizations, 3708 West Brooks Place, Sioux Falls, SD 57106; tel. 605/361–2281; FAX. 605/361–5175; David R. Hewett, President and CEO

TENNESSEE: Tennessee Hospital Association, 500 Interstate Boulevard, South, Nashville, TN 37210; tel. 615/256–8240; FAX. 615/242–4803; Craig A. Becker, President

TEXAS: Texas Hospital Association, 1108 Lavaca, Suite 700, P.O. Box 679010, Austin, TX 78768-9010; tel. 512/465–1000; FAX. 512/465–1090; Dan Stultz, M.D., FACP, FACHE

Dallas-Fort Worth Hospital Council, 250 Decker Drive, Irving, TX 75062; tel. 972/719–4900; FAX. 972/719–4009; W. Stephen Love, President/CEO

Greater San Antonio Hospital Council, 7500 US Highway 90 West, AT&T Building, Suite 200, San Antonio, TX 78227-4023; tel. 210/233–5828; FAX. 210/820–3888; William Dean Rasco, FACHE, President and CEO

UTAH: Utah Hospitals and Health Systems Association, 2180 South 1300 East, Suite 440, Salt Lake City, UT 84106-2843; tel. 801/486–9915; FAX. 801/486–0882; Joseph M. Krella, FACHE President/CEO

VERMONT: Vermont Association of Hospitals and Health Systems, 148 Main Street, Montpelier, VT 05602; tel. 802/223–3461; FAX. 802/223–0364; Beatrice Grause, President and CEO

VIRGINIA: Virginia Hospital & Healthcare Association, 4200 Inslake Drive, Glen Allen, VA 23060; tel. 804/965–1227; FAX. 804/965–0475; Laurens Sartoris, President

WASHINGTON: Washington State Hospital Association, 300 Elliott Avenue/ West, Suite 300, Seattle, WA 98119-4118; tel. 206/281–7211; FAX. 206/283–6122; Leo F. Greenawalt, President and CEO

WEST VIRGINIA: West Virginia Hospital Association, 100 Association Drive, Charleston, WV 25311-1571; tel. 304/344–9744; FAX. 304/344–9745; Joseph M. Letnaunchyn, President & CEO

WISCONSIN: Wisconsin Hospital Association, 5510 Research Park Dr., P.O.Box 259038, Madison, WI 53725-9038; tel. 608/274–1820; FAX. 608/274–8554; Stephen Brenton, President

WYOMING: Wyoming Hospital Association, P.O. Box 249, Cheyenne, WY 82003; tel. 307/632–9344; FAX. 307/632–9347; Dan Perdue, President

U.S. Associated Areas

PUERTO RICO: Puerto Rico Hospital Association, Officina 101-103, Villa Nevarez Professional Center, Centro Commercial Villa Nevarez, San Juan, PR 00927; tel. 787/764–0290; FAX. 787/753–9748; Alfonso Vazguez, Executive Vice President

Canada

NEW BRUNSWICK: New Brunswick Healthcare Association, 861 Woodstock Road, Fredericton, NB E3B 7R7; tel. 506/451–0760; FAX. 506/451–0760; Norah Wilson, Acting Executive Director

NOVA SCOTIA: Nova Scotia Association of Health Organizations, Bedford Professional Centre, 2 Dartmouth Road, Bedford, NS B4A-2K7; tel. 902/832–8500; FAX. 902/832–8505; Mary Lee, President and CEO

ONTARIO: Catholic Health Association of Canada, 1247 Kilborn Place, Ottawa, ON K1H-6K9; tel. 613/731–7148; FAX. 613/731–7797; Gerard Lewis, President & CEO

Ontario Hospital Association, 200 Front Street, W., Suite 2800, Toronto, ON M5V-3L1; tel. 416/205–1452; FAX. 416/205–1310; Tom Closson, President & CEO

PRINCE EDWARD ISLAND: Health Association of PEI, Inc., 10 Pownal Street, Charlottetown, PEI C1A-3V6; tel. 902/368–3901; FAX. 902/368–3231; Ken Ezeard, Executive Director

SASKATCHEWAN: Saskatchewan Association of Health Organizations, 600-2002 Victoria Ave., Regina, SK S4P-0R7; tel. 306/347–5500; FAX. 306/525–1960; Susan Antosh, President and CEO

Hospital Licensure Agencies

Information for the following list of state hospital licensure agencies was obtained directly from the agencies.

United States

ALABAMA: Alabama Department of Public Health, Division of Health Care Facilities, The RSA Tower, Sixth Floor, P.O. Box 303017, Montgomery, AL 36130-3017; tel. 334/206–5366; FAX. 334/206–5088; Rick Harris, Director of Health Provider Standards

ALASKA: Health Facilities Licensing and Certification, Division of Public Health, Alaska Department of Health and Social Services, 619 E. Ship Creek Ave., Suite 232, Anchorage, AK 99501; tel. 907/334–2483; FAX. 907/269–3646; Jane Urbanovsky, Certification & Licensing Section Chief

ARIZONA: Arizona Department of Health Services, Division of Licensing Services/Office of Medical Facilities, 150 N. 18th Avenue, Suite 450, Phoenix, AZ 85007; tel. 602/364–3030; FAX. 602/364–4764; Kathy McCanna, Program Manager

ARKANSAS: Division of Health Facility Services, Arkansas Department of Health, 5800 West 10th Street, Suite 400, Little Rock, AR 72204-9916; tel. 501/661–2201; FAX. 501/661–2165; Connie Melton, Section Chief

CALIFORNIA: State of California/CDPH/CHCQ, P.O. Box 997413, Sacramento, CA 95899-7413; tel. 916/440–7360; FAX. 916/552–8758; Kathleen Billingsley, Deputy Director

COLORADO: Health Facilities Division, Colorado Department of Public Health and Environment, 4300 Cherry Creek Drive, S., Denver, CO 80246-1530; tel. 303/692–2800; FAX. 303/753–6214; Howard Roitman, Director

CONNECTICUT: Department of Public Health, Health Care Systems Branch, 410 Capitol Avenue, MS 12HCS, P.O. Box 340308, Hartford, CT 06134-0308; tel. 860/509–7407; FAX. 860/509–7539; Wendy Furniss, RNC, MS, Branch Chief

DELAWARE: Department of Health and Social Services, Office of Health Facilities Licensing and Certification, 2055 Limestone Road, Suite 200, Wilmington, DE 19808; tel. 302/995–8521; FAX. 302/995–8529; Roseann Sapp, Office Manager

FLORIDA: Agency for Health Care Administration, Division of Health Facility Regulation, Hospital and Outpatient Services Unit, Mail Stop 31, 2727 Mahan Drive, Tallahassee, FL 32308; tel. 850/487–2717; FAX. 850/922–4351; Laura MacLafflerty, Unit Manager

GEORGIA: Health Care Section, Office of Regulatory Services, Georgia Department of Human Resources, Two Peachtree Street, N.W., Room 33-250, Atlanta, GA 30303-3142; tel. 404/657–5550; FAX. 404/657–8934; Carol Zafiratos, Director, Health Care Section

HAWAII: Hawaii Department of Health, Office of Health Care Assurance, P.O. Box 3378, Honolulu, HI 96801-3378; tel. 808/586–4080; FAX. 808/586–4090

IDAHO: Bureau of Facility Standards, Department of Health and Welfare, P.O. Box 83720, Boise, ID 83720-0036; tel. 208/334–6626; FAX. 208/364–1888; Sylvia Creswell or Nicole Wisenor, Co-Supervisors - Non-Long Term Care

ILLINOIS: Division of Health Care Facilities and Programs, Illinois Department of Public Health, 525 West Jefferson Street, Springfield, IL 62761-0001; tel. 217/782–7412; FAX. 217/782–0382; William A. Bell, Acting Deputy Director

INDIANA: Division of Acute Care, Indiana State Department of Health, Two North Meridian Street, Indianapolis, IN 46204; tel. 317/233–7472; FAX. 317/233–7157; Mary Azbill, Director

IOWA: Health Facilities Division, Iowa Department of Inspections and Appeals, Lucas State Office Building, 321 East 12th Street, Des Moines, IA 50319-0083; tel. 515/281–4115; FAX. 515/242–5022; David Werning, Public Information Officer

KANSAS: Kansas Department of Health and Environment, Bureau of Child Care &Health Facilities, 1000 Southwest Jackson, Suite 200, Topeka, KS 66612-1365; tel. 785/296–0131; FAX. 785/291–3419; Charles Moore, Director of Medical Facilities and Support

KENTUCKY: Division of Healthcare Facilities and Services, Cabinet for Health and Family Services, 275 East Main Street, 5E-A, Frankfort, KY 40621; tel. 502/564–7963; FAX. 502/564–6546; Robert Hester, Acting Director

LOUISIANA: Health Standards Section, Louisiana Department of Health and Hospitals, P.O. Box 3767, Baton Rouge, LA 70821; tel. 225/342–0415; FAX. 225/342–5292; Erin Rabalais, RN, Manager

MAINE: Division of Licensing and Certification, Department of Human Services, State House, Station 11, Augusta, ME 04333; tel. 207/287–9300; FAX. 207/287–9304; Catherin Cobb, Director

MASSACHUSETTS: Massachusetts Department of Public Health, Division of Health Care Quality, 99 Chauncy Street, Boston, MA 02111-1703; tel. 617/753–8000; FAX. 617/753–8095; Paul I. Dreyer, Ph.D., Director

MICHIGAN: Division of Licensing and Certification, Michigan Department of Community Health, Bureau of Health Systems, P.O. Box 30664, Lansing, MI 48909; tel. 517/241–4160; FAX. 517/241–3354; Kenneth T. Longton, Director

MINNESOTA: Minnesota Department of Health, Compliance Monitoring Division, Golden Rule Building, 85 East 7th Place, St. Paul, MN 55164-0899; tel. 651/201–3707; FAX. 651/201–3702; Darcy Miner, Director

MISSISSIPPI: Bureau of Health Facilities Licensure and Certification, Mississippi State Department of Health, P.O. Box 1700, Jackson, MS 39215; tel. 601/364–1100; FAX. 601/364–5054; Marilynn Winborne, Director

MISSOURI: Bureau of Health Services Regulation, Missouri Department of Health and Senior Services, P.O. Box 570, Jefferson City, MO 65102; tel. 573/751–6303; FAX. 573/526–3621; Terry Wenkel, Healthcare Regulatory Supervisor

MONTANA: Division of Quality Assurance, Department of Public Health and Human Services, 2401 Colonial Drive, P.O. Box 202953, Helena, MT 59620-2953; tel. 406/444–2676; FAX. 406/444–1742; Roy Kemp, Deputy Administrator

NEBRASKA: Nebraska Department of Health & Human Services Regulation and Licensure, Licensure Unit, Division of Public Health, 301 Centennial Mall, S., P.O. Box 94986, Lincoln, NE 68509-4986; tel. 402/471–4362; FAX. 402/471–0555; Joann Erickson, Administrator

NEVADA: Bureau of Licensure and Certification, Nevada Health Division, 1550 East College Parkway, Suite 158, Carson City, NV 89706-7921; tel. 775/687–4475; FAX. 775/687–6588; Pamela S. Graham BS, RN, LNC Bureau Chief

NEW HAMPSHIRE: Bureau of Health Facilities Administration, Office of Operations Support, Licensure and Regulation, 129 Pleasant Street, Brown Building, Concord, NH 03301; tel. 603/271–4967; FAX. 603/271–8617; Robert Ehlers, Bureau Chief

NEW JERSEY: New Jersey Department of Health and Senior Services, Certificate of Need and Health Care Facility Licensure, P.O. Box 358, Trenton, NJ 08625-0358; tel. 609/292–8773; FAX. 609/292–3780; John A. Calabria, Director

NEW MEXICO: New Mexico Department of Health, Health Facility Licensing and Certification, 2040 S. Pacheco Street, 2nd Floor, Santa Fe, NM 87505; tel. 505/476–9028; FAX. 505/476–9075; Sandra Cole, Bureau Chief

NEW YORK: New York State Department of Health, Centralized Hospital Intake Program, 433 River Street, Suite 303, Troy, NY 12180

NORTH CAROLINA: Division of Facility Services, Acute and Home Care, Licensure and Certification Section, Department of Health and Human Services, 2712 Mail Service Center, Raleigh, NC 27699-2712; tel. 919/855–4620; FAX. 919/715–3073; Azzie Conley, Section Chief

NORTH DAKOTA: North Dakota Department of Health, Health Resources Section, 600 East Boulevard Avenue, Department 301, Bismarck, ND 58505-0200; tel. 701/328–2352; FAX. 701/328–1890; Darleen Bartz, Chief- Health Resources Section

OHIO: Ohio Department of Health, Division of Quality Assurance, Bureau of Information & Operational Support-Hospital Registration, 246 N. High St., Columbus, OH 43215-2412; tel. 614/644–7238; FAX. 614/466–8692; Christine Allen, Health Information Administrator

OKLAHOMA: State Department of Health, 1000 Northeast 10th, Oklahoma City, OK 73117; tel. 405/271–6576; FAX. 405/271–1308

OREGON: Health Care Licensure and Certification, Department of Human Services, 800 Northeast Oregon Street, Suite 305, Portland, OR 97232; tel. 971/673–0546; FAX. 971/673–0556; Ron Prinslow, Manager

PENNSYLVANIA: Division of Acute and Ambulatory Care Facilities, Pennsylvania Department of Health, Division of Acute and Ambulatory Care, Health & Welfare Bldg Room 532, Harrisburg, PA 17120; tel. 717/783–8980; FAX. 717/705–6663; Sandra Knoble, Director

RHODE ISLAND: Rhode Island Department of Health, Office of Facilities Regulation, 3 Capitol Hill, Room 306, Providence, RI 02908-5097; tel. 401/222–2566; FAX. 401/222–3999; Raymond Rusin, Chief

SOUTH CAROLINA: Department of Health and Environmental Control, Division of Health Licensing, 2600 Bull Street, Columbia, SC 29201; tel. 803/545–4370; FAX. 803/545–4212; Dennis Gibbs, Director, Division of Health Licensing

SOUTH DAKOTA: Office of Health Care Facilities Licensure and Certification, State Department of Health, Licensure and Certification, 615 E. 4th Street, Pierre, SD 57501-1700; tel. 605/773–3356; FAX. 605/773–6667; Robert Stahl, Administrator

TENNESSEE: Tennessee Department of Health, Division of Health Care Facilities, 227 French Landing, Suite 501, Heritage Place Metro Center, Nashville, TN 37243; tel. 615/741–7221; FAX. 615/741–7051; Ann R. Thompson, RN, BSN, MBA Licensure Director

TEXAS: Texas Department of State Health Services, Facility Licensing Group, Mail Code: 2835, P.O. Box 149347, Austin, TX 78756-3199; tel. 512/834–6650; FAX. 512/834–4714; Linda R. Porter, LCSW Manager

UTAH: Utah State Department of Health, Bureau of Health Facility Licensing, Certification, and Resident Assessment, Box 144103, Salt Lake City, UT 84114-4103; tel. 801/538–6158; FAX. 801/538–6163; Allan Elkins, Director

VERMONT: Health Improvement, Vermont Department of Health, 108 Cherry Street, P.O. Box 70, Burlington, VT 05402; tel. 802/863–7606; FAX. 802/651–1634; Ellen B. Thompson, Planning Chief

VIRGINIA: Office of Licensure and Certification, Virginia Department of Health, 9960 Mayland Drive, Suite 401, Richmond, VA 23233; tel. 804/367–2102; FAX. 804/527–4502; Christopher Durrer, Director

WASHINGTON: Office of Health Care SurveyFacilities and Services Licensing, Washington Department of Health, 310 Israel Road SE, P.O. Box 47852, Olympia, WA 98504-7852; tel. 360/236–2916; FAX. 360/236–2901; Craig McLaughlin, Executive Director

WEST VIRGINIA: Office of Health Facility Licensure and Certification, West Virginia Department of Health and Human Resources, 1 Davis Square, Suite 101, Charleston, WV 25301-1799; tel. 304/558–0585; FAX. 304/558–5607; John M. Wilkinson, Director

WISCONSIN: Division of Quality Assurance, Department of Health and Family Services, One West Wilson Street, P.O. Box 2969, Madison, WI 53701-2969; tel. 608/267–7185; FAX. 608/267–0352; Otis Woods, Administrator

WYOMING: Wyoming Department of Health, Office of Healthcare Licensing and Surveys, 400 Qwest Bldg., 6101 N. Yellowstone Rd., Cheyenne, WY 82002; tel. 307/777–7123; FAX. 307/777–7127; Jean McLean, Manager

Medical and Nursing Licensure Agencies

The following information is based on information provided by state government entities and the agencies themselves.

United States

ALABAMA

Alabama Board of Nursing, RSA Plaza, 770 Washington Ave., Suite 250, Montgomery, AL 36104; tel. 800/656–5318; FAX. 334/242–4360; N. Genell Lee, RN, M.S.N. JD, Executive Officer

Alabama State Board of Medical Examiners, 848 Washington Avenue, P.O. Box 946, Montgomery, AL 36101-0946; tel. 334/242–4116; FAX. 334/242–4155; Larry D. Dixon, Executive Director

ALASKA

Alaska Board of Nursing, Division of Corporations, Business, and Professional Licensing, PO Box 110806, Juneau, AK 99811-0806; tel. 907/465–2534; FAX. 907/465–2974; Rick Urion, Director

Alaska State Medical Board, 550 West Seventh Ave., Suite 1500, Anchorage, AK 99501; tel. 907/269–8163; FAX. 907/269–8196; Leslie A. Gallant, Executive Administrator

ARIZONA

Arizona Board of Osteopathic Examiners in Medicine and Surgery, 9535 E. Doubletree Ranch Road, Scottsdale, AZ 85258; tel. 480/657–7703; FAX. 480/657–7715; Jack Confer, Executive Director

Arizona Medical Board, 9545 E. Doubletree Ranch Road, Scottsdale, AZ 85258; tel. 877/255–2212; FAX. 480/551–2704; Lisa S. Wynn, Executive Director

Arizona State Board of Nursing, 4747 N. 7th Street, Suite 200, Phoenix, AZ 85014-3653; tel. 602/889–5150; FAX. 602/889–5155; Karen Hardy, RN, MSN, Board President

ARKANSAS

Arkansas State Board of Nursing, University Tower Building, 1123 South University Avenue, Little Rock, AR 72204-1619; tel. 501/686–2700; FAX. 501/686–2714; Faith A. Fields, M.S.N., RN, Executive Director

Arkansas State Medical Board, 2100 Riverfront Drive, Little Rock, AR 72202; tel. 501/296–1802; FAX. 501/603–3555; Trent P. Pierce, M.D., Chairman

CALIFORNIA

California Board of Registered Nursing, 1625 North Market Blvd, Suite N217, Sacramento, CA 95834-1924; tel. 916/322–3350; FAX. 916/574–7697; Ruth Ann Terry, MPH, RN, Executive Officer

Medical Board of California, 2005 Evergreen Street, Suite 1200, Sacramento, CA 95815; tel. 916/263–2382; FAX. 916/263–2944; Barbara Johnston, Executive Director

COLORADO

Colorado State Board of Medical Examiners, 1560 Broadway, Suite 1300, Denver, CO 80202-5140; tel. 303/894–7690; FAX. 303/894–7692; Cheryl Hara, Program Director

Colorado State Board of Nursing, 1560 Broadway, Suite 1350, Denver, CO 80202; tel. 303/894–2430; FAX. 303/894–2821; Rosemary McCool, Division Director

CONNECTICUT

Connecticut Board of Examiners for Nursing, Department of Public Health, 410 Capitol Avenue, MS #13PHO, P.O. Box 340308, Hartford, CT 06134-0308; tel. 860/509–7624; FAX. 860/509–7553; Janice Wojick, Board Liaison

Connecticut Department of Public Health, 410 Capitol Avenue, MS #12 APP, P.O. Box 340308, Hartford, CT 06134-0308; tel. 860/509–7101; FAX. 860/509–8457; J. Robert Galvin, M.D., M.P.H., M.B.A, Commissioner

DELAWARE

Delaware Board of Medical Practice, Cannon Building, 861 Silver Lake Boulevard, Suite 203, Dover, DE 19904; tel. 302/744–4500; FAX. 302/739–2711; James Collin, Executive Director

Delaware Board of Nursing, 861 Silver Lake Boulevard, Suite 203, Dover, DE 19904; tel. 302/744–4500; FAX. 302/739–2712; David C. Mangler, M.S., RN, Executive Director

DISTRICT OF COLUMBIA

District of Columbia Board of Medicine, 717 14th St. NW, Suite 600, Washington, DC 20005; tel. 202/724–8800; FAX. 202/724–8677; James R. Granger, Jr., Executive Director

FLORIDA

Florida Board of Medicine, 4052 Bald Cypress Way, Bin #C03, Tallahassee, FL 32399-3253; tel. 850/245–4131; FAX. 850/488–0596; Larry G. McPherson, Jr., J.D., Board Director

Florida Board of Nursing, Capital Circle Office Center, 4052 Bald Cypress Way, Bin C02, Tallahassee, FL 32399-3257; tel. 850/245–4125; FAX. 850/245–4172; Rick Garcia, MS, RN, CCM, Executive Director

Florida Board of Osteopathic Medicine, 4052 Bald Cypress Way, Bin #C-06, Tallahassee, FL 32399-3256; tel. 850/245–4161; FAX. 850/921–6184; Christy Robinson, POA

GEORGIA

Georgia Board of Nursing, 237 Coliseum Drive, Macon, GA 31217-3858; tel. 478/207–2440; FAX. 478/207–1354; Mrs. Linda Herren, RN, CRNA, President

Georgia Composite State Board of Medical Examiners, 2 Peachtree Street, N.W., 36th Floor, Atlanta, GA 30303-3465; tel. 404/656–3913; FAX. 404/656–9723; LaSharn Hughes, MBA, Executive Director

HAWAII

Hawaii Board of Medical Examiners, Department of Commerce and Consumer Affairs, 335 Merchant Street, Room 301, Honolulu, HI 96813; tel. 808/586–3000; Constance Cabral, Executive Officer

Hawaii Board of Nursing, Professional and Vocational Licensing Division, P.O. Box 3469, Honolulu, HI 96801; tel. 808/586–3000; Kathy Yokouchi, MBA, BBA, Executive Officer

IDAHO

Idaho State Board of Medicine, P.O. Box 83720, Boise, ID 83720-0058; tel. 208/327–7000; FAX. 208/327–7005; Nancy Kerr, Executive Director

Idaho State Board of Nursing, 280 North 8th Street, Suite 210, P.O. Box 83720, Boise, ID 83720-0061; tel. 208/334–3110; FAX. 208/334–3262; Sandra Evans, MA. Ed., RN Executive Director

ILLINOIS

Illinois Department of Financial and Professional Regulation, Division of Professional Regulation, 320 West Washington Street, 3rd Floor, Springfield, IL 62786; tel. 217/785–0800; FAX. 217/782–7645; Daniel E. Bluthardt, Director

Illinois Department of Professional Regulation, James R. Thompson Center, 100 West Randolph Street, Chicago, IL 60601; tel. 312/814–2715; FAX. 312/814–5392; Michele Bromberg, MSN, APN, BC, Nursing Coordinator

INDIANA

Indiana Professional Licensing Agency, Medical Licensing Board of Indiana, Indiana State Board of Nursing, 402 West Washington, Room W072, Indianapolis, IN 46204; tel. 317/232–2960; FAX. 317/233–4236; Frances L. Kelly, Executive Director

Indiana State Board of Nursing, Health Professions Bureau, 402 West Washington, Room W072, Indianapolis, IN 46204; tel. 317/234–2043; FAX. 317/233–4236; Sean Gorman, Board Director

IOWA

Iowa Board of Medicine, 400 S.W. 8th Street, Suite C, Des Moines, IA 50309-4686; tel. 515/281–5171; FAX. 515/242–5908; Ann E. Mowery, Ph.D., Executive Director

Iowa Board of Nursing, Riverpoint Business Park, 400 S.W. 8th Street, Des Moines, IA 50309-4685; tel. 515/281–3255; FAX. 515/281–4825; Lorinda K. Inman, RN, M.S.N., Executive Director

KANSAS

Kansas Board of Healing Arts, 235 SW Topeka Blvd., Topeka, KS 66603-3068; tel. 913/296–7413; FAX. 913/296–0852; Lawrence T. Buening, Jr., Executive Director

Kansas State Board of Nursing, Landon State Office Building, 900 SW Jackson, Topeka, KS 66612-1230; tel. 785/296–4929; FAX. 785/296–3929; Mary Blubaugh MSN, RN, Executive Administrator

KENTUCKY

Kentucky Board of Medical Licensure, The Hurstbourne Office Park, 310 Whittington Parkway, Suite 1B, Louisville, KY 40222; tel. 502/429–7150; FAX. 502/429–7158; Preston P. Nunnelley, M.D., President

Kentucky Board of Nursing, 312 Whittington Parkway, Suite 300, Louisville, KY 40222-2042; tel. 502/429–3300; FAX. 502/696–3936; Charlotte F. Beason, Executive Director

LOUISIANA

Louisiana State Board of Medical Examiners, 630 Camp Street, New Orleans, LA 70130; tel. 504/568–6820; FAX. 504/568–8893; Robert L. Marier, M.D., Executive Director

Louisiana State Board of Nursing, 17373 Perkins Road, Baton Rouge, LA 70810; tel. 225/755–7500; FAX. 225/755–7580; Barbara L. Morvant, MN, RN, Executive Director

Louisiana State Board of Practical Nurse Examiners, 3421 N. Causeway Boulevard, Suite 505, Metairie, LA 70002; tel. 504/838–5791; FAX. 504/838–5279; Claire Glaviano, BSN, MN, RN, Executive Director

MAINE

Maine Board of Licensure in Medicine, 161 Capitol Street, 137 State House Station, Augusta, ME 04333-0137; tel. 207/287–3601; FAX. 207/287–6590; Randal C. Manning, Executive Director

Maine Board of Osteopathic Licensure, 142 State House Station, 161 Capitol Street, Augusta, ME 04333-0142; tel. 207/287–2480; FAX. 207/287–3015; Susan E. Strout, Executive Secretary

Maine State Board of Nursing, 161 Capitol St., 158 State House Station, Augusta, ME 04333-0158; tel. 207/287–1133; FAX. 207/287–1149; Myra A. Broadway, JD, MS, RN, Executive Director

MARYLAND

Maryland Board of Nursing, 4140 Patterson Avenue, Baltimore, MD 21215-2254; tel. 410/585–1900; FAX. 410/358–3530; Patricia A. Noble, MSN, RN, Executive Director

Maryland Board of Physicians, 4201 Patterson Avenue, 4th Floor, P.O. Box 2571, Baltimore, MD 21215-0095; tel. 800/492–6836; FAX. 410/358–2252; C.Irving Pinder, Jr., Executive Director

MASSACHUSETTS

Commonwealth of MassachusettsBoard of Registration in Medicine, 560 Harrison Avenue, Suite G-4, Boston, MA 02118; tel. 617/654–9800; FAX. 617/451–9568; Nancy Achin Audesse, Executive Director

MICHIGAN

Michigan Board of Medicine, 611 West Ottawa Street, First Floor, P.O. Box 30670, Lansing, MI 48909; tel. 517/335–0918; FAX. 517/373–2179

Michigan Board of Nursing, Department of Community Health, 611 West Ottawa Street, P.O. Box 30670, Lansing, MI 48909; tel. 517/335–0918; FAX. 517/373–2179

Michigan Board of Osteopathic Medicine and Surgery, 611 West Ottawa Street, First Floor, P.O. Box 30670, Lansing, MI 48909; tel. 517/335–0918; FAX. 517/373–2179

MINNESOTA

Minnesota Board of Medical Practice, 2829 University Avenue, S.E., Suite 500, Minneapolis, MN 55414-3246; tel. 612/617–2149; FAX. 612/617–2166; Robert A. Leach, Executive Director

Minnesota Board of Nursing, 2829 University Avenue, S.E., Suite 200, Minneapolis, MN 55414-3253; tel. 612/617–2270; FAX. 612/617–2190; Shirley A. Brekken, RN, MS, Executive Director

MISSISSIPPI

Mississippi Board of Nursing, 1935 Lakeland Drive, Suite B, Jackson, MS 39216-5014; tel. 601/944–4826; FAX. 601/364–2352; Melinda E. Rush, DSN, FNP, Executive Director

Mississippi State Board of Medical Licensure, 1867 Crane Ridge Drive, Suite 200-B, Jackson, MS 39216; tel. 601/987–3079; FAX. 601/987–4159; H. Vann Craig, M.D., Executive Director

MISSOURI

Missouri State Board of Nursing, 3605 Missouri Boulevard, P.O. Box 656, Jefferson City, MO 65102; tel. 573/751–0681; FAX. 573/751–0075; Lori Scheidt, Executive Director

Missouri State Board of Registration for the Healing Arts, 3605 Missouri Boulevard, P.O. Box 4, Jefferson City, MO 65109; tel. 573/751–0098; FAX. 573/751–3166; Tina Steinman, Executive Director

MONTANA

Montana Board of Medical Examiners, 301 S. Park Avenue 4th Floor, P.O. Box 200513, Helena, MT 59620-0513; tel. 406/841–2364; FAX. 406/841–2305; Jeannie Worsech, Executive Secretary

Montana State Board of Nursing, 301 South Park, 4th Floor, P.O. Box 200513, Helena, MT 59620-0513; tel. 406/841–2342; FAX. 406/841–2305; Barb Swehla, Executive Director

NEBRASKA

Nebraska Board of Medicine and Surgery, 301 Centennial Mall, S., P.O. Box 94986, Lincoln, NE 68509-4986; tel. 402/471–2118; FAX. 402/471–3577; Becky Wisell, Executive Director

NEVADA

Nevada State Board of Medical Examiners, P.O. Box 7238, 1105 Terminal Way, Reno, NV 85022144; tel. 775/688–2559; FAX. 775/688–2321; Drennan A. Clark, JD, Executive Director

Nevada State Board of Nursing, 5011 Meadowood Mall Way, Suite 300, Reno, NV 89502; tel. 775/688–2620; FAX. 775/688–2628; Debra Scott, Executive Director

Nevada State Board of Osteopathic Medicine, 2860 East Flamingo Road, Suite D, Las Vegas, NV 89121-5270; tel. 702/732–2147; FAX. 702/732–2079; Catryna Kelly, Executive Administrator

NEW HAMPSHIRE

New Hampshire Board of Medicine, Two Industrial Park Drive #8, Concord, NH 03301; tel. 603/271–1203; FAX. 603/271–6702; Penny Taylor, Administrator

NH Board of Nursing, 21 S. Fruit S, Suite 16, Concord, NH 03301-2431; tel. 603/271–2323; FAX. 603/271–6605; Margaret Walker, Ed.D., RN, Executive Director

NEW JERSEY

New Jersey Board of Nursing, 124 Halsey St, Newark, NJ 07102; tel. 973/504–6430; FAX. 973/648–3481; George Hebert, RN, MA, Executive Director

New Jersey State Board of Medical Examiners, P.O. Box 183, Trenton, NJ 08625-0183; tel. 609/826–7100; FAX. 609/826–7117; William V. Roeder, JD, Executive Director

NEW MEXICO

New Mexico Board of Osteopathic Medical Examiners, 2550 Cerrillos Rd., 2nd Floor, Santa Fe, NM 87505; tel. 505/476–4604; FAX. 505/476–4645; Liz Z. Montoya, Board Administrator

New Mexico Medical Board, 2055 S. Pacheco #400, Santa Fe, NM 87505; tel. 505/476–2220; FAX. 505/476–7237; Lynn S. Hart, Executive Director

State of New Mexico Board of Nursing, 6301 Indian School NE Suite,710, Albuquerque, NM 87110; tel. 505/841–8340; FAX. 505/841–8347; Allison Kozeliski, Executive Director

NEW YORK

New York State Board for Nursing, NY State Education Department, Office of the Professions, Division of Professional Licensing Services, Nurse Practitioner Unit, Albany, NY 12234-1000; tel. 518/474–3817; FAX. 518/474–3706; Barbara Zittel, Ph.D., RN, Executive Secretary

New York State Division of Professional Licensing Services, Office of the Professions, State Education Building, 89 Washington Avenue, 2nd Floor North, Albany, NY 12234-1000; tel. 518/474–3817; FAX. 518/474–1449; Tony Lofrumento, Director of Professional Licensing

NORTH CAROLINA

North Carolina Board of Nursing, P.O. Box 2129, Raleigh, NC 27602-2129; tel. 919/782–3211; FAX. 919/781–9461; Mary Polly Johnson, RN, MSN, FAAN, Executive Director

North Carolina Medical Board, 1203 Front Street, Raleigh, NC 27609; tel. 919/326–1100; FAX. 919/326–0036; David Henderson, Executive Director

NORTH DAKOTA

North Dakota Board of Nursing, 919 South Seventh Street, Suite 504, Bismarck, ND 58504-5881; tel. 701/328–9777; FAX. 701/328–9785; Constance Kalanek, Ph D., RN, Executive Director

North Dakota State Board of Medical Examiners, 418 East Broadway Avenue, Bismarck, ND 58501; tel. 701/328–6500; FAX. 701/328–6505; Duane Houdek, J.D. - Executive Secretary

OHIO

Ohio Board of Nursing, 17 South High Street, Suite 400, Columbus, OH 43215-7410; tel. 614/466–3947; FAX. 614/466–0388; Betsy J. Houchen, JD, RN, MS, Executive Director

State Medical Board of Ohio, 30 E. Broad Street, 3rd Floor, Columbus, OH 43215-6127; tel. 614/728–3673; FAX. 614/728–5946; Richard A. Whitehouse, Esq., Executive Director

OKLAHOMA

Oklahoma Board of Nursing, 2915 North Classen Boulevard, Suite 524, Oklahoma City, OK 73106; tel. 405/962–1800; FAX. 405/962–1821; Kimberly Glazier, M.Ed., RN, Executive Director

Oklahoma State Board of Medical Licensure and Supervision, 5104 North Francis, Suite C, Oklahoma City, OK 73118, Oklahoma City, OK 73154-0256; tel. 405/848–6841; FAX. 405/848–8240; Lyle Kelsey, Executive Director

Oklahoma State Board of Osteopathic Examiners, 4848 North Lincoln Boulevard, Suite 100, Oklahoma City, OK 73105-3321; tel. 405/528–8625; Deborah J. Bruce, Executive Director

OREGON

Oregon Medical Board, 1500 S.W. 1st Avenue, Suite 620, Portland, OR 97201-5847; tel. 917/673–2700; FAX. 917/673–2670; Holly Mercer, JD, RN, Executive Director

Oregon State Board of Nursing, 17938 S.W. Upper Boones Jerry Road, Portland, OR 97224-7012; tel. 971/673–0685; FAX. 971/673–0684; Holly Mercer, Executive Director

PENNSYLVANIA

Pennsylvania State Board of Medicine, P.O. Box 2649, Harrisburg, PA 17105-2649; tel. 717/783–1400; FAX. 717/787–7769; Tammy Radel, Administrator

Pennsylvania State Board of Nursing, P.O. Box 2649, Harrisburg, PA 17105-2649; tel. 717/783–7142; FAX. 717/783–0822; Executive Secretary

Pennsylvania State Board of Osteopathic Medicine, P.O. Box 2649, Harrisburg, PA 17105-2649; tel. 717/783–4858; FAX. 717/787–7769; Gina Bittner, Administrative Assistant

Quality Insights of Pennsylvania, Commerce Court, 2601 Market Place Street, Suite 320, Harrisburg, PA 17110; tel. 717/671–5425; John C. Wiesendanger, CEO

RHODE ISLAND

Rhode Island Board of Medical Licensure & Discipline, 3 Capitol Hill, Room 205, Providence, RI 02908-5097; tel. 401/222–3855; FAX. 401/222–2158; David R. Gifford, M.D., MPH, Chief Administrative Officer

Rhode Island Board of Nurse Registration and Nursing Education, 3 Capitol Hill, Room 105, Providence, RI 02908-5097; tel. 401/222–5570; FAX. 401/222–3352; Pamela L. McCue, RN, MS, Director

SOUTH CAROLINA

Department of Labor, Licensing and Regulation, State Board of Nursing for South Carolina, P.O. Box 12367, Columbia, SC 29211-2367; tel. 803/896–4550; FAX. 803/896–4525; Joan Bainer, Administrator

South Carolina Department of Labor, Licensing and Regulation, Board of Medical Examiners, Synergy Business Park, Kingstree Building, 110 Centerview Drive, Suite 202, Columbia, S.C. 29210, Columbia, SC 29210; tel. 803/896–4500; FAX. 803/896–4515; Bruce Duke, Administrator

SOUTH DAKOTA

South Dakota Board of Medical and Osteopathic Examiners, 125 S. Main Avenue, Sioux Falls, SD 57104; tel. 605/367–7781; FAX. 605/367–7786; Margaret B. Hansen, PA-C, MPAS, Executive Director

South Dakota Board of Nursing, 4305 South Louise Avenue, Suite 201, Sioux Falls, SD 57106; tel. 605/362–2760; FAX. 605/362–2768; Gloria Damgaard, Executive Director

TENNESSEE

Tennessee Board of Medical Examiners, 227 French Landing, Suite 300, Heritage Place Metro Center, Nashville, TN 37243; tel. 800/778–4123; FAX. 615/253–4484; Mitchell Mutter, M.D., President

Tennessee Board of Nursing, 227 French Landing Suite 300, Heritage Place Metro Center, Nashville, TN 37243; tel. 800/778–4123; FAX. 615/741–7899; Elizabeth J. Lund, MSN, RN, Executive Director

Tennessee State Board of Osteopathic Examination, Cordell Hull Building, 1st Floor, 425 Fifth Avenue, N., Nashville, TN 37247-1010; tel. 800/778–4123; FAX. 615/253–4484; Rosemarie Otto, Executive Director

TEXAS

Texas Board of Nursing, 333 Guadalupe, Suite 3-460, Austin, TX 78701; tel. 512/305–7400; FAX. 512/305–7401; Katherine A. Thomas, M.N., R.N., Executive Director

Texas Board of Vocational Nurse Examiners, William P. Hobby Building, 333 Guadalupe Street, #3-460, Austin, TX 78701; tel. 512/305–7400; FAX. 512/305–7401; Katherine Thomas, MN, RN, Executive Director

Texas State Board of Medical Examiners, 333 Guadalupe, Tower Three, Suite 610, P.O. Box 2018, Austin, TX 78768-2018; tel. 512/305–7010; FAX. 512/305–7008; Donald W. Patrick, MD, JD, Executive Director

UTAH

Utah Physicians Licensing Board, Division of Occupational and Professional Licensure, Heber M. Wells Building, First Floor, 160 East 300 South, Salt Lake City, UT 84114-6741; tel. 801/530–6621; FAX. 801/530–6511; Noel Taxin, Bureau Manager

Utah State Board of Nursing, 160 East 300 South, Box 146741, Salt Lake City, UT 84114-6741; tel. 801/530–6628; FAX. 801/530–6511; F. David Stanley, Director

VERMONT

Vermont Board of Nursing, National Life Building, North, 2nd Floor, Montpelier, VT 05620-3402; tel. 802/828–2396; FAX. 802/828–2484; Mary Botter, Ph.D., RN, Executive Director

Vermont Board of Osteopathic Physicians and Surgeons, Office of Professional Regulation, National Life Building, North Floor 2, Montpelier, VT 05620-3402; tel. 802/828–1134; FAX. 802/828–2465; Kara Shangraw, Administrative Assistant

VIRGINIA

Virginia Board of Medicine, Perimeter Center, 9960 Mayland Drive, Richmond, VA 232332; tel. 804/367–4600; FAX. 804/527–4426; William L. Harp, M.D., Executive Director

Virginia Board of Nursing, Perimeter Center, 9960 Mayland Drive, Richmond, VA 23233-1463; tel. 804/367–4555; FAX. 804/527–4455; Jay P. Douglas, R.N., M.S.M., C.S.A.C., Executive Director

WASHINGTON

Washington State Board of Osteopathic Medicine and Surgery, Department of Health, 310 Israel Rd, SE, P.O.Box 47866, Olympia, WA 98504-7866; tel. 360/236–4943; FAX. 360/236–2406; Jessica Burris, Licensing Program Representative

Washington State Department of Health, Health Professions Quality Assurance Commission, P.O. Box 47866, Olympia, WA 98504-7865; tel. 360/236–4788; FAX. 360/236–4768; Beverly Teeter, Program Manager

Washington State Nursing Care Quality Assurance Commission, Department of Health, Point Plaza East, 310 Israel Rd. SE, Tumwater, WA 98501; tel. 360/236–4700; FAX. 360/236–4738; Paula Meyer, RN, M.S.N., Executive Director

Section C

WEST VIRGINIA

West Virginia Board of Examiners for Registered Professional Nurses, 101 Dee Drive, Suite 102, Charleston, WV 25311-1620; tel. 304/558–3596; FAX. 304/558–3666; Laura S. Rhodes, RN, M.S.N., Executive Director

West Virginia Board of Osteopathy, 334 Penco Road, Weirton, WV 26062; tel. 304/723–4638; FAX. 304/723–6723; Cheryl D. Schreiber, Executive Secretary

West Virginia State Board of Examiners for Licensed Practical Nurses, 101 Dee Drive, Suite 100, Charleston, WV 25311; tel. 304/558–3572; FAX. 304/558–4367; Lanette Anderson, MSN, JD, RN, Executive Director

WISCONSIN

Wisconsin Department of Regulation and Licensing, 1400 East Washington Avenue, Room 178, P.O. Box 8935, Madison, WI 53708-8935; tel. 608/266–2112; FAX. 608/267–3816; Kimberly Nania, Ph.D, Administrator, Board Services

Wisconsin Medical Examining Board, 1400 East Washington Avenue, Zip 53702, P.O. Box 8935, Madison, WI 53704; tel. 608/266–8098; FAX. 608/267–3816; Tom Ryan

WYOMING

Wyoming Board of Medicine, 320 West 25th Street, Suite 103, Cheyenne, WY 82002; tel. 307/778–7053; FAX. 307/778–2069; Deborah Gillette, Executive Assistant

Wyoming State Board of Nursing, 1810 Pioneer Avenue, Cheyenne, WY 82002; tel. 307/777–7601; FAX. 307/777–3519; Mary Beth Stepans, Ph.D., RN, Interim Executive Director

U.S. Associated Areas

GUAM

Guam Board of Medical Examiners, Health Professional Licensing Office, 123 Chalan Kareta South Route 10, Mangilao, GU 969136304; tel. 671/735–7406; FAX. 671/735–7413; MaryLou Loualhati, Acting Administrator

Guam Board of Nurse ExaminersDepartment of Public Health and Social Services, 123 Chalan Kareta, South Route 10, Mangilao, GU 96923; tel. 671/475–0251; FAX. 671/477–4733; Teofila P. Cruz, RN, M.S., Administrator

PUERTO RICO

Puerto Rico Board of Medical Examiners, P.O. Box 13969, San Juan, PR 00908; tel. 787/782–8937; FAX. 787/706–0304; Ivonne M. Fernandez Colon, Executive Director

Canada

ALBERTA

College of Physicians and Surgeons of Alberta, Suite 2700, 10020 100th Street, N.W., Edmonton, AB; tel. 780/423–4764; FAX. 780/420–0651; Trevor Theman, Registrar

MANITOBA

College of Physicians and Surgeons of Manitoba, 1000-1661 Portage Avenue, Winnipeg, MB R3J 3T7; tel. 204/774–4344; FAX. 204/774–0750; William D.B. Pope, M.D., Registrar

NEW BRUNSWICK

College of Physicians and Surgeons of New Brunswick, One Hampton Road, Suite 300, Rothesay, NB E2E 5K8; tel. 506/849–5050; FAX. 506/849–5069; Dr. Ed Schollenberg, Registrar

NOVA SCOTIA

College of Physicians and Surgeons of Nova Scotia, Office of the Registrar, Sentry Place, Suite 300, 1559 Brunswick Street, Halifax, NS B3J 2G1; tel. 902/422–5823; FAX. 902/422–5035; Dr. Cameron Little, Registrar and CEO

PRINCE EDWARD ISLAND

College of Physicians and Surgeons of Prince Edward Island, 199 Grafton Street, Charlottetown, PE C1A 1L2; tel. 902/566–3861; FAX. 902/566–3986; C.A. Moyse, M.D., Registrar

QUEBEC

College des medecins du Quebec, 2170, boul. Rene-Levesque Ouest, Montreal, PQ H3H 2T8; tel. 514/933–4441; FAX. 514/933–3112; Yves Robert, M.D., Secretary

SASKATCHEWAN

College of Physicians and Surgeons of Saskatchewan, 500 321A 21st Street, E., Saskatoon, SK; tel. 306/244–7355; FAX. 306/244–0090; Dennis Kendel, M.D., Registrar

Quality Improvement Organizations

The following list of QIOs was obtained from the agencies themselves and the Centers for Medicare and Medicaid Services, Quality Improvement Organization programs.

United States

ALABAMA: Alabama Quality Assurance Foundation, Two Perimeter Park, S., Suite 200 West, Birmingham, AL 35243-2337; tel. 205/970–1600; FAX. 205/970–1616; Susan B. Holmes, CFO

ALASKA: Mountain-Pacific Quality Health, 4241 B Street, Suite 303, Anchorage, AK 99503; tel. 907/561–3202; FAX. 907/561–3204; Sharon Stiassny, Office Director

ARIZONA: Health Services Advisory Group, Inc., 1600 E. Northern Avenue, Suite 100, Phoenix, AZ 85020; tel. 602/264–6382; FAX. 602/241–0757; Herbert S. Rigberg, CEO

ARKANSAS: Arkansas Foundation for Medical Care, Inc., 401 W. Capitol, Suite 450, Little Rock, AR 72201; tel. 501/212–8600; FAX. 501/244–2101; Melissa Masingill, Assistant Vice President, Communications

CALIFORNIA: Lumetra, One Sansome Street, San Francisco, CA 94104; tel. 415/677–2000; FAX. 415/677–2195; Jo Ellen H. Ross, President and CEO

COLORADO: Colorado Foundation for Medical Care, 23 Inverness Way East, Suite 100, Englewood, CO 8015708; tel. 303/695–3300; FAX. 303/659–3350; Arja P. Adair, Jr., President and CEO

CONNECTICUT: Qualidigm, 100 Roscommon Drive, Suite 200, Middletown, CT 06457; tel. 860/632–2008; FAX. 860/632–5865; Marcia K. Petrillo, Chief Executive Officer

DELAWARE: Quality Insights of Delaware, Baynard Building Suite 100, 3411 Silverside Rd, Wilmington, DE 19810-4812; tel. 302/478–3600; FAX. 302/478–3873; John C. Wiesendanger, CEO

DISTRICT OF COLUMBIA: Delmarva Foundation for Medical Care, Inc., 2175 K Street, NW, Suite 250, Washington, DC 20037; tel. 202/293–9650; FAX. 202/293–3253; Christian E. Jensen, MD, MPH, President & CEO

FLORIDA: FMQAI, 5201 W. Kennedy Blvd. Suite 900, Tampa, FL 33609; tel. 813/354–9111; FAX. 813/354–1319; Logan Malone, Ed.D, Chief Executive Officer

GEORGIA: Georgia Medical Care Foundation, 1455 Lincoln Parkway, Suite 800, Atlanta, GA 30346; tel. 404/982–0411; FAX. 404/982–7584; Dennis White, Chief Executive Officer

HAWAII: Mountain-Pacific Quality Health Foundation, 1360 South Beretania Street, Suite 501, Honolulu, HI 96814; tel. 808/545–2550; FAX. 808/440–6030; Dee Dee Nelson, Director of Hawaii Office

IDAHO: Qualis Health of Idaho Office, 720 Park Boulevard, Suite 120, Boise, ID 83712-7756; tel. 208/343–4617; FAX. 208/343–4705; Jonathan R. Sugarman MD, MPH, Chief Executive Officer

ILLINOIS: Illinois Foundation for Quality Healthcare, 2625 Butterfield Road, Suite 102E, Oak Brook, IL 60523; tel. 630/571–5540; FAX. 630/571–5611; Don Lovasz, CEO

INDIANA: Health Care Excel, Incorporated, 2629 Waterfront Parkway East Drive, Suite 200, Indianapolis, IN 46214; tel. 317/347–4500; FAX. 317/347–4567; Sharon Smith, Chief Executive Officer

IOWA: Iowa Foundation for Medical Care, 6000 Westown Parkway, West Des Moines, IA 50266-7771; tel. 515/223–2900; FAX. 515/273–8888; Don Lovasz, CEO

KANSAS: The Kansas Foundation for Medical Care, Inc., 2947 Southwest Wanamaker Drive, Topeka, KS 66614; tel. 785/273–2552; FAX. 785/273–0737; Larry Pitman, President and CEO

KENTUCKY: Health Care Excel of Kentucky Incorporated, 1941 Bishop Lane, Suite 400, Louisville, KY 40218; tel. 505/454–5112; FAX. 502/454–5113; Sharon Smith, Chief Executive Officer

LOUISIANA: Louisiana Health Care Review, Inc., 8591 United Plaza Blvd Suite 270, Baton Rouge, LA 70809; tel. 225/926–6353; FAX. 225/923–0957; Gary Curtis, Chief Executive Officer

MAINE: Northeast Health Care Quality (ME), (see New Hampshire), 15 Old Rollinsford Road, Suite 302, Dover, NH, ME; tel. 603/842–8225; FAX. 603/749–1195; Robert A. Aurilio, CEO

MARYLAND: Delmarva Foundation for Medical Care, Inc., 9240 Centreville Road, Easton, MD 21601; tel. 410/822–0697; FAX. 410/822–9572; Christian E. Jensen, MD, MPH, President & CEO

MASSACHUSETTS: MassPro, 245 Winter Street, Waltham, MA 02154-1231; tel. 781/890–0011; FAX. 781/487–0083; Jeffery M. East, President and CEO

MICHIGAN: MPRO, 22670 Haggerty Rd, Suite 100, Farmington Hills, MI 48335-2611; tel. 248/465–7300; FAX. 248/465–7428; Robert J. Yellan, President/CEO

MINNESOTA: Stratis Health, 2901 Metro Drive, Suite 400, Bloomington, MN 55425; tel. 952/854–3306; FAX. 952/853–8503; Jennifer Lundblad, Ph.D, MBA, CEO

MISSISSIPPI: Information & Quality Healthcare, Renaissance Place, 385B Highland Colony Parkway, Suite 504, Ridgeland, MS 39157; tel. 601/957–1575; FAX. 601/956–1713; James McIlwain, M.D., President

MISSOURI: Primaris, 200 N. Keene Street, Columbia, MO 65201; tel. 573/817–8300; FAX. 573/817–8330; Richard A. Royer, Chief Executive Officer

MONTANA: Mountain-Pacific Quality Health Foundation, 3404 Cooney Drive, Helena, MT 59602; tel. 406/443–4020; FAX. 406/443–4585; Janice Connors, CEO

NEBRASKA: CIMRO of Nebraska, 1230 O Street, Suite 120, Lincoln, NE 68508; tel. 402/476–1399; FAX. 402/476–1335; Greg Schieke, MBA

NEVADA: HealthInsight, 6830 W. Oquendo Road Suite 102, Las Vegas, NV 89118; tel. 702/385–9933; FAX. 702/385–4586; Marc Bennett, President & CEO

NEW HAMPSHIRE: Northeast Health Care Quality Foundation, 15 Old Rollinsford Road, Suite 302, Dover, NH 03820-2830; tel. 603/749–1641; FAX. 603/749–1195; Robert A. Aurilio, CEO

NEW JERSEY: Healthcare Quality Strategies, Inc., 557 Cranbury Road, Suite 21, East Brunswick, NJ 08816; tel. 732/238–5570; FAX. 732/238–7766; Martin P. Margolies, Chief Executive Officer

NEW MEXICO: New Mexico Medical Review Association, (NMMRA), 5801 Osuna RD NE, Suite 200, Albuquerque, NM 87109; tel. 505/998–9898; FAX. 505/998–9899; Don F. Seelinger, MD, President

NEW YORK: IPRO, 1979 Marcus Avenue, First Floor, Lake Success, NY 11042-1002; tel. 516/326–7767; FAX. 516/326–7791; Theodore O. Will, Chief Executive Officer

NORTH CAROLINA: Carolinas Center for Medical Excellence, 100 Regency Forest Drive, Suite 200, Cary, NC 27518-8598; tel. 919/380–9860; FAX. 919/380–7637; Charles Riddick, CEO

NORTH DAKOTA: North Dakota Health Care Review Inc., 800 31st Avenue S.W., Minot, ND 58701; tel. 701/852–4231; FAX. 701/838–6009; David Remillard, Chief Executive Officer

OHIO: Ohio KePRO, Inc., Rock Run Center, 5700 Lombardo Center Drive, Seven Hills, OH 44131; tel. 216/447-9604; FAX. 216/447–7925; Joseph Dougher, CEO

OKLAHOMA: Oklahoma Foundation for Medical Quality, Inc., 14000 Quail Springs Parkway, Suite 400, Oklahoma City, OK 73134; tel. 405/840–2891; FAX. 405/840–1343; Jim L. Williams, President and CEO

OREGON: Acumentra Health, 2020 S.W. 4th Avenue, Suite 520, Portland, OR 97201-4960; tel. 503/279–0100; FAX. 503/279–0190; Jon Mitchell, FACHE, President and CEO

PENNSYLVANIA: KEPRO, Inc., 777 East Park Drive, Harrisburg, PA 17111; tel. 717/564–8288; FAX. 717/564–3862; Joseph Dougher, CEO

RHODE ISLAND: Rhode Island Quality Partners, Inc., 235 Promenade St., Suite 500, Providence, RI 02908; tel. 401/528–3200; FAX. 401/528–3210; John Keimig, Executive Director

SOUTH CAROLINA: The Carolinas Center for Medical Excellence, 246 Stoneridge Dr, Suite 200, Columbia, SC 29210; tel. 803/251–2215; FAX. 803/255–0897; Melinda Postal, Director of Communications

SOUTH DAKOTA: South Dakota Foundation for Medical Care, 2600 West 49th Street, Suite 300, Sioux Falls, SD 57105; tel. 605/336–3505; FAX. 605/373–0580; Mark Hoven, Chief Executive Officer

TENNESSEE: Q Source, 3175 Lenox Park Boulevard, Suite 309, Memphis, TN 38115; tel. 901/682–0381; FAX. 901/761–3786; Dawn Fitzgerald, CEO

TEXAS: Texas Medical Foundation, Health Quality Institute, Bridgepoint 1, Suite 300, 5918 West Courtyard Drive, Austin, TX 78730-5036; tel. 512/329–6610; FAX. 512/327–7159

UTAH: Health Insight, 348 East 4500 South, Suite 300, Salt Lake City, UT 84107; tel. 801/892–0155; FAX. 801/892–0160; Marc Bennett, President and CEO

VERMONT: Northeast Health Care Quality (VT)(see New Hampshire), 15 Old Rollinsford Road, Suite 302, Dover, NH, VT; tel. 603/842–8225; FAX. 603/749–1195; Robert A. Aurilio, CEO

VIRGINIA: Virginia Health Quality Center, 4510 Cox Road, Suite 400, Glen Allen, VA 23060; tel. 804/289–5320; FAX. 804/289–5324; Donald A. Glozer, MHA, CHE, President & CEO

WASHINGTON: Qualis Health, 10700 Meridian Avenue, N., Suite 100, Seattle, WA 98133-9075; tel. 206/364–9700; FAX. 206/368–2419; Jonathan Sugarman, MD, MPH, President and Chief Executive Officer

WEST VIRGINIA: West Virginia Medical Institute, Inc., 3001 Chesterfield Avenue, Charleston, WV 25304; tel. 304/346–9864; FAX. 304/346–9863; John Wiesendanger, MHA, Chief Executive Officer

WISCONSIN: MetaStar, Inc., 2909 Landmark Place, Madison, WI 53713; tel. 608/274–1940; FAX. 608/274–5008; Greg E. Simmons, President and CEO

WYOMING: Mountain-Pacific Quality Health Foundation, 2206 Dell Range Blvd., Suite G, Cheyenne, WY 82009; tel. 307/637–8162; FAX. 307/637–8163

U.S. Associated Areas

PUERTO RICO: Quality Improvement Professional Research Organization, Mercantil Plaza Building, 2 Ponce de Leon Ave., San Juan, PR 00918-1696; tel. 787/641–1240; FAX. 787/641–1248; Jose Robles, Chief Executive Officer

VIRGIN ISLANDS: Virgin Islands Medical Institute, Inc., 1AD Estate Diamond Ruby, P.O. Box 5989, Christiansted, VI 00823-5989; tel. 340/712–2400; FAX. 340/712–2449; Jill S. Doran, Chief Executive Officer

Section C

State Health Planning and Development Agencies

The following is a list of state health planning and development agencies. The information was obtained from the agencies themselves. For information about other state agencies and organizations that fulfill many of the same functions, contact the state or metropolitan hospital associations.

United States

ALABAMA: State Health Planning and Development Agency, 100 North Union Street, Suite 870, Montgomery, AL 36103-3025; tel. 334/242–4103; FAX. 334/242–4113; Alva Lambert, Executive Director

ALASKA: Facilities and Planning Section, Department of Health and Social Services, P.O. Box 110650, Juneau, AK 99811-0650; tel. 907/465–1870; FAX. 907/465–2499; Arnold Liebelt, Section Chief

ARIZONA: Arizona Department of Health ServicesDivision of Public Health Services, 150 North 18th Avenue, Phoenix, AZ 85007; tel. 602/542–1023; FAX. 602/364–3445; Susan Gerard, Director

CALIFORNIA: Healthcare Workforce, Development Division, 400 R Street, Room 330, Sacramento, CA 95811; tel. 916/326–3700; FAX. 916/322–2588; Angela L. Minniefield, M.P.A., Deputy Director

COLORADO: Colorado Department of Public Health and Environment, Primary Care Office, 4300 Cherry Creek Drive, S., Denver, CO 80246-1530; tel. 303/692–2000; FAX. 303/758–3448; James B. Martin, Executive Director

CONNECTICUT: Connecticut Department of Public Health, Planning Branch, 410 Capitol Avenue, MS# 13 PBA, Hartford, CT 06134-0308; tel. 860/509–7218; FAX. 860/509–7227; Meg Hooper, MPA, Chief

DELAWARE: Bureau of Health Planning and Resources Management, Department of Health and Social Services, 417 Federal Street, Dover, DE 19901; tel. 302/739–4776; FAX. 302/741–2970; Judith A. Chaconas, Director

DISTRICT OF COLUMBIA: District Of Columbia Department Of Health, 825 North Capital Street, N.E., Second Floor, Washington, DC 20002; tel. 202/671–5000; FAX. 202/442–4795; Dr. Pierre Vigilance, Acting Director, Department of Health

GEORGIA: Georgia Department of Community Health, 2 Peachtree Street, NW, 34th Floor, Suite 102, Atlanta, GA 30303-3159; tel. 404/657–7198; FAX. 404/656–0655; Clyde Reese, Director, Division Of Health Planning

HAWAII: Hawaii State Health Planning and Development Agency, 1177 Alakea Street, Suite 402, Honolulu, HI 96813; tel. 808/587–0788; FAX. 808/587–0783; David Sakamoto, M.D. Administrator

IDAHO: Bureau of Vital Records and Health Statistics, Division of Health, Idaho Department of Health and Welfare, 450 West State Street, First Floor, P.O. Box 83720, Boise, ID 83720-0036; tel. 208/334–5976; FAX. 208/332–7260; James Aydelotte, Bureau Chief

ILLINOIS: Illinois Department of Public Health, Division of Patient Safety & Quality, 525 West Jefferson, Second Floor, Springfield, IL 62761; tel. 217/782–6235; FAX. 217/785–4308; Mary Driscoll, Chief, Division of Safety & Quality

INDIANA: Indiana State Department of Health, Primary Care Office, Two North Meridian Street, Suite Eight-B, Indianapolis, IN 46204-3003; tel. 317/233–7546; FAX. 317/233–7761; Ann M. Alley, Primary Care Office Director

IOWA: Iowa Department of Public Health, Lucas State Office Building, 321 E. 12th Street, Des Moines, IA 50319-0075; tel. 515/281–4348; FAX. 515/281–4535; Louise Lex, Ph.D., Healthy Iowans 2010 Coordinator

KANSAS: Kansas Health Policy Authority, Rm 900-N, Landon State Office Bldg., 900 SW Jackson St., Topeka, KS 66612-1251; tel. 785/296–8585; FAX. 785/368–7180; Doug Farmer, Director of State Employee Health Benefits

MAINE: Office of Rural Health and Primary Care, MeCDC, Department of Health and Human Services, 286 Water Street, Augusta, ME 04333-0011; tel. 207/287–5524; FAX. 207/287–5431; Charles Dwyer, Office of Rural Health & Primary Care

MARYLAND: Maryland Health Care Commission, 4160 Patterson Avenue, Baltimore, MD 21215-2299; tel. 410/764–3460; FAX. 410/385–1311; Dr. Rex W. Cowdry, M.D., Executive Director

MISSISSIPPI: Mississippi State Department of Health, Office of Health Policy and Planning, 570 East Woodrow Wilson, P.O. Box 1700, Jackson, MS 39215-1700; tel. 601/576–7874; FAX. 601/576–7530; Rachel Pittman, Chief

MISSOURI: Missouri Department of Health and Senior Services, 912 Wildwood, P.O. Box 570, Jefferson City, MO 65102; tel. 573/751–6001; FAX. 573/751–6041; Jane Drummond, Director

MONTANA: Health Resources Division, Department of Public Health and Human Services, Cogswell Building, 1400 Broadway, Room A206, Helena, MT 59620; tel. 406/444–4458; Mary Dalton, Administrator

NEBRASKA: Nebraska Health and Human Services, Finance and Support, Research and Performance Measurement, P.O. Box 95026, Lincoln, NE 68509-5026; tel. 402/471–3121; FAX. 402/471–9449; Christine Z. Peterson, CEO

NEVADA: Nevada Department of Health and Human Services, State Health Division, Bureau of Health Planning and Statistics, 4150 Technology Way, Suite 104, Carson City, NV 89706; tel. 775/684–4218; FAX. 775/684–4156; Luana J. Ritch, Ph.D., Bureau Chief

NEW HAMPSHIRE: Office of Health Services Planning and Review, 29 Hazen Drive, Concord, NH 03301-6527; tel. 603/271–4606; FAX. 603/271–4141; Cindy Carrier, Managing Analyst

NEW JERSEY: New Jersey Department of Health and Senior Services, Certificate of Need and Health Care Facility Licensure, P.O. Box 358, Trenton, NJ 08625-0358; tel. 609/292–8773; FAX. 609/292–3780; John A. Calabria, Director

NEW MEXICO: New Mexico Health Policy Commission, 2055 S. Pacheco Street, Suite 200, Santa Fe, NM 87505; tel. 505/827–6201; FAX. 505/424–3222; Liz Stefanics, Agency Director

NEW YORK: New York State Department of Health, Division of Planning, Policy and Resource Development, Corning Tower, Suite 1495, Empire State Plaza, Albany, NY 12237; tel. 518/474–2011; Richard F. Daines, M.D., Commissioner

NORTH CAROLINA: Medical Facilities Planning Section, 2701 Mail Service Center, Raleigh, NC 27699-2701; tel. 919/855–3865; FAX. 919/733–4413; Lee Hoffman, CON Director

NORTH DAKOTA: North Dakota Department of Health, Office of Community Health, 600 East Boulevard Avenue, Dept 301, Bismarck, ND 58505-0200; tel. 701/328–2333; FAX. 701/328–2036; Mary Ann Foss, Director of Community Health

OKLAHOMA: Oklahoma State Department of Health, Healthcare Information, 1000 Northeast 10th Street, Oklahoma City, OK 73117-1299; tel. 405/271–6225; FAX. 405/271–9061; Kelly Baker, Director of Center for Health Statistics

PENNSYLVANIA: Bureau of Health Planning, Pennsylvania Department of Health, Health and Welfare Building, Room 1033, Harrisburg, PA 17120; tel. 717/772–5298; FAX. 717/705–6525; Martin Raniowski, Director

RHODE ISLAND: Rhode Island Department of Health, Three Capitol Hill, Providence, RI 02908; tel. 401/222–2231; FAX. 401/222–6548; David R. Gifford, MD, MPH, Director

SOUTH CAROLINA: DHEC, Division of Planning and Certificate of Need, 2600 Bull Street, Columbia, SC 29201; tel. 803/545–4200; FAX. 803/545–4579; Les Shelton, Senior Planner

SOUTH DAKOTA: South Dakota Department of Health, Division of Administration, 600 East Capitol Avenue, Pierre, SD 57501-2536; tel. 605/773–3361; FAX. 605/773–5683; Laurie Gill, Director, Division of Administration

TENNESSEE: Policy, Planning & Assessment (PPA), Tennessee Department of Health, Cordell Hull Building, 4th Floor, Nashville, TN 37243; tel. 615/532–6566; FAX. 615/253–1688; Marquette Lewis, Director, Health Statistics

TEXAS: Texas Statewide Health Coordinating Council, Center for Health Statistics, Mail Code 1898, Texas Department of State Health Services, Austin, TX 78714-9347; tel. 512/458–7261; FAX. 512/458–7344; Connie Turney, SHCC Project Coordinator

VERMONT: Division of Health Care Administration, Department of Banking Insurance, Securities, and Health Care Administration, 89 Main Street, Montpelier, VT 05620-3601; tel. 802/828–2900; FAX. 802/828–2949; Jennifer Garson, Certificate of Need Specialist

VIRGINIA: Virginia Department of Health, Division of Certificate of Public Need, 9960 Maryland Drive, Suite 401, Richmond, VA 23233; tel. 804/367–2126; FAX. 804/527–4501; Erik O. Bodin, III Director of the Division of Certificate of Public Need

WASHINGTON: Washington State Board of Health, 101 Israel Road SE, P.O. Box 47990, Olympia, WA 98504-7990; tel. 360/236–4100; FAX. 360/236–4088; Craig McLaughlin, MJ, Executive Director

WEST VIRGINIA: West Virginia Health Care Authority, 100 Dee Drive, Charleston, WV 25311-1600; tel. 304/558–7000; FAX. 304/558–7001; Sonia D. Chambers, Chair

WYOMING: Department of Health, Office of Rural Health, 6101 Yellowstone Rd., Suite 510, Cheyenne, WY 82002; tel. 307/777–7293; FAX. 307/777–8545; Sharla Allen, Interim Manager

State and Provincial Government Agencies

The following list includes state departments of health, and their subagencies as well as such independent agencies as those for children's services, insurance, mental health, and vocational rehabilitation. The information was obtained directly from the agencies. Additional licensing agencies are listed in Section C under Medical and Nursing Licensure Agencies and Hospital Licensure Agencies.

United States

ALABAMA

The Honorable Robert Riley, Governor, 334/242-7100

Health

Alabama Department of Public Health, Bureau Of Family Health Services, The RSA Tower, P.O. Box 303017, Montgomery, AL 36130–3017; tel. 334/206–2940; FAX. 334/206–2059; Thomas M. Miller, M.D., MPH, Director

Department of Public Health, The RSA Tower, Suite 1552, P.O. Box 303017, Montgomery, AL 36130–3017; tel. 334/206–5200; FAX. 334/206–2008; Donald E. Williamson, M.D., State Health Officer

Insurance

Department of Insurance, 201 Monroe Street, Suite 1700, Montgomery, AL 36130; tel. 334/241–4101; FAX. 334/241–4192; David Parsons, Commissioner

Social Services

Alabama Medicaid Agency, 501 Dexter Avenue, P.O. Box 5624, Montgomery, AL 36103–5624; tel. 334/242–5500; FAX. 334/242–5097; Carol A. Steckel, Commissioner

Department of Human Resources, Gordon Persons Building, 50 Ripley Street, Montgomery, AL 36104; tel. 334/242–1160; FAX. 334/242–0198; Page B. Walley, Ph.D., Commissioner

Department of Rehabilitation Services, 2129 East South Boulevard, Montgomery, AL 36116; tel. 800/441–7607; FAX. 334/281–1973; Steve Shivers, Commissioner

Other

State Department of Education, Gordon Persons Building, P.O. Box 302101, Montgomery, AL 36130–2101; tel. 334/242–9700; FAX. 334/242–9708; Ed Richardson, Superintendent

ALASKA

The Honorable Sarah Palin, Governor, 907/465–3500

Health

Division of Behavioral Health, 3601 C. St. # 878, Anchorage, AK 99503; tel. 907/269–3600; FAX. 907/269–3623; Melissa Witzler Stone, Director

Health Facilities Licensing and Certification, 4730 Business Park Boulevard, Suite 18, Anchorage, AK 99503–7137; tel. 907/334–2483; FAX. 907/561–3011; Shelbert Larsen, Administrator

Social Services

Department Health and Social Services, Division of Behavioral Health, P.O. Box 110620, Juneau, AK 99811–0620; tel. 907/465–3370; FAX. 907/465–2268

Department of Health and Social Services, 350 Main Street, Room 404, P.O. Box 110601, Juneau, AK 99811–0601; tel. 907/465–3030; FAX. 907/465–3068; Karleen K. Jackson, Commissioner

Division of Administrative Services, Department of Health and Social Services, P.O. Box 110650, Juneau, AK 99811–0650; tel. 907/465–1630; FAX. 907/465–2499; Janet E. Clarke, Director

Division of Health Care Services, 4501 Business Park Blvd., Suite 24, Anchorage, AK 99503–7167; tel. 907/465–3355; FAX. 907/465–2204; William J. Streur, Deputy Commissioner

Office of Children's Services, P.O. Box 110630, Juneau, AK 99811; tel. 907/465–3191; FAX. 907/465–2091; Tammy Sandoval, Deputy Commissioner

State of Alaska Division of Vocational Rehabilitation, 801 West 10th Street, Suite A, Juneau, AK 99801–1894; tel. 907/465–2814; FAX. 907/465–2856; Cheryl A. Walsh, Director

State of Alaska, Department of Health and Social Services, 350 Main Street, Room 404, P.O. Box 110601, Juneau, AK 99811–0601; tel. 907/465–3030; FAX. 907/465–3068; Kurt West, Project Director – Regulations

Other

Department of Education & Early Development, 801 West 10th Street, Suite 200, Juneau, AK 99801–1894; tel. 907/465–2887; FAX. 907/465–2713; Conchita McKnight, Program Assistant

ARIZONA

The Honorable Janet Napolitano, Governor, 602/542–4331

Health

Arizona Department of Health Services, 150 N. 18th Ave, Suite 500, Phoenix, AZ 85007; tel. 602/542–1027; FAX. 602/542–1062; Susan Gerard, Director

Arizona Department of Health Services, Division of Licensing Services, 150 N. 18th Ave., Suite 510, Phoenix, AZ 85007; tel. 602/364–3064; FAX. 602/364–4808; Mary Wiley, Assistant Director

Arizona Department of Health Services, Division of Public Health, Bureau of Epidemiology and Disease Control Services, 3815 North Black Canyon Highway, Phoenix, AZ 85015; tel. 602/230–5808; FAX. 602/230–5959; Lee A. Bland, Bureau Chief

Social Services

Bureau of Community and Family Health Services, 2927 N. 35th Avenue, Suite 100, Phoenix, AZ 85017; tel. 602/542–1223; FAX. 602/542–1265; Raul V. Munoz, MPH, Bureau Chief

Division of Behavioral Health Services, Arizona Department of Health Services, 150 N. 18th Ave, Ste 200, Phoenix, AZ 85007; tel. 602/364–4558; FAX. 602/364–4570; Eddy Broadway, Deputy Director

Office for Children with Special Health Care Needs, OCSACN, 150 N. 18th Avenue, Suite 330, Phoenix, AZ 85007; tel. 602/542–1860; FAX. 602/542–2589; Joan Agostinelli, Chief

Rehabilitation Services Administration (930A), 1789 West Jefferson, Second Floor Northwest, Site Code 930 A, Phoenix, AZ 85007; tel. 602/542–3332; FAX. 602/542–3778; Katharine M. Levandowsky, Administrator

Other

Arizona Department of Environmental Quality, 1110 W. Washington Street, Phoenix, AZ 85007; tel. 602/771–2300; FAX. 602/771–2218; Stephen A. Owens, Director

Department of Economic Security, Site Code 010A, P.O. Box 6123, Phoenix, AZ 85005; tel. 602/542–5678; FAX. 602/542–5339; Tracy L. Wareing, Director

ARKANSAS

The Honorable Mike Beebe, Governor, 501/682–2345

Health

Arkansas Department of Health, Agency Leadership Team, 4815 West Markham, Slot 55, Little Rock, AR 72205; tel. 501/661–2238; FAX. 501/661–2308; Fay Boozman, M.D., Director

Children's Medical Service, Title V Children with Special Healthcare Needs, Donaghey Plaza South, Seventh and Main Streets, Little Rock, AR 72203; tel. 501/682–2277; FAX. 501/682–8247; Nancy Holder, Program Administrator

Division of Health Facility Services, Department of Health, 500 West 10th Street, Suite 400, Little Rock, AR 72203–1437; tel. 501/661–2201; FAX. 501/661–2165; Connie Melton, Section Chief

Division of Medical Services, P.O. Box 1437, Slot S401, Little Rock, AR 72201–1437; tel. 501/682–8292; FAX. 501/682–1197; Roy Jeffus, Director

Social Services

Arkansas Department of Health and Human Services, P.O. Box 1437, Little Rock, AR 72203–1437; tel. 501/682–8650; FAX. 501/682–6836; John Selig, DHHS Director

Arkansas Division of Behavioral Health Services, Arkansas State Hospital, 4313 West Markham, Little Rock, AR 72205–4096; tel. 501/686–9000; FAX. 501/686–9182; Jay Bradford, Director

Arkansas Rehabilitation Services, 1616 Brookwood, P.O. Box 3781, Little Rock, AR 72203; tel. 501/296–1616; FAX. 501/296–1141; Robert P Trevino, Commissioner

Bureau of Alcohol & Drug Abuse Prevention, Freeway Medical Center, Suite 907, 5800 West 10th Street, Little Rock, AR 72204; tel. 501/280–4501; FAX. 501/280–4532; Gary Horton, Team Leader

Division of Aging and Adult Services, P.O. Box 1437, Slot S530, Little Rock, AR 72203–1437; tel. 501/682–2441; FAX. 501/682–8155; Herb Sanderson, Director

Office of Long–Term Care, New Donaghey Plaza South, 7th & Main Street, Little Rock, AR 72203–8059; tel. 501/682–8487; FAX. 501/682–1197; Carol Shockley, Director

Preparedness & Response Branch, Arkansas Department of Health, 4815 West Markham Street, Slot 41, Little Rock, AR 72205–3867; tel. 501/661–2292; FAX. 501/280–4140; Renee Patrick, Associate Chief

CALIFORNIA

The Honorable Arnold Schwarzenegger, Governor, 916/445–2841

Health

California Department of Public Health, P.O. Box 997377, MS 0500, Sacramento, CA 95899–7377; tel. 916/558–1700; Dr. Mark Horton, Director

Department of Developmental Services, 1600 Ninth Street, Suite 240, MS 2–13, Sacramento, CA 95814; tel. 916/654–1897; FAX. 916/654–2167; Terri Delgadillo, Director

Department of Health Services, P.O.Box 997413, MS 0000, Sacramento, CA 95899–7413; tel. 916/440–7400; Sandra Shewry, Director

Licensing

Board of Vocational Nursing and Psychiatric Technicians, 2535 Capitol Oaks Drive, Suite 205, Sacramento, CA 95833; tel. 916/263–7800; FAX. 916/263–7859; Teresa Bello–Jones, JD, M.S.N., RN, Executive Officer

Social Services

CA Health And Human Services Agency, Office of the Secretary, 1600 Ninth Street, Suite 460, Sacramento, CA 95814; tel. 916/654–3454; FAX. 916/654–3343; Lynn Froelic, BSO

California Department of Social Services, Public Inquiry and Response Unit, 744 P Street, Sacramento, CA 95814; tel. 916/651–8848; FAX. 916/651–8866

California Health and Human Services Agency, Office of the Secretary, 1600 Ninth Street, Suite 460, Sacramento, CA 95814; tel. 916/654–3454; FAX. 916/654–3342; Lynn Froelick, Business Services Officer

Community Resources Development Section, California Department of Rehabilitation, 2000 Evergreen Street, Sacramento, CA 95815; tel. 916/263–7374; FAX. 916/263–7456; Kent Thompson, Chief

Department of Alcohol and Drug Programs, 1700 K Street, Sacramento, CA 95811; tel. 916/445–1943; FAX. 916/323–5873; Renee Zito, Director

COLORADO

The Honorable Bill Ritter, Governor, 303/866–2471

Health

Colorado Department of Public Health and Environment, 4300 Cherry Creek Drive, S., Denver, CO 80246–1530; tel. 303/692–2011; FAX. 303/691–7702; James B. Martin, Executive Director

Department of Health Care Policy and Financing, 1570 Grant Street, Denver, CO 80203–1818; tel. 303/866–2868; FAX. 303/866–4411; Stephen C. Tool, Executive Director

Insurance

Division of Insurance, 1560 Broadway, Suite 850, Denver, CO 80202; tel. 303/894–7499; FAX. 303/894–7455; Marcy Morrison, Commissioner

Licensing

Department of Regulatory Agencies, 1560 Broadway, Suite 1550, Denver, CO 80202; tel. 303/894–7855; FAX. 303/894–7885; D. Rico Munn, Executive Director

Social Services

Alcohol and Drug Abuse Division, Colorado Department of Human Services, 4055 S. Lowell Blvd., Denver, CO 80236; tel. 323/866–7480; FAX. 303/866–7481; Janet Wood, Director

Behavioral Health Services, Colorado Department of Human Sciences, Divisions of Mental Health and Alcohol and Drug Abuse, 3824 West Princeton Circle, Denver, CO 80236; tel. 303/866–7400; FAX. 303/866–7428; Janet Wood, Director

Department of Human Services, 1575 Sherman Street, Eighth Floor, Denver, CO 80203; tel. 303/866–5700; FAX. 303/866–4740; Karen L. Beye, Executive Director

CONNECTICUT

The Honorable M. Jodi Rell, Governor, 800/406–1527

Health

Department of Public Health, 410 Capitol Avenue, Mail Stop 12APP, Hartford, CT 06134–0308; tel. 860/509–7590; FAX. 860/509–8457; Jennifer Filippone, Chief Practitioner, Licensing and Investigations

Department of Public Health, Division of Health Systems Regulation, 410 Capitol Avenue, Mail Stop 12HSR, Hartford, CT 06134–0308; tel. 860/509–7407; FAX. 860/509–7539; Valerie Bryan, R.N., S.N.C.

Insurance

Connecticut Department, P.O. Box 816, Hartford, CT 06142–0816; tel. 860/297–3862; FAX. 860/297–3941; Mary Ellen Breault, Director, Life and Health Division

Licensing

Connecticut Board of Examiners for NursingDepartment of Public Health – MS#12APP, Applications and Examinations, 410 Capitol Avenue, P.O. Box 340308, Hartford, CT 06134–0308; tel. 860/509–7603; FAX. 860/509–8457; Janice Wojick, Board Liaison

Social Services

Aging Services Division (State Unit on Aging), Department of Social Services, 25 Sigourney Street, Hartford, CT 06106–5033; tel. 860/424–5277; FAX. 860/424–5301; Pamela A Giannini, MSW, Director

Department of Social Services, 25 Sigourney Street, Hartford, CT 06106; tel. 860/424–5053; FAX. 860/424–5057; Michael P. Starkowski, Commissioner

State Department of Mental Health and Addiction Services, 410 Capitol Avenue, P.O. Box 341431, Hartford, CT 06134; tel. 860/418–7000; FAX. 860/418–6691; Thomas A. Kirk, Jr., Ph.D., Commissioner

Other

Department of Education, 165 Capitol Avenue, Hartford, CT 06106; tel. 203/566–5061; FAX. 203/566–8964

DELAWARE

The Honorable Ruth Ann Minner, Governor, 302/744–4101

Health

Delaware Office of Emergency Medical Services, Blue Hen Corporate Center, 655 South Bay Road, Dover, DE 19901; tel. 302/739–4710; FAX. 302/739–2352; Bill Stevenson, EMS Director

Delaware Public Health Laboratory, P.O. Box 1047, Smyrna, DE 19977–1047; tel. 302/653–2870; FAX. 302/653–2877; Deputy Director

Division of Public Health, Jesse Cooper Building, 417 Federal Street, Dover, DE 19901; tel. 302/744–4700; FAX. 302/739–6659; Barbara Jarrell, Director Deputy, Chief Operating Officer

Division of Public Health, Community Health Care Access Section, Jesse S. Cooper Building, 417 Federal Street, Dover, DE 19903; tel. 302/744–4700; FAX. 302/739–6653; Jacqueline J. Christman, M.D., Section Administrator

Licensing

Department of Health and Social Services, Office of Health Facilities Licensing and Certification, 2055 Limestone Road, Suite 200, Wilmington, DE 19808; tel. 302/995–8521; FAX. 302/995–8529; Roseann Sapp, Office Manager

Social Services

Delaware Psychiatric Center, Division of Substance Abuse and Mental Health, 1901 North DuPont Highway, New Castle, DE 19720; tel. 302/255–2700; FAX. 302/255–4417; Husam E. Abdallah, Hospital Director

Department of Health and Social Services, 1901 North DuPont Highway, Main Administration Building, New Castle, DE 19720; tel. 302/255–9040; FAX. 302/255–4429; Vincent Meconi, Cabinet Secretary

Department of Labor, Division of Vocational Rehabilitation, 4425 North Market Street, P.O. Box 9969, Wilmington, DE 19809–0969; tel. 302/761–8275; FAX. 302/761–6611; Andrea Guest, Director

Division of Medicaid and Medical Assistance, The Lewis Building, P.O. Box 906, New Castle, DE 19720; tel. 302/255–9500; FAX. 302/255–4454; Harry Hill, Director

Division of Services for Aging and Adults with Physical Disabilities, 1901 North DuPont Highway, 2nd Floor Annex, New Castle, DE 19720; tel. 302/255–9390; FAX. 302/255–4445; Allan Zaback, Director

Family Health Services, Division of Public Health, P.O. Box 637, Dover, DE 19903; tel. 302/744–4553; FAX. 302/739–6653; Joan Powell, MPA, Director

DISTRICT OF COLUMBIA

Governor Swithboard, 202/727–1000

Social Services

Rehabilitation Services Administration, 810 First Street, N.E., 10th Floor, Washington, DC 20002; tel. 202/442–8663; FAX. 202/442–8742; Elizabeth B. Parker, Administrator

FLORIDA

The Honorable Charlie Crist, Governor, 850/488–2272

Health

Children's Medical Services, 4052 Bald Cypress Way, Bin A–06, Tallahassee, FL 32399–1700; tel. 850/245–4200; FAX. 904/488–3813; Phyllis Sloyer, RN, PhD, Division Director, CMS

Department of Health, State Surgeon General, 4052 Bald Cypress Way, Bin #A00, Tallahassee, FL 32399–1701; tel. 850/245–4321; FAX. 850/922–9453; Ana Viamonte Ros, M.D., M.P.H.

Licensing

Agency for Health Care Administration, Division of Health Quality Assurance, 2727 Mahan Drive, Tallahassee, FL 32308; tel. 850/414–9796; FAX. 850/487–6240; Elizabeth Dudek, Deputy Secretary

Social Services

Adult Services, 1317 Winewood Boulevard, Building 6, Room 366, Tallahassee, FL 32399–0700; tel. 850/488–2881; FAX. 850/922–4193; Mr. Chris Shoemaker, Deputy Director, Adult Services

Agency for Workforce Innovation, 107 East Madison Street, 100 Caldwell Building, Tallahassee, FL 32399–4120; tel. 850/245–7105; FAX. 850/921–3223; Monesia T. Brown, Director

Department of Children and Families, Mental Health Program Office, 1317 Winewood Boulevard, Tallahassee, FL 32399–0700; tel. 904/488–8304; FAX. 904/487–2239

Division of Vocational Rehabilitation, 2002 Old St. Augustine Road, Building A, Tallahassee, FL 32301–4862; tel. 850/245–3400; FAX. 850/245–3316; Bill Palmer, Director

Health Facility Regulation, Agency for Health Care Administration, MS 28A, 2727 Mahan Drive, Tallahassee, FL 32308; tel. 850/922–0791; FAX. 850/413–7955; Jeff Gregg, Chief

GEORGIA

The Honorable Sonny Perdue, Governor, 404/656–1776

Health

Division of Public Health, Two Peachtree Street, NW, Suite 15–470, Atlanta, GA 30303–3682; tel. 404/657–2700; FAX. 404/657–6709; Stuart T. Brown, M.D., Director

Insurance

Office of Commissioner of Insurance, Two Martin Luther King, Jr. Drive, Seventh Floor, West Tower, Floyd Build, Atlanta, GA 30334; tel. 404/656–2056; FAX. 404/656–4030; John W. Oxendine, Commissioner of Insurance

Licensing

Bright From The Start Georgia Department of Early Care and Learning, 10 Park Place South, Suite 600, Atlanta, GA 30303; tel. 404/657–5562; FAX. 404/657–8936; Justine Strickland, Assistant Commissioner for Child Care Policy

Diagnostic Services Unit, Health Care Section, Office of Regulatory Services, Two Peachtree Street, N.W., 33rd Floor, Room 250, Atlanta, GA 30303–3142; tel. 404/657–5447; FAX. 404/657–5442; Jeannie Arnold, Program Director, Diagnostic Services

Social Services

Department of Human Resources, Two Peachtree N.W., Suite 29.250, Atlanta, GA 30303–3142; tel. 404/656–5680; FAX. 404/651–8669; B.J. Walker, Commissioner

Department of Human Resources, Division of Mental Health, Developmental Disabilities & Addictive Diseases, Two Peachtree Street, NW., 22–224, Atlanta, GA 30303–3171; tel. 404/657–2252; FAX. 404/657–1137; Gwendolyn B. Skinner, Director

Department of Human Resources, Office of Regulatory Services, Health Care Section, Two Peachtree Street, N.W., Suite 33.250, Atlanta, GA 30303–3142; tel. 404/657–5550; FAX. 404/657–8934; Carol Zafiratos, Director of the HCS

Office of Regulatory Services, Georgia Department of Human Resources, Two Peachtree Street, N.W., Room 32–415, Atlanta, GA 30303–3142; tel. 404/657–5700; FAX. 404/657–5708; Sharon E. Dougherty, Director

Personal Care Home Program Office of Regulatory Services, Department of Human Resources, Two Peachtree Street, 31st Floor, Suite 31.447, Atlanta, GA 30303–3167; tel. 404/657–4076; FAX. 404/657–3655; Victoria L. Flynn, Director

Rehabilitation Services of the Georgia, Department of Labor, 148 Andrew Young International Blvd., NE, Suite 510 Sussex Place, Atlanta, GA 30303–1751; tel. 404/232–3910; FAX. 404/232–3912; Peggy D. Rosser, Assistant Commissioner

HAWAII

The Honorable Linda Lingle, Governor, 808/586–0034

Health

Adult Mental Health Division, P.O. Box 3378, Honolulu, HI 96801–3378; tel. 808/586–4688; FAX. 808/586–4745; Thomas W. Hester, M.D., Chief

Communicable Disease Division, P.O. Box 3378, Honolulu, HI 96801; tel. 808/586–4580; FAX. 808/586–7409; Paul V. Effler, M.D., M.P.H., State Epidemiologist

Dental Health Division, 1700 Lanakila Avenue, Suite 203, Honolulu, HI 96817–2199; tel. 808/832–5700; FAX. 808/832–5722; Mark H.K. Greer, D.M.D., MPH, Chief

Hawaii Department of Health, P.O. Box 3378, Honolulu, HI 96801; tel. 808/586–4401; FAX. 808/586–4368; Chiyome L. Fukino, M.D., Director

Licensing

Department of Health/Office of Health Care Assurance, Licensing and Certification, P.O. Box 3378, Honolulu, HI 96801–3378; tel. 808/586–4080; FAX. 808/586–4090; Chief

Social Services

Alcohol and Drug Abuse Division, Department of Health, State of Hawaii, 601 Kamokila Blvd., Room 360, Kapolei, HI 96707; tel. 808/692–7506; FAX. 808/692–7521; Keith Yamamoto, Division Chief

Department of Human Services, Med–QUEST Division, P.O. Box 700190, Kapolei, HI 96709–0190; tel. 808/692–8050; FAX. 808/692–8155; Lois Lee, Acting Med–Quest Administrator

Department of Labor and Industrial Relations, Disability Compensation Division, P.O. Box 3769, Honolulu, HI 96812; tel. 808/586–9151; FAX. 808/586–9219; Gary S. Hamada, Administrator

Family Health Services Division, Hawaii State Department of Health, 1250 Punchbowl Street, Room 216, Honolulu, HI 96813; tel. 808/586–4122; FAX. 808/586–9303; Loretta J. Fuddy, A.C.S.W., M.P.H

Vocational Rehabilitation, 601 Kamokila Blvd, Room 515, Kapolei, HI 96707; tel. 808/692–7715; FAX. 808/692–7727; Neil Shim, Administrator

IDAHO

The Honorable C.L. "Butch" Otter, Governor, 208/334-2100

Health

Bureau of Emergency Medical Services, 590 West Washington Street, Boise, ID 83702–0036; tel. 208/334–4000; FAX. 208/334–4015; Dia Gainor, Bureau Chief

Bureau of Vital Records and Health Statistics, Division of Health, Idaho Dept. of Health and Welfare, 450 West State, First Floor, P.O. Box 83720, Boise, ID 83720–0036; tel. 208/334–5976; FAX. 208/332–7260; James Aydelotte, Bureau Chief

Insurance

Department of Insurance, 700 West State Street, Third Floor, P.O. Box 83720, Boise, ID 83720–0043; tel. 208/334–4250; FAX. 208/334–4398; Bill Deal, Director

Licensing

Bureau of Facility Standards, Department of Health and Welfare, P.O. Box 83720, Boise, ID 83720–0036; tel. 208/334–6626; FAX. 208/364–1888; Debby Ransom, RN, RHIT, Bureau Chief

Social Services

Department of Health and Welfare, Division of Health, 450 West State, Fourth Floor, P.O. Box 83720, Boise, ID 83720–0036; tel. 208/334–6996; FAX. 208/334–6581; Jane Smith, Administrator

Department of Health and Welfare Division of Behavioral Health, Substance Use Disorder Bureau, 450 West State, 3rd Floor, P.O. Box 83720, Boise, ID 83720–0036; tel. 208/334–5756; FAX. 208/332–7305; Bethany Gadzinski, Chief

Vocational Rehabilitation, Len B. Jordan Building, 650 West State, Room 150, P.O. Box 83720, Boise, ID 83720–0096; tel. 208/334–3390; FAX. 208/334–5305; Michael Graham, Administrator

Other

Idaho State Bureau of Laboratories, 2220 Old Penitentiary Road, Boise, ID 83712; tel. 208/334–2235; FAX. 208/334–2382; Richard F. Hudson, Ph.D., Chief

ILLINOIS

The Honorable Rod Blagojevich, Governor, 217/782-6830

Health

Illinois Department of Public Health, 535 West Jefferson Street, Springfield, IL 62761; tel. 217/557–2556; FAX. 217/557–3497; Damon T. Arnold, M.D., MPH, Director

Illinois Department of Public Health, Office of Health Care Regulation, 525 West Jefferson Street, 5th floor, Springfield, IL 62761–0001; tel. 217/782–2913; FAX. 217/524–6292; William A. Bell, Acting Deputy Director

Illinois Department of Public Health, Office of Health Protection, 525 West Jefferson Street, Springfield, IL 62761; tel. 217/782–3984; FAX. 217/524–0802; Tom Hughes, Deputy Director

Illinois Department of Public Health, Office of Statistics Policy, Planning & Statistics, 525 West Jefferson Street, Springfield, IL 62761; tel. 217/785–2040; FAX. 217/785–4308; David Carvalho, Deputy Director

Illinois Department of Public Health Laboratories, 825 North Rutledge Street, P.O. Box 19435, Springfield, IL 62794–9435; tel. 217/782–6562; FAX. 217/524–7924; Bernard T. Johnson, State Laboratory Director

Illinois Department of Public Health, Office of Health Care Regulation, Bureau of Hospitals and Ambulatory Services, 525 West Jefferson Street, Fourth Floor, Springfield, IL 62761; tel. 217/782–7412; FAX. 217/782–0382; Catherine M. Stokes, Assistant Deputy Director

Insurance

Department of Financial & Professional Regulation, Division of Insurance, 320 West Washington Street, Fourth Floor, Springfield, IL 62767; tel. 217/782–4515; FAX. 217/782–5020; Michael T. McRaith, Director

Social Services

Department of Healthcare and Family Services, 201 South Grand Avenue, E., Springfield, IL 62763–0001; tel. 217/782–1200; FAX. 217/524–7979; Barry S. Maram, Director

Division of Specialized Care for Children, University of Illinois, (Illinois' Title V Program for Children with Special Health Care Needs), 2815 West Washington, Suite 300, Springfield, IL 62794–9481; tel. 217/793–2340; FAX. 217/793–0773; Charles N. Onufer, M.D., Director

Office of Finance and Administration, 535 West Jefferson Street, Springfield, IL 62761; tel. 217/785–2033; FAX. 217/782–3987; Gary Robinson, Deputy Director

INDIANA

The Honorable Mitch Daniels, Governor, 317/232-4567

Health

Children's Special Health Care Services, Indiana State Department of Health, Two North Meridian Street, Section 7B, Indianapolis, IN 46204; tel. 317/233–9247; FAX. 317/233–1342; Edward M. Bloom, Director

Indiana State Department of Health, Division of Acute Care, Two North Meridian Street, Indianapolis, IN 46204; tel. 317/233–7474; FAX. 317/233–7157; Mary Azbill, Director

Insurance

Department of Insurance, 311 West Washington Street, Suite 300, Indianapolis, IN 46204; tel. 317/232–2406; FAX. 317/232–5251; John R. Kissling, Jr., Chief Deputy Commissioner

Social Services

Division of Long Term Care, Two North Meridian Street, Section 4–B, Indianapolis, IN 46204; tel. 317/233–7442; FAX. 317/233–7322; Suzanne Hornstein, Director

Indiana Family and Social Services Administration, 402 West Washington Street, P.O. Box 7083, Indianapolis, IN 46207–7083; tel. 317/233–4454; FAX. 317/233–4693; Cheryl G. Sullivan, Secretary

Indiana Family and Social Services Administration, Division of Mental Health and Addiction, Indiana Government Center–South, W353, 402 West Washington Street, Indianapolis, IN 46204; tel. 317/232–7800; FAX. 317/233–3472; Cathy Boggs, Director

Indiana Family and Social Services Administration, Office of Medicaid Policy and Planning, Indiana Government Center–South, 402 West Washington, Indianapolis, IN 46204–2739; tel. 317/234–2407; FAX. 317/233–4693; Jeffrey M. Wells, M.D., MBA, Director of Medicaid

Maternal and Children's Special Health Care Services, Indiana State Department of Health, Two North Meridian Street, Section 7C, Indianapolis, IN 46204; tel. 317/233–1252; FAX. 317/233–1342; Edward M. Bloom, Director

IOWA

The Honorable Chet Culver, Governor, 515/281-5211

Health

Division Health Promotion and Chronic Disease Prevention, Iowa Department of Public Health, Lucas State Office Building, Fourth Floor, Des Moines, IA 50319; tel. 515/281–3104; FAX. 515/242–6384; Julie McMahon

Iowa Department of Public Health, Lucas State Office Building, 321 E. 12th Street, Des Moines, IA 50319–0075; tel. 515/281–8474; FAX. 515/281–4958; Tom Newton, Director

Insurance

Division of Insurance, 330 E. Maple, Des Moines, IA 50319–0065; tel. 515/281–5705; FAX. 515/281–3059; Susan E. Voss, Commissioner

Licensing

Department of Inspection and Appeals, Division of Health Facilities, Lucas State Office Building, Des Moines, IA 50319; tel. 515/281–4115; FAX. 515/242–5022; J. Bennett, Administrator

Social Services

Child Health Specialty Clinics, 247 Center For Disabilities & Development, Iowa City, IA 52242–1011; tel. 319/356–1117; FAX. 319/356–3715; Brian Wilkes, Co-Director and Chief Administrative Officer

Department of Human Services, Hoover State Office Building, 1305 E. Walnut, Des Moines, IA 50319; tel. 515/281–5452; FAX. 515/281–4980; Director

Division of Health Promotion, Prevention, and Addictive Behaviors, Lucas State Office Building – 4th Floor, 321 East 12th Street, Des Moines, IA 50319–0075; tel. 515/281–7689; FAX. 515/281–4535; Janet Zwick, Director

Division of Mental Health and Disability Services, 1305 E. Walnut Street, Hoover Building, Des Moines, IA 50319–0114; tel. 515/281–7277; FAX. 515/242–6036; Allen W. Parks, Ed.D., MPH, Division Administrator

Governor's Office of Drug Control Policy, 401 SW 7th, Suite N, Des Moines, IA 50309; tel. 515/242–6391; FAX. 515/242–6390; Dale Woolery, Associate Director

Iowa Department of Elder Affairs, Jessie Parker Building, 510 E 12th Street, Des Moines, IA 50319–9025; tel. 515/725–3333; FAX. 515/725–3300; John McCalley, Director

Other

Department of Education, Iowa Vocational Rehabilitation Services, 510 East 12th Street, Des Moines, IA 50319; tel. 515/281–6731; FAX. 515/281–4703; Stephen A. Wooderson, Administrator

KANSAS

The Honorable Kathleen Sebelius, Governor, 785/296-3232

Health

Kansas Department of Health and Environment, Curtis Building, 1000 S.W. Jackson, Topeka, KS 66612–1368; tel. 913/296–0461; FAX. 913/368–6368; Roderick Bremby, Secretary, Kansas Health and Environment

Insurance

Kansas Insurance Department, 420 Southwest Ninth, Topeka, KS 66612; tel. 785/296–3071; FAX. 785/296–2283; Sandy Praeger, Commissioner of Insurance

Kansas Insurance Department, Accident and Health Division, 420 Southwest Ninth, Topeka, KS 66612; tel. 785/296–7850; FAX. 785/291–3034; Jay J. Rogers, Director of Accident and Health

Social Services

Division of Health Care Policy, Docking State Office Building, Fifth Floor–N, Topeka, KS 66612; tel. 913/296–3773; FAX. 913/296–6142; J. Lyn Entrikin Goering, Assistant Secretary

Kansas Department of Health and Environment, Bureau of Child Care and Health Facilities, 1000 Southwest Jackson, Suite 200, Topeka, KS 66612–1365; tel. 913/296–1240; FAX. 913/291–3419; Charles Moore, Director of Medical Facilities and Survey Support

Kansas Health Policy Authority, Landon State Office Building, 900 Southwest Jackson, Topeka, KS 66612; tel. 785/296–3981; FAX. 785/296–4813; Dr. Andrew Allison, Medicaid Director

Kansas Rehabilitation Services, 3640 SW Topeka Blvd., Suite 150, Topeka, KS 66611–2373; tel. 785/267–5301; FAX. 785/267–0263; Dale Barnum, Director

State Department of Social and Rehabilitation Services, Economic & Employment Support, Docking State Office Building, 915 SW Harrison, Topeka, KS 66612–1505; tel. 785/296–3349; FAX. 913/296–6960; Bobbi Mariani, Director

KENTUCKY

The Honorable Stephen L. Beshear, Governor, 502/564-2611

Health

Commission for Children with Special Health Care Needs, 982 Eastern Parkway, Louisville, KY 40217; tel. 502/595–4459; FAX. 502/595–4673; Eric Friedlander, Executive Director

Department For Mental Health/Mental Retardation Services, 100 Fair Oaks Lane, Frankfort, KY 40621–0001; tel. 502/564–4527; FAX. 502/564–5478; John M. Burt, Ed.D., Commissioner

Department for Public Health, Cabinet for Health & Family Services, 275 East Main Street, Mail Stop HSIGWA, Frankfort, KY 40621; tel. 502/564–3970; FAX. 502/564–9377; William D. Hacker, MD. FAAP, CPE, Commissioner

Division of Certificate of Need, 275 East Main Street, 3C–B, Frankfort, KY 40621; tel. 502/564–9589; FAX. 502/564–0302; Shane P. O'Donley, Director

Health Data Section, Office of Vital Statistics, 275 East Main Street, HS2E–D, Frankfort, KY 40621; tel. 502/564–2757; FAX. 502/564–4015; George Robertson, Manager

Insurance

Office of Insurance, Division of Health Policy and Managed Care, 215 West Main Street, P.O. Box 517, Frankfort, KY 40602; tel. 502/564–6088; FAX. 502/564–2728; Gary M. Smith, Associate Director

Licensing

Division of Long Term Care, Office of Inspector General, CHS Building, Fifth Floor, E, 275 East Main Street – 5EA, Frankfort, KY 40621; tel. 502/564–7963; FAX. 502/564–6546; Robert Hester, Acting Director

Social Services

Department for Community Based Services, 3W–A, 275 East Main Street, Frankfort, KY 40621; tel. 502/564–3703; FAX. 502/564–6907; Patricia R. Wilson, Commissioner

Department for Medicaid Services, 275 East Main Street, 6WA, Frankfort, KY 40621; tel. 502/564–4321; FAX. 502/564–0509; Elizabeth A. Johnson, Commissioner

Department of Vocational Rehabilitation, 209 St. Clair Street, Frankfort, KY 40601; tel. 502/564–4440; FAX. 502/564–6745; Ralph Clark, Executive Director

LOUISIANA

The Honorable Bobby Jindal, Governor, 225/342–7015

Health

Louisiana State University Health Sciences Center, Health Care Services Division–Medical Center of LA at New Orleans, 2021 Perdido Street, New Orleans, LA 70112–1352; tel. 504/903–8514; FAX. 504/903–2837; Dwayne A. Thomas, M.D., M.M.M., CEO

Louisiana State University Medical Center, Health Care Services Division, 8550 United Plaza Boulevard, Fourth Floor, Baton Rouge, LA 70809; tel. 504/922–0490; FAX. 504/922–2259; Cary M. Dougherty, Jr., Chief Operating Officer

Insurance

Department of Insurance, P.O. Box 94214, Baton Rouge, LA 70804; tel. 225/342–5900; FAX. 225/342–3078; James J. Donelon, Commissioner

Social Services

Office for Addictive Disorders, P.O. Box 2790, Baton Rouge, LA 70821–2790; tel. 225/342–6717; FAX. 225/342–3875; Michael Duffy, Assistant Secretary

Office of Community Services, P.O. Box 3318, Baton Rouge, LA 70821; tel. 225/342–2297; FAX. 225/342–2268; Marketa Garner Gautreau, Assistant Secretary

Office of Family Support, 755 N. Third St. Room 324, P.O. Box 94065, Baton Rouge, LA 70804–9065; tel. 225/342–3950; FAX. 225/219–9399; Mr. Adren O. Wilson, Assistant Secretary

Other

LA Dept. Of Health and Hospital Office of the Secretary, P.O. Box 629, Baton Rouge, LA 70821–0629; tel. 225/342–9500; FAX. 225/342–5568; Alan Levine

MAINE

The Honorable John E. Baldacci, Governor, 207/287–3531

Health

Maine Center for Disease Control and Prevention, Department of Health and Human Services, 11 State House Station, 286 Water Street, Augusta, ME 04333–0011; tel. 207/287–8016; FAX. 207/287–9058; Dora Anne Mills, M.D., MPH, Director

Insurance

Bureau of Insurance, Department of Professional and Financial Regulation, 34 State House Station, Augusta, ME 04333; tel. 207/624–8494; FAX. 207/624–8599; Glenn Griswold, Director CHCD

Licensing

Department of Professional and Financial Regulation, 35 State House Station, Augusta, ME 04333; tel. 207/624–8511; FAX. 207/624–8595

Maine Department of Human Services, Division of Licensing and Regulatory Services, State House Station 11, 41 Anthony Avenue, Augusta, ME 04333; tel. 207/287–9300; FAX. 207/287–9304; Catherine Cobb, Director

Social Services

Bureau of Rehabilitation Services, 150 State House Station, Augusta, ME 04333–0150; tel. 800/698–4440; FAX. 207/287–5292; Jill Duson

Bureau of Rehabilitation Services, Division of Deafness, 150 State House Station, Augusta, ME 04333–0150; tel. 207/623–7958; FAX. 207/287–5292; John G. Shattuck, Director

Department of Health and Human Services, 11 State House Station, Augusta, ME 04333–0011; tel. 207/287–3707; FAX. 207/287–3005; Brenda M Harvey, Commissioner

Department of Human Services, Bureau of Medical Services, State House, Station 11, Augusta, ME 04333; tel. 207/287–2674; FAX. 207/287–2675; Christine Zukas–Lessard, Acting Director

Division for the Blind and Visually Impaired, 150 State House Station, Augusta, ME 04333–0150; tel. 207/624–5950; FAX. 207/624–5980; Harold Lewis, Director

Office of Elder Services, 442 Civic Center Dr., 11 State House Station, Augusta, ME 04333; tel. 207/287–9200; FAX. 207/287–9229; Catherine Cobb, Acting Director

MARYLAND

The Honorable Martin O'Malley, Governor, 410/974–3901

Health

Community and Public Health Administration, 201 West Preston Street, Baltimore, MD 21201; tel. 410/767–5300; FAX. 410/333–7106; Russell Moy, M.D., Director

Department of Health and Mental Hygiene, 201 West Preston Street, Suite 500, Baltimore, MD 21201; tel. 410/767–6500; FAX. 410/767–6489; John M. Colmers, Secretary

Insurance

Maryland Insurance Administration, 525 St. Paul Place, Baltimore, MD 21202; tel. 800/492–6116; FAX. 410/468–2020; Ralph S. Tyler, Insurance Commissioner

Licensing

Office of Health Care Quality, Bland Bryant Building, Spring Grove Center, 55 Wade Avenue, Catonsville, MD 21228; tel. 410/402–8002; FAX. 410/402–8211; Wendy Kronmiller, Director

Social Services

Alcohol and Drug Abuse Administration, 55 Wade Avenue, Catonsville, MD 21228; tel. 410/402–8610; FAX. 410/402–8601; Peter F. Luongo, Ph.D., Director

Community Health Administration, Maryland Dept of Health and Mental Hygiene, 201 West Preston Street, Baltimore, MD 21201; tel. 410/767–6742; FAX. 410/333–5995; Diane L. Matuszak, MD, MPH, Director

Developmental Disabilities Administration, 201 West Preston Street, 4th Floor, Baltimore, MD 21201; tel. 410/767–5600; FAX. 410/767–5850; Diane K. Coughlin, Director

Division of Rehabilitation Services, 2301 Argonne Drive, Baltimore, MD 21218–1696; tel. 410/554–9385; FAX. 410/554–9412; Robert A. Burns, Assistant State Superintendent

Mental Hygiene Administration, State of Maryland, Dix Building Spring Grove Hospital Center, 55 Wade Avenue, Catonsville, MD 21228; tel. 410/402–8452; FAX. 410/402–8441; Brian Hepburn, M.D., Executive Director

Social Services Administration, 311 West Saratoga Street, Fifth Floor, Baltimore, MD 21201; tel. 410/767–7684; FAX. 410/333–0127; C. White, Deputy Executive Director

Other

Laboratories Administration, 201 West Preston Street, Baltimore, MD 21201; tel. 410/767–6100; FAX. 410/333–5403; John M. DeBoy, Dr. P.H.

Maryland Department of the Environment, Office of Environmental Health Coordination, 2500 Broening Highway, Baltimore, MD 21224; tel. 410/631–3851; FAX. 410/631–4112; Tom Allen, Director

Maryland State Department of Education, 200 West Baltimore Street, Baltimore, MD 21201–1595; tel. 410/767–0100; FAX. 410/333–6033; Nancy S. Grasmick, State Superintendent of Schools

Office of Planning and Capital Financing, Maryland State Dept. Of Health and Mental Hygiene Office of Planning and Capital Financing, 201 West Preston Street, room 535, Baltimore, MD 21201; tel. 410/767–6816; FAX. 410/333–5608; Elizabeth G. Barnard, Director

MASSACHUSETTS

The Honorable Deval Patrick, Governor, 617/725–4000

Health

Bureau of Environmental Health, Massachusetts Department of Public Health, 250 Washington Street, Seventh Floor, Boston, MA 02108; tel. 617/624–5757; FAX. 617/624–5777; Suzanne K. Condon, Associate Commissioner, Director – BEH

Bureau of Health Information, Research and Evaluation, Massachusetts Department of Public Health, 250 Washington Street, Sixth Floor, Boston, MA 02108–4619; tel. 617/624–5613; FAX. 617/624–5698; Gerald O'Keefe, Director

Bureau of Health Quality Management, Massachusetts Department of Public Health, 250 Washington Street, Boston, MA 02108–4619; tel. 617/624–5280; FAX. 617/624–5046; Nancy Ridley, Assistant Commissioner

Department of Transitional Assistance, 600 Washington Street, Boston, MA 02111; tel. 617/348–8402; FAX. 617/348–8575; Claire McIntire, Commissioner

Insurance

Division of Insurance, One South Station, Boston, MA 02110–2208; tel. 617/521–7794; FAX. 617/521–7773; Julianne M. Bowler, Commissioner

Licensing

Division of Health Care Quality, Massachusetts Department of Public Health, 99 Chauncy Street, 2nd Floor, Boston, MA 02111; tel. 617/753–8000; FAX. 617/753–8095; Paul I. Dreyer, Ph.D., Director

Social Services

Massachusetts Commission For The Blind, 48 Boylston Street, Boston, MA 02116–4718; tel. 617/727–5550; FAX. 617/626–7685; Janet Labreck, Commissioner

Massachusetts Department of Mental Health, Central Office, 25 Stanford Street, Boston, MA 02114; tel. 617/626–8123; FAX. 617/626–8131; Barbara A. Leadholm, Commissioner

Massachusetts Department of Public Health, Bureau of Substance Abuse, 250 Washington Street, 3rd Floor, Boston, MA 02108–4619; tel. 617/624–5151; FAX. 617/624–5185; Michael Botticelli

Massachusetts Rehabilitation Commission, Fort Point Place, 27 Wormwood Street, Boston, MA 02210–1606; tel. 617/204–3600; FAX. 617/727–1354; Elmer C. Bartels, Commissioner

MICHIGAN

The Honorable Jennifer M. Granholm, Governor, 517/373–3400

Health

Medical Services Administration, 400 South Pine, P.O. Box 30037, Lansing, MI 48909; tel. 517/241–7882; FAX. 517/335–5007; Paul Reinhart, Deputy Director

Public Health Administration, Michigan Department of Community Health, 201 Townsend, Lansing, MI 48913; tel. 517/335–8024; FAX. 517/335–9032; Jean Chabut, Deputy Director for Public Health

Licensing

Department of Labor and Economic Growth, Office of Financial and Insurance Regulation, 611 West Ottawa, 3rd Floor, P.O. Box 30220, Lansing, MI 48909–7720; tel. 877/999–6442; FAX. 517/335–4978; Ken Ross, Commissioner

Division of Licensing and Certification, 3500 North Logan Street, Lansing, MI 48909; tel. 517/335–8505; Nancy Graham, Supervisor

Managed Care Plan Division, Michigan Department of Community Health, P.O. Box 30479, Lansing, MI 48909; tel. 517/241–7933; FAX. 517/241–5713; Cheryl Bupp Director

Social Services

Department of Labor and Economic Growth, Michigan Rehabilitation Services, Box 30010, Lansing, MI 48909; tel. 517/373–3390; Jaye N. Shamsiddeen, Director

Michigan Department of Community Health, Health Policy Regulation & Professions Administration, 201 Townsend Street, Capitol View Building, Lansing, MI 48913; tel. 517/373–2559; FAX. 517/241–1200; Deputy Director

Office of Drug Control Policy, Michigan Department of Community Health, Lewis Cass Building, 320 S. Walnut St, Lansing, MI 48913; tel. 517/373–4700; FAX. 517/335–2121; Doris R. Gellert, Bureau Director

Office of Drug Control Policy, Michigan Department of Community Health, 320 S. Walnut Street, 5th Floor, Lansing, MI 48913; tel. 517/373–4700; FAX. 517/335–3090; Yvonne Blackmond, Director

Office of Health and Human Services, State Budget Office, Michigan Department of Management and Budget, George W. Romney Building, Box 30026, Lansing, MI 48909; tel. 517/373–1076; FAX. 517/335–1521; Charles Overbey, Director

Office of Services to the Aging, P.O. Box 30676, Lansing, MI 48909; tel. 517/373–8230; FAX. 517/373–4092

Other

Department of Education, Office of School Support Services, Coordinated School, School Health & Safety Programs, P.O. Box 30008, Lansing, MI 48909; tel. 517/241–4292; FAX. 517/373–1233; Kim Kovalchick, Consultant, CSHSP

Michigan Department of Community Health, Bureau of Health Professions, Box 30670, Lansing, MI 48909; tel. 517/373–8068; FAX. 517/241–3082; Melanie Brim, Director

Michigan Department of Community Health, Laboratories, Laboratory Improvement Section, P.O. Box 30664, Lansing, MI 48909; tel. 517/241–2648; FAX. 517/241–3354; Pamela Diebolt, Chief

Michigan Department of Human Services, 235 South Grand Avenue, P.O. Box 30037, Lansing, MI 48909; tel. 517/373–2035; FAX. 517/335–6101; Marianne Udow, Director

MINNESOTA

The Honorable Tim Pawlenty, Governor, 651/296–3391

Health

Division of Environmental Health, 625 North Robert Street, P.O. Box 64975, St. Paul, MN 55164–0975; tel. 651/201–4675; FAX. 651/201–4752; John Linc Stine, Director

Minnesota Department of Health, Compliance Monitoring Division, 85 East 7th Place, P.O. Box 64882, St. Paul, MN 55164–0882; tel. 651/201–3707; FAX. 651/215–9695; Darcy Miner, Division Director

Minnesota e–Health Initiative Advisory Committee, 85 East Seventh Place, Suite 300, St. Paul, MN 55164–0882; tel. 651/201–5508; FAX. 651/201–3830; Bill Brand, Deputy Director

Public Health Laboratory Division, Minnesota Department of Health, 601 Robert Street, N., P.O. Box 64899, St. Paul, MN 55164–0899; tel. 651/201–5256; FAX. 651/201–5064; Joanne M. Bartkus, Ph.D., Director

Social Services

Minnesota Department of Health, Division of Community and Family Health, Golden Rule Building, Suite 500, 85 East Seventh Place, Zip 55101, St. Paul, MN 55164–0882; tel. 651/296–9720; FAX. 651/215–8953; Mary Sheehan, Director

Minnesota Department of Health, Division of Disease Prevention and Control, 625 Robert Street N., P.O. Box 64975, St. Paul, MN 55764–0975; tel. 651/201–5414; FAX. 651/201–5743; Ruth Lynfield, State Epidemiologist

Minnesota Department of Human Services, Executive Office, P.O. 64998, St. Paul, MN 55164–0998; tel. 651/431–2907; FAX. 651/431–7443; Cal Ludeman, Commissioner

Rehabilitation Services Branch, Minnesota Department of Employment and Economic Development, 332 Minnesota Street, 1st National Bank Building, #E200, St. Paul, MN 55101; tel. 651/259–7345; FAX. 651/297–5159; Kimberley Peck, Director

MISSISSIPPI

The Honorable Haley Barbour, Governor, 601/359–3150

Health

Department of Health, P.O. Box 1700, Jackson, MS 32915–1700; tel. 601/576–7634; FAX. 601/576–7931; Brian W. Amy, MD, MHA, MPH

Health Planning and Resources Development Division, Mississippi State Department of Health, Osborne Building, 570 East Woodrow Wilson, Jackson, MS 39215–1700; tel. 601/576–7874; FAX. 601/576–7530; Rachel Pittman, Chief

Health Statistics, Mississippi State Department of Health, Health Statistics, Box 1700, Jackson, MS 39215–1700; tel. 601/576–7960; FAX. 601/576–7505; Judy T. Moulder, Director

Mississippi State Department of Health, P.O. Box 1700, Jackson, MS 32915–1700; tel. 601/576–7951; FAX. 601/576–7823; Kaye Bender, RN, PH.D, Deputy State Health Officer

Office of Environmental Health, Mississippi State Department of Health, 120 Osborne Building, P.O. Box 1700, Jackson, MS 32915–1700; tel. 601/576–7680; FAX. 601/576–7270; Rick Herrington, Director

Licensing

Bureau of Health Facilities Licensure and Certification, Mississippi State Department of Health, P.O. Box 1700, Jackson, MS 39215; tel. 601/364–1100; FAX. 601/364–5054; Marilynn Winborne, Director

Social Services

Children's Medical Program, MS State Department of Health, P.O. Box 1700, Jackson, MS 39215–1700; tel. 601/987–3965; FAX. 601/987–5560; Lawrence (Larry) Clark, Director

Department of Mental Health, 1101 Robert E. Lee Building, 239 N. Lamar St., Jackson, MS 39201; tel. 601/359–1288; FAX. 601/359–6295; Edwin C. LeGrand, Director

Mississippi Department of Human Services, P.O. Box 352, Jackson, MS 39205–0352; tel. 601/359–4457; FAX. 601/359–4477; Donald R. Taylor, Executive Director

State Department of Rehabilitation Services, P.O. Box 1698, Jackson, MS 39215–1698; tel. 601/853–5100; FAX. 601/853–5205; H.S. McMillan, Executive Director

Other

State Epidemiologist, 570 E. Woodrow Wilson, P.O Box 1700, Jackson, MS 32915–1700; tel. 601/576–7725; FAX. 601/576–7497; Mary Currier, M.D., MPH

MISSOURI

The Honorable Matt Blunt, Governor, 573/751–3222

Health

Department of Health and Senior Services, P.O. Box 570, Jefferson City, MO 65102; tel. 573/751–6001; FAX. 573/751–6041; Jane Drummond, Director

Missouri Department of Health – Bureau of Special Health Care Needs, 930 Wildwood Drive, P.O. Box 570, Jefferson City, MO 65102; tel. 573/751–6246; FAX. 314/751–6237; Gary Harbison, Chief

Missouri Department of Health and Senior Services, Bureau of Health Informatics, Box 570, Jefferson City, MO 65102; tel. 573/751–6272; FAX. 573/526–4102; Susan Elder, Chief

Insurance

Department of Insurance, Financial Institutions & Professional Registration, P.O. Box 690, Jefferson City, MO 65102; tel. 314/751–4126; FAX. 314/751–1165; Doug Ommen, Director

Licensing

Bureau of Health Services Regulation, Missouri Department of Health and Senior Services, P.O.Box 570, Jefferson City, MO 65102; tel. 573/751–6303; FAX. 573/526–3621; Dean Linneman, Section Administrator

Social Services

Department of Mental Health, 1706 East Elm Street, P.O. Box 687, Jefferson City, MO 65102; tel. 573/751–4122; FAX. 573/526–7926; Keith Schafer, Director

Life and Health Section, Missouri Department of Insurance, P.O. Box 690, Jefferson City, MO 65102; tel. 573/751–4363; FAX. 573/526–6075; John S. Korte, Manager

Missouri Division of Vocational Rehabilitation, 3024 DuPont Circle, Jefferson City, MO 65109–0525; tel. 573/751–3251; FAX. 314/751–1441; C. Jeanne Loyd, Assistant Commissioner

Other

Department of Elementary and Secondary Education, 205 Jefferson, P.O. Box 480, Jefferson City, MO 65102; tel. 573/751–4212; FAX. 573/751–1179; Dr. D. Kent King, Commissioner of Education

Division of Community and Public Health, P.O. Box 570, Jefferson City, MO 65102–0570; tel. 573/751–6252; FAX. 573/526–5348; Glenda R. Miller, Director

MONTANA

The Honorable Brian Schweitzer, Governor, 406/444–3111

Health

Health Resources Division, Montana Department of Public Health and Human Services, 1400 Broadway, P.O. Box 202951, Helena, MT 59620–2951; tel. 406/444–4540; FAX. 406/444–1861; Mary Dalton, Administrator

Licensing

Quality Assurance Division, Department of Public Health and Human Services, Certification Bureau, 2401 Colonial Drive, 2nd Floor, P.O. Box 202953, Helena, MT 59620–2953; tel. 406/444–2099; FAX. 406/444–3456; Marjorie VanderAarde, Chief

Social Services

Aging Services, Senior and Long Term Care Division, Department of Public Health and Human Services, 111 Sanders, P.O. Box 4210, Helena, MT 59604; tel. 406/444–4676; FAX. 406/444–7743; Kelly Moorse, State Long Term Care Ombudsman

Child and Family Services Division, P.O. Box 8005, Helena, MT 59604–8005; tel. 406/444–5902; FAX. 406/444–5956; Hank Hudson, Administrator

Disability Services Division, P.O. Box 4210, Helena, MT 59604; tel. 406/444–2590; FAX. 406/444–3632; Joe A. Mathews, Administrator

Family and Community Health Bureau, Department of Public Health & Human Services, W. F. Cogswell Building, Helena, MT 59620; tel. 406/444–4740; FAX. 406/444–2606; JoAnn Walsh Dotson, RN MSN, Bureau Chief

Montana Department of Public Health and Human Services, 111 North Sanders, P.O. Box 4210, Helena, MT 59604; tel. 406/444–5622; FAX. 406/444–1970; Joan Miles, Director

NEBRASKA

The Honorable Dave Heineman, Governor, 402/471–2244

Licensing

Nebraska Department of Health and Human Services Regulation and Licensure, Credentialing Division, 301 Centennial Mall, South 3rd Floor, P.O. Box 94986, Lincoln, NE 68509–4986; tel. 402/471–2115; FAX. 402/471–3557; Helen L. Meeks, Administrator

Office of Public Health, 301 Centennial Mall, S., P.O. Box 95007, Lincoln, NE 68509; tel. 402/471–0146; FAX. 402/471–8259; David Palm, Ph.D., Director

Social Services

Department of Health and Human Services – Division of Public Health, Certificate of Need Program, P.O. Box 94986, Lincoln, NE 68509; tel. 402/471–4963; FAX. 402/471–3577; Claire Titus, Program Manager

Lifespan Health Services, Nebraska Department of Health and Human Services, Regulation and Licensure, 301 Centennial Mall South, P.O. Box 95026, Lincoln, NE 68509–5007; tel. 402/471–3980; FAX. 402/471–7049; Paula Eurek, Unit Administrator

Nebraska Department of Health & Human Services, Division of Public Health, 301 Centennial Mall South, P.O. Box 95007, Lincoln, NE 68509–5007; tel. 402/471–3121; FAX. 402/471–9449; Joann Schaefer, MD, Director and Chief Medical Officer

Nebraska Department of Health and Human Services, 301 Centennial Mall, South., P.O. Box 95026, Lincoln, NE 68509–5026; tel. 402/471–9433; FAX. 402/471–9449; Chris Peterson, CEO

Nebraska Department of Health and Human Services, Services, 301 Centennial Mall, S., P.O. Box 95044, Lincoln, NE 95007; tel. 402/471–0191; FAX. 402/471–8259; Sue Medinger, Administrator

Nebraska Department of Health and Human Services, Special Services for Children and Adults, 301 Centennial Mall, S., P.O. Box 95044, Lincoln, NE 68509–5044; tel. 402/471–9345; FAX. 402/471–6352; Mary Jo Iwan, Administrator

Nebraska Health and Human Services, Finance and Support Medicaid Division, 301 Centennial Mall, S., P.O. Box 95026, Lincoln, NE 68509; tel. 402/471–9362; FAX. 402/471–9455; Cec Brady, Deputy Administrator

Section C

Other

Department of Education, Vocational Rehabilitation, 301 Centennial Mall, S., P.O. Box 94987, Lincoln, NE 68509; tel. 402/471–3644; FAX. 402/471–0788; Frank Lloyd, Assistant Commissioner

NEVADA

The Honorable Jim Gibbons, Governor, 775/684–5670

Health

Bureau of Health Planning and Statistics, Nevada State Health Division, 505 East King Street, Room 102, Carson City, NV 89701–4749; tel. 775/684–4155; FAX. 775/684–4156; Emil DeJan, Chief

Children With Special Health Care Needs Program, Nevada State Health Division, Bureau of Family Health Services, 3527 Goni Rd., Suite 108, Carson City, NV 89706; tel. 775/684–4285; FAX. 775/684–5840; Gloria Deyhle, MCH Nurse Consultant

Division of Mental Health and Developmental Services, 4126 Technology Way, Suite 201, Carson City, NV 89706; tel. 775/684–5943; FAX. 775/684–5966; Dr. Harold Cook, Administrator

Nevada Division of Health, 4150 Technology Way, Suite 300, Carson City, NV 89706; tel. 775/684–4200; FAX. 775/684–4211; Richard Whitley, Administrator

Nevada State Health Division, Bureau of Community Health Services, 3656 Research Way, Suite 32, Carson City, NV 89706; tel. 775/687–6944; FAX. 775/687–7693; Mary D. Sassi, Bureau Chief

Nevada State Health Laboratory, 1660 North Virginia Street, Reno, NV 89503; tel. 702/688–1335; FAX. 702/688–1460; Arthur F. DiSalvo, M.D., Director

Insurance

Division of Insurance, 788 Fairview Drive, Suite 300, Carson City, NV 89701; tel. 775/687–4270; FAX. 775/687–3937; Alice A. Molasky-Arman, Commissioner

Licensing

Bureau of Licensure and Certification, Nevada Health Division, 1550 East College Parkway, Suite 158, Carson City, NV 89706–7921; tel. 775/687–4475; FAX. 775/687–6588; Pamela S. Graham BS, RN, LNC Bureau Chief

Social Services

Department of Health and Human Services, 4126 Technology Way, 1st Floor, Room 100, Carson City, NV 89706–2009; tel. 775/684–4000; FAX. 775/684–4010; Michael J. Willden, Director

Division of Health Care Financing & Policy, 1100 East William Street, Suite 101, Carson City, NV 89701; tel. 775/684–3677; FAX. 775/687–3893; Charles Duarte, Administrator

Division of Health Care Financing and Policy–Medicaid, 1100 E. William Street, Suite 102, Carson City, NV 89701; tel. 775/684–3600; FAX. 775/687–3893; Mary Wherry, MS, RN, Deputy Administrator

Rehabilitation Division, 1370 S. Curry Street, Carson City, NV 89703; tel. 775/684–4040; FAX. 775/684–4184; Michael T. Coleman Ed.D, Administrator

NEW HAMPSHIRE

The Honorable John Lynch, Governor, 603/271–2121

Health

Department of Health and Human Services, Six Hazen Drive, Concord, NH 03301–6527; tel. 603/271–8560; FAX. 603/271–8705; William J. Kassler, M.D., MPH, State Medical Director

Department of Health and Human Services, 129 Pleasant St., Concord, NH 03301–6527; tel. 603/271–8560; FAX. 603/271–7912; Clint J. Koenig M.D., MA, MSPH, Interim Director

Division of Public Health Services, Dept. of Health and Human Services, 29 Hazen Drive, Concord, NH 03301; tel. 603/271–4501; FAX. 603/271–4827; Maryann Cooney, Director

NH Department of Health and Human Services, Office of The Commissioner, 129 Pleasant Street, Brown Building, Concord, NH 03301–3857; tel. 603/271–4602; FAX. 603/271–4912; Kathleen G. Sgambati, Deputy Commissioner

Insurance

New Hampshire Insurance Department, 21 South Fruit Street, Suite 14, Concord, NH 03301; tel. 603/271–2261; FAX. 603/271–1406; Roger A. Sevigny, Insurance Commissioner

State of New Hampshire, Insurance Department, Examination Division, 56 Old Suncook Road, Concord, NH 03301–5151; tel. 603/271–2241; FAX. 603/271–1406; Thomas S. Burke, Director

Licensing

Office of Program Support, Licensing and Regulation, Health Facilities Administration, 129 Pleasant Street, Concord, NH 03301; tel. 603/271–4607; FAX. 603/271–4968; Theresa Jarvis, Bureau Chief

Social Services

Bureau of Behavioral Health, State Office Park, S., 105 Pleasant Street, Concord, NH 03301; tel. 603/271–5000; FAX. 603/271–5058; Erik G. Riera, Bureau Administrator

New Hampshire Department of Health and Human Services, Division of Public Health Services, 29 Hazen Drive, Concord, NH 03301; tel. 603/271–4496; FAX. 603/271–0545; Donna Severance, Administrator

Vocational Rehabilitation Division, 101 Pleasant Street, Concord, NH 03301–3860; tel. 603/271–3494; FAX. 603/271–1953; Dr. Lyonel B. Tracy, Commissioner

Other

Department of Environmental Services, 29 Hazen Drive, P.O. Box 95, Concord, NH 03301; tel. 603/271–3503; FAX. 603/271–2867; Michael P. Nolin, Commissioner

State Department of Education, 101 Pleasant Street, State Office Park, South, Concord, NH 03301; tel. 603/271–3494; FAX. 603/271–1953; Lyonel B. Tracy

NEW JERSEY

The Honorable Jon Corzine, Governor, 609/292–6000

Health

Division of Health Facilities Evaluation & Licensing, P.O. Box 358, Trenton, NJ 08625; tel. 609/341–3005; FAX. 609/292–3780; John A. Calabria, Director & Alison Gibson, Director

New Jersey Department of Health and Senior Services, Certificate of Need and Healthcare Facility Licensure, P.O. Box 360, Trenton, NJ 08625–0358; tel. 609/292–8773; FAX. 609/292–3780; John A. Calabria, Director

Office of Managed Care, New Jersey State Department of Banking and Insurance Valuation Bureau, P.O. Box 325, Trenton, NJ 08625; tel. 609/292–5427; FAX. 609/633–0527; Holly Gaenzle, Assistant Chief

Licensing

Division of Consumer Affairs, 124 Halsey Street, P.O. Box 45027, Newark, NJ 07101; tel. 201/504–6534; FAX. 201/648–3538

Social Services

Department of Law and Public Safety, P.O. Box 080, 25 Market Street, Trenton, NJ 08625; tel. 609/292–8740; FAX. 609/292–3508; Anne Milgram, Attorney General

Division of Family Development, 6 Quakerbridge Plaza, Trenton, NJ 08625–0716; tel. 609/588–2401; FAX. 609/588–3369; Pearl Elias, Acting Director

Division of Family Health Services, 50 East State Street, P.O. Box 364, Trenton, NJ 08625; tel. 609/292–4043; FAX. 609/292–9599; Celeste Andriot-Wood, Assistant Commissioner

Maternal, Child and Community Health, New Jersey Department of Health and Senior Services, 50 East State Street,, P.O. Box 364, Trenton, NJ 08625–0364; tel. 609/984–1384; FAX. 609/292–3580; Dr. Linda Jones-Hicks, Director of MCCH

N.J. Department of Health and Senior Services, Division Of Health Facilities Evaluation & Licensing, P.O. Box 367, Trenton, NJ 08625; tel. 609/633–8977; FAX. 609/633–9060; William Conroy, Assistant Commissioner

New Jersey Department of Health and Senior Services, Office of the Commissioner, P.O. Box 360, Trenton, NJ 08625–0360; tel. 609/292–7837; FAX. 609/292–0053; Heather Howard, State Commissioner of Health and Senior Services

NEW MEXICO

The Honorable Bill Richardson, Governor, 505/476-2200

Health

Department of Health, P.O. Box 26110, Santa Fe, NM 87502–6110; tel. 505/827–2613; FAX. 505/827–2530; Patricia T. Montoya, Secretary

Public Health Division, New Mexico Department of Health, P.O. Box 26110, Santa Fe, NM 87502–6110; tel. 505/827–2389; FAX. 505/827–2329; Joyce Naseyowma – Chalam, Director

Insurance

New Mexico Department of Insurance, P.O. Drawer 1269, Santa Fe, NM 87504–1269; tel. 505/827–4601; FAX. 505/827–4734; Helen Hordes, Manager, Life and Health Forms Division

Public Regulation Commission, P.O. Box 1269, Santa Fe, NM 87504–1269; tel. 505/827–4299; FAX. 505/476–0326; Eric P. Serna, Superintendent of Insurance

Social Services

Division of Vocational Rehabilitation, 435 St. Michaels Drive, Building D, Santa Fe, NM 87505; tel. 505/954–8511; FAX. 505/954–8562; Gary Beene, Assistant Secretary for Division of Vocational Rehabilitation

Human Services Department, P.O. Box 2348, Santa Fe, NM 87504–2348; tel. 505/827–7750; FAX. 505/827–6286; Pamela S. Hyde, Secretary

Income Support Division, P.O. Box 2348, Santa Fe, NM 87504–2348; tel. 505/827–7250; FAX. 505/827–7203; Myrna L. Vigil, Administrator

Protective Services Division, P.O. Box 5160, Santa Fe, NM 87502–5160; tel. 505/827–8400; FAX. 505/827–8480; Merry Ortiz Y Pino, Director

Other

Public Education Dept., Education Building Jerry Apodaca Education Bldg., 300 Don Gaspar, Santa Fe, NM 87501–2786; tel. 505/827–5800; FAX. 505/827–6520; Dr. Veronica C. Garcia, Sec. Of Education

NEW YORK

The Honorable David Paterson, Governor, Governor, 518/474–7516

Health

New York State Department of Health, Empire State Plaza, Corning Tower, Room 1495, Albany, NY 12237; tel. 518/474–2011; FAX. 518/474–5450; Dr. Richard F. Daines M.D., Commissioner of Health

New York State Department of Health, Office of Health Insurance Programs, Empire State Plaza, Corning Tower, Room 1466, Albany, NY 12237; tel. 518/474–8646; FAX. 518/486–6852; Deborah Bachrach, Deputy Commissioner – Office of Health Insurance Programs

New York State Department of HealthDivision of Managed Care and Program Evaluation, Room 2001 Corning Tower Building, Empire State Plaza, Albany, NY 12237; tel. 518/474–5737; FAX. 518/474–5738; Vallencia Lloyd, Deputy Director

Office of Clinical Affairs, New York State Department of Health OHSM, Corning Tower Room 1815, Albany, NY 12237; tel. 518/402–5914; FAX. 518/402–5902; Nancy Barhydt, Dr.P.H., RN, Director

Licensing

New York State Board for Medicine, 89 Washington Avenue, West Wing 2nd Floor, Albany, NY 12234; tel. 518/474–3841; FAX. 518/486–4846; Thomas J. Monahan, Executive Secretary

Social Services

New York State Office of Alcoholism and Substance Abuse Services, 1450 Western Avenue, Albany, NY 12203; tel. 518/457–2061; FAX. 518/457–5474; Shari Noonan, Acting Commissioner

New York State Office of Mental Health, 44 Holland Avenue, Albany, NY 12229; tel. 518/474–4403; FAX. 518/474–2149; Michael F. Hogan, Ph.D., Commissioner

Office of Mental Retardation and Developmental Disabilities, 44 Holland Avenue, Albany, NY 12229; tel. 518/473–1997; FAX. 518/473–1271; Diana Jones Ritter, Commissioner

Other

Bureau of Project Management, New York State Department of Health, 433 River Street, Suite 303, Troy, NY 12180–2299; tel. 518/402–0911; FAX. 518/402–0931; Diane M. Smith, Acting Director

Office of Health Systems Management, Tower Building, Empire State Plaza, Room 1415, Albany, NY 12237–0701; tel. 518/474–7028; FAX. 518/486–2564; James W. Clyne, Jr., Deputy Commissioner, Office of Health Systems Mgmt

Wadsworth Center for Laboratories and Research, Clinical Lab Evaluatioan, P.O. Box 509, Empire State Plaza, Albany, NY 12201–0509; tel. 518/474–7592; FAX. 518/474–3439; Lawrence S. Sturman, M.D., Ph.D., Director

NORTH CAROLINA
The Honorable Michael Easley, Governor, 919/733–5811

Health

Department of Health and Human Services, 2001 Mail Service Center, Raleigh, NC 27699–2001; tel. 919/733–4534; FAX. 919/715–4645; Dempsy Benton, Secretary

Department of Health and Human Services, Division of Facility Services, 2701 Mail Service Center, Raleigh, NC 27699–2701; tel. 919/855–3750; FAX. 919/733–2757; Robert J. Fitzgerald, Director

Insurance

Department of Insurance, 1201 Mail Service Center, Raleigh, NC 27699–1201; tel. 919/807–6750; FAX. 919/733–0085; James E. Long, Commissioner

Social Services

Division of Medical Assistance, 2501Mail Service Center, Raleigh, NC 27699–2501; tel. 919/855–4100; FAX. 919/733–6608; Allen Dobson, Jr. MD Assistant Secretary for Health Policy/Medical Assist.

Division of Mental Health, Developmental Disabilities and Substance Abuse Services, 3001 Mail Service Center, Raleigh, NC 27699–3001; tel. 919/733–7011; FAX. 919/508–0951; Michael Moseley, Director

Division of Vocational Rehabilitation Services, 2801 Mail Service Center, Raleigh, NC 27699–2801; tel. 919/855–3500; FAX. 919/733–7968; Linda Harrington, Director

NORTH DAKOTA
The Honorable John Hoeven, Governor, 701/328–2200

Health

Children's Special Health Services, Department of Human Services, State Capitol, 600 East Boulevard Avenue, Dept 325, Bismarck, ND 58505–0269; tel. 701/328–2436; FAX. 701/328–1645; Tamara Gallup–Millner, Unit Director

Medical Services Division, North Dakota Department of Human Services, 600 East Boulevard Avenue, Dept 325, Bismarck, ND 58505–0250; tel. 701/328–2321; FAX. 701/328–1544; Maggie D. Anderson, Director

North Dakota Department of Health, Health Resources Section, 600 East Boulevard Avenue, Department 301, Bismarck, ND 58505–0200; tel. 701/328–2352; FAX. 701/328–1890; Darleen Bartz, Chief– Health Resources Section

State Department of Health, 600 East Boulevard Avenue, Bismarck, ND 58505–0200; tel. 701/328–2372; FAX. 701/328–4727; Londa Rodahl, Administrative Assistant

Insurance

North Dakota Department of Insurance, State Capitol, 600 East Boulevard, 5th Floor, Bismarck, ND 58505–0320; tel. 701/328–2440; FAX. 701/328–4880; Adam Hamm, Commissioner

Social Services

Division of Developmental Disabilities, Department of Human Services, 1237 W. Divide Avenue, Suite 1A, Bismarck, ND 58501; tel. 701/328–8930; FAX. 701/328–8969; Jo Anne Hoesel, Director

Division of Family Health, North Dakota Department of Health, State Capitol, 600 East Boulevard Avenue, Bismarck, ND 58505–0200; tel. 701/328–2493; FAX. 701/328–1412; Kim Senn, Director

Division of Mental Health and Substance Abuse Services, 1237 W. Divide Avenue, Suite 1c, Bismarck, ND 58501–1208; tel. 701/328–8920; FAX. 701/328–8969; JoAnne Hoesel, Director

Economic Assistance Policy Division, North Dakota Department of Human Services, 600 East Boulevard Avenue Dept 325, Bismarck, ND 58505–0250; tel. 701/328–2332; FAX. 701/328–1060; Carol K. Olson, Executive Director

Other

Facility Management Division, Office of Management and Budget, 600 East Boulevard, Ave, Dept 130, State Capitol, Bismarck, ND 58505–0130; tel. 701/328–2471; FAX. 701/328–3230; Curt Zimmerman, Director, Facility Management

Program and Policy, State Capitol, 600 East Boulevard Avenue Dept 325, Bismarck, ND 58505–0265; tel. 701/328–2310; FAX. 701/328–2359; Carol K. Olson, Executive Director

OHIO
The Honorable Ted Strickland, Governor, 614/466–3555

Health

Office of Product Regulation and Actuarial Services, 2100 Stella Court, Columbus, OH 43215–1067; tel. 614/644–3315; FAX. 614/728–5238; Teresa Reedus, Senior Contract Analyst

Ohio Department of Health, 246 North High Street, P.O. Box 118, Columbus, OH 43216–0118; tel. 614/466–3543; FAX. 614/644–0085; Alvin Jackson, MD, Director

Ohio Department of Health, Bureau of Community Health Care Facilities & Services, 246 North High Street, P.O. Box 118, Columbus, OH 43216–0118; tel. 614/995–7466; FAX. 614/387–2763; Roy Croy, Bureau Chief, Health Planning Administrator

Ohio Department of Health –Division of Prevention, 246 North High Street, Columbus, OH 43216–0118; tel. 614/466–0302; FAX. 614/564–2410; Steve Wagner, Assistant Chief

Insurance

Department of Insurance, 2100 Stella Court, Columbus, OH 43215–1067; tel. 614/719–1589; FAX. 614/644–3743; Mary Jo Hudson, Director

Licensing

Division of Quality Assurance, Ohio Department of Health, 246 North High Street, Columbus, OH 43216–0118; tel. 614/466–7857; FAX. 614/644–0208; Rebecca S. Maust, Chief, Division of Quality Assurance

Social Services

Bureau of Disability Determination, P.O. Box 359001, Columbus, OH 43235–9001; tel. 614/438–1545; FAX. 614/438–1504; Kathleen Johnson, Director

Department of Mental Health, 30 East Broad Street, Eighth Floor, Columbus, OH 43266–0414; tel. 614/466–2596; FAX. 614/752–9453; Michael F. Hogan, Ph.D., Director

Department of Mental Retardation and Developmental Disability, 1810 Sullivan Avenue, Columbus, OH 43223–0415; tel. 614/466–0129; FAX. 614/644–5013; Kenneth Ritchey, Director

Division of Family and Community Health Services, Ohio Department of Health, 246 North High Street, Columbus, OH 43215; tel. 614/466–3263; FAX. 614/728–9163; Karen Hughes, MPH, Chief

Ohio Department Jobs Family Services, Office of Ohio Health Plans, P.O. Box 182709, Columbus, OH 43218–2709; tel. 614/466–4443; FAX. 614/752–3986; John R. Corlett, Medicaid Director

Ohio Department of Alcohol and Drug Addiction Services, 280 Plaza, 280 North High Street, 12th Floor, Columbus, OH 43215–2550; tel. 614/466–3445; FAX. 614/752–8645; Gary Q. Tester, Director

Ohio Department of Human Services, 30 East Broad Street, 32nd Floor, Columbus, OH 43215–3414; tel. 614/466–6282; FAX. 614/466–2815; Barbara Riley, Director

Ohio Rehabilitation Services Commission, Bureau of Services for the Visually Impaired, 400 East Campus View Boulevard, SW3, Columbus, OH 43235–4604; tel. 614/438–1438; FAX. 614/438–1257; Mike Hanes, Director

Ohio Rehabilitation Services Commission, Bureau of Vocational Rehabilitation, 400 East Campus View Boulevard (SW3), Columbus, OH 43235–4604; tel. 614/438–1210; FAX. 614/438–1257; Katherine A. Brown, Ph.D.

Other

Bureau of Plan Operations, 30 East Broad Street, 31st Floor, Columbus, OH 43266–0423; tel. 614/466–2365; FAX. 614/752–7701; Sheila J. Fuji, Bureau Chief

OKLAHOMA
The Honorable Brad Henry, Governor, 405/521–2342

Health

Oklahoma Health Care Authority, 4545 North Lincoln Boulevard, Suite 124, Oklahoma City, OK 73105; tel. 405/522–7300; FAX. 405/530–3227; Mike Fogarty, Chief Executive Officer

Oklahoma State Department of HealthProtective Health Services, Medical Facilities Service, 1000 Northeast 10th Street, Oklahoma City, OK 73117–1299; tel. 405/271–6576; FAX. 405/271–1308; Tom Welin, Chief, Medical Facilities

Public Health Laboratory Services, 1000 Northeast 10th, Oklahoma City, OK 73117–1299; tel. 405/271–5070; FAX. 405/271–4850; Garry L. McKee, Ph.D., Chief

State Department of Health, 1000 Northeast 10th, Oklahoma City, OK 73117–1299; tel. 405/271–5600; FAX. 405/271–3431

State Department of Health, Nursing Service, 1000 Northeast 10th Street, Oklahoma City, OK 73117–1299; tel. 405/271–5183; FAX. 405/271–1897; Diana Pistole, MPH, RN

State Department of Health, Special Health Services, 1000 Northeast 10th, Oklahoma City, OK 73117–1299; tel. 405/271–4200; FAX. 405/271–2632; Brent E. VanMeter, Deputy Commissioner

Social Services

Aging Services Division, Oklahoma Department of Human Services, Sheperd Mall 2401 NW. 23rd, Ste. 40, Oklahoma City, OK 73107–2422; tel. 405/521–2327; FAX. 405/521–2086; Lance Robertson, Director

Department of Mental Health and Substance Abuse Services, 1200 N.E., 13th Street,, Oklahoma City, OK 73152–3277; tel. 405/522–3877; FAX. 405/522–0637; Rand Baker, Interim Commissioner

Oklahoma State Department of Health, Family Health Services, 1000 Northeast 10th Street, Oklahoma City, OK 73117–1299; tel. 405/271–8172; FAX. 405/271–3632; Edd D. Rhoades, M.D., MPH, Deputy Commissioner

Rehabilitation Services, 3535 Northwest 58th Street, Suite 500, Oklahoma City, OK 73112–4815; tel. 405/951–3400; FAX. 405/951–3529; Linda Parker, Director

OREGON
The Honorable Ted Kulongoski, Governor, 503/378–3111

Licensing

Department of Consumer and Business Services/Oregon, Insurance Division, PO Box 14480, Salem, OR 97301–0405; tel. 503/947–7216; FAX. 503/378–4351; Shelley Bain, Senior Policy Analyst

Oregon Health Services, Health Care Licensure and Certification, 800 Northeast Oregon Street, Suite 305, Portland, OR 97323; tel. 971/673–0546; FAX. 971/673–0556; Ron Prinslow, Manager

Social Services

Addiction and Mental Health Division, 500 Summer St. NE E86, Salem, OR 97301–1118; tel. 503/945–9704; FAX. 503/373–7327; Robert E. Nikkel, MSW, Assistant Director, DHS

Child Development and Rehabilitation Center, Oregon Health Sciences University, Box 574, Portland, OR 97207; tel. 503/494–8362; FAX. 503/494–6868; Clifford J. Sells, M.D., Director

Children, Adults & Families, 500 Summer Street, N.E ., E–62, Salem, OR 97301–1067; tel. 503/945–5600; FAX. 503/373–7032; Brian M. Johnson, Assistant Director

Department of Human Services, Community Human Services, Office of Vocational Rehabilitation Services, 500 Summer Street N.E. E–87, Salem, OR 97301–1120; tel. 503/945–6201; FAX. 503/947–5010; Stephanie Parrish Taylor, Administrator

Other

Oregon State Public Health Laboratory, P.O. Box 275, Portland, OR 97207–0275; tel. 503/693–4100; FAX. 503/693–5602; Michael R. Skeels, Ph.D., MPH

PENNSYLVANIA
The Honorable Edward G. Rendell, Governor, 717/787–2500

Health

Bureau of Health Planning, Pennsylvania Department of Health, Health and Welfare Building, Room 1033, 7th and Forester Streets, Harrisburg, PA 17120; tel. 717/772–5298; FAX. 717/705–6525; Joseph B. May, Director

Department of Health, Bureau of Laboratories, P.O. Box 500, Exton, PA 19341–0500; tel. 610/280–3464; FAX. 610/594–9972; Dr. Nancy Warren, Director

Division of Acute and Ambulatory Care, Pennsylvania Department of Health, Health and Welfare Building, Room 532, Harrisburg, PA 17120; tel. 717/783–8980; FAX. 717/705–6663

Pennsylvania Department of Health, Health and Welfare Building, Suite 802, Harrisburg, PA 17120; tel. 717/787–6436; FAX. 717/787–0191; Calvin B. Johnson, M.D., M.P.H., Secretary

Pennsylvania Department of Health, Division Home Health, 132 Kline Plaza, Suite A, Harrisburg, PA 17104; tel. 717/783–1379; FAX. 717/772–0232; Jan Staloski, Director

Pennsylvania Department of Health, Public Health Programs, 809 Health and Welfare Building, Harrisburg, PA 17120; tel. 717/787–9857; Stephen H. Suroviec, Deputy Secy. for Health Promotion & Disease Prevention

Insurance

Pennsylvania Insurance Department, 1326 Strawberry Square, Harrisburg, PA 17120; tel. 717/783–0442; FAX. 717/772–1969; Joel Ario, Acting Insurance Commissioner

Pennsylvania Insurance Department, Office of Rate and Policy Regulation, 1311 Strawberry Square, Harrisburg, PA 17120; tel. 717/783–5079; FAX. 717/787–8555; Gregory Martino, Deputy Insurance Commissioner

Licensing

Bureau of Facility Licensure and Certification, Health and Welfare Building, Room 932, Harrisburg, PA 17120; tel. 717/787–8015; FAX. 717/787–1491; Sandra M. Knobb, Acting Bureau Director

Pennsylvania Department of Health, Quality Assurance, 7th & Forster Streets, Harrisburg, PA 17120; tel. 717/783–1078; FAX. 717/525–5506; Stacy Mitchell, Acting Deputy Secretary

Social Services

Office of Children, Youth, and Families, Department of Public Welfare, P.O. Box 2675, Harrisburg, PA 17105–2675; tel. 717/787–4756; FAX. 717/787–0414; Richard J. Gold, Deputy Secretary

Office of Income Maintenance, Health and Welfare Building, Room 432, P.O. Box 2675, Harrisburg, PA 17105–2675; tel. 717/783–3063; FAX. 717/787–6765; Linda T. Blachette, Deputy Secretary

Office of Mental Health and Substance Abuse Services, P.O. Box 2675, Harrisburg, PA 17105; tel. 717/787–6443; FAX. 717/787–5394; Joan L. Erney, J.D., Deputy Secretary

Office of Vocational Rehabilitation, 1521 North Sixth Street, Harrisburg, PA 17102–2913; tel. 717/787–7312; FAX. 717/772–1629; William A. Gannon, Executive Director

Pennsylvania Department of Health, Bureau of Drug and Alcohol Programs, 02 Kline Plaza, Harrisburg, PA 17104; tel. 717/783–8200; FAX. 717/787–6285; Gene R. Boyle, Director

Pennsylvania Department of Public Welfare, Office of Medical Assistance Programs, Health and Welfare Building, Room 515, Harrisburg, PA 17120; tel. 717/787–1870; FAX. 717/787–4639; David S. Feinberg, Deputy Secretary

Other

Division of Laboratory Improvement, Bureau of Laboratories, 110 Pickering Way, Lionville, PA 19353; tel. 610/280–3464; FAX. 610/594–9763; Joseph W. Gasiewski, Director

RHODE ISLAND

The Honorable Don Carcieri, Governor, 401/222–2080

Health

Department of Health, Three Capitol Hill, Providence, RI 02908–5097; tel. 401/277–2231; FAX. 401/277–6548; Barbara A. DeBuono, M.D., MPH, Director, Health

Rhode Island Department of Health, Three Capitol Hill, Room 401, Providence, RI 02908–5097; tel. 401/222–2231; FAX. 401/222–6548; William J. Waters, Jr., Ph.D., Deputy Director

Rhode Island Department of Health, Division of Family Health, Three Capitol Hill, Room 302, Providence, RI 02908–5097; tel. 401/222–2312; FAX. 401/222–1442; William H. Hollinshead, M.D., MPH, Medical Director

Rhode Island Department of Health, Office of Health Systems Development, Three Capitol Hill, Providence, RI 02908–5097; tel. 401/222–2788; FAX. 401/273–4350; Michael K. Dexter, Chief

Rhode Island Department of Human Services, Division of Health Care Quality, Financing, and Purchasing, 600 New London Avenue, Cranston, RI 02920; tel. 401/464–5274; John Young, Associate Director

Insurance

Division of Insurance, 233 Richmond Street, Suite 233, Providence, RI 02903–4233; tel. 401/277–2223; FAX. 401/751–4887; Charles P. Kwolek, Jr., CPA, Associate Director, Supervisor

Licensing

Division of Professional Regulation, Rhode Island Department of Health, Three Capitol Hill, Suite 104, Providence, RI 02908–5097; tel. 401/222–2827; FAX. 401/222–1272; Russell J. Spaight, Administrator

Social Services

Office of Rehabilitation Services, 40 Fountain Street, Providence, RI 02903; tel. 401/421–7005; FAX. 401/222–3574; Steve Brunero, Acting Administrator

Rhode Island Department of Health, Office of Facilities Regulation, 3 Capitol Hill, Room 306, Providence, RI 02908–5097; tel. 401/222–2566; FAX. 401/222–3999; Raymond Rusin, Chief

Rhode Island Department of Human Division of Health Care Quality, Financing and Purchasing, 600 New London Avenue, Cranston, RI 02920; tel. 401/464–3575; FAX. 401/464–6338; John Young, Deputy Director

Rhode Island Department of Mental Health, Retardation and Hospitals, Barry Hall, 14 Harrington Road, Cranston, RI 02920; tel. 401/462–3201; FAX. 401/462–3204; Ellen Nelson, Ph.D., Director

Other

Department of Business RegulationOffice of the Health Insurance Commissioner, 233 Richmond Street, Suite 237, Providence, RI 02903–4237; tel. 401/222–5424; FAX. 401/222–6098; Christopher F. Koller, Health Insurance Commissioner

SOUTH CAROLINA

The Honorable Mark Sanford, Governor, 803/734–2100

Health

Bureau of Maternal and Child Health, South Carolina Department of Health and Environmental Control, Mill/Jarrett Complex, Box 101106, Columbia, SC 29211; tel. 803/898–3780; FAX. 803/898–2065; Brenda Y. Martin, RNC, MN, CNAA, Bureau Director

Department of Health and Environmental Control, 2600 Bull Street, Columbia, SC 29201; tel. 803/898–3300; FAX. 803/898–3323; C. Earl Hunter, Commissioner

Department of Health and Human Services, 1801 Main Street, P.O. Box 8206, Columbia, SC 29202–8206; tel. 803/898–2500; FAX. 803/255–8235; Emma Forkner, Director

Division of Preventive and Personal Health, South Carolina Department of Health and Environmental Control, 2600 Bull Street, Columbia, SC 29201; tel. 803/737–4040; FAX. 803/737–4036; Mick Henry, Division Chief

SC. DHEC Health Services Deputy Area, 2600 Bull Street, Columbia, SC 29201; tel. 803/898–0307; FAX. 803/898–0588; Richard L. Hatfield, Assistant Deputy Commissioner Public Health Services

Licensing

Department of Health and Environmental Control, Division of Health Licensing, 2600 Bull Street, Columbia, SC 29201; tel. 803/545–4370; FAX. 803/545–4212; Dennis Gibbs, Director, Division of Health Licensing

Social Services

Bureau of Drug Control, South Carolina Department of Health and Environmental Control, 2600 Bull Street, Columbia, SC 29201; tel. 803/896–0636; FAX. 803/896–0625; Wilbur L. Harling, Director

LLR SC Board of Nursing, 110 Centerview Drive, Suite 202, Columbia, SC 29210; tel. 803/896–4550; FAX. 803/896–4525; Joan K. Bainer, RN, MN, CNA BC, Board Administrator

South Carolina Commission for the Blind, P.O. Box 79, Columbia, SC 29202–0079; tel. 803/898–8822; FAX. 803/898–8852

South Carolina Department of Alcohol and Other Drug Abuse Services, 101 Executive Park Boulevard, Columbia, SC 29202; tel. 803/896–5555; FAX. 803/896–5557; W. Lee Catoe, Director

South Carolina Department of Disabilities and Special Needs, 3440 Harden Street Extension, P.O. Box 4706, Columbia, SC 29240; tel. 803/898–9769; FAX. 803/898–9656; Stan Butkus, PhD, State Director

South Carolina Department of Health and Environmental Control, Bureau Community Health & Chronic Disease Prevention, 1777 St. Julian Place, Columbia, SC 29204; tel. 803/545–4481; FAX. 803/545–4921; Michael D. Byrd, Ph.D., MPH, LMSW

South Carolina Department of Health and Human Services, Office of Senior and Long Term Care Services, 1801 Main Street, P.O. Box 8206, Columbia, SC 29202–8206; tel. 803/898–2500; FAX. 803/898–4515; Elizabeth M. Fuller, Deputy Director – Officer

South Carolina Department of Social Services, P.O. Box 1520, Columbia, SC 29202; tel. 803/898–7360; FAX. 803/898–7277; Kathleen M. Hayes, Ph.D.

State Department of Mental Health, 2414 Bull Street, P.O. Box 485, Columbia, SC 29202; tel. 803/898–8319; FAX. 803/898–8586; John H. Magill, State Director

Vocational Rehabilitation Department, 1410 Boston Avenue, P.O. Box 15, West Columbia, SC 29171–0015; tel. 803/896–6504; FAX. 803/896–6510; Larry C. Bryant, Commissioner

Other

SCDHEC Bureau of Laboratories, 8231 Parklane Road, Columbia, SC 29223; tel. 803/896–0800; FAX. 803/896–0983; Dr. Arthur Wozniak, Bureau Chief

SOUTH DAKOTA

The Honorable Mike Rounds, Governor, 605/773–3212

Health

Division of Developmental Disabilities, Hillsview Plaza, E. Highway 34, c/o 500 East Capitol, Pierre, SD 57501–5070; tel. 605/773–3438; FAX. 605/773–7562; Wanda Seiler, Director

Division of Health Systems Development and Regulation, South Dakota Department of Health, HayesBuilding, 600 East Capitol, Pierre, SD 57501; tel. 605/773–3361; FAX. 605/773–5683; Thomas Martinec, Division Director

South Dakota Department of Health, 600 East Capitol, Pierre, SD 57501–2536; tel. 605/773–3361; FAX. 605/773–5683; Doneen B. Hollingsworth, Secretary of Health

South Dakota Department of Health, Division of Health and Medical Services, 615 East Fourth Street, Pierre, SD 57501; tel. 605/773–3737; FAX. 605/773–5942; Gail Gray, Director

Licensing

Office of Health Care Facilities Licensure and Certification, State Department of Health, 615 E. Fourth Street, Pierre, SD 57501; tel. 605/773–3356; FAX. 605/773–6667; Robert J. Stahl, Administrator

Social Services

Department of Human Services, East Highway 34, Hillsview Plaza, c/o 500 East Capitol, Pierre, SD 57501; tel. 605/773–5990; FAX. 605/773–5483; John N. Jones, Secretary

Department of Social Services, 700 Governors Drive, Pierre, SD 57501–2291; tel. 605/773–3165; FAX. 605/773–4855; Deborah K. Bowman, Secretary

Division of Alcohol and Drug Abuse, 3800 East Highway 34, Hillsview Plaza, Pierre, SD 57501; tel. 605/773–3123; FAX. 605/773–7076; Gilbert Sudbeck, Director

Division of Medical Services, 700 Governor's Drive, Pierre, SD 57501–2291; tel. 605/773–3495; FAX. 605/773–5246; Larry Iversen, Director

TENNESSEE

The Honorable Phil Bredesen, Governor, 615/741–2001

Health

Department of Health, Cordell Hull Building, 3rd Floor, 425 Fifth Avenue, N., Nashville, TN 37247–0101; tel. 615/741–3111; FAX. 615/741–2491; Susan R. Cooper, MSN, RN, Commissioner

Licensing

Board for Licensing Health Care Facilities, 227 French Landing, Suite 501, Heritage Place Metro Center, Nashville, TN 37243; tel. 615/741–7221; FAX. 615/741–7051; Jere Younger, Certification Director

Department of Health, Bureau of Health Licensure and Regulation, Cordell Hull Building, 425 Fifth Avenue, N., Nashville, TN 37247–0501; tel. 615/741–8402; FAX. 615/741–5542; Judy Eads, Assistant Commissioner

Tennessee Medical Laboratory Board, 227 French Landing, Suite 300, Heritage Place MetroCenter, Nashville, TN 37247; tel. 615/532–5128; FAX. 615/741–7698; Lynda S. England, Director

Social Services

Bureau of Alcohol and Drug Abuse Services – TN Dept. of Health, Cordell Hull Building, 425 Fifth Avenue North, Nashville, TN 37247–4401; tel. 615/741–1921; FAX. 615/532–2419; Stephanie W. Perry, M.D., Assistant Commissioner

Department of Children's Services, Program Operations, 3712 Middlebrook Pk., Knoxville, TN 37921; tel. 865/594–7101; FAX. 865/637–8824; Cathy R. Smith, Assistant Commissioner, Department

Division of Rehabilitation Services, Citizens Plaza State Office Building, 15th Floor, Nashville, TN 37248–0060; tel. 615/313–4714; FAX. 615/741–4165; Andrea L. Cooper, Assistant Commissioner

Medicaid/TennCare, 729 Church Street, Nashville, TN 37247–6501; tel. 615/741–0213; FAX. 615/741–0882; Manny Martins, Deputy Commissioner

Tennessee Commission on Aging and Disability, 500 Deaderick Street, Suite 825, Nashville, TN 37243–0860; tel. 615/741–2056; FAX. 615/741–2056; Richard M. Hann, Executive Director

Tennessee Department of Mental Health and Developmental Disabilities, Cordell Hull Building, 3rd floor, 425 Fifth Avenue, N, Nashville, TN 37243–0675; tel. 615/532–6500; FAX. 615/532–6514; Virginia Trotter Betts, Commissioner

Tennessee Rehabilitation Center, 460 Ninth Avenue, Smyrna, TN 37167; tel. 615/459–6811; FAX. 615/355–1373; David Holmes, Superintendent

Other

Bureau of Administrative Services, Tennessee Department of Health, Andrew Johnson Tower, Tenth Floor, Nashville, TN 37243; tel. 615/741–3151; FAX. 615/253–1998; Eugene Neubert Assistant Commissioner

TEXAS

The Honorable Rick Perry, Governor, 512/463–2000

Health

Department of State Health Services, State Hospital Section, 909 West 45th Street, MC: 2023, Austin, TX 78751; tel. 512/206–4616; FAX. 512/206–5089; Tex Killion, Deputy Medical Director for Administration

Health & Human Services Commission, 4900 N. Lamar, 4th Floor, Austin, TX 78751; tel. 512/424–6517; FAX. 512/424–6585; Randy P. Washington, Deputy Commissioner, Health Care

Specialized Health Services Section, Department of State Health Services, 1100 West 49th Street, Austin, TX 78756; tel. 512/458–7700; FAX. 512/458–7264; L. Jann Melton–Kissel

Texas Department of State Health, 1100 West 49th Street, Austin, TX 78756; tel. 512/458–7375; FAX. 512/458–7477; David L. Lakey, MD, Commissioner

Texas Department of State Health Services, Center For Health Statistics, 1100 West 49th Street, Austin, TX 78756; tel. 512/458–7261; FAX. 512/458–7344; Ramdas Menon, Ph.D., Director

Texas Department of State Health Services, Patient Quality Care Unit, 1100 West 49th Street, Austin, TX 78756; tel. 512/834–6650; FAX. 512/834–6653; Derek Jakovich, Manager

Insurance

Texas Department of Insurance, P.O. Box 149104, Mail Code 106–1A, Austin, TX 78714–9104; tel. 512/322–3401; FAX. 512/322–3552; Ana M. Smith–Daley, Deputy Commissioner, Life/Health Division

UTAH

The Honorable Jon Huntsman, Jr., Governor, 801/538–1000

Health

Utah Department of Health, P.O. Box 14100, Salt Lake City, UT 84114–1000; tel. 801/538–6111; FAX. 801/538–6306; Rod L. Betit, Executive Director

Utah Department of Health, Community and Family Health Services Division, P.O. Box 142001, Salt Lake City, UT 84114–2001; tel. 801/538–6901; FAX. 801/538–6591; George Delavan, M.D., Director

Utah Department of Health, Division of Epidemiology and Laboratories, 46 North Medical Drive, Salt Lake City, UT 84113; tel. 801/584–8400; FAX. 801/584–8486; Patrick F. Luedtke, MD, MPH, Director

Utah Department of Health, Office of Primary Care and Rural Health, P.O. Box 142005, Salt Lake City, UT 84114–2005; tel. 801/538–6113; FAX. 801/538–6387; Don Beckwith, Manager

Utah Department of Health – Bureau of Health, Facility Licensing, Certification and Resident Assessment, Box 144103, Salt Lake City, UT 84114–4103; tel. 801/538–6158; FAX. 801/538–6163; Allan Elkins, Director

Insurance

Insurance Department, State Office Building, Suite 3110, Salt Lake City, UT 84114; tel. 801/538–3800; FAX. 801/538–3829; D. Kent Michie, Insurance Commissioner

Licensing

Division of Occupational and Professional Licensing, Heber M. Wells Building, 160 East 300 South, Salt Lake City, UT 84114–6741; tel. 801/530–6628; FAX. 801/530–6511; F. David Stanley, Division Director

Social Services

Department of Human Services, 120 North 200 West #319, Salt Lake City, UT 84103; tel. 801/538–4001; FAX. 801/538–4016; Lisa–Michele Church, Executive Director

Division of Aging and Adult Services, 120 North 200 West, Room 325, Salt Lake City, UT 84103; tel. 801/538–3910; FAX. 801/538–4395; Alan K. Ormsby

Division of Child and Family Services, 120 North. 200 W., Suite 225, Salt Lake City, UT 84103; tel. 801/538–4100; FAX. 801/538–3993; Duane Betournay, Director

Division of Health Care Financing (Utah Medicaid), P.O. Box 144102, Salt Lake City, UT 84114–4102; tel. 801/538–6406; FAX. 801/538–6099; Michael Hales, Director

Division of Services for People With Disabilities, 120 North 200 West, Suite 411, Salt Lake City, UT 84103; tel. 801/538–4200; FAX. 801/538–4279; George Kelner Ph.D

Utah Division of Substance Abuse, 120 North 200 West, Room 209, Salt Lake City, UT 84103; tel. 801/538–3939; FAX. 801/538–9892; Randall W. Bachman, M. Ed.

Utah State Office of Rehabilitation, 250 East 500 South, P.O.Box 1444200, Salt Lake City, UT 84114–4200; tel. 801/538–7530; FAX. 801/538–7522; Donald R. Uchida, Executive Director

Youth Corrections, P.O. Box 45500, Salt Lake City, UT 84145–0500; tel. 801/538–4330; FAX. 801/538–4334; Gary K. Dalton, Director

Other

Department of Environmental Quality, 168 No 1950 West, Salt Lake City, UT 84116; tel. 801/536–4400; FAX. 801/536–0061; Dianne R. Nielson, Ph.D., Executive Director

VERMONT

The Honorable James H. Douglas, Governor, 802/828–3333

Health

Department of Health, Division of Mental Health, 108 Cherry Street, P.O. Box 70, Burlington, VT 05401; tel. 802/951–1258; Susan W. Besio, PhD, Commissioner

Department of Mental Health, P.O. Box 70, Burlington, VT 05402; tel. 802/652–2000; FAX. 802/652–2005; Michael Hartman, Commissioner

Environmental Health Office, 108 Cherry Street, P.O. Box 70, Burlington, VT 05402; tel. 802/863–7220; FAX. 802/863–7425; Austin Sumner, MD, MPH, State Epidemiologist for Non–Infectious Disease

Vermont Department of Health, 108 Cherry Street, P.O. Box 70, Burlington, VT 05402; tel. 802/863–7280; FAX. 802/863–7425; Paul E. Jarris, MD., MBA, Commissioner

Vermont Department of Health, Division of Community Public Health, 108 Cherry Street, P.O. Box 70, Burlington, VT 05402–0070; tel. 802/863–7347; FAX. 802/863–7229; Patricia Berry, Director

Vermont Department of Health, Division of Health Surveillance, 108 Cherry Street, P.O. Box 70, Burlington, VT 05402; tel. 802/863–7494; FAX. 802/652–4157; William K. Apao, Ph.D., Director of Health Surveillance

Vermont Department of Health, Division of Health Surveillance, Public Health Statistics, 108 Cherry Street, P.O. Box 70, Burlington, VT 05402–0070; tel. 802/863–7300; FAX. 802/865–7701; Peggy Brozicevic, Research and Statistics Chief

Vermont Department of Health Laboratory, 195 Colchester Avenue, P.O. Box 1125, Burlington, VT 05402–1125; tel. 802/863–7335; FAX. 802/863–7632; Mary Colotti, MS, Director

Insurance

Department of Banking, Insurance, Securities & Health Care Adm., 89 Main Street, Montpelier, VT 05620–3101; tel. 802/828–3301; FAX. 802/828–2896; Paulette J. Thabault, Commissioner

Licensing

Licensing and Protection, Ladd Hall, 103 South Main Street, Waterbury, VT 05671–2306; tel. 802/241–2345; FAX. 802/241–2358; Laine Lucenti, Director

Vermont Department of Disabilities Aging and Independent Living, Division of Licensing and Protection, Ladd Hall, 103 South Main Street, Waterbury, VT 05671–2306; tel. 802/241–2345; FAX. 802/241–2358; Frances L. Keeler, RN, MSN, DBA, Director

Social Services

Agency of Human Services, 103 South Main Street, Waterbury, VT 05676; tel. 802/241–2220; FAX. 802/241–2979; Cornelius Hogan, Secretary

Department for Children and Families, 103 South Main Street, Osgood Building 3rd floor, Waterbury, VT 05671–2401; tel. 802/241–2100; FAX. 802/241–2980; James L. Morse, Commissioner

Department of Social Welfare, 103 South Main Street, Waterbury, VT 05671–1201; tel. 802/241–2853; FAX. 802/241–2830; M. Jane Kitchel, Commissioner

Division of Alcohol and Drug Abuse Programs, 108 Cherry Street, Burlington, VT 05401; tel. 802/951–1258; FAX. 802/951–1275; Barbara Cimaglio, Deputy Commissioner

Office of Vermont Health Access/Medicaid, 312 Hurricane Lane, Suite 201, Williston, VT 05495; tel. 802/879–5900; FAX. 802/879–5919; Joshua Slen, Director

Vocational Rehabilitation Division, 103 South Main Street, Waterbury, VT 05671–2303; tel. 802/241–2186; FAX. 802/241–3359; Diane P. Dalmasse, Director

VIRGINIA

The Honorable Tim Kaine, Governor, 804/786–2211

Health

Virginia Department of Health, P.O. Box 2448, Richmond, VA 23218; tel. 804/864–7001; FAX. 804/864–7022; Robert B. Stroube, M.D., MPH, State Health Commissioner

Insurance

Bureau of Insurance, Virginia State Corporation Commission, P.O. Box 1157, Richmond, VA 23218; tel. 804/371–9691; FAX. 804/371–9944; Life and Health Consumer Services Section

State Corporation Commission Bureau of Insurance, Company Licensing and Regulatory Compliance Section, P.O. Box 1157, Richmond, VA 23209; tel. 904/371–9636; FAX. 904/371–9396; Andy Delbridge, Supervisor

State Corporation Commission–Bureau of Insurance, P.O. Box 1157, Richmond, VA 23218; tel. 804/371–9869; FAX. 804/371–9511; Douglas C. Stolte, Deputy Insurance Commissioner

Licensing

Office of Licensure and Certification, Virginia Department of Health, 9960 Maryland Drive, Suite 401, Richmond, VA 23233; tel. 804/367–2102; FAX. 804/527–4502; Chris Durrer, Director

Social Services

Children with Special Health Care Needs Program, 109 Governor Street, Eighth Floor, Richmond, VA 23218; tel. 804/864–7706; FAX. 804/846–7723; Nancy R. Bullock, RN, MPH, Director

Department for the Aging, 1610 Forest Avenue, Suite 100, Richmond, VA 23229; tel. 804/662–9333; FAX. 804/662–9354; Linda Nablo, Commissioner

Department of Medical Assistance Services, 600 East Broad Street, Suite 1300, Richmond, VA 23219; tel. 804/786–8099; FAX. 804/371–4981; Patrick W. Finnerty, Director

Department of Mental Health, Mental Retardation and Substance Abuse Services, 1220 Bank Street, P.O. Box 1797, Richmond, VA 23218–1797; tel. 804/786–3921; FAX. 804/371–6638; James S. Reinhard, M.D., Commissioner

Department of Rehabilitative Services, 8004 Franklin Farms Drive, Richmond, VA 23229; tel. 804/662–7000; FAX. 804/662–9532; James A. Rothrock, Commissioner

Division of Women's and Infants' Health, 109 Governor Street, P.O. Box 2448, Richmond, VA 23218–2448; tel. 804/864–7750; FAX. 804/864–7771; Joan Corder–Mabe, RNC, M.S., WHNP, Director

Virginia Department of Social Services, 7 N. 8th Street, Richmond, VA 23219–1949; tel. 804/726–7000; FAX. 804/726–7015; Anthony Conyers, Jr., Commissioner

WASHINGTON

The Honorable Christine Gregoire, Governor, 360/902–4111

Health

Department of Health, Facilities and Services Licensing, P.O. Box 47852, Olympia, WA 98504–7852; tel. 206/705–6652; FAX. 206/705–6654; Kathy Stout, Director

Department of Health, Office of Emergency Medical Services and Trauma System, P.O. Box 47853, Olympia, WA 98504–7853; tel. 360/236–2828; FAX. 360/236–2830; Janet Kastl, Director

Insurance

Office of the Insurance Commissioner, Insurance Building, P.O. Box 40258, Olympia, WA 98504–0258; tel. 360/725–7100; FAX. 360/586–3535; Mike Kreidler, Insurance Commissioner

Licensing

Health Systems Quality Assurance, Department of Health, 310 Israel Rd. SE, Mail Stop 47850, Tumwater, WA 98504–7850; tel. 360/236–4600; FAX. 360/236–4626; Laurie Jinkins, Assistant Secretary

Social Services

Division of Alcohol and Substance Abuse, P.O. Box 45330, Mail Stop 45330, Olympia, WA 98504–5330; tel. 360/725–3700; FAX. 360/438–8078; Doug Allen, Director

Division of Vocational Rehabilitation, P.O. Box 45340, Olympia, WA 98504–5340; tel. 360/725–3636; FAX. 360/438–8007; Lynnae Ruttledge, Director

Health and Recovery Services Administration, P.O. Box 45502, Olympia, WA 98504–5502; tel. 360/725–1863; FAX. 360/586–9551; Doug Porter, Assistant Secretary

State Department of Social and Health Services, P.O. Box 45502, Olympia, WA 98504–5502; tel. 360/725–1863; FAX. 360/586–9551; Douglas Porter, Assistant Secretary

Other

Washington State Nursing Care Quality Assurance Commission, 310 Isreal Road, P.O. Box 47864, Tumwater, WA 98504–7864; tel. 360/236–4713; FAX. 360/236–4738; Paula R. Meyer, MSN, Executive Director

WEST VIRGINIA

The Honorable Joe Manchin III, Governor, 304/558–2000

Health

Bureau for Public Health, 350 Capitol Street, Room 702, Charleston, WV 25301; tel. 304/558–2971; FAX. 304/558–1035; Chris Curtis, M.P.H., Acting Commissioner

Children with Special Health Care Needs Program, 350 Capitol Street, Room 427, Charleston, WV 25301; tel. 304/558–5388; FAX. 304/558–2866; Cathy Capps–Amburgey, Director

Department of Health and Human Resources, Capitol Complex, Building Three, Room 206, Charleston, WV 25305; tel. 304/558–0684; FAX. 304/558–1130; Martha Yeager Walker, Cabinet Secretary

Office of Community and Rural Health Services, Bureau for Public Health, 350 Capitol Street, Room 515, Charleston, WV 25301–3716; tel. 304/558–3210; FAX. 504/558–1437

Office of Environmental Health Services, Capitol and Washington Streets, 1 Davis Square, Charleston, WV 25301–1798; tel. 304/558–2981; FAX. 304/558–1291; Barbara S. Taylor

West Virginia Department of Health and Human Resources, Division of Primary Care, 350 Capitol Street, Room 515, Charleston, WV 25301–3716; tel. 304/558–4007; FAX. 304/558–1437; Nancy Bazzle, Director

Insurance

Office of the West Virginia Insurance Commissioner, 1124 Smith Street, Charleston, WV 25301; tel. 304/558–2100; FAX. 304/558–1365; J. Leah Cooper, Director, Chief Examiner

West Virginia Offices of the Insurance Commissioner, P.O. Box 50540, Charleston, WV 25305–0540; tel. 304/558–3354; FAX. 304/558–0412; Jane L. Cline, Commissioner

Licensing

Office of Chief Medical Examiner, State of West Virginia, 701 Jefferson Road, South Charles, WV 25309; tel. 304/558–3920; FAX. 304/558–7886; James A. Kaplan, M.D., Chief Medical Examiner

Office of Health Facility Licensure and Certification, West Virginia Department of Health and Human Resources, 1 Davis Square, Suite 101, Charleston, WV 25301–1799; tel. 304/558–0585; FAX. 304/558–5607; John M. Wilkinson, Director

Social Services

Division of Rehabilitation Services, P.O. Box 50890, State Capitol Complex, Charleston, WV 25305–0890; tel. 304/766–4985; FAX. 304/766–4956; Sonja School, Manager, WV Rehabilitation Hospital

Division on Alcoholism and Drug Abuse, 350 Capitol Street, Room 350, Charleston, WV 25305; tel. 304/558–2276; FAX. 304/558–1008; Stephen S. Mason, Director

WISCONSIN

The Honorable Jim Doyle, Governor, 608/266–1212

Health

Bureau of Health Information and Policy, P.O. Box 309, Madison, WI 53701–0309; tel. 608/266–1371; FAX. 608/261–4972; John Kiesow, State Registrar

Bureau of Health ServicesWisconsin Department of Correction, P.O. Box 7925, Madison, WI 53707–7925; tel. 608/240–5120; FAX. 608/240–3311; James Greer, Bureau Director of Health Services

Division of Public Health, P.O. Box 2659, Madison, WI 53701–2659; tel. 608/266–1251; FAX. 608/267–2832; Sheri Johnson PhD, Administrator

Insurance

Office of the Commissioner of Insurance, 125 S. Webster St., P.O. Box 7873, Madison, WI 53707–7873; tel. 608/266–3585; FAX. 608/266–9935; Eileen Mallow, Assistant Deputy Commissioner

Licensing

State of Wisconsin, Department of Regulation and Licensing, 1400 East Washington Avenue, P.O. Box 8935, Madison, WI 53708–8935; tel. 608/266–2112; FAX. 608/267–3816

Social Services

Department of Health and Family Services, P.O. Box 7850, Madison, WI 53707–7850; tel. 608/266–9622; FAX. 608/266–7882; Kerin R. Hayden, Secretary

Division for Learning Support: Equity and Advocacy, Wisconsin Department of Public Instruction, 125 South Webster Street, P.O. Box 7841, Madison, WI 53707–7841; tel. 608/266–1649; FAX. 608/267–3746; Carolyn S. Taylor, Assistant State Superintendent

Division of Health Care Access and Accountability (Wisconsin Medicaid), One West Wilson Street, Room 350, P.O. Box 309, Madison, WI 53701–0309; tel. 608/266–8922; FAX. 608/266–1096; Jason A. Helgerson, Administrator

Division of Vocational Rehabilitation, P.O. Box 7852, Madison, WI 53707–7852; tel. 608/261–0050; FAX. 608/266–1133; Charlene Dwyer, Administrator

Other

State Department of Public Instruction, 125 South Webster Street, P.O. Box 7841, Madison, WI 53707–7841; tel. 608/266–1771; FAX. 608/267–1052; Elizabeth Burmaster, State Superintendent

WYOMING

The Honorable Dave Freudenthal, Governor, 307/777–7434

Health

Children's Special Health, Wyoming Department of Health, 6101 N. Yellowstone Rd., Suite 420, Cheyenne, WY 82002; tel. 307/777–7941; FAX. 307/777–7215; Paul Ramirez, CHS Program Manager

Department of Health, 401 Hathaway Building, Cheyenne, WY 82002; tel. 307/777–7656; FAX. 307/777–7439

Mental Health and Substance Abuse Division, 6101 Yellowstone Road, Suite 220, Cheyenne, WY 82002–0480; tel. 307/777–7094; FAX. 307/777–5580; Mary Flanderka, Administrator for Community Services and Prevention

Wyoming Department of Health, Community & Family Health Division, 4020 House Avenue, Cheyenne, WY 82002; tel. 307/777–6004; FAX. 307/777–3617; Molly Bruner, MSN,RNC, Administrator

Licensing

Health Facilities Licensing, Department of Health, Metropolitan Bank Building, Eighth Floor, Cheyenne, WY 82002; tel. 307/777–7123; FAX. 307/777–5970; Charlie Simineo, Program Manager

Social Services

Department of Family Services, Hathaway Building, Third Floor, 2300 Capitol Avenue, Cheyenne, WY 82002–0490; tel. 307/777–7561; FAX. 307/777–7747; Tony Lewis, Director

Division of Vocational Rehabilitation, Herschler Building, Room 1100, Cheyenne, WY 82002; tel. 307/777–7386; FAX. 307/777–5939; Jim McIntosh, Administrator

Wyoming Department of Health, Aging Division, 6101 Yellowstone Road, Suite 259B, Cheyenne, WY 82002; tel. 800/442–2766; FAX. 307/777–5340; Beverly Morrow, Administrator

Wyoming Department of Health–Health Care Financing, Office of Medicaid, 6101 Yellowstone Rd., Suite 210, Cheyenne, WY 82002; tel. 307/777–5081; FAX. 307/777–6964; Renee Props, Facilities Manager

U.S. Associated Areas

GUAM

Social Services

Department of Public Health and Social Services, P.O. Box 2816, Hagatna, GU 96932; tel. 671/735–7102; FAX. 671/734–5910; Peter John D. Camacho, MPH, Acting Director

Division of Public Welfare, #123 Chalan Kareta, Mangilao, GU 969136304; tel. 671/735–7274; FAX. 671/734–7015; Lydia D. Enorio, Acting Chief HAS

PUERTO RICO

Health

Dental Health, Building A–Medical Center, P.O. Box 70184, San Juan, PR 00936; tel. 787/274–7842; FAX. 787/274–6859; Wanda Urbiztondo, D.M.D., MPH, Oral Health Coordinator

Department of Health, Secretary ship for Preventive Medicine and Family Health, Pan–American Health Org., Call Box 70184, San Juan, PR 00936; tel. 787/274–7698; FAX. 787/250–1119; Dr. Raul G. Castellanos Bran, Director, Division of FAA

Environmental Health, Department of Health, Building A, Psiq Hospital, Box 70184, San Juan, PR 00936–0184; tel. 7872747796; FAX. 787/274–7814; Alfredo Casta Velez, Assistant Secretary, Environmental Health

Mental Health and Anti Addiction Services, P.O. Box 21414, San Juan, PR 00928–1414; tel. 787/764–3795; FAX. 787/765–5888; Jose L. Galarza Arbona, MD, MPH

Puerto Rico Department of Health, Building A – Medical Center, Call Box 70184, San Juan, PR 00936–8184; tel. 787/274–6822; FAX. 787/767–8341; Rosa Perez–Perdomo, MD, MPH, PhD, Secretary of Health

Social Services

Department of Family, Call Box 11398, San Juan, PR 00910–1398; tel. 787/294–4900; FAX. 787/294–0732; Felix Matos, Ph.D., Secretary

Puerto Rico Vocational Rehabilitation Administration, Department of Labor and Human Resources, PO Box 191118, San Juan, PR 00919–1118; tel. 707/727–0445; FAX. 787/728–8070; Mrs. Dorcas Hernandez–Arroyo, MRC/CRC Administrator

Other

Department of Health for the Commonwealth of Puerto Rico, Building A–Medical Center, Call Box 70184, San Juan, PR 00936; tel. 809/274–7604; FAX. 809/250–6547; Jr. Johnny V. Rullan, MD, FACPH, Secretary of Health

VIRGIN ISLANDS

Health

Department of Health, Division of Financial Services, Knud Hansen Complex, St. Thomas, VI 00802; tel. 809/774–3171; FAX. 809/777–5120; Alphonse J. Stalliard, Deputy Commissioner

Division of Environmental Health, John Moorehead Complex, Charlotte Amalie, St. Thomas, VI 00802; tel. 340/774–9000; FAX. 340/715–5140; Leonard Reed, Director

Division of Hospitals and Medical Services, Roy Lester Schneider Hospital, 9048 Sugar Estate, St. Thomas, VI 00802; tel. 340/776–8311; FAX. 340/714–6340; Maureen G. Venzen, MPA, Vice President Administration

Prevention, Health, Promotion and Protection, Department of Health, Charles Harwood Hospital, 3500 Richmond Christiansted, St. Croix, VI 00820–4300; tel. 340/773–1311; FAX. 340/773–1376; Vivian J. Ebbesen–Fludd, RN, BSN, MS, Commissioner

Virgin Islands Department of Health, St. Thomas Hospital, St. Thomas, VI 00802; tel. 809/774–0117; FAX. 809/777–4001; Ralph A. de Chabert, M.D., Acting Commissioner

Social Services

Department of HealthDivision of Mental Health, Alcoholism and Drug Dependency Services, Department of Health, Barbel Plaza South, 1st Floor, St. Thomas, VI 00802; tel. 340/774–4888; FAX. 340/774–4701; Ray Fonseca, Acting Director

Disabilities and Vocational Rehabilitation Services, Department of Human Services, Knud Hansen Complex–Building A, 1303 Hospital Ground, St. Thomas, VI 00802; tel. 809/774–0930; FAX. 809/774–3466; Beverly C. Plaskett, Administrator

Division of Maternal and Child Health Services, Virgin Islands Department of Health, #31012 Vitaraco Park, Estate Golden Park, St. Croix, VI 00820; tel. 340/773–9924; FAX. 340/713/9928; Mavis Matthew, MD, MPH Director

Office of the CommissionerDepartment of Human Services, Knud Hansen Complex, Building A, St. Thomas, VI 00802; tel. 340/774–1166; FAX. 340/774–3466; Christopher E. Finch, Commissioner

Canada

ALBERTA

Social Services

Department of Family and Social Services, 109 Street and 97 Avenue, Edmonton, AB T5K 2B6; tel. 403/427–2606; FAX. 403/427–0954; Dr. Lyle Oberg, Minister

MANITOBA

Health

Department of Health, 302 Legislative Building, Winnipeg, MB R3C 0V8; tel. 204/945–3731; FAX. 204/945–0441; Honourable Theresa Oswald, Minister

Social Services

Department of Manitoba Family Services and Housing, 450 Broadway, Room 357 Legislative Building, Winnipeg, MB R3C 0V8; tel. 204/945–4173; FAX. 204/945–5149; Honourable Drew Caldwell

NEWFOUNDLAND

Health

Department of Health and Community Services, Confederation Building (West Block), P.O. Box 8700, St. John's, NF A1B 4J6; tel. 709/729–3124; FAX. 709/729–0121; Ross Wiseman, Minister, Health and Community Services

NOVA SCOTIA

Health

Department of Health, P.O. Box 488, Halifax, NS B3J 2R8; tel. 902/424–3377; FAX. 902/424–0559; Chris d'Entremont

PRINCE EDWARD ISLAND

Social Services

Department of Health and Social Services, Sullivan Building, Second Floor, P.O. Box 2000, Charlottetown, PE C1A 7N8; tel. 902/368–4930; FAX. 902/368–4969; The Honorable Walter A. McEwen, Q.C./Minister

QUEBEC

Social Services

Ministry of Health and Social Services, Ministere de la Sante et des Services Sociaux, Quebec, PQ G1S 2M1; tel. 418/643–3160; FAX. 418/644–4534; Jean Rochon, Minister

SASKATCHEWAN

Health

Department of Health, 3475 Albert Street, Third Floor, Regina, SK S4S 6X6; tel. 306/787–3696; FAX. 306/787–8310; Minister, The Hon. Len Taylor

State Government Agencies for Managed Care Organizations

Information for the following list was obtained directly from the agencies.

United States

ALABAMA: Department of Insurance, 201 Monroe Street, Suite 1700, Montgomery, AL 36104; tel. 334/269–3550; FAX. 334/241–4192; Walter Bell, Commissioner

ALASKA: Alaska Division of Insurance, P.O. Box 110805, Juneau, AK 99811-0805; tel. 907/465–2515; FAX. 907/465–3422; Linda Hall, Director

ARIZONA: Arizona Department of Insurance, 2910 North 44th Street, Suite 210, Phoenix, AZ 85018-7269; tel. 602/364–2393; FAX. 602/364–2175; Christina Urias, Director of Insurance

ARKANSAS: Arkansas Insurance Department, 1200 West Third Street, Little Rock, AR 72201-1904; tel. 501/371–2600; FAX. 501/371–2618; Julie Benafield Bowman, Insurance Commissioner

CALIFORNIA: Department of Corporations, 320 West 4th Street, Suite 750, Los Angeles, CA 90013-2344; tel. 213/576–7500; FAX. 213/576–7660; Preston DuFauchard, Commissioner

COLORADO: Department of Regulatory Agencies, Colorado Division of Insurance, 1560 Broadway, Suite 850, Denver, CO 80202; tel. 303/894–7499; FAX. 303/894–7455; Marcy Morrison, Commissioner

CONNECTICUT: State of Connecticut, Insurance Department, Life & Health Division, P.O. Box 816, Hartford, CT 06142-0816; tel. 860/297–3862; FAX. 860/297–3941; Mary Ellen Breault, Director, Life & Health

DELAWARE: Delaware Department of Insurance, 841 Silver Lake Blvd., Dover, DE 19904; tel. 302/674–7300; Consumer Department

DISTRICT OF COLUMBIA: District of Columbia Department of Insurance and Securities and Banking, 810 1st Street NE, Suite 701, Washington, DC 20002; tel. 202/727–8000; FAX. 202/535–1196; Thomas E. Hampton, Commissioner

FLORIDA: Florida Department of Financial Services, Office of Insurance Regulation, 200 East Gaines Street, Tallahassee, FL 32399-0300; tel. 850/413–3140; FAX. 850/488–7061; Kevin M. McCarty, Commissioner

GEORGIA: Georgia Insurance and Safety Fire Commission, Life and Health Division, Two Martin Luther King, Jr. Drive, West Tower, Suite 704, Atlanta, GA 30334; tel. 404/656–2085; FAX. 404/657–8542; John Oxendine, Commissioner

HAWAII: State of Hawaii Department of Labor and Industrial Relations, Disability Compensation Division, P.O. Box 3769, Honolulu, HI 96812; tel. 808/586–9151; FAX. 808/586–9219; Gary S. Hamada, Administrator

IDAHO: Idaho Department of Insurance, 700 West State Street, Third Floor, P.O. Box 83720, Boise, ID 83720-0042; tel. 208/334–4250; FAX. 208/334–4398; Joan Krosch, Health Care Policy/Program Specialist

ILLINOIS: Illinois Department of Financial and Professional Regulation, Division of Insurance, 320 West Washington Street, Springfield, IL 62767-0001; tel. 217/782–4515; FAX. 217/782–5020; Michael T. McRaith, Director

INDIANA: Indiana Department of Insurance Company Compliance Division, Accident/Health Product Lines, 311 West Washington Street, Suite 300, Indianapolis, IN 46204; tel. 317/232–5695; FAX. 317/232–5251; Carol Cutter, Chief Deputy Commissioner for Health and Legislative Affairs

IOWA: Iowa Department of Commerce, Division of Insurance, 330 Maple, Des Moines, IA 50319-0065; tel. 515/281–5705; FAX. 515/281–3059; Susan E. Voss, Commissioner

KENTUCKY: Office of Insurance, Health Insurance Policy and Managed Care Division, 215 West Main Street, P.O. Box 517, Frankfort, KY 40601; tel. 502/564–6088; FAX. 502/564–2728; Gary M. Smith, Assistant Director

LOUISIANA: Louisiana Department of Insurance, Attn: Company Licensing Division, P.O. Box 94214, Baton Rouge, LA 70804; tel. 225/219–0620; FAX. 225/219–9322; Mike Boutwell, Director of Company Licensing

MAINE: Department of Professional and Financial Regulation, Bureau of Insurance, #34 State House Station, Augusta, ME 04333-0334; tel. 207/624–8416; FAX. 207/624–8599; Michael F. McGonigle, Senior Insurance Analyst

MASSACHUSETTS: Commonwealth of Massachusetts Division of Insurance, 1 South Station, 5th Floor, Boston, MA 02110-2208; tel. 617/521–7794; FAX. 617/521–7575; Nonnie Burnes, Commissioner

MICHIGAN: Department of Labor & Economic Growth, Office of Financial and Insurance Regulation, P.O. Box 30220, Lansing, MI 48909-7979; tel. 517/373–0220; FAX. 517/335–4978; Keith W. Cooley, Director

MISSISSIPPI: Mississippi Department of Insurance, P.O. Box 79, Jackson, MS 39205; tel. 601/359–3577; FAX. 601/359–2474; J. Mark Haire, Special Assistant Attorney General

MISSOURI: Department of Insurance, Division of Market Regulation, Managed Care Section, P.O. Box 690, Jefferson City, MO 65102; tel. 573/526–4106; FAX. 573/526–6075; Molly White, Managed Care Supervisor

MONTANA: Montana State Auditor, Insurance Department, 840 Helena Avenue, Helena, MT 59601; tel. 406/444–2040; FAX. 406/444–3497; Steve Matthews, Chief Examiner

NEBRASKA: Nebraska Department of Insurance, 941 O Street, Suite 400, Lincoln, NE 68508-3639; tel. 402/471–2201; FAX. 402/471–4610; Ann M. Frohman, Director

NEVADA: Nevada Division of Insurance, 788 Fairview Drive, Suite 300, Carson City, NV 89701; tel. 775/687–4270; FAX. 775/687–3937; Alice A. Molasky-Arman, Esq., Commissioner

NEW HAMPSHIRE: Department of Health and Human Services, Office of Community and Public Health, Medicaid Administration Bureau, 29 Hazen Drive, Concord, NH 03301-6521; tel. 603/271–4501; FAX. 603/271–4827; Dr. José T. Montero, Director

NEW JERSEY: Department of Human Services, Division of Medical Services & Managed Care, P.O. Box 360, Trenton, NJ 08625-0360; tel. 609/984–7281; John R. Guhl, Director

NEW MEXICO: Public Regulation Commission, Insurance Division, P.O. Box 1269, Santa Fe, NM 87504-1269; tel. 505/827–4297; FAX. 505/827–4734; Morris J. Chavez, Superintendent of Insurance

NEW YORK: The Bureau of Managed Care Certification and Surveillance, Empire State Plaza, Corning Tower, Room 1911, Albany, NY 12237; tel. 518/474–5515; FAX. 518/473–3583

NORTH CAROLINA: North Carolina Department of Insurance, Financial Evaluation Division, 1201 Mail Service Center, Raleigh, NC 27699-1201; tel. 919/733–2205; FAX. 919/715–7490; Jackie Obusek, Assistant Chief Financial Analyst

NORTH DAKOTA: North Dakota Department of Insurance, State Capitol, 5th Floor, 600 East Boulevard Avenue, Bismarck, ND 58505-0320; tel. 701/328–2440; FAX. 701/328–4880; Adam Hamm, Commissioner

OHIO: The Ohio Department of Insurance, Office of Life, Health, and Managed Care, 50 W. Town Street, Third Floor, Suite 300, Columbus, OH 43215; tel. 614/644–2661; FAX. 614/728–5238; Kay Thompson, Chief, Health Division

OKLAHOMA: Oklahoma State Department of Health, 1000 Northeast 10th Street, Oklahoma City, OK 73117-1299; tel. 405/271–6868; FAX. 405/271–7360; James Joslin, Chief, Human Resource Development Services (HRDS)

OREGON: Department of Consumer and Business Services, Insurance Division, P.O. Box14480, Salem, OR 97309-0405; tel. 503/947–7980; FAX. 503/378–4351; Cory Stresinger, Commissioner

PENNSYLVANIA: Pennsylvania Insurance Department, Office of Corporate and Financial Regulation, Bureau of Company Licensing and Financial Analysis, Company Licensing Division, 1345 Strawberry Square, Harrisburg, PA 17120; tel. 717/787–2735; FAX. 717/787–8557; Robert E. Brackbill, Chief of Company Licensing Division

RHODE ISLAND: Department of Business Regulation, Insurance Regulation Division, 233 Richmond Street, Suite 233, Providence, RI 02903-4233; tel. 401/222–2223; FAX. 401/222–5475; Joseph Torti III, Associate Director & Superintendent

SOUTH CAROLINA: South Carolina Department of Insurance, Office of Financial Analysis, 1201 Main St. Street, Suite 1000, Capitol Center, Columbia, SC 29201; tel. 803/737–6221; FAX. 803/737–6232; Timothy W. Campbell, Chief Financial Analyst

TENNESSEE: Department of Commerce and Insurance, 500 James Robertson Parkway, Nashville, TN 37243-1135; tel. 615/741–6796; FAX. 615/532–2798; Phil Blusteon, Examiner

TEXAS: Texas Department of Insurance, Mail Code 103-6A, P.O. Box 149104, Austin, TX 78714-9104; tel. 512/322–4266; FAX. 512/490–1013; Margaret Lazaretti, Deputy Commissioner

UTAH: Utah Insurance Department, State Office Building, Room 3110, Salt Lake City, UT 84114-6901; tel. 801/538–3800; FAX. 801/538–3829; Jilane Whitby, Information Specialist

VERMONT: Department of Banking, Insurance and Securities, Division of Healthcare Administration, 89 Main Street, Drawer 20, Montpelier, VT 05620-2706; tel. 802/828–2900; FAX. 802/828–2949

VIRGINIA: State Corporation Commission, Bureau of Insurance, P.O. Box 1157, Richmond, VA 23218; tel. 804/371–9901; FAX. 804/371–9511; Connie Doung, Senior Financial Analyst

WASHINGTON: Office of the Insurance Commissioner, Insurance Building, P.O. Box 40255, Olympia, WA 98504-0255; tel. 360/664–8002; FAX. 360/586–3535; Sharlene Bowman, Manager, Health Care

WEST VIRGINIA: West Virginia Offices of the Insurance Commissioner, Attention: Financial Conditions Division, P.O. Box 50540, 1124 Smith Street, Charleston, WV 25305-0540; tel. 304/558–2100; FAX. 304/558–1365; Jane L. Cline, Insurance Commissioner

WISCONSIN: Office of the Commissioner of Insurance, 125 S. Webster Street, P.O. Box 7873, Madison, WI 53707-7873; tel. 608/266–3585; FAX. 608/266–9935; Sean Dillweg, Commissioner

WYOMING: State of Wyoming Department of Insurance, 106 E. Sixth Avenue, Cheyenne, WY 82002; tel. 307/777–7401; FAX. 307/777–2446; Ken Vines, Commissioner

U.S. Associated Areas

GUAM: Department of Public Health and Social Services, Government of Guam, 123 Chalan Kareta Route 10, Mangilao, GU 96923; tel. 671/735–7102; FAX. 671/734–5910; Peter John D. Camacho, MPH, Acting Director

PUERTO RICO: Aurea Lopez, Chief Examiner, Office of the Commissioner of Insurance, B5 Calle Tabonuco, Suite 216, PMB 356, Guaynabo, PR 00968–3029; tel. 787/304–8686; FAX. 787/273–6082; Aurea Lopez, Chief Examiner

State Government Agencies for FASC's

Information for the following list was obtained directly from the agencies. Hospital based ambulatory surgery centers are listed in Section A of AHA Guide and are identified by Facility Code F8 and F79.

United States

ALABAMA
Alabama Department of Public Health, Division of Licensure and Certification, The RSA Tower, 201Monroe Street, Montgomery, AL 36130-3017; tel. 334/206–5366; FAX. 334/206–5219; Rick Harris, Director

ARIZONA
Arizona Department of Health Services, 150 N. 18th Ave, Phoenix, AZ 85007; tel. 602/542–1001; FAX. 602/542–0883; Susan Gerard, Director

ARKANSAS
Department of Health, Health Facility Services, 5800 West 10th Street, Suite 400, Little Rock, AR 72204-9916; tel. 501/661–2201; FAX. 501/661–2165; Connie Melton, Section Chief

CALIFORNIA
Department of Public Health, Licensing and Certification Program, 1615 Capitol Ave, P.O. Box 997413, Sacramento, CA 95899-7413; tel. 916/324–6630; FAX. 916/552–3693; Kathleen Billingsly, Deputy Director

COLORADO
Department of Public Health and Environment, Health Facilities and Emergency Medical Services Division, 4300 Cherry Creek Drive South, Denver, CO 80246-1530; tel. 303/692–2800; FAX. 303/753–6214; James B. Martin, Executive Director

CONNECTICUT
Department of Public Health, Healthcare Systems Branch, 410 Capital Avenue, MS#12HCS, Hartford, CT 06134-0308; tel. 860/509–7406; FAX. 860/509–7539; Wendy Furniss, R.N.C., M.S., Branch Chief, Healthcare Systems Branch

DELAWARE
Department of Health and Social Services, Office of Health Facilities, Licensing and Certification, 2055 Limestone Road, Suite 200, Wilmington, DE 19808; tel. 302/995–8521; FAX. 302/995–8529; Roseann Sapp, Office Manager

DISTRICT OF COLUMBIA
District of Columbia Department of Health, Health Regulation Licensing Administration, 717 14th Street, NW, Suite 600, Washington, DC 20005; tel. 202/442–5888; FAX. 202/442–9430; Patricia Van Buran, Administrator

FLORIDA
Division of Health Quality Assurance, Agency for Health Care Administration, Hospital and Outpatient Services Unit, 2727 Mahan Drive, Mail stop # 31, Tallahassee, FL 32308-5407; tel. 850/487–2717; FAX. 850/922–4351; Laura MacLafferty, Unit Manager

GEORGIA
Health Care Section- Georgia Department. of Human Resources, Office of Regulatory Services, Two Peachtree Street, N.W., Atlanta, GA 30303-3142; tel. 404/657–5550; FAX. 404/657–8934; Carol Zafiratos, Director-Healthcare Section

HAWAII
Hawaii Department of Health, Office of Health Care Assurance, P.O. Box 3378, Honolulu, HI 96801; tel. 808/586–4080; FAX. 808/586–4090; Susan Jackson, Deputy Director of Health

IDAHO
Bureau of Facility Standards, Department of Health and Welfare, P.O. Box 83720, Boise, ID 83720-0036; tel. 208/334–6626; FAX. 208/364–1888; Sylvia Creswell, Supervisor-Non Long Term Care

ILLINOIS
Illinois Department of Public Health, Office of Health Care Regulation, 525 West Jefferson Street, 5th Floor, Springfield, IL 62761-0001; tel. 217/782–2913; FAX. 217/524–6292; William A. Bell, Acting Deputy Director

INDIANA
Indiana State Department of Health, Division of Acute Care, Two North Meridian Street, 4/A, Indianapolis, IN 46204; tel. 317/233–7474; FAX. 317/233–7157; Mary Azbill, Director

IOWA
Health Facilities Division, Iowa Department of Inspection and Appeals, Lucas State Office Building, 321 East 12th Street, Des Moines, IA 50019-0083; tel. 515/281–4115; FAX. 515/242–5022; Mary Spracklin, Medicare Services Bureau Chief

KANSAS
Kansas Department of Health and Environment, Bureau of Child Care and Health Facilities, 1000 SW Jackson Suite 200, Topeka, KS 66612-1365; tel. 785/296–0131; FAX. 785/291–3419; Charles Moore, Director of Medical Facilities

KENTUCKY
Cabinet for Health and Family Services, Division of Health Care Facilities and Services, 275 East Main, 5E-A, Frankfort, KY 40621; tel. 502/564–7963; FAX. 502/564–6546; Robert Hester, Acting Director

LOUISIANA
Louisiana Department of Health and Hospitals, Bureau of Health Services Financing-Health Standards Section, P.O. Box 3767, Baton Rouge, LA 70821; tel. 225/342–4997; FAX. 225/342–5292; Erin Rabalais, Manager, Health Standards Section

MAINE
Division of Licensing and Regulatory Services, Department of Health and Human Services, 41 Anthony Ave, 11 State House Station, Augusta, ME 04333; tel. 207/287–9300; FAX. 207/287–9304; Louis Dorogi, Assistant Director

MARYLAND
Maryland Department of Health and Mental Hygiene, Licensing and Certification, 201 West Preston Street, Baltimore, MD 21201; tel. 410/402–8452; FAX. 410/402–8211; Brian Hepburn, M.D., Executive Director

MASSACHUSETTS
Department of Public Health, Division of Health Care Quality, 99 Chauncy Street, Boston, MA 02111-1703; tel. 617/753–8000; FAX. 617/753–8095; Paul Dreyer, Director

MICHIGAN
Department of Community Health, Division of Licensing and Certification, P.O. Box 30664, Lansing, MI 48909; tel. 517/241–2629; FAX. 517/241–3354; Kenneth T. Longton, Director

MINNESOTA
Minnesota Department of Health, Compliance Monitoring Division, Licensing and Certification Program, P.O. Box 64975, St. Paul, MN 55164-0975; tel. 651/201–4101; FAX. 651/215–8709; Carol Hirschfeld, Program Assurance Unit

MISSISSIPPI
MS State Department of Health, Bureau of Health Facilities, Licensure & Certification, P.O. Box 1700, Jackson, MS 39215; tel. 601/364–1108; FAX. 601/364–5054; Marilynn Winborne, Bureau Director

MISSOURI
Missouri Department of Health and Senior ServicesBureau of Health Services Regulation, P.O. Box 570, Jefferson City, MO 65102; tel. 573/751–6303; FAX. 573/526–3621; Terry Wenkel, Health Care Regulatory Supervisor

MONTANA
Quality Assurance Division, Department of Public Health and Human Services, 2401 Colonial Drive, 2nd Floor, P.O. Box 202953, Helena, MT 59620-2953; tel. 406/444–2099; FAX. 406/444–3456; Jeff Buska, Division Administrator

NEBRASKA
Nebraska Department of Health and Human Services Division of Public Health, Licensure Unit, 301 Centennial Mall, S. 3rd Floor, P.O. Box 94986, Lincoln, NE 68509-4986; tel. 402/471–2115; FAX. 402/471–3577; Helen L. Meeks, Licensure Unit Administrator

NEVADA
Bureau of Licensure and Certification, Nevada Health Division, 1550 East College Parkway, Suite 158, Carson City, NV 89706-7921; tel. 775/687–4475; FAX. 775/687–6588; Pamela S. Graham BS, RN, LNC Bureau Chief

NEW HAMPSHIRE
New Hampshire Department of Health and Human Services, NH DHHS Office of Business Operations, 129 Pleasant Street, Concord, NH 03301; tel. 603/271–4333; FAX. 603/271–4232; James Fredyma, Director, Business Operations

NEW JERSEY
New Jersey Department of Health and Senior Services, Certificate of Need and Healthcare Facility Licensure, P.O. Box 358, Trenton, NJ 08625-0358; tel. 609/292–5960; FAX. 609/292–3780; John A. Calabria, Director

NEW MEXICO
Department of Health and Environment, Health Facility Licensing and Certification Bureau, 2040 South Pacheco, 2nd Floor, Room 413, Santa Fe, NM 87505; tel. 505/476–9025; FAX. 505/476–9026; Sandra Cole, Bureau Chief

NORTH CAROLINA
North Carolina Division of Health Service Regulation, Acute and Home Care Licensure and Certification Section, 2711 Mail Service Center, Raleigh, NC 27699-2711; tel. 919/855–4620; FAX. 919/715–3073; Azzie Conley, Section Chief

NORTH DAKOTA
North Dakota Department of Health, Health Resources Section, 600 East Boulevard Avenue, Department 301, Bismarck, ND 58505-0200; tel. 701/328–2352; FAX. 701/328–1890; Darleen Bartz, Chief- Health Resources Section

OHIO
Division of Quality Assurance, Ohio Department of Health, 246 North High Street, Columbus, OH 43215; tel. 614/466–7857; FAX. 614/644–0208; Rebecca Maust, Chief, Division of Quality Assurance

OKLAHOMA
Oklahoma State Department of Health, Protective Health Services, Medical Facilities Service, 1000 Northeast 10th Street, Oklahoma City, OK 73117-1299; tel. 405/271–6576; FAX. 405/271–1308; Tom Welin, Chief, Medical Facilities

OREGON
Health Care Licensure and Certification, Oregon Department of Human Services, 800 Northeast Oregon Street, Suite 305, Portland, OR 97232; tel. 971/673–0546; FAX. 971/673–0556; Ron Prinslow, Manager

PENNSYLVANIA
Bureau of Quality Assurance, Division of Acute and Ambulatory Care Facilities, Health and Welfare Building, Room 532, Harrisburg, PA 17120; tel. 717/783–8980; FAX. 717/705–6663; Sandra Knoble, Director

RHODE ISLAND
Rhode Island Department of Health, Office of Facilities Regulation, 3 Capitol Hill, Room 306, Providence, RI 02908-5097; tel. 401/222–2566; FAX. 401/222–3999; Raymond Rusin, Chief

SOUTH CAROLINA
Department of Health and Environmental Control, Division of Health Licensing, SCDHEC, 2600 Bull Street, Columbia, SC 29201; tel. 803/545–4370; FAX. 803/545–4212; Dennis Gibbs, Director

SOUTH DAKOTA

Department of Health, Office of Licensure and Certification, 615 East 4th Street, Pierre, SD 57501; tel. 605/773–3356; FAX. 605/773–6667; Bob Stahl, Program Administrator

TENNESSEE

Department of Health, Division of Health Care Facilities, 227 French Landing Ste. 501, Heritage Place Metro Center, Nashville, TN 37243; tel. 615/741–7300; FAX. 615/741–7051; Shirley A. Jones, ASAB

TEXAS

Texas Department of State Health Services, Facility Licensing Group, P.O. Box 149347, Austin, TX 78714; tel. 512/834–6646; FAX. 512/834–4514; Linda Porter, Manager

UTAH

Utah Department of Health, Bureau of Licensing, P.O. Box 142003, Salt Lake City, UT 84114-2003; tel. 801/538–6158; FAX. 801/538–6163; Allan Elkins, Director

VERMONT

Department of Disabilities, Aging & Independent Living, Division of Licensing and Protection, 103 South Main Street, Waterbury, VT 05671; tel. 802/241–2345; FAX. 802/241–2358; Fran Keeler, Director

VIRGINIA

Virginia Department of Health, Office of Licensure & Certification, 9960 Maryland Drive, Suite 401, Richmond, VA 23233; tel. 804/367–2102; FAX. 804/527–4502; Christopher Durrer, Director

WASHINGTON

Washington Department of Health, Facilities and Services Licensing, 310 Israel Road, SE, Point Plaza East Building, Tumwater, WA 98504; tel. 360/236–2900; FAX. 360/236–2901; Byron R. Plan, Executive Manager

WEST VIRGINIA

Office of Health Facility Licensure and Certification, West Virginia Division of Health, 1 Davis Square, Suite 101, Charleston, WV 25301-3718; tel. 304/558–1500; FAX. 304/558–2515; Anita Barnhouse, Program Manager II

WISCONSIN

Division of Quality Assurance, Department of Health and Family Services, P.O. Box 2969, Madison, WI 53701-2969; tel. 608/267–7185; FAX. 608/267–0352; Otis Woods, Administrator

WYOMING

Wyoming Department of Health, Office of Healthcare Licensing and Surveys, 400 Qwest Bldg., 6101 N. Yellowstone Rd., Cheyenne, WY 82002; tel. 307/777–7123; FAX. 307/777–7127; Jean McLean, Manager

U.S. Associated Areas

PUERTO RICO

Department of Health Commonwealth of Puerto Rico, Departamento de Salud, P. O. Box 70184, San Juan, PR 00936–0184; tel. 787/274–7676; FAX. 787/250–6547; Carmen Feliciano de Melecio, M.D., Secretary of Health

Freestanding Ambulatory Surgery Centers

The following list of freestanding ambulatory surgery centers was developed with the assistance of state government agencies and the individual facilities listed.

Hospital based ambulatory surgery centers are listed in section A of the AHA Guide and are identified by Facility Code F8 and F79.

We present this list simply as a convenient directory. Inclusion or omission of any organization's name indicates neither approval nor disapproval by Health Forum LLC, an American Hospital Association company.

United States

ALABAMA

American Surgery Centers of Alabama, d/b/a American Surgery Center, 2802 Ross Clark Circle, S.W., Dothan, AL 36301; tel. 334/793–3411; FAX. 334/712–0227; Carlotta McCallister, Administrator

Baptist Surgery Center, 2035 East South Boulevard, Montgomery, AL 36111-0000; tel. 334/286–3180; FAX. 334/286–3381; Kay Catliffe, Nurse Manager

Birmingham Endoscopy Center, Inc., 2621 19th Street, South, Homewood, AL 35209; tel. 205/271–8200; Kathy Houton, RN, Administrator

Birmingham Outpatient Surgery Center, Ltd., d/b/ a HealthSouth Outpatient Center, 2720 University Boulevard, Birmingham, AL 35233; tel. 205/933–0050; FAX. 205/933–8212; Jackie Harrison, RN, Administrator

Columbia Surgicare of Mobile, 2890 Dauphin Street, Mobile, AL 36606; tel. 334/473–2020; FAX. 334/478–6737; Sandy Bunch, Administrator

Dauphin West Surgery Center, 3701 Dauphin Street, Mobile, AL 36608; tel. 334/341–3405; FAX. 334/341–3404; James L. Spires, Executive Director

Decatur Ambulatory Surgery Center, 2828 Highway 31, S., Decatur, AL 35603; tel. 256/340–1212; FAX. 256/340–0252; Andrew Hetrick, Administrator

Dothan Surgery Center, 1450 Ross Clark Circle, S.E., Suite 4, Dothan, AL 36301; tel. 334/793–3442; FAX. 334/793–3318; Denise Harrington, Clinic Administrator

Florence Surgery Center, L.P., 103 Helton Court, Florence, AL 35630; tel. 256/760–0672; FAX. 256/766–4547; Pam Watson, Administrator

Gadsden Surgery Center, 418 South Fifth Street, Gadsden, AL 35901; tel. 256/543–1253; FAX. 256/543–1260; Harriet Willoughby, Administrator

HealthSouth Surgical Center of Tuscaloosa, 1400 McFarland Boulevard, N., Tuscaloosa, AL 35406; tel. 205/345–5500; Jeff Hayes, Administrator

Huntsville Endoscopy Center, Inc., 119 Longwood Drive, Huntsville, AL 35801; tel. 256/533–6488; FAX. 256/533–6495; Michael W. Brown, M.D.

Medplex Outpatient Medical Centers, Inc., 4511 Southlake Parkway, Birmingham, AL 35422; tel. 205/985–4398; FAX. 205/985–4486; Dawn Ousley, RN, Administrator

Montgomery Eye Surgery Center, 2752 Zelda Road, Montgomery, AL 36106; tel. 334/270–9677; FAX. 334/213–0622; Chris Green, Center Director

Montgomery Surgical Center, 855 East South Boulevard, Montgomery, AL 36116; tel. 334/284–9600; FAX. 334/284–4233; Linda Westhoff, Interim Administrator

Outpatient Services East, Inc., 52 Medical Park Drive, E., Suite 305, Birmingham, AL 35235; tel. 205/838–3874; FAX. 205/838–6181; James E. Stidham, President and CEO

The Kirklin Clinic, 2000 Sixth Avenue, S., Birmingham, AL 35233; tel. 205/801–8000; Nancy E. Dunlap, COO

The Surgery Center of Huntsville, 721 Madison Street, Huntsville, AL 35801; tel. 205/533–4888; FAX. 205/532–9510; William Sammons, Chief Executive Officer

Tuscaloosa Endoscopy Center, 100 Rice Mine Road, N, Suite E, Tuscaloosa, AL 35406; tel. 205/345–0010; FAX. 205/752–1175; A. B. Reddy, M.D., Medical Director

ALASKA

Alaska Women's Health Services, Inc., 4115 Lake Otis Parkway, Anchorage, AK 99508; tel. 907/563–7228; FAX. 907/563–6278; Ellen Cowgill, Administrative Director

Geneva Woods Surgical Center, 3730 Rhone Circle, Suite 100, Anchorage, AK 99508; tel. 907/562–4764; FAX. 907/561–8519; Barbara Cope, Administrator

Pacific Cataract & Laser Institute, 1600 "A" Street, Suite 200, Anchorage, AK 99501; tel. 907/272–2423; FAX. 907/272–2428

ARIZONA

32nd Street Outpatient Surgery Center, 2501 North 32nd Street, Phoenix, AZ 85008; tel. 602/957–6799; FAX. 602/957–0172; Gary W. Hall, M.D., President

A.I.M.S. Outpatient Surgery, 3636 Stockton Hill Road, Kingman, AZ 86401; tel. 602/757–3636; FAX. 602/757–7224; Bill Margita

Adobe Plastic Surgery, 2585 North Wyatt Drive, Tucson, AZ 85712; tel. 602/322–5295; FAX. 602/325–7763; Lucricia Banks, Administrator

Aesthetic Reconstructive Associates, P.C., 5410 N. Scottsdale Road, Suite E200, Paradise Valley, AZ 85253; tel. 480/994–3996; FAX. 480/994–3997; Martin L. Johnson, M.D.

Arizona Diagnostic and Surgical Center, 545 North Mesa Drive, Mesa, AZ 85201; tel. 602/461–4407; FAX. 602/461–4401; David Milton, Administrator

Arizona Medical Clinic, Ltd., 13640 North Plaza Del Rio Boulevard, Peoria, AZ 85381; tel. 602/876–3800; Jan Kaplan, Director, Operations

Arizona Surgical Arts, Inc., 1245 North Wilmot Road, Tucson, AZ 85712; tel. 520/296–7550; FAX. 520/298–5415; Robert M. Dryden, M.D.

Banner Baywood Surgicenter, 6424 East Broadway Road, Suite 102, Mesa, AZ 85206; tel. 480/641–9292; Christine Casto, RN, Administrator

Barnet Dulaney Eye Center, 825 20th Avenue, Safford, AZ 85546; tel. 602/428–6930; FAX. 602/428–7272; Beth Curtis, RN

Barnet Dulaney Perkin Eye Center, 1375 West 16th Street, Yuma, AZ 85364; tel. 602/955–1000; FAX. 602/508–4744; Imelda Kelly, Director of Nursing

Barnet Dulaney Perkins Eye Center, 4800 N. 22nd Street, Phoenix, AZ 85016; tel. 602/955–1000; FAX. 602/508–4700; Ronald W. Barnet, M.D.

Carriker Eye Center, 6425 North 16th Street, Phoenix, AZ 85016; tel. 602/274–1703; FAX. 602/274–3216; Richard G. Carriker, M.D.

CIGNA Healthplan of Arizona, Outpatient Surgery, 755 East McDowell Road, Phoenix, AZ 85006; tel. 602/271–5207; Karen A. Miller, Administrator

Cochise Eye and Laser, PC, 2445 East Wilcox Drive, Sierra Vista, AZ 85635; tel. 520/458–8131; FAX. 520/458–0422; Sheree H. Christian, Administrator

Cottonwood Day Surgery Center, Inc., 55 South Sixth Street, Cottonwood, AZ 86326; tel. 928/634–5118; FAX. 928/634–8522; Linda Davis, Administrator

Desert Mountain Surgicenter, 7776 Pointe Parkway West, Suite 135, Phoenix, AZ 85044; tel. 602/431–8500; FAX. 602/431–1677; David M. Creech, M.D.

Desert Samaritan Surgicenter, 1500 South Dobson Road, Suite 101, Mesa, AZ 85202; tel. 602/835–3590; FAX. 480/835–8774; Brenda Mastopietro, Administrator

Eye Institute at Boswell, 10541 West Thunderbird Boulevard, Sun City, AZ 85351; tel. 602/933–3402; FAX. 602/972–5014; Jan Zellmann, Administrator

Fifty-Ninth Avenue Surgical Facility, Ltd., 8608 North 59th Avenue, Glendale, AZ 85302; tel. 623/934–3211; FAX. 623/930–1891; Mark Gorman, Administrator

Fishkind and Bakewell Eye Care and Surgery Center, 5599 North Oracle Road, Tucson, AZ 85704; tel. 520/293–6740; FAX. 520/293–6771; Kathleen A. Brown, Surgery Center Supervisor

Footcare Surgi Center, 10249 West Thunderbird, Suite 100, Sun City, AZ 85351; tel. 623/979–4466; FAX. 623/933–8354; Gary N. Friedlander, D.P.M.

Footcare Surgi Center of Northern Arizona, 10 West Columbus Avenue, Flagstaff, AZ 86001; tel. 928/774–4191; Dr. Edward L. Wiebe

Good Samaritan Surgicenter, 1111 B East McDowell Road, Phoenix, AZ 85006; tel. 602/239–2776; FAX. 602/239–5352; Brenda Mastopietro, Administrator

Grimm Eye Clinic and Cataract Institute, P.C., 1502 North Tucson Boulevard, Tucson, AZ 85716; tel. 520/326–4321; FAX. 520/326–4736; Stephen F. Grimm, M.D., President

Havasu Foot and Ankle Surgi-Center, 90 Riviera Drive, Lake Havasu, AZ 86403; tel. 928/855–7800; FAX. 928/855–5392; Robert Novack, D.P.M., Director

Kokopelli Eye Care, P.C., 2820 North Glassford Hill Road, Suite 106, Prescott Valley, AZ 86314; tel. 928/775–5605; FAX. 928/722–4999; Barbie Elias

Kokopelli Eye Care, P.C., 412 Whipple St., Prescott, AZ 86301; tel. 928/771–9000; FAX. 928/771–9460; Barbie Elias

Mayo Clinic Scottsdale Ambulatory Surgery Center, 13400 East Shea Boulevard, Scottsdale, AZ 85259; tel. 602/342–2419; FAX. 602/342–2414; Karen A. Biel, Administrator

Metro Surgery Center, L.P., 3131 West Peoria Avenue, Phoenix, AZ 85029; tel. 602/375–1083; FAX. 602/789–6833; Diane Elmore, Administrator

Mohave Surgery Center, Inc., 1919 Florence Avenue, Kingman, AZ 86401; tel. 928/753–5454; FAX. 928/753–7790; Lorrie Waits, Administrator

Nogales Medical Clinic Outpatient Surgery, 480 North Morley Avenue, Nogales, AZ 85621; tel. 520/287–2726; Imogene A. Bell, Administrator

Outpatient Surgical Care, Ltd., 1530 West Glendale, Suite 105, Phoenix, AZ 85021; tel. 602/995–3395; FAX. 602/995–1853; Steven Perlmutter, M.D., Medical Director

Outpatient Surgical Center, 456 North Mesa Drive, Mesa, AZ 85201; tel. 602/464–8000; FAX. 602/969–7107; Maddie Dauernheim, Administrator

Phoenix Eye Surgical Center, L.L.C., 5133 North Central Avenue, Suite 100, Phoenix, AZ 85012; tel. 602/279–2434; FAX. 602/279–6475; Sharon Stulstao, Administrator

Physicians Surgery Center of Tempe, 1940 East Southern Avenue, Tempe, AZ 85282; tel. 602/820–7101; FAX. 602/820–9291; Susan Vitort, Administrator

Prescott Outpatient Surgery Center, Inc., 815 Ainsworth Drive, Prescott, AZ 86301; tel. 602/778–9770; Gail Reidhead, Administrative Director

Prescott Urocenter, Ltd., 811 Ainsworth, Suite 101, Prescott, AZ 86301; tel. 520/771–5282; FAX. 520/771–5283; Jeffrey Sanwick

Scottsdale Eye Surgery Center, P.C., 3320 North Miller Road, Scottsdale, AZ 85251; tel. 480/429–0700; FAX. 480/429–1700; Joyce Schweikert, Administrator

Southwestern Eye Center, 1055 S. Stapley, Mesa, AZ 85204; tel. 480/833–9100; FAX. 480/833–6000; Penny Gold, RN

Southwestern Eye Center-Casa Grande, 560 N. Camino Meccado, Suite 1, Casa Grande, AZ 85222; tel. 520/426–9224; FAX. 520/426–1554; Ellen Lopez. RN, Director of Surgical Services

Southwestern Eye Center-Yuma, 2179 West 24th Street, Yuma, AZ 85364; tel. 520/726–4120; FAX. 520/341–0315; Lance K. Wozniak, M.D.

Southwestern Eye Surgicenter-Nogales, 1815 North Mastick Way, Nogales, AZ 85621; tel. 520/761–3533; Pat Bray, Administrator

Summit Surgery & Recovery Care Center, 1485 N. Turquoise Drive, #100, Flagstaff, AZ 86001; tel. 928/214–3211; FAX. 928/214–3219; Jantina Wilson, Administrator

Sun City Endoscopy Center, Inc., 13203 North 103rd Avenue, Suite C 3, Sun City, AZ 85351; tel. 623/972–5083; FAX. 623/523–0505; Jagdish Patel, M.D.

Surgery Center of Peoria, 13260 North 94th Drive, Suite 301, Peoria, AZ 85381; tel. 623/933–2900; FAX. 623/933–0017; Kay Potter, Administrator

Surgi-Care, 5115 North Central Avenue, Phoenix, AZ 85012; tel. 602/264–1818; FAX. 602/264–2172; Ellison F. Herro, M.D., Administrator

Swagel Wootton Eye Center, 220 South 63rd Street, Mesa, AZ 85206; tel. 602/641–3937; FAX. 602/924–5096; S. Joyce Graham

T.A.S.I. Surgery Center, 5585 North Oracle Road, Suite B, Tucson, AZ 85704; tel. 520/293–4730; FAX. 520/293–7561; John A. Pierce, M.D., Medical Director

Tempe Surgical Center, Inc., 2000 East Southern Avenue, Suite 106, Tempe, AZ 85282; tel. 602/838–9313; Richard F. Pavese, M.D.

Thunderbird Samaritan Surgicenter, 5555 B West Thunderbird Road, Glendale, AZ 85306-4622; tel. 602/588–5475; FAX. 602/588–5472; Diane Elmore, RN, Administrator

Valley Outpatient Surgery Center, 160 West University Drive #1, Mesa, AZ 85201; tel. 602/835–7373; FAX. 602/969–7981; Craig R. Cassidy, D.O., President

Vital Sight P.C., dba Eye Institute of Southern Arizona, 5632 East Fifth Street, Tucson, AZ 85711; tel. 520/790–8888; FAX. 520/790–1427; Marci Hill, Administrator

Warner Park Surgery Center, 604 West Warner Road, Building A, Chandler, AZ 85225; tel. 480/899–2571; FAX. 480/899–4263; Marlene Bell

White Mountain Ambulatory Surgery Center, 2650 East Show Low Lake Road, Suite Two, Show Low, AZ 85901; tel. 908/537–4240; William J. Waldo

Yuma Outpatient Surgery Center, L.P., dba HealthSouth Yuma Surgery Center, 2475 South Avenue A, Suite B, Yuma, AZ 85364; tel. 928/726–6910; FAX. 928/726–7423; Stephen Renfro, Facility Administrator

ARKANSAS

Arkansas Endoscopy Center, P.A., 9501 Lile Drive, Suite 100, Little Rock, AR 72205; tel. 501/224–9100; FAX. 501/224–0420; Ronald D. Hardin, M.D.

Arkansas Surgery and Endoscopy Center, 4800 Hazel Street, Pine Bluff, AR 71603; tel. 870/536–4800; FAX. 870/534–5535; Syed Samad, M.D., FACP, FACG

Arkansas Surgery Center, 10 Hospital Circle, Batesville, AR 72501; tel. 870/793–4040; FAX. 870/793–5649; Ronald L. Lowery, M.D., Administrator

Boozman-Hof Eye Surgery and Laser Center, LLC, 3737 West Walnut Street, P.O. Box 1353, Rogers, AR 72757-1353; tel. 501/246–1751; FAX. 501/631–2702; Donna R. Acord, Director

Cooper Clinic Ambulatory Surgery Center, 6801 Rogers Avenue, P.O. Box 3528, Fort Smith, AR 72903; tel. 501/452–2077; FAX. 501/452–4425; Jerry Stewart, M.D, Administrator

Doctors Surgery Center PA, 303 West Polk Ave, Suite B, West Memphis, AR 72301; tel. 501/732–2100; Doris Davis, Administrator

Endoscopy Center of Hot Springs, 151 McGowan Court, Hot Springs, AR 71913; tel. 501/623–4101; FAX. 501/623–0103; Barbara Hulsey, Administrator

H. Lewis Pearson Eye Institute, 3211 Surger Hill Road, Texarkana, AR 71854-9265; tel. 501/772–4440; FAX. 501/772–7190; James Loomis, Comptroller

James Trice, M.D., P.A., d/b/a Digestive Disease Center, 7005 South Hazel Street, Pine Bluff, AR 71603; tel. 870/536–3070; FAX. 870/536–3171; Louis Trice, Administrator

Little Rock Diagnostic Clinic ASC, 10001 Lile Drive, Little Rock, AR 72205; tel. 501/227–8000; Roger J. St. Onge, Administrator

Little Rock Surgery Center, 8820 Knoedl Court, Little Rock, AR 72205; tel. 501/224–6767; FAX. 501/224–8203; Patricia Reedy, Administrator

Lowery Medical/Surgical Eye Center, P.A., 105 Central Avenue, Searcy, AR 72143; tel. 501/268–7154; FAX. 501/268–9071; Benjamin R. Lowery, M.D., Administrator

North Hills Gastroenterology Endoscopy Center, Inc., 3344 North Futrall Drive, Fayetteville, AR 72703; tel. 501/582–7280; FAX. 510/582–7279; William C. Martin, M.D.

Novamed Surgery Center of Jonesboro, d/b/a Eye Surgery Center of Arkansas, 601 East Matthews, Jonesboro, AR 72401; tel. 870/935–6396; FAX. 870/935–4063; Tracy Gholson, Director

Ozark Eye Center, 360 Highway Five North, Mountain Home, AR 72653; tel. 870/425–2277; Cheryl Pearman, Administrator

Physicians' Surgery Center of Fayetteville, 3873 North Parkview Drive, Suite One, Fayetteville, AR 72703; tel. 479/527–0050; FAX. 479/582–1338; Russ Greene R.N. Administrator

South Arkansas Surgery Center, 4310 South Mulberry, Pine Bluff, AR 71603; tel. 501/535–5719; Tammy L. Studdard, Administrator

The Gastro-Intestinal Center, 405 North University, Little Rock, AR 72205; tel. 501/663–1074; FAX. 501/663–0906; James G. Dunlap, Administrator

CALIFORNIA

Los Gatos Surgical Center, 15195 National Avenue, Suite 100, Los Gatos, CA 95032; tel. 408/356–0454; FAX. 408/358–3924; Kate O'Connor, MBA

Advanced Surgery Center, 5771 North Fresno Street, Suite 101, Fresno, CA 93710; tel. 559/448–9900; FAX. 559/448–9546; B. David Singh M.D., Administrator

Aestheticare Outpatient Surgery Center, 30260 Rancho Viejo Road, San Juan Capistrano, CA 92675; tel. 949/661–1700; FAX. 949/661–4321; Ronald E. Moser, M.D.

Alliance Surgery Center, P.O. Box 22680, Long Beach, CA 90801-5680; tel. 562/446–2229; FAX. 562/446–2239; Judy Hopkins - Chief Operation Officer

Ambulatory Surgical Center of Southern California, Gastroentrology Diagnostic Center, 880 South Atlantic Boulevard G-10, Monterey Park, CA 91754; tel. 213/483–9072; FAX. 213/483–9086; Zelman Weingaren, M.D.

Ambulatory Surgical Center of Zeiter Eye, 117 North San Joaquin Street, Stockton, CA 95202; tel. 209/466–5566; FAX. 209/466–0535; Erin McCarthy/Office Manager

Ambulatory Surgical Center, Inc., 14400 Bear Valley Road, Suite 201, Victorville, CA 92392; tel. 760/951–5162; FAX. 818/985–0055; Garey L. Weber, D.P.M., Administrator

Antelope Valley Surgery Center, 44301 North Lorimer Avenue, Lancaster, CA 93534; tel. 661/940–1112; FAX. 661/940–6856; Cindy J. Casanova, Business Office Manager

Apple Valley Surgery Center, 18122 Outer Highway 18, Apple Valley, CA 92307; tel. 760/946–1170; FAX. 760/946–2646; Jason Barker, Administrator

Arlington Podiatry Surgery Center, 7310 Magnolia Avenue, Riverside, CA 92504; tel. 951/354–8787; FAX. 951/354–0350; James A. De Silva, Administrator

Associates Outpatient Surgery Center, 2128 Eureka Way, Redding, CA 96001; tel. 916/246–9737; FAX. 916/246–4052; Jesse M. Kramer, M.D., Administrator

Bakersfield Endoscopy Center, 1408 Commercial Way, Bakersfield, CA 93309; tel. 661/327–4455; FAX. 661/633–5484; Ramesh Gupta, M.D., Medical Director

Bedford Outpatient Surgery Center, 436 North Bedford, Suite 101, Beverly Hills, CA 90210; tel. 310/777–8820; FAX. 310/777–8890; Patricia Adams, RN,PHD, Director of Nursing

Beverly Hills Ambulatory Surgery Center, Inc., 9201 Sunset Boulevard, Suite 405, Los Angeles, CA 90069; tel. 310/887–1730; FAX. 310/887–1734; Amgad Awad, Administrator

Beverly Hills Outpatient Surgery Center, 250 North Robertson Boulevard, Suite 104, Los Angeles, CA 90211; tel. 310/273–9255; FAX. 310/273–6167; Peter Golden, M.D., Medical Director

Blackhawk Surgery Center, Inc., 4165 Blackhawk Plaza Circle, Suite 195, Danville, CA 94506; tel. 510/736–7881; Molly Healy, Administrator

Bolsa Out-Patient Surgery Center, 10362 Bolsa Avenue, Suite 100, Westminster, CA 92683; tel. 714/775–5690; FAX. 714/775–7405; CO D. L. PHAM, FACOG, M.D., Medical Director

Bonaventure Surgery Center, 221 North Jackson Avenue, San Jose, CA 95116; tel. 408/729–2848; FAX. 408/729–2880; Virginia Field, RN, MBA, Director

Brockton Surgical Center, 5905 Brockton Avenue, Suite B, Riverside, CA 92506; tel. 909/686–5373; FAX. 909/778–9064; Michael N. Durrant, D.P.M., MPH/Donald G. Vogt, D.P.M.

Camden Surgery Center of Beverly Hills, 414 North Camden Drive, Suite 800, Beverly Hills, CA 90210; tel. 310/859–3991; FAX. 310/859–7126; Yvette L. Lee Administrator

Center for Surgery of Encinitas, 477 North El Camino Real, Suite C-100, Encinitas, CA 92024; tel. 760/942–8800; FAX. 760/942–0106; Chris Clinton, RN, CASC Administrator

Channel Islands Surgicenter, 2300 Wankel Way, Oxnard, CA 93030; tel. 805/485–1908; FAX. 805/485–5767; Mary K. Fish, Administrator

Charles S. Nicholson III D.D.S, 820 34th Street, Suite 201, Bakersfield, CA 93301; tel. 805/327–7878; Charles Nicholson III, Administrator

Children's Surgery Center, 744 Fifty-Second Street, Oakland, CA 94609; tel. 510/428–3133; FAX. 510/450–5606; Terry Hawes, Administrator

Columbia Surgicenter of South Bay, 23500 Madison Street, Torrance, CA 90505; tel. 310/539–5120; Debra Saxton

Columbia West Hills Surgical Center, 7240 Medical Center Drive, West Hills, CA 91307; tel. 818/226–9151; FAX. 818/226–6171; Christine Sherman, Administrator

Community Surgery Centre, 17190 Bernado Center Drive, Suite 100, San Diego, CA 92128; tel. 619/675–3270; FAX. 619/675–3260; Regina S. Boore, B.S.N., M.S.

Crown Valley Surgicenter, 26921 Crown Valley Parkway, Suite 110, Mission Viejo, CA 92691; tel. 949/348–7252; FAX. 949/348–7246; Maurice Chammas, M.D., Administrator

Cypress Outpatient Surgical Center, Inc., 1665 Dominican Way, Suite 120, Santa Cruz, CA 95065; tel. 831/476–6943; FAX. 831/476–1473; Patricia Cunnane, Administrator

Cypress Surgery Center, 842 South Akers St., Visalia, CA 93277; tel. 559/740–4094; FAX. 559/740–4100; Cheryl Curcin, RN, CNOR Administrator

Del Rey Surgery Center, 4640 Admiralty Way, Suite 1020, Marina Del Re, CA 90292; tel. 310/305–7570; Lee Estes, Administrator

Digestive Disease Center, 24411 Health Center Drive, Suite 450, Laguna Hills, CA 92653; tel. 949/586–9386; FAX. 949/586–0864; Robert Dyer, Medical Director

Downey Surgery Center, 8555 East Florence Avenue, Downey, CA 90240; tel. 310/923–9784; Marisol Magana, Administrator

E. N. T. Facial Surgery Center, 1351 East Spruce, Fresno, CA 93720; tel. 209/432–3724; FAX. 209/432–8579; JoAnn LoForti, RN, MS, Division of Nursing

El Mirador Surgical Center, 1180 North Indian Canyon Drive, Suite 110, Palm Springs, CA 92262; tel. 760/416–4600; FAX. 760/416–4668; Carol Ann Campbell, RN, CNDR

Endoscopy Center of Chula Vista, 681 Third Avenue, Suite B, Chula Vista, CA 91910; tel. 619/425–2150; Robert Penner, M.D., Administrator

Endoscopy Center of Southern California, 2336 Santa Monica Boulevard, Suite 204, Santa Monica, CA 90404; tel. 310/453–4477; FAX. 310/453–4811; Richard F. Corlin M.D.

Endoscopy Center of the Central Coast, 77 Casa Street, Suite 106, San Luis Obis, CA 93405; tel. 805/541–1021; FAX. 805/541–3142; Sue McMillan, Nurse Manager

Escondido Surgery Center, 343 East Second Avenue, Escondido, CA 92025; tel. 760/480–6606; FAX. 760/480–6671; L. Richard Greenstein, M.D., Medical Director

Eye Center of Northern California, 6500 Fairmount Avenue, Suite Two, El Cerrito, CA 94530; tel. 510/525–2600; FAX. 510/524–1887; William Ellis

Eye Life Institute, 6283 Clark Road, Suite Seven, Paradise, CA 95969; tel. 916/877–2020; FAX. 916/877–4641; Almary Hivale, RN, Administrator

Eye Surgery Center of Southern California, Inc./ Med. Group, DBA: Tri-City Surgery Center, 2023 West Vista Way, Suite E, Vista, CA 92083; tel. 760/941–8152; FAX. 760/941–8967; Daniel Lee, DDS, Medical Director

Eye Surgery Center of the Desert, 39700 Bob Hope Drive, Suite 111, Rancho Mirage, CA 92270; tel. 760/340–3937; FAX. 760/340–1940; Timothy D. Milauskas, Administrator

Feather River Surgery Center, 370 Del Norte Avenue, Yuba City, CA 95991; tel. 916/751–4800; FAX. 916/751–4884; Ann Perry, Administrator

Foothill Ambulatory Surgery Center, 1030 East Foothill Boulevard, Suite 101B, Upland, CA 91786; tel. 909/981–5859; FAX. 909/981–8293; Montra M. Kanok, M.D.

Fort Sutter Surgery Center, 2801 K Street, Suite 525, Sacramento, CA 95816; tel. 916/733–5017; FAX. 916/733–8738; Bill Davis, Administrator

Fremont Surgery Center, 2675 Stevenson Boulevard-South, Fremont, CA 94538; tel. 510/793–4987; FAX. 510/793–5084; Debi Ford, RN, Director of Nursing

GastroDiagnostics, A Medical Group, 1140 West La Veta, Suite 550, Orange, CA 92868; tel. 714/835–5100; FAX. 714/835–5567; Stephanie Quinn, Administrator

Glendale Eye Surgery Center, 607 North Central, Suite 103, Glendale, CA 91203; tel. 818/956–1010; FAX. 818/543–6083; Richard Wires, M.D.

Golden Triangle Surgicenter, 25405 Hancock Avenue, Suite 103, Murrieta, CA 92562; tel. 909/698–4670; FAX. 909/698–4675; Ella Stockstill, Administrator

Greater Long Beach Endoscopy Center, 2880 Atlantic Avenue, Suite 180, Long Beach, CA 90806; tel. 562/426–2606; FAX. 562/426–5866; Andrea Campbell, Business Office Manager

Greater Sacramento Surgery Center, 2288 Auburn Boulevard, Suite 201, Sacramento, CA 95821; tel. 916/929–7229; FAX. 916/929–2590; Susan Brunone, MHS, Administrator

Grossmont Plaza Surgery Center, 5525 Grossmont Center Drive, La Mesa, CA 91942; tel. 619/644–4561; Chris Ekern, Manager

Halcyon Laser and Surgery Center, Inc., 303 South Halcyon Road, Arroyo Grande, CA 93420; tel. 805/489–8254; FAX. 805/474–1997; Michelle Mele, Administrator

Harbor-UCLA Medical Foundation, Inc., Ambulatory Surgery Center, 21840 South Normandie Avenue, Suite 700, Torrance, CA 90502; tel. 310/222–5189; Lee Scher, RN, Administrator

HealthSouth Arcadia Outpatient Surgery, Inc., 614 West Duarte Road, Arcadia, CA 91007; tel. 626/445–4714; FAX. 626/445–1701; Sara Lamm, Administrator

HealthSouth Forest Surgery Center, 2110 Forest Avenue, San Jose, CA 95128; tel. 408/297–3432; FAX. 408/298–3338; Camille Magamon RN

HealthSouth Grossmont Surgery Center, 8881 Fletcher Parkway, Suite 100, La Mesa, CA 91942; tel. 619/698–0930; FAX. 619/698–3093; Administrator

HealthSouth North Coast Surgery Center, 3903 Waring Road, Oceanside, CA 92056; tel. 760/940–0997; FAX. 760/940–0407; Donna Danley, Administrator

HealthSouth Surgery Center, 75 Scripts Drive, Sacramento, CA 95825; tel. 916/929–9431; FAX. 916/929–0132; Deanne Conner, Administrator

HealthSouth Surgery Center of Auburn, 3123 Professional Drive, Suite 100, Auburn, CA 95603; tel. 530/888–8899; FAX. 530/888–1464; Fran Thompson, Administrator

HealthSouth Surgery Center-Scripps, 75 Scripps Drive, Sacramento, CA 95825; tel. 916/929–9431; FAX. 916/929–0132; Jodean Lake, Administrator

HealthSouth Surgery Center-Solano, 991 Nut Tree Road, Suite 100, Vacaville, CA 95687; tel. 707/447–5400; FAX. 707/447–2356; Debra Winslow, Administrator

Hemet Endoscopy Center, 1003 East Florida Avenue, Suite 104, Hemet, CA 92543; tel. 951/652–2252; FAX. 951/652–3173; Milan S. Chakrabarty, M.D.

Hemet Healthcare Surgicenter, 301 North San Jacinto Avenue, Hemet, CA 92543; tel. 909/765–1717; FAX. 909/765–1716; Josh Hoffner, Business Office Manager

Hi-Desert Surgery Center, 18002 Outer Highway 18, Apple Valley, CA 92307; tel. 619/242–5505; FAX. 619/242–3502; Venkat R. Vangala, M.D.

High Desert Endoscopy, 18523 Corwin Road, Suite H2, Apple Valley, CA 92307; tel. 760/242–3000; FAX. 760/242–1802; Raman S. Poola, M.D., Administrator

Hope Square Surgical Center, 39700 Bob Hope Drive, Suite 301, Rancho Mirage, CA 92270; tel. 760/346–7696; FAX. 760/776–1069; Pat Finley, RN, MBA, CASC, Administrator

Huntington Outpatient Surgery Center, 797 South Fair Oaks Avenue, Pasadena, CA 91105; tel. 626/535–2434; FAX. 626/535–2430; Robin Waldvogel, Medical Director

Imperial Valley Surgery Center, 608 G Street, Brawley, CA 92227; tel. 619/344–1101; FAX. 619/344–4985; Vida C. Baron, M.D., Administrator

Inland Endoscopy Center, Inc., d/b/a Mountain View Surgery Center, 10408 Industrial Circle, Redlands, CA 92374; tel. 909/796–7803; FAX. 909/796–0614; Khushal Stanisai

Inland Surgery Center, 1620 Laurel Avenue, Redlands, CA 92373; tel. 909/793–4701; FAX. 909/792–6397; Debra Eisner, Facility Administrator

Inland Surgery Center, 361 North San Jacinto, Hemet, CA 92543; tel. 909/652–4343; FAX. 909/765–6036; Barratt Phillips MD.

Irvine Multi-Specialty Surgical Care, 4900 Barranca Parkway, Suite 104, Irvine, CA 92604-8603; tel. 714/726–0677; FAX. 714/726–0678; Lauren Parrott, B.S, Administrator

Kaiser Ambulatory Surgical Center, 2025 Morse Avenue, Sacramento, CA 95825; tel. 916/973–7675; FAX. 916/973–7786; Richard R. Stading, RN, MSHA., A.S.C. Manager

Kaiser Ambulatory Surgical Center, 10725 International Drive, Rancho Cordov, CA 95670; tel. 916/631–2000; FAX. 916/631–2013; Steven Metzger, RN, Manager

Kaiser Permanente Medical Facility-Stockton, 7373 West Lane, Stockton, CA 95210; tel. 209/476–3300; Jose R. Rivera, Administrator

La Jolla Gastroenterology Medical Group, Inc., Endoscopy Center, 9850 Genesee Avenue, Suite 980, La Jolla, CA 92037; tel. 858/453–7525; FAX. 858/453–5753; Dr. David Roseman

La Veta Surgical Center, an Office of Healthsouth, 725 West La Veta, Suite 270, Orange, CA 92868; tel. 714/744–0900; FAX. 714/744–0283; Lisa Allen, Administrator

Laser Surgery Center, LTD., 2021 Ygnacio Valley Road, Building H-102, Walnut Creek, CA 94598; tel. 925/944–9400; FAX. 925/947–2160; Michele McKinley, Administrator

Lassen Surgery Center, 103 Fair Drive, P.O. Box 1150, Susanville, CA 96130; tel. 530/257–7772; FAX. 530/257–2939; Kim Liebert, Medical Staff Coordinator

Lodi Outpatient Surgical Center, 521 South Ham Lane, Suite F, Lodi, CA 95242; tel. 209/333–0905; FAX. 209/333–0219; Marklin E. Brown, Administrator, CFO

Loma Linda, Ambulatory Surgical Center, Podiatry Corp, 11332 Mountain View Avenue, Suite A, Loma Linda, CA 92354; tel. 909/796–3707; FAX. 909/796–3709; Mariam Amiri, D.P.M., Administrator

Los Altos Surgery Center, 795 Altos Oaks Drive, Los Altos, CA 94024; tel. 650/209–1100; Harry Mittelman, M.D.

Los Robles Surgicenter, 2190 Lynn Road, Suite 100, Thousand Oaks, CA 91360; tel. 805/497–3737; FAX. 805/373–8878; Le Anne Schai, Administrative Director

M/S Surgery Center, LLC, 3510 Martin Luther King Boulevard, Lynwood, CA 90262; tel. 310/635–7550; FAX. 310/603–8749; John H. Shammas, M.D., Medical Director

Madison Park Surgery and Laser Center, 3445 Pacific Coast Highway, Suite 250, Torrance, CA 90505; tel. 310/530–2900; FAX. 310/891–0367; John Abrams

Magnolia Plastic Surgery Center, 10694 Magnolia Avenue, Riverside, CA 92505; tel. 909/358–1445; FAX. 909/688–2803; Alexander Carli

Marin Ophthalmic Surgery Center, 901 E Street, Suite 270, San Rafael, CA 94901; tel. 415/454–2112; FAX. 415/454–6542; Vicki Wininger, RN Clinical Director

Martel Eye Surgical Center, 11216 Trinity River, Rancho Cordov, CA 95670; tel. 916/635–6161; FAX. 916/635–5145; Joseph Martel, M.D.

McHenry Surgery Center, 1524 McHenry Street, Suite 240, Modesto, CA 95350; tel. 209/576–2900; FAX. 209/575–5815; Syd Fuentes, RN, Director

Medical Arts Ambulatory Surgery Center, 205 South West Street, Suite B, Visalia, CA 93291; tel. 209/625–9601; FAX. 209/625–3124; Thomas F. Mitts, M.D., Administrator

Medical Plaza Orthopedic Surgery Center, 1301 20th Street, Suite 140, Santa Monica, CA 90404; tel. 310/315–0333; FAX. 310/315–0341; Trish Fowler, Director Surgical Services

Merced Ambulatory Endoscopy Center, 750 West Olive Avenue, Suite 107A, Merced, CA 95348; tel. 209/384–3116; FAX. 209/384–0878; Vijaya Tangella, Administrator

Mercy Surgical and Diagnostic Center, 3303 North M Street, Merced, CA 95348; tel. 209/384–3533; FAX. 209/383–5047; Lynda Pitts, Administrator

Mission Ambulatory Surgicenter, 26730 Crown Valley Parkway, First Floor, Mission Viejo, CA 92691; tel. 949/364–2201; FAX. 949/364–5372; Mary Parker, Administrator

Mission Valley Surgery Center, 39263 Mission Boulevard, Fremont, CA 94539; tel. 510/796–4500; FAX. 510/796–4573; Sarb S. Hundal, M.D.

Modesto Surgery Center, Inc., 400 East Orangeburg Avenue, Suite One, Modesto, CA 95350; tel. 209/526–3000; FAX. 209/526–3133; Dr. Greg Tesluk, Administrator

Monterey Peninsula Surgery Center, LLC., 966 Cass Street, Suite 210, Monterey, CA 93940; tel. 831/372–2169; FAX. 408/372–6323; David J. Ogimachi, Administrator

Napa Surgery Center, 3444 Valle Verde Drive, Napa, CA 94558; tel. 707/252–9669; FAX. 707/257–3328; Eric Grigsby, M.D., Managing Partner

Newport Beach Orange Coast Endoscopy Center, 1525 Superior Avenue, Suite 114, Newport Beach, CA 92663; tel. 949/646–6999; FAX. 949/646–9699; Donald Abraham

Newport Beach Surgery Center, 361 Hospital Road, Suite 124, Newport Beach, CA 92663; tel. 714/631–0988; FAX. 714/631–2036; Eric Reints, Administrator

Newport Surgery Institute, 360 San Miguel Drive, Suite 406, Newport Beach, CA 92660; tel. 949/759–0995; Suzanne Tavenner, Office Manager

North Anaheim Surgicenter, 1154 North Euclid, Anaheim, CA 92801; tel. 714/635–6272; FAX. 714/635–0943; Jeanette Rasmussen, Administrator

Optima Ophthalmic Medical Associates, Inc., 1237 B Street, Hayward, CA 94541-2977; tel. 510/886–3937; FAX. 510/886–6304; Kelly Best, Office Manager

Orange County Institute of Gastroenterology and Endoscopy, 26732 Crown Valley Parkway, Suite 241, Mission Viejo, CA 92691; tel. 949/364–2611; FAX. 949/364–0226; Dina Moatazedi, Office Manager

Out-Patient Surgery Center, 17752 Beach Boulevard, Huntington Beach, CA 92647; tel. 714/842–1426; FAX. 714/847–1503; Madelyn Tinkler, Administrator

Outpatient Care Surgery Center South, 5225 Kearny Villa Way, Suite 110, San Diego, CA 92123; tel. 619/278–1611; FAX. 619/278–5853; Ronald Gertsch, M.D.

Outpatient Surgery Center of Point Loma, 3434 Midway Drive, Suite 1008, San Diego, CA 92110; tel. 619/223–0910; FAX. 619/221–4456; David M. Kupfer, M.D., Medical Director

Pacific Eye Institute, 555 North 13th Avenue, Upland, CA 91786; tel. 909/982–8846; FAX. 909/982–4007; Robert Fabricant, M.D., FACS, Medical Director

Pacific Hills Surgery Center, Inc., 24022 Calle De La Plata, Suite 180, Laguna Hills, CA 92653; tel. 714/951–9470; FAX. 714/951–9478; George Sexton, Administrator

Pacific Surgicenter, Inc., 1301 20th Street, Suite 470, Santa Monica, CA 90404; tel. 310/315–0222; FAX. 310/828–8852; Randi Ogilvie- Manager

Palm Desert Ambulatory Surgery Center, 73-345 Highway 111, Palm Desert, CA 92260; tel. 619/346–4780; FAX. 619/340–4650; S. C. Shah, M.D., Administrator

Paul L. Archambeau, M.D., Inc., Ambulatory Surgery Center, 380 Tesconi Court, Santa Rosa, CA 95401; tel. 707/544–3375; FAX. 707/544–0808; Paul L. Archambeau, M.D., Administrator

Petaluma Surgicenter, 1400 Professional Drive, Suite 102, Petaluma, CA 94954; tel. 707/763–9325; FAX. 707/769–0751; Ronald M. La Vigna, D.P.M. Manager

Physician's Surgery Center, 901 Campus Drive, Suite 102, Daly City, CA 94015; tel. 650/991–2000; FAX. 650/755–8638; Stuart Katz, FACHE, Administrator

Physicians Plaza Surgical Center, 6000 Physicians Boulevard, Bakersfield, CA 93301; tel. 661/322–4744; FAX. 661/322–2938; Terri Waller, Administrator

Plastic and Reconstructive Surgery Center, 1387 Santa Rita Road, Pleasanton, CA 94566; tel. 925/462–3700; FAX. 510/462–4681; Ronald Iverson, Administrator

Plaza Surgical Center, Inc., 168 North Brent Street, Suite 403B, Ventura, CA 93003; tel. 805/643–5438; FAX. 805/643–1625; Dale P. Armstrong, M.D.

Podiatric Surgery Center, 255 North Gilbert, Suite B, Hemet, CA 92543; tel. 909/925–2186; FAX. 909/925–4947; Robert Drake, D.P.M., Administrator

Section C

Premiere Surgery Center, Inc., 700 West El Norte Parkway, Escondido, CA 92026; tel. 760/738–7830; FAX. 760/738–7834; R. K. Massengill, M.D., President

Providence Ambulatory Surgical Center, 1310 West Stewart Drive, Suite 310, Orange, CA 92668; tel. 714/771–6363; FAX. 714/771–0754; Harrell E. Robinson, M.D., President

Providence Holy Cross Surgery Center, 11550 Indian Hills Road, Suite 160, Mission Hills, CA 91345; tel. 818/256–2100; FAX. 818/256–2156; Dale Bowman, Administrator

Pueblo Nuevo Aesthetic and Reconstructive Surgery, 1334 Nelson Avenue, Modesto, CA 95350; tel. 209/524–9904; FAX. 209/524–4101; Diane Payne, Administrator

Redlands Dental Surgery Center, 1180 Nevada Street, Suite 100, Redlands, CA 92374; tel. 909/335–0474; FAX. 909/335–0477; Russell O. Seheult, D.D.S.

Richburg Valley Eye Institute Ambulatory Surgical Center, 1680 East Herndon Avenue, Fresno, CA 93720; tel. 209/432–4200; FAX. 209/432–0147; Frederick Richburg, M.D., Administrator

Riverside Medical Clinic Surgery Center, 7160 Brockton Avenue, Riverside, CA 92506; tel. 951/782–3801; FAX. 951/328–9742; Diego A. Galvez-Ramirez, MBA, Service Area Director

Sacramento Eye Surgicenter, 3150 J Street, Sacramento, CA 95816; tel. 916/444–7052; FAX. 916/446–1145; Kim Russell, ASC Director

Sacramento Midtown Endoscopy Center, 3941 J Street, Suite 460, Sacramento, CA 95819; tel. 916/733–6940; FAX. 916/733–6934; Gautam Gandhi, MD

Saddleback Eye Center, 23161 Moulton Parkway, Laguna Hills, CA 92653; tel. 949/951–4641; FAX. 949/951–4601; Linda Riley, Administrator

Saddleback Valley Outpatient Surgery, 24302 Paseo De Valencia, Laguna Hills, CA 92653; tel. 949/472–0244; FAX. 949/472–0380; Brian FitzGerald, Administrator

Salinas Surgery Center, 955-A Blanco Circle, Salinas, CA 93901; tel. 831/753–5800; FAX. 831/753–5808; Christine Gallagher, Executive Director

San Diego Endoscopy Center, A Partnership, 4033 Third Avenue, Suite 106, San Diego, CA 92103; tel. 619/291–6064; FAX. 619/291–3078; John D. Goodman, M.D.

San Diego Outpatient Surgical Center, 770 Washington Street, Suite 101, San Diego, CA 92103; tel. 619/299–9530; FAX. 619/296–5386; Carla G. Ramirez, Administrator

San Francisco Surgi Center, 1635 Divisidero Street, Suite 200, San Francisco, CA 94115; tel. 415/346–1218; FAX. 415/346–2930; Judith Mulligan, Administrator

San Gabriel Valley Surgical Center, 1250 South Sunset Avenue, Suite 100, West Covina, CA 91790; tel. 626/960–6623; FAX. 626/962–4341; Susan Raub, Administrator

San Joaquin Laser Surgery Center, 1805 North California Street, # 101A, Stockton, CA 95204; tel. 209/948–3241; FAX. 209/948–8009; Susan Ford, Administrator

San Leandro Surgery Center, 15035 East 14th Street, San Leandro, CA 94578; tel. 510/276–2800; FAX. 510/276–2890; Sheila L. Cook, Executive Director

Sani Eye Surgery Center, 1315 Las Tablas Road, Templeton, CA 93465; tel. 805/434–2533; FAX. 805/434–3037; Karim Rasheed, M.D., Director

Santa Cruz Surgery Center, 3003 Paul Sweet Road, Santa Cruz, CA 95065; tel. 408/462–5512; FAX. 408/462–2451; Mary Ann Dunlap, RN

Santa Monica Surgery and Laser Center, 2001 Santa Monica Boulevard, Suite 1288W, Santa Monica, CA 90404; tel. 310/829–2005; FAX. 310/453–9201; Cindy Schlaak, RN, Administrator

Sebastopol Ambulatory Surgery Center, 6880 Palm Avenue, Sebastopol, CA 95472; tel. 707/823–7628; FAX. 707/823–1521; Edward J. Boland, Administrator

Shepard Surgical Center, 1418 East Main Street, Suite 110, Santa Maria, CA 93454-4806; tel. 805/614–7005; FAX. 805/614–7006; Dennis D. Shepard, M.D.

Sierra Surgery Center Inc., 6153 North Thesta, Fresno, CA 93710; tel. 559/432–2757; FAX. 559/432–3556; John F. Burnett, M.D., Owner and President

Sierra Vista Medical Pavilion Ambulatory Surgery, 77 Casa Street, Suite 203, San Luis Obis, CA 93405; tel. 805/544–6471; FAX. 805/544–4913; James W. Thornton, M.D., Administrator

Solis Surgical Arts Center, 4940 Van Nuys Boulevard, Suite 105, Sherman Oaks, CA 91403; tel. 818/787–1144; Dr. H. William Gottschalk, Administrator

Sonora Eye Surgery Center, 940 Sylva Lane, Suite G, Sonora, CA 95370; tel. 209/532–2020; FAX. 209/532–1687; Desiree Torres, RN, Surgery Administrator

South Coast Laser Center, 3420 Bristol Street, Suite 701, Costa Mesa, CA 92626; tel. 714/957–0272; FAX. 714/641–2020; Michael R. Rose, M.D., Medical Director

Southern California Surgery Center, 7305 Pacific Boulevard, Huntington Pa, CA 90255; tel. 213/584–8222; Amgad A. Awad, Administrator

Southland Endoscopy Center, 949 East Calhoun Place, Suite B, Hemet, CA 92543; tel. 909/929–1177; FAX. 909/765–9111; Sreenivasa R. Nakka, M.D., F.A.C.P.

Southwest Surgical Center, Health South, 201 New Stine Road, Suite 130, Bakersfield, CA 93309; tel. 661/396–8900; FAX. 661/397–2929; Linda Bloomquist, Administrator

St. Joseph Surgery and Laser Center, Inc., d/b/a St. Mary And Joseph Surgery And Laser Center, Inc., 436 South Glassell Street, Orange, CA 92866; tel. 714/633–9566; FAX. 714/633–5193; Kathleen Ruper, Administrator

Starpoint Health, 19000 Macarthur Blvd., #450, Irvine, CA 92612; tel. 949/705–5100; FAX. 949/985–0055; Eric D. Friedlander, CEO

Surgecenter of Palo Alto, 795 El Camino Real, Palo Alto, CA 94301; tel. 650/324–1832; FAX. 650/330–4520; Margo Mynderse - Isola, Chief Executive Officer

Surgery Center, 1111 Sonoma Avenue, Lower Level, Santa Rosa, CA 95405; tel. 707/578–4100; FAX. 707/578–7997; Ken Alban, Administrator

Surgery Center of San Buena Ventura, 3525 Loma Vista Road, Suite 13, Ventura, CA 93003; tel. 805/641–6434; FAX. 805/641–6437; Chris Behm, Administrator

Surgery Center of Santa Monica, 2121 Wilshire Boulevard, Suite 201, Santa Monica, CA 90403; tel. 310/264–7300; Bill Aronis, Administrator

Surgical Eye Care Center, 655 Laguna Drive, Carlsbad, CA 92008; tel. 760/729–7101; FAX. 760/729–7106; Lisa Barron, Administrator

Surgitek Outpatient Center, Inc., 460 North Greenfield Avenue, Suite Eight, Hanford, CA 93230; tel. 209/582–0238; Wiley Elick, Owner, Administrator

Sutter Alhambra Surgery Center, 1201 Alhambra Boulevard, Suite 110, Sacramento, CA 95816; tel. 916/733–8222; FAX. 916/733–8224; Ken Schwam, Administrator

Sutter North Procedure Center, 550 B Street, Yuba City, CA 95991; tel. 530/749–3653; FAX. 530/749–3493; Deborah Smith, Ancillary Services Director

The Beverly Hills Center for Special Surgery, 1125 South Beverly Drive, Suite 505, Los Angeles, CA 90035; tel. 310/277–6780; Alina Pnini, Administrator

The Center for Endoscopy, 3921 Waring Road, Suite B, Oceanside, CA 92056; tel. 760/940–6300; FAX. 760/940–8074; Barbara Bockover, RN, Administrator

The Centre for Plastic Surgery, 401 East Highland Avenue, Suite 352, San Bernardino, CA 92404; tel. 909/883–8686; FAX. 909/881–6537; Dennis K. Anderson, Administrator

The Endoscopy Center, 870 Shasta Street, Suite 200, Yuba City, CA 95991; tel. 530/671–3636; Floyd V. Burton, M.D.

The Endoscopy Center of the South Bay, 23560 Madison Street, Suite 109, Torrance, CA 90505; tel. 310/325–6331; FAX. 310/325–6335; Jerome Cohen M.D., Medical Director

The Eye Surgery Center (Colton), 1900 East Washington Street, Colton, CA 92324; tel. 909/825–8002; FAX. 909/422–8905; Melissa Goins, RN, Director

The Eye Surgery Center of Northern California, 5959 Greenback Lane Suite 310, Citrus Height, CA 95621; tel. 916/723–7400; FAX. 916/723–4449; Terre Lamb, Manager

The Montebello Surgery Center, 229 East Beverly Boulevard, Montebello, CA 90640; tel. 213/728–7998; FAX. 323/728–5041; Millie Kelly, Administrator

The Palos Verdes Ambulatory Surgery Medical Center, 3400 West Lomita Boulevard, Suite 307A, Torrance, CA 90505; tel. 310/539–5888; FAX. 310/517–9916; Christine Petti, M.D., Medical Director

The Plastic Surgery Center, 95 Scripps Drive, Sacramento, CA 95825; tel. 916/929–1833; FAX. 916/929–4962; John Murphy, Administrator

The San Luis Obispo Surgery Center, 1304-C Ella Street, San Luis Obis, CA 93401; tel. 805/544–7874; FAX. 805/544–6057; Judy Shapaziar, RN, Administrator

The Specialists Surgery Center, 2450 Martin Road, Fairfield, CA 94533; tel. 707/427–6233; FAX. 707/427–6255; Ann Karg, Executive Director

The Surgery Center Of Riverside, INC, 8990 Garfield, Suite One, Riverside, CA 92503; tel. 951/785–5421; FAX. 951/785–0130

The Surgery Center, A HealthSouth Surgery Center, 3875 Telegraph Avenue, Oakland, CA 94609; tel. 510/547–2244; FAX. 510/547–6637; Ann Banchero, Administrator

The Valley Endoscopy Center, 18425 Burbank Boulevard, Suite 525, Tarzana, CA 91356; tel. 818/708–6050; FAX. 818/708–6055; Christine Scoggins, RN, Clinical Director

Third Street Surgery Center, 420 East Third Street, Suite 110, Los Angeles, CA 90013; tel. 213/617–9194; FAX. 213/617–0605; David L. Nicolas, RN

Thousand Oaks Endoscopy Center, 227 West Janss Road, Suite 240, Thousand Oaks, CA 91360; tel. 805/371–0455; FAX. 805/371–0459; Hector Caballero, M.D., Administrator

Time Surgical Facility, 720 North Tustin Avenue, Suite 202, Santa Ana, CA 92705; tel. 714/972–1811; Denise Reale, Administrator

Torrance Surgicenter, 22410 Hawthorne Boulevard, Suite Three, Torrance, CA 90505; tel. 310/373–2238; FAX. 310/373–8238; Lindon KenKawahara, M.D., Medical Director

Truxtun Surgery Center, Inc., 4260 Truxtun Avenue, Suite 120, Bakersfield, CA 93309; tel. 661/327–3636; Mary Moesler, AOM

Twin Cities Surgicenter, Inc., 812 Fourth Street, Suite A, Marysville, CA 95901; tel. 916/741–3937; FAX. 916/743–0427; Karen M. Wasilenko, CASC Administrator

University Ambulatory Surgery Center, 8929 University Center Lane, Suite 103, San Diego, CA 92122; tel. 858/554–0220; FAX. 858/554–0458; Eileen Smith, Administrator

Upland Outpatient Surgical Center, Inc., 1330 San Bernardino Road #F, Upland, CA 91786; tel. 909/981–8755; FAX. 909/981–9462; Brian Olson, Administrator

Valencia Outpatient Surgical Center Partners, L.P., d/b/a Valencia Surgical Center, 24355 Lyons Avenue, Suite 120, Santa Clarita, CA 91321; tel. 661/255–6644; FAX. 661/255–7653; Nina Turner, Administrative Director

Ventura Out-Patient Surgery, Inc., 3555 Loma Vista Road, Suite 204, Ventura, CA 93003; tel. 805/653–5460; FAX. 805/653–1470; Brian D. Brantner, M.D.

Visalia Center for Ambulatory Medicine and Surgery, 111 East Noble Avenue, Visalia, CA 93277; tel. 559/739–8383; FAX. 559/739–7929; Renda Liden, Administrator

Wardlow Surgery Center, 200 West Wardlow Road, Long Beach, CA 90806; tel. 310/424–3574; FAX. 310/490–0329; Marisol Magana, Administrator

Washington Outpatient Surgery Center, 2299 Mowry Avenue, First Floor, Fremont, CA 94538; tel. 510/791–5374; FAX. 510/790–8916; Dr. Jeffery Stuart Medical Director

West Valley Surgery Center, 3803 South Bascom Avenue, Suite 106, Campbell, CA 95008; tel. 408/559–4886; FAX. 408/559–4908; Annette Wunderlich, RN, Administrator

Westlake Eye Surgery Center, 2900 Townsgate Road, Suite 201, Westlake Village, CA 91361; tel. 805/496–6789; FAX. 805/494–8392; John Darin, M.D., Medical Director

Woodward Park Surgicenter, 7055 North Fresno Street, Suite 100, Fresno, CA 93720; tel. 559/449–9977; FAX. 559/449–9350; Dee Patrick, RN, BHA, Administrator

COLORADO

Aurora Surgery Center LTD, 1300 S. Potomac Street, #122, Aurora, CO 80012; tel. 303/363–8646; FAX. 303/363–8689; Rosalie Bodenhomer, Administrator

Avista Surgery Center, 2525 Fourth Street, Lower Level, Boulder, CO 80304; tel. 303/443–3672; John Sackett, Administrator

Boulder Medical Center, P C, 2750 Broadway, Boulder, CO 80304; tel. 303/440–3000; Mr. Bradford McKane, Administrator

Centennial Medical Plaza, a Division of HCA-Health one, 14200 East Arapahoe Road, Centennial, CO 80112; tel. 303/699–3000; FAX. 303/699–3152; Mary Beth Savory, Administrator

Center for Reproductive Surgery, 799 East Hampden Avenue, Suite 300, Englewood, CO 80110; tel. 303/788–8300; FAX. 303/788–8310; Dr. William Schoolcraft, Administrator

Centrum Surgical Center, 8200 East Belleview, Suite 300, East Tower, Greenwood Village, CO 80111; tel. 303/290–0600; FAX. 303/290–6359; David Parrott, Administrator

Colorado Outpatient Eye Surgical Center, 2480 South Downing, Suite G-20, Denver, CO 80210; tel. 303/777–7303; FAX. 303/282–0266; Sherrie Addante, RN, ASC Director

Colorado Springs Eye Surgery Center, 2920 North Cascade Avenue, Colorado Springs, CO 80907; tel. 719/636–5054; FAX. 719/520–3576; Dr. Robert Foerster, Medical Director

Colorado Springs Health Partners Ambulatory Surgery Unit, 209 South Nevada Avenue, Colorado Springs, CO 80903; tel. 719/475–7700; FAX. 719/538–2999; Ms. Joan Compton, VP Operations

Colorado Springs Surgery CenterAn Affiliate of SCA, 1615 Medical Center Point, Colorado Springs, CO 80907; tel. 719/635–7740; FAX. 719/635–7750; Gina Lovejoy, Administrator

Denver Eye Surgery Center, Inc., 13772 Denver West Parkway, Building 55, Suite 120, Golden, CO 80401; tel. 303/273–8770; Larry W. Kreider, M.D., Chief of Surgery

Denver Midtown Surgery Center, 1919 East 18th Avenue, Denver, CO 80206; tel. 303/322–3993; FAX. 303/322–7329; Lisa Cross, Administrator

Dishler Laser Institute, 8400 East Prentice Avenue, Suite 1200, Greenwood Village, CO 80111; tel. 303/793–3000; FAX. 303/793–3008; Jon Dishler, M.D., President

Durango Surgicenter, LLC, 316 Sawyer Drive, Durango, CO 81303; tel. 970/259–3818; FAX. 970/259–9553; D.J. Winder, M.D., Administrator

Eye Center of Northern Colorado Surgery Center, 1725 E. Prospect Ave., Fort Collins, CO 80525; tel. 970/221–2222; FAX. 970/221–2223; Carol Wittmer, Administrator

Eye Surgery Center of Colorado, P.C., 8403 Bryant Street, Westminster, CO 80031; tel. 303/426–4810; FAX. 303/426–8708; William G. Self, Jr., M.D., Administrator

Foot Surgery Center of Northern Colorado, 1355 Riverside Ave., #B, Fort Collins, CO 80524; tel. 970/484–4620; FAX. 970/407–1194; Linda Kunkel, RN, Nurse Administrator

HealthSouth Aurora Surgery Center, Ltd., 13701 Mississippi Avenue, Suite 200, Aurora, CO 80012; tel. 303/363–8646; FAX. 303/363–8689; Rosalie Warrington, RN, Administrator

HealthSouth Denver West Surgery Center, 13952 Denver West Parkway, Building 53, Suite 100, Golden, CO 80401; tel. 303/271–1112; FAX. 303/271–1117; Ms. Lisa Austin, Administrator

Kaiser Permanente Ambulatory Surgery Center, 2045 Franklin Street, Denver, CO 80205; tel. 303/764–4444; Rosemarie Polemi, Director

Lakewood Surgical Center, 2201 Wadsworth Boulevard, Lakewood, CO 80215; tel. 303/234–0445; FAX. 303/232–7182; Connie Holtz, Administrator

Littleton Day Surgery Center, 8381 South Park Lane, Littleton, CO 80120; tel. 303/795–2244; FAX. 303/795–5965; Judy Rich, Administrator

North Denver Endoscopy Center., 10001 North Washington, Thornton, CO 80229; tel. 303/252–0083; FAX. 303/252–9095; Craig J. Bakken, Administrator

Orthopedic Center of the Rockies Ambulatory Surgery Center, 2500 East Prospect Road, Fort Collins, CO 80525; tel. 970/493–4010; FAX. 970/419–7151; Yvonne Bochmer, RN, BSN, Director of Surgical Operations

Park Meadows Outpatient Surgery, 7430 Park Meadows Drive #300, Lonetree, CO 80124; tel. 303/706–1100; FAX. 303/662–8484; Charlene A. Sherwood, Practice Administrator

Peak One Surgery Center, LLC, 350 Peak One Drive, P.O. Box 4460, Frisco, CO 80443; tel. 303/668–1458; FAX. 970/668–6677; Lisa Austin, Administrator

Pikes Peak Endoscopy & Surgery Center, 1699 Medical Center Pt., Colorado Springs, CO 80907; tel. 719/632–7101; FAX. 719/632–4468; Rebecca Gooding, CEO

Pueblo Surgery Center, 25 Montebello Road, Pueblo, CO 81001; tel. 719/544–1600; FAX. 719/544–2599; Jennifer Arellano, Administrator

South Denver Endoscopy Center, Inc., 499 East Hampden Avenue, Suite 430, Englewood, CO 80110; tel. 303/874–0350; Dr. Dan Hruza, Medical Director

Spring Creek Surgery Center, Spring Creek Medical Park, 2001 South Shields Street, Building H, Su, Fort Collins, CO 80526; tel. 970/221–9363; FAX. 970/221–9636; Natalie Coubrough, Facility Administrator

Surgery Center of Fort Collins, 1100 East Prospect Road, Fort Collins, CO 80525; tel. 970/494–4800; FAX. 970/493–2380; Ross Alexander, Administrator

Surgicenter of the San Luis Valley Medical, P.C., 2115 Stuart, Alamosa, CO 81101; tel. 719/589–8010; FAX. 719/589–8112; Lori Ann Snow, RN., Supervisor

Western Rockies Surgery Center, Inc., 1000 Wellington Avenue, Grand Junction, CO 81501; tel. 970/243–9000; FAX. 970/245–4936; Carol Ann Campbell, RN, CNOR Surgery Center Administrator

CONNECTICUT

Bridgeport Surgical Center, 4920 Main Street, Bridgeport, CT 06606; tel. 203/374–1515; FAX. 203/374–4702; Anthony German, Administrative Director

Connecticut Foot Surgery Center, 318 New Haven Avenue, Milford, CT 06460; tel. 203/882–0065; FAX. 203/882–0248; Martin Pressman, D.P.M., Administrator

Connecticut Surgical Center, 81 Gillett Street, Hartford, CT 06105; tel. 203/247–5555; FAX. 203/249–5860; Margaret Rubino, President

Danbury Surgical Center, 73 Sandpit Road, Suite 101, Danbury, CT 06810; tel. 203/743–2400; Bernard A. Kershner, President

HealthSouth Surgery Center of Hartford, 100 Retreat Avenue, Hartford, CT 06106; tel. 860/549–7970; FAX. 860/247–4121; Theresa Klimczyk, Administrative Director

Johnson Surgery Center, 148 Hazard Avenue, P.O. Box 1151, Enfield, CT 06083; tel. 860/763–7650; FAX. 860/763–7675; Anthony T. Valente, Vice President

Middlesex Surgical Center, 530 Saybrook Road, Middletown, CT 06457; tel. 203/343–0400; FAX. 203/343–0396; Louise DeChesser, RN, CNOR, M.S.

Naugatuck Valley Surgical Center, Ltd., 160 Robbins Street, Waterbury, CT 06708; tel. 203/755–6663; FAX. 203/756–9645; Bernard A. Kershner, President

Stamford Surgical Center, 32 Strawberry Hill Court, Stamford, CT 06902; tel. 203/276–6196; FAX. 213/359–6341; Steven P. Oster, Executive Director Ambulatory Services

Waterbury Outpatient Surgical Center, 87 Grandview Avenue, Waterbury, CT 06708; tel. 203/574–2020; Nancy Noll, Administrator

Woman's Surgical Center, 40 Temple Street, New Haven, CT 06510; tel. 203/624–3080; Bruce I. Fisher, Administrator

Yale-New Haven Ambulatory Services Corporation, d/b/a Temple Surgical Center, 60 Temple Street, New Haven, CT 06510; tel. 203/624–6008; Alvin D. Greenberg, M.D., Administrator

DELAWARE

Bayview Endoscopy Center, Inc., 1539 Savannah Road, Lewes, DE 19958; tel. 302/644–0455; FAX. 302/645–5214; Harry J. Anagnostakos, D.O., President

Central Delaware Endoscopy Unit, 644 South Queen Street, Suite 105, Dover, DE 19904; tel. 302/677–1617; FAX. 302/677–1669; William M. Kaplan, M.D., Medical Director

Central Delaware Surgery Center, 100 Scull Terrace, Dover, DE 19901; tel. 302/735–8290; Paul Francisco, Administrator

Endoscopy Center of Delaware, Inc., 1090 Old Churchman's Road, Newark, DE 19713; tel. 302/892–2710; FAX. 302/892–2715; Jean-Marie M. Taylor, Administrator

Eye Care of Delaware Cataract and Laser Center, 4102 Ogletown/Stanton Road, Suite 1, Newark, DE 19713; tel. 302/454–8802; FAX. 302/454–8801; Jane Baker, Officer Manager

Limestone Medical Center, Inc., 1941 Limestone Road, Suite 113, Wilmington, DE 19808; tel. 302/633–9873; FAX. 302/992–0563; Thomas E. Mulhern, MBA, CASC Executive Director

DISTRICT OF COLUMBIA

Center for Ambulatory Surgery, Inc., 1145 19th Street, N.W., Suite 850, Washington, DC 20036; tel. 202/223–9040; FAX. 202/223–9047; William Heron, M.D., Medical Director

Planned Parenthood of Metropolitan Washington, D.C., Schumacher Center, 1108 16th Street, N.W., Washington, DC 20036; tel. 202/347–8512; FAX. 202/347–0281; Carin Johnson, Center Manager

Premier Surgery Center of D.C., 6323 Georgia Avenue, N.W., Suite 200, Washington, DC 20011; tel. 202/291–0126; FAX. 202/291–0126; Lenora Hollaway, RN, Administrative Director

The Endoscopy Center of Washington, DC, L.P., 2021 K Street, N.W., Suite T-115, Washington, DC 20006; tel. 202/775–8692; FAX. 202/463–1165; Debra Jay RN, Center Director

FLORIDA

Aesthetic Cosmetic Surgery Center, Inc, 598 Sterthaus Avenue, Ormond Beach, FL 32174; tel. 904/673–2262; FAX. 904/677–3808; Bonnie Dantoni, RN, D.D.N.

Aker-Kasten Eye Center, 1445 Northwest Boca Raton Boulevard, Boca Raton, FL 33432; tel. 561/338–7722; FAX. 561/338–7785; Kim Harrington, Administrator

All Saints Surgery Center, 11377 Cortez Boulevard, Brooksville, FL 34613; tel. 352/597–3060; FAX. 352/597–3077; Teresa Wiley-Director Of Nursing

Alpha Ambulatory Surgery, Inc., 2160 Capital Circle, N.E., Tallahassee, FL 32308; tel. 904/385–0033; FAX. 904/422–0201; Jaunita Legree, R.N., Administrator

Ambulatory Surgery Center, 4500 East Fletcher Avenue, Tampa, FL 33613; tel. 813/977–8550; FAX. 813/977–7941; Donna Durden, Administrator

Ambulatory Surgery Center of Brevard, 719 East New Haven Avenue, Melbourne, FL 32901; tel. 321/726–4106; FAX. 321/728–3001; Norm Gagnon, General Manager

Ambulatory Surgery Center/Bradenton, 5817 21st Avenue, W., Bradenton, FL 34209; tel. 813/794–0379; J. Leikensohn, M.D., Medical Director

Ambulatory Surgical Care, 1045 North Courtenay Parkway, Merritt Island, FL 32953; tel. 321/452–4448; FAX. 321/452–4533; Robyn Allard, RN, Administrator

Ambulatory Surgical Center of Central Florida, Inc., 801 North Stone Street, Deland, FL 32720; tel. 904/734–4431; FAX. 904/738–1045; Albert C. Neumann, M.D., Medical Director

Ambulatory Surgical Facility of South Florida, LTD-East, 4470 Sheridan Street, Hollywood, FL 33021; tel. 305/962–3210; FAX. 305/962–3466; Carl T. Waskiewicz, Executive Director and Administrator

Atlantic Surgery Center, 541 Health Boulevard, Daytona Beach, FL 32114; tel. 386/239–0021; FAX. 386/258–4144; Linda Boyum RN, BSN, LHRM, Director

Atlantic Surgery Center, A HealthSouth Facility, 1707 South 25th Street, Fort Pierce, FL 34947; tel. 772/464–8900; FAX. 561/464–1104; Michele Weinberg, Business Office Manager

Atlantic Surgical Center, Inc., 150 Southwest 12th Avenue, Suite 450, Pompano Beach, FL 33069; tel. 954/941–3369; FAX. 954/941–8470; Brad Stetter, Chief Executive Officer

Ayers Surgery Center, 720 Southwest Second Avenue, Suite 101, Gainesville, FL 32601; tel. 904/338–7100; FAX. 904/338–7102; Barbara Hyder, RN, Nurse Manager

Barkley Surgicenter, 63 Barkley Circle, Suite 104, Fort Myers, FL 33907; tel. 941/275–8452; FAX. 941/275–1969; Kerri Gantt LHRM, CMM, Administrative Director

Bayfront Same Day Surgery Center, LLC, 603 Seventh Street South, St. Petersburg, FL 33701; tel. 727/563–7906; FAX. 727/553–7880; Jatin Motiwal, Director

Belleair Surgery Center, 1130 Ponce de Leon Boulevard, Clearwater, FL 33756; tel. 813/581–4800; FAX. 813/585–0319; Ann Rockwood, Administrator

Beraja Healthcare Corp., 2550 Douglas Road, Coral Gables, FL 33134; tel. 305/357–1711; FAX. 305/357–1701; Margarita Caffe, R.N., D.O.N.

Bethesda Outpatient Surgery Center, LLC, 10301 Hagen Ranch Road, Suite 520, Boynton Beach, FL 33437; tel. 561/374–5550; FAX. 561/374–9977; Maddie Linder, RN, Director of Surgical Services

Boca Raton Outpatient Surgery and Laser Center, 501 Glades Road, Boca Raton, FL 33432; tel. 561/362–4400; FAX. 561/362–4440; Karen Raiano, Administrator

Boynton Beach ASC, LLC, Boynton Beach ASC. LLC, 1717-1799 Woolbright Road, Boynton Beach, FL 33426; tel. 516/737–8031; FAX. 561/736–5062; Lily Lee, Administrator

Section C

Brandon Surgery Center, 711 South Parsons, Brandon, FL 33511; tel. 813/654–7771; FAX. 813/654–3347; Timothy D. Block, M.P.A., Administrator and CEO

Brevard Surgery Center, 665 Apollo Boulevard, Melbourne, FL 32901; tel. 321/984–0300; FAX. 321/984–0032; Terrie Greco, Surgical Director

Cape Surgery Center, 1941 Waldemere Street, Sarasota, FL 34239-3555; tel. 941/917–1900; FAX. 941/917–2356; Sharon Tolhurst, RN, MBA, Administrator

Center for Digestive Health and Pain Management, 12700 Creekside Lane, Suite 202, P.O. Box 33906, Fort Myers, FL 33919; tel. 941/489–4454; FAX. 941/489–2114; Vivian DiCarlo, RN, Nursing Director

Center for Special Surgery, 4650 Fourth Street, N., St. Petersburg, FL 33703; tel. 727/527–1919; FAX. 727/527–0714; Jan Silinsky, Administrator

Central Florida Eye Institute, 3133 Southwest 32nd Avenue, Ocala, FL 34474; tel. 352/237–8400; FAX. 352/237–7190; Thomas L. Croley, M.D.

Citrus Endoscopy and Surgery Center, 6412 West Gulf to Lake Highway, Crystal River, FL 34429; tel. 352/563–0662; FAX. 352/563–2961

Citrus Surgery Center, 110 North Lecanto Highway, Lecanto, FL 34461; tel. 352/527–1825; FAX. 352/527–1827; Ann M. Downs, Facility Administrator

Clearwater Endoscopy Center, 401 Corbett Street, Suite 220, Clearwater, FL 33756; tel. 727/443–0100; FAX. 727/461–4893; Nancy Wheeling RN, LHRM Administrator

Cleveland Clinic Florida, 3000 West Cypress Creek Road, Fort Lauderdale, FL 33309

Collier Surgery Center, 800 Goodlette Road, N., Suite 120, Naples, FL 34104; tel. 239/262–5757; FAX. 239/262–6073; David W. Douglas, Administrator

Columbia Florida Surgery Center, 180 Boston Avenue, Altamonte Springs, FL 32701; tel. 407/830–0573; FAX. 407/830–4373; Anne Hutcheson, Administrator

Columbia Surgery Center, 3901 University Boulevard #111, Jacksonville, FL 32216; tel. 904/448–1948; Debbie Overton-Raines, Administrator

Coral View Surgery Center, 8390 West Flager, Suite 216, Miami, FL 33144; tel. 305/226–5574; Ruben Paradela, CEO

Cortez Foot Surgery Center, PA, 1800 Cortez Road, W., Suite B, Bradenton, FL 34207; tel. 941/758–4608; FAX. 941/758–4438; Connie Bulculfine, Administrator

Countryside Surgery Center, 3291 North McMullen Booth Road, Clearwater, FL 33761; tel. 727/725–5800; FAX. 727/797–4002; Karen Nelson, Administrator

DeLand Surgery Center, 651 West Plymouth Avenue, Deland, FL 32720; tel. 386/738–6811; FAX. 386/822–4316; Lynette Knight, Administrator

Dermatologic and Cosmetic Surgery Center, L.C., 2668 Swamp Cabbage Court, Fort Myers, FL 33901; tel. 239/275–7546; FAX. 239/275–5074; Charles Eby, M.D.

Doctors Surgery Center, 921 North Main Street, Kissimmee, FL 34744; tel. 407/933–7800; FAX. 407/933–0564; Roschelle Cutte, Administrator

Endoscopy Center of Ocala, Inc., 1160 Southeast 18th Place, Ocala, FL 34471; tel. 352/732–8905; FAX. 352/732–2661; Fay McCrocklin, RN, Nurse Manager

Endoscopy Center of Sarasota, 1435 Osprey Avenue, Suite 100, Sarasota, FL 34239; tel. 941/366–4475; FAX. 941/366–4390; Pam Copeland, RN, Administrator

Eye Care and Surgery Center of Ft. Lauderdale, 2540 Northeast Ninth Street, Ft. Lauderdale, FL 33304; tel. 954/561–3533; FAX. 954/565–9706; Jane M. Beatly, Administrator

Eye Surgery and Laser Center, 4120 Del Prado Boulevard, Cape Coral, FL 33904; tel. 239/542–4068; FAX. 239/542–0704; Deborah Hughes, RN, BSN, CNOR, Risk Manager Designee

Eye Surgery and Laser Center, LLC, 409 Avenue K, S.E., Winter Haven, FL 33880; tel. 863/299–8574; FAX. 863/294–8305; Jane Dempsey, RN, Center Director

Eye Surgicenter, 2521 Northwest 41st Street, Gainesville, FL 32606; tel. 352/377–7733; FAX. 352/377–9577; William A. Newsome, M.D.

Faculty Clinic, Inc., 653 West Eighth Street, Jacksonville, FL 32209; tel. 904/350–6708

Florida Eye Clinic Ambulatory Surgical Center, 160 Boston Avenue, Altamonte Springs, FL 32701; tel. 407/834–7776; FAX. 407/834–2478; Genevieve Parm, Chief Executive Officer

Florida Eye Institute Surgicenter, L.L.C, 2750 Indian River Boulevard, Vero Beach, FL 32960; tel. 772/569–9500; FAX. 772/569–9507; Mary Lynne MacDonald, Administrator

Florida Medical Clinic Special Procedures Center, 38135 Market Square, Zephyrhills, FL 33542; tel. 813/780–8266; FAX. 813/715–4150; Melissa LoParco, RN, Manager

Forest Oaks Ambulatory Surgical Center, Inc., 7320 Forest Oaks Boulevard, Spring Hill, FL 34606; tel. 352/683–5666; Thomas D. Stelnicki, D.P.M.

Foundation for Advanced Eye Care, 3737 Pine Island Road, Sunrise, FL 33351; tel. 305/572–5888; Wayne Bizer, D.O. Medical Director

Gaskins Eye Care and Surgery Center, 2335 Ninth Street, N., Suite 304, Naples, FL 34103; tel. 239/263–7750; Cindy Gaskins, RN, M.S.N., R.M.

Gulf Coast Surgery Center, 411 Second Street, E., Bradenton, FL 34208; tel. 941/746–1121; FAX. 941/746–7816; Carlene Bailey, RN, Administrator

Gulfcoast Surgery Center, 12132 Cortez Boulevard, Brooksville, FL 34613; tel. 352/596–0744; Fawzi Soliman, M.D.

Gulfshore Endoscopy Center, 1064 Goodletter Road, Naples, FL 33940

HealthSouth Emerald Coast Surgery Center, 995 Northwest Mar Walt Drive, Fort Walton Beach, FL 32547; tel. 850/863–7887; FAX. 850/863–4955; Karen Payne, Administrator

HealthSouth Indian River Surgery Center, 1200 37th Street, Vero Beach, FL 32960; tel. 407/770–5600; FAX. 407/770–1793; Regina Ludicke, Clinical Administrator

HealthSouth Medical Partners Surgery Center, 4545 Emerson Expressway, Jacksonville, FL 32207; tel. 904/399–2600; Debbie Loeffler, Administrator

HealthSouth Orlando Center for Outpatient Surgery, 1405 South Orange Avenue, Suite 400, Orlando, FL 32806; tel. 407/426–8331; FAX. 407/425–9582

HealthSouth St. Petersburg Surgery Center, 539 Pasadena Avenue, S., St. Petersburg, FL 33707; tel. 727/345–8337; FAX. 727/347–4675; Ruth McConnell, Administrator

Holiday Surgery Center, 1109 U.S. Highway 19, Suite B, Holiday, FL 34691; tel. 727/934–5705; FAX. 727/937–3756; David Wall, Practice Administrator

Jacksonville Surgery Center, 7021 A.C. Skinner Parkway, Jacksonville, FL 32256; tel. 904/281–0021; FAX. 904/281–0988; Katherine Anderson, RN, B.S.N., Center Director

Kissimmee Surgery Center, 2275 North Central Avenue, Kissimmee, FL 34741; tel. 407/870–0573; FAX. 407/870–1859; Lou Warmijak, Administrator

Lake Surgery and Endoscopy Center, 8100 CR 44 LEG A, Leesburg, FL 34788; tel. 352/323–1995; FAX. 352/323–1691; Marie Free, RN, BSN, Nurse Administrator

Lee County Center for Foot and Ankle Surgery, Inc., 12734 Kenwood Lane, Suite 44, Fort Myers, FL 33907; tel. 941/936–2454; FAX. 941/936–1974; Sandra Desai, D.P.M.

Leesburg Regional Day Surgery Center, 601 East Dixie Avenue, Plaza 501, Leesburg, FL 34748; tel. 904/365–0700; FAX. 904/365–0758; Renae Vaughn, RN, B.S.N., CNOR, Clinical Director

Lifeline Endoscopy Center, 665 Del Prado Boulevard, Cape Coral, FL 33990; tel. 239/772–8892; FAX. 239/574–6262; Tamara Rosso, Center Director

Martin Memorial SurgiCenter, 509 Riverside Drive, Suite 100, Stuart, FL 34994; tel. 772/223–5920; FAX. 772/288–5820

Martin Memorial Surgicenter at St. Lucie West, 1095 Northwest St. Lucie West Boulevard, Port St. Lucie, FL 34986; tel. 561/223–5945; FAX. 561/223–6862; Charles S. Immordino, RN, Director, Clinical Operation

Mayo Clinic Jacksonville Ambulatory Surgery Center for G.I., 4500 San Pablo Road, Jacksonville, FL 32224; tel. 904/223–2000; Patricia Sayles, ASC for GI Coordinator

Medical Development Corporation of Pasco County, 7315 Hudson Avenue, Hudson, FL 34667; tel. 727/868–9563; FAX. 727/869–9563; Dawn M. Ernst, Director, Nursing

Medivision of Northern Palm Beach County, 2889 10th Avenue, N., Suite 201, Lake Worth, FL 33461; tel. 407/969–0139; FAX. 407/642–1167; Denise Brower, Administrator

Melbourne Surgery Center, 1340 Medical Park Drive, Suite 101, Melbourne, FL 32901; tel. 321/729–9493; FAX. 321/768–6043; Kim St. Amand, Administrator and CEO

Merritt Island Surgery Center, 220 North Sykes Creek Parkway, Suite 101, Merritt Island, FL 32953; tel. 321/459–0015; FAX. 321/459–2291; Cynthia Johnson, Administrator

Miami Eye Center, 619 Northwest 12th Avenue, Miami, FL 33136; tel. 305/326–0260; FAX. 305/326–1907; Edward C. Gelber, M.D., F.A.C.S.

Mid Florida Surgery Center, 17564 West Highway 441, Mt. Dora, FL 32757; tel. 352/735–4100; FAX. 352/735–2444; Patsy Lentz, RN, Administrative Director

Montgomery Eye Center, 700 Neapolitan Way, Naples, FL 34103; tel. 239/261–8383; FAX. 239/261–8443; Jay E. Montgomery, Administrator

Mullis Eye Institute, Inc., 1600 Jenks Avenue, Panama City, FL 32405; tel. 904/763–6666; FAX. 904/763–6665; Colette Smith, RN, Director

Naples Day Surgery North, 11161 Health Park Boulevard, Naples, FL 34110; tel. 239/598–3111; FAX. 239/598–1707; Thomas C. Buckley, Executive Director

New Port Richey Surgery Center, 5415 Gulf Drive, New Port Rich, FL 34652; tel. 727/848–0446; FAX. 727/842–3166; Sandra McFarland, RN, Administrator

Newgate Surgery Center, Inc., 5200 Tamiami Trail, Suite 202, Naples, FL 34103; tel. 239/263–6766; FAX. 239/263–3320; Dr. R. Crane

North County Surgicenter, 4000 Burns Road, Palm Beach, FL 33410; tel. 561/626–6446; FAX. 561/626–7244; Victoria Giraldo, Business Manager

North Florida Surgery Center, 4600 North Davis, Pensacola, FL 32503; tel. 904/494–0048; FAX. 904/494–0065; D. M. Whitehead, Administrator and CEO

North Florida Surgery Center, 256 Professional Glen, Lake City, FL 32025; tel. 386/758–8937; FAX. 386/755–2169; Angela Kohlhepp, Administrator

North Florida Surgical Pavilion, 6705 Northwest 10th Place, Gainesville, FL 32605; tel. 352/333–4555; FAX. 352/333–4569; Susan Roland, Administrative Director

Northwest Florida Surgery Center, 767 Airport Road, Panama City, FL 32405; tel. 850/747–0400; FAX. 850/913–9744; Ron Samuelian, Chief Executive Officer

Oakwater Surgical Center, Inc., 3885 Oakwater Circle, Suite B, Orlando, FL 32806; tel. 407/438–9533; FAX. 407/438–9542; Karen Keith, RN, BSN, Administrator

One Day Surgery, Inc., 1715 Southeast Tiffany Avenue, Port St. Lucie, FL 34952; tel. 772/335–7005; FAX. 772/335–3394; Diane DelRosario, Administrator

Orange Park Surgery Center, 2050 Professional Center Drive, Orange Park, FL 32073; tel. 904/272–2550; FAX. 904/272–7911; Michele K. Cook, RN, Administrator

Orlando Surgery Center II, LTD., 2000 North Orange Avenue, Orlando, FL 32804; tel. 407/897–2000; FAX. 407/894–7802; Gwe H. Travis, RS, BS, Administrator

Outpatient Surgical Services, Ltd., 301 Northwest 82nd Avenue, Plantation, FL 33324; tel. 954/693–8600; FAX. 954/424–1966; Randy L. Huffman, Administrator

Pal-Med Same Day Surgery, 6950 West 20th Avenue, Hialeah, FL 33016; tel. 305/821–0079; FAX. 305/558–7494; Mario Machado, RN, Director

Palm Beach Eye Clinic, 130 Butler Street, West Palm Beach, FL 33407; tel. 561/832–6113; FAX. 561/833–3003; Andre J. Golino, M.D.

Palm Beach Lakes Surgery Center, 2047 Palm Beach Lakes Boulevard, West Palm Beach, FL 33409; tel. 561/296–1330; FAX. 561/296–1350; Jonathan Cutler DPM, Manager

Parkside Surgery Center, 2731 Park Street, Jacksonville, FL 32205; tel. 904/389–1077; FAX. 904/338–9016; David Manning, Administrator

Pasco Surgery Center, 5923 Seventh Street, Zephyrhills, FL 33539; tel. 813/782–2143; FAX. 813/788–6011; Mary LePiere, Center Director

Physician's Surgical Care Center, 2056 Aloma Avenue, Winter Park, FL 32792; tel. 407/647–5100; FAX. 407/647–1966

Physicians Ambulatory Surgery Center, 300 Clyde Morris Boulevard, Suite B, Ormond Beach, FL 32174; tel. 386/672–1080; FAX. 386/672–8628; Joel M. Wilder, RN, Administrator

Physicians Surgery Center, Ltd., DBA Lee Island Coast Surgery Center, 4035 Evans Avenue, Fort Myers, FL 33901; tel. 941/939–7375; FAX. 941/275–5248; Michael Pankey, RN, Administrator

Rand Surgical Pavilion Corp., Five West Sample Road, Pompano Beach, FL 33064; tel. 954/782–1700; FAX. 954/782–7490; Deborah Rand, Administrator

Reed Centre for Ambulatory Urological Surgery, 1111 Kane Concourse, Suite 311, Bay Harbor, FL 33154; tel. 305/865–2000

Same-Day Surgicenter of Orlando, 88 West Kaley Street, Orlando, FL 32806; tel. 407/423–0573; FAX. 407/841–3872; Deborah Herdman, Administrator

Samuel Wells Surgicenter, Inc., 3599 University Boulevard, S., Suite 604, Jacksonville, FL 32216; tel. 904/399–0905; FAX. 904/346–0757; Faye T. Evans, Risk Manager

Santa Lucia Surgical Center Inc., 2441 Southwest 37th Avenue, Miami, FL 33145; tel. 305/442–0066; FAX. 305/445–6896

Sarasota Surgery Center, 983 South Beneva Road, Sarasota, FL 34232; tel. 941/365–5355; FAX. 941/953–7080; Administrator

Seven Springs Surgery Center, Inc., 2024 Seven Springs Boulevard, New Port Richey, FL 34655; tel. 727/376–7000; FAX. 727/375–8944; Kathleen M. Geiger, RN, Surgery Director

Southwest Florida Endoscopy Center, 5050 Mason Corbin Court, Ft. Myers, FL 33907; tel. 239/275–6678; FAX. 239/275–5216; Jansi Prabakaran, MD, Administrator

Southwest Florida Institute of Ambulatory Surgery, 3700 Central Avenue, Suite Two, Ft. Myers, FL 33901; tel. 239/275–0665; FAX. 239/275–0503; Susan Hanzevack, Executive Director

Specialty Surgery Of Ocala, LLC, 3201 Southwest 34th Street, Ocala, FL 34474; tel. 352/237–3387; FAX. 352/861–4208; Raymond J. Mencal, Administrator

St. Augustine Endoscopy Center, 212 Southpark Circle, East, St. Augustine, FL 32086; tel. 904/824–6108; FAX. 904/823–9613; Santiago A. Rosado, M.d., FACP, FACG, President

St. John's Surgery Center, Inc., 8901 Conference Drive, Fort Myers, FL 33919; tel. 941/481–8833; FAX. 941/481–7898; Linda Pavletich, RN, Administrator

St. Lucy's Outpatient Surgery Center, 21275 Olean Boulevard, Port Charlotte, FL 33952; tel. 941/625–1325; FAX. 941/255–6985; Barb DeMarco RN, DON, Administrator

St. Luke's Outpatient Surgery Center - Satellite, 4500 San Pablo Road, Jacksonville, FL 32224; tel. 904/953–0100; FAX. 904/953–0019; Carla Pats, Manager

St. Luke's Surgical Center, 43309 U.S. Highway 19, N., P.O. Box 5000, Tarpon Spring, FL 34688-5000; tel. 813/938–2020; FAX. 813/938–5606; Glenn S. Wolfson, M.D., Medical Director

Suncoast Eye Center, Eye Surgery Institute, 14003 Lakeshore Boulevard, Hudson, FL 34667; tel. 727/868–9442; FAX. 727/862–6210; Lawrence A. Seigel, M.D., P.A., Medical Director

Suncoast Medical Clinic,LLC, 601 Seventh Street, S., St. Petersburg, FL 33701; tel. 727/894–1818; FAX. 727/824–7177; Cheryl Macurdy, Director of Clinical Service

Suncoast Skin Surgery Clinic, 4519 U.S. Highway 19, New Port Richey, FL 34652; tel. 813/849–8922; FAX. 813/841–7553; Bethany Carvallo, Administrator

Sunrise Surgical Center, 110 Yorktowne Drive, Daytona Beach, FL 32119; tel. 904/788–6696; FAX. 904/788–2219; Carolyn Teal

Surgery Center at Coral Springs, 967 University Drive, Coral Springs, FL 33071; tel. 954/341–5553; FAX. 954/344–7054; Barb Wegener, Administrator

Surgery Center at St. Andrews, Inc., 1350 East Venice Avenue, Venice, FL 34285; tel. 941/488–2030; FAX. 941/484–2010; Laura Hendershott, Business Office Supervisor

Surgery Center of Jupiter, Inc., 102 Coastal Way, Jupiter, FL 33477; tel. 561/747–1111; FAX. 560/747–4151; Monroe N. Benaim, M.D., Medical Director

Surgery Center of North Florida, Inc., 6520 Northwest Ninth Boulevard, Gainsville, FL 32615; tel. 352/331–7987; FAX. 352/331–2787; Joy Ingram, Administrator

Surgery Center of Stuart, 2096 Southeast Ocean Boulevard, Stuart, FL 34996; tel. 561/223–0174; FAX. 561/223–0946; Charles Immordino, RN, Administrator

Surgical Center of Central Florida, 3601 South Highlands Avenue, Sebring, FL 33870; tel. 863/382–7500; FAX. 863/385–7332; Sharon Keiber, RN, Administrator

Surgical Licensed Ward, 110 West Underwood Street, Suite B, Orlando, FL 32806; tel. 407/648–9151; FAX. 407/426–7017; William Hughes, Administrator

Surgical Park Center, Ltd., 9100 Southwest 87th Avenue, Miami, FL 33176; tel. 305/271–9100; FAX. 305/270–8527; Mike Casanova, Administrator

Surgicare Center, Inc., 4101 Evans Avenue, Ft. Myers, FL 33901; tel. 239/939–3456; FAX. 239/939–1164; Sharon A. Sileno, Director of Nursing

Tallahassee Endoscopy Center, 2400 Miccosukee Road, Tallahassee, FL 32308; tel. 850/877–2105; FAX. 850/942–1761; Noel Withers, Administrator

Tallahassee Outpatient Surgery Center, Inc., 3334 Capital Medical Boulevard, Suite 500, Tallahassee, FL 32308; tel. 904/877–4688; FAX. 904/877–0368; Judi Cleckner RN, Administrator

Tallahassee Single Day Surgery, 1661 Phillips Road, Tallahassee, FL 32308; tel. 850/878–5165; FAX. 850/942–5545; Elizabeth Trikardos, Director of Nursing

Tampa Bay Surgery Center, 11811 North Dale Mabry Hwy, Tampa, FL 33618; tel. 813/961–8500; FAX. 813/265–2564; Jay L. Rosen, M.D., Executive Director

Tampa Eye Surgery Center, 4302 North Gomez, Tampa, FL 33607; tel. 813/870–6330; FAX. 813/871–3956; Beverly Martin, Administrator

Tampa Outpatient Surgical Facility, 5013 North Armenia Avenue, Tampa, FL 33603; tel. 813/875–0562; FAX. 813/871–5236; Maureen F. Martin RN, CASC

The Aesthetic Plastic Surgery Center, 135 San Marco Drive, Venice, FL 34285; tel. 941/484–6836; FAX. 941/484–9690; Linda Martin, Administrative Director

The Endoscopy Center, 4810 North Davis Highway, Pensacola, FL 32503; tel. 850/474–8988; FAX. 850/478–9903; Alice Cartee, Administrator

The Endoscopy Center of Naples, 150 Tamiami Trail, N., Suite One, Naples, FL 34102; tel. 941/262–8306; FAX. 941/262–3179; Marjorie Venditti, Billing Office Manager

The Endoscopy Center, Inc., 5101 Southwest 8th Street, Miami, FL 33134; tel. 305/461–1881; Regina Dhanani, Center Director

The Eye Associates Surgery Center, 6002 Pointe West Boulevard, Bradenton, FL 34209; tel. 941/792–2020; FAX. 941/792–2832; Linda Colson, RN, Director

The Gastrointestinal Center of Hialeah, INC, 135 West 49th Street, Hialeah, FL 33012; tel. 305/825–1487; FAX. 305/825–9731; Omar Escalona, Administrator

The Ocala Eye Surgery Center, 3330 Southwest 33rd Road, Ocala, FL 34474; tel. 352/873–9311; FAX. 352/873–9652; Jeanne Thompson, RN, CRNO Administrator

The Sarasota Ophthalmology, ASC, LLC, dba Center for Advanced Eye Surgery, 3920 Bee Ridge Road Building F, Suite C, Sarasota, FL 34233; tel. 941/925–0000; FAX. 941/927–2726; Darice Downs, RN, LHRM,Center Director

The Sheridan Surgery Center, 95 Bulldog Boulevard, Suite 104, Melbourne, FL 32901; tel. 321/952–9800; FAX. 321/952–7889; Anne Latorra, Director

The Surgery Center of Coral Gables, LLC., 1097 S.W. Le Jeune Road, Miami, FL 33134; tel. 305/461–1300; Laura Lilburn, RN, CNOR, Center Director

Total Surgery Center, 130 Tamiami Trail, Suite 210, Naples, FL 34102; tel. 239/434–4118; FAX. 239/434–6343; Mary Boedeker, Administrator

Treasure Coast Center for Surgery, 1411 East Ocean Boulevard, Stuart, FL 34996; tel. 772/286–8028; FAX. 772/283–6628; Andrea Day, Business Office Manager

University Surgical Center, 7251 University Boulevard, Suite 100, Winter Park, FL 32792; tel. 407/677–0066; FAX. 407/677–4199; Laura Hofma, MBA, RHIA, CASC, Administrator

Urological Ambulatory Surgery Center, Inc., 1812 North Mills Avenue, Orlando, FL 32803; tel. 407/992–2640; FAX. 407/897–2290; William Hamiger, Administrator

Venice HealthPark Surgery Center, 1283 Jacaranda Boulevard, Venice, FL 34292; tel. 941/497–5660; FAX. 941/492–3942; Kermit Knight, CASC Administrator

Venture Ambulatory Surgery Center, 16853 Northeast Second Avenue, Suite 400, North Miami Beach, FL 33162; tel. 305/652–2999; FAX. 305/652–8156; Lali Perez, RN, B.S.N., Center Director

Vero Eye Center, 70 Royal Palm Pointe, Vero Beach, FL 32960; tel. 772/569–6600; FAX. 772/569–5341; E.S. Branigan, III, M.D.

Volusia Endoscopy & Surgery Center, Inc., 550 Memorial Circle, Suite G, Ormond Beach, FL 32174; tel. 386/672–0017; FAX. 386/672–6732; Susan K. Amon, RN, DON LHCRM

Waterside Ambulatory Surgical Center, Inc., 2001 North Flagler Drive, West Palm Beach, FL 33407; tel. 561/659–6543; FAX. 561/659–3533; Lisa Bolognini, Admin. Director

GEORGIA

Advanced Aesthetics Plastic Surgery Center, 874 Lanier Ave. West, One Prestige Park, Fayetteville, GA 30124; tel. 770/603–6000; FAX. 770/603–7064; Paul D. Feldman, President

Advanced Surgery Center of Georgia, 220 Hospital Road, Canton, GA 30114; tel. 770/479–2202; FAX. 770/479–6666; Judith Grady, Administrator

Aesthetic Laser & Surgery Facility, 416 Gordon Ave., Thomasville, GA 31792-6644; tel. 229/228–7200; FAX. 229/228–5193; G. Courtney Houston, M.D., Medical Director

Aestheticare Surgicenter, P.C., 975 Johnson Ferry Road, Suite 160, Atlanta, GA 30342; tel. 404/303–7542; FAX. 404/531–0649; Sharon A. Pesselato, Director

Affinity Outpatient Services, 2224 US Highway 41 North, Tifton, GA 31794; tel. 912/391–4299; FAX. 912/391–4291; Barry L. Cutts, Administrator

Albany Surgery Center, LLP, 531 Seventh Avenue, Albany, GA 31701; tel. 229/883–3535; FAX. 229/883–3783; Stephen M. Wilder, D.P.M., Medical Director

Ambulatory Foot and Leg Surgical Center, 1650 Mulkey Road, Austell, GA 30106; tel. 770/941–3633; FAX. 770/944–9038; Douglas Elleby, D.P.M., CEO

Ambulatory Laser and Surgery Center, 425 Forest Parkway, Suite 103, Forest Park, GA 30297-2135; tel. 404/363–1087; FAX. 404/363–9951; Dr. Paul A. Colon, Medical Director

Athens Plastic Surgery Center, 2325 Prince Avenue, Athens, GA 30606; tel. 706/546–0280; FAX. 404/548–0258; Stephen B. Lober, M.D., Administrator

Atlanta Aesthetic Surgery Center, Inc., 4200 Northside Parkway, Building Eight, Atlanta, GA 30327; tel. 404/233–3833; FAX. 404/233–8447; Debbie Clotfelter, Administrator

Atlanta Endoscopy Center, LTD, 2665 North Decatur Road, Suite 545, Decatur, GA 30033; tel. 404/297–5000; FAX. 404/296–9890; Kevin Mussared RN Clinical Coordinator

Atlanta Eye Surgery Center, P.C., 3200 Downwood Circle, NW, Suite 200, Atlanta, GA 30327; tel. 404/355–8721; Walter G. Elliott, Administrator

Atlanta Outpatient Peachtree Dunwoody Center, 5505 Peachtree-Dunwoody Road, Suite 150, Atlanta, GA 30342; tel. 404/847–0893; FAX. 404/843–8664; Janie Ellison, Administrator

Atlanta Surgi-Center, Inc., 1113 Spring Street, Atlanta, GA 30309; tel. 404/892–8608; FAX. 404/892–8143; Toni P. Hawkins, Administrator

Atlanta Women's Medical Center, Inc., 235 West Wieuca Road, Atlanta, GA 30342; tel. 404/257–0057; FAX. 404/257–1245; Golda Melnik, Administrator

Augusta Plastic Surgery Center, Inc., 1348 Walton Way, Suite 6300, Augusta, GA 30901-2772; tel. 706/724–5611; FAX. 706/724–5435; Sandy Woodward, Administrator

Augusta Surgical Center, 915 Russell Street, Augusta, GA 30904-4115; tel. 706/738–4925; FAX. 706/738–7224; Jeff Simless, Administrator

Brunswick Endoscopy Center, 3217 4th Street, Brunswick, GA 31520-3759; tel. 912/267–1802; FAX. 912/267–0061; Rita Warren, Administrator

Center for Plastic Surgery, Inc., 365 East Paces Ferry Road, Atlanta, GA 30305; tel. 404/814–1100; FAX. 404/814–0015; Dr. Vincent Zubowicz, Medical Director

Clayton Outpatient Surgical Center, Inc., 6911 Tara Boulevard, Jonesboro, GA 30236; tel. 770/477–9535; FAX. 770/471–7826; Renee Grimsley, Administrator

Section C

Cobb Foot and Leg Surgery Center, 792 Church Street, Suite 102, Marietta, GA 30060; tel. 770/422–9864; FAX. 770/984–0303; Glyn Lewis, Administrator

Coliseum Same Day Surgery, 340 Hospital Drive, P.O. Box 6154, Macon, GA 31208; tel. 912/742–1403; FAX. 912/742–1671; Lenore Sell, Administrator

Columbia Augusta Surgical Center, 915 Russell Street, Augusta, GA 30904; tel. 706/738–4925; FAX. 706/738–7224; Beryl Barrett, RN, Administrator

Columbus Women's Health Organization, Inc., 3850 Rosemont Drive, Columbus, GA 31901; tel. 706/323–8363

Decatur Urological Clinic-Ambulatory Surgery Center, Inc., 428 Winn Court, Decatur, GA 30030; tel. 404/298–0217; FAX. 404/299–5178; Sabrina Jones, Office Manager

DeKalb Endoscopy Center, 2675 North Decatur Road, Suite 506, Decatur, GA 30033; tel. 404/299–1679; FAX. 404/508–7558; Mark A. Stern, M.D

Dennis Surgery Center, Inc., 3193 Howell Mill Road, Suite 215, Atlanta, GA 30327; tel. 404/355–1312; FAX. 404/352–2798; Valerie Garrett, Administrator

Dunwoody Outpatient Surgicenter, Inc., 4553 North Shallowford Road, Suite 60C, Atlanta, GA 30338; tel. 770/455–1983; FAX. 770/457–2823; Janet Davies, Administrator

Endoscopy Center of Columbus, Inc, 1130 Talbotton Road, Columbus, GA 31904-8745; tel. 706/327–0700; FAX. 706/327–0757; Jean Patterson, RN, Administrator

Endoscopy Center of Southeast Georgia, Inc., 200 Maple Drive, P.O. Box 1367, Vidalia, GA 30474; tel. 912/538–1003; FAX. 912/537–9843; Dixie Calhoun, RN, Administrator

Evans Surgery Center, 635 Ronald Reagan Drive, Evans, GA 30809; tel. 706/868–3110; FAX. 706/868–3156; Sharon Gelinas, Administrator

Feminist Women's Health Center, 1924 Cliff Valley Way, Atlanta, GA 30329; tel. 404/728–7900; FAX. 404/728–7907; Emily Mason, Clinical Director

G.I. Endoscopy Center, 6555 Professional Place, Suite B, Riverdale, GA 30274; tel. 770/692–0100; FAX. 770/692–6190; Aruna Jaya Prakash, Administrator

Gainesville Surgery Center, 1945 Beverly Road, Gainesville, GA 30501-2034; tel. 770/287–1500; Karen Fankhauser, Administrator

Gastrointestinal Endoscopy of Gwinnett, 600 Professional Drive, Suite 130, Lawrenceville, GA 30045; tel. 770/995–7989; FAX. 770/339–8646; Betsy Roberts, Practice Manager

Georgia Lithotripsy Center, 120 Trinity Place, Athens, GA 30607; tel. 404/543–2718; David C. Allen, M.D., Administrator

Georgia Surgical Centers - South, 541 Forest Parkway, Suite 14, Forest Park, GA 30297-6110; tel. 404/366–5652; Trudy Hunley, Administrator

Golden Isles Surgical Center, Inc., 2916 Glynn Avenue, Brunswick, GA 31530; tel. 912/265–3210; FAX. 912/265–1481; J. Brooker, Office Manager

Gwinnet Endoscopy Center, 758 Old Norcross Road, Suite 250, Lawrenceville, GA 30045; tel. 770/682–7220; FAX. 770/338–0510; Kerry H. King, M.D., Medical Director

HealthSouth Surgery Center of Atlanta, 1140 Hammond Drive, Building F, Suite 6100, Atlanta, GA 30328; tel. 770/551–9944; FAX. 770/551–8826; Mary Hardwick, Administrator

HealthSouth Surgery Center of Gwinnett, 2131 Fountain Drive, Snellville, GA 30078; tel. 770/979–8200; FAX. 770/979–1327; Holly Kouts, Administrator

Kramer Professional Building, 215 Clairemont Avenue, Decatur, GA 30030; tel. 404/373–2529; FAX. 404/373–1655; Jerald N. Kramer, D.P.M., President

Marietta Surgical Center, Ambulatory Surgery Division, HCA, The Health Company, 780 Canton Road, Suite 100, Marietta, GA 30060; tel. 770/422–1579; FAX. 770/428–4861; Faith Wheeler, RNCNOR, QA/Risk Manager

Medical Eye Associates, Inc., 1429 Oglethorpe Street, Macon, GA 31201; tel. 478/743–7061; FAX. 478/743–6296; Diane Vaughn, Practice Manager

Midtown Urology Surgical Center, 128 North Avenue, N.E., Suite 100, Atlanta, GA 30308; tel. 404/881–0966; FAX. 404/874–5902; Jenelle E. Foote, M.D., Medical Director

North Atlanta Endoscopy Center, 5555 Peachtree-Dunwoody Road, Suite G70, Atlanta, GA 30342-1703; tel. 404/843–0500; Phyllis Pritchett, Administrator

North Atlanta Head and Neck Surgery Center, LLC., 980 Johnson Ferry Road, Northside Doctors Centre, Atlanta, GA 30342; tel. 404/843–9171; FAX. 404/250–1881; Pradeep K. Snha, M.D.,PhD

North Georgia Endoscopy Center, Inc., 320 Hospital Road, Canton, GA 30114; tel. 770/479–5535; FAX. 770/479–8821; Kevin V. Kellogg, Administrator

North Georgia Outpatient Surgery Center, 795 Red Bud Road, Calhoun, GA 30701; tel. 706/629–1852; FAX. 706/629–8004; Herbert E. Kosmahl, President

North Oak Ambulatory Surgical Center, 2718 North Oak Street, Valdosta, GA 31602; tel. 229/242–3668; FAX. 229/253–8666; T.E. Pitts, D.P.M.

Northeast Georgia Plastic Surgery Center, 1296 Sims Street, Gainesville, GA 30501; tel. 770/534–1856; FAX. 770/531–0355; Sam Richwine, Medical Director

Northlake Endoscopy Center, 1459 Montreal Road, Suite 204, Tucker, GA 30084; tel. 770/939–4721; FAX. 770/939–1187; Ellen Burney, Administrator

Northside Foot and Ankle Outpatient Surgical Center, 3415 Holcomb Bridge Road, Norcross, GA 30092; tel. 770/449–1122; FAX. 770/242–8709; Steven T. Arminio, DPM, Administrator

Northside Women's Clinic, Inc., 3543 Chamblee-Dunwoody Road, Atlanta, GA 30341; tel. 770/455–4210; FAX. 770/451–9529; James W. Gay, M.D., Administrator

Novamed Surgery Center Of Columbus, GA, 7351 Old Moon Road, Columbus, GA 31909; tel. 706/221–2721; FAX. 706/221–2754; Nancy Beth Pedersen, RN ASC Director

Outpatient Center for Foot Surgery, Inc., 730 South Eighth Street, Suite B, Griffin, GA 30224; tel. 770/228–6644; FAX. 770/228–5769; Mark Henson, Administrator

Paces Plastic Surgery Center, Inc., 3200 Downwood Circle, Suite 640, Atlanta, GA 30327; tel. 404/351–0051; FAX. 404/351–0632; Linda Neal, Administrator

Parkwood Ambulatory Surgical Center, 2605 Parkwood Drive, Brunswick, GA 31520; tel. 912/265–4766; FAX. 912/267–9857; Louise Shaw, RN

Piedmont Surgery Center, 4660 Riverside Park Boulevard, Macon, GA 31210; tel. 912/471–6300; Mikell Peed, Administrator

Planned Parenthood of Reproductive Health Services, 1289 Broad Street, Augusta, GA 30911; tel. 706/724–5557; FAX. 706/724–5293; Vanetta D. King, Center Manager

Pulliam Ambulatory Surgical Center, 4167 Hospital Drive, Covington, GA 30015, P.O. Box 469, Covington, GA 30015; tel. 404/786–1234; M.M. Pulliam, P.C., Medical Director

Resurgens Surgical Center, 5671 Peachtree Dunwoody Road, Suite 800, Atlanta, GA 30342; tel. 404/531–8532; Leslie Mattson, RN Administrator

Roswell Ambulatory Surgery Center, 1250 Upper Hembree Road, Ste. A, Roswell, GA 30076; tel. 770/663–8011; FAX. 770/754–9820; Dr. Glyn Lewis, Administrator

Savannah Medical Clinic, 120 East 34th Street, Savannah, GA 31401; tel. 912/236–1603; FAX. 912/236–1605; William Knorr, M.D., Administrator

Savannah Outpatient Foot And Ankle Surgery Center, 310 Eisenhower Drive, Suite Seven B, Savannah, GA 31406; tel. 912/356–8440; FAX. 912/356–8439; Susan Brown, RN Administrator

Savannah Plastic Surgicenter, 7208 Hodgson Memorial, Suite 505, Savannah, GA 31406; tel. 912/351–5050; FAX. 912/351–5051; Scott W. Vann MD

Statesboro Ambulatory Surgery Center, 95 Bel-Air Drive, Statesboro, GA 30461-6879; tel. 912/489–6519; FAX. 912/764–7882; Luane L. Jordan, RN

Surgery Center At Mount Zion, 4000 Corporate Center Drive, Suite 100, Morrow, GA 30260-1407; tel. 770/960–2701; FAX. 770/960–2702; Linda Simmons, Administrator

The Emory Clinic Ambulatory Surgery Center, 1365 Clifton Road, N.E., Atlanta, GA 30322; tel. 404/778–5000; W. Mike Mason, Administrator

The Foot Surgery Center, 2520 Windy Hill Road, Suite 105, Marietta, GA 30067; tel. 770/952–0868; Donna L. Cowan, Nurse Administrator

The Rome Surgery Center, 16 John Maddox Drive, Rome, GA 30165; tel. 706/802–3727; FAX. 706/802–3883; Neal Jochimsen, Administrator

Tifton Endoscopy Center, Inc., 1111 E. 20th Street, Tifton, GA 31794-3668; tel. 229/382–9338; FAX. 229/382–4282; Linda Ingram, RN, Nursing Administrator

HAWAII

Aloha Surgical Center, 239 Hoohana Street, Kahului, HI 96732; tel. 808/893–0578; FAX. 808/893–0580; Russell T. Stodd, M.D., Medical Director

Big Island Endoscopy Center, LLC, 64-5188 Kinohou Street, Kamuela, HI 96743; tel. 808/887–0600; FAX. 808/887–6699; Aulii Delenia, Administrator

Cataract and Vision Center of Hawaii, 1712 Liliha Street, Suite 400, Honolulu, HI 96817; tel. 808/524–1010; FAX. 808/531–1030; Worldster Lee, M.D., Director

Hawaii Endoscopy Center, LLC, 2226 Liliha Street, Suite 307, Honolulu, HI 96817; tel. 808/531–5823; FAX. 808/531–5819; James Willie, Administrator

Hawaiian Eye Surgicenter, 606 Kilani Avenue, Wahiawa, HI 96786; tel. 808/622–2645; FAX. 808/621–2082; Christopher M. Tortora, M.D., Surgeon, Director

Hilo Community Surgery Center, 82 Pu'uhonu Place, Suite 100, Hilo, HI 96720; tel. 808/969–9669; FAX. 808/969–9608; Allan S. Takase, MD, Administrator

Kaiser Honolulu Clinic, 1010 Pensacola Street, Honolulu, HI 96814; tel. 808/545–2950; FAX. 808/597–2249; Jonathan Ganz, Administrator

Kaiser Wailuku Clinic, 80 Mahalani Street, Wailuku, HI 96793; tel. 808/243–6112; FAX. 808/243–6609; Martha Turner, Director

Surgicare of Hawaii, an affiliate of S.C.S., 550 South Beretania Street, Suite 700, Honolulu, HI 96813; tel. 808/528–2511; FAX. 808/526–0651; Kare Klungreseter, Administrator

The Endoscopy Center, 134 Pu'uhou Way, Hilo, HI 96720; tel. 808/935–1956; FAX. 808/935–7657; Jody Montell, Administrator

The Surgical Suites, LLC, 1100 Ward Avenue, Suite 1001, Honolulu, HI 96814; tel. 808/531–0127; FAX. 808/531–0455; Carlos Omphroy, M.D., President

IDAHO

Addison Surgery Center, 191 Addison Avenue, Twin Falls, ID 83301; tel. 208/734–5993; FAX. 208/734–5993; David A. Blackmer, D.P.M., President

Boise Gastroenterology Associates, P.A., Idaho Endoscopy Center, 6259 W. Emerald Street, Boise, ID 83704; tel. 208/489–1900; FAX. 208/375–5286; Robb F. Gibson, M.D., President

Coeur D'Alene Foot and Ankle Surgery Center, 101 Ironwood Drive, Suite 131, Coeur D'Alene, ID 83814; tel. 208/666–0814; Stephen A. Isham, D.P.M., Chairman, Board of Directors

Coeur D'Alene Surgery Center, 2121 Ironwood Center Drive, Coeur D'Alene, ID 83814; tel. 208/765–9059; FAX. 208/664–9998; Peter C. Jones, M.D., President

Emerald Surgical Center, 811 North Liberty, Boise, ID 83704; tel. 208/323–4522; FAX. 208/321–9585; William Evans, Administrator

Idaho Ambucare Center, Inc., 4400 Flamingo Ave., Nampa, ID 83686; tel. 208/288–4750; FAX. 208/288–4765; Gary Botimer, Administrator

Idaho Eye Surgicenter, 2025 East 17th Street, Idaho Falls, ID 83404; tel. 208/524–2025; FAX. 208/529–1924; Bradley P. Garnder, M.D.

Idaho Falls Surgical Center, 1945 East 17th Street, Idaho Falls, ID 83404; tel. 208/529–1945; FAX. 208/529–1961; Steven V. Klippert, M.D., CEO

Idaho Foot Surgery Center, 1540 Elk Creek Drive, Idaho Falls, ID 83401; tel. 208/529–8393; FAX. 208/529–8078; Bruce G. Tolman, D.P.M., Facility Director

Jefferson Day Surgery Center, 220 West Jefferson, Boise, ID 83702; tel. 208/343–3802; FAX. 208/343–9161; William Stano, President

Millenium Surgery Center, 1828 S. Millenium Way, Meridian, ID 83642; tel. 208/381–0262; FAX. 208/429–8575; Shane Ricks, Administrator

North Idaho Cataract and Laser Center, Inc., 1814 Lincoln Way, Coeur D'Alene, ID 83814; tel. 208/667–2531; FAX. 208/765–9385; Karen Sines, Administrator

Pacific Cataract and Laser Institute, 250 Bobwhite Court, Suite 100, Boise, ID 83706-3983; tel. 208/385–7576; FAX. 208/385–0050; Lisa Brady, Site Manager

Snake River Endoscopy Center, 141 Morrison St., Twin Falls, ID 83301; tel. 208/732–3030; FAX. 208/733–8970; Karen R. Butler, Nurse Manager
Surgicare Center of Idaho, L.L.C., 360 East Mallard Drive, Suite 125, Boise, ID 83706; tel. 208/336–8700; FAX. 208/426–0902; Mark Hollingshead, Medical Director
The Surgery Center, 115 Falls Avenue, W., P.O. Box 1864, Twin Falls, ID 83303-1864; tel. 208/733–1662; FAX. 208/734–3632; Larry Maxwell, M.D., Administrator

ILLINOIS

25 East Same Day Surgery, 25 East Washington, Suite 300, Chicago, IL 60602; tel. 312/726–3329; FAX. 312/726–3823; Patricia Wamsley, CASC, Administrator
A.C.U. Health Center, LTD., 736 York Road, Hinsdale, IL 60521; tel. 630/794–0645; FAX. 630/794–0169; Lisa Shyne, Executive Director
Able Health Center, Ltd., 1640 Arlington Heights Road, Suite 110, Arlington Heights, IL 60004; tel. 847/255–7400; FAX. 847/398–4585
Access Health Center, Ltd., 1700 75th Street, Downers Grove, IL 60516; tel. 630/964–0000; FAX. 630/964–0047; Lisa Shyne, Director
ACU Health Center, Ltd., 736 N. York Rd., Hinsdale, IL 60521; tel. 630/794–0645; FAX. 630/794–0169; Vera Schmidt, Chief of Operations
Advantage Health Care, LTD., 203 E. Irving Park Road, Wood Dale, IL 60191; tel. 630/595–1515; FAX. 630/595–9097; Lynn Henricks, Administrator
Albany Medical Surgical Center, 5086 North Elston, Chicago, IL 60630; tel. 312/725–0200; FAX. 312/725–6152; Diana Lammon, Administrator
Ambulatory Surgicenter of Downers Grove, Ltd., 4333 Main Street, Downers Grove, IL 60515; tel. 630/322–9451; FAX. 630/322–9455; Inga Ferdkoff, M.D., Administrator
American Women's Medical Center, 2744 North Western, Chicago, IL 60647; tel. 773/772–7726; FAX. 773/772–3696; Jan Barton, M.D., Administrator
AmSurg/Columbia HCA, 330 North Madison Street, Joliet, IL 60435; tel. 815/744–3000; FAX. 815/744–7916; Anne M. Cole, Administrator
Arlington Health Center, Ltd., 1640 Arlington Heights Road, Suite 210, Arlington Heights, IL 60004; tel. 847/255–7474
Bel-Clair Ambulatory Surgical Treatment Center, 325 West Lincoln, Belleville, IL 62220; tel. 618/235–2299; FAX. 618/235–2556; David Horace, Administrator
Carle Surgicenter, 1702 South Mattis Avenue, Champaign, IL 61821; tel. 217/326–2030; Julie Root, RN, Administrator
Children's Pediatric Specialty Services In Westchester, 2301 Enterprise Drive, Westchester, IL 60154; tel. 708/836–4800; FAX. 708/836–4805; Grace Doherty, Director, Satellite Services
CMP Surgicenter, Ltd, 3412 West Fullerton Avenue, Chicago, IL 60647; tel. 773/235–8000; FAX. 773/235–7018; Carlos G. Baldoceda, M.D., Medical Director
Columbia Surgicare-North Michigan Avenue, L.P., 60 East Delaware, 15th Floor, Chicago, IL 60611; tel. 312/440–5100; FAX. 312/440–5114; Barbara Villa, Administrator
Community Health and Emergency Services, 13245 Kessler Road, P.O. Box 233, Cairo, IL 62914; tel. 618/734–4400; FAX. 618/734–9046; Frederick L. Bernstein, Chief Executive Officer
Dimensions Medical Center, Ltd., 1455 East Golf Road, Suite 108, Des Plaines, IL 60016; tel. 847/390–9300; FAX. 847/390–0001; Vera Schmidt, Administrator
Dreyer Ambulatory Surgery Center, 1221 North Highland Avenue, Aurora, IL 60506; tel. 630/264–8400; FAX. 630/264–8402; Josie Nash, RN, BSN, Administrator
Eastland Medical Plaza SurgiCenter, LLC, 1505 Eastland Drive, Suite 180, Bloomington, IL 61701; tel. 309/662–2500; FAX. 309/662–7143; Brenda Cyrulik, Manager
Edwardsville Ambulatory Surgical Center, LLC, 12, Ginger Creek Parkway, Glen Carbon, IL 62034; tel. 618/656–8200; FAX. 618/656–8204; Michelle Looney, Director of Operations
Effingham Ambulatory Surgical Treatment Center, LTD., 904 West Temple Street, Effingham, IL 62401; tel. 217/342–1234; FAX. 217/342–1230; Leanne Fish, RN, CNOR, Administrator
Elmwood Park Same Day Surgery Center, 1614 North Harlem Avenue, Elmwood Park, IL 60607; tel. 708/452–5000; FAX. 708/452–5588; K. Rainone, Administrator
Foot and Ankle Surgical Center, Ltd., 1455 Golf Road, Suite 131, Des Plaines, IL 60016; tel. 847/390–7666; Lowell S. Weil, DPM, FACHS, Medical Director
Golf Surgical Center, 8901 Golf Road, Des Plaines, IL 60016; tel. 847/299–2273; FAX. 847/299–2297; John B. Kinzer, M.D., Executive Director
Hawthorn Surgery Center, 1900 Hollister Drive, Suite 100, Libertyville, IL 60048; tel. 847/367–8100; FAX. 847/367–8335; Dr. Gary Rippberger, Administrator
HealthSouth Surgery Center of Belleville, 28 North 64th Street, Belleville, IL 62223; tel. 618/398–5705; FAX. 618/398–5764; Diane Joiner, RN, Administrator
HealthSouth Surgery Center of Southern Illinois, P.O. Box 1729, 806 N. Treas, Marion, IL 62959; tel. 618/993–2113; FAX. 618/993–2041; Linda Bickers, RN, Administrator
Hinsdale Surgical Center, LLC, 908 North Elm Street, Suite 401, Hinsdale, IL 60521; tel. 630/325–5035; FAX. 630/325–5134; Shirley E. Zemansky, RN, Executive Director
Hope Clinic for Women, Ltd., 1602 21st Street, Granite City, IL 62040; tel. 800/844–3130; FAX. 615/451–9092; Sally Burgess, MBA, Executive Director
Illinois Eye Surgeons Cataract Surgery, 3990 North Illinois Street, Belleville, IL 62221; tel. 618/235–3100; Nancy Mueth, Administrator
Ingalls Same Day Surgery, 6701 West 159th Street, Tinley Park, IL 60477; tel. 708/429–0222; FAX. 708/429–0293; John Czech, Administrator
Loyola Ambulatory Surgery Center at Oakbrook, One South 224 Summit Avenue, Suite 201, Oakbrook Terrace, IL 60181; tel. 630/916–7088; Geoff Abbott, Administrator
LP Central Community Halth Centre, 355 East Fifth Ave., P.O. Box 68, Clifton, IL 60927; tel. 815/694–2392; Steve Wilder, Administrator
Midwest Center for Day Surgery, 3811 Highland Avenue, Downers Grove, IL 60515; tel. 630/852–9300; FAX. 630/852–7773; Ronald P. Ladniak, Administrator
Midwest Eye Center, S.C., 1700 East West Road, Calumet City, IL 60409; tel. 708/891–3330; FAX. 708/891–0904; Afzal Ahmad, M.D., Administrator
Naperville Surgical Centre, 1263 Rickert Drive, Naperville, IL 60540; tel. 630/305–3300; FAX. 630/305–3301; Ronald P. Ladniak
North Shore Endoscopy Center, 101 South Waukegan Road, Suite 980, Lake Bluff, IL 60044; tel. 847/604–8700; FAX. 847/604–8711; Everett P. Kirch, M.D., Administrator
North Shore Same Day Surgicenter, 815 Howard Street, Evanston, IL 60202; tel. 847/869–8500; FAX. 847/869–0028; Edward Atkins, M.D., Medical Director
Northern Illinois Women's Center, Ltd., 1400 Broadway Street, Suite 201, Rockford, IL 61104; tel. 815/963–4101; FAX. 815/963–6122; Meg Larkin, Administrator
Northwest Community Day Surgery Center, 675 West Kirchoff Road, Arlington Heights, IL 60005; tel. 874/618–7075; FAX. 874/618–7069; Meaghan Reshoft, Director
Northwest Surgicare, 1100 West Central Road, Arlington Heights, IL 60005; tel. 847/259–3080; FAX. 847/259–3190; Karolynn Wela-Kuecker, RN, Administrator
Nova Med Eye Surgery Center of Maryville, L.L.C., 12 Maryville Professional Park Drive, Maryville, IL 62062; tel. 618/288–7483; Sarah Davis, Administrator
Novamed Center for Reconstructive Surgery- Oak Lawn, 6311 West 95th Street, Oak Lawn, IL 60453; tel. 708/499–3355; FAX. 708/425–5654; Carmen Hollimon, Administrator
NovaMed Surgery Center River Forest, LLC, 7427 Lake Street, River Forest, IL 60305; tel. 708/488–1300; FAX. 708/771–7321; Troy Litch,, RN, BSHA, Regional Director
Oak Brook Surgical Centre, Inc., 2425 West 22nd Street, Suite 101, Oak Brook, IL 60523; tel. 630/990–2212; FAX. 630/990–3130; George H. Olsen, Administrator
Oak Park Eye Center, S.C., 7055-61 West North Avenue, Oak Park, IL 60302; tel. 708/848–1182; FAX. 708/848–5033; James L. McCarthy, M.D., Administrator
Orthopedic Institute of Illinois Ambulatory Surgery Center, 303 North Kumpf Boulevard, Peoria, IL 61605; tel. 309/676–5559; FAX. 309/676–5045; Donna Adair, Administrator
Palos Surgicenter, 7340 West College Drive, Palos Heights, IL 60463; tel. 708/361–3233; FAX. 708/361–4876; Thomas Holecek, Administrator
Peoria Ambulatory Surgery Center, 4909 North Glen Park Place, Peoria, IL 61614; tel. 309/691–9069; FAX. 309/691–9286; Cynthia J. Leisinger, MBA,CASC, Director of Surgical Services
Peoria Day Surgery Center, 7309 North Knoxville, Peoria, IL 61614; tel. 309/692–9210; FAX. 309/693–6472; Wanda Spacht, RN, Nursing Administrator
Physicians' Surgery Center, 2601 West Main Street, Carbondale, IL 62901; tel. 618/549–5361; FAX. 618/457–7890; Susan Hankins, RN, CNOR
Physicians' Surgical Center, LTD., 311 West Lincoln, Suite 300, Belleville, IL 62220; tel. 618/233–7077; FAX. 618/233–2814; Mary Frances Soltys, RN, Nurse Manager
Planned Parenthood of East Central Illinois, 302 East Stoughton Street, Champaign, IL 61820; tel. 217/359–8022; FAX. 217/359–2683; Robin Beach, Vice President & COO
Quad City Ambulatory Surgery Center, 520 Valley View Drive, Suite 300, Moline, IL 61265; tel. 309/762–1952; FAX. 309/762–3642; Gloria Catlett, RN, Administrative Manager
Quad City Endoscopy, LLC, 2525 24th Street, Suite 104, Rock Island, IL 61201; tel. 309/788–5624; FAX. 309/788–5668
Regional Surgicenter, Ltd., 545 Valley View Drive, Moline, IL 61265; tel. 309/762–5560; FAX. 309/762–7351; Kay Wynn, Administrator
Resurrection Health Care Surgery Center, 3101 North Harlem Avenue, Chicago, IL 60634; tel. 773/889–2000; FAX. 773/745–5522; Sandra Ankebrant, Executive Director
River North Same Day Surgery, One East Erie, Suite 300, Chicago, IL 60611; tel. 312/649–3939; FAX. 312/649–5747; Judith Courtney, RN Administrator
Rockford Ambulatory Surgery Center, 1016 Featherstone Drive, Rockford, IL 61107; tel. 815/226–3300; FAX. 815/226–9990; Dr. Steven Gunderson, CEO/Medical Director
Rockford Endoscopy Center, 401 Roxbury Road, Rockford, IL 61107; tel. 815/397–7340; FAX. 815/397–7388; Nancy Garry, Administrator
Rogers Park One Day Surgery Center, 7616 North Paulina, Chicago, IL 60626; tel. 773/761–0500; FAX. 773/761–0500; Jerry Ruffino, RN Nurse Administrator
Southwestern Medical Center, LLC, dba Magna Surgical Center, 9831 South Western Avenue, Chicago, IL 60643; tel. 312/445–9696; FAX. 312/445–9590; Teri Kerns, Facility Manager
Spiritus Dei Eye Surgery Center, 7600 West College Drive, Palos Heights, IL 60463; tel. 708/361–0010; Audrey Schmidt-Annerino, Administrator
Springfield Clinic Ambulatory Surgery and Endoscopy Center, 1025 South Seventh Street, Springfield, IL 62794-9248; tel. 217/528–7541; FAX. 217/527–8956; Ginny Timke
SureVision Surgery & Laser Center-Northshore, 3034 West Peterson Avenue, Chicago, IL 60659; tel. 773/973–7432; FAX. 773/973–1119; MaryAnn Lassiter, Administrator
Surgicare Center, Inc., 333 Dixie Highway, Chicago Heights, IL 60411; tel. 708/754–4890; FAX. 708/709–6242; Dolores Stam, RN - Supervisor
Surgicore, Inc., 10547 South Ewing Avenue, Chicago, IL 60617; tel. 773/221–1690; Michael A. Wood, DPM, Medical Director
The Center for Orthopedic Medicine, LLC, d/b/a The Center For Outpatient Medicine, 2502-B East Empire Street, Bloomington, IL 61704; tel. 309/662–6120; FAX. 309/661–0060; Sarah Gardner, Business Director
The Center for Surgery, 475 East Diehl Road, Naperville, IL 60563-1253; tel. 630/505–7733; FAX. 630/505–0656; Eric Myers, Administrator
The Surgery Center of Centrailia, 1045 Martin Luther King Jr. Drive, Centralia, IL 62801; tel. 618/532–3110; FAX. 618/532–7226; Ghulam Merchant, M.D., Medical Director
Valley Ambulatory Surgery Center and Valley Medical Inn, 2210 Dean Street, St. Charles, IL 60175; tel. 630/584–9800; FAX. 630/584–9805; Deborah Lee Crook, R.N., Administrator
Women's Aid Clinic, 4751 West Touhy Avenue, Lincolnwood, IL 60712-2212; tel. 847/676–2428; Iris Schneider

INDIANA

Aesthetic Surgery Center, 13590 N. Meridian, Carmel, IN 46032; tel. 317/846–0846; FAX. 317/846–0722; William H. Beeson, M.D., Medical Director

Section C

Ambulatory Care Center, LLC, 300 Circle Front Drive, Evansville, IN 47715; tel. 812/475–1800; FAX. 812/475–1801; Andrea Jarvis, Controller
Ambulatory Care Center, LLC d/b/a, 1125 Professional Boulevard, Evansville, IN 47714; tel. 812/475–1000; FAX. 812/475–1001; Andrea Jarvis, Controller
Calumet Surgery Center, 7847 Calumet Avenue, Munster, IN 46321-1296; tel. 219/836–5102; FAX. 219/836–4496; Denise Cheek, RN Administrator
Central Indiana Surgery Center, 9002 North Meridian, Lower Level, Indianapolis, IN 46260; tel. 317/846–9906; FAX. 317/846–9949; William E. Whitson, M.D., Medical Director
Columbus Surgery Center, 940 North Marr Road, Suite B, Columbus, IN 47201; tel. 812/372–1370; FAX. 812/373–9526; Marcy Ross, R.N.
Digestive Health Center, 1120 AAA Way, Suite A, Carmel, IN 46032-3210; tel. 317/848–5494; FAX. 317/575–0392; Daniel J. Stout, M.D., President
Dupont Ambulatory Surgery Center, 2510 East Dupont Road, Suite 130, Fort Wayne, IN 46825; tel. 219/489–8785; FAX. 219/489–2148; Rick C. Trego, Administrator
Evansville Surgery Center, 520 Mary Street, Evansville, IN 47710; tel. 812/433–3166; FAX. 812/433–3176; Cathy Head RN, BS, MHA, CASO Administrator
Foot and Ankle Surgery Center, Inc., 1950 West 86th Street, Suite 105, Indianapolis, IN 46260; tel. 317/334–0232; FAX. 317/334–0268; Anthony E. Miller, D.P.M., Administrator
Fort Wayne Cardiology Outpatient Catheterization Laboratory, 1819 Carew Street, Fort Wayne, IN 46805; tel. 260/481–4896; FAX. 260/481–4814; Douglas W. Martin, RN, MBA, Director of Clinical Operations
Fort Wayne Ophthalmic Surgical Center, 321 East Wayne Street, Ft. Wayne, IN 46802-2713; tel. 260/422–5976; FAX. 260/969–1041; J. Rex Parent, M.D., Chief Executive Officer
Fort Wayne Orthopaedics LLC, 7601 West Jefferson Boulevard, Fort Wayne, IN 46804-4133; tel. 260/436–8383; FAX. 260/436–8477; Robert D. Bergstrom, COO
Gastrointestinal Endoscopy Center, 801 St. Mary's Drive, Suite 110 West, Evansville, IN 47714; tel. 812/477–6103; FAX. 812/477–4897; Butch Moors, CPA, Administrator
Grand Park Surgical Center, 1479 East 84th Place, Merrillville, IN 46410; tel. 219/738–2828; FAX. 219/756–3349; Chris Macarthy, Administrator
Grossnickle Eye Surgery Center, Inc., 2251 DuBois Drive, Warsaw, IN 46580-3292; tel. 574/269–3777; FAX. 574/371–4697; Diana Ostrom, R.N., Clinical Administrator
Illiana Surgery & Medical Center, 701 Superior Avenue, Munster, IN 46321; tel. 219/924–1300; FAX. 219/922–4810; Virgil Villaflor, Executive Director
Illiana Surgery Center Of Merrillville, 315 W. 89th Ave., Merrillville, IN 46410-2904; tel. 219/757–5275; FAX. 219/757–5290; Mike Baker, COO
IMA Endoscopy Surgicenter, P.C., 8895 Broadway, Merrillville, IN 46410; tel. 219/736–4660; FAX. 219/736–4663; Dawn Bailey, Administrator
Indiana Eye Clinic, 30 North Emerson Avenue, Greenwood, IN 46143-9760; tel. 317/881–3937; FAX. 317/887–4008; Charles O. McCormick, M.D., Administrator
Indiana Surgery Center, 1550 East County Line Road, Suite 100, Indianapolis, IN 46227; tel. 317/621–7600; FAX. 317/621–7606; Peggy Davidson, Administrator
Indiana Surgery Center - North, 8040 Clearvista Parkway, Suite 150, Indianapolis, IN 46256; tel. 317/621–2000; FAX. 317/621–2005; Shannon Arrendale, RN, MBA, Executive Director
Indianapolis Endoscopy Center, 7353 East 21st Street, Indianapolis, IN 46219; tel. 317/353–2232; FAX. 317/353–2522; Kathy Anderson
Meridian Endoscopy Center, 1801 North Senate, Suite 400, Indianapolis, IN 46202; tel. 317/962–5660; FAX. 317/962–2346; Robert J. Whitmore, Executive Director
Meridian Plastic Surgery Center, 170 West 106th Street, Indianapolis, IN 46290-1004; tel. 317/575–0336; FAX. 317/571–8667; Joann Jones, RN, Director
MHC Surgical Center Associates, Inc., d/b/a Broadwest Surgical Center, 315 West 89th Avenue, Merrillville, IN 46410-2904; tel. 219/757–5275; FAX. 219/757–5290; Melvin Lichtenfeld, P.D., Administrator
Michiana Endoscopy Center, LLC, 53830 Generation Drive, South Bend, IN 46635; tel. 219/271–0893; FAX. 219/271–1285; David Mark, M.D., CEO
Midwest Surgery Centers, Inc., 650 Surgery Center Drive, Terre Haute, IN 47802; tel. 812/232–8325; FAX. 812/234–8385; Brenda R. Stallop, Corporate Manager
Muncie Ambulatory Surgicenter, LLC, 200 North Tillotson Avenue, Muncie, IN 47304-3988; tel. 765/286–8888; FAX. 765/747–7962; Jeffrey S. Rapkin, M.D., Medical Director
Munster Same Day Surgery Center, 761 Forty Fifth Avenue, Suite 116, Munster, IN 46321; tel. 219/924–3090; FAX. 219/924–2161
North Meridian Surgery Center, 10601 North Meridian Street, Suite 100, Indianapolis, IN 46290; tel. 317/574–5400; FAX. 317/575–0173; Julie Berzins, Director/CEO
Northeast Indiana Endoscopy Center, 7900 West Jefferson Boulevard, Suite 200, Fort Wayne, IN 46804; tel. 206/969–7181; FAX. 260/969–7182; Jerry Steele, Administrator
Northside Cardiac Cath Lab, 8333 Naab Road, Suite 180, Indianapolis, IN 46260; tel. 317/338–9001; FAX. 317/338–9045; Cecilia Culp RN, Director
NovaMed Inc., 8514 Broadway, Merrillville, IN 46410; tel. 219/756–5010; FAX. 219/736–5106; Seurina Vinovich, Director
Oakview Surgical Center, Inc., 120 E. 18th St., Rochester, IN 46975; tel. 574/224–7500; FAX. 574/223–3057; Laurence C. Rogers, D.P.M., Administrator
Outpatient Surgery Center of Indiana, LLP, 711 Gardner Drive, Marion, IN 46952; tel. 317/664–2000; FAX. 317/668–6797; Dixie Hewitt, RN, Director
Premier Surgery Center, 1333 Maycrest Drive, Fort Wayne, IN 46805-5478; tel. 260/423–3339; FAX. 260/423–6344; Becky Trimbur, Executive Director
Richmond Surgery Center, 1900 Chester Boulevard, Richmond, IN 47374; tel. 765/966–1776; FAX. 765/962–1191; Lynn Greene, RN, Nurse Manager
Riverpointe Surgery Center, 500 Arcade Avenue, Suite 100, Elkhart, IN 46514-2459; tel. 574/522–9505; FAX. 574/296–6484; John Cloyd, PhD, Executive Director
Sagamore Surgical Services, Inc., 2320 Concord Road, Suite B, Lafayette, IN 47909; tel. 765/474–7854; FAX. 765/474–1317; Carol Blanar, Administrator
South Bend Clinic Surgicenter, 211 North Eddy Street, P.O. Box 1755, South Bend, IN 46634-4061; tel. 574/237–9366; FAX. 574/237–9363; Paul J. Meyer, Executive Director
Southern Indiana Surgery Center, 2800 Rex Grossman Boulevard, Bloomington, IN 47403; tel. 812/333–8969; FAX. 812/335–2309; Miriam Malone, RN, B.S.N., Executive Director
Surgery Center of Eye Specialists, 1901 North Meridian Street, Indianapolis, IN 46202; tel. 317/925–2200; FAX. 317/921–6614; Dan Bradford, Administrator
Surgery Center of Southeastern Indiana, Inc., 999 N. Michigan Ave., Greensburg, IN 47240; tel. 812/663–3222; FAX. 812/663–3622; Deanna Borgman, RN, DON
Surgery Center Plus, 7430 North Shadeland Avenue, Suite 100, Indianapolis, IN 46250-2025; tel. 317/841–8005; FAX. 317/577–7538; James Hansen, Administrator
Surgery ONE, 5052 North Clinton, Fort Wayne, IN 46825-5822; tel. 219/482–5194; FAX. 219/482–5686; Debra McCarter, Director
Surgical Care Center, Inc., 8103 Clearvista Parkway, Indianapolis, IN 46256-4600; tel. 317/842–5173; FAX. 317/570–7429; Janelle Gray, RN, Director
Surgical Center of New Albany, 2201 Green Valley Road, New Albany, IN 47150-4648; tel. 812/949–1223; FAX. 812/945–4765; Tamara E. Jones, B.S.N., Administrator
Surgicare, 2907 McIntire Drive, Suite C, Bloomington, IN 47403; tel. 812/339–8000; FAX. 812/339–2524; Rhonda Jacobs, RN, Administrator
Surgicare of Jeffersonville, 1305 Wall Street, Suite 101, Jeffersonville, IN 47130-3898; tel. 812/288–9674; FAX. 812/283–6955; Marsha Parker, Administrator
The Endoscopy Center, 8051 South Emerson, Suite 150, Indianapolis, IN 46237; tel. 317/865–2955; FAX. 317/865–2952; John Murphy, Administrator
The Indiana Hand Center, 8501 Harcourt Road, P.O. Box 80434, Indianapolis, IN 46260-0434; tel. 317/875–9105; FAX. 317/875–8638; Valeria M. Wareham, Chief Operating Officer
Unity Surgery Center, 1011 West Second Street, Bloomington, IN 47403-2216; tel. 812/334–1213; FAX. 812/333–5039; Michael D. Bishop, M.D., CEO
Valley Cataract and Laser Institute, Inc., dba Valley Surgery Center, 220 East Virginia, Evansville, IN 47711; tel. 812/435–1600; FAX. 812/435–1603; Lisa J. Gossman-Werner, Facility Administrator
Valparaiso Physician and Surgery Center, 1700 Pointe Drive, Valparaiso, IN 46383; tel. 219/531–5000; FAX. 219/531–5010; Lilly Veljovic, RN, Manager
Welborn Clinic Surgery Center, 421 Chestnut Street, Evansville, IN 47713; tel. 812/426–9412; Claudia R. Earnest, Administrator
Williams Eye Surgery Center, 6836 Hohman Avenue, Hammond, IN 46324; tel. 219/937–5063; FAX. 219/937–5068; Renee Peters, Administrator

IOWA

Iowa Endoscopy Center, 1378 NW124th Street, Clive, IA 50325; tel. 515/288–6097; FAX. 515/288–8335; Veryl Kroon, CEO
Iowa Eye Institute, P.C., 1721 West 18th Street, P.O. Box 420, Spencer, IA 51301; tel. 712/262–8878; FAX. 712/262–8807; Dennis D. Gordy, M.D., Administrator
Jones Eye Clinic, 4405 Hamilton Boulevard, Sioux City, IA 51104-1140; tel. 712/239–3937; FAX. 712/239–4946; Charles E. Jones, M.D., Medical Director
Mississippi Valley Surgery Center, L.C., 3400 Dexter Court, Suite 200, Davenport, IA 52807; tel. 563/344–6600; FAX. 563/344–6699; John B. Dooley, Administrator
Spring Park Surgery Center, LLC, 3319 Spring Street, Suite 202-A, Davenport, IA 52807; tel. 563/355–6236; FAX. 563/359–6347; David Rohlf, Medical Director
Surgery Center of Des Moines, 717 Lyon Street, Des Moines, IA 50312; tel. 515/266–3140; FAX. 515/266–3073; Bridget Weaver, RN, Administrator

KANSAS

Cotton-O'Neil Clinic Endoscopy Center, 823 Southwest Mulvane Street, Suite 375, Topeka, KS 66606-1679; tel. 785/354–0538; FAX. 785/368–0735; Irene Hasenbank, RN, Director
Emporia Ambulatory Surgery Center, 2528 West 15th Avenue, Emporia, KS 66801-6102; tel. 602/343–2233; J. E. Bosiljevac, M.D., Administrator
Endoscopic Services, P.A., 1431 South Bluffview Street, Suite 215, Wichita, KS 67218-3000; tel. 316/687–0234; FAX. 316/687–0360; Jace Hyder, M.D.
Endoscopy and Surgery Center of Topeka, L.P., 2200 Southwest Sixth Avenue, Suite 103, Topeka, KS 66606-1707; tel. 913/354–1254; FAX. 913/354–1255; Ashraf M. Sufi, M.D., Medical Director
Hutchinson Clinic Ambulatory Surgery Center, 2205 North Waldron, Hutchinson, KS 67502; tel. 620/728–2700; FAX. 620/728–2728; Mary Wood, Director
Kansas Surgery & Recovery Center, 2770 N. Webb Road, Wichita, KS 67226; tel. 316/634–0090; FAX. 316/634–0005
Newton Surgery Center, 800 Medical Center Drive, Newton, KS 67114-3761; tel. 316/283–4400; FAX. 316/283–6606; Joyce Hartner RN, BA, CNOR Director
Ochsner Eye Medical/Associated Eye Surgical Center, 1100 North Topeka Street, Wichita, KS 67214-2810; tel. 316/263–6273; FAX. 316/263–5568; Bruce B. Ochsner, Medical Director
Surgicare of Wichita, Inc., 810 North Lorraine, Wichita, KS 67214-4841; tel. 316/685–2207; FAX. 316/685–2861; Robert J. Kozicki, Administrator
Team Vision Surgery Center East, 6100 East Central Street, Suite Six, Wichita, KS 67208-4237; tel. 316/681–2020; FAX. 316/684–4939; Judy Brown, Director of Nursing
Team Vision Surgery Center West, 834 North Socora, Suite One, Wichita, KS 67212-3238; tel. 316/681–2020; FAX. 316/684–4939; Susan Wade, Administrative Director
Topeka Single Day Surgery, 823 Southwest Mulvane Street, Suite 101, Topeka, KS 66606-1679; tel. 913/354–8737; FAX. 913/354–1440; Linda Daniel, Executive Director
Wichita Clinic DaySurgery, 1947 Founders' Circle, Wichita, KS 67206; tel. 316/613–4934; Yvonne Nutsch RN, Manager

KENTUCKY

Ambulatory Surgery Center, 2831 Lone Oak Road, Paducah, KY 42003; tel. 270/554–8373; FAX. 270/554–8987; Laxmaiah Manchikanti, M.D.

Asethetic Plastic Surgery Institute of Louisville, LLC, d/b/a Louisville Surgery Center, 444 S. First St., Suite 201, Louisville, KY 40202; tel. 502/238–2861; FAX. 502/238–2897; Amy McKiernan, Director of Nursing

Baptist-Physicians' Surgery Center, 1720 Nicholasville Rd, Lexington, KY 40503; tel. 859/260–7000; Robert Ramey, Administrator

Bluegrass Surgery & Laser Center, 1400 Poplar Level Road, Suite 1, Louisville, KY 40217; tel. 502/637–4800; FAX. 502/637–1550; Mary H. Ricci, RN, Administrator

Center For Surgical Care, 7575 U.S. 42, Florence, KY 41042; tel. 606/283–6050; FAX. 606/283–6060; Jenny Brallier, RN Nurse Manager

Center For Surgical Care, 7575 Us 42, Florence, KY 41042; tel. 859/283–6050; FAX. 859/283–6046; Steven P. Magary

Commonwealth Eye Surgery Center, 2353 Alexandria Dr., Suite 350, Lexington, KY 40504; tel. 859/224–2655; R. Aric Myers, Administrator

Commonwealth Urology PSC ASC, 1760 Nicholasville Rd, Suite 301, Lexington, KY 40503; tel. 859/277–5766; Maryagnes Little, Administrator

Cumberland Valley Surgical Center, 275 Hwy 770, Corbin, KY 40729; tel. 606/261–7874; Alfred Smith, Administrator

Dermatology Associates Of KY, PSC, 250 Fountain Court, Lexington, KY 40509; tel. 859/263–4444; Kathy Kesheimer, Administrator

Downing - McPeak Surgery Center, 1507 Bravo Boulevard, Glasgow, KY 42141; tel. 270/651–2181; FAX. 270/651–2183; Sheila Dishman, Administrator

Dupont Surgery Center, 4004 Dupont Circle, Louisville, KY 40207; tel. 502/896–6428; FAX. 502/893–5270; Sherry Oeswein, Administrator

E.M.W. Women's Surgical Center, 138 West Market Street, Louisville, KY 40202; tel. 502/589–2124; FAX. 502/589–1588; Anne Ahola, Executive Director

Eyecare Network, Ltd, 1360 Medical Park Dr, Maysville, KY 41056; tel. 606/759–5341; Bryan Prater, Administrator

Healthsouth Lexington Surgery Center, 1451 Harrodsburg Rd, Suite 102, Lexington, KY 40504; tel. 859/276–2525; Dianna Bennett, Administrator

Healthsouth Louisville Surgery Center, 614 E Chestnut St, Louisville, KY 40202; tel. 502/589–9488; Vanessa McDermott, Administrator

Healthsouth Somerset Surgery Center, 353 Bogle St., Suite 101, Somerset, KY 42503; tel. 606/679–9322; Kathy Turner, Administrator

HealthSouth Surgery Center of Louisville, 4005 DuPont Circle, Paducah, KY 40207; tel. 502/897–7401; FAX. 502/897–5652; Sheila S. Boros, Administrator

HealthSouth Surgical Center of Elizabethtown, 108 Financial Drive, Elizabethtown, KY 42701; tel. 270/737–5200; FAX. 270/737–2422

Jewish Hospital Medical Center East, 3920 Dutchman's Lane, Louisville, KY 40207; tel. 502/259–6003; FAX. 502/259–6111; Shelley Neal, Administrator

Kentucky Surgery Center, 240 Fountain Court, Lexington, KY 40509; tel. 859/278–1460; FAX. 859/278–0115; Kelvin Hanger, Administrator

Lake Cumberland Surgery Center, 301 Langdon St., Somerset, KY 42501; tel. 606/678–9688; FAX. 606/679–7479; Brandon Dugger, Administrator

Lexington Clinic, 1221 South Broadway, Lexington, KY 40504; tel. 606/258–4000; Kathleen Whitlow, Administrator

Louisville Endoscopy Center, 1400 Poplar Level Road, Suite 2, Louisville, KY 40217; tel. 502/636–2003; FAX. 502/636–4032; Mary H. Ricci, RN, Administrator

Louisville Surgery Center, 614 East Chestnut Street, Louisville, KY 40202; tel. 502/589–9488; FAX. 502/589–9928; Vanessa McDermott, Administrator

Mangat-KUY Plastic Surgery Center, 133 Barnwood Drive, Edgewood, KY 41017; tel. 859/331–9600; FAX. 859/578–3321; Linda Robinson, Administrator

Muhlenberg Surgery Center, 1008 Medical Center Dr, Suite A, Powderly, KY 42367; tel. 270/338–9653; Susan Hust, Administrator

Patient First Digestive Disease Center, 340 Thomas More Parkway, Suite 160B, Crestview, KY 41017; tel. 859/331–6466; Gail Hynko, Site Manager

PCN Surgical Suites, 6400 Dutchmans Parkway, Suite 60, Louisville, KY 40205; tel. 502/897–3500; FAX. 502/897–3755; Elmer Dunbar, Administrator

Somerset Surgery Center, 353 Bogle Street, Suite 101, Somerset, KY 42501; tel. 606/679–9322; FAX. 606/678–2666; Kathy Turner, Administrator

Stone Road Surgery Center, 280 Pasadena Dr, Lexington, KY 40503; tel. 859/278–1316; Ballard Wright, Administrator

Surgicare, 225 Medical Center Drive, Suite 105, Paducah, KY 42003; tel. 270/441–4500; FAX. 270/441–4577; Nancy Edwards, Director

The Eye Surgery Center of Paducah, 100 Medical Center Drive, P.O. Box 8269, Paducah, KY 42002-8269; tel. 502/442–1024; FAX. 502/442–1001; Kelly Harris, RN, Administrator

The Pain Treatment Center Inc. d/b/a Stone Road Surgery Center, 280 Pasadena Drive, Lexington, KY 40503; tel. 859/278–1316; FAX. 859/276–3847; Heather Loy, CEO

Tri-State Digestive Disorder Center Ambulatory Surgery Center, 425 Centre View Blvd, Crestview Hills, KY 41017; tel. 859/341–3575; FAX. 859/341–5701; Ross McHenry, M.D.

LOUISIANA

Acadiana Surgery Center, Inc., 2309 East Main Street, Suite 102, New Iberia, LA 70560; tel. 337/364–9680; FAX. 337/364–9689; Dana W. Stokes, RN. Director of Nurses

Alexandria Laser and Surgery Center, 4100 Parliament Drive, Alexandria, LA 71303; tel. 318/487–8342; FAX. 318/487–9942; Martina Anders, RN., Center Director

Ambulatory Eye Surgery Center of Louisiana, 3900 Veterans Boulevard, Suite 100, Metairie, LA 70002; tel. 504/455–1550; FAX. 504/455–2011; Judy Dufrechou RN, Director

Brass Surgery Center, 5328 Didesse Drive, Baton Rouge, LA 70808; tel. 225/766–1718; FAX. 225/766–1225; Derald W. Smith, Administrator

Broussard Surgery Institute, 1250 Pecanland Road, Suite E-1, Monroe, LA 71203; tel. 318/387–2015; FAX. 318/387–2097; Gerald Broussard, M.D., Administrator

Central Louisiana Ambulatory Surgical Center, 651 North Bolton Ave, Alexandria, LA 71301; tel. 318/443–3511; FAX. 318/443–5628; Louise Barker, RN, CEO

Colonnade Surgery, 555 South Ryan Street, Lake Charles, LA 70601; tel. 337/439–6226; FAX. 337/436–6223; Nellie Rideaux, Administrative Assistant

Columbia Greater New Orleans Surgery Center, 3434 Houma Boulevard, Suite 300, Metairie, LA 70006; tel. 504/454–2017; FAX. 530/869–5348; Penny A. Nichols, Administrator

Eye Care and Surgery Center, 10423 Old Hammond Highway, Baton Rouge, LA 70816; tel. 504/923–0960; FAX. 504/923–2419; M. Brian Roper

Foot Surgery Center of Shreveport, 9308 Mansfield Road, Suite 300, Shreveport, LA 71118; tel. 318/686–9622; Richard Havens, D.P.M., Administrator

Gamble Ambulatory Surgery Center, 2601 Line Avenue, Suite B, Shreveport, LA 71104; tel. 318/424–3291; Michael Drews, D.P.M., Administrator

Green Clinic Surgery Center, 1200 South Farmerville Street, Ruston, LA 71270; tel. 318/255–3690; FAX. 318/251–6116; Glenn Scott, Executive Director

HealthSouth Surgi-Center of Baton Rouge, 5222 Brittany Drive, Baton Rouge, LA 70808; tel. 225/767–5636; FAX. 225/215–3477; Denise T. Fortenberry, Administrator

Hedgewood Surgical Center, 2427 St. Charles Avenue, New Orleans, LA 70130; tel. 504/895–7642; FAX. 504/895–0728; Sally Carpenter, RN

Houma Outpatient Surgery Center, Ltd., 3717 Houma Boulevard, Suite 300, Metairie, LA 70006; tel. 504/456–1515; FAX. 504/454–3810; Landon Tucker, Administrator

Houma Surgi Center, Inc., 1020 School Street, Houma, LA 70360; tel. 985/868–4320; FAX. 985/868–3617; Pat Hitt, RN Assistant Administrator

LaHaye Eye and Ambulatory Surgical Center, 4313 I-49 S. Service Rd., Opelousas, LA 70570; tel. 337/942–2024; FAX. 337/948–8869; Douglas C. Mankin, Administrator

LaHaye Total Eye Care, 201 Rue Iberville, Suite 800, Lafayette, LA 70508; tel. 337/235–2149; Bridget Ray

Lake Charles Medical-Surgical Clinic, 501 South Ryan, Lake Charles, LA 70601; tel. 337/433–8400; FAX. 337/433–7350; Carolyn Spikes, Administrator of Endoscopy

Laser and Surgery Center of Acadiana, 514 St. Landry Street, Lafayette, LA 70506; tel. 337/234–2020; FAX. 318/234–8230; Barbara L. Azar, Administrator

Laser and Surgery Center of the South, 1101 Audubon Avenue, Suite S-Four, Thibodaux, LA 70301; tel. 504/447–7258; FAX. 504/446–7614; Nate Graff, Administrator

Louisiana Endoscopy Center, Inc., 9103 Jefferson Highway, Baton Rouge, LA 70809; tel. 225/927–0970; FAX. 225/706–0160; Albert Hart, IV, Administrator

LSU Eye Surgery Center, 2020 Gravier Street, Suite B, New Orleans, LA 70112; tel. 504/412–1590; FAX. 504/472–1268; W. L. Blackwell, Chief Executive Officer

Magnolia Surgical Facility, 3939 Houma Boulevard, Suite 216, Metairie, LA 70006; tel. 504/455–7771; FAX. 504/885–5063; Melissa Johnson, Administrator, Medical Director

MGA-GI Diagnostic and Therapeutic Center, 1111 Medical Center Boulevard, Suite 450, Marrero, LA 70072; tel. 504/349–6310; FAX. 504/349–6444; Thomas D. McCaffery, Jr., President

MGA-GI Diagnostic and Therapeutic Center, 2633 Napoleon Avenue, Suite 707, New Orleans, LA 70115; tel. 504/896–8680; FAX. 504/896–8699; Thomas D. McCaffery, Jr., President

Northeast Louisiana Surgery Center, 3101 Kilpatrick Boulevard, Monroe, LA 71201; tel. 318/322–5506; FAX. 318/322–5916; David G. Gardner, President

Ochsner Clinic-Center for Cosmetic Surgery, 1514 Jefferson Highway, Fifth Floor, New Orleans, LA 70121; tel. 504/842–3950; FAX. 504/842–5003; Rachel Franz, RN, B.S.N., Manager

Omega Hospital, LLC, 2525 Severn Avenue, Metairie, LA 70001; tel. 504/832–4200; FAX. 504/832–4209; Deborah Scnenck, Administrator

Outpatient Eye Surgery Center, 4324 Veterans Boulevard, Metairie, LA 70006; tel. 504/455–4046; FAX. 504/455–9890; Cheryl Crouse, RN, Administrator

Physicians Surgery Center, 218 Corporate Drive, Houma, LA 70360; tel. 504/853–1390; FAX. 504/853–1470; Connie K. Martin, Administrator

Saints Streets Lafayette General Ambulatory Endoscopy Center Inc., 201 St. Patrick Street, Suite 202, Lafayette, LA 70506; tel. 337/269–6062; FAX. 337/233–8065; Stephen G. Abshire, M.D., Administrator

Shreveport Endoscopy Center, A.M.C., 3217 Mabel Street, P.O. Box 37045, Shreveport, LA 71133-7045; tel. 318/631–0072; FAX. 318/631–9688; Linda Ray, Administrator

Shreveport Surgery Center, 745 Olive Street, Suite 100, Shreveport, LA 71104; tel. 318/227–1163; FAX. 318/227–0413; Mary Jones, Administrator

Surgery Center, Inc., 1101 South College Road, Suite 100, Lafayette, LA 70503; tel. 337/233–8603; FAX. 337/234–0341; Russell J. Arceneaux, Administrator

Surginet Outpatient Surgery, LLC, 101 La Rue France, Suite 400, Lafayette, LA 70508; tel. 318/269–9828; FAX. 318/269–9823; Millissa R. Coco, Administrator

The Endoscopy Center of Monroe, 316 South Sixth Street, Monroe, LA 71201; tel. 318/325–2649; FAX. 318/325–0717; Andy W. Waldo, Administrator

The Outpatient Surgery Center for Sight, 7732 Goodwood Blvd., Ste D., Baton Rouge, LA 70806; tel. 225/925–2031; FAX. 225/924–2809; Connie Commons

The Surgery Suite, 103 Medical Center Drive, Slidell, LA 70461; tel. 985/646–4466; FAX. 985/646–5699; Allison F. Maestri, RN, Administrator

Urology Specialty and Surgery Center, 234 South Ryan Street, Lake Charles, LA 70601; tel. 337/433–5282; FAX. 337/433–1159; Shari Davis, Administrator

West Monroe Endoscopy Center, 102 Thomas Road, Suite 506, West Monroe, LA 71291; tel. 318/388–8878; FAX. 318/388–8870; C.B. Dunn, Jr. M.D.

Young Eye Surgery Center, Inc., 204 North Magdalen Square, Abbeville, LA 70510; tel. 318/893–4452; FAX. 318/893–7870; Virginia Y. Hebert, Administrator

MAINE

Acadia Medical Arts Ambulatory Surgical Suite, 404 State Street, Bangor, ME 04401; tel. 207/990–0928; Jordan J. Shubert, M.D., President

Eyecare Medical Group, 53 Sewall Street, Portland, ME 04102; tel. 207/773–6336; FAX. 207/773–7034; William S. Holt, M.D., President

Maine Eye Center, P.A., 15 Lowell Street, Portland, ME 04102; tel. 207/774–8277; FAX. 207/871–1415; Frank Read, M.D., Director

Northern Maine Ambulatory Endoscopy Center, 11 Martin Street, P.O. Box 748, Presque Isle, ME 04769-0151; tel. 207/764–2482; FAX. 207/764–1569; Devin McHalten, Administrator

Orthopaedic Associates of Portland, P.A., 33 Sewall Street, Portland, ME 04102; tel. 207/828–2100; FAX. 207/828–2190; Linda M. Ruterbories, ASU Director

Vision Care Of Maine-Ardostook,LLC, 173 Academy Street, Presque Isle, ME 04769; tel. 207/764–0376; FAX. 207/764–7612; Craig W. Young, M.D., Director

Western Avenue Day Surgery Center, a/k/a Plastic and Hand Surgical Associates, P.A., 244 Western Avenue, South Portland, ME 04106; tel. 207/775–3446; FAX. 207/879–1646; Jean J. Labelle, M.D., President

MARYLAND

Albert Shoumer, D.P.M., Dundalk Professional Center, 40 South Dundalk Avenue, Dundalk, MD 21222; tel. 410/282–6434; FAX. 410/284–4636; Darleen Grupp, Office Manager

Albert Shoumer, D.P.M., 1645 Liberty Road, Eldersburg, MD 21784; tel. 310/795–2889

Ambulatory Endoscopy Center of Maryland, Inc., 7350 Van Dusen Road, Suite 230, Laurel, MD 20707; tel. 301/498–5500; FAX. 301/604–5956; Kim Wilson RN, Center Director

Ambulatory Plastic Surgery Center Associates, CHTD, 9715 Medical Center Drive, Suite 315, Rockville, MD 20850; tel. 301/738–9137; FAX. 301/738–7920; Mary Vincent, Office Manager

American Podiatric Surgery, 10236 River Road, Potomac, MD 20854; tel. 301/983–9873; FAX. 301/299–3985; Amy Meehan, Administrator

Anne Arundel Gastroenterology Associates, 703 Giddings Avenue, Suite M, Annapolis, MD 21401; tel. 410/224–2116; Gary M. Evans, Administrator

Baltimore Ambulatory Center for Endoscopy, 19 Fontana Lane, Suite 104, Baltimore, MD 21237; tel. 410/574–7776; FAX. 410/574–9038; Dr. J. Khan, Medical Director

Baltimore Podiatry Group, 5205 East Drive, Suite I, Arbutus, MD 21227; tel. 410/247–5333; Neil Scheffler, D.P.M., President

Baltimore Washington Eye Center, 200 Hospital Drive, Suite 600, Glen Burnie, MD 21061; tel. 410/766–3937; FAX. 410/761–4386; Kris Morgan, ASC Coordinator

Bayside Surgical Center, Inc., 8023 Ritchie Highway, Pasadena, MD 21122; tel. 410/761–4190; FAX. 410/761–0265; Sheila Freeze, Office Manager

Beitler, Samuel D., D.P.M. Ambulatory Surgery Center, Glen Burnie Podiatric Surgery Center, 795 Aquahart Road, Suite 125, Glen Burnie, MD 21061; tel. 410/768–0702; FAX. 410/768–0649; Samuel D. Beitler, D.P.M.

Bel Air Ambulatory Surgical Center, LLC, 2007 Rock Spring Road, Lower Level, Forest Hill, MD 21050; tel. 410/879–2474; FAX. 410/879–8194; Karen Askew, RN, Nurse Manager

Belcrest Surgery Center, 6505 Belcrest Road, Suite One, Hyattsville, MD 20782; tel. 301/699–5900; FAX. 301/699–9297; Mark H. Sugar, D.P.M., Director

Bethesda Ambulatory Surgical Center, 5620 Shields Dr., Bethesda, MD 20817; tel. 301/530–4181; FAX. 301/530–4373; John Lydon, D.P.M., Administrator

Center for Oral & Maxillofacial Surgery, 1212 York Road, Suite A201, Lutherville, MD 21093; tel. 410/337–7755; FAX. 410/337–7922; Laurie Kolmer, Office Manager

Chesapeake Ambulatory Surgery Center, LLC, 8028 Governor Ritchie Highway, Suite 100, Pasadena, MD 21122; tel. 410/768–5800; FAX. 410/768–5806; Ira J. Gottlieb, D.P.M., Owner, Administrator

Chesapeake Surgery Center, 145 East Carroll Street, Salisbury, MD 21801; tel. 410/548–1108; FAX. 410/548–2607; Joseph G. Walters, PA-C Administrative Director

Clinical Associates, 515 Fairmont Avenue, Suite 500, Towson, MD 21286; tel. 410/494–1335

Cumberland Valley Surgical Center, LLC, 1110 Professional Court, Hagerstown, MD 21740; tel. 240/420–5559; Stacey Taylor, RN, BSN, Administrator, CASC

D/B/A Maryland Outpatient Foot Surgery Center, Dennis M. Weber D.P.M., 4701 Randolph Road, Suite 115, Rockville, MD 20852; tel. 301/770–5741; FAX. 301/468–1093; Dennis M. Weber, D.P.M., Director

De Leonibus and Palmer, L.L.C., A.S.C., MedSurg Foot Center, 2086 Generals Highway, Suite 101, Annapolis, MD 21401; tel. 410/266–7666; FAX. 410/266–7703; Courtney Palmer, DPM

Digestive Disease Consultant of Frederick, 915 Toll House Avenue, Suite 201, Frederick, MD 21701; tel. 301/662–7822; James A. Frizzell, M.D.

Dimensions Surgery Center, 14999 Health Center Drive, Bowie, MD 20716; tel. 301/809–2000; FAX. 301/464–3572; Joan McHale, Director of Operations

Dr. Michael K. Schwartz, D.D.S., P.A., 723 South Charles Street, Baltimore, MD 21230; tel. 410/727–4886

Dulaney Eye Institute, 901 Dulaney Valley Road, Towson, MD 21204; tel. 410/583–1000; FAX. 410/583–4718; Andrea Hyatt, CASC, Administrator

Dundalk Ambulatory Surgery Center, 1123 Merritt Boulevard, Baltimore, MD 21222; tel. 410/282–6666; FAX. 410/282–0357; Pam Green, Office Manager

Easton Foot Center, 8579 Commerce Drive, Suite 100A, Easton, MD 21061; tel. 410/822–0645

Eye Surgery Center of Ophthalmology Associates, L.L.C., 10755 Falls Road, Suite 110B, Lutherville, MD 21093; tel. 410/583–2808; FAX. 410/583–2814; Amina C. Barnes, Operating Manager

Eye Surgical Center Associates of Baltimore, dba The Surgicenter at Towson, 1122 Kenilworth Drive, Suite 18, Towson, MD 21204; tel. 410/321–4400; FAX. 410/321–4909; Susanne Varmer, RN, Director of Nursing

Facial Plastic Surgicenter, Ltd., 1838 Greene Tree Road, Baltimore, MD 21208; tel. 410/486–3400; FAX. 410/486–0092; Ira D. Papel, M.D., President

Flaum, Martin/Rockville Ambulatory Surgical Center, LLC, 50 West Edmonston Drive, Suite 306, Rockville, MD 20852; tel. 301/340–8666; FAX. 301/340–7448; Martin C. Flaum, Owner

Foot and Ankle Associates d/b/a, Kensington Surgery Center, 10901 Connecticut Avenue, Suite 200, Kensington, MD 20895; tel. 301/949–2000; FAX. 301/949–2002; Dr. Gene Mirkin

Foot Care Associates Ambulatory Care Center at Joppa Foot Care, 2316 East Joppa Road, Baltimore, MD 21234; tel. 410/882–5100

Footer, Ronald, D.P.M., P.A., 16220 Frederick Avenue, Suite 200, Gaithersburg, MD 20877; tel. 301/948–2995; FAX. 301/948–6056; Maryrose Hanks, Office Manager

Four Corners Ambulatory Surgical Center, LLC, Dr. Gary A. Lieberman, PA, 10101 Lorain Avenue, Silver Spring, MD 20901; tel. 301/681–8400; FAX. 301/681–3339; Gayle Rickert, Administrator

Frederick Surgical Center, 915 Toll House Avenue, Suite 103, Frederick, MD 21701; tel. 301/694–3400; FAX. 301/694–3620; Marjorie Blouin, Administrator & Director of Surgical Services

Gastrointestinal Diagnostic Center, 4660 Wilkens Avenue, Suite 302, Baltimore, MD 21229; tel. 410/242–3636; FAX. 410/242–4404; Mary C . Harrison, Business Manager

Gehris, Heroy and Associates of Lutherville, 1212 York Road, Suite 201B, Lutherville, MD 21093; tel. 410/821–6130; James H. Heroy III, Administrator

Giardina and Glubo, P.A., 4660 Wilkens Avenue, Baltimore, MD 21229; tel. 410/242–7066; FAX. 410/242–4126; Eileen Giardina, RN

Gynemed Surgi-Center, 17 Fontana Lane, Suite 201, Baltimore, MD 21237; tel. 410/686–8220; FAX. 410/391–0943; David O'Neil, M.D.

Hamilton Foot Care Associates ASC, 5508 Harford Road, Baltimore, MD 21214; tel. 410/426–5508

Harford County Ambulatory Surgery Center, 1952-A Pulaski Highway, Edgewood, MD 21040; tel. 410/538–7000; FAX. 410/679–4291; Ms. Kim Merrill, RN, BN, Nurse Administrator

Harford Endoscopy Center, LLC, Two North Avenue, Suite 102, Belair, MD 21014; tel. 410/838–6345; FAX. 410/838–1595; Sherry Adkins, Center Director

HealthSouth St. Agnes Surgery Center of Ellicott City, 2850 North Ridge Road, Ellicott City, MD 21043; tel. 410/461–1600; FAX. 410/750–7615; Melaine Medura Faculty Administrator

Johns Hopkins Plastic Surgery Associates, JHOC 8, 601 North Caroline Street, Baltimore, MD 21287; tel. 410/955–6897; FAX. 410/614–1296

Kaiser-Permanente-Kensington, 10810 Connecticut Avenue, Kensington, MD 20895; tel. 301/929–7275; FAX. 301/929–7577; Wanda McCulley, RN, Administrator

Kenneth Margolis, M.D., P.A., Ambulatory Endoscopy Surgical Center, 9101 Franklin Square Drive, Suite 213, Baltimore, MD 21237; tel. 410/687–0202; FAX. 410/687–0985; Jo Ann Smith, Office Manager

Lake Forest Ambulatory Surgical Center, 702 Russell Avenue, Gaithersburg, MD 20877; tel. 301/948–3668; FAX. 301/926–7787

Laser Surgery Center, Inc., 484A Ritchie Highway, Severna Park, MD 21146; tel. 410/544–4600; FAX. 410/544–0997; Gerri Taylor, Office Manager

Laurel Ambulatory Surgery Center, 2401 Brandermill Blvd, Suite 340, Gambrills, MD 21054; tel. 410/451–3206; FAX. 410/451–3207; Lance Caffiero, Administrator

Laurel Foot and Ankle Surgery Center Inc., 14440 Cherry Lane Court, Suite 104, Laurel, MD 20707; tel. 301/953–3668; Dr. Frank Smith, Administrator

Maclean, Kishel, Applestein, M.D., A.S.C., 11085 Little Patuxent Parkway, Columbia, MD 21044; tel. 410/997–1930

Maple Springs Ambulatory Surgery Center, 10810 Darnstown Road, Suite 101, Gaithersburg, MD 20878; tel. 301/762–3338; FAX. 301/762–1585; Dr. Stuart Snyder, PA, President

Maryland Endoscopy Center, L.L.C., 100 West Road, Suite 115, Towson, MD 21204; tel. 410/494–0144; FAX. 410/494–0147; Irma Haak, R.N., Nurse Manager

Maryland Kidney Stone Center/AKSM, 6115 Falls Road, LL-a, Baltimore, MD 21209; tel. 410/377–2622; FAX. 410/377–4410; Walter Weinstein, Regional Manager

Maryland Urology Surgicenters, LLC, 6830 Hospital Drive, Suite 204, Baltimore, MD 21237; tel. 410/391–6131; FAX. 410/391–6144; Dr. William Dowling, Head Doctor

Metropolitan Ambulatory Urologic Institute LLC, 7759 Belle Point Drive, Greenbelt, MD 20770; tel. 301/474–5583; FAX. 301/474–5742; Kristy Browning CRNA, Manager

Michetti, Michael, Dr. of District Heights, 6400 Marlboro Pike, District Heights., MD 20747; tel. 301/736–6900

Mid Shore Surgical Eye & Laser Center, 8420 Ocean Gateway, Suite One, Easton, MD 21601; tel. 410/822–0424; FAX. 410/822–2283; Cheryl Schmitt, RN

Montgomery Endoscopy Center P.A., Montgomery Gastroenterology P.A., 12012 Veirs Mill Road, Wheaton, MD 20906; tel. 301/942–3550; FAX. 301/933–3621; Howard Goldberg, M.D., A.S.C Director

Montgomery Surgical Center, 46 West Gude Drive, Rockville, MD 20850; tel. 301/424–6901; FAX. 301/294–7847; Patti Hartsfield, Administrator

Moulsdale, Murphy, Siegelbaum and Lerner, 7505 Osler Drive, Suite 508, Towson, MD 21204; tel. 410/296–0166; FAX. 410/828–7275

North Arundel Plastic Surgery Specialists, A89 Ritchie Highway, Building C, 2nd Floor, Severna Park, MD 21146; tel. 410/841–5355; FAX. 410/841–6589; Ajia S. Layman, Administrator

Parris-Castoro Eye & Laser Center, 620 Boulton Street, Bel Air, MD 21014; tel. 410/836–7010; FAX. 410/399–8427; Michael Grasham, ASC Administrator

Plastic Surgery Specialists, 2448 Holly Avenue, Suite 400, Annapolis, MD 21401; tel. 410/841–5355; FAX. 410/841–6589; Ajia S. Layman, Administrator

Plaza Ambulatory Surgical Center, 6506 Reisterstown Road, Suite 501, Baltimore, MD 21215; tel. 410/764–7044; Dr. Brian Kashan, Administrator

Podiatry Associates, P.A., 9712 Bel Air Road, Baltimore, MD 21236; tel. 410/574–6060; FAX. 410/256–2727; Stanley Book

Podiatry Associates, P.A., One North Main Street, Bel Air, MD 21014; tel. 410/879–1212; FAX. 410/893–1081

Podiatry Associates, P.A., 6569 North Charles Street, Suite 702, Towson, MD 21204; tel. 410/828–5420; FAX. 410/828–1663; Stan Book, Billing Manager

Podiatry Associates, P.A., Charter Professional Center, 10700 Charter Drive, Suite 300, Columbia, MD 21044; tel. 410/730–0970; FAX. 410/730–0161; Dr. Boyd, Capello, Ritter, Podiatrist
Podiatry Group, P.A. of Annapolis, 139 Old Solomons Island Road, Suite C, Annapolis, MD 21401; tel. 410/224–4448; FAX. 410/841–5200; Kate Pearson, Administrator
Prince George's Ambulatory Care Center/ Endoscopy Suites, Inc., 6001 Landover Road, Suite One, Cheverly, MD 20785; tel. 301/773–3900; FAX. 301/773–7869; Jeannette Figueroa, Administrator
Prince George's Multi-Specialty Surgery Centre, Inc., 8700 Central Avenue, Suite 106, Landover, MD 20785; tel. 301/808–9298; FAX. 301/499–1266; Douglas Hallgren, Administrator
Queen Anne Surgery Center, 2108 DiDonato Drive, Chester, MD 21619; tel. 410/643–7207; FAX. 410/643–9274; Lisa Parks, Administrator
River Reach Outpatient Surgery Center, 790 Governor Ritchie Highway, Suite E-35, Severna Park, MD 21146; tel. 410/544–2487; FAX. 410/544–1872; Pat Hofmeier, Administrator
Riverside Ambulatory Surgery Center, 560 Riverside Drive, Suite A-101, Salisbury, MD 21801; tel. 410/749–0121; FAX. 410/749–6807; Patricia Timmons, PMAC, Administrator
Rivertowne Surgery Center, 6196 Oxon Hill Road, Suite 650, Oxon Hill, MD 20745; tel. 301/839–7499; FAX. 301/839–8726; Deborah Arminio, Administrator
Robinwood Surgery Center, LLC, 11110 Medical Campus Road, Suite 200, Hagerstown, MD 21742; tel. 301/714–4300; FAX. 301/714–4324; Lana Gladhill, Director
Roger J. Oldham, M.D., Ambulatory Surgery Center, LLC, Bethesda Surgery Center, 10215 Fernwood Road, Suite 412, Bethesda, MD 20817; tel. 301/530–6100; Janet Scanlon
Rotunda Ambulatory Surgery Center, 711 West 40th Street, Suite 410, Baltimore, MD 21211; tel. 410/889–4885; FAX. 410/889–2497; Theresa Steele, Administrator
Saint Mary's Multispecialty Surgery Center, Inc., Route 235 and Chancellors Run Road, Suite 15, P.O. Box 1310, California, MD 20619; tel. 301/862–3984; FAX. 301/862–3335; Douglas H. Hallgren, Administrator
Spector, Adam, D.P.M., Ambulatory Surgery Center, 2730 University Blvd. W., Suite 1000, Wheaton, MD 20902; tel. 301/949–3668; FAX. 301/949–8833; Adam Spector, D.P.M., Administrator
Suburban Endoscopy Center, L.L.C., 10215 Fernwood Road, Suite 206, Bethesda, MD 20817; tel. 301/530–2800; FAX. 301/530–9560
Summit Ambulatory Surgery Center, Ambulatory Surgery Center, 1001 Pine Heights Avenue, Suite 104, Baltimore, MD 21229; tel. 410/644–0929; Narang Ashok, Administrator
SurgiCenter of Baltimore, LLP, 23 Crossroads Drive, Suite 100, Owings Mills, MD 21117; tel. 410/356–0300; FAX. 410/356–7507; Rosemary L. Lambie, RN, Administrator
The Adult and Pediatric Urology Surgery Center of MD, 3455 Wilkens Avenue, Suite 100, Baltimore, MD 21229; tel. 410/646–0330; FAX. 410/644–6182; Bridget Mastrounni, Practice Administrator
The Ambulatory Urosurgical Center, 401 East Jefferson Street, Suite 105, Rockville, MD 20850; tel. 301/309–8219; FAX. 301/309–9370; Bernadette Noel, RN, Administrative Director
The Endoscopy Center, 7402 York Road, Suite 101, Towson, MD 21204; tel. 410/494–0156; FAX. 410/828–1706; Barry Gendason, General Manager
The Friendship Ambulatory Surgery Center, P.C., 5550 Friendship Boulevard, Suite 270, Chevy Chase, MD 20815; tel. 301/215–7347; FAX. 301/215–7345; Anthony Ruffin, Administrator/Dr. Mary Craddock, Medical Director
Total Foot Care Surgery Center, Inc., 7525 Greenway Center Drive, Suite 112, Greenbelt, MD 20770; tel. 301/345–4087; FAX. 301/345–0482; Kathi Reinhart, Office Manager
W.G.. Armiger, P.A., d/b/a Chesapeake Plastic Surgery Associates, 1421 South Caton Avenue, Suite 203, Baltimore, MD 21227; tel. 410/646–3226; FAX. 410/644–2134; William G. Armiger, M.D., Director
Waldorf Endoscopy Center, 11340 Pembroke Square, Suite 202, Waldorf, MD 20603; tel. 310/638–5354; FAX. 301/843–5184; Denise Moran Center Director
Washington Surgi Center, 6228 Oxon Hill Road, Oxon Hill, MD 20745; tel. 301/839–0770; FAX. 301/839–1350; Dr. Othman A. Baban
Western Maryland Eye Surgical Center, 1003 West Seventh Street, Suite 400, Frederick, MD 21701; tel. 301/662–3721; FAX. 301/698–8164

MASSACHUSETTS

Andover Surgery Center, LP, 138 Haverhill Street, Andover, MA 01810; tel. 508/475–2880; FAX. 508/475–9562; Nancy Aucoin, Executive Director
Boston Center for Ambulatory Surgery, Inc., 170 Commonwealth Avenue, Boston, MA 02116; tel. 617/267–0710; FAX. 617/236–8704; Philip J. Gaven, MBA, Administrator
Boston Eye Surgery & Laser Center, P.C., 50 Stanford Street, Boston, MA 02114; tel. 617/723–2015; FAX. 617/723–7787; Sheila M. Harney, Business Manager
Boston University Eye Assoc., Inc., 90 New State Highway, Raynham, MA 02767; tel. 508/822–8839; FAX. 508/880–3616; Judith A. Orsie, RNBSN, Director of Surgical Services
Cataract and Laser Center West, LLC., 171 Interstate Drive, West Springfield, MA 01089; tel. 413/737–5500; FAX. 413/732–3514; Robert E. Dempsey, Jr, Administrator
Cataract and Laser Center, Inc., 333 Elm Street, Dedham, MA 02026; tel. 781/326–3800; FAX. 728/326–2120; John Dunne, Administrator
Cosmetic Surgery Center, 68 Camp Street, Hyannis, MA 02601; tel. 508/775–7026; FAX. 508/771–0499; Laura Norkatis, Office Manager
HealthSouth Maple Surgery Center, 298 Carew Street, Springfield, MA 01104; tel. 413/739–9668; FAX. 413/781–3652; Kathleen S. Loomis, RN, Facility Administrator
New England Eye Surgery Center, 696 Main Street, Weymouth, MA 02190; tel. 617/331–3820; FAX. 617/331–1076; Kenneth Camerota
New England Surgicare, One Brookline Place, Suite 201, Brookline, MA 02146; tel. 617/730–9650; Gratia S. Chase, RN, Administrator
Northeast Ambulatory Center, Three Woodland Road, Suite 321, Stoneham, MA 02180; tel. 781/665–5233; FAX. 781/662–4878; Anil Kumar M.D., Medical Director
Plymouth Laser and Surgical Center, 40 Industrial Park Road, Plymouth, MA 02360; tel. 508/746–8600; FAX. 508/747–0824; Kathleen Murphy, Administrator
Same Day SurgiClinic, 272 Stanley Street, Fall River, MA 02720; tel. 508/672–2290; FAX. 508/679–3766; Steven Pimental, Business Manager
Surgery Center of Waltham, 130 2nd Avenue, Waltham, MA 02451; tel. 781/434–6500; FAX. 781/434–6501; Alan S. Penzias, Director of Surgery
The Eye Center LLC, 61 Lincoln St, Suite 305, Lincoln Medical Center Building, Framingham, MA 01702; tel. 508/620–0017; Mona Bhan M.D., or Lawrence Rand M.D.
Worcester Surgical Center, Inc., 300 Grove Street, Worcester, MA 01650; tel. 508/754–0700; FAX. 508/831–9989; Andy H. Poritz, M.D., Professional Services Director

MICHIGAN

Balian Eye Center, 432 West University Drive, Rochester, MI 48307; tel. 248/651–6122; FAX. 248/651–4825; E. Mike Raphtis, M.D.
Birth Control Center, Inc., 2783 Fourteen Mile Road, Sterling Heights, MI 48310; tel. 810/939–4000; Armen Vartanian, Administrator
Centre for Plastic Surgery, 426 Michigan Street, N.E., Suite 300, Grand Rapids, MI 49503; tel. 616/454–1256; FAX. 616/454–0308; Daniel Reeder, Administrator
Community Surgical Center, 30671 Stephenson Highway, Madison Height, MI 48071; tel. 810/588–8000; FAX. 810/588–9140; C. J. Yanos, Administrator
East Michigan Surgery Center, 701 South Ballenger, Flint, MI 48532; tel. 810/238–3603; FAX. 810/767–5194; Lucy Marshall, Administrator
Eastside Endoscopy Center, 28963 Little Mack, Suite 103, St. Clair Shores, MI 48081; tel. 586/447–5115; FAX. 586/774–6091; Beth Miller, Administrator
Endoscopy and Surgery Center at Woodbridge Hills, 7901 Angling Road, Portage, MI 49024; tel. 269/324–8406; FAX. 269/324–8476; Renee Langeland, M.S.N., RN, Administrator
Glascco Ambulatory Surgery Center, 1707 West Lake Lansing Road, Lansing, MI 48912; tel. 517/267–0033; FAX. 517/267–0430; Michael Falatko, CEO
Health Care Midwest Surgery Center, 125 West Walnut, Kalamazoo, MI 49007; tel. 616/343–1381; Gregor W. Blix, M.D., Medical Director
Hemorrhoid Clinics of America, 22000 Greenfield Road, Oak Park, MI 48237; tel. 248/967–4140; FAX. 248/967–0745; Max Ali, M.D., President
Henry Ford Hospital Fairlane Center, 19401 Hubbard Drive, Dearborn, MI 48126; tel. 313/593–8100; Jay Zerwekh, Administrator
Henry Ford Medical Center, 6777 West Maple Road, West Bloomfield, MI 48322; tel. 248/661–4100; FAX. 248/661–6494; Sally Bertonia, Administrative Manager
Henry Ford Medical Center-Lakeside Ambulatory Surgery, 14500 Hall Road, Sterling Heights, MI 48313; tel. 810/247–2680; FAX. 810/247–2682; Mary Vidaurri, Ph.D., Regional Administrator
Holland Eye Clinic, 999 South Washington, Holland, MI 49423; tel. 616/396–2316; FAX. 616/396–0085; Kristine Curtis, Assistant Administrator
John Michael Garrett, M.D., 1301 Carpenter Avenue, Iron Mountain, MI 49801; tel. 906/774–1404; FAX. 906/774–8132; Susan Brunnette, RN, ASC Supervisor
M.D. Surgicenter, 375 Barclay Circle, Rochester Hill, MI 48307; tel. 810/852–3636; FAX. 810/852–3631; Robert Swartz, Administrator
Metropolitan Eye Center, 21711 Greater Mack Avenue, St. Clair Shores, MI 48080; tel. 586/774–0343; FAX. 586/777–2214; James W. Klein, M.D., Director
Michigan Center for Outpatient Ocular Surgery, 33080 Utica Road, P.O. Box 26010, Fraser, MI 48026; tel. 810/296–7250; FAX. 810/296–0276; Norbert P. Czajkowski, M.D., Director
Midwest Health Center, 5050 Schaefer Avenue, Dearborn, MI 48126; tel. 313/581–5500; FAX. 313/581–6013; Mark B. Saffer, M.D., President and CEO
North Oakland ASC, LLC, 1305 North Oakland Boulevard, Waterford, MI 48327; tel. 248/666–5552; FAX. 248/666–5508; Mary Becker, Director
Oakland Surgi Center, Inc., 2820 Crooks Road, Suite 200, Rochester Hills, MI 48309; tel. 248/852–7484; FAX. 248/852–4279; Beverly Huffman, CMM, Administrator
Park Eye and Surgicenter, 5014 Villa Linde Parkway, Flint, MI 48532
Planned Parenthood League, Inc., 25932 Dequindre, Warren, MI 48091; tel. 810/758–2100; FAX. 810/758–2104; Carrie Haneckow, Administrator
Planned Parenthood of Mid-Michigan Alliance, 3100 Professional Drive, P.O. Box 3673, Ann Arbor, MI 48106-3673; tel. 734/973–0710; FAX. 734/973–0595; Danielle Terry
Planned Parenthood of South Central Michigan, 4201 West Michigan Avenue, Kalamazoo, MI 49006-5833; tel. 269/372–1205; FAX. 269/372–1279; Rev. Mark Pawlowski, CEO
Somerset Surgery Center, P.C., 1565 West Big Beaver Road, Building F, Troy, MI 48084; tel. 248/649–7343; FAX. 248/643–0999; Frank A. Nesi, M.D., Medical Director
Southgate Surgery Center, 14050 Dix-Toledo Road, Southgate, MI 48195; tel. 734/281–0100; FAX. 734/281–7447; Linda Phillips, RN, Administrator
Spectrum Health Surgical Center, 1000 East Paris S.E., Suite 100, Grand Rapids, MI 49546; tel. 616/285–1822; FAX. 616/285–1850; Deb Williams, Senior Manager
St. John Surgery Center, 21000 12 Mile Road, St. Clair Shores, MI 48081; tel. 810/447–5015; FAX. 810/447–5012; Cheri Dendy, Administrator
St. Mary's Ambulatory Care Center, 4599 Towne Centre, Saginaw, MI 48604; tel. 517/797–3000; FAX. 517/797–3010; Lori Jurgens, Director
Superior Endoscopy Center/U P Digestive Disease Associates, P.C., 1414 West Fair Avenue, Suite 135, Marquette, MI 49855; tel. 906/226–6025; FAX. 906/226–5366; Kristine Gorsalitz, RN, Director of Nursing
Surgery Center of Michigan, 44650 Delco Boulevard, Sterling Heights, MI 48313; tel. 586/254–3391; FAX. 586/254–3344; Jay Novetsky, M.D., Medical Director
Surgical Care Center of Michigan, 750 East Beltline, N.E., Grand Rapids, MI 49525; tel. 616/940–3600; FAX. 616/954–0216; Kris Kilgore, RN, B.S.N, Administrative Director
The Berry Center LLC, 28500 Orchard Lake Road, Suite100, Farmington Hills, MI 48334; tel. 248/851–6767; FAX. 248/851–2077; Aaron Betel, Medical Director

MINNESOTA

Centennial Lakes Surgery Center, 7373 France Avenue, S., Suite 404, Edina, MN 55435; tel. 952/832-9360; FAX. 952/832-5079; Pamela Spohn, Administrator

Children's West, 6050 Clearwater Drive, Minnetonka, MN 55343; tel. 612/930-8600; FAX. 612/930-8650; Lynn Goodenough, Director

Innovis Health, LLC, 125 Frazee Street East, Detroit Lakes, MN 56501; tel. 218/844-2300; FAX. 218/844-2445; Linda L. Walz, Division Manager

Landmark Surgery Center, 17 West Exchange Street, Suite 222, St. Paul, MN 55102; tel. 651/842-5468; FAX. 651/842-5491; Jayne Baker, RN Clinical Nurse Manager

Maplewood Surgery Center, 1655 Beam Ave., Maplewood, MN 55109; tel. 612/232-7780; Sandra Todd, Administrator

Midwest Surgery Centers, 2080 Woodwinds Drive, Woodbury, MN 55125; tel. 651/642-1106; FAX. 651/642-9837; H. Joseph Drannen, Administrator

St. Cloud Surgical Center, 1526 Northway Drive, St. Cloud, MN 56303; tel. 320/251-8385; FAX. 320/251-1267; Jeanette I. Stack, Administrator

WestHealth, Inc., 2855 Campus Drive, Plymouth, MN 55441; tel. 763/577-7120; FAX. 763/577-7130; Kurt Neil, Executive Officer

Willmar Surgery Center, 1320 South First Street, Willmar, MN 56201; tel. 320/235-6506; FAX. 320/235-7069; Harley Pakola, Medical Director

MISSISSIPPI

Ambu-Care Outpatient Surgery Center, 6204 North State Street, Jackson, MS 39213; tel. 601/956-3251; FAX. 601/957-8456; Frank McCune, M.D., Administrator

Better Living Clinic Endoscopy Center, 3000 Halls Ferry Road, Vicksburg, MS 39180; tel. 601/638-9800; FAX. 601/638-9808; Barbara Neal, Office Manager

Cedar Lake Surgery Center, 1720 B Medical Park Drive, Biloxi, MS 39532; tel. 228/702-2000; FAX. 228/702-2019; Michael Gossman, Administrator

Columbus Endoscopy Center, Inc., 600 Leigh Drive, Columbus, MS 39705; tel. 662/327-7525; FAX. 662/243-2252; Melanie Taylor, Administrator

East Mississippi Endoscopic Center, LLC, 1926 23rd Ave, Meridian, MS 39302; tel. 601/485-1131; FAX. 601/485-1336; Crystal Bowler, Director

Endoscopy Center of North Mississippi, 1206 Office Park Drive, Oxford, MS 38655; tel. 662/234-9888; FAX. 662/234-9872; Roger Franck, Administrator

ENT and Facial Plastic Surgery, P.A., DBA Head & Neck Surgery Center, LLC., 107 Millsaps Drive, P.O. Box 17829, Hattiesburg, MS 39402; tel. 601/268-5131; FAX. 601/268-5138; Ronny Johnson, Administrator

Eye Surgical Center of Mississippi, LLC, 1053 River Oaks Drive, Flowood, MS 39232; tel. 601/969-1430; FAX. 601/709-2117; Dr. Brannon Aden, Administrator

Gastrointestinal Association Endoscopy, 1405 North State Street, Third Floor, Jackson, MS 39205; tel. 601/354-1234; FAX. 601/352-4882; Diane Winsner, Administrator

Gulf Coast Outpatient Surgery Center, 2781 C T Switzer Sr Drive, Suite 101, Biloxi, MS 39531; tel. 228/594-2900; FAX. 228/594-2901; Diane Farris, Administrator

Gulf South Outpatient Center, 1206 31st Avenue, P.O. Box 1778, Gulfport, MS 39501; tel. 228/864-0008; FAX. 228/863-1747; Jason V. Smith, M.D., President

Gulfport Outpatient Surgical Center, 1240 Broad Avenue, Gulfport, MS 39501; tel. 228/868-1120; FAX. 228/864-0265; William Peaks, Administrator

Gulfport Surgery Center, 1300 Broad Ave, Gulfport, MS 39501; tel. 228/575-2200; FAX. 228/575-2249; William Hertzog, Administrator

Healthsouth Surgicare of Jackson, 760 Lakeland Drive, Jackson, MS 39216; tel. 601/362-8700; FAX. 601/362-6349; Don Thomas, Administrator

Jackson Eye Institute & ASC, 2500 Lakeland Drive, Suite B, Flowood, MS 39208; tel. 601/933-1197; FAX. 601/939-6823; Dr. James Bruce, Administrator

Laurel Surgery and Endoscopy Center, LLC, 1710 West 12th Street, Laurel, MS 39440; tel. 601/369-2021; FAX. 601/369-2022; Heather Zadrozny, Administrator

Lowery A. Woodall Outpatient Surgery Facility, 105 South 28th Avenue, Hattiesburg, MS 39401; tel. 601/579-3400; FAX. 601/264-2025; Tommy Thornton, Administrator

MAE Physicians Surgery Center, LLC, 1190 North State Street, Suite 102, Jackson, MS 39202; tel. 601/968-1790; FAX. 601/292-4531; Carla Glaze, Administrator

Magnolia Regional Health Center Surgery Center, 401 Alcorn Drive, Corinth, MS 38834; tel. 662/293-2000; FAX. 662/287-3562; Angela Jackson, Administrator

Meridian Surgery Center, 2100 13 Street, Meridian, MS 39301; tel. 601/485-4443; FAX. 601/485-9060; Debbi Funck, Administrator

Mississippi Coast Endoscopy & ASC, 2406 Catalpa Ave, Pascagoula, MS 39567; tel. 228/696-0818; FAX. 228/696-0893; Mary Lynn, Administrator

Mississippi Surgical Center, 1421 North State Street, Suite 101, Jackson, MS 39202; tel. 601/353-8000; Judy Gray, Administrator

New Gulf Coast Surgery Center, LLC, 3882 Bienville Blvd, Ocean Springs, MS 39564; tel. 228/872-0400; FAX. 228/818-5538; Donna Griggs, CNO, Administrator

North Mississippi Surgery Center, LLC, 589 Garfield, Tupelo, MS 38801; tel. 662/377-4700; FAX. 662/377-3101; Beth Taylor, RN, Clinical Manager

Ocean Springs Surgical & Endoscopy Center, 3301 Bienville Blvd, Ocean Springs, MS 39564; tel. 228/872-8854; FAX. 228/872-0265; Mary Lynn, Administrator

Oxford Surgery Center, 499 Azalea Drive, Oxford, MS 38655; tel. 662/234-7979; FAX. 662/234-7079; Karry Allen, Administrator

Pain Treatment Center, LLC, 106 Asbury Circle, Hattiesburg, MS 39402; tel. 601/268-8698; FAX. 601/296-3049; Tracey Oden, Administrator

Southern Eye Center of Excellence, 1420 South 28th Avenue, Hattiesburg, MS 39402; tel. 601/264-3937; FAX. 601/264-5930; Lynn McMahan, M.D., Medical Director

MISSOURI

Auburn Surgery Center, Inc., 300 South Mount Auburn Road, Suite 200, Cape Girardeau, MO 63703; tel. 573/332-7881; FAX. 573/332-7176; Tammy Hobby, Administrator

Cape Girardeau Outpatient Surgery Center, 1429 Mount Auburn Road, Cape Girardeau, MO 63701; tel. 573/335-9175; FAX. 573/335-2392; Mary S. Vickery, RN, Administrator

Cataract and Glaucoma Outpatient Surgicenter, 7220 Watson Road, St. Louis, MO 63119; tel. 314/352-5500; Stanley C. Becker, M.D.

CMMP Surgical Center, 1705 Christy Drive, Suite 100, Jefferson City, MO 65101; tel. 573/635-7022; FAX. 573/635-7029; Angela R. Erosenko, Administrator

Creekwood Surgery Center, 211 Northeast 54th Street, Suite 100, Kansas City, MO 64118; tel. 816/455-4214; FAX. 816/455-4216; Melissa Waibel, Administrator

Creve Coeur Surgery Center, LLC, dba City Place Surgery Center, LLC 845 N. New Ballas Ct., Suite 100, Creve Coeur, MO 63141; tel. 314/872-7100; FAX. 314/872-9176; Carolyn Hollowood, Administrator, RN,BSN,CASC

Doctors' Park Surgery, Inc., 30 Doctors' Park, Cape Girardeau, MO 63703; tel. 573/334-9606; FAX. 573/334-9608; Ronald G. Wittmer, President

Eye Surgery Center-The Cliffs, 4801 Cliff Avenue, Suite 101, Independence, MO 64055; tel. 816/478-4400; FAX. 816/478-8240; Jacki Wyrick, RN, B.S.N., Direct of Nursing

G.I. Diagnostics, Inc., 4321 Washington, Suite 5700, Kansas City, MO 64111; tel. 816/561-2000; FAX. 816/931-7559; Craig B. Reeves, Administrator

HealthSouth Surgery Center of West County, 1130 Town and Country Commons, Chesterfield, MO 63017; tel. 314/394-0698; FAX. 314/394-7493; Sandi Baber RN, Administrator

NovaMed Eye Surgery Center (Plaza) L.L.C., 4321 Washington, Suite 6001, Kansas City, MO 64111; tel. 816/753-6511; FAX. 816/753-6513; Ann Israel, ASC Director

NovaMed Eye Surgery Center of North county, d/b/a Cataract Surgery Center, 900 North Highway 67 (Lindbergh), Florissant, MO 63031; tel. 314/838-0321; FAX. 314/838-6532; Karen L. Bell, RN, ASC Director

Outpatient Surgery Center, 450 North New Ballas Road, Suite 103, St. Louis, MO 63141; tel. 314/991-0776; FAX. 314/991-3076; Raymond Mangrich, Administrator

South County Outpatient Surgery Center, 13303 Tesson Ferry Road, St. Louis, MO 63128; tel. 314/842-3200; FAX. 314/525-0198; Ellen Kluesner, Administrator

Surgery Center of Springfield, L.P., 1350 East Woodhurst Drive, Springfield, MO 65804; tel. 417/887-5243; FAX. 417/887-6507; Joyce Gillespie, Administrator

Surgery Center of St. Joseph, 3201 Ashland Avenue, Suite C & D, St. Joseph, MO 64506; tel. 816/279-0079; FAX. 816/364-1100; Colleen Sweet, Nurse Manager

Surgicenter of Kansas City, LLC, 1800 East Meyer Boulevard, Kansas City, MO 64132; tel. 816/523-0100; FAX. 816/995-3190; Cynthia Clark, RN, MBA, CNOR, Administrator

The Endoscopy Center, 3800 South Whitney, Independence, MO 64055; tel. 816/478-4887; FAX. 816/478-7140; Jean Thompson, FACMPE Administrator

The Endoscopy Center II, 5330 North Oak Trafficway, Suite 100, Kansas City, MO 64118; tel. 816/478-4887; FAX. 816/478-7140; Jean Thompson, Administrator

The Tobin Eye Institute, 3902 Sherman Avenue, St. Joseph, MO 64506; tel. 816/279-1363; FAX. 816/233-8936; Jennifer Houston, RN, Director of Nursing and Operations

Tri County Surgery Center, LP, 1111 East Sixth Street, Washington, MO 63090; tel. 636/239-1766; FAX. 636/239-2964; Ellen Kluesner, Administrator

MONTANA

Billings Cataract and Laser Surgicenter, 1221 North 26th Street, Billings, MT 59101; tel. 406/252-5681; FAX. 406/252-5025; Brenda Emerick, Business Manager

Montana Surgical Center, Inc., 840 South Montana, Butte, MT 59701; tel. 406/782-2391; Charles Harris, Manager

Northern Rockies Surgery Center, 940 North 30th Street, Billings, MT 59101; tel. 406/248-7186; FAX. 406/248-6889; Karen Fillner, Administrator

Rocky Mountain Eye Surgery Center, 700 West Kent, Missoula, MT 59801; tel. 406/543-8179; Darlene Timmerhoff, Administrator

Same Day Surgery Center, Inc., 300 North Wilson, Suite 600F, Bozeman, MT 59715; tel. 406/586-1956; Sandra Converse, Clinical Director

The Eye Surgicenter, 2475 Village Lane, Suite 202, Billings, MT 59102; tel. 406/252-6608; FAX. 406/252-6600; Cheri Salthe, Office Manager

NEBRASKA

Aesthetic Surgical Images, P.C., 8900 West Dodge Road, Omaha, NE 68114; tel. 402/390-0100; FAX. 402/390-2711; Rita Petersen, Administrator

Anis Eye Institute, P.C., 1500 South 48th Street, Suite 610, Lincoln, NE 68506; tel. 402/483-4448; FAX. 402/483-4750; Dr. Aziz Y. Anis

Bergan Mercy Surgical Center, 11704 West Center Road, Omaha, NE 68124; tel. 402/333-3111; Richard A. Hachten III

Lincoln Surgical Center, 1710 South 70th, Suite 200, Lincoln, NE 68506; tel. 402/484-9090; FAX. 402/483-0476; Robin Linnafelter, Administrator

Omaha Ambulatory Surgery Center, 825 North 90th Street, Omaha, NE 68114; tel. 402/397-1180; Liza Grasz RN, DON

Omaha Surgical Center, 8051 West Center Road, Omaha, NE 68124; tel. 402/391-3333; James Quinn, M.D., Administrator

Omega Surgery Centers, LLC, 11606 Nicholas Street, Suite 200, Omaha, NE 68154; tel. 402/493-2020; FAX. 402/493-8987; Dr. Robert S. Vandervort, Administrator

The Nebraska Eye Surgical Center, 1500 S. 48th Street, Suite 612, Lincoln, NE 68506; tel. 402/483-4448; FAX. 402/483-4750; Aziz Anis, M.D., Administrator

The Urology Center, P.C., 111 1/2 South 90th Street, Omaha, NE 68114; tel. 402/397-9800; Laura Forehead, Administrator

Tobin Eye Institute, 4151 E Street, Omaha, NE 68107; tel. 402/731-1363; FAX. 402/731-3292; Jenny Caniglia, LPN Facility Director

NEVADA

Ambulatory Surgery Center of Nevada, 4631 E. Charleston Blvd., Las Vegas, NV 89104; tel. 702/438-8417; Neal A. Marek, Administrator

American Surgery Center of Las Vegas, 2575 Lindell Road, Las Vegas, NV 89102; tel. 702/367-7874; FAX. 702/227-6055; Cynthia Butt, Center Director

Carson Endoscopy Center, 707 North Minnesota, Carson City, NV 89703; tel. 775/884-8818; FAX. 775/884-4569; Jay M. Coller, Executive Director

Carson Valley Ambulatory Surgery Center, 1107 Highway 395, Gardnerville, NV 89410; tel. 775/782–1595; FAX. 775/782–1592; Laura D. Strong, Director
Columbia Sunrise Flamingo Surgery Center, 2565 East Flamingo Road, Las Vegas, NV 89121; tel. 702/697–7900; FAX. 702/697–5383; Mia Alfonso, Business Manager
Columbia Sunrise Surgical Center-Sahara, 2401 Paseo Del Prado, Las Vegas, NV 89102; tel. 702/362–7874; FAX. 702/362–3567; Stephanie Finkelstein, Administrator
Digestive Disease Center, 2136 East Desert Inn Road, Suite B, Las Vegas, NV 89109; tel. 702/734–0075; FAX. 702/734–3912; Osama Haikal, M.D., Administrator
Digestive Health Center, 5250 Kietzke Lane, Reno, NV 89511; tel. 775/829–8855; FAX. 775/829–3752; Theresa Brandt, Center Director
Endoscopy Center of Southern Nevada, LLC, 700 Shadow Lane, Suite 165B, Las Vegas, NV 89106; tel. 702/382–8101; FAX. 702/382–4641; Dipak K. Desai, Administrator
Eye Surgery Center of Nevada, 3839 North Carson Street, Carson City, NV 89706; tel. 702/882–3950; FAX. 708/882–1726; Michael J. Fischer, M.D., Administrator
Foot Surgery Center of Northern Nevada, 1300 East Plumb Lane, Suite A, Reno, NV 89502; tel. 702/829–8066; FAX. 702/829–8069; Dr. Frank M. Davis, Jr., Administrator
Ford Center for Foot Surgery, 2321 Pyramid Way, Sparks, NV 89431; tel. 702/331–1919; FAX. 702/331–2008; Dr. L. Bruce Ford, Administrator
Gastrointestinal Diagnostic Clinic, 3196 South Maryland Parkway, Suite 207, Las Vegas, NV 89109; tel. 702/369–3400; Enrique Lacayo, MD, Administrator
Las Vegas Surgicare, Ltd., 870 South Rancho Drive, Las Vegas, NV 89106; tel. 702/870–2090; FAX. 702/870–5468; Kathy King, Administrator
Shepherd Eye Surgicenter, 3575 Pecos McLeod, Las Vegas, NV 89121; tel. 702/731–2088; FAX. 702/734–7836; Christina Kennelley, Administrator
Sierra Center for Foot Surgery, 1801 North Carson, Suite B, Carson City, NV 89701; tel. 702/882–1441; FAX. 702/882–6844; H. Kim Bean, D.P.M., Administrator
Sierra Surgery And Imaging, 1400 Medical Parkway, Carson City, NV 89703; tel. 775/883–1700; FAX. 775/883–8905; Joan P. Lapham, MBA, Executive Director
SMA Surgery Center, 2450 West Charleston, Las Vegas, NV 89102; tel. 702/877–8660; FAX. 702/877–5180; Steve Evans, M.D., Medical Director
Valley View Surgery Center, 1330 Valley View Boulevard, Las Vegas, NV 89102; tel. 702/870–7101; FAX. 702/870–7118; Shelia Donnell, Administrator

NEW HAMPSHIRE

Ambulatory Surgery Center, 100 Hitchcock Way, Manchester, NH 03104; tel. 603/695–1800; FAX. 603/629–1730; Patricia Bonchard, Clinical Manager, ASC
Bedford Ambulatory Surgical Center, 11 Washington Place, Bedford, NH 03110; tel. 603/622–3670; FAX. 603/626–9750; Laurie T. Roderiques, CRNFA, Nurse Director
Clinic Surgery Center (The), 253 Pleasant Street, Concord, NH 03301; tel. 603/226–2200; Kevin Appleton, Administrator
Dr. O'Connell's Pain Care Centers, Inc., Pinewood Medical Center, 255 Route 108, Somersworth, NH 03878; tel. 603/692–3166; FAX. 603/692–3168; Tom Barnes, BA Administrator
Dunning Street Ambulatory Care Center, Seven Dunning Street, Claremont, NH 03743; tel. 603/543–3501; Jyl Bradley, Administrator
Elliot One Day Surgery Center, One Elliot Way, Manchester, NH 03103; tel. 603/627–4889; FAX. 603/663–5900; MaryBeth Jenkins, RN,MS, Director
Nashua Eye Surgery Center, Inc., Five Coliseum Avenue, Nashua, NH 03063; tel. 603/882–9800; FAX. 603/882–0556; Paul O'Leary, Administrator
Orthopaedic Surgery Center, 264 Pleasant Street, Concord, NH 03301; tel. 603/228–7211; FAX. 603/228–7192; Donna Quinn, Administrator
Salem Surgery Center, 32 Stiles Road, Salem, NH 03079; tel. 603/898–3610; FAX. 603/890–3313; Cynthia C. Fortune, Director

NEW JERSEY

A Center for Advanced Surgery, Three Winslow Place, Paramus, NJ 07652; tel. 201/843–9390; FAX. 201/843–0591; Marc L. Reichman, Director of Administration
Affiliated Ambulatory Surgery PA, 182 South Street, Suite One, Morristown, NJ 07960; tel. 973/267–0300; FAX. 973/984–2670; Sylvia Wexler, Administrator
Arthur W. Perry, M.D., FACS Plastic Surgery Center, 3055 Route 27, Franklin Park, NJ 08823; tel. 732/422–9600; FAX. 732/422–9606; Arthur W. Perry, M.D., Director
Associated Surgeon of Northern New Jersey, 25 Rockwood Place, Englewood, NJ 07631; tel. 201/567–3999; FAX. 201/567–9288
Atlantic Surgery Center, LLC, 279 Third Avenue, Suite 105, Long Branch, NJ 07740; tel. 732/222–7373; FAX. 732/571–9212; Daniel B. Goldberg, M.D., President
Atrium Surgery Center, Inc., 195 Route 46, Suite 202, Mine Hill, NJ 07803; tel. 201/989–5185; FAX. 201/328–4097; Jennifer Rand, RN, CNOR, President
Bergen Gastroenterology, 466 Old Hook Road, Suite One, Emerson, NJ 07630; tel. 201/967–8221; FAX. 201/967–0340; Robert Ein, M.D., President
Bergen-Passaic Cataract Surgery and Laser Center, Inc., 19-21 Fair Lawn Avenue, Fair Lawn, NJ 07410; tel. 201/794–8444; FAX. 201/794–1615; Caroline B. Ivanovski-Hauser, Project Manager
Berkeley Heights Eye Group, PA, Summit Eye Group, 369 Springfield Avenue, Berkeley Heights, NJ 07922; tel. 908/464–4600; FAX. 908/464–4737; Elizabeth Way, RN, Administrator
Burlington County Internal Medicine, 651 John F Kennedy Way, Willingboro, NJ 08046; tel. 609/871–7070; FAX. 609/835–4510; Toni McNeil, Administrator
Campus Eye Group, 1700 Whitehorse Hamilton Square Road, Suite A, Hamilton Square, NJ 08690; tel. 609/587–2020; FAX. 609/588–9545; Denise Agness, O.D., Office Manager
Cataract and Laser Institute, PA, 101 Prospect Street, Suite 102, Lakewood, NJ 08701; tel. 908/367–0699; FAX. 908/367–0937
Center for Special Surgery, 104 Lincoln Avenue, Hawthorne, NJ 07506; tel. 973/427–6800; FAX. 973/427–9602; John Tauber, Business Administrator
Clifton Surgery Center, 1117 Route 46 East Suite 303, Clifton, NJ 07013; tel. 973/779–7210; FAX. 973/779–7387; Ramon Silen, M.D., President and Medical Director
Drs. Scherl, Chessler, Zingler, Spinnell, PA, 1555 Center Avenue, Fort Lee, NJ 07024; tel. 201/945–6564; FAX. 201/461–9038; Lynn A. Sculley, Practice Administrator
Endo-Surgi Center, 1201 Morris Avenue, Union, NJ 07083; tel. 908/686–0066; FAX. 908/686–5388; Sharon DeMato, Administrator
Endo-Surgi Center of Old Bridge, 42 Throckmorton Lane, Old Bridge, NJ 08857; tel. 732/679–8808; Sharon DeMato, Executive Director
Endo/Surgical Center of New Jersey, 999 Clifton Avenue, Clifton, NJ 07013; tel. 201/777–3938; FAX. 201/777–6738; Ellen Tummillo RN, CGRN, Director of Nursing
Englewood Endoscopic Associates, 420 Grand Avenue, Englewood, NJ 07631; tel. 201/569–7044; FAX. 201/569–1999; Carmen Rivera, Office Manager
Essex Eye Surgery and Laser Center, 1460 Broad Street, Bloomfield, NJ 07003; tel. 973/338–5566; FAX. 973/338–0753; Joyce Mazur, Director Patient Accounts
Essex Surgical, LLC, 776 Northfield Ave., West Orange, NJ 07052; tel. 973/324–2300; FAX. 973/324–1421; George C. Peck, Jr., M.D.
Eye Institute of Essex Surgeye Center, 50 Newark Avenue, Belleville, NJ 07109; tel. 973/751–6060; FAX. 973/450–1464; Eileen Beltramba, Administrator
Eye Physician of Sussex County Surgical Center, 183 High Street, Newton, NJ 07860; tel. 973/383–6345; FAX. 973/383–0032; Patricia Fowler, RN
Eye Surgery Princeton, 419 North Harrison Street, Princeton, NJ 08540; tel. 609/921–9437; FAX. 609/921–0277; Richard H. Wong, M.D., Medical Director
Freehold Ent, d/b/a Face to Face, Patriots Park, 222 Schanck Road, Freehold, NJ 07728; tel. 908/431–1666; FAX. 908/431–1665
Gastroenterology Diagnosis Northern New Jersey, 205 Browertown Road, Suite 102, West Paterson, NJ 07424; tel. 973/890–4780; FAX. 973/890–1097; Kathy Shadiack, Administrative Director
Hand Surgery and Rehabilitation Center of New Jersey, P.A., 5000 Sagemore Drive, Suite 103, Marlton, NJ 08053; tel. 856/983–4263; FAX. 856/983–9362; Tina Hunt, Administrator
HealthSouth Surgical Center of South Jersey, 130 Gaither Drive, Suite 160, Mount Laurel, NJ 08054; tel. 856/722–7000; FAX. 856/722–8962; Eleanor O. Peschko, Administrator
Horizon Laser and Eye Surgery Center, 9701 Ventnor Avenue, Suite 301, Margate City, NJ 08402; tel. 609/822–7171; FAX. 609/822–3211; Suzanne D. Bruno, Administrator
Hunterdon Center for Surgery, LLC T/A Surgery Today, 121 Highway 31, Suite 1300, Flemington, NJ 08822; tel. 908/806–7017; FAX. 908/806–2838; Saleha Faruqi, M.D., Medical Director
James Street Surgical Suite, 261 James Street, Suite 3E, Morristown, NJ 07960; tel. 973/267–7181; FAX. 973/267–3656; Jeannette Villano RN, Director of Nursing
Mediplex Surgery Center, 98 James Street, Suite 108, Edison, NJ 08820-3998; tel. 732/632–1600; FAX. 732/632–1678; Janet Kovacs, Director
Mid Atlantic Eye Center, 70 East Front Street, Red Bank, NJ 07701; tel. 732/741–0858; FAX. 732/219–0180; Walter J. Kahn, M.D.
Newark Mini-Surgi Site, Inc., 145 Roseville Avenue, Newark, NJ 07107; tel. 201/485–3300; FAX. 201/485–2404; Monica Chomsky
North Jersey Center for Surgery, 39 Newton Sparta Road, Newton, NJ 07860; tel. 973/383–0153; FAX. 973/300–9002; Bruno J. Casatelli, D.P.M., Administrator
Northern New Jersey Eye Institute, 71 Second Street, South Orange, NJ 07079; tel. 973/763–2203; FAX. 973/763–5207; Shirley Vitale, Practice Administrator
Northwest Jersey Ambulatory Surgery Center, 350 Sparta Avenue, Building A, Sparta, NJ 07871; tel. 973/729–8580; FAX. 973/729–2344; D. Crowley, RN, MSN, ASC Supervisor
Ocean County Eye Associates, P.C., 18 Mule Road, Toms River, NJ 08755
Ocean Surgical Pavilion, Inc., 1907 Highway 35, Suite Nine, Oakhurst, NJ 07755; tel. 732/517–8885; FAX. 732/517–0304; Laura Lewis, RN
Ophthalmic Physicians of Monmouth, 733 North Beers Street, Holmdel, NJ 07733; tel. 732/739–0707; FAX. 732/739–8533; Renee Sharkey, RN, Surgical Coordinator
Pavonia Surgery Center, Inc., 600 Pavonia Avenue, Fourth Floor, Jersey City, NJ 07306; tel. 201/216–1700; FAX. 201/216–1800; William H. Constad, M.D., President
Princeton Orthopaedic Associates, P.A., 727 State Road, Princeton, NJ 08540; tel. 609/924–8131; FAX. 609/924–8532; William G. Hyncik, Jr., Executive Director
Princeton Surgical Center, Inc., 281 Witherspoon Street, Third Floor, Princeton, NJ 08542; tel. 609/497–4380; FAX. 609/497–4986; James Demetriades, Administrative Director
Retina Consultants Surgery Center, 39 Sycamore Avenue, Little Silver, NJ 07739; tel. 732/530–7730; FAX. 732/530–3837
Ridgedale Surgery Center, 14 Ridgedale Avenue, Suite 120, Cedar Knolls, NJ 07927; tel. 973/605–5151; FAX. 973/605–1208; Rosalind Silber, Office Administrator
Ridgewood Ambulatory Surgery Center, 1200 Ridgewood Avenue, Ridgewood, NJ 07450; tel. 201/444–4499; FAX. 201/612–8114
Robert Wood Johnson Surgery Center, 561 Cranbury Road, East Brunswick, NJ 08816; tel. 908/390–4300; FAX. 908/390–4405; Evelyn Tornquist, Office Manager
Roseland Surgery Center, 556 Eagle Rock Avenue, Roseland, NJ 07068; tel. 201/226–1717; FAX. 201/403–9034; Joseph Brandspiegel, Executive Director
Saddle Brook Surgicenter, Inc., 289 Market Street, Saddle Brook, NJ 07663; tel. 201/843–4444; FAX. 201/368–2817; Dr. Ronald Sollitto, President and CEO
Seashore Ambulatory Surgery Center, 1907 New Road, Northfield, NJ 08225; tel. 609/645–8884; FAX. 609/645–9780; Kathleen Clark, Administrator
Somerset Eye Institute, P.C., 562 Easton Avenue, Somerset, NJ 08873; tel. 732/828–5900; FAX. 732/828–3327; Suzanne Eileen SoSardo, Business Manager

Somerset Surgical Center, P.A., 1081 Route 22 West, Suite 201, Bridgewater, NJ 08807; tel. 908/575–0020; FAX. 908/575–1515; Ileana Pustai, Administrator and Colleen Relay, Business Manager

South Jersey Endoscopy Center, 17 West Red Bank Avenue, Suite 302, Woodbury, NJ 08096; tel. 856/848–4464; FAX. 856/848–8706; Barbara Fargnoli, Billing Manager

South Jersey Surgicenter, 2835 South Delsea Drive, Vineland, NJ 08360; tel. 856/696–0020; FAX. 856/205–0300; Susy Olmeda, Administrative Coordinator

Summit Surgical Center, LLC, 110 Carnie Boulevard, Voorhees, NJ 08043; tel. 856/325–5813; FAX. 856/325–5858; Phyllis Schlichtmann, Director of Patient Care

Surgery Center of Cherry Hill, 408 Route 70 East, Cherry Hill, NJ 08034; tel. 856/354–1600; FAX. 856/429–7555; Gina Marone RN, MSN, Administrator

Surgicare of Central Jersey, Inc., 40 Stirling Road, Watchung, NJ 07060; tel. 908/769–8000; FAX. 908/668–3139; Marion Jenkins, Executive Director

Surgicare Surgical Associates of Fair Lawn, LLC, 1501 Broadway, Route 4 West, Suite One and Three, Fairlawn, NJ 07410; tel. 201/703–8487; FAX. 201/791–6585; John H. Hajjar, M.D., Member

Teaneck Gastroenterology and Endoscopy Center, 1086 Teaneck Road, Suite Three B, Teaneck, NJ 07666; tel. 201/837–9636; FAX. 201/837–9544; Mia D. Oliver, Manager

The Endoscopy Center of Red Bank, 365 Broad Street, Red Bank, NJ 07701; tel. 732/842–4294; FAX. 732/842–3854; Elizabeth Boyle, Provider Relations or Joan Halvey, Office Manager

The Endoscopy Center of South Jersey, 2791 South Delsea Drive, South Vinelan, NJ 08360; tel. 609/691–1400; FAX. 609/691–7117; Richard Wagar, Assistant Director

The Eye Care Center, 500 West Main Street, Freehold, NJ 07728; tel. 908/462–8707; FAX. 908/462–1296; Dale A. Ingram, Administrator

The New Jersey Eye Center, 1 North Washington Avenue, Bergenfield, NJ 07621; tel. 201/384–7333; FAX. 201/384–2564; James Dello Russo

The Surgical Center at South Jersey Eye Physicians, P.A., 509 South Lenola Road,Suite 11B, Moorestown, NJ 08057; tel. 856/234–0258; FAX. 609/727–0064; Elizabeth Hanley, RN

NEW MEXICO

Alamogordo Eye Clinic and Surgical Center, 1124 10th Street, Alamogordo, NM 88310; tel. 505/434–1200; FAX. 505/437–3947; Cindy Buttram, RN

Eye Care Surgery, 105 North Coronado Avenue, Espanola, NM 87532; tel. 505/753–7391; FAX. 505/753–2749; Dr. Gary Puro

HealthSouth Albuquerque Surgery Center, 1720 Wyoming Boulevard, N.E., Albuquerque, NM 87112; tel. 505/292–9200; FAX. 505/292–1398; Terry Sanchez, Administrator

Lazaro Eye Surgical Center, 1131 Mall Drive, Las Cruces, NM 88011; tel. 505/522–7676; Corine B. Lazaro, M.D., Administrator

Northside Presbyterian, P.O. Box 26666, 5901 Harper Drive, NE, Albuquerque, NM 87125; tel. 505/291–2114; FAX. 505/291–2983; Karin Vantiunen

The Endoscopy Center of Santa Fe, 1650 Hospital Drive, Suite 900, Santa Fe, NM 87505; tel. 505/988–3373; FAX. 505/984–1858; Jim Howlett, Administrator

NEW YORK

Ambulatory Surgery Center of Brooklyn, 313 43rd Street, Brooklyn, NY 11232; tel. 718/369–1900; FAX. 718/965–4157; Frank A. Mazzagatti, Ph.D., Vice President of Operations & Administrator

Ambulatory Surgery Center of Greater New York, Inc., 1101 Pelham Parkway, N., Bronx, NY 10469; tel. 718/515–3500; FAX. 718/655–1795; Joanne McLaughlin, Administrator

Brook Plaza Ambulatory Surgical Center, 1901 Utica Avenue, Brooklyn, NY 11234; tel. 718/629–5590; FAX. 718/629–2833; Steven Ackerman, CEO

Brooklyn Eye Surgery Center, LLC, 1301 Avenue J, Brooklyn, NY 11230; tel. 718/688–3937; FAX. 718/692–4456; Yafa L. Shevlin, Administrator

Buffalo Ambulatory Surgery Center, 3095 Harlem Road, Cheektowaga, NY 14225; tel. 716/896–3815; FAX. 716/896–3015; Dorothy L. Zimdahl, RN, B.S., CNOR, CASC, Administrator

Central New York Eye Center, 22 Green Street, Poughkeepsie, NY 12601; tel. 845/471–3720; FAX. 845/471–9516; Kim M. Quick, R.N., CRNO, COE

Day-Op Center of Long Island, Inc., 110 Willis Avenue, Mineola, NY 11501; tel. 516/294–0030; FAX. 516/294–0228; Juliette LaRegina, Administrator

Fifth Avenue Surgery Center, 1049 Fifth Avenue, New York, NY 10028; tel. 212/772–6667; FAX. 212/988–8018; Charles J. Raab, CEO

Harrison Center Outpatient Surgery, 5700 Genesee Street, Suite 11, Camillus, NY 13031; tel. 315/701–9378; FAX. 315/701–0871; Margaret M. Alteri, Administrator/CEO

Harrison Center Outpatient Surgery, Inc., 550 Harrison Street, Suite 230, Syracuse, NY 13202; tel. 315/472–4424; FAX. 315/475–8056; Margaret M. Alteri, Administrator and CEO

Kingston Ambulatory Surgical Center, LLC, 40 Hurley Avenue, Suite 13, Kingston, NY 12401; tel. 845/338–4777; FAX. 845/339–7339; Kathleen Keily, Administrator

Lattimore Community Surgicenter, 125 Lattimore Road, Rochester, NY 14620; tel. 585/473–9000; FAX. 585/697–3519; Peter G. Varlan, Administrator

Long Island Surgi-Center, 1895 Walt Whitman Road, Melville, NY 11747; tel. 516/293–9700; FAX. 516/293–1018; Ronald Perrone M.D.

Millard Fillmore Ambulatory Surgery Center, 215 Klein Road, Williamsville, NY 14221; tel. 716/568–6100; FAX. 716/568–6166; Joel C. Farwell, Business Manager

Nassau Center for Ambulatory Surgery, Inc., dba Garden City SurgiCenter, 400 Endo Boulevard, NY 11530; tel. 516/832–8504; FAX. 516/228–9429; Carol Stahl, Administrator

New York Institute for Same Day Surgery, Inc., 99 Dutch Hill Plaza, Orangeburg, NY 10962; tel. 845/359–9000; FAX. 845/359–1495; Lisa A. Bloise, COA Operations Director

North Shore Surgi Center, Inc., 989 West Jericho Turnpike, Smithtown, NY 11787; tel. 631/864–7100; FAX. 631/864–7129; George Seaman, CEO

Our Lady of Victory Surgery Center, 6300 Powers Road, Orchard Park, NY 14127; tel. 716/667–3222; FAX. 716/667–3120; Dana M. Mata, Administrative Director

Queens Surgi-Center, 83-40 Woodhaven Boulevard, Glendale, NY 11385; tel. 718/849–8700; FAX. 718/849–6523; Adce Abadir, Administrator

Queens Surgical Community Center, 46-04 31st Avenue, Long Island C, NY 11103; tel. 718/545–5050; FAX. 718/721–8709; Mr. Misk, Partner

Same Day Surgery of Latham, Inc., Seven Century Hill Drive, Latham, NY 12110; tel. 518/785–5741; FAX. 518/785–8134; Jennifer L. Allen, RN, BSN, OR, Coordinator

The Mackool Eye Institute, 31-27 41st Street, Astoria, NY 11103; tel. 718/728–3400; FAX. 718/721–7562

Westfall Surgery Center, LLP, 1065 Senator Keating Boulevard, Rochester, NY 14618; tel. 585/256–1330; FAX. 585/256–3823; Gary J. Scott, Administrative Director

NORTH CAROLINA

Asheboro Endoscopy Center, 700 Sunset Avenue, P.O. Box 4830, Asheboro, NC 27203; tel. 336/625–0305; FAX. 336/625–9941; Vickie Whitaker, RN, Clinical Director

Blue Ridge Day Surgery Center, 2308 Wesvill Court, Raleigh, NC 27607; tel. 919/781–4311; FAX. 919/781–0625; Marshall Cox III, RN Administrator

Caromont Specialty Surgery, 2511 Court Drive, Gastonia, NC 28054; tel. 704/671–5600; FAX. 704/671–5650; Mike Smith, Manager

Carteret Surgery Center, 3714 Guardian Avenue, Morehead City, NC 28557; tel. 252/247–0314; FAX. 252/247–2031; Kim Blaine, Business Manager

Chapel Hill Surgical Center, 109 Conner Drive, Suite 1201, Chapel Hill, NC 27514; tel. 919/968–0611; FAX. 919/967–8637; Gary S. Berger, M.D., President

Charlotte Surgery Center, 2825 Randolph Road, Charlotte, NC 28211; tel. 704/377–1647; FAX. 704/358–8267; Connie M. Wilson, Administrator

Cleveland Ambulatory Services, 1100 North Lafayette Street, Shelby, NC 28150; tel. 704/482–1331; FAX. 704/482–4833; John Reynolds, MD, Clinical Director

Craven Surgery Center, 630 McCarthy Blvd, P.O. Box 12446, New Bern, NC 28561; tel. 252/633–2000; FAX. 252/633–9045; Joseph Hageman, RN, Executive Director

Eye Surgery and Laser Clinic, 500 Lake Concord Road, N.E., Concord, NC 28025; tel. 704/782–1127; FAX. 704/782–1207; Clayton Bonnett, Administrator

Eye Surgery Center of Shelby, 1622 East Marion Street, Shelby, NC 28150; tel. 704/482–2020; FAX. 704/482–7707; Frank T. Hannah, M.D., Medical Director

Fayetteville Ambulatory Surgery Center, 1781 Metromedical Drive, Fayetteville, NC 28304; tel. 910/323–1647; FAX. 910/323–4142; John T. Henley, Jr., M.D., Medical Director

Goldsboro Endoscopy Center, Inc., 2705 Medical Office Place, Goldsboro, NC 27534; tel. 919/580–9111; FAX. 919/580–0988; Venkata C. Motaparthy, M.D., Chief Executive Officer

Hawthorne Surgical Center, 1999 South Hawthorne Road, Winston-Salem, NC 27103; tel. 910/718–6800; FAX. 910/718–6847; Teresa L. Carter, Facility Director

HealthSouth Surgecenter of Wilson, 1709 Medical Park Drive, Wilson, NC 27893; tel. 919/237–5649; Phyllis S. Renfrow, Administrator

HealthSouth Surgery Center of Charlotte, 2825 Randolph Rd., Charlotte, NC 28211; tel. 704/377–1647; Connie M. Wilson, Administrator

HealthSouth Surgery Center of Hickory, L.P., 27 13th Avenue, N.E., Hickory, NC 28601; tel. 704/328–1493; FAX. 704/322–6097; Kevin Deal, RN, Administrator

High Point Surgery Center, 600 Lindsay Street, P.O. Box 2476, High Point, NC 27261; tel. 336/878–6068; FAX. 336/878–6111; Joan D. White, Administrative Director

Iredell Head, Neck and Ear Ambulatory Surgery Center, Inc., 707 Bryant Street, Statesville, NC 28677; tel. 704/873–5224; FAX. 704/873–5984; Angie Kerr, Office Manager

Iredell Surgical Center, 1720 Davie Avenue, Statesville, NC 28677; tel. 704/871–0081; FAX. 704/871–0086; Glenda Tallent, MBA, Administrator

Medivision, Inc., 2170 Midland Road, P.O. Box 1938, Southern Pine, NC 28387; tel. 910/295–1221; FAX. 910/295–0512; Kathy Stout, RN, Administrator

Piedmont Gastroenterology Center, Inc., 1901 South Hawthorne Road, Suite 308, Winston-Salem, NC 27103; tel. 910/760–4340; FAX. 919/765–2869; Charles H. Hauser, Administrator

Plastic Surgery Center of North Carolina, Inc., 2901 Maplewood Avenue, Winston-Salem, NC 27103; tel. 336/768–6210; FAX. 336/768–6236; Melba Edwards, Administrator

Raleigh Plastic Surgery Center, Inc., 1112 Dresser Court, Raleigh, NC 27609; tel. 919/872–2616; FAX. 919/872–2771; Nancy Nicoll O'Neil, Administrator

Raleigh Women's Health Organization, Inc., 3613 Haworth Drive, Raleigh, NC 27609; tel. 919/783–0444; FAX. 919/781–8432; Susan Hill, President

Regional Medical Services Surgery Center, 5200 North Croatan Highway, Kitty Hawk, NC 27949; tel. 252/261–9000; FAX. 919/261–4329; Yvonne Burdick, Executive Director

Southern Eye Associates, P.A., Ophthalmic Surgery Center, 2801 Blue Ridge Road, Suite 200, Raleigh, NC 27607; tel. 919/571–0081; Kathryn Levari, Director of Clinical Services

Surgery Center of Morganton Eye Physicians, P.A., 335 East Parker Road, Morganton, NC 28655; tel. 704/433–6225; L. A. Raynor, M.D., Medical Director

Surgical Eye Center, 3312 Battleground Avenue, Greensboro, NC 27410; tel. 336/282–8330; FAX. 336/282–2625; Trudy Wester, Center Director

SurgiCare of Jacksonville, 166 Memorial Court, Jacksonville, NC 28546; tel. 910/353–9565; FAX. 919/353–5497; Takey Crist, Medical Director

SurgiCenter of Wilson, 209 Richards Street, Wilson, NC 27893; tel. 919/237–5649; FAX. 919/237–4977; Phyllis Renfrow, President

Surgicenter Services of Pitt, Inc., 102 Bethesda Drive, Greenville, NC 27834; tel. 919/847–7700; FAX. 919/847–7784; Anna M. Weaver, President

The Endoscopy Center, 191 Biltmore Avenue, Asheville, NC 28801; tel. 704/254–0881; Michael Grier, M.D.

WHA Medical Clinic, PLLC, 1202 Medical Center Drive, Wilmington, NC 28401; tel. 910/341–3433; Diane A. Atkinson, Executive Director

Wilmington SurgCare, 1801 South 17th Street, Wilmington, NC 28401; tel. 910/763–4555; FAX. 910/332–8920; James Shafer, Facility Administrator

Wilson OB-GYN, 2500 Horton Boulevard, Zip 27893, P.O. Box 7639, Wilson, NC 27895; tel. 919/206–1000; FAX. 919/237–0704; Daniel P. Michalak, M.D., Administrator

NORTH DAKOTA

Bismarck Surgical Associates, 600 N. 9th Street, Bismarck, ND 58501; tel. 701/221–2299; FAX. 701/221–3239; Dr. Atlas Boutrous, Administrator

Centennial Medical Center, 1500 24th Avenue, S.W., Minot, ND 58702; tel. 701/852–0777; Dr. Manuel Neto, Administrator

Dakota Clinic Ltd Endoscopy, 1702 S. University Drive, Fargo, ND 58108; tel. 701/280–8900; Curt Noyes-Chief Operating Officer

Dakota Surgery & Laser Center, 430 E. Sweet Avenue, Bismarck, ND 58504; tel. 701/222–4900; FAX. 701/222–4999; Charles R. Volk, Administrator

Day Surgery-Wahpeton, 275 South 11th Street, Wahpeton, ND 58075; tel. 701/642–2000; FAX. 701/671–4106; Jeffery A. Cook, Administrator

FM Endoscopy Center, 4344 20th Ave SW, Fargo, ND 58103; tel. 701/371–5094; Rodney Ludwig, Administrator

Great Plains Clinic Surgery Center, 33 Ninth Street, W., Dickinson, ND 58601; tel. 701/483–6017; FAX. 701/483–5018; Mark Grove, Administrator

Institute For Lower Back Care, 4344 20th Ave SW, Fargo, ND 58103; tel. 701/297–0817; Panjin Sivanna, MD, Administrator

Institute for Special Surgery, 2301 25th Street, Fargo, ND 58103; tel. 702/271–1045; FAX. 702/271–1044; Timothy Haugen, Administrator

Lamb Plastic Surgery Center, 1507 S University Dr, Fargo, ND 58103; tel. 701/237–9592; Donald Lamb, MD, Administrator

Laser and Surger Center, 4344 20th Ave S, Fargo, ND 58103; tel. 701/277–7200; Steve Bagan, MD, Administrator

Mid Dakota Clinic Surgicenter, 401 N 9th St., Bismarck, ND 58501; tel. 701/530–6010; FAX. 701/530–5996; Marlene Sapa, Administrator

North Dakota Surgery Center, 3035 Demers Ave., Grand Forks, ND 58201; tel. 701/775–3151; FAX. 701/775–3153; Ross J. Gonitzke, Administrator

Northern Plains Surgery Center, 44 4th St S, Fargo, ND 58103; tel. 701/232–9200; Ron Flag, Administrator

St. Alexius Same Day Surgery Center, 810 East Rosser, Bismarck, ND 58501; tel. 701/530–5000; Sandy Gerving, Director

Trinity Community Clinic-Western Dakota, 1102 Main, Williston, ND 58801; tel. 701/572–7711; FAX. 701/572–2283; Mary E. Banta, Administrator

Trinity Health-MA Same Day Surgery, 400 E Burdick Expwy, Suite 400, Minot, ND 58702; tel. 701/857–7000; Renda Wilson, Administrator

OHIO

Advanced Cosmetic and Laser Surgery Center, Inc., 2200 Philadelphia Drive, Suite 651, Dayton, OH 45406; tel. 937/278–0809; FAX. 937/278–3590

Akron Endoscopy Center, 1037 North Main Street, Suite B, Akron, OH 44310; tel. 330/940–3000; FAX. 330/940–3675; Nicole King, RN, Center Director

Amend Center for Eye Surgery, 5939 Colerain Avenue, Cincinnati, OH 45239; tel. 513/923–3900; FAX. 513/923–3012

Austintown Surgery, 45 North Canfield-Niles Road, Youngstown, OH 44515; tel. 330/792–2722; FAX. 330/792–9482; Vicki Merrick, Administrator

Bloomberg Eye Center, 1651 West Main Street, Newark, OH 43055; tel. 614/522–3937; FAX. 614/522–0063; Judy Mackey, Director of Corp. Services

Cincinnati Eye Institute and Ambulatory Surgery Center, 1945 CEI Drive, Cincinnati, OH 45242; tel. 513/984–5133; FAX. 513/984–4240; Clyde Bell, President

Cincinnati Foot Clinic, Inc., 8111 Cheviot Road, Cincinnati, OH 45247; tel. 513/385–6946; Robert Hayman, M.D., President

Columbus Eye Surgery Center, 5965 East Broad Street, Suite 460, Columbus, OH 43213; tel. 614/751–4080; FAX. 614/751–4092; Toni Van Horn, Executive Director

Consultants in Gastroenterology, Inc., 5900 Landerbrook Dr., Suite 195, Mayfield Heights, OH 44124; tel. 440/461–2550; FAX. 440/461–5319; Karen Wahl, Manager

Consultants in Gastroenterology, Inc., 7530 Fredle Dr., Concord, OH 44077; tel. 440/942–7909; FAX. 440/942–7846; Kare Wahl, Manager

Crystal Clinic Surgery Center, 3975 Embassy Parkway, Suite 202, Akron, OH 44313; tel. 330/668–4085; FAX. 330/668–2624; Katherine L. McNeal, RN, Administrator

Dayton Ear, Nose and Throat Surgeons, Inc., 7076 Corporate Way, Centerville, OH 45459; tel. 937/434–0555; FAX. 937/434–7413; Jana White, Administrator

Digestivecare Endoscopy Unit, 75 Sylvania Drive, Beavercreek, OH 45440; tel. 937/320–5050; FAX. 937/320–5060; Craig Penno, Administrator

Endoscopy Center of Dayton LTD, 4200 Indian Ripple Road, Beavercreek, OH 45440; tel. 937/427–1680; FAX. 937/427–9081; Tamme Hafer, Practice Administrator

Endoscopy Center West, 3654 Werk Road, Cincinnati, OH 45248; tel. 513/451–6001; FAX. 513/451–7310; Lorrie Johnson, Administrator

Eye Institute of Northwestern Ohio, Inc., 3509 Briarfield Blvd, Maumee, OH 43537; tel. 419/865–3866; FAX. 419/865–3451; Carol R. Kollarits, M.D., President

Eye Surgery Center of Wooster, 3519 Friendsville Road, Wooster, OH 44691; tel. 330/345–6371; FAX. 330/345–8029; Michelle Morrison, Director

Facial Surgery Center, 1130 Congress Avenue, Glendale, OH 45246; tel. 513/772–2442; FAX. 513/772–2844; Joseph J. Moravec, M.D., Medical Director

Fairview Hospital Surgery Center, 850 Columbia Road, Westlake, OH 44145; tel. 216/808–4000; FAX. 216/808–4010; Michelle Padden, RN, Administrator

Firas Atassi, M.D. Outpatient Surgery Center, 34500 Center Ridge Road, North Ridgeville, OH 33039; tel. 216/327–2414

Gastroenterology Associates, Inc., 4665 Belpar Street, NW, P.O. Box 36329, Canton, OH 44735; tel. 330/493–1480; FAX. 330/493–6805; Rachelle Willis, Endoscopy Nurse Manager

Gastroenterology Specialists, Inc., 2726 Fulton Drive, N.W., Canton, OH 44718; tel. 330/455–5011; FAX. 330/588–7127; Faith M. Thigpen, RN

HealthSouth Endoscopy West, 1930 State Route 59, Kent, OH 44240; tel. 216/677–3292; FAX. 330/677–3624; Laurie Simon, Office Manager

Heritage Surgical Associates of Cincinnati, d/b/a Healthsouth Surgery Center of Cincinnati, 2925 Vernon Place, Suite 101, Cincinnati, OH 45219; tel. 513/872–4541; FAX. 513/872–4558; Patti Murphy, RN, Director

Kunesh Eye Surgery Center, 2601 Far Hills Avenue, Dayton, OH 45419-1665; tel. 937/298–1093; FAX. 937/298–6344; Lucy Helmers, Administrator

Midwest Eye Center, 119 West Kemper Road, Cincinnati, OH 45246; tel. 513/671–6112; FAX. 513/671–6386; Lorrie Walters, Business Office Supervisor

Midwest Eye Surgery Center, 4452 Eastgate Boulevard, Suite 305, Cincinnati, OH 45245; tel. 513/752–5700; FAX. 513/752–5716; Holly Schwab, RN, Surgery Manager

North Coast Endoscopy, Inc., 9500 Mentor Avenue, Suite 380, Mentor, OH 44060; tel. 440/352–9400; FAX. 440/352–9407; Ahmad Ascha, M.D.

North Shore Endoscopy Center, 850 Columbia Road, Suite 200, Westlake, OH 44145; tel. 440/808–1212; FAX. 440/808–0321; Christine St.George-Gray, RN, BSN, Operations Manager

Ohio Eye Associates, Eye Surgery & Laser Center, 466 South Trimble Road, Mansfield, OH 44906; tel. 419/756–8000; FAX. 419/756–7100; Thomas F. Marquardt, Administrator

Ohio Gastroenterology Group, Inc., Endoscopy Center, 777 West State Street, Suite 402, Columbus, OH 43222; tel. 614/221–7431; FAX. 614/341–2401; Jean Yarletts, RN, B.S.N.

Optivue Vision, 2740 Navarre Avenue, Oregon, OH 43616; tel. 419/697–3616; FAX. 419/697–3637; Karen R. Hess, RN, LMT, O.R. Manager

Parkway Surgery Center, Ltd., 3500 Executive Parkway, Toledo, OH 43606; tel. 419/531–8349; FAX. 419/531–6833; Richard I. Tapper, MD, Medical Executive Director

Ross Park Surgical Services, One Ross Park, Steubenville, OH 43952; tel. 614/282–4790; Kathy Lemasters, RN, Manager

Sandusky Surgeons, Inc., 1221 Hayes Avenue, Sandusky, OH 44870; tel. 419/625–1374; William A. Schuchardt, MD. President

Sidney Foot and Ankle Center, 1000 Michigan, Sidney, OH 45365; tel. 937/492–1211; FAX. 937/492–6557; Norma Polasky, Administrative Director

Stoneridge Endoscopy Center, 3900 Stoneridge Lane, Dublin, OH 43017; tel. 614/889–5001; FAX. 614/889–5913; Cheryl Miller, Clinic Manager

Surgery Alliance Ltd., 975 Sawburg Avenue, Alliance, OH 44601; tel. 330/821–7997; FAX. 330/821–7295; Hazel Thomas, Administrator

Taylor Station Surgery Center, 275 Taylor Station Road, Columbus, OH 43213; tel. 614/751–4466; FAX. 614/751–4474; Julie Bernard, Director

The Endoscopy Center, 3439 Granite Circle, Toledo, OH 43617; tel. 419/843–7993; FAX. 419/841–7789; Alice Horner, R.N. Nurse Manager

The LCA Center for Surgery, 7840 Montgomery Road, Cincinnati, OH 45236; tel. 513/792–9099; FAX. 513/792–5634; Rene Fischer, President and CEO

The Surgery Center, 19250 East Bagley Road, Middleburg Heights, OH 44130; tel. 440/826–3240; FAX. 440/826–3250; Barb Draves, CASC, Administrator

The Surgery Center At Southwoods, LLC, 7525 California Avenue, Youngstown, OH 44512; tel. 330/758–1954; FAX. 330/758–3254

The Surgical Center of East Liverpool, 16480 St. Clair Avenue, P.O. Box 2640, East Liverpool, OH 43920; tel. 330/386–9000; FAX. 330/386–1255; Joseph P. Sitarik D.O., Medical Director

Tippecanoe Endoscopy, Inc., 1210 Boardman Canfield Road, Youngstown, OH 44512; tel. 330/726–0132; FAX. 330/726–2571; Mary Amorn, RN, Administrator

Toledo Clinic, Inc., 4235 Secor Road, Toledo, OH 43623; tel. 419/473–3561; FAX. 419/472–0838; Roberta Reichle, Administrator

Toledo Community Lithotripter Center, 3158 West Central Avenue, Toledo, OH 43606; tel. 419/531–3538; FAX. 419/531–2807; Kelly Noward, Director

Tri-State Centers, For Sight Surgery Center, 8044 Montgomery Road, Suite 155, Cincinnati, OH 45236; tel. 513/791–7967; FAX. 513/791–1473; Jo Slocum RN, BSN, Administrator

Wright Surgery Center, 1611 South Green Road, Suite 124, South Euclid, OH 44121; tel. 216/382–1868; FAX. 216/382–0584; Sheryl Ontell-Silverman, MD, PhD, Medical Director

Zeeba Ambulatory Surgery Center, 29017 Cedar Road, Lyndhurst, OH 44124; tel. 440/460–8000; FAX. 440/460–4225; Franklin Keathley, Administrator

OKLAHOMA

Ambulatory Surgery Associates, 6160 South Yale Avenue, Tulsa, OK 74136; tel. 918/495–2625; FAX. 918/497–3259; Kathy Helberg, RN, Director

Central Oklahoma Ambulatory Surgical Center, Inc., 3301 Northwest 63rd Street, Oklahoma City, OK 73116; tel. 405/842–9732; FAX. 405/842–9771; Paul Silverstein, M.D., Administrator

Columbia Surgicare of Tulsa, 4415 South Harvard Avenue, Suite 100, Tulsa, OK 74135; tel. 918/742–2502; FAX. 918/745–9750; Dirk Foxworthy, Administrator

Eastern Oklahoma Surgery Center, L. L. C., 5020 East 68th Street, Tulsa, OK 74136; tel. 918/492–1539; FAX. 918/494–8683; Linda Taylor, RN Supervisor

Great Plains Ambulatory Surgery Center, 5404 West Lee Boulevard, Suite 100, Lawton, OK 73505; tel. 580/536–7533; FAX. 580/536–7535; Donald Garrett, M.D., Medical Director

Heritage Eye Surgicenter of Oklahoma, 6922 South Western, Oklahoma City, OK 73139; tel. 405/636–1508; FAX. 405/636–1239; Edward D. Glinski, D.O., MBA, Administrator

McGee Eye Surgery Center, 1000 North Lincoln, Suite 150, Oklahoma City, OK 73104; tel. 405/232–8696; FAX. 405/235–4023; Glenda Woodside, Administrator

Medical Plaza Endoscopy Unit, 1125 North Porter, Suite 304, Norman, OK 73071; tel. 405/360–2799; FAX. 405/447–0321; Philip C. Bird, M.D.

Oklahoma Surgicare, 4317 W. Memorial Road, Oklahoma City, OK 73134; tel. 405/755–6240; FAX. 405/752–1819; Lindie Slater, Administrator

Orthopedic Associates Ambulatory Surgery Center, Inc., 3301 Northwest 50th Street, Oklahoma City, OK 73112; tel. 405/947–5610; FAX. 405/948–5166; Carolyn Moles, RN, Director

Outpatient Surgical Center of Ponca City, 400 Fairview, Suite 50, Ponca City, OK 74601; tel. 580/762–0695; FAX. 580/765–9406; Steffi Cowan, Operations Manager

Physicians Surgical Center, 805 East Robinson, Norman, OK 73071-6610; tel. 405/364–9789; FAX. 405/366–8081; Sandra Vaughn, RN, Administrator

Southern Oklahoma Surgical Center, Inc., 2412 North Commerce, Ardmore, OK 73401; tel. 580/226–5000; FAX. 580/226–5035; Ann Willis, RN, Administrator

Southern Plains Ambulatory Surgery Center, 2222 Iowa Avenue, P.O. Box 1069, Chickasha, OK 73023; tel. 405/224–8111; FAX. 405/222–9557; Gary Gaspaid, Executive Director

Southwest Ambulatory Surgery Center, LLC, 8125 South Walker Avenue, Oklahoma City, OK 73139; tel. 405/631–1015; FAX. 405/631–1050; Anthony L. Cruse, D.O., Medical Director

Surgery Center of South Oklahoma City, 100 Southeast 59th Street, Oklahoma City, OK 73109; tel. 405/634–9300; FAX. 405/634–8300; Larry Smith, Administrator

The Cataract Center of Lawton, 4214 Southwest Lee Boulevard, Lawton, OK 73505; tel. 405/353–5860; Stephen W. Gilkeson, Executive Administrator

Three Rivers Surgery Center, 3800 West Okmulgee, Muskogee, OK 74401; tel. 918/682–9899; FAX. 918/687–0786; Doug Blessen, Chief Executive Officer

Tower Day Surgery, 1044 Southwest 44th Street, Suite 100, Oklahoma City, OK 73109; tel. 405/636–1701; FAX. 405/636–4314; Marie Smith, RN, Director of Nursing

Triad Eye Medical Clinic and Cataract Institute, 6140 South Memorial, Tulsa, OK 74133; tel. 918/252–2020; FAX. 918/252–7466; Marc L. Abel, D.O., Medical Director

OREGON

Aesthetic Breast and Cosmetic Surgery Center, 10201 Southeast Main, Suite 20, Portland, OR 97216; tel. 503/253–3458; FAX. 503/253–0856; Ronald V. DeMars, M.D., Administrator

Center for Cosmetic and Plastic Surgery, 1353 East McAndrews Road, Medford, OR 97504; tel. 541/770–6776; FAX. 541/770–5791; Robert M. Jensen, M.D., Administrator

Eye Surgery Center, 2925 Siskiyou Boulevard, Medford, OR 97504; tel. 541/779–2020; FAX. 541/770–6838; Loren R. Barrus, M.D., Administrator

Eye Surgery Institute, 813 S.W. Highland Ave., Redmond, OR 97756; tel. 541/548–7170; FAX. 541/548–3842; Sara Harvey, Administrator

Futures Outpatient Surgical Center, Inc., 1849 Northwest Kearney, Suite 302, Portland, OR 97209; tel. 503/224–0723; FAX. 503/224–0722; Bryce E. Potter, M.D., Principal

GI Endoscopy Center, 2560 N.W. Medical Park Drive, Roseburg, OR 97470; tel. 541/673–2046; FAX. 541/673–0454; Ruth E. Harpole, RN, Administrator

Lovejoy Surgicenter, Inc., 933 Northwest 25th Avenue, Portland, OR 97210; tel. 503/221–1870; FAX. 503/221–1488; Kayla Reich, Administrator

McKenzie Surgery Center, 940 Country Club Road, Eugene, OR 97401; tel. 541/344–2600; FAX. 541/344–3317; Lynn M. Stapes, RN, Administrator

North Bend Medical Center, Inc., 1900 Woodland Drive, Coos Bay, OR 97420; tel. 541/267–5151; FAX. 541/266–4501; J. Peter Johnson, CEO

Ontario Surgery Center, 251 S.W. 19th Street, Ontario, OR 97914; tel. 541/889–3198; FAX. 541/889–3904; Jeffrey C. Pitts, M.D., Administrator

Oregon Cataract and Laser Institute, 2700 Southeast 14th Avenue, Albany, OR 97321; tel. 503/928–1666; Darrell Genstler, M.D., Administrator

Oregon Eye Surgery Center, Inc., 1550 Oak Street, Eugene, OR 97401; tel. 541/683–8771; FAX. 541/484–4993; Virginia Pecora, RN, Administrator

The Oregon Clinic Gastroenterology Division Gresham Office, 24900 Southeast Stark, Suite 205, Gresham, OR 97030; tel. 503/661–2000; FAX. 503/661–2001; Jeffrey S. Albaugh, M.D., Administrator

The Portland Clinic Surgical Center, 800 Southwest 13th Avenue, Portland, OR 97205; tel. 503/221–0161; FAX. 503/221–4451; J. Michael Schwab, CEO

Tigard Surgery Center, 13240 Southwest Pacific Highway, Suite 200, Tigard, OR 97223; tel. 503/639–6571; FAX. 503/624–6037; Ivan L. Bakos, M.D., Administrator

Willamette Valley Eye SurgiCenter, 2001 Commercial Street, S.E., Salem, OR 97302; tel. 503/363–1500; FAX. 503/588–2028; Gordon Miller, M.D., Administrator

PENNSYLVANIA

Abington Surgical Center, 2701 Blair Mill Road, Suite 35, Willow Grove, PA 19090; tel. 215/443–8505; FAX. 215/957–0565; Stanley E. Grissinger, MBA, CHE, Executive Director

Aestique Ambulatory Surgical Center, One Aesthetic Way, Greensburg, PA 15601; tel. 724/832–7555; FAX. 724/832–7568; Theodore A. Lazzaro, M.D., Medical Director

Delaware Valley Laser Surgery Institute(Nevyas Eye Associates), Two Bala Plaza, Pl 33, Bala Cynwd, PA 19004; tel. 215/668–2847; FAX. 215/668–1509; Herbert J. Nevyas, M.D., Medical Director

Dermatologic SurgiCenter, 1200 Locust Street, Philadelphia, PA 19107; tel. 215/546–3666; FAX. 215/546–6060; Anthony V. Benedetto, D.O., FACP, Medical Director

Dermatologic SurgiCenter, 2221 Garrett Rd., Drexel Hill, PA 19026; tel. 610/623–5885; FAX. 610/623–7276; Anthony V. Benedetto, D.O., FACP, Medical Director

Digestive Disease Institute, 899 Poplar Church Road, Camp Hill, PA 17011; tel. 717/763–1239; FAX. 717/763–9854; Iris Garman, Administrator

Fairgrounds Surgical Center, 400 North 17th Street, Suite 300, Allentown, PA 18104; tel. 610/821–2020; FAX. 610/821–2016; Darlene G. Hinkle/ Debi Baker, Co-Administrative Directors

Fort Washington Surgery Center, 467 Pennsylvania Avenue, Fort Washington, PA 19034; tel. 215/628–4300; FAX. 215/628–4253; Charles Pappas, M. D.

HealthSouth Scranton Surgery and Laser Center, 425 Adams Street, Scranton, PA 18510; tel. 717/348–1114; FAX. 717/347–4351; Marion Smith, Administrative Director

HealthSouth Surgery Center of Lancaster, 217 Harrisburg Avenue, Suite 103, Lancaster, PA 17603; tel. 717/295–2500; FAX. 717/295–4898; Joanne Hettel, Administrator

John A. Zitelli, M.D., P.C., Ambulatory Surgery Facility, 5200 Centre Avenue, Suite 303, Pittsburgh, PA 15232; tel. 412/681–9400; FAX. 412/681–5240; John A. Zitelli, M.D.

Kremer Laser Eye Center, 200 Mall Boulevard, King of Prussia, PA 19406; tel. 610/337–1580; FAX. 610/337–1153; Tara Hopewell, RN

Lebanon Outpatient Surgical Center, L.P., 830 Tuck Street, Lebanon, PA 17042; tel. 717/228–1620; FAX. 717/228–1642; Anita Gingrich Fuhrman, RN, B.S., CASC, Director

Lowry SurgiCenter, 1115 Lowry Avenue, Jeannette, PA 15644; tel. 412/527–2885; FAX. 412/527–6885; K. Diddle, M.D., Medical Director

Mt. Lebanon Surgical Center, Professional Office Building, 1050 Bower Hill Road, Suite 102, Pittsburgh, PA 15243; tel. 412/563–6808; FAX. 412/563–6857; Patricia Strosnider, Director, Nursing

Mt. Pleasant Surgery Center, 200 Bessemer Road, Mt. Pleasant, PA 15666; tel. 724/547–5432; FAX. 724/547–2435; Brian Konieczny, Administrative Director

NEI Ambulatory Surgery Center Inc., P.C., 204 Mifflin Avenue, Scranton, PA 18503; tel. 570/342–3145; FAX. 570/342–3136; Mary Ann Labas, RN, ASC Supervisor

North Shore Surgi-Center, Two Allegheny Center, Suite 530, Pittsburgh, PA 15212-5493; tel. 412/231–0200; FAX. 412/231–0613; Jack Demos, M.D., FACS

Northwood Surgery Center, 3729 Easton-Nazareth Highway, Easton, PA 18045; tel. 610/559–7110; FAX. 610/559–7317; Chitu Patel, Administrator

Ophthalmology Laser and Surgery Center, Inc., 92 Tuscarora Street, Harrisburg, PA 17104; tel. 717/233–2020; FAX. 717/233–0825

Paoli Surgery Center, One Industrial Boulevard, Paoli, PA 19301; tel. 610/408–0822; FAX. 610/408–9933; Caryl Berlin, Facility Manager

Pennsylvania Eye Surgery Center, 4100 Linglestown Road, Harrisburg, PA 17112; tel. 717/657–2020; FAX. 717/657–2071; Jill Stileler, RN, Director, Surgical Services

Pocono Ambulatory Surgery Center, One Veterans Place, Stroudsburg, PA 18360; tel. 570/421–4978; Mary P. Hayden RN, B.S.,CASC, Administrative Director

Shadyside Surgi-Center, Inc., 5727 Centre Avenue, Pittsburgh, PA 15206; tel. 412/363–6626; FAX. 412/363–7008; Susan M. Katch, RN, Director

Southwestern Ambulatory Surgery Center, 500 Lewis Run Road, Suite 202, Pittsburgh, PA 15122; tel. 412/469–6964; FAX. 412/469–6948; Pamela Wrobleski, CRNA, M.P.M., CASC Administrator

Southwestern Pennsylvania Eye Surgery Center, 750 East Beau Street, Washington, PA 15301; tel. 412/228–7477; FAX. 412/228–6271; Mary Roth, RN, Clinical Director

Surgical Center of York, 1750 Fifth Avenue, P.O. Box 290, York, PA 17405; tel. 717/843–7613; FAX. 717/849–5662; James Van Etten, Administrative Director

Surgical Eye Institute of Western Pennsylvania, 618 Monongahela Avenue, Glassport, PA 15045; tel. 412/664–7874; FAX. 412/673–5720; Shirley A. Smith, RN

The Surgery Center of Chester County, Suite 100, 460 Creamery Way, Oaklands Corporate Center, Exton, PA 19341-2533; tel. 610/594–8900; FAX. 610/594–8907; Lorraine Gambol, Manager

The SurgiCenter at Ligonier, 221 West Main Street, Ligonier, PA 15658; tel. 724/238–9573; FAX. 724/238–4709; Kim Kenney-Ciarimboli, Ambulatory Services Director

UPMC Monroeville Surgery Center, 125 Daugherty Drive, Monroeville, PA 15146-2749; tel. 412/374–9385; FAX. 412/374–9490; Carol Fiske Boumbouras, CMSC, Administrative Assistant, Medical Staff Mgr.

Valley Surgery Center, 1130 Highway 315, Wilkes-Barre, PA 18702; tel. 570/821–2830; FAX. 570/823–7921; Patricia Williams, Administrator

West Shore Endoscopy Center, 423 North 21st Street, Camp Hill, PA 17011; tel. 717/975–2430; FAX. 717/730–2158; Lisa Scichitano, R.N., B.S.N., Administrator

Wills Surgery Center of Bucks County, 401 North York Road, Warminster, PA 18974; tel. 215/443–3022; FAX. 215/443–5859; JoAnn Quinn, Director, Nursing

RHODE ISLAND

Bayside Endoscopy Center, 33 Staniford Street, Providence, RI 02905; tel. 401/274–1810; FAX. 401/273–9689; Nicholas Califano, M.D., Administrator

Ocean State Endoscopy, 148 West River Street, Providence, RI 02904; tel. 401/274–1260; Joel Spellun, M.D.

St. James Surgery Center, 444 Quaker Lane, Warwick, RI 02886; tel. 401/384–6537; FAX. 401/384–6541; Paul S. Koch, M.D., Medical Director

Wayland Square Surgicare, 17 Seekonk Street, Providence, RI 02906; tel. 401/453–3311; FAX. 401/351–1280; Ann Dugan, Administrator

Women's Medical Center, 1725 Broad Street, Cranston, RI 02905; tel. 401/467–9111; FAX. 401/461–1390; Nancy Ganem, Administrator

SOUTH CAROLINA

Ambulatory Eye Surgery and Laser Center, Inc., 9297 Medical Plaza Drive, Charleston, SC 29406; tel. 803/572–2888; Margaret A. Thompson

AnMed Health Medicus Surgery Center, LLC, 107 Professional Court, P.O. Box 1886, Anderson, SC 29622-1886; tel. 864/225–1933; FAX. 864/716–7965; Angela Kay, RN, Administrator

Bay Microsurgical Unit, Inc., 1200 Highmarket St., Georgetown, SC 29440; tel. 843/546–8421; FAX. 843/546–1173; Janet Spring, Director of Nursing

Bearwood Ambulatory Surgery Center, 3031 Highway 81, N., Anderson, SC 29621; tel. 864/226–0837; FAX. 864/226–8367; Kathy D. Gibson, R.N., Administrator

Charleston Plastic Surgery Center, Inc., 261 Calhoun St., Ste. 200, Charleston, SC 29401; tel. 843/722–1985; FAX. 843/722–4840; Linda Crosby, Office Manager

Columbia Gastrointestinal Endoscopy Center, 2739 Laurel Street, Suite One-B, Columbia, SC 29240; tel. 803/254–9588; FAX. 803/931–8085; Cindy Sease, R.N., Administrator

Columbia Surgery Center, Inc., 338 Harbison Boulevard, Columbia, SC 29212; tel. 803/732–6180; FAX. 803/732–6563; Vickie H. Ott, Administrator

Cross Creek Surgery Center of Greenville Hospital System, Nine Doctors Drive, Crosscreek Medical Park, Greenville, SC 29605; tel. 803/455–8400; Barbara Callahan, Administrator

Greenville Endoscopy Center, Inc., 317 St. Francis Drive, Suite 150, Greenville, SC 29601; tel. 864/232–7338; FAX. 864/240–8140; Rebecca K. Swoyer, Administrator
Greenville Surgery Center, Five Memorial Medical Court, Greenville, SC 29605; tel. 864/295–3067; FAX. 864/295–3096; Angela Kay, Administrator
HealthSouth Surgery Center of Charleston, 2690 Lake Park Drive, North Charles, SC 29406; tel. 803/764–0992; FAX. 803/764–3187; Rosina Feagin, RN, M.S.N., Administrator
Patewood Surgery Center, LLC, 10 Enterprise Boulevard, Suite 104, Greenville, SC 29615; tel. 803/458–7141; FAX. 803/676–9116; Mary Jane Knottek, RN, B.S.N., CNOR, Clinical Nurse
Pee Dee Ambulatory Surgery Center, 602 Cheves, P.O. Box F-17, Florence, SC 29506; tel. 803/669–3822; Joseph J. McEvoy, Administrator
Roper West Ashley Surgery Center, 18 Farmfield Avenue, Charleston, SC 29407; tel. 843/763–3763; FAX. 843/763–3721; Maria I. Sample, Administrator
Spartanburg Urology Surgicenter, L.P., 391 Serpentine Drive, Suite 330, Spartanburg, SC 29303; tel. 864/585–2002; FAX. 864/585–3300; Rick Sizemore, RN, OR Director
The Greenwood Endoscopy Center, 103 Liner Drive, Greenwood, SC 29646; tel. 803/227–3838; FAX. 803/227–6116; A. A. Ramage, M.D., Administrator
Trident Surgery Center, 9313 Medical Plaza Drive, Suite 102, Charleston, SC 29406; tel. 803/797–8992; FAX. 803/797–4094; Leah J. Dawson, Administrator

SOUTH DAKOTA

Black Hills Regional Eye Surgery Center, 2800 Third Street, Rapid City, SD 57701-7394; tel. 605/341–2000; FAX. 605/341–0278; Richard B. Hanafin, Executive Director
Jones Eye Clinic, 3801 South Elmwood Avenue, Sioux Falls, SD 57105-6565; tel. 605/336–3142; FAX. 605/334–0737; Charles E. Jones, M.D.
Mallard Pointe Surgical Center, 1201 Mickelson Drive, Watertown, SD 57201-7100; tel. 605/882–4743; FAX. 605/882–6064; Mary Petersen, Administrative Director
Medical Associates Clinic Surgery Center, 772 East Dakota, Pierre, SD 57501-3399; tel. 605/945–5210; FAX. 605/224–2217; Michael Pfeifer, Administrator
Sioux Falls Surgical Center, 910 East 20th Street, Sioux Falls, SD 57105-1012; tel. 605/334–6730; FAX. 605/334–8096; Donald A. Schellpfeffer, M.D., Ph.D., Medical Director
Spearfish Surgery Center, LLC, 1316 10th Street, Spearfish, SD 57783-1530; tel. 605/642–3113; FAX. 605/642–3117; Peggy O'Sullivan, Director of Nursing
Women's Health Services, Ltd., 909 South Miller, Mitchell, SD 57301; tel. 605/995–8040; FAX. 605/995–8043; Sheri Trudeau, CNP, Clinic Director

TENNESSEE

Atrium Memorial Surgical Center, 1949 Gunbarrel Road, Suite 290, Chattanooga, TN 37421; tel. 615/495–3550; FAX. 615/495–3580; Sandy Proctor, Administrator
Bristol Surgery Center, 350 Blountville Highway, Suite 108, Bristol, TN 37620; tel. 423/844–6120; FAX. 423/844–6119; Karen Williams,GCHC,MPH,NHA,CHES Administrator
Cataract Surgery Center, 825 Ridge Lake Blvd, Suite 200, Memphis, TN 38120-9411; tel. 901/360–8081; FAX. 901/368–3822
Chattanooga Surgery Center, 400 North Holtzclaw Avenue, Chattanooga, TN 37404; tel. 423/698–6871; FAX. 423/622–8993; K.D. Ratchford, Administrator
Clarksville Endoscopy Center, 132 Hillcrest Drive, Clarksville, TN 37043; tel. 931/552–0180; FAX. 931/572–0915
Columbia Endoscopy Center, Inc., 1510 1/2 Hatcher Lane, Columbia, TN 38401; tel. 615/381–7818; FAX. 615/381–5625; Dianne Roberts, RN, Head Nurse
Columbia Sullins Surgery Center, 2761 Sullins Street, Knoxville, TN 37919; tel. 423/522–2949; FAX. 423/637–3259; Tina Shelby-Kahl, Assistant Administrator
D D C Surgery Center, Nine Physicians Drive, Jackson, TN 38305; tel. 731/661–0086; FAX. 731/661–9783; Kelly Joyce, Clinical Director
East Memphis Surgery Center, 80 Humphreys Center Drive, Suite 101, Memphis, TN 38120; tel. 901/747–3233; FAX. 901/747–3230; Cathy Gilland, RN, Facility Administrator
Endoscopy Center of Kingsport, d/b/a Sullivan Digestive Center, 2204 Pavilion Drive, Kingsport, TN 37660; tel. 423/392–6100; FAX. 423/392–6159; Penny Lloyd, Administrator
Endoscopy Center of Northeast Tennessee, 310 State of Franklin Road, Suite 202, Johnson City, TN 37604; tel. 615/929–7111
Eye Surgery Center of East Tennessee, 1124 Weisgarber Road, Suite 110, Knoxville, TN 37909; tel. 423/588–1037; FAX. 423/909–9104; Pat Pullen, RN
Eye Surgery Center of Middle Tennessee, Parkview Tower, Suite 900, 210 25th Avenue, N., Nashville, TN 37203; tel. 615/327–2244; FAX. 615/327–9254; Stephen J. Molnar, Jr., Executive Administrator
Fort Sanders West Outpatient Surgery Center, Ltd., 210 Fort Sanders West Boulevard, Knoxville, TN 37922; tel. 865/531–5200; FAX. 865/531–5043; Leslie Irwin, Vice President
Franklin Surgery Center at MedCore, 2105 Edward Curd Lane, Franklin, TN 37067; tel. 615/794–7320
G. Baker Hubbard Ambulatory Surgery Center, 616 West Forest Avenue, Jackson, TN 38301; tel. 731/422–0330; FAX. 731/422–0478
Germantown Ambulatory Surgical Center, Inc., 7499 Poplar Pike, Germantown, TN 38138; tel. 901/756–5474; FAX. 901/756–5292
HealthSouth Nashville Surgery Center, 1717 Patterson Street, Nashville, TN 37203; tel. 615/329–1888; FAX. 615/329–0179; Lori Seymore, Administrator
HealthSouth Surgery Center of Clarksville, 121 Hillcrest Drive, Clarksville, TN 37043; tel. 931/552–9992; Jennifer Hines, Administrator
Knoxville Center for Reproductive Health, 1547 West Clinch Avenue, Knoxville, TN 37916; tel. 865/637–3861; FAX. 865/637–0222; Kim Denison, Director
Knoxville Surgery Center, 9300 Park West Boulevard, Knoxville, TN 37923; tel. 615/691–2725; FAX. 615/691–3090; Ranae Thompson, RN, Facility Administrator
Lebanon HMA Surgical Center, 1414 Baddour Parkway, Lebanon, TN 37087; tel. 615/444–8944; FAX. 615/444–8994; Sylvia Black, Clinical Director
LeBonheur East Surgery Center, L.P., 786 Estate Place, Memphis, TN 38120; tel. 901/287–4100; FAX. 901/287–4140; Sherrye Crone, Administrative Director, Carol Langston, Asst. Director
Lisa Ross Birth & Women's Center, Inc, Maternity Center of East Tennessee (formerly), 1925-B Ailor Avenue, Knoxville, TN 37921; tel. 865/524–4422; FAX. 865/523–3687; Linda Cole, CNM Executive Director
Mays & Schnapp Pain Clinic and Rehabilitation Center, 55 Humphreys Center Drive, Suite 200, Memphis, TN 38120; tel. 901/747–0040; FAX. 901/747–0042; Theresa A. Lewis, Administrator Assistant
Memphis Center for Reproductive Health, 1462 Poplar Avenue, Memphis, TN 38104; tel. 901/274–3550; FAX. 901/274–3551; Mary J. Frank, Executive Director
Memphis Eye and Cataract Ambulatory Surgery Center, 6485 Poplar Avenue, Memphis, TN 38119; tel. 901/767–3937
Memphis Gastroenterology Endoscopy Center, 8000 Wolf River Blvd, #200, Germantown, TN 38138-1727; tel. 901/747–3630; FAX. 901/747–4039; Sylvia Hawkins, RN, Compliance Manager
Memphis Regional Gamma Knife Center, 1265 Union Avenue, Memphis, TN 38104; tel. 901/726–6444; FAX. 901/726–6145
Memphis Regional Planned Parenthood, Inc., 1407 Union Avenue, Third Floor, Memphis, TN 38104; tel. 901/725–1717; Ellen Ruby - Markie, Chief Executive Officer
Memphis Surgery Center, 1044 Cresthaven Road, Memphis, TN 38119; tel. 901/682–1516; FAX. 901/682–1545; Jane Almon RN, CNOR, Facility Administrator
Mid-State Endoscopy Center, 2010 Church Street, Suite 420, Nashville, TN 37203; tel. 615/329–2141; FAX. 615/321–0522; Allan H. Bailey, M.D., Medical Director
Nashville Endoscopy Center, 300 20th N., Eighth Floor, Nashville, TN 37203; tel. 615/284–1335; FAX. 615/284–1316; Marie DeBolt, RNMSN Nurse Manager
Nashville Gastrointestinal Endoscopy Center, 4230 Harding Road, Suite 309, Nashville, TN 37205; tel. 615/383–0165; FAX. 615/292–4657; Ron E. Pruitt, M.D.
Northridge Surgery Center, 647 Myatt Drive, Madison, TN 37115; tel. 615/868–8942; FAX. 615/860–3820; Melba Willis, Administrator
Ophthalmic Ambulatory Surgery Center, P.C., 342 22nd Street, Nashville, TN 37203; tel. 615/327–2001; FAX. 615/327–2069; Alec Dryden, Administrator
Oral Facial Surgery Center, 322 22nd Avenue, N., Nashville, TN 37203; tel. 615/321–6160; FAX. 615/327–9612; Shea Love, Administrator
Ridge Lake Ambulatory Surgery Center, 825 Ridge Lake Boulevard, Memphis, TN 38119; tel. 901/685–2200
Shea Ear Clinic, 6133 Poplar Pike, Memphis, TN 38119; tel. 901/761–9720; FAX. 901/763–4400; John J. Shea Jr., MD, President
Southern Endoscopy Center, 397 Wallace Road, Suite 407, Nashville, TN 37211; tel. 615/832–5530; FAX. 615/832–5713; Robert W. Herring, Jr., M.D., Medical Director
St. Thomas Medical Group Endoscopy Center, 4230 Harding Road, Suite 400, Nashville, TN 37205; tel. 615/297–2700; Jeff May RN, Center Director
Surgical Services, P.C., 604 South Main Street, Sweetwater, TN 37874; tel. 423/337–4508; FAX. 423/337–4588
Surgicenter Of Murfreesboro Medical Clinic, P.A., 1004 North Highland Avenue, Murfreesboro, TN 37130; tel. 615/867–8160; FAX. 615/876–7876; Sandy Gordon, Coordinator
Tennessee Endoscopy Center, 1706 East Lamar Alexander Parkway, Maryville, TN 37804; tel. 615/983–0073; FAX. 615/984–1731; Craig Jarvis, M.D., Administrator
The Cookeville Surgery Center, 100 West Fourth Street, Suite 100, Cookeville, TN 38501; tel. 931/526–8115; FAX. 931/526–7619; Jeanie McGinnis, RN Administrator
The Endoscopy Center, 801 Weisgarber Road, Suite 100, Knoxville, TN 37909, Knoxville, TN 37950-9002; tel. 615/588–5121; Gayle Mahan, Office Manager
The Endoscopy Center of Centennial, L.P., 2400 Patterson Street, Suite 515, Nashville, TN 37203; tel. 615/327–2111; FAX. 615/327–9292; Donna Crumley, RN, B.S., MBA, Endoscopy Administrator
The Eye Surgery Center Oak Ridge, 90 Vermont Avenue, Oak Ridge, TN 37830; tel. 865/482–8894; FAX. 865/481–8349; Regina Harkleroad, Director of Nursing
Urology Surgery Center, L.P., 2801 Charlotte Avenue, Nashville, TN 37209; tel. 615/250–9200; FAX. 615/250–9251; Mark Flora, M.D., Chairman
Van Dyke Ambulatory Surgery Center, 1024 Kelley Drive, Paris, TN 38242; tel. 901/642–5003; FAX. 901/642–8756; John T. VanDyck III, M.D., Owner
Volunteer Women's Medical Clinic, 313 Concord Street, Knoxville, TN 37919; tel. 865/522–5173; FAX. 865/522–9907; Elizabeth Fraley-Dumas, Clinical Director
Wesberry Surgery Center, 2900 South Perkins Road, Memphis, TN 38118-3237; tel. 901/362–3100; FAX. 901/362–3372; Jesse Wesberry, Jr., M.D., President
Wesley Ophthalmic Plastic Surgery Center, 250 25th Avenue North, Suite 213, Nashville, TN 37203; tel. 615/329–3624; Janie Stucker, RN, Director

TEXAS

Las Colinas Surgery Center, 4255 North Macarthur Boulevard, Irving, TX 75038; tel. 214/257–0144; FAX. 214/258–0436; Michael Scott, Administrator
Abilene Cataract and Refractive Surgery Center, 2120 Antilley Road, Abilene, TX 79606; tel. 325/695–2020; FAX. 325/695–2326; Paul B. Thomas M.D. Medical Director
Abilene Endoscopy Center, 1249 Ambler Avenue, Abilene, TX 79601; tel. 325/677–2626; FAX. 325/677–6835; Gary Roark, M.D., Medical Director
Amarillo Cataract and Eye Surgery Center, Inc., 7310 Fleming Avenue, Amarillo, TX 79106; tel. 806/354–8891; FAX. 806/354–2591; Carol A. Pearson, Director
Ambulatory Urological Surgery Center, Inc., 1149 Ambler, Abilene, TX 79601; tel. 915/676–3557; FAX. 915/673–2143; Angela X. Young, RN, Manager
American Surgery Centers of South Texas, LTD, 7810 Louis Pasteur, Suite 100, San Antonio, TX 78229; tel. 210/692–0218; FAX. 210/692–7980; Letty Herrera, Administrator
Bailey Square Surgical Center, Ltd., 1111 West 34th Street, Austin, TX 78705; tel. 512/454–6753; FAX. 512/454–4314; Rod Seidel, Administrator

Bay Area Endoscopy Center, 444 FM 1959, Houston, TX 77034; tel. 281/481–9400; FAX. 281/481–9490; N.S. Bala, Medical Director
Bay Area Surgicare Center, 502 Medical Center Boulevard, Webster, TX 77598; tel. 281/332–2433; FAX. 281/332–0619; Carol Simons, Administrator
Baylor SurgiCare, 3920 Worth Street, Dallas, TX 75246; tel. 214/820–2581; FAX. 214/820–7484; Robin Shaw, Administrative Director
Baylor Surgicare at Valley View, 5744 LBJ Freeway, Suite 200, Dallas, TX 75240; tel. 972/490–4333; FAX. 972/991–1649; Gina Schilthuis, RN, Administrator
Brazosport Eye Institute, 103 Parking Way, P.O. Box 369, Lake Jackson, TX 77566; tel. 979/297–2961; FAX. 979/297–2395; Frank J. Grady, M.D., Ph.D., FACS, Director
Central Texas Day Surgery Center, L.P., 1817 Southwest Dodgen, Loop, Temple, TX 76502; tel. 817/773–7785; FAX. 817/773–9333; Debby Meyer, Director
Coastal Bend Ambulatory Surgical Center, 900 Morgan, Corpus Christ, TX 78404; tel. 361/888–4288; FAX. 361/888–4786; Barbara VandenBout, Administrator
Columbia Physicians DaySurgery Center, 3930 Crutcher Street, Dallas, TX 75246; tel. 214/827–0760; FAX. 214/827–0944; Robin Shaw, RN, Administrator
Conroe Surgery Center, 1501 River Pointe Dr., Suite 200, Conroe, TX 77304; tel. 936/760–3443; FAX. 936/760–1322; Kathy Schutz, RN, B.S.N., CASC, Facility Administrator
Covenant Surgicenter, Ltd., 2301 Quaker Avenue, Lubbock, TX 79410; tel. 806/725–8801; FAX. 806/725–8820; Elizabeth Hawronsky, Director
Crystal Outpatient Surgery Center, Inc., 215 Oak Drive, S., Suite J, Lake Jackson, TX 77566; tel. 409/299–6118; FAX. 409/299–1007; R. Scott Yarish, M.D., Administrator
Cy-Fair Surgery Center, 11250 Fallbrook Drive, Houston, TX 77065; tel. 713/955–7194; FAX. 713/890–0895; Sonja Christmas, Administrator
Dallas DaySurgery of Texas LTD., 411 North Washington, Suite 5400, Dallas, TX 75246; tel. 214/821–8613; Henry S. Byrd, President
Dallas Ophthalmology Center, Inc., 4633 North Central Expressway, Suite 310, Dallas, TX 75205; tel. 214/520–7600; FAX. 214/528–6522; Susan Points, RN, Administrator
DeHaven Surgical Center, 1424 East Front Street, Tyler, TX 75702; tel. 903/595–4144; FAX. 903/595–6821; Terri McDougal, RN, Administrator
Doctors' Surgery Center, Inc., 5300 North Street, Nacogdoches, TX 75965; tel. 936/569–8278; FAX. 936/569–0275; Robert P. Lehmann, M.D., Director
East El Paso Surgery Center, 7835 Corral Drive, El Paso, TX 79915; tel. 915/595–3353; FAX. 915/595–6796; Laura Ice, Administrator
East Side Surgery Center, Inc., 10918 East Freeway, Houston, TX 77029; tel. 713/451–4299; FAX. 713/451–4383; Vicky Mizell, Administrator
East Texas Eye Associates Surgery Center, 1306 Frank Avenue, Lufkin, TX 75904; tel. 409/634–8381; Jo Ann O'Neill, C.O.T., Administrator
El Paso Institute of Eye Surgery, Inc., 1717 North Brown Street, Building #3, El Paso, TX 79902; tel. 915/544–0526; FAX. 915/544–2877; Esther A. Calderon, Administrator
Elm Place Ambulatory Surgical Center, 2217 South Danville Drive, Abilene, TX 79605; tel. 325/695–0600; FAX. 325/695–3908; Rebecca Laird, RN, or Verna Brister, Office Manager
Endoscopy Center of Dallas, Ambulatory Endoscopy Clinic of Dallas, 6390 LBJ Freeway, Suite 200, Dallas, TX 75240; tel. 972/934–3691; FAX. 972/934–3694; Jeane Suggs, Administrator
Facial Plastic and Cosmetic Surgical Center, 6300 Humana Plaza, Suite 475, Abilene, TX 79606; tel. 915/695–3630; FAX. 915/695–3633; Howard A. Tobin, M.D., FACS, Medical Director
Fort Worth Endoscopy Center, 900 W. Magnolia Street, Suite 101, Fort Worth, TX 76104; tel. 817/332–6500; Jenny Hunter, Administrator
Forth Worth Surgery Center, 2001 West Rosedale, Fort Worth, TX 76104; tel. 817/877–4777; David Yodge, Administrator
Foundation Surgery Center of Dickinson, 3810 Hughes Court, Dickinson, TX 77539; tel. 713/337–7001; FAX. 713/337–7091; Paul Bolling, Administrator
Garland Surgery Center L.P., 777 Walter Reed Boulevard, Suite 105, Garland, TX 75042; tel. 214/494–2400; FAX. 214/494–3873; Dan Nicholson, President
Gastroenterology Consultants Outpatient Surgical Center, 8214 Wurzbach, San Antonio, TX 78229; tel. 210/614–1234; FAX. 210/614–7749; Bonnie Draude, B.S.N., RN, C.G.RN, Clinical Manager
Gastrointestinal Endoscopy Center Number Two, LTD, 1600 Coit Road, Suite 401A, Plano, TX 75075; tel. 214/867–0019; Brian Cooley, M.D., Administrator
Gonzaba Surgical Center, 720 Pleasanton Road, San Antonio, TX 78214; tel. 210/921–3826; FAX. 210/921–3825; William Gonzaba, M.D., Chief Executive Officer
Good Shepard Ambulatory Surgical Center, Ltd., 703 East Marshall Avenue, Suite 2000, Longview, TX 75601-5563; tel. 903/315–5300; FAX. 903/315–5301; Marion Benson, VP/ Executive Director
Gramercy Outpatient Surgery Center, LTD, 2727 Gramercy, Houston, TX 77025; tel. 713/660–6900; FAX. 713/660–0704; Anita Gill, RN, Clinical Director
Greenville Surgery Center, 7150 Greenville Avenue, Suite 200, Dallas, TX 75231; tel. 214/891–0466; FAX. 214/739–4702; Christine Locke, RN, Administrator
HealthSouth Arlington Day Surgery, 918 North Davis Street, Arlington, TX 76012; tel. 817/860–9933; FAX. 817/860–2314; Diane Wood, RN, Administrator
HealthSouth Northeast Surgery Center, 18929 Highway 59, Humble, TX 77338; tel. 713/446–4053; Holly Reems, R.N.
HealthSouth Surgery Center of Beaumont, 3050 Liberty, Beaumont, TX 77702; tel. 409/835–3535; FAX. 409/835–6005; Tammie Clodfelter, Administrator
HealthSouth Waco Surgery Center, 2911 Herring, Waco, TX 76708; tel. 817/755–4430; FAX. 817/755–4590; Connie Allen, RN, Administrator
Heart of Texas Outpatient Cataract Center, 100 South Park Drive, Brownwood, TX 76801; tel. 325/643–3561; Larry Smith, CRNA, Administrator
Heritage Surgery Center, 1501 Redbud Blvd., McKinney, TX 75069; tel. 972/548–0771; FAX. 972/562–2300; Rudolf Churner, M.D., Administrator
Howerton Surgical Center, 2610 I.H. 35 South, Austin, TX 78704-5703; tel. 512/443–9715; FAX. 512/443–9845; Ernest E. Howerton, M.D., Administrator
Key Whitman Surgery Center, 2801 Lemmon Avenue, Suite 400, Dallas, TX 75204; tel. 214/754–0000; FAX. 214/754–0079; Jeffrey Whitman, M.D.
Lufkin Endoscopy Center, 317 Gaslight Boulevard, Lufkin, TX 75904; tel. 936/634–3713; FAX. 936/634–8136; Bhagvan R. Malladi, M.D., Administrator
Medical City Dallas Ambulatory Surgery Center, 7777 Forest Lane, Suite C-150, Dallas, TX 75230; tel. 972/566–6171; FAX. 972/566–2502; Vickie Roberts, Administrator
Medical Mall Surgery Center, Inc., 1665 Antilley Road, Suite 170, Abilene, TX 79606; tel. 325/692–6694; FAX. 325/691–1568; Daniel Brewer, RN
Metroplex Ambulatory Surgical Center, 2717 Osler Drive, Suite 102, Grand Prairie, TX 75051; tel. 972/647–6272; FAX. 972/660–1822; Glenda Daniels, RN, Director
Metroplex Surgicare, 1600 Central Drive, Suite 180, Bedford, TX 76022; tel. 817/571–1999; FAX. 817/571–1220; Richard Smith, Administrator
Mid-Town Surgical Center, LLP, 2105 Jackson Street, Suite 200, Houston, TX 77003; tel. 713/571–8141; FAX. 713/571–8184; Louis Varela, M.D.
North Carrier Surgicenter, 517 North Carrier Parkway, Suite A, Grand Prairie, TX 75050-5494; tel. 972/264–0533; FAX. 972/262–5974; Abraham F. Syrquin, M.D., Medical Director
North Dallas Surgicare, 375 Municipal Drive, Suite 214, Richardson, TX 75080; tel. 214/918–9400; FAX. 214/918–9749; Mike Kelley, Administrator
North Texas Surgi-Center, 917 Midwestern Parkway, E., Wichita Falls, TX 76302; tel. 940/767–7273; FAX. 940/723–9059; Barbara Dawson, Administrator
Northeast Texas Surgical Center, 1801 Galleria Oaks Drive, Texarkana, TX 75503; tel. 903/792–2108; FAX. 903/792–0606; Kelly Pugh, Business Office Manager
Park Central Surgical Center, 12200 Park Central Drive, Third Floor, Dallas, TX 75251; tel. 972/661–0505; FAX. 972/661–5511; Molly Paulose, Administrator
Physicians SurgiCenter of Houston True Results, 7515 South Main Street, Suite 800, Houston, TX 77030; tel. 713/799–9990; FAX. 713/796–1142; Patsy Mitchusson, RN, MBA, CASC, Administrator
Plano Ambulatory Surgery Associates, L.P., d/b/a Surgery Center of Plano, 1620 Coit Road, Plano, TX 75075-7799; tel. 972/519–1100; DeWayne Hodges, Administrator
Plaza Day Surgery, 909 Ninth Avenue, Fort Worth, TX 76104-3986; tel. 817/336–6060; FAX. 817/339–2329; Deborah Pelton RN, Administrator
Port Arthur Day Surgery Center, 3449 Gates Boulevard, Port Arthur, TX 77642; tel. 409/983–6144; Vicki Clark, Administrative Director
Premier Ambulatory Surgery of Austin, dba South Austin Surgery Center, 4207 James Casey, Suite 203, Austin, TX 78745; tel. 512/440–7894; FAX. 512/440–1932; Patricia Philbin, Executive Director
Q Plus Outpatient Surgery Center, 2507 Medical Row, Suite 101, Grand Prairie, TX 75051; tel. 972/647–8520; FAX. 972/336–0488; James L. Grace Administrator
Rio Grande Surgery Center, 1809 South Cynthia, McAllen, TX 78503; tel. 956/618–4402; FAX. 956/618–4174; Nelda C. Pence, RN, CNOR Administrator
San Antonio Digestive Disease Endoscopy Center, 1804 Northeast Loop 410, Suite 101, San Antonio, TX 78217; tel. 210/828–8400; FAX. 210/828–8648; Rebecca Trevino, RN, Clinical Director
San Antonio Gastroenterology Endoscopy Center, 520 Euclid Avenue, San Antonio, TX 78212; tel. 210/271–0606; FAX. 210/271–0180; Ernesto Guerra, M.D.
San Antonio Surgery Center, Inc.DBA The Center for Special Surgery, 21 Spurs Lane, Sub-Level 100, San Antonio, TX 78240; tel. 210/614–0187; FAX. 210/692–7757; Eric Day, Administrator
South Plains Endoscopy Center, 3610 24th Street, Lubbock, TX 79410; tel. 806/797–1015; Pat S. Wheeler, Administrator
South Texas Eye Surgicenter, Inc., 4406 North Laurent, Victoria, TX 77901; tel. 800/352–5928; Robert T. McMahon, M.D., Chief Executive Officer
Southwest Endoscopy Center, 11803 South Freeway, Suite 115, Fort Worth, TX 76115; tel. 817/293–9292; FAX. 817/551–0616; Esther Cruz, MA/Office Manager
Surgery Center of Duncanville, 1018 East Wheatland Road, Duncanville, TX 75116; tel. 972/296–6912; FAX. 972/296–6912; David Gross, Administrator
Surgery Center of Texas, 155 East Loop 338, Suite 500, Odessa, TX 79762; tel. 432/367–3906; FAX. 432/367–3895; Libby Palma, Administrator
SurgEyeCare, Inc., 5421 La Sierra Drive, Dallas, TX 75231; tel. 214/361–1443; FAX. 214/691–3299; Sandra J. Yankee, Administrator
Surgical and Diagnostic Center, Inc., 729 Bedford Euless Road West 100, Hurst, TX 76053; tel. 817/282–6905; FAX. 817/285–8114; Cynessa Whaley, RN, Director of Surgical Services
Surgical Center of El Paso, 1815 North Stanton, El Paso, TX 79902; tel. 915/533–8412; FAX. 915/542–0367; Raymond Sainz, Administrator
Surgicare of Travis Centre, Inc., 6655 Travis, Suite 200, Houston, TX 77030; tel. 713/526–5100; FAX. 713/520–1782; Sherri Bronikowski, Administrator
Surgicenter of San Antonio, L.P., 5290 Medical Drive, San Antonio, TX 78229; tel. 210/614–0187; FAX. 210/692–7757; Ann Mueller, Executive Director
Texarkana Surgery Center, 5404 Summerhill Road, Texarkana, TX 75503; tel. 903/793–4872; FAX. 903/794–6300; Kimble Hatridge, Administrator
Texoma Outpatient Surgery Center, Inc., 1712 Eleventh Street, Wichita Falls, TX 76301; tel. 940/723–2499; FAX. 940/923–2497; Tracy Youngblood, Administrator
The Cataract Center of East Texas, 802 Turtle Creek Drive, Tyler, TX 75701; tel. 903/595–4333; FAX. 903/535–9845; Emmitte Hall, RN, Administrator
The Center for Sight, P.A., 2 Medical Center Boulevard, Lufkin, TX 75904-3175; tel. 936/634–8434; Richard J. Ruckman, M.D.
The Endoscopy Center of Southeast Texas, 950 North 14th Street,#200, Beaumont, TX 77702; tel. 409/833–5555; FAX. 409/833–9911; Jackie Sullivan, RN Center Director

The Ocular Surgery Center, Inc., 1100 North Main Avenue, San Antonio, TX 78212; tel. 210/222–2154; FAX. 512/222–0706; Jane Wilson, Administrator
The Surgery Center of Mesquite, 2690 North Galloway Avenue, Mesquite, TX 75150; tel. 972/279–8100; FAX. 972/279–3300; Susan Erickson, Administrator
The Surgery Center of the Woodlands, 1441 Woodstead Court, Suite 100, The Woodlands, TX 77380; tel. 281/363–0058; FAX. 281/363–0450; Susan Olis, Administrator
Urological Surgery Center of Fort Worth, 418 South Henderson, Fort Worth, TX 76104; tel. 817/338–4637; FAX. 817/335–5421; Charles Bamberger, M.D.
Valley Endoscopy Center, LLP, 3101 South 77 Sunshine Strip, Suite B, Harlingen, TX 78550; tel. 956/421–2324; FAX. 956/421–5791; Oral James MD/ Lou Valenzela RN Center Director
Vista Surgical Center West, 2500 Fondren, Suite 350, Houston, TX 77063; tel. 713/782–8279; FAX. 713/782–3139; Diana Hastings, RN, CNOR - Clinical Director
Weslace Eye Surgery Center of the Rio Grande Valley, 1402 East Sixth Street, Weslaco, TX 78596; tel. 210/968–6155; FAX. 210/968–8291; Dora Gutierrez, Administrator
West Houston Surgicare, 970 Campbell Road, Houston, TX 77024-2804; tel. 713/461–3547; FAX. 713/722–8921; Charles Mattea, Administrator
WestPark Surgery Center, 130 South Central Expressway, McKinney, TX 75070; tel. 214/542–9382; FAX. 214/548–5303; Debbie Taylor
Wilson Surgicenter, 4315 28th Street, Lubbock, TX 79410; tel. 806/792–2104; Bill W. Wilson, M.D., Chief Executive Officer

UTAH

Central Utah Surgical Center, 1067 North 500 West, Provo, UT 84604; tel. 801/374–0354; FAX. 801/717–2364; Jill Andrews, RN, BSN, CNOR, Administrator
HealthSouth Provo Surgical Center, 585 North 500 West, Provo, UT 84601; tel. 801/375–0983; Ken Armstrong, Administrator
Institute of Facial and Cosmetic Surgery, 5929 Fashion Boulevard, Salt Lake City, UT 84107; tel. 801/261–3637; FAX. 801/261–4096; Dr. Brent D. Kennedy, Director
Intermountain Surgical Center, 359 Eighth Avenue, Salt Lake City, UT 84103; tel. 801/321–3200; FAX. 801/321–3035; Joan W. Lelis, Administrative Director
Salt Lake Endoscopy Center, 24 South 1100 East, Salt Lake City, UT 84102; tel. 801/355–2987; FAX. 801/531–9704; Cher Struck, Office Manager
Salt Lake Surgical Center, 617 East 3900 South, Salt Lake City, UT 84107; tel. 801/261–3141; FAX. 801/268–2599; Robyn Archer, Administrator
St. George Surgical Center, 676 South Bluff Street, St. George, UT 84770; tel. 435/673–8080; FAX. 435/673–0096; Terrill Dick, Administrator
St. Mark's Outpatient Surgery Center, 1250 East 3900 South, Suite 100, Salt Lake City, UT 84124; tel. 801/262–0358; FAX. 801/262–0901; Marjorie Kimes, Administrator
The SurgiCare Center of Utah, 755 East 3900 South, Salt Lake City, UT 84107; tel. 801/266–2283; FAX. 801/268–6151; Edward Barber, Administrator
Wasatch Endoscopy, 1220 East 3900 South, Suite 1B, Salt Lake City, UT 84124; tel. 801/281–3657; Lynnie Marietta, Clinical Coordinator
Wasatch Surgery Center, 555 South Foothill Boulevard, Salt Lake City, UT 84112; tel. 801/581–7782; FAX. 801/581–8962; Karen Ipson, Administrator, Manager

VIRGINIA

Ambulatory Surgery Center, 844 Kempsville Road, Norfolk, VA 23502; tel. 757/466–6900; FAX. 757/466–6313; Darleen S. Anderson, Site Administrator
Blue Ridge Surgery Center, 1802 Braeburn Drive, Salem, VA 24153; tel. 540/772–3601; FAX. 540/725–4543; Kay D'Ardenne, Administrator
Columbia Fairfax Surgical Center, 10730 Main Street, Fairfax, VA 22030; tel. 703/691–0670; Sharon B. Johnson, Chief Executive Officer
CountrySide Ambulatory Surgery Center, Four Pidgeon Hill Drive, Sterling, VA 20165; tel. 703/444–6060; FAX. 703/444–2278; Deborah F. Arminio, RN, Director
Fredericksburg Ambulatory Surgery Center, 1201 Sam Perry Blvd., Suite 101, Fredericksburg, VA 22401; tel. 540/741–7000; FAX. 540/899–6893; Jeane Bullock, Administrator
Hanover Outpatient Center, 7016 Lee Park Road, Mechanicsville, VA 23111; tel. 804/730–9000; FAX. 804/730–1460; Valene S. Rice, RN, Director
Kaiser Permanente Falls Church Ambulatory Surgery Center, 201 North Washington Street, Falls Church, VA 22046; tel. 703/531–1623; FAX. 703/536–1400; Eileen Field, Director, ASC
Lakeview Medical Center, Inc., 2000 Meade Parkway, Suffolk, VA 23424; tel. 757/934–9433; FAX. 757/934–9497; Michael B. Stout, Executive Director
Novamed Surgery Center of Richmond, LLC, 2010 Bremo Road, Suite 132, Richmond, VA 23226; tel. 804/285–0680; FAX. 804/285–3441; Patricia Lampman, Director
Piedmont Day Surgery Center, Inc., 1040 Main Street, P.O. Box 1360, Danville, VA 24543-1360; tel. 434/792–1433; FAX. 434/797–2807; Joseph M. Carlone, MD President
Riverside Surgery Center-Warwick, 12420 Warwick Boulevard, Building 3, Newport News, VA 23606; tel. 804/594–2796; FAX. 804/594–3911; M. Caroline Martin, Executive Vice President
Surgi Center of Central Virginia, Inc., 12 Chatham Heights Rd, Fredericksburg, VA 22405; tel. 703/371–5349; FAX. 703/373–1745; William A. Keeney, Facility Administrator
Surgi-Center of Winchester, Inc., 1860 Amherst Street, P.O. Box 2660, Winchester, VA 22604; tel. 540/536–8934; FAX. 540/536–8936; Nelson N. Isenhower, M.D., Medical Director
Tuckahoe Surgery Center, Inc., 8919 Three Chopt Road, Richmond, VA 23229; tel. 804/285–4763; FAX. 804/288–8946; Sandra W. Pearson, Administrator
Urosurgical Center of Richmond, 9105 Stony Point Dr, Richmond, VA 23235; tel. 804/330–9105; FAX. 804/560–0914; Terry W. Coffey, Administrator
Urosurgical Center of Richmond-North, 8228 Meadowbridge Road, Mechanicsville, VA 23116; tel. 804/730–5023; FAX. 804/746–4015; Terry W. Coffey, Administrator
Virginia Ambulatory Surgery,Inc., 337-15th Street, S.W., Charlottesville, VA 22903; tel. 434/951–4600; FAX. 434/817–8465; Gerry Dobrasz, Administrator
Virginia Beach Ambulatory Surgery Center, 1700 Will-o-Wisp Drive, Virginia Beach, VA 23454; tel. 757/496–6400; FAX. 757/496–3137; Renee Woodford, M.D.
Virginia Eye Institute/Eye Surgeons of Richmond, Inc., 400 Westhampton Station, Richmond, VA 23226; tel. 804/287–4200; FAX. 804/287–4210; Jane Broadbent, Marketing Director
Virginia Heart Institute, LTD., 205 North Hamilton Street, Richmond, VA 23221; tel. 804/359–9265; FAX. 804/358–0317; Charles L. Baird, Jr., M.D., Director
Woodburn Surgery Center, 3289 Woodburn Road, Suite 100, Annandale, VA 22003; tel. 703/207–7520; Jolene Tornabeni, Senior Vice President, Administrator

WASHINGTON

Aesthetic Eye Associates, P.S. ASC, 625 4th Avenue, Suite 302, Kirkland, WA 98033; tel. 425/216–7200; FAX. 425/216–7272; Janet Jordan, Administrator
Auburn Outpatient Surgery Center, 101 Second Street, N.E., Auburn, WA 98002; tel. 253/833–6241; FAX. 253/833–4113; Nancy Juhlin, MD, Medical Director
Bel-Red Ambulatory Surgical Facility, 1260 116th Ave., NE, #110, Bellevue, WA 98004; tel. 425/455–7225; FAX. 425/455–0045; Jan Zemplenyi, M.D., Director
Cascade Valley Arlington Surgery Center, 875 Wesley Street, Suite 160, Arlington, WA 98223; tel. 360/435–6969; FAX. 360/435–1068
Central Washington Cataract Surgery, 1450 North 16th Avenue, Building J, Yakima, WA 98902; tel. 509/457–5000; FAX. 509/457–6498
Central Washington Surgicare, 307 South 12th Avenue, Suite Nine, Yakima, WA 98902; tel. 509/248–4900; FAX. 509/248–0609
Covington Day Surgery Center, 17700 Southeast 272nd Street, Kent, WA 98042; tel. 206/639–8302; FAX. 206/639–8301; Victoria Fitzpatrick, B.S.N., Director
Edmonds Surgery Center, 21229 84th Avenue W., Edmonds, WA 98026; tel. 206/775–1505; FAX. 206/775–9078; Mark A. Kuzel, D.P.M., F.A.C.F.S
Evergreen Endoscopy Center, 11800 NE 128th Street, Suite 100, Kirkland, WA 98034; tel. 425/899–4500; FAX. 425/899–4510; Cathy Richardson, Office Manager
Evergreen Eye Surgery Center, 34719 Sixth Avenue South, Federal Way, WA 98003; tel. 253/874–3969; FAX. 253/661–7383; Richard A. Boudreau, Administrator
Eye Surgery Center Northwest, South 842 Cowley, Suite 3, Spokane, WA 99202; tel. 509/747–6358; FAX. 509/747–1348; Michael H. Cunningham, M.D., President
First Hill Surgery Center, 515 Minor Avenue, Suite 130, Seattle, WA 98104; tel. 206/682–6103; FAX. 206/682–3511; Debbie Perdue, Director
Good Samaritan Surgery Center, 1322 Third Street S.E., Suite 100, Puyallup, WA 98372; tel. 253/697–5700; FAX. 253/840–2352; William Rinker, MD, Medical Director
Kruger Clinic Day Surgery, 21600 Highway 99, Suite 150, Edmonds, WA 98026; tel. 425/774–2636; FAX. 425/774–2688; Marilyn Degan, Director
Lomas Surgery Center, 17800 Talbot Road, S., Renton, WA 98055; tel. 425/255–0986; FAX. 425/271–5703; Marilyn Kritzer - Administrator
Madrona Medical Group, ASC, 4545 Cordata Parkway, Bellingham, WA 98226; tel. 360/738–2200; FAX. 360/752–5677; Sandy Mellott, Clinical Services Director
Minor & James Medical, PLLC, 515 Minor Avenue, Suite 200, Seattle, WA 98104; tel. 206/386–9500; FAX. 206/576–3807; Jody Burnell, RN, ASC Supervisor
Monroe Foot Care Associates Ambulatory Surgery Center, 14692 179th Avenue, S.E., Suite 300, Monroe, WA 98272; tel. 206/794–1266; Dr. Brunsman, Medical Director
Moses Lake Surgery Center, 840 East Hill Avenue, Moses Lake, WA 98837; tel. 509/764–6400; FAX. 509/764–6464; Larry Poff, RN, BSN, Mgr ASC
North Cascade ENT and Facial Plastic Surgery, 111 South 13th Street, Mount Vernon, WA 98273; tel. 360/336–2178; Alex O'Dell, Business Administrator
North Kitsap Ambulatory Surgical Center Pacific Surgery Center, DBA Pacific Surgery Center, 20669 Bond Road, N.E., Poulsbo, WA 98370; tel. 360/779–6527; FAX. 360/697–2743; Susan Simons, RN, Administrator
Northwest Center for Plastic and Reconstructive Surgery, 16259 Sylvester Road, S.W., Suite 302, Seattle, WA 98166; tel. 206/241–5400; FAX. 206/241–8591; Sindi Miller, Office Manager
Northwest Gastroenterology, d/b/a Northwest Endoscopy, 2930 Squalicum Parkway, Suite 202, Bellingham, WA 98225; tel. 360/734–1420; FAX. 360/734–8748; Sandra Vander Yacht, Manager
Northwest Nasal Sinus Center, 10330 Meridan Avenue, N., Suite 240, Seattle, WA 98133; tel. 206/525–2525; FAX. 206/525–0346; Rick Fischer, Business Administrator
Northwest Nasal Sinus Center, 3100 Carillon Point, Kirkland, WA 98033; tel. 206/525–2525; FAX. 206/525–0346; Rick Fischer, Business Administrator
Northwest Surgery Center, 1920 100th Street, S.E., Everett, WA 98208; tel. 425/316–3700; FAX. 425/316–6881; Chris Vance, President
Northwest Surgery Center, Inc., West 123 Francis, Spokane, WA 99205; tel. 509/483–9363; FAX. 509/483–0355; Douglas P. Romney
NW Center for Corrective Jaw Surgery, 550 16th Avenue, Suite 303, Seattle, WA 98122; tel. 206/324–6570; FAX. 206/324–9936; Dotti Miller, Practice Manager
Olympia Outpatient Surgery Center, 205 Lilly Road, NE, Suite D, Olympia, WA 98506; tel. 360/412–1281; FAX. 360/491–7902; Robert Kugel, M.D., Director
Olympic Ambulatory Surgery Center, Inc., 2613 Wheaton Way, Bremerton, WA 98310; tel. 206/479–5990; FAX. 360/479–0948; Dori Robinson, Administrator
Olympic Plastic Surgery Suite, 2600 Cherry Avenue, Suite 201, Bremerton, WA 98310; tel. 360/415–0762; Suzanne Fletcher, Administrator
Pacific Cataract and Laser Institute, 2517 Northeast Kresky, Chehalis, WA 98532; tel. 206/748–8632; Debbie Eldredge, Vice President and COO
Pacific Cataract and Laser Institute, 10500 Northeast Eighth Street, Suite 1650, Bellevue, WA 98004-4332; tel. 425/462–7664; FAX. 425/462–6429; Maynard Pohl, O.D., Clinical Director

Section C

Pacific Cataract and Laser Institute, 8200 West Grandridge, Kennewick, WA 99336; FAX. 360/748–4007; Debbie Eldredge, Vice President and COO
Pacific NW Facial Plastic Ambulatory Surgery Center, 600 Broadway, Suite 280, Seattle, WA 98122; tel. 206/386–3550; FAX. 206/386–3553; Sherry Gizewski, Practice Manager
Parkway Surgical Center, 2940 Squalicum Parkway, Suite 204, Bellingham, WA 98225; tel. 206/676–8350; FAX. 206/676–8351; Orville Vandergriend, M.D., Administrator
Physicians Eye Surgical Center, 3930 Hoyt Avenue, Everett, WA 98201; tel. 206/259–2020; Ms. Mello Johnson, Administrator
Plastic Surgicenter of Olympia, 400 Lilly Road, N.E., Building Four, Olympia, WA 98506; tel. 360/456–4400; FAX. 360/491–7619; Wayne L. Dickason, M.D.
Redmond Foot Care Associates, ASC, 16146 Cleveland Street, Redmond, WA 98052; tel. 206/885–7004
Rockwood Clinic, d/b/a Gastrointestinal Endoscopy Unit, Sacred Heart Doctor's Building, West 105 Eighth Avenue, Spokane, WA 99204; tel. 509/838–2531; FAX. 509/455–8828; Kevin Sweeney, Administrator
Rockwood Clinic, PS, East 400 Fifth Avenue, Spokane, WA 99202; tel. 509/838–2531; FAX. 509/455–5315; Kevin D. Sweeney, M.D., CEO/ President
Seattle Endoscopy Center, 11027 Meridian Avenue, N., Suite 100, Seattle, WA 98133; tel. 206/365–4492; FAX. 206/368–3456; Mary Beth Philips, BSN,RN, CGRN, Manager
Seattle Hand Surgery Group, P.C., 600 Broadway, Suite 440, Seattle, WA 98122; tel. 206/292–6252; FAX. 206/292–7893; Tamiko Gandy, Administrator
Seattle Plastic Surgery Center, 600 Broadway, Suite 320, Seattle, WA 98122; tel. 206/324–1120; FAX. 206/720–0800; Doris Sevedge, Manager
Seattle Surgery Center, Columbus Pavilion, 900 Terry Avenue, Third Floor, Seattle, WA 98104-1240; tel. 206/382–1021; FAX. 206/332–9369; Jim Sapienza, FACHE, CEO
Sequim Same Day Surgery, 777 North Fifth Avenue, Sequim, WA 98382; tel. 360/582–2632; FAX. 360/582–2631; Tammy Paolini, Surgical Technician
South Hill Ambulatory Surgical Center, South 3028 Grand Boulevard, Spokane, WA 99203; tel. 509/747–0279; FAX. 509/747–3220; Borys Markewych
Spokane Digestive Disease Center, 105 West Eighth Avenue, Suite 6010, Spokane, WA 99204-2318; tel. 509/838–5950; FAX. 509/838–5961; Michelle Avenger, RN, CGRN, Director
Spokane Surgery Center, North 1120 Pines Road, Spokane, WA 99206; tel. 509/928–1990; FAX. 509/928–2933; Stewart P. Brim, D.P.M.
St. Mark's Micro Surgical Center, Inc., 502 South M Street, Tacoma, WA 98405; tel. 206/627–8266; Roy Baker, Chief Executive Officer
Stanley M. Jackson, M.D. and Phillip C. Klerney, M.D., Cosmetic and Plastic Surgery, 105 27th Avenue, S.E., Puyallup, WA 98374; tel. 253/848–8110; FAX. 253/845–3561; Jane Hafer, LDN, Clinical Manager
Surgery Center Of Spokane, 205 N. University #4, Spokane, WA 99206; tel. 509/922–3199; Dr. Jacqueline Borbol
Tacoma Ambulatory Surgery Center, 1112 Sixth Avenue, Suite 100, Tacoma, WA 98405; tel. 253/272–3916; FAX. 253/627–1713; Deborah Gist, Clinical Director
Tacoma Endoscopy Center, 1112 Sixth Avenue, Suite 200, Tacoma, WA 98405; tel. 253/272–8664; FAX. 253/627–7880; John G. Carrougher, M.D., Medical Director
Tacoma Specialty ASU, 209 Martin Luther King Jr. Way, Tacoma, WA 98405; tel. 253/596–3590; Linda Shirley, Manager
The Eastside Endoscopy Center, L.L.C., A Physicians Endoscopy Partnered Facility, 1135 116th Ave NE Suite 570, Bellevue, WA 98004-3049; tel. 425/451–7335; FAX. 425/451–1226; Michelle Steele, CGRN, Nurse Administrator
The Plastic SurgiCentre, Inc., 535 South Pine Street, Spokane, WA 99202; tel. 509/623–2160; FAX. 509/623–1135; Pamala Silvers, RN, Manager
The Polyclinic, Inc., 1145 Broadway, Seattle, WA 98122; tel. 206/329–1760
Valley Outpatient Surgery Center, North 1414 Houk Road, Suite 204, Spokane, WA 99216; tel. 509/922–0362; FAX. 509/927–8316; Joel San Nicholas, Administrator
Virginia Mason Federal Way, 33501 First Way South, Federal Way, WA 98003; tel. 253/874–1699; FAX. 253/874–1709; Margaret Brewer
Virginia Mason-Issaquah, 100 Northeast Gilman Boulevard, Issaquah, WA 98027; tel. 425/557–8000; Bobbie Eatmon, Director Ambulatory Services
Washington Centre for Reproductive Medicine, ASC, 1370 116th Avenue, N.E., Suite 202, Bellevue, WA 98004; tel. 425/462–6100; FAX. 425/635–0742; Dr. James Kustin, Medical Director
Washington Orthopedic Center, Inc., PS, 1900 Cooks Hill Road, Centralia, WA 98531; tel. 360/736–2889; Dondi Sahlinger, OR Manager
Wenatchee Valley Clinic/Cascade Surgery Center, 820 North Chelan, Wenatchee, WA 98801; tel. 509/663–8711; FAX. 509/665–2309; Dr. Don Paugh, Chief, Cascade Surgery Center
Whidbey SurgiCare, 31775-SR 20, Suite A Two, Oak Harbor, WA 98277-2334; tel. 360/679–3117; FAX. 360/679–3118; Stephen T. Miller, DPM, Medical Director

WEST VIRGINIA
Anwar Eye Center, 1500 Lafayette Avenue, Moundsville, WV 26041; tel. 304/845–0908; FAX. 304/845–1250; M. F. Anwar, M.D.
Cabell Huntington Surgery Center, 1201 Hal Greer Boulevard, Huntington, WV 25701; tel. 304/523–1885; FAX. 304/523–8942; Lexa Woodyard, Administrator
Cook Eye Surgery Center, 1300 Third Avenue, Huntington, WV 25701; tel. 304/522–1802; FAX. 304/529–6752; David W. Cook, M.D., President
Day Surgery Center, 4701 Maccorkle Ave, Charleston, WV 25304; tel. 304/925–9300
Greenbrier Clinic Surgery Center, Inc, 320 W. Main Street, White Sulphur Spring, WV 24986; tel. 304/536–4870; Leta Morgan, Administrator
Jerry N. Black, M.D., Surgical Suite, 10 Amalia Drive, Suite 3C, Buckhannon, WV 26201; tel. 304/472–2100; FAX. 304/472–2118; Jerry N. Black, M.D., Medical Director
Kanawha Valley Surgi-Center, 4803 MacCorkle Avenue, S.E., Charleston, WV 25304; tel. 304/925–6390; FAX. 304/925–7931; Gorli Harish, M.D., Medical Director
Surgical Eye Center of Morgantown, 1299 Pineview Drive, Morgantown, WV 26505; tel. 304/598–5755; Heather Huffman, Administrator
Tri State Surgical Center, LLC, 1006 Tavern Road, Martinsburg, WV 25401; tel. 304/267–0556; Stacey Ferguson, Administrator

WISCONSIN
Aurora Health Center, 10400 75th Street, Kenosha, WI 53142; tel. 414/697–6907; FAX. 414/697–3022; Thomas M. Warsocki, Administrator
Bay Lake Surgery Outpatient Surgery Center, Inc., 1843 Michigan Street, P.O. Box 678, Sturgeon Bay, WI 54235; tel. 414/746–1070; FAX. 414/746–1072; Michael Herlache, Administrator
BayCare Surgery Center, 2253 West Mason, P.O. Box 33227, Green Bay, WI 54303-0102; tel. 920/592–9100; FAX. 920/497–8056; Tammy Kruegger, Executive Director
Green Bay Surgical Center, Ltd., 704 South Webster Avenue, Green Bay, WI 54301; tel. 920/432–7433; FAX. 920/432–6003; Herbert F. Sandmire, M.D., Medical Director, Administrator
Menomonee Falls Ambulatory Surgery Center, W180 N8045 Town Hall Road, Menomonee Falls, WI 53051; tel. 262/250–0950; FAX. 262/250–0955; Dianne Wallace, Executive Director
North Shore Surgical Center, 7007 North Range Line Road, Milwaukee, WI 53209; tel. 414/352–3341; FAX. 414/352–3218; Helen Kowalski, Executive Director
Northwest Surgery Center, 2300 North Mayfair Road, Wauwatosa, WI 53226; tel. 414/257–3322; Nancy Jones, Administrator
Riverview Surgery Center, 616 North Washington Street, Janesville, WI 53545; tel. 608/758–7300; FAX. 608/758–1050; Lynn Jenkins, Director
St. Mary's Dean Ventures Surgery Centers, 800 South Brooks Street, Madison, WI 53715; tel. 608/259–3510; FAX. 608/255–1272; Lynn Jenkins, Director
Surgicenter of Greater Milwaukee, 3223 South 103rd Street, Milwaukee, WI 53227; tel. 414/328–5800; FAX. 414/328–5805; Denise Augustin, President
Surgicenter of Racine, Ltd., 5802 Washington Avenue, Racine, WI 53406; tel. 262/886–9100; FAX. 262/886–9130; Dennis J. Kontra, Administrator
Wauwatosa Surgery Center, 10900 West Potter Road, Wauwatosa, WI 53226-3424; tel. 414/774–9227; FAX. 414/774–0957; Cathy Logue, Administrator

WYOMING
Gem City Bone and Joint Surgery Center, 1909 Vista Drive, Laramie, WY 82070; tel. 307/745–8851; FAX. 307/742–8851; Trent Kaufman, Admin. Director
Wyoming Outpatient Services, 5050 Powderhouse Road, Cheyenne, WY 82009; tel. 307/634–1311; FAX. 307/638–6820; Cindy Stolz, Reception/ OCC Med Supervisor
Yellowstone Surgery Center, LLC., 5201 Yellowstone Road, Cheyenne, WY 82009; tel. 307/635–7070; FAX. 307/632–9920; Deborah Wright, Office Administrator

U.S. Associated Areas

PUERTO RICO
ASC Espanola Clinic, Box 490, La Quinta, Mayaguez, PR 00681; tel. 787/832–2094
Cirugia Ambulatoria y Centro de Diagnostico y Tratamiento de S, Box 486, San Sebastian, PR 00755; tel. 809/896–1850
Clinica de Cirugia Ambulatoria de Puerto Rico, Box 3748, Mayaguez, PR 00681; tel. 787/833–4400; FAX. 787/265–6621; Roberto Ruiz, Administrator
Instituto Cirugia Plastica Del Oeste, 165 Este Mendez Vigo Street, Mayaguez, PR 00680; tel. 787/833–3248; FAX. 787/831–4400; Oscar Vargas, M.D., Medical Director
Instituto Quirurgico De Un Dia - Dr. Pila, P.O. Box 331910, Ponce, PR 00733–1910; tel. 787/848–5600; FAX. 787/841–1085; Mrs. Joselyn Irizarry RN, Supervisor
OJOS, Eye Surgery Specialists of P.R.L.L.C., Hipodromo Street 809, Santurce, PR 00909; tel. 787/721–8330; FAX. 787/722–3222; Maria Delos A. Tirado, Administrator
San Juan Medical Plaza, 150 De Diego Avenue, Baldorioty Corner, San Juan, PR 00907; tel. 787/977–7575; FAX. 787/977–7587; Roberto Ruiz, MHSA Administrator
Southern SurgiCenter, Edificio Parra Office 201, Ponce, PR 00717-1320; tel. 787/841–0303; FAX. 787/841–0387; Mr. Roberto Rentas, MHSA

Section C

State Government Agencies for Freestanding Hospices

Information for the following list was obtained directly from the agencies. For a complete list of hospital based hospice programs please refer to Section A of AHA Guide. In Section A hospice program are identified by Facility Code F42.

United States

ALABAMA
Alabama Department of Public Health, Division of Licensure and Certification, 201 Monroe Street, Suite 600, Montgomery, AL 36130; tel. 334/206–5300; FAX. 334/206–5366; Rick Harris, Bureau Director

ALASKA
Alaska Division of Public Health, Section of Certification and Licensing, 619 E. Ship Creek Ave, Suite 232, Anchorage, AK 99501; tel. 907/269–3640; FAX. 907/269–3640; Jane Urbansky, Certification & Licensing Section Chief

ARIZONA
Arizona Department of Health Services, Medical Facilities, 150 North 18th Ave., Suite 450, Phoenix, AZ 85007; tel. 602/364–3030; FAX. 602/364–4764; Mary Wiley, Assistant Director

ARKANSAS
Department of Health, Health Facility Services, 5800 West 10th, Suite 400, Little Rock, AR 72204-9916; tel. 501/661–2201; FAX. 501/661–2165; Connie Melton, Section Chief

CALIFORNIA
California Department of Public Health, Center for Healthcare Quality, 1615 Capital Avenue, MS 0512, P.O. Box 997377, Sacramento, CA 95899-7377; tel. 916/324–6630; FAX. 916/552–8988; Kathleen J. Billingsley, R.N., Deputy Director

COLORADO
Colorado Department of Public Health and Environment, Health Facilities Division - Hospices, 4300 Cherry Creek Drive South, Denver, CO 80246-1530; tel. 303/692–2800; FAX. 303/753–6214; James B. Martin, Executive Director

CONNECTICUT
Department of Public Health, Health Care Systems Branch, 410 Capital Avenue, MS 12HCS, P.O. Box 340308, Hartford, CT 06134-0308; tel. 860/509–7400; FAX. 860/509–7538; Wendy Furniss, RNC, MS, Branch Chief

DELAWARE
Department of Health and Social Services, Office of Health Facilities Licensing and Certification, 2055 Limestone Road, Suite 200, Wilmington, DE 19808; tel. 302/995–8521; FAX. 302/995–8529; Roseann Sapp, Office Manager

DISTRICT OF COLUMBIA
District of Columbia Department of Health, Health Regulation Licensing Administration, 717 14th Street, NW, Suite 600, Washington, DC 20005; tel. 202/422–5888; FAX. 202/442–9430; Patrice Van Buran, Administrator

FLORIDA
Florida Agency for Health Care Administration, Division of Health Quality Assurance, Bureau of Health Facility Regulation, Home Care Unit - Mail Stop # 34, 2727 Mahan Drive, Tallahassee, FL 32308-5407; tel. 850/414–6010; FAX. 850/922–9374; Anne Menard, Unit Manager

GEORGIA
Health Care Section - Georgia Dept. of Human Resources, Office of Regulatory Services, Two Peachtree Street, N.W., Atlanta, GA 30303-3142; tel. 404/657–5700; FAX. 404/657–5708; Sharon Dougherty, Director

HAWAII
Department of Health, Licensing and Certification, Office Health Care Assurance, P.O. Box 3378, Honolulu, HI 96801; tel. 808/586–4080; FAX. 808/586–4090

IDAHO
Bureau of Facility Standards, Department of Health and Welfare, P.O. Box 83720, Boise, ID 83720-0036; tel. 208/334–6626; FAX. 208/364–1888; Sylvia Cresell or Nicole Winsenor, Co-Supervisors - Non Long Term Care

ILLINOIS
Illinois Department of Public Health, Office of Health Care Regulation, Bureau of Hospitals and Ambulatory Services, 525 West Jefferson Street, 4th Floor, Springfield, IL 62761-0001; tel. 217/782–7412; FAX. 217/782–0382; William A. Bell, Acting Deputy Director

INDIANA
Indiana State Department of Health, Division of Acute Care, Two North Meridian Street, Indianapolis, IN 46204; tel. 317/233–7474; FAX. 317/233–7157; Mary Azbill, Director

IOWA
Iowa Department of Inspections and Appeals, Health Facilities Division, Lucas State Office Building, 321 East 12th Street, Des Moines, IA 50319-0083; tel. 515/281–7102; FAX. 515/242–6863; Dean Lerner, Director

KANSAS
Department of Health and Environment, Bureau of Child Care and Health Facilities, 1000 Southwest Jackson, Suite 200, Topeka, KS 66612-1365; tel. 785/296–1240; FAX. 785/291–3419; Charles Moore, Director of Medical Facilities

KENTUCKY
Cabinet for Health and Family Services, Division of Health Care Facilities and Services, 275 East Main Street, Fifth Floor East, Frankfort, KY 40621; tel. 502/564–7963; FAX. 502/564–6546; Robert Hester, Acting Director

LOUISIANA
Department of Health and Hospitals, Bureau of Health Services, Health Standards Section Licensing Unit, 500 Laurel Street, Suite 100, P.O. Box 3767, Baton Rouge, LA 70821; tel. 225/342–0138; FAX. 225/342–5292; Erin Rabalais, RN Manager

MAINE
Division of Licensing and Regulatory Services, Department of Human Services, State House, Station 11, Augusta, ME 04333; tel. 207/287–9300; FAX. 207/287–9304; Anne Flanagan, Assistant Director

MARYLAND
Maryland Department of Health and Mental Hygiene, Mental Hygiene Administration, Spring Grove Hospital Center, 55 Wade Avenue, Cantonville, MD 21228; tel. 410/402–8452; FAX. 410/402–8301; Brian Hepburn, M.D., Executive Director

MASSACHUSETTS
Massachusetts Department of Public Health, Division of Health Care Quality, 99 Chauncy St., 2nd Floor, Boston, MA 02111-1703; tel. 617/753–8000; FAX. 617/753–8095; Paul I. Dreyer, Ph.D. Director

MICHIGAN
Michigan Department of Community Health, Division of Licensing and Certification, P.O. Box 30664, Lansing, MI 48909; tel. 517/241–3829; FAX. 517/241–3354; Kenneth T. Longton, Director

MINNESOTA
Department of Health, Division of Compliance Monitoring, Licensing and Certification Program, 85 East Seventh Place, Suite 220, St. Paul, MN 55164-0900; tel. 651/201–4101; FAX. 651/215–9697; Linda Tallaksen, Supervisor, Program Assurance Unit

MISSISSIPPI
Mississippi State Department of Health, Bureau of Health Facilities, Licensure and Certification, P.O. Box 1700, Jackson, MS 39215; tel. 601/364–1100; FAX. 601/364–5054; Marilynn Windborne, Director

MISSOURI
Bureau of Home Care and Rehabilitative Standards, Missouri Department of Health of Senior Services, P.O. Box 570, Jefferson City, MO 65102-6336; tel. 573/751–6336; FAX. 573/751–6315; Lisa Coots, RN, Administrator

NEBRASKA
Nebraska Department of Health and Human Services Regulation and Licensure, Licensing & Regulatory Affairs, 301 Centennial Mall, South, 3rd Floor., P.O. Box 94986, Lincoln, NE 68509-4986; tel. 402/471–3651; FAX. 402/471–0555; Marcia Cederdahl, RN, Section Administrator

NEVADA
Nevada State Health Division, Bureau of Licensure and Certification, 1550 East College Parkway, Suite 158, Carson City, NV 89706-7921; tel. 775/687–4475; FAX. 775/687–6588; Lisa Jones, Chief

NEW HAMPSHIRE
NH DHHS Office of Program Support, Bureau of Health Facilities Administration, 129 Pleasant Street, Concord, NH 03301-3857; tel. 603/271–4592; FAX. 603/271–4968; Nicholas A. Toumpas, Commissioner

NEW JERSEY
New Jersey Department of Health and Senior Services, Division, Certificate of Need and Acute Care Licensure, P.O. Box 358, Trenton, NJ 08625; tel. 609/292–8773; FAX. 609/292–3780; John A. Calabria, Director

NEW MEXICO
Department of Health, Division of Health Improvement, Health Facility Licensing and Certification, 2040 S. Pacheco St., Santa Fe, NM 87505; tel. 505/476–9007; FAX. 505/476–9075; Sandra Cole, Bureau Chief

NEW YORK
New York State Department of Health, Office of Health Care Quality & Safety, Corning Tower, Empire State Plaza, Albany, NY 12237; tel. 518/402–5733; Anna D. Colello, Director, Regulatory Compliance

NORTH CAROLINA
Department of Human Resources, Division of Health Service Regulation, 1205 Umstead Drive, Raleigh, NC 27603; tel. 919/855–4620; FAX. 919/715–3073; Azzie Y. Conley, Chief, Acute & Home Care Licensure and Certification

NORTH DAKOTA
North Dakota Department of Health, Health Resources Section, 600 East Boulevard Avenue, Department 301, Bismarck, ND 58505-0200; tel. 701/328–2352; FAX. 701/328–1890; Darleen Bartz, Chief- Health Resources Section

OHIO
Division of Quality Assurance, Ohio Department of Health, 246 North High Street, Columbus, OH 43266-0588; tel. 614/466–7857; FAX. 614/644–0208; Rebecca Maust, Chief, Division of Quality Assurance

OKLAHOMA
Oklahoma State Department of Health, Protective Health Services, Medical Facilities Service, 1000 Northeast 10th Street, Oklahoma City, OK 73117-1299; tel. 405/271–6576; FAX. 405/271–1308; Tom Welin, Chief, Medical Facilities

OREGON
Health Care Licensing and Certification, Department of Human Services, 800 Northeast Oregon Street, Suite 305, Portland, OR 97232; tel. 971/673–0546; FAX. 971/673–0556; Ron Prinslow, Manager

PENNSYLVANIA
Department of Health, Division of Home Health, 132 Kline Plaza, Suite A, Harrisburg, PA 17104; tel. 717/783–1379; FAX. 717/772–0232; Cindy Boyne, Director

RHODE ISLAND
Rhode Island Department of Health, Division of Facilities Regulation, 3 Capitol Hill, Room 306, Providence, RI 02908-5097; tel. 401/222–2566; FAX. 401/222–6542; Chief of Facilities Regulation

SOUTH CAROLINA
Department of Health and Environmental Control, Division of Health Insurance Benefit, 2600 Bull Street, Columbia, SC 29201; tel. 803/545–4293; FAX. 803/545–4292; Mary Jo Roue, Division Director

SOUTH DAKOTA
Department of Health, Office of Licensure and Certification, 615 East 4th Street, Pierre, SD 57501-1700; tel. 605/773–3356; FAX. 605/773–6667; Bob Stahl, Program Administrator

TENNESSEE
Department of Health, Division of Health Care Facilities, 227 French Landing Suite 501, Heritage Place Metro Center, Nashville, TN 37243; tel. 615/741–7300; FAX. 615/741–7051; Shirley Jones, ASA III

TEXAS
Texas Department of State Health Services, Facility Licensing Group (MC 2835), PO Box 149347, Austin, TX 78714-9347; tel. 512/458–7375; FAX. 512/458–7477; David L. Lakey, M.D., Commissioner

UTAH
Utah Department of Health, Bureau of Health Facility Licensure, P.O. Box 144103, Salt Lake City, UT 84114-4103; tel. 801/538–6158; FAX. 801/538–6163; Allan Elkins, Director

VERMONT
Hospice and Palliative Care, Council of Vermont, 10 Maine Street, Montpelier, VT 05602; tel. 802/229–0579; FAX. 802/223–6218; Virginia L. Fry, Executive Director

VIRGINIA
Virginia Department of Health, Office of Licensure & Certification, 9960 Maryland Drive, Suite 401, Richmond, VA 23233; tel. 804/367–2102; FAX. 804/257–4502; Christopher Durrer, Director

WASHINGTON
Washington State Department of Health, Facilities and Services Licensing, PO Box 47990, Olympia, WA 98504-7852; tel. 360/236–4106; FAX. 360/236–4088; Craig McLaughlin, M.J., Executive Director

WEST VIRGINIA
Office of Health Facility Licensure and Certification, West Virginia Department of Health, 1 Davis Square, Suite 101, Charleston, WV 25301-1799; tel. 304/558–0585; FAX. 304/558–5607; John M. Wilkinson, Director

WISCONSIN
Division of Quality Assurance, Division of Supportive Living, P.O. Box 2969, Madison, WI 53701-2969; tel. 608/267–7185; FAX. 608/267–0352; Otis Woods, Administrator

WYOMING
Wyoming Department of Health, Community and Public Health Division, 6101 Yellowstone Road, Suite 420, Room #33, Cheyenne, WY 82002; tel. 307/777–6004; FAX. 307/777–3617; Molly M. Bruner, MSN, RNC, Administrator

U.S. Associated Areas

PUERTO RICO
Puerto Rico Department of Health, Building A - Medical Center, Call Box 70184, San Juan, PR 00936–0184; tel. 787/274–6822; FAX. 787/767–8341; Rosa Perez-Perdomo, MD, MPH, PhD, Secretary of Health

Joint Commission Accredited Freestanding Long–Term Care Organizations

The accredited freestanding long–term care organizations listed have been accredited as of April, 2008 by the Joint Commission on Accreditation of Healthcare Organizations by decision of the Accreditation Committee of the Board of Commissioners.

The organizations listed here have been found to be in compliance with the Joint Commission standards for long–term care organizations, as found in the Comprehensive Accreditation Manual for the Long–Term Care Organizations.

Please refer to section A of the AHA Guide for information on hospitals with Long–Term Care services. These hospitals are identified by Facility Code 117. In section A, those hospitals identified by Approval Code 1 are Joint Commission accredited.

We present this list simply as a convenient directory. Inclusion or omission of any organization's name indicates neither approval nor disapproval by Health Forum LLC, an American Hospital Association company.

United States

ALABAMA

Central Alabama Veterans Health Care System, 215 Perry Hill Road, Montgomery, AL 36109; tel. 334/272–4670; FAX. 334/260–4143; Dr. Robert W Ratliff

East Alabama Medical Center, 2000 Pepperell Parkway, Opelika, AL 36801-5422; tel. 334/749–3411; FAX. 334/528–3280; Mr. Terry Andrus

Fayette Medical Center, P.O. Drawer 710, Fayette, AL 35555; tel. 205/932–5966; FAX. 205/932–1260; Mr. Barry S. Cochran

Marion Regional Medical Center, Inc., 1256 Military Street South, Hamilton, AL 35570; tel. 205/921–6200; FAX. 205/921–6210; Mr. Donald Jones

Mercy Medical, A Corporation, PO Box 1090, Daphne, AL 36526-1090; tel. 334/626–2694; FAX. 334/626–0315; Ms. Mary Kay Polys

Mercy Medical-Mobile, 3712 Dauphin Street, Mobile, AL 36608; tel. 215/621–4452; FAX. 215/621–4499; Ms. Mary Kay Polys

Tuscaloosa VA Medical Center, 3701 Loop Road East, Tuscaloosa, AL 35404; tel. 205/554–2000; FAX. 205/554–2034

ALASKA

Fairbanks Memorial Hospital /Denali Center, 1650 Cowles Street, Fairbanks, AK 99701-5998; tel. 907/458–5300; FAX. 907/458–5324; Mr. Michael K. Powers

Ketchikan General Hospital, 3100 Tongass Avenue, Ketchikan, AK 99901; tel. 907/225–5171; FAX. 907/228–8322; Mr. Patrick Branco

Norton Sound Regional Hospital, PO Box 966, Nome, AK 99762; tel. 907/443–3311; FAX. 907/443–4538; Mr. Trevor Colby

ARIZONA

Carl T. Hayden VA Medical Center, 650 East Indian School Road, Phoenix, AZ 85012-1892; tel. 602/277–5551; FAX. 602/222–6488; Mr. Donald F. Moore

Citadel Care Center, 5121 East Broadway Road, Mesa, AZ 85206; tel. 480/832–5555; FAX. 480/924–0090; Ms. Molly Bischoff

Desert Cove Nursing Center, 1750 West Frye Road, Chandler, AZ 85224; tel. 480/899–0641; FAX. 480/899–1785

Glendale Care Center, 4704 West Diana Avenue, Glendale, AZ 85302; tel. 623/247–3949; FAX. 623/930–1104; Ms. Debra Kiesner

Heritage Health Care Center, 1300 South Street, Globe, AZ 85501; tel. 928/425–3118; FAX. 928/425–0707; Mr. Greg George LeCheminant

La Canada Care Center, 7970 North LaCanada Dr., Tucson, AZ 85704; tel. 520/797–1191; FAX. 520/742–3437

Las Fuentes Care Center, 1045 Scott Drive, Prescott, AZ 86301; tel. 928/778–9603; FAX. 928/778–5909

Life Care Center at South Mountain, 8008 South Jesse Owens Parkway, Phoenix, AZ 85040; tel. 602/243–2780; FAX. 602/243–7079; Mr. Dennis Graf

Life Care Center of North Glendale, 13620 North 55th Avenue, Glendale, AZ 85304; tel. 602/843–8433; FAX. 602/588–1056; Mr. Gary Davis

Life Care Center of Paradise Valley, 4065 East Bell Road, Phoenix, AZ 85032; tel. 602/867–0212; FAX. 602/867–0321; Ms. Sadie Speer

Life Care Center of Scottsdale, 9494 East Becker Lane, Scottsdale, AZ 85260; tel. 480/860–6396; FAX. 480/391–9699

Life Care Center of Sierra Vista, 2305 East Wilcox Drive, Sierra Vista, AZ 85635; tel. 520/458–1050; FAX. 520/458–6944; Mr. Matthew D Ham

Life Care Center of Tucson, 6211 North LaCholla Boulevard, Tucson, AZ 85741; tel. 520/575–0900; FAX. 520/575–0483; Mrs. Ellen K. Cote

Life Care Center of Yuma, 2450 South 19th Avenue, Yuma, AZ 85364; tel. 928/344–0425; FAX. 928/344–3015

Mi Casa Nursing Center, 330 S. Pinnule Circle, Mesa, AZ 85206; tel. 480/981–0687; FAX. 480/396–5011; Mr. Robert Tunila

Mountain View Care Center, 1313 West Magee Road, Tucson, AZ 85704; tel. 520/797–2600; FAX. 520/797–3100; Mrs. Maria Jesus Montion

Northern Arizona VA Health Care System, 500 Highway 89 North, Prescott, AZ 86313; tel. 928/445–4860; FAX. 928/776–6098; Ms. Susan A. Angell

Payson Care Center, 107 East Lone Pine Drive, Payson, AZ 85541; tel. 928/474–6896; FAX. 928/474–6997; Mr. Brian Hackerott

Scottsdale Heritage Court, 3339 N. Drinkwater Blvd, Scottsdale, AZ 85251; tel. 480/949–5400; FAX. 480/949–9467; Ms. Lisa Maria Harrison

Southern Arizona VA Health Care System, 3601 South Sixth Avenue, Tucson, AZ 85723; tel. 520/629–1821; FAX. 520/629–1820; Mr. Jonathan H. Gardner

Sun Grove Village Care Center, 20625 N. Lake Pleasant Road, Peoria, AZ 85382; tel. 623/566–0642; FAX. 623/566–1512; Mr. Adam Utan

ARKANSAS

Baptist Health Medical Center - Little Rock, 9601 Interstate 630, Exit 7, Little Rock, AR 72205-7299; tel. 501/202–2000; FAX. 501/202–1434; Mr. Doug Weeks

Central Arkansas Veterans Healthcare System, 4300 West Seventh Street (00/LR), Little Rock, AR 72205; tel. 501/257–5314; FAX. 501/257–5305; Mr. Michael R. Winn

CALIFORNIA

Alta Los Angeles Hospitals, Inc., 4081 East Olympic Boulevard, Los Angeles, CA 90023; tel. 323/881–2600; FAX. 323/261–0809; Mr. Al Souza

Anaheim General Hospital, 3350 West Ball Road, Anaheim, CA 92804; tel. 714/220–4500; FAX. 714/821–6537; Dr. Josh D Luke

Bel Tooren Villa Convalescent Hospital, 16910 Woodruff Avenue, Bellflower, CA 90706; tel. 562/867–1761; FAX. 562/867–1571; Mr. Ed Cayetano

California Special Care Center, Inc., 8787 Center Drive, La Mesa, CA 91942; tel. 619/460–4444; FAX. 619/460–6341; Mr. John Jimenez

CareMeridian - Oxnard, 18-A Journey, Suite 200, Aliso Viejo, CA 92656; tel. 949/263–6630; FAX. 949/261–0457; Ms. Sherri L Medina

CareMeridian - Artesia, 18-A Journey, Suite 200, Aliso Viejo, CA 92656; tel. 949/263–6630; FAX. 949/261–0457; Ms. Sherri L Medina

CareMeridian - Cowan Heights, 18-A Journey, Suite 200, Aliso Viejo, CA 92656; tel. 949/263–6630; FAX. 949/261–0457; Ms. Sherri L Medina

CareMeridian - Elk Grove, 18-A Journey, Suite 200, Aliso Viejo, CA 92656-3317; tel. 949/263–6630; FAX. 949/261–0457; Ms. Sherri L Medina

CareMeridian - Fairfax, 18-A Journey, Suite 200, Aliso Viejo, CA 92656; tel. 949/263–6630; FAX. 949/261–0457; Ms. Sherri L Medina

CareMeridian - Fresno County - Fresno, 18-A Journey, Suite 200, Aliso Viejo, CA 92656; tel. 949/263–6630; FAX. 949/261–0457; Mr. Jim Ashby

CareMeridian - La Habra Heights, 18-A Journey, Suite 200, Aliso Viejo, CA 92656-3317; tel. 949/263–6630; FAX. 949/261–0457; Ms. Sherri L Medina

CareMeridian - San Martin, 18-A Journey, Suite 200, Aliso Viejo, CA 92656; tel. 949/263–6630; FAX. 949/261–0457; Ms. Sherri L Medina

CareMeridian -Escondido, 18-A Journey, Suite 200, Aliso Viejo, CA 92656-3317; tel. 949/263–6630; FAX. 949/261–0457; Ms. Sherri L Medina

CareMeridian-Las Vegas, 18-A Journey, Suite 200, Aliso Viejo, CA 92656; tel. 949/263–6630; FAX. 949/261–0457; Mr. Jim Ashby

CareMeridian-Santiago Canyon, 18-A Journey, Suite 200, Aliso Viejo, CA 92656; tel. 949/263–6630; FAX. 949/261–0457; Ms. Sherri L Medina

CHW Dominican Hospital, 1555 Soquel Drive, Santa Cruz, CA 95065; tel. 831/462–7700; FAX. 831/462–7555; Dr. Nanette Mickiewicz

Coastal Communities Hospital, 2701 South Bristol Street, Santa Ana, CA 92704; tel. 714/754–5454; FAX. 714/754–5556; Mr. Craig Myers

Community Hospital of the Monterey Peninsula, PO Box HH, Monterey, CA 93942; tel. 831/625–4553; FAX. 831/625–4877; Dr. Steven J Packer

East Los Angeles Doctors Hospital, 4060 East Whittier Boulevard, Los Angeles, CA 90023; tel. 323/268–5514; FAX. 323/260–4274; Mrs. Araceli Lonergan

El Camino Hospital, 2500 Grant Road, Mountain View, CA 94040; tel. 650/940–7000; FAX. 650/988–7862; Mr. Kenneth Graham

Encino-Tarzana Regional Medical Center, 18321 Clark Street, Tarzana, CA 91356-3501; tel. 818/708–5254; FAX. 818/708–5382; Mr. Dale Surowitz

Fallbrook Hospital Corporation, 624 East Elder Street, Fallbrook, CA 92028-3099; tel. 760/728–1191; FAX. 760/723–0863; Mr. Larry W. Payton

Fresno Community Hospital & Medical Center, PO Box 1232, Fresno, CA 93715-1232; tel. 559/459–6000; FAX. 559/459–2798; Mr. Jack Chubb

Goleta Valley Cottage Hospital, PO Box 6306, Santa Barbara, CA 93160-6306; tel. 805/967–3411; FAX. 805/681–6437; Mr. Steven Fellows

Hazel Hawkins Memorial Hospital, 911 Sunset Drive, Hollister, CA 95023; tel. 831/637–5711; FAX. 831/636–2668; Mr. Ken S Underwood

Hemet Valley Medical Center, 1117 East Devonshire Avenue, Hemet, CA 92543; tel. 951/652–2811; FAX. 951/765–4711; Mrs. Annette Greenwood

Hemet Valley Medical Center, 1117 East Devonshire Avenue, Hemet, CA 92543; tel. 951/652–2811; FAX. 951/765–4711; Mrs. Annette Greenwood

Hi Desert Medical Center, 6601 White Feather Road, Joshua Tree, CA 92252; tel. 760/366–6260; FAX. 760/366–6251; Mr. Micheal Barry

Hollenbeck Palms, 573 South Boyle Avenue, Los Angeles, CA 90033; tel. 323/263–6195; FAX. 323/268–8610; Mr. Morris Shockley

Hollywood Presbyterian Medical Center, 1300 North Vermont Avenue, Los Angeles, CA 90027; tel. 323/413–3000; FAX. 323/660–0446; Mr. Jeff Nelson

Imperial Convalescent Center, 11926 La Mirada Boulevard, La Mirada, CA 90638; tel. 562/943–7156; FAX. 562/947–6084; Mr. Rob Takami

Kaiser Foundation Hospital - Manteca, 1777 West Yosemite Avenue, Manteca, CA 95337; tel. 209/825–3700; FAX. 209/825–3524; Mr. Corwin N Harper

La Habra Convalescent Hospital, 1233 West La Habra Boulevard, La Habra, CA 90631; tel. 562/691–0781; FAX. 562/694–2279; Mr. Daniel Husband

Lake Forest Nursing Center, 25652 Old Trabuco Road, Lake Forest, CA 92630; tel. 949/380–9380; FAX. 949/380–1499

Life Care Center Corona, 2600 South Main Street, Corona, CA 92882; tel. 951/736–4700; FAX. 951/736–4999; Ms. Sharron Clark

Life Care Center of Escondido, 1980 Felicita Road, Escondido, CA 92025; tel. 760/741–6109; FAX. 760/741–5237

Life Care Center of Vista, 304 North Melrose Drive, Vista, CA 92083; tel. 760/724–8222; FAX. 760/724–8038; Mr. Robert Lorenzo

Lompoc Valley Medical Center, 508 East Hickory Avenue, Lompoc, CA 93436; tel. 805/737–3301; FAX. 805/737–3326; Mr. James J. Raggio

Los Robles Hospital and Medical Center, 215 West Janss Road, Thousand Oaks, CA 91360; tel. 805/370–4421; FAX. 805/370–4666; Mr. Jim Sherman

Magnolia Special Care Center, 635 South Magnolia, El Cajon, CA 92020; tel. 619/442–8826; FAX. 619/442–0288

Marian Medical Center, 1400 East Church Street, Santa Maria, CA 93454; tel. 805/739–3000; FAX. 805/739–3060; Mr. Charles J. Cova

Mercy General Hospital, 4001 J Street, Sacramento, CA 95819; tel. 916/453–4545; FAX. 916/453–4587; Mr. Denny Powell

Mercy Medical Center Mt. Shasta, 914 Pine Street, Mount Shasta, CA 96067; tel. 530/926–6111; FAX. 530/926–0517; Mr. Chuck Gersdorf

Methodist Hospital of Sacramento, 7500 Hospital Drive, Sacramento, CA 95823; tel. 916/423–3000; FAX. 916/689–2959; Mr. Tim Moran

Metropolitan State Hospital, 11401 South Bloomfield Avenue, Norwalk, CA 90650; tel. 562/863–7011; FAX. 562/651–4546; Ms. Sharon Smith Nevins

Mills-Peninsula Health Services, 1783 El Camino Real, Burlingame, CA 94010; tel. 650/696–5270; FAX. 650/696–5279; Mr. Robert W Merwin

Mirada Hills Rehabilitation and Convalescent Hospital, 12200 La Mirada Boulevard, La Mirada, CA 90638; tel. 562/947–8691; FAX. 562/943–1073

Motion Picture and Television Fund Hospital, 23388 Mulholland Drive, Woodland Hills, CA 91364; tel. 818/876–1888; FAX. 818/225–1359; Dr. David Tillman

North Walk Villa Convalescent Hospital, 12350 Rosecrans Avenue, Norwalk, CA 90650; tel. 562/921–6624; FAX. 562/404–8778; Mr. Michael Kremer

Oak Valley District Hospital, 350 South Oak Avenue, Oakdale, CA 95361; tel. 209/847–3011; FAX. 209/848–4122; Mr. John Friel

Orangegrove Rehabilitation Hospital, 12332 Garden Grove Boulevard, Garden Grove, CA 92843; tel. 714/534–1041; FAX. 714/534–7921; Mrs. Nelia de la Merced Yonzon

Pacifica Nursing and Rehabilitation Center, 385 Esplanade Avenue, Pacifica, CA 94044; tel. 650/993–5576; FAX. 650/359–0405; Mr. Brian Ramos

Palomar Medical Center, 555 East Valley Parkway, Escondido, CA 92025; tel. 760/739–3104; FAX. 760/739–3107; Mr. Gerald Bracht

Pomerado Hospital, 15615 Pomerado Road, Poway, CA 92064; tel. 858/613–4710; FAX. 858/613–4764; Mr. Steve Gold

Rady Children's Hospital San Diego, 3020 Children's Way, MC 5069, San Diego, CA 92123-4282; tel. 858/576–1700; FAX. 858/966–8538; Ms. Kathleen Sellick

Reche Canyon Rehabilitation and Health Care Center, 1350 Reche Canyon Road, Colton, CA 92324; tel. 909/370–4411; FAX. 909/370–1846; Mr. Fred Frank

Rimrock Villa Convalescent Hospital, 27555 Rimrock Road, Barstow, CA 92311; tel. 760/252–2515; FAX. 760/252–1572; Ms. Mary Lou Miller

Saint Francis Memorial Hospital, 900 Hyde Street, San Francisco, CA 94109; tel. 415/353–6000; FAX. 415/353–6177; Mr. Thomas Hennessy

San Francisco General Hospital Medical Center, 1001 Potrero Avenue, San Francisco, CA 94110; tel. 415/206–4294; FAX. 415/206–3747; Ms. Gene Marie O'Connell

San Francisco VA Medical Center, 4150 Clement Street, San Francisco, CA 94121; tel. 415/750–2014; FAX. 415/750–2185; Ms. Sheila M Cullen

San Gabriel Valley Medical Center, 438 West Las Tunas Drive, San Gabriel, CA 91776; tel. 626/289–5454; FAX. 626/570–6555; Mr. Makoto Nakayama

Seton Medical Center, 1900 Sullivan Avenue, Daly City, CA 94015; tel. 650/992–4000; FAX. 650/991–6024; Ms. Bernadette Smith

Sharp Chula Vista Medical Center, 751 Medical Center Court, Chula Vista, CA 91911-6699; tel. 619/482–3664; FAX. 619/482–3535; Mr. Chris Boyd

Sharp Coronado Hospital, 250 Prospect Place, Coronado, CA 92118; tel. 619/522–3700; FAX. 619/522–3777; Ms. Marcia K. Hall

Sharp Grossmont Hospital, 5555 Grossmont Center Drive, La Mesa, CA 91942; tel. 619/740–4179; FAX. 619/461–7191; Ms. Michele Tarbet

Sharp Memorial Hospital, 7901 Frost Street, San Diego, CA 92123; tel. 858/939–3400; FAX. 858/939–3514; Mr. Tim Smith

South Coast Medical Center, 31872 Coast Highway, Laguna Beach, CA 92651; tel. 949/499–1311; FAX. 949/499–5789; Mr. Bruce Christian

St. John's Pleasant Valley Hospital, 1600 N. Rose Ave, Oxnard, CA 93030; tel. 805/988–2750; FAX. 805/981–4466; Mr. Jerry Conway

St. Joseph's Medical Center of Stockton, 1800 North California Street, Stockton, CA 95204; tel. 209/467–6512; FAX. 209/461–3299; Mr. Donald J Wiley

St. Jude Medical Center, 101 East Valencia Mesa Drive, Fullerton, CA 92835; tel. 714/992–3000; FAX. 714/447–6565; Mr. Robert J Fraschetti

St. Mary's Medical Center, 450 Stanyan Street, San Francisco, CA 94117; tel. 415/668–1000; FAX. 415/668–4531; Mr. Ken Steele

St. Mary's Medical Center, 450 Stanyan Street, San Francisco, CA 94117; tel. 415/668–1000; FAX. 415/668–4531; Mr. Ken Steele

Sun City Convalescent Center, 27600 Encanto Drive, Sun City, CA 92586; tel. 951/679–6858; FAX. 951/679–0399; Mr. Rodger Groves

The Cloisters of La Jolla, 7160 Fay Avenue, La Jolla, CA 92037; tel. 858/459–4361; FAX. 858/459–1386; Ms. Cheryl Thompson

The Cloisters of Mission Hills, 3680 Reynard Way, San Diego, CA 92103; tel. 619/297–4484; FAX. 619/297–4490; Ms. Katherine Oh

Totally Kids Specialty Healthcare, 1720 Mountain View Avenue, Loma Linda, CA 92354; tel. 909/796–6915; FAX. 909/799–6205; Mr. Doug Padgett

VA Central California Health Care System, 2615 East Clinton Avenue, Fresno, CA 93703; tel. 559/225–6100; FAX. 559/228–6903; Mr. Alan S Perry

VA Greater Los Angeles Healthcare System, 11301 Wilshire Boulevard, Los Angeles, CA 90073; tel. 310/268–3132; FAX. 310/268–3494; Mr. Charles M Dorman

VA Loma Linda Healthcare System, 11201 Benton Street, Loma Linda, CA 92357; tel. 909/583–6002; FAX. 909/422–3107; Mr. Dean R Stordahl

VA Long Beach Health Care System, 5901 East Seventh Street, Long Beach, CA 90822; tel. 562/826–5400; FAX. 562/826–5906; Mr. Ronald Norby

VA Northern California Health Care System, 150 Muir Road, Martinez, CA 94553-4668; tel. 925/372–2010; FAX. 925/372–2020; Dr. Brian J O'Neill

VA Palo Alto Health Care System, 3801 Miranda Avenue, Palo Alto, CA 94304; tel. 650/493–5000; FAX. 650/849–0117; Ms. Elizabeth Joyce Freeman

VA San Diego Healthcare System, 3350 La Jolla Village Drive, San Diego, CA 92161; tel. 858/552–8585; FAX. 858/552–7509; Mr. Gary J. Rossio

Verdugo Hills Hospital, 1812 Verdugo Boulevard, Glendale, CA 91208; tel. 818/790–7100; FAX. 818/952–4616; Mr. Leonard LaBella

Whittier Hospital Medical Center, 9080 Colima Road, Whittier, CA 90605-1898; tel. 562/907–1540; FAX. 562/693–6811; Mr. Howard Ternes

COLORADO

Arkansas Valley Regional Medical Center, 1100 Carson Avenue, La Junta, CO 81050; tel. 719/383–6001; FAX. 719/383–6005; Mr. Lynn Crowell

Berkley Manor Care Center, 735 South Locust Street, Denver, CO 80224; tel. 303/320–4377; FAX. 303/355–6289; Ms. Dawn Brown

Briarwood Health Care Center, 1440 Vine St., Denver, CO 80206; tel. 303/399–0350; FAX. 303/399–4276; Mr. Gary Kotz

Canon Lodge Care Center, 905 Harding Avenue, Canon City, CO 81212; tel. 719/275–4106; FAX. 719/275–2895; Ms. Ann Maloney

Columbine Manor Care Center, 530 W 16th st., Salida, CO 81201; tel. 719/539–6112; FAX. 719/539–6510; Ms. Lisa A Forsyth

Evergreen Nursing Home, 1991 Carroll Avenue, Alamosa, CO 81101; tel. 719/589–4951; FAX. 719/589–5651; Mrs. Barbara Fransen

Exempla Lutheran Medical Center, 8300 West 38th Avenue, Wheat Ridge, CO 80033; tel. 303/425–2979; FAX. 303/425–8537; Mr. Robert H. Malte

Garden Terrace Alzheimer's Center of Excellence, 1600 South Potomac Street, Aurora, CO 80012; tel. 303/750–8418; FAX. 303/750–0021

Grand Junction Veterans Affairs Medical Center, 2121 North Avenue, Grand Junction, CO 81501; tel. 970/242–0731; FAX. 970/244–1303; Dr. Michael Murphy

Hallmark Nursing Center, 3701 West Radcliff Avenue, Denver, CO 80236; tel. 303/794–6484; FAX. 303/797–8781; Ms. Anne Deines

Heritage Park Care Center, 1200 Village Road, Carbondale, CO 81623; tel. 970/963–1500; FAX. 970/963–3703; Mr. Patrick Raab

Life Care Center of Aurora, 14101 East Evans Avenue, Aurora, CO 80014; tel. 303/751–2000; FAX. 303/751–0026; Ms. Angie Herrera

Life Care Center of Colorado Springs, 2490 International Circle, Colorado Springs, CO 80910; tel. 719/630–8888; FAX. 719/634–3908; Ms. Debra Welker

Life Care Center of Evergreen, 2987 Bergen Peak Drive, Evergreen, CO 80439; tel. 303/674–4500; FAX. 303/674–8436; Mr. Treg Warnsholz

Life Care Center of Greeley, 4800 25th Street, Greeley, CO 80634; tel. 970/330–6400; FAX. 970/506–1370

Life Care Center of Littleton, 1500 W. Mineral Avenue, Littleton, CO 80120; tel. 303/795–7300; FAX. 303/795–6210; Mrs. Erin E. Cook

Life Care Center of Longmont, 2451 Pratt Street, Longmont, CO 80501; tel. 303/776–5000; FAX. 303/776–7661; Mr. Stephen DeBelle

Life Care Center of Pueblo, 2118 Chatalet Lane, Pueblo, CO 81005; tel. 719/564–2000; FAX. 719/564–7741; Mr. Stanley J Murdoch

Life Care Center of Westminster, 7751 Zenobia Court, Westminster, CO 80030; tel. 303/412–9121; FAX. 303/412–9187; Ms. Aletha Shawver

San Luis Care Center, 240 Craft Drive, Alamosa, CO 81101; tel. 719/589–9081; FAX. 719/589–9083; Ms. Mikel Barr

University Park Care Center, 945 Desert Flower Boulevard, Pueblo, CO 81001; tel. 719/545–5321; FAX. 719/545–0096; Ms. Barbara Strombeck

VA Eastern Colorado Healthcare System, 1055 Clermont St, Denver, CO 80220; tel. 303/399–8020; FAX. 303/393–2861; Mrs. Lynette A. Roff

Valley View Villa, 815 Fremont Ave., Fort Morgan, CO 80701; tel. 970/867–8261; FAX. 970/867–2652

Villa Manor Care Center, 7950 W. Mississippi Ave., Lakewood, CO 80226; tel. 303/986–4511; FAX. 303/986–0828; Ms. Nancy Emerick

Western Hills Health Care Center, 1625 Carr Street, Lakewood, CO 80214; tel. 303/232–6881; FAX. 303/232–1927; Ms. DeAnn Cure

CONNECTICUT

Aaron Manor Nursing & Rehabilitation Center, 3 South Wig Hill Road, Chester, CT 06412; tel. 860/526–5316; FAX. 860/526–2436; Dr. Robert Sbriglio

Ashlar of Newtown, 139 Toddy Hill Road, Newtown, CT 06470; tel. 203/426–5847; FAX. 203/364–3156; Mr. Thomas M. Gutner

Astoria Park, 725 Park Avenue, Bridgeport, CT 06604; tel. 203/366–3653; FAX. 203/333–6974; Mr. Donald L. Franco

Beechwood Rehabilitation and Nursing Center, 31 Vauxhall Street, New London, CT 06320; tel. 860/442–4363; FAX. 860/447–3749; Mr. William G. White
Bel-Air Manor Nursing and Rehabilitation Center, 256 New Britain Avenue, Newington, CT 06111; tel. 860/666–5689; FAX. 860/666–7046; Mr. Robert Sbriglio
Branford Hills Health Care Center, 189 Alps Road, Branford, CT 06405; tel. 203/481–6221; FAX. 203/483–1893; Mr. Stephen J. Shelton
Brittany Farms Health Center, 400 Brittany Farms Road, New Britain, CT 06053; tel. 860/224–3111; FAX. 860/229–0066; Mr. David Crandall
Brook Hollow Health Care Center, LLC, 55 Kondracki Lane, Wallingford, CT 06492; tel. 203/265–6771; FAX. 203/284–3883; Mr. Stuart Lindeman
Cedar Lane Rehabilitation and Health Care Center, 128 Cedar Avenue, Waterbury, CT 06705; tel. 203/757–9271; FAX. 203/757–2988; Ms. Christine Fitzgerald
Cheshire House Nursing and Rehabilitation Center, 3396 East Main Street, Waterbury, CT 06705; tel. 203/754–2161; FAX. 203/756–2293
Evergreen Health Care Center, PO Box 549, Stafford Springs, CT 06076; tel. 860/684–6341; FAX. 860/684–0881; Mr. Scott L. Ziskin
Filosa Convalescent Home, Inc., & Hancock Hall, 31 Staples Street, Danbury, CT 06811; tel. 203/794–9466; FAX. 203/791–2613; Dr. Frank D. Malone
Golden Hill Health Care Center, 2028 Bridgeport Avenue, Milford, CT 06460; tel. 203/877–0371; FAX. 203/882–8760; Ms. Mary J. Grabell
Greentree Manor Nursing and Rehabilitation Center, 4 Greentree Drive, Waterford, CT 06385; tel. 860/442–0647; FAX. 860/439–0821; Mr. Kenneth S. Kopchik
Hartford Hospital, 80 Seymour Street, Hartford, CT 06102-5037; tel. 860/545–2100; FAX. 860/545–3622; Mr. John Meehan
Hebrew Health Care, Inc., One Abrahms Boulevard, West Hartford, CT 06117-1525; tel. 860/523–3800; FAX. 860/523–3949; Ms. Bonnie B. Gauthier
Hilltop Health Center, 126 Ford Street, Ansonia, CT 06401; tel. 203/736–1100; FAX. 203/736–1101; Mr. Aldo Napoletano
Jerome Home, 975 Corbin Avenue, New Britain, CT 06052; tel. 860/229–3707; FAX. 860/229–4785; Ms. Lisa Connolly
Jewish Home for the Aged, Inc., 169 Davenport Avenue, New Haven, CT 06519; tel. 203/789–1650; FAX. 203/787–0071; Mrs. Beth Goldstein
Laurel Woods, Inc., 451 North High Street, East Haven, CT 06512; tel. 203/466–6850; FAX. 203/466–6852; Mr. Robert M. Mislow
Lord Chamberlain Nursing and Rehabilitation Center, 7003 Main Street, Stratford, CT 06614; tel. 203/375–5894; FAX. 203/375–1199; Mr. Martin Sbriglio
Mansfield Center for Nursing and Rehabilitation, 100 Warren Circle, Mansfield, CT 06268; tel. 860/487–2300; FAX. 860/487–0022; Mr. Alan Green
Masonic Healthcare Center, PO Box 70, Wallingford, CT 06492; tel. 203/679–5900; FAX. 203/679–6459; Mr. William Piper
Meriden Center, 845 Paddock Avenue, Meriden, CT 06450; tel. 203/238–2645; FAX. 203/238–7376; Ms. Linda P. Garcia
Meridian Manor Corporation, 1132 Meriden Road, Waterbury, CT 06705; tel. 203/757–1228; FAX. 203/757–4531; Ms. Sheila C. Smith
Montowese Health and Rehabilitation Center, Inc., 163 Quinnipiac Avenue, North Haven, CT 06473; tel. 203/624–3303; FAX. 203/787–9243; Mr. Farooq H. Khan
Mystic Manor Nursing & Rehabilitation Center, 475 High Street, Mystic, CT 06355-1707; tel. 860/536–6070; FAX. 860/536–9480; Mr. Kenneth Kopchik
Odd Fellows Home of Connecticut, 235 Lestertown Road, Groton, CT 06340; tel. 860/445–7478; FAX. 860/445–9575; Mr. James K. Malloy
Salmon Brook Center, 72 Salmon Brook Drive, Glastonbury, CT 06033; tel. 860/633–5244; FAX. 860/657–2360; Mr. Trevor Kinney
Seabury Retirement Community, 200 Seabury Drive, Bloomfield, CT 06002; tel. 860/286–0243; FAX. 860/242–4552; Mr. John S. Mobley
Sharon Health Care Center, PO Box 1268, Sharon, CT 06069; tel. 860/364–1002; FAX. 860/364–0237; Mr. Robert L. Clapp
Sister Anne Virginie Grimes Health Care, 1354 Chapel Street, New Haven, CT 06511; tel. 203/867–8300; FAX. 203/867–8370; Mr. John Tarutis
Skyview Center, 35 Marc Drive, Wallingford, CT 06492; tel. 203/265–0981; FAX. 203/284–1759; Mr. Jeffery E. Turner
Southington Care Center, 45 Meriden Avenue, Southington, CT 06489; tel. 860/621–9559; FAX. 860/628–9366; MP David M Santoro
Subacute Center of Bristol, 23 Fair Street, Forestville, CT 06010; tel. 860/589–2923; FAX. 860/589–3148; Mr. Stuart D. Lindeman
The Elim Park Baptist Home, Inc., 140 Cook Hill Road, Cheshire, CT 06410; tel. 203/272–3547; FAX. 203/250–6258; Mr. Ronald Dischinger
The Glendale Center, 4 Hazel Avenue, Naugatuck, CT 06770; tel. 203/723–1456; FAX. 203/723–0242; Mrs. Giovanna A. Griffin
VA Connecticut Healthcare System, 950 Campbell Avenue, West Haven, CT 06516; tel. 203/932–5711; FAX. 203/937–3823; Mr. Roger Johnson
Walnut Hill Care Center, 55 Grand Street, New Britain, CT 06052; tel. 860/223–3617; FAX. 860/229–1820; Mr. David Bond
Waveny Care Center, 3 Farm Road, New Canaan, CT 06840; tel. 203/594–5200; FAX. 203/594–5327; Ms. Heather Neff
Wolcott View Manor, Inc., PO Box 6192, Wolcott, CT 06716; tel. 203/879–8066; FAX. 203/879–8072; Mr. James E. Cleary
Woodlake at Tolland (ECHN Eldercare Services), 26 Shenipsit Lake Road, Tolland, CT 06084; tel. 860/872–2999; FAX. 860/872–1848; Mr. Peter Karl
Yale University Health Services, P.O. Box 208237, New Haven, CT 06520; tel. 203/432–4096; FAX. 203/432–8053; Dr. Paul Genecin

DELAWARE

Christiana Care - Wilmington Hospital, PO Box 1668, Wilmington, DE 19899; tel. 302/428–2570; FAX. 302/428–2540; Dr. Robert J Laskowski
VA Medical Center, 1601 Kirkwood Highway, Wilmington, DE 19805; tel. 302/994–2511; FAX. 202/633–5591; Mr. Charles M Dorman

DISTRICT OF COLUMBIA

Armed Forces Retirement Home-Washington, 3700 North Capitol Street, NW, Washington, DC 20011-8400; tel. 202/730–3323; FAX. 202/730–3407; Dr. Linda Rader
Providence Hospital, 1150 Varnum Street, Northeast, Washington, DC 20017; tel. 202/269–7000; FAX. 202/269–7892; Mr. Julius D. Spears
Specialty Hospital of Washing-Hadley, LLC, 4601 Martin Luther King Jr. Avenue, Southwest, Washington, DC 20032; tel. 202/574–5770; FAX. 202/373–5906; Mr. Irving B. Sawyers
The Washington Home and Community Hospices, 3720 Upton Street NW, Washington, DC 20016-2299; tel. 202/895–2600; FAX. 202/966–5241
VA Medical Center, 50 Irving Street, Northwest, Washington, DC 20422; tel. 202/745–8000; FAX. 202/745–8530; Mr. Fernando O. Rivera

FLORIDA

Baptist Hospital, Inc., PO Box 17500, Pensacola, FL 32522; tel. 850/469–2313; FAX. 850/469–2307; Mr. Mark Faulkner
Bay Pines VA Healthcare System, PO Box 5005, Bay Pines, FL 33744; tel. 727/398–6661; FAX. 727/398–9442; Mr. Wallace M. Hopkins
Bon Secours Maria Manor Nursing & Rehabilitation Center, 10300 4th Street North, Saint Petersburg, FL 33716; tel. 727/576–1025; FAX. 727/576–1447
Centre Pointe Health and Rehab, 2255 Centerville Road, Tallahassee, FL 32308; tel. 850/386–4054; FAX. 850/422–3206
Darcy Hall of Life Care, 2170 Palm Beach Lakes Blvd., West Palm Beach, FL 33409; tel. 561/683–3333; FAX. 561/683–1752; Mr. Kris Berntsen
Holy Cross Hospital Ministries, 4725 North Federal Highway, Fort Lauderdale, FL 33308; tel. 954/771–8000; FAX. 954/351–5947; Mr. John C. Johnson
Jackson Plaza Nursing and Rehabilitation Center, 1861 Northwest 8th Avenue, Miami, FL 33136; tel. 305/347–3380; FAX. 305/347–3388; Ms. Terry G. Escobar
James A. Haley Veterans' Hospital, 13000 Bruce B. Downs Boulevard, Tampa, FL 33612; tel. 813/972–2000; FAX. 813/979–3693; Mr. Stephen M. Lucas
Jupiter Medical Center, 1210 South Old Dixie Highway, Jupiter, FL 33458; tel. 561/747–2234; FAX. 561/745–5788; Mr. Paul Dell Uomo
Lakeside Health Center, 2501 Australian Avenue, West Palm Beach, FL 33407; tel. 561/655–7780; FAX. 561/655–9894
Life Care Center of Jacksonville, 4813 Lenoir Avenue, Jacksonville, FL 32216; tel. 904/332–4546; FAX. 904/332–4548; Ms. Patricia A. Hammond
Life Care Center at Inverrary, 4300 Rock Island Road, Lauderhill, FL 33319; tel. 954/485–6144; FAX. 954/485–6406; Mr. Kenneth Nichols
Life Care Center at Wells Crossing, 355 Crossing Boulevard, Orange Park, FL 32073; tel. 904/264–1950; FAX. 904/264–6574
Life Care Center of Altamonte Springs, 989 Orienta Avenue, Altamonte Springs, FL 32701; tel. 407/831–3446; FAX. 407/831–2820; Mr. Joseph Jicha
Life Care Center of Citrus County, 3325 Jerwayne Lane, Lecanto, FL 34461; tel. 352/746–4434; FAX. 352/746–7022; Mr. Lenny Ow
Life Care Center of Estero, 3850 Williams Road, Estero, FL 33928; tel. 239/495–4000; FAX. 239/495–1981; Mr. James Michael Breuler
Life Care Center of Hilliard, 3756 W. 3rd Street, Hilliard, FL 32046; tel. 904/845–3988; FAX. 904/845–7414; Mr. Tim Hall
Life Care Center of Melbourne, 606 East Sheridan Road, Melbourne, FL 32901; tel. 321/727–0984; FAX. 321/727–3606
Life Care Center of New Port Richey, 7400 Trouble Creek Rd., New Port Richey, FL 34653; tel. 727/375–2999; FAX. 727/569–1667; Ms. Kimberly Smith
Life Care Center of Ocala, 2800 Southwest 41st Street, Ocala, FL 34474; tel. 352/873–7570; FAX. 352/873–7112; Ms. Janice Cericola
Life Care Center of Orange Park, 2145 Kingsely Avenue, Orange Park, FL 32073; tel. 904/272–2424; FAX. 904/272–0013; Mr. John Driggers
Life Care Center of Orlando, 3211 Rouse Road, Orlando, FL 32817; tel. 407/281–1070; FAX. 407/281–1001; Mrs. Laura J Haraburda
Life Care Center of Palm Bay, 175 Villa Nueva Avenue, Palm Bay, FL 32907; tel. 321/952–1818; FAX. 321/952–1113; Ms. Nancy S. McGoldrick
Life Care Center of Port St. Lucie, 3720 SE Jennings Road, Port Saint Lucie, FL 34952; tel. 772/398–8080; FAX. 772/398–9365; Ms. Alison Graziani
Life Care Center of Punta Gorda, 450 Shreve Street, Punta Gorda, FL 33950; tel. 941/639–8771; FAX. 941/639–3422; Mr. Bruce Freeman
Life Care Center of Sarasota, 8104 Tuttle Avenue, Sarasota, FL 34243; tel. 941/360–6411; FAX. 941/360–6499; Mrs. Nina K Willingham
Life Care Center of Winter Haven, 1510 Cypress Gardens Boulevard, Winter Haven, FL 33884; tel. 863/318–8646; FAX. 863/318–1382; Mr. Ralph M Jacobs
Miami Jewish Home & Hospital for the Aged, 5200 Northeast 2nd Avenue, Miami, FL 33137; tel. 305/751–8626; FAX. 305/759–1689; Mr. Fred Stock
Miami VA Healthcare System, 1201 NW 16th Street, Miami, FL 33125; tel. 305/575–7000; FAX. 305/575–3266; Ms. Mary D Berrocal
North Florida/South Georgia Veterans Health System, 1601 Southwest Archer Road, Gainesville, FL 32608-1197; tel. 352/376–1611; FAX. 352/374–6116; Mr. Thomas A Cappello
Shands Jacksonville Medical Center, 655 West Eighth Street, Jacksonville, FL 32209; tel. 904/244–3002; FAX. 904/244–7732; Mr. Jim Burkhart
St. Anne's Nursing Center, 11855 Quail Roost Drive, Miami, FL 33177; tel. 305/252–4000; FAX. 305/969–6752; Mr. Ian MacBradt
St. Catherine's Rehab Hospital/Villa Maria Nursing Center, 1050 N.E. 125th Street, Miami, FL 33161; tel. 305/891–8850; FAX. 305/891–3361; Mr. James Reiss
St. John's Rehabilitation Hospital and Nursing Center, 3075 Northwest 35th Avenue, Lauderdale Lakes, FL 33311; tel. 954/739–6233; FAX. 954/733–9579; Ms. Diane A. Dube
Sunrise Health and Rehabilitation Center, 4800 Nob Hill Road, Sunrise, FL 33351; tel. 954/577–3600; FAX. 954/577–3640; Ms. Virginia Roper

Tallahassee Memorial HealthCare, Inc., 1300 Miccosukee Road, Tallahassee, FL 32308; tel. 850/431–5380; FAX. 850/431–5883; Mr. G Mark O'Bryant
The Gardens Court, 3803 PGA Boulevard, Palm Beach Gardens, FL 33410; tel. 561/626–1125; FAX. 561/626–3334
VA Medical Center - West Palm Beach, Florida, 7305 N. Military Trail, West Palm Beach, FL 33410-6400; tel. 561/422–8600; FAX. 561/422–6707; Ms. Charleen R. Szabo

GEORGIA
Appling HealthCare System, PO BOX 2070, Baxley, GA 31513; tel. 912/367–9841; FAX. 912/367–1272; Mr. Dale Spell
Bacon County Hospital and Health System, PO Drawer 1987, Alma, GA 31510-0987; tel. 912/632–8961; FAX. 912/632–5000; Mrs. Cindy R. Turner
Camellia Gardens of Life Care, 804 South Broad Street, Thomasville, GA 31792; tel. 229/226–0076; FAX. 229/228–9798; Mrs. Vicki Cooper
Central State Hospital, 620 Broad St, Milledgeville, GA 31062; tel. 478/445–4128; FAX. 478/445–6034; Mr. Marvin Bailey
Crisp Regional Hospital, Inc., PO Box 5007, Cordele, GA 31010; tel. 229/276–3320; FAX. 229/276–3108; Mr. D. Wayne Martin
Dogwood Health and Rehabilitation, 7560 Butner Road, Fairburn, GA 30213; tel. 770/306–7878; FAX. 770/306–7779; Mr. Neil L. Pruitt
Early Memorial Hospital and Nursing Home, 11740 Columbia Road, Blakely, GA 39823; tel. 229/723–4241; FAX. 229/723–2930; Ms. Robin Rau
East Central Regional Hospital, P.O. Box 1299, Gracewood, GA 30812-1299; tel. 706/790–2030; FAX. 706/790–2025; Mr. Stephen T. Smith
Effingham Hospital, PO Box 386, Springfield, GA 31329; tel. 912/754–6451; FAX. 912/754–9901; Mrs. Norma J Morgan
Emanuel Medical Center, PO Box 879, Swainsboro, GA 30401; tel. 478/289–1100; FAX. 478/289–1300; Mr. Len Daugherty
Family Life Enrichment Center, Inc., PO Box 10, High Shoals, GA 30645; tel. 706/769–7738; FAX. 706/769–5944; Ms. Magda D. Bennett
Georgia Regional Hospital at Atlanta, PO Box 37047, Decatur, GA 30034-0407; tel. 404/243–2100; FAX. 404/212–4621
Georgia War Veterans Home, 2249 Vinson Highway, Milledgeville, GA 31061; tel. 478/445–4516; FAX. 478/445–1701; Mr. H. Morris Graybeal
Georgia War Veterans Nursing Home, 1101 15th Street, Augusta, GA 30901; tel. 706/721–2531; FAX. 706/721–3892; Mr. Charles Esposito
Grady Health System, 80 Jesse Hill, Jr., Drive, S.E., Atlanta, GA 30303; tel. 404/616–5243; FAX. 404/616–1768
Gwinnett Hospital System, Inc., PO Box 348, Lawrenceville, GA 30046; tel. 678/442–4306; FAX. 770/682–2257; Mr. Phillip Wolfe
Henry Medical Center, 1133 Eagle's Landing Parkway, Stockbridge, GA 30281-5099; tel. 678/604–1000; FAX. 770/506–1320; Mr. Charles F Scott
Hutcheson Medical Center, 100 Gross Crescent Circle, Fort Oglethorpe, GA 30742; tel. 706/858–2000; FAX. 706/858–2578; Mr. Charles Stewart
Irwin County Hospital, 710 North Irwin Avenue, Ocilla, GA 31774; tel. 229/468–3800; FAX. 229/468–3973; Ms. Sue Spivey
John D. Archbold Memorial Hospital, Gordon Avenue at Mimosa Drive, Thomasville, GA 31792; tel. 229/228–2000; FAX. 229/228–8591; Mr. J. Perry Mustian
Liberty Regional Medical Center, PO Box 919, Hinesville, GA 31310; tel. 912/369–9400; FAX. 912/877–9438; Mr. H. Scott Kroell
Life Care Center of Gwinnett, 3850 Safehaven Drive, Lawrenceville, GA 30044; tel. 770/923–0005; FAX. 770/279–7067; Ms. Regina Louis
Life Care Center of Lawrenceville, 210 Collins Industrial Way, Lawrenceville, GA 30045; tel. 678/442–0777; FAX. 678/442–9777; Mr. Bart Walker
Louis Smith Memorial Hospital, 852 West Thigpen Avenue, Lakeland, GA 31635; tel. 229/482–8440; FAX. 229/482–8539; Mr. Neil Ginty
Meadows Regional Medical Center, Inc., 1703 Meadows Lane, Vidalia, GA 30474; tel. 912/537–8921; FAX. 912/538–5333; Mr. Alan Kent
Memorial Hospital of Adel, 706 North Parrish Avenue, Adel, GA 31620; tel. 229/896–8000; FAX. 229/896–8001; Mr. Bill Hawley
Mitchell County Hospital, PO Box 639, Camilla, GA 31730; tel. 229/336–5284; FAX. 229/336–4682; Adm. Mark Kimball
North Georgia Medical Center, PO Box 2239, Ellijay, GA 30540; tel. 706/276–4741; FAX. 706/276–3698; Mr. Jeffrey M Dunn
Quinton Memorial Health Care and Rehabilitation Center, 1114 Burleyson Road, Dalton, GA 30720; tel. 706/226–4642; FAX. 706/226–9785; Mr. Dennis Stout
Regency Park Health Care Center, 1212 Broadrick Drive, Dalton, GA 30720; tel. 706/270–8008; FAX. 706/270–8248; Mr. Steve Fromm
Ridgewood Manor Nursing Home, 1110 Burleyson Road, Dalton, GA 30720; tel. 706/226–1021; FAX. 706/278–0619; Mr. Gregg W. Martin
Sadie G. Mays Health and Rehabilitation Center, 1821 Anderson Avenue, NW, Atlanta, GA 30314; tel. 404/794–2477; FAX. 404/799–9876; Mr. Charles Robinson
Satilla Regional Medical Center, 410 Darling Avenue, Waycross, GA 31501; tel. 912/287–3030; FAX. 912/287–2505; Mr. Robert M Trimm
Southland Nursing Home, Inc., 151 Wisdom Road, Peachtree City, GA 30269; tel. 770/631–9000; FAX. 770/487–2788; Mr. Gary Massengale
The Hospital Authority of Habersham County, PO Box 37, Demorest, GA 30535; tel. 706/754–3113; FAX. 706/754–7300; Mr. C. Richard Dwozan
VA Medical Center, 1 Freedom Way, Augusta, GA 30904; tel. 706/733–0188; FAX. 706/823–3934; Ms. Rebecca J Wiley
VA Medical Center - Atlanta, 1670 Clairmont Road, Decatur, GA 30033; tel. 404/728–7601; FAX. 404/728–7794; Mr. James A. Clark
VA Medical Center - Carl Vinson, 1826 Veterans Boulevard, Dublin, GA 31021; tel. 478/277–2701; FAX. 478/277–2789; Ms. Kelly O Duke
Wood Dale Health Care Center, 1102 Burleyson Road, Dalton, GA 30720; tel. 706/226–1285; FAX. 706/226–6877; Mr. Jon Renegar

HAWAII
Hale Anuenue Restorative Care Center, 1333 Waianuenue Avenue, Hilo, HI 96720; tel. 808/961–6644; FAX. 808/961–6630; Mr. Ivan S Yamamoto
Ka Puna Wai Ola, 91-575 Farrington Highway, Kapolei, HI 96707; tel. 808/674–9262; FAX. 808/674–8481; Ms. Kerry Pitcher
Kona Community Hospital, 79-1019 Haukapila Street, Kealakekua, HI 96750; tel. 808/322–9311; FAX. 808/322–4488; Mr. Donald Lewis
Life Care Center of Hilo, 944 West Kawailani Street, Hilo, HI 96720; tel. 808/959–9151; FAX. 808/959–6202; Mr. Fred Horwitz
Life Care Center of Kona, 78-6957 Kamehameha III Road, Kailua Kona, HI 96740; tel. 808/322–2790; FAX. 808/324–1750; Mr. Raymond Marks
VA Pacific Islands Health Care System, 459 Patterson Road, Honolulu, HI 96819-1522; tel. 808/433–0100; FAX. 808/433–0390; Dr. James E. Hastings

IDAHO
Bingham Memorial Hospital and Extended Care Facility, 98 Poplar Street, Blackfoot, ID 83221; tel. 208/785–3804; FAX. 208/785–3806; Mr. Louis D. Kraml
Bridgeview Estates, 1828 Bridgeview Boulevard, Twin Falls, ID 83301; tel. 208/736–3933; FAX. 208/736–3941; Ms. Lori Bentzler
Life Care Center of Coeur d'Alene, 500 West Aqua Avenue, Coeur D Alene, ID 83815; tel. 208/762–1122; Mr. Mark Scroggin
Life Care Center of Idaho Falls, 2725 East 17th Street, Idaho Falls, ID 83406; tel. 208/529–4567; FAX. 208/529–4304; Ms. Renee L. Mai
Life Care Center of Lewiston, 325 Warner Drive, Lewiston, ID 83501; tel. 208/798–8500; FAX. 208/798–8530; Mr. Dan Knapp
Life Care Center of Sandpoint, 1125 North Division Street, Sandpoint, ID 83864; tel. 208/265–9299; FAX. 208/265–9710; Ms. Irene Michael
Life Care Center of Treasure Valley, 502 North Kimball Place, Boise, ID 83704; tel. 208/377–1900; FAX. 208/377–1905; Ms. Natalie Peterson
State Hospital South, PO Box 400, Blackfoot, ID 83221; tel. 208/785–1200; FAX. 208/785–8448; Mr. Tracy J. Farnsworth
VA Medical Center, 500 West Fort Street, Boise, ID 83702-4598; tel. 208/422–1100; FAX. 208/422–1157; Mr. DeWayne Hamlin
Valley View Retirement Community, 1130 N Allumbaugh Street, Boise, ID 83704; tel. 208/322–0311; FAX. 208/327–1050; Mr. Brian Weaver

ILLINOIS
Advocate South Suburban Hospital, 17800 South Kedzie Avenue, Hazel Crest, IL 60429; tel. 708/213–3000; FAX. 708/213–0100; Ms. Ann M Errichetti
Alden - Des Plaines Skilled Nursing and Rehabilitation, 1221 East Golf Road, Des Plaines, IL 60016; tel. 847/768–1300; FAX. 847/768–1668; Mr. Floyd A. Schlossberg
Alden Estates of Evanston, 2520 Gross Point Road, Evanston, IL 60201; tel. 847/328–6000; FAX. 847/328–6166; Mr. Floyd A Schlossberg
Alden North Shore Rehabilitation Health Care Ctr, 5050 West Touhy Avenue, Skokie, IL 60077; tel. 847/679–6100; FAX. 847/679–3822; Mr. Floyd A. Schlossberg
Alden Rehabilitation and Health Care Center/ Orland Park, 16450 South 97th Avenue, Orland Park, IL 60462; tel. 708/403–6500; FAX. 708/873–9774; Mr. Floyd A. Schlossberg
Alden-Lakeland Rehabilitation and Health Care Center, 820 West Lawrence Avenue, Chicago, IL 60640; tel. 773/769–2570; FAX. 773/769–1551; Mr. Floyd A. Schlossberg
Anna Hospital Corporation, 517 North Main, Anna, IL 62906; tel. 618/833–4511; FAX. 618/833–4183; Mr. James R. Farris
ASTA Care Center, 300 West Lowell, Pontiac, IL 61764; tel. 815/842–1181; FAX. 815/842–3406; Mr. Michael Gillman
ASTA Care Center of Elgin, 134 North McLean Boulevard, Elgin, IL 60123; tel. 847/742–8822; FAX. 847/742–6629; Dr. Michael Gillman
Brentwood North Health Care Center, 3705 Deerfield Road, Riverwoods, IL 60015; tel. 847/947–9000; FAX. 847/947–9005
Burgess Square Healthcare Centre, 5801 South Cass Avenue, Westmont, IL 60559; tel. 630/971–2645; FAX. 630/969–7166; Ms. Jacqueline L. Mason
Crawford Memorial Hospital, 1000 North Allen Street, Robinson, IL 62454; tel. 618/544–3131; FAX. 618/546–2442; Mr. Don Annis
Decatur Memorial Hospital, 2300 North Edward Street, Decatur, IL 62526; tel. 217/876–2106; FAX. 217/876–2125; Mr. Kenneth L Smithmier
DuPage Convalescent Center, 400 North County Farm Road, Wheaton, IL 60187; tel. 630/784–4200; FAX. 630/668–9633; Ms. Beth Welch
Edward Hines Jr. VA Hospital, PO Box 5000, Hines, IL 60141-5000; tel. 708/202–5609; FAX. 708/202–2506; Mr. Nathan L Geraths
Elmhurst Memorial Hospital, 200 Berteau Avenue, Elmhurst, IL 60126; tel. 630/833–1400; FAX. 630/782–7801; Mr. Leo F Fronza
Evergreen Healthcare Center, 10124 South Kedzie Avenue, Evergreen Park, IL 60805; tel. 708/907–7000; FAX. 708/907–7003; Ms. Judy Dabertin
Fairfield Memorial Hospital Association, 303 Northwest 11th Street, Fairfield, IL 62837; tel. 618/847–8333; FAX. 618/847–8387; Ms. Katherine J. Bunting
Forest Villa Nursing and Rehabilitation Center, LLC, 6840 West Touhy Avenue, Niles, IL 60714; tel. 847/647–6400; FAX. 847/647–1539; Mr. Barry Carr
GlenBridge Nursing and Rehabilitation Centre, Ltd, 8333 West Golf Road, Niles, IL 60714; tel. 847/966–9190; FAX. 847/966–4455; Mrs. Nancy J. Crutcher
Glencrest Nursing and Rehabilitation Centre, 2451 West Touhy Avenue, Chicago, IL 60645; tel. 773/338–6800; FAX. 773/338–1166; Mr. William Pfeiffer
GlenShire Nursing and Rehabilitation Centre, Ltd., 22660 South Cicero Avenue, Richton Park, IL 60471; tel. 708/747–6120; FAX. 708/747–7066; Mr. Dave Zaruba
Glenview Terrace Nursing Center, 1511 Greenwood Road, Glenview, IL 60026; tel. 847/729–9090; FAX. 847/729–9135; Mr. Mark Hollander
Glenview Terrace Nursing Center, 1511 Greenwood Road, Glenview, IL 60026; tel. 847/729–9090; FAX. 847/729–9135; Mr. Mark Hollander
Graham Hospital, 210 West Walnut Street, Canton, IL 61520; tel. 309/647–5240; FAX. 309/649–5101; Mr. Robert Senneff
Graham Hospital, 210 West Walnut Street, Canton, IL 61520; tel. 309/647–5240; FAX. 309/649–5101; Mr. Robert Senneff

Greek American Rehabilitation and Care Center, 220 N 1st Street, Wheeling, IL 60090; tel. 847/459–8700; FAX. 847/465–9957; Mrs. Eleni Ifantis
Hammond Henry Hospital, 600 N. College Avenue, Geneseo, IL 61254-1099; tel. 309/944–6431; FAX. 309/944–9229; Mr. Bradley Solberg
Hillsboro Area Hospital Inc, 1200 East Tremont Street, Hillsboro, IL 62049; tel. 217/532–6111; FAX. 217/532–4414; Mr. Rex Brown
Hoopeston Community Memorial Hospital and Nursing Home, 701 East Orange Street, Hoopeston, IL 60942-1871; tel. 217/283–5531; FAX. 217/283–6458; Mr. David Elliott
Jesse Brown VA Medical Center, 820 South Damen Avenue, Chicago, IL 60612; tel. 312/569–6101; FAX. 312/569–6188; Mr. James S Jones
Lake Forest Hospital, 660 North Westmoreland Road, Lake Forest, IL 60045; tel. 847/234–5600; FAX. 847/535–7846; Mr. Thomas J. McAfee
Lake Shore HealthCare and Rehabilitation Centre, 7200 North Sheridan Road, Chicago, IL 60626; tel. 773/973–7200; FAX. 773/338–9373; Mr. James R Farlee
MacNeal Hospital, 3249 South Oak Park Avenue, Berwyn, IL 60402; tel. 708/783–9100; FAX. 708/783–3489; Mr. Brian Lemon
ManorCare Health Services - Arlington Heights, 715 West Central Road, Arlington Heights, IL 60005; tel. 847/392–2020; FAX. 847/392–0174; Ms. Theresa Smelser
ManorCare Health Services - Elk Grove Village, 1920 Nerge Road, Elk Grove Village, IL 60007; tel. 847/301–0550; FAX. 847/301–0013; Mr. Brian Gross
ManorCare Health Services - Hinsdale, 600 West Ogden Avenue, Hinsdale, IL 60521; tel. 630/325–9630; FAX. 630/325–9648; Mr. John F Vrba
ManorCare Health Services - Naperville, 200 Martin Avenue, Naperville, IL 60540; tel. 630/355–4111; FAX. 630/355–7602; Ms. Diane Lube
ManorCare Health Services - Northbrook, 3300 Milwaukee Avenue, Northbrook, IL 60062; tel. 847/795–9700; FAX. 847/795–9600; Ms. Eliana Casella
ManorCare Health Services - South Holland, 2145 E 170th Street, South Holland, IL 60473; tel. 708/895–3255; FAX. 708/895–3315; Ms. Kimberly Saggese
ManorCare Health Services-Oak Lawn East, 9401 South Kostner Avenue, Oak Lawn, IL 60453; tel. 708/423–7882; FAX. 708/423–7947; Ms. Karen Petyko
ManorCare Health Services-Westmont, 512 East Ogden Avenue, Westmont, IL 60559; tel. 630/323–4400; FAX. 630/323–4583
Memorial Medical Center, 527 South Street, Woodstock, IL 60098; tel. 815/759–4259; FAX. 815/759–4568; Mr. Michael Eesley
Mercy Harvard Hospital, PO Box 850, Harvard, IL 60033; tel. 815/943–5431; FAX. 815/943–0659; Ms. Sue Ripsch
North Chicago VA Medical Center, 3001 Green Bay Road, North Chicago, IL 60064; tel. 224/610–3700; FAX. 224/610–3727; Mr. Patrick L Sullivan
Oakton Pavilion Health Care Facility, 1660 Oakton Place, Des Plaines, IL 60018; tel. 847/299–5588; FAX. 847/493–6525; Mr. Jay Lewkowitz
Red Bud Regional Hospital, LLC, 325 Spring Street, Red Bud, IL 62278; tel. 618/282–3831; FAX. 618/282–6101; Mr. Robert C Honeycutt
Regency Healthcare and Rehabilitation Centre, 6631 North Milwaukee Avenue, Niles, IL 60714; tel. 847/647–7444; FAX. 847/647–6403; Mr. Benjamin Rogow
Renaissance at Hillside, 4600 North Frontage Road, Hillside, IL 60162; tel. 708/544–9933; FAX. 708/493–1192; Mr. Gerry Jenich
Rest Haven Illiana Christian Convalescent Home, 13259 South Central Avenue, Palos Heights, IL 60463; tel. 708/597–1000; FAX. 708/389–9990
Rest Haven South, 16300 South Wausau Avenue, South Holland, IL 60473; tel. 708/596–5500; FAX. 708/596–5527; Ms. Evelyn B. Hanna
Rest Haven West Christian Skilled Nursing Center, 3450 Saratoga Avenue, Downers Grove, IL 60515; tel. 630/969–2900; FAX. 630/969–2148; Ms. Jacquelyn L Terpstra
Rosewood Care Center Inc. of Northbrook, 4101 Lake Cook Road, Northbrook, IL 60062; tel. 847/562–1770; FAX. 847/562–1909; Mr. Larry Vander Maten
Sherman West Court, 1950 Larkin Avenue, Elgin, IL 60123; tel. 847/742–7070; FAX. 847/742–7248; Mr. Joseph McManus
St. John's Hospital, 800 East Carpenter Street, Springfield, IL 62769; tel. 217/544–6464; FAX. 217/535–3989
St. Joseph's Hospital, 1515 Main Street, Highland, IL 62249; tel. 618/654–7421; FAX. 618/654–2012; Mr. Claudio Fort
St. Mary's Hospital, 111 Spring Street, Streator, IL 61364; tel. 815/673–2311; FAX. 815/673–4621; Ms. Sharon Timmons
Taylorville Memorial Hospital, 201 East Pleasant, Taylorville, IL 62568; tel. 217/824–3331; FAX. 217/824–1608
The Abington of Glenview, 3901 Glenview Road, Glenview, IL 60025; tel. 847/729–0000; FAX. 847/729–1552; Ms. Barbara Lyons
The Carlton at the Lake, Inc., 725 West Montrose Avenue, Chicago, IL 60613; tel. 773/929–1700; FAX. 773/929–3068; Mrs. Rose Marie Betz
The Claremont Rehab and Living Center, 150 North Weiland Road, Buffalo Grove, IL 60089; tel. 847/465–0200; FAX. 847/465–0400; Ms. Rupal Mistry
Trinity Medical Center, 2701 17th Street, Rock Island, IL 61201; tel. 309/779–2200; FAX. 309/779–2303; Mr. Kevin Vermeer
VA - Illiana Health Care System, 1900 East Main Street, Danville, IL 61832; tel. 217/554–5082; FAX. 217/554–4904; Mr. Daniel D Hendee
VA Medical Center, 2401 West Main Street, Marion, IL 62959; tel. 618/997–5311; FAX. 618/993–4155
Warren Barr Pavilion, 66 West Oak Street, Chicago, IL 60610; tel. 312/705–5100; FAX. 312/337–5041; Mrs. Judy Dabertin
Whitehall North, 300 Waukegan Road, Deerfield, IL 60015-4988; tel. 847/945–4600; FAX. 847/945–6492; Mr. Mark Hollaner

INDIANA
Community Hospital of Anderson and Madison County, 1515 North Madison Avenue, Anderson, IN 46011; tel. 765/298–4242; FAX. 765/298–5848; Dr. William Vanness
Deaconess Hospital, 600 Mary Street, Evansville, IN 47747; tel. 812/450–5000; FAX. 812/450–3437; Mr. Harry Smith
Gibson General Hospital, Inc., 1808 Sherman Drive, Princeton, IN 47670; tel. 812/385–9221; FAX. 812/385–9323; Mr. Emmett Schuster
Green Valley Care Center, 3118 Green Valley Road, New Albany, IN 47150; tel. 812/945–2341; FAX. 812/945–0089
Hammond Whiting Care Center, 1000 114th Street, Whiting, IN 46394; tel. 219/659–2770; FAX. 219/659–2803; Ms. Caryn G Moore
Heritage Healthcare, 3401 Soldiers Home Road, West Lafayette, IN 47906; tel. 765/463–1541; FAX. 765/497–0687; Ms. Raelene Wing
La Porte Regional Health System, Inc., PO Box 250, La Porte, IN 46350; tel. 219/325–4664; FAX. 219/326–2015; Mr. Michael E. Haley
Life Care Center of Fort Wayne, 1649 Spy Run Ave., Fort Wayne, IN 46805; tel. 260/422–8520; FAX. 260/422–9345
Life Care Center of LaGrange, 0770 N 075 E, Lagrange, IN 46761; tel. 260/463–7445; FAX. 260/463–7282; Ms. Patricia A Ward
Life Care Center of Michigan City, 802 US Highway 20 East, Michigan City, IN 46360; tel. 219/872–7251; FAX. 219/874–8571; Ms. Peg Mark
Life Care Center of Rochester, 827 West 13th Street, Rochester, IN 46975; tel. 574/223–4331; FAX. 574/223–4172; Mr. Gregg Fuller
Life Care Center of Valparaiso, 3405 Campbell Road, Valparaiso, IN 46385; tel. 219/462–1023; FAX. 219/477–4439; Ms. Amber Janeczko
Life Care Center of Willows, 1000 Elizabeth Street, Valparaiso, IN 46383; tel. 219/464–4858; FAX. 219/477–4746; Mr. Michael Baran
Mitchell Manor, PO Box 338, Mitchell, IN 47446; tel. 812/849–2221; FAX. 812/849–6971; Mr. Joe Cox
Parkview Care Center, 2819 North St. Joseph Avenue, Evansville, IN 47712; tel. 812/424–2941; FAX. 812/423–6230; Ms. Connie Kirwer
Rensselaer Care Center, 1309 East Grace Street, Rensselaer, IN 47978; tel. 219/866–4181; FAX. 219/866–3292; Ms. Paula Powers
Saint John's Health System, 2015 Jackson Street, Anderson, IN 46016; tel. 765/646–8373; FAX. 765/646–8504
The Altenheim Community, 3525 East Hanna Avenue, Indianapolis, IN 46237; tel. 317/788–4261; FAX. 317/781–4512; Mr. Randy Hornstein
The Lane House, 1000 Lane Avenue, Crawfordsville, IN 47933; tel. 765/362–0007; FAX. 765/362–4168; Mrs. Cynthia Stevens
The Woodlands, 3820 W Jackson Street, Muncie, IN 47304; tel. 765/289–3451; FAX. 765/289–3480; Mr. Duane Ott
VA Northern Indiana Health Care System, 2121 Lake Avenue, Fort Wayne, IN 46805; tel. 260/460–1310; FAX. 260/460–1336; Ms. Cathi Spivey-Paul
Wishard Health Services, 1001 West Tenth Street, Indianapolis, IN 46202; tel. 317/639–6671; FAX. 317/630–7678; Dr. Lisa E. Harris

IOWA
Covenant Medical Center-Wheaton Franciscan Healthcare, 3421 West 9th Street, Waterloo, IA 50702; tel. 319/272–8000; FAX. 319/272–7313; Mr. Jack Dusenbery
Mercy Medical Center, 250 Mercy Drive, Dubuque, IA 52001; tel. 563/589–8000; FAX. 563/589–8073; Mr. Russell M. Knight
VA Central Iowa Health Care System, 3600 30th Street, Des Moines, IA 50310-5774; tel. 515/699–5850; FAX. 515/699–5862; Mr. Donald C. Cooper

KANSAS
Garden Terrace at Overland Park, 7541 Switzer Rd., Overland, KS 66214; tel. 913/631–2273; FAX. 913/631–7154; Ms. Debra L Biehl
Life Care Center of Andover, 621 West 21st Street, Andover, KS 67002; tel. 316/733–1349; FAX. 316/733–0919
Life Care Center of Burlington, 601 Cross Street, Burlington, KS 66839; tel. 620/364–2117; FAX. 620/364–2013; Mr. Michael Pelzer
Life Care Center of Kansas City, 3231 N. 61st Street, Kansas City, KS 66104; tel. 913/299–1770; FAX. 913/299–1539; Ms. Lisa M Kolman
Life Care Center of Osawatomie, 1615 Parker Street - Box 159, Osawatomie, KS 66064; tel. 913/755–4165; FAX. 913/755–1976; Mr. Thomas Cameron Hodges
Life Care Center of Seneca, 512 Community Dr., Seneca, KS 66538; tel. 785/336–3528; FAX. 785/336–3621
Life Care Center of Wichita, 622 North Edgemoor, Wichita, KS 67208; tel. 316/686–5100; FAX. 316/686–3993; Ms. Bonnie Jackson
Robert J. Dole VA Medical Center, 5500 East Kellogg, Wichita, KS 67218; tel. 316/651–3601; FAX. 316/651–3666; Mr. Thomas J. Sanders
VA Eastern Kansas Health Care System, 2200 SW Gage, Topeka, KS 66622; tel. 785/350–3111; FAX. 785/350–4336; Ms. Marie L. Weldon

KENTUCKY
Appalachian Regional Healthcare, 260 Hospital Drive, South Williamson, KY 41503; tel. 606/237–1700; FAX. 606/237–1701; Mr. Timothy Hatfield
Bureau of Prisons - FMC Lexington, 3301 Leestown Road, Lexington, KY 40511-8799; tel. 859/255–6812; FAX. 859/253–8876
Highlands of Ft. Thomas, 960 Highland Avenue, Fort Thomas, KY 41075; tel. 859/572–0660; FAX. 859/572–0950; Mr. Barry N. Bortz
J. J. Jordan Geriatric Center, 270 East Clayton Lane, Louisa, KY 41230; tel. 606/638–4586; FAX. 606/638–0367; Mr. David McKenzie
Kindred Hospitals Limited Partnership, 1313 St. Anthony Place, Louisville, KY 40204; tel. 502/587–7001; FAX. 502/587–0060; Mr. Ron Cronen
Lancaster Medical Investors, LLC, 308 West Maple Avenue, Lancaster, KY 40444; tel. 859/792–6844; FAX. 859/792–1806; Mr. Tom Davis
Laurel Creek Health Care Center, 1033 North Highway 11, Manchester, KY 40962; tel. 606/598–6163; FAX. 606/598–6164; Mrs. Clara Benge
Life Care Center of Bardstown, 120 Life Care Way, Bardstown, KY 40004; tel. 502/348–4220; FAX. 502/349–0900
Life Care Center of LaCenter, 252 W. 5th Street, La Center, KY 42056; tel. 270/665–5681; FAX. 270/665–9766; Ms. Ginger Atkins
Life Care Center of Morehead, PO Box 884, Morehead, KY 40351; tel. 606/784–7518; FAX. 606/784–7619; Mr. Kevin Trent

Mountain View Health Care, PO Box 650, Elkhorn City, KY 41522; tel. 606/754–4134; FAX. 606/754–5704; Ms. Sharon K Hall

Murray-Calloway County Hospital, 803 Poplar Street, Murray, KY 42071-2432; tel. 270/762–1102; FAX. 270/767–3600; Mr. Keith Bailey

Nicholas County Hospital / Johnson Mathers Nursing Home, PO Box 232, Carlisle, KY 40311; tel. 859/289–7181; FAX. 859/289–7510; Ms. Doris Ecton

Owensboro Medical Health System, 811 East Parrish Avenue, Owensboro, KY 42303; tel. 270/688–2000; FAX. 270/688–2124; Dr. Jeffrey Barber

Parkview Nursing and Rehabilitation Center, 544 Lone Oak Road, Paducah, KY 42003; tel. 270/443–6543; FAX. 502/442–3312; Ms. Lori Moberly

Pineville Community Hospital Association, Inc., 850 Riverview Avenue, Pineville, KY 40977; tel. 606/337–3051; FAX. 606/337–4284; Mr. Milton Brooks

Rockcastle Hospital and Respiratory Care Center, Inc., 145 Newcomb Avenue P.O. Box 1310, Mount Vernon, KY 40456; tel. 606/256–2195; FAX. 606/256–3232; Mr. Stephen A Estes

The Medical Center, PO Box 90010, Bowling Green, KY 42102-9010; tel. 270/745–1000; FAX. 270/842–0765; Ms. Connie D Smith

The St. Luke Hospitals, Inc., 85 North Grand Avenue, Fort Thomas, KY 41075; tel. 859/572–3100; FAX. 859/572–2349; Ms. Nancy Kremer

VA Medical Center, 1101 Veterans Drive, Lexington, KY 40502-2236; tel. 859/233–4511; FAX. 859/281–4911; Mrs. Sandy J. Nielsen

VillaSpring Healthcare Center, 630 Viox Drive, Erlanger, KY 41018; tel. 859/727–6700; FAX. 859/727–6710; Mr. Barry Bortz

Western Baptist Hospital, 2501 Kentucky Avenue, Paducah, KY 42003-3200; tel. 270/575–2100; FAX. 270/575–2217; Mr. Larry O Barton

LOUISIANA

East Jefferson General Hospital, 4200 Houma Boulevard, Metairie, LA 70006; tel. 504/454–4000; FAX. 504/454–5299; Dr. Mark J. Peters

Franciscan Missionaries of Our Lady Health System, 4200 Essen Lane, Baton Rouge, LA 70809; tel. 225/765–8866; FAX. 225/765–8305

Lane Regional Medical Center, 6300 Main Street, Zachary, LA 70791; tel. 225/658–4303; FAX. 225/658–4287; Mr. Randall M Olson

National Hansen's Disease Programs, 1770 Physicians Park Drive, Baton Rouge, LA 70816; tel. 225/756–3700; FAX. 225/756–3819; Dr. James L Krahenbuhl

Southeast Louisiana Veterans Healthcare System, P.O. Box 61011, New Orleans, LA 70161-1011; tel. 504/556–7300; FAX. 504/589–5956; Ms. Julie Catellier

Trinity Neurologic Rehabilitation Center, LLC, 1400 Lindberg Drive, Slidell, LA 70458; tel. 985/641–4985; FAX. 985/646–0793; Mr. Patrick Foret

VA Medical Center, PO Box 69004, Alexandria, LA 71306; tel. 318/473–0010; FAX. 318/483–5091; Ms. Barbara C. Watkins

MAINE

Northern Maine Medical Center, 194 East Main Street, Fort Kent, ME 04743; tel. 207/834–3155; FAX. 207/834–2949; Mr. Martin Bernstein

Togus VA Medical Center, 1 VA Center, Augusta, ME 04330; tel. 207/623–8411; FAX. 207/623–5792; Mr. Brian G. Stiller

MARYLAND

Calvert Memorial Hospital, 100 Hospital Road, Prince Frederick, MD 20678; tel. 410/535–8239; FAX. 410/535–8174; Mr. James J. Xinis

Deer's Head Center, PO Box 2018, Salisbury, MD 21802-2018; tel. 410/543–4000; FAX. 410/543–4004; Mrs. Sandra K. Smith

Fox Chase Rehabilitation and Nursing Center, 2015 East West Highway, Silver Spring, MD 20910; tel. 301/587–2400; FAX. 301/587–2404; Ms. Jean A Raiche

Gladys Spellman Specialty Hospital and Nursing Center, 2900 Mercy Lane, Cheverly, MD 20785; tel. 301/618–2010; FAX. 301/772–7689; Mr. Stewart R. Seitz

Jewish Convalescent and Nursing Home, 7920 Scotts Level Road, Baltimore, MD 21208; tel. 410/521–3600; FAX. 410/521–0892; Mr. Ron Rothstein

Johns Hopkins Bayview Medical Center, 4940 Eastern Avenue, Baltimore, MD 21224-2780; tel. 410/550–0120; FAX. 410/550–7996; Mr. Gregory F Schaffer

Levindale Hebrew Geriatric Center and Hospital, 2434 West Belvedere Avenue, Baltimore, MD 21215; tel. 410/466–8700; FAX. 410/601–2700; Mr. Ronald Rothstein

Potomac Valley Nursing Facilities Inc., 1235 Potomac Valley Road, Rockville, MD 20850; tel. 301/762–0700; FAX. 301/294–3293; Mrs. Leah T Bowden

Southern Maryland Hospital Center, 7503 Surratts Road, Clinton, MD 20735; tel. 301/868–8000; FAX. 301/877–1938; Mr. Michael J Chiaramonte

St. Elizabeth Rehabilitation and Nursing Center, 3320 Benson Avenue, Baltimore, MD 21227; tel. 410/644–7100; FAX. 410/646–6541; Ms. Christine L Mour

VA Maryland Health Care System, 10 North Greene Street, Baltimore, MD 21201; tel. 410/605–7000; FAX. 410/605–7832; Mr. Dennis H. Smith

Western Maryland Hospital Center, 1500 Pennsylvania Avenue, Hagerstown, MD 21742-3194; tel. 301/745–4200; FAX. 301/791–4450; Ms. Cynthia M. Pellegrino

MASSACHUSETTS

Abbott House, 28 Essex Street, Lynn, MA 01902; tel. 781/595–5500; FAX. 781/595–3624; Ms. Michele Desmarais

Aberjona Nursing Center, Inc., 184 Swanton Street, Winchester, MA 01890; tel. 781/729–9370; FAX. 781/994–1683; Ms. Joy Gucciardi

Alden Court Nursing Care and Rehabilitation Center, 389 Alden Road, Fairhaven, MA 02719; tel. 508/991–8600; FAX. 508/992–3708; Mr. Brad Truini

Alliance Health, Inc., 804 Pleasant Street, Brockton, MA 02301-3055; tel. 508/583–6000; FAX. 508/580–2468; Mr. John G Soule

Alliance HealthCare Center at Braintree, 175 Grove Street, Braintree, MA 02184; tel. 781/848–2050; FAX. 781/794–0141; Ms. Mary Kilcommons

Amesbury Village, LLC, 22 Maple Street, Amesbury, MA 01913; tel. 978/388–4682; FAX. 978/388–6979; Mr. Mark L Carroll

Apple Valley Nursing and Rehabilitation Center, 400 Groton Road, Ayer, MA 01432; tel. 978/772–1704; FAX. 978/772–1708; Mr. Mark R. Laroche

Autumn Village, LLC, 25 Oriol Drive, Worcester, MA 01605; tel. 508/852–3330; FAX. 508/595–1055; Mr. Mark Carroll

Avery Manor, 100 West Street, Needham Heights, MA 02494; tel. 781/234–6300; FAX. 781/234–6381; Ms. AnnMarie Jaworski

Bay Path Rehabilitation & Nursing Center, 308 Kingstown Way, Duxbury, MA 02332; tel. 781/585–5561; FAX. 781/585–1481; Mrs. Marianne Welch-Martinez

Baypointe Rehabilitation and Skilled Care Center, 50 Christy Place, Brockton, MA 02301; tel. 508/580–6800; FAX. 508/587–6633; Mr. Jim Morris

Bear Hill Nursing Center at Wakefield, 11 North Street, Stoneham, MA 02180; tel. 781/438–8515; FAX. 781/279–4730; Mr. William E. Ring

Beaumont Rehabilitation & Skilled Nursing Center, 3 Vision Drive, Route 9 West, Natick, MA 01760; tel. 508/655–3344; FAX. 508/655–9702; Mr. William McGinley

Beaumont Rehabilitation and Nursing Center at Northborough, 238 West Main Street, Northborough, MA 01532; tel. 508/393–2368; FAX. 508/393–3870; Mr. Phil LaCasse

Beaumont Rehabilitation and Skilled Nursing Center, Three Lyman Street, Westborough, MA 01581; tel. 508/366–9933; FAX. 508/898–3931; Mr. Paul J. O'Connell

Beaumont Rehabilitation and Skilled Nursing Center, PO Box 935, Northbridge, MA 01534-0935; tel. 508/234–9771; FAX. 508/234–2635; Mr. Andrew Salmon

Belmont Manor Nursing Center, 34 Agassiz Avenue, Belmont, MA 02478; tel. 617/489–1200; FAX. 617/489–0855; Mr. Stewart A. Karger

Beverly Healthcare Birchwood Care Center, 1199 John Fitch Highway, Fitchburg, MA 01420; tel. 978/345–0146; FAX. 978/345–4053; Mr. Gary J. Leger

Blaire House of Milford, 20 Claflin Street, Milford, MA 01757; tel. 508/473–1272; FAX. 508/634–3943; Ms. Deborah Klock

Blaire House of Tewksbury, 10 Erlin Terrace, Tewksbury, MA 01876; tel. 978/851–3121; FAX. 978/640–0981; Mr. Frank C. Romano

Blueberry Hill Skilled Nursing and Rehabilitation Center, 75 Brimbal Avenue, Beverly, MA 01915; tel. 978/927–2020; FAX. 978/922–4643

Bolton Manor Nursing and Rehabilitation Center, 400 Bolton Street, Marlborough, MA 01752; tel. 508/481–6123; FAX. 508/481–6130; Mr. Thomas Sullivan

Bostonian Nursing Care and Rehabilitation Center, 337 Neponset Ave, Dorchester, MA 02122; tel. 617/265–2350; FAX. 617/265–0577; Mr. Thomas Lynch

Bourne Manor Extended Care Facility, 146 MacArthur Boulevard, Bourne, MA 02532; tel. 508/759–8880; FAX. 508/759–8883; Ms. Linda Valenzano

Braemoor Rehabilitation and Nursing Center, Inc., 34 North Pearl Street, Brockton, MA 02301; tel. 508/586–3696; FAX. 508/584–0470; Mr. Michael J Roland

Braintree Landing Rehabilitation and Skilled Nursing Center, 95 Commercial Street, Braintree, MA 02184; tel. 781/848–3678; FAX. 781/356–8559; Mr. Philip F. Quillard

Braintree Manor Rehabilitation and Nursing Center, 1102 Washington Street, Braintree, MA 02184; tel. 781/848–3100; FAX. 781/849–6487; Mr. David Johnson

Braintree Manor Rehabilitation and Nursing Center, 1102 Washington Street, Braintree, MA 02184; tel. 781/848–3100; FAX. 781/849–6487; Mr. David Johnson

Briarwood Healthcare Nursing Center, 150 Lincoln Street, Needham, MA 02492; tel. 781/449–4040; FAX. 781/449–4129; Mr. Walter M. Collins

Brookline Health Care Center, 99 Park Street, Brookline, MA 02446; tel. 617/731–1050; FAX. 617/731–6516; Mr. Kurt Wheaton

Buckley HealthCare Center, 95 Laurel Street, Greenfield, MA 01301; tel. 413/774–3143; FAX. 413/772–0478; Ms. Edin Barone

Calvin Coolidge Nursing & Rehabilitation Center, 548 Elm Street, Northampton, MA 01060; tel. 413/586–3150; FAX. 413/584–7720; Mr. John Crotty

Cambridge Public Health Commission, 1493 Cambridge Street, Cambridge, MA 02139; tel. 617/665–1001; FAX. 617/665–1003; Mr. Dennis Keefe

Cape Heritage A Radius Healthcare Center, 37 Route 6A, Sandwich, MA 02563; tel. 508/888–8222; FAX. 508/888–5583; Mr. Emmanuel Freddura

Cape Regency, A Radius HealthCare Center, 120 South Main Street, Centerville, MA 02632; tel. 508/778–1835; FAX. 508/771–7411; Ms. Daniele Breault

Caritas St. Elizabeth's Medical Center of Boston, Inc., 736 Cambridge Street, Boston, MA 02135; tel. 617/789–3000; FAX. 617/562–7588; Mr. Christopher O'Connor

Caritas St. Elizabeth's Medical Center of Boston, Inc., 736 Cambridge Street, Boston, MA 02135; tel. 617/789–3000; FAX. 617/562–7588; Mr. Christopher O'Connor

Catholic Memorial Home, Inc., 2446 Highland Avenue, Fall River, MA 02720-4599; tel. 508/679–0011; FAX. 508/672–5858; Rev. Edmund J. Fitzgerald

Cedar Hill Healthcare Center, 49 Thomas Patten Drive, Randolph, MA 02368; tel. 781/961–1160; FAX. 781/963–5744; Mr. John Fredette

Charlene Manor Extended Care Facility, 130 Colrain Road, Greenfield, MA 01301; tel. 413/774–3724; FAX. 413/774–7390

Charlwell House, 305 Walpole Street, Norwood, MA 02062; tel. 781/762–7700; FAX. 781/255–0387; Mr. Kenneth Kelley

Christopher House of Worcester, Inc., 10 Mary Scano Drive, Worcester, MA 01605; tel. 508/754–3800; FAX. 508/755–2502; Mr. Walter V Ohanian

Clark House at Fox Hill Village, 30 Longwood Drive, Westwood, MA 02090; tel. 781/326–5652; FAX. 781/326–4034; Mr. Chris Wasel

Clifton Rehabilitative Nursing Center, 500 Wilbur Avenue, Somerset, MA 02725; tel. 508/675–7589; FAX. 508/672–7422; Ms. Andrea Greenwood-Syron

Colonial Rehabilitation and Nursing Center, 125 Broad Street, Weymouth, MA 02188; tel. 781/337–3121; FAX. 781/337–9831; Mr. Stephen Kelly

Concord Health Care Center, 57 Old Road to Nine Acre Corner, Concord, MA 01742; tel. 978/371–3400; FAX. 978/371–3406; Mr. Scott Dickinson

Concord Health Care Center, 57 Old Road to Nine Acre Corner, Concord, MA 01742; tel. 978/371–3400; FAX. 978/371–3406; Mr. Scott Dickinson

Coolidge House Nursing Care Center - Genesis ElderCare, 30 Webster Street, Brookline, MA 02446; tel. 617/734–2300; FAX. 617/232–1131; Ms. Christine Battisti-Kane

Copley at Stoughton Nursing Care Center, 380 Sumner Street, Stoughton, MA 02072; tel. 781/341–2300; FAX. 781/341–2402; Ms. Doreen Ledoux

Country Estates Nursing, LLC, 1200 Suffield Street, Agawam, MA 01001; tel. 413/789–2200; FAX. 413/789–2269; Mr. Jeffrey Graham

Country Rehabilitation and Nursing Center, 180 Low Street, Newburyport, MA 01950; tel. 978/465–5361; FAX. 978/462–5607; Mr. Edward Stewart

Courtyard Nursing Care Center, 200 Governors Avenue, Medford, MA 02155; tel. 781/391–5400; FAX. 781/391–4254; Ms. Allison B Hughan

D'Youville Senior Care, Inc., 981 Varnum Avenue, Lowell, MA 01854; tel. 978/569–1000; FAX. 978/453–3561; Ms. Naomi M. Prendergast

Dartmouth House Nursing Home, Inc., 567 Dartmouth Street, South Dartmouth, MA 02748; tel. 508/997–7787; FAX. 508/997–5598

Den Mar Rehabilitation and Nursing Center, 44 South Street, Rockport, MA 01966; tel. 978/546–6311; FAX. 978/546–9185; Mrs. Christine Marek

Deutsches Altenheim Inc., 2222 Centre Street, West Roxbury, MA 02132; tel. 617/325–1230; FAX. 617/323–7523; Mr. Gregory Karr

Devereux House Nursing Home, 39 Lafayette Street, Marblehead, MA 01945-1997; tel. 781/631–6120; FAX. 781/631–6122; Mrs. Erin Mondello

Eagle Pond Rehabilitation and Living Center, PO Box 208, South Dennis, MA 02660; tel. 508/385–6034; FAX. 508/385–3533; Mr. Paul J Marchwat

East Longmeadow Skilled Nursing Center, 305 Maple Street, East Longmeadow, MA 01028; tel. 413/525–6361; FAX. 413/525–6456; Mr. Patrick Arguin

Eastpointe Rehabilitation and Skilled Care Center, 255 Central Avenue, Chelsea, MA 02150; tel. 617/884–5700; FAX. 617/884–7005; Mr. Richard M Augeri

Edgar P. Benjamin Healthcare Center, 120 Fisher Avenue, Boston, MA 02120; tel. 617/738–1500; FAX. 617/738–6560; Ms. Myrna E. Wynn

Edith Nourse Rogers Memorial Veterans Hospital, 200 Springs Road, Bedford, MA 01730; tel. 781/687–3080; FAX. 781/687–3553; Mr. George R. Poulin

Emerson Village, LLC, 59 Coolidge Hill Road, Watertown, MA 02472-2884; tel. 617/924–1130; FAX. 617/924–5215

EPOCH Senior Healthcare of Brewster, 873 Harwich Road, Brewster, MA 02631; tel. 508/896–7046; FAX. 508/896–4820; Ms. Maureen Kalivas

EPOCH Senior Healthcare of Harwich, 111 Headwaters Drive, Harwich, MA 02645-1726; tel. 508/430–1717; FAX. 508/432–1809; Mrs. Karen Lee Wadlow

EPOCH Senior Healthcare of Melrose, 15 Green Street, Melrose, MA 02176; tel. 781/665–3950; FAX. 781/665–9059; Ms. Bonnie Jean McLean

EPOCH Senior Healthcare of Sharon, 259 Norwood Street, Sharon, MA 02067; tel. 781/784–6781; FAX. 781/784–4023; Ms. Kim Sciacca

EPOCH Senior Healthcare of Weston, 75 Norumbega Road, Weston, MA 02493; tel. 781/891–6100; FAX. 781/891–0109; Mr. Adam Goldman

EPOCH Senior Living, Inc., 51 Sawyer Road, Waltham, MA 02453; tel. 781/891–0777; Dr. Ellen Alperen

Essex Park Rehabilitation & Nursing Center, 265 Essex Street, Beverly, MA 01915; tel. 978/927–3260; FAX. 978/922–8347; Ms. Pat Devereaux

Essex Pavilion, LLC, 876 Falmouth Road, Hyannis, MA 02601; tel. 508/775–6663; FAX. 508/778–9891; Ms. Mary E. Benoit

Everett Nursing and Rehabilitation Center, 289 Elm Street, Everett, MA 02149; tel. 617/387–6560; FAX. 617/387–2885; Mr. Tim Connor

Fairhaven Healthcare Center, 476 Varnum Avenue, Lowell, MA 01854; tel. 978/458–3388; FAX. 978/454–7772; Ms. Joanne M. Shaw

Fairview Commons Nursing & Rehabilitation Center, 151 Christian Hill Road, Great Barrington, MA 01230; tel. 413/528–4560; FAX. 413/528–5691; Ms. Deborah Richardson

Farren Care Center, Inc., 340 Montague City Road, Turners Falls, MA 01376; tel. 413/774–3111; FAX. 413/774–7049; Mr. Christopher J McLaughlin

Federal Bureau of Prisons Federal Medical Center Devens, PO Box 880, Ayer, MA 01432; tel. 978/796–1000; FAX. 978/796–1511; Ms. Carolyn A. Sabol

Forestview Nursing Home of Wareham, 50 Indian Neck Road, Wareham, MA 02571; tel. 508/295–6264; FAX. 508/295–3484; Ms. Michelle Brown

Forestview Nursing Home of Wareham, 50 Indian Neck Road, Wareham, MA 02571; tel. 508/295–6264; FAX. 508/295–3484; Ms. Michelle Brown

Franklin Skilled Nursing & Rehab. Center LLC, 130 Chestnut Street, Franklin, MA 02038; tel. 508/528–4600; FAX. 508/528–7976; Adm. Kevin Diehl

Geriatric Authority of Milford Nursing and Rehabilitation Center, 1 Countryside Drive, Milford, MA 01757; tel. 508/473–0435; FAX. 508/473–9755; Mr. Barry Chiler

Glen Ridge Nursing Care Center, 120 Murray Street, Medford, MA 02155; tel. 781/391–0800; FAX. 781/391–9127; Mr. Robert M. Hayes

Goddard House, 201 S. Huntington Avenue, Jamaica Plain, MA 02130; tel. 617/522–3080; FAX. 617/524–1578; Mr. Kevin Comick

Golden Living Center - Chestnut Hill, 188 Florence Street, Chestnut Hill, MA 02467; tel. 617/332–4730; FAX. 617/969–6592

Golden Living Center - Plymouth, 19 Obery Street, Plymouth, MA 02360; tel. 508/747–4790; FAX. 508/746–3880; Mr. Robert Eisenstein

Great Barrington Rehab & Nursing Center, 148 Maple Ave., Great Barrington, MA 01230; tel. 413/528–3320; FAX. 413/528–2302; Ms. Katie Coburn

Greycliff at Cape Ann, 272 Washington Street, Gloucester, MA 01930; tel. 978/281–0333; FAX. 978/281–8985; Mr. Michael T. Corbett

Grosvenor Park Nursing Center, Inc., 7 Loring Hills Avenue, Salem, MA 01970; tel. 978/741–5700; FAX. 978/745–8888; Ms. Nancy Escalada

Guardian Center, Inc., 888 North Main Street, Brockton, MA 02301; tel. 508/587–6556; FAX. 508/588–1694; Ms. Denise Riley Okun

Hallmark Nursing and Rehabilitation Center, 1123 Rockdale Avenue, New Bedford, MA 02740; tel. 508/997–7448; FAX. 508/992–3006

Hammersmith House Nursing Care Center, 73 Chestnut Street, Saugus, MA 01906; tel. 781/233–8123; FAX. 781/231–2918

Hancock Park Rehabilitation and Nursing Center, 164 Parkingway, Quincy, MA 02169; tel. 617/773–4222; FAX. 617/773–1115; Mr. Richard Coughlin

Hannah Duston Healthcare Center, 126 Monument Street, Haverhill, MA 01832; tel. 978/373–1747; FAX. 978/373–5277; Mr. Leo Curtin

Harbor House Rehabilitation and Nursing Center, 11 Condito Road, Hingham, MA 02043; tel. 781/749–4774; FAX. 781/749–6881; Ms. Susan Jessup

Harborlights Rehabilitation and Nursing Center, 804 East 7th Street, South Boston, MA 02127; tel. 617/268–8968; FAX. 617/268–4616; Mr. Paul Shannon

Harborside Healthcare Danvers Twin Oaks, 63 Locust Street, Danvers, MA 01923; tel. 978/777–0011; FAX. 978/774–2886; Mr. Gary C DiPietro

Harborside Healthcare Falmouth Rehabilitation and Nursing, 359 Jones Road, Falmouth, MA 02540; tel. 508/457–9000; FAX. 508/548–6903; Mr. John L Bonfardeci

Harborside Healthcare-Mashpee, 161 Falmouth Road, Mashpee, MA 02649; tel. 508/477–2490; FAX. 508/477–9656; Mr. Robert David Theroux

Harrington House Nursing and Rehabilitation Center, 160 Main Street, Walpole, MA 02081; tel. 508/660–3080; FAX. 508/660–1634; Mr. Anthony D Lacke

Hathaway Manor, ECF, 863 Hathaway Road, New Bedford, MA 02740; tel. 508/996–6763; FAX. 508/996–8596; Mr. Paul Marois

Hellenic Rehabilitation and Nursing Center, 601 Sherman Street, Canton, MA 02021-2053; tel. 781/828–7450; FAX. 781/828–0244; Mr. Brian Hurley

Heritage Hall East Center, 464 Main Street, Agawam, MA 01001; tel. 413/821–0753; FAX. 413/789–1099; Mr. Bryan Morgan Rossano

Heritage Hall North, 55 Cooper Street, Agawam, MA 01001; tel. 413/821–0751; FAX. 413/789–4739; Ms. Elizabeth Stroshine

Heritage Hall South, 65 Cooper Street, Agawam, MA 01001; tel. 413/786–8000; FAX. 413/306–6401; Mr. Ira Schoenberger

Heritage Hall West - Genesis HealthCare, 61 Cooper Street, Agawam, MA 01001; tel. 413/786–8000; FAX. 413/786–5066; Ms. Pamela Klapproth

Heritage Nursing Care Center, 841 Merrimack Street, Lowell, MA 01854; tel. 978/459–0546; FAX. 978/970–0715; Ms. Elizabeth Rozzi

Highgate Manor, 10 CareMatrix Drive, Dedham, MA 02026; tel. 781/461–9663; FAX. 781/461–9680

Highlander Nursing LLC, 1748 Highland Avenue, Fall River, MA 02720; tel. 508/730–1070; FAX. 508/730–2033; Mr. Kenneth Persinko

Hillcrest Commons, 169 Valentine Road, Pittsfield, MA 01201; tel. 413/445–2300; FAX. 413/445–2306; Mr. William Kittler

Hillcrest Nursing Center, 94 Summer Street, Fitchburg, MA 01420; tel. 978/343–3530; FAX. 978/343–6473

Holy Trinity Nursing and Rehabilitation Center, 300 Barber Avenue, Worcester, MA 01606; tel. 508/852–1000; FAX. 508/854–1622; Ms. Karen Laganelli

Holyoke Rehabilitation Center, 260 Easthampton Road, Holyoke, MA 01040; tel. 413/538–9733; FAX. 413/538–9919; Mr. Kevin Breslin

JAC S OPS IV inc, 184 Mansfield Avenue, Norton, MA 02766; tel. 508/285–7745; FAX. 508/285–5541; Mr. Jefferey Aframe

Jewish Geriatric Services, Inc, 770 Converse Street, Longmeadow, MA 01106; tel. 413/567–3949; FAX. 413/567–0175; Mr. Alan Rosenfeld

Jewish Healthcare Center, Inc., 629 Salisbury Street, Worcester, MA 01609; tel. 508/798–8653; FAX. 508/753–2668; Mr. Steven Willens

Jewish Rehabilitation Center for Aged of the North Shore, 330 Paradise Road, Swampscott, MA 01907; tel. 781/598–5310; FAX. 781/581–8021; Mr. Stephen H Neff

JML Care Center, Inc., 184 Ter Heun Drive, Falmouth, MA 02540-2503; tel. 508/457–4621; FAX. 508/457–1218; Mr. Charles Peterman

John Scott House Rehabilitation and Nursing Center, 233 Middle Street, Braintree, MA 02184; tel. 781/843–1860; FAX. 781/843–8834; Mr. Thomas D. Nolan

Kimball Farms Nursing Care Center, 40 Sunset Avenue, Lenox, MA 01240; tel. 413/637–5011; FAX. 413/637–0421; Ms. Sandy Shepard

Knollwood Nursing Center, 87 Briarwood Circle, Worcester, MA 01606; tel. 508/853–6910; FAX. 508/856–0112; Mr. Paul Bowler

Lanessa Extended Care, 751 School Street, Webster, MA 01570; tel. 508/949–1334; FAX. 508/943–6628; Mrs. Joanne M. Bruell

Laurel Lake Health and Rehabilitation, LLC, 620 Laurel Street, Lee, MA 01238; tel. 413/243–2010; FAX. 413/243–4288; Mr. Dan Larouche

Ledgewood Rehabilitation and Skilled Nursing Center, 87 Herrick Street, Beverly, MA 01915; tel. 978/921–1392; FAX. 978/927–8627; Ms. Laurie A Roberto

Leo P. LaChance Center for Rehabilitation and Nursing, 59 Eastwood Circle, Gardner, MA 01440; tel. 978/632–8776; FAX. 978/632–5048; Mr. Dennis P. Lopata

Lexington Health Care Center, 178 Lowell St., Lexington, MA 02420; tel. 781/862–7400; FAX. 781/862–3332; Mr. Michael Flaherty

Life Care Center of Acton, One Great Road, Acton, MA 01720; tel. 978/263–9101; FAX. 978/263–3278; Mr. Mark P Presutti

Life Care Center of Attleboro, 969 Park Street, Attleboro, MA 02703; tel. 508/222–4182; FAX. 508/226–0457; Mr. Patrick O'Connor

Life Care Center of Auburn, 14 Masonic Circle, Auburn, MA 01501; tel. 508/832–4800; FAX. 508/832–0631; Mr. James A. Nugent

Life Care Center of Leominster, 370 West Street, Leominster, MA 01453; tel. 978/537–0771; FAX. 978/534–0824

Life Care Center of Merrimack Valley, 80 Boston Road, North Billerica, MA 01862; tel. 978/667–2166; FAX. 978/670–5625; Ms. Colleen Lovering

Life Care Center of Nashoba Valley, 191 Foster Street, Littleton, MA 01460; tel. 978/486–3512; FAX. 978/486–8850; Ms. Ellen Levinson

Life Care Center of Plymouth, 94 Obery Street, Plymouth, MA 02360; tel. 508/747–9800; FAX. 508/747–2278; Ms. Mary M Schroeder
Life Care Center of Raynham, 546 South Street East, Raynham, MA 02767; tel. 508/821–5700; FAX. 508/821–5780; Mr. Michael Gallagher
Life Care Center of Stoneham, 25 Woodland Road, Stoneham, MA 02180; tel. 781/662–2545; FAX. 781/662–7775
Life Care Center of the North Shore, 111 Birch Street, Lynn, MA 01902; tel. 781/592–9667; FAX. 781/599–6590; Mr. Joseph Deveau
Life Care Center of the South Shore, PO Box 830, Scituate, MA 02066; tel. 781/545–1370; FAX. 781/545–2198; Mr. Geoff Rauch
Life Care Center of West Bridgewater, 765 West Center Street, West Bridgewater, MA 02379; tel. 508/580–4400; FAX. 508/580–2412; Mr. Alan J. Richman
Life Care Center of Wilbraham, 2399 Boston Road, Wilbraham, MA 01095; tel. 413/596–3111; FAX. 413/596–9072; Mr. Andrew Hastie
Linda Manor Extended Care Facility, 349 Haydenville Road, Leeds, MA 01053; tel. 413/586–7700; FAX. 413/586–8137; Ms. Michelle Wuest
Lowell Health Care Center, 19 Varnum Street, Lowell, MA 01850; tel. 978/454–5644; FAX. 978/459–6520; Mr. Mark O'Flaherty
Madonna Manor, Inc., 85 North Washington Street, North Attleboro, MA 02760; tel. 508/699–2740; FAX. 508/699–0481; Rev. Edmund J Fitzgerald
Marian Manor, Inc., 33 Summer Street, Taunton, MA 02780; tel. 508/822–4885; FAX. 508/880–3386; Rev. Edmund J. Fitzgerald
Marina Bay Skilled Nursing and Rehabilitation Center, 2 Seaport Drive, Quincy, MA 02171; tel. 617/769–5100; FAX. 617/786–8812; Ms. Rosemary McLaughlin
Maristhill Nursing & Rehabilitation Center, 66 Newton Street, Waltham, MA 02453; tel. 781/893–0240; FAX. 781/894–6330; Ms. Carolyn Fenn
Marlborough Hills Healthcare Center, 121 Northboro Road, East, Marlborough, MA 01752; tel. 508/485–4040; FAX. 508/481–5585; Mr. Michael Lincoln
Mary Ann Morse Nursing and Rehabilitation Center, 45 Union Street, Natick, MA 01760; tel. 508/650–9003; FAX. 508/650–9209; Ms. Lisa Kubiak
Mary Lyon Nursing and Rehabilitation Center, 34 Main Street, Hampden, MA 01036; tel. 413/566–5511; FAX. 413/566–8488; Mr. Steven J Tyer
Masconomet Healthcare Center, 123 High Street, Topsfield, MA 01983-1926; tel. 978/887–7002; FAX. 978/887–4093; Dr. Alfred L Arcidi
Masonic Home, Inc., PO Box 1000, Charlton, MA 01507-1000; tel. 508/248–7344; FAX. 508/248–0119; Mr. David C. Turner
Mayflower Place Nursing and Rehabilitation Center, 579 Buck Island Road, W Yarmouth, MA 02673; tel. 508/957–7007; FAX. 508/790–8116; Ms. Cathy S Sawyer
Meadow Green Nursing and Rehabilitation Center, 45 Woburn Street, Waltham, MA 02452; tel. 781/899–8600; FAX. 781/899–3124; Mr. David L. Bell
Medway Country Manor Skilled Nursing and Rehabilitation, 115 Holliston Street, Medway, MA 02053; tel. 508/533–6634; FAX. 508/533–7048; Mr. John Peters
Millbury Health Care Center, 312 Millbury Avenue, Millbury, MA 01527; tel. 508/793–0088; FAX. 508/793–1671; Mr. Scott Bullock
Milton Health Care, 1200 Brush Hill Road, Milton, MA 02186; tel. 617/333–0600; FAX. 617/361–8175; Mr. Rob Grady
Mount Saint Vincent Care Center, 35 Holy Family Road, Holyoke, MA 01040; tel. 413/532–3246; FAX. 413/532–0309; Mr. Christopher McLaughlin
Mt. Greylock Extended Care Facility, 1000 North Street, Pittsfield, MA 01201; tel. 413/499–7186; FAX. 413/499–3086; Mrs. Maria T. Craft
Nemasket Healthcare Center, 314 Marion Road, Middleboro, MA 02346; tel. 508/947–8632; FAX. 508/947–9600; Dr. Alfred L. Arcidi
Neville Center at Fresh Pond for Nursing and Rehabilitation, 640 Concord Ave., Cambridge, MA 02138; tel. 617/430–0600; FAX. 617/497–4447; Adm. Gregory Karr
New Bedford Health Care Center, 221 Fitzgerald Drive, New Bedford, MA 02745; tel. 508/996–4600; FAX. 508/998–3047; Mr. Albert E Crabtree
New Bedford Jewish Convalescent Home, Inc., 200 Hawthorn Street, New Bedford, MA 02740; tel. 508/997–9314; FAX. 508/996–3664; Mrs. Carol A Trudeau
New Bedford Operating Co. LLC, 4586 Acushnet Avenue, New Bedford, MA 02745; tel. 508/998–1188; FAX. 508/985–0287; Mr. John H Keeney
New England Pediatric Care, 78 Boston Road, North Billerica, MA 01862; tel. 978/667–5123; FAX. 978/663–5154; Ms. Ellen J. O'Gorman
Newton Health Care Center, 2101 Washington Street, Newton Lower Falls, MA 02462; tel. 617/969–4660; FAX. 617/964–4622; Mr. Daniel Straus
North Adams Commons, 175 Franklin Street, North Adams, MA 01247; tel. 413/664–4041; FAX. 413/664–1027; Ms. Sandra Cunningham
North End Rehabilitation & Nursing Center, 70 Fulton Street, Boston, MA 02109; tel. 617/726–9701; FAX. 617/726–9911; Mr. Justin D Verge
Northampton VA Medical Center, 421 North Main Street, Leeds, MA 01053-9764; tel. 413/584–4040; FAX. 413/582–3121; Ms. Mary A Dowling
Oak Knoll Healthcare Center, 9 Arbetter Drive, Framingham, MA 01701; tel. 508/877–3300; FAX. 508/788–0079; Ms. Kimberly Grasso
Oakwood Rehabilitation and Nursing Center, 11 Pontiac Avenue, Webster, MA 01570; tel. 508/943–3889; FAX. 508/949–6125; Mr. George Mercier
Our Lady's Haven of Fairhaven, Inc., 71 Center Street, Fairhaven, MA 02719; tel. 508/999–4561; FAX. 508/997–0254; Rev. Edmund J Fitzgerald
Palm Manor Nursing Center, 40 Parkhurst Road, Chelmsford, MA 01824; tel. 978/256–3151; FAX. 978/250–4942; Ms. Andrea Rathbone
Park Avenue Nursing and Rehabilitation Center, 146 Park Avenue, Arlington, MA 02476; tel. 781/648–9530; FAX. 781/646–3668; Mr. John J. Alessandroni
Parsons Hill Nursing and Rehabiltation Center, 1350 Main Street, Worcester, MA 01603; tel. 508/791–4200; FAX. 508/459–4567; Mr. Rick Kravetz
Peabody Glen Health Care Center, 199 Andover Street, Peabody, MA 01960; tel. 978/531–0772; FAX. 978/532–4134
Pilgrim Rehabilitation and Skilled Nursing Center, 96 Forest Street, Peabody, MA 01960-3907; tel. 978/532–0303; FAX. 978/531–6112; Mrs. Tara Gibney
Poet's Seat Health Care Center, 359 High Street, Greenfield, MA 01301; tel. 413/774–6318; FAX. 413/773–0060; Mr. Patrick McManus
Prescott House, 140 Prescott Street, North Andover, MA 01845; tel. 978/685–8086; FAX. 978/687–2665; Mr. Chris Sintros
Presentation Nursing and Rehabilitation Center, 10 Bellamy Street, Brighton, MA 02135; tel. 617/782–8113; FAX. 617/787–7775; Mr. Tim Churchill
Providence Care Center of Lenox, 320 Pittsfield Road, Lenox, MA 01240; tel. 413/637–2660; FAX. 413/637–3085; Mr. Robert Post
Quabbin Valley Healthcare, 821 Daniel Shays Highway, Athol, MA 01331; tel. 978/249–3717; FAX. 978/575–1431
Queen Anne Nursing Home, Inc., 50 Recreation Park Drive, Hingham, MA 02043; tel. 781/749–4982; FAX. 781/740–4283; Mrs. Kristen Lundin
Quincy Rehabilitation and Nursing Center, 11 McGrath Highway, Quincy, MA 02169-5311; tel. 617/479–2820; FAX. 617/471–5226; Mr. Armand Traino
Radius Healthcare Center at Danvers, 56 Liberty Street, Danvers, MA 01923; tel. 978/777–2700; FAX. 978/777–2372; Mr. Scott Stone
Radius HealthCare Center at Millbury, 29 Main Street, Millbury, MA 01527; tel. 508/865–6106; FAX. 508/865–3944; Mrs. Joann McCarron
Radius HealthCare Center at Southbridge, 84 Chapin Street Suite 84, Southbridge, MA 01550; tel. 508/765–9133; FAX. 508/765–9228; Mr. Paul Knutsen
Radius HealthCare Center at Worcester, 119 Providence Street, Worcester, MA 01604; tel. 508/860–5000; FAX. 508/860–5109; Mr. Daniel Mitchell
Radius Mayflower Operating LLC, 123 South Street, Plymouth, MA 02360; tel. 508/746–4343; FAX. 508/732–0160; Mr. Matt Muratore
Radius Northwood HealthCare Center, 1010 Varnum Avenue, Lowell, MA 01854; tel. 978/458–8773; FAX. 978/458–6366; Mr. Jim Dillon
Redstone Rehabilitation and Nursing Center, 135 Benton Drive, East Longmeadow, MA 01028; tel. 413/525–3336; FAX. 413/525–9814; Mr. Michael Rivers
Redstone Rehabilitation and Nursing Center, 135 Benton Drive, East Longmeadow, MA 01028; tel. 413/525–3336; FAX. 413/525–9814; Mr. Michael Rivers
Renaissance Manor of Westfield, 37 Feeding Hills Road, Westfield, MA 01085; tel. 413/568–2341; FAX. 413/572–1226; Mr. Michael Stroetzel
Ring HealthCare Center, 215 Bicentennial Highway, Springfield, MA 01118; tel. 413/796–7511; FAX. 413/783–4020; Mr. Steven J Tyer
River Terrace Healthcare, 1675 Main Street, Lancaster, MA 01523; tel. 978/365–4537; FAX. 978/365–4546; Mr. John Danforth
Rosewood Nursing and Rehabilitation Center, 22 Johnson Street, Peabody, MA 01960; tel. 978/535–8700; FAX. 978/535–2300; Mr. Paul B. Mahoney
Royal Nursing Center, 545 Main Street, Falmouth, MA 02540; tel. 508/548–3800; FAX. 508/548–6936; Mr. James Mamary
Sachem Skilled Nursing and Rehab Center, 66 Central Street, East Bridgewater, MA 02333; tel. 508/378–7227
Sacred Heart Home, Inc., 359 Summer Street, New Bedford, MA 02740; tel. 508/996–6751; FAX. 508/992–3145; Rev. Edmund J. Fitzgerald
Sancta Maria Nursing Facility, 799 Concord Avenue, Cambridge, MA 02138; tel. 617/868–2200; FAX. 617/864–2801; Sister Mary Mark Pizzotti
Sarah S. Brayton Nursing Care Center, 4901 North Main Street, Fall River, MA 02720; tel. 508/675–1001; FAX. 508/675–1088; Adm. Jeffrey A Govoni
Seacoast Nursing and Rehabilitation Center, 292 Washington Street, Gloucester, MA 01930; tel. 978/283–0300; FAX. 978/281–6774; Mr. Stan Trocki
Senior Residential Care/South Hadley, LLC, 573 Granby Road, South Hadley, MA 01075; tel. 413/532–2200; FAX. 413/534–8796; Mr. Scott Schuster
Shaughnessy - Kaplan Rehabilitation Hospital, Dove Avenue, Salem, MA 01970; tel. 978/825–8500; FAX. 978/741–1967; Ms. Maureen Banks
Sherrill House, Inc., 135 South Huntington Avenue, Boston, MA 02130; tel. 617/731–2400; FAX. 617/731–8671; Mr. Patrick Stapleton
Sippican Healthcare Center, 15 Mill Street, Marion, MA 02738; tel. 508/748–3830; FAX. 508/748–3834; Dr. Alfred L Arcidi
Soldiers' Home in Holyoke, 110 Cherry Street, Holyoke, MA 01040; tel. 413/532–9475; FAX. 413/538–7968; Mr. Michael J. Pasterczyk
Somerset Ridge Nursing Center, 455 Brayton Ave., Somerset, MA 02725; tel. 508/679–2240; FAX. 508/679–2983; Mr. Gilbert C Reis
Southeast Rehabilitation and Nursing Center, 184 Lincoln Street, North Easton, MA 02356; tel. 508/238–7053; FAX. 508/238–7049; Ms. Patrick Sheehan
Southpointe Rehabilitation and Skilled Care Center, 100 Amity Street, Fall River, MA 02721; tel. 508/675–2500; FAX. 508/675–8874; Mr. Barry Freid
Southwood at Norwell Nursing Center, 501 Cordwainer Drive, Norwell, MA 02061; tel. 781/982–7450; FAX. 781/982–7451; Mr. Richard H. Starr
Springfield Park View Hospital, LLC, 1400 State Street, Springfield, MA 01109; tel. 413/726–6700; FAX. 413/726–6704
St. Camillus Health Center, 447 Hill Street, Whitinsville, MA 01588; tel. 508/234–7306; FAX. 508/234–7597; Mr. William Graves
Sterling Healthcare Center, 18 Dana Hill Road, Sterling, MA 01564; tel. 978/422–5111; FAX. 978/422–5925; Ms. Rosemary Carlson
Sudbury Pines Extended Care Facility, 642 Boston Post Road, Sudbury, MA 01776; tel. 978/443–9000; FAX. 978/443–9510; Ms. Roberta C. Henderson
SunBridge Care and Rehabilitation for Milford, 10 Veterans Memorial Drive, Milford, MA 01757; tel. 508/473–6414; FAX. 508/473–9974; Mr. Michael Isabella

SunBridge Healthcare Corporation, PO Box 720 20 North Maple Street, Hadley, MA 01035; tel. 413/584–5057; FAX. 413/584–3736; Ms. Karen Crafa
Sweet Brook Transitional Care and Living Centers, 1561 Cold Spring Road, Williamstown, MA 01267; tel. 413/458–8127; FAX. 413/458–8209; Ms. Susan Gancarz
The Boston Center For Rehabilitative & Subacute Care, 1245 Centre Street, Roslindale, MA 02131; tel. 617/325–5400; FAX. 617/363–9971; Ms. Christine Reilly
The Eliot Health Care Center, 168 W. Central Street, Natick, MA 01760; tel. 508/655–1000; FAX. 508/655–5838; Ms. Joyce Sears-Whitbeck
The Ellis Nursing and Rehabilitation Center, 135 Ellis Avenue, Norwood, MA 02062; tel. 781/762–6880; FAX. 781/769–0482; Mr. Anthony A Franchi
The Goddard Rehabilitation and Nursing Center, 909 Sumner Street, Stoughton, MA 02072; tel. 781/297–8200; FAX. 781/297–8615; Ms. Diane Dickerman
The Highlands, 335 Nichols Road, Fitchburg, MA 01420; tel. 978/343–4411; FAX. 978/343–5370; Mr. Jeff Martin
The Lafayette Convalescent Home, 25 Lafayette Street, Marblehead, MA 01945; tel. 781/631–4535; FAX. 781/631–6400; Mr. George Barbuzzi
The Meadows Skilled Nursing and Rehabilitation Center, 111 Huntoon Memorial Highway, Rochdale, MA 01542; tel. 508/892–4858; FAX. 508/892–4857; Mr. Gerald Shaffer
The Neuro-Rehabilitation Center at Middleboro, 23 Isaac Street, Middleboro, MA 02346-2080; tel. 508/947–9295; FAX. 508/947–7974
The Oaks Nursing Center, 4525 Acushnet Avenue, New Bedford, MA 02745; tel. 508/998–7807; FAX. 508/998–8865; Mr. Robert G. Noonan
The Oxford, 689 Main Street, Haverhill, MA 01830; tel. 978/373–1131; FAX. 978/373–3074; Mr. John Holt
Tower Hill Center for Health and Rehabilitation, One Meadowbrook Way, Canton, MA 02021; tel. 781/961–5600; FAX. 781/961–5688; Mrs. Jennifer Conley
Town & Country Nursing Center, 259 Baldwin Avenue, Lowell, MA 01851; tel. 978/454–5438; FAX. 978/970–3692; Mr. Norman Michaud
University Commons Nursing Care Center, 378 Plantation Street, Worcester, MA 01605; tel. 508/755–7300; FAX. 508/799–9907; Mr. James V Divver
VA Boston Healthcare System, 1400 VFW Parkway, West Roxbury, MA 02132; tel. 617/323–7700; FAX. 857/203–5500; Mr. Michael M. Lawson
Waban Health Skilled Nursing and Rehabilitation, 20 Kinmonth Road, Newton, MA 02468; tel. 617/332–8481; FAX. 617/332–8959; Mr. James Sullivan
Wachusett Extended Care Facility, 56 Boyden Road, Holden, MA 01520; tel. 508/829–5555; FAX. 508/829–1221; Ms. Sandra L Bauer Mahoney
Walden Rehabilitation and Nursing Center, 785 Main Street, Concord, MA 01742; tel. 978/369–6889; FAX. 978/369–8392; Ms. Phoebe Loyer
We Do Care, Inc. dba Carlyle House, 342 Winter Street, Framingham, MA 01702; tel. 508/879–6100; FAX. 508/872–1253; Mr. J. Dennis Morgan
Webster Manor, 745 School Street, Webster, MA 01570; tel. 508/949–0644; FAX. 508/949–0647; Mr. Michael B. Lincoln
Westborough Health Care Center, 5 Colonial Drive, Westborough, MA 01581; tel. 508/366–9131; FAX. 508/836–3869; Mr. David Morrall
Westford House, 3 Park Drive, Westford, MA 01886; tel. 978/392–1144; FAX. 978/392–0032; Mr. Donald Schwarz
Weymouth Health Care Center, 64 Performance Drive, Weymouth, MA 02189; tel. 781/340–9800; FAX. 781/340–1771; Ms. Lisa Marie Coppola
Willow Manor Genesis ElderCare, 30 Princeton Boulevard, Lowell, MA 01851; tel. 978/454–8086; FAX. 978/453–9772; Mr. Frank J McGuire
Willowood of Williamstown, 25 Adams Road, Williamstown, MA 01267; tel. 413/458–2111; FAX. 413/458–4907; Mr. J. Michael Rivers
Wilmington Health Care Center, 750 Woburn Street, Wilmington, MA 01887; tel. 978/988–0888; FAX. 978/658–6470; Ms. Joanne H. Carbone
Winchester Nursing Center, Inc, 223 Swanton Street, Winchester, MA 01890; tel. 781/729–9595; FAX. 781/721–2966; Ms. Shelley S. King
Windsor Skilled Nursing and Rehabilitation Center, 265 North Main Street, South Yarmouth, MA 02664; tel. 508/394–3514; FAX. 508/394–9360; Mr. Thomas P. Coffey
Wingate at Andover, 80 Andover Street, Andover, MA 01810; tel. 978/470–3434; FAX. 978/470–0098; Ms. Diane Tessier
Wingate at Brighton, Inc., 100 North Beacon Street, Boston, MA 02134; tel. 617/787–2300; FAX. 617/787–1539
Wingate at East Longmeadow Rehabilitative & Skilled Nursing, 32 Chestnut Street, East Longmeadow, MA 01028; tel. 413/525–1893; FAX. 413/525–8261; Mr. Steven Tyer
Wingate at Needham, 589 Highland Avenue, Needham, MA 02492; tel. 781/455–9090; FAX. 781/455–9012; Mr. Stephen Davis
Wingate at Reading, 1364 Main Street, Reading, MA 01867; tel. 781/942–1210; FAX. 781/942–7251; Ms. Anne L. Pelrine
Wingate at Silver Lake, 17 Chipman Way, Kingston, MA 02364; tel. 781/585–4100; FAX. 781/585–1651; Ms. Elinor Black
Wingate at Sudbury, Inc., 136 Boston Post Road, Sudbury, MA 01776; tel. 978/443–2722; FAX. 978/443–2711; Mr. Steven J. Tyer
Wingate at West Springfield, 42 Prospect Avenue, West Springfield, MA 01089; tel. 413/733–3151; FAX. 413/731–9984; Mr. Steven J Tyer
Wingate at Wilbraham, 9 Maple Street, Wilbraham, MA 01095; tel. 413/596–2411; FAX. 413/599–1738; Mr. Steven Tyer
Woodbriar of Wilmington Rehab and Skilled Nursing Center, 90 West Street, Wilmington, MA 01887; tel. 978/658–2700; FAX. 978/657–0015; Mr. Dennis S Sargent
Worcester Skilled Care Center, 59 Acton Street, Worcester, MA 01604; tel. 508/791–3147; FAX. 508/753–6267; Mr. Joel R Stevens

MICHIGAN
Aleda E. Lutz VA Medical Ctr., 1500 Weiss Street, Saginaw, MI 48602; tel. 989/497–2500; FAX. 989/791–2428; Mr. Gabriel Perez
Chippewa County War Memorial Hospital, Inc, 500 Osborn Boulevard, Sault Sainte Marie, MI 49783; tel. 906/635–4460; FAX. 906/635–4467; Mr. David Jahn
Father Murray Nursing Center, 8444 Engleman, Center Line, MI 48015; tel. 586/755–2400; FAX. 586/757–8657; Mr. Michael C Richards
Helen Newberry Joy Hospital, 502 West Harrie Street, Newberry, MI 49868; tel. 906/293–9222; FAX. 906/293–9208; Mr. Wayne Hellerstedt
John D. Dingell VA Medical Center, 4646 John R, Detroit, MI 48201; tel. 313/576–1000; FAX. 313/576–1191
Life Care Center of Plainwell, 320 Brigham Street, Plainwell, MI 49080; tel. 269/688–9805; FAX. 269/685–8542; Ms. Linda Potter
Maple Manor Rehab Center, 3999 Venoy Road, Wayne, MI 48184; tel. 734/727–0440; FAX. 734/727–0441; Dr. Stella Evangelista
Marlette Regional Hospital, PO Box 307, Marlette, MI 48453-0307; tel. 989/635–4000; FAX. 989/635–5358; Mr. David S McEwen
Rivergate Health Care Center, 14041 Pennsylvania Road, Riverview, MI 48192; tel. 734/284–7200; FAX. 734/284–9027; Ms. Regina Casabal
Rivergate Terrace, 14141 Pennsylvania Road, Riverview, MI 48192; tel. 734/284–8000; FAX. 734/284–0333; Mr. John Polturanus
Special Tree NeuroCare Center, 39000 Chase Road, Romulus, MI 48174; tel. 734/941–1142; FAX. 734/941–7522; Ms. Cathy A Blevins
Spectrum Health United Memorial, 615 South Bower Street, Greenville, MI 48838; tel. 616/225–6409; FAX. 616/397–3184; Mr. Paul Bonis
St. John Senior Community, 18300 East Warren Avenue, Detroit, MI 48224; tel. 313/343–8000; FAX. 313/343–8959; Ms. Julie Kaslly
VA Ann Arbor Healthcare System, 2215 Fuller Road, Ann Arbor, MI 48105; tel. 734/769–7100; FAX. 734/769–7148; Ms. Lou Ann Atkins
VA Medical Center, 325 East H Street, Iron Mountain, MI 49801; tel. 906/774–3300; FAX. 906/779–3188; Mr. Michael J Murphy
VA Medical Center, 5500 Armstrong Road, Battle Creek, MI 49015; tel. 269/966–5600; FAX. 269/223–6046; Mr. Tony Zapata

MINNESOTA
Bureau of Prisons - FMC Rochester, PO Box 4600, Rochester, MN 55903; tel. 507/287–0674; FAX. 507/287–9601; Mr. Duke Terrell
Fairmont Medical Center - Mayo Health System, 800 Medical Center Drive, Fairmont, MN 56031; tel. 507/238–8100; FAX. 507/238–8686; Dr. Barbara L Allen
Lake City Medical Center-Mayo Health System, 500 West Grant Street, Lake City, MN 55041; tel. 651/345–3321; FAX. 651/345–1182; Dr. Thomas J. Witt
St. Cloud VA Medical Center, 4801 8th Street North, Saint Cloud, MN 56303; tel. 320/255–6480; FAX. 320/255–6426; Mr. Barry I Bahl
VA Medical Center - Minneapolis, One Veterans Drive, Minneapolis, MN 55417; tel. 612/725–2000; FAX. 612/725–2049; Mr. Steve Kleinglass

MISSISSIPPI
Mississippi State Hospital, PO Box 157-A, Whitfield, MS 39193-0157; tel. 601/351–8000; FAX. 601/351–8326; Mr. James G. Chastain
North Mississippi Medical Center, Inc., 830 South Gloster Street, Tupelo, MS 38801; tel. 662/377–3837; FAX. 662/377–2348; Mr. Charles D Stokes
Pontotoc Health Services, Inc., PO Box 790, Pontotoc, MS 38863-0790; tel. 662/488–7670; FAX. 662/488–7675
VA Gulf Coast Veterans Health Care System, 400 Veterans Avenue, Biloxi, MS 39531; tel. 228/523–4206; FAX. 228/523–4996; Mr. Charles Sepich
VA Medical Center - G. V. (Sonny) Montgomery, 1500 East Woodrow Wilson Avenue, Jackson, MS 39216; tel. 601/364–1201; FAX. 601/364–1359; Mr. Richard J Baltz
Webster Health Services, Inc., 70 Medical Plaza, Eupora, MS 39744; tel. 662/258–9341; FAX. 662/258–9291; Mr. Bob Jones

MISSOURI
Barnes-Jewish Hospital, 4905 Forest Park, Mailstop 90-75-501, Saint Louis, MO 63108; tel. 314/747–3000; FAX. 314/454–5302; Dr. Andrew A. Ziskind
Bethesda Health Group, Inc Bethesda Southgate, 1630 Des Peres Road, Saint Louis, MO 63131; tel. 314/846–2000; FAX. 314/800–1961; Mr. John W. Rowe
Bethesda Health Group, Inc dba Bethesda Meadow, 1630 Des Peres Road, Saint Louis, MO 63131; tel. 636/227–3431; FAX. 314/800–1961; Mr. John W. Rowe
Bethesda Health Group, Inc. dba Bethesda Dilworth, 1630 Des Peres Road, Saint Louis, MO 63131; tel. 314/968–5460; FAX. 314/968–5253; Mr. John W. Rowe
Excelsior Springs City Hospital, 1700 Rainbow Boulevard, Excelsior Springs, MO 64024; tel. 816/630–6091; FAX. 816/629–2713; Ms. Sally S Nance
Harry S. Truman Memorial Veterans' Hospital, 800 Hospital Drive, Columbia, MO 65201; tel. 573/814–6000; FAX. 573/814–6600; Mrs. Sallie Houser-Hanfelder
John J. Pershing VA Medical Center, 1500 North Westwood Boulevard, Poplar Bluff, MO 63901; tel. 573/686–4151; FAX. 573/778–4699; Ms. Nancy C. Arnold
Lester E. Cox Medical Centers, 1423 North Jefferson Avenue, Springfield, MO 65802; tel. 417/269–3000; FAX. 417/269–4104; Mr. Robert H Bezanson
Life Care Center of Waynesville, 700 Birch Lane, Waynesville, MO 65583; tel. 573/774–6456; FAX. 573/774–6778; Adm. MaryAnn Bonomolo
Life Care Center of Bridgeton, 12145 Bridge Square Dr., Bridgeton, MO 63044; tel. 314/298–7444; FAX. 314/298–7456; Ms. Deborah Bland
Life Care Center of Brookfield, 315 Hunt Street, Brookfield, MO 64628; tel. 660/258–3367; FAX. 660/258–3903; Mr. Michael K Young
Life Care Center of Cape Girardeau, 2852 Independence Street, Cape Girardeau, MO 63703; tel. 573/335–2086; FAX. 573/335–2398; Ms. Margaret Green
Life Care Center of Carrollton, 300 Life Care Lane, Carrollton, MO 64633; tel. 660/542–0155; FAX. 660/542–0032; Mrs. Lynn Hayes
Life Care Center of Grandview, 6301 East 125th Street, Grandview, MO 64030; tel. 816/765–7714; FAX. 816/765–5272; Mr. Jerry Lindenbaum

Life Care Center of Saint Louis, 3520 Chouteau Avenue, Saint Louis, MO 63129; tel. 314/771–2100; FAX. 314/771–7667; Ms. Arlen Davidson
Life Care Center of Sullivan, 875 Dunsford Drive, Sullivan, MO 63080; tel. 573/468–3128; FAX. 573/860–3196; Ms. Luana Indelicato
Northwood Hills Care Center LLC, PO Box 187, Humansville, MO 65674; tel. 417/754–2208; FAX. 417/754–8092; Mr. Bobby Frank Reed
The Westchester House, 550 White Road, Chesterfield, MO 63017; tel. 314/469–1200; FAX. 314/469–7512; Ms. Kristin Shambro
Truman Medical Center, 2301 Holmes Street, Kansas City, MO 64108; tel. 816/404–1000; FAX. 816/404–0572; Mr. John Bluford
U.S. Medical Center for Federal Prisoners, 1900 West Sunshine Street, Springfield, MO 65807; tel. 417/862–7041; FAX. 417/837–1721; Mr. Marty C Anderson
VA Medical Center, 915 North Grand Boulevard, Saint Louis, MO 63106; tel. 314/289–7020; FAX. 314/289–7602; Mr. Glen E Struchtemeyer

MONTANA
VA Montana Healthcare System, 1892 Williams St, Fort Harrison, MT 59636; tel. 406/447–7910; FAX. 406/447–7991; Mr. Joseph M. Underkofler

NEBRASKA
Life Care Center of Elkhorn, 20275 Hopper Street, Elkhorn, NE 68022; tel. 402/289–2572; FAX. 402/289–0925; Ms. Judy Sealer
Life Care Center of Omaha, 6032 Ville De Sante Drive, Omaha, NE 68104; tel. 402/571–6770; FAX. 402/571–6273; Ms. Kathy Scheele
VA Nebraska-Western Iowa Health Care System, 4101 Woolworth Avenue, Omaha, NE 68105; tel. 402/449–0600; FAX. 402/449–0684; Mr. Al Washko

NEVADA
Life Care Center of Las Vegas, 6151 Vegas Drive, Las Vegas, NV 89108; tel. 702/648–4900; FAX. 702/648–5227; Ms. Jeni A Terwilliger
Life Care Center of Paradise Valley, 2325 East Harmon, Las Vegas, NV 89119; tel. 702/798–7990; FAX. 702/798–9910; Ms. Jeni Terwilliger
Life Care Center of Reno, 445 West Holcomb Lane, Reno, NV 89511; tel. 775/851–0123; FAX. 775/851–3754; Ms. Machelle Harris
VA Sierra Nevada Health Care System, 1000 Locust Street, Reno, NV 89502-2597; tel. 775/786–7200; FAX. 775/328–1447; Dr. Kurt W. Schlegelmilch

NEW HAMPSHIRE
Good Shepherd Healthcare Center, 20 Plantation Drive, Jaffrey, NH 03452; tel. 603/532–8762; FAX. 603/532–6057; Mrs. Ann E. Nunn
Mount Carmel Healthcare Center, 235 Myrtle Street, Manchester, NH 03104; tel. 603/627–3811; FAX. 603/626–4696; Mr. Ted J. Purdy
Rochester Manor, 40 Whitehall Road, Rochester, NH 03867; tel. 603/332–7711; FAX. 603/332–0854; Ms. Mary P Flynn
Saint Ann Healthcare Center, 195 Dover Point Road, Dover, NH 03820; tel. 603/742–2612; FAX. 603/743–3055; Mrs. Karyn J. Partin
Saint Francis Rehabilitation and Nursing Center, 406 Court Street, Laconia, NH 03246; tel. 603/524–0466; FAX. 603/527–0884; Mrs. Brenda Lynn Buttrick
Saint Teresa Healthcare Center, 519 Bridge Street, Manchester, NH 03104; tel. 603/668–2373; FAX. 603/668–0059; Mr. Joe Bohunicky
Saint Vincent de Paul Healthcare Center, 29 Providence Avenue, Berlin, NH 03570; tel. 603/752–1820; FAX. 603/752–5766; Mrs. Louise L. Marquis
VA Medical Center, 718 Smyth Road, Manchester, NH 03104-4098; tel. 603/624–4366; FAX. 603/626–6576

NEW JERSEY
Absecon Manor Nursing and Rehabilitation Center, 1020 Pitney Road, Absecon, NJ 08201; tel. 609/646–5400; FAX. 609/645–9125; Ms. Tara Mullineaux
Bacharach Institute for Rehabilitation, PO Box 723, Pomona, NJ 08240-0723; tel. 609/748–5460; FAX. 609/652–7487; Dr. Richard Kathrins
Bartley Healthcare Nursing and Rehabilitation, 175 Bartley Road, Jackson, NJ 08527; tel. 732/370–4700; FAX. 732/370–8872; Mr. Philip Scalo
Bergen Regional Medical Center, 230 East Ridgewood Avenue, Paramus, NJ 07652; tel. 201/967–4000; FAX. 201/967–4014; Ms. Susan Mendelowitz
Bey Lea Village Care Center, 1351 Old Freehold Road, Toms River, NJ 08753-2795; tel. 732/240–0090; FAX. 732/244–8551; Mr. Mike Norbury
Camden County Health Services Center, 20 N. Woodbury Turnersville Road, Blackwood, NJ 08012; tel. 856/374–6500; FAX. 856/374–6520; Mr. Kevin Halpern
Daughters of Miriam Center, 155 Hazel Street, Clifton, NJ 07015; tel. 973/772–3700; FAX. 973/253–5389; Mr. Frank DaSilva
Forest Hill Healthcare Center, Inc., 497 Mount Prospect Ave., Newark, NJ 07104; tel. 973/482–5000; FAX. 973/482–6500; Dr. Richard G Stefanacci
Forkidcare LLC, 1304 Laurel Oak Road, Voorhees, NJ 08043; tel. 856/346–3300; FAX. 856/435–4223; Mr. Scott L. Goldberg
Franklin Care Center, 433 Hackensack Avenue, 8th Floor, Hackensack, NJ 07601; tel. 732/821–8000; FAX. 732/821–9253; Adm. John Pilek
Gateway Care Center, LLC, 139 Grant Avenue, Eatontown, NJ 07724; tel. 732/542–4700; FAX. 732/935–7509; Mr. Jonathan Rosenberg
Green Acres Manor, 1931 Lakewood Road, Route 9, Toms River, NJ 08755; tel. 732/286–2323; FAX. 732/240–4985; Ms. Maria Lapid
Hamilton Plaza Nursing and Rehabilitation Center, 56 Hamilton Avenue, Passaic, NJ 07055; tel. 973/773–7070; FAX. 973/773–3171; Mr. Stuart Lindeman
Innova Health and Rehab, 3718 Church Road, Mount Laurel, NJ 08054; tel. 856/235–7100; FAX. 856/235–6813; Ms. Dina Sottile
Jersey Shore Convalescent Center, 2050 Sixth Avenue, Neptune, NJ 07753-6197; tel. 732/774–8300; FAX. 732/774–0908; Mrs. Mary Lou Browning
JFK Hartwyck at Cedar Brook, 1340 Park Avenue, Plainfield, NJ 07060; tel. 908/754–3100; FAX. 908/754–3418; Ms. Aimee Allen
JFK Hartwyck at Edison Estates, 10 Brunswick Avenue, Edison, NJ 08817; tel. 732/985–1500; FAX. 732/572–3399; Ms. Renee Lake
JFK Hartwyck at Oak Tree Nrsg, Convalescent, & Rehab Center, 2048 Oak Tree Road, Edison, NJ 08820; tel. 732/906–2100; FAX. 732/321–9217; Ms. Dawn A Giakas
Kennedy Memorial Hospitals - University Medical Center, 1099 White Horse Road, Voorhees, NJ 08043; tel. 856/566–5200; FAX. 856/566–5277
Laurelton Village, 475 Jack Martin Boulevard, Brick, NJ 08724; tel. 732/458–6600; FAX. 732/458–2674; Mr. Ray Medina
Linwood Care Center, New Road and Central Avenue, Linwood, NJ 08221; tel. 609/927–6131; FAX. 609/927–5899; Ms. Leonora Dwyer
Mainland Manor Nursing and Rehabilitation Center, PO Box 1309, Pleasantville, NJ 08232; tel. 609/646–6900; FAX. 609/645–3799; Ms. Linda M Gatier
McCarrick Care Center, 15 Dellwood Lane, Somerset, NJ 08873; tel. 732/545–4200; FAX. 732/846–1089; Mr. James F Caron
Medford Care Center, 185 Tuckerton Road, Medford, NJ 08055; tel. 856/983–8500; FAX. 856/983–8965; Ms. Sandy Lowden
Morristown Memorial Hospital, 100 Madison Avenue, Morristown, NJ 07962-1956; tel. 973/971–5450; FAX. 973/290–7010; Dr. Joanne Conroy
Neptune Rehabilitation and Care Center, 101 Walnut Street, Neptune, NJ 07753; tel. 732/774–3550; FAX. 732/775–7534; Mr. Ray Medina
Princeton HealthCare System, 253 Witherspoon Street, Princeton, NJ 08540; tel. 609/497–4000; FAX. 609/497–4459; Mr. Barry S Rabner
Prospect Heights Care Center, 336 Prospect Avenue, Hackensack, NJ 07601; tel. 201/678–1800; FAX. 201/678–5811; Mr. Steve Schilsky
Regent Care Center, 50 Polifly Road, Hackensack, NJ 07601; tel. 201/646–1166; FAX. 201/487–3835
Robert Wood Johnson University Hospital at Rahway, 865 Stone Street, Rahway, NJ 07065; tel. 732/499–6050; FAX. 732/499–6337; Mr. Kirk C Tice
Seacrest Village Nursing and Rehabilitation Center, PO Box 1480, Little Egg Harbor Twp, NJ 08087; tel. 609/296–9292; FAX. 609/296–0508; Mr. Brian T Holloway
South Mountain Healthcare and Rehabilitation Center, 2385 Springfield Avenue, Vauxhall, NJ 07088-1046; tel. 908/688–3400; FAX. 908/687–4736; Mr. Jacob Frommer
St. Joseph's Hospital and Medical Center, 703 Main Street, Paterson, NJ 07503; tel. 973/754–2098; FAX. 973/754–2857; Mr. William McDonald
St. Lawrence Rehabilitation Center, 2381 Lawrenceville Road, Lawrenceville, NJ 08648; tel. 609/896–9500; FAX. 609/844–0648; Mr. Charles L. Brennan
The Manor, 689 West Main Street, Freehold, NJ 07728; tel. 732/431–5200; FAX. 732/409–2446; Mr. John Gribbin
The Pope John Paul II Pavilion at Saint Mary's Life Center, 135 South Center Street, Orange, NJ 07050; tel. 973/266–3202; FAX. 973/266–3094; Ms. Diane King
VA New Jersey Health Care System, 385 Tremont Avenue, Director's Office (00), East Orange, NJ 07018; tel. 973/676–1000; FAX. 973/676–4226; Mr. Kenneth H. Mizrach
Virtua Health, Inc., 401 Route 73 North, 50 Lake Center Drive, Suite 402, Marlton, NJ 08053; tel. 856/355–0070; FAX. 856/355–6468; Mr. Richard P Miller
Wayne View Care Center, 2020 Route 23 North, Wayne, NJ 07470; tel. 973/305–8400; FAX. 973/694–0006; Mr. Vincent Tufariello
West Caldwell Care Center, 165 Fairfield Avenue, West Caldwell, NJ 07006; tel. 973/226–1100; FAX. 973/226–5993; Mr. Michael P Duffy
Whiting Healthcare Center, 3000 Hilltop Road, Whiting, NJ 08759; tel. 732/849–4400; FAX. 732/849–4698; Mr. Gary Pizzichillo
Willow Creek Rehabilitation and Care Center, 1165 Easton Avenue, Somerset, NJ 08873; tel. 732/246–4100; FAX. 732/246–3926; Ms. Allyson Brown

NEW MEXICO
Deming Hospital Corporation, 900 W Ash Street, Deming, NM 88030; tel. 505/546–5800; Mr. John Gallagher
Life Care Center of Farmington, 1101 West Murray Drive, Farmington, NM 87401; tel. 505/326–1600; Mr. John Snyder
New Mexico Behavioral Health Institute at Las Vegas, 3695 Hot Springs Boulevard, Las Vegas, NM 87701; tel. 505/454–2201; FAX. 505/454–2211; Mr. Steve M Martinez
New Mexico State Veteran's Home, 992 South Broadway, Truth Or Consequences, NM 87901; tel. 505/894–4200; FAX. 505/894–4270; Mrs. Lori Montgomery
New Mexico VA Health Care System, 1501 San Pedro Drive SE, Albuquerque, NM 87108; tel. 505/265–1711; FAX. 505/256–2855; Mr. George Marnell

NEW YORK
Alice Hyde Medical Center, P.O. Box 729, Malone, NY 12953; tel. 518/483–3000; FAX. 518/481–2540; Mr. John Johnson
Bainbridge Nursing and Rehabilitation Center, 3518 Bainbridge Avenue, Bronx, NY 10467; tel. 718/655–1991; FAX. 718/655–8585; Mr. James K Ryan
Carthage Area Hospital, 1001 West Street, Carthage, NY 13619; tel. 315/493–1005; FAX. 315/493–4231; Mr. Walter Becker
Casa Promesa, Residential Health Care Facility, Inc., 308 East 175th Street, Bronx, NY 10457; tel. 718/960–7600; FAX. 718/901–1118; Mr. Ruben A. Medina
Catskill Regional Medical Center, PO Box 800, Harris, NY 12742-0800; tel. 845/794–3300; FAX. 845/794–5078; Mr. Steven Ruwoldt
Coler-Goldwater Specialty Hospital and Nursing Facility, 1 Main Street Roosevelt Island, New York, NY 10044-0052; tel. 212/318–8000; FAX. 212/318–4370; Mr. Claude Ritman
DeWitt Rehabilitation and Nursing Center, 211 East 79th Street, New York, NY 10021; tel. 212/879–1600; FAX. 212/988–3103; Mr. Saunders Preiss
Dr. Susan Smith McKinney Nursing/Rehabilitation Center, 594 Albany Avenue, Brooklyn, NY 11203; tel. 718/245–7170; FAX. 718/245–7060; Adm. Peola V Small
Dumont Masonic Home, 676 Pelham Road, New Rochelle, NY 10805; tel. 914/632–9600; FAX. 914/632–9247; Mr. Robert S. Bardach

East Haven Nursing and Rehab Center, 2323 Eastchester Road, Bronx, NY 10469; tel. 718/655–2848; FAX. 718/515–8249; Mr. Joseph Brachfeld
Four Seasons Nursing and Rehabilitation Center, 1555 Rockaway Parkway, Brooklyn, NY 11236; tel. 718/927–6300; FAX. 718/927–6301; Mr. Barry Friedman
Golden Gate Rehabilitation and Health Care Center, LLC.GG, 191 Bradley Avenue, Staten Island, NY 10314; tel. 718/698–8800; FAX. 718/698–5536
Good Samaritan Hospital Medical Center, 1000 Montauk Highway, West Islip, NY 11795; tel. 631/376–4001; FAX. 631/376–4208; Mr. Richard J. Murphy
Gouverneur Nursing Facility, 227 Madison Street, New York, NY 10002; tel. 212/238–7800; FAX. 212/238–7760; Mr. Mendel Hagler
Grace Plaza Nursing and Rehabilitation Center, 15 St. Paul's Place, Great Neck, NY 11021; tel. 516/466–3001; FAX. 516/466–5790; Ms. Martha Sweet
Greater Harlem Nursing Home, 30 West 138th Street, New York, NY 10037; tel. 212/690–7400; FAX. 212/690–8763; Ms. Reita Fuller
Helen and Michael Schaffer Extended Care Center, 16 Guion Place, New Rochelle, NY 10802; tel. 914/632–5000; FAX. 914/637–1117; Mr. John R Spicer
Helen Hayes Hospital, Route 9, West, West Haverstraw, NY 10993; tel. 845/786–4000; FAX. 845/947–0036; Ms. Magdalena Ramirez
Hillside Manor Rehabilitation and Extended Care Center, LLC, 182-15 Hillside Avenue, Jamaica, NY 11432; tel. 718/291–8200; FAX. 718/262–8651; Ms. Judith Dicker
Hudson Valley Rehabilitation and Extended Care Center, 260 Vineyard Avenue, Highland, NY 12528; tel. 845/691–7201; FAX. 845/691–7201; Mr. Donald D. Aldrige
Isabella Geriatric Center, 515 Audubon Avenue, New York, NY 10040; tel. 212/342–9300; FAX. 212/927–4592; Mr. Mark Kator
James J Peters Bronx VA Medical Center, 130 West Kingsbridge Road, Bronx, NY 10468; tel. 718/584–9000; FAX. 718/741–4269; Ms. MaryAnn Musumeci
Kaleida Health, 100 High Street, Buffalo, NY 14203; tel. 716/859–5600; FAX. 716/859–1530; Mr. James Kaskie
Kateri Residence, 150 Riverside Drive, New York, NY 10024; tel. 646/505–3500; FAX. 212/873–0658; Mr. Lascelles L Bond
Kingsbrook Jewish Medical Center, 585 Schenectady Avenue, Brooklyn, NY 11203; tel. 718/604–5000; FAX. 718/604–5740; Dr. Linda Brady
Laconia Nursing Home, Inc., 1050 East 230th Street, Bronx, NY 10466; tel. 718/654–5875; FAX. 718/405–5958; Mr. Barry Braunstein
Long Beach Medical Center, 455 East Bay Drive, Long Beach, NY 11561; tel. 516/897–1208; FAX. 516/897–1214; Mr. Douglas L. Melzer
M.J.G. Nursing Home Company, Inc., 4915 Tenth Avenue, Brooklyn, NY 11219; tel. 718/851–3700; FAX. 718/851–5936; Mr. Eli S Feldman
Margaret Tietz Nursing and Rehabilitation Center, 164-11 Chapin Parkway, Jamaica, NY 11432; tel. 718/298–7800; FAX. 718/262–8839; Mr. Kenneth M. Brown
Medina Memorial Health Care System, 200 Ohio Street, Medina, NY 14103; tel. 585/798–2000; FAX. 585/798–8107; Mr. James E. Sinner
Menorah Home and Hospital for the Aged and Infirm, Inc., 1516 Oriental Boulevard, Brooklyn, NY 11235; tel. 718/646–4441; FAX. 718/615–6381; Mr. Eli Feldman
Morningside House Nursing Home Company, Inc., 1000 Pelham Parkway, Bronx, NY 10461; tel. 718/409–8200; FAX. 718/828–2697; Dr. William T Smith
Morris Park Nursing Home, 1235 Pelham Parkway North, Bronx, NY 10469; tel. 718/231–4300; FAX. 718/881–3534; Mr. Morris Berkowitz
Mosholu Parkway Nursing and Rehabilitation Center, 3356 Perry Avenue, Bronx, NY 10467; tel. 718/655–3568; FAX. 718/547–8295; Mr. Isaac Shapiro
Nassau Health Care Corporation, 2201 Hempstead Turnpike, East Meadow, NY 11554; tel. 516/572–4877; FAX. 516/572–5793; Mr. Arthur A. Gianelli
North Shore University Hospital Stern Family Center for Extended Care and Rehabilatation, 330 Community Drive, Manhasset, NY 11030; tel. 516/562–8070; FAX. 516/562–8064; Mr. Michael Dowling
Northern Manhattan Rehabilitation & Nursing Cntr, 116 East 125th Street, New York, NY 10035; tel. 212/426–1284; FAX. 212/426–1297; Ms. Verna Fitzpatrick
Northwoods Rehabilitation and Extended Care Facility at Troy, 100 New Turnpike Road, Troy, NY 12182; tel. 518/235–1410; FAX. 518/235–1632; Mr. Raymond Klocek
Oceanview Nursing & Rehabilitation Center, 315 Beach 9th Street, Far Rockaway, NY 11691; tel. 718/471–6000; FAX. 718/327–8980; Mr. Louis Wolcowitz
Orzac Center for Extended Care and Rehabilitation, 900 Franklin Ave, Valley Stream, NY 11580; tel. 516/256–6502; FAX. 516/256–6601; Ms. Barbara Southard
Our Lady of Consolation Nursing & Rehabilitative Care Center, 111 Beach Drive, West Islip, NY 11795; tel. 631/587–1600; FAX. 631/587–5960; Mr. Dennis J Verzi
Parker Jewish Institute for Health Care and Rehabilitation, 271-11 76th Avenue, New Hyde Park, NY 11040-1433; tel. 718/289–2100; FAX. 718/289–2323; Mr. Michael N. Rosenblut
Peninsula Center for Extended Care and Rehabilitation, 50-15 Beach Channel Drive, Far Rockaway, NY 11691; tel. 718/734–2000; FAX. 718/734–2274; Mrs. Janet Miele-Powers
Providence Rest, 3304 Waterbury Avenue, Bronx, NY 10465; tel. 718/931–3000; FAX. 718/863–0185; Sister Seline Mary Flores
Queens Boulevard Extended Care Facility, 61-11 Queens Boulevard, Woodside, NY 11377; tel. 718/205–0288; FAX. 718/205–0667; Mr. Kenneth Gordon
Rome Memorial Hospital, 1500 North James Street, Rome, NY 13440; tel. 315/338–7000; FAX. 315/338–7533; Mrs. Darlene A. Burns
Samuel S. Stratton VA Medical Center, 113 Holland Avenue, Albany, NY 12208; tel. 518/626–5000; FAX. 518/626–6953; Ms. Mary-Ellen Piche
Sarah Neuman Center for Healthcare and Rehabilitation, 845 Palmer Avenue, Mamaroneck, NY 10543; tel. 914/698–6005; FAX. 914/777–6105; Ms. Rita Morgan
Sea View Hospital Rehabilitation Center and Home, 460 Brielle Avenue, Staten Island, NY 10314; tel. 718/317–3000; FAX. 718/351–7898; Mr. Angelo Mascia
Seacrest Health Care Center, 3035 W. 24th Street, Brooklyn, NY 11224; tel. 718/372–4500; FAX. 718/372–4579; Ms. Evelyn Jones
Shore View Nursing Home, 2865 Brighton 3rd Street, Brooklyn, NY 11235; tel. 718/891–4400; FAX. 718/891–5031; Mr. Howard M Small
Shorefront Jewish Geriatric Center, 3015 West 29th Street, Brooklyn, NY 11224; tel. 718/266–5700; FAX. 718/265–1471; Mr. Eli S Feldman
St. James Healthcare Center, 275 Moriches Road, St James, NY 11780; tel. 631/862–8000; FAX. 631/862–6456; Mr. William J St. George
St. Joseph's Hospital, 127 South Broadway, Yonkers, NY 10701; tel. 914/378–7839; FAX. 914/965–4838; Mr. Michael J. Spicer
Summit Park Hospital and Nursing Care Center, 50 Sanitorium Road, Pomona, NY 10970; tel. 845/364–2700; FAX. 845/364–2708; Mr. Richard J. Maloney
The Jewish Home and Hospital - Bronx Division, 100 West Kingsbridge Road, Bronx, NY 10468; tel. 718/410–1851; FAX. 718/410–1323; Mr. Kenneth J. Sherman
The Jewish Home and Hospital Lifecare System, 120 West 106 Street, New York, NY 10025; tel. 212/870–4901; FAX. 212/870–5718; Ms. Audrey Weiner
The Silvercrest Center for Nursing and Rehabilitation, 144-45 87th Avenue, Briarwood, NY 11435; tel. 718/480–4026; FAX. 718/480–4028; Mr. Cosmo J. LaCosta
The Wayne Center for Nursing & Rehabilitation, 3530 Wayne Avenue, Bronx, NY 10467; tel. 718/655–1700; FAX. 718/515–5650; Mrs. Miriam Socorro Velez-Thompson
United Hebrew Geriatric Center, 60 Willow Drive, New Rochelle, NY 10805; tel. 914/632–2804; FAX. 914/654–1087; Ms. Rita C. Mabli
Upstate New York VA Health Care Network at Canandaigua, 400 Fort Hill Avenue, Canandaigua, NY 14424; tel. 585/394–2000; FAX. 585/393–8328; Mr. Craig S Howard
VA Healthcare Network Upstate New York at Bath, 76 Veterans Avenue, Bath, NY 14810; tel. 607/664–4000; FAX. 607/664–4861; Mr. David J West
VA Healthcare Network Upstate New York at Syracuse, 800 Irving Avenue, Syracuse, NY 13210; tel. 315/425–4400; FAX. 315/425–2425; Mr. James P Cody
VA Hudson Valley Health Care System, Route 9A, Montrose, NY 10548; tel. 914/737–4400; FAX. 914/788–4244; Mr. Michael A Sabo
VA Medical Center Northport, 79 Middleville Road, Northport, NY 11768; tel. 631/261–4400; FAX. 631/544–5313; Mr. Gerald F. Culliton
VA New York Harbor Health Care System, 800 Poly Place, Brooklyn, NY 11209; tel. 718/630–3521; FAX. 718/630–2840; Mr. John J Donnellan
VA Western New York Health Care System, 3495 Bailey Avenue, Buffalo, NY 14215; tel. 716/862–8529; FAX. 716/862–8533; Mr. Michael S. Finegan
Victory Memorial Hospital / Skilled Nursing Center, 699 92nd Street, Brooklyn, NY 11228; tel. 718/567–1234; FAX. 718/567–1002; Dr. Vincent Calamia
Waterview Nursing Care Center, 119-15 27th Avenue, Flushing, NY 11354; tel. 718/461–5000; FAX. 718/321–1984; Mr. Anthony J Restaino
Wingate at Dutchess, Inc., 3 Summit Court, Fishkill, NY 12524; tel. 845/896–1500; FAX. 845/897–2289; Mr. Clayton M. Harbby
Wingate at Saint Francis, L.L.C., 10 Hastings Drive, Beacon, NY 12508; tel. 845/440–1600; FAX. 845/831–2865; Mr. Christopher Johnson
Wingate at Ulster, One Wingate Way, Highland, NY 12528; tel. 845/691–6800; FAX. 845/691–7063; Mr. Joseph Murabito

NORTH CAROLINA

Alamance Regional Medical Center, Inc., PO Box 202, Burlington, NC 27216-0202; tel. 336/538–7450; FAX. 336/538–7425; Mr. John Currin
Blowing Rock Hospital and Davant Extended Care Facility, PO Box 148, Blowing Rock, NC 28605-0148; tel. 828/295–3136; FAX. 828/295–5277; Mr. Timothy R. Ford
Carolinas Medical Center - Union, PO Box 5003, Monroe, NC 28111; tel. 704/283–3100; FAX. 704/296–4175; Mr. John Sullivan
Cleveland Pines Nursing Center, 1404 North LaFayette Street, Shelby, NC 28150; tel. 704/480–0128; FAX. 704/480–2238; Ms. Charlotte F Young
ECH- Chowan, Inc., PO Box 629, Edenton, NC 27932; tel. 252/482–8451; FAX. 919/482–6435; Mr. Jeffrey Sackrison
FirstHealth Richmond Memorial Hospital, 925 Long Drive, Rockingham, NC 28379; tel. 910/417–3641; FAX. 910/417–3909; Mr. John J. Jackson
GGNSC Tarboro LLC, 1000 Western Blvd., Tarboro, NC 27886; tel. 252/823–0401; FAX. 252/823–1819; Mrs. Effie E Webb
Granville Health System, 1010 College Street, Oxford, NC 27565; tel. 919/690–3418; FAX. 919/690–3400; Dr. L Lee Isley
Highlands - Cashiers Hospital, Inc., PO Drawer 190, Highlands, NC 28741-0190; tel. 828/526–1200; FAX. 828/526–1226; Mr. Ken Shull
Iredell Memorial Hospital, Incorporated, PO Box 1828, Statesville, NC 28687-1828; tel. 704/878–4500; FAX. 704/872–7924; Mr. Ed Rush
Lenoir Memorial Hospital, Inc., PO Drawer 1678, Kinston, NC 28503-1678; tel. 252/522–7000; FAX. 252/522–7596; Mr. Gary E Black
Life Care Center of Banner Elk, PO Box 2199, Banner Elk, NC 28604; tel. 828/898–5136; FAX. 828/898–8426; Mr. Brian Hutchison
Life Care Center of Hendersonville, 400 Thompson Street, Hendersonville, NC 28792; tel. 828/697–4348; FAX. 828/696–1668; Ms. Michelle Morrow
Margaret R. Pardee Memorial Hospital, 800 North Justice Street, Hendersonville, NC 28791; tel. 828/696–4660; FAX. 828/696–1128; Mr. Kristopher Hoce
Person Memorial Hospital, 615 Ridge Road, Roxboro, NC 27573; tel. 336/599–2121; FAX. 336/503–5765; Mr. V Otis Wilson
Sampson Regional Medical Center, PO Box 260, Clinton, NC 28329; tel. 910/592–8511; FAX. 910/590–2321; Mr. Lee Pridgen

Southeastern Regional Medical Center, PO Box 1408, Lumberton, NC 28359; tel. 910/671–5860; FAX. 910/671–5200; Mrs. Joann Anderson
Stokes-Reynolds Memorial Hospital, Inc., PO Box 10, Danbury, NC 27016; tel. 336/593–2831; FAX. 336/593–5350; Mr. Lance Labine
United Veteran Services of North Carolina, 214 Cochran Avenue, Fayetteville, NC 28301; tel. 910/482–4131; FAX. 910/822–0979; Mr. Neil L. Pruitt
VA Medical Center, 508 Fulton Street, Durham, NC 27705; tel. 919/286–0411; FAX. 919/286–6805; Mr. Ralph T Gigliotti
VA Medical Center, 2300 Ramsey Street, Fayetteville, NC 28301; tel. 910/822–7091; FAX. 910/822–7927; Mr. Bruce C Triplett
Veteran's Affairs Medical Center, 1100 Tunnel Road, Asheville, NC 28805; tel. 828/298–7911; FAX. 828/299–5846; Dr. Susan Pendergrass
W. G. (Bill) Hefner VA Medical Center, 1601 Brenner Avenue, Salisbury, NC 28144; tel. 704/638–9000; FAX. 704/638–3835; Mrs. Carolyn L. Adams

NORTH DAKOTA

VA Medical Center, 2101 Elm Street North, Fargo, ND 58102; tel. 701/239–3241; FAX. 701/237–3705; Mr. Robert P McDivitt

OHIO

Arlington Court Nursing and Rehabilitation Center, 1605 NW Professional Plaza, Columbus, OH 43220; tel. 614/451–5677; FAX. 614/451–8096; Mr. Blue Johnson
Aultman Hospital, 2600 Sixth Street SW, Canton, OH 44710; tel. 330/438–6352; FAX. 330/438–6356; Mr. Ed Roth
Broadview Multi-Care Center, 5520 Broadview Road, Parma, OH 44134; tel. 216/749–4010; FAX. 216/778–6860; Mr. Harold Shachter
Chapel Hill Community, 12200 Strausser Road, Canal Fulton, OH 44614; tel. 330/854–4177; FAX. 330/854–1824; Mrs. Susan Strutner
Cleveland Clinic, 9500 Euclid Avenue, Mailstop W-15, Cleveland, OH 44195; tel. 216/444–2200; FAX. 216/445–9470; Dr. Delos Cosgrove
Coshocton County Memorial Hospital, 1460 Orange Street, Coshocton, OH 43812; tel. 740/623–4348; FAX. 740/623–4350; Mr. Gregory M. Nowak
DaySpring of Miami Valley Health Care Center and Rehab, 8001 Dayton-Springfield Road, Fairborn, OH 45324; tel. 937/864–5800; FAX. 937/864–2595; Mr. Barry N Bortz
Deupree Health Center, 3939 Erie Avenue, Cincinnati, OH 45208; tel. 513/561–6363; FAX. 513/561–2064; Mr. R. Douglas Spitler
Drake Center, Inc., 151 West Galbraith Road, Cincinnati, OH 45216; tel. 513/948–2500; FAX. 513/948–2501; Dr. Karen Bankston
East Ohio Regional Hospital, 90 North Fourth Street, Martins Ferry, OH 43935; tel. 740/633–1100; FAX. 740/633–4512; Mr. Brian K. Felici
Eastgatespring Health Care Center and Rehabilitation, 4400 Gleneste Withamsville Rd, Cincinnati, OH 45245; tel. 513/752–3710; FAX. 513/753–7603; Mr. Barry N Bortz
Euclid Hospital, 18901 Lake Shore Boulevard, Euclid, OH 44119; tel. 216/531–9000; FAX. 216/692–7425; Mr. Robert Stall
Fairhaven Community, 850 Marseilles Street, Upper Sandusky, OH 43351; tel. 419/294–4973; FAX. 419/294–4975; Mr. Dan Miller
Franciscan Care Center of Sylvania, 4111 North Holland Sylvania Road, Toledo, OH 43623; tel. 419/882–6582; FAX. 419/885–1422; Mr. Shawn T Litten
Fulton County Health Center, 725 South Shoop Avenue, Wauseon, OH 43567; tel. 419/335–2015; FAX. 419/330–2602; Mr. E. Dean Beck
Graceworks Lutheran Services, 6430 Inner Mission Way, Dayton, OH 45459; tel. 937/436–6924; FAX. 937/436–7024; Mr. Willis O Serr
Hocking Valley Community Hospital, PO Box 966, Logan, OH 43138; tel. 740/380–8000; FAX. 740/385–9771; Mrs. LeeAnn Lucas-Helber
Hospitality Homes East, 1301 North Monroe Drive, Xenia, OH 45385; tel. 937/372–4495; FAX. 937/372–8038; Mr. Tony D. Deaton
Lakewood Hospital Association, 14519 Detroit Avenue, Lakewood, OH 44107; tel. 216/521–4200; FAX. 216/529–7161; Mr. Jack Gustin
Life Care Center of Elyria, 1212 South Abbe Road, Elyria, OH 44035; tel. 440/365–5200; FAX. 440/365–5266; Mr. Douglas R McDermott
Life Care Center of Medina, 2400 Columbia Road, Medina, OH 44256; tel. 330/483–3131; FAX. 330/483–3132; Mr. Steve Wolf
Louis Stokes, Cleveland VA Medical Center, 10701 East Boulevard, Cleveland, OH 44106; tel. 216/231–3456; FAX. 216/231–3460; Mr. William D Montague
Marjorie P. Lee Care Center, 3550 Shaw Avenue, Cincinnati, OH 45208; tel. 513/871–2090; FAX. 513/533–5096; Mr. R. Douglas Spitler
Mayfair Village Nursing Care Center, 3000 Bethel Road, Columbus, OH 43220; tel. 614/889–6320; FAX. 614/889–7532; Ms. Julie M Klein
Montefiore, One David N. Myers Parkway, Beachwood, OH 44122; tel. 216/910–2200; FAX. 216/910–2699; Ms. Arlene Manross
Ohio Valley Manor Nursing and Rehabilitation Center, 5280 Routes 62 and 68, Ripley, OH 45167; tel. 937/392–4318; FAX. 937/392–4599; Mr. George W Balz
Oregon Health Investors Co., 2841 Munding Drive, Oregon, OH 43616; tel. 419/697–4100; FAX. 419/697–4101; Mr. Bruce Daskal
Parkside Villa, 7040 Hepburn Road, Middleburg Heights, OH 44130; tel. 440/260–7626; FAX. 440/260–5957; Ms. Amy Kraynak
Parkvue Health Care Center, 3800 Boardwalk Boulevard, Sandusky, OH 44870; tel. 419/621–1900; FAX. 419/621–1121; Mr. Kenneth Keller
Parma Community General Hospital, 7007 Powers Boulevard, Parma, OH 44129; tel. 440/743–3000; FAX. 440/743–4386; Ms. Patricia A. Ruflin
Pleasant Lake Villa, 7260 Ridge Road, Parma, OH 44129; tel. 440/842–2273; FAX. 440/842–5809; Mr. James Taylor
Providence Care Center, 2025 Hayes Avenue, Sandusky, OH 44870; tel. 419/627–2273; FAX. 419/627–5588; Mr. Stacy Scott Terrell
Riverview Community, 5999 Bender Road, Cincinnati, OH 45233; tel. 513/922–1440; FAX. 513/922–2927; Mrs. Leigh Deaton
Rosary Care Center, 6832 Convent Blvd., Sylvania, OH 43560; tel. 419/824–3600; FAX. 419/824–3931
SEM Haven Health and Residential Care Center, 225 Cleveland Avenue, Milford, OH 45150; tel. 513/248–1270; FAX. 513/248–0318; Ms. Barbara Wolf
St. Leonard Health Care Center, 8100 Clyo Road, Centerville, OH 45458; tel. 937/439–7119; FAX. 937/439–7165; Mr. Timothy C. Dressman
The Oakridge Home, 26520 Center Ridge Road, Westlake, OH 44145; tel. 440/871–3030; FAX. 440/871–3036
The Ohio Eastern Star Health Care Center, 1451 Gambier Road, Mount Vernon, OH 43050; tel. 740/397–1706; FAX. 740/392–1662; Ms. Zandra L. Smith
The Village at St. Edward Nursing Care, 3131 Smith Road, Fairlawn, OH 44333-2697; tel. 330/666–1183; FAX. 330/666–2721; Mr. John J Hennelly
Trinity Community of Beavercreek, 3218 Indian Ripple Road, Dayton, OH 45440; tel. 937/426–8481; FAX. 937/426–3043; Ms. Laura M Farrell
Trinity Health System, 380 Summit Avenue, Steubenville, OH 43952; tel. 740/283–7212; FAX. 740/283–7104; Mr. Fred B Brower
VA Healthcare System of Ohio - Cincinnati Campus, 3200 Vine Street, Cincinnati, OH 45220; tel. 513/861–3100; FAX. 513/475–6525; Ms. Linda Smith
VA Medical Center - Chillicothe, 17273 State Route 104, Chillicothe, OH 45601; tel. 740/773–1141; FAX. 740/772–7102; Mr. Jeffrey T. Gering
VA Medical Center - Dayton Campus, 4100 West 3rd Street, Dayton, OH 45428; tel. 937/268–6511; FAX. 937/262–2179; Mr. Guy B. Richardson
Wickliffe Country Place, 1919 Bishop Road, Wickliffe, OH 44092; tel. 440/944–9400; FAX. 440/944–0955; Mr. Ed Husbands

OKLAHOMA

Department of Veterans Affairs Medical Center, 921 Northeast 13th Street, Oklahoma City, OK 73104; tel. 405/270–5194; FAX. 405/552–4364; Mr. David Wood

OREGON

Life Care Center of Coos Bay, 2890 Ocean Boulevard, Coos Bay, OR 97420; tel. 541/267–5433; Ms. Mardi Robers
Life Care Center of McMinnville, 1309 East 27th Street, McMinnville, OR 97128; tel. 503/472–4678; FAX. 503/435–2203; Mr. John Wakeman
Life Care Center Valley West Health Care Center, 2300 Warren Street, Eugene, OR 97405; tel. 541/686–2828; FAX. 541/686–9093; Ms. Marilyn Goodsell
Portland VA Medical Center, PO Box 1034, Portland, OR 97207; tel. 503/273–5267; FAX. 503/273–5319; Dr. James Tuchschmidt
VA Roseburg Healthcare System, 913 NW Garden Valley Boulevard, Roseburg, OR 97470; tel. 541/440–1000; FAX. 541/440–1225; Ms. Susan Yeager

PENNSYLVANIA

Albert Einstein Medical Center, 5501 Old York Road, Philadelphia, PA 19141; tel. 215/456–7890; FAX. 215/456–6242; Ms. A. Susan Bernini
Angela Jane Pavilion, 8410 Roosevelt Boulevard, Philadelphia, PA 19152; tel. 215/708–1200; FAX. 215/708–5057; Ms. Rosemary Valentine
Barclay Friends, 700 North Franklin Street, West Chester, PA 19380; tel. 610/696–5211; FAX. 610/918–3405; Ms. Carol J. Hanson
Berwick Hospital Center, 701 East 16th Street, Berwick, PA 18603; tel. 570/759–5000; FAX. 570/759–3473
Charles Cole Memorial Hospital, 1001 East Second Street, Coudersport, PA 16915; tel. 814/274–5347; FAX. 814/274–0884; Mr. Edward C. Pitchford
Erie VA Medical Center, 135 East 38th Street, Erie, PA 16504; tel. 814/868–8661; FAX. 814/860–2135; Dr. Michael D Adelman
Fellowship Community, 3000 Fellowship Drive, Whitehall, PA 18052; tel. 610/799–3000; FAX. 610/799–2878; Mr. Robert Zentz
Fox Subacute at Clara Burke, 251 Stenton Avenue, Plymouth Meeting, PA 19462; tel. 610/828–2272; FAX. 484/342–4146; Mr. James M Foulke
Fox Subacute Center, 2644 Bristol Road, Warrington, PA 18976; tel. 215/343–2700; FAX. 215/343–8761; Mr. James Foulke
Gnaden Huetten Memorial Hospital, 211 North 12th Street, Lehighton, PA 18235-1195; tel. 610/377–1300; FAX. 610/377–7920; Mr. Andrew E Harris
Good Shepherd Rehabilitation Hospital, 850 S. Fifth Street, Allentown, PA 18103-3295; tel. 610/776–3133; FAX. 610/776–3503; Ms. Sara T Gammon
Hickory House Nursing Home, 3120 Horseshoe Pike, Honey Brook, PA 19344; tel. 610/273–2915; FAX. 610/273–9399; Ms. Mary E Magner
Holland-Glen, 412 South York Road, Hatboro, PA 19040; tel. 215/441–1178; FAX. 215/441–1184; Mr. William Schlacter
Holy Redeemer Health System, 1648 Huntingdon Pike, Meadowbrook, PA 19046; tel. 215/938–3202; FAX. 215/938–3822; Mr. Michael B. Laign
Lankenau Hospital, 100 Lancaster Ave., Wynnewood, PA 19096; tel. 610/645–2000; FAX. 610/645–8007; Ms. Elaine Thompson
Lebanon VA Medical Center, 1700 South Lincoln Avenue, Lebanon, PA 17042; tel. 717/272–6621; FAX. 717/228–5907; Mr. Robert W. Callahan
Lock Haven Hospital and Extended Care Unit, 24 Cree Drive, Lock Haven, PA 17745; tel. 570/893–5000; FAX. 570/893–5172
Nazareth Hospital, 2601 Holme Avenue, Philadelphia, PA 19152-2096; tel. 215/335–6000; FAX. 215/335–6303; Ms. Christina Fitz-Patrick
Philadelphia Nursing Home, 2100 W. Girard Avenue, Philadelphia, PA 19130; tel. 215/685–0800; FAX. 215/685–0846; Mrs. Mary K Hess
Philadelphia VA Medical Center, University and Woodland Avenues, Philadelphia, PA 19104; tel. 215/823–5857; FAX. 215/823–6010; Mr. Richard S Citron
Presbyterian Medical Center of the UPHS, 39th and Market Street, Philadelphia, PA 19104; tel. 215/662–8260; FAX. 215/662–9662; Ms. Michele M Volpe
River's Edge Nursing and Rehabilitation Center, 9501 State Road, Philadelphia, PA 19114; tel. 215/632–5700; FAX. 215/632–4029; Ms. Andrea Naticchione
Rockhill Mennonite Community, 3250 State Road, Sellersville, PA 18960; tel. 215/257–2751; FAX. 215/257–7390; Mr. Steve Breidigan
Saint Agnes Continuing Care Center, 1900 South Broad Street, Philadelphia, PA 19145; tel. 215/339–4220; FAX. 215/339–0482; Mrs. Maryann Papa
South Mountain Restoration Center, 10058 South Mountain Road, South Mountain, PA 17261-0999; tel. 717/749–3121; FAX. 717/749–4071; Mr. J. Michael Hogarth

St. Luke's Miners Memorial Hospital, 360 West Ruddle Street, Coaldale, PA 18218-0067; tel. 570/645–8229; FAX. 570/645–8875; Mr. William J. Crossin

The Commons at Squirrel Hill, 2025 Wightman Street, Pittsburgh, PA 15217; tel. 412/421–8443; FAX. 412/422–4994; Ms. Peggy Means

UPMC Horizon, 110 North Main Street, Greenville, PA 16125; tel. 724/588–2100; FAX. 724/588–2289; Mr. Joel P. Yuhas

VA Medical Center, 1400 Black Horse Hill Road, Coatesville, PA 19320-2097; tel. 610/384–7711; FAX. 610/383–0293; Mr. Gary W. Devansky

VA Medical Center, 325 New Castle Road, Butler, PA 16001-2480; tel. 800/362–8262; FAX. 724/282–4408; Ms. Patricia Nealon

VA Medical Center, 1111 East End Boulevard, Wilkes Barre, PA 18711; tel. 570/821–7204; FAX. 570/821–7296; Ms. Janice M Boss

VA Medical Center - James E. Van Zandt, 2907 Pleasant Valley Boulevard, Altoona, PA 16602-4377; tel. 814/943–8164; FAX. 814/940–7871

VA Pittsburgh Healthcare System, University Drive, Pittsburgh, PA 15240; tel. 412/365–4058; FAX. 412/365–4059; Mrs. Terry Gerigk Wolf

Westmoreland Hospital, 532 West Pittsburgh Street, Greensburg, PA 15601; tel. 724/832–5050; FAX. 724/832–5051; Mr. David S Gallatin

RHODE ISLAND

Cedar Crest Sub Acute & Rehabilitation Centre, 125 Scituate Avenue, Cranston, RI 02921; tel. 401/944–8500; FAX. 401/944–5162; Ms. Susan K Whipple

Cherry Hill Manor, 2 Cherry Hill Road, Johnston, RI 02919; tel. 401/231–3102; FAX. 401/232–5520; Mr. David Jasinski

EPOCH SL 1, Inc/EPOCH Senior Healthcare on Blackstone Blvd, 353 Blackstone Boulevard, Providence, RI 02906; tel. 401/273–6565; FAX. 401/273–6568; Mr. Rodney Gonsalves

Evergreen House Health Center, One Evergreen Drive, East Providence, RI 02914; tel. 401/438–3250; FAX. 401/438–4813; Ms. Deborah Ready

Golden Crest Nursing Centre, 100 Smithfield Road, North Providence, RI 02904; tel. 401/353–1710; FAX. 401/353–1618; Mr. Paul Pezzelli

Heatherwood Nursing & Rehabilitation Center, 398 Bellevue Ave, Newport, RI 02840; tel. 401/849–6600; FAX. 401/367–0090; Ms. Cindy Macioci

Kent Regency Genesis Health Care, 660 Commonwealth Avenue, Warwick, RI 02886; tel. 401/739–4241; FAX. 401/732–3358; Ms. Stella C. Moran

Oak Hill Nursing and Rehabilitation Center, 544 Pleasant Street, Pawtucket, RI 02860; tel. 401/725–8888; FAX. 401/722–8560; Mr. Scott M Sanborn

Overlook Nursing & Rehabilitation Center, PO Box 152, Pascoag, RI 02859; tel. 401/568–2549; FAX. 401/568–6085; Mr. Harold H. Kenoian

Roger Williams Medical Center, 825 Chalkstone Avenue, Providence, RI 02908; tel. 401/456–2043; FAX. 401/456–2029; Mr. Kenneth Belcher

Ryan Health Center, Inc., 80 Morgan Avenue, Johnston, RI 02919; tel. 401/944–7800; FAX. 401/944–6037; Mr. David Ryan

South County Nursing and Subacute Center, 740 Oak Hill Road, North Kingstown, RI 02852; tel. 401/294–4545; FAX. 401/295–7650; Mr. Donald E. Woods

Westerly Health Center, 280 High Street, Westerly, RI 02891; tel. 401/348–0020; FAX. 401/596–9783; Mr. David Ryan

Woonsocket Health and Rehabilitation Center, 262 Poplar Street, Woonsocket, RI 02895; tel. 401/765–2100; FAX. 401/232–7275; Ms. Norma M Pezzelli

SOUTH CAROLINA

Bamberg County Memorial Hospital and Nursing Center, PO Drawer 507, Bamberg, SC 29003; tel. 803/245–6228; FAX. 803/245–6213; Mr. Warren E Hammett

C. M. Tucker, Jr. Nursing Care Center, 2200 Harden Street, Columbia, SC 29203; tel. 803/737–5301; FAX. 803/737–5364; Mr. John H Mcgill

Life Care Center of Charleston, 2600 Elms Plantation Boulevard, North Charleston, SC 29406; tel. 843/764–3500; FAX. 843/569–7222; Ms. Beth A Cliett

Life Care Center of Columbia, 2514 Faraway Drive, Columbia, SC 29223; tel. 803/865–1999; FAX. 803/865–0759

Life Care Center of Hilton Head, 120 Lamotte Drive, Hilton Head Island, SC 29926; tel. 843/681–6006; FAX. 843/681–2853; Mr. Jim Hardy

Oconee Memorial Hospital, 298 Memorial Drive, Seneca, SC 29672; tel. 864/885–7780; FAX. 864/885–7782; Ms. Jeanne L Ward

Ralph H. Johnson VA Medical Center, 109 Bee Street, Charleston, SC 29401-5799; tel. 843/577–5011; FAX. 843/937–6100; Mr. John E Barilich

William Jennings Bryan Dorn VA Medical Center, 6439 Garners Ferry Road, Columbia, SC 29209; tel. 803/776–4000; FAX. 803/695–6739; Mr. Brian Heckert

SOUTH DAKOTA

Royal C. Johnson Veterans Memorial Hospital,Sioux Falls VAMC, PO Box 5046, Sioux Falls, SD 57117; tel. 605/336–3230; FAX. 605/333–6872; Mr. Paul D Bockelman

VA Black Hills Health Care System-Fort Meade-Hot Springs, SD, 113 Comanche Road, Fort Meade, SD 57741; tel. 605/720–7170; FAX. 605/720–7171; Mr. Peter P Henry

TENNESSEE

Baptist Hospital of Cocke County, 435 Second Street, Newport, TN 37821; tel. 423/625–2200; FAX. 423/625–2215; Dr. Patricia Ketterman

Baptist Memorial Hospital, 6019 Walnut Grove Road, Memphis, TN 38120; tel. 901/226–0505; FAX. 901/226–5618; Mr. Jason Little

Christian Care Center of Cheatham County, 2501 River Road, Ashland City, TN 37015; tel. 615/792–4948; FAX. 615/746–7685; Ms. Suzanne M Hendrickson

Christian Care Center of Springfield, LLC, 704 5th Avenue E, Springfield, TN 37172; tel. 615/384–7977; FAX. 615/382–1023; Ms. Lucy Townsend

Colonial Hills Nursing Center, 2034 Cochran Road, Maryville, TN 37803; tel. 865/982–6161; FAX. 865/982–6930; Mr. Rick Sharpe

Durham-Hensley Health and Rehab., 55 Nursing Home Road, Chuckey, TN 37641; tel. 423/257–6761; FAX. 423/257–4936; Ms. Kathie Ball

Fort Sanders Regional Medical Center, 1901 Clinch Avenue, Knoxville, TN 37916; tel. 865/541–1100; FAX. 865/541–1262; Mr. Keith Altshuler

Fort Sanders Sevier Medical Center, 709 Middle Creek Road, Sevierville, TN 37862; tel. 865/429–6618; FAX. 865/429–6595; Ms. Ellen F. Wilhoit

Hardin Medical Center, 935 Wayne Rd., Savannah, TN 38372; tel. 731/926–8121; FAX. 731/926–8303; Ms. Charlotte C Burns

Hickman Community Hospital, 135 East Swan Street, Centerville, TN 37033; tel. 931/729–4271; FAX. 931/729–4612; Mr. Jack M Keller

Ivy Hall Nursing Home, 301 Watauga Avenue, Elizabethton, TN 37643; tel. 423/542–6512; FAX. 423/542–9311; Adm. Judy DeLoach

Jackson-Madison County General Hospital, 708 West Forest Avenue, Jackson, TN 38301; tel. 731/425–5000; FAX. 731/425–6684; Mr. Richard Parks

Lakebridge Medical Investors, LLC, 115 Woodlawn Drive, Johnson City, TN 37604; tel. 423/975–0095; FAX. 423/928–0358; Mrs. Nyda Bays

Life Care Center of Chattanooga, 455 N. Highland Park Ave, Chattanooga, TN 37404; tel. 423/698–5494; FAX. 423/622–4484; Mr. Randal Rouse

Life Care Center of Elizabethton, 1641 Hwy 19E Bypass, Elizabethton, TN 37643; tel. 423/542–4133; FAX. 423/542–3874

Life Care Center of Athens, PO Box 786, Athens, TN 37371-0786; tel. 423/754–8181; FAX. 423/745–9257; Mr. Wallace Stutts

Life Care Center of Bruceton, PO Box 137, Bruceton, TN 38317; tel. 731/586–2061; FAX. 731/586–2047; Mr. Walter E. Weingarten

Life Care Center of Centerville, 112 Old Dickson Road, Centerville, TN 37033; tel. 931/729–4236; FAX. 931/729–5489; Mrs. Latessa Morris

Life Care Center of Cleveland, 3530 Keith Street NW, Cleveland, TN 37312; tel. 423/476–3254; FAX. 423/476–5974

Life Care Center of Collegedale, PO Box 658, Collegedale, TN 37315; tel. 423/396–2182; FAX. 423/396–3420; Ms. Carla K Youngberg

Life Care Center of Columbia, 841 W. James Campbell Blvd., Columbia, TN 38401; tel. 931/388–5035; FAX. 931/380–9213; Ms. Andrea Craig

Life Care Center of Copper Basin, PO Box 518, Ducktown, TN 37326-0518; tel. 423/496–3245; FAX. 423/496–1906; Mr. Brian Hackerott

Life Care Center of East Ridge, 1500 Fincher Avenue, East Ridge, TN 37412; tel. 423/894–1254; FAX. 423/499–8616; Mr. Doyle Love

Life Care Center of Gray, 791 Old Gray Station Road, Gray, TN 37615; tel. 423/477–7146; FAX. 423/477–2311; Mr. Brian Scott Woods

Life Care Center of Greeneville, 725 Crum Street, Greeneville, TN 37743; tel. 423/639–8131; FAX. 423/639–4742; Ms. Jennifer Solomon

Life Care Center of Jefferson City, 336 W Old Andrew Johnson Hwy, Jefferson City, TN 37760; tel. 865/475–6097; FAX. 865/475–5236; Mrs. Laurah Meade Branam

Life Care Center of Missionary Ridge, 708 Dwight Ave, Chattanooga, TN 37406; tel. 423/622–4301; FAX. 423/622–1331; Mr. Harold Wetherbee

Life Care Center of Morgan County, 419 South Kingston Street, Wartburg, TN 37887; tel. 423/346–6691; FAX. 423/346–7031; Mr. Douglas Clanton

Life Care Center of Morristown, 501 West Economy Road, Morristown, TN 37814; tel. 423/581–5435; FAX. 423/587–1056; Ms. Amanda Cochran

Life Care Center of Red Bank, 1020 Runyan Drive, Chattanooga, TN 37405; tel. 423/473–5553; FAX. 423/339–8332; Mr. Guy Crosson

Life Care Center of Sparta, 508 Mose Drive, Sparta, TN 38583; tel. 931/738–9430; FAX. 931/738–9455; Ms. Kimberly D Parrish

Life Care Center of Tullahoma, 1715 No. Jackson Street, Tullahoma, TN 37388; tel. 931/455–8557; FAX. 931/393–2406; Mr. Kenneth Eisele

Lynchburg Nursing Center, 40 Nursing Home Road, Lynchburg, TN 37352; tel. 931/759–6000; FAX. 931/759–6003; Ms. Jane M. Edwards

Methodist Healthcare, 1211 Union Avenue, Memphis, TN 38104; tel. 901/516–0702; FAX. 901/516–0699; Mr. Gary S. Shorb

Ridgeview Terrace of Life Care, PO Box 26, Rutledge, TN 37861; tel. 865/828–5295; FAX. 865/828–5592; Ms. Karen L Bourgeois

Roan Highlands Nursing Center, 146 Buck Creek Road, Roan Mountain, TN 37687; tel. 423/772–0161; FAX. 423/772–3481; Mrs. Joy Powers

Sweetwater Nursing Center, Inc., 978 Highway 11S, Sweetwater, TN 37874; tel. 423/337–6631; FAX. 423/337–3801; Adm. Jeffrey Walter Scott

The Heritage Center, 1026 McFarland Street, Morristown, TN 37814; tel. 423/581–5100; FAX. 423/587–4649; Mr. Robert Breeden

VA Medical Center - James H. Quillen, PO Box 4000, Mountain Home, TN 37684; tel. 423/926–1171; FAX. 423/979–3572; Ms. Charlene S. Ehret

VA Tennessee Valley Healthcare System, 1310 24th Avenue South, Nashville, TN 37212-2637; tel. 615/327–4751; FAX. 615/321–6350; Mr. Juan Morales

TEXAS

Alameda Oaks Nursing Center, 1101 South Alameda, Corpus Christi, TX 78404; tel. 361/882–2711; FAX. 361/882–9527; Ms. Alicia Nieto

Amarillo VA Health Care System, 6010 Amarillo Boulevard, West, Amarillo, TX 79106; tel. 806/355–9703; FAX. 806/354–7807; Mr. Byron K. Jaqua

Central Texas Veterans Health Care System, 1901 Veterans Memorial Drive, Temple, TX 76504; tel. 254/743–2306; FAX. 254/743–2388; Mr. Bruce A Gordon

CHRISTUS Spohn Hospital Alice, 2500 East Main Street, Alice, TX 78332; tel. 361/661–8000; FAX. 361/661–8073; Mr. Mark Casanova

Fort Worth Nursing and Rehabilitation Center, 1000 6th Avenue, Fort Worth, TX 76104; tel. 817/336–2586; FAX. 817/336–6620; Mr. John Tubbs

Garden Terrace Alzheimer's Center of Excellence, 7500 Oakmont Boulevard, Fort Worth, TX 76132; tel. 817/346–8080; FAX. 817/346–9191; Ms. Gloria Bautista

Garden Terrace Alzheimer's Center of Excellence, 7887 Cambridge Street, Houston, TX 77054; tel. 713/796–2777; FAX. 713/796–2772; Ms. Carol C Pritchett

Glen Rose Medical Center Foundation, PO Box 2099, Glen Rose, TX 76043; tel. 254/897–2215; FAX. 254/897–1427; Mr. Gary A. Marks

Haltom Convalescent Center, 2936 Markum Drive, Haltom City, TX 76117; tel. 817/831–0545; FAX. 817/831–3051; Ms. Diana Russell
Life Care Center of Plano, 3800 West Park Boulevard, Plano, TX 75075; tel. 972/612–1700; FAX. 972/612–2233; Ms. Kimberly Hannan
Memorial Hermann Southwest Hospital, 7600 Beechnut, Houston, TX 77074; tel. 713/776–5111; FAX. 713/776–5652; Ms. Sonja Hagel
Memorial Hospital, 224 East Second Street, Dumas, TX 79029; tel. 806/935–7171; FAX. 806/935–6578; Ms. Yvonne Blue
Michael E. DeBakey VA Medical Center, 2002 Holcombe Boulevard, Houston, TX 77030; tel. 713/794–7100; FAX. 713/794–7038; Mr. Edgar L Tucker
North Texas VA Health Care System, 4500 South Lancaster Road, Dallas, TX 75216; tel. 202/273–8334; FAX. 202/273–9030; Mr. Joseph M Dalpiaz
Renaissance Park Multi-Care Center, 4252 Bryant Irvin Road, Fort Worth, TX 76109; tel. 817/738–2975; FAX. 817/731–7002
San Jacinto Methodist Hospital, 4401 Garth Road, Baytown, TX 77521; tel. 281/420–8765; FAX. 281/420–8852
Scott and White Memorial Hospital and Scott, Scott, Sherwood and Brindley Foundation, 2401 South 31st Street, Temple, TX 76508; tel. 254/724–1912; FAX. 254/724–0866; Dr. Alfred B Knight
South Texas Veterans Health Care System, 7400 Merton Minter Boulevard, San Antonio, TX 78229-4404; tel. 210/617–5205; FAX. 210/949–3670; Mr. Andrew M Welch
The Methodist Hospital, 6565 Fannin Street, Houston, TX 77030; tel. 713/790–3311; FAX. 713/790–2605; Mr. Ron Girotto
The Vosswood Nursing Center, 815 South Voss Road, Houston, TX 77057; tel. 713/827–0883; FAX. 713/827–0914
West Texas VA Health Care System, 300 Veterans Boulevard, Big Spring, TX 79720; tel. 432/263–7361; FAX. 432/264–4878; Mr. Michael Bell
Wooldridge Place Nursing Center, 7352 Wooldridge Rd., Corpus Christi, TX 78414; tel. 361/991–9633; FAX. 361/991–5948; Ms. Nancy Foster

UTAH

CHRISTUS Health Utah, 451 Bishop Federal Lane, Salt Lake City, UT 84115-2295; tel. 801/487–7557; FAX. 801/487–1112; Mr. Galen K Ewer
Garden Terrace Alzheimer's Center of Excellence, 1201 East 4500 South, Salt Lake City, UT 84117; tel. 801/261–3664; FAX. 801/261–3691; Mr. Ric Toomer
Life Care Center of Bountiful, 460 West 2600 South, Bountiful, UT 84010; tel. 801/295–3135; FAX. 801/295–2143
Sunshine Terrace Foundation, Inc., 225 North 200 West, Logan, UT 84321-3805; tel. 435/752–0411; FAX. 435/752–1318; Mr. David L. Seria

VERMONT

Bennington Health and Rehabilitation Center, 2 Blackberry Lane, Bennington, VT 05201; tel. 802/442–8525; FAX. 802/442–7225; Ms. Wendy Beatty
Berlin Health and Rehabilitation Center, 98 Hospitality Drive, Barre, VT 05641; tel. 802/229–0308; FAX. 802/223–4864; Mr. John Grimes
Burlington Health and Rehabilitation Center, 300 Pearl Street, Burlington, VT 05401; tel. 802/658–4200; FAX. 802/863–8016; Ms. Ursula Margazano
Rowan Court Health and Rehabilitation Center, 378 Prospect Street, Barre, VT 05641; tel. 802/476–4166; FAX. 802/476–5679; Ms. Candice Roy
St. Johnsbury Health and Rehab Center, 1248 Hospital Drive, Saint Johnsbury, VT 05819; tel. 802/748–8757; FAX. 802/748–6503; Mr. Edward Baker
SVHC Centers for Living and Rehabilitation, 160 Hospital Drive, Bennington, VT 05201; tel. 802/447–1547; FAX. 802/447–5482; Ms. Susan Kane

VIRGINIA

Augusta Medical Center, PO Box 1000, Fishersville, VA 22939; tel. 540/332–4800; FAX. 540/332–4809; Ms. Mary N. Mannix
Bedford Memorial Hospital, PO Box 688, Bedford, VA 24523; tel. 540/586–2441; FAX. 540/586–6563; Mr. William J. Flattery
Community Memorial Healthcenter, PO Box 90, South Hill, VA 23970-0090; tel. 434/447–3151; FAX. 434/774–2401; Mr. W. Scott Burnette
Eastern State Hospital, PO Box 8791, Williamsburg, VA 23187-8791; tel. 757/253–5562; FAX. 757/253–5184; Mr. John M Favret
Health Care Center at Lucy Corr Village, PO Drawer 170, Chesterfield, VA 23832; tel. 804/748–1511; FAX. 804/796–6285; Ms. Leigh Robbins
Hiram W. Davis Medical Center, PO Box 4030, Petersburg, VA 23803; tel. 804/524–7344; FAX. 804/524–7148; Mr. David A. Rosenquist
Iliff Nursing and Rehabilitation Center, 8000 Iliff Drive, Dunn Loring, VA 22027; tel. 703/560–1000; FAX. 703/280–0406; Mr. Stuart Lindeman
Inova Cameron Glen Care Center, 1800 Cameron Glen Drive, Reston, VA 20190; tel. 703/834–5800; FAX. 703/834–5851; Ms. Elissa Clark
Inova Commonwealth Care Center, 4315 Chain Bridge Road, Fairfax, VA 22030; tel. 703/934–5000; FAX. 703/934–5098; Mr. Chris Gardner
Inova Loudoun Hospital, PO Box 6000, Leesburg, VA 20177-0600; tel. 703/858–6000; FAX. 703/858–6610; Mr. Randall Kelley
James River Convalescent Center, 540 Aberthaw Avenue, Newport News, VA 23601; tel. 757/595–2273; FAX. 757/595–2271; Mr. Jeffrey L Mendelsohn
Life Care Center of New Market, 315 East Lee Highway, New Market, VA 22844; tel. 540/740–8041; FAX. 540/740–8757; Ms. Deanne Craft
Mountain View Regional Medical Center, 310 Third Street, NE, Norton, VA 24273; tel. 276/679–9100; FAX. 276/679–1926; Mr. David L Brash
Salem VA Medical Center, 1970 Roanoke Boulevard, Salem, VA 24153; tel. 540/982–2463; FAX. 540/224–1966; Mr. John E. Patrick
Smyth County Community Hospital, PO Box 880, Marion, VA 24354; tel. 276/782–1234; FAX. 276/782–1328; Mrs. Lindy P White
Southampton Memorial Hospital, PO Box 817, Franklin, VA 23851-0817; tel. 757/569–6128; FAX. 757/569–6390; Mr. David W Fuller
VA Medical Center, 100 Emancipation Drive, Hampton, VA 23667; tel. 757/722–9961; FAX. 757/728–3169; Ms. Wanda Mims
VA Medical Center - Hunter Holmes McGuire, 1201 Broad Rock Boulevard, Richmond, VA 23249; tel. 804/675–5756; FAX. 804/675–5319; Mr. Michael B. Phaup
Warren Memorial Hospital, 1000 Shenandoah Avenue, Front Royal, VA 22630; tel. 540/636–0299; FAX. 540/636–0258; Mr. Patrick B Nolan

WASHINGTON

Alderwood Manor, 3600 East Hartson Avenue, Spokane, WA 99202; tel. 509/535–2071; FAX. 509/536–7741; Ms. Donna Casey
Cascade Park Care Center, 801 SE Park Crest Avenue, Vancouver, WA 98683; tel. 360/260–2200; FAX. 360/260–9829; Ms. Shannon L Smith
Cottesmore of Life Care, 2909 14th Avenue NW, Gig Harbor, WA 98335; tel. 253/851–5433; FAX. 253/851–6924; Mr. Jeron Walker
Garden Terrace Alzheimers Center of Excellence, 491 S 338th Street, Federal Way, WA 98003; tel. 253/661–2226; FAX. 253/661–2327; Ms. Martha A Bol
Hallmark Manor, 32300 1st Ave. South, Federal Way, WA 98003; tel. 253/874–3580; FAX. 253/874–0258; Mr. Roger Joice
Islands Convalescent Center, 660 Spring street, Friday Harbor, WA 98250; tel. 360/378–2117; FAX. 360/378–5700; Mr. Rusty Pollock
Jonathan M. Wainwright Memorial VA Medical Center, 77 Wainwright Drive, Walla Walla, WA 99362; tel. 509/525–5200; FAX. 509/527–3452; Mrs. Sharon M Helman
Kah Tai Care Center, 751 Kearney Street, Port Townsend, WA 98368; tel. 360/385–3555; FAX. 360/385–7409; Ms. Holly Shepherd
Lake Vue Gardens Convalescent Center, 10101 Northeast 120th Street, Kirkland, WA 98034; tel. 425/823–2323; FAX. 425/821–2892; Ms. Nancy Butner
Life Care Center of Mount Vernon, 2120 East Division Street, Mount Vernon, WA 98274; tel. 360/424–4258; FAX. 360/428–5825; Ms. Patricia Schumacher
Life Care Center of Bothell, 707 228th Street Southwest, Bothell, WA 98021; tel. 425/481–8500; FAX. 425/487–2804; Ms. Erin Doss
Life Care Center of Burien, 1031 Southwest 130th Street, Burien, WA 98146; tel. 206/242–3213; FAX. 206/242–0528; Ms. Stephanie Bonanzino
Life Care Center of Federal Way, 1045 S. 308th Street, Federal Way, WA 98003; tel. 253/946–2273; FAX. 253/946–1596; Mr. Johnathan Owens
Life Care Center of Kennewick, 1508 W. Seventh Avenue, Kennewick, WA 99336; tel. 509/586–9185; FAX. 509/586–3544; Mr. Don Werner
Life Care Center of Port Orchard, 2031 Pottery Avenue, Port Orchard, WA 98366; tel. 360/876–8035; FAX. 360/895–0975; Mr. Mike Jacobs
Life Care Center of Puyallup, 511 10th Avenue S.E., Puyallup, WA 98372; tel. 253/845–7566; FAX. 253/845–3386; Mr. Kevin Scott Fletcher
Life Care Center of Skagit Valley, 1462 West SR 20, Sedro Woolley, WA 98284; tel. 360/856–6867; FAX. 360/856–2526; Mr. Mike McCormick
Life Care Center of West Seattle, 4700 SW Admiral Way, Seattle, WA 98116; tel. 206/935–2480; FAX. 206/937–8064; Mr. Ward Tappero
Linden Grove Health Care Center, 400 29th Street NE, Puyallup, WA 98372; tel. 253/840–4400; FAX. 253/840–6733; Mr. Jarom David Eberhard
Marysville Care Center, 1821 Grove Street, Marysville, WA 98270; tel. 360/659–3926; FAX. 360/658–0555; Ms. Tresa Johnson
Ocean View Convalescent Center, 211 Pioneer Road West, Long Beach, WA 98631; tel. 360/642–3123; FAX. 360/642–8536; Mr. Mark Harebottle
Ritzville Medical Investors,Inc., 506 South Jackson Street, Ritzville, WA 99169; tel. 509/659–1600; FAX. 509/659–1317; Ms. Kathy L Gillis
VA Medical Center, North 4815 Assembly Street, Spokane, WA 99205; tel. 509/434–7000; FAX. 509/434–7100; Dr. Nirmala Rozario
VA Puget Sound Health Care System, 1660 South Columbian Way (S-002-QI), Seattle, WA 98108-1597; tel. 206/764–2353; FAX. 206/764–2250; Mr. Stan Q Johnson

WEST VIRGINIA

Appalachian Regional Healthcare, Inc., PO Box 940, Hinton, WV 25951; tel. 304/466–1000; FAX. 304/466–2939; Mr. Wes Dangerfield
Camden-Clark Memorial Hospital, PO Box 718, Parkersburg, WV 26102; tel. 304/424–2420; FAX. 304/424–2906; Mr. Mike King
Pleasant Valley Hospital, 2520 Valley Drive, Point Pleasant, WV 25550; tel. 304/675–4340; FAX. 304/675–5243; Mr. Alvin R. Lawson
VA Medical Center, 200 Veterans Avenue, Beckley, WV 25801; tel. 304/255–2121; FAX. 304/256–5165; Ms. Karin L. McGraw
VA Medical Center, 510 Butler Avenue, Martinsburg, WV 25405; tel. 304/263–0811; FAX. 304/262–4881; Mr. Pedro Garcia
VA Medical Center - Louis A. Johnson, 1 Medical Center Drive, Clarksburg, WV 26301; tel. 304/623–3461; FAX. 304/623–7660; Mr. William E. Cox

WISCONSIN

Barron Memorial Medical Ctr., Inc. / Mayo Health System, 1222 East Woodland Avenue, Barron, WI 54812; tel. 715/537–3186; FAX. 715/537–9951; Mrs. Rita Sullivan
Bloomer Memorial Medical Center, 1501 Thompson Street, Bloomer, WI 54724; tel. 715/568–2000; FAX. 715/568–6129; Ms. Colleen Skold
Clement J. Zablocki VA Medical Center, 5000 West National Avenue, Milwaukee, WI 53295-1000; tel. 414/384–2000; FAX. 414/382–5370
Divine Savior Healthcare, Inc., PO Box 387, Portage, WI 53901; tel. 608/742–4131; FAX. 608/742–6098; Mr. Michael T. Decker
Franciscan Skemp Medical Center - Arcadia Hospital, 464 South St. Joseph Avenue, Arcadia, WI 54612; tel. 608/323–3341; FAX. 608/323–3694; Ms. Darlene Feltes
Mercy Health System Corporation, PO Box 5003, Janesville, WI 53547-5003; tel. 608/756–6625; FAX. 608/756–6168; Mr. Javon R. Bea
Osseo Medical Center, 13025 8th Street, Osseo, WI 54758; tel. 715/597–6418; FAX. 715/597–6250; Mr. Michael Ryan
Southwest Health Center, Inc., 1400 East Side Road, Platteville, WI 53818; tel. 608/348–2331; FAX. 608/342–4713; Ms. Anne K Klawiter

Upland Hills Health, Inc., 800 Compassion Way, Dodgeville, WI 53533; tel. 608/930–8000; FAX. 608/930–7250; Ms. Phyllis Fritsch

VA Medical Center - Great Lakes Health Care System, 500 East Veterans Street, Tomah, WI 54660; tel. 608/372–3971; FAX. 608/372–1654; Mr. Jerald Molnar

WYOMING

Campbell County Memorial Hospital, PO Box 3011, Gillette, WY 82717; tel. 307/688–1000; FAX. 307/688–1570; Mr. Robert Allen Morasko

Life Care Center of Casper, 4041 South Poplar Street, Casper, WY 82601; tel. 307/266–0000; FAX. 307/234–8934; Ms. Sara Delahoyde

Life Care Center of Cheyenne, 1330 Prairie Avenue, Cheyenne, WY 82009; tel. 307/778–8997; FAX. 307/778–2912; Mr. Derek Schmidt

Sheridan VA Medical Center, 1898 Fort Road, Sheridan, WY 82801; tel. 307/672–3473; FAX. 307/672–1639; Ms. Debra L Hirschman

St. John's Medical Center, PO Box 428, Jackson, WY 83001; tel. 307/733–3636; FAX. 307/739–7522; Mr. James Schuessler

VA Medical Center, 2360 East Pershing Boulevard, Cheyenne, WY 82001; tel. 307/778–7550; FAX. 307/778–7336; Dr. David M Kilpatrick

Westview Health Care Center, 1990 West Loucks, Sheridan, WY 82801; tel. 307/672–9789; FAX. 307/673–1079

U.S. Associated Areas

PUERTO RICO

VA Caribbean Healthcare System, P.O. Box 2713, San Juan, PR 00921-3201; tel. 787/641–7582; FAX. 787/641–4557; Dr. Rafael E. Ramirez-Gonzalez

Joint Commission Accredited Freestanding Behavioral Health Care Organizations

The accredited freestanding mental health care organizations listed have been accredited as of April, 2008 by the Joint Commission on Accreditation of Healthcare Organizations by decision of the Accreditation Committee of the Board of Commissioners.

The organizations listed here have been found to be in compliance with the Joint Commissions standards for Accreditation Manual for Mental Health, Chemical Dependency, and Mental Retardation/Development Disabilities Services.

Please refer to section A of the AHA Guide for information on hospitals with inpatient and/or outpatient services. These hospitals are identified by Facility Codes F88, F89, F90, F91, F92, F93, F94, and F95. In section A, those hospitals identified by Approval Code 1 are Joint Commission accredited.

We present this list simply as a convenient directory. Inclusion or omission of any organization's name indicates neither approval nor disapproval by Health Forum LLC, an American Hospital Association company.

United States

ALABAMA

Alabama Clinical Schools, Inc, P.O. Box 100968, Birmingham, AL 35210; tel. 205/836–9923; FAX. 205/836–9483; Mr. Ed Mehollin

AltaPointe Health Systems, Inc., 5750-A Southland Drive, Mobile, AL 36693; tel. 251/450–5901; FAX. 251/666–7537; Mr. J. Tuerk Schlesinger

***Birmingham Health Care,** P.O. Box 11523, Birmingham, AL 35202; tel. 205/212–5600; FAX. 205/212–5650; Mr. Jonathan Dunning

***Bradford Health Services - Huntsville Lodge,** 1600 Browns Ferry Road, Madison, AL 35758; tel. 256/461–7272; FAX. 256/464–9618; Mr. Robert S. Hinds

***Bradford Health Services - Warrior Lodge,** PO Box 129, Warrior, AL 35180; tel. 205/647–1945; FAX. 205/244–3483; Mr. Roy M. Ramsey

Glenwood, Inc., 150 Glenwood Lane, Birmingham, AL 35242; tel. 205/969–2880; FAX. 205/969–0611; Ms. D. Lee Yount

***Greater Mobile-Washington County MH/MR Board, Inc.,** 2400 Gordon Smith Drive, Mobile, AL 36617; tel. 251/450–5901; FAX. 251/666–7537; Mr. Tuerk Schlesinger

Magnolia Creek RTCED, 645 Crenshaw Road, Columbiana, AL 35051; tel. 205/678–4373; Mr. James L. Palmer

Pathway, Inc., P.O. Box 311206, Enterprise, AL 36331; tel. 334/894–5591; FAX. 334/894–5264; Mr. Norman G. Hemp

ALASKA

Alaska Children's Services Inc., 4600 Abbott Road, Anchorage, AK 99507-4314; tel. 907/346–2101; FAX. 907/348–9230; Mr. James E. Maley

Providence Adolescent Residential Treatment Program, 3400 East 20th, Anchorage, AK 99508; tel. 907/272–2148; FAX. 907/272–2169; Ms. Susan Humphrey-Barnett

ARIZONA

A New Leaf, PO Drawer 5860, Mesa, AZ 85211-5860; tel. 480/969–4024; FAX. 480/969–0039; Mr. Michael T. Hughes

***Academy of Eastern Arizona,** 522 Mission Lane, Holbrook, AZ 86025; tel. 928/524–9777; Mr. Faron Taylor

ANASAZI Foundation, 1424 S. Stapley Dr., Mesa, AZ 85204; tel. 480/892–7403; FAX. 480/892–6701; Mr. Micheal Merchant

***Chandler Valley Hope,** PO Box 1839, Chandler, AZ 85244-1839; tel. 602/899–3335; FAX. 602/899–3335; Dr. Kenneth C. Gregoire

***Community Counseling Centers, Inc.,** 105 North Fifth Avenue, Holbrook, AZ 86025; tel. 928/524–6701; FAX. 928/524–3068; Dr. Robert Wilderman

***Desert Visions Youth Wellness Center,** PO Box 458, Sacaton, AZ 85247; tel. 888/431–4096; FAX. 520/562–3415; Mr. Reuben Howard

Devereux/Arizona - Richard L. Raskin Treatment Network, 11000 N Scottsdale Rd, Ste 260, Scottsdale, AZ 85254; tel. 480/998–2920; FAX. 480/443–5587; Mrs. Lane Martin-Barker

***Helping Associates, Inc.,** 1901 North Trekell Road, Ste A, Casa Grande, AZ 85222; tel. 520/836–1029; FAX. 520/836–6733

***Horizon Human Services, Inc.,** 210 East Cottonwood Lane, Casa Grande, AZ 85222; tel. 520/836–1688; FAX. 520/421–2708; Mr. Norman E. Mudd

***Little Colorado Behavioral Health Centers,** PO Box 579, St Johns, AZ 85936; tel. 928/337–4301; FAX. 928/337–2269; Mr. Michael T. Downs

Magellan Health Services of Arizona, Inc., 4129 E Van Buren St Suite 250, Phoenix, AZ 85008; tel. 602/652–5881; FAX. 888/290–1282; Dr. Chris Carson

***Main Street Diagnostics, LLC,** 636 N.Main Street, Cottonwood, AZ 86326; tel. 928/639–4440; FAX. 928/639–3924; Mr. Steve Estes

Mingus Mountain Estate Residential Center, Inc., PO Box 26485, Prescott Valley, AZ 86312; tel. 602/335–2000; FAX. 602/249–1311; Mr. Chris A. Banken

***Mohave Mental Health Clinic, Inc.,** 1743 Sycamore Avenue, Kingman, AZ 86401; tel. 928/757–8111; FAX. 928/757–3256; Mr. B.W. Brown

Parc Place, 2190 North Grace Boulevard, Chandler, AZ 85225; tel. 480/917–9301; FAX. 480/917–0503; Mr. Michael Puthoff

***Pinal Hispanic Council,** 712 North Main Street, Eloy, AZ 85231; tel. 520/466–7765; FAX. 520/466–4475; Mr. Ralph Varela

Recovery Innovations of Arizona, Inc., 2701 N. 16th Street, Suite 316, Phoenix, AZ 85006; tel. 602/650–1212; FAX. 602/650–1616; Mr. Eugene Johnson

Remuda Ranch, One East Apache Street, Wickenburg, AZ 85390; tel. 928/684–3913; FAX. 928/684–4594; Mr. Ward E. Keller

Rosewood Ranch L.P., 36075 South Rincon Road, Wickenburg, AZ 85390; tel. 928/684–9594; FAX. 520/684–9562; Ms. Michelle Klinedinst

Sierra Tucson, Inc., 39580 S. Lago del Oro Parkway, Tucson, AZ 85739; tel. 520/624–4000; FAX. 520/825–3523; Mr. Keith P. Arnold

Southern Arizona Mental Health Corporation, 2502 North Dodge Boulevard, Suite 190, Tucson, AZ 85716; tel. 520/617–0043; FAX. 520/617–1608; Ms. Carol Little

***St. Luke's Behavioral Hospital L.P.,** 1800 East Van Buren, Phoenix, AZ 85006; tel. 602/251–8808; FAX. 602/251–8707

***Superstition Mountain Mental Health Center, Inc.,** PO Box 3160, Apache Junction, AZ 85217-3160; tel. 480/288–5328; FAX. 480/288–5339

***the EXCEL group,** 3250A E. 40th Street, Yuma, AZ 85365; tel. 928/341–0335; FAX. 928/329–8950; Mrs. Carol A. Carr

***The Guidance Center, Inc.,** 2187 North Vickey Street, Flagstaff, AZ 86004; tel. 928/527–1899; FAX. 928/714–6480; Mrs. Linda Cowan

***The Meadows of Wickenburg, Inc.,** 1655 North Tegner, Wickenburg, AZ 85390; tel. 928/684–3926; FAX. 928/684–1143; Mr. Robert Fulton

The New Foundation, PO Box 3828, Scottsdale, AZ 85257; tel. 480/945–3302; FAX. 480/945–9308; Mrs. Jewel D. Owens

Three Springs Sierra Vista, 4120 East Ramsey Road, Hereford, AZ 85615; tel. 520/378–6466; FAX. 520/378–6553; Mr. Kris Heindel

Touchstone Behavioral Health, 6153 West Olive Avenue, Ste 1, Glendale, AZ 85302; tel. 623/930–8705; FAX. 623/930–8752; Mr. Timothy Dunst

***Verde Valley Guidance Clinic, Inc.,** 8 East Cottonwood Street, Cottonwood, AZ 86326; tel. 928/634–2236; FAX. 928/634–8960; Mr. Robert D. Cartia

***West Yavapai Guidance Clinic,** 505 South Cortez Street, Prescott, AZ 86303; tel. 520/445–5211; FAX. 520/445–9522; Mr. Larry D. Green

Youth Development Institute, 1830 East Roosevelt Street, Phoenix, AZ 85006; tel. 602/254–0884; FAX. 602/258–4033; Mr. David J. Cocoros

ARKANSAS

Amicare of Arkansas, 4253 Crossover Road, Fayetteville, AR 72703; tel. 479/587–1408; FAX. 479/587–1085

Boeckmann Consulting, Inc., 2022 East Broadway, Forrest City, AR 72335; tel. 870/494–4600; FAX. 870/494–4607; Mrs. Jeannie Boeckmann

Brighter Futures Behavioral, 1217 Hwy. 367 North, Newport, AR 72112; tel. 870/523–9300; FAX. 870/523–9301; Mr. Johnny White

Centers for Youth and Families, P.O. Box 251970, Little Rock, AR 72225-1970; tel. 501/666–8686; FAX. 501/666–0891; Mr. Doug Stadter

Clinical Neuropsych, PA, 1201 Fleming Ave, Jonesboro, AR 72401; tel. 870/933–5174; FAX. 870/933–5235; Dr. Daniel Johnson

Community Counseling Services, Inc., 125 Don's Way, Hot Springs National Park, AR 71913; tel. 501/624–7111; FAX. 501/620–5203; Dr. Donald G. Martin

Cornerstone Community Counseling Corp., 106 East Third Street, Imboden, AR 72434; tel. 870/869–1500; FAX. 870/869–1500; Mrs. Brenda Marie Ray

Counseling and Education Center, Inc., 406 Pecan Street, Helena, AR 72342; tel. 870/338–8447; FAX. 870/338–8048; Ms. Gracie Giles-Gonner

Delta Counseling Associates, Inc., 790 Roberts Drive, Monticello, AR 71655; tel. 870/367–9732; FAX. 870/367–2363; Mr. Michael Walsh

Delta Family Health and Fitness Center for Children, Inc., 103 South Elm, Hamburg, AR 71646; tel. 870/853–4224; FAX. 870/853–4457; Mr. Maxwell Dean Hill

Families, Inc. of Arkansas, 4508 Stadium Blvd., Jonesboro, AR 72404; tel. 870/933–6886; FAX. 870/933–9395; Ms. Joy Davis

***Gilead Family Resource Center, Inc.,** 515 Holly Street, McGehee, AR 71654; tel. 870/222–4500; FAX. 870/222–4505

Habilitation Centers, Inc., PO Box 727, Fordyce, AR 71742; tel. 870/352–8203; FAX. 870/352–5311; Mrs. Margaret Stept

Hope Behavioral Health Care, P.O. Box 176, Cherokee Village, AR 72525; tel. 479/409–7913; Dr. Paul Bokker

Life Strategies Counseling, Inc., 1217 Stone Street, Jonesboro, AR 72401; tel. 870/972–1268; FAX. 870/934–0847; Dr. William Wolters

Life Strategies of Arkansas, LLC, 203 West Bond Street, West Memphis, AR 72301; tel. 870/732–1878; FAX. 870/732–2427; Mr. Rick R. Draper

Living Hope Southeast, LLC, 100 South University, Suite 401, Little Rock, AR 72205; tel. 501/663–5473; FAX. 501/801–1816; Mr. Mike Grundy

Maxus, Inc., PO Box 315, Warm Springs, AR 72478; tel. 870/647–2541; FAX. 870/647–2337; Mr. Ted Suhl

*Indicates organization is a Joint Commission accredited Chemical Dependency organization.

Section C

***Ozark Counseling Services, Inc,** PO Box 1776, Mountain Home, AR 72654-1776; tel. 870/425–6901; FAX. 870/425–0263; Dr. Mark Clark

***Ozark Guidance Center, Inc.,** PO Box 6430, Springdale, AR 72766-6430; tel. 479/750–2020; FAX. 479/751–2964

The Lord's Ranch Behavioral Health Care System, Inc., 1033 Old Burr Road, Warm Springs, AR 72478; tel. 870/647–2541; FAX. 870/647–2337; Mr. Ted E. Suhl

Therapeutic Family Services, Inc., 600 Main Street, Hot Springs National Park, AR 71913; tel. 501/321–8200; FAX. 501/321–8202; Mr. Birkes Williams

Timber Ridge Ranch NeuroRestorative Center, PO Box 208, Benton, AR 72018; tel. 501/594–5211; FAX. 501/594–5236; Mr. Rob McDaniel

***UAMS-Substance Abuse Treatment Clinic,** 4301 West Markham Street Slot # 554, Little Rock, AR 72205-4096; tel. 501/686–5483; FAX. 501/686–8154; Dr. G. Richard Smith

United Methodist Children's Home Inc., PO Box 56050, Little Rock, AR 72215; tel. 501/661–0720; FAX. 501/664–3702; Mr. William A. Altom

***University of Arkansas for Medical Sciences,** 4301 West Markham Street, Mail Slot 554, Little Rock, AR 72205; tel. 501/686–5483; FAX. 501/686–8154; Dr. G. Richard Smith

Youth Home, Inc., 20400 Colonel Glenn Road, Little Rock, AR 72210-5323; tel. 501/821–5500; FAX. 501/821–5580; Ms. Beth Cartwright

CALIFORNIA

Abundant Life and Adolescent Growth, Inc., 6055 East Washington Boulevard, Suite 240, Commerce, CA 90040; tel. 323/722–8950; FAX. 323/722–8952; Dr. Joilyn Holmes

***Action Family Counseling, Inc.,** 26893 Bouquet Canyon Road, Suite C-134, Santa Clarita, CA 91350; tel. 661/297–9716; FAX. 661/297–9701; Mr. Cary Quashen

***AltaMed Health Services Corporation,** 500 Citadel Drive Suite 490, Los Angeles, CA 90040; tel. 323/889–7307; FAX. 323/889–7843; Mr. Castulo de la Rocha

Aspen Achievement Academy, 17777 Center Court Drive, Suite 300, Cerritos, CA 90703; tel. 562/467–5509; FAX. 562/402–7036; Mr. Gilbert Hallows

***Berkeley Addiction Treatment Services, Inc.,** 2975 Sacramento Street, Berkeley, CA 94702; tel. 510/644–0200; FAX. 510/644–2044; Ms. Matonia Williams

***Betty Ford Center,** 39000 Bob Hope Drive, Rancho Mirage, CA 92270; tel. 760/773–4100; FAX. 760/346–6961; Mr. John T. Schwarzlose

Broad Horizons, PO Box 1920, Ramona, CA 92065; tel. 760/789–7060; FAX. 760/789–4062; Dr. E. Kent McIntyre

***California Institution for Women,** P.O. Box 6000, Corona, CA 92878-6000; tel. 909/597–1771; FAX. 909/606–4905; Dr. Jacqueline Long

College Hospital, 10802 College Place, Cerritos, CA 90703; tel. 562/924–9581; FAX. 562/924–6523; Mr. Stephen Witt

***Cornerstone of Southern California,** 13682 Yorba Street, Tustin, CA 92780; tel. 714/730–5399; FAX. 714/730–3505; Ms. Lynda klinger

***CRC Health Corporation - eGetgoing,** 20400 Stevens Creek Blvd, Suite 600, Cupertino, CA 95014; tel. 866/435–7999; FAX. 408/918–2256; Dr. Barry Karlin

***El Dorado Community Service Centers,** 5200 San Gabriel Place, Ste. B & C, Pico Rivera, CA 90660; tel. 562/222–1322; FAX. 562/222–1322; Dr. Stan Sharma

***Fort Help Methadone Program,** 915 Bryant Street, San Francisco, CA 94103; tel. 415/777–9953; FAX. 415/777–4717; Dr. Stan Sharma

***HAART- Oakland,** 10850 MacArthur Boulevard Suite 200, Oakland, CA 94605; tel. 510/875–2300; FAX. 510/875–2310; Ms. Anne Branch

***HAART-Hayward,** 20094 Mission Boulevard, Hayward, CA 94541; tel. 510/727–9755; FAX. 510/727–9761; Ms. Anne Branch

Hathaway-Sycamores Child and Family Services, 210 S DeLacey Ave, Ste 110, Pasadena, CA 91105; tel. 626/395–7100; FAX. 626/395–7270; Mr. William P. Martone

***Impact Drug and Alcohol Treatment Center,** PO Box 93607, Pasadena, CA 91103; tel. 626/798–0884; FAX. 626/798–6970; Mr. James M Stillwell

***J. Cole Recovery Homes,** 1408 A Street, Antioch, CA 94509; tel. 925/978–2873; FAX. 925/757–0411; Mr. Jesse L. Cole

Oak Grove Institute, 24275 Jefferson Avenue, Murrieta, CA 92562; tel. 951/677–5599; FAX. 951/698–0461; Ms. Tamara L. Wilson

***Opioid Replacement Treatment Program, Dept of Veterans Affairs,** 2505 West 14th Street, Oakland Army Base, Oakland, CA 94607; tel. 510/587–3434; FAX. 510/587–3420; Dr. Matthew Moore

***OTP Los Angeles Ambulatory Care Center,** 351 East Temple Street, Los Angeles, CA 90012; tel. 310/268–3132; FAX. 213/253–5149; Dr. Susan C. Rosenbluth

***R House, Inc.,** P.O. Box 2587, Santa Rosa, CA 95405; tel. 707/571–2215; FAX. 707/526–9672; Ms. Mimi G. Donohue

River Oak Center for Children, 5030 El Camino Rd, Carmichael, CA 95608; tel. 916/609–5100; FAX. 916/609–5105; Dr. Mary Hargrave

***San Mateo Medical Center Methadone Treatment Program,** 795 Willow Road, Building #332, Menlo Park, CA 94025; tel. 650/578–7190; FAX. 650/324–4149; Dr. Sang-ick Chang

***Sepulveda CA VAH Opioid Treatment Program,** 16111 Plummer Street, Bldg 62, Sepulveda, CA 91343; tel. 310/268–3132; FAX. 818/895–5883; Dr. Susan C. Rosenbluth

***Sharp Vista Pacifica,** 7989 Linda Vista Road, San Diego, CA 92111; tel. 858/637–6920; FAX. 858/637–6959

Solano Psychiatric Health Facility, PO Box 2866, Fairfield, CA 94533; tel. 707/784–2130; FAX. 707/435–2139; Ms. Stacey Calhoun

***Spencer Recovery Centers, Inc.,** PO Box 118, Monrovia, CA 91017; tel. 949/376–3705; FAX. 949/376–6862; Mr. Christopher C. Spencer

***Tarzana Treatment Centers, Inc.,** 18646 Oxnard Street, Tarzana, CA 91356; tel. 818/654–3815; FAX. 818/996–3051; Mr. Scott Taylor

The Discovery Adolescent Program, 4136 Ann Arbor Road, Lakewood, CA 90712; tel. 562/425–6918; FAX. 562/981–0809; Dr. Craig M. Brown

***Twin Town Treatment Centers,** 4388 E. Katella Ave, Los Alamitos, CA 90720; tel. 562/594–8844; FAX. 562/493–1280; Mr. David Lisonbee

***VAMC-San Francisco Substance Abuse Treatment Clinic,** 4150 Clement Street, Bldg 1, San Francisco, CA 94121; tel. 415/750–2050; FAX. 415/750–2152; Dr. Peter Banys

Vista Del Mar Child and Family Services, 3200 Motor Avenue, Los Angeles, CA 90034; tel. 310/836–1223; FAX. 310/204–4134; Dr. Elias Lefferman

***West Los Angeles Drug Treatment Services,** 11301 Wilshire Blvd, Bldg 257C, Los Angeles, CA 90073; tel. 310/268–3132; FAX. 310/268–4774; Dr. Susan C. Rosenbluth

***West Oakland Health Council,** 700 Adeline Street, Oakland, CA 94607; tel. 510/835–9610; FAX. 510/835–9610; Dr. Robert Cooper

***Westside Community Mental Health, Inc.,** 1301 Pierce Street, San Francisco, CA 94115; tel. 415/563–8200; FAX. 415/563–5985; Dr. Abner Boles

COLORADO

***Adolescent and Family Institute of Colorado, Inc.,** 10001 West 32nd Avenue, Wheat Ridge, CO 80033; tel. 303/238–1231; FAX. 303/238–0500; Dr. Alex M. Panio

Colorado Boys Ranch, PO Box 681, La Junta, CO 81050; tel. 719/384–5981; FAX. 719/384–8119; Mr. Charles M. Thompson

***Denver Health and Hospital Authority,** 777 Bannock Street, Unit 9, Denver, CO 80204; tel. 303/436–5690; FAX. 303/436–3327; Mrs. Patricia Gabow

Devereux Cleo Wallace, 8405 Church Ranch Blvd, Westminster, CO 80021; tel. 303/466–7391; FAX. 303/466–0904; Mr. Bentley Smith

El Pueblo Boys' & Girls' Ranch, Inc., One El Pueblo Ranch Way, Pueblo, CO 81006; tel. 719/544–7496; FAX. 719/544–7705; Ms. Patty A. Erjavec

Forest Heights Lodge, PO Box 789, Evergreen, CO 80437-0789; tel. 303/674–6681; FAX. 303/674–6805; Ms. Linda Clefisch

***Parker Valley Hope,** PO Box 670, Parker, CO 80134; tel. 303/841–7857; FAX. 303/841–6526; Dr. Kenneth C. Gregoire

***Pikes Peak Mental Health,** 220 Ruskin Drive, Colorado Springs, CO 80910; tel. 719/572–6100; FAX. 719/572–6195; Mr. Morris Roth

Southern Peaks Regional Treatment Center, 700 Four Mile Parkway, Canon City, CO 81212; tel. 719/276–7511; FAX. 719/276–6961; Mr. Dan Zarecky

CONNECTICUT

***Alcohol and Drug Recovery Centers, Inc.,** 500 Blue Hills Avenue, 6th Floor Administration, Hartford, CT 06112; tel. 860/714–3701; FAX. 860/714–8974; Dr. Ronald C. Fleming

***Blue Hills Substance Abuse Services,** 525 Russell Road, Newington, CT 06111; tel. 860/666–7665; FAX. 860/666–7642; Ms. Brenda Thorington

Capitol Region Mental Health Center, 500 Vine Street, Hartford, CT 06112; tel. 860/297–0903; FAX. 860/297–0914; Ms. Karen Evertson

***Community Health Resources, Inc.,** 995 Day Hill Road, Windsor, CT 06095; tel. 860/731–5522; FAX. 860/731–5536; Ms. Heather M. Gates

***Community Mental Health Affiliates, Inc.,** 29 Russell Street, New Britain, CT 06052; tel. 860/826–1358; FAX. 860/229–6575

***Community Renewal Team,** 555 Windsor Street, Hartford, CT 06120; tel. 860/560–5784; FAX. 860/527–3305; Ms. Magadalena Rodriguez

***Connecticut Valley Hospital-Addiction Services Div.-Merritt,** PO Box 351, Middletown, CT 06457-7023; tel. 860/262–5887; FAX. 860/268–5895; Mr. Luis B. Perez

Inter-Community Mental Health Group, Inc., 281 Main Street, East Hartford, CT 06118; tel. 860/569–5625; FAX. 860/569–5925; Ms. Kimberly L. Beauregard

Klingberg Family Centers, Inc., 370 Linwood Street, New Britain, CT 06052; tel. 860/224–9113; FAX. 860/826–1739; Ms. Rosemarie Burton

***New Era Rehabilitation Center,** 3851 Main Street, 2nd floor, Bridgeport, CT 06606; tel. 203/372–3333; FAX. 203/374–7515; Dr. Ebenezer A. Kolade

***Opiate Treatment Program, VA Connecticut Heathcare System,** 950 Campbell Avenue, Bldg 36, West Haven, CT 06516; tel. 203/932–5711; FAX. 203/937–3478; Dr. Kishorchandra Gonsai

***Perception Programs, Inc.,** PO Box 407, Willimantic, CT 06226; tel. 860/450–7122; FAX. 860/450–7127; Ms. Linda Mastrianni

River Valley Services, PO Box 351, Middletown, CT 06457; tel. 860/262–5200; FAX. 860/262–5203; Mr. Howard Reid

***Rushford Center, Inc.,** 384 Pratt Street, Meriden, CT 06450; tel. 203/235–1792; FAX. 203/634–2799; Mr. Jeffrey L. Walter

***Saint Francis Hospital & Medical Center - 8 West Unit,** 500 Blue Hills Avenue, Hartford, CT 06112; tel. 860/714–2333; FAX. 860/714–2971; Mr. Christopher M. Dadlez

***Silver Hill Hospital,** 208 Valley Road, New Canaan, CT 06840; tel. 203/801–2297; FAX. 203/966–9336; Dr. Sigurd H. Ackerman

***South Central Rehabilitation Center,** 232 Cedar Street, New Haven, CT 06519; tel. 203/503–3356; FAX. 203/503–3370; Mr. Cornell Scott

***Southwest Connecticut Mental Health System,** 97 Middle Street, Bridgeport, CT 06604; tel. 203/579–7368; FAX. 203/579–6305; Mr. James M. Pisciotta

***State of Connecticut DMHAS - Southeastern Mental Health Authority,** 401 West Thames Street, Bldg. 301, Norwich, CT 06360; tel. 860/859–4674; FAX. 860/859–4790; Mr. William J. Newkirk

***Stonington Behavioral Health, Inc.,** 234A Bank Street, New London, CT 06320; tel. 860/439–6005; FAX. 860/439–6008; Mr. William A. Aniskovich

***The Children's Center of Hamden, Inc.,** 1400 Whitney Avenue, Hamden, CT 06517; tel. 203/248–2116; FAX. 203/248–9339; Mr. Anthony DelMastro

The Wellspring Foundation, Inc., 21 Arch Bridge Road, Bethlehem, CT 06751; tel. 203/266–8000; FAX. 203/266–8030; Mr. Harvey I. Newman

***The Wheeler Clinic,** 91 Northwest Drive, Plainville, CT 06062; tel. 860/793–3500; FAX. 860/793–3520; Dr. David J. Berkowitz

*Indicates organization is a Joint Commission accredited Chemical Dependency organization.

*United Services, Inc., Post Office Box 839, Dayville, CT 06241; tel. 860/774–2020; FAX. 860/774–0826; Ms. Diane L. Manning
Western Connecticut Mental Health Network, 55 West Main Street, Suite 410, Waterbury, CT 06702; tel. 203/805–6400; FAX. 203/805–6432; Ms. Colette Anderson

DELAWARE
*Brandywine Counseling, Inc, Lancaster, 2713 Lancaster Avenue, Wilmington, DE 19805; tel. 302/656–2348; FAX. 302/656–0746; Ms. Sara T. Allshouse
*Brandywine Counseling, Inc., 2814 West Second Street, Wilmington, DE 19805; tel. 302/472–0381; FAX. 302/472–0392; Ms. Sara T. Allshouse
*Brandywine Counseling, Inc., South Chapel, 24 Brookhill Drive, Newark, DE 19702; tel. 302/454–3020; FAX. 302/454–0298; Ms. Sara T. Allshouse
*Connections Community Support Programs, Inc., 500 West 10th Street, Wilmington, DE 19801; tel. 302/984–3380; FAX. 302/984–3324; Ms. Catherine Devaney McKay
Delaware Guidance Services for Children and Youth, Inc., 1213 Delaware Avenue, Wilmington, DE 19806; tel. 302/652–3948; FAX. 302/652–8297; Mr. Bruce Kelsey
*Gateway Foundation Delaware City Treatment Center, P.O. Box 547, Delaware City, DE 19706; tel. 312/663–1130; FAX. 312/663–0504; Mr. Michael Darcy
*SODAT - Delaware, Inc., 625 N. Orange Street, Wilmington, DE 19801; tel. 302/656–4044; FAX. 302/656–3439; Mr. Eric Saul
*Thresholds, Inc., 526-D North DuPont Highway, Georgetown, DE 19947; tel. 302/856–1835; FAX. 302/856–1764; Mr. Bruce R. Lorenz

DISTRICT OF COLUMBIA
*Department of Veterans Affairs, Substance Abuse Rehab Program, 50 Irving Street, Northwest, Washington, DC 20422; tel. 202/745–8564; FAX. 202/745–8530; Dr. Stephen Deutsch
McClendon Center, 1313 New York Avenue, NW, Washington, DC 20005; tel. 202/737–6191; FAX. 202/737–2316; Mr. Richard E. Davis
*Psychiatric Institute of Washington, 4228 Wisconsin Avenue, NW, Washington, DC 20016; tel. 202/885–5600; FAX. 202/966–7374; Mr. Ken Courage
The Episcopal Center for Children, 5901 Utah Avenue, NW, Washington, DC 20015-1616; tel. 202/363–1333; FAX. 202/537–5044; Mr. Alan C. Korz

FLORIDA
Alternate Family Care, Inc., 10001 W Oakland Park Blvd, Suite 302, Sunrise, FL 33351; tel. 954/746–5200; FAX. 954/746–5217; Dr. David Ferguson
*Alternative Treatment International, Inc., 2919 Northfield Drive, Tarpon Springs, FL 34688; tel. 800/897–8060; FAX. 727/461–3651; Ms. Julia Stewart
*American Therapeutic Corp., 1801 NE 2nd Avenue, Miami, FL 33132; tel. 305/371–5777; FAX. 305/371–6007; Ms. Marianella Valera
*Apalachee Center, Inc., 2634-J Capital Circle NE, Tallahassee, FL 32308; tel. 850/523–3333; FAX. 850/523–3434; Mr. Ronald P. Kirkland
Awakenings Community Mental Health Center, 2281 SW 27th Ave., Miami, FL 33145; tel. 305/860–5727; FAX. 305/860–9355; Dr. Mari Cazares
Bayview Center for Mental Health, Inc., 111 NW 183rd Street, 5th Fl., Miami Gardens, FL 33169; tel. 305/892–4600; FAX. 305/893–1224; Mr. James R. Sleeper
*Beachcomber Rehab, Inc., 4493 North Ocean Boulevard, Delray Beach, FL 33483; tel. 561/276–6226; FAX. 561/265–1349; Mr. Joseph R Bryan
*Behavioral Health of the Palm Beaches, Inc., 3153 Canada Court, Lake Worth, FL 33461; tel. 561/615–6664; FAX. 561/615–4042; Mr. Donald Mullaney
Behavioral Support Services, 315 N. Lakemont Avenue, Winter Park, FL 32792; tel. 407/831–6412; FAX. 407/830–8413
*Broward Addiction Recovery Division, 115 S. Andrews Avenue Suite 318, Fort Lauderdale, FL 33301; tel. 954/357–5444; FAX. 954/357–5468; Mr. Paul Jaquith
Broward County/Human Services Dept/Family Success Administrative Division, 115 S Andrews Ave, Ste 303, Fort Lauderdale, FL 33301; tel. 954/357–6367; FAX. 954/357–5468; Mr. Fredrick J. Murry
*Central Florida Treatment Center - Ft. Pierce Clinic, 1302 Lawnwood Circle, Suite B, Fort Pierce, FL 34950; tel. 772/468–6800; FAX. 772/464–3800; Mrs. Carol S. Ball
*Central Florida Treatment Centers, 7 North Cocoa Boulevard, Cocoa, FL 32922; tel. 321/631–4578; FAX. 321/631–1640; Ms. Carol S. Ball
*Central Florida Treatment Centers - Orlando, 1800 West Colonial Drive, Orlando, FL 32804; tel. 407/843–0041; FAX. 407/481–7078; Mrs. Carol Ball
*Central Florida Treatment Centers - Palm Bay, 2198 Harris Avenue, Palm Bay, FL 32905; tel. 321/951–9750; FAX. 321/951–9765; Mrs. Carol Ball
*CFSATC, Inc., 3155 Lake Worth Road Suite #2, Lake Worth, FL 33461; tel. 561/439–8440; FAX. 561/439–8229; Mrs. Carol Ball
*Chautauqua Offices of Psychotherapy & Evaluation, 3686 US Highway 331 South, Defuniak Springs, FL 32435; tel. 850/892–8035; FAX. 850/892–8074; Ms. Rachel R. Gillis
*Choices Recovery Center, 606 North US Highway 1, Fort Pierce, FL 34950; tel. 772/460–5053; FAX. 772/460–5054; Mr. David Agnolucci
*Coastal Behavioral Healthcare, Inc., 1565 State Street, Sarasota, FL 34236; tel. 941/927–8900; FAX. 941/927–6315; Dr. Jerry Thompson
*Comprehensive Psychiatric Center, 9735 East Fern Street, Miami, FL 33157; tel. 305/238–5121; FAX. 305/238–8140; Dr. Roberto Ruiz
*Comprehensive Psychiatric Center North, 240 Northwest 183rd Street, Miami, FL 33169; tel. 305/651–2332; FAX. 305/651–1173; Dr. Roberto Ruiz
*Comprehensive Psychiatric Center-Central, 4790 N. W. 7th Street Suite 101 & 102, Miami, FL 33126; tel. 305/238–5121; FAX. 305/529–5824; Dr. Roberto Ruiz
*Dade Family Counseling Community Mental Health Center, 4343 West Flagler Street Suite 100, Miami, FL 33134; tel. 305/774–9570; FAX. 305/774–9573; Mrs. Maria E. Fields
*David Lawrence Center, 6075 Golden Gate Parkway, Naples, FL 34116; tel. 239/455–8500; FAX. 239/455–6561; Mr. David C. Schimmel
*Destination Hope, Inc., 6555 NW 9th Ave. Suite 214, Fort Lauderdale, FL 33309; tel. 954/771–2091; FAX. 954/771–2098; Mr. Ben Brafmam
*Fair Oaks Pavilion at Delray Medical Center, 5352 Linton Boulevard, Delray Beach, FL 33484; tel. 561/495–3278; FAX. 561/495–3467; Mr. Robert Krieger
*Fairwinds Treatment Center, 1569 S Fort Harrison Avenue, Clearwater, FL 33756; tel. 727/449–0300; FAX. 727/446–1022; Mr. Mazhar K. Al-Abed
*Family Resource Center of South Florida, Inc., 155 South Miami Ave. 4th Fl, Miami, FL 33130-1617; tel. 305/374–6006; FAX. 305/374–6112; Dr. Oren Wunderman
*Florida Center for Recovery, 3451 West Midway Road, Fort Pierce, FL 34981; tel. 772/460–2777; FAX. 772/460–2771; Mr. Jack Hamilton
Florida Institute for Neurologic Rehabilitation, Inc, PO Box 1348, Wauchula, FL 33873; tel. 863/773–2857; FAX. 941/773–2041; Mr. Joseph Brennick
*Focus Healthcare of Florida, 5960 Southwest 106th Avenue, Cooper City, FL 33328; tel. 954/680–2700; FAX. 954/680–9941
*G&G Holistic Addiction Treatment Inc., 1590 NE 162nd Street Suite 200, North Miami Beach, FL 33162; tel. 305/945–8384; FAX. 305/957–7076; Mr. Jerry Goldfarb
Green Cross Health Systems, Inc., 2645 Douglas Road, Suite 601, Miami, FL 33133; tel. 305/443–9990; FAX. 305/443–9493; Dr. Miguel A. Nunez
Gulf Coast Treatment Center, 1015 Mar Walt Drive, Fort Walton Beach, FL 32547; tel. 850/863–4160; FAX. 850/863–8576; Mr. Jeffrey M. Kaplan
*Hanley Center, 5200 East Avenue, West Palm Beach, FL 33407; tel. 561/841–1000; FAX. 561/841–1100; Mr. Terry Allen
*HealthCare Connection of Tampa, Inc., 825 West Linebaugh Avenue, Tampa, FL 33612; tel. 813/931–5560; FAX. 813/932–4960; Mr. Jess Loven
*Hendry Glades Mental Health Clinic, Inc., 601 West Alverdez Avenue, Clewiston, FL 33440; tel. 863/983–1423; FAX. 863/983–1426
Homestead Behavioral Health Clinic, 654 NE 9th Place, Homestead, FL 33030; tel. 305/248–3488; FAX. 305/248–3499; Mrs. Aidelyn Lopez
*Jackson North Community Mental Health Center, 20201 NW 37th Ave, Miami, FL 33056; tel. 786/466–2701; FAX. 786/466–2748; Mrs. Melida Akiti
*John's Place, Inc., 315 SE 11th Street, Fort Lauderdale, FL 33316; tel. 954/463–9590; FAX. 954/463–9794; Mr. John Cates
La Amistad Behavioral Health Services, 1650 Park Avenue North, Maitland, FL 32751; tel. 407/647–0660; FAX. 407/647–0099; Ms. Vickie Lewis
Lakeside Alternatives, Inc., 434 West Kennedy Boulevard, Orlando, FL 32810; tel. 407/875–3700; FAX. 407/667–6195; Mr. Jerry Kassab
*Lakeview Health Systems, LLC, 8889 Corporate Square Court, Jacksonville, FL 32216; tel. 904/727–6455; FAX. 904/855–4364; Mrs. Joanne Telmosse
*LifeStream Behavioral Center, PO Box 491000, Leesburg, FL 34749-1000; tel. 352/315–7500; FAX. 352/360–6595; Mr. Jonathan M. Cherry
*Lighthouse CMHC, 1704 NW 7th Street, Miami, FL 33125; tel. 305/541–2600; FAX. 305/541–2222; Mr. Alex Menendez
*Manatee Glens Corporation, PO Box 9478, Bradenton, FL 34206-9478; tel. 941/782–4299; FAX. 941/782–4301; Ms. Mary Ruiz
Manatee Palms Youth Services, 4480 51st Street West, Bradenton, FL 34210; tel. 941/792–2222; FAX. 941/761–1632; Mr. David Guymon
Mental Health Care, Inc., 5707 North 22nd Street, Tampa, FL 33610; tel. 813/272–2244; FAX. 813/272–3766; Mr. Julian I. Rice
National Deaf Academy, LLC, 19650 US Highway 441, Mount Dora, FL 32757; tel. 352/735–9500; FAX. 352/735–4939; Mr. Stephen P. Fahey
*New Era Health Center, 9600 Southwest 8th Street Suite 1, Miami, FL 33174; tel. 305/559–8838; FAX. 305/559–6608; Mr. Enrique A. Garcia
New Life Community Mental Center, Inc., 1690 North West 19 Terrace, Miami, FL 33125; tel. 305/325–8620; FAX. 305/549–7229; Ms. Jennifer Stevens
Northside Mental Health Center, 12512 Bruce B. Downs Boulevard, Tampa, FL 33612-9209; tel. 813/977–8700; FAX. 813/971–2029; Ms. Marsha L Brown
*Oakwood Center of the Palm Beaches, Inc., 1041 45th Street, West Palm Beach, FL 33407; tel. 561/383–8000; FAX. 561/514–1995; Dr. Linda C. DePiano
Parent's Information and Resource Center, Inc., 817 North Dixie Highway, Pompano Beach, FL 33060; tel. 954/785–8285; FAX. 954/784–2756; Mrs. Janet V. Ward
*PB Institute Partners Limited Partnership, 1017 N. Olive Avenue, West Palm Beach, FL 33401; tel. 800/433–5098; FAX. 561/655–5327; Mr. Ron Dawe
Peace River Center for Personal Development, Inc., P.O. Box 1559, Bartow, FL 33831-1559; tel. 863/534–7020; FAX. 863/534–7028; Ms. Mary Lu Kiley
Personal Enrichment through Mental Health Services, Inc., 11254 58th Street North, Pinellas Park, FL 33782; tel. 727/545–6477; FAX. 727/545–6526; Mr. Thomas C. Wedekind
*RBHS & MHRC & MHCJ, PO Box 19249, Jacksonville, FL 32245-9249; tel. 904/743–1883; FAX. 904/743–5109; Dr. Robert Sommers
*Recovery First, Inc., 5844 Sterling Road, Hollywood, FL 33020; tel. 954/981–4545; FAX. 954/735–6033; Mr. James Davis
*Reflections Wellness Center, Inc., 5753 Miami Lakes Drive East, Miami Lakes, FL 33014; tel. 305/403–0006; FAX. 305/403–0007; Dr. Leonel E. Mesa
South County Mental Health Center, Inc., 16158 South Military Trail, Delray Beach, FL 33484; tel. 561/637–1004; FAX. 561/495–7975; Dr. Joseph S. Speicher

*Indicates organization is a Joint Commission accredited Chemical Dependency organization.

Section C

SP Behavioral,LLC, 11301 SE Tequesta Terrace, Tequesta, FL 33469; tel. 561/744–0211; FAX. 561/575–1445; Dr. John W. Thompson

***Stepping Stones,** 4825 N Dixie Highway, Oakland Park, FL 33334; tel. 954/489–2580; FAX. 954/491–4193; Mrs. Joanne Telmosse

***Sunrise Detoxification Center, LLC,** 3185 Boutwell Road, Lake Worth, FL 33461; tel. 561/533–0074; FAX. 561/533–8077; Mr. Jeffrey G. Gorin

Tampa Bay Academy, 12012 Boyette Road, Riverview, FL 33569; tel. 813/677–6700; FAX. 813/671–3145; Mr. Stephen Albrecht

***Ten Broeck Ocala,** 3130 SW 27th Avenue, Ocala, FL 34474; tel. 352/671–3130; FAX. 352/861–3134; Mr. James E. Ledbetter

***The Centers,** 5664 SW 60th Ave, Ocala, FL 34474; tel. 352/291–5456; FAX. 352/291–5581; Mr. Russell Rasco

***The Centre for Women, Inc.,** 305 South Hyde Park Avenue, Tampa, FL 33606; tel. 813/251–8437; FAX. 813/253–2081; Ms. Beth Ficquette

The Devereux Foundation, Inc., 5850 T. G. Lee Blvd, Suite 400, Orlando, FL 32822; tel. 407/362–9210; FAX. 407/816–6481; Mr. Michael C Becker

***The Recovery Place, Inc.,** 3100 E. Commercial Blvd., Fort Lauderdale, FL 33308; tel. 954/200–8308; FAX. 954/200–8320; Mr. John Cates

***The Village South, Inc.,** 3180 Biscayne Boulevard, Miami, FL 33137; tel. 305/573–3784; FAX. 305/576–1348; Mr. Frank Rabbito

***The Watershed at Clear Lake,** 200 Congress Park Drive, Suite 100, Delray Beach, FL 33445; tel. 561/361–6608; FAX. 561/860–8275; Mr. Chris Crosby

***The Watershed Treatment Programs,** 200 Congress Park Drive, #100, Delray Beach, FL 33445; tel. 561/361–6608; FAX. 561/860–8275; Mr. Chris Crosby

***The Watershed Treatment Programs, Boca Raton FL- OTP,** 200 Congress Park Dr. Suite 100, Delray Beach, FL 33445; tel. 561/361–6608; FAX. 561/860–8275; Mr. Christopher Crosby

***The Willough at Naples,** 9001 Tamiami Trail East, Naples, FL 34113; tel. 941/775–4500; FAX. 941/793–0534; Mr. James O'Shea

***Transitions Recovery Program,** 1928 Northeast 154th Street, North Miami, FL 33162; tel. 305/949–9001; FAX. 305/945–6074; Mr. Lee Barchan

***Treatment Resources of Margate, Inc.,** 5100 Coconut Creek Parkway, Margate, FL 33063; tel. 954/917–3334; FAX. 954/917–9369; Ms. Bea Redlich

***Treatment Solutions of South Florida, Inc.,** 1421 Southeast 4th Avenue, Suite D, Fort Lauderdale, FL 33316; tel. 954/463–2810; FAX. 954/463–2817; Mr. Augustine J. Crocco

***Turning Point of Tampa, Inc.,** 6227 Sheldon Road, Tampa, FL 33615; tel. 813/882–3003; FAX. 813/885–6974; Ms. Robin Piper

***UMC Wekiva Springs, Inc.,** 3947 Salisbury Road, Jacksonville, FL 32216; tel. 904/296–3533; FAX. 904/296–3536; Mr. Paul Andrews

University Behavioral Center, 2500 Discovery Drive, Orlando, FL 32826; tel. 407/281–7000; FAX. 407/282–7012

Volunteers of America of Florida, Inc., 1205 East 8th Avenue, Tampa, FL 33605; tel. 813/282–1525; FAX. 813/287–8831; Ms. Kathryn E. Spearman

GEORGIA

***Albany Area Community Service Board,** PO Box 1988, Albany, GA 31702; tel. 229/430–4005; FAX. 229/430–6651; Mrs. Faye Holt

***AmericanWork, Inc.,** PO Box 20664, Saint Simons Island, GA 31522; tel. 912/638–0350; FAX. 912/638–9030; Mr. Ken Whiddon

Central State Hospital, 620 Broad St, Milledgeville, GA 31062; tel. 478/445–4128; FAX. 478/445–6034; Mr. Marvin Bailey

Chanan Foundation, INC, 6470 Cedar Mountain Road, Douglasville, GA 30134; tel. 678/715–8891; FAX. 770/489–6517; Mr. Lon Bell

Coastal Harbor Treatment Center, 1150 Cornell Avenue, Savannah, GA 31406; tel. 912/354–3911; FAX. 912/355–1336; Mr. Raymond Frederick Heckerman

Devereux Georgia Treatment Network, PO Box 1688, Kennesaw, GA 30144-8688; tel. 678/303–2665; FAX. 770/423–1679; Mr. Mario Bolivar

***DM & ADR, Inc.,** 1710 Commerce Road, Athens, GA 30607; tel. 706/552–0688; FAX. 706/552–0608; Ms. Ali McCorkle

***Fulton County Dept of MHDDAD,** 115 MLK, Jr., Drive, Suite 277, Atlanta, GA 30303; tel. 404/730–0230; FAX. 404/730–0341; Dr. Barbara J Lattimore

***Gateway Behavioral Health Services,** 1000 Commisioners Drive, Darien, GA 31305; tel. 912/437–7300; FAX. 912/437–9483; Dr. Frank A. Bonati

***Georgia Pines Community Service Board,** 1102 Smith Avenue Suite K, Thomasville, GA 31799; tel. 229/225–4335; FAX. 229/225–4374; Mr. Robert H. Jones

***Georgia Psychological Services,** PO Box 211626, Augusta, GA 30917-1626; tel. 706/210–3066; FAX. 706/210–8703; Mr. David W. Proefrock

***Grady Health System-Drug Dependence Unit,** 48-50 Coca Cola Place, Atlanta, GA 30303-3043; tel. 404/616–3970; FAX. 404/616–3978; Ms. Pamela Stephenson

Inner Harbour, Ltd., 4685 Dorsett Shoals Road, Douglasville, GA 30135; tel. 770/942–2391; FAX. 770/489–0406; Mr. Ronald Scroggy

Laurel Heights Hospital, 934 Briarcliff Road, Northeast, Atlanta, GA 30306; tel. 404/888–7860; FAX. 404/872–5088; Ms. Gloria Choo

Macon Behavioral Health System, 3500 Riverside Drive, Macon, GA 31210; tel. 478/477–3829; FAX. 478/477–4642

***McIntosh Trail MH/MR/SA Community Service Board,** PO Box 1320, Griffin, GA 30224; tel. 770/358–8250; FAX. 770/229–3223; Ms. Pam McCollum

***Metro Atlanta Recovery Residences, Inc.,** PO Box 48349, Atlanta, GA 30342; tel. 678/805–5100; FAX. 770/216–9398; Mr. Guerry Dyes

Murphy Harpst Children's Centers, 740 Fletcher Street, Cedartown, GA 30125; tel. 770/748–1500; FAX. 770/749–1094; Ms. Joanne G. Simmons

***Ogeechee Behavioral Health Services,** PO Box 1259, Swainsboro, GA 30401; tel. 478/289–2522; FAX. 478/289–2544; Mrs. Victoria Richbourg

***Opiate Agonist Treatment Therapy Clinic,** 1670 Clairmont Road, Decatur, GA 30033; tel. 404/321–6111; FAX. 404/329–4643; Dr. Jennifer Casarella

Ridge Creek, Inc., 830 Hidden Lake Road, Dahlonega, GA 30533; tel. 706/867–1720; FAX. 706/864–5826; Dr. Leonard Buccellato

Skyland Trail, 1903 North Druid Hills Road, Atlanta, GA 30319; tel. 404/315–8333; FAX. 404/315–9838; Mrs. Elizabeth E. Finnerty

***Southside Behavioral Lifestyle Enrichment Center,** 2685 Metropolitan Parkway, Suite C, Atlanta, GA 30315; tel. 404/627–1385; FAX. 404/564–6990; Dr. Robert E. Williams

***Sylvanus Memorial Treatment Centers, Inc.,** 734 Hospital Road, Commerce, GA 30529; tel. 706/335–5180; FAX. 706/335–5217; Mr. William W. Read

***Talbott Recovery Campus,** 5448 Yorktowne Drive, Atlanta, GA 30349; tel. 770/994–0185; FAX. 770/997–8230; Mr. Benjamin H. Underwood

***Turning Point Hospital,** PO Box 1177, Moultrie, GA 31768; tel. 229/985–4815; FAX. 229/891–2198; Mr. Ben Marion

***Willingway Hospital,** 311 Jones Mill Road, Statesboro, GA 30458; tel. 912/764–6236; FAX. 912/764–7063; Mr. Jimmy Mooney

HAWAII

Benchmark Behavioral Health Systems - Pearl City, P.O Box 1196, Pearl City, HI 96782; tel. 808/454–1411; FAX. 808/454–0659; Mr. Ryan B. Marendiuk

IDAHO

Ascent, 1 Ruby Creek Road, Naples, ID 83847; tel. 208/267–3626; FAX. 208/267–2295; Mrs. Trilby Hoover

Project Patch, PO Box 450, Garden Valley, ID 83622; tel. 503/653–8086; FAX. 503/653–8265; Mr. Tom Sanford

ILLINOIS

***Advocate Addiction Treatment Program,** 1775 Dempster Street, 10 South, Park Ridge, IL 60068; tel. 847/795–3900; FAX. 847/795–3901; Dr. James Dan

Alexian Center for Mental Health, 3350 Salt Creek Lane, #114, Arlington Heights, IL 60005; tel. 847/952–7460; FAX. 847/222–1754; Mr. Denis Ferguson

Allendale Association, PO Box 1088, Lake Villa, IL 60046; tel. 847/356–2351; FAX. 847/356–2393; Ms. Mary Shahbazian

***Arlington Center for Recovery,** 1655 South Arlington Heights Road, Suite 200, Arlington Heights, IL 60005; tel. 847/427–9680; FAX. 847/427–9561; Mr. Tim Fellers

Beacon Therapeutic Diagnostic and Treatment Center, 1912 West 103rd Street, Chicago, IL 60643; tel. 773/298–1243; FAX. 773/298–1078; Ms. Susan Reyna-Guerrero

***Ben Gordon Center,** 12 Health Services Drive, Dekalb, IL 60115; tel. 815/756–4875; FAX. 815/756–5161; Mr. Michael D. Flora

Camelot Schools, LLC, 1150 North River Road, 300 Quigley Bldg., Des Plaines, IL 60016; tel. 847/391–8000; FAX. 847/391–8001

***CAP of Downers Grove,** 4954 South Main Street, Downers Grove, IL 60515; tel. 630/810–0186; FAX. 630/810–0179; Dr. Ernest Rose

***Center for Addictive Problems,** 609 North Wells Street, Chicago, IL 60610; tel. 312/266–0404; FAX. 312/266–8169; Dr. Ernest Rose

Center on Deafness, 3444 Dundee Road, Northbrook, IL 60062; tel. 847/559–0110; FAX. 847/559–8199; Dr. Bonita Simon

***Central Illinois Center for the Treatment of Addiction,** 228 Northeast Jefferson, Peoria, IL 61654; tel. 309/671–8000; FAX. 309/671–4695; Mr. Michael G. Boyle

***Chestnut Health Systems,** 1003 Martin Luther King Drive, Bloomington, IL 61701; tel. 309/827–6026; FAX. 309/820–1386; Mr. Russell J. Hagen

***Chicago Lakeshore Hospital,** 4840 North Marine Drive, Chicago, IL 60640; tel. 773/878–9700; FAX. 773/904–4607; Mr. C. Alan Eaks

Coles County Mental Health Association, Inc., 750 Broadway Avenue East, Mattoon, IL 61938; tel. 217/234–6405; FAX. 217/235–0632; Mrs. Lynette Ashmore

***Community Counseling Centers of Chicago,** 4740 North Clark Street, Chicago, IL 60640; tel. 773/765–0810; FAX. 773/769–0344; Dr. Anthony A. Kopera

***Comprehensive Mental Health Center of St. Clair County,** 3911 State Street, East Saint Louis, IL 62205; tel. 618/482–7330; FAX. 618/482–4351; Mrs. Marsha R. Johnson

***Cornell Interventions - DuPage,** 11 S 250 Route 83, Hinsdale, IL 60521; tel. 630/325–5050; FAX. 630/325–9130; Ms. JoAnne Marks

***Cornell Interventions - Woodridge,** 2221 64th Street, Woodridge, IL 60517; tel. 630/968–6477; FAX. 630/968–8945

***Cornell Interventions East St. Louis,** 302 North 5thStreet, East Saint Louis, IL 62201; tel. 618/271–4542; FAX. 618/271–5975; Mr. Don Otis

***Cornell Interventions Life Works,** 1611 Jefferson Street, Joliet, IL 60435; tel. 815/730–7521; FAX. 815/730–7524; Ms. Karen Monroe

***Cornell Interventions Southwood,** 5701 South Wood Street, Chicago, IL 60636; tel. 773/737–4600; FAX. 773/737–5790; Mr. Walter Carlson

***Counseling Center of Lake View,** 3225 North Sheffield Avenue, Chicago, IL 60657; tel. 773/549–5886; FAX. 773/549–3265; Mr. Norman J. Groetzinger

DuPage County Health Dept./ Mental Health Services, 111 North County Farm Road, Wheaton, IL 60187; tel. 630/682–7400; FAX. 630/690–5282; Ms. Maureen McHugh

***Edward Hines Jr VA Hospital / Drug Dependency Treatment Center,** PO Box 5000, Hines, IL 60141; tel. 708/202–8387; FAX. 708/202–7217; Dr. David Barthwell

Family Alliance, Inc., 2028 N. Seminary Ave., Woodstock, IL 60098; tel. 815/338–3590; FAX. 815/337–4406; Mrs. Carol Louise

***Family Guidance Centers, Inc.,** 751 Aurora Avenue, Aurora, IL 60505; tel. 630/801–0017; FAX. 630/801–0018; Dr. Larry Kroll

***Family Guidance Centers, Inc.,** 310 West Chicago Avenue, Chicago, IL 60610; tel. 312/943–6545; FAX. 312/943–9430; Dr. Larry Kroll

***Family Guidance Centers, Inc.,** 484 Lee Street, Des Plaines, IL 60016; tel. 847/827–7517; FAX. 847/827–2707; Dr. Larry Kroll

***Family Service and Community Mental Health Center/McHenry,** 4100 Veterans Parkway, McHenry, IL 60050; tel. 815/363–3105; FAX. 815/385–8127; Mr. Robert M. Martens

*Indicates organization is a Joint Commission accredited Chemical Dependency organization.

FHN Family Counseling Center, 414 W. Stephenson St., Freeport, IL 61032; tel. 815/599–7337; FAX. 815/599–7397; Mr. Daniel E. Neal

***Garfield Counseling Center, Inc.,** 4132 West Madison, Chicago, IL 60624; tel. 773/533–0433; FAX. 773/533–1448; Mr. Richard E. Shelton

***Gateway Foundation Inc.,** 55 East Jackson Blvd, Suite 1500, Chicago, IL 60604; tel. 312/663–1130; FAX. 312/663–0504; Mr. Michael Darcy

***Heartland Human Services,** PO Box 1047, Effingham, IL 62401; tel. 217/347–7179; FAX. 217/342–6971; Ms. Cheryl Compton

***Human Service Center,** PO Box 1346, Peoria, IL 61654-1346; tel. 309/671–8000; FAX. 309/671–4695; Mr. Michael G. Boyle

Janet Wattles Center, Inc., 526 West State Street, Rockford, IL 61101; tel. 815/968–9300; FAX. 815/968–5314; Mr. Frank H. Ware

***Jesse Brown Opioid Addiction Treatment Program (OTP) VA,** 820 South Damen Avenue (Independence Hall), Chicago, IL 60612; tel. 312/569–6101; FAX. 312/569–6188

Kenneth Young Center, 1001 Rohlwing Road, Elk Grove Village, IL 60007; tel. 847/524–8800; FAX. 847/524–8824; Mr. Mitchell Bruski

***Lake County Health Department / Behavioral Health Services,** 3012 Grand Avenue, Waukegan, IL 60085; tel. 847/377–8299; FAX. 847/336–1517; Mr. Dale W. Galassie

***Leyden Family Service and Mental Health Center,** 10001 West Grand Avenue, Franklin Park, IL 60131; tel. 847/451–0330; FAX. 847/451–1652; Mr. Dennis P. Vaccaro

***McHenry County Youth Service Bureau,** 101 South Jefferson Street, Woodstock, IL 60098; tel. 815/338–7360; FAX. 815/337–5510; Ms. Susan H. Krause

Mental Health and Deafness Resources, Inc., 614 Anthony Trail, Northbrook, IL 60062; tel. 847/509–8260; FAX. 847/509–8157; Ms. Patricia A Scherer

Mental Health Center of Champaign County, Inc., 1801 Fox Drive, Champaign, IL 61820; tel. 217/398–8080; FAX. 217/398–0172; Ms. Sheila Ferguson

***Mercy Hospital and Medical Center,** 2525 S. Michigan Ave., Chicago, IL 60616; tel. 312/567–2000; FAX. 312/567–6575; Sister Sheila Lyne, RSM

***Michael Reese Hospital - OTP,** 2929 South Ellis Avenue, Chicago, IL 60616; tel. 312/791–3545; FAX. 312/791–3927; Dr. Enrique Beckmann

***North Central Behavioral Health Systems, Inc.,** PO Box 1488, La Salle, IL 61301; tel. 815/223–0160; FAX. 815/223–1634; Mr. Donald P. Miskowiec

***Northwest Community Hospital Youth Center,** 901 Kirchoff Road, Arlington Heights, IL 60005; tel. 847/618–1000; FAX. 847/618–5009; Mr. Bruce K. Crowther

***P.H.A.S.E. Inc., Methadone Treatment Program,** 516 Green Street, Rockford, IL 61102; tel. 815/966–1285; FAX. 815/490–1051; Mr. Gary Halbach

***PEER Services, Inc.,** 906 Davis Street, Evanston, IL 60201; tel. 847/492–1778; FAX. 847/492–0320; Ms. Kate Mahoney

***ProCare Centers,** 1820 South 25th Avenue, Broadview, IL 60153; tel. 708/338–3806; FAX. 708/681–1289; Mr. Frank Perham

Rosecrance, Inc., 1601 University Drive, Rockford, IL 61107; tel. 815/391–1000; FAX. 815/391–5041; Mr. Philip W. Eaton

***Sangamon Menard Alcoholism and Drugs Council,** 120 North 11th Street, Springfield, IL 62703-1002; tel. 217/544–9858; FAX. 217/544–0223; Mr. Stephen J. Knox

***Sinnissippi Centers, Inc.,** 325 Illinois Route 2, Dixon, IL 61021; tel. 815/284–6611; FAX. 815/284–6642; Mr. James R. Sarver

***South Shore Hospital,** 8012 S. Crandon Avenue, Chicago, IL 60617; tel. 773/356–5200; FAX. 773/768–8154; Mr. Jesus M. Ong

***Southeastern Illinois Counseling Centers, Inc.,** Drawer M, Olney, IL 62450; tel. 618/395–4306; FAX. 618/395–4507; Mr. Glenn Jackson

***Tazwood Mental Health Center, Inc.,** 3248 Vandever Ave., Pekin, IL 61554; tel. 309/347–5579; FAX. 309/347–4264; Mr. Michael Polson

The Ecker Center for Mental Health, 1845 Grandstand Place, Elgin, IL 60123; tel. 847/695–0484; FAX. 847/695–1265; Ms. Karen Beyer

***The South Suburban Council on Alcoholism and Substance Abuse,** 1909 Cheker Square, East Hazel Crest, IL 60429; tel. 708/647–3333; FAX. 708/647–3399; Mr. Allen Sandusky

***The Women's Treatment Center,** 140 N. Ashland Avenue, Chicago, IL 60607; tel. 312/850–0050; FAX. 312/850–9095; Dr. Jewell Oates

***Timberline Knolls, LLC,** 40 Timberline Drive, Lemont, IL 60439; tel. 630/257–9600; FAX. 630/257–9708

***Triangle Center Methadone Clinic,** 120 North 11th Street, Springfield, IL 62703; tel. 217/544–9858; FAX. 217/544–0223; Mr. Stephen J. Knox

INDIANA

Adult and Child Mental Health Center, Inc., 8320 Madison Avenue, Indianapolis, IN 46227; tel. 317/882–5122; FAX. 317/859–5308; Mr. A. Robert Dunbar

***BehaviorCorp, Inc.,** 697 Pro-Med Lane, Carmel, IN 46032-5323; tel. 317/587–0500; FAX. 317/574–1234; Mr. Larry L. Burch

***Center for Behavioral Health,** 645 South Rogers Street, Bloomington, IN 47403; tel. 812/339–1691; FAX. 812/337–2438; Dr. Dennis P. Morrison

Columbus Behavioral Center for Children and Adolescents, 2223 Poshard Drive, Columbus, IN 47203; tel. 812/376–1711; FAX. 812/376–0801; Mrs. Kelly Ulreich

***Community Mental Health Center, Inc.,** 285 Bielby Road, Lawrenceburg, IN 47025; tel. 812/537–1302; FAX. 812/537–0194; Mr. Joseph D. Stephens

***Cummins Behavioral Health Systems, Inc.,** 6655 East US 36, Avon, IN 46123; tel. 317/272–6361; FAX. 317/272–3331; Ms. Ann Borders

Evansville Psychiatric Children's Center, 3300 East Morgan Avenue, Evansville, IN 47715; tel. 812/477–6436; FAX. 812/474–4247; Mrs. Lottie Cook

***Fairbanks Hospital, Inc.,** 8102 Clearvista Parkway, Indianapolis, IN 46256-4698; tel. 317/849–8222; FAX. 317/849–1455; Ms. Helene M. Cross

***Family & Children's Ctr. Counseling & Development Services,** 611 Lincoln Way East, South Bend, IN 46601; tel. 574/232–2255; FAX. 574/287–9377; Mr. Bruce L. Greenberg

***Four County Comprehensive Mental Health, Inc.,** 1015 Michigan Avenue, Logansport, IN 46947; tel. 574/722–5151; FAX. 574/722–9523; Mr. Lawrence R. Ulrich

Ft Wayne Children's Home of United Church of Christ, Inc, 2525 Lake Avenue, Fort Wayne, IN 46805-5457; tel. 260/484–4153; FAX. 260/484–2337; Mr. Randall J. Rider

***Grant-Blackford Mental Health, Inc.,** 505 Wabash Avenue, Marion, IN 46952; tel. 765/662–3971; FAX. 765/662–7480; Mr. Paul G. Kuczora

***Hamilton Center, Inc,** PO Box 4323, Terre Haute, IN 47804-0323; tel. 812/231–8323; FAX. 812/231–8411; Mr. Galen Goode

***LifeSpring, Inc.,** 460 Spring Street, Jeffersonville, IN 47130; tel. 812/280–2080; FAX. 812/206–1229; Dr. Terry L. Stawar

***Madison Center, Inc.,** PO Box 80, South Bend, IN 46624; tel. 574/234–0061; FAX. 574/234–0670; Mr. Jack Roberts

***Meridian Services, Corp.,** 240 North Tillotson Avenue, Muncie, IN 47304; tel. 765/288–1928; FAX. 765/741–0310; Mr. Hank A. Milius

Michiana Behavioral Health Center, 1800 North Oak Road, Plymouth, IN 46563; tel. 574/936–3784; FAX. 574/935–9076; Mr. Bryan Lett

***Oaklawn Psychiatric Center, Inc.,** PO Box 809 330 Lakeview Drive, Goshen, IN 46527-0809; tel. 574/533–1234; FAX. 574/537–2673; Ms. Laurie N. Nafziger

Options Treatment Center, 5602 Caito Drive, Indianapolis, IN 46226; tel. 317/544–4340; FAX. 317/544–4353; Ms. Roxane Harcourt

***Quinco Behavioral Health Systems,** 720 N. Marr Rd., Columbus, IN 47201; tel. 812/348–7449; FAX. 812/376–4875; Dr. Robert J Williams

R.T.C. Resource Acquisition Corporation, 1404 South State, Indianapolis, IN 46203; tel. 317/783–4003; FAX. 317/780–4810; Mr. Jeff Catlett

Resolute Acquisition Corporation, 320 North Tibbs, Indianapolis, IN 46222; tel. 317/630–5215; FAX. 317/630–5223; Ms. Lisa Machado

***Richard L. Roudebush VAMC Opioid Substitution Clinic,** 1481 West 10th Street, Bldg 1, Indianapolis, IN 46202; tel. 317/554–0000; FAX. 317/554–0012; Dr. Sean O'Connor

***Riverside Hospital,** PO Box 80, South Bend, IN 46624; tel. 574/234–0061; FAX. 574/234–0670; Mr. Jack Roberts

***Southlake Community Mental Health Center, Inc.,** 8555 Taft Street, Merrillville, IN 46410-6199; tel. 219/769–4005; FAX. 219/769–2508; Mr. Bob Krumwied

***Southwestern Indiana Mental Health Center, Inc.,** 415 Mulberry Street, Evansville, IN 47713-1298; tel. 812/436–4231; FAX. 812/422–7558; Mr. John K. Browning

***Tara Treatment Center, Inc.,** 6231 South US 31, Franklin, IN 46131; tel. 812/526–2611; FAX. 812/526–9949; Ms. Theresa Stratton

***The Center for Mental Health, Inc.,** PO Box 1258, Anderson, IN 46015; tel. 765/649–8161; FAX. 765/641–8238; Mr. C. Richard DeHaven

The Children's Campus, Inc., 1411 Lincoln Way West, Mishawaka, IN 46544-1690; tel. 574/259–5666; FAX. 574/255–6179; Ms. Kris Ermeti

The Midwest Center for Youth and Families, PO Box 669, Kouts, IN 46347; tel. 219/766–2999; FAX. 219/766–2998; Mr. Michael Perry

***The Otis R. Bowen Center for Human Services, Inc.,** PO Box 497, Warsaw, IN 46581-0497; tel. 574/267–7169; FAX. 574/269–3995; Mr. Kurt Carlson

***Tri-City Community Mental Health Center, Inc.,** 3903 Indianapolis Boulevard, East Chicago, IN 46312; tel. 219/392–6010; FAX. 219/392–6998; Mr. Robert Krumwied

***Wabash Valley Hospital, Inc.,** 2900 North River Road, West Lafayette, IN 47906; tel. 765/463–2555; FAX. 765/497–3960; Mr. Rick Crawley

Willowglen Academy - Indiana, Inc., 308 East 21st Avenue, Gary, IN 46407; tel. 219/886–1320; FAX. 219/886–1319; Mr. Leonard F. Dziubla

***Wishard Health Services,** 850 N. Meridian, Indianapolis, IN 46204; tel. 317/655–2255; FAX. 317/630–7678; Mrs. Margie Payne

IOWA

Boys and Girls Home and Family Services, Inc., 2101 Court Street, Sioux City, IA 51104; tel. 712/293–4700; FAX. 712/293–4800; Mr. Robert P Sheehan

Hillcrest Family Services, 2005 Asbury Road, Dubuque, IA 52001; tel. 563/583–7357; FAX. 563/583–7026; Mr. Gary L. Gansemer

***Orchard Place,** 925 Southwest Porter Avenue, Des Moines, IA 50315; tel. 515/285–6781; FAX. 515/287–9695; Mr. Brock Wolff

Woodward Academy, 1251 334th St., Woodward, IA 50276; tel. 515/438–3481; FAX. 515/438–3489; Mr. Bill Dean

KANSAS

***Atchison Valley Hope,** PO Box 312, Atchison, KS 66002; tel. 913/367–1618; FAX. 913/367–6224; Dr. Kenneth C. Gregoire

Camelot of Kansas, 2050 West 11th Street, Wichita, KS 67203; tel. 949/887–7713; Mr. Bob Lysek

***Kansas City Metro Methadone Program,** MS 4015, 3901 Rainbow Boulevard, Kansas City, KS 66160-7341; tel. 913/588–6493; FAX. 913/588–8094; Dr. William F. Gabrielli

KVC Behavioral HealthCare, Inc., 21350 W. 153 Street, Olathe, KS 66061; tel. 913/322–4900; Mr. B. Wayne Sims

***Marillac Center,** 8000 W. 127th Street, Overland Park, KS 66213; tel. 816/508–3300; FAX. 816/508–3321; Mr. Mark S. Richards

***Norton Valley Hope,** PO Box 510, Norton, KS 67654; tel. 785/877–5101; FAX. 785/877–3903; Dr. Kenneth C. Gregoire

***Saint Francis Community Services, Inc.,** 509 East Elm Street, Salina, KS 67401; tel. 785/825–0541; FAX. 785/825–2502; Rev. Edward W. Fellhauer

***United Methodist Youthville, Inc.,** 4505 E 47th Street South, Wichita, KS 67210; tel. 316/529–9100; FAX. 316/529–9351; Mrs. Shelley A. Duncan

*Indicates organization is a Joint Commission accredited Chemical Dependency organization.

KENTUCKY

*****Adanta Behavioral Health Services,** 259 Parkers Mill Road, Somerset, KY 42501; tel. 606/679–4782; FAX. 606/678–5296; Ms. Cathy Epperson

*****Bluegrass Regional Mental Health & Narcotics Addiction Program,** 1351 Newtown Pike, Lexington, KY 40511; tel. 859/253–1686; FAX. 859/255–4866; Mr. Joseph A Toy

Central State ICF/MR, 10510 LaGrange Road, Louisville, KY 40223; tel. 502/253–7311; FAX. 502/253–7335; Ms. Deborah Zech

*****Cumberland River Regional MH/MR Board, Inc.,** PO Box 568, Corbin, KY 40702; tel. 606/528–7010; FAX. 606/528–5401; Mr. Danny Jones

*****NorthKey Community Care,** PO Box 2680, Covington, KY 41012; tel. 859/578–3233; FAX. 859/578–3259; Dr. Edward G. Muntel

*****Recovery Works Drug & Alcohol Rehabilitation Center,** 3107 Cincinnati Road, Georgetown, KY 40324; tel. 502/570–9313; FAX. 502/867–7978; Mr. Matt Amos Rice

*****Seven Counties Services, Inc.,** 101 West Muhammad Ali Blvd, Louisville, KY 40202; tel. 502/589–8600; FAX. 502/589–8614; Dr. Howard F Bracco

Spectrum Care Academy, Inc., PO Box 911, Columbia, KY 42728; tel. 270/384–6444; FAX. 270/384–9126; Dr. Ben Arnold

Sunrise Children's Services, 300 Hope Street, Ministry Support Center, Mount Washington, KY 40047; tel. 502/538–1000; FAX. 502/254–0110; Dr. William K. Smithwick

LOUISIANA

*****Acadia Vermilion Hospital,** 2520 North University Avenue, Lafayette, LA 70507; tel. 337/234–5614; FAX. 337/210–1197; Mr. Craig Juengling

*****Addiction Recovery Resources of New Orleans,** 4836 Wabash Street, Suite 202, Metairie, LA 70001; tel. 504/780–2766; FAX. 504/780–9699; Ms. Tricia B. Mogg

*****DRD New Orleans Medical Clinic,** 417 S. Johnson Street, New Orleans, LA 70112; tel. 816/357–2461; FAX. 816/370–2242; Mr. Andrew Love

Jennings Behavioral Health, 619 North Main Street, Jennings, LA 70546; tel. 337/824–4300; FAX. 337/824–4315; Ms. Tehjan Martin

Lifecare Psychiatric Services, 170 Industrial Parkway, Lafayette, LA 70508; tel. 337/262–8672; FAX. 337/262–8676; Mr. Harry Cicero

OASIS Integrated Medical Services, LLC, 820 Jordan Street Suite 306, Shreveport, LA 71101; tel. 318/678–8880; FAX. 318/678–8886; Ms. Jacqueline Abrams Danzell

Positive Choices Counseling Services, Inc., 1644 Carter Street, Suite 2, Vidalia, LA 71373; tel. 318/336–4700; FAX. 318/336–4777; Mr. Edward J. Brown

Success Counseling Services-North, 1504 Barksdale Blvd., Bossier City, LA 71111; tel. 318/222–4299; FAX. 318/425–2696; Ms. Donnalee Ammons

MAINE

*****Acadia Hospital - Narcotic Treatment Program,** PO Box 422, Bangor, ME 04402-0422; tel. 207/973–6100; FAX. 207/973–6109; Ms. Dorothy E. Hill

*****Cap Quality Care, Inc.,** 1 Delta Drive, Suite A, Westbrook, ME 04092; tel. 207/856–7227; FAX. 207/856–2112; Mrs. Noa Shinderman

*****Mercy Recovery Center,** 40 Park Road, Westbrook, ME 04092; tel. 207/857–8085; FAX. 207/857–8077; Mrs. Eileen F. Skinner

MARYLAND

*****Addiction Treatment Services of Hopkins Bayview,** 5510 Nathan Shock Drive, Suite 1500, Baltimore, MD 21224; tel. 410/550–0028; FAX. 410/550–2957; Mr. Gregory Schaffer

*****Ashley, Inc.,** 800 Tydings Lane, Havre De Grace, MD 21078; tel. 410/273–6600; FAX. 410/272–5617; Mr. Mark Hushen

*****Awakenings,** 2 West Aylesbury Road, Timonium, MD 21093; tel. 410/561–9591; FAX. 410/560–1082; Dr. Sheldon D. Glass

*****Baltimore Behavioral Health, Inc.,** 1001 W Pratt Street/201 S. Arlington, Baltimore, MD 21223; tel. 410/962–7180; FAX. 410/962–7194; Mr. William Kris Hathaway

*****Behavioral Pharmacology Research Unit,** 5510 Nathan Shock Drive, Baltimore, MD 21224; tel. 410/550–0035; FAX. 410/550–0030; Mr. Gregory Schaffer

*****Bon Secours Hospital Baltimore, Inc.,** 2000 West Baltimore Street, Baltimore, MD 21223; tel. 410/362–3011; FAX. 410/362–3578; Dr. Samuel L. Ross

*****Bon Secours New Hope Treatment Center,** 2401 West Baltimore Street, Baltimore, MD 21223; tel. 410/945–7706; FAX. 410/945–8767; Dr. Samuel L. Ross

*****Bon Secours' ADAPT Cares,** 2000 W Baltimore Street, Baltimore, MD 21223; tel. 410/383–4995; FAX. 410/669–5179; Dr. Samuel Ross

Brook Lane Health Services, PO Box 1945, Hagerstown, MD 21742-1945; tel. 301/733–0330; FAX. 301/733–4038; Mr. R. Lynn Rushing

*****Center for Addiction Medicine,** 827 Linden Avenue, Baltimore, MD 21201; tel. 410/225–8240; FAX. 410/225–8209; Dr. Michael Hayes

*****Chase Brexton Health Services, Inc.,** 1001 Cathedral Street, Baltimore, MD 21201; tel. 410/545–4481; FAX. 410/234–0537; Mr. David H. Shippee

*****Daybreak Rehabilitation Center,** 2490 Giles Road, Baltimore, MD 21225; tel. 410/396–1646; FAX. 410/396–2903; Dr. Sheldon D. Glass

*****Druid Heights Treatment and Counseling Center, Inc.,** 2009 Druid Hill Avenue, Baltimore, MD 21217; tel. 410/669–0475; FAX. 410/669–3681; Ms. Barbara Bostick-Hunt

*****Frederick County Health Dept. /Substance Abuse Services,** 300-B Scholl's Lane, Frederick, MD 21701; tel. 301/694–1775; FAX. 301/694–1803; Dr. Barbara Brookmyer

*****Glass Substance Abuse Program, Inc.,** 821 North Eutaw Street, Baltimore, MD 21202; tel. 410/225–9185; FAX. 410/225–7964; Dr. Sheldon D. Glass

House of the Good Shepherd of the City of Baltimore, 4100 Maple Avenue, Baltimore, MD 21227; tel. 410/247–2770; FAX. 410/247–1635; Dr. Trudy Turner

*****Hudson Health Services, Inc.,** PO Box 1096, Salisbury, MD 21802-1096; tel. 410/219–9000; FAX. 410/742–7048

Jewish Family Services, Inc., 5750 Park Heights Avenue, Baltimore, MD 21215; tel. 410/843–7409; FAX. 410/664–0551; Ms. Barbara Levy Gradet

John L. Gildner Regional Institute for Children & Adolescents, 15000 Broschart Road, Rockville, MD 20850; tel. 301/251–6800; FAX. 301/309–9004; Mr. Thomas E. Pukalski

Maple Shade Youth & Family Services, Inc., 23704 Ocean Gateway, Mardela Springs, MD 21837; tel. 410/742–7400; FAX. 410/742–6452; Ms. Jarvia L. Fishell

*****Maryland Treatment Centers, Inc.,** PO Box 136, Emmitsburg, MD 21727; tel. 301/447–2361; FAX. 301/447–6504; Ms. Mary A. Roby

*****MBA - Cherry Hill,** 2490 Giles Road, Baltimore, MD 21225; tel. 410/225–9185; FAX. 410/225–7964; Dr. Sheldon D. Glass

*****Methadone for Business Achievers (MBA),** 821 North Eutaw Street, Baltimore, MD 21201; tel. 410/225–9185; FAX. 410/225–7964; Dr. Sheldon D. Glass

*****Methadone for Business Achievers - Timonium,** 2 West Aylesbury Road, Timonium, MD 21093; tel. 410/561–9591; FAX. 410/225–7964; Dr. Sheldon D. Glass

*****Mid-Atlantic Treatment Services, Inc.,** 2100 North Charles Street, Baltimore, MD 21218; tel. 410/752–6505; FAX. 410/385–1237; Ms. Barbara Q. McKenna

*****Partners in Recovery,** 6525 North Charles Street, Gibson Bldg., Baltimore, MD 21204; tel. 410/296–2268; FAX. 410/938–3555; Ms. Marcia Ellis

*****Pathways,** 2620 Riva Road, Annapolis, MD 21401; tel. 410/573–5400; FAX. 410/573–5401; Mrs. Helen K Reines

Potomac Ridge Behavioral Health System - Eastern Shore, 821 Fieldcrest Road, Cambridge, MD 21613; tel. 410/221–0288; FAX. 410/228–7496

*****Prince George's County Health Department,** 1701 McCormick Drive, Suite 230, Upper Marlboro, MD 20772; tel. 301/883–7903; FAX. 301/883–7881

*****Prince George's County Health Dept/Northern Region Treatment,** 1701 McCormick Drive, Largo, MD 20774; tel. 301/883–7853; FAX. 301/883–7881; Dr. Donald W. Shell

*****Reflective Treatment Center,** 301 N Gay Street, Baltimore, MD 21202; tel. 410/752–3500; FAX. 410/752–6922; Dr. Marie J. Washington

Regional Institute for Children and Adolescents-Baltimore, 605 South Chapel Gate Lane, Baltimore, MD 21229; tel. 410/368–7800; FAX. 410/368–7886; Ms. Penny Makris

RICA - Southern Maryland, 9400 Surratts Road, Cheltenham, MD 20623; tel. 301/372–1800; FAX. 301/372–1906; Ms. Mary Sheperd

Saint Luke Institute, 8901 New Hampshire Avenue, Silver Spring, MD 20903; tel. 301/445–7970; FAX. 301/422–5400; Rev. Stephen J. Rossetti

*****Sinai Hospital Addictions Recovery Program,** 2401 West Belvedere Avenue, Baltimore, MD 21215; tel. 410/601–5355; FAX. 410/601–6281; Mr. Neil Meltzer

*****The Johns Hopkins Hospital Drug Abuse Program,** 600 North Wolfe Street, Baltimore, MD 21287; tel. 410/955–5000; FAX. 410/955–0856; Mr. Ron R. Peterson

*****Tuerk House, Inc.,** PO Box 31419, Baltimore, MD 21216-6119; tel. 410/233–0684; FAX. 410/947–8707; Dr. John E. Hickey

*****VA Maryland Health Care System Opioid Treatment Program,** 10 North Greene Street, Baltimore, MD 21201; tel. 410/605–7410; FAX. 410/605–7931; Dr. Joseph Liberto

Villa Maria Continuum, 2300 Dulaney Valley Road, Timonium, MD 21093; tel. 410/252–4700; FAX. 410/252–3040; Mr. Mark Greenberg

*****Wicomico County Health Department,** 108 East Main Street, Salisbury, MD 21801; tel. 410/742–3784; FAX. 410/543–6680; Mrs. Lori Brewster

Woodbourne Center, Inc., 1301 Woodbourne Avenue, Baltimore, MD 21239; tel. 410/433–1000; FAX. 410/435–4745; Dr. Stanley E. Weinstein

*****Worcester County Health Department,** PO Box 249, Snow Hill, MD 21863; tel. 410/632–1100; FAX. 410/632–0906; Ms. Deborah Goeller

MASSACHUSETTS

*****AdCare Hospital of Worcester, Inc.,** 107 Lincoln Street, Worcester, MA 01605-2499; tel. 508/799–9000; FAX. 508/795–0224; Mr. David W. Hillis

Austen Riggs Center, 25 Main Street, Stockbridge, MA 01262-0962; tel. 413/298–5511; FAX. 413/298–4020; Dr. Edward R. Shapiro

*****Baldpate Hospital,** 83 Baldpate Road, Georgetown, MA 01833; tel. 978/352–2131; FAX. 978/352–6755; Ms. Lucille M. Batal

*****Bournewood Hospital (Detoxification Program),** 300 South Street, Chestnut Hill, MA 02467; tel. 617/469–0300; FAX. 617/469–5013; Dr. Nasir A. Khan

Bridgewater State Hospital, 20 Administration Road, Bridgewater, MA 02324; tel. 508/279–4500; FAX. 508/279–3192; Ms. Karin T. Bergeron

Brockton Multi Service Center, 165 Quincy Street, Brockton, MA 02302; tel. 508/897–2000; FAX. 508/897–2075; Mr. Richard Jobin

Cape Cod and Islands Community Mental Health Center, 830 County Road, Pocasset, MA 02559; tel. 508/564–9626; FAX. 508/564–9700; Mr. Stephen Jochim

*****Carlson Recovery Center,** 471 Chestnut, Springfield, MA 01199; tel. 413/794–3971; FAX. 413/794–0532; Mr. Mark R. Tolosky

Centerpoint, PO Box 374, Tewksbury, MA 01876; tel. 978/858–3776; FAX. 978/858–3494; Ms. Carolyn F. Ingalls

Chauncy Hall Academy, PO Box 732, Westborough, MA 01581; tel. 508/898–3280; FAX. 508/836–5512; Mr. Steven Hahn

Cohannet Academy, 60 Hodges Avenue - Goss 3, Taunton, MA 02780; tel. 508/977–3730; FAX. 508/824–7528; Mr. Bryan Lary

*****Dimock Community Foundation, Inc. - OTP,** 55 Dimock Street, Roxbury, MA 02119; tel. 617/442–8800; FAX. 617/445–0091; Ms. RuthEllen Fitch

Doctor Franklin Perkins School, 971 Main Street, Lancaster, MA 01523; tel. 978/365–7376; FAX. 978/368–8861; Dr. Charles P. Conroy

Dr. John C. Corrigan Mental Health Center, 49 Hillside Street, Fall River, MA 02720; tel. 508/235–7200; FAX. 508/235–7346; Mr. Steven Figueiredo

*****Gosnold, Inc.,** 200 Ter Heun Drive, Falmouth, MA 02540; tel. 508/540–6550; FAX. 508/540–7480; Mr. Raymond V Tamasi

*Indicates organization is a Joint Commission accredited Chemical Dependency organization.

*High Point Treatment Center, 940 Belmont Street Building # 60, Brockton, MA 02301; tel. 508/584–9210; FAX. 508/584–9520; Mr. Daniel S. Mumbauer

*High Point Treatment Center, Inc., 1233 State Road, Plymouth, MA 02360; tel. 508/224–7701; FAX. 508/224–2845; Mr. Daniel S. Mumbauer

*High Point Treatment Center, Inc. (OTP), 100 North Front Street, New Bedford, MA 02740; tel. 774/628–1000; FAX. 774/628–1099; Mr. Daniel Mumbauer

Hillcrest Educational Centers, Inc., PO Box 4699, Pittsfield, MA 01202; tel. 413/499–7924; FAX. 413/445–2693; Mr. Gerard E. Burke

Laurel Hill Inn, Ltd., PO Box 368, Medford, MA 02155-0004; tel. 781/396–1116; FAX. 781/391–8820; Mr. William H. McDonald

*Lowell Community Health Center Behavioral Health Services, 365 East Street, Tewksbury, MA 01876; tel. 978/858–0533; FAX. 978/858–0473; Ms. Dorcas Grigg-Saito

*McLean Hospital Alcohol & Drug Abuse Treatment Program, 115 Mill Street, Belmont, MA 02478; tel. 617/855–3450; FAX. 617/855–3536; Dr. Scott L. Rauch

*Mercy Medical Center - MMTP, 227 Mill Street, Springfield, MA 01102; tel. 413/539–2400; FAX. 413/493–2768; Mr. Vincent J. McCorkle

*Mercy Medical Center - MMTP & Inpatient Detox Program, 1233 Main Street, Holyoke, MA 01040; tel. 413/539–2950; FAX. 413/493–2768; Mr. Vincent J McCorkle

Metro Boston Mental Health Units, 25 Staniford Street, Boston, MA 02114; tel. 617/626–8510; FAX. 617/626–8515; Dr. Mary Louise White

Quincy Mental Health Center, 460 Quincy Avenue, Quincy, MA 02169; tel. 617/626–9003; FAX. 617/770–2953; Mr. Paul Davidson

*SSTAR (Detoxification Program), 386 Stanley Street, Fall River, MA 02720; tel. 508/324–3500; FAX. 508/676–5671; Ms. Nancy E. Paull

*St. Anne's Hospital Lifeline Program, 795 Middle Street, Fall River, MA 02721; tel. 508/675–0131; FAX. 508/235–5053; Mr. Robert Guyon

The Three Rivers Treatment Program, 26 Ridgewood Terrace, Springfield, MA 01105; tel. 413/733–4032; FAX. 413/733–4130; Mr. Andrew Pollock

The Whitney Academy, Inc., PO Box 619, East Freetown, MA 02717; tel. 508/763–3737; FAX. 508/763–4200; Mr. George E. Harmon

University of Massachusetts Medical School, Transitions IRTP, 305 Belmont Street, 7th Flr C, Worcester, MA 01604; tel. 508/856–1455; FAX. 508/856–1435; Dr. Michael Collins

*VA Boston Healthcare System Drug Dependence Treatment Center, 1400 VFW Parkway, West Roxbury, MA 02132; tel. 617/323–7700; FAX. 857/203–5500

Wild Acre Inns, Inc., 108 Pleasant Street, Arlington, MA 02476; tel. 781/643–0643; FAX. 781/648–2937; Dr. Bernard S. Yudowitz

MICHIGAN

*ACAC, Inc., 3949 Sparks Drive SE Suite 103, Grand Rapids, MI 49546; tel. 616/957–5850; FAX. 616/957–5853; Mr. Michael R. Durco

*Access Behavioral Healthcare, LLC, 42189 E. Ann Arbor Road, Plymouth, MI 48170; tel. 734/453–5603; FAX. 734/453–5621; Mr. Donald Warner

*Apex Behavioral Health, PLLC, 1547 S. Wayne Rd., Westland, MI 48186; tel. 734/729–3133; FAX. 734/729–3130; Mr. Thomas Johnson

*Arbor Circle Corporation, 1115 Ball Avenue, Grand Rapids, MI 49505; tel. 616/456–7775; FAX. 616/456–8568; Mr. Jack Greenfield

Bay-Arenac Behavioral Health, 201 Mulholland, Bay City, MI 48708; tel. 989/895–2300; FAX. 989/895–2357; Mr. Robert Blackford

Beacon Specialized Living Services, 555 Railroad Street P.O. 69, Bangor, MI 49013; tel. 269/427–8400; FAX. 269/427–6027; Mr. Ken Ratzlaff

*Brighton Hospital, 12851 Grand River, Brighton, MI 48116; tel. 810/227–1211; FAX. 810/227–1869; Ms. Denise Bertin-Epp

C.W. Enterprises LLC, 32743 23 Mile Road, New Baltimore, MI 48047; tel. 586/716–0980; FAX. 586/716–0985; Dr. Cherie C. Whiting

*Catholic Services of Macomb, Inc., P.O. Box 380290, Clinton Township, MI 48038; tel. 586/416–2300; FAX. 586/416–2311; Mr. Thomas J. Reed

Children's Home of Detroit, 900 Cook Road, Grosse Pointe, MI 48236; tel. 313/886–0800; FAX. 313/417–3549; Dr. William Steele

*Community Care Services, 26184 West Outer Drive, Lincoln Park, MI 48146; tel. 313/389–7525; FAX. 313/389–7515; Mr. William P. Walsh

Community Mental Health for Central Michigan, 301 South Crapo, Suite 100, Mount Pleasant, MI 48858; tel. 989/772–5938; FAX. 989/773–1968; Ms. Linda Kaufmann

Comprehensive Psychiatric Services, PC, 28800 Orchard Lake Rd, Ste 250, Farmington Hills, MI 48334; tel. 248/932–2500; FAX. 248/932–2506; Dr. Saul Z. Forman

*Counseling & Evaluation, P.L.L.C., 53950 Van Dyke Avenue, Suite 210 B, Shelby Township, MI 48316; tel. 586/781–8400; FAX. 586/781–8300; Mr. Leo M. Szalma

Cruz Clinic, 17177 North Laurel Park Drive, Suite 131, Livonia, MI 48152; tel. 734/462–3210; FAX. 734/462–1024; Dr. Victor M. Cruz

*Deaf Options, 220 Bagley, Suite 600, Detroit, MI 48226-1420; tel. 313/961–8120; FAX. 313/961–9168; Mrs. Reichelle P. Tucker

DeLano Clinic, 1722 Shaffer Street, Suite 3, Kalamazoo, MI 49048; tel. 269/226–5695; FAX. 269/226–5606

*Delta Family Clinic South, 6201 Miller Road, Suite A, Swartz Creek, MI 48473; tel. 810/630–1152; FAX. 810/630–9107; Dr. Gerard R. Williams

*Department of Human Services - Gratiot Clinic, 3506 Gratiot Clinic, Detroit, MI 48207; tel. 313/887–6760; FAX. 313/852–4847; Mr. Octavius Sapp

*Department of Human Services, Herman Kiefer Hospital, Bldg 5, 8809 John C. Lodge, Detroit, MI 48202; tel. 313/887–6737; FAX. 313/852–5500; Mr. Octavius Sapp

Genesys Practice Partners, Inc., 3495 Center Road, Burton, MI 48519; tel. 810/424–2400; FAX. 810/579–7222; Mr. Paul Garson

*Growth Works Incorporated, PO Box 6115, Plymouth, MI 48170-0115; tel. 734/455–4095; FAX. 734/455–1254; Mr. Dale F. Yagiela

*Hegira Programs, Inc., 8623 N Wayne Road, Suite 200, Westland, MI 48185; tel. 734/458–4601; FAX. 734/458–4611; Mr. Edward L. Forry

*Horizon Treatment Services, LLC, 17117 W. 9 Mile Rd., Suite 646, Southfield, MI 48075; tel. 248/423–1728; FAX. 248/423–1734; Mr/Mrs Monique A. Smith

Huron Valley Consultation Center, Inc., 2750 South State Street, Ann Arbor, MI 48104; tel. 734/662–6300; FAX. 734/662–3365; Mr. Alex Martinez

Integro, llc, 1200 N West Avenue, Suite 300, Jackson, MI 49202; tel. 517/789–1234; FAX. 517/784–7040; Mrs. Marilyn Meadowcroft

Karalee & Associates, P.C., 1308 South Main Street, Plymouth, MI 48170; tel. 734/451–3440; FAX. 734/451–8720; Dr. Karen J. Maier

*Lapeer County Health Department, 1800 Imlay City Road, Lapeer, MI 48446; tel. 810/667–0243; FAX. 810/245–5676; Ms. Stephanie Simmons

*Latino Family Services, Inc., 3815 West Fort Street, Detroit, MI 48216; tel. 313/841–7380; FAX. 313/841–3730; Ms. Alicia Villarreal

Lenawee Community Mental Health Authority, 1040 S. Winter St., Ste.#1022, Adrian, MI 49221; tel. 517/263–8905; FAX. 517/263–7616; Mr. Roger Myers

Livingston County Community Mental Health Authority, 2280 East Grand River, Howell, MI 48843; tel. 517/546–4126; FAX. 517/546–1300; Mr. Angus Miller

*Meridian Professional Psychological Consultants, PC, 5031 Park Lake Road, East Lansing, MI 48823; tel. 517/332–0811; FAX. 517/332–4452; Dr. Thomas S. Gunnings

*Metro East Substance Abuse Treatment Corporation, PO Box 13408, Detroit, MI 48213; tel. 313/371–0055; FAX. 313/371–1409; Mr. Leslie B. Carroll

Metro Emergency Services, Inc., 224 Highland Avenue, Highland Park, MI 48203-3405; tel. 313/867–0111; FAX. 313/867–0208; Mr. Jon P. Rutherford

*Michigan Behavior Medicine, 625 East Big Beaver, Suite 101, Troy, MI 48083; tel. 248/740–9360; Dr. Kalappurackal Chacko Joseph

Michigan Psychiatric & Behavioral Associates, P.C., 690 South Trumbull Street, Bay City, MI 48708; tel. 989/922–4900; FAX. 989/922–4911; Dr. Kishore B. Kondapaneni

Monroe Community Mental Health Authority, P.O. Box 726, Monroe, MI 48161-0726; tel. 734/243–7340; FAX. 734/243–5564; Ms. Jane S. Terwilliger

*Motivational Empowerment Counseling Center and Associates, 7845 Middlebelt Rd., Romulus, MI 48174; tel. 734/721–0900; FAX. 734/721–0909; Mr. Roderick D. Peterson

*Nardin Park Recovery Center, 9605 Grand River, Detroit, MI 48204; tel. 313/834–5930; FAX. 313/834–4541; Mrs. Annie B Scott

New Center Community Mental Health Services, 2051 West Grand Boulevard, Detroit, MI 48208; tel. 313/961–3200; FAX. 313/961–3769; Ms. Roberta V. Sanders

*Oakland Psychological Clinic, P.C., 2550 South Telegraph Road Suite 250, Bloomfield Hills, MI 48302; tel. 248/322–0003; FAX. 248/322–0006; Dr. Barry H. Tigay

*Opioid Treatment Program - John D. Dingell VA Medical Center, 4646 John R. Street, Detroit, MI 48201; tel. 313/576–4644; FAX. 313/576–1091; Dr. John Grabowski

*Quality Behavioral Health, Inc., 751 East Grand Boulevard, Detroit, MI 48207; tel. 313/922–2222; FAX. 313/922–8771; Mr. Naveed V. Syed

*Rainbow Center of Michigan (Monroe), 14733 South Telegraph Road, Monroe, MI 48161; tel. 313/865–1580; FAX. 313/865–1582; Ms. Winnifred Griffin

*Rainbow Center of Michigan Inc, 12501 Hamilton Avenue, Highland Park, MI 48203; tel. 313/865–1580; FAX. 313/865–1582; Ms. Winnifred Griffin

*Redford Counseling Center, 25945 West Seven Mile Road, Redford, MI 48240; tel. 313/535–6560; FAX. 313/535–5266; Ms. JoAnn Sadler

*River's Bend, P.C., 33975 Dequindre, Suite 5, Troy, MI 48083; tel. 248/585–3239; FAX. 248/616–9759; Mr. Bruce Goldberg

Rose Hill Center, Inc., 5130 Rose Hill Boulevard, Holly, MI 48442; tel. 248/634–5530; FAX. 248/634–7754; Mr. Daniel J. Kelly

Shiawassee County Community Mental Health Authority, PO Box 428, Owosso, MI 48867; tel. 989/723–6791; FAX. 989/723–0761

*Star Center, Inc., 13575 Lesure, Detroit, MI 48227; tel. 313/493–4410; FAX. 313/493–4415; Ms. Lucila S. Ryder

Summit Pointe, 140 West Michigan Avenue, Battle Creek, MI 49017; tel. 616/966–1460; FAX. 616/966–2844; Mr. Ervin R. Brinker

Taylor Psychological Clinic, PC, 1172 Robert T. Longway Blvd, Flint, MI 48503; tel. 810/232–8466; FAX. 810/232–0041; Dr. Maxwell F. Taylor

*The Guidance Center, 13101 Allen Road, Southgate, MI 48195; tel. 734/785–7700; FAX. 734/287–1661; Mr. Leroy A. Lott

The Montcalm Center for Behavioral Health, 611 North State Street, Stanton, MI 48888; tel. 989/831–7520; FAX. 989/831–7578; Mr. Robert Brown

*The Salvation Army Turning Point Programs, 72 Sheldon Boulevard, S.E., Grand Rapids, MI 49503; tel. 616/742–0351; FAX. 616/742–0370; Mr. Dale Wanty

*Treatment Works, 2722 East Michigan Ave. Suite 104, Lansing, MI 48912; tel. 517/332–9000; FAX. 517/332–1670; Ms. Karen Moore

Tuscola Behavioral Health Systems, PO Box 239, Caro, MI 48723; tel. 989/673–6191; FAX. 517/673–1596; Ms. Sharon Beals

*Ultimate Solutions, 29240 Buckingham, Suite 11, Livonia, MI 48154; tel. 734/513–2800; FAX. 734/513–3606; Dr. Verona W. Morton

*Washtenaw County Community Supports and Treatment Services, 2140 East Ellsworth Road, Ann Arbor, MI 48108; tel. 734/544–3000; FAX. 734/544–6732; Ms. Donna Sabourin

MINNESOTA

Andrew Residence, 1215 South 9th Street, Minneapolis, MN 55404; tel. 612/333–0111; FAX. 612/338–1734; Ms. Karen Foy

*Community Addiction Recovery Enterprise, 3301 Seventh Avenue North, Anoka, MN 55303; tel. 651/431–5020; FAX. 763/712–4037; Mr. Mike Tessneer

*Indicates organization is a Joint Commission accredited Chemical Dependency organization.

***Community Addiction Recovery Enterprise - Willmar OTP,** 1705 16th Street NE, Willmar, MN 56201; tel. 320/231–5356; FAX. 320/231–5923; Mr. Mike Tessneer

***Hazelden Foundation, Recovery Services Division,** PO Box 11, Center City, MN 55012; tel. 612/257–4000; FAX. 612/213–4738; Ms. Ellen Breyer

***Hennepin Faculty Associates Addiction Medicine Program,** 914 South Eighth St. (D131), Minneapolis, MN 55404; tel. 612/347–0950; FAX. 612/347–0955; Mr. Larry Fosbury

Minnesota Security Hospital, 2100 Sheppard Drive, St Peter, MN 56082; tel. 507/931–7128; FAX. 507/931–7711; Mr. Mike Tessneer

***New Beginnings at Waverly, LLC,** 109 North Shore Drive, Waverly, MN 55390-9743; tel. 763/658–5800; FAX. 763/658–4128; Mr. Clelland P. Gilchrist

***St. Joseph's Hospital Chemical Dependency Unit,** 69 West Exchange Street, Saint Paul, MN 55102; tel. 651/232–3300; Mr. Tim Hansen

***Veterans Affairs Medical Center Outpatient Methadone Program,** One Veterans Drive, Minneapolis, MN 55417; tel. 612/725–2228; FAX. 612/970–5891; Dr. Zaheer Aslam

MISSISSIPPI

***CARES Center, Inc.,** 402 Wesley Avenue, Jackson, MS 39202; tel. 601/352–7784; FAX. 601/360–0585; Mr. Christopher M Cherney

***COPAC, Inc.,** 3949 Highway 43 North, Brandon, MS 39047; tel. 601/829–2500; FAX. 601/829–4278; Dr. J. Stacy Hughes

Diamond Grove Center for Children and Adolescents, PO Box 848, Louisville, MS 39339; tel. 662/779–0119; FAX. 662/779–0126; Mr. Patrick Swoopes

Millcreek of Pontotoc, PO Box 619, Pontotoc, MS 38863; tel. 662/488–8878; FAX. 662/488–8767; Dr. Matt Wiltshire

PSI Crossings, 5000 Highway 39 North, Meridian, MS 39301; tel. 601/483–5452; FAX. 601/581–9944; Mr. Bill Patterson

Rehabilitation Centers, Inc., PO Box 1160, Magee, MS 39111; tel. 601/849–4221; FAX. 601/849–6427; Ms. Margaret Stept

Saint Francis Community Services, Inc., PO Drawer 640, Picayune, MS 39466; tel. 785/825–0541; FAX. 785/825–2012; Rev. Edward W. Fellhauer

Specialized Treatment Facility, 14426 James Bond Road, Gulfport, MS 39503; tel. 228/328–6000; FAX. 228/328–6035; Ms. Anastasia "Stacy" Garnett Miller

MISSOURI

***Alternative Behavioral Care,** P.O. Box 67, Saint Peters, MO 63376; tel. 636/477–6111; FAX. 636/477–6111; Ms. Cynthia Kay Duga

Amicare of Missouri LLC, PO Box 4067, Waynesville, MO 65583; tel. 573/774–5353; FAX. 573/774–2192; Mr. Michael S. Talmo

BJC Behavioral Health, 1430 Olive Street - Suite 400, Saint Louis, MO 63103; tel. 314/206–3712; FAX. 314/206–3721; Mr. Mark E. Stansberry

***Boonville Valley Hope,** PO Box 398, Boonville, MO 65233; tel. 660/882–6547; FAX. 660/882–2391; Dr. Kenneth C. Gregoire

Boys Town of Missouri, Inc., 13160 County Rd 3610, Saint James, MO 65559; tel. 573/265–3251; FAX. 573/265–8571; Mr. Vincent Hillyer

***Centrec Care, Inc.,** 1030 Woodcrest Terrace Drive; suite 206, Saint Louis, MO 63141; tel. 314/205–8068; FAX. 314/469–4507; Dr. Mohammed A. Kabir

Child Advocacy Services Center Inc., 2 East 59th Street, Kansas City, MO 64113-2116; tel. 816/363–1898; FAX. 816/822–7711; Mr. Alan Murray

Cottonwood Residential Treatment Center, 1025 N. Sprigg, Cape Girardeau, MO 63701; tel. 573/290–5888; FAX. 573/290–5895; Ms. Karen Adams

***DRD Columbia Medical Clinic,** 1415 Paris Road, Columbia, MO 65201; tel. 573/449–8338; FAX. 573/499–3878; Mr. Andrew Love

***DRD Kansas City Medical Clinic,** 723 East 18th Street, Kansas City, MO 64108; tel. 816/283–3877; FAX. 816/283–3310; Mr. Andrew Love

***DRD Springfield Medical Clinic,** 404 East Battlefield Street, Springfield, MO 65807; tel. 417/865–8045; FAX. 417/865–1007; Mr. Andrew Love

Epworth Children and Family Services, 110 North Elm Avenue, Saint Louis, MO 63119; tel. 314/961–5718; FAX. 314/961–3503; Mr. Kevin Drollinger

***Northland Family Counseling Center, Inc.,** 429 Northeast 69 Highway, Kansas City, MO 64119; tel. 816/452–8777; FAX. 816/452–8795; Mr. Maurice L. Cummings

***Premier Care of New Mexico,** P. O. Box 220, Sullivan, MO 63080; tel. 573/860–2273; FAX. 573/860–6227; Mr. Charlie Feese

***Provident,** 2650 Olive Street, Saint Louis, MO 63103; tel. 314/371–6500; FAX. 314/371–6510; Ms. Kathleen E. Buescher

***St. Louis VA Medical Center - Opioid Treatment Program,** 915 North Grand Boulevard, Saint Louis, MO 63106; tel. 314/289–7020; FAX. 314/289–7096; Dr. Stephen Gaioni

The Salvation Army Children's Shelter, 101 W Linwood, Kansas City, MO 64111; tel. 816/285–2480; FAX. 816/303–0183; Lt.Col Theodore Dalberg

MONTANA

Acadia Montana, 55 Basin Creek Road, Butte, MT 59701; tel. 406/494–4183; FAX. 406/494–5869

Intermountain, 500 South Lamborn, Helena, MT 59601; tel. 406/442–7920; FAX. 406/442–7949; Mr. Jim FitzGerald

Montana Academy, 9705 Lost Prairie Road, Marion, MT 59925; tel. 406/858–2339; FAX. 406/858–2356; Dr. John Santa

***Rocky Mountain Treatment Center,** 920 Fourth Avenue North, Great Falls, MT 59401; tel. 406/727–8832; FAX. 406/727–8172; Dr. Raphael (Monty) E. Kuka PH.D.

Shodair Children's Hospital, PO Box 5539, Helena, MT 59604; tel. 406/444–7500; FAX. 406/444–7588; Mr. John P. Casey

NEBRASKA

***BAART Community Healthcare, Inc,** 1941 S. 42nd Street, Suite 210, Omaha, NE 68105; tel. 402/595–1703; FAX. 402/595–1704; Dr. Todd Stull

***Behavioral Health Specialists, Inc.,** 600 South 13th Street, Norfolk, NE 68701; tel. 402/370–3140; FAX. 402/370–3373; Ms. Connie Barnes

***Blue Valley Mental Health Center, Inc.,** 1123 North 9th Street, Beatrice, NE 68310; tel. 402/228–3386; FAX. 402/228–2004; Mr. Jonathan Day

Developmental Services of Nebraska, Inc., 5701 Thompson Creek Blvd, Suite 200, Lincoln, NE 68516; tel. 402/435–2800; FAX. 402/435–8801; Mr. Scott Lefevre

Epworth Village, Inc., PO Box 503, York, NE 68467-0503; tel. 402/362–3353; FAX. 402/362–3248; Mr. Thomas G McBride

Father Flanagan's Boys' Home, 13603 Flanagan Boulevard, Boys Town, NE 68010; tel. 402/498–3090; FAX. 402/498–1925; Rev. Fr. Steven E. Boes

***Hastings Regional Center,** PO Box 579, Hastings, NE 68902-0579; tel. 402/462–1971; FAX. 402/460–3144; Mr. William R. Gibson

Lincoln Lancaster County Child Guidance Center, 2444 'O' Street, Lincoln, NE 68510; tel. 402/475–7666; FAX. 402/476–9623; Dr. Carol Crumpacker

***O'Neill Valley Hope,** 1421 North 10th Street, O' Neill, NE 68763; tel. 402/336–3747; FAX. 402/336–3096; Dr. Kenneth C. Gregoire

OMNI Behavioral Health, 5115 F Street, Omaha, NE 68117; tel. 402/397–9866; FAX. 402/397–1404; Dr. William E. Reay

Uta Halee Girls Village, 10625 Calhoun Road, Omaha, NE 68112; tel. 402/457–1300; FAX. 402/453–8410; Mr. Denis D McCarville

NEVADA

Desert Willow Treatment Center, 6171 W Charleston Boulevard, Building #17, Las Vegas, NV 89146; tel. 702/486–8900; FAX. 702/486–6307; Dr. Linda K. Santangelo

***Las Vegas Recovery Center,** 3371 N. Buffalo Drive, Las Vegas, NV 89129; tel. 702/515–1374; FAX. 702/658–5670; Mr. Stuart P. Smith

***New Frontier Treatment Center,** 165 North Carson Street, Fallon, NV 89406; tel. 775/423–1412; FAX. 775/423–4054; Mrs. Lana K. Henderson

NEW HAMPSHIRE

Community Council of Nashua, NH, 7 Prospect Street, Nashua, NH 03060; tel. 603/889–6147; FAX. 603/598–7135; Dr. Hisham Hafez

Lakeview NeuroRehabilitation Center, 244 Highwatch Road, Effingham, NH 03882; tel. 603/539–7451; FAX. 603/539–8888; Mr. David Armstrong

***Southern New Hampshire Medical Center/ Pregnant Women's Meth,** PO Box 2014, Nashua, NH 03061-2014; tel. 603/577–2709; FAX. 603/577–2772; Mr. Thomas Wilhelmsen

NEW JERSEY

AtlantiCare Behavioral Health, 2511 Fire Road, Unit B10 Bellevue Commons, Egg Harbor Township, NJ 08234; tel. 609/645–7600; FAX. 609/646–5725; Mr. Ted Stryker

Bancroft Rehabilitation Services, 425 East Kings Highway Hopkins Lane, Haddonfield, NJ 08033-0018; tel. 856/429–0010; FAX. 856/429–1613; Ms. Toni Pergolin

***Bayonne Community Mental Health Center,** 601 Broadway, Bayonne, NJ 07002; tel. 201/339–9200; FAX. 201/339–7842; Mr. Joseph M Kadian

***Bonnie Brae,** 3415 Valley Road, P. O. Box 825, Liberty Corner, NJ 07938-0825; tel. 908/647–0800; FAX. 908/647–5021; Mr. William M. Powers

***Camden Treatment Associates, LLC,** 424-32 Market Street, Camden, NJ 08102; tel. 856/338–1811; FAX. 856/338–1753; Mrs. Michelle Norquest

***Cape Counseling Services,** 217 N. Main Street Suite 2, Cape May Court House, NJ 08210; tel. 609/463–0014; FAX. 609/463–8671; Mr. Gregory Speed

Care Plus NJ, Inc., 610 Valley Health Plaza, Paramus, NJ 07652; tel. 201/265–8200; FAX. 201/265–3543; Mr. Joseph A. Masciandaro

***Carrier Clinic,** PO Box 147, Belle Mead, NJ 08502-0147; tel. 908/281–1381; FAX. 908/281–1673; Mr. C. Richard Sarle

***Catholic Charities - Diocese of Metuchen,** 319 Maple Street, Perth Amboy, NJ 08861; tel. 732/324–8200; FAX. 732/826–3549; Ms. Marianne Majewski

***CPC Behavioral Healthcare, Inc,** 10 Industrial Way, Eatontown, NJ 07724; tel. 732/935–2220; FAX. 732/389–3207; Mr. John Mans

***Delaware Valley Medical Inc,** P O Box 8697, Collingswood, NJ 08108; tel. 856/665–5100; FAX. 856/665–5212; Mr. Christopher G. Bass

***Drug Dependence Treatment Program-VANJHCS-East Orange Campus,** 385 Tremont Avenue. Bldg 15, East Orange, NJ 07018; tel. 973/676–1000; FAX. 973/395–7122; Dr. Miklos Losonczy

Ewing Residential Treatment Center, 1610 Stuyvesant Avenue, Trenton, NJ 08618; tel. 609/530–3350; FAX. 609/530–3467; Mr. William J. May

***High Focus Centers,** 47 Maple Street, Suite 404, Summit, NJ 07901; tel. 908/363–1023; FAX. 908/363–1030; Dr. David Nyman

***Khaleidoscope Health Care, Inc.,** Jones and Associates-111 Wayne Street, Jersey City, NJ 07302; tel. 201/451–5425; FAX. 201/451–7499; Mr. Larry M. Ali Blake

***Liberty Behavioral Management, Inc.,** 19 Spear Road, Ramsey, NJ 07446; tel. 201/236–8880; FAX. 201/236–9117; Mr. Patrick G. Carrese

***Mt. Carmel Guild Behavioral Healthcare System,** 1160 Raymond Boulevard, Newark, NJ 07102; tel. 973/690–3606; FAX. 973/690–3601; Ms. Anita Holland

***New Street Treatment Associates,** 57-59 New Street, Irvington, NJ 07111; tel. 973/373–2010; FAX. 973/373–1245; Ms. Janet Ramos

***Ocean Medical Services, Inc,** 2001 Route 37 East, Toms River, NJ 08753; tel. 732/288–9322; FAX. 732/288–9264; Mr. Christopher Bass

***Organization for Recovery, Inc,** P.O. Box 827, Plainfield, NJ 07061; tel. 908/769–4700; FAX. 908/769–8812; Mr. Brian J. Rafferty

***Raritan Bay Medical Center - Methadone Program,** 530 New Brunswick Avenue, Perth Amboy, NJ 08861; tel. 732/442–3700; FAX. 732/442–9006; Mr. Michael D'Agnes

***Recovery Services of New Jersey, Inc.,** 5034 Atlantic Avenue, Mays Landing, NJ 08330; tel. 609/625–4900; FAX. 609/625–8034; Dr. Kenneth R. Sandler

*Indicates organization is a Joint Commission accredited Chemical Dependency organization.

Richard Hall Community Mental Health Center, 500 North Bridge Street, Bridgewater, NJ 08807; tel. 908/725–2800; FAX. 908/725–1394; Mr. Michael J. Frost

Saint Barnabas Behavioral Health Center, Inc., 1691 US Highway 9, CN 2025, Toms River, NJ 08754; tel. 732/914–1688; FAX. 732/914–3854; Mr. Joe Hicks

***South Jersey Drug Treatment,** 162 Sunny Slope Drive, Bridgeton, NJ 08302; tel. 856/455–5441; FAX. 856/455–0505; Adm. Anatoli Redka

***St. Joseph's Hospital and Medical Center,** 703 Main Street, Paterson, NJ 07503; tel. 973/754–2098; FAX. 973/754–2857; Mr. William McDonald

***The Lester A. Drenk Behavioral Health Center, Inc.,** 1289 Route 38 West, Suite 203, Hainesport, NJ 08036; tel. 609/267–5656; FAX. 609/267–8892; Mr. Harry Marmorstein

UCPC Behavioral Health Care, 117-119 Roosevelt Avenue, Plainfield, NJ 07060; tel. 908/756–6870; FAX. 908/756–5566; Ms. Marcyann E. Sosnoski

UMDNJ - University Behavioral HealthCare, PO Box 1392, Piscataway, NJ 08855-1392; tel. 732/235–5500; FAX. 732/235–4594; Mr. Christopher Kosseff

Vineland Children's Residential Treatment Center, 2000 Maple Avenue, Vineland, NJ 08361; tel. 856/696–6620; FAX. 856/696–6847; Mr. Robert Fiorini

***Warren Medical Services, Inc,** 590 Marshall Street, Phillipsburg, NJ 08865; tel. 908/387–0003; FAX. 908/387–0005; Mr. Gary D. Gavornik

Willowglen Academy New Jersey, Inc., 4 Gail Court, Suite 1, Sparta, NJ 07871; tel. 973/579–3700; FAX. 973/579–1786; Mr. Leonard F. Dziubla

Woodbridge Child Diagnostic and Treatment Center, 15 Paddock Street, Avenel, NJ 07001; tel. 732/499–5050; FAX. 732/815–4874; Mr. Gregory J. Love

***Youth Consultation Service,** 284 Broadway, Newark, NJ 07104; tel. 973/482–8411; FAX. 973/482–5325; Mr. Richard Mingoia

NEW MEXICO

***Desert Hills of New Mexico,** 5310 Sequoia Northwest, Albuquerque, NM 87120; tel. 505/836–7330; FAX. 505/836–7424; Ms. Carol Bickelman

E L Rocky Mountain Management & Services, LLC, 712 Rencher, Clovis, NM 88101; tel. 505/762–6091; FAX. 505/742–0209; Mr. Eugene D. Lovato

Sequoyah Adolescent Treatment Center, 3405 W Pan American Freeway NE, Albuquerque, NM 87107; tel. 505/222–0375; FAX. 505/222–0301

***University of New Mexico Health Sciences Center,** 2450 Alamo SE, Albuquerque, NM 87102; tel. 505/272–2121; FAX. 505/272–1827; Mr. Steve McKernan

NEW YORK

***A.R.E.B.A.-Casriel, Inc,** 555 West 57th Street, New York, NY 10019; tel. 212/376–1810; FAX. 212/843–5040; Mr. Steven J. Yohay

***Acute Chemical Dependency Detox Unit - Kings County,** 606 Winthrop Street, Brooklyn, NY 11203; tel. 718/245–3901; FAX. 718/953–1316; Ms. Jean Leon

***Adolescent Development Program,** 525 East 68th Street, Box 437, New York, NY 10065; tel. 212/305–8000; FAX. 212/305–8012; Dr. Herbert Pardes

***Adult Services Clinic,** 525 East 68th Street, Box 437, New York, NY 10065; tel. 212/305–8000; FAX. 212/305–8012; Dr. Herbert Pardes

***Arms Acres,** 75 Seminary Hill Road, Carmel, NY 10512; tel. 845/225–3400; FAX. 845/225–0596; Ms. Patrice Wallace-Moore

August Aichhorn R.T.F., 23 West 106th Street, New York, NY 10025; tel. 212/316–9353; FAX. 212/662–2755; Dr. Michael A. Pawel

Baker Victory Services, Inc., 780 Ridge Road, Lackawanna, NY 14218; tel. 716/828–9515; FAX. 716/828-9503; Mr. James J. Casion

***Bellevue Hospital Center Chemi Dependency Medically Detox,** 462 First Avenue, New York, NY 10016; tel. 212/562–4132; FAX. 212/562–4036; Ms. Lynda Curtis

***Beth Israel Medical Center,** 1-9 Nathan Perlman Place, New York, NY 10003; tel. 212/844–1929; FAX. 212/420–2004; Dr. David J. Shulkin

***Beth Israel Medical Center MMTP - Gouverneur Clinic,** 109-11 Delancey Street, New York, NY 10002; tel. 212/420–2086; FAX. 212/979–0925; Mr. Patti Juliana

***Beth Israel Medical Center MMTP - Harlem 6/7,** 103 East 125th Street, 2nd Flr, New York, NY 10035; tel. 212/774–3260; FAX. 212/876–5862; Mrs. Patti Juliana

***Beth Israel Medical Center MMTP - Marie Nyswander Clinic,** 160 Water Street, New York, NY 10038; tel. 212/247–7180; FAX. 212/315–3919; Mrs. Patti Juliana

***Beth Israel Medical Center MMTP - Vincent P Dole,** 25 - 12th Street, Brooklyn, NY 11215; tel. 718/965–7900; FAX. 718/965–1114; Ms. Patti Juliana

***Beth Israel Medical Center MMTP Clinic,** 429 Second Avenue, New York, NY 10010; tel. 212/844–1929; FAX. 212/420–2798; Ms. Patti Juliana

***Beth Israel Medical Center MMTP Clinic,** 435 Second Avenue, 3rd Floor, New York, NY 10010; tel. 212/726–6824; FAX. 212/696–0677; Ms. Patti Juliana

***Beth Israel Medical Center MMTP Clinic 8D,** 140 West 125th Street, 6th Flr, New York, NY 10027; tel. 212/864–0904; FAX. 212/865–6128; Mrs. Patti Juliana

***Beth Israel Medical Center MMTP Cumberland Clinic,** 100 Flatbush Avenue, Brooklyn, NY 11217; tel. 718/237–9600; FAX. 718/875–0967; Ms. Patti Juliana

***Beth Israel Medical Center MMTP Harlem 3,** 103 East 125th Street, 8th Flr, New York, NY 10003; tel. 212/774–3230; FAX. 212/987–0484; Ms. Patti Juliana

***Beth Israel Medical Center MMTP Harlem Clinic 1,** First Avenue & 16th Street, New York, NY 10003; tel. 212/774–3210; FAX. 212/722–6234; Mrs. Patti Juliana

***Beth Israel Medical Center MMTP Harlem Clinic 2,** 103 East 125th Street, 4th Flr, New York, NY 10035; tel. 212/774–3200; FAX. 212/996–3502; Mrs. Patti Juliana

***Beth Israel Medical Center MMTP Harlem Clinic 8,** 140 West 125h Street, 6th Flr, New York, NY 10027; tel. 212/864–8177; FAX. 212/866–5741; Mrs. Patti Juliana

***Beth Israel Medical Center MMTP, Avenue A Clinic,** 26 Avenue A, New York, NY 10009; tel. 212/420–2078; FAX. 212/982–6990; Ms. Patti Juliana

***Beth Israel Medical Center MMTP-St Vincent's,** 201 West 13th Street, New York, NY 10011; tel. 212/420–2015; FAX. 212/675–1028; Ms. Patti Juliana

***Bon Secours Community Hospital - OTP,** 160 East Main St., Port Jervis, NY 12771; tel. 845/368–5302; FAX. 845/368–5937; Ms. Leah Cerkvenik

***Bronx Veterans Administration Medical Center Substance Abuse,** 130 W Kingsbridge Rd, Ward 5B, Bronx, NY 10468; tel. 718/584–9000; FAX. 718/741–4269; Dr. Michael Scimeca

***Bronx-Lebanon Hospital Center - MMTP/Keep,** 1650 Selwyn Avenue Suite 3A, Bronx, NY 10457; tel. 718/503–7750; FAX. 718/503–7751; Mr. Miguel A. Fuentes

***Cabrini Medical Center,** 227 E 19th Street, 13th Floor - Chemical Dependency Unit, New York, NY 10003; tel. 212/995–6000; FAX. 212/995–6568; Dr. Ron Gade

***Canton-Potsdam Hospital - Opioid Treatment Program,** 50 Leroy St., Potsdam, NY 13676; tel. 315/265–3300; FAX. 315/261–6422; Mrs. Marlinda L. LaValley

***Carnegie Hill Institute,** 116 East 92nd Street, New York, NY 10128; tel. 212/289–7166; FAX. 212/831–6433; Dr. Harvey D Karkus

***Coney Island Hospital - Acute Care Addictions Program,** 2601 Ocean Parkway, Brooklyn, NY 11235; tel. 718/616–3000; FAX. 718/616–4439; Mr. Peter N. Wolf

***Conifer Park, Inc.,** 79 Glenridge Road, Glenville, NY 12302; tel. 518/399–6446; FAX. 518/952–8228; Mr. Patrick Carrese

***Crouse Hospital Methadone Maintenance Treatment Program,** 410 South Crouse Avenue, Syracuse, NY 13210; tel. 315/470–8300; FAX. 315/470–8309; Dr. Paul Kronenberg

***Drug Treatment & Education Cen North Shore Univ Hospital,** 400 Community Drive, Manhasset, NY 11030; tel. 516/562–3010; FAX. 516/562–3996; Mr. Michael Dowling

***Elmhurst Hospital Center Methadone Treatment Program,** 79-01 Broadway, 2nd Floor, Annex O, Elmhurst, NY 11373; tel. 718/334–1638; FAX. 719/334–1810; Mr. Chris D. Constantino

***Erie County Medical Center,** 462 Grider Street, Buffalo, NY 14215; tel. 716/898–3000; FAX. 716/898–5178; Mr. Michael A. Young

***Flushing Hospital Medical Center / Chemical Dependency Unit,** 45th Avenue at Parsons Blvd, Flushing, NY 11355; tel. 718/670–5918; FAX. 718/670–3077; Mr. David P. Rosen

***Good Samaritan Hospital - OTP,** 255 Lafayette Avenue, Suffern, NY 10901; tel. 845/368–5302; FAX. 845/368–5937; Mr. Michael Schnieders

***Gracie Square Hospital - OTP,** 420 East 76th Street, New York, NY 10021; tel. 212/434–5322; FAX. 212/434–5373; Mr. Frank Bruno

***Harlem Hospital Center Chemical Dependence Detoxification Unit,** 506 Lenox Ave, New York, NY 10037; tel. 212/939–1340; FAX. 212/939–8300; Dr. John M. Palmer

***Harlem Hospital Center MMTP,** 264 West 118th Street, New York, NY 10026; tel. 212/939–1340; FAX. 212/939–8300; Dr. John Palmer

***Hudson Valley Hospital Center M.M.T.P.,** 1980 Crompond Road, Cortlandt Manor, NY 10567; tel. 914/737–6117; FAX. 914/737–6973; Mr. John C. Federspiel

***Interfaith Medical Center Substance Abuse Detoxification,** 1545 Atlantic Avenue, 6th Floor, Brooklyn, NY 11213; tel. 718/613–4001; FAX. 718/613–4101; Mr. Edward J. Glicksman

***Jacobi Medical Center Chemical Dependence/ Medically Detoxification,** 1400 Pelham Parkway, Bronx, NY 10461; tel. 718/918–5322; FAX. 718/918–7071; Mr. William Walsh

***Long Beach Medical Center M.M.T.P.,** 455 East Bay Drive, Long Beach, NY 11561; tel. 516/897–1330; FAX. 516/897–1149; Mr. Douglas Melzer

***Long Island Center for Recovery Inc.,** 320 West Montauk Highway, Hampton Bays, NY 11946; tel. 631/728–3100; FAX. 631/728–9075; Mr. Jack Hamilton

***Long Island Jewish Medical Center - M.M.T.P.,** 75-59 263rd Street, Glen Oaks, NY 11004; tel. 718/470–8285; FAX. 718/470–6248; Mr. Michael J. Dowling

***Lutheran Medical Center (Acute Care Addiction Program),** 150 55th Street, Brooklyn, NY 11220; tel. 718/630–7363; FAX. 718/630–6549; Ms. Wendy Z. Goldstein

***Mary Immaculate Hospital Clinic, MMTP,** 147-20 Archer Avenue, Jamaica, NY 11435; tel. 718/291–1888; FAX. 718/291–0557; Mr. Dominick J. Gio

***Mary Immaculate Hospital K.E.E.P,** 147-18 Archer Avenue, Jamaica, NY 11435; tel. 718/291–1888; FAX. 718/291–0557; Mr. Dominick J. Gio

***Medically Managed Inpatient Detoxification,** 2 Park Avenue, Yonkers, NY 10703; tel. 914/964–7383; FAX. 914/964–7704; Mr. Jim Foy

***Methadone Treatment Program,** 600 Albany Avenue, Brooklyn, NY 11203; tel. 718/245–3901; FAX. 718/953–1316; Ms. Jean G. Leon

***Metropolitan Correctional Center - New York / OTP,** 150 Park Row, New York, NY 10007; tel. 646/836–6300; FAX. 646/836–7703; Mr. James N. Cross

***Metropolitan Hospital Center Detoxification Unit,** 1901 First Avenue, New York, NY 10029; tel. 212/423–7554; FAX. 212/423–7974; Miss Meryl Weinberg

***Montefiore Medical Center - SATP,** 111 East 210th Street, Bronx, NY 10467; tel. 718/920–2001; FAX. 718/652–2161; Dr. Spencer Foreman

***Montefiore Medical Center - SATP - OTP - Unit III,** 2005 Jerome Avenue, 1st Floor, Bronx, NY 10467; tel. 718/583–0600; Dr. Spencer Foreman

***Narco Freedom Inc. MMTP,** 250 Grand Concourse, Bronx, NY 10451; tel. 718/292–2240; FAX. 718/292–3030; Mr. Alan Brand

***Narco Freedom, Inc.-Bridge Plaza MMTP,** 37-18 34th Street, Long Island City, NY 11101; tel. 718/292–2240; FAX. 718/292–3030; Mr. Alan Brand

*Indicates organization is a Joint Commission accredited Chemical Dependency organization.

*Nassau County Dept. Methadone Maintenance Treatment Program, NUMC, 2201 Hempstead Turnpike Building K, East Meadow, NY 11554; tel. 516/572–5906; FAX. 516/572–6777; Ms. Christine Hunter
*North General Hospital - MMTP Program, 1879 Madison Avenue, New York, NY 10035; tel. 212/423–4000; FAX. 212/423–1454; Dr. Samuel J. Daniel
*Pathways - St. Louise, 209 Niagara Street, Buffalo, NY 14201; tel. 716/856–8411; FAX. 716/856–1909; Mr. Peter U. Bergmann
*Pathways, Sisters of Charity Hospital, 158 Holden Street, Buffalo, NY 14214; tel. 716/862–1000; FAX. 716/862–1877; Mr. Peter U Bergmann
*PROMESA Methadone Treatment Program, 1776 Clay Ave, Bronx, NY 10457; tel. 718/960–7601; FAX. 718/583–5529; Mr. Ruben A. Medina
*Quannacut at Eastern Long Island Hospital, 201 Manor Place, Greenport, NY 11944; tel. 631/477–1000; FAX. 631/477–1746; Mr. Paul J. Connor
*Queens Hospital Center Inpatient Detox Unit, 82-68 164 Street, Jamaica, NY 11434; tel. 718/883–2222; FAX. 718/883–6235; Mr. Antonio D. Martin
Rochester Mental Health Center, 490 East Ridge Road, Rochester, NY 14621; tel. 585/922–2500; FAX. 585/922–2664; Mr. Mark Clement
*Rochester Pathways, Sisters of Charity Hospital, 435 East Henrietta Road, Rochester, NY 14607; tel. 585/424–6580; FAX. 585/424–6609; Mr. Peter U. Bergmann
*SBH Chemical Dependence Methadone Substance Abuse Treatment, 4535-39 Third Avenue, Bronx, NY 10457; tel. 718/960–6170; FAX. 718/960–3618; Dr. Scott Cooper
*SBH Chemical Dependence-Medically Managed, 183rd Street and Third Avenue, Bronx, NY 10457; tel. 718/960–6170; FAX. 718/960–3618; Dr. Scott Cooper
*Seafield Center, Inc., 7 Seafield Lane, Westhampton Beach, NY 11978; tel. 631/288–1122; FAX. 631/288–1638; Mr. John C. Haley
*Sound Shore Medical Center, 16 Guion Place, New Rochelle, NY 10802; tel. 914/632–5000; FAX. 914/637–1976; Mr. John R Spicer
*South Oaks Hospital, 400 Sunrise Highway, Amityville, NY 11701; tel. 631/608–5108; FAX. 631/264–5259; Mr. Robert Detor
*St. John's Episcopal Hospital, 327 Beach 19th Street, Far Rockaway, NY 11691; tel. 718/869–7320; FAX. 718/869–7089; Mr. John Gupta
*St. Johns Riverside Hospital M.M.T.P., 70 Ashburton Avenue, 2nd Floor, Yonkers, NY 10701; tel. 914/964–4000; FAX. 914/965–4812; Mr. Jim Foy
*St. Joseph's Hospital - MMTP, 8 Guion Street, 1st Floor, Yonkers, NY 10701; tel. 914/378–7000; FAX. 914/965–0912; Mr. Michael Spicer
*St. Joseph's Villa of Rochester, 3300 Dewey Avenue, Rochester, NY 14616; tel. 585/865–1550; FAX. 585/865–5219; Mr. Roger C. Battaglia
*St. Lukes - Roosevelt Hospital Center - Clark 6, 1111 Amsterdam Ave, New York, NY 10025; tel. 212/523–4000; FAX. 212/523–8790; Mr. FranK Cracolici
*St. Lukes-Roosevelt Hospital - Inpatient Rehab Unit / MMTP, 1000 Tenth Avenue, New York, NY 10019; tel. 212/523–6881; FAX. 212/523–8057; Dr. Petros Levounis
*St. Mary's Hospital at Amsterdam - OTP, 427 Guy Park Avenue, Amsterdam, NY 12010; tel. 518/841–7101; FAX. 518/842–0107; Mr. Victor F. Giulianelli
*St. Vincent Midtown Hospital, 415 West 51st Street, New York, NY 10019; tel. 212/459–8402; FAX. 212/459–8127; Mr. Leonard Walsh
*Staten Island Univ Hospital (Canarsie M.M.T.P. Clinic), 376 Seguine Avenue, Staten Island, NY 10309; tel. 718/226–9000; FAX. 718/226–2826; Mr. Anthony Ferreri
*Staten Island Univ Hospital (Coney Island M.M.T.P. Clinic), 375 Seguine Avenue, Staten Island, NY 10309; tel. 718/226–9000; FAX. 718/226–2826; Mr. Anthony Ferreri
*Staten Island Univ Hospital (Princess Bay M.M.T.P. Clinic), 392 Seguine Avenue, Staten Island, NY 10309; tel. 718/226–9000; FAX. 718/226–2826; Mr. Anthony C. Ferreri
*Staten Island Univ Hospital (Stapleton M.M.T.P. Clinic), 376 Seguine Avenue, Staten Island, NY 10309; tel. 718/226–9000; FAX. 718/226–2826; Mr. Anthony C. Ferreri
*Staten Island Univ Hospital Inpatient Chemical Dependence Detox Unit, 375 Seguine Avenue, Staten Island, NY 10305; tel. 718/226–9000; FAX. 718/226–2826; Mr. Anthony Ferreri
Stony Lodge Hospital, Inc., PO Box 1250, Briarcliff Manor, NY 10510; tel. 914/941–7400; FAX. 914/941–4102; Mr. Kevin F. Czipo
*Strong Memorial Hospital - MMTC - Dept of Psychiatry, 601 Elmwood Avenue, Rochester, NY 14642; tel. 585/275–5489; FAX. 585/756–0221; Mr. Steven Goldstein
*Stuyvesant Square Chemical Dependency Outpatient Detox, 1-9 Nathan Perlman Place, New York, NY 10003; tel. 212/420–4220; FAX. 212/844–1454; Dr. David J. Shulkin
*Suffolk County Department of Health - East End Clinic, 300 Center Drive, Riverhead, NY 11901; tel. 631/852–2680; FAX. 631/852–2674; Mr. Thomas MacGilvray
*Suffolk County Department of Health - Hauppauge Clinic, 200 Wireless Blvd, Hauppauge, NY 11788; tel. 631/853–7373; FAX. 631/853–7376; Mr. Thomas O. MacGilvray
*Suffolk County Department of Health - North County Complex, P O Box 6100 Building 151 North County Complex, Hauppauge, NY 11788; tel. 631/853–6410; FAX. 631/853–6413; Mr. Thomas O. MacGilvray
*Suffolk County Dept. of Health, Huntington Methadone Clinic, P O Box 6100 Building 159 North County Complex, Hauppauge, NY 11788; tel. 631/854–4400; FAX. 631/854–4411; Mr. Thomas MacGilvray
*Summit Park Hospital, 50 Sanitorium Road, Pomona, NY 10970; tel. 845/364–2378; FAX. 845/364–2381; Ms. Mary Ann Walsh-Tozer
*SVCMCNY, 275 North St, Harrison, NY 10528; tel. 718/485–3400; FAX. 718/922–5496; Dr. Brian Fitzsimmons
*The Astor Home for Children, PO Box 5005, Rhinebeck, NY 12572-5005; tel. 845/871–1000; FAX. 845/876–2020; Dr. James McGuirk
*The Brooklyn Hospital Center Parkside Drug Detox Program, 121 DeKalb Avenue, Brooklyn, NY 11201; tel. 718/250–8005; FAX. 718/625–4109; Mr. Samuel Lehrfield
The Children's Home RTF, Inc., 638 Squirrel Hill Road, Chenango Forks, NY 13746; tel. 607/656–9004; FAX. 607/656–9076; Ms. Karen Wright
*The Guidance Center Chemical Dependency Treatment Center, 70 Grand Street, New Rochelle, NY 10801; tel. 914/636–4440; FAX. 914/632–8822; Ms. Amy Gelles
The House of the Good Shepherd, 1550 Champlin Avenue, Utica, NY 13502; tel. 315/235–7600; FAX. 315/235–7609; Mr. William F. Holicky
*The Kingston Hospital Methadone Treatment Program, 2 Barbarossa Lane, Kingston, NY 12401; tel. 845/943–6022; FAX. 845/943–6092; Mr. Allen Nace
*The Mount Vernon Hospital Methadone Maintenance Program, 3 South 6th Avenue, 3rd Floor, Mount Vernon, NY 10550; tel. 914/664–8000; FAX. 914/668–2113; Mr. John R. Spicer
*The Turning Point - Detox Unit Saint Francis Hospital, 11 Hastings Drive, Beacon, NY 12508; tel. 845/838–4405; FAX. 845/831–8131; Mr. Robert Savage
*United Health Services Hospitals, 33-57 Harrison Street, Johnson City, NY 13790; tel. 607/763–6130; FAX. 607/763–6789; Mr. Matthew Salanger
*VA New York Harbor Healthcare System - BK OTP, 800 Poly Place, Brooklyn, NY 11209; tel. 718/836–6600; FAX. 718/630–3513; Dr. Eric Peselow
*VA New York Harbor Healthcare System - OTP, 437 West 16th Street, New York, NY 10011; tel. 212/462–4461; FAX. 212/462–4405; Dr. Paul Casadonte
*West Midtown Medical Group - OTP, 505 Eighth Avenue, 10th Floor, New York, NY 10018; tel. 212/736–5900; FAX. 212/643–1441; Mr. Andrew Schorr
*White Plains Hospital Center, Davis Avenue at East Post Road, White Plains, NY 10601; tel. 914/681–2800; FAX. 914/681–2850; Mr. Jon B. Schandler
*Whitney M. Young, Jr. MMTP, 4-10 Dewitt Street, Albany, NY 12207; tel. 518/463–3882; FAX. 518/455–8806; Mr. Jamed D. Sinkoff
*Woodhull Medical & Mental Health Medically Managed Detoxification, 760 Broadway, Units 8-300 and 9-300, Brooklyn, NY 11206; tel. 718/963–5959; FAX. 718/630–3031; Ms. Iris R. Jimenez-Hernandez

NORTH CAROLINA

Alexander Youth Network, PO Box 220632, Charlotte, NC 28222-9979; tel. 704/366–8712; FAX. 704/362–8464; Mr. N.Craig Bass
*Alpha Omega Health, Inc., 5950 Six Forks Road, Raleigh, NC 27609; tel. 919/844–1008; FAX. 919/844–0042; Mr. John K. Horne
*Fellowship Hall, Inc., PO Box 13890, Greensboro, NC 27415; tel. 336/621–3381; FAX. 336/621–7513; Mr. Rodney Battles
Grandfather Home for Children, P. O. Box 98, Banner Elk, NC 28604; tel. 828/898–5465; FAX. 828/898–8513; Mr. James Swinkola
*Julian F. Keith Alcohol and Drug Abuse Treatment Center, 201 Tabernacle Road, Black Mountain, NC 28711; tel. 828/669–3402; FAX. 828/669–3451; Mr. William Douglas Baker
KidsPeace Foster Care and Family Services, 3109 Poplarwood Court, Suite 310, Raleigh, NC 27604; tel. 919/872–6447; FAX. 919/872–6671; Dr. Lorrie Henderson
Old Vineyard Youth Services, 3637 Old Vineyard Road, Winston Salem, NC 27104-4842; tel. 336/794–3550; FAX. 336/794–3545; Mr. Wesley Mason
*R. J. Blackley, MD-Alcohol & Drug Abuse Treatment Center, 1003 12th Street, Butner, NC 27509-1626; tel. 919/575–7229; FAX. 919/575–7643; Dr. Stephen Oxley
Timber Ridge Treatment Center, P O Box 259, Gold Hill, NC 28071; tel. 704/279–1199; FAX. 704/279–7668; Mr. Thomas A. R. Hibbert
*Unity Healing Center, PO Box 201, Cherokee, NC 28719; tel. 828/497–3958; FAX. 828/497–6826; Ms. Hillane Lambert
*Wilmington Treatment Center, Inc., 2520 Troy Drive, Wilmington, NC 28401; tel. 910/762–2727; FAX. 910/762–7923; Mr. Charles Sharp

OHIO

Access Ohio, 2 Miranova Place, Columbus, OH 43215; tel. 614/225–0400; FAX. 614/225–0401; Dr. John A. Johnson
*Akron Drug Abuse Clinic - Community Health Center, 725 East Market Street, Akron, OH 44305; tel. 330/434–4141; FAX. 330/996–5142; Mr. Theodore P. Ziegler
*Akron-Urban Minority Alcoholism Drug Abuse Outreach, 665 W Market Street, Akron, OH 44303; tel. 330/379–3467; FAX. 330/379–3465; Dr. Janice T. Mercier Wade
Beech Brook, 3737 Lander Road, Cleveland, OH 44124; tel. 216/831–2255; FAX. 216/831–1442; Ms. Debra Rex
*Behavioral Connections of Wood County, Inc., Post Office Box 29, Bowling Green, OH 43402; tel. 419/352–5387; FAX. 419/352–3430; Dr. Richard M. Goldberg
*Bellefaire Jewish Children's Bureau, 22001 Fairmount Boulevard, Shaker Heights, OH 44118; tel. 216/932–2800; FAX. 216/932–6704; Dr. Adam G. Jacobs
*Catholic Charities, 7911 Detroit Ave, Cleveland, OH 44102; tel. 440/843–5582; FAX. 440/843–1626; Mr. Thomas W. Woll
*Center for Chemical Addictions Treatment, 830 Ezzard Charles Drive, Cincinnati, OH 45214; tel. 513/381–6672; FAX. 513/381–6080; Ms. Sandra L. Kuehn
Child Guidance & Family Solutions, 312 Locust Street, Akron, OH 44302; tel. 330/762–0591; FAX. 330/258–0931; Ms. Elaine Harlin
*Cleveland Clinic, 9500 Euclid Ave. W-15, Cleveland, OH 44195; tel. 216/444–2200; Dr. Delos Cosgrove
Community Behavioral Health Center, 3355 Richmond Road, 225-A, Beachwood, OH 44122; tel. 216/831–1494; FAX. 216/831–9931; Mr. Arun Kumar Chattree
*Community Behavioral Health, Inc, 520 Eaton Ave, Hamilton, OH 45013; tel. 513/785–4784; FAX. 513/785–4789; Mrs. Jean Glowka

*Indicates organization is a Joint Commission accredited Chemical Dependency organization.

*Community Counseling Center of Ashtabula County, 2801 C Court, Ashtabula, OH 44004; tel. 440/998–4210; FAX. 440/998–6489; Mr. Dale Brinker
*Community Health Center, 725 East Market Street, Akron, OH 44305; tel. 330/434–4141; FAX. 330/434–7125; Mr. Theodore P. Ziegler
*Comprehensive Addiction Service Systems, Inc., 2465 Collingwood Blvd., Toledo, OH 43620; tel. 419/241–8827; FAX. 419/321–6834; Mr. William Sanford
Comprehensive Psychiatry Specialists, 955 Windham Court, Suite 2, Boardman, OH 44512; tel. 330/884–1900; FAX. 330/884–1928
*Connecting Point, 1212 Cherry Street, Toledo, OH 43608; tel. 419/243–6326; FAX. 419/243–6346; Mr. Jeff Deckebach
*Cornell Abraxas, 2775 State Route 39, Shelby, OH 44875; tel. 419/747–3322; FAX. 419/747–3504; Mr. Leonard J. Kirby
*Crisis Intervention and Recovery Center, Inc., 832 McKinley Avenue NW, Canton, OH 44703; tel. 330/452–9812; FAX. 330/430–1288; Dr. Bernard S Jesiolowski
*Dept., of Veterans Affairs-Dayton Campus Opioid Treatment, 4100 W Third Street, Bldg 302, Dayton, OH 45428; tel. 937/268–6511; FAX. 937/267–5386; Dr. Alberto Rincon-Belzres
Far West Center, 29133 Health Campus Drive, Westlake, OH 44145; tel. 440/835–6212; FAX. 440/899–4394; Ms. Helen M. (Kelly) Dylag
Fox Run Hospital, 67670 Traco Drive, Saint Clairsville, OH 43950; tel. 740/695–2131; FAX. 740/695–7158; Ms. Karen Maxwell
*Glenbeigh, PO Box 298, Rock Creek, OH 44084-0298; tel. 440/563–3400; FAX. 440/563–9661; Ms. Pat Weston-Hall
Harbor Behavioral Healthcare, 4334 Secor Road, Toledo, OH 43623-4234; tel. 419/475–4449; FAX. 419/479–3230; Mr. Dale E. Shreve
*Interval Brotherhood Homes, Inc., 3445 South Main Street, Akron, OH 44319; tel. 330/644–4095; FAX. 330/645–2031; Rev. Samuel R Ciccolini
*Lincoln Behavioral Healthcare, 880 E Indianola Ave, Youngstown, OH 44502; tel. 330/783–5242; FAX. 330/788–3428; Mrs. Robin Vaccar
Maumee Valley Guidance Center, 211 Biede Ave., Defiance, OH 43512; tel. 419/782–8856; FAX. 419/784–4506; Mr. William Bierie
*Methadone Maintenance Program, Substance Abuse,Mental Health, 10701 East Blvd, Room H127, Cleveland, OH 44106; tel. 440/526–3030; FAX. 440/546–2705
NECCO Center, 115 Private Road 977, Pedro, OH 45659; tel. 740/534–1386; FAX. 740/534–0577; Mr. Randy O'Donnell
*Neil Kennedy Recovery Clinic, 2151 Rush Boulevard, Youngstown, OH 44507; tel. 330/744–1181; FAX. 330/740–2849; Mr. Gerald V. Carter
*New Directions, Inc., 30800 Chagrin Boulevard, Cleveland, OH 44124; tel. 216/591–0324; FAX. 216/591–1243; Mr. Michael E. Matoney
*Opiate Substitution Services - SUDEP, CVAMC, 3200 Vine Street, Cincinnati, OH 45220; tel. 513/861–3100; FAX. 513/475–6525; Dr. Show W. Lin
Phoenix Rising Behavorial Healthcare And Recovery, Inc., 1930 Fremont Pl Sw, Canton, OH 44706; tel. 330/455–5950; FAX. 330/455–5960; Ms. Lisa K Grubbs
Portage Path Behavioral Health, 340 South Broadway, Akron, OH 44308; tel. 330/376–6144; FAX. 330/253–5248; Mr. Jerome T. Kraker
*PsyCare, Inc., 2980 Belmont Avenue, Youngstown, OH 44505; tel. 330/759–2310; FAX. 330/759–0018; Dr. Douglas C. Darnall
Rakesh Ranjan MD and Associates, Inc., 3690 Orange Place, Suite 330, Beachwood, OH 44122; tel. 216/464–5200; FAX. 216/464–5208; Dr. Rakesh Ranjan
*Ravenwood Mental Health Center, 12557 Ravenwood Drive, Chardon, OH 44024; tel. 440/285–3568; FAX. 440/285–4552; Mr. David A. Boyle
*Rescue Mental Health Services, 3350 Collingwood Boulevard, Toledo, OH 43610; tel. 419/255–9585; FAX. 419/255–2801; Ms. Janet Eppard
Shaker Clinic, LLC, 20600 Chagrin Blvd. Suite 620, Shaker Heights, OH 44122; tel. 216/751–4762; FAX. 216/751–5894; Mrs. Roxanne Jividen
*Southeast, Inc., 16 West Long Street, Columbus, OH 43215; tel. 614/225–0980; FAX. 614/225–0986; Mr. William F. Lee
Specialty Care Counseling Services, Ltd, 2000 East Market Street, Warren, OH 44483; tel. 330/399–1221; FAX. 330/399–1205; Mrs. Nivine S. Sedra
*Stella Maris, Inc., 1320 Washington Avenue, Cleveland, OH 44113; tel. 216/781–0550; FAX. 216/781–7501; Mrs. Margaret A. Roche
*Substance Abuse Services, Inc., 1832 Adams Street, Toledo, OH 43604; tel. 419/241–8827; FAX. 419/243–1505; Mr. William Sanford
*The Buckeye Ranch, Inc., 5665 Hoover Road, Grove City, OH 43123; tel. 614/875–2371; FAX. 614/871–6487; Mr. Richard E. Rieser
*The Crossroads Center, 311 Martin Luther King Drive, Cincinnati, OH 45219-3116; tel. 513/475–5300; FAX. 513/281–1645; LtCmdr Jacqueline P. Butler
The Woods at Parkside, 349 Olde Ridenour Road, Columbus, OH 43230; tel. 614/471–2552; FAX. 614/337–3124; Mr. Jim O'Shea
Unison Behavioral Health Group, PO Box 10015, Toledo, OH 43699-0015; tel. 419/242–9577; FAX. 419/321–6913; Mrs. Courtney Weiss
*Wood County Children's Services Association, PO Box 738, Bowling Green, OH 43402; tel. 419/352–7588; FAX. 419/354–4977; Mr. Timothy K Scherer
Zepf Community Mental Health Center, Inc., 6605 West Central Avenue, Toledo, OH 43617; tel. 419/841–7701; FAX. 419/843–6431; Ms. Jennifer Moses

OKLAHOMA

BetterLife Counseling Services, Inc., 6801 South Western, Suite #108, Oklahoma City, OK 73139; tel. 405/632–0029; FAX. 405/632–0057; Mr. Isaac O Olorunnisomo
*Broadway House, Inc, 221 Second Avenue NW, Ardmore, OK 73401; tel. 580/226–3252; FAX. 580/226–3849; Ms. Wadonna Wells
Brookhaven Hospital, 201 South Garnett Road, Tulsa, OK 74128-1800; tel. 918/438–4257; FAX. 918/438–8016; Dr. Rolf B. Gainer
Carl Albert Community Mental Health Center, PO Box 579, McAlester, OK 74502; tel. 918/426–7800; FAX. 918/426–5526; Ms. Margaret Bradford
Cedar Ridge, 6501 NE 50th Street, Oklahoma City, OK 73141; tel. 405/605–6111; FAX. 405/424–0457; Mr. John Holter
Choices Institute, 529 N. Grand, Enid, OK 73701; tel. 580/234–8880; FAX. 580/234–8891; Ms. Joyce Carter Bean
*Cornerstone Clinical Services, Inc., P.O. Box 36, Clinton, OK 73601; tel. 580/595–7000; FAX. 580/595–7005; Mr. Darrell Eugene Smith
*Cushing Valley Hope, PO Box 472, Cushing, OK 74023-0472; tel. 918/225–1736; FAX. 918/225–7742; Dr. Kenneth C. Gregoire
Discovery Uttuwah LLC, 118 So. Main, Wagoner, OK 74467; tel. 918/485–1573; FAX. 580/922–3437; Ms. Sue Billups
Jim Taliaferro Community Mental Health Center, 602 SW 38th st, Lawton, OK 73505; tel. 580/248–5780; FAX. 580/248–3610; Mr. Jim Regan
Land Of Hope, RT 1 Box 85, Prague, OK 74864; tel. 580/310–4164; Mrs. Mary Ann Thornton
*Northwest Center for Behavioral Health (NCBH), 1222 10th Street, Suite 211, Woodward, OK 73801; tel. 580/256–8615; FAX. 580/256–8609; Mrs. Trudy Hoffman
Oklahoma Counseling Services, Inc., 3104 South Elm Place Suite M, Broken Arrow, OK 74012; tel. 918/286–2535; FAX. 918/286–7693; Mr. Michael E. Crawford
Oklahoma Forensic Center, PO Box 69, Vinita, OK 74301-0069; tel. 918/256–7841; FAX. 918/256–4491; Mr. William T. Burkett
Oklahoma Youth Center, 320 12th Avenue Northeast, Norman, OK 73071; tel. 405/573–3821; FAX. 405/573–8256
Parkside, Inc., 1620 East 12th Street, Tulsa, OK 74120; tel. 918/582–2131; FAX. 918/588–8822; Ms. Debra Moore
Positive Changes, 744 S.E. 25th Street, Oklahoma City, OK 73129; tel. 405/636–1463; FAX. 405/635–8417; Mrs. Laura C. Balliett-Box
Professional Counseling Solutions, 102 North 9th Street, Frederick, OK 73542; tel. 580/335–3320; FAX. 580/335–7433; Ms. Debbie Morey
Restorative Counseling Services, Inc, 937 SW 89th Street suite B, Oklahoma City, OK 73139; tel. 405/601–2154; FAX. 405/601–5359; Ms. Gina M. Pazzaglia-Filkins
Solutions for Life Counseling Services, 309 W. Cherokee, Enid, OK 73701; tel. 580/234–4700; FAX. 580/234–4727; Mrs. Kathy E. Andrews
South Oklahoma City Counseling Clinic, 1145 W. I-240 Service Rd. Bldg E, Ste 200, Oklahoma City, OK 73139; tel. 405/850–2063; FAX. 405/879–2925; Mr. Doug Baker
Southeastern Psychiatric Services, P.O. Box 1589, McAlester, OK 74502; tel. 918/423–3700; FAX. 918/423–3712; Dr. R.T. Bowden
SouthWest Counseling Services, PLLC, 1029 Circle Dr, Clinton, OK 73601; tel. 580/331–9449; FAX. 580/765–3419; Mr. William L. Walker
Southwest Foster Care Of Oklahoma, 4801 North Classen Blvd Suite 135, Oklahoma City, OK 73118; tel. 405/848–0011; FAX. 405/848–2111; Mr. Jack Lewis
*Substance Abuse Treatment Center, OKC VAMC, 921 NE 13th St, Bldg 1, 116C, Oklahoma City, OK 73104; tel. 405/270–5194; FAX. 405/270–1583; Dr. Gita Pujari
The Camelot School - Oklahoma, 3301 North Martin Luther King Avenue, Oklahoma City, OK 73111; tel. 405/548–1280; FAX. 405/548–1299
Tulsa Center for Behavioral Health, 2323 South Harvard, Tulsa, OK 74114; tel. 918/293–2140; FAX. 918/712–7164; Ms. Leah Price
Volunteers of America of Oklahoma, Inc., 4012 East 35th Street, Tulsa, OK 74135; tel. 918/749–6668; FAX. 918/748–8814; Mr. John Selph
Willow Crest Hospital, Inc., 130 A Street SouthWest, Miami, OK 74354; tel. 918/542–1836; FAX. 918/542–8730; Mrs. Anne G. Anthony
YCO Clinton, Inc., 2250 W. Modelle, Clinton, OK 73601; tel. 405/222–8167; Mr. Robert Lobato

OREGON

*Catherine Freer Wilderness Therapy Expeditions, PO Box 1064, Albany, OR 97321; tel. 541/926–7252; FAX. 541/812–0116; Dr. Robert Cooley
ChristieCare, PO Box 368, Marylhurst, OR 97036; tel. 503/635–3416; FAX. 503/697–6932; Ms. Lynne Saxton
*CODA, Inc., 1027 E. Burnside, Portland, OR 97214-1328; tel. 503/236–2290; FAX. 503/239–8407; Mr. Timothy T. Hartnett
Kerr Youth and Family Center, 722 Northeast 162nd Avenue, Portland, OR 97230; tel. 503/255–4205; FAX. 503/255–5095; Mr. Christopher J. Krenk
Northwest Behavioral Healthcare Services, 18000 Southeast Webster Road, Gladstone, OR 97027; tel. 503/722–4470; FAX. 503/722–4410; Mr. Daniel Mahler
Pendleton Academies, 622 Airport Road, Pendleton, OR 97801; tel. 541/276–0057; FAX. 541/276–1704; Ms. Mary Moore Suever
*Portland VA Medical Center Opiate Treatment Program, 3710 SW US Hospital Road, Building 100, Portland, OR 97207; tel. 503/220–8262; FAX. 503/220–3457; Dr. Peter Benson
*Serenity Lane, 2133 Centennial Plaza, Eugene, OR 97401; tel. 541/284–8629; FAX. 541/485–8484; Mr. Peter J. Asmuth
Southern Oregon Adolescent Study and Treatment Center, 715 SW Ramsey Avenue, Grants Pass, OR 97527; tel. 541/956–4943; FAX. 541/956–5463; Mr. Robert E. Lieberman
Trillium Family Services, 3415 SE Powell Blvd, Portland, OR 97202; tel. 503/234–9591; FAX. 503/205–0189; Mr. Kim Scott
*VA Southern Oregon Rehabilitation Center and Clinics, 8495 Crater Lake Highway, White City, OR 97503; tel. 541/830–3515; FAX. 541/830–3500; Dr. Max E. McIntosh

PENNSYLVANIA

*Adelphoi Village, Inc., 1119 Village Way, Latrobe, PA 15650; tel. 724/520–1111; FAX. 724/520–1878; Mr. Larry Breitenstein
Associates in Counseling & Child Guidance, 272 East Connelly Boulevard, Sharon, PA 16146; tel. 724/983–1381; FAX. 724/983–8260; Mr. Shayen A George
Beacon Light Behavioral Health Systems, 800 East Main Street, Bradford, PA 16701; tel. 814/362–5250; FAX. 814/362–2185; Mr. Thomas E Urban

*Indicates organization is a Joint Commission accredited Chemical Dependency organization.

Bethesda Children's Home, 15667 State Highway 86, Meadville, PA 16335; tel. 814/724–7510; FAX. 814/724–6237; Mr. Gene Wisinski

***Bowling Green Brandywine,** PO Box 787, Kennett Square, PA 19348; tel. 610/268–3588; FAX. 610/268–2334; Mrs. Lisa M. Olander

Child Guidance Resource Centers, 2000 Old West Chester Pike, Havertown, PA 19083; tel. 484/454–8700; FAX. 484/454–8706; Mr. Brad Barry

Children's Aid Home Programs of Somerset County, Inc., PO Box 1195, Somerset, PA 15501; tel. 814/443–1637; FAX. 814/445–8481; Mr. Robert C. Miller

Children's BehavioralHealth, Inc., 203 College Park Plaza, Johnstown, PA 15904; tel. 814/262–0768; FAX. 814/262–0795; Mr. George V. Kelly

Children's Service Center of Wyoming Valley, Inc., 335 South Franklin Street, Wilkes Barre, PA 18702; tel. 570/825–6425; FAX. 570/301–3330; Ms. Patricia Finan

***Choices Recovery Program,** 307 Laird Street, Plains, PA 18705; tel. 570/552–3700; FAX. 570/552–3705; Mr. Joseph Knecht

CHOR Youth & Family Services, Inc., 1010 Centre Avenue, Reading, PA 19601-1498; tel. 610/478–8266; FAX. 610/478–8094; Mr. Vince Lasorsa

***Clear Brook, Inc.,** 1003 Wyoming Avenue, Forty Fort, PA 18704; tel. 570/288–6692; FAX. 570/288–2574; Dr. Nicholas F. Colangelo

***Cornell Abraxas,** 429 West 6th Street, Erie, PA 16507; tel. 814/459–0618; FAX. 814/459–0682; Mr. Jim Torok

***Cornell Abraxas I,** PO Box 59, Marienville, PA 16239; tel. 814/927–6615; FAX. 814/927–8560; Mr. James E. Newsome

***Crozer Chester Medical Center-Community Hospital of Chester,** One Medical Center Blvd., Chester, PA 19013; tel. 610/447–2000; FAX. 610/447–6121; Ms. Joan K. Richards

Devereux Beneto Center, 655 Sugartown Road, PO Box 297, Malvern, PA 19355-0297; tel. 484/595–6733; FAX. 610/296–5866; Mr. Walter Grono

Diversified Treatment Alternatives, Inc., 148 Fairfield Road, Lewisburg, PA 17837; tel. 570/523–3457; FAX. 570/524–4849; Mr. Timothy J. Kelleher

***Dolminis Methadone Clinic,** 2 Sellers Drive, Altoona, PA 16601; tel. 814/940–0407; FAX. 814/940–0411; Mr. Jonathan Wolf

***Eagleville Hospital,** 100 Eagleville Road, PO Box 45, Eagleville, PA 19408-0045; tel. 610/539–6000; FAX. 610/539–9314; Mrs. Maureen King Pollock

***Foundations Medical Services,** 124 Hollywood Dr. Bantam Commons Bld 2, Butler, PA 16001; tel. 724/431–2006; FAX. 724/431–2003; Mr. Jonathan Wolf

***Gateway Rehabilitation Center / Genesis Division,** 100 Moffett Run Road, Aliquippa, PA 15001; tel. 412/766–8700; FAX. 412/747–0398; Dr. Kenneth S. Ramsey

Glade Run Lutheran Services, PO Box 70, Zelienople, PA 16063-0070; tel. 724/452–4453; FAX. 724/452–6576; Dr. Charles T. Lockwood

***Greenbriar Treatment Center,** 800 Manor Drive, Washington, PA 15301; tel. 724/225–9700; FAX. 724/225–9764; Ms. Mary G. Banaszak

Hoffman Homes, Inc., PO Box 4777, Gettysburg, PA 17325; tel. 717/359–7148; FAX. 717/359–2606; Mr. George Sepic

***Holcomb Behavioral Health Systems,** 835 Springdale Drive Suite 100, Exton, PA 19341; tel. 610/363–1488; FAX. 610/363–8273; Mr. William DiFabio

International Latino Women's Congress /Tree of Life Behavioral Services, 6404 Roosevelt Blvd. Suite 1 - C, Philadelphia, PA 19149; tel. 215/533–5433; FAX. 215/533–5432; Ms. Ada L. Tuleja

***Kensington Hospital Outpatient Treatment Program & Non-Hospital Detoxification Unit,** 136 West Diamond Street, Philadelphia, PA 19122; tel. 215/426–8100; FAX. 215/965–2344; Ms. Eileen Hause

***KidsPeace National Centers Inc.,** 5300 KidsPeace Drive, Orefield, PA 18069-9101; tel. 610/799–8000; FAX. 610/799–8001; Mr. Lorrie Henderson

***Kirkbride Center,** 111 North 49th Street, Philadelphia, PA 19139; tel. 215/471–2600; FAX. 215/471–2897; Ms. Rose Diottavio

***Livengrin Foundation, Inc.,** 4833 Hulmeville Road, Bensalem, PA 19020-3099; tel. 215/638–5200; FAX. 215/638–2603; Mr. Richard M. Pine

***Marworth,** PO Box 36, Waverly, PA 18471; tel. 570/563–1112; FAX. 570/563–2711; Mr. James J. Dougherty

***Mercy Catholic Medical Center/Mercy Hospital of Philadelphia,** 501 South 54th Street, Philadelphia, PA 19143; tel. 215/748–9300; FAX. 215/748–9709; Ms. Kathryn Conallen

***Mirmont Treatment Center,** 100 Yearsley Mill Road, Media, PA 19063-5593; tel. 610/744–1400; FAX. 610/744–1406; Mr. Thomas F. Cain

***Narcotic Addict Rehabilitation Program of Thomas Jefferson University,** South 21st St & Washington Ave, Philadelphia, PA 19146; tel. 215/735–5979; FAX. 215/503–2850; Dr. Stephen Weinstein

***NATP of Western Psychiatric Institute & Clinic of UPMC P-S,** 6714 Kelly Street, Pittsburgh, PA 15208; tel. 412/246–6806; FAX. 412/246–6810; Ms. Elizabeth Concordia

***New Day Behavioral Healthcare, Inc.,** 333 N. Oxford Valley Rd. Suite 601, Fairless Hills, PA 19030; tel. 215/949–2255; FAX. 215/949–2590

New Vitae, Inc. Partial Hospital Program & Outpatient Clinic, 16 South Main Street, Quakertown, PA 18951; tel. 215/538–3403; FAX. 215/538–3402; Mr. Adam Devlin

***NorthEast Treatment Centers,** 499 North 5th Street, Suite A, Philadelphia, PA 19123; tel. 215/451–7000; FAX. 215/451–7110; Mr. Terence McSherry

Nulton Diagnostic and Treatment Center, PC, 214 College Park Plaza, Johnstown, PA 15904; tel. 814/262–0025; FAX. 814/266–2880; Dr. Larry J. Nulton

Paoletta Psychological Services, 456 N Pitt St., Mercer, PA 16137; tel. 724/662–7202; FAX. 724/662–7208; Miss Dawn R. Hanaway

Perseus House, Inc., 1511 Peach Street, Erie, PA 16501; tel. 814/480–5900; FAX. 814/454–8670; Mr. A. Mark Amendola

***Philadelphia VA Medical Center Opioid Treatment Program,** University and Woodland Aves, Building 7, Philadelphia, PA 19104; tel. 215/823–5857; FAX. 215/823–6007; Mr. Richard S. Citron

Presbyterian Children's Village Services, 452 South Roberts Road, Rosemont, PA 19010; tel. 610/525–5400; FAX. 610/525–8396; Mrs. Darlene Hewett

***Progressive Medical Specialists, Inc.,** 2453 West Pike Road, Houston, PA 15342; tel. 724/873–5655; FAX. 724/873–5656; Ms. Annamarie Roberto

***Progressive Medical Specialists, Inc.,** 2900 Smallman Street, Pittsburgh, PA 15201; tel. 412/391–6384; FAX. 412/391–7882; Ms. Annamaire Roberto

Psychiatric Care Systems, PC, 110 Hidden Valley Road, McMurray, PA 15317; tel. 724/941–4070; FAX. 724/941–5083; Dr. Oscar Urrea

***Pyramid Healthcare, Inc.,** P.O. Box 1153, Altoona, PA 16603; tel. 814/940–0407; FAX. 814/940–0411; Mr. Jonathan Wolf

***RHJ Medical Center, Inc.,** RR 1, Box 224, Hunker, PA 15639; tel. 724/696–9600; FAX. 724/696–9500; Mrs. Kathleen A. Jones

Saint John Vianney Center, 151 Woodbine Road, Downingtown, PA 19335; tel. 610/269–2600; FAX. 610/873–8028; Mr. Thomas F. Dugan

Sarah A. Reed Children's Center, 2445 West 34th Street, Erie, PA 16506; tel. 814/838–1954; FAX. 814/835–2196; Mr. James Mando

Shawnee Academy, River Road, Minisink Hills, PA 18341; tel. 570/420–8601; FAX. 570/420–8609; Mr. Aldo Cavalli

Silver Springs - Martin Luther School, 512 West Township Line Road, Plymouth Meeting, PA 19462-1001; tel. 610/825–4440; FAX. 610/825–7989; Ms. Ruth W. Bartelt

***St. Joseph's Hospital Detoxification/ Rehabilitation,** 16th and Giard Avenue, Philadelphia, PA 19130; tel. 215/787–2000; FAX. 215/787–2525; Ms. Catherine Kutzler

St. Michael's School, Box 370 Hoban Heights, Tunkhannock, PA 18657; tel. 570/388–6155; FAX. 570/388–4069; Mr. Andrew M. Varzaly

***Stairways Behavioral Health,** 138 East 26th Street, Erie, PA 16504; tel. 814/453–5806; FAX. 814/453–4757; Mr. William F. McCarthy

SummitQuest Academy, PO Box 729, Ephrata, PA 17522; tel. 717/859–4100; FAX. 717/859–2734; Mr. Steven Palmer

The Bradley Center, Inc., 5180 Campbells Run Road, Pittsburgh, PA 15205; tel. 412/788–8219; FAX. 412/788–8215; Ms. Lisa Fox

The Bridge, 8400 Pine Road, Philadelphia, PA 19111; tel. 215/342–5000; FAX. 215/342–7709; Mr. Michael Ogden

***The Goldman Clinic,** 8th Street and Girard Avenue, Philadelphia, PA 19122; tel. 215/787–2000; FAX. 215/787–2310; Ms. Marlene D-Walsh

The Renfrew Centers, Inc., 475 Spring Lane, Philadelphia, PA 19128; tel. 215/482–5353; FAX. 215/482–1761; Mr. Samuel E. Menaged

***Thomas Jefferson University - Family Center,** 1201 Chestnut Street, Philadelphia, PA 19107; tel. 215/955–1951; FAX. 215/568–6414; Dr. Karol A. Kaltenbach

***TODAY, Inc.,** PO Box 908, Newtown, PA 18940; tel. 215/968–4713; FAX. 215/968–8742; Dr. John E Howell

***Universal Recovery Foundation,** 2001 Providence Avenue, Chester, PA 19013; tel. 610/876–9000; FAX. 610/876–5441; Dr. Michael Salazar

***UPMC Presbyterian Shadyside,** 200 Lothrop Street, Pittsburgh, PA 15213; tel. 412/647–8788; FAX. 412/647–5551; Mr. John Innocenti

***VA Medical Center - (SATU/OTP),** 1400 Blackhorse Hill Road, Coatesville, PA 19320; tel. 610/384–7711; FAX. 610/380–4324; Dr. Gary Devansky

***Valley Forge Medical Center & Hospital/OTP,** 1033 West Germantown Pike, Norristown, PA 19403; tel. 610/539–8500; FAX. 610/539–0910; Ms. Marian Colcher

***VAPHS - CTAD-OPIOID SUBSTITUTION THERAPY CLINIC,** 7180 Highland Drive, Bldg 4-1W, Pittsburgh, PA 15206; tel. 412/365–5010; FAX. 412/365–5009; Dr. Steve D. Forman

VisionQuest - Western Pennsylvania, 352 Marshalton Thorndale Road, Downingtown, PA 19335; tel. 800/433–4362; Mr. Kenn Capper

VisionQuest Guided Centering Program at South Mountain Lodge, 352 Marshalton Thorndale Road, Downingtown, PA 19335; tel. 800/433–4362; FAX. 717/749–3146; Mr. Gerry Fox

Warwick House, Inc., 1460 Meetinghouse Rd., Warminster, PA 18974; tel. 215/491–7404; FAX. 215/491–7405; Mr. Kenneth W. Brownell

***White Deer Run Inc.,** 360 White Deer Run Road, Allenwood, PA 17810; tel. 800/255–2335; FAX. 570/538–5303; Mr. Joseph Procopio

Wordsworth, 3905 Ford Road, Philadelphia, PA 19131; tel. 215/452–5170; FAX. 215/473–1854; Mr. Michael A. Davis

RHODE ISLAND

Alternatives, 350 Duncan Drive, Providence, RI 02906; tel. 401/453–4742; FAX. 401/453–2508

***Butler Hospital Alcohol and Drug Treatment Services,** 345 Blackstone Boulevard, Providence, RI 02906; tel. 401/455–6220; FAX. 401/455–6300; Dr. Patricia R. Recupero

***East Bay Center,** 2 Old County Road, Barrington, RI 02806; tel. 401/437–8844; FAX. 401/438–1957; Mr. Robert Crossley

***Gateway Healthcare, Inc.,** 249 Roosevelt Avenue, Pawtucket, RI 02860; tel. 401/724–8400; FAX. 401/724–8488; Mr. Richard H. Leclerc

Newport County Community Mental Health Center, Inc., 127 Johnnycake Hill Road, Middletown, RI 02842; tel. 401/846–1213; FAX. 401/848–9151; Mr. J. Clement Cicilline

***Providence VA Opioid Treatment Program,** 830 Chalkstone Avenue, Bldg 1, Providence, RI 02908; tel. 401/273–7100; FAX. 410/457–1401; Dr. Robert G. Johnston

***South Shore Mental Health Center, Inc.,** P.O. Box 899, Charlestown, RI 02813; tel. 401/364–7705; FAX. 401/364–9104; Mr. Wm. Michael Johnson

***SSTAR of Rhode Island,** 1950 Tower Hill Road, North Kingstown, RI 02852; tel. 401/294–6160; FAX. 401/295–2513; Ms. Nancy E. Paull

***The Providence Center,** 528 North Main Street, Providence, RI 02904; tel. 401/528–0123; FAX. 401/528–0124; Dr. Dale Klatzker

*Indicates organization is a Joint Commission accredited Chemical Dependency organization.

SOUTH CAROLINA

*__Lighthouse Care Center of Conway,__ 152 Waccamaw Medical Park Dr., Conway, SC 29526; tel. 843/347–8871; FAX. 843/234–6100; Mr. Francis Sauvageau

New Hope Treatment Centers, Inc., 7515 Northside Drive, Suite 200, North Charleston, SC 29420; tel. 843/851–5010; FAX. 843/851–5020; Mr. Jay S. Orvin

Palmetto Pee Dee Behavioral Health, LLC, 601B Gregg Avenue, Florence, SC 29502; tel. 843/667–0644; FAX. 843/669–5127; Ms. Denise Johnson

The Pines Residential Treatment Center-Charleston Campus, 225 Midland Parkway, Summerville, SC 29485; tel. 803/791–9918; FAX. 843/419–1211; Mr. Andy Hanner

Three Rivers Residential Treatment | Midlands Campus, 200 Ermine Road, West Columbia, SC 29170; tel. 803/791–9918; FAX. 803/926–5925; Mr. Jeff Barnett

SOUTH DAKOTA

Black Hills Children's Home, 24100 South Rockerville Road, Rapid City, SD 57701; tel. 605/334–6004; FAX. 605/335–2776; Mr. Dennis Daugaard

Sioux Falls Children's Home, PO Box 1749, Sioux Falls, SD 57101-1749; tel. 605/334–6004; FAX. 605/335–2776; Mr. Dennis Daugaard

TENNESSEE

Advanced Horizons, 6685 Quince Road Suite 124, Memphis, TN 38119; tel. 901/624–3581; FAX. 901/757–3830; Mr. Stan Caummisar

Agency for Youth and Family Development, 1071 Millins Station Rd, Memphis, TN 38134; tel. 901/387–5840; FAX. 901/387–5739; Dr. Gerald Jerome Jordan

*__Brookhaven Retreat,__ 1016 I.C. King Rd., Seymour, TN 37865; tel. 865/573–3656; FAX. 865/573–3655; Ms. Jacqueline Ann Dawes

*__Buffalo Valley, Inc.,__ PO Box 879, Hohenwald, TN 38462; tel. 931/796–5427; FAX. 931/796–5124; Mr. Jerry T. Risner

*__Child & Family Tennessee,__ 901 East Summit Hill Drive, Knoxville, TN 37915; tel. 865/524–7483; FAX. 865/521–4205; Ms. Kathryn R. O'Day

Compass Intervention Center, LLC, 7900 Lowrance Road, Memphis, TN 38125; tel. 901/758–2002; FAX. 901/758–2156; Mr. Nashon I. McPherson

*__Cornerstone of Recovery, Inc.,__ 1214 Topside Road, Louisville, TN 37777; tel. 865/970–7747; FAX. 865/681–2266; Mr. Dan R. Caldwell

*__Council for Alcohol and Drug Abuse Services, Inc.,__ PO Box 4797, Chattanooga, TN 37405; tel. 423/756–7644; FAX. 423/756–7646; Dr. Paul Fuchcar

Counseling and Consultation Services, Inc., P.O. Box 278, Limestone, TN 37681; tel. 423/257–6054; FAX. 423/257–6975; Mr. Thomas R. Herington

*__Cumberland Heights Foundation, Inc.,__ PO Box 90727, Nashville, TN 37209; tel. 615/352–1757; FAX. 615/353–4325; Mr. James B. Moore

Daybreak Treatment Center and Specialized School, 2262 Germantown Road South, Germantown, TN 38138; tel. 901/753–4300; FAX. 901/751–8105; Ms. Tina C. Mills

Dickson Recovery Center, LLC, 222 Church Street, Dickson, TN 37055; tel. 615/405–9453; Mr. John Jackson

*__DRD Knoxville Medical Clinic,__ 626 Bernard Street, Knoxville, TN 37921; tel. 865/522–0161; FAX. 865/521–7920; Mr. Andrew Love

*__DRD Medical Clinic - Central,__ 412 Citico Street, Knoxville, TN 37921; tel. 865/522–0661; Mr. Andrew Love

First Hospital Corporation of Chattanooga, 7351 Standifer Gap Road, Chattanooga, TN 37421; tel. 423/499–9007; FAX. 423/499–9757; Mrs. Stephanie Elaine Austin

*__Focus Healthcare,__ 7429 Shallowford Road, Chattanooga, TN 37421; tel. 423/308–2560; FAX. 423/308–6567

Foothills Care, Inc., 404 North Kentucky Street, Kingston, TN 37763; tel. 865/376–3464; FAX. 865/376–3433; Mr. James Pedigo

*__Pathways of Tennessee, Inc.,__ 238 Summar Drive, Jackson, TN 38301; tel. 731/935–8200; FAX. 731/935–8327; Mrs. Pam Henson

Reflections Treatment Agency, 6628 Central Avenue Pike, Knoxville, TN 37912; tel. 865/219–9444; FAX. 865/219–9555; Mr. James Slattery

Ridgeview Psychiatric Hospital and Center, Inc., 240 West Tyrone Road, Oak Ridge, TN 37830; tel. 865/482–1076; FAX. 865/481–6164; Mr. Robert Benning

The Camelot Schools,LLC, 183 Fiddlers Lane, Kingston, TN 37763; tel. 865/376–2296; FAX. 865/376–1850

The Fit For Life Transformation Center For Women, 110 Timbercreek Drive, Cordova, TN 38018; tel. 901/755–0099; Mr. Neil Smith

The Oak Plains Academy, 1751 Oak Plains Road, Ashland City, TN 37015; tel. 931/362–4723; FAX. 931/362–4248; Mr. Matt Ours

Youth Villages, 3320 Brother Blvd, Memphis, TN 38133; tel. 901/251–5000; FAX. 901/251–5001; Mr. Patrick W. Lawler

TEXAS

*__Addiction and Psychotherapy Services,__ 2824 South Congress Avenue, Austin, TX 78704; tel. 512/444–5092; FAX. 512/444–5099; Dr. Heinz Aeschbach

*__Alternatives Centre for Behavioral Health,__ 5001 Alabama Street, El Paso, TX 79930; tel. 915/565–4800; FAX. 915/565–3163; Ms. Carol J Anderson

Austin Child Guidance Center, 810 West 45th Street, Austin, TX 78751; tel. 512/451–2242; FAX. 512/454–9204; Dr. Donald J. Zappone

*__Austin Travis County MHMR Methadone Maintenance Program,__ 1631 A East 2nd Street, Austin, TX 78702; tel. 512/472–6261; FAX. 512/472–5857; Mr. David Evans

*__Bay Area Care Center, Inc,__ 3138 S. Alameda Suite B, Corpus Christi, TX 78404; tel. 361/882–9602; FAX. 361/882–9604; Mr. Tone Johnson

*__Burke Center,__ 4101 South Medford Drive, Lufkin, TX 75901; tel. 936/639–1141; FAX. 936/634–8601; Ms. Susan Rushing

Canyon Lakes Residential Treatment Center, 2402 Canyon Lake Drive, Lubbock, TX 79415; tel. 806/762–5782; FAX. 806/762–0838; Dr. Ray H. Brown

Cedar Crest Hospital and RTC, 3500 South I-H 35, Belton, TX 76513; tel. 254/939–2100; FAX. 254/939–2334; Mr. Steve Rublee

CONTINUUM, 3003 South Loop West, Suite 475, Houston, TX 77054-1301; tel. 713/383–0888; FAX. 713/383–0895; Dr. Barbara Ann Candley

*__DebLin Health Concepts and Associates, Inc.,__ P. O. Box 550769, Houston, TX 77255-0769; tel. 713/686–9194; FAX. 713/686–9413; Ms. Debra R. Jackson

*__East Texas Clinic,__ PO Box 9486, Longview, TX 75608; tel. 903/759–4966; FAX. 903/759–3414; Ms. Diane Stalnaker

Family Services of Greater Houston, 3815 Montrose Boulevard, Suite 200, Houston, TX 77006; tel. 713/868–4466; FAX. 713/868–2619; Ms. Nyla K. Woods

Five Oaks Achievement Center, P.O. Box 1249, New Ulm, TX 78950; tel. 979/992–3791; FAX. 979/992–2828; Mr. Jerry Craig Bibb

*__Grapevine Valley Hope,__ 2300 William D. Tate Avenue, Grapevine, TX 76051; tel. 817/424–1305; FAX. 817/424–1327; Dr. Kenneth C. Gregoire

*__HCI of Denison,__ 2301 S. Austin Avenue Unit 3, Denison, TX 75020; tel. 903/464–0727; FAX. 903/464–0737; Mr. Andrew Love

*__Huntsville Clinic, Inc.,__ 829 10th Street, Huntsville, TX 77320; tel. 936/291–9172; FAX. 936/291–7156; Ms. Stacey R. Harris

InnerWisdom, Inc., 1325 La Concha Lane, Houston, TX 77054; tel. 713/592–9292; FAX. 713/592–9296; Ms. JoAnne Mandel

*__Johnnie M. Hawkins LAMP Clinic,__ 431 Fulton, Fort Worth, TX 76104; tel. 817/336–3754; FAX. 817/336–0651; Dr. Sidarth Wakhlu

*__La Hacienda Treatment Center,__ PO Box 1, Hunt, TX 78024; tel. 830/238–4222; FAX. 830/238–4070; Mr. Arthur VanDivier

Meridell Achievement Center, PO Box 87, Liberty Hill, TX 78642; tel. 512/515–2100; FAX. 512/515–6710; Ms. Gail Oberta

*__Meth-Laam,__ 3204 Ennis Street, Houston, TX 77004; tel. 713/526–2441; FAX. 713/522–9362; Mr. Earnest Gibson

*__Michael E. DeBakey VA MC Opioid Treatment Program,__ 2002 Holcombe Blvd, Bldg 100, Houston, TX 77030; tel. 713/794–7100; FAX. 713/794–7854; Ms. Margaret L. Landrum

*__Montrose Counseling Center, Inc.,__ 401 Branard, 2nd Floor, Houston, TX 77006; tel. 713/529–0037; FAX. 713/526–4367; Dr. Ann J. Robison

*__New Dimensions,__ 1345 Space Park, Suite C, Houston, TX 77058; tel. 281/333–2284; FAX. 281/333–0221; Mr. George R. Brazzel

*__Nexus Recovery Center, Inc.,__ 8733 La Prada, Dallas, TX 75228; tel. 214/321–0156; FAX. 214/321–3096; Ms. Becca Crowell

Nueces County MHMR Community Center, 1630 South Brownlee Street, Corpus Christi, TX 78404; tel. 361/886–6900; FAX. 361/883–5842; Mrs. Diane Staley

*__Pasadena Substance Abuse Clinic, Inc,__ 1645 Pasadena Boulevard, Pasadena, TX 77502; tel. 713/473–1405; FAX. 713/473–3779; Ms. Nighat Shaheen

*__River Oaks Academy Day Hospital,__ 10600 Richmond Avenue, Houston, TX 77042; tel. 713/783–7200; FAX. 713/783–7286; Mr. Louis Valdes

*__RR Recovery, LLC,__ 2501 Taylor Street, Wichita Falls, TX 76309; tel. 940/761–3034; FAX. 943/761–3074; Mr. Raul Domingo Ruelas

*__Sabine Valley Regional MHMR Center,__ PO BX 6800, Longview, TX 75601; tel. 903/237–2323; FAX. 903/234–1639; Mr. Inman White

*__Serenity Foundation of Texas,__ 1546 North 2nd Street, Abilene, TX 79601; tel. 325/673–6489; FAX. 325/673–1794; Mr. Richard L. Spalding

Shiloh Treatment Center, Inc., 3926 Bahler Avenue, Manvel, TX 77578; tel. 281/489–1290; FAX. 281/489–0167; Mr. Clay D. Hill

*__Shoreline, Inc.,__ PO Box 68, Taft, TX 78390; tel. 361/528–3356; FAX. 361/528–3249; Dr. Sharel Zacharias

Southwest Mental Health Center, 8535 Tom Slick Drive, San Antonio, TX 78229; tel. 210/616–0300; FAX. 210/692–1266; Mr. Frederick W. Hines

*__Spindletop MHMR Services,__ PO Box 3846, Beaumont, TX 77704; tel. 409/839–1000; FAX. 409/784–5521; Dr. N. Charles Harris

*__Starlite Recovery Center,__ PO Box 317, Center Point, TX 78010-0317; tel. 830/292–0148; FAX. 830/634–2532

*__Summer Sky, Inc.,__ 1100 McCart Street, Stephenville, TX 76401; tel. 254/968–2907; FAX. 254/968–4509; Ms. Nicole Conlan

Sundance Behavioral Healthcare, Inc., 2707 Airport Freeway, Fort Worth, TX 76111-2333; tel. 817/222–9191; FAX. 817/222–9797; Dr. Puskoor Kumar

*__Sundown Ranch, Inc.,__ 3120 Van Zandt County Road #2318, Canton, TX 75103; tel. 903/479–3933; FAX. 903/479–3999; Mr. Robert H. Power

Texas San Marcos Treatment Center, LP, 120 Bert Brown Road, San Marcos, TX 78666; tel. 512/396–8500; FAX. 512/754–3883; Ms. Cassie Schmidt

*__Texoma Treatment Clinic - OTP,__ 1615 Kemp Street, Wichita Falls, TX 76309; tel. 214/346–3821; FAX. 214/276–7702; Mr. Andy Love

*__The Anchor Behavioral Health Centers,__ 6585 S. FM 183, Evant, TX 76525; tel. 254/471–5709; FAX. 254/471–5710; Mr. Bob Wilson

The Oaks Treatment Center, 1407 West Stassney Lane, Austin, TX 78745; tel. 512/464–0200; FAX. 512/464–0444; Dr. Edgar E. Prettyman

*__The Patrician Movement,__ 222 East Mitchell Street, San Antonio, TX 78210; tel. 210/532–3126; FAX. 210/534–3779; Dr. Patrick M. Clancey

*__VA North Texas Health Care System / Opioid Replacement Clinic,__ 4500 Lancaster Road, Bldg 71B, Dallas, TX 75216; tel. 214/857–0513; FAX. 214/857–0506; Dr. Cemal Unverdi

Waco Center for Youth, 3501 North 19th Street, Waco, TX 76708; tel. 254/756–2171; FAX. 254/745–5398; Mr. Eddie Greenfield

Whispering Hills Achievement Center, 4110 FM 609, Flatonia, TX 78941; tel. 361/865–3083; FAX. 361/865–3316; Mrs. Loueva H. Hatfield

UTAH

Benchmark Behavioral Health Systems, 592 West 1350 South, Woods Cross, UT 84087; tel. 801/299–5300; FAX. 801/296–2163; Mr. Barry Woodward

Blue Mountain Family Center / Wilderness Quest, PO Box 2878, Salt Lake City, UT 84110-2878; tel. 435/587–2801; FAX. 435/587–3164; Dr. Cory Reich

*Indicates organization is a Joint Commission accredited Chemical Dependency organization.

Center for Change, 1790 North State Street, Orem, UT 84057; tel. 801/224–8255; FAX. 801/224–8301; Dr. Michael E. Berrett
***Cinnamon Hills Youth Crisis Center,** 770 East St. George Boulevard, Saint George, UT 84770; tel. 435/674–0984; FAX. 435/674–0114; Mr. Jim Downey
***Cirque Lodge,** 1240 East 800 North, Orem, UT 84097; tel. 801/222–9200; FAX. 801/222–0112; Mr. Gary Fisher
Heritage Schools Inc, 5600 N Heritage School Drive, Provo, UT 84604; tel. 801/226–4600; FAX. 801/226–4696; Mr. Glen Zaugg
***Highland Ridge Hospital,** 7309 South 180 West, Midvale, UT 84047; tel. 801/569–2153; FAX. 801/567–9006; Mr. Robert Beatty
Hightop Ranch School, PO Box 440029, Koosharem, UT 84744; tel. 435/638–7411; FAX. 435/638–7511; Mr. Justin Sorenson
***Integrity House,** 465 W. 1600 N., Cedar City, UT 84720; tel. 435/586–8336; FAX. 435/865–6806; Mrs. Phyllis J. Charles
Island View Residential Treatment Center, 2650 West 2700 South, Syracuse, UT 84075; tel. 801/773–0200; FAX. 801/773–0208; Dr. Jared U. Balmer
Kids Behavioral Health of Utah Inc., 5899 West Rivendell Drive, West Jordan, UT 84088; tel. 801/561–3377; FAX. 801/569–3274; Mr. R. Michael Rowley
Solacium - New Haven, Post Office Box 50238, Provo, UT 84605; tel. 801/794–1218; FAX. 801/794–1223; Mr. Val Christensen
Sorenson's Ranch School, Inc., Box 440219, Koosharem, UT 84744; tel. 435/638–7318; FAX. 435/638–7582; Mr. Shane Sorenson
Telos Residential Treatment, PO Box 537, Orem, UT 84059; tel. 801/426–8800; FAX. 801/426–8825; Mr. Craig LaMont
UHS of Provo Canyon, Inc, 1350 E 750 North, Orem, UT 84097; tel. 801/227–2000; FAX. 801/229–1043; Mr. Jeremy Cottle
UHS of Salt Lake City, LLC, 1144 West 3300 South, South Salt Lake, UT 84119; tel. 801/433–2900; FAX. 801/433–2999; Mr. James Bailey
UT-TEX, Inc., PO Box 69, Magna, UT 84044; tel. 801/250–9762; FAX. 801/250–8483; Mr. H. Matthew Dixon
Youth Care of Utah, Inc., PO Box 909, Draper, UT 84020; tel. 801/572–6989; FAX. 801/572–8220; Ms. Trina Packard
Youthtrack - Utah, PO Box 887, Brigham City, UT 84302; tel. 435/723–1799; FAX. 435/723–2521; Mr. Scott Stringam

VERMONT
***Brattleboro Retreat,** Anna Marsh Lane, Brattleboro, VT 05302; tel. 802/257–7785; FAX. 802/258–3792; Mr. Robert E Simpson
***Health Care & Rehabilitation Services of Southeastern Vermont,** 390 River Street, Springfield, VT 05156; tel. 802/463–3294; FAX. 802/463–1204; Ms. Judith Poole Hayward

VIRGINIA
Alice C. Tyler Village of Childhelp East, 23164 Dragoon Road, Lignum, VA 22726; tel. 540/399–1926; FAX. 540/399–9730; Mr. John Bachand
***Carilion New River Valley Medical Ctr.- Methadone Short Term,** PO Box 5, Radford, VA 24143; tel. 540/731–2000; FAX. 540/633–4559; Mr. Donald B. Halliwill
Commonwealth Center for Children and Adolescents, P.O. Box 4000, Staunton, VA 24402-4000; tel. 540/332–2100; FAX. 540/332–2202; Mr. William J. Tuell
Ed Murphy & Associates, PO Box 35, Bumpass, VA 23024; tel. 540/872–4545; FAX. 540/872–4546; Mr. Ed J. Murphy
***Family Counseling Center for Recovery,** 4906 Radford Avenue, Richmond, VA 23230; tel. 804/354–1996; FAX. 804/354–5516; Mr. Charles R. Adcock
***Galax Treatment Center, dba, Life Center of Galax,** 111 Town Hollow Road, Cedar Bluff, VA 24609; tel. 540/963–3554; FAX. 540/963–4653; Ms. Tina R. Bullins
***Galax Treatment Center, Inc.,** PO Box 27, Galax, VA 24333; tel. 540/236–2994; FAX. 540/236–8821; Ms. Tina R. Bullins
Graydon Manor, 801 Children's Center Road, SW, Leesburg, VA 20175; tel. 703/777–3485; FAX. 703/777–4887; Mr. Bernard J. Haberlein
Hallmark Youthcare - Richmond, 12800 West Creek Parkway, Richmond, VA 23238; tel. 804/784–2200; FAX. 804/784–5331; Mr. Scott Cook
***Inova Comprehensive Addiction Treatment Services (CATS),** 3300 Gallows Road, Falls Church, VA 22042; tel. 703/776–7777; FAX. 703/776–7799; Mr. Douglas P. Cropper
***Inova Kellar Center,** 11204 Waples Mill Road, Fairfax, VA 22030-2522; tel. 703/218–8500; FAX. 703/359–0463; Dr. Richard Leichtweis
Keystone Newport News Youth Center, 17579 Warwick Boulevard, Newport News, VA 23603; tel. 757/888–0400; FAX. 757/888–0359; Mr. Robert Lehmann
Liberty Point Health Care, 1110 Montgomery Ave., Staunton, VA 24401; tel. 540/213–0450; FAX. 540/213–0456; Mr. Christopher Ruble
Marion Correctional Treatment Center, PO Box 1027, Marion, VA 24354-1027; tel. 276/783–7154; FAX. 276/783–2862; Mr. Kenneth L Osborne
***Mount Regis Center,** 405 Kimball Avenue, Salem, VA 24153; tel. 540/389–4761; FAX. 540/389–6539; Ms. Gail S. Basham
North Spring Behavioral Healthcare, 42009 Victory Lane, Leesburg, VA 20176; tel. 703/777–0800; FAX. 703/777–6970; Mr. Scott Zeiter
***Poplar Springs Hospital,** PO Box 3060, Petersburg, VA 23805; tel. 804/733–6874; FAX. 804/861–0076; Mr. Richard Clark
Remuda Ranch Center for Eating Disorders East, Inc., 20500 Remuda Drive, Milford, VA 22514; tel. 804/632–5600; FAX. 804/632–1242; Ms. Sallie Hershkowitz
***Snowden at Fredericksburg,** 1200 Sam Perry Boulevard, Fredericksburg, VA 22401; tel. 540/741–3900; FAX. 540/741–3918
The Barry Robinson Center, 443 Kempsville Road, Norfolk, VA 23502; tel. 757/455–6100; FAX. 757/455–6127; Dr. Patrick J. Bateman
The Pines Residential Treatment Center, 825 Crawford Parkway, Portsmouth, VA 23704; tel. 757/393–0061; FAX. 757/391–6750
***VA Medical Center - Methadone Maintenance Program,** 1201 Broad Rock Boulevard, SATP Inpatient Unit 1F, Richmond, VA 23249; tel. 804/675–5000; FAX. 804/675–5451
***Virginia Treatment Center, Inc.,** 3208 Hershberger Road, Roanoke, VA 24017; tel. 540/336–5248; FAX. 540/366–5211; Ms. Tina R. Bullins
Whisper Ridge Behavioral Health System, 2101 Arlington Boulevard, Charlottesville, VA 22903; tel. 434/977–1523; FAX. 434/977–5274; Mr. Taylor Davis
***Williamsburg Place,** 5477 Mooretown Road, Williamsburg, VA 23188; tel. 757/565–0106; FAX. 757/565–0620; Ms. Stephanie Loebs

WASHINGTON
***American Lake Opioid Treatment Program,** American Lake Drive, Bldg 61, Tacoma, WA 98493; tel. 206/762–1010; FAX. 206/764–2293; Dr. Andrew J. Saxon
***Central Washington Comprehensive Mental Health,** 402 South Fourth Avenue, Yakima, WA 98902; tel. 509/575–4084; FAX. 509/575–4811; Mr. Rick Weaver
Grant Mental Healthcare, PO Box 1057, Moses Lake, WA 98837; tel. 509/765–9239; FAX. 509/765–1582; Ms. Sherri M. Taylor
Pearl Street Center / Comprehensive Mental Health, 815 South Pearl Street, Tacoma, WA 98465; tel. 253/396–5930; FAX. 253/566–2252; Dr. Michael K. Laederich
Seattle Children's Home, Inc., 2142 Tenth Avenue West, Seattle, WA 98119; tel. 206/283–3300; FAX. 206/284–7843; Dr. Gena Palm
***Seattle Opioid Treatment Program,** 1660 S Columbian Way, Bldg 24, Seattle, WA 98108; tel. 206/764–2782; FAX. 206/764–2293; Dr. Andrew Saxon
***Sound Mental Health,** 1600 East Olive Street, Seattle, WA 98122; tel. 206/302–2200; FAX. 206/302–2210; Mr. David Stone
Tamarack Center, 2901 W Ft. George Wright Drive, Spokane, WA 99224; tel. 509/326–8100; FAX. 509/326–9358; Mr. Tim Davis
***Valley Cities Counseling & Consultation,** 2704 I Street NE, Auburn, WA 98002; tel. 253/833–7444; FAX. 253/833–0480; Ms. Faith Richie

WEST VIRGINIA
Elkins Mountain Schools, 100 Bell Street, Elkins, WV 26241; tel. 304/637–8000; FAX. 304/636–4694; Ms. Carolyn J. Pingley
***Olympic Center - Preston, Inc.,** PO Box 158, Kingwood, WV 26537; tel. 304/329–2400; FAX. 304/329–2405; Ms. Arlene Glover

WISCONSIN
***Aurora Psychiatric Hospital,** 1220 Dewey Avenue, Wauwatosa, WI 53213; tel. 414/454–6600; FAX. 414/454–6450; Mr. Peter Carlson
***Cadott Medical Center, SC - Methadone Program,** PO Box 69, Cadott, WI 54727; tel. 715/289–4221; FAX. 715/289–3534; Dr. Clifford T. Bowe
***Gundersen Lutheran Medical Center, Inc.- Methadone Maintenance,** 1910 South Avenue, La Crosse, WI 54601; tel. 608/782–7300; FAX. 608/775–4410; Dr. Jeffrey Thompson
***Libertas Treatment Center,** 1701 Dousman Street, Green Bay, WI 54303; tel. 920/498–8600; FAX. 920/496–2027; Mr. David B. Fish

WYOMING
Cathedral Home for Children, PO Box 520, Laramie, WY 82073; tel. 307/745–8997; FAX. 307/742–6146; Ms. Robin J. Haas
Normative Services, Inc., 5 Lane Lane, Sheridan, WY 82801; tel. 307/674–6878; FAX. 307/674–7781; Mr. Cal Furnish
St. Joseph's Children's Home, PO Box 1117, Torrington, WY 82240; tel. 307/532–4197; FAX. 307/532–8405; Mr. Robert C. Mayor
***Wyoming Recovery, LLC,** 231 South Wilson, Casper, WY 82601; tel. 307/265–3791; FAX. 307/265–4480; Ms. Carolyn Toews

U.S. Associated Areas

APO/AE
Installation Management Command - Europe, IMCOM-EUROPE, Atten IMEU-HRD,Unit 29353 Box 200, APO, AE 09014; tel. 011–496–2215; FAX. 011–496–2215; Dr. Robert S. McCollum

PUERTO RICO
Clinica Interdisciplinaria de Psiquiatria Avanzada, 650 Lloveras St Cond Centro Plaza Suite 101, San Juan, PR 00909-2113; tel. 787/721–4020; FAX. 787/721–4555; Dr. Carlos A. Caban
Instituto Latinoamericano, Inc., Carretera # 2 M239 Villa Caparra, Guaynabo, PR 00966; tel. 787/792–8383; FAX. 787/792–8778; Dr. Rafael Padro-Castro
Instituto Psicoterapeutico de Puerto Rico, PO Box 367221, San Juan, PR 00936–7221; tel. 787/753–9515; FAX. 787/753–8327; Dr. Alberto Varela

VIRGIN ISLANDS
Division of Mental Health, Alcoholism & Drug Dependency Service, 3500 Richmond, Christiansted, VI 00820; tel. 340/773–1992; FAX. 340/773–7900

*Indicates organization is a Joint Commission accredited Chemical Dependency organization.

Abbreviations Used in the AHA Guide

AB, Army Base
ACSW, Academy of Certified Social Workers
AEC, Atomic Energy Commission
AFB, Air Force Base
AHA, American Hospital Association
AK, Alaska
AL, Alabama
AODA, Alcohol and Other Drug Abuse
APO, Army Post Office
AR, Arkansas
A.R.T., Accredited Record Technician
A.S.C., Ambulatory Surgical Center
A.T.C., Alcoholism Treatment Center
Ave., Avenue
AZ, Arizona

B.A., Bachelor of Arts
B.B.A., Bachelor of Business Administration
B.C., British Columbia
Blvd., Boulevard
B.S., Bachelor of Science
B.S.Ed., Bachelor of Science in Education
B.S.H.S., Bachelor of Science in Health Studies
B.S.N., Bachelor of Science in Nursing
B.S.W., Bachelor of Science and Social Worker
CA, California; Controller of Accounts

C.A.A.D.A.C., Certified Alcohol and Drug Abuse Counselor
CAC, Certified Alcoholism Counselor
CAE, Certified Association Executive
CAP, College of American Pathologists
CAPA, Certified Ambulatory Post Anesthesia
C.A.S., Certificate of Advanced Study
CCDC, Certified Chemical Dependency Counselor
C.D., Commander of the Order of Distinction
CDR, Commander
CDS, Chemical Dependency Specialist
CFACHE, Certified Fellow American College of Healthcare Executives
CFRE, Certified Fund Raising Executive
C.G., Certified Gastroenterology
CHC, Certified Health Consultant
CHE, Certified Healthcare Executive
C.L.D., Clinical Laboratory Director
CLU, Certified Life Underwriter, Chartered Life Underwriter
CMA, Certified Medical Assistant
C.M.H.A., Certified Mental Health Administrator
CNHA, Certified Nursing Home Administrator
CNM, Certified Nurse Midwife
CNOR, Certified Operating Room Nurse
C.N.S., Clinical Nurse Specialist
CO, Colorado; Commanding Officer
COA, Certified Ophthalmic Assistant
COMT, Commandant
C.O.M.T., Certified Ophthalmic Medical Technician
Conv., Conventions
Corp., Corporation; Corporate
C.O.T., Certified Ophthalmic Technician
CPA, Certified Public Accountant
C.P.H.Q., Certified Professional in Health Care Quality
CPM, Certified Public Manager
CRNA, Certified Registered Nurse Anesthetist
CRNH, Certified Registered Nurse Hospice
C.S.J.B, Catholic Saint John the Baptist
CSW, Certified Social Worker
CT, Connecticut
CWO, Chief Warrant Officer

D.B.A., Doctor of Business Administration
DC, District of Columbia
D.D., Doctor of Divinity
D.D.S., Doctor of Dental Surgery
DE, Delaware
Diet, Dietitian; Dietary; Dietetics
D.M.D., Doctor of Dental Medicine
D.MIN., Doctor of Ministry
D.O., Doctor of Osteopathic Medicine and Surgery, Doctor of Osteopathy
DPA, Doctorate Public Administration
D.P.M., Doctor of Podiatric Medicine
Dr., Drive
Dr.P.h., Doctor of Public Health
D.Sc., Doctor of Science
D.S.W., Doctor of Social Welfare
D.V.M., Doctor of Veterinary Medicine

E., East
Ed.D., Doctor of Education
Ed.S., Specialist in Education
ENS, Ensign
Esq., Esquire
Expwy., Expressway
ext., extension

FAAN, Fellow of the American Academy of Nursing
FACATA, Fellow of the American College of Addiction Treatment Administrators
FACHE, Fellow of the American College of Healthcare Executives
FACMGA, Fellow of the American College of Medical Group Administrators
FACP, Fellow of the American College of Physicians
FACS, Fellow of the American College of Surgeons
FAX, Facsimile
FL, Florida
FPO, Fleet Post Office
FRCPSC, Fellow of the Royal College of Physicians and Surgeons of Canada
FT, Full-time

GA, Georgia
Govt., Government; Governmental

HHS, Department of Health and Human Services
HI, Hawaii
HM, Helmsman
HMO, Health Maintenance Organization
Hon., Honorable; Honorary
H.S.A., Health System Administrator
Hts., Heights
Hwy., Highway

IA, Iowa
ID, Idaho
IL, Illinois
IN, Indiana
Inc., Incorporated

J.D., Doctor of Law
J.P., Justice of the Peace
Jr., Junior

KS, Kansas
KY, Kentucky

LA, Louisiana
LCDR, Lieutenant Commander
LCSW, Licensed Certified Social Worker
L.H.D., Doctor of Humanities
L.I.S.W., Licensed Independent Social Worker
LL.D., Doctor of Laws
L.L.P., Limited Licensed Practitioner
L.M.H.C., Licensed Master of Health Care
L.M.S.W., Licensed Master of Social Work
L.N.H.A., Licensed Nursing Home Administrator
L.P.C., Licensed Professional Counselor
LPN, Licensed Practical Nurse
L.P.N., Licensed Practical Nurse
L.S.W., Licensed Social Worker
Lt., Lieutenant
LTC, Lieutenant Colonel
Ltd., Limited
LT.GEN., Lieutenant General
LTJG, Lieutenant (junior grade)

MA, Massachusetts
M.A., Master of Arts
Maj., Major
M.B., Bachelor of Medicine
M.B.A., Masters of Business Administration
MC, Medical Corps; Marine Corps
M.C., Member of Congress
MD, Maryland
M.D., Doctor of Medicine
ME, Maine
M.Ed., Master of Education
MFCC, Marriage/Family/Child Counselor
MHA, Mental Health Association
M.H.S., Masters in Health Science; Masters in Human Service
MI, Michigan
MM, Masters of Management
MN, Minnesota
M.N., Master of Nursing
MO, Missouri
M.P.A., Master of Public Administration; Master Public Affairs
M.P.H., Master of Public Health
M.P.S., Master of Professional Studies; Master of Public Science
MS, Mississippi
M.S., Master of Science
MSC, Medical Service Corps
M.S.D., Doctor of Medical Science
MSHSA, Master of Science Health Service Administration
M.S.N., Master of Science in Nursing
M.S.P.H., Master of Science in Public Health
M.S.S.W., Master of Science in Social Work
M.S.W., Master of Social Work
MT, Montana
Mt., Mount

N., North
NC, North Carolina
N.C.A.D.C., National Certification of Alcohol and Drug Counselors
ND, North Dakota
NE, Nebraska
NH, New Hampshire
NHA, National Hearing Association; Nursing Home Administrator
NJ, New Jersey
NM, New Mexico
NPA, National Perinatal Association
NV, Nevada
NY, New York

OCN, Oncology Certified Nurse
O.D., Doctor of Optometry
O.F.M., Order Franciscan Monks, Order of Friars Minor
OH, Ohio
OK, Oklahoma
OR, Oregon
O.R., Operating Room
O.R.S., Operating Room Supervisor
OSF, Order of St. Francis

PA, Pennsylvania
P.A., Professional Association
P.C., Professional Corporation
Pharm.D., Doctor of Pharmacy
Ph.B., Bachelor of Philosophy
Ph.D., Doctor of Philosophy
PHS, Public Health Service
Pkwy., Parkway
Pl., Place
PR, Puerto Rico
PS, Professional Services
PSRO, Professional Standards Review Organization

RADM, Rear Admiral
RD, Rural Delivery
Rd., Road
R.F.D., Rural Free Delivery
RI, Rhode Island
R.M., Risk Manager
RN, Registered Nurse
RNC, Republican National Committee; Registered Nurse or Board Certified
R.Ph., Registered Pharmacist
RRA, Registered Record Administrator
R.S.M., Religious Sisters of Mercy
Rte., Route

S., South
SC, South Carolina
S.C., Surgery Center
SCAC, Senior Certified Addiction Counselor
Sc.D., Doctor of Science
Sci., Science, Scientific
SD, South Dakota
SHCC, Statewide Health Coordinating Council
Sgt., Sergeant
SNA, Surgical Nursing Assistant
SNF, Skilled Nursing Facility
Sq., Square
Sr., Senior, Sister
St., Saint, Street
Sta., Station
Ste., Saint; Suite

Tel., Telephone
Terr., Terrace
TN, Tennessee
Tpke, Turnpike
Twp., Township
TX, Texas

USA, United States Army
USAF, United States Air Force
USMC, United States Marine Corps
USN, United States Navy
USPHS, United States Public Health Service
UT, Utah

VA, Virginia
VADM, Vice Admiral
VI, Virgin Islands
Vlg., Village
VT, Vermont

W., West
WA, Washington
WI, Wisconsin
WV, West Virginia
WY, Wyoming

Index

Notes

Notes

Notes

Notes